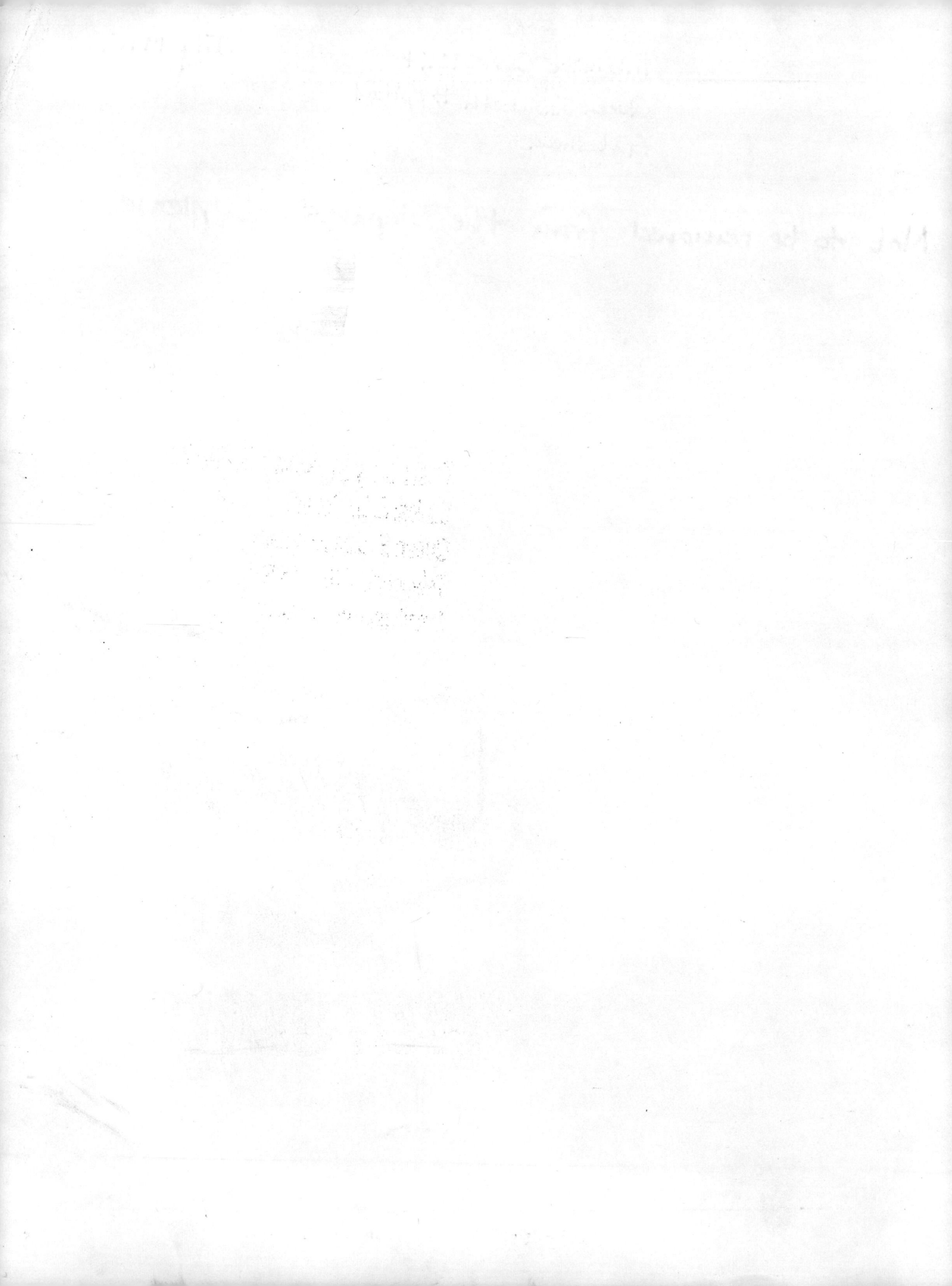

Critical Care Nursing

JOHN M. CLOCHESY, RN, MS, CS, FCCM
Instructor, Acute and Critical Care Nursing
Frances Payne Bolton School of Nursing
Case Western Reserve University
Cleveland, Ohio

CHRISTINE BREU, RN, MN, CNAA
Associate Executive Director/Nursing
Humana Hospital Suburban
Louisville, Kentucky

SUZETTE CARDIN, RN, MS, CCRN, CNAA
Nurse Manager
Cardiac Care Unit/Cardiac Observation Unit
UCLA Medical Center
Los Angeles, California

ELLEN B. RUDY, RN, PhD, FAAN
Dean, School of Nursing
University of Pittsburgh
Pittsburgh, Pennsylvania

ALICE A. WHITTAKER, RN, MS
Instructor
Creighton University
Mary Lanning Campus
Hastings, Nebraska

Critical Care Nursing

W. B. SAUNDERS COMPANY
Harcourt Brace Jovanovich, Inc.
Philadelphia London Toronto Montreal Sydney Tokyo

W. B. SAUNDERS COMPANY
Harcourt Brace Jovanovich, Inc.

The Curtis Center
Independence Square West
Philadelphia, Pennsylvania 19106

Library of Congress Cataloging-in-Publication Data

Critical care nursing/[edited by] John M. Clochesy . . . [et al.].

p.   cm.

ISBN 0–7216–2856–7

1. Intensive care nursing.   I. Clochesy, John M.
    [DNLM: 1. Critical Care—nurses' instruction. WY 154
    C93332]

RT120.I5C743 1993   610.73′61—dc20

DNLM/DLC   92–11666

Critical Care Nursing   ISBN 0–7216–2856–7

Printed in the United States of America.

Last digit is the print number: 9   8   7   6   5   4   3   2   1

Contributors

THOMAS S. AHRENS, RN, DNS, CCRN
Clinical Nurse Specialist, Critical Care, Barnes
Hospital, St. Louis, Missouri
Respiratory Monitoring

CYNTHIA L. ALLEN, RN, MSN
Staff Nurse, Cardiovascular ICU, Emory University
Hospital, Atlanta, Georgia
Patients with Sepsis

CAROL F. BAKER, RN, PhD
Assistant Professor, Ohio State University,
Columbus, Ohio
Acid-Base Physiology

RITA M. BARDEN, RN, MSN, CCRN
Instructor, ADN Program, Southwestern College,
Chula Vista, California
Patients with Hypertension

MARILYN ROSSMAN BARTUCCI, RN, MSN, CS,
CCTC
Clinical Instructor, Medical-Surgical Nursing, Case
Western Reserve University, Frances Payne Bolton
School of Nursing; Head Nurse Manager,
Transplant Center, University Hospitals of
Cleveland, Cleveland, Ohio
Organ Donation

MARIA BEASLEY DIXON, RN, MS
Clinical Nurse Specialist, SICU/Trauma Unit,
UCI Medical Center, Orange, California
Patients with Vascular Emergencies

CHRISTINE BREU, RN, MN, CNAA
Director of Nursing, Humana Hospital Suburban,
Louisville, Kentucky
Editor of Sections 2, 5, 8

TERESA L. BRITT, RN, MS
Case Manager Supervisor, Carle
Clinical Studies, Champaign, Illinois
Elderly Patients

S. DANIELLE BROWN, RN, MS, CCRN
Clinical Nurse Specialist, Ballard Community
Hospital, Seattle, Washington
*Patients with Disorders of the Thyroid and
Neurohypophysis*

RANDY M. CAINE, RN, EdD, CS, CCRN
Professor of Nursing, California State University,
Long Beach, Long Beach, California
Patients with Burns

VICTOR G. CAMPBELL, RN, PhD
Assistant Professor, Ohio State University,
Columbus, Ohio
Neurophysiology

MARY M. CANOBBIO, RN, MN, MPH
Cardiovascular Clinical Specialist, Assistant Clinical
Professor, UCLA School of Nursing, Los Angeles,
California
Patients with Congenital Heart Defects

SUZETTE CARDIN, RN, MS, CCRN
Nurse Manager, Cardiac Care Unit/Cardiac
Observation Unit, UCLA Medical Center, Los
Angeles, California
***Editor of Sections 3, 4, 12; *** *Patients with
Cardiomyopathies*

KATHLEEN McMAHON CASEY, RN, MEd, MA
National Clinical Director, HIV Care Program,
Critical Care America, Westborough, Massachusetts
Patients with HIV-Related Disease and AIDS

LUCINDA H. CAVE, RN, MSN
Formerly Clinical Nurse Specialist, University
Hospitals of Cleveland, Cleveland, Ohio
Patients with HIV-Related Disease and AIDS

SUZANNE CLARK, RN, MSN, MA, CS
Clinical Nurse Specialist, Department of Psychiatry,
Kaiser Permanente Foundation, Los Angeles,
California
Psychosocial Needs of Critically Ill Patients

JOHN M. CLOCHESY, RN, MS, CS, FCCM
Instructor, Acute and Critical Care Nursing, Frances
Payne Bolton School of Nursing, Case Western
Reserve University, Cleveland, Ohio
Editor of Sections 1, 9, 13; Patients with Sepsis

BERNICE COLEMAN, RN, MSN, CCRN
Clinical Nurse Specialist, Cardiovascular Surgery,
Patient Care Services, Cedars-Sinai Medical Center,
Los Angeles, California
Patients Undergoing Cardiac Surgery

PATRICIA McCALL COMOSS, RN, BS, FAACVPR
Nursing Enrichment Consultants, Inc., Harrisburg,
Pennsylvania
*Optimizing Patient Recovery (Inpatient Cardiac
Rehabilitation)*

PATRIA E. CONSTANCIA, RN, MN
Clinical Nurse Specialist, Adult Cardiothoracic
Surgery, Department of Cardiodiagnostics, UCLA
Medical Center, Los Angeles, California
Patient Education

DIANE COOPER, RN, MN
Assistant Dean of Student Affairs, UCLA School of
Nursing, Los Angeles, California
Patients with Obstructive Pulmonary Disease

BARBARA J. DALY, RN, MSN, FAAN
Assistant Director of Nursing, University Hospitals
of Cleveland, Cleveland, Ohio
Ethics in Critical Care

JOANNE M. DISCH, RN, PhD, FAAN
Senior Associate Director/Director of Nursing,
University of Minnesota Hospital and Clinic,
Minneapolis, Minnesota
Effect of the Economic Environment on Patient Care

PETER R. DOYLE, BS, RCP, RRT
Clinical Specialist, Puritan Bennett Group,
Carlsbad, California
Advances in Mechanical Ventilation

DIANE K. DRESSLER, RN, MSN, CCTC
Clinical Cardiac Transplant Coordinator, Midwest
Heart Surgery Institute, Ltd., Milwaukee,
Wisconsin
Hematologic Physiology; Patients with Coagulopathies

ELAINE L. ENGER, RN, MS
Clinical Director, Midwest Heart Research
Foundation, Lombard, Illinois; Adjunct Facility,
University of Illinois at Chicago, Chicago, Illinois
Patients with Adult Respiratory Distress Syndrome

DeANN M. ENGLERT, RN, MN, CNSN
Nurse Manager, Caremark, Inc., Houston, Texas
Patients with Gastrointestinal Bleeding

JULIE FLEURY, RN, PhD
Postdoctoral Fellow, University of Arizona College
of Nursing, Tucson, Arizona
Patients with Coronary Artery Disease

DORRIE K. FONTAINE, RN, DNSc, CCRN
Assistant Professor and Coordinator,
Trauma/Critical Care Nursing, University of
Maryland School of Nursing, Baltimore, Maryland
Effect of Sensory Alterations

GERALDINE M. GOOSEN, RN, PhD
Assistant Professor and Director, Critical Care
Graduate Program, University of Texas Medical
Branch, Galveston, Texas
Patients with Pain

STACEY B. GROSS, RN, MS, CCRN, CS
Clinical Nurse Specialist, Cardiothoracic Surgery,
Boston University Medical Center, University
Hospital, Boston, Massachusetts
Patients Undergoing Cardiac Surgery

GINNY WACKER GUIDO, RN, JD
University of Texas Health Science Center School of
Nursing, Houston, Texas
Legal Issues in Critical Care

JAN L. HAWTHORNE, RN, MSN, OCN
Oncology Clinical Nurse Specialist, University
Hospitals of Cleveland; Clinical Faculty, Frances
Payne Bolton School of Nursing, Case Western
Reserve University, Cleveland, Ohio
Immunocompromised Patients

MARGARET HEITKEMPER, RN, PhD
Professor, Department of Physiological Nursing,
University of Washington, Seattle, Washington
Gastrointestinal Physiology

ELIZABETH A. HENNEMAN, RN, MS, CCRN
Clinical Nurse Specialist, UCLA Medical Center,
Los Angeles, California
Patients with Acute Respiratory Failure

KATHRYN HENNESSY, RN, MS, CNSN
Northwest Gastroenterologists, SC, Arlington
Heights, Illinois
Patients with Acute Pancreatitis

MAIREAD HICKEY, RN, PhD
Yale School of Nursing, New Haven, Connecticut
Psychosocial Needs of Families

BECKY J. HULL, RN, MS
Perinatal Clinical Nurse Specialist, University
Medical Center, Tucson, Arizona
Patients with Obstetric Crises

LUCILLE T. KADOTA, RN, MN, CCRN
Nurse Practitioner, Surgery Center, UCLA Medical
Plaza, Los Angeles, California
Hemodynamic Monitoring

MARCIA L. KEEN, RN, MSN, PhD CANDIDATE
Director of Clinical Research, Fresenius USA,
Concord, California
Patients with Fluid and Electrolyte Disturbances

KATHY KIGERL, RN, MN
Department Director, Perinatal Services, Henry
Mayo Newhall Memorial Hospital, Valencia,
California
Patients with Disorders of Glucose Metabolism

CHRISTINE RESTIFO KRAAY, BSN, MSN
Intracranial Pressure Monitoring

MARY COUGHLAN LAVIERI, RN, MS, CCRN
Clinical Nurse III, Surgical Intensive Unit, Beth
Israel Hospital, Boston, Massachusetts
Patients Undergoing Cardiac Surgery

NANCY D. LEFCOURT, RN, MSN, CCRN
Former Clinical Nurse Specialist, Burn Center, UCI
Medical Center, Orange, California
Patients with Burns

BRIAN D. LEHR, RN, ND
Staff Nurse, Department of Veterans Affairs
Medical Center, Louisville, Kentucky
Consultant for Nursing Care Plans

NORLEE K. MANLEY, RN, BSN, CD
Deputy Director, Veterans Addiction Recovery
Center, Department of Veterans Affairs Medical
Center, Cleveland, Ohio
Patients with Chemical Dependency

LINDA K. MENZEL, RN, PhD(c), CCRN
Doctoral Candidate, Case Western Reserve
University, Cleveland, Ohio
ECG Interpretation

CAROLYN L. MURDAUGH, RN, PhD, CCRN
Associate Professor, University of Arizona College
of Nursing, Tucson, Arizona
Patients with Coronary Artery Disease

MARTY NASON, BSN, MN
Executive Director, The Wellness Community–
Valley/Ventura, Westlake Village, California
Psychosocial Needs of Critical Care Staff

SUSAN JOY NELSON, RN, MN, CCRN
Senior Analyst, Blue Shield of California, Medical
Protcol Development, Canoga Park, California
Patients After Near Drowning

DONNA C. OWEN, RN, PhD
Assistant Professor, Emory University, Atlanta,
Georgia
Physiologic Response to Infection

PATRICIA PESCHMAN, RN, MS
Renal Clinical Nurse Specialist, Abbott
Northwestern Hospital, Minneapolis, Minnesota
Renal Physiology

PAULA RABINOWITZ, RN, MSN
Adjunct Instructor, Kent State University, Kent,
Ohio; Director of Nursing, Behavioral Health,
Robinson Memorial Hospital, Ravenna, Ohio
Patients with Chemical Dependency

VIRGINIA A. RAHR, RN
University of Texas School of Nursing, Galveston,
Texas
Patients with Pain

BARBARA RIEGEL, RN, DNSc, CS
Adjunct Facility, School of Nursing, San Diego
State University; Clinical Researcher, Critical Care
Division, Sharp Memorial Hospital, San Diego,
California
Patients with Myocardial Infarction

JUNE HART ROMEO, RN, BSN, MAEd,
PhD Candidate
Adjunct Faculty, Cleveland State University; Nurse
Clinician, Department of Veterans Affairs Medical
Center, Cleveland, Ohio
Patients with Craniotomies

MARCIA E. ROSTAD, RN, MS, NS
Nursing Administration, University Medical Center,
Tucson, Arizona
Patients with Oncologic Emergencies

ELLEN B. RUDY, RN, PhD, FAAN
Dean, School of Nursing, University of Pittsburgh,
Pittsburgh, Pennsylvania
Editor of Sections 6, 11, 15; Brain Death

SUSAN D. RUPPERT, RN, PhD(c), MSN, CCRN
Assistant Professor, The University of Texas Health
Science Center at Houston School of Nursing,
Houston, Texas
Patients with Gastrointestinal Bleeding

SHELLEY RUZEVICH, RN
Nurse Clinician, Circulatory Support, UCLA
Medical Center, Los Angeles, California
Cardiac Assist Devices

CATHERINE J. RYAN, RN, MS, CCRN
Clinical Nurse Specialist—Critical Care, Alexian
Brothers Medical Center, Elk Grove Village, Illinois
Patients with Pulmonary Infections

MICHAEL A. SALATKA, JD, MPH
Cleveland, Ohio
Effect of Occupational Hazards

LINDA H. SCHAKENBACH, RN, MSN, CCRN, CS
Clinical Nurse Specialist, Fairfax Hospital, Falls
Church, Virginia
Patients with Valvular Disease

JUDY SELFRIDGE, RN, MSN, CEM, MICN
Clinical Nurse Specialist, Emergency Department,
St. Mary Medical Center, Long Beach, California
Patients with Trauma

MARY CUSELLA SELLER, RN, MSN, CS
Clinical Nurse Specialist, John Muir Hospital,
Walnut Creek, California
Physiologic Response to Infection

SHEILA SANNING SHEA, RN, MSN, CEN
Clinical Nurse Specialist, Department of Emergency
Medicine, St. Mary Medical Center, Long Beach,
California
Patients with Trauma

VERNA MEDINA SITZER, RN, MN, CCRN
Clinical Nurse Specialist, MICU/CCU, Sharp
Memorial Hospital, San Diego, California
Effect of Communication Patterns

PHYLITA SKOV, RN, MS
Assistant Clinical Professor, Department of
Physiological Nursing, University of California, San
Francisco, San Francisco, California
Cardiovascular Anatomy and Physiology

SUSAN L. SMITH, RN, MN, CCRN
Associate Professor, Emory University School of
Nursing; Clinical Nurse Specialist, Liver

Transplantation, Emory University Hospital,
Atlanta, Georgia
Patients with Liver Dysfunction

GARY SPARGER, RN, MSN, CEN, MICN
Late Coordinator, Trauma/Emergency CNS
Program, California State University, Long Beach,
Long Beach, California
Patients with Trauma

KATHLEEN S. STONE, RN, PhD, RN
Professor, Ohio State University, Columbus, Ohio
Respiratory Physiology

NANCY A. STOTTS, RN, EdD
Associate Professor, University of California, San
Francisco; Clinical Associate, Medical Center at the
University of California, San Francisco, San
Francisco, California
Wound Healing

JEREMIAH SUHL, MD
Pulmonary Disease and Critical Care Medicine,
Lexington Clinic, Lexington, Kentucky
Patients with Shock

NANCY L. SZAFLARSKI, RN, MS, CCRN, FCCM
Doctoral Student, Department of Physiological
Nursing, University of California, San Francisco,
San Francisco, California
Immobility Phenomena in Critically Ill Adults

KATHRYN SABO THOMPSON, RN, MSN
Project Leader, Special Care Unit, University
Hospitals of Cleveland, Cleveland, Ohio
Patients with Guillain-Barré Syndrome

PATRICIA L. VASKA, RN, MSN, CCRN
Cardiovascular Surgery Clinical Nurse Specialist,
Sioux Valley Hospital, Sioux Falls, South Dakota
Cardiovascular Anatomy and Physiology

CONNIE A. WALLECK, RN, MS, CNRN, FCCM
Adjunct Assistant Professor, SUNY Health Science
Center at Syracuse, School of Nursing; Senior
Associate Director of Nursing, University Hospital,
SUNY Health Science Center at Syracuse, Syracuse,
New York
Patients with Head Injury and Brain Dysfunction;
Patients with Spinal Cord Injury

UNA E. WESTFALL
Associate Professor, Department of Adult Health
and Illness, School of Nursing, Oregon Health
Sciences University, Portland, Oregon
Gastrointestinal Physiology

JoANNE D. WHITNEY, RN, PhD
Assistant Professor, University of Washington,
Seattle, Washington
Wound Healing

CHRISTINA M. WHITNEY-RAINBOLT, RN, MSN
Adjunct Assistant Professor, Montana State
University, Bozeman, Montana
Patients with Cerebral Vascular Disorders

ALICE A. WHITTAKER, RN, MS, CCRN
Instructor, Creighton University, Mary Lanning
Campus, Hastings, Nebraska
Editor of Sections 7, 10, 14, 15; *Patients with Acute
Renal Failure*

DONNA J. WILSON, RN, RRT
Pulmonary Clinical Nurse Specialist, Nursing
Department, Memorial Sloan-Kettering Cancer
Center, New York, New York
Chronic Ventilator-Dependent Patients

GINGER SCHAFER WLODY, RN, MS, FCCM
Assistant Clinical Professor, UCLA School of
Nursing; Director of Quality Management,
Department of Veterans Affairs Medical Center,
Wadsworth Division, Los Angeles, California
Preventing Post-anesthesia Complications

JOHN WRIGHT, BS, RRT
Assistant Director of Respiratory Therapy, UCLA
Medical Center, Los Angeles, California
Advances in Mechanical Ventilation

SYLVIA YARIAN, RN, MSN
Hemodialysis Research Nurse, Davies Medical
Center, San Francisco, California
Patients with End-Stage Renal Disease

GARY YOSHIHARA, BA, RRT, RCP
Clinical Supervisor, Huntington Memorial Hospital,
Pasadena, California
Advances in Mechanical Ventilation

Foreword

Over the last three decades, the specialty of critical care and the profession of nursing have interacted in some very important ways. Clearly, critical care, as a nursing specialty, has had an important impact on the profession. The first of these effects is related to nursing's image. When critical care evolved in the late 1960s, nurses working in intensive care units (ICUs) developed a knowledge level and confidence rarely seen in the hospital setting. The patients that nurses cared for in the ICUs were physiologically unstable and, often, desperately ill. Nurses in these early units were technically proficient and highly knowledgeable clinicians. Medical house staff learned from them. Families and patients were grateful for their competence and compassion. Over the years, the image of nursing has been greatly enhanced by critical care nurses who often have embodied the best of our profession to the public.

Second, the relationship between medicine and nursing was (and still is) positively affected by the specialty of critical care. An intensive care unit is an arena where nurses and physicians must work collaboratively, in an atmosphere of mutual respect, or patient care is tragically compromised. Since economic competition usually is not at issue (as opposed to specialties such as obstetrics and midwifery or anesthesia), the incentives to develop productive working relationships have resulted in numerous collaborative efforts at the local and national level, as well as at the bedside. Joint position statements between medicine and nursing (e.g., the American Association of Critical-Care Nurses and the Society of Critical Care Medicine), joint educational efforts, and numerous liason activities on national committees all reflect the positive nature of physician-nurse collaboration within the specialty.

A final sphere of influence for critical care nurses is in the area of nursing science. Nurses specializing in critical care are highly proficient in the medical model. They need to understand the physiology and pathophysiology of the organ systems and be able to respond quickly and intelligently to subtle alterations in a critically ill patient. In fact, part of the respect accorded to nurses by physicians in those early days of critical care was based on the knowledge that critical care nurses had in the science of medicine.

Critical care nurses' comfort with and appreciation for the medical model have led to important discussions within the nursing community. In the nursing diagnosis movement, it is critical care nurses who have demanded that the movement's leaders consider physiologic problems and distinguish how these might be different than medical diagnoses. They have grappled with how to merge the medical model, a model that has provided the framework for their practice in the ICU, with models that are unique to nursing. They have continued to ask how nursing models, which are often conceptually clear in a setting that emphasizes health prevention or rehabilitation, can be applied to the patient with multisystem failure.

Critical care is a highly interdisciplinary specialty. ICU nurses need to be able to communicate with other members of the health team in a meaningful way. They have demanded of nurse theorists that the nursing models and diagnoses currently being proposed and tested be conceptually clear; easy to understand by professionals outside of nursing; and meaningful in the setting of an acute, catastrophic illness. I believe that these demands help keep the nursing profession honest and, ultimately, will result in nursing frameworks that are more cogent to practice.

In summary, the specialty of critical care has positively influenced nursing's image, enhanced the collaborative relationships between physicians and nurses, and positively influenced the development of nursing theory. But how has nursing influenced critical care?

By definition, nursing is concerned with human responses to illness. The patients who require care in an intensive care unit are frequently sustained by a potpourri of machinery. As every ICU nurse can attest, there are times when such individuals seem remotely human. It's hard to imagine them inhabiting a life outside of the ICU cubicle, dressed, going to work, surrounded by family and friends. In the ICU, they are a collection of organs operating at a submaximal level. Nusing's orientation to care rather than cure has continued to be a humanizing force in the ICU. By focusing on patient responses, ICU nurses treat not only a patient's renal failure but also the confusion and fear that results from severe electrolyte disturbance. Intensive care nurses move beyond the technical demands of patient care to care for the individual who is often frightened and confused. Their preparation and identity as nurses helps ICU nurses to see patients as the individuals they are—not just a collection of body systems.

Nursing also has a focus of care that goes beyond the patient to the family system. The profession's commitment to the family as our unit of care (rather than just the patient) helps remind busy ICU nurses that when they spend time supporting distraught family members, they are performing just as critical a function as when they are assessing the hemodynamic status of a patient and titrating drugs. The orientation of our profession helps remind us that both are valuable functions. We are constantly enriched by this reminder.

This reference text constitutes an important contribution to critical care literature. It provides nurses, both students and experienced clinicians, with the latest information on critical care practice. It will be an invaluable reference to nurses who need to know the latest scientific data on which to base their clinical decision-making.

I also believe that this text stands as an excellent example of the "philosophical marriage" of nursing and the speciality of critical care. It reflects the integration of medical and nursing knowledge that makes the most sense in the setting of an intensive care unit. The book is organized by body systems, and the authors have integrated nursing care, and the data that contribute to the science of that care, throughout their discussions. The editors have also included sections that reflect the unique perspective of nursing. For example, no matter what organ systems are affected, critically ill patients suffer from mobility restrictions. They experience sensory deprivation or sensory overload. They struggle to communicate, despite endotracheal tubes, tracheostomies, sedation, and fatigue. They feel frightened, powerless, and confused. None of these problems are described within the medical model, and yet often they constitute the patient's biggest challenge to recovery. It is nurses' empathetic and compassionate caring that often makes the difference in a patient's recovery. It is also nurses' knowledge translated into clinical decisions that saves lives. This text covers these aspects.

This text is a suberb compilation of the latest biologic, social, behavioral, and nursing knowledge related to the critically ill. It is an important source book for nursing students and for critical care nurses who, despite having many years of experience in the ICU, always strive to learn more.

KATHLEEN DRACUP
Professor
School of Nursing
University of California
Los Angeles

Preface

The focus of critical care nursing is to provide care for patients who are experiencing a life-threatening or potentially life-threatening illness or injury. The nursing care that is provided is intended to restore health, alleviate suffering and pain, and preserve the rights and dignity of individuals. In cases where life is no longer possible, critical care nurses assist patients to a humane and dignified death. In caring for critically ill patients, nurses continuously observe and monitor the patients for physiologic and psychological alterations, plan and carry out interventions that compensate for altered body functioning, and recognize both complications and improvements in response to therapeutic modalities.

With advances in biomedical technology, diagnostic procedures, and clinical therapeutics, critically ill patients are treated in a complex and highly charged milieu. Providing competent nursing care to critically ill patients requires that critical care nurses have a broad knowledge base, demonstrate expert clinical and decision-making skills, and share a commitment to nursing's ethical and professional values.

KNOWLEDGE FOR CRITICAL CARE NURSING

The practice base for critical care nursing requires knowledge from the biologic, behavioral, social, and nursing domains. This knowledge is not static and thus requires a life-long commitment to learning. Critical care nursing requires a thorough understanding of the relatedness of the body systems, including the reciprocal relationship between the physiologic, psychological, social, and spiritual dimensions of the person, as well as an understanding of the dynamic nature of the life process.

Knowledge, the elusive goal of education, can be gained through a variety of formal and informal means, and requires the recognition that it belongs only to those who seek it out. The purpose of this book is to share knowledge from critical care experts with those students and practitioners who wish to broaden their knowledge base. For the most part, the book is organized according to body systems. While some will lament this as not uniquely nursing, it is, nonetheless, the universally accepted organization given to the human body, and is one that critical care nurses are most familiar with and use in their practice.

Within critical care, the perspective of nursing comes not in isolating nursing from the other disciplines. Rather, it arises from the application of knowledge from other disciplines in conjunction with knowledge from nursing science in a way that recognizes the wholeness of the individual, provides care and comfort to the critically ill patient, and continually seeks new ways to expand knowledge.

PRACTICE OF CRITICAL CARE NURSING

Nursing is a practice discipline, and as such, the profession is judged by the care it provides to patients and the value that society places on that care. In the specialty of critical care nursing, clinical competency focuses on the ability to detect and respond to life-threatening situations in an effective, ethical, and humane manner.

Critically ill patients are particularly vulnerable because of the disease states that put them at physiologic, psychological, and pharmacologic risk. These risks to the patient's integrity are compounded by the environment in which care is delivered. The fast-paced, labor-intensive environment, while life-saving in its technology and vigilance, makes nursing an essential element in coupling care with compassion.

As we move from replacing heart valves to transplanting entire hearts, nurses learn new ways of treating old problems and are introduced to new technologies that replace old ones. The stresses inherent within this environment require the critical care nurse to create a compassionate, humanistic, and flexible approach to care. This care, which provides support to patients, families, and colleagues, is predicated on a respect for the dignity, value, and rights of each individual person.

Critical care nurses who strive to improve their clinical practice will seek new experiences, expand their knowledge base, and take responsibility for their practice decisions. The practice of critical care nursing requires continual growth of the individual nurse, both professionally and intellectually. In addition, autonomy over practice decisions and accountability for the care delivered are required. Because of the continued advancements in biomedical technology and their impact on patients, critical care nursing remains challenging and ever-changing.

COMMITMENT TO CRITICAL CARE NURSING

As nursing seeks to promote its professional values, so too must the practitioners portray a commitment to these values. Within critical care nursing, there is a commitment to quality patient care for all those entrusted to our care; a level of personal conduct that respects personal worth and ensures compassion for others; a recognition of the ethical responsibilities of care; and an appreciation of the collaborative nature of critical care. These values can be expressed both personally and professionally, but can only be strengthened as we become a coherent whole within our profession.

As with other commitments in life, a commitment to the professional values of critical care nursing is strengthened as experienced nurses help the novices, as service and education develop collaborative ties, and as individual nurses mature and develop within their professional roles.

As editors of this book for critical care nurses, it is our hope that each of you share our belief in the need to continually update your knowledge base, evaluate your practice skill, and reaffirm your commitment to critical care nursing. The contributors to this book join us in striving for a continued productive future in critical care nursing.

JOHN CLOCHESY
CHRISTINE BREU
SUZETTE CARDIN
ELLEN RUDY
ALICE WHITTAKER

Contents

S·E·C·T·I·O·N

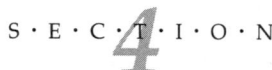

Cardiovascular System, 229

S·E·C·T·I·O·N

5

Pulmonary System, 485

S·E·C·T·I·O·N

6

Nervous System, 641

S·E·C·T·I·O·N

7

Renal System, 827

S·E·C·T·I·O·N 10
Hematologic System, 1045

S·E·C·T·I·O·N 11
Immune System, 1073

S·E·C·T·I·O·N
12
Integumentary System, 1165

S·E·C·T·I·O·N
13
Multisystem Disorders, 1217

S · E · C · T · I · O · N
14
Special Clinical Situations, 1301

S · E · C · T · I · O · N
15
Advocacy, 1373

Environments of Care

1

Effect of the Economic Environment on Patient Care

Joanne Disch

During the past 10 years, a revolution has been launched within the health care industry. The source of this revolution was the institution of prospective reimbursement through Diagnosis-Related Groups (DRGs). Not since the emergence of Medicare and Medicaid in the 1960s has there been such a force for change in health care. However, as far-reaching as the use of DRGs has proved to be, they represent only the tip of the iceberg. Massive changes even more pervasive than the use of DRGs are unfolding within health care.

This chapter presents a framework within which to view not only the emergence of DRGs but also the extensive changes now occurring in the American health care system. In addition, an evaluation of the impact of the prospective reimbursement system to this point is offered, and finally, implications for nurses practicing within this system are highlighted.

BACKGROUND FOR CHANGE

Assumptions Have Changed. Although a tremendous transformation has occurred in the production and distribution of health care services within the past 10 years, much of the current picture can be understood by focusing on three major changes. The first of these is that basic assumptions underlying the health care industry have changed. Assumptions are perceptions of reality that, to the extent that they are true, offer help in examining situations and determining courses of action. To the extent that they are false, however, they lead to wrong conclusions and result in lost time and energy. Up to this point our health care system has operated under certain assumptions, which have now changed.

The first assumption was that equal health care for all was a major priority. Interwoven into the American tradition is a sense of democracy, equality, justice, and fairness arising from the belief that all men are created equal and no one person is better than another. This tradition is based on humanitarian principles:

To each person according to fair opportunity

To each person according to basic needs

To each person according to individual needs

From this philosophy comes the belief that no individual should be either granted or denied benefits for factors over which he has no control. Because health is a societal priority, society should help individuals who need assistance in attaining it. Therefore, everyone should have equal access to the same level of health care. Those who are least advantaged or whose basic needs are most in jeopardy may require special assistance to reach the point of equal care. But a certain level of health care for all citizens is the goal.

A second assumption underlying our approach to health care has been that we have unlimited resources, especially for priorities like health care and social welfare. We as a nation have access to bright people, adequate financial resources, a sense of dedication, and new technologies. Advertisements on television and in the print media proclaim, "What mankind can dream, technology can achieve."

3

A third assumption closely linked to the second has been that, although perhaps our resources are not unlimited, health care is such a high priority that a major portion of our country's resources should be devoted to providing it.

Why have these assumptions changed? Four reasons might be offered. In some ways, health care has been too successful. Knowledge and research have enabled us to save infants who previously would have died, to prolong life of seriously ill patients far beyond expectations, to extend the life of the elderly, to develop therapies and equipment for the replacement of almost all body parts, and to use disposable medical supplies almost exclusively to save time and enhance convenience. Societal expectations about the elements constituting even baseline care have now been raised.

A second factor that has caused a rethinking of our underlying assumptions is the tremendous rise in the cost of providing care. In 1950, health care expenditures totalled $10.8 billion; in 1989, that rose to $604 billion, which equals 11.6% of our Gross National Product and, incidentally, an average of $2354 spent for every person in the United States (Levit et al., 1991; Division of National Cost Estimates, 1987) (Fig. 1–1).

A third factor forcing a reexamination of basic assumptions is the emergence of other national non-health related priorities that clamored for attention. Other equally pressing concerns demanded funds: education for children, food for the hungry, housing for the indigent, national defense.

A fourth factor was the growing suspicion that, in spite of the incredible financial outlay for the health care sector, the return on the investment was inadequate. A poll commissioned by the Robert Wood Johnson Foundation in 1982 found that access to health care was woefully inadequate: One in eight Americans had serious difficulty in obtaining medical treatment, and one in nine had no regular source of health care. Of most concern was the finding that 1 million families had at least one family member who had been refused care for financial reasons (Aday et al., 1984). At present, approximately 31 million Americans receive no financial assistance for medical care expenses (Moyer, 1989).

In short, with the increasing cost of health care came the realization that neither quality of care nor access to care was improving accordingly. Perceptions about realistic health goals and capabilities were challenged. Financial considerations forced changes in the basic assumptions underlying health care and the emergence of new ones. These new assumptions have been made operable by policy makers:

1. Health care is a priority but only one of many.
2. The cost of health care must be brought into line.
3. A change in the system of health care delivery is necessary.

The Goal for Health Care Is Cost-Containment. The second major change affecting the health care industry in the United States is the institution of a new goal: cost-containment. Prior to the enactment of prospective payment legislation, hospitals were able to pursue a number of goals—among them, augmenting the status of the hospital, expanding the range of services, serving as a community resource, offering optimal quality care, maximizing output. Most institutions pursued several goals; occasionally cost-minimization was one of them.

However, the focus has changed. Hospitals are now vitally concerned about the costs of the care they provide because the mechanism for reimbursement has changed. Through a prospective reimbursement methodology, hospitals are paid a standardized amount according to patient diagnosis and other selected variables. If the hospital spends less on a patient's hospitalization, it essentially keeps the balance; if costs exceed the standardized amount, the hospital incurs a debt. Consequently, there is now great incentive to:

Decrease the length of patient stay

Increase the hospital's mix of patients for whom reimbursement is profitable

Increase the turnover of patients

Decrease the costs of providing care

DRGs have provided an incentive and a mechanism

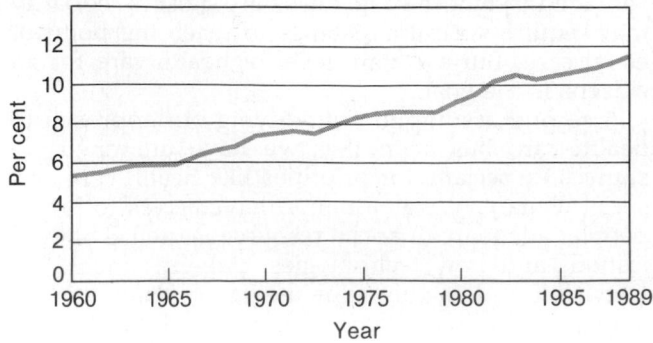

National Health Expenditures as Percentage of Gross National Product, 1960–1989

FIGURE 1–1. National health expenditures as percentage of Gross National Product, 1960–1989. (From Levit, K. R., Lazenby, H. C., Letach, S. W., and Cowan, C. A. (1991). National health care spending, 1989. *Health Affairs*, 10(1), 117–130.)

by which hospitals and other providers have been encouraged to control the costs of health care. But they are not an end in themselves.

Man is a clever animal who will discover new tools. A fatal error could be to think tools are the solution.

JOHN HESS

A Competitive Health Care Market Has Been Established. Just as DRGs are not an end in themselves, neither is cost-containment for hospitals. The new direction in the health care industry is toward a more competitive environment. A competitive market is one in which there are many buyers and sellers of a service or product. Both buyers and sellers are involved in a transaction, and negotiation centers around the price or cost of the service. Both buyers and sellers have some sensitivity to the cost, i.e., there is some financial stake or benefit in the decisions made by each. Finally, buyers are actively involved in choosing among alternatives, which implies that there are alternatives from which to choose. In other words, barriers to practice must be eliminated, and qualified providers must have equal access to the system.

An example serves to illustrate how a competitive market works. A woman planning to have a child today is usually able to select from several alternatives, for instance, a birthing center, home birth, or a hospital maternity ward. For the delivery, she can be assisted by a nurse midwife or an obstetrician. In choosing among alternatives, the woman probably considers such factors as her previous experience with and beliefs about childbirth, her health and that of the baby, the services offered by the different providers, and the cost of the care. Possibly other considerations might be part of the decision, as they are when any purchase is made—for example, the personality of the provider, the confidence he or she inspires, the concern expressed about the mother's worries, or the availability of financial support. The choice one mother makes is often very different from that made by another mother. But the existence of choices is one of the benefits of a competitive system.

Contrast this scenario with the health care system in place prior to the advent of prospective reimbursement. Physicians (obstetricians in this example) were the gatekeepers of the system, acting as agents for the mother, making decisions about the kind or form of childbirth to be used, the need for or extent of anesthesia, the setting. In addition, they controlled the choice of other caregivers who might be utilized. Alternative choices were rarely available, partly because of restrictive barriers that prevented other caregivers from giving care that directly competed with the care provided by physicians but also because of ignorance by the public about the existence of these alternative caregivers. Until recently, bans on advertising were in place to keep the public ignorant of other choices. Neither physicians nor patients were motivated to seek cost-effective therapies. Many patients were protected from the cost of care by extensive, almost total insurance coverage. Physicians, too, were protected from concerns about the cost of care by comprehensive third-party reimbursement. Consequently, a health care system was in place that (1) was driven by physicians as both major providers of care and decision makers, and (2) was insensitive to the costs being generated. Naturally, in this kind of system patients wanted the best because they need not be concerned about paying for it, and physicians wanted to use the best and the latest equipment, which saved their time and protected them from malpractice claims. Physicians also wanted quality through good results, but if there were two ways to achieve the same quality endpoint, little motivation existed to select the less expensive method, particularly if the other therapy were faster, newer, or more innovative.

Proponents of competition cite several advantages. First, competition involves all parties directly in the medical transaction. Individuals who participate actively in a transaction are believed to better represent their wishes and demands than if an intermediary is used. Second, individuals who are actively involved are more price conscious. If they have a stake in the outcome, people are more likely to be alert and at least somewhat informed, to identify, question, and possibly eliminate unnecessary services whether they are patients seeking care or physicians providing it. Research shows that when individuals have a financial incentive, they do choose more judiciously: In one study, those patients who had to pay a portion of their medical bills out of pocket made one-third fewer ambulatory visits and were hospitalized one-third less often (Free medical care, 1984).

Obviously, there are negative possibilities with this kind of system. An increase in price consciousness may overcorrect the problem and may lead to excesses in the opposite direction, such as individuals failing to seek needed care or waiting until the current problem becomes more serious, requiring even more resources to correct. Also, in a competitive system there may be a failure to distinguish between low prices due to efficiency and low prices due to poor quality. There may be trimming or outright slashing of needed resources. Finally, in a system such as this an unequal burden may be placed on those most needing assistance. If needed services are cut under the guise of efficiency, those least able to fend for themselves may be severely affected.

In general, a movement has evolved toward greater choices and options, toward increased participation by consumers of health care, and toward a concern for cost. Barriers that limit certain practitioners from offering legitimate services are coming down. Whereas previously a major portion of health care was directed by physicians in hospitals, now care is being provided by alternative providers. Tremendously innovative and creative changes have been made.

THE CURRENT ECONOMIC ENVIRONMENT

Although the objective of the health care revolution has been clear—to contain costs without significantly compromising quality—the results have been less clear. Certainly there has been an increased focus on the cost of care, but has less money or resources been spent? A competitive market suggests that a number of changes in the way health care is produced and distributed need to be made, but have these changes been realized? Satisfaction with health care is a function of several factors, among them expectations of care and access to it, but in what ways have the level of care and general access changed?

According to economic theory, in a competitive environment, certain predictable changes should occur: (1) new providers of a service emerge, some of whom represent creative alternatives to the traditional delivery pattern; (2) providers compete on the cost of producing the service, encouraging efficiency and cost-effectiveness; (3) consumers participate more actively in decision making related to the service, choosing among alternatives at least partially on the basis of price; and (4) marketing and advertising of services increase. This section presents findings from studies that have examined the impact of recent changes in the health care system on several key variables, among them the cost of care, the utilization of health care services, the distribution of and access to health care, and the quality of care. Based on an analysis of current trends, future directions for a health care focus are outlined.

Impact of Prospective Reimbursement on Hospitals

Between 1983 and 1987, more than 45,000 beds were removed from service (American Hospital Association, 1987). During that time 128 urban hospitals and 116 rural facilities closed their doors, compared with 73 and 47 hospitals, respectively, during the years between 1980 and 1983 (McCarthy, 1988).

The financial impact of the prospective reimbursement system on hospitals is equivocal. For example, in 1986, average Medicare margins were 8.2%, but one-third of the country's hospitals lost money on Medicare patients. Conversely, approximately 25% of hospitals enjoyed profits in excess of 12.7% (Prospective Payment Assessment Commission, 1988). What has seemed to emerge is a situation in which hospitals are differentially affected by a variety of factors, among them size, location, fiscal pressure, and ownership (Hadley et al., 1989).

The potential impact on teaching hospitals is of particular interest. Although costs are higher for these institutions, some studies have suggested that cost differences between teaching and non-teaching hospitals are due to the increased number of diagnostic tests or DRG coding peculiarities, rather than to differences in underlying patient case mix (Goldfarb and Coffey, 1987; Frick et al., 1985; Jones, 1985). Interestingly, in the first year of prospective reimbursement, major teaching hospitals also enjoyed "excess revenues" of 23% (Health Care Financing Administration, 1985). For the next few years, these hospitals continued to experience profits higher than those of other hospitals (Pear, 1988). This trend has begun to change as Congress seeks to reduce the payments to these institutions.

Costs of Health Care

Since 1980, spending for medical care has more than doubled, reaching $604 billion in 1989 (Cantor et al., 1991). Each year since 1985, both hospital spending and health care costs in general have risen faster than the preceding year (Levit et al., 1991) (Table 1–1). Although in a competitive health care environment, costs of health care would be expected to either decrease or level out, this has not consistently been the finding. Although some studies have found that costs have decreased (Melnick and Zwanziger, 1988; McCusker et al., 1988), some researchers have found that costs were higher in competitive markets. For example, in a study of 5732 United States hospitals, Robinson and Luft (1987) found that in markets with more than 10 neighboring hospitals, cost per admission was 26% higher and the average cost per patient in hospitals was 15% higher than in areas where there were fewer hospitals.

A few hypotheses have been put forth to explain the variability in findings. First, it may be that hospitals are competing but not on the basis of price. McLaughlin (1988) differentiates price competition from "rivalry," in which hospitals compete on the basis of services offered or quality provided. Competition in this type of market could potentially increase costs. Second, depending on how costs are defined, there may be differences in whether they are increasing or decreasing. For example, if length of stay is decreasing, average cost per day would be expected to rise, whereas cost per admission could conceivably decrease. Finkler and colleagues (1988) found that as length of stay decreased, the extent and cost of resource use also decreased, in many cases at a proportionately greater rate, such as with supplies and respiratory therapy. A third possible explanation for the variability in findings related to the cost of health care is that there may be a shift toward outpatient care such that hospital costs may be growing less rapidly but overall health care costs continue their exponential rise.

Delivery Patterns of Health Care

Since the advent of prospective reimbursement, hospital admissions for patients over 65 years of age

TABLE 1–1. National Health Expenditures, 1960–1989*

Spending Category	1960	1970	1980	1985	1986	1987	1988	1989
National health expenditures	$27.1	$74.4	$249.1	$420.1	$452.3	$492.5	$544.0	$604.1
Health services and supplies	25.4	69.1	237.8	404.7	436.3	475.2	524.1	583.5
Personal health care	23.9	64.9	218.3	367.2	398.2	436.7	480.0	530.7
Hospital care	9.3	27.9	102.4	167.9	179.4	193.8	211.7	232.8
Physician services	5.3	13.6	41.9	74.0	82.1	93.0	105.1	117.6
Dentist services	2.0	4.7	14.4	23.3	24.7	27.1	29.4	31.4
Other professional services	0.6	1.5	8.7	16.6	18.6	21.2	23.8	27.0
Home health care	0.0	0.1	1.3	3.8	4.0	4.1	4.5	5.4
Drugs and other nondurable medical products	4.2	8.8	20.1	32.3	35.6	38.7	41.5	44.6
Vision products and other durable medical products	0.8	2.0	5.0	8.4	9.5	10.7	12.0	13.5
Nursing home care	1.0	4.9	20.0	34.1	36.7	39.8	42.8	47.9
Other personal health care	0.7	1.4	4.6	6.8	7.6	8.3	9.3	10.5
Program administration and net cost of private insurance	1.2	2.8	12.2	25.2	24.7	23.9	27.9	35.3
Government public health	0.4	1.4	7.2	12.3	13.5	14.7	16.2	17.5
Research and construction	1.7	5.3	11.3	15.4	16.0	17.3	19.8	20.6
Research	0.7	2.0	5.4	7.8	8.5	9.0	10.3	11.0
Construction	1.0	3.4	5.8	7.6	7.4	8.2	9.5	9.6
National health expenditures as percent of GNP	5.3%	7.3%	9.1%	10.5%	10.7%	10.9%	11.2%	11.6%
National health expenditures per capita (dollars)	$143	$346	$1,059	$1,700	$1,813	$1,955	$2,139	$2,354

*National health expenditures, aggregate and average annual growth, selected calendar years 1960–1989, billions of dollars.
Note: Per capita figures are derived using July 1 Social Security area population estimates.
(From Levit, K. R., Lazenby, H. C., Letach, S. W., and Cowan, C. A. (1991). National health care spending, 1989. *Health Affairs,* 10(1), 117–130.)

have declined. In addition, the length of stay for the elderly, previously 10.2 days in 1982, decreased to 8.9 days in 1987 (American Hospital Association, 1987). The percentage of patients using intensive care units (ICUs) and coronary care units (CCUs) dropped significantly for Medicare patients during the period 1980 to 1984, as did the preoperative and postoperative lengths of stay for these patients (DesHarnais et al., 1987).

During the past 10 years, a significant shift to outpatient care has occurred. From 1981 to 1985 the number of outpatient visits increased from 220.9 million to 243.4 million (Managed care, 1986). Moreover, spending for ambulatory services has also grown: up 5.4% from 1977 to 1983, and up 8.6% from 1983 to 1987 (Levit and Freeland, 1988). In particular, the use of ambulatory surgery has seen tremendous growth. In 1980, 16% of hospital operations were performed in outpatient settings; by 1986, that figure had increased to 40% (Prospective Payment Assessment Commission, 1987). This growth in outpatient care has essentially offset the savings obtained from declines in the growth of inpatient services. Consequently, the net result has been that health care costs have continued their upward spiral.

Although health maintenance organizations (HMOs) were in existence prior to the emergence of the prospective reimbursement system they have certainly benefited from the move to a more competitive environment. Membership in HMOs has more than doubled, from 9.1 million Americans in 1980 to approximately 21 million in 1985. In certain areas of the country, the growth rate has been spectacular.

In the Twin Cities area, 42% of the population belongs to an HMO (Managed care, 1986).

In addition to HMOs, other alternative settings for health care delivery have emerged, as would be expected in a more competitive environment. Skilled nursing facilities, urgent care centers, freestanding emergency centers, home health care agencies—these and others are representative of the opportunities that are presently available in a competitive health care market.

Access to Health Care

Currently, it is estimated that 31 million Americans have no insurance or other financial coverage for health care, although some researchers would say that the figure is closer to 36 million if one counts persons eligible only for VA benefits among the uninsured (Moyer, 1989).

Reported earlier in this chapter were findings from a Robert Wood Johnson Foundation study, conducted in 1982, that reflected problems with access to health care. This study was conducted prior to the implementation of the prospective reimbursement system. Since then, two national studies have found some areas of improvement over the 1982 survey, but a number of areas of concern remain.

A repetition of the 1982 study was conducted in 1986 (Freeman et al., 1987). This study involved telephone interviews with 10,130 people in the

United States, representing the population at large. Certain groups were oversampled, such as those with chronic and serious illnesses. Six findings were found to be of particular significance:

1. The overall use of medical care by Americans declined. The percentage of Americans who were hospitalized during the previous year declined 22%; visits to physicians decreased from 81% of Americans in the year prior to the 1982 survey to 67% in the year prior to the 1986 survey; the percentage of patients without a usual source of care increased from 11% to 18%.

2. Access to medical care for poor, minorities, and uninsured persons decreased. In general, physician visits for low-income adults decreased by 30% between 1982 and 1986. For those in poor health, visit rates decreased by 8%; for the nonpoor in poor health, visit rates increased by 42%. There was a difference of 33% between physician visit rates of black Americans in ill health and those of whites.

3. The hospitalization rate for these disadvantaged groups decreased but not at a rate greater than that found in the general population. However, given the higher rate of poor health among these groups, the hospitalization rate may be less than would be warranted by patient condition.

4. Significant underuse of medical care occurred. One in six Americans with diagnosed serious chronic illness did not see a physician during the year, nor did one in seven pregnant women early in their pregnancies, nor one in five hypertensive patients. Additionally, 41% of patients with one or more of five serious symptoms did not see or tell a physician about them.

5. One positive change reported was that differences in the use of medical care between rural and urban residents seem to have decreased. Certain rural and urban residents still have some difficulty in finding access to health care, but major improvements have apparently occurred.

6. Satisfaction with physician and inpatient hospital care remains high.

A second study, reported in the New England Journal of Medicine, generally affirmed these findings but found in addition that the elderly actually had better access to health care than most other groups, even those who were nonpoor, insured, and working (Hayward et al., 1988). Medicare provided general assistance to the elderly, and their perceived vulnerability enhanced their ability to obtain supplemental coverage. The researchers found that the group that seemed most at risk comprised those individuals who were younger, low-income, uninsured, and nonwhite.

Consumer Role in Cost-Containment

A major component of a competitive health care system is that both buyers and sellers have a financial incentive to be concerned about the cost of care. Changes that would be expected to reflect this increased participation in controlling health care costs include increased use of insurance deductibles and co-insurance and increased employer intervention in health care costs. One study of 1185 firms in 1984 demonstrated that companies were changing their cost-management strategies in an attempt to limit costs (Hewitt Associates, 1985). For example, in 1982, 39% of insurance plans required a front-end deductible for inpatient hospital charges, whereas 63% did so in 1984. Conversely, in 1982 67% of insurance plans paid all hospital charges for first-day coverage of the hospital stay versus 42% in 1984.

Employers were also involved in new practices designed to influence decision making regarding necessary hospital and medical care. In 1982, 2% of firms required preadmission utilization review; in 1984 that figure had increased to 26%. Perhaps of greater significance was the fact that in 1982 no firms mandated a second surgical opinion or paid the full cost for one; in 1984, 28% of firms required a second surgical opinion, and 53% paid the full cost.

Personnel Shortages

In addition to affecting the accessibility and quality of health care for Americans, the prospective reimbursement system has been associated with changes in the quantity and type of personnel utilized. Although these relationships are not necessarily causal, the establishment of a cost-conscious environment has predictably influenced the delivery of health care and preferred providers.

From fiscal year 1983 through 1987, the number of full-time equivalent (FTE) staff members in hospitals was reduced by almost 114,000 (American Hospital Association, 1987). However, the number of FTE positions for registered nurses (RNs) per 1000 adjusted patient days increased 18% between 1983 and 1986, building upon an increase of 11.7% between 1980 and 1983. Moreover, nurses as a percentage of total hospital nursing personnel increased to 58% in 1986, compared with 46% in 1979 and only 33% in 1968 (Aiken, 1988). On the other hand, the number of licensed practical nurse (LPN) FTE positions *decreased* 15% between 1983 and 1986; during the period 1980 to 1983, the number of these positions stayed essentially flat (Examination, 1988). The combination of an increased number of RN vacancies and a tendency to substitute RNs for LPNs strongly suggests an increased demand by employers for the services of nurses. Many have postulated that this demand was largely due to the fact that RN salaries were comparatively low, and it was preferable to use the relatively less expensive, flexible nurse for health care. Coupled with the fact that patient acuity and new technology required increased numbers of skilled nurses, the demand for nurses increased.

Quality of Health Care

Perhaps the most uncertain effect of prospective reimbursement is the impact exerted on the quality of care. Part of this uncertainty is related to the difficulty of defining which elements of care are to be evaluated as contributing to quality. Certainly the absence of complications or untoward changes is important. A number of studies suggest that changes in the financing of health care have had relatively little effect on this aspect of patient care (Lave et al., 1988; DesHarnais, Chesney and Fleming, 1988; DesHarnais et al., 1987). Other studies point out some unacceptable consequences that have been associated with the change toward a prospective reimbursement system (Fitzgerald et al., 1987; Linn and Robinson, 1988).

To the extent that length of stay has decreased and patients are spending less time in hospitals, care could be improved. Additionally, elimination of unnecessary tests and diagnostic procedures could decrease the exposure of patients to potentially dangerous events. On the other hand, if patients are deferring care and waiting longer before presenting themselves for necessary treatment, health status could be jeopardized. It is generally accepted that cost-containment and high-quality outcomes are not mutually exclusive; rather, it has been shown that efficiency and elimination of duplicate services can actually improve health care outcomes (Longest, 1978; Singer et al., 1983).

After almost a decade of experience with prospective reimbursement, many economists, health care providers, and payors are calling for further reform (Iglehart, 1991; Pauly et al., 1991). For example, 91% of *Fortune 500* CEOs participating in a survey indicated that fundamental changes or complete rebuilding of the health care system is needed (Cantor et al., 1991). Similarly, in polls of Americans, the vast majority have expressed the same views (Blendon, 1989; Blendon and Taylor, 1989). Concerns that have been expressed include (1) the continuing increase in health care costs; (2) the lack of access by so many Americans to health care services; (3) the inability of many Americans, even those who are insured, to afford sufficient health care coverage; and (4) increasing concerns about the quality, effectiveness, and equity of health care. Initiatives such as national health insurance, consumer copayment, and managed care will be among those debated for effecting needed change.

IMPLICATIONS FOR NURSING PRACTICE

Trends—like horses—are easier to ride in the direction they're already going.

The trend within health care is toward more competition and a business orientation for health care delivery. Care must be delivered as always with a concern for quality but now in a cost-effective manner as well. Diers (1982) posed the definitive question: "How can I say that what I do makes a person feel better and improves his health status while saving money for the patient and the whole system?" Several implications for nurses emerge: (1) Care must be delivered with a focus on quality and resource use; (2) new knowledge, skills, and abilities must be developed; and (3) nurses must become adept at promoting nursing care as a cost-effective alternative. The economic principle of cost-minimization provides a framework for directing this effort.

Economic theory for firms that want to minimize costs—whether they be hospitals, garages, record stores, or whatever—suggests that each input should contribute the same amount to the final output or product per dollar spent on that input. Inputs can be considered as anything needed to produce the hospital's product (e.g., personnel, equipment, supplies, or unit structure). What a nurse contributes to the overall hospital product or specific product line should be in proportion to the cost of that nurse, just as a nursing assistant's contribution to output should be proportional to the cost of using the assistant. Hospitals, as cost-minimizers, will use inputs as long as the inputs contribute an amount proportional to their cost. When the inputs being considered are employees, wages are the essential component of the cost.

The equation in Figure 1–2 depicts this relationship. For a firm to be able to minimize costs, the marginal product (MP) or contribution to output of the first worker on the left (e.g., a nurse) must be proportional to the cost of that worker in the same ratio that the MP of another worker (e.g., a nursing assistant) is proportional to the cost of hiring that worker. This is not to say that nurses and assistants contribute the same amount or should receive the same wages or cost the same to use. Rather, a ratio should exist between an input's contribution to output, in this example an employee, and the cost to the institution of using that employee. This equation implies that a nurse will be valued, paid, and used according to a perception of his or her relative productivity and relative cost.

For nurses, then, there are four challenges:

1. To determine nursing's product
2. To calculate nursing's cost
3. To enhance one's own marginal product
4. To clearly communicate what nursing offers

These strategies will be reviewed in more depth in the following section.

$$\frac{\text{MP (nurse)}}{\$} = \frac{\text{MP (nursing assistant)}}{\$}$$

FIGURE 1–2. Principle of cost-minimization. MP, marginal product.

Determine Nursing's Product in the Unit and Institution. Listed here are a number of questions that need to be asked and explored. What is the service that nurses currently provide? What are nurses currently doing? What outcomes or products are they achieving, congruent with the hospital's mission and goals? What resources are being used? What resources are needed? What *could* nurses be doing? Are nurses engaged in nursing or non-nursing tasks? Could other caregivers be more appropriately used to free up nurses to do nursing and thus increase the nurse's marginal product, the contribution to output? On the other hand, could nurses appropriately assume additional responsibilities consistent with patient care needs? Over the years, a number of tasks and responsibilities have been given to other caregivers, most notably technicians. Could nurses realistically incorporate some of these activities and still maintain high-quality care, thus eliminating the need for certain workers and saving money for the institution?

Determine Both the Costs and Revenue Generated Through Nursing Services. Both the costs of nursing care and the revenue generated by nurses providing measurable services with specific outcomes should be calculated. To carry out this strategy, facts, data, research, and statistics are needed—*data* to reflect a particular unit's acuity level and thereby support the need for the present staff mix with no reductions; *figures* that show how many fewer complications there are on a unit when nurses deliver care rather than technicians; *statistics* that show how much faster a patient is discharged when nurses do preoperative teaching; *research results* that indicate that nurses in a primary nursing system deliver care more efficiently than nurses in a team system; *answers from patient questionnaires* indicating that patients experience greater satisfaction and will choose the hospital more frequently if care is visibly coordinated by a registered nurse. In short, in what measurable ways do nurses influence health care so that the costs of using professional nursing staff can be balanced against the positive outcomes realized?

Enhance the Individual Nurse's Marginal Product. An individual's marginal product or value to an organization is influenced by a number of factors, among them education, experience, interpersonal skills, and relevant knowledge of the task at hand. Given that new goals within the health care system include decreasing the length of patient stay and use of resources and increasing the number of admissions, particularly for patients for whom financial reimbursement is optimal, the development of certain skills and knowledge bases is especially important. Among health care professionals, nurses have already developed skills in a number of necessary areas: functioning as a team member; understanding the organization; conducting quick, accurate assessments and acting rapidly upon them; relating effec-

tively with a variety of people; skillfully helping patients learn to care for themselves; making the most of scarce resources.

In addition, there are other qualities that can be nurtured, preparing nurses to compete successfully within the current health care environment. First, a nurse with *specialized skills* or *knowledge* will be highly valued. Regarding specialization, factors linked with efficient performance include experience, familiarity, and practice. Nurses who work with a consistent patient population are able to develop skills, gain proficiency, and achieve certain outcomes more consistently. Consequently, the nurse who offers experience or expertise in an area in which the hospital needs help, and who can articulate the expected value of that expertise, is the nurse who will be valued and retained. Consider a situation in which only one nurse can be retained: the nurse who has developed expertise in preoperative teaching and whose patients go home 2 days earlier, or the nurse who haphazardly carries out teaching and whose patients stay an average of an extra day, costing the hospital thousands of dollars. Whom would you choose?

A final comment: The types of special knowledge, skills, or abilities acquired by nurses can be very diverse. Knowledge of a particular patient population, cultivation of skills in certain patient or organizational practices, an ability to interact effectively with a wide variety of people, even serving as an outstanding generalist who pulls everything together—these and many other areas of competency can be developed into an example of specialized mastery.

A second quality of nurses that can be fostered is *flexibility*. Because of the rapid changes occurring within the health care system, individuals who are able to respond quickly and adapt readily are particularly valuable. Those who bemoan change, struggle to maintain the status quo, or resist the inevitable are not helpful. Moreover, individuals who emphasize why changes should not occur rather than how we can make them happen are particularly unhelpful.

The reassignment of nurses to other patient care areas underscores this issue. Because of the impact of the nursing shortage on many hospitals, the reassignment of staff to provide adequate patient care has experienced a resurgence. This option for matching nursing resources to patient care needs poses problems but has been utilized by a number of institutions rather than closing beds or using agency nurses. Nursing staff are rarely enthused by this practice, but it can be handled in ways so that nursing frustration is minimized and satisfactory patient care is ensured, for example, with preplanning, a fair system of assignment, adequate orientation, and sufficient support. One factor that particularly influences the situation is the attitude of flexibility and cooperation generated by the nursing staff. Again, a spirit of flexibility, a willingness to look at options, and a "can-do" spirit are especially valued today.

Diversification is another quality that adds to an

individual nurse's value or contribution. Diversification refers to the process whereby an individual or organization extends its effort into new activities. During the past several years hospitals and other health care agencies have developed new product lines or entered new fields in an attempt to strengthen their financial positions. Similarly, individuals also can diversify, acquiring new skills or broadening their capabilities. Within nursing, there have been a number of subspecialties that have expanded their sphere of influence. For example, operating room nurses have become perioperative nurses, indicating that these nurses are skilled in the care of patients not only during surgery but before and immediately after surgery as well. Another example can be seen from the name change of the journal of the Nurses' Association of the American College of Obstetricians and Gynecologists (NAACOG). Formerly, the title was the Journal of Obstetrical and Gynecological Nursing; today, the title is Journal of Obstetrical, Gynecological and Neonatal Nursing. With that name change, the journal indicated that it encompassed and was relevant to a larger readership.

Similarly, individual nurses can look for opportunities to diversify and thus expand their competency and value. For example, oncology nurses are skilled in the care of patients with cancer. Many of these nurses have also developed proficiency in pain management. Although that skill is certainly integral to the care of cancer patients, there are a number of other patients within the hospital or outpatient setting for whom this knowledge and skill would also be beneficial. An oncology nurse who could also demonstrate and promote the fact that she could provide specialized care for other patients in pain would be especially valuable.

Accountability is the final factor to be discussed here. The health care industry is moving toward a system in which recognition of the contributions of individuals and an emphasis on outcomes are requisites. Relman (1988) suggested that the health care industry has gone through two revolutions and currently is in the midst of a third: the era of assessment and accountability. During the past few years, surveys reporting hospital morbidity and mortality statistics have emerged. Currently being developed are comparisons of individual physician performance, looking at outcomes such as the number of patient complications and length of stay. Also in place are new standards developed by the Joint Commission on the Accreditation of Healthcare Organizations that direct hospitals to develop systems for the tracking of individual nurses and patient care outcomes. Patient care systems such as primary nursing and nurses who are comfortable with the accountability required will do well in the current health care environment.

Communicate Clearly What Nurses and Nursing Accomplish. A final strategy is to communicate clearly to relevant publics and markets what it is that nurses offer. Through formal mechanisms, such as the publication of standards, the creation of marketing approaches, the revision of state nurse practice acts, and the incorporation of nursing into organizational decision-making bodies, among others, the perception of nurses' contributions and their impact can be shaped and shared. Perhaps of greater importance, however, is the use of informal or direct mechanisms of communication between caregiver and patient.

Individual efforts by nurses to communicate clearly to patients and their families the services offered by nurses are essential strategies. Recipients of nursing care must be able to identify clearly what they received from professional nursing services and what difference these services made. This can take the form of verbal communications, written brochures or pamphlets, posters, or separate tabulation of the costs of nursing services on patients' bills. In other words, any mechanism that highlights the contributions of nurses to patient care outcomes is a potential source of education.

The easiest and often the most overlooked mechanism is the verbal exchange between the patient (or family) and the nurse. Every interaction with a patient provides an opportunity for the nurse to point out his or her contributions: for example, "Today I will be working with you to teach you how to check your blood pressure so that you can monitor it at home," or, "I am responsible for helping you learn how to change these dressings so that you can get home as quickly as possible," or, "The reason I am checking this incision is to evaluate its status and make sure no complications develop." Too often, patients perceive nursing, when they notice it at all, as an expected benefit of health care; this benefit needs to be pulled out and highlighted.

CONCLUSION

Health care delivery has changed irrevocably. The trend now is toward a business orientation, the goal being to balance quality and cost-effectiveness. For nurses to compete effectively at this time, new knowledge and skills must be learned and new abilities developed. Moreover, an understanding of the pervasive changes occurring within the health care system must be gained so that the nurse can anticipate further changes and modify practice accordingly.

References

Aday, L. A., Fleming, G. V., and Andersen, R. (1984). *Access to medical care in the U.S.: Who has it, who doesn't.* Chicago: Pluribus Press.

Aiken, L. (1988). Assuring the delivery of quality patient care. In State of the Science Invitational Conference, *Nursing resources and the delivery of patient care.* Washington, DC: National Center for Nursing Research, NIH Publ No 89–3008.

American Hospital Association (1987). *National hospital panel survey reports, year ending September 1972 through year ending September 1987.* Chicago: Author.

Blendon, R. J. (1989). Three systems: A comparative survey. *Health Management Quarterly,* 5, 2–10.

Blendon, R. J., and Taylor, H. (1989). View on health care: Public opinion in three nations. *Health Affairs,* 8 (1), 149–157.

Cantor, J. B., Barrand, N. L., Desonia, R. A., et al. (1991). Business leaders' views on American health care. *Health Affairs,* 10 (1), 98–106.

DesHarnais, S., Chesney, J., and Fleming, S. (1988). Trends and regional variations in hospital utilization and quality during the first two years of the prospective payment system. *Inquiry,* 25 (3), 374–382.

DesHarnais, S., Chesney, J., and Fleming, S. (1988). Trends and regional variations in hospital utilization and quality during the first two years of the prospective payment system. *Inquiry,* 24 (1), 7–16.

Examination of the relationship between Medicare prospective payment and the nursing shortage (1988). *Nursing Economics,* 6 (6), 317–318.

Finkler, S. A., Brooten, D., and Brown, L. (1988). Utilization of inpatient services under shortened lengths of stay: A neonatal case example. *Inquiry,* 25, 271–280.

Fitzgerald, J. F., Fagan, L. F., Tierney, W. M., et al. (1987). Changing patterns of hip fracture care before and after implementation of the prospective payment system. *Journal of the American Medical Association,* 258, 218–221.

Free medical care has little effect on health: Rand study (1984). *Hospitals,* 58 (1), 29.

Freeman, H. E., Blendon, R. J., Aiken, L. H., et al. (1987). Americans report on their access to health care. *Health Affairs,* 6, 6–18.

Frick, A. P., Martin, S. G., and Schwartz, M. (1985). Case-mix and cost differences between teaching and nonteaching hospitals. *Medical Care,* 23, 283–295.

Goldfarb, M. G., and Coffey, R. M. (1987). Case-mix differences between teaching and non-teaching hospitals. *Inquiry,* 24 (1), 68–84.

Hadley, J., Zuckerman, S., and Feder, J. (1989). Profits and fiscal pressure in the prospective payment system: Their impacts on hospitals. *Inquiry,* 26 (3), 354–365.

Hayward, R. A., Shapiro, M. R., Freemand, H. E., et al. (1988). Inequities in health services among insured Americans. *New England Journal of Medicine,* 318 (23), 1507–1512.

Health Care Financing Administration (1985). Report to Congress: Impact of the Medicare hospital patient system, 1985 annual report. HCFA Publication No. 03251. Baltimore, MD: Department of Health and Human Services.

Hewitt Associates (1985). Company Practice In Health Care Cost Management—1984.

HMO penetration in the largest metropolitan areas (1991). *Penn Market Report,* 3, 4.

Iglehart, J. K. (1991). Health care and American business: One CEO's view. *Health Affairs,* 10 (1), 76–86.

Jones, K. R. (1985). Predicting hospital charge and stay variation. *Medical Care,* 23, 220–235.

Lave, J. R., Frank, R. G., Taube, C., et al. (1988). The early effects of Medicare's prospective payment system on psychiatry. *Inquiry,* 25 (3), 354–363.

Levit, K. R., and Freeland, M. S. (1988). DataWatch: National medical care spending. *Health Affairs,* 7 (5), 124–136.

Levit, K. R., Lazenby, H. C., Letsch, S. W., and Cowan, C. A. (1991). National health care spending, 1989. *Health Affairs,* 10 (1), 117–130.

Linn, B. S., and Robinson, D. S. (1988). The possible impact of DRGs on nutritional status of patients having surgery for cancer of the head and neck. *Journal of the American Medical Association,* 260 (4), 514–518.

Longest, B. B. (1978). Hospital services: An empirical analysis of their quality-cost relationship. *Hospital and Health Services Administration,* 23, 20–27.

Managed care: Will it push providers against the wall? (1986). *Hospitals,* October 5, 66–71.

McCarthy, C. M. (1988). DRGs—five years later. *New England Journal of Medicine,* 318 (25), 1683–1686.

McCusker, J., Stoddard, A. M., and Sorensen, A. A. (1988). Do HMOs reduce hospitalization of terminal cancer patients? *Inquiry,* 25, 263–270.

McLaughlin, C. G. (1988). Market responses to HMOs: Price competition or rivalry? *Inquiry,* 25, 207–218.

Melnick, G. A., and Zwanziger, J. (1988). Hospital behavior under competition and cost-containment policies: The California experience, 1980–1985. *Journal of the American Medical Association,* 260 (18), 2669–2675.

Moyer, M. E. (1989). A revised look at the number of uninsured Americans. *Health Affairs,* 8 (2), 102–110.

Pauly, M., Danzon, P., Feldstein, P., and Hoff, J. (1991). A plan for "responsible national health insurance." *Health Affairs,* 10 (1), 5–25.

Pear, R. (1988). Hospitals' Medicare profits drop: Decline may curb access to care. *New York Times,* A1.

Prospective Payment Assessment Commission (1987). Medicare prospective payment and the American health care system: report to the Congress. Washington, DC: U.S. Government Printing Office.

Prospective Payment Assessment Commission (1988). Annual Report: Medicare prospective payment system. Washington, DC: U.S. Government Printing Office.

Relman, A. S. (1988). Assessment and accountability: The third revolution in medical care. *New England Journal of Medicine,* 319 (18), 1220–1222.

Robinson, J. C. and Luft, H. S. (1987). Competition and the cost of hospital care, 1972–1982. *Journal of the American Medical Association,* 257, 3241–3245.

Singer, D. E., Carr, P. L., Mulley, A. G., et al. (1983). Rationing intensive care—physician responses to a resource shortage. *New England Journal of Medicine,* 309 (19), 1155–1160.

2

Effect of Sensory Alterations

Dorrie K. Fontaine

The technologic critical care environment offers numerous benefits to the critically ill patient including increased survival, rapid identification of complications, and prompt intervention, which often achieves dramatic results. These well-recognized benefits are attended by several physical and psychosocial burdens imposed by the environment that have been of interest to many researchers in a variety of disciplines. The sensory alterations of accompanying immobility, pain, and noise are well documented. Indeed, despite modern advances, the intensive care unit (ICU) has been referred to as "both psychologically and physically a very unkind environment" (Bryan-Brown, 1986). In order to maximize patient benefit and minimize physical and psychosocial distress, the critical care nurse manipulates and controls the environment. This can only be accomplished if the nurse has a keen awareness of the impact of the sensory technical environment on the critically ill patient.

Critical care units are characterized by a triumph of life-saving high technology, which lends a space-age appearance to even the smallest ICU. Brightly lit, frequently windowless units are often noticed by infrequent visitors to appear noisy, hustling, crowded, and tense. In fact, ICUs are noisy (Hilton, 1985; Woods and Falk, 1974), communication is not always therapeutic (Noble, 1979), and specific patient behaviors detrimental to recovery and caused in part by the environment, such as sleep deprivation, are frequently not diagnosed by the health care team.

The purpose of this chapter is to describe the sensory-perceptual alterations common to patients in critical care settings. Environmental stressors that create excessive stimuli such as noise or reduced stimuli such as immobility will be examined. Research evidence suggesting that various stressors are detrimental to patient outcomes will be explored. A common consequence of multiple sensory-perceptual alterations is sleep pattern disturbance, and this will

be reviewed in depth. Nursing therapies directed toward minimizing the psychophysiologic effects of the critical care setting are reviewed with recommendations for practice and further research.

PSYCHOPHYSICAL ENVIRONMENT OF CRITICAL CARE UNITS

A central theme throughout the nursing literature is the impact of person-environment interaction on health and illness (Meleis, 1985). The environment as a key concept in critical care nursing is depicted in the model shown in Figure 2–1 (American Association of Critical-Care Nurses, 1986). Three levels are depicted in this model: (1) the direct interactive nurse-patient environment, (2) the resource environment in terms of supplies and patient safety, and (3) the institutional administrative setting. The psychophysical environment within the dashed lines of the center circles demonstrates the continuous interchange between the nurse and the patient including the totality of sensory stimuli received by the critically ill patient. It is the immediate sensory environment that is the focus of this chapter.

An encompassing definition of environment includes the myriad aspects that surround an individual or a group, with emphasis on continuous interaction between the person and the environment. According to Dossey and colleagues (1988), the environment "may be physical, social, psychological, cultural, or spiritual; [it] includes external and internal animate and inanimate objects, seen and unseen vibrations and frequencies, climate, and not yet understood energy patterns." The critical care environment contains all these aspects, with noise, drugs, communication patterns, temperature, and potentially unknown factors affecting how a patient ultimately perceives and responds to the clinical setting.

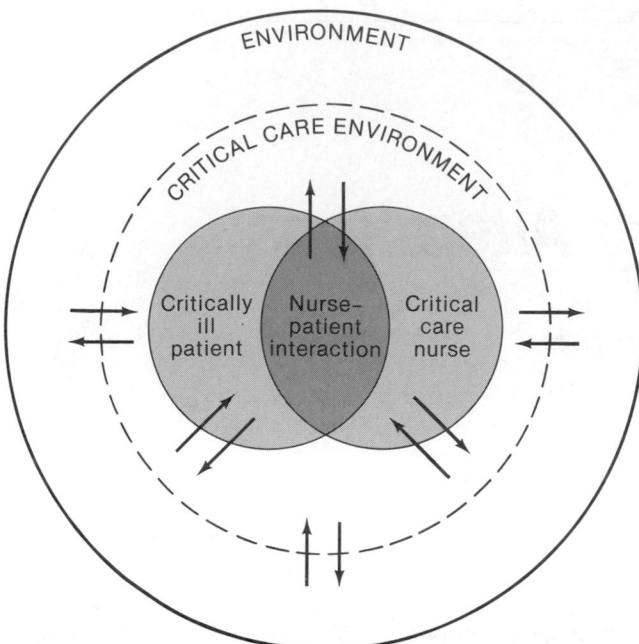

FIGURE 2–1. The critical care environment. (Redrawn from AACN, *Scope of critical care nursing practice*, AACN Position Statement, 1986.)

An environmental focus in nursing is a legacy from Nightingale (1859), who first warned of the potential physical, personal, and cognitive effects of the environment on the ill person. The need for adequate ventilation and protection from "cruel" noise and offensive odors (effluvia) are all presented in *Notes on Nursing*. Nursing therapeutics that promote, maintain, or change the environment for the benefit of the patient are the focus of increasing attention (Meleis, 1985). Evidence is accumulating that the therapeutic environment provided by the nurse brings about positive patient outcomes. One example is the work of Holden-Lund (1988), who identified a nursing environmental therapy that may have implications for wound healing in critical care.

Physical Features of the Environment

The central features of critical care units that make up the physical environment are related primarily to the surveillance function for which ICUs were first developed. Beds may be close together, creating little privacy but permitting ready observation of more than one patient by the nurse. Monitoring equipment and ventilators surround the critically ill patient with the unique tones and intensity of various continuous or intermittent alarms. Typically, these generate dissonance when sounding together. Noises from equipment are accompanied by often tense, shouted conversation, hurried footsteps, or the sound of running water. Visually, the continuous lighting, which produces an absence of time cues, accompanied by the distortion of viewing all caregivers by

gazing upward 2 or more feet, contributes to altered time and space perceptions by the patient. The physical environment thus created may be perceived by the individual in varying ways ranging from reassurance to terror.

Psychosocial Features of the Environment

The emotional tone of a critical care unit is determined by its physical configuration, degree of family access, and, to a great extent, the communication patterns of the critical care team. The physical configuration of most units leads to limited personal space for the patient and frequent loss of control over all space due to health team spatial invasions. Territorial dominance struggles that create tension between nurses, physicians, patients, and families can occur (Gowan, 1979). This factor is typified by the restricted access of the family and significant others to the patient, a central feature of the psychosocial environment in all critical care settings that is undergoing serious debate (Bay et al., 1988; Heater, 1985). Perhaps Viner (1985) identified the emotional climate of critical care best when stating that the critically ill patient lives in a narrowly circumscribed world acutely aware and at the mercy of the mood and tone set by all caregivers.

IMPACT OF THE CRITICAL CARE ENVIRONMENT

The impact of the critical care environment on the patient is best considered in terms of a psychophysiologic framework that considers the interaction among physiologic, personal, and cognitive patient responses. Physiologic responses are those characteristic biologic actions common to all individuals; the metabolism of nutrients and the sympathoadrenal stress reaction are examples. Personal responses include the affective, feeling aspects of the person and account for his or her unique value system. Patterns of thinking and communicating characterize the cognitive responses of individuals. The complex pattern of patient responses to the environment are inherently integrated, with sensation and perception playing fundamental roles. Patient response to noise well demonstrates this integration. Perception of sound as noise causes personal discomfort and may lead to physiologic vasoconstriction and elevated blood pressure (Kryter, 1985).

The environment may be perceived by the patient as frightening due to the physical and psychosocial features described. In the critical care setting, psychological factors such as fear or anxiety can worsen physiologic instability through stimulation of neurohormonal messengers in the brain (Dossey et al., 1988). Although psychological turmoil may not always be revealed by the critically ill (Easton and MacKenzie, 1988), researchers have identified multiple stressors reported by ICU patients. Many of these are related to sensory alterations.

Environmental Stressors in the Critical Care Unit

The combination of a painful, life-threatening illness, an uncertain outcome, and the closeness of strangers caring for intimate bodily processes creates the context in which environmental stressors must be viewed. It is not surprising that since the advent of critical care units, patients report a variety of noxious stimuli during their stay in an ICU (Dracup, 1988). Nonetheless, it is useful to consider the following paradox: Although the patient and family are often reassured by the close surveillance opportunities allowed by the ICU, the environment also creates numerous stressful phenomena. Indeed, patients and their families are known to experience "transfer anxiety" when recovery necessitates a less intense level of care despite the adverse effects reported by patients during the critical care stay (Urban, 1988). These stressors are important because many could be better anticipated and controlled by the critical care team.

Table 2–1 identifies the major environmental stressors reported by critically ill patients in two studies. The researchers investigated a total of 48 surgical ICU patients using a Q sort technique or an environmental stressor scale (Ballard, 1981; Wilson, 1987). The sensory alterations caused by immobilization and pain caused the highest stress in both studies. Themes of isolation, noise, crowding, altered lighting, and time loss all involve sensory alterations. In a study of 59 patients' recollections of their critical care experience, pain and sleeplessness were the major stressors identified (Simpson et al., 1989).

The degree to which an environmental feature

TABLE 2–1. *Environmental Stressors Reported by Patients in Critical Care Units*

Being tied down by tubes/ Not being able to move freely*
Being in pain*
Being thirsty*
Being on a ventilator/ Having to wear an oxygen mask*
Frequent interruptions of sleep*
Missing your spouse
Seeing family and friends for only a few minutes each day
Not being able to sleep
Having too many tubes
Not knowing when to expect things will be done to you
Losing track of time
Having doctors and nurses talk about you rather than to you
Too much noise
Having no privacy
Too much light

*Top 10 stressors common to both studies.
Data from Ballard (1981) and Wilson (1987).

---

causes arousal and discomfort to the patient resulting in psychophysiologic effects is determined by the processes of sensation and perception. An interesting example is conversation at the patient's bedside, considered a potential stressor in critical care (Mitchell and Mauss, 1978; Noble, 1979; Johnson et al., 1989). Johnson and colleagues (1989) re-examined the finding of Mitchell and Mauss (1978) that conversation about a neurologically impaired patient's condition at his bedside elevated intracranial pressure (ICP). Johnson and colleagues reported the effects on ICP of two types of conversation between nurses at the bedside of the head-injured patient—one a social conversation and the other a discussion of the patient's condition. Results demonstrated no significant difference between conversations; however, individual differences in response to conversation were noted, and ICP was significantly lower during the social conversation compared with the patient's baseline ICP. The researchers recommended careful scrutiny of all bedside conversations and further examination of the effects of conversation and other environmental factors on ICP.

The critical care patient has a driving need to make sense of and order the environment in order to adapt to it. This is demonstrated by the patient who strives to touch and examine his endotracheal tube, pulmonary artery catheter, or dressings. Critically ill patients interpret the environment based on the raw data of sensory exposure. These data come from the sensory modalities: visual, auditory, tactile, gustatory, and kinesthetic. Defining reality in order to make sense of the surrounding stimuli is the purpose of perception. However, many patients have alterations in their sensory-perceptual equipment that endanger their ability to understand the environment fully. In addition, the cues in the sensory environment itself may serve to confuse and cloud even the patient who is cognitively intact. The nature of sensory perception itself is first briefly considered.

THE NATURE OF SENSORY PERCEPTION

Critical attributes for receiving and processing sensory information include a stimulus, intact sensory receptors, intact neural pathways, and adequate processing by the brain to assign meaning to the stimuli (DiMinno and Ozuna, 1987). The neural pathways involve the reticular formation (RF), a network of neurons extending from the lower brain to the thalamus in the diencephalon. The reticular activating system (RAS) is an area within the RF that has a neurophysiologic role in cortical arousal. The RF, along with the thalamus and hypothalamus, collects sensory information. A stimulus of a given intensity is necessary to stimulate a healthy RAS; without adequate individual stimulation, boredom, restlessness, or drowsiness may occur (DiMinno and Ozuna, 1987).

Perception occurs when the sensory input is received, decoded, and analyzed by the cerebral cortex. Characteristics of perception can be summarized as follows: Perception is a universal and individual process; it is interactive and continuous and has maturational and developmental features (Thompson et al., 1986). The critically ill patient has a unique view of the world of the ICU depending on age, previous experience, and severity of illness. The nurse strives to understand individual impressions of the critical care environment from the patient's psychophysiologic responses.

An optimal sensory stimulation level for each individual is unknown. At what precise point adequacy of sensory stimuli moves toward monotony, a condition of sensory deprivation, or noise, a condition of sensory overload, is also an unknown. Sensory alterations in critical care typically span the continuum from deprivation to overload. Of interest to the clinician is the fact that both conditions demonstrate psychophysiologic effects (Kryter, 1985; Zubek, 1969).

ALTERATIONS IN SENSORY PERCEPTION DUE TO CRITICAL ILLNESS

Critically ill patients may experience a wide range of potential alterations in sensory perception. Some are due to the nature of the critical illness, whereas others arise from the therapeutically and socially restricted environment. In the first category, injury to the sense organs themselves may occur, as in a patient with multiple traumatic injuries creating blindness or with massive facial fractures causing altered smell and taste. The patient who survives a traumatic ruptured aorta may experience paraplegia and an altered kinesthetic sense. Obviously, any damage to the brain, such as occurs with head injury or a cerebrovascular accident, will lead to altered reception of stimuli. All patients with endotracheal tubes used for mechanical ventilation experience unpleasant stimuli such as gagging and frustration with communication (Gries and Fernsler, 1988).

The therapeutic critical care environment, with its varying degrees of overload and deprivation of stimuli, presents a sensory challenge to the patient. Social isolation and immobility alone can create perceptual distortions. Externally, noise, odors, and lack of space all bombard the senses. Internally, the polypharmacy of critical care, experienced by most patients, and potential electrolyte imbalances all tend to promote sensory distortion. The environment itself, with its monotonous though loud sounds, as well as the lack of a usual pattern of stimulation from family, friends, work, and recreation, adds to the reduced sensory input. Patients with restricted movement due to pain, traction, equipment, or the injury itself experience a positional deprivation due to immobility.

In summary, an alteration in sensory perception may occur due to an unfamiliar environment, altered sensory reception, chemical alterations such as electrolyte imbalance or drugs, and extreme anxiety or panic, which will narrow perceptual fields (Thompson et al., 1986). Anxiety, an important area for creative calming nursing interventions, is under increasing study. In this regard, the concept of patient control has been investigated in terms of sensory input. A focus on patient control has several implications in critical care, especially for mediating the sensory stimuli of noise and pain.

Patient Control of Sensory Stimuli

Patients interact with the environment, responding to stimuli and attempting to seek or avoid that which is pleasurable or noxious, respectively. Such interaction may be difficult in the critical care setting, where patient control is uncommon. Patients lose situational control over many impinging stimuli, of which noise and pain are paramount.

Topf (1984) described a framework suggesting that perceived control and exercised control of an aversive environmental effect such as noise could decrease reactivity and the damaging psychophysiologic response to this stimulus. Exercised control is the ability to regulate intended outcomes, whereas perceived control refers to an expectation of having the ability to make decisions to achieve desirable outcomes (Topf, 1984). A similar hypothesis of control has been used to investigate patient-controlled analgesia (PCA) in several patient populations (Giuffre et al., 1988). Many nursing therapeutics addressing sensory alterations are currently based on the concept of patient control and should promote recovery in the critically ill (Riegel, 1989).

NURSING DIAGNOSIS: SENSORY-PERCEPTUAL ALTERATIONS

Sensory-perceptual alterations, as defined by the North American Nursing Diagnosis Association (NANDA), are considered a "state in which an individual experiences a change in the amount or patterning of incoming stimuli accompanied by a diminished, exaggerated, distorted, or impaired response to such stimuli" (McLane, 1987). Alterations may be of a visual, auditory, kinesthetic, gustatory, tactile, or olfactory nature. Table 2–2 lists the major and minor defining characteristics approved for clinical testing.

Sensory-Perceptual Alterations in the Critically Ill: Overview of Research

Patients undergoing open heart surgery were one of the first critical care groups believed to experience

TABLE 2–2. Defining Characteristics of the Nursing Diagnosis: Sensory-Perceptual Alterations

Major Defining Characteristics
Disoriented in time, in place, or with persons
Altered abstraction
Altered conceptualization
Change in problem-solving abilities
Reported or measured change in sensory acuity
Change in behavior pattern
Anxiety
Apathy
Change in usual response to stimuli
Indication of body-image alteration
Restlessness
Irritability
Altered communication patterns

Minor Defining Characteristics
Complaint of fatigue
Alteration in posture
Change in muscular tensions
Inappropriate responses
Hallucinations

From McLane, A. M. (Ed.). (1987). *Classification of nursing diagnoses: Proceedings of the seventh conference* (p. 501). St. Louis: C. V. Mosby.

transient sensory-perceptual alterations. Findings of studies of these patients suggest that multiple factors may be involved including unit design, cardiac by-pass pump time, 24-hour nursing care interruptions, and drugs. Little conclusive evidence points to one stressor over another in precipitating the unique psychological disturbance that has become known as "ICU psychosis." Nursing research has continued to identify several perceptual distortions that may be experienced by more than 50% of critically ill patients.

In interviewing 38 patients in a surgical ICU, Wilson (1987) identified a 58% incidence of transient delirium or impaired psychological response (IPR). The instrument used to measure psychological status examined orientation, cognitive function and memory, hallucinations, illusions, and delusions and had been used in previous research. Patient perception of stressors was also examined. Patients who had an IPR were more likely to state that noise, losing track of time, being talked about rather than to, and multiple examinations were highly stressful. This finding supports the concept that sensory impingement in critical care situations can have adverse psychological effects. Patients often hesitate to mention sensory changes to the nurse because they believe that they would be labeled "crazy" and that no one else experiences bizarre dreams.

Easton and MacKenzie (1988) interviewed 10 surgical ICU patients using a semistructured interview guide to elicit specific information about the nature and incidence of the illusions, hallucinations, or delusions they experienced. Patients were interviewed after transfer from the unit. As in the study by Wilson (1987), 50% of the patients experienced psychological reactions such as delusions and nightmares. Patients experienced distorted perceptions

related to space ships, buildings rotating, feelings of persecution, and a fear of falling.

Medical research in the form of case reports has also supported the existence of transient sensory-perceptual changes during critical care. In a case report written by a physician-patient, Viner (1985) noted the presence of dreams and delusions after being on a ventilator for over 30 days in an ICU. The "putt-putt" sound of the water in the ventilator tubing caused him to remark, "I got to know John F. Kennedy very well as we sat in the bottom of PT boat 109." Other dreams and fantasies were related to the lack of privacy and the fear that werewolves would eat the blood stains on the sheet.

When critical care patients demonstrate any abnormal behavior, the label frequently applied to the condition is "ICU psychosis." Cassem (1989) cautions that often this diagnosis is one of convenience and fixing the blame on the sensory environment may limit a thorough search for other causative factors. The etiology of delirium in patients with ICU psychosis is typically unknown, and external and internal stressors must be examined. Drugs, lack of sleep, and sensory monotony are all potential contributing factors, especially drugs.

The polypharmacy of critical care is life-saving in many instances. However, the critically ill patient may pay a psychological price for the therapeutic effects of many needed drugs. Table 2–3 identifies the medications that have been previously linked to delirium in patient care.

As the research demonstrates, not all patients experience psychological disruptions while in the critical care setting. Why some experience perceptual alterations and others escape them is an important question. Factors associated with ICU psychosis include sleep deprivation (Helton et al., 1980), unit design without windows (Keep, 1977), and multiple other variables. Figure 2–2 shows numerous mechanisms that have been proposed for psychosis in the critical care setting; most require further investigation. The concept of hardiness may help to explain individual patient protection against perceptual alterations (Riegel, 1989). The perception of control over the situation is an important component of hardiness that is of increasing interest to researchers.

Prior to suggesting specific therapeutic interventions for mediating sensory-perceptual alterations, the two common categories of sensory alteration will be reviewed. Sensory deprivation of some senses often accompanies sensory bombardment of others. An example is the immobilized elderly multiple trauma patient with a pelvic external fixator device who is forced to listen to loud rock music from the nurse's station. Although the distinction between deprivation and overload is often arbitrary, the important factor remains patient perception. In this example, sensory deprivation results from immobility and overload occurs secondary to the undesirable noise.

TABLE 2–3. Drugs Associated with Delirium and Other Psychiatric Symptoms

Antiarrhythmics	Cimetidine, ranitidine
Diisopropamide	Digitalis preparations
Lidocaine	Disulfiram, metronidazole
Mexilitine	Dopamine agonists (central)
Procainamide	Amantadine
Quinidine	Bromocriptine
Tocainide	Levodopa
Antibiotics	Ergotamine
Aminoglycosides	GABA agonists
Amodioquin	Benzodiazepines
Amphotericin	Baclofen
Cephalosporins	Immunosuppressives
Chloramphenicol	Procarbazine
Chloroquine	L-Asparaginase
Colistin	Methotrexate (high dose)
Ethambutol	5-Azacytidine
Gentamicin	Cytosine arabinoside (high dose)
Isoniazid	Vincristine
Rifampin	Vinblastine
Sulfonamides	5-Fluorouracil
Tetracyclines	Hexamethylmelamine
Ticarcillin	DTIC
Vancomycin	Aminoglutethimide
Anticholinergics	Tamoxifen
Atropine	Lithium
Scopolamine	Metrizamide
Tricyclic antidepressants: amitriptyline, protriptyline,	Monoamine oxidase inhibitors
imipramine, desipramine, nortriptyline, trimipramine,	Isoniazid
maprotiline	Phenelzine
Trihexyphenidyl	Procarbazine
Benztropine	Narcotic analgesics
Diphenhydramine	Meperidine (Normeperidine)
Thioridazine	Pentazocine
Eye and nose drops	Nonsteroidal anti-inflammatory drugs
Anticonvulsants	Ibuprofen
Phenytoin	Indomethacin
Antihypertensives	Naproxen
Captopril	Sulindac
Clonidine	Podophyllin (topical)
Methyldopa	Steroids, ACTH
Reserpine	Sympathomimetics
Antiviral agents	Amphetamine
Acyclovir	Cocaine
Interferon	Ephedrine
Barbiturates	Phenylephrine
Benzodiazepines	Phenylpropanolamine
Beta-blockers	Aminophylline
Propranolol	Theophylline
Timolol	

From Cassem, N. H. (1989). Psychiatric problems of the critically ill patient. In W. C. Shoemaker, S. Ayres, A. Grenvik, et al. (Eds.), *Textbook of critical care* (2nd ed., p. 1406). Philadelphia: W. B. Saunders.

SENSORY DEPRIVATION

Sensory deprivation refers to a reduction in the amount or intensity of sensory stimulation (Jackson and Ellis, 1971; Goldberger, 1966). Perceptual isolation, in contrast, refers to a severe reduction in the patterning or meaningfulness of sensory stimuli. Some relate sensory deprivation to the uniqueness of each individual by defining it as a reduction in sensory stimulation below the individual's tolerance level (DiMinno and Ozuna, 1987).

Prior to the 1950s, anecdotal reports of solitary sailors, polar inhabitants, or prisoners were the sole source of data on nonexperimental sensory depriva-

tion experiences (Goldberger, 1966). With some impetus from the space program, by 1969 there were at least 20 major centers investigating experimental sensory deprivation (Zubek, 1969). These researchers assisted in identifying the potentially damaging physiologic and cognitive effects of sensory deprivation and the personality variables associated with it in healthy volunteers. A variety of auditory, visual, and cognitive changes were noted to occur depending upon the intensity and duration of the deprivation and subject motivational factors.

Jackson and Ellis (1971) categorized the phenomena associated with the majority of experimental and clinical sensory deprivation reports as follows:

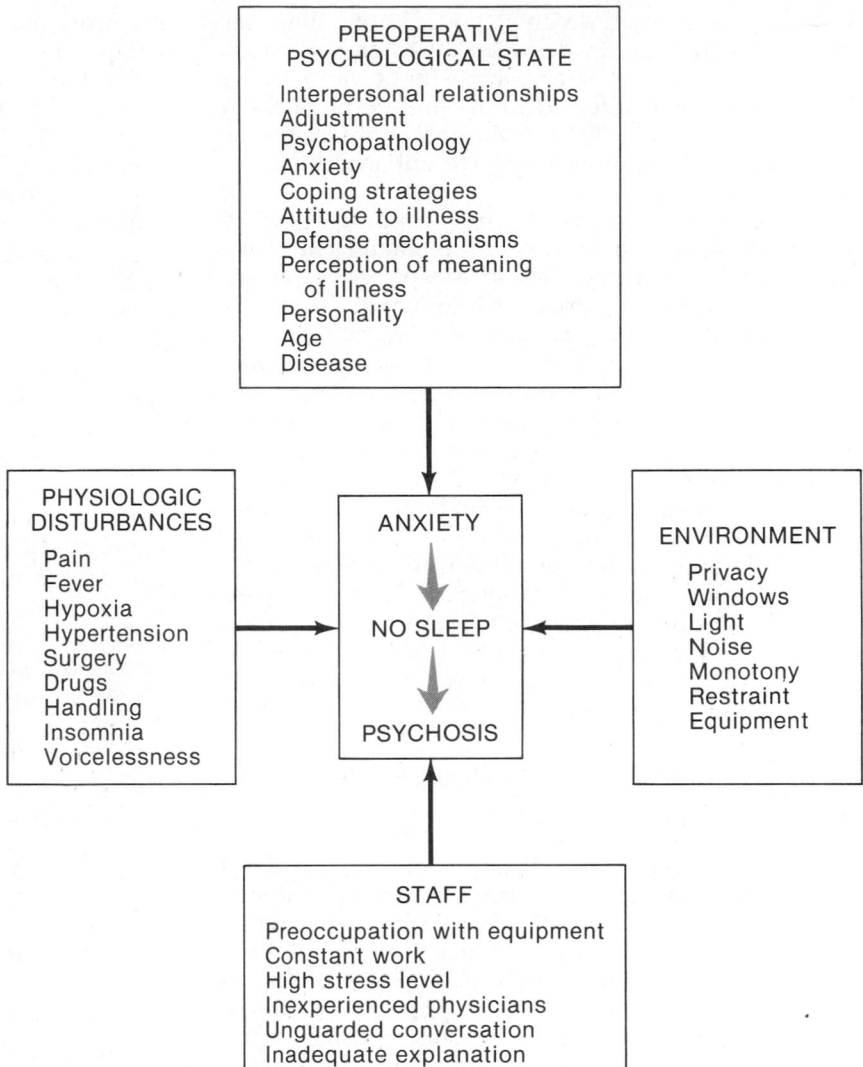

FIGURE 2–2. Intrinsic and extrinsic factors combine to cause sleeplessness and anxiety in the ICU patient. (Redrawn from Cousins, M. J., and Phillips, G. D. (1984). Sleep, pain, and sedation. In W. C. Shoemaker, W. L. Thompson, and P. R. Holbrook (Eds.), *Textbook of critical care.* Philadelphia: W. B. Saunders, p. 798.)

(1) perceptual—mild images to hallucinations; (2) cognitive—difficulty thinking or paying attention; (3) emotional—fear, depression, or anxiety; (4) motor—impaired fine or gross coordination; (5) somatic—galvanic skin response or catecholamine changes; and (6) other behaviors, such as noncompliance. Of these, the first two categories of experience are most frequently reported. However, individual responses to the deprivation experience are emphasized.

Clinical sensory deprivation has been less systematically studied than experimental deprivation. However, eye surgery patients have been an important prototype patient group that has contributed to our knowledge of sensory alterations (Jackson and Ellis, 1971). These patients experienced phenomena similar to those just described. Factors related to sensory alterations were believed to be the eye patching itself, the recumbent position, age, drugs, and the unfamiliar environment. The difficulty in interpreting clinical sensory deprivation studies is that they rarely encompass deprivation alone but may include sensory overload as well (Worrell, 1977). For example,

the surgical patient may experience sensory deprivation due to immobility and sensory overload due to intense pain. Methodical identification of variables for the clinical study of sensory deprivation has been a challenge.

Immobility and Sensory Deprivation

Alterations in mobility produce sensory-perceptual changes even in healthy individuals. The recumbent position alters perception, and when forced due to critical illness or injury, free movement is restricted, leading to dependence and loss of control (Barry, 1979). Individuals restricted to bedrest, even for brief periods of time, may develop sensory-perceptual alterations (Downs, 1974). In Downs' (1974) classic research, 20% of 180 healthy adults who experienced bedrest for nearly 3 hours in a laboratory simulation of a hospital room reported sensory distortions. Various audio tapes were used to simulate half-heard hospital conversations. Sensory distortions included hallucinations, mini-dreams, and altered time perception. The subjects described various sensations: visual, auditory, olfactory, kinesthetic, and tactile. These have been referred to as "indeterminate sensory experiences" (ISEs). Minimal human contact causing social isolation may have enhanced the sensory alterations.

In a clinical, noncritical care setting, Bolin (1974) identified sleep and dream pattern changes in a small group of immobilized orthopedic patients. An immobilized patient experiences minimal and restricted visual input and may be unable to receive the necessary feedback that would help to orient his body and its parts in relation to the environment (Scanlon-Schilpp and Robinson, 1988). The spinal cord–injured patient on a Stryker frame is an example of a person whose perceptual world may be limited to the floor, the ceiling, and whatever peripheral vision provides. The majority of critically ill patients begin their ICU stay on bedrest and thus experience the sensory restrictions of that position. Sensory perceptions of critical care patients who are cared for in an increasing variety of specialty beds, such as the Kinetic Roto Rest, the Mediscus low air loss beds, and others are unknown.

Neuromuscular Blocking Agents and Sensory Deprivation

Perhaps the ultimate example of sensory deprivation in a critical care setting is the patient who is receiving neuromuscular blocking agents. These commonly used drugs (pancuronium bromide [Pavulon], metocurine iodide [Metubine Iodide], or vecuronium bromide [Norcuron]) create widespread systemic paralysis without accompanying central nervous system depression. Sedatives and narcotics are thus required. Neuromuscular blocking agents are increasingly used in the management of acute respiratory insufficiency in critical care settings to better control ventilation.

Several reports indicate that patients receiving this type of drug therapy remember feeling isolated and alone, not sure if they were alive or dead (Parker et al., 1984; Schnaper, 1975; Vitello-Cicciu, 1984). Patients report a desire to be touched and to be called by name. Contact with reality would seem to assist in counteracting the severe sensory deprivation and perceptual monotony reported by this patient group. Conversations of staff at the bedside are recalled by these patients and can be a major source of anxiety. One patient vividly recalled hearing a nurse remark on the futility of further treatment for the patient because she was to "die anyway" (Schnaper, 1975). Examples such as this provide the reason for all caregivers to engage in therapeutic bedside conversation.

Time Alteration and Sensory Deprivation

Critically ill patients lose track of time because the constant fluorescent lights create a confused day-night orientation (Kleck, 1984). Time is an important component of the environment because it allows individuals to make adjustments and establish contact with and ultimately control their environment (Snyder, 1985). Research has determined that the perception of time passing can be affected by emotions, temperature, or immobility (Snyder, 1985). Patients in critical care settings may have a greatly distorted sense of time due to fever, medications, or continuous bedrest.

Individuals are equipped with a biologic clock that sets a unique pattern for endocrine, temperature, and sleep-wake cycles, among others. In the altered hospital environment, numerous internal rhythms shift out of phase with external cues, or zeitgebers, that normally assist in synchronizing circadian rhythms (Felton, 1987). To judge time accurately, a constant source of invariable stimuli such as physiologic body rhythms and interaction with the environment is needed (Felton, 1987). The environment should be consistent and familiar, which is not possible in typical hospital settings. Nurses can use a knowledge of chronobiology to help synchronize patients' unique biologic rhythms (Snyder, 1985). Timing of drug administration and independent nursing activities such as scheduling of relaxation techniques may have superior outcomes when patient rhythms are taken into account.

Windowless Units and Sensory Deprivation

Environmental designers in critical care units often recommend strategic placement of windows (Ulrich, 1984), a recommendation that is not always feasible in older recovery rooms or critical care units. Windowless units may result in memory alterations, delusions, and hallucinations. In a study comparing the mental status of 72 former patients in an ICU with windows with that of 78 patients in a windowless unit, Keep and associates (1980) identified twice the presence of delusions and hallucinations in the windowless unit group. Nearly 25% of the patients could not remember anything about their critical care stay, which is similar to Schnaper's (1975) finding of amnesia in multiple trauma patients. However, those with intact memory reported distorted visual images, feelings of persecution, depersonalization, and "out of body" experiences.

Increasing evidence supports the existence of detrimental sensory-perceptual alterations in an environment with no view to the outside. Although the presence of a hospital window helps to ensure that the patient at least has a sense of day and night, one unique report suggests that some scenery may have greater healing potential than others. A total of 46 surgical patients in two groups were studied, one group facing a brown brick wall and the other with a view of deciduous trees. The tree-view patients

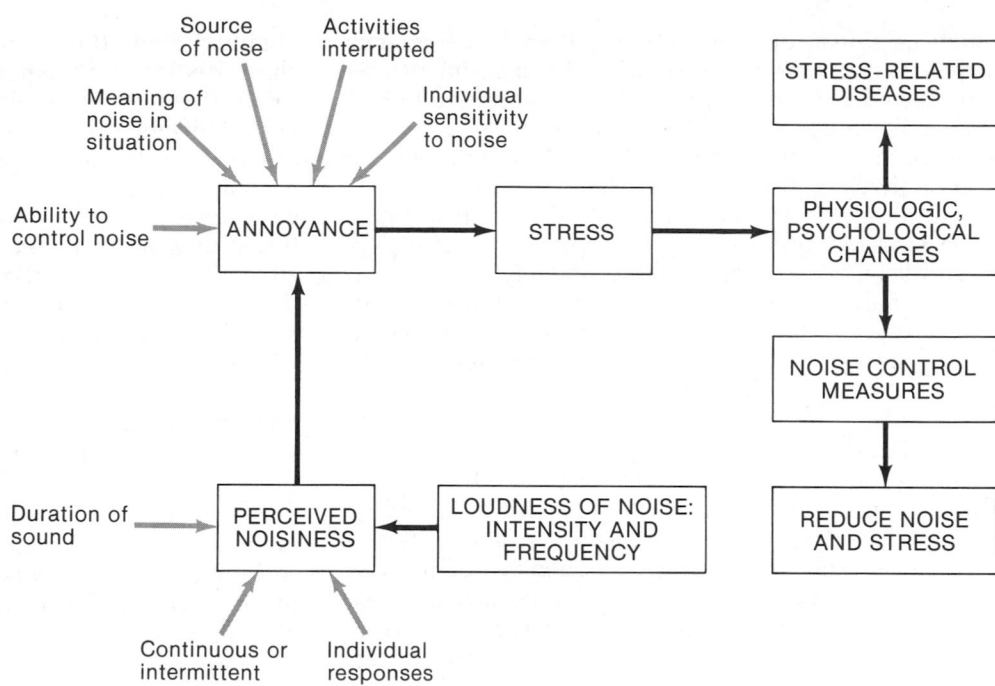

FIGURE 2–3. Relationship between characteristics of noise and human response. (Reprinted from *Critical Care Quarterly*, Vol. 6, No. 4, p. 72, with permission of Aspen Publishers, Inc., © 1983.)

received significantly less narcotic than the wall-view group postoperatively. Being able to look out a window at a natural scene rather than a more monotonous one may decrease patient requirements for medication and length of hospital stay (Ulrich, 1984). Further research on the effects of other potentially therapeutic views such as posters or paintings in windowless units is needed.

SENSORY OVERLOAD

Sensory overload is defined as a marked increase in the intensity of stimuli at greater than normal levels or simultaneous multisensory experiences (Baker, 1984). At its most damaging, sensory overload promotes patient hypervigilance in the critical care setting due to continuous arousal. Escape from fear, anxiety, or pain through sleep is often not possible. Noise is implicated most often and has been extensively studied. However, pain is probably the best known stressor causing sensory overload in the critical care patient. The combination of pain and a noisy environment serves only to increase patient perception of pain.

In the critical care setting sensory overload is the most important immediate perception of the infrequent visitor and the patient. Health care professionals may become desensitized over time so that the impinging multisensory stimuli are not cognitively processed but become background. However, patients remain in the unit 24 hours a day, whereas the health care team and visitors come and go.

Noise and Sensory Overload

Noise or unwanted sound can be considered as an audible acoustic energy that adversely affects physiologic or psychological well-being (Kryter, 1985). Individual perceptions of a sound constitute the uniqueness of noise. Noise pollution in the hospital environment, especially critical care areas, has been well documented (Hilton, 1985; Redding et al., 1977; Woods and Falk, 1974). According to Hilton (1985), noise is an important sensory stressor in hospitals because it may impede healing.

A model of the relationship of noise and human response is depicted in Figure 2–3. The physiologic response approximates the stress response initiated when sound is perceived as annoying (Baker, 1984). The physical effects of noise consist of general physiologic overarousal, demonstrated by increased respiratory rate, peripheral blood vessel vasoconstriction, minimum heart rate change, adrenal gland secretions, and elevated levels of blood cortisol and cholesterol (Kryter, 1985). A startle effect may initiate the autonomic and endocrine response. Cognitive functioning may be affected when noise competes with nonauditory stimuli in the environment (Kryter, 1985). As decibel levels rise, noise in the environment affects the cognitive and perceptual ability of healthy individuals (Hansell, 1984).

The meaningfulness of the sound is a critical variable for the patient. Stress occurs when the sound is annoying or its meaning uncertain. Critical care patients often struggle cognitively to make sense of the sounds they hear. Smith (1986) determined that it was more restful to listen to patterned audio input, such as music or taped stories, than to experience ambient environmental sounds. The experiment was conducted with 120 healthy subjects confined to bed in a laboratory setting. Examination of an intervention such as patterned sound in severely ill patients needs investigation.

Although hospitalized patients complain of noise as a stressor, little is known about the precise psychophysiologic response of the severely ill patient to noise. Baker (1984) suggests that individuals with cardiovascular disease may be more susceptible to noise stressors. Other patient groups sensitive to noise need to be identified.

Sound has frequency and intensity. Frequency is measured in cycles per second (Hz), and normal hearing covers the 20 to 2000 Hz range. Intensity is the loudness of a sound (Woods and Falk, 1974). Sound is measured in decibel (dB) units on the A scale to closely approximate frequencies of the human ear. Decibels are one-tenth of a bel and increase exponentially. For example, a 10-dB(A) noise sounds twice as loud as a 1-dB(A) noise (Baker 1984; Kryter, 1985).

Sound Levels in Critical Care Units

Researchers have identified the high levels of noise in critical care settings. Table 2–4 summarizes data

TABLE 2–4. Noise Levels in the Critical Care Setting

Noise Source	Intensity dB(A)
Equipment	
Ventilator (at HOB)	60–65
Ventilator alarm at 20 feet	71–76
Cardiac alarm (at HOB)	71
Ice machine dispensing ice	62–64
Radio (at HOB)	64–68
Oxygen by mask	63
Treatments	
Chest percussion	83
Patient weighed	60–64
Putting HOB up	68–78
Endotracheal suction	70
Obtaining vital signs	60–68
Environment	
Garbage cans moved	48–83
Things thrown into garbage can	67–80
Water running	44–70
Voice over intercom	60–70
Toilet flushed	44–60
Telephone ringing (at 6 feet)	60–65
Squeaking chair	76
Telephone ringing (at 10 feet)	67
Staff conversation at bedside	63
Rattling side rails	80
Computer printer	70–72
Patient crying out	80

HOB = head of bed.
Adapted from Baker (1984); Hilton (1985); Redding, Hargest, and Minsky (1977); Woods and Falk (1974).

obtained from the work of several researchers on clinical noise. Most equipment produces noise close to 70 db(A), which is the level at which annoyance occurs (Baker, 1984). Sleep occurs best at levels below 35 dB(A). To gain perspective on these noise levels, normal ambient living room noise is 30 to 40 dB(A), conversational voices are heard at 60 dB(A), heavy traffic or a noisy restaurant produces sound in the 70 to 80 dB(A) range (Baker, 1984), and a pneumatic drill at a distance of 50 feet has a decibel level of 80 dB(A) (Redding et al., 1977).

Hilton (1985) compared the level of sound in four ICUs and two general care units. Continuous dB(A) level recordings were made for 24 hours, and observations of the sources of sound were made for briefer periods. Continuous sound recorded in the open heart recovery room and ICU in the larger hospital ranged between 48.5 and 68.5 dB(A), even at night. Although some patients were not concerned about the noise level, others were highly upset. Communication by staff at the bedside was loud. This finding supports other research suggesting that staff communication is not only noisy but often nontherapeutic as well (Noble, 1979). Importantly, Hilton noted that several sounds can be greatly diminished. Turning the bell down on telephones decreases the noise level from 70 to 60 dB(A), while closing a patient's door in the ICU can decrease noise by 15 dB(A).

Woods and Falk (1974) investigated noise levels in a seven-bed acute care unit and a 17-bed recovery room. Noise levels were consistently related to the number of personnel present. The mean noise level for each area was consistently greater than 50 dB(A), whether measured during the day or at night. Incidental findings of this study revealed that a domino effect often occurred in which one patient might cry out and all others were aroused, one after another.

Although several studies report that noise from staff is particularly disturbing (Noble, 1982), others identify noise from mechanical equipment as most annoying (Snyder-Halpern, 1985). The latter study investigated healthy subjects' perception of their sleep during a quiet condition and a taped ICU noise condition in a laboratory setting. Undisputed is the claim that critical care settings are noisy 24 hours a day, and much of the noise can be controlled through staff behavior and equipment adjustments.

Critical care nurses are known to become desensitized to environmental stimuli. Lindenmuth and colleagues (1980) investigated the effects of environmental stimuli on critical care nurses acting as patients in an ICU bed for 1½ hours. Perceptions were similar to those reported by patients with noise from alarms on monitors and ventilators found to be bothersome. Feelings of loneliness and immobility were experienced, along with the perception of time as slowing down. These authors advocated a plan to sensitize critical care nurses to environmental stimuli, a concept that may be especially important with the widespread institution of 12-hour shifts.

NURSING THERAPEUTICS FOR SENSORY-PERCEPTUAL ALTERATIONS

Numerous nursing therapies addressing sensory alterations in the critically ill have been described in the literature. Several of these can be considered collaborative interventions with medicine; many more are in the realm of independent nursing strategy. All of the therapies suggested can be usefully categorized as: (1) surveillance, (2) shielding, or (3) modification.

Surveillance

Monitoring of the patient-environment interface is an initial nursing strategy. The critically ill patient and the environment are assessed separately, and the quality of the interaction is determined based on these findings. The patient should be assessed for the critical attributes of sensory perception, with any alterations noted. Function of all sensory modalities needs to be carefully assessed along with the ability to process information (Scanlon-Schilpp and Robinson, 1988).

Patient perception of the environment is evaluated by means of direct questions related to the stressors previously identified by researchers (see Table 2–1). How stressful is immobility in this patient? How supportive is the family and what is the patient's psychophysiologic response when family members visit? (Bay et al., 1988). Patient characteristics obtained from the patient or family and recorded on the data base are useful in suggesting avenues for further assessment. For example, patients with significant drug histories may have problems with forced dependency and loss of control in the critical care unit. They may also experience perceptual distortions and loss of reality due to the effects of withdrawal.

Knowledge of a usual coping pattern for any critically ill patient is useful in planning therapy to mediate sensory alterations. Dealing with special populations such as children (Betz, 1982) or elderly persons in critical care units requires a knowledge of the developmental level and stressors unique to that age group in critical care.

Surveillance for environmental effects ensures that the critical care nurse question the patient about noise perception, time perception, and distracting or annoying environmental factors that can potentially be manipulated. The view that the patient has from his or her particular corner of the critical care setting should be identified and analyzed in terms of lighting, privacy, and monotony.

Surveillance of the sensory environment to sensitize the nurse to potential negative effects is recommended (Snyder-Halpern, 1985). One technique that assists the critical care staff in increasing sensitivity to environmental overload is to place a tape recorder

close to the patient's ear to record environmental sounds for 1 to 2 hours. This allows a close approximation to the reality of noise in the ICU as the patient receives it. Reviewing the taped sounds of the critical care unit later at a staff meeting is a good learning opportunity whether the nurse is a novice, an advanced beginner, or an expert in critical care practice.

Dossey and colleagues (1988) recommend the following environmental exercise for nurses to deal with our increasing technologic environment:

At different times during the day, close your eyes and take a few moments to listen carefully to all sounds in your environment. Jot down the many different sounds you hear, noting which are distracting or disturbing noises. Become aware of all the sounds that you ordinarily hear, such as the air conditioner, radios and televisions, the hum of fluorescent lights, the beeping and buzzing of hospital machinery, or the incessant MUSAK that some institutions play over the speaker system. Notice new smells, feelings or temperature, etc. There will be many sounds, smells, and sensations of which you may not have previously been aware.

This exercise may be suggested to nurses when they are introduced to a new critical care practice setting and repeated at intervals of weeks to months.

Finally, monitoring of the patient-environment interaction includes assessment of the patient for any sensory and perceptual disturbances reported in the literature. For example, patients should be asked about any dreams or altered feelings. They should be encouraged in a nonjudgmental way to identify unusual sensations (Bolin, 1974; MacKinnon-Kesler, 1983; Worrell, 1977). Wakeful patients may confess to a fear of falling asleep and experiencing nightmares. Critical care patients need to be assured that these are common transient experiences and encouraged to discuss them; ICU patients may erroneously believe they have become psychologically ill (Easton and MacKenzie, 1988). Multiple trauma patients need to be assessed for hyperalertness, survivor guilt, and other behaviors classified as the post-traumatic stress disorder (Scanlon-Schilpp and Robinson, 1988). Wilson (1987) advocates frequent use of a mental status examination to document disorientation, hallucinations, illusions, delusions, or paranoia.

Shielding

The nursing therapy of shielding refers to protection of the critically ill patient from the aversive effects of the critical care environment. Shielding the patient physically through noise abatement and psychologically from nontherapeutic bedside conversation are good examples. Recommendations for protection of the patient from noise range from simply closing the patient's door when possible (Hilton, 1985) to developing strict guidelines on new equipment noise. The critical care nurse who successfully uses shielding has a keen awareness of the environment and sensitively screens out potentially harmful elements based on knowledge of unique patient characteristics. Some patients are more sensitive to cold, to odors, or to a loud radio.

Providing orientation to reality is a protective nursing therapy. Addressing the patient by name, interpreting stimuli in the environment, and assisting in clarifying reality are useful in restoring or maintaining sensory-perceptual function (Thompson et al., 1986).

Modification

Modification involves numerous independent interventions to restructure the patient's external and internal environment. Family visiting periods, use of earphones or television, dim lighting at night, possibly a window, and use of calendars and clocks are all examples of modifying the external environment to overcome the damaging effects of sensory alterations. The nurse manipulates the sensory environment by altering the patient's position at frequent intervals and moving him or her to a chair or instituting ambulation as early as possible.

Allowing and encouraging patient control is difficult for some critical care nurses. Evidence that outcomes improve when the patient perceives himself in control and exercises control needs to be further explored using the areas of pain, noise, and sleep. Establishing an effective communication link between the patient and the nurse is an initial measure needed to determine mutual goals. More attention needs to be focused on the precise way in which nurses determine the needs of critically ill patients. Patients claim that they experience much stress because of an inability to communicate. The work of Stovsky and associates (1988) in investigating patient and nurse satisfaction with different methods of communication needs to be continued in examining several populations in critical care settings.

Closely related to patient control is the use of family visiting in critical care settings. Nurses are rethinking some of the past restrictions on visiting. Certainly pediatric critical care nurses are way ahead of adult critical care nurses in family-focused care in many settings (Betz, 1982). More work documenting the effects of family visits on the psychophysiologic response of patients is needed.

Modification of the physical environment to limit noise can be accomplished in many ways ranging from turning equipment alarms away from the patient's ear to making complete structural changes in a new unit (Hilton, 1987; Hansell, 1984). Brewer (1985) recommended several features for an "ideal" critical care unit. Many recently constructed or renovated critical care units have taken at least some of these design features into account. Such features include (1) spacious, attractively decorated private rooms with outside windows and window coverings, variable lighting, adequate storage, a clock and calendar easily visible from the patient's bed, adjustable bedside monitors, accurate individually controlled thermostats, and television or radio; (2) nursing work stations separate from but convenient to patient rooms; (3) utility rooms separate from the general unit for noise and odor control; (4) separate but convenient conference rooms for staff reports, breaks, and family conferences; and (5) volume control for equipment and dimmers for lighting. Private rooms and outside windows have been shown to mediate the environmental load on the patient and promote more timely recovery. It is essential that critical care nurses collaborate early with other disciplines when any blueprint designs for new units are generated.

Last but just as important, manipulation and modification of the patient's internal psychophysiologic environment is a priority. Nursing therapies range from collaborative ones, such as the administration of various medications that may ease pain and promote rest, to independent actions such as the judicious use of nontraditional approaches to helping the patient cope in a stressful environment. These include relaxation techniques, guided imagery, music therapy, and others (Dossey et al., 1988). Research investigating patient outcomes in critical care settings, not just in medical-surgical patients (Holden-Lund, 1988), needs to be undertaken. Paradoxic reactions to drugs intended to relax and calm patients need to be quickly identified (Worrell, 1977). Evaluation and documentation of the effectiveness of all therapies directed at mediating the patient's internal environment are needed.

The strongest impact of the environment, whether due to sensory overload or sensory deprivation, is exerted on the normal sleep pattern of a critically ill patient. Sleep disturbance has intrigued researchers since the inception of ICUs, with the discipline of nursing providing much of the widely cited research literature. This chapter on sensory alterations concludes with a discussion of the nursing diagnosis of sleep pattern disturbance and nursing interventions for this universal phenomenon.

SLEEP AND REST DISTURBANCES IN THE CRITICAL CARE UNIT

Critically ill patients have difficulty meeting their need for sleep and rest in the intensive care environment. Although the precise psychophysiologic effects of sleep deprivation are controversial, there is no dispute about the severe sleep disruption that routinely occurs in the hospital setting, especially in critical care units (Aurell and Elmquist, 1985; Helton et al., 1980; Hilton, 1976). Beginning with the classic work of Dlin and colleagues in 1971, sleep problems of the critically ill have often been noted. However, studies that critically examine activities that promote sleep and rest that would benefit the critically ill, as recommended by an AACN Delphi Study of research priorities in critical care nursing, are noticeably absent (Lewandowski and Kositsky, 1983).

Complicating the sleep and rest problem is the fact that the critical care team may view sleep disruption as an expected and uncontrollable aspect of patient care and therefore place a low priority on sleep promotion activities. This attitude directly conflicts with the nurse's accepted role of manipulating the environment to promote healing. Despite controversies over the consequences of sleep deprivation (Naitoh et al., 1990; Parkes, 1985), increasing support for the possibility of patient harm due to sleep pattern disturbance cannot be ignored.

Evidence suggests that sleep disruption may lead to depressed ventilation (White et al., 1983), decreased immunocompetence (Palmblad et al., 1979), increased pain perception (Phillips and Cousins, 1986), and the confusional syndrome of ICU psychosis (Helton et al., 1980). In addition to patients' own complaints that sleep disturbance is a major stressor during their ICU stay, many of the potential problems of sleep pattern disturbance may worsen patient psychophysiologic status. For example, weaning the patient from a ventilator, healing difficult wounds, and limiting confusion in the critically ill patient may all be greatly assisted by a rested patient, one who is at least achieving some complete sleep cycles.

Physiology of Sleep

Sleep is referred to as a "soft area" in physiologic research due to the many gaps in our present knowledge of sleep mechanisms and other biochemical aspects of sleep (Karnofsky, 1986). Much of what is known about sleep is less than 40 years old, and even the question of the function of sleep remains elusive. Sleep researchers have identified the stages of sleep and several neurochemical regulators of sleep, and have proposed sleep factors, hypnogenic areas, and immune modulators for sleep (Gaillard, 1990; Institute of Medicine, 1990; Parkes, 1985).

The field of sleep research is flourishing. Sleep is a complex multidimensional process that is cyclical, reversible, and characterized by a comparative decrease in the levels of cortical vigilance (Hartman, 1973; Koella, 1978). Sleep can be measured by behavioral observation, subjective reports, and physiologic monitoring. However, the only method that accurately detects specific sleep stages is polysomnography (PSG), in which simultaneous electroencephalograms (EEGs), electro-oculograms (EOGs), and electromyograms (EMGs) are made. These cortical tracings emerge from intense brain activity during sleep, which is not the passive state previously assumed.

STRUCTURES OF SLEEP AND NEUROTRANSMITTERS

Primary brain areas implicated in sleep and wakefulness include the locus ceruleus, the raphe nuclei, and the hippocampus (Robinson, 1986). Numerous neurotransmitters have been implicated in the regulation of vigilance (Wauquier et al., 1985). Those most examined are serotonin (5-HT), norepinephrine, and acetylcholine, although researchers continue to identify biologic substances with potential sleep generation capabilities (Gaillard, 1990). The importance of neurotransmitter interaction in the sleep-organizing apparatus is well recognized, but the patterns of integration continue to be investigated.

Specific neurotransmitters that are more easily measured have been linked to anatomic sites within the brain. These substances can be characterized as vigilance enhancers, which promote wakefulness, or vigilance suppressors, which elicit sleep (Koella, 1985). Nonrapid eye movement (NREM) sleep stages 1 through 4 was purportedly under the control of serotonin, but this theory has been abandoned (Institute of Medicine, 1990). According to Gaillard (1990), serotonin may be important throughout the sleep-wake cycle for the synthesis and use of unknown sleep-promoting factors. Rapid eye movement (REM) sleep, characterized by intense activation of the central nervous system, is mediated by acetylcholine from the hippocampus. During REM sleep, acetylcholine is released by the caudate nucleus at the same level as during the awake state. The vigilant awake state is under the control of the norepinephrine adrenergic system, which discharges from the locus ceruleus. It is the interaction among and modulation of these neurotransmitters that permits the well-established progression of sleep and waking stages.

Descent into the various stages of sleep is more complex than this brief review of neurotransmitters permits. Researchers are beginning to discover the integral network of many hypnogenic systems, and specific sleep factors such as factor S or delta sleep-inducing peptides have been isolated in animals. (Gaillard, 1990). Other substances under study include gamma-aminobutyric acid (GABA), dopamine, and various hypnogenic peptides.

SLEEP ARCHITECTURE

Sleep is categorized into five stages based on the polysomnographic criteria of the EEG, EOG, and EMG: stages 1 through 4 NREM sleep and REM sleep. An individual progresses from the drowsy state of stage 1 sleep through the slow-wave sleep (SWS) of stages 3 and 4. Stage REM sleep is reached by recycling through stage 2, in which the young adult spends 50% of the night. Table 2–5 depicts the characteristics of each sleep stage as developed by a consensus of sleep researchers. The mean time percentage spent by young adults in each stage is also presented, based on normative data from the University of Florida (Williams et al., 1974).

TABLE 2–5. Sleep Characteristics and Percentage of Time Spent in Each Sleep Stage in Young Adulthood

Stage	Sleep Characteristics	Percentage of Sleep Time for Men Aged 20 to 29
Awake	Alpha activity 8–13 Hz or mixed-frequency EEG; high tonic EMG; eye blinks on EOG	1.26
1	Low-voltage, mixed-frequency EEG; EOG shows slow rolling eye movements	4.44
2	Sleep spindles on EEG (12–14 Hz) and K complexes	45.54
3	At least 20 to 50% of the sleep record (30-second epoch) contains delta waves of 2–4 Hz and 75 microvolts	6.21
4	Greater than 50% of the sleep record contains delta waves of 75 microvolts	14.55
REM	Low-voltage, mixed-frequency EEG; episodic eye movements on EOG; low-amplitude EMG	28.00

Abbreviations: EEG, electroencephalography; EMG, electromyography; EOG, electro-oculography; Hz, hertz.

Data from Rechtschaffen, A., and Kales, A. (Eds.) (1968). *A manual of standardized terminology, techniques, and scoring system for sleep stages of human subjects.* Bethesda, MD: U.S. Department of Health, Education, and Welfare; and Williams, R. L., Karacan, I., and Hursch, C. J. (1974). *Electroencephalography (EEG) of human sleep: Clinical applications.* New York: John Wiley & Sons.

Sleep Measurement

Since nurses make decisions about sleep promotion activities based on their assessment of the quality and quantity of a patient's sleep, it is important to consider the components of sleep measurement. Nurses often represent a patient's sleep with the ubiquitous comment "Patient appears to be sleeping" documented in the patient record. The measurement of sleep patterns reflects the complexity of sleep. To show the multidimensionality of sleep clearly, sleep measurement instruments can be categorized as follows: physiologic, objective, and subjective (Beck, 1988; Johns, 1971; Richards, 1987). When possible, sleep assessment measures should provide a sense of the quality of sleep and not quantity alone.

Physiologic sleep measurement instruments include the polysomnograph, in which EEG, EOG, and EMG tracings are recorded simultaneously. This is the only scientific measure of sleep in which precise sleep stages can be discerned and is primarily a research or diagnostic tool. Objective sleep measures include the nurse's estimate of a patient's sleep through observation of a combination of the following: (1) respiratory pattern, (2) movement, (3) possibly monitored heart rate and blood pressure changes, and (4) lack of arousal to environmental stimuli. Several researchers have used a sleep estimate form to document observable behaviors (Aurell and Elmqvist, 1985; McFadden and Giblin, 1971; Woods, 1972). The frequency of observation is a concern because infrequent observations may miss either awakenings or a return to sleep. These instruments have been used solely for research purposes. Other physiologic and observable measures are critiqued by Johns (1971) and Richards (1987).

A third category of sleep measures is the subjective one, in which patients examine their own perceptions of sleep quality. Patients assess the quality of their sleep based on sleep latency, or the time it takes to fall asleep; the number of awakenings experienced or disrupted sleep; and the total sleep time. Delayed sleep onset is often cited by patients as contributing to poor quality sleep. A patient may be lying awake with eyes closed but feeling anxious, fearful, or in pain. Robinson (1986) pointed out that insomnia can be induced through stress by shunting tryptophan away from the serotonin pathway. This would create long sleep latencies or difficulty in returning to sleep once interrupted.

Several subjective instruments use either a questionnaire approach (Parsons and Ver Beek, 1982) or a visual analogue scale. The Richards Campbell Sleep Questionnaire (Richards, 1987) and the Verran/Snyder-Halpern Sleep Tool (Snyder-Halpern and Verran, 1987) are examples of visual analogue scales that have been tested in critical care settings (Fontaine, 1989). At present there is no one instrument that will reliably and validly assess a critical care patient's sleep that is feasible in all settings and with all patients.

Comparison of nursing observations and polysomnographic (PSG) data reveals inconsistent findings. Nurses consistently overestimated the sleep time of ICU patients in a study comparing all-night PSG recordings of sleep stages and nursing observations made at 5-minute intervals (Aurell and Elmqvist, 1985). The reliability and validity of the sleep observation measure were not reported. Other research using a reliable sleep observation tool with specific criteria demonstrated good correlation with PSG data for wake after sleep onset in 20 trauma patients in an ICU setting (Fontaine, 1989). Because of the difficulty of observing sleep accurately, several researchers examined "potential sleep cycles" by noting periods when patients were undisturbed (Helton et al., 1980).

Measuring sleep in an accurate, noninvasive, and unobtrusive manner in critical care patients can be problematic. It is a mistake to assume that just leaving the patient undisturbed will guarantee sleep. Therefore, when an opportunity to sleep is provided, it is essential to examine what the patient does with the chance to sleep. A combination of nursing observation of sleep and eliciting the patient's perception of his sleep quality should be used.

Sleep Research in Critical Care

The sleep patterns of a variety of cardiac and other patients in critical care have been studied in critical care settings with the same general finding. Table 2–6 lists most of the sleep research studies that have been done in critical care for the past two decades. Greatly disturbed sleep occurred in patients in all studies whether measured by PSG recordings, nursing observations, or patient perception.

Sleep fragmentation leading to altered sleep architecture is noted in any study using PSG monitoring in the critical care unit. Sleep cycles are rarely completed, and there is a noted absence of REM sleep. Even when patients do fall asleep, they may awaken as often as a mean of 50 times per night (Richards and Bairnsfather, 1988). Of interest were two reports that at least 40% to 60% of sleep time was found to occur during the day (Aurell and Elmqvist, 1985; Hilton, 1976). Sleeping during the day may be explained by the widespread occurrence of sleep deprivation. Noise, the stress of injury, frequent interruptions, and pain were believed to contribute to sleep disruption. Noise levels often demonstrate little difference between day and night (Hilton, 1985).

In addition to environmental stimuli, numerous medications are known to disrupt sleep in the critically ill. Many patients in the studies listed in Table 2–6 probably received sleep-altering drugs. Narcotic analgesics often head the list, with morphine quantitatively decreasing stages 3 and 4 sleep and REM sleep (Sanford, 1988). Various barbiturates and hypnotics may also depress certain sleep stages. Hypnotics in critical care settings require further evaluation. The polypharmacy of critical care makes it increasingly difficult to examine any one drug's ef-

fects on sleep pattern. Patient perception thus becomes of great importance in evaluating sleep promotion using pharmacotherapy.

To demonstrate the extent of sleep disruption in young adult trauma patients in an ICU setting, Figure 2–4 depicts comparisons of the percentage of time spent in each sleep stage for an ICU group of patients (Fontaine, 1989) and for healthy young adults in a laboratory setting (Williams et al., 1974). Major features of sleep in the ICU group include a greatly increased wake time and stage 1 sleep with reduced amounts of REM sleep.

Although the literature contains numerous prescriptions for promoting sleep (Brewer, 1985; Sanford, 1988), few have been tested in the critical care setting.

NURSING THERAPEUTICS FOR SLEEP PATTERN DISTURBANCE

Sleep probably holds unknown healing powers that critical care nurses should strive to harness. Of interest is the substantial number of independent nursing interventions for the nursing diagnosis of sleep pattern disturbance. Sleep promotion in critical care is very much a nursing role. Selected strategies for sleep promotion are identified in Table 2–7. The therapeutic intervention categories are designed to assist in keeping the goal and patient outcomes clearly in mind.

Surveillance activities are designed to assess specific patient characteristics or behaviors and to make the nursing diagnosis. Obtaining a sleep history and documenting sleep-wake times on the flow sheet are important surveillance activities. Patients who will spend days to weeks in the critical care unit are at greatest risk of experiencing sleep deprivation and are the primary patients for whom sleep time documentation should be a priority.

Shielding interventions attempt to protect the pa-

TABLE 2–6. Overview of Sleep Research in Critical Care

Year	Author/Title	Subjects
1971	McFadden and Giblin. Sleep deprivation in patients having open heart surgery	4 open heart surgery patients
1972	Woods. Patterns of sleep in postcardiotomy patients	4 open heart surgery patients
1972	Walker. Amount of uninterrupted time for sleep and rest during the first, second, and third postoperative days in a teaching hospital	4 open heart surgery patients
1976	Hilton. Quantity and quality of patients' sleep and sleep-disturbing factors in a respiratory ICU	10 respiratory ICU patients
1978	Broughton and Baron. Sleep patterns in the intensive care unit and on the ward after acute myocardial infarction	12 myocardial infarction patients
1979	Dohno et al. Some aspects of sleep disturbance in coronary patients	42 coronary care patients
1980	Helton, Gordon, and Nunnery. Correlation between sleep deprivation and the intensive care unit syndrome	62 critical care patients
1985	Aurell and Elmqvist. Sleep in the surgical ICU: Continuous polygraphic recording of sleep in nine patients receiving postoperative care	9 surgical ICU patients
1988	Richards and Bairnsfather. Night sleep patterns in the critical care unit	10 medical ICU patients
1989	Fontaine. Measurement of nocturnal sleep patterns in trauma patients	20 multisystem trauma patients

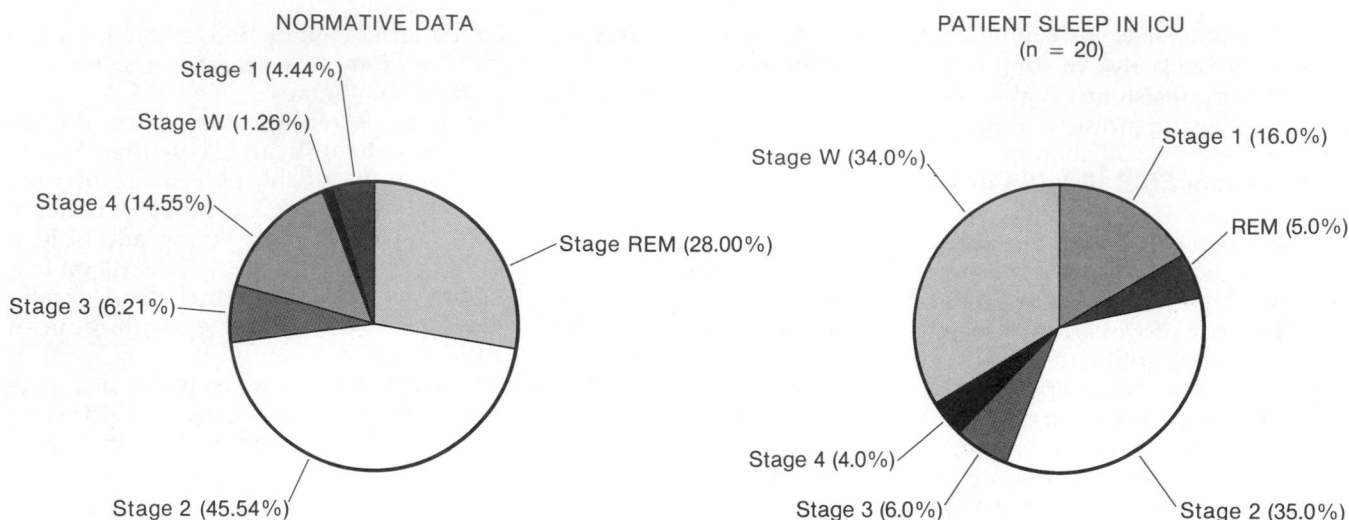

FIGURE 2–4. Comparison of trauma patients' sleep in ICU (data from Fontaine, 1989) with normative sleep data for early adult males. (Redrawn from Williams, R. L., Karacan I., and Hursch, C. J. (1974). *Electroencephalography (EEG) of human sleep: Clinical applications.* New York: John Wiley & Sons.)

tient from the aversive effects of the environment. Finally, modification as a nursing therapeutic strategy focuses on two areas, changing the external environment through activities such as noise abatement, and realigning the internal environment through the use of independent actions such as

---

TABLE 2–7. Strategies to Promote Sleep

Surveillance

Obtain and use sleep history to plan care.
Assess quality and quantity of sleep using appropriate methods.
Document sleep/wake time for all high-risk patients.
Monitor patient for psychophysiologic signs of sleep deprivation.
Determine if sleep occurs during the limited opportunity provided.

Shielding

Increase nurses' sensitivity to sounds and lights in the ICU.
Prevent excessive lights and noise from alarms and limit staff conversation.
Evaluate the need for nursing care interruptions.
Use a nursing care plan to individualize and block sleep times.
Allow an opportunity for uninterrupted sleep time during day and night.
Promote comfortable positioning of the patient for sleep.
Explain environmental sounds and provide other information to lower patient anxiety.

Modification

Provide adequate pain relief and evaluate continuous analgesia or epidural anesthesia for promoting effective sleep.
Include backrubs and patient's own presleep routine.
Use relaxation techniques and imagery or music therapy.
Administer hypnotics according to patient protocol and evaluate their effectiveness.
Maximize patient privacy through the use of curtains and doors.
Post sign at designated sleep times—**Patient Sleeping.**
Provide large clocks and natural lighting.
Evaluate bed for comfort and sleep quality.
Ease visitor restrictions if this encourages patient to sleep.

From Fontaine, D. K. (1987). Sleep deprivation in the critical care unit. *Critical Care Nursing Currents,* 5(4), p 22. Reprinted with permission from Ross Laboratories.

relaxation techniques or collaborative approaches using medications. These overlap with activities suggested for modification of sensory alterations.

Whether or not to interfere with a patient's sleep to change wound dressings or initiate chest physiotherapy is at times a collaborative nursing decision with the medical team. More likely, the nursing care plan reflects the priority the nurse places on sleep promotion by giving sleep and rest a prominent role alongside physiologic interventions. The nurse uses clinical decision-making skills to determine if a 5 A.M. bath is in the patient's best interests or the interests of the nursing staff. Novice nurses who are socialized into a critical care unit need to identify quickly the priority of rest and sleep along with continuous surveillance. In the future, increasing sophistication of monitoring equipment will permit even further physiologic assessment without disturbing the patient.

All sleep-promoting interventions need to be studied to determine the effectiveness of each for the different critical care populations. Of special interest is the investigation of pain control and sleep quality in critically ill patients. With advances in pain management, such as patient-controlled analgesia, studies examining the effect of pain management on sleep patterns are a high priority. Exploration of sleep patterns is needed in patients with differing environmental configurations, in various specialty beds, and after independent nursing interventions for relaxation.

SUMMARY

The common sensory alterations identified in the critically ill were the focus of this chapter. Immobility, altered time perception, and the use of neuromuscular blocking agents are several areas in which patients are at risk of experiencing sensory deprivation. The consistently high noise levels in critical care settings make noise a universal sensory overload phenomenon. Collaborative and independent nursing therapeutics addressing the sensory-perceptual alterations were recommended. In addition, sleep pattern disturbances, the ultimate consequence of environmental intrusion in critical care, was reviewed with suggestions for independent nursing strategies and further needed research. The uniqueness of these patient problems in critical care settings centers not only on their universal nature in critical care but also on the importance of independent nursing therapies in mediating the effects of an aversive critical care environment. The critically ill patient requires a nurse who can truly "tame the technology" (Jennett, 1984) in the critical care setting and create the necessary healing environment.

References

American Association of Critical-Care Nurses (1986). *Scope of critical care nursing practice* (AACN position statement, Newport Beach, CA).

Aurell, J., and Elmqvist, D. (1985). Sleep in the surgical intensive care unit: Continuous polygraphic recording of sleep in nine patients receiving postoperative care. *British Medical Journal*, 290, 1029–1032.

Baker, C. (1984). Sensory overload and noise in the ICU: Sources of environmental stress. *Critical Care Quarterly*, 6 (4), 66–80.

Ballard, K. S. (1981). Identification of environmental stressors for patients in a surgical intensive care unit. *Issues in Mental Health Nursing*, 3, 89–108.

Barry, M. J. (1979). Sensory alterations, overload, and underload: Making a nursing diagnosis. In M. S. Kennedy and G. M. Pfeifer (Eds.), *Current practice in nursing care of the adult: Issues and concepts* (pp. 33–45). St. Louis: C. V. Mosby.

Bay, E. J., Kupferschmidt, B., Opperwal, B. J., et al. (1988). Effect of the family visit on the patient's mental status. *Focus on Critical Care*, 15 (1), 10–16.

Beck, S. L. (1988). Measuring sleep. In M. Frank-Stromborg (Ed.), *Instruments for clinical nursing research* (pp. 255–267). Norwalk, CT: Appleton & Lange.

Betz, C. L. (1982). Sensory disturbances among children in the ICU. *Dimensions of Critical Care Nursing*. 1 (3), 145–151.

Bolin, R. H. (1974). Sensory deprivation: An overview. *Nursing Forum*, 13 (3), 240–258.

Brewer, M. J. (1985). To sleep or not to sleep: The consequences of sleep deprivation. *Critical Care Nurse*, 5 (6), 35–41.

Broughton, R., and Baron, R. (1978). Sleep patterns in the intensive care unit and on the ward after acute myocardial infarction. *Electroencephalography and Clinical Neurophysiology*, 45, 348–360.

Bryan-Brown, C. W. (1986). Development of pain management in critical care. In M. J. Cousins and G. D. Phillips (Ed.), *Acute pain management* (pp. 1–19). New York: Churchill Livingstone.

Cassem, N. H. (1989). Psychiatric problems of the critically ill patient. In W. C. Shoemaker, S. Ayres, A. Grenvik, et al. (Eds.), *Textbook of critical care* (2nd ed., pp. 1404–1414). Philadelphia: W. B. Saunders.

Cousins, M. J., and Phillips, G. D. (1984). Sleep, pain, and sedation. In W. C. Shoemaker, W. L. Thompson, and P. R. Holbrook (Eds.), *Textbook of critical care* (pp. 787–801). Philadelphia: W. B. Saunders.

DiMinno, M., and Ozuna, J. H. (1987). Sensory overload and sensory deprivation. In W. J. Phipps, B. C. Long, and N. F. Woods (Eds.), *Medical-surgical nursing concepts and clinical practice* (3rd ed., pp. 397–407). St. Louis: C. V. Mosby.

Dlin, B. M., Rosen, H., Dickstein, K., et al. (1971). The problems of sleep and rest in the intensive care unit. *Psychosomatics*, 12 (3), 155–163.

Dohno, S., Paskewitz, D. A., Lynch, J. J., et al. (1979). Some aspects of sleep disturbance in coronary patients. *Perceptual and Motor Skills*, 48, 199–205.

Dossey, B. M., Keegan, L., Guzzetta, C. E., et al. (1988). *Holistic nursing: A handbook for practice*. Rockville, MD: Aspen Publishers.

Downs, F. (1974). Bedrest and sensory disturbances. *American Journal of Nursing*, 74, 434–438.

Dracup, K. (1988). Are critical care units hazardous to health? *Applied Nursing Research*, 1, 14–21.

Easton, C., and MacKenzie, F. (1988). Sensory-perceptual alterations: Delirium in the intensive care unit. *Heart & Lung*, 17, 229–235.

Felton, G. (1987). Human biologic rhythms. In J. J. Fitzpatrick, and R. L. Taunton (Eds.), *Annual review of nursing research* (pp. 45–77). New York: Springer.

Fontaine, D. K. (1987). Sleep deprivation in the critical care unit. *Critical Care Nursing Currents*, 5 (4), 19–24.

Fontaine, D. K. (1989). Measurement of nocturnal sleep patterns in trauma patients. *Heart and Lung*, 18 (4), 402–410.

Gaillard, J. M. (1990). Neurotransmitters and sleep pharmacology. In M. J. Thorpy (Ed.), *Handbook of sleep disorders* (pp. 55–76). New York: Marcel Dekker.

Giuffre, M., Keane, A., Hatfield, S. M., et al. (1988). Patient controlled analgesia in clinical pain research management. *Nursing Research*, 37, 254–255.

Goldberger, L. (1966). Experimental isolation: An overview. *American Journal of Psychiatry*, 122, 774–782.

Gowan, N. J. (1979). The perceptual world of the intensive care unit: An overview of some environmental considerations in the helping relationship. *Heart & Lung*, 8, 340–344.

Gries, M. L., and Fernsler, J. (1988). Patient perceptions of the mechanical ventilation experience. *Focus on Critical Care*, 15 (2), 52–59.

Hansell, H. N. (1984). The behavior effects of noise on man: The patient with "intensive care unit psychosis." *Heart & Lung*, 13, 59–65.

Hartman, E. (1973). *The functions of sleep*. New Haven, CT: Yale University Press.

Heater, B. S. (1985). Nursing responsibilities in changing visiting restrictions in the intensive care unit. *Heart & Lung*, 14, 181–186.

Helton, M. C., Gordon, S. H., and Nunnery, S. L. (1980). The correlation between sleep deprivation and the intensive care unit syndrome. *Heart & Lung*, 9, 464–468.

Hilton, B. A. (1976). Quantity and quality of patients' sleep and sleep-disturbing factors in a respiratory intensive care unit. *Journal of Advanced Nursing*, 1, 453–468.

Hilton, B. A. (1985). Noise in acute patient care areas. *Research in Nursing and Health*, 8, 283–291.

Hilton, B. A. (1987). The hospital racket: How noisy is your unit? *American Journal of Nursing*, 87, 59–61.

Holden-Lund, C. (1988). Effects of relaxation with guided imagery on surgical stress and wound healing. *Research in Nursing and Health*, 11, 235–244.

Institute of Medicine. (1990). *Basic sleep research*. Washington, DC: National Academy Press.

Jackson, C. W., and Ellis, R. (1971). Sensory deprivation as a field of study. *Nursing Research*, 20, 46–54.

Jennett, B. (1984). *High technology medicine: Benefits and burdens*. London: The Nuffield Provincial Hospitals Trust.

Johns, M. W. (1971). Methods for assessing human sleep. *Archives of Internal Medicine*, 127, 484–492.

Johnson, S. M., Omery, A., and Nikas, D. (1989). Effects of conversation on intracranial pressure in comatose patients. *Heart & Lung*, 18, 56–63.

Karnofsky, M. L. (1986). Progress in sleep. *New England Journal of Medicine*, 315, 1026–1028.

Keep, P. J. (1977). Stimulus deprivation in windowless rooms. *Anaesthesia*, 32, 598–602.

Keep, P. J., James, J., and Inman, M. (1980). Windows in the intensive therapy unit. *Anaesthesia*, 35 (3), 256–262.

Kleck, H. G. (1984). ICU syndrome: Onset, manifestations, treatment, stressors, and prevention. *Critical Care Quarterly*, 6, 21–28.

Koella, W. P. (1978). Vigilance: A concept and its neurophysiological and biochemical implications. In P. Passouant, and I. Oswald (Eds.), *Pharmacology of the states of alertness* (pp. 171–178). Oxford, England: Pergamon Press.

Koella, W. P. (1985). Organization of sleep. In D. J. McGinty, R. Drucker-Colin, A. Morrison, et al. (Eds.), *Brain mechanisms of sleep*. New York: Raven Press.

Kryter, K. D. (1985). *The effects of noise on man* (2nd ed.). Menlo Park, CA: Academic Press.

Lewandowski, L. A., and Kositsky, A. M. (1983). Research priorities for critical care nursing. *Heart & Lung*, 12, 35–44.

Lindenmuth, J. E., Breu, C. S., and Malooley, J. A. (1980). Sensory overload. *American Journal of Nursing*, 80, 1456–1458.

MacKinnon-Kesler, S. (1983). Maximizing your ICU patient's sensory and perceptual environment. *Canadian Nurse*, 79 (5), 41–45.

McFadden, E. H., and Giblin, E. C. (1971). Sleep deprivation in patients having open heart surgery. *Nursing Research*, 20, 249–254.

McLane, A. M. (Ed.). (1987). *Classification of nursing diagnoses: Proceedings of the seventh conference*. St. Louis: C. V. Mosby.

Meleis, A. I. (1985). *Theoretical nursing: Development and progress*. Philadelphia: J. B. Lippincott.

Mitchell, P., and Mauss, N. (1978). Relationships of patient/nurse activity to intracranial pressure variations: A pilot study. *Nursing Research*, 27, 4–10.

Naitoh, P., Kelly, T. L., and Englund, C. (1990). Health effects of sleep deprivation. *Occupational Medicine*, 5, 209–237.

Nightingale, F. (1859). *Notes on nursing*. London: Harrison & Sons.

Noble, M. A. (1979). Communication in the ICU: Therapeutic or disturbing? *Nursing Outlook*, 27, 195–198.

Noble, M. A. (Ed.). (1982). *The ICU environment: Directions for nursing*. Reston, VA: Reston Publishing.

Palmblad, J., Petrini, B., Wasserman, J., et al. (1979). Lymphocyte and granulocyte reactions during sleep deprivation. *Psychosomatic Medicine*, 41, 273–277.

Parker, M. M., Schubert, W., Shelhamer, J. H., et al. (1984). Perceptions of a critically ill patient experiencing paralysis in an ICU. *Critical Care Medicine*, 12, 69–71.

Parkes, J. D. (1985). *Sleep and its disorders*. Philadelphia: W. B. Saunders.

Parsons, L. C., and Ver Beek, D. (1982). Sleep-awake patterns following cerebral concussion. *Nursing Research*, 31, 260–264.

Phillips, G. D., and Cousins, M. J. (1986). Neurological mechanisms of pain and the relationship of pain, anxiety, and sleep. In M. J. Cousins and G. D. Phillips (Eds.), *Acute pain management* (pp. 21–48). New York: Churchill Livingstone.

Rechtschaffen, A., and Kales, A. (Eds.). (1968). *A manual of standardized terminology, techniques, and scoring system for sleep stages of human subjects*. Bethesda, MD: U.S. Department of Health, Education, and Welfare.

Redding, J. S., Hargest, T. S., and Minsky, S. H. (1977). How noisy is intensive care? *Critical Care Medicine*, 5, 275–276.

Richards, K. C. (1987). Techniques for measurement of sleep in critical care. *Focus on Critical Care*, 14, 34–40.

Richards, K. C., and Bairnsfather, L. (1988). A description of night sleep patterns in the critical care unit. *Heart & Lung*, 17, 35–42.

Riegel, B. (1989). Stressors of critically ill patients. In B. Riegel, and D. Ehrenreich (Eds.), *Psychological aspects of critical care* (pp. 17–30). Rockville, MD: Aspen Publishers.

Robinson, C. (1986). Impaired sleep. In V. K. Carrieri, A. M. Lindsey, and C. M. West (Eds.), *Pathophysiological phenomena in nursing: Human responses to illness* (pp. 390–417). Philadelphia: W. B. Saunders.

Sanford, S. J. (1988). Sleep in the critically ill patient. In M. R. Kinney, D. R. Packa, and S. B. Dunbar (Eds.), *AACN'S clinical reference for critical-care nursing* (2nd ed., pp. 399–413). New York: McGraw Hill.

Scanlon-Schilpp, A. M., and Robinson, L. (1988). Psychosocial responses of the human spirit: The journey of trauma. In V. D. Cardona, P. D. Hurn, P. J. B. Mason, et al. (Eds.), *Trauma nursing from resuscitation through rehabilitation* (pp. 184–203). Philadelphia: W. B. Saunders.

Schnaper, N. (1975). The psychological implications of severe trauma—emotional sequelae to unconsciousness. *Journal of Trauma*, 15, 94–98.

Simpson, T. F., Armstrong, S., and Mitchell, P. (1989). American Association of Critical-Care Nurses Demonstration Project: Patients' recollections of critical care. *Heart & Lung*, 18, 325–332.

Smith, M. J. (1986). Human-environment process: A test of Rogers' principle of integrality. *Advances in Nursing Science*, 9 (1), 21–28.

Snyder, M. (1985). *Independent nursing interventions*. New York: John Wiley & Sons.

Snyder-Halpern, R. (1985). The effect of critical care unit noise on patient sleep cycles. *Critical Care Quarterly*, 7 (4), 41–50.

Snyder-Halpern, R., and Verran, J. (1987). Instrumentation to describe subjective sleep characteristics in healthy subjects. *Research in Nursing and Health*, 10 (3), 155–163.

Stovsky, B., Rudy, E., and Dragonette, P. (1988). Comparison of two types of communication methods used after cardiac surgery with patients with endotracheal tubes. *Heart & Lung*, 17, 281–289.

Thompson, J. M., McFarland, G. K., Hirsch, J. E., et al. (1986). *Clinical nursing*. St. Louis: C. V. Mosby.

Topf, M. (1984). A framework for research on aversive physical aspects of the environment. *Research in Nursing and Health*, 7, 35–42.

Ulrich, R. S. (1984). View through a window may influence recovery from surgery. *Science*, 224, 420–421.

Urban, N. (1988). Responses to the environment. In M. R. Kinney, D. R. Packa, and S. B. Dunbar (Eds.), *AACN'S clinical reference for critical-care nursing* (2nd ed., pp. 96–112). New York: McGraw Hill.

Viner, E. D. (1985). Life at the other end of the endotracheal tube: A physician's personal view of critical illness. *Progress in Critical Care Medicine*, 2, 3–13.

Vitello-Cicciu, J. M. (1984). Recalled perceptions of patients administered pancuronium bromide. *Focus on Critical Care*, 11 (1), 30–35.

Walker, B. B. (1972). The postsurgery heart patient: Amount of uninterrupted time for sleep and rest during the first, second, and third postoperative days in a teaching hospital. *Nursing Research*, 21, 164–169.

Wauquier, A., Monti, J. M., Gaillard, J. M., et al. (1985). *Sleep neurotransmitters and neuromodulators*. New York: Raven Press.

White, D. P., Douglas, N. J., Pickett, C. K., et al. (1983). Sleep deprivation and the control of ventilation. *American Review of Respiratory Diseases*, 128, 984–986.

Williams R. L., Karacan, I., and Hursch, C. J. (1974). *Electroencephalography (EEG) of human sleep: Clinical applications*. New York: John Wiley & Sons.

Wilson, V. S. (1987). Identification of stressors related to patients' psychologic responses to the surgical intensive care unit. *Heart & Lung*, 16, 267–273.

Woods, N. F. (1972). Patterns of sleep in postcardiotomy patients. *Nursing Research*, 21, 347–352.

Woods, N. F., and Falk, S. A. (1974). Noise stimuli in the acute care area. *Nursing Research*, 23, 144–150.

Worrell, J. D. (1977). Nursing implications in the care of the patient experiencing sensory deprivation. In K. C. Kintzel (Ed.), *Advanced concepts in clinical nursing* (2nd ed., pp. 618–638). Philadelphia: J. B. Lippincott.

Zubek, J. P. (Ed.) (1969). *Sensory deprivation: Fifteen years of research*. New York: Appleton-Century-Crofts.

3

Immobility Phenomena in Critically Ill Adults

Nancy L. Szaflarski

Mobility is a fundamental characteristic of man and is vital to independence. Mobility serves to promote physical fitness, prevent disability, and slow the onset of degenerative processes. Maintenance of optimal health requires a proper balance of rest, sleep, exercise, and time in an upright position. The upright, standing position serves to trigger physiologic responses that counteract gravity effects and maintain a state of homeostasis. Even at rest, the healthy adult normally turns or changes position an average of every 11.6 minutes, emphasizing the important role of mobility in life (Milazzo and Resh, 1981). This standard of movement has been defined as the "minimal physiological mobility requirement."

Bedrest has been traditionally used as a cornerstone, therapeutic measure for critically ill patients. Its benefits result mainly from decreasing oxygen consumption ($\dot{V}O_2$), preventing or reducing trauma to a body part, and allowing energy resources to be directed toward healing. Numerous studies have examined the physiologic and psychological consequences of bedrest. The bulk of these studies were conducted during the 1960s and 1970s for the United States space program because bedrest was used as an analogue of weightlessness. Clinical studies have further defined the pathophysiologic consequences of bedrest, and these have highlighted the use of bedrest as a double-edged sword.

Immobility is a disuse phenomenon that evokes physiologic, psychological, and psychosocial effects that are interrelated. The stimulus for this akinetic phenomenon in critically ill adults is bedrest. The prevalence of bedrest in this population approaches nearly 100%. An observation of any critical care unit will reveal adults confined to bed in supine, Trendelenburg, lateral recumbent, and Fowler positions. Few studies have defined the length and degree of immobility in critically ill patients. Chulay and colleagues (1982) found that 9 of 18 university hospitals required 24 hours of supine bedrest for patients recovering from coronary artery bypass surgery during their immediate postoperative period.

The reasons for immobility in critically ill adults are listed in Table 3–1. The increased use of sophisticated technology has had a major impact on im-

---

TABLE 3–1. Reasons for Immobility in Critically Ill Adults

Therapeutic Gain

1. Decrease $\dot{V}O_2$ and carbon dioxide production (refractory hypoxemic-hypercarbic respiratory failure; acute myocardial infarction; congestive heart failure)
2. Attain and maintain cardiopulmonary stability (cardiopulmonary arrest; postarrest states; postcardiopulmonary bypass; shock states; severe burns; intra-aortic and pulmonary artery balloon pumping)
3. Promote healing or minimize trauma (intracranial bleeding; disseminated intravascular coagulation; aortic or arterial graft approximations; large wounds with questionable tensile strengths; burns; acute spinal cord injuries; acute stroke)
4. Maintenance of spinal or bone alignment (acute spinal cord injuries, orthopedic fractures)

Safety

1. Altered mental states (coma; confusion; postanesthesia states; sedation or narcotization)
2. Maintenance of intravascular access lines and associated drug or fluid infusions
3. Secure provision for artificial airways and ventilatory modes
4. Provision for accurate invasive monitoring and therapy (hemodynamic and intracranial pressure lines; oximetry or capnography; intra-aortic and pulmonary artery balloon pumping; transesophageal echocardiography)
5. Altered motor or sensory function (generalized weakness; stroke; peripheral neuropathies; neuromuscular blockade; paralysis)

posing supine immobilization in critically ill adults (Chulay et al., 1982; Tyler, 1984). The length of immobilization is nearly directly proportional to the length of stay in the intensive care unit (ICU), since many patients are not fully ambulatory upon discharge from the ICU.

The high morbidity rate associated with immobility is related to the length of immobilization. Although studies of healthy young adults have demonstrated the presence of significant physiologic changes from bedrest within as few as 3 to 4 days (Chobanian et al., 1974; Greenleaf, 1982; Lamb et al., 1965), the occurrence of pathophysiologic changes is associated with longer immobilization periods. Critically ill patients with long-term disease processes such as multisystem failure, Guillain-Barré syndrome, adult respiratory distress syndrome (ARDS), and sepsis are at greater risk for morbidity than are elective postoperative patients who are subjected to a 1- or 2-day recovery period. Factors associated with increased risk of morbidity from immobilization in critically ill adults are listed in Table 3–2. The signs and symptoms of complications resulting from immobility may not be fully apparent at the time of discharge from the ICU because many patients remain on bedrest and have not begun the remobilization process.

Major forms of morbidity resulting from immobility include infection, sepsis, muscle atrophy, pressure sores, respiratory failure, thromboembolism, and pulmonary embolism. Such morbidity results in increased length of ICU or hospital stay, increased caregiver and equipment costs, and increased duration and extent of suffering for the patient. The critical care nurse can play a major role in preventing these complications by understanding the physiologic, pathophysiologic, and psychological effects of immobility. ■

PHYSIOLOGIC AND PATHOPHYSIOLOGIC EFFECTS OF IMMOBILITY

Many of the physiologic effects induced by immobility occur immediately as a recumbent position is achieved. Other physiologic and pathophysiologic effects are associated with longer periods of immobility. An appreciation of the time course of the effects is essential to project potential complications.

Cardiovascular Effects

FLUID SHIFTS

When an individual moves from an upright to a supine position, central fluid shifts occur. Eleven per cent of total blood volume is shifted from the legs to other parts of the body (Rubin, 1988). Of this shifted volume, 78% is directed to the thorax and 20% to the head and neck (Rubin, 1988). These shifts result

TABLE 3–2. Risk Factors Associated with Complications of Immobility in Critically Ill Adults

Length and degree of immobility
Past medical history (peripheral vascular disease, DVT, PE, decubiti, pneumonia)
Altered motor or sensory function
Altered level of consciousness
Incontinence
Poor nutrition
Advancing age
Obesity
Altered skin integrity
Present infection
Extensive surgery
Significant sustained hypotension
Hypoxemia
Altered immunocompetence
Malignancy
Exogenous steroid administration

Abbreviations: DVT, deep venous thrombosis; PE, pulmonary embolism.

in an increased central venous pressure, left ventricular end-diastolic pressure, and stroke volume. A successful adaptation to the supine position activates volume receptors and renal and hormonal mechanisms to produce a diuresis. This diuresis results in a reduction of plasma volume, total blood volume, and end-diastolic filling pressures and volumes and is independent of total fluid intake. Plasma volume losses occur during short periods of bedrest but then level off and do not regain normal levels. Losses of 6% to 15% of plasma volume have been associated with bedrest (Dietrick et al., 1948; Johnson et al., 1971; Saltin et al., 1968; Stremel et al., 1976). Total blood volume losses parallel plasma volume losses but are not as great (Winslow, 1985). Dietrick and colleagues (1948) reported a decline in total blood volume averaging 5.4% in a classic study of four normal men on 6 to 7 weeks of bedrest. If bedrest continues, the initial decrease in extracellular volume is restored by an increase in interstitial volume, although plasma volume remains low.

PHYSICAL WORK CAPACITY

Prolonged bedrest results in cardiovascular deconditioning as reflected in a decreased physical work capacity and orthostatic intolerance (Blomquist and Stone, 1983; Chobanian et al., 1974; Saltin et al., 1968; Taylor et al., 1949). Increases of resting heart rates of 4 to 15 beats per minute have been reported with prolonged bedrest (Dietrick et al., 1948; Miller et al., 1964, 1965; Saltin et al., 1968; Taylor et al., 1949). Cardiovascular deconditioning effects from bedrest can also be quantified by a measure of physical working capacity known as maximal or peak $\dot{V}_{O_2}$ (oxygen uptake). Peak oxygen uptake is the maximal rate at which oxygen can be delivered to the tissues during periods of exhaustive isotonic exercise. It is the product of the maximal cardiac output and the maximal arteriovenous oxygen difference. Maximal

$\dot{V}O_2$ is a well-recognized measure of cardiopulmonary fitness, maximal aerobic capacity, and deconditioning adaptation of bedridden subjects (Greenleaf, 1982). Significant decreases of 13% to 46% in maximal $\dot{V}O_2$ after prolonged bedrest were found to occur in men during treadmill testing after 3 to 4 weeks of bedrest (Miller et al., 1965; Saltin et al., 1968; Taylor et al., 1949). Convertino and associates (1977) demonstrated proportional deterioration in maximal $\dot{V}O_2$ following 14 to 17 days of bedrest in young healthy women (-9.7%, $p < .01$) and young healthy men (-9.1%, $p < .05$). Saltin et al. (1968) found that the decrease in maximal $\dot{V}O_2$ associated with prolonged bedrest was primarily related to a decrease in stroke volume.

ORTHOSTATIC CAPACITY

When a normal adult assumes the erect position from a supine position, approximately 500 mL of blood shifts largely from the intrathoracic cardiovascular compartment to the lower parts of the body. This loss of blood volume from the thorax decreases venous return, stroke volume, cardiac output, and arterial pressure. Neurovascular stretch receptors located in the carotid arteries and aorta and in the walls of the heart are stimulated by a lack of stretch. Their activation results in increased heart rate, increased myocardial contractility, vasoconstriction, and antidiuresis, which maintain arterial pressure and adequate perfusion pressure to the vital organs. Movement of the lower extremities in an erect position causes skeletal muscle contraction, which exerts pressure against the veins and lymph vessels in the legs. Such movement aids in increasing venous return in the presence of competent venous valves.

Orthostatic hypotension occurs in individuals placed on bedrest (Dietrick et al., 1949; Miller et al., 1964, 1965; Vogt et al., 1966). Orthostatic intolerance has been reported to occur after as little as 6 hours of bedrest (McCally et al., 1968). The sudden development of hypotension, weakness, faintness, or dizziness in a recumbent patient who is placed upright is explained by two contributing factors. Neurovascular reflexes have become dormant during the period of bedrest despite adequate epinephrine output. The peripheral vessels thus fail to constrict appropriately in response to the stress. The general loss of muscle tone that occurs with bedrest also depresses the normal venopressor mechanism, resulting in venous pooling of blood in the dependent lower extremities (Olson, 1967). The compensatory tachycardia that usually occurs is evoked to sustain cerebral perfusion pressure. Chobanian and co-workers (1974) reported significant decreases in cardiac output and stroke volume during upright tilt in normal subjects after bedrest. Increases in heart rate during tilt in this study averaged 13% before bedrest, 32% after 3 days of bedrest, 62% after 1 week, and 89% after 3 weeks of bedrest. Occasionally individuals have been reported to exhibit a bradycardic response to the falling blood pressure of orthostasis (Chobanian et al., 1974; Fareeduddin and Abelmann, 1969). The ability of the cardiovascular system to respond appropriately to the upright posture is regained slowly after resumption of activity. Taylor and colleagues (1949) reported that more than 5 weeks were needed to regain appropriate reflexes in healthy young men who had been subjected to up to 21 days of bedrest.

VENOUS FLOW

Due to the decreased use of leg muscles associated with bedrest, the frequency and strength of skeletal muscle contractions are decreased, resulting in unaided venous blood return. Decreased venous flow results in venous blood pooling and stasis in the lower extremities. This phenomenon alone may result in venous thrombosis. Damage to the venous intima also may occur with bedrest when a flaccid leg is subjected to sustained pressure from a supporting surface or another body part (Roberts, 1987). Intimal damage of veins has been a well-recognized contributory factor in the development of thrombophlebitis. Hypercoagulability due to associated decreases in plasma volume with immobility also predisposes to thrombophlebitis. These three risk factors—venous stasis, intimal damage, and hypercoagulability—comprise Virchow's triad.

Critically ill patients should be considered as being at high risk for deep vein thrombosis (DVT) based solely on the prevalence and extent of their immobility. Immobility has been defined as a prime risk factor in the development of venous stasis and DVT (Coon et al., 1987; Pingleton, 1985). Plate and associates (1986) reported that prolonged immobility was the most frequent etiologic factor for acute iliofemoral venous thrombosis in 25% of 128 medical-surgical patients. Other factors, identified in Table 3–3, elicit one or more arms of Virchow's triad in predisposing to DVT (Coon et al., 1987; Fahey, 1984; Pingleton, 1985). The frequent synergism of these risk factors in critically ill adults places most such patients at high risk for this complication.

Although the major complication of DVT is pulmonary embolism, it is important to note that DVT may also result in recurrent venous thrombosis and the post-phlebitic syndrome. Venous hypertension

---

TABLE 3–3. Risk Factors for Deep Venous Thrombosis in Critically Ill Adults

Immobilization
Major abdominal or orthopedic surgery
Nonsurgical trauma
Advancing age (>40 years)
Obesity
Cardiopulmonary disease
Past medical history (DVT, PE, leg trauma)
Pregnancy or parturition
Malignancy
Altered coagulation (thrombocytosis, polycythemia vera)

Abbreviations: DVT, deep venous thrombosis; PE, pulmonary embolism.

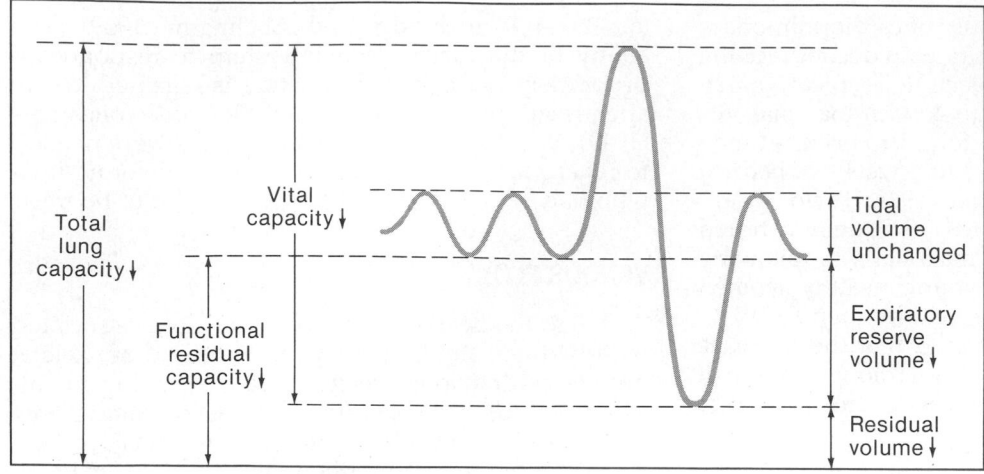

FIGURE 3–1. Effect of supine position on lung volumes and capacities in normal lungs.

is present with DVT. As lysis of the clot occurs, subsequent recanalization of the vein may cause destruction of valves in deep and communicating veins. Chronic venous insufficiency may result, causing chronic leg pain, edema, and stasis ulceration. Even when DVT is clinically silent, the post-phlebitic syndrome may result (Coon et al., 1987).

Pulmonary Effects

LUNG VOLUMES

Upon assuming a recumbent position, all lung volumes decrease except for tidal volume (Fig. 3–1). Residual volume and functional residual capacity (FRC) are decreased due to the increase in intrathoracic blood volume associated with recumbency. Recumbency-induced diaphragmatic elevation secondary to the gravitational redistribution of the abdominal contents also reduces FRC. Blair and Hickam (1955) found that the mean FRC ranged from 3.3 liters in the sitting position to 3.79 liters in the standing position to 2.69 liters in the recumbent position in normal subjects. Normal subjects placed in the supine position have shown decreases in FRC of 30% (Craig et al., 1971). Marini and associates (1984) reported a mean fall in FRC of only 3.5% when patients with chronic air flow obstruction changed from upright to seated to supine positions.

The clinical relevance of changing lung volumes and capacities with the supine and lateral recumbent positions is dependent upon the newly altered relationship between the closing volume and FRC. The FRC needs to be greater than the closing volume in order to keep airways open. If the closing volume is greater than the FRC, some alveoli will be closed, thus creating areas of ventilation-perfusion ($\dot{V}/\dot{Q}$) mismatch in the lung. The sensitivity of closing volumes to changes in posture and overall higher closing volumes have been associated with obese and older adults (Don et al., 1971).

VENTILATION-PERFUSION RELATIONSHIPS

In the upright, normal lung, ventilation and perfusion both increase from the upper to the lower areas of the lung (Fig. 3–2). Perfusion is greater in the bases due to the profound influence of gravitational forces sequestering greater blood flow. Although there is less lung expansion in the bases due to the weight of the lung, ventilation remains greatest in the bases in the upright position due to less negative intrapleural pressures, which are determined by gravitational forces and the weight of the lung. Since increases in perfusion are greater than increases in ventilation down the lung in the upright position, $\dot{V}/\dot{Q}$ ratios decrease from the lung apex to the lung base.

Assumption of the supine, lateral recumbent, or prone position causes a redistribution of ventilation and perfusion in the lung. The dependent lung portion in the supine position becomes the dorsal

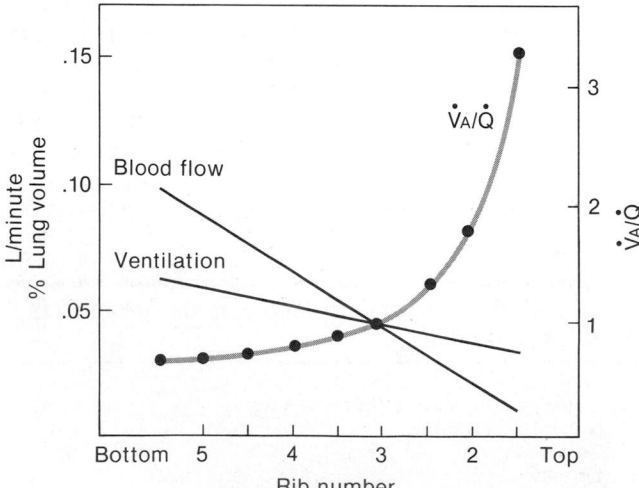

FIGURE 3–2. Ventilation and blood flow distribution in the upright, normal lung. Although ventilation and blood flow both increase down the lung, perfusion increases remain greatest. The ventilation-perfusion ratios ($\dot{V}/\dot{Q}$) thus decrease from apex to base. (Redrawn from West, J. B. (1977). *Ventilation/blood flow and gas exchange* (3rd ed.). Oxford: Blackwell.)

portion of the lung; in a lateral recumbent position it becomes the lung portion that meets the supporting surface; and in a prone position it becomes the anterior lung region. Changes in V̇/Q̇ ratios in the supine position have resulted in impaired gas exchange in individuals from 35 to 61 years of age (Don et al., 1971). Cardus (1967) reported decreases in the partial pressure of oxygen in arterial blood (Pa_{O_2}) and increases in the alveolar-arterial oxygen difference in normal young men who were subjected to 7 days of bedrest and permitted to turn at will.

Factors impairing ventilation in patients on bedrest may also contribute to altered V̇/Q̇ relationships. Restriction of chest excursion and diaphragmatic descent can occur with abdominal distention, abdominal or chest binders, use of pharmacologic agents, and a slumped sitting position, which is a common sight in an ICU. The effects of anesthesia on decreasing diaphragmatic excursion, FRC, and diaphragmatic activity for 24 hours after surgery are also well-known factors in impairing ventilation in immobilized patients (Ford et al., 1983; Froese and Bryan, 1974).

ATELECTASIS AND PNEUMONIA

Atelectasis is a known consequence of prolonged bedrest. Due to weakened thoracic muscles, decreased ciliary movement in the tracheobronchial tree, and impaired cough mechanisms, respiratory secretions may easily accumulate in dependent lung areas and block bronchioles. Lung gas distal to these blockages is absorbed, resulting in alveolar collapse. Decreased surfactant production due to decreases in regional blood flow has also been implicated in the development of atelectasis (Memmer and Kozier, 1987). The stasis and pooling of pulmonary secretions can lead to hypostatic pneumonia and may create an excellent medium for bacterial growth. The confounding factors of dehydration and use of anticholinergic drugs in immobile patients may result in secretions that are thick, tenacious, and hard to raise. The clinical consequence of atelectasis and pneumonia is hypoxemia due to low V̇/Q̇ units and intrapulmonary shunting.

Pennington (1987) reported a rate of nosocomial pneumonia as high as 20% in patients in a respiratory ICU. Yannelli and Gurevich (1988) have defined the major risk factor of nosocomial pneumonia in critically ill patients as endotracheal intubation because host defenses are bypassed with this therapeutic adjunct. Pennington (1987) found a four times greater incidence of nosocomial pneumonia in intubated patients than in those who were not. Other risk factors for critically ill patients identified by Yannelli and Gurevich (1988) included the presence of nasogastric tubes, assisted ventilation, immunosuppression, impaired mental status, antibiotic usage, surgical procedures, and gastric or oropharyngeal aspiration. Immobility as a factor in predisposing critically ill adults to nosocomial pneumonia has not been independently defined or controlled for. Since most ICU patients are on bedrest, the factor of immobility remains implied in the identified risk factors.

ASPIRATION

Elpern et al. (1987) reported an overall 77% aspiration rate in a study of 31 critically ill intubated adults. A risk factor for aspiration identified in this study was the flat or head-down position, which was a potential cause of retrograde movement of gastroesophageal contents. Subjects placed in these positions were limited in number in this study, limiting the statistical inference of this finding. Elpern and colleagues (1987) also found that the head-up position in these 31 intubated patients did not prove beneficial in protecting against aspiration because the aspiration rate was 27% in this subgroup. The assumption that a Fowler's position protects the airway from aspiration may indeed not be thoroughly true. The major clinical consequences of aspiration are noscomial pneumonia, chemical pneumonitis, acute lung injury, hypoxemia, and mechanical obstruction. The volume and pH of the aspirate are critical factors in determining the patient's clinical response to aspiration.

PULMONARY EMBOLISM

The release, travel, and lodging of a venous thrombus into a lobar artery or distal arterial branch in the lung can occur in an immobile, critically ill patient without warning. Occasionally associated with no prior symptoms or signs, pulmonary embolism represents a serious, often fatal, complication. Pulmonary embolism occurs in approximately 50% of patients with documented DVT (Gallus and Hirsh, 1976; Kakker et al., 1969; Morrell and Dunhill, 1968). Pingleton and associates (1981) reported a 13% incidence of pulmonary embolism over a period of 1 year in respiratory ICU patients who received no prophylaxis. A 27% incidence was discovered by Neuhaus and co-workers (1978) in respiratory ICU patients at autopsy. Significant and fatal emboli originate as thrombi in the iliofemoral veins (Kakkar et al., 1969; Morrell and Dunhill, 1968).

The clinical consequences of pulmonary embolism depend upon the percentage of the pulmonary vascular bed that is occluded. Acute pulmonary hypertension usually results when greater than 50% of the pulmonary vascular bed is occluded (Roberts, 1987). The result of the embolus is a decrease in the cross-sectional area of the lung vasculature, resulting in increases in pulmonary artery pressures, pulmonary vascular resistance, and right ventricular (RV) workload. Shock may result due to acute RV failure secondary to the acute increase in afterload to the right ventricle. The stimulation of intrapulmonary receptors in the alveolar-capillary wall may produce dyspnea. Dyspnea also may result from severe arterial hypoxemia, which has been reported in 85% to 90% of critically ill patients experiencing a pulmonary embolism (Roberts, 1987). Hypoxemia occurring during a massive pulmonary embolism is related to overperfusion of the nonembolized lung, resulting in low $\dot{V}/\dot{Q}$ units that cause pulmonary shunting. Increases in dead space ventilation develop due to areas of high $\dot{V}/\dot{Q}$ units created by poor or absent pulmonary perfusion.

Gastrointestinal Effects

CONSTIPATION

Immobility contributes to the development of constipation due to several factors. Overall skeletal muscle weakness can affect the primary muscles of elimination (the diaphragm, abdominals, and levator ani), which may result in a decrease in expulsive power secondary to the loss of ability to increase intra-abdominal pressure. Loss of the defecation reflex may occur if patients fail to defecate when the reflexes are excited. If ignored, these reflexes will become weaker over time. The use of a bedpan is often refused or is nonproductive of stool due to its uncomfortableness and forced, unnatural position. Patients may repeatedly postpone using the bedpan due to the embarrassment, lack of privacy, and dependence on others (Memmer and Kozier, 1987). Such postponement suppresses the defecation reflex and results in greater water absorption from the stool in the colon. Hardened and dry stool in the colon may lead to fecal impaction, resulting in partial or complete mechanical obstruction of the colon. Colonic contractures may result in excessive intraluminal pressures whereby liquid stool may be forced around the impaction and expelled as a ribbon of diarrhea or a fecal-colored smear (Memmer and Kozier, 1987). If the impaction is not effectively treated, mechanical bowel obstruction may result in impaired bowel circulation secondary to intraluminal compression of the mesenteric vessels, abdominal distention, impaired fluid and substrate absorption, and venous thrombi formation secondary to large abdominal vein compression resulting from increased abdominal pressure (Leithauser, 1946; Olson, 1967).

In contrast to constipation associated with immobility is the reported incidence of diarrhea in critically ill patients, which has been reported to be as high as 41% (Kelly et al., 1983). Often due to enteral feedings, the enhanced gut motility may serve to prevent impaction or confound a pre-existing impaction or obstruction.

Urinary Effects

The human kidney and urinary bladder are anatomically designed to function optimally in an erect position (Figs. 3–3A and 3–4A). Erect positions allow a majority of urine to flow out of the renal pelvis because the hilus emerges from the medial aspect of the kidney. A minimal amount of urine is left in the dependent calyces. The urethra is the dependent path for urine flow in an erect position.

URINARY STASIS

Supine positions result in the renal pelvis filling with urine before urine can be expressed into the ureter. The result is urinary stasis (Fig. 3–3B). Urinary stasis provides a focus for bacterial growth and renal calculus formation. Accumulation of urine in the dependent portion of the urinary bladder in a supine position potentially results in a medium for bacterial growth, urinary retention, and urinary incontinence (Fig. 3–4B). Bladder distention may result, inhibiting the urge to void due to chronic stretching of the bladder and loss of bladder tone.

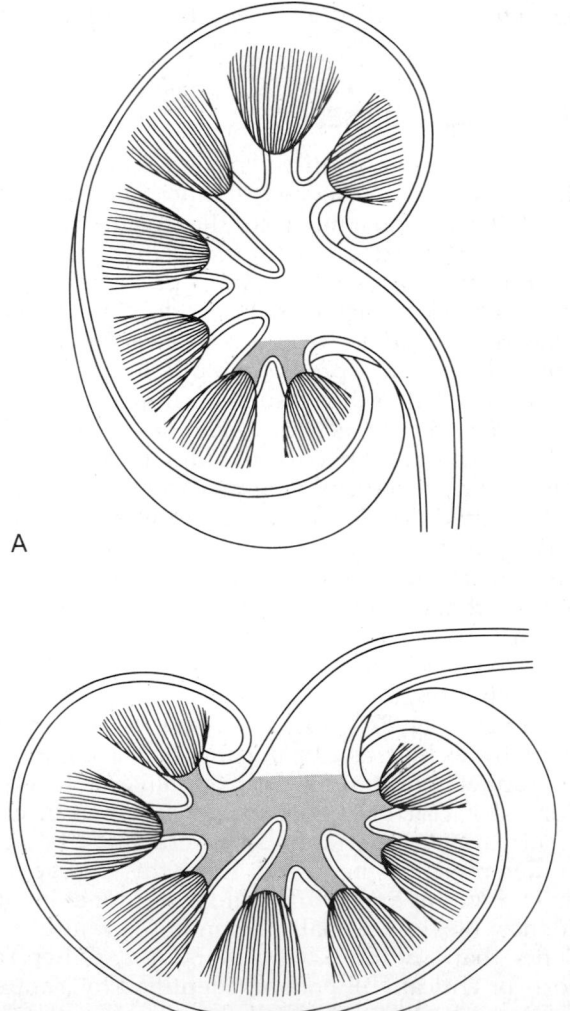

A

B

FIGURE 3–3. Urinary stasis in the kidney. *A,* Upright, standing position. *B,* Supine position. (Redrawn from *Fundamentals of Nursing,* Fourth Edition, by Kozier, Erb, and Olivieri (Redwood City, CA: Addison-Wesley Nursing, 1991), p. 846. Reprinted by permission.)

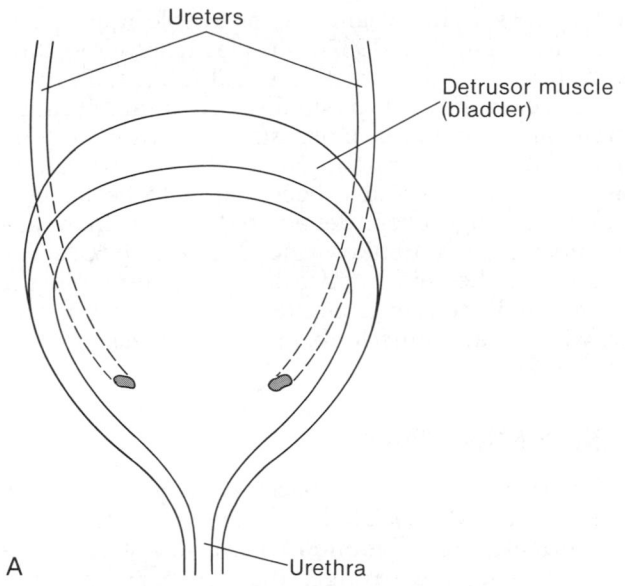

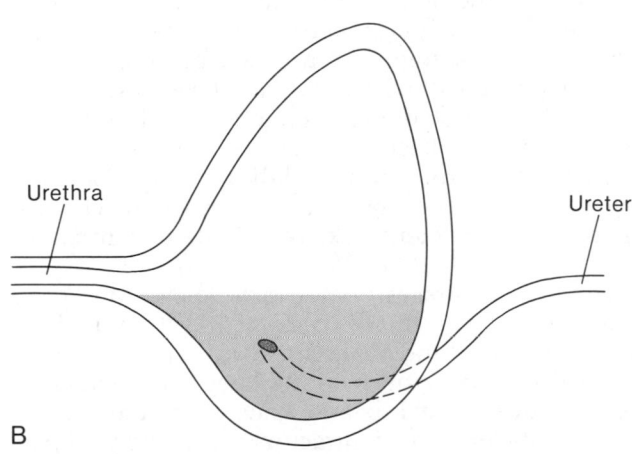

FIGURE 3–4. Urinary stasis in the urinary bladder. *A,* Upright, standing position. *B,* Supine position. (Redrawn from *Fundamentals of Nursing,* Fourth Edition, by Kozier, Erb, and Olivieri (Redwood City, CA: Addison-Wesley Nursing, 1991), p. 847. Reprinted by permission.)

Some involuntary urinary incontinence may also occur with considerable distention. The process of voiding in bed is also inhibited by the difficulty of relaxing the perineal muscles and the external sphincter and by ignoring the sensation to void.

URINARY MINERAL EXCRETION

Upon assuming a supine position, circulatory blood volume is increased, which normally evokes a diuresis and a natriuresis in order to maintain a normal plasma concentration. Bedrest also affects urinary calcium excretion owing to the hypercalcemia that results from bone disuse. Hwang and associates (1988) reported increases in mean urinary calcium and phosphorus excretion during the first week of bedrest; these increases were sustained throughout 5 weeks of bedrest in normal subjects. Due to this

increased urinary load, calcium deposits may occur in the renal pelvis or bladder, leading to nephrolithiasis and potentially to postrenal failure. Hematuria, dull flank pain, backache, and severe bouts of coliclike pain with nausea and vomiting are classic signs and symptoms of urinary stones. Four factors favor the precipitation of calcium salts in the kidney or bladder: urinary stasis, hypercalciuria, hyperphosphaturia, and alkaline urine (Dietrick et al., 1948; Johnson, 1974; Olson, 1967; O'Neill, 1981). Increased urine alkalinity occurs with immobility due to fewer acid end-products of metabolism. Increases in urine pH cause calcium salts to precipitate. The incidence of nephrolithiasis has been reported to be as high as 15% to 30% in individuals immobilized for extended periods (Mitchell, 1981) and is clearly higher than in other studied populations (Dietrick et al., 1948).

URINARY TRACT INFECTION

Factors favoring the development of urinary tract infections (UTIs) associated with immobility include urinary stasis, bladder distention, increased urinary alkalinization, nephrolithiasis, the presence of an indwelling urinary catheter, and host susceptibility. Stasis and alkaline urine provide a susceptible medium for bacterial growth. Urinary retention with distention along with nephrolithiasis may cause minute tears in the mucosal lining of the urinary tract, providing routes for infection. Bacteriuria has been reported in 50% of patients requiring indwelling urinary catheters for more than 7 to 10 days (Stamm, 1986).

Urinary tract infections are a frequent source of nosocomial infections in critically ill patients. Nosocomial bacteriuria usually represents urinary tract colonization in hospitalized patients (Yannelli and Gurevich, 1988). The most serious complication that can arise from bacteriuria in immobilized patients is urosepsis.

Metabolic Effects

HYPERCALCEMIA AND HYPERCALCIURIA

Immobility results in increased calcium excretion from bones due to the removal of weight-bearing forces from the long bones rather than to inactivity (Issekutz et al., 1966). Osteoblastic activity decreases in all weight-bearing bones subjected to bedrest, and osteolytic activity increases, resulting in osteoporosis and hypercalcemia (Maynard, 1986). Normally this leads to hypercalciuria and an eventual return to normal serum calcium levels. Dietrick et al. (1948) reported that hypercalciuria occurred after 2 to 3 days of bedrest in normal subjects; the level rose gradually and peaked at 4 to 5 weeks of bedrest. The calcium content of urine doubled during 6 to 7 weeks of bedrest in normal subjects. Hypercalciuria has been associated with prolonged immobility in all age groups (Stewart et al., 1982).

The incidence of immobilization hypercalcemia has been reported to range from 10.8% to 23.6% in spinal cord–injured patients (Maynard, 1986; Nand and Goldschmidt, 1976). Clinically significant hypercalcemia also occurs in patients with fractures of the lower limbs and pelvis (Henke et al., 1975; Pezeshki and Brooker, 1977; VanZuiden et al., 1982) and in patients with the Guillain-Barré syndrome (Evans et al., 1984; Meythaler et al., 1986). Weissman and colleagues (1983) reported a case of hypercalcemia and hypercalciuria in a 50-year-old critically ill patient requiring prolonged immobility.

GLUCOSE-INSULIN INTOLERANCE

Physical inactivity has been reported to alter glucose homeostasis in humans (Vernikos-Danellis et al., 1976). Glucose intolerance has been positively related to the length of bedrest (Blotner, 1945; Buhr, 1963). Increasing levels of serum insulin are thus required to maintain normal glucose levels (Lipman et al., 1970; Vernikos-Danellis et al., 1976). The mechanisms explaining the unresponsiveness of glucose to hyperinsulinemia remain unclear. One theory focuses on the existence of insulin inhibitors altering cellular membrane function. Restoration of normal glucose tolerance after activity was resumed occurred in 7 to 14 days in persons subjected to bedrest without exercise (Lipman et al., 1970).

Musculoskeletal Effects

BONE LOSS

Weight-bearing is a critical factor in the normal functioning of osteoblasts and osteoclasts. Loss of longitudinal pressure on the long bones results in decreased osteoblastic activity. Osteoclasts continue to destroy bone matrix even in lieu of increased osteoblastic activity, which results in bone demineralization and decreased bone density. Short-term immobility results in hypercalciuria in the first 2 days of bedrest (Dietrick et al., 1948; Greenleaf et al., 1977), which usually does not present significant problems. During continued bedrest, total body calcium losses have been estimated at 0.5% per month (Rubin, 1988). Demineralization continues with bedrest despite the amount of dietary calcium consumed (Memmer and Kozier, 1987). The porous, soft bones characteristic of disuse osteoporosis may result in bone pain, bone fractures, or nephrolithiasis (O'Neill, 1981).

MUSCLE ATROPHY

One of the most obvious effects of prolonged immobility is muscle atrophy. Muscle atrophy is the loss of actual muscle mass and results in a decrease

of the cross-sectional area of the whole muscle (St. Pierre and Gardiner, 1987). Muscle atrophy resulting from disuse leads to weakness and fatigue. The rate of muscle atrophy is rapid in the early immobilization phase and continues more slowly with long-term immobility (Summers and Hines, 1951). The rate of muscle atrophy has also been found to be faster if the muscle has been denervated rather than just immobilized (Domonkos and Heiner, 1965). The muscles of the thigh and calf usually undergo the greatest reduction in circumference during immobility, with the arm muscles being affected least (Greenleaf, 1982).

JOINT CONTRACTURES

Decrease in skeletal muscle activity along with muscle atrophy associated with immobility may limit the normal range of motion (ROM) of a joint. Since flexor muscles are stronger than extensor muscles, joints often remain in a flexed position in bed. If exercise of the joints does not occur, the flexor muscles become permanently shortened, and the joint becomes stiffened in a flexed position. A contracture may result when fibrofatty tissue proliferates within the immobile joint (Enneking and Horowitz, 1972), forming adhesions and maturing as scar tissue. Impairment of the normal gliding motion between collagen fibrils and abnormalities of the mechanical properties of ligaments also contribute to contracture formation (Frank et al., 1984).

Common contracture sites include the hip, knee, and plantar flexor of the ankle. Critically ill patients who are placed and maintained in varying degrees of the Fowler position with the knees elevated are at risk of developing hip and knee contractures. The reversibility of joint contractures is heavily dependent on their course of development.

PERIPHERAL NERVE INJURY

The immobile patient who is on bedrest is at risk of ulnar nerve injury secondary to compression resulting from improper positioning techniques. Due to the anatomic relationship of the ulnar nerve to structures around the elbow, supination of the forearm in a supine position frees the nerve from external compression at the cubital tunnel (Fig. 3–5A). Pronation of the forearm in a supine position, however, traps the ulnar nerve in the cubital tunnel (Fig. 3–5B). Flexion of the elbow adds an additional 11 to 24 mm Hg of pressure on the ulnar nerve (Pechan and Julis, 1975).

Chuman (1985) found that ulnar nerve compression occurred in 23% of a patient population composed of orthopedic, neurologic, neurosurgical, and rehabilitative patients who were on bedrest for a minimum of 12 hours per day for 3 consecutive days. Identified risk factors for ulnar nerve compression in this study included diabetes mellitus, bedrest for greater than 22 hours per day, injury or pathology of the wrist or elbow, alcoholism, family history of nerve damage, and an age of 50 years or more.

Integumentary Effects

PRESSURE SORES

Being confined to bed implies that a patient will incur any damage resulting from the pressure of his body against the supporting surface and from the friction and shearing effects that occur with confined movement. Integumentary damage resulting from immobility is an iatrogenic complication in the ICU and is often casually accepted as a normal result of prolonged bedrest. The term "pressure sore" is used to describe integumentary damage on any body surface that is related to immobility and that results from the forces of pressure, friction, shearing, or moisture.

Pressure remains the primary cause of pressure sores (Maklebust, 1987). Perpendicular forces exerted by gravity on any skin surface must exceed mean capillary pressures in the skin in order to produce tissue ischemia and necrosis (Larsen et al., 1979). Normal pressure gradients in the capillary arteriolar limb have been reported as 32 mm Hg and as 12 mm Hg in the venous capillary limb (Reuler and Cooney, 1981). Pressures exceeding these levels in the arteriolar capillary limb will lead to lymphatic occlusion, increased interstitial fluid pressure, and filtration of fluid from the capillaries, resulting in edema and tissue ischemia (Burn et al., 1987). Factors affecting the critical arteriolar closing pressure are skin pressure, systemic hypotension, vascular shunting, and shock.

Development of pressure sores is dependent on a time-pressure relationship (Dinsdale, 1973; Koziak,

TABLE 3–4. Classification of Severity of Pressure Sores

Stage 1	Redness of skin after alleviation of pressure. Skin remains intact, although bruising, swelling, or vesicle formation may be present.
Stage 2	Skin breakdown with exposure of dermis and subcutaneous fat. Serous drainage may be present.
Stage 3	Extension of tissue disruption into subcutaneous fat, muscle, or fascia. Necrosis or infection may be evident.
Stage 4	Extension of tissue disruption into bone. Necrosis, infection, or eschar is often evident.

1959). The higher the pressure, the less time is needed for necrosis to occur (Brooks and Duncan, 1940). Dinsdale (1974) reported that a constant pressure of 70 mm Hg applied for more than 2 hours produced irreversible tissue damage.

After a skin surface has been compressed, the skin immediately appears blanched due to decreased local blood flow. Reactive hyperemia normally then results as a compensatory measure to enhance blood flow to the compromised area and to decrease the risk of microvascular thrombosis. If the skin remains reddened after the pressure source has been removed, tissue damage can be inferred. The severity of pressure sores has been described according to four standard stages (Table 3–4).

Pressure is not equally distributed across the skin surface in any position in bed. Pressure is often concentrated over the bony prominences, where a cone-shaped pressure gradient develops (Fig. 3–6). Generation of this type of gradient results in compression of the soft tissues that lie between the skin and the bony prominence (Reuler and Cooney, 1981). Although redness may be visible on the skin surface, the damage caused to the underlying tissues from this process may not be clinically evident. Brunner and Suddarth (1986) reported that 75% of all pressure sores were located at weight-bearing bony promi-

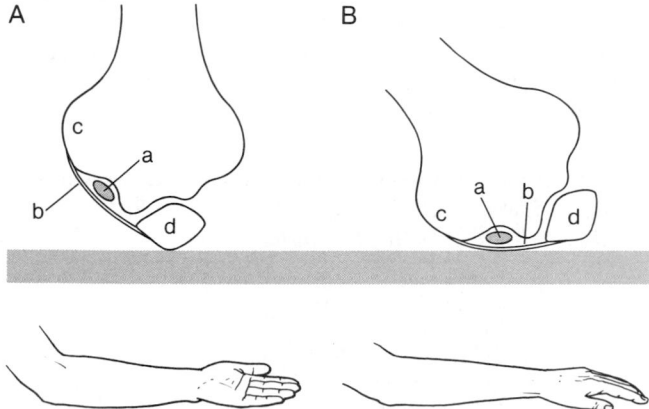

FIGURE 3–5. Relationship of ulnar nerve (a), arcuate ligament (b), medial epicondyle (c), and olecranon process of ulna (d). The arcuate ligament normally holds the ulnar nerve within the cubital tunnel. A, The supine position with the forearm supinated keeps the cubital tunnel free of external pressure. B, The supine position with the forearm pronated creates external pressure at the cubital tunnel that may result in ulnar nerve injury. (Redrawn from Chuman, M. A. (1985). *Journal of Neurosurgical Nursing, 17,* 339.)

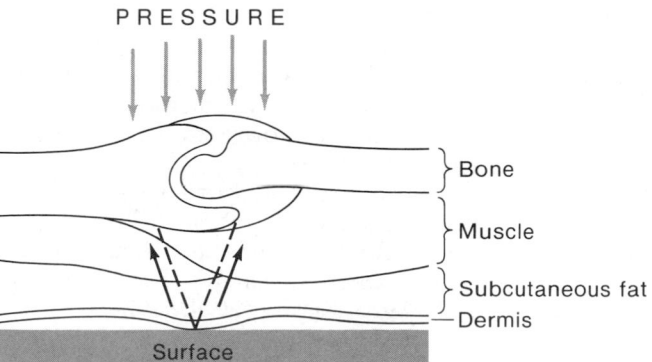

FIGURE 3–6. The creation of a cone-shaped pressure gradient between the skin's surface and the underlying bony prominence. The full extent of soft tissue damage may not appear at the skin surface because the base of the cone resides on the bone surface. (Reproduced, with permission, from: Reuler, J. B., and Cooney, T. G. *Annals of Internal Medicine,* 1981, Vol. 94, p. 662.)

nences. Ninety-six per cent of all pressure sores occur in the lower half of the human body (Reuler and Cooney, 1981). Common sites prone to pressure ulceration include the sacrum, coccygeal areas, ischial tuberosities, greater trochanters, lateral malleoli, medial and lateral condyles of the tibia, and the heels. Figure 3–7 delineates common pressure sites in a variety of bedrest positions.

Friction is the force created when two surfaces in contact with each other move in opposite directions. Skin friction results in the removal of the protective stratum corneum, leading to potential skin breakdown. Pulling rather than lifting patients up in bed remains the classic source of friction frequently experienced by critically ill patients. Continuous, spontaneous skeletal muscle motion due to seizures, agitation, or combativeness may also contribute to friction from bed surfaces or restraining devices in critically ill adults.

Shearing forces are created by a combination of friction and pressure. Shearing occurs commonly when a bedridden patient slumps toward the foot of the bed after being placed in a Fowler's position. As the body slides down, pressure is created on the sacral tissues. At the same time, friction is created between the posterior sacral skin and tissues and the bed surface. Stretching and angulation of blood vessels may occur and may result in dermal damage.

Moisture contributes to skin maceration because it softens the epidermal tissue and decreases its tensile strength. In the critically ill adult on bedrest, moisture accumulation may result from perspiration, fecal or urinary incontinence, or wound drainage. Norton and associates (1962) identified incontinence as the single most reliable predictor of the development of pressure sores. Allman and co-workers (1986) also found that fecal soiling was a major risk factor for the development of pressure sores in hospitalized patients.

Table 3–5 identifies major risk factors that have been implicated in pressure sore development (Allman et al., 1986; Braden and Bergstrom, 1987; Brunner and Suddarth, 1986; Feustel, 1982; Gosnell, 1987; Hotter, 1982; Maklebust, 1987; Stotts, 1987). Although many of these factors operate independently in predicting the development of pressure sores, the synergistic action of two or more factors cannot be overlooked because so many of them are present in critically ill patients.

Clinical complications of pressure sores include infections, sepsis, and osteomyelitis. Polymicrobial wound infections tend to result that frequently involve obligate anaerobes, particularly *Bacteroides fragilis* (Galpin et al., 1976; Rissing et al., 1974).

Psychological Effects

SENSORY-PERCEPTUAL ALTERATIONS

Conscious, critically ill patients who are immobile may experience a state of waiting. Waiting is the perceived process of the passage of time (Smith, 1975). Waiting may lead to hypervigilance and the overestimation of time. Because of the perceived "dragging of time," the nonoptimal stimulation of the ICU environment, and the lack of patient-structured activities, the patient may become unable to maintain temporal integrity.

The ICU environment is often the stimulus for sensory and perceptual changes in the immobilized patient. The underload and overload of auditory, visual, olfactory, kinesthetic, and tactile sensory experiences can lead to aberrant processing of perceived thoughts and sensations. The presence of restraints and side rails along with the ceiling and dependent view that accompanies a recumbent position may restrict the field of vision. Social isolation may occur due to restricted visiting hours and decreased interpersonal contact. Other factors contributing to the development of ICU psychosis resulting from sensory alterations include communication impairments (Ballard, 1981; Belitz, 1983), sleep deprivation (Belitz, 1983; Hansell, 1984; Helton et al., 1980), and pharmacologic agents (Belitz, 1983).

Sensory-perceptual alterations become manifest as states of confusion, disorientation, restlessness, incoherency, and anxiety or fear along with hallucinations, delusions, and illusions. This symptomatology has frequently been described in the literature by use of the term ICU psychosis or ICU delirium. Estimates of the incidence of ICU psychosis range from 12.5% to 38% in conscious patients admitted to critical care settings (Belitz, 1983).

ALTERED BODY IMAGE

Mobility allows individuals to exercise and maintain control over their environment. Body image is formed from the level of independence that one chooses to maintain. Immobility affects body image because bed confinement gravely alters independence (Baird, 1985; Christian, 1982; Olson, 1967). Body image disturbances may result in intense feelings of inferiority, anxiety, withdrawal, self-destructive behavior, anger, despair, or noncompliance with

TABLE 3–5. Major Risk Factors for Pressure Sore Development in Critically Ill Adults

Immobilization
Altered mental status
Incontinence
Length of hospitalization
Altered motor or sensory function
Advancing age (>40 years)
Altered cardiac output
Orthopedic fractures
Altered nutritional status
  Cachexia or obesity
  Hypoalbuminemia
  Dehydration or edema
  Anemia
Exogenous corticosteroids

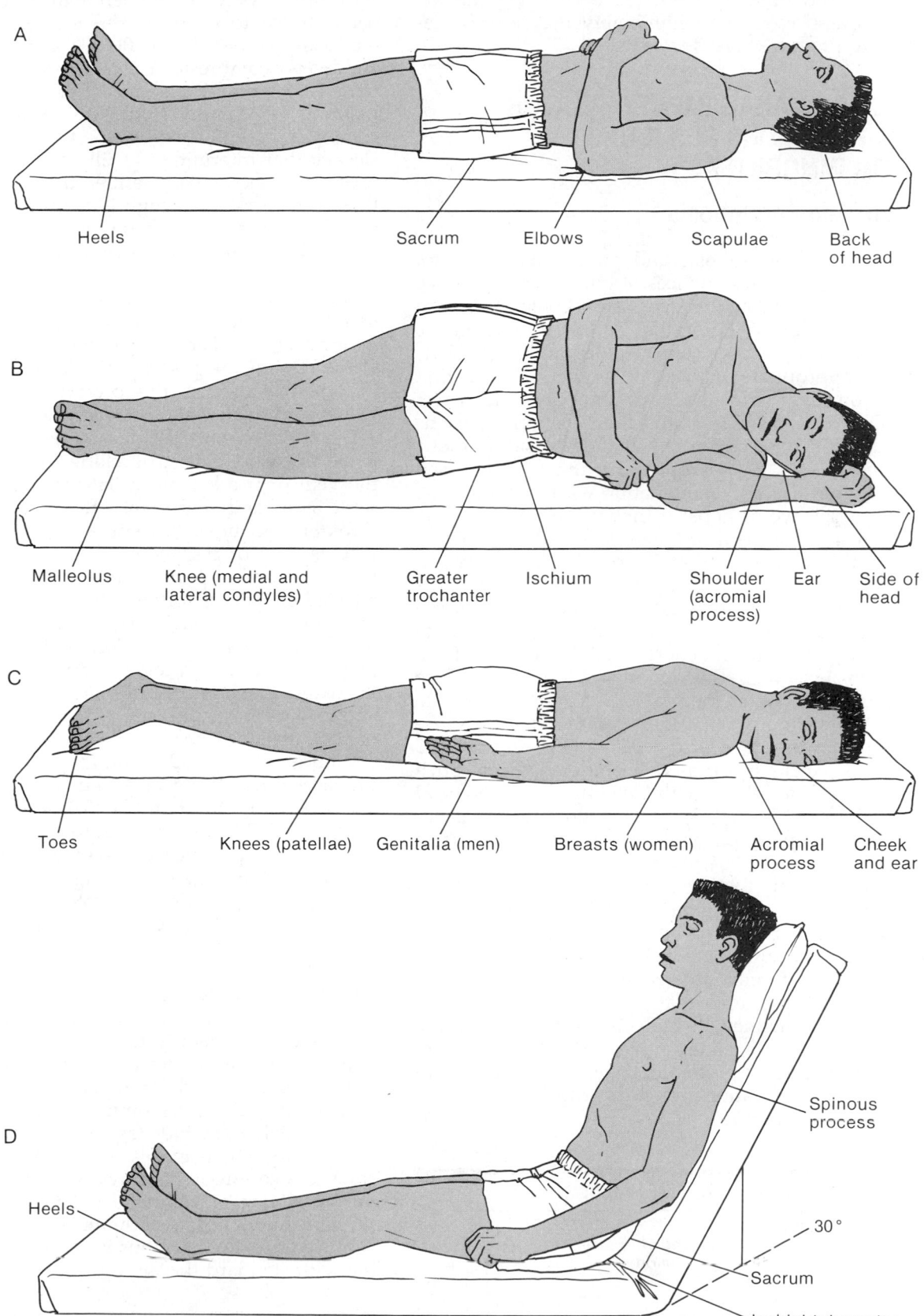

FIGURE 3–7. Body areas susceptible to pressure, friction, and shearing forces. *A,* Supine position. *B,* Lateral position. *C,* Prone position. *D,* Fowler position. (Redrawn from *Fundamentals of Nursing,* Fourth Edition, by Kozier, Erb, and Olivieri (Redwood City, CA: Addison-Wesley Nursing, 1991), p. 850. Reprinted by permission.)

medical and nursing regimens. Body image disturbances associated with immobility may also be related to pressure sore development.

MEDICAL MANAGEMENT OF MAJOR COMPLICATIONS RESULTING FROM IMMOBILITY

Deep Vein Thrombosis

Deep vein thrombosis and pulmonary embolism are two major consequences of immobility that have been highlighted as the two easiest consequences to prevent. Acknowledging that 50% of thrombi in the iliofemoral venous system will embolize (Kakkar, 1969), appropriate management goals should first focus on identifying which patients are at high risk for DVT (see Table 3–3) and then start prophylactic therapy for those patients. Table 3–6 lists the various alternatives to DVT prophylaxis that can be used independently or in combination with each other.

The objective of heparin therapy in DVT prophylaxis is to arrest the thrombotic process by enhancing the inhibitory action of antithrombin III on factor X. Low-dose heparin therapy has been found to be efficacious in preventing DVT in a variety of medical diseases (Belch et al., 1981; Halkin et al., 1982). Cade (1982) reported a reduction in DVT incidence from 30% to 12% with the administration of low-dose heparin therapy in a medical ICU. Moser and Fedullo (1983) and Pingleton (1985) recommended low-dose heparin as prophylaxis for all medical-surgical ICU patients except those at risk of hemorrhage. Such patients include those with bleeding disorders, head injury, general trauma, and severe hypertension. Low-dose heparin prophylaxis has not been reported to increase upper gastrointestinal bleeding episodes (Pingleton et al., 1981) but does slightly increase the risk of wound hematoma in surgical patients (Coon et al., 1987). Standard adult doses are 5000 units administered subcutaneously every 8 to 12 hours. Such doses do not require monitoring of clotting times. Anticoagulants may also be used in an adjusted-dose regimen in high-risk patients in whom fixed low doses are ineffective. Adjusted-dose heparin or warfarin (Coumadin) requires frequent monitoring of coagulation times in order to ensure its efficacy and safety.

TABLE 3–6. Measures for DVT Prophylaxis

Anticoagulants
   Fixed low-dose heparin
   Adjusted-dose heparin
   Warfarin
Early mobilization
Intermittent pneumatic compression
Graduated compression elastic stockings
Active or passive leg exercises
Intravenous Dextran

Compressive forces applied to the lower limbs have been shown to decrease the incidence of DVT by increasing venous blood flow (Caprini et al., 1983). Graduated compression elastic stockings and intermittent pneumatic compression boots represent methods of compression. Intermittent pneumatic compression (IPC) involves the wearing of plastic leg sleeves that intermittently fill with air and decompress in a sequential manner that enhances blood flow in the calf and thigh. An advantage of IPC is that it is associated with rare complications and can become the best choice of prophylaxis in patients at hemorrhagic risk.

Dextran may be used to prevent DVT because of its effects on decreasing blood viscosity and platelet adhesiveness and enhancing fibrinolysis (Coon et al., 1987). Disadvantages of this intravenous therapy include the cost of the product, associated fluid volume overloads, and increased tendency to bleed.

Development of DVT may remain clinically silent if the thrombus fails to occlude the inner lumen of the vein or if adequate collateral circulation is present. Signs and symptoms often develop when the thrombus occludes the entire lumen and impedes venous flow or creates an inflammatory process of the vessel wall or perivascular tissue. Swelling of the affected limb occurs often with an associated increase in circumference distal to the occlusion and increased temperature. Pain and tenderness in the calf or thigh may be present with fever and malaise. Evidence of Homans sign should be cautiously weighted because its presence has not been reliable in defining states of DVT (Fahey, 1984).

Clinical signs and symptoms alone have not proved sufficiently reliable to diagnose DVT (Hull et al., 1977, 1981; Moser and LeMoine, 1981). Diagnostic tests for DVT include venography, Doppler ultrasonography, impedance plethysmography (IPG), and ^{125}I-labeled fibrinogen scanning. A diagnostic accuracy rate of approximately 95% has been reported when IPG and Doppler ultrasonography are used in conjunction (Fahey, 1984).

The treatment of DVT revolves around the use of adjusted-dose anticoagulants to prevent enlargement of existing thrombi and their migration. Contraindications to this therapy include hemorrhagic risk in patients who are critically ill with diseases such as acute liver failure, disseminated intravascular coagulopathy (DIC), or bleeding dyscrasias. Other treatment modalities include leg elevation, thrombectomy (if the thrombus is in a large vessel), and the use of compressive forces. Prophylactic treatment to minimize the risk of pulmonary embolism from DVT through inferior cava clipping or screening may be considered if the thrombus is large and is not resolving with standard therapy.

Pulmonary Embolism

The migration of a venous thrombus to the lung may result in absent or dramatic clinical signs and symptoms depending upon the percentage of pulmonary vasculature that is obstructed. Table 3–7 lists the common subjective signs and symptoms of pulmonary embolism (PE). McCaffree (1978) reported an incidence of dyspnea of 81% and an incidence of pleuritic chest pain of 72% in patients experiencing a pulmonary embolism. It is important to note that subjective symptoms are frequently masked in critically ill adults due to depression of the level of consciousness. Tachypnea and tachycardia are frequent objective findings with incidences of 90% to 100% and 60% to 75%, respectively (Roberts, 1987). Development of the symptomatology of right ventricular heart failure secondary to an acute and substantial increase in pulmonary vascular resistance may signal the presence of a massive PE and greatly narrows the time span available for treatment initiation.

Because the clinical signs and symptoms of PE are often confused with those of other states, laboratory methods are often used to confirm or rule out the diagnosis. Pulmonary angiography is the most definitive test for this diagnosis, but it is often difficult to perform if the patient is unstable from the event. Ventilation and perfusion lung scans, chest radiography, IPG, contrast venography, and the radioactive fibrinogen test can aid in the medical diagnosis.

The goals of medical therapy for PE are to lyse existing large thromboemboli and to prevent new ones from forming. Fibrinolytic therapy is indicated for massive PEs that evoke severe systemic hypotension or that obstruct greater than 50% of the pulmonary vascular bed (Moser and Fedullo, 1983). Intravenous urokinase and streptokinase cause rapid lysis and prolong thrombin times. Frequent, intermittent laboratory measurements of coagulation are indicated to detect uncontrolled fibrinolysis. Contraindications to fibrinolytic therapy include defective hemostasis, tumor, infarction, trauma, severe hypertension, pregnancy, surgery, or an intra-arterial diagnostic procedure performed within the past 10 days. Pulmonary embolectomy may be performed on critically ill patients if the embolism is massive and is not responsive to standard therapy.

Infection

Medical management of infections resulting from immobility revolves around timely diagnosis, obtainment of culture data, and institution and optimalization of antimicrobial therapy. Pneumonia, UTI, and infection of pressure sores are prevalent disorders that can lead to associated bacteremias and septicemias.

Immobilization Hypercalcemia

The diagnosis of immobilization hypercalcemia is made only after exclusion of other causes for it are ruled out. High serum calcium levels may be associated with hypercalciuria (>200 mg of urinary calcium per 24 hours) and depressed neuromuscular excitability resulting in nausea, vomiting, constipation, anorexia, or fecal impaction (Maynard, 1986). Other signs may be orthostatic hypotension, cardiac irregularities, and seizures. Treatment modalities include vigorous hydration with intravenous saline, furosemide to decrease sodium loads, oral phosphate administration, mithramycin, and calcitonin.

NURSING MANAGEMENT OF PHENOMENA RESULTING FROM IMMOBILITY

The focus of care of the immobilized patient is on prevention. Prevention of complications results in significant cost savings to the patient and family, the multidisciplinary team, and the health care system. An astute awareness of and vigilance for early symptomatology may also expedite the application of preventive and therapeutic measures.

Impaired Physical Mobility

Impaired physical mobility in critically ill adults is associated with several etiologic factors. Of primary prevalence is immobility induced by bedrest for safety or therapeutic gain. Pre-existing joint contrac-

---

TABLE 3–7. Clinical Signs and Symptoms of Pulmonary Embolism

Subjective
Dyspnea
Pleuritic chest pain
Anxiety
Syncope

Objective
General
  Tachypnea
  Tachycardia
  Confusion
  Cough
  Hemoptysis
  Diaphoresis
Cardiopulmonary
  Hypoxemia
  Systemic hypotension
  Jugular venous distention
  Split second heart sound
  Dysrhythmias (atrial flutter or fibrillation)
  Right axis deviation
  Enlarged or peaked P waves on electrocardiogram
  Peaked or inverted T waves in chest leads
  Incomplete or complete right bundle branch block
  Increased pulmonary artery pressures
  Increased pulmonary vascular resistance
  Increased central venous pressure
  Normal or decreased cardiac output
  Presence of thrombophlebitis

tures, muscle atrophy, and bone loss may also lead to further constraints on mobility.

The defining characteristics of joint contractures include stiffness or discomfort on joint movement, limited range of motion, and joint swelling or redness. Muscle atrophy results in a decreased circumference of the involved muscle group, decreased strength and tolerance for exercise, impaired coordination of the involved muscle group, and a reluctance to move. Bone loss may be inferred from hypercalcemia and hypercalciuria and may be represented by bone pain when resumption of weight-bearing activities occur.

Nursing strategies to prevent or to treat these effects revolve around proper body positioning, exercises, and weight-bearing activities. Correct body alignment ensures that body joints are placed in their most functional position. The supine position, which is often unavoidable for extended periods of time in critically ill adults, predisposes patients to external hip rotation and footdrop. The use of trochanter rolls strategically positioned at the crest of the ilium to the midthigh assists in proper hip positioning. The use of footboards, high-top tennis shoes, or foot splints helps to prevent footdrop if the patient is positioned correctly in bed. A trapeze bar may be added to assist certain patients in self-movement. The purposeful and intelligent selection of positioning schedules needs to be individualized to meet restrictions on turning unstable patients.

Isotonic and isometric exercises assist in preventing or minimizing joint contractures or neuromuscular degeneration and aid in promoting venous return. Since isotonic exercises result in constant tension and a shortening of the muscle, they will maintain or increase muscle strength and mass and joint mobility. Isotonic exercises while on bedrest can be accomplished through active range of motion (ROM) exercises in which the patient moves each joint through its complete range of motion. Passive ROM exercises will maintain joint mobility but are of no value in maintaining muscle strength (Brower and Hicks, 1972). Regardless of which type of ROM is performed, these exercises should be performed to the point of slight resistance but never to the extent of producing discomfort. Range of motion exercises should be performed for the neck, shoulder, elbows, wrist, fingers, ankles, and feet in a systematic sequence a minimum of four times a day.

Isometric exercises generate tension by muscle groups' opposing one another while the muscle length remains constant. Muscle groups are alternatively contracted and relaxed. These exercises can be performed on casted extremities because no joint movement is required. Major muscle groups involved in walking such as the quadriceps, lower abdominals, femoris, and gluteals can be maintained with such exercises if they are done regularly. Caution must be used when considering an isometric exercise schedule for critically ill adults because adverse cardiovascular changes can occur. Blood pressure changes are especially prevalent in people with hypertension.

Assessment of blood pressure is thus predicated before, during and after isometric exercise (Chrysant, 1978). The associated hypertension is felt to be so significant that the chances of myocardial compromise or cardiovascular accident are increased (Lentz, 1981).

Weight-bearing activities are critical in preventing extensive calcium loss from bone in long-term ICU patients. Standing and ambulating remain the only forms of weight-bearing for ICU patients. Contemporary ICU beds presently lack the design feature of a reverse Trendelenburg position that would allow an adult to weight-bear against a sturdy foot surface. Emphasis thus should be placed on early and frequent mobilization because studies have shown that standing for 3 hours per day provides sufficient gravitational stress to decrease calcium bone loss (Issekutz et al., 1966). Expected outcomes of impaired physical mobility are focused on the maintenance of muscle mass and strength, joint mobility, and absence of bone pain upon rising.

Altered Skin Integrity

A combination of pressure, shearing, friction, and moisture may be factors causing changes in skin integrity in the immobile adult. The presence of hyperemia on the skin surface over a pressure point that lasts longer than 30 seconds may be the first sign of altered circulation. Tenderness, edema, vesiculation, local warmth, decreased skin turgor, and a failure of the skin to blanche with finger pressure are parameters indicating a stage 1 pressure sore. A break in the skin surface may overlie a large undermining defect in the soft tissue due to cone-shaped pressure gradients. Closed and open skin sores should be observed for their location, size (length, width, and depth), shape, color, odor, and associated drainage. The integument should be fully inspected minimally every 4 to 8 hours in critically ill patients. All deviations should be documented according to the standard classification listed in Table 3–4.

A key approach to preventing pressure sores lies in the prediction of their occurrence in high-risk patients admitted to the ICU. Although nursing research focusing on prediction in critically ill adults is nonexistent, significant risk factor assessment tools have been developed and studied in medical, surgical, and geriatric populations. Although many of these tools need further refinement and testing for predictive validity, their defined risk factors have been identified consistently and have proved useful in critically ill adult populations.

The classic instrument used to predict pressure sore risk is the Norton scale (Norton et al., 1962), which was developed using geriatric hospital patients. It is composed of five risk factors (Table 3–8), which are rated independently and then summed for a total score. Total scores of 14 or greater indicate high-risk candidates. Norton and colleagues (1962)

TABLE 3–8. Norton Scale of Pressure Sore Risk

General Physical Condition		Mental State		Activity		Mobility		Incontinence	
Good	4	Alert	4	Ambulatory	4	Full	4	Absent	4
Fair	3	Apathetic	3	Walks with help	3	Slightly limited	3	Occasional	3
Poor	2	Confused	2	Chairbound	2	Very limited	2	Usually urinary	2
Very bad	1	Stuporous	1	Bedfast	1	Immobile	1	Double	1

From Norton, D., McLaren, R., and Exton-Smith, A. N. (1962). *An investigtion of geriatric nursing problems in hospitals.* London: Churchill Livingstone.

reported a high linear relationship between scores and the actual incidence of pressure sores. Goldstone and Goldstone (1982) reported a high degree of accuracy using the Norton scale in a more recent study. Stotts (1988) found that pressure sores were not predicted at the time of hospital admission using

TABLE 3–9. Prevention and Treatment Strategies for Pressure Sores According to Their Effect on External Factors

Pressure
Static
  Flotation gel pads
  Foam, convoluted mattresses
  Pillows or foam wedges
  Elbow or heel protectors
  Wrinkle-free foundation
  Appropriate restraint application
Dynamic
  Manual positioning regimens
  Air-fluidized bed
  Low airloss bed
  Oscillating bed
  Alternating pressure mattress

Friction
Turning sheets
Sheepskin
Appropriate restraint application
Transfer aids
Trapeze
Sedation for continuous motion
Air-fluidized bed
Low airloss bed
Oscillating bed

Shearing
Lifting or turning sheets
Footboards
Sheepskins
Transfer aids
Heel or elbow protector pads
Trapeze
Sedation for continuous motion
Appropriate restraint application
Air-fluidized bed
Low airloss bed
Oscillating bed

Moisture
Sheepskin
Skin hygiene
Linen changes
Air-fluidized bed
Low airloss bed
Containment of urine or feces (condom catheter, indwelling urinary or rectal catheter, fecal incontinence bag)

a modified form of the Norton scale in elective cardiovascular and neurosurgical patients.

Other risk assessment tools include those published by Gosnell (1973), Gruis and Innes (1976), Williams (1973), and Bergstrom and colleagues (1987). The risk factors of mental status, incontinence, mobility, activity, nutritional status, and physical condition are common elements of these tools. Regardless of which tool may be used, the process of systematically evaluating patients against set high-risk parameters is invaluable in the identification process and in prescribing costly preventive and therapeutic modalities.

The goal of preventive and therapeutic strategies for pressure sores is to alleviate or minimize their external causes and to maintain optimal skin integrity. Table 3–9 lists interventions in relation to their effects on the external factors of pressure, friction, shearing, and moisture.

Turning regimens should be developed based on individual curtailments in repositioning critically ill adults. Limitations on turning are often related to traction, unilateral lung disease, inaccuracies associated with invasive and noninvasive monitoring, and cardiopulmonary instability. Although major turns may be contraindicated, modified turns or small shifts in body position can change pressure points. The frequency of repositioning should be determined based upon skin assessment and on the comfort levels of the individual patient. The classic standard of turning patients every 1 to 2 hours may not be adequate in patients at high risk.

Pillow bridging along with heel and elbow protectors can be used to relieve pressure over bony prominences without requiring major changes in position. Adjunctive static devices such as flotation gel pads and foam mattresses may be used to distribute pressure over large areas.

The use of a new generation of dynamic beds has assisted in the prevention and treatment of pressure sores in critically ill adults. Air-fluidized, oscillating, and low airloss beds have been successfully used with a variety of high-risk patients. Air-fluidized beds operate on the principle of minimizing pressure, friction, moisture, and shearing forces. Thousands of silicon-coated glass beads are suspended in the bed by the pressurized flow of warm air through the beads (Fig. 3–8). Such fluidization improves capillary blood flow to the skin by minimizing external pressures over bony prominences and keeping them

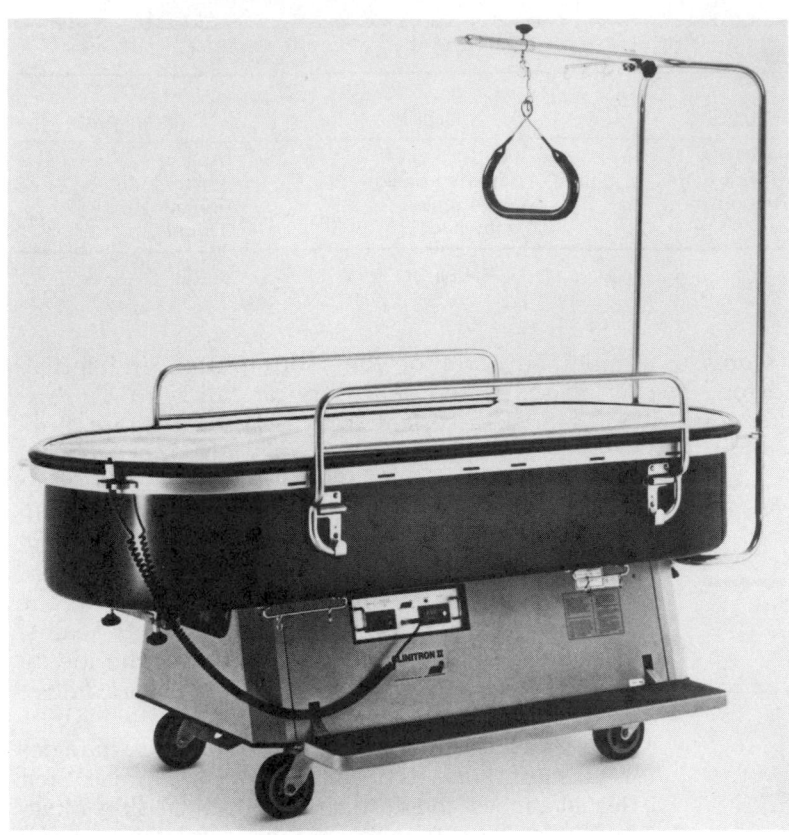

FIGURE 3–8. CLINITRON® Air Fluidized Therapy Unit. (Courtesy of Support Systems International, Inc. Reprinted by permission.)

lower than capillary filling pressures (Lucke and Jarlsberg, 1985). The use of a polyfilament polyester filter sheet separates the patient from the beads and minimizes friction and shearing forces because the sheet is loose and moves freely. Drainage or exudates that penetrate the filter sheet clump with the glass beads, encrust and then fall to the bottom of the bed into a filter. Healing of pressure sores in hospitalized patients using air-fluidized therapy was shown to be greater than that observed in patients placed on conventional beds (Allman et al., 1987). In this study greater improvement was seen in patients who had larger pressure sores.

Features of air-fluidized beds include the quick conversion of the fluidized beads to a solid medium, which assists in attaining a hard surface for cardiopulmonary resuscitation (CPR). The bed design does not allow the head of the bed to be raised or lowered electrically. Foam supports are used to attain degrees of Fowler's position. Bed controls allow for adjustments in temperature of air flow. Concerns about aerosolization of microorganisms due to air flow through the filter sheet have recently been shown to be an insignificant problem if the beds are maintained as intended (Vesley et al., 1986; Bolyard et al., 1987).

Oscillating beds provide perpetual motion for the critically ill adult unless the motion is suppressed. Pressure forces are thus reduced. Shearing and friction are also decreased due to the qualities of the contact surface and the supported alignment of the patient. The most well-studied oscillating bed is the

Kinetic Treatment Table (Fig. 3–9). The Kinetic Treatment Table™ (Kinetic Concepts) is designed to position patients through an arc of 124 degrees every 3.5 minutes. Such rotation is roughly equivalent to approximately 200 to 300 turns every 24 hours if the bed is allowed to rotate most the time. Comparing this figure to the typical 12 manual turns that are standard in a 24-hour period, it is evident that superior turning can be achieved with this bed. The slow rotation speed (0.5 degree per second) of the bed prevents sleep and vestibular disturbances. Other features of the bed allow achievement of Trendelenburg and reverse Trendelenburg positions, rapid positioning for CPR, accurate weights, full joint exercises, access to thoracic, cervical, and rectal regions, and traction including cervical halo systems. The Kinetic Treatment Table™ has a silent motor and a radiolucent table surface. Chest drainage, ventilator tubing, and invasive intravascular and intracranial monitoring are easily accommodated.

Patients with cardiovascular instability and spinal cord injury with continued pain at the site of injury are not candidates for kinetic therapy. Patients who show signs and symptoms of claustrophobia due to the confinement of the bed's safety straps and securing pads are also not candidates. Diarrhea is a relative contraindication for kinetic therapy because the bed enhances gut motility.

Low airloss beds use electricity to alternate currents of air to regulate and redistribute pressures against the body surface. Such regulation allows less than 25

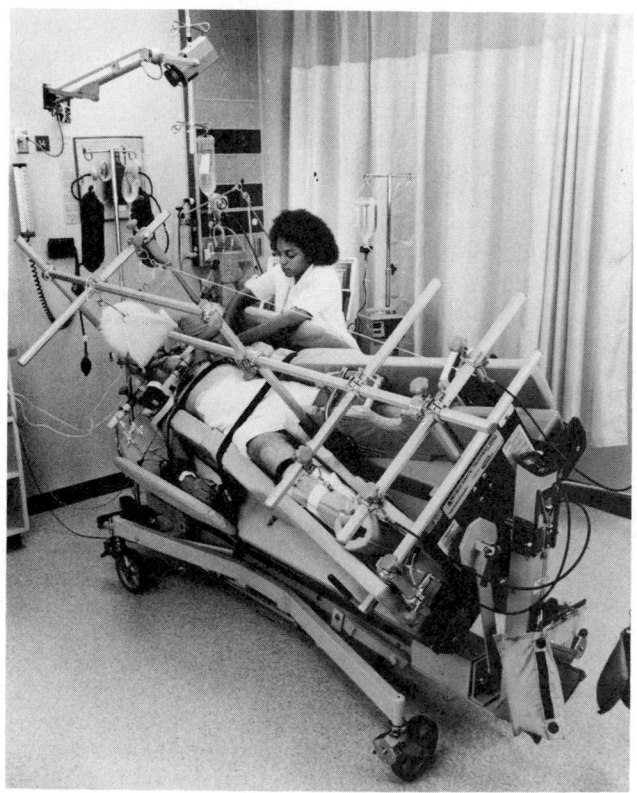

FIGURE 3–9. Kinetic Treatment Table™. (Courtesy of Kinetic Concepts, Inc. Reprinted by permission.)

mm Hg of pressure to be applied on any given body surface. The pressure in the compartmental air sacs is individualized to the patient's distributed weight (Fig. 3–10). Features of many low airloss beds include rapid deflation of the air sacs for CPR institution, underbed scales, transport battery, hand controls for

positioning, foot support cushions, and breathable underpads for fecal or urinary incontinence. Most low airloss beds use a low-shear, breathable, waterproof sheet over the air sacs. Such features provide a low friction and shearing interface that allows moisture control. Fine pores in the air sacs and cover sheet prevent aerosolization of bacteria that may accumulate.

A recent technologic advance is the development of an oscillating bed with low airloss characteristics. The BioDyne™ bed provides side-to-side rotation with continuous air suspension (Fig. 3–11). The bed design minimizes all causative forces of pressure sores.

The prevention and treatment of pressure sores are critically dependent on the optimal maintenance of the skin state. Interventions that enhance systemic oxygenation and perfusion and eliminate or minimize peripheral edema and anemia are key internal factors in preventing and healing sores. Provision of adequate nutrition to the intact or damaged skin requires protein and calorie intake along with iron, ascorbic acid, and zinc supplements. Critically ill adults often have protein-calorie malnutrition on hospital admission. Nutritional problems often encountered in critically ill adults center around fluid restrictions, organ failure, limited enteral or central venous access, depressed level of consciousness, and impaired absorption by shrunken intestinal villi secondary to prolonged parenteral feedings (Echenique et al., 1982). The need to attain and maintain adequate visceral protein stores and a positive nitrogen balance to optimize skin nutrition is a challenge.

The aim of skin care is to keep the surface clean but not too dry or too moist. Skin should be patted dry but not rubbed to minimize shearing and friction effects. Gentle skin massage may be done only after

FIGURE 3–10. FLEXICAIR® MC3 Low Airloss Therapy Unit. (Courtesy of Support Systems International, Inc. Reprinted by permission.)

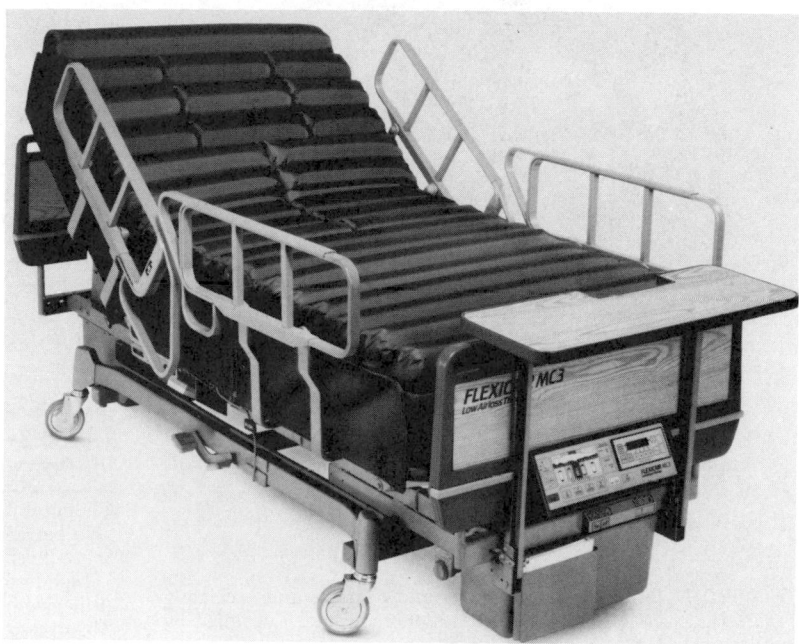

reactive hyperemia has dissipated. Massaging skin surfaces that remain reddened should not be done because underlying tissue damage is often present. Massage may only create further tissue damage.

Since fecal incontinence is a major risk factor for pressure sore development, the use of a soft, rubber-tipped rectal catheter to drain liquid stool may assist in the prevention or treatment of sores. Channick and associates (1988) examined the short-term effects of rectal tubes in 142 ICU patients. Tubes were inserted to help decrease soiling in 92% of the patients and to assist in healing pressure sores in 9%. The mean duration of tube placement was 3.3 days. No complications were identified in this study even when the balloon on the catheter tip was inflated to assist in containing stool. It was also reported that no patient developed a pressure sore with a rectal tube in place. Although the long-term effects of rectal tubes have not been researched in ICU patients, the rectal tube remains a common and useful adjunct in the care of patients with diarrhea.

Because pressure sores differ little from other types of wounds, the general principles of wound healing and care are applicable and are discussed in Chapter

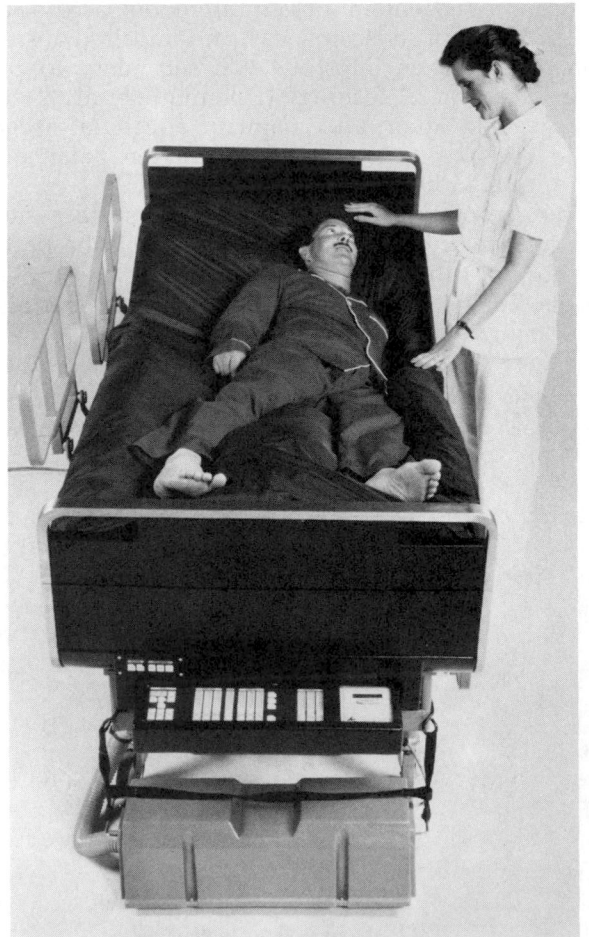

FIGURE 3–11. BioDyne® bed featuring low airloss and oscillating characteristics. (Courtesy of Kinetic Concepts, Inc. Reprinted by permission.)

55. A variety of skin care products and wound coverings are available to assist in the healing of various stages of pressure sores (Table 3–10). Surgical débridement may be necessary to treat extensive and infected sores to remove devitalized tissue, which otherwise may slow healing, delay granulation, and promote infection.

The expected outcomes for altered skin integrity are healed pressure sores, absence of infected sores, absence of further skin breakdown, and evidence of adequate nutritional intake.

Impaired Gas Exchange

Etiologic factors for impaired gas exchange in immobilized patients include pulmonary embolism, aspiration pneumonitis, hypostatic pneumonia, atelectasis, and alveolar hypoventilation. General symptomatology includes the development of confusion, dyspnea, tachypnea, labored breathing with accessory muscle use, and cyanosis. Abnormal breath sounds, depression in Pa_{O_2} and oxygen saturation values, and elevation of partial pressures of arterial carbon dioxide (Pa_{CO_2}) may be present. Depression of cough, gag, or swallow reflexes or inadequate minute ventilation may be found in patients with blunted reflexes secondary to anesthesia, intravenous muscle relaxants, or narcotic or sedative effects. The abrupt onset of dyspnea, hypoxemia, tachypnea, or complaints of pleuritic chest pain are classic findings of pulmonary embolism.

Astute surveillance for and reporting of depression of gag, swallow, and cough reflexes in patients with altered levels of consciousness is the key in preventing aspiration. Frequent assessment of nasogastric tube patency and gastric residuals associated with enteral feedings are necessary as well as ongoing abdominal assessments for distention and stool frequency. It should be remembered that positioning a patient who is receiving enteral feedings in a semi-Fowler's position is standard care but does not thoroughly guarantee prevention of aspiration.

Monitoring for alveolar hypoventilation in immobile patients is based on clinical signs and symptoms but is ultimately focused on the Pa_{CO_2}. Intermittent arterial blood gases or continual, noninvasive monitoring of end-tidal carbon dioxide in intubated patients is essential in patients receiving muscle relaxants or large or frequent doses of intravenous sedatives or narcotics. Optimal maintenance of arti-

---

TABLE 3–10. Common Skin and Wound Care Products for Pressure Sores

Chemical débriding agents (Elase; Travase; Santyl)
Skin barriers (Karaya powder; Stomadhesive)
Self-adhesive, nonabsorbing transparent films (OpSite; Tegaderm)
Adhesive hydrocolloid wafers (Duoderm)
Absorptive hydrophilic beads or granules (Debrisan; Duoderm)

ficial ventilation occurs with the trending of Pa_{CO_2} values.

The simple measures of turning, coughing, and deep breathing are used to prevent and treat the etiologic factors of impaired gas exchange. The use of standard body positions can enhance gas exchange by optimizing $\dot{V}/\dot{Q}$ matching in the lung. Dependent areas of normal lung tissue receive more blood flow due to gravitational effects and more ventilation due to the increased weight from the lung tissue. A knowledge of the location of lung disease is essential in order to provide optimal positioning. The lateral decubitus position has proven to be very effective in increasing Pa_{O_2} in patients with unilateral lung disease. Placing the "good lung down" has consistently resulted in improved oxygenation in these patients (Zack et al., 1974; Remolina et al., 1981; Seaton et al., 1979). The upright or Fowler's position has traditionally been used to decrease the effect of abdominal pressure on diaphragmatic excursion and to increase FRC. Prone positioning has been used less frequently in critically ill patients because of the difficulty associated in maneuvering patients with complex invasive technology and because of hindrances in providing timely resuscitative measures. The prone position, however, has been demonstrated to be very beneficial in patients with bilateral lung disease due to the associated increase in FRC from the displacement of abdominal contents (Piehl and Brown, 1976; Douglas et al., 1977). The benefit of the Trendelenburg position has been demonstrated in patients with bilateral lower lobe disease (Regnier et al., 1981).

Chulay and associates (1982) demonstrated that manual turning every 2 hours in the first 24 hours of the postoperative period of patients undergoing coronary artery bypass grafting (CABG) decreased ICU length of stay by 32% (p <.025). The time course of postoperative fever was also significantly altered in this study. The control group in this study was not turned for the 24-hour study period.

Other studies have attempted to define the effect of the Kinetic Treatment Table on pulmonary complications in immobilized critically ill patients. A recent randomized, prospective study examined 65 immobilized critically ill patients who either were placed on conventional beds and turned every 2 hours or placed on Kinetic Treatment Tables and rotated approximately 50% of the time (Gentilello et al., 1988). The total incidence of significant atelectasis and pneumonia was higher in the control group (66%) than in the treatment group (33%, p <.01). Other variables between the two groups such as severity of ARDS, ventilator requirements, levels of positive end-expiratory pressures, and high inspired oxygen concentrations were not statistically significant.

Because supplemental oxygen and artificial ventilation are frequently used in the treatment of impaired gas exchange, nursing interventions include monitoring for the adequacy of these treatments through arterial blood gases, pulse oximetry, and capnography. Expected outcomes of treatment for impaired gas exchange include a minimal Pa_{O_2} of 65 mm Hg, a minimal arterial oxygen saturation of 94%, eucarbia, spontaneous breathing, eupnea, and normal breath sounds.

Altered Tissue Perfusion

Tissue perfusion to the pulmonary bed may be impaired by pulmonary embolism. The focus of nursing care should be placed on preventing this event through DVT prophylaxis. Insertion of intravenous devices in the lower extremities should be avoided at all costs due to their significant association with DVT. Active or passive plantar flexion and dorsiflexion should be performed frequently to enhance venous return, although the effect remains temporary. The use of high compressive, elastic stockings will assist in venous return if the correct size is used and if they do not cause banding effects. Removal of these stockings for approximately 30 minutes every 8 hours allows capillary filling to occur in superficial veins and allows time for skin care. The appropriate application of IPC boots is also critical to their intended benefits. Protective leg positioning should also be monitored to prevent impaired venous return from leg crossing. The efficacy of the Kinetic Treatment Table in preventing DVT remains unknown because research needs to be replicated in large, diverse, critically ill populations. Initial evidence from a study of 15 acute spinal cord–injured patients showed that the table may be helpful in DVT prophylaxis (Becker et al., 1987).

Nursing interventions in the care of patients with DVT center on monitoring for the adequacy of intravenous full-dose heparin therapy with partial thromboplastin time. Bleeding complications associated with this therapy need to be monitored and reported. The circumference, color, sensation, and vascularity of the affected and nonaffected extremity are assessed frequently. Leg elevation may be beneficial if venous return is not impeded by hip flexion. Acute surveillance for the sudden development of symptoms and signs of pulmonary embolism is essential.

Nursing interventions for the patient sustaining a pulmonary embolism revolve around providing adequate oxygen transport, surveillance for and adequate pharmacologic support for right ventricular heart failure and systemic hypotension, management of anxiety, and monitoring for uncontrolled fibrinolysis associated with intravenous fibrinolytic therapy. Expected outcomes of interventions for altered pulmonary tissue perfusion include a Pa_{O_2} of >65 mm Hg, an arterial oxygen saturation of >94%, absence of signs of DVT, normalized right ventricular function, and normotension.

Activity Intolerance

Intolerance of activity in patients immobilized for long periods of time results from decreases in maximal $\dot{V}O_2$ and from sluggish neurovascular reflexes. Signs and symptoms of intolerance in resting supine positions may be evident only as increases in resting heart rates. Upon rising, patients often develop dizziness, lightheadedness, tachycardia, hypotension, and narrowed pulse pressures secondary due to decreases in stroke volume.

The effects of isotonic exercises performed while on bedrest on maximal $\dot{V}O_2$ have been variable. A decrease in exercise tolerance in persons who performed daily supine exercise while on bedrest was found to be similar to a decrease in subjects who performed no exercise (Miller et al., 1965). Supine maximal $\dot{V}O_2$ was also found to be significantly decreased after 14 days of bedrest in subjects who performed no exercise or static or dynamic exercise (Stremel et al., 1976). Although supine exercise does not clearly prevent cardiovascular deconditioning, it can assist in maintaining some degree of exercise capacity. Considering the other benefits of isotonic exercise, construction of an isotonic exercise plan for critically ill adults should be considered if such exercise is not contraindicated.

Supine exercise has been reported to be ineffective in preventing orthostatic intolerance (Winslow, 1985). Prevention of orthostatic hypotension centers on repositioning patients from horizontal to vertical positions frequently in order to provide sufficient stimulus to neurovascular reflexes. As patients who have been immobile and supine for long periods become mobile, safety precautions need to be taken. Supine vital signs are taken to compare values. Factors that can increase orthostatic intolerance should be noted such as vasodilatory drugs and fever. Gradual increases in vertical positions should be made only in the absence of significant orthostasis. Expected outcomes of interventions for activity intolerance include an absence of orthostatic signs, appropriate increases in heart rate with increased activity, lessening complaints of tiredness or exhaustion upon rising or ambulating, and progressive distances and times associated with ambulation.

Potential for Infection

Hypostatic pneumonia and UTI are the two leading infections in the immobile critically ill patient. Pneumonia is represented by fever, chills, chest radiologic changes, positive sputum cultures, and a change in the color and consistency of tracheal secretions. Signs and symptoms of a UTI are fever, chills, urinary frequency, dysuria, increased urine turbidity, malaise, hematuria, and a positive urine culture (>100,000 colonies of bacteria per mL of urine).

Institution of aggressive pulmonary toileting is essential in preventing and treating pneumonias. Coughing, deep breathing, incentive spirometry, appropriate antimicrobial therapy, turning regimens, and tracheobronchial suctioning are critical, as are good handwashing techniques of caregivers.

Urinary tract infections can be prevented by minimizing the urinary stasis that occurs with supine positions. Indwelling urinary catheters are often placed in critically ill adults. Such insertion requires good handwashing, sterile insertion, and provision of a closed urinary drainage system with adequate gravity flow. Since urine often becomes colonized after placement of indwelling catheters, emphasis should be placed on discontinuing the catheter as soon as possible. Dietary methods of acidifying the urine should be implemented if feasible to decrease the risk of UTI.

Potential for Injury

All too frequently critically ill patients are confused, agitated, or combative from a variety of causes. Physical restraint, pharmacologic interventions, and behavioral modifications are frequently used as management strategies to maintain needed immobility. The correct or incorrect application of soft and hard restraints may lead to joint dislocation, peripheral nerve injury, impaired circulation distal to limb restraints, and skin blisters, abrasions, or pressure sores. Judicious use of restraints in the agitated patient should be coupled with appropriate pharmacologic sedation to prevent enhanced combativeness due to the sensation of lack of control induced by restraints. Monitoring restraint sites for skin integrity, adequate circulation, and joint alignment should be performed often, especially if the patient remains physically active in bed.

Inappropriate positioning of arms may lead to ulnar nerve compression and altered motor and sensory function. Paresthesia, hypesthesia, hypalgia, analgesia, and muscle weakness associated with elbow flexion are diagnostic of ulnar nerve compression (Chuman, 1985). Purposeful positioning of the arms in a supinated state in the supine position is critical to prevent this complication.

Altered Bowel Elimination: Constipation

Bedrest can be a major etiologic factor in the development of constipation, which can lead to fecal impaction. Complaints of anorexia, headache, nausea, and dizziness may accompany signs of irritability, insomnia, flatulence, straining with defecation, dehydration, abdominal distention, and hard dry stool. A rock-hard mass palpated in the abdomen associated with fecal-colored smears or a ribbon of diarrhea is a classic sign of fecal impaction.

Management strategies for constipation are aimed at increasing dietary fiber, increasing activity, and increasing fluid intake if tolerated. Bran, cereals, fresh fruits, and whole-wheat bread have a high fiber content that possesses hydrophobic bulking properties. Psyllium hydrophobic mucilloid (Metamucil, Hydrocil) may also be used for this purpose. Stool softeners may be effective in lowering the surface tension of stool and allowing water and fat to enter the fecal mass. Chemical stimulants such as bisacodyl (Dulcolax) increase colonic activity, which may prove effective in increasing peristalsis. Saline cathartics such as milk of magnesia and sodium phosphate-biphosphate (Fleet's) compounds may be used for their osmotic effects. Increasing activity levels should be stressed if feasible because of the beneficial effect of activity on peristalsis. Treatment of fecal impaction is often digital removal coupled with a combination of the above measures.

Monitoring for the frequency, amount, color, and consistency of stool is basic to prevent constipation. The quantity of stool should be evaluated based on whether the critically ill adult is being fed enterally or parenterally. Expected outcomes of treatment measures for the enterally fed patient with altered bowel elimination are soft, formed stool, absence of straining with defecation, adequate appetite, and a soft, nondistended abdomen.

Incontinence

Altered level of consciousness, bedrest, use of pharmacologic agents, and use of restraints are major etiologic factors in urinary and fecal incontinence in the immobile patient. Signs and symptoms of urinary retention, which may precede urinary incontinence, are a distended bladder, lower abdominal discomfort, and restlessness. Management of retention may simply involve establishing a voiding regimen with the patient or using intermittent urinary catheterization or an indwelling catheter. Monitoring for signs and symptoms of UTI and catheter patency as well as intermittent cleansing around the insertion site of the indwelling catheter are essential.

The use of a soft, rubber-tipped rectal tube to manage liquid fecal incontinence may prove advantageous in monitoring output and preventing pressure sores. If the balloon on the tip of the rectal tube needs to be inflated with air to seal stool contents effectively, balloon volume and pressure as well as appropriate deflation must be monitored to avoid potential complications. Nursing care also involves exploring the reason for the diarrhea. Expected outcomes of management of incontinence are focused on the absence of complications of treatment modalities, absence of pressure sores, and regained continence.

Sensory-Perceptual Alterations

Bedrest in an ICU environment restricts sensory input and proprioception but also often simultaneously exposes the patient to sensory overload. Boredom, anxiety, tension, inability to concentrate, somatic complaints, and auditory and visual illusions and hallucinations may develop, leading to depression and hostility. Sensory-perceptual alterations related to sensory overload have been referred to as ICU psychosis (Easton and MacKenzie, 1988). This reversible state often begins between the third and seventh day after ICU admission and clears by itself within 48 hours of ICU discharge (Ballard, 1981).

Management goals are directed toward decreasing excessive and inappropriate sensory stimulation such as noise, light, pain, tactile stimulation, and excessive numbers of caregivers and providing adequate rest, sleep, and sedation. Time and spatial orientation, family socialization, and use of sensory aids should be implemented and planned appropriately. Preoperative interviewing for patients undergoing elective surgery should be conducted if feasible because it has been found to decrease the incidence of postoperative delirium by 50% (Kornfeld et al., 1974). Management strategies for sensory-perceptual alterations are discussed in detail in Chapter 2.

Disturbance in Self-Concept: Body Image

Dependency is implied with bedrest. Nearly all normal role functions are curtailed by bedrest, and a reliance on caregivers is prevalent. Kornfeld and associates (1974) found that dominant, active patients who demonstrated high self-confidence and competitive qualities failed to tolerate the dependent, immobilized role well. Coupled with the lack of intellectual stimulation, the sick role, and the stresses of illness, altered body image may occur, becoming manifest through anger, despair, weeping, excessive dependence on caregivers, and general deterioration in problem-solving and decision-making abilities. Management strategies should be aimed at establishing a trusting nurse-patient relationship in which expression of feelings about dependency may be confidently shared. Promotion of social interaction along with construction of a mutually agreed upon plan to promote self-care and control over bedside activities are key interventions. Expected outcomes of such interventions are the resumption of role-related responsibilities, stated confidence toward the reconstruction of an altered body image, and exhibited desire to control body functions and bedside activities.

Diversional Activity Deficit

The monotony of confinement may give rise to boredom, lack of motivation, depression, restlessness, anger, or a flat affect. The creative construction of a plan based on the patient's interests and hobbies should include the use of a wide variety of media, diversified visitors, and a varied care routine. Time set aside exclusively for intellectual discussion as well as for sharing of feelings should be planned for.

Outcome criteria include active participation in diversional activities and suppression of symptoms.

SUMMARY

The prevalence of immobility in critically ill adults makes it an important phenomenon that can have monumental effects on patients' physical and emotional suffering and on caregiver, hospital, and equipment costs. The construction and execution of a plan by the critical care nurse that predicts patients at high risk, reduces modifiable risk factors, and effectively treats incurred complications are essential. Initiation by the critical care nurse to reinstitute mobilization as soon as possible in critically ill adults is important and remains the most cost-effective and simple plan to avoid the complications of immobility. Communication of the plan and collaboration with other members of the multidisciplinary ICU team will help to decrease the effects of a phenomenon that potentially affects every critically ill adult.

References

Allman, R. M., Walker, J. M., Hart, M. K., et al. (1987). Air-fluidized beds or conventional therapy for pressure sores. *Annals of Internal Medicine*, 107, 641–648.

Allman, R. M., Laprade, C. A., Noel, L. B., et al. (1986). Pressure sores among hospitalized patients. *Annals of Internal Medicine*, 105, 337–342.

Baird, S. E. (1985). Development of a nursing assessment tool to diagnose altered body image in immobilized patients. *Orthopedic Nursing*, 4, 47–54.

Ballard, K. S. (1981). Identification of environmental stressors for patients in a surgical intensive care unit. *Issues in Mental Health Nursing*, 3, 89–108.

Becker, D. M., Gonzalez, M., Gentili, A., et al. (1987). Prevention of deep vein thrombosis in patients with acute spinal cord injury: Use of rotating treatment tables. *Neurosurgery*, 20, 675–677.

Belch, J. J., Low, G. D., Ward, A. G., et al. (1981). Prevention of deep vein thrombi in medical patients by low dose heparin. *Scottish Medical Journal*, 26, 115–117.

Belitz, J. (1983). Minimizing the psychological complications of patients who require mechanical ventilation. *Critical Care Nurse*, 3, 42–46.

Bennett-Canclini, S. (1985). The Kinetic Treatment Table: A new approach to bedrest. *Orthopaedic Nursing*, 4, 61–70.

Bergstrom, N., Broden, B. J., Laguzza, A., et al. (1987). The Braden scale for predicting pressure sore risk. *Nursing Research*, 36, 205–210.

Blair, E., and Hickam, J. B. (1955). The effect of changes in body position on lung volumes and intrapulmonary gas mixing on normal subjects. *Journal of Clinical Investigation*, 34, 383–389.

Blomquist, C. G., and Stone, H. L. (1983). Cardiovascular adjustments to gravitational stress. In J. T. Shepherd and F. M. Abboud (Eds.), *Handbook of physiology* (pp. 1025–1063). Bethesda: American Physiological Society.

Blotner, H. (1945). Effect of prolonged inactivity on tolerance of sugar. *Archives of Internal Medicine*, 75, 39–44.

Bolyard, E. A., Townsend, T. R., and Horan, T. (1987). Airborne contamination associated with in-use air-fluidized beds: A descriptive study. *American Journal of Infection Control*, 15, 75–78.

Braden, B., and Bergstrom, N. (1987). A conceptual schema for the study of the etiology of pressure sores. *Rehabilitation Nursing*, 12, 8–12.

Brooks, B., and Duncan, G. W. (1940). Effects of pressure on tissues. *Archives of Surgery*, 40, 696–709.

Brower, P., and Hicks, D. (1972). Maintaining muscle function in patients on bedrest. *American Journal of Nursing*, 72, 1250–1253.

Brunner, L., and Suddarth, D. (1986). Rehabilitation concepts. In L. Brunner and D. Suddarth (Eds.), *Manual of nursing practice* (pp. 51–73.). Philadelphia: J. B. Lippincott.

Buhr, P. A. (1963). On the influence of prolonged bodily inactivity on the blood sugar curves after oral glucose loading. *Helvetica Medica Acta*, 30, 156–175.

Burn, F. D., Johnson, J., and Ellis, N. (1987). Managing decubiti ulcers. *Hospital Therapy*, 12, 67–75.

Cade, J. F. (1982). High risk of the critically ill for venous thromboembolism. *Critical Care Medicine*, 7, 448–450.

Caprini, J. A., Chucker, J. L., Zuckerman, L., Vagher, et al. (1983). Thrombosis prophylaxis using external compression. *Surgery, Gynecology, and Obstetrics*, 156, 599–604.

Cardus, D. (1967). Oxygen alveolar-arterial tension differences after 10 days recumbency in man. *Journal of Applied Physiology*, 23, 934–937.

Channick, R., Curley, F. J., and Irwin, R. S. (1988). Indications for and complications of rectal tube use in critically ill patients. *Journal of Intensive Care Medicine*, 3, 321–323.

Chobanian, A. V., Lille, R. D., Tercyak, A., et al. (1974). The metabolic and hemodynamic effects of prolonged bedrest in normal subjects. *Circulation*, 49, 551–559.

Christian, B. J. (1982). Immobilization. In C. Norris (Ed.), *Psychological aspects in concept classification in nursing*. Rockville, Maryland: Aspen Systems.

Chrysant, S. (1978). Hemodynamic effects of isometric exercise in normotensive subjects. *Angiology*, 29, 379–385.

Chulay, M., Brown, J., and Summer, W. (1982). Effect of postoperative immobilization after coronary artery bypass surgery. *Critical Care Medicine*, 10, 176–179.

Chuman, M. A. (1985). Risk factors associated with ulnar nerve compression in bedridden patients. *Journal of Neurosurgical Nursing*, 17, 338–342.

Coe, S. W. (1954). Cardiac work and the chair treatment of acute coronary thrombosis. *Annals of Internal Medicine*, 40, 42–47.

Convertino, V. A., Stremel, R. W., Bernauer, E. M., et al. (1977). Cardiorespiratory responses to exercise after bedrest in men and women. *Acta Astronautica*, 4, 895–905.

Coon, W. W., Hirsh, J., and Rubin, L. J. (1987). Preventing deep vein thrombosis. *Patient Care*, 21, 82–90.

Craig, D. B., Wahba, W. M., and Don, H. F. (1971). Airway clearance and lung volumes in surgical positions. *Canadian Anaesthetists Society Journal*, 18, 92–99.

Dietrick, J. E., Whedon, G. W., and Shorr, E. (1948). Effects of immobilization upon various metabolic and physiologic functions of normal men. *American Journal of Medicine*, 4, 3–36.

Dinsdale, S. M. (1974). Decubitus ulcers: Role of pressure and friction in causation. *Archives of Physical Medicine and Rehabilitation*, 55, 147–152.

Dinsdale, S. M. (1973). Decubitus ulcers in swine: Light and electron microscopy study of pathogenesis. *Archives of Physical Medicine and Rehabilitation*, 54, 51–56.

Domonkos, J., and Herr, L. (1965). Effect of denervation and immobilization on carbohydrate metabolism in tonic and tetanic muscles: Glycogen metabolism. *Acta Physiologica Hungarica*, 28, 227–236.

Don, H. F., Craig, D. B., Wahba, W. M., et al. (1971). The measurement of gas trapped in the lungs at functional residual capacity and the effects of posture. *Anesthesiology*, 35, 582–590.

Douglas, W. W., Rehder, K., Beynen, F. M., et al. (1977). Improved oxygenation in patients with acute respiratory failure: The prone position. *American Review of Respiratory Disease*, 115, 559–566.

Downs, F. S. (1974). Bedrest and sensory disturbances. *American Journal of Nursing*, 74, 434–439.

Easton, C., and MacKenzie, F. (1988). Sensory-perceptual alterations: Delirium in the intensive care unit. *Heart and Lung*, 17, 229–235.

Echenique, M. M., Bistrian, B. R., and Blackburn, G. L. (1982). Theory and techniques of nutritional support in the intensive care unit. *Critical Care Medicine*, 10, 546–549.

Elpern, E. H., Jacobs, E. R., and Bone, R. C. (1987). Incidence of aspiration in tracheally intubated adults. *Heart and Lung, 16,* 527–531.

Enneking, W. F., and Horowitz, M. (1972). The intraarticular effects of immobility on the human knee. *Journal of Bone and Joint Surgery, 54A,* 973.

Evans, R. A., Bridgeman, M., and Hills, E. (1984). Immobilization hypercalcemia. *Mineral and Electrolyte Metabolism, 10,* 244–248.

Fahey, V. A. (1984). An in-depth look at deep vein thrombosis. *Nursing 84, 14,* 35–41.

Fareeduddin, K., and Abelman, W. H. (1969). Impaired orthostatic tolerance after bedrest in patients with myocardial infarction. *New England Journal of Medicine, 280,* 345.

Feustel, D. E. (1982). Pressure sore prevention. *Nursing 82, 82,* 78–83.

Ford, G. T., Whitelaw, W. A., Rosenal, T. W., et al. (1983). Diaphragm function after upper abdominal surgery in humans. *American Review of Respiratory Disease, 127,* 431–436.

Frank, C., Akeson, W. H., Woo, S. L., et al. (1984). Physiology and therapeutic value of passive joint motion. *Clinical Orthopaedics and Related Research, 185,* 113–125.

Froese, A. B., and Bryan, A. C. (1974). Effects of anesthesia and paralysis on diaphragmatic mechanics in man. *Anesthesiology, 41,* 242–255.

Gallus, A. S., and Hirsh, J. (1976). Treatment of venous thromboembolic disease. *Seminars in Thrombosis and Hemostasis, 2,* 291–331.

Galpin, J. E., Chow, A. W., Boyer, A. S., et al. (1976). Sepsis associated with decubitus ulcers. *American Journal of Medicine, 61,* 346–350.

Gentilello, L., Thompson, D. A., Tonnesen, A. S., et al. (1988). Effect of a rotating bed on the incidence of pulmonary complications in critically ill patients. *Critical Care Medicine, 16(8),* 783–786.

Goldstone, L. A., and Goldstone, J. (1982). The Norton score: An early warning of pressure sores. *Journal of Advanced Nursing, 7,* 419–426.

Gosnell, D. J. (1987). Assessment and evaluation of pressure sores. *Nursing Clinics of North America, 22,* 399–416.

Gosnell, D. J. (1973). An assessment tool to identify pressure sores. *Nursing Research, 22,* 55–59.

Greenleaf, J. E. (1982). Physiological consequences of reduced physical activity during bedrest. *Exercise and Sport Sciences Reviews, 10,* 84–119.

Greenleaf, J. E., Bernauer, E. M., Jukos, I. T., et al. (1977). Effects of exercise on fluid exchange and body composition in man during 14-day bedrest. *Journal of Applied Physiology, 43,* 126–132.

Gruis, M. L., and Innes, B. (1976). Assessment: Essential to prevent pressure sores. *American Journal of Nursing, 76,* 1762–1764.

Halkin, H., Goldbert, J., Modan, M., et al. (1982). Reduction of mortality in general medical in-patients by low-dose heparin prophylaxis. *Annals of Internal Medicine, 96,* 561–565.

Hansel, H. N. (1984). The behavioral effects of noise on man: The patient with ICU psychosis. *Heart & Lung, 13,* 59–65.

Helton, M. C., Gordon, S. H., and Nunnery, S. L. (1980). The correlation between sleep deprivation and the ICU syndrome. *Heart & Lung, 9,* 464–469.

Henke, J. A., Thompson, N. W., and Kaufer, H. (1975). Immobilization hypercalcemia crises. *Archives of Surgery, 110,* 321–323.

Hotter, A. N. (1982). Physiologic aspects and clinical implications of wound healing. *Heart & Lung, 11,* 522–530.

Hull, R., Hirsh, J., Sackett, D. L., et al. (1981). Cost effectiveness of clinical diagnosis, venography, and non-invasive testing in patients with symptomatic deep vein thrombosis. *New England Journal of Medicine, 301,* 1561–1567.

Hull, R., Hirsh, J., Sackett, D. L., et al. (1977). Combined use of leg scanning and impedance plethysmography in suspected venous thrombosis. *New England Journal of Medicine, 296,* 1497–1500.

Hwang, T. I., Hill, K., Schneider, V., et al. (1988). Effect of prolonged bedrest on the propensity for renal stone formation. *Journal of Clinical Endocrinology and Metabolism, 66,* 109–112.

Issekutz, B., Blizzard, J. J., Birkhead, N. C., et al. (1966). Effect of prolonged bedrest on urinary calcium output. *Journal of Applied Physiology, 21,* 1013–1020.

Johnson, P. C. (1974). How does the human body adapt to conditions of weightlessness, and are the changes reversible? *American Scientist, 72,* 495.

Johnson, P. C., Driscoll, T. B., and Carpenter, N. R. (1971). Vascular and extravascular fluid changes during six days of bedrest. *Aerospace Medicine, 42,* 875–878.

Kakkar, V. V., Flank, C., and Howe, C. T. (1969). Natural history of postoperative deep vein thrombosis. *Lancet, 2,* 230–233.

Kelly, T. W., Patrick, M. R., and Hillman, K. M. (1983). Study of diarrhea in critically ill patients. *Critical Care Medicine, 11,* 7–9.

Kornfeld, D. S., Heller, S. S., Frank, K. A., et al. (1974). Personality and psychological factors in postcardiotomy delirium. *Archives of General Psychiatry, 31,* 249–253.

Koziak, M. (1959). Etiology and pathology of ischemic ulcers. *Archives of Physical Medicine Rehabilitation, 40,* 62–69.

Lamb, L., Stevens, P., and Johnson, R. (1965). Hypokinesia secondary to chair rest from four to ten days. *Aerospace Medicine, 36,* 755–763.

Larsen, B., Holstein, P., and Lassen, N. A. (1979). On the pathogenesis of bedsores. *Journal of Plastic Reconstruction Surgery, 13,* 347.

Leithauser, D. J. (1946). *Early ambulation and related procedures in surgical management.* Springfield, IL: Charles C Thomas.

Lentz, M. (1981). Selected aspects of deconditioning secondary to immobilization. *Nursing Clinics of North America, 16,* 729–736.

Lipman, R. L., Schnure, J. J., Bradley, E. M., et al. (1970). Impairment of peripheral glucose utilization in normal subjects by prolonged bedrest. *Journal of Laboratory and Clinical Medicine, 76,* 221.

Lucke, K., and Jarlsberg, C. (1985). How is the air-fluidized bed best used? *American Journal of Nursing, 85,* 1338–1340.

Maklebust, J. (1987). Pressure ulcers: Etiology and prevention. *Nursing Clinics of North American, 22,* 359–377.

Marini, J. J., Tyler, M. L., Hudson, L. D., et al. (1984). Influence of head-dependent positions on lung volumes and oxygen saturation in chronic airflow obstruction. *American Review of Respiratory Disease, 129,* 101–105.

Maynard, F. M. (1986). Immobilization hypercalcemia following spinal cord injury. *Archives of Physical Medicine and Rehabilitation, 67,* 41–43.

McCaffree, R. (1978). Pulmonary embolism: Diagnosis, treatment, and prevention. *Medical Times, 106,* 49.

McCally, M., Pohl, S. A., and Samson, P. A. (1968). Relative effectiveness of selected flight deconditioning countermeasures. *Aerospace Medicine, 39,* 722.

Memmer, M. K., and Kozier, B. (1987). Mobility and immobility. In B. Kozier and G. Erb (Eds.), *Fundamentals of nursing: Concepts and procedures* (pp. 964–1025). Menlo Park: Addison-Wesley.

Meythaler, J. M., Korkor, A. B., Nanda, T., et al. (1986). Immobilization hypercalcemia associated with Landry-Guillain-Barré syndrome. *Archives of Internal Medicine, 146,* 1567–1571.

Milazzo, V., and Resh, C. (1981). Kinetic nursing—a new approach to the problems of immobility. *Journal of Neurosurgical Nursing, 14,* 120–124.

Miller, P. B., Johnson, R. L., and Lamb, L. E. (1965). Effects of moderate physical exercise during four weeks of bedrest on circulatory functions in man. *Aerospace Medicine, 36,* 1077.

Miller, P. B., Hartman, B. O., and Johnson, R. L. (1964). Modification of the effects of bedrest upon circulatory functions in man. *Aerospace Medicine, 35,* 931.

Mitchell, P. H. (1981). Motor status. In P. H. Mitchell and A. Lonstau (Eds.), *Concepts basic to nursing* (pp. 343–390). New York: McGraw-Hill.

Morrell, M. P., and Dunhill, M. S. (1968). The postmortem incidence of pulmonary embolism in a hospital population. *British Journal of Surgery, 55,* 347.

Moser, K. M., and Fedullo, P. F. (1983). Venous thromboembolism (part I). *Chest, 83,* 117–121.

Moser, K. M., and Fedullo, P. F. (1983). Venous thromboembolism (part II). *Chest, 83,* 256–260.

Moser, K. M., and LeMoine, J. R. (1981). Is emboli risk conditional by location of deep vein thrombosis? *Annals of Internal Medicine, 94,* 439–444.

Nand, S., and Goldschmidt, J. W. (1976). Hypercalcemia and hypercalciuria in young patients with spinal cord injury. *Archives of Physical Medicine and Rehabilitation, 57,* 553.

Neuhaus, A., Bentz, R. R., and Weg, J. C. (1978). Pulmonary embolism in respiratory failure. *Chest*, 73, 464–465.

Norton, D., McLaren, R., and Exton-Smith, A. N. (1962). *An investigation of geriatric nursing problems in hospitals*. Edinburgh: Churchill Livingstone.

Olson, E. V. (1967). The effects of immobility. *American Journal of Nursing*, 67, 780–796.

O'Neill, R. H. (1981). Problems associated with disuse syndromes—including the integument. In I. L. Beland and J. Y. Passos (Eds.), *Clinical nursing: Pathophysiologic and psychosocial approaches* (pp. 1107–1123). New York: Macmillan.

Pechan, J., and Julis, I. (1975). The pressure measurement in the ulnar nerve: Contribution to the pathophysiology of the carpal tunnel syndrome. *Journal of Biomechanics*, 8, 75–79.

Pennington, J. (1987). Hospital-acquired pneumonias. In P. R. Wenzel (Ed.), *Prevention and control of nosocomial infections* (pp. 321–334). Baltimore: Williams & Wilkins.

Pezeshki, C., and Brooker, A. F. (1977). Immobilization hypercalcemia: Report of two cases transmitted with calcitonin. *Journal of Bone and Joint Surgery*, American, volume 59, 971–973.

Piehl, M. A., and Brown, R. S. (1976). Use of extreme position changes in acute respiratory failure. *Critical Care Medicine*, 4, 13–14.

Pingleton, S. K. (1985). Thromboembolism and bleeding disorders in the critically ill patient. *Respiratory Care*, 30, 481–486.

Pingleton, S. K., Bone, R. C., Pingleton, W. W., et al. (1981). Prevention of pulmonary embolism in a respiratory intensive care unit. *Chest*, 79, 647–650.

Plate, G., Einarsson, E., and Eklof, B. (1986). Etiologic spectrum in acute iliofemoral venous thrombosis. *International Angiology*, 5, 59–64.

Regnier, B., Prokocimer, P., and Wolfe, M. (1981). Influence of position in unilateral lung disease. *New England Journal of Medicine*, 305, 287.

Remolina, C., Khan, A. U., Santiago, T. V., et al. (1981). Positional hypoxemia in unilateral lung disease. *New England Journal of Medicine*, 304, 523–525.

Reuler, J. B., and Cooney, T. G. (1981). The pressure sore: Pathophysiology and principles of management. *Annals of Internal Medicine*, 94, 661–666.

Rissing, J. P., Crowder, J. G., Dunfee, T., et al. (1974). Bacteroides bacteremia from decubitus ulcers. *Southern Medical Journal*, 67, 1179–1182.

Roberts, S. L. (1987). Pulmonary tissue perfusion altered: emboli. *Heart & Lung*, 16, 128–137.

Rubin, M. (1988). The physiology of bedrest. *American Journal of Nursing*, 88, 50–56.

Saltin, B., Blomquist, G., and Mitchell, J. H. (1968). Response to exercise after bedrest and after training: A longitudinal study of adaptive changes in oxygen transport and body composition. *Circulation*, 38, 1–78.

Seaton, D., Lapp, N. L., and Morgan, K. C. (1979). Effect of body position on gas exchange after thoracotomy. *Thorax*, 34, 518–522.

Seiler, W. O., and Stahelin, H. B. (1985). Decubitus ulcers: Preventive techniques for the elderly patient. *Geriatrics*, 40, 53–60.

Smith, M. J. (1975). Changes in judgment of duration: With different patterns of auditory information for individuals confined to bed. *Nursing Research*, 24, 93–98.

Stamm, W. (1986). Nosocomial urinary tract infections. In J. K. Bennett and P. S. Brachman (Eds.), *Hospital infections* (pp. 375–384). New York: Little, Brown.

Stewart, A. F., Adler, M., and Byers, C. M. (1982). Calcium homeostasis in immobility: An example of resorptive hypercalciuria. *New England Journal of Medicine*, 306, 1136.

Stotts, N. A. (1988). Predicting pressure ulcer development in surgical patients. *Heart & Lung*, 17, 641–647.

Stotts, N. A. (1987). Age-specific characteristics of patients who develop pressure ulcers in the tertiary-care setting. *Nursing Clinics of North America*, 22, 391–398.

St. Pierre, D., and Gardiner, P. F. (1987). The effect of immobility and exercise on muscle function: A review. *Physiotherapy Canada*, 39, 24–36.

Stremel, R. W., Convertino, V. A., and Bernauer, E. M. (1976). Cardiorespiratory deconditioning with static and dynamic exercise during bedrest. *Journal of Applied Physiology*, 41, 905.

Summers, T. B., and Hines, H. M. (1951). Effect of immobility in various positions upon the weight and strength of skeletal muscles. *Archives of Physical Medicine*, 32, 142–145.

Taylor, H. L., Henschel, A., and Brozek, J. (1949). Effects of bedrest on cardiovascular function and work performance. *Journal of Applied Physiology*, 2, 223.

Tyler, M. L. (1984). The respiratory effects of body positioning and immobility. *Respiratory Care*, 29, 472–481.

Van Zuiden, L., Anquist, K. A., and Schachar, N. (1982). Immobilization hypercalcemia. *Canadian Journal of Surgery*, 25, 647–649.

Vernikos-Danellis, J., Leach, C. S., Winget, C. M., et al. (1976). Changes in glucose, insulin, and growth hormone levels associated with bedrest. *Aviation, Space, and Environmental Medicine*, 47, 583–587.

Vesley, D., Hankinson, S. E., and Lauer, J. L. (1986). Microbial survival and dissemination associated with an air-fluidized therapy unit. *American Journal of Infection Control*, 14, 35–40.

Vogt, F. B., Mack, P. B., and Johnson, P. C. (1966). Tilt table response and blood volume changes associated with 30 days of recumbency. *Aerospace Medicine*, 37, 771.

Weissman, C., Askanazi, J., Hyman, A. I., et al. (1983). Hypercalcemia and hypercalciuria in a critically ill patient. *Critical Care Medicine*, 11, 576–578.

West, J. B. (1985). *Respiratory physiology—The essentials*. Baltimore: Williams & Wilkins.

Williams, A. (1973). A study of factors contributing to skin breakdown. *Nursing Research*, 22, 238–243.

Winslow, E. H. (1985). Cardiovascular consequences of bedrest. *Heart & Lung*, 14, 236–246.

Wood, M. (1977). Clinical sensory deprivation: A comparative study of patients in single care and two-bedrooms. *Journal of Nursing Administration*, 7, 28–32.

Yannelli, B., and Gurevich, I. (1988). Infection in critical care. *Heart & Lung*, 17, 596–600.

Zack, M. B., Pontoppidan, H., and Kazemmi, A. (1974). The effect of lateral positions on gas exchange in pulmonary disease. *American Review of Respiratory Disease*, 110, 49–55.

4

Effect of Communication Patterns

Verna Medina Sitzer

The critical care environment is an enormous arena in which communication occurs constantly. The intensity of care required by critically ill patients necessitates effective communication between members of the health care team and the patient-family unit. Effective communication implies that both verbal and nonverbal means of communication are understood and that the interaction results in a positive experience or outcome. This chapter presents components of the communication process, elements that enhance as well as interfere with communication, and strategies to overcome communication barriers in the critical care unit.

COMMUNICATION PROCESS

Interpersonal communication involves the transfer of information between two or more people. It is the concurrent process of sending messages, receiving messages, and obtaining immediate feedback (De-Vito, 1980). The roles of sender and receiver are both assumed by each individual. The sender generates and delivers information in the form of a code, a process referred to as encoding. The receiver accepts and interprets the information delivered in a process referred to as decoding. For communication to occur, messages must be sent and received, or encoded and decoded. Messages conveyed serve as stimuli for the receiver. They may be verbal, nonverbal, or written. In response to the stimulus or message, the receiver generates and conveys a message back to the sender. Thus, the receiver becomes the sender and so on. Participants in the communication process both send and receive messages at the same time. The messages received in response to information conveyed is called feedback. Feedback may take the form of verbal or nonverbal cues and may be positive or negative. Feedback enables communicators to judge the effectiveness of interactions and to adjust their behavior accordingly. Communication is a continuous circular process whereby every message is influenced by the messages preceding it (Fig. 4–1).

Communication is affected by the attitudes, feelings, beliefs, and values of both sender and receiver as well as by the context in which the interaction

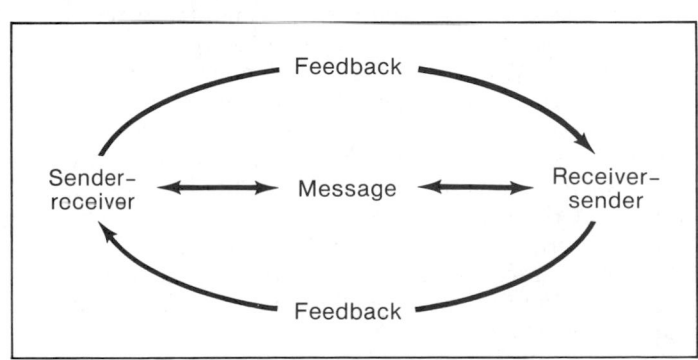

FIGURE 4–1. Communication process within a context.

occurs. These elements constantly interact during the communication process and serve as reference points for interpretation of messages. The sender and the receiver are influenced by each other, and both are influenced by the context in which the interaction takes place. For example, communication that occurs between the nurse and a patient in the hectic critical care environment will certainly be different from communication that occurs between the patient and his family in his own home.

An important aspect of communication is that one cannot choose not to communicate. Although one may not be aware of it, body positioning, facial expressions, gestures, silence, and even body odors communicate a message. Choosing not to respond in a communication interaction is itself a response. Another aspect of communication is that it is irreversible. Once a message is conveyed it cannot be retrieved.

COMMUNICATION CHANNELS

A channel is a route of communication. Messages received involve the use of our senses—visual, auditory, kinesthetic, olfactory, and gustatory. Messages conveyed involve verbal and written language and nonverbal language such as gestures, facial expressions, and body positioning. Communication interactions usually involve a combination of these channels. The more channels used, the clearer the message transmission and reception.

Visual Channel. Vision is one of the most important senses used for communication. Observation of a person's eyes, lips, facial expressions, body movements, and other facets in a communication interaction can provide significant information about behavior and attitude. In communicating with patients in the critical care unit, nurses frequently focus on body language to provide clues to the patient's feelings. For example, facial expressions and guarding movements can alert the nurse to the patient's pain or distress. In addition, much of the physiologic information obtained from the patient is observed and interpreted through the visual channel.

The visual pathway begins with light rays entering each eye and striking the retina. Light rays entering from the peripheral or temporal field hit the nasal region of the retina, and those entering from the nasal field strike the temporal region of the retina. From each retina visual impulses are transmitted by way of nerve fibers in the optic nerve. Nerve fibers from the nasal region of the both retinas cross at the optic chiasm and continue with nerve fibers from the temporal regions (which do not cross), forming optic tracts. The optic tracts terminate in the thalamic areas of the brain, and visual impulses are then carried by means of optic radiations to the visual center in the occipital cortex.

The crossing of nerve fibers in the optic chiasm results in transmission of visual impulses from the same half of each retina along one side of the pathway to the visual cortex. Lesions or injury affecting the visual pathway can result in blindness of specific visual fields (Fig. 4–2). Injury to the retina or optic nerve on one side of the pathway will result in total blindness of the eye on the same side of the lesion (unilateral blindness). Injury to the optic chiasm will result in partial blindness affecting only the temporal fields of both eyes (bitemporal hemianopsia). Injury to the optic tract or radiation on one side of the visual pathway will result in partial blindness affecting the temporal field of the same side and the nasal field of the opposite side (homonymous hemianopsia). These visual defects are commonly associated with visual pathway injuries. However, depending on the area of injury and extent of involvement, other visual field defects can occur including quadrantic defects and cortical blindness. Cortical blindness may occur with injury to the visual area of the cerebral cortex, such as may occur with an air embolus, and result in either short-term or permanent blindness.

It is essential for the critical care nurse to possess knowledge of the visual pathway and the effects of various lesions in order to detect potential or actual visual field defects and to develop appropriate communication stategies.

Auditory Channel. Listening is another important component of communication. Messages sent verbally must be accurately received or heard before true meaning is assigned. True meaning is that which is congruent with the sender's meaning. Listening is an active process that necessitates attention, concentration, and supportive use of body language to hear what is being said and to understand it. It is important to hear all aspects of speech such as tone, pitch, speed, and volume, not just the words. By careful listening, critical care nurses can not only obtain important and useful information about the patient but also detect hidden concerns, fears, anxieties, and needs.

Sounds in the environment are conducted inward toward auditory receptors in the inner ear by way of sound waves, vibrations, and pressure waves. Sound waves traverse the external ear to reach the tympanic membrane, where they are converted to vibrations. These vibrations are then relayed to the inner ear, where they are converted to pressure waves. In the cochlea, pressure waves stimulate the sensory receptors (hair cells), which are innervated by the vestibulocochlear nerve. With the stimulation of the vestibulocochlear nerve (cranial nerve VIII), sound impulses are carried to the auditory center in the temporal lobe.

A hearing impairment exists when sounds are unable to reach the inner ear or when the neural mechanism responsible for transmitting impulses to the brain has been damaged. A conductive hearing loss is present when sound waves are unable to

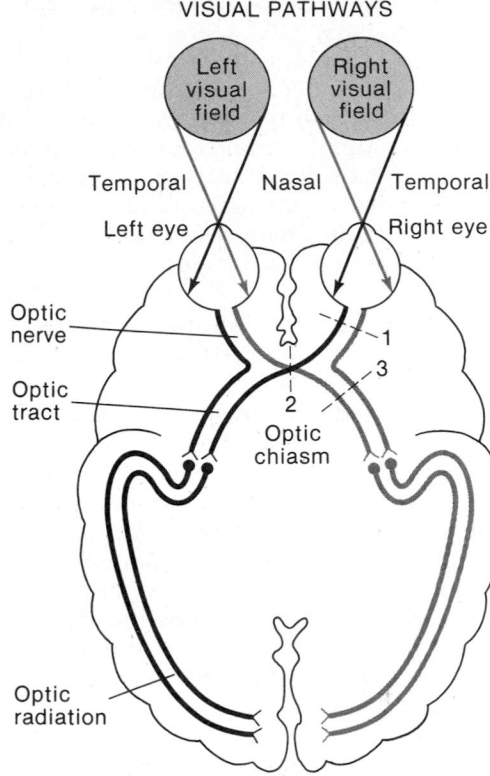

VISUAL PATHWAYS

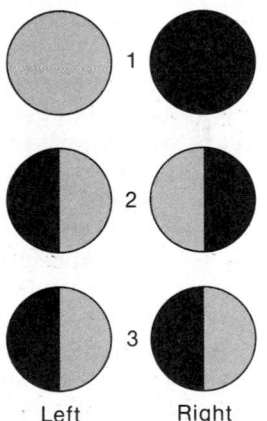

BLACKENED FIELD INDICATES
AREA OF NO VISION

Left   Right

FIGURE 4–2. Visual field defects. (Redrawn from Bates, B. (1991). *A guide to physical examination* (5th ed., p. 198). Philadelphia: J. B. Lippincott.)

reach the middle ear. This condition may be due to trauma, obstruction, or infection and rarely results in deafness. A sensorineural hearing loss results when the inner ear (hair cells) or neural pathway is damaged, in which case, impulses do not reach the auditory center. Conditions that can cause a sensorineural loss include trauma, anoxia, and toxic medications such as aminoglycosides and loop diuretics. Damage to the hair cells and nerve tissue of the inner ear usually produces permanent deafness. Another type of hearing loss occurs with aging. Presbycusis is the gradual hearing loss that results from degenerative processes.

Kinesthetic Channel. Significant information can be obtained and communicated through touch. Touch is an important aspect of nursing practice. Critical care nurses and other health care professionals use casual touch to administer care and needed therapeutic procedures to their patients. This privilege is granted to nurses and physicians by nature of their role in the institution. However, touch can also be used as a channel for communicating feelings of concern, support, and empathy and for developing a therapeutic relationship. Therapeutic touch, the laying on of hands with the intent to heal, has been used by some to relieve anxiety and pain and to facilitate healing (Heidt, 1981; Keller and Bzdek, 1986; Clement, 1986).

Touch receptors are located superficially on the skin surface. Sensory information such as touch, temperature, pain, and pressure are conveyed to the thalamus and cerebral cortex through either the spinothalamic or dorsal tract in the spinal cord, Lesions that interfere with the conduction of sensory impulses to the brain may result in an inability to experience sensations such as touch.

Output Channels. Messages received through each of the channels are processed in specific areas of the brain. After messages have been integrated, ideas are generated and a response is made. There are two important speech centers in the brain, Broca's area and Wernicke's area. The left hemisphere of the brain is usually dominant for speech functions. Broca's area, located in the frontal lobe, is the motor speech area that controls the movements of the tongue, lips, and vocal cords that are responsible for speech. It also directs and coordinates the muscles involved in writing. Wernicke's area, located in the temporal lobe, is important for the comprehension of spoken or written language.

Injury to these areas can have a profound impact on a person's ability to communicate. Aphasia is the loss or impairment of the ability to communicate through speech by expression or comprehension or both. Focal brain injury such as a cerebrovascular accident or a hemorrhage affecting Broca's area will result in loss of speech and is termed expressive aphasia. Language comprehension remains intact; however, speech is usually slow and unintelligible. Receptive aphasia, or loss of language comprehension, occurs with injury to Wernicke's area. Speech may be fluent, but the content is usually unorganized. Global aphasia may occur when several areas in the dominant hemisphere are damaged. Dysarthria is a group of speech disorders resulting from damage to or poor coordination of the speech muscles. The resulting speech pattern is slow and slurred. The ability to swallow may also be affected. Damage to Broca's or Wernicke's area and other areas of the brain will significantly affect a patient's ability to communicate through speech, writing, and gestures.

Body language refers to the way a person uses his or her body position or movements as a means of communication. It involves posture, gestures, facial movements, and other forms of nonverbal expressions. Body language often accompanies verbal communication. For example, "yes" is often accompanied by nodding the head up and down. However, body language may also contradict what is being said or felt, as in a patient who says he is fine but appears restless, and is often used in place of speech, as with the intubated patient. Body language in itself is a good indicator of how a person is feeling.

Eye contact, body posture, and appearance are forms of body language that play an important part in the communication process. The use and interpretation of eye contact is a cultural variable that must be explored before appropriate meaning can be assigned. Avoidance of eye contact during a communication interaction may indicate feelings of shame, fear, or low self-worth. It can be used to maintain distance, prevent an interaction from occurring, or halt a present interaction. Posture can help nurses determine a patient's feelings. For example, a slouched position may indicate lack of energy or motivation, whereas a rigid, tense posture may indicate pain or fear. Appearance also provides clues to the patient's feelings. An unkempt appearance may suggest lack of energy, motivation, or even depression. It is important to note when body language is incongruent with spoken words. Critical care nurses must skillfully interpret and validate the patient's communications to understand the intended meaning.

ESSENTIAL ELEMENTS FOR EFFECTIVE COMMUNICATION

Thus far, the communication process and the channels through which messages are relayed have been presented. Equally important in the communication process are elements that can enhance communication interactions. These include trust, active listening, empathy, and the use of touch.

Trust. The communication interaction between a patient or his family and the nurse is enhanced when a trusting relationship is established. Trust is reliance on, belief in, and confidence in another without doubt. In the critical care unit, patients are bombarded with new information and requests to make decisions about their illness and treatment options. Without a trusting relationship, the patient may be faced with uncertainty, fear, and inability to make decisions. The patient may also manifest anger and withdrawal. A common misconception of health care professionals is that patients and their families trust automatically when a relationship is begun. Trust develops over time. It occurs when repeated interactions have a positive or significant impact on the patient.

The critical care nurse must develop trust through open and honest communication. Establishing a trusting relationship in the critical care setting is often difficult because of the numerous and varying kinds of personnel involved in a patient's care. A nurse's work schedule and shift rotation can interfere with progression through the orientation, working, and termination phases of developing a relationship with patients and their families. In the orientation phase, the relationship is superficial. Rapport is developed as the nurse gathers important information about the patient and plans his nursing care. Information is also gathered from and given to the patient's family about the patient's illness, prognosis, and treatment plan. It is during the working phase that the critical care nurse and the patient feel enough ease with each other to share their feelings. Focus is placed on the patient's needs and concerns. The nurse intervenes to help the patient and his family to cope, adapt, or achieve comfort. In most instances, the critical care nurse is unable to terminate her relationship with the patient properly. This may be due to staffing arrangements or the sudden transfer of the patient to surgery or another service. A rapid, unexpected end to a therapeutic, trusting relationship may affect a patient's sense of trust in future relationships.

Active Listening. Effective communication occurs when one listens with understanding (Rogers and Roethlisberger, 1952). To listen with understanding implies placing one's self in the other person's mind set; to see and feel from the other person's point of view. The critical care nurse is actively listening to her patient when she is able to hear and derive meaning from what is being said. Active listening can be demonstrated by restating and verifying the statements and feelings conveyed by the patient. Active listening requires hard work and energy on the part of the nurse. To achieve the goal of accurate understanding, the nurse must listen to her patient with a mind free of distractions and biases. Active listening also requires a keen awareness of nonverbal behavior and integration of that behavior with unspoken words. Active listening is an essential ingredient for effective communication.

Empathy. Empathy is a process whereby an individual attempts to think and feel like another individual (Northouse, 1979). The critical care nurse who practices empathy places herself in the patient's shoes and experiences that patient's situation from his point of view rather than her own. This is done in an attempt to understand fully what the patient is communicating and to best meet the patient's needs. To practice empathy is to maintain one's identity while feeling with another, to be objective while at the same time offering support and understanding. Empathy differs from sympathy in that the latter involves relinquishing one's identity. To sympathize is to feel sorry for the other, to be subjective and to offer pity. Empathetic understanding is understanding with the patient, not about him. The use of empathy promotes effective communication by fostering trust, acceptance, and understanding.

Touch. Touch is a positive commodity that is satisfying and necessary for physical and mental development (Weirs, 1979). In an interpersonal interaction, touch is given meaning by its quality. In the highly technical arena of intensive care, critical care nurses and physicians are constantly touching patients. The nature of health care delivery necessitates access to a patient's body for examination, treatment, and provision of hygenic measures. Touch in these situations is usually task-oriented or proce-

dural. Procedural touch occurs during most nursing procedures. Expressive touch is a form of contact that is spontaneously directed toward improving communication (Pearce, 1988). Some nurses may feel uncomfortable or hesitant to provide expressive touch to their patients, fearing that they may be misinterpreted. This behavior may be due to cultural or social influences or past experiences. The assimilation of touch into one's nursing practice is risky when one is not sure how the patient will react. However, the benefits that touch can bring to an interpersonal interaction outweigh the risks involved. If possible, the nurse should first assess the patient's desire for and ability to be comforted by touch to avoid miscommunication.

Expressive or caring touch is used outside routine nursing procedures. This form of touch is used to convey concern, empathy, and closeness. It is also employed to comfort, support, and reassure patients in physical or psychological pain. For the unconscious or blind patient, it increases awareness that someone is present. For the patient or family in distress, it facilitates expression of feelings. For touch to be effective, its meaning must be accurately conveyed. The nurse must feel comfortable in using touch as a communicative channel. Verbal and other nonverbal forms of communication may be used to augment the use of touch. The critical care environment, with all its technologic wonders, diverts the nurse's time and attention away from the patient. Critical care nurses can counterbalance this highly technical environment by providing personalized care with the use of touch (Sinclair, 1988). The effectiveness of expressive touch lies with the nurse's ease in providing it and the patient's comfort in receiving it.

COMMUNICATION BARRIERS

The continuous nature of communication is theoretical. In actuality, a breakdown in communication can occur at any point in the communication process. Such a breakdown may be due to a number of reasons, too many for this chapter to discuss. It is sufficient to say, however, that anything that interferes with message transmission forms a barrier to communication and results in a communication breakdown. For effective communication to occur in the critical care setting, barriers common to this arena must be recognized and overcome.

Physical Factors. Communication deficits resulting from injury to the speech centers in the brain have been discussed previously. Depending on the extent of injury to the speech centers, inability to communicate may be permanent or transitory. Transitory alterations in communication usually occur when mentation is affected such as occurs with medications, hypoxia, or electrolyte imbalances. In the critical care unit, it is more commonly due to intubation or tracheostomy.

Intubation or tracheostomy is established to provide a patient with an airway or to facilitate mechanical ventilation. The presence of an artificial airway interferes with the patient's ability to communicate by affecting the vocal cords. Intubated patients rely on gestures or writing to communicate their needs to the nurse. This communicative technique is often thwarted when wrist restraints are used, invasive lines are present, or when the patient is weak. Understanding an intubated patient's attempts to communicate is a challenging responsibility that must be undertaken by the critical care nurse.

One study revealed a lack of communication between intubated patients and nurses (Salyer and Stuart, 1985). Interestingly, a lack of patient-initiated interaction was found. In this study, positive actions by either the nurse or the patient tended to result in positive reactions. Likewise, negative actions tended to yield negative reactions. However, in one-third of positive interactions initiated by patients, the nurses tended to respond negatively. Silence was the most common nurse action-reaction during administration of nursing care that elicited a negative patient response. This study points out the need for critical care nurses to communicate with their patients in an empathetic manner.

The challenge of communicating effectively with intubated patients is heightened when patients are placed on neuromuscular blocking agents to achieve adequate ventilation. In this situation, the patient is unable to communicate at all. Furthermore, these patients are usually sedated to blunt their perception and to decrease the fear and anxiety of not being able to move. Although the patient is paralyzed, he remains conscious with intact auditory and kinesthetic abilities. It is not unusual for the critical care nurse to bypass communication with patients paralyzed in this way, treating them as if they were unconscious.

Environmental Factors. The special characteristics of the critical care unit often create communication barriers. Specifically, these include lack of privacy, high noise levels, use of technical language, and rigid routines.

The patient's privacy is often violated in the critical care setting. The patient's body is subjected to numerous examinations and procedures by health care workers who may or may not have an established relationship with the patient. This characteristic is especially evident in teaching hospitals, where the care of patients is provided by all members of the health care team. "Rounds" are held within the various units, where every bedside becomes a conference room for open discussion and examination of patients. A patient's disease, treatment, and prognosis are discussed with other members of the health care team around the unit, in elevators, and in cafeterias, often without sensitivity to the presence of other patients, visitors, and other personnel. Careless treatment of privileged information and poor regard for patient privacy can lead to misinterpretation on the part of the patient or reluctance to disclose information to health care providers. Respect for a patient's privacy, especially with regard to personal information, significantly influences the effectiveness of communication interactions.

A considerable amount of information exists on the effect of noise on patients (Hansell, 1984). Noise is anything that interferes with effective transmission of messages. Visual distractions, unintelligible writing, offensive odors, and biases all constitute "noise." In the critical care unit noise often comprises the sounds of beeping monitors, alarms, ventilators, and staff conversations. Critical care nurses have become accustomed to such noises and do not recognize them as potential barriers to communication. The bustling environment, high-tech machines, and rigid routines of the unit tend to make staff lose sight of the patient as a thinking, feeling individual. Although nurses spend much of their time at patient bedsides, much of their attention is focused on technical competence. Technologic advances have greatly assisted in the delivery of health care. However, this increased focus on the physiologic aspects of care has left the patient's psychological and emotional needs unattended.

The patient in the critical care unit, on the other hand, may be overwhelmed with and fearful of the unfamiliar sights and sounds to such an extent that his sensory-perceptual abilities become distorted or impaired. "ICU psychosis" and other similar syndromes have been extensively documented in the literature.[11, 12] The high-tech aspects of the equipment and procedures can make a patient sense the urgency of the nurse's actions, causing him subsequently to minimize or refrain from communicating his needs. Similarly, the nurse may feel too busy to provide time for therapeutic communication. Developing a keen awareness of "noise" in the critical care unit can assist a nurse in controlling or reducing its impact on critically ill patients. To start with, nurses can attempt to lower the tone of their voices and limit their personal conversations around the bedside.

Technical language specific to a particular field such as medicine is referred to as jargon. For the health care professional, jargon is part of everyday language and conversation. For the patient, highly technical language is perceived as foreign and serves to distance him and his family from the communication interaction. Without appropriate explanations in "lay" terms that the patient can understand clearly, communication may be fraught with misinterpretations and misconceptions. Critical care nurses should consciously examine their communication with patients to determine their use of jargon. They should be astute in noting a patient's or family's nonverbal cues indicating a lack of understanding and quick to adjust the level of communication. Most important, nurses should encourage patients and their families to ask questions.

The patient and his visitors are frequently reminded of the hospital's policies and routines. The monitoring of vital signs, provision of hygienic measures, scheduling of procedures, and maintenance of visiting hours are part of the hospital routine and are often inflexible. As much as possible, traditional practices should be arranged to promote effective communication interactions. Environmental barriers must be prevented from interfering with the communication process. A proper climate for clear transmission of messages, careful listening, and thoughtful discussion should be established.

Sociocultural Factors. Sociocultural barriers that can influence communication between patients and nurses include differences in culture, language, and race. Culture is the sum of all experiences past and present that provide criteria against which choices and decisions are made. Each patient is a unique individual, possessing a different value system and cultural background. Cultural differences result in various patient behaviors and communication styles. In an interpersonal interaction, cultural diversity influences the display of emotions, the use and interpretation of eye contact and touch, and the person in the family who should be spoken to for proper respect. Variables such as these must be explored by the sensitive nurse to prevent breakdowns in communication.

The cultural needs of a patient and his family must be identified for effective communication to occur. Routinely, these include the language spoken by the patient, food preferences, religious affiliation, and other cultural practices. It is important to note also the family structure and role relationships, decision-making practices, beliefs about health and illness, and expectations for the hospitalization. These additional factors can influence a patient's response to treatment and his compliance. Cultural needs are determined to avoid ethnocentrism and stereotyping (Parfitt, 1988). Ethnocentrism is the belief that one's own culture is superior to that of another. The nurse who conveys such a belief is unaccepting of a patient's individuality. The patient who perceives this attitude may be unwilling or reluctant to share meaningful and useful information. It is essential that the nurse demonstrate an attitude of acceptance and the belief that no culture is superior to another to facilitate communication.

The possession of preconceived ideas about a patient's cultural pattern or group can severely affect communication and can lead to misguided interventions. Stereotyping occurs when a person believes that all members of a particular group are the same. The tendency to label ethnic groups based on frequently observed reactions to certain situations is not uncommon and impairs effective communication. Due to past or present experiences or beliefs, the nurse may possess a certain attitude toward a particular group that surfaces upon contact with a member of that group. This tendency is evident in nurses'

opinions of hospitalized patients in terms of "good" versus "problem" patients. "Good" patients tend to be quiet, nondemanding, and cooperative. "Difficult" patients, defined in a survey of 73 nurses, are "demanding, complaining, frustrating, time-consuming, requesting, frequently calling, manipulative, female, impolite, unreasonable or uncooperative" (Podraskey and Sexton, 1988). The nurse's reaction and response to these types of patients may be based on such false assumptions. Critical care nurses should consciously treat every patient as an individual with a set of unique characteristics and experiences. The common tendency to judge, evaluate, approve, or disapprove messages exchanged in an interpersonal interaction is a major barrier to communication (Rogers and Roethlisberger, 1952).

Communicating with culturally diverse patients in the critical care unit is a challenging responsibility for all nurses. When a language barrier is present, this challenge is intensified. Patients who are unable to speak the dominant language may not effectively communicate their needs. The nurse may find it very difficult to interpret what the patient is trying to convey. This can lead to feelings of fear and anxiety by the patient and frustration by the nurse. Critical care nurses should use trained interpreters to facilitate communication with patients who cannot speak or understand the dominant language. Family members may be used when necessary but with caution because the potential for misinterpretation exists. When an interpreter is not available, the nurse must use her creativity in communicating with the patient. The use of nonverbal behaviors, pictures, and demonstration can be helpful. It should not be forgotten that nonverbal messages often give clues to how one is feeling. Nurses must be sensitive to their own behaviors when using this technique.

Psychological Factors. Anxiety, fear, and loneliness are feelings of patients that can affect the communication interaction. Such feelings arise when patients experience unexpected illnesses, sensations, life-threatening conditions, environmental changes, and role changes. Ironically, critically ill patients must attempt to cope with these feelings when they are least capable of doing so. The critical care nurse is in the best position to alleviate or reduce these feelings by interpreting the environment and providing information to the patient.

Anxiety and fear are feelings that arise when a perceived threat is present. Anxiety differs from fear in that the latter is more tangible and easier to identify. Anxiety is a state of mind that exists when one's sense of well-being is threatened. There are various levels of anxiety that can significantly affect a person's ability to communicate effectively. Mild anxiety is experienced frequently in day-to-day life. It improves one's functioning by motivating, preparing, and sharpening the senses and perceptions. An individual experiencing mild anxiety tends to solve problems more effectively. Moderate anxiety limits one's perceptual field to such a degree that one's problem-solving ability is lessened. Severe anxiety occurs when stress is intense. A person in this state can focus on only one detail (relieving anxiety) due to limited attention and perception. Panic, the most destructive level of anxiety, impairs an individual's perceptual ability to a point where effective communication and functioning are disabled.

Critical illness and hospitalization in a critical care unit can often precipitate feelings of loneliness in a patient. Loneliness should not be confused with social isolation because the former is not an imposed condition; rather, it is a disheartened awareness of being alone. Loneliness creates physical and psychological pain and anxiety for the patient (Buchda, 1957). This pain may be due to the threat of illness on life or to separation from loved ones and familiar surroundings. A patient experiencing loneliness may appear quiet and withdrawn or may display tearfulness or restlessness. Feelings of anxiety may be present, arising from a fear of being lonely.

Anxiety, fear, and loneliness are feelings that may be felt alone or in combination with each other. The critical care nurse should recognize situations that can precipitate and behaviors that indicate the presence of such feelings in order to plan and develop proper strategies to alleviate them. Whenever possible, the precipitating stressor should be identified and either reduced or eliminated. Understanding the different levels of anxiety and their resultant effects can allow the nurse to intervene at an early stage. Patients should be encouraged to express their concerns to decrease their feelings of anxiety, fear, or loneliness. Nurses should attempt to reduce these feelings by providing time, support, reassurance, and personalized care. The family should be encouraged to visit and participate in the patient's care. Minimizing and controlling the stressful feelings of a patient can facilitate effective communication interactions.

INTERVENTIONS THAT IMPROVE COMMUNICATION

Communicating with the Patient and the Family. Communicating effectively with the patient and his family is a challenge faced by critical care nurses on a daily basis. The presence of physical, environmental, sociocultural, and psychological barriers can affect the quality of messages exchanged in a communication interaction. Nurses must possess the necessary skills to promote an environment conducive to the mutual sharing of information.

The patient with a visual defect, particularly homonymous hemianopsia, may not be aware of his defect or the potential problems that may occur. The critical care nurse can detect a visual deficit by assessing whether the patient has had problems colliding with objects or people and by observing his performance of daily activities and his reactions to movement around him. For example, the patient may eat from only one side of the plate or respond to the nurse or visitor on only one side of the bed. A patient with homonymous hemianopsia or right hemiplegia should be taught to compensate for the visual defect by turning his head. This allows the patient to use the intact visual fields of each eye. Family members should be taught to announce their presence and approach the patient on the unaffected side. Essential objects, such as a clock or calendar, should be placed in the field of vision that is unaffected. The patient with a left hemiplegia may have more difficulty in compensating for his visual defect because of an altered visual perception. Such a patient may not see or deny seeing objects on his left side. In this case, the nurse must provide the patient with step-by-step verbal guidance during an activity. Detailed explanations may be necessary, especially if the patient is completely blind. Auditory and kinesthetic channels should also be used to augment communication.

Critical care patients with an auditory deficit will face serious problems unless caring and sensitive strategies for communication are established. A lack of understanding of the methods used to communicate with these patients may lead to poor communication and omission of explanations. The nurse must assess the extent of the patient's hearing disorder, ability to understand, and the presence of such capabilities as use of sign language and lip-reading. It is also important to ascertain the patient's reading and writing ability. Sounds help to orient a person to his surroundings. The deaf patient relies on visual input to cue in on the environment and on personal interactions. If the patient has a hearing aid and requires glasses, these aids must be readily available at all times and their use encouraged.

Patients should be clearly identified as having a hearing deficit so that caregivers can be alerted and prepared. This may include placing a sign at the patient's bedside and writing it in the care plan. The deaf patient's reliance on the visual channel necessitates face-to-face communication. If the patient can lip read, short and simple words should be used. Illustrations and written material are helpful when detailed explanations and teaching are needed. Writing material or a communication board should be placed within reach of the patient. An interpreter or family member skilled in sign language should be used whenever possible to assist in the communication process. Awareness of one's own nonverbal messages is important when communicating with a deaf patient. Since the patient is unable to process auditory stimuli such as the tone, pitch, and volume of verbal language, the critical care nurse must use her body actions to convey concern and reassurance. Touch is an excellent channel for communicating these qualities.

Aphasia, often resulting from a stroke, poses a significant communication challenge for the critical care nurse. Aphasia is a frightening experience for the patient, who is unable to express or understand thoughts and ideas. It is imperative that the nurse provide support and information to these patients and their families. Speech patterns should be discussed to alleviate feelings of anger, frustration, and anxiety. Creative approaches are essential to facilitate communication in these patients.

Assessment of aphasia begins with identifying the patient's ability to communicate. The nurse should engage the patient in conversation to determine his speech and language skills such as fluency, difficulty in finding words, and difficulty in building grammatically correct sentences (Boykin, 1984). Comprehension can be assessed by asking the patient to repeat words and sentences and to carry out motor commands. It is also important to assess the patient's understanding of written language. Some aphasic patients are unable to understand words but do well with pictures and diagrams. To facilitate communication with these patients, nurses must create an environment of support and concern. They should interact with the patient face to face, speak slowly, use simple words, phrases, and diagrams, and refrain from jumping from topic to topic. Environmental distractions should be also be limited. The nurse must be patient enough to allow sufficient time for the patient to respond.

The nurse caring for an aphasic patient must realize that it is not the mechanical production of speech that is affected but the mental processes that control formulation and comprehension of language. The patient with expressive aphasia will have good understanding but problematic speech. Such a patient may have difficulty in finding words or may use certain words and phrases repeatedly. He may construct sentences using only key words (telegraphic speech). The nurse should acknowledge the patient's difficulty, provide reassurance, and promote verbalization. The patient can be encouraged to use simple nouns and verbs. Visual aids and models can assist the patient in communicating his needs. Patients who have extreme difficulty with verbal expression may find writing more manageable. For these patients writing materials should be readily available. Gesturing may be the form of communication used by some patients. Nurses must skillfully interpret the meaning of the various gestures and verify them with the patient by asking questions that require a yes or no answer. The patient and his family should be taught to use these communication strategies.

The patient with receptive aphasia, on the other hand, will have poor understanding of verbal or written speech and therefore will also have expressive difficulties, which he may be unaware of. The patient may substitute words on the basis of sound or meaning, speak with little regard for content, produce inappropriate words, or express himself in an exaggerated manner. He may understand and express himself better in writing than through speech. The nurse caring for a receptive aphasic patient should speak slowly and clearly, use simple sentences, and repeat instructions or questions. Use of compound commands such as asking the patient to raise his right arm, pick up the pencil, and write on the pad should be avoided. Tasks should be delineated step by step or one at a time. The use of nonverbal language such as facial expressions and gestures can be useful in communicating with these patients.

A variety of communication methods can be used with intubated patients. When a patient is electively intubated or when intubation is anticipated, the nurse should discuss and establish in advance the communication difficulties that may arise and what patient-preferred alternative communication methods should be used. In most instances, intubation is performed emergently, leaving little time to prepare the patient. Nevertheless, the patient and the nurse should determine a reliable method of communication. A helpful start is to establish a pattern of yes and no responses, such as one eye blink for yes and two blinks for no. With this system, information can be gathered when questions are appropriately phrased. Any patient movement will suffice provided that it can be used consistently and without fatigue (Easton, 1988). Writing material, picture boards, or magic slates should be used by the patient if and when he is able to do so. A communication board with illustrations, words, and letters of the alphabet can facilitate communication and reduce frustration for the patient and the nurse (Fig. 4–3). Every attempt must be made by the nurse to interpret the patient's verbal and nonverbal messages. Establishing a communication plan with the patient and sharing it with the family can enhance the communication process.

Communication with patients given paralyzing agents must not cease. It is not uncommon for nurses to treat these patients as if they were comatose and incapable of feeling and sensing. Since consciousness, hearing, and feeling remain intact in these patients, critical care nurses must continue to provide sensitive and caring communication with them. The patient should be provided with explanations about his care and with frequent orientation to his surroundings. He must be reassured about his situation and the nature of his paralysis. Touch should be used to link him to his environment. The family should be encouraged to touch and communicate with their loved one.

Communicating with Members of the Health Care Team. Much of the information presented on barriers to communication also pertains to communication between members of the health care team. For example, noise levels, unit routines, cultural differences, language barriers, and anxiety can influence the effectiveness of communication between a nurse and a physician or between a nurse and another nurse. Effective communication between these team members is vital to ensure the quality of patient care.

Critical care nurses are frequently the first to learn of or obtain significant information about the patient. This information must be communicated to the ap-

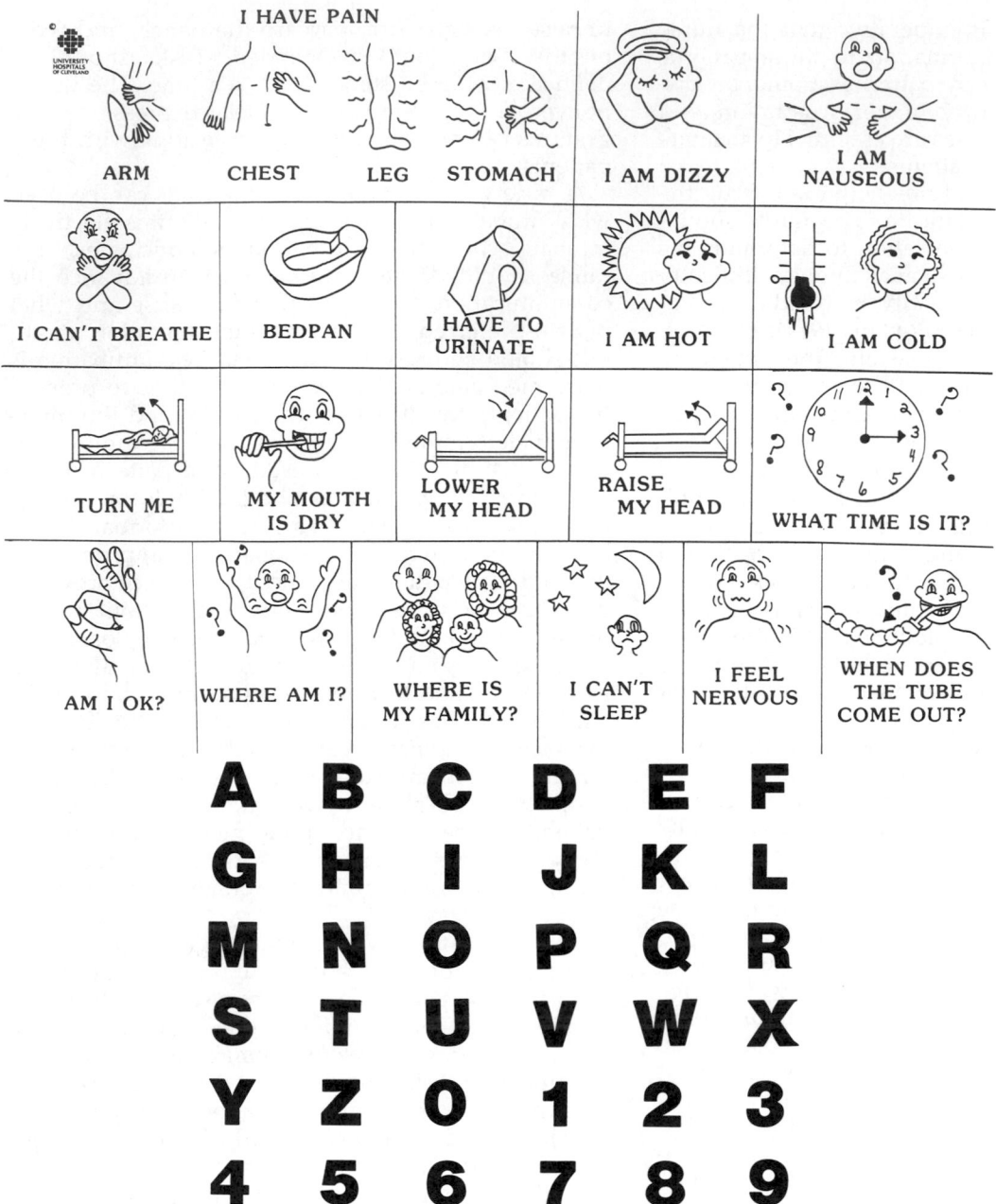

FIGURE 4–3. Communication board. (Courtesy of the University Hospitals of Cleveland.)

propriate persons to facilitate treatment and to evaluate the patient's health status. Communication between the critical care nurse and a physician may often be tense because important information about a patient is not communicated to one or the other. This tension may stem from differences about their relationship with each other. Traditionally, the relationship between physician and nurse has been one of authority and subordination. Nurses have long been viewed as handmaidens to physicians. With the increased autonomy, responsibility, and educational preparation of nurses, this view is changing rapidly. Nurses and physicians are now gaining acceptance of their collaborative roles in providing patient care.

SUMMARY

This chapter presents aspects of the communication process that are useful for critical care nurses as they provide care to critically ill patients, speak with family members, and work with other members of the health care team. The components of the communication process, such as messages conveyed through various sensory channels, and the essential elements of effective communication including trust, active listening, empathy, and touch are discussed in order to highlight the factors that enhance effective communication. Barriers to communication that may be physical, psychological, environmental, or sociocultural in nature also need to be recognized. Finally, specific interventions to improve communication with patients, families, and other members of the health care team are provided as strategies to assist the critical care nurse in the intensive care unit, where challenges to communication occur every day.

References

Boykin, G. V. (1984). Strategies for increasing communication with the dysphagic patient. *Dimensions of Critical Care Nursing,* 3 (5), 279–287.

Buchda, V. L. (1987). Loneliness in critically ill adults. *Dimensions of Critical Care Nursing,* 6 (6), 335–340.

Clement, J. M. (1986). Caring and touching as nursing interventions. In C. Hudak, et al. (Eds.), *Critical care nursing: A holistic approach* (4th ed., pp. 33–42). Philadelphia: J. B. Lippincott.

DeVito, J. A. (1980). *The interpersonal communication book* (2nd ed.). New York: Harper & Row.

Easton, J. (1988). Alternative communication for patients in intensive care. *Intensive Care Nursing,* 4, 47–55.

Gowan, N. J. (1979). The perceptual world of the intensive care unit: An overview of some environmental considerations in the helping relationship. *Heart & Lung,* 8 (2), 340–344.

Hansell, H. N. (1984). The behavioral effects of noise on man: The patient with "intensive care unit psychosis." *Heart & Lung,* 13, 59–65.

Heidt, P. (1981). Effect of therapeutic touch on anxiety level of hospitalized patients. *Nursing Research,* 30 (1), 32–37.

Keller, E., and Bzdek, V. (1986). Effects of therapeutic touch on tension headache pain. *Nursing Research,* 35 (2), 101–105.

Northouse, P. G. (1979). Interpersonal trust and empathy in nurse-nurse relationships. *Nursing Research,* 28 (6), 365–368.

Parfitt, B. A. (1988). Cultural assessment in the intensive care unit. *Intensive Care Nursing,* 4 (3), 124–127.

Pearce, J. (1988). The power of touch. *Nursing Times,* 15 (84), 26–29.

Podrasky, D. L., and Sexton, D. L. (1988). Nurses' reactions to difficult patients. *Image,* 20 (1), 16–21.

Rogers, C. R., and Roethlisberger, F. J. (1952). Barriers and gateways to communication. *Harvard Business Review,* 30 (4), 28–34.

Salyer, J., and Stuart, B. J. (1985). Nurse-patient interaction in the intensive care unit. *Heart & Lung,* 14 (1), 20–24.

Sinclair, V. (1988). High technology in critical care: Implications for nursing's role and practice. *Focus,* 15 (4), 36–41.

Weiss, S. J. (1979). The language of touch. *Nursing Research,* 28 (2), 76–80.

5

Effect of Occupational Hazards

Michael A. Salatka

Critical care nurses are exposed to a variety of biologic, physical, chemical, ergonomic, and psychosocial hazards in the hospital environment. There is increasing concern among all health care professionals about the transmission of blood and air-borne pathogens, musculoskeletal injury, toxic chemicals, radiation, noise, and chemical dependency. Nurses must be aware of the potential hazards they face and preventive strategies that are effective.

INFECTIOUS HAZARDS

There is a potentially high risk of acquiring infectious diseases in the critical care unit. Potential infections may be transmitted by blood or body fluids, by droplets in the air, or by direct contact. Blood-borne pathogens of major concern include human immunodeficiency virus (HIV), hepatitis B virus (HBV), and hepatitis C virus. Infections transmitted by air-borne particles include cytomegalovirus (CMV), tuberculosis (TB), and meningococcal disease. Direct contact with secretions infected with herpes simplex virus produces herpetic whitlow. Adherence to strict procedures involving body substance isolation (BSI) minimizes the risk of occupational exposure to infectious agents.

The risk of acquiring infection from exposure to blood and body fluids varies. It is estimated that 10% to 20% of health care workers are seropositive (anti-HBs) for hepatitis B (Patterson et al., 1985). The risk of seroconversion following exposure to blood from HIV-infected patients is less than 1% (Gurevich, 1989; CDC, 1988, 1989; Marcus, 1988; Wormser et al., 1984; Allen and Curran, 1988; Kuhls et al., 1987; McCray, 1986; Henderson et al., 1986; Hirsch et al., 1985; Weiss et al., 1985). The prevalence of hepatitis C among health care workers is unknown because no diagnostic tests have been available (Dienstag, 1980; Hoofnagle et al., 1977).

Methods of minimizing exposure to blood and body fluids are known as universal precautions or BSI. Since the infection status of patients is usually unknown, all patients should be considered potential carriers of HIV, HBV, and other blood-borne pathogens. Recommendations from the Centers for Disease Control (CDC, 1989) for health care professionals who are likely to have percutaneous or mucous-membrane exposure to blood or body fluids include:

1. Proper handling and disposal of needles or other sharp instruments
2. Use of gloves, masks, gowns, or eyewear when direct contact, aerosolization, or splashing of blood and body fluids is likely
3. Immediate washing of hands and other skin surfaces after contamination with blood or body fluids
4. Use of effective germicides for cleaning spills of blood or body fluids (1:10 dilution of household bleach).

Special attention should be given to proper handling and disposal of needles because the incidence of needle-stick injury remains high among nurses (Jackson et al., 1986; Wormser et al., 1984; McCormick and Maki, 1981; Reed et al., 1980). Table 5–1 lists situations during which potential needle-stick injuries occur most frequently. Needles should never be recapped, bent, or separated from the syringe. Impervious receptacles for needle-disposal should be conveniently placed as close to the bedside as possible.

Data on CMV seroconversion among nurses working in pediatric intensive care units are similar to those seen in the general population, ranging from 3.3% to 7.7% per year (Brady, 1986; Yeager, 1975; Dworsky et al., 1983; Ahlfors et al., 1981; Balfour and Balfour, 1986). The hepatitis B virus is a potentially unrecognizable source of infection for critical care nurses because asymptomatic carriers remain infectious. The risk of acquiring HBV infection following a puncture from a contaminated needle ranges from 6% to 30%.

Two types of vaccines are effective in preventing hepatitis B. One is plasma-derived, and the other is a recombinant vaccine. Use of the plasma-derived vaccine is restricted to dialysis patients, other immunocompromised persons, and those with a known allergy to yeast. Pre-exposure vaccination is recommended for all health care and public safety workers due to their risk of exposure to blood or body fluids (Centers for Disease Control, 1990).

MUSCULOSKELETAL INJURIES

Back pain occurs frequently among nurses despite their training and experience. The frustration and discomfort of back pain decreases patient care efficiency. Determining the cause in individual cases is complex because nurses perform many activities that lead to musculoskeletal strain. Since the continuum of symptoms ranges from minor to severe pain, it is difficult to characterize back injury. Most injuries involve the lumbar muscle group.

Results from a number of back pain studies conducted during the past 15 years show an annual prevalence rate of 400 to 500 injuries per 1000 nurses at risk (Buckle, 1987). Strains and sprains of the lower back account for 50% of all musculoskeletal disorders among American workers (Williamson et al., 1988). Back injuries result in more lost time and wages among nurses who provide bedside care than any other single injury.

The annual cost to employers in the United States for workers' compensation claims involving back injury is estimated at between $2.7 and $4.6 billion (Jensen, 1987). Nationally, musculoskeletal injuries cost approximately $20 billion per year in lost productivity, medical care, compensation, and disability (Omenn and Morris, 1984). The true expense to an individual and organization cannot be assessed easily because other, less tangible costs include psychological trauma from physical pain, fear of recurring back injury, and anxiety about the financial obligations due to loss of work.

Nursing is unique because the occupation involves lifting and transferring human beings rather than inanimate objects. As Harber and associates (1985) point out, the human body is not a compact mass, and patients are unpredictable. Sudden resisting movements are common in critical care. The proper technique for lifting or transferring a patient may depend on patient size, available staffing, or accessible equipment. Nurses must assess each individual patient separately to minimize the risk of back injury, especially during patient transfers.

Conditions that predispose nurses to musculoskeletal injury can be classified into two major categories: nurse characteristics and hospital environment (Feldman, 1986). Table 5–2 summarizes the factors in these two categories that increase the risk of back injury. Nurse characteristics are divided into three subgroups: physical, emotional, and preferential. Preferential characteristics include activities that nurses perform on their own volition. The categories and subgroups are not mutually exclusive. For example, stress caused by inadequate staffing may cause fatigue, which in turn may produce carelessness.

Physical characteristics such as leg length or heredity cannot be changed. However, emotional and preferential characteristics of nurses can be modified or alleviated to reduce the risk of back injury. Char-

---

TABLE 5–1. Potential Situations for Needle-Stick Injury

Carelessness
  Inattentiveness or distractions
  Fatigue
  Stress
Recapping needles after use
Disposal of used needles or receptacles
Administration of parenteral medications
Drawing blood
Failure to ensure adequate restraint of uncooperative patients
Drawing medications from ampules or vials
Cleaning trays after procedures
Working in minimally lighted areas
Inadequate staffing
Handling linens or trash containing uncapped needles
Lack of experience or technique with needles and syringes

TABLE 5–2. Nurse and Hospital Environment Factors that Increase the Risk of Back Injury

Nurse	Hospital Environment
Physical	Decreased staffing
Weak abdominal and lumbar muscles	Inaccessible lifting devices
Poor posture	Static actions
Unequal leg length	Stress
Decreased proprioception	Inadequate storage space for equipment and furniture
Hereditary back problems	Uncooperative patients
Headache	Non-patient transfer activities
Fatigue	Leg, head, and elbow clearance
Obesity or poor nutrition	Workstation design
Lifestyle	Equipment design
Smoking, drug use, inadequate exercise	Weight of "portable" equipment
Emotional	Working surface height
Stress	Presence of tubes or catheters on patient
Lack of motivation	
Job dissatisfaction	
Preferential	
Ignoring physical limitations	
Not soliciting assistance from patient or co-workers	
Lack of training and experience with lifting and transfer techniques and devices	
Carelessness	
Restrictive clothing	
Risk-taking behavior	

acteristics of the work environment cannot always be altered as effectively as the personal characteristics of the nurse. For example, the height of the bed influences the working posture of the nurse. The optimal bed height for a nurse's performance of routine procedures is usually higher than the desired height for the patient (Pheasant, 1987). Patient comfort and safety may be compromised if a nurse adjusts the bed height to provide protection from back strain. Bed height will be different for each nurse depending on the procedure to be performed and the height of the nurse. Maintaining ergonomically correct equipment for each nurse at any given time is problematic, especially when more than one nurse is assigned to a patient.

Patient contact activities in critical care frequently require nurses to maintain an awkward, stressful posture for an extended period of time. In an observational study, Harber and colleagues (1987) found that 78% of static actions were performed in a squatting or semisquatting position. These actions may be particularly stressful on the lower back because the same muscle groups are involved throughout the activity.

It is important to recognize and develop ways to minimize stressful postures. Methods for minimizing low back pain are listed in Table 5–3. A combination of personal and environmental modifications should be implemented to be effective. No single method will completely prevent or control low back pain.

Nurses are not selected by physical ability, and job strength requirements are rarely addressed in critical care. Conducting pre-employment strength tests to determine whether the nurse can perform strenuous nursing tasks is feasible (Keyserling et al., 1980). Patient assignments could then be matched according to the physical strength of the nurse.

TABLE 5–3. Methods for Minimizing Low Back Injury

Personal

Strengthen abdominal and lumbar muscles through regular exercise
Maintain good posture
Maintain proper nutrition
Solicit assistance from co-workers and patients
Use mechanical devices for lifting
Review knowledge of proper lifting techniques
Alleviate risk-taking behaviors
Wear nonrestrictive clothing
Lift no more than 35% of your body weight or less
Raise or lower beds to facilitate good posture
Minimize stress

Environmental

Design workplace layout using ergonomic principles
Provide adequate staffing
Conduct pre-employment strength testing and evaluation
Make lifting devices accessible
Conduct regular in-service training addressing static actions
Consult a nursing ergonomic specialist
Redesign storage areas
Maintain clear paths for walking and moving furniture or equipment
Install nonslippery floor surfaces

Because the number of low back injuries among nurses has not shown any appreciable decline, researchers question the effectiveness of training programs that focus on safe lifting procedures (Harber et al., 1985, 1987a and b; Stubbs et al., 1983; Snook et al., 1978). As Cato and colleagues (1989) point out, perhaps training programs are more effective when used in conjunction with ergonomic job analysis and job-specific training.

Traditional techniques for lifting may not be best for all nurses because they do not use the lumbar muscle group and completely ignore the principles of leverage with balance. Consistent use of the lumbar muscles in synchronization with other muscle groups increases strength and reduces the risk of injury (Owen, 1980). Training programs should provide information on correct postures to minimize muscle strain, exercises to strengthen the back, and proper lifting techniques. A well-trained "nursing ergonomic consultant" who is sensitive to each nurse's physical ability could provide services and assistance to individuals who are at risk of low back injury (Harbor et al., 1985).

Although patient comfort and safety are the highest priorities in hospital care, nurses should be encouraged to develop an understanding of basic ergonomic concepts and to analyze their own safety at the bedside and work station. Personal habits are not easily modified, but an awareness and effort to maintain a safe environment in the workplace is important. Efforts should be made to minimize back injury away from the workplace as well. Application of these principles will reduce musculoskeletal injury, increase productivity, improve health and safety, and provide a higher quality of patient care.

CHEMICAL HAZARDS

There are a variety of chemicals, including many therapeutic agents, in the critical care setting that may pose a hazard to nurses. Nearly 400,000 cancer patients received therapy with cytotoxic drugs in 1986 (Williamson et al., 1988). Some of these patients required care for septic complications. Aerosolized drugs used to treat infections in neonates and persons with HIV infection may cause birth defects. Pregnant women should avoid ribavirin. Because so many unknown factors are associated with these agents, nurses should minimize contact with all potential chemical hazards. Antineoplastic agents may enter humans inadvertently through inhalation, ingestion, or absorption through unprotected skin. These agents have carcinogenic potential (Valanis and Shortridge, 1987; Valanis et al., 1984; Crudi et al., 1982; Reich, 1981). All nurses should wear gloves when handling potentially hazardous drugs. Strict adherence to body substance isolation precautions will help prevent exposure to drugs and their metabolites in body fluids, including urine.

RADIATION HAZARDS

Portable radiography and fluoroscopy are routine bedside procedures in critical care. Radiation exposure carries the potential for both short-term and long-term biologic effects. Familiarity with the types and sources of radiation, the maximum permissible doses for occupational exposure, and ways in which the risk of exposure to ionizing radiation can be minimized will protect nurses from harmful biologic effects.

When atoms and molecules undergo change, energy is released in the form of heat or light. This energy is referred to as radiation. The three common forms of radiation used in hospitals are alpha particles, beta particles, and gamma rays (x-rays). Alpha particles travel only inches in the air and are stopped by healthy skin tissue. Beta particles may travel several feet before they are absorbed by a thin piece of metal or wood. Gamma rays travel hundreds of feet and have great penetrating power (Fig. 5–1).

The penetrating ability of each type of radiation varies. Harmful effects to human tissue result largely from the energy absorbed by the cells (Bomberger and Dannenfelser, 1984). The amount of energy absorbed or deposited in human tissue determines the total biologic effect. The rem (roentgen equivalent

man or mammal) is the unit that represents the biologic dose used to estimate potential damage caused by radiation.

There are three potential sources of scattered radiation in the critical care environment: portable x-ray equipment, fluoroscopic equipment, and diagnostic or therapeutic radionuclides. Scattered or "secondary" radiation occurs after the primary radiation beam or application passes through matter. All x-ray and fluoroscopic examinations generate some scattered radiation. Alpha, beta, and gamma rays exist in the isotopes used for external and internal radiation treatments. The amount of secondary radiation emitted by patients receiving radionuclide therapy depends on the organ in which it is localized, the dosage, the elapsed time after injection, patient size, and the distance from the patient (Jankowski, 1984). Critical care nurses should pay particular attention to the levels of secondary radiation received from patients who receive radionuclides because the number of hours they spend in individual patient contact is greater than the time needed in other units in the hospital. The body fluids of patients who have received injections of radioactive substances contain significant amounts of radioactivity. Compliance with BSI procedures is crucial.

The National Council on Radiation Protection and Measurements (NCRPM) establishes maximum permissible dose (MPD) levels of radiation for occupational exposure. The current recommendation is 5000 mrem per year for employees who are likely to be exposed to ionizing radiation during the course of their work (National Council on Radiation Protection and Measurements, 1980). According to the Code of Federal Regulations (CFR), radiation dosimetry badges are required when nurses receive doses in excess of 1250 mrem every 3 months.

Actively proliferating cells, such as the gonads, are highly sensitive to radiation. Teratogenic or carcinogenic effects may occur when an embryo, fetus, or male germ cell is irradiated. Studies show that ionizing radiation damages the gonads, alters genetic material, reduces fertility, and induces spontaneous abortion (Hunt, 1978).

Female nurses represent the largest number of potentially pregnant women exposed to low-level radiation (Burks et al., 1982). Ninety-seven per cent of the 1.5 million registered nurses licensed in the United States are women (Maraldo and Solomon, 1986). Nurses of childbearing age must be aware of the hazards of radiation because there is increased potential for damage to a developing embryo during the first month of pregnancy. This is especially important because women generally do not realize they are pregnant at this stage of fetal development. The Nuclear Regulatory Commission standards recommend that pregnant women do not receive more than 500 mrem of radiation during gestation.

Exposure to scattered radiation can be minimized in three ways: by *time*, by *distance*, and by *shielding*. Protection from secondary radiation can be enhanced by completing nursing procedures in the shortest

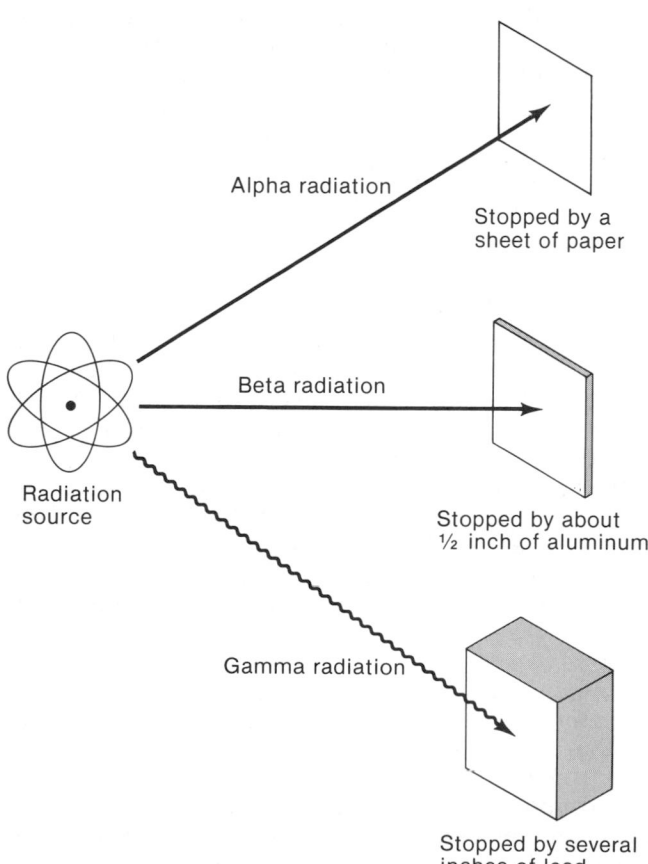

Alpha radiation

Stopped by a sheet of paper

Beta radiation

Stopped by about ½ inch of aluminum

Radiation source

Gamma radiation

Stopped by several inches of lead

FIGURE 5–1. Relative penetrating power of alpha, beta, and gamma radiation.

possible time without compromising good clinical practice. Penetrable radiation rapidly decreases as the distance from the source increases. For example, a single film taken by a portable x-ray machine at 1 meter will produce approximately 0.06 mrem of scattered radiation. At 2 meters the amount is indistinguishable from background radiation existing in the natural environment (Herman et al., 1980).

The third method of minimizing exposure to secondary radiation is the use of protective shielding. Lead screens or aprons 5 mm in lead-equivalent thickness should be used during x-rays and fluoroscopy to protect the gonads. Protective shielding is particularly important when working with patients who have received radiopharmaceuticals. Leaded glasses and a thyroid shield are recommended during procedures involving elevated levels of radiation such as angioplasty (Patterson et al., 1985).

Further epidemiologic studies on the effects of long-term occupational exposure to ionizing radiation are needed. Until more data are available, pocket dosimeters and film badges for monitoring exposure to radiation should be used by nurses who are likely to receive more than 1250 mrem in a 3-month period. Radiation safety committees should periodically monitor nurses for proper radiation safety techniques. Radiation safety should be included in hospital orientation programs for new staff and should be reviewed annually for all employees. Finally, hospital policies regarding the use of radioactive substances and equipment should be reviewed and revised to include methods for minimizing radiologic hazards to staff.

NOISE

Prolonged exposure to noise can be distracting and can prohibit mental concentration. Psychological responses to noise include increased annoyance and irritability, impaired judgment, and altered perception (Hilton, 1987). Controlling noise in the critical care environment will help to minimize fatigue and reduce errors. Factors that influence the impact of noise on nurses include the intensity or loudness of the sound, type of sound, distance from the source, frequency and duration of exposure, individual perception of sound, stress level, and age.

The decibel (dB) is used to express the sound level associated with noise measurement. The Occupational Safety and Health Administration (OSHA) standard for permissible exposure to noise is 90 dB during an 8-hour shift (Code of Federal Regulations, 1980). The International Noise Council recommends that sound levels in patient care areas not exceed 45 dB during the day and 20 dB at night (Hansell, 1984).

Background noise occurs in most work environments. Critical care areas, however, are remarkably loud. One study reported that sound levels in four critical care units were as high as 77 dB, which is comparable to a hospital cafeteria at noon (Redding

---

TABLE 5–4. Sources of Noise in the Critical Care Unit

Equipment or Alarms
Ventilators
Monitor alarms
Chest drainage systems
Special therapy beds
Infusion pumps
Intra-aortic balloon pumps
Suction machines
Cooling blankets
Cooling fans in computers and monitoring equipment

Extraneous Sound
Telephones
Televisions and radios
Doors
Intercoms and pagers
Sinks and toilets
Refrigerators
Ice machines
Bedrails
Squeaking equipment (chairs, drawers, carts)
Personnel activity (rustling papers, binders)

People
Staff conversations
Patients coughing or retching
Visitors

---

et al., 1977). Other studies have reported sound levels greater than 50 dB over a 24-hour period, with a number of noises exceeding 70 dB (Hilton, 1987; Hansell, 1984). Noise levels of this magnitude increase the tendency for nurses to become desensitized to noise levels in the critical care environment. (Lindenmuth et al., 1980). Table 5–4 lists the most frequent sources of noise in critical care units.

Elimination or reduction of unnecessary sources of noise is essential. Increasing nurses' sensitivity to the level of noise on the unit will help to develop appropriate interventions to decrease or control unwanted sound. Everyone should be encouraged to speak softly. Patients report that staff conversations and activity are the most disturbing noise (Hansell, 1984). Discussions among nurses and other hospital staff can generate sound levels as high as 90 dB (Hilton, 1987). Normal conversational tones measure between 56 and 60 dB. As Hilton (1987) points out, whispering may be appropriate at night. Conversations between staff should be limited to patient care concerns, especially at the bedside. A system of constant reminders, such as signs near areas of concentrated noise, may be helpful (Lindenmuth et al., 1980).

Noise can also be reduced by introducing sound-absorbing materials into the architectural design of the unit. Carpeted walls and floors in the nursing station and patient care areas will have a dramatic effect on reducing noise. Each unit should have a soundproof section in which nurses and physicians can confer or spend break periods without disturbing patients (Dracup, 1988). Utility rooms with sinks, refrigerators, and ice machines should be partitioned separately from patient care areas. Alarm parameters should be set appropriately to avoid false alarms. Nurses must take an active role in developing effective strategies to reduce noise. Strict compliance with the standards of occupational exposure to noise will enhance awareness of noise reduction among the staff. Nurses should be responsible for evaluating and purchasing equipment such as ventilators, monitors, and balloon pumps. Equipment that produces excess noise can be modified by the manufacturer to meet noise reduction standards. Nursing consultants should assist in the development of plans for construction or remodeling of critical care units (Dracup, 1988).

Suppression of noise is an important element of occupational safety and health in the critical care environment. Nurses and other hospital staff must develop an appreciation for a quiet working environment. Keeping the noise level as low as reasonably possible is advantageous to nurses and beneficial to patients.

CHEMICAL DEPENDENCY

Chemical dependency occurs among workers in every occupation. Nurses are exposed to constant stress and human suffering. They also have easy access to narcotics and other drugs. Although there are no reliable estimates of the number of nurses who suffer from chemical dependency, the problem of chemical dependency is surfacing more frequently. The costs to society of chemical dependency include increased use of health insurance benefits, decreased productivity, increased absenteeism, poor patient relations, reduced staff morale, poor judgment, and increased mistakes or accidents. Mistakes or accidents often lead to litigation and damage to the reputations of both the organization and the nurse. Drugs that may be abused include cocaine, marijuana, alcohol, narcotics, amphetamines, and tranquilizers. Nurses should be observant of colleagues who may display signs of chemical dependency or impairment and should refer them to the peer counseling program run by the nurses' association or employee assistance program at the hospital.

CONCLUSION

Nurses must examine the hazards in the critical care work environment. An awareness of hazards and nurses' perceptions of their causes and solutions set the stage for developing appropriate occupational safety programs. Nurses with research skills and a familiarity with the tasks, procedures, and physical environment of the critical care unit have an opportunity to study and contribute to the understanding of occupational hazards and ways to prevent them (Jensen, 1987).

References

Ahlfors, K., Ivarsson S.-A., Johnsson, T., et al. (1981). Risk of cytomegalovirus infection in nurses and congenital infection in their offspring. *Acta Paediatrica Scandinavica, 70,* 819–823.

Allen, J. R., and Curran, J. W. (1988). Prevention of AIDS and HIV infection: Needs and priorities for epidemiologic research. *American Journal of Public Health, 78,* 381–386.

Balfour, C. L., and Balfour, H. H. (1986). Cytomegalovirus is not an occupational risk for nurses in renal transplant and neonatal units. *Journal of the American Medical Association, 256,* 1909–1914.

Bomberger, A. S., and Dannenfelser, B. A. (1984) *Radiation and health.* Rockville MD: Aspen Publishers.

Brady, M. T. (1986). Cytomegalovirus infections: Occupational risk for health professionals. *American Journal of Infection Control, 14,* 197–203.

Buckle, P. (1987). Epidemiological aspects of back pain within the nursing profession. *International Journal of Nursing Studies, 24,* 319–324.

Burks, J., Griffith, P., McCormick, K., et al. (1982). Radiation exposure to nursing personnel from patients receiving diagnostic radionuclides. *Heart & Lung, 11,* 217–220.

Cato, C., Olson, D. K., and Studer, M. (1989). Incidence, prevalence, and variables associated with low back pain in staff nurses. *AAOHN Journal, 37,* 321–327.

Centers for Disease Control. (1987). Recommendations for prevention of HIV transmission in health-care settings. *Morbidity and Mortality Weekly Report, 36,* 1S–18S.

Centers for Disease Control. (1988). Update: Universal precautions for prevention of transmission of human immunodeficiency virus, hepatitis B virus, and other bloodborne pathogens in health-care settings. *Morbidity and Mortality Weekly Report, 37,* 377–388.

Centers for Disease Control. (1989). Guidelines for prevention of transmission of human immunodeficiency virus and hepatitis B virus to health-care and public-safety workers. *Morbidity and Mortality Weekly Report, 38,* 3–37.

Centers for Disease Control. (1990). Protection against viral hepatitis. Recommendations of the Immunization Practices Advisory Committee (ACIP). *Morbidity and Mortality Weekly Report, 39* (RR-2), 10–16.

Code of Federal Regulations. (1980). Vol. 29, Part 19–10.95.

Crudi, C., Stephens, B., and Maier, P. (1982). Possible occupational hazards associated with the preparation and administration of antineoplastic agents. *National Intravenous Therapy Association, 5,* 264–266.

Dienstag, J. L. (1980). Non-A, non-B hepatitis. *Advances in Internal Medicine, 26,* 187–233.

Dracup, K. (1988). Are critical care units hazardous to health? *Applied Nursing Research, 1,* 14–21.

Dworsky, M. E., Welch, D., Cassady, G., et al. (1983). Occupational risk for primary cytomegalovirus infection among pediatric health-care workers. *New England Journal of Medicine, 309,* 950–953.

Feldman, R. (1986). Hospital injuries. *Occupational Health and Safety, 55,* 12–17.

Gurevich, I. (1989). Acquired immunodeficiency syndrome: Realistic concerns and appropriate precautions. *Heart & Lung, 18,* 107–112.

Hansell, H. N. (1984). The behavioral effects of noise on man: The patient with intensive care unit psychosis. *Heart & Lung, 13,* 59–65.

Harber, P., Billet, E., Gutowski, M., et al. (1985). Occupational low-back pain in hospital nurses. *Journal of Occupational Medicine, 27,* 518–524.

Harber, P., Billet, E., Lew, M., et al. (1987a). Importance of non-patient transfer activities in nursing-related back pain: I. Questionnaire survey. *Journal of Occupational Medicine, 29,* 967–970.

Harber, P., Billet, E., Shimozaki, S., et al. (1988). Occupational back pain of nurses: Special problems and prevention. *Applied Ergonomics, 19,* 219–224.

Harber, P., Shimozaki, S., Gardner, G., et al. (1987b). Importance of non-patient transfer activities in nursing-related back pain:

II. Observational study and implications. *Journal of Occupational Medicine*, 29, 971–974.

Henderson, D. K., Saah, A. J., Zak, B. J., et al. (1986). Risk of nosocomial infection with human T-cell lymphotropic virus type III/lymphadenopathy-associated virus in a large cohort of intensively exposed health care workers. *Annals of Internal Medicine*, 104, 644–647.

Herman, M. W., Patrick, J., and Tabrisky, J. (1980). A comparative study of scattered radiation levels from 80-kVp and 240-kVp x-rays in the surgical intensive care unit. *Radiology*, 137, 552–553.

Hilton, A. (1987). The hospital racket: How noisy is your unit? *American Journal of Nursing*, 87, 59–61.

Hirsch, M. S., Wormser, G. P., Schooley, R. T., et al. (1985). Risk of nosocomial infection with human T-cell lymphotropic virus III (HTLV III). *New England Journal of Medicine*, 312, 1–4.

Hoofnagle, J. H., Gerety, R. J., Tabor, E., et al. (1977). Transmission of non-A, non-B hepatitis. *Annals of Internal Medicine*, 87, 14–20.

Hunt, V. (1978). Occupational radiation exposure of women workers. *Preventive Medicine*, 7, 294–310.

Jackson, M. M., Dechairo, D. C., and Gardner, D. F. (1986). Perceptions and beliefs of nursing and medical personnel about needle-stick handling practices and needlestick injuries. *American Journal of Infection Control*, 14, 1–10.

Jankowski, C. (1984). Radiation exposure of nurses in a coronary care unit. *Heart & Lung*, 13, 55–58.

Jensen, R. (1987). Disabling back injuries among nursing personnel: Research needs and justification. *Research in Nursing and Health*, 10, 29–38.

Keyserling, W. M., Herrin, G. D., and Chaffin, D. B. (1980). Isometric strength testing as a means to controlling medical incidents on strenuous jobs. *Journal of Occupational Medicine*, 22, 332–336.

Kuhls, T. L., Viker, S., Parris, N. B., et al. (1987). Occupational risk of HIV, HBV, and HSV-2 infections in health care personnel caring for AIDS patients. *American Journal of Public Health*, 77, 1306–1309.

Lindenmuth, J. E., Breu, C. S., and Malooley, J. A. (1980). Sensory overload. *American Journal of Nursing*, 8, 1456–1458.

Maraldo, P., and Soloman, S. (1986). Talking points. New York: National League for Nursing.

Marcus, R. (1988). CDC cooperative needlestick study group. Surveillance of health-care workers exposed to blood from patients infected with human immunodeficiency virus. *New England Journal of Medicine*, 319, 1118–1123.

McCormick, R. D., and Maki, D. G. (1981). Epidemiology of needle-stick injuries in hospital personnel. *American Journal of Medicine*, 70, 928–932.

McCray, E. (1986). Occupational risk of the acquired immunodeficiency syndrome among health care workers. *New England Journal of Medicine*, 314, 1127–1132.

National Council on Radiation Protection and Measurements. (1980). Basic radiation protection criteria. NCRP Report No. 39, Washington D.C.

Omenn, G., and Morris, S. (1984). Occupational hazards to health care workers: Report on a conference. *American Journal of Industrial Medicine*, 6, 134–135.

Owen, B. (1980). How to avoid that aching back. *American Journal of Nursing*, 80, 894–897.

Owen, B., and Damron, C. (1984). Personal characteristics and back injury among hospital nursing personnel. *Research in Nursing and Health*, 7, 305–313.

Patterson, W. B., Craven, D. E., Schwartz, D. A., et al. (1985). Occupational hazards to hospital personnel. *Annals of Internal Medicine*, 102, 658–680.

Pheasant, S. (1987). Some anthropometric aspects of workstation design. *International Journal of Nursing Studies*, 24, 291–298.

Redding, J. S., Hargest, T. S., and Minsky, S. H. (1977). How noisy is intensive care? *Critical Care Medicine*, 5, 275–276.

Reed, J. S., Anderson, A. C., and Hodges, G. R. (1980). Needlestick and puncture wounds: Definition of the problem. *American Journal of Infection Control*, 8, 101–106.

Reich, S. (1981). Antineoplastic agents as potential carcinogens: Are nurses and pharmacists at risk? *Cancer Nursing*, 4, 500–502.

Scott, E. (1979). Radiation protection for nurses. *Nursing Times*, 75, 441–445.

Snook, S. H., Campanelli, R. A., and Hart, J. W. (1978). A study of three preventive approaches to low back injury. *Journal of Occupational Medicine*, 20, 478–481.

Stubbs, D. A., Buckle, P. W., Hudson, M. P., et al. (1983). Back pain in the nursing profession: II. The effectiveness of training. *Ergonomics*, 26, 767–779.

U.S. Nuclear Regulatory Commission (1980). 10 CFR 20.202.

Valanis, B., and Shortridge, L. (1987). Self protective practices of nurses handling antineoplastic drugs. *Oncology Nursing Forum*, 14, 23–27.

Valanis, B., Shortridge, L., Hertzberg, V. (1984). Acute symptoms and occupational exposure of nurses to antineoplastic drugs. *Oncology Nursing Forum*, 11 (Suppl.), 78–93.

Weiss, S. H., Saxinger, C., Rechtman, D., et al. (1985). HTLV-III infection among health care workers. *Journal of the American Medical Association*, 254, 2089–2093.

Williamson, K., Turner, J., Brown, K., et al. (1988). Occupational health hazards for nurses—Part II. *Image*, 20, 162–168.

Wormser, G. P., Joline, C., and Duncanson, F. (1984). Needlestick injuries during the care of patients with AIDS. *New England Journal of Medicine*, 310, 1461–1462.

Yeager, A. S. (1975). Longitudinal, serological study of cytomegalovirus infections in nurses and in personnel without patient contact. *Journal of Clinical Microbiology*, 2, 448–452.

2

Psychosocial Problems

CHAPTER

6

Psychosocial Needs of Critically Ill Patients

Suzanne Clark

The Critical Care Nurse shall gather pertinent physical, social, psychological, and spiritual data from the patient, significant others, and other health team members.

AMERICAN ASSOCIATION OF CRITICAL-CARE NURSES
Standards for Nursing Care of the Critically Ill

MEETING PSYCHOSOCIAL NEEDS IN CRITICAL CARE: THE CHALLENGE

Patients with diseases or traumatic injuries that lead to admission to a critical care unit almost always face severe disruptions in a previously balanced existence. The patient responds to the challenges created by the illness, the treatment, and the environment to regain some sense of equilibrium. Nurses interact with patients and their situations in ways that assist them to regain control and to integrate the experience into their lives.

The Standards for Nursing Care developed by the American Association of Critical-Care Nurses clearly support a holistic approach to the care of the critically ill patient. A holistic approach is based on the premise that disease is never the result of one causative agent or condition but rather the result of a complex interplay between people and their physical, emotional, cultural, social, and spiritual situations. To care optimally for patients, nurses must assess all aspects of the patient's response to his or her illness and hospitalization, identify the physiologic and psychosocial concerns that may influence the patient's course, and use a variety of interventions targeted to the specific problems identified.

This chapter will discuss the forces that may inhibit or facilitate a holistic approach, a framework for critical care nurses to use in identifying psychosocial

needs, and specific interventions that can be used to meet those needs. One primary nursing diagnosis will be addressed throughout, Ineffective Coping.

FORCES THAT INHIBIT A HOLISTIC APPROACH

Traditional Views of Health and Medicine

Current mainstream beliefs about health and disease can be traced to the mechanistic model of the person developed in the seventeenth and eighteenth centuries (Benner and Wrubel, 1989). In this view, body and mind are separate, and disease is defined as a malfunction at the molecular level. This view does not provide solutions to the experience of illness that engulfs individuals and affects their lives.

The following example may serve to illustrate the limitations of this stance.

CASE HISTORY

An 82-year-old woman with ovarian cancer was treated successfully with surgery but was unable to eat and refused all attempts to entice her. She was fatigued and ready to die. In the physician's experience people did not die from this type of cancer, in this stage, with no evidence of metastasis. The woman's daughter and granddaughter spent most of their visits with the patient trying to get her to eat and deflecting her comments about dying. The patient's subsequent death surprised everyone because "her cancer wasn't advanced enough for her to die yet." The nurse, who had also focused her interventions on trying to get the patient to eat, felt that she had failed because the patient died. Had the nurse used a more holistic approach, the patient and family might have been able to talk more directly about their feelings and might have received care and comfort in this situation. The nurse could have had a different yardstick by which to measure her success. In this situation, the caregivers and the family viewed death as the end result of pathology at the molecular level rather than as a complex response to physiologic, psychological, and spiritual factors (Lynch and Convey, 1979; Lynch, 1977; Krantz and Glas, 1984).

Technology

Caring for the whole person in the highly charged setting of the critical care unit has become more difficult (MacKellaig, 1987). Machines are available to maintain and extend life in the presence of organ failure. Sophisticated computerized and automated monitoring systems provide minute-to-minute data on multiple physiologic responses. Some treatment decisions are even made by machines that can monitor parameters, analyze the data, and administer the correct dose of medication. These explosive advances in technology may free nurses from their former repetitive tasks but also create significant challenges for nurses, who must now manage both patients and machines (Sinclair, 1988). The plethora of equipment may not only create a mechanistic, dehumanizing atmosphere but also build a physical barrier that prevents meaningful patient-nurse contact.

Ethical Dilemmas

Life-saving and life-extending therapies used to improve short-term survival may create increasing numbers of highly dependent, critically ill patients who have little hope of long-term survival. Nurses may feel that the patient and the family need help in accepting the inevitable downward spiral of the disease process but cannot work against the medical goal of cure at all costs. These situations create ethical dilemmas for which there is no right answer. Consequently, nurses may retreat from the patient to protect themselves from their feelings of frustration and despair. Patients may have a difficult time in meeting their psychosocial needs when nurses feel that they must withdraw for their own protection.

Nursing Shortage

According to a survey of 200 randomly selected hospitals conducted from January to April, 1988, as many as 125,000 critical care nurses are needed to fill existing vacancies. By 1990, a 42% to 90% increase in critical care nurses was needed (American Association of Critical-Care Nurses, 1988). Shortages in nursing staff lead to increased overtime and the use of outside supplementary personnel. Increased over-

time by nurses taxes their personal resources and leaves them little energy to meet the psychological needs created by a critical illness. The use of supplemental personnel means that patients are cared for by nurses who are often transient. They may not have time to develop the type of nurse-patient relationship necessary to identify and meet complex psychosocial needs.

Current Economic Pressures

Diagnosis-related groupings (DRGs) is a prospective payment system that was established by the federal government to try to stop the spiraling costs of health care that are incurred in part by increased use of technology, wastefulness in the system, the practice of defensive medicine, and the profits taken by suppliers and users of medical products (Wilson, 1988). Under this system, hospitals are reimbursed a set amount for certain types of illnesses, no matter what the actual cost to the hospital. Although adjustments can be made in extreme circumstances, the system is set up to decrease spending and dramatically reduce the amount of money that is spent on health care. Hospital administrators are being forced to control expenditures and may try to replace professional staff with ancillary personnel (Wilson, 1988). This could leave the remaining professional nurses responsible for greater numbers of patients. The ability to provide individualized care in this atmosphere could be more difficult.

In summary, multiple forces in health care and the critical care environment work together to deter nurses from attending to the psychosocial needs of patients.

FORCES THAT FACILITATE A HOLISTIC APPROACH

Behavioral Medicine

A major force supporting a holistic approach is the recent interest in the relationship of genetic, biologic, psychological, sociocultural, and ecologic factors to physical health and disease. Increasing numbers of researchers in the fields of neurophysiology, neuropsychology, and neuroimmunology strive to find the connecting links between psychological and biologic responses.

Research linking psychosocial factors has taken many directions: the impact of sociocultural factors on the etiology of disease; personality and behavioral patterns and their impact on disease onset and outcomes; the effect of exposure to stress and disease onset; the impact of stress on the immune system; the individual resources that mediate the stress-illness connection; and behavioral interventions that influence a person's response to illness and treatment. These directions have been influenced by, among other things, the fact that researchers are unable to explain in a conclusive way why some people become ill and others remain well even when they have been exposed to the same pathogens (Gentry, 1984). These studies formalize and add credence to what any experienced nurse already knows: that the course of illness is heavily influenced by the individual's psychological and social milieu.

Refining of Nursing Theory

The formation of nursing as a discipline is taking place through the development of models for nursing practice. Central to most nursing models is the complexity of stressors that affect healthy and full functioning (Leininger, 1986). The domain of nursing practice is not only disease, which is pathologic change at the cellular, tissue, and organ levels, but also the individual human responses to disease (American Nurses Association, 1980).

More than any other group of helping professionals involved in the care of people experiencing illness, nurses are encouraged to direct their attention to the totality of the illness experience, integrating the relationship between the disease and the experience of being sick (Benner and Wrubel, 1989; Riehl and Rog, 1974). The profession's current approach to diagnostic categories includes problems arising from the realms of the physiologic (ineffective airway clearance, alteration in cardiac output), the psychological (anxiety, ineffective coping), and the spiritual (spiritual distress). The variety of these categories reinforces the holistic nature of nursing practice.

Nursing Process

Using a systematic approach to problem identification and the generation of solutions is an important tool in ensuring that all pertinent problems are identified and addressed. This logical step-by-step approach begins with a complete assessment, including data from the biopsychosocial areas. Following the assessment, the nurse should be able to identify nursing diagnoses that are consistent with the data gathered. For each diagnosis, specific goals can be formulated using input from the patient. Nurses can then plan interventions that are (1) scientifically sound, based on theory from the basic sciences and current nursing research; (2) acceptable to and feasible for the patient and family; and (3) practical within the existing system of care (Clark, 1988).

Balancing Inhibiting and Facilitating Forces

The most important relationships in the critical care setting are between nurses and patients. Nurses spend more time with the patient than any other caregiver. They are responsible for the environment in which the patient is cared for, identifying and mitigating unsafe and harmful stimuli. They carefully assess physiologic parameters to maintain or achieve homeostasis. They implement physicians' plans of care and alert them to rapidly changing situations that need their attention. They anticipate problems and respond as first-line defenses in life-threatening emergencies.

At the same time, in order to put nursing theory into practice, nurses must practice in a holistic way, considering data from the psychological, cultural, and spiritual realms to formulate successful nursing interventions. Each nurse, as she or he works with each patient, must find a way through the maze of equipment and the stress of nursing in today's environment to develop a therapeutic relationship that combines technical proficiency with caring. This process comprises a complex interplay of rational and intuitive thinking that often takes years to refine (Benner, 1984).

How can nurses develop the level of expertise that allows them to practice holistically and intuitively, combining technical proficiency and caring almost effortlessly? In terms of understanding and meeting psychosocial needs, it means having a framework that charts the territory of human responses to illness and directs the nurse's attention to specific patient behaviors (Visitainer, 1986). One of the most useful frameworks for understanding the psychosocial needs and responses of critically ill patients is the stress-coping framework developed primarily by Richard Lazarus (1966).

STRESS-COPING FRAMEWORK (Fig. 6–1)

Stressors

Stressors are situational demands that disrupt smooth functioning and interfere with understood meanings in one's life by challenging one's world view and values (Benner and Wrubel, 1989; Scott et al., 1980; Jacobson, 1983; Moos and Tsu, 1979). Some stressors are recognized almost universally because of commonly held beliefs and goals. Threats of death or pain are two such stressors. Other conditions are seen as stressful only by certain individuals whose idiosyncratic meanings are disrupted.

Cognitive Appraisal

Central to Lazarus' stress and coping theory is the cognitive process of appraisal. With regard to stressors, people ask themselves, "What is happening or going to happen?" and "How bad (or good) can it be?" (Lazarus and Folkman, 1984). These questions are not necessarily clear and deliberate but rather automatic and rapid and may be outside the person's

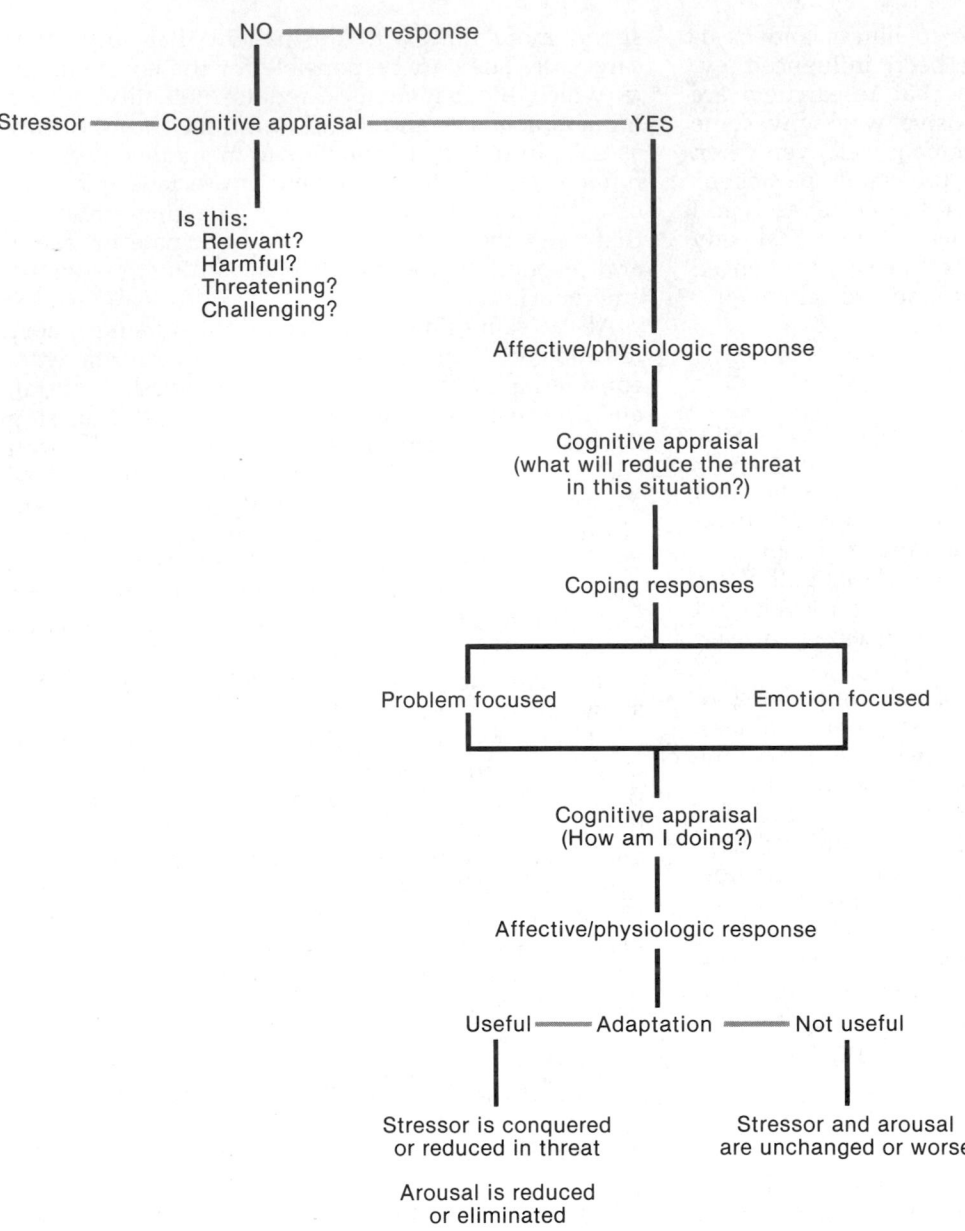

FIGURE 6-1. Stress-coping framework. (From Lazarus, R.S. (1966). *Psychological stress and the nursing process.* New York: McGraw-Hill, Inc. With permission.)

awareness. This evaluation of the situation is primary to the concept of stress and coping and explains individual variation in responses to situations of apparently objective danger, such as an earthquake or admission to a critical care unit.

How the individual appraises a stressor is influenced by his past experiences, cognitive and emotional development, personal traits, philosophy of life, and the type of coping responses available to him. Appraisal of threat is also dependent on how much is at stake for the individual.

Finally, the perception of a stressor as threatening will depend on how dangerous the threat appears to be in relation to the individual's feeling of competence to intervene. The relationship between the size of the threat and the individual's perception of resources is known as the threat-resource ratio (Lazarus and Folkman, 1984).

Affective or Physiologic Response

If the answer to the question, "How bad can this be?" confirms that something terrible is happening or about to happen, the person generally experiences feelings of threat or vulnerability as well as some physiologic response. This mind-body connection is the "fight or flight" reaction, the body's stress response (Selye, 1956; Pollock, 1984). This reaction can be activated by a variety of sources including biologic sources, such as infection, trauma, and drugs; environmental sources, such as noise, heat, and cold; and psychological sources, such as fear, anxiety, loss, and change in life circumstances. The response to these stressors is a complex interaction between hormonal and neurologic factors that influences the function of specific organs. For example, an increase in circulating epinephrine and norepinephrine as well as the release of mineralocorticoids triggers major cardiovascular effects. The resulting increase in heart rate, vasoconstriction, myocardial contractility, and sodium and water retention all serve to increase myocardial oxygen consumption and the work of the heart. These responses are relevant to any critically ill patient because of the link between emotional reactions, physiologic response, and significant cardiac dysrhythmias (Lown et al., 1980). Emotional stress has also been implicated in platelet aggregation in the small vessels of the heart, suggesting a relationship between acute myocardial infarction and severe stress that results from catecholamine release (Haft and Arkel, 1976).

Other potentially deleterious effects of the stress response are related to immunologic changes. Although current thinking about the relationship between behavior and the immune system is far from definitive, research with animals demonstrates a causal relationship between stress and susceptibility to disease. Behavioral factors can affect both cell-mediated and hormonal immunity through the release of corticosteroids and catecholamines, which in turn inhibit immune responses (Borysenko and Borysenko, 1982).

There is also some evidence in humans that exposure to severe stressors that overpower an individual's coping ability can lead to immunosuppressive changes (Lock, 1982; Ader and Cohen, 1984). Also, the direct effects of the cortisol that is released during the stress response can retard wound healing. The inflammatory response can be blocked, granulation response and antibody formation are inhibited, and the supply of oxygen and nutrients to the wound site is limited by peripheral vasoconstriction (DeVillier, 1984). Inhibited wound healing can increase the length of the recovery period and hospital stay, contributing to feelings of hopelessness in the patient, which may further inhibit the immune response.

Affective disturbance may be experienced in a variety of ways. Feelings of turmoil, agitation, anxiety, fear, depression, helplessness, hopelessness, worthlessness, or frustration are common responses (Weisman, 1987).

Nurses cannot directly experience a person's perceptual and appraisal processes. Rather, nurses see the affective and physiologic responses in their patients and recognize them as the end result of a response to a threat. The observed physiologic responses and dysphoric feelings are clues to the fact that something is wrong and needs to be assessed further.

Coping Responses

Most individuals who perceive conditions as threatening to their psychological equilibrium will attempt to restore some sort of balance in their lives.

Feelings of vulnerability and physiologic responses lead the involved person to question what will reduce the threat given the circumstances and known resources. Again, this question is not necessarily conscious but occurs almost automatically and instantaneously in stressful circumstances. People evaluate the threat-resource ratio and make their best attempt to cope with or master the demands that are felt to be straining or overtaking their usual resources. Coping is an ongoing process of cognitive and behavioral efforts to manage internal or external demands that are seen to be taxing or exceeding one's personal resources (Lazarus and Folkman, 1984).

Coping behaviors can be problem focused, directed toward the stressor in some way, or emotion focused, directed toward mitigating or altering one's emotional response (Benner and Wrubel, 1989; Lazarus, 1966; Weisman, 1987). Problem-focused options include:

1. Gathering more information
2. Identifying alternative solutions
3. Letting someone else solve the problem
4. Talking the problem over with others who have had the same problem
5. Consciously deciding to do nothing

Some types of emotion-focused coping are:

1. Practicing relaxation techniques
2. Altering the way one thinks about a situation
3. Making light of a situation
4. Putting the problem out of one's mind
5. Using drugs and food
6. Becoming angry or depressed

Some forms of coping have elements of both approaches. Gathering information can be a way to solve problems as well as a way to support a decision already made or add to feelings of control (Lazarus and Folkman, 1984). The use of defense mechanisms, which are primarily unconscious mental processes, is also a way to control anxiety and internal conflict and is a form of emotion-focused coping.

Coping is a process that occurs over time with ongoing reappraisal of the situation and personal responses until adaptation or neutralization of the stressor occurs (Scott et al., 1980).

STRESS-COPING FRAMEWORK: PLANNING NURSING CARE

The stress-coping model provides a unified way of approaching the challenge of meeting the psychosocial needs of critically ill patients. Nurses can identify appropriate interventions and approaches by understanding the relationships of the model's components to each other and how they combine to influence a patient's ability to cope (Clark, 1988).

Identifying and Reducing Known Stressors for Critically Ill Patients

One of the ways in which nurses can make an impact on patients' responses to being sick is to identify stressors inherent in the critical care setting and the illness experience and either remove them when possible or lessen their impact if complete elimination is not realistic.

A critical illness involving hospitalization in a critical care unit by itself creates predictable stressors (Beglinger, 1983; Moos and Tsu, 1979; Keily, 1972). Pain, separation from the usual support systems, and fear and anxiety related to death are all aspects of an illness that can lead to feelings of vulnerability. The critical care environment itself can lead to decompensation and ineffective coping.

UNIVERSAL STRESSORS

Pain

A major stressor for critically ill patients is the experience of or the threat of pain (Ballard, 1981; Jones et al., 1979). Because of the physiologic and psychological ramifications of pain, it is important for nurses to attend to it.

Autonomic nervous system responses to acute pain include increased heart rate, blood pressure, and depth and rate of respirations (Puntillo, 1988). These responses can result in pulmonary and cardiovascular complications. Intolerable pain may lead to depression or suicidal ideation. Pain contributes to feelings of powerlessness and increases susceptibility to other stressors that might otherwise be tolerated.

There are three major independent nursing approaches that are important in the control of pain: relaxation techniques, information sharing, and a commitment to pain relief.

Relaxation Techniques. The relaxation response provides opposition to the sympathetic nervous response. It includes a decrease in heart rate, oxygen consumption, respiratory rate, and muscle tension (Benson, 1975). In one study a very simple relaxation technique was used: The patient was instructed to lower the jaw, keep the tongue quiet in the bottom of the mouth, relax the lips, breathe slowly and rhythmically in an inhale, exhale, and rest pattern, and refrain mentally from forming words. The experimental group used the technique during postoperative ambulation. This group reported less pain and used less narcotics in the first 24-hour period after surgery (Flaherty and Fitzpatrick, 1978).

Relaxation techniques such as the one used above are relatively easy to explain and use. They are not meant to replace analgesia administration but rather serve as an adjunct to pharmacologic interventions. These techniques not only reduce pain but also increase feelings of personal control in a situation that offers few opportunities for self-management.

Helping patients cope with pain is an example of a combined problem-focused and emotion-focused intervention.

Information Sharing. Radwin (1987), in a summary article on patients with acute pain, cites several studies that demonstrate that patients who learn about the potential pain and discomfort of upcoming procedures as well as methods to reduce pain experience less subjective pain. In some cases, patients have been able to decrease the amount of analgesia used and even the length of the hospital stay. Teaching patients about the procedural and sensory components of upcoming treatments can reduce pain as well as increase feelings of self-control and is an example of facilitating problem-focused coping.

Holistic Approach. Patients who have been cared for by nurses who approach patients holistically have also experienced more pain relief than control group patients who were given only routine pain medications (Radwin, 1987). Interventions employed in the holistic approach included

■ Identifying pain relief as a mutual goal
■ Addressing all physical and psychological factors that might be contributing to the pain
■ Offering alternatives for pain control such as analgesia, relaxation, or distraction
■ Allowing the patient to chose among alternatives whenever possible

Attending to pain addresses several points in the stress-coping cycle. It decreases the size of the threat while at the same time increasing feelings of control and confidence in one's ability to cope. It provides a problem-oriented coping strategy that may at the same time increase feelings of self-esteem and confidence. It may decrease the sympathetic nervous system response to pain, thus influencing the physiologic response to stress. It may make other stressors more tolerable. Although life-threatening events or hemodynamic instability may compete with nurses' attention, helping patients cope with pain can have far-reaching implications for patient care outcomes.

Separation From Support Systems

The connection between social networks and illness is not entirely clear, but there is supporting evidence that disrupted social networks can contribute to disease processes. Support systems may in some way serve as buffers between risk factors and disease. Disrupted social ties may in fact be a risk factor or an etiologic agent. It is possible that disrupted social connections affect resistance to disease, increasing an individual's vulnerability to a wide range of pathologic processes (Syme, 1984).

One study in postmyocardial infarction patients showed that patients with perceived life stress and little social support had four times the risk of sudden cardiac death than patients with lower levels of perceived stress and greater social connectedness (Ruberman et al., 1984). Another study indicated that men with myocardial infarctions who experienced difficulty in communicating with friends and family had an elevated risk of sudden death (Ruberman et al., 1983).

Nurses have done research on the connection between social support and patient outcomes. For example, when family members were taught simple orientation techniques to use with post–open heart surgery patients, the patients in the experimental group had fewer symptoms of postcardiotomy psychosis (Chatham, 1978). Patients who were transferred from the critical care unit (CCU) with family support showed reduced levels of stress and cardiovascular complications (Schwartz and Brenner, 1979).

Despite the fact that families can often be a source of increased tension for staff (Dunkel and Eisendrath, 1983), nurses need to find ways to maintain these important connections in their patients' lives. A Spouse Care Plan (Breu and Dracups, 1978), for example, can help to maintain important supportive relationships for the patient (Table 6–1). Spouses who experienced these interventions showed fewer symptoms of crisis. Presumably, spouses who are more in control can be more helpful to their family members who are ill.

Incorporating families in the plan of care may positively affect the disease process, the patient's feelings of self-esteem, and the family's ability to cope, and these may in turn affect the nurse's stress level and the smooth functioning of the unit.

Anxiety and Fear Related to Death

When facing a life-threatening illness, patients confront the reality of death and characteristically experience intense anxiety, which triggers profound defensive behavior. Interventions that are appropriate to help the patient adapt to this threat include giving information, providing hope, helping to maintain relationships with family, and allowing the patient to talk about his or her feelings. The type of intervention and support needed depends on the type of dying pattern: uncertain death at an uncertain time, certain death at an unknown time, or certain death at a known time (Glaser and Straus, 1968).

For some patients, such as those with uncomplicated myocardial infarctions, the possibility of death

TABLE 6–1. Spouse Care Plan

Orient the spouse to the environment
Arrange for a nurse to call the spouse at home once per shift
Take the spouse away from the bedside to talk for fifteen
  minutes per shift about specific concerns
Make the spouse feel welcome
Allow flexible visiting

is present but not certain. In these cases, rehabilitative interventions are usually emphasized. Patients, families, and staff use education about postdischarge life-style changes as a way of coping with the uncertain prognosis.

There is a greater possibility of death for patients who are experiencing acute exacerbations of a chronic illness. Nurses are often uncertain as to whether interventions should be directed toward plans for living or for dying (Marocchio, 1982). It is helpful for patients to talk about the full range of their feelings, both the possibility of death and the potential for survival. This helps them to talk about their fears while at the same time supporting their hope for recovery.

For patients for whom there is no hope for survival, death will occur within a specified period of time. Some patients will be too exhausted to share their feelings at this time. Others may have to need to find meaning and purpose in their experience. Nurses can assess a patient's readiness to talk about his or her feelings by asking open-ended questions such as: "What is your understanding of what is happening to you?" or, "How are you feeling about what is happening to you?" Patients' responses will reflect their readiness to grieve actively.

Environmental Stressors: Noise

Acute care settings are particularly stressful because of, among other things, excess noise (Zimmerman, 1988). Noise is an important stressor because it is related to a startle response that elicits increases in heart rate, metabolism, and overall oxygen consumption. It is also an important factor in sleep disruption and consequent episodes of delirium (Hansell, 1984; Easton and MacKenzie, 1988). In a study conducted by Helton and colleagues (1980) a 33% increase in mental status changes occurred in patients who were rated as severely sleep deprived.

In studies done in acute care settings, the noise levels were consistently above the limits set by the International Noise Council (Bentley et al., 1977). Noise comes from two primary sources—equipment and staff. One study showed that noise levels in the critical care unit were comparable to the hospital's cafeteria at noon and slightly less noisy than the boiler room (Redding et al., 1977). Another study concluded that the noise levels produced by conversations between nursing and medical personnel were louder than those made by equipment (Woods and Falk, 1974).

Noise is an important environmental stressor that can interfere with sleep and rest and lead to perceptual alterations that contribute to increased anxiety and physiologic response. It is also a stressor that can be easily attended to and altered by nursing personnel.

Disease-Specific Stressors

One of the most important questions to ask when assessing a patient's coping response is, What is it that the patient must cope with? Each disease poses unique threats, follows a relatively predictable course, makes certain demands on patient and family, and creates particular limitations and possibilities.

The behavioral responses and coping strategies used by the patient depend in large part on the situational demands created by this illness trajectory. A person coping with the acute onset of an illness for the first time will respond differently than a patient who has an acute exacerbation of a chronic illness. For example, the symptoms may be more frightening because the patient already understands their implications, or they may be less frightening because the patient is familiar with them. Different phases of an illness present different challenges. The period between the appearance of symptoms and the diagnosis presents multiple ambiguities. During the treatment phase, patients may have more knowledge of the implications and potential outcomes of the illness. At first, patients must cope with uncertainty, whereas later they must cope with the reality of the illness. If the illness has remissions and exacerbations or downward spirals, patients must learn to balance wellness with illness, hope with despair.

Recent trends in nursing research demonstrate an interest in identifying those aspects of specific situations that patients rate as stressors. For example, transfer away from a coronary care unit has been identified as a difficult aspect of the illness experience. Patients experience increased feelings of anxiety and an increase in cardiovascular complications including reinfarction and fatal dysrhythmias near the time of the transfer (Schwartz and Brenner, 1979; Klein et al., 1968; Toth, 1980). Structured preparation for the transfer, including specific information (Toth, 1980) and the use of family support (Schwartz and Brenner, 1979) have been shown to reduce the physiologic indicators of the stress response.

Other important studies have attempted to identify, from the patient's point of view, the factors that need adaptation by the patient. Researchers have looked at the incidence and severity of stressors associated with coronary artery bypass surgery (Carr and Powers, 1986; Stanton et al., 1984). One study showed that there were significant differences between the nurse and the patient in the perception of stress. Stress for both hospital- and illness-related items was rated significantly higher by the nurse than by the patient (Carr and Powers, 1986). Using interviews with patients who had been mechanically ventilated, another study revealed the specific stressors associated with that experience (Gries and Fernsler, 1988).

Anticipatory guidance to reduce the impact of specific stressors is one important intervention that can be used by nurses. Interestingly, however, in the study just mentioned of patients undergoing mechanical ventilation, most patients were unable to recall specific nursing interventions that were done. Those that were recalled were reassuring words, just the presence of the nurse, and a caring manner.

Studies like these help nurses understand the patient experience and allow them to plan their interventions accordingly.

Expert nurses have an awareness of the expected and serve as guides for patients, making what is strange and frightening more approachable (Benner and Wrubel, 1989). They can provide a road map for patients to help them anticipate and plan for known stressors. This is one of the many ways in which nurses can incorporate research into their practice.

ASSESSMENTS AND INTERVENTIONS RELATED TO COGNITIVE APPRAISAL

Understanding the Patient's Perspective

An individual's appraisal of a situation is the major determinant of what is and what is not stressful. Nurses demonstrate understanding of the concept of individual appraisal of stressors when they are willing to accept the patient's perception of the threat. For example, alterations in appearance will not be as threatening to an individual in whom attractiveness is not a prime source of self-esteem or identity. This is an example of how individual values determine stressors.

A heart transplant candidate who viewed the heart as a repository for the soul found the idea of using another's heart more stressful than another candidate who viewed the heart as a mechanical pump. This is an example of how an individual's belief system determines what is stressful.

A patient who is generally mistrustful of others will experience more stress at having to place himself in the care of strangers than someone who is generally trustful. There is also some evidence that patients who feel that they can and should be able to have some impact on the surrounding circumstances may experience a more stressful response to hospitalization than patients who do not have as high a need for control (Topf, 1984). This is an example of how an individual's personality style can influence his appraisal of the stress inherent in some situations.

The most important intervention that nurses can use in understanding a patient's perspective is empathetic listening, which is the ability to hear the patient's perception of his or her situation completely without offering advice or solutions. Many nurses feel uncomfortable working with a patient's psychosocial needs because they are unsure of what to say. In actuality, it is more important to hear what the patient has to say. The skill that is most important is knowing how to help people express their concerns fully, thus validating their perceptions and reactions. In this way, nurses provide an opportunity for patients to express their fears and concerns, and this by itself may be enough to decrease anxiety and its corresponding physiologic reactivity (Tables 6–2 and 6–3).

Another reason for allowing patients to express

TABLE 6–2. Assessment Questions to Identify a Patient's Perception

What do you think is the matter with you?
What does it mean to you that you have a _____ (valve replacement)?
What does it feel like to use the word _____ (tumor)?
What do you think may have caused this to happen?
Do you think you are making progress?
Are you worried about any long-term effects?

From Bilodeau, C. B. (1981). In C. V. Kenner, C. E. Guggetta, and B. M. Dorsey (Eds.), *Critical care nursing: Body-mind-spirit.* Boston: Little, Brown.

their perceptions fully is to identify misconceptions that can be corrected based on the nurse's experience with the specific illness. For example, if a patient with a colostomy expresses concerns about loss of sexual function and vitality, the nurse can assist in redefining the situation based on her or his reality-based experience with other patients (Lindquist, 1986). By assisting the patient to redefine the situation, the nurse can be a source of hope and strength. By helping patients identify the meaning the situation holds for them, nurses can help patients move from generalized concerns that may be overwhelming to specific concerns that may be more manageable.

Alterations in Cognitive Function

The ability to perceive and interpret reality accurately is vital to coping effectively. Neurologic and metabolic changes leading to delirium can distort perception, sensation, and thinking, thus interfering with effective coping responses. This perceptual distortion is known as delirium or "ICU psychosis." At the very least, delirium is anxiety-producing for the patient and the family. Delirium marked by paranoid ideation and hallucinations can be life-threatening if patients pull out important intravenous lines or other equipment and attempt to get out of bed. Anxiety, agitation, and combativeness can induce life-threatening dysrhythmias, wound dehiscence, and orthopedic injuries. Many factors can contribute to this response: metabolic factors such as pain, hemodynamic instability, electrolyte imbalance, sepsis, pharmaceuticals, and history of drug abuse; environmental factors such as noise, sleep deprivation, frightening atmosphere, and absence of windows; psychological factors such as anxiety, fear, and lack of control.

Some of the behavioral changes accompanying delirium can be mistaken for ineffective coping responses. Patients may become restless, listless, irritable, depressed, anxious, combative, and incoherent. They may refuse to answer questions or demonstrate alterations in intellectual capacity and memory. They may become defensive and paranoid. They may experience delusions, illusions, and hallucinations. A case example illustrates the importance

of a methodical approach to assessing changes in behavior.

CASE HISTORY

Mr. G. had a long-standing history of restrictive cardiomyopathy resulting in symptoms of right-sided heart failure, severe ascites, liver engorgement, and cardiac cachexia. He was admitted to the hospital for evaluation for a cardiac transplant. The transplant team was uncertain about the patient's medical suitability. They had vacillated, telling the patient at one point that he was a candidate and then withdrawing that decision when new data about him came to light. The patient was placed in the very difficult position of waiting for further evaluation before a third and final decision was made.

One night when the nurse went to administer his routine medication, Mr. G. was lethargic and refused to respond to her questions. The nurse thought that he was becoming depressed about the uncertainty of his situation. Her interventions included explanations and comfort measures, but as the night wore on the patient became angry and uncooperative, trying to get out of bed without assistance. When he fell and was incontinent the nurse restrained him to prevent further incident. She felt frustrated that no intervention had helped to calm him. In the morning, his blood ammonia level was tested and was found to be toxic. Treatment to reduce the blood ammonia was started, and 3 days later the patient's behavior returned to normal. The behavioral changes noted in this patient were ascribed to psychological causes and diagnosed as ineffective coping responses.

An estimated 12.5% to 38% of conscious patients admitted to critical care units experience delirium that may be terrifying to the patient and may be unrecognized by the nurse (Easton and MacKenzie, 1988). Assessing delirium is difficult because the most common effects seen are anxiety, fear, and depression, alone or in combination. Also, many patients may be aware that something is wrong and are afraid they are going crazy. They may try to hide the alteration from themselves and others by denying

TABLE 6–3. Therapeutic and Nontherapeutic Communication Techniques

Therapeutic Techniques	Nontherapeutic Techniques
Develop caring, nonjudgmental relationship that will allow for the expression of feelings	*Passing judgment* on behavior or feelings: "Most patients don't get this anxious."
Open-ended questions: "What is your understanding of what the doctor has told you?"	*Giving advice:* "You should make your husband stop smoking now."
Reflection of thoughts or feelings: "It sounds as if you are really worried"; or, "It sounds as if you've been thinking about hurting yourself."	*Give false reassurance:* "I'm sure everything will turn out just fine."

Data from Gorman, L. M., Sultan, D., and Luna-Raines, M. (1989). *Psychosocial nursing handbook for the nonpsychiatric nurse* (pp. 8–9). © 1989, the Williams & Wilkins Co., Baltimore.

any problem or withdrawing to prevent detection (Murray, 1987). Important symptoms to be noted are disorientation as to time, place, and person; failure to recognize family members; perceptual illusions (mistaking environmental stimuli such as hearing the hissing of the oxygen valve as whispering); paranoid ideation; and hallucinations (perceiving environmental stimuli when there are none) (Sadler, 1979).

Interventions that may prevent delirium from occurring include a preadmission visit by the intensive care unit (ICU) nurse to patients with planned admissions. One study demonstrated a 50% reduction in delirium in patients who participated in a preoperative interview (Kornfeld, 1979). Patients should be told about the possibility of delirium and given brief explanations and assurances as well as instructions to inform nurses of any unusual sensations or thoughts. The importance of providing adequate rest and sleep and controlling pain as preventive measures has already been discussed.

ASSESSMENT OF AND INTERVENTIONS FOR AFFECTIVE OR PHYSIOLOGIC AROUSAL

As discussed earlier, nurses can intervene in the stress-coping cycle at the point of Cognitive Appraisal. Nurses can also intervene by working directly to correct the physiologic and emotional arousal states that result when a threat is recognized.

Fight or Flight Response

Physiologic arousal can cause increases in oxygen consumption, heart rate, lethal dysrhythmias, blood pressure, respiratory rate, fatigue, and irritability. As discussed in the earlier section on pain, the relaxation response has been shown to counter these effects by producing an opposing response that includes decreases in oxygen consumption, respiratory rate, and heart rate. The relaxation response generally involves four elements: a comfortable position, a quiet environment, concentration on one's breathing, and a passive attitude (Clark, 1988). The use of a physiologic monitoring device to give the patient immediate information about the state of relaxation is called biofeedback. Often, special time is set aside to teach patients these techniques and allow time for practice (Melville, 1987; Miller, 1985; Acosta, 1988). However, the critical care unit is not the ideal atmosphere for helping patients to achieve a state of relaxation. But the following example illustrates how an expert nurse was able to incorporate this technique into her care.

CASE HISTORY

A patient who had been admitted to the CCU with acute chest pain started to have ventricular irritability. He had multifocal premature ventricular contractions (PVCs) and runs of ventricular tachycardia (VT). Eventually, despite maximum doses of lidocaine, his heart rhythm deteriorated to the point of ventricular fibrillation. A "code" was called, and he was successfully resuscitated. However, his monitor continued to show extreme ventricular irritability. The patient lay awake and alert in his bed, surrounded by nurses and doctors nervously eyeing his monitor and talking about what to do next. A nurse went to the patient's side, took his hand, got his attention, and helped him to concentrate on his breathing, guiding him to inhale through his nose and exhale slowly through his mouth. He visibly relaxed, his body became less tense, he focused his attention on the nurse and participated in the rhythmic breathing. While this was taking place, another nurse had hung a different intravenous antiarrhythmic medication. After several minutes, the patient's rhythm returned to a regular sinus pattern, and the physicians thought that they had made the right treatment decision regarding the medication. But using a holistic model, the nurse also played an important role in this successful ending (Gomez and Gomez, 1984). Her attention to the patient as a biopsychosocial being prompted her intervention and allowed the patient to participate in his own treatment. Even in highly charged situations, nurses who have a commitment to holistic care will find ways to practice it.

Anxiety and Fear

Although patients can respond to threats to their physical safety in a variety of ways, a common response is one of fear and anxiety. These are closely linked emotions that differ only in terms of cause. Fear is a response to an identified stressor such as impending surgery, possible death, pain, and diagnostic procedures. Anxiety is characterized by feelings of dread, worry, and apprehension that cannot be specifically linked to an external cause. For example, a patient who has never acknowledged dependency needs may feel extremely uncomfortable at the prospect of placing himself in the care of others but will be unaware that this is the issue that is causing distress. Anxiety can range from vague feelings of edginess to feelings of uncontrolled terror and panic.

MILD ANXIETY

Some anxiety is an expected response to illness and in its more mild form may actually stimulate a coping response by increasing alertness and motivating learning or change. Signs and symptoms may include statements from the patient that he or she is worried, anxious, nervous, and so on; increases in pulse, blood pressure, and respirations; and narrowed focus of attention. Nursing interventions for patients experiencing this level of anxiety include encouraging the patient to talk about specific concerns and providing realistic information to assist with problem solving.

MODERATE ANXIETY

Anxiety at a moderate level may decrease a patient's ability to take in information and communicate needs. Patients may ask the same questions repeatedly. Providing more information at this time may contribute to the feeling of being overwhelmed. The patient may be acutely aware of the uncomfortable physiologic response that can occur with anxiety. Certainly, medication with a mild anxiolytic would be appropriate to assist the patient to regain control. Staying with the patient and providing reassurance may also help him to regain control.

SEVERE ANXIETY

Severe anxiety or panic seems resistant to efforts to change it made by either the individual or the environment. Patients have little ability to withstand the level of discomfort they are experiencing. They have an extremely narrow focus of attention, are unable to take in information or solve problems, may have difficulty in concentrating, and may have distorted perceptions. This level of anxiety impairs the ability to cope, may lead to extremes of withdrawal or avoidance, and disrupts all normal functioning.

Although pharmacologic intervention with short-acting benzodiazepines is appropriate in these situations, the approach to the patient is also critical. Patients experiencing extreme anxiety generally cannot respond to rational explanations and information because cognitive function is seriously impaired. A more helpful approach is to speak softly and simply and to indicate a willingness to be with the patient. These patients should not be left alone because they may harm themselves either purposefully or inadvertently. It is important to transmit feelings of calm and being in control of the situation so that the patient feels that someone is in charge while he cannot be. Do not attempt to engage the patient in problem-solving behavior until you know that he is certain that you fully understand his fears and concerns, and the ability to attend to explanations has returned.

Hopelessness

Feelings of helplessness and lowered self-esteem that seem to be a natural response to the threats posed by a critical illness can contribute to feelings of hopelessness. It is important to help patients combat these feelings because they can contribute to a lack of participation in treatment and therefore to increased complications. A major contributor to feelings of hopelessness is the patient's perception that her or his condition is at a standstill and that there is nothing she or he can do to get well. Nurses can provide hope by normalizing the experience by assuring patients that much of the weakness and fatigue they are experiencing is a normal response to

illness and prolonged bedrest. It is also important to anticipate setbacks and let the patient know that progress is rarely a steady uphill climb.

Nurses can assist patients to set small goals that are realistic and attainable. Many patients want to leap past the day-to-day discomfort of gradually regaining strength and function; they have unrealistic expectations about what they can actually do. By setting small goals in consultation with the patient and then pointing out the small steps that are achieved, the nurse can provide hope that things are in fact improving. By helping patients recognize the signs of progress, nurses instill hope while at the same time increasing the patient's feelings of control and self-esteem.

SUPPORTING ADAPTIVE COPING RESPONSES AND DEFENSE MECHANISMS

Another goal of nursing interventions is to support effective coping responses. More research is being done to identify exactly what patients do in certain situations to help them manage their uncomfortable reactions and which of these responses are most effective.

Problem-Focused and Emotion-Focused Coping

Recent studies have looked at specific situations in order to identify exactly what patients do to cope (Nyamathi, 1987; King, 1985; Sutherland, 1988), and several broad generalizations about coping can be made:

- Most people in complex situations use a combination of problem-focused and emotion-focused coping responses.
- Coping responses can change from one encounter to another and over time.
- Coping behaviors that work well in one phase of the illness may not be useful in another phase.
- Coping depends on the stake that the individual has in the stressor.
- The coping process depends on the patient's appraisal of what can and cannot be done; if an individual believes that something can be done, problem-focused coping will be used, but if he feels that nothing can be done, emotion-focused coping predominates.

The above information supports the idea that there may not be a "right" way to cope and that nurses must see the patient's attempts to cope as the best he can do at a given point in time. Attempts to change a particular coping behavior must be done carefully and with the knowledge that behavior change takes time and a commitment to change on the part of the patient.

In a recent study of patients undergoing cardiac catheterization (Watkins et al., 1986), patients were divided into groups depending on whether they used a "monitoring" or "blunting" approach to stressful circumstances. Monitors generally use intellectualization and information gathering, whereas blunters prefer to diminish the psychological effect of the stressor. Patients received two types of information about the catheterization experience—either procedural information only or a combination of procedural information and descriptions of the sensations that were frequently experienced. The results indicated that:

1. Monitors who received procedural and sensation information reported less anxiety than monitors who received procedural information only. Monitors had lower levels of anxiety and psychophysiologic arousal if they were provided with procedural as well as sensation information.

2. Blunters who received procedural plus sensation information experienced higher levels of anxiety than when they received procedural information only. Blunters had lower levels of anxiety and psychophysiologic arousal if they were provided with procedural information only.

This study emphasizes that nursing interventions that are taken for granted such as preprocedural teaching, if not individualized, may interfere with the coping behaviors used by patients and may actually lead to increased arousal.

As nurses try to evaluate the effectiveness of coping responses of critically ill patients who are responding to often overwhelming threats to body, ego, and social situation, the most important question to ask is: Does this behavior work for this person, at this time, in this context? Coping can only be judged in terms of its consequences for an individual in terms of his or her ability to maintain adequate social relationships, keep feelings of anxiety at a manageable level, and minimize the effects of the stressor on physical well-being (Lazarus and Folkman, 1984) (Table 6–4).

For example, patients who experience symptoms but deny them and delay seeking treatment are coping ineffectively because the behavior has implications for their physical well-being. One patient experiencing crushing chest pain while riding his bicycle turned around and rode back home rather than seeking help. On the other hand, patients who use denial to control their anxiety about the meaning of their symptoms but seek out and participate in treatment are still coping effectively even though they are not able to face the problem directly. Patients who get angry to avoid feelings of powerlessness but are able to talk about their feelings with caregivers are coping effectively. Patients who direct their anger toward caregivers as if they rather than the situation were the source of the stress cut themselves off from

TABLE 6–4. Patient Care Plan for Ineffective Coping

Defining Characteristics	Interventions
Patient states that he is unable to cope	Identify potential organic causes of behavior
Stressor appears greater than available resources	1. Assess orientation to time/place/person
Use of behaviors that are destructive to self or others: aggression; suicide; use of alcohol or drugs	2. Assess memory for recent events and immediate recall
Unable to solve problems	3. Observe for altered perceptions
Use of defense mechanisms that interfere with getting treatment or support	4. Assess thought processes
	5. Confer with MD regarding diagnostic tests
	During high levels of anxiety, give short, simple explanations
	Develop caring nonjudgmental relationship through use of effective communication skills that will
	1. Encourage expression of feelings
	2. Allow development of alternative perceptions of the event that promote evaluation of the stressor into manageable terms
	3. Allow reassessment of the situation without making patient feel discounted
	Set limits on unacceptable behavior
	Develop support system
	1. Involve mental health professional to assess and treat acute confusional states, major depression, suicide risk
	If present and helpful, involve significant others
	Develop own support system to help cope with own reactions to difficult patients

Reprinted from p. 202 of *Psychological aspects of critical care nursing* by B. Reigel and D. Ehrenreich (Eds.), with permission of Aspen Publishers, Inc., © 1989.

support and are coping ineffectively. However, the need to defend oneself against the painful feelings initiated by the stressors of illness is universal, and people make do with whatever tools they have to achieve the greatest level of peace and functioning during the crisis (Groves and Kucharski, 1987).

Sometimes coping involves the use of defense mechanisms that are unconscious psychological processes used to control feelings of intense anxiety. They are not directed toward problem solving but instead help to deceive the person about the actual threat. Defense mechanisms permit a person to take in only as much reality as he feels equipped to handle and serve to keep anxiety at tolerable levels.

Some defenses are more costly than others in terms of effects on well-being, social interaction, and morale. Vaillant (1976) constructed a theoretical hierarchy of ego defenses that may help caregivers understand the degree of threat a person may be experiencing. The more primitive or regressive the defense mechanism, the higher the degree of threat (Groves and Kucharski, 1987).

Primitive Defenses

The least effective mechanisms are those that alter reality for the person using them but seem "crazy" to others. Distortion involving delusions and hallucinations to reshape reality to meet internal needs is an example of this level of defense. These defenses are very difficult to change and respond best to medication and removal of the stressor rather than to therapeutic interactions. Although the patient who is using this level of defense may be frightening to work with because his behavior is so bizarre, nurses can see that the behavior is not directed at them, and they generally do not get caught in defensive responses to such patients.

Immature Defenses

Immature mechanisms are used by normal children or adults who have regressed to earlier behavior patterns. These mechanisms may decrease anxiety for the person using them but generally create feelings of annoyance and irritation in the people around them. Three examples of this level of defense are (1) projection, attributing one's own unacceptable feelings to others; (2) passive-aggressive behavior, covertly expressing hostility while appearing to be compliant; and (3) acting-out, the direct expression of impulses. These behaviors are often deeply ingrained and inflexible but are amenable to change by prolonged relationships with caring and mature individuals who are willing to develop a therapeutic relationship.

Patients using immature defense mechanisms are often the most frustrating to work with because their affect and behavior cause negative reactions in the people who care for them. For example, one of the most difficult patients to care for is the one who uses acting-out and anger to gain control. This angry response is not the same as rational anger, which is a response to the external situation and is expressed directly in order to create constructive change. Rather, this type of anger is characterized by verbal threats, physical aggression, and hostility and is connected more to internal threats than to external reality. This type of behavior often sets up an automatic defensive reaction in the nurse that, although understandable, escalates the patient's anger and usually leads to a no-win power struggle (Minarik and Leavitt, 1988).

Interventions that are most likely to succeed in these cases include a nondefensive acceptance of the situation from the patient's point of view and a sincere effort to discover what can be done to alleviate the situation. Allowing the patient to express anger fully without offering resistance eliminates the patient's need to continue escalating his behavior to make sure she or he is understood.

Different approaches are appropriate for the different ways people express anger (Leavitt, 1982). When anger is expressed passively, as when patients pull out lines or deliberately spill food or water, an attempt should be made to look for the underlying intention so that the concerns can be expressed more directly. If anger is expressed directly, it is better to focus on the factor in the situation that caused the anger rather than on the anger itself. If anger is expressed in a destructive and hostile manner, the nurse should calmly set limits on the unacceptable behavior without cutting off the anger. Setting limits makes the environment safe but should not be a way for the nurse to express his or her own anger (Minarik and Leavitt, 1988).

The most important approach for nurses to take with all patients using immature defense mechanisms is first to recognize their own reactions and accept them as normal rather than as an indication of personal inadequacy. Once nurses can monitor their own reactions, they can begin to work with the patient's behavior in a problem-solving way. These patients are troublesome to the whole staff and generate feelings of frustration and of wanting to flee. Often, a consultant not directly involved in the situation is necessary to help sort through the various feelings and develop a reasonable plan.

Neurotic Defenses

Neurotic defenses are common and can be seen in most healthy adults, especially at times of acute stress. Examples of this type of defense mechanism are (1) displacement, the focusing on less threatening aspects of a situation, and (2) intellectualization, the avoidance of the emotional components of a situation.

Patients who use neurotic defenses can be very rewarding to work with. If their behavior is the result of regression due to the immediate situation rather than to rigidly held beliefs, it is amenable to dramatic change with even brief therapeutic interactions that help them identify the underlying source of the anxiety. For example, some patients who have had spinal cord injuries begin to make sexual jokes and treat the nursing staff as sexual objects. If nurses understand that this behavior is a response to an underlying anxiety related to sexual performance they can help the patient by acknowledging the behavior and wondering out loud if he is having some concerns about this area. This type of confrontation must be done within the context of a therapeutic relationship based on trust, which permits the patient to acknowledge the underlying anxiety that the defensive behavior was intended to mask.

It is important for nurses to remember that defense mechanisms are neither "bad" nor "good" but are the person's best available method for containing feelings of anxiety. They serve a useful purpose and should be left in place unless they can be replaced by something else that will be useful to the patient. Also, defense mechanisms are unconscious and may not be specifically intended to create negative reactions in others, although that is often the end result (Clark, 1988). Approaching patients with these concepts in mind helps nurses to cope more effectively with patients' upsetting affects and behaviors.

THE PREREQUISITE FOR NURSING INTERVENTIONS: A CARING RELATIONSHIP

The relationship that is formed between the patient and the nurse is the vehicle through which all other interventions take place and is based on caring. Caring is essential for effective nursing practice. It causes the nurse to notice subtle changes in the patient's condition and identify what needs to be done. Caring makes the nurse notice which interventions work and which do not. Caring sets up the conditions of trust that allow the one cared for to use the help that is offered (Benner and Wrubel, 1989).

How do nurses convey that they care about patients? Caring is demonstrated by interventions that meet the treatment needs of patients (instrumental activities) as well as by those that are more psychologically oriented (expressive functions). Patients and family members rank instrumental activities as most important to feeling cared for, whereas nurses rank meeting expressive needs as most important to caring. Patients perceive that nurses who know what they are doing, know how to give shots, know when to call the physician, give treatments on time, are well organized, answer questions clearly, and provide information are demonstrating caring (Brown, 1986; Cronin and Harrison, 1988). However, nurses ranked the following behaviors as important caring activities: allowing expression of feelings, realizing that the patient knows himself best, listening to the patient, touching the patient for comfort, and perceiving patient needs as important (Larson, 1987; Mayer, 1986).

What accounts for this discrepancy? Caring is always understood within the context of the situation. When a swift and accurate intervention is necessary, that is what the patient will perceive as caring. When technical actions are *not* called for, psychologically directed activities will be perceived as caring (Benner and Wrubel, 1989).

One implication of these differences in perception is that patients must first feel safe and have confidence in the nurses caring for them. Once that goal is achieved, the expressive nursing activities become more prominent in the patient's awareness. Another important implication is that nurses cannot assume that their well-intentioned acts of what they consider caring will be experienced as such by patients expecting something else (Brown, 1986).

However, just as one cannot split the mind-body connection, neither can instrumental and expressive nursing functions be considered separately. Nursing care, even technical functions, delivered in a noncaring manner has important implications for patients and health. Nursing care that was perceived as distancing was described in the following terms: too casual an attitude; the nurse just doing a job; not using eye contact; treating patients as objects; being rough and in a hurry; not listening; not responding; being stiff, starchy, insensitive, irritated, or defensive. As a result of these noncaring behaviors, patients felt humiliated, out-of-control, and frightened. Patients felt that being cared for by nurses with these behaviors could slow the process of recovery and leave patients feeling hopeless. Others felt that noncaring relationships added to their stress and depleted energy that could be used for healing (Drew, 1986; Reimaen, 1986).

On the other hand, nurses who were perceived as caring were described as concerned about what happened, liking their work, using eye contact, physically relaxed, matter-of-fact about messes, and not in a hurry. Almost any action was seen as caring if it was not done in a hurry. Patients who received care from these nurses felt more confident, more in control, and more relaxed. They felt that some form of energy was passed from the caregiver to them and that this energy contributed to their healing and recovery (Drew, 1986). As one patient explained, "The nurses came in and they talked to me and hugged me because they knew about my problem. And it seemed like I started getting better right away, right then" (Brown, 1986).

SUMMARY

The stress-coping model seeks to identify aspects of the patient care situation that need to be attended to. Expert nurses learn to assess the different components of the model almost automatically and decide intuitively what intervention would best serve the patient. They weave technical activities into an intricate pattern with expressive actions. Every contact with the patient is purposeful and goal-directed in terms of understanding the stressors affecting the patient, the patient's cognitive appraisal process, the affective and physiologic responses, and the effectiveness of the coping strategies used by the patient.

Meeting the psychosocial needs of critically ill patients is not something that nurses do when they have a few extra minutes but rather is a consistent commitment to a holistic approach to patient care. Nurses who learn to integrate these components into an intuitive whole and meet both the physical and psychosocial needs of their patients are the expert nurses who exemplify the goals, values, and beliefs of the profession.

References

Acosta, F. (1988). Biofeedback and progressive relaxation in weaning the anxious patient from the ventilator: A brief report. *Heart and Lung*, 17, 299–301.

Ader, R., and Cohen, N. (1984). Behavior and the immune system. In W. D. Gentry (Ed.), *Handbook of behavioral medicine* (pp. 117–173). New York: Guilford Press.

American Association of Critical-Care Nurses (1981). *Standards for nursing care of the critically ill*, (p. 64). Reston, VA: Reston Publishing Co.

American Association of Critical-Care Nurses (1988). *AACN News*, August.

American Nurses Association (1980). *Nursing: A social policy statement*. Kansas City, MO.

Ballard, K. (1981). Identification of environmental stressors for patients in a surgical intensive care unit. *Issues in Mental Health Nursing*, 3, 89–108.

Beglinger, J. E. (1983). Coping tasks in critical care. *Dimensions in Critical Care Nursing*, 2 (2), 80–89.

Benner, P. (1984). *From novice to expert: Excellence and power in clinical nursing practice*. Menlo Park, CA: Addison-Wesley.

Benner, P., and Wrubel, J. (1989). The primacy of caring: Stress and coping in health and illness, (p. 30). Menlo Park, CA: Addison-Wesley.

Benson, H. (1975). *The relaxation response*. New York: Avon Books.

Bentley, S., Murphy, F., and Dudley, H. (1977). Perceived noise in surgical wards and in intensive care areas: An objective analysis. *British Medical Journal*, 2, 1503.

Bilodeau, C. B. (1981). Psychologic aspects. In C. V. Kenner, C. E. Guzzetta, and B. M. Dossey (Eds.), *Critical care nursing: Body-mind-spirit*. Boston: Little, Brown.

Borysenko, M., and Borysenko, J. (1982). Stress, behavior and immunity: Animal models and mediating mechanisms. *General Hospital Psychiatry*, 4, 59–67.

Breu, C., and Dracup, K. (1978). Helping spouses of critically ill patients. *American Journal of Nursing*, 78, 50.

Brown, L. (1986). The experience of care: Patient perspectives. *Topics in Clinical Nursing*, 8 (2), 56–62.

Carr, J. A., and Powers, M. J. (1986). Stressors associated with coronary bypass surgery. *Nursing Research*, 35, 243–246.

Chatham, M. A. (1978). The effect of family involvement on patients' manifestations of post-cardiotomy psychosis. *Heart and Lung*, 7, 995.

Clark, S. (1988). Ineffective coping patient and family. In L. Kern (Ed.), *Cardiac critical care nursing* (p. 293). Rockville, MD: Aspen Press.

Clark, S. (1988). Intervention. In R. Hathaway (Ed.), *Nursing care of the critically ill surgical patient*. Frederick, MD: Aspen Press.

Clark, S. (1988). Preoperative phase: Intervention. In R. G. Hathaway (Ed.), *Nursing care of the critically ill surgical patient*. Rockville, MD: Aspen Press.

Clark, S. (1989). Transplantation. In B. Riegel, and D. Ehrenreich (Eds.), *Psychological aspects of critical care nursing*. Rockville, MD: Aspen Press.

Cronin, S. N., and Harrison, B. (1988). Importance of nurse caring behaviors as perceived by patients after myocardial infarction. *Heart and Lung*, 17, 374–380.

DeVillier, B. (1984). Physiology of stress: Cellular healing. *Critical Care Quarterly*, 6 (4), 15–20.

Drew, N. (1986). Exclusion and confirmation: A phenomenology of patients' experiences with caregivers. *Image*, 18 (2), 39–43.

Dunkel, J., and Eisendrath, S. (1983). Families in the intensive care unit: Their effect on staff. *Heart and Lung*, 12, 258.

Easton, C., and MacKenzie, F. (1988). Sensory-perceptual alterations: Delirium in the intensive care unit. *Heart and Lung*, 17, 229–235.

Flaherty, G. G., and Fitzpatrick, J. J. (1978). Relaxation techniques to increase comfort level in postoperative patients: A preliminary study. *Nursing Research*, 27, 352.

Gentry, W. D. (1984). Behavioral medicine: A new research paradigm. In W. D. Gentry (Ed.), *Handbook of behavioral medicine*. New York: Guilford Press.

Glaser, B. G., and Straus, A. L. (1968). *A time for dying*. Chicago: Adeline.

Gomez, G. E., and Gomez, E. A. (1984). Sudden death: Biopsychosocial factors. *Heart and Lung*, 13, 389–394.

Gorman, L. M., Sultan, D., and Luna-Raines, M. (1989). *Psychosocial nursing handbook for the non-psychiatric nurse* (pp. 8–9). Baltimore: Williams & Wilkins.

Gries, M. L., and Fernsler, J. (1988). Patient perceptions of the mechanical ventilation experience. *Focus on Critical Care*, 15 (2), 52–59.

Groves, J. E., and Kucharski, A. (1987). Brief psychotherapy. In T. P. Hackett, and N. H. Cassem (Eds.), *Massachusetts General Hospital handbook of general hospital psychiatry* (p. 322). Littleton, MA: PSG Publishing.

Haft, J. I., and Arkel, Y. S. (1976). Effect of emotional stress on platelet aggregation in humans. *Chest*, 70, 501–505.

Hansell, H. N. (1984). The behavioral effects of noise on man: The patient with "intensive care unit psychosis." *Heart and Lung*, 13, 59–65.

Helton, M. C., Gordon, S. H., and Nunnery, S. L. (1980). The correlation between sleep deprivation and the intensive care unit syndrome. *Heart and Lung*, 9, 464.

Jacobson, S. F. (1983). An overview of coping. In S. F. Jacobson, and H. M. McGrath (Eds.), *Nurses under stress* (pp. 26–46). New York: John Wiley and Sons.

Jones, J., Hoggart, B., Withey, J., et al. (1979). What patients say: A study of reactions to an intensive care unit. *Intensive Care Medicine*, 5, 89–92.

Keily, W. F. (1972). Coping with severe illness. *Advances in Psychosomatic Medicine*, 8, 105–118.

King, K. B. (1985). Measurement of coping strategies, concerns, and emotional response in patients undergoing coronary bypass grafting. *Heart and Lung*, 14, 579–586.

Klein, R. F., Kliner V. A., and Zites, D. P. (1968). Transfer from a coronary care unit: Some adverse responses. *Archives of Internal Medicine*, 122, 104.

Kornfeld, D. S., Heller, S. S., Frank, K. A., et al. (1979). Personality and psychological factors in postcardiotomy delirium. *Archives of General Psychiatry*, 31, 249–253.

Krantz, D. S., and Glas, D. C. (1984). Personality, behavior patterns, and physical illness: Conceptual and methodological issues. In W. D. Gentry (Ed.), *Handbook of behavioral medicine* (pp. 38–86). New York: Guilford Press.

Larson, P. J. (1987). Comparison of cancer patients' and professional nurses' perceptions of important nurse caring behaviors. *Heart and Lung*, 16, 187–192.

Lazarus, R. S. (1966). *Psychological stress and the coping process*. New York: McGraw-Hill.

Lazarus, R. S., and Folkman, S. (1984). Coping and adaptation. In W. D. Gentry (Ed.), *Handbook of behavioral medicine* (p. 291). New York: Guilford Press.

Lazarus, R. S., and Folkman, S. (1984). *Stress, appraisal, and coping*. New York: Springer.

Leavitt, M. B. (1982). *Families at risk: Primary prevention in nursing practice*. Boston: Little, Brown.

Leininger, M. (1986). Care facilitation and resistance factors in the culture of nursing. *Topics in Clinical Nursing*, 8 (2), 1–12.

Lindquist, R. D. (1986). Providing patient opportunities to increase control. *Dimensions in Critical Care Nursing*, 5, 304–309.

Lock, S. E. (1982). Stress, adaptation and immunity: Studies in humans. *General Hospital Psychiatry*, 4, 49–58.

Lown, B., Regis, A. D., Reich, P., et al. (1980). Psychophysiologic factors in sudden cardiac death. *American Journal of Psychiatry*, 137, 1325–1335.

Lynch, J. J. (1977). *The broken heart*. New York: Basic Books.

Lynch, J. J., and Convey, W. H. (1979). Loneliness, disease, and death: Alternative approaches. *Psychosomatics*, 20, 702–708.

MacKellaig, J. M. (1987). A study of the psychological effects of intensive care with particular emphasis on patients in isolation. *Intensive Care Nursing*, 2, 176–185.

Marocchio, B. (1982). *Living while dying*. Bowie, MD: Robert J. Brady.

Mayer, D. K. (1986). Cancer patients' and families' perceptions of nursing care behaviors. *Topics in Clinical Nursing*, 8(2), 63–69.

Melville, S. B. (1987). Relaxation techniques in acute myocardial infarction: The theoretic rationale. *Focus on Critical Care,* 14 (1), 9–11.

Miller, B. K. (1985). Teaching biofeedback techniques in critical care. *Dimensions of Critical Care Nursing,* 4, 314–318.

Minarik, P., and Leavitt, M. (1988). The angry, demanding, hostile response. In B. Reigel, and D. Ehrenreich (Eds.), *Psychological aspects of critical care nursing.* Rockville, MD: Aspen Press.

Moos, R. H., and Tsu, V. S. (1979). The crisis of physical illness: An overview. In R. Moos (Ed.), *Coping with physical illness.* New York: Plenum Medical Book.

Murray, G. B. (1987). Confusion, delirium, and dementia. In T. P. Hackett, and N. H. Cassem (Eds.), *Massachusetts General Hospital handbook of general hospital psychiatry.* Littleton, MA: PSG Publishing.

Nyamathi, A. (1987). Coping response of spouses of MI patients and of hemodialysis patients as measured by the Jalowiec Coping Scale. *Journal of Cardiovascular Nursing,* 2, 67–74.

Pollock, S. E. (1984). The stress response. *Critical Care Quarterly,* 6 (4), 1–14.

Puntillo, K. A. (1988). The phenomenon of pain and critical care nursing. *Heart and Lung,* 17, 262–271.

Radwin, L. E. (1987). Autonomous nursing interventions for treating the patient in acute pain: A standard. *Heart and Lung,* 16, 258–265.

Redding, J. S., Hargest, T. S., and Minsky, S. H. (1977). How noisy is intensive care? *Critical Care Medicine,* 5, 275.

Reimaen, D. J. (1986). Noncaring and caring in the clinical setting: Patients' descriptions. *Topics in Clinical Nursing,* 8 (2), 30–36.

Riehl, J. P., and Roy, C. (1974). *Conceptual models for nursing practice.* New York: Appleton-Century-Crofts.

Ruberman, W., Weinblatt, E., Goldberg, J. D., et al. (1983). Education, psychosocial stress and sudden cardiac death. *Journal of Chronic Diseases,* 36, 151.

Ruberman, W., Weinblatt, E., Goldberg, J. D., et al. (1984). Psychosocial influences on mortality after myocardial infarction. *New England Journal of Medicine,* 311, 552.

Sadler, P. D. (1979). Nursing assessment of postcardiotomy delirium. *Heart and Lung,* 8, 745–750.

Scott, D. W., Oberst, M. T., and Dropkin, M. J. (1980). A stress-coping model. *Advances in Nursing Science,* 3 (1), 9–23.

Schwartz, L. P., and Brenner, Z. R. (1979). Critical care unit transfer: Reducing stress through nursing interventions. *Heart and Lung,* 8, 540.

Selye, H. (1956). *The stress of life.* New York: McGraw-Hill.

Sinclair, V. (1988). High technology in critical care: Implications for nursing's role and practice. *Focus on Critical Care,* 15 (4), 36–41.

Stanton, B. A., Jenkins, D., Savageau, J. A., et al. (1984). Perceived adequacy of patient education and fears and adjustments after cardiac surgery. *Heart and Lung,* 13, 525–530.

Sutherland, S. (1988). Burned adolescents' descriptions of their coping strategies. *Heart and Lung,* 17, 150–157.

Syme, S. L. (1984). Sociocultural factors in disease etiology. In W. D. Gentry (Ed.), *Handbook of behavioral medicine* (pp. 13–37). New York: Guilford Press.

Topf, M. (1984). A framework for research on aversive physical aspects of the environment. *Research in Nursing and Health,* 7, 35.

Toth, J. C. (1980). Effect of structured preparation for transfer on patient anxiety on leaving coronary care unit. *Nursing Research,* 29, 28.

Vaillant, G. E. (1976). Theoretical hierarchy of adaptive ego mechanisms. *Archives of General Psychiatry,* 24, 535–545.

Visintainer, M. A. (1986). The nature of knowledge and theory in nursing. *Image,* 18 (2), 32–38.

Watkins, L. O., Weaver, L., and Odegaard, V. (1986). Preparation for cardiac catheterization: Tailoring the content of instruction to coping style. *Heart and Lung,* 15, 382–389.

Weisman, A. D. (1987). Coping with illness. In T. P. Hackett, and N. H. Cassem (Eds.), *Massachusetts General Hospital handbook of general hospital psychiatry.* Littleton, MA: PSG Publishing.

Wilson, T. A. (1988). Nursing megatrends induced by diagnosis-related groups. *Focus on Critical Care,* 15 (3), 55–61.

Woods, N. F., and Falk, S. A. (1974). Noise stimuli in the acute care area. *Nursing Research,* 23, 144.

Zimmerman, L. M., Pierson, M. A., and Marker, J. (1988). Effects of music on patient anxiety in coronary care units. *Heart and Lung,* 17, 560–566.

7

Psychosocial Needs of Families

Mairead Hickey

Most people are members of a family. The purpose of the family is to provide an environment that supports and meets the needs of family members. Family members are bound by affection, loyalty, caring, and trust. They have the capacity to assume new roles and adjust the basic family structure as necessary to meet the needs of individual family members.

When a family member experiences a crisis, the family actively helps the member in need. Thus, when a family member is critically ill and is hospitalized, the family feels responsible for helping the ill person. It is ironic, however, that during a critical illness and hospitalization of a family member, the family is usually physically separated from the sick family member. During hospitalization, families are ambivalent; on the one hand, they are relieved that the loved one is receiving the best care possible, but on the other hand, they sense a loss of control over what is happening to their sick family member.

Families' functional abilities are threatened by the critical illness of a family member. Families must rely on their internal and external supports and resources to maintain or restore their equilibrium during the crisis of critical illness. The health care system provides the supports and resources to help the critically ill patient during a crisis, but who helps the family at this time?

This chapter will use crisis theory as a framework for building an understanding of what families experience during the critical illness of a family member. Research that has been conducted on the needs of families of critically ill patients will be reviewed and will serve as the basis for suggestions for an intervention plan for families of critically ill patients. One primary nursing diagnosis will be addressed throughout the chapter, that of potential ineffective family coping.

FAMILY THEORY

The family has been defined in a traditional sense as a small social system made up of individuals related to each other by strong reciprocal affection and loyalties and comprising a permanent "household" that persists over years and decades. Members enter the family through birth, adoption, or marriage and leave only through death (Terkelsen, 1980).

This definition is no longer adequate when considering families in the modern industrialized world. Modern families are characterized by their small size, lack of roots, flexible structure, and geographic distance from the nuclear family. Members of a modern family must often rely on family members *not* bound by marriage, birth, or adoption to provide the support that was once considered solely within the role of the traditional family. The definition of the modern family should include the interactive and supportive nature of members within the family unit; however, membership in a family should not be limited by relationships formed by blood, adoption, or marriage.

The *structure* of the modern family is flexible and changes as new members enter and old members leave or as members' roles and responsibilities change. The underlying *function* or *purpose* of the family remains constant as its structure changes. The purpose of the family is to adjust and change as necessary to support the survival and developmental needs of members while maintaining the identity of the family (Epperson, 1977). When the family structure changes to meet the needs of members, the family's equilibrium is threatened, and the family structure is vulnerable to crisis states. The family's ability to maintain its equilibrium during change is dependent upon how well the family can realistically interpret the situation, utilize the available resources and supports, and employ coping behaviors.

CRISIS THEORY

Individuals normally function in a state of equilibrium. They maintain this state by using appropriate coping behaviors and problem-solving techniques to meet their needs. In a state of crisis, these normal coping behaviors and problem-solving techniques are no longer effective enough to maintain equilibrium (Rapoport, 1969). This situation is different from that of a noncrisis state, in which individuals are able to use coping behaviors successfully to deal with the problems at hand.

Caplan (1964) defined *crisis* as an upset in a steady state. It occurs when people face obstacles that threaten their life goals and that are insurmountable through utilization of their customary coping mechanisms and problem-solving techniques (Aguilera and Messick, 1982). More specifically, crisis is a result of three interrelated circumstances. First, a hazardous event which poses a threat to an individual or family must exist. Second, the hazardous event is perceived by an individual or family as similar to other prior events that caused conflict. Third, the individual's or family's normal coping mechanisms are ineffective in dealing with the threat (Rapoport, 1969).

According to Caplan (1964), there are four phases in a crisis. Initially, individuals experience a rise in tension associated with unusual and perhaps disorganized behavior when routine problem-solving techniques are employed. In the second phase, more tension and discomfort are felt as coping behaviors are found to be unsuccessful. There is a further increase in tension that seems to mobilize additional internal or external resources in the third phase. In the fourth phase, if the threat persists, individuals face more disorganization or further crisis. During each phase, individuals attempt to restore equilibrium by employing coping behaviors to deal with the imposed threat.

In her studies on families in crises, Epperson (1977) identified six phases that families go through before they can reorganize and restore equilibrium. Phase one, *high anxiety,* is characterized by acute physical anxiety such as physical agitation, fainting, tightened muscles, and gastrointestinal upset. This phase may last from a few minutes to several hours. *Denial* is exhibited in phase two and serves as a coping behavior that softens any bad news that the family may receive. Usually this phase lasts until the time the family sees the patient. The third phase comprises *anger* on the part of families, followed by *guilt and sorrow* in the fourth phase. Families are saddened by the tragedy and feel guilty that they did not do something to prevent it. *Grief* is experienced in the fifth phase when families sense the impending loss of their family member that may result from the

critical illness. In the sixth and last phase *reconciliation* takes place after families have gone through the earlier phases and are ready to cope with and adapt to the stress at hand.

Not all individuals or families, when faced with the same stressful event, will be in crisis. However, some events that typically precipitate crisis states for most people are death, critical illness, or other situations that trigger grief and bereavement (Rapoport, 1969). When crises do occur they can be self-limiting, lasting anywhere from 4 to 6 weeks (Caplan, 1964). During crises, individuals seek resolution and will eventually resume functioning at the same level or at a higher or lower level than that existing before the crisis event.

The high tension and anxiety states of crises often cause individuals to feel helpless, hopeless, and powerless. They are easily confused and unable to concentrate on details. Their perceptions of reality and normal daily events may even be distorted. Rapoport (1969) suggested, however, that growth can occur during this period of confusion and disorganization. Crises may be the catalysts for people or families to change old behaviors and adopt new ones. People may also be more receptive to therapeutic intervention during crisis situations than during noncrisis periods.

Types of Crises

There are certain inevitable events in the course of our lives that can be described as hazardous enough to generate crises. These events can be classified into two categories, situational crises and maturational crises. *Situational crises* result from stressful events that are unexpected, occur without warning, and threaten the individual's equilibrium. Accidents, physical illness, bankruptcy, and divorce are examples of potential situational crises. They require immediate adjustment responses to restore equilibrium. *Maturational crises,* on the other hand, are considered normal processes of growth and development and occur at specific times in life; examples are birth, marriage, adolescence, and death. Maturational crises usually evolve over time and allow gradual adjustment by the individual over time. Although usually not disrupted, the individual's equilibrium is also vulnerable during maturational crises.

Duvall (1967) identified specific stages in a family's growth and development when the family potentially faces maturational crises. Table 7–1 outlines these stages. During any of these stages, the equilibrium of the family may be disrupted if the family members do not have the coping behaviors and problem-solving techniques necessary to adapt to these developmental demands. If a situational crisis occurs during a maturational crisis, family equilibrium will be greatly threatened.

TABLE 7–1. Eight Stages of Family Life Cycle When Maturational Crises Are Imminent

1. Beginning families (married couple without children)
2. Childbearing families (oldest child, birth to 30 months)
3. Families with preschool children (oldest child, 30 months to 6 years)
4. Families with school children (oldest child, 6 to 13 years)
5. Families with teenagers (oldest child, 13 to 20 years)
6. Families as launching centers (first child gone to last child leaving home)
7. Families in the middle years (empty nest to retirement)
8. Aging families (retirement to death of both spouses)

Adapted from Duvall, E. M. (1967). *Family development.* Philadelphia: J. B. Lippincott.

Factors Affecting the Family's Vulnerability to Crisis

A family's vulnerability to crises is determined by three factors. These factors are the family's perception of the event, their available situational supports, and the type and availability of their coping mechanisms (Aguilera and Messick, 1982).

Perception of the Event. If the event is perceived realistically, there is a realistic awareness of it, and the associated feelings of stress are usually appropriate. Coping behaviors and problem-solving strategies will probably ameliorate the effect of the threat. If the event is perceived unrealistically, however, coping and problem-solving techniques will probably be ineffective. Critical care nurses have a responsibility to provide family members with the information necessary to understand the situation at hand realistically.

For example, consider Mr. Smith, who was admitted to the coronary care unit with the diagnosis of an anterior myocardial infarction. His family received information about his condition, and as a result, their perceptions of his diagnosis and hospitalization were accurate. When families perceive the crisis situation accurately, they usually employ coping mechanisms that help them function during the crisis and restore equilibrium. When families perceive a crisis situation inaccurately, they employ coping mechanisms that are not appropriate for the crisis at hand and as a result will have difficulty in restoring their equilibrium.

Situational Supports. Throughout life, individuals and families use a variety of situational supports to maintain or restore equilibrium. Situational supports refer to those persons, places, or things in the environment that assist individuals or families to solve the problems at hand. The availability and quality of situational supports, as well as the ways in which individuals use them during stressful events, will affect how well individuals or families cope during a crisis. Critical care nurses must assist family members to find and utilize adequate situational supports and coping behaviors during crises.

Again, in the example of Mr. Smith, the Smith family routinely utilized the services of clergy when they faced crisis situations. If this situational support were not available to Mr. Smith's family, they would have to find and use other situational supports, which may not be as effective in helping them deal with the crisis.

Coping Mechanisms. Coping mechanisms differ from person to person and from family to family. Most individuals and families have a limited repertoire of coping behaviors from which to draw during stressful situations. If a coping behavior that had always been successful in the past is no longer effective, new coping behaviors will need to be utilized to thwart the crisis. Equilibrium is greatly threatened when the coping behavior employed is unsuccessful in helping individuals deal with the crisis.

Crisis Intervention

Crisis intervention refers to the process whereby health professionals mediate the crisis situation by assisting the individual or family to mobilize those coping behaviors and situational supports that will help them deal with the threat at hand. Crisis intervention is aimed at resolving the immediate crisis and restoring individuals to their precrisis level of function (Aguilera and Messick, 1982).

There are many strategies or techniques that can be considered as crisis interventions. Caplan (1964) suggested the following process of crisis intervention:

1. Assess the individual or family in crisis and offer help.
2. Help the individual or family choose healthy coping behaviors by providing them with accurate, reality-based information about the crisis situation.
3. Support the individual or family during their negative, nonproductive feelings.
4. Encourage the individual or family to communicate with family, friends, and professionals if they need to ventilate their feelings and concerns.
5. Provide anticipatory guidance so that the individual or family will learn from this experience and will be better prepared to deal with similar situations in the future.

Aguilera and Messick (1982) also identified four basic steps in the crisis intervention process that resemble the steps of the nursing process:

1. Assess the individual or family and their problem.
2. Plan a therapeutic intervention.
3. Implement the therapeutic intervention.
4. Assess the resolution of the crisis and provide anticipatory guidance.

Regardless of which strategy is employed, the essential message is that individuals and families often need assistance to restore their equilibrium during a crisis. The critical care nurse has an integral role in identifying families in crisis and in planning and providing or coordinating the interventions necessary to resolve the crisis.

CRITICAL ILLNESS AS A CRISIS FOR THE FAMILY

Since the family unit is the sum of its members, when one member becomes critically ill, the whole family is affected. Critical illness threatens the family's most basic function, the support of the basic survival needs of family members. Families react automatically to the critical illness of a family member in a manner that will be least disruptive and upsetting to the family's structure and the sick family member. They employ a variety of coping behaviors to alleviate the crisis of critical illness (Herz, 1980).

Critical Illness As a Crisis

Rapoport (1969) identified critical illness as a hazard that would almost inevitably induce a crisis state in families regardless of their coping skills. When family members are critically ill, families may be immobilized by panic, shock, helplessness, or disbelief (Braulin et al., 1982; Gardner and Stewart, 1978; Skelton and Dominian, 1973). Families often feel anxiety about the prognosis of the patient along with guilt and resentment about the effect of the critical illness on their structure and function.

Hospitalization of a critically ill family member is stressful for the entire family. First, the critical care environment with its sights, smells, and sounds provides a source of discomfort for the family. The sight of a critically ill family member, often unresponsive and connected to many tubes and machines, is overwhelming for families (Miles and Carter, 1982; Roberts, 1976; Williams and Rice, 1977). Another aspect that is stressful for families is the fact that they must depend on strangers to care for their loved one. Gardner and Stewart (1978) suggested that families see themselves as helpless and powerless and unable to help the patient during this time.

Families rely on receiving frequent informative reports about their loved one and become distressed by poor communication with staff (Miles and Carter, 1982). Information and communication contribute to the realism with which families perceive the illness of their family member. Since families do not process information well during crises, they have difficulty in comprehending information that is highly technical or is presented too rapidly.

Another factor that may be stressful to families is the way critical illness and hospitalization affect their ability to function. As Breu and Dracup (1978) described in their study of interventions to help spouses of critically ill patients, drastic role reversals by wives of myocardial infarction patients contributed to an intense sense of loss and stress.

Considering the family's feelings of helplessness and powerlessness during the critical illness of a family member, it is not surprising that they have a heightened need to be with or near the patient. Visiting policies and practices that restrict the frequency and length of time families can visit their sick relative also contribute to the stressfulness of the event.

Family's Response to Critical Illness

Hill (1969) separated the family's reaction to critical illness into three phases. An initial period of denial is usually followed by a period of cognitive confusion, anxiety, and even resentment toward the sick member, leading eventually to a period of recovery and reorganization. Mailick (1979) also suggested that critical illness can be divided into three phases, during which the family must master certain tasks by utilizing coping behaviors. The first set of tasks is associated with the onset of illness, the *diagnostic phase;* the second set of tasks is associated with *adjustment and adaptation* to the critical illness and its potential long-term effects; and the last task deals with the *resolution of the event* through either cure, remission, or death (Table 7–2).

Diagnostic Phase. Families must employ various coping behaviors to deal with the period of uncertainty when a diagnosis is being formulated. They face the fears and fantasies of not knowing what may be wrong and guilt about not being able to help the sick family member. During this time families may respond to crisis with poor communication skills, decreased productivity and creativity, and disorganized behavior.

Adjustment and Adaptation Phase. When the diagnostic phase ends and the family has dealt with its demands, they must then deal with the tasks associated with the potential long-term effects of the critical illness of a family member. New coping behaviors may or may not need to be employed during

---

TABLE 7–2. Three Phases of Hospitalization for Families of Critically Ill Patients

1. Diagnostic phase
2. Adjustment and adaptation phase
3. Resolution of the critical illness phase

Data from Mailick (1979).

this phase. Families must deal with their feelings of powerlessness, fear, guilt, and ambivalence, which are associated with the patient's suffering and pain. They must also learn how to deal with the attitudes and behaviors of health care workers and often must learn to assume an active role in planning any future care for the patient (Moos and Tsu, 1977). Family members strive to create a partnership with the health care team at this time. Another task for families during this phase is managing any role shifts that occur or may need to occur so that the responsibilities, once assumed by the sick member, will be reassigned within the family (Mailick, 1979).

Resolution of the Event. The cessation of illness may occur as a result of cure, remission, or death. If cure is experienced, families will strive to reassume their pre-illness function. In death, families will need to "work through" the loss. They may have difficult tasks to master during remission when they face the ambivalence of the joy associated with remission along with the fear of recurrence. They need to open themselves to the patient while realizing this may be only a temporary effort.

Some families, however, are unable to cope with the stress of critical illness. They may be overwhelmed by the threat to their equilibrium and may employ coping mechanisms that do not support the overall function of the family. The degree to which critical illness will disrupt family equilibrium will depend on many factors: the family's stage in the life cycle, the nature of the illness, the openness of the family, the family's perception of the event, the situational supports available and utilized by the family, and the coping mechanisms utilized by the family (Herz, 1980; Barrett, 1974) (Table 7–3).

The Stage of the Family in the Life Cycle. Families have different goals and expectations during different stages of their life cycles. For example, the critical illness of an elderly family member who has already achieved his personal goals and met his family responsibilities would cause less disruption for the family than the illness of a family member who is in the prime of life and holds a major role within the family structure. Critical illness may be more expected and accepted in the later phases of the life cycle and may cause less disruption than in the earlier phases. Although children have very little responsibility in the family unit, their illness may cause

---

TABLE 7–3. Factors That Affect Families' Susceptibility to Crisis During Critical Illness

> Family's stage in life cycle
> Nature of critical illness
> Openness of the family system
> Family's perception of the critical illness
> Availability to family of situational supports
> Coping mechanisms used by family

Data from Herz, 1980; Barrell, 1974.

---

serious familial disruption because children are often viewed as emotional extensions of the parents (Herz, 1980).

The Nature of Critical Illness. Critical illness can be sudden or expected and may or may not include periods of exacerbations and remissions. Both sudden and expected critical illnesses have the potential to disrupt the family structure and function. A critical illness with a sudden onset gives the family little or no time to prepare for the crisis. Families often experience shock and disbelief on hearing the news of a sudden illness, and disorganization in family structure and function may follow. Expected and long-term critical illness, on the other hand, usually contributes to fewer feelings of shock and disbelief and to more emotional and physical exhaustion among family members. Both types of critical illness pose threats to the family and require major adjustments and the use of familiar coping behaviors to restore equilibrium.

The Openness of the Family System. Family members who are able to express their thoughts and feelings to each other and yet stay nonreactive to the emotional intensity of the situation appear to do best during crises. However, if crisis situations persist over time, it is difficult for any family to stay nonreactive in the face of long-term stress (Herz, 1980).

Perceptions of the Event and Situational Supports. As mentioned earlier, the family's ability to perceive the situation realistically and employ situational supports affects the amount of disequilibrium they will experience during a crisis.

Coping Behaviors. Families may employ a variety of coping behaviors during the critical illness of a family member. Although they may seem unusual to an unrelated observer, these behaviors are usually essential to the family's success in maintaining or restoring equilibrium. Coping behaviors allow the family to repress the excessive threats of a situation and focus on what can be mastered (Murphy et al., 1962). Some coping behaviors frequently employed by families of critically ill patients are initial immobilization, withdrawal, focusing, intellectualization, and sensitivity toward self (Lewandowski, 1980; Sedgewick, 1975).

Initial Immobilization. Sometimes, when first seeing a hospitalized critically ill patient, family members may appear immobilized as they stand at the foot of the sick relative's bed. This is a strategy that enables family members to "defuse" the initial impact of the situation, allowing them to mobilize their internal resources to provide support to the critically ill family member. Immobilization is employed initially when visiting a critically ill family member; it is rarely utilized on subsequent visits.

Withdrawal. Family members may need to "withdraw" emotionally or physically from the crisis of

TABLE 7–4. Families' Coping Behaviors and Reactions to Critical Illness

Initial immobilization
Withdrawal
Focusing
Intellectualization
Sensitivity toward self
Reduced ability to concentrate and utilize incoming information
Reduced ability to make decisions and solve problems
Decreased sense of personal effectiveness
Decreased sensitivity to or awareness of the environment

Data from Lewandowski, 1980; Sedgwick, 1975.

the critical illness of a family member in order to maintain their equilibrium. Withdrawal is not usually an effective long-term coping behavior because the individuals using it literally remove themselves from the situation at hand without applying any problem-solving techniques to the crisis. If withdrawal is employed over the long term, family members will not deal well with the crisis because they will not see or use the supports necessary to alleviate the crisis.

Focusing. Family members may "focus" on something other than the critically ill patient because it may be easier to focus on equipment or a piece of bed linen that needs changing than to deal with the patient and his serious condition and unstable prognosis. Focusing allows family members to control the amount of information about the patient they deal with at any given time.

Intellectualization. Intellectualization occurs when family members direct their attention toward objective "facts" about the patient's status rather than toward subjective knowledge of the patient's experiences or feelings. When employing intellectualization, family members seek and discuss information about such things as the date of surgery, the length of the surgical procedure, or how long the patient's situation should last; information that is more sensory in nature is avoided.

Sensitivity Toward Self. In the presence of a relative's critical illness, family members may direct their attention inward toward themselves and their own needs. When visiting their critically ill family member, they may become preoccupied with their own ailments. Although this may appear to be an insensitive reaction, it may provide family members with enough diversion to restore and maintain their equilibrium.

Families' Reactions to Critical Illness. In addition to these coping behaviors, families experience different reactions to critical illness, as listed in Table 7–4. These reactions are typical reactions to any stressful situation. Families usually have a *reduced ability to concentrate and utilize incoming information.* They also have a *decreased ability to make decisions and solve problems.* At a time when they are usually inundated with information about the patient, the critical care

unit, and the upcoming tests and procedures and are required to make decisions that may seriously affect the lives of both the patient and themselves, they may be least equipped to do so.

Family members also report a *decreased sense of personal effectiveness* and feel a loss of control in their family member's experience. They would benefit by helping the patient in some way, perhaps by rubbing his back or feeding him (Molter, 1976; Daley, 1984). As family members confront the critical illness of a family member, they also experience a *decreased sensitivity to or awareness of the environment.* This may explain why they may be found standing in the hallway blocking the normal traffic flow in the critical care unit, or why they may "camp out" in the waiting room, apparently insensitive to the needs of other families waiting there.

These coping behaviors and normal responses to stress provide insight into the reasons why families of critically ill patients behave the way they do during the crisis of critical illness. It is important that nurses *understand* these behaviors rather than *judge* them as appropriate or inappropriate because it is usually these coping behaviors and responses to stress that help families restore equilibrium. Only if a behavior is obviously detrimental to the patient, family, or other patients and their families should it be modified with the help and support of the nursing staff.

NEEDS OF FAMILIES OF CRITICALLY ILL PATIENTS

In addition to many anecdotal reports that address the nature of crisis in critical illness for families and their responses to it, several empiric studies have described or explored the needs of families of critically ill patients (Bedsworth, 1982; Bouman, 1984; Boykoff, 1986; Breu and Dracup, 1978; Brown, 1976; Chavez and Faber, 1987; Daley, 1984; Dracup and Breu, 1978; Fuller and Foster, 1982; Geary, 1974; Gilliss, 1984; Hampe, 1975; Hentinen, 1983; Leske, 1986; Mayou, 1978; Molter, 1979; Mongiardi et al, 1987; Norris and Grove, 1986; Nyamathi, 1987; Pike, 1984; Rodgers, 1983; Stillwell, 1984; Williams, 1978). These studies have reported common themes that were consistently identified by families as their needs during the critical illness of family members (Table 7–5). The themes are the need for hope, the need for information, the need to be with the patient, the

TABLE 7–5. Needs of Families of Critically Ill Patients

For hope
For information
To be with the patient
To be helpful to the patient
To believe hospital personnel care about the patient
Personal needs

need to be helpful to the patient, the need to believe that personnel care about the patient, and the personal needs of family members.

The Need for Hope

The importance of the need for *hope* has been consistently emphasized by families during the critical illness of a family member. During a crisis, when individuals sense a loss of control over the situation, hopelessness is a common reaction. The term "hope," however, has not been defined in these studies, and therefore nurses can only surmise how families interpreted hope in these reports. Family members may interpret hope as a "hope" that the sick relative will get better. This interpretation may contribute to an unmet need if the ill person's condition does not improve.

If, however, hope reflects a more spiritual notion that fate is not predetermined and that the patient's emotional and physiologic responses to critical illness are influenced by the care that is provided, then the word hope may refer to the family's hope that the patient is comfortable during the illness, that he is receiving the best possible care, and that either a comfortable recovery or death will follow. Critical care nurses can foster this sense of hope in families of critically ill patients by assuring them that patients are receiving the best possible care. Nurses who demonstrate sensitivity and caring and who respect the patients' best interests may also provide a sense of hope to families.

The Need for Information

Families repeatedly identified the need for information about their family member's condition as very important. At a time when families feel physically isolated from their sick relative, information provides them with a sense of control and may relieve some of their anxieties. It is essential that families have realistic perceptions of the illness so that they can employ the coping behaviors necessary to restore their equilibrium.

Family members are not necessarily selective in the information they seek about their loved one. They want any information they can acquire. Their interests range from information about the diagnosis and prognosis to more trivial information about how the patient ate or slept. Family members often feel guilty because they are not able to provide care for the patient. They may believe that if they stay informed about their relative's condition, they are indirectly providing care by evaluating whether he is progressing as they believe he should.

Research has reported that family members want honest, current information. They do not want to be surprised by a change in their relative's condition when they visit, and they do not want to fear that information is being withheld from them. They actively solicit information about the patient from anyone who can provide it. They may also actively seek information from many sources until they receive indications that realistically or unrealistically suggest that the patient is improving (Roberts, 1976).

Although family members seek and often seem even to demand information, their ability to comprehend and process it is usually impaired because of the emotional and cognitive disruption that results from their crisis situation. For this reason, it is important to provide information that is simple and nontechnical. Written information about routine hospital services and unit policies is usually an appropriate method of communication because family members can read this information when they are emotionally and cognitively ready to do so.

Nurses may find it helpful to establish family representatives who can be contacted at least daily with information about the patient. The family representative will then communicate with the rest of the family, decreasing the number of family members inquiring about the patient's general condition.

The Need to Be with the Patient

Family members also report a need to be with the patient, especially during the admission and diagnosis phases of hospitalization. They are usually not prepared for this unfamiliar experience and receive more comfort by seeing their relative in person than by relying on reports from staff who are strangers to both the patient and the family.

When family members are in crisis, they do not always think clearly, and if they are not permitted to see their sick relative they may imagine a scenario far worse than the one that really exists. Limited or infrequent visiting policies such as 10 minutes per hour or two to three visits per day may lead to more anxiety and more confusion within the family. Since family visits are usually beneficial to both patients and families, traditional restrictive visiting practices during the crisis of critical illness should be exchanged for more lenient policies.

It is important to assess the patient's and family's physiologic and emotional responses to family visits to evaluate the risk-benefit ratio of family visits for the patient and family. It must be remembered, however, that the patient is a member of the family and as such is able to deal with and even receive comfort from the family's behavior during visits no matter how atypical such behavior may seem to the staff. As the patient's condition becomes more stable and as family members become more familiar with the staff and hospital routines, they may need to be with the patient less frequently than during the initial phase of hospitalization.

The Need to Be Helpful

It is not surprising that families need to believe they are helping their critically ill family member. Normally, during a crisis family members come to the aid of family members in need. However, during the crisis of critical illness, family members are usually unable to offer and provide the help they believe to be an important part of their role. This feeling of helplessness adds to their sense of ineffectiveness during crisis.

During a crisis, individuals have difficulty in mastering new or difficult tasks. Therefore, during the crisis of critical illness it is appropriate for family members to help patients with fairly simple routine tasks that are important to the patient. Family members can be taught or encouraged to feed the patient, wash his face, or turn his pillow. If the patient's condition stabilizes and if family members are able to master more difficult tasks, nurses can assess the feasibility of teaching family members to perform such tasks as administering backrubs, recording hourly drainage, or helping the patient change his position. Family members may need to be reminded that they are also contributing to the care of the patient by taking care of matters at home, coordinating attendance at family-staff meetings, and meeting with resources such as social services or chaplain services, which may assist the family to cope during the crisis.

The Need to Believe That Staff Care About the Patient

Family members are forced to relinquish their caring and supportive role when their critically ill family member is hospitalized. It is difficult for families to think that strangers are caring for their loved one. If they believe that the staff care and are genuinely concerned about their relative, they can deal with the hospitalization more easily. Although most nurses pride themselves on the way they care and assume an advocacy role for their patients, they may want to convey this message purposely to families to put families more at ease during the hospitalization.

Personal Needs of Family

Family members also have a need for emotional support during the critical illness of a family member. They do not perceive nursing staff as being responsible for helping them meet these needs, however, because they believe that nurses should direct their energies toward the care of patients. In light of these emotional needs, critical care nurses can assume the responsibility for assessing the adequacy of the family's ability to function during the crisis and for providing or coordinating the necessary services to help families restore their equilibrium.

NURSING RESPONSIBILITIES WITH FAMILIES OF CRITICALLY ILL PATIENTS

This chapter has identified the following major points:

- Families function primarily to support their members.
- Critical illnesses of family members may present a crisis situation for the family.
- Families respond to the crisis of critical illness by employing a variety of coping mechanisms to restore their equilibrium.
- The event of a critical illness can be divided into three distinct phases, each with specific needs and tasks for families.
- Family members have specific needs of their own during the critical illness of a loved one.

The first priority of nursing care must be directed toward meeting the most basic survival needs of the patient. The patient, however, even during a critical illness does not exist in a vacuum. He is still a member of a family, and he acts and reacts not only as an individual but also as a family member (Brandt, 1984).

In light of the major points reviewed in this chapter, the nursing diagnosis that most appropriately directs nursing care for families of critically ill patients throughout the entire hospitalization is "potential ineffective family coping related to the critical illness of a family member." The overall goal of this nursing diagnosis is that families, with the support of nursing and other support services, will employ the coping behaviors necessary to restore and maintain their equilibrium during the critical illness of a family member. To plan interventions for this diagnosis, nurses must first compile a family history from which individualized family plans can be formulated and implemented.

Family History

To assess, understand, and even predict the family's behavior during the crisis of critical illness, a comprehensive family history should be obtained to provide data about the structure and function of the family, its religious affiliations, previous coping behaviors during stressful situations, prior experiences with critical illness and hospitalization, and their

TABLE 7–6. Nursing Intervention Plan for Families of Critically Ill Patients

Nursing Diagnosis: Potential Ineffective Family Coping Related to the Critical Illness of a Family Member

Phase I: Admission to Hospital/Diagnostic Phase	Phase II: Adjustment/Adaptation Phase	Phase III: Resolution Phase

1. *Assess the family structure and function:*
  a. Obtain initial family history data
  b. Establish a temporary family contact person
	1. *Assess the family structure and function:*
	  a. Complete the family history
	  b. Assess the family's structure, function, and coping behaviors realizing they are essential to the family's restoration of equilibrium
	  c. Establish a family contact person
		1. *Assess the family structure and function:*
		  a. Assess the effectiveness of the family's role changes on family function
		  b. Evaluate staff-family communication patterns

2. *Provide* simple, nontechnical, essential *information* to the family about the patient's condition and what to expect to see and sense upon entering the critical care unit and seeing the ill person
Provide written information about:
  a. Visiting policies
  b. When and how to call the critical care unit about the patient's condition
  c. The name of the patient's nurse and doctor
  d. The location of the cafeteria, family waiting room, restrooms, and telephones
  e. Parking, food, and lodging in the hospital vicinity
	2. *Provide information* to the family about the patient's diagnosis, prognosis, and course of treatment to minimize their anxiety and to assist them to have a realistic perception of the critical illness of the family member
	  a. Contact a family member in person or by telephone at least once daily about the patient's condition and course of treatment
	  b. Inform family of available supports (financial, social, group, etc.)
	  c. Direct family to appropriate hospital departments (social services, clergy) as necessary
		2. *Provide information* to the family about the same items as in phases 1 and 2, community resources, financial services, and future course of treatment for patient
		  a. Predict, with family, the difficulties or probable events that may be encountered during resolution
		  b. Discuss realistic long-term goals for patient

3. Allow the *family to spend time* with the patient
  a. Assess the family's need to be with the patient and establish a visitation plan that meets the patient's and family's needs
  b. Accompany the family members to visit the patient
  c. Respect the coping behaviors and responses (immobilization, intellectualization, denial, focusing, etc.) of the family and intervene *only* if the behavior is detrimental to the family or patient
  d. Assist family members to be near or to touch the patient if they wish
  e. Encourage family members to talk to the patient
	3. Allow the *family to spend time* with the patient
	  a. Assess the patient's and family's needs for visitation
	  b. Provide visitation periods according to the patient's and family's needs
		3. Allow the *family to spend time* with the patient (as in phases 1 and 2)

4. Allow the *family to be helpful* to the patient by assuring the family that their visits will help the patient to be more comfortable in an unfamiliar environment	4. Allow the *family to be helpful* by suggesting small tasks that they may perform (if they wish) to make the patient comfortable (cool cloth on forehead; mouth care; feeding, etc.)	4. Allow the *family to be helpful* to the patient (as in phases 1 and 2)
		  a. Provide information so that families can participate in more patient care activities (if they wish)
		  b. Point out to the family how they are helping the patient

5. Provide *hope* for the family by explaining how the patient will be monitored closely and will receive highly skilled care in the critical care unit	5. Provide *hope* for the family
	  a. Continue to inform the family that the patient is receiving highly qualified care
	  b. If the patient's condition is improving, stress such improvement
	  c. If the patient's condition is very serious and probably will not improve, stress the care that *is* being provided to the patient
		5. Provide *hope* for the family as in phases 1 and 2

6. Convey the *staff's caring attitude* about the patient to the family
  a. Identify the nurse who will care for the patient
  b. Reassure the family that every measure will be taken to make the patient as comfortable as possible
  c. Convey the nurse's patient advocacy role to the family
	6. Convey the *staff's caring attitude* about the patient to the family as in phase 1	6. Convey the *staff's caring attitude* about the patient to the family as in phases 1 and 2

7. Support the *personal needs* of the family
  a. Respect the coping behaviors of the family
  b. Guide the family to make well-informed decisions about the patient and the family during the initial admission to the hospital. (This may include decisions about treatment for the patient; decisions about whether to contact other family members about the critically ill patient; decisions about whether to leave the hospital to get rest, etc.)
	7. Support the *personal needs* of the family
	  a. Respect the coping behaviors of the family
	  b. Allow family members to ventilate their emotions and concerns
	  c. Foster acceptance, comfort, and support from health professionals
	  d. Coordinate services of support personnel such as clergy, social service, etc.
	  e. Commend the family on their ability to function during this event
		7. Support the *personal needs* of the family as in phases 1 and 2

beliefs and values toward health and disease. Because of the crisis situation and the stress imposed on the family, it may be necessary to spread the collection of data for the family history over an extended period of time, perhaps during the first 48 hours after the patient's admission to the critical care unit. After these initial data are collected, periodic follow-up family assessments should be performed to evaluate how well the family is functioning.

Nursing Interventions

The nursing interventions for the nursing diagnosis "potential ineffective family coping related to the critical illness of a family member" should be specific for the individual family's needs and should focus on the needs of families during the three phases of the critical illness experience. Table 7–6 outlines the nursing interventions for this nursing diagnosis during the three phases of hospitalization.

SUMMARY

Nursing has made great strides during the past 15 years in acknowledging the role of families and their needs during the critical illness of a family member. Research reports and anecdotal accounts on the effect of critical illness on families provide a body of data from which nursing interventions for families of critically ill patients can be developed. If nurses expand their concept of the patient as an individual in a bed to that of a member of a family, they will expand their roles to assist families to cope and function during the critical illness of a family member (Craven and Sharp, 1972).

References

Aguilera, D. C., and Messick, J. M. (1982). *Crisis intervention, theory and methodology*. St. Louis: C. V. Mosby.
Barrett, L. M. (1974). Crisis intervention: Partnership in problem solving. *Nursing Clinics of North America*, 9 (1), 5–16.
Bedsworth, J. A., and Molen, M. T. (1982). Psychological stress in spouses of patients with myocardial infarctions. *Heart and Lung*, 11 (5), 450–456.
Bouman, C. C. (1984). Identifying priority concerns of families of ill patients. *Dimensions of Critical Care Nursing*, 3 (5), 313–319.
Boykoff, S. L. (1986). Visitation needs reported by patients with cardiac disease and their families. *Heart and Lung*, 15 (6), 573–578.
Brandt, M. A. (1984). Consider the patient part of a family. *Nursing Forum*, 21 (1), 12–23.
Braulin, J. L. D., Rook, J., and Sills, G. M. (1982). Families in crisis: The impact of trauma. *Critical Care Quarterly*, 5 (3), 38–46.
Breu, C., and Dracup, K. (1978). Helping the spouses of critically ill patients. *American Journal of Nursing*, 78 (1), 50–53.
Brown, A. J. (1976). Effect of family visits on the blood pressure and heart rate of patients in the coronary care unit. *Heart and Lung*, 5 (2), 291–296.
Caplan, G. (1964). *Principles of preventive psychiatry*. New York: Basic Books.
Chavez, C. W., and Faber, L. (1987). Effect of an education-orientation program on family members who visit their significant other in the intensive care unit. *Heart and Lung*, 16 (1), 92–99.
Craven, R., and Sharp, B. H. (1972). The effects of illness on family functions. *Nursing Forum*, 11 (2), 187–193.
Daley, L. (1984). The perceived immediate needs of families with relatives in the intensive care setting. *Heart and Lung*, 13 (2), 231–237.
Danis, M., Jarr, S., Southerland, L. I., et al. (1987). A comparison of patient, family, and nurse evaluations of the usefulness of intensive care. *Critical Care Medicine*, 15 (2), 138–143.
Dracup, K. A., and Breu, C. S. (1978). Using nursing research findings to meet the needs of grieving spouses. *Nursing Research*, 27 (4), 212–216.
Duvall, E. M. (1967). *Family development*. New York: J. B. Lippincott.
Epperson, M. M. (1977). Families in sudden crisis: Process and intervention in a critical care center. *Social Work in Health Care*, 2 (3), 265–273.
Fuller, B. F., and Foster, J. M. (1982). The effects of family/friend visits vs. staff interaction on stress/arousal of surgical intensive care patients. *Heart and Lung*, 11 (5), 457–463.
Gardner, D., and Stewart, N. (1978). Staff involvement with families of patients in critical care units. *Heart and Lung*, 7 (1), 105–110.
Geary, M. C. (1974). An exploratory study of families of seriously ill patients. Unpublished Master's Thesis, Yale University School of Nursing.
Gilliss, C. L. (1984). Reducing family stress during and after coronary artery bypass surgery. *Nursing Clinics of North America*, 19 (1), 103–112.
Hampe, S. D. (1975). Needs of the grieving spouse in a hospital setting. *Nursing Research*, 24 (2), 113–120.
Hentinen, M. (1983). Need for instruction and support of the wives of patients with myocardial infarction. *Journal of Advanced Nursing*, 8 (6), 519–524.
Herz, F. (1980). The impact of death and serious illness on the family life cycle. In E. A. Carter and M. McGoldrick (Eds.), *The family life cycle*. New York: Gardner Press.
Hill, R. (1969). Generic features of families under stress. In H. J. Parad (Ed.), *Crisis intervention*. New York: Family Service Association of America.
Leske, J. S. (1986). Needs of relatives of critically ill patients: A follow-up. *Heart and Lung*, 15 (2), 189–193.
Lewandowski, L. A. (1980). Stresses and coping styles of parents of children undergoing open-heart surgery. *Critical Care Quarterly*, 3 (1), 75–84.
Mailick, M. (1979). The impact of severe illness on the individual and family: An overview. *Social Work in Health Care*, 6, 117–128.
Mayou, R. (1978). The psychological and social effects of myocardial infarction on wives. *British Medical Journal*, 1, 699–701.
Miles, M. S., and Carter, M. C. (1982). Sources of parental stress in pediatric intensive care units. *Child Health Care*, 11 (2), 65–69.
Molter, N. C. (1979). Needs of relatives of critically ill patients: A descriptive study. *Heart and Lung*, 8 (2), 332–339.
Mongiardi, F., Payman, B. C., and Hawthorn, P. (1987). The needs of relatives of patients admitted to the coronary care unit. *Intensive Care Nursing*, 3, 67–70.
Moos, R., and Tsu, V. D. (1977). The crisis of physical illness: An overview. In R. Moos (Ed.), *Coping with physical illness*. New York: Plenum Medical Book.
Murphy, L. B., et al. (1962). *The widening world of childhood: Paths toward mastery*. New York: Basic Books.
Norris, L. O., and Grove, S. K. (1986). Investigation of selected psychosocial needs of family members of critically ill adult patients. *Heart and Lung*, 15 (2), 194–199.
Nyamathi, A. M. (1987). The coping responses of female spouses of patients with myocardial infarction. *Heart and Lung*, 16 (1), 86–92.
Pike, A. W. (1984). The effects of information about the intensive

care environment on the distress levels of families of critically ill patients. Unpublished Master's Thesis, Yale University School of Nursing.

Rapoport, L. (1969). The state of crisis: Some theoretical considerations. In H. J. Parad (Ed.), *Crisis intervention.* New York: Family Service Association of America.

Roberts, S. L. (1976). *Behavioral concepts and the critically ill patient.* Englewood Cliffs, NJ: Prentice-Hall.

Rodgers, C. D. (1983). Needs of relatives of cardiac surgery patients during the critical care phase. *Focus on Critical Care,* 10 (5), 50–55.

Sedgwick, R. (1975). Psychological responses to stress. *Journal of Psychiatric Nursing,* 13, 20–23.

Skelton, M., and Dominian, J. (1973). Psychological stress in wives of patients with myocardial infarction. *British Medical Journal,* 8, 101–103.

Stillwell, S. B. (1984). Importance of visiting needs as perceived by family members of patients in the intensive care unit. *Heart and Lung,* 13 (3), 238–242.

Terkelson, K. G. (1980). Toward a theory of the family life cycle. In E. A. Carter and M. McGoldrick (Eds.), *The family life cycle.* New York: Gardner Press.

Williams, A. (1978). Perceptions of nursing care: Effects of written and verbal instructional methods on families of head injury patients. *Heart and Lung,* 7 (2), 306–312.

Williams, C. C., and Rice, D. G. (1977). The intensive care unit: Social work intervention with families of critically ill patients. *Social Work in Health Care,* 2 (4), 391–398.

8

Psychosocial Needs of Critical Care Staff

Marty Nason

Intensive-care settings reveal humanity at its best and at its worst. This is as true for the staff as it is for the patients. We who serve in intensive-care settings in a true sense risk our own lives in these settings . . . our feelings, our self-esteem, our self-respect. By risking these daily we grow; by avoiding the risk we must face the dehumanization of ourselves or of our patients. It is a challenge too great to be borne alone.

(CASSEM AND HACKETT, 1975)

This chapter acknowledges the incredible complexity of the critical care system in which nurses find themselves and the impact upon the psyche of the critical care nurse (CCN). An analysis of the research performed, the views of experts in stress and burnout, and identification of the psychosocial needs of CCNs are presented. The latter half of this chapter deals with specific strategies to promote satisfaction of these needs.

STRESS

Stress Theory

Stress is not necessarily bad. It is an integral part of life. Major stress or crisis causes us to draw upon adaptive resources we never thought we had. We can gain strength from and *grow* from stress. We experience the growth of competence and the joy of triumph over adversity. Children who are protected from stress are more vulnerable to stress later because they have not learned coping skills that are needed for day-to-day living. A stress-free life could be very boring and have negative effects upon health. Indeed, people often seek stress, taking high risks such as mountain climbing and sky diving. Normal excite-

ment and pleasurable emotions may involve stress and tension and are often exhilarating. This type of stress (called eustress) is important and healthy provided that it is followed by a "relaxation rebound" that is, after being "wound up" the body returns to a normal level of functioning and does not carry tension beyond the time it is necessary.

Definitions of Stress

Experts have generated many definitions of stress. Selye, a pioneer in stress research, defined stress as "the nonspecific response of the body to any demand made upon it" (Selye, 1975). He found that during emergency situations the body reacts with a stress-alarm response by increasing the heart rate, muscle tension, blood pressure, and other physiologic changes that rally the body in preparedness for action. These reactions are helpful in crisis situations, but when the alarm response is maintained over a long time, a person's health can deteriorate.

One way of looking at stress has been in terms of "stressors" or stimuli. Events impinging upon a person (external stressors), include such things as interruptions and noise, whereas conditions arising within a person (internal stressors) include things such as hunger. Another approach is to view stress as change. Stressors may be changes affecting large numbers of persons such as floods, earthquakes, and war, or changes affecting one or a few persons such as the death of a loved one, life-threatening or incapacitating illness, being laid off from work, or divorce. Holmes and Rahe (1967) developed a social readjustment rating scale, which indicated that the total number of life changes is related to stress and the potential for becoming ill. Some researchers maintain that any change, positive or negative, is stressful.

Lazarus and Folkman (1984) expanded the definition of stress to include "daily hassles," those stressful experiences that arise from roles in daily living. Research now indicates that although daily hassles are far less dramatic than major changes in life such as divorce or bereavement, they may be even more important. For CCNs, daily hassles can be incomplete or illegible orders, lost laboratory values, a hostile and insecure physician or intern, visitors' demands, frequent phone interruptions, and malfunctioning or unavailable equipment.

Stressors arise from the physical environment, from social interactions, from organizations, and from our own self-talk. A small work space, no windows in a work area, traffic on freeways, and crowding are examples of *physical-environmental stressors*. *Social stressors* include angry or aggressive people, the need to give or receive negative feedback, ungrateful patients, and frightened and anxious families. Some *organizational stressors* are unclear role expectations and role conflict, interdisciplinary or interdepartmental conflicts, inadequate staffing, or unclear work priorities. Probably the most common contributor to stress resides not in the external environment but within the CCN. This "self-talk" refers to the self-imposed demands placed on ourselves in the form of "shoulds," "musts," "ought to's," and our own professional and personal "myths" or performance expectations (Steinmetz et al., 1980).

For this chapter, psychological stress is defined as *a relationship between the person and the environment that is appraised by the person as taxing or exceeding his or her resources and endangering his or her well-being* (Lazarus and Folkman, 1984).

PERCEIVED STRESS

Certain environmental demands and pressures seem to produce stress in everyone. But individuals differ in their sensitivity and vulnerability to certain types of events as well in their interpretations and reactions to them. For example, when confronted with a demanding patient, one person responds with anger, another with anxiety or guilt, and still others feel challenged rather than threatened. Likewise, one nurse handles an insult by ignoring it, another cries, and a third grows angry and plans revenge. To understand variations among individuals in comparable conditions, one must take into account the thinking (cognitive) processes that intervene between the encounter and the reaction.

Many CCNs believe that other people and the events in their lives cause them to feel the way they do. But how a CCN acts and feels depends on the way she *thinks* or talks to herself about the event (stressor). CCNs make a mental evaluation of how an event is going to affect them, whether it will be irrelevant, benign-positive, or stressful. A stressful appraisal can be one of *harm/loss, threat, or challenge.*

Harm/loss refers to the damage or loss a person has already sustained, threat refers to anticipated harm or loss, and challenge refers to events that hold the possibility for mastery or gain. Frequently, CCNs can judge an event to be both a threat and a challenge (Lazarus and Folkman, 1984).

In a study by Oskins (1979), 79 Intensive Care Unit (ICU) nurses rated 12 narratives as stressful or nonstressful and identified them as a challenge or a threat. All 12 narratives were seen as stressful, but the same events were seen as challenging by some nurses and as threatening by others. This discrepancy was explained by the fact that what each person feels depends on that individual's perception and appraisal of the situation, not on the situation itself. Stress is a personal response to a unique or personal interpretation of events. This concept implies that one way to manage stress is to change one's thinking or interpretation about an event. It can be "reframed" or interpreted in a different way. For example, a CCN can look at change as a chance to learn and grow—an opportunity, not a crisis. CCNs feel different when they view change as a catastrophe and when they see it as an opportunity. The difference in interpretation makes one feeling response unpleasant and the other pleasant.

Stressors for Critical Care Nurses

Studies of ICU nurses affirm that critical care units consistently present a highly stressful working environment for even the best-prepared CCN (Table 8–1). Some of these stresses include communication conflicts with physicians and nursing administrators, understaffing, heavy work load, constant threat of death or disability, personal insecurity, unpleasant sights and smells, and moral and ethical problems (Anderson and Basteyns, 1981; Gray-Toft and Anderson, 1983; Huckabay and Jagla, 1979; Jacobson, 1978; Hay and Oken, 1972; Duxbury et al., 1984; Keane et al., 1985; Stehle, 1981).

Notable research has been done by Claus and Bailey (1980). In a stress survey of 1794 ICU nurses they found that the major stressors, in order, were interpersonal conflict, management of the unit, nature of direct patient care, inadequate knowledge and skill, physical work environment, life events, and lack of rewards.

TABLE 8–1. Stresses for Critical Care Nurses

Conflicts with physicians
Conflicts with hospital or nursing administration
Inadequate staff or inadequate licensed staff
Moral and ethical dilemmas
Personal insecurity
Threat of patient morbidity and mortality
Inadequate knowledge or skill
Physical work environment
Lack of rewards
Interpersonal conflict

Claus and Bailey (1980) also found that nurse-physician problems were the most intense and frequently cited interpersonal stressors. These problems involved lack of a collegial relationship (e.g., disregard for nurses' opinions, suggestions, observations, and questions). Stress intensified when the nurse perceived that patient management was ineffective or incorrect. Nurses described being blamed for failing to inform physicians of pertinent facts, and being ignored or ridiculed for overstepping the boundaries of their role when they did inform them. Other stressors were incongruity of orders and conflicting communication lines when a patient had several physicians, unavailability of the physician, and being "caught in the middle" when the patient received inadequate information about the diagnosis or prognosis.

Interpersonal problems were abundant between nurses as well. Nurse-nurse problems consisted of continuous competition and lack of camaraderie between staff nurses of equal rank. Anxious new nurses must earn acceptance by their peers; nurses who ask too many questions are often viewed as incompetent. Nurse-supervisor problems caused additional stress rather than support because of a "bureaucratic value system" and inability of the immediate supervisor to provide positive feedback (Claus and Bailey, 1980).

Stressors identified by Claus and Bailey related to management of the unit included insensitivity of administration to the physical, emotional, or intellectual demands of the ICU as reflected by inadequate numbers of staff and incompetent or poorly trained staff and float nurses.

The nature of direct patient care, the third greatest source of stress described by Claus and Bailey, included emergencies and the constant potential for crisis, unnecessary prolongation of patients' lives, philosophical and moral dilemmas, inability to meet both the patient's and the family's psychological needs, and the death and dying of special patients (those perceived as having a good life potential or those to whom the nurse had become especially attached) and children. Numerous investigations have corroborated the findings of Claus and Bailey.

Contact with dying patients, people in pain, and people with a questionable quality of life (i.e., those on life-support machines for months at a time) is a threat to the nurse's own sense of body integrity and boundaries. Dying patients can arouse feelings about one's own death or the death of one's loved ones. The goals of providing patient comfort and dignity may be in conflict with the realities of providing highly technical care. CCNs are often involved in what Hay and Oken (1972) refer to as "intimacy with the frightening, repulsive, and forbidden."

Nurses are often the recipients of negative emotions felt by distraught and anxious patients and families. Families may want immediate answers to questions, may act out their fear, may be unable to accept limits, make frequent phone calls and visits, and are too anxious to "hear" explanations. These behaviors require a great deal of patience and un-derstanding to handle. Providing supportive care for them can be an added stressor for the nurse (Cassem and Hackett, 1975; Hay and Oken, 1972).

The research validating and delineating the stressors of critical care points to the need for CCNs to be experts in stress management. An examination of the various ways of conceptualizing stress has been presented. This information increases our understanding of stress, an initial step in managing it. Research into the concept of burnout provides additional information about the needs of CCNs.

BURNOUT

"Burnout" is a word used in space rocketry to refer to the moment when the rocket's fuel is exhausted and the engine's flame goes out. Storlie (1979) describes burnout as the "collapse of the human spirit." CCNs are vulnerable to burnout owing to the stressors that have been previously described. Investigations of burnout among CCNs have documented moderate degrees of burnout (Bartz and Maloney, 1986; Nason, 1988). The cost of burnout is high, affecting the individual CCN, the institution, and the patient. Awareness of the signs and symptoms of burnout will facilitate early identification of the existence of the problem and appropriate intervention. Signs and symptoms of burnout are listed in Table 8–2.

The Burnout Syndrome

Burnout is conceptualized by Maslach (1982) as "a syndrome of emotional exhaustion, depersonaliza-

---

TABLE 8–2. Signs and Symptoms of Burnout

Individual
Physical health
  Backache
  Upset stomach
  Nervousness
  Headache
  Fatigue
  Difficulty sleeping
  Loss of appetite
Mental health
  Hopelessness (and suicidal potential)
  Alcohol and prescription drug use
  Interpersonal conflict

Organizational
Absenteeism
High turnover
Intrastaff conflict
Declining work quality
Tardiness
Low morale
Requests for transfer
Declining productivity

Patient
Serious clinical mistakes
Patient neglect
Dehumanized care

Data from Jones, 1981; Pines, 1983.

tion, and reduced personal accomplishment that can occur among individuals who do 'people work' of some kind. It is a response to the chronic emotional strain of dealing extensively with other human beings, particularly when they are troubled or having problems." The unique feature of this type of job stress is that it arises from the social interaction between helper and recipient.

Central to burnout is a pattern of overinvolvement and a sense of being overwhelmed by the emotional demands of clients. The response to this is a feeling of *emotional exhaustion* or of feeling drained, used up, and without a source of replenishment (Maslach, 1982). Caregivers may achieve relief from emotional exhaustion by reducing their involvement with others. Contact with patients can become minimal. Detachment protects the caregiver from the strain of close involvement with others, but it can evolve into feelings of indifference to patients' needs and cold, impersonal administration of care, Development of this callous and dehumanized response is the second aspect of Maslach's concept of burnout, *depersonalization*. Depersonalization may be manifested by some individuals as a literal shutting out of other people, not only clients but also co-workers, friends, and family.

Negative feelings about clients and people in general can extend to one's feelings about oneself. This is characteristic of Maslach's third aspect of burnout, feelings of *reduced personal accomplishment*. Helpers feel guilty about the way they are treating clients, realizing that they are becoming cold and callous. A sense of inadequacy and failure ensues. Self-esteem is reduced, and depression may occur.

Individuals are more likely to attribute burnout to themselves if they feel that their reaction is unique and is not shared by others. There is often a tendency to hide one's true feelings and pretend that everything is all right. This facade leads others to conclude erroneously that they are alone in their distress. A downward spiral is set in motion. Feelings of failure lead to shame and further hiding of one's feelings. This isolation cuts one off from the potentially valuable support of peers. Lost are the benefits of validation of feelings and reality-testing that co-workers can provide.

Factors Contributing to Burnout

Maslach (1982) conceptualized burnout as a function of the stresses engendered by involvement with patients and family, by the job setting, and by personal characteristics. She cited work overload, role conflict, powerlessness, conflict between the real and the ideal, unrealistic expectations by self and others, lack of positive feedback, disproportionate focus on the negative, and lack of support and positive feedback from supervision and administration as some of the factors contributing to burnout. Additional factors are the stress engendered by work-

ing with patients and families with intense feelings and reactions to the threat of illness and hospitalization, the need to face death, and being the recipient of projected negative feelings. All of these factors described by Maslach are consistent with the stressors identified in the research of critical care nursing stress described earlier.

THE WORK SETTING AS A SOURCE OF BURNOUT

In addition to the stressors previously described, certain characteristics of the work setting contribute to burnout. Job settings that produce burnout are associated with *overload* (Maslach, 1982). This is a crucial factor today, as CCNs are challenged to work more effectively than ever with sicker patients and diminishing resources and support. Unremitting *intensity* of patient contact is another contributant to burnout. The more hours the nurse spends in direct, unrelieved contact with the patient, the greater the risk of burnout (Maslach, 1982).

When helpers lack a sense of *control* over the care they are providing, burnout is high. Lack of control can be due to rigid prescriptions about how a job is to be done or denial of input by staff on policies and decisions that directly affect them. Lack of control occurs when a person has no opportunity to take a break or leave a stressful situation; is given responsibility beyond his or her abilities; or feels forced to stay in a stressful, unpleasant situation for economic reasons.

In critical care situations, nurses frequently perceive their lack of control over the outcomes of their efforts to maintain life or to allow a peaceful death. The resulting helplessness contributes to a sense of anger and frustration and may promote feelings of failure and ineffectiveness.

Role conflict and unrealistic expectations are prevalent owing to the diverse opinions within and outside the profession about the nurse's role. There is a paradoxic expectation by both nurses and others that the CCN should maintain objectivity, sound judgment, and firmness and at the same time be professionally intimate, emotionally available, empathetic, patient, nurturing, and supportive.

PERSONAL CHARACTERISTICS AS A SOURCE OF BURNOUT

Individual factors determine how each person handles sources of emotional stress and help to explain why one person experiences burnout in a particular work setting while another does not. Demographic data reveal that men and women are fairly similar in their experience of burnout. Burnout is greatest for younger people and tends to develop within the first 2 years of practice. The burnout-prone person appears to be characterized by nonassertiveness, difficulty in setting limits, lack of self-confidence, dependence upon others for validation of worth, and a

TABLE 8–3. Psychosocial Needs of Staff

Balance between eustress and negative stress
Perception of control over one's work and work environment
Fulfilling roles or relationships in addition to the role as a critical
    care nurse
Expression and validation of negative feelings that arise as a
    result of the nature of critical care nursing
A well developed sense of "child"—and ability to play and see
    humor in situations
Separation between work and personal life
Recognition from patients, peers, institutions, and other
    members of the health care team
Sense of achievement as a critical care nurse
Balance between being emotionally available and overinvolved
    (intellectual empathy)
Realistic daily work goals
Restorative time (adequate work breaks, vacation, hobbies)
Social support

strong need to be liked and approved of by others. There is such a strong need to achieve that all else is sacrificed (Maslach, 1982). Single or divorced status and childlessness are demographic factors associated with higher rates of burnout. White people tend to be more likely to burn out than blacks (Maslach, 1982).

Relationship Between Stress and Burnout

Recent investigations have attempted to identify factors that buffer the effects of stress on CCNs. Studies indicate that the leadership style of the head nurse (Duxbury et al., 1984) and the existence of a social support network (Suls, 1982) tend to buffer the effects of stress and hence may prevent burnout. Kobasa et al. (1982) identified a "hardiness personality" that may be related to burnout resistance. Hardiness is characterized by a sense of commitment, the ability to exercise internal control, and a tendency to seek challenge or novelty. One study showed that CCNs who were characterized as hardy experienced lower levels of burnout than CCNs rated lower in this construct (Keane et al., 1985). However, other researchers found that hardiness did not appear to prevent high levels of job stress from leading to high levels of burnout (McCranie et al., 1987).

The analysis of stress and burnout presented thus far clearly demonstrates that CCNs are at high risk for stress and burnout. But burnout is not inevitable. The focus of the remaining sections of the chapter is on how to maintain health. One way to maintain wellness among CCNs is to aim to meet their psychosocial needs. These needs are listed in Table 8–3. The causes of burnout are multifaceted, and hence prevention and treatment must be approached by the individual, the profession, and the system (critical care unit or hospital) in which the CCN works. The next section discusses strategies for CCNs to care for themselves and for each other and for man-

agers to care for CCNs. Using a team approach, CCNs can effectively manage stress and prevent burnout.

CARING FOR ONESELF

Although stress and burnout are professional problems, they must be confronted and handled by each nurse individually. The purpose of this section is to identify ways in which CCNs can cope with job-related stress, prevent or reduce burnout, satisfy their own psychosocial needs, and increase the enjoyment of nursing. Meeting the demands of critical care nursing without falling victim to burnout can best be done by people who are strong, both in body and spirit, and who make sure they stay that way. Thus, taking care of oneself is an essential prerequisite for taking care of others. Perhaps the first and most important step is acquiring the belief that it is all right to take care of oneself. CCNs are accustomed to taking care of others and, like many nurses, may be uncomfortable with the idea of making their own needs a priority. To thrive in nursing, however, CCNs must make a special effort to take care of themselves (Table 8–4).

Set Realistic Goals

Nurses often strive to achieve noble ideals such as "making a difference" or "helping people." But noble ideals are vague and abstract, making it difficult to tell if they are achieved. Also, noble ideals do not guide the direction of daily work. Ideals should not be abandoned but instead translated into concrete subgoals that are clearly possible to achieve. CCNs can start by making a list of specific accomplishments to aim for on a given day, during a given month, and for the year. The goals must be *specific* and *realistic*. CCNs can use them to measure their progress and achieve a sense of accomplishment.

Setting realistic goals involves recognizing one's personal limitations as well as abilities. For example, it is not realistic for a new CCN to expect to be as efficient as a 10-year veteran. Also, the limitations of

TABLE 8–4. Strategies for Caring for Oneself

Set realistic goals
Break away
Take things less personally
Accentuate the positive
Seek out positive feedback
Develop self-knowledge
Use relaxation techniques
Exercise
Develop a life away from work
Use decompression activities
Assess coping style
Learn assertion techniques
Seek professional help

available staff and the job setting are important considerations in setting realistic goals. If the unit has eight patients and seven of the eight are unstable patients on ventilators and some of the staff are inexperienced, nursing goals will be very basic.

Break Away

Critical care nurses often find it impossible to leave a patient's bedside. Unfortunately, this becomes a daily routine. The importance of getting away from the bedside and the critical care unit cannot be overestimated. CCNs need to work hard to get peer and management consensus about the importance of taking breaks *away* from the unit and of making breaks a necessity, not a luxury.

Constructive use of breaks for emotional recharging involves leaving the work area to go for a walk, read a book, listen to music, play cards, visit with a friend, or plan a dinner. Nurses should not use breaks for catching up on paperwork, making a telephone call, or doing other chores. Gains that come from working around the clock are lost in reduced efficiency, energy, and patience and an increase in errors and poor judgment.

Mini-breaks are also helpful. Simply walking away from the bedside or angry doctor for 1 minute with the excuse of getting a chart or linen gives one time to cool off. This pause lets one slow down, regain calm, stop a situation that is getting out of hand, and start all over again.

It is important to not overdo overtime. Learning to say "no" is an essential technique in taking care of oneself. There may be times when CCNs need to withdraw completely by taking a "mental health day" or a long lunch, if staffing permits.

CCNs can get away from intense patient contact by doing technical work such as stocking shelves, working on the time schedule, or passing medications and asking for a break away from a stressful patient when it is needed. This requires team work, placing value on one another's mental health, and being able to acknowledge limitations to oneself and peers.

Take Things Less Personally

When CCNs feel overinvolved, that is, feel a patient's problems as if they were their own or react to negative comments as personal insults, it is helpful to try to look at the situation in more abstract and intellectual terms. The ability to practice intellectual rather than emotional empathy is a valuable coping skill. Intellectual empathy occurs when one understands intellectually another person's feelings but does not experience the same feelings. Emotional empathy occurs when one feels the other person's pain as if it were one's own. One can be empathetic and understanding without emotionally taking on

patients' problems and feelings. This ability does not come easily but can be acquired with conscious effort.

Accentuate the Positive

One of the factors contributing to burnout is dealing exclusively with people who are very ill and in crisis. Actively emphasizing what is good, pleasant, or satisfying about a nurse's contact with others helps to balance this negative focus in a helping relationship. CCNs can pay more attention to their accomplishments, even the minor ones such as sharing a joke, having an interesting conversation, or helping someone with directions. They may deliberately include some positive moments in their people contact. By reevaluating their work, they may find positive aspects in it that they had not previously recognized.

CCNs can consider how they might include some positive moments in their people contact at work. What part of the job, no matter how small, gave a good feeling this week? They might try taking 10 minutes to think about all the good things that happened during the day and record at least one of them in a private journal with the date.

Seek Out Positive Feedback

Positive feedback helps to build the CCN's vulnerable self-esteem and sense of personal accomplishment. Seeking out positive feedback rather than passively waiting for it can be done by asking for strokes. Most CCNs are unaccustomed to asking for positive feedback, but they might try the following: "If this helps you (makes you feel better) I would appreciate it if you would tell me"; "Let me know if this works out"; or "I can do a better job for you if I know what you like about my work (as well as what you dislike)."

The CCN can ask herself: "Who gives me positive feedback at work; who would I like to hear it from; how can I 'ask' for it; who gave me positive feedback this week; would my response encourage more positive feedback or less; did I give any of my peers positive feedback this week?"

Critical care nurses can get positive feedback by creating opportunities to see their successes. They can do this by asking patients to stop by the ICU to say good-by, to send a picture of themselves taken in their homes doing something they like to do, or to write them a note. These photos and letters can be posted on a bulletin board or kept in a scrapbook. Or the fruits of their labor can be seen by encouraging favorite patients to stop by the unit when coming back to the clinic, telling them this is something they can do to help the nurses. Seeing a recovered patient enjoying life, who was pulled back from the brink of death with the help of CCNs, can give them a great deal of satisfaction and enhance their feelings of personal accomplishment. Also, nurses can visit patients when they have transferred out of the ICU.

Involving oneself in positive experiences outside the primary area of work helps balance the negative aspects of work. CCNs can benefit by being with people who are healthy, happy, and free of major problems, people for whom life is going well. CCNs should actively seek out these people and relationships. If CCNs examine some of their personal relationships, they may find that they, like many nurses, are also "caretakers" in their private lives. Are their friends and families a source of nurturance and rejuvenation or do they drain them?

Another way to counterbalance the negative and sad aspects of the job is to moonlight in an area other than nursing. One CCN helped balance her job by working one day a week in an antique store. If CCNs need to supplement their hours, they might work in something like the newborn nursery or spend 1 month working with healthy children as a camp nurse.

Develop Self-knowledge

The ability to be introspective and to understand oneself is critical for coping with burnout and stress. The first step in knowing what action to take is to know what is being felt and why. Tuning in to one's inner feelings and being sensitive to personal reactions and the underlying reasons for them are ways of promoting self-knowledge. Self-analysis should be constructive—a way of acknowledging strengths, limitations, and learning from mistakes.

Self-understanding begins with self-observation. The CCN can ask, What am I feeling? When, where, and with whom? What am I doing in response to that feeling? Keeping a log is an effective way of discovering patterns of emotional stress (Table 8–5). This log should be kept on a daily basis for the entire day including time at home as well as at work. The record should be made for 2 weeks and then examined for patterns of emotional response, possible causes, and styles of coping. The nurse may see that anxiety arises whenever he or she deals with older people or authority figures. Or perhaps irritability peaks in the late morning regardless of the situation.

Information gained from this stress record may help one begin to answer such questions as "Why am I feeling this way? What could I do about it that would be better than what I am now doing?" The nurse can choose coping techniques based on self-awareness that fits personal needs within a particular situation.

It is normal to have strong emotional reactions to certain patients. Some patients may be reminders of a friend or relative. Other patients' behavior may be distasteful or may conflict with the nurse's value system. Recognizing and dealing with one's own feelings helps decrease emotional exhaustion.

Trying to find ways to express feelings verbally is another way of reducing stress. Writing feelings down in a diary, talking into a tape recorder, and talking to a supportive colleague or friend are helpful. These techniques force the nurse to articulate and give shape to what may at first be vague and confusing feelings. Also, articulating one's feelings helps to "blow off steam" and release emotional energy.

Use Relaxation Techniques

Relaxation is an effective coping technique in situations that are stressful and cannot be changed. Relaxation exercises are helpful in two general ways: One is to reduce or prevent the physical symptoms of stress (tense muscles, especially in the neck, increased blood pressure, and upset stomach "tied up in knots"). The second reason is to help reduce anxiety to a more manageable level. Many individuals become so anxious in thinking about or approaching certain situations that they are unable to use other (problem-focused) techniques until their anxiety is reduced.

There are many forms of relaxation techniques including meditation, biofeedback, and imagery. No matter which is chosen, the key to achieving effectiveness is practice. By setting aside time every day to practice the procedures, they become second nature.

CCNs can use relaxation techniques during lunch or coffee breaks to refresh themselves. Relaxation techniques can be helpful just before a stressful event, such as assisting a new Cardiology Fellow insert a pulmonary artery catheter. They can be done

---

TABLE 8–5. Daily Log of Stress and Tension Patterns

What Are the Physical Signs of Stress?					
What Time of Day Do They Occur?					
Where Do They Occur? What Am I Doing? Who Am I With?					
What Thoughts or Feelings Do I Have?					
What Did I Do in Response to the Stress?					

almost anywhere at any time (sitting or standing, between patients, waiting in line). A tape recorder in the car or purse makes it possible to listen to relaxation tapes while commuting to or from work. Through practice of the longer relaxation exercises, one will acquire the ability to elicit the relaxation response within seconds by simply taking a slow deep breath and telling oneself "to relax." This instant relaxation is helpful when one feels tension building up. CCNs can develop cuing systems to remind themselves to use this technique (for example, any time they become impatient over having to wait). Relaxation exercises and instructions for visualization or imagery can be found in a variety of books and tapes listed at the end of this chapter.

Imagery (also called visualization) is like taking an imaginary vacation or daydreaming for relaxation purposes. One can begin with a progressive relaxation exercise or by taking a deep breath and slowly exhaling. The person then imagines being in a special place that is peaceful and pleasant for her or him. She pictures herself in a passive role with no people. She recreates the scene with all the sensations associated with it. All senses are involved; one smells the fragrance associated with that place, feels the warm sun, hears the wind blowing in the trees, sees the bright-colored flowers. One stays in this restful place for 5 to 15 minutes. The benefits will last far beyond the 15 minutes it takes.

Exercise

The fight or flight reaction with its adrenalin rush was adaptive for survival in earlier times when one could actually fight or flee. However, physical aggression is not appropriate today. Swallowing the feelings of anger and frustration is acceptable in our modern society but can be very harmful for one's body. CCNs need to find ways to dissipate the energy of arousal through activity. The activity does not have to be related to the perceived threat. Exercise can help reduce the level of catecholamines in the system, which increases with stress, and prevent the harmful effects of prolonged physiologic arousal.

CCNs should learn what different types of exercise programs are available in their area. They should consult their doctor to obtain guidance to avoid injuries or complications with exercise if they are over 35, have never seriously exercised, or have a chronic illness. CCNs should establish an exercise routine, choose exercises or sports they enjoy, and find a companion to make it more pleasant. An exercise class can be created before, during, or after work. They should set realistic goals and work slowly to achieve them. Care should be taken about creating competition. Creative activities such as dance, Tai Chi, and other expressive movements are other possible choices.

Develop a Life Away From Work

What do CCNs do when they are not at work? What are they besides their job title? A life outside of work can offset the emotional strain of work and help to "recharge their batteries." Their nonworking hours need to be not just an *absence* of work but rather a *presence* of something else. If a CCN's whole world is work, then her world is more likely to fall apart when problems arise on the job.

The first step in strengthening one's private life is to protect it from encroachments by work. CCNs need to set clear boundaries between job and home. This means that when they leave the job, they really leave it, psychologically as well as physically. Keeping the job out of home life is easier said than done. Pieces of private time are taken over by work every time the day's problems are reviewed at home, when work is taken home to do in the evening or on weekends, during overtime, or when the nurse is "on call."

Bringing home the emotional turmoil of the job is perhaps the most insidious way to let work run into private life. It is hard to put a stop to recurring thoughts and unresolved feelings and to avoid venting them on the nearest target. Decompression activities help, as does a cooling-off period of an hour or so once the nurse is home. During this time the rule is "nothing negative." Whatever is talked about with friends, spouse, or children must be pleasant or interesting. This ensures a pleasant time with the people the nurse cares about most. Problems become less immediate and less intense, and perhaps less important, as the CCN gains some distance from them.

Mini-vacations are a good idea. These can be accomplished by filling private time with activities that provide a diversion from job tensions, provide positive experiences with other people, and boost one's sense of competence and self-esteem.

CCNs should include people contact in their leisure time. Successes in their personal relationships can be an effective antidote to feelings of frustration or failure in their professional contacts. "I could not ease my client's troubles today, but I did make my spouse feel happy (or friend, neighbor, child, parent)." Personal strength often comes from strong social supports. Research shows that people who are part of a solid social support network are better able to cope with physical ills and psychological problems.

Use Decompression Activities

People working in an environment of high emotional pressure need to decompress—to get completely out of that high-pressure environment before moving into the "normal pressure" of their private lives. Decompression refers to some activity that occurs between working and nonworking times and allows one to unwind, relax, and leave the job behind before getting fully involved with family and friends.

Activities that contrast sharply with the CCN's work routine are helpful. Because in nursing there is emphasis on problem-solving and intellectual skills, decompression activities should avoid mental exertion. Nursing involves people contact, so CCNs might choose solitary decompression activities in which they can find peace, quiet, and time for themselves. Their decompression activities should be self-indulgent and give them some privacy. Activities that help them slow down help counteract the pace of critical care. They may just sit and relax in their car for a few minutes before going home or unwind in a spa or bubble bath. Other suggestions are reading a romance novel, window shopping, gardening, painting, taking photographs, gourmet cooking, or having a massage.

Assess Coping Style

Coping is what a person does or thinks to manage feeling harmed, threatened, or challenged (Lazarus and Folkman, 1984). Coping can be directed at managing or altering the problem causing the distress *(problem-focused coping)* or at regulating one's emotional response to the problem *(emotion-focused coping)*. Problem-focused coping involves defining the problem, generating alternative solutions, weighing the alternatives in terms of their costs and benefits, choosing among them, and acting.

The following examples illustrate emotion-focused coping and compares the results of the coping attempts of two nurses. A patient's wife is expressing anger. The CCN can respond by taking some deep breaths and giving self-comforting messages that the wife is not really angry *at her* but is angry and frightened because of her mate's sudden heart attack. This helps reduce emotional distress and allows the nurse to direct her attention toward problem-focused coping skills. The CCN can decide to use active listening to convey empathy and yet not get involved in the family member's stress cycle.

Another nurse might handle the situation in a different manner. To reduce her emotional distress she walks away (avoidance), but the irate and emotionally distraught woman is still going to be there. If the nurse takes this time to cool down and think, this technique will facilitate problem-focused coping. If, however, she does nothing more, the woman may go to the hospital administrator and complain about the poor nursing care.

Many sources of stress cannot be mastered. It is a helpful strategy for the CCN to ask herself whether the stressor can or cannot be changed and then to use techniques to minimize the emotional distress caused by stressors in the latter category. Effective coping under these conditions is that which allows the CCN to tolerate, minimize, accept, or ignore what cannot be mastered. Often physical environ-

mental stressors cannot be avoided; the CCN is stuck in the unit and cannot get away for a break. But he can use relaxation exercises or imagery, imagining he is in more pleasant surroundings. Assertion training is very effective for social stressors. Negative self-talk can be handled by learning new ways to talk to oneself. Organizational stressors may require intervention at many different levels. Managing this type of stress consists of working with others to change some of these stressors, or coping with them if they cannot be changed.

Learn Assertion Techniques

Interpersonal stress was ranked as the number one stressor in many CCN studies. Do CCNs have differences of opinion with their supervisors or physicians? Do they have difficulty in giving negative feedback to peers or people they supervise? Do they have difficulty in dealing with aggressive or passive people? Do they avoid conflicts with peers or superiors or subordinates? Do they have unsettled conflicts with the people they work with? Stress occurs when individuals are not able to express themselves appropriately or effectively and as a result feel angry at the other person or at themselves for holding "it" in or inappropriately blurting "it" out, "it" being the statements they wished they had said, if they had only been true to themselves and had had the self-confidence to state, diplomatically but firmly, what they believe.

Nurses may be subassertive because of what is called the "compassion trap" (Adams, 1971), a trap exclusive to women who feel that they exist to serve others and must provide tenderness and compassion to all people at all times. Nurses may be particularly susceptible to this trap because meeting the needs of others is the essence of nursing.

Assertiveness is a skill that can be learned with training and practice. Assertion is "behavior which enables a person to act in his own best interests, to stand up for himself **without** undue anxiety, to express honest feelings **com**fortably, and to exercise personal rights without **denying** the rights of others" (Alberti and Emmons, 1978). Acquiring assertiveness skills may be the most important thing that CCNs can do for themselves as nurses. Using socially acceptable ways to express their concerns and frustrations can do much to reduce feelings of helplessness and powerlessness.

Assertion can be learned from books and workshops, but the most effective learning takes place in a group where there are opportunities to play roles, to practice, and to share the results of their attempts to be assertive in the real world.

Seek Professional Help

If a CCN is feeling extremely depressed or finds herself engaging in self-destructive behaviors (substance abuse) or simply feels that she is having trouble coping, the benefits of counseling may be considered. Often short-term therapy (6 to 8 weeks) can reduce emotional distress and turn the burnout–stressed out syndrome around. Clinical nurse specialists in psychiatry or mental health and other mental health professionals are potential resources. Help is available from personnel assistance programs and in the private sector. Most health insurance companies pay for these services.

CARING FOR ONE ANOTHER

Friends and spouses can provide many things, but often the people who are best able to provide job-related help and support are co-workers. Their power to help handle stress and burnout should not be underestimated. Support from co-workers can come from professional support groups or staff meetings, or it may be informal (i.e., talking over lunch or during breaks, or socializing after working hours).

Peers can do something about the source of stress by, for example, rescuing a fellow CCN from a difficult situation, or by giving direct aid (such as providing assistance when a client is particularly rude or threatening), or by teaching a peer how to handle a certain problem. They might take over for a peer temporarily, allowing the person to withdraw from an upsetting situation. Peers can also provide comfort and emotional support by listening empathetically. They have a special understanding because they are familiar with the situation and have a similar status and perspective.

Peers can help by providing a new perspective on a problem. They may be able to express the thoughts and feelings that a fellow CCN finds uncomfortable to say. Co-workers can help to analyze feelings and provide insight into reactions.

Peers can provide a basis for personal comparison. This is particularly helpful when a CCN is not sure of the appropriateness of his or her reactions. "Is it normal to feel this way? Am I overreacting? Am I the only one who feels like this?" By talking to co-workers CCNs may often discover that they are not alone and that their feelings are indeed shared by others. This helps to prevent blaming oneself.

Peers can also tell a CCN if they are good at their work. The most important (and perhaps) only source of praise, compliments, and recognition for doing a job well may be a fellow worker. Peers are able to evaluate what a CCN has done and can give immediate and meaningful feedback. However, to get positive feedback from peers, CCNs may have to ask for it. The best way for a CCN to get feedback is first to give positive feedback to peers noticing all the things they do well and telling them so.

Jokes and laughter can reduce emotional strain by making a situation seem less serious, less frightening, and less overwhelming. Humor injects a positive element and lifts everyone's spirits. But humor must

be used carefully to avoid laughing at or putting other people down.

CCNs can get away from work more completely during breaks by talking with co-workers about topics other than work such as movies, vacations, or the weekend football game.

STRATEGIES FOR MANAGEMENT

Behavioral patterns that contribute to burnout and specific interventions that can be made by individuals to reduce the pressures they are under have been discussed earlier. But this is only half of the equation. Certain changes in the organizational climate may be critical in preventing burnout. We will focus on these changes in this section—more detailed material on organizational strategies that can reduce stress and prevent burnout is given by Lachman (1983).

The effects of burnout (high turnover and absenteeism, antagonism in group process, errors, lack of cooperation and initiative) interfere with obtaining the goals of the institution and can create daily hassles for the manager. Often the most valuable employees fall victim to burnout. For the sake of the patient, the staff, and the institution it behooves the manager to examine the current climate critically, identify any damaging aspects, and make needed changes. Management or institutional strategies for handling burnout include mechanisms that empower and support nurses; provide for ventilation of feelings, open two-directional communication, flexible leaves and support services, and training programs that develop interpersonal skills; and clarify roles and lines of authority (Table 8–6).

Empower Staff

It is imperative to find ways to give staff control over their work and the environment. CCNs experience high performance demands and an intense sense of personal responsibility for patients. Yet frequently they have little personal control over their environment, and the lines of authority are ambiguous. Because their personal style may be weak and unassertive, CCNs may feel trapped by other people's demands. The work environment may have

TABLE 8–6. Strategies Used by Managers in Reducing Staff Stress

Empower the staff
Support the staff
Offer support groups
Sharpen interpersonal skills
Take care of yourself
Develop the team
Be a staff advocate
Provide feedback
Encourage use of humor

created a belief among nurses that it is hopeless to change things; they may have a sense of "learned helplessness" (Seligman, 1975).

Ways to empower staff include participative management with the active involvement of staff in planning and decision-making. Decentralization is another way to empower staff; decentralization allows nurses and managers to try new ideas and implement change without the need for an elaborate approval process involving layers of hierarchy. Inclusion of nurses on hospital-wide committees and on committees directly affecting critical care also gives CCNs mechanisms for personal power.

Communication needs to flow two ways. Managers need to indicate a desire for upward communication by what they say and, more important, by what they do: Seeking out staff input and acting on this input is one way; other ways are being open and *actively listening* to what staff say; asking questions to clarify; seriously considering staff suggestions; acting upon staff input by bringing it to the attention of upper management and committee meetings; and getting back to the staff with the results. A manager's behavior must reinforce the belief that what the staff think is important. A manager may communicate this verbally: "Thank you; that is important. I am glad you brought this problem to my attention. I will bring it up at the next critical care meeting."

Support Staff

Managerial support can be put into operation in a number of ways. The stresses experienced by CCNs and the variety of emotional responses to them can be acknowledged and validated. Staff can be encouraged to practice the strategies described for the individual and to develop balance in their work and life. It should be recognized that staff will be trying new behaviors that may feel uncomfortable. They may fall short of success in their attempts to develop new ways of interacting with their peers, physicians, and managers. Managers need to be patient and supportive of the staff's attempts to grow. Policies making personal time sacrosanct and limiting the amount of overtime permitted should be made, as should provisions for taking breaks away from the unit.

Staff meetings to ventilate and define problems are helpful. All must recognize that conflict is inevitable and should not be avoided; it can be used as an opportunity for growth. Outside help to resolve conflicts may be necessary. Work assignments may need to be changed to provide increased satisfaction. Managers should distribute frustrating and unpleasant tasks as equitably as possible. In a staffing crisis, managers may help with patient care to communicate their support. An additional benefit of participating in patient care is that it helps managers take on the perspective of the staff. Managers should rotate nurses out of the ICU when they need a break from

the pressure. Facilitating the sharing of responsibility for patient care through collaboration with liaison nurses, psychiatrists, social workers, and pastoral counselors lessens the burden of individual responsibility.

Offer Support Groups

A powerful way in which managers can communicate their care and concern for their staff is by establishing and encouraging participation in support groups. Support groups provide a sanctioned outlet for negative feelings generated by the nature of the work and interactions with peers, patients, physicians, and families. Support groups provide an opportunity to share, clarify, and validate feelings; explore work-related stresses and experiences; solve problems, and learn from others how to handle stress more effectively. Isolated nurses may realize that they are not alone and can gain support from one another. The group process enhances feelings of belonging and self-esteem.

Psychiatric mental health clinical nurse specialists are ideal choices as leaders of support groups and can provide ongoing consultation to management and staff nurses. Because they are nurses themselves, they often have a deep understanding of nursing issues that other mental health professionals may not have. Mental health specialists can help with difficult patients, interstaff conflicts, and intrastaff conflicts and can increase managers' awareness and responsiveness to the psychosocial needs of the staff.

Sharpen Interpersonal Skills

Managers may need to attend workshops or study assertiveness, conflict resolution, and group process. Competence with interpersonal skills is a major necessity for manager and staff, and they can be learned.

Take Care of Yourself

Managers are not immune to emotional exhaustion and feelings of demoralization. Unyielding daily exposure to stress may result in a negative perception of staff, distancing of themselves, and treatment of staff in a depersonalized manner. Others may be the first to notice this trend. Managers should heed what others tell them about their own signs of burnout and take care of themselves. See the earlier discussion of individual strategies.

Develop the Team

Cohesive teams do not just happen. Specific actions can be taken by management to establish conditions that enhance teamwork and reward people for playing their part on the team. The reader is referred to the excellent article by Callaway (1986), which describes in detail the steps a nurse manager can take to develop a strong team.

Be a Staff Advocate

Managers can work for adequate staffing with well-prepared CCNs, flexible scheduling, good salaries, and state-of-the-art equipment. Institutional policies that support nurse role definition and a sense of professional worth and that allow nurses to be creative, flexible, and resourceful rather than restrained should be encouraged.

Provide Feedback

Burnout research shows that nurses need feedback from their supervisors about their job performance. Managers' feedback tells the staff how well they are doing, where they can improve, and that their work is appreciated and valued. To be helpful, feedback should be as specific as possible (e.g., "You were very kind and patient with Mr. Jones' family the other night when they were so upset" rather than, "You are doing a good job"). When negative feedback is needed, it should be phrased in constructive ways that show the nurse how to improve. Feedback should be given at the time of the occurrence and not "saved" for the next evaluation.

Managers can be creative in finding ways to make positive feedback happen, such as a bulletin board with "success stories," photos, and thank you cards. They can recognize increasing competence and patient care rendered beyond the usual and customary—care reflecting creativity, unusual effort, or collaboration. For example, a letter from the Director of Nurses letting a nurse know how much her or his efforts were appreciated can be a morale booster. Specific examples of how she or he has helped patients, families, and colleagues can be included. Managers can work for a Nurse Recognition Day on which peers vote for an outstanding nurse. Winners can be honored, have a day off with pay, and be awarded a premium parking spot for a month marked by the notation "Outstanding Nurse" painted on the curb. Managers can write up special "incident reports" of excellent performance to recognize a job well done. These should be circulated through the administrative hierarchy, just as a negative incident report would be, and kept in the personnel file. Managers should be sure to reward examples of positive behavior upon which their staff needs to improve such as teamwork.

Encourage Use of Humor

Victor Borge once said "Laughter is the shortest distance between two people." Finding the funny side of the daily routine improves morale, builds a sense of teamwork, and keeps work fun. Humor helps one handle the problems that cannot be controlled or solved. A well-placed laugh can bring staff out of the stress cycle and return them to productive problem-solving. Humor can help managers reframe stress into an opportunity and can defuse anger. Managers are encouraged to take time to laugh and smile daily on the job. Trying to see the humor in their daily hassles will help them keep a healthy perspective. They should take their job and responsibilities seriously but themselves lightly. They should strive to be able to take a joke; laughing at themselves and the work situation will make it easier for others to do the same in the face of their problems. By cultivating humorous statements they can use in talking to themselves, managers can break the stress cycle. Laughter is contagious and so is negativism; the manager can greatly influence the dominance of either.

SUMMARY

This chapter has focused on identifying and meeting the psychosocial needs of the critical care staff. Results of research in stress and burnout have validated the evidence that the frustrations and difficulties experienced by CCNs are universal. The distress felt by CCNs is not the result of inadequacy but is due to the complex social system of the critical care unit and hospital setting and to the nature of the caregiving experience. This chapter has delineated some of the contributors to stress and burnout, including individual behavior patterns in response to these stresses and the work environment. It has offered strategies for modifying both. It is evident that decreasing stress and burnout takes a collaborative effort on the part of CCNs, their colleagues, and their managers.

References

Adams, M. (1971). The compassion trap. In Gornick, V., and Moran, B. K. (Eds.), *Woman in sexist society: Studies in power and powerlessness*. New York: Basic Books.
Alberti, R. E., and Emmons, M. L. (1978). *Your perfect right: A guide to assertive behavior.* San Louis Opispo, CA: Impact Publishers.
Anderson, C. A., and Basteyns, M. (1981). Stress and the critical care nurse reaffirmed. *Journal of Nursing Administration*, 1, 31–34.
Bartz, C., and Maloney, J. (1986). Burnout among intensive care nurses. *Research in Nursing and Health*, 9, 147–153.
Callaway, J. (1986). Developing a cohesive team in a critical care unit. *Nursing Management*, 17, 34B–34F.
Cassem, N. H., and Hackett, T. P. (1975). Stress on the nurse and therapist in the intensive-care unit and the coronary-care unit. *Heart and Lung*, 4, 252–259.
Claus, K. E., and Bailey, J. T. (1980). *Living with stress and promoting well-being*. St. Louis: C. V. Mosby.
Duxbury, M., Armstrong, G., Drew, D., et al. (1984). Head nurse leadership style with staff nurse burnout and job satisfaction in neonatal intensive care units. *Nursing Research*, 33, 97–101.

Gray-Toft, P., and Anderson, J. (1983). A hospital staff support program: Design and evaluation. *International Journal of Nursing Studies, 20,* 137–147.

Hay, D., and Oken, D. (1972). The psychological stresses of intensive care unit nursing. *Psychosomatic Medicine, 34,* 109–118.

Holmes, T. H., and Rahe, R. H. (1967). The social readjustment rating scale. *Journal of Psychosomatic Research, 11,* 213–218.

Huckabay, L. D., and Jagla, B. (1979). Nurses' stress factors in the intensive care unit. *Journal of Nursing Administration, 9,* 21–26.

Jacobson, S. (1978). Stressful situations for neonatal intensive care unit nurses. *American Journal of Maternal-Child, 3,* 144–150.

Jones, J. W. (1981). Attitudinal correlates of employee theft of drugs and hospital supplies among nursing personnel. *Nursing Research, 30,* 349–351.

Keane, A., Ducette, J., and Adler, D. (1985). Stress in ICU and non-ICU nurses. *Nursing Research, 34,* 231–236.

Kobasa, S., Maddi, S., and Kahn, S. (1982). Hardiness and health: A prospective study. *Journal of Personality and Social Psychology, 1,* 168–177.

Lachman, V. D. (1983). *Stress management: A manual for nurses.* New York: Grune & Stratton.

Lazarus, R. S., and Folkman, S. (1984). *Stress, appraisal, and coping.* New York: Springer.

Maslach, C. (1982). *Burnout—The cost of caring.* Englewood-Cliffs: Prentice-Hall.

McCranie, E. W., Lambert, V. A., and Lambert, C. E. (1987). Work stress, hardiness, and burnout among hospital staff nurses. *Nursing Research, 36,* 374–378.

Nason, M. C. (1988). The impact of support groups on burnout in critical care nurses (in press).

Oskins, S. L. (1979). Identification of situational stressors and coping methods by intensive care nurses. *Heart & Lung, 8,* 953–960.

Pines, A. (1983). On burnout and the buffering effects of social support. In Farber, B. A. (Ed.), *Stress and burnout in the human service professions.* New York: Pergamon Press.

Seligman, M. E. P. (1975). *Helplessness.* San Francisco: W. H. Freeman.

Selye, H. (1975). *Stress without distress.* New York: Signet.

Stehle, J. L. (1981). Critical care nursing stress: The findings revisited. *Nursing Research, 30,* 182–188.

Steinmetz, J., Blankenship, J., Brown, L., et al. (1980). *Managing stress before it manages you.* Menlo Park: Bull Publishing.

Storlie, F. J. (1979). Burnout: The elaboration of a concept. *American Journal of Nursing, 19,* 2108–2111.

Suls, J. (1982). Social support, interpersonal relations, and health: Benefits and liabilities. In Sanders, G. S., and Suls, J. (Eds.), *Social psychology of health and illness.* Hillsdale, NJ: Lawrence Erlbaum Associates.

Bibliography

American Academy of Nursing, Task Force on Nursing Practice in Hospitals. (1983). *Magnet hospitals: Attraction and retention of professional nurses.* Kansas City: American Nurses' Association.

Buechler, D. (1985). Help for the burned-out nurse? *Nursing Outlook, 4,* 181–185.

Chenevert, M. (1985). *Pro-nurse handbook.* St. Louis: C. V. Mosby.

Cronin-Stubbs, D., and Rooks, C. A. (1985). The stress, social support, and burnout of critical care nurses: The results of research. *Heart & Lung, 14,* 31–39.

Cronin-Stubbs, D., and Schaffner, J. W. (1985). Professional impairment: Strategies for managing the troubled nurse. *Nursing Administration Quarterly, 9,* 44–54.

Dolan, S. N. (1987). The relationship between burnout and job satisfaction in nurses. *Journal of Advanced Nursing, 12,* 3–12.

Dubovsky, S. L., Getto, C. J., Gross, S. A., et al. (1977). Impact on nursing care and mortality: Psychiatrists on the coronary care unit. *Psychosomatics, 18,* 18–27.

Forsyth, D. M., and Cannady, N. J. (1981). Preventing and alleviating staff burnout through a group. *Journal of Psychosocial Nursing and Mental Health Services, 19,* 35–39.

Freudenberger, H. J. (1981). *Burnout: How to beat the high cost of success.* New York: Bantam Books.

Friedman, E. H. (1982). Stress and ICU: A ten-year reappraisal. *Heart and Lung, 11,* 26–28.

Hagenmaster, J. N. (1983). Job stress vs. nurse burnout: Are you caught in the middle? *Occupational Health Nursing, 31,* 38–40.

Harris, J. S. (1984). Stressors and stress in critical care. Home study program. *Critical Care Nurse, 4,* 84–96.

Kramer, M., and Schmalenber, C. E. (1976). Conflict: The cutting edge of growth. *Journal of Nursing Administration, 6,* 19–25.

Lachman, V. D. (1983). *Stress management: A manual for nurses.* New York: Grune & Stratton.

Maslach, C., and Jackson, S. (1982). Burnout in health professions: A social psychological analysis. In Sanders, G., and Suls, J. (Eds.), *Social psychology of health and illness* (pp. 227–251). Hillsdale, NJ: Lawrence Erlbaum Associates.

McConnell, E. A. (1982). *Burnout in the nursing profession.* St. Louis: C. V. Mosby.

Norbeck, J. A. (1985). Types and sources of social support for managing job stress in critical care nursing. *Nursing Research, 34,* 225–230.

Pelletier, K. (1977). *Mind as healer, mind as slayer.* New York: Delacorte.

Pines, A., Aronson, E., and Kafry, D. (1981). *Burnout.* New York: Free Press.

Pines, A. M., and Kanner, A. D. (1982). Nurses' burnout: Lack of positive conditions and presence of negative conditions as two independent sources of stress. *Journal of Psychosomatic Nursing and Mental Health Services, 20,* 30–35.

Pines, A., and Maslach, C. (1978). Characteristics of staff burnout in mental health settings. *Hospital and Community Psychiatry, 29,* 233–237.

Randolph, G. (1979). The yin and yang of clinical practice. *Topics in Clinical Nursing, 1,* 221–231.

Scully, R. (1983). The work setting support group: A means of preventing burnout. In Farber, B. A. (Ed.), *Stress and burnout in the human service professions.* New York: Pergamon Press.

Stone, G. L., Jebsen, P., Walk, P., et al. (1984). Identification of stress and coping skills within a critical care setting. *Western Journal of Nursing Research, 6,* 201–211.

Monitoring and Technology

C · H · A · P · T · E · R

9

ECG Interpretation

Linda K. Menzel

During the last 10 years our knowledge and understanding of the conduction system and dysrhythmias have grown immensely. New information on cardiac cell physiology and His bundle electrocardiography as well as other methods has made the study of the electrocardiogram increasingly interesting and complex. With this growth of knowledge has come an increase in responsibility for critical care nurses. The nurse is no longer responsible only for the interpretation of simple dysrhythmias as may have been the case in the late 1960s and early 1970s. Nurses now have increased responsibility and are challenged to interpret ischemia, infarction, and axis deviation as well as more complex dysrhythmias. The 1990s will be an exciting time for critical care nurses as they work collaboratively with their medical colleagues.

This chapter focuses on interpretation of the electrocardiogram (ECG) as it relates to axis deviation, coronary artery disease, and complex dysrhythmias. The chapter begins with a discussion of the conduction system and normal cardiac electrophysiology and continues on to interpretation of the 12-lead ECG and dysrhythmias.

NURSING DIAGNOSES

A number of nursing diagnoses may be relevant to the individual patient with cardiac dysrhythmias. Some of these are diagnoses that nurses can treat independently, particularly those relating to the individual's ability to cope with the stress and uncertainty of his condition and the critical care environment. Other diagnoses are related to the person's physiologic response to the medical diagnosis and belong in the interdependent dimension. These interdependent interventions will require close monitoring and early detection by the nurse and authori-

zation to initiate treatment. For example, the patient receiving vasodilators to decrease afterload must be monitored for hypotension and signs of decreased tissue perfusion.

Decreased cardiac output and altered tissue perfusion are two common physiologic nursing diagnoses that should be anticipated and quickly identified in critical care patients. Both diagnoses are frequently pertinent in patients who have alterations in myocardial perfusion with electrocardiographic changes and dysrhythmias.

Decreased Cardiac Output

Decreased cardiac output is a state in which the amount of blood pumped by an individual's heart is so reduced that it is inadequate to meet the needs of the body's tissues (Carroll-Johnson, 1989). Major defining characteristics identified by the North American Nursing Diagnosis Association (NANDA, 1989) include variations in blood pressure readings; dysrhythmias; fatigue; jugular venous distention; color changes in skin and mucous membranes; oliguria; decreased peripheral pulses; cold, clammy skin; rales; dyspnea; orthopnea; and restlessness.

Cardiac output is the product of heart rate and stroke volume. Heart rate is frequently affected by altered conduction and dysrhythmias. A decrease in heart rate may cause inadequate perfusion if there is not a concurrent increase in stroke volume. Tachycardias may not allow time for ventricular filling. Likewise, the absence of atrial contractions (the "atrial kick") in rhythms such as atrial fibrillation may result in decreased ventricular filling. Maintaining an adequate cardiac output should be the utmost priority in patients with dysrhythmias. A supraventricular rhythm with a rapid rate is as potentially detrimental to a particular patient as a ventricular rhythm, especially if the patient has preexisting heart disease.

Decreased Tissue Perfusion

Altered tissue perfusion is the state in which an individual experiences a decrease in nutrition and oxygenation at the cellular level due to a deficit in capillary blood supply (Carroll-Johnson, 1989). Identifying characteristics suggesting an acute state of decreased peripheral tissue perfusion include cold skin temperature, pale or blue skin color, and decreased capillary refill. Decreased cerebral perfusion, for example, may result in confusion, restlessness, or other changes in the level of consciousness. A decrease in tissue perfusion in the cardiac patient may be seen as primary or secondary. A primary decrease in myocardial tissue perfusion occurs when there is inadequate blood flow to the myocardium. The potential for a secondary decrease in peripheral perfusion occurs when the myocardial damage has been so extensive that it results in pump failure. Dysrhythmias and electrocardiographic changes have the potential to cause decreased tissue perfusion through decreased cardiac output.

ANATOMY AND PHYSIOLOGY

The conduction system of the heart is composed of the sinus node, the atrioventricular (AV) node, and the His-Purkinje system, which is in turn composed of the bundle of His, the right and left bundle branches, and the Purkinje fibers (Fig. 9–1).

The normal cardiac cycle begins with an impulse propagated in the sinus node. The impulse is conducted rapidly through the atria by internodal pathways to the AV node, where it slows to allow time for ventricular filling. The impulse then continues down through the bundle of His and spreads rapidly

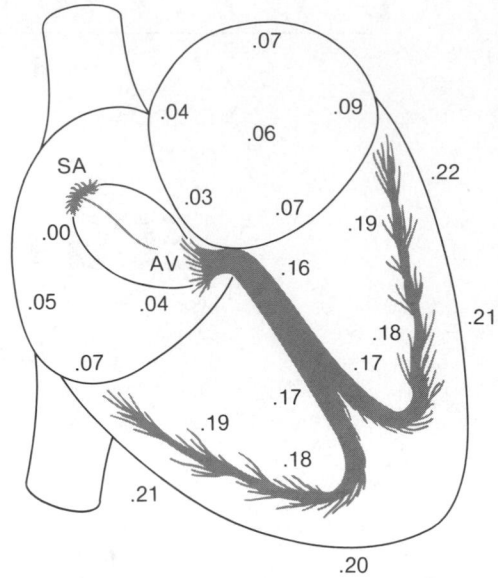

FIGURE 9–2. Transmission of the cardiac impulse through the heart, showing the time of appearance (in fractions of a second) of the impulse in different parts of the heart. (Redrawn from Guyton, A. C. (1991). *Textbook of medical physiology* (8th ed., p. 114). Philadelphia: W. B. Saunders.)

through the bundle branches to the Purkinje fibers and ventricular myocardium (Fig. 9–2).

Sinus Node

The sinus node (SA node), first identified by Keith and Flack in 1907, is located in the posterior aspect of the right atrium at the junction of the superior vena cava and the body of the right atrium. The SA node is elliptically shaped with a cross section of 2 to 3 mm and a length that varies from 15 to 30 mm (Thalen, 1981). Its blood supply arises from the right coronary artery in 55% of individuals and from the left circumflex in the remaining population. The sinus

FIGURE 9–1. The conduction system. (Figure from PRINCIPLES OF HUMAN ANATOMY, 4th edition, by Gerald J. Tortora. Copyright © 1986 by Leonard Dank, 1986 by Biological Sciences Textbooks, Inc. Reprinted by permission of HarperCollins Publishers.)

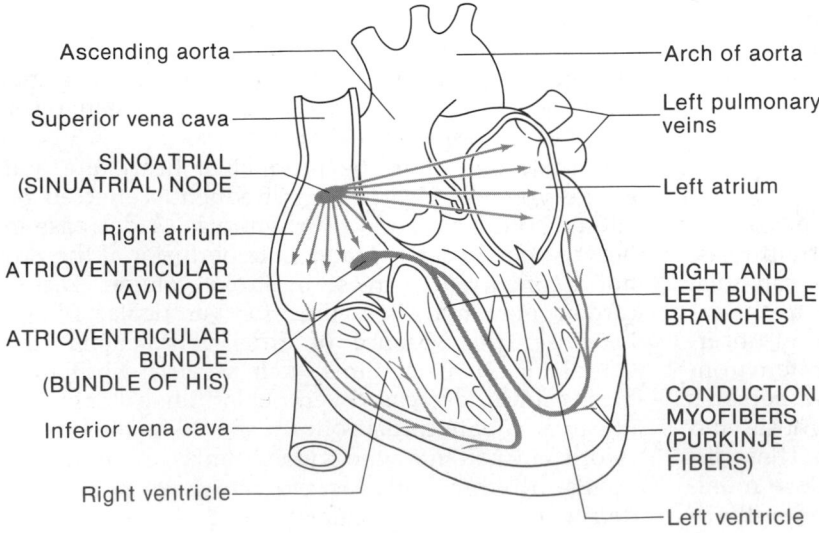

Ascending aorta

Superior vena cava

SINOATRIAL (SINUATRIAL) NODE

Right atrium

ATRIOVENTRICULAR (AV) NODE

ATRIOVENTRICULAR BUNDLE (BUNDLE OF HIS)

Inferior vena cava

Right ventricle

Arch of aorta

Left pulmonary veins

Left atrium

RIGHT AND LEFT BUNDLE BRANCHES

CONDUCTION MYOFIBERS (PURKINJE FIBERS)

Left ventricle

node is the normal pacemaker of the heart and has an intrinsic rate of approximately 60 to 100 beats per minute.

Internodal Tracts

The impulse from the sinus node passes to the AV node by three pathways: the anterior, middle, and posterior tracts. The anterior internodal pathway begins at the anterior margin of the sinus node and curves anteriorly around the superior vena cava to enter the anterior interatrial band, called Bachmann's bundle. This bundle is the preferential pathway to the left atrium. The middle internodal tract begins at the superior and posterior margins of the sinus node and travels behind the superior vena cava to the crest of the interatrial septum, where a few strands continue to the left atrium, but the bulk of fibers descend in the interatrial septum to the superior margin of the AV node. The posterior internodal tract begins at the posterior margin of the sinus node, travels posteriorly around the superior vena cava into the interatrial septum above the coronary sinus, and joins the posterior portion of the AV node (Braunwald, 1988). Destruction of one or more of these pathways during surgery seems to be associated with a higher incidence of postoperative dysrhythmias, and some evidence seems to exist that these pathways could form important components of the route taken by the circus movements of atrial flutter (Thalen, 1981).

The AV Node

The AV node is located on the floor of the right atrium anterior to the coronary sinus. The node is a flat elliptical structure about 3 mm wide and 6 mm long and is located in the endocardial surface of the right side of the interatrial septum just anterior to the ostium of the coronary sinus and directly above the insertion of the septal leaflet of the tricuspid valve. Hoffman and Cranefield (1960) divided the AV node electrophysiologically into three parts according to the action potentials and response to electrical and chemical stimulation demonstrated by the cells in the three regions: (1) the upper junctional area (AN region), (2) the middle nodal area (N region), and (3) the lower junctional area (NH region) (Fig. 9–3).

The upper and lower junctional areas contain cells that depolarize rapidly and demonstrate automaticity. The middle nodal area contains cells that depolarize slowly, conduct slowly, lack automaticity, and are difficult to stimulate electrically. The artery supplying the AV node arises from the right coronary artery in about 86% of individuals, from the left coronary artery in 12%, and from both arteries in 2% (Lipman et al., 1984).

The AV node has two separate conduction path-

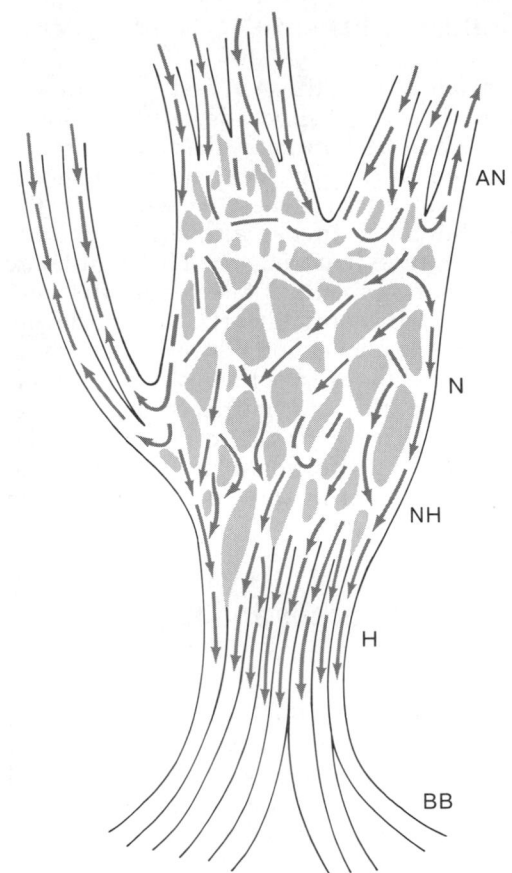

FIGURE 9–3. The AV junction. *Abbreviations:* AN, atrionodal; N, nodal; NH, nodal–His; H, bundle of His; BB, bundle branches. (Redrawn from Sherf, L., and James, T. N. (1972). *American Journal of Cardiology,* 29, 529.)

ways, called alpha and beta, each with distinct electrophysiologic features. The alpha pathway has slower conduction and a shorter refractory period. The beta pathway has faster conduction and a longer refractory period. Impulses originating from the sinus node normally travel along the beta pathway because of its faster conduction (Fig. 9–4).

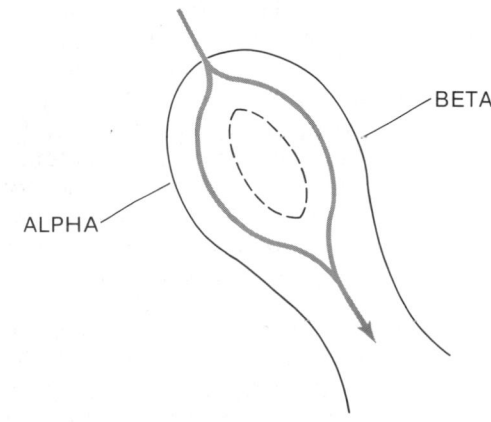

FIGURE 9–4. Normal conduction through fast and slow pathways of the AV node.

The Bundle of His

The distal end of the AV node continues as the bundle of His and is approximately 2 cm long in the adult. The bundle penetrates the central fibrous body and proceeds anteriorly, descending toward the intraventricular septum, where it divides into the right and left bundle branches and finally the Purkinje system. Impulses entering the His bundle are conducted rapidly—six times faster than through myocardial tissue. In normal hearts, the bundle of His is the sole muscle connection between the atria and the ventricles. Pathologic problems of the central fibrous body or of the tricuspid, mitral, or aortic valves may affect the AV node or the common bundle. Any dysfunction of this portion of the conducting system may affect the coordinated functioning of the atria and ventricles.

The Bundle Branches and Purkinje System

The bundle of His divides into the right and left bundle branches. The right bundle branch (RBB) is a stalk of fibers that extends down the right side of the ventricular septum until it reaches the anterior papillary muscle at the apex of the right ventricle. There it divides into smaller branches, joining the Purkinje system and spreading out over the free right ventricular wall and adjacent septum. The right bundle is close to the endocardial surface along two-thirds of its length (proximal third and distal third) and is therefore vulnerable to slight pressure changes on the intracavitary portion of the right side of the ventricular septum. Because of its length, thinness, location, and single blood supply, the right bundle branch is more frequently involved in conduction delays or conduction block.

The main trunk of the left bundle branch (LBB) is narrow and widens prior to branching into the anterior (superior) division and the posterior (inferior) division. The anterior fascicle is long and thin and lies below the aortic valve in the left ventricular outflow tract. Its size and location as well as its single blood supply make it the next most vulnerable branch after the right bundle branch. The posterior division is much thicker and shorter and extends along the septum toward the inferior and posterior surfaces of the left ventricle. With its double blood supply from the left anterior descending coronary artery and posterior branch of the right coronary artery, it is much less vulnerable to disease, and therefore a block affecting the posterior division has greater prognostic significance. Many individuals have an additional fascicle of the left bundle branch that supplies the septum (Marriott, 1988). This little known fascicle was depicted by Tawara as early as 1906 and has been found to originate either from the common left bundle or from the anterior or posterior fascicle (Marriott and Conover, 1989). Histopatho-logic studies have noted this midseptal addition in 33 of 49 normal hearts (Demoulin and Kulbertus, 1972).

Blood Supply to Conducting Tissues

Blood supply to the conduction system comes from the coronary arteries, which are located behind the cusps of the aortic valve. The right coronary artery (RCA) leaves the right aortic sinus and descends in the right atrioventricular groove curving posteriorly at the acute margin of the right ventricle. The main left coronary artery (LCA) arises from the upper portion of the left aortic sinus, passing behind the right ventricular outflow tract before bifurcating into the left anterior descending (LAD) and circumflex branches. Figure 9–5 illustrates circulation to the anterior and posterior surfaces of the heart in greater detail.

The terms "dominant" and "preponderance" are often used when referring to the coronary arteries. These terms relate to the vessel, either the right coronary artery or the left coronary artery (usually the left circumflex), that supplies the posterior diaphragmatic portion of the intraventricular septum and the diaphragmatic surface of the left ventricle (Schlesinger, 1940). The right coronary artery is dominant in 77% to 90% of human hearts (Baroldi and Scomazzoni, 1967; James, 1961). Table 9–1 provides a comprehensive list of the patterns of circulation to the conduction system.

Frink and James (1973) studied the blood supply to the bundle of His and proximal conduction system in 10 normal hearts, and although their sample was small, it provides helpful information on the blood supply to the conduction system. These researchers found that the bundle of His was supplied by the AV nodal artery and the septal branch of the LAD in nine cases. The RBB and anterior fascicle of the LBB were supplied by the septal branch of the LAD in nine cases, five of which also received some blood from the AV nodal artery. The posterior fascicle of the LBB was supplied by the septal branch of the LAD in five cases, four of which also received some blood from the AV nodal artery. The AV nodal artery alone supplied the RBB in one case, the anterior fascicle in one case, and the posterior fascicle in five cases. The reader is referred to Braunwald (1988) for a comprehensive discussion of this subject.

Innervation of Conducting Tissues

The heart is supplied with both sympathetic and parasympathetic nerves (Fig. 9–6). Parasympathetic innervation of the heart is transmitted via the vagus nerve. The parasympathetic system has its greatest influence on the SA and AV nodes and atrial muscle, which represents the primary distribution of the parasympathetic fibers within the heart (Guyton, 1991). Stimulation of the parasympathetic system

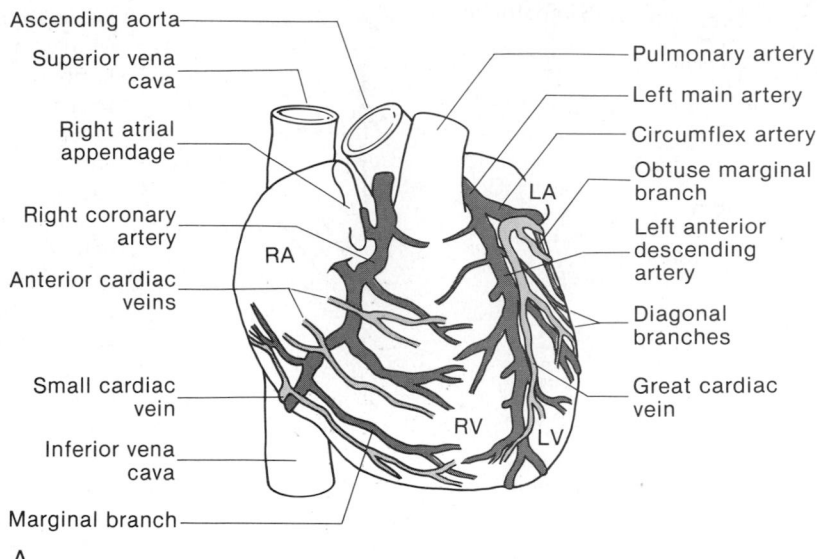

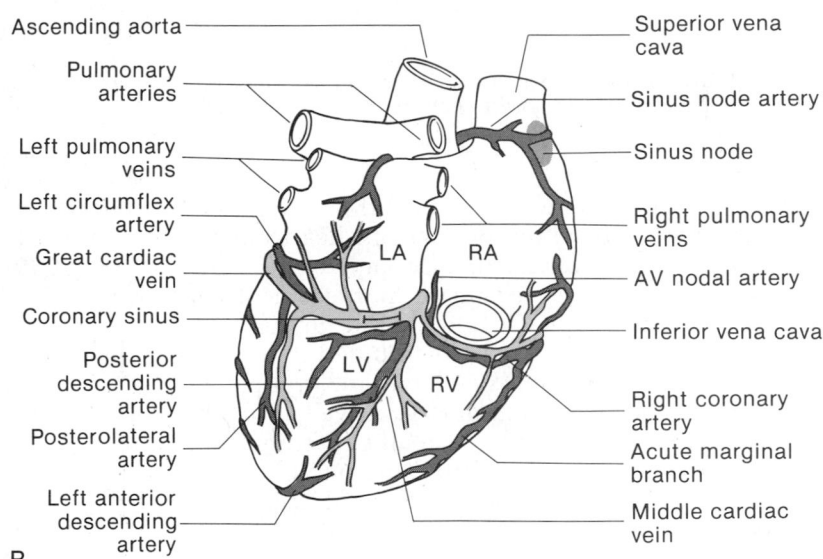

FIGURE 9–5. *A*, Principal arteries and veins on the anterior surface of the heart. Part of the right atrial appendage has been resected. The left coronary artery arises from the left coronary aortic sinus behind the pulmonary trunk. *B*, Principal arteries and veins on the inferior-posterior surfaces of the heart. This schematic drawing illustrates the heart tilted upward at a nonphysiologic angle; normally, little of the inferior cardiac surface is visible posteriorly. The right coronary artery is shown to cross the crux and to supply the atrioventricular node. The artery to the sinus node in this figure arises from the right coronary artery. *Abbreviations:* RA, right atrium; RV, right ventricle; LA, left atrium; LV, left ventricle. (Redrawn from Halpenny, J. (1989). Functional clinical anatomy. In Underhill, S., Woods, S., Sivarajan, E., and Halpenny, C. (Eds.), *Cardiac nursing* (2nd ed., p. 22). Philadelphia: J. B. Lippincott. Previously adapted from Walmsley, R., and Watson, H. (1978). *Clinical anatomy of the heart* (p. 205). New York: Churchill Livingstone.)

TABLE 9–1. Circulation to the Conduction System

Structure	RCA	LAD	LCA
SA node	55%	—	45%
Right atrium	55%	—	45%
Left atrium	—	—	Predominantly
AV node	90%	—	10%
Bundle of His	90%	—	10%
Septum	—	Predominantly	Occasionally
RBB	Occasionally	Predominantly	—
Left anterior fascicle	Occasionally	Predominantly	—
Left posterior fascicle			
Right ventricle			
Anterior wall	Predominantly	Occasionally	—
Posterior wall	90%	—	10%
Left ventricle			
inferior	Predominantly	—	—
anterior	—	Predominantly	—
lateral	—	—	Predominantly
posterior	Predominantly	Occasionally	Predominantly
apex	Occasionally	Predominantly	Occasionally

Abbreviations: RCA, right coronary artery; LAD, left anterior descending artery; LCA, left coronary artery; RBB, right bundle branch; AV node, atrioventricular node.

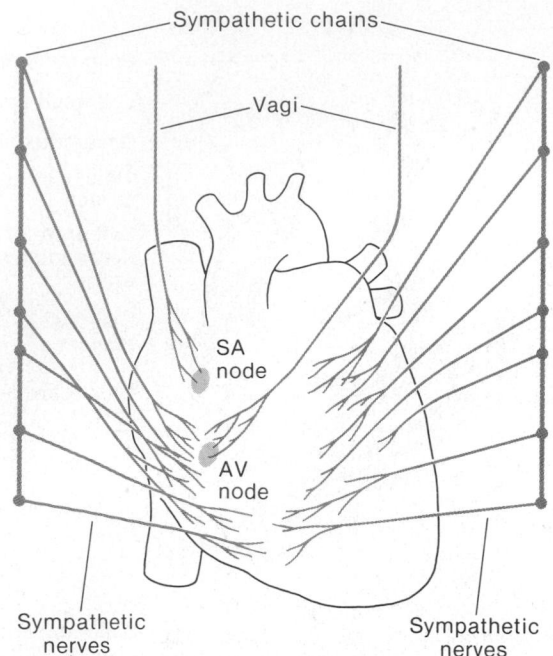

FIGURE 9–6. The cardiac nerves. (Redrawn from Guyton, A. C. (1991). *Textbook of medical physiology* (8th ed., p. 107). Philadelphia: W. B. Saunders.)

causes acetylcholine to be released from vagal nerve endings with a resulting decrease in heart rate and decrease in rate of conduction through the AV node.

Sympathetic nerves originate in the spinal cord between the first thoracic and second lumbar vertebrae. Sympathetic nerves are distributed to the same areas as parasympathetic fibers but are strongly represented in the ventricular muscle as well as in other parts of the heart. With sympathetic stimulation, norepinephrine is released from the nerve endings, resulting in increases in heart rate, contractility, and speed of conduction through the AV node.

ELECTROPHYSIOLOGY

Electrical activity in the heart precedes and initiates mechanical contraction and relaxation. Electrophysiologic events are regulated by the sarcolemma, the cell membrane, which functions as a cell insulator preventing leakage of the electrical charge. Gates in this membrane open in response to changes in the electrical current, allowing movement of ions. These gates are composed of protein or protein-lipid complexes positioned within the phospholipid sarcolemma. Other proteins within the sarcolemma have special pumping functions. The sodium-potassium (Na-K) ATPase pump activates ATP and moves sodium out of the cell and potassium into the cell against concentration gradients (Berne and Levy, 1989).

An action potential is the change in electrical activity that initiates muscular contraction. Action potentials result from changes in the ionic permea-

bility of the cell membrane to such ions as sodium (Na^+), potassium (K^+), and calcium (Ca^{2+}). The concentration gradient of these ions across the semipermeable membrane of the cardiac cell provides an electrochemical basis for the development of the cardiac action potential. Intracellular potassium is 30 times more concentrated inside the cell, whereas sodium is 30 times more concentrated outside the cell. This concentration difference is actively brought about by the outer limiting cell membrane, which possesses an active ion exchange pump: the ATP-dependent Na-K ion pump (Viersma, 1981). This concentration gradient permits the cell to act as a capacitor and to store electrical energy.

The resting cell membrane is relatively permeable to potassium but much less so to sodium and calcium (Fig. 9–7). The difference in permeability promotes a net diffusion of potassium out of the cell. Many of the remaining anions, such as proteins and phosphates, are unable to diffuse out with potassium and cause the interior of the cell to become electronegative while the exterior is positive. This electrical gradient across the cell membrane at rest is called the transmembrane resting potential (TRP) and measures approximately -70 to -90 millivolts (mV) in cardiac cells, depending on their location in the heart. This negativity is partly maintained by the sodium-potassium pump, which moves three sodium ions out of the cell in exchange for two potassium ions (Katz, 1977).

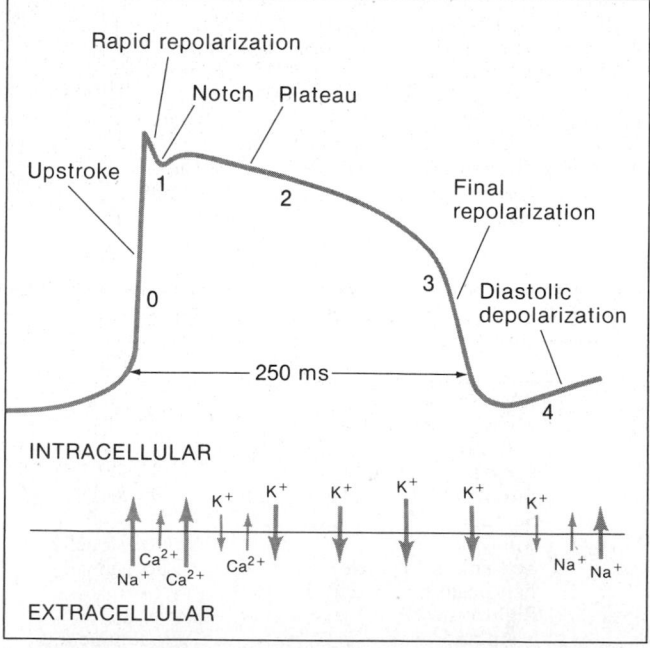

FIGURE 9–7. Schematic illustration of major ionic movements during a Purkinje cell action potential. (Redrawn from Ten Eick, R. E., et al. (1981). Ventricular dysrhythmia: Membrane basis. *Progress in Cardiovascular Disease, 24* (2), 159; Fozzard, J. A., and Gibbons, W. R. (1973). Action potential and contraction of heart muscle. *American Journal of Cardiology, 31,* 183; Underhill, Woods, Sivarajan Froelicher, and Halpenny (1989). *Cardiac nursing* (2nd ed.). Philadelphia: J. B. Lippincott.)

The action potential of pacemaker cells consists of five phases:

Phase 0, rapid depolarization

Phase 1, a brief, rapid period of repolarization

Phase 2, the plateau phase of repolarization

Phase 3, the end of repolarization in which the membrane potential returns to resting potential

Phase 4, resting membrane potential

Cell membrane permeability changes when the cell receives a sufficiently strong stimulus. The stimulus may be electrical, chemical (as in hypoxia), or mechanical (as in chamber dilatation) (Guyton, 1991). With the change in membrane permeability, sodium influx occurs into the cell through "fast sodium channels" in the cell membrane (also known as "fast-response" action potentials). The inside of the cell changes from −90 to about +30 mV. This reversal of the membrane polarity is the so-called overshoot of the cardiac action potential. This rapid depolarization comprises phase 0 and is responsible for the QRS complex on the electrocardiogram. Because the ionic balance has been disturbed, an attempt to balance the charges occurs, and potassium moves out of the cell, completing the terminal phase of depolarization. The inside of the cell becomes positive in relation to the outside. Also during phase 0, the threshold potential for calcium is reached, and calcium begins flowing into the cell through "calcium-sodium channels" (also called "slow channels") (Guyton, 1991) and will continue to do so until the end of phase 2. The overshoot is immediately followed by repolarization, which occurs in three rapid stages as the transmembrane potential returns to the resting state (Fig. 9–8).

Phase 1 signifies inactivation of the fast sodium channels. The fast sodium channels close, and potassium begins to move out of the cell. The slight downward trend is thought to be due to the inward flow of a small amount of negatively charged chloride ions and the efflux of potassium ions (Braunwald, 1988). During phase 2, the plateau phase, there is an influx mainly of calcium, but sodium also diffuses into the cell through slow channels. This influx maintains a prolonged period of depolarization. Calcium ions entering the muscle during this action potential play an important role in the muscle contractile process. The plateau phase is represented on the ECG by the ST segment. During phase 3, the slow channels close and the influx of calcium and sodium ceases. The cell membrane becomes more permeable to potassium, which then diffuses out of the cell, reestablishing the cell's electronegative state.

FIGURE 9–8. Transmembrane potential in the resting, depolarized, and repolarized states. (Redrawn from Lipman, B. S., Dunn, M., and Massie, E. (1984). *Clinical electrocardiography* (7th ed., p. 35). Chicago: Year Book Medical Publishers.)

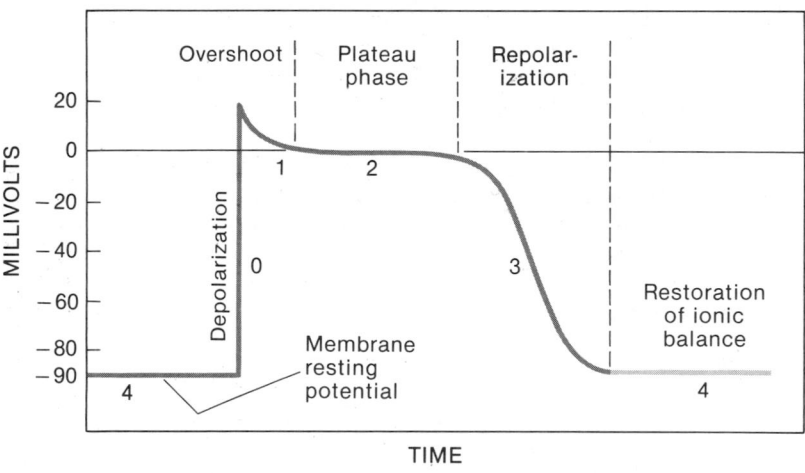

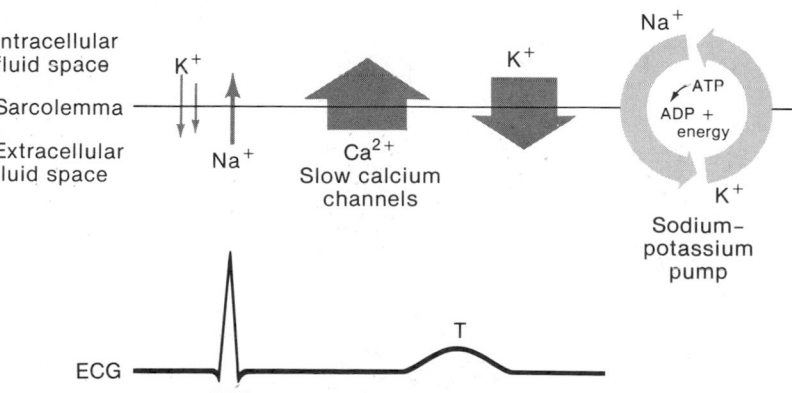

Phase 3 correlates with the T wave on the ECG. At the end of phase 3, distribution of sodium and potassium ions is reversed from the normal resting state. Therefore, in phase 4, the Na^+/K^+ pump is activated, sodium is actively transported out of the cell, and potassium is transported back into the cell.

Automaticity

The action potential of the pacemaker cell differs from the action potential of the myofibril. In the myofibril, the muscle cell, the potential remains at phase 4 until the membrane is reactivated by another stimulus. In contrast, pacemaker cells that have automaticity are unstable and show an upward drifting of phase 4 that results in spontaneous depolarization when the level of electrical activity falls to a certain critical point. The pacemaker cells, located in the sinoatrial node, the distal part of the AV node, and the His-Purkinje network, are capable of spontaneous depolarization and are responsible for the rhythmicity of the heart. Cells in the SA node have the fastest intrinsic rate (60 to 100) and therefore the fastest rate of rise in phase 4, followed by cells just distal to the AV node in the bundle of His. Ventricular cells have the slowest rate of rise in phase 4 and produce a slower rate (less than 40). Both the SA node and the AV node have a slow channel mechanism. The action potential of cells in the sinus node is shown in Figure 9–9. The maximum resting potential of -60 to -70 mV (Guyton, 1991) is substantially less than the -85 to -95 mV characteristic of the ventricular fiber. As the potential reaches approximately 40 mV, the threshold for sodium influx is reached, and the cell suddenly undergoes rapid and full depolarization, or phase 0. Thus, the sinus cell displays automaticity, which is thought to be due to the inherent leakiness of the SA nodal fibers to sodium ions. Phase 0 is slower, and the phase 2 plateau is absent as phase 2 merges gradually into

phase 3. Phase 4 is again established, completing the process of repolarization.

The automatic firing of all pacemaker cells is controlled primarily by the autonomic nervous system. Sympathetic stimulation causes a steepening of phase 4 by increasing the permeability of the fiber membrane to sodium and calcium, resulting in an increased heart rate. Parasympathetic stimulation decreases the "resting" membrane potential of the SA nodal fibers to a level more negative than the normal value, for example, to -65 to -75 mV rather than the normal level of -55 to -60 mV (Guyton, 1991). Thus, the upward drift of the resting membrane potential caused by sodium leakage requires a much longer time to reach the threshold potential for excitation.

Changes in cellular environment with relation to K^+, pH, P_{O_2}, and Ca^{2+} also have a secondary effect on the rate of firing of automatic fibers.

Overdrive suppression is a concept related to automaticity. The automaticity of pacemaker cells becomes depressed after a period of excitation at a high frequency. The SA node with its faster intrinsic rate normally suppresses the automaticity of other potential pacemaker cells, such as those in the Purkinje system. If the SA node should fail, as in a Stokes-Adams attack, a new pacemaker in the Purkinje system may take over but not for 5 to 30 seconds (Guyton, 1991). This period of time is required before the Purkinje fibers can become self-excitatory because of their previous suppression by the SA node. Likewise, if an ectopic atrial focus takes over the rhythm for a certain time period and then suddenly terminates, the SA node might remain quiescent for a short period of time because of overdrive suppression.

The mechanism for overdrive suppression is uncertain. A reasonable hypothesis is based on the activity of the membrane pump, which actively extrudes sodium from the cell in partial exchange for potassium. Sodium enters the cell during depolari-

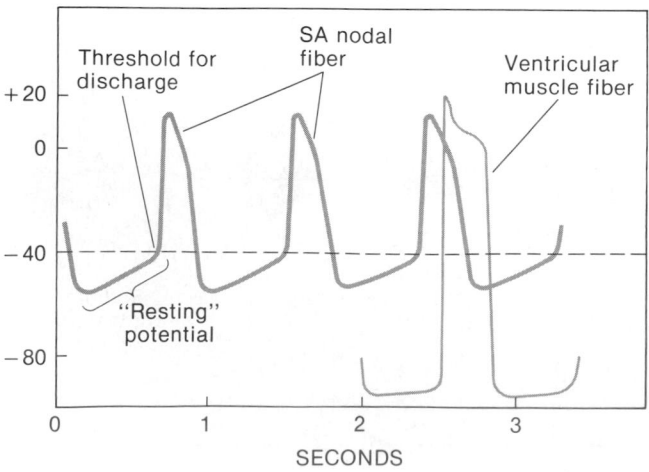

FIGURE 9–9. Action potential of SA nodal fiber and ventricular muscle fiber. (Redrawn from Guyton, A. C. (1991). *Textbook of medical physiology* (8th ed., p. 112). Philadelphia: W. B. Saunders.)

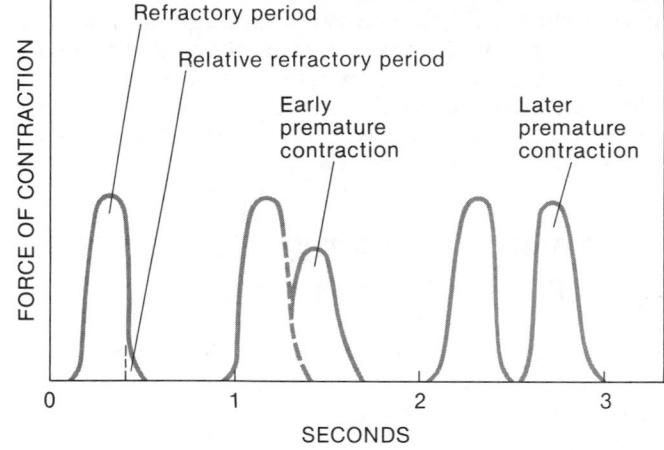

FIGURE 9–10. Contraction of the heart with durations of the refractory period and the relative refractory period, the effect of an early premature contraction, and the effect of a later premature contraction. (Redrawn from Guyton, A. C. (1991). *Textbook of medical physiology* (8th ed., p. 100). Philadelphia: W. B. Saunders.)

zation. The faster the heart rate, the more sodium enters each minute. Under conditions of overdrive, the sodium pump becomes more active in the process of extruding this larger quantity of sodium from the cell interior. The quantity of sodium extruded by the pump exceeds the quantity of potassium that enters the cell. This enhanced activity of the pump results in some hyperpolarization of the cell, since there is a net loss of positive ions from the inside of the cell. Because of hyperpolarization of the cell, the pacemaker potential requires more time to reach the threshold. It has been postulated that, when overdrive suppression suddenly ceases, the sodium pump continues to operate at an accelerated rate for some time, causing an excessive extrusion of sodium that opposes the gradual depolarization of the pacemaker cell during phase 4 and suppresses the intrinsic automaticity temporarily (Berne and Levy, 1988).

Refractory Periods

Cardiac muscle, like all excitable tissue, is refractory to restimulation during the action potential. Specifically, the heart is refractory from phase 0 until almost the end of phase 3 of the action potential.

The total refractory period is divided into two smaller periods: absolute and relative. From the beginning of depolarization with phase 0 and through phases 1 and 2 of repolarization, the heart is in a state of absolute refractoriness. Once a cell has been depolarized, it cannot respond to another stimulus regardless of its strength until the cell is repolarized to a value of approximately −50 mV. The absolute refractory period correlates with the beginning of the QRS complex, includes the ST segment, and terminates just below the beginning of the T wave on the ECG. Phase 3, when the cell returns to a transmembrane potential of approximately −60 mV to −85 mV, is known as the relative refractory period. Phase 3 correlates with the T wave on the ECG. A relatively strong stimulus may evoke a response if it is applied during this phase, but conduction of impulses is slower than in fully repolarized fibers. If an ectopic focus fires during this vulnerable period (R-on-T phenomenon), lethal dysrhythmias may occur. Figure 9–10 illustrates the durations of the refractory period and the relative refractory period, the effect of an early premature contraction, and the effect of a later premature contraction.

The supernormal period is the terminal part of phase 3 just before the cell returns to its resting potential (Fig. 9–11). During this period the cell may

FIGURE 9–11. The various refractory periods during an action potential. *Abbreviations:* ARP, absolute refractory period; ERP, effective refractory period; RRP, relative refractory period; SNP, supernormal refractory period; FRT, full recovery time. (Redrawn from Hoffman, B. F., and Cranefield, P. F. (1960). *Electrophysiology of the heart.* New York: McGraw-Hill.)

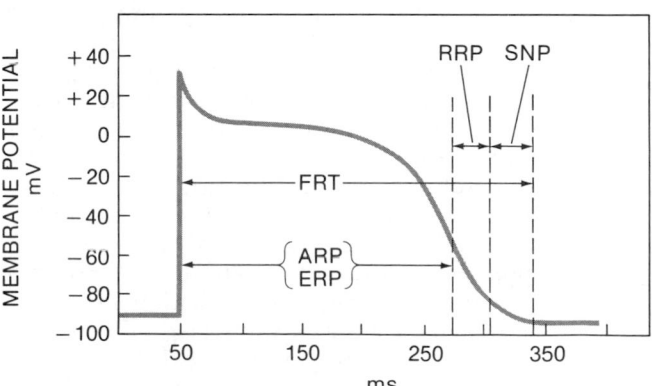

respond to a weaker stimulus than normal. At this point, the cell has recovered enough so that an adequate number of fast sodium channels are available, but the membrane potential is closer to threshold than if the cell had achieved full repolarization. This period corresponds to the terminal portion of the T wave and the U wave.

INTERPRETATION OF THE ELECTROCARDIOGRAM

The electrocardiogram is a simple, inexpensive, and noninvasive graphic recording of the electrical activity of the heart that is invaluable in the diagnosis of many cardiovascular diseases. It records only activity of the myocardial cells, the muscle cells of the heart. Pacemaker cells (such as those in the SA node) and conducting cells (such as those in Bachmann's bundle in the atrium) conduct impulses too rapidly to be picked up by the ECG.

The ECG records the direction and magnitude of the electrical current produced by the heart. During depolarization and repolarization, current flows in many directions at once. The ECG records the resultant forces at each moment in time by averaging these individual forces into a single vector. If all of the instantaneous resultant vectors occurring during one cycle were added together, their sum would represent the average magnitude and direction of ventricular depolarization. The mean QRS axis that we determine on the standard ECG is the average direction of this sum.

The ECG is made up of 12 leads, each viewing the heart from a different perspective. Each lead is made up of two electrodes, one designated as positive and the other negative (as is the case with the bipolar leads I, II, and II) or one designated as positive and the other as a reference point (as is the case with the unipolar leads aVR, aVL, and aVF). This is done automatically by the ECG machine with the positive electrode being designated arbitrarily. If an imaginary line were drawn from the negative to the positive lead, or from the reference point to the positive lead, this line would be the axis of the lead. It is necessary to memorize which electrode is positive and which is negative in each lead to correctly interpret the ECG.

Leads are joined by wires that pass through the galvanometer of the electrocardiograph. These electrodes are placed at specific sites on the body, and the leads are named according to the body sites. Currents generated by the heart cause certain deflections on the ECG according to how they relate to the axis of the lead. A depolarization wave moving toward a positive lead will create an upright, positive complex on the ECG (Fig. 9–12). A depolarization wave moving away from a positive lead will create a downward, negative complex on the ECG (Fig. 9–13). A depolarization wave that moves toward and

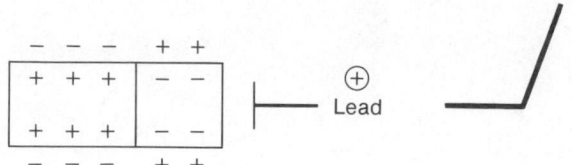

FIGURE 9–12. Depolarization wave toward a positive lead.

then passes the positive lead creates a complex that is biphasic or half positive and half negative (Fig. 9–14).

The Limb Leads

The limb leads, composed of three standard (I, II, and II) and three augmented leads (aVR, aVL, and aVF), view the heart in a vertical, or frontal, plane. To make up the limb leads, electrodes are placed on the arms and the legs and attached to cables connected to the ECG machine. The electrode at the right leg is consistently the ground, or neutralizing, electrode, whereas the left leg is consistently positive in leads in which it is involved. In lead I, the negative electrode is on the right arm and the positive electrode is on the left arm. In lead II, the negative electrode is on the right arm and the positive electrode is on the left leg. In lead III, the negative electrode is on the left arm and the positive electrode is on the left leg (Fig. 9–15).

The same electrodes are used to record the unipolar leads aVR, aVL, and aVF. In these leads, one electrode is chosen to be positive, and all the others are averaged to make a common negative electrode halfway between the two negative limbs. The electrical forces recorded in the unipolar leads are small; they are, therefore, augmented, which is designated by the prefix "a"—aVR, aVL, aVF. The positive electrode of aVR is on the right arm. The positive electrode of aVL is on the left arm, and the positive electrode of aVF is toward the feet (Fig. 9–16).

Willem Einthoven first introduced the three bipolar limb leads in 1902. Einthoven's law states that the complex in lead II is equal to the sum of the complexes in leads I and III. The three leads may be transposed into an equilateral triangle called the Einthoven triangle in Figure 9–17A. Visualizing the heart in the center of the triangle is helpful in

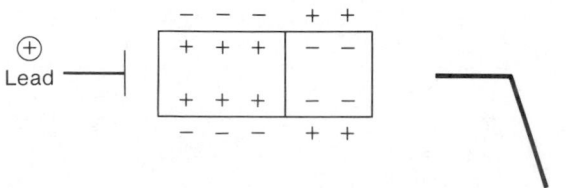

FIGURE 9–13. Depolarization wave moving away from a positive lead.

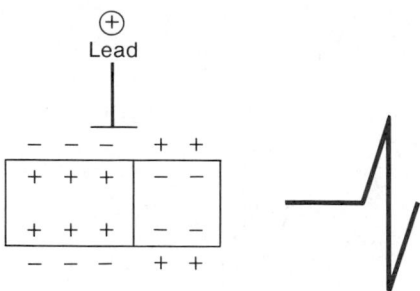

FIGURE 9–14. Biphasic complex.

determining its relationship to the directions of current and in visualizing the QRS complex in each lead. The sum of its forces is directed down and toward the left because of the greater mass and electrical force of the left ventricle. The small arrows (Fig. 9–17B) show the magnitude and direction of the many vectors, whereas the large arrow shows the summation or average orientation of these forces. This summation of forces in the ventricles is called the QRS axis. Although the QRS axis is of primary importance, the axis of the P and T waves can also be calculated.

With the heart in the middle of each of these leads, it is apparent why the QRS appears as it does in each lead in the normal heart (Fig. 9–18). In lead I, the ventricular forces are moving toward the positive electrode, so the QRS complex has a mostly positive deflection. Remember, however, that ventricular depolarization begins with septal depolarization, which occurs from left to right, causing an initial movement toward the negative electrode and resulting in a small Q wave in several leads. This septal Q is seen in leads aVL, I, V_5, V_6, and sometimes in lead III. General characteristics of this nonpathologic Q wave are that the wave must be less than 0.04 second wide and of low amplitude, with a depth of less than 25% of the height of the preceding R wave (Marriott, 1988).

In lead II, the ventricular forces travel more directly toward the positive electrode than in all other leads. Because the normal atrial forces also travel toward the positive electrode, the P wave is also upright. In

contrast, in aVR, when atrial forces flow directly away from the positive electrode, the P wave is negative. Negative Ps in lead II should cause one to suspect that electrodes have been incorrectly applied.

The Precordial Leads

The precordial leads (also known as chest leads or V leads) record the heart's activity in the horizontal plane. The electrodes are placed in the intercostal spaces, identified in Figure 9–19. The correct positions are identified by palpating the intercostal spaces. To find V_1, palpate the second intercostal space, which is slightly down and to the right from the angle of Louis, and continue to palpate down two more intercostal spaces. This will be the fourth intercostal space on the right side of the sternum (the sternal border). From this point, the rest of the precordial leads can be placed in the following locations:

V_1, fourth intercostal space (4ICS) at the right sternal border (RSB)

V_2, 4ICS at the left sternal border (LSB)

V_3, midway between V_2 and V_4

V_4, 5ICS at the midclavicular line (MCL)

V_5, 5ICS at the anterior axillary line

V_6, 5ICS at the midaxillary line

Occasionally additional precordial leads may be necessary, as in patients with congenital heart disease or right ventricular infarction. Leads on the right side of the chest are placed by palpating the right side of the chest for the landmarks described earlier. These areas should be marked on the patient's chest upon admission to the critical care unit to ensure consistent placement and subsequent accurate interpretation of the ECG. Too often, application of leads is a haphazard procedure, making day-to-day comparison of a patient's electrocardiogram a difficult task.

Each of the precordial leads views ventricular depolarization from a different perspective (Fig. 9–20).

FIGURE 9–15. Three standard limb leads.

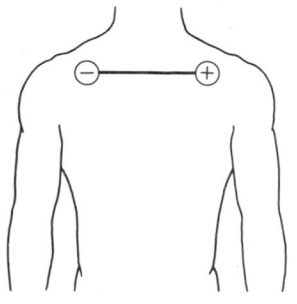
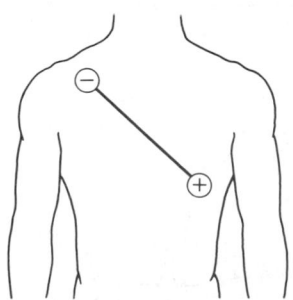
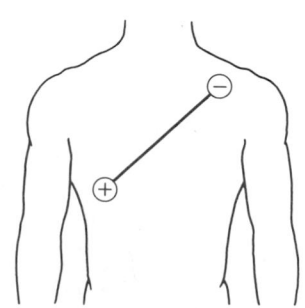

I   II   III

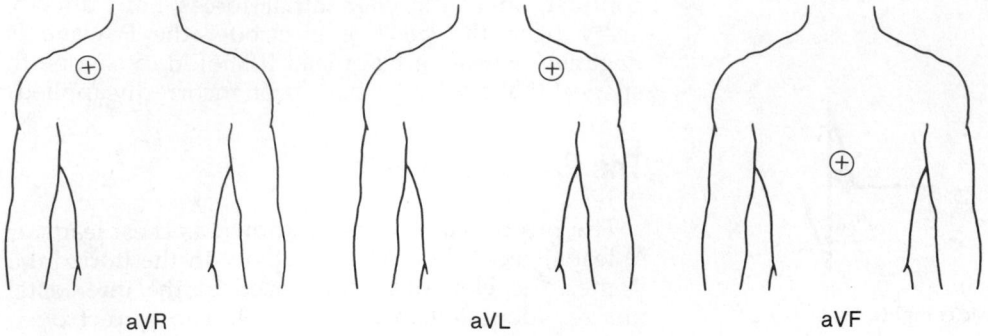

aVR   aVL   aVF

FIGURE 9–16. Three augmented leads.

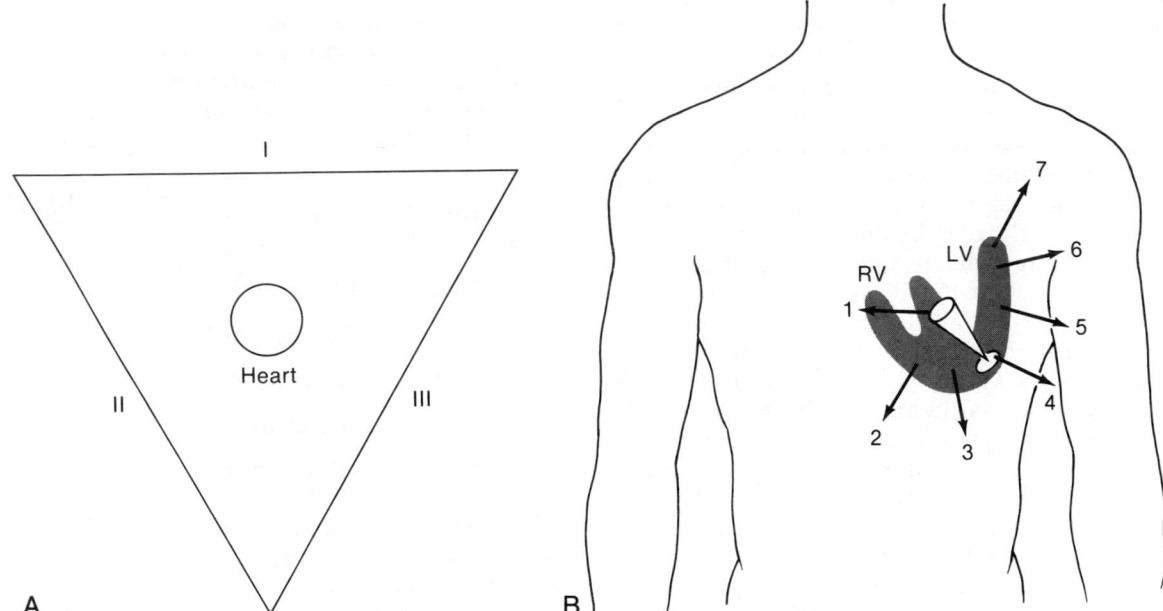

A   B

FIGURE 9–17. *A,* Einthoven triangle. *B,* QRS axis.

FIGURE 9–18. QRS in each lead.

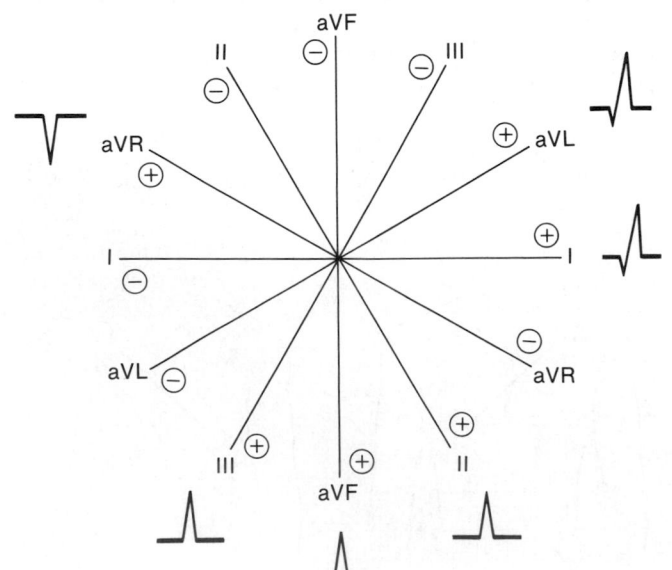

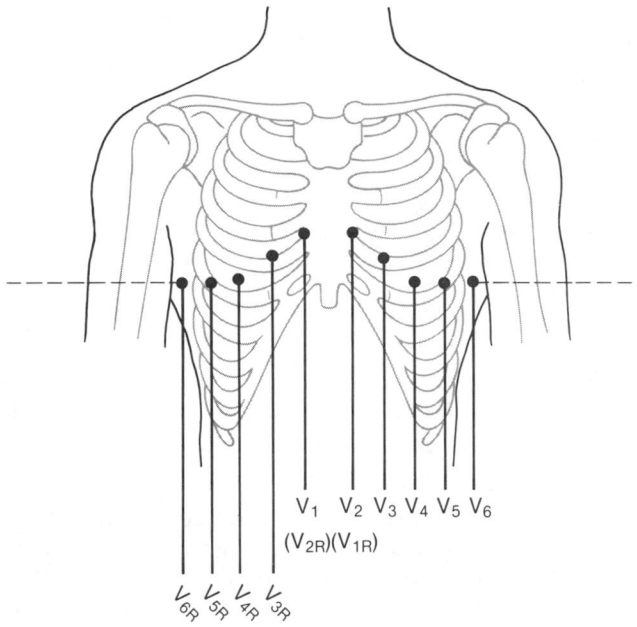

FIGURE 9–19. Precordial leads.

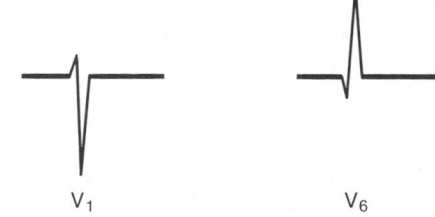

FIGURE 9–20. Ventricular depolarization in the precordial leads.

Lead V_1 lies over the right ventricle and "sees" the wave of septal depolarization coming toward it initially before it turns and travels in the opposite direction. Thus, lead V_1 has a small R wave and a deep S wave and is primarily a negative complex. This may be denoted by $_r$S.

The opposite is true in V_6. Initially, the ventricular depolarization wave (septal depolarization) moves away from the positive lead in V_6, and then the majority of forces move directly toward the lead as the lateral ventricular wall depolarizes. This creates a QRS with a small Q (a "septal" Q) wave and a tall R wave.

Applying the preceding information, one can see how and why the QRS evolves from V_1 to V_6. This change in the QRS complex across the precordium is called "R wave progression" and is an indication of a normal myocardium (Fig. 9–21). Leads V_3 and V_4 are called the "transition zone." This is where the predominantly QRS deflections in leads V_1 and V_2 become predominantly more positive. Usually one of these leads is biphasic, as is V_3 in Figure 9–19. A transition complex (RS) in lead V_1 or V_2 indicates early transition, whereas a biphasic complex in V_5 or V_6 represents late transition (Abedin and Conner, 1989).

Monitoring Leads

Any of the leads above may be used to monitor the patient in the critical care unit if the monitoring equipment has the capability. Lead II has frequently been the lead of choice because of the easy visibility of P waves. However, there is good evidence that lead V_1 and sometimes V_6 provide more information. Marriott has advocated the use of a modified V_1, MCL_1, for years (1983, 1988). This lead is a modified version of V_1 in which the positive electrode is in the V_1 position at the fourth right intercostal space, and the negative electrode is on the left arm (or left shoulder area). The ground lead may be placed anywhere but is usually at the right shoulder.

To obtain an MCL_6 lead, the positive electrode is at the V_6 position with the negative lead at the left shoulder and the ground at the right shoulder. MCL_1 and MCL_6 are useful in detecting bundle branch blocks, differentiating right and left ventricular premature beats, and differentiating ventricular beats from aberrantly conducted beats (Fig. 9–22). See Table 9–2 for a summary of the advantages of the various ECG monitoring leads.

Axis Determination

The ECG records the mean vector, which is the sum of electrical potentials as well as mean magnitude, direction, and polarity, as discussed earlier. A vector can be drawn for the P wave, the QRS complex, and the T wave. Each vector is constantly changing and precise calculation is complicated, requiring the use of frequent plotting with a vectorcardiogram. For clinical purposes with most patients, the ECG is sufficient to determine the general orientation of this vector, which normally points left-

FIGURE 9–21. R wave progression.

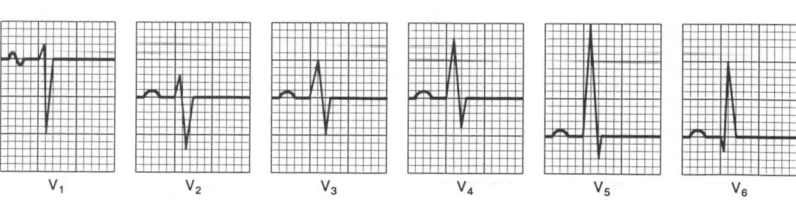

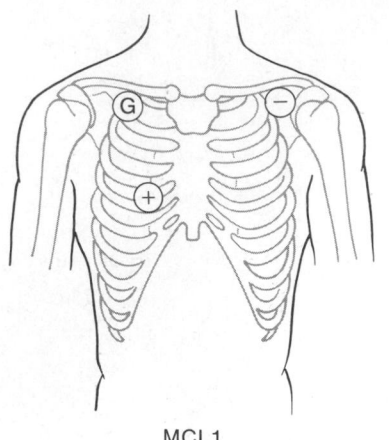
MCL1

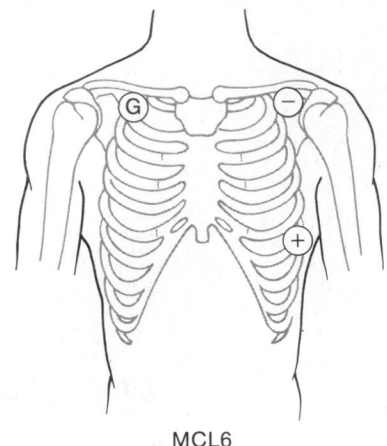
MCL6

FIGURE 9–22. Monitoring leads of MCL₁ and MCL₆.

ward and inferiorly, somewhere between the left shoulder and just below the right hip (Conover, 1988). An ability to determine ventricular ectopy from ventricular aberrancy and in diagnosing hemiblock is important for the critical care nurse.

The QRS axis changes normally with age and may vary with chest size. During infancy and childhood the axis is more rightward or inferior but becomes more leftward or horizontal throughout life (Ziegler, 1951). Individuals with a long thin chest tend to have a QRS that is more vertical or rightward, and those with a thick, wide chest will have a leftward, more horizontal axis. The QRS axis may be altered abnormally by pathology as shown in Table 9–3.

The hexaxial reference system is used in discussing and determining axis. It is enclosed within a circle with the positive and negative ends of each of the frontal leads labeled and the degrees of a 360 degree circle identified (Fig. 9–23). Each end of a lead corresponds to a particular degree on the hexaxial reference system.

Using the quadrant method, normal axis is between 0 and +90 degrees. Left axis deviation (LAD) is between 0 degrees and −90 degrees, while right axis deviation (RAD) is between +90 and +180 degrees. The area between −90 and ±180 is called indeterminate, extreme right, or extreme left axis and must be resolved by methods to be discussed (Marriott, 1983).

The QRS vector is determined from the ECG by projecting the magnitude, direction, and polarity of the QRS deflection in the ECG lead onto its axis lead in the hexaxial reference system. If the majority of the QRS deflection in the lead is positive (above the baseline), the vector points toward the positive end of that axis lead. If the majority of the deflection is negative (below the baseline), the vector points toward the negative end of that axis lead in the hexaxial reference system. If the QRS is biphasic (equally positive and negative), the vector will be perpendicular to that axis lead in the reference system.

Several rules are helpful in determining axis. First, the largest deflection in an ECG lead projects a vector that is parallel to its corresponding axis lead. Conversely, the smallest or most biphasic QRS deflection in a lead projects a vector that is perpendicular to its corresponding axis lead.

There are several ways to determine axis. One of the quickest is to simply look at leads I and aVF. If the QRS complex is positive in leads I and aVF, the QRS axis must be normal. The positive end of lead I

TABLE 9–2. Advantages of Electrocardiographic Leads

Lead	Advantages
MCL₁ (modified V₁), MCL₆ (modified V₆)	1. Allows distinction between (a) left ventricular and right ventricular ectopy, and (b) left ventricular and right ventricular artificial pacing 2. Allows distinction between right and left bundle branch block 3. Allows distinction between aberration and ectopy 4. Assists in diagnoses that require well-formed P waves 5. Apex of the heart is not covered by an electrode and is clear for auscultation and defibrillation without electrode interference
M3	1. Allows identification of retrograde P waves.
Lead II	1. Assists in the diagnosis of hemiblock

From Marriott, H.J.L. and Fogg, E. (1970). Constant monitoring for cardiac dysrhythmias and block. *Modern Concepts of Cardiovascular Disease,* 39 (6), 103–108. By permission of the American Heart Association, Inc.

TABLE 9–3. Causes of Axis Deviation

Left	Right
Normal variation	Normal variation
Extensive inferior MI	Lateral MI
Left anterior hemiblock	Left posterior hemiblock
WPW syndrome	Right bundle branch block
Hyperkalemia	Emphysema
Emphysema	Right ventricular hypertrophy
Mechanical shifts—ascites, pregnancy, tumors	WPW syndrome
Left bundle branch block	Ventricular ectopic rhythms
Left ventricular hypertrophy	Left ventricular pacing
Older age	
Ventricular ectopic rhythms	

Abbreviations: MI, myocardial infarction; WPW, Wolff-Parkinson-White.

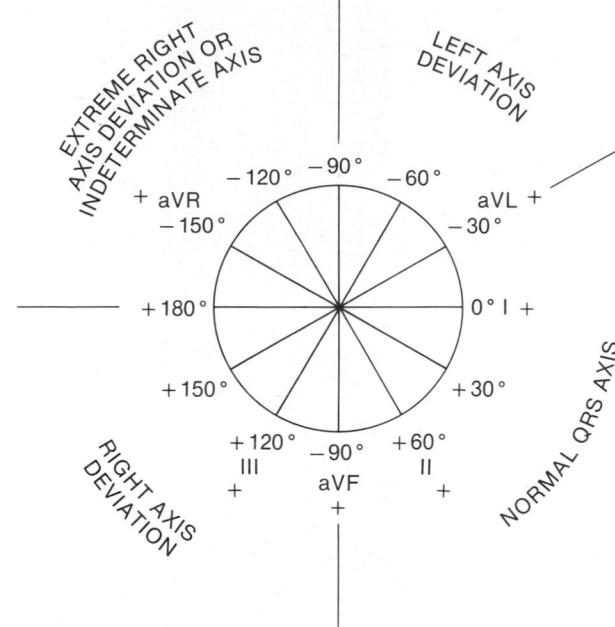

FIGURE 9–23. Hexaxial reference system.

is at 0 degrees. A complex is positive in lead I if the wave of depolarization is coming toward it. This information alone tells us that the vector is between −90 degrees and +90 degrees.

The positive end of aVF is at +90 degrees. The complex will be positive if the wave of depolarization is coming toward it, indicating that the mean vector for the lead is between 0 degrees and 180 degrees. Therefore, if the QRS complex is positive in both lead I and aVF, the mean QRS vector is somewhere between 0 and +90 degrees in the normal range. Figure 9–24 illustrates axis deviations in leads I and aVF.

A more interesting and exact method, although time-consuming, of determining axis is to draw the hexaxial reference system on graph paper and plot several of the leads on the system (Fig. 9–25). For instance, in the following ECG, the complex in lead II has a positive deflection of 5 mm and a negative deflection of 0 mm, the sum of the deflection is +5 mm. This +5 mm can be plotted on the positive end

of lead II as in Figure 9–26 and a line drawn through it that is perpendicular to lead II. Then, another lead can be looked for on the ECG and the same thing done, for example, lead III in Figure 9–26. If it is plotted and another line drawn through it that is perpendicular to lead III, the place where these two lines intersect is the mean QRS vector. A line is then drawn from the intersection through the center of the hexaxial center. In this situation, the vector is about +50 degrees. If the rule above applies, the lead perpendicular to this vector should be isoelectric. The lead closest to being perpendicular in this example is lead aVL, and it is indeed isoelectric. This vector is closest to lead II, which, following the rule, has the biggest positive deflection of all six leads.

Rotation

The discussion of axis relates only to the QRS vector in the frontal plane. When the vector is deter-

FIGURE 9–24. Axis deviation in leads 1 and aVF.

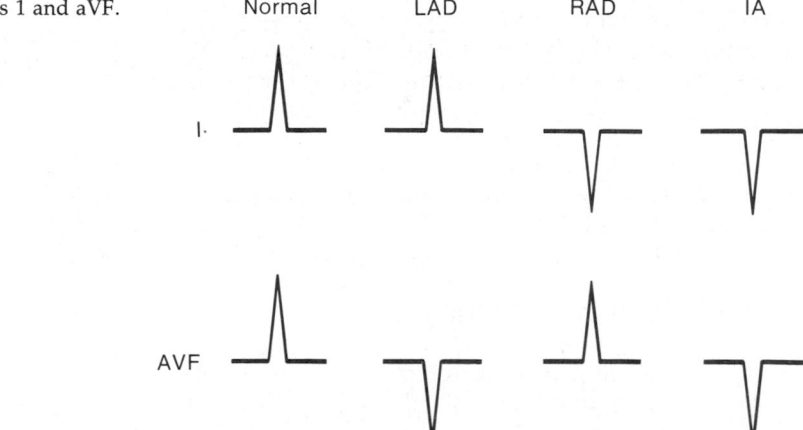

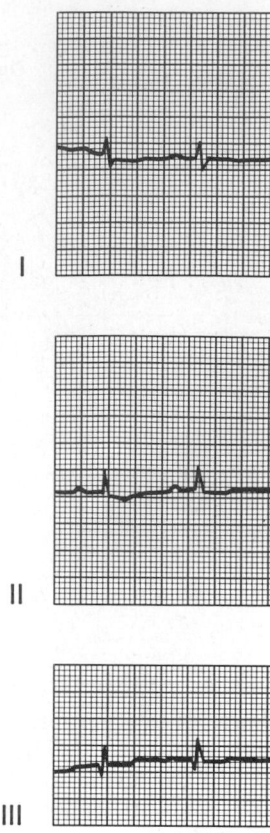

FIGURE 9–25. Hexaxial reference system in various leads.

ventricular hypertrophy (LVH), left axis deviation may occur because the mean vector is pulled even more to the left than usual. Left axis deviation beyond −15 degrees is often seen, but the predominant feature of left ventricular hypertrophy is an increased R wave amplitude in leads overlying the left ventricle and an increased S wave amplitude in leads overlying the right ventricle. Thaler (1988) suggests the following useful criteria in the precordial leads:

- The R wave amplitude in lead V_5 or V_6 plus the S wave amplitude in lead V_1 or V_2 exceeds 35 mm
- The R wave amplitude in V_5 exceeds 26 mm
- The R wave amplitude in V_6 exceeds 18 mm
- The R wave amplitude in V_6 exceeds the R wave amplitude in V_5.

The more positive the criteria, the greater the possibility that the patient has left ventricular hypertrophy (Fig. 9–28). Generally, with left ventricular hypertrophy, the normal dominance of the left ventricle is exaggerated, and tall R waves become taller and deep S waves become deeper (Marriott, 1988).

Look for evidence of left ventricular hypertrophy in patients with hypertension, aortic valvular disorders, mitral valve insufficiency, and any conditions that lead to pressure or volume overload of the left ventricle.

Right Ventricular Hypertrophy

In patients with right ventricular hypertrophy the normal dominance of the left ventricle is upset, and there is a change in the normal precordial pattern: R

mined in the horizontal plane it is called rotation. Cardiac rotation is conventionally expressed as if one were looking up at the heart from the pelvis. It is determined by looking at the precordial leads and noting whether the transitional zone (where the R and S waves are approximately equal in size as discussed earlier) occurs at V_3 and V_4, as it does normally, or if it occurs at a different time. Normally, the interventricular septum is positioned under the center of the sternum, so that lead V_1 is to the right of the septum and is located over the right ventricle. Lead V_2 is located over the interventricular septum and may reflect either the right ventricle or the left ventricle. If the transition occurs early, in V_1 or V_2, the rotation is counterclockwise. If it occurs later in V_5 or V_6, the rotation is clockwise. See Figure 9–27. The top figure shows an observer lying on the ground, viewing someone's heart. The six V leads show normal R wave progression. In the bottom figure, the V leads show a delayed transition occurring at V_5 and V_6. Clockwise rotation describes a delayed transition zone, and counterclockwise rotation an early transition.

Left Ventricular Hypertrophy

An understanding of axis determination is useful in determining hypertrophy on the ECG. With left

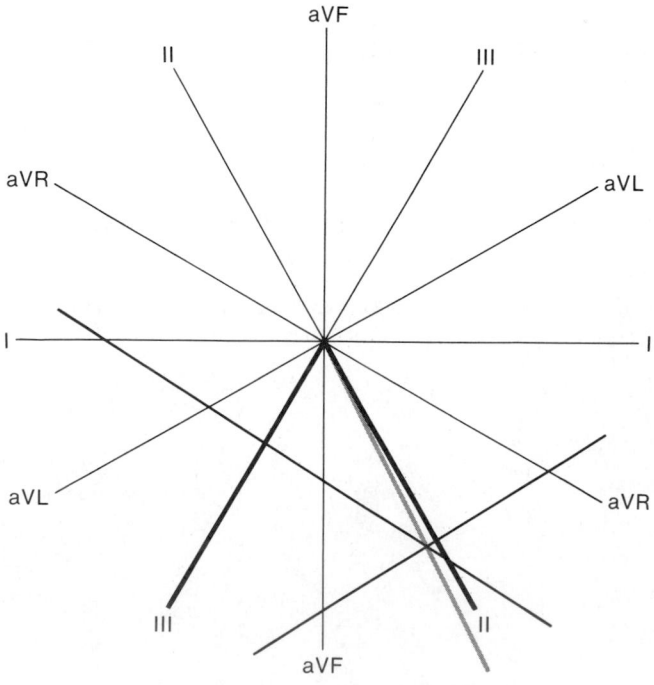

FIGURE 9–26. Determining QRS vector.

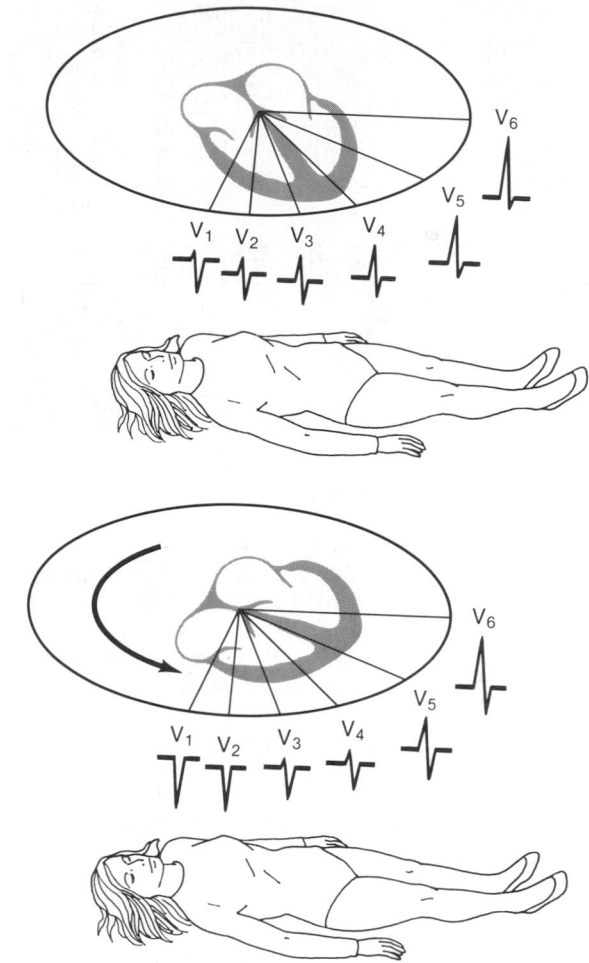

FIGURE 9–27. Cardiac rotation. The top figure shows an observer lying on the ground, viewing someone's heart. The six V leads are illustrated, showing normal R wave progression. In the bottom figure, the six V leads show a delayed transition zone occurring at V_5/V_6. This situation is created by keeping the V leads where they are but rotating the heart clockwise (as perceived by our supine figure). Clockwise rotation moves the septum, where transition occurs, into the territory of leads V_5 and V_6. Similarly, counterclockwise rotation would move the transition zone into the territory of V_1/V_2. (Redrawn from Thaler, M. S. (1988). *The only EKG book you'll ever need* (p. 73). Philadelphia: J. B. Lippincott.)

waves assume prominence in the right precordial leads while deepening S waves develop in the left precordial leads (Fig. 9–29). Other criteria for determining right ventricular hypertrophy include:

■ Reversal of the precordial pattern with tall R waves over the right precordium (V_1 and V_2) and deep S waves over the left precordium (V_5 and V_6); or RS across the precordium

FIGURE 9–28. Left ventricular hypertrophy. (Redrawn from Goldman, M. J. (1986). *Principles of clinical electrocardiography* (p. 194). Los Altos, CA: Lange Medical Publications.)

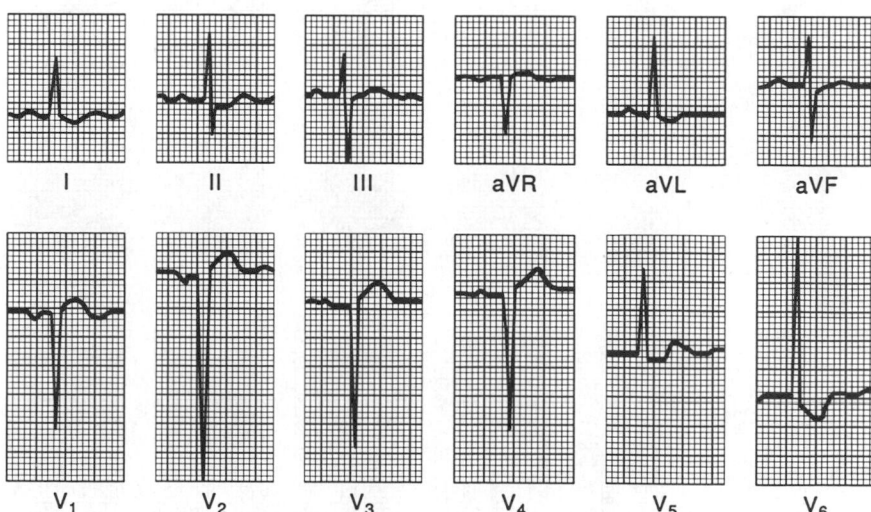

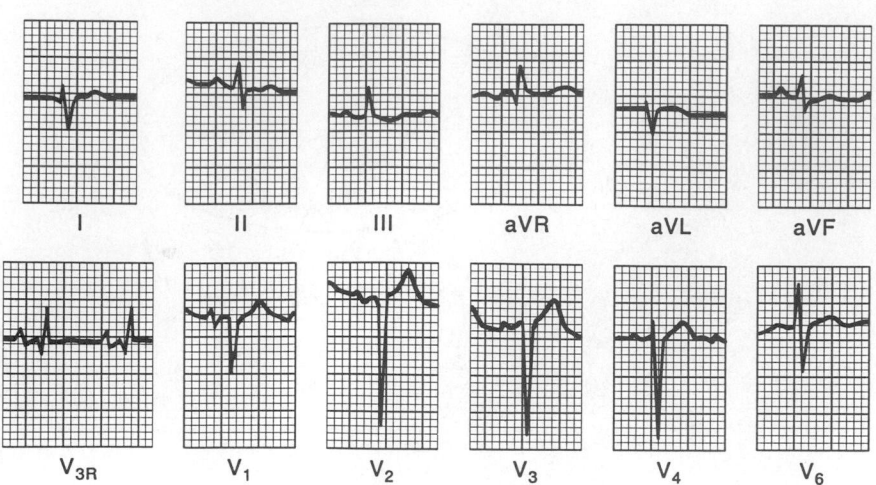

FIGURE 9–29. Right ventricular hypertrophy. (Redrawn from Goldman, M. J. (1986). *Principles of clinical electrocardiography* (p. 103). Los Altos, CA: Lange Medical Publications.)

- QRS interval within normal limits
- Late intrinsicoid* deflection in leads V_1 and V_2
- Right axis deviation (Marriott, 1988).

Right ventricular hypertrophy can be caused by abnormalities of the pulmonary valve, conditions causing pulmonary hypertension, and congenital lesions that overload the right ventricle.

---

*A "late intrinsicoid deflection" refers to a downstroke (or S wave) recorded on a clinical, rather than direct epicardial, lead that is delayed longer than 0.02 second in V_1 and 0.04 second in V_6 (Marriott, 1988).

Atrial Hypertrophy

The normal P wave is gently rounded, less than 0.12 second in duration, and should not exceed 2.5 mm in amplitude in any lead. The first part of the P wave represents right atrial depolarization, whereas the second part of it reflects left atrial depolarization.

In right atrial hypertrophy, the first portion of the P wave increases in amplitude to 3 mm or greater, especially in leads II, III, and aVF, where P waves are most pronounced, and the axis of the P wave may swing rightward of +90 degrees (Fig. 9–30A).

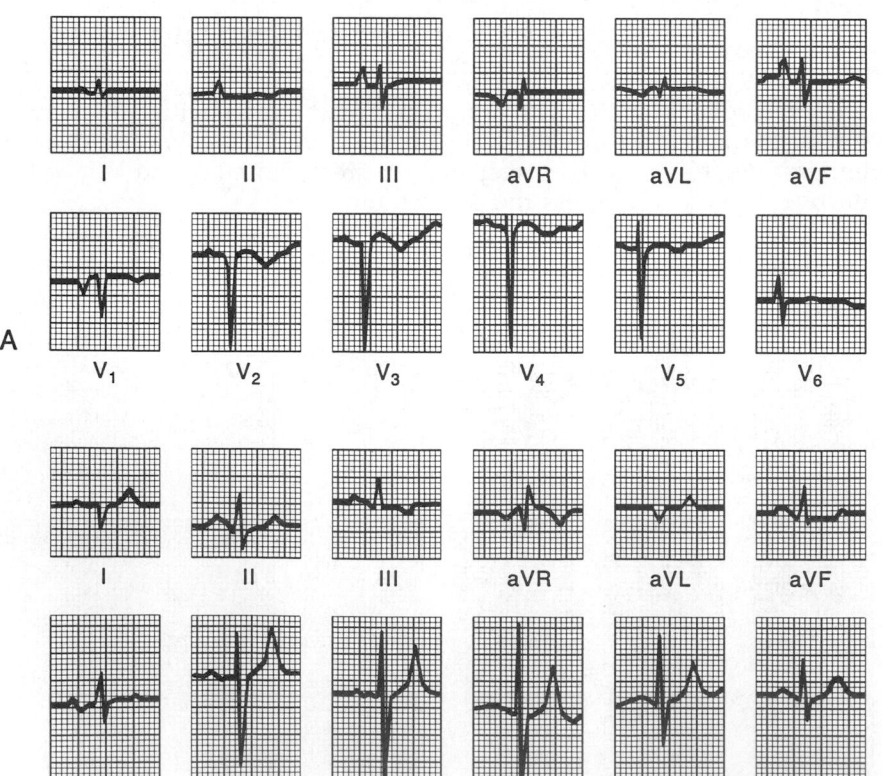

FIGURE 9–30. *A*, Right atrial enlargement. *B*, Left atrial enlargement. (Redrawn from Goldman, M. J. (1986). *Principles of clinical electrocardiography* (pp. 87 and 88). Los Altos, CA: Lange Medical Publications.)

The duration of the P wave usually remains normal. Right atrial hypertrophy is sometimes referred to as P pulmonale because of its association with pulmonary disease.

In left atrial hypertrophy, the P wave is often widened to 0.12 second and is notched, and the second portion of the P wave may increase in amplitude (Fig. 9–30B). The large native P deflection in V_1 represents the depolarization forces traveling posteriorly in the larger left atrium (Lipman and Lipman, 1987). Left atrial hypertrophy is often referred to as P mitrale because it is associated with mitral valve disease.

ELECTROCARDIOGRAPHIC CHANGES WITH CORONARY ARTERY DISEASE

Myocardial Infarction

Myocardial infarction (MI) causes permanent damage to the myocardium and characteristic ECG changes in the T wave, ST segment, and QRS complex. T wave changes are the first to occur and indicate myocardial ischemia. Within minutes after the initial decrease in blood supply to the myocardium, T waves become peaked, or hyperacute (Shamroth, 1984), indicating the presence of severe subendocardial ischemia (Fig. 9–31). These changes are probably due to leakage of intracellular potassium from damaged muscle cells into the extracellular spaces (Goldman, 1986). They are frequently missed because they last for only minutes to several hours and may have disappeared by the time the first ECG is taken.

If ischemia persists, ST segment elevation occurs representing myocardial injury (Fig. 9–32). This is often the first change noted. During evolution of the MI, the ST segments return to baseline, and an inverted T wave that remains on the ECG indefinitely is seen. The T waves of myocardial ischemia are inverted symmetrically, with a gentle downslope and rapid upstroke. This inverted T wave may remain on the ECG for an indefinite period of time during the healing process. Normal ST segments are isoelectric, beginning at the end of the QRS complex at the J point (the junction between the end of the QRS complex and beginning of the ST segment). They may be normally elevated 1 mm in the frontal leads

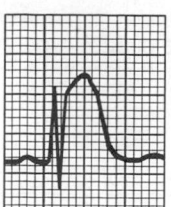

FIGURE 9–32. ST segment elevation.

and up to 2 mm in the horizontal leads. ST elevation with myocardial infarction may be confused with J point elevation of "early repolarization" that occurs with young healthy individuals and has no pathologic implications. In J point elevation, the T wave maintains its independent waveform (Thaler, 1988). With myocardial disease, ST segments are bowed upward and tend to merge imperceptibly with the T wave. Although the pathophysiology of ST segment elevation is not certain, it is known that intracellular potassium leaks from injured tissue. Because the resting potential of myocardial cells depends on the ratio of intracellular to extracellular potassium, this leakage of potassium is thought to alter the baseline of the ECG and thus the ST segment following depolarization (Scheidt, 1986).

Q waves have traditionally been considered a sign of necrosis associated with transmural myocardial infarctions and have been explained using the "electrical window" concept (Fig. 9–33). If an area of myocardium is severely damaged, it is unable to depolarize and repolarize normally. This necrotic area is like a window to the electrode placed over it, which "allows" visualization of the electromotive forces moving away from it through the rest of the heart. These forces produce a negative deflection, a Q wave, in this electrode. These Q waves should be 0.03 second or more compared with normal "septal" Q waves, as previously described.

It has been general knowledge until recently that Q waves on the ECG indicated a transmural infarction (an infarction through the full thickness of the muscle), whereas an absence of Q waves indicated a subendocardial infarction (an infarction of only the subendocardial portion of the muscle). We now know, based on pathology reports, that infarctions found to be transmural can occur in the absence of Q waves on the ECG, whereas those found to be nontransmural may be associated with the appearance of new Q waves (Sullivan et al., 1978). Table 9–4 illustrates the frequency of Q waves in transmural

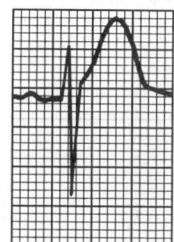

FIGURE 9–31. Peaked T wave.

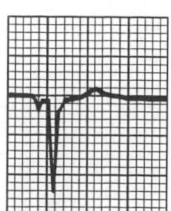

FIGURE 9–33. Q wave.

TABLE 9–4. Incidence of Q Waves in 100 Infarctions

	Transmural	Subendocardial
Number	55	45
Q waves	67%	30%
ST–T changes	33%	70%

From Antaloczy, A. (1987). *Journal of Electrocardiology*, 20, 72. © 1987, Churchill Livingstone, New York.

TABLE 9–5. Indicative and Reciprocal Changes with Myocardial Infarctions (MIs)

Site	Indicative	Reciprocal
Inferior	II, III, aVF	I, aVL, V leads
Anteroseptal	V_1–V_3	II, III, AVF
Anterolateral	I, aVL, V_4–V_6	II, III, aVF
Extensive anterior	I, aVL, V_1–V_6	II, III, aVF, posterior chest
Posterior	V_7–V_9*	V_1 (tall R)

*These are leads placed directly over the left posterior chest in the fifth intercostal space beginning at the left posterior axillary line.

and subendocardial MIs in a series of 100 patients. Subsequently, infarctions should be described as either Q wave or non–Q wave on the basis of serial ECG evaluations. In most patients with Q wave infarctions, the infarction will probably, but not necessarily, be transmural.

The changes just described are indicative changes recorded in the leads overlying the area of damage. Changes are also recorded on the ECG in the leads overlying the opposite side of the heart called reciprocal changes. Just as there is an absence of electromotive forces during depolarization and repolarization in the damaged part of the myocardium, so there is a relative gain in forces directed away from the inert area (Marriott, 1983) that are assessed by other electrodes. Those electrodes will register on the ECG a mirror image of the damaged area. For example, reciprocal changes that would be recorded opposite a Q wave, elevated ST segments, and inverted T waves would be an increase in the R wave, depressed ST segments, and tall upright T waves. Table 9–5 indicates where indicative and reciprocal changes occur with different types of MIs.

Anterior Wall Myocardial Infarctions. In an anterior wall myocardial infarction, damage results from the occlusion of the left coronary artery. The left main artery divides into the left anterior descending artery, which supplies the anteroseptal portion of the left circumflex artery, which in turn supplies the lateral wall of the left ventricle. ECG changes with anterior wall myocardial infarctions occur in the precordial leads and leads I and aVL, whereas reciprocal changes develop in leads II, III, and aVF (Fig. 9–34). Changes that are seen across the precordial leads from V_1 to V_6 and in leads I and aVL indicate

an extensive anterior MI or anterolateral infarction, whereas changes seen only in leads V_1 to V_4 indicate an anteroseptal MI.

The nurse may anticipate problems with pump failure and with the conduction system because the left coronary artery supplies large areas of the left ventricular musculature as well as the right and left bundle branches and the anterior two-thirds of the ventricular septum. If conduction disturbances occur, they represent an extensive loss of myocardium and may indicate a poor prognosis. Mobitz type II block is the form of second degree block most frequently seen in patients with anterior MIs. AV sequential pacing can be used to improve cardiac performance in some patients but does not improve prognosis (Brugada and Wellens, 1986). Mortality is related to extensive myocardial damage and pump failure.

Inferior Wall Myocardial Infarctions. An inferior myocardial infarction may be caused by occlusion of either the right coronary artery or a dominant left circumflex coronary artery. Less commonly, it may be caused by occlusion of a very long descending anterior coronary artery supplying the distal aspect of the left ventricular apex and the distal part of the inferior wall. Indicative changes occur in leads II, III, and aVF (Fig. 9–35). When the infarction results from involvement of the left circumflex artery, there is likely to be ST segment elevation in at least one of the lateral leads (aVL, V_5, or V_6) with no reciprocal ST segment depression in lead I (Bairey et al., 1987). A prominent Q wave in lead III is found in inferior

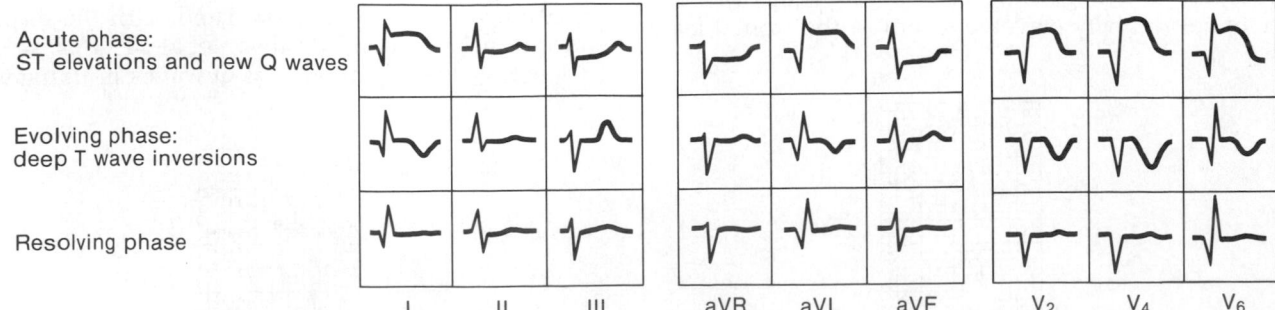

Acute phase: ST elevations and new Q waves								
Evolving phase: deep T wave inversions								
Resolving phase								
I	II	III	aVR	aVL	aVF	V_2	V_4	V_6

FIGURE 9–34. Anterior wall MI. (Reproduced by permission from: Goldberger, A. L., and Goldberger, E. *Clinical electrocardiography* (p. 90). St. Louis, 1981, The C. V. Mosby Co.)

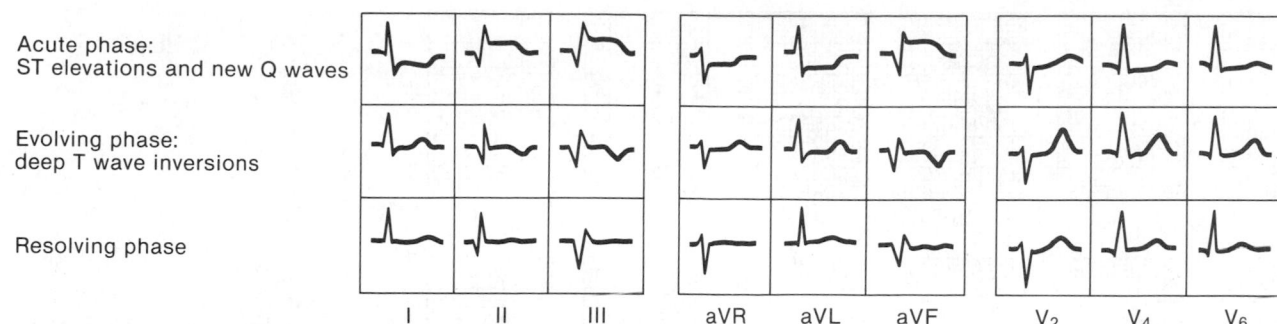

Acute phase:
ST elevations and new Q waves

Evolving phase:
deep T wave inversions

Resolving phase

    I   II   III   aVR   aVL   aVF V_2 V_4 V_6

FIGURE 9–35. Inferior wall MI. (Reproduced by permission from: Goldberger, A. L., and Goldberger, E. *Clinical electrocardiography* (p. 90). St. Louis, 1981, The C. V. Mosby Co.)

infarctions but must be differentiated from a normal Q wave that may occur in that lead. Deep inspiration will usually cause a positional Q wave to disappear or to decrease, whereas the Q wave occurring with an infarction will be unchanged (Evans, 1951).

Although most Q waves that develop during an infarction persist for a lifetime, this is not true with inferior infarctions. In as many as 50% of patients with inferior MIs the criteria for detection of significant Q waves are lost (Thaler, 1988).

The right coronary artery usually supplies the SA and AV nodes, the bundle of His, and the posterior third of the septum as well as a portion of the posteroinferior division of the left bundle as discussed earlier. Occlusion of the artery causes ischemia of the SA and AV nodes and is commonly associated with sinus bradycardia and Mobitz type I (Wenckebach) block. The timing of AV block in patients with inferior MIs has significance. Block occurring very early after onset of chest pain is caused by increased vagal tone rather than ischemia and is accompanied by sinus bradycardia. When block develops later in the course of the MI, it is caused by ischemia, and atropine does not affect the conduction disturbance (Brugada and Wellens, 1986).

Pacing is not usually recommended in patients with inferior MIs but may be necessary when the escape rhythm is slow or is associated with symptoms, or when AV block worsens the patient's hemodynamic condition. Tans and Lie (1976) and Braat (1984) found that all patients surviving inferior MIs were discharged from the hospital with 1:1 conduc-tion regardless of the degree of AV block experienced during the MI.

Posterior Wall Myocardial Infarctions. A posterior infarction involves the posterior surface of the heart and often occurs in association with inferior or lateral MIs. AV block may occur because a branch of the posterior descending artery is also a branch of the artery that supplies the AV node in most cases. In the normal 12-lead ECG, no leads are placed directly over the posterior wall and diagnosis depends upon detecting reciprocal changes in leads V_1 and V_2—ST segment depression and tall R waves (Fig. 9–36). Tall symmetric T waves will appear in these leads later. An abnormally tall R wave in V_1 in an adult is defined as an R:S ratio greater than 1 or an R duration of 0.03 second or greater (Goldman, 1986). One must differentiate a posterior infarction from right ventricular hypertrophy, which also has a large R wave in V_1. The presence or absence of right axis deviation is the distinguishing characteristic, since a right axis deviation is not present in the posterior leads.

Right Ventricular Myocardial Infarctions. It has been noted that 40% of all patients with inferior wall myocardial infarctions also have a right ventricular myocardial infarction that results from proximal occlusion of the right coronary artery before the take-off of the major right ventricular branch (Brugada and Wellens, 1986). This right ventricular MI is manifested by ST segment elevation of at least 1 mm in the right precordial leads V_{4R} and V_{5R}. According

FIGURE 9–36. Posterior wall MI. (Redrawn from Marriott, H. J. L. (1988). *Practical electrocardiography* (p. 442). © 1988, The Williams & Wilkins Co., Baltimore.)

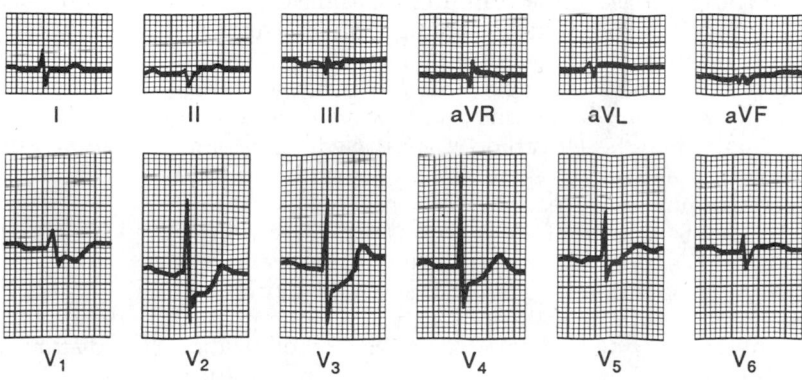

    I   II   III   aVR   aVL   aVF

    V_1 V_2 V_3 V_4 V_5 V_6

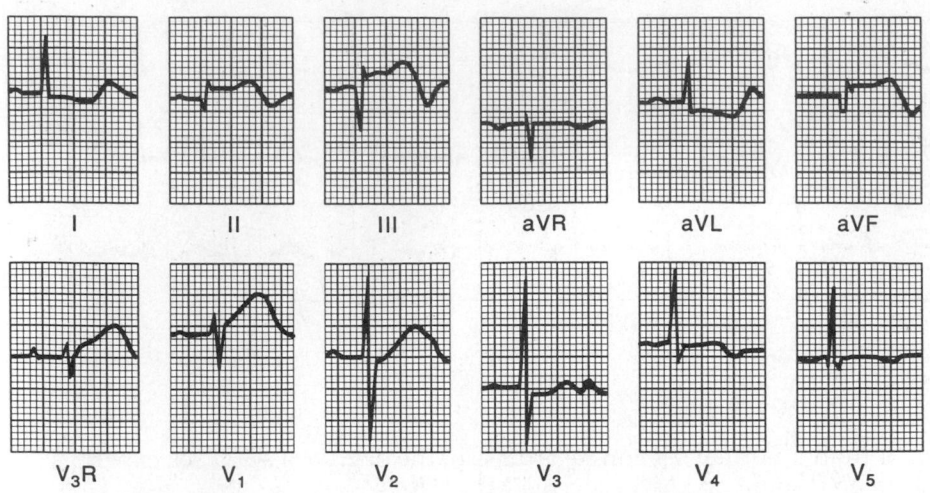

I   II   III   aVR   aVL   aVF

V₃R   V₁   V₂   V₃   V₄   V₅

FIGURE 9–37. Right ventricular MI. (Reproduced by permission from: Goldberger, A. L. *Myocardial infarction* (p. 316). St. Louis, 1984, The C. V. Mosby Co.)

to data compiled by Braat (1984), the chance of observing ST segment elevation in the right precordial leads sharply decreases 8 hours or more after onset of chest pain. It is therefore important to record a right chest lead (V_{4R}) on admission to the critical care unit and with daily ECGs. When a right ventricular infarction occurs in conjunction with an inferior MI there is an increased possibility of AV nodal conduction disturbance (48% versus 13% in patients without right ventricular infarction) (Braat, 1984). Therefore, the recording of right precordial leads is helpful not only in identifying right ventricular involvement during an acute inferior MI but also in predicting the development of conduction disturbances and in identifying the coronary artery responsible for the acute inferior MI (Fig. 9–37).

Atrial Infarctions. Atrial infarctions usually accompany inferior myocardial infarctions. They should be suspected when atrial dysrhythmias occur. Other clues include abnormal P wave contour, PR segment displacement, especially PR segment depression with atrial dysrhythmias, elevation of the PR segment in the left chest leads with reciprocal depression in the right chest leads, or elevation in lead I with reciprocal depression in lead III (Liu, 1961).

Myocardial Ischemia

Myocardial ischemia (angina, coronary insufficiency) refers to reversible changes in the myocardium resulting from a temporary decrease in blood supply. On the ECG these changes produce transitory ST segment deviations and T wave changes. ST segments may be elevated or depressed. As a practical rule, a tracing taken directly over the injured myocardium will record ST segment elevations, whereas ST segment depression results if normal muscle lies between the injured muscle and the electrode (Goldman, 1986). ST segment depression is the most typical pattern. T waves may be peaked or inverted owing to a delay in phase 3 repolarization in the affected area of the heart. The mean vector is

directed away from the ischemic area, so that leads oriented to the surface of the ischemic area will reflect inverted T waves, whereas leads oriented to the opposite or healthy surface will reflect upright T waves (Shamroth, 1984). The T wave of myocardial ischemia is characterized by symmetry and increased narrowness.

One variant form of angina characterized by chest pain that usually occurs at rest and accompanies ST segment elevation is called Prinzmetal angina. Prinzmetal and associates (1959) demonstrated that the chemical behavior of the myocardial areas showing the ST segment elevation differs from that of areas showing ST segment depression with other types of angina and that ST segment elevation represents a more severe degree of oxygen lack than does ST segment depression. ST segments are elevated owing to a reduction in coronary blood flow in the epicardial half of the myocardium (Lipman et al., 1984) (Fig. 9–38).

Extensive studies during the past decade have demonstrated a definite relationship between chest pain and the underlying coronary artery spasm (Chahine, 1979; Meller et al., 1976). Although most of these patients have significant atherosclerotic lesions in their coronary arteries, the spasm appears to play the crucial role that results in their symptoms (Raizner and Chahine, 1979). Prinzmetal angina is more likely to be associated with various types of dysrhythmias and conduction defects than typical angina (Sokolow and McIlroy, 1981). It also has a well-established relationship with torsades de pointes (Krikler and Curry, 1976). For these reasons, it may be useful to monitor the patient in a lead that displays the ST segment elevation so that changes can be quickly visualized and interventions taken.

Dysrhythmogenesis

A dysrhythmia is any abnormality in heart rate, regularity, or site of origin of the cardiac impulse or a disturbance in the conduction of that impulse such that the normal sequence of activation of atria and

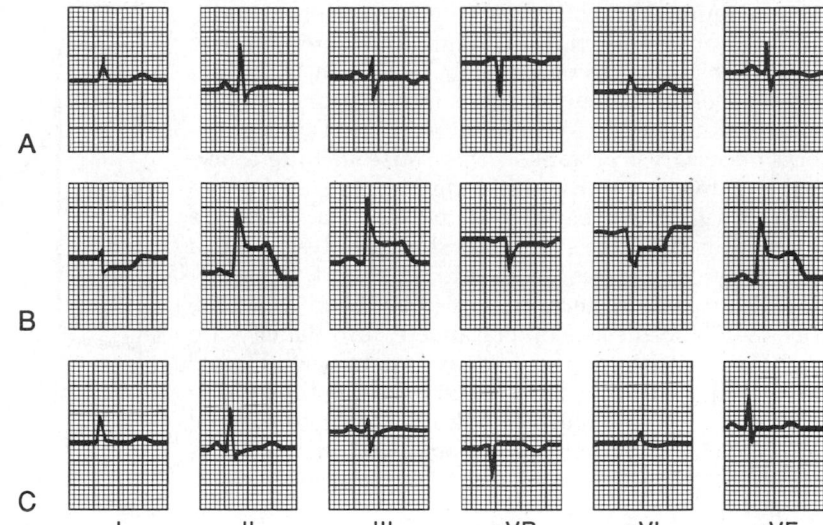

FIGURE 9–38. Prinzmetal angina. *A,* The baseline ECG shows nonspecific inferior ST–T changes. *B,* With chest pain, the marked ST segment elevations occur in leads II, III, and aVF, and there are reciprocal ST depressions in leads I and aVL. *C,* Return of ST segments to baseline. (Reproduced by permission from: Goldberger, A. L. *Myocardial infarction* (p. 151). St. Louis, 1989, The C. V. Mosby Co.)

ventricles is altered (Wit et al., 1974). Thus, the basic mechanisms of cardiac dysrhythmias are abnormalities of impulse generation or impulse conduction, or a combination of both. See Table 9–6.

Abnormal impulse formation results from localized changes in ionic currents, which flow across the membranes of single cells or groups of cells (Wit and Rosen, 1984). It results from normal or enhanced automaticity and triggered activity.

Automaticity, the ability to initiate spontaneous action potentials, is a normal property of some cardiac cells, as discussed earlier. The basis of normal automaticity is a slow fall in the membrane potential during phase 4 of the action potential. This decrease in membrane potential reflects a gradual shift in the

balance between the inward and outward current components in the direction of net inward current (Wit, 1984). The sinus node, normally the controlling pacemaker, both excites and inhibits other potentially automatic cells elsewhere in the heart. If it should fail because of sick sinus syndrome or be suppressed secondary to ischemia, pacemaker cells in the AV node or Purkinjie fibers usually generate impulses.

Dysrhythmias may occur because of enhanced automaticity outside the sinus node. Working atrial and ventricular myocardial cells do not normally show spontaneous diastolic depolarization. If, however, the resting potential of these cells is reduced to less than about −60 mV, spontaneous diastolic depolarization may occur, causing repetitive impulse initia-

TABLE 9–6. Mechanisms for Dysrhythmias

I Abnormal Impulse Generation	II Abnormal Impulse Conduction	III Simultaneous Abnormalities of Impulse Generation and Conduction
A. Normal automatic mechanism 　1. Abnormal rate 　　a. Tachycardia 　　b. Bradycardia 　2. Abnormal rhythm 　　a. Premature impulses 　　b. Delayed impulses 　　c. Absent impulses B. Abnormal automatic mechanism 　1. Phase 4 depolarization at low 　　membrane potential 　2. Oscillatory depolarizations at low 　　membrane potential preceding 　　upstroke C. Triggered activity 　1. Early afterdepolarizations 　2. Delayed afterdepolarizations 　3. Oscillatory depolarizations at low 　　membrane potentials following 　　action potential upstroke	A. Slowing and block 　1. Sinoatrial block 　2. Atrioventricular block 　3. His bundle block 　4. Bundle branch block B. Unidirectional block and reentry 　1. Random reentry 　　a. Atrial muscle 　　b. Ventricular muscle 　2. Ordered reentry 　　a. Sinoatrial node and junction 　　b. AV node and junction 　　c. His-Purkinje system 　　d. Purkinje fiber-muscle junction 　　e. Abnormal AV connection (WPW) 　3. Summation and inhibition C. Conduction block and reflection	A. Phase 4 depolarization and impaired 　conduction 　1. Specialized cardiac fibers B. Parasystole

Abbreviation: WPW, Wolff-Parkinson-White syndrome.
From Hoffman, B. F., and Rosen, M. R. (1981). *Circulation Research,* 49, 2. By permission of the American Heart Association, Inc.

tion (Cranefield, 1975; Katzung and Morgenstern, 1977). Such a reduction in membrane potential may be the result of hyperkalemia, ischemia, hypoxia, chamber enlargement, digitalis intoxication, or other factors (Katz, 1977; Wit and Rosen, 1981). ECG criteria necessary to establish this cause include a normal P–R interval of the initiating impulse, and sameness of all P waves of the tachycardia (they are different from sinus P waves). The dysrhythmia gradually accelerates after initiation and gradually decelerates before termination (Josephson and Kastor, 1977). Examples of enhanced automaticity are multifocal atrial tachycardia and paroxysmal atrial tachycardia with block secondary to digitalis toxicity (Marriott, 1983). Conditions that promote abnormal automaticity include hypoxia, acidosis, alkalosis, hypokalemia, hypocalcemia, and catecholamine administration.

Triggered Activity

Recent studies on abnormal electrical activity of the Purkinje fibers and on electrical activity of fibers in the AV valves and coronary sinus (Wit and Cranefield, 1976, 1977) have led to the concept of triggered activity. Triggered dysrhythmias are depolarizations that occur after an initiating action potential. An afterdepolarization is a depolarization that occurs during or after repolarization of the beat immediately preceding it. In other words, triggered activity requires an initiating action potential before one or more additional abnormal impulses are generated. Only if the afterdepolarization achieves threshold potential does triggered activity result. Cells that exhibit this mechanism, once excited, give rise to two or more action potentials or a long run of repetitive responses (Hurst, 1986).

Depolarizing afterpotentials that cause triggered activity may be one of two types: early and delayed. Early afterdepolarizations usually occur during repolarization of an action potential that has been initiated from a high level of membrane potential, usually between -75 and -90 mV (Josephson and Wellens, 1984) (Fig. 9–39).

The membrane potential during the early afterdepolarization reaches threshold potential for activation of the slow calcium channels. Dysrhythmias that may be seen with early afterdepolarization are bigeminal rhythms with fixed coupling and paroxysms of tachycardia in which the first beat has the same coupling interval as the other couplets (Rosen, 1986). Early afterdepolarizations leading to triggered activity in isolated cardiac preparations may be caused by factors that are present in the heart in situ under pathologic conditions such as hypoxia and high P_{CO_2} (Brooks et al., 1955). Drugs used clinically, such as sotolol, may prolong the time course for repolarization and cause early afterdepolarizations and triggered activity (Wit, 1984). However, according to Josephson and Wellens (1984), interventions that

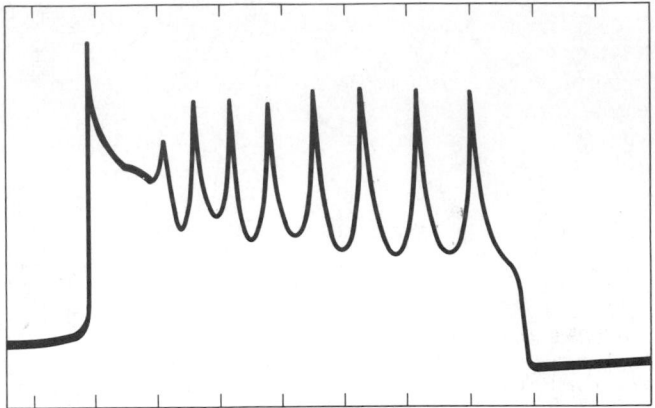

FIGURE 9–39. Early afterdepolarization and repetitive activity in canine cardiac Purkinje fiber. The maximum diastolic potential was -87 mV. A "burst" of rhythmic activity arising from a low level of membrane potential occurred during repolarization of the action potential. The slow responses during this burst peaked near 0 mV. Time marks occur at 1-second intervals. (Redrawn from Wit, A. L., Cranefield, P. R., and Gadsby, D. C. (1980). Triggered activity. In Zipes, D. P., Bailey, J. C., and Elharrar, V. (Eds.), *The slow inward current cardiac arrhythmias.* The Hague: Martinus Nijhoff.)

increase the time course of repolarization favor the occurrence of early afterdepolarizations.

Delayed afterdepolarizations occur after completion of phase 3 repolarization. When the afterdepolarization is large enough to bring the membrane potential to threshold, a triggered impulse arises, followed by an afterdepolarization. Delayed afterdepolarizations occur under conditions in which there are large increases in intracellular calcium (Kass et al., 1978).

Hurst (1986) provides other distinctive features of triggered activity:

1. There is a tendency toward a gradually increasing rate.
2. Triggered activity is usually observed at fast rates, in contrast to reentry, which is more common at slow rates.
3. Overdrive pacing results in acceleration of the rate of activity (in contrast to reentry, which is generally terminated or unaffected by overdrive pacing).
4. The number of triggered responses appears to be directly related to the basic cycle length of pacing.
5. Triggered activity can be promptly suppressed by verapamil, whereas reentry seems to be resistant to verapamil.

Delayed afterdepolarizations occur under conditions in which there are large increases in intracellular calcium. Digitalis toxicity is one condition associated with delayed afterdepolarizations. Digitalis inhibits the sodium-potassium pump, leading to an increase in intracellular sodium, which is then exchanged for calcium by a sodium-calcium exchange mechanism (Josephson and Wellens, 1984). Most delayed afterdepolarizations induced by digitalis are reduced in amplitude or abolished by agents that block the slow inward channels (Rosen and Danilo, 1980). Dysrhythmias common to digitalis toxicity that may result from triggered activity are atrial tachycardia, junctional tachycardia, and ventricular tachycardia.

IMPULSE CONDUCTION

Abnormalities of impulse conduction are probably more common as a basis for dysrhythmias than abnormal impulse formation. Abnormalities of conduction are due to conduction block, reentry, or reflection.

Decremental Conduction

Decremental conduction is the slowing of the conduction velocity of an impulse by the AV node as it travels from the atria to the ventricle. In the AV fibers the amplitude of the action potential and the rate of depolarization decrease progressively from cell to cell so that the resulting stimulus becomes weaker as it is propagated (Alpert, 1980). The impulse may fade out completely when the strength of the stimulus proximally becomes insufficient to elicit a response in the distal fibers even if they are still excitable. Decremental conduction normally occurs in areas of the heart where resting potentials are low and upstroke of the action potential is dependent on slow calcium channels as in the SA and AV nodes. It can also occur in areas where opening of the fast sodium channels is impaired by ischemia, disease, or drugs. These areas are partly depolarized, resulting in inactivation of some sodium channels, which reduces action potential amplitude and the rate of rise of phase 0, thus decreasing conduction velocity (Jacobson, 1983). Decremental conduction is responsible not only for normal slowing of the impulse in the AV node but also for the prolonged AV conduction time of early atrial premature beats. An accentuation of the normal decremental conduction time through the AV node is the probable explanation of first degree AV block. Mobitz type I block (Wenckebach phenomenon) has been attributed to decremental conduction in the AV node. In Mobitz type II block the conduction disturbance is situated in the more peripheral ramifications of the AV conduction system. The mechanism is probably a transient but complete decrement of conduction in both bundle branches, or in one bundle branch if the other is already blocked (Friedman, 1985). See Figure 9–40.

Reentry

Reentry occurs when an impulse, rather than dying out after completely activating the heart, continues to excite the atria or ventricles after the refractory period. In other words, the impulse depolarizes an

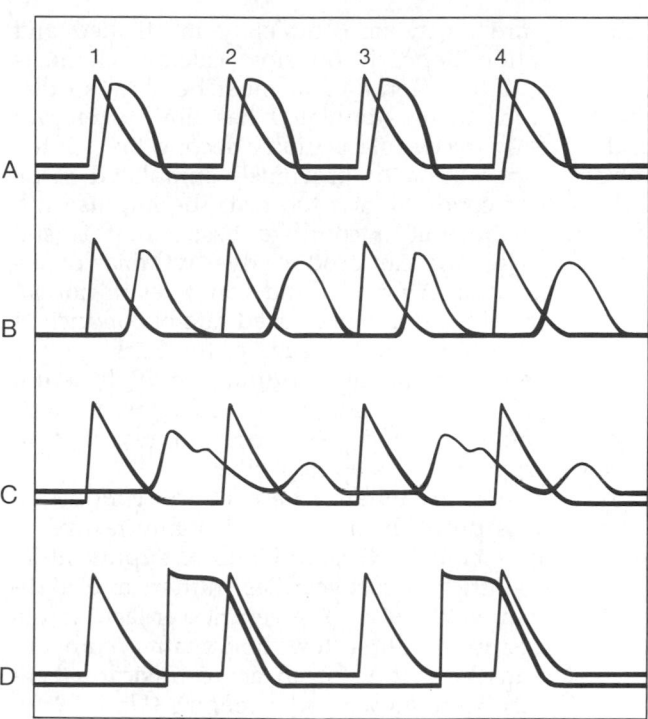

FIGURE 9–40. Tracings of transmembrane action potentials recorded from a single fiber of the atrium and from fibers of the AV node and His bundle, showing decremental conduction during a sustained supraventricular tachycardia. *A,* Atrium and atrial margin of the node. *B,* Atrium and middle node. *C,* Atrium and lower node. *D,* Atrium and His bundle. The same atrial fiber was employed in all records. Note that during the second and fourth beats, the abortive responses in the lower node fail to produce a His bundle response. This is 2:1 AV heart block resulting from complete decrement of beats 2 and 4 within the node. Beats 2 and 4 also are concealed responses. Note the relative loss of resting membrane potential from the fibers in the middle and lower nodal areas, panels *B* and *C.* The resting potential of fibers in the His bundle, panel *D,* is normal. (Redrawn from Hoffman, B., Cranefield, P., and Wallace, A. G. (1966). Physiological basis of cardiac arrhythmias (II). *Modern Concepts of Cardiovascular Disease,* 35, 108. By permission of the American Heart Association, Inc.)

area of the myocardium and then is able to reenter the same area to depolarize it again. Hoffman and Rosen (1981) have subdivided reentry into random reentry and ordered reentry. Random reentry is most often associated with atrial or ventricular fibrillation, whereas ordered reentry can cause most other types of dysrhythmias. The main distinction between the two is that during random reentry propagation occurs over reentrant pathways that continuously change their size and location with time, whereas ordered reentry implies a relatively fixed reentrant pathway.

Several conditions are necessary for the occurrence of reentrant dysrhythmias. First, there must be an available circuit with more than one possible route for impulse transmission. There must be a unidirectional block in one route that allows the impulse to be conducted in one direction through an area but not in the opposite direction. Such areas of depressed conduction can occur in ischemic fibers with low threshold resting potentials (TRPs) where sodium channels are partly or completely inactivated and depolarization depends on slow calcium channels (Jacobson, 1983). Conduction must be slow so that the first area to be stimulated has time to recover and be ready for depolarization a second time. If the refractory period of the previously stimulated tissue is long or if conduction is too fast, the impulse will die out because it encounters tissue that is still refractory. Reentry can produce dysrhythmias occurring in the atria, AV node, and ventricles in normal and abnormal hearts. A decreased rate of conduction frequently results from blockage of the Purkinje system, ischemia of the myocardium, or high serum potassium levels, among many other factors. A shortened refractory period may occur in response to various drugs, such as epinephrine.

Reentry may occur anywhere in the conduction system. It is probably the cause of many tachydysrhythmias, including various kinds of supraventricular and ventricular tachycardias, flutter, and fibrillation (Braunwald, 1988). The ventricular tachycardia that occurs in the first few hours after coronary occlusion in the setting of an acute myocardial infarction has been shown to be reentry (Han, 1969), and that occurring at 24 hours is thought to be abnormal automaticity (Conover, 1988). Reentry is the mechanism for supraventricular dysrhythmias due to Wolff-Parkinson-White (WPW) syndrome involving the normal conducting pathway and the accessory pathway. Tachydysrhythmias due to reentry require an initiating beat. In the case of ventricular tachycardia, the initiating beat may be a sinus or supraventricular impulse that is conducted normally until it reaches a bifurcation, which is usually located in ventricular Purkinje tissue. The impulse activates the ventricles and then reenters the ventricular conduction system to reactivate them. It may or may not be conducted in a retrograde fashion to activate the atria. The initiating beat is normal in appearance, whereas the following "reentered" beat is wide and bizarre-looking because the reentry process has taken place entirely within the ventricle. This phenomenon is known as a fixed coupling interval (Alpert, 1980). Circuits in long tracts such as WPW tachycardias or the fascicular divisions of the left bundle branch are termed macroreentry, whereas reentry in small fibers in the AV node or a distal Purkinje circuit is called microreentry.

Reflection

Reflection is a form of reentry in which the two potential conducting pathways are parallel rather than branching off a single conduction pathway (Fig. 9–41). Although both pathways may be depressed, an impulse may be conducted through one, however slowly. At some point, it may turn and move retrogradely through the other fiber back to its origin. If normal myocardium has completely repolarized, the impulse will be conducted onward to produce a premature contraction. Reflection occurs potentially

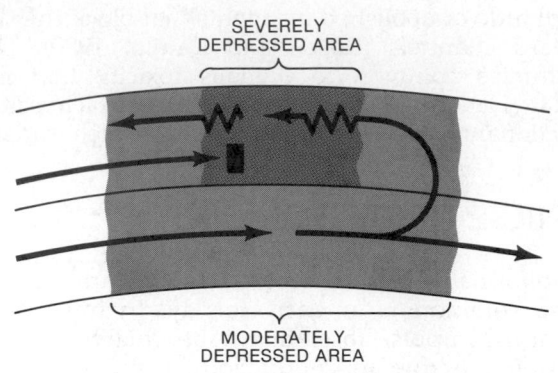

FIGURE 9–41. Reflection.

in Purkinje fibers or myocardial muscle tissue. This model of ectopic impulse formation has been suggested in some instances of parasystolic pacemaker activity (Hurst, 1986).

WIDE QRS COMPLEXES: DIFFERENTIATING SUPRAVENTRICULAR AND VENTRICULAR RHYTHMS

Supraventricular impulses may be conducted through the ventricles in an altered or abnormal fashion, resulting in wide, bizarre QRS complexes that are difficult to distinguish from ventricular-initiated ectopic impulses. There are three main causes for wide QRS complexes that look like ventricular ectopic beats but originate from supraventricular sites: (1) bundle branch block, (2) preexcitation syndromes, and (3) aberrant ventricular conduction. Each of these rhythm variations will be discussed in this section.

Bundle Branch Blocks

Conduction defects or intraventricular block may occur in the ventricular conducting system below the bundle of His as the result of ischemia or degeneration of conducting tissue. A block may occur in the right bundle branch (RBB), left bundle branch (LBB), left anterior fascicle (LAF), or left posterior fascicle (LPF), causing abnormal ventricular depolarization. Block in the bundle branches causes the QRS to be prolonged, whereas block in one of the fascicles of the left bundle causes a QRS with a shift in axis but a normal duration. When an intraventricular block is indicated by a wide QRS complex but lacks specific features of either right bundle branch block (RBBB) or left bundle branch block (LBBB), it is called an intraventricular conduction defect.

Normally, impulses from the sinus node, atrium, and AV node proceed through the common bundle of His and then down both left and right bundle branches to the Purkinje fibers, causing simultaneous ventricular depolarization. Conduction is rapid due

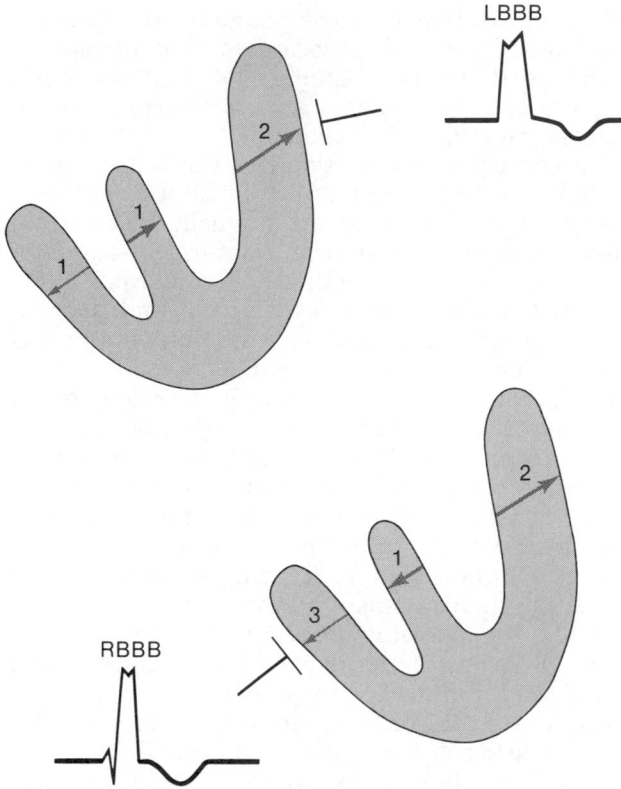

FIGURE 9–42. Sequence of ventricular activation in bundle branch block (BBB). In left bundle branch block (LBBB) (*upper diagram*), the septum is activated (1) exclusively from the right side at the same time that the free wall of the right ventricle (1) is activated. The meager forces of the free wall are overshadowed by the much stronger septal forces. Once the septum and the right ventricle have been depolarized, the left ventricle alone remains and the direction of its activation (2) is similar to that of the septum; hence the complex of LBBB tends to be monophasic and is upright in V₆. In right BBB (*lower diagram*), the septum is first activated, as in the normal heart, from the left side (1); a moment later, activation begins in the left ventricular free wall (2) but, since septal forces are simultaneously spreading in the opposite direction, the free wall deflection (S wave in V₁) is dwarfed. Once the septum and left ventricular free wall have been depolarized, all that is left is the right ventricular free wall. Its feeble forces now are unopposed, and so write the largest deflection of the ventricular complex (R′ in V₁). (Redrawn from Marriott, H. J. L. (1988). *Practical electrocardiography* (p. 67). Baltimore: Williams & Wilkins.)

to the character of the action potential of their specialized cells, their large size, their more or less parallel alignment, and their relatively sparse branching. Bundle branch blocks alter this normal progression of depolarization, causing the ventricles to de-

FIGURE 9–43. Right bundle branch block. (Redrawn from Marriott, H. J. L. (1988). *Practical electrocardiography* (p. 68). © 1988, The Williams & Wilkins Co., Baltimore.)

polarize one after the other because the impulses must travel through muscle tissue rather than through specialized conductile tissue. This delayed conduction lengthens the QRS to 0.12 second or greater in duration.

Leads V₁ and V₆ are the best leads to use in diagnosing bundle branch block and recording ventricular activation time because of their placement over the right (V₁) and left (V₆) ventricles (Fig. 9–42).

RIGHT BUNDLE BRANCH BLOCK

The right bundle branch is a long thin stem, descending along the right ventricular surface of the septum to the right ventricular apex and then sweeping upward along the lateral endocardial wall. The right bundle has a longer refractory period than the left bundle, and because of its thin structure it is more vulnerable to pathologic factors. Blood supply to the right bundle branch comes from the septal perforating branches of the left anterior descending coronary artery, which supplies the anterior surface of the left ventricle.

RBBB is most commonly caused by degeneration of the conducting system, causing fibrosis and interruption of the conduction fibers and ischemic heart disease in the anterior septum. It may be accompanied by rapid heart rates because of its longer refractory period, and it also frequently accompanies supraventricular premature contractions, as will be discussed later.

Electrocardiographic Features of RBBB. V₁ is the best diagnostic lead for the determination of RBBB. V₁ normally shows a small R wave, reflective of septal depolarization, followed by a deep S wave, reflecting the depolarization of the left ventricle. Left ventricular depolarization, because of its size, normally obscures right ventricular depolarization. In RBBB, septal depolarization proceeds normally through the septum and left ventricle, and the right ventricle is depolarized by forces coming from the left ventricle through cells in the intraventricular septum (see Fig. 9–43 for the sequences of ventricular activation in right and left bundle branch blocks). This normal septal depolarization causes the normal small r from septal depolarization to be present followed by an S wave from left ventricular depolarization and a late right ventricular depolarization,

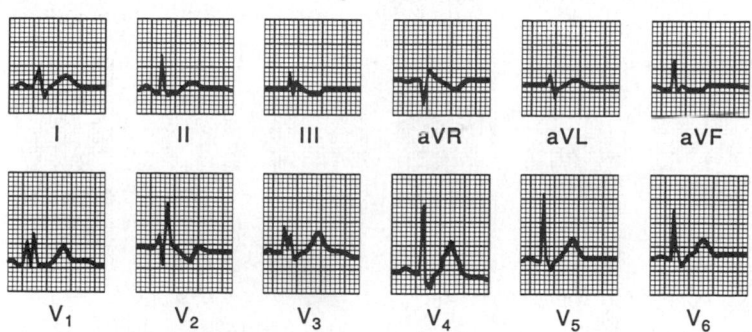

I	II	III	aVR	aVL	aVF
V₁	V₂	V₃	V₄	V₅	V₆

which, now unopposed, causes the electrical axis of current to swing sharply back to the right and inscribe a second R wave, called R prime (R') on the ECG in V_1. In V_6, late right ventricular depolarization inscribes reciprocal late deep S waves. If septal forces are lost, as in anteroseptal MI, the small R in V_1 and the small q in V_6 will not be present. Because the initial activation of the septum is normal, RBBB does not obscure the pattern of anterior myocardial infarction. In summary, the distinguishing features of RBBB include

- A wide or slurred S wave in leads V_5 and V_6
- ST-T changes indicating abnormal ventricular depolarization and repolarization
- Late onset of intrinsicoid deflection in leads V_1 and V_2 (greater than .04 second; this represents delayed onset of right ventricular activation (Lipman and Lipman, 1986)
- QRS equal to or greater than 0.12 second (an RBBB configuration with a QRS narrower than 0.12 second is called an incomplete RBBB)
- A triphasic rSR' QRS configuration (this pattern may be altered by MI, ischemia, or hemiblock)

There will always be a late R wave no matter what the initial deflection appears to be.

An rSr' with a QRS of 0.10 or 0.11 has been called an incomplete right bundle branch block in the past. It is questionable whether anatomically there is such a thing as an incomplete block. Terms such as "borderline" or "incomplete" may be used within quotation marks to indicate that the diagnosis is only a description of the ECG.

LEFT BUNDLE BRANCH BLOCK

Whereas the right bundle branch is a more direct extension of the His bundle, the left bundle branch arises almost perpendicularly from the common bundle (Fig. 9–44). It almost immediately subdivides into the left anterior and posterior fascicles.

Hypertension is the most common cause of left bundle branch block (LBBB). The next most common causes are anteroseptal myocardial infarction and aortic stenosis. It may also be encountered in patients with cardiomyopathy, myocarditis, and other congenital heart diseases (Chung, 1983). When LBBB occurs acutely it is almost always due to an acute anteroseptal myocardial infarction.

The consequences of complete LBBB are similar but opposite to those of RBBB. In LBBB, right ventricular depolarization occurs normally followed by activation of the septum from right to left, and later activation of the left ventricle. The normal initial activation of the septum is disturbed, and the first part of the QRS is altered, causing normal septal Q waves in left chest leads to disappear.

The QRS complex has the same general orientation as in normal depolarization, although it is wide and bizarre in appearance (see Figure 9–44 for the sequence of ventricular activation in bundle branch block). Thus, the main current is directed leftward, away from lead V_1 (causing a deep S wave in that lead) and toward lead V_6 (causing a tall R wave in that lead). There are many variations in the shape of the QRS. The following are commonly seen: notches in the QRS complex, unusually high voltage, either deep S waves in lead V_1, V_2, or V_3, or tall R waves in lead I, aVL, V_5, or V_6. There may be very small R waves in leads V_1 through V_3 and some delay in the time elapsing from onset of the QRS to its peak amplitude, manifested as a less steep upstroke of the initial portion of the QRS (Scheidt, 1986). This initial upstroke has been called the "intrinsicoid deflection." A delayed intrinsicoid deflection is a feature of LBBB.

Left Bundle Branch Block and Myocardial Infarction. It appears to be common knowledge that a myocardial infarction cannot be diagnosed in the presence of a left bundle branch block. LBBB is capable of masking Q waves of infarction because the initial septal vector is directed from right to left, and the infarct is inscribed during the latter part of the QRS complex after septal activation is complete. Subsequently, a Q wave cannot be registered except when there is extensive septal infarction (Braunwald, 1988). As Marriott (1988) puts it, "The reputation for

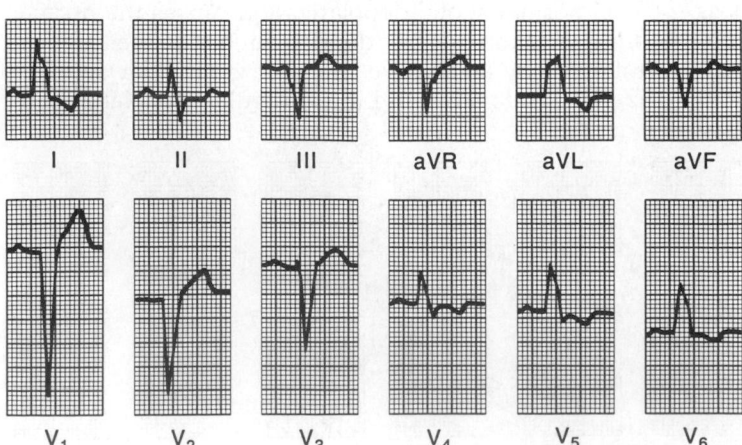

I   II   III   aVR   aVL   aVF

V_1 V_2 V_3 V_4 V_5 V_6

FIGURE 9–44. Left bundle branch block. (Redrawn from Marriott, H. J. L. (1988). *Practical electrocardiography* (p. 68). © 1988, The Williams & Wilkins Co., Baltimore.)

difficulty resides in the fact that myocardial infarction and LBBB have opposing designs on the QRS complex—they produce a tug-of-war on the QRS-writing stylus, and sometimes one and sometimes the other wins.'' In the presence of LBBB, one must look for disproportionate ST-T displacement (elevation or depression) and loss of the normal ST segment concavity or convexity. An infarction will cause more exaggerated ST segment elevation than could be explained solely by an LBBB. The evolution of ECG changes accompanying an MI provides further evidence that the changes are the result of an MI and not merely LBBB. By concentrating on the ST-T displacement, about two-thirds of infarctions can be recognized (Marriott, 1988).

In summary, distinguishing features of an LBBB include:

- QRS duration greater than .12 second
- RSR' in I, aVL, V_5, and V_6
- Wide or slurred S wave in V_1 and V_2 (representing late activation of the left ventricle)
- ST-T wave changes (downsloping ST segment and inverted T wave) in I, aVL, V_5, and V_6
- Late onset of intrinsicoid deflection in V_5 and V_6 (greater than .06 second; representing delayed onset of left ventricular activation) (Lipman and Lipman, 1986).

Hemiblocks

Block may occur in the left main bundle before it bifurcates into the fascicles, or it may occur in one or all of the fascicles. Although there are three fascicles, it is useful as far as ECG interpretation is concerned to discuss the fascicles as if there were only the anterior and posterior ones, since the septal branch exerts little influence on the frontal plane axis. Subsequently, a block of one of the two branches of the left bundle is called a hemiblock. It should be noted that when one refers to monofascicular, bifascicular, or trifascicular block, one is referring to block in one, two, or all of the branches of the right bundle branch, the left anterior branch (also called the left anterosuperior branch), and the left posterior branch (also called the left posteroinferior branch).

Hemiblocks do not cause a prolonged QRS complex because the spread of electrical activity into the blocked areas is rapid enough. The QRS is generally of normal shape, without unusual notching, delayed upstroke, or ST segment or T wave abnormalities. The major effect that hemiblocks have on the ECG is axis deviation.

LEFT ANTERIOR HEMIBLOCK

The anterior fascicle of the left bundle is long and thin and supplies the anterior and superior portions of the left ventricle. It lies superiorly and laterally to

the left posterior fascicle. Blood supply to the anterior fascicle comes from the left anterior descending artery, which also supplies the right bundle. Because this branch lies in close approximation to the right bundle branch, these two fascicles are often injured simultaneously (Fig. 9–45). The anterior fascicle is thought to be the most vulnerable structure of the conduction system because of its anatomic location in the hemodynamically turbulent aortic area, its size and length, and its single blood supply. A block of the anterosuperior division of the left bundle is called a left anterior hemiblock. With left anterior hemiblock, conduction down the left anterior fascicle is blocked, and the impulse subsequently rushes down the left posterior fascicle to the interior surface of the heart. The impulse is conducted superiorly and to the left, causing left axis deviation, inscribing tall positive R waves in the left lateral leads (lead I) and deep S waves in inferior leads II and aVF. This results in left axis deviation of between 0 and 90 degrees. Remember that axis deviation is derived from the limb leads. As was discussed earlier, the simplest method to determine axis is to look at the QRS complexes in leads I and aVF. With left axis deviation, the QRS complex is positive in lead I and negative in aVF.

The left anterior descending artery supplies the

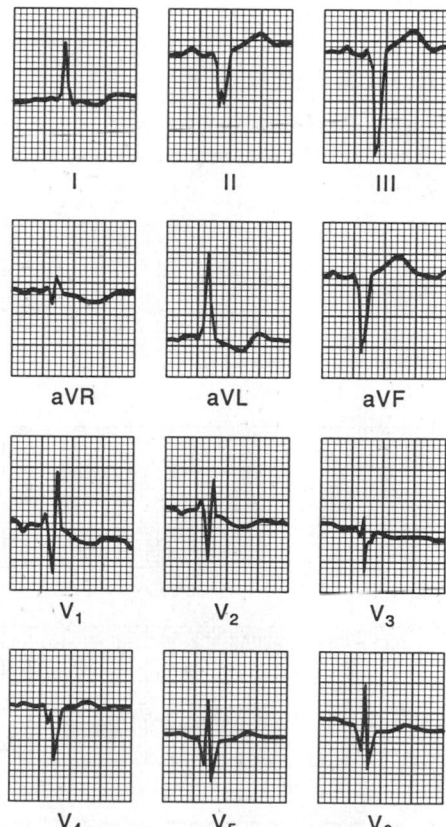

FIGURE 9–45. Bifascicular block (RBBB + anterior hemiblock) in a patient with acute anterior wall MI. Note the abnormal left axis deviation. (Reproduced by permission from: Conover, M. *Understanding electrocardiography* (p. 298). St. Louis, 1988, The C. V. Mosby Co.)

right bundle branch as well as the left anterior fascicle. Therefore, right bundle branch block and blockage of the left anterior fascicle that produces a left anterior hemiblock are usually associated with extensive anteroseptal infarction. The development of RBBB in patients with anterior or anteroseptal myocardial infarctions has prognostic significance. In a study of 1200 patients (Lie et al., 1976), 612 patients had anterior myocardial infarctions. Of these, 70 developed right bundle branch block, 8 developed left bundle branch block, and 13 had pre-existing bundle branch blocks. Patients with RBBB had an inpatient mortality of 71%, those with LBBB 21%, and patients with pre-existing bundle branch block had a mortality of 28%. Mortality in patients without conduction disturbances was 14%. Thus, acquired right bundle branch block has a very poor prognosis due to extensive loss of myocardium during anterior myocardial infarction.

Disagreement exists about the use of permanent pacing in patients who develop conduction disturbances during the acute phase of anterior myocardial infarction. Some authors recommend permanent pacing in patients who develop complete AV block during the acute phase of the MI. Others recommend permanent pacing in survivors of anterior myocardial infarction only when AV block persists or a high-degree AV block is recurrent (Brugada and Wellens, 1986).

LEFT POSTERIOR HEMIBLOCK

The posterior fascicle of the left bundle is short and wide and supplies the posterior and inferior portions of the left ventricle through a fanlike array of conducting fibers. The blood supply to the posterior fascicle is from the right and left coronary arteries. It is the least vulnerable fascicle due to its size and its dual blood supply. In left posterior hemiblock, the impulse travels down the left anterior fascicle, causing ventricular myocardial depolarization to occur in a superior-to-inferior and a left-to-right direction. The axis of depolarization is directed downward and rightward, inscribing tall R waves in leads II and aVF and deep S waves in aVL. The result is right axis deviation (or an electrical axis of between +90 and +180 degrees.

Left posterior hemiblock is seen in diseased hearts, usually in combination with RBBB, whereas left anterior hemiblock may be seen in normal as well as diseased hearts (Fig. 9–46). Other potential causes of axis deviation (i.e., chronic lung disease, ventricular hypertrophy) must be ruled out before one diagnoses right or left hemiblock from the ECG.

Monitoring Implications with Conduction Defects

The foregoing information has implications for monitoring patients in critical care units. The patient who has an RBBB should be monitored in lead II to observe for left anterior hemiblock. If a left anterior or posterior hemiblock is present, the patient should be monitored for the development of RBBB in lead V_1 or MCL_1. If bifascicular block is present (i.e., RBBB plus left anterior hemiblock or left posterior hemiblock), the patient should be monitored closely for

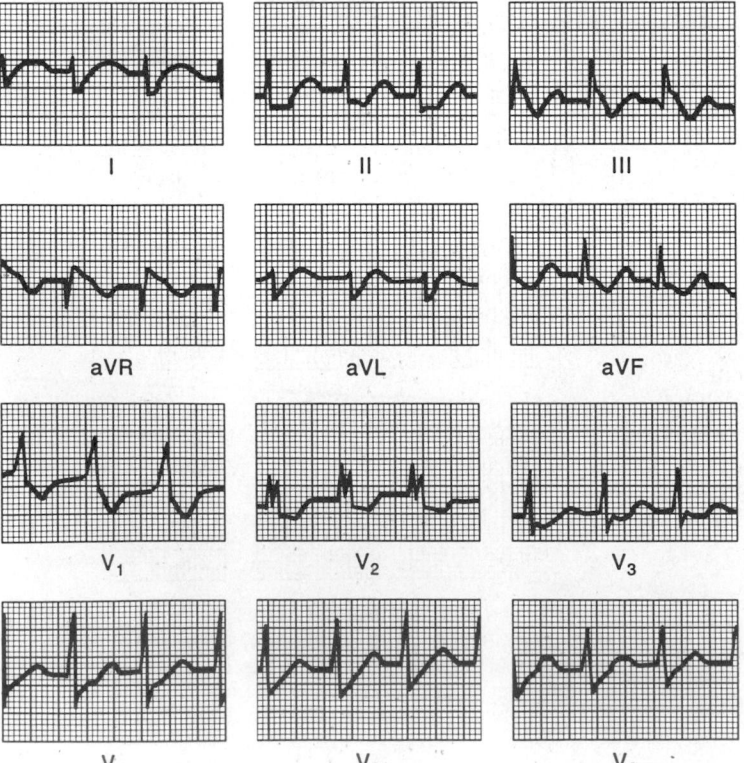

I II III

aVR aVL aVF

V_1 V_2 V_3

V_4 V_5 V_6

FIGURE 9–46. Bifascicular block (RBBB + posterior hemiblock) in a patient with an old inferior wall and evolving anterior wall MI. Note the abnormal right axis deviation. (Reproduced by permission from: Conover, M. *Understanding electrocardiography* (p. 297). St. Louis, 1988, The C. V. Mosby Co.)

other conduction disturbance (AV block) in the lead that shows the most obvious P waves and QRS complexes.

PREEXCITATION SYNDROMES

"Preexcitation" is a name given to syndromes that permit the ventricles to depolarize earlier than would be possible if an impulse had been conducted through the normal AV conduction system to the ventricles. A number of different accessory pathways have been discovered that allow impulses to bypass the AV node and arrive in the ventricle ahead of time or to be conducted through the AV node in an accelerated fashion through special pathways. These pathways are remnants of embryonic stages of development when the atria and ventricles formed an anatomic and electrical continuum across the length of the primitive heart. Between 33 and 37 days after conception these fibers merge into the AV node with its specialized properties. When these accessory pathways persist, they may be found in otherwise normal hearts or may be associated with mitral valve prolapse and various congenital disorders.

There are four types of accessory pathways or syndromes discussed in the literature: Wolff-Parkinson-White syndrome, Lown-Ganong-Levine syndrome, Mahaim fibers, and the concealed unidirectional retrograde accessory pathway. In Wolff-Parkinson-White (WPW) syndrome the bypass pathway is the bundle of Kent that connects either the right or left atria and ventricles (Fig. 9–47).

WPW is the most common preexcitation syndrome and is characterized by a short PR interval, a delta wave, and a wide QRS complex. In Lown-Ganong-

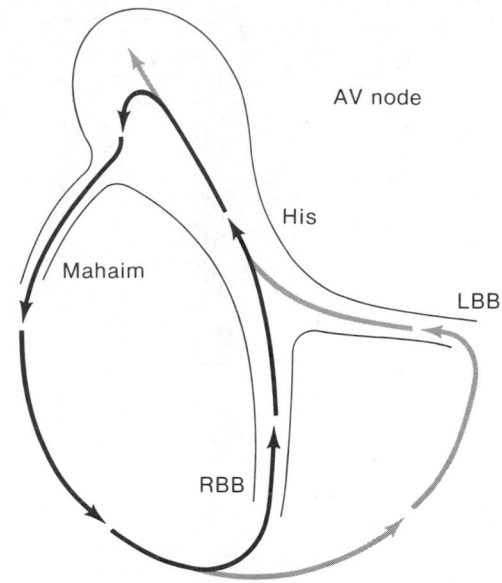

FIGURE 9–48. Mahaim fibers. (Redrawn from Gallagher, J. J., Smith, W. M., Kasall, J. H., et al. (1989). Role of Mahaim fibers in cardiac arrhythmias in man. *Circulation*, 64, 176. By permission of the American Heart Association, Inc.)

Levine syndrome the accessory pathway is the James fibers; the pathway originates in the atrial myocardium, inserting into the bundle of His or into the right and left bundle branches, thereby bypassing the AV node. ECG features include a short PR interval, absence of a delta wave, and a normal QRS complex.

Another preexcitation syndrome, although unnamed, involves the Mahaim fibers, which may pass from the AV node or the His-Purkinje system to the ventricular myocardium (Mahaim, 1947) (Fig. 9–48). Conduction through Mahaim fibers generates a normal PR interval, a delta wave, and a wide QRS complex. The most recent accessory tract to be identified is designated as a "concealed unidirectional retrograde accessory pathway" (CURAP) because it does not produce a characteristic pattern at normal sinus rates (Fig. 9–49). This pathway is embedded in the left free wall of the heart, is unidirectional, and conducts exclusively in a retrograde fashion in 95% of the cases (Ross, 1984). Its most preferred concealed reentrant circuit consists of the AV node, the His bundle, the left bundle branch (or right bundle branch when the left bundle is blocked), a unidirectional accessory pathway, and the left atrium. Clues to the diagnosis of CURAP include rates greater than 200 per minute, inverted P waves following QRS complexes in lead I, atrial flutter or atrial fibrillation during paroxysmal SVT, and a decrease in the tachycardia rate with left bundle branch block. CURAP has proved to be the second most common cause of reentrant supraventricular tachycardia (Ross, 1984). The remainder of this section will be devoted to a discussion of WPW as the most commonly occurring preexcitation syndrome.

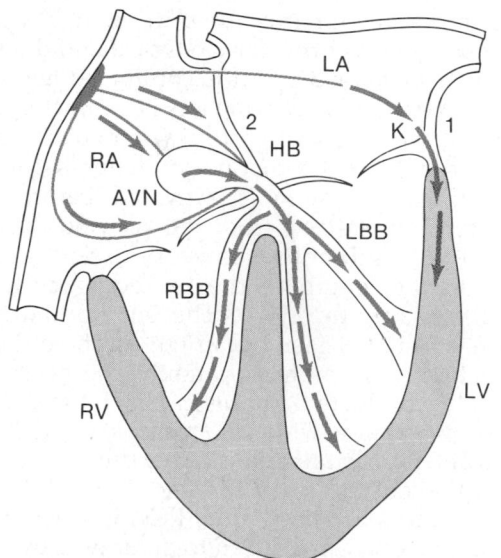

FIGURE 9–47. Wolff-Parkinson-White syndrome conduction pathway. (Redrawn from Horowitz, L. N., and Josephson, M. E. (1980). *Practical Cardiology*, 6 (3), 129–141.)

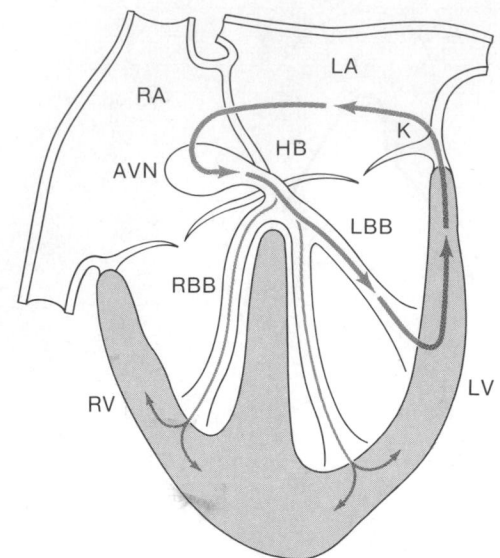

FIGURE 9–49. Concealed retrograde conduction pathway. (Redrawn from Horowitz, L. N., and Josephson, M. E. (1980). *Practical Cardiology*, 6 (3), 129–141.)

Wolff-Parkinson-White Syndrome

WPW is the most common of the preexcitation syndromes. Connections between the atria and ventricles were described by Kent as early as 1893, but it was not until the early 1940s that accessory AV connections were confirmed on autopsy. The syndrome occurs in 0.5% to 2% of the population, and paroxysmal atrial dysrhythmias occur in half of affected individuals (Sokolow and McIlroy, 1981)

In WPW the bypass pathway may occur between the right atrium and right ventricle or between the left atrium and left ventricle. The anomalous fibers may be inserted either on the intraventricular septum or on the outer (or parietal) wall of the ventricle (Phillips, 1980). WPW characteristically causes several changes on the ECG as outlined earlier. First, the PR interval is shortened to less than 0.12 second because the impulse has bypassed the AV node. Second, the QRS is usually wider than normal because of the premature activation of the ventricles.

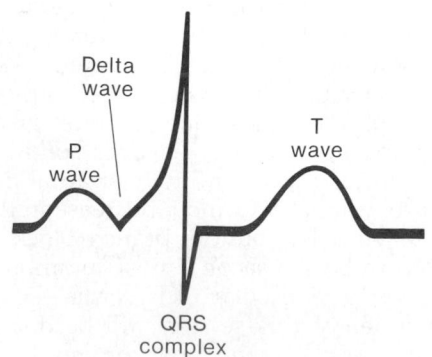

FIGURE 9–50. Slurred upstroke of the QRS (delta wave).

Actually, the QRS complex in WPW represents a fusion beat because most of the ventricle is activated via the normal conducting pathways and only a small portion is depolarized early via the bundle of Kent. This small portion that depolarizes early causes a characteristic initial upstroke on the ECG called a delta wave (Fig. 9–50). This wave may be present in only a few leads.

There are two types of WPW: type A and type B. In type A the accessory pathway connects the free wall of the left atrium to the left ventricle. Lead V_1 usually has a wide QRS that is upright with inverted T waves and depressed ST segments, somewhat resembling a right bundle branch block or right ventricular hypertrophy. Such a pattern can be anticipated when one considers that the left ventricle depolarizes first and then spreads anteriorly to the right ventricle. Type B involves an accessory pathway connecting the right atrium to the right ventricle. It is recognized by a negative QRS complex in V_1 from ventricular depolarization that is anterior to posterior, thereby resembling a left bundle branch block.

Accessory pathways are significant clinically because they provide parallel pathways to facilitate reentry rhythms. In normal sinus rhythm, impulses descend down both pathways, and the resulting beat is a fusion beat. If a premature supraventricular beat finds one pathway refractory, the impulse proceeds in antegrade fashion down one path and returns retrogradely via the other. The reentrant dysrhythmia is dependent upon opposing dual pathways composed exclusively of AV nodal tissue (Ross, 1984). Approximately 40% of supraventricular tachycardias (SVT) are related to accessory tracts.

Aberrancy

It is important for the nurse to be able to differentiate between ventricular tachycardia and a supraventricular tachycardia that is conducted aberrantly. Aberrant ventricular conduction is characterized by prolonged spread of a supraventricular impulse through the ventricles that occurs when a portion of the conduction system is activated before it has completely repolarized from the previous depolarization. The length of the refractory period is directly related to the length of the preceding cycle (R–R interval) (Shamroth, 1984). The left bundle branch repolarizes slightly faster than the right, so the right bundle branch is more commonly the cause of an aberrantly conducted impulse. His bundle studies have shown that a wide rSR′ complex without previous RBBB is aberrant and is rarely due to ventricular ectopy (Wellens et al., 1978).

Correct interpretation of the ECG is essential. The following criteria can be used to determine the source of wide, bizarre QRS complexes (Fig. 9–51). Ventricular rhythms originate in the ventricle and so are not preceded by a premature P wave. If a P wave is

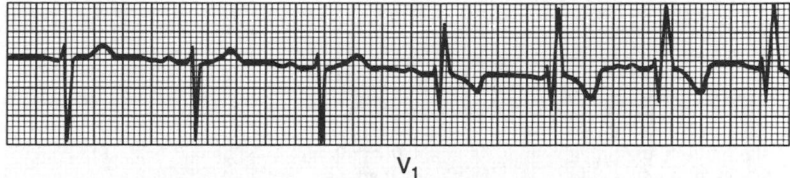

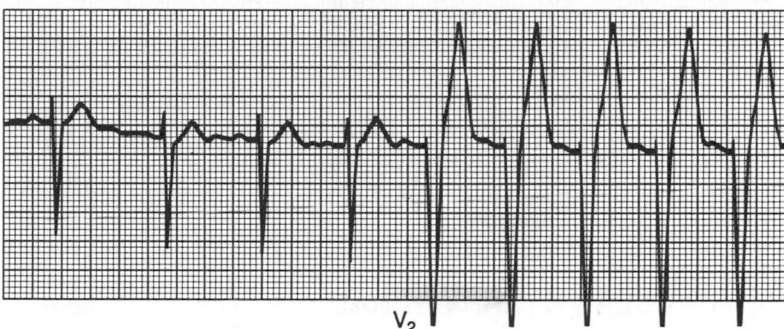

FIGURE 9–51. Aberrant ventricular conduction in two different leads. (Reproduced by permission from: Marriott, H. J. L., and Conover, M. *Advanced concepts in arrhythmias.* St. Louis, 1989, The C. V. Mosby Co.)

present, it will occur on time or may be fused with the premature ventricular complex. The QRS duration is usually wide (0.12 second or greater), and the impulse is usually followed by a compensatory pause. Wellens and associates (1978) suggest that the QRS has a left axis deviation greater than −30 degrees and that there may be fusion beats and sinus capture beats. The QRS morphology in V_1 (or MCL_1) is an RS or RSr', while the QRS morphology in V_6 is a qR or QS, and the R:S ratio is less than 1.

Supraventricular rhythms may be preceded by a premature P wave, which may be hidden in the preceding T wave, and the QRS complex may be narrower than 0.12 second. (Junctional aberrancies are probably the most difficult beats to differentiate from ventricular premature beats because they may not be preceded by a P wave.)

Because it is usually the right bundle branch that causes the prolonged intraventricular conduction with premature beats, supraventricular aberrant beats usually have an RBBB configuration when the patient is monitored with MCL_1.

One method of differentiating between supraventricular and ventricular dysrhythmias is the electrophysiologic study (EPS). The EPS is an intracardiac recording of the electrical activity of the heart that, as well as differentiating the origin of dysrhythmias, is used to identify characteristics of dysrhythmias and to evaluate the efficacy of antidysrhythmic therapies such as drugs, pacing, and surgical interventions. The procedure is performed in a cardiac catheterization laboratory and involves introducing catheters similar to pacing catheters into the heart via veins (usually the femoral, brachial, or basilic veins, or a femoral or basilic if left ventricular stimulation is necessary). The catheter tips are positioned at specific sites along the conduction pathway or chamber wall—usually the high right atrium, the bundle of His, and the right ventricular apex. Sometimes the electrode may be positioned at a reentrant pathway within the ventricle. Recordings are made of intervals of the surface ECG (P–R, QRS, Q–T, R–

R) and on the intracardiac ECG (PA, AH, and H–V). Ventricular tachycardia may be induced by rapid atrial or ventricular pacing or by delivering atrial or ventricular extrasystoles during a paced or spontaneous rhythm. Each extrasystole is delivered slightly earlier in the refractory period in an attempt to find the crucial point of stimulating tachycardia (Douglas, 1985). When tachycardia is induced, its characteristics are noted and compared with ECGs taken during previous episodes of spontaneous ventricular tachycardia. The bundle of His ECG is also inspected for the relationship between atrial and ventricular depolarization.

Electrophysiologic studies are valuable in differentiating supraventricular aberrant rhythms from ventricular tachycardia. According to Frankl and Greenspon (1983), the ability to reproduce ventricular tachycardia with EPS strongly suggests a reentrant mechanism in the ventricle.

Ashman phenomenon, commonly seen in atrial fibrillation, is another example of aberrant conduction. It is seen when a wide, aberrantly conducted supraventricular beat occurs after a QRS complex that is preceded by a long pause (Fig. 9–52). The bundle branches reset their rate of repolarization according to the length of the preceding beat. It the preceding beat occurred a relatively long time ago, repolarization is slower after that beat. If a supraventricular impulse passes through the AV node before repolarization is complete, that beat will be conducted aberrantly, producing a wide, bizarre QRS complex. In Figure 9–52, the sixth beat looks like a premature ventricular contraction but is probably an aberrant beat because it occurs after a long-short cycle.

The value of Ashman phenomenon in atrial fibrillation is controversial, however. According to Marriott and Conover (1988), because of concealed conduction one never knows from the surface ECG exactly when a bundle branch is activated. According to these authors, if an aberrant beat ends a long-short cycle sequence during atrial fibrillation, it may

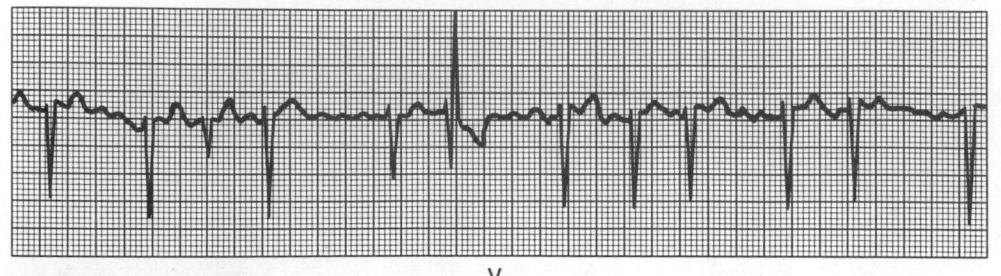

V₁

FIGURE 9–52. Ashman phenomenon. (Reproduced by permission from: Marriott, H. J. L., and Conover, M. *Advanced concepts in arrhythmias.* St. Louis, 1989, The C. V. Mosby Co..)

be because of refractoriness of a bundle branch secondary to concealed conduction into it rather than because of changes in the length of the ventricular cycle.

VENTRICULAR DYSRHYTHMIAS

Historically, critical care nurses have been aware of the need to monitor patients closely for ventricular dysrhythmias and to treat patients either prophylactically during the first few days after a myocardial infarction or when the following usual criteria are observed: greater than 5 beats per minute or beats that are multiform, repetitive (3 or more in a row), and occur early in the cardiac cycle (R on phenomenon). It was previously thought that these signs warned of ventricular fibrillation. More recently, doubts have been cast upon the concept of "warning dysrhythmias" (Campbell et al., 1981). Investigations have shown that as many as 50% of patients with ventricular fibrillation during acute MI may not exhibit such warning ventricular premature beats. Warning dysrhythmias may occur relatively infrequently in a given patient or may occur only seconds before fibrillation is seen. Conversely, warning dysrhythmias may develop in as many as 50% of patients who do not go on to ventricular fibrillation (Antman

and Rutherford, 1986). In view of these facts, and the fact that lidocaine, to be effective, must be given at a dose of 3 mg per minute for 24 hours (Lie et al., 1974), many clinicians now believe that lidocaine may be administered more selectively. Analysis of pooled data from several studies suggests that certain patients may benefit more than others from lidocaine prophylaxis (Horwitz and Feinstein, 1981; Goldman and Batsford, 1980; DeSilva et al., 1981). Patients who are 40 to 50 years of age with no previous history of congestive heart failure or acute MI and who are admitted early after onset of chest pain are at high risk for ventricular fibrillation and should therefore receive lidocaine prophylaxis (Antman and Rutherford, 1986). In elderly patients aged 70 and above, the risk of ventricular fibrillation appears to be reduced, especially if they are admitted to the critical care unit late after the onset of chest pain and the risk of lidocaine toxicity appears to be increased. Subsequently, cautious administration of lidocaine is advised (Antman and Rutherford, 1986).

Torsades de Pointes

Torsades de pointes, a form of ventricular tachycardia, occurs in the presence of Q–T prolongation (Fig. 9–53). It is frequently prefibrillatory and appears

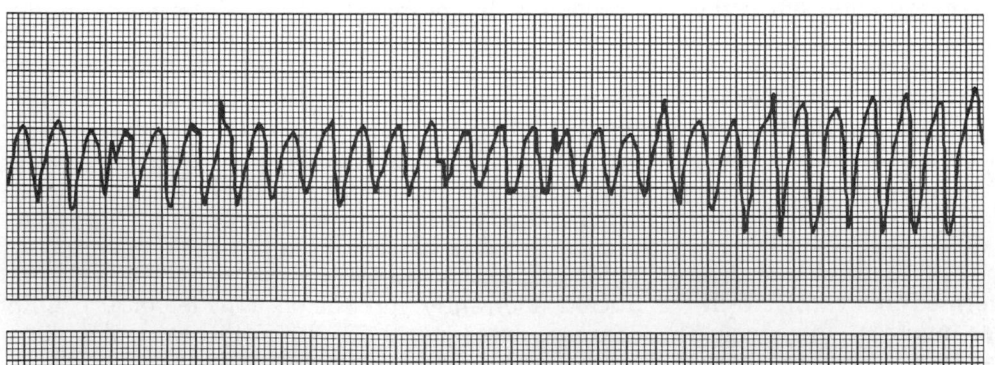

FIGURE 9–53. Torsades de pointes.

to be transitional between conventional ventricular tachycardia and ventricular fibrillation (Smith and Gallagher, 1980). Its mechanism is probably a form of reentry (Horwitz, 1981), although others have proposed multiple competing activation sites as a mechanism (Bardy, 1983).

Characteristics of torsades de pointes include:

- Irregular rhythm
- Wide QRS complex
- Polymorphism
- QRS configuration twists about the isoelectric point, changing axis every 5 to 20 beats (i.e., QRS changes from an upright complex to isoelectric to downward)
- Heart rate greater than 150 and sometimes greater than 200 beats per minute.

In many cases, the twisting of the QRS configuration is apparent only in certain ECG leads, and therefore, a 12-lead ECG should record the dysrhythmia. Torsades de pointes is usually associated with a long QT interval during periods of normal sinus rhythm.

Torsades de pointes is caused by acquired or congenital conditions and is associated with a prolonged Q–T interval. Acquired mechanisms that prolong the Q–T interval include: type I antidysrhythmic drugs (quinidine, procainamide, disopyramide), psychotropic drugs, electrolyte abnormalities (hypomagnesemia, hypokalemia, hypocalcemia), insecticide poisoning, and liquid protein diets. It is often associated with bradycardia, especially when due to AV block, and it has been associated with Prinzmetal's angina (Krikler and Curry, 1976). Congenital conditions associated with torsades de pointes include the autosomal recessive Jervell and Lange-Nielsen syndrome with accompanying deafness and the autosomal dominant Romano-Ward syndrome without deafness. Torsades de pointes may be provoked by stress-induced sudden changes of sympathetic tone, although the evidence of such a triggering mechanism is not always present or readily producible. Treatment includes removal of the predisposing cause as well as the use of isoproterenol to increase heart rate and shorten the Q–T interval, propranolol, phenytoin, and a pacemaker. Some patients with recurrent uncontrolled episodes may require a left stellate ganglionectomy as well as an implantable cardioverter-defibrillator.

Monitoring the Q–T Interval

The Q–T interval is an important measurement in the routine monitoring of patients in critical care units. The normal value for the Q–T interval depends on heart rate. As heart rate increases, the Q–T interval shortens. As heart rate decreases, the Q–T interval lengthens. The normal upper limit for the Q–T interval in heart rates increasing from 60 to 100 beats per minute diminishes from 0.40 to 0.34 second for males and 0.44 to 0.34 second for females (Braunwald, 1988). The formula used to correct the Q–T interval for heart rate is:

$$QTc = Q{-}T \, / \, R{-}R$$

where Q–T is the Q–T interval measured from the beginning of the QRS complex to the end of the T wave. The R–R interval is the time between two successive R waves measured. Most authors agree that a QTc exceeding 0.44 second is prolonged and should be reported.

The nurse should suspect potential torsades de pointes when the usual treatments, lidocaine and procainamide, are not effective in treating ventricular dysrhythmias. A family and personal history should be obtained from the patient, with a focus on history of syncope or transient palpitations, medication use, and exposure to insecticides.

Correct diagnosis of this form as of other forms of ventricular tachycardia is critical. If the rhythm is torsades de pointes and the patient receives the usual medications (lidocaine, procainamide, quinidine), his condition will worsen. Similarly, if the rhythm is ventricular tachycardia and is mistaken for supraventricular tachycardia with aberrancy, verapamil may be given; verapamil has been associated with profound hypotension and increased mortality when used in the setting of ventricular tachycardia (Steward et al., 1986).

PARADYSRHYTHMIAS: PARASYSTOLE AND AV DISSOCIATION

A paradysrhythmia is an abnormal rhythm in which two pacemakers discharge independently of each other (Fig. 9–54). One pacemaker is usually the SA node and the activity of the other pacemaker does not disturb the conduction of the normal sinus impulse. There are two types of paradysrhythmias: parasystole and AV dissociation.

Parasystole

In parasystole, one pacemaker is in the SA node and the second is an ectopic site. The dominant pacemaker coexists with, but never discharges or is discharged by, the second pacemaker. The second

FIGURE 9–54. Parasystole. (Redrawn from Phillips, R., and Feeney, M. (1990). *The cardiac rhythms* (3rd ed.). Philadelphia: W. B. Saunders.)

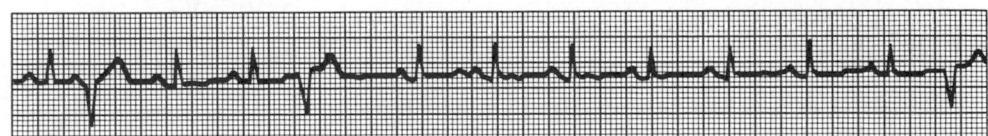

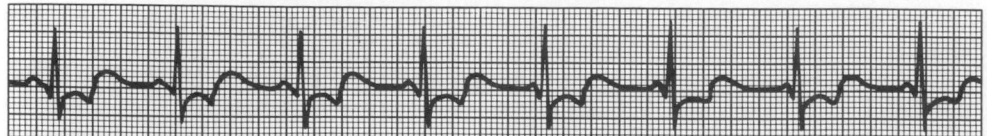

FIGURE **9–55.** AV dissociation. (Redrawn from Phillips, R., and Feeney, M. (1990). *The cardiac rhythms* (3rd ed). Philadelphia: W. B. Saunders.)

pacemaker may or may not be faster than the sinus node but somehow is prevented from taking over control of the heart by a "protective entrance" block (Goldman, 1986). Similarly, an "exit" block occurs when an impulse does not emerge from its origin. Therefore, entrance blocks keep impulses from the primary pacemaker (i.e., the SA node) from invading and resetting the ectopic focus, and exit blocks limit the number of impulses propagated from the regularly firing ectopic pacemaker.

This dysrhythmia is most commonly seen in association with organic heart disease but has been found to be relatively benign. It is common with patients with heart transplants who have an atrial parasystole resulting from SA node impulse formation and atrial activation from the donor heart and the recipient's residual SA node and atria. Obviously, the P wave that results from depolarization of the recipient's own residual atria never captures the ventricle.

ECG criteria for parasystole are:

1. There is no constant relationship between the sinus beat and the ectopic beat; the coupling interval usually varies more than 0.8 second (Medina, 1981).
2. The time interval between ectopic beats is constant or an exact multiple of a common denominator (the least common denominator will represent the actual rate of discharge of the ectopic focus).
3. Fusion beats representing depolarization from both sites are commonly seen.
4. The QRS configuration of the parasystolic beat is unchanging (Lipman and Lipman, 1987).

The most common type of parasystole is one in which the slower ectopic center (often the ventricle) competes with the SA node. Ventricles are depolarized by one or the other pacemaker depending upon the refractoriness of the AV node and ventricles at that moment. The slower ectopic center produces a QRS that looks like an ectopic beat. The less common form of parasystole is one in which the rate of impulse formation of the ectopic focus is more rapid than that of the SA node. This pacemaker does not take over control of the heart because of an exit block, which prevents some of the ectopic impulses from leaving their site of origin (Goldman, 1986).

Recognizing parasystole requires a long rhythm strip to calculate the interectopic intervals and absence of fixed coupling.

AV Dissociation

AV dissociation is a paradysrhythmia in which the atria and ventricles are beating independently, i.e.,

dissociated (Fig. 9–55). As such, it is a generic term that may be applied to any rhythm in which the atria and ventricles are activated independently, for example, ventricular tachycardia. The dominant pacemaker is in the AV junction or below and controls ventricular activation, while another pacemaker, in the SA node or atria, controls the atria. This situation results either from suppression of the SA node, as may occur secondarily to vagal stimulation or drug therapy, or from increased automaticity of the junctional tissue.

AV dissociation may be complete or incomplete. If it is incomplete, impulses from the SA node arrive at the AV junction, which is nonrefractory, and so the impulse is conducted through to the ventricles. In complete AV dissociation, the AV node is refractory from the dominant junctional pacemaker, and impulses from the SA node cannot be conducted.

On the ECG, P waves bear no relationship to the QRS complexes. When the sinus rhythm is slower than the ventricular rhythm, the P to P intervals will be longer than the R to R intervals. As the result, the P waves overtake the QRS complexes, and the P–R interval becomes progressively shorter. The P wave then becomes superimposed on the QRS complex and eventually occurs after the QRS complex. When the P wave falls sufficiently far beyond the QRS complex, the sinus impulse is conducted to the ventricles, resulting in a captured ventricular beat.

SUMMARY

This chapter has discussed the interpretation of the electrocardiogram as it relates to coronary artery disease, axis deviation, and complex dysrhythmias. Our knowledge base of the conduction system and dysrhythmias has grown considerably in the last 10 to 15 years. This knowledge has increased the complexity of critical care nursing as well as nurses' responsibility for the early detection and recognition of alterations in normal cardiac rhythms. Whether employed in large medical centers or small community hospitals, nurses must be able to combine rapid ECG interpretation with astute assessment skills in anticipating and forestalling life-threatening situations in their patients.

References

Abedin, A., and Conner, R. (1989). *12 lead ECG interpretation: the self-assessment approach.* Philadelphia: W. B. Saunders.
Alpert, M. (1980). *Cardiac arrhythmias: A bedside guide to diagnosis and treatment.* Chicago: Year Book Medical Publishers.

Antaloczy, A. (1987). Correlation of electrocardiographic and pathologic findings in 100 cases of Q and ST myocardial infarcts. *Journal of Electrocardiography*, 20, 72.

Antman, E. M., and Rutherford, J. D. (1986). *Coronary care medicine: a practical approach*. Boston: Martinus Nijhoff.

Bairey, C. N., Shah, P. K., Lew, A. S., et al. (1987). Electrocardiographic differentiation of occlusion of the left circumflex versus the right coronary artery as a cause of acute inferior myocardial infarction. *Journal of Cardiology*, 60, 456.

Bardy, G. H. (1983) A mechanism of torsades de pointes in a canine model. *Circulation*, 67, 52.

Baroldi, G., and Scomazzoni, G. (1967). *Coronary circulation in the normal and pathologic heart*. Washington, D.C., Office of the Surgeon General.

Berne, R. M., and Levy, M. N. (1988). *Physiology*. St. Louis: C. V. Mosby.

Braat, W. H. J. G. (1984). *Right ventricular infarction*. Thesis. University of Limburg, Maastricht.

Braunwald, E. (1988). *Heart disease: A textbook of cardiovascular medicine* (3rd ed.). Philadelphia: W. B. Saunders.

Brooks, C., Hoffman, E. E., and Orias, O. (1955). *Excitability of the heart*. New York: Grune & Stratton.

Brugada, P., and Wellens, H. J. J. (1986). How to approach conduction disturbances. In E. Andries and R. Stroobandt (Eds.), *Clinical arrhythmias for the clinical cardiologist*. New York: Excerpta Medica.

Campbell, R. W., Murry, A., and Julian, D. G. (1981). Ventricular arrhythmias in the first twelve hours of acute myocardial infarction. *British Heart Journal*, 46, 351.

Carroll-Johnson, R. M. (1989). *Classification of nursing diagnosis: Proceedings of the eighth conference*. Philadelphia: J. B. Lippincott.

Chahine, R. A. (1979). Prinzmetal's variant angina: A syndrome apart or another clinical presentation of atheromatous heart disease. *Archives of Internal Medicine*, 139, 26.

Chung, E. K. (1983). *Principles of cardiac arrhythmias*. Baltimore: Williams & Wilkins.

Conover, M. (1988). *Understanding electrocardiography*. St. Louis: C. V. Mosby.

Cranefield, P. F. (1975). *The conduction of the cardiac impulse: The slow response and cardiac arrhythmias*. Mt. Kisco, NY: Futura Press.

DiSilva, R. A., Lown, B., Hennekens, C. H., et al. (1981). Lidocaine prophylaxis in acute myocardial infarction: An evaluation of randomized trials. *Lancet*, 1, 855–858.

Douglas, M. K. (1985). The use of electrophysiologic studies in the management of recurrent ventricular tachyarrhythmias. In M. Douglas and J. Shinn (Eds.), *Advances in cardiovascular nursing*. Rockville, MD: Aspen.

Evans, W. (1951). The effect of deep breathing on lead III of the electrocardiogram. *British Heart Journal*, 13, 457.

Frankl, W. S., and Greenspon, A. J. (1983). Electrophysiologic testing: Clinical applications. *Cardiovascular Clinics*, 3, 301–319.

Friedman, H. (1985). *Diagnostic electrocardiography and vector cardiography*. New York: McGraw-Hill.

Frink, R. J., and James, T. N. (1973). Normal blood supply to the His bundle and proximal bundle branches. *Circulation*, 47, 8.

Gilcrest, I. C., et al. (1981). Left bundle branch block eliminates Q waves of inferior infarction: Confirmation by ventriculography. *American Journal of Noninvasive Cardiology*, 1, 206.

Goldberger, A. (1984). *Myocardial infarction: Electrocardiographic differential diagnosis*. St. Louis: C. V. Mosby.

Goldman, M. J. (1986). *Principles of clinical electrocardiography*. Los Altos, CA: Lange Medical Publications.

Goldman, L., and Batsford, W. P. (1986). Risk-benefit stratification as a guide to lidocaine prophylaxis of primary ventricular fibrillation in acute myocardial infarction: An analytic review. *Yale Journal of Biological Medicine*, 52, 455–466.

Guyton, A. (1991). *Textbook of medical physiology* (8th ed). Philadelphia: W. B. Saunders.

Han, J. (1969). Mechanics of ventricular arrhythmias associated with myocardial infarction. *American Journal of Cardiology*, 24, 800.

Hoffman, B., and Cranefield, P. (1960). *Electrophysiology of the heart*. New York: McGraw-Hill.

Hoffman, B., and Rosen, M. (1981). Cellular mechanisms for cardiac arrhythmias. *Circulation Research*, 49, 1–15.

Horwitz, L. N. (1981). Torsade de pointes: electrophysiologic studies in patients without transient pharmacologic or metabolic abnormalities. *Circulation*, 57, 431.

Horwitz, R. I., and Feinstein, A. R. (1981). Improved observational method for studying therapeutic efficacy. Suggestive evidence that lidocaine prophylaxis prevents death in acute myocardial infarction. *Journal of the American Medical Association*, 246, 2455–2459.

Hurst, J. W. (1986). *The heart: Arteries and veins* (6th ed.). New York: McGraw-Hill.

Jacobson, C. (1983). Interpretation of complex arrhythmias. In S. Woods (Ed.), *Cardiovascular critical care nursing*. New York: Churchill Livingstone.

James, T. N. (1961). *Anatomy of the coronary arteries*. New York: Paul B. Hoeber.

Josephson, M., and Kastor, J. (1977). Supraventricular tachycardia: Mechanism and management. *Annals of Internal Medicine*, 87, 346–358.

Josephson, M., and Wellens, H. (1984). *Tachycardias: Mechanisms, diagnosis and treatment*. Philadelphia: Lea & Febiger.

Kass, R., Tsien, R., and Weingart, R. (1978). Ionic basis of transient inward current induced by strophanthidin in cardiac Purkinje fibers. *Journal of Physiology* (London), 281, 209.

Katz, A. M. (1977). *Physiology of the heart*. New York: Raven Press.

Katzung, B., and Morgenstern, J. (1977). Effects of extracellular potassium on ventricular automaticity and evidence for a pacemaker current in mammalian ventricular myocardium. *Circulation Research*, 40, 105.

Krikler, D. M., and Curry, P. V. (1976). Torsade de pointes, an atypical ventricular tachycardia. *British Heart Journal*, 38, 117.

Lie, K. I., Wellens, H. J. J., and Schuilenburg, R. M. (1976). Bundle branch block in acute myocardial infarction. In H. J. J. Wellens, K. I. Lie, and M. J. Janse (Eds.), *The conduction system of the heart*. Leiden: Stenfert Kroese.

Lie, K., Wellens, H. J. J., van Capelle, F., et al. (1974). Lidocaine in the prevention of primary ventricular fibrillation. *New England Journal of Medicine*, 291, 1324.

Lipman, B. S., Dunn, M., and Massie, E. (1984). *Clinical electrocardiography*. Chicago: Year Book Medical Publishers.

Lipman, B. C., and Lipman, B. S. (1987). *ECG pocket guide*. Chicago: Year Book Medical Publishers.

Liu, C. K. (1961). Atrial infarction of the heart. *Circulation*, 23, 331.

Mahaim, I. (1949). Kent's fibers and the A-V paraspecific conduction through the upper connections of the bundle of His-Tarawa. *American Heart Journal*, 33, 651.

Marriott, H. J. (1983). *Practical electrocardiography* (7th ed.). Baltimore: Williams & Wilkins.

Marriott, H. J. (1988). *Practical electrocardiography* (8th ed.). Baltimore: Williams & Wilkins.

Marriott, H. J., and Conover, M. B. (1989). *Advanced Concepts in Arrhythmias* (2nd ed). St. Louis: C. V. Mosby.

Medine, R. (1981). Supraventricular arrhythmias. In J. Nieveen (Ed.), *Arrhythmias of the heart*. Oxford: Excerpta Medica.

Meller, J., Pichard, A., and Dack, S. (1976). Coronary arterial spasm in Prinzmetal's angina: A proven hypothesis. *American Journal of Cardiology*, 37, 938.

Phillips, R., and Feeney, M. (1990). *The cardiac rhythms* (3rd ed). Philadelphia: W. B. Saunders.

Prinzmetal, M., Ekmekci, A., Toyoshima, H., et al. (1959). Angina pectoris: III. Demonstration of a chemical origin of ST deviation in classic angina pectoris, its variant form, early myocardial infarction, and some noncardiac conditions. *American Journal of Cardiology*, 3, 276.

Raizner, A. E., and Chahine, R. A. (1979). The treatment of Prinzetal's variant angina with coronary bypass surgery. In J. W. Hurst (Ed.), *Update II to the heart*. New York: McGraw-Hill.

Rosen, M. (1986). Is the response to programmed electrical stimulation diagnostic of mechanisms for arrhythmias? *Circulation* (Suppl. II), 73, 18–37.

Rosen, M., and Danilo, P. (1980). Effects of tetrodotoxin, lidocaine, verapamil, and AHR-266 on ouabain-induced delayed afterdepolarizations in canine Purkinje fibers. *Circulation Research*, 46, 117–124.

Ross, J. H. (1984). Embryonic myocardial remnants and dual

pathway conduction: Management of related reentrant supraventricular tachycardia. *Critical Care Nurse, 4*(2), 78–85.

Scheidt, S. (1986). *Basic electrocardiology.* West Caldwell, NJ: Ciba-Geigy Pharmaceuticals.

Schlesinger, M. J. (1940). Relation of anatomic pattern to pathologic conditions of coronary arteries. *Archives of Pathology, 30,* 403.

Shamroth, L. (1984). *The electrocardiology of coronary artery disease.* Oxford: Blackwell Scientific Publications.

Smith, W. M., and Gallagher, J. J. (1980). Les torsades de pointes: An unusual ventricular arrhythmia. *Annals of Internal Medicine, 93,* 578–584.

Sokolow, M., and McIlroy, M. B. (1981). *Clinical cardiology.* Los Altos, CA: Lange Medical Publications.

Steward, R. B., Bardy, G. H., and Green, H. L. (1986). Wide complex tachycardia: Misdiagnosis and outcome after emergent therapy. *Annals of Internal Medicine, 104,* 766–771.

Sullivan, W., Vlodaver, A., Tuna, N., et al. (1978). Correlation of electrocardiographic and pathologic findings in healed myocardial infarctions. *American Journal of Cardiology, 42,* 724–732.

Tans, A. C., and Lie, K. I. (1976). A-V nodal block in acute myocardial infarction. In H. J. J. Wellens, K. I. Lie, and M. J. Janse (Eds.), *The conduction system of the heart.* Leiden: Stenfert Kroese.

Thalen, H. J. T. (1981). Anatomy of the conduction system of the human heart. In J. Nieveen (Ed.), *Arrhythmias of the heart.* Oxford: Excerpta Medica.

Thaler, M. S. (1988). *The only EKG book you'll ever need.* Philadelphia: J. B. Lippincott.

Viersma, J. W. (1981). Electrophysiology of impulse formation and conduction. In J. Nieveen (Ed.), *Arrhythmias of the heart* (pp. 14–22). Oxford: Excerpta Medica.

Viersma, J. W. (1981). Treatment of ventricular arrhythmias. In J. Nieveen (Ed.), *Arrhythmias of the heart* (pp. 136–145). Oxford: Excerpta Medica.

Wit, A. (1984). Cellular electrophysiologic mechanisms of cardiac arrhythmias. *Annals of the New York Academy of Sciences, 432,* 1–15.

Wit, A. L., and Cranefield, P. F. (1976). Triggered activity in cardiac muscle fibers of the simian mitral valve. *Circulation Research, 38,* 85–98.

Wit, A. L., and Cranefield, P. F. (1977). Triggered and automatic activity in the canine coronary sinus. *Circulation Research, 41,* 435–445.

Wit, A., and Rosen, M. (1981). Cellular electrophysiology of cardiac arrhythmias. I. Arrhythmias caused by abnormal impulse generation. *Modern Concepts of Cardiovascular Disease, 50,* 1–6.

Wit, A., and Rosen, M. (1984). Cellular electrophysiology of cardiac arrhythmias. In M. E. Josephson and H. Wellens (Eds.), *Tachycardias: Mechanisms, diagnosis, and treatment.* Philadelphia: Lea & Febiger.

Wit, A., Rosen, M., and Hoffman, F. (1974). Electrophysiology and pharmacology of cardiac arrhythmias II. Relationship of normal and abnormal electrical activity of cardiac fibers to the genesis of arrhythmias. *American Heart Journal, 88,* 515.

Ziegler, R. F. (1951). *Electrocardiographic studies in normal infants and children.* Springfield, IL: Charles C. Thomas.

10

Hemodynamic Monitoring

Lucille T. Kadota

Hemodynamic monitoring is an integral part of managing physiologically unstable patients. This chapter will discuss hemodynamic pressure recorders and the monitoring of central venous pressure, intra-arterial pressure, pulmonary artery pressure, and cardiac output and will conclude with the clinical implications of hemodynamic data.

HEMODYNAMIC PRESSURE RECORDERS

The three basic components of a hemodynamic biomedical recorder are (1) a transducer to detect pressure changes, (2) an amplifier to increase the magnitude of the transducer signals, and (3) a system monitor with a recorder or oscilloscope to display the signal. A transducer detects pressure changes and transmits these signals to the system monitor, which converts the signals into electrical energy. The recorder then displays the signals in digital and graphic form.

Most hemodynamic monitors have the capacity to present hemodynamic pressures by digital display, graphic form on the oscilloscope, and by graphic form on a paper printout. There are different protocols for recording hemodynamic pressures. The key factor is consistent application among clinicians of whatever protocol is used for the interpretation of the waveforms. Changes in pressures can then be attributed to actual changes in the patient's condition, either as a result of therapy or as a consequence of the underlying disease process, and not to different measurement methods. This is particularly important because of the variation in waveforms caused by the respiratory cycle, dysrhythmias, valvular insufficiency, mechanical ventilation, and catheter fling.

The three procedures that are performed at the start of hemodynamic monitoring and every 4 to 12 hours thereafter (and more often as needed) are positioning of the transducer at the phlebostatic axis, setting the zero reference, and electrical calibration. The transducer is positioned at the phlebostatic axis to negate the effect of hydrostatic forces on the observed hemodynamic pressures. The phlebostatic axis is located at the intersection of the transverse plane through the fourth intercostal space adjacent to the sternum and the frontal plane midway between the posterior surface of the body and the base of the xiphoid process (Fig. 10–1) (Bartz et al., 1988; Windsor and Burch, 1945). The phlebostatic axis should be marked on the patient with a washable felt pen and a leveler used to ensure consistent measurement technique. Falsely high pressures will result if the transducer is below the phlebostatic axis, and, conversely, falsely low pressures will result if the transducer is above the phlebostatic axis.

The zero-reference is set to negate the force (approximately 760 mm Hg) exerted by the atmosphere so that only the pressures within the heart or vessel are recorded. Pressure transducers are affected by changes in temperature that result in a drift away from the zero baseline. Electrical calibration yields a known pressure value within the monitor, and in some monitors electrical calibration is done by simply pressing the calibration button on the system monitor. Performance of the zero-reference and calibration procedure at least two to three times per day can correct baseline drift.

Performance of the above three procedures may occasionally result in pressures that are markedly different from the last readings recorded by the nurse on the previous shift. The pressure difference may be due to repositioning of the transducer at the phlebostatic axis, zeroing, recalibration, different method of measuring the waveform, or an actual change in the patient's condition. A standard protocol will minimize differences due to the way wave-

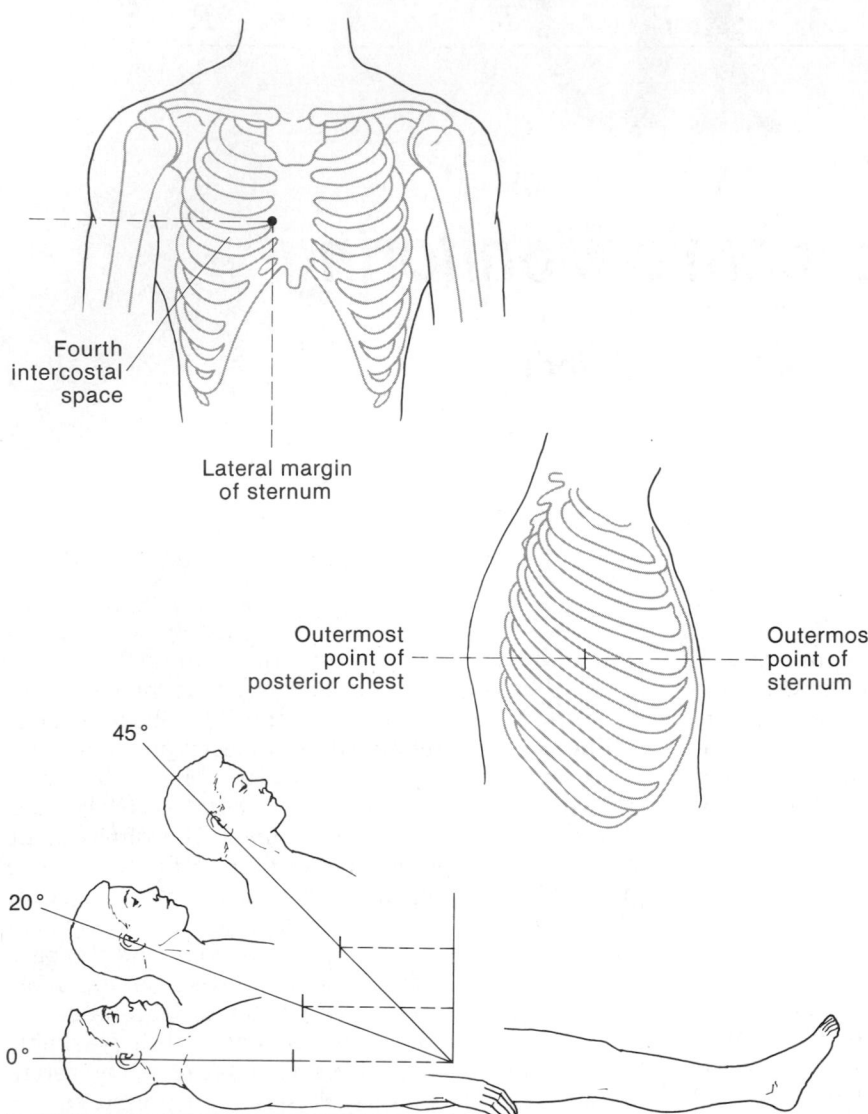

FIGURE 10–1. Phlebostatic axis. The phlebostatic axis is located at the intersection of the transverse plane through the fourth intercostal space adjacent to the sternum and the frontal plane midway between the posterior surface of the body and the base of the xiphoid process. (Redrawn from Shinn, J. A., et al. (1979). *Heart & Lung*, 8(2)322–327; Gardner, P. E., and Woods, S. L. (1989). Hemodynamic monitoring. In S. L. Underhill, S. L. Woods, E. S. S. Froelicher, and C. J. Halpenny, (Eds.), *Cardiac nursing* (2nd ed., p. 452). Philadelphia: J. B. Lippincott.

forms are measured. A dual-channel tracing (electrocardiogram and pulmonary artery, pulmonary artery wedge, or right atrial pressure) may facilitate identification of atypical waveforms because waveform morphology is more easily identified when timed with the electrocardiogram.

The first set of readings taken by a nurse may be measured prior to zeroing and recalibration and the second set of readings measured after zeroing and recalibration. This will permit comparison of readings done by different nurses, and by the same nurse before and after zeroing and recalibration. In addition, mounting a paper printout on the chart during each shift with the date, time, scale, and exact location of the part of the waveform where the measurement was taken can help to maintain consistency, particularly when one is faced with unusual waveforms. The paper printout should include waveforms recorded during at least three respiratory cycles to document clearly the variability resulting from inspiration and expiration (Fig. 10–2).

CENTRAL VENOUS PRESSURE MONITORING

Catheterization of the inferior vena cava with a ureteral catheter inserted in the thigh was first reported by Bleichroeder in 1905. Twenty-four years later, Forssman catheterized his own right atrium with a ureteral catheter inserted in a left antecubital vein (Steckelberg et al., 1979). Today, central venous pressure (CVP) monitoring is indicated when the patient's condition requires information about right ventricular function or blood volume as reflected by central venous return.

The central venous pressure corresponds to the right atrial pressure and reflects the end-diastolic pressure in the right ventricle when the tricuspid valve is open. The CVP is equivalent to the right atrial pressure measured by the pulmonary artery catheter. The mean right atrial pressure is recorded. The determinants of the CVP are blood volume, vascular tone, and right ventricular function.

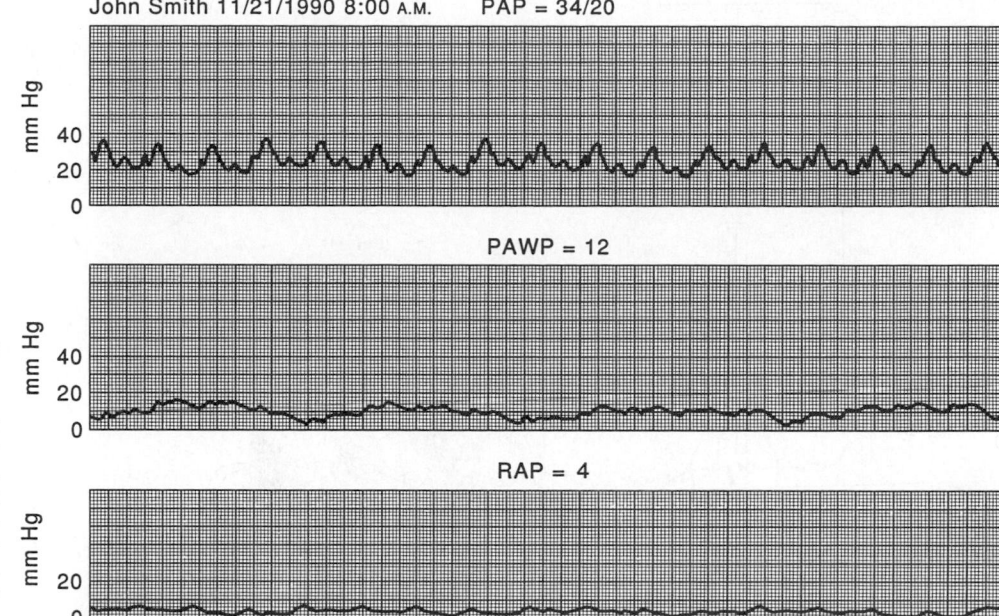

John Smith 11/21/1990 8:00 A.M.   PAP = 34/20

PAWP = 12

RAP = 4

FIGURE 10–2. Documentation of hemodynamic monitoring should include a paper printout of the waveforms recorded over at least three respiratory cycles to display the variability due to inspiration and expiration. The printout should include the patient's name, date, time of measurement, scale, and exact location on the waveform where the measurement was taken.

The physician is responsible for obtaining informed consent from the patient and for inserting the CVP catheter. The nurse is responsible for setting up the CVP line, calibration, monitoring vital signs, and observing for potential complications.

Insertion sites include the antecubital veins (medial basilic or lateral cephalic), the internal or external jugular vein, or the subclavian vein. Catheter insertion is a sterile procedure, and a mask should be worn. The insertion site is shaved and cleansed, and lidocaine is used for local anesthesia. The catheter is inserted into the vein with the catheter tip in the right atrium or in the superior vena cava just above the right atrium, and the proximal end of the catheter is attached to a manometer or pressure transducer monitoring system. The catheter is then sutured to the skin and a sterile occlusive dressing applied according to institutional protocol. Catheter patency is maintained with a pressurized tubing system that delivers approximately 3 ml of flush solution (1 unit of heparin/mL 5% dextrose or 0.9% saline) or another type of intravenous solution. Intravenous fluids should be kept at a low "to keep vein open" rate (approximately 5 to 10 mL/hour) until catheter placement is confirmed by fluoroscopy or chest x-ray. Details of equipment, insertion technique, maintenance, and troubleshooting that may be helpful for critical care orientation have been published (Daily and Schroeder, 1989, Millar et al., 1980, Yacone, 1987).

The potential complications of CVP monitoring are laceration of the vein, pneumothorax (with subclavian or jugular vein insertion), hydrothorax, hemothorax, brachial plexus injury, dysrhythmias, right ventricular perforation, emboli, thrombosis, thrombophlebitis, or infection (Daly et al., 1975; Millar et al., 1980; Yacone, 1987).

Measurement Guidelines

Although it is preferable to measure the CVP with the patient in the same position to minimize sources of variability, reproducible measurements may be obtained with the patient lying supine or sitting with the head rest elevated (Eckstein, 1972; Daily, 1972; Driver, 1972; Windsor and Burch, 1945). The transducer must have its zero-reference point at the patient's phlebostatic axis. At least 5 minutes should elapse after a patient changes position before measurements are performed. The procedure for measuring the CVP with a manometer is described in Figure 10–3.

Measurements obtained with a manometer are expressed in centimeters of water. The unit of measurement is millimeters of mercury for pressures recorded by the transducer system monitor connected to a pressurized transducer tubing set. One millimeter of mercury is equivalent to 1.36 cm of water (mercury is 13.6 times as heavy as water [Price and Fox, 1987]). Centimeters of water may be converted to millimeters of mercury by the formula:

$$\frac{x \text{ cm } H_2O}{1.36} = y \text{ mm Hg}$$

where x = the measurement of CVP in cm H_2O; 1.36 = the conversion factor; y = the measurement of CVP in mm Hg.

CVP can also be measured using a pressure transducer. The unit of measure in this case is millimeters of mercury, which may be converted to centimeters of water by the formula:

$$y \text{ mm Hg} \times 1.36 = x \text{ cm } H_2O$$

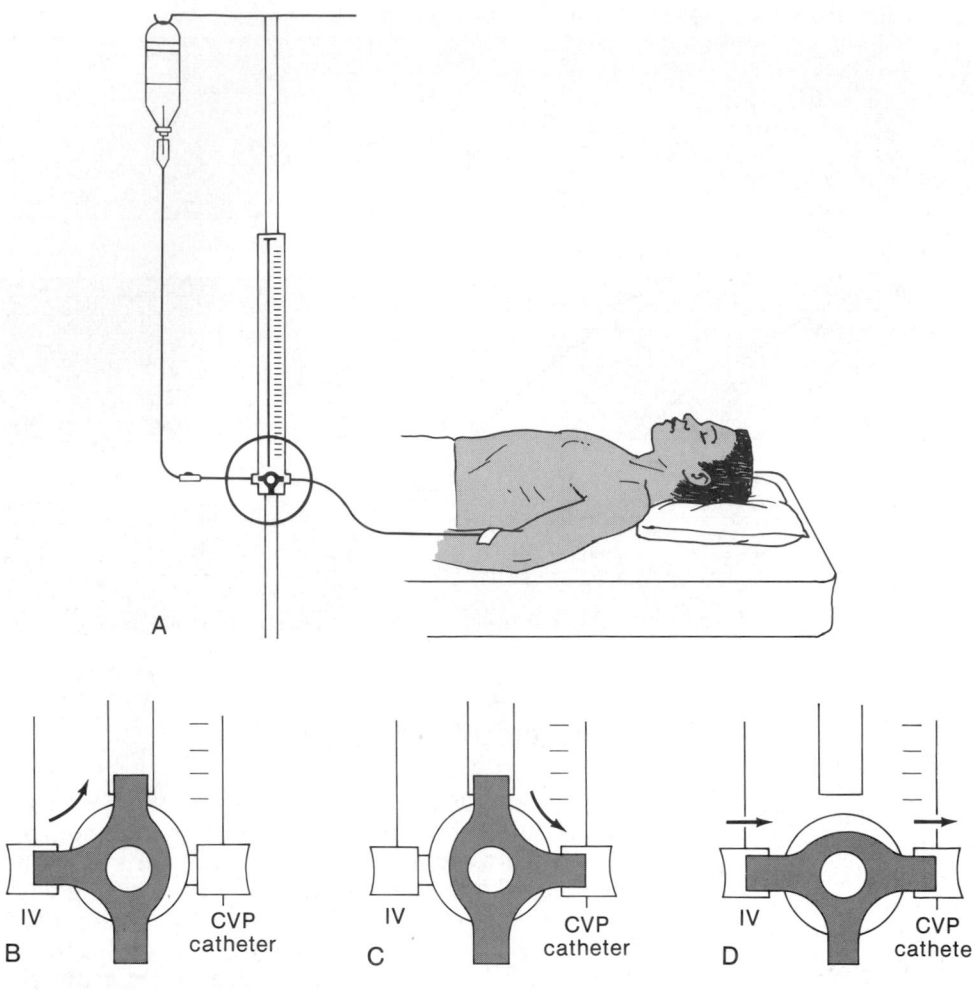

FIGURE 10-3. Central venous pressure measurement procedure using a manometer. *A*, Position the zero line of the manometer at the patient's phlebostatic axis. *B*, Turn the stopcock to let the fluid flow from the intravenous bag to the manometer. Fill the manometer to a level above the patient's expected central venous pressure (CVP). *C*, Turn the stopcock to stop the flow of the intravenous fluid from the intravenous bag such that the fluid now flows from the manometer to the patient. The CVP is measured after the fluid in the manometer stabilizes. *D*, Turn the stopcock to let the fluid flow from the intravenous bag to the patient at a low "to keep vein open" rate (approximately 5 to 10 mL/ hour). (Redrawn by permission from Daily, E. K., and Schroeder, J. S., *Techniques in bedside hemodynamic monitoring* (4th ed.). St. Louis, 1989, The C. V. Mosby Co.)

Clinical Interpretation

The normal range of CVP is 4 to 7 cm of water (−1 to 7 mm Hg)(Gowen, 1973). A CVP waveform with fluctuations due to respiratory variation is presented in Figure 10–4.

The possible interpretations of normal, elevated, and low CVP are presented in Table 10–1.

The CVP is one measurement of right heart hemodynamics. The CVP must be interpreted with caution in patients with coronary atherosclerosis, elevated pulmonary vascular resistance, and valvular disease because normal right and left ventricular function should not be assumed. In these situations, CVP monitoring yields accurate information only about the right heart and may be seriously misleading if the measurements are extrapolated for the evaluation of left heart hemodynamics. (Forrester et al., 1971).

Blood Sampling

The CVP catheter can be used to obtain blood samples for laboratory tests. Reliable plasma glucose, sodium, and potassium levels have been obtained from a multiple-lumen central venous catheter (Anderson et al., 1988).

INTRA-ARTERIAL PRESSURE MONITORING

One of the earliest instruments for the measurement of intra-arterial pressure was devised in 1733 by English scientist and clergyman Hales. He inserted a brass rod into the carotid artery of a mare and connected the rod to a goose trachea, which was in turn attached to a glass manometer that measured the height of the column of blood (Morton, 1980).

Intra-arterial monitoring permits direct measurement of the systemic blood pressure and is the standard against which indirect methods of measurement are compared. Clinically significant differences may occur when blood pressure measurements obtained by palpation or auscultation are compared with intra-arterial blood pressure measurements (Rebenson-Piano et al., 1987), particularly in hemodynamically unstable patients and patients with vascular disease. In general, the intra-arterial pressure will be more accurate than blood pressures obtained by palpation or auscultation. One exception may

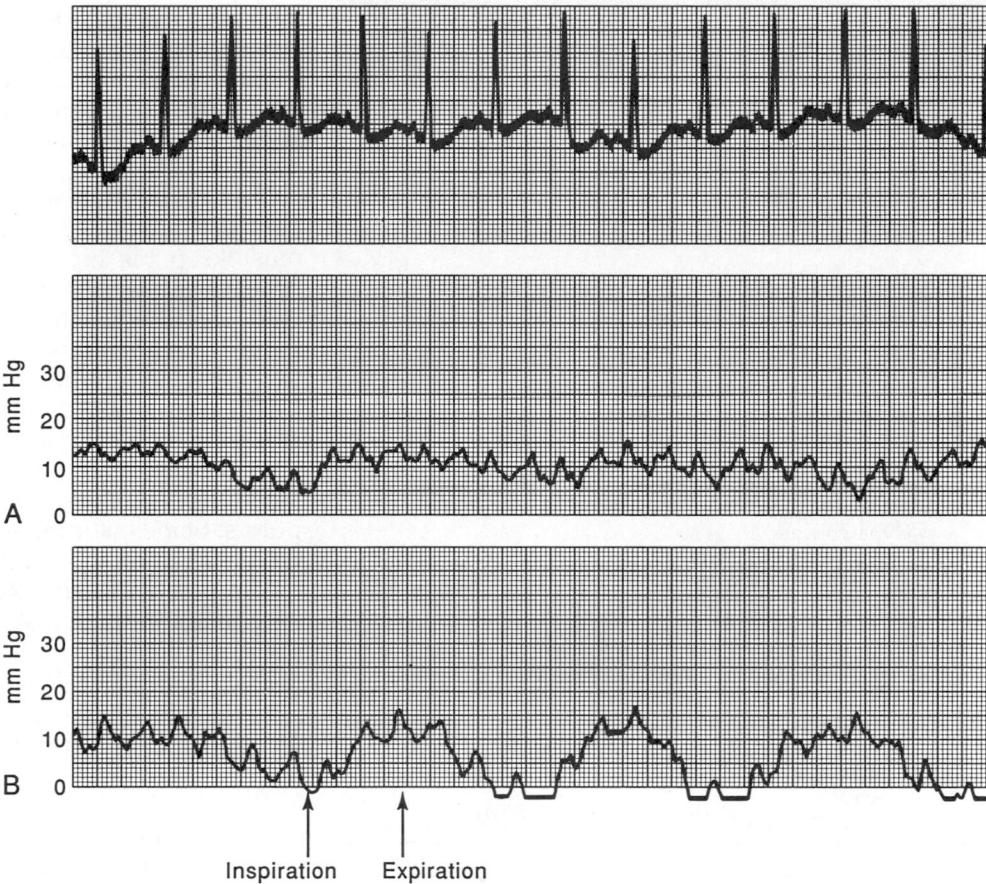

FIGURE 10–4. Central venous pressure waveform. *A,* Central venous pressure waveform with simultaneous electrocardiogram. *B,* Central venous pressure waveform with marked respiratory variation in the same patient.

Inspiration   Expiration

occur if the catheter is in a relatively small vessel like the radial artery in patients with marked peripheral vasoconstriction. For these patients, cannulation of more central locations such as the brachial artery or femoral artery may provide more accurate pressure readings (Chatterjee, 1985). Another exception occurs if a clot forms at the catheter tip and results in a dampened waveform. The indications for intra-arterial monitoring are hemodynamic instability, need to obtain frequent arterial blood gas samples, and the need to avoid traumatizing vessels for repeated blood samples.

The radial artery is a common site for cannulation because of the good collateral circulation provided by the ulnar artery (in most patients) and its accessibility and ease of maintenance. Alternate sites for intra-arterial monitoring are the brachial, axillary, femoral, and dorsalis pedis arteries (VanRiper and VanRiper, 1987).

The physician is responsible for obtaining informed consent from the patient and for inserting the arterial catheter. The nurse is responsible for setting up the arterial line, calibration, monitoring vital signs, obtaining blood samples, and observing for potential complications.

The modified Allen test (Allen, 1929; Gelberman and Blasingame, 1981; Millam, 1988) is performed to assess the adequacy of circulation to the hand prior to cannulation of the radial artery. The radial and ulnar arteries are compressed simultaneously with the clinician's thumbs or fingers. The patient is instructed to open and close his fist several times; the patient's hand should appear blanched. The pressure over the radial artery is released and the patient's hand observed for reactive hyperemia, which should be completed within 6 seconds if there is adequate circulation. This procedure is repeated, releasing the pressure over the ulnar artery while maintaining pressure over the radial artery.

Some physicians prefer to stabilize the wrist with an armboard so that the wrist is slightly hyperextended. The insertion site is then cleansed. The over-the-needle catheter (usually 20-gauge for the radial artery) is inserted at a 15- to 45-degree angle (Millam, 1988). When there is a blood return, the inner stylet is removed, and the pressure tubing is attached to the catheter hub. Aspiration of the deadspace volume between the catheter tip and the hub may be done to remove any air bubbles prior to flushing the catheter. Visualization of the arterial waveform on the oscilloscope will confirm proper placement (Fig. 10–5).

The pressurized transducer tubing system will deliver 3 to 5 mL of heparinized flush solution per hour to maintain catheter patency. If the waveform is dampened, the catheter tip may be lodged against the artery wall. Retracting the catheter slightly usually resolves this problem. The catheter is then se-

TABLE 10–1. Clinical Implications of Normal, Elevated, and Low Central Venous Pressures

Normal central venous pressure (−1 to 7 mm Hg)
 Normovolemic
 Acute left ventricular failure
High central venous pressure (>7 mm Hg)
 Normovolemia
  Right-sided heart failure
  Chronic biventricular failure
  Left to right shunt
  Pericardial disease
  Vasopressor medications
  Restless patient
  Tachypnea
  Chronic obstructive pulmonary disease
  Superior vena cava compression
  Pulmonic stenosis
  Pulmonary embolus
  Positive pressure ventilation
  Pneumothorax
 Hypervolemia
  Fluid overload
 Hypovolemia with severe cardiac decompensation
Low central venous pressure (<−1 mm Hg)
 Hypovolemia
  Dehydration
  Hemorrhage
  Diarrhea
  Peritonitis
 Hypervolemia with profound vasodilation
 Vasodilation
  Sepsis
  Vasodilator medications

Data from Daily and Schroeder (1989).

cured to the skin, and a sterile dressing is applied. The cannulation site should be inspected daily for erythema, drainage, bruising, or increasing radial girth and neurovascular checks made to the hand. The assessment should involve comparison of the cannulated extremity with the opposite extremity.

Cannulation of the femoral artery may be done in patients with severe hypotension, peripheral vasoconstriction, cardiac failure, or upper extremity trauma, or in those requiring intra-arterial pressure monitoring after percutaneous transluminal coronary angioplasty. A higher risk of contamination is associated with femoral artery cannulation. Detection and control of bleeding is relatively more difficult with bleeding into the groin than in the arms. The patient must keep his hip in straight alignment, and the head of the bed should not be elevated more than 30 degrees. When turning the patient, the patient's entire body should be kept in straight alignment with the nurse supporting the patient's back and hip. Circulation to the lower extremities is monitored by assessing skin color and temperature, observing patient discomfort (pain, tingling, or numbness), and palpating the dorsalis pedis and posterior tibialis pulses. Some institutional protocols include checking the blood pressure in the calf by Doppler technique.

The potential complications of intra-arterial pressure monitoring are listed in Table 10–2.

Measurement Guidelines

The blood pressure obtained from the arterial catheter should be compared to the blood pressure obtained by sphygmomanometer at least two to three times a day or more often as needed. In stable cardiac patients with radial or pedal artery catheters, the mean arterial pressure can be obtained with the patient in the supine or semi-Fowler's position using either the right atrium or the tip of the intra-arterial catheter site as the reference point for calibration. However, in unstable patients or in situations where therapy is based on the mean arterial pressure, the

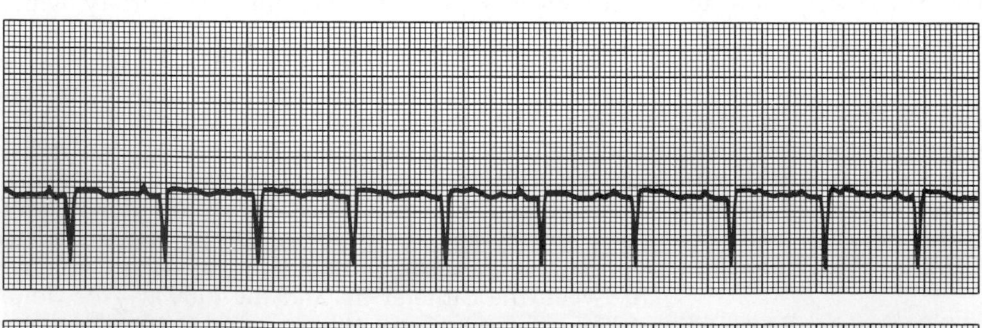
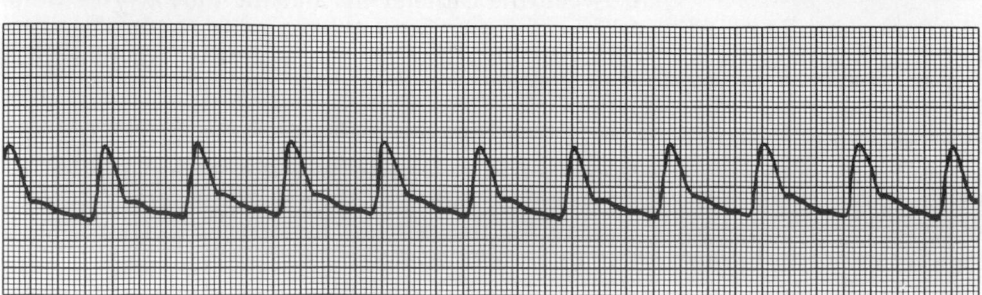

FIGURE 10–5. Intra-arterial pressure waveform with simultaneous electrocardiogram.

TABLE 10–2. Potential Complications of Intra-Arterial Pressure Monitoring

Hematoma
Ecchymosis
Purpura
Bleeding
Sclerosis
Thrombosis
Infection
Peripheral embolization
Ischemia
Distal vascular insufficiency
Arterial occlusion

same position and reference point should be used. In such patients, use of the supine position and the right atrium as the reference point may be more convenient for the nurse and more comfortable for the patient because these patients often have both an arterial catheter as well as a pulmonary artery catheter (Rebenson-Piano and Kirchhoff, 1983).

Blood Sampling

The arterial catheter makes it possible to obtain blood specimens without further traumatizing the patient. The need for arterial blood gas tests in patients with ventilatory problems makes the indwelling catheter invaluable. Traditionally, a blood gas sample is obtained 10 to 30 minutes after making a change in ventilator settings. Preliminary research suggests that homeostasis occurs sooner and that it may not be necessary to wait as long as 30 minutes (Schuch and Price, 1987). Aspiration of approximately two and one half times the deadspace volume of the arterial tubing between the indwelling catheter and the first stopcock provides blood gas results comparable to those obtained from direct arterial puncture (Molter, 1983). As a general guideline, the clinician may aspirate until the blood at the stopcock closest to the patient looks red and thick, indicating that the flush solution is not diluting the blood sample.

The use of arterial catheters for obtaining samples for coagulation studies is controversial because contamination of the laboratory specimen by the heparinized flush solution can result in falsely high partial thromboplastin (PTT) and thrombin time (TT) values (Cannon et al., 1985; Gregersen et al., 1987; Kajs, 1986; Molyneaux et al., 1987; Pryor, 1983; Rakowski et al., 1987). Studies indicate that accurate prothrombin time (PT), TT, and PTT results can be obtained from samples taken from arterial catheters in some patients. However, it has not been established how many milliliters of fluid should be withdrawn to clear the heparinized flush solution adequately from the deadspace between the arterial catheter tip and the syringe port where the blood specimen is collected (Cannon et al., 1985; Gregersen et al., 1987; Pryor, 1983). The actual volume discarded depends on the

distance of the stopcock from the indwelling catheter. Approximately 5 to 10 times the deadspace volume (3.3 to 4.8 mL) (Merenstein, 1971; Molyneaux et al., 1987; Rakowski et al., 1987) seems to be an adequate volume to discard, although one study (Cannon et al., 1985) showed good correlation after discarding only 2 mL from an arterial line with a deadspace volume of 1 mL between the catheter tip and syringe port.

Of great concern are abnormally high PTT and TT values in a minority of patients due to contamination of the specimen with heparin from the flush solution (Gregersen et al., 1987; Pryor, 1983). The consequence of an abnormally high PTT value on a sample drawn from a heparinized catheter is that the PTT would have to be redone on a fresh sample because one would not know if the result was due to heparin contamination or excessive heparin therapy. The delay in making clinical decisions and the cost of repeating laboratory tests may, in the opinion of some clinicians, not be in the patient's best interests compared to the discomfort caused by venipuncture. The reality of the patient's experience in the intensive care unit, however, is one of pain and bruising due to multiple venipunctures and arterial blood samplings.

Venipuncture remains the standard method against which other methods of blood draws for coagulation studies are compared (Kajs, 1986). One potential alternative in patients requiring short-term (less than 72 hours) intra-arterial monitoring is the use of nonheparinized flush solutions (Hook et al., 1987). Another alternative may be to obtain the blood sample for the PT, PTT, and TT last when multiple blood tests are done. This would result in 10 to 20 mL of blood being withdrawn before the blood samples for coagulation studies are obtained. This area of research needs further investigation, particularly in patients receiving continuous intravenous infusions of heparin.

PULMONARY ARTERY PRESSURE MONITORING

Catheterization of the heart had its origins in the mid-nineteenth century, when glass tubes or flexible probes were inserted in animal hearts (Cournand, 1975). In 1929 Forssman inserted a 4 French ureteral catheter through a vein in his left cubital fossa and into his heart (Steckelberg et al., 1979). The landmark paper by Swan and Ganz and their colleagues (1970) described a 5 French balloon-tipped polyvinyl chloride catheter that could be safely used to catheterize the heart in man. The subsequent addition of pacing capabilities, continuous mixed venous oxygen saturation (Sv_{O_2}) monitoring (Martin et al., 1973), and an extra proximal port for drug infusion expanded the utility of the pulmonary artery catheter.

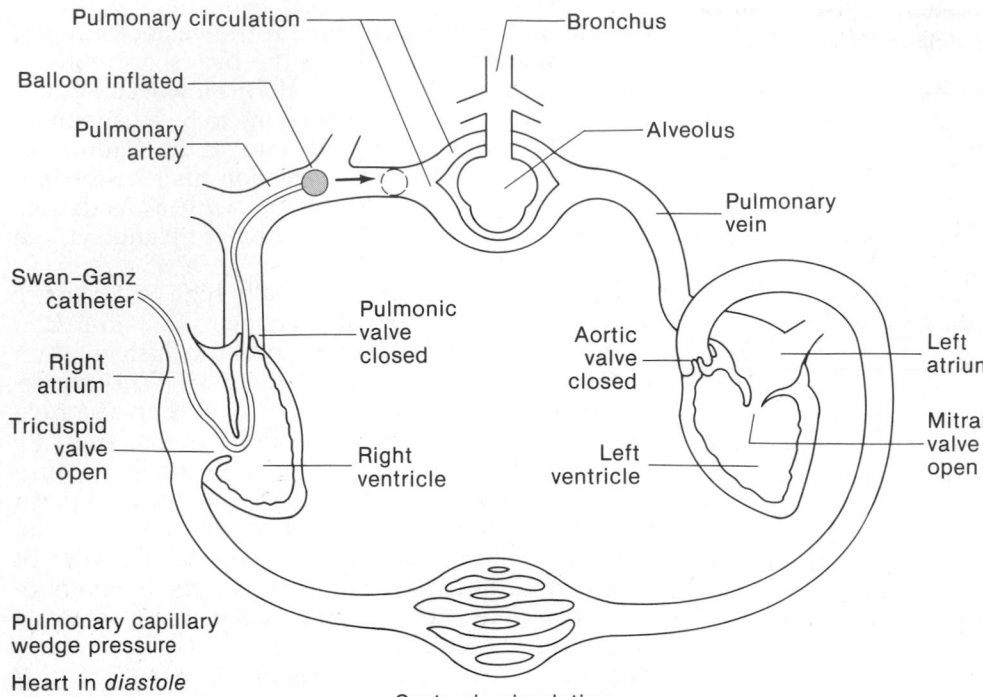

FIGURE 10–6. The pulmonary artery diastolic pressure and the pulmonary artery wedge pressure reflect left ventricular end-diastolic pressure during diastole because there are no closed valves between the pulmonary vascular bed, left atrium, and left ventricle. (Redrawn from Baxter Healthcare Corporation. *Understanding hemodynamic measurements made with the Swan-Ganz catheter.* © 1982 Baxter Healthcare Corporation. All rights reserved. Swan-Ganz® catheter manufactured by the Edwards Critical-Care Division of Baxter Healthcare Corporation; trademarks are registered trademarks of Baxter.)

TABLE 10–3. Indications for Pulmonary Artery Catheter Monitoring

Medical
    Complicated acute myocardial infarction
    Right ventricular infarction
    Perforated ventricular septum
    Mitral regurgitation
    Cardiac tamponade
    Dilated cardiomyopathy
    End-stage cardiac failure
    Constrictive pericarditis
    Acute pulmonary edema
    Intra-aortic balloon support
    Pulmonary embolus
    Pulmonary hypertension
    Cor pulmonale with pneumonia
    Adult respiratory distress syndrome
    Shock
        Hypovolemia
        Cardiogenic
        Septic
    Acute renal failure
    Dialysis
    Complex fluid management (severe burns and sepsis)
    Drug intoxication
    High-risk obstetrical patients
        Preexisting cardiac disease
        Toxemia
        Abruptio placentae
Surgical
    Cardiac surgery
        Valve replacement (multiple, elderly)
        Severe associated pulmonary disease (mitral stenosis)
    Coronary artery bypass grafting
        Ventricular aneurysm resection
        Preoperative congestive heart failure
    High-risk patients
        Elderly with preexisting cardiac disease
        Extensive intra-abdominal operations

The purpose of hemodynamic monitoring is to aid in the establishment of a diagnosis, guide and optimize therapy, and provide prognostic information (Gore et al., 1985; Matthay and Chatterjee, 1988). The value of pulmonary artery catheter monitoring is that a single catheter placed in the right heart can measure pressures directly in the right heart and indirectly from the left heart. The physiologic basis for this is that during diastole, there are no closed valves between the pulmonary vascular bed, left atrium, and left ventricle. These form a common chamber, and in patients with normal pulmonary vasculature and normal mitral valve and left ventricular function, the pulmonary artery diastolic pressure (PAD) and the pulmonary artery wedge pressure (PAWP) reflect the left ventricular end-diastolic pressure (Fig. 10–6) (Falicov and Resnekov, 1970; Forrester et al., 1976; Jenkins et al., 1970; Scheinman et al., 1973; Kaltman et al., 1966). The left ventricular end-diastolic pressure is an important measure for evaluating left ventricular function and prognosis, which in turn have a major role in determining which therapy (usually pharmacologic) will best help the patient. In patients with coronary artery disease, equal right and left ventricular function cannot be assumed because the amount of function depends on the area that is diseased. The indications for pulmonary artery catheter monitoring are presented in Table 10–3.

The physician is responsible for obtaining informed consent from the patient, inserting the pulmonary artery catheter, repositioning the catheter as needed, and removing the catheter. The nurse is responsible for setting up the pressure tubing and transducer system monitor, calibration, monitoring vital signs, and observing for potential complications. In some institutions, nurses may reposition and remove the pulmonary artery catheter.

Catheter Models

The four catheter models in use today are described below. Illustrations of the catheter models are presented in Figure 10–7. Physicians may insert a catheter introducer with a sideport that can be used for infusing medications and obtaining blood samples.

Triple Lumen Thermodilution Catheter. This 7

French catheter has a thermistor near the tip of the catheter. One lumen terminates in the right atrium and is used for measuring right atrial pressure (RAP) and cardiac output. The second lumen terminates in the pulmonary artery and is used for measuring pulmonary artery pressure (PAP). The third lumen also terminates in the pulmonary artery and is used to measure the PAWP. The PAWP is obtained by using a syringe to inflate the balloon-tipped port with up to 1.5 mL of air.

Quadruple Lumen Thermodilution Catheter. This 7.5 French catheter has the features of the triple

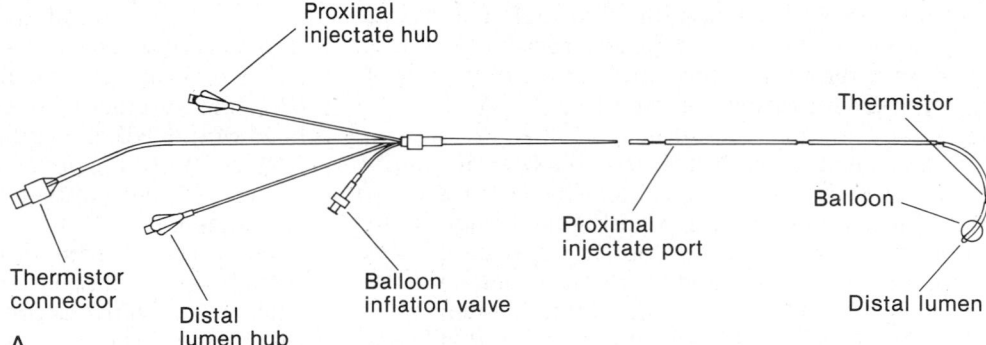

FIGURE 10–7. Types of pulmonary artery catheters. *A,* Triple lumen catheter. *B,* Quadruple lumen catheter. *C,* Oximetry catheter. (Redrawn from Baxter Healthcare Corporation. All rights reserved.)

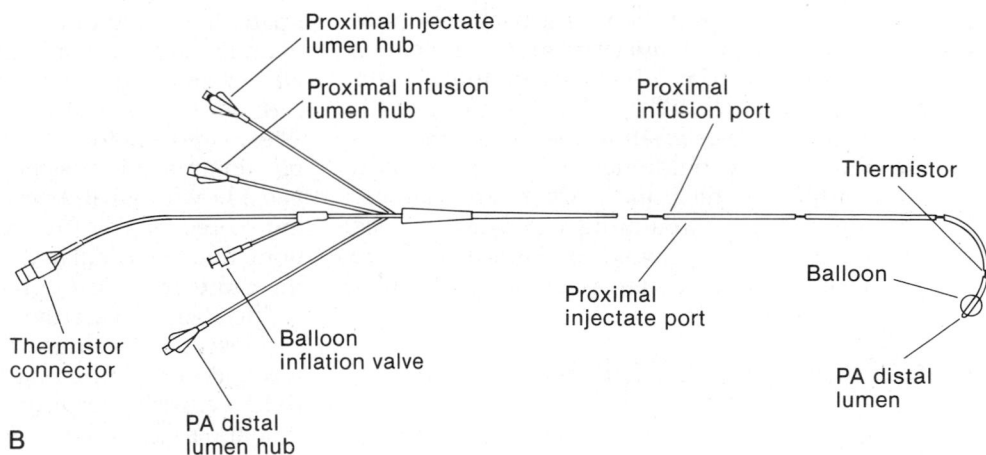

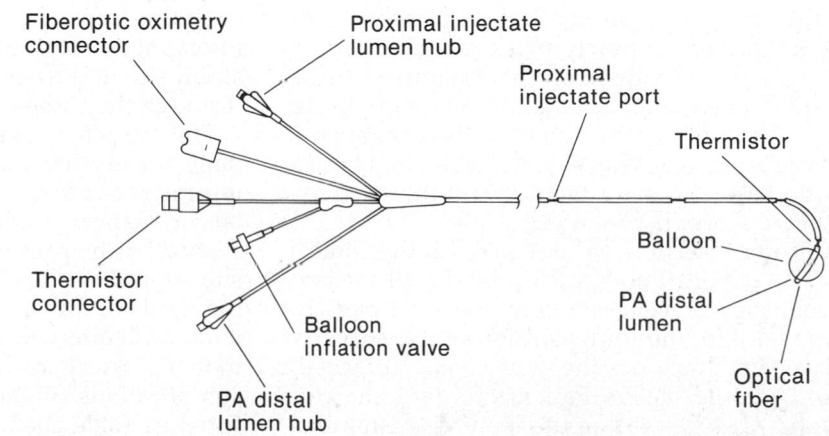

lumen catheter with an additional proximal port that may be used to administer fluids and medication.

Pacing Thermodilution Catheter. One model has three ring electrodes for atrial pacing and two ring electrodes for bipolar right ventricular pacing. Some clinicians may prefer not to inflate the balloon to obtain the PAWP to minimize the risk of either the ring electrodes or the pacing wire losing contact with the endocardium.

Another model has an additional lumen through which a 2 French bipolar pacing wire can be inserted into the right ventricle. If this model is utilized but the pacing wire is not inserted, lumen patency can be maintained with standard intravenous solutions (5% dextrose or 0.9% sodium chloride). The pulmonary artery catheter with pacing capability is indicated as a temporary measure until a more reliable pacing catheter can be inserted (Guzy, 1986).

Mixed Venous Oxygen Saturation Thermodilution Catheter. This catheter includes the features of the triple lumen model with an additional lumen for the fiberoptic filaments and an optical connector. Mixed venous oxygen saturation monitoring utilizes reflection spectrophotometry. A fiberoptic filament transmits light of selected wavelengths through the pulmonary artery catheter and out through the catheter tip in the pulmonary artery. A second fiberoptic filament transmits the reflected light back to a photodetector in the optical module, and the venous saturation is displayed at a bedside module (Baxter Healthcare Corporation, 1987; White, 1987a and b). The blood sample for calibrating the Sv_{O_2} catheter is obtained through the pulmonary artery port. Indications for utilizing the pulmonary artery catheter with continuous Sv_{O_2} monitoring capability are the need to evaluate the response to therapy and the need to check the adequacy of tissue oxygenation.

Contraindications and Cautions

Although there are no known absolute contraindications, relative contraindications are recurrent sepsis or a hypercoagulable state. The electrocardiogram should be closely monitored in patients with complete left bundle branch block because of the increased risk of complete heart block; some of these patients may need a pacemaker inserted prior to insertion of the pulmonary artery catheter. Patients with Wolff-Parkinson-White syndrome and Ebstein malformation are at risk for tachydysrhythmias (Baxter Healthcare Corporation, 1982).

The choice of insertion site depends on the clinical needs of the patient and the skill of the physician. The internal jugular vein is a common site, particularly for patients undergoing cardiothoracic surgery. Alternative sites include the subclavian, brachial, basilic, and femoral veins. Patients undergoing cardiac catheterization or percutaneous transluminal coronary angioplasty sometimes have a pulmonary artery catheter inserted through the femoral vein for short-term monitoring. Catheter position should be confirmed by fluoroscopy or by a chest x-ray.

Measurement Guidelines

Reliable PAP and PAWP measurements have been obtained in patients positioned either supine or with the head of the bed elevated at 20 degrees (Woods et al., 1980), 45 degrees (Woods and Mansfield, 1976), or 70 degrees (Prakash et al., 1973). Clinically insignificant changes in the PAP and PAWP measurements have been obtained with the patient in the right and left lateral decubitus positions with the transducer placed at the fourth intercostal space in the midaxillary line (Kennedy et al., 1984). Reliable CVP measurements have been obtained with the head of the bed elevated at 15 degrees or 30 degrees (Driver, 1972). However, in some patients significant changes in measurements occur when their position is changed.

The precise landmark on the pressure monitoring transducer set that is leveled at the patient's phlebostatic axis varies according to the particular brand that is used. The physician advances the pulmonary artery catheter until the RAP waveform appears on the oscilloscope. The balloon is then inflated with air up to the maximum volume recommended by the manufacturer (1.5 mL in one model). The distinct waveforms (Fig. 10–8) that appear during passage through the right atrium, right ventricle, pulmonary artery, and finally into the pulmonary artery wedge position make it possible to insert the catheter at the bedside without fluoroscopy. The patient should be monitored closely for premature ventricular contractions and ventricular tachycardia during passage of the catheter tip through the right ventricle.

The PAP waveform should remain visible on the oscilloscope because the catheter may become wedged in the pulmonary artery or slip back into the right ventricle, leaving the patient at risk for pulmonary infarction or ventricular dysrhythmias. An attempt to dislodge the catheter should be made by having the patient cough, breathe deeply, or change position (supine to lateral or vice versa). If these interventions do not dislodge the catheter, the physician should be notified to withdraw the catheter to dislodge the catheter tip.

The catheter insertion site should be inspected daily for erythema, drainage, or swelling. Swelling is sometimes seen in the arm when the brachial or basilic vein is used due to reduced venous return caused by the presence of the catheter. The insertion site should be cleansed and a sterile occlusive dressing applied. Table 10–4 presents the potential problems and intervention strategies applicable to pulmonary artery catheter monitoring. The potential complications of the pulmonary artery catheter are listed in Table 10–5.

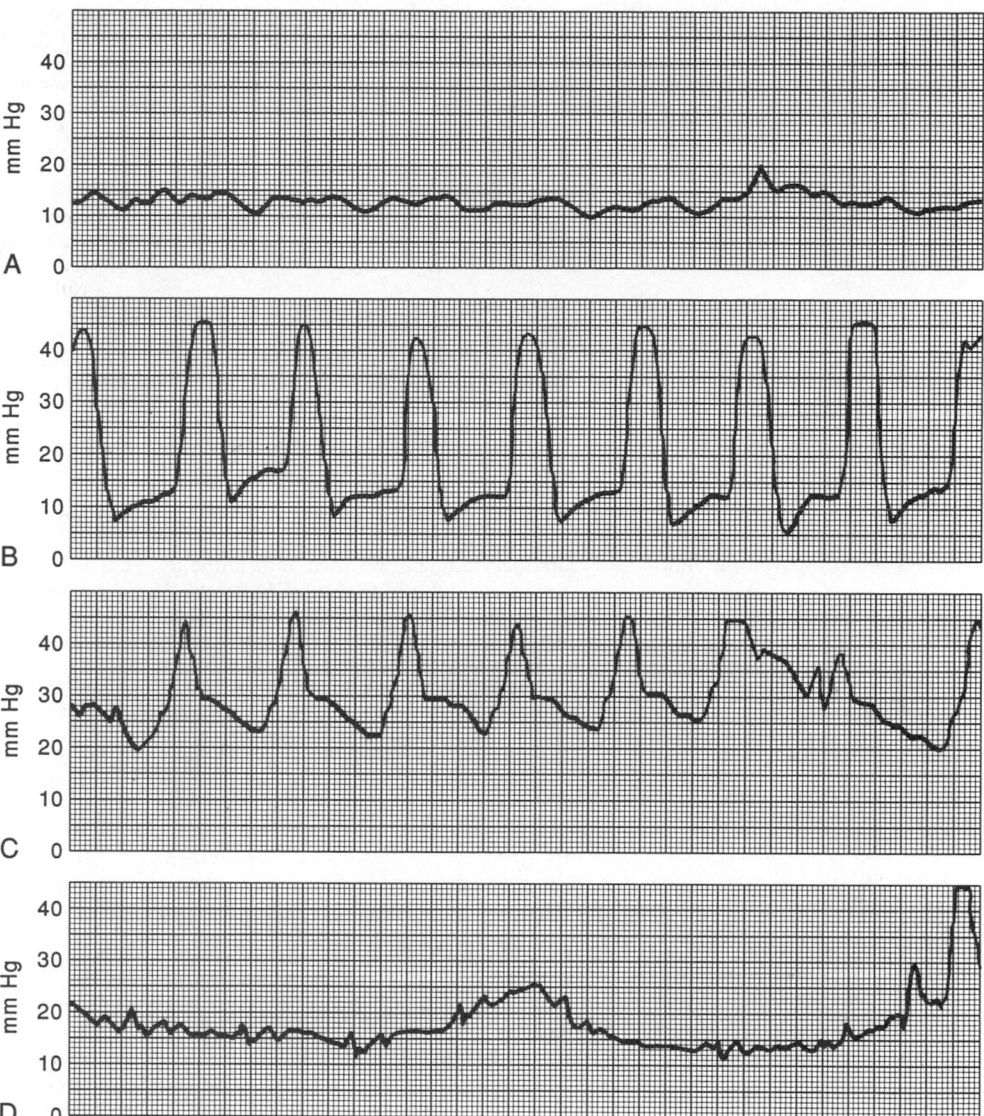

FIGURE 10–8. Waveforms observed during insertion of a pulmonary artery catheter. *A,* Right atrial pressure. *B,* Right ventricular pressure. *C,* Pulmonary artery pressure. *D,* Pulmonary artery wedge pressure.

Right Atrial Pressure. Right atrial pressure (RAP) reflects right ventricular diastolic pressure because the open tricuspid valve permits direct communication between both chambers. The normal RAP is −1 to 7 mm Hg. The RAP has a, c, and v waves and an x and y descent (Fig. 10–9, *I*). The a wave reflects atrial systole and occurs approximately at the time of the QRS complex. The x descent occurs as atrial pressure drops following atrial systole. The c wave reflects closure of the tricuspid valve as it bulges into the right atrium after ventricular contraction. The v wave reflects the increase in atrial pressure during ventricular systole and occurs at the time of the T wave. The y descent reflects the drop in atrial pressure as the blood flows through the tricuspid valve. The mean RAP is recorded.

Right atrial pressure is elevated in the presence of right ventricular failure, tricuspid regurgitation and stenosis, pericardial tamponade, and fluid overload (Forrester et al., 1976) and reduced in the presence of hypovolemia or vasodilation. Right atrial pressure does not reflect right ventricular filling pressure when there is elevated intrapericardial pressure or acute right ventricular dilation (Chatterjee, 1985).

Right Ventricular Pressure. The six components of the right ventricular pressure (RVP) are isovolumetric contraction, rapid ejection, reduced ejection, volumetric relaxation, early diastole, and atrial systole (Fig. 10–9, *II*). The normal RVP is 15 to 25 systole/0 to 8 mm Hg diastole. If the catheter slips back into the right ventricle, the balloon should be inflated to float the catheter tip back to the pulmonary artery because of the risk of ventricular ectopy and trauma. The physician should be notified immediately to reposition the catheter.

Pulmonary Artery Pressure. The components of the PAP are peak systolic pressure, dicrotic notch, and diastole (Fig. 10–9, *III*). The normal PAP is 15 to

TABLE 10–4. Potential Problems and Intervention Strategies for Pulmonary Artery Catheter Monitoring

Problem	Cause	Intervention
No waveform appears on oscilloscope	Cable disconnected	Secure all cable connections
	Stopcock turned off to the patient	Turn stopcock to open the catheter to the transducer
	Kink in catheter	Check for kinks in the exposed portion of the catheter, particularly near the introducer, and straighten catheter
	Clot in catheter	Aspirate catheter and irrigate. Do not irrigate catheter if no fluid is aspirated.
		May need to replace catheter
		Use continuous flush with heparin in 0.9% sodium chloride 1 unit/mL
	Faulty transducer	Replace transducer
Dampened waveform		
All pressures dampened	Insufficient inflation of pressure bag	Inflate pressure bag to 300 mm Hg
	Leak in pressure bag due to faulty valve or defective bladder	Replace pressure bag
	Air bubble in pressure monitoring set	Thoroughly prime pressure monitoring set
	Incorrect calibration or gain control	Recalibrate and adjust gain
Dampened RA waveform only	Gradual clotting of proximal lumen due to stopcock not being returned to the proper position after performing cardiac output measurement, administering medication, or withdrawing blood	Position stopcock to keep the flush system open to the catheter
Dampened PA and PCWP waveform only	Gradual clotting of distal lumen	Use continuous flush system with heparin in 0.9% sodium chloride 1 unit/mL
		Rapidly flush lumen after obtaining blood
	Catheter tip occluded by balloon or lodged against the wall of the pulmonary artery	Deflate balloon and slowly flush lumen with heparinized solution
		Chest x-ray can confirm catheter position
		Physician may need to withdraw the catheter 1–2 cm
Marked change in all pressures	Incorrect calibration. This may occur when patients are moved from one area to another	Recalibrate
	Recalibration; for example, at the change of shift when a different nurse commences monitoring of the patient	The oncoming nurse may take the first set of readings prior to the zeroing and recalibration procedure and compare these to the last readings taken by the outgoing nurse. The oncoming nurse may then zero and calibrate the equipment and compare readings obtained after this procedure to the first set of readings obtained. This will permit comparison of readings between nurses and by the same nurse before and after zeroing and recalibration
	Baseline drift	
	Different method of measuring waveforms	Establish standard protocol to be utilized by all personnel involved in hemodynamic monitoring
		Mount a paper printout in the patient's medical record of the RA, PA, and PCWP waveforms over three respiratory cycles. Label the printout with the patient's name, date, time, scale, and mark the location where the measurements were taken
Right ventricular waveform appears on the oscilloscope	Catheter drifted back into the right ventricle	Notify the physician to advance the catheter. Observe closely for ventricular dysrhythmias and have lidocaine available

25 systole/8 to 15 mm Hg diastole. The pulmonary artery systolic pressure is usually equal to the right ventricular systolic pressure. However, the pulmonary artery diastolic pressure is higher than the right ventricular diastolic pressure because of the closure of the pulmonic valve. The dicrotic notch reflects closure of the pulmonic valve. The pulmonary artery end-diastolic pressure usually correlates with the PAWP when the pulmonary vascular resistance (PVR) is normal. In these patients, the pulmonary artery diastolic pressure may be substituted for the PAWP when the catheter cannot be wedged. However, when the PVR is elevated, the pulmonary artery diastolic pressure will be higher than the PAWP; this

TABLE 10–4. Potential Problems and Intervention Strategies for Pulmonary Artery Catheter Monitoring *Continued*

Problem	Cause	Intervention
Increased frequency of premature ventricular contractions	Catheter may be flipping in and out of the right ventricle or may have drifted back and remained in the right ventricle	Notify the physician to reposition the catheter. Keep lidocaine available
Noise or fling in pressure waveform	Excessive catheter movement (fling), particularly in the pulmonary artery	Notify physician because catheter may need to be repositioned. Avoid excessive catheter length in the ventricle
Unable to obtain PCWP	Catheter not advanced far enough into the pulmonary artery	Notify physician to advance the catheter
No resistance to injection of air into the balloon port. Syringe plunger does not spontaneously slide back after attempted inflation	Ruptured balloon	Slide lock on the balloon port to the closed position. Do not attempt further inflations
Volume of air needed to inflate balloon is less than was needed for initial flotation	Catheter migrated to a distal pulmonary vessel close to the wedge position	Notify physician because catheter may need to be withdrawn
PCWP waveform remains on the oscilloscope	Catheter migrated distally and lodged in a vessel	Attempt to dislodge catheter by having the patient cough, breathe deeply, or change position. Notify physician to withdraw catheter to dislodge the catheter tip. Observe chest x-ray for pulmonary infiltrates
	Balloon left inflated	Let balloon deflate spontaneously after each PCWP measurement by disconnecting the syringe or by letting the syringe plunger slide back Do not pull back on plunger
Bleeding from catheter or pressure tubing	Leak in the pressure monitoring set	Tighten all connections Check inflation pressure of pressure bag Flush system
Bleeding from insertion site	Improper anchor or vessel trauma	Inspect insertion site Notify physician Anchor catheter Apply pressure to site until bleeding stops
Pain at insertion site	Pain during the first few hours after insertion may be due to the local anesthetic wearing off	Analgesia as prescribed
	Local inflammation or infection	Use aseptic technique for insertion and removal Perform daily inspection of insertion site with application of topical antibiotic and sterile dressing May need to remove catheter Exudate and catheter tip may be sent for culture, particularly if patient is febrile
	Excessive motion due to inadequate anchoring of catheter	Anchor catheter
Infection	Contamination during insertion or through stopcocks	Use sterile technique Physician may remove catheter and prescribe antibiotics Cap all stopcock ports Change flush solution every 24 hours Change tubing every 24 to 48 hours

Abbreviations: RA, right atrium; PA, pulmonary artery; PCWP, pulmonary capillary wedge pressure.
Data from Armstrong and Baigrie (1980); Daily and Schroeder (1989); Gardner and Woods (1989).

may occur in patients with pulmonary hypertension and adult respiratory distress syndrome. The pulmonary artery diastolic pressure may not reflect left ventricular end-diastolic pressure when there is left ventricular dysfunction such as mitral stenosis or decreased ventricular compliance (Bouchard et al., 1971; Falicov and Resnekov, 1970; Rahimtoola et al., 1972).

Cyclic changes in the PAP are caused by changes in intrathoracic pressure during the respiratory cycle. In spontaneously breathing patients, the PAP waveform will dip to its lowest point during inspiration. These changes may become more marked in patients with pulmonary disease, heart failure, or hypovolemia, or in those on mechanical ventilation. In some of these patients there may be a paradoxical increase

TABLE 10–5. Potential Complications of the Pulmonary Artery Catheter

Complications associated with insertion and advancement
  Vascular damage (venous and arterial)
  Hematoma
  Infection
  Local thrombus
  Premature atrial contractions
  Premature ventricular contrations
  Ventricular fibrillation
  Complete heart block
  Right bundle branch block
Complications associated with an indwelling pulmonary artery
    catheter
  Thrombosis
  Bacteremia
  Endocarditis
  Valve rupture
  Pneumothorax
  Pulmonary embolus
  Pulmonary infarction
  Pulmonary artery rupture and hemorrhage
  Pulmonary infiltrates

in PAP on inspiration (Fig. 10–10). The PAP is measured at the end-expiration phase of the respiratory cycle. This corresponds to the diastolic and systolic pressure that exists immediately preceding the lowest point in the tracing during one respiratory cycle (or the highest point if inspiration results in a paradoxical increase in pressure) (Fig. 10–11). The patient's breathing pattern should be observed simultaneously with the tracing on the monitor or paper printout.

Catheter fling (Fig. 10–12) will result in artifact, making it difficult to determine the PAP accurately. The catheter should be repositioned; one possible cause is excessive catheter length in the right ventricle. If the problem cannot be corrected, one possible solution is to use the digital output to obtain a mean pressure.

Pulmonary Artery Wedge Pressure. The PAWP, measured on the right side of the heart, reflects the left ventricular filling pressure because during diastole the pulmonary venous bed and left ventricle are in direct communication (Fig. 10–6) (Forrester et al., 1976). The normal PAWP is 6 to 12 mm Hg. The PAWP is obtained by slowly inflating the balloon (approximately 0.8 to 1.5 mL) until a wedge tracing appears on the recorder or until the maximum volume recommended by the manufacturer has been injected.

The a wave reflects atrial contraction (see Fig. 10–9, *IV*). The x descent reflects a pressure drop during late diastole when the atria are relaxed and the ventricles are filled. The c wave occurs as the mitral valve closes and bulges back into the atrium after ventricular contraction. The y descent reflects the drop in atrial pressure when the mitral valve opens. The v wave occurs when the mitral valve bulges back into the left atrium during systole.

There are certain diseases in which the PAWP does not reflect left ventricular filling pressure. These diseases include mitral stenosis and regurgitation, left atrial myxoma, ball valve thrombus, cor triatriatum, pulmonary veno-occlusive disease, total anomalous pulmonary venous drainage, cardiac tamponade, and acute right ventricular dilation resulting from right ventricular infarction, massive pulmonary embolism, and acute severe tricuspid regurgitation (Chatterjee, 1985). In the presence of decreased left ventricular compliance or marked atrial contribution to ventricular filling, the left ventricular end-diastolic pressure may be as much as 20 mm Hg higher than the PAWP or the mean left ventricular diastolic pressure (Forrester et al., 1976).

In most patients the average PAWP is recorded. The value of the average PAWP is usually similar to the pulmonary artery diastolic pressure. However, if a patient has mitral regurgitation, the v wave will be prominent, and two pressures should be recorded: the PAWP measured without the v wave and the PAWP measured with the v wave (Fig. 10–13). Although the volume of air used for lung inflation in patients receiving mechanical ventilation can affect pulmonary blood flow and pulmonary artery wedge pressures (Murao and Rodbard, 1971), the difference in PAWP measured with patients on and off intermittent positive pressure ventilation is not clinically significant (Shinn et al., 1979). It is not necessary to disconnect patients from ventilators during the measurement of the PAWP.

The PAWP may be used as an index of left ventricular volume because of its direct relationship to diastolic myocardial fiber stretch. Starling's law of the heart states that the energy of contraction is a function of the length of the muscle fiber (Forrester et al., 1976; Starling, 1918). When the PAWP is between 6 and 20 mm Hg, it usually correlates closely with the mean left atrial and left ventricular diastolic pressures. However, the PAWP may not equal left ventricular end-diastolic pressure because the mitral valve begins to close before the start of ventricular systole.

During balloon inflation, the injection of 0.8 to 1.0 mL of air should be adequate to obtain a PAWP. The waveform on the oscilloscope should be observed so that the minimum volume of air needed to wedge the balloon is used. If the PAWP waveform continues to rise while the balloon is inflated and the tracing dampens, overwedging has occurred (Fig. 10–14). This falsely high pressure may be due to the pressure from an overinflated balloon (Baxter Healthcare Corporation, 1982). The balloon should be deflated. Reinflation may be attempted after the PAP is visualized on the oscilloscope. Overinflation will increase the risk of balloon rupture, air emboli, and loss of PAWP monitoring capability. If the catheter remains in the wedge position after deflating the balloon, the patient should be asked to cough and breathe deeply, or change position. The physician must be notified immediately if the catheter remains wedged because the physician will need to pull back on the catheter

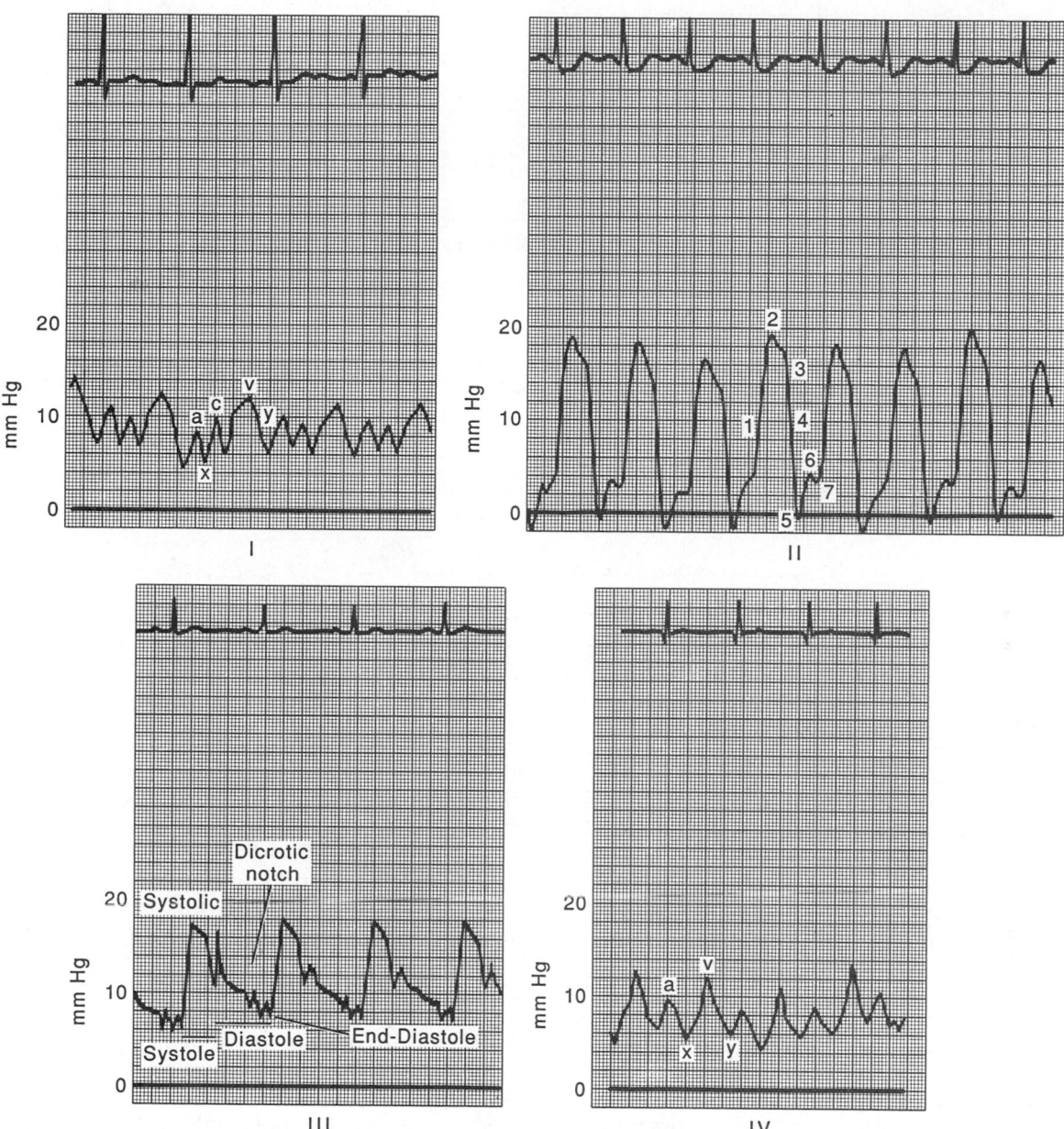

FIGURE 10–9. *I,* Right atrial pressure waveform. *II,* Right ventricular waveform (1 = isovolumetric contraction; 2 = rapid ejection; 3 = reduced ejection; 4 = volumetric relaxation; 5 = early diastole; 6 = atrial systole; 7 = end-diastole). *III,* Pulmonary artery waveform. *IV,* Pulmonary artery wedge pressure waveform. a, a wave indicates atrial systole; c, c wave represents the movement of the atrioventricular (AV) valve toward the atrium during valve closure; v, v wave represents filling of the right atrium during ventricular systole with bulging of the AV valve into the atrium; x, the descent following the a wave represents the decline in presence during atrial relaxation; y, the descent following the v wave represents the opening of the AV valve, allowing blood flow into the ventricle. (Redrawn by permission from Daily, E. K. and Schroeder, J. S. *Techniques in bedside hemodynamic monitoring* (4th ed.). St. Louis, 1989, The C. V. Mosby Co.)

to dislodge it to prevent pulmonary infarction. The catheter should be withdrawn 2 to 3 cm at a time until a pulmonary artery tracing is visualized. When the balloon is reinflated with near maximum balloon volume, the PAWP waveform should appear. If the balloon volume needed to obtain the PAWP is much less than near the maximum, the tip of the catheter is too far into the pulmonary artery. The balloon should be deflated and the catheter pulled back.

Blood Sampling

The pulmonary artery catheter can be used for obtaining blood for laboratory tests (Bodai and Holcroft, 1983). The right atrial port should be used instead of the pulmonary artery port to minimize the risk of falsely high results if saline, dextrose, potassium, or other electrolytes are being centrally in-

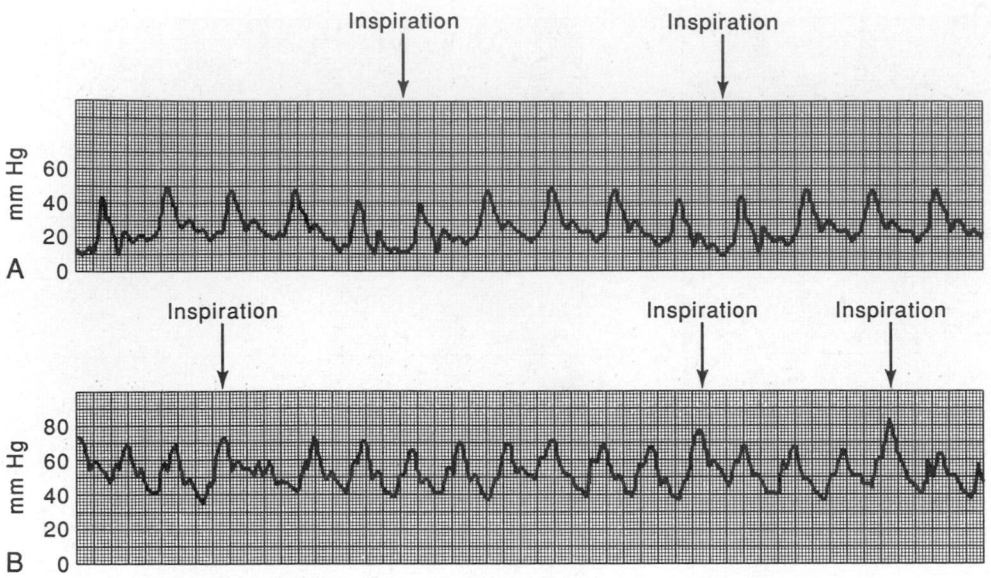

FIGURE 10–10. Pulmonary artery pressure waveform with respiratory variation. *A,* Patient with spontaneous respiration shows typical decrease in pressure during inspiration. *B,* Patient receiving mechanical ventilation shows increase in pressure during inspiration.

fused. However, if aspiration from the right atrial port is not possible, samples may be obtained from the pulmonary artery port. It is usually necessary to stop fluids infusing through the side port of the catheter introducer during aspiration because this fluid is entering the right atrium. However, great caution must be taken if vasoactive drugs such as nitroprusside, nitroglycerin, and dopamine are being centrally infused. Patients on such medications often have an intra-arterial catheter, and it is preferable to obtain blood specimens from the arterial catheter if the vasoactive drugs are being centrally infused.

Approximately 3 mL of infusate should be aspirated and discarded before the blood sample is drawn. Because existing research is inconclusive, more research is needed to determine the optimal discard volume for laboratory tests, particularly for coagulation studies. The blood should be aspirated slowly to prevent hemolysis. Slow and steady aspiration is also important when obtaining a mixed venous oxygen sample from the pulmonary artery port to avoid withdrawing arterialized blood (Bodai and Holcroft, 1983).

CARDIAC OUTPUT MEASUREMENTS

Investigators in the mid-1800s broadly estimated the stroke volume in man to range from 45 to 200 mL per beat (Fick, 1870; Hoff and Scott, 1948; Stewart, 1897). Fick, Stewart, Hamilton, Fegler, and Ganz developed the theoretical framework and instrumentation that laid the foundation for the accurate determination of cardiac output and stroke volume in man by the thermodilution method (Fegler, 1954, 1957; Fick, 1870; Ganz et al., 1971; Hamilton et al., 1928, 1932, 1948; Stewart, 1893, 1897, 1921). The accuracy, validity, and reliability of the thermodilution method has been established during the past 35 years (Kadota, 1985).

The theory upon which the validity of the thermodilution method is based is the law of conservation of mass. The Fick principle, an application of the law of conservation of mass, is the hypothesis on which the direct Fick method and the dye dilution method are based, and these in turn are the standards against which the thermodilution method is

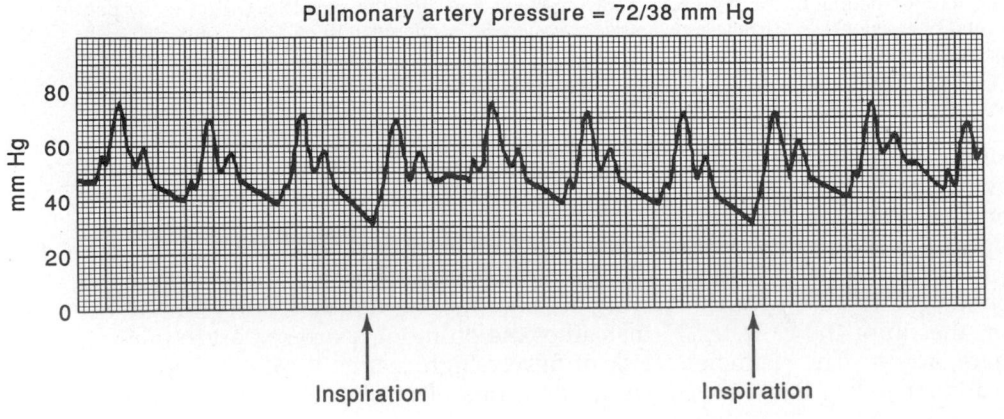

Pulmonary artery pressure = 72/38 mm Hg

FIGURE 10–11. The pulmonary artery pressure is measured at end-expiration.

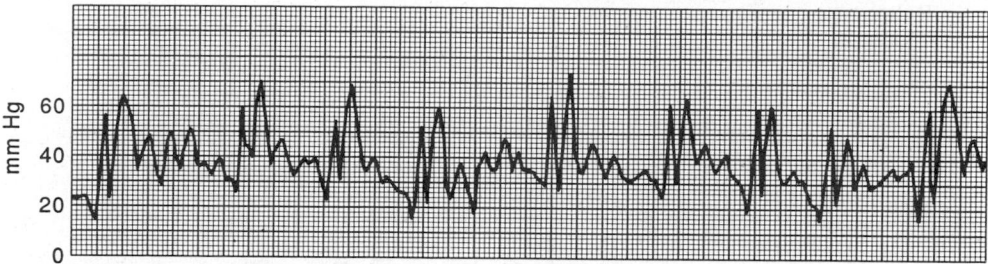

FIGURE 10–12. Pulmonary artery pressure waveform with catheter fling.

compared. The Fick principle states that flow, measured per unit of time, is equal to the amount of an indicator substance introduced to the flow in that same unit of time divided by the difference in the concentration of the indicator substance before and after the point of entry (Fick, 1870).

Direct Fick Method

Current application of the Fick principle involves calculation of the cardiac output (Berne and Levy, 1986):

$$Q = V_{O_2}/Cpv_{O_2} - Cpa_{O_2}$$

where Q = cardiac output in liters/minute; V_{O_2} = oxygen consumption (mL/minute); Cpv_{O_2} = oxygen content (O_2/mL blood) in the pulmonary vein; Cpa_{O_2} = oxygen content (O_2/mL blood) in the pulmonary artery. By this method, oxygen serves as the indicator substance, and the flow is the amount of blood passing through the pulmonary capillary beds per unit of time. The oxygen consumption is the net rate of the amount of oxygen that the pulmonary capillaries extract from the alveoli. The arterial oxygen content is the concentration of oxygen (mL) per milliliter of blood in the pulmonary vein. The venous oxygen content is the concentration of oxygen (mL) per milliliter of blood in the pulmonary artery. In clinical practice, the direct Fick method involves taking blood samples from a peripheral artery and the right ventricle or pulmonary artery to obtain the values for arterial oxygen content and venous oxygen content, respectively. The oxygen consumption is measured by having the patient breathe through a

valve system that allows the separate collection of expired air. The oxygen concentration in the expired air is subtracted from the oxygen concentration in the inspired air to obtain the value for the oxygen consumption.

Dye Method

The dye dilution method involves the injection of a known quantity and concentration of indocyanine green into the bloodstream. Flow and volume are calculated by measuring the dye concentration at a point downstream at selected time intervals. The cardiac output is equal to the area under the exponential indicator dilution curve. Although the dye dilution method is less cumbersome than the direct Fick method in the clinical setting, this method does involve the problem of dye recirculation, which may cause inaccuracies in subsequent measurements and requires arterial blood sampling.

Thermodilution Method*

Fegler (1954) published the first study using the thermodilution method to measure cardiac output. Ganz and associates (1971) stated the principle of thermodilution cardiac output measurement:

A known amount of a cold indicator is injected into the superior vena cava or upper right atrium, and the resultant change in blood temperature detected in the pulmonary artery. The cardiac output is inversely proportional to the fall in temperature.

*From Kadota, L. T. (1985). *Heart & Lung*, 14(6), 605.

FIGURE 10–13. Pulmonary artery wedge pressure showing the v wave in a patient with mitral regurgitation.

Pulmonary artery wedge pressure without v wave = 16 mm Hg
Pulmonary artery wedge pressure with v wave = 22 mm Hg

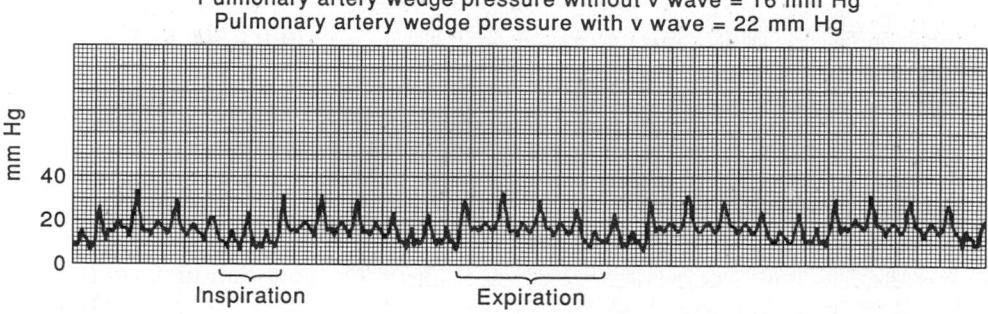

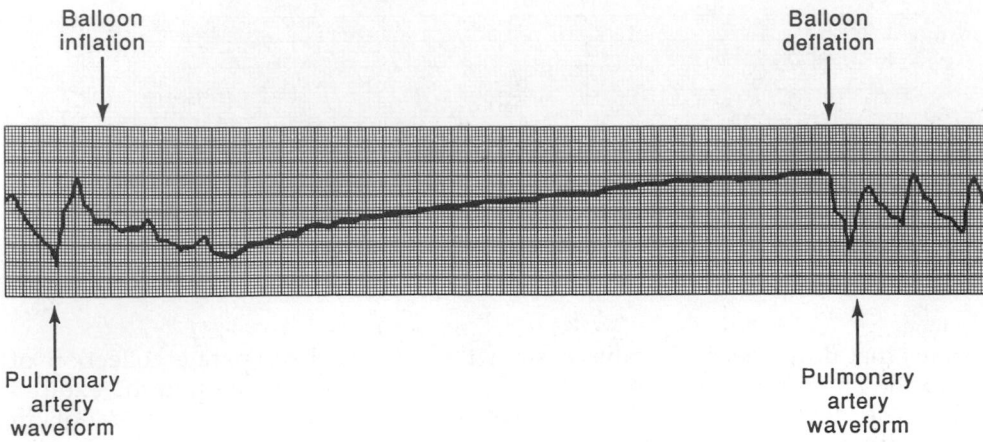

Balloon inflation

Balloon deflation

Pulmonary artery waveform

Pulmonary artery waveform

FIGURE 10–14. Overwedging of the pulmonary artery catheter during balloon inflation.

Stewart-Hamilton Equation

The thermodilution method required modification of the Stewart-Hamilton equation by substituting the specific gravity and the specific heat of both blood and injectate for the particle concentration that was used in the formula for the dye method:

$$CO_{TD} = \frac{(V_I)(T_B - T_I)(S_I)(C_I)(60)(T_C)}{(S_B)(C_B)\int_0^\infty \Delta T_B (t)\, dt}$$

where CO_{TD} = cardiac output by thermodilution (L/min); V_I = volume of injectate (mL); T_B = blood temperature (°C); T_I = injectate temperature (°C); S_I = specific gravity of injectate; C_I = specific heat of injectate; 60 = number of seconds per minute; C_T = correction factor; S_B = specific gravity of blood; C_B = specific heat of blood; and $\int_0^\infty \Delta T_B (t)\, dt$ = integral of blood temperature change (degrees Centigrade minus seconds) (Baxter Healthcare Corporation, 1977; Forrester et al., 1972). The specific gravity of blood, 5% dextrose, and 0.9% saline are 1.045, 1.018, and 1.005, respectively. Values for the specific heat of these substances are, accordingly, 0.87, 0.965, and 0.997 (Ganz and Swan, 1972). When 5% dextrose is used, $(S_I)(C_I)/(S_B)(C_B)$ equals 1.08; the value is 1.10 when 0.9% saline is used. The measured cardiac output will be 2% lower when saline is used as the injectate instead of dextrose (Baxter Healthcare Corporation, 1983). A change in the hematocrit from 52% to 30% alters the value of $(S_I)(C_I)/(S_B)(C_B)$ from 1.013 to 1.07 (Meisner et al., 1974).

The computation constant is the value obtained by the calculation $(V_I)(S_I)(C_I)(60)(C_T)/(S_B)(C_B)$. It is entered into the cardiac output computer prior to bolus delivery. The computer continuously monitors the difference between the temperature of the blood and injectate. After bolus delivery, the computer integrates the resulting thermodilution curve until the descending slope is 30% of the peak value (Fig. 10–15). The area of the thermodilution curve that is excluded at the 30% cutoff point is integrated back into the computer by amplification of the dilution signal. The cardiac output is determined by the ratio of the computation constant to the final integrated value (Baxter Healthcare Corporation, 1977).

A correction factor is necessary to account for the loss of thermal indicator due to the time required to deliver the injectate, the length of the catheter within the patient's vein, and the temperature of the patient's blood:

$$C_T = \frac{T_B - T_{IM}}{T_B - T_I}$$

where C_T = correction factor; T_B = blood temperature (°C); T_{IM} = mean temperature (°C) of injectate delivered to the right atrium; and T_I = injectate temperature (°C) prior to injection (Forrester et al., 1972). The correction factor is 0.837 when 10 mL of iced 5% dextrose is used (Baxter Healthcare Corporation, 1977).

Injectate

Ten milliliters of iced (0–5°C) 5% dextrose is commonly used as the injectate. An alternative solution is 0.9% saline. The rationale for using iced injectate is to increase the signal-to-noise ratio (Ganz and Swan, 1972). Studies have demonstrated that room temperature injectate correlates well with the dye dilution method (Evonuk et al., 1961) and with iced injectate (Elkayam et al., 1981; Hruby and Woods,

FIGURE 10–15. Thermodilution cardiac output curve.

1982; Killpack et al., 1981; Larson and Woods, 1982; Shellock and Riedinger, 1983; Swinney et al., 1981). Iced injectate may be preferable to room temperature injectate in patients with poor forward blood flow, such as those with right ventricular failure, tricuspid stenosis, or tricuspid regurgitation. These conditions make it difficult to get accurate cardiac output measurements, but the larger signal-to-noise ratio obtained with iced injectate may improve the estimates obtained with the thermodilution method. Injectate volumes of 1 to 5 mL may be used in infants and children (Freed and Keane, 1978; Mathur et al., 1976; Wyse et al., 1975), and volumes of 5 to 10 mL may be used in adults (Enghoff and Sjogren, 1973). The smaller volume should be considered in fluid-restricted patients. If the actual volume of the delivered injectate is less than it should be, or if the injectate temperature is warmer than the temperature recorded by the temperature probe, falsely high cardiac output measurements will result (Baxter Healthcare Corporation, 1983; Reininger and Troy, 1976). The closed injectate delivery system correlates well with the 10-mL prefilled syringes of iced 5% dextrose solution (Gardner et al., 1987).

The closed system injectate delivery system eliminates the need to uncap the stopcock on the pulmonary artery catheter, thus minimizing the risk of contamination. Although no difference in contamination rates between the closed system and prefilled capped syringes was found in one study, the closed system seemed to be more convenient for nurses to use (Yonkman and Hamory, 1988).

Measurement Guidelines

At the present time, insufficient data exist to determine whether trends in a patient's hemodynamics or response to therapeutic interventions can be accurately monitored if cardiac output measurements are done with the patient in a sidelying or elevated backrest position instead of in the standard supine position. One study found that accurate measurements using 10 mL of room temperature 5% dextrose injectate may be obtained with the patient in either a supine position or in 45-degree backrest elevation (Shenkman and Kasprow, 1988). Three other studies (Doering and Dracup, 1988; Grose et al., 1981; Whitman et al., 1982), however, noted clinically significant changes in some of the subjects. More research is needed because these patients are often sleep deprived, due in part to frequent awakenings for repositioning when hemodynamic measurements are done.

Electronic averaging of the blood temperature prior to injection and rapid delivery of the injectate minimizes variability caused by the physiologic responses to dysrhythmias, emotional stimuli, and changes in venous return caused by positional changes and the respiratory cycle. Accurate measurements are obtained when the bolus is delivered within 4 seconds

with firm, steady pressure. Measurements are unreliable when the bolus lasts 8 seconds or longer (Enghoff and Sjogren, 1973), and falsely low cardiac output measurements will result. Although some studies (Dizon et al., 1977; Nelson and Houtchens, 1982) have demonstrated improved reproducibility of sequential cardiac output measurements when automatic injectors were used instead of manual injections, a clinically significant improvement has not yet been adequately demonstrated to justify the additional equipment (Manifold, 1984; Riedinger and Shellock, 1984). The manual injection method remains acceptable for clinical practice.

Proper measurement technique is important to minimize thermal loss. When measurements are taken with iced injectate, approximately 45 to 60 minutes should be allowed for the prefilled syringes to equilibrate with the ice bath (Levett and Replogle, 1979); less than 10 to 15 minutes are needed for the closed injectate system. Thermal indicator loss begins from the time the injectate is removed from the ice bath and continues as the injectate flows past the pulmonary artery thermistor. It is estimated that 17% of thermal indicator in 10 mL of 0°C 5% dextrose is lost before the injectate enters the central circulation (Sorensen et al., 1976). Loss of thermal indicator is demonstrated by the tendency of the first in a series of injections to produce the highest cardiac output measurement (Kadota, 1986; Wong et al., 1978). Wong and colleagues (1978) concluded that the temperature gradient between the indicator and the extravascular segment of the catheter did not plateau until the third injection, resulting in an overestimation of cardiac output by 3% to 12%. However, one study noted that the loss of thermal indicator in the central circulation is clinically insignificant when the thermistor is in the pulmonary artery (Pavek et al., 1964). In addition, the correction factor in the Stewart-Hamilton formula partially compensates for thermal loss by taking into account the time required to deliver the injectate, the length of the catheter within the patient's vein, and the temperature of the patient's blood. The bolus must be delivered within 30 seconds of removal from the ice bath (Levett and Replogle, 1979) because an error of 2.86% in cardiac output occurs for each degree of variance in the blood-injectate thermal gradient (Powner, 1975). Falsely high cardiac output measurements are avoided when there is minimal handling of the syringe barrel (Levett and Replogle, 1979; Powner, 1975). There is disagreement over whether injection of the bolus should be timed with a particular phase of the respiratory cycle (Armengol et al., 1982; Baxter Healthcare Corporation, 1983; Jansen et al., 1981; Levett and Replogle, 1979; Riedinger and Shellock, 1984; Snyder and Powner, 1982; Wise et al., 1981; Woods et al., 1976). Jansen and co-workers (1981) mapped out the cyclic variations in cardiac output through the respiratory cycle and concluded that end-expiration is the best time to inject the bolus for the left side of the heart; the authors concluded that the data did not reveal a satisfactory moment for timing bolus delivery for the right side of the heart when different levels of positive end-expiratory pressure were used. The cyclic variations in cardiac output for both the left and right sides of the heart are similar to the cyclic variations seen in pulmonary artery pressure waveforms measured at end-expiration. It is important to consider a method that will be consistent and sensitive in detecting trends in a patient's hemodynamic status to permit evaluation of therapeutic interventions. Armengol and co-workers (1982) reported that the standard error of cardiac output measurements taken at random points during the respiratory cycle is 9.8% compared to 5.1% when measurements are timed at end-expiration. The recommendation to time the injection of the bolus at the end-expiratory phase of the respiratory cycle appears to be the method that is best suited for the clinical setting (Armengol et al., 1982; Levett and Replogle, 1979; Stevens et al., 1985).

Cardiac output decreases with intermittent positive pressure ventilation, continuous positive pressure ventilation, and positive end-expiratory airway pressure (PEEP) because of the increase in airway and intrapleural pressure, (Grenvik, 1966; Jardin et al., 1981; Lamy et al., 1973; Qvist et al., 1975; Rankin et al., 1981), although some patients may have a paradoxical increase (Powers et al., 1973). The patient should not be disconnected from the ventilator for cardiac output measurements. Hemodynamic monitoring and serial arterial blood gases can guide the clinician in optimizing the patient's cardiovascular and pulmonary status.

Studies (Samet et al., 1966a and b) have demonstrated that the indicator dilution method provides clinically acceptable estimates of cardiac output in patients with mitral and aortic insufficiency if the downslope of the initial thermodilution curve permits semilogarithmic extrapolation. The thermodilution method has been shown to provide accurate measurements in the presence of pulmonary insufficiency due to pulmonary stenosis or atresia (Beyer et al., 1977). Prosthetic cardiac valves yield a dilution curve with a steep downslope that makes it possible to use the Stewart-Hamilton formula (Carey and Hughes, 1969). In patients with enlarged hearts and a low stroke volume or those in cardiogenic shock, the injectate may sometimes take more than 20 seconds to travel from the right atrium to the pulmonary artery thermistor. The cardiac output computer may not be able to process the delay in the onset of the thermodilution curve and the delay in the termination of the curve. In this instance, the "delay START" injection technique may be necessary to measure cardiac output. The details of this technique are described in the cardiac output computer operations manual (Baxter Healthcare Corporation, 1983).

On rare occasions, the proximal port of the pulmonary artery catheter, which is used to deliver the injectate, may no longer be patent because of a blood clot. Reasonably accurate cardiac output measurements using iced 5% dextrose may be made by using the side port of the catheter introducer (Lee and Stevens, 1985). It may also be possible to make accurate measurements through the venous infusion port of one type of pulmonary artery catheter (Model 93A–831–7.5F, Baxter Healthcare Corporation) if the proximal port is no longer patent. Critically ill patients often have multiple central infusions, particularly since the development of catheter introducers that have a side port that provides an additional access site. Research is needed to determine the maximum central infusion rate that will still permit clinicians to obtain accurate cardiac output measurements because large volumes of room temperature solutions infusing through or alongside the pulmonary artery thermodilution catheter will lead to an overestimation of cardiac output. It is possible to stop central infusions prior to taking cardiac output measurements to avoid the problem of catheter cool down and dilution of the central blood flow. Unstable patients, however, must be closely observed if the central infusions are momentarily stopped, particularly if vasopressor or vasodilator medications are infusing through these ports.

The standard protocol for measuring cardiac output by the thermodilution method involves taking the average of three sequential measurements (Millar et al., 1980). The rationale for averaging multiple measurements is based on the dynamic biologic factors and technical limitations of the thermodilution method that influence reproducibility. Technical and biologic variance accounts for approximately 4% to 10% of the variability among sequential measurements (Singh et al., 1970; Swan, 1990; Weil, 1977). Variations of 10% or more from previous measurements, assuming proper technique and steady state conditions, indicate a change in cardiac output (Swan, 1990). The data from the study by Wong and associates (1978) suggested that the standard protocol should be modified so that the first in a series of measurements be discarded as a falsely high reading because of thermal loss. It is not recommended that single cardiac output measurements be used to interpret trends in a patient's hemodynamic status because variations of 15% to 25% may occur (Bilfinger et al., 1982; Stetz et al., 1982). Triplicate determinations provide clinically acceptable data (Forrester et al., 1972). Although quadruplicate measurements may reduce the error further, such a protocol may be best reserved for use in research (Rubin et al., 1982) because the volume of injectate may become a significant factor in the fluid status of unstable patients in renal failure who are undergoing simultaneous preload and afterload reduction.

The final step in cardiac output measurement is to calculate the cardiac index using the Dubois body surface area nomogram (Fig. 10–16) to standardize the cardiac output to the size of the patient.

In patients with acute myocardial infarction, a cardiac index of 2.7 to 4.3 liters/minute/m² is normal, 2.2 to 2.7 liters/minute/m² indicates subclinical depression, 1.8 to 2.2 liters/minute/m² reflects the onset of clinical hypoperfusion, and less than 1.8 liters/minute/m² reflects cardiogenic shock (Forrester et al., 1976). A high cardiac output is seen in patients with septic shock, anemia, or hyperthyroidism and in some with acute myocardial infarction (Swan and Ganz, 1975).

CLINICAL APPLICATION

The hemodynamic data obtained from the pulmonary artery catheter and cardiac output measurements aid in the diagnosis, evaluation, and estimation of prognosis in patients with heart disease. The data from the pulmonary artery catheter should always be used in conjunction with the medical history and physical assessment of the patient to treat the patient as a whole, not just the numbers.

Diagnosis

The relationship between intracardiac pressures and characteristic changes in waveform morphology permit the diagnosis of certain cardiac diseases. Tricuspid insufficiency may be diagnosed by the presence of large v waves in the right atrial pressure waveform. Mitral regurgitation may result in large v waves in the pulmonary artery wedge pressure waveform due to the backflow of blood through the incompetent valve during systole.

Pericardial tamponade may be diagnosed when the right atrial pressure is elevated and equal diastolic measurements are obtained from the right atrium, right ventricle, pulmonary artery, and pulmonary artery wedge pressure (Forrester et al., 1976). The PAP is elevated when the pulmonary vascular resistance is high (chronic lung disease, pulmonary embolism, or pulmonary hypertension) or when pulmonary blood flow is increased (ventricular septal defect) (Forrester et al., 1976).

Evaluation

Heart function is optimal when there is a balance between myocardial oxygen demand and myocardial oxygen supply. The determinants of cardiac output are preload, afterload, contractility, and heart rate. Therapy can be implemented to affect each of the determinants of cardiac output to achieve optimum heart function. The following discussion will examine each of the determinants of cardiac output and the specific therapies used for hemodynamically compromised patients.

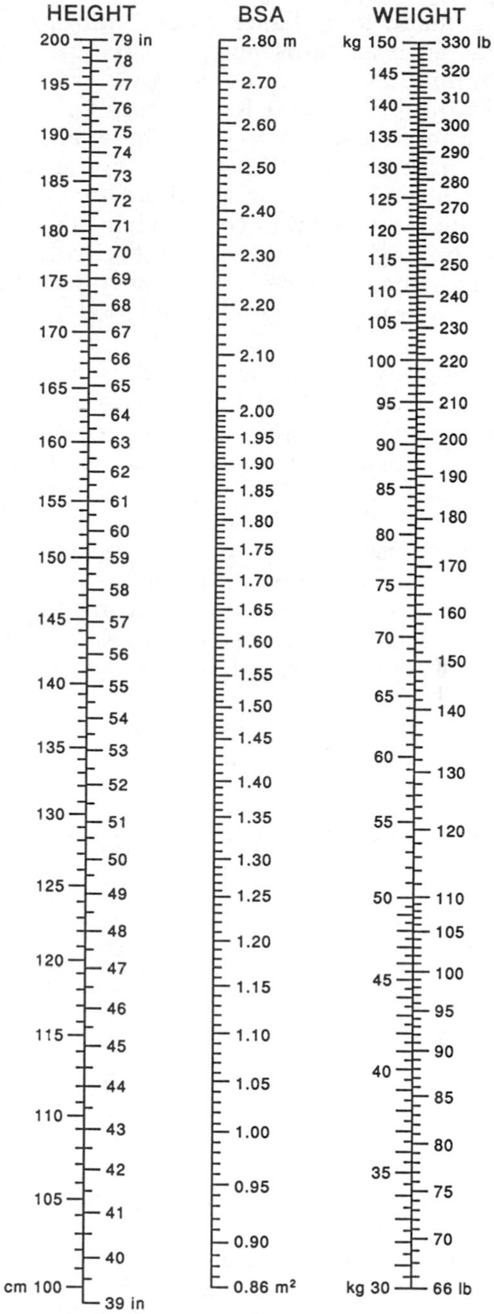

Preload. Preload is defined as the volume or pressure generated at end-diastole. In the clinical setting preload is measured by the PAWP. The PAWP can be used to monitor the relative extent of pulmonary congestion, from no congestion (PAWP = 6 to 12 mm Hg) to pulmonary edema (PAWP = >30 mm Hg). The PAWP is elevated when there is an in-

FIGURE 10–16. Body surface area nomogram from the formula of Dubois. Calculating the body surface area: 1. Find the height (in inches or centimeters) of the individual on the scale on the left. 2. Find the weight (in pounds or kilograms) of the individual on the scale on the right. 3. Connect these points with a ruler. 4. The body surface area is at the point where the ruler crosses the scale in the middle. (Redrawn from Grossman, W. (Ed.) (1986). *Cardiac catheterization and angiography* (3rd ed.). Philadelphia: Lea & Febiger.)

creased blood volume in the left ventricle, which reflects a reduced ejection fraction. This may be due to decreased left ventricular compliance or acute mitral insufficiency. The PAWP can also be used to evaluate the effectiveness of interventions to relieve pulmonary congestion. Medications that decrease preload include diuretics, nitroglycerin, morphine sulfate, and, to a lesser extent, nitroprusside. A diuretic such as furosemide can reduce the PAWP within minutes by venous dilation. A further reduction in the PAWP and RAP occurs within an hour when diuresis commences (Dikshit et al., 1973). The PAWP may be low (PAWP = <6 mm Hg) when there is a fluid deficit due to dehydration, excessive diuresing, or bleeding. The mechanism used to increase preload is to increase the circulating blood volume, which may be accomplished by administering normal saline or transfusing blood.

Afterload. Afterload is defined as the impedance to the ejection of blood from the ventricle. It is the resistance that the ventricle must overcome to eject blood in a forward direction. The two determinants of afterload are (1) the volume and mass of blood ejected from the ventricle, and (2) the compliance and total cross sectional area of the vascular space into which the blood is ejected. In the clinical setting, right ventricular afterload is measured by the pulmonary vascular resistance (PVR), and left ventricular afterload is measured by the systemic vascular resistance (SVR).

The normal value for PVR is 150 to 250 dynes/sec/cm^{-5}. The PVR is calculated by the formula:

$$PVR\ (dynes/sec/cm^{-5}) = \frac{MPAP - PAWP}{CO} \times 80$$

where MPAP = mean pulmonary artery pressure (mm Hg); PAWP = pulmonary artery wedge pressure (mm Hg); and CO = cardiac output (liters/minute).

The MPAP is calculated by the formula:

$$MPAP = \frac{[(PAD)(2)] + PAS}{3}$$

where PAD = pulmonary artery diastolic pressure and PAS = pulmonary artery systolic pressure.

Pulmonary hypertension, reflected by an elevated PVR, occurs when disease alters the determinants of pulmonary vascular pressure. Primary pulmonary hypertension is the diagnosis given when the etiology of the elevated PVR is unknown. Secondary pulmonary hypertension is the diagnosis given when the etiology is known. Cardiac diseases that may result in an elevated PVR are (1) increased left atrial pressure due to left ventricular failure, and (2) increased pulmonary blood flow due to an atrial or ventricular septal defect. Pulmonary diseases that may result in an elevated PVR are (1) obstruction that occurs in patients with massive pulmonary emboli or thrombosis, (2) obliteration that occurs in severe emphysema, and (3) vasoconstriction that occurs in the pulmonary arterioles in response to alveolar hypoxia. The pulmonary vasculature reacts less to neural and pharmacologic stimuli than the systemic vasculature. This makes it difficult to de-

velop effective therapy for pulmonary hypertension. One medication that may reduce the pulmonary vascular resistance through vasodilation is a prostaglandin, alprostadil. Alprostadil is administered as a continuous intravenous infusion at 0.05 to 0.05 μg/kg/minute in adult patients. Patients should be monitored for hypotension and flushing.

The normal value for the SVR is 1000 to 1300 dynes/sec/cm^{-5}. The SVR is calculated by the formula:

$$SVR\ (dynes/sec/cm^{-5}) = \frac{MAP - RAP}{CO} \times 80$$

where MAP = mean arterial pressure (mm Hg); RAP = right atrial pressure (mm Hg); and CO = cardiac output (liters/minute). The MAP is calculated by the formula:

$$MAP = \frac{[(ADP)(2)] + (ASP)}{3}$$

where ADP = arterial diastolic pressure; and ASP = arterial systolic pressure.

A high SVR (greater than 1300 dynes/sec/cm^{-5}) may reflect psychological stress or left ventricular failure. A low SVR (less than 600 dynes/sec/cm^{-5}) may reflect septic shock or excessive administration of afterload reduction medications. Medications that decrease the SVR include nitroprusside, hydralazine, and captopril. Dobutamine may also be used to decrease the SVR by increasing the cardiac output. Medications that increase the SVR include dopamine, epinephrine, norepinephrine, and phenylephrine.

In patients with a high PAWP and a low cardiac output, vasodilators such as nitroprusside can improve ventricular function (Chatterjee et al., 1973) by reducing the force that the left ventricle has to generate to eject blood. This is reflected in an increased cardiac output, increased systemic blood pressure in hypotensive patients, and a reduction of an abnormally high SVR. In the failing heart, cardiac output may be augmented with dobutamine or dopamine and nitroprusside. The rationale for combining dopamine and nitroprusside is to increase cardiac output by the positive inotropic effect of dopamine and the afterload reduction effect of nitroprusside (Dracup et al., 1981). In contrast, patients with right ventricular infarction require elevated right filling pressures in order to maintain an adequate cardiac output.

Contractility. Contractility is the third determinant of cardiac output. Contractility is defined as the ability to shorten and develop tension. It is not possible at the present time to measure contractility directly in the clinical setting. Positive inotropic agents include caffeine, digitalis, dobutamine, dopamine, epinephrine, isoproterenol, and norepinephrine. Negative inotropic agents include hypoxia, hypercapnia, acidosis, esmolol, propranolol, quinidine, procainamide, and barbiturates.

Heart Rate. The fourth determinant of cardiac output is heart rate. The normal heart rate in an adult at rest is 60 to 100 beats/minute. An elevated heart rate increases myocardial demand and reduces the diastolic phase of the cardiac cycle when the coronary arteries are being filled. Treatment includes resolving the underlying cause of the elevated heart rate (for example, antibiotics and antipyretics for sepsis and sedation for excessive anxiety). The heart rate may also be decreased in patients with heart disease by medications such as digitalis, propranolol, and verapamil. Lower heart rates usually result in a compensatory increase in stroke volume. An extremely low heart rate that causes hemodynamic instability may be increased by administering atropine or isoproternol, or by inserting a pacemaker.

Stroke Volume. The stroke volume is the average volume of blood ejected per cardiac contraction. The normal stroke volume depends on the patient's size and level of activity. In an adult at rest, the normal stroke volume is 60 to 130 mL/contraction. The stroke volume is calculated by the formula:

$$SV = \frac{CO}{HR}$$

where SV = stroke volume; HR = heart rate.

Stroke Volume Index. This is calculated to permit the comparison of the stroke volume in people of different sizes. The normal stroke volume index in an adult at rest is 40 to 50 mL/contraction/m^2 body surface area. The stroke volume index is calculated by the formula:

$$SI = \frac{SV}{BSA}$$

where SI = stroke index; BSA = body surface area (square meter).

Left Ventricular Stroke Work. This value is used to estimate the functional capability of the left ventricle. The normal left ventricular stroke work (LVSW) is 60 to 80 g. An elevated LVSW is seen in patients with hypervolemia or hypertension. A low LVSW is seen in patients with left ventricular failure, acute myocardial infarction, aortic stenosis, septic shock, or cardiogenic shock. The LVSW is calculated by the formula:

$$(SV)(MAP - PAWP)(0.0136)$$

where 0.0136 = constant that converts stroke work units into gm.

Right Ventricular Stroke Work. This value is used to estimate the functional capability of the right ventricle. The normal right ventricular stroke work (RVSW) is 10 to 15 g. An elevated RVSW is seen in patients with hypervolemia and pulmonary embolism with cor pulmonale. A decreased RVSW is seen in patients with right ventricular failure, severe cor pulmonale, ventricular septal defect, or right ventricular infarction. The formula for the RVSW is:

$$(SV)(MPAP = CVP)(0.0136)$$

where CVP = central venous pressure. The right atrial pressure may be substituted for the CVP.

Mixed Venous Oxygen Saturation. Mixed venous oxygen saturation (Sv_{O_2}) reflects the adequacy of the oxygen supply relative to the oxygen demand at the tissue level. The normal value for Sv_{O_2} is 60% to 80%. A normal value may indicate that the tissues are being adequately perfused but does not indicate whether compensatory mechanisms are being used to maintain perfusion. For example, a patient may have a normal Sv_{O_2} because an increased cardiac output is compensating for an inadequate blood supply. Table 10–6 presents the possible causes of abnormally high or low Sv_{O_2} values.

The range of normal values for hemodynamic parameters is summarized in Table 10–7.

Prognosis

Forrester et al. (1976) developed a classification for estimating short-term mortality in patients with acute myocardial infarction based on clinical and hemodynamic data (Table 10–8). The underlying pathophysiology of subsets II, III, and IV reflect the increasing severity of left ventricular failure that may occur after an acute myocardial infarction. This type

TABLE 10–6. Interpretation of Sv_{O_2} Monitoring Values

High Sv_{O_2} (>80%)			
↑ **Oxygen Delivery**	↓ **Oxygen Demand**	**Interference in Oxygen Diffusion**	**Technical Problem**
↑ FI_{O_2} Hyperoxia	Hypothermia Anesthesia	Cyanide toxicity	Wedged PA catheter

Low Sv_{O_2} (<80%)	
↓ **Oxygen Delivery**	↑ **Oxygen Demand**
↓ Hemoglobin due to anemia, hemorrhage ↓ Sa_{O_2} due to hypoxia, suctioning ↓ Cardiac output due to hypovolemia, shock	Hyperthermia Pain Shivering Seizures Stress

TABLE 10–7. Range of Normal Values for Hemodynamic Parameters

Parameter	Normal Values
Mean right atrial pressure	–1–7 mm Hg
	4–7 cm H_2O
Right ventricle pressure	
Systolic	15–25 mm Hg
Diastolic	0–8 mm Hg
Pulmonary artery pressure	
Systolic	15–25 mm Hg
Diastolic	8–15 mm Hg
Mean	10–20 mm Hg
Mean pulmonary artery wedge pressure	6–12 mm Hg
Mean arterial pressure	80–95 mm Hg
Systemic vascular resistance	1000–1300 dynes/sec/cm^{-5}
Pulmonary vascular resistance	150–250 dynes/sec/cm^{-5}
Cardiac output	4–8 liters/minute
Cardiac index	2.5–4.5 liters/m^2 body surface area
Stroke volume	60–130 mL/contraction
Stroke volume index	40–50 mL/contraction/ m^2 body surface area
Left ventricular stroke work	60–80 gm/contraction
Right ventricular stroke work	10–15 gm/contraction
Mixed venous oxygen saturation	60–80%

of prognostic classification can provide guidance in making medical and nursing decisions about therapy and for providing patient and family support.

SUMMARY

During the past 20 years hemodynamic monitoring has become an important aid in the diagnosis, evaluation, and estimation of prognosis in critically ill patients. Expansion of the capabilities of the pulmonary artery catheter to include pacing, continuous Sv_{O_2} monitoring, and additional access for administration of medications through central infusions has broadened the nursing responsibilities for these patients. One of the research challenges facing clinicians is the refinement of measurement protocols to maximize patient comfort while maintaining a high level of accuracy. These catheters provide an inval-

TABLE 10–8. Clinical and Hemodynamic Subsets in Patients with Acute Myocardial Infarction

Subset	Pulmonary Congestion (PAWP = >18 mm Hg)	Peripheral Hypoperfusion (Cardiac Index <2.2 liters/minute/m^2 BSA)	% Mortality
I	–	–	3
II	+	–	9
III	–	+	23
IV	+	+	51

Abbreviations: PAWP, pulmonary artery wedge pressure; BSA, body surface area.

Reprinted, by permission, from the New England Journal of Medicine, 295, 1356–1362, 1976.

uable means of evaluating nursing and medical interventions to provide optimal patient care.

References

Hemodynamic Pressure Recorders

Bartz, B, Maroun, C., and Underhill, S. (1988) Differences in midanteroposterior level and midaxillary level in patients with a range of chest configurations (Abstract). *Heart & Lung*, 17 (3), 308.

Daily, E. K., and Schroeder, J. S. (1989). *Techniques in bedside hemodynamic monitoring* (4th ed.). St. Louis: C. V. Mosby.

Windsor, T., and Burch, G. E. (1945). Phlebostatic axis and phlebostatic level, reference levels for venous pressure measurements in man. *Proceedings of the Society for Experimental Biology and Medicine*, 58 (2), 165–169.

Central Venous Pressure Monitoring

Anderson, H. L., Underhill, S. L., Fine, J. S., et al. (1988). Reliable plasma glucose, sodium, and potassium measurement from a multiple-lumen central venous catheter with concurrent infusion of total parenteral nutrition solution (Abstract). *Heart and Lung*, 17 (3), 302.

Daily, E. K., and Schroeder, J. S. (1989). *Techniques in bedside hemodynamic monitoring* (4th ed.). St. Louis: C. V. Mosby.

Daily, P. O. (1972). Position of patient for central venous pressure measurements. *American Medical Association Journal*, 219 (9), 1223.

Daly, J. M., Ziegler, B., and Dudrick, S. J. (1975). Central venous catheterization. *American Journal of Nursing*, 5 (5), 820–824.

Driver, C. E. (1972). The effect of elevating the head of the patient's bed while obtaining the central venous pressure measurement. *Circulation*, 46 (4, Suppl. II), II–241.

Eckstein, J. W. (1972). Position of patient for central venous pressure measurements. *American Medical Association Journal*, 219 (9), 1223.

Forrester, J. S., Diamond, G., McHugh, T. J., et al. (1971). Filling pressures in the right and left sides of the heart in acute myocardial infarction. *New England Journal of Medicine*, 285 (4), 190–193.

Gowen, G. F. (1973). Interpretation of central venous pressure. *Surgical Clinics of North America*, 53 (3), 649–656.

Guyton, A. C., and Jones, C. E. (1973). Central venous pressure: physiological significance and clinical implications. *American Heart Journal*, 86 (4), 431–437.

Haughey, B. (1978). CVP lines: Monitoring and maintaining. *American Journal of Nursing*, 78 (4), 635–638.

Millar, S., Sampson, L. K., Soukup, M., et al. (Eds.). (1980). *Methods in critical care*. Philadelphia: W. B. Saunders.

Price, M. S., and Fox, J. D. (1987). *Hemodynamic monitoring in critical care*. Rockville, MD: Aspen Publishers.

Steckelberg, J. M., Vlietstra, R. E., Ludwig, J., et al. (1979). Werner Forssman (1904–1979) and his unusual success story. *Mayo Clinic Proceedings*, 54 (11), 746–748.

Yacone, L. A. (1987). Monitoring central venous pressure. In G. O. Darovic (Ed.), *Hemodynamic monitoring: Invasive and noninvasive clinical application*. Philadelphia: W. B. Saunders.

Windsor, T., and Burch, G. E. (1945). Phlebostatic axis and phlebostatic level, reference levels for venous pressure measurements in man. *Proceedings of the Society for Experimental Biology and Medicine*, 58 (2), 165–169.

Intra-arterial Pressure

Abbott, N., Walrath, J. M., and Scanlon-Trump, E. (1983). Infection related to physiologic monitoring venous and arterial catheters. *Heart & Lung*, 12 (1), 28–34.

Allen, E. V. (1929). Thromboangiitis obliterans: Methods of diagnosis of chronic occlusive arterial lesions distal to the wrist with illustrative cases. *American Journal of the Medical Sciences*, 178 (1), 237–244.

Bedford, R. F. (1977). Radial arterial function following percutaneous cannulation with 18- and 20-gauge catheters. *Anesthesiology*, 47 (1), 37–39.

Bedford, R. F., and Wollman, H. (1973). Complications of percutaneous radial artery cannulation: An objective prospective study in man. *Anesthesiology*, 38 (3), 228–236.

Brown, A. E., Sweeney, D. B., and Lumley, J. (1969). Percutaneous radial artery cannulation. *Anaesthesia*, 24 (4), 532–536.

Cannon, K., Mitchell, K. A., and Fabian, T. C. (1985). Prospective randomized evaluation of two methods of drawing coagulation studies from heparinized arterial lines. *Heart & Lung*, 14 (4), 392–395.

Chatterjee, K. (1985). Bedside hemodynamic monitoring in the cardiac care unit. In A. N. Brest (Ed.), *Cardiovascular clinics*, Philadelphia: F. A. Davis.

Daily, E. K., and Schroeder, J. S. (1989). *Techniques in bedside hemodynamic monitoring* (4th ed.). St. Louis: C. V. Mosby.

Downs, J. B., Rackstein, A. D., Klein, E. F., Jr., et al. (1973). Hazards of radial-artery catheterization. *Anesthesiology*, 38 (3), 283–286.

Gelberman, R. H., and Blasingame, J. P. (1981). The timed Allen test. *The Journal of Trauma*, 21 (6), 477–479.

Gregersen, R. A., Underhill, S. L., Detter, J. C., et al. (1987). Accurate coagulation studies from heparinized radial artery catheters. *Heart & Lung*, 16 (6, Pt 1), 686–693.

Hook, M. L., Reuling J., Luettgen, M. L., et al. (1987). Comparison of the patency of arterial lines maintained with heparinized and nonheparinized solutions. *Heart & Lung*, 16 (6, Pt. 1), 693–699.

Jones, R. M., Hill, A. B., Nahrwold, M. L., et al. (1981). The effect of method of radial artery cannulation on postcannulation blood flow and thrombus formation. *Anesthesiology*, 55 (1), 76–78.

Kajs, M. (1986). Comparison of coagulation values obtained by traditional venipuncture and intra-arterial line methods. *Heart & Lung*, 15 (6), 622–627.

Kaye, W. (1983). Invasive monitoring techniques: Arterial cannulation, bedside pulmonary artery catheterization, and arterial puncture. *Heart & Lung*. 12 (4), 395–427.

Merenstein, G. B. (1971). Heparinized catheters and coagulation studies. *Journal of Pediatrics*, 79 (1), 117–119.

Millam, D. A. (1988). Mastering arterial punctures. *American Journal of Nursing*, 88 (9), 1213–1224.

Molter, N. (1983). Arterial blood gas analysis: A study of sampling techniques from indwelling arterial catheter systems (Abstract). *Heart & Lung*, 12 (4), 428.

Molyneaux, R. D., Jr., Papciak, B., and Rorem, D. A. (1987). Coagulation studies and the indwelling heparinized catheter. *Heart & Lung*, 16 (1), 20–23.

Morton, B. C. (1980). Basic equipment requirements. In P. W. Armstrong, and R. S. Baigre, (Eds.), *Hemodynamic monitoring in the critically ill*. Hagerstown, MD: Harper & Row.

Pryor, A. C. (1983). The intra-arterial line: A site for obtaining coagulation studies. *Heart & Lung*, 12 (6), 586–590.

Rakowski, A. C., Tonneson, A. S., Bracey, A., et al. (1987). Minimum discard volume from arterial catheters to obtain coagulation studies free of heparin effect. *Heart & Lung*, 16 (6, Pt. 1), 699–705.

Rebenson-Piano, M., Holm, K., and Powers, M. (1987). An examination of the differences that occur between direct and indirect blood pressure measurement. *Heart & Lung*, 16 (3), 285–294.

Rebenson-Piano, M., and Kirchhoff, K. T. (1983). Mean arterial pressure: Readings in two positions and with two reference points (Abstract). *Heart & Lung*, 12 (4), 431.

Schuch, C. S., and Price, J. G. (1987). Determination of time required for blood gas homeostasis in the intubated post-open-heart surgery adult after a ventilator change. *Heart & Lung*, 16 (4), 364–370.

Spaccavento, L. J., and Hawley, H. B. (1982). Infections associated with intra-arterial lines. *Heart & Lung*, 11 (2), 118–122.

VanRiper, J., and VanRiper, S. (1987). Arterial pressure monitoring. In G. O. Darovic (Ed.), *Hemodynamic monitoring: Invasive and noninvasive clinical application*. Philadelphia: W. B. Saunders.

Pulmonary Artery Pressure Monitoring

Applefeld, J. J., Caruthers, T. E., Reno, D. J., et al. (1978). Assessment of the sterility of long-term cardiac catheterization using the thermodilution Swan-Ganz catheter. *Chest*, 74 (4), 377–380.

Armstrong, P. W., and Baigrie, R. S. (1980). Strategy for troubleshooting problems in hemodynamic monitoring. In P. W. Armstrong and R. S. Baigrie (Eds.), *Hemodynamic monitoring in the critically ill*. Hagerstown, MD: Harper & Row.

Baxter Healthcare Corporation. (1982). *Understanding hemodynamic measurements made with the Swan-Ganz catheter*. Santa Ana, CA: Baxter Healthcare Corporation.

Baxter Healthcare Corporation. (1987). *Understanding continuous mixed venous oxygen saturation (Sv_{O_2}) monitoring with the Swan-Ganz oximetry TD system*. Santa Ana, CA: Baxter Healthcare Corporation.

Bodai, B. I., and Holcroft, J. W. (1983). (Letter to the editor.) *Heart & Lung*. 12 (3), 329.

Bouchard, R. J., Gault, J. H., and Ross, J., Jr. (1971). Evaluation of pulmonary arterial end-diastolic pressure as an estimate of left ventricular end-diastolic pressure in patients with normal and abnormal left ventricular performance. *Circulation*, 46 (6), 1072–1079.

Boyd, K. D., Thomas, S. J., Gold, J., et al. (1983). A prospective study of complications of pulmonary artery catheterizations in 500 consecutive patients. *Chest*, 84 (3), 245–249.

Bustin, D. (1986). *Hemodynamic monitoring for critical care*. Norwalk, T: Appleton-Century-Crofts.

Caruthers, T. E., Reno, D. J., and Civetta, J. M. (1979). Implications of positive blood cultures associated with Swan-Ganz catheters (Abstract). *Critical Care Medicine*, 7 (3), 135.

Chatterjee, K. (1985). Bedside hemodynamic monitoring in the cardiac care unit. In A. N. Brest (Ed.), *Cardiovascular clinics* (pp. 253–268). Philadelphia: F. A. Davis.

Chatterjee, K., Parmley, W. W., Ganz, W., et al. (1973). Hemodynamic and metabolic responses to vasodilator therapy in acute myocardial infarction. *Circulation*, 48 (6), 1183–1193.

Cournand, A. (1975). *Cardiac catheterization: Development of the technique, its contributions to experimental medicine, and its initial applications in man*. Uppsala, Sweden: Almqvist & Wiksell.

Daily, E. K., and Schroeder, J. S. (1989). *Techniques in bedside hemodynamic monitoring* (4th ed.). St. Louis: C. V. Mosby.

Dikshit, K., Vyden, J. K., Forrester, J. S., et al. (1973). Renal and extrarenal hemodynamic effects of furosemide in congestive heart failure after acute myocardial infarction. *New England Journal of Medicine*, 288 (21), 1087–1090.

Dracup, K. A., Breu, C. S., and Tillisch, J. H. (1981). The physiologic basis for combined nitroprusside-dopamine therapy in post-myocardial infarction heart failure. *Heart & Lung*, 10 (1), 114–120.

Driver, C. E. (1972). The effect of elevating the head of the patient's bed while obtaining central venous pressure measurement (Abstract). *Circulation*, 46 (4, Suppl. II), II–241.

Etling, T., and Reno, D. (1978). Septicemia rates using Swan-Ganz catheters: Influence of duration of catheterization (Abstract). *Critical Care Medicine*, 6 (2), 129.

Falicov, R. E., and Resnekov, L. (1970). Relationship of the pulmonary artery end-diastolic pressure to the left ventricular end-diastolic and mean filling pressures in patients with and without left ventricular dysfunction. *Circulation*, 42 (1), 65–73.

Fields, A. I. (1970). Invasive hemodynamic monitoring in children. *Clinics in Chest Medicine*, 8 (4), 611–618.

Forrester, J. S., Diamond, G., Chatterjee, K., et al. (1976). Medical therapy of acute myocardial infarction by application of hemodynamic subsets (Pt. 1). *New England Journal of Medicine*, 295 (24), 1356–1362.

Foote, G. A., Schabel, S. I., and Hodges, M. (1974). Pulmonary complications of the flow-directed balloon-tipped catheter. *New England Journal of Medicine*, 290 (17), 927–931.

Gardner P. E., and Woods, S. L. (1989). Hemodynamic monitoring. In S. L. Underhill, S. L. Woods, E. S. S. Froelicher, et al. (Eds.), *Cardiac nursing* (2nd ed.). Philadelphia: J. B. Lippincott.

Gore, J. M., Alpert, J. S., Benotti, J. R., et al. (1985). *Handbook of hemodynamic monitoring*. Boston: Little, Brown.

Greene, J. F., Fitzwater, J. E., and Clemmer, T. P. (1975). Septic endocarditis and indwelling pulmonary artery catheters. *American Medical Association Journal*, 233 (8), 891–892.

Guzy, P. M. (1986). Emergency cardiac pacing. *Emergency Medicine Clinics of North America*, 4 (4), 745–759.

Jenkins, B. S., Bradley, R. D., and Branthwaite, M. A. (1970). Evaluation of pulmonary arterial end-diastolic pressure as an indirect estimate of left atrial mean pressure. *Circulation*, 42 (1), 75–78.

Kaltman, A. J., Herbert, W. H., Conroy, R. J., et al. (1966). The gradient in pressure across the pulmonary vascular bed during diastole. *Circulation*, 34 (3), 377–384.

Kennedy, G. T., Bryant, A., and Crawford, M. H. (1984). The effect of lateral body positioning measurements of pulmonary artery and pulmonary artery wedge pressures. *Heart & Lung*, 13 (2), 155–158.

Lemen, R., Jones, J. G., and Cowan, G. (1975). A mechanism of pulmonary artery perforation by Swan-Ganz catheters (Letter). *New England Journal of Medicine*, 292 (4), 211.

Matthay, M. A., and Chatterjee, K. (1988). Bedside catheterization of the pulmonary artery: Risks compared with benefits. *Annals of Internal Medicine*, 109 (10), 826–834.

Martin, W. E., Cheung, P. W., Johnson, C. C., et al. (1973). Continuous monitoring of mixed venous oxygen saturation in man. *Anesthesia and Analgesia*, 52 (5), 784–793.

McLoud, T. C., and Putman, C. E. (1975). Radiology of the Swan-Ganz catheter and associated pulmonary complications. *Radiology*, 116 (1), 19–22.

Murao, H., and Rodbard, S. (1971). Effects of ventilation on pulmonary arterial flow and vascular conductance. *American Heart Journal*, 81 (1), 69–79.

Nichols, W. W., Nicholes, M. A., and Barbour, H. (1979). Complications associated with balloon-tipped, flow-directed catheters. *Heart & Lung*, 8 (3), 503–506.

Price, M. S., and Fox, J. D. (1987). *Hemodynamic monitoring in critical care.* Rockville, MD: Aspen Publishers.

Prakash, R., Parmley, W. W., Dikshit, K., et al. (1973). Hemodynamic effects of postural changes in patients with acute myocardial infarction. *Chest*, 64 (1), 7–9.

Rahimtoola, S. H., Loeb, H. S., Ehsani, A., et al. (1972). Relationship of pulmonary artery to left ventricular diastolic pressures in acute myocardial infarction. *Circulation*, 46 (2), 283–290.

Scheinman, M., Evans, G. T., Weiss, A., et al. (1973). Relationship between pulmonary artery end-diastolic pressure and left ventricular filling pressure in patients in shock. *Circulation*, 47 (2), 317–324.

Shinn, J. A., Woods, S. L., and Huseby, J. S. (1979). Effect of intermittent positive pressure ventilation upon pulmonary artery and pulmonary capillary wedge pressures in acutely ill patients. *Heart & Lung*, 8 (2), 322–327.

Sise, M. J., Hollingsworth, P., Brimm, J. E., et al. (1981). Complications of the flow-directed pulmonary artery catheter: A prospective analysis in 219 patients. *Critical Care Medicine*, 9 (4), 315–318.

Starling, E. H. (1918). *The Linacre lecture on the law of the heart.* London: Longmans, Green.

Steckelberg, J. M., Vlietstra, R. E., Ludwig, J., et al. (1979). Werner Forssman (1904–1979) and his unusual success story. *Mayo Clinic Proceedings*, 54 (11), 746–748.

Swan, H. J. C. (1990). Monitoring the seriously ill patient with heart disease (including use of Swan-Ganz catheter). In J. W. Hurst, R. C. Schlant, C. E. Rackley, et al. (Eds.), *The heart, arteries, and veins* (7th ed., pp. 2072–2077). New York: McGraw-Hill.

Swan, H. J. C., and Ganz, W. (1982). Measurement of right atrial and pulmonary arterial pressures and cardiac output: clinical application of hemodynamic monitoring. *Advances in Internal Medicine*, 27, 453–473.

Swan, H. J. C., Ganz, W., Forrester, J., et al. (1970). Catheterization of the heart in man with use of a flow-directed balloon-tipped catheter. *New England Journal of Medicine*, 283 (9), 447–451.

Weinstein, R. A., Stamm, W. E., Kramer, L., et al. (1976). Pressure monitoring devices: Overlooked source of nosocomial infection. *American Medical Association Journal*, 236 (8), 936–938.

White, K. M. (1987a). Continuous monitoring of mixed venous oxygen saturation (Sv$_{O_2}$): A new assessment tool in critical care nursing (Part I). *Cardiovascular Nursing*, 23 (1), 1–6.

White, K. M. (1987). Continuous monitoring of mixed venous oxygen saturation (Sv$_{O_2}$): A new assessment tool in critical care nursing (Part II). *Cardiovascular Nursing*, 23 (2), 7–12.

Woods, S. L., Laurent, D. J., Grose, B. L., et al. (1980). Effect of backrest position on pulmonary artery pressures in acutely ill patients (Abstract). *Circulation*, 62 (4), III–184.

Woods, S. L., and Mansfield, L. W. (1976). Effect of body position upon pulmonary artery and pulmonary capillary wedge pressures in noncritically ill patients. *Heart & Lung*, 5 (1), 83–90.

Cardiac Output Measurements

Armengol, J., Man, G. C. W., Balsys, A. J., et al. (1982). Effects of the respiratory cycle on cardiac output measurements: Reproducibility of data enhanced by timing the thermodilution injections in dogs. *Critical Care Medicine*, 9 (12), 852–854.

Baxter Healthcare Corporation. (1977). *Cardiac output computer operations and field manual 9520.* Santa Ana, CA: Baxter Healthcare Corporation.

Baxter Healthcare Corporation. (1983). *Model 9520 and 9520A cardiac output computer operations and troubleshooting manual.* Santa Ana, CA: Baxter Healthcare Corporation.

Berne, R. M., and Levy, M. H. (1986). *Cardiovascular physiology* (5th ed.). St. Louis: C. V. Mosby.

Beyer, J., Lamberti, J. J., and Replogle, R. L. (1977). Validity of thermodilution cardiac output determination in the presence of pulmonary insufficiency. *Thoraxchirurgie Vaskulaere Chirurgie*, 35 (1), 40–44.

Bilfinger, T. V., Lin, C., and Anagnostopoulos, C. E. (1982). In vitro determination of accuracy of cardiac output measurements by thermal dilution. *Journal of Surgical Research*, 33 (5), 409–414.

Carey, J. S., and Hughes, R. K. (1969). Cardiac output: clinical monitoring and management. *Annals of Thoracic Surgery*, 7 (2), 150–176.

Dizon, C. T., Gezari, W. A., Barash, P. G., et al. (1977). Hand held thermodilution cardiac output injector. *Critical Care Medicine*, 5 (4), 210–212.

Doering, L., and Dracup, K. (1988). Comparisons of cardiac output in supine and lateral positions. *Nursing Research*, 37 (2), 114–118.

Elkayam, U., Mumford, M., Tobis, J., et al. (1981). Thermodilution cardiac output determination: The effect of injectate volume and temperature on accuracy and reproducibility (Abstract). *Clinical Research*, 29 (2), 188A.

Enghof, E., and Sjogren, S. (1973). Thermal dilution for measurement of cardiac output in the pulmonary artery in man in relation to choice of indicator volume and injection time. *Upsala Journal of Medical Sciences*, 78 (1), 33–37.

Evonuk, E., Imig, C. J., Greenfield, W., et al. (1961). Cardiac output measured by thermal dilution of room temperature injectate. *Journal of Applied Physiology*, 16 (2), 271–275.

Fegler, G. (1954). Measurement of cardiac output in anaesthetized animals by a thermo-dilution method. *Quarterly Journal of Experimental Physiology and Cognate Medical Sciences*, 39 (3), 153–164.

Fegler, G. (1957). The reliability of the thermodilution method for determination of the cardiac output and the blood flow in central veins. *Quarterly Journal of Experimental Physiology and Cognate Medical Sciences*, 42 (3), 254–266.

Fick, A. (1870). Über die Messung des Blutquantums in der Herzventrikeln. Verhandl d phys-med Ges zu Wurzberg, 2, 16. In H. E. Hoff and H. J. Scott (Eds) (1948), Physiology. *New England Journal of Medicine*, 239 (4), 120–126.

Forrester, J. S., Diamond, G., Chatterjee, K., et al. (1976). Medical therapy of acute myocardial infarction by application of hemodynamic subsets (Pt. 1). *New England Journal of Medicine*, 295 (24), 1356–1362.

Forrester, J. S., Ganz, W., Diamond, G., et al. (1972). Thermodilution cardiac output determination with a single flow-directed catheter. *American Heart Journal*, 83 (3), 306–311.

Freed, M. D., and Keane, J. F. (1978). Cardiac output measured by thermodilution in infants and children. *Journal of Pediatrics*, 92 (1), 39–42.

Ganz, W., Donoso, R., Marcus, H., et al. (1971). A new technique for measurement of cardiac output by thermodilution in man. *American Journal of Cardiology*, 27 (4), 392–396.

Ganz, W., and Swan, H. J. C. (1972). Measurement of blood flow by thermodilution. *American Journal of Cardiology*, 29 (2), 241–246.

Gardner, P. E., Monat, L. A., and Woods, S. L. (1987). Accuracy of the closed injectate delivery system in measuring thermodilution cardiac output. *Heart & Lung*, 16 (5), 552–561.

Grenvik, A. (1966). Respiratory, circulatory and metabolic effects of respirator treatment. *Acta Anaesthesiologica Scandinavica*, Supplement 19, 7–152.

Grose, B. L., Woods, S. L., and Laurent, D. J. (1981). Effect of backrest position on cardiac output measured by thermodilution method in acutely ill patients. *Heart & Lung*, 10 (4), 661–665.

Grossman, W. (Ed.). (1986). *Cardiac catheterization and angiography* (3rd ed.). Philadelphia: Lea & Febiger.

Hamilton, W. F., Moore, J. W., Kinsman, J. M., et al. (1928). Simultaneous determination of the pulmonary and systemic circulation times in man and of a figure related to the cardiac output. *American Journal of Physiology*, 84 (2), 338–344.

Hamilton, W. F., Moore, J. W., Kinsman, J. M., et al. (1932). Studies on the circulation. IV. Further analysis of the injection method and of changes in hemodynamics under physiological and pathological conditions. *American Journal of Physiology*, 99 (3), 534–551.

Hamilton, W. F., Riley, R. L., Attyah, A. M., et al. (1948). Comparison of the Fick and dye injection methods of measuring cardiac output in man. *American Journal of Physiology*, 153 (2), 309–311.

Hoff, H. E., and Scott, H. J. (1948). Physiology. *New England Journal of Medicine*, 239 (4), 120–126.

Hruby, I. M., and Woods, S. L. (1983). Effect of injectate temperature on measurement of thermodilution cardiac output in cardiac surgical patients (Abstract). *Circulation*, 68 (Suppl. III), III–222.

Jansen, J. R. C., Schreuder, J. J., Bogard, J. M., et al. (1981). Thermodilution technique for measurement of cardiac output during artificial ventilation. *Journal of Applied Physiology*, 50 (3), 584–591.

Jardin, F., Farcot, J., Boisante, L., et al. (1981). Influence of positive end-expiratory pressure on left ventricular performance. *New England Journal of Medicine*, 304 (7), 387–392.

Kadota, L. T. (1985). Theory and application of thermodilution cardiac output measurement: a review. *Heart & Lung*, 14 (6), 605–614.

Kadota, L. T. (1986). Reproducibility of thermodilution cardiac output measurements, *Heart & Lung*, 15 (6), 618–622.

Killpack, A. K., Davidson, L. J., Woods, S. L., et al. (1981). Effect of injectate volume and temperature on measurement of thermodilution cardiac output in acutely ill patients (Abstract). *Circulation*, 64 (Suppl. IV), IV–165.

Lamy, M., Deghislage, J., Lamalle, D., et al. (1973). Hemodynamic effects of intermittent or continuous positive-pressure breathing in man. *Acta Anaesthesiologica Belgica*, 24 (3), 270–287.

Larson, C. A., and Woods, S. L. (1982). Effect of injectate volume and temperature on thermodilution cardiac output measurements in acutely ill adults (Abstract). *Circulation*, 66 (Suppl. II), II–98.

Lee, D. W., and Stevens, G. H. (1985). Comparison of thermodilution measurement by injection of the proximal lumen versus side port of the Swan-Ganz catheter. *Heart & Lung*, 14 (2), 126–127.

Levett, J. M., and Replogle, R. L. (1979). Thermodilution cardiac output: A critical analysis and review of the literature. *Journal of Surgical Research*, 27 (6), 392–404.

Manifold, S. (1984). A comparison of two alternate methods for the determination of cardiac output by thermodilution: Automatic vs. manual injections (Abstract). *Heart & Lung*, 13 (3), 304–305.

Mathur, M., Harris, E. A., Yarrow, S., et al. (1976). Measurement of cardiac output by thermodilution in infants and children after open-heart operations. *Journal of Thoracic Cardiovascular Surgery*, 72 (2), 221–225.

Meisner, H., Hagl, S., Heimisch, W., et al. (1974). Evaluation of the thermodilution method for measurement of cardiac output after open-heart surgery. *Annals of Thoracic Surgery*, 18 (5), 504–515.

Millar, S., Sampson, L. K., Soukup, M., et al. (Eds.). (1980). *Methods in critical care*. Philadelphia: W. B. Saunders.

Nelson, L. D., and Houtchens, B. A. (1982). Automatic versus manual injections for thermodilution cardiac output measurements. *Critical Care Medicine*, 10 (3), 190–192.

Pavek, K., Boska, D., Selecky, E., et al. (1964). Measurement of cardiac output by thermodilution with constant rate injection of indicator. *Circulation Research*, 15 (4), 311–319.

Powers, S. R., Jr., Mannal, R., Neclerio, M., et al. (1973). Physiologic consequences of positive end expiratory pressure (PEEP) ventilation. *Annals of Surgery*, 178 (3), 265–271.

Powner, D. J. (1975). Thermodilution technic for cardiac output (Letter). *New England Journal of Medicine*, 293 (23), 1210–1211.

Qvist, J., Pontoppidan, H., Wilson, R. S., et al. (1975). Hemodynamic responses to mechanical ventilation with PEEP. *Anesthesiology*, 42 (1), 45–55.

Rankin, J. S., Olsen, C. O., Tyson, G. S., et al. (1981). Effects of airway pressure on cardiac function in intact dogs and man (Abstract). *Circulation*, 64 (Suppl. IV), IV–251.

Reininger, E. J., and Troy, B. L. (1976). Error in thermodilution cardiac output caused by variation in syringe volume. *Catheterization and Cardiovascular Diagnosis*, 2 (4), 415–417.

Riedinger, M. S., and Shellock, F. G. (1984). Technical aspects of the thermodilution method for measuring cardiac output. *Heart & Lung*, 13 (3), 215–221.

Rubin, S. A., Siemienczuk, D., Prause, J., et al. (1982). Accuracy of cardiac output, oxygen uptake, and arteriovenous oxygen difference at rest, during exercise, and after vasodilator therapy in patients with severe, chronic heart failure. *American Journal of Cardiology*, 50 (5), 973–978.

Samet, P., Bernstein, W. H., and Castillo, C. (1966). Validity of indicator dilution determination of cardiac output in patients with mitral regurgitation. *Circulation*, 33 (3), 410–416.

Samet, P., Castillo, C., and Bernstein, W. H. (1966). Validity of indicator dilution determination of cardiac output in patients with aortic regurgitation. *Circulation*, 34 (4), 609–610.

Shellock, F., and Riedinger, M. S. (1983). Reproducibility and accuracy of using room temperature versus ice temperature injectate for thermodilution cardiac output determination. *Heart & Lung*, 12 (2), 175–176.

Shenkman, E., and Kasprow, M. (1988). Effect of backrest position on cardiac output determinations (Abstract). *Heart & Lung*, 17 (3), 308–309.

Singh, R., Ranieri, A. J., Jr., Vest, H. R., et al. (1970). Simultaneous determinations of cardiac output by thermal dilution, fiberoptic and dye dilution methods. *American Journal of Cardiology*, 25 (5), 579–587.

Snyder, J. V., and Powner, D. J. (1982). Effects of mechanical ventilation on the measurement of cardiac output by thermodilution. *Critical Care Medicine*, 10 (10), 677–682.

Sorensen, M. B., Bille-Brahe, N. E., and Engell, H. C. (1976). Cardiac output measurement by thermal dilution. *Annals of Surgery*, 183 (1), 67–71.

Stetz, C. W., Miller, R. G., Kelly, G. E., et al. (1982). Reliability of the thermodilution method in the determination of cardiac output in clinical practice. *American Review of Respiratory Disease*, 126 (6), 1001–1004.

Stevens, J. H., Raffin, T. A., Mihm, F. G., et al. (1985). Thermodilution cardiac output measurement: effect of the respiratory cycle on its reproducibility. *American Medical Association Journal*, 253 (15), 2240–2242.

Stewart, G. N. (1893). Researches on the circulation time in organs and on the influences which affect it. I. Preliminary paper. *Journal of Physiology*, 15 (4), 1–89.

Stewart, G. N. (1897). Researches on the circulation time in organs and the influences which affect it. IV. The output of the heart. *Journal of Physiology*, 22 (3), 158–183.

Stewart, G. N. (1921). The output of the heart in dogs. *American Journal of Physiology*, 57 (1), 27–50.

Swan, H. J. C. (1990). Techniques of monitoring the seriously ill patient with heart disease (including use of Swan-Ganz catheter). In J. W. Hurst, R. C. Schlant, C. E. Rackley, et al. (Eds.), *The heart, arteries and veins* (7th ed.). New York: McGraw Hill.

Swan, H. J. C., and Ganz, W. (1975). Use of balloon flotation catheters in critically ill patients. *Surgical Clinics of North America*, 55 (3), 501–520.

Swan, H. J. C., Ganz, W., Forrester, J., et al. (1970). Catheterization of the heart in man with use of a flow-directed balloon-tipped catheter. *New England Journal of Medicine* 283 (9), 447–451.

Swinney, R. S., Davenport, M. W., Wagers, P. W., et al. (1981). Iced versus room temperature injectate for thermal dilution cardiac output (Abstract). *Critical Care Medicine,* 8 (4), 265.

Weil, M. H. (1977). Measurement of cardiac output (Editorial). *Critical Care Medicine,* 5 (2), 117–119.

Whitman, G. R., Howaniak, D. L., and Verga, T. S. (1982). Comparison of cardiac output measurements in 20-degree supine and 20-degree right and left lateral recumbent positions (Abstract). *Heart & Lung,* 11 (3), 256–257.

Wise, R. A., Robotham, J. L., Bromberger-Barnea, B., et al. (1981). Effect of PEEP on left ventricular function in right heart-bypassed dogs. *Journal of Applied Physiology,* 51 (3), 541–546.

Wong, M., Skulsky, A., and Moon, E. (1978). Loss of indicator in the thermodilution technique. *Catheterization and Cardiovascular Diagnosis,* 4 (1), 103–109.

Woods, M., Scott, R. N., and Harken, A. H. (1976). Practical considerations for the use of a pulmonary artery thermistor catheter. *Surgery,* 79 (4), 469–475.

Wyse, S. D., Pfitzner, J., Rees, A., et al. (1975). Measurement of cardiac output by thermal dilution in infants and children. *Thorax,* 30 (3), 262–265.

Yonkman, C. A., and Hamory, B. H. (1988). Sterility and efficiency of two methods of cardiac output determination: closed loop and capped syringe methods. *Heart & Lung,* 17 (2), 121–128.

Cardiac Assist Devices

Shelley Ruzevich

The first effort at mechanical support of the circulation was made in the 1950s with the development of cardiopulmonary bypass (CPB) (Gibbon, 1954; Kirklin et al., 1955). This initial discovery lead to further attempts to support the circulation for extended periods of time, which proved to be generally unsuccessful (Zapoh et al., 1979; Cooley et al., 1969). The development of the intra-aortic balloon pump (IABP) aided in the reduction of postcardiotomy mortality (Moulopoulos et al., 1962; Clauss et al., 1961; Kantrowitz et al., 1969). Since that time the IABP has gained widespread recognition in the treatment of patients with low cardiac output conditions (McEnany et al., 1978; Bolooki, 1984). However, many patients with severe cardiogenic shock remained unresponsive to IABP therapy because it is capable of supplying only a limited amount of support. The need for a more complete form of assistance was recognized. Subsequently, several groups began utilizing ventricular assist devices (VAD), which could be implanted for extended periods of time (Farrar et al., 1988; Pennington et al., 1988; Portner et al., 1983). By the mid-1980s, the majority of experience with VADs was with the postcardiotomy population (Farrar et al., 1988; Ruzevich et al., 1987; Pae et al., 1990). Recently, the scarcity of donor hearts has led many groups to recognize the role of VADs as a bridge to cardiac transplantation (Farrar et al., 1988; Pennington et al., 1988; Portner et al., 1983).

To date several types of mechanical assistance are available depending on the extent of support that is required. These devices include the IABP, VADs (centrifugal, pneumatic, pulsatile, and electrical pulsatile), and extracorporeal membrane oxygenation (ECMO). Device selection is dependent upon the patient's clinical status, device availability to the institution, type of ventricular failure, and expected outcome. Categories of patients requiring the devices include postcardiotomy patients, patients suffering from acute cardiogenic shock, and patients who are being bridged to cardiac transplantation. This chapter is designed to acquaint the nurse with the different types of support available and the nursing care of patients requiring this support.

CENTRIFUGAL ASSIST DEVICES

Low cost and easy insertion have made centrifugal pumps popular in the field of circulatory support (Table 11–1). One type is the Biomedicus (Eden Prairie) vortex pump, which allows right atrial to pulmonary artery (right ventricular [RV]) assist and left atrium to aorta or left ventricular apex to aorta (left ventricular [LV]) assist (Fig. 11–1). Biopump heads are available in either a 50-mL pediatric or 80-mL adult size. A series of rotating cones will speed up and spin the blood during its course between the inlet and outlet points of the pump head, where rotational energy is recovered in the form of pressure-slow work (Fig. 11–2). The pressure created by the pump facilitates blood movement. While operating

TABLE 11–1. Centrifugal Pumps

Advantages
Ready availability
Inexpensive
No size limitations
Easy to insert
Capable of biventricular support
Allows for either atrial or ventricular apex cannulation
Not viewed as investigational

Disadvantages
Limited mobility
Increased incidence of thrombus formation
Anticoagulation usually required
Does not provide pulsatile flow
Requires constant surveillance

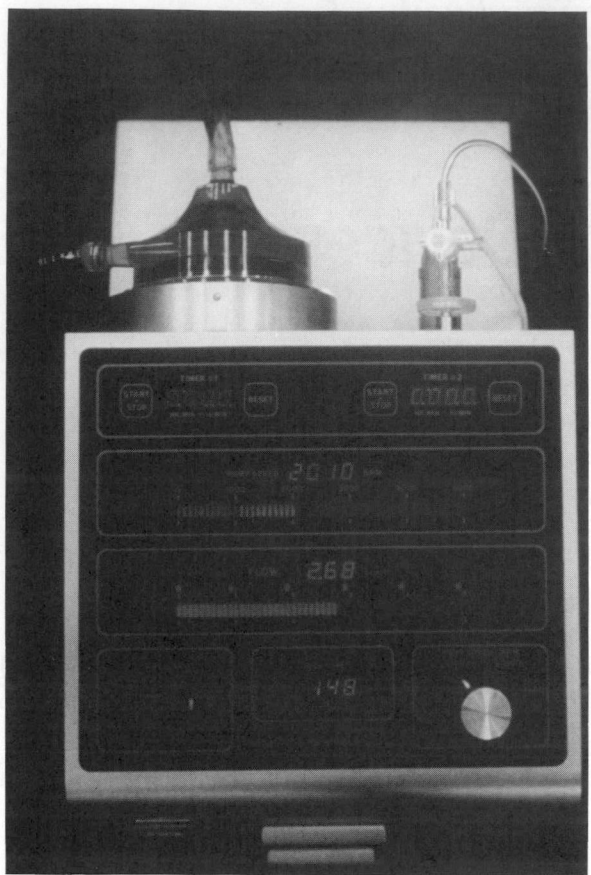

FIGURE 11–1. Biomedicus centrifugal vortex pump and console.

at a given steady speed, the biopump generates a nearly constant pressure over a wide range of flow rates. Magnets within the pump head housing approximate magnets in the drive console. When these magnets revolve, the ones within the pump head housing begin to rotate. Most investigators use standard cardiopulmonary bypass cannulas for connection to the device (Pennington and McBride, 1987).

The majority of institutions utilizing a centrifugal pump use some form of anticoagulation therapy (Pennington et al., 1982). However, it has been demonstrated that there is safety against thrombus formation without the need for anticoagulation (Magovern et al., 1985), but there is limited information about long-term support (greater than 14 days) with this type of pump. Frequently, pump heads need to be changed in the event of thrombus. The current policy is to check the pump head every 8 hours for signs of thrombus. This is accomplished by clamping the inflow and outflow lines and turning the pump off. The head can then be removed from the magnet and inspected; the entire procedure can be done in less than 2 to 3 minutes. Also at this time the flow probe may be recalibrated for better accuracy. This type of procedure is done only by perfusionists or those trained in device management.

EXTERNAL PULSATILE DEVICES

The Pierce-Donachy Ventricular Assist Pump (Thoratec Incorporated, Berkeley, CA) is an external pulsatile device (Fig. 11–3). This system is composed of cannulas, a pump, and a drive and control console. The cannulas provide communication between the patient's own heart and the mechanical device. Cannulation sites include right atrium to pulmonary artery for right ventricular assistance, and left atrium to aorta or left ventricular apex to aorta for left ventricular assistance. The pump is a sac-type pneumatic device with four components:

1. A polysulfone housing, which is the covering of the device
2. The polyurethane blood sac, which provides a highly smooth antithrombolytic surface to inhibit blood coagulation. The sac has a stroke volume of 65 mL with an ejection fraction of 75%
3. Inflow and outflow mechanical valves
4. A sensing instrument (Hall effect switch), which provides information to the pump for regulation of flow (Pennington et al., 1988; Gaines et al., 1985).

The control console is electrically powered and is capable of three different modes of operation: fixed rate mode, fill-to-empty volume mode, and an ECG synchronization mode (Farrar et al., 1986).

The pump has three different modes of operation:

1. Fixed rate mode. This mode operates independent from the heart. The pumps are set at a fixed number of beats per minute. This type of control is

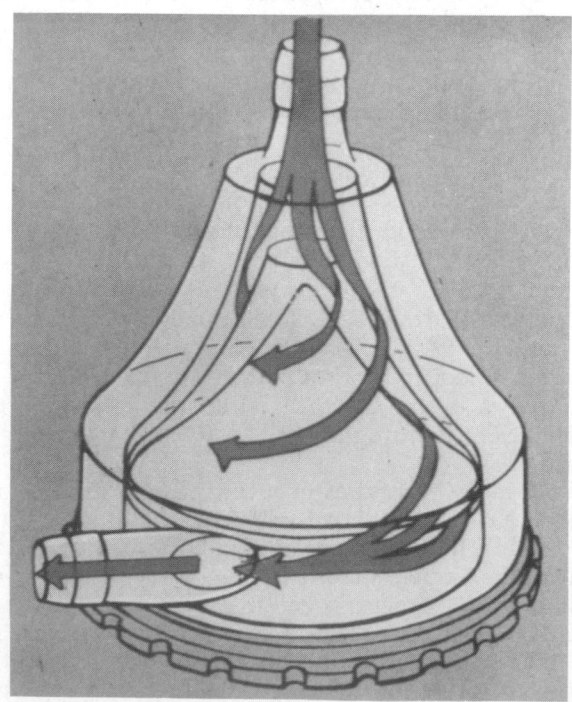

FIGURE 11–2. Biomedicus cone showing direction of blood flow.

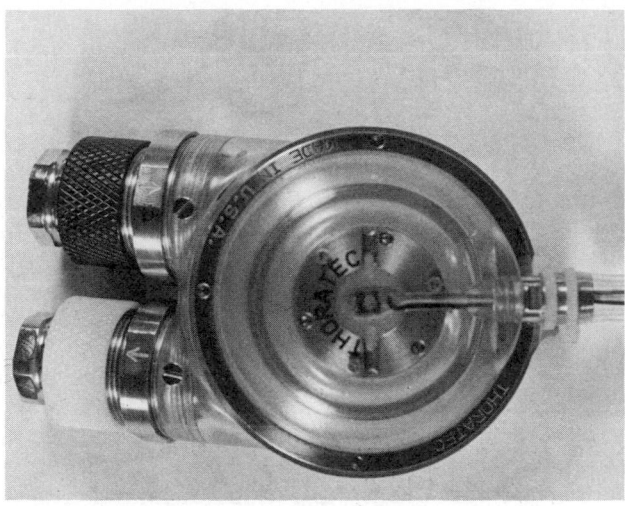

FIGURE 11-3. Pierce-Donachy Ventricular Assist Pump.

often used for initiation to and weaning from the device.

2. Fill-to-empty volume mode. This mode allows the pump to empty as soon as the blood sac is filled. The speed with which the pump is filled with blood determines the rate at which it will operate. This mode also operates independent of the heart.

3. ECG synchronized mode. The device is synchronized to the natural heart by detecting the R wave of the QRS complex and emptying at the occurrence of each QRS complex. This mode does not ensure full filling and emptying of the assist device.

The Pierce-Donachy pump has been used in the clinical setting for several years by various institutions (Farrar et al., 1988; Pennington et al., 1988). It has proved to be safe and successful in the treatment of patients experiencing cardiogenic shock. (Farrar et al., 1988; Pennington et al., 1988; Pae et al., 1990). It has also been used successfully in the treatment of postcardiotomy patients and as a bridge to transplantation. It allows patients to be ambulatory and has successfully supported them for periods of more than 80 days (Reedy et al., 1989). The advantages and disadvantages of this type of device are listed in Table 11-2.

TABLE 11-2. External Pulsatile Pump

Advantages
Is capable of providing biventricular support (using two pumps)
ICU nurse can be trained to manage pump
Allows for either atrial or apex cannulation
Has a proven safety record for long-term support
Moderate expense
Smaller size requirements than the implantable devices

Disadvantages
Requires an investigational device evaluation
Moderate cost
Need to implant a second device in the event of biventricular failure

---

TABLE 11-3. Implantable Pump

Advantages
Implantable, lower infection rate
Proven low risk of thrombus formation
Allows increased mobility

Disadvantages
Investigational device evaluation required
Expensive
Provides only univentricular support
Can be more difficult to insert than external devices
Apex cannulation only

IMPLANTABLE ASSIST DEVICES

Some advantages in the use of implantable systems are the decreased chance for infection, improved mobility, and more intact body image. Disadvantages are the need for LV apical cannulation and the limitation on LV support (Table 11-3). This type of cannulation usually limits the patient to cardiac transplantation because a part of the myocardium is removed during LV placement. A second device must be implanted or pharmacologic support used if right ventricular failure occurs. There are two implantable systems available today, the Heartmate 1000 IP and the Novacor Left Ventricular Assist System.

The Heartmate pump (Thermo Cardiosystems, Inc.) is designed to provide either pneumatic or electrical action (Fig. 11-4). The device contains a pusher plate design incorporating a biomer diaphragm. Twenty-millimeter Dacron grafts form the outflow conduit, whereas the inlet conduit is 19 mm. Twenty-five-millimeter porcine xenograft tissue valves are positioned in both inlet and outlet conduits. The pump is capable of an 80-mL stroke volume. A Dacron-covered pneumatic driveline connects the pump to a small console. The blood pump is implanted in the abdomen with left ventricular

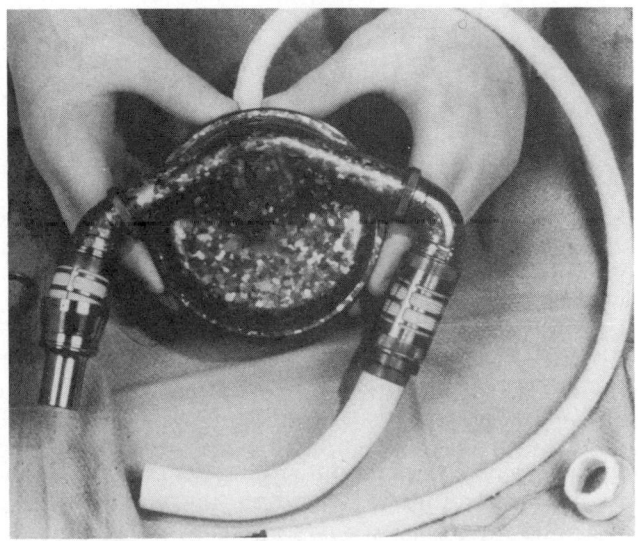

FIGURE 11-4. Heartmate 1000 IP Implantable System.

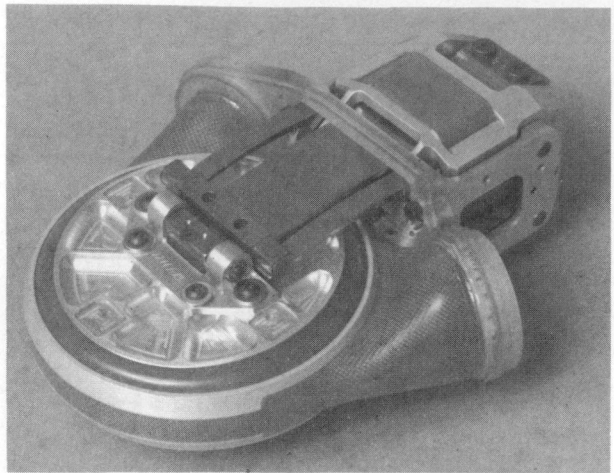

FIGURE 11–5. Novacor Left Ventricular Assist System. (Courtesy of Novacor Division, Baxter Healthcare Corporation.)

apex (inflow to pump) and ascending aorta (outflow from pump) cannulation. The drive console allows for three modes of operation: fixed-rate nonsynchronous mode, automatic pump on full mode; various pump rates with patient's cardiac output; and external mode, in which pumping is synchronized with an external trigger, such as an R wave on the ECG or a defibrillator synchronization pulse (Nakatani et al., 1989). These types of control modes were also explained in the previous section.

The Novacor Model 100 Left Ventricular Assist System (LVAS) (Baxter Corporation, Oakland, CA) consists of a balanced solenoid energy converter, dual pusher-plate, sac-type blood pump, and a microprocessor-based control and monitoring console. The energy converter and blood pump are encapsulated in a fiberglass/epoxy resin shell (Fig. 11–5), with Dacron conduits connecting the pump to the left ventricular apex (inflow to pump) and the ascending aorta (outflow from pump). A percutaneous extension cable connects the energy converter to the extracorporeal control console. All tissue- or blood-contacting surfaces are biocompatible. The blood pump consists of a seamless, smooth-surfaced polyurethane sac bonded to dual symmetrically opposed pusher plates and to a light weight housing that incorporates the valve fittings. The blood pump is designed to provide optimal flow patterns to reduce stasis of blood flow, risk of thrombus formation, and hemolysis. The use of two pusher plates instead of one results in reduced sac deformation and improved flex life as well as improved flow characteristics throughout the pumping cycle. Twenty-one-millimeter Carpentier-Edwards pericardial bioprosthetic valves with modified mounting flanges are used to allow unidirectional blood flow through the pump (Starnes et al., 1988). The console has three modes of operation: fill-to-empty, ECG synchronization, and fixed rate. The longest period for which a patient has been successfully bridged is 370 days.

EXTRACORPOREAL MEMBRANE OXYGENATION

The first multicenter evaluation of extracorporeal membrane oxygenation (ECMO) in the 1970s was generally unfavorable (Zapoh et al., 1979). This study involved using ECMO for the treatment of respiratory failure. However, there were documented reports of its success in the treatment of pediatric cardiac failure (Hill et al., 1972; Bartlett et al., 1974; Soeter et al., 1973). Since that time, ECMO has become an acceptable means of supporting pediatric patients in postcardiotomy shock. Unfortunately, it is one of the few types of support available to children. On the other hand, ECMO in adults is poorly tolerated over long periods of time (Pennington et al., 1984) (Table 11–4).

The ECMO perfusion circuit in Figure 11–6 resembles the one developed by Bartlett (Bartlett and Gazzaniga, 1978). It consists of a Scimed Membrane Lung (Scimed, Inc., Minneapolis), a Biopump (Biomedicus, Inc., Eden Prairie, MN), and a heat exchange connected together by polyvinyl chloride tubing. Ninety-five per cent of the institutions utilizing ECMO use Roller pumps, and the remaining 5% use a Biopump (Allison et al., in press). The membrane lung is connected to gas sources (oxygen and carbon dioxide) through a gas mixer, which allows appropriate changes in gas flow. The heat exchanger is connected to a circulating water heater usually set at 38°C. Line pressures are continuously monitored before and after the membrane lung (Kanter et al., 1987). Cannulation can be performed through the femoral vessels (Fig. 11–7) or chest for cardiac support. To date, ECMO remains the support method of choice in the treatment of biventricular failure in children (Pennington et al., 1989).

CANNULATION

The type of cannulation is decided by the surgeon at the time of implantation of the device. This decision is dependent upon the type of support required, the expected treatment outcome of the patient (recovery versus transplantation), and the condition of the patient's heart at the time of implantation.

TABLE 11–4. Extracorporeal Membrane Oxygenation

Advantages
Rapid resuscitation
Biventricular support
Allows time for further evaluation
Provides respiratory support

Disadvantages
Continuous anticoagulation
Increased rate of complications (thrombus, infection, bleeding)
Poorly tolerated for longer than 24 hours in adults
Nonpulsatile flow

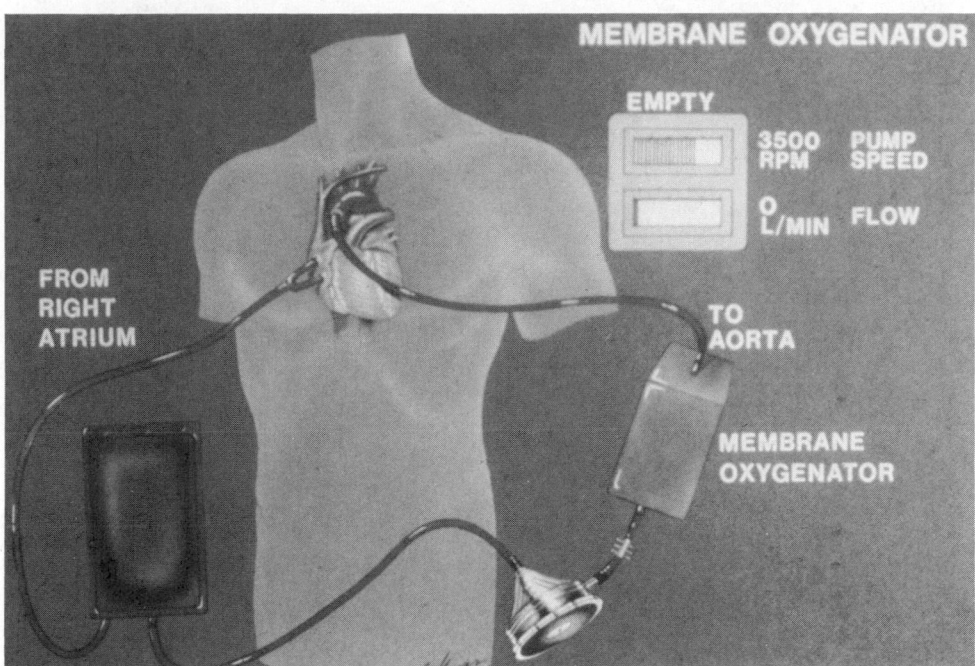

FIGURE 11–6. Extracorporeal membrane oxygenation (ECMO) perfusion circuit showing chest cannulation.

Atrial

With atrial cannulation, the inflow cannula is placed in the atrium to provide removal of blood from the heart to the assist device. The outflow cannula is sutured to the side of the aorta in left ventricular assist (Fig. 11–8) or to the pulmonary artery in right ventricular assist (Fig. 11–9) to facilitate return of the blood to the body. This type of support is preferred if the heart is expected to recover because it is easier technically and less injurious to the myocardium (Swartz and Pennington, 1985; LaForge et al., 1985). The disadvantage is that the left atrium may not be accessible due to scarring from previous surgeries or the danger of compressing saphenous vein grafts. Figure 11–10 shows biventricular support utilizing atrial cannulation.

Ventricular

In patients being bridged to transplantation, left ventricular cannulation is the method of choice. This allows for total decompression of the ventricle while preserving the atria for attachment during transplantation (Swartz and Pennington, 1985; LaForge et al., 1985). When biventricular assistance is required, a right ventricular assist device (RVAD) is placed with cannulation to the right atrium and pulmonary artery. The right ventricle is not used for cannulation due to its size. The disadvantages of ventricular cannulation include (1) it requires multiple sutures for fixation, (2) it damages an already impaired ventricle, and (3) it places the heart in a position that does not allow for exposure of the posterior surface (Swartz and Pennington, 1985; LaForge et al., 1985).

NURSING CARE

Many institutions utilize perfusionists or a team consisting of nurses, perfusionists, engineers, and doctors to monitor the devices while in use (Swartz et al., 1989). Due to limitations in staffing or case loads that require perfusionists to be elsewhere, quite frequently management of these patients becomes dependent upon the bedside nurse. The nurse should be familiar with the device, acquire a knowledge of its function and safety requirements, and be able to recognize complications associated with its use. There are two categories of complications: device-related complications and complications related to the patient.

Device-Related Complications

Hemolysis. Hemolysis is the destruction of red blood cells, which may be detected by blood in the urine or hemolyzed blood specimens. Hemolysis may also be accompanied by bleeding and hyperkalemia, which are late indicators. It should be determined whether the hemolysis is related to cardiopulmonary bypass, blood transfusions, or the VAD itself. Frequently, patients requiring a VAD have already undergone long bypass times for surgical repair and device implantation. Since bleeding is the most common patient complication, multiple blood transfusions may have been given. If the hemolysis occurs during the immediate postoperative period, the cause is most likely due to cardiopulmonary bypass and should clear. Hemolysis that occurs 3 to 4 days postoperatively or has not cleared is usually associated with the device. In this case, drive pressures or

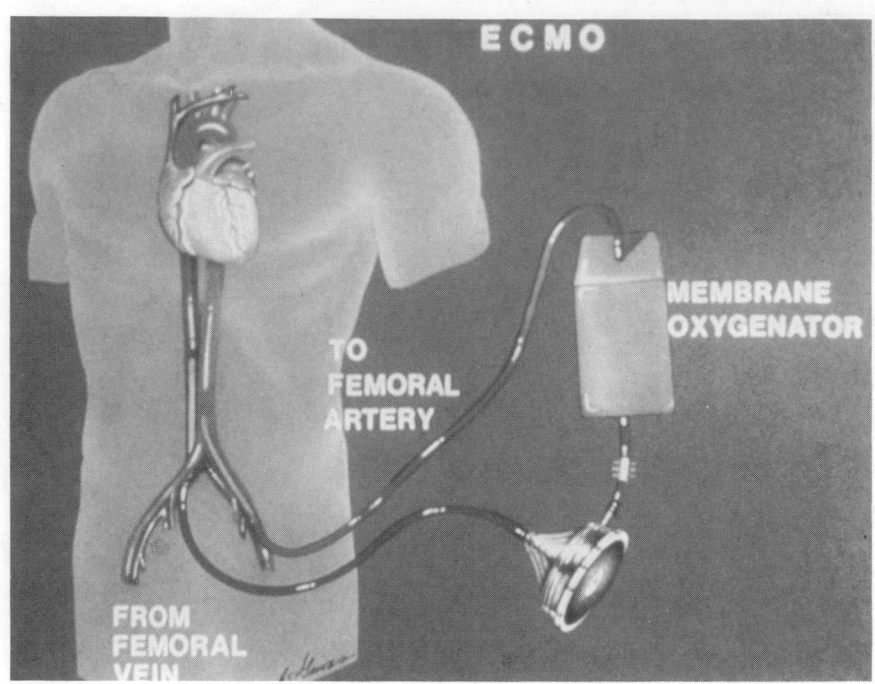

FIGURE 11–7. Extracorporeal membrane oxygenation (ECMO) perfusion circuit showing femoral cannulation.

the revolutions per minute (RPMs) of the device should be decreased. One way of detecting hemolysis is to measure daily serum hemoglobin. An elevated serum hemoglobin may be indicative of hemolysis.

Thromboembolism. The presence of artificial surfaces, mechanical valves, and pumping chambers may potentiate thrombus formation. High flows, maintenance of a high-pressure system, and complete emptying of the VAD may assist in preventing thrombus formation. The nurse should observe the

cannulas for kinks or disconnections. ECMO requires anticoagulation with heparin. Hourly activated clotting times (ACT) should be performed to allow timely manipulation of the dosage. The nurse should be aware of the ACT limits and the amount of heparin being administered. Overanticoagulation may result in bleeding, whereas inadequate anticoagulation may result in thrombus formation. If there is an increase in the mediastinal chest tube drainage or a noticeable oozing from the cannulation sites and incisions, the ACT may need to be set at a lower limit until the

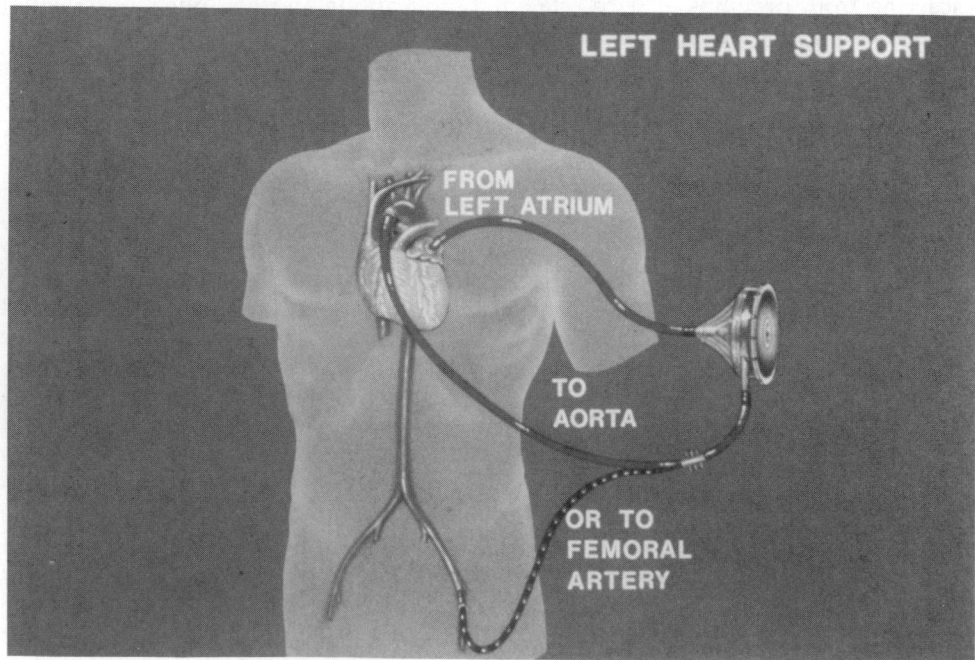

FIGURE 11–8. Left ventricular support using left atrial to aorta cannulation.

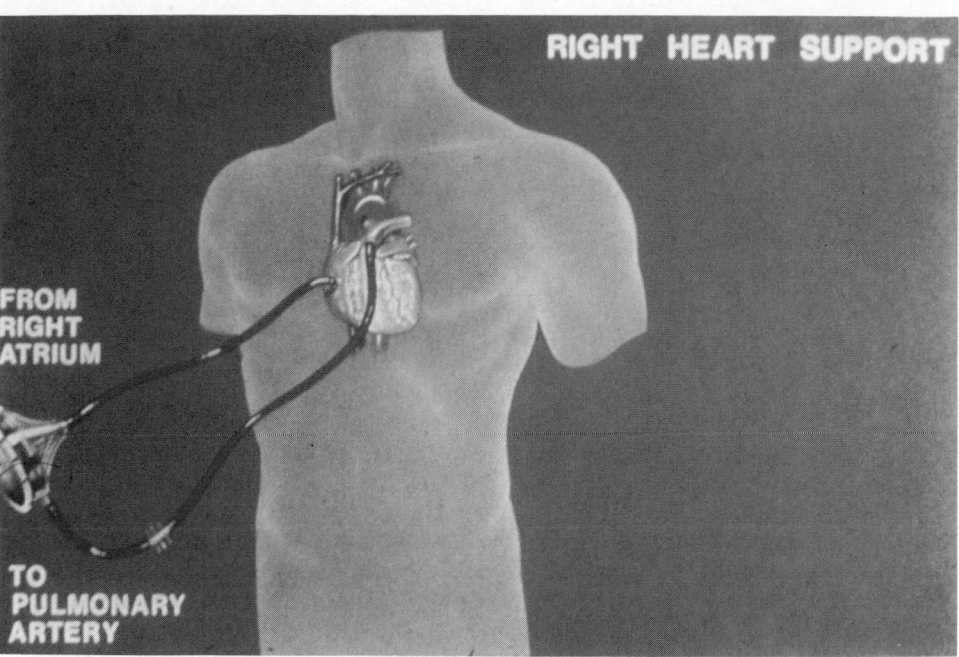

FIGURE 11–9. Right ventricular support using right atrial to pulmonary artery cannulation.

bleeding is controlled. An antithrombolytic agent such as dextran can be started until heparin can be used safely. Once the patient has been extubated he or she may be switched to a regimen of warfarin Coumadin (maintaining the partial thromboplastin time at one and one half times normal) and Persantine, 100 mg three times a day (Reedy et al., 1989)

Mechanical Failure. Backup equipment should be available at all times, and the nurse should be aware of its location in case of an emergency. If mechanical failure of the external components of the device occurs, the device should to be switched immediately

to the reserve console. Physicians and circulatory team members should be notified to ensure proper connection and adjustment. Mechanical failure can and does occur, but with proper safety techniques complications to the patient may be avoided.

Patient Complications

Biventricular Failure. Biventricular failure is described as an increase in the atrial pressure of the unassisted ventricle with a corresponding decrease in cardiac output. This results in poor pump filling

FIGURE 11–10. Biventricular support using atrial cannulation.

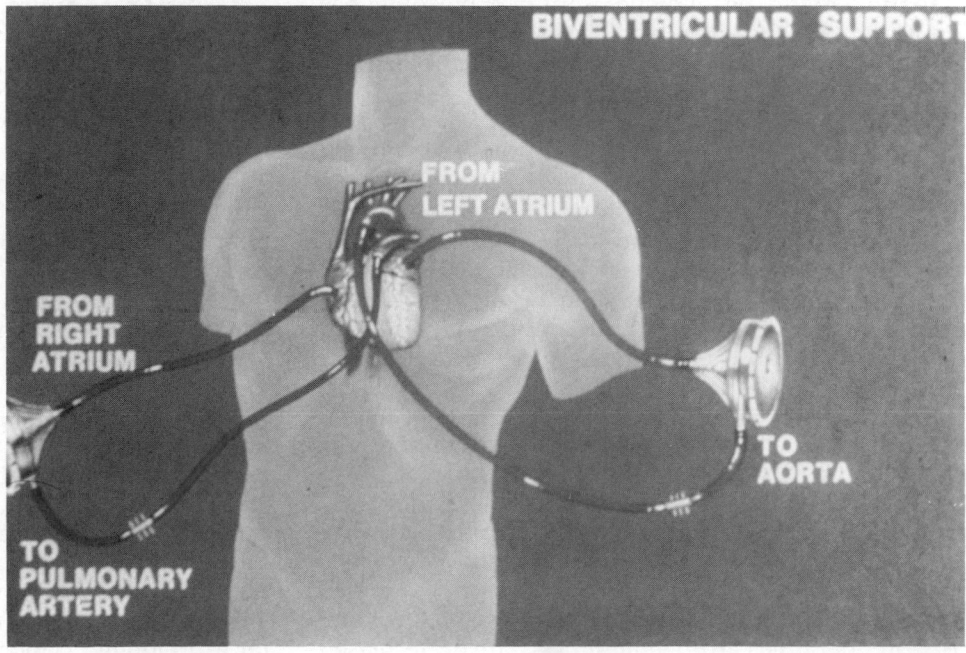

and low output of the assist device. Biventricular failure occurs because the unassisted ventricle has to handle the output from the mechanical device as well as any cardiac output from the patient's natural heart. This may occur in the operating room upon implantation of the device or later during the postoperative period. In either case, the problem cannot be treated lightly. Inotropic support with dopamine, amnirone, isoproterenol, or prostaglandin E have proved to be beneficial (Pierce, 1979; Pennington et al., 1985) If the failing ventricle does not improve, a second device should be implanted to assist that ventricle as well. In the event of left ventricular failure in a patient with an RVAD, pulmonary congestion and increased left atrial pressure develop, possibly leading to pulmonary edema and lengthening the amount of time the patient is intubated. During implantation of an RVAD an intra-aortic balloon pump may be inserted to assist the left ventricle and, ideally, deter any further development of failure.

Bleeding. Due to the prolonged bypass times and multiple insertion sites required for implantation of the VAD, postoperative bleeding is common. The current standard is to have six units of packed red blood cells available while the device is implanted. Coagulation studies (including partial thromboplastin time [PTT], prothrombin time [PT], thrombin time, fibrinogen, and platelet count) are checked every 6 hours while the patient is actively bleeding and then daily. Hourly ACTs are obtained in those patients receiving heparin. Any abnormalities in these results should be treated immediately. A platelet count below 100,000/mm^3 should be corrected by the administration of platelets. Fresh frozen plasma can be given to correct coagulation abnormalities. Administration of anticoagulation agents such as heparin should be avoided until the bleeding has subsided. Washed red blood cells are preferred instead of directly infused shed mediastinal blood. At the termination of cardiopulmonary bypass, heparin is reversed with protamine. Hemostatic agents such as Surgi-cel, bone wax, and fibrin glue have proved to be beneficial for persistent oozing prior to closing the chest. The use of cryoprecipitate and vitamin K should be discouraged due to the high risk of clot formation in the device itself (Ruzevich et al., 1988). A skin closure is used for patients who are bleeding excessively to avoid a cardiac tamponade situation. The sternum can then be closed when the device is removed or when the bleeding has stabilized. If the patient is to be supported for long periods of time it is ideal to close the sternum so that extubation may be accomplished.

Renal Failure. If the patient has experienced prolonged hypotension and decreased blood flow to the kidneys, acute tubular necrosis, a form of renal failure, may occur. The renal failure may result from the preoperative cardiogenic shock state or decreased perfusion following surgery (Kanter et al., 1987). A urine output of 1 mL/kg/hour is the goal. Serum electrolytes, blood urea nitrogen, and creatinine values should be obtained and compared daily. Daily weight and accurate intake and output values should be recorded. Daily chest x-rays are advisable to aid in the diagnosis of fluid overload. Progressive renal failure may be treated with dialysis or hemofiltration but can prove to be irreversible. Patients who develop renal failure during assistance can be at higher risk for secondary complications such as infection (Ruzevich et al., 1988).

Infection. Prevention is the key to minimizing infection. Patients with a VAD may be potential candidates for systemic and local infections due to their pre- and postoperative debility. Invasion with multiple intravascular monitoring lines and device-related conduits cross the skin barrier and increase the risk of infection. Strict aseptic technique in handwashing and dressing changes should be observed. Some institutions prefer the use of povidone-iodine spray for insertion sites and avoid the use of ointment because it is harder to remove with each dressing change (Reedy et al., 1989; Ruzevich et al., 1988). Prophylactic antibiotic coverage is recommended but should be discontinued after 4 days if there is no clinical evidence of infection. Fever and leukocytosis are good indicators of infection. Blood, urine, sputum, and wounds are routinely cultured if the patient has a temperature greater than 38.3°C. Antifungal oral solutions such as nystatin are advisable to prevent fungal infections in the mouth. Such treatment can be advantageous because it is believed that these patients develop some degree of immunosuppression as soon as 48 hours after VAD placement (Termuhlen et al., 1989).

Respiratory Failure. In the past, prolonged intubation of patients with a VAD led to respiratory complications (Hill et al., 1983). Today, patients are being extubated sooner, decreasing their chances of developing these complications. It is advisable to suction these patients every 1 to 2 hours if they are intubated and perform chest physical therapy every 4 hours. Daily chest x-rays aid in the prevention and treatment of future complications. Vigorous pulmonary toilet needs to be continued to prevent the need for re-intubation. Extubation allows greater freedom and enables the patient to ambulate.

Support Measures. Initiation of total parenteral nutritional support is recommended within 48 hours of VAD insertion, and administration of at least 3000 calories a day should be attempted (Reedy et al., 1989; Ruzevich et al., 1988). If the patient can be extubated the diet can be advanced as tolerated. Proper nutrition can aid in decreasing the risk of infection and assist in wound healing. Air mattresses are advisable because the patient may remain in bed for a prolonged period of time. Once vital signs are stable, turning every 2 hours is initiated. Passive range of motion exercises can be performed at the bedside. Once the patient is awake and hemodynamically stable, sitting in a chair is feasible without harm to the device. Thereafter, ambulation can be encouraged and has been demonstrated to be safe without presenting a risk to function of the device (Reedy et al., 1990).

The physical and mechanical side effects and implications of the presence of VADs were found to be greater than the emotional complications in a recent psychological study conducted on VAD patients (Ruzevich et al., 1990). Patient comfort may be maintained through the use of pain medications as needed. One important finding from this study is the benefit gained from patient and family teaching. It is important that the family be kept up to date daily on the patient's condition and care. It is also important to recognize each patient's individuality and to ensure that their emotional needs are met as well as their physical needs. Lenient visiting hours encouraging family interaction are advisable and beneficial. These patients may require support for long periods of time, and their psychological outlook can greatly influence their clinical course. A team approach has been found to be very successful in covering all aspects of the patient's care (Swartz et al., 1989). This approach will allow input from various staff members, including intensive care nurses, dietitians, physical and occupational therapists, social workers, psychiatric liaison, and pastoral care. This study further revealed that 80% of those surveyed would recommend an assist device to someone who needed one, and 67% of the patients would agree to a second implant if it were necessary. These results demonstrate that despite the fact that patients were connected to mechanical support they viewed their experience as a positive one. Many patients see this device as a second chance at life and feel fortunate to have this technology available to them.

SUMMARY

Temporary mechanical support of the circulation has proven to be successful in the treatment of reversible cardiac damage (Swartz and Pennington 1985; Gaines et al., 1985). The ability of an injured myocardium to recover is much better than was once thought. Long-term survivors can now return to a New York Heart Association class I cardiac status (Ruzevich et al., 1987). For this reason, more institutions are becoming interested in the use of mechanical support. The scarcity of donor organs and the number of cardiogenic shock patients who are unresponsive to conventional therapy has also furthered this interest. This increased interest has led to advances in the treatment or prevention of complications associated with mechanical assist devices. Major complications such as biventricular failure, bleeding, and infection are being treated more effec-

tively and with lower morbidity and mortality as experience grows. Irreversible cardiac damage remains a major cause of death but can be avoided if the patient qualifies for cardiac transplantation. It is hoped that with more patients, improved protocols, and multi-institutional studies the remaining problems can be solved. Mechanical support has become an acceptable and successful means of supporting patients experiencing cardiac failure that is refractory to other forms of therapy.

References

Allison, P. L., Kuruz, M., Graves, D. F., et al. (in press). Devices and monitoring during neonatal ECMO: Survey results. *Perfusion.*

Bartlett, R. H., and Gazzaniga, A. B. (1978). Extracorporeal circulation for cardiopulmonary failure. In R. H. Bartlett (Ed.), *Current problems in surgery.* (Vol. 15). Chicago, Year Book Medical Publishers.

Bartlett, R. H., Gazzaniga, A. B., Fong, S. W., et al. (1974). Prolonged extracorporeal membrane cardiopulmonary support in man. *Journal of Thoracic and Cardiovascular Surgery, 68,* 918–932.

Bolooki, H. (1984). *Clinical application of intra-aortic balloon pump* (2nd ed.). Mt. Kisco, NY: Futura.

Clauss, R. H., Birtwell, W. C., Albertal, G. (1961). Assisted circulation 1. The arterial counter-pulsator. *Journal of Thoracic and Cardiovascular Surgery, 41,* 447.

Cooley, D. A., Liotta, D., Hallman, G. L., et al. (1969). Orthotopic cardiac prosthesis for two-staged cardiac replacement. *American Journal of Cardiology, 24,* 723–730.

Drinkwater, D. C., and Laks, H. (1988). Clinical experience with centrifugal pump ventricular support at UCLA Medical Center. *ASAIO Transactions, 34,* 505–508.

Farrar, D. J., Compton, P. G., Lawson, J. H., et al. (1986). Control modes of a clinical assist device. *Engineering and Biology* IEEEP, 19–25.

Farrar, D. J., Hill D. H., Gray L. A., et al. (1988). Heterotopic prosthetic ventricles as a bridge to cardiac transplantation. A multicenter study in 29 patients. *New England Journal of Medicine, 318,* 333–340.

Gaines, W. E., Pierce W. S., Donachy, J. H., et al. (1985). The Pennsylvania State University paracorporeal ventricular assist pump: Optimal methods of use. *World Journal of Surgery, 9,* 47–54.

Gibbon, J. H., Jr. (1954). Application for a mechanical heart and lung apparatus to cardiac surgery. *Minneapolis Medicine, 37,* 171.

Hill, J. D., De Leval, M. R., Fallat, R. J. (1972). Acute respiratory insufficiency: Treatment with prolonged extracorporeal membrane oxygenation. *Journal of Thoracic and Cardiovascular Surgery 64,* 551–662.

Hill, J. D., Farrar, D. J., Compton, P., et al. (1983). Present and future of ventricular support systems for acute and chronic end-stage heart disease. *Journal of Heart Transplantation, 3,* 30–37.

Kanter, K. R., Pennington, D. G., Weber, T. R., et al. (1987). Extracorporeal membrane oxygenation for post-operative cardiac support in children. *Journal of Thoracic and Cardiovascular Surgery 93,* 27–35.

Kanter, K. R., Swartz, M. T., Pennington, D. G., et al. (1987). Renal failure in patients with ventricular assist devices. *ASAIO Journal, 10,* 426–428.

Kantrowitz, A., Krakauer, J. S., Rosenbaum, A., et al. (1969). Phase-shift balloon pumping in medically refractory cardiogenic shock. Results in 27 patients. *Archives of Surgery, 99,* 739–743.

Kirklin, J. W., Dushane, J. W., Patrick, R. T., et al. (1955). Intracardiac surgery with the aid of a mechanical pumpoxygenator (Gibbon type): Report of eight cases. *Proceedings of the Staff Meetings, Mayo Clinic, 30,* 201–206.

LaForge, C. G., Schoen, F. J., Monreld, R. G., et al. (1985). Left-atrium-to-aorta versus left ventricular-to-aorta bypass: The Lewis and anrep effects. *ASAIO Journal* 8, 191–204.

Magovern, G. J., Park, S. B., and Maher, T. D. (1985). Use of a centrifugal pump without anticoagulation for post-op LV assist. *World Journal of Surgery,* 9, 25–36.

McEnany, M. T., Kay H. R., Buckely, J. M., et al. (1978). Clinical experience with intra-aortic balloon pump in 728 patients. *Circulation* 58 (Suppl. I), I-124–I-132.

Moulopoulos, S. D., Topaz, S., and Kolff, W. J. (1962). Balloon pumping (with carbon dioxide) in the aorta: Mechanical assistance to the failing circulation. *American Heart Journal,* 63, 669–675.

Nakataki, T., Frazier, O. H., and McGee, M. G. (1989). Extended support prior to cardiac transplant: Using a left ventricular assist device with textured blood-contracting surfaces. Paper presented at the Meeting of the International Society for Artificial Organs, Sapporo, Japan.

Pae, W. E., Rosenberg, G., Donachy, J. H., et al. (1990). Mechanical circulatory assistance for postoperative cardiogenic shock. A three year experience. *ASAIO Transactions* 26, 256–260.

Pennington, D. G., Kanter, K. R., McBride, L. R., et al. (1988). Seven years experience with the Pierce-Donacy ventricular assist device. *Journal of Thoracic and Cardiovascular Surgery,* 96, 901–911.

Pennington, D. G., and McBride, L. R. (1987). The use of mechanical support devices in heart transplant recipients In P. D. Myerowitz (Ed.), *Heart transplantation,* pp. 357–387. Mt.Kisco, NY: Futura.

Pennington, D. G., Merjavy, J. P., Codd, J. E., et al. (1984). Extracorporeal membrane oxygenation for patients with cardiogenic shock. *Circulation* 70 (Suppl I), 130–137.

Pennington, D. G., Merjavy, J. P., Swartz, M. T., et al. (1982). Clinical experience with a centrifugal pump ventricular assist device. *ASAIO Transactions* 28, 9395.

Pennington, D. G., Merjavy, S. P., Swartz, M. T., et al. (1985). The importance of biventricular failure in patients with post-operative cardiogenic shock. *Annals of Thoracic Surgery* 39, 16–21.

Pennington, D. G., Swartz, M. T., Ruzevich, S. A., et al. (1989). In R. H. Anderson (Ed.), *Perspectives in pediatric cardiology* (Vol. 2, pp. 296–301). Mt. Kisco, NY: Futura.

Pierce, W. S. (1979). Clinical left ventricular bypass: Problems of pump inflow obstruction and right ventricular failure. *ASAIO Journal,* 1, 1–9.

Portner, P. M., Oyer, P. E., Jassawatta, J. S., et al. (1983). An alternative in end-stage heart disease: Long term ventricular assistance. *Journal of Heart Transplantation,* 3, 4759.

Reedy, J. E., Ruzevich, S. A., Swartz, M. T., et al. (1989). Nursing care of a patient requiring prolonged mechanical circulatory support. *Progress in Cardiovascular Nursing,* 4, 1–9.

Reedy, J. E., Ruzevich, S. A., Vitali, L. J., et al. (1990). Nursing care of the ambulatory patient with a mechanical assist device. *Journal of Heart Transplantation,* 9, 97–105.

Ruzevich, S. A., Pennington, D. G., Kanter, K. R., et al. (1987). Long-term follow-up Study of Survivors of Post-cardiotomy Circulatory Support. *ASAIO* 10, 177–181.

Ruzevich, S. A., Swartz, M. T., and Pennington, D. G. (1988). Nursing care of the patient with a pneumatic ventricular assist device. *Heart & Lung,* 17, 399–406.

Ruzevich, S. A., Swartz, M. T., Reedy, J. E., (1990). Retrospective analysis of the psychological effects of mechanical circulatory support. *Journal of Heart Transplantation,* 9, 209–212.

Soeter, J. R., Mamiya, R. T., Sprague, A. Y., et al. (1973). Prolonged extracorporeal oxygenation for cardiorespiratory failure after tetralogy correction. *Journal of Thoracic and Cardiovascular Surgery,* 66, 214.

Starnes, V. A., Oyer, P. E., Portner, P. M., et al. (1988). Isolated left ventricular assist as bridge to cardiac transplantation. *Journal of Thoracic and Cardiovascular Surgery* 96, 62–71.

Swartz, M. T., and Pennington, D. G. (1985). Use of a ventricular assist device in postcardiotomy shock. *Journal of Clinical Engineering,* 10, 241–249.

Swartz, M. T., Ruzevich, S. A., Reedy, J. E., et al. (1989). Team approach to circulatory support. *Critical Care Nursing Clinics of North America* 1 (3), 479–484.

Termuhlen, D. F., Pennington, D. G., Roodman, S. T., et al. (1989). T-cells in ventricular assist device patients. *Circulation* 80, 174–182.

Zapoh, W. M., Snider, M. T., Hill, J. D., et al. (1979). Extracorporeal membrane oxygenation in severe respiratory failure. A randomized prospective study. *Journal of the American Medical Association,* 242, 2193–2196.

C · H · A · P · T · E · R
12

Respiratory Monitoring

Tom Ahrens

Concepts in pulmonary critical care are at the center of much of the assessment and treatments administered in current Intensive Care Units (ICUs). Although it is unrealistic to discuss all aspects of pulmonary critical care in one chapter, the major aspects that are encountered on a daily basis will be presented. The key aspects of pulmonary critical care involve concepts relating to oxygenation and gas exchange. The goal of this chapter is to present the fundamentals of oxygenation and gas exchange while simultaneously exploring more advanced applications of these concepts. Blood gas and hemodynamic analysis will be emphasized as the mechanism through which more advanced aspects of pulmonary critical care are applied.

Two features are included in the presentation of oxygenation and gas exchange: first, the separation of oxygenation from gas exchange is emphasized, and second, the interaction of other organ systems on oxygenation and gas exchange is recognized. Through analysis of more advanced aspects of oxygenation and gas exchange, critical care nurses can increase their ability to make more sophisticated assessments and interventions in the patient with acute pulmonary disturbances. Practical examples are included to assist the nurse with the interpretation of clinical data.

OXYGENATION COMPONENTS

Cellular oxygenation is a combination of adequate oxygen transport relative to cellular oxygen consumption. Assessment of oxygenation must account for each facet of oxygenation. Employing each component also helps to avoid the use of components that are not as important. For example, the partial pressure of arterial oxygen (Pa_{O_2}) plays a role in oxygenation by aiding oxygen transport. This role is not as important, however, as the other factors in oxygenation. Clinically, the Pa_{O_2} has a tendency to be inappropriately applied in the assessment of oxygenation. Some clinicians believe that if the Pa_{O_2} is adequate, oxygen transport is adequate. Actually, the Pa_{O_2} is poorly correlated with cellular oxygenation. The role of the Pa_{O_2} and other components of oxygenation must be clearly understood to apply each component appropriately in an oxygenation assessment.

Determinants of Oxygenation

Oxygenation is determined by five factors, four of which are involved in oxygen transport. To determine how important any one parameter is in an oxygenation assessment, the factors in oxygen transport (D_{O_2}) must be considered. The main factors in oxygen transport, in order of importance, are cardiac output (CO_2), hemoglobin (Hgb), hemoglobin saturation (Sa_{O_2}), and Pa_{O_2}. The fifth factor in oxygenation is cellular oxygen consumption. Normal values for each of the components are listed in Table 12–1.

Oxygen transport is measured by the following equation:

TABLE 12–1. Normal Components of Oxygenation

Oxygen transport	600–1000 cc/minute 500–600 mL/minute/m²
Oxygen consumption	120–160 mL/minute/m² 3–4 cc/minute/kg
Oxygen extraction	0.25–0.35%
Cardiac output	4–8 liters/minute 2.5–4 liters/minute/m²
Hemoglobin	12–16 g/dL
Sa_{O_2}	>0.90
Pa_{O_2}	60–100 mm Hg

$$O_2 \text{ transport} = \text{cardiac output} \times \text{oxygen content (Ca}_{O_2}) \times 10$$

where 10 is a conversion factor to change Ca_{O_2} measurement from deciliters to liters. Cardiac output, as seen by this equation, accounts for at least 50% of oxygen transport; Ca_{O_2} accounts for the other 50%. Three factors comprise Ca_{O_2}—Hgb, Sa_{O_2}, and Pa_{O_2}. Ca_{O_2} is calculated by the following equation:

$$Ca_{O_2} = Hgb \times 1.34 \times Sa_{O_2} + (0.003 \times Pa_{O_2})$$

The 1.34 is the amount of oxygen maximally carried by Hgb if all oxygen sites of Hgb are occupied (Bunn and Forget, 1986). The 0.003 is the oxygen solubility coefficient. The oxygen solubility coefficient is used to determine how much oxygen is being transported by the Pa_{O_2}. Hgb accounts for the majority of Ca_{O_2}, with Sa_{O_2} and Pa_{O_2} playing smaller roles. Two case examples will illustrate the different roles of Hgb, Sa_{O_2}, and Pa_{O_2} in determination of Ca_{O_2}.

CASE HISTORIES

Case 1. An 80-year-old male patient was admitted to the ICU with pneumonia. The initial blood gas determination was listed at 8 A.M. The fraction of inspired oxygen (FI_{O_2}) was increased at this time. Later in the morning, the patient had an episode of hematemesis. Repeat blood gas and Hgb measurements demonstrated the values listed at 10 A.M. The FI_{O_2} was again increased at this time. A second episode of hematemesis occurred at 12:30 P.M. A repeat blood gas and Hgb were obtained at 1 P.M. From these data, at which time did the patient have the best arterial oxygen content?

Time	8 A.M.	10 A.M.	1 P.M.
Pa_{O_2} mm Hg	56	87	111
Hgb g/dL	15	12	10
Sa_{O_2}%	0.88	0.96	0.98
FI_{O_2}	0.21	0.30	0.40

Ca_{O_2} Computation

8 A.M. $Ca_{O_2} = 15 \times 1.34 \times 0.88 + (0.003 \times 56) =$
                 17.7   + 0.168   = 17.868 cc/dL

10 A.M. $Ca_{O_2} = 12 \times 1.34 \times 0.96 + (0.003 \times 87) =$
                 15.5   + 0.261   = 15.79 cc/dL

1 P.M. $Ca_{O_2} = 10 \times 1.34 \times 0.98 + (0.003 \times 111) =$
                 13.1   0.333   = 13.43 cc/dL

These calculations demonstrate two important points. First is the significance of Hgb in determining Ca_{O_2}. Eight o'clock was the point at which the patient had the highest oxygen content due to the high Hgb level at this time. The second important point is the minimal contribution of Pa_{O_2} levels to oxygen transport. When the Pa_{O_2} was highest, at 1 P.M., the Ca_{O_2} was at its lowest. Pa_{O_2} and Ca_{O_2} are not linearly related. Shoemaker (1989) has demonstrated in several subgroups of patients (i.e., those with sepsis, trauma, or adult respiratory distress syndrome (ARDS) that the Pa_{O_2} not only has a weak correlation with oxygenation but also has little clinical value in identifying survivors as opposed to nonsurvivors. To further illustrate the small contribution of Pa_{O_2} to Ca_{O_2}, note the minimal change in Ca_{O_2} that occurs if the contribution of the Pa_{O_2} is removed:

	With PaO2	Without PaO2
8 A.M.	17.868 cc/dL	17.7 cc/dL
10 A.M.	15.79 cc/dL	15.5 cc/dL
1 P.M.	13.42 cc/dL	13.1 cc/dL

The clinical implications of the above computations are easy to apply. Pa_{O_2} levels should not be used as a primary tool in the assessment of oxygenation. A common clinical error is to assume that oxygen transport is adequate if the Pa_{O_2} is normal. It is important to avoid this pitfall. The Pa_{O_2} is a minor contributor to oxygen transport; cardiac output and Hgb levels are far more important. The following case illustrates the importance of cardiac output and Hgb compared with Pa_{O_2}.

Case 2. Assume that you are the charge nurse and would like to teach a new orientee one aspect of prioritizing important physiologic data, in this case, oxygen transport. The three patients listed below are in your unit. Which of these three patients would be prioritized as being the most threatened in regard to oxygen transport?

	Patient 1	Patient 2	Patient 3
Pa_{O_2} mm Hg	91	53	160
Hgb g/dL	12	12	10
Sa_{O_2}	0.96	0.85	0.99
CO liters/minute	4.5	6	3

Oxygen transport for each patient:

Pt. 1 $4.5 \times 15.7 \times 10 = 707$ cc/minute
Pt. 2 $6 \times 13.8 \times 10 = 830$ cc/minute
Pt. 3 $3 \times 13.7 \times 10 = 412$ cc/minute

If the Pa_{O_2} were the only assessment tool used to assess oxygenation, the third patient would have been assumed to be adequate. Actually, his oxygen transport level is dangerously low. In the second patient, although Pa_{O_2} levels are lower than desirable, oxygen levels are adequate, and the patient is in no immediate danger from hypoxia. In teaching the new orientee, the charge nurse would emphasize that the person most at risk is the third patient. As long as the limitations of the clinical application of Pa_{O_2} are understood, appropriate use of Pa_{O_2} in assessing oxygenation is possible.

The value of the Pa_{O_2} in assessing oxygenation does not rest in how much oxygen is carried by Pa_{O_2}. The Pa_{O_2} does have a value, however, in that one can estimate Sa_{O_2} levels from given Pa_{O_2} values. The Sa_{O_2} indicates how much Hgb is carrying oxygen. A Sa_{O_2} level of 0.90 indicates that Hgb is carrying 90% of all the oxygen it is capable of carrying. Pa_{O_2} levels are related to Sa_{O_2} levels according to the oxyhemoglobin dissociation curve. As seen in Figure 12–1, Pa_{O_2} levels are related to Sa_{O_2} values and can be used to predict Sa_{O_2} values. At Pa_{O_2} levels in excess of 60 mm Hg, Sa_{O_2} values are greater than 0.90. Pa_{O_2} levels higher than this will contribute to a slight but not substantial increase in Sa_{O_2}. For example, a Pa_{O_2} value of 100 mm Hg will have a Sa_{O_2} value of 0.98, whereas a Pa_{O_2} of 60 mm Hg has a saturation value of 0.90. Because Sa_{O_2} does not increase substantially after a Pa_{O_2} of 60 mm Hg is reached, Pa_{O_2} levels of 60 mm Hg or higher are clinically acceptable.

On the other hand, if the partial pressure of oxygen (P_{O_2}) falls to less than 60 mm Hg, Hgb rapidly loses its ability to carry oxygen. From Figure 12–1, a P_{O_2} of 40 mm Hg is associated with a S_{O_2} of 0.75. If the P_{O_2} falls to

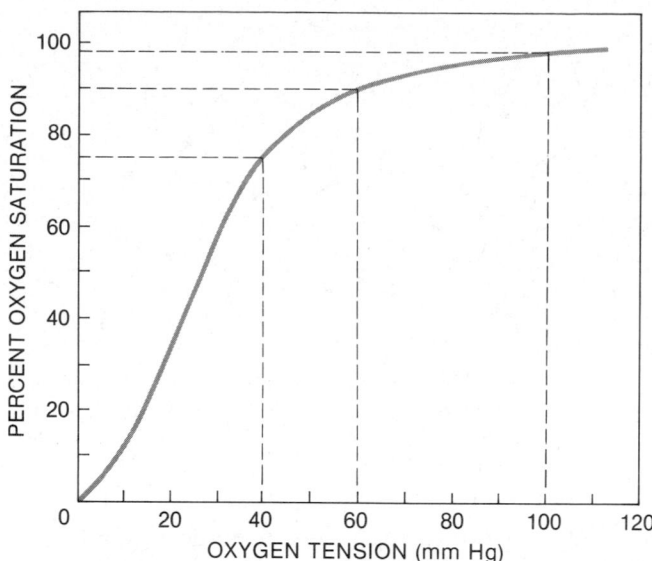

FIGURE 12–1. Oxyhemoglobin dissociation curve.

Oxygen transport at 2 A.M.:
$$5 \times (1.34 \times 13 \times 0.91) \times 10 = 793 \text{ cc/minute}$$

Oxygen transport at 5 A.M.:
$$3.5 \times (1.34 \times 13 \times 0.92) \times 10 = 561 \text{ cc/minute}$$

The best time to have administered oxygen therapy would have been at 5 A.M. because of the overall diminished oxygen transport seen at this time. Increasing the $F_{I_{O_2}}$ and therefore the Pa_{O_2} would not address the major problem but would offer a small improvement in oxygenation until the cardiac output could be improved.

Oximetry

With the advent of pulse oximetry (Sp_{O_2}), the need to use Pa_{O_2} values to estimate Sa_{O_2} levels has diminished markedly. However, understanding how to apply pulse oximetry depends on understanding oxygen transport. Because oximetry estimates Sa_{O_2} values, its use in assessing oxygen transport is limited. Pulse oximetry detects neither Hgb or cardiac output, and, as such, it reveals little about oxygen transport. Sa_{O_2} levels are very useful in determining changes in lung function (intrapulmonary shunting) and in altering oxygen therapy. Sa_{O_2} values are potentially very useful in appropriate circumstances. A brief review of the principles of pulse oximetry will help to illustrate the basis of the use of Sa_{O_2} values.

Two common clinical applications of oximetry exist: one is invasive and measures venous hemoglobin saturation (Sv_{O_2}), and the other is noninvasive and estimates arterial saturation (Sa_{O_2}). Venous oximetry is related more to oxygenation and pulse oximetry more to intrapulmonary shunting. In addition, the principles of measurement used in oximetry rely on either an absorptive or a reflectance component. New developments in oximetry are occurring and will be in place by the time this text is published. For example, noninvasive pulse oximetry will shift its focus away from specific locations such as the finger or ear to applications virtually anywhere on the body. Forehead oximetry has already been studied and is an example of a future application of oximetry principles (Cheng et al., 1988).

Oxyhemoglobin

Regardless of the application or of the use of reflectance or absorptive principles, the underlying theory remains the same. The key principle in oximetry is the different properties of absorption of light between oxyhemoglobin and reduced hemoglobin (or deoxyhemoglobin). Two other common types of hemoglobin exist, methemoglobin (MetHgb) and carboxyhemoglobin (COHgb), and although there are instances in which these values are important, the present explanation will focus on oxyhemoglobin. Generally, oxyhemoglobin is the value of interest

27 mm Hg, S_{O_2} is near 0.50. The rapid decrease in oxygen-carrying capacity of Hgb as the P_{O_2} drops to less than 60 mm Hg highlights the clinical significance of P_{O_2} levels. From the point of view of oxygenation, maintaining the P_{O_2} value in excess of 60 mm Hg will provide satisfactory hemoglobin saturation levels. Levels in excess of 60 mm Hg will generally provide little further improvement in oxygen transport. For example, in a patient who is admitted with a diagnosis of rule out myocardial infarction, who has no evidence of left ventricular failure, and in whom room air blood gases indicate Pa_{O_2} values greater than 60 mm Hg, the addition of oxygen therapy will probably not increase oxygen transport to any substantial degree.

There is one exception to increasing the Pa_{O_2} value when it is higher than 60 mm Hg. When a patient has a low Hgb or a low cardiac output level, improving the Pa_{O_2} value may produce a small improvement in oxygen transport that could be clinically important. In a patient with a low Hgb, oxygen therapy may slightly improve oxygen transport until a transfusion can be initiated. Similarly, in a patient with a low cardiac output, the addition of oxygen therapy may provide a small boost to oxygen transport until the cardiac output can be augmented. The following case example helps to illustrate this point.

Case 3. A 62-year-old woman was admitted with the diagnosis of chronic asthma. Because of a hypotensive episode in the emergency room a few hours earlier, a pulmonary artery catheter was inserted in the ICU. Initial data were listed at 2 A.M. During the night, she developed chest pain, and an electrocardiogram (ECG) revealed a probable anterior myocardial infarction (MI). Further data were presented at 5 A.M. From these two sets of data, at which time would an increase in oxygen therapy have been most useful?

	2 A.M.	5 A.M.
Pa_{O_2}	63	70
Sa_{O_2}	.91	.92
Hgb	13	13
$F_{I_{O_2}}$	.21	.30
CO	5	3.5

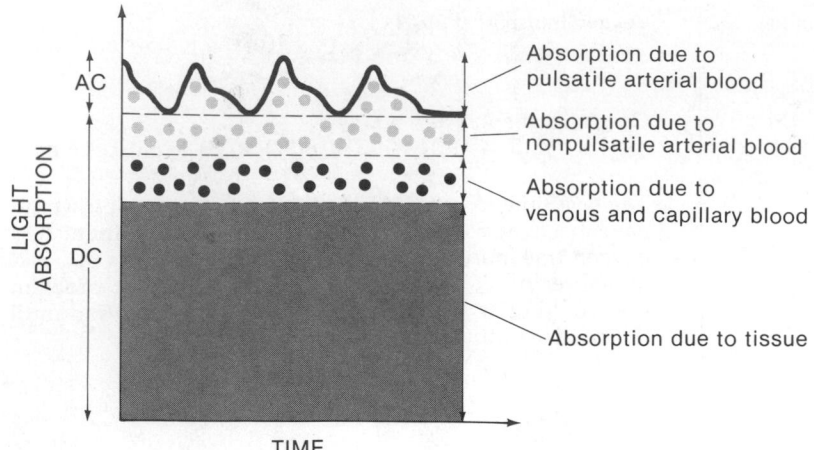

FIGURE 12–2. Factors affecting light transmission through tissue. (Redrawn from Tremper, K. K., and Barker, S. J. (1989). Pulse Oximetry. *Anesthesiology,* 70(1), 98–101.)

with a few clinical exceptions. For example, in patients with smoke inhalation an elevation in COHgb occurs that will decrease the reliability of pulse oximeters in accurately estimating oxyhemoglobin because the pulse oximeter cannot measure COHgb. Because COHgb is assumed to be oxyhemoglobin by the pulse oximeter, the oxyhemoglobin value will be overestimated by the pulse oximeter. High COHgb levels will reduce the oxyhemoglobin value, but the pulse oximeter will not detect the reduction in oxyhemoglobin.

Sa_{O_2} indicates arterial oxyhemoglobin values, and Sv_{O_2} refers to venous oxyhemoglobin. Oxyhemoglobin is identified through oximetry by measuring two lights (red and infrared) emitted by light-emitting diodes (LEDs). If reflectance oximetry is used, the amount of light reflecting back to the measurement source is measured (e.g., venous oximetry in a pulmonary artery catheter). If absorptive oximetry is used, the amount of light passing through a tissue is measured (e.g., pulse oximetry).

Two light wavelengths are employed to measure oxyhemoglobin and reduced hemoglobin (deoxyhemoglobin). Four wavelengths are required to measure other types of hemoglobins (Barker and Tremper, 1987). Oximetry in the clinical setting employs the two-wavelength system. Failure to measure the other types of hemoglobin can present clinical problems, which will be illustrated later.

The two sources of light, red and infrared, used to measure oxyhemoglobin and reduced hemoglobin have different wavelengths. Red light is emitted at a wavelength of 660 nm, and infrared light is emitted at 940 nm (Millikan, 1942). Red light flows through oxyhemoglobin but is absorbed by reduced hemoglobin. Infrared light is absorbed by oxyhemoglobin but flows through reduced hemoglobin. By noting the ratio of the difference in the light that passes through a tissue or is reflected, the amount of oxyhemoglobin and deoxyhemoglobin can be estimated. Red light (660 nm) is considered the numerator of the ratio, infrared light the denominator (940 nm). The ratio is low when oxyhemoglobin values are high (Stasic, 1986). The low ratio results from the fact that more red light reaches the light sensor, indicating a higher oxyhemoglobin level. More infrared light passing through indicates a higher level of deoxyhemoglobin and is reflected in a high red-infrared ratio.

One obvious concern in shining a light through a tissue is the potential for tissue other than hemoglobin to absorb the light. Pulse oximetry circumvents this problem by measuring the red-infrared light ratio only during maximal light absorption, which occurs during pulsation of arterial blood into the tissue. Other tissues that could absorb light, i.e., muscle, fat, connective tissue, and venous and capillary blood, are part of the baseline absorptive components that must be avoided (Fig. 12–2). When the tissue bed expands due to arterial pulsation, there is an expansion in the amount of light that passes through the tissue (Tremper and Barker, 1989). By sensing light only during the period of maximal absorption, the influence of other components is reduced.

Clinical Application of Pulse Oximetry

A second point regarding pulse oximetry is helpful in applying the values in the clinical setting. Pulse oximetry measures hemoglobin saturation based on the following equation:

$$\frac{Hgb_{O_2}}{Hgb_{O_2} + Hb}$$

where Hgb_{O_2} = oxyhemoglobin, and Hb = reduced hemoglobin.

This form of hemoglobin measurement is referred to as functional hemoglobin saturation. Other forms of hemoglobin, i.e., carboxyhemoglobin and methemoglobin, are not measured. To measure other common types of hemoglobins, the following equation would be necessary:

$$\frac{Hgb_{O_2}}{Hgb_{O_2} + Hb + COHgb + MetHgb}$$

where MetHgb = methemoglobin, and COHgb = carboxyhemoglobin.

The result is that the value displayed on the pulse oximeter is higher than the value of the measurement of all hemoglobins. Measurement of all hemoglobin saturation is referred to as fractional measurement, such as is performed with a laboratory co-oximeter. Clinicians must not compare the Sa_{O_2} values obtained from the oximeter to laboratory oxyhemoglobin values unless the above formula is also applied to the laboratory values. MetHgb and COHgb levels, when combined, usually comprise less than 3% of the total hemoglobin. Based on the combined amounts of MetHgb and CoHgb measuring about 3% of the total, the Sp_{O_2} (pulse oximeter) value usually is about 3% (or more) higher than the actual Sa_{O_2}. The only way to validate this estimate is to obtain a fractional hemoglobin saturation and compare the values according to the formulas given earlier. This should be done at least once before using the Sp_{O_2} to safely trend the Sa_{O_2}.

The value of measuring Sa_{O_2} from pulse oximetry data centers around two key components, the continuous measurement of Sa_{O_2} and the assessment of intrapulmonary shunting, Qs/Qt. As noted earlier, Sa_{O_2} does not reveal as much about oxygen transport as does hemoglobin or cardiac output. Maintaining Sp_{O_2} values in excess of 0.93 generally will mean that Sa_{O_2} values are higher than 0.90, a value which is adequate for most situations involving oxygen transport.

Use of Sp_{O_2} for assessing Qs/Qt is of value either as an assessment tool or to avoid having to measure blood gases while $F_{I_{O_2}}$ levels are being reduced. When using Sp_{O_2} for assessing Qs/Qt, the clinician watches for changes in Sp_{O_2} while the $F_{I_{O_2}}$ remains unchanged. If the Sp_{O_2} falls while the $F_{I_{O_2}}$ is unchanged, Qs/Qt may be worsening. A falling Sp_{O_2} that is not due to a change in Qs/Qt may occur if the Sv_{O_2} is decreased (Ahrens and Rutherford, 1987).

The most practical use of Sp_{O_2} is in continually monitoring the patient during $F_{I_{O_2}}$ changes while avoiding the need to measure blood gases. As a guide, $F_{I_{O_2}}$ levels can be reduced or increased until a desired Sp_{O_2} (usually 0.93) is reached. The following case study illustrates the use of the Sp_{O_2} in $F_{I_{O_2}}$ manipulation.

CASE HISTORY

Case 4. A 62-year-old man was admitted to your unit following coronary bypass graft surgery. His initial blood gas values and Sp_{O_2} indicated the following:

Pa_{O_2}	390	Pa_{CO_2}	37
Sp_{O_2}	1.00	pH	7.41
$F_{I_{O_2}}$	1.00		

Your unit has a policy of reducing the $F_{I_{O_2}}$ by 0.20 and drawing a sample for blood gas determination at each reduction. The $F_{I_{O_2}}$ is reduced until a Pa_{O_2}

value of below 100 but over 80 is reached. This policy generally requires three blood gas samples to reach a $F_{I_{O_2}}$ value of 0.40. How could Sp_{O_2} values avoid the need for these blood gas samples?

The answer is to lower the $F_{I_{O_2}}$ by 0.20 (or another level) until the Sp_{O_2} is 0.93 or higher. Generally, no blood gas samples would need to be obtained during this time to assess Sa_{O_2} or Pa_{O_2} as long as the only change occurred in the $F_{I_{O_2}}$.

Several research studies have demonstrated the value of Sp_{O_2} in manipulating the $F_{I_{O_2}}$, particularly in the postoperative setting (Niehoff et al., 1988; King and Simon, 1987). The use of Sp_{O_2} in tapering $F_{I_{O_2}}$ values is of clinical value in that the cost of blood gas determinations can be avoided while improving assessment through the continuous monitoring of patients during the manipulation. Also, in the patient without an arterial line, the pain of the arterial puncture is avoided.

ASSESSMENT OF OXYGEN TRANSPORT AND CONSUMPTION

With the exception of the Sv_{O_2}, none of the components of oxygen transport presented so far take into account oxygen consumption. Without understanding the oxygen consumption rates of the cells, the adequacy of oxygen transport can never be known. The concept of comparing oxygen transport with oxygen consumption is at the heart of an accurate assessment of oxygenation.

Oxygen Consumption

Values for oxygen consumption (V_{O_2}) are not always available unless ready access to exhaled gases or mixed venous oxygen values are present. Two common methods exist to measure V_{O_2}, neither of which are difficult, but each presents practical problems. The first method is the use of exhaled gas analysis, and the second the use of an indirect application of the Fick equation.

Measurement of V_{O_2} through exhaled gas analysis is based on the following simplified formula (several formulas account more accurately for other gases, but this method is simple and relatively accurate):

$$V_{O_2} = V_E \times (F_{I_{O_2}} - F_{E_{O_2}})$$

where V_E = minute ventilation (liters/minute or cc/minute); $F_{I_{O_2}}$ = fraction of inspired oxygen; $F_{E_{O_2}}$ = fraction of expired oxygen. For example, if the $F_{I_{O_2}}$ is 0.40, $F_{E_{O_2}}$ is 0.35, and V_E is 5 LPM (or 5000 cc/minute), then:

$$V_{O_2} = 5000 \times (0.40 - 0.35) = 250 \text{ cc/minute}$$

The problem with exhaled gas analysis centers mainly on the difficulty of obtaining accurate inspired and expired oxygen levels. Technically, sample collection may be difficult. Evidence also exists that FI_{O_2} values in excess of 50% may not be accurately utilized in computing V_{O_2} (Ultman and Bursztein, 1981). This obviously limits application in critical care settings.

The second method for measuring oxygen consumption employs the Fick equation. The formula employed is:

$$V_{O_2} = CO \times (Ca_{O_2} - Cv_{O_2}) \times 10$$

As an example, assume a cardiac output of 5 LPM, Ca_{O_2} of 15, and Cv_{O_2} of 11. The V_{O_2} would be:

$$V_{O_2} = 5 \times (15 - 11) \times 10 = 200 \text{ cc/minute}$$

This method has been demonstrated to correlate closely with measured oxygen consumption by exhaled gas analysis (Liggett et al., 1987).

Nurses in critical care units should be familiar with one of the above methods in order to make a more complete assessment of oxygenation. The exhaled gas method is more accurate and less invasive but has more technical problems. The indirect Fick equation method requires Sv_{O_2} values and is therefore invasive, yet many patients already have Sv_{O_2} values available if a pulmonary artery catheter is present.

Oxygen Balance

Actual measurement of cellular oxygenation is not possible at this time. To measure the adequacy of oxygenation of the cells, many parameters that are not readily measured at the bedside are necessary. Factors affecting mitochondrial use of oxygen include substrate availability, especially carbohydrates, intercapillary distance, diffusion capabilities of oxygen, tissue P_{O_2} and oxygen gradients between cells and capillaries, and the adequacy of electron transfer systems. However, instead of measuring these aspects of oxygenation, a more global method of assessment is used clinically. The primary method of assessment involves a comparison of oxygen transport parameters against oxygen consumption. Such a comparison has distinct limitations but can provide approximate estimates of the adequacy of cellular oxygenation.

Three methods are commonly used to compare oxygen transport with oxygen consumption. None of these methods can be accomplished noninvasively at the present time. These methods include oxygen extraction analysis, Sv_{O_2} monitoring, and lactate level measurements.

Oxygen Extraction. Oxygen extraction (O_{2e}) is obtained by dividing oxygen consumption by oxygen transport. Normal oxygen extraction is approximately 25%. In other words, 25% of all oxygen transported is removed from hemoglobin by the cells. For example, if the oxygen transport was 1000 cc and the

V_{O_2} 250 cc, the extraction rate would be 250/1000 = 25%.

The following examples help to illustrate the value of oxygen extraction. Note that in the first patient below, a normal Ca_{O_2} is present. However, with a low cardiac output and a normal oxygen consumption, cellular oxygenation may be threatened. In the second patient, a low Ca_{O_2} is present with a normal cardiac output and normal V_{O_2}. The low Ca_{O_2} threatens oxygenation. In the third example, normal Ca_{O_2} and CO are present, but a high V_{O_2} threatens oxygenation.

	Patient 1	Patient 2	Patient 3
Pa_{O_2}	75	90	65
Sa_{O_2}	0.93	0.96	0.91
Hgb	13	8	14
CO	3	4.5	5
Ca_{O_2}	16.2	10.3	17.1
D_{O_2}	486	463	855
V_{O_2}	245	210	375
Wt (kg)	70	60	70
O_{2e}	0.50	0.45	0.44

Extraction rates become clinically significant as they increase. Although the upper limits tolerated by humans are unknown, empirical evidence suggests that extraction rates in the 40% range may indicate disturbances in cellular oxygenation. The point at which humans reach a dangerous cellular imbalance of oxygen is not clear, although some studies suggest that humans can tolerate oxygen extraction ratios as high as 0.80 (Cain, 1983). It should not be assumed that all patients can achieve extraction rates at this level, however; Shoemaker and Appel (1985) have demonstrated that patients with sepsis have increased mortality at levels as low as the high 0.30s. A more useful way to apply oxygen extraction rates clinically is to note the trend in extraction. As extraction rates increase, cellular oxygenation is being threatened.

Two factors complicate the use of oxygen extraction rates. One is the apparent dependence of V_{O_2} on D_{O_2} at critically low levels of adequate oxygen balance. Several studies have indicated that, as D_{O_2} falls, V_{O_2} may fall in similar proportions (Danek et al., 1980; Gutierrez and Pohil, 1986). If this is true, V_{O_2} falls as D_{O_2} decreases. The dependence of V_{O_2} on oxygen delivery emphasizes the need to track oxygen extraction trends rather than noting absolute values of O_{2e}. As O_{2e} increases, the clinician should search for methods of increasing oxygen transport or decreasing V_{O_2}. A stable O_{2e} does not, however, necessarily mean that oxygenation is adequate or stable. The clinician must continue to track all parameters of oxygenation.

The second limiting feature of the assessment of oxygen extraction is the difference between oxygen consumption and oxygen demand. Oxygen consumption of the cells differs from oxygen demand of the cells. In patients with disturbances in cellular utilization of oxygen, oxygen consumption may decrease, although demand for oxygen is high. Unfortunately, measurement of oxygen consumption is easier than that of oxygen demand. When utilizing oxygen extraction rates, simultaneous use of lactate levels may also be helpful to reflect anaerobic metabolism and oxygen demand. Methods of making lactate measurements are presented later in this chapter.

Sv_{O_2} Monitoring and Analysis. Oxygen extraction can be estimated without performing all the above measurements with Sv_{O_2} analysis. Sv_{O_2} analysis applies theoretical principles to estimate the balance between oxygen transport and consumption. Sv_{O_2} values, normally between 0.60 and 0.75, trend oxygen extraction. If, for example, oxygen transport decreases without decreasing oxygen consumption, more oxygen will be extracted from Hgb to maintain cellular oxygen levels. The result of the increased extraction of oxygen from the Hgb is a reduction in hemoglobin saturation. The Sv_{O_2} can therefore, be used as an estimate of the adequacy of the balance between oxygen transport and oxygen consumption. Many articles have been written on Sv_{O_2} monitoring, and the reader is referred to these for more introductory material on this subject (White, 1984; Schweiss, 1987). One important point of Sv_{O_2} monitoring that is frequently overlooked is the ability of Sv_{O_2} levels to reflect the adequacy of treatment, as illustrated in the following case study.

CASE HISTORY

Case 5. A 73-year-old man was admitted with a diagnosis of congestive heart failure. A fiberoptic pulmonary artery catheter was placed to aid in assessment. At 4 P.M., the low cardiac output and high pulmonary capillary wedge pressure (PCWP) were used as the basis for starting dobutamine at 3 μg/kg per minute. Based on the change in cardiac index and PCWP that occurred between 4 P.M. and 5 P.M., was the change adequate?

	4 P.M. (dobutamine started)	5 P.M.
Pa_{O_2}	69	72
Sa_{O_2}	0.92	0.92
Hgb	12	12
Cardiac output	3.4	4.0
Cardiac index	2.1	2.5
PCWP	21	18
Sv_{O_2}	0.52	0.54

Although a subsequent increase in cardiac output was noted, the Sv_{O_2} did not substantially increase. The increase in CO apparently was not enough to change oxygenation substantially.

The Sv_{O_2} can be used in several ways to estimate the adequacy of oxygenation. The most common use is to note trends in Sv_{O_2}. If Sv_{O_2} is trending downward, investigation into the components of oxygen transport and consumption to locate a potential disturbance is necessary. If the trend is upward, the patient may be improving provided no technical problems exist. A second use of Sv_{O_2} monitoring is as a catastrophic warning. Because Sv_{O_2} monitoring can be continuous in patients requiring the use of fiberoptic pulmonary artery catheters, early warnings of severe derangements in oxygenation can be obtained more easily than with any other method of oxygenation monitoring. A third, less common use, is illustrated in Case 5, given above. Sv_{O_2} monitoring can be used as a means of determining the adequacy of therapies in hemodynamics, oxygen, and positive end-expiratory pressure or continuous positive airway pressure therapy and ventilator adjustments. The ability of Sv_{O_2} to aid in treatment assessment is the area of its highest potential.

The disadvantages of Sv_{O_2} monitoring center on the technical problems involved in fiberoptic monitoring and the occurrence of physiologic situations that cause unexpected Sv_{O_2} values. Technically, Sv_{O_2} catheters are reliable, but problems can be experienced in operation. Most of the nursing interventions necessary to correct these problems can be found in the service manuals provided by each manufacturer. Of the three current companies that manufacture Sv_{O_2} catheters, Abbott's Oximetrix Opticath has been demonstrated to be more clinically reliable (Gettinger et al., 1987). Technologic improvements made by the manufacturers are continually reducing the technical problems associated with each catheter, and accuracies associated with each manufacturer need to be assessed frequently. By the time this chapter is published, further changes may have occurred.

Physiologically, Sv_{O_2} monitoring can be misleading in two circumstances. First, in patients with sepsis, precapillary sphincter closure secondary to mechanisms such as endotoxin release cause arterial blood to bypass the cells and empty directly into the veins. The result is high Sv_{O_2} values (generally higher than 75%) that do not reflect cellular oxygenation. Caution in interpreting high Sv_{O_2} values is necessary. If the Sv_{O_2} is higher than 75%, the clinician must decide whether the value is possible, whether a technical problem exists, or whether a potential for pericapillary shunting is present, i.e., the patient may be septic. The second circumstance is again related to the dependence of V_{O_2} on D_{O_2}. If V_{O_2} is correlated with D_{O_2}, as currently thought, Sv_{O_2} will lose its ability to predict cellular oxygenation as V_{O_2} changes with D_{O_2}.

One factor that can also be used to assess oxygenation is venous P_{O_2} values (Pv_{O_2}). Although the arterial P_{O_2} does not contribute substantially to oxygen transport, venous oxygen tensions can be used to highlight the driving pressure that forces oxygen into the cells. As the venous P_{O_2} decreases, the pressure driving oxygen into the cells is diminishing. The potential for loss of cellular oxygen will increase as the Pv_{O_2} falls (Synder and Pinsky, 1987). As a guideline, if the Pv_{O_2} falls less than 30 mm Hg, the potential for cellular hypoxia increases at a faster rate. From a clinical perspective, keeping the Pv_{O_2} higher than

30 mm Hg may be helpful in protecting cellular oxygenation.

Lactate Levels. A third method of measuring cellular oxygenation is to measure lactic acid levels. Normal lactate levels are between 1 and 2 mmol. The potential advantage of using lactate levels is that they reflect a more accurate chemical picture of cellular oxygenation. Normal lactate use can be understood by reviewing substrate metabolism patterns.

To generate energy, carbohydrates must be available to allow fats and proteins to enter the Kreb cycle. Both fats and protein can be catabolized only through the Kreb cycle and oxidative phosphorylation, a process that requires the presence of oxygen to act as the final electron acceptor from the hydrogen electron removed from each substrate. Carbohydrates serve to process fats and proteins through the generation of pyruvate. In the absence of oxygen, pyruvate cannot aid in the processing of other substrates. Without oxygen, carbohydrates form increasing amounts of lactate, an anaerobic method of generating energy, although this process is much less efficient in terms of generating energy (Kruse and Carlson, 1987). Because the only substrate capable of producing energy without oxygen is carbohydrates, and normal carbohydrate stores are less than 1000 Kcal (one-half of one day's normal energy requirement), anaerobic metabolism is only a short-term solution to oxygen deprivation.

Lactate levels have a potential clinical use in predicting survival. Since the 1960s the literature has included references to the correlation of lactate levels with survival (Peretz et al., 1965). These early studies indicated that lactate levels in excess of 4 mmol/liter were associated with much higher mortality levels, with only 11% survival in some cases. Lactate levels are not, however, without limitations in predicting outcome. The ability to clear lactate from the blood may be a better indicator of survival than the notation of lactate acid levels alone (Broder and Weil, 1964). The use of lactate levels as a predictor of outcome requires further analysis at this time. Lactate levels may best be used as a means of confirmation of cellular hypoxia in conjunction with other aspects of oxygenation. As lactate levels start to rise over 2 mmol/liter, the potential for anaerobic metabolism may be increasing. If the lactate level is rising, the clinician should examine oxygen transport and consumption parameters.

The advantage of measuring lactate is that it reflects cellular oxygenation disturbances with more certainty than other methods. If lactate levels are rising, there is an excellent possibility of an imbalance in cellular oxygenation. Although there are other reasons for lactate increases, the most common and significant reason in the critically ill population is an oxygen deficit.

Lactate levels do not necessarily correlate with other parameters of oxygenation, such as Sv_{O_2} and D_{O_2} (Astiz et al., 1988). The reasons for this are not well understood but may be related to variations in individual metabolic needs or regional perfusion problems. The important point is that, in a patient with a threatened oxygenation status, as many variables should be examined as possible to determine whether a trend of worsening oxygenation can be established.

The disadvantage of lactate levels is the lag time between cellular lactate generation and serum values. Levels below 2 mmol/liter do not necessarily indicate normal oxygenation because they do not rule out regional or beginning oxygenation imbalances (Mizock, 1987). By the time the cellular lactate level corresponds to the serum level, several minutes (possibly longer in underperfused areas) may have passed. On the other hand, if cellular lactate levels are returning to normal, the serum value will not immediately reflect this change. Although increases in lactate levels indicate that a problem with oxygenation exists, these increases are not as time specific as other parameters of oxygenation. Interpretation of lactate levels is an important part of oxygenation assessments but should not be used to reflect immediate assessment of oxygenation.

There is no perfect method of assessing oxygenation at this time. Some advances can be seen in the application of computer technology to the utilization of simultaneous parameters, such as Sp_{O_2} and Sv_{O_2}, to allow more continuous assessment of the components of oxygenation (Rasanen et al., 1987). What is still needed, however, is an easy to apply, continuous, and rapid means of reflecting cellular oxygenation. Newer techniques such as positron emission tomography are being developed that should aid in more sophisticated assessment of cellular oxygenation. Until such techniques are fully developed, assessment of oxygenation must depend on combining the components of oxygenation, centering on the aspects of oxygen transport and consumption.

Pa_{O_2} AND INTRAPULMONARY SHUNTING

Although the Pa_{O_2} is limited in assessing oxygen transport, it can be used to estimate one of the parameters of lung function. Intrapulmonary shunting (Qs/Qt), the main cause of clinical hypoxemia, can be estimated by noting the discrepancy between alveolar (PA_{O_2}) and arterial (Pa_{O_2}) oxygen levels.

Normal intrapulmonary shunts are small, generally less than 5% of the total pulmonary blood flow. Intrapulmonary shunting, defined as blood passing through underventilated alveoli, is illustrated in Figure 12–3. As intrapulmonary shunting increases, the work on the heart and respiratory muscles also increases. Cardiac work increases because an increase in cardiac output is necessary to compensate for the decreased oxygen exchange resulting from reduced alveolar function. Respiratory work increases in an

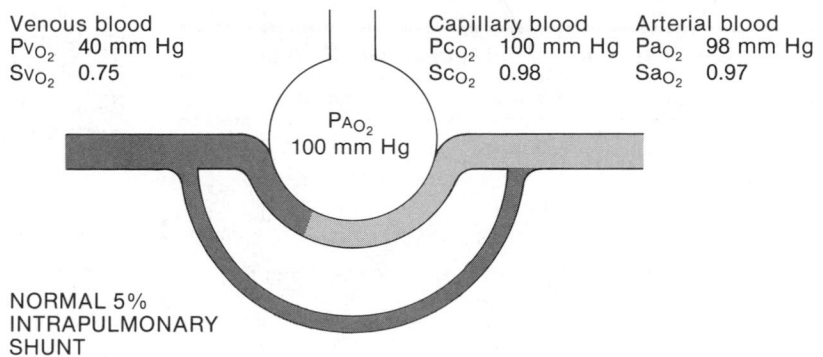

Venous blood
Pv_{O_2} 40 mm Hg
Sv_{O_2} 0.75

PA_{O_2}
100 mm Hg

Capillary blood   Arterial blood
Pc_{O_2} 100 mm Hg Pa_{O_2} 98 mm Hg
Sc_{O_2} 0.98 Sa_{O_2} 0.97

NORMAL 5%
INTRAPULMONARY
SHUNT

FIGURE 12–3. Normal intrapulmonary shunt. (Copyright 1987, American Journal of Nursing Company. Reprinted from American Journal of Nursing, 1987, 87(3), 337A–340H. Used with permission. All rights reserved.)

Pv_{O_2}—Partial pressure of oxygen in the veins
Sv_{O_2}—Hemoglobin saturation with oxygen in the veins
Pc_{O_2}—Partial pressure of oxygen in the capillaries
Sc_{O_2}—Hemoglobin saturation with oxygen in the capillaries
Pa_{O_2}—Partial pressure of oxygen in the arteries
Sa_{O_2}—Hemoglobin saturation in the arteries
PA_{O_2}—Partial pressure of oxygen in the alveoli

attempt to compensate and to provide increased alveolar ventilation to functioning alveoli.

Clinically, intrapulmonary shunting does not present significant problems until the shunt fraction climbs higher than 15%. Near 15% shunt values, the patient will be experiencing marked increases in the work of breathing and in myocardial oxygen consumption. At levels higher than 30%, the work of maintaining alveolar ventilation may require mechanical ventilation (West, 1985).

Estimates of Qs/Qt can be useful clinically to track progress or deterioration in clinical situations. Several methods exist that either measure or attempt to estimate intrapulmonary shunting. The key to estimating the size of the intrapulmonary shunt is the concept that alveolar oxygen levels are the primary determinant of arterial levels. Normally, venous blood in the pulmonary circulation is exposed to alveoli with immediate equilibration of alveolar/blood oxygen tensions. Arterial levels should, in theory, equal alveolar levels. The major reason that arterial levels do not equal alveolar levels is alveoli are malfunctioning. Venous blood passing through non-functioning alveoli create a mixture of venous and arterial blood. The result is a decreased Pa_{O_2}.

Intrapulmonary shunting can be measured by employing the shunt formula:

$$Qs/Qt = \frac{Cc_{O_2} - Ca_{O_2}}{Cc_{O_2} - Cv_{O_2}}$$

This formula is the most accurate estimate of Qs/Qt, although it has two obvious drawbacks. The most obvious is the need for a pulmonary artery catheter to obtain the Cv_{O_2} value. The second is the assumption that end-capillary oxygen values for the calculation of Cc_{O_2} will be the same as alveolar oxygen values. The primary problem with the use of the

classic shunt equation listed above is its limited practicality in patients without pulmonary artery (PA) catheters. Because of this limitation, several other methods of estimating Qs/Qt have been proposed. Included in these estimates are the alveolar/arterial gradient, arterial/alveolar ratio, Pa_{O_2}/Fi_{O_2} ratio, and the respiratory index. Each of these has its own strengths and weaknesses. They are all based on a comparison of the difference between alveolar and arterial oxygen values in an attempt to approximate Qs/Qt easily. Table 12–2 presents the formulas and normal values for each of these estimates of Qs/Qt.

Other methods for estimating Qs/Qt exist that attempt to utilize more data than the oxygen tension indices. The clinical shunt equation, which uses an assumed $Ca_{O_2} - Cv_{O_2}$ value of 3.5 cc/DL, has the potential to be more accurate than the oxygen tension indices (Cane et al., 1988). Another promising technique is possible in patients in whom both Sp_{O_2} and Sv_{O_2} values exist. Through computer integration of simultaneous changes in both Sp_{O_2} and Sv_{O_2}, an improved accuracy in estimating Qs/Qt is possible (Rasanen et al., 1987). If an institution has the technologic ability to employ integration of data, more accurate assessments are likely. Critical care nurses should learn the capabilities of their institution in order to explore the potential to calculate more sophisticated estimates of parameters such as Qs/Qt.

The primary advantage of using oxygen tension indices as opposed to the other techniques of measuring Qs/Qt is the ability to apply the indices easily and to use them in all patients with blood gas values. It is crucial to keep in mind that the oxygen tension indices are guidelines rather than exact values for estimating Qs/Qt. Due to the ease of use of oxygen tension indices, practical illustrations of Qs/Qt tracking will be explained through common clinical situations.

TABLE 12–2. Estimates of Intrapulmonary Shunting

Estimate Measure	Formula	Normal Value
Pa_{O_2}/FI_{O_2} ratio	$\dfrac{Pa_{O_2}}{FIO_2}$	Greater than 300
Arterial/alveolar ratio	$\dfrac{Pa_{O_2}}{PA_{O_2}}$	Greater than 60%
Alveolar-arterial gradient	$PA_{O_2} - Pa_{O_2}$	0–20 mm Hg
Respiratory index	$\dfrac{PA_{O_2} - Pa_{O_2}}{Pa_{O_2}}$	<1
O_2 content index	$\dfrac{Cc_{O_2} - Ca_{O_2}}{(Cc_{O_2} - Ca_{O_2}) + 3.5}$	<5%

where PA_{O_2} = alveolar oxygen tension; PA_{O_2} is obtained by the following equation

$$FI_{O_2} (Pb - H_2O) - Pa_{CO_2}/RQ$$

where FI_{O_2} = fraction of inspired oxygen
Pb = barometric pressure (approximately 760 mm Hg at sea level)
H_2O = alveolar water vapor pressure (47 mm Hg)
Pa_{CO_2} = partial pressure of arterial carbon dioxide
RQ = respiratory quotient (normally 0.8)

Clinical Applications of Qs/Qt

Of the oxygen tension indices, the alveolar-to-arterial (A-a) gradient is the most inaccurate of the estimated values, yet surprisingly it is the most frequently cited. The arterial-to-alveolar (a/A) ratio is one of the oldest methods of estimating Qs/Qt and has demonstrated clinical utility in several studies (Gilbert and Keighley, 1974). Although the a/A ratio has limitations (Covelli et al., 1983), it can be applied under many conditions (Gilbert et al., 1979). The a/A ratio will be presented here as a satisfactory means of estimating Qs/Qt with the understanding that other methods can also be used with similar accuracy.

In order to apply the arterial-to-alveolar ratio, the alveolar level must be calculated. Alveolar oxygen levels can be computed by the alveolar air equation:

$$PA_{O_2} = FI_{O_2} (PB \times P_{H2O}) - Pa_{CO_2}/r$$

This equation can be simplified by allowing the following assumptions: (1) PB (barometric pressure) is 760; (2) H_2O (water vapor pressure) is 47; (3) r (respiratory quotient) is 0.8. These assumptions are generally accurate at sea level. If these assumptions are allowed, then the equation is calculated:

$$PA_{O_2} = FI_{O_2} (713) - Pa_{CO_2}/0.8$$

The alveolar oxygen tension on room air (FI_{O_2} of 0.21) could be calculated as follows (assume a normal Pa_{CO_2} of 40):

$$PA_{O_2} = 0.21 (713) - 40/0.8 = 100 \text{ mm Hg}$$

Normally, arterial levels differ only slightly from alveolar levels. If the acceptable Pa_{O_2} level is 60 to 100 mm Hg, the normal a/A ratio on room air would be between 0.60 and 1.00:

	Pa_{O_2} 60	Pa_{O_2} 100
PA_{O_2}	100	100
a/A	0.60	1.00

As long as the a/A ratio is over 0.60, the intrapulmonary shunt is small. If the shunt increases, the a/A ratio decreases. The lower the a/A ratio, the worse the patient's pulmonary status. The following examples will illustrate applications of the a/A ratio to clinical settings.

CASE HISTORIES

Case 6. Assume that a patient has returned from the operating room (OR) on 100% oxygen. He has the following blood gases: Pa_{O_2}, 470; Pa_{CO_2}, 40. Should his FI_{O_2} be lowered slowly or quickly? The alveolar oxygen level is: PA_{O_2} = 1.00 (713) − 40/0.8 = 663. The patient has an a/A ratio of 0.71 (470/663), which is within the normal range. His intrapulmonary shunt is so small that oxygen therapy is probably unnecessary. For this patient, the oxygen level probably could be reduced markedly and he would still maintain Pa_{O_2} levels higher than 60 mm Hg.

Case 7. A patient with a 40% face mask in place receives a meal. He has a Pa_{O_2} of 88, and a Pa_{CO_2} of 35. Can you allow him to remove his mask to eat without replacing it with a nasal cannula? The alveolar oxygen level is: 0.40(713) − 35/0.8 = 241. The a/A ratio is 0.37 (88/241). The ratio is well below normal limits, indicating substantial intrapulmonary shunting. The patient would therefore require supplemental oxygen even while eating to avoid Pa_{O_2} levels of less than 60.

Case 8. A patient experiences an FI_{O_2} change from 50% to 30%. His blood gases change as follows:

	FI_{O_2} 0.50	FI_{O_2} 0.30
Pa_{O_2}	110	68
Pa_{CO_2}	39	41

Based on the change in FI_{O_2}, did the lung function change? In the first reading, the a/A ratio is 0.36 (110/307). In the second, the ratio is 0.42 (68/163). Lung function appears to be practically unchanged, although the a/A ratio is slightly improved.

The use of estimates of Qs/Qt can guide assessment of clinical changes relative to lung function. These estimates are not to be assumed to be as accurate as the actual measurement of Qs/Qt. Several limitations of the a/A ratio (and other estimates of Qs/Qt) are present, and the clinician should be aware of these to apply the a/A ratio safely. One limitation is the effect of the Sv_{O_2} on the Pa_{O_2}. When Qs/Qt is large, changes in Sv_{O_2} are more likely to change Pa_{O_2} values (Fig. 12–4). Subsequently, the a/A ratio may change without a change in Qs/Qt. If the patient has an unstable oxygenation status with a potential for reductions in Sv_{O_2}, a/A ratios should be used more cautiously.

A second limitation is that small changes in the a/A ratio may not have significant meaning. For example, if the a/A ratio changes from 0.35 to 0.39, this change generally does not indicate a substantial change in lung function. The a/A ratio should change by greater than 5% before any assumption of change in Qs/Qt has occurred. How much the a/A ratio should change before it indicates a clinically significant change in Qs/Qt requires further research. In addition, although a normal a/A ratio may be as low as 0.60, a higher ratio than 0.60 should be allowed when using the a/A ratio to estimate what level of Fi_{O_2} support should be used. Because the a/A ratio estimates Qs/Qt and is not "rock" stable, a safety margin should be allowed when applying the ratio to change Fi_{O_2} support. For example, if the a/A ratio is near 0.60, oxygen support is probably unnecessary. Yet to allow for a safety margin, a reduction in the Fi_{O_2} to 0.24 to 0.28 would be more clinically acceptable. This would avoid a situation in which the a/A ratio might change and not predict a fall in the Pa_{O_2} to less than 60 mm Hg.

It is important when using estimates of Qs/Qt to acknowledge that they are just estimates, not replacements for Qs/Qt measurements. If one can measure Qs/Qt, as is possible with continuous Sv_{O_2} and Sa_{O_2}

monitoring, the actual Qs/Qt should be measured. In the absence of Qs/Qt measurements, techniques such as the a/A ratio can be used to approximate Qs/Qt.

V_D/V_T APPLICATION

The Pa_{CO_2} value can be used to estimate a second aspect of lung function in much the same way as Pa_{O_2} is used to estimate Qs/Qt. Pa_{CO_2}, in conjunction with other respiratory parameters, can be used to estimate deadspace to tidal volume ratio (V_D/V_T). In addition, actual measurement of deadspace can be done if exhaled gases and volumes are present. This next section will describe the methods used to estimate V_D/V_T from Pa_{CO_2} values and respiratory parameters and will review ways to measure V_D/V_T from exhaled gases.

The normal amount of deadspace (the amount of inspired air not participating in gas exchange) is usually 25% to 35% of each breath or tidal volume (V_T). Two types of deadspace exist, anatomic and physiologic. Anatomic deadspace is the amount of air that will not reach gas-exchanging units due to the anatomy of the lung. For example, airways as low as the terminial bronchioles contain air that cannot participate in alveolar gas exchange. Physiologic deadspace is anatomic deadspace plus any increase in inspired volume that cannot participate in gas exchange. For example, if a patient develops a pulmonary embolism, no blood will perfuse the

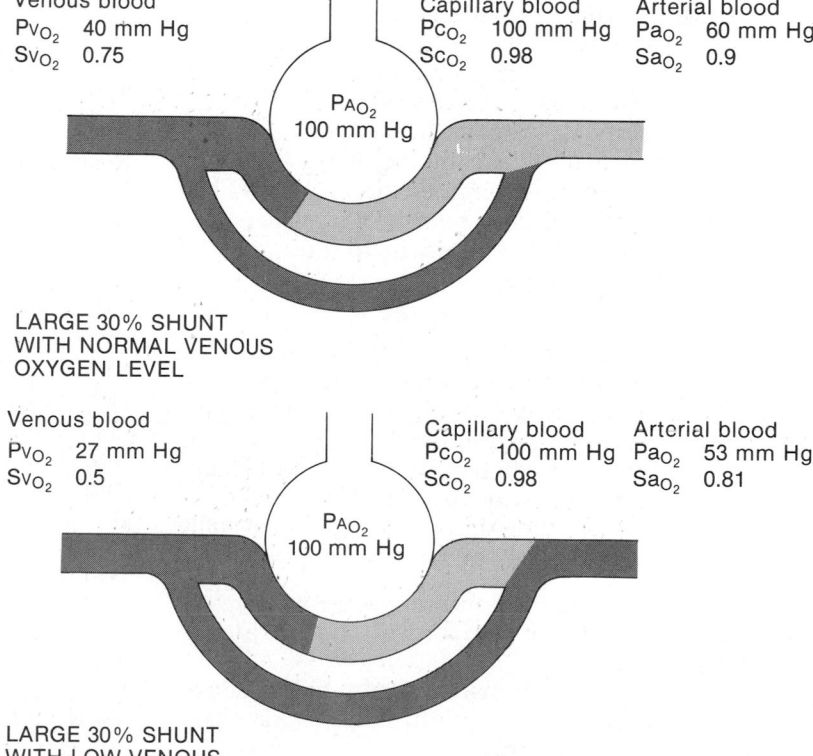

FIGURE 12–4. Effect of Sv_{O_2} on Pa_{O_2}. (Copyright 1987, American Journal of Nursing Company. Reprinted from American Journal of Nursing, 1987, 87(3), 337A–340H. Used with permission. All rights reserved.)

affected area of functioning alveoli. The affected area now does not participate in gas exchange and adds to the deadspace volume. The deadspace volume that is of interest to clinicians is the physiologic deadspace.

An understanding of deadspace is important because of the impact of increased deadspace on respiratory effort. As deadspace increases, the work of breathing increases. Increased work of breathing occurs as increased volumes of air are necessary to reach functioning alveoli. If a part of the alveolar area cannot participate in gas exchange, more air must be brought to alveoli that are in contact with functioning pulmonary capillaries. Unfortunately, as a person inspires, part of the air inspired still goes to the lung unit that is not in contact with functioning alveoli. To increase the volume of air to the functioning alveoli, overall ventilation (minute ventilation) must increase. The net result is increased work of breathing proportional to the degree of deadspace.

Pa_{CO_2} is maintained at normal levels as long as adequate alveolar ventilation (VA) is maintained. Pa_{CO_2} falls if excessive alveolar ventilation occurs relative to carbon dioxide production (V_{CO_2}). Pa_{CO_2} values rise if alveolar ventilation is inadequate compared to V_{CO_2} or if pulmonary blood flow falls. Clinically, a rise in Pa_{CO_2} has more serious implications because a rise in Pa_{CO_2} values can bring about an acute respiratory acidosis, producing a simultaneous systemic acidosis. Because of the role of Pa_{CO_2} in reflecting alveolar ventilation, it can be used to estimate deadspace volume.

Under ordinary circumstances, if minute ventilation (VE) is within normal limits (5 to 10 liters/minute, Pa_{CO_2} is also normal provided VD is normal. The combination of normal VD and normal VE will result in adequate alveolar ventilation (VA). Changes in Pa_{CO_2} levels can usually be traced to the factors affecting VA, such as changes in VD. As a practical aid, VE can be measured by a spirometer or estimated by noting a change in respiratory rate or depth. The following examples of changes in Pa_{CO_2} values and the influence of VD/VT will aid in identification of the cause of Pa_{CO_2} changes.

Decreased Pa_{CO_2} Levels and VD/VT. When the Pa_{CO_2} falls below normal levels (less than 35 mm Hg), VA and VE must be increased. In such circumstances, VD is usually normal or minimally increased. It is important to note that when VE is elevated and Pa_{CO_2} is decreased, pulmonary dysfunction is generally not a problem. The cause of the low Pa_{CO_2} can usually be narrowed to the following factors:

1. Factors affecting the voluntary control of breathing, such as anxiety or fear, causing an increase in breathing
2. Compensatory response to a metabolic acidosis
3. Excessive ventilation due to inappropriate mechanical ventilation settings
4. Neurologic injury at the brainstem level

Low Pa_{CO_2} levels are not usually dangerous in themselves. They are, however, guides to other problems. Whenever a respiratory alkalosis exists, a search for the problem causing excessive work of breathing should be made. Correction of the problem will correct the abnormal Pa_{CO_2}.

Physical assessment is helpful in the clinical assessment of deadspace. VE is the most helpful tool in assessing deadspace noninvasively. However, measurement of VE is not always practical. Assessment of respiratory rate and tidal volume (depth of breathing) can be used as a substitute for VE measurement, yet inaccuracies can occur. For example, a patient with a rapid respiratory rate may not have an increased VE if the VT is reduced. Or, a rapid respiratory rate may not lower the Pa_{CO_2} if the VD/VT has increased. Therefore, if a patient is breathing rapidly or deeply, he may or may not be hyperventilating (lowering the Pa_{CO_2}), depending on the VD/VT. If the deadspace is large, the patient with a rapid respiratory rate may actually be hypoventilating. Without blood gas measurement to determine Pa_{CO_2} levels and deadspace, a patient breathing rapidly should be identified as tachypneic, not hyperventilating.

Increased Pa_{CO_2} Levels. Increased Pa_{CO_2} levels occur only when alveolar ventilation is inadequate or when decreased pulmonary perfusion occurs. Such a situation could occur in the presence of the following factors:

1. Medication-induced brainstem depression
2. Increased deadspace ventilation
   a. Pulmonary emboli
   b. Chronic lung disease
3. Severe hypovolemia
4. Cardiopulmonary resuscitation (reflecting loss of pulmonary perfusion)

Respiratory acidosis is always significant because it indicates inadequate alveolar air movement. It becomes more serious, however, when the increased Pa_{CO_2} occurs suddenly without renal compensation. In this situation, the respiratory impairment is of recent origin and implies acute respiratory embarrassment. If the Pa_{CO_2} rises and produces a pH less than 7.25, intubation should be considered, particularly in light of a decreasing level of consciousness.

Identifying the cause of the increased CO_2 retention involves a search for any reason for respiratory depression or loss of pulmonary blood flow. If respiratory depression or loss of blood flow is not likely, then increased deadspace is the likely cause. Even without an identifiable cause of respiratory depression, the reason for an increase in Pa_{CO_2} level can be determined by a knowledge of the Pa_{CO_2} level and VE. When both the Pa_{CO_2} and VE are increased, VD must also be increased because normally an increased VE would lower the Pa_{CO_2}. In addition, an increased VD can be identified even if the Pa_{CO_2} is normal, provided the VE is increased.

If the Pa_{CO_2} is increased but V_E is low, V_D/V_T is probably normal. The cause of the increased Pa_{CO_2} is respiratory depression. The Pa_{CO_2} has increased simply because of reduced alveolar ventilation.

CASE HISTORIES

To help illustrate these concepts, the following specific cases are presented.

Case 9. A 42-year-old woman was in your unit postoperatively after a colon resection. She was breathing rapidly and appeared anxious. You obtain a blood gas determination and the following respiratory parameters. From the information presented here, what is the likely cause of the increased work of breathing?

Pa_{CO_2} (mm Hg)	20
Pa_{O_2} (mm Hg)	92
$F_{I_{O_2}}$	0.21
V_E (LPM)	15
RR (bpm)	30
V_T (cc)	500

The Pa_{CO_2} is low secondary to an increased V_E. The V_D/V_T is probably normal because the Pa_{CO_2} is expected to decrease with an increase in V_E. One of the reasons listed earlier that increase V_E without pulmonary dysfunction must be present. In this case, anxiety or pain is a potential cause.

Case 10. A 52-year-old man was admitted to your unit after an abdominal aortic aneurysm repair. Shortly after admission to the unit, he was extubated. During your postextubation assessment, you note that he is difficult to wake and responds only to vigorous stimuli. You obtain a set of blood gas levels and respiratory parameters as follows:

Pa_{CO_2} (mm Hg)	55
pH	7.28
Pa_{O_2} (mm Hg)	100
$F_{I_{O_2}}$	0.30
V_E (LPM)	3
RR (bpm)	15
V_T (cc)	200

In this patient, the Pa_{CO_2} is high due to a low V_E. The V_D/V_T is probably normal because the Pa_{CO_2} is expected to rise if the V_E is inadequate. The cause of the increased Pa_{CO_2} may be respiratory depression. Perhaps the anesthetic has not been completely eliminated. Reintubation should be considered.

Case 11. A 65-year-old man with a diagnosis of chronic obstructive pulmonary disease (COPD) was in your unit. He had no immediate distress, although he had complained of shortness of breath in the emergency room. His admitting blood gas levels and respiratory parameters are as follows:

Pa_{CO_2} (mm Hg)	70
pH	7.35
Pa_{O_2} (mm Hg)	67
$F_{I_{O_2}}$	0.28
V_E (LPM)	13
RR (bpm)	30
V_T (cc)	433

The Pa_{CO_2} in this patient was increased along with the V_E. The cause is most likely an increased V_D or a reduction in pulmonary blood flow. Because the patient has a compensated respiratory acidosis, the problem is more likely chronic. The chronic nature of the problem probably reflects an increased V_D secondary to the lung disease. Problems of reduced blood flow tend to be short term in nature.

Case 12. A 32-year-old woman was admitted to the unit complaining of shortness of breath and right-sided chest pain. She had the following blood gas levels and respiratory parameters.

Pa_{CO_2} (mm Hg)	40
pH	7.38
Pa_{O_2} (mm Hg)	89
$F_{I_{O_2}}$	.40
V_E (LPM)	16
RR (bpm)	32
V_T (cc)	500

This patient had a normal Pa_{CO_2} with an increased V_E. Either the V_D is increased or the pulmonary perfusion is reduced if the Pa_{CO_2} is normal in the presence of an increased V_E. In this patient, the increased V_E without a corresponding fall in the Pa_{CO_2} is of concern. A problem with pulmonary blood flow (pulmonary embolus) causing a large deadspace is likely in this person.

Exhaled Gas Analysis

Estimation of V_D and arterial P_{CO_2} has been made more accurate by the use of exhaled gas analyzers, specifically capnography (carbon dioxide waveform) analysis. Technically, CO_2 is measured by either mass spectrometry or infrared analysis (Stock, 1988). Mass spectrometry requires the aspiration of exhaled gas samples for analysis by a mass spectrometer. Infrared analysis requires a sample chamber and gas analyzer attached to part of the expired circuit (usually the exhalation tubing in the ventilation circuit). Each technique has advantages and limitations, although both can be used with generally accurate results.

The theory of analyzing exhaled CO_2 is based on two factors—first, the CO_2 elimination pattern during exhalation, and second, the total percentage of CO_2 eliminated during exhalation. The CO_2 elimination pattern makes possible the prediction of arterial CO_2 values, and the total percentage of CO_2 exhaled makes deadspace analysis feasible. Examples of the clinical application of each of these factors will help to illustrate the theoretical principles of exhaled gas analysis.

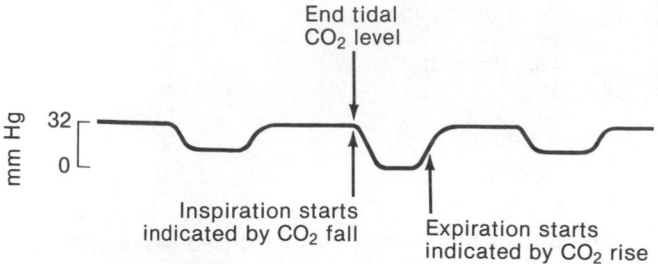

FIGURE 12–5. Tracing of capnogram.

END-TIDAL CARBON DIOXIDE ($P_{ET_{CO_2}}$) ANALYSIS

During exhalation, the initial percentage of CO_2 is minimal. As gas from the alveoli enter the larger airways, the percentage of CO_2 increases until the end of exhalation. At this point, the percentage of CO_2 approximates alveolar levels. An example of the exhaled CO_2 waveform is shown in Figure 12–5. The near-alveolar levels allow a useful clinical application, i.e., prediction of arterial CO_2 values. Since alveolar and arterial CO_2 values are similar, samples of exhaled CO_2 at the end of exhalation can provide approximate Pa_{CO_2} values.

The $P_{ET_{CO_2}}$ is usually lower than Pa_{CO_2} levels. If the $P_{ET_{CO_2}}$ is 30 mm Hg, the Pa_{CO_2} is higher than 30 mm Hg. How much higher depends on several factors, primarily pulmonary blood flow. Under normal circumstances (normal pulmonary blood flow), $P_{ET_{CO_2}}$ does not vary from Pa_{CO_2} by more than several millimeters of mercury. Unfortunately, in critical care settings, the assumptions for $P_{ET_{CO_2}}$/Pa_{CO_2} correlations are not always met. This means that the clinician needs to apply data from $P_{ET_{CO_2}}$ analysis in conjunction with other clinical data before making judgments based on $P_{ET_{CO_2}}$ changes.

The use of $P_{ET_{CO_2}}$, despite its limitations, has several clinical applications. The primary benefit of exhaled gas analysis is the continuous evaluation of alveolar ventilation. Reliance on blood gas levels is markedly reduced, providing both an economic (reduction in cost) and patient (reduction in pain) advantage. The value of $P_{ET_{CO_2}}$ analysis centers on assessments that are useful in monitoring Pa_{CO_2} changes. $P_{ET_{CO_2}}$ analysis is commonly used for monitoring during spontaneous breathing (weaning) trials, ventilator changes, cardiopulmonary resuscitation, endotracheal intubation, and deadspace analysis.

During weaning and ventilator changes, the $P_{ET_{CO_2}}$ can be used as a marker for observing acceptable Pa_{CO_2} values. If the $P_{ET_{CO_2}}$ increases during weaning, a blood gas determination may be necessary to determine the extent of the developing respiratory acidosis. The value of $P_{ET_{CO_2}}$ lies in its capability for constant monitoring and early identification of problems in alveolar ventilation.

Endotracheal intubation can be confirmed by noting the capnograph waveform. Esophogeal intubations do not produce CO_2 waveforms. Avoidance of

dangerous situations in which esophogeal intubations may occur offers a strong advantage to any unit in which endotracheal intubations are common. $P_{ET_{CO_2}}$ analysis has been so useful in this area that many anesthesia departments are now equipped with mass spectrometers, partly to assess CO_2 waveforms to avoid esophageal intubations.

Exhaled CO_2 has been described as useful in determining the adequacy of CPR (Weil et al., 1985). The principle applied in CPR is similar to the effect of pulmonary blood flow on $P_{ET_{CO_2}}$. Weil and associates (1985) noted that the mixed venous P_{CO_2} value increased during CPR, possibly indicating diminished pulmonary blood flow and resulting in inadequate clearance of CO_2. Weil's group postulated that the adequacy of CPR could be determined by noting the capnograph results. If blood flow is adequate, a good capnograph is produced. If CPR is inadequate, the capnograph will accurately and quickly illustrate the problem.

Exhaled gas analysis is also helpful in reading end-expiration tracings during hemodynamic waveform analysis. The point at which inspiration begins (end-exhalation) can be noted by a drop in the CO_2 waveform. The point just before the drop in CO_2 level can be used to identify end-exhalation. Through this technique, inspiratory artifact in pulmonary artery tracings can be avoided relatively easily (Fig. 12–6).

DEADSPACE ANALYSIS WITH EXHALED CARBON DIOXIDE

Deadspace data can be obtained using mixed exhaled CO_2 values combined with $P_{ET_{CO_2}}$ values to yield noninvasive assessment of V_D. In practical terms, the mixed exhaled P_{CO_2} values are better applied with Pa_{CO_2} values, but $P_{ET_{CO_2}}$ can be used as a substitute to provide continuous $\dot{V}_D$ analysis. If a patient develops a problem that may change the deadspace volume, i.e., a pulmonary embolus, the use of exhaled gas analysis can detect the problem earlier than all other clinical measurements commonly used. The formula for measuring V_D/V_T is:

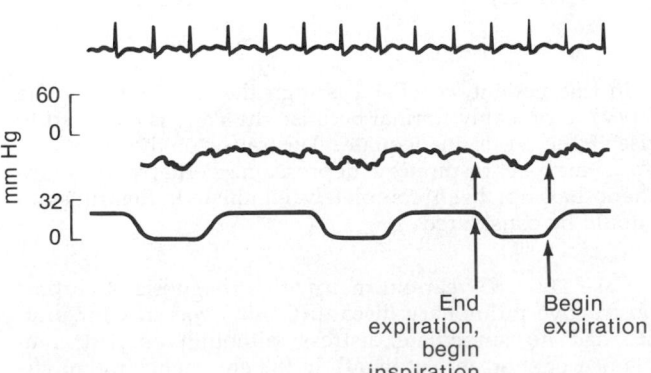

FIGURE 12–6. Use of capnogram in hemodynamic waveform analysis to identify end-exhalation.

$$\frac{Pa_{CO_2}}{Pa_{CO_2} - PE_{CO_2}}$$

The prime advantage of all exhaled gas analysis methods is the speed with which assessments can be made in regard to pulmonary gas exchange and blood flow. Questions exist about the cost effectiveness of these applications, and these can only be answered through further research. Empirically, exhaled gas analysis appears to have several specific and practical applications.

SUMMARY

Assessment of oxygenation and ventilation requires possession of substantial understanding of cardiopulmonary principles. The nurse must be able to distinguish oxygenation from intrapulmonary shunting and differentiate alveolar ventilation from oxygenation. To further the accomplishment of these skills, this chapter has presented concepts in oxygenation (i.e., oxygen transport and consumption), intrapulmonary shunting estimates, deadspace analysis, and exhaled gas analysis. Material necessary to expand one's knowledge of basic physiologic concepts and make more advanced assessments of oxygenation and ventilation has been presented.

References

Ahrens, T. S., and Rutherford, K. (1987). The new pulmonary math: Applying the a/A ratio. *American Journal of Nursing*, 87 (3), 337A–340H.

Astiz, M. E., Rachow, E. C., Kaufman, B., et al. (1988) Relationship of oxygen delivery and mixed venous oxygenation to lactic acidosis in patients with sepsis and acute myocardial infarction. *Critical Care Medicine*, 16 (7), 655–658.

Barker, S. J., and Tremper, K. K. (1987). Pulse oximetry: Applications and limitations. *International Anesthesiology Clinics*, 25 (3), 155–175.

Broder, G., and Weil, M. H. (1964). Excess lactate: An index of reversibility of shock in human patients. *Science*, 143, 1457–1459.

Bunn, H. F., and Forget, B. G. (1986). *Hemoglobin: Molecular, genetics, and clinical aspects*. Philadelphia: W. B. Saunders.

Cain, S. M. (1983). Peripheral oxygen uptake in health and disease. *Clinics in Chest Medicine*, 4, 139–148.

Cane, R. D., Shapiro, B. A., Templin, R., et al. (1988). Unreliability of oxygen derived tension based indices in reflecting intrapulmonary shunting in critically ill patients. *Critical Care Medicine*, 16 (12), 1243–1245.

Cheng, E. Y., Hopwood, M. B., and Kay, J. (1988). Forehead pulse oximetry compared with finger pulse oximetry and arterial blood gas measurement. *Journal of Clinical Monitoring*, 4 (3), 223–226.

Coveli, H. D., Nessan, V. J., and Tuttle, W. K. (1983). Oxygen derived variables in acute respiratory failure. *Critical Care Medicine*, 11 (8), 646–649.

Danek, S. J., Lynch, J. P., Weg, J. G., et al. (1980). The dependence of oxygen uptake on oxygen delivery in the acute respiratory distress syndrome. *American Review of Respiratory Disease*, 122, 387–395.

Gettinger, A., DeTraglia, M. C., and Glass, P. D. (1987). In vivo comparison of two mixed venous saturation catheters. *Anesthesiology*, 66, 373–375.

Gilbert, R., Auchincloss, J. H., Kuppinger, M., et al. (1979). Stability of the arterial/alveolar oxygen partial pressure ratio. *Critical Care Medicine*, 7 (6), 267–271.

Gilbert, R., and Keighley, J. F. (1974). The arterial/alveolar oxygen tension ratio. *American Review of Respiratory Disease*, 109, 144.

Gutierrez, G., and Pohil, R. (1986). Oxygen consumption is linearly related to O_2 supply in critically ill patients. *Journal of Critical Care*, 1 (1), 45–53.

King, T., and Simon, R. H. (1987). Pulse oximetry for tapering supplemental oxygen in hospitalized patients. *Chest*, 92 (4), 713–716.

Kruse, J. A., and Carlson, R. W. (1987). Lactate metabolism. *Critical Care Clinics*, 5 (4), 725–746.

Liggett, S. B., St. John, R. E., and Lefrak, S. S. (1986). Determination of resting energy expenditure utilizing the thermodilution pulmonary artery catheter. *Chest*, 91 (4), 562–566.

Millikan, G. A. (1942). The oximeter, an instrument for measuring continuously the oxygen saturation of arterial blood in man. *Review of Scientific Instruments*, 13, 434–444.

Mizock, B. A. (1987). Controversies in lactic acidosis. Implications in critically ill patients. *Journal of the American Medical Association*, 258 (4), 497–501.

Niehoff, J., DelGuercio, C., LaMorte, W., et al. (1988). Efficacy of pulse oximetry and capnometry in postoperative ventilatory weaning. *Critical Care Medicine*, 16, 701–705.

Peretz, D. I., Scott, H. M., Duff, J., et al. (1965). The significance of lactic acidemia in the shock syndrome. *Annals of the New York Academy of Sciences*, 119, 1133–1141.

Rasanen, J., Downs, J. B., Malec, D. J., et al. (1987). Estimation of oxygen utilization by dual oximetry. *Annals of Surgery*, 206 (5), 621–623.

Schweiss, J. F. (1987). Mixed venous hemoglobin saturation: Theory and application. *International Anesthesiology Clinics*, 25 (3), 113–136.

Shoemaker, W. C. (1989). Pathophysiology and fluid management of postoperative and post-traumatic ARDS. In W. C. Shoemaker, et al. (Eds.), *Textbook of critical care* (2nd ed., pp. 615–635). Philadelphia: W. B. Saunders.

Shoemaker, W. C., and Appel, P. L. (1985). Pathophysiology in adult respiratory distress syndrome following sepsis and surgical operations. *Critical Care Medicine*, 13, 166.

Stasic, A. F. (1986). Continuous evaluation of oxygenation and ventilation. In D. D. Civetta, and D. D. Taylor (Eds.), *Critical care*. Philadelphia: W. B. Saunders.

Stock, M. C. (1988). Noninvasive carbon dioxide monitoring. *Critical Care Clinics*, 4 (3), 511–526.

Synder, J. V., and Pinsky, M. R. (1987). *Oxygen transport in the critically ill*. Chicago: Year Book Medical Publishers.

Tremper, K. K., and Barker, S. J. (1989). Pulse oximetry. *Anesthesiology*, 70 (1), 98–108.

Ultman, J. S., and Bursztein, S. (1981). Analysis of error in determination of respiratory gas exchange at varying FI_{O_2}. *Journal of Applied Physiology*, 50 (1) 210–216.

Weil, M. H., Bisera, J., and Trevino, R. P., et al. (1985). Cardiac output and end-tidal carbon dioxide. *Critical Care Medicine*, 13, 907.

West, J. B. (1985). *Ventilation—Blood flow and gas exchange*. Boston: Blackwell Scientific Publications.

White, K. M. (1984). Completing the hemodynamic picture: Sv_{O_2}. *Heart & Lung*, 14 (3), 113–136.

Intracranial Pressure Monitoring

Christine R. Kraay

Intracranial pressure (ICP) is a dynamic process that is influenced by physiologic variables that affect the volume within the intracranial compartment. The major components of intracranial volume include the cerebrospinal fluid, intracranial blood volume, and brain tissue. The equilibrium pressure generated by the total volume within the confines of the intracranial compartment is referred to as the ICP. This pressure can be measured in the ventricles, in the subarachnoid, subdural, or epidural space, or in the brain parenchymal tissue. Normal intracranial pressure is between 0 and 15 mm Hg (Ricci, 1984; Saul, 1986). ICP values may vary slightly depending on the site of ICP monitoring, the location of the intracranial pathology, and the monitoring equipment utilized. Continuous ICP monitoring can serve as a guide for the diagnosis and continuing management of patients with increased ICP. The pathophysiologic basis of increased ICP as well as related assessment parameters will be reviewed in this chapter before the many techniques of ICP monitoring are described.

PHYSIOLOGY OF INTRACRANIAL PRESSURE

Intracranial Volume Relationships

In a normal adult, the total intracranial volume is approximately 1900 mL (Ricci, 1984). This volume includes the cerebrospinal fluid (CSF; approximately 10%), brain tissue with its associated intra- and extracellular fluid (approximately 80%), and the cerebral blood volume (CBV) contained within the venous, capillary, and arterial vessels (approximately

10%) (Hickey, 1986; Ricci, 1984; Rockoff and Kennedy, 1988). Changes in volume of any one of these components, if uncompensated for, will influence the ICP.

Observations relating to the intracranial volume relationships of the brain and blood volume were first reported in the late eighteenth and early nineteenth centuries by Alexander Monro and George Kellie. During the nineteenth and twentieth centuries the contribution of the CSF to intracranial volume was appreciated, and a greater understanding of the interrelationships among the brain, blood, and CSF volumes and their effects on ICP was achieved. The key principles governing the relationships between these volumes and changes in ICP have been referred to as the modified Monro-Kellie doctrine and can be summarized by the following points. The intracranial space is nearly constant in volume with essentially noncompressible contents (Langfitt, 1990). The intracranial components, including the blood, brain matter, and CSF, fill the skull to capacity. If any one of these components increases in volume, there must be a compensatory decrease in another for the overall volume to remain constant; otherwise, there will be an increase in ICP.

These principles apply primarily to rigid, fused skulls. In certain situations the intracranial space has a limited ability to respond to an increased volume by expansion of the skull, for example, in the infant before the sutures of the skull have fused, or in the patient with a skull fracture.

Physiologic Compensatory Response to Volume Changes

The first potential compensatory response to the need to accommodate increased volume is a reduction in the volume of the intracranial CSF. This occurs primarily through displacement or shunting of CSF from the intracranial space to the spinal subarachnoid space. Reduction in total CSF volume may also be achieved by increasing reabsorption of CSF through the arachnoid villi (Rockoff and Kennedy, 1988). CSF production, in most situations, is not significantly affected by volume or pressure changes except in severe cases, when cerebral blood flow is compromised (Sklar et al., 1980; Ward et al., 1987).

Another method of compensation involves displacement of the low-pressure venous blood volume out of the intracranial compartment (Rockoff and Kennedy, 1988). The ability of this response to compensate for an increase in volume is limited, however, by the relatively low volume of venous blood. At some point, the compensatory mechanisms involving CSF and blood volume will be exhausted, and ICP will begin to rise (Fig. 13–1).

FACTORS INFLUENCING ABILITY TO COMPENSATE

Many factors can influence the effectiveness of this intracranial compensation. These factors include the rate of expansion of the mass, the location of the mass or volume in the intracranial compartment, impairment of CSF dynamics, and brain compliance (Ricci, 1984).

Rate of Expansion in Intracranial Volume. An increase in volume that occurs over a long period of time can be compensated for more completely than a rapid increase of the same volume. For example, a patient with an acute epidural hematoma may develop markedly increased intracranial pressure, whereas a patient with a slowly growing brain tumor of similar size may have a normal or slightly increased ICP.

Location of Mass or Lesion. The location of the mass lesion can also influence the ability of the brain to compensate for a change in volume within the intracranial compartment. Intracranial lesions at different sites may result in direct or indirect obstruction of CSF pathways through distortion of brain tissue, limiting the compensatory mechanism of CSF displacement (Langfitt, 1990). For example, a large tumor of the third ventricle, in addition to increasing brain volume, may obstruct normal CSF circulation, resulting in increased ICP with minimal compensatory ability.

Impaired CSF Drainage or Reabsorption. CSF drainage and reabsorption can also be limited by obstruction or inflammation of the arachnoid villi. A complication of subarachnoid hemorrhage is hydrocephalus resulting from blood obstructing the arachnoid villi. CNS infections such as meningitis may also result in increased ICP due to inflammation of the meningeal layers and secondary obstruction of the arachnoid villi (Rockoff and Kennedy, 1988).

COMPLIANCE

Compliance (C) refers to the ratio of the change (Δ) in volume (V) to the resulting change in pressure (P). It is a measure of the amount of "give" in the system (Langfitt, 1990). When compliance is high, larger volume changes can occur without causing a significant change in ICP. Conversely, when compliance is low, any small increase in intracranial volume results in a marked increase in intracranial pressure. The following formula represents this relationship:

$$C = \frac{\Delta V}{\Delta P}$$

In the clinical setting, compliance testing can be

FIGURE 13–1. Physiologic compensatory response to intracranial volume changes. In this figure, "volume mass" indicates any additional volume in the intracranial compartment that is not normally present. This may include additional brain tissue, blood, or CSF volume. (Redrawn from Ward, J.D., et al. (1981). Intracranial pressure, head injuries, subarachnoid hemorrhage, non-surgical coma, and brain tumors. In W.C. Shoemaker and W.L. Thompson (Eds.), *Critical care, state of the art* (Vol. II, p. 2). Fullerton, CA: Society of Critical Care Medicine.)

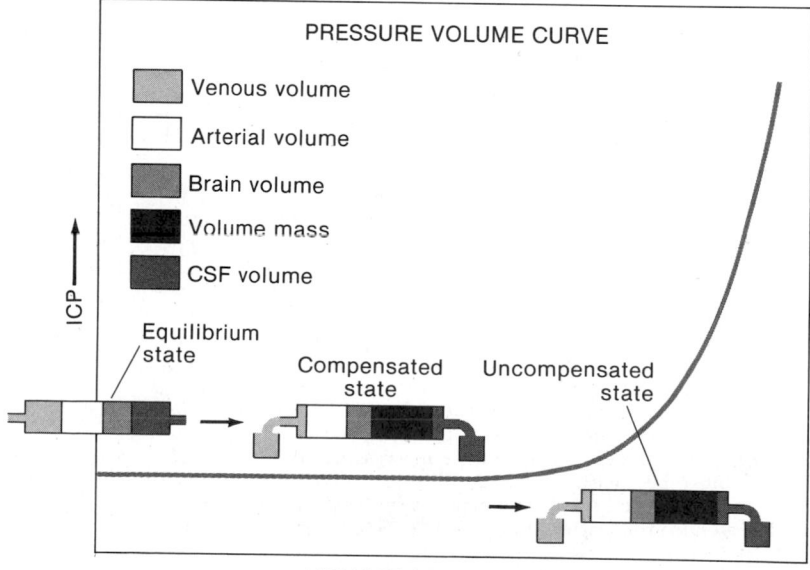

PRESSURE VOLUME CURVE

- Venous volume
- Arterial volume
- Brain volume
- Volume mass
- CSF volume

ICP

Equilibrium state

Compensated state

Uncompensated state

VOLUME OF MASS ⟶

performed by a physician utilizing the technique described in Figure 13–2.

Elastance is the inverse of compliance and describes the amount of resistance offered to expansion of the mass (Langfitt, 1990). A diagrammatic representation of this pressure volume relationship is included in Figure 13–1. As illustrated in the initial portion of the curve, a small increase in volume does not result in an increase in pressure because compensatory mechanisms are effective and compliance is high. When the compensatory mechanisms are exhausted and compliance decreases, any addition in volume will result in a sharp increase in pressure. The precise shape of the curve and the point at which an additional increase in volume results in a sharp increase in pressure varies with the individual patient and the pathophysiologic condition.

Cerebral Blood Flow

The brain demands a constant supply of oxygen, glucose, and other metabolic substrates for cellular oxygenation and metabolism in the brain. An understanding of the factors that influence cerebral blood

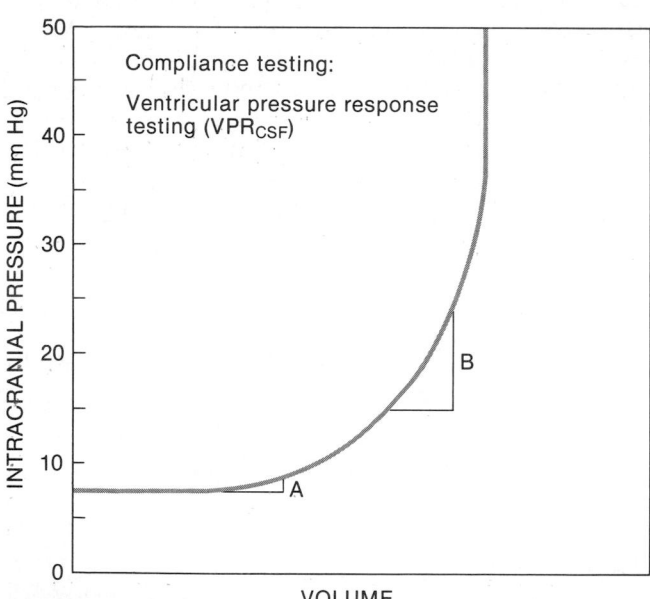

FIGURE 13–2. Compliance testing: (1) A baseline ICP reading is obtained and recorded.* (2) 1 mL of sterile saline is injected into the ventricular catheter within 1 second. (3) ICP readings are then obtained.* (4) Interpretation of data is based on the change in ICP in response to additional 1 mL of volume. If the resulting pressure change is less than or equal to 4 mm Hg *(A)*, compliance is high and functional compensatory mechanisms are present. If there is an increase in ICP greater than 4 mm Hg *(B)*, this is indicative of low compliance and poor compensatory reserve (Pollack-Latham, 1987).

Note: It is recommended that a test dose of 0.2 mL of sterile normal saline be injected prior to the complete 1-mL injection (Hickey, 1986). If there is no change in pressure, the additional 0.8 mL may be quickly injected. This precaution will prevent unnecessary pressure spikes in a patient with very low compliance.

(Redrawn from Pollack-Latham, C. L. (1987). *Critical Care Nurse*, 7(5), 40–51.)

flow is essential because an increase in cerebral blood flow results in an increase in cerebral blood volume and an increased ICP. Variables that have a significant effect on cerebral blood flow include the following: metabolic demands of the brain, the influence of ICP reflected in the cerebral perfusion pressure, and the influence of arterial blood gas parameters and systemic blood pressure on autoregulatory mechanisms.

METABOLIC DEMANDS

The first variable, metabolic demands, is determined by the relative neuronal activity in the brain (Ward et al., 1987). Cerebral blood flow varies with the functional activity level of the brain, and blood flow increases as activity increases. In conditions in which metabolic demands are increased, such as during seizure activity or febrile episodes, there is a corresponding increase in cerebral blood flow. Conditions that decrease metabolic demands and thus cerebral blood flow include barbiturate therapy and hypothermia.

CEREBRAL PERFUSION PRESSURE

Cerebral perfusion pressure (CPP) is a calculated value that may be used as a guide in reflecting the adequacy of cerebral blood flow. This value incorporates the influence of ICP on cerebral blood flow and is calculated by subtracting the mean ICP from the mean arterial pressure (MAP). For example, a patient with a MAP of 90 and an ICP of 10 would have a CPP of 80. An example of how this calculated value is obtained is shown by this equation:

$$MAP\ (90) - ICP\ (10) = CPP\ (80)$$

A normal range for CPP is approximately 70 to 100 mm Hg (Smith, 1983; Rockoff and Kennedy, 1988). A CPP of at least 50 to 60 mm Hg is necessary for adequate cerebral perfusion. Ischemia and neuronal death may be seen when CPP falls below 30 to 40 mm Hg (Jennet et al., 1970). A word of caution is in order when assessing the CPP of head-injured patients. These patients may appear to maintain an adequate CPP (>50 mm Hg) by calculations based on MAP and ICP; however, this may not reflect problems with inadequate perfusion to regions of the brain that have been injured. For this reason, in head-injured patients, adequate cerebral perfusion cannot be ensured for all regions of the brain based solely on the calculation of cerebral perfusion pressure values.

AUTOREGULATION

Autoregulation refers to the ability to maintain a relatively constant cerebral blood flow (CBF) over a wide range of CPP, arterial blood pressures, and metabolic conditions. Autoregulatory control is achieved by initiating a change in cerebral vascular resistance, which regulates cerebral blood flow in the absence of severe brain injury.

Metabolic Autoregulation. Metabolic autoregulation maintains a relatively constant CBF with Pa_{O_2} greater than 50 mm Hg. Profound hypoxia or Pa_{O_2} less than 50 mm Hg will result in cerebral vasodilation and increased CBF (Rockoff and Kennedy, 1988). Cerebral blood flow is very sensitive to changes in P_{CO_2}. From approximately 20 to 80 mm Hg, cerebral vasodilation occurs, and CBF increases with an increasing P_{CO_2} (Rockoff and Kennedy, 1988). In contrast, a decreased P_{CO_2} results in vasoconstriction and decreased cerebral blood volume. This is the basis for therapeutic hyperventilation of a patient with increased ICP to maintain a P_{CO_2} of between 25 and 35 mm Hg.

Pressure Autoregulation. Cerebral blood flow is constant in healthy adults with a MAP ranging from approximately 60 to 160 mm Hg and a CPP of between 50 and 150 mm Hg due to pressure autoregulatory mechanisms maintained in part through control of arteriolar resistance (Rockoff and Kennedy, 1988). As perfusion pressure decreases, cerebral vessels dilate to maintain a relatively constant cerebral blood flow. When perfusion pressure increases, cerebral vasoconstriction occurs, and cerebral blood flow is maintained within a normal range. With a MAP of less than 60 or greater than 160 mm Hg, or a CPP of less than 50 or greater than 150 mm Hg, autoregulation may cease to function, and cerebral blood flow may become passively dependent on changes in systemic arterial pressure (Rockoff and Kennedy, 1988). If this pathologic state begins, an increase in MAP will result in increased cerebral blood flow, increased cerebral blood volume, and further increases in ICP. As the MAP falls to less than 60 mm Hg, cerebral blood flow will continue to decrease, resulting in eventual neuronal hypoxia and cell death.

ETIOLOGY OF INCREASED INTRACRANIAL PRESSURE

Multiple etiologies and pathophysiologic conditions are associated with increased intracranial pressure (Table 13–1). Many of these are discussed in detail in Chapters 32, 33, and 37 in this text. To facilitate an understanding of the primary mechanisms resulting in increased ICP, the more common etiologies and general conditions associated with increased ICP will be reviewed in relation to their potential effects on increases in brain volume, blood volume, or the volume of CSF. Various conditions associated with increased ICP have more than one mechanism through which the increase in ICP can occur. For example, mechanisms resulting in increased ICP associated with a brain tumor may be the mass effect (increased brain tissue volume), cer-

TABLE 13–1. Factors Associated with Increased Intracranial Pressure

Influence on Intracranial Volume	Associated Factors
Increased total brain volume	Mass lesions 　Brain tumors 　Intracranial hematomas 　Abscesses Cerebral edema
Increased intravascular blood volume	Cerebral vasodilation 　Hypoxia, hypercapnia 　Increased metabolic demands 　Drug effect Venous outflow obstruction 　Head position 　　Hyperextension, flexion, rotation 　Circumferential ties around neck 　Positive end-expiratory pressure 　　(PEEP) 　Valsalva maneuver Other 　Endotracheal suctioning
Increased cerebrospinal fluid volume	Increased CSF production 　Choroid plexus papilloma Decreased CSF reabsorption 　Communicating hydrocephalus CSF outflow obstruction 　Obstructive hydrocephalus

ebral edema (increased brain tissue volume), obstruction to cerebrospinal fluid circulation (increased CSF), and even increased blood volume varying with the vascularity of the tumor.

Increases in Total Brain Tissue Volume

Mass Lesions. Increases in brain tissue volume can result from a number of conditions. Neoplasms, including primary brain tumors, as well as metastatic tumors, produce a mass effect resulting in an increase in total brain volume. Space-occupying mass lesions may result from any subdural, epidural, or intracerebral hematoma that may occur spontaneously or as a result of head trauma. A cyst, abscess, or any other space-occupying lesion may also result in increased intracranial pressure.

Cerebral Edema. Cerebral edema refers to an abnormal accumulation of water or fluid in the intracellular space or extracellular space that results in an increase in brain tissue volume. This edema can be vasogenic, cytotoxic, or interstitial. The specific types of cerebral edema are further discussed in Chapter 32 of this text.

Increased Intravascular Blood Volume

Venous Outflow Obstruction. Increased intrathoracic or intra-abdominal pressures may result in impaired venous return from the intracranial compartment. Because there are no valves in the central venous system, this pressure is transmitted through the great veins, resulting in impaired venous return. The Valsalva maneuver, coughing, vomiting, or positive end-expiratory pressure (PEEP) may cause this phenomenon. Additional research has also demonstrated that hyperextension or hyperflexion of the head may cause compression or extrinsic pressure on the great veins of the neck resulting in venous engorgement and decreased venous return from the intracranial compartment (Boortz-Marx, 1985; Parsons and Wilson, 1984).

Cerebral Vasodilation. Cerebral vasodilation results in increased cerebral blood volume and increased ICP. As described previously, hypoventilation leading to increasing P_{CO_2} results in cerebral vasodilation. Hypoxia also results in vasodilation if the Pa_{O_2} is less than 50 to 60 mm Hg. In addition, certain anesthetic agents such as halothane, ketamine, and nitrous oxide result in cerebral vasodilation and thus should be avoided in patients at risk of increased ICP (Eichelberger, 1985). Nitroprusside also may cause vasodilation and should be used with caution in patients at risk for increased ICP (Nikas, 1991).

Increased Volume of Cerebrospinal Fluid

Conditions that affect CSF production, absorption, and circulation may also result in increased ICP. A choroid plexus papilloma may result in increased CSF production, although this condition is rare. Subarachnoid hemorrhage or inflammatory meningitis may result in obstruction of the arachnoid villi leading to decreased CSF reabsorption and communicating hydrocephalus. Any condition that obstructs the normal CSF circulation pathway may result in noncommunicating or obstructive hydrocephalus and increased ICP due to increased CSF volume in one location.

NEUROLOGIC ASSESSMENT

In any patient with known or suspected increased intracranial pressure, the neurologic examination is an essential component of patient management. Although ICP monitoring is the most precise method of assessing ICP, it is not practical or feasible in all patients. If ICP monitoring is implemented, the data from the neurologic assessment will supplement the data obtained with ICP monitoring. The presenting signs and symptoms will vary with the location of the mass or lesion, the degree of intracranial compensation, and the effect of the lesion on cerebral perfusion pressure or brain tissue distortion. Many of the neurologic signs and symptoms associated with increased ICP are not due to increased ICP alone but to distortion and shifting of brain tissue in response to the underlying lesion. Signs and symptoms that may be indicative of increasing ICP include decreased level of consciousness, headache, vomiting, papilledema, pupillary dysfunction or visual abnormalities, motor or sensory dysfunction, and alterations in vital signs or respiratory patterns. Although any of these signs and symptoms may alert the caregiver to the possibility of increased ICP, the presence or progression of these signs and symptoms does not always indicate or parallel an increasing ICP.

Potential Signs and Symptoms Associated with Increased Intracranial Pressure

Decreased Level of Consciousness. Change in the level of consciousness is considered to be one of the most sensitive, reliable, and earliest indicators of neurologic deterioration (Rudy, 1984). This change may be caused by interference with functioning of the reticular activating system at the level of the diencephalon or high midbrain. Decreased level of consciousness may also be due to cerebral hypoxia secondary to decreased cerebral blood flow. Early changes reflecting a decreased level of consciousness may include confusion, restlessness, or lethargy. As the patient's condition deteriorates, these symptoms may progress to eventual coma. The Glasgow Coma Scale is an assessment tool that has become widely used to describe and document consistently changes in the level of consciousness. It is essential to identify very subtle changes in the level of consciousness as early as possible.

Headache. Headache has been an associated symptom of increased intracranial pressure. The pain-sensitive structures within the intracranial compartment include the middle meningeal artery and its branches, the large arteries at the base of the brain, the sinuses and bridging veins, and the dura at the base of the cranial fossae (Langfitt, 1990). Headache that occurs with increased intracranial pressure is generally due to displacement or traction on bridging cerebral vessels, stretching of the arteries, and pressure on the dura at the base of the skull. The headache is generally reported to be most severe on awakening in the morning (Langfitt, 1990). Nurses should recognize the request for pain medication by patients with intracranial pathology to be a potential indication of increasing ICP. A careful neurologic assessment should be done when these patients report headache pain.

Pupillary Changes. Pupillary changes in patients with increased ICP are a reflection of tissue shifts, which may result in compression of the oculomotor nerve (cranial nerve III) or distortion of the midbrain. When pupillary changes occur they are often associated with high ICPs of greater than 28 to 34 mm Hg, or they may be a relatively late sign of increasing ICP (Rockoff and Kennedy, 1983). However, pupillary changes have been reported in patients with intracranial pressure as low as 14 mm Hg, depending on the location of the lesion, and they are especially common in patients with middle fossa or medial temporal lobe lesions, which may cause early midbrain or oculomotor nerve compression (Marshall et al., 1986; Ropper, 1985).

Motor Function Changes. In the earlier stages of increased ICP, hemiparesis may develop contralateral to the intracranial mass due to pressure on the motor tracts. In the later stages, hemiplegia, decortication, or decerebration may occur as a result of increasing pressure on the brainstem (Hickey, 1986).

Papilledema. Papilledema is edema of the optic disc resulting from compression on the optic nerve that may be seen in patients with increased ICP (Langfitt, 1990). It may be detected during the ophthalmoscopic evaluation of the patient. It appears as a blurring of the disc margins due to engorgement and swelling of the disc vessels and elevation of the disc margins. Papilledema is generally a late sign of increased ICP. It is not seen in all patients but may be one of the first signs of increased ICP in patients in whom increased ICP has developed gradually (Hickey, 1986).

Vital Sign Changes. Abnormalities of respiratory rate and rhythm may be the first change in vital signs in a patient with increased ICP. These respiratory changes may not be evident, however, until several hours after an increase in ICP, and the specific respiratory pattern changes do not correlate consistently with increasing ICP (Ropper, 1985).

The Cushing response of bradycardia, increasing systolic pressure, and widening pulse pressure has been associated with increasing ICP. This mechanism is felt to be one of the body's final compensatory mechanisms to maintain adequate cerebral blood flow. In recent studies this response has been reported as a late sign of increasing ICP and has been reported in less than 30% of patients with increased ICP (Ropper, 1985; Marshall et al., 1978). In the final decompensatory stages of increased ICP, hypotension and tachycardia may be observed.

Although the neurologic assessment is very important in the patient with or at risk of increased ICP, it is often unreliable as an early indicator of this condition. These findings support the role of direct ICP monitoring as an important tool in the early detection and management of increased ICP.

INTRACRANIAL PRESSURE MONITORING

In 1960 Lundberg published the results of his experience with ICP monitoring utilizing a ventricular catheter in a series of 143 patients with a variety of neurosurgical problems (Lundberg, 1960). This report has been cited as a major landmark in our understanding of the clinical significance of ICP monitoring as well as in establishing the safety and feasibility of ICP monitoring (Barnett and Chapman, 1988). Since 1960, many new methods of ICP monitoring have been introduced. The indications for and the many techniques used for ICP monitoring will be reviewed next, focusing on the advantages and disadvantages of each technique.

Indications for ICP Monitoring

Many neurologic disorders place patients at risk for development of increased ICP. This, in addition to the fact that neurologic signs and symptoms alone may be unreliable indicators of increased ICP, has warranted consideration of ICP monitoring in patients who have evidence of or are at significant risk for the development of increased ICP. ICP monitoring, however, is not indicated for every patient. Although complications related to ICP monitoring are infrequent, monitoring does carry some degree of risk. Many authorities, therefore, have addressed the question of which patients require ICP monitoring. Some state simply that ICP monitoring should be used when the risks of not monitoring outweigh the risks of monitoring (Ward et al., 1987). More objective indications include disease processes that are known to be associated with a significant incidence of intracranial hypertension and are amenable to medical therapies. Additional indications include situations in which the neurologic examination is either ineffective, insensitive, or equivocal, as in the pavulonized or paralyzed patient. Finally, in patients who exhibit clinical signs of increased ICP, ICP monitoring serves as a method for documenting clinical suspicion and evaluating the effectiveness of therapy (Ward et al., 1987).

Rockoff and Kennedy (1988) suggest that the intracranial dynamics of many of the conditions that can result in increased ICP should be considered in deciding which patients require ICP monitoring. Chronic slow changes in ICP are better tolerated than acute changes. Pressure equilibrium or high but equal pressures on both sides of the tentorium, as in communicating hydrocephalus or pseudotumor cerebri, are better tolerated than unequal transtentorial pressures, as with a mass lesion that can result in herniation. In a young child, open fontanelles and separated sutures may delay some of the deleterious effects of increased ICP (Rockoff and Kennedy, 1988).

Features that are strongly associated with intracranial hypertension in head-injured patients include lesions visible on computed tomography (CT) scan at the time of admission as well as two or more of the following features in patients with no visible lesion on admission: age greater than 40 years, systolic blood pressure under 90 mm Hg, and motor posturing (Narayan et al., 1982). Some authorities have found a correlation between a low Glasgow Coma Scale score (<7) and intracranial hypertension (Bruce et al., 1977), whereas others have not found this correlation (Narayan et al., 1982).

In summary, the decision to monitor ICP is not based on one set of absolute criteria. It is a subjective decision made by the physician based on the patient's history, clinical diagnosis, presentation, and plan of therapy.

Techniques for Measurement of Intracranial Pressure

ICP monitoring systems most commonly used today involve the use of a sensor or transducer to pick up mechanical (pressure) impulses and convert them to electrical impulses. In addition, a monitor or recording device, preferably with an oscilloscopic display, is required to convert these impulses into visible signals. ICP is usually measured in the supratentorial space with potential sites for ICP monitoring being the lateral ventricles, the subarachnoid, subdural, or epidural space, or the brain parenchymal tissue (Fig. 13–3). Ideally, all of these pressures should be approximately the same. However, with certain pathophysiologic conditions there may be slight variations in values depending on the location of the monitoring device. Normal intracranial pressure varies from 0 to 15 mm Hg.

BASIC SYSTEMS FOR ICP MONITORING

Before each of the available ICP monitoring devices is described, it is helpful to understand the two primary categories of ICP monitoring devices. The first group includes those devices that utilize fluid or hydrostatic coupling to transmit the reflected ICP to an extracranial transducer. This group includes the traditional ventricular catheters, subarachnoid bolts or screws, and the subdural catheters. The second group includes monitoring devices that directly monitor ICP using an intracranial membrane or transducer. These intracranial transducers use such things as fiberoptics, pneumatic systems, or intracranial strain gauges to transmit pressures. ICP may be monitored in any of the potential intracranial locations according to the specific device utilized.

PRINCIPLES OF CALIBRATION OF INTRACRANIAL PRESSURE MONITORING SYSTEMS

ICP is a relative value, obtained in reference to atmospheric pressure. The point at which the atmospheric reference is made is referred to as the "zero" point. The technique of referencing the transducer to atmospheric pressure is referred to as "zeroing the transducer." For fluid-coupled systems utilizing external transducers, hydrostatic forces dictate that the position of the transducer when the reference is made as well as when readings are obtained must remain constant in relation to a specific point on the patient's head. For intracranial pressure monitoring, this reference point is the inferred anatomic level of the foramen of Monro. Some clinicians identify this site as a point lateral to the outer canthus of the eye or the top of the ear, whereas others utilize the external auditory meatus as a reference point (Barnett and Chapman, 1988). Whichever point is used, consistency is essential when fluid-coupled systems are used because a 1.38-cm variation in the reference point can result in a 1-mm Hg change in the measured pressure due to hydrostatic effects (Barnett and Chapman, 1988). Any change in the height of the patient's head in respect to the transducer requires the transducer to be leveled to the anatomic reference point and ideally zeroed to atmospheric pressure prior to obtaining readings to ensure the highest accuracy.

In ICP monitoring systems utilizing intracranial transducers that do not depend on fluid-coupling effects, the atmospheric reference point is constant at the position of the transducer. Since the transducer is in the catheter tip, repeated leveling to an external site is not necessary. In using intracranial transducers, this zero point may be defined in reference to atmospheric pressure either prior to insertion of the device, or, with some monitors, "in vivo" calibration may be performed. The ability to reference the transducer to atmosphere in vivo ensures the greatest accuracy over time because the atmospheric reference can be recalibrated periodically during ICP monitoring. If in vivo calibration is not possible, the transducer is referenced once to atmospheric pressure prior to insertion. In this situation there is, however, no method of assessing for any slight drift

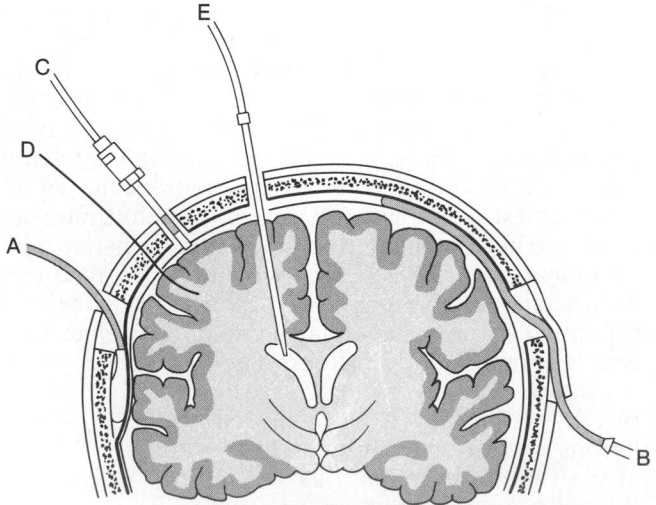

FIGURE 13–3. Coronal section of brain showing potential sites for placement of ICP monitoring devices. *A,* Epidural. *B,* Subdural. *C,* Subarachnoid. *D,* Intraparenchymal. *E,* Intraventricular.

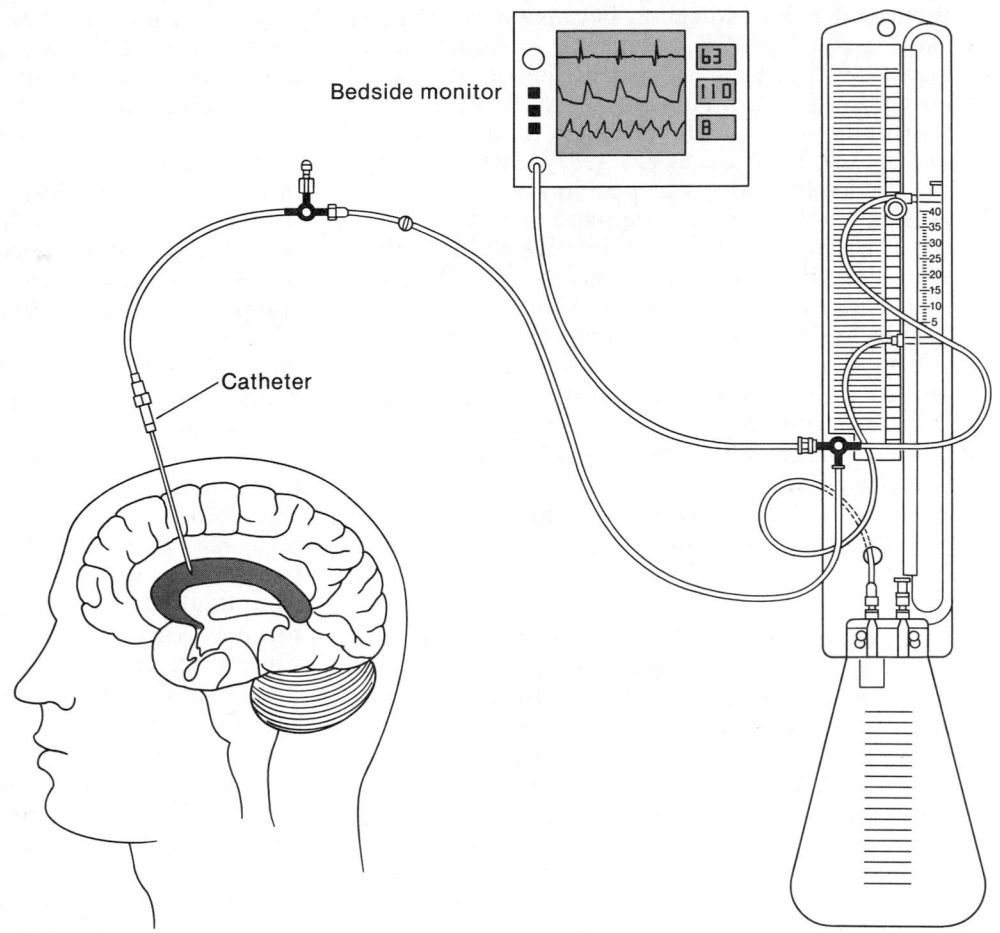

Bedside monitor

Catheter

FIGURE 13–4. Intraventricular catheter attached to closed system for ICP monitoring and CSF drainage.

or variation of the atmospheric reference following insertion.

EXTERNAL TRANSDUCER SYSTEMS

Devices that couple ICP to an external transducer system through a fluid-filled pressure tubing have been commonly used as ICP monitoring devices. Advantages of this type of a system include simplicity, low cost, familiarity, and compatibility with existing monitoring equipment.

Ventricular Catheter. The ventricular catheter was the first device utilized for ICP monitoring (Lundberg, 1960). It has been proved to be clinically reliable and accurate and is the current standard against which other methods are compared (Barnett and Chapman, 1988; Ward et al., 1987). The intraventricular catheter is a soft catheter made of radiopaque Silastic. A wire stylet is introduced into the catheter while it is being inserted to stiffen the catheter. The stylet is then removed following insertion. The catheter is inserted through a twist drill hole through the skull, usually into the anterior horn of the lateral ventricle in the nondominant hemisphere (Silverberg, 1985). Placement of the catheter is guided by

anatomic landmarks and is confirmed by the drainage of CSF and the presence of an appropriate ICP waveform on the monitor. Some institutions utilize a method of tunneling the catheter from the point of exit from the skull to a different point of exit from the scalp in an effort to reduce the incidence of infection (Friedman and Vries, 1980). Following insertion, the catheter is connected to a closed fluid-filled system. There are many systems available with similar basic features. These include a proximal stopcock or sampling port and a more distal stopcock that allows communication with either an external transducer for ICP monitoring or a collection system for CSF drainage (Fig. 13–4). Accuracy in ICP readings is ensured by using the shortest possible length of tubing between the catheter and the transducer and eliminating air bubbles in the system.

Advantages of the ventricular catheter include accuracy, reliability, and the capability to therapeutically drain CSF and control ICP. It can also be used for CSF sampling, for insertion of contrast medium in diagnostic studies, and for compliance testing. An additional advantage is its capability of being zeroed as necessary to avoid inaccurate ICP values due to drift of the zero reference point.

Disadvantages of the ventricular catheter include

an increased risk of infection because it is the most invasive method of ICP monitoring. Insertion of the ventricular catheter also carries the risk of intracranial hemorrhage. The catheter may be difficult to insert in a patient with small ventricles or a significant intracranial shift (Ward et al., 1987). The sensitivity of this device to changes in position of the patient's head is also a relative disadvantage of this system.

Of particular importance in the care of the patient with an intraventricular catheter is the need to maintain a closed system and the need to use meticulous technique in caring for the system to minimize risk of infection. If CSF specimens are obtained, a well-controlled protocol for collection of these specimens is essential. This includes maintaining sterile technique and collecting the specimens by passive flow, preventing negative pressure against the ventricles. Details of the maintenance and monitoring of a ventricular drainage system are discussed later in this chapter.

Subarachnoid Bolt or Screw. A less invasive technique using a fluid-coupled system is the subarachnoid bolt or screw (Fig. 13–5). There are many variations of this device, most of which use a hollow metal shaft or screw that is threaded at one end (Landy and Villanueva, 1984; Vries et al., 1973). The insertion site is generally in the frontal area over the nondominant hemisphere. The landmarks for the ventricular catheter may be utilized in some situations, allowing for use of this site if a ventricular catheter is needed later (Barnett and Chapman, 1988). The screw or bolt is inserted through a one-quarter inch twist drill hole in the skull until it protrudes through the dura into the subarachnoid space (Ward et al., 1987). The proximal end of the screw lies in direct communication with the subarachnoid space.

After insertion, the hollow screw or bolt is hydrostatically coupled to a fluid-filled tubing, a stopcock, and an external transducer.

The advantages of this device are its simplicity as well as its relative ease and speed of insertion. This device can be utilized in patients with small, shifted, or collapsed ventricles. In addition, it is less invasive than the ventricular catheter, and there is no disruption of the brain parenchyma. These factors contribute to a decreased risk of infection and hemorrhage compared with the ventricular catheter.

Disadvantages of the subarachnoid bolt or screw include decreased reliability and accuracy of ICP measurements due to possible "microleaks" in the system or obstruction of the device by blood or edematous brain tissue (Vries et al., 1973). Some of these problems can be identified by dampened ICP waveforms. Despite the fact that the risk of infection is decreased compared with the ventricular catheter, there still remains a risk of infection. CSF drainage from the bolt or screw is not recommended because this may result in occlusion of the device. In addition, compliance testing cannot be performed with this device. Some previously designed metallic screws, specifically ferrous compounds, were not totally compatible with magnetic resonance (MR) imaging because of the strong magnetic field (Barnett and Chapman, 1988). It is, therefore, important to know the composition of the bolt being used and whether it is MR compatible.

Troubleshooting of the system includes checking all connections for potential leaks that may contribute to dampened waveforms. Obstructions may be cleared from the system by the physician with intermittent flushes of 0.1 mL of preservative-free saline or other antibiotic flush solution (Barnett and Chapman, 1988).

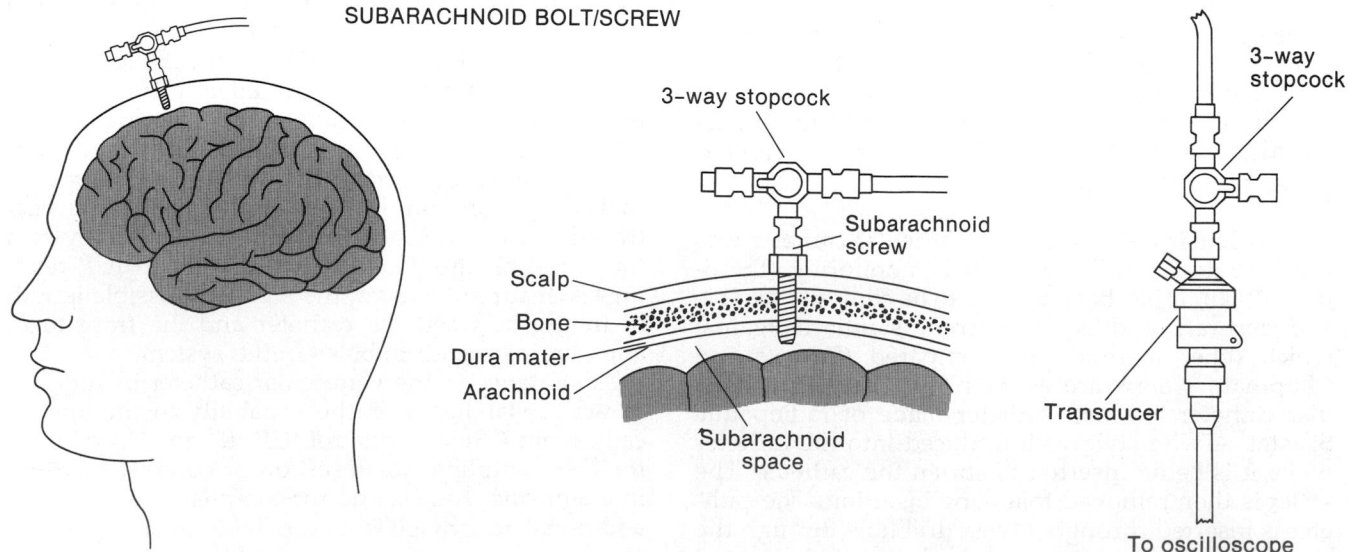

FIGURE 13–5. Subarachnoid bolt pressure monitoring. The subarachnoid bolt is inserted through a burr hole in the skull and is attached to a transducer and oscilloscope for continuous ICP monitoring. (Redrawn by permission from Rudy, E. *Advanced neurological and neurosurgical nursing.* St. Louis, 1984, The C.V. Mosby Co.)

Subdural Catheters. Another method of monitoring ICP through an external transducer involves the use of a catheter placed in the subdural space. Various types of catheters have been placed in the subdural space including red rubber catheters or ventricular catheters, which are then fluid-coupled to a transducer system. Wilkinson (1977) described the use of a ribbon-shaped Silastic catheter with a distal indented cavity or cup on one surface that faces the arachnoid membrane of the brain and communicates with a saline-filled lumen (Fig. 13–6). This catheter is called a subdural cup catheter and has been primarily designed for use following a craniotomy, although it can also be inserted through a burr hole (Wilkinson, 1977). The design of the catheter allows it to be passed through a subcutaneous scalp incision and tunneled to a location away from the point of entry into the subdural space (Wilkinson, 1977). Following insertion, this catheter is then connected to fluid-filled pressure tubing and a transducer.

Advantages of this type of catheter include the fact that it is one of the least invasive methods for ICP monitoring and results in a very low incidence of complications of infection or hemorrhage. The device itself is relatively inexpensive and can be used with most currently available electronic pressure transducers in critical care settings.

Disadvantages of this catheter include the fact that small leaks or air in the system or obstruction of the catheter lumen may cause a dampened waveform and inaccurate readings, which are generally lower than the true ICP. In addition, CSF drainage and compliance testing are not possible.

To maintain this system, Wilkinson (1977) recommends that a small amount of sterile solution (0.1 to 0.25 mL) be injected at 2-hour intervals through a stopcock to replace any fluid leakage from the distal cup. This practice is controversial and in some institutions may be performed only by a physician. If this

practice is followed, a closed system should be maintained to prevent possible contamination. A closed system utilizing a series of stopcocks, an attached reservoir containing flush solution, and a 1-mL Luer lock syringe utilized for injecting the solution has been recommended by some institutions (Price, 1981; Smith, 1987). To obtain accurate readings the system should be zeroed and calibrated frequently.

INTRACRANIAL TRANSDUCER SYSTEMS

The direct hydrostatic coupling of the intracranial space with an external transducer common to each of the ICP monitoring techniques described so far has some principal disadvantages. These include increased risk of infection through the fluid-filled column and the potential for inaccurate ICP readings due to factors that can interrupt the fluid column. In addition, the need to level the transducer and zero the system with any change in position of the patient's head relative to the transducer is a disadvantage. To avoid these problems, a variety of instruments have been designed that utilize an intracranial transducer system.

Fiberoptic Monitoring Devices. A fiberoptic transducer-tipped disposable catheter is available for ICP monitoring. This type of catheter uses sophisticated fiberoptic technology, which receives information from a transducer located in the tip of the catheter. Within the transducer, movement of a mirrored diaphragm in response to pressure is sensed by light fibers (Hollingsworth-Fridlund et al., 1988). This information is converted into a signal in the amplifier connector, which is based on a precalibrated relationship between the amount of reflected light and the corresponding ICP (Fig. 13–7). The appropriate ICP value is then displayed on a compatible digital monitor. The monitor can "interface with conventional bedside monitoring systems for oscilloscopic display

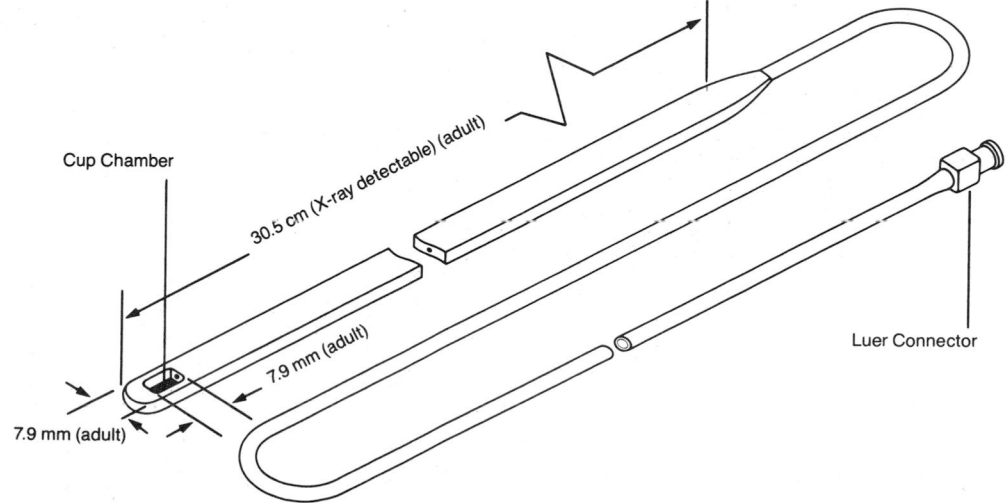

FIGURE 13–6. Subdural cup catheter. This catheter is hydrostatically coupled to an external transducer for use as an ICP monitoring device. The distal portion of the device is ribbon shaped with a central lumen connected to an indented cup near the tip. The proximal tube ends in a Luer connector. When the catheter is in place, the open side of the cup communicates with the arachnoid membrane. (By permission of Cordis Corporation, Miami, FL.)

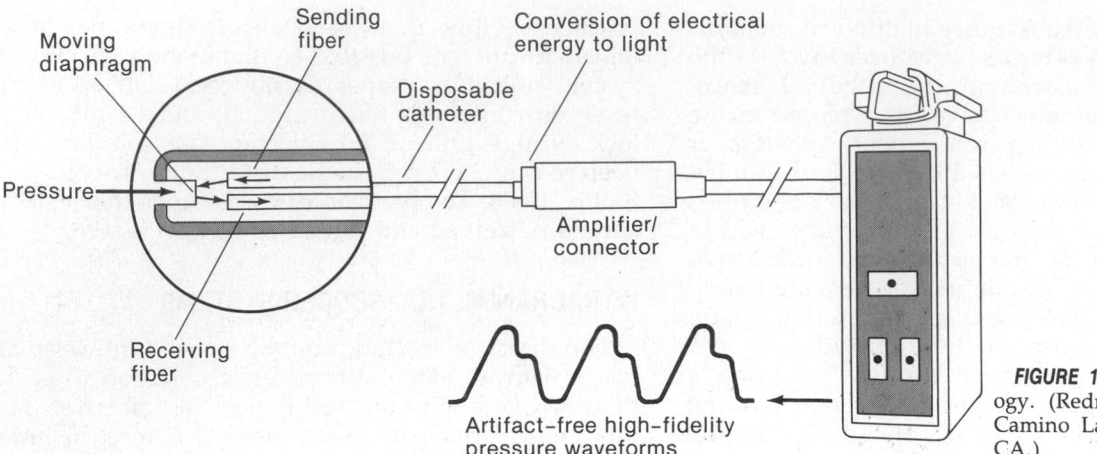

FIGURE 13–7. Fiberoptic technology. (Redrawn by permission of Camino Laboratories, San Diego, CA.)

and paper readout of the waveform and pressure value (Hollingsworth-Fridlund et al., 1988).

This fiberoptic catheter has been utilized for ICP monitoring at various locations including intraventricular, subarachnoid, subdural, and intraparenchymal sites. With intraventricular pressure monitoring, the fiberoptic-tipped catheter is inserted into a ventriculostomy catheter up to the point at which there is a sharp angular bend in the ventricular catheter. A Y-connector at the proximal end of the catheter allows CSF drainage through one port and ICP monitoring through the other (Fig. 13–8) (Hollingsworth-Fridlund et al., 1988).

The fiberoptic transducer-tipped catheter can also be inserted through a subarachnoid bolt with the tip of the catheter extending just slightly beyond the tip of the bolt in the subarachnoid space (Fig. 13–9). The bolt is inserted through a twist drill hole, which is made in either the left or right prefrontal areas. After penetration of the inner table of the skull, the drill is removed, and the hole is irrigated with normal saline.

The bolt is then screwed in manually. At this point, a stylet is inserted through the bolt to clear any debris, and the hole is again irrigated with normal saline. The catheter is zeroed, passed through the bolt approximately 1 cm beyond the end of the bolt, and then secured to the bolt by tightening a compression cap.

If brain parenchymal pressure monitoring is to be utilized, a fiberoptic catheter may be inserted through the meningeal layers and advanced a few centimeters into the brain parenchyma. This type of device can be inserted through a subarachnoid bolt using a technique similar to the one described above.

A transducer-tipped fiberoptic catheter eliminates the problems of dampening waveforms due to catheter occlusion or air bubble entrapment. Because the system is not fluid-coupled, it is not necessary to irrigate the system due to dampening waveforms, and this may reduce the risk of infection (Narayan et al., 1987). A more detailed waveform with less artifact has also been reported (Narayan et al., 1987).

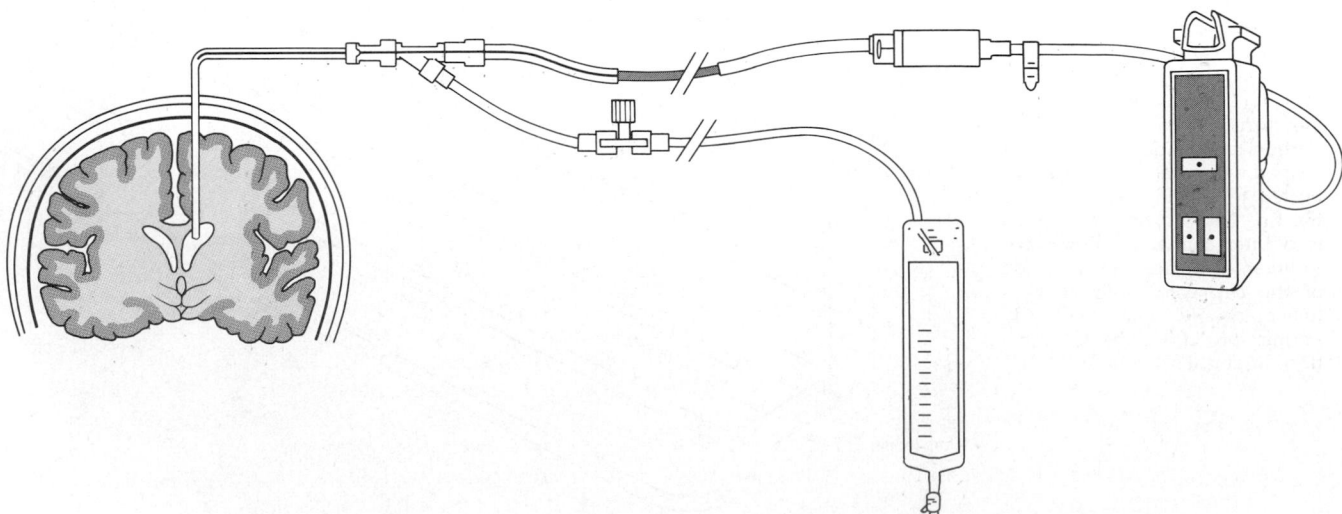

FIGURE 13–8. Ventricular fiberoptic catheter. A Y-connector is attached to the system at the proximal end to allow for CSF drainage via one port and ICP monitoring on the other. (Redrawn by permission of Camino Laboratories, San Diego, CA.)

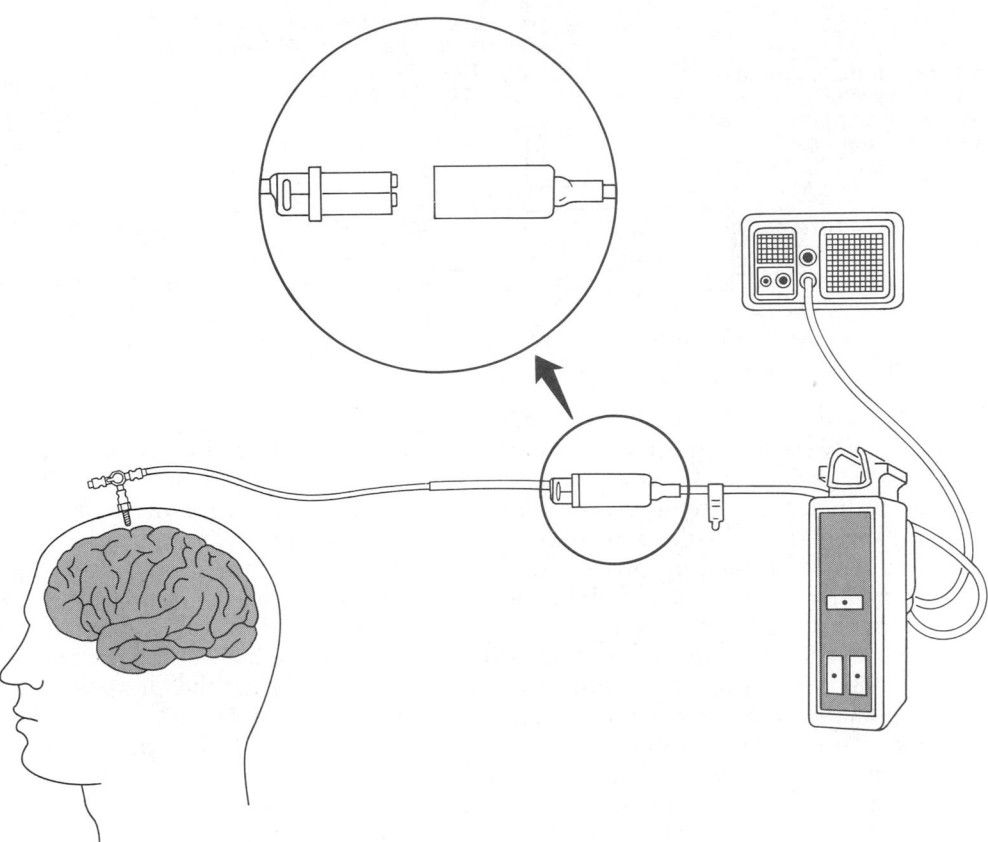

FIGURE 13–9. Subarachnoid bolt monitoring utilizing a fiberoptic transducer-tipped catheter. Circular enlargement illustrates adjoining connections of catheter and preamplifier cable. (Redrawn by permission of Camino Laboratories, San Diego, CA.)

Because the transducer lies in the catheter tip, the zero point relative to atmospheric pressure is independent of the patient's position. Continuous ICP readings may also be obtained during patient transport with a battery-powered monitor. The ability of the fiberoptic catheter to be utilized in various monitoring locations is an additional advantage.

A specific advantage of the intraventricular monitoring technique is its capability for monitoring ICP and draining CSF. Advantages of the intraparenchymal location include the capability for insertion of this monitor in patients with compressed or distorted ventricles while maintaining accurate readings (Narayan et al., 1987; Sundberg et al., 1987).

Disadvantages of the fiberoptic transducer-tipped catheter include the expense of the catheters and the initial expense involved in the purchase of the cable and compatible monitor compared to the expense of fluid-coupled monitoring devices. In addition, the catheter is only capable of being zeroed to an atmospheric reference prior to insertion and cannot be rezeroed once in place. It is therefore not possible to check for drift; however, those who have utilized the system report a stable zero baseline with minimal drift (Hollingsworth-Fridlund et al., 1988; Narayan et al., 1987). Another potential disadvantage of the catheter is the risk of fiberoptic breakage due to inadvertent bending of the catheter (Ostrup et al., 1987). If fiberoptic breakage occurs, there is a signal on the monitor that will alert the caregiver. However, as those working with the catheters and equipment

become increasingly familiar with the equipment, fiberoptic breakage has not been reported to be a significant problem (Ostrup et al., 1987).

Other Intracranial Transducer Systems. Other methods that have been developed to monitor ICP using some type of intracranial transducer include electrical transducers as well as pneumatic flow systems and sensors. The electrical transducers house a strain gauge transducer in the catheter tip. ICP is sensed by the face of the tip sensor in a classic transducer manner (Fig. 13–10). The catheter that contains the transducer is connected to an adaptor cable that can be attached to any standard bedside monitor for continuous display of the ICP waveform (Barnett and Chapman, 1988). This catheter was designed and approved in the United States for use in monitoring epidural pressure. However, investigators outside the United States have reported reliable readings obtained in the subdural space (Barlow et al., 1986). This device may be inserted surgically or through a burr hole; it can be done in the operating room, ICU, or emergency room. To zero or reference the transducer to atmospheric pressure once the catheter is in place, approximately 0.3 cc of air is injected into the catheter. This equalizes the atmospheric pressure across the transducer, allowing a zero reference to be obtained.

Another recently developed ICP monitoring device utilizes a pneumatic flow system to obtain ICP pressure values (Marcotty and Levin, 1984). With this system there is a small sensor plenum in the catheter

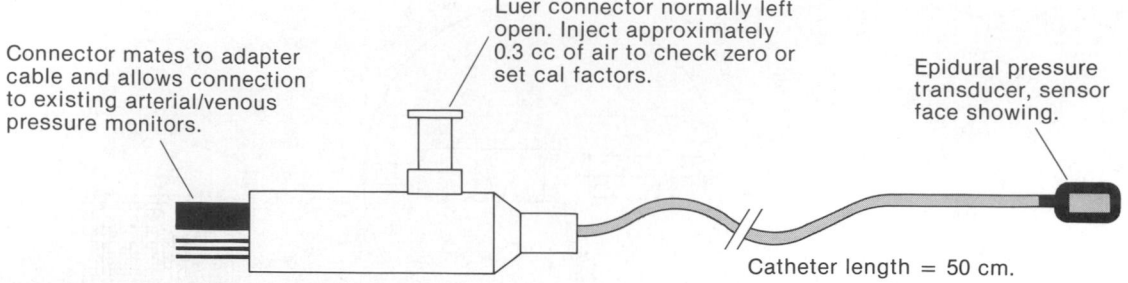

Connector mates to adapter cable and allows connection to existing arterial/venous pressure monitors.

Luer connector normally left open. Inject approximately 0.3 cc of air to check zero or set cal factors.

Epidural pressure transducer, sensor face showing.

Catheter length = 50 cm.

FIGURE 13–10. Electrical epidural transducer system. (Redrawn by permission of Medical Measurements, Inc., Hackensack, NJ.)

tip that is covered on one side by a pressure-sensitive membrane. Air flows into this sensor plenum at a predetermined rate. Any increase in pressure against the membrane as a result of increased ICP will affect the air flow in the plenum by closing off the air flow at an exhaust port. Pressure then increases within the plenum to overcome the pressure against the membrane and reestablish air flow (Marcotty and Levin, 1984). The pressure required to maintain air flow is calculated to represent ICP and is displayed on the compatible monitor (Marcotty and Levin, 1984). This system represents a modification of the design of a previously used counterpressure system (Levin, 1977; Barnett and Chapman, 1988). This earlier system was designed to be placed in the epidural space through a burr hole in a place where the dura had been carefully stripped (Marcotty and Levin, 1984).

The advantages of these monitoring devices are that they are relatively quick and easy to insert, especially when small or shifted ventricles are present. Because there is no penetration of the dura when they are placed epidurally, the risk of infection is low. In addition, in vivo calibration or zero point referencing is possible after insertion of the electrical transducer (Barlow et al., 1986). The pneumatic system has an automatic in vivo calibration feature (Marcotty and Levin, 1984). Additional advantages include those common to all intracranial transducer systems in which the disadvantages of fluid-coupled systems are eliminated.

One disadvantage is that inaccurate placement of the sensor, especially if the dura is not carefully freed from the skull, may result in inaccurate ICP readings (Marcotty and Levin, 1984). In addition, CSF sampling and drainage are not possible. These monitoring devices do carry a risk of rupture of the intracranial membrane with a resulting air leak (Gentleman and Mendelow, 1986). With electrical transducers, fracture of the electrical connections due to stress is a possibility (Gentleman and Mendelow, 1986). As with other intracranial transducer systems, the cost of the individual catheters and other necessary equipment compared with hydrostatically coupled monitoring devices may be seen as another disadvantage.

Telemetric Devices. With the successful use of intracranial transducers that have a low incidence of infection, recent efforts have been directed toward development of an ICP monitoring instrument that could be internalized and could remain in place for an unlimited period. Examples of patients who might benefit from this type of monitoring include those with communicating hydrocephalus or pseudotumor cerebri in whom increased ICP is a constant possibility. Although these devices are still considered to be in the process of evolution, some are currently available for use. The source of power and the method of transmission used in the currently available devices vary. Some use detection of radioactive source activity, and others use detection of resonant frequency in passive resonant circuits to detect changes in ICP.

In the future use of these products, advantages include long-term measurement of ICP with minimal incidence of infection. These devices will also allow ICP to be checked noninvasively on an outpatient basis in patients with shunts with nonspecific symptoms.

The greatest disadvantage reported to date with the use of these devices is the incidence of significant drift, resulting in decreased reliability of pressure readings (Barnett and Chapman, 1988). Readings that were lower than readings made by direct measurement, especially in patients with increased ICP, have been reported (Minns and Shaw, 1986). Certain designs have been introduced that allow for in vivo calibration and zero point determination, and these may result in increased accuracy and reliability (Zervas et al., 1977). Another reported disadvantage is that some systems are incompatible with MR imaging (Barnett and Chapman, 1988).

INTRACRANIAL PRESSURE WAVEFORMS

Oscilloscopic display of ICP waveforms has been considered important in the analysis of ICP. The initial work on ICP monitoring, in which ICP waveforms were described, was done by Lundberg in 1960 using ventricular catheters (Lundberg, 1960). The configuration of the ICP waveform results from the transmission of systolic and diastolic arterial pressures from the cerebrovascular system and choroid plexus (capillaries within the ventricles) to the CSF

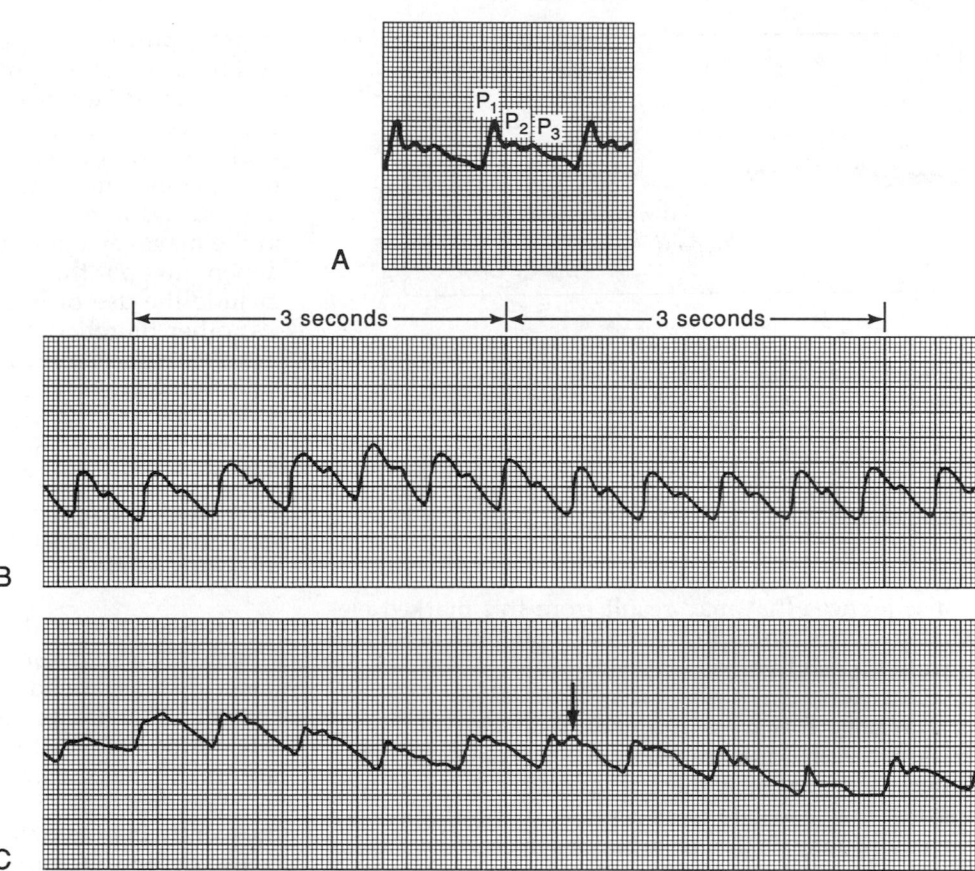

FIGURE 13–11. Normal intracranial pressure waveforms. *A*, ICP pulse wave with three main components: P_1, P_2, and P_3. The clarity of the three distinct waves will vary with the type of ICP monitoring device utilized and the calibration range of the bedside monitor. *B*, Waveform obtained from fluid-coupled intraventricular catheter. Calibration range is 0–50 mm Hg. *C*, ICP waveform obtained from ventriculostomy catheter. Arrow illustrates elevation of P_2 in relationship to P_1 secondary to increased ICP in a patient with ICPs ranging from 20 mm Hg to 40 mm Hg.

in the ventricular and subarachnoid spaces. On close analysis, the ICP waveform has three or more peaks (Fig. 13–11). The large initial peak, P_1, the percussion wave, results from transmission of arterial pressure from the choroid plexus (Cardoso et al., 1983), has a sharp peak, and is relatively constant in amplitude. The second peak, P_2, generated by venous pressure, is referred to as the tidal wave. It is more variable in shape and amplitude and ends in the dicrotic notch. Following the dicrotic notch is the third wave, the dicrotic wave, which is also felt to be generated by venous pressure (Castel and Cohadon, 1976). After the dicrotic wave the pressure usually tapers down to its diastolic position, although occasionally a few more peaks may be observed due to retrograde venous pulsations (Cardoso et al., 1983; Germon, 1988). The exact appearance of the waveform and the ability to detect the waveform peaks will vary with the type of ICP monitoring device being used.

When caring for a patient with an ICP monitor it is important to document and compare ICP waveforms to confirm the accuracy of values and to observe for dampening of the waveform. In addition, certain changes in the configuration of the normal ICP waveform have been correlated with actual or future elevations in ICP or decreased compliance (Germon, 1988). When ICP waveforms were studied, it was found that an elevation of the P_2 component of the waveform that was equal to or higher than the P_1 component might reflect a state of decreased compliance (Cardoso et al., 1983; Germon, 1988).

Monitors that are capable of providing trends of ICP values over time or that allow slow strip chart recording can also provide valuable information about the patient. The three types of abnormal ICP waveforms that can most readily be identified on a slow strip chart recorder are the A, B, and C waveforms (Fig. 13–12).

A Waves (Plateau Waves). A waves, also called plateau waves, occur during elevations of ICP to 50 to 100 mm Hg and last from 5 to 20 minutes (Lundberg, 1960). These abnormal waveforms have been correlated with falls in cerebral perfusion pressure due to decreased arterial blood pressure and decreased intracranial compliance (Rosner and Becker, 1984). The decrease in perfusion pressure serves as a stimulus for an intact autoregulatory response of cerebral vasodilation, which results in further increases in ICP (Rosner and Becker, 1984). Clinical

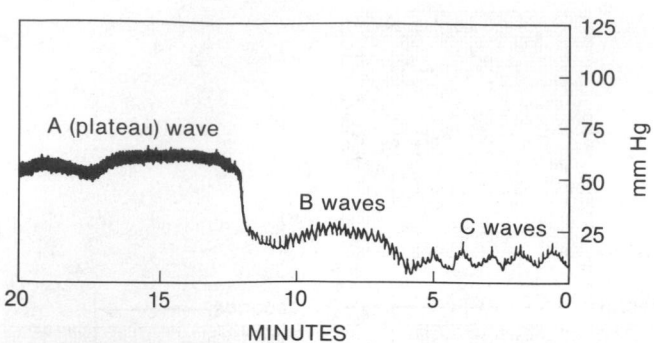

FIGURE 13–12. Abnormal intracranial pressure waves. Composite drawing of pressure waves that may be recorded over time with a slow strip chart recorder, including A (plateau) waves, B waves, and C waves. Note that this type of recording is used to illustrate trends in ICP over time. (Redrawn from Holloway, N.M. (1988). *Nursing care of the critically ill adult* (3rd ed.). Menlo Park, CA: Addison-Wesley.)

consequences that may result from this marked elevation in ICP include decreased cerebral perfusion and brain cell hypoxia.

B Waves. B waves are defined as sharp rhythmic pressure variations occurring at a frequency of 0.5 to 2.0/minute in which the ICP averages 20 to 40 mm Hg but may oscillate to as high as 50 mm Hg. These variations may be due to variations in cerebrovascular resistance or pressure within the cerebral vasculature bed (Lundberg, 1960) and are influenced by changes in ventilation as well as arterial pressure (Price, 1981).

C Waves. C waves are transient rhythmic waves that occur every 4 to 8 minutes and raise ICP to as high as 20 mm Hg (Lundberg, 1960). C waves have been associated with variations in ventilation and arterial pressure (Pollack-Latham, 1987). The clinical significance of these waves is unknown.

MANAGEMENT OF INTRACRANIAL HYPERTENSION

Intracranial hypertension is defined as a sustained elevation of ICP greater than 15 to 20 mm Hg (Langfitt, 1990). There is, however, no absolute pressure value that indicates a need for treatment. Guidelines provided in the literature state that the decision to initiate treatment should be based on the neurologic condition of the brain, the rapidity with which the ICP is rising, the underlying pathophysiologic condition resulting in increased ICP, and the estimated cerebral perfusion pressure (Ward et al., 1987). Results of the neurologic examination also are used as an indicator; however, many patients do not show evidence of neurologic deterioration until ICP has become markedly elevated.

The initial goal for management of patients with increased ICP is to control intracranial hypertension,

thereby preventing secondary cerebral ischemia. In addition, the underlying cause of intracranial hypertension must be treated and further increases in ICP prevented. Strategies for accomplishment of these goals involve a collaborative effort and include carefully planned medical management and skilled nursing interventions. The major medical interventions in the management of intracranial hypertension vary depending on the underlying condition but may include the use of hyperventilation, osmotic diuretics, other diuretics, fluid restriction, corticosteroids, blood pressure control, and, in extreme situations, barbiturate therapy. The specific management of conditions associated with increased ICP and possible surgical interventions are presented in Chapter 32 of this text. Cerebrospinal fluid drainage through a ventriculostomy is a surgical intervention that may be utilized to control ICP and will be reviewed in the following section.

Cerebrospinal Fluid Drainage. As described previously, ICP monitoring with a ventricular catheter has a distinct advantage in that it allows for some control of ICP by its capability of draining CSF. This intervention allows for rapid reduction of ICP and is the treatment of choice when increased ICP is due to hydrocephalus. When CSF drainage is utilized, the ventricular catheter is connected to an external collecting and measuring system by pressure tubing and a series of stopcocks. One stopcock may be used for intermittent ICP monitoring, if an external transducer is used, by connecting a transducer dome to this port. The other stopcocks may be used for injecting medications, sampling CSF, testing volume pressure response, or intermittently flushing the ventriculostomy if necessary.

CSF drainage is regulated or controlled by adjusting the height of the drainage system relative to a reference point on the patient. This reference point is often the inferred anatomic level of the foramen of Monro or the level at the top of the ear or the outer canthus of the eye. The height of the fluid column in the pressure tubing above this reference point creates a hydrostatic pressure that opposes the intracranial pressure. To increase or decrease this hydrostatic pressure, the height of the highest point of the drainage system may be raised or lowered in relation to the reference point on the patient. If the drainage system is raised, CSF drainage will decrease. In this situation, greater intracranial pressure is necessary to overcome the pressure created by the height of the fluid column. When the highest point of the drainage system is lowered, the hydrostatic pressure created by the fluid column is also decreased, and CSF drainage will occur more rapidly.

In an average adult, cerebrospinal fluid is normally produced at a rate of 20 to 30 mL/hour with approximately 90 to 150 mL of CSF circulating between the ventricles and the subarachnoid space at any one time if the normal mechanisms for CSF reabsorption are functional (Rockoff and Kennedy, 1988). This basic physiologic understanding is important when monitoring CSF drainage. Too rapid drainage of CSF may result in ventricular collapse. Therefore, it is generally recommended that CSF be drained in a controlled manner against a positive back pressure, which corresponds to a predetermined ICP (Deardon, 1986). Such a procedure can be accomplished by maintaining the drainage system at a specified height, e.g., 10 cm above the top of the ear. To decrease the risk of complications, a pressure-regulated valve may be placed in line with the tubing going to the drainage system. This technique allows close regulation of CSF pressure and decreases the chance of too rapid CSF drainage (Mapstone and Ratcheson, 1985). It also retards retrograde travel of bacteria from the closed drainage system (Mapstone and Ratcheson, 1985).

To minimize the risk of infection, every effort should be made to maintain a closed system. Some preassembled closed drainage systems are currently available. In addition, sterile technique is essential whenever the system is entered.

NURSING DIAGNOSES AND INTERVENTIONS

Potential for Alteration in Cerebral Tissue Perfusion Related to Increased Intracranial Pressure

In providing nursing care to a patient with or at risk of increased ICP, many nursing interventions can be implemented independently. Defining characteristics for the patient with a potential for alteration in cerebral tissue perfusion include an actually measured ICP of greater than 15 mm Hg or signs or symptoms of decreasing cerebral tissue perfusion. These signs or symptoms may include an alteration in the level of consciousness or other changes in the neurologic status of the patient. Nursing goals should be directed toward supporting the patient's functional abilities, which may be compromised as a result of decreased cerebral tissue perfusion, and preventing further increases in ICP. ICP should ideally be maintained between 0 and 15 mm Hg, and cerebral perfusion pressure should be maintained at greater than or equal to 50 mm Hg.

One limiting factor in this diagnosis is the inability to actually measure cerebral tissue perfusion as well as the lack of correlation between neurologic signs and symptoms and decreasing tissue perfusion. In addition, many nursing interventions are directed toward identifying patients at risk of sharp increases in ICP and preventing these increases before they occur. Mitchell (1986) has proposed the nursing diagnosis "decreased intracranial adaptive capacity" to replace "alteration in cerebral tissue perfusion." In recent research she has been able to define some

characteristics that may be present prior to these sudden increases in ICP that may help to guide nursing interventions.

Several nursing interventions that influence ICP have been reported and will be discussed in this section. Potential interventions that can be instituted in caring for the patient with, or at risk for, increased ICP are listed at the end of the chapter.

Patient Positioning and Turning. Maintaining the head of bed elevation at approximately 30 to 45 degrees in most situations has been found to result in decreased ICP. Some investigators, however, have found that the optimal position for the head of the bed varies between patients and should be determined on an individual basis (Ropper et al., 1982). The recommended position is generally ordered by physicians and should be maintained as consistently as possible. Nursing implications are to constantly assess and document changes in ICP in relation to the head of bed elevation.

Turning the head position 90 degrees to the extreme left or right results in increases in ICP ranging from 5 to 20 mm Hg (Lipe and Mitchell, 1980). This pressure increase is felt to be due to obstruction of venous outflow and should be avoided.

Turning the patient in bed may also result in increases in ICP, although this finding is inconsistent. Patients in whom this pattern is identified should be instructed to allow the nurse to turn them passively, avoiding isometric contractions and the Valsalva maneuver, which result in increased ICP (Mitchell, 1980). Hip flexion has been found to produce significant increases in ICP (Boortz-Marx, 1985).

The use of oscillating beds that rotate from side to side was studied to assess the effect on ICP (Gonzales-Aires et al., 1983). It was found that changes in bed position from extreme left to right and supine did not result in significant changes in ICP (Gonzales-Aires et al., 1983). This study supported the finding that raised ICP should not limit the use of oscillating beds in appropriate patients.

Securing of Endotracheal Tubes. Securing an endotracheal tube with a circumferential tie around the neck can potentially result in increased ICP by obstructing venous outflow. Thus, noncircumferential taping of endotracheal tubes is preferred in patients with or at risk of intracranial hypertension.

Endotracheal Suctioning. Because hypoxia or hypercapnia can result in cerebral vasodilation and increased ICP and because stimulation may increase ICP, the potential for increased ICP resulting from endotracheal suctioning has been a nursing concern. In a literature review of investigations related to endotracheal suctioning and intracranial pressure, it was concluded that endotracheal suctioning may produce transient but significant increases in ICP, which quickly return to baseline in patients with a baseline ICP of less than 20 mm Hg (Rudy et al.,

1986). In such patients this transient elevation was of no consequence. In patients with an ICP of greater than 20 mm Hg, however, any further increases in ICP might have significant deleterious effects (Rudy et al., 1986).

Nursing interventions to minimize the negative effects associated with endotracheal suctioning include manually hyperventilating the patient with 100% O_2 for 20 to 30 seconds prior to suctioning. In addition, duration of the time of suctioning should be less than 10 seconds with each attempt (Parsons and Shogan, 1984). In additional investigations, intravenous lidocaine administered prior to suctioning was found to prevent intracranial hypertension effectively during periods of endotracheal suctioning (Donegan and Bedford, 1980; Yano et al., 1986). Although this practice is not utilized routinely, it may be considered in patients at particularly high risk for marked increases in ICP with endotracheal suctioning.

Environmental Stimuli or Touch. Current research has demonstrated that the effects of certain environmental stimuli may result in either increased or decreased ICP. Conversations about the patient's condition at the bedside may elevate ICP (Boortz-Marx, 1985; Mitchell and Mauss, 1978; Lundberg, 1960). In addition, Bruya (1981) and Mitchell and co-workers (1985) found that the presence of family members and gentle touching or stroking of the patient by family members can produce significant decreases in ICP. Walleck (1987) summarized the findings of studies related to nursing interventions and ICP. She reported that "there appears to be a cumulative effect on ICP when activities are clumped together, but if CPP remains at 50 mm Hg or greater, any nursing activity can be safely performed" (Walleck, 1987).

Potential for Infection Related to ICP Monitoring

Although ICP monitoring has been recognized as a valuable tool in the diagnosis and management of intracranial hypertension, the risk of complications associated with such monitoring has been a significant concern with all types of ICP monitoring. A brief summary of some of the variables influencing the incidence of infection and interventions used to decrease the incidence of infection will be reviewed.

Type of ICP Monitor. Ventricular catheters fluid-coupled to external transducers are associated with the overall highest incidence of infection. Research on the incidence of ventriculostomy-related infections has ranged from less than 1% when the catheter is percutaneously tunneled under the scalp (Friedman and Vries, 1980) to approximately 21.9% (Aucoin et al., 1986), with an average of approximately 9% at 5 days of ICP monitoring (Mayhall et al., 1984). The fluid-coupled subarachnoid bolt has been associated with the lowest incidence of infection, ranging from no reported infection (Smith, 1987) to a 7.5% incidence that included the complications of wound infection and osteomyelitis (Aucoin et al., 1986).

Intracranial transducer systems and infection rates have not been studied in as much detail; however, it appears that the more invasive monitoring devices are associated with a higher incidence of infection. In addition, because system irrigation is not needed and a static fluid column is not present, it has been suggested that these factors may reduce the risk of infection with internal transducer systems (Narayan et al., 1987; Hollingsworth-Fridlund et al., 1988).

Length of ICP Monitoring. Studies of ICP monitoring have reported a correlation between the incidence of infection and the duration of ICP monitoring. The incidence of infection has been reported to be very low if the monitoring device is in place less than 72 hours. In a study of 255 patients with fluid-coupled ICP monitoring devices, only two cases of infection were reported if the ICP monitoring device was in place for less than 72 hours (Aucoin et al., 1986). A significantly higher rate of infection was associated with the use of fluid-coupled devices when the ICP monitor remained in place 5 days or longer (Aucoin et al., 1986; Mayhall et al., 1984).

Use of Prophylactic Antibiotics. Many institutions use prophylactic antibiotic administration in an effort to decrease the incidence of infection during ICP monitoring. The most frequently used prophylactic antibiotics include nafcillin, cephalothin, and gentamicin, although many others are used as well. A decrease in the incidence of infection with the prophylactic use of antibiotics during ICP monitoring has been reported (Aucoin et al., 1986; Wyler and Kelly, 1972); however, data from other studies of infection associated with ICP monitoring have not supported this correlation (Mayhall et al., 1984).

Utilization of Antibiotic Flush Solution. Many fluid-coupled ICP monitoring systems require the use of a flush solution to maintain patency. Intermittent flushes (every 2 to 3 hours) with 0.1 to 0.3 mL of sterile saline or an antibiotic flush solution such as bacitracin or gentamicin can prevent occlusion of these devices with blood or brain tissue. An increased incidence of infection, however, has been associated with flushing of ICP monitoring devices (Aucoin et al., 1986; Mayhall et al., 1984). One study reported an 18.6% incidence of infection when a bacitracin flush solution was utilized in contrast to a 5.7% incidence of infection without the use of a flush solution (Aucoin et al., 1986). If the decision is made to utilize an intermittent flush the principle of maintaining a closed system is very important.

Additional Nursing Implications in Prevention of Infection. In any patient with an ICP monitoring device in place one of the most important variables influencing the rate of infection is the technique of the caregiver working with the system. Strict attention to maintaining aseptic technique in routine use of the system and sterile technique whenever the system is opened cannot be overemphasized. It has been documented that the use of in-line stopcocks in many ICP monitoring methods may increase the incidence of infection (McArthur et al., 1975). To prevent contamination of the stopcock, a T-piece connector or rubber sampling port that is routinely cleansed with bacteriacidal solution before the system is entered may be utilized (Jones and Cayard, 1982).

A consistent recommendation for the frequency of dressing changes over ICP monitoring sites has not been made. In following the recommendations made by individual institutions, sterile technique should be maintained.

CSF Samples. When a patient has a ventriculostomy catheter in place, it is possible to sample CSF specimens daily and to send them for culture and sensitivity testing, for glucose and protein evalua-

tion, and for cell counts to monitor the patient carefully for any evidence of infection. In some institutions CSF sampling is performed by nurses with specialized education, whereas in others it is the responsibility of the physician. CSF samples can be obtained from a ventriculostomy by using a rubber sampling port at a stopcock site. Correct technique for CSF sampling includes first cleansing the sampling port carefully several times with povidone-iodine (Betadine) solution. Specimens may then be obtained by either allowing passive flow through a needle inserted into the sampling port, which drains from the ventricle, or by turning the proximal stopcock to the patient off and withdrawing a small amount (approximately 3 mL) of CSF from the distal tubing using a 25-gauge needle and syringe. In sampling CSF, undue pressure created by aspirating against the ventricles must be avoided because this could result in aspiration of brain tissue or ventricular collapse. The techniques described prevent opening the system and may decrease the incidence of infection. When CSF samples are obtained, the nurse should be aware of the results and should report any evidence of infection immediately.

ncp nursing care plan

NURSING DIAGNOSIS AND INTERVENTIONS IN INTRACRANIAL PRESSURE MONITORING

1. Nursing Diagnosis: Potential for decreased cerebral tissue perfusion related to increased ICP

Outcome Criteria	Nursing Interventions
1. Intracranial pressure (ICP) will be maintained within the normal limits of 0–15 mm Hg. 2. Cerebral perfusion pressure (CPP) will be maintained at a level of 50 mm Hg or greater. 3. Patient will not exhibit signs or symptoms of neurologic deterioration related to decreased cerebral perfusion.	1. Assess and document the neurologic status of the patient every 1–4 hours and prn, especially associated with any increases in intracranial pressure. 2. Obtain ICP readings consistently according to recommendations for specific type of ICP monitoring device to ensure accurate ICP readings. 3. Document and record ICP values and assess response in ICP to various therapeutic interventions and nursing measures. 4. Document ICP waveform (if possible based on type of ICP monitoring device). Assess for wide amplitude tracing (Mitchell, 1988) or an elevation of P_2 in relationship to P_1 (Germon, 1988), which may be indicative of decreasing compliance. 5. Position patient with head maintained in a neutral position avoiding extreme flexion or hyperextension of neck or rotation of the head. 6. When turning and positioning a conscious patient, instruct the patient to allow the nurse to turn him or her passively and to avoid Valsalva maneuver or isometric contractions, which may increase ICP. Avoid position with marked degree of hip flexion. 7. Maintain open, unobstructed airway. 8. If patient is intubated with an endotracheal tube, the tube should be secured noncircumferentially with tape. Circumferential ties around the patient's neck may result in obstruction of venous return. 9. When endotracheal suctioning is performed, hyperventilate the patient with 100% oxygen for 20–30 seconds prior to suctioning and limit the duration of suctioning with each attempt to less than 10 seconds. Attempt to reduce coughing with endotracheal suctioning when possible. 10. Decrease environmental stimuli and activity near the patient's bedside. Avoid unnecessary conversation regarding the patient's condition at the bedside. 11. Avoid extreme elevations in body temperature. Utilize antipyretics or other nonpharmacologic measures as ordered to maintain normothermia. 12. Prevent constipation or straining at stool, which may result in a Valsalva maneuver and increased ICP. Assess and document bowel status and maintain regular bowel regimen.

Nursing Care Plan continued on following page

2. Nursing Diagnosis: Potential for infection related to ICP monitoring	
Outcome Criteria	**Nursing Interventions**
Patient will remain free of signs or symptoms of infection related to intracranial pressure monitoring as evidenced by absence of fever, negative cerebrospinal fluid cultures (if obtained), and no evidence of redness, swelling, or drainage from ICP monitoring site.	1. Maintain sterile technique during ICP monitor insertion, whenever the ICP monitor system is opened to air, and with ICP monitor dressing changes. 2. Minimize use of intermittent flushing methods for fluid-coupled ICP monitoring devices. 3. Document and be aware of length of time that ICP monitoring device is in place and communicate this information to physicians in an effort to limit the length of time device is in place to less than 5 days if possible. 4. Maintain a closed system, minimizing the number of times any piece of the system is opened, which may decrease infection. 5. Assess ICP monitor dressing site for any signs of CSF leakage or drainage. Notify physician if this is noted. 6. When an intraventricular catheter is in place, obtain CSF specimens if ordered according to protocol established by institution, utilizing sterile technique and following results of CSF cultures.

SUMMARY

This chapter has provided a brief overview of the pathophysiologic basis of increased intracranial pressure as well as pertinent assessment parameters in caring for a patient with actual or potential increased ICP. In addition, the importance of ICP monitoring as an adjunctive measure in the assessment and management of increased intracranial pressure was presented. The various techniques for ICP monitoring, including the basic principles involved in the use of a fluid-coupled external transducer versus an internal transducer system were reviewed. Although the advantages and disadvantages of each monitoring technique were presented, no one system that is optimal in every situation has been developed. In 1960 Lundberg presented criteria for an ideal ICP monitoring technique that still serves as standards referred to in an effort to develop an optimal system for ICP monitoring. These criteria include:

1. The technique should cause as little trauma to intracranial structures as possible.
2. It should involve a negligible risk of infection.
3. CSF leakage around the monitor should not be possible.
4. Recording of ICP pressures should be possible during various diagnostic and therapeutic measures without disturbing the care and comfort of the patient.
5. The apparatus should be easy to handle, reliable, and reasonably foolproof.

Although all these standards may not consistently be attained, great progress has been made in the design and maintenance of ICP monitoring systems. The specific techniques utilized in each situation will vary with the monitoring capabilities of the institution, the pathophysiologic condition of the patient, and the risks and benefits of each technique available in a particular situation. The nurse caring for the patient with an intracranial pressure monitoring device must use this information to facilitate an understanding of the basic monitoring techniques and should continue to update and expand his or her knowledge in this highly dynamic area of ICP monitoring.

With increased use of ICP monitoring, there is a great potential to study many of the common interventions used to control intracranial hypertension and their effect on ICP. The generation of nursing research based on observations of response of ICP to various nursing interventions as well as specific nursing interventions to maintain ICP monitoring devices and prevent infection are areas with great potential.

References

Aucoin, P.J., Kotilainen, H.R., Gantz, N.M., et al. (1986). Intracranial pressure monitors: Epidemiological study of risk factors and infections. *American Journal of Medicine*, 80, 369–376.

Barlow, P., Mendelow, A.D., Rowan, J.O., et al. (1986). Clinical evaluation of the Gaeltec ICT/b pressure transducer placed subdurally. In J.D. Miller, G.M. Teasdale, J.O. Rowan, et al. (Eds.), *Intracranial pressure VI* (pp. 181–183). Berlin: Springer-Verlag.

Barnett, G.H., and Chapman, P.H. (1988). Insertion and care of intracranial pressure monitoring devices. In A.J. Ropper and S.F. Kennedy (Eds.), *Neurological and neurosurgical intensive care* (2nd ed.), pp. 43–55. Rockville, MD: Aspen Publishers.

Boortz-Marx, R. (1985). Factors affecting intracranial pressure: A descriptive study. *Journal of Neurosurgical Nursing*, 17(2), 89–94.

Bruce, D.A., Berman, W.A., and Schut, L. (1977). Cerebrospinal fluid pressure monitoring in children: Physiology, pathology and clinical usefulness. *Advances in Pediatrics*, 24, 233–290.

Bruya, M.A. (1981). Planned periods of rest in the intensive care unit: Nursing care activities and intracranial pressure. *Journal of Neurosurgical Nursing*, 13(4), 184–193.

Cammermeyer, M., and Appeldorn, C. (Eds.) (1990). *Core curriculum for neuroscience nursing*. Chicago: Chicago Press. American Association of Neuroscience Nurses.

Castel, J., and Cohadon, F. (1976). The pattern of cerebral pulse. In J.W. Beks, D.A. Bosch, and M. Brock (Eds.), *ICP III* (pp. 305–307). New York: Springer.

Cardoso, E.R., Rowan, J.O., and Galbraith, S. (1983). Analysis of cerebrospinal fluid pulse wave in intracranial pressure. *Journal of Neurosurgery*, 59, 817–821.

Deardon, N.M. (1986). Management of raised intracranial pressure after severe head injury. *British Journal of Hospital Medicine*, 36(2), 94–100.

Donegan, M.F., and Bedford, R.F. (1980). Intravenously administered lidocaine prevents intracranial hypertension during endotracheal suctioning. *Anesthesiology*, 52, 516–518.

Eichelberger, J. (1985). Clinical monitoring of brain dynamics. *Journal of the American Association of Nurse Anesthetists*, 53(4), 342–352.

Friedman, W.A., and Vries, J.K. (1980). Percutaneous tunnel ventriculostomy. *Journal of Neurosurgery*, 53, 662–665.

Gentleman, D., and Mendelow, A.D. (1986). Intracranial rupture of a pressure monitoring transducer: Technical note. *Neurosurgery*, 19, 91–92.

Germon, K. (1988). Interpretation of ICP pulse waves to determine intracerebral compliance. *Journal of Neuroscience Nursing*, 20(6), 344–349.

Gonzalez-Aries, S.M., Goldberg, M.L., Baumgartner, R., et al. (1983). Analysis of the effect of kinetic therapy on intracranial pressure in comatose neurosurgical patients. *Neurosurgery*, 13(6), 654–656.

Hickey, J.V. (1986). *The clinical practice of neurological and neurosurgical nursing* (2nd ed.). Philadelphia: J.B. Lippincott.

Hollingsworth-Fridlund, P., Vos, H., and Daily, E. (1988). Use of fiber-optic pressure transducer for intracranial pressure measurements: A preliminary report. *Heart & Lung*, 17(2), 111–120.

Holloway, N.M. (1988). *Nursing care of the critically ill adult*. Menlo Park, CA: Addison-Wesley.

Jennet, W.B., Harper, A.M., Miller, J.D., et al. (1970). Relation between cerebral blood flow and cerebral perfusion pressure. *British Journal of Surgery*, 390, 57(5).

Jones, C., and Cayard, C. (1982). Care of ICP monitoring devices: A nursing responsibility. *Journal of Neurosurgical Nursing*, 14(5), 255–261.

Landy, H.J., and Villanueva, P.A. (1984). An improved subarachnoid screw for intracranial pressure monitoring. *Journal of Neurosurgery*, 61, 606–608.

Langfitt, T.W. (1990). Increased intracranial pressure and the cerebral circulation. In J.R. Youmans (Ed.), *Neurological surgery* (3rd ed.). Philadelphia, W.B. Saunders.

Levin, A.B. (1977). The use of a fiberoptic intracranial pressure in clinical practice. *Neurosurgery*, 1(3), 266–271.

Lipe, H.P., and Mitchell, P.H. (1980). Positioning the patient with intracranial hypertension: How turning and head rotation affect the internal jugular vein. *Heart & Lung*, 9, 1031–1037.

Lundberg, N. (1960). Continuous recording and control of ventricular fluid pressure in neurosurgical practice. *Acta Psychiatrica et Neurologica Scandinavica*, 36 (Suppl. 149), 1–193.

Mapstone, T.B., and Ratcheson, R.A. (1985). Techniques of ventricular puncture. In R.H. Wilkins and S.S. Rengachary (Eds.), *Neurosurgery*, New York: McGraw Hill.

Marcotty, S.F., and Levin, A.B. (1984). A new approach in epidural intracranial pressure monitoring. *Journal of Neurosurgical Nursing*, 16(1), 54–59.

Marshall, L.F., Cotten, J.M., Bowers-Marshall, S., et al. (1986). Pupillary abnormalities, elevated intracranial pressure and mass lesion location. In J.D. Miller, G.M. Teasdale, J.O. Rowan, et al. (Eds.), *Intracranial pressure VI* (pp. 656–660). Berlin: Springer-Verlag.

Marshall, L.F., Smith, R.W., and Shapiro, H.M. (1978). The influence of diurnal rhythms in patients with intracranial hypertension: Implications for management. *Neurosurgery*, 2, 100–101.

Mayhall, C.G., Archer, N.H., Lamb, V., et al. (1984). Ventriculostomy related infections. *New England Journal of Medicine*, 310(9), 553–559.

McArthur, B.J., Hargiss, C., and Schoenknecht, F.D. (1975). Stopcock contamination in an ICU. *American Journal of Nursing*, 75, 96.

McNamara, M., and Quinn, C. (1981). Epidural intracranial pressure monitoring: Theory and clinical application. *Journal of Neurosurgical Nursing*, 13(5), 267–281.

Minns, R.A., and Shaw, J.F. (1986). Clinical evaluation of the Cosman ICP Telesensor in children. In J.D. Miller, G.M. Teasdale, J.O. Rowan, et al. (Eds.), *Intracranial pressure VI* (pp. 222–225). Berlin: Springer-Verlag.

Mitchell, P.H. (1980). Intracranial hypertension: Implications of research for nursing care. *Journal of Neurosurgical Nursing*, 12(3), 145–154.

Mitchell, P.H. (1986). Decreased adaptive capacity, intracranial: A proposal for a nursing diagnosis. *Journal of Neuroscience Nursing*, 18(4), 170–175.

Mitchell, P.H. (1988). Decreased behavioral arousal. In P.W. Mitchell, L.C. Hodges, M. Muwaswes, et al. (Eds.), *AANN's neuroscience nursing*. Norwalk, CT: Appleton & Lange.

Mitchell, P.H., Habermann-Little, B., Johnson, F., et al. (1985). Critically ill children: The importance of touch in a high-technology environment. *Nursing Administration Quarterly*, 9(4), 38–46.

Mitchell, P.H., and Mauss, N.K. (1978). Relationship of patient-nurse activity to intracranial pressure variations: A pilot study. *Nursing Research*, 27, 4–10.

Narayan, R., Bray, R.S., Robertson, C.S., et al. (1987). *Experience with a new fiberoptic device for intracranial pressure monitoring*. Presented at the annual meeting of the American Association of Neurological Surgeons, May, 1987, Dallas, Texas.

Narayan, R.K., Kishore, P.R., Becker, D.P., et al. (1982). Intracranial pressure: To monitor or not to monitor? *Journal of Neurosurgery*, 56, 650–659.

Nikas, D.L. (1991). The neurological system. In J.G. Alspach (Ed.), *AACN core curriculum for critical care nursing* (4th ed). Philadelphia: W.B. Saunders.

Ostrup, R.C., Luerssen, T.G., Marshall, L.F., et al. (1987). Continuous monitoring of intracranial pressure with a miniaturized fiberoptic device. *Journal of Neurosurgery*, 67, 206–209.

Parsons, L.C., and Shogan, J.S. (1984). The effects of the endotracheal tube suctioning/manual hyperventilation procedure on patients with severe closed head injuries. *Heart & Lung*, 13(4), 372–380.

Parsons, L.C., and Wilson, M.M. (1984). Cerebrovascular status of severe closed head injured patients following passive position changes. *Nursing Research*, 33(2), 68–75.

Pollack-Latham, C.L. (1987). Intracranial pressure monitoring: Part I. Physiological principles. *Critical Care Nurse*, 7(5), 40–51.

Price, M.P. (1981). Significance of intracranial pressure waveform. *Journal of Neurosurgical Nursing*, 13(2), 202–206.

Roberts, P.A., Fullenwider, C., Stevens, F.A., et al. (1983). Experimental and clinical experience with new solid state intracranial pressure monitor with in vivo zero capability. In S. Ishii, H. Nagai, and M. Brock (Eds.), *Intracranial pressure V* (pp. 104–105). Berlin: Springer-Verlag.

Rockoff, M., and Kennedy, S. (1988). Physiology and clinical aspects of raised intracranial pressure. In A.H. Ropper and S.F. Kennedy (Eds.), *Neurological and neurosurgical intensive care* (pp. 9–21). Rockville, MD: Aspen Publishers.

Ropper, A.H. (1985). Fundamental clinical aspects of increased intracranial pressure: Monitoring and treatment. In R.J. Henning, and D. Jackson (Eds.), *Critical care neurology and neurosurgery*. New York: Praeger Special Studies.

Ropper, A.H., O'Rourke, D., and Kennedy, S.K. (1982). Head position, intracranial pressure and compliance. *Neurology*, 32, 1288–1291.

Rosner, M.J., and Becker, D.P. (1984). Origin and evolution of plateau waves. *Journal of Neurosurgery*, 60(2), 312–324.

Rudy, E.B. (1984). *Advanced neurological and neurosurgical nursing*. St. Louis: C.V. Mosby.

Rudy, E.B., Baun, M., Stone, K., et al. (1986). The relationship between endotracheal suctioning and changes in intracranial pressure: A review of the literature. *Heart & Lung*, 15(5), 488–494.

Saul, T.G. (1986). Is ICP monitoring worthwhile? *Clinical neurosurgery: Proceedings of the Congress of Neurological Surgeons* (pp. 560–571). Baltimore: Williams & Wilkins.

Silverberg, G.D. (1985). Intracranial pressure monitoring. In R.H. Wilkins, and S. Rengachary (Eds.), *Neurosurgery*. New York: McGraw Hill.

Sklar, F., Reisch, J. Ealshvili, I., et al. (1980). Effects of cerebrospinal fluid formation: Nonsteady-state measurements in dogs. *American Journal of Physiology*, 239, R277–R284.

Smith, K.A. (1987). Head trauma: Comparison of infection rates for different methods of intracranial pressure monitoring. *Journal of Neuroscience Nursing*, 19(6), 310–314.

Smith, S. (1983). Continuous intracranial pressure monitoring:

Implications and applications for critical care. *Critical Care Nurse,* 42–51.

Sundbarg, G., Nordstrom, C., Messeter, K., et al. (1987). A comparison of intraparenchymatous and intraventricular pressure recording in clinical practice. *Journal of Neurosurgery, 67,* 841–845.

Vries, J.K., Becker, D.P., and Young, H.F. (1973). A subarachnoid bolt for monitoring intracranial pressure. *Journal of Neurosurgery, 39,* 416–419.

Walleck, C.A. (1987). Intracranial hypertension: Interventions and outcomes. *Critical Care Quarterly,* 10(1), 45–57.

Ward, J.D., et al. (1981). Intracranial pressure, head injuries, subarachnoid hemorrhage, nonsurgical coma and brain tumors. In W.C. Shoemaker, and W.L. Thompson (Eds.), *Critical care state of the art* (p. 2). Fullerton, CA: Society of Critical Care Medicine.

Ward, J.D., Moulton, R.J., Muizelaar, J.P., et al. (1987). Cerebral homeostasis and protection. In F.P. Wirth and R.A. Ratcheson (Eds.), *Neurosurgical critical care* (pp. 187–213). Baltimore: Williams & Wilkins.

Wilkinson, H.A. (1977). The intracranial pressure-monitoring cup catheter: Technical note. *Neurosurgery,* 1(2), 139–141.

Wyler, A.R., and Kelly, W.A. (1972). Use of antibiotics with external ventriculostomies. *Journal of Neurosurgery, 37,* 185–187.

Yano, M., Nishiyama, H., Yokota, H., et al. (1986). Effect of lidocaine on ICP response to endotracheal suctioning. *Anesthesiology, 64,* 651–653.

Zervas, N.T., Cosman, E.R., and Cosman, B.J. (1977). A pressure-balanced radio-telemetry system for the measurement of intracranial pressure. *Journal of Neurosurgery, 47,* 899–911.

Cardiovascular System

14

Cardiovascular Anatomy and Physiology

Phylita Skov
Patricia L. Vaska

OVERVIEW

The Heart and Circulation

The purpose of the cardiovascular system is to supply nutrients to cells and remove metabolic waste products. The system is composed of two coordinated pumps—the right side of the heart (the right atria and ventricle) and the left side of the heart (the left atria and ventricle)—and two circulations—the pulmonary circulation, between the right side of the heart and the left side of the heart; and the systemic circulation, between the left and right sides of the heart (Fig. 14–1).

The right and left atria are thin-walled chambers that serve primarily as reservoirs for blood returning to the heart from the systemic and pulmonary circulations (Guyton, 1991). A weak atrial contraction at the end of ventricular diastole provides 10% to 15% of the ventricular end-diastolic volume, the "atrial kick," in normal hearts. The atria are divided by a septum that continues inferiorly to become the membranous portion of the intraventricular septum that divides the two ventricles. During ventricular diastole (relaxation), blood flows through the atrioventricular valves, the tricuspid valve in the right side of the heart and the mitral valve in the left side of the heart, into the respective ventricles. During ventricular systole (contraction), blood is pumped through the semilunar valves, the pulmonic valve in the right side of the heart and the aortic valve in the left side of the heart, to the pulmonary artery and the aorta.

The pulmonary vasculature is relatively short and broad and has minimal resistance to flow. In contrast to the pulmonary system, the systemic vessels are longer and have a higher resistance. Left-sided pressures are relatively high in comparison with right-sided pressures. The arteries distribute blood to the microcirculation, where exchange of nutrients and waste products occurs. The systemic veins return deoxygenated blood to the right atrium, and the pulmonary veins return oxygenated blood to the left atrium (Cohn, 1985; Rhoades and Pflanzer, 1989).

Oxygen saturation of blood leaving the left side of the heart is approximately 95% and oxygen saturation of venous blood returning to the right side of the heart is approximately 75% at rest. Thus, in one circuit, at rest, approximately 25% of available oxygen is extracted by the tissues. Clinically, left-sided cardiac oxygen saturation is measured as arterial oxygen saturation, and right-sided cardiac oxygen saturation is measured as mixed venous oxygen saturation (Sv_{O_2}) from a pulmonary artery catheter, or, less accurately, from the right atrium because total mixing of venous blood occurs in the right ventricle, and right atrial samples may not be homogeneous. Mixed venous oxygen saturation is an overall measure of the adequacy of cardiopulmonary function in relation to tissue demand. In addition, oxygen content, oxygen delivery, and oxygen demand can be calculated (Shoemaker et al., 1988).

The circulatory system is composed of arteries, arterioles, capillaries, venules, and veins that branch going away from the heart and coalesce coming toward the heart. As the total cross-sectional area of the system increases, the rate of flow decreases, and conversely, as the cross-sectional area decreases, the rate of flow increases. The aorta and major arteries are conductance vessels, and no nutrient exchange

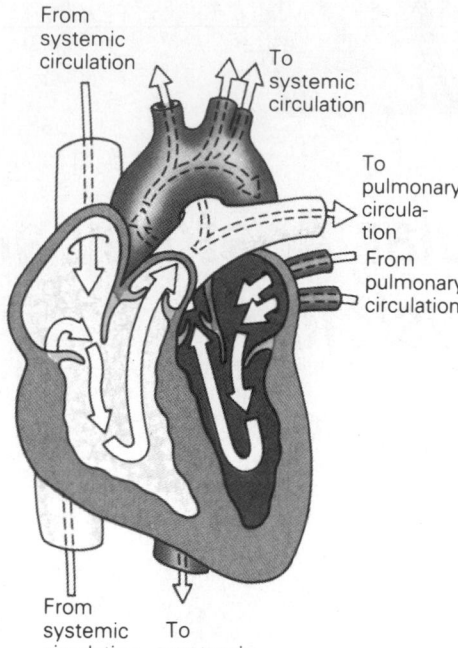

From systemic circulation

To systemic circulation

To pulmonary circulation

From pulmonary circulation

From systemic circulation

To systemic circulation

FIGURE 14–1. Overview of the heart. The direction of blood flow through the chambers of the heart and the major vessels leading into and out of the heart are indicated by the arrows. (Figure from HUMAN PHYSIOLOGY, Second Edition, by R. Rhoades and R. Pflanzer, copyright © 1992 by Saunders College Publishing, reprinted by permission of the publisher.)

occurs. The arterioles are the primary regulators of resistance. Nutrient exchange occurs at the capillary level. The veins are capacitance vessels and serve as reservoirs for blood volume. In the systemic circuit the total cardiac output is divided among the various organs according to local demand and due to changes in arteriolar resistance. The pulmonary system receives the total cardiac output (Cohn, 1985).

Physical Properties of the System

Concepts of pressure, resistance, flow, and compliance are essential to an understanding of the cardiovascular system and will be briefly reviewed (Table 14–1). These concepts will be applied in subsequent discussions.

Pressure. The driving pressure is the difference in pressure between two points in the circuit that drives flow from high pressure to low pressure. For example, the driving pressure for the systemic circuit is the pressure difference (ΔP) between the mean arterial pressure (MAP) and the mean right arterial pressure (RAP). The driving pressure for the pulmonary circuit is the difference between mean pulmonary artery pressure (PA) and the mean left atrial pressure (LA), or the pulmonary capillary wedge pressure (PCWP). The transmural pressure (P_{tm}) is the difference across the wall between the inside of a vessel or a cardiac chamber and the outside.

Resistance. The resistance to flow is directly proportional to the length of the vessel (1) and the viscosity (η) of the fluid and inversely proportional to the fourth power of the radius of the vessel (r^4).

The length of the vascular system does not change appreciably in any given individual. The primary determinant of the viscosity of blood is the hematocrit, and within the normal range hematocrit does not significantly alter the viscosity. At hematocrits

---

TABLE 14–1. Equations Defining Pressure, Flow (Ohm's Law), Resistance (Poiseuille's Law), and Compliance

Pressure across a vessel:

$$\Delta P = P_1 - P_2$$

where   P = Pressure across the vessel
   P_1 = Pressure at the proximal end
   P_2 = Pressure at the distal end

Ohm's law for calculation of flow through a vessel:

$$\dot{Q} = \frac{\Delta P}{R}$$

where $\dot{Q}$ = Flow
   ΔP = Pressure difference between the two ends of the vessel
   R = Resistance

Poiseuille's law for the relationship between flow, pressure, and resistance:

$$\dot{Q} = \frac{\pi \Delta P r^4}{8 \eta l}$$

where $\dot{Q}$ = Flow
   ΔP = Pressure difference between the ends of the vessel
   η = Blood viscosity
   r = Radius of the vessel
   l = Length of the vessel

Compliance:

$$\text{Compliance} = \frac{\text{Increase in volume}}{\text{Increase in pressure}}$$

above 60% viscosity increases, and at hematocrits below 15% viscosity decreases. The primary determinant of resistance in the body is the radius of the blood vessels, particularly the arterioles (note that the radius is raised to the fourth power in the equation defining Poiseuille's law [see Table 14–1]). Resistance increases as the vessels become more constricted and decreases as vessels dilate.

Flow. Flow ($\dot{Q}$) in the system is directly proportional to the driving pressure and inversely proportional to resistance. Clinically, flow and driving pressure can be measured, and resistance can be calculated by the equations given in Table 14–2.

Compliance. The compliance (C) of a distensible container such as the heart and blood vessels is the relationship between change in volume (ΔV) and change in pressure (ΔP) within the container. When compliance is low, the container is stiffer or less distensible and the pressure change is greater for any given volume put into the container. When compliance is high the container is easily distensible and the pressure change is less for any given volume. For example, in heart failure, in which compliance is decreased, the change in intraventricular pressure is greater for any given volume put into the ventricle than it is in a normal heart (Goerke and Mines, 1988).

TABLE 14–2. Clinical Equations for Calculation of Pressure and Resistance

Mean arterial pressure:

$$MAP = \frac{2DP + SP}{3}$$

where MAP = Mean arterial pressure
DP = Diastolic pressure
SP = Systolic pressure

Mean pulmonary artery pressure:

$$PAM = \frac{2PAD + PAS}{3}$$

where PAM = Pulmonary artery mean pressure
PAD = Pulmonary artery diastolic pressure
PS = Pulmonary artery systolic pressure

Systemic vascular resistance:

$$SVR = \frac{MAP - CVP}{CO} \times 80$$

where SVR = Systemic vascular resistance
MAP = Mean arterial pressure
CVP = Central venous pressure
CO = Cardiac output

Pulmonary vascular resistance:

$$PVR = \frac{PAM - PCWP}{CO} \times 80$$

where PVR = Pulmonary vascular resistance
PAM = Pulmonary mean pressure
PCWP = Pulmonary capillary wedge pressure
CO = Cardiac output

Wall Tension. Tension (T) in the walls of the heart or blood vessels is described by LaPlace's law, which relates the transmural pressure (P_{tm}) and the radius (r) of the structure to the wall thickness (Th) such that T = P × r/2Th. Wall tension is a major determinant of oxygen consumption. The larger the internal pressure and the larger the radius of the structure in relation to the wall thickness, the greater the oxygen demand. This concept has important implications in relation to cardiac compensatory mechanisms. An increased pressure load on the ventricle, such as occurs with hypertension or aortic stenosis, increases the wall thickness to maintain oxygen consumption at normal levels for the weight of the ventricular muscle. In a failing heart that is dilated, oxygen demand is increased simply by virtue of the increase in ventricular radius and pressure (Goerke and Mines, 1988).

The Heart

The heart hangs in the chest from the great vessels (Fig. 14–2). Anatomically, the right atrium and ventricle are anterior structures, and the left atrium and ventricle are primarily posterior structures. The heart is surrounded by the fibrous pericardium, which protects the heart and, to a degree, limits acute overdistention of the cardiac chambers.

Cardiac Skeleton and Musculature. The cardiac skeleton is a fibrous zone surrounding the valves and separating the atria and the ventricles. Atrial muscle fibers originate and insert on this fibrous skeleton. The atrial muscle fibers are composed of two layers: Deep fibers within each atria shorten toward the atrioventricular (AV) valves, propelling blood into the ventricle, and superficial fibers that pass across both atria produce lateral constriction of the atria and coordinated contraction between them (Little and Little, 1985).

The ventricular wall is composed of three layers—the epicardium lying outermost, the myocardium in the middle, and the endocardium, which lines the ventricular chamber. The area next to the myocardium, the subendocardium, is the area at greatest risk of ischemia. Ventricular muscle fibers arise from the fibrous skeleton, the root of the aorta, and the root of the pulmonary artery. Each ventricle is formed from a mass of interlocking, nested fibers that change orientation as they pass from the epicardium through the myocardium to the endocardium. During contraction this arrangement produces both circumferential and longitudinal compression of the ventricular chamber and propels blood into the great vessels. There are some fibers that surround both ventricles as well (Streeter et al, 1969).

The left ventricle, which is conically shaped, is much thicker than the right ventricle and contracts with a wringing motion that forcefully propels blood into the aorta. The right ventricle wraps around the

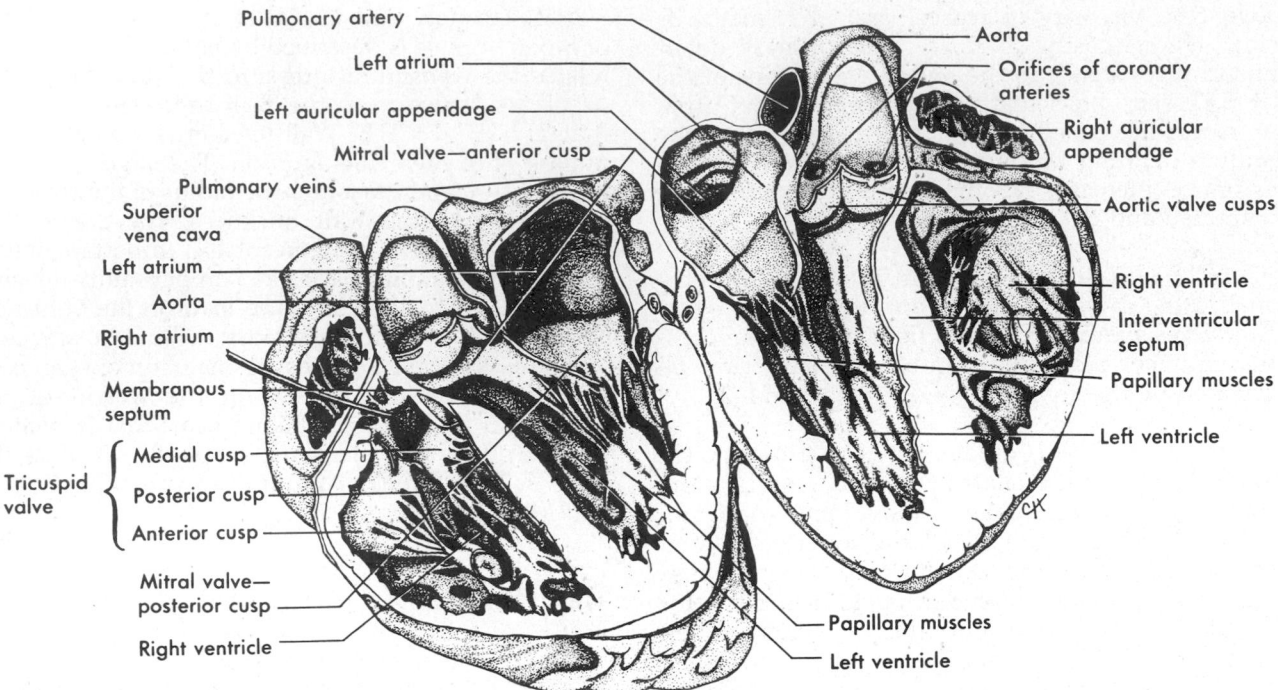

FIGURE 14–2. Drawing of a heart split perpendicular to the interventricular septum to illustrate the anatomic relationships of the leaflets of the atrioventricular (AV) and aortic valves. (Reproduced by permission from: Berne, R., and Levy, M. *Cardiovascular physiology* (5th ed). St. Louis, 1986, The C. V. Mosby Co.)

convex intraventricular septum, is crescent-shaped, and contracts with a bellows motion that effectively pumps large volumes of blood into the low-pressure pulmonary circuit. The intraventricular septum is both structurally and functionally more a part of the left ventricle than the right; however, deformation of the septum occurs with abnormal loading conditions in either ventricle, and thus impaired function in one ventricle will affect function in the other ventricle (Halpenny and Bond, 1989).

The Valves. The valve leaflets are a cartilaginous, avascular matrix with a covering of endothelium. Many mechanisms have been proposed to explain valve motion. Most evidence suggests that the opening and closing motions of the cardiac valves are passive and are due to differences in pressure between the cardiac chambers or between the chamber and the respective great vessel. The atrioventricular valves, the two-leaflet mitral valve, and the three-leaflet tricuspid valve are complicated structures (Fig. 14–2). The atrial wall, the annulus, the papillary muscles, and the chordae tendineae are all involved in closure and competency of the valve during ventricular systole. As the ventricle contracts and the pressure exceeds that of the atria, the leaflets begin to close. With a long ventricular filling time (P–R interval greater than 0.18), atrial pressure falls below ventricular pressure due to atrial relaxation, and valve closure may begin before the onset of ventricular systole (Cohn, 1985). Narrowing of the annulus with the decrease in ventricular chamber size assists coaptation of the leaflets. Contraction of the papillary

muscles maintains tension on the chordae and prevents eversion of the leaflets into the atria. Additionally, chordae from one papillary muscle insert on both leaflets, thus providing some assistance to both leaflets.

The semilunar valves, comprising the aortic and pulmonic valves, have three cusps that allow them to open maximally with ventricular ejection. During ejection, the aortic valve leaflets are held away from the aortic wall by turbulent flow in the sinus of Valsalva and do not obstruct the coronary ostia. During ventricular diastole, reversal of flow in the great arteries catches the cusps and closes the valves.

The Coronary Arteries. The coronary arteries arise in the aortic root just above the aortic valve and run in the epicardial layer. They give off penetrating branches that provide blood to the myocardium (Fig. 14–3). Unlike flow in other arteries in the body, the majority of coronary blood flow occurs during ventricular diastole. Thus, the perfusion pressure for the coronary arteries is the aortic diastolic pressure minus the intracavitary diastolic pressure. The subendocardium is most distant from the major epicardial vessels and most affected by intracavitary pressure and is at greatest risk for ischemia.

The major epicardial vessels (Fig. 14–4) are the right coronary artery and the left main coronary artery, which divides into the left anterior descending branch and the circumflex branch. The right coronary artery runs laterally and posteriorly, in the atrioventricular sulcus between the right atrium and the right ventricle. The acute marginal branches perfuse the

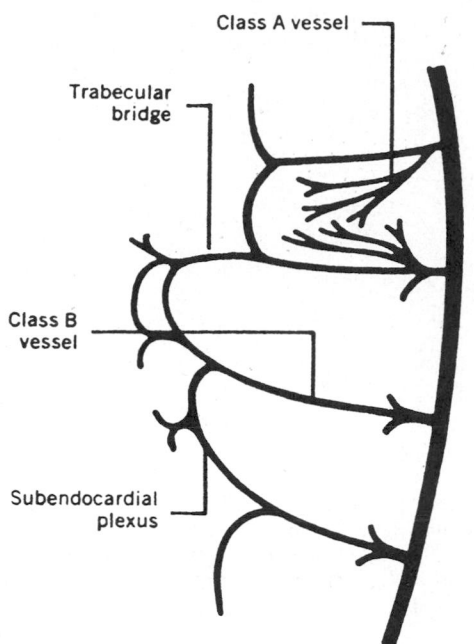

FIGURE 14-3. Anatomy of the normal coronary circulation. (From Gorlin, R., and Herman, M. (1972). Angina pectoris: A physiologic update. In R. Gorlin (Ed.), *Coronary artery disease.* Morris Plains, NJ: Warner-Chilcott Laboratories.)

right ventricular free wall. Posteriorly, in most of the population, the right coronary artery turns downward in the posterior interventricular sulcus and becomes the posterior descending artery, which perfuses the posterior third of the intraventricular septum and a portion of the posterior left ventricle.

The left main coronary artery is very short and branches into the left anterior descending and the circumflex arteries. The left anterior descending runs inferiorly in the anterior interventricular sulcus and branches into septal perforators that perfuse the anterior two-thirds of the intraventricular septum and most of the conduction system. Diagonal branches perfuse the anterior and lateral walls of the left ventricle. The circumflex turns posteriorly in the atrioventricular sulcus and, with its major branches, the obtuse marginals, perfuses the posterior portion of the left ventricle. Deoxygenated blood returns through the cardiac veins and the coronary sinus to the right atrium (Hurst et al., 1990; Little and Little 1985).

The Conduction System. The conduction system is composed of the sinus (sinoatrial [SA]) node, the atrial internodal tracts, the atrioventricular (AV) node, the common bundle, the left and right bundle branches, and the Purkinje fibers (Fig. 14–5). Normally, a cell or cells in the SA node reaches threshold first, and this stimulus then spreads to other cells via low-resistance pathways, intercalated discs, and gap junctions. This wave of excitation spreads throughout the atria from cell to cell and to the AV node through specialized conduction pathways. In the AV node the rate of conductance of the impulse is slowed (decremental conduction), allowing time for mechanical contraction in the atria and final filling of the ventricles before ventricular contraction begins. From the AV node the impulse moves into the common bundle, the only normal conductive pathway between the atria and the ventricles, and then to the left and right bundle branches, the Purkinje fibers, and then from cell to cell. The ventricle depolarizes from the endocardium to the epicardium. However, unlike other types of cells, it does not repolarize in the same direction. It repolarizes from

FIGURE 14-4. Diagram showing location of major coronary arteries and veins on anterior *(top)* and posterior *(bottom)* surfaces of the heart. (From Little, R., and Little, W. (1985). *Physiology of the heart and circulation.* Chicago: Year Book Medical Publishers.)

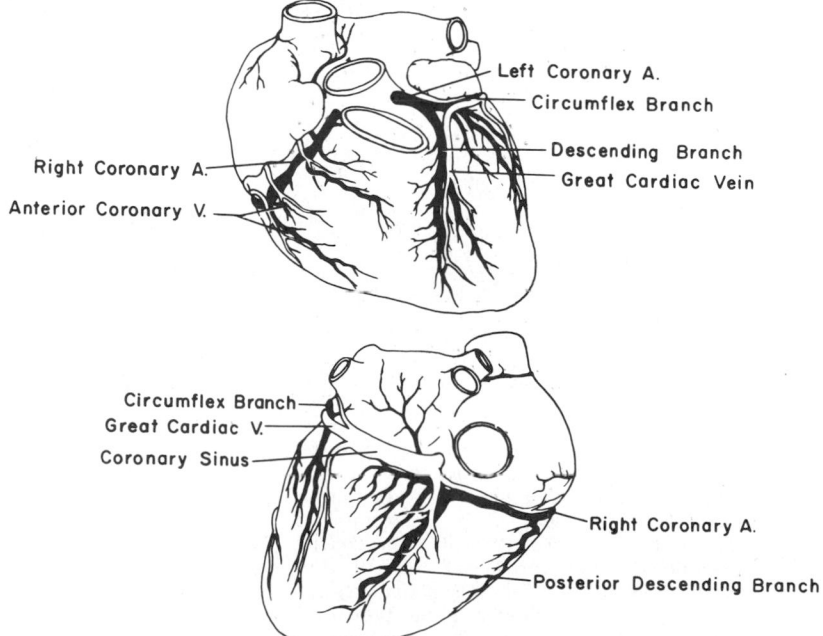

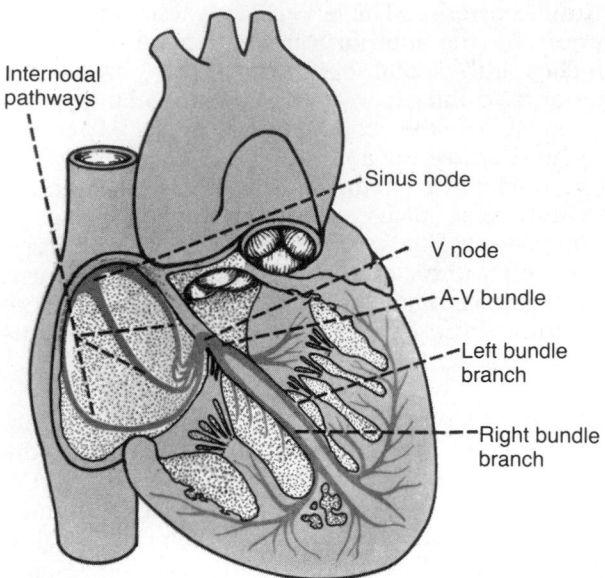

Internodal pathways

Sinus node

V node

A-V bundle

Left bundle branch

Right bundle branch

FIGURE 14–5. The sinus node and the Purkinje system of the heart showing also the AV node, the atrial internodal pathways, and the ventricular bundle branches. (From Guyton, A. (1991). *Textbook of medical physiology* (8th ed.). Philadelphia: W. B. Saunders.)

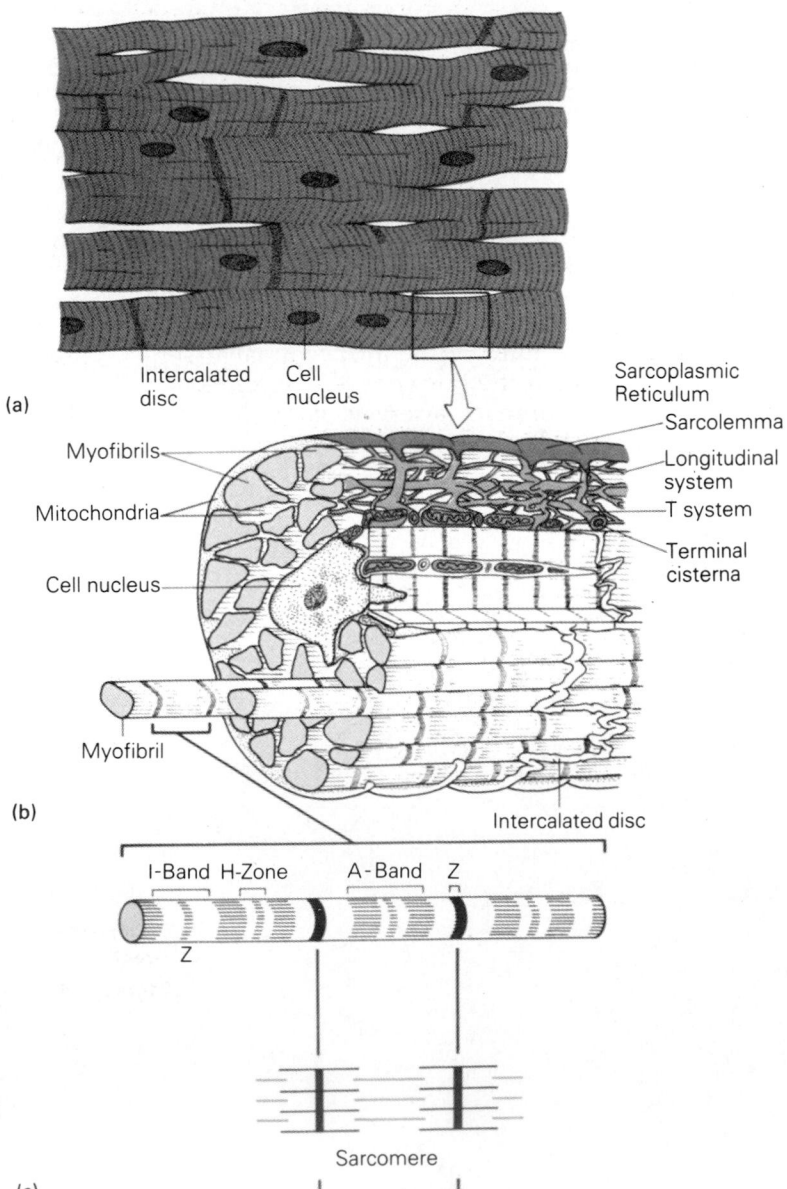

(a)

Intercalated disc   Cell nucleus

Sarcoplasmic Reticulum

Sarcolemma

Myofibrils

Mitochondria

Cell nucleus

Longitudinal system

T system

Terminal cisterna

Myofibril

(b)

Intercalated disc

I-Band   H-Zone   A-Band   Z

Z

Sarcomere

(c)

FIGURE 14–6. Structure of cardiac muscle. *A,* The cells of the muscle are small and sometimes branched, and they attach end to end. *B,* Seen at higher magnification, bundles of myofibrils run the length of the muscle, and a sarcoplasmic reticulum and T system, which function much as they do in skeletal muscle, are present. *C,* The sarcomere is organized in the same way that it is in skeletal muscle. (Modified from Braunwald, E., Ross, J., and Sonnenblick, E. H. (1968). *Mechanism of contraction of the normal and failing heart.* Boston: Little, Brown. In Rhoades, R., and Pflanzer, R. (1989). *Human physiology.* Philadelphia: Saunders College Publishing.)

the epicardium to the endocardium. The reason for this is unclear but is thought to be due to the stresses placed on the endocardium by the increased intra-cavitary pressure and decreased blood flow to the endocardium that occurs during ventricular systole (Bayés De Luna, 1987).

Ultrastructure and Mechanisms of Contraction

Ultrastructure. Cardiac muscle (Fig. 14–6) is a syncytium, a multinucleated mass of protoplasm formed by a secondary union of separate cells that acts as a single unit. Cardiac muscle fibers are the cells of the heart. They are joined by a specialized, thickened portion of the cell membrane called the intercalated disc. The intercalated disc allows the contractile force of one cell to be transmitted to the next. In addition, a specialized area within the inter-calated disc called the nexus is a low-resistance pathway that allows rapid conduction of impulses between adjacent cardiac cells. It is thought that within the nexus there is an area where the mem-branes of adjoining cells are in extremely close phys-ical proximity and that some exchange of ions may occur that enhances conduction (Cohn, 1985; Bond, 1989).

Molecular Basis of Contraction. Each cardiac cell, or fiber, contains multiple myofibrils made up of repeating sarcomeres that are longitudinally joined (Fig. 14–7). The sarcomeres are the functional units of the cardiac muscle fiber. They contain thin bands of the protein actin and thick bands of the protein myosin in an alternating arrangement (Fig. 14–7). Actin filaments are anchored at each end of the sarcomere at the z-lines and extend toward the center of the sarcomere but do not meet. At rest, the actin-binding sites for myosin are covered by long chains of tropomyosin that are held in place by troponin.

The myosin fibrils extend from the center of the sarcomere toward, but not to, the Z-lines. Following electrical excitation, globular projections on the myosin fibers form cross-bridges between the myosin and actin fibers. There are no globular heads in the middle of the myosin filaments, and therefore con-nection between myosin and actin cannot occur in the very middle of the sarcomere. The filaments do not shorten themselves but slide past each other, thus shortening the fiber. At very long and very short fiber lengths the number of cross-bridges that can be attached is reduced, thus limiting the force of contraction.

The T system is composed of the T tubules and the sarcoplasmic reticulum (see Fig. 14–6). The T tubules are invaginations of the cell membrane (sarcolemma) that are in direct contact with the extracellular fluid, allowing rapid transmission of the action potential to each of the myofibrils within the cardiac cell so that they contract together. As in other areas of the cell membrane, there are voltage-gated ionic channels and active transport systems as well as receptors for

FIGURE 14–7. A structure of the myofilaments. *A,* The actin filaments are made up of two chains of action monomers twisted one half-turn for every seven monomers. The regulatory protein troponin (composed of three subunits) is associated with the fibrous protein tropomyosin, which extends along a group of seven monomers in the filament. *B,* Struc-ture of the individual myosin molecules. The myosin molecules are assembled into a two-ended filament with their heads protruding out to form cross-bridges and their tail portions forming the main body of the filament. *C,* Diagram showing how myosin and actin filaments are arranged in a sarcomere. (Figure from HUMAN PHYSIOLOGY, Second Edition, by R. Rhoades and R. Pflanzer, copyright © 1992 by Saun-ders College Publishing, reprinted by permission of the publisher.)

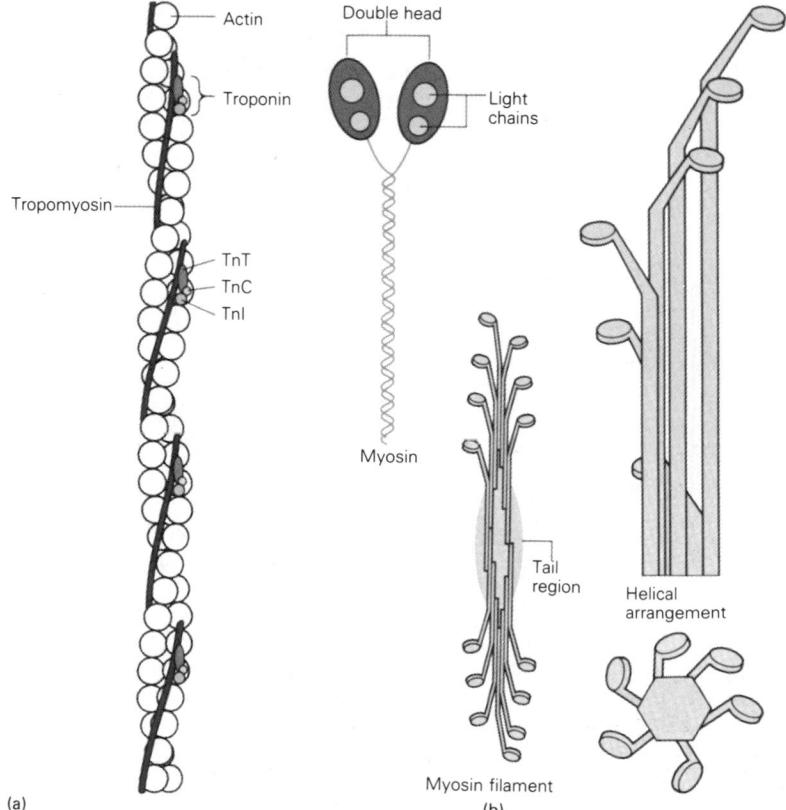

(a)

(b)

neurotransmitters and hormones (Rhoades and Pflanzer, 1989; Braunwald et al., 1976.)

The sarcoplasmic reticulum is an intracellular structure that surrounds the myofibrils and is in close proximity with the T tubules. It is thought to be the primary source of calcium for muscle contraction. The membrane of this organelle is also supplied with active transport systems and receptor sites (Stern et al., 1988).

There is no direct physical connection between the T tubules and the sarcoplasmic reticulum, but there is thought to be a "coupling process," a voltage-gated channel for calcium and possibly other ions. It is thought that when an action potential occurs, the gate is opened, and calcium entering the sarcoplasmic reticulum from the T tubule triggers the release of calcium from the sarcoplasmic reticulum to the cytosol. The quantity and rate of calcium movement is influenced by neurotransmitter and hormonal receptors (Cohn, 1985).

Excitation-Contraction Coupling. This is the sequence of events, initiated by an action potential, that increases the availability of calcium and allows cross-bridging to occur. In the relaxed state, the active binding sites for myosin on the actin chains are covered, or inhibited, by tropomyosin. In the myosin head, the enzyme ATPase splits adenosine triphosphate (ATP) to adenosine diphosphate (ADP) and organic phosphate, providing the energy to be used as soon as the active binding sites on the actin chains become available.

The action potential propagated down the T tubule increases calcium diffusion from the interstitial fluid to the cytosol and also triggers release of calcium from the sarcoplasmic reticulum to the cytosol (Fig. 14–8). The calcium (up to four ions) binds with troponin, which alters the configuration of tropo-

myosin and exposes the active binding sites on the actin chain. The myosin head attaches to the actin site and swivels toward the center of the sarcomere, pulling the actin filaments past and resulting in fiber shortening. ADP and inorganic phosphate are released from the myosin head, and a binding site for ATP on the myosin head is exposed. The binding of ATP to this site breaks the connection with actin, and the myosin head returns to its original position. Myosin ATPase again splits the ATP, and the myosin head attaches to another binding site. This process is repeated many times during a single contraction and continues as long as ATP and calcium are available and active binding sites on the actin chains are exposed.

During relaxation, active calcium pumps in the membrane of the sarcoplasmic reticulum and the T tubules remove calcium from the cytosol, and calcium is released by troponin. Tropomyosin returns to its previous configuration, and the active binding sites on the actin chain are covered. In addition, calcium returns to the T tubules through the sodium-calcium exchange mechanism (Ruegg, 1986).

Cytosolic calcium concentration, the rate of calcium exchange, and the resting fiber length determine the number of cross-bridges that can attach, the strength and rate of contraction, and the rate and degree of relaxation. In a normal individual at rest, the cytosolic calcium concentration is relatively low, not all of the troponin molecules are fully activated, and not all of the binding sites on the actin chain are uncovered. In addition, fiber length is relatively short, and the actin and myosin chains are not optimally aligned for the occurrence of maximum cross-bridging. Thus, there is a contractile reserve that can be used to increase the rate and force of contraction when required by metabolic demands.

For example, sympathetic stimulation increases

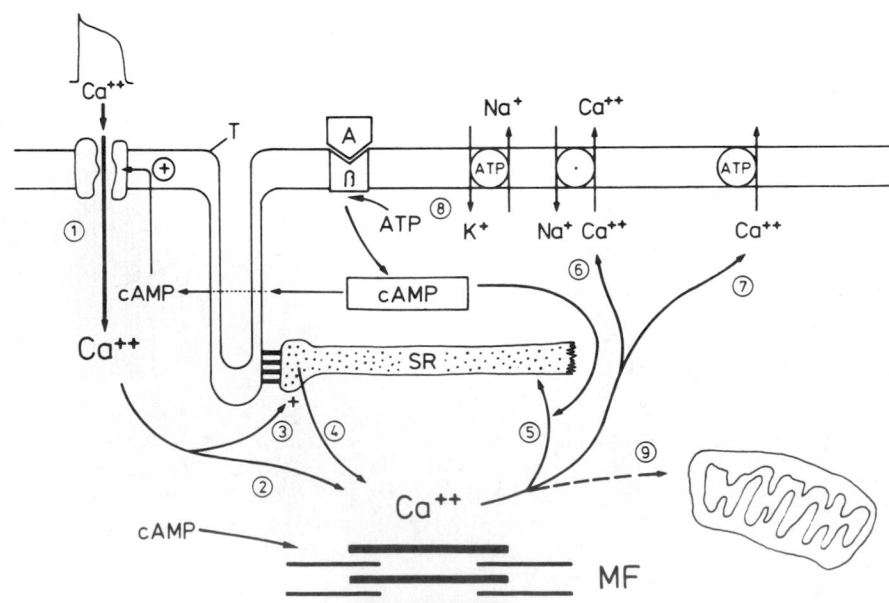

FIGURE 14–8. Calcium movements in mammalian cardiac muscle. *1*, Ca^{2+} influx through hypothetical cyclic AMP regulated calcium channel. *2*, Calcium action on myofilaments. *3*, Calcium triggering of Ca^{2+} release from sarcoplasmic reticulum (SR). *4*, Calcium release from SR. *5*, Calcium reuptake into SR. *6*, Calcium extrusion from cell by Na–Ca exchange. *7*, Calcium extrusion by active membrane pump. *8*, Na–K pump. *9*, Mitochondrial calcium uptake. *Abbreviations: MF*, myofilaments; *T*, transverse tubule; *A*, agonist binding to beta-adrenergic receptor. Calcium-channel regulation by alpha-adrenergic receptors is not shown. (Adapted from Ruegg, J. (1988). *Calcium in muscle activation.* Berlin: Springer-Verlag; in Milnor, W. (1990). *Cardiovascular physiology.* New York: Oxford University Press.) (Reproduced from Ruegg, with permission of Springer-Verlag.)

both the amount of calcium that enters the cell and the rate of active transport through receptor-mediated channels. Thus, both the strength of the contraction and the rate of contraction and relaxation are increased. Conversely, drugs that block calcium channels produce a negative inotropic effect and slow the rate of fiber shortening and relaxation (Noble, 1987).

In cardiac failure, fibers are stretched, and the number of cross-bridges that can attach are decreased, and therefore the force of contraction is decreased. Additionally, in chronic heart failure the number of beta receptors is reduced (down-regulation), decreasing receptor-mediated calcium transport and further impairing contractile function and the ability to raise cardiac output to meet metabolic demands. If cardiac failure is due to ischemia, the amount of calcium removed from the cytosol is also decreased, which impairs relaxation and decreases ventricular compliance (Yancy and Firth, 1988).

ELECTRICAL ACTIVITY OF THE HEART
Resting Membrane Potential

In cardiac cells, as in other cells in the body, there is a concentration gradient across the cell membrane for sodium, potassium, calcium, and other ions that is determined by the permeability of the membrane to each ion, its electrical charge, and the functioning of active ionic pumps in the cell membrane. Movement of ions across the cell membrane occurs both passively down the electrochemical gradient and through energy-requiring ionic pumps in the cell membrane that actively transport specific ions against the electrochemical gradients. It must be noted that the ionic exchanges discussed in the following sections involve only a small amount of the total ionic composition of the cell and the extracelullar fluid.

Membrane Permeability. It has been proposed that the permeability of the cell membrane for specific ions is controlled by gates in the cell membrane that open and close in response to electrical stimulation and other factors. These voltage-gated channels open and close within specific voltage ranges. For example, gates that allow rapid sodium influx are activated at about −70 millivolts (mV), whereas slow inward calcium and sodium channels are activated at −40 to −30 mV (Guyton, 1991; Milnor, 1990).

Electrochemical Gradients. In the resting state the cell membrane is permeable to potassium and minimally permeable to sodium. Potassium slowly leaks out of the cell down its concentration gradient, leaving behind negatively charged proteins and other substances. The movement of potassium ions out of the cell is limited by the increasing negativity inside the cell. The diffusion gradient for potassium is counterbalanced by the electrical gradient, and equilibrium is reached when inward and outward move-

ment of potassium is equal. If the membrane were permeable only to potassium this would establish a resting membrane potential of −95 mV, which is slightly more negative than the actual resting potential in the Purkinje fibers and ventricular cells of about −90mV. However, the membrane is also slightly permeable to the influx of sodium and calcium, and a true equilibrium is not reached (Goerke and Mines, 1988).

Active Transport. In addition to passive movement of ions due to electrochemical gradients, membrane potential is maintained by active transport of ions across the membrane by energy-requiring pumps (see Fig. 14–8). The sodium–potassium ATPase pump operates in such a way that two potassium ions are exchanged for three sodium ions, resulting in a net loss of positive ions within the cell and intracellular negativity (Vassalle, 1987). The sodium–calcium exchange system in the cell membrane uses electrochemical energy to transport two sodium ions into the cell for one calcium ion transported out of the cell during the resting phase (McGuigan and Blatter, 1987). The calcium ATPase pump moves calcium out of the cell as well as into the sarcoplasmic reticulum from the cytosol during recovery (McGuigan and Blatter, 1987).

These mechanisms establish and maintain the resting membrane potential. An electrical stimulus or other conditions that alter these mechanisms allows the cell to become more positive until it reaches threshold, when depolarization continues.

Action Potential

Ventricular Action Potential. At rest, potassium channels are open, and potassium is conducted out of the cell, establishing the resting membrane potential (Fig. 14–9). With excitation of the membrane in phase 0, fast sodium channels open, there is a rapid influx of sodium into the cell and a slowing of potassium efflux out of the cell, and the membrane potential rises to +30. In phase 1, the fast inward sodium channels close, and potassium efflux continues at a slower rate, bringing the membrane potential to approximately 0. In phase 2, the plateau phase, slow inward sodium and calcium channels open, the influx of these ions matches the outward flow of potassium, and the membrane remains depolarized. The influx of calcium participates in the cross-bridging of actin and myosin and mechanical contraction and also triggers the release of calcium from the sarcoplasmic reticulum for this process. In phase 3 the slow sodium and calcium channels close, and potassium conductance increases to the level of the resting state. The efflux of potassium then returns the membrane to the resting membrane potential, and the sodium–potassium ATPase pump is activated. During phases 0, 1, and 2 the cell is absolutely refractory. It is not polarized and cannot accept another stimulus. As the membrane potential is re-

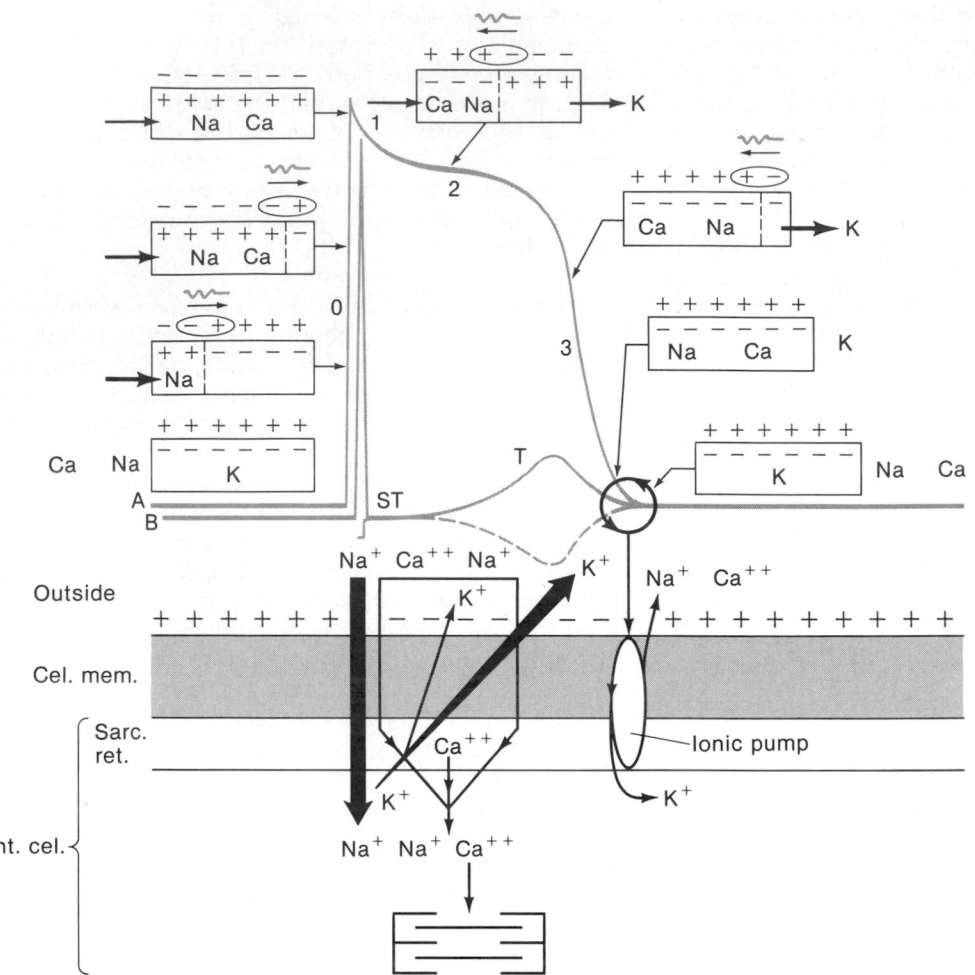

FIGURE 14–9. Diagram of the electronic correlation in a contractile cell. Cel. mem., cell membrane; sarc. ret., sarcoplasmic reticulum; int. cel., intracellular. (From Bayés De Luna, A. (1987). *Textbook of clinical electrocardiography.* Dordrecht: Martinus-Nijhoff. Reproduced with permission of Kluwer Academic Press.)

stored during phase 3, the cell becomes relatively refractory—that is, it can be stimulated but requires a stronger stimulus. At the end of phase 3 there is a supernormal period during which a very small stimulus will elicit an action potential.

Sinus Node Action Potential. The action potential in the sinus node varies from that of the ventricle and Purkinje fibers in several ways (Fig. 14–10). The maximum resting potential is only -55 to -60 mV. At this level, fast sodium channels are inactivated, and the rise in phase 0 is slower due to the opening of slow sodium and calcium channels. There is no plateau phase. Sodium and calcium channels become inactivated, and potassium channels open, allowing repolarization to occur.

The spontaneous rise of phase 4 of the sinus node action potential to threshold is the basis of the property of automaticity in the heart. That is, an action potential can be initiated without an outside stimulus. The ionic shifts that produce this spontaneous diastolic depolarization are somewhat controversial. During phase 4 there may be a slow decrease in the rate of outward potassium conductance that limits the amount of negativity that builds up in the cell, allowing the membrane potential to rise to threshold or an increase in inward sodium and cal-

cium flux that would have the same effect, or both (Cohn, 1985; Guyton, 1991). The cell reaches threshold and depolarizes, initiating depolarization for the entire heart, and the cycle starts over.

The rate of rise of phase 4 in automatic cells is affected by neurotransmitters, thus altering heart rate as well as conduction velocities within the conduction system (Fig. 14–11). Afferent parasympathetic fibers from the vagus nerve innervate primarily the conduction system at the SA and AV nodes. There are few parasympathetic afferents to the ventricle or the ventricular muscle fibers. Parasympathetic stimulation releases the neurotransmitter acetylcholine, causing the resting membrane potential to be more negative, that is, further from threshold, slowing the

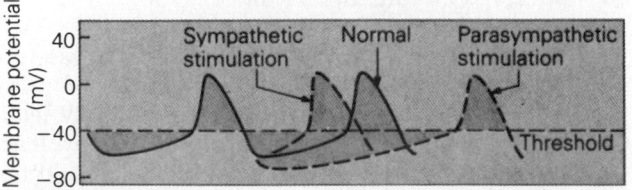

FIGURE 14–10. Effect of autonomic nerve activity on spontaneous depolarization of the sinus node. (Figure from HUMAN PHYSIOLOGY, Second Edition, by R. Rhoades and R. Pflanzer, copyright © 1992 by Saunders College Publishing, reprinted by permission of the publisher.)

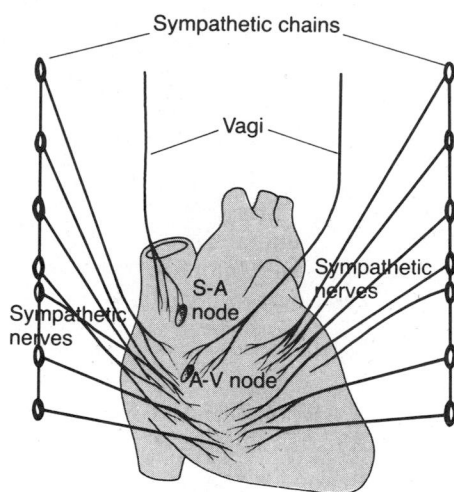

FIGURE 14–11. The cardiac nerves. (From Guyton, A. (1991). *Textbook of medical physiology* (8th ed.). Philadelphia: W. B. Saunders.)

rate of conduction in the AV node and slowing the rate of spontaneous depolarization in phase 4. It does this by maintaining the rate of potassium conductance and slowing sodium conductance. The effect of this is that it takes longer for the cell to rise to threshold and fire and longer for the stimulus to reach and be conducted through the AV node. Extreme stimulation, such as occurs with carotid sinus massage, may block conduction at the AV node altogether. Normally, parasympathetic tone predominates at rest, and the resting heart rate is 80 beats/minute as opposed to the basic unregulated rate of 100 to 120 beats/minute.

Norepinephrine increases membrane permeability to calcium, increasing the rate of rise of phase 4 to threshold and also increasing the velocity of conduction. It acts along the entire excitation pathway and on contractile muscle cells as well.

CARDIAC PUMPING

The Cardiac Cycle

The relationship of electrical events, mechanical events, and blood flow that occur during each heart beat within the heart itself and in the major vessels is depicted in Figure 14–12. Electrical events are clinically evaluated by the electrocardiogram (ECG) and by electrophysiologic studies.

Arterial and atrial pressures can be monitored at the bedside, and inferences are made about volume and flow. Measurement of ventricular volumes and pressures usually requires diagnostic procedures such as echocardiography or cardiac catheterization; however, a pulmonary artery catheter capable of measuring right ventricular volumes at the bedside has recently become available (Hurford and Zapol, 1988). A clear understanding of the cardiac cycle is essential for clinical assessment of normal and abnormal heart sounds and interpretation of other clinical findings.

The cardiac cycle is divided into two major phases, ventricular systole and ventricular diastole. Atrial systole occurs during late ventricular diastole. Electrical events precede mechanical events due to the time required for the biochemical processes previously described. Mechanical contraction begins in the middle of the QRS complex, and electrical repolarization, the T wave on the ECG, occurs during ventricular ejection. The same events occur on the right side of the heart but at lower pressures due to the lower resistance of the pulmonary circuit.

Ventricular Systole. Following excitation, the muscle begins to contract. When the ventricular pressure exceeds the pressure in the atria, which occurs almost immediately, the atrioventricular valves close, producing the first heart sound (S_1). At this time the pressure in the ventricle is less than that in the aorta and the pulmonary artery, and the semilunar valves remain closed. Tension continues to increase in the muscle, increasing the intraventricular pressure. Because all the valves are closed there is no change in volume, and this is called isovolumetric contraction. During this phase of systole, 90% of myocardial oxygen consumption occurs. The ventricle shortens from base to apex, becoming more spherical, the AV valves bulge into the atria, producing the c wave in the atrial and jugular venous waveforms, and the chordae tendineae tense to prevent eversion of the leaflets into the atria. Continuing increases in ventricular muscle tension pull down on the atrial floor, increasing atrial size and decreasing atrial pressure, as evidenced by the x descent in the atrial and jugular venous wave forms.

When the ventricular pressure exceeds the diastolic pressure in the receiving vessels, the aorta and the pulmonary artery, the semilunar valves open, and rapid ejection occurs. Peak ejection produces systolic pressure in the receiving vessel. During ejection, ventricular fibers shorten circumferentially as well as longitudinally, wall thickness increases, and chamber size decreases. The atria continue to fill during ventricular ejection, and the increase in pressure produces the v wave in the atrial and jugular venous waveforms.

As the ventricle empties, the volume ejected decreases, and the pressure in the ventricle and the receiving vessels falls. At the end of ejection, reversal of flow catches the cusps of the semilunar valves, closing them and producing the second heart sound (S_2) and the dicrotic notch in the arterial waveforms. Aortic pressure declines to the diastolic level as blood runs off into the periphery. Volume left in the ventricle at the end of systole is called the end-systolic volume (ESV) or residual volume and is increased in patients with heart failure. The ESV is a reserve volume that with increased vigor of contraction can be used to increase cardiac output in the healthy heart.

Ventricular Diastole. The ventricle continues to relax with all the valves closed, and there is no

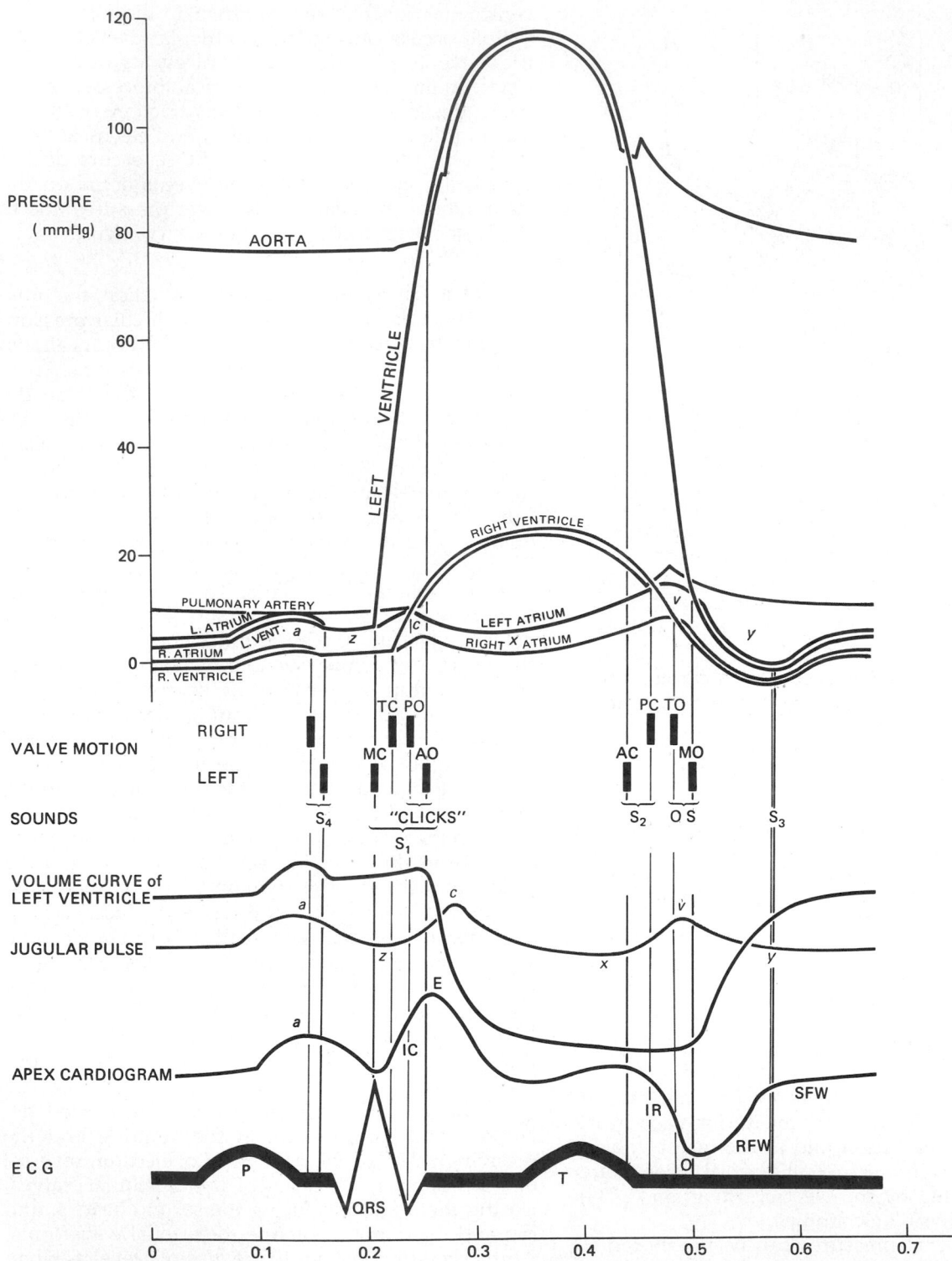

FIGURE 14–12. Diagram of the cardiac cycle, showing the pressure curves of the great vessels and cardiac chambers, valvular events and heart sounds, left ventricular volume curve, jugular pulse wave, apex cardiogram (Sanborn piezo crystal), and the electrocardiogram. For illustrative purposes, the time intervals between the valvular events have been modified and the z point has been prolonged. *Valve motion:* MC, mitral component of the first heart sound; MO, mitral valve opening; TC, tricuspid component of the first heart sound; TO, tricuspid valve opening; AC, aortic component of the second heart sound; AO, aortic valve opening; PC, pulmonic valve component of the second heart sound; PO, pulmonic valve opening; OS, opening snap of atrioventricular valves. *Apex cardiogram:* IC, isovolumic or isovolumetric (isochoric) contraction wave; IR, isovolumic or isovolumetric (isochoric) relaxation wave; O, opening of mitral valve; RFW, rapid-filling wave; SFW, slow-filling wave. (From Hurst, J., et al. (Ed.) (1978). *The heart, arteries and veins* (7th ed.). Copyright © 1978 by McGraw-Hill, Inc. Used by permission of McGraw-Hill Book Company.)

change in volume during isovolumetric relaxation. When the pressure in the ventricles falls below that in the atria, the AV valves open, and blood that returned to the atria during ventricular systole rushes into the ventricle during the phase of rapid ventricular filling. This is seen as the y descent in the atrial and jugular venous waveforms. Normally, the ventricle continues to relax during this period, and ventricular pressure continues to decline rapidly despite the inrush of blood. A third heart sound (S_3) may be produced at this time if the heart is already overfilled or poorly compliant. At the end of the rapid filling phase, the ventricle has completed relaxation, and the slow filling phase begins as the ventricle is distended by blood that continues to return to the heart. This is seen as an increase in pressure in the ventricular waveform.

At end-diastole, atrial depolarization (the P wave in the ECG) and subsequent contraction of the atria provide the final component of ventricular filling. This is seen as the a wave in the atrial, jugular venous, and ventricular pressure waveforms. In a normal heart this atrial kick provides 10% to 15% of the ventricular end-diastolic volume (EDV). However, if ventricular compliance is decreased, as in patients with heart failure, or if the heart rate is rapid, limiting diastolic filling time, the atrial kick may provide 30% to 40% of the ventricular end-diastolic volume. The propulsion of blood into the ventricle by atrial contraction may produce a fourth heart sound (S_4) if the ventricle is poorly compliant.

The amount of blood ejected per beat is the stroke volume and is the EDV minus the ESV. The normal value at rest is about 75 mL. The stroke volume expressed as a percentage of EDV is called the ejection fraction and is a measure of global ventricular function, that is, the percentage of the EDV that is ejected per beat. A normal ejection fraction is 67%. Ejection fractions below 40% are considered to represent a clinically significant reduction in myocardial function (Cohn, 1985; Little and Little, 1985).

Another way of depicting the changes in pressure and volume that occur during the cardiac cycle is the pressure-volume loop (Fig. 14–13). Ventricular systole begins at the lower right corner with mitral valve closure producing S_1, followed by isovolumetric contraction. When the pressure in the ventricle exceeds that in the aorta, the aortic valve opens, and the stroke volume is ejected. At end-ejection, the aortic valve closes, producing S_2, and isovolumetric relaxation begins. When the pressure in the relaxing ventricle becomes lower than that in the atria, the mitral valve opens, and rapid filling ensues. Slow filling continues with a gradual rise in ventricular pressure until atrial contraction produces the final EDV, and the cycle starts over. The area enclosed in the diagram in Figure 14–13 is representative of cardiac work during that heartbeat (Goerke and Mines, 1988).

The end-diastolic and end-systolic pressure volume relationships reflect the interactions between the

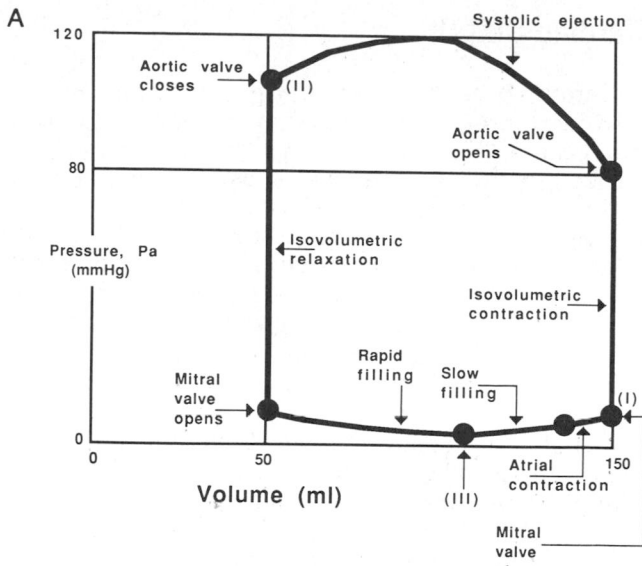

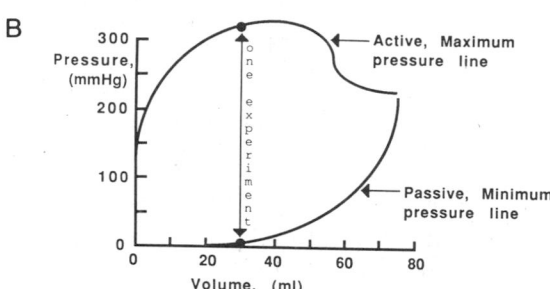

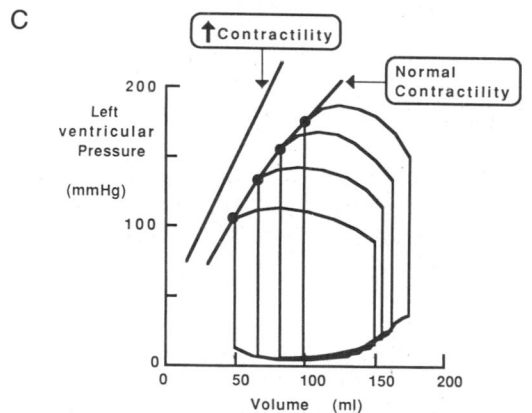

FIGURE 14–13. *A,* Left ventricular pressure–volume diagram. *B,* Isovolumetric contractions of a dog heart at different volumes. (From F. H. Starling's Linacre Lecture.) *C,* Contractility as defined by plots of end-systolic points. (From Goerke, J., and Mines, A. (1988). *Cardiovascular physiology.* New York: Raven Press.)

heart and the circulation. The end-diastolic pressure volume point is determined by the compliance of the ventricle and the amount of venous return. The end-systolic point is determined by the resistance in the vascular system and the contractile state of the myocardium. Plots of the end-systolic pressure volume points in successive heart beats (Fig. 14–13) demonstrate the contractile function of the heart (Katz, 1988).

Cardiac Output

Cardiac output (CO) is the product of heart rate (HR) and stroke volume (SV) or the amount ejected per beat (CO = HR × SV). The determinants of stroke volume are the end-diastolic fiber tension (preload), the tension developed in the myocardium during ejection (afterload), and the contractile state of the myocardium exclusive of preload (contractility). The ability to contract is a property of muscle and is independent of loading conditions. However, changes in loading conditions or inotropic state will alter the rate and force of contraction.

Preload, the Length-Tension Relationship. In isolated muscle strips the force and rate of fiber shortening depend on the resting length of the fiber. The greater the length, within physiologic limits, the more forceful the contraction. Fiber length cannot be directly determined in the intact heart. Starling demonstrated, however, that the same relationship exists between ventricular end-diastolic volume and fiber length (Fig. 14–14). An increase in volume or preload intrinsically increases the force of contraction and the stroke volume if all other parameters are held constant. Conversely, a decrease in preload decreases the force of contraction and the stroke volume. Figure 14–15 demonstrates the major factors that influence preload. These include venous tone, the pumping action of skeletal muscle, atrial contraction, total blood volume, body position, and intrathoracic and intrapericardial pressure. The preload reserve is the increase in volume that will increase stroke volume and provide a higher cardiac output to meet increases in tissue demand. This mechanism allows the heart to adapt to changes in venous return and maintains equality between the outputs of the right and left sides of the heart. At low and excessively high volumes (short and very long fiber lengths) cross-

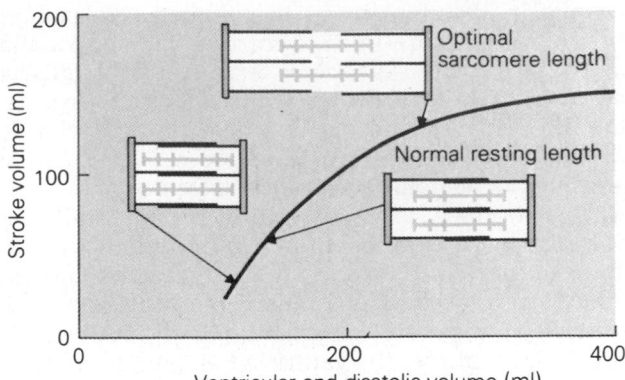

FIGURE 14–14. Frank-Starling law of the heart. This graph illustrates the relationship between stroke volume and changes in ventricular end-diastolic volume. The insets showing, diagrammatic sarcomeres, illustrate the relationship between end-diastolic volume and myofilament overlap. At normal resting ventricular volumes, sarcomere length is less than the optimal length for contraction. (Figure from HUMAN PHYSIOLOGY, Second Edition, by R. Rhoades and R. Pflanzer, copyright © 1992 by Saunders College Publishing, reprinted by permission of the publisher.)

bridging of myosin and actin filaments is impaired, and the force of contraction is limited (Braunwald et al., 1976; Rhodes and Pflanzer, 1989).

At the bedside, pressures are measured rather than volumes. Because the AV valves are open during diastole, the atrial pressures are representative of ventricular diastolic pressures. Thus, the clinical measure of right ventricular preload is the right atrial pressure or central venous pressure, and the measure of left ventricular preload is the left atrial pressure or pulmonary capillary wedge pressure. In a normal ventricle a change in pressure reflects a change in volume. However, if ventricular compliance is altered, changes in pressure reflect changes in ventricular volume less accurately. For example, ischemia or hypertrophy decreases ventricular compliance, and a relatively small change in ventricular volume may produce a large change in pressure.

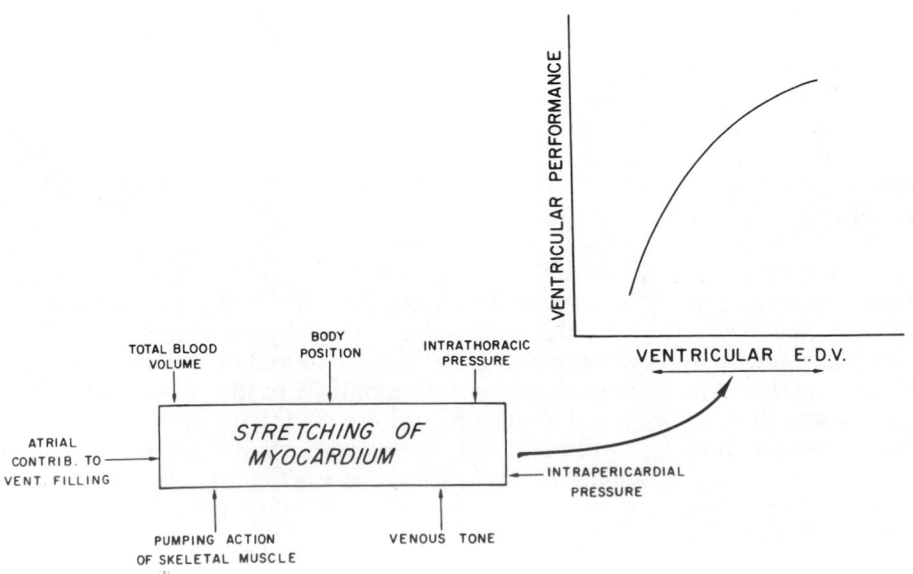

FIGURE 14–15. *Top, right,* Diagram of a Frank-Starling curve, relating ventricular end-diastolic volume (EDV) to ventricular performance. *Bottom, left,* Major influences that determine the degree of stretching of the myocardium, that is, the magnitude of the EDV. (From Braunwald, E., Ross, J., and Sonnenblick, E. (1976). *Mechanisms of contraction of the normal and failing heart* (2nd ed.). Boston: Little, Brown.)

Afterload, the Force-Velocity Relationship. In isolated muscle strips at a fixed length the force generated by the muscle and the rate of fiber shortening are determined by the load on the muscle. If the load is very heavy, exceptional force is required for the fibers to shorten. If the load is light, less force is required to lift the weight. Afterload in the intact heart is the force per unit of cross-sectional area in the ventricular wall once fiber shortening has begun (Cohn, 1985). The forces opposing fiber shortening in the ventricular wall include ventricular size and shape (the law of La Place), aortic impedance, and systemic vascular resistance.

The larger the end-diastolic volume, the larger the intraventricular pressure that must be overcome before fiber shortening can actually begin (and hence a longer isovolumetric contraction exists). The larger the radius of the ventricle in relation to wall thickness, the more oxygen is consumed. Thus, the level of preload contributes to the force of the afterload and to the level of myocardial oxygen consumption.

Aortic impedance is the stiffness of the aortic wall and the inertia of the column of blood in the aorta that must be overcome before ejection can begin. The more compliant the aorta, the more easily it will stretch during ventricular ejection and the less force the ventricle must generate.

Vascular resistance, the degree of constriction (radius) of the arterioles, is the major variable determining afterload and is a function of local tissue demands, the level of autonomic stimulation, and the level of circulating catecholamines. This factor can be calculated clinically if cardiac output, end-diastolic pressure or filling pressure, and output pressure are known (SVR = MAP − RAP/CO).

When all other variables are held constant (EDV, contractility, and heart rate), an increase in afterload either increases cardiac work to maintain stroke volume or decreases stroke volume and thus cardiac output (Fig. 14–16). In the normal heart, a sudden increase in afterload decreases the stroke volume, which increases the end-systolic volume and thus the preload for the next beat. This increases the contractility of subsequent beats through the Starling mechanism and maintains cardiac output in the face

of increased afterload but does so at increased metabolic cost.

An increase in ventricular wall thickness occurs with aging, probably due to the increase in afterload resulting from the structural and functional changes in the aorta, which will be discussed later. Capillary growth may not be adequate to supply the increase in muscle mass, and therefore the individual may be at risk for ischemia even in the presence of normal coronary vessels.

Contractility. Contractility is the effect of extrinsic influences on the rate and force of fiber shortening exclusive of fiber length (Fig. 14–17). Norepinephrine and epinephrine increase the rate of calcium movement into the cytosol during excitation (through cAMP) and back into the sarcoplasmic reticulum and thus increase both the force and rate of contraction and relaxation. Metabolic imbalances, depressant drugs, and loss of myocardium will impair the contractile function of the ventricle (Braunwald et al., 1976).

Heart Rate. An increase in the heart rate at the same stroke volume increases cardiac output within limits. At rates greater than 160 to 180 beats/minute the diastolic filling time shortens, decreasing the end-diastolic volume, and this reserve mechanism begins to impair the effectiveness of the preload reserve mechanism. Increased heart rate is the primary mechanism in infants for increasing cardiac output because the ventricle has more fibrous and fewer contractile elements than the adult heart; it is stiffer and less responsive to increasing preload. Thus, infants are said to be preload limited and heart rate dependent.

Maximum achievable heart rate decreases with age for any given level of exercise, possibly due to diminished adrenergic responsiveness. The balance between catecholamine effect, increased heart rate, and increased rate of contraction and relaxation (Ca^{2+} movement) may become competitive with rather than additive to the preload reserve mechanism. Figure 14–18 summarizes the relationship of the factors that determine cardiac output.

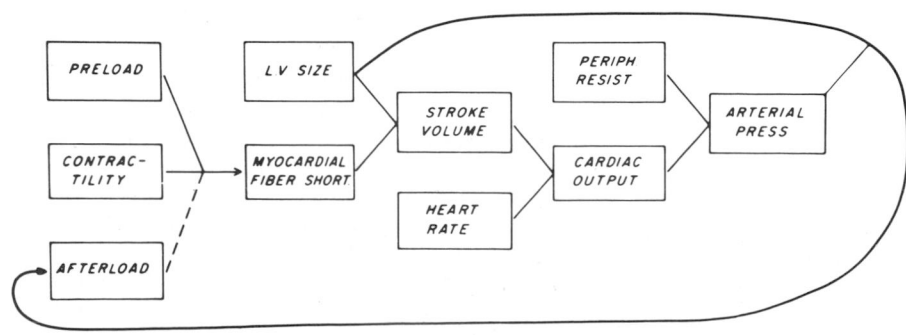

FIGURE 14–16. Schema of interactions between various components that regulate cardiac activity. Solid lines indicate an increasing effect; broken line represents a depressing effect. Note that left ventricular (LV) size is a determinant of both stroke volume and afterload. (From Braunwald, E., Ross, J, and Sonnenblick, E. (1976). *Mechanisms of contraction of the normal and failing heart* (2nd ed.). Boston: Little, Brown.)

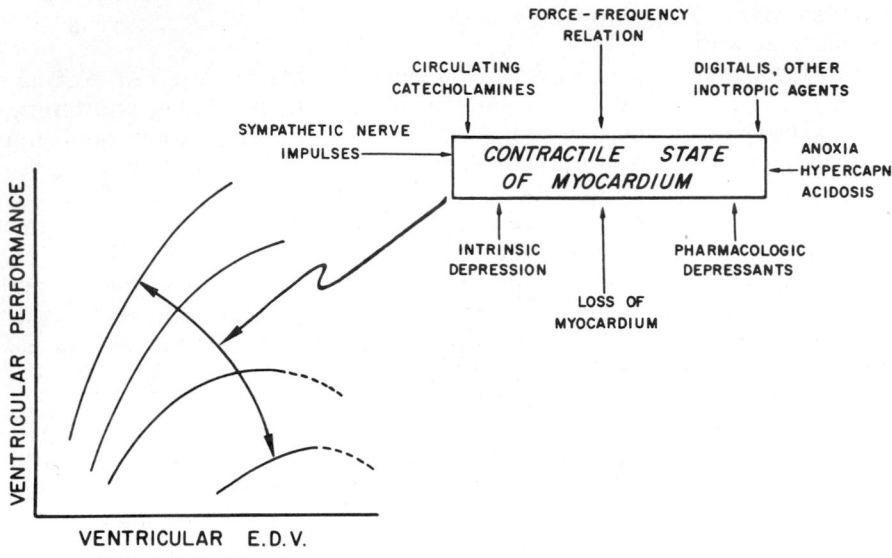

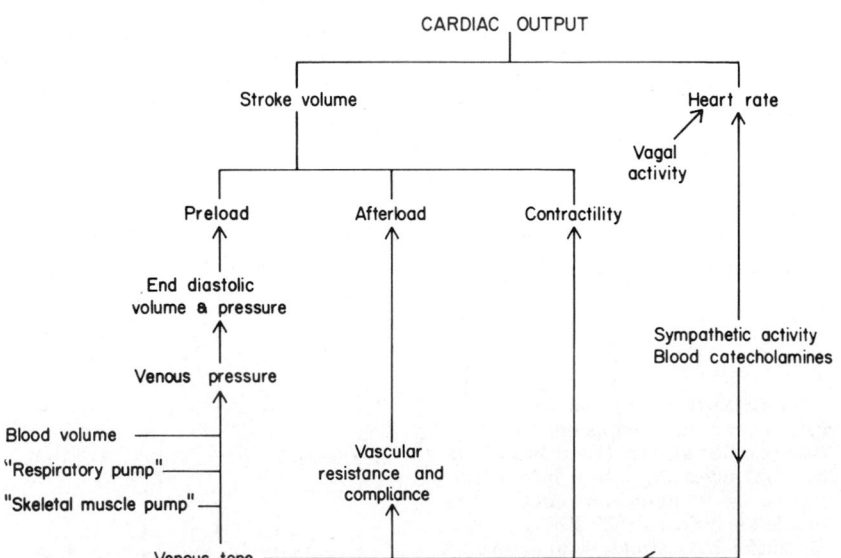

FIGURE 14–17. *Top, right,* Diagram showing the major influences that elevate or depress the contractile state of the myocardium. *Bottom, left,* The way in which alterations in the contractile state of the myocardium affect the level of ventricular performance at any given level of ventricular end-diastolic volume. (From Braunwald, E., Ross, J., and Sonnenblick, E. (1976). *Mechanisms of contraction of the normal and failing heart.* (2nd ed.). Boston: Little, Brown.)

FIGURE 14–18. Major factors determining cardiac output. (From Vander, A., Sherman, J., and Luciano, D. (1990). *Human physiology. The mechanisms of body function.* Reproduced with permission of McGraw-Hill, Inc.)

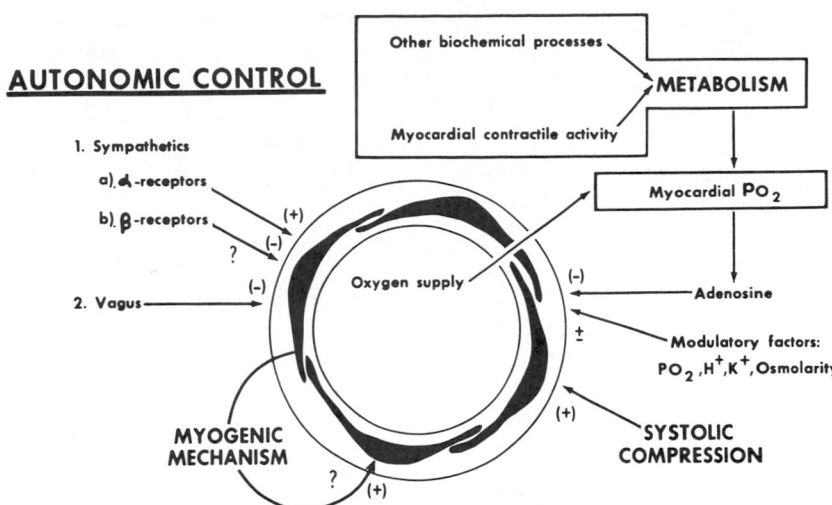

FIGURE 14–19. Factors increasing (+) or decreasing (−) coronary vascular resistance. (From Rubio, R., and Berne, F. M. (1975). *Progress in cardiovascular diseases* 18, 120.)

Control of the Coronary Circulation

At rest the myocardium extracts most of the available oxygen, so that an increase in oxygen demand can only be met by an increase in coronary flow. The coronary system is autoregulatory between perfusion pressures of approximately 50 mm Hg and 160 mm Hg. That is, local factors regulating resistance also regulate flow. Below a perfusion pressure of 50 mm Hg the vessels become maximally dilated, and flow becomes totally pressure dependent.

A variety of factors influence coronary vascular resistance (Fig. 14–19), the most important being local metabolic conditions. A decrease in oxygen delivery such as systemic hypoxia or obstruction of the large epicardial vessels, or an increase in tissue oxygen demand produces vasodilation either globally or locally. The mechanism for this vasodilation is unclear but is thought to be related to the release of adenosine from the myocardial cells (Berne and Levy, 1986). In addition, parasympathetic stimulation and beta-receptor stimulation may dilate the large epicardial vessels and some of the major branches. It is controversial whether these stimuli have a significant effect on the intramyocardial vessels. Increased resistance occurs primarily from systolic compression and alpha-adrenergic stimulation. The effect of myogenic response and vascular constriction secondary to a large distending pressure remains controversial in the coronary circulation.

Determinants of Myocardial Oxygen Consumption. The primary determinants of myocardial oxygen demand are the intramyocardial wall tension, which is related to pressure, volume, and wall thickness (law of La Place); the state of myocardial contractility, which is related to adrenergic and cholinergic stimulation; and the heart rate. Minor determinants of oxygen consumption are the resting metabolic rate, myocardial fiber shortening (ejection), and energy available for the activation of contraction (Cohn, 1985).

SYSTEMIC CIRCULATION

Structure

Histology. Blood vessels are composed of three layers—the intima, the media, and the adventitia. The intima is composed of a single layer of endothelial cells lining the lumen of the vessels and a basement membrane. The media is composed of collagen, elastin, and smooth muscle cells. The relative quantities and arrangement of these components influence the compliance, elastic recoil, and resistance of the vessel. The adventitia is the outermost layer of loosely meshed connective tissue. Blood supply to the outer two-thirds of the vessel wall comes from a special network of vessels, the vasa vasorum. The inner third of the vessel wall receives oxygen from diffusion of the blood in the vessels. At the place where these two oxygen supplies meet the vessel wall is at the greatest risk of ischemia.

The Arterial System. The aorta and major arteries are conduits and pressure reservoirs. No nutrient exchange with tissues occurs in these vessels, which distribute blood throughout the system. The media of the intrathoracic arteries contains more elastin and fewer smooth muscle cells than the media of the more peripheral arteries and the arterioles. Volume ejected into the aorta during ventricular systole distends the wall. Elastic recoil of the aorta during ventricular diastole continues to propel blood through the system and maintains diastolic pressure in the system (Windkessel effect).

Arterial pressures measured clinically reflect two components, aortic compliance and cardiac function. Aortic compliance (Fig. 14–20) decreases with age due to thickening of the intima and media resulting from increasing collagen and smooth muscle cell proliferation. Thus, for any given stroke volume the peak aortic pressure will be higher in the elderly than in the middle-aged adult. Clinically, this result is seen as isolated systolic hypertension in the el-

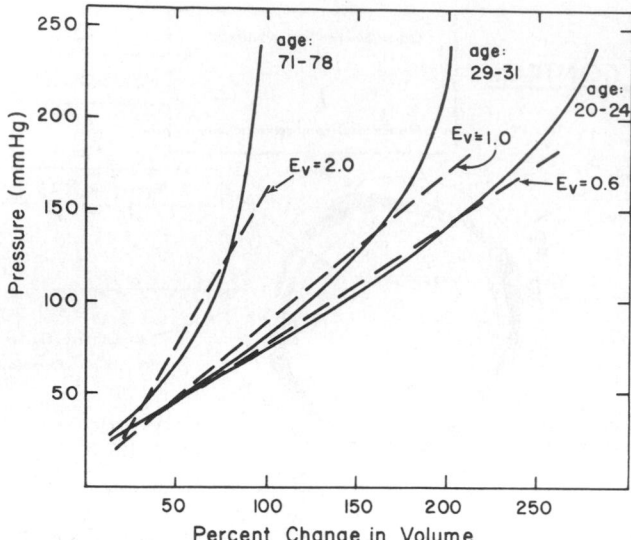

FIGURE 14-20. Static volume-pressure curves of aorta determined for different age groups. Each of these curves can be approximated by a linear relationship *(dashed lines)* within the physiologic pressure range (50 to 175 mm Hg). E, volume elasticity. (Modified from Hallock, P., and Benson, IC (1937). *Journal of Clinical Investigation,* 16, 595; from Little, R., and Little, W. (1985). *Physiology of the heart and circulation.* Chicago: Year Book Medical Publishers.)

derly. Although this is considered part of normal aging, it also increases the risk of cerebral vascular accident. By age 85 the aorta is an almost rigid tube. Thinning and fragmentation of elastin fibers decrease elastic recoil, and dilatation occurs as a compensatory respose to accommodate the same stroke volume in a more rigid space. Decreased recoil reduces the contribution to forward flow, and the amount of blood in the aorta at end-diastole increases the impedance or afterload to the left ventricle (Welsh, 1987).

During intra-aortic balloon pumping (IABP) the peak pressure achieved by the diastolic inflation of the balloon in the aorta is affected by the compliance of the aorta as well as by the size of the balloon in relation to the size of the aorta and the ventricular and balloon stroke volumes (Quaal, 1984).

The Microcirculation. The microcirculation is composed of arterioles, metarterioles, capillaries, and venules (Fig. 14–21). This is the functional unit of the circulation where nutrients are delivered to the tissues and waste products are removed.

Arterioles are resistance vessels. The media contains less collagen and elastin and more smooth muscle cells than does the media of the aorta. Many arterioles branch from each artery and have a smaller radius and a higher resistance. Significant change in the radius of the arteriole is produced by constriction or relaxation of the vascular smooth muscle in response to various stimuli, and thus the arterioles are the primary regulators of changes in resistance. Additionally, the increase in total cross-sectional area as a result of branching results in a reduced rate of flow.

Capillaries are the nutrient vessels. Many capillaries branch from each arteriole, and the total cross-sectional area again increases, thus decreasing further the rate of flow. This slow flow rate allows time

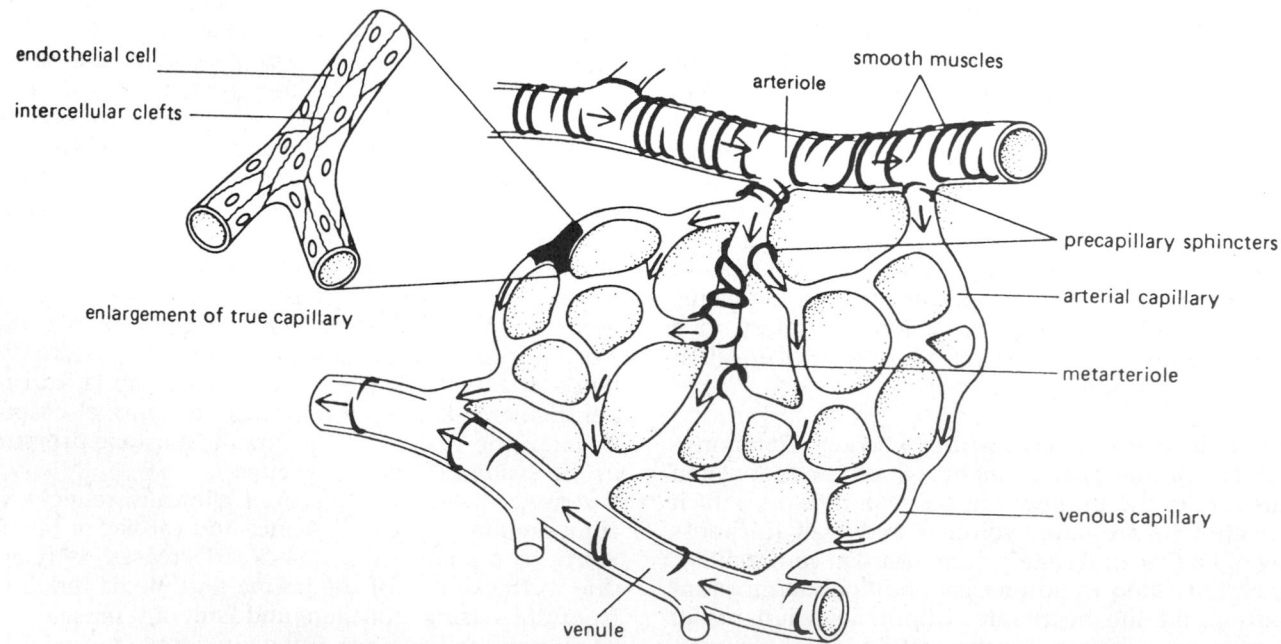

FIGURE 14-21. Diagram of microcirculation. Note the absence of smooth muscle in the true capillaries. (Adapted from E. E. Chaffee and I. M. Lytle (1980). *Basic physiology and anatomy* (4th ed.). Philadelphia. J. B. Lippincott; In Vander, A., Sherman, J., and Luciano, D. (1990). *Human physiology. The mechanisms of body function* (5th ed.). Copyright © 1990 by McGraw-Hill Inc. Used by permission of McGraw-Hill Book Company.)

for exchange of nutrients to occur within the tissues. Capillary walls are one cell thick and contain no smooth muscle cells. Nutrients diffuse through gap junctions or are actively transported to the interstitial fluid and then to the cells from the arterial end of the capillary. Interstitial fluid and waste products reenter the capillary at the venous end or are removed by the lymphatics. Precapillary sphincters control flow through individual capillary beds depending on tissue demand. During times of low demand, some blood bypasses the true capillaries through the metarterioles and enters the venules directly. Venules contain a small amount of smooth muscle but less than that in the arterioles. As venules coalesce, the cross-sectional area decreases, and the rate of flow begins to increase.

Veins are capacitance vessels. Vein walls have some smooth muscle but less than that in arteries. They are larger in diameter and therefore have a larger total cross-sectional area. The rate of flow is slower and the pressure is lower because the walls are more compliant. Approximately 60% of the total blood volume is found in the venous circuit at rest. As the veins coalesce at the inferior and superior vena cavae, the rates of flow and pressure increase but remain below aortic rates.

The pulmonary circulation also branches into arteries, arterioles, capillaries, venules, and veins. However, the vessels are shorter and have a larger radius, a relatively high elastin content, a more fragmented arrangement, and fewer smooth muscle cells. The pulmonary artery carries deoxygenated blood, and the pulmonary veins carry oxygenated blood.

Arterial Pressure

Systolic and Diastolic Blood Pressure. The maximum blood pressure at peak ejection is called the systolic pressure. It is a function of the volume ejected and the compliance of the aorta (Fig. 14–22). Only one-third of the stroke volume leaves the arteries during systole, and the rest of the stroke volume must be accommodated by stretching of the aorta and the major arteries during systole.

Diastolic pressure is the minimum pressure just before ejection begins. It is primarily a function of the systemic vascular resistance and elastic recoil. Systolic and diastolic pressures are considered important primarily as the upper and lower limits of the mean arterial pressure rather than as independent values (Berne and Levy, 1986; O'Rourke, 1982).

Mean Arterial Pressure. The mean perfusion pressure for the tissues is called the mean arterial pressure (MAP). It is from the systolic and diastolic blood pressures in the aorta and major arteries during any given cardiac cycle (see Table 14–2). The MAP is dependent only on the elastic properties of the arterial walls and the mean blood volume in the arterial

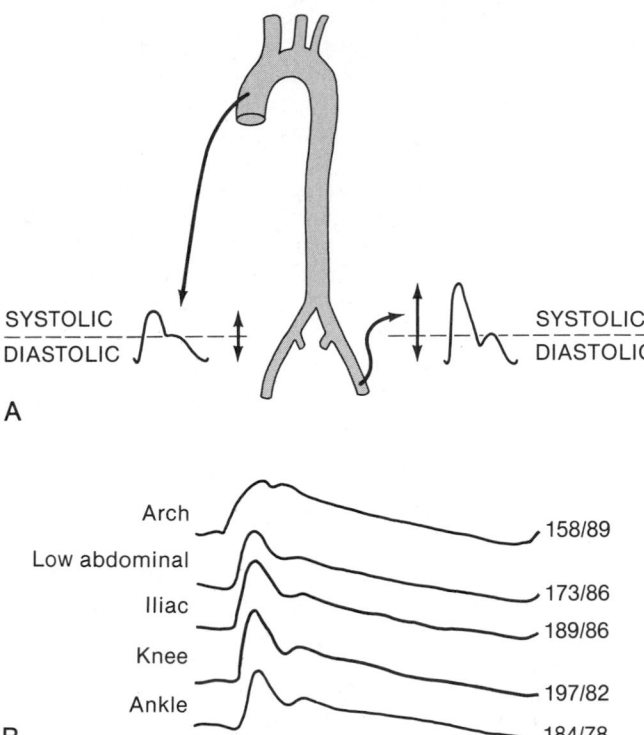

FIGURE 14–22. *A* and *B*, The propagation of the arterial pressure trace down the arterial tree. (*A* from O'Rourke, M. (1982). *Arterial function in health and disease.* Edinburgh: Churchill Livingstone; *B* from Remington, J. W., and O'Brien, L. J. (1970). *American Journal of Physiology, 218,* 437.)

tree. The arterial volume is contingent upon the rate of inflow from the heart into the arteries (cardiac output) and the rate of outflow from the arteries through the capillaries (peripheral runoff). When the rate of inflow exceeds the rate of outflow, the MAP increases due to stretch of the arterial walls. When peripheral runoff exceeds cardiac output, the MAP decreases. The MAP remains constant when the rate of arterial inflow equals arterial outflow (cardiac output equals peripheral runoff). Clearly, if the arteries are poorly distensible and cannot accommodate an increased inflow or decreased outflow by stretching, the MAP will rise even further. Therefore, the only factors that determine MAP are cardiac output and peripheral resistance (Berne and Levy, 1986).

Pulse Pressure. Pulse pressure is the difference between the systolic and diastolic pressures and is a function of stroke volume and the distensibility of the aorta. The speed of systolic ejection also determines the pulse pressure but is less important than the ratio of stroke volume to aortic compliance (Guyton, 1991).

During systole, a large volume of blood is ejected into the aorta. This volume generally exceeds the peripheral runoff and is called the stroke volume. By introducing the maximum volume into the aorta, a peak pressure is obtained. This is the systolic pressure. As stated earlier, the diastolic pressure is dependent upon the SVR, which is a measure of aortic compliance. Because the pulse pressure is the difference between the systolic and diastolic pressures, it is easy to see why it is dependent upon the stroke volume and aortic compliance.

Arterial Pressure Curves. The transmission of pressure as it is propagated from the aorta to the peripheral arteries produces a characteristic waveform (see Fig. 14–22). The stretch of the aorta and its branches is substantially faster than the actual forward movement of blood and is responsible for the peripheral pulse (Berne ad Levy, 1986).

The initial sharp upstroke of the arterial waveform is due to the rapid ejection period of the heart. It is followed by a slower rise to the peak of the curve, the apex of which is the systolic pressure. The waveform then acutely declines, but the descent is briskly interrupted by a sharp notch, called the incisura in an aortic waveform and the dicrotic notch in a peripheral waveform. The incisura results from the abrupt closure of the aortic valve at the onset of diastole, which causes a temporary rebound of blood into the aorta. Following the dicrotic notch, there is an exponential diastolic decline in the waveform that culminates in the diastolic pressure.

The arterial waveform subtly changes as it is propagated from the aortic arch to the distal peripheral arteries (Fig. 14–22). The vascular distensibility varies inversely with the velocity of transmission of the pressure wave. Because vascular capacitance decreases in the distal periphery, the velocity of transmission increases incrementally along the path. There are four changes in the configuration of the arterial waveform associated with distal measurements in the arterial tree: (1) There is a delay in the rapid upslope portion of the waveform; (2) the incisura and other high-frequency portions of the waveform dampen; (3) the peak systolic pressure narrows and culminates at a higher level (systolic pressures can be 25 to 40 mm Hg higher at the dorsalis pedal artery than in the aorta); and (4) a hump may develop at the diastolic portion of the waveform (Berne and Levy, 1986; O'Rourke, 1982; Guyton, 1991). The magnitude of the changes in waveform from the aorta to the distal periphery are less pronounced in elderly patients, particularly those with atherosclerosis (Berne and Levy, 1986). This difference results from (1) backward reflection of the pressure wave; (2) tapering due to progression of the wave from larger to smaller arteries; (3) resonance of the sine waves that compose the waveform; and (4) changes in transmission velocity due to decreased capacitance (Berne and Levy, 1986).

Local Acute Control of Blood Pressure

Because there is a finite amount of blood in the body, it is impossible for equal amounts of blood to be circulated to every tissue in the body and still meet the metabolic needs of each tissue. Different tissues have different needs at any given time, and the body is able to deliver increased amounts of nutrients to those tissues based upon local needs. Hence the concept of autoregulation. Acute local control of the circulation occurs within seconds to minutes and has a limited duration of action.

The Metabolic Theory of Autoregulation. The metabolic theory of autoregulation simply states that blood flow is controlled by local metabolic needs. When the tissues have increased metabolic needs, vasodilation occurs. Conversely, when metabolic requirements are low, vasoconstriction occurs, thus allowing adequate distribution of the blood volume.

The vasodilator theory states that increased metabolic activity causes local formation of vasodilator substances such as adenosine, carbon dioxide, lactic acid, hydrogen ions, and bradykinin. These substances have a direct dilatory effect on the precapillary sphincters, metarterioles, and arterioles. Research suggests that tissue hypoxia is directly responsible for the release of these vasodilating substances (Guyton, 1991). The problem with this theory is that even excessive amounts of any one of these substances do not elicit profound vasodilation in the laboratory (Berne and Levy, 1986).

The oxygen demand theory states that oxygen deficiency in tissues causes vasodilation. This theory is based on the knowledge that oxygen is required to maintain vascular tone (smooth muscle contraction) and that a lack of it, caused by increased metabolic activity, allows the vascular smooth muscle to dilate (Guyton, 1991). Berne and Levy (1986) state, however, that there is no correlation between oxygen tension and arteriolar radius over a wide range of oxygen concentrations when oxygen tension is directly measured at points of resistance. They support the idea that metabolic control is probably exerted by a mechanism combining parts of the vasodilatory theory and the oxygen demand theory.

When blood flow to a vascular bed is abruptly obstructed, release of the obstruction causes a surplus blood flow that continues for minutes to hours. This surplus blood flow, called reactive hyperemia, declines to the preocclusion level gradually (O'Rourke, 1982; Berne and Levy, 1986). Active hyperemia is the term given to excess blood flow to tissues at the period of increased demand. These phenomena stress the relationship between metabolic requirements and nutrient delivery.

The myogenic theory states that vascular smooth muscle contracts and dilates in response to changes in tension. According to this theory, a decrease in mean arterial pressure reduces arteriolar tone, thus allowing increased flow to the area (Garfein, 1990). Below a MAP of 50 mm Hg, arterioles are maximally dilated and flow is totally pressure dependent. This fact is important in both the coronary and peripheral circulations when obstruction from atherosclerosis or thrombus exists. Conversely, an increase in MAP increases arteriolar tone, decreases radius, and increases resistance. Arterial hypertension is thus minimally transmitted to capillary beds (Nichols and O'Rourke, 1990).

Humoral Regulation of Blood Flow

Humoral factors that affect blood flow include the local substances discussed earlier as well as hormones and other products that are manufactured by the body or absorbed by it. The discussion of humoral factors is based on their effect on the vascular smooth muscle.

Vasoconstrictors. Sympathetic stimulation causes direct release of norepinephrine from the nerve fibers. The adrenal medulla secretes epinephrine and norepinephrine, which circulate and cause profound vasoconstriction. Angiotensin II is one of the most powerful vasoconstricting substances known to man and causes a profound increase in the SVR, thus increasing the arterial blood pressure. The role of angiotensin in blood pressure control will be discussed in more detail later. Vasopressin, or antidiuretic hormone (ADH), is an even more powerful vasoconstrictor than angiotensin. Its release from the posterior pituitary gland, however, occurs in such minute amounts that it has relatively insignificant effects on blood pressure control.

Vasodilators. Bradykinin, a byproduct of kallikrein, produces intense vasodilation and increased capillary permeability. The role of bradykinin is primarily important in the regulation of blood flow to inflamed tissues. Serotonin, which is present in the intestinal tissues and platelets, has both vasodilating and vasoconstricting properties. It has minimal effect on the systemic regulation of blood flow. Histamine, derived from mast cells and released in response to allergy or inflammation, is a powerful vasodilator and also causes capillary leakage. Unlike bradykinin, histamine can produce severe hypotension, such as that resulting from an anaphylactic reaction. Prostaglandins present exciting possibilities for therapeutics because of their potent vasodilatory effects. Prostaglandin E infusions are currently being used to treat refractory pulmonary hypertension.

Nervous System Regulation of Blood Pressure

Nervous input to blood pressure regulation operates globally rather than locally. It can redistribute blood flow within the body and affects inotropy and chronotropy of the heart itself. The nervous system exerts extremely rapid control of blood pressure.

Autonomic Nervous System. The autonomic nervous system (AN) regulates both sympathetic and parasympathetic functions (Fig. 14–23). Parasympa-

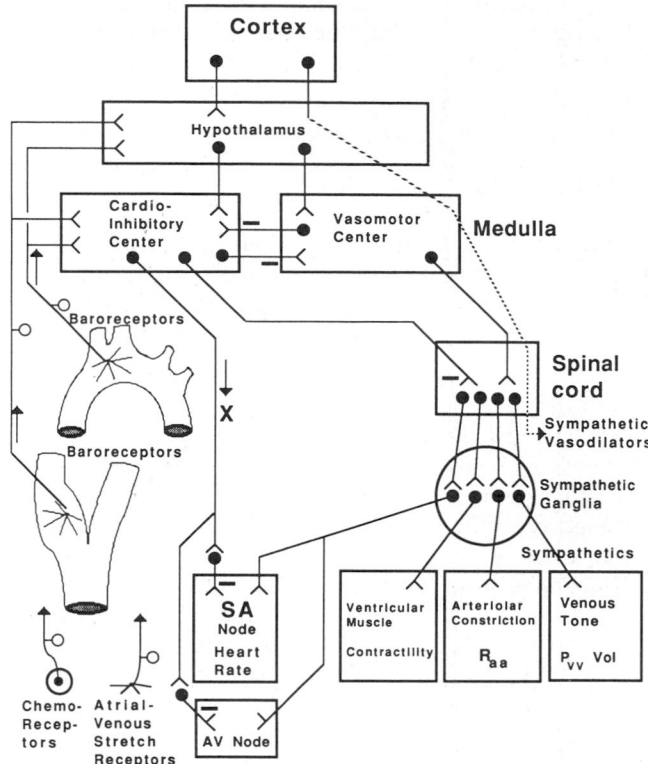

FIGURE 14–23. Autonomic control of circulation. (From Goerke, J., and Mines, A. (1988). *Cardiovascular physiology*. New York: Raven Press.)

thetic stimulation occurs primarily through the vagus nerve and inhibits heart rate and contractility. Its effects on peripheral blood pressure control are negligible.

The sympathetic nervous system (SNS) affects both the heart and the vascular smooth muscle. Cardiac inotropy and chronotropy are increased by SNS stimulation. A myriad of vasoconstrictor fibers and a minimal number of vasodilatory fibers are inherent in the nerves of the SNS. It is through the wide distribution of the vasoconstrictor fibers that the SNS exerts its powerful effects on the systemic blood pressure.

The vasomotor center of the medulla is composed of three major areas. The vasoconstrictor area secretes norepinephrine, which stimulates the vasoconstrictor fibers of the SNS. The vasodilator area of the vasomotor center works by inhibiting vasoconstriction. Sympathetic vasoconstrictor tone is maintained under normal conditions by continuous slow firing of the vasoconstrictor area. The sensory area of the vasomotor center is predominantly a reflex center. It receives impulses from the vagus and glossopharyngeal nerves and responds by stimulating the vasoconstrictor or vasodilatory fibers of the SNS according to need (Guyton, 1991; Vander et al., 1990).

The higher centers of the brain also affect vasomotor control. The pons, mesencephalon, diencephalon, hypothalamus, and regions of the cerebral cortex can stimulate or depress activity of the vasomotor center of the medulla (Guyton, 1991). A vasovagal response that causes hypotension, bradycardia, and fainting can be elicited by emotional upset, thus demonstrating higher nervous controls on the systemic blood flow.

SNS Rapid Control of the Blood Pressure

Extremely rapid increases in blood pressure can be elicited by the SNS. Three principal responses occur as a result of stimulation of the entire vasoconstrictor and cardioaccelerator areas of the vasomotor centers:

1. SVR is increased by generalized arteriolar constriction.
2. Venous return is increased by constriction of the venous system.
3. Heart rate and strength of contractions are increased (Guyton, 1991).

Baroreceptor Control Mechanism. Baroreceptors in the aortic arch, atria, large arteries, and veins respond to a decrease in stretch, mean pressure, or pulse pressure by decreasing their rate of firing (Fig. 14–23). The sensory area of the vasomotor center responds by increasing SNS output and decreasing parasympathetic nervous system (PNS) output through the efferent neurons. The immediate response is an increase in venous tone, which increases return to the heart and also increases end-diastolic volume and cardiac output through the Starling mechanism. Increased arteriolar tone maintains central pressure and redistributes blood flow to the most vital organs. Increased heart rate and contractility maintain cardiac output despite increase in resistance (Berne and Levy, 1986).

CNS Ischemic Response. When ischemia occurs in the vasomotor center, neurons in the medulla itself are stimulated and elicit a powerful vasoconstrictor response. Systemic blood pressure peaks. It is hypothesized that carbon dioxide and other metabolic byproducts accumulate in the local tissues of the vasomotor center and are responsible for the profound excitatory response of the center, much like a local control mechanism that has significant systemic effects (Guyton, 1991).

Long-Term Regulation of Blood Flow

Long-term control of blood flow occurs primarily through activation of the renin-angiotensin system or through changes in tissue vascularity. Pressure diuresis and natriuresis by the kidneys also aid in long-term regulation of blood pressure.

Renin-Angiotensin System. (Fig. 14–24). The juxtaglomerular cells of the kidney produce, store, and secrete a substance called renin. A decrease in renal blood flow causes the release of renin, which enzy-

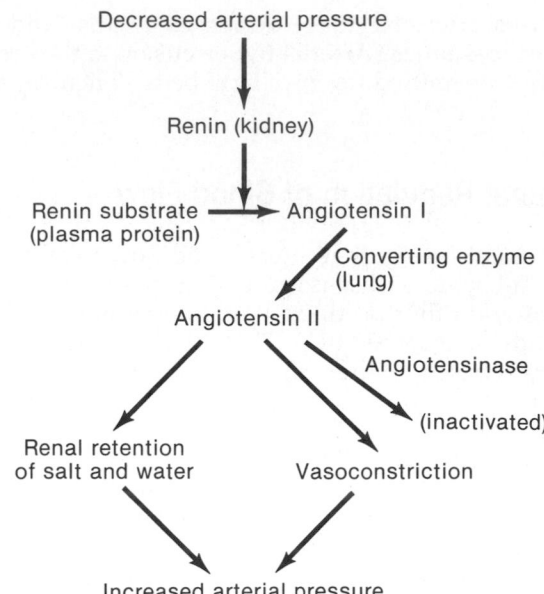

FIGURE 14–24. The renin-angiotensin constrictor mechanisms for arterial pressure control. (From Guyton, A. C. (1991). *Textbook of medical physiology.* (8th ed.). Philadelphia: W. B. Saunders.)

matically acts on angiotensinogen to release angiotensin I. The cleft of two amino acids from angiotensin I results in the formation of angiotensin II, the potent vasoconstrictor substance referred to earlier. Angiotensin II has two major effects that cause the arterial pressure to increase. The first and most rapid effect is generalized vasoconstriction. The second effect is a decrease in sodium and water excretion from the kidneys. Salt and water retention increase the blood volume, thus increasing the blood pressure. Although the renal action of angiotensin II takes longer to increase the arteriolar pressure, it has longer term effects than the vasoconstrictor action.

Changes in Tissue Vascularity. Prolonged hypotension (<60 mm Hg) can cause reconstruction of the vasculature in the affected tissues. Reconstruction can take the form of actual changes in the physical structure of the vessels or the development of new vessels (development of collateral circulation). Angiogenesis, the development of new blood vessels, occurs in response to stimulatory factors released from ischemic tissue, rapidly growing tissues, or tissues with an extremely high metabolic activity (Nichols and O'Rourke, 1990).

Specific substances responsible for initiating angiogenesis include endothelial cell growth factor, fibroblast growth factor, and angiogenin. These angiogenic factors cause new vessels to germinate from existing venules and capillaries. Dissolution of the basement membrane of the endothelial cells is followed by brisk multiplication of new endothelial cells that grow out of the originating vessel in cordlike fashion. The cords form a tube that attaches to a tube from another originating vessel, and a capillary loop develops that allows blood to flow through it.

Continued blood flow stimulates smooth muscle proliferation inside the tube wall, creating a new arteriole (Guyton, 1991).

Volume Retention by the Kidney. Through SNS stimulation and aldosterone secretion from the adrenal medulla, and augmented by atrial receptors, the kidney retains sodium and therefore water. Potassium is excreted. Atrial receptors stimulate ADH release, which results in water retention independently of sodium. This is an effective method of increasing blood volume and is beneficial in hemorrhage. However, if the low-flow state results from pump failure, this additional volume may be detrimental. If cardiac fibers are already stretched beyond their optimum length, additional preload further impairs their contractile function, and heart failure worsens. The normal reserve mechanism now contributes to the pathology.

Additionally, in cardiac failure there is a chronic elevation of serum catecholamines. Thus, a portion of the reserves is used to maintain the cardiac output at rest, resulting in less reserve available to increase cardiac output in the presence of increased metabolic requirements. Clinically, the decreased reserve is evidenced as decreased exercise tolerance and impaired functional ability.

Capillary Dynamics

Solute Diffusion. Solutes move across the capillary wall down their concentration gradient. Lipid-soluble substances such as oxygen and carbon dioxide are transported through the cells. Other substances move through intercellular junctions, and some are transported through pinocytic vesicles and other passive transport mechanisms. The concentration gradient of the solutes is altered by the rate of blood flow. The faster the flow, the greater the solute washout and the lower the concentration. Large molecules such as proteins, primarily albumin, are too large to filter across the wall and must be actively transported.

Filtration of Fluid. Because the capillary wall is freely permeable to water, the amount of fluid filtered across the wall depends on the balance between the pressure within the capillary and the pressure in the interstitium. The hydrostatic pressure within the capillary is the result of blood pressure at the capillary level and is about 30 mm Hg. The tissue hydrostatic pressure is very low and in some tissues is negative. The oncotic pressure in the capillary is high and is mostly the result of intravascular albumin. The interstitial oncotic pressure is quite small. Thus, the primary balance is the difference between the hydrostatic pressure favoring filtration out of the capillary and the oncotic pressure favoring reabsorption. A drop in pressure across the capillary results from a

loss of fluid within the capillary; therefore, in many capillaries there is filtration at the arterial end and reabsorption at the venous end. Fluid that is not reabsorbed and macromolecules are removed from the interstitium by the lymphatics (Guyton, 1991).

The Starling hypothesis describes the mechanism of transcapillary fluid and solute exchange as a function of (1) the hydrostatic pressure gradient (microvascular pressure minus perimicrovascular pressure) and (2) the protein osmotic pressure gradient (plasma protein osmotic pressure minus perimicrovascular protein osmotic pressure). Normally, the sum of the forces of microvascular pressure, perimicrovascular pressure, and perimicrovascular protein osmotic pressure favoring outward movement is slightly greater than plasma protein osmotic pressure. Thus, there is a slight net fluid movement into the tissue spaces that is equaled by lymph flow returning this fluid to the vascular system. Specific values for each of these factors may vary among tissues. The combination of the net rate of filtration per millimeters of mercury (the hydraulic conductance) and the surface area perfused is called the filtration coefficient. In addition, capillary membranes are not totally impermeable to proteins, as the above relationships suggest. The osmotic reflection coefficient expresses the degree of protein permeability and is one if the capillary is totally impermeable and zero if the capillary is totally permeable. Thus the Starling equation is:

$$\text{Fluid movement} = k[(P_c + \pi_i) - (P_i + \pi_p)]$$

where P_c = capillary hydrostatic pressure, P_i = interstitial fluid hydrostatic pressure, π_p = plasma protein oncotic pressure, π_i = interstitial fluid oncotic pressure, and K = filtration constant for the capillary membrane. When the algebraic sum is positive, filtration occurs. When the algebraic sum is negative, absorption occurs (Berne and Levy, 1986).

The filtration coefficient and osmotic reflection coefficient for individual tissues and organ system barriers are related to the capillary ultrastructure and its responsiveness to hormonal influences. The presence, type, and number of intercellular junctions, pinocytic vesicles, transendothelial channels, and the structure of the basement membrane affect the rate and degree of edema formation in various tissues. Pinocytic vesicles and transendothelial channels are modes of molecular transport through the cells. Their presence in large numbers increases the filtration coefficient in that tissue. For example, in the hepatic sinusoids, intercellular junctions are quite loose, and the osmotic reflection coefficient approaches zero. Pulmonary capillaries are moderately leaky to proteins, those in skeletal muscle are less so, and in cerebral capillaries the osmotic reflection coefficient approaches one. In general, more sites exist for fluid and solute movement on the venous end of the capillary than on the arterial end.

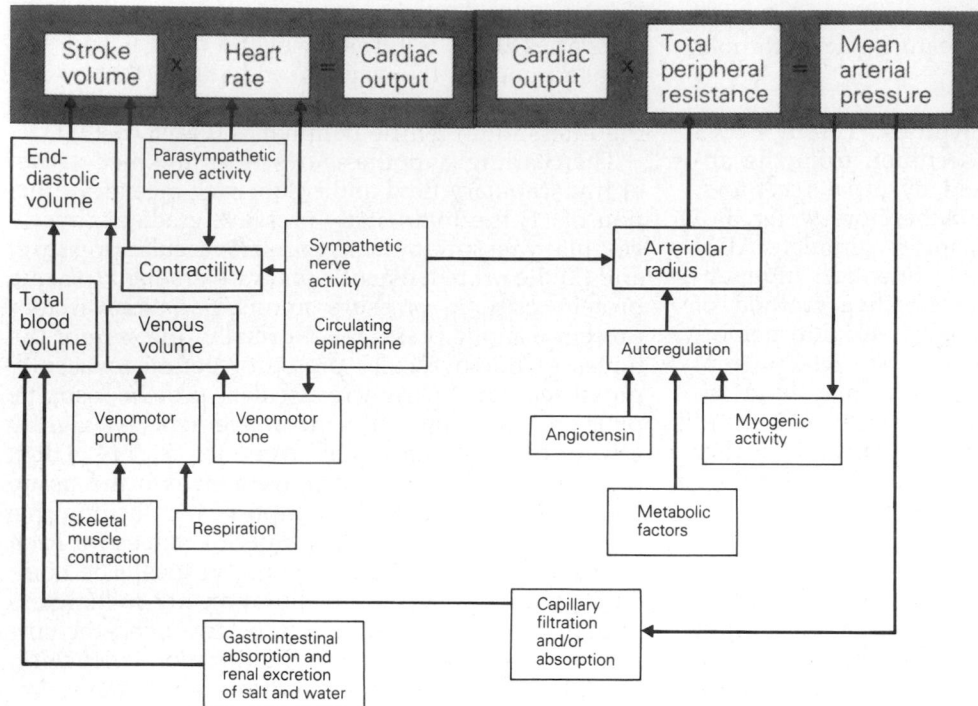

FIGURE 14–25. Summary of the factors that can alter cardiac output and arterial pressure. (Figure from HUMAN PHYSIOLOGY, Second Edition, by R. Rhoades and R. Pflanzer, copyright © 1992 by Saunders College Publishing, reprinted by permission of the publisher.)

INTEGRATION OF CENTRAL AND PERIPHERAL FACTORS IN CARDIAC OUTPUT CONTROL

Cardiac output is a function of preload, afterload, heart rate, and contractility. Each of these factors is determined by a myriad of peripheral, central, and intracardiac components (Fig. 14–25). This section will examine cardiac output control as a result of the integration of each of these influences.

Preload

Venous Return. Stroke volume is governed by the inotropic ability of the heart and the capability of the peripheral circulation to return blood to the heart. The latter is referred to as venous return. Most alterations in cardiac output in the normal heart are due to changes in venous return. In the absence of heart failure, augmentation of contractility (i.e., through pharmaceutical infusions) has a minimal effect on increasing the cardiac output. Modifications of venous return (i.e., through volume or position), however, contribute to relatively large changes in the cardiac output (Braunwald and Ross, 1979).

Venous constriction has a profound effect on improving venous return and hence cardiac output. Even marked venous constriction has a minimal effect on the total SVR because the venous system is so compliant (Braunwald and Ross, 1979). This is important because reduction in total SVR is probably

the most influential factor in increasing cardiac output.

Total Blood Volume. Massive or rapid reduction of the total blood volume causes the stroke volume to decline. However, decreases in cardiac output are barely perceptible with gradual reductions or with loss of less than 15% of the total blood volume (Braunwald and Ross, 1979).

Distribution of Blood Volume. Distribution of blood volume between the intrathoracic and extrathoracic compartments exerts control over the ventricular end-diastolic volume. Factors that contribute to this distribution are delineated as follows (Braunwald et al., 1988). Body position affects blood distribution due to gravitational forces. While in a supine position, the blood pools in the lower limbs. The Trendelenburg position increases the venous return, thus increasing cardiac output. Military antishock trousers (MAST) increase venous return through the same mechanism.

Normally, the intrathoracic pressure becomes negative during inspiration. This acts as a vacuum to assist in displacing more blood volume into the intrathoracic cavity. Positive pressure ventilation reverses this phenomenon and can decrease venous return by itself. Combined with positive end-expiratory pressure (PEEP), cardiac output can be severely embarrassed.

Increased intrapericardial pressure, such as occurs with pericardial effusion, reduces cardiac filling (preload). Complete circulatory collapse can result from significant increases in intrapericardial pressure; cardiac tamponade is the classic clinical condition that results from the increase in pressure.

Venous tone is dependent upon a variety of nervous and humoral factors. The benefits of venoconstriction in augmenting preload were discussed earlier. Venoconstriction can be caused by SNS stimulation, muscular exercise, anxiety, deep respiration, and marked hypotension. Medications that can cause venoconstriction include sympathomimetic agents and cardiac glycosides. Venodilation can be caused by ganglionic blockers and nitrates and can cause extrathoracic pooling (Braunwald and Ross, 1979).

Afterload

Stroke volume, a determinant of cardiac output, is dependent upon the degree of ventricular fiber shortening that occurs during systole. It is inversely proportional to afterload. Afterload is chiefly determined by aortic impedance and SVR. Myocardial fiber shortening is reduced with elevations in SVR, and therefore contractility and cardiac output are also decreased (Braunwald and Ross, 1979).

The key determinants of afterload are SVR, the physical characteristics of the arterial tree (i.e., atherosclerosis), and the volume of blood ejected. SVR is the most easily modified of these factors and is influenced by many diverse humoral, neural, and extrinsic factors. Hypertension, obstruction to ejection (i.e., by aortic stenosis), hypothermia, and SNS stimulation profoundly increase SVR. Acidosis, hyperthermia, aortic incompetence, and many pharmaceutical agents reduce SVR and hence afterload.

Contractility

Contractility, also known as inotropy, influences cardiac output independent of preload or afterload. Inotropy refers to the myocardial force-velocity length relationship and the level of ventricular performance at end-diastolic volume (Braunwald et al., 1988).

SNS Activity. Sympathetic stimulation increases cardiac contractility through excitation of the superior, middle, and inferior cardiac nerves and the paravertebral sympathetic chain (Berne and Levy, 1986). Increased inotropy is a result of direct release of norepinephrine into the cardiac tissue (Braunwald and Ross, 1979).

Humoral Factors. Circulating catecholamines released by the adrenal medulla, nerve impulses, and extracardiac ganglia augment inotropy. Although circulating catecholamines are slower to stimulate contractility than intracardiac norepinephrine, they are important in chronic conditions (Braunwald and Ross, 1979).

Exogenous Inotropic Agents. Cardiac glycosides, caffeine, sypathomimetic agents, theophylline, and glucagon all have positive inotropic effects.

Depressants. Cardiac contractility can be depressed by physiologic and pharmacologic agents. These factors include anoxia, ischemia, acidemia, beta-adrenergic blockade, anesthetics, and barbiturates.

Loss of Contractile Mass. Myocardial infarction results in a loss of functional cardiac muscle. Global ventricular performance (contractility) is thus impaired.

Heart Rate

Alterations in heart rate, called chronotropy, can have positive or negative effects on cardiac output (Fig. 14–25). Because cardiac output is a function of stroke volume times heart rate, it is easy to see how increased heart rate can improve cardiac output. Improved cardiac output can be achieved only as long as the diastolic volume of the heart remains constant (Braunwald et al., 1988). Extremely rapid or prolonged tachycardia, however, can reduce the diastolic filling time and thus reduce diastolic volume. In this case, cardiac output is reduced by tachycardia.

SUMMARY

This chapter reviews the physical properties of the cardiovascular system and the ultrastructure and mechanisms of contractions. The electrical activity of the heart is described. The mechanical and clinical features of cardiac pumping are delineated. The structure and control of the systemic circulation is discussed. In the discussion of the integration of control of peripheral factors in cardiac output, how the body strives to maintain homeostasis and the mechanisms that it uses to achieve the steady state are reviewed.

References

Bayés De Luna, A. (1987). *Textbook of clinical electrocardiography.* Dordrecht: Martinus-Nijoff.

Berne, R., and Levy, M. (1986). *Cardiovascular physiology* (5th ed). St. Louis: C.V. Mosby.

Bond, E. (1989). Physiology of the heart. In S. Underhill, S. Woods, E. Froelicher et al. (Eds.), *Cardiac Nursing* (pp. 44–56). Philadelphia: J. B. Lippincott.

Braunwald, E., Ross, J., and Sonnenblick, E. (1976). *Mechanisms of contraction of the normal and failing heart* (2nd ed.). Boston: Little, Brown.

Braunwald, E., and Ross, J. (1979). Control of cardiac performance. In R. Berne, N. Sperelakis, and S. Geyer (Eds.), *Handbook of physiology: The cardiovascular system* (pp. 533–580). Bethesda, MD. American Physiological Society.

Braunwald, E., Sonnenblick, E., and Ross, J. (1988). Mechanisms of cardiac contraction and relaxation. In E. Braunwald (Ed.), *Heart disease* (3rd ed., pp. 383–425). Philadelphia: W. B. Saunders.

Cohn, P. (1985). *Clinical cardiovascular physiology*. Philadelphia: W. B. Saunders.

Garfein, O. (1990). *Current concepts in cardiovascular physiology*. San Diego: Academic Press.

Goerke, J. and Mines, A. (1988). *Cardiovascular physiology*. New York: Raven Press.

Guyton, A. (1991). *Textbook of medical physiology* (8th ed.). Philadelphia: W. B. Saunders.

Halpenny C., and Bond, E. (1989). Cardiac anatomy. In S. Underhill, S. Woods, E. Froelicher, et al. (Eds.), *Cardiac Nursing*. Philadelphia: J. B. Lippincott.

Hurford, W., and Zapol, W. (1988). The right ventricle and critical illness: A review of anatomy, physiology, and clinical evaluation of its function. *Intensive Care Medicine*. 14, 448–457.

Hurst, J., Logue, R., and Wenger, N. (1990). *The heart, arteries and veins*. (2nd ed.). New York: McGraw-Hill.

Katz, A. (1988). Influence of altered inotropy and lusitropy on ventricular pressure-volume loops. *Journal of the American College of Cardiology*, 11, 438–445.

Little, R., and Little, W. (1985). *Physiology of the heart and circulation*. Chicago: Year Book.

McGuigan, J., and Blatter, L. (1987). Sodium/calcium exchange in ventricular muscle. *Experentia*, 43, 1140–1145.

Milnor, W. (1990). *Cardiovascular physiology*. New York: Oxford University Press.

Nichols, W., and O'Rourke, M. (1990). *McDonald's blood flow in arteries* (3rd ed.). Philadelphia: Lea & Febiger.

Noble, D. (1987). Experimental and theoretical work on excitation and excitation-contraction coupling in the heart. *Experientia*, 43, 1146–1149.

O'Rourke, M. (1982). *Arterial function in health and disease*. Edinburgh: Churchill Livingstone.

Rhoades, R., and Pflanzer, R. (1989). *Human physiology*. Philadelphia: Saunders College Publishing.

Ruegg, J. (1986). *Calcium in muscle activation*. Berlin: Springer-Verlag.

Shoemaker, W., Appel, P., Kram, H., et al. (1988). Multicomponent noninvasive monitoring of circulatory function. *Critical Care Medicine*, 16, 482–490.

Stern, M., Capogrossi, M., and Lakatta, E. (1988). Spontaneous calcium release from the sarcoplasmic reticulum in myocardial cells: Mechanisms and consequences. *Cell Calcium*, 9, 247–256.

Streeter, D., Spotnitz, H., and Patel, D. (1969). Fiber orientation in the canine left ventricle during diastole and systole. *Circulation Research*, 24, 339–347.

Quaal, S. (1984). *Comprehensive intra-aortic balloon pumping*. St. Louis: C. V. Mosby.

Vander, A., Sherman, J., and Luciano, D. (1990). *Human physiology: The mechanisms of body function* (5th ed.). New York: McGraw-Hill.

Vassalle, M. (1987). Contribution of the Na/K-pump to the membrane potential. *Experientia* 43, 1135–1140.

Walsh, R. (1987). Cardiovascular effects of the aging process. *The American Journal of Medicine*, 82 (Suppl. 1B), 34–40.

Yancy, C., and Firth, B. (1988). Congestive heart failure. *Disease-a-month*, 34, 473–536.

15

Patients with Coronary Artery Disease

Julie Fleury
Carolyn Murdaugh

ATHEROSCLEROSIS: THE LESION OF CORONARY ARTERY DISEASE

Atherosclerosis is a pathologic condition of the arteries clinically manifested as cardiovascular disease, the major cause of death in the industrialized world. Coronary artery disease and cerebrovascular disease, both of which are atherosclerotic diseases, cause more death, disability, and economic loss in the United States than any other disease (American Heart Association, 1988a).

Natural History

The lesions of atherosclerosis occur mainly in the intima, the innermost layer of the artery wall. However, secondary changes can be found in the media or middle layer as well. Over a period of years these lesions progress and undergo changes that lead to serious clinical consequences. More precise accounts of the sequential changes that may take place have been difficult due to the inability to sample human arteries at various time intervals. Until recently, the changes were construed from lesions obtained at autopsies or surgical procedures, or extrapolated from animal studies. In the last few years information on atherosclerotic progression has been obtained through serial imaging of arterial lesions, most commonly by angiography. In addition, ultrasound and magnetic resonance arterial imaging are being used

The authors wish to acknowledge the assistance of Robert O'Rourke, M.D., in the preparation of this manuscript.

to augment angiography, especially for examination of the aortoiliac and peripheral vessels.

Three characteristic lesions of atherosclerosis have been identified: the fatty streak, the fibrous plaque, and the complicated lesion. The fatty streak, the earliest lesion, begins in early childhood. The fatty streak is a grossly flat, lipid-rich lesion consisting of both macrophages and some smooth muscle. Fatty streaks are found in the aorta shortly after birth and in most children over 1 year of age in all populations. They increase in number between the ages of 8 and 18 years. Fatty streaks appear in the coronary arteries around age 15 and increase in these vessels through the third decade (Ross, 1986). Fatty streaks are yellowish in appearance due to extensive lipid deposits. They cause little or no obstruction and do not produce any clinical effects. By themselves, fatty streaks are considered benign. Whether or not fatty streaks are the precursors of fibrous plaques and atherosclerosis has not been resolved.

In industrialized nations, such as the United States, more advanced lesions called fibrous plaques begin to develop in the coronary arteries after 20 years of age. They are grossly white in appearance and become elevated so they may protrude into the lumen of the artery. The lesions are composed of increased intimal smooth muscle cells surrounded by connective tissue matrix. The smooth muscle cells may form a fibrous cap due to the accumulation of intracellular and extracellular lipids and deposition of connective tissue. Beneath the fibrous cap the lesions contain smooth muscle and macrophages that contain lipid droplets surrounded by connective tissue. Beneath these cells there may be an area of necrotic debris, cholesterol crystals, and calcification. Smooth muscle–rich fibrous plaques are often found at the same anatomic sites in coronary and extracranial cerebral arteries where fatty streaks were found early in life (Stacy, 1983). This finding suggests that fibrous plaques are derived from fatty streaks that have continued the process of cell proliferation, lipid accumulation, and connective tissue formation.

Advanced or complicated lesions occur over the age of 30 when fibrous plaques undergo complex changes and increase in frequency. The fibrous plaques become vascularized, and the necrotic lipid-rich core increases in size and may become calcified. The intimal surface of the lesion may disintegrate and ulcerate, allowing thrombi to form on the surface of the plaque. The thrombi may further increase the size of the plaque and reduce the lumen of the artery, resulting in a reduction in blood flow (ischemia) or occlusion of an artery (necrosis). Clinical symptoms occur as a result of the ischemia or necrosis and are manifested as myocardial infarction, stroke, aortic aneurysm, and gangrene of the extremities.

Pathogenesis

Over the years several theories have been developed to describe the etiology and pathogenesis of atherosclerosis. Two theories that have received the most attention are the response to injury hypothesis and the lipid-lipoprotein hypothesis (Ross, 1986; Ross et al., 1984). Four principal cells are involved in both theories: endothelium, smooth muscle, platelets, and monocytes.

Response to Injury Hypothesis. The response to injury hypothesis postulates that injury occurs to the endothelial cells. The injury may be due to such factors as chronic hypercholesterolemia, increased shear stress from blood flow at bifurcations in arteries, hypertension, and chemical toxins found in cigarette smoke that change the nature of the permeability barrier of the endothelial cells.

Endothelial cells, functionally active components of the intima, perform two vital functions. The cells normally form a permeability barrier that functions to control the passage of molecules from the plasma into the artery wall. Second, the endothelium forms a thromboresistant surface that promotes the continuous flow of blood by producing a heparin-like surface proteoglycan and synthesizing prostacycline (prostaglandin I_2, PGI_2). Prostacyclin, a potent vasodilator, is also a potent inhibitor of platelet aggregation.

Injury to the endothelium results in an immediate platelet response. Platelets begin to adhere to the subendothelial layer at the site of injury. They aggregate and release their granule contents. Platelets contain several mitogens, one of which is of interest in atherosclerosis: platelet-derived growth factor (PDGF). PDGF can bind to connective tissue at sites of endothelial injury to attract smooth muscle cells from the media into the intima. PDGF induces

smooth muscle migration and proliferation. Within 3 to 5 days after platelets release their contents, smooth muscle cells have been shown to migrate from the media into the intima of the artery, inducing proliferation of these smooth muscle cells. According to the hypothesis, if the injury and the tissue response is a self-limited event and the integrity of the endothelium is restored, the lesion may be capable of regressing. For example, endothelial injury occurs when a balloon catheter is placed in an artery. However, endothelial cells regenerate slowly. In young monkeys complete regeneration of the endothelium can take as long as 9 months (Ross, 1986). If the injury is of long-standing or is chronically repeated, the lesions may continue to progress to advanced plaques with clinical consequences. An example of a long-standing injury is the chronic elevation of low-density lipoproteins (LDL), also called chronic hypercholesteremia.

Faggiotto and colleagues' (1984) research sheds light on the response to injury hypothesis. They studied the effects of chronic hypercholesterolemia lasting from 12 days to 13 months in 40 pigtail monkeys. Within 12 days, hypercholesterolemia with LDL levels between 300 and 1000 mg/dL were obtained, and monocytes were observed attached to the endothelial surface throughout the arterial tree. These monocytes seemed to be in the process of migrating between endothelial cells into the intima. Within 1 month many monocytes had begun to accumulate lipid and take on the appearance of foam cells.

During the next 3 months the lesions began to resemble fatty streaks consisting of two to three layers of foam cells. Foam cells derive their name from the intracellular lipid accumulation. Their relation to atherogenesis remains debatable. According to one viewpoint, foam cells are intimal smooth muscle cells that have been transformed by the accumulation of lipids that have been inadequately metabolized by the cells. The second theory is that foam cells are wandering blood monocytes that have entered the artery wall after engulfing lipid-containing debris. Depending on the viewpoint, foam cells may either be passive or play an important role in the genesis of atherosclerosis.

After 4 months of hypercholesterolemia, breaks occurred between the endothelial cells separating the fatty streaks. The breaks resulted in retraction of the endothelium, providing opportunity for platelet adherence, aggregation, and release of PDGF. During the next 2 months smooth muscle proliferation lesions of atherosclerosis appeared. The observations of Fagiotto and Ross (1984) support other studies that have reported that smooth muscle proliferation lesions of atherosclerosis are preceded by endothelial injury in the form of breaks in the endothelium, exposure of macrophages, and platelet interactions.

Lipogenic Hypothesis. The lipogenic hypothesis is associated with elevations of plasma LDL. Low-density lipoproteins, the major cholesterol-transporting lipoproteins, transport cholesterol and phospholipid to the peripheral cells. Thus, LDL are the major carriers for entry of cholesterol into tissues. Elevated levels of LDL may induce injury to the endothelial lining of the artery by infiltrating the intima from the blood.

Brown and Goldstein's (1984) work has contributed knowledge about the interaction of LDL with cells. They demonstrated that human cells possess specific receptors on their surface membranes that bind LDL with high affinity. This "LDL pathway" is part of a complex biochemical pathway that regulates the uptake, storage, and synthesis of cholesterol by the cell. The number of receptors is adjusted to provide the cell with enough cholesterol to meet its functional needs. Thus, the cholesterol needs of the cell determine LDL receptor synthesis, or the number of LDL receptors available for binding LDL. If LDL receptors are abnormally decreased or missing, the cell cannot gain adequate access to LDL, leading to high plasma LDL concentrations. For example, in familial hypercholesterolemia LDL receptors are either reduced or lacking.

Whether LDL are elevated due to a defect in the LDL receptor or other genetic or environmental factors, cholesterol esters are ultimately deposited in the arterial wall due to endothelial injury. Injury results from exposure of the endothelium to the high LDL levels. Smooth muscle cells take up the excess LDL and become foam cells. Thus, the above process repeats itself.

In summary, the mechanisms of atherosclerosis are much better understood than they were 10 years ago. Most researchers agree that endothelial injury and dysfunction are key events in the initiation of atherosclerosis. Changes in endothelial function result in a change in the interaction between the artery and the blood cellular elements. Such functional changes promote the entry of monocyte-derived macrophages to the intima, lipid accumulation, and smooth muscle proliferation. Over time, these events produce the vascular lesions of atherosclerosis.

ATHEROGENIC RISK FACTORS

Several risk factors have been linked to the presence of atherosclerosis. Age, male gender, hypertension, cigarette smoking, elevated serum cholesterol levels, and diabetes mellitus have all been positively correlated with atherosclerotic lesions (Criqui, 1986). Reduction or elimination of these risk factors has also been linked to a reduced death rate from coronary artery disease (CAD) and stroke and regression of the atherosclerotic lesions (Blankenhorn et al., 1988; Nash, 1988). Although most of the evidence for regression has been described in animal experimental models, such evidence is also accumulating in humans. In both animal and human angiographic studies, a reduction in the major risk factors has resulted in reduced morbidity and mortality from coronary atherosclerosis. Because of the importance of risk factor reduction in the prevention of atherosclerotic heart disease, each risk factor will be discussed in detail. In addition, interventions that reduce or eliminate the risk factor will be described.

Age

The risk for CAD rises sharply with age in all populations that have been studied. In the United States, CAD becomes evident when adults enter their 40s. The incidence reaches substantial proportions beyond age 45 in men and age 55 in women (Kannel et al., 1984). The rate of increase in CAD mortality is linear for men, whereas in women the rate of increase is relatively slow prior to menopause. However, the rate of increase rises rapidly in postmenopausal women. Women lag behind men by 10 years or more in the occurrence of CAD, but the gap narrows with advancing age.

Questions raised in relation to aging and CAD revolve around the role of life style versus the aging of the vascular system. In other words, does the "wear and tear" of aging produce atherosclerosis? Or does a lifetime spent in the presence of risk factors contribute to the atherosclerotic process? Researchers are continuing to attempt to answer these questions. The recent declines in the death rate due to coronary heart disease are thought to be partially related to widespread changes in life style and improvements in healthy behavior. Thus, evidence is accumulating that life style plays a significant role in the development of atherosclerosis. The exact role of the aging process in the development of CAD is currently unknown (Kreisberg and Kasim, 1987).

Gender

Men continue to have a much higher incidence of CAD than women at all ages. The age-adjusted death rates for CAD in men are twice as high as they are for women in the United States. For sudden coronary death, women have the same mortality rates as men 15 years younger (Jenkins, 1985). In spite of the differences between men and women, CAD is the number two cause of death in women over age 40 and the number one cause of death in women after age 60 (American Heart Association, 1988a). Debate continues on the reasons for the differences in mortality between men and women. Evidence implicating the menopause in the loss of protection against CAD has been inconsistent (Murdaugh and O'Rourke, 1988). Other biologic or life-style differences may play a role, but they have not been identified.

Family History

Both genes and environment predispose family members to CAD. For example, a person's smoking status, level of cholesterol, and dietary sodium intake are determined to a large degree by the shared family environment. Such risk factors tend to cluster within families.

The role of genetic factors in atherosclerosis is difficult to evaluate because of the clustering of other risk factors. However, certain inherited disorders are known to predispose a person to premature CAD. In homozygous familial hypercholesterolemia, myocardial infarction often occurs in the second decade of life (Hamley, 1981). Three-quarters of heterozygous parents are dead from CAD by age 60.

Other risk factors in families may suggest an increased susceptibility to CAD. For example, gout, hypertension, and diabetes mellitus need aggressive correction in families with known histories of CAD before age 55. In such families, the family history needs to be evaluated and all relatives screened. Interventions can be initiated for those identified to be at high risk for CAD.

Hypertension

Hypertension is one of the most potent risk factors for all cardiovascular complications. Elevated blood pressure is the major factor underlying strokes and a major factor for heart attacks and death from both of these events. The risk of cardiovascular complications increases continuously with increasing levels of both systolic blood pressure and diastolic pressure. Hypertension is defined as a diastolic blood pressure of 90 mm Hg and above. Of the 60 million Americans with hypertension, 75% have mild hypertension, or diastolic blood pressures between 90 and 105 mm Hg. The term "mild" refers only to the degree of elevation and is no indication of the seriousness of the condition because persons with mild hypertension are at considerably higher risk of morbidity and mortality (National Heart, Lung, Blood Institute, 1988). Both systolic and diastolic blood pressure are related to cardiovascular risk. Hypertensive persons have twice the incidence of peripheral vascular disease, sudden death, coronary heart disease, and myocardial infarction and four times the incidence of stroke as those with normal blood pressure (Kannel et al., 1985).

The clinical complications of hypertension result from either a direct pathologic effect on the vasculature or promotion of the atherogenic process. Atherosclerotic complications include CAD, myocardial infarction, and peripheral vascular disease. The relationship between hypertension and atherosclerosis has been studied mainly in animal models. Findings from animal, population, and postmortem studies conclude that hypertension serves as a stimulus for the development of CAD in persons with high levels

of circulating lipoproteins (Leitshuh and Chobanian, 1987). The reader is referred to Chapter 22 for a detailed discussion of hypertension.

Cigarette Smoking

Cigarette smoking is the most important known modifiable risk factor for CAD. Deaths from coronary artery disease related to cigarette smoking are three times higher than deaths from lung cancer (Kannel et al., 1984). In almost all studies a dose-response gradient has been documented between the number of cigarettes smoked daily and the incidence of coronary heart disease. In other words, death rates increase with the number of cigarettes smoked. Those who quit smoking have lower death rates than persons who continue to smoke. In addition, cigarette smoking acts synergistically with other risk factors to greatly increase the risk for coronary heart disease. For example, smoking and the concurrent use of oral contraceptives greatly increases the risk of coronary heart disease in women compared to the risk in those who neither smoke nor use oral contraceptives.

Over 4000 substances have been identified in cigarette smoke; some are toxic, mutagenic, carcinogenic, and pharmacologically active (Holbrook et al., 1984). Such diverse biologic effects shed light on the adverse consequences of smoking. The addictive properties of nicotine, one of the substances identified, is considered to be responsible for the failure to quit smoking. Nicotine crosses the blood–brain barrier and is distributed throughout the brain. Most of the effects of nicotine on the central nervous system are due to direct actions on brain receptors (Clark, 1987). Nicotine excites nicotinic receptors in the spinal cord, autonomic ganglia, and adrenal medulla.

Smoking a cigarette activates the central nervous system. Transient cardiovascular responses in healthy people include an increased heart rate and blood pressure, cardiac stroke volume and output, and coronary blood flow. In addition, peripheral cutaneous vasoconstriction and increased muscle blood flow occur due to the release of vasopressin. Concentrations of free fatty acids, glycerol, and lactate are increased.

Carbon monoxide from cigarette smoke also produces cardiovascular effects. Carbon monoxide binds to hemoprotein such as hemoglobin. Cigarette smokers have carboxyhemoglobin levels that are five times greater than those of nonsmokers (Holbrook et al., 1984). Thus, the oxygen-carrying capacity of the blood is reduced.

The link between cigarette smoking and atherosclerosis is thought to be mediated through the response to injury hypothesis. Carbon monoxide may produce hypoxia of the intima and increase endothelial permeability. In addition, nicotine may exert a toxic effect on the endothelium. In animal studies repeated endothelial injury has resulted from hypoxia and the effects of nicotine from cigarette smoking (Zimmerman and McGeachie, 1987).

Cigarette smoking facilitates the development of thrombosis. Increased platelet aggregation, increased platelet adhesiveness, shortened platelet survival, decreased clotting times, and an increased hematocrit have been recorded in smokers. Tobacco smoke may reduce the production of prostacyclin (PGI_2, the potent inhibitor of platelet aggregation. Nicotine may be the agent responsible (Zimmerman and McGeachie, 1987). In animal studies cardiac automaticity is increased, and the threshold for ventricular fibrillation is lowered. These effects may account for the increased risk of sudden death observed in cigarette smokers.

The adverse effects of "involuntary" smoking on healthy adults and children were first published in 1986. Involuntary smoking occurs when nonsmokers are exposed to cigarette smoke in an enclosed environment. The sidestream smoke has higher concentrations of carbon monoxide and many toxic and carcinogenic substances as well (Fielding and Phenow, 1988). In a review of 15 studies of involuntary smoking, an increased risk of lung cancer was found in 10 nonsmokers married to smokers. However, many of the studies that examined the relationships between involuntary smoking and lung cancer had defects. Four studies undertaken since 1981 have addressed some of the earlier design problems and supported the results of the earlier studies: Involuntary smoking is associated with an increased risk of lung cancer in nonsmokers. Although additional studies are needed, evidence is accumulating to support the carcinogenic effects of passive or sidestream smoke on nonsmokers. In addition, high mortality rates from cardiovascular disease have been observed in persons who have lived with smokers (Fielding and Phenow, 1988). However, no causal relationship has been proved.

Nicotine Substitution Therapy. Nicotine is known to be the dependence-producing substance in tobacco. As previously mentioned, nicotine easily crosses the blood–brain barrier to affect both mood and cognitive function. Benowitz (1988) provides considerable evidence to substantiate nicotine dependence in humans. For this reason, nicotine substitution therapy, using nicotine gum, has been a successful pharmacologic approach to smoking cessation. Each piece of gum contains 2 mg of nicotine. When the nicotine gum is used regularly throughout the day, the levels of nicotine average one-third to two-thirds of the levels observed with smoking. Gum containing 4 mg of nicotine is available in Europe. Studies indicate that the higher level is more effective in highly dependent smokers.

Nicotine gum is most effective when used as one component of a comprehensive smoking-cessation program. The gum reduces nicotine-withdrawal symptoms and provides a substitute oral activity. After the patient decides to quit smoking, the gum must be made available. The patient is instructed to chew the gum for 20 to 30 minutes whenever the urge to smoke arises. Up to 30 pieces of gum per day may be chewed. Most persons chew 10 to 15 pieces per day. They need to be told to chew slowly until a taste or tingling is experienced. The effects of the nicotine will not occur as rapidly as they do with cigarette smoking, but chewing will reduce withdrawal effects.

Side effects of nicotine gum may occur and include sore throat, tired jaws, hiccups, palpitations, nausea, and other gastrointestinal symptoms. Patients need to be encouraged to chew more slowly if side effects are reported. No studies have been reported on the safety of the gum for persons with diagnosed CAD or hypertension.

Nursing Management. Despite knowledge of the adverse health consequences of smoking, one-third of the adults in the United States continue to smoke. Increased numbers of smokers continue to be noted among young women between the ages of 15 and 24. Thus, school-, hospital-, and community-based interventions need to begin with making smokers aware of the consequences of smoking as the first step. Next, motivation to stop must be increased by providing incentives to stop. Smokers need to be taught strategies for stopping. During smoking cessation programs both role models and emotional support must be provided. In addition, long-term support is necessary to help maintain the change in behavior.

Preventing relapse remains the primary challenge in smoking cessation programs. In patients who have sustained a myocardial infarction, 40% had resumed smoking 6 months after they had stopped, and almost 50% smoked at a 3- to 5-year follow-up (Havik and Maeland, 1988). These relapse rates are consistent with those seen in other studies in which 30% to 50% of patients have resumed smoking at 6 months.

Several relapse-prevention strategies have been developed (Marlatt and Gordon, 1985). Skill training to learn to identify and cope with situations in which relapse is likely to occur, identification of potentially self-defeating beliefs and expectations about smoking, and acknowledgement and acceptance of "slips" are three such interventions. Despite these and other relapse-prevention strategies, a high rate of relapse is noted in behaviorally oriented programs at the 6 months follow-up (Kamarck and Lichtenstein, 1988; Curry et al., 1988).

Elevated Blood Cholesterol

Dietary lipids are one of the most important agents responsible for the high incidence of atherosclerotic disease in industrially developed parts of the world. A significant positive association has been demonstrated between ingestion of dietary cholesterol and plasma cholesterol levels and the incidence of CAD within population groups. Results from the trial organized by the Lipid Research Clinics Program (1984) demonstrated a causal relationship between the plasma lipoprotein profile, cholesterol levels, and morbidity and mortality from coronary atherosclerosis.

Longitudinal studies such as the Framingham Study and the Seven Country Study clearly demonstrate that individuals with clinical CAD have higher levels of cholesterol than individuals without clinical symptoms. Prospective studies of individuals within a population have shown that serum cholesterol levels predict the future occurrence of morbidity and mortality due to CAD. For persons with cholesterol values in the top 10% of the population, the risk of CAD mortality is four times as high as the risk in the bottom 10% of the population.

Lowering cholesterol levels has been shown to reduce the incidence of CAD events. The results of clinical trials indicate that dietary intervention is as effective in preventing recurrent myocardial infarction and death in patients with diagnosed CAD as it is in primary prevention. Although the direct evidence is strongest in middle-aged men with high initial cholesterol levels, epidemiologic observations and animal experiments also support the generalization that reducing total and LDL cholesterol levels is likely to reduce CAD incidence in younger and older men, in women, and in individuals with more moderate elevations of cholesterol.

Classification of Lipoproteins. Cholesterol is a naturally occurring lipid component of cell membranes and a precursor of bile acids and steroid hormones. In addition, cholesterol is the predominant lipid constituent of the atherosclerotic lesion. Cholesterol travels in the circulation in spherical particles that contain both lipids and proteins called lipoproteins.

Three major classes of lipoproteins can be measured in the serum of a fasting individual: very low density lipoproteins (VLDL), low-density lipoproteins (LDL), and high-density lipoproteins (HDL). LDL are the primary atherogenic lipoprotein and contain approximately 60% of the total cholesterol. LDL levels are inversely correlated with risk for CAD. VLDL, which are largely composed of triglycerides, contain 10% to 15% of the total serum cholesterol. Thus, serum cholesterol is highest in the low-density lipoprotein fraction, and serum triglyceride is greatest in the VLDL fraction. The VLDL fraction transports the majority of endogenous triglycerides and may be related to CAD incidence through its association with reduced HDL, diabetes, and obesity. VLDL are also precursors of LDL.

Because most of the cholesterol in the serum is found in the LDL, the concentration of total cholesterol is closely correlated with the concentration of LDL cholesterol. Although LDL cholesterol offers more precision in determining individual risk and is

preferred in clinical decisions about interventions to lower blood cholesterol, total cholesterol levels can be used in initial serum lipid evaluation. Serum HDL levels reflect the process of cholesterol removal from the peripheral tissues to the liver for degradation. Higher levels of HDL tend to facilitate the process of cholesterol removal from the body. Thus, the ratio of HDL to cholesterol is also significant in assessing cardiovascular risk.

Classification of Patients. The National Heart, Lung, and Blood Institute (NHLBI) recommends measurement of serum total cholesterol in all adults 20 years of age and over at least once every 5 years (1987). Optimal serum cholesterol values for American adults should not exceed 200 mg/dL. Patients with an optimal blood cholesterol level should be provided with educational materials designed to maintain blood cholesterol levels below 200 mg/dL and reduce associated risk factors. These patients are advised to have another serum cholesterol test within 5 years. Serum cholesterol levels measuring 200 to 239 mg/dL are classified as "borderline high blood cholesterol." These patients are given dietary and associated risk factor modification guidelines designed to lower their serum cholesterol level and are rechecked annually. Individuals who have diagnosed CAD or two associated nonlipid risk factors need to be tested for serum LDL cholesterol levels. Cholesterol levels of 240 mg/dL and above are classified as "high blood cholesterol." All patients with high blood cholesterol levels need to be tested for the serum level of LDL cholesterol. In addition to total blood cholesterol levels, the level of LDL cholesterol serves as a key index for clinical decision-making in instituting cholesterol-lowering therapy. Desirable LDL cholesterol levels are 130 mg/dL and below. Levels of LDL cholesterol of 160 mg/dL or greater are classified as "high-risk LDL cholesterol," and those 130 to 159 mg/dL are classified as "borderline high-risk LDL cholesterol." Patients with borderline high-risk LDL cholesterol are advised to follow a fat-modified diet and are reevaluated annually. Patients with diagnosed CAD or two associated nonlipid risk factors and all patients in the high-risk cholesterol group are evaluated annually and advised to enter a cholesterol-lowering treatment program.

The relationship between serum cholesterol level and CAD is considered linear. The 240 mg/dL cutpoint for total serum cholesterol is a level at which CAD risk is almost double that at 200 mg/dL (National Heart, Lung and Blood Institute, 1987). Patients with cholesterol levels at or above 240 mg/dL have a sufficiently high risk to warrant evaluation and treatment. Cholesterol testing must be viewed as one component of a comprehensive risk factor evaluation that includes assessment of nonlipid risk factors such as hypertension, cigarette smoking, diabetes mellitus, obesity, and a history of CAD in the patient or premature CAD in family members.

Dietary Management. Reduction of serum cholesterol begins with dietary therapy. Although the overall goal of treatment is to lower the LDL cholesterol level, the aim of dietary therapy is to lower total cholesterol levels. If the goal of normalizing plasma cholesterol levels is not fully achieved with dietary management, pharmacologic therapy must be instituted. However, continued dietary management can reduce the drug dosage, lessening the occurrence of drug side effects.

Dietary guidelines recommended by the National Cholesterol Education Program (1988) suggest a two-step program designed to reduce progressively the intake of saturated fatty acids and cholesterol and eliminate excess total calories. This diet provides an intake of total fat less than 30% of calories, saturated fatty acids of less than 10% of calories, and cholesterol of less than 300 mg/day. Serum cholesterol levels need to be measured at 4 to 6 weeks and at 3 months after starting the Step-One diet. If the goals of therapy are not achieved on the Step-One diet by 3 months, the Step-Two diet is implemented. The Step-Two diet calls for a further reduction in saturated fatty acid intake to less than 7% of calories and cholesterol intake to less than 200 mg/day.

The degree of reduction of LDL cholesterol levels that can be achieved by dietary therapy depends on the dietary habits of the patient before starting the diet and patient adherence to dietary modifications. Changing a typical American diet to the Step-One diet could reduce cholesterol levels on the average by 30 to 40 mg/dL. Advancing to the Step-Two diet can be expected to cause a further decline of approximately 15 mg/dL in cholesterol levels. Most of the decrease in total blood cholesterol will occur in the LDL cholesterol fraction.

Cholesterol reduction can be achieved by dietary therapy alone in many high-risk patients. Persons without high LDL cholesterol levels or severe dyslipidemias should be continued on dietary therapy for at least 6 months before considering drug therapy. Modification of associated risk factors such as obesity, sedentary life style, and smoking should be maintained throughout cholesterol-lowering therapy. If the goals of LDL cholesterol reduction are met by diet modification, long-term monitoring is indicated. If reduction of LDL cholesterol is not achieved, lipid-lowering drugs are considered along with continued dietary intervention.

Pharmacologic Management. Patients whose LDL cholesterol levels remain high despite adequate dietary therapy are considered for drug treatment. However, a minimum of 3 months of dietary therapy is required to provide a baseline for evaluating the efficacy of pharmacologic therapy. According to the National Cholesterol Education Program Expert Panel (1988), LDL cholesterol levels at which to consider drug therapy are 190 mg/dL or higher in patients without diagnosed CAD or at least two associated CAD risk factors, and 160 mg/dL or greater in patients with diagnosed CAD or two associated CAD risk factors.

Treatment goals for pharmacologic therapy are the same as those used for dietary therapy. Both treatment modalities attempt to achieve LDL cholesterol levels of less than 160 mg/dL in patients without diagnosed CAD or two associated CAD risk factors, or LDL cholesterol levels of less than 130 mg/dL in patients with diagnosed CAD or two associated CAD risk factors.

A summary of the major cholesterol-lowering drugs is presented in Table 15–1. Guidelines established by the National Cholesterol Education Program (1988) recommend the bile acid sequestrants and nicotinic acid as first-choice drugs for treatment of elevated levels of LDL. Both drugs are effective in lowering LDL cholesterol and have been found to lower CAD risk. Both are generally safe for long-term use. Nicotinic acid is the drug of choice for patients with triglyceride levels of greater than 250 mg/dL because it lowers LDL cholesterol without exacerbating the hypertriglyceridemia. Administration of bile acid sequestrants may increase hepatic VLDL production and increase the plasma concentration of triglycerides. Bile acid sequestrants are thus contraindicated as single-drug therapy in patients with hypertriglyceridemia.

Lovastatin, an HMG CoA reductase inhibitor, has recently been approved by the Food and Drug Administration (FDA) for marketing. Its long-term safety and effects on CAD risk have not been established. Lovastatin is effective in lowering LDL cholesterol levels and produces a slight reduction in serum triglyceride levels.

Gemfibrozil and probucol belong to the category of fibric acids. The fibric acids have not been approved by the FDA but are currently in wide use. Although gemfibrozil has been approved for treatment of hypertriglyceridemia, results of the Helsinki Heart Study (Frick et al., 1987) indicate that the drug is also effective for the treatment of hypercholesterolemia. Fibric acids appear to lower serum levels of VLDL and LDL and raise HDL cholesterol levels. Thus, the net effect is to reduce the total cholesterol-HDL cholesterol ratio.

Nursing Management. The management of hyperlipidemia must incorporate a multifaceted approach composed of dietary modification, weight loss, exercise, and drug therapy. For maximum reduction of CAD morbidity and mortality, all modifiable risk factors must be addressed. The overall objective in cholesterol reduction is to implement an individualized program leading to permanent life-style changes with self-management as the central focus. Both dietary and pharmacologic therapy require long-term behavioral changes. Adherence to life-style changes may be increased through a combination of education and behavior modification strategies.

Initially, the patient must recognize and accept personal responsibility for making life-style changes and must understand the rationale for the recommended changes. This phase includes assessment of

TABLE 15–1. Summary of the Major Cholesterol-Lowering Drugs

Drug	LDL Cholesterol Lowering (%)	Primary Actions	Side Effects	Maximum Dose
Cholestyramine Colestipol (Questran Colestid)	15–30	Bile acid sequestrant Binds bile acids in the intestinal lumen Increased hepatic synthesis of bile acids from cholesterol	Alters absorption of other drugs; increases triglyceride levels; upper and lower gastrointestinal symptoms are dose dependent	24 g/day 30 g/day
Nicotinic acid (Niacin)	15–30 Raises HDL levels	Decreases hepatic production of VLDL and production of LDL-cholesterol	Hyperuricemia; hyperglycemia; liver function abnormalities; upper gastrointestinal symptoms; flushing	3 g/day
Lovastatin	25–45	Competitive inhibitor of the limiting enzyme in cholesterol biosynthesis (HGM CoA reductase)	Liver function abnormalities; lens opacities; gastrointestinal and hepatic symptoms; muscle pain	80 mg/day
Gemfibrozil Clofibrate Fenofibrate Bezafibrate (Lopid, Atrinud-S)	5–15 Raises HDL levels	Fibric acid derivative; initially used for triglyceride reduction	Increases LDL-cholesterol in hypertriglyceridemic patients; gastrointestinal symptoms; liver function abnormalities; potentiates oral anticoagulants	1200 mg/day
Probucol	10–15	May inhibit oxidation and tissue deposition of LDL cholesterol. Increases LDL catabolism	Lowers LDL cholesterol; prolongs Q–T interval; diarrhea, nausea abdominal pain	1 g/day

Data from National Cholesterol Education Program Expert Panel. (1988). *Archives of Internal Medicine,* 148, 36–69.

the patient's current level of knowledge, awareness of the need for change, available support systems, perceived barriers to life-style change, and level of motivation.

The patient must be assisted in identifying and prioritizing problem areas related to dietary modification and associated risk factor reduction. The use of a food record may help to identify environmental cues associated with overeating. Specific short- and long-term goals should be established related to the problem areas identified. Behavioral change needs to be implemented over time, with easier changes introduced first to increase feelings of success. Patients are encouraged to monitor their own progress in relation to the problem areas identified and goals set. Monitoring of blood lipid levels and weight loss and gain and analysis of food records will help in evaluating patient progress.

The institution of pharmacologic therapy must include patient education about the goals of drug treatment and the expected side effects of the medication. Side effects may occur with all cholesterol-lowering drugs and need to be reported to the nurse or physician. The need for a long-term commitment to pharmacologic therapy is emphasized. Dietary modification must be maintained even after drug therapy is implemented.

Diabetes Mellitus

Diabetes mellitus affects between 8 and 10 million Americans. Approximately 12% of those over 65 have diabetes mellitus. It is one of the leading causes of disability in those over 45 years of age (Hopper and Schechtman, 1985). Coronary artery disease represents the ultimate cause of death in more than half of diabetic patients and tends to occur at an earlier age and with greater severity than in the nondiabetic population (Nesto and Kowalchuk, 1986).

Accelerated atherosclerosis is a major complication of diabetes mellitus. Accelerated atherogenesis may be related to factors such as hyperglycemia, hyperinsulinemia, and plasma lipid abnormalities, all of which are common in diabetics (Laakso et al., 1986). Hyperglycemia is considered an independent risk factor in the development of CAD in diabetics. Increased blood glucose is associated with increased plasma lipid levels (Sosenko et al., 1980), elevated mean systolic and diastolic blood pressures, and a higher mean body mass. Accelerated atherosclerosis in patients with diabetes mellitus indicates an alteration in both lipid and lipoprotein metabolism (Sevior and Elkeles, 1985). Elevation of VLDL concentrations occur frequently in insulin-dependent diabetics, resulting in increased total plasma cholesterol and triglyceride levels (Kannel, 1985). Comparisons of lipid values for diabetic and nondiabetic individuals have shown elevated cholesterol levels in diabetics. Increased fasting blood glucose levels among diabetics are associated with significant increases in all lipid components except HDL cholesterol (Ohlson et al., 1986).

The relationship between glycemic control and plasma cholesterol and triglyceride levels may be significant in altering the predicted risk of CAD in noninsulin-dependent diabetics (West et al., 1983; Ruderman and Haudenschild, 1984). Although both male and female noninsulin-dependent diabetics have lower HDL cholesterol levels than nondiabetic controls, the relative decrease is greater for women (Walden et al., 1984). One explanation of the loss of premenopausal protection from microvascular disease in women may lie in the differing effect of diabetes upon HDL cholesterol in the two sexes. Improved glycemic control may influence the course of CAD directly by diminishing such risk factors as hypercholesterolemia, increased LDL cholesterol, decreased HDL cholesterol, and increased plasma triglycerides (Ruderman and Haudenschild, 1984).

Another potential risk factor for CAD in the diabetic is the level of circulating insulin. Hyperinsulinemia promotes ischemic vascular disease and is a risk factor independent of the blood glucose level, plasma cholesterol, and blood pressure (Ruderman and Haudenschild, 1984). Because the precursor stages of type II diabetes are characterized by hyperinsulinemia, subjects may be exposed to increased circulating insulin levels over time. Hyperinsulinemia is prevalent in type II diabetics secondary to insulin resistance related to obesity.

Nursing Management. Because the control of hyperglycemia alone does not appear to reduce the risk of macrovascular sequelae in persons with diabetes mellitus, attention must be directed toward the management of associated cardiovascular risk factors. Risk reduction in the diabetic patient must begin with an assessment of patient needs and education related to the diabetic process and the role of associated risk factors. As with all life-style changes, priorities must be identified by the patient, including both short- and long-term goals. The nurse serves as a partner in assisting the patient to meet the set goals and evaluating his or her progress toward future goals.

The primary factor in reduction of cardiovascular risk is dietary control. In diabetic individuals, caloric restriction combined with intake alteration can significantly decrease plasma insulin, triglycerides, total cholesterol, VLDL cholesterol, and elevated blood pressure, increase HDL cholesterol levels, and aid in glycemic control (Ruderman and Haudenschild, 1984). Current American Diabetes Association guidelines for dietary modification urge reduction in saturated fat and cholesterol intake and increased intake of dietary fiber and complex carbohydrates. These recommendations parallel those of the American Heart Association (1988a) for prevention of CAD in the general population.

In addition, education and intervention for the diabetic patient must include a reduction of caloric intake to reduce the risk of CAD due to obesity. The increased risk of CAD in obese individuals may be due to its association with atherogenic factors such as hypertension, hypercholesterolemia, hypertriglyceridemia, and hyperinsulinemia. Type II diabetics have a higher incidence of obesity than nondiabetics in the same population. Because atherogenic vascular disease is more prevalent in diabetics who have gained weight in adult life, the reversal or prevention of obesity by caloric restriction may reduce the incidence of a number of atherogenic risk factors.

Sedentary Life Style

Data from several epidemiologic studies suggest that populations with habitual physical activity have decreased mortality from atherosclerotic coronary artery disease. Paffenberger and associates' (1978) study of Harvard alumni showed that exercise was inversely related to cardiovascular mortality. A trend toward reduced mortality was seen as physical activity increased. The Framingham data showed improved cardiovascular and CAD mortality rates with increased physical activity at all ages including the elderly. Similarly, the level of physical fitness in women has been associated with a more protective lipid profile, lower blood pressure, and less cigarette smoking (Blackburn and Jacobs, 1988).

Physiologic benefits of regular physical activity are related to increased HDL cholesterol levels (Superko et al., 1985), reduction in blood pressure (Tipton, 1984), increased cardiovascular functional capacity (Astrand and Rodahl, 1977), increased myoglobin, decreased myocardial oxygen demand, lowered plasma insulin levels with improved glucose tolerance (Schneider et al., 1986), and a decrease in platelet adhesiveness (Sarajas, 1976) and fibrolytic activity (Schneider et al., 1986). The protective effect of physical activity is seen at all ages. In patients with diagnosed CAD, preanginal exercise levels and stress tolerance are increased even with low-intensity exercise.

Nursing Management. Prudent physical activity incorporates regular moderate physical exercise such as exercising three times a week aerobically for 30 minutes to a level of 75% to 85% of maximal capacity. The goal of exercise is to increase or maintain functional capacity, which is accomplished by aerobic endurance activity.

Reports from cardiac exercise programs reveal that, on the average, half of the patients who start a program never finish. In studies of exercise adherence, dropout rates range from 20% to 60% with the lowest attrition occurring during the first 3 months of a program and the highest after 48 months (Oldridge, 1986). Fifty per cent of the dropout occurs between 6 and 12 months after starting both supervised and unsupervised exercise programs. A number of factors frequently associated with nonadherence to exercise programs have been identified. The most frequently reported factor associated with dropout is smoking. Smoking patterns are indicative of an individual's general adherence to a healthy life style. Blue collar occupations are another frequently cited factor in nonadherence with regular exercise. Blue collar workers may have less knowledge of their disease process and less frequently utilize health care services in general (Oldridge, 1984). Patients who are inactive in their leisure time also tend to have a higher dropout rate. Overweight participants (Dishman and Gettman, 1980) and those with angina (Shepard, 1985) have lower adherence rates.

Psychosocially, a primary factor predictive of nonadherence is lack of support from a significant other. Unless encouragement and ongoing support are provided, adherence to prescribed regimens will decrease. In addition to the support of others, individual motivation to initiate and sustain healthy behavior is essential in making successful life-style modifications.

Nursing interventions to increase adherence to exercise programs must begin with an assessment of the patient's existing level of physical activity, knowledge level, perceived barriers to exercise, available support systems, and level of motivation. The patient must establish exercise as a personal priority to achieve success. The advantages of exercise in reducing cardiovascular risk should be emphasized in patient education.

A mutually agreeable plan of exercise must be established including both short- and long-term exercise goals. Small, flexible goals established by the patient may increase feelings of success and achievement. Emphasis should be placed on time- rather than distance-oriented goals (Ice, 1985). Rewards are planned in advance as a reinforcement for goals achieved.

The first component addressed is the type of exercise to be performed. The exercise program should fit the needs and desires of the patient whenever possible (Martin and Dubert, 1984). Exercise conditioning will produce changes in the aerobic system only if the mode of activity is aerobic. Aerobic exercise refers to rhythmic, continuous exercise that maintains isometric muscle contractions and increases the efficient intake of oxygen by the body. Such exercises include walking, running, cycling, and swimming. The intensity of exercise performed refers to the energy expenditure required per minute to perform the exercise. Heart rate is usually used to estimate the intensity of exercise. The intensity of conditioning should be 65% to 90% of maximal heart rate (American College of Sports Medicine, 1986). The exercise pace is increased gradually to minimize injury. The patient is instructed on pulse-taking techniques and the effect of pharmacologic agents on heart rate, and a training heart rate is established. The patient is instructed to stop exercise if the heart rate exceeds the maximum, at the onset of chest pain, with an irregular heart rate, or with the occurrence of palpitations. The duration of exercise is at least 5 minutes per session initially and is adjusted for intensity as the patient becomes more comfortable with his new life style. Each exercise session is performed three to five times each week. Even high-intensity exercise must be performed more than twice

a week to gain aerobic benefits (American College of Sports Medicine, 1986). In developing any exercise program, basic exercise principles and safety measures during exercise are emphasized.

Obesity

Obesity is considered the most prevalent and potentially controllable health problem in the United States today. More than 30% of the adult population in this country is more than 20% overweight, and this figure continues to increase. Obesity is best defined as an excess of relative body fat content, or a body mass index (weight/height) greater than 20% above ideal.

The association between obesity and premature atherosclerotic coronary artery disease, increased angina pectoris, and increased mortality, particularly by sudden death, is well known. Data suggest that the degree of obesity may be an independent risk factor, especially in women (Hubert et al., 1983). The effects of increased weight are many: increased serum lipids and blood pressure, increased blood volume and resting cardiac output, elevated left ventricular filling time at rest or during exercise, diminished left ventricular chamber compliance, and increased pulmonary and systemic vascular resistance. Obesity also adversely affects the cardiovascular risk profile and increases atherogenesis through impaired glucose tolerance, increased plasma uric acid levels, elevated LDL cholesterol levels, decreased HDL cholesterol levels, and elevated serum triglyceride levels (Tyroler, 1980).

Promotion of Life-Style Change. The predominant rationale for the control of obesity is that obesity adversely affects the cardiovascular risk profile and accentuates atherosclerosis. Weight reduction lessens cardiac work and thereby decreases angina pectoris: Weight reduction improves exercise tolerance and exerts a favorable effect on blood pressure, glucose intolerance, plasma uric acid level, and the HDL–total cholesterol ratio. It is therefore an effective approach to reduction of multiple atherogenic risk factors.

In overweight individuals, weight loss will reduce both plasma cholesterol and serum triglycerides. Reduction in cholesterol and triglycerides is partly due to dietary modifications involving decreased intake of total fat and saturated fat but is also a physiologic response to weight reduction. Weight reduction by means of a diet low in saturated fat and cholesterol lowers the risk of coronary heart disease by decreasing multiple atherogenic risk factors except smoking. Although no confirmatory evidence from intervention studies is available, dietary management of obesity is recommended because weight reduction is beneficial as a component of multifactoral risk reduction and life-style change.

Nursing Management. In order to minimize the risk of CAD, individuals need to attain and maintain an optimal body weight. Evaluation and management of obesity is important because of its relationship to other cardiovascular risk factors. Minor defining characteristics related to obesity include dietary intake in excess of metabolic requirements, sedentary activity patterns, and undesirable eating patterns.

As with management of associated cardiovascular risk factors, the patient must make the commitment to changing the eating behavior before it can be modified. Behavior modification, group therapy, and self-directed change technique may be used. A program of weight reduction must begin with education related to cardiovascular risk associated with excess body weight and measures available to reduce weight. Health teaching must include nutrition, exercise, and stress management techniques. The nurse must work with the patient to assess the patient's level of knowledge, available support systems and level of motivation. The goal of appropriate body weight is more easily attained if the nurse helps the client to establish a diet related to dietary intake through the use of a food diary and to identify mutually agreeable areas for behavior modification. Once trends have been identified, both short- and long-term goals for weight reduction should be set. The patient's family should be involved in the planning phase to ensure support for proposed changes. In addition, nonfood rewards should be established for attainment of increments of weight loss.

Throughout the weight loss process the nurse must provide positive reinforcement and encourage self-reinforcement on the part of the patient. Reinforcement of positive behavior serves to enhance self-esteem and increases the likelihood of permanent behavior change. A gradual dietary modification may be most beneficial in ensuring long-term weight loss. Weight loss can be maintained through eating well-balanced, calorie-controlled meals. The goal is a long-term commitment to a change in eating habits that will serve as one component in multifactoral risk reduction.

Oral Contraceptives

Oral contraceptive use is associated with an increased incidence of cardiovascular disease. The risk of myocardial infarction in women users of oral contraceptives with no predisposing medical conditions is related to age and the presence of other risk factors. Women younger than 40 who suffer a myocardial infarction have almost always been cigarette smokers (Rosenberg et al., 1983; Salonen, 1982). Use of oral contraceptives in women over age 40 is associated with an increased risk of myocardial infarction, particularly if other risk factors and long-term use are associated. The incidence of stroke or thromboembolism is increased with oral contraceptive use at all ages compared to nonusers.

Oral contraceptives have an effect on other risk factors, because of their effects on lipid metabolism and blood pressure. Total serum cholesterol, triglycerides, and LDL cholesterol values are increased, and HDL cholesterol is decreased (Powell et al., 1984; Russel-Briefel et al., 1982). The magnitude of the lipid changes are dependent on the estrogen and progestogen content of the oral contraceptive, in addition to age, weight, and smoking history (Powell et al., 1984). Blood pressure levels, both systolic and diastolic, are increased slightly in oral contraceptive users (Meade, 1982). The risk of hypertension may be three to six times greater in oral contraceptive users than in nonusers depending on the oral contraceptive formulation. Glucose tolerance is also decreased in oral contraceptive users, especially in women with a family history of diabetes. Cigarette smoking in users of oral contraceptives increases the risk of myocardial infarction in premenopausal women. In studies of women smokers aged 35 years or older who used oral contraceptives, the relative risk of myocardial infarction has been estimated to be 4 to 20 times that of nonusers who have never smoked. One study found that the increased risk of myocardial infarction remained after discontinuance of oral contraceptives for 5 years or more (Lapidus et al., 1985).

Since the mid-1970s the estrogen and progestogen dosages in oral contraceptives have been decreased based on the relationship of these two hormones to coronary heart disease risks in oral contraceptive users. Although prescribing practices have improved since the 1970s, data from the National Health and Nutrition Examination Survey (NHANES II) indicate that many young women oral contraceptive users are at increased risk for the development of coronary heart disease (Russel-Briefel et al., 1982). Clinicians have the responsibility not only to screen and detect risk factors in oral contraceptive users but also to monitor and intervene appropriately to reduce or eliminate any major risk factors for coronary heart disease in young women of childbearing age.

Menopause and Noncontraceptive Estrogen Replacement

The differences in incidence of coronary heart disease between men and women decrease with advancing age, and menopause has been thought to be a relevant factor. A twofold increase in mortality from CAD was noted among postmenopausal women in the Framingham Study. Cigarette smoking, hypertension, and elevated serum cholesterol levels were present in women who sustained a myocardial infarction. In another report of CAD in women, smoking and elevated serum lipid values were more common in women with menopause before age 45 than in women who experienced a later menopause (Lindquist and Bengtsson, 1982). Cross-sectional evidence indicates that women who smoke cigarettes tend to experience natural menopause 1 to 2 years earlier than nonsmokers. (Cross-sectional research refers to data collection at only one point in time as opposed to longitudinal research.)

The incidence of CAD in women who undergo menopause prematurely is not consistent. Surgical menopause increased the relative risk for coronary heart disease to 7.2 in women under the age of 35 years. An increased incidence of coronary heart disease has also been reported in women in whom natural menopause occurs prematurely compared with age-matched premenopausal women. However, risk for ischemic heart disease was not increased in women with premature menopause in a 12-year follow-up of women in Göteborg, Sweden (Lapidus et al., 1985). The discrepant results do not permit any conclusions concerning the relationship between premature menopause and coronary heart disease.

Estrogen replacement in postmenopausal women has been advocated because of the increased incidence of coronary heart disease following menopause. However, controversy concerning the association between noncontraceptive estrogen treatment and risk of coronary heart disease continues to exist. Evidence is now accumulating to suggest that the use of noncontraceptive estrogens by postmenopausal women is not associated with an increased risk of myocardial infarction and may possibly provide a protective effect (Stampfer et al., 1988). Two studies have shown an increased risk of cardiovascular disease (Wilson et al., 1985; Petitti et al., 1979). Women in the Framingham Study who were taking estrogens had a higher risk of coronary disease. The Framingham data included patients with unrecognized myocardial infarctions, and the sample was older. Among the oldest women in the study, estrogen replacement was first prescribed after the age of 60 years in contrast to perimenopausal prescriptions in young women. Thus, all age groups were not homogeneous for estrogen replacement. Wilson and colleagues (1985) reanalyzed their data using an approach taken in another study and reported no relation between estrogen use and cardiovascular disease in younger women. However, a strong positive relationship was noted in women 60 years and older. Methodologic differences in the studies may account for the controversial results and need attention in further research.

The effect of estrogen replacement on lipids is thought to explain some of the protective effects. Estrogens both raise HDL and lower LDL cholesterol (LaRosa, 1985). Progestogens are prescribed in combination with estrogens because of the otherwise increased risk of endometrial cancer. Since progestogens have an adverse effect on plasma lipoproteins, the positive effect of estrogen may be neutralized in women taking both drugs.

Type A Behavior Pattern

The type A or coronary-prone behavior pattern is described as a style of behavior that emerges when a person is challenged or blocked by an environmental circumstance (Jenkins, 1988). The behavior is characterized by competitiveness, a sense of urgency, easily provoked hostility, impatience, and concentration on self-selected goals to the exclusion of other aspects of the environment. Type A behavior is not the same as stress.

The relationship between type A behavior pattern and coronary heart disease morbidity and mortality continues to be debated. Most recently Ragland and Brand (1988) reported a lower mortality rate among type A than in type B subjects. However, letters to the editor in a later journal (Friedman et al., 1988) discuss the major inconsistencies and limitations of Ragland and Brand's findings. Thus, authors continue to discuss the potential role of the type A behavior pattern in coronary heart disease. Recent evidence indicates that anger and hostility may be more important components (Williams, 1987). However, more research is needed to clarify which components are related to an increased risk for coronary heart disease.

MYOCARDIAL ISCHEMIA

Pathogenesis

Myocardial ischemia stems from an imbalance between myocardial oxygen requirements and oxygen availability. The imbalance can be due to either a decrease in coronary blood flow (supply) or a disproportionate increase in myocardial oxygen requirements (demand). Decreased coronary blood flow is most commonly due to atherosclerosis in the coronary arteries. However, myocardial ischemia can also result from nonatherosclerotic disease. For example, congenital anomalies of the coronary arteries, hereditary metabolic disorders, and systemic collagen vascular disease may produce chronic myocardial ischemia (Chatterjee, 1990). Increased myocardial oxygen requirements may precipitate myocardial ischemia in valvular heart disease or hypertrophic cardiomyopathy because demand may exceed the capacity to supply oxygen to the myocardium. Recently, vasoconstriction (spasm) of the coronary arteries has also been found to be a cause of myocardial ischemia.

Under normal conditions myocardial metabolic demands closely parallel coronary blood flow. Ischemia is avoided by a careful matching of blood flow to metabolism. Even in a resting state, the cardiac muscle extracts 65% to 75% of available oxygen. Thus, augmenting coronary blood flow is the principal means of increasing the oxygen supply. In the presence of coronary atherosclerosis increased demands for blood flow cannot be met, and ischemia results.

Because the major cause of myocardial ischemia is decreased blood flow (supply), emphasis is usually placed on the supply side of the oxygen supply–demand ratio. Under normal hemodynamic conditions coronary blood flow is distributed uniformly. The amount of coronary blood flow during diastole is usually several times greater than that during systole. Thus, satisfactory regulation of the transmural distribution of coronary blood flow is maintained until the vessels become maximally dilated. However, with progressive obstruction of a large coronary artery with atherosclerotic lesions, adequate flow is maintained in the epicardial (outer myocardial) layers but is insufficient to the subendocardial layers of the heart. Thus, the onset of myocardial ischemia is dependent on the pathophysiologic mechanisms in the subendocardium (Factor and Kirk, 1986).

Several metabolic changes occur in myocardial cells during ischemic episodes. Oxygen diffuses from the capillaries to the mitochondria in the myocardial cells. Ischemia occurs when the concentration of oxygen falls below a critical level in the mitochondria. Within 15 seconds of ischemia there is an acceleration of glycolysis and lactate production from anaerobic metabolic reactions, which leads to a fall in intracellular pH. The altered pH leads to changes in the interaction between calcium and the contractile proteins (actin-myosin), resulting in impaired myocardial contractile function (Alpert, 1984; Kawaniski and Rahimtoola, 1987). Ischemia results in cessation of myocardial contraction in the affected zones of the myocardium. Diastolic myocardial function is also impaired because the ischemic cells do not completely relax, as noted by increased ventricular stiffness. This stiffness in turn increases ventricular diastolic pressures.

As noted earlier, left ventricular wall abnormalities occur early in the ischemic episode. These changes are followed by electrocardiographic (ECG) abnormalities and the development of symptoms. The commonly observed ECG changes are ST segment depression or elevation and dysrhythmias due to electrical excitability (Fig. 15-1). Patient symptoms include angina, acute dyspnea, or sudden death.

Investigations have recently focused on the importance of free radicals in the pathophysiology of ischemia. As ischemic tissues are reperfused, molecular oxygen is reintroduced. The oxygen molecule interacts with byproducts of the ischemia to form oxygen-derived free radicals, including the superoxide anion, the hydroxy radical, and hydrogen peroxide. These free radicals can react with various cell components such as unsaturated fatty acids. In turn, loss of membrane permeability and loss of enzyme activity occur, resulting in further damage to the myocardial cells. Enzymes that are present react with the free radicals to prevent further cell damage. These enzymes are termed "free radical scavengers" (Werns et al., 1986; Shlafer et al., 1982).

Clinical, angiographic, and pathologic evidence indicates that an alteration in the integrity of the atherosclerotic plaque is the underlying mechanism of acute coronary ischemia. Endothelial and smooth muscle cells maintain the homeostasis of the vessel wall. Stable states are achieved following injury in

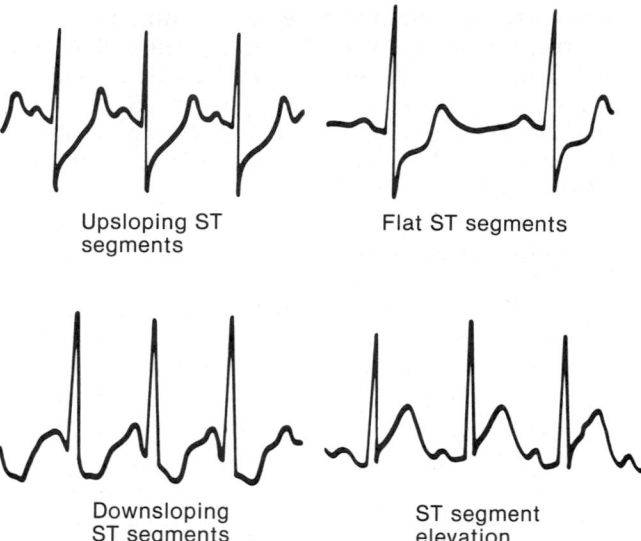

Upsloping ST segments   Flat ST segments

Downsloping ST segments   ST segment elevation

FIGURE 15–1. Family of ST segment changes seen with ischemia. (From Parmley, O., and Chatterjee, K. (1988). *Cardiology vol. 1: Physiology, pharmacology, diagnoses.* Philadelphia: J. B. Lippincott.)

that the vessel is able to maintain blood flow. However, injury enables the atherosclerotic plaque to form. Raised plaques consist of a pool of fatty material covered by a cap of fibrous tissue. The fibrous cap may crack, resulting in either rapid plaque progression or hemorrhage into the plaque. These cracks are also referred to as intimal fissures, breaks, tears, ulcers, and ruptures. The clinical manifestations, i.e., angina or infarction, depend on the severity of impaired flow, the presence and extent of impaired flow, and the presence and extent of collateral flow (Cowley et al., 1989; Falk, 1989). The clinical spectrum of ischemic heart disease includes asymptomatic CAD, the anginal syndromes, myocardial infarction, and sudden death.

Noninvasive Diagnosis

Recent experimental studies have delineated the sequence of metabolic, mechanical, hemodynamic, and electrocardiographic abnormalities resulting from inadequate coronary blood flow to contracting ventricular myocardium (Erickson and Thaulow, 1984). The occurrence of these abnormalities in the presence of myocardial ischemia forms the basis for noninvasive diagnostic testing for coronary artery disease (American College of Sports Medicine, 1986).

In using noninvasive testing it is important to consider the sensitivity, percentage of true positive results, and specificity and percentage of true negative results for each test; the quality of the laboratory available for performing the study; the cost of the procedure; and whether or not a positive test will alter the decision-making process. Using Bayes theorem, the post-test odds of a disease being present are equal to pretest odds times the odds that the results of the test are true (Shulman, 1984). For example, the odds of CAD being the cause of atypical chest pain in a 35-year-old woman with no risk factors are less than 5%. After a positive ECG exercise test with ST segment depression, the odds are still less than 20%, and in such a case a false-positive exercise ECG result is likely.

ELECTROCARDIOGRAPHY

The ECG recorded with the patient at rest may show abnormalities due to a prior myocardial infarction, left ventricular hypertrophy, or other cardiac disease. However, the resting ECG is normal or nonspecific in up to 50% of patients with chronic exertional angina. In patients with angina occurring at rest, ECG abnormalities such as ST-T wave depression, bundle branch block, or dysrhythmias occurring during a painful episode will often lead to the correct diagnosis of CAD. However, rest angina often occurs without ECG changes.

Exercise ECG Testing. ECG monitoring during graded bicycle or treadmill exercise testing is the most commonly used noninvasive method used for identifying patients likely to have CAD or likely to be at high risk. High-risk patients are those who have severe myocardial ischemia at a low workload (Weiner et al., 1987; Bruce et al., 1980). Many exercise ECG protocols exist. All are based on increasing the myocardial oxygen demand at 3-minute intervals by altering the workload progressively; the incremental increases in heart rate and systolic blood pressure result in augmented myocardial oxygen demands that eventually cannot be met because of a compromised coronary blood flow reserve.

The sensitivity of exercise ECG recording improves with 12-lead ECG monitoring. The test reaches peak sensitivity for identifying patients with coronary artery stenosis when at least 85% of predicted maximal heart rate is attained during exercise and is most accurate in patients with a normal resting ECG and no other reasons for ST segment depression during exercise such as hypokalemia or digitalis therapy. In most studies, the sensitivity of 1-mm ST segment depression beyond baseline during exercise has been about 70% with a specificity of 90% (Weiner et al., 1979; Chaitman et al., 1978; Bruce et al., 1980).

Exercise ECG testing is generally considered useful for (1) diagnoses of coronary artery disease in male patients with atypical symptoms of myocardial ischemia; (2) assessment of the functional capacity and prognosis in patients with known CAD; and (3) evaluation of patients with symptoms consistent with recurrent exercise-induced cardiac dysrhythmias. The specificity of exercise-induced ST segment changes in women with atypical or typical angina has been lower than that in men, producing more false-positive results. Endpoints during exercise testing of importance include ST segment depression, a suboptimal rise or actual fall in the systolic blood pressure, exercise-induced ventricular dysrhythmias, chest pain with or without ECG changes, exercise-induced conduction abnormalities, failure to increase heart rate, and clinical signs of congestive heart failure.

Ambulatory ECG Recordings. Initially used primarily for dysrhythmia detection and documentation in symptomatic patients, ambulatory ECG recorders are now used commonly to demonstrate ST segment alterations in patients with symptomatic or asymptomatic myocardial ischemia (Knoebel et al., 1989). Improvements in the low-frequency response of the detection, playback, and recorder components of the necessary equipment have increased the utilization of the ambulatory ECG for providing accurate information concerning ST segment shifts during normal activity. However, the use of only two ECG leads, the multiple causes of ST segment depression, and the lesser amount of physical activity compared to exercise testing results in a poor sensitivity and specificity of ambulatory ECG recording for the diagnosis of CAD.

Ambulatory ECG recordings are useful for detecting ST segment elevation, often with dysrhythmias, in patients with variant (Prinzmetal) angina due to coronary artery spasm. This diagnostic method is less valuable in patients with other ischemic syndromes, including asymptomatic myocardial ischemia.

An American College of Cardiology–American Heart Association Committee (Brook, 1989) has published *Guidelines for Ambulatory ECG Recordings.* Indications are graded as useful and reliable (class I), commonly used but controversial (class II), or not useful (class III). Table 15–2 summarizes the indications for ambulatory ECG monitoring.

EXERCISE TESTING WITH THALLIUM-201 IMAGING

Myocardial perfusion imaging with thallium-201 (^{201}Tl) has been widely applied in the clinical assessment of patients with known or suspected CAD. The

---

TABLE 15–2. Indications for Ambulatory Electrocardiography in Detecting Ischemia in Patients with Chest Pain

Class I	Chest pain suggestive of Prinzmetal (variant) angina
Class II	Symptomatic patients unable to be tested by treadmill or bicycle
Class III	Chest pain classic for angina *with* one or more risk factors
	or
	Atypical chest pain *with* one or more risk factors
	or
	Atypical chest pain with no risk factors

Modified with permission from the American College of Cardiology (Journal of the American College of Cardiology), 1989, 13:249.

amount of ^{201}Tl extracted by the myocardium is dependent on regional coronary blood flow (Fig. 15–2). Myocardial uptake in the absence of CAD is relatively homogeneous on assessment by gamma camera imaging (Dehmer, 1987; Beller, 1985).

However, after its initial extraction, ^{201}Tl does not remain fixed within the myocardial cells, and there is a continuous exchange between myocardial thallium and thallium that was initially distributed into the systemic blood pool. Thus, redistribution of ^{201}Tl is defined as the total or partial resolution of myocardial defects that are detected 5 to 20 minutes after intravenous [201]Tl. Defect disappearance or partial improvement is determined by obtaining delayed images 3 to 4 hours after the initial injection of [201]Tl. Thus, initial thallium defects following intravenous injection of the isotope near the end of exercise that are improved 3 hours later usually indicate reversible ischemia. In contrast, persistent thallium defects during exercise and several hours later usually indicate old or recent irreversible myocardial damage.

The sensitivity and specificity of exercise ^{201}Tl scintigraphy for identifying myocardial ischemia averages 85% and 90%, respectively (Ritchie et al., 1978). Therefore, the accuracy of ^{201}Tl exercise studies generally has been superior to that of ECG exercise tests, but the experience of the observer is an important factor. In addition, myocardial perfusion imaging costs several times more than standard exercise testing.

The use of ^{201}Tl exercise imaging has been beneficial in patients demonstrating nonspecific ST segment depression, left ventricular hypertrophy, or preexcitation conduction patterns, digitalis therapy, or metabolic abnormalities that may render inconclusive results with standard ECG exercise testing. Thallium-201 scintigraphy may also provide useful information about patients who cannot exercise to at least 85% of their age-predicted maximum heart rate. Most recently, intravenous dipyridamole, which dilates the large coronary arteries, has been used to distribute myocardial blood flow away from areas of reversible myocardial ischemia as an intervention for demonstrating areas of thallium redistribution in patients unable to perform sufficient exercise for exercise thallium imaging (Boucher et al., 1985).

RADIONUCLIDE VENTRICULOGRAPHY

This radionuclide technique utilizes technetium bound to red blood cells for "blood pool" imaging with ECG-gated left ventricular time-activity curves obtained from summed cardiac cycle data at points from end-diastole to end-systole (Beller, 1985) (Fig. 15–3). Gamma camera imaging is performed at rest and during the last 2 minutes of exercise, and the global left ventricular ejection fraction is determined from end-diastolic counts minus end-systolic counts divided by end-diastolic counts. Regional wall motion can also be assessed by careful review of the cine-film format of the radionuclide ventriculogram (RVG).

The normal response to exercise has been defined as an absolute increment of at least 5% in the left ventricular ejection fraction *without* the development of a new wall motion abnormality. Failure to increase the left ventricular ejection fraction on RVG has a sensitivity similar to (85% to 90%) that of ^{201}Tl exercise imaging but much less specificity (60% to 76%) (Borer et al., 1979; Caldwell et al., 1979; Rozawski et al., 1983). An abnormal ejection fraction response occurs in many elderly patients, women without heart disease, patients with depressed cardiac function due to valvular heart disease or cardiomyopathy, and

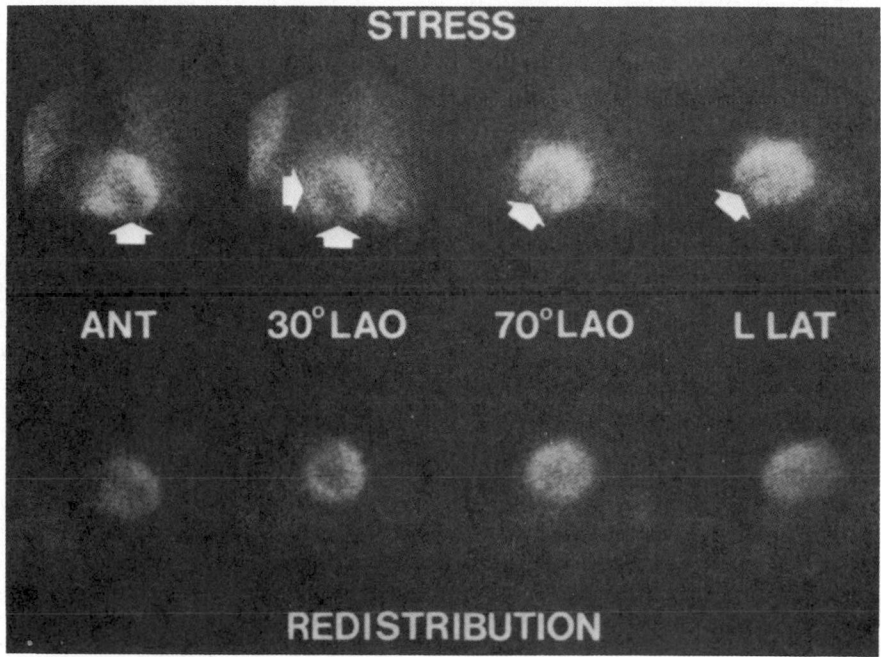

FIGURE 15–2. Myocardial perfusion scintigraphy with thallium-201 in a patient with 90% stenosis of the left anterior descending artery along with less severe stenosis involving the left circumflex system. A large reversible perfusion defect involving the anteroseptal and apical segments of the left ventricle is seen best on the 30-degree LAO immediate postexercise image *(arrows).* The defect is not present on redistribution imaging 4 hours later *(lower panel)* because it is due to transiently increased lung uptake on the immediate postexercise images *(upper panel). Abbreviations:* ANT, anterior; 30 LAO, 30 degrees left anterior oblique; 70 LAO, 70 degree left anterior oblique; LLAT, left lateral. (From Braunwald, E. (1988). *Heart disease: Textbook of cardiovascular medicine* (3rd ed). Philadelphia: W. B. Saunders.)

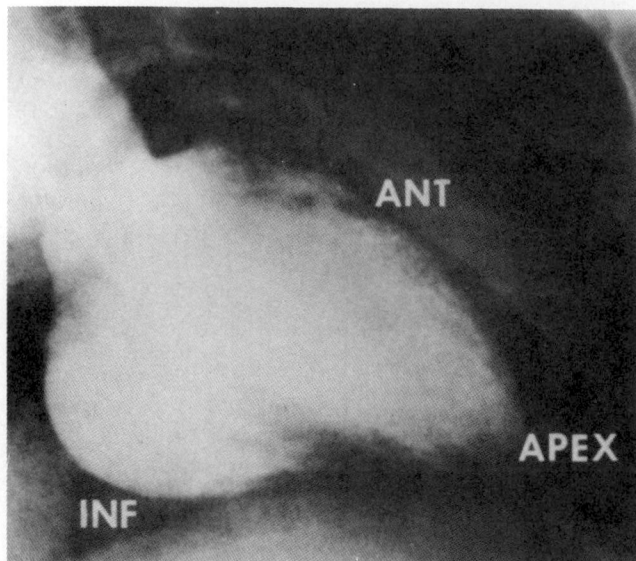

FIGURE 15–3. A 30-degree right anterior oblique (ROA) projection of the end-diastolic frame of a left ventriculogram. Anterior *(ANT)*, apical *(APEX)*, and inferior *(INF)* segments of the left ventricle are demonstrated in this view. (From Parmley, O., and Chatterjee, K. (1988): *Cardiology vol 1: Physiology, pharmacology, diagnoses.* Philadelphia: J. B. Lippincott.)

hypertensive patients. The demonstration of a new wall motion abnormality during exercise is less sensitive (65% to 76%) but more specific (95%) for a diagnosis of coronary heart disease. Table 15–3 compares the usefulness of ^{201}Tl exercise imaging and exercise RVG in the detection of myocardial ischemia.

EXERCISE ECHOCARDIOGRAPHY

In the past several years exercise echocardiography has been used with increasing frequency to assess total and regional left ventricular function to detect abnormalities resulting from myocardial ischemia (Fig. 15–4). In subjects with excellent two-dimensional echocardiographic images, the reported sensitivity and specificity are similar to those characteristic of radionuclide ventriculography and better than those of exercise ECG testing (Crawford et al., 1984). However, not all patients have adequate echocardiographic images during bicycle exercise. Images suitable for quantitating left ventricular ejection fraction during bicycle exercise can be obtained in 75% of patients and for qualitative assessment of left ventricular wall motion in 85%. The use of early post-treadmill exercise two-dimensional echocardiography is being evaluated in several medical centers and thus far has resulted in a slight decrease in the sensitivity for detecting CAD.

OTHER NONINVASIVE METHODS

The physical examination, especially during an episode of chest pain, the standard chest radiographs, and cardiac fluoroscopic studies may provide indirect or direct evidence of CAD. In the absence of other obvious cardiac diseases, certain findings such as a new fourth heart sound, a palpable left ventricular wall motion abnormality, or a transient murmur of mitral regurgitation suggest that ischemia is the cause of the chest pain.

The most common use of the chest roentgenogram is in the evaluation of left ventricular failure. Increased pulmonary vascular markings often indicate pulmonary venous hypertension due to left ventricular diastolic dysfunction related to CAD or other causes of left ventricular disease.

Although used infrequently other than during cardiac catheterization, cardiac fluoroscopy is extremely useful for detecting coronary artery calcification. The sensitivity and specificity of coronary artery calcification for significant coronary artery stenosis has varied between 40% and 76% for specificity and between 78% and 85% for specificity (Margolis et al., 1980). However, the presence of severe coronary artery stenosis does not indicate whether or not myocardial ischemia is a result of the coronary atherosclerosis that is present.

Invasive Diagnosis

CARDIAC CATHETERIZATION

Although noninvasive techniques assume an important role in assessment of cardiovascular disease, cardiac catheterization with coronary angiography remains the most definitive procedure for the evaluation and diagnosis of coronary disease. Cardiac catheterization is a combined hemodynamic and angiographic procedure performed for a diagnostic assessment of the presence and extent of coronary artery disease. The procedure consists of the introduction of a catheter into the vascular system and heart to obtain hemodynamic measurements, draw blood samples, or inject radiographic indicators. The

TABLE 15–3. Comparison of Thallium-201 and Exercise Radionuclide Ventriculography

^{201}Tl is preferable:
1. In the presence of certain dysrhythmias (e.g., atrial fibrillation, frequent premature beats) that may interfere with ability to properly "gate" the blood pool scan
2. When presence of CAD needs to be assessed in a patient who may have exercise-induced LV dysfunction for some other reason (e.g., hypertension)
3. When the LV ejection fraction is severely depressed at rest

Exercise radionuclide ventriculography is preferable
1. When a measurement of LV ejection fraction is also necessary
2. When extraneous factors could cause the impression of decreased or heterogeneous myocardial uptake (e.g., large breasts, mastectomy, left pleural effusion, pacemaker hardware)
3. When right ventricular function must also be assessed

Abbreviations: LV, left ventricular.

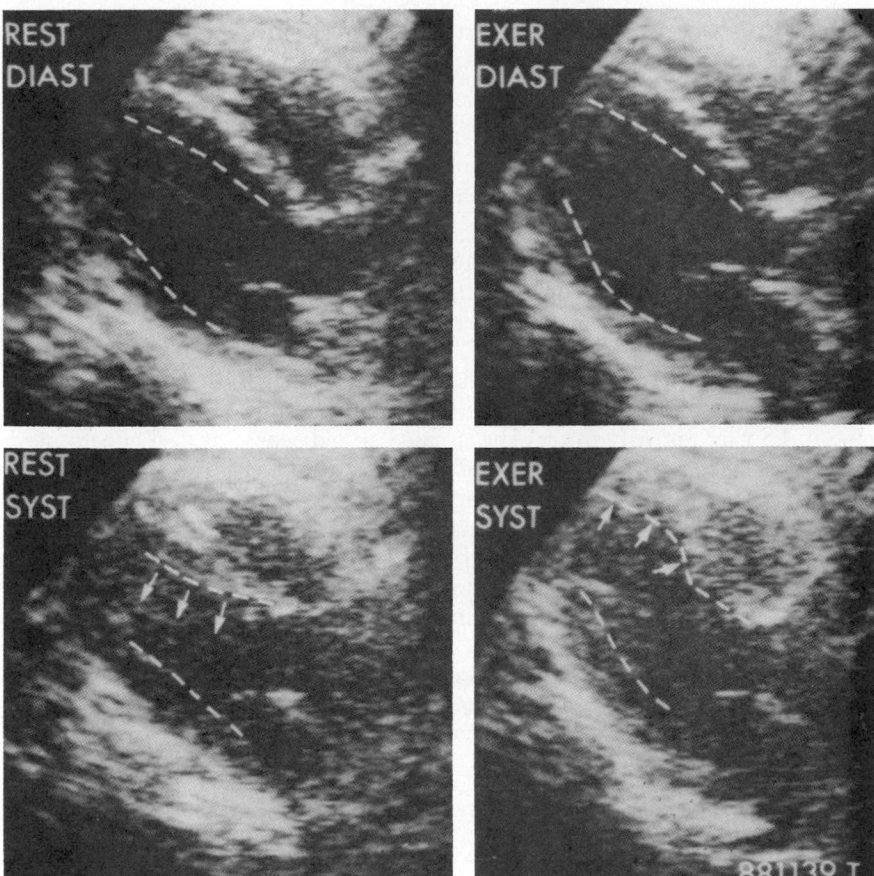

FIGURE 15–4. Resting and immediate postexercise echocardiograms of a patient with an obstruction in the left anterior descending coronary artery. At rest, the septal motion is normal *(arrows) (REST, SYST)*. (From Felgenbaum, H. (1986). *Echocardiogaphy* (4th ed.). Philadelphia: Lea & Febiger.)

goals of cardiac catheterization are (1) to define cardiovascular anatomy; (2) document the existence of known or suspected conditions; (3) compare catheterizations to evaluate increased severity of known conditions; (4) explore the possibility of associated conditions that may result from primary cardiac disease; (5) detect intracardiac shunts; and (6) carry out medical or presurgical evaluation. Cardiac catheterization is indicated in preparation for all cardiac surgical procedures. Combined right and left catheterization is now the most widely used approach.

With current levels of safety, there are relatively few contraindications to cardiac catheterization. Acute myocardial infarction, drug toxicities, and controllable dysrhythmias are examples of conditions that need to be managed prior to catheterization. Cardiac catheterization is contraindicated in patients whose cardiac diagnosis is certain but in whom cardiac surgery must be deferred because of debilitating illness, massive obesity, or severe cardiomegaly. Anticoagulation as a contraindication is debatable. Some investigators have reported an increase in hemorrhages and other complications in patients receiving anticoagulants, whereas others believe that anticoagulants are safe and at times beneficial.

During catheterization, several strategies are used to obtain data on cardiac pressures, output, oxygenation, and the integrity of the cardiac structures. The progress of the catheter in both right and left heart catheterizations is followed by fluoroscopy and pressure measurement.

Right heart catheterization involves the insertion of a catheter into either the femoral or the antecubital vein. The catheter is then floated to the right atrium through the right ventricle and into the pulmonary artery. Conduction irritability may occur as the catheter tip passes through the right ventricle. Hemodynamic measurements are obtained within each chamber and the pulmonary artery. Phasic and mean pulmonary artery tracings are recorded in the main pulmonary artery. When withdrawal tracings from the pulmonary artery are obtained, blood samples are taken from each chamber. Radiographic contrast material may also be injected for x-ray films. Right heart catheterization is beneficial in the evaluation of right heart pressures, sampling of blood oxygen content of right heart chambers for detection of a left-to-right shunt, assessment of tricuspid and pulmonic valves, and evaluation of mitral valve stenosis or insufficiency by the transseptal approach. A Swan-Ganz catheter may also be inserted to determine left heart function indirectly through measurement of the pulmonary artery wedge pressure.

Left heart catheterization is usually carried out in combination with right heart studies. Left heart catheterization has come to be widely used in all forms of heart disease affecting the left heart, mitral and aortic valve disease, coronary artery disease, and cardiomyopathy.

Direct data on left heart function may be obtained through either a transseptal puncture from the right atrium across the foramen ovale or retrograde passage of a catheter in the brachial or femoral artery up the aorta and across the aortic valve into the left ventricle. As in right heart catheterization, hemodynamic pressure readings are obtained, blood samples are withdrawn, and contrast material may be injected for x-ray films.

Left heart catheterization is a diagnostic procedure used to evaluate pressures in the left atrium, ventricle, and aorta; identify mitral and aortic valve disease; determine left ventricular contractility; identify cardiac shunts; and measure cardiac output. Pre- and postcatheterization nursing interventions must be focused toward meeting the psychological and physical needs of the patient. Related nursing diagnoses and interventions are presented in Table 15–4.

CORONARY ANGIOGRAPHY

Angiocardiography has played a major role in the clinical assessment of cardiac lesions during the last 20 years. The use of image intensifiers and cineangiography has greatly increased the use of angiography in the diagnosis and evaluation of coronary heart disease. Coronary angiography is an extremely important procedure that is indicated in all patients with CAD in whom surgical treatment is contemplated. Specifically, coronary angiography is indicated in those individuals who manifest the following:

1. Unstable angina pectoris
2. Prolonged chest pain due to myocardial ischemia without objective signs of myocardial infarction
3. Myocardial infarction with repeated incidence of chest pain
4. Stable angina in whom a stress electrocardiogram or thallium myocardial perfusion scan suggests high-risk coronary artery disease

TABLE 15–4. Invasive Cardiac Procedures

Nursing Diagnoses	Related Nursing Interventions
Knowledge deficit pre- and post-procedure	1. Implement relevant teaching plan 2. Provide a description of sensations patient may experience and equipment used during and after procedure 3. Include family members in both pre- and post-procedure teaching
Anxiety	1. Encourage verbalization of patient and family concerns 2. Clarify misconceptions, reinforce explanations 3. Instruct and encourage relaxation techniques 4. Administer analgesics and sedatives as ordered 5. Encourage self-care and family participation as appropriate
Impaired tissue integrity	1. Instruct patient not to move affected extremity; maintain immobilization according to protocol 2. Maintain and monitor occlusive dressing at femoral puncture site 3. Report signs of swelling, bleeding, or hematoma formation at the puncture site
Altered tissue perfusion, peripheral	1. Monitor and report signs of inadequate peripheral perfusion: a. Decreased or absent pulses b. Limb coolness c. Limb pallor or cyanosis 2. Instruct patient to notify the nurse for coolness, numbness, or paresthesias distal to insertion site 3. Implement thromboembolitic prevention measures: a. Protect patient from potential injury due to oral care, shaving b. Monitor and report appropriate laboratory values, prothrombin time, partial thromboplastin time
Potential for fluid volume deficit related to osmotic diuresis of hypertonic contrast media; possible bleeding from insertion site	1. Administer IV fluids per order 2. Record patient intake and output 3. Instruct patient as to the need for increased fluid intake 4. Encourage oral fluid intake a. Offer fluids frequently b. Keep water pitcher at the bedside within patient reach
Potential for alteration in cardiac output, related to complications of invasive procedures	1. Report findings of initial cardiovascular assessment: a. Monitor ECG continuously. Note ECG rate and rhythm. Compare with preprocedure ECG b. Check pulse for rate, rhythm and volume c. Compare apical and radial pulses, rate pulse defects d. Auscultate for S_3, S_4 murmurs 2. Evaluate circulatory pressure and volume Note preprocedure blood pressure and trends following procedure 3. Report symptoms of myocardial ischemia Note location of pain, pattern and relief methods 4. Monitor and report changes in neurologic status

5. Stable angina when revascularization surgery or angioplasty is contemplated

6. Atypical chest pain when diagnostic tests have failed to clarify the diagnosis

7. Angina and valvular heart disease to delineate the coronary anatomy and establish the mechanism of angina

8. Variant angina with ST elevation or depression during angina to determine presence of coronary artery stenosis

9. A diagnosis of variant angina suspected but not documented by noninvasive studies

As a special procedure during cardiac catheterization, coronary angiography allows visualization of cardiac structures through use of contrast agents and x-ray films taken from various projections (Fig. 15–5). The procedure involves inserting a catheter into the femoral artery and passing it under fluoroscopic control to the desired vessel. Coronary angiography can be performed using either the direct brachial approach or the percutaneous femoral approach. Using the direct approach, a single catheter is manipulated to achieve selective catheterization of both the left and right coronary arteries. During passage of the catheter from the subclavian artery to the aortic arch, the patient may be asked to shrug the shoulders, turn the head to the left, or take a deep breath to assist passage of the catheter. With the percutaneous femoral approach, two preformed catheters are used for catheterization of the right and left coronary arteries. The catheters are guided to the distal aortic arch over a Teflon-coated guidewire, the guide is then withdrawn, and the catheter is filled with contrast medium and guided to the appropriate artery.

Assessment of CAD involves evaluation of both the coronary vasculature and left ventricular function. The first step in evaluating the coronary angiogram is determining whether the coronaries are unobstructed and free of lesions. Each major artery is traced along its entire length, and branches and collaterals are noted and evaluated for irregularities or narrowing. When occlusion is present, the degree of disease and the suitability of the artery for revascularization are of primary concern. Lesions are often graded on a percentage basis reflecting the decrease in lumen diameter. Coronary arteriography provides not only an anatomic map of the coronary arteries, including the site and severity of stenotic lesions, but also the characteristics of distal vessels in terms of size, presence of atherosclerotic disease, mass of myocardium served, index of differential coronary flow, identification of collateral vessels, and an estimate of their functional importance.

Left ventriculography provides a visual analysis of wall motion. Ventricular systolic and diastolic volume and ejection fraction can be calculated. Correlation of the coronary arteriogram and left ventriculogram permits identification of stenotic and potentially bypassable arteries that serve viable myocardium. Augmenting left ventricular contraction by the use of nitrates, catecholamines, or post-extrasystolic beats may permit the identification of left ventricular wall segments that have the potential for improved function following revascularization surgery. In patients who have undergone surgery previously, the patency of grafts and the status of native coronary arteries can be ascertained.

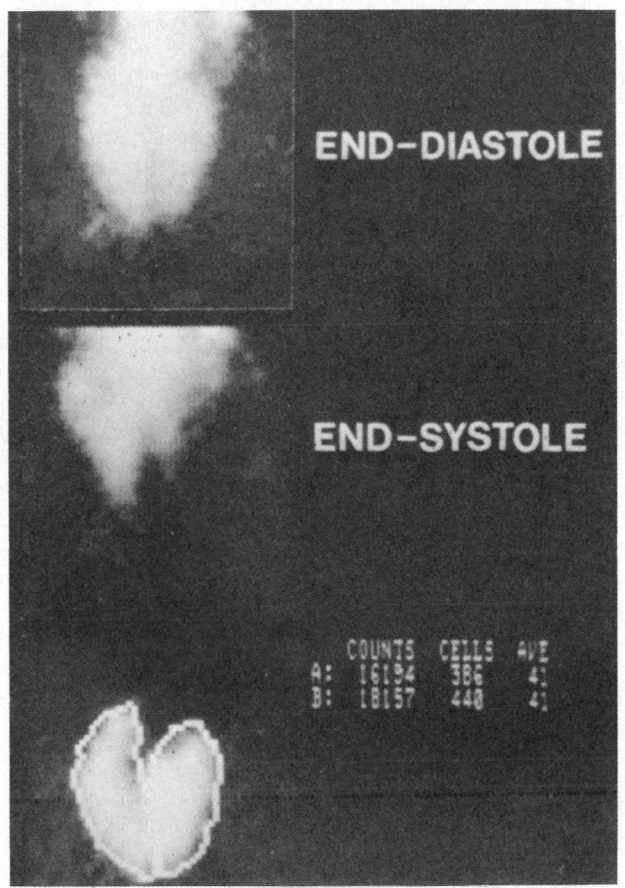

FIGURE 15–5. Equilibrium (gated) radionuclide angiocardiogram of a patient with coronary artery disease and normal ventricular performance at rest. Images were obtained in the 45-degree modified left anterior oblique projection. The end-diastolic image demonstrates vigorous and uniform contraction of the left and right ventricles, which are at the right and left side of image, respectively. The stroke volume image *(lower panel)* has uniformly high activity throughout the right and left ventricle, indicating normal ejection of blood from both ventricular cavities. (From Braunwald, E. (1988). *Heart disease: A textbook of cardiovascular medicine* (3rd ed). Philadelphia: W. B. Saunders.)

Evaluation of myocardial function is an important part of the evaluation of coronary artery disease. Patterns of ventricular contraction and the ejection fraction are determined during angiography. Because the ejection fraction represents the ratio of the stroke volume to the end-diastolic volume, a decreasing ejection fraction may represent either a decrease in stroke volume or an increase in end-diastolic volume. The latter situation represents the compensatory mechanism for maintaining cardiac output as myocardial function decreases. Thus, the ejection fraction is a reflection of the degree to which contraction abnormalities have compromised myocardial performance.

In patients with stable angina, the incidence of single-, double-, and triple-vessel coronary artery disease is approximately the same. Abnormalities of left ventricular wall motion can be detected by contrast ventriculography in approximately 60% of patients with chronic ischemic heart disease. Intervention ventriculography may be performed in these patients to differentiate between scar tissue and reversibly ischemic myocardial segments. In some patients with chronic ischemic heart disease, a contrast left ventriculogram also reveals mitral regurgitation.

For those patients with unstable angina, single- and multiple-vessel disease also occurs with approximately equal frequency. However, the incidence of single-vessel disease is higher in patients with recent onset of angina. Left main coronary artery stenosis is more frequent in patients with unstable angina, the left anterior descending coronary artery being the most frequently affected vessel. Less developed collateral circulation has been observed in patients with unstable angina than in those with chronic stable angina.

In patients with a diagnosis of variant angina, coronary arteriography reveals fixed proximal stenosis involving at least one major coronary artery in the majority of patients, although in some patients angiographically detectable atherosclerotic lesions are absent. In patients with suspected variant angina, provocation of coronary artery spasm is required to confirm the diagnosis. Ergonovine, methacholine, and hyperventilation have been used to provoke coronary artery spasm. However, unless the provoked coronary artery spasm is accompanied by the patient's usual chest pain, along with ECG changes indicating myocardial ischemia, the diagnosis of variant angina is not established.

Pre- and postprocedure nursing diagnoses and related interventions are similar to those described under cardiac catheterization.

Angina Pectoris

Angina pectoris is a symptom of myocardial ischemia resulting from an imbalance between oxygen supply and demand, as previously described. The mechanisms of myocardial ischemia may vary in different circumstances, and, as a result, the clinical manifestations also change. An imbalance between myocardial oxygen supply and demand can occur either from a primary decrease in coronary blood flow or from a disproportionate increase in myocardial oxygen requirements. The capacity to increase coronary blood flow to the increase in myocardial oxygen demand is limited in CAD, resulting in myocardial ischemia whenever this reserve for myocardial perfusion is exceeded. Ischemia also results from a primary decrease in oxygen supply due to coronary artery vasospasm, which may occur at the point of a

coronary lesion or in otherwise normal coronary arteries.

Angina can be classified as chronic exertional, variant (Prinzmetal), or unstable. Chronic exertional angina is associated with a characteristic onset, duration, location, radiation, and quality of pain. Variant angina is not typically associated with these characteristic findings. Unstable angina signifies a recent change in frequency, intensity, duration, or character of pain and may signify impending infarction.

Obstructive CAD is the most common cause of chronic ischemic heart disease. In the great majority of patients with chronic exertional angina, resting coronary blood flow is proportional to myocardial oxygen consumption (MVO_2) at rest, indicating that stenotic resistance and the resistance of the distal coronary vascular bed, which promotes coronary blood flow to meet the need for increased MVO_2, are equal. Although vasodilation increases blood flow to potentially ischemic myocardial zones, the increase in flow for a given increase in demand is progressively lessened as the degree of stenosis increases, resulting in relative myocardial ischemia. In patients with stable angina, the level of activity that precipitates angina is usually predictable. The extent of physical activity that precipitates angina appears to be inversely related to the severity but not necessarily to the extent of coronary artery lesions.

Chest discomfort produced by exertion and relieved by rest is most frequently diagnosed as exertional angina by the history alone. Chronic exertional angina may also occur postprandially due to an increase in gastrointestinal oxygen consumption both during and after a large meal. In addition, digestion requires increased cardiac output, which increases myocardial oxygen demands, resulting in anginal pain. Emotional tension has also been identified as a precursor of angina. Chest discomfort due to emotional stress tends to last longer than that produced by physical stress because emotional responses are not as easily limited as activity. For the patient with coronary atherosclerosis who cannot increase coronary blood flow, smoking tobacco will further increase myocardial workload, resulting in angina. This effect may be worsened by the presence of carboxyhemoglobin in the blood due to smoking.

VARIANT OR PRINZMETAL ANGINA

When myocardial ischemia occurs in the presence of normal coronary arteries, a number of pathologic conditions should be considered. If coronary artery spasm is demonstrated, variant angina, also known as Prinzmetal angina, is the most likely diagnosis. Although acute episodes of myocardial ischemia can result from coronary artery embolism, myocardial ischemia is a rare sequela.

Variant angina is characterized by cyclically recurrent angina at rest, usually unrelated to effort. The chest discomfort of Prinzmetal angina is similar to but of longer duration than that of chronic exertional angina. It appears to be cyclic, frequently occurring at the same time every day, most often on arising or in the early morning. The patient may also complain of palpitations, syncope, or bradycardia during the peak of discomfort. Classic anginal pain is usually not brought on by exertion but may be relieved by rest and nitroglycerin.

The primary mechanism of variant angina is a spontaneous decrease in coronary blood flow unrelated to changes in MVO_2. Coronary sinus venous oxygen content tends to decrease, suggesting a decrease in coronary blood flow. Angiographic studies have documented the presence of transient complete or incomplete, localized or diffuse narrowing of the epicardial coronary arteries (coronary artery spasm) causing interruption of blood flow to the myocardium during variant angina. The mechanism for the focal or diffuse spasm of the coronary arteries is unknown. Many patients with variant angina also have fixed obstructive coronary lesions of varying severity. The sites of coronary artery spasm may vary, although they most frequently occur at or in the vicinity of atherosclerotic lesions.

UNSTABLE ANGINA

Unstable angina is characterized clinically by angina of changing character, duration and intensity in patients with either a history of stable angina or a recent onset of angina. Discrete single or multiple episodes or prolonged rest angina are important features of the clinical profile. The quality, location, and radiation of chest pain in patients with unstable angina are similar to those in patients with stable or variant angina, but the duration is usually longer, and the intensity may be more severe. Unstable angina is frequently not completely relieved by nitroglycerin.

The mechanisms of spontaneous rest angina are unclear and may have multiple causes. The systemic hemodynamic changes preceding, during, and following unstable angina suggest that different mechanisms operate in different patients. A spontaneous reduction in coronary blood flow rather than an increase in MVO_2 appears to be the principal mechanism of rest angina in these patients.

The frequency of coronary artery spasm in the occurrence of rest angina in patients with unstable angina remains undetermined. Mechanical obstruction at the site of atherosclerotic lesions due to platelet or fibrin thrombi formation has been considered. Coronary arteriographic studies have demonstrated the presence of severe fixed atherosclerotic coronary artery lesions in many patients with unstable angina and the presence of thrombus in the affected coronary artery. These findings provide a basis for the use of antiplatelet drugs or thrombolytic agents in the management of unstable angina.

Physical Examination. Physical examination of a patient with ischemic heart disease may yield normal findings or may reveal risk factors for CAD. Detection of hypertension or peripheral vascular disease may strengthen the suspicion of ischemic heart disease because there is a higher prevalence of atherosclerotic disease in these patients. Cardiac examination may reveal manifestations and sequelae of ischemic heart disease as well as causes of angina other than CAD. An S_4 and S_3 gallop is present in some patients with CAD. During exercise-induced angina or spontaneous angina, these physical findings are frequently present. Paradoxical (reversed) splitting of the second heart sound can occur transiently during an anginal attack. Transient depression of pump function and a prolonged left ventricular ejection time appear to be the mechanisms. The murmur of mitral regurgitation can be detected in patients with chronic ischemic heart disease and a previous myocardial infarction. Papillary muscle dysfunction is the most frequent cause, but left ventricular dilatation may also be contributory.

History. The patient history alone is a powerful diagnostic tool because it will modify the utility of many of the diagnostic tests and guide the choice of subsequent procedures. The character, location, and radiation of angina are similar in the different clinical syndromes. The location of pain is most frequently retrosternal but can be left pectoral or epigastric. Radiation is common and usually occurs down the medial aspect of the left arm. Radiation can also occur to both arms, throat, lower jaw, back, and epigastrium.

The duration, precipitating factors, and clinical presentations of anginal states may differ. In patients with chronic exertional angina, the duration of pain is usually brief, and pain is precipitated by physical activity and relieved by cessation of activity. The intensity of discomfort is extremely variable and may be relieved by rest and the use of nitroglycerin. In variant angina, severe, often prolonged, chest pain occurs in the absence of precipitating factors such as exercise and stress. Anginal pain appears to be cyclical and may be relieved by nitroglycerin. The patient may also complain of palpitations, syncope, or bradycardia during the peak of discomfort. Unstable angina is characterized by pain of changing character, duration, and intensity at rest. However, the duration may be prolonged, and pain may be severe. Relief of pain in response to nitroglycerin is incomplete.

Precipitating factors must be evaluated for an accurate determination of angina. Analysis of the mode of relief of chest discomfort is also helpful in the diagnosis of angina pectoris. The typical anginal episode dissipates gradually over a period of minutes, usually as a result of cessation of the activity that precipitated it. Angina pectoris also begins gradually and reaches its maximum intensity over a period of minutes. Relief of anginal pain in response to nitroglycerin is also a helpful diagnostic clue.

TABLE 15–5. Nitrates for Anginal Therapy: Dosage, Duration, Side Effects

Drug	Dosage/Formulation	Onset	Duration	Side Effects
Nitrostat	0.3–0.6 mg sublingual tablets	30 seconds	15–30 minutes	Headache Flushing Tachycardia
Nitrobid	2.5 mg 3 times/day sustained release capsules	1 hour	2–4 hours	Dizziness
Nitro-SA	2.5 mg 2 times/day sustained release capsules	1 hour	2–4 hours	Reflex tachycardia
Nitrol ointment	½–2 inches topically	1 hour	6–24 hours	Contact dermatitis
Isosorbid dinitrate (Isordil)	2.5–10 mg every 3 hours sublingual tablets	5 minutes	1–2 hours	Headache Flushing Dizziness Tachycardia

Nonpharmacologic Management. Management of a patient with ischemic heart disease will incorporate modification of risk factors for coronary atherosclerosis with nursing interventions to prevent adverse consequences of myocardial ischemia. Life-style changes may provide symptomatic relief or retard or reverse the atherosclerotic process. Thus, treatment of hypertension, hyperlipidemia, obesity, diabetes, and elimination of the use of cigarettes are part of the routine management of patients with ischemic heart disease. Physical exercise has been advocated for select patients with ischemic heart disease to decrease the complications of CAD.

In addition to modification of risk factors for coronary atherosclerosis, the treatment of angina and other manifestations of myocardial ischemia is based on reducing MVO_2 and increasing coronary blood flow to the potentially ischemic myocardium in order to restore the balance between myocardial oxygen supply and demand.

Pharmacologic Management. The basic goal in the pharmacologic management of angina is to reduce factors that increase myocardial oxygen demand and improve those that impinge on oxygen supply, depending on the underlying pathologic mechanism. Patients with CAD have relied on the use of pharmacologic agents to prevent and control anginal symptoms. Traditional therapy has centered on the use of nitroglycerin and nitrates for prevention and relief of anginal attacks. Beta-adrenergic blocking agents, calcium channel blockers, and antiplatelet therapies are now used in the treatment of angina.

Nitrates. Nitrates are the most common medications used to treat patients with angina pectoris. Nitroglycerin and nitrates are direct-acting, smooth muscle relaxants and cause vasodilation of the peripheral vascular bed. Peripheral vasodilation with nitrate therapy reduces MVO_2 through a reduction in cardiac preload and afterload. Nitrates dilate venous capacitance vessels, which results in decreased venous return to the heart and decreased left ventricular diastolic volume and pressure or preload. There is a reflex-mediated increase in heart rate and contractility. Arteriolar dilatation reduces systemic vascular resistance, or afterload. This further reduces left ventricular end-diastolic pressure and allows enhanced cardiac output. Decreased arterial pressure and left ventricular volume are associated with decreased left ventricular wall tension and resulting decreased MVO_2.

Nitrate therapy exerts its beneficial effects primarily by decreasing MVO_2 in patients with fixed obstructive coronary artery disease and coronary vasospasm. Increases in regional coronary blood flow and myocardial perfusion are associated with relief of angina. However, evidence suggests that it is the systemic vasodilating effects of nitrates that produce relief of anginal symptoms. The combined administration of nitrates and beta-adrenergic blocking drugs may further reduce the frequency of anginal episodes. Beta blockers may also block the reflex tachycardia, which is a potential side effect of nitrate therapy.

Sublingual nitroglycerin is the drug of choice for treatment of acute angina. Sublingual nitroglycerin may be taken prophylactically before activities likely to cause angina. Oral nitrates can increase the activity threshold for anginal symptoms and reduce the incidence of anginal attacks. Topical nitroglycerin allows daily application of medication. Absorption through the skin allows distribution of the medication. Absorption through the skin allows distribution of the medication without inactivation by the liver. Table 15–5 reviews the dosage and effects of the most commonly used nitrates.

Beta-Adrenergic Blocking Agents. Beta blockers inhibit response to adrenergic stimuli by competitively blocking adrenergic receptors. These drugs may selectively block beta-1 adrenergic receptors in the myocardium or both the myocardial beta-1 receptors and beta-2 receptors of bronchial and vascular smooth muscle. Beta blockers are classified as selective or nonselective according to their relative abilities to bind to the different beta receptors. Drugs with an affinity for beta-1 receptors such as atenolol and metoprolol are considered cardioselective because of the predominance of beta-1 receptors in the myocardium. When used in low doses, beta-1 selective blocking agents inhibit cardiac beta-1 receptors, but have little influence on bronchial and vascular beta-2 receptors. However, at higher doses beta-1 selective blocking agents will also block beta-2 receptors, leading to increased airway resistance and the potential for bronchospasm.

Beta-blocking drugs are used for the prevention and relief of cardiac ischemia because of their ability to decrease heart rate, blood pressure, and cardiac contractility. Beta blockers, as a class, act by reducing myocardial oxygen utilization. This is accomplished through both negative inotropic and chronotropic actions produced by blockade of the cardiac beta-1 receptors. Thus, beneficial effects are related to a decrease in MVO_2. Reduced heart rate, contractility, and systemic blood pressure at any level of activity account for the reduced oxygen requirements. A decreased frequency of anginal attacks combined with a reduction in nitrate dosage and increased exercise tolerance has been noted.

Some beta-blocking drugs reduce myocardial oxygen demands through differential effects on coronary vascular resistance in both relatively ischemic and nonischemic myocardial segments. Because beta blockers reduce heart rate, diastolic filling time is lengthened, and coronary artery perfusion is improved. Beta blockers have also reduced abnormally increased platelet aggregability in patients with angina pectoris and increased tissue oxygen delivery through a rightward shift of the oxygen-hemoglobin dissociation curve.

Beta blockers are primarily beneficial for the relief of angina due to a decrease in myocardial oxygen demand. Research on the use of beta blockers in the treatment of chronic angina has shown a reduction in both coronary events and mortality (Goldman and Pitchard, 1983). Thus, beta blockers have not proved effective in treatment of anginal states due to coronary vasospasm.

Beta-adrenergic blocking drugs may cause fatigue, weakness, depression, gastrointestinal upset, and nightmares. As a result of beta-1 receptor blockade, bradycardia, heart block, heart failure, and hypotension may occur. In patients with impaired left ventricular function, congestive heart failure may occur or may be intensified, a side effect that can be reduced by the use of digitalis or diuretics.

Beta-2 receptor blockade may cause bronchospasm in patients with underlying obstructive lung disease. Inhibition of beta receptors may precipitate vasoconstriction, hyperglycemia, or hypoglycemia in diabetic patients. Coronary vasoconstriction may be intensified by beta-adrenergic blockade with propranolol (Kern et al., 1983). Propranolol is contraindicated in patients with Prinzmetal angina due to its role in prolonging episodes of myocardial ischemia. Withdrawal symptoms have been documented when beta-blocker therapy is abruptly discontinued. Beta-blocker therapy should be tapered to avoid acute ischemic episodes (Brodde, 1986).

Eight beta blockers are available for the treatment of angina pectoris (see Table 15–6 for a description of the most commonly used beta blockers). One group of beta blockers with intrinsic stimulating activity causes both blockade and stimulation of beta

receptors. These drugs cause less beta antagonism, producing less reduction in resting heart rate and atrioventricular conduction and contractility at rest while blocking the effects of exercise on these parameters. Thus, a beta blocker with intrinsic stimulating activity is as effective as a beta blocker without this mechanism in reducing the normally increased heart rate and blood pressure response to exercise. Beta blockers with intrinsic stimulating activity may be of value in patients with resting bradycardia, peripheral vascular disease, or obstructive lung disease.

Calcium Channel Blockers. Drugs that inhibit the flow of calcium ions across cellular membranes (calcium channel blocking drugs) have emerged as an important addition to the pharmacologic therapy of anginal syndromes. Calcium channel blocking drugs are effective because of their ability to cause direct increases in coronary blood flow and myocardial perfusion as well as decreases in myocardial oxygen requirements. Calcium channel blocking drugs also inhibit calcium entry to the smooth muscles of the peripheral vascular bed. Blockage of calcium inflow in smooth muscle cells by calcium channel blocking agents thus decreases arterial vascular resistance. Heart rate may also decrease with the use of some calcium channel blocking agents. Vasodilation of the coronary arteries provides an increase in coronary blood flow and oxygen supply. Arteriolar vasodilation in peripheral circulation produces a reduction in afterload and reduces myocardial oxygen demand.

Calcium channel blocking agents may also increase coronary blood flow through direct mechanisms. Calcium channel blocking agents currently in use can cause dilatation of the epicardial coronary arteries, thus preventing and relieving angina due to vasospasm. Thus, coronary blood flow may increase. Three calcium channel blocking agents are approved for the treatment of angina. These agents differ in their effects on peripheral and coronary vasodilation, sinus node automaticity, atrioventricular (AV) node conduction, and myocardial contractility.

The beneficial effects of calcium channel blocking agents in the treatment of angina result from their ability to reduce myocardial oxygen needs secondary to afterload reduction and to increase coronary blood flow secondary to dilating action on the coronary vascular bed. Nifedipine is the most potent vasodilator among the calcium channel blocking agents.

Both verapamil and diltiazem reduce heart rate and AV node conduction, which may result in sinus bradycardia, sinus arrest, and AV block. Nifedipine does not alter AV node conduction, may cause an increase in heart rate due to potent peripheral vasodilation (Antman et al., 1980), and is the drug of choice in patients with sinus or AV node disease.

All calcium channel blocking agents depress myocardial contractility to some degree and thus have the potential to precipitate congestive heart failure. Verapamil is the most potent negative inotrope and should be avoided in patients with depressed left ventricular function (Stone et al., 1980). Left ventricular function may improve with the use of nifedipine

TABLE 15–6. Beta-Adrenergic Blockers: Dosage, Effects, Nursing Diagnoses

Drug	Maintenance Dosage	Metabolism	Cardioselective	Side Effects	Contraindications	Drug Interactions	Nursing Diagnoses
Nadolol	80–120 mg	Renal	No	Cardiovascular: bradycardia, peripheral vascular, insufficiency Central nervous system: dizziness, fatigue Gastrointestinal: nausea, vomiting, diarrhea, constipation	Sinus bradycardia Cardiogenic shock Cardiac failure Bronchospasm	Diuretic and hypotensive drugs: additive effect Antidysrhythmic drugs: additive effect Neuromuscular blocking drugs: potentiate Antimuscarinic drugs: counteract Sympathomimetic drugs: antagonize	Altered potential for health maintenance Alteration in cardiac output: decreased Potential for injury Altered thought processes Alteration in bowel elimination Activity intolerance Sleep pattern disturbance
Timilol maleate	Increased to 20–40 mg daily Administered in two doses	Liver	No	Cardiovascular: hypotension, dysrhythmia, atrioventricular/ sinoatrial block Central nervous system: see under Nadolol Gastrointestinal: see under Nadolol Pulmonary: rales, bronchospasm, dyspnea	See under Nadolol	Cardiovascular drugs: potentiate Nonsteroidal anti-inflammatory drugs: antagonize	See under Nadolol Impaired gas exchange
Propranolol	160–480 mg daily, 120–160 mg daily extended release capsules	Liver	No	Gastrointestinal: see under Nadolol Central nervous system: see under Nadolol Cardiovascular: see under Nadolol; pulmonary edema Dermatologic: rash Hematologic: eosinophilia, elevated BUN	See under Nadolol	See under Nadolol Cimetidine: reduces drug clearance	See under Nadolol Impaired gas exchange Impaired skin integrity Potential for injury
Labetalol hydrochloride	IV: 40–80 mg at 10-min intervals PO: 200 mg initially followed in 6–12 hours Increase every 2–3 days at 100-mg twice a day increments	Liver	No	Cardiovascular: hypotension, congestive heart failure, precipitation or exacerbation Central nervous system: see under Nadolol Gastrointestinal: see under Nadolol Respiratory: nasal congestion Genitourinary: ejaculatory failure, urinary retention Dermatologic: rashes	See under Nadolol	See under Nadolol Cimetidine: reduces drug clearance Glutethimide: decreases bioavailability Halothane: hypotensive effect Nitroglycerin: antagonizes reflex tachycardia Tricyclic antidepressants: increased tremors	See Nadolol Tissue perfusion altered Impaired peripheral gas exchange
Pindolol	10–30 mg two or three times a day	Liver	No	Cardiovascular: see under Nadolol Central nervous system: see under Nadolol Gastrointestinal: see under Nadolol; elevated SGOT; elevated SGPT; muscle and leg cramps	See under Nadolol	See under Nadolol Digoxin: transient decrease in serum digoxin levels	See under Nadolol Alteration in comfort, pain

TABLE 15–7. Calcium Channel Blocking Agents: Dosage, Effects, Nursing Diagnoses

Drug/Diagnosis	Maintenance Dosage	Metabolism	Side Effects	Contraindications	Drug Interactions	Nursing Diagnosis
Nifedipine Angina: Prinzmetal Variant Chronic Stable	30–60 mg daily in 3 divided doses	Liver	Cardiovascular: dizziness, headache, flushing, lightheadedness, hypotension, peripheral edema Central nervous system: shakiness, mood changes, weakness Gastrointestinal: nausea, diarrhea, constipation Pulmonary: dyspnea, wheeze, cough	Hypersensitivity	Beta blockers: anginal exacerbation, hypotension, congestive heart failure Fentanyl: hypertension Digoxin: increase serum concentrations Hypotensive drugs: potentiate	Alteration in cardiac output: decreased Activity intolerance Potential for injury Potential for injury Altered tissue perfusion Impaired peripheral gas exchange Alteration in bowel elimination Alteration in thought process Ineffective airway clearance
Verapamil Angina: Prinzmetal Variant chronic Stable	240–480 mg daily in 3–4 divided doses	Liver	Cardiovascular: bradycardia, heart block, congestive heart failure, hypotension Gastrointestinal: nausea, constipation	Left ventricular dysfunction	See under nifedipine Antidysrhythmic drugs: potentiate hypotension	See under Nifedipine

related to its afterload reduction properties. Table 15–7 reviews the calcium channel blocking agents.

Combination Drug Therapy. The hemodynamic properties of nitroglycerin and calcium channel blocking drugs suggest that combination therapy might be useful. The choice of pharmacologic therapy is determined by the pathophysiologic mechanism causing the angina, the severity of the angina, concomitant medical conditions, and side effects of medical therapy. Combination therapy may serve to reduce potential side effects of one class of drugs or work to enhance the oxygen supply and demand ratio.

The combination of a beta blocker and a calcium channel blocker is superior to either drug used alone for the treatment of angina. However, in combining beta blockers and both verapamil and diltiazem caution should be used because severe left ventricular dysfunction may result (Packer et al., 1982).

Platelet Antiaggregants. Platelet aggregation and platelet-derived vasoactive substances have been implicated in the occurrence of ischemic episodes and anginal symptoms. Mechanisms involved include (1) alterations in arterial blood flow due to vasospasm or transient platelet obstruction; (2) release of platelet emboli as an initiating event in sudden cardiac death; and (3) acute arterial thrombotic occlusion (Frishman and Miller, 1986).

Currently, the first-generation platelet antiaggregants aspirin, sulfinpyrazone, and dipyridamole have been the most widely used and evaluated drugs in controlling platelets by pharmacologic therapy. Drugs that modify platelet integrity perform by (1) inhibiting the arachidonic acid pathway; (2) altering platelet cyclic AMP levels; (3) inhibiting thrombin formation; and (4) modifying platelet behavior. Table 15–8 describes the varying effects of the most common platelet antiaggregants. Both aspirin and other nonsteroidal anti-inflammatory compounds act on the arachidonate pathway by inhibiting its main enzymes. Platelet aggregation is blocked by competitive inactivation of cyclo-oxygenase, which converts arachidonic acid to indoperoxides. This process leads to the formation of regulatory prostaglandins.

TABLE 15–8. Platelet Antiaggregants

Drug	Inhibits Aggregation	Prolongs Bleeding Time	Prolongs Platelet Survival	Duration of Effect
Aspirin	+ +	+ +	−	1 week
Calcium channel blockers	+ +	+ +	−	24 hours
Dipyridamole	−	−	+ +	6 hours
Ibuprofen	+ +	+ +	−	6 hours
Indomethacin	+ +	+ +	−	24 hours
Propranolol	+ +	−	−	24 hours
Prostacyclin	+ +	+ +	+ +	10 minutes
Sulfinpyrazone	+	−	+ +	6 hours
Thromboxone A_2 synthesis inhibitors	+ +	+ +	+ +	24 hours

Adapted from Frishman, W. H., and Miller, K. P. (1986). *Current Problems in Cardiology,* 11 (2), 71–136.

Aspirin acts on platelets by reducing occlusion of small vessels by platelet aggregates. Ingestion of 325 mg of aspirin will inhibit thromboxane A_2 synthesis and platelet aggregation for approximately 48 hours (Preston et al., 1981). Cyclo-oxygenase is inhibited for approximately 1 week. Care should be taken when administering aspirin in combination with other oral anticoagulants because of the additive effects. In addition, chronic aspirin administration may lead to hyperuricemia or an elevated blood urea nitrogen.

Unlike aspirin, sulfinpyrazone competitively inhibits cyclo-oxygenase and therefore has reversible side effects. In therapeutic doses of 400 to 800 mg daily, bleeding time is not prolonged, and platelet aggregation is not affected. Sulfinpyrazone has an additive effect when administered with oral anticoagulants and may produce an increase in hypoglycemia when used with hypoglycemic agents. Due to uricosuric mechanisms, fluid intake must be sufficient to support urinary output and avoid potential uric acid nephropathy. The uricosuric action of sulfinpyrazone is antagonized by aspirin and other salicylates.

Imidazole compounds are selective in platelet inhibition. They inhibit thromboxane synthetase, the enzyme responsible for the synthesis of thromboxane A_2 but not of active prostaglandins. Selective inhibition of thromboxane synthetase may provide an increase in the amount of prostaglandin endoperoxide available for conversion to prostacyclin.

Pharmacologic agents that increase cyclic AMP levels inhibit platelet adhesion and aggregation. Cyclic AMP is increased by stimulation of adenylate cyclase and by blockage of platelet phosphodiesterase, which breaks down cyclic AMP. Dipyridamole is an inhibitor of platelet phosphodiesterase, an enzyme responsible for the conversion of adenosine triphosphate (ATP) to adenosine diphosphate (ADP). By blocking this conversion, dipyridamole potentiates increased cyclic AMP formation and impairs platelet aggregation. Dipyridamole also lengthens platelet survival and inhibits platelet adhesion to the damaged endothelium, thereby reducing thrombus formation at the sites of injury. Prostacyclin also serves to increase cyclic AMP levels, leading to inhibition of platelet adhesion, release reaction, and aggregation. Dipyridamole is administered in 50-mg doses three times each day. This drug is generally free of toxicity or drug interactions. Potential side effects include gastric distress and headaches.

Antianginal Drugs as Platelet Antiaggregants. Nitroglycerin and nitrates inhibit platelet arachidonate metabolism through direct antiplatelet mechanisms and increased prostacyclin synthesis (Mehta and Mehta, 1980). Both direct antiplatelet effects and prostacyclin synthesis mechanisms are dose-dependent. Beta-adrenergic blocking agents such as propranolol have been shown to reduce platelet aggregability in doses sufficient to improve exercise tolerance. Propranolol binds to the platelet membrane and may serve to both inhibit phospholipase and decrease thromboxane A_2 formation and release.

Calcium channel blocking agents function as platelet antiaggregants through a variety of mechanisms. Diltiazem inhibits ADP formation as well as collagen and arachidonate acid–induced platelet aggregation. Nifedipine inhibits epinephrine-induced platelet aggregation through inhibition of thromboxane receptors. Verapamil both inhibits membrane alpha-adrenergic receptors and blocks intraplatelet calcium influx.

Invasive Management
Coronary Artery Angioplasty. Percutaneous transluminal coronary angioplasty (PTCA) has been established as an effective method for both improving symptoms and ameliorating the metabolic, hemodynamic, and functional consequences of myocardial ischemia in selected patients. Angioplasty decreases or eliminates resistance at the site of coronary artery stenosis and enhances blood flow to ischemic myocardial segments. Thus increased coronary perfusion rather than decreased MVO_2 is the mechanism causing the beneficial aspects of angioplasty.

The rationale behind PTCA is that of increasing the luminar diameter of the diseased vessel. This goal is achieved through the application of a lateral force against the vessel wall by means of a distensible balloon-tipped catheter. Compression of the atherosclerotic lesion by the balloon causes a localized injury to the involved vessel. Consequent to the localized injury, histologic changes occur that promote vessel dilation. Platelet aggregation at the site of injury triggers the release of prostacyclin, a potent vasodilator. The platelets also release thromboxane, which initiates thrombus formation. Phagocytosis, retraction, and incorporation at the injury site lead to the removal of fibrous debris. In conjunction with plaque mobilization, endothelialization at the injury site often occurs, contributing to dilatation of the arterial lumen.

Technique. Coronary angioplasty involves the introduction of an outer guiding catheter and a double-lumen dilatation catheter into either the femoral or the brachial artery. The catheter is guided through the ascending aorta and into the ostium of the right or left coronary artery (Fig. 15–6). Advancement of the catheter as well as visualization of the stenotic vessel is enhanced through angiography. When the correct position is ensured, the balloon-tipped dilating catheter is inserted through the guiding catheter and into the artery's stenotic area. Continuous pressure monitoring reveals blockage of the coronary artery ostium and permits measurement of the pressure gradient across the lesion.

The number of balloon inflations, inflation time, and balloon size are relative to the coronary vessel involved, the degree of stenosis, and the occurrence of ischemic symptoms during the procedure. Balloon inflations are repeated at intervals that allow interim recovery until reductions in the pressure gradient are

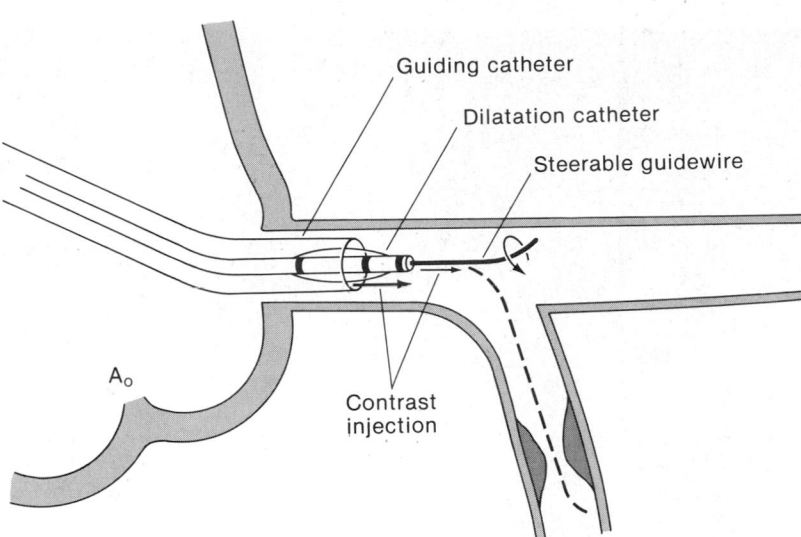

FIGURE 15–6. Movable guidewire dilation system. The dilatation catheter is shown here at the end of a large (No. 8 or 9 French, 2.7- or 3.0-mm) guiding catheter, which is positioned at the ostium of the involved vessel. The soft, yet steerable, guidewire is then advanced through the central lumen of the dilatation catheter and directed through and beyond the target lesion. The position of this guidewire relative to coronary branches and lesions can be revealed by contrast injection through the guiding catheter or through the central lumen of the dilatation catheter. Once the guidewire has been successfully positioned, it serves as a "track" over which the dilatation catheter itself can be advanced. (Redrawn from Baim, D. S., and Faxon, D. P. (1986). In Grossman, W. (Ed.), *Cardiac catheterization and angiography* (3rd ed.). Philadelphia: Lea & Febiger.)

not apparent or until the gradient falls below 16 mm Hg (Block et al., 1981). With successful dilatation, the balloon catheter is removed after a period of observation, and a repeat angiogram is performed. If residual obstruction is noted, the lesion is recrossed, and additional inflations are performed. When the procedure is completed, the inner cannulas are secured within the femoral sheaths, and the patient is transported to the critical care unit.

Patient Selection. Patient eligibility for both initial and repeat PTCA has been established on the basis of clinical and morphologic considerations. Clinical factors associated with reduced procedural risk and successful dilatation include the presence of well-defined, limiting ischemic symptoms and ischemic symptoms of short duration (Gruentzig and Meier, 1983). In addition, the eligibility of the patient for potential coronary artery bypass surgery must also be considered (Hall and Morris, 1984).

Isolated, discrete single-vessel disease remains the classic angiographic indication for PTCA (Hall and Greuntiz, 1983). In patients with single-vessel disease, PTCA best treats fixed, noncalcified lesions in the proximal two-thirds of the coronary circulation that are accessible for dilatation. Stenosis of the left mainstream artery is considered unacceptable for dilatation because of associated procedural complications (Cumberland, 1985; Hall and Gruentzig, 1984).

Although repeat PTCA can be performed safely in the majority of patients with restenosis, screening for eligibility in this population is of primary importance. Repeat PTCA should be considered carefully for high-risk patients such as those with left anterior descending artery lesions, a time interval of less than 3 months between the first and second PTCA procedures, diabetes mellitus, and the presence of multiple lesions (Deligonaul et al., 1989).

A subset of patients with double-vessel disease may also be considered as candidates for PTCA. Selection in this group corresponds to the criteria used for single-vessel disease and excludes patients with high-risk lesions at either vessel site.

In selected patients who have undergone coronary artery bypass grafting, PTCA may be used as an alternative to additional surgery. Angiographic indications for PTCA in this population include vessels jeopardized by graft closure, lesions distal to implanted grafts, lesions proximal to patent grafts but compromising collateral flow, and distal anastomoses (Hall et al., 1984).

Results. The primary goal of PTCA is the successful dilation of involved coronary arteries as evidenced by angiography (Fig. 15–7). Reduced pressure gradients across the arterial narrowing and the relief of ischemic symptoms are also considered essential (Shillinger, 1983). The effectiveness of PTCA in achieving these goals has been documented in patients with both stable and unstable angina pectoris (Kent et al., 1985; Mabin et al., 1985). The long-term efficacy of PTCA in patients with coronary artery disease has been established, with follow-up periods of up to 8 years (Gruentzig et al., 1987). The confirmation of improved ventricular performance and increased functional capacity following PTCA has been demonstrated by myocardial scintigraphy (Kent et al., 1982) as well as by serial exercise testing (Meier et al., 1983). Studies examining diastolic function following PTCA have shown improved filling at rest after successful dilatation (Bonow et al., 1982). In examining the clinical expression of improved functional capacity, patient benefits have been identified in both employment and recreation patterns following successful dilatation (Holmes et al., 1983).

Although the majority of patients continue to demonstrate sustained angiographic and clinical improvement after successful dilatation, a number of patients will evidence recurrent stenosis; however, restenosis rarely occurs after 9 months (Renkin et al., 1983). The basis for recurrent disease is not known but may reflect fibrocellular proliferation that exceeds the corrective effects of angioplasty. Restenosis is usually

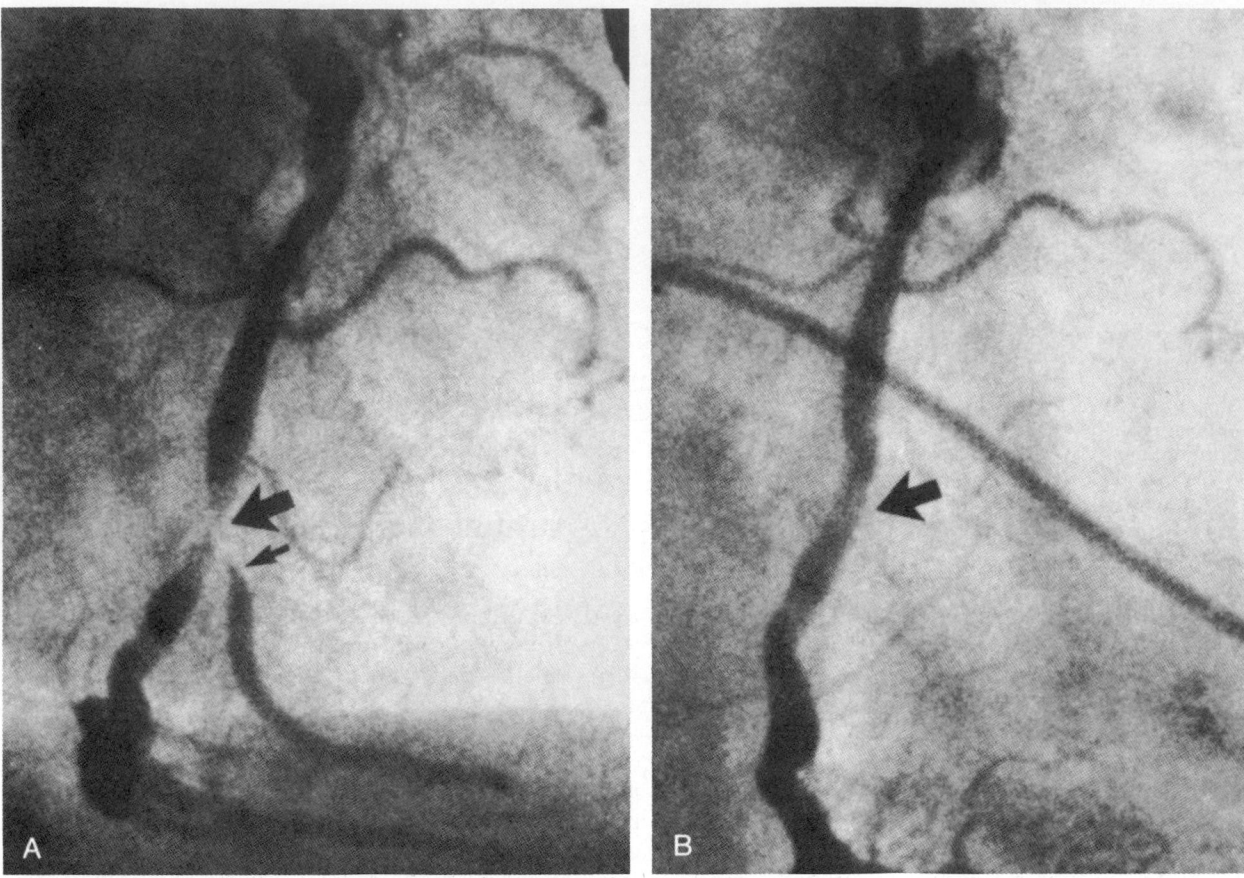

FIGURE 15–7. The "snowplow" effect. *A* shows severe stenosis of the midportion of the right coronary artery *(large arrow)*, from which a proximally diseased right ventricular branch *(small arrow)* originates. After PTCA *(B)*, dilatation of the right coronary lesion has been achieved at the expense of occlusion of the right ventricular side branch. (From Baim, D. S. (1983). In Petersdorf, R. G., et al., (Eds.), *Harrison's principles of internal medicine*, Update VI. New York, McGraw-Hill, with permission.)

manifested as recurrent angina appearing 2 to 4 months following successful dilatation (Renkin et al., 1983). Repeat dilatation can be performed in selected patients with a high success rate (Scholl et al., 1981) and a low complication rate (Gruentzig et al., 1981).

Recurrence rates following successful angioplasty have not been established. Potential reasons are the lack of a standard definition of recurrence as well as the difficulty of achieving angiographic follow up.

As an alternative to repeat dilatation following PTCA, Sigwart and associates (1987) developed an intravascular mechanical support with the goal of reducing arterial restenosis and closure following angioplasty. The intravascular stent consists of a self-expandable, stainless steel mesh that can be implanted nonsurgically in the coronary or peripheral arteries. The self-expanding stent is delivered percutaneously by a guiding system to the site of stenosis. Following an inner balloon inflation, the stent is secured against the vessel wall. The use of thrombolytic or long-term anticoagulant therapy will vary with institutional protocols.

Although a number of stent prototypes are currently available, the principles of deliverability, versatility, and biocompatibility will determine the clin-

ical success of the stent. The use of stents in iliac and coronary arteries has demonstrated their safety and effectiveness in the short term. Their use in vein grafts and venous lesions has been reported (Mullins et al., 1988). The precise indications for the use of intravascular stents in the future will only be defined following the completion of prospective clinical trials.

Potential Risks. Since 1976, coronary angioplasty has undergone many refinements with resulting reductions in procedural morbidity and mortality. Mortality associated with dilatation in single-vessel disease is approximately 1% (Dorros et al., 1983). An increased risk of mortality has been identified in women, patients over 60 years of age, and patients who have had coronary bypass grafting (Dorros et al., 1981).

The most frequent major complication of PTCA is coronary artery dissection as a result of localized trauma. Reported in approximately 5% of patients, acute reduction in coronary blood flow may be manifested as prolonged angina or coronary occlusion leading to infarction (Holmes et al., 1988). Additional bases for myocardial ischemia include coronary artery spasm, coronary embolization, and intimal trauma. Associated minor complications include bradycardia, ventricular fibrillation, hypotension, and vascular complications including hematoma formation and retroperitoneal blood loss.

Pre- and postangioplasty nursing interventions are similar to those described for the patient undergoing cardiac catheterization. Nursing diagnosis and interventions specific to PTCA are presented in Table 15–4.

Laser Angioplasty

The use of laser radiation is currently being investigated as an adjunct to PTCA and coronary bypass surgery in the revascularization of occluded vessels. The laser is a monochromatic and coherent light amplification stimulated by the emission of radiation. The suitability of laser radiation for use in opening coronary and peripheral atherosclerotic plaque obstructions is based on the ability to transmit the laser through an optical fiber, to direct it precisely, and to use it for tissue photocoagulation and on its capability for selective absorption.

The total amount of energy delivered by a laser is defined by the pulse duration and strength of the radiation wavelength utilized. The degree of laser penetration of atherosclerotic plaque depends on the beam focus, the total energy delivered, and the duration of exposure, as well as the density and absorptive characteristics of the atherosclerotic tissue.

The composition of the tissue that is receiving the laser energy determines the distribution of that energy within the tissue (Fox, 1986). When the laser is directed at tissue, the tissue may reflect, absorb, transmit, or scatter the light. Atherosclerotic plaque, which may have a homogeneous or a heterogeneous composition, has an unpredictable absorption pattern. Fibrous areas of plaque or calcified plaque will have different absorption characteristics than primarily lipid-containing lesions.

There are three types of lasers currently being used for medical purposes, the carbon dioxide (CO_2) laser, the argon laser, and the neodymium-yttrium-aluminum garnet (Nd:YAG) laser. The infrared wavelength emitted by the CO_2 laser is well absorbed by the water in plasma and in red blood cells. This property makes the CO_2 laser less efficient for vaporizing tissues through a water or blood medium because the majority of laser energy is absorbed by the fluid. Argon laser radiation is poorly absorbed by water but is well absorbed by hemoglobin, making it suitable for use in revascularization. The Nd-YAG laser's wavelength is partially absorbed by water in plasma and in red blood cells but remains effective in vaporizing tissue through a fluid medium.

Several recent investigations have demonstrated the ability of lasers to penetrate and affect the vaporization of atherosclerotic plaque. Laser recanalization of obstructed vessels can be approached in two ways. In most approaches laser energy is passed through a semiflexible laser fiber using a percutaneous transluminal approach, but some clinicians use direct laser application in laser-assisted endarterectomy.

From the time the laser was shown to be effective in removing coronary atherosclerotic obstruction in cadaver hearts (Lee et al., 1981), attempts have been made to apply laser technology to the clinical setting. The laser has been used to vaporize coronary obstruction during bypass surgery (Choy et al., 1984; Lee et al., 1986; Lee et al., 1986) and to widen stenotic arteries during PTCA (Lee et al., 1985; Sanborn et al., 1987). Despite these efforts, laser revascularization has demonstrated technical limitations including difficulty in resecting a significant volume of atherosclerotic plaque and a high frequency of vessel perforation (Lawrence et al., 1987).

In response to these complications, the hot-tipped laser was developed and has been proved effective in vaporizing coronary and peripheral atherosclerotic plaque obstructions (Lee et al., 1987). The laser catheter consists of an optical fiber attached to a metal cap with a central extruding guidewire tip. This single unit allows easy placement inside the coronary artery and control of plaque vaporization. The use of a laser-heated thermal cap results in removal of a greater volume of plaque and has the mechanical effect of a smoother intimal surface. Thermal smoothing and compression of the intimal surface serve to improve intraluminal geometry, reduce blood flow turbulence, and possibly reduce reocclusion rates. The hot-tipped laser may also be used to facilitate placement of the balloon angioplasty catheter, to increase dilatation of the stenotic arterial lumen, and to ablate atherosclerotic obstruction during coronary bypass surgery (Lee et al., 1987).

Although the use of lasers in the recanalization of obstructed vessels has demonstrated benefits, the majority of animal and clinical studies have concentrated on the acute effects of the laser on the arterial wall. Long-term complications such as aneurysm formation, accelerated atherosclerosis, and intimal hyperplasia must be considered in determining the efficacy of the laser.

The nursing care of the laser angioplasty patient is comparable to that of the patient who has undergone PTCA. Pre- and postprocedure interventions specific to laser angioplasty are presented in Table 15–4.

Coronary Artery Bypass Surgery

Coronary artery bypass surgery is performed to relieve the symptoms of myocardial ischemia by revascularizing the myocardium. The procedure is not indicated for relief of myocardial ischemia that is not manifested by angina unless a left main coronary lesion has been documented by angiography. (See Chapter 20 for a detailed discussion of surgery.)

Asymptomatic Ischemia

Myocardial ischemia may be manifested as angina, asymptomatic ischemia, dysrhythmias, dyspnea, myocardial infarction, or sudden death. Asymptomatic or "silent" myocardial ischemia is defined as objective evidence of myocardial ischemia without angina or other signals such as dyspnea, exhaustion, or cardiac dysrhythmias (Epstein et al., 1988). Objective evidence means documentation of ischemia by ECG, radionuclide studies, or angiographic studies. The increasing ability to detect myocardial ischemia independent of the patient's complaints of pain (angina) focuses attention on the diagnosis and treatment of myocardial ischemia instead of on angina pectoris (Kawaniski and Rahimtoola, 1987). However, it must be noted that the understanding of the pathophysiology, diagnosis, prognosis, and treatment of silent ischemia is incomplete at present.

PATHOPHYSIOLOGY

The distinction between asymptomatic and symptomatic (i.e., angina) ischemia is currently thought to be due to a difference in the duration and severity of myocardial ischemia or to a difference in the perception of pain (Maseri, 1987). As described earlier, the onset of myocardial ischemia initiates cellular events that are manifested sequentially depending on the duration and severity of the ischemia. Changes in the electrocardiogram occur before the onset of angina, indicating that duration and severity of ischemia determine the manifestations of angina. Both animal and human observations have validated the sequential nature of ischemic changes (Bishop et al., 1974; Nesto and Kowalchuk, 1987). Abnormalities of left ventricular function are detected first; ECG abnormalities occur next, and the development of angina occurs even later and inconsistently.

The second consideration in the distinction between asymptomatic and symptomatic ischemia is related to the mechanism of pain perception. Recent studies provide evidence of differences in pain perceptions between groups of patients with silent and painful ischemia (Droste and Roskamm, 1983; Glazier et al., 1987). However, the roles of pain perception, threshold, nociceptive pathways, and endorphin-related systems are too incompletely understood to make any concrete statements in relation to asymptomatic pain at present.

DIAGNOSIS

Asymptomatic myocardial ischemia may be detected by electrocardiographic ST wave changes during continuous ambulatory ECG recordings or exercise testing; by transient myocardial perfusion abnormalities using ^{201}Tl myocardial imaging, or by the demonstration of abnormal left ventricular systolic function with two-dimensional echocardiography or radionuclide ventriculography. The sensitivity, specificity, and predictive accuracy of the above methods have yet to be determined. Needless to say, highly specific tests are needed in asymptomatic patients.

Ambulatory ECG monitoring is one of the most commonly used tests to detect asymptomatic ische-

mia. As many as 80% of patients with severe angina have documented episodes of asymptomatic ischemia. In some studies between 75% and 90% of documented episodes of ST segment depression are silent (Selwyn et al., 1978). In patients with CAD, 4.3 to 5.5 episodes of asymptomatic ischemia have been documented in a 24-hour period. Thus, extended monitoring is necessary to detect and quantify asymptomatic ischemia (Gottlieb et al., 1988).

However, ambulatory monitoring has disadvantages as well as advantages (Knoebel et al., 1989). The routine use of ambulatory ECG recordings cannot be justified in most asymptomatic patients, especially if less than two cardiovascular risk factors are present, due to the high incidence of false-positive ST segment shifts. Second, technical problems in the detection of ST segment changes exist despite the application of computer analysis.

Exercise ECG testing is considered a valuable diagnostic test for asymptomatic ischemia despite its limitations. Often thallium myocardial perfusion imaging is used with an exercise ECG. Almost all patients who have episodes of asymptomatic myocardial ischemia on ambulatory ECG monitoring have a positive exercise test (Deedwanian et al., 1989). In patients who have a high likelihood of having CAD, the exercise test is likely to be positive for myocardial ischemia even in the absence of chest pain.

Because abnormal left ventricular wall function is one of the early manifestations of myocardial ischemia, methods of assessing wall motion abnormalities are useful diagnostic tests for asymptomatic myocardial ischemia. However, the value of exercise radionuclide ventriculography is unknown currently due to technical problems and the lack of sensitivity in detecting ischemia in asymptomatic patients. The value of exercise echocardiography is similarly unknown due to the greater likelihood of false-positive tests in an asymptomatic group.

PROGNOSIS

Three different groups of persons with asymptomatic ischemia have been described (Cohn, 1987). The first includes patients with isolated asymptomatic ischemia without evidence of painful angina. These people are asymptomatic for ischemic heart disease. The second group consists of patients with asymptomatic ischemia occurring at rest or during exercise testing. These persons have CAD or coronary spasm or both. The third group is composed of patients who have suffered a myocardial infarction. The incidence of silent ischemia in this group ranges from 30% to 70%.

In the Framingham Study 25% of myocardial infarctions were detected only on routine ECG examinations, and half of these patients were totally free of symptoms (Kannel and Abbott, 1984). Men over the age of 60 had a higher proportion of unrecognized infarctions than men under age 60. Women had a higher proportion of unrecognized infarctions than men. In addition, an increased severity of hypertension was associated with a higher number of unrecognized infarctions, indicating that individuals with unrecognized infarctions are at as much risk for complications and sudden death as those with recognized infarctions. Thus, a similar treatment approach is warranted for persons with asymptomatic myocardial infarction (Kannel, 1987).

In patients with isolated asymptomatic myocardial ischemia the yearly mortality rate is less than 1% per year, but the morbidity is greatly increased, with 6% to 10% of patients developing angina or myocardial infarction per year (Gottlieb et al., 1988; Alpert, 1984; American College of Sports Medicine, 1986).

In patients with a recent myocardial infarction or unstable angina, the existence of asymptomatic myocardial ischemia has the same poor prognostic significance as recurrent angina (American College of Sports Medicine, 1986; Antman et al., 1980; Astrand and Rodahl, 1977). It is an indication for aggressive assessment of the extent of coronary artery disease and its effect on left ventricular function and for appropriate medical therapy or revascularization procedures, depending on findings.

The presence of multiple episodes of asymptomatic ischemia in patients with chronic exertional angina is associated with an unfavorable morbidity and mortality (Beller, 1985; Benowitz, 1988). In one recent study the number of deaths, myocardial infarctions, episodes of unstable angina, and revascularization for progressive symptoms were frequent in 49 patients with stable coronary artery disease and asymptomatic ischemic on ambulatory ECG recordings compared to similar patients without evidence of myocardial ischemia. However, all patients in the study had positive ECG exercise tests for myocardial ischemia and might have been candidates for earlier aggressive antianginal therapy.

MEDICAL MANAGEMENT

The treatment for asymptomatic myocardial ischemia is the same as that for symptomatic ischemia. The goal of therapy is to eliminate or reduce the episodes of asymptomatic ischemia. Management begins with reduction of the major cardiovascular risk factors, i.e., smoking, hypertension, and hypercholesterolemia. Elimination of these risk factors is supported by the effect of these factors on the development of atherosclerosis, as discussed earlier.

Pharmacologic antianginal therapy is warranted by the evidence indicating that episodes of asymptomatic ischemia are reduced in frequency and duration when patients are treated with such medications. Pharmacologic trials with nitrates, calcium channel blockers, and beta blockers have all been effective in patients with both angina and episodes of asymptomatic ischemia (Shell, 1985; Quyyumi et al., 1984; Crawford, 1989). However, no data are currently available on the benefits of therapy directed primarily at asymptomatic ischemia.

The role of coronary bypass surgery or percutaneous transluminal coronary angioplasty in the treatment of asymptomatic ischemia has not been established. However, guidelines have been established to assist in making decisions about surgery. For example, asymptomatic patients with positive exercise test results who have left main coronary artery obstruction are candidates for coronary bypass surgery, as are asymptomatic patients with triple-vessel disease who exhibit greater than 1.5-mm ST segment displacement on exercise ECG (European Coronary Surgery Study Group, 1982). Asymptomatic patients with double-vessel disease with one of the obstructions located in the proximal portion of the left anterior descending artery who exhibit greater than 1.5-mm ST segment displacement on exercise ECG are candidates for coronary angioplasty, as are asymptomatic patients with single-vessel disease who have a positive exercise ECG test results (Hurst et al., 1986).

Nursing Management

The primary concern of the critical care nurse is to provide symptomatic relief to the patient with ischemic heart disease. Nursing care in the acute situation is focused on reducing or eliminating myocardial ischemia, whether symptomatic or asymptomatic. In chronic anginal states the nurse provides assistance in life-style change and risk factor modification.

ALTERATION IN COMFORT: PAIN

Pain is the predominant symptom in an ischemic attack. Pain experienced during an anginal attack may cause the release of endogenous catecholamines, which stimulate heart rate, contractility, and systemic vasoconstriction. Thus, the experience of anginal pain will increase myocardial oxygen demand. In stenotic vessels the oxygen demand may increase beyond the heart's ability to increase supply, leading to potential myocardial damage. Patient education related to pharmacologic therapy, stress reduction techniques, activity limitation, and emergency medical procedures is essential to help the patient reduce both pain and myocardial damage during an ischemic event.

ANXIETY/FEAR

Patients with angina often manifest fear related to anginal pain. They frequently associate the occurrence of chest discomfort with impending death. Anticipated limitation in activity or life-style changes may also increase anxiety and fear. Anxiety and fearfulness increase sympathetic nervous system responses and elevate serum catecholamines, leading to increased MVO_2 and increased severity of anginal symptoms. The critical care nurse intervenes to reduce anxiety in both the patient and family members.

This can be accomplished both through treatment of anginal discomfort and by maintaining a caring, reassuring attitude. The nurse should encourage verbalization of fears by both the patient and the family and provide clear instructions on ways to reduce anginal pain. Normal cardiac function, pathophysiology related to disease processes, and the role of pharmacologic therapy in relieving anginal symptoms are important topics to be reviewed in the educational sessions. Goals should be set related to activity and life-style changes to guide the patient and family members.

Stress reduction techniques may assist the patient in preventing or minimizing anginal episodes and may help to reduce atherosclerotic progression. The physiologic benefit to be derived by stress management is a reduction in MVO_2 and a lessening of myocardial ischemia. Such measures are viewed as an adjunct to traditional therapy. Methods include relaxation responses such as meditation, autogenic training, progressive relaxation, and use of biofeedback techniques.

KNOWLEDGE DEFICIT

Prior to instituting a teaching plan, the critical care nurse assesses both the patient and family reaction to the diagnosis of myocardial ischemia and its implications. Educational programs focus on an awareness of precipitating factors, pharmacologic therapy, and cardiovascular risk factor modification. The nurse can assist patients to identify specific situations that precipitate anginal attacks so that they can learn to modify, avoid, or react in a more positive way. The use of a diary that records time, onset, duration, and events associated with anginal pain may reveal patterns of anginal occurrence due to both physical and emotional stressors.

Adherence to the prescribed drug regimen including the use of prophylactic and anginal-onset nitroglycerin is important in limiting both anginal pain and myocardial damage due to ischemia. The nurse should instruct the patient and family on the action, dose, and side effects of medications including specific side effects that require medical intervention. Dosage schedules are designed to meet patient needs whenever possible. Risk factor modification efforts include the use of mutual goal setting combined with a supportive and nonjudgmental attitude on the part of the nurse. Education focuses on means to achieve goals to modify risk factors to limit the underlying process of myocardial ischemia.

POTENTIAL /ACTUAL ACTIVITY INTOLERANCE

Exercise and certain activities may increase ischemia in the patient with angina by producing a further imbalance in oxygen supply and demand. Thus, activity must be specifically prescribed to produce benefits and prevent complications. Both patient and family need to understand activity restrictions and the rationale for such restrictions. Patients with stable angina may perform activity as tolerated. Walking is a recommended form of exercise. Prolonged physical training in patients with angina has produced a reduced pressure rate both at rest and at work, reduced frequency and intensity of angina, and improved exercise tolerance. Patients with unstable angina may need to limit activity to prevent progression of myocardial ischemia. Activity levels are adjusted for any change in patient status.

Education related to activity progression and goal setting includes education about the use of prophylactic nitroglycerin and about limiting, pacing, and timing physical activity. An awareness of safety measures in activity progression is essential both to relieve patient anxiety and achieve exercise goals. Sexual activity is discussed with both the patient and the partner. For patients with stable angina, maintenance of sexual activity is encouraged. Patients with unstable angina may resume sexual activity following stabilization of angina.

NONADHERENCE

The goal of primary and secondary prevention of myocardial ischemia is to develop the best possible therapeutic regimen to modify risk factors associated with life style for each individual and to enhance adherence to that regimen once it has been established. For the success of primary and secondary programs, individuals must adhere to their regimens as part of ongoing life-style change. Therefore, all efforts must be made to understand the factors involved in adherence behavior, and plans must be made to incorporate motivational interventions whenever possible.

The process of developing nursing interventions to increase adherence to proposed life-style change begins with an assessment of the likelihood of early attrition for each patient. Data on physical and psychosocial status as well as present life-style habits and available support systems may provide indications of potential compliance. In addition, an exploration of the relative value of health to the individual, perception of control over health outcome, and potential barriers to initiating and sustaining health behaviors are needed to provide a basis for individualized program planning. Analysis of assessment data will assist in identifying individual motivational levels and areas that may require intervention. Intervention strategies that meet the needs of the individual patient are more likely to increase motivation to initiate and adhere to recommended life-style change.

Because both initiation and maintenance of behavioral changes are essential in primary and secondary prevention, both external and internal motivational interventions need to be planned. Interventions to improve adherence involve breaking down barriers and motivating the individual by reinforcing positive health behaviors extrinsically and intrinsically. Extrinsic motivational strategies include reducing perceived barriers to life-style change through (1) education specifying cardiovascular risk reduction techniques that can be individually controlled; (2) increased involvement of supportive others in the rehabilitative process; and (3) collaborative decision making related to health goals and desired health outcomes. Intrinsic motivation may provide the basis for long-term life-style changes. Ultimately, adherence to risk-reducing behavior must be self-regulated by the individual, not through continued reliance on the health professional (Dishman, 1984). Intrinsically oriented nursing interventions include (1) allowing the individual to determine his own health-related goals; (2) involving the individual in decision-making and development of specific actions toward achievement of health-related goals; and (3) emphasizing individual responsibility and self-directedness in undertaking risk-reducing health behaviors.

In summary, each individual requires individualized intervention strategies. Emphasis is placed on assisting the client to make informed decisions, including supportive others in the behavior modification process and identifying and implementing solutions to barriers that may impede health-related goal attainment.

SUDDEN DEATH

Sudden cardiac death (SCD) is defined as an unexpected, witnessed death of an apparently healthy person resulting from cardiac dysfunction and occurring within 6 hours of the onset of new symptoms. This definition does not include persons who have had a recent acute onset of heart disease but does include persons with known coronary artery disease if their condition is considered stable (Ruskin et al., 1990).

More than 300,000 sudden coronary deaths occur each year, representing one-half of the annual coronary mortality. In a prospective study of men aged 35 to 74, Greenburgh and Dwyer (1982) found that the incidence of sudden death increased with age in both men and women. Sudden coronary death occurs in women at only one-fourth the rate seen in men, and the occurrence in women lags behind that of men by 20 years. Sudden death occurs more frequently in men with an average age of 60 years. At any age, in either sex, those who are especially vulnerable can be identified from their coronary risk profile. The presence of CAD is by far the most common indicator of sudden cardiac death. In attempting to define the candidate for sudden death, emphasis must be placed on CAD and its precursors.

Pathophysiology

The atherosclerotic coronary artery plaque is the most frequent pathologic (postmortem) finding in cases of sudden death. Ventricular fibrillation is the leading cause of cardiac arrest in sudden death victims. It is believed to be triggered by ischemia due to coronary vascular changes leading to electrical instability of the myocardium. Most episodes of sudden cardiac death are not initiated by acute myocardial infarction.

The major cardiac risk factors are commonly present in victims of sudden cardiac deaths, namely, hypertension, hypercholesterolemia, or a history of cigarette smoking. In the Framingham Study every man who died suddenly before age 65 was a cigarette smoker (Cobb et al., 1983). Hypertension was present in nearly one-fourth of the victims and left ventricular hypertrophy was present in one-fifth of these men.

Four major characteristics are associated with an increased risk of sudden death: (1) ventricular electrical instability, (2) extensive coronary artery narrowing, (3) abnormal left ventricular function, and (4) electrocardiographic conduction and repolarization abnormalities (Cobb et al., 1983). Ventricular ectopic activity in persons with atherosclerotic heart disease is predictive of sudden cardiac death in 78% to 95% of patients, especially complex ventricular ectopy. It is important to note that ventricular ectopic activity by itself has little prognostic importance in persons without atherosclerotic heart disease. Patients who develop sudden cardiac death typically have severe coronary artery narrowing in two or three coronary arteries. Left ventricular dysfunction and congestive heart failure are associated with ventricular dysrhythmias, indicating a possible interaction between ventricular dysfunction and ventricular arrhythmias. Impairment of left ventricular function is reflected by the systolic ejection fraction. Last, electrocardiographic abnormalities include prolongation of Q–T intervals and ST-T changes.

Data from the Framingham Study indicate a threefold increased risk of sudden death in subjects with ventricular premature contractions compared with those who do not exhibit them on a standard electrocardiogram at rest. However, virtually all patients with ventricular premature contractions who died suddenly also had other abnormalities such as left ventricular hypertrophy, ventricular conduction disturbances, or cardiovascular disease history.

Definitive mechanisms of ventricular fibrillation have not been established. However, it is well established that nonuniform cardiac recovery properties reduce the threshold for ventricular fibrillation. A variety of states including ischemia and sympathetic stimulation will increase the degree of inequality of refractory periods in ventricular muscle.

Ventricular tachycardia can result from several causes, but the predominant theory involves reentry. Reentry is a self-perpetuating tachydysrhythmia frequently associated with hemodynamic collapse and subsequent degeneration to ventricular fibrillation (see Chap. 9). In the reentry mechanism, one of the ventricular pathways may be refractory or may conduct more slowly than an adjacent pathway. The impulse is temporarily slowed but conducts normally through adjacent areas. When the impulse arrives at the previously refractory branch it may find it excitable, thus allowing retrograde conduction. This type of dysrhythmia is frequently found in individuals with a unidirectional block in one limb of the conduction pathway (see Chap. 9). Blocks such as this may occur in individuals with congenitally deformed conduction systems (Braunwald et al., 1987) or diseased, ischemic hearts.

Virtually everyone with premature contractions who dies suddenly has evidence of an ischemic myocardium, usually with other electrocardiographic abnormalities. Persons with overt CAD are at a fourfold increased risk of sudden death but only because of a greater incidence of coronary attacks.

Ventricular dysrhythmias that are related to myocardial ischemia may be due to the effects of hypoxia, pH changes, and anaerobic metabolism on the electrical properties of cardiac fibers (see Chap. 9). An abnormal "slow response" action potential of the myocardial cells induced by calcium, potassium, and catecholamine release may be one cause of ventricular fibrillation in sudden cardiac death.

The prevalence of ventricular premature beats is greater in men and increases with age, with the presence of other electrocardiographically demonstrated ischemic abnormalities, and with the severity of the coronary risk profile. Angiographic study in coronary patients indicates that a higher prevalence and a more severe grade of ventricular premature contractions exist in patients with multivessel coronary artery disease than in those with only one vessel involved. Thus, ventricular premature contractions, particularly when frequent or complex, often serve as an indicator of severe cardiac disease and left ventricular dysfunction.

Pharmacologic Management

Antidysrhythmic drug therapy is always the first line of defense against recurrent ventricular dysrhythmias. Antidysrhythmic drugs suppress ventricular dysrhythmias by (1) altering the conductivity of myocardial tissue, (2) altering the refractory period of myocardial tissue, and (3) increasing myocardial electrical activity.

Antidysrhythmic drugs are classified according to their effects on cardiac muscle action potential (Table 15–9). Class I drugs interfere directly with depolarization and repolarization of the cardiac muscle. This class of drugs is effective in treating recurrent ventricular dysrhythmias due to abnormal automaticity or reentry mechanisms. Drugs are subclassified according to their effects on action potential duration as follows: IA, prolongation; IB, shortening; IC, no effect. These drugs have little effect on QRS width or QRS interval as seen on electrocardiograms. Class II drugs produce antisympathetic effects. Beta-blocking drugs have been shown to control ventricular dysrhythmias associated with exercise or adrenergic

stimulation. These drugs are used to treat angina associated with an ischemic myocardium rather than sustained ventricular dysrhythmias. Class III drugs markedly prolong the duration of the action potential. This effect has been successful in treatment of resistant ventricular dysrhythmias. Electrophysiologic effects are QRS widening and Q–T prolongation. Class IV drugs, the calcium antagonists, affect the slow inward depolarizing current in the sinoatrial and atrioventricular nodes. These drugs are used in the treatment of angina pectoris as well as supraventricular tachycardias that use the AV node as part of the reentrant circuit. Calcium antagonists are ineffective in treating recurrent ventricular dysrhythmias.

Patients receiving antidysrhythmic drug therapy must be monitored for signs of intolerance, toxicity, increases of intolerance, increases in ventricular ectopic activity, and changes in P–R, QRS, and Q–T intervals. Serum drug levels must also be monitored and toxic or subtherapeutic levels identified. Potential nursing diagnoses for these patients are listed in Table 15–10.

Nonpharmacologic Management

Occasionally an individual will have a dysrhythmia that is resistant to all medications tested. In this event, other treatment modalities are indicated. Intraoperative mapping with endocardial resection of the site of dysrhythmia origination is one possibility. Surgical intervention, intended to excise the focus or interrupt reentrant conduction, is used to abolish dysrhythmias or increase drug manageability.

Currently, antitachycardia pacemakers are being evaluated for efficacy in patients who have had one or more episodes of sustained ventricular tachycardia with hemodynamic collapse and who have failed to respond to antidysrhythmic pharmacologic therapy as evaluated by electrophysiologic testing (Fisher et al., 1988). The automatic implantable cardioverter defibrillator (AICD), detects and terminates life-threatening ventricular dysrhythmias. It is a small monitor generator that is surgically implanted in the left upper quadrant of the abdomen (Fig. 15–8). Electrodes surgically placed on and within the heart continuously sense electrical conduction. If electrical activity occurs that is interpreted by the AICD as ventricular tachycardia or fibrillation, it delivers a small electric shock directly to the heart to convert the dysrhythmia. The survival rate of patients with recurrent ventricular dysrhythmias treated with antidysrhythmic drugs or surgical intervention without AICD ranges from 34% to 74%. One-year survival rates of patients treated with AICD alone or in combination with antidysrhythmic drug therapy and surgery is 97% (Kelly et al., 1988).

Intraoperative mapping is a technique wherein the electrical activity of the epicardial or endocardial surface of the myocardium is recorded with delineation of impulse origination and sequence conduc-

TABLE 15–9. Antidysrhythmic Drugs: Dosage and Effects

Drug/Class	Maintenance Dosage/ Therapeutic Level	Metabolism	Major Effects	Side Effects
Lidocaine (Class I)	IV bolus: 50–100 mg constant infusion of 2–4 mg/minute. Therapeutic serum level: 1.5–4.0 mg/mL	Liver	↓ Automaticity ↓ Refractory period ↓ Repolarization ECG: No change in QRS or Q–T intervals	Cardiovascular: bradycardia Central nervous system: drowsiness, irritability, tinnitus, focal seizures, weakness, visual disturbances Gastrointestinal: diarrhea, nausea/vomiting
Tocainide (Class I)	PO: 400–600 mg every 8 hours after loading dose	Liver	See under Lidocaine	See under Lidocaine
Quinidine (Class I)	PO: 200–400 mg each 4–6 hours. Therapeutic serum level: 3–6 mg/mL	Liver/Kidney	↓ Automaticity ↓ Conductivity ↑ Repolarization ECG: prolonged Q–T interval; widened QRS interval	Cardiovascular: sinus arrest, sinoatrial block, ventricular fibrillation, hypotension Central nervous system: blurred vision Gastrointestinal: diarrhea, anorexia Hematologic: thrombocytopenia
Procainamide (Class IA)	PO: 1 g initially; 350–500 mg every 4–6 hours. Therapeutic serum level: 4–8 mg/mL	Liver/Kidney	↑ Repolarization ↓ Automaticity ↓ Conductivity ECG: prolonged P–R, Q–T, QRS intervals	Cardiovascular: heart block, ventricular fibrillation, hypotension Central nervous system: insomnia, weakness, depression Gastrointestinal: anorexia, nausea/vomiting Hematologic: agranulocytosis
Flecainide, encainide, lorcainide (Class I)	PO: 100–200 mg twice daily. Therapeutic serum level: 0.2–1 µg/mL	Liver/Kidney	↓ Conductivity ECG: prolonged QRS interval	Cardiovascular: may worsen dysrhythmias Central nervous system: dizziness, blurred vision, headache Gastrointestinal: nausea
Mexilitine (Class I)	PO: 600 mg loading dose; 500–1000 mg daily	Liver	See under Lidocaine	See under Lidocaine
Disopyramide (Norpace) (Class I)	PO: 200–400 mg loading dose; 100–200 mg every 6 hours		↓ Automaticity ↓ Conductivity ↑ Refractory period ECG: prolonged Q–T interval	Cardiovascular: hypotension, heart block, heart failure Central nervous system: dry mouth, blurred vision, headache, fatigue, aggravation of glaucoma Genitourinary: urinary retention
Propranolol (Class II)	IV: 1 mg/minute to 5–7 mg PO: 10–200 mg two to three times a day	Liver	↓ Heart rate ↓ Contractility ↓ Automaticity ↓ Conductivity ↑ AV node ↓ Refractory period ECG: no effect on QRS or Q–T intervals	Cardiovascular: hypotension, bradycardia, congestive heart failure, heart block Central nervous system: dizziness, fatigue, insomnia, depression Gastrointestinal: diarrhea, nausea, cramping, hyperglycemia/hypoglycemia
Amiodarone (Class III)	600–800 mg each day for 1–2 weeks Loading dose: 200–600 mg daily		↑ Refractory period ↑ Repolarization	Cardiovascular: hypotension, AV block, bradycardia Dermatologic: photosensitivity, rash
Bretylium (Class III)	IV: 5–10 mg/kg repeat 1–2 hours; 5 mg/kg every 6–8 hours 1–2 mg/minute drip		↑ Ventricular refractory period ↑ Ventricular fibrillation threshold ECG: prolongation of QRS and Q–T intervals	Cardiovascular: hypotension Gastrointestinal: vomiting/nausea
Verapamil (Class IV)	PO: 480–640 mg/day divided dose	Kidney	↓ AV node conduction ↓ Automaticity ↑ Refractory period	Cardiovascular: hypotension, bradycardia, AV block, asystole Central nervous system: headache, dizziness

TABLE 15–10. Potential Nursing Diagnoses: Patients on Antidysrhythmic Therapy

Health Management

Health maintenance, altered due to regimen complexity.
Knowledge deficit of pharmacologic therapy. Noncompliance with medical regimen

Cardiovascular Function

Altered cardiac output: decreased
Altered tissue perfusion: peripheral
Potential activity intolerance

Central Nervous System Function

Potential for injury
Altered thought processes
Anxiety
Sleep pattern disturbance

Pulmonary Function

Impaired gas exchange

Gastrointestinal Function

Alteration in bowel elimination: diarrhea
Urinary retention
Altered nutrition: less than body requirements

---

tion. In this way, areas of electrically diseased tissue are identified. Surgical treatment for ventricular dysrhythmias provides elimination of those areas of diseased myocardium that are responsible for recurrent ventricular tachycardia through endocardial resection.

Additional measures that may be used to prevent death or disability from sudden cardiac death episodes include cardiac resuscitation from ventricular fibrillation through community emergency medical aid units and through education of lay persons (including school children) in cardiopulmonary resuscitation (CPR). Multifactorial intervention programs that include exercise conditioning and modification of cardiovascular risk factors may also serve to decrease sudden cardiac death by decreasing the incidence of ischemic events due to coronary heart disease.

Nursing Management

The prevention of sudden cardiac death begins with identifying persons at risk. Once these persons are identified, nursing interventions can be implemented to assist in preventing the occurrence or recurrence of sudden cardiac death in persons who have been successfully resuscitated. The following discussion is directed toward management of patients and families who have survived a sudden death experience.

ANXIETY/FEAR

Survivors of sudden cardiac death may manifest fear, anger, anxiety, or depression (Haggerty et al.,

1983). Patients may be anxious or fearful for many reasons. For many, the near-death occurrence may be the first experience with the reality of their own mortality. Patients and their families commonly fear recurrence of cardiac arrest and the effects of their illness on their future and level of functioning. Patients may be fearful of the real or imagined discomfort associated with diagnostic procedures or repeated defibrillations.

Assessing the source of the patient's fears is appropriate when it is combined with problem-solving or education to address verbalized concerns. Anxiety may be reduced by ensuring that the patient and family have an understanding of the plan of care, adequate situational support, and realistic short-term goals. In addition, reassurance that heart rhythm and status are being closely monitored and that emergency measures are available may reduce the anxiety related to recurrence of arrest.

KNOWLEDGE DEFICIT

Knowledge deficit in sudden cardiac death survivors may be related to the events leading to and following dysrhythmic events, pharmacologic therapy, and possible surgical intervention. Initially, the critical care nurse assesses the patient and family's readiness to learn about the disease process and diagnostic plan. Education begins as soon as the patient's condition permits. Attempts should be made to include the family in as many teaching sessions as possible. Education includes cardiac anatomy and normal function of cardiac conduction, dysrhythmic symptoms, associated pathophysiologic processes, and pharmacologic or surgical treatment to prevent recurrence. The purpose, associated sensory experiences, significance, and care following diagnostic tests are reviewed with the patient and family.

NONADHERENCE

Adherence to the prescribed drug regimen is crucial for effective control of dysrhythmias. Instruct the patient and family on the action, dosage, and side effects of medications. Specific symptoms that require medical intervention are outlined. Emphasis is placed on the importance of the dosage interval of the medications to maintain therapeutic blood levels of the drug. Designing a dosage schedule that fits the patient's life style may assist the patient in adhering to the drug regimen.

Similarly, the patient and family are instructed about possible surgical interventions, the expected outcome of surgery, pharmacologic therapy, and the plan and goals of care. Postoperative testing may include an electrophysiologic study to test for the presence of inducible ventricular dysrhythmias as well as a submaximal stress test.

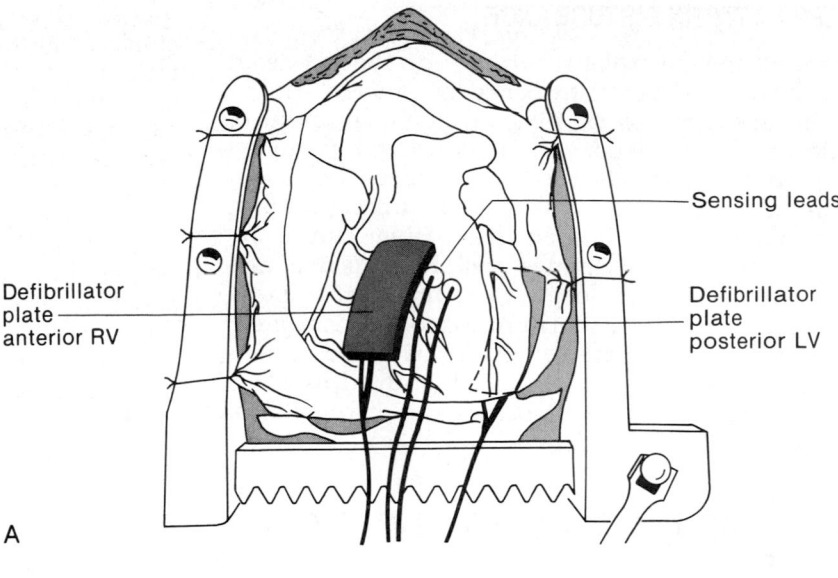

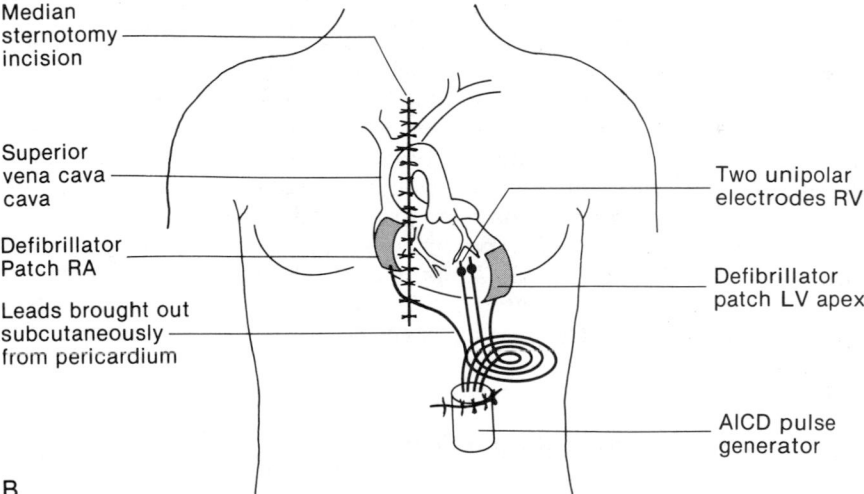

FIGURE 15–8. Methods of automatic cardioverter-defibrillator implantation. *A,* By way of a median sternotomy. Two epicardial sensing leads are shown on the anterior right ventricle. The anodal patch is placed on the anterior right ventricle (RV) and the cathodal patch on the posterolateral left ventricular (LV) wall. *B,* Implantation with the generator in a left upper quadrant subcutaneous pocket. *Abbreviations:* LV, left ventricle; R, right; RA, right atrium; Sup, superior. (Redrawn with permission from the American College of Cardiology (Journal of the American College of Cardiology), Vol. 9, pp 1349–1356, 1987.)

ALTERATION IN THOUGHT PROCESSES

Frequently patients display varying degrees of memory loss and neurologic deficit after sudden cardiac death resuscitation. These changes are caused by anoxic brain injury sustained during the arrest. A change in mental status is frightening to both the patient and the family. Acceptance of the hospitalization and sudden illness becomes even more difficult under these circumstances. The patient and family need to be reassured that the transient anoxic encephalopathy usually disappears within approximately 2 weeks of the injury. The critical care nurse assists the patient and family to cope with the experience by facilitating discussion of the arrest and verbalization of feelings related to the event.

In addition to anoxic encephalopathy, class IV drugs may cause transient confusion. Decreasing drug dosage or stopping the drug will alleviate the problem. Patient safety during periods of confusion is maintained through frequent reorientation to per-

son, place, and time, protective restraints as necessary, and assistance with ambulation and activities of daily life.

ACTIVITY INTOLERANCE (ACTUAL OR POTENTIAL)

Survivors of sudden cardiac death may experience decreased activity tolerance manifested by fatigue or weakness. Activity intolerance may be attributable to decreased cardiac output related to CAD processes or the use of antidysrhythmic agents. In addition, surgical intervention may limit progressive ambulation. Monitored patient activity is encouraged as tolerated with frequent rest periods. The critical care nurse is alert for situations such as orthostatic hypotension, hypoxia, and dysrhythmias. Assistance in performing activities of daily life is provided. The frequency of activity needs to be maintained while activity duration and intensity are modified to suit the patient's tolerance.

SLEEP PATTERN DISTURBANCE

Fear of the potential recurrence of sudden-death may lead to sleep disturbance in sudden cardiac death survivors (Rossi, 1984). Patients complain of difficulty falling asleep, early awakening, interrupted sleep, and fatigue. The nurse encourages the patient to discuss fears related to sleep or disturbing dreams. If the patient is monitored, the patient can be reassured that dysrhythmias will be detected and treated even during sleep. An environment conducive to normal sleep patterns needs to be maintained, even in the critical care setting. Pharmacologic therapy also needs to be reviewed and adjusted as appropriate because beta blockers and other antidysrhythmics can induce sleep disturbances.

PREVENTION OF CORONARY ARTERY DISEASE

During the last 15 years a steady decline in mortality from CAD has occurred in western countries. The decline has been attributed both to advances in the diagnosis and treatment of this disease and to the institution of primary and secondary preventive measures. Recent studies suggest that modification of cardiac risk factors is feasible in clinical practice, and risk factor reduction may be associated with halting the progression and possibly regression of atherosclerosis (Mancia, 1988). Thus, modification of risk factors must be considered an important therapeutic component of the management of ischemic heart disease.

Evidence for Primary Prevention

Although both total cholesterol and LDL cholesterol can be reduced by an appropriate diet, research done to date has shown little correlation between reduced dietary fat intake and plasma cholesterol level in primary prevention of CAD. Thus, the results of studies in which plasma cholesterol is modified by drug treatment as a primary preventive measure must be examined. The use of plasma cholesterol—lowering drugs has demonstrated efficacy in primary prevention of CAD. In individuals with hypercholesterolemia studied at the National Heart, Lung, and Blood Institute (Levy et al., 1984), cholestyramine therapy appeared to retard the development of coronary atherosclerosis as measured by coronary angiography. Results of the Coronary Primary Prevention Trial (Lipid Research Clinics Program, 1984) demonstrated a 24% decrease in coronary mortality and a 19% decrease in nonfatal myocardial infarction with a combined modification of dietary and cholestyramine therapy compared with dietary modification alone. Coronary arteriography performed before and after 5 years of treatment suggested a reduction in progression of atherosclerotic lesions with choles-

tyramine therapy. In the Helinski Heart Study (Frick et al., 1987) reductions in total cholesterol and non-HDL cholesterol and an increase in serum HDL cholesterol was observed with daily use of gemfibrozil. In a 5-year follow-up study, statistically significant differences in nonfatal myocardial infarctions were noted in subjects who received gemfibrozil compared to those receiving a placebo.

Additional measures that are gaining attention in primary prevention are the use of antiplatelet agents and fish oil derivatives. Low-dose aspirin, Persantine, and the consumption of cold water oily fish reduce platelet aggregation, and fish oil may also decrease plasma cholesterol and triglyceride levels. Marine fatty acids, particularly from cold water fish, contain omega-3 fatty acids, predominantly ucosapentaenoic and docasahexaenoic acids. Consumption of omega-3 fatty acids has produced changes in both plasma fatty acid and platelet composition (Phillipson et al., 1985; Fehily et al., 1983; Thargren and Gustafson, 1981). Such changes are consistent with favorable lipid profiles, prolonged bleeding times, and decreased platelet aggregation. The addition of cold water fish several times a week to the diet may be beneficial in prevention of coronary artery disease. However, the use of fish oil supplements is considered drug therapy. Investigation of long-term efficacy and toxicity of supplements is needed before general use is recommended.

Antiplatelet agents such as aspirin and dipyridamole alone or in combination have shown varied results in the primary prevention of CAD. Data from the American Heart Association (1988b) showed a 47% reduction in the risk of total myocardial infarction in a trial test group receiving 325 mg of aspirin every other day. However, due to sampling limitations the results may not be generalizable.

Evidence for Secondary Prevention

The goal of secondary prevention is to slow the progression and perhaps reverse clinically manifest atherosclerosis. In the most limited sense, secondary prevention refers to a decrease in the incidence of subsequent cardiac events in patients with known CAD. Secondary prevention is initiated during hospitalization or a cardiac rehabilitation program when the patient and family are ready to assimilate educational content. Rehabilitation begins with attempts to minimize deconditioning and restore the patient's confidence in his ability to maintain the activities of daily life. Further rehabilitative measures are designed to modify risk-producing behaviors, retard disease progression, and improve exercise tolerance.

The traditional coronary risk factors appear to play a lesser role in determining individual prognosis in persons with CAD, and the benefits of secondary prevention are less well established. However, secondary preventive efforts may play a role in causing regression or delay of atherosclerotic plaque (Vliestra et al., 1980).

As in primary prevention, smoking cessation and alteration of serum lipid levels provide the most consistent evidence of benefit in secondary prevention. Results of the Coronary Drug Project (Schlant, 1982) demonstrated that cigarette smoking and hypercholesterolemia increased the risk of coronary events in men who had recovered from myocardial infarction. Regular physical activity and increased levels of serum HDL cholesterol were associated with a decrease in 5-year mortality levels (Berge et al., 1982). Avoidance of cigarette smoking has produced the most consistent individual benefit in established CAD (Mulcahy, 1983). Smoking cessation lowers the risk of fatal and nonfatal reinfarction, sudden coronary death, and total mortality by 20% to 50%, particularly in the first 5 years postinfarction (Aberg et al., 1983; Daley et al., 1983).

In the Cholesterol-Lowering Atherosclerosis Study (Blankenhorn et al., 1987) a combination of cholestyramine and niacin was used to achieve reduction in plasma cholesterol levels in patients with documented CAD. Blankenhorn and colleagues' research supports the concept that drug-induced lowering of plasma cholesterol may retard coronary atherogenesis, thereby reducing the risk of coronary heart disease. However, due to the limited number of secondary prevention clinical trials, the decision to institute cholesterol-lowering drug therapy must be made on an individual basis. Currently, no documentation of reduced mortality or evaluation of long-term drug toxicity or drug interactions with this form of therapy is available.

Clinical trials using beta-adrenergic blocking drugs administered to patients after a myocardial infarction have shown a 26% to 39% reduction in mortality (Beta Blocker Heart Attack Research Group, 1982; Norwegian Multicenter Study Group, 1981) up to 3 years postinfarction.

A comprehensive approach to coronary risk management appears to be most effective for patients with symptomatic CAD. Emphasis must be placed on avoidance of cigarette smoking, reduction of dietary intake of cholesterol, saturated fat, sodium, and total calories, and initiation and maintenance of a program of regular physical activity.

nursing care plan

PATIENTS WITH CORONARY ARTERY DISEASE

1. Altered comfort: pain related to:
Myocardial ischemia and/or injury

Outcome Criteria	Nursing Interventions
Patient will verbalize relief of anginal pain within 1 hour of admission. Patient will not display further signs or symptoms of pain.	Provide education regarding pharmacologic relief. Prevent occurrence of pain through teaching stress reduction techniques, activity limitation, and emergency medical procedures.

2. Anxiety related to:
Anginal pain, impending death, limitations in activity and/or life-style changes

Outcome Criteria	Nursing Interventions
Patient will verbalize anxiety/fear and usual coping behaviors. Anxiety/fear will be reduced through use of effective coping mechanisms.	Encourage verbalization of fears of both patients and families. Provide clear instructions on ways to reduce anginal pain. Review normal cardiac function, pathophysiology related to the disease process, and the role of pharmacologic therapy in relieving anginal symptoms. Set mutual goals with patient and family related to activity and life-style changes. Provide adjunctive relaxation techniques to reduce stress such as meditation, autogenic training, progressive relaxation, and biofeedback.

Nursing Care Plan continued on following page

3. Knowledge deficit related to:
Diagnosis of myocardial ischemia

Outcome Criteria	*Nursing Interventions*

Patient and family will describe factors that precipitate anginal attacks.
Patient and family will describe the action, dosage, schedule, and side effects of cardiac medications.
Patient and family will identify risk factors of coronary artery disease and develop a plan to modify life style as able.
	Assess patient and family reaction to diagnosis of myocardial ischemia and its implications.
	Provide education about precipitating factors, pharmacologic therapy, and risk factor modification:
	    Assist patients to identify specific situations that precipitate anginal attacks.
	    Consider use of a diary that records time, onset, duration, and events associated with anginal pain.
	    Instruct patient and family about the action, dosage, and side effects of medications, including side effects that require medical intervention.
	    Use mutual goal setting and a supportive, nonjudgmental attitude when achieving risk factor modification goals.

4. Activity intolerance related to:
Myocardial ischemia

Outcome Criteria	*Nursing Interventions*
Activity will be conducted at a level promoting optimal cardiac function while preventing complications.	Provide patient and family with specific activity restrictions and rationale. Provide education about the prophylactic use of nitroglycerin and about limiting, pacing, and timing of physical activity.

5. Nonadherence related to:
Ongoing life-style changes and risk factor modification

Outcome Criteria	*Nursing Interventions*

Patient will identify modifiable risk factors and life-style changes necessary to prevent myocardial ischemia.
Patient and family will engage in necessary life-style changes and risk factor modification on a permanent basis.
	Assess likelihood of early attrition.
	Explore the relative value of health, perception of control over health outcome, and potential barriers to initiating and sustaining health behaviors.
	Incorporate motivational interventions to reduce perceived barriers to life-style changes whenever possible:
	    Extrinsic: Education specifying easily controlled cardiovascular risk reduction techniques; increased involvement of supportive others in the rehabilitation process; and collaborative decision-making related to health goals and desired health outcomes.
	    Intrinsic: Allow individual to determine his or her own health-related goals: involve the individual in decision-making and development of specific actions toward achievement of health-related goals; emphasize individual responsibility and self-directedness in undertaking risk-reducing health behaviors.

SUDDEN CARDIAC DEATH

1. Anxiety/fear related to:
Survival of sudden cardiac death

Outcome Criteria	*Nursing Interventions*
Patient will verbalize anxiety/fear. Patient will report increase in comfort through effective use of coping behaviors.	Assess source(s) of patient's fear. Ensure that patient and family have an understanding of the plan of care, adequate emotional supports, and realistic short-term goals. Reassure patient and family that heart rhythm and hemodynamic status are being closely monitored and that a team to provide emergency care measures is close at hand.

2. Knowledge deficit related to:
Survival of sudden cardiac death

Outcome Criteria	*Nursing Interventions*
Patient and family will describe normal heart function, pathologic process, symptoms of dysrhythmias, and related treatment.	Assess the patient and family's readiness to learn about the disease process and diagnostic plan. Teach the patient and family normal heart anatomy and impulse conduction, dysrhythmic symptoms, associated pathologic process, and pharmacologic or surgical treatment. Review purpose, associated sensory experiences, significance, and care following diagnostic tests such as electrophysiologic studies and cardiac mapping.

3. Nonadherence related to:
Prescribed drug regimen

Outcome Criteria	Nursing Interventions
Patient will demonstrate correct use of prescribed medications.	Instruct patient and family about the action, dose and frequency, and side effects of medications. Outline specific symptoms that require medical intervention. Emphasize the importance of timing of medication doses. Collaborate in designing a medication dose/time schedule that fits the patient's life-style. Teach patient and family about the plan and goals of care, including pharmacologic therapy and possible surgical interventions and their expected outcomes.

4. Altered thought processes related to:
Memory loss and neurologic deficits following resuscitation from sudden cardiac death

Outcome Criteria	Nursing Interventions
Patient will demonstrate optimal use of cognition. Patient will remain free of injury during hospitalization.	Reassure patient and family that the transient anoxic encephalopathy usually disappears within 2 weeks of the neurologic insult (cardiac arrest). Facilitate discussion of the arrest and verbalization of feelings. Reorient the patient to person, place, and time frequently. Use clock and calendar at bedside. Assist with ambulation and activities of daily living. Encourage and monitor activity. Allow for frequent rest periods. Monitor for orthostatic hypotension, hypoxemia, and dysrhythmias.

5. Sleep pattern disturbance related to:
Fear of recurrence of sudden cardiac death

Outcome Criteria	Nursing Interventions
Patient will describe factors and feelings that hinder sleep. Patient will resume usual sleep patterns.	Encourage patient to discuss fears. Reassure patient that he or she will be monitored during sleep. Maintain environment conducive to sleep—quiet, minimal lighting.

SUMMARY

Although CAD continues to be the number one cause of disability and death in the western world, a steady decline has been observed during the past 10 to 15 years. The decrease has been attributed to better diagnosis and treatment and primary preventive efforts through elimination or reduction of risk factors. Advanced technology and pharmacology for the treatment of CAD have imposed new responsibilities on the critical care nurse. In addition, the challenge of promoting sustained life-style change to reduce or eliminate atherogenic risk factors has not been met. Thus, nurses in critical care continue to be faced with the need to assimilate new data and to apply this knowledge to the care of the patient with CAD.

References

Abela G. S., Cohen D., Feldman R. L. Use of laser radiation to recanalize stenosed arteries in a live animal model (Abstract). *Circulation,* 66 (Suppl 12), 366.
Aberg, A., Bergstrand, R., Johansson, S., et al. (1983). Cessation of smoking after myocardial infarction—effects on mortality after 10 years. *British Heart Journal,* 49, 416–422.
Abula, G. S., Conti, C. R., Normann, S., et al. (1984). A new model for investigation of transluminal recanalization: Human atherosclerotic coronary artery xenografts. *American Journal of Cardiology,* 54, 208–205.
Alpert, J. S. (1984). *Pathophysiology of the cardiovascular system* (pp. 211–216). Boston: Little, Brown.
American College of Sports Medicine (1986). *Guidelines for exercise testing and prescriptions.* Philadelphia: Lea & Febiger.
American Heart Association (1988a). *Heart facts.* Dallas: AHA National Center.
American Heart Association (1988b). Position statement: Physicians' Health Study report on aspirin. *Circulation,* 77 (6), 1447A.
Antman, E. M., Stone, P. H., Muller, J. E., et al. (1980). Calcium channel blocking agents in the treatment of cardiovascular disorders. Part I: Basic and clinical electrophysiological effects. *Annals of Internal Medicine,* 93, 875–885.
Astrand, P., and Rodahl, K. (1977). *Textbook of work physiology.* New York: McGraw-Hill.
Beller, G. (1985). Nuclear cardiology: Current indications and clinical usefulness. *Current Problems in Cardiology,* 10, 1–48.
Benowitz, N. L. (1988). Pharmacologic aspects of cigarette smoking and nicotine addiction. *New England Journal of Medicine,* 319, (20), 1318–1330.
Berge, K., Carner, P., Hairline, S., et al. (1982). High density lipoprotein cholesterol and prognosis after myocardial infarction. *Circulation,* 66, 1176.
Berman, D. S., Rozauski, A., and Knoebel, S. B. (1987). The detection of silent ischemia: Caution and precaution. *Circulation,* 75, 101–105.
Beta-Blocker Heart Attack Research Group (1982). A randomized trial of propranolol in patients with acute myocardial infarction: I. Mortality results. *Journal of the American Medical Association,* 247, 1707.
Bishop, V. S., Kasper, R. L., Barnes, G. E., et al. (1974). Left ventricular function during acute regional myocardial ischemia in the conscious dog. *Journal of Applied Physiology,* 37, 785.
Blackburn, H., and Jacobs, D. R. (1988). Physical activity and the

risk of coronary heart disease. *New England Journal of Medicine,* 319 (18), 1217–1219.

Blankenhorn, D. H., Nessim, S., Johnson, S., et al. (1987). Beneficial effects of combined colestipol-niacin therapy on coronary atherosclerosis and coronary venous bypass grafts. *Journal of the American Medical Association* 257, 3233–3240.

Block, P. C., Myler, R. K., Sretzer, S., et al. (1981). Morphology after transluminal angioplasty in human beings. *New England Journal of Medicine,* 305, 382.

Bonow, R. O., Kent, K. M., Rosing, D. R., et al. (1982). Improved left ventricular diastolic filling in patients with coronary artery disease after percutaneous coronary angioplasty. *Circulation,* 66, 1159.

Borer, J. S., Kurt, K. M., Bachanach, S. L., et al. (1979). Sensitivity, specificity and predictive accuracy of radionuclide cineangiography during exercise in patients with coronary artery disease. *Circulation,* 60, 572–580.

Boucher, C. A., Brewster, D. C., Darling, R. C., et al. (1985). Determination of cardiac risk before peripheral vascular surgery: Use of dipyridamole thallium imaging to select patients for considerations of preoperative coronary angiography and myocardial revascularization. *New England Journal of Medicine,* 312, 389–394.

Braunwald, E., Isselbacker, K. J., Petersdorf, R. G., et al. (Eds.) (1987). *Harrison's principles of internal medicine* (11th ed.). New York: McGraw-Hill.

Brodde, O. E. (1986). Molecular pharmacology of beta adrenoceptors. *Journal of Cardiovascular Pharmacology,* 8 (Suppl. 4), 516–520.

Brook, H. L. (1989). Electrocardiography: 100 diagnostic criteria. Guidelines of the American College of Cardiology Committee on Electrocardiography. Chicago: Year Book Medical Publishers.

Brown, M. S., and Goldstein, J. L. (1984). How LDL receptors influence cholesterol and atherosclerosis. *Scientific American,* 251 (5), 58–66.

Bruce, R. A., DeRoven, T. A., Hossack, K. R., et al. (1980). Value of maximal exercise tests in risk assessment of primary coronary heart disease events in healthy men: Five years experience at the Seattle Heart Watch Study. *American Journal of Cardiology,* 46, 377–378.

Caldwell, J., Sorenson, S., Ritchie, J., et al. (1979). Exercise radionuclide ventriculography and thallium imaging: Comparison of sensitivity and specificity. *American Journal of Cardiology,* 43, 432–438.

Chaitman, B. R., Bourassa, M. G., Wagniant, P., et al. (1978). Improved efficiency of treadmill exercise testing using a multiple lead ECG system and basic hemodynamic response. *Circulation,* 57, 71–79.

Chatterjie, K. (1990). Ischemia heart disease. In J. Stein (Ed.), *Internal medicine* (3rd ed). Boston: Little, Brown.

Choy, D. S. J., Stertzer, S. H., Myler, R. V., et al. (1984). Human coronary laser recanalization. *Clinical Cardiology,* 7 (7), 377–381.

Clark, P. B. (1987). Nicotine and smoking: A perspective from animal studies. *Psychopharmacology,* 92, 135–143.

Cobb, L. A., Hallstrom, A. P., Weaver, W. D., et al. (1983). Considerations in the long-term management of survivors of cardiac arrest. *Annals of New York Academy of Sciences.*

Cohn, P. F. (1987). Silent myocardial ischemia: Present status. *Modern Concepts in Cardiovascular Disease,* 56, 1–5.

Cowley, M. J., DiSciascio, G., Rehr, G. B., et al. (1989). Angiographic observations and clinical relevance of coronary thrombosis in unstable angina pectoris. *American Journal of Cardiology,* 63, 108E–113E.

Crawford, M. H., Petru, M. A., Amon, K., et al. (1984). Comparative value of 2-D echocardiography and radionuclide angiography for quantitating changes in left ventricular performance during exercise limited by angina pectoris. *American Journal of Cardiology,* 53, 42–47.

Crawford, M. H. (in press). Theoretical considerations in the use of calcium entry blockers in silent myocardial ischemia. *Circulation,* 80, IV74–IV77.

Criqui, M. H. (1986). Epidemiology of atherosclerosis: An updated overview. *American Journal of Cardiology,* 57, 18C–23C.

Cumberland, D. C. (1985). The current status of percutaneous coronary angioplasty. *Acta Radiologicia,* 26, 497.

Curry, S. J., Marlott, G. A., Gordin, J., et al. (1988). A comparison of alternative theoretical approaches to smoking cessation and relapse. *Health Psychology,* 7(6), 545–556.

Daley, E., Mulcahy, R., Daly, L., et al. (1983). Long term effect on mortality of stopping smoking after unstable angina or myocardial infarction. *British Heart Journal,* 49, 42–43.

David, P., Walters, D., Scholl, J., et al. (1982). Percutaneous transluminal coronary angioplasty in patients with variant angina. *Circulation,* 66, 695.

Deedwanian, P., Carbajal, E., Nelson, J., et al. (1989). Silent ischemia during daily life as an independent predictor of survival in stable angina (Abstract). *Journal of American College of Cardiology,* 13, 3A.

Dehmer, G. J. (1987). Angina pectoris: Diagnosis, treatment and prognosis. *Current Problems in Cardiology,* 12, 215–281.

Deligonaul, U., Vandormael, M., Kern, M. J., et al. (1989). Repeat coronary angioplasty for restenosis: Results and predictors for follow-up clinical events. *American Heart Journal,* 117, 997.

Dishman, R. (1984). Motivation and exercise adherence. In J. M. Silva, and R. S. Weinberg (Eds.), *Psychological foundations of sport.* Champaign, IL: Human Kinetics.

Dishman, R., and Gettman, L. R. (1980). Psychological influences on exercise adherence. *Journal of Sports Psychology,* 2, 295–310.

Dorros, G., Gowley, M., Simpson, J., et al. (1983). Percutaneous transluminal coronary angioplasty: Report of complications from the National Heart, Lung and Blood Institute PTCA Registry. *Circulation,* 67(4), 723–730.

Droste, C., and Roskamm, H. (1983). Experimental pain measurement in patients with asymptomatic myocardial ischemia. *Journal of the American College of Cardiology,* 1, 940.

Dunnington, C. S., and Finkelmeier, B. A. (1988). Psychological support of the survivor of sudden coronary death. *Journal of Cardiovascular Nursing,* 3(1), 33–46.

Epstein, S. E., Quyyumi, A. A., and Bonow, R. O. (1988). Myocardial ischemia—silent or symptomatic. *New England Journal of Medicine,* 318, 1038–1043.

Erickson, J., and Thaulow, E. (1984). Follow-up of patients with asymptomatic myocardial ischemia. In W. Ruthauser, and H. Roskamm (Eds.), *Silent myocardial ischemia.* Berlin: Springer-Verlag.

European Coronary Surgery Group (1982). Long-term results of prospective randomized study of coronary artery bypass surgery in stable angina pectoris. *Lancet,* 27, 1173–1176.

Factor, S. M., and Kirk, E. S. (1986). Pathophysiology of myocardial ischemia. In J. W. Hurst (Ed.), *The heart* (pp. 856–881). New York: McGraw-Hill.

Fagiotto, A., Ross, R., and Harker, L. (1984). Studies of hypercholesteremia in the nonhuman primate. I. Changes that lead to fatty streak formation. *Arteriosclerosis,* 4, 323.

Fagiotto, A., and Ross, R. (1984). Studies of hypercholesteremia in the nonhuman primate. II. Fatty streak conversion to fibrous plaque. *Arteriosclerosis,* 4, 341.

Falk, E. (1989). Morphologic features of unstable atherthrombic plaques underlying acute coronary syndromes. *American Journal of Cardiology,* 63, 114E–120E.

Fehily, A., Burr, M., Phillips, N., et al. (1983). The effect of fatty fish on plasma lipid and lipoprotein concentrations. *American Journal of Clinical Nutrition,* 38, 349–351.

Fielding, J. E., and Phenow, K. J. (1988). Health effects of involuntary smoking. *New England Journal of Medicine,* 319 (22), 1452–1459.

Fisher, J., Kim, S., and Mercando, A. (1988). Electrical devises for the treatment of arrhythmias. *American Journal of Cardiology,* 61, 45A–57A.

Fox, J. (1986). Laser coronary angioplasty, *Journal of Cardiovascular Nursing,* 1, 57.

Frick, M., Elo, O., Happa, K., et al. (1987). Helinski Heart Study: Primary prevention trial with Gemfibrozil in middle-aged men with dyslipidemia. *New England Journal of Medicine,* 317 (20), 1237–1245.

Friedman, M., Powell, L. H., La Croix, A. Z., et al. (1988). Type A behavior and mortality from coronary heart disease (letter to the editor). *New England Journal of Medicine,* 319 (2), 114–116

Frishman, W. H., and Miller, K. P. (1986). Platelets and antiplatelet activity in ischemic heart disease. *Current Problems in Cardiology,* 11 (2), 71–136.

Gerrity, R. G., Loop, F. D., Golding, L. A., et al. (1983). Arterial response to laser operation for removal of atherosclerotic plaques. *Journal of Thoracic Cardiovascular Surgery*, 85, 409.

Glazier, J. J., Chierchia, S., Brown, M. J., et al. (1987). Importance of generalized defective perception of painful stimuli as a cause of silent myocardial ischemia in chronic stable angina pectoris. *American Journal of Cardiology*, 58, 667–702.

Goldman, G. J., and Pichard, A. D. (1983). The natural history of coronary artery disease: Does medical therapy improve the prognosis? *Progress in Cardiovascular Disease*, 25, 513.

Gottlieb, S. O., Weisfeldt, M. L., Onyang, P., et al. (1986). Silent ischemia as a marker for early unfavorable outcomes in patients with unstable angina. *New England Journal of Medicine*, 314, 1214–1219.

Gottlieb, S. O., Gottlieb, S. H., Achutt, S. C., et al. (1988). Silent ischemia on Holter monitoring predicts mortality in high risk post-infarction patients. *Journal of the American Medical Association*, 259 (19), 1030–1035.

Greenburgh, H. M., and Dwyer, E. M. (Eds.) (1982). Sudden coronary death. *Annals of the New York Academy of Sciences*, 382, 3.

Gruentzig, A., King, S. B., Schlumpf, M., et al. (1987). Long-term follow-up after transluminal coronary angioplasty. *New England Journal of Medicine*, 316, 1127–1132.

Gruentzig, A., Knudson, M., and Schlumpf, M. (1981). Repeated coronary angioplasty (PTCA) after recurrence of stenosis. *Circulation*, 64 (Suppl. 4), 108.

Gruentzig, A., and Meier, B. (1983). Percutaneous transluminal coronary angioplasty. The first five years and future. *International Journal of Cardiology*, 2, 319.

Haggerty, J. J., Burkett, M. B., and Foster, J. R., et al. (1983). Psychological dysfunction in patients surviving ventricular tachycardia or ventricular fibrillation (abstract). *Circulation*, 68 (Suppl. 3), 108.

Hall, D. P., Corozo, O., Douglass, J. S., et al. (1984). Percutaneous transluminal coronary angioplasty in patients with prior coronary bypass surgery. *International Journal of Cardiology*, 6, 645.

Hall, D. P., and Gruentzig, A. (1984). Selection of patients for percutaneous coronary angioplasty—current procedures and future directions. *American Journal of Cardiology*, 142 (1), 13.

Hall, D. P., and Morris, D. C. (1984). Coronary disease in the elderly. In J. W. Hurst (Ed.), *Clinical essays on the heart* (Vol. 3, p. 3). New York: McGraw Hill.

Hall, P., and Gruentzig, A. (1983). Percutaneous transluminal coronary angioplasty. The first five years and future. *International Journal of Cardiology*, 2, 319.

Hamly, R. I. (1981). Hereditary aspects of coronary artery disease. *American Heart Journal*, 101, 639.

Havik, O. E., and Maeland, J. G. (1988). Changes in smoking behavior after a myocardial infarction. *Health Psychology* 7 (5), 403–420.

Health and Public Policy Committee: American College of Physicians (1983). Percutaneous transluminal angioplasty. *Internal Medicine*, 99, 864.

Hjermann, I., Velve, B. K., Decker, J. R., and Phillips, R. D. (1981). Effect of diet and smoking intervention of the incidence of coronary heart disease. Report from the Oslo Study Group of a Randomized Trial in Healthy Men. *Lancet*, 2, 1303–1310.

Holbrook, J. H., Grundy, S. M., Hennekens, C. H., et al. (1984). Cigarette smoking and heart disease. *Circulation*, 70 (6), 1114A–1116A.

Holmes, D. R., Holbukov, R., and Vliestra, R. E. (1988). Comparison of complications during PTCA in the NHLBI PTCA registry. *Journal of the American College of Cardiology*, 12, 1149–1155.

Holmes, D. R., Vliestra, R. E., Mock, M. B., et al. (1983). Employment and recreation patterns in patients treated by percutaneous transluminal coronary angioplasty: A multicenter study. *American Journal of Cardiology*, 52, 710.

Hopper, S., and Schechtman, K. (1985). Factors associated with diabetic control and utilization patterns in a low income older adult population. *Patient Education and Counseling*, 1, 275–288.

Hubert, H. B., Feinleib, M., McNamara, P. M., et al. (1983). Obesity as an independent risk factor for cardiovascular disease: A 25-year follow-up of participants in the Framingham Heart Study. *Circulation*, 67, 968.

Hurst, J. W., King, S. B., Friesinger, G. C., et al. (1986). Atherosclerotic coronary heart disease: Recognition, prognosis, and treatment. In J. W. Hurst, (Ed.), *The heart* (6th ed., pp. 882–1008). New York: McGraw Hill.

Ice, R. (1985). Long term compliance. *Physical Therapy*, 65, 1832–1839.

Jenkins, C. D. (1988). Epidemiology of cardiovascular disease. *Journal of Consulting and Clinical Psychology*, 56 (3), 324–332.

Jenkins, C. D. (1985). The epidemiology of sudden death. In R. E. Beamish, P. K. Singal, and N. S. Dhalla (Eds.), *Stress and heart disease* (pp. 17–43). Boston: Nijhoff.

Kamarck, T. W., and Lichtenstein, E. (1988). Program adherence and coping strategies as predictors of success in a smoking treatment program. *Health Psychology*, 7 (6), 557–574.

Kannel, W. B. (1985). Lipids, diabetes and coronary heart disease. *American Heart Journal*, 110, 1100–1106.

Kannel, W. B. (1987). Prevalence and clinical aspects of unrecognized myocardial infarction and sudden unexpected death. *Circulation*, 75 (Suppl. II), II, 4–5.

Kannel, W. B., and Abbott, R. D. (1984). Incidence and prognosis of unrecognized myocardial infarction: An update on the Framingham Study. *New England Journal of Medicine*, 311, 1144–1147.

Kannel, W. B., Dannenberg, A. L., and Abbott, R. D. (1985). Unrecognized myocardial infarction and hypertension. *American Heart Journal*, 109, 581–584.

Kannel, W. B., Doyle, J. T., Ostfeld, A. M., et al. (1984). Optimal resources for primary prevention of atherosclerotic disease. *Circulation*, 70 (1), 157A–205A.

Kawaniski, D. T., and Rahimtoola, S. H. (1987). Silent myocardial ischemia. *Current Problems in Cardiology*, 12 (9), 511–566.

Kelly, P., Cannon, D., and Garan, H. (1988). The automatic implantable cardioverter/defibrillator: Efficacy, complications, survival in patients with malignant ventricular arrhythmias. *Journal of the American College of Cardiology*, 11, 1278.

Kent, K. M., Bentivoglio, L. G., and Block, P. C. (1984). Long-term efficacy of percutaneous transluminal coronary angioplasty: Report from the Heart, Lung, and Blood Institute PTCA Registry. *American Journal of Cardiology*, 53, 27C.

Kent, K. M., Bentivoglio, L. G., Block, P. C., et al. (1982). Percutaneous transluminal coronary angioplasty: Report from the Registry of the National Heart, Lung and Blood Institute. *American Journal of Cardiology*, 1, 1268.

Kern, M. J., Ganz, P., Horowitz, J., et al. (1983). Potentiation of coronary vasoconstriction by beta adrenergic blockade. *Circulation*, 67, 1178.

Knoebel, S. B., Crawford, M. H., Dunn, M. I., et al. (1989). American College of Cardiology, American Heart Association Task Force Report: Guidelines for ambulatory electrocardiography. *Journal of the American College of Cardiology*, 13, 249–258.

Kreisberg, R., and Kasim, S. (1987). Cholesterol metabolism and aging. *American Journal of Medicine*, 82 (Suppl. 1B), 54–59.

Laakso, M., Pyrolala, K., Sarlund, H., et al. (1986). Lipids and lipoprotein abnormalities associated with CHD in patients with insulin dependent diabetes mellitus. *Arteriosclerosis*, 6, 679–684.

Lapidus, L., Bengtsson, C., and Lindquist, O. (1985). Menopausal age and risk of cardiovascular disease and death: A 12 year follow-up study of participants in women in Goteberg, Sweden. *Acta Obstetricia et Gynecolica Scandinavica*, 130 (Supp.), 37–41.

LaRosa, J. C. (1985). Effect of estrogen replacement therapy on lipids: Implications for cardiovascular risks. *Journal of Reproductive Medicine*, 30 (Suppl. 10), 811–813.

Lawrence, P. F., Kercher, J. M., Dries, D. J., et al. (1987). Endoscopic laser resection of atherosclerotic plaque in a live animal model. A preliminary report on some technical difficulties. *Journal of Vascular Surgery*, (5), 470–475.

Lee, G., Chan, M. C., Ikeda, R. M., et al. (1985). Applicability of laser to assist coronary balloon angioplasty. *American Heart Journal*, 110, 1233.

Lee, G., Chan, M. C., Rink, D. L., et al. (1987). Coronary revascularization by a new coaxially guided laser-heated metal cap system. *American Heart Journal*, 113, 1507.

Lee, G., Garcia, J. M., Chan, M. C., et al. (1986a). Clinically successful long-term coronary recanalization. *American Heart Journal*, 112, 1323.

Lee, G., Ikeda, R. M., Chan, M. C., et al. (1985). Limitations, risks and complications of laser recanalization: A cautious approach warranted. *American Journal of Cardiology,* 56, 181.

Lee, G., Ikeda, R. M., Kozina, J., et al. (1981). Laser dissolution of coronary atherosclerotic obstruction. *American Heart Journal,* 102, 1074.

Lee, G., Reis, R. L., Chan, M. C., et al. (1986b). Clinical laser recanalization of coronary obstruction—angioscopic and angiographic documentation, *Chest,* 90, 770.

Lee, G., Sommerhaug, R. B., Argenal, A., et al. (1987). Clinical laser revascularization of coronary obstruction with the coaxial-guided laser-heated metal cap catheter. *American Heart Journal,* 114, 1524–1526.

Leitshuh, M., and Chobanian, A. (1987). Vascular changes in hypertension. *Medical Clinics of North America,* 71 (5), 827–846.

Levy, R. I., Brensike, J. F., Epstein, S., et al. (1984). Influence of changes in lipid values induced by cholestryamine and diet on progression of CAD: Results of the NHLBI type II coronary intervention study. *Circulation,* 69, 325–337.

Lindquist, O., and Bengtsson, C. (1979). Menopausal age in relation to smoking. *Acta Medica Scandinavica,* 205, 73–77.

Lipid Research Clinics Program (1984). The Lipid Research Clinics Coronary Primary Prevention Trial Results I. Reduction in incidence of coronary heart disease. *Journal of the American Medical Association,* 251, 351–364.

Mabin, T. A., Holmes, D. R., Smith, H. C., et al. (1985). Intracoronary thrombus: Role in coronary occlusion complicating percutaneous transluminal angioplasty. *Journal of the American College of Cardiology,* 5, 198–202.

Malun, T. A., Holmes, D. R., Smith, H. C., et al. (1983). Long-term follow up after percutaneous transluminal coronary angioplasty (PTCA). *Circulation,* 68 (Suppl. 3), 97.

Mancia, G. (1988). Opening remarks: The need to manage risk factors of coronary heart disease. *American Heart Journal,* 115, 240–241.

Margolis, J. R., Chen, J. T. T., Kong, Y., et al. (1980). The diagnostic and prognostic significance of coronary artery calcifications. *Radiology,* 137, 609–616.

Marlatt, G. A., and Gordon, J. R. (Eds.) (1985). *Relapse prevention: Maintenance strategies in the treatment of addictive behaviors.* New York: Guilford.

Martin, J. E., and Dubert, P. M. (1984). Behavioral management strategies for improving health and fitness. *Journal of Cardiac Rehabilitation,* 4, 200–208.

Maseri, A. (1987). Role of coronary artery spasm in symptomatic and silent myocardial ischemia. *Journal of American College of Cardiology,* 9, 249–256.

Meade, T. W. (1982). Effects of progestogens on the cardiovascular system. *American Journal of Obstetrics and Gynecology,* 142, 776–780.

Mehta, J., and Mehta, P. (1980). Comparative effects of nitroprusside and nitroglycerine on platelet aggregation in patients with heart failure. *Journal of Cardiovascular Pharmacology,* 2, 25.

Meier, B., Gruentzig, A., Siegenthaler, W. E., et al. (1983). Long-term exercise performance after percutaneous coronary angioplasty and coronary artery bypass grafting. *Circulation,* 68, 796.

Mulcahy, R. (1983). Influence of cigarette smoking on morbidity and mortality after myocardial infarction. *British Heart Journal,* 49, 410–415.

Mullins, C. E., O'Laughlin, M. P., Vick, G. W., et al. (1988). Implantation of balloon-expandable intravascular grafts by catheterization in pulmonary arteries and systemic veins. *Circulation,* 77 (1), 188–199.

Murdaugh, C. L., and O'Rourke, R. A. (1988). Coronary heart disease in women: Special considerations. *Current Problems in Cardiology,* 13 (2), 79–156.

Nash, D. T. (1988). Prospects for regression of human atherosclerosis. *Cardiovascular Reviews and Reports,* December, 42–45.

National Cholesterol Education Program Expert Panel (1988). Report of the National Cholesterol Education Program Expert Panel on Detection, Evaluation and Treatment of High Blood Cholesterol in Adults. *Archives of Internal Medicine,* 148, 36–69.

National Heart, Lung, Blood Institute (1987). *High blood cholesterol in adults.* Bethesda, MD: NHLBI, National Cholesterol Education Program.

National Heart, Lung, Blood Institute (1988). *The 1988 report of the Joint National Committee on Detection, Evaluation and Treatment of High Blood Pressure.* Washington, DC: U.S. Department of Health and Human Services, NIH Publication No. 88-1088.

Nesto, R. W., and Kowalchuk, G. J. (1987). The ischemic cascade: Temporal sequence of hemodynamic, electrocardiographic and symptomatic expressions of ischemia. *American Journal of Cardiology,* 57, 23C–29C.

Norwegian Multicenter Study Group (1981). Timolol induced reduction in mortality and reinfarction in patients surviving acute myocardial infarction. *New England Journal of Medicine,* 304, 801.

Ohlson, L., Svardusudd, K., Welin, L., et al. (1986). Fasting blood glucose and risk of coronary heart disease, stroke, and all-cause mortality: A 17-year follow-up study of men born in 1913. *Diabetic Medicine,* 3, 33–37.

Oldridge, N. B. (1984). Compliance and drop-out in cardiac rehabilitation. *Journal of Cardiac Rehabilitation,* 7, 166–177.

Oldridge, N. B. (1986). Cardiac rehabilitation, self-responsibility and quality of life. *Journal of Cardiopulmonary Rehabilitation,* 6, 153–156.

Packer, M., Meller, J., Medina, N., et al. (1982). Hemodynamic consequences of combined beta adrenergic and slow calcium channel blockade in man. *Circulation,* 65, 660.

Paffenbarger, R. S., Wing, A. L., and Hyde, R. T. (1978). Physical activity as an index of heart attack in Harvard alumni. *American Journal of Epidemiology,* 1, 69–71.

Petitti, D. B., Wingard, J., Pellegren, F., et al. (1979). Risk of vascular disease in women: Smoking, oral contraceptives, noncontraceptive estrogens, and other factors. *Journal of the American Medical Association,* 242, 1150–1154.

Phillipson, B., Rothrock, D., Connor, W., et al. (1985). Reduction of plasma lipids, lipoproteins and apoproteins by dietary fish oils in patients with hypertriglyceredemia. *New England Journal of Medicine,* 312, 1210–1216.

Powell, M. G., Hedlin, A. M., Cerkus, I., et al. (1984). Effects of oral contraceptives on lipoprotein lipids: Prospective study. *Obstetrics and Gynecology,* 63, 764–770.

Preston, F. E., Whipps, S., Jackson, C. A., et al. (1981). Inhibition of prostacyclin and platelet thromboxane A_2 after low dose aspirin. *New England Journal of Medicine,* 304, 76.

Quyyumi, A. A., Wright, C., and Mockus, L. (1984). Effect of partial against activity in beta-blockers in severe angina pectoris: A double-blind comparison of pindolol and atenolol. *British Medical Journal,* 289, 951.

Ragland, D. R., and Brand, R. J. (1988). Type A behavior and mortality from coronary heart disease. *New England Journal of Medicine,* 318, (2), 65–69.

Renkin, J., David, P. R., Dangoisse, V., et al. (1983). Coronary angiographic results 6 and 18 months after successful percutaneous transluminal coronary angioplasty in 53 consecutive patients. *Circulation,* 68 (Suppl. 3), 314.

Ritchie, J. L., Zaret, B. L., Strauss, H. W., et al. (1978). Myocardial imaging with Thallium-201: A multicenter study in patients with angina pectoris or acute myocardial infarction. *American Journal of Cardiology,* 42, 345–350.

Rosenberg, M., Miller, D. R., Kaufman, D. W., et al. (1983). Myocardial infarction in women under 50 years of age. *Journal of the American Medical Association,* 250, 2801–2806.

Ross, R. (1986). The pathogenesis of atherosclerosis—An update. *New England Journal of Medicine,* 314, (8), 488–500.

Ross, R., Faggioto, A., Bowen-Pope, D., et al. (1984). The role of endothelial injury and platelet and macrophage interactions in atherosclerosis. *Circulation,* 70 (Suppl. 3), III-77–III-82.

Rossi, L. (1984). Nursing care for survivors of sudden cardiac death. *Nursing Clinics of North America,* 19, 411–425.

Rozawski, A., Diamong, G. A., Bennan, E., et al. (1983). The declining specificity of exercise radionuclide ventriculography. *New England Journal of Medicine,* 309, 518–522.

Ruderman, N. B., and Haudenschild, C. (1984). Diabetes as an atherogenic factor. *Progress in Cardiovascular Disease,* 26, 373–412.

Ruskin, J. N., McGovern, B., and Garan, H. (1990). Sudden death. In J. H. Stein (Ed.), *Internal medicine* (3rd edition). Boston: Little, Brown.

Russel-Briefel, R., Ezzati, T., Fulwood, R., et al. (1982). Cardiovascular risk status and oral contraceptive use: United States, 1976–80. *Preventive Medicine, 15,* 352–362.

Salonen, J. L. (1982). Oral contraceptives, smoking, and risk of MI in young women: A longitudinal population study in eastern Finland. *Acta Medica Scandinavica, 212,* 141–144.

Sanborn, T. A., Faxon, D. P., Kellett, M. A., et al. (1987). Percutaneous coronary laser thermal angioplasty with a metallic capped fiber. *Journal of American Cardiology, 9,* 104A.

Sarajas, H. (1976). Reaction patterns of blood platelets in exercise. *Advances in Cardiology, 18,* 176–195.

Scheuer, J., and Brachfeld, N. (1968). Coronary insufficiency: Relations between hemodynamic, electrical and biochemical parameters. *Circulation Research, 18,* 178–185.

Schlant, R., and Coronary Drug Project Research Group (1982). The natural history of coronary artery disease: Prognostic factors after recovery from myocardial infarction in 2789 men. In the 5-year findings of the Coronary Drug Project. *Circulation, 66,* 401–414.

Schneider, S., Vitus, A., and Ruderman, N. (1986). Atherosclerosis and physical activity. *Diabetes/Metabolism Reviews, 1,* 513–553.

Scholl, J. M., David, P. R., Chaitman, J., et al. (1981). Recurrence of stenosis following percutaneous transluminal angioplasty. *Circulation, 64* (Suppl. 4), 193.

Selwyn, A. P., Fox, K., and Eves, M. (1978). Myocardial ischemia in patients with frequent angina pectoris. *British Medical Journal, 2,* 1594.

Sevior, P. W., and Elkeles, R. S. (1985). Necrobiosis lipoidica in two diabetic sisters. *Clinical and Experimental Dermatology, 10* (2), 159–161.

Shell, W. E. (1985). Mechanisms and therapy of silent myocardial ischemia and the effect of transdermal nitroglycerin. *American Journal of Cardiology, 56,* 231.

Shepard, R. J. (1985). Physical activity and quality of life. *Quality of Life and Cardiovascular Care, 1,* 40–44.

Shlafer, M., Kane, P. F., Wiggins, V. Y., et al. (1982). Possible role for cytotoxic oxygen metabolites in the pathogenesis of cardiac ischemic injury. *Circulation, 66* (Suppl. 2), 185–192.

Shillinger, F. L. (1983). Percutaneous transluminal coronary angioplasty. *Heart & Lung, 12,* 46.

Shulman, P. (1984). Bayes theorem—A review. In S. P. Glasser (Ed.). Symposium on clinical exercise testing. *Cardiology Clinics, 2,* 309.

Sigwart, U., Puel, J., Mirkovitch, V., et al. (1987). Intravascular stents to prevent occlusion and restenosis after transluminal angioplasty. *New England Journal of Medicine, 316,* 701–706.

Sosenko, J. M., Breslow, J. L., and Miettinen, O. S. (1980). Hyperglycemia and plasma lipid levels: A prospective study of young insulin-dependent diabetic patients. *New England Journal of Medicine, 302,* 650–654.

Stacy, H. L. (1983). Evolution of atherosclerotic plaques in the coronary arteries of young adults (Abstract). *Arteriosclerosis, 3,* 471a.

Stampfer, M. J., Willett, W. C., Colditz, G. A., et al. (1988). A prospective study of past use of oral contraceptive agents and risk of cardiovascular disease. *New England Journal of Medicine, 319,* 1313–1317.

Stone, P. H., Antman, E. M., Muller, J. E., et al. (1980). Calcium channel blocking agents in the treatment of cardiovascular disorders. Part II: Hemodynamic effects and clinical applications. *Annals of Internal Medicine, 93,* 875–885.

Superko, H., Haskell, W., and Wood, P. (1985). Modification of plasma cholesterol through exercise: Rationale and recommendations. *Postgraduate Medicine, 78,* 64–75.

Thargren, M., and Gustafson, A. (1981). Effects of 11-week increase in dietary ercosapentaenoic acid on bleeding time, lipids and platelet aggregation. *Lancet, 2,* 1190–1193.

Tipton, C. (1984). Exercise training and hypertension. *Exercise Sport Science Review, 12,* 245–306.

Tyroler, H. A. (Ed.) (1980). Epidemiology of plasma high-density lipoprotein cholesterol levels. The Lipid Research Clinics Program Prevalence Study. *Circulation, 62* (Suppl. 4, Part 2), 1.

Vliestra, R., et al. (1980). Risk factors and coronary artery disease: A report from the coronary artery surgery study (CASS). *Circulation, 60,* 254.

Walden, C. E., Knopp, R. H., Wahl, P. W., et al. (1984). Sex differences in the effect of diabetes mellitus on lipoprotein triglyceride and cholesterol concentration. *New England Journal of Medicine, 311,* 953–959.

Weiner, D. A., Ryan, T. J., McCabe, C. H., et al. (1979). Exercise stress testing correlations among history of angina, ST-segment response and prevalence of coronary artery disease in the Coronary Artery Surgical Study. *New England Journal of Medicine, 301,* 230–235.

Weiner, D. A., Ryan, T. J., McCabe, C. H., et al. (1987). Significance of silent myocardial during exercise testing in patients with silent ischemia. *American Journal of Cardiology, 59,* 725–729.

Werns, S. W., Shea, M. J., and Lucchesi, B. R. (1986). Free radicals and myocardial injury: Pharmacologic implications. *Circulation, 74,* 1–5.

West, K. M., Ahiya, M. S., Bennett, P. H., et al. (1983). The role of circulating glucose and triglyceride concentrations and their interactions with other "risk factors" as determinants of arterial disease in nine diabetic population samples from the WHO multinational study. *Diabetes Care, 6,* 361–369.

Wilber, D. J., Garan, H., and Kelley, E. (1988). Out of hospital cardiac arrest: Role of electrophysiologic testing in the prediction of long-term outcomes. *New England Journal of Medicine, 318,* 19–24.

Williams, R. (1987). Psychologic factors in coronary artery disease: Epidemiologic evidence. *Circulation, 76* (Suppl. 1), 1-117–1-123.

Wilson, P., Garrison, R., and Castelli, W. (1985). Postmenopausal estrogen use, cigarette smoking and cardiovascular morbidity in women over 50. *New England Journal of Medicine, 313,* 1038–1043.

Zimmerman, M., and McGeachie, J. (1987). The effect of nicotine on aortic endothelium. *Atherosclerosis, 63,* 33–41.

16

Patients with Myocardial Infarction

Barbara Riegel

Acute myocardial infarction (AMI) remains the primary cause of mortality in the United States today. Cardiovascular disease accounts for approximately 45% of all deaths. Over 1.5 million people experience AMI each year, and more than a third of these die. A significant (>300,000) number of deaths occur before patients reach the hospital, a statistic inflated beyond necessity because of denial and delay by the patient (American Heart Association, 1991).

Almost 5 million AMI victims are still living (American Heart Association, 1991) and must learn to cope with chronic coronary artery disease (CAD). Recovery from AMI is difficult; as many as 88% of the patients experience emotional distress and family turmoil after AMI (Doehrman, 1977; Razin, 1982). Many patients fail to return to work when physiologically capable of doing so (Brown and Munford, 1983–1984; Cay et al., 1972; Razin, 1982). Most AMI patients do not return to their previous levels of sexual activity (Razin, 1982). The monetary cost is also high. It is estimated that cardiovascular disease will cost our society over $101 billion in 1991 including fees for professional services, hospital and nursing home facilities, medications, and lost occupational income (American Heart Association, 1991).

The incidence of AMI increases with age. In men, AMI is uncommon before the age of 40 years, but 45% of all events occur before age 65 (American Heart Association, 1991). CAD is the leading cause of death in women (Murdaugh, 1990); one in three women has some form of cardiovascular disease and 73% of acute events occur after age 65 (American Heart Association, 1991). Most events occur later in life, perhaps due to a protective effect of estrogen (Murdaugh, 1990). This difference in age of onset

creates the mistaken impression that CAD is a disease of males.

This chapter describes AMI as an evolving, dynamic event occurring over hours or days. This health crisis has significant physiologic sequelae and long-term psychological implications. Clinical presentation, physical assessment, and diagnostic findings are described following a discussion of the pathophysiology. Medical and nursing management techniques are aimed at early identification of physiologic changes with the goal of limiting infarct size through maintenance of balance between myocardial oxygen supply and demand. Psychological adjustment is facilitated through early mobilization, control of symptoms, and stress reduction techniques such as patient education.

PATHOPHYSIOLOGY
Acute Event

As discussed in Chapter 15, coronary artery disease refers to a progressive accumulation of plaque on the arterial wall or intima. The hemodynamic significance of plaques is not usually apparent until 70% of the arterial cross-sectional area has been compromised. At that time symptoms may result during times of increased myocardial oxygen demand (e.g., exertion, a heavy meal, anxiety) because of inadequate oxygen supply.

Until recently, AMI was thought to occur when the atheromatous plaque grew large enough to totally occlude the coronary artery. It is now recognized that physiologic events cause disruption of the intima covering the plaque (Davies and Thomas, 1985).

Thrombosis forms (DeWood et al., 1980), coronary covering the plaque (Davies and Thomas, 1985). spasm may occur, and blood flow to that area of the heart ceases. Infarction results from the mechanical obstruction caused by thrombosis, plaque rupture, dissection, and sometimes spasm.

The events triggering plaque disruption and thrombus formation are not yet fully understood, but two major theories have been proposed. Constantinides (1966) first suggested that forces within the arterial lumen such as increased arterial pressure cause hemorrhage into the plaque. More recently, Barger and associates (1984) suggested the opposite mechanism, i.e., that rupture of the abnormal vaso vasorum within an atherosclerotic plaque may extend into the lumen. Whichever sequence of events is correct, myocardial damage results from physical blockage of the lumen with thrombus in 80% to 90% of cases (DeWood et al., 1980). Thrombosis is more likely to occur in the presence of severe atherosclerotic narrowing, coronary spasm brought on by plaque rupture, or hypercoagulability (Muller and Tofler, 1988).

Information from the Multicenter Investigation of Limitation of Infarct Size (MILIS) provided some clues about the events precipitating infarction (Rude and MILIS Study Group, 1985). Their data, supported by evidence from other studies, demonstrate that AMI is most likely to occur between 6 A.M. and noon. Muller and Tofler (1988) suggest that plaque rupture may be associated with the morning rise in systemic arterial pressure of 20 to 30 mm Hg or increases in coronary vascular tone associated with normal circadian rhythm. Thrombus formation may be related to elevated plasma epinephrine and norepinephrine levels that accompany assumption of the upright posture upon awakening. Sympathetic stimulation may increase platelet aggregability. Other natural processes associated with awakening and arising that may predispose to thrombus formation include low fibrinolytic activity, high hematocrit and blood viscosity, and increased heparin metabolism in patients receiving heparin infusion (Muller and Tofler, 1988) (Fig. 16–1).

Collateral Circulation

One major factor influencing the incidence and severity of AMI is the presence of collateral coronary circulation. Piek and Becker (1988) found that the amount of collateral vessel development determined whether an AMI involved only the subendocardium or the entire transmural area. Further, ventricular function following AMI is influenced by the extent of the collateral vessels (Rentrop et al., 1988).

Factors influencing collateral vessel development have been a mystery. In a recent study of 29 CAD patients, Rentrop and colleagues (1988) found that hemodynamically important coronary artery occlusions were associated with functional collateral vessels. All patients with narrowing of more than 70% had collateral vessels capable of maintaining circulation to the jeopardized myocardium, while most with coronary stenoses of less than 70% did not have collateral vessels. Further, collateral function was directly related to the severity of stenosis; more severely narrowed arteries had more functional collaterals.

These data have important clinical implications. Patients experiencing coronary occlusion in an artery with less than 70% narrowing probably have no collateral support and therefore suffer severe infarction, hemodynamic compromise, and potential death. Patients with less severe disease in whom total coronary occlusion develops as a complication of percutaneous transluminal coronary angioplasty (PTCA) are at more risk than patients with narrowings of more than 70% (Epstein, 1988).

The time available for beneficial reperfusion following occlusion is also influenced by the presence of collateral vessels. Patients with more than 70% narrowing may tolerate coronary occlusion without transmural infarction and hemodynamic compromise longer than patients with occlusion of a less severe stenosis. Epstein (1988) notes that these data also explain why sudden cardiac death and left ventricular aneurysm occur so commonly when AMI is the first symptom of CAD.

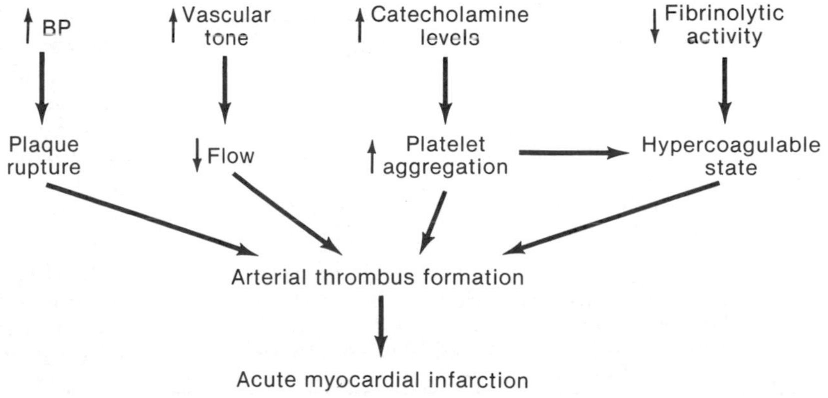

FIGURE 16–1. Potentially adverse physiologic changes occurring in the morning. (Redrawn by permission of The New England Journal of Medicine, *313*:1315, 1985.)

Evolution of Acute Myocardial Infarction

Thus far, AMI has been described as an acute event following chronic atherosclerotic plaque formation involving plaque rupture and thrombus formation that occludes blood flow in the coronary artery. Circadian periodicity data suggest that changes in blood pressure, coronary tone, and coagulability may be associated with sudden occlusion. Collateral circulation, with its potential to protect against dire outcomes, develops over time in response to hemodynamically significant narrowing.

Occlusion of a coronary artery may cause a full-thickness, transmural AMI or a non–Q wave, nontransmural (formerly called subendocardial) AMI. Transmural AMI results most frequently from total arterial occlusion. Nontransmural AMI occurs during incomplete occlusion or early spontaneous thrombolysis, secondary to illnesses that increase oxygen demand suddenly, e.g., pulmonary embolism (Pasternak et al., 1988), and in the presence of collateral circulation (Piek and Becker, 1988).

Coronary arterial occlusion most frequently results in necrosis of an area of the left ventricle or septum. (See Table 16–1 for the site of AMI typically associated with occlusion of specific coronary arteries.) Interestingly, about two-thirds of all left ventricular transmural infarcts also involve the right ventricle (RV) (Anderson et al., 1987). Isolated right ventricular AMI occurs in only 3% to 5% of cases, perhaps because of lower RV oxygen demands, enhanced collateral circulation, and a thinner RV wall, which allows nutrients to be derived from blood in the RV chamber. Situations in which RV oxygen demands are increased, as in chronic lung failure or right ventricular hypertrophy, are associated with right ventricular AMI. Atrial infarction occurs in 7% to 17% of left ventricular (LV) infarcts, usually involving the thin right atrial appendage (Pasternak et al., 1988).

Left ventricular function and prognosis are usually worse after anterior compared with posterior infarcts of equal size. The poor prognosis following anterior AMI may be due to different involvement of the RV and LV walls. Autopsy data suggest that posterior infarcts typically involve the RV more than anterior infarcts; anterior infarcts involve more of the major pump, the LV. Therefore, anterior infarcts compromise cardiac output and negatively affect prognosis more than posterior infarcts (Anderson et al., 1987).

Total occlusion of a coronary artery does not always result in AMI. Collateral circulation (Piek and Becker, 1988; Rentrop et al., 1988), level of myocardial metabolism, rate of occlusive development, quantity of myocardium supplied by the vessel (Pasternak et al., 1988), and the presence and location of other stenoses (Rentrop et al., 1988) all influence the evolution of AMI. For instance, occlusions of the right coronary artery (RCA) or the mid or distal left anterior descending (LAD) artery are less likely to cause severe left ventricular dysfunction than occlusions of the proximal LAD (Rentrop et al., 1988). A few (<5%) AMI occur in the absence of any significant atherosclerotic obstruction, perhaps due to embolus or prolonged spasm (Pasternak et al., 1988). Cocaine use has also been shown to cause AMI (Cregler and Mark, 1985).

Blockage of a coronary artery produces ischemia immediately. Ischemia is defined as oxygen deprivation accompanied by inadequate removal of metabolites because of inadequate perfusion (Braunwald and Sobel, 1988). Ischemia results from an actual decrease in blood flow (oxygen supply) or an increase in oxygen demand when supply is fixed. When blockage is total, infarction evolves over approximately 3 hours (Ritchie et al., 1988), although the anatomic and hemodynamic factors previously mentioned may slow the process. Edema and color changes in the heart are evident 6 hours after occlusion. A decrease in wall thickness is evident 8 to 10 days following the acute event due to necrotic tissue removal by mononuclear cells (Pasternak et al., 1988).

Infarct extension refers to early recurrence and occurs within the first 10 days in approximately 10% of AMI patients (Rude and MILIS Study Group, 1985). Infarct expansion refers to ventricular remodeling, an event that occurs in approximately 50% of transmural infarcts in the early weeks (Pasterak et al., 1988). This remodeling process causes changes in left ventricular size, shape, and wall thickness that increase the size of the infarct. Expansion seems to be related to preinfarction wall thickness and may be the cause of myocardial rupture. Left ventricular aneurysm occurs in 12% to 15% of patients who survive AMI (Pasternak et al., 1988), especially in patients with poor collateral circulation (Forman et al., 1986). Firm scar tissue forms from the periphery of the necrotic area into the center within 2 to 3 months.

Systolic function of the LV is altered immediately following the acute event because of abnormal contraction patterns of the damaged myocardium. Significant diastolic dysfunction occurs even in patients without significant LV systolic dysfunction (Seals et al., 1988). Ejection fraction is reduced when more

---

TABLE 16–1. Typical Site of Infarction According to Occluded Coronary Artery

Left anterior descending coronary artery
    Anterior left ventricle
    Apical left ventricle
    Ventricular septum
    Anterolateral left ventricle
    Left ventricular papillary muscles
    Inferoapical left ventricular wall
Left circumflex artery
    Lateral left ventricle
    Inferoposterior left ventricle
Right coronary artery
    Inferoposterior left ventricle
    Inferior septum
    Posteromedial left ventricular papillary muscles
    Portions of the right ventricle

than 10% of the LV contracts abnormally. Left ventricular end-diastolic pressure (LVEDP) and volume are elevated when 15% of the LV is involved. When 20% to 25% of the LV contracts abnormally, congestive heart failure results. Cardiogenic shock and often death accompany loss of 40% or more of functional LV (Pasternak et al., 1988). Dilation of the LV is an early compensatory mechanism in patients with left ventricular failure (LVF) (Seals et al., 1988). LV dilation facilitates cardiac emptying initially, conserving myocardial oxygen consumption (MVO_2) but eventually increases MVO_2. Some improvement in wall motion occurs with healing because of scarring and stiffness unless infarct extension occurs.

Limitation of Infarct Size

Data relating the percentage of LV involvement to ejection fraction demonstrate that infarct size is directly associated with prognosis and quality of life. Fifty per cent of AMI patients with large infarcts and severe heart failure (ejection fraction <30%) die within 5 years (Shah et al., 1980). Patients with a poor ejection fraction have little energy for the activities of daily living. Therefore, limitation of infarct size, not merely prevention of complications, is the goal of AMI patient care.

Limitation of infarct size is achieved primarily by maintaining a balance of myocardial oxygen supply and demand during the evolution of the acute event. Interventions designed to increase oxygen supply are most effective in limiting infarct size. Minimizing oxygen demand can delay the evolution of the infarct until more definitive interventions can be implemented (Genton and Sobel, 1987).

Myocardial oxygen supply is limited by coronary blood flow, oxygen content of arterial blood, and the amount of oxygen extracted from blood by the heart (Karliner, 1981). Coronary blood flow is the most important of these factors because a high percentage of oxygen is normally extracted through the coronary

circulation. The myocardium requires a blood flow of 60 to 90 mL/minute per 100 g of heart tissue (Braunwald and Sobel, 1988) and consumes 8 to 10 mL of oxygen/minute per 100 g of oxygen under basal conditions, an amount that can increase several times during exercise (Berne and Levy, 1986). Little additional oxygen is available for extraction from cardiac venous blood (Berne and Levy, 1986). The oxygen-carrying capacity of the blood cannot be increased significantly unless considerable hypoxemia is present (Karliner, 1981).

Myocardial oxygen demand is determined by wall tension, contractility, and heart rate. Ventricular wall tension is influenced by heart size, or preload, and left ventricular systolic pressure, or afterload. Preload is defined as the rest fiber length (Lakatta, 1987) due to the volume of blood in the ventricles at the end of diastole, immediately prior to systole (Lewis, 1983). Afterload is defined as the tension, force, or stress acting on ventricular fibers after the onset of shortening during systole (Braunwald et al., 1988). Afterload is strongly influenced by and often inaccurately thought to be synonymous with arterial pressure or systemic vascular resistance (SVR).

The degree of myocardial fiber shortening or contractility influences myocardial oxygen demand to the same extent as wall tension (Braunwald and Sobel, 1988). Lakatta (1987) notes that contractility and preload can no longer theoretically be considered independent determinants of myocardial performance because contraction depends on fiber length and varies throughout contraction as fiber length varies.

Heart rate also influences myocardial oxygen requirements. Heart rate is a function of heart size. The optimum frequency of heart rate at which contraction efficiency is ideal can be estimated for any heart size (Levine, 1987). Increases in heart rate increase myocardial oxygen consumption by increasing both the frequency of wall tension development and contractility (Braunwald and Sobel, 1988) (Fig. 16–2).

Methods of limiting infarct size focus on increasing

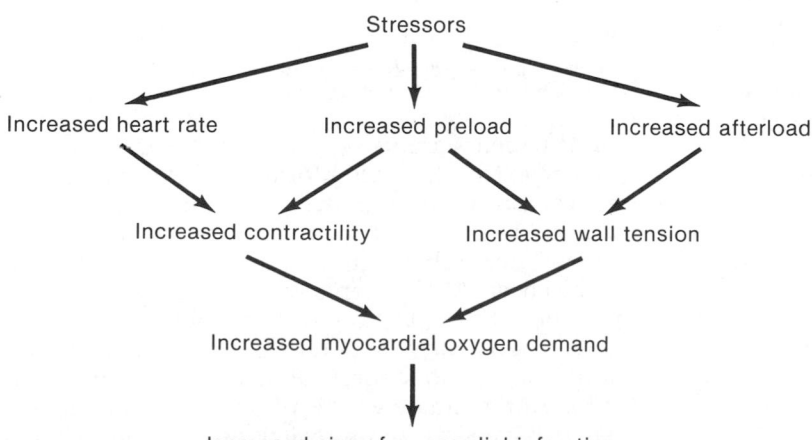

FIGURE 16–2. Effect of physiologic and psychological stressors on myocardial oxygen demand. Myocardial oxygen demand is determined by wall tension—a function of preload and afterload—contractility, and heart rate.

the oxygen supply by increasing the flow of well-oxygenated blood through the coronary arteries. Techniques that decrease myocardial oxygen demand include optimizing preload and contractility, and decreasing afterload and heart rate.

CLINICAL PRESENTATION

A significant proportion (20% to 60%) of AMI patients experience a prodromal period prior to infarction. This prodrome is usually characterized by classic angina pectoris that is unrelieved by rest or limitations on activity. According to Pasternak and colleagues (1988), patients experiencing a prodrome can be divided into thirds based on the length of the prodrome:

■ One-third have symptoms for 1 to 4 weeks prior.
■ One-third have symptoms for a week or less.
■ One-third have symptoms for less than 24 hours.

Chest pain of variable intensity is the most common presenting symptom of the AMI patient. According to Uretsky and colleagues (1977), 73% to 99% of AMI patients have chest pain. Hofgren and associates (1988) found that patients with larger infarcts required significantly ($p < .01$) more morphine sulfate during the first 3 hours of hospitalization. These data suggest that the severity of pain may predict infarct size and prognosis, a conclusion supported by earlier findings of Ledwich and Mondragon (1980).

Most AMI patients describe the chest pain as severe and intolerable, lasting more than 30 minutes and sometimes hours. Adjectives used to describe the pain of AMI are listed in Table 16–2. The pain of AMI is usually similar in character to that of an individual's preinfarction angina pectoris; therefore, it is helpful to determine what the patient's angina is usually like.

Although the pain of AMI is typically retrosternal, it often involves the entire thorax, particularly the left anterior chest. It may radiate down the ulnar aspect of the left arm, causing tingling or numbness in the wrist, hand, or fingers. Atypical chest pain

---

TABLE 16–2. Adjectives Used to Describe the Pain of Acute Myocardial Infarction

Boring
Burning
Choking
Compressing
Constricting
Crushing
Heavy
Knifelike
Oppressive
Squeezing
Stabbing
Tightness
Viselike

---

involves the shoulders, upper extremities, neck, jaw, teeth, and interscapular region.

The pain of angina pectoris and AMI is due to stimulation of nerve endings in ischemic or injured myocardium (Malliani and Lombardi, 1982). Necrotic tissue is not painful; pain indicates that viable myocardium is present. Pain that is referred to the left arm, for instance, probably reflects excitation of afferent sympathetic and vagal fibers (Malliani, 1986).

Many patients describe their discomfort as "indigestion," associating epigastric symptoms with a gastrointestinal disorder. Approximately 50% of AMI patients experience symptoms of nausea and vomiting along with the pain, probably due to vagal stimulation or bradycardia and hypotension due to activation of the Bezold-Jarisch reflex (Braunwald and Sobel, 1988). Nausea and vomiting are especially common in patients with inferior wall infarction. Other associated symptoms include diaphoresis, pallor, weakness, diarrhea, palpitations, shortness of breath, dizziness, and a sense of impending doom. Inferior infarction is occasionally associated with hiccups, which are thought to be due to diaphragmatic irritation. Syncope is reported rarely (Hofgren et al., 1988).

Approximately 20% to 60% of infarctions are unrecognized because there are no symptoms ("silent") or because the symptoms are not recognized as infarction. Pasternak and colleagues (1988) suggest that about 30% of infarcts are truly silent and may be associated with diabetes mellitus or hypertension. Deanfield and colleagues (1983) found that 73% of ischemic attacks occurring during activities of daily living were silent. Falcone and co-workers (1988) found that 48% of 108 patients with documented CAD had silent ischemia during exercise testing. Electrical dental stimulation of the same 108 subjects revealed that the majority (71%) of the silent ischemia group did not experience dental pain, even at maximal stimulation, a response significantly different ($p < .0005$) from the subjects in the exercise-induced chest pain group. These data suggest that a generalized hyposensitivity to pain may partly explain the occurrence of silent myocardial ischemia.

PHYSICAL ASSESSMENT

AMI patients are usually anxious, distressed, restless, and extremely uncomfortable. Facial expressions may communicate anguish, suffering, and perhaps fear. A clenched fist held against the chest is a common nonverbal sign of chest pain, as is massaging the chest. AMI patients with pain may shift about in the bed, trying to find a comfortable position.

Vital signs vary depending on the site of the infarct, size, and degree of left ventricular failure (LVF). Approximately 50% of patients with inferior infarcts have signs of an overriding parasympathetic response with hypotension or bradycardia; about 50% of those with anterior infarcts have a sympathetic response with hypertension or tachycardia (Pasternak et al., 1988). It may be difficult to discern whether the etiology of hypotension is inferior infarction or impending cardiogenic shock; other physical findings discussed below may help to make the distinction. Hypertension due to sympathetic stimulation during AMI rarely exceeds 200/110 (Pasternak et al., 1988).

Most AMI patients with uncomplicated illness are normotensive and have sinus tachycardia at 100–110 beats/minute. Tachycardia may lower stroke volume and cause a slight decrease in systolic blood pressure (BP) and a rise in diastolic BP. The heart rate returns to normal after pain and anxiety are relieved. Premature ventricular contractions (PVCs) are common, occurring in more than 95% of AMI patients (Pasternak et al., 1988).

Fever due to tissue necrosis is common and may reach 101° to 102°F rectally. Fever begins 24 to 48 hours after AMI onset and returns to normal within 7 or 8 days. Respiratory rate may be elevated during pain or anxiety or because of LVF. This finding may be masked by the respiratory depression caused by opiates. Patients with LVF and sympathetic stimulation may be frankly dyspneic and may complain of suffocating. Frothy, pink sputum indicates impending pulmonary edema.

Jugular venous pressure (JVP) elevation results from right heart diastolic pressure elevation such as occurs with extensive RV infarct involvement. JVP is usually normal in AMI patients, but abnormalities may warn of impending complications. For instance, a prominent "a" wave in the jugular venous pulse contour is evidence of pulmonary hypertension, which may be caused by LVF or decreased left ventricular compliance. Moist crackles heard during lung auscultation also suggest LVF or decreased left ventricular compliance and can be used to estimate prognosis (Table 16–3). Ischemia or rupture of the right ventricular papillary muscle causes tricuspid insufficiency, which causes a tall "v" wave in the jugular venous pulse. Assessment of jugular venous pressure and pulse contour are essential in the differential diagnosis of hypotension. Hypotension with flat neck veins suggests parasympathetic stimulation associated with inferior infarcts or hypovolemia rather than cardiogenic shock.

Cardiac auscultation often reveals muffled heart sounds that become clearer as healing progresses. A fourth heart sound (S_4) immediately preceding the first heart sound is almost universal and is heard best between the left sternal border and the apex. The S_4 reflects atrial contraction and is heard because the left atrium is contracting against a noncompliant left ventricle with an elevated left ventricular end-diastolic pressure (LVEDP).

A third heart sound (S_3) is heard in patients with large transmural infarcts and extensive LV dysfunction, or with mitral regurgitation due to papillary muscle dysfunction, or with a ventricular septal defect. An S_3 is heard best at the apex with the patient in the left lateral recumbent position and is accentuated when the patient coughs. Coughing makes an S_3 more pronounced by raising pulmonary venous pressure and heart rate. These hemodynamic changes accentuate an S_3 when the ventricle is unable to accommodate the volume of LV inflow occurring during the rapid filling phase of diastole (Walsh and O'Rourke, 1981). The combination of an S_3 and an S_4, or "gallop" rhythm, is heard best at the apex and, again, may be accentuated by coughing. A third heart sound and a gallop rhythm are prognostic indicators of a severe infarction.

An uncomplicated AMI is not usually associated with a murmur, although papillary muscle dysfunction may cause a transient or persistent systolic mitral regurgitation murmur. Rupture of the head of a papillary muscle causes a prominent holosystolic murmur that should be reported to the physician immediately. The murmur is heard best at the apex, may radiate to the axilla, and may be accompanied by a thrill. A systolic murmur, heard best along the left and right sternal borders, suggests rupture of the interventricular septum.

Transient pericardial friction rubs occur in 7% to 20% of AMI patients and are more common in transmural infarcts (Pasternak et al., 1988). Friction rubs are heard best along the left sternal border during the second or third day following an anterior or inferoposterior transmural infarct. Rubs may be

---

TABLE 16–3. Killip Classification of Patients with Acute Myocardial Infarction

	Definition	Patients with Acute Myocardial Infarction Admitted to CCU in This Category (%)	Approximate Mortality (%)*
Class I	Absence of rales over the lung fields and absence of S_3	30–40	8
Class II	Rales over 50% or less of the lung fields or the presence of an S_3	30–50	30
Class III	Rales over more than 50% of the lung fields (frequently pulmonary edema)	5–10	44
Class IV	Shock	10	80–100

*Estimated mortality in the 1960s. Mortality still rises with increased class, although the values in each class are lower today than in the 1960s.
Adapted from Killip, T., and Kimball, J. T. (1967). *American Journal of Cardiology*, 20, 457; from Braunwald, E. B. (Ed.) (1988). *Heart Disease: A Textbook of Cardiovascular Medicine* (3rd ed.). Philadelphia, W.B. Saunders.

heard during the first day or as late as 2 weeks following the acute event. An extensive infarct may cause a loud and persistent friction rub that lasts for several days.

Abdominal examination may reveal hepatomegaly in patients with right ventricular failure due to right ventricular infarct or prolonged LVF. Hepatomegaly indicates a poor prognosis. Peripheral edema suggests chronic right ventricular failure. Following bedrest, edema can be noted in the sacrum and scrotum, not the ankles.

Cardiogenic Shock

Cardiogenic shock occurs in about 10% of AMI patients and is associated with a mortality of 85% to 100% that has not improved during the past 30 years (Killip and Kimball, 1967; Weil et al., 1988). The onset and severity of cardiogenic shock are directly associated with the amount of damaged myocardium. The majority of patients with shock have lost approximately 40% of the left ventricular pump function (Weil et al., 1988).

The physical presentation of AMI patients with cardiogenic shock differs from that of stable AMI patients. These patients usually lie listlessly, moving little because of lack of energy. The face is pale, and the skin is cool and clammy with a bluish, mottled appearance. Peripheral cyanosis of the nailbeds or the perioral area may be evident. The patient may

be anxious or fearful. Poor cerebral perfusion may cause confusion or disorientation.

Blood pressure with cardiogenic shock is, by definition, 90 mm Hg systolic or lower. Respiratory rate is normal. JVP is elevated. Pulsus alternans may be evident on carotid pulse palpation. Invasive hemodynamic monitoring is essential for these patients. Prognosis can be estimated using arterial blood lactate levels (a byproduct of anaerobic metabolism), cardiac output or stroke work, and arterial pressure, in that order (Weil et al., 1988). According to Afifi and colleagues (1974), the following findings are associated with mortality approaching 100%:

- Lactate levels exceeding 4 mM/liter
- Cardiac index of less than 2.2 liters/minute/m²
- Arterial resistance of greater than 2000 dyne/seconds/cm^{-5}
- Left ventricular filling pressure of greater than 18 mm Hg
- Mean arterial pressure of less than 60 mm Hg after fluid challenge

LABORATORY FINDINGS

Three enzymes are released into the blood during AMI: creatine kinase (CK), lactic dehydrogenase (LDH), and (serum) glutamic oxaloacetic transferase (SGOT). Of these, CK is by far the most specific and useful enzyme; SGOT is rarely used today. Table 16–4 summarizes the times of initial elevation, peak,

---

TABLE 16–4. Elevation Times and False-Positive Results Associated with Cardiac Enzymes

Enzyme	Initial	Peak	Return to Baseline	Causes of False-Positive Results
Creatine kinase (CK)	4–8 hr	8–58 hr Average 24 hr	3–4 days	Muscle disease Alcohol intoxication Diabetes mellitus Skeletal muscle trauma Vigorous exercise Convulsions Intramuscular injections Thoracic outlet syndrome Pulmonary embolism Hypothyroidism
Lactic dehydrogenase (LDH)	24–48 hr	3–6 days	8–14 days	Hemolysis Leukemia Liver disease Hepatic congestion Renal disease Neoplasms Pulmonary embolism Myocarditis Skeletal muscle disease Shock
Serum glutamic oxaloacetic transaminase (SGOT)	8–12 hr	18–36 hr	3–4 days	Primary liver disease Hepatic congestion Skeletal muscle disease Intramuscular injections Pulmonary embolism Shock Pericarditis

return to normal, and conditions causing false-positive elevations of the three enzymes discussed.

Creatine kinase, formerly creatinine phosphokinase (CPK), is composed of three isoenzymes: MM, found in both skeletal and cardiac muscle; BB, found in brain and kidney; and MB, found in cardiac muscle. MB-CK is the primary diagnostic enzyme for AMI. It should be noted that small amounts of MB-CK are found in the small intestines, tongue, diaphragm, uterus, and prostate. Therefore, trauma or surgery to any of these organs as well as strenuous exercise or cardiopulmonary resuscitation may cause elevations of MB-CK that do not signify AMI. Total CK values normally range from 40 to 180 IU/liter, lower for females. Isoenzyme MB-CK levels should be less than 5% when analyzed by standard methods, or up to 3.7 IU/liter using radioimmunometric assay (RIA). Minor elevations of MB-CK without subsequent diagnosis of AMI may indicate ischemia or microinfarctions (Pasternak et al., 1988). Peak CK elevations vary greatly and are probably due to dynamic infarct evolution. Peak CK values occur earlier than expected following spontaneous or therapeutic thrombolysis, making estimation of infarct size difficult. Cox and colleagues (1987) suggest that early peak MB-CK values indicate a subset of high-risk patients who have residual jeopardized myocardium. In the near future, isoforms of MB-CK will become generally available; these isoforms will allow diagnosis of AMI within minutes.

Isoenzymes of LDH, (LDH$_{1-5}$), have also been identified. The heart contains primarily LDH$_1$; if LDH$_1$ is higher than LDH$_{2-5}$ in a nonhemolyzed sample, a cardiac process is probably occurring.

Other laboratory abnormalities associated with AMI include hyperglycemia and myoglobinemia. Lipid levels are altered by stress, intravenous glucose, and recumbency. Cholesterol and triglyceride analyses should be deferred until approximately 8 weeks following AMI (Smith, 1987). Erythrocyte sedimentation rate (ESR) is frequently elevated, as is the white blood count (WBC). WBC elevations may be due to tissue necrosis or adrenal glucocorticoids released during the stress response. Hematocrit increases due to hemoconcentration.

DIAGNOSTIC PROCEDURES

Electrocardiographic Findings

The electrocardiogram (ECG) can contribute useful information to the diagnosis of AMI. However, a wide variety of conditions mimic infarction (Table 16–5), thereby limiting the specificity of the ECG. Factors such as extent of injury, age and site of the infarction, conduction defects, previous injury, acute pericarditis, electrolyte imbalance, and cardioreactive medications affect the ECG and also limit its usefulness in the diagnosis of AMI (Pasternak et al., 1988). AMI is best diagnosed using a combination of clinical

TABLE 16–5. Conditions Mimicking Infarction on Electrocardiograms

Ventricular hypertrophy
Conduction disturbances
Wolff-Parkinson-White syndrome
Dilated or hypertrophic cardiomyopathy
Myocarditis
Pneumothorax
Pulmonary embolism
Traumatic heart disease
Intracranial hemorrhage
Hyperkalemia
Pericarditis
Early repolarization
Ventricular aneurysm
Prinzmetal angina

Data from Pasternak et al., 1988; Fisch, 1988.

findings including the ECG but relying primarily on enzyme changes.

T wave changes occur with ischemia. With injury to the myocardium, ST segment displacement occurs. Cellular death results in persistent Q waves. Transient Q waves may be caused by angina pectoris or electrolyte imbalance (Pasternak et al., 1988). Serial tracings are diagnostic of AMI in only slightly more than 50% of patients (Fisch, 1988). The first ECGs taken following the onset of symptoms in 40% to 50% of AMI patients may be either normal or have the following nonspecific abnormalities:

■ Subtle ST and T wave changes
■ Isolated T wave abnormalities
■ Transient normalization of T, ST, or QRS changes
■ Masking of conduction defects (Fisch, 1988)

The classic ECG pattern of AMI includes abnormalities of the T wave that progress to ST segment elevation in the leads facing the injured area and reciprocal ST depression in the opposite leads. The QRS amplitude decreases and evolves into a QS pattern. Q waves appear immediately, within hours, or perhaps not for days. Q waves are thought to represent electrically inert myocardium that fails to contribute to the normal electrical forces of contracting myocardium as measured by vector (Fisch, 1988). Q waves had been thought to occur in only transmural infarcts, but approximately 50% of nontransmural infarcts are now known to have Q waves (Fisch, 1988). Non–Q wave patterns suggest that the damage has not involved the entire transmural wall. ECG findings typical of occlusion of specific coronary arteries are listed in Table 16–6.

The site and type (transmural versus nontransmural) of infarct have prognostic significance. In a study of 471 first AMI patients, Stone and associates (1988) found that anterior infarcts were substantially larger and were associated with lower LV ejection fractions, a higher incidence of heart failure, and more ectopy, in-hospital deaths, and total cumulative cardiac mortality compared to patients with inferior AMIs. Patients with Q wave patterns had larger

TABLE 16–6. Sites of Infarcts and Corresponding Electrocardiographic Changes

Septum: V_1, V_2
Anterior wall: V_3, V_4
Anteroseptal surface: V_{1-6}
Lateral wall: I, aV_1, V_6
Anterolateral wall: I, aV_1, V_{3-6}
Extensive anterior infarct: I, aV_1, V_{1-6}
High lateral wall: I, aV_1
Inferior wall: II, III, aVF
Anteroinferior or apical wall: II, III, aV_1, and one or more V_{1-4}
Posterior wall: prominent R wave in V_1 or V_2

Data from Fisch, C. (1988). In E. B. Braunwald (Ed.), *Heart disease: A textbook of cardiovascular medicine* (3rd ed., pp. 180–222). Philadelphia: W. B. Saunders.

infarcts, lower ejection fractions, and a higher incidence of heart failure and in-hospital deaths compared to patients with non–Q wave infarcts. Those with anterior infarcts had a poorer prognosis regardless of infarct type (Q wave versus non–Q wave). The better prognosis of patients with inferior AMIs may be due to involvement of the right ventricle and therefore less LV pump impairment.

Right ventricular infarcts are difficult to diagnose because electrical signals of the relatively thin muscle mass are usually dominated by changes in the left ventricle. ST segment elevation in V_1 and the right precordial leads V_{3R} through V_{6R} (Pasternak et al., 1988), especially V_{4R} (Fisch, 1988), may be seen with small inferior infarctions. Atrial infarctions should be suspected with changes in the PR segment or contour of the P wave. Abnormal atrial rhythms such as atrial flutter, atrial fibrillation, wandering atrial pacemaker, or atrioventricular (AV) nodal rhythms also suggest atrial infarction (Pasternak et al., 1988).

Dysrhythmias are extremely common following AMI. It has been estimated that 72% to 96% of coronary care patients experience dysrhythmias (Pasternak et al., 1988). The incidence is highest in patients seen early following the onset of symptoms. Ventricular ectopy is found in 57% of AMI patients and therefore is the most common dysrhythmia associated with AMI. About half of patients with ventricular tachycardia (VT) develop ventricular fibrillation (VF); 40% of those with R-on-T phenomenon develop VF (Norris and Singh, 1982).

Sinus bradycardia (SB) is also very common in the early stages of AMI; 25% to 40% of AMI patients have SB within the first hour of symptoms (O'Doherty et al., 1983). Sinus tachycardia is seen in 41% of AMI patients (Norris and Singh, 1982). Sinus tachycardia is always a symptom, not a primary dysrhythmia. Conditions causing sinus tachycardia, e.g., pain, anxiety, fever, hypotension, medications, and dehydration, should be suspected and treated.

Particular conduction disturbances and dysrhythmias should be suspected based on the site of infarction. First and second degree heart block, type I, are common, transient, and self-limiting effects of infe-

rior infarction. Mobitz type II second degree heart block is a rare but serious complication of anterior infarcts. Bradycardia is more common in inferoposterior infarcts than in anterior ones. Sinus tachycardia is common in patients with anterior AMI. Ventricular tachycardia occurs with equal frequency in inferior and anterior infarcts but is less common in patients with nontransmural AMI.

Clinical lore suggests that AMI patients experience dysrhythmias most commonly during sleep. In a review of the literature, Landis (1988) found that both NREM and REM* sleep states were associated with increased ectopy and angina episodes in cardiac patients. Rhythm disturbances were most common in cardiac patients with neurologic abnormalities and sleep apnea syndromes. No typical pattern of dysrhythmias during sleep has been found.

Radiographic Findings

The chest x-ray is useful in diagnosing heart failure or cardiomegaly in patients with AMI. However, pulmonary vascular markings due to LVF do not appear immediately. Evidence of pulmonary edema on a chest x-ray is found approximately 12 hours after left ventricular filling pressures rise. Further, pulmonary vascular markings may still be found on x-rays after pulmonary edema has been treated successfully because accumulated fluid takes a day or two to be reabsorbed. Cardiomegaly is evidence of impaired ventricular function and suggests a prior AMI or chronic disease causing left ventricular dilation such as aortic or mitral regurgitation or cardiomyopathy.

Cardiac Imaging

A variety of techniques are used to visualize cardiac structures noninvasively. Only the techniques used commonly today and those with great potential for the future are mentioned here.

ECHOCARDIOGRAPHY

M-mode echocardiography is useful for assessing function of the posterior left ventricular wall and the interventricular septum; small segments of the anterior wall also can be visualized. This type of echocardiography is effective in diagnosing abnormal left ventricular wall motion, LVF, and pericardial effusions.

Two-dimensional echocardiography can be used to visualize a much larger portion of the left ventricle than M-mode. Two-dimensional techniques can be used to diagnose abnormal regional wall motion, especially in patients with transmural infarctions. Estimates of left ventricular wall function obtained from two-dimensional echocardiograms correlate well with those obtained during angiography (Pasternak et al., 1988). AMI diagnostic specificity with

---

*NREM, non–rapid eye movement; REM, rapid eye movement.

two-dimensional echocardiography is poor, however, because both ischemic and infarcted myocardium contract poorly.

Two-dimensional echocardiography is useful in the diagnosis of mechanical complications of AMI including:

- Left ventricular aneurysm and pseudoaneurysm
- Ventricular septal defect
- Mitral regurgitation
- Myocardial rupture
- Papillary muscle or chordae tendineae rupture
- Pericardial effusion
- Left ventricular thrombus (Pasternak et al., 1988)

The addition of color Doppler to the two-dimensional echocardiogram can provide quantification of flow, cardiac output, shunts, mitral and tricuspid regurgitation, and ventricular septal defects.

RADIONUCLIDE ANGIOGRAPHY

Technetium-99m pyrophosphate is the substance currently used to detect a recent AMI using radionuclide angiography. Pyrophosphate binds to free calcium in the necrotic myocardium, resulting in a "hot spot" showing the area of infarct (Gawlinski, 1988). If the test is performed within a week after AMI it is extremely accurate as a method of diagnosing a transmural infarct. The scan reverts to normal within a week after the event.

PERFUSION SCINTIGRAPHY

First pass imaging of the LV following injection of technetium-99m allows calculation of the ejection fraction without the need for cardiac catheterization. Subsequent information can be gained during the same or a separate procedure by gated cardiac blood pool imaging. In multiple gated acquisition (MUGA) scanning, motion films are generated that allow evaluation of regional wall motion and ejection fraction. MUGA can also be performed during exercise for evaluation of changes in cardiac function and ejection fraction (Gawlinski, 1988).

MAGNETIC RESONANCE IMAGING

Magnetic resonance imaging (MRI), formerly called nuclear magnetic resonance, is a noninvasive technique that produces high-resolution tomographic and three-dimensional images. These images provide information about cardiac structure and blood flow (Fahey and Riegel, 1989). Although not commonly used for this purpose, MRI can detect, localize, and size an infarct. Future applications of MRI may include judging the severity of ischemia and myocardial perfusion as well as the transition from ischemia to injury. MRI can be used to quantify chamber size and identify jeopardized myocardium, evaluate segmental wall motion, detect abnormalities such as edema, fibrosis, wall thinning, and hypertrophy (Gawlinski, 1988; Higgins, 1988).

POSITRON EMISSION TOMOGRAPHY

At this time positron emission tomographic (PET) scanning is primarily a research tool used to assess regional perfusion and myocardial metabolism noninvasively through direct measurement of fuel uptake and use. This procedure has advantages compared to conventional radionuclide studies, which allow assessment of only perfusion and cardiac performance.

PET scanning can localize and facilitate understanding of ischemia in discrete areas of myocardium resulting from an imbalance of oxygen supply and demand (Holman, 1988). During normal aerobic myocardial metabolism, free fatty acids are the energy substrate. The amount of free fatty acids that are metabolized is proportional to increases in MVO_2. Therefore, measures of free fatty acid metabolism can provide information about MVO_2 during ischemia. Glucose is utilized by the heart as an energy substrate during anaerobic metabolism or when high glucose levels are present. Measures of myocardial glucose uptake may allow prediction of ischemic myocardium viability (Gawlinski, 1988). PET can also provide information about both the size and extent of infarction.

Cardiac Catheterization

Cardiac catheterization with angiography is frequently performed following AMI to determine the extent of underlying coronary atherosclerosis that is amenable to definitive intervention. Candidates for PTCA or surgical intervention require angiographic evidence of the site and severity of plaques in the coronary arteries. The incidence of complications associated with the procedure is extremely low, varying according to patient characteristics, e.g., age, infarct size, hemodynamic profile, time since infarct, and experience of the cardiologist. Contraindications to the procedure are few; ventricular irritability increases risk and interferes with the quality of the test (Grossman and Barry, 1988). A prothrombin time of more than 15 seconds increases the risk of bleeding. Conditions requiring correction prior to catheterization include digitalis toxicity, severe hypertension, fever, severe LVF, gastrointestinal bleeding, anemia, renal failure, and electrolyte imbalance (Grossman and Barry, 1988). Allergic reactions to radiographic dye can be prevented by administration of diphenhydramine (Benadryl), cimetidine, or hydroxyzine pamoate (Vistaril). Patients with known dye allergy need pretreatment with methylprednisolone 14 and 2 hours prior to the procedure.

Low Level Exercise Testing

Following AMI low level exercise treadmill testing may be performed to assess the risk of early return to former activities. Patients are exercised at low work levels such as modified treadmill stages zero and one-half until 70% to 75% of their maximum heart rate or effort intolerance is achieved. Results are evaluated on the basis of ischemia, dysrhythmias, and exercise tolerance (Sheffield, 1988).

MEDICAL MANAGEMENT

Recent Changes in Management of AMI Patients

Treatment of AMI patients has changed radically in the past decade. Until recently, patients with CAD were managed primarily with pharmaceutical agents. AMI was treated conservatively in the coronary care unit with the goal of preventing complications (Riegel, 1986). Today, patients with suspected CAD often undergo diagnostic cardiac catheterization so that definitive therapy such as PTCA, atherectomy, or coronary artery bypass graft (CABG) surgery can be performed before infarction occurs. AMI patients who present at the hospital within a few hours after the onset of chest pain usually receive thrombolytic agents. They may undergo revascularization prior to discharge. Nursing care has also changed. Patients are no longer fed and restricted to bed for days on end (Riegel, 1988a).

AMI patients are being discharged earlier. Hlatky and colleagues (1988) documented, in a national survey of 1065 physicians, that stays in the coronary care unit have decreased from an average of 4.5 days in 1970 to 2.8 days in 1987. Patients were formerly hospitalized for 3 weeks but are now discharged in 9 days. Topol and associates (1988) suggest that hospital discharge at 3 days is safe and cost effective for patients with uncomplicated AMI.

Changes are also evident in the procedures and medications offered for treatment of uncomplicated AMI. Hlatky and associates (1988) documented that an exercise ECG is performed prior to hospital discharge or soon after in 72% of patients, and 81% of patients under the age of 45 years undergo angiography. Thrombolysis is used by 64% of physicians surveyed in approximately a quarter of their AMI patients.

Immediate thrombolytic therapy and early coronary angiography is now recommended in preference to the traditional conservative treatment of patients with suspected AMI (Kennedy et al., 1988). Schulman and colleagues (1988) found that coronary angiography after an AMI provided information about LAD coronary artery stenoses, ejection fraction, and segments at risk that predicted recurrent coronary events in the subsequent 5 years. These data support the need for aggressive intervention to prevent subsequent catastrophes in patients experiencing AMI. Appropriate timing of interventions is essential. In a postmorten study of 43 matched pairs of hearts, Cowan and Reichenbach (1989) found that reperfusion implemented within 3 hours of symptoms was related to accelerated healing. However, reperfusion begun after more than 4 hours was associated with significantly more hemorrhage and necrosis.

Conservative Medical Management

In spite of the recent trend toward aggressive interventional measures, some patients warrant conservative therapy with purely pharmacologic modalities. Nitrates and beta blockers have been shown to limit infarct size effectively, but only when treatment is implemented early, i.e., preferably within 4 to 6 hours.

NITRATES

Nitrates are potent vasodilators that act primarily on the capacitance circulation. Venous dilatation occurs at low plasma concentrations; arterial and then arteriolar or resistance vessel dilatation occurs at higher concentrations (Imhof et al., 1980). Nitrates have been shown to decrease dysrhythmias and death in patients with heart failure, to enhance myocardial perfusion, and to limit infarct size as measured by peak CK levels. These beneficial effects occur, however, only when care is taken to avoid hemodynamic changes that increase myocardial oxygen demand. Hemodynamic effects include decreased pulmonary artery wedge pressure and left ventricular end-diastolic and end-systolic volumes. Decreases in preload decrease cardiac output, potentially causing reflex tachycardia. Nitrates also decrease systemic arterial pressure and afterload, which may result in hypotension. Tachycardia and hypotension can both increase infarct size.

In patients with AMI with a systolic BP of greater than 95 mm Hg, nitrates can be used to decrease ischemia, lessen pain, and facilitate cardiac output by decreasing resistance to ejection or afterload. Nitrates are effective in the treatment of heart failure and pulmonary edema because of their beneficial effects on cardiac output.

Long-acting nitrates should be avoided in acute care of patients with AMI because of the potentially prolonged harmful effects on hemodynamics. One or two tablets of sublingual nitroglycerin should be administered to those with pain and an adequate BP. Patients with an inferior or right ventricular infarct should receive nitroglycerin only with extreme caution because of the potential for sudden and extreme hypotension due to inadequate preload. Severe hypotension and tachycardia due to nitrates can be treated with postural changes or reversed with intravenous atropine.

Intravenous nitroglycerin may be administered to decrease ischemia and control symptoms. One dosing protocol suggests that therapy begin with 10 μg/minute, followed by stepwise increases of the same dose (Pasternak et al., 1988) up to a maximum of approximately 200 to 250 μg/minute. Frequent monitoring of vital signs facilitates immediate detection of hypotension or tachycardia. Weaning from nitroglycerin is typically done by decreasing the dose 10 μg/minute every 10 minutes and watching for signs of angina or ST segment changes. Continued administration of intravenous nitroglycerin may result in signs of alcohol intoxication because ethanol is a common dilutant for commercial preparations (Pasternak et al., 1988). Nitrates can oxidize hemoglobin to methemoglobin, a compound that is ineffective in carrying oxygen. The major symptom of methemoglobinemia is pallor that is unimproved with oxygen therapy. Other nonspecific symptoms include dyspnea, headache, fatigue, and dizziness. A venous blood sample will appear chocolate brown even after being shaken in air (Rosenthal and Braunwald, 1988).

BETA-ADRENORECEPTOR BLOCKERS

Beta blockers have been shown to interrupt evolving infarcts, limit infarct size as measured by CK levels, and decrease the incidence of ventricular dysrhythmias (Pasternak et al., 1988). These agents are effective in reducing ischemic pain, presumably because of changes in cardiac index, stroke index, heart rate, BP, tension-time index, and free fatty acid production, all of which affect myocardial oxygen consumption. Beta blockers are recommended for patients with tachycardia and hypertension because they lower pulse rate and BP. Beta blockers are contraindicated in patients with heart failure, hypotension, bradycardia, heart block, and bronchial asthma.

One protocol recommends metoprolol in three 5-mg intravenous boluses for AMI. Following each bolus, vital signs must be assessed for 2 to 5 minutes. Any heart rate of less than 60 beats minute or a BP of less than 100 mm Hg signals the end of the protocol. If, after three boluses, the patient is hemodynamically stable 6 to 8 hours later, 50 mg of metoprolol is given orally. If the patient is still hemodynamically stable a day later, metoprolol 100 mg is given twice a day. Patients treated with beta blockers should be assessed routinely for the following signs, which may warrant drug discontinuation:

- PR interval of greater than 0.24 second
- Second or third degree heart block
- Rales in more than one-third of the lung fields
- Wheezes
- Heart rate of less than 50 beats/minute
- Systolic BP of less than 90 mm Hg
- Pulmonary artery wedge pressure of more than 20

OTHER AGENTS

A variety of other agents have been suggested as potentially effective in limiting infarct size. An ac-cumulation of intracellular calcium causes cellular dysfunction and death (Genton and Sobel, 1987). Therefore, the effect of calcium channel blockers on infarct size has been studied. Several investigators have shown that neither nifedipine or verapamil are effective in limiting infarct size (Muller et al., 1984; Roberts, 1987). Animal studies suggest that diltiazem facilitates collateral perfusion, relieves vasospasm in ischemic areas, and protects myocytes (Genton and Sobel, 1987). Diltiazem was found to prevent reinfarction over a 2-week period (p < .03) in a study of 576 patients with AMI (Roberts, 1987). At this time, only diltiazem is recommended to prevent reinfarction and severe angina after non–Q wave infarction (Roberts, 1989).

Glucose-insulin-potassium (GIK) has been debated as therapy for AMI for decades. However, little research has been done to document its effectiveness. GIK has been shown to lower plasma concentrations of free fatty acids, which in turn decreases myocardial oxygen consumption and improves ventricular performance (Pasternak et al., 1988). To date, however, no prospective randomized trials evaluating the effects of GIK on infarct size have been performed.

Glucocorticoids have been studied in treatment of AMI because of their known anti-inflammatory effects. However, a series of studies documented that steroids increase infarct size and elevate MB-CK levels. Bulkley and Roberts (1974) found a high incidence of ventricular rupture and mortality thought to be caused by steroid inhibition of healing. Corticosteroids and the nonsteroidal anti-inflammatory agents such as ibuprofen and indomethacin are contraindicated following AMI (Pasternak et al., 1988). Aspirin is not contraindicated and in fact is advocated to prevent reinfarction because of its antiplatelet activity and subsequent effect on thrombus formation.

AGGRESSIVE MEDICAL MANAGEMENT

Thrombolysis

The most effective treatment for limiting infarct size is thrombolysis (Genton and Sobel, 1987; Pasternak et al., 1988; Ross, 1988). Because 80% to 90% of AMI are the result of thrombus (DeWood et al., 1980), early reperfusion of ischemic and jeopardized myocardium can supply needed oxygen to the threatened myocardium if it is implemented early following the onset of symptoms. Washout of noxious metabolites is thought to occur during reperfusion (Genton and Sobel, 1987), although there is some evidence that reperfusion injury results from free radicals that are not eliminated (Quaal, 1986).

The largest clinical trial to date (the GISSI trial [Gruppo Italiano, 1987]) of thrombolysis with streptokinase compared to standard therapy in 11,806 patients with AMI demonstrated significant reduction in mortality when thrombolysis was implemented within 6 hours of symptoms. The earlier therapy was implemented, the lower the mortality. When streptokinase was administered within 1 hour of symptoms, premature mortality was decreased by 50%. The best results were found in patients

■ Less than 65 years of age
■ Experiencing an anterior AMI
■ Experiencing their first AMI
■ Rated low risk on the Killip scale

A recent 12-month follow-up of 98% of these patients demonstrated that the significant differences in mortality noted between the streptokinase and control groups were maintained a year later (Gruppo Italiano, 1987).

As the GISSI trial and others have demonstrated, the time elapsed between intervention and the onset of symptoms is very important because the age of the thrombus affects its ability to be lysed. Recanalization can be achieved in 75% of patients treated with a thrombolytic agent within 1 hour (Genton and Sobel, 1987). Although most authors advocate the institution of thrombolytic therapy within 3 hours of symptoms (Genton and Sobel, 1987; Ritchie et al., 1988), later thrombolysis is harmful (Cowan and Reichenbach, 1989), useless, or beneficial in preventing early recurrence, stuttering infarctions, or infarct extension (Genton and Sobel, 1987). Further research in this area is needed.

Reperfusion is not without risk. Even with recanalization, the no-reflow phenomenon may occur when cellular edema due to ischemia prevents restoration of flow at the microvascular level. Reperfusion can accentuate this swelling and inhibit oxygenation of ischemic myocardium (Pasternak et al., 1988). Cellular reperfusion injury may also occur due to oxygen-free radicals (Bodwell, 1989). It is now recognized that the reintroduction of oxygen to previously anoxic myocardium initiates a series of biochemical reactions resulting in the production of superoxide anion, a potent cytotoxic oxygen-free radical. Oxygen-free radical scavengers are presently being investigated as a means of stopping the cellular destruction associated with reperfusion.

Dysrhythmias are common with reperfusion. Premature ventricular contractions are so common that they are thought to represent markers of successful reperfusion. Other dysrhythmias include sinus bradycardia, especially with inferior AMI, accelerated idioventricular rhythm, or VT. Conversely, ventricular dysrhythmias or heart block secondary to ischemia may improve following reperfusion of ischemic myocardium (Pasternak et al., 1988).

Accelerated idioventricular rhythm or ventricular tachycardia may occur without warning. Therefore, prophylactic lidocaine is frequently begun when intravenous administration of the thrombolytic agent is started. The need for intravenous antidysrhythmic agents complicates patient care, necessitating three intravenous lines for (1) the thrombolytic agent, (2) heparin, and (3) other agents such as lidocaine.

Some centers recommend piggybacking lidocaine, nitroglycerin, and heparin.

At this time three major thrombolytic agents are available in the United States: streptokinase, urokinase, and tissue plasminogen activator (t-PA). Controversy continues regarding which agent is superior in regard to reperfusion rate, reocclusion rate, synergism with PTCA, complication rate, and mortality reduction. Although t-PA was initially thought to be superior in reperfusion rate, streptokinase has been shown to be equivalent in effectiveness and less expensive. Reocclusion occurs in 9% to 13% of all patients undergoing thrombolysis regardless of the agent used (Ross, 1988).

Another controversy in thrombolysis is whether intracoronary administration is superior to the intravenous route. At this time intravenous administration is advocated because it allows early administration without the delay inherent in catheterization, it can be given in a variety of locations (e.g., in the ambulance), and the cost is significantly lower than that of intracoronary administration. Further, newer agents, which are extremely effective when given intravenously, may soon make intracoronary thrombolysis obsolete except in patients undergoing angiography for other reasons. See Table 16–7 for nursing care guidelines for t-PA administration. Table 16–8 lists current contraindications for thrombolytic administration; these contraindications are at present being re-evaluated.

Angioplasty in Acute Myocardial Infarction

Since it was first used to dilate coronary stenoses in 1977, percutaneous transluminal coronary angioplasty has become one of the most commonly performed procedures in the treatment of CAD. It is estimated that 400,000 PTCAs/year will be performed in the early 1990s (Ross, 1988).

Controversy exists about the timing of PTCA following AMI. PTCA has been advocated as immediate primary therapy to open the occluded vessel or as an adjunct to thrombolysis, performed either immediately or following lysis by 1 to 3 days. Early reperfusion using only PTCA has been found to be about 90% effective, a rate comparable to or better than that recorded for thrombolysis (Ross, 1989). But PTCA performed immediately after AMI runs the risk of initiating vessel occlusion due to dissection, spasm, subintimal hematoma, or propagation of thrombus from vessel wall trauma (Pasternak et al., 1988). The rate of restenosis following thrombolysis is similar to that seen with immediate thrombolysis with PTCA (Ross, 1988; Simoons et al., 1988). The percentage of restenosis occurring within the first year after PTCA is similar to that seen in patients undergoing PTCA for treatment of AMI (30%) and those undergoing elective PTCA (27%) (Califf et al.,

TABLE 16–7. Nursing Care Guidelines for Intravenous Tissue Plasminogen Activator (t-PA)

1. Identify suitable patients in the emergency department or intensive care unit (ICU) and contact the attending cardiologist immediately. If no answer is received within 5 minutes, repeat the call. Rationale: Thrombolysis must be administered as soon as possible to limit infarct size.
2. Screen for contraindications to thrombolytic therapy (see Table 16–8). Rationale: This action may avoid a complication.
3. Suitable candidates need three vascular access lines begun with a minimum of excess punctures; adequate hemostasis of unused puncture sites is essential. Rationale: Three lines are needed for t-PA, heparin, and other drugs such as lidocaine. Excess bleeding may occur due to the thrombolytic agent if hemostasis is not adequate.
4. Total creative kinase (CK) and CK-MB should be drawn just prior to beginning t-PA infusion and every 6 hours for 24 hours. An electrocardiogram (ECG) should be documented prior to beginning the infusion, at the end of t-PA infusion, 1 hour later, and every 8 hours for 24 hours. Repeat the ECG if chest pain or dysrhythmias recur. Rationale: These diagnostic tests are used to demonstrate reperfusion, reocclusion, and myocardial ischemia or damage.
5. Lidocaine 1.5 mg/kg bolus should be administered prophylactically when t-PA is begun and followed by a 0.75 mg/kg bolus 15 minutes later. A 2 mg/minute drip should be started following the initial bolus. Adjust dosages as necessary based on age, liver function, perfusion status, and allergic history. Rationale: Reperfusion dysrhythmias frequently occur without warning.
6. Heparin therapy is begun 1 hour after t-PA is started. Administer a 5000-unit intravenous bolus and infuse heparin at the dose needed to keep the partial thromboplastin time (PTT) between 50 and 80 seconds. Continue heparin infusion for 24 to 48 hours. Although the PTT will be higher during the first 24 hours following t-PA therapy, the heparin should not be discontinued unless frank bleeding occurs. Rationale: t-PA dissolves thrombus; heparin prevents the recurrence of thrombus formation and reocclusion.
7. Monitor for complications during and following t-PA infusion. During infusion, dysrhythmias not prevented by prophylactic lidocaine should be anticipated and treated if serious or symptomatic. Avoid cardiopulmonary resuscitation if possible. Following infusion, minor oozing at the venipuncture sites and gingival bleeding are common. Gingival bleeding must be distinguished from gastric hemorrhage. New onset back or leg pain (retroperitoneal bleeding) or a change in mental status (cerebral bleeding) indicates a need to stop t-PA and heparin infusions, draw blood for determination of coagulation parameters, and contact the physician immediately. Reocclusion or reinfarction often occurs in the first few days, suggesting the need for adequate anticoagulation. Monitor PTT closely. Rationale: Serious complications require vigilance.

1989). Interestingly, patients who have been catheterized immediately following the onset of symptoms and again a few days later have been found to have less residual stenosis over time even without treatment beyond initial thrombolysis (Ross, 1988). These data suggest that PTCA should be delayed for a few days following AMI unless thrombolysis has failed.

Most patients experiencing AMI should probably not be discharged home without further evaluation and intervention if necessary. For instance, the GISSI (1987) trial showed that the rates of postinfarction ischemia and in-hospital reinfarction are twice as high in patients following successful lysis compared to those receiving standard therapy. These data suggest that the myocardium preserved by thrombolysis is still at risk and requires a definitive mode of intervention such as PTCA or bypass surgery.

The current recommendation is that intravenous thrombolysis be administered immediately following the onset of symptoms. Catheterization and potential PTCA should be performed prior to hospital discharge. Any recurrence of symptoms following patient stabilization, e.g., return of chest pain following 2 hours or more of a stable period, requires immediate catheterization (Ross, 1988). This is an area of active medical research, and these recommendations may change as more is learned.

TABLE 16–8. Contraindications to Thrombolytic Therapy

Recent hemorrhage or active internal bleeding
History of cerebrovascular accident
Recent major surgery, especially intracranial or intraspinal within 2 months
Intracranial neoplasm, arteriovenous malformation, or aneurysm
Known bleeding diathesis
Severe uncontrolled hypertension
   Systolic BP >180 mm Hg or
   Diastolic BP >110 mm Hg
Gastrointestinal or genitourinary bleeding within 10 days
Recent trauma, especially intracranial or intraspinal trauma within 2 months, including cardiopulmonary resuscitation
Valvular thrombus
Acute pericarditis
Subacute bacterial endocarditis
Hemostatic defects (e.g., severe hepatic or renal disease)
Pregnancy or recent delivery
Organ biopsy
Diabetic hemorrhagic retinopathy
Septic thrombophlebitis
Advanced age (i.e., >75 years)
Current treatment with oral anticoagulants

Data from Quaal, 1986.

Emergent Surgical Revascularization

As with other methods designed to limit infarct size, surgical reperfusion of patients with AMI must be accomplished within 4 to 6 hours after the onset of symptoms if jeopardized myocardium is to be saved. CABG performed after 6 hours is contraindicated for uncomplicated transmural infarcts because it causes hemorrhage into the area of infarct (Pasternak et al., 1988). The logistics of getting the patient to the hospital, through coronary angiography, under anesthesia, on cardiopulmonary bypass, and surgically revascularized within 6 hours are formidable. Therefore, widespread use of CABG as a treatment for AMI is doubtful (Genton and Sobel, 1987).

Appropriate candidates for surgical reperfusion for AMI include hospitalized patients who have been catheterized recently and suffer an infarct. Some stable AMI patients who have received thrombolysis may benefit more from CABG than PTCA prior to discharge. Silverstein (1987) reported on three methods of coronary sinus intervention that have been effective in treating patients with myocardial ischemia:

- Pressure-controlled intermittent coronary sinus occlusion
- Synchronized retroperfusion
- Retroinfusion of pharmacologic agents

These interventions are still experimental but hold promise for future surgical treatment of AMI.

NURSING MANAGEMENT

Specific collaborative and independent nursing interventions used in the care of patients with AMI have been alluded to throughout this chapter. Further nursing interventions will be summarized under the appropriate nursing diagnoses.

Alteration in Comfort: Pain

Pain is the most common symptom of AMI. Physiologic response patterns to stressors such as pain depend on the aversiveness, intensity, controllability, novelty, and ambiguity of the situation. Pain of AMI is aversive, uncontrollable, and intense. It is usually a new experience for the patient that has an ambiguous meaning; "Will I die?" This type of situation typically produces a pattern of sympathetic nervous system arousal with increases in BP, heart rate, and cardiac output, skeletal muscle vasodilation, and secretion of both epinephrine and norepinephrine from the adrenal medulla, and cortisol from the adrenal cortex (McCabe and Schneiderman, 1984). Zaleska and Ceremuzynski (1980) documented increases in norepinephrine and epinephrine during acute coronary pain lasting an average of 3 hours.

Epinephrine levels were higher than those of norepinephrine, suggesting that cardiac pain is associated with anxiety (McCabe and Schneiderman, 1984).

Stimulation of the sympathetic nervous system causes physiologic changes that increase myocardial oxygen demand and may extend infarct size. Therefore, pain relief is a primary focus of nursing care for these patients. Intravenous narcotic analgesics should be administered until total pain relief is achieved. Following administration of morphine sulfate, the drug of choice for pain of AMI, maximal respiratory depression occurs within 7 minutes and may last for 4 or 5 hours (Riegel, 1985). Hypotension following morphine administration can be treated by placing the patient in the supine position. Elevation of the feet may be necessary if systolic BP declines lower than 100 mm Hg.

Administration of supplemental oxygen may relieve pain in hypoxemic individuals by augmenting the oxygen supply to ischemic tissues. However, high-flow oxygen therapy has been shown to increase heart rate (Rawles and Kenmure, 1976), systemic vascular resistance, and arterial pressure (Kenmure et al., 1968), which could potentially extend infarct size. Measures potentiating analgesia such as a confident attitude, a quiet environment (Riegel, 1985), and relaxation techniques (Altice and Jamison, 1989) are appropriate independent nursing interventions.

Patients should be instructed to notify the nurse immediately if discomfort returns. In a study of patients with AMI in the coronary care unit, Schneider (1987) found through interviews that 14 of 19 patients had experienced discomfort that they had not reported. The primary reason for not reporting chest pain was that it was not considered severe enough to report. Other reasons included a wish not to bother staff or complain, a desire to see if the pain would subside on its own ("It was nothing I couldn't stand"), and misunderstanding of the need to report chest pain ("They asked me to tell about chest pain; I had a burning in my upper chest and in my arms"). This small study has important implications for practice. When beginning a shift the nurse should question each patient with AMI about the character of his or her discomfort or angina. The patient should then be instructed to inform the nurse of any recurrence of any of those symptoms. Explaining that these symptoms can increase the work of the heart can motivate patients to report symptoms rapidly.

Activity Intolerance

Activity intolerance is defined as a state in which the individual experiences an inability to endure or tolerate an increase in activity (Carpenito, 1983). Patients with AMI may experience activity intolerance because of pain, alterations in vital signs (i.e., hypotension or tachycardia), or even a short period of bedrest. Activity intolerance due to pain, medications, or illness states should be noted so that stimulation that accentuates the tachycardia or hypotension is avoided. Activity intolerance due to unnecessary immobility must be avoided by cautious activity as soon as pain is controlled.

Orthostatic intolerance becomes more severe the longer a patient is on bedrest, but tachycardia and narrowed pulse pressure can occur after only 6 hours in the supine position (Chobanian et al., 1974). These physiologic responses are more pronounced in the elderly and those receiving vasodilators.

Low energy level activities can be used to counteract the physiologic effects of immobility (Winslow et al., 1985). A variety of activities such as bathing, toileting, transfer, bedmaking (Lane and Winslow, 1987), and positioning have been studied in cardiac and normal subjects (Riegel, 1988a). Most of these studies are one of a kind and use small samples, and generalizations based on these data therefore have limited value. One consistent finding, however, is that none of these activities requires more than a minimal energy expenditure. Thus, typical activities of daily living are appropriate for most AMI patients.

Appropriate short-term activity goals include using the bedside commode, feeding self, and assisting with the bath on the first day after admission for an AMI. On the second day, most patients will be able to sit in the chair and bathe themselves from the sink or basin. On the third day, the patient with an uncomplicated AMI can usually sit in the chair for various periods of time. Most are discharged from the coronary care unit on day two or three. During the fourth day the typical patient is walking in the halls and taking either a shower or a tub bath (Riegel, 1988a).

Factors that influence the response to activity include medications, age, size of the infarct, vital signs, fluid balance, anxiety, body weight, time on bedrest, presence of varicosities, environmental temperature, and time elapsed since other exertion (e.g., meals). Response to activity can be evaluated using the Borg Perceived Exertion Scale (Noble, 1983) or the rate pressure product (RPP). The product of heart rate multiplied by systolic blood pressure correlates well with myocardial oxygen consumption (Gobel et al., 1978). Activity should be terminated for any of the following reasons:

- Complaints of angina
- Generalized fatigue
- Shortness of breath
- Dizziness or lightheadedness
- Unsteady gait
- Heart rate increase greater than 120 beats/minute
- ST segment depression of greater than 1.5 mm
- Drop in systolic blood pressure below the resting level or failure to rise with activity
- Significant dysrhythmias such as PVCs in excess of 10/minute, couplets, or R-on-T phenomenon (Alteri, 1984)

Alteration in Cardiac Output

Injured or ischemic myocardium contracts poorly, thereby decreasing cardiac output. Reduced cardiac output results in increases in left ventricular end-systolic volume and pressure, pulmonary vascular congestion, and hypotension (BP equals cardiac output times peripheral resistance). Clinically, the patient may show signs of poor cerebral perfusion, or urinary output of less than 30 mL/hour. Direct hemodynamic monitoring reveals decreases in cardiac output and increases in pulmonary artery wedge pressure. Hypotension may be due to hypovolemia or excess vagotonia. Hypotension due to hypovolemia will be accentuated by diuretics.

A variety of pharmacologic agents are typically prescribed during the early stages of AMI to augment cardiac output. Others are avoided because of their effects on heart rate, BP, or contractility, i.e., MVO_2. Sodium nitroprusside, a potent vasodilator, is commonly prescribed to increase stroke volume and cardiac output in patients with LVF. Any increases in myocardial oxygen demand due to increases in contractility are offset by decreases in arteriolar resistance and afterload, pulmonary artery wedge pressure, and frequency of ectopic beats. Intravenous nitroglycerin is also used to augment cardiac output by decreasing afterload and optimizing preload in patients with heart failure.

Digitalis administration in the early stages of AMI is still debated because (1) it increases MVO_2 in normal hearts through enhanced contractility, (2) its beneficial effects are not evident immediately after AMI, and (3) dysrhythmias may be accentuated in hypokalemic patients (Pasternak et al., 1988). However, in failing hearts, digitalis decreases wall tension, thereby decreasing MVO_2. At this time, digoxin in patients with AMI is reserved for those with moderate degrees of LVF. Supraventricular dysrhythmias are effectively treated with digoxin.

Dobutamine and dopamine are positive inotropic agents that are useful for patients with decreases in cardiac output. Both drugs are potent inotropic agents; dobutamine has slightly less positive chronotropic effects. Both drugs are administered intravenously and require careful monitoring of systemic arterial pressure, pulmonary artery or pulmonary artery wedge pressure, and cardiac output.

Amrinone is a noncatecholamine, inotropic, and vasodilating agent recommended for decreases in cardiac output. Milrinone is a related agent still in the investigational stage. In patients with LVF after AMI, amrinone increases cardiac output and reduces pulmonary artery wedge pressure and afterload. Milrinone does not increase MVO_2, nor does it exacerbate angina and dysrhythmias. Tachycardia occurs in only high doses (Pasternak et al., 1988).

Angiotensin-converting enzyme (ACE) inhibitors, e.g., captopril, are used to increase cardiac output. ACE inhibitors are not direct-acting inotropic agents;

rather they decrease afterload by inhibiting vasoconstriction due to angiotensin II. Preload is also decreased through inhibition of sodium retention. Decreases in afterload and preload increase cardiac output and decrease the work of the heart (Hartshorn and Brundage, 1989).

Agents that should be avoided in the care of AMI patients include isoproterenol, atropine, norepinephrine, and metaraminol (Pasternak et al., 1988). Isoproterenol is a potent cardiac stimulant that increases $M\dot{V}O_2$ through its effects on contractility. Atropine increases $M\dot{V}O_2$ through augmentation of heart rate. The catecholamine norepinephrine and the stimulant metaraminol are reserved for emergency situations because of their peripheral vasoconstrictor (afterload) and cardiac contractility effects, which increase $M\dot{V}O_2$.

Counterpulsation with the intra-aortic balloon pump (IABP) is another intervention used to treat decreases in cardiac output following AMI. Phased pulsations augment coronary perfusion pressure during diastole and deflation throughout systole to facilitate ventricular emptying. In this way, the IABP augments oxygen supply and decreases oxygen demand by minimizing afterload. The IABP is used primarily in treatment of hemodynamically unstable patients, particularly those in cardiogenic shock (Marchetta and Stennis, 1988).

Dysrhythmia control is another method of augmenting cardiac output. Tachydysrhythmias decrease cardiac output by limiting the time available for ventricular filling; bradydysrhythmias decrease cardiac output because of the slowed heart rate. Tachydsyrhythmias may increase infarct size by increasing heart rate. Although slow rhythms may decrease cardiac output, the slowest rate compatible with cerebral and renal perfusion is recommended. A wide variety of antidysrhythmic agents are available to treat atrial and ventricular dysrhythmias. Dysrhythmias may, however, be a symptom of other treatable conditions such as hypokalemia, hypovolemia, and hypoxemia.

Ineffective Individual and Family Coping

The stressfulness of the critical care environment has been the subject of much research in recent years. Regardless of the type of critically ill patient studied, stressors identified include limited mobility and control necessitated by treatment; pain; sleep interruptions; and lack of knowledge and understanding of the illness and its treatment (Riegel, 1988b). Patients with AMI specifically fear early death and the impact of serious illness on their finances, family roles, life style, and sexuality (Miller, 1988). Threats to self-identity are common in these patients, who are typically middle-aged males.

Patients differ in their ability to cope with critical illness and hospitalization, probably based on differences in cognitive interpretation and perception of events (Lazarus and Folkman, 1984). As noted earlier, situations that are novel, ambiguous, intense, uncontrollable, and aversive cause stimulation of the sympathetic nervous system, producing physiologic effects that increase $M\dot{V}O_2$. For this reason as well as for humanitarian, caring concerns, patients at risk for ineffective coping should be identified as soon as possible so that interventions can be implemented early before physiologic and psychological detriment occurs.

Dependable pain relief is one intervention that may build trust and facilitate coping with the stress of admission to the coronary care unit. Early mobilization can support self-esteem as well as prevent the hazards of immobility. Answering questions and teaching patients what to expect are simple but powerful interventions that may decrease the ambiguity, uncontrollability, and aversiveness of coronary care unit admission.

Families are also at risk for ineffective coping because critical illness in a loved one is a major life stressor. Major stressors facing families of critically ill patients include potential death of a mate, loss of a healthy mate, potential recurrence of the event, financial insecurity, new roles within the family unit, change in one's own life goals or motives, change in responsibility for care of dependents in household, and strange hospital environment (Riegel, 1988c).

Family coping can be facilitated by meeting the family's primary needs for hope, information, and the knowledge that hospital personnel really care about the patient (Riegel, 1988c). Nurses can be encouraging, providing honest information that focuses on potential positive outcomes. Information also decreases the novelty, ambiguity, uncontrollability, intensity, and aversiveness of coronary care unit admission. Families can be reassured that they will be contacted immediately if the patient's condition changes. Liberalizing visiting hours, whenever possible, may decrease the novelty, intensity, and uncontrollability of the coronary care unit and relax both patients and their families. Family members should be encouraged to rest, eat well, and exercise to conserve energy and promote relaxation.

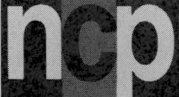 **nursing care plan**

1. Altered comfort, related to:
   Myocardial ischemia and anxiety

Outcome Criteria	Nursing Interventions
Patient will verbalize relief from pain. Myocardial oxygen demand will decrease and/or oxygen supply will increase to meet demand without symptoms of ischemia.	Assess quantity and quality of pain. Instruct patient to notify nurse if discomfort or pain returns. Administer intravenous narcotics as needed. Provide quiet environment and relaxation techniques to potentiate analgesia. Convey confident attitude. Administer supplemental oxygen as needed.

2. Activity intolerance related to:
   Pain
   Hypotension/tachycardia
   Medications
   Illness state
   Immobility

Outcome Criteria	Nursing Interventions

Patient will gradually resume activities of daily living without experiencing symptoms of intolerance.	Avoid stimulation that accelerates tachycardia or hypotension.
	Encourage patient to participate in activities of daily living:
	  1st day after admission: Use bedside commode, feed self, assist with bath.
	  2nd day: Sit in chair, bathe self from sink.
	  3rd day: Sit in chair for various periods of time.
	  4th day: Shower or tub bath, ambulate in halls.

3. Altered cardiac output related to:
   Injured or ischemic myocardium

Outcome Criteria	Nursing Interventions
Cardiac output will be maintained at an asymptomatic level.	Administer medications as needed: nitroprusside, digoxin, dobutamine, dopamine, amrinone or milrinone, and angiotensin-converting enzyme inhibitors. Avoid isoproterenol, atropine, norepinephrine, and metaraminol. Control dysrhythmias with medications. Administer counterpulsation with intra-aortic balloon if patient is hemodynamically unstable.

4. Ineffective individual and family coping related to:
   Critical care environment
   Fear of early death
   Financial concerns
   Family roles
   Life-style changes
   Sexuality
   Threatened self-identity

Outcome Criteria	Nursing Interventions
Patient and family will not experience psychological and physiologic effects of failure to cope.	Provide dependable pain relief. Encourage early mobilization. Provide information and answer patient's questions. Provide and facilitate hope, information, and knowledge that members of the health care team care. Provide honest, encouraging information while focusing on positive outcomes. Obtain family telephone numbers and reassure them that they will be contacted regarding changes in the patient's condition. Liberalize visiting hours whenever possible. Encourage family members to get rest, proper nutrition, and exercise.

SUMMARY

The prognosis for patients experiencing acute myocardial infarction is far brighter today than it was even a decade ago. A wide variety of diagnostic tools and treatment modalities are now readily available. The philosophy of early, aggressive intervention is becoming more commonplace, even in small community hospitals. Collaborative nursing interventions such as medication administration and independent interventions such as activity management and stress reduction are potent tools for increasing myocardial oxygen supply while minimizing oxygen demand. Nurses who understand these interventions designed to limit infarct size can benefit their patients by influencing both medical and nursing care.

References

Afifi, A.A., Chang, P.C., Liu, V.Y., et al. (1974). Prognostic indexes in acute myocardial infarction complicated by shock. *American Journal of Cardiology*, 33, 826.

Alteri, C.A. (1984). The patient with myocardial infarction: Rest prescriptions for activities of daily living. *Heart & Lung*, 13, 355.

Altice, N.L.F., and Jamison, G.B. (1989). Myocardial infarction: Interventions to facilitate pain management. *Journal of Cardiovascular Nursing*, 3 (4), 49–56.

American Heart Association (1991). *1991 Heart and Stroke Facts*. Dallas, TX: American Heart Association.

Anderson, H.R., Falk, E., and Nielsen, D. (1987). Right ventricular infarction: Frequency, size and topography in coronary heart disease: A prospective study comprising 107 consecutive autopsies from a coronary care unit. *Journal of the American College of Cardiology*, 10 (6), 1223–1232.

Barger, A.C., Beeuwkes, R., III, Lainey, L.L., et al. (1984). Hypothesis: Vasa vasorum and neovascularization of human coronary arteries. *New England Journal of Medicine*, 310, 175.

Berne, R.B., and Levy, M.N. (1986). *Cardiovascular physiology* (5th ed.). St. Louis: C.V. Mosby.

Bodwell, W. (1989). Ischemia, reperfusion, and reperfusion injury: Role of oxygen free radicals and oxygen free radical scavengers. *Journal of Cardiovascular Nursing* 4 (1), 25–32.

Braunwald, E.B., and Sobel, B.E. (1988). Coronary blood flow and myocardial ischemia. In E.B. Braunwald (Ed.), *Heart disease: A textbook of cardiovascular medicine* (3rd ed.). Philadelphia: W.B. Saunders.

Braunwald, E.B., Sonnenblick, E.H., and Ross, J. (1988). Mechanisms of cardiac contraction and relaxation. In E.B. Braunwald (Ed.), *Heart disease: A textbook of cardiovascular medicine* (3rd ed.). Philadelphia: W.B. Saunders.

Brown, M.A., and Munford, A. (1983–1984). Rehabilitation of post MI depression and psychological invalidism: A pilot study. *International Journal of Psychiatry in Medicine*, 13 (4), 291–298.

Bulkley, B.H., and Roberts, W.C. (1974). Steroid therapy during acute myocardial infarction: A cause of delayed healing and of ventricular aneurysm. *American Journal of Medicine*, 56, 244.

Califf, R.M., George, B.S., Candela, R.J., et al. (1989). Immediate and deferred angioplasty after acute myocardial infarction: Long-term angiographic follow-up (Abstract 1903). *Circulation* (Suppl.) 80 (4), pII–478.

Carpenito, L.J. (Ed.). (1983). *Nursing diagnosis: Application to clinical practice*. Philadelphia: J.B. Lippincott.

Cay, E.L., Vetter, N., Philip, A.E., et al. (1972). Psychological status during recovery from an acute attack. *Journal of Psychosomatic Research*, 16, 425–435.

Chobanian, A. (1974). The metabolic and hemodynamic effects of prolonged bed rest in normal subjects. *Circulation*, 49, 551.

Constantinides, P. (1966). Plaque fissure in human coronary thrombosis. *Journal of Atherosclerotic Research*, 1, 1.

Cowan, M.J., and Reichenbach, D.D. (1989). Cellular response of the evolving myocardial infarction after therapeutic coronary artery reperfusion. (Abstract 0040). *Circulation* (Suppl.) 80 (4), pII–10.

Cox, D.A., Stone, P.H., Muller, J.E., et al. (1987). Prognostic implications of an early peak in plasma MB creatine kinase in patients with acute myocardial infarction. *Journal of the American College of Cardiology*, 10 (5), 979–990.

Cregler, L.L., and Mark, H. (1985). Relation of acute myocardial infarction to cocaine abuse. *American Journal of Cardiology*, 56, 793.

Davies, M.J., and Thomas, A.C. (1985). Plaque fissuring—the cause of acute myocardial infarction, sudden ischemic death, and crescendo angina. *British Heart Journal*, 53, 363.

Deanfield, J.E., Selwyn, A.P., and Chierchia, S. (1983). Myocardial ischaemia during daily life in patients with stable angina: Its relation to symptoms and heart rate changes. *Lancet*, 2, 753–758.

DeWood, M.A., Spores, J., Notske, R., et al. (1980). Prevalence of total coronary occlusion during the early hours of transmural myocardial infarction. *New England Journal of Medicine*, 303, 897.

Doehrman, S.R. (1977). Psycho-social aspects of recovery from coronary heart disease: A review. *Social Science and Medicine*, 11, 199–218.

Epstein, S.E. (1988). Influence of stenosis severity of coronary collateral development and importance of collaterals in maintaining left ventricular function during acute coronary occlusion. *American Journal of Cardiology*, 61 (10), 866–868.

Fahey, V., and Riegel, B. (1989). Advances in diagnostic testing for vascular disease. *Cardiovascular Nursing*, 25 (3), 13–18.

Falcone, C., Sconocchia, R., Guasti, L., et al. (1988). Dental pain threshold and angina pectoris in patients with coronary artery disease. *Journal of the American College of Cardiology*, 12 (2), 348–352.

Fisch, C. (1988). Electrocardiography and vectorcardiography. In E.B. Braunwald (Ed.), *Heart disease: A textbook of cardiovascular medicine* (3rd ed., pp. 180–222). Philadelphia: W.B. Saunders.

Forman, M.D., Collins, H.W., Kipelman, H.A., et al. (1986). Determinants of left ventricular aneurysm formation after anterior myocardial infarction: A clinical and angiographic study. *Journal of the American College of Cardiology*, 8, 1256.

Gawlinski, A. (1988). New diagnostic techniques. In L. Kern (Ed.), *Cardiac critical care nursing* (pp. 33–57). Rockville, MD: Aspen Publishers.

Genton, R.E., and Sobel, B.E. (1987). Early intervention for interruption of acute myocardial infarction. *Modern Concepts of Cardiovascular Disease*, 56 (7), 35–41.

Gobel, F.L., Nordstrom, L.A., Nelson, R.R., et al. (1978). The rate-pressure-product as an index of myocardial oxygen consumption during exercise in patients with angina pectoris. *Circulation*, 57, 549.

Grossman, W., and Barry, W.H. (1988). Cardiac catheterization. In E.B. Braunwald (Ed.), *Heart disease: A textbook of cardiovascular medicine* (3rd ed.). Philadelphia: W.B. Saunders.

Gruppo Italiano per lo Studio della Streptochinasi nell'Infarto Miocardico. (1987). Long-term effects of intravenous thrombolysis in acute myocardial infarction: Final report of the GISSI study. *Lancet*, 2, 871–874.

Hartshorn, J., and Brundage, D. (1989). Angiotensin converting enzyme inhibitors. *Journal of Cardiovascular Nursing*, 3 (2), 79–82.

Higgins, C.B. (1988). Newer cardiac imaging techniques: Digital subtraction angiography, computed tomography, magnetic resonance imaging. In E.B. Braunwald (Ed.), *Heart disease: A textbook of cardiovascular medicine* (3rd ed.). Philadelphia: W.B. Saunders.

Hlatky, M.A., Cotugno, H.E., Mark, D.B., et al. (1988). Trends in physician management of uncomplicated myocardial infarction, 1970–1987. *American Journal of Cardiology* 61 (8), 515–518.

Hofgren, K., Bondestam, E., Johansson, F.G., et al. (1988). Initial pain course and delay to hospital admission in relation to myocardial infarct size. *Heart & Lung*, 17 (3), 274–280.

Holman, B.L. (1988). Nuclear cardiology. In E.B. Braunwald (Ed.), *Heart disease: A textbook of cardiovascular medicine* (3rd ed.). Philadelphia: W.B. Saunders.

Imhof, P.R., Ott, B., Frankhauser, P., et al. (1980). Differences in nitroglycerin dose-response in the venous and arterial beds. *European Journal of Clinical Pharmacology*, 18, 455–460.

Karliner, J.S. (1981). Congestive heart failure: Pathophysiology and Treatment. In J.S. Karliner, and G. Gregoratos (Eds.), *Coronary care* (pp. 449–470). New York: Churchill Livingstone.

Kenmure, A.C.F., Murdoch, W.R., Beattie, A.D., et al. (1968). Circulatory and metabolic effects of oxygen in myocardial infarction. *British Medical Journal*, 4, 360.

Kennedy, J.W., Atkins, J.M., Goldstein, S., et al. (1988). Recent changes in management of acute myocardial infarction: Implications for emergency care physicians. *Journal of the American College of Cardiology*, 11 (2), 446–449.

Killip, T., and Kimball, J.T. (1967). Treatment of myocardial infarction in a coronary care unit. A two year experience with 250 patients. *American Journal of Cardiology*, 20, 457.

Lakatta, E.G. (1987). Starling's law of the heart is explained by an intimate interaction of muscle length and myofilament calcium activation. *Journal of the American College of Cardiology* 10 (5), 1157–1164.

Landis, C.A. (1988). Arrhythmias and sleep pattern disturbances in cardiac patients. *Progress in Cardiovascular Nursing*, 3 (3), 73–80.

Lane, L.D., and Winslow, E.H. (1987). Oxygen consumption, cardiovascular response, and perceived exertion in healthy adults during rest, occupied bedmaking, and unoccupied bedmaking activity. *Cardiovascular Nursing*, 23 (6), 31–36.

Lazarus, R., and Folkman, S. (1984). *Stress appraisal and coping*. New York: Springer.

Ledwich, J.R., and Mondragon, G.A. (1980). Chest pain duration in myocardial infarction. *Journal of the American Medical Association*, 244 (19), 2172–2174.

Levine, H.J. (1987). Optimum heart rate of large failing hearts. *American Journal of Cardiology*, 61 (8), 633–636.

Lewis, K.M. (1983). Review of functional cardiovascular anatomy and physiology. In C.R. Michaelson (Ed.). *Congestive heart failure*. St. Louis: C.V. Mosby.

Malliani, A., and Lombardi, F. (1982). Consideration of the fundamental mechanisms eliciting cardiac pain. *American Heart Journal*, 103, 575–578.

Malliani, A. (1986). The elusive link between transient myocardial ischemia and pain. *Circulation*, 73, 201.

Marchetta, S., and Stennis, E. (1988). Ventricular assist devices: Applications for critical care. *Journal of Cardiovascular Nursing*, 2 (2), 39–55.

McCabe, P.M., and Schneiderman, N. (1984). Psychophysiologic reactions to stress. In J.T. Tapp, and N. Schneiderman (Eds.), *Behavioral medicine: The biopsychosocial approach*. Hillsdale, NJ: Erlbaum.

Miller, N. (1988). Acute myocardial infarction. In B. Riegel, and D. Ehrenreich (Eds.), *Psychological aspects of critical care nursing*. Rockville, MD: Aspen.

Muller, J.E., and Tofler, G.E. (1988). Circadian variation in onset of cardiovascular disease. In E. Braunwald (Ed.), *Heart disease: Update*. Philadelphia: W.B. Saunders. 13–24.

Muller, J.E., Morrison, J., Stone, P.H., et al. (1984). Nifedipine therapy for patients with threatened and acute myocardial infarction: A randomized, double-blind, placebo-controlled comparison. *Circulation*, 69, 740.

Murdaugh, C. (1990). CAD in women. *Journal of Cardiovascular Nursing*, 4 (4), 35–50.

Noble, B.J., et al. (1983). A category-ratio perceived exertion scale: Relationship to blood and muscle lactates and heart rate. *Medical Science Sports and Exercise*, 15, 523.

Norris, R.M., and Singh, B.N. (1982). Arrhythmias in acute myocardial infarction. In R.M. Norris (Ed.), *Myocardial infarction. Its presentation, pathogenesis and treatment* (p. 55). Edinburgh: Churchill Livingstone.

O'Doherty, M., Tayler, D.I., Quinn, E., et al. (1983). Five hundred patients with myocardial infarction monitored within one hour of symptoms. *British Medical Journal*, 286, 1405.

Pasternak, R.C., Braunwald, E.B., and Sobel, B.E. (1988). Acute myocardial infarction. In E.B. Braunwald (Ed.), *Heart disease: A textbook of cardiovascular medicine* (3rd ed.). Philadelphia: W.B. Saunders.

Piek, J.J., and Becker, A.E. (1988). Collateral blood supply to the myocardium at risk in human myocardial infarction: A quantitative postmortem assessment. *Journal of the American College of Cardiology*, 11 (6), 1290–1296.

Quaal, S. (1986). Thrombolytic therapy: An overview. *Journal of Cardiovascular Nursing*, 1 (1), 45–56.

Rawles, J.M., and Kenmure, A.C.F. (1976). Controlled trial of oxygen in uncomplicated myocardial infarction. *British Medical Journal*, 1, 1121.

Razin, A.M. (1982). Psychosocial intervention in coronary artery disease: A review. *Psychosomatic Medicine*, 44 (4), 363–387.

Rentrop, K.P., Thornton, J.C., Feit, F., et al. (1988). Determinants and protective potential of coronary arterial collaterals as assessed by an angioplasty model. *American Journal of Cardiology*, 61 (10), 677–684.

Riegel, B. (1985). The role of nursing in limiting infarct size. *Heart & Lung*, 14 (3), 247–254.

Riegel, B. (1986). History of treatment of coronary artery disease. *Journal of Cardiovascular Nursing*, 1 (1), vii–viii.

Riegel, B. (1988a). Acute myocardial infarction: Nursing interventions to optimize oxygen supply and demand. In L. Kern (Ed.), *Cardiac critical care nursing* (pp. 59–60). Rockville, MD: Aspen.

Riegel, B. (1988b). Patient responses to critical illness. In B. Riegel and D. Ehrenreich (Eds.), *Psychological aspects of critical care nursing*. Rockville, MD: Aspen.

Riegel, B. (1988c). Family responses to critical illness. In B. Riegel, and D. Ehrenreich (Eds.), *Psychological aspects of critical care nursing*. Rockville, MD: Aspen.

Ritchie, J.L., Cerqueira, M., Maynard, C., et al. (1988). Ventricular function and infarct size: The Western Washington Intravenous Streptokinase in Myocardial Infarction trial. *Journal of the American College of Cardiology*, 11 (4), 689–697.

Roberts, R. (1987). Results of calcium trials in management of acute myocardial infarction. Presented at the American College of Cardiology Conference, Snowmass, CO.

Roberts, R. (1989). Calcium antagonists in prevention of reinfarction. Presented at the American College of Cardiology Conference, Snowmass, CO.

Rosenthal, D.S., and Braunwald, E.B. (1988). Hematological-oncological disorders and heart disease. In E.B. Braunwald (Ed.), *Heart disease: A textbook of cardiovascular medicine* (3rd ed.) Philadelphia: W.B. Saunders.

Ross, A.M. (1988). Thrombolysis and angioplasty in acute myocardial infarction—1988. Presented at the American College of Cardiology Conference: Future Directions in Interventional Cardiology, September 16–18, Santa Barbara, CA.

Ross, A.M. (1989). TIMI, TAMI, ISSIS, GISSI: The role of PTCA in myocardial infarction. Presented at the American College of Cardiology Conference, Snowmass, CO.

Rude, R.E., and the MILIS Study Group (1985). Myocardial infarct extension: Incidence and clinical significance in MILIS. *Circulation* (Suppl. 3), 72, 55.

Schneider, A.C. (1987). Unreported chest pain in a coronary care unit. *Focus on Critical Care*, 14 (5), 21–25.

Schulman, S.P., Achuff, S.C., Griffith, L.C., et al. (1988). Prognostic cardiac catheterization variables in survivors of acute myocardial infarction: A five year prospective study. *Journal of the American College of Cardiology*, 11 (6), 1164–1172.

Seals, A.A., Pratt, C.M., Mahmarian, J.J., et al. (1988). Relation of left ventricular dilation during acute myocardial infarction to systolic performance, diastolic dysfunction, infarct size and location. *American Journal of Cardiology*, 61 (4), 224–229.

Shah, P., Pichler, M., Berman, D.S., et al. (1980). Left ventricular ejection fraction determined by radionuclide ventriculography in early stages of first transmural myocardial infarction. *American Journal of Cardiology*, 45, 542.

Sheffield, L.T. (1988). Exercise stress testing. In E.B. Braunwald (Ed.), *Heart disease: A textbook of cardiovascular medicine* (3rd ed., pp. 223–241). Philadelphia: W.B. Saunders.

Silverstein, B.A. (1987). New dimensions in myocardial protection: Coronary sinus interventions. *Critical Care Nursing Quarterly*, 9 (4), 40–52.

Simoons, M.L., Arnold, A.E., Betriu, A., et al. (1988). Thrombolysis with tissue plasminogen activator in acute myocardial infarction: No additional benefit from immediate percutaneous coronary angioplasty. *Lancet*, 1, 197–203.

Smith, A. (1987). Physiology, diagnosis, and life-style modifications for hyperlipidemia. *Journal of Cardiovascular Nursing, 1* (4), 15–27.

Stone, P.H., Raabe, D.S., Jaffe, A.S., et al. (1988). Prognostic significance of location and type of myocardial infarction: Independent adverse outcome associated with anterior location. *Journal of the American College of Cardiology, 11* (3), 453–463.

Topol, E.J., Burek, K., O'Neill, W.W., et al. (1988). Early hospital discharge 3 days after myocardial infarction: A randomized, controlled clinical trial in the era of reperfusion. *Journal of the American College of Cardiology, 11* (2) (Suppl A), 27A.

Uretsky, B.F., Farquhar, D.S., Berezin, A.F., et al. (1977). Symptomatic myocardial infarction without chest pain: Prevalence and clinical course. *American Journal of Cardiology, 40*, 498–503.

Walsh, R.A., and O'Rourke, R.A. (1981). The physical examination in uncomplicated and complicated myocardial infarction. In J.S. Karliner, and G. Gregoratos (Eds.), *Coronary care.* New York: Churchill Livingstone.

Weil, M.H., von Planta, M., and Rackow, E.C. (1988). Acute circulatory failure (shock). In E.B. Braunwald (Ed.), *Heart disease: A textbook of cardiovascular medicine* (3rd ed., pp. 561–580). Philadelphia: W.B. Saunders.

Winslow, E.H., Lane, L., and Gaffney, A. (1985). Oxygen uptake and cardiovascular responses in control adults and acute myocardial infarction patients during bathing. *Nursing Research, 34*, 164.

Zaleska, T., and Ceremuzynski, L. (1980). Metabolic alterations during and after termination of coronary pain in myocardial infarction. *European Journal of Cardiology, 11*, 201–213.

17

Patients with Valvular Disease

Linda H. Schakenbach

PATHOPHYSIOLOGY: OVERVIEW

The heart moves blood throughout the body via the vascular system. Within the heart, unidirectional blood flow is maintained by valves. Diseases affecting or damaging the cardiac valves impair the heart's ability to maintain an effective cardiac output.

The atrioventricular (AV) valves are located between the atria and the ventricles. The valve on the right side of the heart has three leaflets and is called the tricuspid valve. The valve on the left side of the heart has two leaflets and is called the mitral valve. Both atrioventricular valves are complex structures of leaflets with tendinous filaments at the inferior free edges. The other end of these filaments, the chordae tendineae, are attached to the papillary muscles. The papillary muscles arise from the ventricular wall. When pressure in the atrium exceeds ventricular pressure, the atrioventricular valve opens and blood flows from the atrium to the ventricle. When pressure in the ventricle exceeds pressure in the atrium, the atrioventricular valve closes, and blood cannot flow back into the atrium.

A second set of valves, the semilunar valves, are located in the ventricular outflow tracts. The valve between the right ventricle and the pulmonary artery is the pulmonic valve. The valve between the left ventricle and the aorta is the aortic valve. Both semilunar valves have three leaflets called cusps. The semilunar valves do not have chordae tendineae or papillary muscles. The pulmonic and aortic valves also open and close in response to pressure changes. When ventricular pressure exceeds arterial pressure, the valve opens, and blood flows from the ventricle to the artery. When pressure in the artery is higher than ventricular pressure, the semilunar valve closes, and blood cannot flow back into the ventricle.

The pathophysiologic consequence of valvular lesions is that unidirectional blood flow is not maintained. The disorders are categorized into two func-

tional types, regurgitation and stenosis. Regurgitation, also called insufficiency, is blood flowing backward across the valve. Effective forward blood flow may eventually diminish while blood volumes and pressures behind the valve increase. Stenosis is a narrowing of the valve and impedance of forward blood flow. Effective forward blood flow requires greater pressures to open the valve and move the blood volume. Eventually, forward blood flow decreases, and blood volumes and pressures behind the valve increase.

Regurgitation and stenosis are not mutually exclusive or limited to a single valve. A valve may be narrowed at the annulus and not able to close at the center of the orifice. Combined regurgitation and stenosis have been reported in all four cardiac valves. Aortic stenosis may cause or be associated with mitral regurgitation or stenosis. Aortic and mitral stenosis are associated with tricuspid stenosis or regurgitation. Aortic regurgitation may precipitate mitral regurgitation. Mitral stenosis or regurgitation may cause or be associated with tricuspid regurgitation. Mitral stenosis has been associated with tricuspid stenosis. Pulmonic stenosis may cause or be associated with tricuspid regurgitation or stenosis. Pulmonic regurgitation may precipitate tricuspid stenosis.

The most characteristic feature of each disease is the murmur. Murmurs are the result of turbulent blood flow. Turbulence may result from blood flowing in an abnormal direction, such as regurgitation. Blood flow turbulence is also created by abnormal or narrowed blood flow tracts, such as vegetations, calcifications or tears of leaflets, thickened or fused chordae tendineae, and constricted valve orifices. Additionally, turbulence may result from thickened or stiffened leaflets that are unable to open or close completely. The leaflets may create even more turbulence by vibrating.

Historically, rheumatic endocarditis has been the

primary etiology of valvular heart disease. The incidence had decreased with better public and medical community awareness and antibiotic therapies. However, in the 1980s a strain of group A streptococci again increased the incidence of rheumatic fever (Markowitz and Kaplan, 1989). Infective endocarditis, myxomatous changes, coronary artery disease, hypertension, and congenital disorders are some of the other etiologies of cardiac valvular disorders. Medical treatment is being prescribed earlier in the course of the lesions. Better, more specific and more frequent monitoring techniques are being utilized for individuals at risk and for those with murmurs. Surgical interventions are being refined and advances made with prostheses. This chapter will review some of the specific characteristics of regurgitation and stenosis of each cardiac valve.

Nursing has a major role in caring for patients who have valvular heart disease. Education and enhancement of coping mechanisms are universally required interventions. Inpatient and outpatient care require nursing expertise. This chapter will review some of the specific characteristics of regurgitation and stenosis of each cardiac valve. Nursing diagnoses for the patient with valvular heart disease will be highlighted.

MITRAL REGURGITATION

Pathophysiology

Structurally, the mitral valve is the most complex heart valve. The four major components are the leaflets, the annulus, the chordae tendineae, and the papillary muscles. Mitral regurgitation results from a malfunction of one or more of the valve's components and may be either acute or chronic. Barlow (1987) and Braunwald (1988) have summarized the malfunctions of the mitral valve's components. Disorders involving the leaflets are common. Acute rheumatic endocarditis often results in transient mitral regurgitation. Of more importance is rheumatic myocarditis that leads to chronic mitral regurgitation (Fig. 17–1). In this disease, one or both of the mitral valve leaflets fibrose and shorten as a result of recurrent inflammation. As a leaflet shortens, it becomes incapable of approximation with the other. The shortened leaflet may also calcify, further impairing its movement for valve closure. Rheumatic endocarditis is also known to fuse either the anterolateral or posteromedial commissure and may rarely fuse both. The fusion is unique in that rather than causing stenosis, the fusion prevents complete closure of the leaflets.

Infective endocarditis, usually bacterial but also viral or fungal in origin, erodes, perforates, clefts, or scars the leaflets. Vegetations resulting from infective endocarditis may prevent leaflet approximation acutely or may become fibrous adhesions between the inferior side of the posterior leaflet and the wall of the left ventricle during healing.

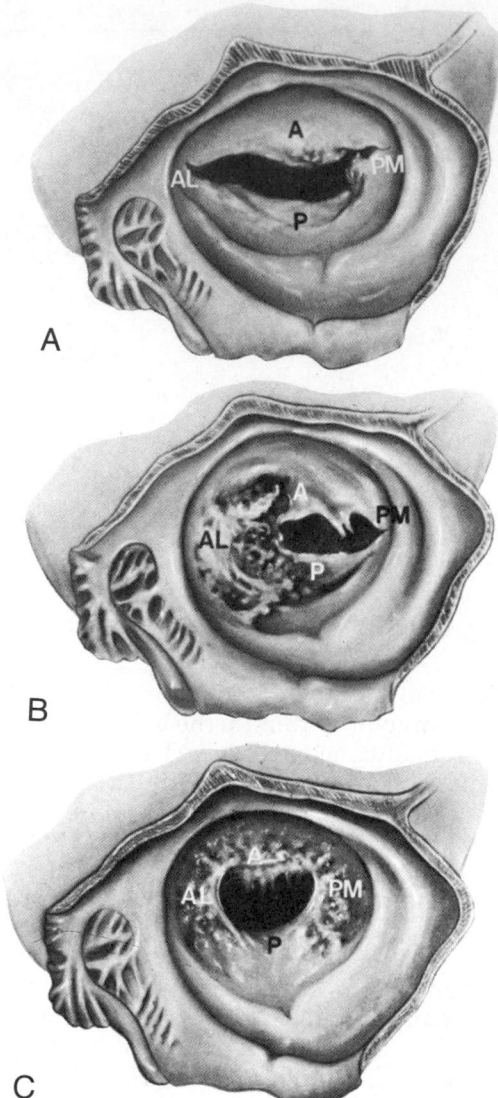

FIGURE 17–1. Anatomic types of rheumatic mitral regurgitation. Each unopened mitral valve viewed from above. In each, A = anterior, P = posterior leaflet of the mitral valve, respectively; AL, PM = anterolateral and posteromedial commissures of the mitral valve. *A,* Intrinsically short leaflets. Commissures essentially unaffected. *B,* Calcification and fusion of anterolateral commissure giving rise to the tear drop type of mitral regurgitation. *C,* Calcification of the leaflets and commissures in continuity, yielding a wedding ring type of mitral regurgitation. Some restriction of the orifice is present, but regurgitation is prominent. (Adapted from Edwards, J. E. (1983). Pathology of mitral incompetence. In M. D. Silver, (Ed.), *Cardiovascular pathophysiology* (vol. 1). New York: Churchill Livingstone. By permission.)

Mitral regurgitation is also the result of myxomatous changes in the leaflets. The central layer of the leaflet, the spongiosa layer, has an overabundance of myxomatous cells. The myxomatous cells spread into the supporting layer of the leaflet, the fibrosa, interfering with the continuity of the layer. The weakened valve thins and stretches, resulting in interchordal hooding and prolapse. Other names for this are "floppy valve," "billowing valve," and "mid-" or "mid-late systolic click" syndromes. As the myxomatous changes progress, the surfaces of the leaflets that make contact with each other fibrose and thicken. Collagenous fibrous tissue develops on the ventricular side of the leaflet in the areas of hooding, thickening the leaflet. Fusion of the commissures and calcification are rare. Regurgitation typically results from severe prolapse causing incompetence of the valve. Myxomatous changes have been identified in the genetic lines of families with both connective tissue disorders, such as Marfan syndrome, and those without connective tissue disorders.

The mitral valve leaflets may produce regurgitation by a variety of rarer causes. The posterior leaflet may adhere to the left ventricular wall as a sequela of the hypereosinophilic syndrome (also known as Loeffler syndrome, disseminated eosinophilic collagen disease, and eosinophilic leukemia). The syndrome begins with a myocarditis that progresses through stages of mural thrombosis and fibrosis, the development of collagen fibers, and finally, endocardial thickening and connective tissue development. The inferior aspect of the posterior leaflet is often incorporated in the mural thrombi of the left ventricular endocardium. As the process continues, the leaflet is held to the ventricular wall, rendering it immobile. Hurler syndrome is similar; large balloon cells enter the normal leaflet tissue, thickening and shortening the leaflet. The leaflet becomes less mobile and cannot approximate with the other leaflet of the mitral valve.

Lupus erythematosus also causes mitral regurgitation by immobilizing the posterior mitral leaflet. Vegetations from the inferior surface of the posterior mitral leaflet become fibrous tethers to the left ventricular wall. Left atrial enlargement pulls the posterior mitral leaflet backward and downward until the leaflet is pulled taut across the left ventricular wall. Asymmetric septal hypertrophy (ASH), also known as idiopathic hypertrophic subaortic stenosis (IHSS), may result in such high ventricular pressure during systole that the anterior leaflet moves away from the posterior leaflet.

Disorders of the mitral valve annulus also cause mitral regurgitation. Conditions such as cardiomyopathies, left ventricular failure, Marfan syndrome, and Hurler syndrome eventually cause left ventricular dilation. The ventricular dilation pulls the mitral valve annulus wider, and eventually the leaflets cannot cover the broader area, causing regurgitation. The annulus may also calcify. Calcification is known to be idiopathic and may be accelerated by systemic hypertension, aortic stenosis, diabetes, Marfan syndrome, Hurler syndrome, and asymmetric septal hypertrophy. The typical mechanism of regurgitation in calcification is a leaflet, usually the posterior leaflet, that becomes immobilized in the calcification or against the ventricular wall. Atypically, the calcification prevents constriction of the annulus with ventricular systole. Rheumatic disease may thicken and stiffen the annulus, also resulting in immobili-

zation of the annulus. The mitral leaflets are not able to approximate across the orifice.

Disorders of the complex chordae tendineae network cause mitral regurgitation. The myxomatous process discussed previously in regard to leaflet disorders also affects the chordae. In the acute stages, the chordae may weaken and occasionally elongate. As the fibrous changes occur, the chordae may rub on the left ventricular wall, causing fibrous deposits to develop on the endocardium. Eventually, the fibrous deposits can fuse with the chordae. The chordae are anchored in the deposits and may impair leaflet closure or rupture. If fibrous deposits do not adhere with the chordae, the weakened chordae may rupture from the normal strain. Ruptured chordae also occur secondary to the rheumatic or bacterial endocarditis and left ventricular dilation processes. Rupture of the chordae may be caused by friction with the septum in asymmetric septal hypertrophy or secondary to hypoxia due to coronary artery disease or myocardial infarction. There are also instances of chordae rupture for which the cause is not known. Abnormally elongated or shortened chordae may be caused by prolapsed leaflets, connective tissue disorders such as Marfan syndrome, and unidentified etiologies. Chordae elongation also occurs as the left ventricle dilates, pulling the papillary muscles down and exerting tension on the chordae. Chordae shortening prevents leaflet closure. Chordae elongation and rupture permit the leaflets to move toward the atrium during systole. All three chordae abnormalities may result in mitral regurgitation.

Papillary muscle disorders are the fourth cause of mitral valve regurgitation. The most common cause of papillary muscle dysfunction is myocardial infarction. A papillary muscle may rupture as a complication of an acute myocardial infarction. When this complication occurs, the posterior medial papillary muscle is usually involved with inferior or inferolateral myocardial infarctions and the anterolateral muscle with lateral or anterolateral myocardial infarctions. Usually rupture of only some of the papillary muscle heads occurs, not the entire muscle. The papillary muscle may not rupture as a consequence of myocardial infarction but may be pulled out of position as the involved ventricular wall necroses and scars. Myocardial infarction and ischemia may impair papillary muscle contraction. Trauma involving the lateral wall or septum of the heart may rupture a papillary muscle.

Mitral regurgitation may also occur in individuals with prosthetic valves. The leaflets, disc, or ball and strut components may fail. Tissue valves may experience changes of the annulus as described with native valves. Any of the prostheses may develop regurgitation at the sewing ring when sutures or tissue fail.

Any cause of mitral regurgitation results in bidirectional blood flow. During diastole, blood flows from the left atrium into the left ventricle. During systole, blood flows back from the left ventricle into

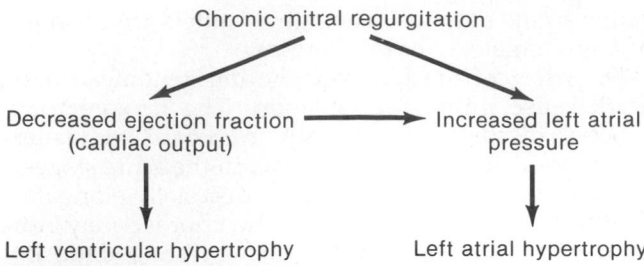

FIGURE 17–2. Pathophysiology of chronic mitral regurgitation. (Adapted from *The Journal of Cardiovascular Nursing*, Vol. 1, No. 3, pp. 1–17, with permission of Aspen Publishers, Inc., © 1987.)

the left atrium. The pathophysiology depends on how quickly the mitral regurgitation develops. Most commonly, mitral regurgitation develops gradually over a period of time. It is known as chronic mitral regurgitation (Fig. 17–2). Some volume of blood flows retrograde from the left ventricle into the left atrium during isovolumetric contraction or ventricular ejection. Depending on the size of the regurgitation orifice and the ventricular pressures, up to 50% of ventricular volume may enter the atrium during isovolumetric contraction, and more flows during ventricular ejection.

Left atrial pressures rise, leading to left atrial hypertrophy and eventually dilation. As the left atrium dilates, it is displaced caudally and posteriorly. The posterior mitral valve leaflet is then stretched across its annulus, shortening the leaflet and compounding the regurgitation process.

The left ventricle also dilates to accommodate the large diastolic blood volume. It hypertrophies in an attempt to maintain systolic pressures and effective stroke volumes through the aortic valve. In chronic mitral regurgitation, the left ventricular mass to volume ratio (preload) is normal. The wall tension (afterload) is often decreased because regurgitation decreases systolic pressure and systolic ventricular radius (Laplace's law). The myofibril energy is therefore able to be expended as increased velocity of contraction, maintaining cardiac output without increasing heart rate or myocardial oxygen consumption. As the left ventricle dilates, however, papillary muscles and chordae tendineae may become stretched or displaced, worsening the regurgitation.

The dilation of both the left atrium and the left ventricle minimizes pulmonary and right heart symptoms. Eventually, the dilation causes atrial and ventricular dysrhythmias, most commonly atrial fibrillation. As the mitral regurgitation and chamber dilations progress, less blood volume displacement or movement occurs. Stagnated blood leads to thrombus formation, especially common in the left atrium, and the potential for emboli. Progression in left ventricular dilation is evidenced as left ventricular failure.

Mitral regurgitation may also be acute, and the pathophysiology of this condition is quite different from that of chronic mitral regurgitation (Fig. 17–3).

The amount of regurgitation, atrial compliance, and ventricular function determine the severity. The atrium and ventricle do not have time to dilate or hypertrophy to compensate for the regurgitation. Blood flows back into the pulmonary and right heart systems. Systemic cardiac output decreases, resulting in increased heart rate and increased systemic vascular resistance. Acute mitral regurgitation may be mild to severe. Mild acute regurgitation may become chronic as the atrium and ventricle begin to dilate and the pathophysiologic events change. Severe acute regurgitation is an emergency situation presenting with acute pulmonary edema of left ventricular failure.

Physical Assessment

The signs and symptoms of mitral regurgitation correspond with the pathophysiology. Chronic mitral regurgitation is often asymptomatic, but signs of the disease are usually found on examination. Acute mitral regurgitation is often very symptomatic, and signs supporting the diagnosis are also found on examination.

The presenting symptoms of chronic mitral regurgitation are often those of left ventricular failure—fatigue, weakness, and dyspnea. Other symptoms are palpitations related to dysrhythmias, orthopnea

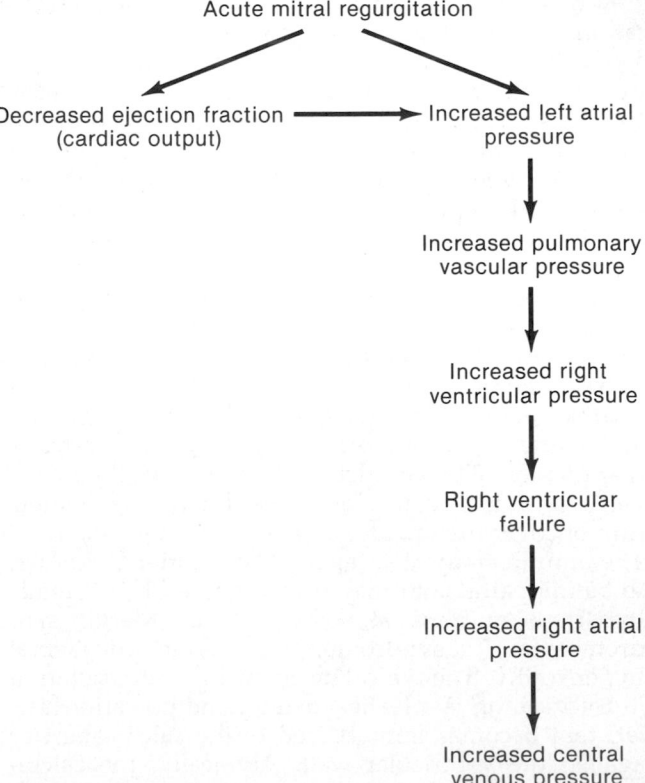

FIGURE 17–3. Pathophysiology of acute mitral regurgitation. (Adapted from *The Journal of Cardiovascular Nursing*, Vol. 1, No. 3, pp. 1–17, with permission of Aspen Publishers, Inc., © 1987.)

and paroxysmal nocturnal dyspnea related to left ventricular failure, as well as atypical chest pains and dysphagia related to the hypertrophied atrium. Ultimately, right heart failure will result in distended jugular veins, peripheral edema, hepatomegaly, and ascites. Occasionally, the presenting symptom is an embolic phenomenon.

Physical examination may reveal a point of maximum impulse that is brisk, hyperdynamic, and displaced caudally and laterally, related to the left ventricular hypertrophy. The atrial hypertrophy may be evidenced by an impulse in the third intercostal space at the left sternal border during systole. (Atrial contractions are usually weak or absent due to atrial fibrillation; the impulse is the jet of regurgitating blood from the left ventricle.) A brisk upstroke may be palpated in the pulse, and the heart rate may be increased or irregular. The blood pressure and pulse pressures are normal until left ventricular failure occurs.

Auscultation at the point of maximum impulse most often reveals a blowing, high-pitched pansystolic murmur. The murmur may radiate into the left axilla or infrascapular areas. When the posterior leaflet is regurgitant, the murmur may radiate up into the aortic valve auscultation area, the base of the neck, or the spine. The murmur may also be late systolic or may be absent. It is the only murmur that does not change intensity with changes in stroke volume. The grade of the murmur does not correlate with the severity of the regurgitation. The first heart sound may be soft because the mitral component is soft or absent. The second heart sound may be widely split because of the shortened left ventricle ejection time. The dilated left ventricle and large atrial blood volume may result in a third heart sound.

Hemodynamic monitoring often demonstrates left atrial pressures below 20 mm Hg with large v waves and steep y descents. Left ventricular stroke volumes are high, usually maintaining a normal cardiac output although some of the stroke volume returns to the left atrium. Cardiac output may also be slightly low. Systemic vascular resistance may be normal or elevated to compensate for a decreased cardiac output. Electrocardiographic monitoring often demonstrates atrial fibrillation but may also show normal sinus rhythm with premature atrial contractions, atrial tachycardia, or atrial flutter. The P wave may widen and notch with atrial hypertrophy. Controlled atrial fibrillation is well tolerated if the ventricle is not dependent on the atrial kick. Some electrocardiograms also demonstrate the increased amplitude or wide QRS and wide T wave characteristic of left ventricular hypertrophy (Dubin, 1974; Marriott, 1988; Schamroth, 1989).

The presenting symptom of acute mitral regurgitation is often pulmonary edema. Other symptoms are severe dyspnea, distended jugular veins, peripheral edema, and shock. Physical examination may reveal a systolic thrill over the left sternal border at the third intercostal space. Blood pressure and pulse

pressure are usually low. Tachycardia and tachypnea are typically present. Auscultation of acute mitral regurgitation reveals a harsh decrescendo early systolic murmur. The murmur may radiate across the precordium, left axilla, back, and left sternal border. The third and fourth heart sounds are usually present.

Hemodynamic monitoring demonstrates elevated left atrial pressures and pulmonary artery wedge pressures as high as 25 to 35 mm Hg or more. Left atrial pressures rise as systemic vascular resistance rises and drops as the resistance decreases. There is a prominent v wave and steep y descent in the atrial tracing. Cardiac output is low. Pulmonary artery pressures, pulmonary vascular resistance, and central venous pressures may be elevated. Electrocardiographic monitoring usually demonstrates sinus tachycardia but can also demonstrate atrial fibrillation.

Laboratory Findings

Blood samples for oxygen saturation studies may be obtained from pulmonary artery catheters at the bedside or in the cardiac catheterization laboratory. Chronic mitral regurgitation often demonstrates low oxygen saturations, whereas normal oxygen saturation is present in acute mitral regurgitation until the left ventricle fails. As left ventricular failure complicates acute mitral regurgitation, pulmonary artery oxygen saturation falls and indicates a poor prognosis (Table 17–1).

Mitral regurgitation caused by an infectious process often increases the total white blood cell count; increased neutrophils, increased band neutrophils, and increased lymphocytes may also be noted. Mitral regurgitation complicating a myocardial infarction can be suspected by elevated creatine phosphokinase (CPK) enzymes and CPK-MB bands or lactic dehydrogenase (LDH_1) greater than LDH_2 within 2 weeks prior to the symptoms of mitral regurgitation.

Diagnostic Procedures

Chest x-rays are commonly performed when diagnosing and monitoring the course of mitral regurgitation. Left ventricular and left atrial enlargement are often seen in chronic mitral regurgitation. Calcification of the annulus may also be seen. The left mainstem bronchus may be elevated by the enlarged left atrium, and Kerley B lines characteristic of interstitial pulmonary edema may be present. Acute mitral regurgitation may or may not demonstrate left ventricular or atrial enlargement but typically presents with pulmonary congestion and edema.

Echocardiograms are another noninvasive technique used to assess patients with mitral regurgitation (Table 17–2). Echocardiograms can diagnose the severity of the lesion and may be used to identify

TABLE 17–1. Laboratory Findings in Valvular Heart Disease

Heart Disease	Sa$_{O_2}$	S$\bar{v}_{O_2}$	Pa$_{O_2}$	WBC	RBC	Platelets	Coagu-lopathies	Liver Enzymes	Blood Cultures	CPK	LDH
MR	Acute, normal; late, decreased; chronic, decreased		Acute, normal; late, decreased	Increased neutrophils,* possibly increased lymphocytes*						If MI, positive MB bands	↑, If MI, LDH$_1$> LDH$_2$
MVP					↓						
MS ⎱	↓**				? ↑			? ↑			
AR ⎰	↓**				? ↓			↑ ***			
AS	↓ with LVF				? ↓						
TR ⎱		↓ with low CO					↑ late	↓ albumin	positive****		
TS ⎰											
PR											
PS											

Abbreviations: Sa$_{O_2}$, oxygen saturation of arterial blood; S$\bar{v}_{O_2}$, oxygen saturation of mixed venous blood; Pa$_{O_2}$, partial pressure of arterial oxygen; MR, mitral regurgitation; MVP, mitral valve prolapse; MS, mitral stenosis; AR, aortic regurgitation; AS, aortic stenosis; TR, tricuspid regurgitation; TS, tricuspid stenosis; PR, pulmonic regurgitation; PS, pulmonic stenosis; LVF, left ventricular failure; WBC, white blood cells; RBC, red blood cells; MI, myocardial infarction; CO, cardiac output; CPK, creatine phosphokinase; LDH, lactic dehydrogenase; *, with an infectious process; **, with pulmonary edema/transudates; ***, with right ventricular failure; ****, with a blood infection; ↑, increased; ↓, decreased.

the etiology of the regurgitation and monitor the progression of the pathophysiology. Color and pulsed Doppler echocardiograms are preferred to M-mode and two-dimensional techniques. Chronic mitral regurgitation will demonstrate enlargement of the left ventricle and atrium as well increased wall motion of these chambers. The jet of regurgitant blood to the atrium may be identified. Mitral valve leaflet thickening and annulus calcification may also be demonstrated. In patients with acute mitral regurgitation, echocardiography can be used to identify an enlarged left ventricle or atrium when it is present, but is most useful for identifying increased systolic wall motions. The etiology of the acute regurgitation, such as flail or perforated leaflets, vegetations, and ruptured chordae or papillary muscles, may be identified on echocardiography. Prosthetic valves may also be evaluated by echocardiography.

Other noninvasive studies are occasionally utilized for investigation of mitral regurgitation. Holter monitoring may help to determine the dysrhythmia type, frequency, and duration. Graded exercise studies

TABLE 17–2. Cardiac Valve Echocardiography

Valve Disease	M-Mode	Two-Dimensional	Pulsed Doppler	Color Doppler
Mitral regurgitation		+	+ + +	+ + + +
Mitral valve prolapse	+	+ +	+ +	+
Mitral stenosis	+ +	+ +	+ +	+ +
Aortic regurgitation	+	+ +	+ + +	+ + +
Aortic stenosis	+	+ +	+ +	+
Tricuspid regurgitation	+	+	+ +	+ +
Tricuspid stenosis	+	+ +	+	+
Pulmonic regurgitation	+	+	+ +	+ +
Pulmonic stenosis		? +	+ +	+ +

Abbreviations: +, somewhat useful; + +, commonly used; + + +, examination of choice; + + + +, especially recommended.

may be used to evaluate functional cardiac reserve in chronic mitral regurgitation. Radionuclide imaging has been used to identify ejection fractions, diastolic and systolic ventricular volumes, and left ventricular function. Cardiac imaging has been used in patients with chronic mitral regurgitation to help determine the timing of surgical interventions. Phonocardiography may be used to demonstrate the diminished first heart sound, accentuation of the murmur with increased afterload (Valsalva maneuver, squatting) and diminished intensity with decreased afterload (amyl nitrate). It is also used to graph the murmur. The phonocardiogram of chronic mitral regurgitation shows a high-frequency and pansystolic murmur. There may be a third heart sound and a mid-diastolic component. Acute mitral regurgitation murmurs are high-frequency, decrescendo sounds that terminate in mid to late systole. Acute mitral regurgitation usually demonstrates third and fourth heart sounds.

The diagnosis and severity of mitral regurgitation is best quantified by cardiac catheterization. Mitral regurgitation is confirmed by a left ventriculogram demonstrating contrast entering the left atrium. The angiogram also provides measurements for determining left ventricular function and left ventricular mass and stress. Cardiac catheterization also provides an opportunity to evaluate the entire cardiac anatomy and identify any other cardiac lesions. In chronic mitral regurgitation, contrast enters the atrium and may not clear for many cardiac cycles. In acute mitral regurgitation, the left atrium and ventricle are often normal in size, and the ventricular contrast medium regurgitates not only to the atrium but also into the pulmonary veins.

Medical Treatment

Chronic mitral regurgitation may not require continuous treatment because there may be no symptoms. Some authorities recommend continuous prophylactic treatment for endocarditis until the patient reaches 30 years of age. Most also recommend specific prophylaxis in these patients for infective endocarditis during dental and surgical procedures (Table 17–3). Symptomatic treatment is utilized on an individual basis. Atrial fibrillation is usually treated with digoxin to slow the ventricular response, and many clinicians believe that anticoagulation minimizes the risk of embolization. Electrical cardiover-

TABLE 17–3. Antibiotic Prophylaxis

For Dental Procedures and Surgery of the Upper Respiratory Tract

1. For most patients: oral amoxicillin	Adults: 3.0 g orally of amoxicillin 1 hour prior to procedure and then 1.5 g 6 hours after initial dose.
2. For those *allergic to amoxicillin/penicillin* (may also be selected for those receiving oral penicillin as continuous rheumatic fever prophylaxis): erythromycin or clindamycin	Adults: 1.0 g orally 2 hours prior to procedure and then 500 mg 6 hours after initial dose.
3. For those patients at *higher risk* of infective endocarditis (especially those with prosthetic heart valves) who are not allergic to penicillin: ampicillin, gentamicin, and amoxicillin	Adults: Ampicillin 2.0 g plus gentamicin 1.5 mg/kg IM or IV, both given 30 minutes before procedure; then amoxicillin 1.5 g orally 6 hours after initial dose.
4. For *higher risk* patients (especially those with prosthetic heart valves) who are *allergic to penicillin*: vancomycin	Adults: Vancomycin 1 g IV over 60 minutes begun 60 minutes before procedure; no repeat dose is necessary.

For Gastrointestinal and Genitourinary Tract Surgery and Instrumentation

1. For most patients: ampicillin, gentamicin, and amoxicillin	Adults: 2.0 g ampicillin IM or IV plus gentamicin 1.5 mg/kg IM or IV given 30 minutes before procedure; followed by amoxicillin 1.5 g, orally 6 hours after initial dose. May repeat once 8 hours later.
2. For patients *allergic to penicillin*: vancomycin plus gentamicin	Adults: 1.0 g vancomycin IV given over 60 minutes plus 1.5 mg/kg gentamicin IM or IV, each given 60 minutes before procedure. Doses may be repeated once 8 hours after initial dose.
3. Oral regimen for minor or repetitive procedures in low-risk patients: amoxicillin	Adults: 3.0 g amoxicillin 1 hour before procedure and 1.5 g 6 hours after initial dose.

Note: In patients with compromised renal function, it may be necessary to modify or omit the second dose of antibiotics. Intramuscular injections may be contraindicated in patients receiving anticoagulants.
Adapted from Dajani, A. S., Bisno, A. L., Chung, K. J. et al., (1990) Prevention of bacterial endocarditis. Recommendations by the American Heart Association, JAMA, 264, 2912–2922. Copyright 1990, American Medical Association.

sion may be utilized for atrial fibrillation of sudden onset or in cases of mild regurgitation or atrial hypertrophy. With the onset of left ventricular failure, digoxin and diuretics are begun to increase contractility and decrease preload. Dietary sodium, fluid, and activity restrictions are recommended. Decreasing afterload to decrease regurgitation and increase aortic flow combined with decreasing preload to minimize left ventricular volume and the size of the mitral orifice may be accomplished with nitrates, hydralazine, prazosin, or captopril. If the signs and symptoms of left ventricular failure cannot be controlled by medical regimens, surgical intervention is considered (see Chap. 20). Some authorities consider performing surgical intervention prior to the appearance of symptoms of left ventricular failure to secure a better prognosis. (Braunwald, 1988; Chung, 1983; McGoon et al., 1986; Sokolow and McIlroy, 1986).

Surgical treatment is based on the underlying pathology as well as the surgeon's opinion and experience. Valvuloplasty (Fig. 17–4) is often a lengthy, complex procedure. When the leaflets have been stretched, such as with prolapse or myxomatous changes, they may be resected. Cleft leaflets may be patched, and retracted leaflets can be extended with prepared pericardium grafts. A dilated or deformed annulus may also be repaired (Fig. 17–5). Annuloplasty with a ring or stent has been used when calcifications are not present (Fig. 17–6).

Short, elongated, or ruptured chordae tendineae may result in mitral regurgitation. Valvuloplasty involves resecting, dividing, or fenestrating shortened or fused chordae. Elongated chordae may be shortened by implanting the superfluous length in its papillary muscle. Ruptured chordae are treated differently depending on which leaflet is involved; however, annuloplasty completes all procedures to correct ruptured chordae. Ruptured chordae of the posterior leaflet are repaired by resecting the leaflet to eliminate the need for the ruptured chordae. The anterior leaflet is repaired by transposing a section of the posterior leaflet with its chordae to the anterior leaflet. The posterior leaflet is then closed. Fused or calcified commissures are another cause of chronic mitral regurgitation. A commissurotomy may be used to correct this lesion by splitting the commissures open to within 2 to 3 mm of the annulus.

Mitral valve replacement is also a treatment for chronic mitral regurgitation. As with valvuloplasty, the best timing for surgery in the course of the disease is difficult to determine. Again, the surgeon's opinions and experience determine the device utilized, but some general guidelines are commonly agreed upon. Calcified and otherwise immobilized leaflets are indications for valve replacement. Mechanical prostheses, the ball-cage and tilt disc, require lifelong anticoagulation. Porcine and bovine xenografts and homografts do not require anticoagulation more than 6 weeks postimplantation unless atrial fibrillation or a large left atrium exist. The xenografts and homografts have smaller effective orifices for the size of their sewing rings. Xenograft

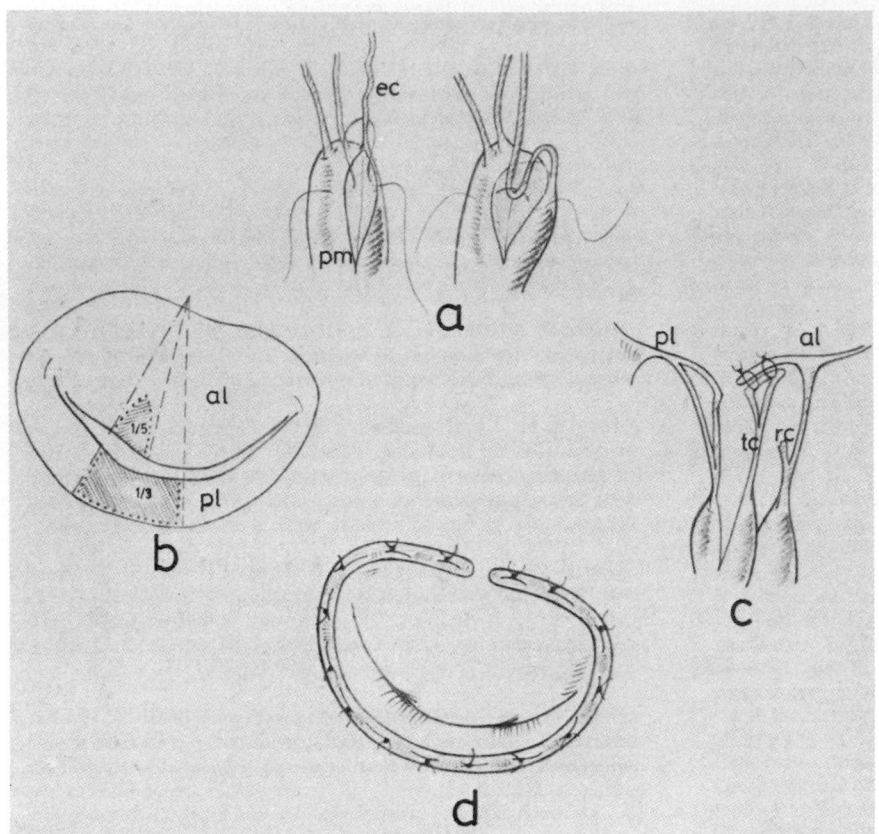

FIGURE 17–4. Techniques of valvuloplasty for correction of mitral regurgitation. *a*, Shortening of elongated chordae tendineae *(ec)* by burying the excessive length into a trench created in the papillary muscle *(pm)*. *b*, Leaflet resection; the two leaflets are resected following the triangular outline indicated. The anterior leaflet *(al)* can only tolerate small resections of up to one-fifth of its free edge, whereas the posterior leaflet *(pl)* is amenable to a much wider resection, of up to one-third of its substance. *c*, Transposition of the chordae tendineae *(tc)* from the posterior leaflet *(pl)* to the anterior leaflet *(al)* to replace ruptured chordae *(rc)*. *d*, Final result after implantation of a Carpentier ring to consolidate the repair and to reshape the annulus. (From Barlow, J. B. (1987). *Perspectives on the mitral valve.* Philadelphia: F. A. Davis.)

and homograft prostheses are considered preferable for children, females of childbearing age, patients over 70 years of age, and those with a history of bleeding (Braunwald, 1988) (Fig. 17–7). If possible, surgical replacement should be postponed until 4 to 6 weeks after a myocardial infarction. Medical management of atrial fibrillation with digoxin and prophylaxis against infective endocarditis should continue postoperatively.

The treatment of acute mitral regurgitation begins with nitroprusside and diuretics to decrease afterload and ventricular diameter to minimize the size of the mitral annulus. An intra-aortic balloon may be utilized to further decrease afterload in patients with severe left ventricular failure. In cases of severe regurgitation, defined as 3 to 4+ on a scale of 1 to 4, with a cardiac index of 1.5 liters/min per m² or greater and an ejection fraction of over 35%, surgical intervention is indicated (Frankel and Brest, 1986). Less severe regurgitation may be managed medically. A common cause of acute mitral regurgitation is elongated or ruptured chordae, which may be repaired as previously described. Mitral valve replacement may also be used to treat acute mitral regurgitation (see Chap. 20).

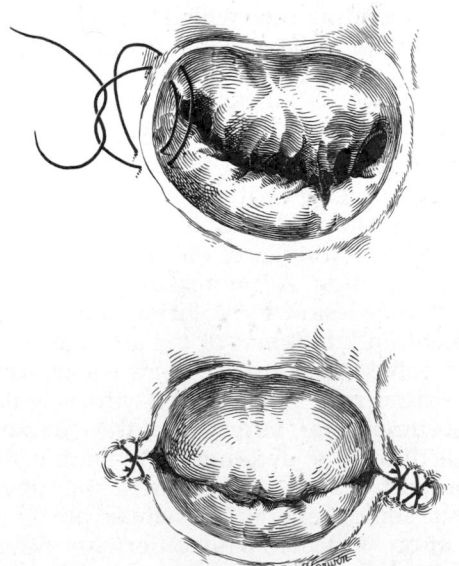

FIGURE 17–5. Commissural plication of the regurgitant mitral valve annulus. (Reproduced by permission from: Starr, A., and Macmanus, Q.: Acquired valvular heart disease. In D. B. Effler, (ed.): *Blades' surgical diseases of the chest* (4th ed). St. Louis, 1978, The C. V. Mosby Co., p. 513.)

MITRAL VALVE PROLAPSE

Pathophysiology

Mitral valve prolapse, also called Barlow syndrome, floppy valve, billowing mitral valve, balloon-

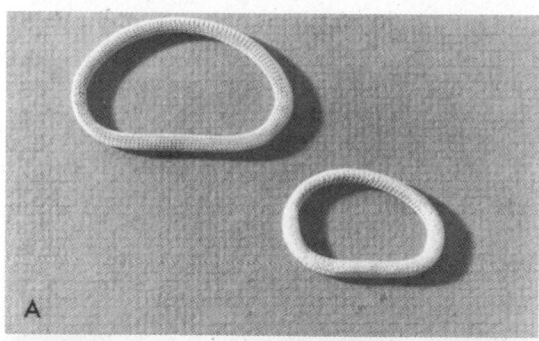
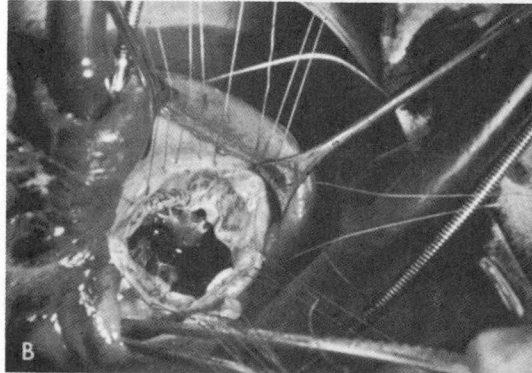
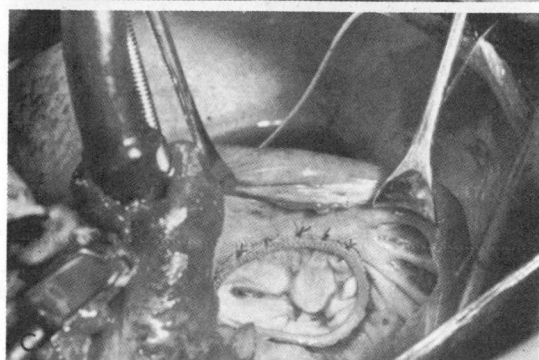

FIGURE 17–6. *A*, Carpentier rings. *B*, Ring being sutured into place. *C*, Completion of Carpentier ring annuloplasty. (From Starr, A. (1976). Acquired disease of the tricuspid valve. In D. C. Sabiston, Jr., and F. C. Spencer (Eds.): *Gibbon's surgery of the chest* (p. 1182). Philadelphia: W. B. Saunders.)

the thoracic cage occur simultaneously. Individuals with mitral valve prolapse have been found to have a high frequency of dysautonomia, narrow anterior-posterior chest diameters, pectus excavatum, and scoliosis. Barlow (1987) and Braunwald (1988) have summarized the etiologies and conditions associated with mitral valve prolapse. As with mitral regurgitation, disorders of the leaflets, annulus, chordae tendineae, or papillary muscle may result in mitral valve prolapse.

The most common cause of mitral valve prolapse is myxomatous changes of the leaflets. A disorder of collagen metabolism results in a proliferation of the spongiosa layer of the leaflet. As the myxomatous cells spread into the fibrous layer of the leaflet, the leaflet stretches and prolapse occurs. The myxomatous changes may be idiopathic and may be associated with connective tissue disorders such as Marfan syndrome, osteogenesis imperfecta, periarteritis nodosa, Duchenne muscular dystrophy, and cardiomyopathy. Leaflets may also be damaged by left atrial myxomas that rub or fall down onto a leaflet. Asymmetric septal hypertrophy, also known as idiopathic hypertrophic subaortic stenosis, often causes anterior leaflet movement, which may in turn precipitate posterior leaflet prolapse. Mitral valve surgery, such as commissurotomies, insufficient leaflet resection, and chordae resection, division, or fenestration, may result in prolapse. Myxomatous changes may also affect the annulus, causing it to dilate, and have also been associated with calcification. The distortion of the annulus may result in mitral valve prolapse.

The third element of the mitral valve structure is the chordae tendineae. The degenerative myxomatous changes that affect the leaflets and annulus also affect the chordae. The central layer of the chordae weakens with the collagen disruption, and the chordae elongate and may rupture. Coronary artery disease and coronary artery spasm may lead to chordae ischemia and rupture. The rheumatic disease process may result in shortened chordae that rupture from prolonged strain. Whatever the cause, the chordae are not able to control the leaflet movement during ventricular systole and prolapse results.

The papillary muscles are the final mitral valve component. Ischemic coronary disease may cause papillary muscle ischemia, papillary muscle head necrosis and rupture, ventricular hypertrophy, cardiomyopathy, and impaired left ventricular wall motion. Malfunction of the papillary muscle impairs the chordae tendineae, and the leaflets prolapse.

Abnormal movement of the mitral valve leaflets may occur during the patient's lifetime with no pathophysiologic changes. Atrial, junctional, and ventricular dysrhythmias may be precipitated by abnormal leaflet movement or by the elevated epinephrine or norepinephrine of dysautonomia. The patient may be at increased risk of bacterial endocarditis and cerebral ischemia. Mitral valve prolapse rarely progresses to mitral regurgitation.

ing mitral cusp, midsystolic click-murmur, redundant cusp syndromes, and numerous other names, is usually a benign lesion. Controversy exists as to the definition of mitral valve prolapse. Some state that it is an abnormal or exaggerated movement of a leaflet into the left atrium during ventricular systole, whereas others believe that there must be dissociation of the leaflets at the commissures and the resultant mitral regurgitation to make a diagnosis of mitral valve prolapse. The incidence of mitral valve prolapse ranges from 4% to 21% of the population (Anderson, 1987; Braunwald, 1988; Cornell, 1985; Frankl and Brest, 1986; Hunt, 1985). In many cases it is inherited as an autosomal dominant trait. Developmentally, the formation of the mitral valve structures, the autonomic nervous system, and the ossification of

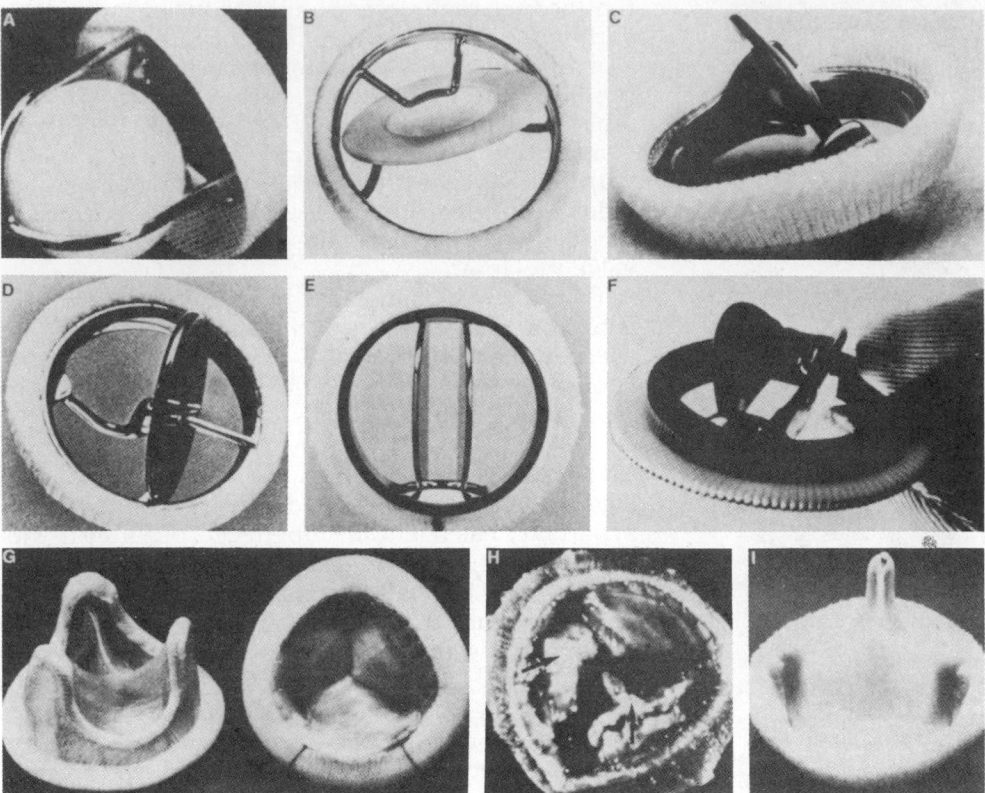

FIGURE 17–7. Prosthetic cardiac valves. *A,* Starr-Edwards ball-cage. *B,* Bjork-Shiley tilting disc. *C,* Omniscience tilting disc. *D,* Medtronic-Hall tilting disc. *E,* St. Jude Medical bileaflet. *F,* Duromedics bileaflet. *G,* Carpentier-Edwards porcine. *H,* Porcine valve removed several years following implantation because of primary valve failure; arrows point to areas of calcification and destruction of leaflets. *I,* Ionescu-Shiley pericardial valve. (Adapted from Braunwald, E. (1988). *Heart disease* (3rd ed.). Philadelphia: W. B. Saunders.)

Physical Assessment

Many patients with mitral valve prolapse have no signs or symptoms of the disorder. In these individuals prolapse is discovered during examination for another reason or at autopsy. Other patients with mitral valve prolapse may be symptomatic, but there are very few physical signs of the condition.

Inspection of the patient may reveal a narrow anterior-posterior chest diameter, pectus excavatum, or scoliosis. Auscultation is usually the most revealing assessment. Mitral valve prolapse is often characterized by a mid or late systolic click heard best between the apex and the lower left sternal border. The click is often heard after the beginning of the carotid pulsation is felt. The timing of the click or clicks (there may be more than one) can be changed using the usual ventricular size and afterload altering procedures. Standing and administration of amyl nitrite, which decrease ventricular size and afterload, cause the click to occur earlier in the cycle. Squatting, isometric exercise, and lying down, which increase ventricular size and afterload, cause the click to occur later in the cycle. Patients with mitral valve prolapse occurring with or because of left ventricular hyper-

trophy, mitral regurgitation, or other pathology will demonstrate signs or symptoms of those disorders as well, such as a laterally displaced point of maximum impulse and a systolic murmur.

Although mitral valve prolapse may not provide many physical signs, patients are often quite symptomatic. The presenting symptoms are usually fatigue, shortness of breath, lightheadedness, dizziness or syncope, palpitations, chest pain or anxiety (Frankl and Brest, 1986). Fatigue has been attributed to exertion and emotional stress, but the patient is often tired regardless of physical or emotional stress and the amount of rest and sleep. Shortness of breath is not correlated with pulmonary function or graded exercise tests. Dyspnea may be correlated with or contribute to the anxiety associated with mitral valve prolapse. Lightheadedness, dizziness, and syncope may be attributed to orthostatic hypotension or dysrhythmias, but this has not always been documented. Palpitations, a frequent complaint, are often correlated with atrial and ventricular dysrhythmias, but not in all cases. Chest pain, which may be typical or atypical, is another common complaint. It responds variably to nitrate treatment in the same patient. The pain is not correlated with physical or emotional stress, is often localized, and diminishes when the patient lies down. The pain may last for seconds or for days. The pathogenesis has not been determined. The final symptom of mitral valve prolapse is anxiety. The poor correlation of symptoms with physical signs of pathology has led to other diagnoses, such as neurosis, in many patients. Anxiety may be correlated with dysrhythmias and orthostatic hypotension. Some have correlated all of the symptoms with dysautonomia. When moving from a supine to a standing position, patients with mitral valve prolapse may experience lightheadedness, dizziness, syncope, palpitations, chest pains, and anxiety. When returning to the supine position, bradycardias may precipitate fatigue and anxiety. To date, there is no universally accepted explanation for the symptoms.

Electrocardiographic monitoring may reveal flattened or inverted T waves in leads II and III and, rarely, a prolonged Q–T interval. Many dysrhythmias may be observed, among them sinus bradycardia, sinus arrest, premature atrial contractions (PACs), atrial tachycardia, atrial fibrillation, first degree atrioventricular block, right bundle branch block, premature ventricular contractions (PVCs), ventricular tachycardia, and ventricular fibrillation.

Laboratory Findings

Blood samples from patients with mitral valve prolapse are usually within normal ranges (see Table 17–1). Some patients have been found to have shortened platelet survival times and a higher incidence of arterial thromboembolism (Dalen and Alpert, 1981).

Diagnostic Procedures

Electrocardiograms may be useful for providing information beyond that of the bedside monitor. The flattening and inversion of the T wave may also be noted in aVF, V_5, and V_6. Many patients with Wolff-Parkinson-White syndrome also demonstrate mitral valve prolapse. ST segment depression may be noted or accentuated by standing. Graded exercise and Holter monitor studies may be useful for detection of dysrhythmias and ST segment depression. ST segment depression may normalize with peak exertion.

Echocardiograms are the primary diagnostic modality for detecting mitral valve prolapse (see Table 17–2). The more recently developed pulsed Doppler and two-dimensional echocardiograms have been used more frequently than M-mode because of their sensitivity, but many still use M-mode echocardiography successfully (Fig. 17–8). The echocardiographic finding is the posterior movement of a leaflet, usually the posterior leaflet but sometimes the anterior leaflet, or both, into the left atrium.

Radionuclide imaging has been utilized to identify false-positive graded exercise studies. Phonocardi-

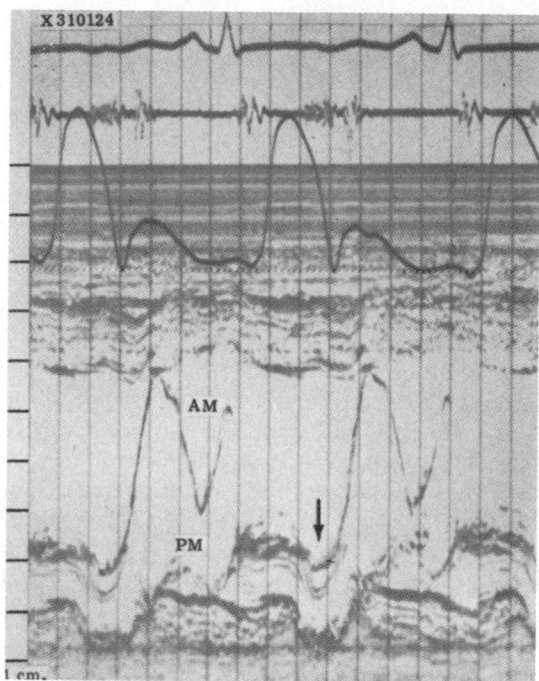

FIGURE 17–8. Echocardiogram of a patient with a prolapsed mitral valve. Note the late systolic posterior motion of the anterior *(AM)* and posterior *(PM)* mitral valve leaflets *(arrow)*. This abnormal motion corresponds with a later systolic murmur as seen on the phonocardiogram. (From Feigenbaum, H. (1986). *Echocardiography*. Philadelphia: Lea & Febiger.)

ograms may demonstrate the systolic click at least 0.14 second after the first heart sound and changing timing with the methods discussed in the Physical Assessment section. Cardiac catheterization may demonstrate prolapse of the posterior leaflet but is not as sensitive to the anterior leaflet. One advantage of the ventriculogram is that it may demonstrate mitral regurgitation and assist with differentiation of chest pain by determining the degree of coronary artery disease. Cardiac catheterization is not usually necessary for the diagnosis or treatment of mitral valve prolapse.

Medical Treatment

The medical therapy for patients with mitral valve prolapse depends on the symptoms and whether or not mitral regurgitation complicates the diagnosis. Many physicians prescribe antibiotic prophylaxis for bacterial endocarditis regardless of whether regurgitation is known or not, and when systolic clicks are auscultated whether or not echocardiographic prolapse can be demonstrated (see Table 17–3).

Dysautonomia may respond to propranolol or barbiturates. Propranolol may decrease fatigue, lightheadedness, dizziness, syncope, palpitations, supraventricular dysrhythmias, ventricular dysrhythmias, chest pain, and anxiety. Dysrhythmias not controlled with propranolol may be treated with quinidine, procainamide, phenytoin, calcium channel blockers, or clonidine. If atrioventricular block progresses to Mobitz II or complete heart block, a temporary or permanent pacemaker may be required. Ventricular tachycardia refractory to other therapies may be treated with stellate ganglion blockers.

Chest pain usually decreases with propranolol. Calcium channel blockers may be added when propranolol does not control the chest pain. Nitrates may decrease preload and therefore ventricular size, exaggerating the prolapse and the ischemia. Nitrates, when used, are used with caution.

Systemic emboli may result from fibrin and platelet deposits on the prolapsed leaflet. Prophylaxis for transient ischemic attacks and embolic strokes is accomplished with aspirin or dipyridamole.

Mitral valve prolapse rarely requires surgical intervention (see Chap. 20). Mitral valve replacement may be necessitated by refractory dysrhythmias, reduced cardiac reserves, severe mitral regurgitation, or incapacitating pain.

MITRAL STENOSIS

Pathophysiology

The most common etiology of mitral stenosis is rheumatic disease. (Mitral stenosis is also the most common sequela of rheumatic disease.) Rheumatic endocarditis results in an inflammatory process or an abnormal valvular blood flow pattern that initiates progressive changes in the leaflets, annulus, chordae tendineae, or papillary muscles.

Aschoff bodies in the left atrial wall suggest ongoing subclinical rheumatic activity. Other researchers have documented structural valve changes related to abnormal blood flow caused by a limited rheumatic insult. The stenotic process continues for years after the initial insult, and many patients cannot identify a rheumatic episode. Many patients do not develop symptoms for 10 years or more.

The rheumatic inflammatory process causes nodules to develop along the edges of the leaflets at the commissures and within the leaflets themselves. The continuing process may result in fusion of the commissures and thickened, stiff leaflets. Calcification of the leaflets and commissure adhesions are common. The rheumatic process or its sequela may also scar, shorten, or fuse the chordae and shorten or scar the papillary muscles. The fused chordae narrow or obliterate the secondary orifices below the mitral valve leaflets. The rheumatic insult stiffens the mitral valve annulus and may eventually lead to its calcification. Other causes of mitral stenosis are congenital deformities of shortened, thick chordae tendinea, a decreased number of chordae, or a single papillary muscle. In these conditions, the leaflets may be thickened but are seldom calcified. Infective bacterial endocarditis may result in the development of large vegetations that occlude the mitral valve orifice.

Large left atrial ball thrombus or tumors may partially or totally occlude the mitral valve at some time during diastole. Metabolic and enzymatic changes such as mucopolysaccharide deposits, carcinoid heart disease, macrophage collection, and reaction to methysergide treatment may also result in thick, stiff leaflets. Valve prostheses may also become thrombosed (Fig. 17–9) or immobilized by pannus.

Mitral stenosis increases impedance of blood flow from the left atrium to the left ventricle. The ensuing pathophysiology is dependent on the degree of obstruction (Fig. 17–10). The normal mitral orifice is 4 to 6 cm², and signs and symptoms may not be noticed

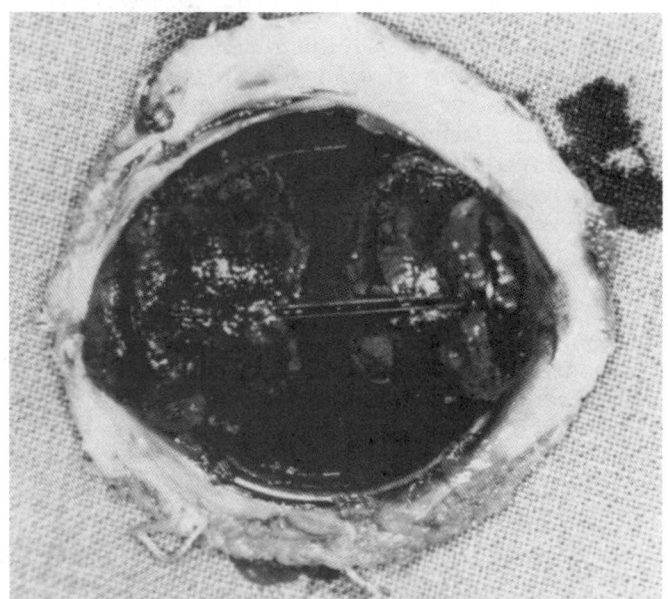

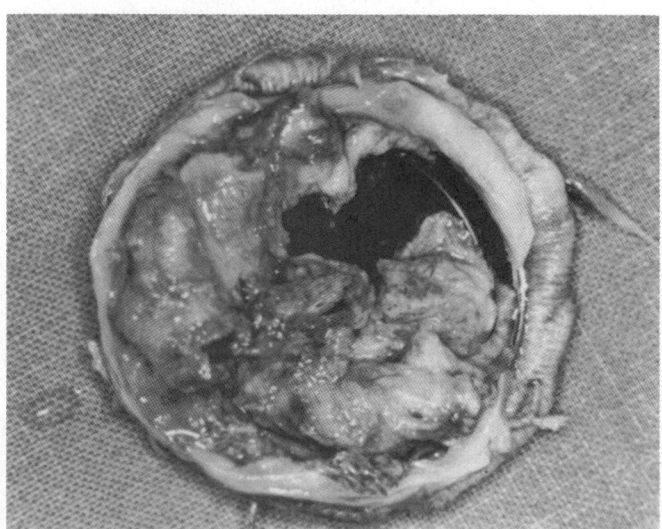

FIGURE 17–9. Thrombosed mechanical prostheses. *Top*, Atrial surface of a St. Jude prosthesis with leaflets immobilized by large clots that appear to originate from the hinge areas. *Bottom*, Thrombosed Medtronic-Hall prosthesis with the disc almost completely covered by a mass of organized blood clot. (From Barlow, J. B. (1987). *Perspectives on the mitral valve.* Philadelphia: F. A. Davis.)

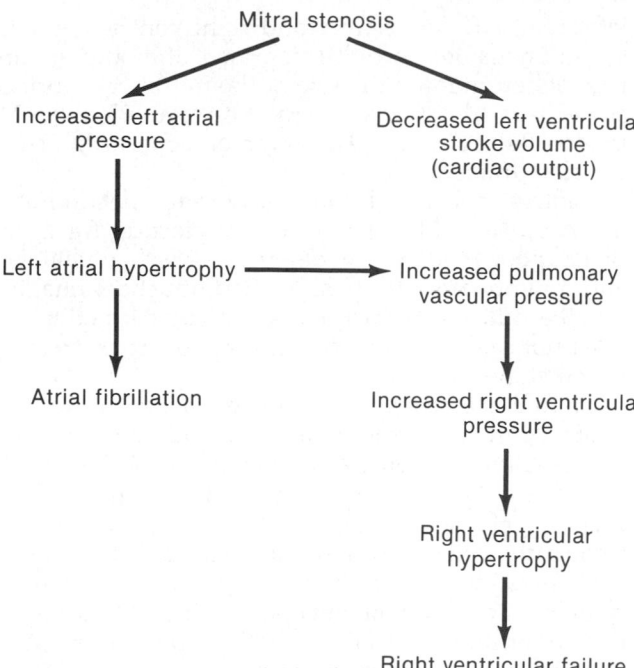

Mitral stenosis

Increased left atrial pressure

Decreased left ventricular stroke volume (cardiac output)

Left atrial hypertrophy ⟶ Increased pulmonary vascular pressure

Atrial fibrillation

Increased right ventricular pressure

Right ventricular hypertrophy

Right ventricular failure

FIGURE 17–10. Pathophysiology of mitral stenosis. (Adapted from *The Journal of Cardiovascular Nursing*, Vol. 1, No. 3, pp. 1–17, with permission of Aspen Publishers, Inc., © 1987.)

until the orifice is 1 to 2 cm². The left atrial blood volume and pressures become elevated, resulting in left atrial hypertrophy. The dilated left atrium often develops atrial fibrillation, and the poor blood flow predisposes the patient to the development of atrial thrombus. The elevated atrial blood volume and pressure are referred back into the pulmonary veins, which distend and thin under the stress. Eventually, the blood volume and pressures are referred into the pulmonary capillaries and arteries. Perivascular and perialveolar transudates stiffen the lung and may lead to pulmonary edema. The entire pulmonary vascular system becomes hyperplastic and hypertrophies. Changes in the pulmonary vascular system increase right ventricular afterload. The right ventricle eventually hypertrophies. In severe mitral stenosis, the right ventricle may fail. Mitral stenosis will decrease preload and eventually stroke volume. The degree of forward failure is dependent on the ability of the heart rate and systemic vascular resistance to compensate for the decreased stroke volume.

Physical Assessment

Dyspnea is the most common presenting symptom of mitral stenosis. The patient may notice the dyspnea with exertion, anxiety, fever, during pregnancy, or when lying supine. Dyspnea may become more severe with the onset of atrial fibrillation. It is related to the pulmonary transudates, which may also be evidenced by hemoptysis. Progression of pulmonary volumes and pressures may cause pulmonary edema.

A careful history may identify a gradually decreasing exercise tolerance and fatigue related to the dyspnea. As the pulmonary pathology progresses, the patient may develop a chronic cough due to the pulmonary congestion. Pulmonary congestion increases the patient's risk of bronchitis, pulmonary embolism, and pulmonary infarction. The distended pulmonary artery has been known to compress the laryngeal nerve against the aorta on rare occasions, causing hoarseness. Pulmonary hypertension has also been manifested as chest pain, associated with dyspnea and responsive to nitroglycerin. No mechanism has been identified for the pain.

Pulmonary symptoms are most common, but there are other symptoms of mitral stenosis. Systemic emboli, especially cerebral emboli, may occur, especially after the onset of atrial fibrillation. Some patients complain of palpitations. Symptoms of right ventricular failure such as peripheral dependent edema, left upper quadrant fullness (hepatic congestion), abdominal enlargement, and cold extremities may be reported. The enlarged left atrium may cause dysphagia.

Inspection of the patient may reveal flushed cheeks in less pigmented patients, called mitral facies. There may be peripheral cyanosis and jugular vein distention. The respiratory rate is increased. These patients are often thin. Palpitation often reveals a normal pulse and point of maximum impulse. The apical impulse may include a tapping vibration of the first heart sound. The left lower sternal and parasternal areas may have a lift if the patient has severe pulmonary hypertension.

Auscultation provides the most revealing assessments. The murmur of mitral stenosis is an early to mid-diastolic, low-pitched rumbling sound heard best at the apex. Turning the patient to the left lateral position facilitates auscultation as does exercise, coughing, and amyl nitrate. There is usually an opening snap prior to the murmur, a high-pitched sound that follows the second heart sound. No opening snap often indicates that both leaflets are immobile. The closer the opening snap to the second heart sound, the more severe the stenosis. The first heart sound is usually loud if the leaflets and chordae are pliable but may be soft if the mitral immobility is severe and the sound is produced primarily by the tricuspid valve. Correlating with the pulmonary symptoms, crackles are commonly found in the lower lung fields, and wheezes may be found if the mitral stenosis has progressed to the stage of chronic coughing.

Hemodynamic monitoring will demonstrate elevated left atrial pressures with an exaggerated a wave and a slow y decent. Pulmonary artery pressures are elevated in more severe mitral stenosis. If mitral stenosis has caused right ventricular failure, central venous pressure will also be elevated, and large a waves and slow y descents may be evident. Cardiac output is usually normal until the orifice is less than 1 cm².

Electrocardiographic monitoring may demonstrate normal sinus rhythm. In lead II a widened notched P wave (P mitrale) may reflect the left atrial hypertrophy. Premature atrial contractions may occur secondary to atrial dilation. Eventually, most patients with mitral stenosis develop atrial fibrillation due to the atrial dilation.

Laboratory Findings

There is seldom any indication of mitral stenosis on laboratory examination of blood (Table 17–1). Red blood cell destruction may be increased across the stenotic valve; after right ventricular failure occurs the liver enzymes may be elevated. Patients with pulmonary edema and possibly those with pulmonary transudates will have decreased oxygen saturation.

Diagnostic Procedures

Electrocardiograms may demonstrate cardiac changes such as the wide (> 0.12 second) notched P waves in leads II, III, and aVF or biphasic P waves with the second portion negative in V_1, which is indicative of left atrial hypertrophy. Right ventricular hypertrophy may cause a right axis deviation, R waves in V_1.

Chest x-rays may demonstrate the left atrial enlargement that may elevate the left mainstem bronchus. Elevated pulmonary pressures cause redistribution of blood flow to the upper lobes of the lung, Kerley B lines in the lung fields, and possibly enlargement of the pulmonary arteries and right ventricle. Calcifications of the mitral valve may be noted. Pulmonary effusions, interstitial edema, and pulmonary edema may also be detected.

Phonocardiograms may be utilized to clarify the aortic component of the second heart sound and the timing of the opening snap. Serial phonocardiograms demonstrating a narrowing of the interval between the two sounds indicate increasing left atrial pressures. Serial recordings demonstrate increased duration of the murmur as the stenosis increases. Apex cardiograms may be utilized to record or track rapid ventricular filling. As mitral stenosis progresses, the rapid filling wave is lost. The intensity of the mitral component of the first heart sound is usually increased, but as the leaflets become less mobile, this sound may also be lost. As pulmonary hypertension develops, the phonocardiogram can demonstrate the increased intensity of the pulmonic component of the second heart sound.

Echocardiograms can confirm the diagnosis of mitral stenosis (see Table 17–2). M-mode echocardiography can demonstrate the thick leaflets and their limited or abnormal movements. M-mode echocardiography can document the rate of diastolic closure of the mitral valve leaflet or annulus calcification, leaflet vegetations, atrial thrombus or myxoma, and left atrial, left ventricular, and right ventricular size. Two-dimensional echocardiograms offer the advantage of determining the size of the mitral valve orifice as well as all of the information provided by M-mode. Pulsed and color Doppler echocardiograms are also utilized.

Contrast and gated pool study radionuclide imaging has been utilized to calculate ejection fractions. Blood pool studies can determine cardiac chamber and pulmonary artery size. Radionuclide imaging may be utilized to track left ventricular function but does not play a major role in diagnosing or treating mitral stenosis.

Graded exercise studies can be utilized to demonstrate a patient's activity tolerance and hemodynamic abnormalities. Exercise studies may be useful to document dysrhythmia control by pharmacologic therapy. However, graded exercise studies are not frequently utilized for patients with mitral stenosis.

Patients with intermittent symptoms or complaints of palpitations may be evaluated with a Holter monitor. Intermittent atrial fibrillation, premature atrial contractions, or other dysrhythmias may be identified by this method. Holter monitoring is another diagnostic modality that is seldomly employed for mitral stenosis.

Cardiac catheterization is primarily utilized to measure the gradient across the mitral valve. Angiography may also be used to determine whether coronary artery disease, mitral regurgitation, or aortic valve lesions are also present. Ventricular wall motion and size may be determined by angiography. Cardiac catheterization is not considered necessary for diagnosing or treating isolated mitral stenosis.

Medical Treatment

Rheumatic endocarditis is treated with penicillin; alternatively, sulfadiazine or erythromycin is prescribed. Sources differ on the length of time for continued prophylaxis with these antibiotics, ranging from continuing until the patient is 30 years of age to continuing for life. The second antibiotic regimen is aimed at preventing infective endocarditis. Prophylaxis for dental and surgical procedures consists of amoxicillin, ampicillin, erythromycin, or clindamycin and may be followed or combined with gentamicin or vancomycin. It is typically a two-dose regimen (see Table 17–3). The third antibiotic regimen is short-course, intermittent treatment for infections as they occur.

Dyspnea and other respiratory symptoms are often treated by limiting activity, maintaining appropriate weight for height, eating a sodium-restricted diet, and taking diuretics such as chlorothiazide, chlorthalidone, or furosemide. In severe cases sedation and hospitalization with bedrest are required. Decreased exercise tolerance and fatigue eventually affect all individuals with mitral stenosis. The limited cardiac reserve usually is the basis for recommending that the patient avoid competitive sports. Many physicians believe that the adrenalin, endorphins, and psychologic factors involved in competitive sports may cause the patient to miss or ignore symptoms. Some patients have found nitroglycerin effective in decreasing pulmonary symptoms because it promotes venous dilation. The decreased right ventricular preload and increased pulmonary venous capacitance caused by nitroglycerin reduce pulmonary congestion, transudates, and edema.

Dysrhythmias are usually atrial, and the first signs of cardiac failure usually are those of right ventricular failure. Either of these signs are treated with digoxin. Dysrhythmias may also be treated with propranolol, quinidine, calcium channel blockers, or cardioversion. Anticoagulation is often prescribed for 2 or 3 weeks prior to attempting cardioversion for longstanding atrial fibrillation. Because of the risk of systemic emboli, the occurrence of left atrial dilation or atrial fibrillation is an indication for anticoagulation with acetylsalicylic acid, warfarin, or dipyridamole. Anemia should be treated by diet, if possible, or otherwise transfusions.

Surgical treatment of mitral stenosis is recommended prior to the occurrence of pulmonary hypertension or right ventricular failure. Valvuloplasty is often attempted. Closed mitral commissurotomy with one or two balloons (Vahanian et al., 1989) or a finger or mechanical dilator (Fig. 17–11) may be attempted, but open commissurotomy is performed more frequently (Fig. 17–12). During open commissurotomy, atrial thrombus may be removed, the left atrial appendage may be amputated to decrease the risk of thrombus formation, fused chordae may be separated, scarred papillary muscles may be split, and some calcium deposits may be removed from

the leaflets and annulus. Some patients benefit from two or three different valvuloplasties. Mitral valve replacement is indicated when valvuloplasty is no longer successful or is not possible due to scarring, calcification, or deformity (see earlier discussion of mitral valve replacement in the section on mitral regurgitation, and Chapter 20). Antibiotic prophylaxis, activity restrictions, diet, diuretics, digoxin, other antidysrhythmics, and anticoagulation therapies are usually resumed after surgical intervention.

AORTIC REGURGITATION

Pathophysiology

Aortic regurgitation may result from disorders of the aortic valve leaflets or disorders of the base of the aorta. Connective tissue disorders of the leaflets or aorta are the most common causes of aortic regurgitation. Myxomatous degeneration begins in the central layer of the leaflet, the spongiosa, or in the tunica media of the aorta. The myxomatous cells spread into the supporting layers of the leaflet or aorta, interrupting its continuity and weakening the structure. The aorta often develops cystic medial necrosis secondary to this process. The weakened leaflets prolapse or tear and the aorta dilates, distorting the annulus of the aortic valve. Conditions associated with myxomatous changes are Marfan syndrome and osteogenesis imperfecta.

The rheumatic disease process also affects the aortic valve. The inflammatory reaction causes fibrosis and contracture of the leaflets (Fig. 17–13). One or more of the shortened leaflets, or cusps, cannot approximate with the others, and blood is able to

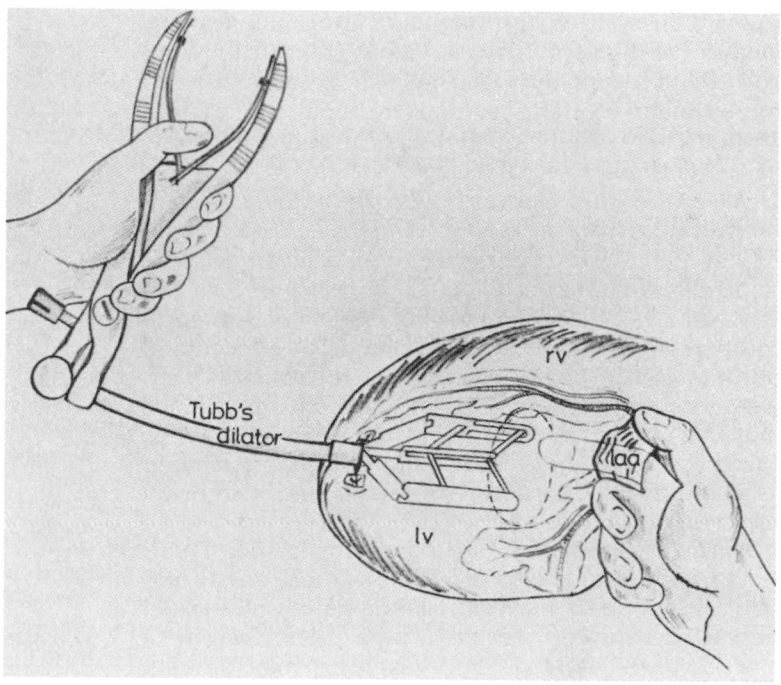

FIGURE 17–11. Technique of closed commissurotomy. An index finger is introduced through the left atrial appendage *(laa)* into the left atrium and helps guide the Tubb dilator, which is introduced via the apex of the left ventricle *(lv)*, through the mitral valve. rv, right ventricle. (From Barlow, J. B. (1987). *Perspectives on the mitral valve.* Philadelphia, F. A. Davis.)

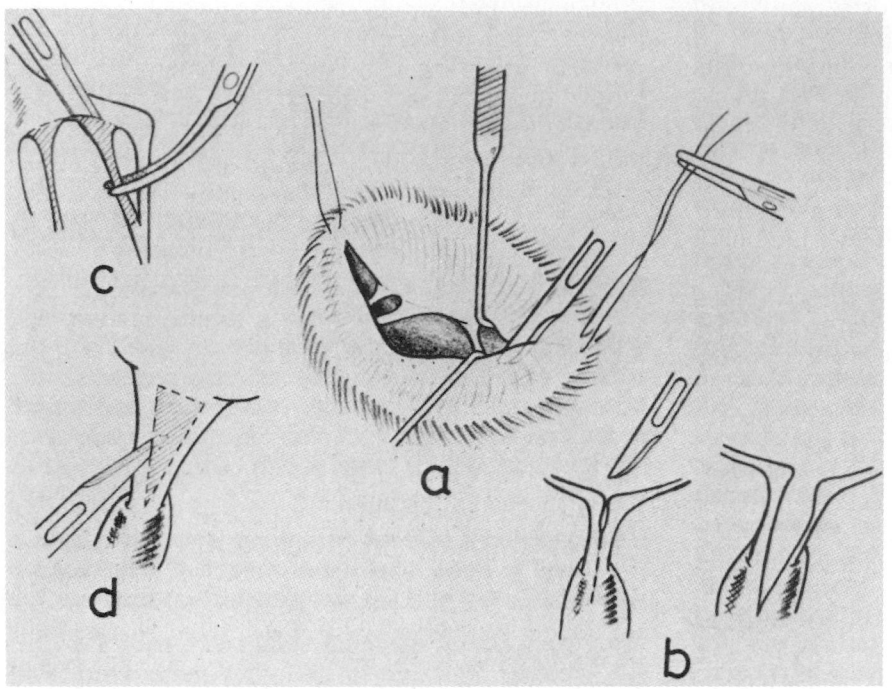

FIGURE 17–12. Technique of open commissurotomy. *a,* Sharp division of the commissures helped by retraction of the free edges of the two leaflets. *b,* When the chordae tendineae and the papillary muscle heads are fused at the commissural level, these are incised longitudinally. *c,* Thickened secondary and basal chordae contribute to the thickening and immobility of the posterior leaflet and are resected thoroughly. *d,* Fused chordae tendineae obstructing the flow of blood are fenestrated by the removal of triangular portions of the fibrosed tissue. (From Barlow, J. B. (1987). *Perspectives on the mitral valve.* Philadelphia: F. A. Davis.)

flow back across the valve. The aortic commissures seldom fuse in the rheumatic process.

Infective endocarditis, usually due to *Staphylococcus aureus* or enterococci, may result in aortic regurgitation. The disease process destroys cusp tissue, resulting in perforations of the cusp or tears along the annulus where the cusp attaches to the aorta. Occasionally, vegetations may prevent complete apposition of the cusps.

Syphilis (Fig. 17–13) and rheumatoid (ankylosing) spondylitis affect both the aorta and the valve. The aorta dilates, separating the leaflets. As the dilation progresses, tension on the cusps causes them to curl toward their base, further separating the leaflets. Dilation of the aorta may also result from a dissecting aortic aneurysm, hypertension, senile dilation, and hypervolemia (often secondary to renal failure). The annulus may also be dilated or distorted from below by a ventricular septal defect. The defect may also weaken the cusp support, distorting the leaflet or permitting prolapse.

Traumatic lesions are another rare cause of aortic regurgitation. Typically, blunt force trauma causes an aortic tear that disrupts the cusp's connection to the aorta. The support of the cusp is weakened and permits prolapse. Direct injury to the valve is rare, but tears in a cusp may occur. Penetrating wounds may lacerate cusps or penetrate the aorta or annulus. Ruptured cusps have been reported after straining, as in childbirth. Aortic valvuloplasty may also result in aortic regurgitation.

Aortic regurgitation may also occur in individuals with prosthetic valves. The leaflets, disk, or ball and strut components may fail. Tissue valves may experience changes of the annulus as described with native valves. Any of the prostheses may develop

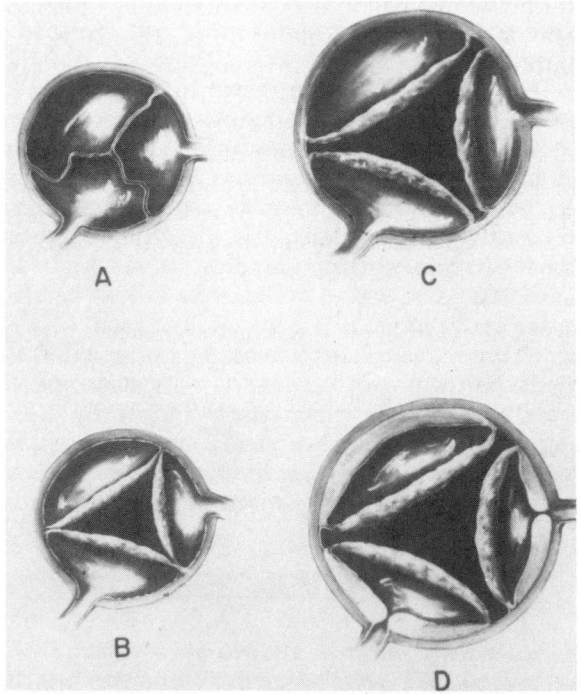

FIGURE 17–13. Variations in the aortic valve. *A,* The normal valve. *B,* Shortening of the cusps characteristic of rheumatic aortic regurgitation. *C,* Dilation of the aorta, as occurs in syphilitic aortitis and other conditions in which dilation is responsible for aortic regurgitation. The main feature results from bowing of the leaflets. Commissural separation is illustrated and may also be present. *D,* In addition to the feature shown in *C,* there is atherosclerosis of the aorta, as occurs in syphilitic aortitis, with consequent coronary ostial narrowing. (From Roberts, W. C. (1973). Valvular, subvalvular and supravalvular aortic stenosis: Morphologic features. In J. E. Edwards (ed.): *Clinical-pathologic correlations #2* (p. 133). Philadelphia: F. A. Davis.)

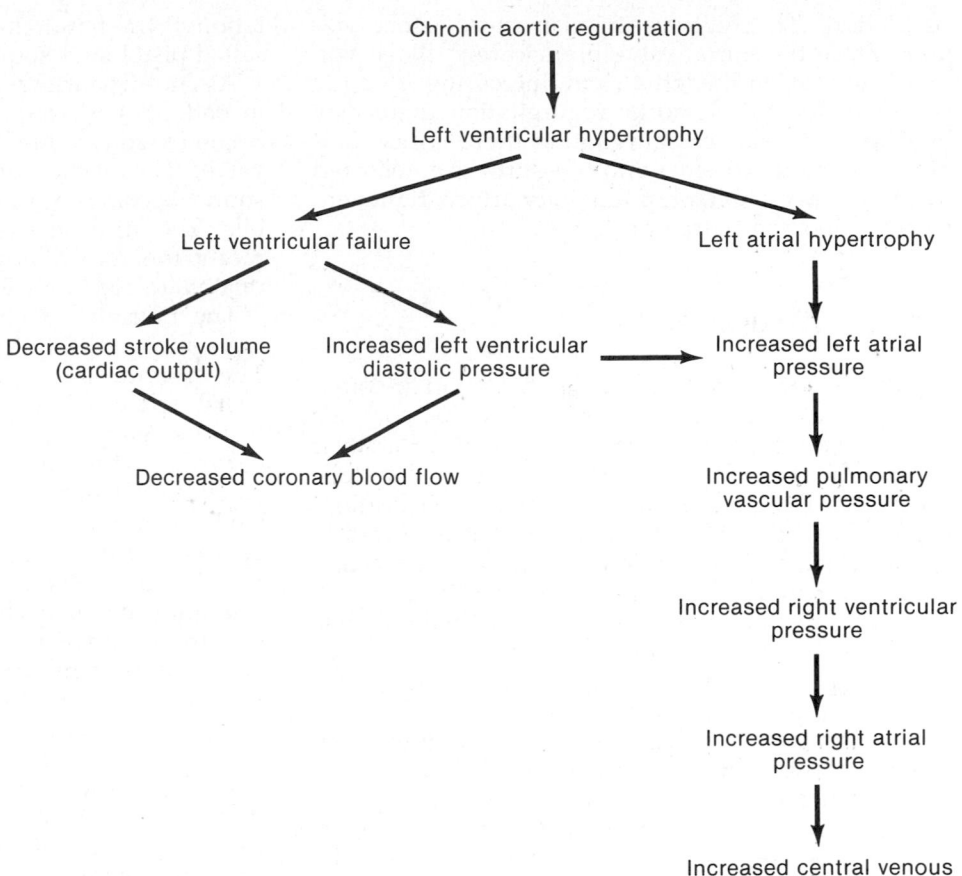

Chronic aortic regurgitation

Left ventricular hypertrophy

Left ventricular failure   Left atrial hypertrophy

Decreased stroke volume   Increased left ventricular   Increased left atrial
(cardiac output)   diastolic pressure   pressure

Decreased coronary blood flow   Increased pulmonary
vascular pressure

Increased right ventricular
pressure

Increased right atrial
pressure

Increased central venous
pressure

FIGURE 17–14. Pathophysiology of chronic aortic regurgitation. (Adapted from *The Journal of Cardiovascular Nursing,* Vol. 1, No. 3, pp. 1–17, with permission of Aspen Publishers, Inc., © 1987.)

regurgitation at the sewing ring when sutures or tissue fail.

Aortic regurgitation may be acute or chronic, but the effect is the same: increased left ventricular volume related to systemic blood flowing back into the left ventricle during diastole. The increased left ventricular end-diastolic volume results in a dilated left ventricle with increased wall tension. The ventricle contracts swiftly and strongly as a result of the increased tension (Starling's law). In chronic aortic regurgitation, the stroke volume increases to maintain the normal forward stroke volume plus the regurgitant volume (Fig. 17–14). The ventricle hypertrophies and thickens, usually maintaining a normal ratio of wall thickness to cavity and size. Eventually, the ventricle with aortic regurgitation fibroses and fails. In acute aortic regurgitation, the ventricle cannot adapt to the increased volume by dilating to the extent required (Fig. 17–15). Ventricular hypertrophy is absent or minimal and the left ventricle fails earlier.

Cardiac output is often maintained in both chronic and acute aortic regurgitation. In the chronic condition, the rapid upstroke and high pressure of systole stimulate the aortic baroreceptors. The reflex dilation of the systemic arteries decreases afterload and minimizes the regurgitant volume. Isotonic exercise causes further vasodilation and an increased heart rate that shortens diastole, thereby decreasing regurgitation. Isometric exercise, cold, and sympathetic

stimulation cause vasoconstriction, which may increase the regurgitation. In the acute condition, the heart rate increases rapidly to maintain cardiac output. The hypertrophied ventricle or tachycardia increases myocardial oxygen demand. Vasodilation decreases diastolic pressure, and tachycardia decreases the time of diastole, thereby decreasing coronary perfusion. Myocardial ischemia may be caused by this mechanism.

Eventually, the left ventricle cannot maintain forward blood flow from the left atrium to the systemic

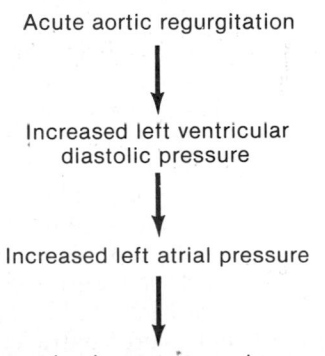

Acute aortic regurgitation

Increased left ventricular
diastolic pressure

Increased left atrial pressure

Increased pulmonary vascular pressure

FIGURE 17–15. Pathophysiology of acute aortic regurgitation. (Adapted from *The Journal of Cardiovascular Nursing,* Vol. 1, No. 3, pp. 1–17, with permission of Aspen Publishers, Inc., © 1987.)

circulation. The high ventricular end-diastolic volumes close the mitral valve prematurely. Blood volume increases in the left atrium, increasing left atrial pressure. In chronic aortic regurgitation there may be dilation; in acute regurgitation there is not. Pulmonary venous volumes and pressures rise, followed by pulmonary capillary, pulmonary artery, right ventricular, and right atrial pressures.

Physical Assessment

Patients with chronic aortic regurgitation are often asymptomatic. Some patients perceive palpitations in the head or neck from the forceful ventricular contractions or pulsations due to the elevated systolic pressures. Others are aware of their heart beating, especially while lying down, a sign that is related to the ventricular hypertrophy. Once left ventricular failure occurs with acute or chronic aortic regurgitation, the most common presenting symptom is dyspnea. Other symptoms of left ventricular failure are fatigue, cough, orthopnea, paroxysmal nocturnal dyspnea, pulmonary edema, and syncope. Myocardial ischemia may precipitate other symptoms such as angina, dysrhythmias, and myocardial infarctions. An unexplained symptom is profuse sweating.

Inspection of the patient with severe aortic regurgitation may reveal a head bob with each systole. Carotid or temporal pulsations may be clearly seen, the uvula may pulsate, and when a glass slide is pressed against the patient's lip or a light is pressed to the fingertip, capillary pulsations of the lip or nailbed may be observed. The point of maximal impulse may be observed laterally and caudally. Pulsations of the left chest may be noted if left ventricular hypertrophy exists. If the aorta is dilated, pulsations may be visible in the second and third intercostal spaces. Patients with acute aortic regurgitation may have pale or acrocyanotic extremities and jugular venous distention.

Palpitation of the carotid pulse demonstrates a distinctive rapid upstroke and downstroke. It has been called the waterhammer or Corrigan pulse. The point of maximum impulse is larger than normal and may actually be diffuse if left ventricular hypertrophy is present. Pulsations of the digital arteries may be palpable, and the hands may be warm and sweaty. Patients with acute or late chronic aortic regurgitation are tachycardic. There may be a carotid thrill if regurgitation is severe. In acute cases, pulsus alternans characteristic of left ventricular failure may be noted, especially in the femoral arteries.

Auscultation of patients with aortic regurgitation can be difficult. The systolic blood pressure may be normal but is often increased. The diastolic blood pressure is low until the left ventricle fails, then it rises. Korotkoff sounds often continue to 0 mm Hg; in these cases the reading should be taken when the sound changes intensity or muffles. The pulse pressure is widened until the left ventricle fails. Auscul-

tation of the femoral artery may reveal brisk sounds called pistol-shot sounds or Traube sign.

As chronic aortic regurgitation progresses and also in patients with acute disease, the first heart sound becomes softer due to early closure of the mitral valve. The aortic component of the second heart sound becomes softer if the leaflets become immobile. The third heart sound may be heard and more rarely the fourth heart sound. When the aorta is dilated an ejection click may be heard.

The murmur of chronic aortic regurgitation is a high-pitched, blowing, decrescendo diastolic sound. The murmur is best heard in the second right intercostal space while the patient is sitting, leaning forward, and exhaling. The duration of the murmur correlates with the severity of the regurgitation. Auscultation should also be done to the left of the sternum and in the third intercostal space. A systolic ejection murmur radiating to the carotids may be heard if the valve is distorted or the aorta dilated. The murmur may be increased by vasopressors, squatting, and isometric exercise and decreased by vasodilators, amyl nitrite, and the Valsalva maneuver. A coarse vibrating sound is usually detected if there is a tear in a cusp or along the annulus.

A second diastolic murmur may be heard at the apex. It is a low-pitched, rumbling sound that is mid-diastolic, holodiastolic, or presystolic. This sound is called the Austin Flint murmur. It is thought to be caused by the regurgitant flow contacting the anterior mitral leaflet and pushing it up into the flow of blood from the left atrium. Another hypothesis is that the regurgitation murmur is referred to the apex through the thorax. The murmur of acute regurgitation is a mid-pitched, short diastolic sound. An Austin Flint murmur is usually heard in mid-diastole. The third heart sound is common. Peripheral arterial sounds are seldom heard.

Laboratory Findings

There are no changes in blood sample values until left ventricular failure affects the pulmonary vasculature (see Table 17–1). Transudates and pulmonary edema will ultimately result in decreased oxygen saturation. The decreased cardiac output leads to acidosis and fluid retention.

Diagnostic Procedures

Chest x-rays may demonstrate the left ventricular hypertrophy characteristic of chronic aortic regurgitation. Dilation of the ascending aorta may be detected. Chronic aortic regurgitation eventually causes left atrial enlargement, which may be evident. Acute and chronic conditions with left ventricular failure will demonstrate pulmonary congestion.

The electrocardiogram usually has a left axis deviation and often tall R waves in V_{4-6} in patients with chronic aortic regurgitation. First degree atrioventricular block is common. Left or right bundle branch blocks and third degree atrioventricular block are also seen. In acute aortic regurgitation nonspecific ST-T wave changes may be seen, and sinus tachycardia is nearly universal.

Echocardiography is used to track the severity of aortic regurgitation (see Table 17–2). In chronic conditions the dilated aorta may be documented. Aortic valve leaflet movement, thickness, and vegetations may be visualized. Left ventricular diameter, wall thickness, and motion can be determined. Tracking the left ventricular end-systolic diameter is often used to determine the best time for surgical intervention. Echocardiography may demonstrate fluttering of the anterior or posterior mitral valve leaflet or the ventricular septum during diastole, caused by the regurgitant blood flow. The size, shape, direction and velocity of the regurgitant jet may be determined by color Doppler. The size of the left atrium can be determined. Patients with acute aortic regurgitation often demonstrate a delayed slow opening of the mitral valve, diastolic anterior mitral valve leaflet or ventricular septal fluttering, and early mitral valve closure. Indications that the aorta has dissected may also be obtained by echocardiography.

Phonocardiography may be most useful for detecting acute aortic regurgitation when tachycardia alters the sounds and shortens diastole. Recorded simultaneously with the electrocardiogram, both components of the first and second heart sounds can be identified. The third heart sound may be depicted. The murmur of aortic regurgitation may be recorded immediately after the aortic component of the second heart sound. In chronic aortic regurgitation, the Austin Flint murmur may also be recorded.

Graded exercise studies may be utilized to document a patient's activity tolerance. Radionuclide studies may be utilized independently or in combination with graded exercise studies. The extent of the regurgitation may be quantified by blood pool imaging, and ejection fractions can be determined.

Cardiac catheterization is employed when surgical intervention is contemplated. The aorta is visualized for dilation and lesions and to determine the degree of regurgitation. Left ventricular pressures, cardiac output, ejection fraction, and regurgitant fraction can be measured and quantified. Left ventricular wall motion is also recorded. The coronary arteries are usually visualized, and coronary artery disease may be evaluated. Right heart catheterization is used to determine pulmonary, right heart, and venous pressures.

Medical Treatment

The signs and symptoms determine the priority of treatment for aortic regurgitation. Antibiotic prophylaxis (see Table 17–3) for endocarditis should be prescribed for patients undergoing all dental and surgical procedures. Amoxicillin is used, and gentamicin or vancomycin may be added to the regimen. Once left ventricular failure develops, treatment may include digitalis, diuretics (hydralazine, furosemide), vasodilators (nitrates, sodium nitroprusside), and a salt-restricted diet. Dysrhythmias should be treated with antidysrhythmics. Isometric exercises and the use of an intra-aortic balloon pump are to be avoided because both increase diastolic pressures and accentuate the regurgitation.

Acute aortic regurgitation usually requires aortic valve surgery at an early stage. Chronic aortic regurgitation may not require valve surgery for many years. The ultimate treatment for both types of aortic regurgitation is usually surgical valve replacement (see Chap. 20). The best time for surgery is prior to the occurrence of significant left ventricular failure. Valvuloplasty may be attempted in a few cases. Torn leaflets or those torn from the annulus may be surgically repaired. The annulus may be narrowed with a stent or by excising a section of the dilated aorta that is dilating the annulus. The majority of surgical procedures consist of total valve replacements. Considerations relating to prostheses are as follows:

1. Mechanical valves (ball-cage or disc) require the patient to take anticoagulants to prevent thrombus formation as long as the valve is in place.
2. Tissue valves (homeografts, xenografts, heterografts, allografts) do not require prolonged anticoagulation, but the leaflets become stiff and sometimes calcify or leak after being exposed to the high-pressure blood flow in the aortic position.
3. The annulus of all valve prostheses and some of the components will create some degree of aortic stenosis (Fig. 17–7). (Refer to the section on mitral regurgitation for criteria for prosthesis selection.)

The aortic valve presents a unique problem compared to the other cardiac valves because of the proximity of the coronary artery ostia. Postoperatively, patients will continue to require antibiotic prophylaxis for endocarditis and may require antidysrhythmics or anticoagulation (warfarin).

AORTIC STENOSIS

Pathophysiology

Aortic stenosis may be caused by idiopathic fibrosis and calcification as an individual ages (Fig. 17–16). The calcification of the leaflets usually begins along the edge of the annulus and slowly moves toward the commissures. Eventually, the leaflet's endothelial layer is injured and becomes fibrous, scarred, and thickened. The aortic valve cusps become less mobile, and the commissures may fuse, narrowing the orifice. Microthrombi may develop on the cusps during and after this process.

Atherosclerotic changes of the aorta or valve may

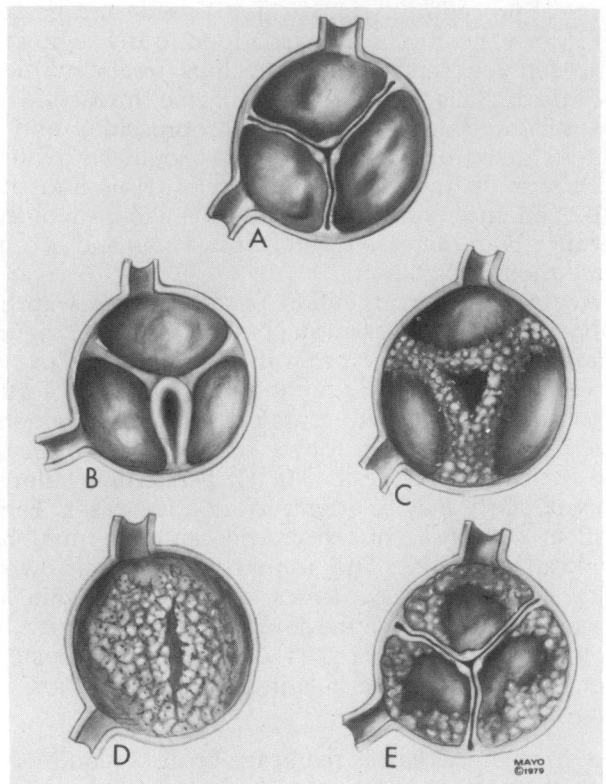

FIGURE 17–16. Types of aortic valve stenosis. *A,* Normal aortic valve. *B,* Congenital aortic stenosis. *C,* Rheumatic aortic stenosis. *D,* Calcific bicuspid aortic stenosis. *E,* Calcific senile aortic stenosis. (From Brandenburg, R. O., et al. (1979). Valvular heart disease: When should the patient be referred? *Practical Cardiology* 5:50. By permission of Mayo Foundation.)

also immobilize the cusps or cause fusion of the commissures. The aortic valve may be immobilized by lipid deposits on the cusps in patients with hyperlipidemia, vegetations of active infection or calcified vegetations due to endocarditis, accumulation of metabolic products due to ochronosis or Fabry disease, and by thrombosis in patients with systemic lupus erythematosus (Hurst, 1986). Stenosis may be caused by a prosthetic valve that has a narrower orifice because of the mechanical annulus. Prosthetic valves also develop calcifications and stiffening and may develop thrombus, vegetations, or pannus.

Rheumatic endocarditis affects the aortic valve and may cause stenosis (Fig. 17–16). The cusps and annulus thicken, stiffen, and calcify. The commissures fuse and calcify. These changes may be a direct result of the inflammatory process or may predispose the valve to the fibrous, calcific process. In this case, the calcifications begin on the free edges of the leaflets.

Stenosis of the ascending aorta or narrowing of the subvalvular outflow tract by fibroelastic membranes (discrete subaortic stenosis) or muscular tissue (asymmetric septal hypertrophy/idiopathic hypertrophic subaortic stenosis, papillary muscle mass) may mimic aortic valve stenosis. Congenital lesions

are a more common cause of aortic stenosis (see Fig. 17–16). The lesions are commonly unicuspid and bicuspid valves or malformed tricuspid valves, and calcification precipitates the symptoms. In many cases, the etiology of aortic stenosis is unknown.

Whatever the etiology, the stenotic aortic valve is typically calcified, decreasing both its mobility and its orifice size. Because the process is gradual, the left ventricle compensates for the increased systolic pressures needed by hypertrophy (Fig. 17–17). The hypertrophied ventricle generates high enough pressures to maintain normal stroke volume and cardiac output for a period of time. The left ventricular hypertrophy eventually elevates left ventricular end-diastolic pressures, increasing the work of the left atrium. The left atrium also hypertrophies. The atrial kick component is maintained (Starling's law). As stenosis continues, the left ventricle begins to fail and dilates. Stroke volume decreases, further increasing left ventricular volume and pressure. Strain on the left atrium develops, resulting in backward failure. The left atrial volume and pressures rise, followed by rises in pulmonary venous, capillary, and arterial pressures and then by right ventricular, atrial, and systemic venous pressures.

The rising left ventricular diastolic pressures inhibit coronary artery perfusion. Ventricular oxygen demand is often increased because of hypertrophy, tachycardia, and the need to work against the increased afterload of stenosis, which prolongs the isovolumetric contraction. The degree of stenosis may limit stroke volume, which cannot be compensated by increased heart rate, so cardiac output falls.

Physical Assessment

Presenting symptoms of aortic stenosis may be dyspnea, angina, or syncope. Usually the patient is asymptomatic for many years. Dyspnea is usually noted on exertion and is an indication of left ventricular failure, either progressive or as a result of atrial fibrillation. Angina (described in the pathology section) may also be related to calcific emboli or concurrent coronary artery disease. Syncope is usually related to exertion and may also be a sign of left ventricular failure or dysrhythmia. Stroke, endocarditis, palpitations, and vision disturbances may also be presenting symptoms.

Inspection usually reveals no abnormal findings. If congestive heart failure is present, jugular vein distention, peripheral edema, and respiratory distress may be noted. Palpation may reveal a slowly rising, sustained pulse, especially at the carotid and brachial arteries (carotid sinus sensitivity should be considered before palpating the carotid). The carotid may also reveal systolic vibrations called the carotid shudder, and, with left ventricular failure, pulsus alternans. The point of maximum impulse is of longer duration than normal and, as the left ventricle dilates, is displaced laterally and caudally. A systolic thrill

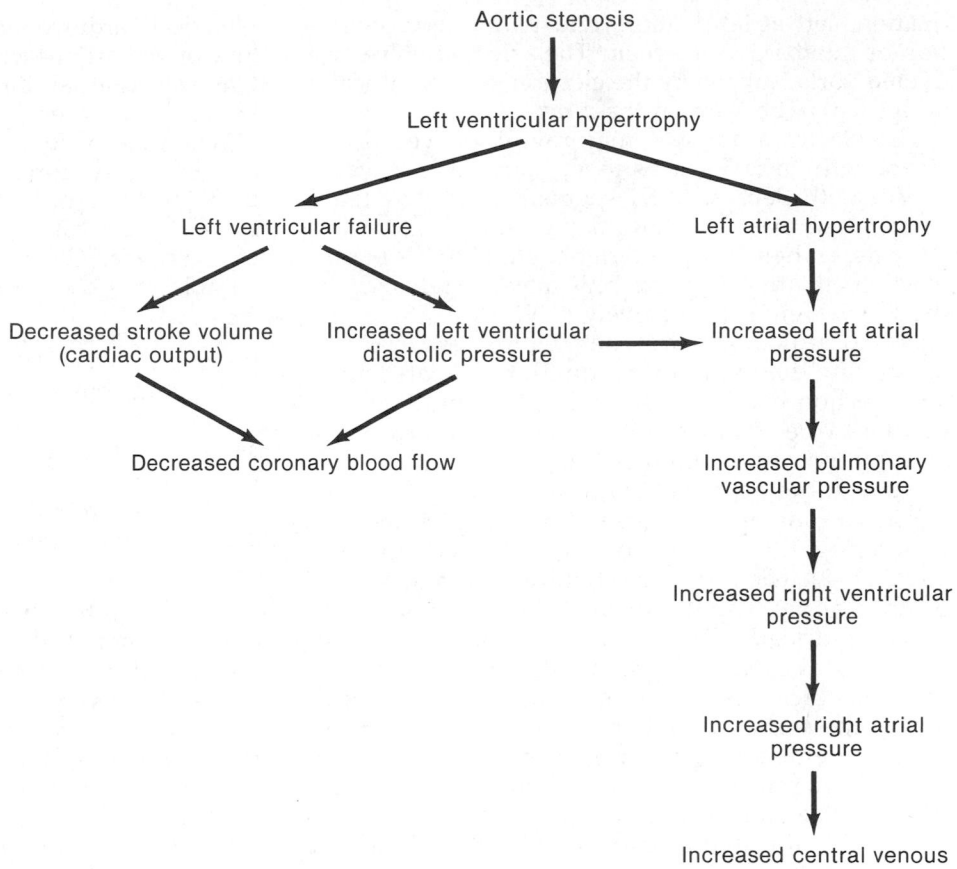

FIGURE 17-17. Pathophysiology of aortic valve stenosis. (Adapted from *The Journal of Cardiovascular Nursing*, Vol. 1, No. 3, pp. 1–17, with permission of Aspen Publishers, Inc., © 1987.)

may be palpable at the second intercostal space on either side of the sternum, especially during exhalation with the patient sitting and leaning forward. If right heart failure has been prolonged, the liver may be palpable.

Auscultation usually reveals a soft first heart sound as the mitral valve closes early. The second heart sound is variable. While the cusps are mobile, the aortic component may be accentuated, but once they are immobile, the aortic component may be absent. The second heart sound is often single or, with left ventricular failure or left bundle branch block, paradoxical. The third and fourth heart sounds are often heard. An aortic ejection click, a high-pitched sound heard best along the left sternal border, may be heard immediately after the first heart sound if the cusps are mobile. The murmur is a harsh, high-pitched, systolic murmur that is crescendo-decrescendo in nature. The murmur is heard best at the right sternal border at the second intercostal space and may radiate to the neck or apex. The murmur will increase with amyl nitrate, squatting, or lying flat. The murmur will decrease with vasopressors, isometric exercise, the Valsalva maneuver, and standing. Other auscultatory findings may be pulmonary crackles with left ventricular failure and changes in blood pressure. The blood pressure usually demonstrates a low systolic combined with a normal diastolic pressure, therefore, a narrowed pulse pressure. When the aorta is calcified, the systolic pressure may be elevated.

The electrocardiogram usually reveals normal sinus rhythm. First degree atrioventricular block, left bundle branch block, and atrial fibrillation may also be evident. Hemodynamic monitoring may reveal high readings and prominent a, c, and v waves in the central venous pressure because of right ventricular failure. The pulmonary artery wedge pressure (PAWP) is usually the first to demonstrate backward failure. PAWP may be elevated and may demonstrate prominent a waves due to left ventricular failure. Pulmonary artery systolic pressures rise; diastolic pressures rise later. Pulmonary vascular resistance may also be elevated. The arterial line waveform may reveal the slow, flat, systolic waveform.

Laboratory Findings

The turbulent blood flow across the stenotic valve may damage red blood cells. Hemolytic anemia is demonstrated by a decreased red blood cell count. The red cell indices will demonstrate normocytic, normochromic red cells. Once left ventricular failure occurs, a decreased arterial oxygen saturation may be found (see Table 17–1).

Diagnostic Procedures

Chest x-rays may be normal with early aortic stenosis. As the left ventricle fails, left ventricular dilation, left atrial dilation, and pulmonary congestion or edema may be seen. The calcified valve or a dilated aorta, caused by the ejection jet of ventricular systole, may be seen on the x-ray.

The electrocardiogram may reveal left ventricular strain with large S waves in V_{1-2} and large R waves in V_{4-6} with depressed ST segments and inverted T waves. Left axis deviation may be noted, as well as left anterior hemiblock and right or left bundle branch block. Left atrial hypertrophy may be reflected by the P wave ending negatively in V_1.

Phonocardiograms can be helpful, especially in identifying the fourth heart sound, first heart sound, and ejection click. The second heart sound components can be demonstrated. The electrocardiogram and phonocardiogram used together can help to determine the degree of aortic stenosis.

Echocardiography is useful in diagnosing and monitoring the progression of aortic stenosis (see Table 17–2). The M-mode echocardiogram may demonstrate aortic cusp thickness and movement as well as left ventricular diameter and wall thickness. Two-dimensional echocardiography may demonstrate the number, thickness, shape, movement, and calcification of the aortic cusps. Left ventricular function can be documented. Doppler echocardiography may be used to determine the pressure gradient between the left ventricle and the aorta.

Radionuclide studies may be utilized to document ventricular function, myocardial perfusion, and left ventricular ejection fraction. Graded exercise studies are seldom attempted because of the risk of peripheral vasodilation, decreasing preload, and increasing heart rate. The resultant decrease in cardiac output and coronary perfusion may result in severe left ventricular failure.

Cardiac catheterization is used for definitive diagnosis of aortic stenosis. A catheter is used to measure left ventricular and aortic pressures. The gradient, systolic blood flow, and valve orifice area can be determined. Ventricular and atrial dimensions, wall thickness, and movement can be observed. The number and shape of the aortic cusps may be demonstrated. The coronary arteries, aorta, and other valves' function can be evaluated as well.

Medical Treatment

The primary medical management of patients with aortic stenosis consists of prophylaxis for endocarditis (see Table 17–3). Amoxicillin is prescribed for all dental and surgical procedures. Gentamicin or ampicillin may be added to the regimen.

Once left ventricular failure develops, digoxin, diuretics (furosemide, hydrochlorothiazide), and low-salt diets may be prescribed to minimize the effects of ventricular failure until surgical repair can be provided. Premature atrial contractions are prophylactically treated with quinidine or disopyramide. Atrial fibrillation is treated with digoxin or quinidine.

Electrical cardioversion is utilized, especially when loss of the atrial kick decreases the cardiac output. Unresolved atrial fibrillation is also an indication for anticoagulant therapy (warfarin, heparin).

When the patient develops left ventricular failure, angina, or syncope or when echocardiography or cardiac catheterization demonstrates significant aortic stenosis, surgical valve replacement is the treatment of choice (see Chap. 20). Factors requiring consideration in regard to prosthetic valves are as follows:

1. Mechanical valves (ball-cage, disc) require continuous anticoagulation.
2. Tissue valves (homeografts, xenografts, heterografts, allografts) do not require prolonged anticoagulation, but the tissue becomes stiff, may calcify, leak or tear.
3. All prosthetic valves create some stenosis because of their annulus and components (see Fig. 17–7).

One- and two-balloon valvuloplasty is also an option, although the disease process continues, and the procedure may result in aortic regurgitation.

Postoperatively, anticoagulation (warfarin and possibly also dipyridamole) is prescribed for all patients for 6 weeks; it is then discontinued if the valve replacement was a tissue valve. Supraventricular dysrhythmias are treated with digoxin. Ventricular dysrhythmias are treated with lidocaine or pronestyl. If dysrhythmias continue beyond 3 postoperative days, pronestyl is continued for 6 weeks. The prophylactic antibiotic regimen should continue as described in Table 17–3.

Subvalvular fibrous membrane and supravalvular aortic stenoses are usually surgically corrected. Subvalvular muscular stenosis is usually treated with propranolol. Surgical intervention is attempted if symptoms persist despite propranolol therapy, but surgical mortality is high.

TRICUSPID REGURGITATION

Pathophysiology

Tricuspid regurgitation is rarely an isolated lesion. Most often, it is a sequela of rheumatic endocarditis (Fig. 17–18) and is highly correlated with mitral stenosis. It is also frequently the result of infectious endocarditis. Tricuspid valve endocarditis often results from drug abuse but also from complications of alcoholism, burns, immunodepression, rheumatic disease, or pulmonary artery catheters (Chan et al., 1989). The inflammatory reaction may result in thickened, shortened leaflets or fused, shortened chordae tendineae. Patients with infectious endocarditis may also develop vegetations that prevent apposition of the leaflets or that perforate the leaflets or chordae. The tricuspid valve annulus may be distorted by right ventricular dilation (Fig. 17–18). Some causes of right ventricular dilation are right ventricular fail-

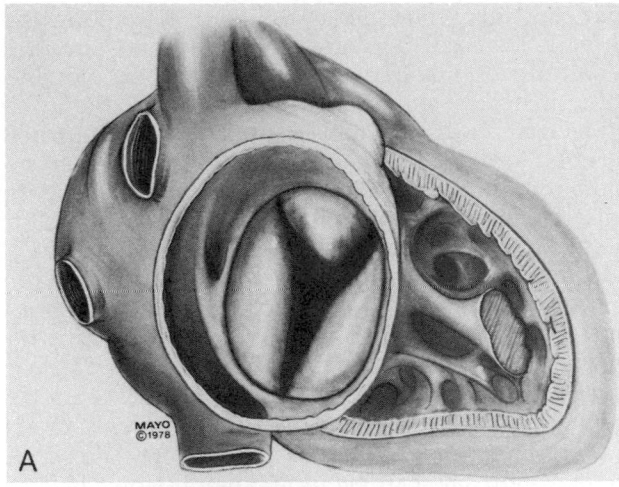
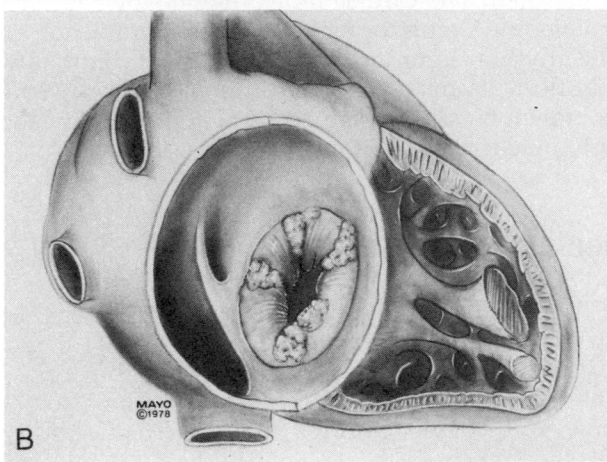

FIGURE 17–18. Types of tricuspid regurgitation. *A,* Functional tricuspid regurgitation secondary to dilation of the right ventricle. *B,* Organic rheumatic tricuspid regurgitation. (Adapted from Brandenburg, R. O., et al. (1979). Valvular heart disease: When should the patient be referred? *Practical Cardiology,* 5:50. By permission of Mayo Foundation.)

ure, pulmonary hypertension, and left ventricular failure. Endomyocardial fibrosis and the carcinoid syndrome result in fibrous tissue development on the ventricular aspects of the leaflets. The fibrous tissue eventually causes adhesions between the leaflets and the right ventricular endocardium, preventing leaflet closure.

The tricuspid valve's papillary muscles may be ischemic, infarcted, or ruptured as a result of coronary artery disease and trauma. The trauma may be blunt (with no symptoms for a number of years) or may result from injury by pacer wires or right heart catheters. The tricuspid valve may develop myxomatous changes in the leaflets, annulus, or chordae tendineae. The central layer of the leaflets, the spongiosa layer, has an overabundance of myxomatous cells. These cells spread into the supporting layer of the leaflet, the fibrosa, interrupting its continuity. The weakened valve stretches and develops interchordeal hooding and prolapse. The surfaces of the leaflets that contact each other fibrose and thicken over time. The thinned, hooded areas develop collagenous fibrous tissue on the ventricular aspect,

thickening the leaflet. The weakening and fibrous processes may also occur in the annulus and chordae. The annulus may become distorted or inflexible. The chordae may stretch or shorten. Myxomatous changes typically result in tricuspid regurgitation secondary to prolapse, usually of the posterior leaflet; the leaflets may also be drawn toward the ventricle and are then not able to approximate.

Right atrial tumors may produce friction on a leaflet, stretching or perforating it. Ebstein anomaly is a congenital cause of tricuspid regurgitation. The posterior and septal leaflets develop abnormally. Some patients' leaflets are attached to the ventricular wall; others originate from the ventricular wall distal to the normal position. The anterior leaflet is usually large and fibrotic. The leaflets may be fused. The chordae and papillary muscles may be shortened or attached to the leaflets abnormally. Other congenital causes typically involve deformed leaflets.

In tricuspid regurgitation blood flows from the right ventricle to the right atrium during systole (Fig. 17–19). The increased right atrial volume increases right atrial pressure. The right atrium hypertrophies and dilates. Central venous volume and pressure increase. Peripheral edema and fluid weight gain progress to hepatomegaly and may cause ascites, intestinal vein distention, and splenomegaly. The dilated atrium typically fibrillates. Tricuspid regurgitation decreases right ventricular output through the pulmonary system and decreases left ventricular output. The right ventricle dilates to accommodate large diastolic volumes and hypertrophies in an attempt to increase output to the pulmonary system. The dilated ventricle may displace chordae or papillary muscles and actually increase the regurgitation.

Physical Assessment

Tricuspid regurgitation may be asymptomatic in many patients, especially if it is an isolated lesion.

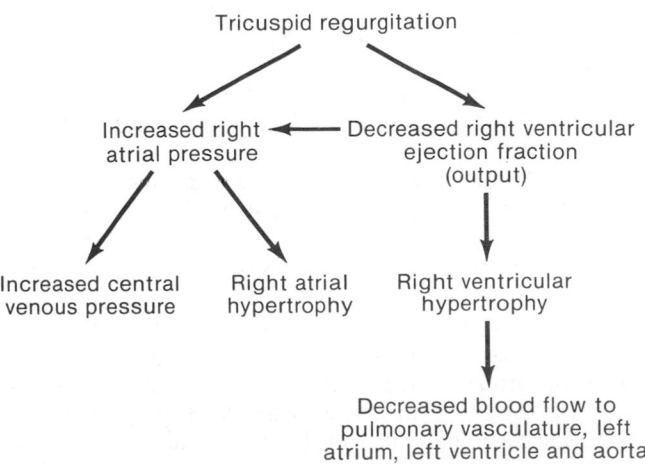

FIGURE 17–19. Pathophysiology of tricuspid regurgitation. (Adapted from *The Journal of Cardiovascular Nursing,* Vol. 1, No. 3, pp. 1–17, with permission of Aspen Publishers, Inc., © 1987.)

Once the right ventricle fails to maintain its cardiac output, signs and symptoms will increase. The initial symptoms of right heart failure are increased venous pressure, peripheral edema, fluid retention and, therefore, weight gain. Some patients can feel the systolic pulsations of the jugular vein. Eventually, hepatomegaly, ascites, and splenomegaly develop. Hepatomegaly may cause abdominal pain. Ascites and venous engorgement may cause anorexia and weight loss. The decreased cardiac output may limit activity tolerance. Low cardiac output or perfusion may cause fatigue and peripheral cyanosis due to desaturated hemoglobin. When tricuspid regurgitation develops as a result of severe left ventricular failure, the pulmonary symptoms of left ventricular failure may decrease or resolve. The patient will have decreased dyspnea, will regain the ability to lie supine, and will have fewer crackles. Tricuspid regurgitation is seldom an isolated lesion, and symptoms of other conditions are often more prominent.

Inspection may reveal jugular neck vein distention. In normal sinus rhythm the a wave has little or no x descent, and the c and v waves merge and are prominent. The c-v wave, also called an s wave, is followed by a brisk y descent. If atrial fibrillation is the rhythm, no a waves are noted, but the c-v wave and y descent remain. There is a positive hepatojugular reflex, and liver pulsations may be noted in the right flank. Eventually, congestion causes cirrhosis of the liver, and pulsations may cease. Anorexia will cause weight loss. The patient may be jaundiced or may demonstrate ascites as right ventricular failure progresses. Water weight gain may then become evident. Peripheral edema is common, and the veins in the extremities may also pulsate. The lips, tongue, face, and nailbeds are the first to develop cyanosis. The lower sternum and lower left sternal border may pulsate as a result of right ventricular hypertrophy, and the lower right sternal border may pulsate as a result of right atrial hypertrophy.

Palpation of the chest often reveals a lower sternal lift. The liver is palpable, and pulsations may be palpable. While the liver is engorged, it is tender, but once it becomes cirrhotic, it is firm and nontender. The pulse is often tachycardiac and will be regular in sinus rhythm and irregularly irregular in atrial fibrillation. Palpation will assist in determining the severity of peripheral edema and in diagnosing ascites. The spleen may be palpated.

On auscultation a normal blood pressure is usually present until cardiac output becomes severely impaired. The first heart sound may be normal if the mitral component is normal and the patient in normal sinus rhythm, or soft, as with atrial fibrillation or an abnormal mitral valve. The second heart sound may be normal, or, if pulmonary hypertension is present, the pulmonary component may be louder. When right bundle branch block coexists, the physiologic splitting of the second heart sound will be widened. A third heart sound is often present, originating from the right ventricle; it is heard best along the lower left sternal border. The third heart sound is louder during inspiration. The murmur is a blowing, high-pitched, systolic sound heard best at the lower left sternal border or xiphoid area. The murmur may be enhanced by inspiration, lying down, exercise, and amyl nitrate. It is decreased by standing and the Valsalva maneuver. The murmur is often difficult to identify because right heart pressures are so low.

Hemodynamic monitoring will demonstrate the central venous pressure waveforms that correspond with the jugular vein pulsations noted during inspection. The a wave may not be present because of atrial fibrillation. In normal sinus rhythm the x descent is small or absent. The c and v waves merge and are large, and the y descent is steep. Pressures are elevated. The cardiac index may be low. Electrocardiographic monitoring may demonstrate normal sinus rhythm, sinus tachycardia, or, most commonly, atrial fibrillation. Incomplete or complete right bundle branch block, premature atrial contractions, and large, notched P waves may be present.

Laboratory Findings

Chronic liver congestion may be evidenced by hypoalbuminemia. In more advanced cases, coagulopathies may be noted. Low cardiac output conditions may cause venous oxygen saturations to fall below 70%. Blood cultures may be positive if an infectious process is active (see Table 17–1).

Diagnostic Procedures

Chest x-rays may demonstrate right atrial, right ventricular, or superior vena cava enlargement. The azygous vein may be distended, and the resulting pleural effusions may be evident. If ascites has developed, the diaphragm will be displaced cephalically.

Fluoroscopy may be employed to identify systolic pulsations of the right atrium and superior vena cava.

Electrocardiograms will provide additional information to that supplied by electrocardiographic monitoring data. The axis can be determined and is usually deviated to the right but may be vertical. Right ventricular hypertrophy may be confirmed by voltage criteria. Right atrial enlargement may be confirmed by Q waves in V_1.

Phonocardiograms may be helpful because right heart sounds are soft, and tricuspid regurgitation may be overshadowed by other cardiac valve lesions. The components of the first heart sound and murmur can be recorded. The second and, if present, the third heart sounds may be documented.

Echocardiography may be of assistance in diagnosing tricuspid regurgitation (see Table 17–2). M-mode can be used to document right atrial and ventricular size, septal movement, vegetations, and, especially in systole, leaflet movement. Two-dimensional echocardiography is used to identify vegetations and, in combination with an intravenous contrast agent, will demonstrate blood flow back and forth across the valve. Doppler echocardiography may also be used.

Right heart cardiac catheterization may be useful. Pressure and wave form recordings can be obtained. Contrast material can be injected into the ventricle, but regurgitation may be created or exaggerated by the catheter crossing the tricuspid valve. Indicator-dilution curves have been more useful. An indicator is injected into the right ventricle, and samples are taken from the right atrium and the femoral artery. The indicator's appearance in atrial samples is quicker or in higher concentrations than in arterial samples and is an indication of tricuspid regurgitation.

Medical Treatment

Medical management of tricuspid regurgitation varies with the symptoms and etiology. Treatment of isolated tricuspid regurgitation is geared to the etiology. Antibiotic treatment and prophylaxis (Table 17–3) for rheumatic disease and for endocarditis during dental and surgical procedures is achieved with amoxicillin. Gentamicin and ampicillin may be added to the regimen. Right ventricular failure is treated with digoxin, diuretics (furosemide, hydrochlorothiazide), vasodilators (nitroglycerin, nitroprusside), low-salt diets, fluid restriction, and activity restriction. Atrial fibrillation is treated with digoxin, quinidine, or electrical cardioversion as well as with anticoagulation (warfarin). Tricuspid regurgitation related to left heart or pulmonary pathology is treated by treating the original cause. Patients with tricuspid endocarditis secondary to substance abuse require treatment for their dependent behavior and personality as well as for the endocarditis.

Surgical intervention is rarely required unless pulmonary artery hypertension is chronic or the leaflets are deformed. Most surgical interventions are associated with mitral valve surgery (see Chap. 20). Two types of valvuloplasty may be performed, plication of the posterior leaflet or narrowing of the annulus. Surgery on the annulus may be comprised of a purse-string suture or a ring/stent. Total valve replacement (see Fig. 17–7) may be done with either mechanical (ball-cage, disc) or tissue (porcine, bovine, human) prostheses. Tissue valve stiffening and calcification do not occur with the low right heart pressures characteristic of tricuspid regurgitation; however, most surgeons use anticoagulation (warfarin, dipyridamole) for all patients because of the slow blood flow in the right heart. Endocarditis prophylaxis is prescribed for life. Digoxin and diuretics may be required for a few months after surgery.

TRICUSPID STENOSIS

Pathophysiology

Tricuspid stenosis is most commonly the result of rheumatic disease. It is usually associated with left heart valve involvement. The inflammatory process results in fibrosing of the leaflets, commissures, and chordae. Most commonly, the commissures fuse (usually the anteroseptal commissure), narrowing the orifice. The chordae thicken, shorten, and fuse. Infectious endocarditis may result in the same changes but is rare in the right heart except among intravenous drug users. In addition, vegetations may occlude part or all of the lumen.

Atrial myxomas or thrombi may occlude the right ventricular inflow channel. Endocardial fibroelastosis and the carcinoid syndrome result in fibrous tissue development on the leaflets, which may fuse the commissures or stiffen the leaflets, decreasing their movement. A form of Ebstein anomaly with fused leaflets may also cause stenosis.

Tricuspid stenosis results in accumulation of blood in the right atrium and in less blood reaching the right ventricle (Fig. 17–20). The increased volume and pressure dilate and hypertrophy the right atrium. The veins entering the atria dilate as the volume of blood backs into the system. Pressures in the venous organs, such as the liver and spleen, rise, and the organs become engorged; peripheral edema is seen. Eventually, the liver fibroses. Decreased right ventricular filling volumes result in decreased cardiac output throughout the pulmonary and systemic circulations.

Physical Assessment

Dyspnea and fatigue are the most common symptoms of tricuspid stenosis. Patients cannot increase their cardiac output with exertion. Dyspnea and fatigue may also be the result of mitral stenosis, which is nearly always present with tricuspid stenosis. The pulmonary symptoms of mitral stenosis

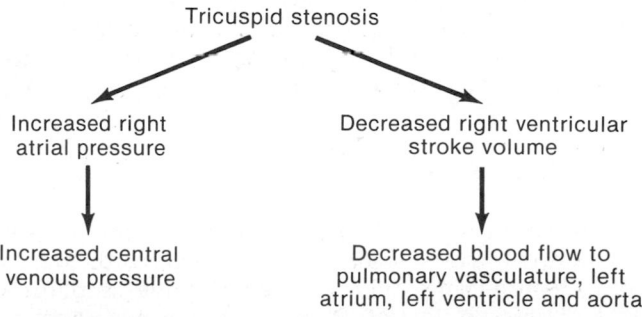

FIGURE 17–20. Pathophysiology of tricuspid stenosis. (Adapted from *The Journal of Cardiovascular Nursing,* Vol. 1, No. 3, pp. 1–17, with permission of Aspen Publishers, Inc., © 1987.)

often decrease as tricuspid stenosis progresses. Other symptoms reported by patients result from venous distention, pulsations of the neck (jugular vein), and abdominal fullness or discomfort (hepatic vein).

Inspection demonstrates jugular vein distention with a slow y descent and, in normal sinus rhythm, a prominent a wave and slow x descent. There is a positive hepatojugular reflex. Peripheral, generalized, or central edema may be observed. The right flank may demonstrate diastolic hepatic pulsations. In advanced stages, cyanosis resulting from low cardiac output and jaundice due to hepatomegaly may cause the skin to have a greenish cast.

Palpation may reveal pulsations at the lower right sternal border due to right atrial hypertrophy. There may also be a diastolic thrill at the lower left sternal border during inspiration.

Auscultation may demonstrate an accentuated first heart sound because the tricuspid valve closure may be intensified. The second heart sound may not demonstrate normal respiratory splitting because right ventricular filling is fixed. The murmur is a rumbling, low-pitched, decrescendo diastolic sound. It is best appreciated at the left sternal border in the fourth intercostal space or lower. The murmur may be increased during inspiration, while lying on the left side or squatting, during isotonic or isometric exercise, while raising the legs, and with amyl nitrate. The murmur is diminished by exhalation and the Valsalva maneuver. Auscultation at the left sternal border at the fourth intercostal space may also demonstrate an opening snap.

Hemodynamic monitoring demonstrates central venous waveforms corresponding with the jugular vein pulsations noted during inspection. Pressures are elevated. The cardiac index may be low, and passing a catheter through the stenotic valve may not be possible. Electrocardiographic monitoring usually demonstrates atrial fibrillation if the cause is rheumatic disease, but normal sinus rhythm may be present if the cause is right sided.

Laboratory Findings

Chronic liver congestion may be evidenced by hypoalbuminemia. In later stages, coagulopathies may be evident. Low cardiac output conditions may cause venous oxygen saturations to fall below 70%. Blood cultures may be positive if an infectious process is active (see Table 17–1).

Diagnostic Procedures

Chest x-rays may demonstrate right atrial or superior vena cava enlargement. Electrocardiograms may demonstrate the increased P wave amplitude and depressed P—R interval (atrial repolarization) characteristic of right atrial hypertrophy. The P wave may be deformed. Phonocardiograms are often very useful for recording the components of the first and second heart sounds as well as the opening snap. The murmur may be better appreciated, especially when other valve lesions are also present.

Echocardiograms may be utilized to identify the movement and thickness of the leaflets (see Table 17–2). M-mode may be able to demonstrate atrial thrombus, leaflet vegetations, calcification, and atrial and ventricular size. Two-dimensional echocardiography may also document the size of the tricuspid valve orifice.

Cardiac catheterization may be used to record pressures simultaneously in the right atrium and ventricle to confirm a gradient. Contrast medium may be injected into the right atrium to visualize the contour of the blood flow tract. Right atrial wall thickness as well as leaflet mobility and thickening may also be visualized. Right atrial pressures and waveforms may be documented.

Medical Treatment

Antibiotic treatment and prophylactic therapy with amoxicillin (see Table 17–3) are prescribed for endocarditis. Gentamicin and ampicillin may be added to the regimen. Symptoms of venous congestion may be treated with low-sodium diet, fluid restriction, diuretics (furosemide, hydrochlorothiazide), and digoxin. Quinidine may be added if atrial fibrillation exists.

Surgical correction of tricuspid stenosis is indicated if the stenosis is severe (see Chap. 20). One- and two-balloon valvuloplasty has been utilized, but may be complicated by tricuspid regurgitation or right bundle branch block. Finger valvulotomies have had limited success and have been complicated by tricuspid regurgitation. Open commissurotomies of either septal leaflet commissure have been successful. Commissurotomy of the anterior-posterior leaflet commissure has been complicated by tricuspid regurgitation. Valve replacement with mechanical (ball-cage, disc) or tissue (porcine, bovine, human) prostheses has been successful (Fig. 17–7). Low blood flow on the right side is an indication for anticoagulation (warfarin, dipyridamole) regardless of what kind of prostheses is used. Tissue valves do not stiffen or calcify in the low-flow, low-pressure environment of the right heart. Endocarditis prophylaxis is continued, and digoxin and diuretics may be continued for a few months after surgery.

PULMONIC REGURGITATION

Pathophysiology

Pulmonic regurgitation is often the result of pulmonary hypertension. The annulus stretches, and the leaflets cannot approximate. The same mechanism of dilation may result from a syphilitic aneu-

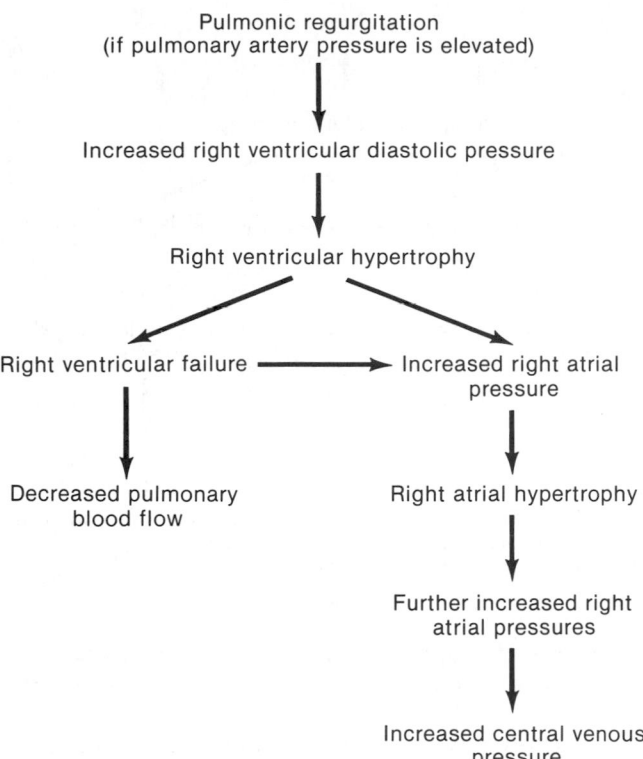

Pulmonic regurgitation
(if pulmonary artery pressure is elevated)

↓

Increased right ventricular diastolic pressure

↓

Right ventricular hypertrophy

Right ventricular failure → Increased right atrial pressure

↓ ↓

Decreased pulmonary blood flow | Right atrial hypertrophy

↓

Further increased right atrial pressures

↓

Increased central venous pressure

FIGURE 17–21. Pathophysiology of pulmonic regurgitation. (Adapted from *The Journal of Cardiovascular Nursing,* Vol. 1, No. 3, pp. 1–17, with permission of Aspen Publishers, Inc., © 1987.)

rysm or an idiopathic or connective tissue abnormality of the pulmonary artery. Regurgitation may be the result of a valvulotomy for pulmonic stenosis. Infective and rheumatic endocarditis and the carcinoid syndrome all result in fibrous plaque formation on the leaflets. The plaques cause contractures of the leaflets, preventing apposition. Pulmonary regurgitation may also be the result of congenitally absent or malformed leaflets.

Pulmonic regurgitation results in blood flowing from the pulmonary artery into the right ventricle during diastole (Fig. 17–21). Right ventricular volume and pressure will increase if pulmonary artery pressures are high. Increased volume and pressure cause the right ventricle to hypertrophy. Right atrial volume and pressure may increase, causing right atrial hypertrophy and increased central venous pressure. If pulmonary artery pressure remains high, the hypertrophied right ventricle may eventually fail. Pulmonary regurgitation with normal or low pulmonary artery pressure seldom produces pathophysiologic changes.

Physical Assessment

Pulmonic regurgitation without pulmonary hypertension is usually asymptomatic and is well tolerated. There are no visible or palpable signs of the condition. The murmur is a blowing, medium-pitched,

crescendo-decrescendo diastolic sound. It is accentuated by inspiration and amyl nitrate. It is heard best at the third or fourth intercostal space of the left sternal border. It follows a short pause after the second heart sound. The second heart sound may be normal, may be more widely split, or may not have a pulmonic component.

Pulmonic regurgitation with pulmonary hypertension may present with signs of right heart failure (weight gain, edema, fatigue, dyspnea) but typically presents with signs and symptoms characteristic of the cause of the pulmonary hypertension. Inspection may rarely reveal distended jugular veins. Palpation of the lower left sternal border may reveal a pulsation characteristic of right ventricular hypertrophy. Palpation of the second intercostal space at the left sternal border may reveal systolic pulsations or the systolic or diastolic thrill of an enlarged pulmonary artery. Auscultation usually reveals a loud second heart sound that is widely split. Third and fourth heart sounds may be found at the fourth intercostal space at the lower left sternal border. A pulmonary artery ejection click may precede the blowing, high-pitched, decrescendo, diastolic murmur. The murmur is heard best at the left mid-sternal border and increases with inspiration or amyl nitrate.

Laboratory Findings

There are no specific laboratory findings for pulmonic regurgitation (see Table 17–1).

Diagnostic Procedures

Chest x-rays of pulmonary regurgitation without pulmonary hypertension may reveal an enlarged pulmonary artery and, more rarely, an enlarged right ventricle. The electrocardiogram may reveal right ventricular diastolic overload with an rSr′ or rsR′ in leads V_1 and V_2.

Chest x-rays of patients with pulmonic regurgitation and pulmonary hypertension usually demonstrate enlargement of the pulmonary artery, right atrium, and right ventricle. The electrocardiogram may reveal right ventricular hypertrophy or right bundle branch block.

Pulmonic regurgitation with and without pulmonary hypertension may be evaluated by other techniques. Phonocardiograms are often useful for differentiating the heart sounds and murmurs. M-mode and two-dimensional echocardiography may demonstrate leaflet movement, vegetations, and ventricular enlargement or hypertrophy. Pulsed and color Doppler echocardiography may identify the regurgitant flow (see Table 17–2). Cardiac catheterization may be utilized to measure pressure gradients or record regurgitation of a contrast material from the pulmonary artery into the right ventricle. Some regurgitation will occur because the catheter traverses the pulmonary valve.

Medical Treatment

The primary treatment of pulmonic regurgitation is prophylaxis for endocarditis (see Table 17–3) with amoxicillin. Gentamicin and ampicillin may be added to the regimen. If right ventricular failure occurs, it is treated with digoxin. Surgical intervention is rarely required for pulmonary regurgitation but may be utilized for individuals with severe right ventricular failure (see Chap. 20). Tissue prostheses (bovine, porcine, human) are preferred to mechanical (ball-cage, disc) prostheses because less thrombus formation (see Fig. 17–7) is associated with their use. Anticoagulants (warfarin, dipyridamole) are then prescribed because the low blood flow of the right heart predisposes all prostheses to thrombus. The low pressures of the right heart do not stiffen or calcify tissue prostheses as in the left heart. Endocarditis prophylaxis is continued, and digoxin may also need to be continued.

PULMONIC STENOSIS

Pathophysiology

Pulmonic stenosis is most commonly a congenital lesion and is frequently associated with atrial or ventricular septal defects and tetralogy of Fallot. The congenital malformation is often leaflets fused at the annulus, leaving a small opening at the center and giving a dome shape to the valve. Another configuration is dysplasia, three shortened, thickened, and immobilized leaflets, the result of an overgrowth of myxomatous tissue.

The rare acquired pulmonic stenosis may result from thickened leaflets and commissural fusion resulting from rheumatic endocarditis or the carcinoid syndrome. Calcific pericarditis may immobilize the leaflets or annulus. Pulmonic calcification also occurs as a sequela to pulmonary hypertension or cardiac or pulmonary tumors; or thrombi may occlude blood flow and mimic pulmonic stenosis.

Pulmonic stenosis causes obstruction to right ventricular systolic ejection (Fig. 17–22). Right ventricular volumes and pressures increase; right ventricular stroke volume decreases. The right ventricle hypertrophies and may dilate. The stiff, hypertrophied right ventricle and elevated diastolic pressures increase the work of the right atrium. Right atrial volumes and pressures rise. The right atrium hypertrophies, and venous volumes and pressures rise. Right ventricular failure may occur.

Physical Assessment

Many individuals have no symptoms and very few signs of pulmonic stenosis. The presenting symptom may be pulsations of the neck, exertional dyspnea or fatigue, dizziness, and syncope. Late symptoms are

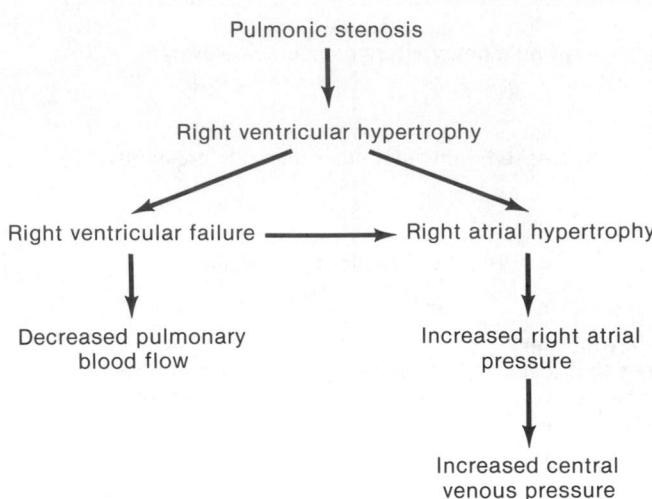

FIGURE 17–22. Pathophysiology of pulmonic stenosis. (Adapted from *The Journal of Cardiovascular Nursing*, Vol. 1, No. 3, pp. 1–17, with permission of Aspen Publishers, Inc., © 1987.)

peripheral edema, ascites, weight gain, cyanosis, and hepatomegaly due to right ventricular failure and angina.

Inspection may identify a round or triangular face, cyanosis, distended neck veins or large jugular vein a waves, and a left parasternal lift. More rarely, clubbing or flushed fingers or toes may be evident. Palpation may identify a left parasternal or subxyphoid pulsation due to right ventricular hypertrophy. A thrill is often found at the second intercostal space at the left sternal border. In the late stages, hepatomegaly, hepatojugular reflex, peripheral edema, and ascites may be found.

Auscultation often identifies the only sign of pulmonic stenosis. The second heart sound eventually softens as the pulmonic component decreases in intensity. The second sound may split on exhalation and widen further during inspiration or may not be audible because of the murmur. An ejection click may be audible at the second intercostal space at the left sternal border as the stenotic valve snaps open. The murmur is often the first sign of pulmonic stenosis. The murmur is a harsh, crescendo-decrescendo, systolic sound heard best in the second intercostal space at the left sternal border. The murmur may radiate along the left sternal border and the neck.

The electrocardiographic monitor usually reveals normal sinus rhythm but may demonstrate supraventricular or ventricular tachycardias and atrioventricular blocks. Hemodynamic monitoring may reveal elevated central venous or right atrial pressures. Swan-Ganz catheters may be difficult to place, but the wave form often demonstrates a slow upstroke.

Laboratory Findings

There are no laboratory findings specific to pulmonic stenosis (see Table 17–1).

Diagnostic Procedures

Chest x-rays typically reveal enlargement of the pulmonary artery's main trunk and left branches. If the right ventricle is enlarged, it may be seen on the x-ray. Occasionally, a calcified valve may also be visualized.

Fluoroscopy may be utilized to demonstrate pulsations of the main and left pulmonary arteries.

Electrocardiograms usually demonstrate right ventricular hypertrophy with incomplete or complete right bundle branch block and right axis deviation. Right atrial enlargement may be seen by upright P waves in V_1.

Phonocardiograms are often helpful to differentiate the aortic and pulmonic components of the second heart sound from the murmur. It can also graph both components of the first heart sound and differentiate the ejection click. The changes in timing and intensity of each sound during inhalation and exhalation can be graphed.

Echocardiograms are not able to demonstrate the pulmonic valve definitively. M-mode cannot visualize the anterior leaflet but can demonstrate atrial contractions and ventricular size and wall motion, which can support the diagnosis. Two-dimensional echocardiography may demonstrate the shape, thickness, and movement of the pulmonic valve leaflets. Vegetations and stenosis may be identified. Ventricular size and wall motion can be determined. Pulsed and color Doppler echocardiograms are utilized to identify flow dynamics.

Cardiac catheterization of the right heart may be used to demonstrate the severity and location of pulmonic stenosis. Central venous, right atrial, and right ventricular pressures may be recorded. Pulmonary pressures may be recorded if the catheter can be maneuvered across the valve and the pressure gradient between the right ventricle and pulmonary artery calculated.

Medical Treatment

The primary treatment of pulmonic stenosis is prophylaxis for endocarditis (see Table 17–3) with amoxicillin. Gentamicin and ampicillin may be added to the regimen. Ventricular or pulmonary thromboses are indications for anticoagulation. Right ventricular failure is an indication for surgical correction (see Chap. 20). Valvuloplasty, valvulotomy, commissurotomy for fused commissures, or excision of leaflets may be performed. Pulmonic regurgitation may result and is often tolerated. Pulmonic valve replacement is rare. Tissue prostheses (bovine, porcine, human) are preferred to mechanical prostheses (ball-cage, disc) because there is less thrombus formation. Anticoagulants (warfarin, dipyridamole) must be prescribed because the low blood flow increases the risk of thrombus formation (see Fig. 17–7). The low flow does not stiffen or calcify tissue prostheses as in the left heart. Endocarditis prophylaxis must continue after any surgical intervention.

ncp nursing care plan

1. **Knowledge deficit of:**
   Diagnosis
   Diet
   Acitivity/rest
   Medications
   Fluids

   Diagnostic/monitoring/treatment regimens
   Complications
   Follow-up
   Unit admitted to
   Genetic factors related to the pathophysiology
   (MR, MVP, MS, AR, AS, TR, TS, PR, PS)

Outcome Criteria	Nursing Interventions
The patient/family will relate an understanding of/demonstrate compliance with The diagnosis The diet Activity/rest guidelines Medication regimen Fluid intake guidelines Diagnostic/monitoring/treatment procedures Complications/deterioration/progression Unit admitted to Follow-up regimens	Describe the cardiac anatomy and physiology. Describe the patient's pathophysiology. (Consult physicians prn.) Describe the ordered diet. Sodium and caffeine restrictions are most common. (Consult dietitian/nutrition support team prn.) Evaluate/discuss the self-selected menu while in the hospital. (Discuss diet as an outpatient.) Assist with or describe activity/rest patterns and activity restrictions. Aerobic exercises and benefits of endorphins may be appropriate. (Consult physical/occupational therapist or exercise physiologist prn.) Evaluate activity tolerance and compliance with activity/rest. Describe medications: name, action, dose, route, frequency/timing, indications, contraindications, side effects, interactions, and any special considerations. Antibiotic prophylaxis should also be taught (see Table 17–3). (Consult pharmacist prn.) Request medication information from the patient each time medications are administered until the patient is proficient with such knowledge. Discuss fluid intake guidelines with the patient if necessary. A 1 kg/2.2 lb weight gain equates with 1 liter fluid volume, therefore establish a regular weight-taking schedule.

Abbreviations: MR, mitral regurgitation; MVP, mitral valve prolapse; MS, mitral stenosis; AR, aortic regurgitation; AS, aortic stenosis; TR, tricuspid regurgitation; TS, tricuspid stenosis; PR, pulmonic regurgitation; PS, pulmonic stenosis.

Nursing Care Plan continued on following page

Describe all procedures to the patient/family (preferably prior to implementation, and performed with the patient's consent).

Evaluate patient/family's assistance with and understanding of procedures. (Consult other members of the heath care team prn.)

Discuss complications and preventive or monitoring measures for complications (i.e., pulse taking, leg exercises, bleeding precautions, signs and symptoms of infection).

Evaluate patient for compliance with precautions for complications.

Discuss follow-up regimens (i.e., visits to physicians, laboratory blood studies, periodic/serial diagnostic procedures, antibiotic prophylaxis).

Discuss caffeine, alcohol, tobacco, cocaine, and other substances as contributors to natural diuresis and to dysrhythmias.

Assess the patient for Potential for Noncompliance.

---

2. Potential for infection related to:
   Endocarditis
   Invasive techniques
   Valvular irregularities

Outcome Criteria	Nursing Interventions
The patient's current infections will be eradicated. The patient will comply with prophylaxis. The patient will not develop endocarditis.	Administer/monitor the effectiveness of antibiotic/antifungal/antiviral medications as ordered. Evaluate the patient's understanding of the treatment regimen (See under Knowledge Deficit). Utilize clean and aseptic techniques as appropriate; utilize universal precautions. Evaluate patient/family's understanding of the signs and symptoms of infection, the prevention precautions, and prophylaxis (See under Knowledge Deficit).

---

3. Decreased cardiac output related to:
   Decreased forward/increased backward blood flow by valvular irregularities
   Atrial fibrillation or other conduction abnormalities
   Fluid volume imbalances
   Increased systemic/pulmonic vascular resistance
   Ventricular hypertrophy with or without dilation
   Dysfunctional valve repairs/prostheses

Outcome Criteria	Nursing Interventions
The patient will be in normal sinus rhythm; there will be no dysrhythmia or conduction abnormality. The patient's capillary refill time will be less than 3 seconds. The patient's urine output will be greater than or equal to 30 mL/hour. The patient will be free of fine crackles and pulmonary edema; bilateral breath sounds are clear. The patient will not demonstrate an S_3 or S_4. The patient will not demonstrate jugular vein distention or peripheral/central edema; no hepatomegaly or splenomegaly. The patient's blood pressure and pulse pressure will be normal for the patient. The patient's pulmonary artery oxygen saturations (Sv_{O_2}) will be greater than or equal to 70%. The patient will deny fatigue, dyspnea, and weakness with and without activity. Patient will maintain/improve activity tolerance. The patient's cardiac index will be greater than 1.5–2.0 liters/m per m². The patient will not experience syncope or angina.	Administer and monitor the effectiveness of antidysrhythmics (digoxin, quinidine, procainamide, disopyramide), afterload-reducing agents (hydralazine, nitroprusside, prazosine, captopril), preload-reducing agents (hydrochlorothiazide, furosemide, nitrates), anticoagulants (heparin, coumarin, acetylsalicylic acid, dipyridamole), and antimicrobial, antifungal, or antiviral medications. Monitor serial ECGs or bedside/telemetry ECGs. Monitor intake and output; establish a routine body weight schedule. Monitor breath sounds and heart sounds on a routine basis. Monitor vital signs, hemodynamic values, and laboratory study results on a routine basis. Monitor the patient's activity tolerance/sleep pattern. Monitor physical assessments paying particular attention to jugular veins, dependent area and abdominal edema, capillary refill time, cyanosis, skin and mucous membrane color/moisture. Assist with electrical cardioversion prn. Assess patient for Potential for Altered Role Performance, Impaired Skin Integrity, Impaired Social Interaction, Noncompliance, Self-Care Deficit, and Sexual Dysfunction.

4. Activity intolerance related to:
   Backward blood flow
   Decreased forward blood flow

Outcome Criteria	Nursing Interventions
The patient will maintain current activity tolerance. The patient will demonstrate activity/rest patterns that prevent dyspnea, tachycardia, and decreased blood pressure. The patient will improve activity tolerance.	Evaluate the patient's knowledge of his or her activity tolerance. Monitor the patient's tolerance of activity/rest patterns. Provide feedback to the patient. Consult cardiac rehabilitation program, exercise physiologist, physical or occupational therapists prn. Discuss aerobic exercise, avoidance of isometric exercise, the need for rest periods, and the correlation of shortness of breath/dyspnea on exertion with left ventricular failure/volume overload.

5. Impaired gas exchange related to:
   Pulmonary congestion
   Decreased pulmonary perfusion

Outcome Criteria	Nursing Interventions
The patient will be able to perform activities of daily living without shortness of breath. The patient will be able to sleep through the night. The patient will have clear bilateral breath sounds. The patient's respiratory rate will be 8–20/minute. The patient will not experience cough or hemoptysis. The patient's arterial oxygen saturations (Sa_{O_2}) will be greater than or equal to 90%. The patient's mixed venous oxygen saturations (Sv_{O_2}) will be greater than or equal to 70%. The patient will deny shortness of breath.	Evaluate the patient's ability to perform activities of daily living and his or her respiratory rate, dyspnea, and sleep pattern. (Consult physical/occupational therapists and exercise physiologists prn.) Auscultate bilateral breath sounds regularly. Monitor fluid balance; teach patient relationship between 1 liter fluid and 1 kg/2.2 lb. (See under Knowledge Deficit.) Monitor activity/rest and dietary compliance. Encourage appropriate weight for height; overweight people produce more carbon dioxide and require more oxygen, thus producing more pulmonary as well as cardiac work. (Consult dietitian/nutrition support teams prn.) Monitor arterial and mixed venous blood gases/oxygen saturation regularly. Discuss sitting, leaning forward, raising arms up and forward over a table, placing hands on knees with the thumbs on the lateral aspects of the leg/fingers on the medial aspects, elevating elbows on a pillow while keeping upper arms along flanks to assist with expanding the apices, as positions that may assist with decreasing shortness of breath. Administer and monitor the effectiveness of diuretics, sedation, and nitroglycerin. (See under Knowledge Deficit for patient education needs.)

6. Altered tissue perfusion related to:
   Decreased forward blood flow
   Thrombus formation and/or emboli

Outcome Criteria	Nursing Interventions
The patient will maintain a capillary refill time of less than or equal to 3 seconds. The patient will not develop a thrombus. The patient will not experience an embolic event.	Assess circulation regularly. Administer/monitor the effectiveness of antidysrhythmic and anticoagulant medications. (Consult pharmacist prn.) Discuss activity/rest/exercise restrictions and recommendations with the patient. (Consult physical/occupational therapist and exercise physiologist prn.) (See under Knowledge Deficit.) Discuss the Homan sign as one mechanism of assessing for leg thrombus formation.

7. Nutrition, more/less than body requirements related to:

Excessive intake	Dysphagia
Decreased activity	Anorexia
Fluid retention	Increased activity
Inadequate intake	Diuretics

Outcome Criteria	Nursing Interventions
The patient will be within the appropriate weight for height range. The patient will demonstrate compliance with eating a well-balanced diet at the appropriate calorie level. The patient will not experience dysphagia/impaired swallowing (enlarged atrium). The patient will retain his or her appetite.	Develop routine body weight–taking schedule (i.e., daily, weekly, monthly). Discuss dietary regimen. (Consult dietitian/nutrition support team prn.) Monitor patient's compliance with diet. Discuss weight's additional effects on the myocardium, the effects of protein catabolism on the myocardium, anorexia, and dysphagia prn. (Consult physician/exercise physiologist/dietitian prn.) Assist patients with dysphagia to find foods/textures that minimize the sensation. Provide counseling to assist the patient in understanding the dysphagia and assist with focusing on aspects of the meal other than dysphagia. Assess patient for potential for impaired swallowing.

Nursing Care Plan continued on following page

8. Disturbance in self-concept: body-image related to:
 The diagnosis
 Monitoring/treatment regimen

Outcome Criteria	Nursing Interventions
The patient will express comfort with his or her lifestyle. The patient will incorporate monitoring/treatment regimen into the desired lifestyle (rather than allowing it to become the patient's lifestyle). The patient will not experience anxiety, fear, hopelessness, impaired adjustment, ineffective individual coping, or powerlessness.	Actively listen to the patient's perceptions of what the diagnosis means to him. Provide factual information. (Consult other members of the health care team prn.) Assist patient to set realistic goals for returning to former lifestyle. Assist patient to incorporate the monitoring/treatment regimen into the lifestyle. Discuss coping mechanisms, support systems, relaxation, biofeedback, counseling Assess patient for potential for anxiety, fear, hopelessness, impaired adjustment, ineffective individual coping, and powerlessness.

9. Potential for injury related to:
 Emboli
 Endocarditis
 Side effects/complications of medications
 Complications of diagnostic/treatment procedures
 Dysrhythmias
 Bleeding, hemolysis
 Progression of the valvular disease process

Outcome Criteria	Nursing Interventions
The patient will not experience any embolic events. The patient will not develop endocarditis. The patient will not experience side effects/complications of medications, diagnostic/treatment procedures. The patient will not experience injury due to the progression of valvular disease.	Discuss valvular pathophysiology, prevention/treatment of complications with the patient (see Table 17–3). (See under Knowledge Deficit.) Administer/monitor the effectiveness of medications. Monitor the laboratory results. Assess for altered tissue perfusion.

10. Altered comfort: pain related to:
 Palpitations
 Decreased coronary artery blood flow
 Pulmonary congestion
 Hepatomegaly
 Splenomegaly

Outcome Criteria	Nursing Interventions
The patient will acknowledge being pain free. The patient will report pain to the health care team as requested. The patient will be able to identify the etiology of the pain. The patient will be able to treat his or her own pain.	Administer and monitor the effectiveness of medications (use caution with nitroglycerin in aortic stenosis). Discuss the pain's characteristics with the patient. Discuss the etiology and treatment of the pain with the patient; consider rest, medications, oxygen, aerobic exercise, relaxation techniques, imagery, meditation, osteopressure (Consult pharmacist, pain specialist/clinic; see under Knowledge Deficit.) Evaluate the effectiveness of the patient's self-administered pain control interventions.

11. Potential for altered family process and/or family coping: potential for growth related to:
 Diagnosis of valvular heart disease
 Outpatient and inpatient visits
 Changes in roles
 Possible changes in life style

Outcome Criteria	Nursing Interventions
The family will maintain/regain their normal family processes. The family will identify and use their support systems. The family will demonstrate appropriate coping techniques.	Actively listen to the family's statement regarding the meaning of the diagnosis/monitoring/treatment to them. Provide factual information. (Consult other members of the health care team prn.) Assist the family to set realistic goals. Assist the family to identify their support systems. (Consult social services/clergy prn.) Assist the family to use appropriate coping techniques.

SUMMARY

This chapter has reviewed some of the specific characteristics of regurgitation and stenosis of each cardiac valve. The primary pathophysiology for each valvular disorder has been discussed in detail; rheumatic endocarditis remains the predominant cause. Signs and symptoms develop because unidirectional blood flow is not maintained. Physical assessment of the patient, including the timing and characteristics of the murmur unique to each valvular condition, was presented. Laboratory analysis was discussed, although it does not usually provide more than supporting data in the diagnosis and tracking of valvular heart disease. Echocardiography was reviewed as the most reliable method of diagnosing and monitoring the progression of many regurgitant and stenotic cardiac valve disorders. Medical treatment is often prescribed for symptoms and does not usually include surgical intervention until late in the course of the disease process. Patients with valvular heart disorders need to be able to manage their chronic disease, and nurses should play a major role in this process. The nursing care plan provided in the chapter can be individualized for specific patients.

References

Alspach, J. G. (Ed.). (1991). Core curriculum for critical care nursing (4th ed.) Philadelphia: W. B. Saunders.

Anderson, U. K. (1987). Mitral valve prolapse: A diagnosis for primary nursing intervention. Journal of Cardiovascular Nursing. 1(3), 41–51.

Aronow, W. S., and Franklin, M. (1987). Diagnosis and treatment of valvular heart disease. Patient Care, 11, 39–60.

Barlow, J. B. (Ed.). (1987). Perspective on the mitral valve. Philadelphia: F. A. Davis.

Berdoff, R. L., Strain, J., Crandall, C., et al. (1989). Pathophysiology of aortic valvuloplasty: Findings after postmortem successful and failed dilation. American Heart Journal, 3, 688–690.

Berne, R. M., and Levy, M. N. (1986). Cardiovascular physiology (5th ed.). St. Louis: C. V. Mosby.

Bourdillon, P. D. V., Hookman, Z. D., Morris, S. N., et al. (1989). Percutaneous balloon valvuloplasty for tricuspid stenosis. American Heart Journal, 117, 492–495.

Braunwald, E. (Ed.). (1988). Heart disease (3rd ed.). Philadelphia: W. B. Saunders.

Cavallo, G. A. O. (1984). The person with valvular heart disease. In C. E. Guzzetta, and B. M. Dorsey (Eds.), Cardiovascular nursing: Bodymind tapestry (pp. 623–658). St. Louis: C. V. Mosby.

Chan P., Ogilby, J. D., and Segal, B. (1989). Tricuspid valve endocarditis. American Heart Journal, 117, 1140–1146.

Chung, E. K. (Ed.). (1983). Quick reference to cardiovascular diseases (2nd ed.). Philadelphia: J. B. Lippincott.

Cohn, L. H., and Gallucci, V. (Eds.). (1982). Cardiac bioprostheses. New York: York Medical Books.

Cohn, P. F., and Wynne, J. (1982). Diagnostic methods in clinical cardiology. Boston: Little, Brown.

Collins, S. M., and Shorton, D. J. (Eds.). (1986). Cardiac imaging and image processing. New York: McGraw-Hill.

Come, P. C. (Ed.). (1985). Diagnostic cardiology: Noninvasive imaging techniques. New York: J. B. Lippincott.

Cornell, L. V. (1985). Mitral valve prolapse syndrome: Etiology and symptomatology. Nurse Practitioner, 10 (4), 25–29, 34.

Dalen, J. E., and Alpert, J. S. (1981). Valvular heart disease. Boston: Little, Brown.

Dajani, A. S., Bisno, A. L., Chung, K. J., et al. (1990). Prevention of bacterial endocarditis: Recommendations by the American Heart Association. Journal of the American Medical Association, 264, 2919–2922.

Dubin, D. (1974). Rapid interpretation of EKG's (3rd ed.). Tampa: Cover Publishing Company.

Feigenbaum, H. (1986). Echocardiography (4th ed.). Philadelphia: Lea & Febiger.

Fowler, N. O. (Ed.). (1980). Cardiac diagnosis and treatment (3rd ed.). Hagerstown: Harper & Row.

Fowler, N. O. (Ed.). (1983). Noninvasive diagnostic methods in cardiology. Philadelphia: F. A. Davis.

Frankl, W. S., and Brest, A. N. (Eds.). (1986). Valvular heart disease: Comprehensive evaluation and management. Philadelphia: F. A. Davis.

Gerson, M. C. (1987). Cardiac nuclear medicine. New York: McGraw-Hill.

Goldenberg, I. F., Pedersen, W., Olson, J., et al. (1989). Percutaneous double balloon valvuloplasty for severe tricuspid stenosis. American Heart Journal, 118, 417–419.

Hunt, A. H. (1985). Mitral valve prolapse: Physical assessment, complications and management. Nurse Practitioner, 10 (4), 15–21.

Hurst, J. W. (Ed.). (1986). The Heart (6th ed.). New York: McGraw-Hill.

Ionescu, M. I., and Cohn, L. H. (Eds.). (1985). Mitral valve disease. London: Butterworths.

Katz, A. M. (1977). Physiology of the heart. New York: Raven.

Krayenbuehl, H. P. (1986). Surgery for mitral regurgitation: Repair versus valve replacement. European Heart Journal, 7, 638–643.

Lamb, J. I., and Carlson, V. R. (Eds.). (1986). Handbook for cardiovascular nursing. Philadelphia: J. B. Lippincott.

Markowitz, M., and Kaplan, E. L. (1989). Reappearance of rheumatic fever. Advances in Pediatrics, 36, 39–65.

Marriott, H. J. L. (1988). Practical electrocardiography (8th ed.). Baltimore: Williams & Wilkins.

McCauley, K. M., Brest, A. N., and McGoon, D. C. (1985). McGoon's cardiac surgery: An interprofessional approach to patient care. Philadelphia: F. A. Davis.

McGoon, M. D., Callahan, M. J., and Gersh, B. J. (1986). Operative timing in chronic valvular heart disease. Applied Cardiology, 14, 19–24.

Orme, E. C., Wray, R. B., Barry, W. H., et al. (1989). Comparison of three techniques of percutaneous balloon aortic valvuloplasty of aortic stenosis in adults. American Heart Journal, 117, 11–17.

Rahimtoola, S. H. (1984). Valvular heart disease: The decision to treat. Hospital Practice, 19 (11), 63–78.

Schakenbach, L. H. (1987). Physiologic dynamics of acquired valvular heart disease. Journal of Cardiovascular Nursing, 1 (3), 1–17.

Schamroth, L. (1989). The 12 lead electrocardiogram. Oxford: Blackwell Scientific Publications.

Seifert, P. C. (1982). Mitral valve replacement. AORN Journal, 36, 959–972.

Sherman, W. J. Hershman, R. Lazzam, C., et al. (1989). Balloon valvuloplasty in adult aortic stenosis: Determinants of clinical outcome. Annals of Internal Medicine, 110, 421–425.

Silver, M. D. (Ed.). (1983). Cardiovascular pathology. New York: Churchill Livingstone.

Smith, N. D., and Abrams, J. (1984). Valvular heart disease of rheumatic origin. Hospital Medicine, 20, 77–117.

Sokolow, M., and McIlroy, M. B. (1986). Clinical cardiology (4th ed.). Norwalk, CT: Appleton-Century-Crofts.

Starek, P. J. K. (1987). Heart valve replacement and reconstruction. Chicago: Year Book.

Swearingen, P. L., Sommers, M. S., and Miller, K. (Eds.). (1988). Manual of critical care. St. Louis: C. V. Mosby.

Vahanian, A., Michel L., Cormier, B. et al. (1989). Results of percutaneous mitral commissurotomy in 200 patients. American Journal of Cardiology, 63, 847–852.

Waller, B. F. (Ed.). (1988). Contemporary issues in cardiovascular pathology. Philadelphia: F. A. Davis.

Zschoche, D. A. (Ed.). (1986). Mosby's comprehensive review of critical care. St. Louis: C. V. Mosby.

18

Patients with Cardiomyopathies

Suzette Cardin

Cardiomyopathy means that the heart as a muscular pump is no longer effective. Pump failure is the result of myocardial disease that results in a structural or functional abnormality of the myocardium. It is caused by the inability of the heart to maintain cardiac outputs within acceptable parameters. Cardiomyopathy is unique in that it can be diagnostically differentiated from hypertensive, congenital, valvular, or pericardial disease (Wynne and Braunwald, 1988).

In 1980 the World Health Organization officially recommended that cardiomyopathy be classified according to its anatomic and pathophysiologic basis. This chapter will review this classification system and discuss the common pathophysiologic abnormalities of dilated, hypertrophic, and restrictive cardiomyopathy (Fig. 18–1). Although hypertrophic and restrictive cardiomyopathy will be included in the preliminary discussion, the primary focus will be on dilated cardiomyopathy.

The similarities among the three types of cardio-myopathies are as follows: (1) The etiology is usually idiopathic or unknown; (2) the myocardium is affected in all three types and may or may not involve the endocardial and pericardial layers; and (3) the disease process is usually one of cardiomegaly and heart failure (Vitello-Cicciu and Johantgen, 1988).

Each category within this classification also has a set of unique characteristics. Dilated cardiomyopathy, which has been previously termed congestive cardiomyopathy, is characterized by excessive dilation of all four cardiac chambers, contractile dysfunction, impaired systolic function, and symptoms of congestive heart failure. Ejection fractions are always below 40% with high cardiac end-systolic volumes. Genetic hypertrophic cardiomyopathy is recognized by inappropriate left ventricular hypertrophy, decreased cardiac output, and outflow obstruction. Restrictive cardiomyopathy is characterized by endocardial scarring or filling of the myocardial muscle mass and subsequent impairment of diastolic filling; this presentation is similar to that of constrictive

THE CARDIOMYOPATHIES

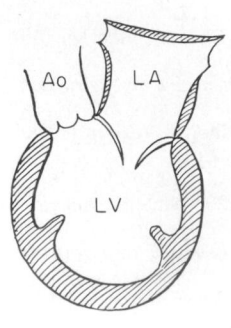
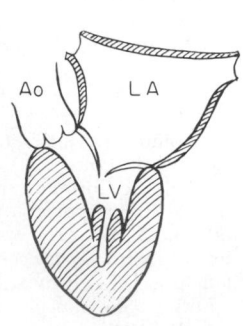
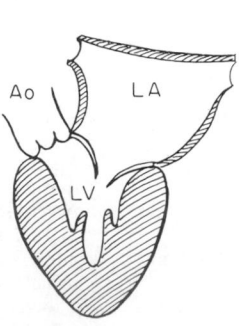

DILATED HYPERTROPHIC RESTRICTIVE

FIGURE 18–1. Pathophysiologic classification of cardiomyopathies. *Abbreviations*: Ao, aorta; LA, left atrium; LV, left ventricle. (From Perloff, J. K. (1988). Introduction to the cardiomyopathies. *Cardiology Clinics*, 6 (2), 185–186.

pericarditis. Restrictive cardiomyopathy is secondary to disease processes such as amyloidosis or a neoplastic process. Ejection fractions are usually below 40%.

The remainder of this chapter will focus on dilated cardiomyopathy, the type of cardiomyopathy in which the greatest strides have been made. With the advent of heart transplantation there is now a reasonable therapeutic option for this population. The current survival rate is 73% for patients with dilated cardiomyopathy who undergo heart transplantation (Imperial et al., 1989). Current nursing and medical management will be discussed. The relationship of the patient and family to the critical care environment and critical care unit will be highlighted. Many patients spend prolonged periods of time in critical care units awaiting their transplant, or they are frequently in and out of congestive heart failure and need medical and nursing care in balancing their hemodynamic parameters.

PATHOPHYSIOLOGY

The disease process of dilated cardiomyopathy is characterized by a profound reduction in left ventricular ejection fraction. Ejection fraction in patients with this condition is always less than 40%, and it is not uncommon for patients to have ejection fractions of 10% to 20% prior to therapy. The deterioration of cardiac output is progressive unless the vicious circle of cardiomyopathy is broken (Fig. 18–2). No specific curative therapy is currently available, but the treatment for dilated cardiomyopathy is guided by the patient's hemodynamic status, the dysrhythmic and embolic risks present, and the potential for heart transplantation (Stevenson and Perloff, 1988). The disease process occurs in approximately 200 patients per 1,000,000 population in the United States (Gillium, 1986). The majority of cases are idiopathic due

TABLE 18–1. The Dilated Cardiomyopathies: Etiologic Classification

1. *Idiopathic*	4. *Metabolic*
2. *Inflammatory*	Nutritional
Infectious	Endocrinologic
Bacterial	Electrolyte abnormalities
Mycobacterial	5. *Familial cardiomyopathy*
Parasitic	Neuromyopathic
Rickettsial	Progressive muscular
Spirochetal	dystrophy
Fungal	Myotonic muscular
Noninfectious	dystrophy
Transplantation rejection	Friedreich ataxia
Autoimmune diseases	Hereditary dilated
Hypersensitivity	cardiomyopathy
reactions	6. *Abnormal coronary*
Peripartum	*microvasculature*
3. *Toxic*	
Ethyl alcohol	
Chemotherapeutic agents	
Catecholamines	

From Stevenson, L. W., and Perloff, J. K. (1988). *Cardiology Clinics*, 6 (2), 187–218.

to the unknown etiology of the disease process (Table 18–1).

ETIOLOGY

Regardless of the etiology dilated cardiomyopathy clinically presents as a pathologic process that interferes with the contractile function of the myocardium. One hypothesis is that there is a decrease in calcium uptake by the mitochondria in the myocardial cell (Cardin and Clark, 1985). The inadequate amount of calcium is then unable to bind with troponin, causing failure of the actin-myosin myofibrils to cross-bridge (Fig. 18–3). The end result is a decrease in contractility, which leads to ineffective global pumping of the left ventricle (Fig. 18–4).

Two theories prevail regarding the etiology of decreased calcium intake. An autoimmune process related to a viral process has been postulated as a first theory. Goodwin (1982) hypothesized that dilated cardiomyopathy is a disease of cellular immunity set up by previous viral infection. Coxsackievirus B titers appear to be higher in patients who present with idiopathic dilated cardiomyopathy. Factor and Sonnenblick (1985) reported that antibodies to coxsackievirus B were found in 30% of patients diagnosed with dilated cardiomyopathy. Casey (1987) suggests that a preexisting genetic disorder of cellular and humoral immunity renders the myocardium more vulnerable to exposure to a virus. Goodwin (1982) further theorized that there are three possible outcomes of an acute episode of myocarditis: complete recovery, acute heart failure, or full recovery followed by a latent period. It is during this latent period that an autoimmune process may develop, resulting in an idiopathic cardiomyopathy months to years later (Wingate, 1984).

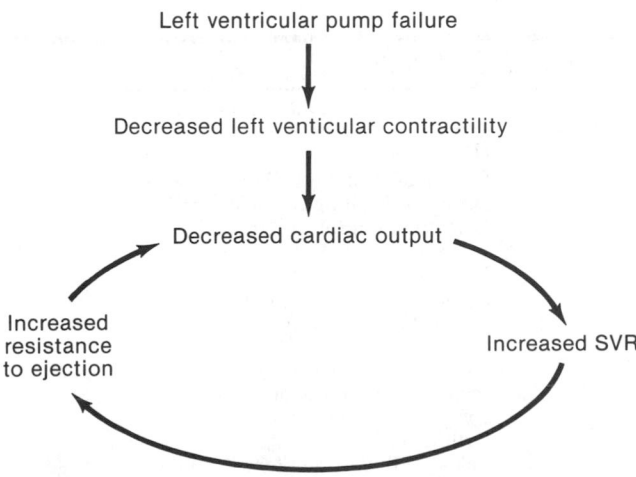

FIGURE 18–2. Vicious circle of cardiomyopathy. SVR, systemic vascular resistance.

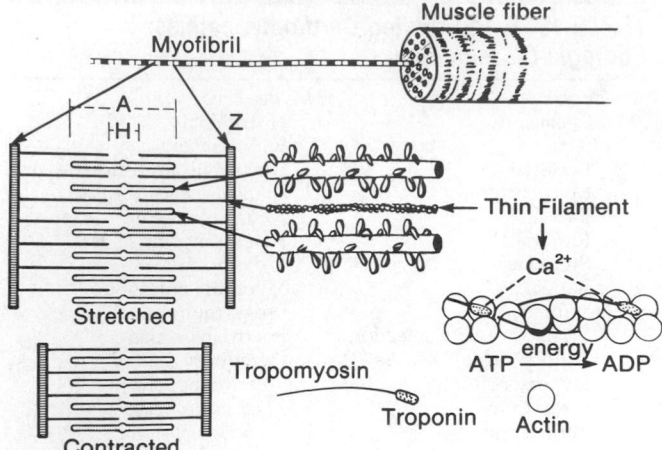

FIGURE 18-3. Structure of the myocardial muscle cell. The myofibrils consist of overlapping thick (myosin) and thin (primarily actin) filaments with cross-bridges between them. The actin of the thin filament is closely bound to two additional proteins—i.e., tropomyosin and troponin complex. During the plateau of the actin potential, Ca^{2+} ions bind with troponin, which triggers the coupling of actin and myosin and the movement of the cross-bridges. Pulled by the cross-bridges, the filaments slide across one another, pulling the Z lines together and causing contraction. (From Smith, J., and Kampine, J. (1984). *Circulatory physiology; the essentials* (2nd ed., p. 73). © 1984, the Williams & Wilkins Co., Baltimore.)

Microvascular spasm is the second theory suggested to explain the initial cause of dilated cardiomyopathy (Casey, 1987). It has been postulated by Factor and Sonnenblick (1985) that a focal transient spasm of small blood vessels causes myocytolytic necrosis leading to scar formation and reactive hypertrophy, leading in turn to cardiomyopathy. The necrotic mitochondria are then unable to participate in the cellular activity of the myocardium. Calcium is unable to be released from the T tubule because energy is not available in the form of ATP to allow the contractile process to begin. This transient spasm of precapillary arterioles could be caused by increased sensitivity to catecholamines or by increased adre-

nergic activity resulting from the virus attacking the myocardium (Casey, 1987).

CLINICAL MANIFESTATIONS

The loss of functioning myocytes in patients with dilated cardiomyopathy causes decreased contractility, dilatation, and increased myocardial oxygen consumption (Casey, 1987). The heart failure characteristic of dilated cardiomyopathy is caused by a severe reduction in ventricular systolic function. The clinical profile is one of both forward or low cardiac output syndrome and backward or pulmonary congestion syndrome (Table 18–2). The clinical profile is one of progressive deterioration, and therapy is aimed at improving the clinical presentation. It is not uncommon for the systolic blood pressure to be between 80 and 90 mm Hg and cardiac outputs to be between 2 and 3 liters/minute. Even without the advantage of invasive hemodynamic monitoring the signs of cardiac failure are to a large extent guided by the cerebral and renal perfusion states of the patient. Changes in the level of consciousness and decreasing urine output are indicative of advancing failure. The majority of clinical manifestations are the result of a low ejection fraction with resultant ventricular and pulmonary congestion. The holosystolic murmur of mitral regurgitation is, for example, a consequence of ventricular enlargement with distortion and variability in filling pressures (Parrillo, 1988).

Traditionally, chest pain is the result of ischemia of the myocardium. Nitroglycerin administered intravenously is the method of choice for prompt relief of ischemic chest pain. The genesis of chest pain in cardiomyopathy is different. Low stroke volume (<80 mL/minute) and increased wall stress decrease subendocardial blood flow and diastolic pressures in the aorta. These events result in the development of chest pain and contribute to the inadequate filling of the coronary arteries. Thus, the goal of therapy is to

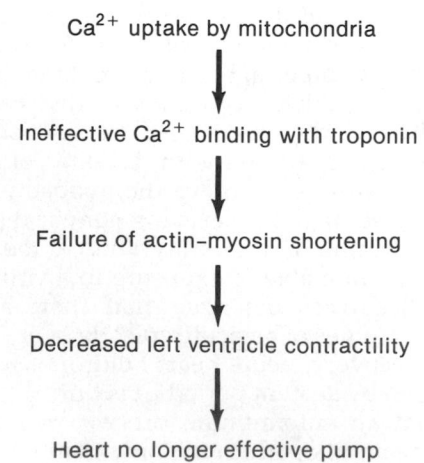

FIGURE 18-4. Physiology of inadequate pumping.

TABLE 18–2. Clinical Profile

Forward failure/low cardiac output
  Fatigue, weakness
  Hypotension
  Peripheral hypoperfusion
  Ischemia resulting in chest pain
  Low urine output
  Altered mental status
  Diffuse sustained PMI
  S_3, S_4 with gallop rhythm
  Holosystolic murmur at apex

Backward failure/pulmonary congestion
  Increased shortness of breath
  Dyspnea on exertion
  Orthopnea
  Rales leading to pulmonary edema
  Systemic or pulmonary emboli
  Right-sided heart failure

TABLE 18–3. Hemodynamic Presentation of Cardiomyopathy

	Normal	Cardiomyopathy
Right atrial pressure	0–8 mm Hg	↑
Systolic pulmonary artery pressure	20–30 mm Hg	↑
Diastolic pulmonary artery pressure	8–12 mm Hg	↑
Pulmonary wedge pressure	5–12 mm Hg	↑
Cardiac output (HRxSV)	4–6 liters/minute	↓
Cardiac index (CO/BSA)	2.5–4.2 liters/minute	↓
Pulmonary vascular resistance	100–300 dynes/cm per second	↑
Systemic vascular resistance	800–1200 dynes/cm per second	↑

increase stroke volume by improving systolic function. Systolic function is enhanced by aggressive use of inotropic agents and by achieving a reduction in afterload. Decreasing systemic vascular resistance (SVR) or afterload decreases the amount of myocardial oxygen consumption (MVO_2) needed to generate an effective stroke volume. The patient is generally classified as New York Heart Association Class IV, and the clinical profile shown in Table 18–2 is present. Usually the patient presents for treatment at this time.

Stevenson and Perloff (1988) contend that there is a state of compensated dysfunction. Stroke volume is initially maintained despite a reduced ejection fraction because the decrease in systolic function is accompanied by an increase in end-systolic and end-diastolic volumes (Stevenson and Perloff, 1988). Gradually the dysfunction progresses to a decompensated state. The clinically dilated ventricle faces a progressive elevation in wall stress and increased MVO_2 consumption, both of which are likely to develop long before peripheral imbalance becomes a significant factor limiting ventricular function (Stevenson and Perloff, 1988). Ventricular dysfunction is further potentiated by increased wall stress and an intrinsically injured myocardium. The hemodynamic presentation is one of a high filling pressure, low output state, and resistance to the ventricle in both sides of the heart (Table 18–3). Systolic blood pressure is usually 80 to 90 mm Hg and is tolerated with no clinical signs or symptoms of hypoperfusion in patients with dilated cardiomyopathy.

The goal of therapy for patients with dilated cardiomyopathy is to achieve symptomatic stability and pulmonary pressures that will allow a reasonable quality of life. Baseline criteria for consideration for a heart transplant include a pulmonary artery systolic pressure of less than 50 mm Hg and a pulmonary vascular resistance (PVR) of less than 250 dynes/sec/cm^{-5}. Reduction in both of these pressures must occur before the patient can be considered for successful heart transplantation. If the pulmonary artery systolic pressure and PVR cannot be reduced through manipulation of preload and afterload

agents, the newly transplanted heart will not tolerate these elevated pressures.

Total hemodynamic goals include titration of intravenous nitroprusside (NTP) followed by use of oral afterload agents such as captopril or hydralazine, plus nitroglycerin (NTG), inotropic agents, and diuretics. Diuretics must be used cautiously in patients with renal failure. Stevenson and Tillisch (1986) advocate pulmonary capillary wedge pressures less than or equal to 15 mm Hg, systemic vascular resistance less than or equal to 1200 dynes/sec/cm^{-5} and systolic blood pressure greater than or equal to 80 mm Hg. Cardiac output is usually maximal when these goals are achieved (Stevenson et al., 1987). Symptomatic status has improved in most patients who have been treated with aggressive unloading therapy and many patients experience increase in exercise tolerance as a result of this therapy (Stevenson et al., 1988).

DIAGNOSTIC FINDINGS

There is no one distinct laboratory test for the diagnosis of dilated cardiomyopathy. It has been called a disease of exclusion because all possibilities are ruled out before a definitive diagnosis is made. The use of intravenous endomyocardial biopsy has become the standard for diagnosis, particularly if there is a viral process component in the patient's history (Fig. 18–5). Table 18–4 lists the common indications for an endomyocardial biopsy. One major

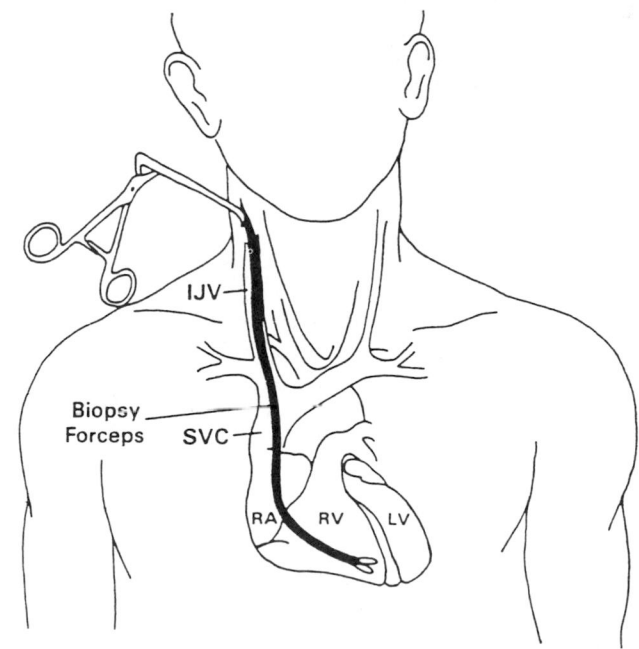

FIGURE 18–5. Transvenous endomyocardial biopsy. *Abbreviations*: IJV, internal jugular vein; SVC, superior vena cava. (From Shoemaker, W. C., et. al. (1989). *Textbook of critical care.* Philadelphia: W. B. Saunders.)

drawback seems to be that because only small portions of the myocardium are sampled for biopsy, the problem could be missed because only a select portion of the myocardium is analyzed. A specific etiology is established in only 20% of cases (Stevenson and Perloff, 1988). Biopsy will show myocardial inflammation, fibrosis, or necrosis or may go unnoticed depending on where the biopsy is done and where in the myocardium the inflammatory process has occurred.

Many diagnostic tests are done to rule out some other myocardial disease process. The critical care nurse caring for these patients needs to be aware of the tremendous need for reassurance of these patients. Each diagnostic procedure will either verify or fail to verify the existence of the disease process of cardiomyopathy. For many patients the only option if such a diagnosis is made is transplantation. The array of tests is therefore crucial to their future.

All patients have chest x-rays. The chest x-ray characteristically shows enlargement of all four chambers of the heart (Fig. 18–6). Left ventricular failure may result in signs of pulmonary venous hypertension as well as interstitial and alveolar edema (Wynne and Braunwald, 1988).

The electrocardiogram (ECG) is nonspecific in dilated cardiomyopathy. When overt failure is present, the underlying rhythm is usually sinus tachycardia. The ECG is rarely normal; there are often nonspecific ST- and T-wave changes, and left ventricular hypertrophy or atrial and ventricular dysrhythmias are present (Unverferth, 1985). Q waves may be present when extreme left ventricular fibrosis is present without discrete myocardial infarction; these Q waves are believed to be due to myonecrosis of the cardiotrophic sinus (Wynne and Braunwald, 1988; Stevenson and Perloff, 1988).

Echocardiography is particularly useful in the diagnosis of dilated cardiomyopathy because it may help to rule out other causes or confirm the diagnosis. M-mode, two-dimensional, or Doppler echocardiography is useful in assessing the degree of impairment of left ventricular function and in excluding concomitant valvular or pericardial disease (Wynne and Braunwald, 1988). M-mode echocardiograms will record dilation of the left ventricle with decreased wall motion and normal wall thickness (Gawlinski, 1988). Two-dimensional echocardiography (Fig. 18–7) is more useful for showing the abnormalities of the right chambers; it also shows that left ventricular function is globally rather than segmentally depressed (Gawlinski, 1988). The main advantages of two-dimensional echocardiography are that real-time imaging is done and endocardial thrombi can be

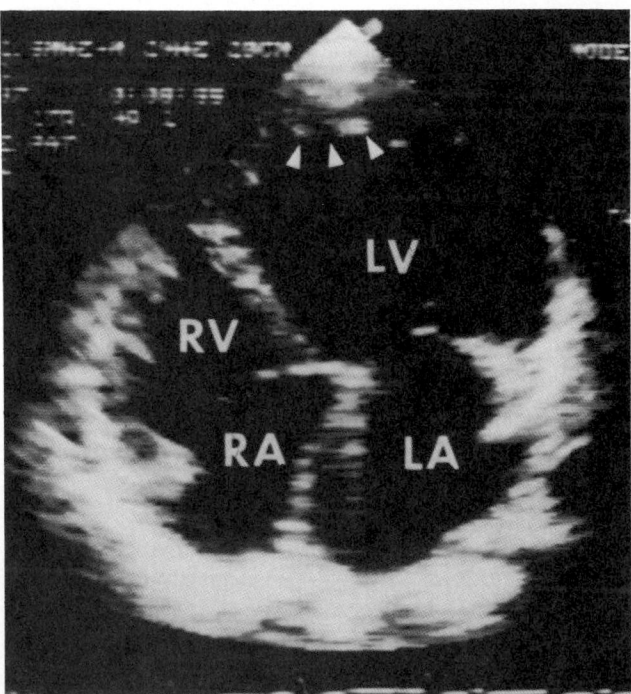

FIGURE 18–7. Apical four-chamber view of the heart showing the large left ventricular *(LV)* cavity of idiopathic dilated cardiomyopathy. Arrowheads identify thrombus attached to the apical endocardium. *Abbreviations*: RV, LV right and left ventricles; RA, LA, right and left atria. (From Stevenson, L. W., and Perloff, J. K. (1988). The dilated cardiomyopathies: Clinical aspects. *Cardiology Clinics*, 6 (2), 187–218.)

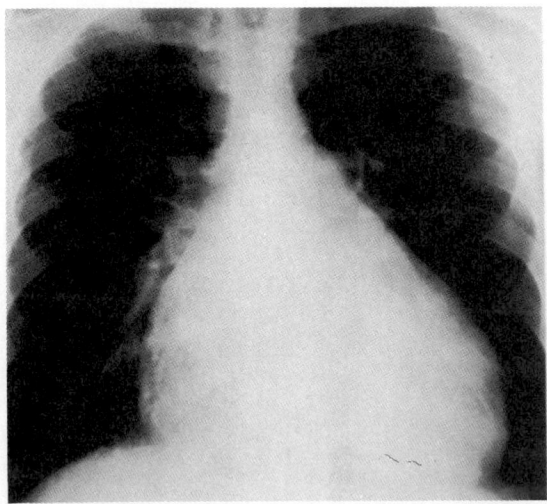

FIGURE 18–6. Chest x-ray of a patient with cardiomyopathy. The left sternal border is enlarged, producing a bottle-like effect. Pulmonary vascularity is within normal limits. (From Stevenson, L. W., and Perloff, J. K. (1988). The dilated cardiomyopathies: Clinical aspects. *Cardiology Clinics*, 6 (2), 187–218.)

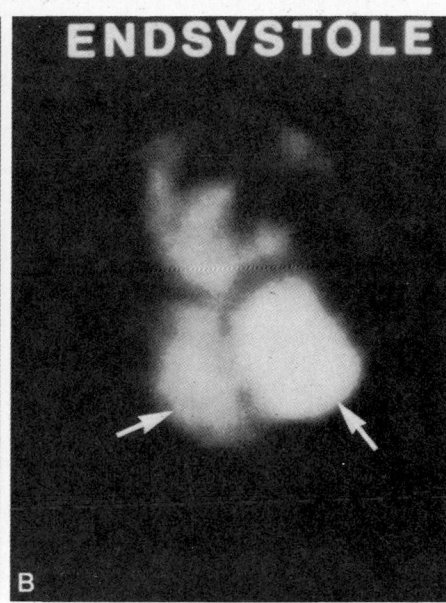

FIGURE 18–8. Technetium-99m equilibrium gated blood pool images in a patient with idiopathic dilated cardiomyopathy. From end-diastole *(A)* to end-systole *(B)*, there is virtually no change in the dimensions of the dilated left ventricle *(LV)* and little change in the right ventricle *(RV).* RA, right atrium; LA, left atrium. (From Stevenson, L. W., and Perloff, J. K. (1988). The dilated cardiomyopathies: Clinical aspects. *Cardiology Clinics,* 6 (2), 187–218.)

visualized. By the time the patient has become symptomatic and scanning is done, the left ventricular ejection fraction is usually less than 30% (Stevenson and Perloff, 1988).

Technetium-99m scintigraphy or radionuclide imaging is also used to define ventricular function and wall motion (Fig. 18–8). Ventricular ejection fraction and end-systolic and end-diastolic volumes are useful in evaluating disease progression and the patient's response to therapy (Vitello-Cicciu and Johantgen, 1988). Wall motion and ventricular function are globally depressed in patients with dilated cardiomyopathy. The ejection fraction is similar to that measured with an echocardiogram. Yamaguchi and Tsuiki (1987) divided 20 of these patients into two groups: those with a segmental wall motion abnormality and those with a diffuse wall motion abnormality. Ejection fractions for both groups measured 33%; however, preload was increased more in the group with a diffuse wall motion abnormality than in the group with a segmental wall motion abnormality ($p < .05$).

Cardiac catheterization with coronary angiography allows direct assessment of the cardiac status. It is particularly useful when other disease possibilities are being ruled out, especially in the presence of unexplained Q waves on the ECG and nonspecific chest pain. Catheterization of the heart reveals elevated volumes and pressures on both sides of the heart, indicating biventricular failure (Vitello-Cicciu and Johantgen, 1988). Left ventriculography demonstrates enlargement of this chamber, typically with a diffuse reduction in wall motion (Wynne and Braunwald, 1988). Compared to coronary artery disease, in which localized wall disorders are prominent, ventriculography in patients with dilated cardiomyopathy will show a more diffuse, global dysfunction (Wynne and Braunwald, 1988). The ejection fraction is reduced and end-systolic volume is

increased as a result of the impairment of left ventricular contractility. Coronary arteriography usually reveals normal vessels and is done to define the presence of the abnormal Q waves described earlier. Wynne and Braunwald (1988) believe that this technique is valuable in patients with Q wave or regional left ventricular wall motion abnormalities on noninvasive testing because these findings may be due to myocardial infarction or extensive localized myocardial fibrosis secondary to severe dilated cardiomyopathy.

MEDICAL MANAGEMENT OF CARDIOMYOPATHY: THERAPY

Therapy for dilated cardiomyopathy is aimed at reducing the amount of work required by the dilated heart and improving the cardiac output of the heart. Therapeutic concerns can be separated into three major categories: (1) the hemodynamic state of the dilated heart; (2) the risk of systemic emboli and ventricular dysrhythmias; and (3) the proper selection of patients for cardiac transplantation.

Hemodynamic Management

The goals of therapy from a hemodynamic standpoint are to augment cardiac output and reduce congestion (Leier, 1985). On the Frank-Starling curve (Fig. 18–9), therapy should be aimed at moving the patient's ventricular function from the low output/congestion portion of the curve upward and to the left, to a position of less congestion and greater systolic function. Hemodynamic management is therefore directed at preload reduction, afterload reduction, and enhanced contractility.

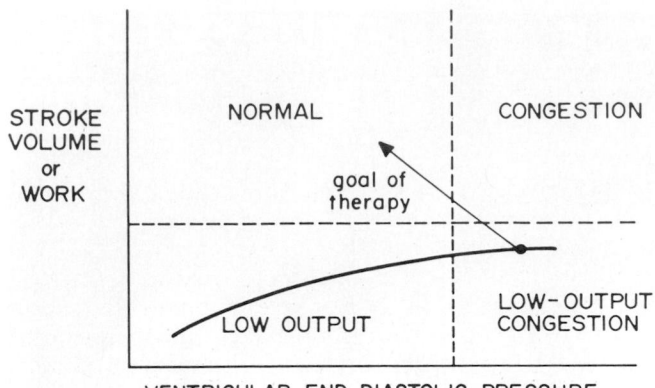

STROKE VOLUME or WORK

NORMAL | CONGESTION

goal of therapy

LOW OUTPUT

LOW-OUTPUT CONGESTION

VENTRICULAR END-DIASTOLIC PRESSURE

FIGURE 18–9. The hemodynamic goals of therapy involve shifting a patient's ventricular function point to a better Frank-Starling curve. (From Leier, C. V. (1988). Treatment of congestive heart failure. In D. V. Unverferth (Ed.), *Dilated cardiomyopathy*. Mount Kisco, NY: Futura Publishing.)

Reducing Preload. Preload reduction is achieved through pharmacologic manipulation and controlled fluid intake; the aim is to decrease intravascular volume, increase venous capacitance, and improve ventricular compliance (Leier, 1985). Diuretic therapy and nitrates are the means used to reduce preload.

Diuretics are the major class of drugs used to reduce intravascular volume. The availability of potent oral diuretics has been a major advance in the medical control of fluid retention in patients with cardiomyopathy (Stevenson and Perloff, 1988). It is still unknown whether diuretics truly prolong life or merely relieve the symptoms of heart failure (Litchtenberg and Schreiber, 1988). Important considerations for diuretic therapy include the site of action of the diuresis, the occurrence of hypokalemia, and the effect of using diuretics in combination with vasodilators and inotropic agents.

The three sites of action of diuretic activity are the distal convoluted tubule, the proximal convoluted tubule, and the collection duct. Table 18–5 summarizes the specific sites of action of the three classes of clinically useful diuretics. In patients in whom the diuretic response is impaired by compromised renal perfusion or intrinsic renal disease, the intermittent addition of a proximal tubular diuretic such as metalazone increases fluid delivery to the distal site of action of the maintenance diuretic (Stevenson and Perloff, 1988). This has been termed "rescue therapy" for patients with otherwise refractory fluid retention. Diuretics are usually given intravenously in the acute phase of cardiomyopathy treatment, and oral therapy is started when optimal hemodynamic therapy has been achieved.

A second concern in preload reduction is the reduced potassium concentration. Unless superimposed renal dysfunction is present, patients with cardiomyopathy are generally hypokalemic because of elevated aldosterone levels and the use of diuretic therapy (Leier, 1985). A brisk and rapid diuresis is intended to reduce intravascular volume while maintaining constant surveillance of the serum potassium level. The goal is to maintain a potassium level of at least 3.5 mEq/liter by means of potassium supplements and the use of potassium-sparing diuretics.

In addition to the traditional methods of diuretic therapy, nitrates are used to achieve further reductions in preload by increasing venous capacitance. Nitrates are now considered one of the standard treatments in the acute and long-term management of heart failure. Nitrates consistently reduce the left ventricular workload by reducing venous return to the heart, lowering pulmonary capillary wedge pressure, and optimizing the Frank-Starling curve (Doyle, 1988). Nitrates also dilate nonstenotic coronary arteries, which can be helpful in patients with ischemic cardiomyopathy.

Nitrate therapy is administered in several ways. Given intravenously, doses of less than 1 mcg/kg/minute will decrease preload, and doses higher than

TABLE 18–5. Three Classes of Clinically Useful Diuretics

Class Name	Dosage range (mg)	Site of Action 1	Site of Action 2	Duration (hr)
Thiazides				
Hydrochlorothiazide	50–100 qd	DCT	PCT	6–12
Chlorthalidone	25–100 qd	DCT		12–18
Chlorthiazide	500–100 qd	DCT		48–72
Metolazone	5–10 qd	DCT	PCT	12–24
Loop				
Furosemide	40–300 bid	Loop	PCT	6–8
Ethacrynic acid	50–100 bid	Loop		6–8
Bumetanide	0.5–5 qd	Loop	PCT	4
Potassium-sparing				
Triamterene	50–150 bid	DCT	CD	12–16
Spironolactone	25–100 bid	DCT	CD	48–72
Amiloride	5–20 qd	DCT	CD	24

Abbreviations: DCT, distal convoluted tubule; PCT, proximal convoluted tubule; CD, collecting duct.
Reprinted from Englemeier, R. S., and O'Connell, J. B. (1988). *Drug therapy in dilated cardiomyopathy and myocarditis*, p. 55, by courtesy of Marcel Dekker, Inc.

1 mcg/kg/minute will produce arterial and venous dilation and in some instances will decrease SVR (Purcell, 1990). Sublingual and oral forms of organic nitrates are well absorbed from the oral and gastrointestinal tracts. Oral nitrate therapy is usually given in the form of isosorbide dinitrate; the dosage can be as high as 120 mg four times a day (Doyle, 1988). Topical nitrates are also utilized in patients with dilated cardiomyopathy, particularly in those who are either edematous or have poor perfusion. Oral preparations seem to be favored over topical agents. Doyle (1988) recommends changing the transdermal patch more frequently than every 24 hours as recommended by the manufacturer. Patients with heart failure generally tolerate nitrates quite well. Excessive preload reduction may occur in some patients who have low end-diastolic pressures and volume and may lead to reduced cardiac output, hypotension, and syncope, which cannot be tolerated for prolonged periods of time in patients with cardiomyopathy (Young and Yusef, 1988).

Reducing Afterload. Afterload reduction improves the systolic function of the failing ventricle by improving forward cardiac output and decreasing ventricular filling pressures. Afterload reduction is accomplished by agents that reduce systemic vascular resistance, generally through arteriolar vasodilation (Leier, 1985). The goal of therapy is the achievement of maximal cardiac output.

The drug of choice for initial afterload reduction is sodium nitroprusside (Nipride). This drug's effectiveness in reducing preload and afterload make it a valuable adjunct in the therapy of low cardiac output syndromes associated with high pulmonary capillary wedge pressure (PCWP) and high SVR (Passmore and Goldstein, 1989). Hemodynamically, nitroprusside decreases PCWP and SVR, leading in turn to increases in cardiac output and stroke volume. Nitroprusside also acts rapidly and can be easily titrated to changing responses in the patient.

Stevenson and Tillisch (1986) advocate use of nitroprusside and diuretics to achieve a PCWP of less than or equal to 15 mm Hg, an SVR of less than or equal to 1200 dynes/sec per cm^{-5}, and a systolic blood pressure of greater than or equal to 80 mm Hg. When these goals are achieved, cardiac output is maximal. Nitroprusside is given in a dosage of 100 mg in 250 mL of 5% dextrose and water and started at 20 mcg/kg/minute, titrating the dose until acceptable hemodynamics are achieved. This result is usually achieved over a 24- to 48-hour period. Oral afterload agents such as captopril or hydralazine are then substituted in higher doses if necessary to maintain acceptable hemodynamics while nitroprusside is tapered (Stevenson and Perloff, 1988).

As described above, the oral agents of choice for afterload reduction are hydralazine and captopril. Hydralazine acts directly on the arterioles to effect relaxation in patients with cardiomyopathy. It produces impressive increases in stroke volume by reducing arteriolar resistance and has no effect or only a modest lowering effect on systemic or pulmonary venous pressure (Bolen and Alderman, 1976; Chatterjee et al., 1980). For a given change in blood pressure, hydralazine increases cardiac output more than nitroprusside or nitrates (Parrillo, 1989). Blockade of the angiotensin I-II converting enzyme is currently one of the most popular approaches used to reduce afterload (Leier, 1985). Inhibition of the renin-angiotensin system reduces afterload or impedance and enhances cardiac performance (Parrillo, 1989). The drug of choice for this result is captopril, and the hemodynamic effects are similar to those achieved with nitroprusside. Captopril also reduces preload; the mechanism for this is unknown, but it has been postulated that it could be due to inhibition of the enzyme that degrades bradykinin, leading to an increase in the circulating level of this potent vasodilator (Parrillo, 1989).

Enhancing Contractility. Improvements in systolic function with increases in stroke volume and cardiac output augment myocardial contractility (Leier, 1985). Positive inotropic agents are the preferred pharmacologic treatment for patients with dilated cardiomyopathy. These drugs include dopamine, dobutamine, and the phosphodiesterase inhibitor, amrinone (Fig. 18–10). The common pathway for augmentation of contractility is enhanced intracellular release and utilization of calcium (Braunwald et al., 1988). Enhanced use of calcium can be accomplished by stimulating the specific beta receptor with either dopamine or dobutamine or by blocking cyclic AMP (cAMP) breakdown with amrinone.

Digoxin has always been mandatory in the treatment of heart failure induced by dilated cardiomyopathy; however, that treatment is now considered controversial. Leya and Gunnar (1988) believe that there is no convincing evidence to support the claim that digoxin plays a useful role in either short-term or long-term treatment when the patient with cardiomyopathy is treated by placing limits on sodium intake and activity and by using diuretics. Digoxin acts specifically on phase four of the action potential and does this by blocking the Na-K-ATPase cycle.

In patients with cardiomyopathy, low-dose dopamine is advocated. A dosage range of 2 to 5 mcg/kg/minute of dopamine stimulates the dopaminergic receptors in the splanchnic and renal vascular beds, producing vasodilation, enhanced blood flow, and diuresis (Dasta and Kirby, 1986; Goldberg, 1972). Cardiac performance is improved by direct stimulation of the beta-adrenergic receptors and indirectly by stimulating the release at the nerve endings of norepinephrine (Goldberg, 1972; Tuttle and Mills, 1975). A dosage range higher than 5 mcg/kg/minute increases the risk of ischemia (Dasta and Leier, 1989). At higher doses, a greater burden is placed on the myocardial tissue secondary to the rise in myocardial oxygen demand incurred by the increase in mean arterial pressure, PCWP, stroke volume, and heart

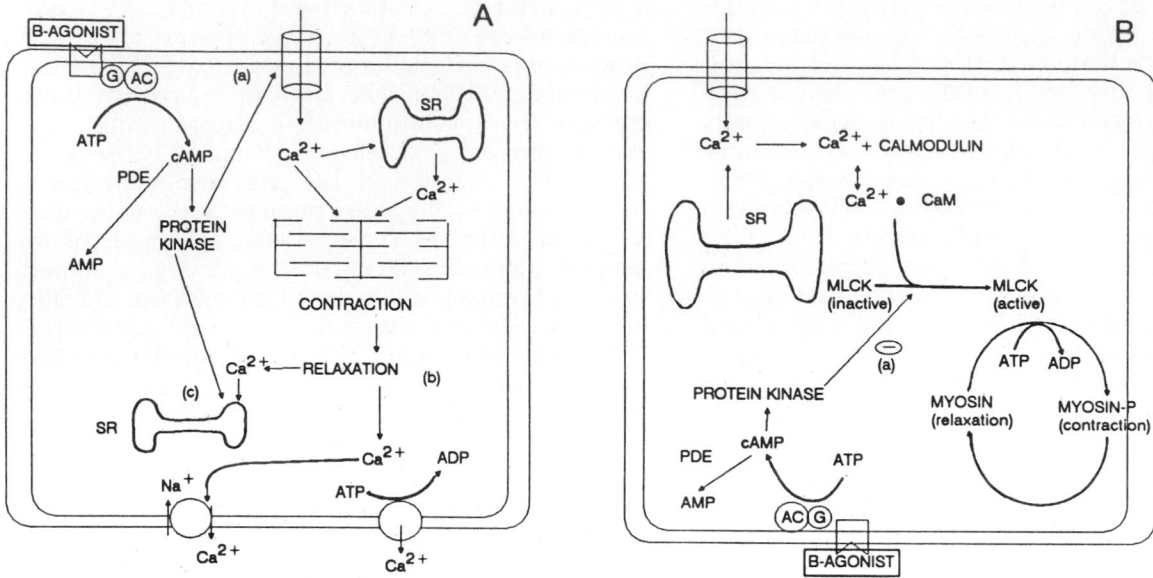

FIGURE 18-10. Influence of cyclic AMP *(cAMP)* on cardiac contraction and on relaxation *(A)* and smooth muscle contraction *(B)*. Agonist binding to B-receptors activates adenylate cyclase *(AC)*, producing cAMP in heart cells. cAMP-dependent protein kinase phosphorylation causes (1) increased influx of Ca^{2+} through cell surface channels *(a)*, resulting in enhanced contractile force; and (2) accelerated uptake of Ca^{2+} into sarcoplasmic reticulum *(SR)*, which facilitates relaxation *(b)* and *(c)*. In smooth muscle cells, Ca^{2+} calmodulin *(CaM)* complex activates myosin light chain kinase *(MLCK)*, thus initiating contraction. cAMP-dependent protein kinase phosphorylates MLCK, making it less sensitive to activation *(a)*. *Abbreviations*: G, G protein; PDE, phosphodiesterase; AMP, adenosine monophosphate; ADP, adenosine diphosphate; ATP, adenosine triphosphate. (From Schwertz, D. W., and Piano, M. R. (1990). New inotropic drugs for treatment of congestive heart failure. *Cardiovascular Nursing*, 26 (2), 7–12. By permission of the American Heart Association, Inc.)

rate. Dopamine usage is therefore restricted to the lower dosage range, especially if cardiomyopathy is secondary to advanced ischemic heart disease. As the disease progresses, if either hemodynamic management or renal perfusion is not achieved, drug tolerance develops. Over the long term this becomes a problem because the dosage must be increased to maintain stability, and the patient then is at risk for an increase in myocardial oxygen consumption.

Dobutamine was first utilized in 1975 to increase cardiac contractility selectively in patients with an altering heart rate or blood pressure (Tuttle and Mills, 1975). In patients with cardiomyopathy, the hemodynamic profile of dobutamine use is characterized by consistent increases in cardiac output and stroke volume, decreases in SVR, PVR, and PCWP with little effect on heart rate or blood pressure (Leier et al., 1978). Dobutamine directly stimulates the beta receptors of the heart, which can over time increase heart rate and the force of contractions. This result is achieved with a dosage in the range of 2 to 10 mcg/kg/minute. Dobutamine, unlike dopamine, has no direct effect on renal perfusion. Enhancement of cardiac output is improved indirectly with dobutamine therapy and can be measured indirectly by PCWP, the presence of clear lungs, and an increase in urine output.

Both dopamine and dobutamine at doses higher than 15 mcg/kg/minute can cause vasoconstriction similar to that seen with stimulation of the alpha receptors. When such doses are required to sustain

the systolic blood pressure, vasodilators (e.g., nitroprusside) may be given to counteract the arterial constriction (Purcell and Holder, 1989). At these doses, Purcell and Holder (1989) also warn of ensuing tachycardia and the development of ectopy. Concurrent usage of dopamine or dobutamine with nitroprusside provides optimal pharmacologic support. The following results are achieved when these two drugs are given in coordination: improved cardiac output, maintenance of mean systolic pressure, enhancement of renal function, and decreased arterial vasoconstriction (Purcell and Holder, 1989).

Amrinone, administered intravenously, is useful in the treatment of cardiomyopathy refractory to the combination of vasodilators, diuretics, and digoxin (Braunwald et al., 1988). Amrinone exerts its inotropic and vasodilating action through phosphodiesterase inhibition, thereby indirectly elevating cAMP and increasing calcium availability (Passmore and Goldstein, 1989). Increased cAMP in cardiac tissue activates a protein kinase that enhances the slow inward current and increases the force of myocardial contractions (Dasta and Leier, 1989). In patients with cardiomyopathy, amrinone improves exercise tolerance and does not adversely affect myocardial oxygen consumption or coronary blood flow (Colucci et al., 1986). Amrinone has been combined with dobutamine for the management of patients with cardiomyopathy and can increase the mean cardiac index (Uretsky et al., 1987).

Intravenous amrinone therapy is initiated with a

bolus of 0.75 mcg/kg given slowly over 3 to 5 minutes. A maintenance dose is continued at 5 mcg/kg/minute, titrated to the desired effect up to 10 mcg/kg/minute. The drug must be mixed with saline to avoid a chemical reaction with glucose (Passmore and Goldstein, 1989). Long-term therapy is associated with increased liver function abnormalities such as platelet dysfunction and an increased incidence of dysrhythmias and thrombocytopenia (Stanley, 1990).

Risk of Embolus Development and Ventricular Dysrhythmias

Once hemodynamic stability has been achieved, attention is directed to the prevention of related complications of the dilated ventricle (Stevenson and Perloff, 1988). Dilation of the left ventricle and a decreased ejection fraction allow stasis of blood to occur in the left ventricle. Both of these factors increase the probability of thrombus formation. Systemic emboli may target the spleen, kidney, or extremities but are most dangerous when they lodge in the cerebral or coronary circulation (Stevenson and Perloff, 1988). Roberts and associates (1987) found that pulmonary emboli may occur or arise from thrombi in the endocardium in up to 50% of patients. In this group of patients, emboli were believed to be the immediate cause of death in 10% of those studied at necropsy (Roberts et al., 1987).

There are currently no controlled studies indicating whether the benefits of anticoagulation exceed the complications if this therapy is administered routinely to all patients with dilated cardiomyopathy (Stevenson and Perloff, 1988). Shabetai (1983) advocates the use of long-term oral anticoagulation for patients with dilated cardiomyopathy who have intracardiac thrombi, a previous history of an embolic event, or atrial fibrillation. Another guideline for anticoagulation therapy for patients with cardiomyopathy is that all patients with ejection fractions of less than 30% or those who have an elevated mean right atrial pressure of more than 7 mm Hg should be anticoagulated with warfarin (Coumadin) (Leier, 1985).

Sudden cardiac death remains a major cause of death in patients with dilated cardiomyopathy. The risk of ventricular dysrhythmias correlates closely with evidence of clinical and hemodynamic deterioration; however, ventricular dysrhythmias appear to be an independent risk factor in early mortality (Stevenson et al., 1987). To date, dysrhythmic drugs have not been shown to decrease mortality (Stevenson, et al., 1988). It is estimated that at least 50% of the patients awaiting cardiac transplant with an ejection fraction of less than 50% will die within a 5-year period (Foster, et al., 1981).

The pathogenesis of dysrhythmias is poorly understood. Underlying ischemic heart disease, wall motion abnormalities, electrolyte imbalances (hypoka-

lemia and hyponatremia), and inotropic therapy may contribute to the high incidence of ventricular dysrhythmias in these patients (Doyle, 1988). Ventricular dysrhythmias in patients with dilated cardiomyopathy may be the result of subendocardial ischemia in the presence of normal coronary arteries. The ischemia may be due to reduced cardiac output/coronary artery perfusion or high left ventricular end-diastolic pressures preventing subendocardial coronary filling. Correction of the ischemia with intravenous nitroglycerin usually terminates the dysrhythmia (Purcell, 1990).

A reasonable approach to treating ventricular dysrhythmias in patients with cardiomyopathy is to limit dysrhythmic therapy to patients who have inducible ventricular tachycardia or symptomatic dysrhythmia, especially those with a family history of sudden death (Stevenson and Perloff, 1988). Low-dose dysrhythmic therapy is utilized. Lower doses are required to avoid toxicity, especially if there is renal or liver dysfunction associated with right-sided heart failure (Purcell, 1990). An example of lower dosage might be lidocaine given at 1 to 2 mg/minute to minimize liver dysfunction and cerebral side effects.

Treatment of patients who are at high risk of development of a fatal dysrhythmia should probably be guided by the patient's response to programmed electrical stimulation. Drugs with strong negative inotropic effects such as disopyramide and flecainide should be avoided. The most promising drug is amiodarone, which is highly selective in suppressing ventricular dysrhythmias and has a negligible negative inotropic effect (DiMarco, 1989). The adverse effects of amiodarone need to be carefully monitored during therapy. Toxicity noted in the pulmonary system, thyroid gland, corneas, and dermatologic system warrants careful surveillance (DiMarco, 1989). The use of implantable defibrillators for patients awaiting transplantation is highly debatable. In some clinical situations they are warranted because of the high incidence of clinical recurrence of ventricular dysrhythmias and sudden death. Because defibrillators are implantable they are recommended as "selective" therapy (Stevenson and Perloff, 1988).

Selection of Candidates for Cardiac Transplantation

Cardiac transplantation has come of age as a reasonable therapeutic option for patients suffering from end-stage dilated cardiomyopathy (Cardin and Clark, 1985). Recent advances have made this option possible (Table 18–6). Patients with few symptoms but with an ejection fraction of less than or equal to 25% are usually offered transplantation to prolong survival (Stevenson and Perloff, 1988). Criteria for patient selection are outlined in Table 18–7. For patients with dilated cardiomyopathy who have had severe symptoms for an extended length of time, survival

TABLE 18–6. Advances in Cardiac Transplantation

Better organ retrieval
Monitoring for allograft rejection
Use of endomyocardial biopsy
Improvements in surgical technique
More efficient organ preservation
Immunosuppressive drug therapy—cyclosporin
Increase in centers doing transplants
Bridge to transplant devices
Expansion of patient selection criteria

after cardiac transplantation is better than survival on intensive medical therapy. Survival is currently 70% to 85% at 1 year and 50% to 60% at 5 years for patients on current immunosuppressive regimens (Stevenson and Perloff, 1988). For patients with severe symptoms that persist despite intensive medical therapy, the quality of life is also clearly improved by cardiac transplantation (Stevenson and Perloff, 1988). Stevenson and Perloff emphasize, however, that for patients who have responded well to medical therapy for heart failure, the quality of life may not be significantly improved by transplantation, which requires them to assume constant vigilance for rejection, infection, medications, and repeated biopsies in exchange for functional capacity, which is still less than normal.

In spite of recent advances in cardiac transplantation, it is not the only option available to patients with dilated cardiomyopathy. Transplantation can be performed only in a few patients due to the shortage of donor hearts. Stevenson and colleagues (1989) studied 50 patients who were transferred from other hospitals for urgent transplantation and received a transplant, and 40 patients who were discharged on oral regimens of vasodilators and diuretics. All were treated with intensive afterload reduction therapy. Both groups were reported to be experiencing the same results, and both reported a better quality of life. With new emphasis placed on medical therapy, the potential may exist for a more effective distribution of limited donor hearts.

COLLABORATIVE MANAGEMENT OF CARDIOMYOPATHY

In the patient with end-stage cardiomyopathy, the goal of nursing is to obtain optimal hemodynamic function for adequate tissue perfusion to enable the patient to carry out his or her daily activities. The goal of medical management is to maximize the patient's level of functioning using the most effective yet simple pharmacologic, dietary, and exercise regimens. To achieve these collaborative goals, the following nursing diagnoses are suggested to help the nurse develop a workable plan for the patient:

1. Alteration in cardiac output related to decreased ventricular function.
2. Alteration in cardiac output related to dysrhythmias.
3. Activity intolerance related to low cardiac output, side effects of medical therapy, extended stay in the hospital, and potential for malnutrition.
4. Potential or actual ineffective coping related to loss of control engendered by a life-threatening illness and complicated medical care.

TABLE 18–7. Criteria for Patient Selection for Heart Transplantation

1. Severe cardiac disease despite tailored medical therapy:
   Cardiomyopathy with unacceptable quality of life
   Unacceptable risk of death within the next year

2. No other reasonable surgical options

3. Patient characteristics:
   Over upper age limit of 55–65 years of age
   Ability to understand and comprehend medical regimen following transplantation

4. Relative contraindications:
   Active infection, particularly respiratory in nature
   Active ulcer disease
   Severe peripheral vascular disease
   Insulin-dependent diabetes with end-organ damage
   Pulmonary vascular resistance over 240 dynes/cm per second
   Pulmonary artery systolic pressure over 60 mm Hg after optimal hemodynamics are reached
   Mean transpulmonary gradient >15 mm Hg
   Creatinine over 2 mg%, creatinine clearance < 50 mL/minute
   Bilirubin over 2.5 mg%
   SGOT twice normal
   History of medical noncompliance with prescribed regimen
   History of refractory alcohol or drug abuse
   Inability to make strong, consistent commitment to transplantation program

Adapted from Stevenson, L. W., and Miller, L. W. (1991). Cardiac transplantation as therapy of heart failure. *Current Problems in Cardiology,* XVI (4), 219–305.

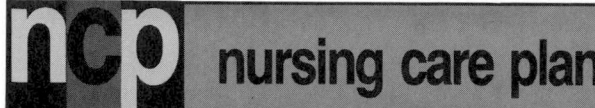

nursing care plan

---

1. Alteration in cardiac output related to decreased ventricular function

---

Outcome Criteria	Nursing Interventions

Patient will have adequate output as evidenced by:
Orientation to person, place, time, and event.
Vital signs within normal limits e.g., systolic blood pressure greater than 80 to 90 mm Hg, heart rate 60 to 120 beats/minute, respiratory rate 16 to 24 breaths/minute.
Hemodynamic function within optimal prescribed parameters, e.g., PCWP less than 15 mm Hg, pulmonary artery pressure (PAP) less than 25/10 mm Hg, right atrial pressure less than 7 mm Hg, SVR less than 1200 dynes/cm per second. Note: PAP and PWCP are read at end-expiration; RA pressure is read as a mean.
Changes in findings on physical assessment are immediately reported and steps are taken to maintain parameters.
Patient will be able to participate in spaced activities.
Hazards of immobility are prevented.

Assessment of cardiac output is achieved by the following nursing actions:
Mental status is assessed every hour and prn.
Vital signs are measured and recorded every hour and prn (every 5 to 15 minutes when changing medications or medication dose).
Hemodynamic measurements are measured and recorded every hour and prn: PAP, PCWP, RA every 5 to 15 minutes and cardiac output (CO) and SVR every 30 to 60 minutes. Vital signs and hemodynamic function are evaluated before and after any medication is given or any dose is changed to ensure appropriate unloading therapy.
Physical assessment measures are performed every 4 to 6 hours and prn, initially every 8 to 12 hours and prn after the unloading regimen is established.
Intake and output are measured every shift and prn.
Daily weight of the patient is recorded.
Medication regimen is started and maintained as indicated and prescribed.
To evaluate medication effects clearly only one drug is changed at a time. The rate at which intravenous medications are titrated varies with the status of the patient. A patient with an acute change in mental status may require medication changes every few minutes as indicated by the rapid onset of the medication's effect.
For fluid-restricted patients it may be necessary to increase the concentration of continuous IV infusions to allow for a decrease in rate—i.e., nitroprusside 100 mg/250 mL; dobutamine 800 mg/250 mL.
Nitroprusside and nitroglycerine are tapered slowly as oral vasodilators and nitrates are added. Tapering is done to maintain optimal hemodynamic function within the parameters as described. Due to the time required to evaluate oral therapy, tapering often requires 2 to 4 days. Oral medications may cause abrupt changes 20 to 60 minutes after administration.
Some patients may not have adequate unloading with oral therapy. These patients may be kept on IV therapy in the ICU. If dopamine or dobutamine is required for renal perfusion, the transplant candidate may go to a telemetry unit to await heart transplantation.
Hemodynamic function is evaluated standing and supine after the patient is on oral therapy and 1 hour after medications have been given. This evaluation is done to check the efficacy of the pharmacologic regimen and to see how it will balance with the patient's daily activities.
Liver and renal function are monitored to evaluate the patient's ability to excrete drugs and to tolerate transplantation. The patient with poor renal function may require acute hemodialysis. The patient with elevated liver function test results may require further reduction of PCWP to decrease liver congestion.
The patient is supported with oxygen therapy.
The patient's visitors and activity are limited as medical condition permits.
Dietary and fluid restrictions are assessed by intake and output, daily weight, and calorie count. The patient is instructed about his or her individual need for dietary or fluid restriction.

---

2. Alteration in cardiac output related to dysrhythmias

Outcome Criteria	Nursing Interventions

To initiate preventive treatment for high-risk patients promptly and to teach the patient and family how to recognize problems and manage the drug regimen.

ECG monitoring is assessed and analyzed for changes and for the occurrence of ectopy.
If changes in intervals or ectopy occur:
Serum potassium levels, oxygenation, and dysrhythmic levels are assessed.
Patient's mental status and vital signs are assessed.
If life-threatening dysrhythmias occur, patient's oxygenation and circulation are supported as per ACLS protocol.
The patient's response to therapy is evaluated.
The occurrence of dysrhythmias is prevented.
Potassium levels are monitored.
Oxygenation via arterial blood gases or pulse oximetry is monitored.
Therapeutic levels of dysrhythmic drugs are monitored.
A quiet environment is provided and care for the patient is carried out in an unhurried manner to facilitate minimizing patient's catecholamine levels.
Vital signs are maintained within acceptable limits for that particular patient when any medication is changed.
The patient is prepared for electrophysiologic study if indicated:
The patient is taught what to expect.
The patient is premedicated as ordered.
Groin or shoulder area is prepared for catheter placement.
The patient and family are taught any information pertinent to the dysrhythmic medications prescribed, including checking the pulse response during an emergency, dealing with anxiety, and what to do if the dysrhythmia occurs.

Nursing Care Plan continued on following page

3. **Activity Intolerance related to:**
   Low cardiac output
   Side effects of medical therapy
   Extended stay in the hospital
   Potential for malnutrition.

Outcome Criteria	Nursing Interventions

The patient will have little or no discomfort, will rest at appropriate intervals, will have no skin breakdown, will have no infection, and understands and cooperates in the nursing care.	Patient's level of comfort is assessed as the patient reports it.
	Signs and symptoms of discomfort are assessed:
	  Signs of skin breakdown are monitored and assessed.
	  Patient's nutritional status and causes of loss of appetite are assessed.
	  Patient's activities or lack of activities are assessed.
	Measures to prevent skin breakdown are instituted.
	  Patient is turned every 2 hours.
	  Active/passive range of motion exercises are performed twice a day.
	  Special bed or bedding is instituted as indicated, i.e., egg crate mattress or air-fluid therapy bed.
	  Patient performs incentive spirometry every 2 hours.
	  Appropriate nutrition is facilitated, i.e., patient is allowed to arrange activities so that he or she is rested at meal times. Patient is helped to choose appetizing foods, and food supplements are given.
	The patient is taught what is being done and why.
	The patient is involved in his or her care whenever possible.

4. **Potential or actual ineffective coping related to the demands of a life-threatening illness and complicated medical care**

Outcome Criteria	Nursing Interventions
The patient will participate in his or her own care. The patient will seek appropriate resources when help is necessary.	The patient's ability to cope with everyday routines is assessed. The patient's comments and questions are documented. The transplant team is consulted when the patient seems to be experiencing difficulty with problem solving. The patient is allowed time to voice concerns and feelings, and anticipate grieving reactions at times. Identify coping mechanisms that have worked for the patient in the past. Support the patient and family in using their style of coping and grieving. Provide flexible visiting hours. Encourage the patient to choose his/her nursing care routines. Provide diversional activities. Promote adequate rest and sleep.

SUMMARY

Care of the patient with cardiomyopathy awaiting transplantation is a challenge for nurses who actively work with these patients. The majority of patients usually present with end-stage cardiac failure and require aggressive nursing and medical care considerations. The nursing diagnoses that were discussed in this chapter represent the goals and interventions that the nurse has to deal with when caring for this particular patient population. A thorough understanding of hemodynamic monitoring and medication regimens are essential for the collaborative care of these patients. Dysrhythmic management is of prime importance to prevent the 50% chance of sudden death in this vulnerable patient population. The nursing diagnoses of alteration in cardiac output, potential for ineffective coping, and activity intolerance are all pertinent in patients awaiting transplantation. It is, however, only with a continual effort made by all services that these patients are successfully cared for until transplantation is achieved or they have achieved maximal benefit from the medical regimen. One does need to remember, however, that not all collaborative efforts are successful, and there are issues that do need to be addressed if the patient does not survive until transplant or is becoming refractory to medical therapy. Collaboration is the key element in the care of these patients and needs to be incorporated into both medical and nursing care of those patients.

References

Bolen, J. L., and Alderman, E. L. (1976). Hemodynamic consequences of afterload reduction in patient with chronic aortic regurgitation. *Circulation*, 53, 879–883.

Braunwald, E., Sonnenblick, E. H., and Ross, J. (1988). Mechanisms of cardiac contraction and relaxation. In E. Braunwald (Ed.), *Heart disease: A textbook of cardiovascular medicine* (pp. 383–425). Philadelphia: W. B. Saunders.

Cardin, S., and Clark, S. (1985). A nursing diagnosis approach to the patient awaiting cardiac transplantation. *Heart & Lung*, 14(5), 499–504.

Casey, P. (1987). Pathophysiology of dilated cardiomyopathy: nursing implications. *Journal of Cardiovascular Nursing*, 2(1), 1–12

Chatterjee, K., Ports, T. A., Brumdage, B. H., et al, (1980). Oral hydralazine in chronic heart failure: sustained beneficial hemodynamic effects. *Annals of Internal Medicine*, 92, 600–604.

Culucci, W. S., Wright, R. F., and Braunwald, E. (1986). New positive inotropic agents in the treatment of congestive failure. Mechanisms of action and recent clinical developments. *New England Journal of Medicine*, 314, 349–358.

Dasta, J. F., and Kirby, R. B. (1986). Pharmacology and therapeutic use of low-dose dopamine. *Pharmacotherapy*, 6, 304–310.

Dasta, J. F., and Leier, C. V. (1989). *Perspectives on inotropic therapy: Continuing rule of dobutamine*. Springfield, NJ: Scientific Therapeutics Information.

DiMarco, J. P. (1989). Antiarrhythmics. In B. Chernow (Ed.), *Essentials of critical care pharmacology* (pp. 168–206). Baltimore: Williams & Wilkins.

Doyle, B. (1988). Nursing challenge: The patient with end-stage heart failure. In L. S. Kern (Ed.), *Cardiac critical care nursing* (pp. 311–362). Rockville, MD: Aspen Publishers.

Factor, S. M., and Sonnenblick, E. D. (1985). Hypothesis: Is congestive cardiomyopathy caused by a hyperreactive myocardial microcirculation (microvascular spasm). *American Journal of Cardiology*, 50(5), 1149–1152.

Fuster, V., Gersh, B. J., Biuliani, E. R., et al. (1981). The natural history of idiopathic cardiomyopathy. *American Journal of Cardiology*, 47, 525.

Gawlinski, A. F. (1988). New diagnostic techniques. In L. S. Kern (Ed.), *Cardiac critical care nursing* (pp 33–58). Rockville, MD: Aspen Publishers.

Gillium, R. F. (1986). Idiopathic cardiomyopathy in the United States 1970–1982. *American Heart Journal*, 111(4), 752–755.

Goldberg, L. I. (1972). Cardiovascular and renal actions of dopamine: Potential clinical applications. *Pharmacology Review*, 24, 1–29.

Goodwin, J. F. (1982). The frontiers of cardiomyopathy. *British Heart Journal*, 48, 1–18.

Hlatky, M., Fleg, J., Hinton, P., et al, (1986). Physician practice in the management of congestive heart failure. *Journal of the American College of Cardiology*, 8, 966–970.

Imperial, F. A., Cordova-Manigbas, L., and Ward, C. R. (1989). Cardiac transplantation. *Critical Care Nursing Clinics of North America*, 1(2), 399–415.

Leier, C. V., Heban, P. T., Huss, P., et al. (1978). Comparative systemic and regional hemodynamic effects of dopamine and dobutamine in patients with cardiomyopathic heart failure. *Circulation*, 58, 466–475.

Leier, C. V. (1985). Treatment of congestive heart failure. In D. V. Unverferth (Ed.), *Dilated cardiomyopathy* (pp. 223–240). Mount Kisco, NY: Futura.

Leya, F. T., and Gunnar, R. M. (1988). Is digitalis beneficial in congestive heart failure secondary to dilated cardiomyopathy? In R. S. Engelmeir and J. B. O'Connell (Eds.), *Drug therapy in dilated cardiomyopathy and myocarditis* (pp. 87–102). New York: Marcel Dekker.

Litchtenberg, R., and Schreiber, R. R. (1988). Diuretic therapy of dilated cardiomyopathy. In R. S. Engelmeier and J. B. O'Connell (Eds.), *Drug therapy in dilated cardiomyopathy and myocarditis* (pp. 49–67). New York: Marcel Dekker.

Parrillo, J. E. (1989). Cardiomyopathies: Pathogenesis and treatment in a critical care environment. In W. C. Shoemaker, S. Ayres, A. Grevik, et al. (Eds.), *Textbook of critical care* (pp. 452–463). Philadelphia: W. B. Saunders.

Passmore, J. M., and Goldstein, R. M. (1989). Acute recognition and management of congestive heart failure. *Critical Care Clinics*, 5(3), 497–532.

Purcell, J. A. (1990). Advances in the treatment of dilated cardiomyopathy. *AACN clinical issues in critical care nursing*, 1(1), 31–45.

Purcell, J. A., and Holder, C. K. (1989). Cardiomyopathy: understanding the problem. *American Journal of Nursing*, 89(1), 57–74B.

Roberts, W. C., Siegel, R. J., and McManus, B. M. (1987). Idiopathic dilated cardiomyopathy: Analysis of 152 necropsy patients. *American Journal of Cardiology*, 60, 1340.

Shabetai, R. (1983). Cardiomyopathy: How far have we come in 25 years, how far yet to go? *Journal of the American College of Cardiology*, 1, 252.

Stanley, R. (1990). Drug therapy of heart failure. *Journal of Cardiovascular Nursing*, 4(3), 17–34.

Stevenson, L. W., Donahue, B. C., Tillisch, J. T., et al., (1987). Urgent priority transplantation: When should it be done? *Journal of Heart Transplantation*, 6, 267–272.

Stevenson, L. W., Dracup, K. A., and Tillisch, J. T. (1989). Efficacy of medical therapy tailored for severe congestive heart failure in patients transferred for urgent cardiac transplantation. *American Journal of Cardiology*, 63, 461–464.

Stevenson, L. W., Fawler, M. B., Schaeder, J. S., et al., (1987). Poor survival of patients with idiopathic cardiomyopathy considered too well for transplantation. *American Journal of Medicine*, 83, 871–876.

Stevenson, L. W., and Miller, L. W. (1991). Cardiac transplantation as therapy for heart failure. *Current Problems in Cardiology, XVI* (4), 219–305.

Stevenson, L. W., and Perloff, J. K. (1988). The dilated cardiomyopathies: Clinical aspects. *Cardiology Clinics*, 6(2), 187–218.

Stevenson, L. W., Sietsema, K. E., Lem, V., et al. (1988). Comparison of exercise capacity in heart failure patients following cardiac transplantation or intensive medical therapy. *Clinical Research*, 36, 115A.

Stevenson, L. W., and Tillisch, J. T. (1986). Maintenance of cardiac output with normal filling pressures in patient with dilated heart failure. *Circulation*, 74, 1303–1308.

Stevenson, W. G., Stevenson, L. W., Weiss, J., et al. (1988). Inducible ventricular arrhythmias and sudden death during vasodilator therapy of severe heart failure. *American Heart Journal*, 116(6), 1447–1454.

Tuttle, R. R., and Mills, J. (1975b). Dobutamine: Development of a new catecholamine to selectively increase cardiac contractility. *Circulation Research*, 36, 185–196.

Unverferth, D. (1985). The diagnosis of dilated cardiomyopathy. In. D. Unverferth (Ed.) Dilated cardiomyopathy. (pp. 9–15). Mt Kisco, NY: Futura Publishing Company.

Uretsky, B. F., Lawless, C. E., Verbalis, J. G., et al. (1987). Combined therapy with dobutamine and amrinone in severe heart failure: Improved hemodynamics and increased activation of the renin-angiotensin system with combined intravenous therapy. *Chest*. 92, 657–662.

Vitello-Cicciu, J., and Johantgen, M. (1988). Cardiomyopathy. In M. R. Kinney, D. R. Packa, and S. R. Dunbar (Eds.), *AACN's clinical reference for critical care nursing* (pp. 681–755). New York: McGraw Hill.

Wingate, S. (1984) Dilated cardiomyopathy, Part I. *Focus on Critical Care*, 11(4), 49–56.

Wynne, J., and Braunwald, E. (1988). The cardiomyopathies and myocarditis. In E. Braunwald (Ed.), *Heart disease* (pp. 1410–1469). Philadelphia: W. B. Saunders.

Yamaguchi, S., and Tsuiki, K. (1987). Wall motion abnormalities in dilated cardiomyopathy. *Cardiology Board Review*, 4(11), 106–115.

Young, J. B., and Yusef, S. (1988). Vasodilator therapy other than angiotensin-converting enzyme inhibition in dilated cardiomyopathy. In R. S. Engelmeier and J. B. O'Connell (Eds.), *Drug therapy in dilated cardiomyopathy and myocarditis* (pp. 103–120). New York: Marcel Dekker.

19

Patients with Congenital Heart Defects

Mary M. Canobbio

Contrary to common belief, congenital heart disease does not remain static after birth but changes both anatomically and physiologically throughout life. Another serious misconception is that with surgical correction, congenital heart disease is "cured." It is now generally accepted that with the exception of a ligated patent ductus, there is no cure for congenital heart disease; the best one can hope for is a good corrective repair that develops little or no clinical residua. But that is not to say that the patient is categorically assured of a lifetime free of concern for late complications. This concept is important because many defects that are benign or are repaired in infancy and childhood evolve into clinically significant disorders in adulthood. In addition, mild defects may be overlooked or misinterpreted in childhood, setting the stage for serious consequences in early or late adulthood.

This chapter is designed to provide the critical care nurse with an overview of congenital heart disease as it currently presents in the adult population. Although an in-depth review of all congenital cardiac defects is beyond the scope of this text, the focus will be on the long-term follow-up of congenital heart disease and the issues that influence 10- and 20-year survival.

ETIOLOGY

There is no single cause of congenital heart malformations; rather, they are the result of a complex interaction between genetic and environmental factors. On the genetic side, cardiac malformations are frequently familial. However, the familial recurrence rate due to single gene mutations or chromosomal abnormalities is small. Nora and Nora (1978) found

that primary genetic factors accounted for only 8% of all cardiac abnormalities. Of the cardiovascular defects that occur as a result of a genetic disorder, some result from either an autosomal recessive or autosomal dominant pattern, which accounts for 3% of all primary genetic disorders, or by chromosomal transmission, which accounts for 5% of all genetic disorders. Holt-Oram syndrome, Noonan syndrome, and Marfan syndrome are examples of autosomal dominant disorders that have a recurrence rate of 50%, whereas Friedreich ataxia and Duchenne muscular dystrophy are neuromuscular defects associated with myocardiopathy and conduction defects that are transmitted via autosomal recessive genes. Chromosomal abnormalities commonly associated with congenital cardiovascular defects include trisomy 21 (Down syndrome), and XO Turner syndrome. Table 19–1 provides a partial listing of congenital heart malformations that may occur as the result of specific genetic disorders. Because chromosomal and single genetic mutations account for less than 10% of all cardiac anomalies, it is more likely that the etiologic element permitting transmission from one generation to the next is multifactorial, meaning that it is the interaction of certain genetic patterns with multiple environmental factors that are responsible for the familial tendency observed in this group of patients (Goldstein and Brown, 1988).

Environmental factors known to contribute to fetal cardiac embryopathy include a variety of teratogens or exposure by the mother to rubella during the first 8 weeks of pregnancy. Altitude at birth also may be a factor contributing to the occurrence of congenital heart disease, particularly patent ductus arteriosus. Teratogens, substances used by the mother during gestation, known to cause congenital cardiac defects include thalidomide ingested during the first trimes-

TABLE 19–1. Partial List of Syndromes Known to Be Associated with Cardiac Malformations

Syndrome	Cardiac Anomaly	Incidence Rate (Approximate Risk) (%)
Chromosomal Defects		
Trisomy 21 (Down syndrome)	Endocardial cushion defects, ASD, VSD, PDA	50
Trisomy 13 (Patau syndrome)	VSD, PDA, double-outlet right ventricle	90
Trisomy 18 (Edward syndrome)	VSD, PDA, PS	99
XO (Turner syndrome)	Coarctation of aorta; aortic stenosis, ASD	35
Nonchromosomal Disorders		
Autosomal Dominant		
Holt-Oram	ASD, VSD	50
Noonan (Male Turner syndrome)	PS, ASD	50
Ehlers-Danlos	Dissecting aneurysm, AV valve regurgitation	50
Marfan	Aortic dilatation and rupture	60–80
Autosomal Recessive		
Cutis laxa	Peripheral pulmonary artery stenosis; pulmonary hypertension	50
Friedreich ataxia	Conduction defects; myocardiomyopathy	50
Laurence-Moon-Biedl	Tetralogy of Fallot, VSD	30
TAR (thrombocytopenia-absent radius)	ASD, tetralogy of Fallot, dextrocaedia	30
Osteogenesis imperfecta	Aortic insufficiency	5–10
Teratogenic Disorders		
Drugs		
Fetal alcohol syndrome	VSD, ASD, PDA, tetralogy of Fallot	25–30
Fetal hydantoin syndrome	Coarctation of aorta; aortic stenosis, PS, PDA	2–3
Fetal trimethadione syndrome	ASD, tetralogy of Fallot, TGA	15–30
Lithium	Ebstein anomaly, tricuspid atresia, ASD	10
Thalidomide	Tetralogy of Fallot, VSD, ASD, truncus arteriosus	5–10
Infections, Maternal		
Maternal rubella	PDA, pulmonic valvular stenosis, ASD, VSD	35
Other		
Maternal lupus erythematosus	Congenital heart block	?
Maternal diabetes	Coarctation of aorta, TGA, VSD	3–5

Abbreviations: ASD, atrial septal defect; VSD, ventricular septal defect; PDA, patent ductus arteriosus; PS, pulmonic stenosis; TGA, transposition of the great arteries.

Modified from Nora, J. J., and Nora, A. (1978). The evolution of specific genetic and environmental counseling in congenital heart disease. *Circulation* 57, 205–213. By permission of the American Heart Association, Inc.

ter, trimethadione, hydantoin, and alcohol. Chronic maternal alcohol abuse contributes to the development of fetal alcohol syndrome, which results in a variety of central nervous system defects (e.g., microcephaly) as well as cardiac anomalies. The most frequently seen defects are those involving the ventricular septum, which have been reported to occur in approximately 30% to 45% of affected infants (Nora and Nora, 1978; Friedman, 1988).

INCIDENCE AND PREVALENCE

Precise incidence rates for congenital heart disease are not available. It is, however, generally accepted that approximately 0.8% of all live births are complicated by some cardiovascular malformation (American Heart Association, 1988a). Unfortunately, this widely quoted figure underestimates the true incidence of congenital heart disease because many defects are undiagnosed at the time of birth. For example, congenital bicuspid aortic valve, which is

reported to be the most frequent congenital anomaly of the heart, often goes unnoticed unless it is associated with another defect or becomes dysfunctional later in life (Roberts, 1970). Even less clear is the actual prevalence rate of corrected and uncorrected congenital heart disease among adults. What is clear, however, is that rapid advances in surgical interventions have increased not only the life expectancy of patients with defects for which natural survival is common but also now permit survival of a large number of patients with defects that were previously fatal in childhood (Laks et al., 1980; Zuberbuhler, 1983). Today, a life expectancy of 10 to 25 years beyond surgical intervention is not uncommon; therefore, a new population of adult cardiac patients is emerging.

Adults with Congenital Heart Disease

Three categories of adults with congenital heart disease (CHD) are emerging. First and most preva-

TABLE 19–2. Natural Survival of Common and Uncommon Defect Forms of Congenital Heart Disease

A. Common congenital cardiac defects in which postpediatric
   survival is expected:
   Functionally normal bicuspid aortic valve
   Congenital valvular aortic stenosis
   Coarctation of the aorta
   Valvular pulmonic stenosis
   Atrial septal defect
   Patent ductus arteriosus
   Ventricular septal defect with pulmonic stenosis
      (Fallot tetralogy)

B. Uncommon congenital cardiac defects in which postpediatric
   survival is expected:
   Situs inversus
   Dextroversion of the heart
   Congenital complete heart block
   Congenitally corrected transposition of the great arteries
   Idiopathic dilatation of the pulmonary trunk
   Subvalvular pulmonic stenosis
   Supravalvular pulmonic stenosis
   Ebstein anomaly of the tricuspid valve
   Congenital pulmonary arteriovenous fistula
   Lutembacher syndrome
   Common atrium
   Congenital coronary arteriovenous fistula
   Congenital aneurysms of the sinus of Valsalva
   Vena caval to left atrial connection
   Congenital pulmonary valve regurgitation
   Primary pulmonary hypertension

C. Common congenital cardiac defects in which postpediatric
   survival is exceptional:
   Ventricular septal defect
   Ventricular septal defect with aortic regurgitation
   Endocardial cushion defect
   Tricuspid atresia
   Complete transposition of the great arteries

D. Uncommon congenital cardiac defects in which postpediatric
   survival is exceptional:
   Anomalous origin of the left coronary artery from pulmonary
      trunk
   Cor triatriatum
   Total anomalous pulmonary venous connection
   Right ventricular origin of both great arteries (double-outlet
      right ventricle)
   Truncus arteriosus
   Single ventricle
   Discrete subvalvular aortic stenosis

Reprinted from *Critical Care Nursing Quarterly*, Vol. 4, No. 3, p. 41, with permission of Aspen Publishers, Inc., © 1981.

lent are adults with surgically corrected CHD. Although precise numbers are unavailable, it has begun to be evident from the centers that report follow-up studies on large populations of adult patients that the numbers are rising (Schaff and Danielson, 1987; McNamara and Latson, 1982). The recently completed *Second Natural History of Congenital Heart Defects* (American Heart Association, 1988b) further documents the fact that 20-year survival of individuals with pulmonic stenosis, ventricular septal defect, and aortic stenosis (with gradients of <50 mm Hg) is now possible following surgical repair.

A second group of adults with CHD are those for whom operative correction has been impossible either because their cardiac anomalies have not been amenable to surgical correction or they have developed pulmonary vascular disease.

The third group of adults with CHD is the small percentage of individuals who have unrecognized or undiagnosed disease. Table 19–2 summarizes both common and uncommon forms of congenital heart defects in which natural survival can be expected or is considered exceptional. Included in this category are patients who may have received palliative treatment in early childhood with the hope of later repair but for a variety of reasons have been lost to follow-up. Larger medical centers have confirmed that a number of cardiac anomalies continue to be detected initially and surgically treated in adulthood (Danielson and McGoon, 1987). To understand what long-term follow-up can be expected, patients can be classified by their functional status rather than by their individual defects (Table 19–3).

Patients in category I are those who have undergone complete repair and have no residual effects. Included in this group are those who have experienced spontaneous closure of a ventricular septal defect (VSD). These patients, who fortunately make up the largest majority of the population of patients with CHD, are asymptomatic and are normal when measured on objective functional tests and evaluation such as exercise tests and echocardiography. Socially, they are able to work, have children, and live well-adjusted lives.

Patients in category II are those with documented residual effects and complications who are either asymptomatic or remain minimally symptomatic for many years and require varying degrees of long-term

TABLE 19–3. Four-Category System for Determining Impact on Quality of Life

Category I: Those who have undergone a complete repair and have no residual effects and are asymptomatic. Their clinical course is stable, they have normal functional capacity, are generally less anxious, and lead normal lives.

Category II: Those who have undergone surgical correction but are left with known residual defects or complications, such as the postoperative coarctation patient who is left with residual hypertension. They may remain asymptomatic for years, but over time develop symptoms because of the residual defect. Their level of social adjustment will vary.

Category III: Those who have undergone corrective procedures for complex cardiac defects. They are similar to patients in category I in that they may have had good to excellent repairs and are asymptomatic, but unlike the patient with a common defect the long-term sequelae of these patients remain unknown.

Category IV: Those who may have undergone previous palliative or corrective procedures but remain symptomatic due to a limited cardiac reserve. Their prognosis is usually poor and their social adjustment may have marked limitations.

Reprinted from *Cardiac Rehabilitation Nursing* by C. Jillings, p. 114, with permission of Aspen Publishers, Inc., © 1988.

follow-up care. Conditions characterizing people in this category include residual hypertension following a coarctectomy, residual mitral regurgitation following closure of an ostium primum atrial septal defect, or a patch leak with residual shunt following closure of a ventricular septal defect (VSD). The prognosis for patients in this category is largely dependent upon the specific type of lesion and the degree of severity of the residual effects. Their level of social adjustment will vary with the degree of functional limitation. Often, they may live several years before the onset of symptoms and not infrequently will require a repeat operation.

A third category of patients includes those who have undergone successful surgical repair but are subject to unknown residual and long-term sequelae after 10 to 20 years. This group includes patients who have undergone repair for complex congenital defects such as single ventricle, tricuspid atresia, and transposition of the great arteries. By objective measurements, these individuals may have achieved a normal functional capacity and are asymptomatic, but they must be carefully monitored to detect the frequent subtle onset of symptoms.

A fourth category of adult patients includes those whose defects remain unrepaired because they either have developed pulmonary hypertension, or have an anatomic arrangement not amenable to correction, or have residual effects that have produced complications that are no longer amenable to surgical intervention. Conditions that characterize this last category include (1) unrepaired defects such as atrial or ventricular septal defects with right to left shunts due to increased pulmonary vascular resistance (commonly referred to as Eisenmenger syndrome—see later discussion), (2) pulmonary atresia with an inadequate supply of pulmonary collaterals for a staged repair, and (3) ventricular failure. The clinical course of this group of patients varies widely. Many patients with Eisenmenger syndrome remain clinically free of symptoms for years and are able to lead relatively normal lives. However, their prognosis is guarded, and they require careful and frequent evaluation. Understandably, the level of social adjustment in this group of patients is hampered by their physical limitations, and they generally require much in the way of emotional support and counseling. They are also the group who may have the greatest difficulty in obtaining health insurance.

FACTORS INFLUENCING LONG-TERM SURVIVAL

In dealing with the adult patient with a congenital heart defect it is important to recognize that survival is influenced by several factors. First, the primary cardiac defect or defects must be considered and the complications, if any, that have developed must be determined. Second, the surgical interventions that may have taken place must be identified. In patients who have undergone previous surgical correction, it is important to consider what postoperative residua and known sequelae are associated with the procedure. Finally, the age at which surgical repair occurred is important.

Primary Defects

Congenital heart defects are frequently described in terms of the presence or absence of cyanosis. Although this is clinically correct, for purposes of understanding the hemodynamic consequences of these defects it is preferable to classify congenital heart defects by the direction and magnitude of pulmonary blood flow (Table 19–4) (Morgan, 1978).

Acyanotic Defects

Normal Pulmonary Blood Flow. Defects such as coarctation of the aorta, aortic stenosis, and pulmonic stenosis cause impairment or obstruction of ventricular outflow. The result creates an increased pressure load on the ventricle, leading to concentric hypertrophy of the wall of the respective chamber. The anatomic location of the obstruction and the severity of the obstructive gradient together dictate the degree of clinical pathology that results. For example, congenital aortic stenosis can occur at the valvular, subvalvular, or supravalvular level of the aortic ring.

TABLE 19–4. Congenital Heart Disease Based Upon the Direction of Pulmonary Blood Flow

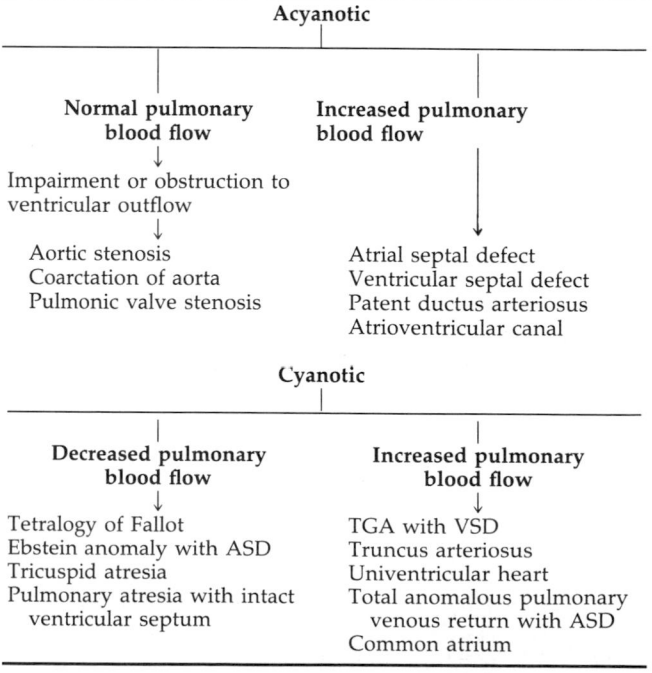

Acyanotic	
Normal pulmonary blood flow	**Increased pulmonary blood flow**
Impairment or obstruction to ventricular outflow	
Aortic stenosis	Atrial septal defect
Coarctation of aorta	Ventricular septal defect
Pulmonic valve stenosis	Patent ductus arteriosus
	Atrioventricular canal

Cyanotic	
Decreased pulmonary blood flow	**Increased pulmonary blood flow**
Tetralogy of Fallot	TGA with VSD
Ebstein anomaly with ASD	Truncus arteriosus
Tricuspid atresia	Univentricular heart
Pulmonary atresia with intact ventricular septum	Total anomalous pulmonary venous return with ASD
	Common atrium

Abbreviations: ASD, atrial septal defect; TGA, transposition of great arteries; VSD, ventricular septal defect.

The most common type is valvular. If it is stenotic from birth, the valve is usually bicuspid, and the valve tissue becomes progressively thickened and fibrotic during childhood and adolescence. Calcification of the valve that does not usually begin until early adulthood results in further restriction in valve mobility and obstruction of left ventricular outflow. The clinical manifestations of aortic stenosis, as with other obstructive lesions, are largely determined by the severity of the valve stenosis and the degree of obstruction it presents. In aortic stenosis, the response of the left ventricle to chronic pressure overload is concentric hypertrophy (Friedman, 1988). In severe forms of obstruction of ventricular outflow, the electrocardiogram (ECG) will show signs of hypertrophy with strain when there is an imbalance between myocardial oxygen supply and demand. As with most cases of persistent increased afterload, dilatation and decompensation occur in the natural progression of the disease process.

Increased Pulmonary Blood Flow. Anomalies that redirect the flow of blood from the left heart back to the right side (l → r), as in atrial septal defect (ASD) or VSD, produce an added burden on the right atria or ventricles and pulmonary vessels. Pathophysiology is largely determined by the size of the defect and the ratio of pulmonary to systemic vascular resistance. For example, a small restrictive VSD may result in little or no increased cardiac or pulmonary workload (Borow and Braunwald, 1988). But when the left to right shunt is large, the additional burden of increased pulmonary blood flow frequently leads to enlargement of the pulmonary artery and thus to pulmonary hypertension. If this situation is left unrepaired, as in the case of a large nonrestrictive VSD, equilibration of systolic pressures in the two ventricles occurs. Pulmonary blood flow is then determined by the ratio of systemic and pulmonary vascular resistance. When pulmonary vascular resistance equals or exceeds that of systemic circulation, a bidirectional or right to left shunt develops.

Cyanotic Defects

Cyanotic lesions represent a shunting of blood from the right heart to the left. They generally result from an abnormal communication between the two circulations, leading to venoarterial mixing. A variety of cardiac anomalies can result in an abnormal connection between the two circulations. The distinguishing feature, however, is whether the anomaly contributes to a decrease or an increase in pulmonary blood flow, and this then becomes the basis for therapeutic interventions.

Decreased Pulmonary Blood Flow. Malformations that lead to shunting of blood away from the lungs generally occur because (1) there is a severe pulmonary obstruction, as in tetralogy of Fallot, tricuspid

atresia, or pulmonary atresia with intact ventricular septum, or (2) the right ventricle is inadequate as a pumping chamber, as in Ebstein anomaly of the tricuspid valve. Clinically, the patient is deeply cyanotic, hypoxic, and easily fatigued. Rarely do any of these defects go undetected. Diagnosed usually in infancy or during early childhood, the majority of adult patients with these defects have undergone definitive intracardiac repair or placement of a surgically created systemic-pulmonary arterial shunt that permits increased pulmonary arterial blood flow with enhanced oxygen saturation. In the latter group of patients, intracardiac repair is still a possibility but only in the absence of pulmonary vascular disease.

Increased Pulmonary Blood Flow. Increased pulmonary blood flow is the result of either common mixing of blood in the atrium (common atrium) or ventricles (single ventricle) or an abnormal communication between the great vessels as in transposition of the great arteries (TGA) with VSD. Excessive pulmonary blood flow generally results in cardiac failure unless a palliative procedure such as pulmonary banding can minimize the amount or unless the patient develops pulmonary vascular disease, which decreases the degree of shunting. Survival to adulthood is possible but generally only with an early palliative procedure followed later by surgical correction.

Surgical Intervention

With few exceptions, surgical intervention is recommended when feasible for the majority of uncorrected congenital heart disorders. But the operative risk and prognosis are largely dependent upon the complexity of the defect, the presence of and severity of associated cardiac symptoms, and the presence or absence of pulmonary hypertension. In the adult patient, surgery for congenital heart disease may have been undertaken as a palliative measure or as a method of physiologic intracardiac repair.

Palliative Procedures. A wide range of palliative procedures has been introduced during the past four decades. These generally serve as a preliminary step toward total intracardiac repair for correctable lesions. For defects that are not reparable, palliative procedures have served as the sole means of survival for patients with defects that would otherwise prove fatal during infancy. Palliative procedures are either shunt operations designed to improve pulmonary blood flow (Fig. 19–1) (Table 19–5) or surgical operations designed to create arteriovenous mixing at the atrial level (Table 19–6).

Of the various systemic to pulmonary artery shunting procedures that have been developed to increase pulmonary blood flow, the earliest and perhaps the most widely used is the Blalock-Taussig anastomosis, which connects the subclavian artery to the pulmo-

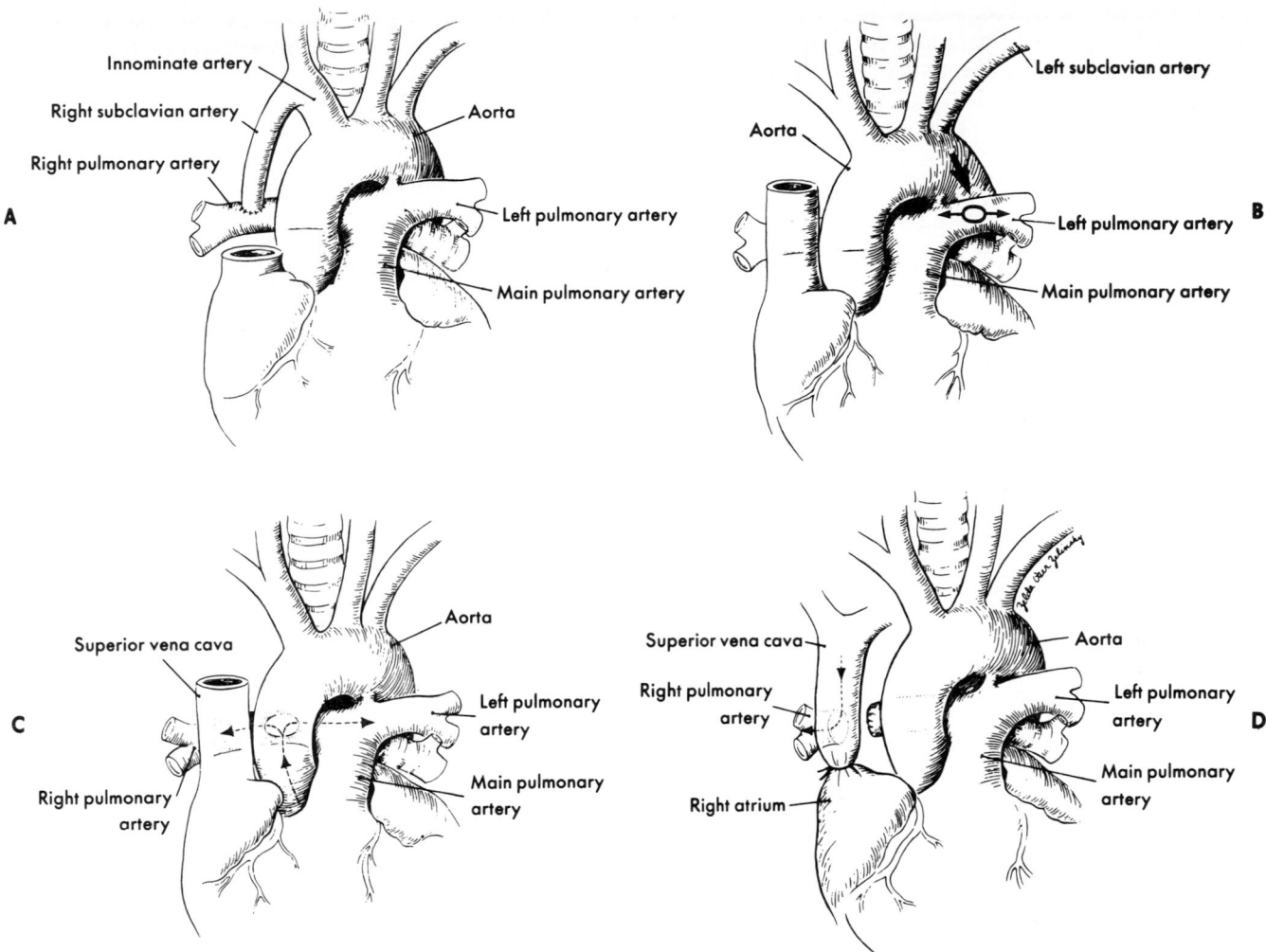

FIGURE 19–1. Shunting procedures used to increase pulmonary artery blood flow. *A,* Blalock-Taussig (BT) shunt; subclavian artery is divided. The proximal portion is brought down, and the end of the subclavian is anastomosed to the pulmonary artery. *B,* Potts anastomosis. The left pulmonary artery is anastomosed to a portion of the left descending aorta. *C,* Waterston-Cooley shunt. A fistula is created between the posterior ascending aorta and the anterior portion of the right pulmonary artery. *D,* Glenn anastomosis. Superior vena cava (SVC) is ligated at its junction with right atrium; the SVC is attached to the right pulmonary artery using Gore-Tex graft. SVC blood is directed to the right pulmonary artery. (Reproduced by permission from: Hazinski: *Nursing care of the critically ill child* (p. 195). St. Louis, 1984, The C. V. Mosby Co.)

nary artery. Introduced more than 35 years ago, it has proved to have one of the highest patency rates and lowest complication rates among shunting procedures (complications include heart failure or development of pulmonary vascular disease). Furthermore, it is generally easier to close at the time of definitive repair (Pacifico and Sand, 1987). Over the years additional shunts have been devised, but several, such as the Potts procedure, have been abandoned due to a tendency toward excessive pulmonary blood flow (von Bermuth et al., 1971).

Surgical procedures designed to promote mixing of blood by creating an atrial septal defect (left to right shunt) include the balloon atrial septostomy (Rashkind procedure) and an atrial septectomy (Blalock-Hanlon technique). These procedures permit a free flow of oxygenated blood to the right atrium, from which location it enters the right ventricle and

pulmonary circulation (Cooley, 1988). Generally performed during the first weeks of life, these procedures are used to palliate transposition of the great arteries with pulmonic stenosis.

The majority of patients, who have undergone these procedures in infancy, have later had corrective or definitive repair. However, a small number reach adulthood with no repairs. These patients usually have limited cardiac reserve, and although most have adjusted to their condition, they are functionally limited (Borow and Braunwald, 1988). As adults, some may still be amenable to surgical repair; however, the development of pulmonary vascular disease or a failing myocardium in some prohibits further surgical intervention.

Corrective Procedures. Since the introduction of intracardiac repair for CHD more than 30 years ago,

TABLE 19–5. Shunting Operations for Congenital Heart Defects: Procedures That Permit Increased Pulmonary Blood Flow by Creating Systemic to Pulmonary Artery Shunt

Shunt	Year Introduced	Description	Morbidity
Blalock-Taussig	1945	Subclavian artery to pulmonary artery	BA (<6%) IE (<6%) Patency (>50%) PVD (1–5%)
Potts	1946	Descending aorta anastomosed side-to-side to left pulmonary artery	PVD (>15%) IE (15%) CHF (38%)
Glenn	1958	Superior vena cava anastomosis to right pulmonary artery	
Modified Blalock-Taussig	1962	Subclavian artery to pulmonary artery using Gore-Tex graft	
Waterston-Cooley	1962–1966	Ascending aorta-to-right pulmonary artery anastomosis	PVD (6%) CHF (26%) Kinking of right pulmonary artery

Abbreviations: BA, brain abscess; IE, infective endocarditis; PVD, pulmonary vascular disease; CHF, congestive heart failure.

the clinical course of patients in whom congenital cardiac anomalies have been corrected has been carefully scrutinized. It is generally agreed that there are few surgical cures for congenital heart disease. In most cases what has been rendered is a definitive repair that has either reestablished anatomic integrity and a normal circulation, or has restored a normal circulation through an artificial inserted conduit or baffle. An example of total correction, which has been available for more than two decades, is the procedure for tetralogy of Fallot. The procedure includes the ligation or takedown of any prior palliative shunts, patch closure of the VSD, and relief of the right ventricular outflow tract obstruction. To accomplish this, one of several techniques is used, infundibular resection, pulmonary valvotomy, or transannular patch, depending upon the amount of outflow obstruction and the degree of pulmonary valve involvement. Results of long-term survival for tetralogy of Fallot have been very favorable. Today, reports

TABLE 19–6. Surgical Palliation for Congenital Heart Disease: Procedures That Permit Arteriovenous Mixing by Creating Left-to-Right Shunts

Procedure	Year Introduced	Description
Blalock-Hanlon atrial septectomy	1948	Entering through a left thoracotomy, incisions are made into the right and left atria and interatrial septum is removed
Rashkind, balloon atrial septostomy	1966	Balloon-tipped catheter passed through inferior vena cava and foramen ovale into left atrium

indicate that survival rates of 85% and 95% for up to 20 years after operation are now possible (Pacifico and Sand, 1987; Fuster et al., 1980).

Another procedure that is now available and typifies the physiologic correction of complex cyanotic defects is the Fontan procedure. Originally described in 1971 (Fontan and Baudet, 1971) for tricuspid atresia, the procedure continues to undergo modifications and is now being used in the treatment of several defects including single ventricle disease and double-inlet ventricles (Humes et al., 1988). The procedure involves closure of the ASD and surgical connection of the right atrium to the pulmonary artery or right ventricle by direct anastomosis (Fig. 19–2A) or by means of a nonvalved conduit (Fig. 19–2B and C). Earlier techniques that included the use of porcine valve conduits have been abandoned because of development of valvular dysfunction and obstruction. Currently, 5- and 10-year survival rates are reported. In one series 5-year survival rates of 87% were reported (Humes et al., 1988). However, during the past decade, two chief concerns in long-term postoperative follow-up of these patients have emerged. First, the effects of chronically elevated right atrial (RA) pressure and systemic venous hypertension on liver function are worrisome, and second, ventricular function appears to be abnormal. Postoperative RA pressures tend to be higher than normal, with means of 14 mm Hg reported in one series (Mair et al., 1985) and 15 mm Hg in another (Laks et al., 1984). Hemodynamic results of left ventricular function have demonstrated subnormal results despite normal functional abilities (Mair et al., 1985; Laks et al., 1984; Shachar et al., 1982). Mair and associates found that ventricular end-diastolic pressures of less than 15 mm Hg were necessary postoperatively if a good clinical result was to occur. Yet pressures of 15 mm Hg or less may still be

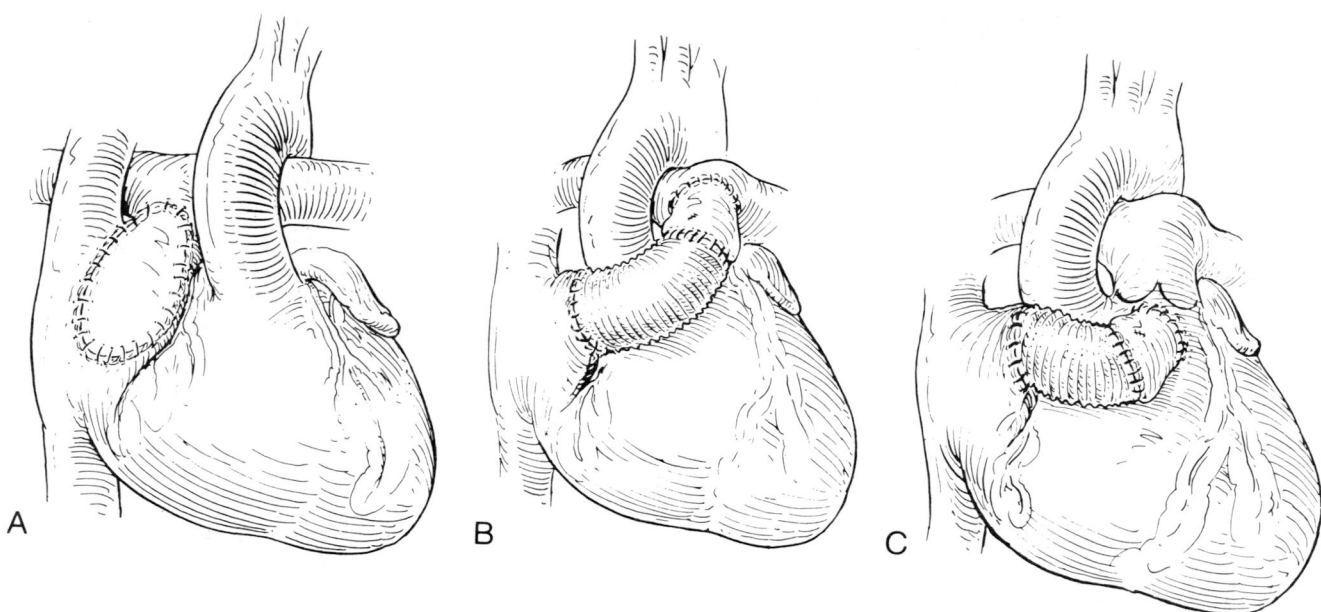

FIGURE 19–2. Fontan procedure. Direct right atrium to pulmonary artery anastomosis. *A,* Direct right atrium to pulmonary artery connection is shown, with augmentation of the anastomosis by a pericardial patch. *B,* Right atrium to left pulmonary artery connection with an aortic homograft supplemented by a synthetic conduit. *C,* Right atrium to right ventricle aortic homograft connection. The atrial and ventricular septal defects are closed. (From Barre, A. E., et al. (1991). *Glenn's thoracic and cardiovascular surgery* (5th ed.). Norwalk, CT: Appleton & Lange.)

misleading, particularly in patients who may have had preoperative ventricular volume loads of more than three times normal.

Therefore, despite the favorable results of many surgical interventions for congenital heart defects, over time it has been determined that a wide range of residual effects ranging from mild to severe can exist. These effects may develop as a direct result of the surgical intervention, such as a residual pulmonic stenosis that exists following repair of tetralogy of Fallot, or they may develop separately and demand reoperation, such as a conduit obstruction associated with the Fontan procedure (Laks et al., 1980; Mair et al., 1985). Furthermore, for many complex defects, the long-term natural sequelae following surgical correction remain unknown.

One area of investigation has been the postoperative myocardium. Studies have shown that, regardless of the site of incision (atrium or ventricle), subendocardial fibroelastosis of the left ventricle is likely to develop because of prolonged pump time, and it is this fibrosis that is responsible for the development of late ventricular dysfunction (Henson et al., 1969; Bharati and Levi, 1983). The long-term effects of ventriculotomy and the subsequent development of scar tissue in the myocardium also have been attributed to development of reentry phenomena leading to ventricular tachycardia and sudden death (Bharati and Levi, 1983). Aneurysm formation at the ventriculotomy site is yet another consideration in the development of postoperative ventricular tachycardia. In addition to effects on the myocardium, the bundle of His and its branches also may be damaged by the effects of ventriculotomy, resec-

tion of obstructive right ventricular muscle, or development of fibrosis. Sinus node dysfunction is a late concern following complex intra-atrial connections such as the Mustard or Senning procedure for TGA, during repair of a sinus venosus atrial septal defect, or following the Fontan repair for tricuspid atresia. Similarly, the atrioventricular (AV) node is at risk during repair of AV septal defects, ventricular septal defects, or tricuspid valve defects. Consequently, postoperative dysrhythmias pose one of the major challenges to long-term survival.

Additional late complications that have been reported as a direct result of the original surgical procedure include development of true or pseudo-aneurysms in the right ventricular outflow tract following the insertion of patches, obstruction of intra-atrial baffles or conduits, and valvular incompetence due to suturing.

Although many of the postoperative problems apparent in this first generation of adult patients may be a reflection of early surgical techniques rather than current ones, only time will tell whether improved intraoperative procedures will be able to decrease or eliminate these complications in long-term follow-up.

Age at Surgery. With respect to the clinical outcome, it is becoming increasingly clear that the best surgical results occur when procedures are undertaken in childhood rather than in adolescence (McNamara and Latson, 1982). This is true for a wide range of defects including ventricular septal defect, tetralogy of Fallot, tricuspid atresia, and single ventricle (Kirklin et al., 1983; Ebert et al., 1984; Mair et al., 1985; Pacifico and Sand, 1987).

In contrast, information about the long-term psychological outcome or emotional adjustment relative to the age of surgery has not been studied as rigorously. To date, the effects of hypothermia, circulatory arrest, and cardiopulmonary bypass (Glasner and Bentovim, 1987) on cognitive and neurologic functioning have been examined. Overall, the clinical findings show that following surgical repair children have intellectual and motor skills that are normal or equal to those of their age-matched counterparts (Glasner and Bentovim, 1987). Less clear, however, is the issue of age of operation and long-term effects on emotional adjustment. From the limited information available, it appears that individuals on whom surgery was performed in late childhood or preadolescence compared with those who underwent repairs before the age of 6 are significantly different in terms of personality traits and dependency. As a whole, they tend to display traits similar to those seen in persons who are chronically ill (Baer et al., 1984). Such information suggests that when some state of invalidism is imposed upon a child during important periods of cognitive, motor, and emotional development, long-term psychological well-being may be impaired.

LONG-TERM COMPLICATIONS ASSOCIATED WITH CONGENITAL HEART DISEASE

Dysrhythmias

As previously mentioned, dysrhythmias occur frequently as a long-term postoperative complication. But they also are a major cause of morbidity and mortality among patients who have had no repair.

McNamara and Latson (1982), in their 25-year postoperative follow-up of five common congenital heart defects (ventricular septal defect, atrial septal defect, patent ductus arteriosus, pulmonary stenosis, and coarctation of the aorta), reported that although most patients were living normal lives, there continued to be a large incidence of residual effects and sequelae, namely, late unexpected dysrhythmias requiring periodic follow-up. The 1988 *Second Natural History Study of Congenital Heart Disease* conducted a 20-year follow-up study that included VSD, pulmonic stenosis, and aortic stenosis. The results of this study showed that although patients were generally in good health, individuals with VSD or aortic stenosis with residual gradients were at greater risk of developing late dysrhythmias (American Heart Association, 1988b).

Dysrhythmias encountered among patients who have had no repairs are often the result of a complication or electrophysiologic instability associated with the primary congenital defect. For example, patients with Ebstein anomaly may present with rapid heart action resulting from supraventricular tachycardia (SVT). These dysrhythmias, which have been reported in 25% to 30% of patients, represent reentrant SVT, atrial fibrillation, and atrial flutter and are not necessarily related to accelerated or anomalous atrioventricular conduction (Ferguson et al., 1986; Perloff, 1987). One variety of Ebstein anomaly is also associated with preexcitation patterns such as Wolff-Parkinson-White (WPW) syndrome, which usually represents a right bypass tract (Perloff, 1987). Several congenital heart anomalies show evidence of atrioventricular conduction abnormalities. For example, first degree AV block is characteristically seen in patients with endocardial cushion defects (such as ostium primum). Atrial fibrillation and flutter are frequently encountered in patients who develop volume overload. Lesions such as atrial septal defect or ventricular septal defect that produce significant left to right shunting will, over time, lead to atrial tachyarrhythmias. Ventricular dysrhythmias are characteristically seen in the setting of long-standing volume overload or ventricular failure as well as in conditions where there has been chronic pressure overload of the left ventricle as seen in aortic valve disease and palliative systemic-pulmonary shunts (Sloss and Ellison, 1987). Ventricular dysrhythmias also are the most probable cause of sudden death in patients who develop the Eisenmenger syndrome (Wood, 1958; Young and Marks, 1971). Table 19–7 presents a listing of several defects and the dysrhythmias associated with them. Thus, with few exceptions, patients with known congenital heart disease should be periodically evaluated for the development of late dysrhythmias.

Infective Endocarditis

Susceptibility to infective endocarditis is an essential concern in the management and long-term follow-up of the adult with congenital heart disease. In certain cases, such as patients with a ligated patent ductus or a secundum ASD, the risk of endocarditis may be decreased or eliminated postoperatively. However, all patients must be carefully evaluated for the presence of residual lesions that will necessitate continued preventive measures for prevention of endocarditis. Recommendations from the American Heart Association have stratified risk levels for prevention of endocarditis into a two-dose antibiotic regimen. In general, patients with anomalies associated with jet formation and vortex shedding are considered at greater risk for developing bacteremia than those with low-pressure, high-flow lesions (Dajani et al., 1990). Individuals with prosthetic valves and other prosthetic material such as conduits and shunts should have lifelong prophylaxis. Table 19–8 can be used as a guide in estimating risk for infective endocarditis in patients with congenital heart disease (Canobbio, 1987).

TABLE 19–7. Electrocardiographic Patterns Associated with Congenital Heart Defects

Cardiac Defect	Atrial Flutter/Fibrillation	Supraventricular Tachycardia	Ventricular Dysrhythmia	Atrioventricular Block	Preexcitation Syndrome	Abnormal P Orientation	Right Atrial Overload	Left Atrial Overload	Left Axis Deviation	Left Bundle Branch Block	Right Bundle Branch Block	Right Ventricular Volume Overload	Right Ventricular Pressure Overload	Left Ventricular Volume Overload	Left Ventricular Pressure Overload	Bi-ventricular Overload	Abnormal Q Waves or Myocardial Infarction Pattern
Atrial septal defect (secundum)	+ +	+	0	+	0	+	+ +	+	0	0	+	+ + +	+	0	0	0	0
Prolapsed mitral valve	+	+	+	0	+	0	0	+	0	0	0	0	0	+	0	0	0
Aortic stenosis	0	0	+	+	0	0	0	+	+	+	0	0	0	0	+ + +	0	0
Hypertrophic cardiomyopathy	+	0	+ +	0	+	0	0	+ +	+ +	+ +	0	0	0	0	+ + +	0	+ +
Pulmonary stenosis	0	0	0	0	0	0	+ +	0	0	0	+	+	+ + +	0	0	0	0
Ventricular septal defect	+	0	0	0	0	0	0	+	+	0	0	0	0	+ + +	0	+	0
Ductus arteriosus	+	0	0	0	0	0	0	+ +	+	+	0	0	0	+ + +	0	0	0
Tetralogy of Fallot	0	0	+	0	0	0	+ +	0	+	0	+	0	+ + +	0	0	+	0
Coarctation of aorta	+	0	0	0	0	0	0	+	+	0	0	0	0	0	+ +	0	0
Eisenmenger syndrome	+	0	+	0	0	0	+ +	0	0	0	+	0	+ + +	0	0	+	0
Atrial septal defect (primum)	+ +	+	0	+ +	0	0	+	+	+ + +	0	+	+ + +	+	+	0	+	0
Corrected transposition*	+	+	0	+ + +	+	0	+	+	+	0	0	0	0	+	+	+	+ + +
Ebstein anomaly	+ +	+ + +	0	+	+ +	0	+ + +	0	+	0	+ + +	+	0	0	0	0	0
Tricuspid atresia	+	+	+	0	0	0	+ + +	+	+ + +	+	0	0	0	+	+	0	+
Coronary artery anomalies	+	0	+ +	0	0	0	0	+ +	+ +	+	0	0	0	+	+	0	+ + +
Transposition of great arteries (postop)	+	+ +	0	+	0	0	+	0	0	0	0	0	+ + +	0	0	0	0

+ + +, Almost always seen (characteristic of defect)
+ +, Commonly seen with defect
+, Sometimes seen with defect (especially with associated defects or advancing age)
0, Rarely seen with defect
*The precordial QRS progression in corrected transposition may mimic left ventricular hypertrophy, usually with S-T abnormalities. True hypertrophy of the left-sided ventricle can occur in corrected transposition from associated left atrioventricular valvular insufficiency, ventricular septal defect, etc.
From Sloss, L. J., and Ellison, R. C. (1987). In W. C. Roberts (Ed.), *Adult congenital heart disease* (2nd ed., p. 168). Philadelphia: F. A. Davis.

Eisenmenger Syndrome

Eisenmenger syndrome occurs as a result of pulmonary vascular resistance (PVR) greater than 800 dynes/second per cm^{-5}. It is associated with decreased oxygen saturation in the systemic circulation, cyanosis, and polycythemia (Canobbio, 1984). Originally described as Eisenmenger complex, which referred to a VSD with a reversed or bidirectional shunt (Fig. 19–3), today the term is applied to a number of shunting defects occurring at the aorticopulmonary, ventricular, or atrial level. These defects are hemodynamically similar in that they characteristically involve persistent increased pulmonary blood flow that over time will produce pulmonary vascular disease of such severity that a bidirectional or right to left shunt occurs. Eisenmenger syndrome generally develops as a consequence of delayed operation or of failure to detect the lesion until adolescence or adulthood, when surgical repair is of little use. Heart and lung transplantation is the only surgical alternative.

Clinically, the most common complaint is effort intolerance probably related to decreased arterial oxygen saturation and, in the later stages, to ventricular dysfunction. Significant clubbing and polycythemia are usually present. Other clinical findings are summarized in Table 19–9. Medical management is directed by the clinical presentation. Polycythemia, a constant feature of cyanotic congenital heart disease, occurs as a compensatory mechanism that maintains adequate oxygen supply to the tissues.

Particular attention must be paid to the use of drugs that lower systemic vascular resistance. Unloading agents such as nitroglycerin are potentially harmful because they can lead to a sudden drop in systemic vascular resistance, reduced stroke volume, and an increase in the right to left shunt, which leads to further increases in cyanosis and tissue hypoxia.

In the natural course of this disorder the patient

TABLE 19–8. Patients at Risk for Infective Endocarditis

No Risk, Prophylaxis Exempt	Low Risk, Oral Prophylaxis	High Risk,* Injectable
Patent ductus arteriosus (ligated)	Repaired tetralogy of Fallot	Aortic valve stenosis, regurgitation
Repaired secundum atrial septal defect	Tricuspid regurgitation	Bicuspid aortic valve
Small ventricular septal defect	Pulmonic valve disease	Ventricular septal defect
Trivial pulmonic valve stenosis	Repaired coarctation of aorta without bicuspid aortic valve	Coarctation of aorta
Repaired ventricular septal defect	Ventricular septal defect, pulmonary hypertension (Eisenmenger complex)	Mitral insufficiency
		Prosthetic valves, conduits
		Systemic to pulmonary shunts
		Previous history of endocarditis

*Oral prophylaxis may be used in some high-risk groups (Dajani et al., 1990).

From Canobbio, M. M. (1987). In W. C. Roberts (Ed.), *Adult congenital heart disease* (2nd ed.). Philadelphia: F. A. Davis.

TABLE 19–9. Physical Findings Common in Patients with Eisenmenger Syndrome

Central cyanosis
Digital clubbing
Normal jugular venous pressure
Normal arterial pulse volume
Right ventricular thrust
Increased pulmonary closure with variable splitting of S_2
Pulmonary ejection click
Pulmonary ejection murmur
Systolic murmur at the lower sternal border

From Canobbio, M. M. (1984). *Nursing Clinics of North America*, 19, 537–545.

becomes increasingly symptomatic after age 30. However, many patients do survive and are able to live reasonably active lives throughout the third, fourth, and fifth decades. Sudden death, presumably from dysrhythmias, is the usual cause of death. Other causes of death include myocardial failure, pulmonary infarction due to arterial thrombosis, and complications of cerebral abscesses and cerebrovas-cular accidents, although the latter are not seen as frequently in older patients (Rosove et al., 1986).

Heart Failure

As in most cases of cardiac failure, heart failure in the adult with congenital heart disease occurs as a result of excessive work load imposed upon the cardiac muscle, usually by structural defects, or by basic changes in myocardial performance. Excessive workload can occur as a result of volume overload created by a large left to right shunt or by defects that lead to valvular insufficiency. Increased work-load also may result from pressure overload of the ventricles, as in lesions causing obstruction to out-flow such as aortic or pulmonic stenosis or coarcta-tion of the aorta. Pressure overload also may occur in lesions causing an obstruction to inflow, such as cor triatriatum or stenosis of the mitral or tricuspid valves (Talner, 1983).

Myocardial performance may be impaired either by changes in the chronotropic state of the heart, as observed with the tachydysrhythmias that can arise as result of a primary defect, or as a consequence of surgical intervention.

The onset of symptoms of cardiac failure in the adult with congenital heart disease is not predictable. Therefore, it is important to continue follow-up on patients who have residual effects, such as volume overload of a ventricle due to patch leak requiring reoperation, if the negative effects of excessive vol-ume and pressure overload are to be avoided.

MEDICAL MANAGEMENT

Although most patients have had surgery in in-fancy or childhood, there are some who require primary surgical repair as adults. In others, reoper-ation may be necessary because of a complication or because symptoms are appearing once again. For example, patients who have undergone aortic val-votomy may again present with clinical signs of severe aortic stenosis. The decision to operate will depend upon several factors, beginning with an

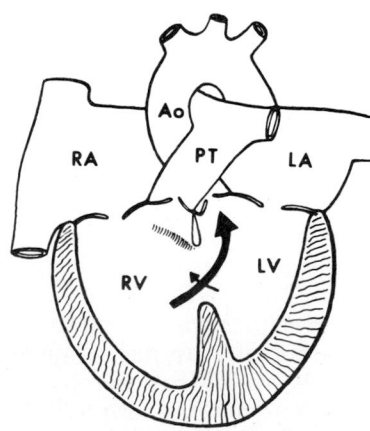

LARGE VSD
HIGH PVR

FIGURE 19–3. Schematic illustration of a large ventricular septal defect with high pulmonary vascular resistance and reversed shunt. (Courtesy of J. K. Perloff, M. D. From Canobbio, M. M. (1984). Eisenmenger syndrome. *Nursing Clinics of North America*, 19, 537–545.)

accurate diagnostic evaluation of the primary defect and its morphology. In addition, careful study of the hemodynamic consequences of many of these disorders is essential. A major concern is the presence of increased pulmonary hypertension, which increases the risk of operation, thereby making it prohibitive. Similarly, evaluation of ventricular function by two-dimensional, Doppler, or color flow echocardiography as well as by angiography offers a basis for determining the feasibility of surgical intervention.

For the patient in whom surgical intervention is not an option, medical therapy is generally directed by the clinical presentation. A brief overview of the most commonly occurring problems observed in this population is presented in this section. For detailed descriptions of therapeutic interventions for previously described complications of dysrhythmias, heart failure, or endocarditis, the reader is referred to other chapters in this text.

Medical treatment of atrial tachydysrhythmias generally consists of pharmacologic agents or electrical cardioversion to control ventricular response. Symptomatic ventricular dysrhythmias require careful monitoring with or without electrophysiologic testing to determine appropriate use of antidysrhythmic agents to suppress the dysrhythmias (Sloss and Ellison, 1987).

The treatment of cardiac failure begins with digitalization, diuretics, and restriction of sodium. However, as left ventricular dysfunction progresses, it frequently becomes necessary to initiate vasodilator therapy to unload the left ventricle by reducing peripheral vascular resistance or promoting systemic venous pooling.

Unique to the population of adults with congenital heart disease is the problem of hematologic management of the cyanotic patient. Cyanotic patients, who have increasing erythrocytosis, are bothered by a variety of complaints such as headaches, muscle and joint pain, fatigue, dizziness, and hemoptysis. These clinical symptoms have been attributed to increased blood viscosity and intravascular red cell aggregation (Rudolph et al., 1953; Rosove et al., 1986). Isovolumetric phlebotomy for excessive erythrocytosis has been shown to be an effective method of reducing red cell volume (Perloff et al., 1988). Indications for phlebotomy are based upon the presence of moderate to severe clinical symptoms in conjunction with a hematocrit of greater than 65%. It must, however, be pointed out that an elevated hematocrit alone is not an appropriate criterion for phlebotomy. Rosove and colleagues (1986) have reported that hematocrits of 69% and 70% are well tolerated without risk of cerebrovascular events. Pharmacologic measures used in response to signs of cardiac failure must be managed carefully because indiscriminate use of certain agents such as diuretics can lead to serious complications. For example, diuretics can contribute to hemoconcentration. Unloading agents can be harmful because they cause a sudden decrease in systemic vascular resistance, reduce the stroke volume, and can increase right to left shunting, which leads to increased cyanosis and tissue hypoxia.

NURSING MANAGEMENT

If nurses are to carry out collaborative and independent nursing actions in the management of the patient with congenital heart disease they must first understand the basic anatomic defect, and be aware of and alert to the potential acute complications associated with the defect, the residual effects of surgical interventions, and any unrepaired defects. For example, failure to recognize the presence of a bicuspid aortic valve increases the risk of the patient developing endocarditis or aortic insufficiency. Similarly, if the nursing staff fails to understand that systemic hypertension may be a long-term postoperative residual finding associated with coarctation of the aorta, this sign may often remain unrecognized. As a consequence, these patients may develop signs and symptoms of heart failure or coronary artery disease (Maron et al., 1973).

Nurses also play an important role in furthering efforts at secondary prevention that must be stressed to patient and family. Nurses must be prepared independently to assess and determine the supportive and health education needs of each patient that will allow him or her to effectively assume responsibility for self care.

Although each congenital heart defect presents with its own list of actual and potential nursing problems, the primary problems observed in the critical care unit arise from the complications of dysrhythmias, cardiac failure, or endocarditis or from the Eisenmenger syndrome. Problems requiring collaborative nursing interventions are listed in Table 19–10. In addition, many of these patients lack a clear understanding of their clinical problem and need for follow-up care. Frequently, adolescents and adults with congenital heart disease are found to be misinformed about their defect and about appropriate activity allowances and limitations. As a result, they may be either inappropriately limited or engaging in strenuous isometric types of activities. For example, patients with a residual postoperative gradient, such as those with aortic stenosis or coarctation of the aorta, may be engaging in activities that require

---

TABLE 19–10. Collaborative and Independent Nursing Diagnoses for Adults with Congenital Heart Disease

Nursing Diagnosis

1. Decreased cardiac output related to mechanical factors (preload, afterload), contractility, or electrical factors (rate, rhythm, conduction)
2. Alteration in fluid volume, excess, related to increased levels of aldosterone sodium retention
3. Activity intolerance related to diminished cardiac reserve versus increased pulmonary vascular resistance

heavy lifting or participating in competitive sports. Emotionally, the level of individual adjustment may vary greatly. In the adult, the psychological consequences of having congenital heart disease may reflect several factors. Among these factors are the complexity of the primary defect, the surgical repair performed, the age at which repair was undertaken, and the physical restrictions imposed upon the individual throughout childhood. The emotional and behavioral reactions of the family also play an important role in the ability of the patient to accept and deal with the consequences of congenital heart disease. Often, in an understandable attempt to protect their young child, parents have been overprotective and may have imposed unnecessarily severe restrictions on physical and social activities. Specific nursing diagnoses for these problems and the appropriate interventions are summarized in the nursing care plan.

ncp nursing care plan

1. Anxiety related to:
Actual or perceived threat to biologic integrity

Outcome Criteria	Nursing Interventions
Patient will exhibit decrease in anxiety level	Assess level of anxiety, noting both verbal and nonverbal expressions; determine primary cause to identify any misconceptions or fears regarding condition. Elicit questions or concerns Probe for and encourage questions, allowing time for expression of feelings; work and assist patient to identify source(s) of anxiety Assess usual coping mechanisms for dealing with stressful events in order to determine if adequate to control anxiety Assist patient to deal realistically with feelings of anxiety, providing alternative methods for dealing with anxiety such as deep breathing techniques, guided imagery, stress relaxation Provide, clarify, and validate information relative to the defect, the clinical condition, and the prognosis Provide positive reinforcement about prognosis. Assist patient in attaining realistic goals and life style Make appropriate referrals for short- or long-term counseling as indicated by anxiety level

2. Ineffective/compromised individual coping:
actual or potential

Outcome Criteria	Nursing Interventions
Patient will exhibit appropriate coping mechanisms	Assess patient's perception of condition; identify any misconceptions, associated guilt, fears; explore history for inappropriate overprotective nature Determine degree of emotional and financial stress placed on patient or family by the patient's condition Assist patient to make use of appropriate support services (e.g., social services, vocational training, counseling, or support groups) Acknowledge and encourage verbalization of feelings; include family in discussions when possible

3. Knowledge deficit

Outcome Criteria	Nursing Interventions

Patient will demonstrate an increased knowledge and understanding regarding disease process	Assess level of understanding to identify any misconceptions regarding defect, allowances, and limitations
	Develop a comprehensive plan that includes any of the following as indicated:
	1. Description of primary defect; provide detailed explanation of defect and any surgical interventions that have taken place
	2. Discuss patient's current functional status, reviewing allowances and limitations as indicated by defect and clinical status
	3. Discuss the importance of need for endocarditis prophylaxis as indicated by defect (see Table 19–8)
	Review level of understanding regarding the following quality of life issues:
	  1. Childbearing; risk of genetic transmission
	  2. For women: contraception, pregnancy
	  3. Insurability
	  4. Employability
	Review any dietary restrictions and medications
	Discuss importance of regular or periodic follow-up

SUMMARY

The foregoing discussion has focused on specific issues that influence the long-term survival of adults with congenital heart disease. Although the majority of patients do well, there is an increasing awareness that many patients will develop late residual effects from an earlier surgical experience. Consequently, the critical care nurse must be able not only to recognize the most commonly occurring problems but also have an understanding of their etiology to provide appropriate care and management.

References

American Heart Association. (1988a). *Heart facts.* Dallas: American Heart Association.

American Heart Association. (1988b). *Report of the second natural history study of congenital heart defects: A 20-year follow-up* (61st Scientific Session). Washington, D. C.: AHA.

Arciniegas, E., Farooki, Z. Q., Hakimi, M., et al. (1982). Classic shunting operations for congenital cyanotic heart defects. *Journal of Thoracic and Cardiovascular Surgery, 84,* 88–96.

Baer, P., Freedman, D. A., and Garson, A. (1984). Long-term psychological follow-up of patients after corrective surgery for tetralogy of Fallot. *Journal of American Academy of Child Psychiatry, 23,* 622–625.

Bharati, S., and Levi, M. (1983). The myocardium, the conduction system and general sequelae after surgery for congenital heart. In M. A. Engle, and J. K. Perloff (Eds.), *Congenital heart disease after surgery* (pp. 247–260). New York: Yorke Medical Books.

Borow, K. M., and Braunwald, E. (1988). Congenital heart disease in the adult. In E. Braunwald (Ed.), *Heart disease: A textbook of cardiovascular medicine* (3rd ed., pp. 976–1008). Philadelphia: W. B. Saunders.

Canobbio, M. M. (1984). The Eisenmenger syndrome. *Nursing Clinics of North America, 19,* 537–554.

Canobbio, M. M. (1987). Counseling the adult with congenital heart disease. In W. C. Roberts (Ed.), *Adult congenital heart disease* (2nd ed., pp. 733–739). Philadelphia: F. A. Davis.

Canobbio, M. M. (1990). *Cardiovascular disorders* (Mosby's Clinical Series). St. Louis: C. V. Mosby.

Cooley, D. A. (1988). Palliative surgery for cyanotic congenital heart disease. *Surgical Clinics of North America, 68,* 477–474.

Dajani, A. S., Bisno, A. L., Chung, K. J., et al. (1990). Prevention of bacterial endocarditis: Recommendations by the American Heart Association. *Journal of the American Medical Association, 264,* 2919–2922.

Danielson, G. K., McGoon, D. (1987). Surgical therapy and results. In W. C. Roberts (Ed.), *Adult congenital heart disease* (2nd ed., pp. 695–715). Philadelphia: F. A. Davis.

Ebert, P. A., Turley, K., and Stanger, P. (1983). Surgery for cyanotic heart disease in the first year of life. *Journal of American College of Cardiology, 1,* 274–277.

Ebert, P. A., Turley, K., Stanger, P., et al. (1984). Surgical treatment of truncus arteriosus in the first 6 months of life. *Annals of Surgery, 200,* 451–454.

Ferguson, T. R., Suping, H., Bland, G., et al. (1986). Four adults with Ebstein's anomaly. *Illinois Medical Journal, 170,* 137–140.

Fontan, F., and Baudet, E. (1971). Surgical repair of tricuspid atresia. *Thorax, 26,* 241–248.

Friedman, W. F. (1988). Congenital heart disease in infancy and childhood. In E. Braunwald (Ed.), *Heart disease: A textbook of cardiovascular medicine* (3rd ed., pp. 896–975). Philadelphia: W. B. Saunders.

Fuster, V., McGoon, D. C., Kennedy, M. A., et al. (1980). Longterm evaluation (12–20 years) of open heart surgery for tetralogy of Fallot. *American Journal of Cardiology, 80,* 635–642.

Glasner, D., and Bentovim, A. (1987). Psychological aspects of congenital heart disease. In R. H. Anderson, Macartney, F. J., Shinbone, E., et al. (Eds.), *Paediatric cardiology* (pp. 1373–1383). London: Churchill-Livingstone.

Goldstein, J. L., and Brown, M. S. (1988). Genetics and cardiovascular disease. In E. Braunwald (Ed.), *Heart disease: A textbook of cardiovascular medicine* (3rd ed., pp. 1617–1649). Philadelphia: W. B. Saunders.

Graham, T. P. (1987). The Eisenmenger reaction and its management. In W. C. Roberts (Ed.), *Adult congenital heart disease* (2nd ed., pp. 567–581). Philadelphia: F. A. Davis.

Henson, D. E., Najafi, R., Callaghan, R., et al. (1969). Myocardial lesions following open-heart surgery. *Archives of Pathology, 88,* 423–430.

Humes, R. A., Mair, D. D., Poster, C. B., et al. (1988). Results of the modified Fontan operation in adults. *American Journal of Cardiology, 61,* 602–604.

Kawabori, I. (1978). Cyanotic congenital heart defects with increased pulmonary blood flow. *Pediatric Clinics of North America, 25,* 777–795.

Kirklin, J. W., Blackstone, E. H., Dirkin, J. K., et al. (1983). Surgical results and protocols in the spectrum of tetralogy of Fallot. *Annals of Surgery, 198,* 251–265.

Laks, H., Millikan, J. C., Perloff, J. K., et al. (1984). Experience with the Fontan procedure. *Journal of Thoracic and Cardiovascular Surgery, 88,* 939–951.

Laks, H., Hellenbrand, W. E., Stansel, H. C., et al. (1980). Repair of complex congenital cardiac defects with the valved conduits. *Surgical Clinics of North America, 60,* 1225–1237.

Mair, D. D., Rice, M. J., Hagler, D. J., et al. (1985). Outcome of the Fontan procedure in patients with tricuspid atresia. *Circulation, 72,* Suppl. II-88–92.

Maron, B. J., Humphries, H. O., Rowe, R. D., et al. (1973). Prognosis of surgically corrected coarctation of the aorta. A 20-year post-operative appraisal. *Circulation, 47,* 19.

McNamara, D. G., and Latson, L. A. (1982). Long-term follow-up of patients with malformations for which definitive surgical repair has been available for 25 years or more. *American Journal of Cardiology, 50,* 560.

Morgan, B. C. (1978). Incidence, etiology, and classification of congenital heart disease. *Pediatric Clinics of North America, 26,* 721–700.

Noonan, J. A. (1978). Association of congenital heart diseases with syndromes or other defects. *Pediatric Clinics of North America, 25,* 797.

Noonan, J. A. (1981). Syndromes associated with cardiac defects. *Cardiovascular Clinics, 11,* 97.

Nora, J. J., and Nora, A. H. (1978). The evolution of specific genetic and environmental counseling in congenital heart disease. *Circulation, 57,* 205–213.

Pacifico, A. D., and Sand, M. E. (1987). Advances in the surgical management of congenital heart disease in infants and children. In D. C. McGoon (Ed.), *Cardiac surgery* (2nd ed., pp. 177–219). Philadelphia: F. A. Davis.

Perloff, J. K. (1973). The pediatric congenital cardiac patient becomes a post-operative adult. *Circulation, 47,* 606–619.

Perloff, J. K. (1987). *The clinical recognition of congenital heart disease* (3rd ed.). Philadelphia: W. B. Saunders.

Perloff, J. K., Rosove, M. H., Child, J. S., et al. (1988). Adults with congenital heart disease: Hematologic management. *Annals of Internal Medicine, 5,* 406–413.

Roberts, W. C. (1970). The congenitally abnormal bicuspid aortic valve—a study of 85 autopsy cases. *American Journal of Cardiology, 26,* 72.

Rosove, M. H., Perloff, J. K., Hocking, W. G., et al. (1986). Chronic hypoxemia and decompensated erythrocytosis in cyanotic congenital heart disease. *Lancet, 2,* 313–315.

Rudolph, A. M., Nadas, A. S., Borges, W. H. (1953). Hematologic adjustment to cyanotic congenital heart disease. *Pediatrics, 11,* 454–464.

Shachar, G., Fuhrman, B. P., Wang, Y., et al. (1982). Rest and exercise hemodynamics after the Fontan procedure. *Circulation, 65,* 1043–1048.

Schaff, H. V., Danielson, G. K. (1987). Advances in surgical management of congenital heart disease in adults. In D. C. McGoon (Ed.), *Cardiac Surgery* (2nd ed., pp. 221–238). Philadelphia: F. A. Davis.

Sloss, L. J., and Ellison, R. C. (1987). Electrocardiographic features. In W. C. Roberts (Ed.), *Adult congenital heart disease* (2nd ed., pp. 167–189). Philadelphia: F. A. Davis.

Talner, N. S. (1983). Heart failure. In F. H. Adams, and G. C. Emmanouilides (Eds.), *Heart disease in infants, children and adolescents.* Baltimore: Williams & Wilkins.

von Bermuth, G., Ritter, D. G., Frye, R. L., et al. (1971). Evaluation of patients with tetralogy of Fallot and Potts anastomosis. *American Journal of Cardiology, 27,* 259–263.

Wood, P. (1958). The Eisenmenger syndrome. *British Heart Journal,* 2, 701.

Young, D., and Marks, H. (1971). Fate of the patient with Eisenmenger syndrome. *American Journal of Cardiology, 28,* 658–669.

Zuberbuhler, J. R. (1983). Symposium on results of the Mustard operation for complete transposition of the great arteries. *American Journal of Cardiology, 51,* 1513–1535.

20

Patients Undergoing Cardiac Surgery

Bernice Coleman
Mary Coughlan Lavieri
Stacey Gross

Surgical treatment for coronary heart disease and valvular disease continues to provide a significant challenge to nurses in the management of these patients. This chapter on cardiac surgical interventions reviews coronary revascularization, valvular disease, cardiopulmonary bypass conduct, myocardial preservation, surgical conduct, and operative correlations of postoperative common problems and presents a common nursing care plan.

The content is presented with a focus upon the current data in these areas. It is hoped that these data will provide nurses with the needed facts to better plan for the "whys" of practice. Likewise, as advances in various areas occur, critical care nurses can appreciate how these innovations can affect the way patients present during the postoperative period and devise the plan of care accordingly.

CORONARY ARTERY BYPASS GRAFT SURGERY

Cardiovascular disease accounts for 45% of all deaths in the United States (American Heart Association, 1991). The prevalence of coronary heart disease (CHD) is alarming, afflicting over 6 million Americans. Coronary heart disease represents the number one cause of death, claiming over 511,050 lives each year. Researchers estimate that this year as many as 1.5 million people will suffer an acute myocardial infarction, and more than one-third will die. Consequently, intensive research efforts have focused not only on identification of the causes and

contributing factors of CHD but also on the best methods of combatting this disease in terms of both prevention and treatment.

During the last decade, a rapid upsurge in technologic and scientific investigations have produced an array of choices for treating the patient with severe coronary atherosclerosis. Coronary revascularization procedures have been redefined to reflect both interventional and surgical approaches. Strides gained in interventional procedures such as percutaneous transluminal coronary angioplasty (PTCA) have provided added versatility in treatment options. At the same time, clinicians are working vigorously to clarify and define which patients will reap the most benefit from each interventional or surgical approach to coronary revascularization.

Surgical revascularization in the form of coronary artery bypass grafting (CABG) remains in the forefront of treatment of coronary heart disease. Approximately 353,000 CABG operations are performed annually in the United States (American Heart Association, 1991). Within the last 3 decades more than 1 million patients have had bypass procedures. Seventy-six per cent of these operations were performed on men, comprising approximately 270,000 men compared with 83,000 women. Fifty per cent of the patients were under the age of 65. Cost expenditure estimates reveal that approximately 6 to 7 billion dollars are spent annually in the treatment of heart disease measured just in direct care services alone (nurse/physician services).

The rationale for performing surgical revascularization or aortocoronary bypass grafting is to restore adequate blood flow or blood supply and to provide nutritional support to the myocardial tissue. A harvested vessel (conduit) is anastomosed between the aortic root and a point distal to the obstructing coronary lesion or stenosis. The restoration of myocardial perfusion aids in preventing further ischemia and in salvaging viable muscle mass and ventricular function.

Historically, the first surgical approach to indirect myocardial revascularization was developed by Vineberg in 1946 (Vineberg, 1946). This technique involved implantation of the internal mammary artery into the myocardial wall in an attempt to facilitate coronary flow through growth of a vascular network. Limited technology affected the ability to evaluate the results of the initial surgical trials. The advent of extracorporeal circulation and selective coronary arteriography in the 1950s and 1960s ignited renewed interest and investigation into the feasibility of performing direct revascularization procedures (Sones and Shirey, 1962). Reports of varied surgical revascularization attempts emerged during the next decade. In 1968, surgical teams led by Dr. Johnson (Milwaukee) and by Drs. Favalaro and Effler (Cleveland) performed the first successful aortocoronary bypass graft procedures using a reversed saphenous vein as the graft material (Favalaro, 1969; Johnson et al., 1969). By 1972, improvements in extracorporeal circulation and cardioplegic techniques made aortocoronary saphenous bypass graft procedures a common method of revascularization.

Indications for Myocardial Revascularization

During the last decade, a number of multicenter clinical investigations have focused attention on patient selection criteria for surgical myocardial revascularization (Table 20–1). Due to the immense cost and large number of CABGs performed each year this operation has become the most studied surgical procedure. In 1980 a task force was established to examine management strategies used for patients

---

TABLE 20–1. Indications for Coronary Artery Bypass Grafting

Chronic stable angina refractory to medical therapy
Significant left main coronary occlusion (>50%)
Triple vessel coronary artery disease
  Left ventricular dysfunction
  Proximal left anterior descending disease (as part of two-vessel disease)
Unstable angina pectoris
Acute myocardial infarction
  Emergent
  Delayed
Intractable ventricular irritability
Left ventricular failure
  Congestive heart failure
  Cardiogenic shock
Percutaneous transluminal coronary angioplasty failure

---

with cardiovascular disease. In March of 1991, as a result of a joint effort of the American College of Cardiology and the American Heart Association, guidelines were released illustrating the recommended indications for CABG (Kirklin et al., 1991). These guidelines represent a framework around which to establish standards for practice and on which to base treatment decisions. The guidelines address which patient populations would obtain the most benefit in terms of relief of angina, survival, and quality of life following CABG. Patients were classified according to severity of disease and, in particular, the most appropriate therapy. With more research emerging regarding revascularization techniques, the question now becomes which mode (interventional versus surgical) will afford the most positive cost-benefit ratio. Consequently, two ongoing trials, the Bypass Angioplasty Revascularization Investigation (BARI) and the Emory Angioplasty/Surgery Trial (EAST), are seeking to examine and compare the differences between CABG and PTCA for selected patients with multivessel coronary artery disease (CAD). Enrollment in the BARI trial ended in July of 1991 with the accumulation of approximately 2400 patients. Follow-up will continue at specified points during a 5-year period. Comparisons among the groups will be analyzed. Evaluation criteria will focus upon left ventricular function, angiographic findings, exercise capacity, return of angina, quality of life, and crossover to CABG. Other investigations, such as the Randomized Interventional Treatment of Angina (RITA) in the United Kingdom, the Coronary Angioplasty versus Bypass Revascularization Investigation (CABRI) in Western Europe, and the German Angioplasty versus Bypass Investigation are being conducted to compare angioplasty to surgery. When the results of these and other trials become available, more conclusive recommendations can be made regarding patient selection and therapeutic choices. Until these data become available, the decision to perform either procedure is based upon clinical findings and patient preference.

At present, chronic angina, left main coronary disease, and acute myocardial infarction are the prime indications for surgical intervention. An increasing number of patients also are referred following failed PTCA. The most significant clinical benefit is derived from relief of symptoms. Conclusive findings reported by several authors demonstrate the effectiveness of CABG in reducing the frequency and severity of anginal pain in 75% to 90% of patients (Braunwald, 1983). Improved survival and longevity have been observed with surgical therapy in patients with left main coronary disease, triple vessel disease, and left ventricular dysfunction. Compared with medical therapy alone, surgery has been found to prolong survival in patients with the greatest risk inclusive of poor ventricular function (Killip et al., 1985). Eight-year survival rates approximate 79% in patients with three-vessel disease compared to 82% in patients with two-vessel disease.

The decision to perform CABG is based upon several factors, foremost among them being the alleviation of symptoms and improved survival. An extensive evaluation of the patient's condition is conducted based upon the history, symptomatology, and results of coronary arteriography. Some centers also include echocardiography and exercise tolerance testing as components in the diagnostic process. Current controversy over the prognostic value and reliability of exercise testing in women has resulted in limited application of this component in potential surgical candidates. The clinical conditions warranting surgical intervention are reviewed here based on current recommendations.

Chronic Stable Angina Pectoris. Chronic angina pectoris that is unresponsive to medical therapy represents the most widely accepted indication for myocardial revascularization. Stable angina is generally characterized as angina occurring with minimal change in frequency, duration, or severity of symptoms. Stable angina categorized as class I to class II occurs in symptomatic patients who have a varying degree or extent of coronary involvement and ventricular dysfunction. Class III to class IV angina is found in patients who are symptomatic and have one or more severe proximal stenoses and clearly demonstrate a poor response to medical therapy. Patients in the latter functional category warrant definitive revascularization. Factors such as disability resulting from anginal symptoms, adverse side effects from medications, and noncompliance with medical treatment justify consideration of surgical intervention in this population of patients.

Initial treatment aimed at controlling anginal pain is achieved through the use of long-acting nitrates, aspirin, beta-adrenergic blocking agents, or calcium channel blockers (Silverman and Grossman, 1984). Failure to alleviate ischemic symptoms following a course of maximum medical therapy warrants surgical consideration. Optimal timing of surgery in patients who have been initially treated medically requires scrupulous evaluation and examination of the nature of the disease process. Evidence from several sources illustrates dramatic relief of pain following surgical intervention. Operative mortality in patients with stable angina ranges from 1% to 3% (Rahimtoola, 1985).

Significant Left Main Coronary Artery Occlusion. Surgical treatment is indicated in patients with severe stenosis of the left main coronary artery. Often, stenosis located within the left main coronary is referred to as the *widow-maker* lesion. Patients with this condition receiving medical treatment alone have demonstrated a diminished prognosis and increased risk of mortality (European Coronary Surgery Study Group [ECSSG], 1982).

A narrowing of greater than 50% of the luminal diameter is considered a significant stenosis (Hurst et al., 1986). Sixty per cent of left main coronary artery lesions are associated with significant disease elsewhere in the coronary vasculature (Chaitman et al., 1981). Commonly, patients exhibit triple vessel disease during angiographic studies. Significant left main stenosis (or stenosis of the proximal left anterior descending artery [LAD]) jeopardizes a large portion of the myocardium because the vascular distribution of these vessels supplies the apex, part of the lateral wall, anterior wall, and two-thirds of the septum. Thus, these patients are at increased risk for acute anterior wall infarction and sudden death (Loop, 1983; Silverman and Grossman, 1984). Prompt surgical intervention in patients with left main disease has been shown to increase their 3-year survival rates to 85% to 90% compared with medical therapy (65% to 69%) (Rahimtoola, 1985; CASS, 1984).

Triple Vessel Coronary Artery Disease. CABG is indicated in patients with high-grade pathoanatomic lesions involving two or more vessels (Rahimtoola, 1985; ECSSG, 1982). Severe coronary artery stenosis, exceeding 70% of the luminal diameter, is classified as significant. Diseased vessels to be grafted must demonstrate adequate perfusion distal to the obstruction indicating a patent peripheral coronary bed. Poor distal flow in vessels with a luminal size of less than 1.0 to 1.5 mm in diameter increases the risk of early thrombosis and limits the feasibility of revascularization to the vessel. The evidence has consistently demonstrated improved survival following CABG in patients with two- and three-vessel disease and normal ventricular function (CASS, 1984; Killip et al., 1985; ECSSG, 1982). Findings from recent investigations have revealed that patients with impaired ventricular function (left ventricular ejection fraction [LVEF] of 16% to 30%) experience an increased survival benefit and a reduction in mortality that is attributed to surgical revascularization (Myers et al., 1989; Killip et al., 1985).

Unstable Angina Pectoris. Patients with unstable angina pectoris represent another subgroup of candidates for CABG surgery. The term unstable angina has been used to describe a number of clinical conditions such as preinfarction angina, crescendo angina, rest angina, and postinfarction angina. Manifestations of anginal pain that escalates in intensity, frequency, or duration and is unrelieved by rest or pharmacologic therapy typically characterize this syndrome. Unstable angina has been associated with a high risk of subsequent ischemic events. Among patients managed medically, approximately 21% of those with new-onset unstable angina experience a myocardial infarction within 8 months. An associated 41% mortality rate has been observed in this group (Eugene et al., 1983; Kaiser et al., 1989).

Increasing frequency and severity of chest pain, angina occurring at night or at rest, and ST-T segment changes on electrocardiography (ECG) during anginal episodes correlate with an increased risk (CASS investigators, 1984). The rationale for surgical intervention in this population is related to the high incidence of myocardial infarction and death. Significant benefit is obtained in patients with prior subendocardial damage, who frequently have a propensity to develop transmural infarctions (Kaiser et al., 1985). The CASS investigation focused on coronary care patients who experienced atypical angina that was unresponsive to pharmacologic therapy. The majority of patients required CABG. The incidence of myocardial infarction in this group (occurring 6 hours to 30 days prior to surgery) was 50%, and approximately 75% of patients were found to have extensive three-vessel disease and some degree of left ventricular dysfunction (Rankin et al., 1984). The operative mortality was 4%, approximately twice that of patients with stable angina (Kaiser et al., 1985). Increased age, left ventricular impairment, left main coronary lesions, and female gender represent the variables having a significant impact upon operative mortality (Kaiser et al., 1989).

Acute Myocardial Infarction. The role of CABG in patients with acute myocardial infarction remains a controversial issue and requires extensive examination of the cost-benefit factors. Multiple therapeutic options exist and provide versatility in the management and support of the patient experiencing an acute event. Use of pharmacologic agents (such as propranolol, nitrates, and sodium nitroprusside), thrombolytic agents, and cardiac-assist devices such as intra-aortic balloon counterpulsation (IABC) represent the various alternative treatment modalities available for patients with acute myocardial infarction. Use of tissue-type plasminogen activator (t-PA), streptokinase (SK), and acylated plasminogen-streptokinase activator complex (APSAC) in the early phases of myocardial injury have been shown to be effective in restoring coronary perfusion to the area in jeopardy (Rentrop, 1985; Geltman, 1987). The efficacy of t-PA administration in re-establishing coronary flow has been recorded as 75% to 85%; efficacy associated with SK ranges from 55% to 65% (Chesebro et al., 1987; Braunwald, 1988; TIMI II, 1989). The incidence of restenosis following these therapies is approximately 17% with both t-PA and SK. Close follow-up is vital to detect recurrent angina or ischemic symptoms warranting further intervention with PTCA or CABG.

The aim of therapy in patients with acute myocardial infarction (AMI) focuses upon interrupting the progressive ischemia and myocardial necrosis. The zone of ischemic tissue (the "twilight zone" surrounding the infarcted region) remains viable for 3 to 6 hours. Theoretically, timely performance of CABG aids in restoration of myocardial perfusion to the jeopardized region and potential salvation of viable muscle mass. Readily accessible and expedient treatment options such as thrombolytic therapy or coronary angioplasty often preclude the performance of immediate surgical revascularization. Thus, CABG is not routinely considered the first therapy of choice in acute myocardial infarction.

The question of when to intervene surgically following AMI remains debatable. Statistics during the last 5 years reveal an increasing trend toward surgery performed early after AMI (Kennedy, et al., 1989). This trend has been attributed to the expanding application of invasive interventional cardiologic techniques as well as to recognition of the potential risks associated with acute infarction. In patients who survive an acute myocardial infarction, the 1-year mortality rates are 10% to 15%; approximately 20% incur significant left ventricular damage (LVEF < 30%) leading to increased risk of death (Kay, 1982; Epstein et al., 1982). Noninvasive testing and angiographic studies are conducted to evaluate the extent of coronary disease, ventricular performance, or any resultant structural anomalies. Recommendations for PTCA or CABG are established based upon test findings and the clinical patient profile. Current guidelines advocate delaying surgery preferably 1 week after an AMI (Kennedy et al., 1989). The incidence of operative mortality is the same whether surgery is performed 8 days or 30 days following an infarction (Kennedy et al., 1989). In patients who remain free from angina or experience mild angina following a myocardial infarction, no significant differences exist in 5-year mortality figures comparing surgical with medical treatment (CASS principal investigators, 1984).

Intractable Ventricular Irritability. Recurrent ventricular irritability due to complications resulting from acute myocardial infarction represents another indication for myocardial revascularization. Left ventricular aneurysm formation following an acute infarction may be the site of electrical instability, which induces reentrant pathways for ventricular dysrhythmias. Symptomatic, persistent dysrhythmias refractory to pharmacologic therapy may increase the risk of sudden cardiac death.

Surgical intervention focuses on interrupting reentrant pathways through myocardial revascularization, myocardial resection of localized infarcted tissue, or excision of a left ventricular aneurysm. The results of such surgical procedures in treating recurrent ventricular dysrhythmias have been variable and inconsistent, with many patients continuing to demonstrate a need for either pharmacologic management with antidysrhythmic agents or placement of the automatic implantable cardioverter/defibrillator (AICD).

Left Ventricular Failure. The efficacy of CABG in the management of left ventricular failure has not been clearly substantiated. In patients with advanced congestive heart failure, the results of myocardial revascularization have been inconsistent and conflicting with regard to improvement in symptoms or survival benefits. Recent clinical studies have illustrated a positive correlation between heart failure and operative risk (Wechsler and Junod, 1989). In patients with depressed left ventricular performance, further insult from cardiopulmonary bypass, inadequate myocardial protection, perioperative infarction, or incomplete revascularization may precipitate cardiac decompensation (Wechsler and Junod, 1989). Most evidence indicates that CABG is of limited value in reversing myocardial damage or ventricular function following extensive loss of muscle mass due to an acute infarction. Patients with congestive heart failure who experience severe angina pectoris are considered candidates for surgery after evaluation of the coronary vasculature, left ventricular wall motion, and cardiac performance. Mechanical assist devices are frequently utilized in the early postoperative period to provide temporary hemodynamic support (Wechsler and Junod, 1989).

Manifestations of congestive heart failure (CHF) may be seen as a complication of acute myocardial infarction. CHF may be precipitated by an acquired ventricular septal defect, acute mitral regurgitation, or ventricular aneurysm (Kay, 1982). Rupture of the intraventricular septum occurs in 1% to 2% of patients with AMI, and survival is about 20% at 2 months following AMI without surgical repair (Kay, 1982). Development of a systolic murmur, congestive heart failure, and severe left ventricular failure warrants immediate evaluation to detect the presence of a ventricular septal defect. Interim stabilization with intra-aortic balloon counterpulsation may be required. Urgent surgical repair is indicated to close the defect, and CABG may be necessary to improve coronary blood flow.

Cardiogenic Shock. When damage from AMI encompasses more than 40% of the left ventricular muscle mass, marked left ventricular failure and cardiogenic shock ensue (Caulfield et al., 1976). Mortality rates range from 85% to 95% with medical therapy alone (Caulfield et al., 1976). Maximum support utilizing mechanical assist devices provides a temporary early means of augmenting systemic perfusion during the acute insult (O'Rourke et al., 1979). Results of CABG upon survival in patients suffering from cardiogenic shock vary. Critical determinants of operative mortality depend upon the extent of left ventricular dysfunction, myocardial damage, and remaining cardiac reserve (Phillips et al., 1983). The availability of expert, seasoned medical and surgical teams combined with appropriate mechanical support, timely diagnosis, and surgical technique has had a significant impact on decreasing the incidence of mortality.

Percutaneous Transluminal Coronary Angioplasty Failure. PTCA has emerged as a viable alternative treatment for selected patients with coronary artery disease. The increasing number of procedures performed and their growing complexity require continuous surgical support and operative backup. Complications such as coronary artery dissection (most common), complete coronary occlusion, dysrhyth-

mias, and unstable angina resulting in acute ischemia occur in 5% of cases, necessitating emergent surgical intervention (Talley et al., 1989). Careful patient selection, refinements in technique, and the use of reperfusion or "bailout" catheters has aided in limiting myocardial damage and reducing mortality (Hinohara et al., 1988). Advancement of reperfusion catheters through the angioplasty sheath beyond the site of occlusion promotes blood flow distal to the stenosis and maintains supply to the ischemic region. Further support utilizing intra-aortic balloon counterpulsation, femoral bypass, and pharmacologic agents such as intracoronary nitroglycerin have been effective in enhancing hemodynamic stability and cardiovascular function (Murphy et al., 1982).

Emergent CABG (defined in most clinical series as operative intervention within 24 hours following PTCA) carries an obvious increased risk of operative death (7% to 11%) and perioperative infarction (29% to 50%) compared to planned elective surgical revascularization (Talley et al., 1989). Initial PTCA trials involved patients with single vessel disease and normal left ventricular function. Emergent CABG undertaken in this patient population revealed little or no added increased operative mortality; the incidence of complications approached 5% in this group. Today, the selection criteria have expanded to include patients with depressed left ventricular function, increased age, left main coronary stenosis, and multivessel disease (Daily, 1989). The presence of one or more of these factors significantly influences the operative outcome, and these factors have been identified as predictors of mortality used to analyze the associated risk of emergent CABG. Complication rates in this patient population approach 28%, prolonging the length of hospital stay (Greene, 1991).

Restenosis rates associated with PTCA for single vessel disease are approximately 20% to 30%; restenosis typically presents within the first 6 months following the initial procedure (Hurst et al., 1986). In patients with multiple lesions, the restenosis rate is higher. Repeat procedures often produce successful results in 70% to 80% of patients (Daily, 1989). Patients with lesions located in the LAD, right coronary artery (RCA), or left circumflex artery (LCX); a post-PTCA translesional gradient of greater than 15 mm Hg; a residual stenosis greater than 30%; and unstable angina incur a higher risk for restenosis at the time of initial angioplasty and at repeat PTCA. Various new techniques utilizing laser balloon angioplasty, intracoronary stents, and atherectomy devices hold promise for preventing restenosis. Yet continued patency and complete revascularization in patients with extensive three-vessel disease remain problematic. Consequently, these patients eventually require surgical intervention to correct coronary hypoperfusion. Current statistics indicate that within 1 year of angioplasty, 85% to 90% of patients maintain freedom from the need to cross over to CABG. Subsequently, 81% of patients are free at 3 years, and 75% to 86% are free at 5 years (O'Keefe, 1990).

Relative Contraindications

Comprehensive patient assessment is crucial to the identification and elucidation of factors influencing the feasibility of surgical revascularization. Technical constraints imposed by anatomic anomalies create considerable problems for the surgeon. Small, narrowed, atheromatous coronary vessels (less than 1.0 to 1.5 mm in diameter) accompanied by diffuse distal disease and poor collateralization may prohibit bypass grafting. An open artery greater than 1 mm in diameter beyond the stenotic lesion must exist. Furthermore, viable myocardial tissue in the area supplied by the recipient vessel must be documented. Lack of a conduit or suitable graft material in patients with severe systemic vascular disease may inhibit revascularization attempts. Aortic root anomalies or severe aortic sclerosis can complicate proximal anastomosis construction, precipitating unsatisfactory results.

Alterations in physiologic and functional states have been used as indicators to determine the relative risk associated with surgery. Left ventricular function has been identified as a significant prognostic indicator of survival and surgical outcome (Gersh et al., 1989). Left ventricular dysfunction (LVEF < 20%) accompanied by cardiomegaly or elevated left ventricular end-diastolic volume incurs an increased risk of associated surgical mortality (Parsonnet et al., 1989). Preexisting pulmonary disease, renal insufficiency, and carotid disease represent incremental risk factors predisposing the patient to postoperative complications (Rich et al., 1988). Age as an isolated factor in itself has not been identified as a significant prognostic indicator (Rich et al., 1988), but a consensus exists that patients over 70 years of age carry a higher risk (Parsonnet et al., 1989). Several reports from septuagenarian and octogenarian studies cite factors such as low body weight, prolonged bypass time, and need for repeated operations as contributing to an increased risk of perioperative complications (Rich et al., 1988).

Selection of Conduits

The saphenous vein and the internal mammary artery (commonly referred to as the internal thoracic artery) are the most commonly used conduits today for myocardial revascularization. Both vessels have been employed successfully, alone or in combination, when multiple bypasses are needed.

The greater saphenous vein, located anterior to the medial malleolus, travels upward to join the common femoral vein at the groin. Exposure of the vessel is accomplished through a continuous incision starting at the ankle. Utilization of the saphenous vein segment below the knee is preferred because of its closer approximation in size (4 to 5 mm in diameter) to that of the coronary arteries. Generally, 15- to 20-cm vein

segments are harvested for each graft. Once the vein has been excised, the tributaries arc ligated. Injection of a heparinized plasmolytic or saline solution gently distends the graft segment to detect the presence of any leaks in the vessel. Extreme care is exercised in handling the vein graft material. Excessive manipulation may result in vasospasm or intimal damage, activating a potential thrombotic process that has been implicated in early graft closure (Baumann, 1981). Prior to aortic anastomosis, vein graft material is placed in a reverse direction to prevent venous valves from impeding the flow of coronary blood. The leg incision is irrigated with antibiotic solution and closed with running nylon or subcuticular sutures (Fig. 20–1).

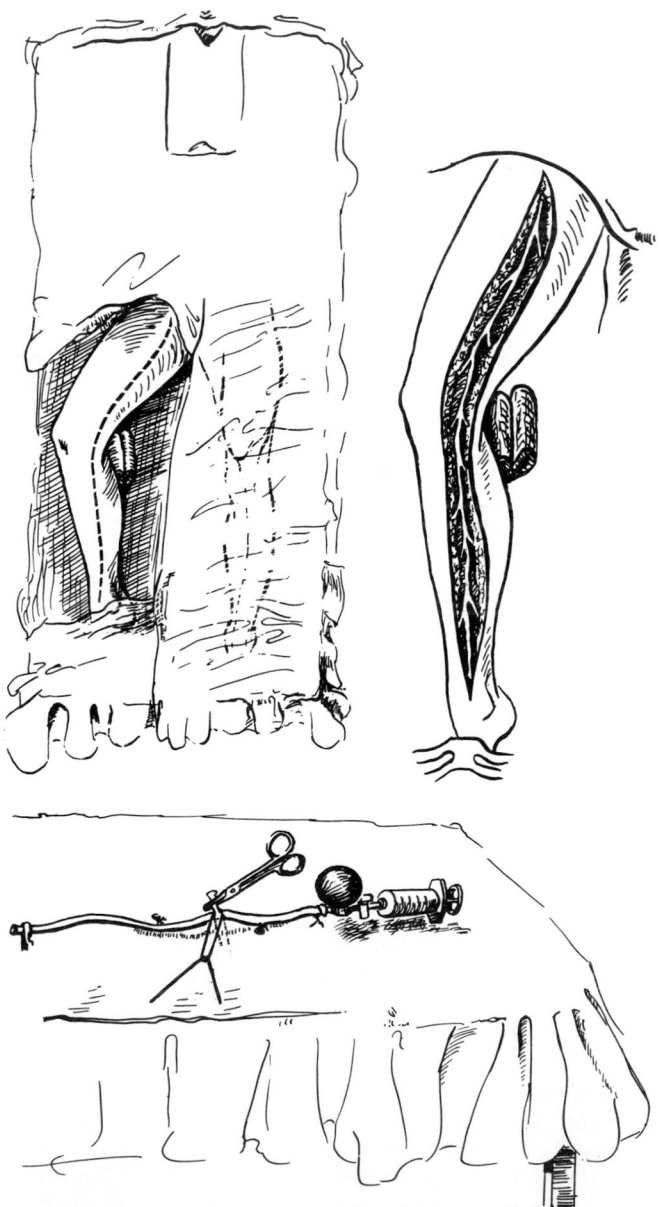

FIGURE 20–1. Harvesting the saphenous vein. (From Dillard, D. H., and Miller, D. W. (1983). *Atlas of cardiac surgery* (Plate XXXI, p. 81). New York: Macmillan.)

The patency rate for saphenous vein grafts at 1 year is 98% but at 10 years falls to 81% (Loop et al., 1986). Use of the saphenous vein graft offers several advantages such as technical ease and flexibility and less time required to dissect and harvest the vessel, both of which aid in decreasing bypass and operative time. Satisfactory flow rates have been demonstrated with the saphenous vein graft due to the lower resistance and large diameter characteristic of venous vessels. Because the saphenous vein is an accessory vein, circulation in the lower extremity is not usually interrupted because of its removal. In patients with preexisting deep venous obstructions, impaired circulation resulting in edema has been found to occur.

The internal mammary artery (IMA) has emerged as the conduit of choice for bypass of the left anterior descending coronary artery (Loop et al., 1986). The internal mammary artery arises from the subclavian artery as the second branch. Located 1 to 2 cm lateral to the sternal border, it descends inferiorly through the diaphragm to become the superior epigastric artery. The IMA, used as a pedicle bypass graft, is left attached proximally to the subclavian artery and is transsected distally for anastomosis to the recipient coronary artery. Due to its diminished diameter below the sixth intercostal space, use of the IMA is limited to bypass of anterior coronary vessels such as the proximal LAD, proximal diagonal, or marginal vessels. The longer length and diameter of the left IMA compared to the right IMA provide increased versatility for bypassing obstructed coronary vessels (Fig. 20–2).

Applications of the IMA have expanded to include use as a free graft. Some authors report increased technical difficulty, inconsistent flow rates, and a propensity for vasospasm as problems associated with use of the IMA as a free graft (Green, 1989). More recent experiences with free grafts have led to improved results and lower attrition rates (Green, 1989). Bilateral grafting offers additional options for patients with poor quality lower extremity vessels or calcific lesions. Use of both internal mammary arteries in younger patients enhances revascularization results, increasing graft longevity and survival (Green, 1989). In women, use of the IMA is particularly advantagous due to the prevalence of small primary vessels (Loop et al., 1989). Some controversy accompanies the use of the IMA in elderly women. However, limited availability of conduits may make the IMA the best choice.

The IMA has demonstrated excellent long-term patency rates approaching 96% at 10 years (Loop et al., 1986). Efforts to explain the increased longevity and durability of the IMA graft have focused on increased prostacyclin synthesis and vasoactive properties inherent within the arterial lumen wall (Chaikhouni et al., 1986). Progression of atherosclerotic disease and subintimal changes appear to be inhibited. The absence of valves minimizes luminal turbulence, reducing the risk of thrombosis and occlusion. Angiographic evaluation has documented

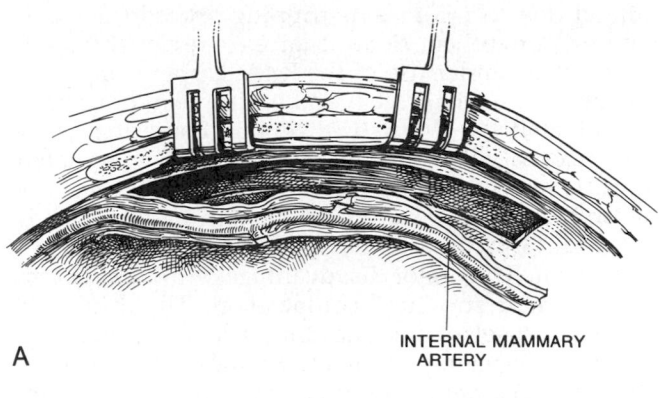

A

INTERNAL MAMMARY
ARTERY

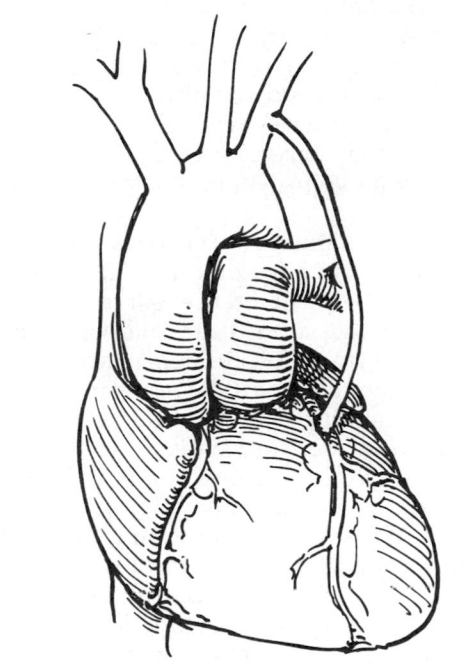

B

FIGURE 20–2. *A*, Dissection of the left internal mammary artery from left sternal wall and surrounding tissue. Use of retractors facilitates optimum visualization. *B*, Aortocoronary bypass of left internal mammary artery to left anterior descending artery. (From Waldhausen, J. A., and Pierce, W. S. (1985). *Surgery of the chest* (5th ed., p. 481). Chicago: Year Book Medical Publishers.)

the ability of the IMA to enlarge in response to increased demand. Flow rates of IMA grafts have been demonstrated to be equivalent to its vein graft counterpart (Green, 1989).

Some of the limitations associated with IMA grafts include the increased operative time needed for retrosternal dissection, bleeding, postoperative chest wall discomfort, and technical difficulties (Jansen and McFadden, 1986). The incidence of postoperative bleeding can be minimized with careful inspection prior to chest closure. Circumstances precluding use of the IMA may occur in patients with a prior mastectomy, a history of chest wall radiation, brachiocephalic disease, or emergent revascularization for myocardial instability (Loop et al., 1989).

Alternative Venous and Arterial Conduits. In some patients the number of available grafts may be limited due to prior vein stripping procedures, varicosities, or other circumstances previously mentioned that hinder use of the IMA. Upper arm veins, namely, the cephalic vein and basilic vein, have been investigated as alternative venous conduits. Location, accessibility, and length of vessels were noted advantages. Compared to the saphenous vein, the internal diameter of the cephalic and basilic veins is less than 3.5 cm, slightly less than optimal for implantation. The major disadvantage of the upper arm veins is their structural composition. The thin walls of these vessels make anastomotic construction and suturing extremely difficult. Studies have demonstrated poor patency rates. Occlusions were evident in 42% to 47% of patients at 2 years. Basilic and cephalic veins appear to develop significant intimal changes by the second or third postoperative year. Other findings indicate a high rate of aneurysm formation within these vessels. Thus, the use of upper extremity veins has not proved to be a reliable alternative.

The internal mammary vein (IMV) represents another potential venous conduit. Clinical experience to date is limited, but French surgeons report that IMV characteristics are similar to those of the saphenous vein in terms of resiliency and size. Initial reports indicate that the IMV appears to be suitable as a venous conduit (Stephan et al., 1990). The IMV is dissected and prepared similarly to the saphenous vein graft. Reports of use of the radial artery as an arterial conduit for coronary bypass grafting emerged in the early 1970s (Foster and Kranc, 1989). On initial evaluation, properties similar to those of the internal mammary were apparent. Luminal size equivalent to that of the coronary vessels, long length, superficial position, and ease of removal represented qualities inherent in a good conduit. However, initial trials using free radial artery grafts revealed significant graft occlusion within 1 year (Foster and Kranc, 1989). A majority of the grafts were found to be completely occluded and stenosed upon repeat angiography. Subsequent studies demonstrated disappointing results, rendering use of the radial artery unsuitable for CABG procedures.

While some researchers examined use of the radial artery, other investigators focused on the feasibility of the splenic artery for myocardial revascularization procedures. The splenic artery as a pedicled artery graft was thought to possess physiologic features similar to that of the IMA. Initial experiences yielded satisfactory results in terms of graft patency. However, preparation and harvesting of this vessel imposed great difficulty, requiring rerouting of the splenic artery from the abdomen through the diaphragm (Foster and Kranc, 1989). A splenectomy was performed concomitantly. Problems with kinking, size, and atherosclerotic lesions precluded continued use of the splenic artery.

Recent attention has focused on use of the right gastroepiploic artery (RGEA) in coronary artery bypass grafting (Mills and Everson, 1989; Suma et al.,

1989; Lytle et al., 1987). The right gastroepiploic artery has been used both as a pedicle graft and as a free graft (Lytle et al., 1987). The RGEA, originating from the anterior superior pancreaticoduodenal artery (Fig. 20–3) is routed upward through the diaphragm to the recipient coronary artery. Initial investigations have yielded mixed results. Because the RGEA is part of an arterial system, researchers have suggested that it may possess physiologic characteristics of increased longevity and patency similar to those of the IMA. The RGEA has been used in patients who have poor quality or absent saphenous veins, diabetes mellitus, or aortic sclerosis (Mills and Everson, 1989). The main disadvantage associated with the RGEA is its entrance into the abdominal cavity, which has significant implications if future abdominal surgery is necessary. Due to the lack of experience with RGEA grafts, information about flow rates and long-term patency remains to be determined. Initial data at 3 months reveal 93% patency

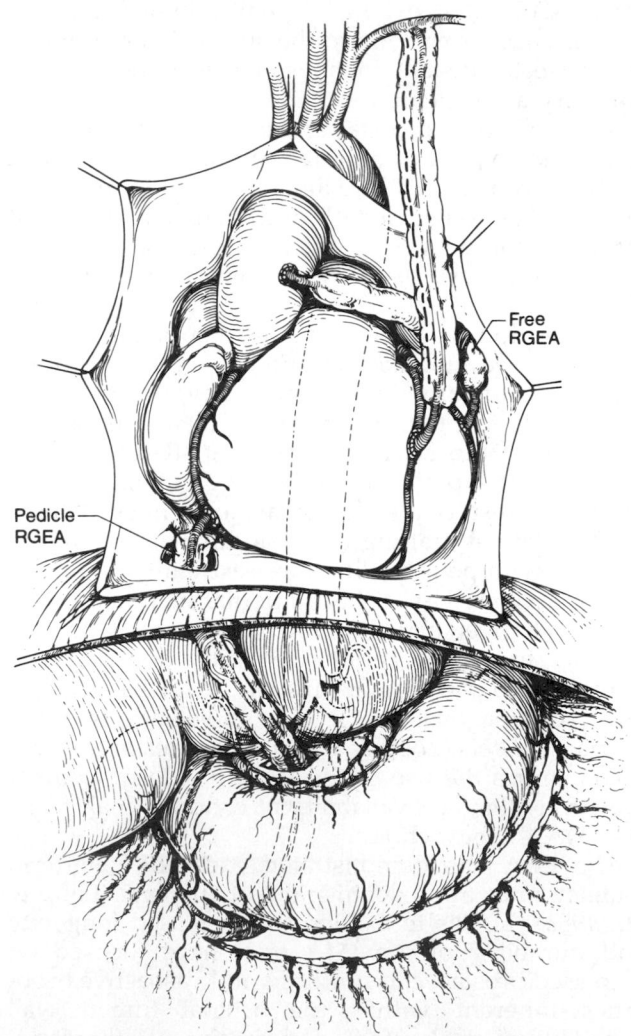

FIGURE 20–3. Right gastroepiploic artery (RGEA) graft to right coronary artery. The RGEA is passed behind the stomach, over the liver, and through the pericardium. (Reprinted with permission from The Society of Thoracic Surgeons, THE ANNALS OF THORACIC SURGERY, Vol 47, 1989, p. 710.)

rates compared to 95% patency rates with IMA grafts (Suma et al., 1989). Further research continues, and other investigators have pursued use of the inferior epigastric artery (IEA) as a potential arterial conduit (Puig et al., 1990). The IEA, originating from the external iliac artery, possesses histologic features similar to those of the IMA. Results with IEA grafts are limited but display promise as clinicians explore other sources of viable conduits.

There have been a few reports regarding the use of synthetic graft material for myocardial revascularization. Polytetrafluoroethylene (PTFE, or Gore-Tex) has been used in most investigations as the graft material. Graft occlusion represents a significant limitation. Two-year patency rates approach only 32% (Foster and Kranc, 1989). Despite the limited experience and exposure, poor results have not provided the clinical application of synthetic grafts.

Results

The results of CABG have been subject to scrutinization by the general public and health care professionals alike. Controversy fuels the debate over the "need" for the vast number of surgical procedures currently being performed. Questions posed address the efficacy of CABG surgery on survival, relief of symptoms, and quality of life. Current research efforts have now refocused upon the comparative outcomes of medical and surgical therapy and on risk factor stratification. Results from several large-scale observational investigations have illustrated the relatively low mortality rates, increased survival, longevity, and improved quality of life associated with coronary artery bypass surgery (Califf et al., 1989).

Operative Mortality. Wide variation exists in reports of operative mortality for patients undergoing CABG. Overall, mortality rates equal 2.7% (with a range of 0.5% to 11%) (Gersh et al., 1989). A changing patient profile accounts for these variations. Despite the increasing severity in patient condition and the complexity of procedure, operative mortality figures have remained relatively stable in recent years. This current trend reflects improvements in surgical technique, perioperative management, myocardial protection, and cardiopulmonary bypass.

Multiple factors influence the surgical outcome. The most significant prognostic indicator of operative mortality in patients with chronic stable angina is left ventricular function (Gersh et al., 1989). Risk of operative mortality has been found to be inversely proportional to left ventricular function. Patients with mild left ventricular dysfunction (LVEF > 50%), moderate left ventricular dysfunction (LVEF = 30% to 50%), and severe left ventricular dysfunction (LVEF < 30%) incur a risk of operative mortality approximating 1.5%, 3.8%, and 6.1%, respectively (Gersh et al., 1989). Operative mortality rates double in patients with unstable angina compared to those with stable angina. Figures range from 1.2% to 8.5% (Kaiser et al., 1989). Attempts to isolate definitive predictors of mortality for patients with unstable angina have been unsuccessful.

Patients undergoing CABG for treatment of recent myocardial infarction incur an increased risk of operative death. The time interval between the acute event and surgery is a significant factor. Patients operated on within 1 week of the event have been found to have the highest mortality (Kennedy et al., 1989). Advanced age, female gender, presence of left main coronary artery disease, and need for emergent operation have been identified as preoperative factors contributing to an increased risk of operative mortality (Kennedy et al., 1989).

Late Survival. Increased longevity and survival is one of the most significant benefits derived from coronary bypass graft surgery (Califf et al., 1989). Approximately 90% of patients are alive 5 years following surgery, and 80% survive 10 years (Kirklin et al., 1989). Comparatively, statistics for patients treated medically reveal an 80% 5-year and a 65% 10-year survival rate (Califf et al., 1989).

Impressive findings from several large-scale studies have helped to provide concrete evidence about the survival benefits of CABG. Many studies focus on survival statistics in certain patient subsets. Previous research has documented improved survival following surgery in patients with left main coronary disease and three-vessel disease with impaired left ventricular function (Takaro et al., 1976; Killip et al., 1985). Duke University investigators reported that this survival benefit extends even to patients considered high risk. In particular, older patients and those with poor left ventricular function or severe angina were found to exhibit the greatest improvement in survival benefits (Califf et al., 1989). The degree of survival benefit correlated proportionally with the severity of symptoms and the presence of a greater number of adverse prognostic indicators. Overall mortality was reduced in patients who were at highest risk for sudden death. Other studies have also noted improved survival benefits in some patients with normal left ventricular function and those with two proximal coronary artery stenoses (Meyers et al., 1989).

Consistent findings indicate that the year in which the operation was performed affects survival (Teoh et al., 1987; Califf et al., 1989). Progressive improvements in surgical results are related to advances in cardiopulmonary bypass procedures, surgical techniques, and perioperative management. Consequently, increased survival benefits have been extended to patients with more complex underlying pathologies.

Incomplete revascularization influences late survival (Loop, 1983). The number of ungrafted diseased vessels increases the risk of developing future ischemic events. Complete revascularization of all major areas with significant stenoses affords the greatest relief of symptoms and improved survival.

Relief of Angina. Relief of angina pectoris gained following CABG clearly represents the outcome of greatest magnitude for patients. In both patient subsets of chronic stable angina and unstable angina, dramatic improvement in chest pain has been noted both subjectively and from graded exercise testing (Kirklin et al., 1989; Kaiser et al., 1989). Nearly, 80% to 90% of CABG patients experience complete relief of symptoms (Kirklin et al., 1989; Kaiser et al., 1989). Consequently, this finding has a significant impact upon the patient's quality of life and return to work. Freedom from disabling anginal symptoms affords patients the opportunity to engage in a more productive life style. As time progresses, the beneficial effects of coronary artery bypass surgery diminish. A lack of consensus is evident among reports of recurrence of symptoms. Seventy to eighty per cent of patients remain pain-free or experience minimal symptoms 7 to 10 years after CABG (Kaiser et al., 1989). Other reports note a significant acceleration of recurrent anginal symptoms after 5 years (Davidson, 1980). These data reflect the difficulty in quantifying subjective pain. Some patients remain asymptomatic despite angiographic evidence denoting severe reocclusion of both native and grafted vessels. Researchers have attributed this phenomenon to the placebo effect of surgery as well as to the possibility of psychological denial or silent ischemia.

Reoperation. A vast increase in the number of reoperations has been observed during the last several years. Reoperation accounts for approximately 15% to 20% of coronary bypass procedures performed (Lytle et al., 1987). Early reintervention within the first year often results from technical problems or conduit viability (Gersh et al., 1989). Young age, nonuse of the internal mammary artery, atherosclerotic disease progression, and recurrence of symptoms comprise the most common indicators for late reoperation (Gersh et al., 1989).

Operative mortality figures associated with reoperation are two to three times higher than those of the first operation. Consequences of aging on multiple organ systems influence the surgical outcome. Studies reveal that patients undergoing reoperation inherently display an increased incidence of left ventricular dysfunction, left main coronary disease, and diabetes (Loop et al., 1983). Increased technical difficulties often prolong the operative time. Perioperative myocardial infarction, respiratory complications, and bleeding are common postoperative sequelae associated with reoperation (Gersh et al., 1989). The potential of atherosclerotic plaque embolization is also a threat.

Overall, results of reoperation have not been as promising or comparable to those seen in primary operations. Redevelopment of angina is common within several years following reoperation. Survival is difficult to predict and must be viewed in the light of preoperative risk factors and susceptibility.

Graft Patency. Graft patency is the pivotal factor that determines the degree of success and the results following CABG surgery. A direct correlation has been established between graft patency and the recurrence of angina, ischemic symptoms, survival, and quality of life (Loop, 1983; Loop et al., 1989).

Excellent long-term patency rates associated with use of the IMA have led to improved 10-year survival rates (Fig. 20–4) approaching 90% (Loop et al., 1989). Survival statistics in patients with normal left ventricular function indicate significant differences between those who received an IMA graft and those who received saphenous vein grafts. Eighty-seven per cent of IMA patients survived 10 years compared to 78% of patients with SV grafts (Loop et al., 1986, 1989). The most dramatic survival difference emerged in patients with impaired left ventricular function. The IMA group experienced a 16% greater 10-year survival compared to the SV group (Loop et al., 1986, 1989) (Fig. 20–5). Significantly fewer myocardial infarctions, fewer reoperations, and longer event-free survival have been observed in patients with IMA grafts (Loop et al., 1986, 1989). Several reports demonstrate that patients who receive an IMA graft to the left anterior descending artery exhibit a reduction in risk of mortality by 0.62 to 0.65 (Loop et al., 1989).

Ten-year patency rates for IMA grafts approach 96% compared with 81% for saphenous vein grafts (Zeff et al., 1988). Saphenous vein grafts are associated with a dramatic attrition rate with time. Approximately 8% to 12% of grafts occlude in the early postoperative period (Fitzgibbon et al., 1986; Grondin et al., 1989). Surgical technique, recipient vessel size, and graft flow rates are factors influencing early vein patency. Angiographic studies performed at 1 year revealed that significant morphologic changes affected 12% to 20% of the vein grafts (Grondin et al., 1989). At 5 years, 20% to 30% of grafts were found

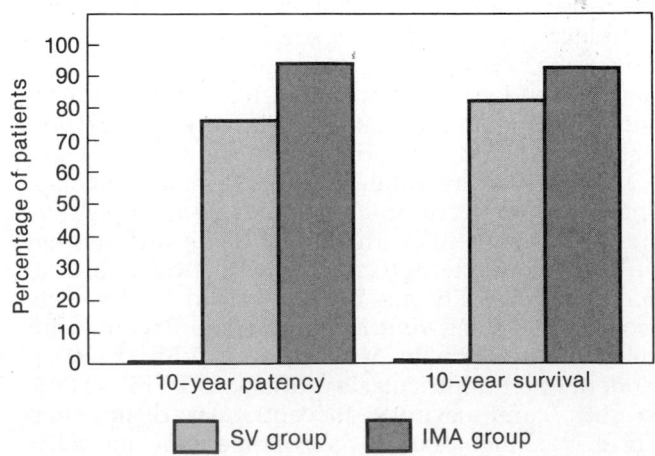

FIGURE 20–4. Comparison of internal mammary artery (IMA) and saphenous vein (SV) grafts.

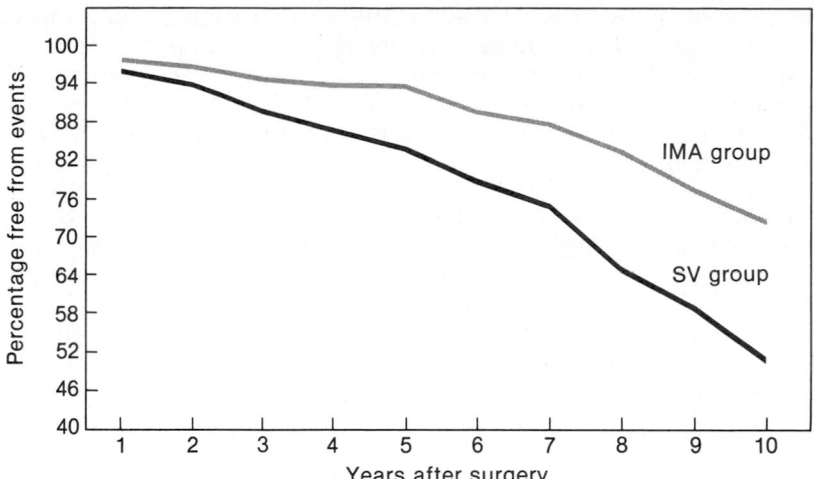

FIGURE 20–5. Occurrence of cardiac events with IMA and SV grafts.

to display impressive narrowing and luminal changes, compromising flow. This rate doubled to approximately 50% at 10 years (Fitzgibbon et al., 1986; Grondin et al., 1989).

Histologic changes occurring within vein grafts are responsible for failure and occlusion. Intimal proliferation and migration of smooth muscle cells precipitate a thickening of the endothelial layer. Platelet deposition and release of thromboxane (a potent vasoconstrictor) further contribute to the development of vein graft atherosclerosis (Goldman et al., 1988). Measures to retard the rapidity and acceleration of atherosclerotic disease have focused on the use of aspirin and dipyridamole. Dipyridamole acts to inhibit platelet aggregation, mural thrombus formation, and thromboxane release (Goldman et al., 1988). Some centers administer dipyridamole 24 to 48 hours preoperatively. Institution of antiplatelet therapy preoperatively and postoperatively has been found to improve early graft patency (Goldman et al., 1988). Emphasis on serum cholesterol and diet warrants continued investigation. Evidence suggests that cholesterol-lowering agents have an important role in potentially limiting both systemic and coronary vein graft atherosclerosis (Grondin et al., 1989).

Prevention of Cardiac Events. The role of CABG surgery in preventing further myocardial injury is difficult to quantify. Patients who have undergone surgery demonstrate greater freedom from cardiac events compared to patients treated medically. The incidence of myocardial infarction approaches 1.1% per year in surgical patients. This figure doubles to 2.6% in medically treated patients. Approximately 77% of CABG patients remain free from ischemic or myocardial injury during the first 5 years, and almost 50% report event-free survival at 10 years (Kirklin et al., 1989). Surgical patients demonstrate a 26% reduction in cardiac-related hospital admissions (Kirklin et al., 1989). This result has a significant impact not only on health care costs but also on the patient's ability to maintain an uninterrupted quality of life, free from hospital admissions.

Quality of Life. Improved quality of life represents one of the most important benefits derived from coronary artery bypass graft surgery. From the patient's perspective, the crucial determinant of operative success hinges on the ability to resume an active and productive life style. Several investigations have focused on patient expectations in regard to postoperative outcome. Patients expectations represent key determinants of recovery. The majority of patients achieved the expected benefits of prolongation of life, prevention of infarct, and improved quality of life at 6 months after surgery (Gortner et al., 1989). However, during the first 6 to 8 weeks, patients frequently report symptoms of decreased activity tolerance, weakness, and fatigue. As time progresses, improved exercise tolerance most often leads to increased participation in daily activities. Increased coronary blood flow is demonstrated on postoperative exercise tolerance testing (Kirklin et al., 1989). Reports of improved left ventricular wall motion and performance postoperatively facilitate increased myocardial work capacity. Patients enjoy greater freedom to participate in physical activity and sexual activity and have fewer and less severe associated symptoms (Gortner et al., 1989). Decreased requirements for medications and reliance on nitrates allows patients greater independence, both physically and psychologically (Gortner et al., 1989).

Patients are encouraged to return to work following successful surgery. The goal of recovery focuses upon return to gainful employment. Wide variations exist in figures depicting patients who return to work postoperatively. It is estimated that 38% to 81% (average 62%) of patients are employed after surgery (Allen, 1990). Preoperative work status is the major predictor of postoperative employment. Some clinicians suggest that patients become accustomed to not working, thus affecting their motivation and physical ability to actualize their work status. Reports indicate that participation in some form of structured cardiac rehabilitation program increases the likelihood of return to work (Gutmann et al., 1982). Patients who returned to work experienced greater degrees of self-worth and self-confidence. Factors such as high income, male age less than 55 years, self-employed status, white-collar work, college education, freedom from symptoms, and good ventricular function were factors predicting return to work (Loop, 1983).

Gender. Until recently, data about results and outcomes associated with CABG procedures were derived primarily from studies composed of males. Limited information was available about recovery in women. Thus, a number of recent investigations have focused on examining the impact of gender upon recovery from surgical revascularization.

Mortality figures are higher for women undergoing coronary bypass surgery than for men. Women incur an operative mortality rate of approximately 4.6% with first CABG compared to 2.6% in men. Reasons explaining an almost 50% higher mortality rate have centered on differences in age and functional class. Women are older, being referred for surgery later in the course of disease, which contributes to a higher preoperative functional class prior to surgery. Other reports have indicated that the predictive accuracy of diagnostic testing (such as exercise testing) has led to a misinterpretation of disease severity. Tobin (1987) noted that when exercise results were abnormal in women with anginal symptoms, recommendations for angiographic study were less likely to occur. Rankin (1990) showed that preoperatively women displayed significantly greater symptoms of dypsnea and hypercholesterolemia and postoperatively had longer intensive care unit stays and mortality rates than men. Factors such as hypertension, diabetes, family history, and smoking were equitable between the sexes.

Long-term survival rates are similar in men and women. However, women demonstrate lowered rates of graft patency. Consequently, more women

develop an increased incidence of anginal symptoms, shortness of breath, and myocardial infarctions. Differences also exist in psychosocial outcomes denoting a correlation between physiologic status and psychologic functioning. Women report decreased levels of postoperative activity compared to men. At 12 to 21 months after surgery, men participate in some form of moderate activity twice as often as women (Stanton et al., 1984). Employment status is closely related to the patient's personal, social, and economic status. Most investigations reveal that fewer women are employed outside the home postoperatively. Several reports have shown that women display less anxiety, anger, and depression postoperatively than men (Rankin, 1990). Figure 20–6 depicts the differences noted between women and men following cardiac surgery. For nurses caring for these patients, knowledge of postoperative differences will assist in planning interventions and providing support to facilitate optimal postoperative recovery and adaptation.

VALVULAR DISEASE

Diseases affecting the cardiac valves often lead to severe functional limitations for patients due to either a stenotic or a regurgitant change in the valve function. Most commonly, the mitral and aortic valves are involved because of the higher pressures generated by the left side of the heart. Tricuspid or pulmonic valve involvement is usually not associated with aortic or mitral valve disease. Typically, progression of either stenotic or regurgitant valvular lesions produces chronic fatigue, dyspnea, palpations, angina, or congestive heart failure. In 1964, the New York Heart Association (NYHA) developed a classification system that describes the functional ability or limitations imposed by heart disease (New York Heart Association, 1964) (Table 20–2). As val-

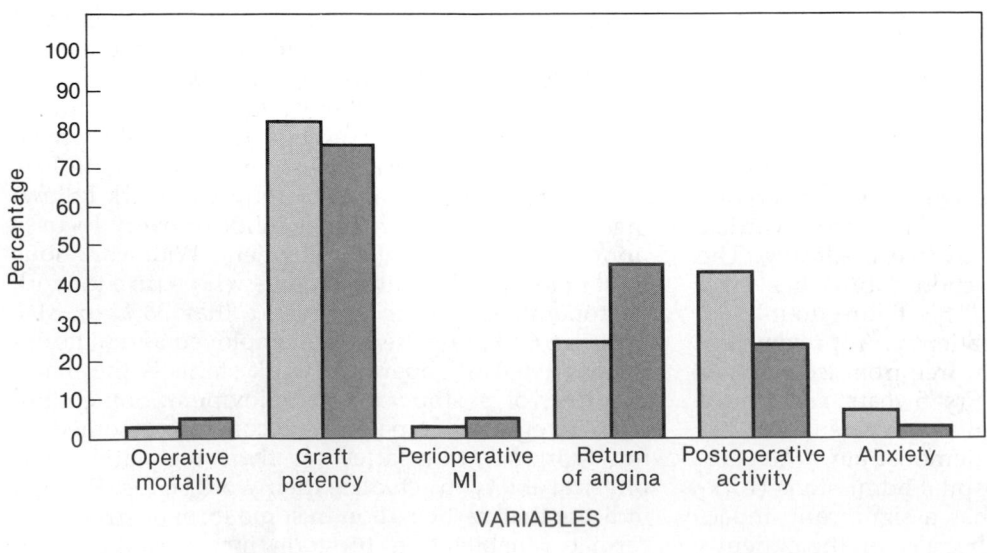

FIGURE 20–6. Comparison of results by gender.

TABLE 20–2. Functional Classification of Patients with Heart Disease

Class I.	Patients with cardiac disease but without resulting limitations on physical activity. Ordinary physical activity does not cause undue fatigue, palpitations, dyspnea, or anginal pain
Class II.	Patients with cardiac disease resulting in slight limitation of physical activity. They are comfortable at rest. Ordinary physical activity results in fatigue, palpitations, dyspnea, or anginal pain
Class III.	Patients with cardiac disease resulting in marked limitation of physical activity. They are comfortable at rest only. Less than ordinary physical activity causes fatigue, palpitations, dyspnea, or angina
Class IV.	Patients with cardiac disease resulting in inability to carry on any physical activity without discomfort. Symptoms of cardiac insufficiency or of the anginal syndrome may be present even at rest. If any physical activity is undertaken, discomfort is increased

From New York Heart Association Criteria Committee (1964). *Nomenclature and criteria for diagnosis of diseases of the heart and great vessels* (6th ed., (pp. 110–114). Boston: Little, Brown.

vular disease worsens, compensatory mechanisms become inadequate, and left ventricular dysfunction increases; medical management then becomes less effective, and surgical repair or valve replacement is indicated.

Advances made in the development of prostheses and reconstructive techniques and the use of cold cardioplegia for myocardial preservation have had a positive influence on the outcomes of valvular surgery. Valve replacement and valve reconstruction have enabled many patients with valvular heart disease to resume activities that they were unable to tolerate prior to surgery. Clinical data support the finding that patients with valvular disease, including the elderly in functional Class III or IV preoperatively, improve by at least one class level within several months after valvular surgery (Stephenson et al., 1978; Tsai et al., 1986).

The etiology, pathophysiology, clinical findings, and indications for surgery for mitral and aortic valve disease will be discussed. Additionally, the types of prosthetic valves and surgical techniques used to repair or replace these values will be reviewed.

Indications for Valve Replacement

Mitral Stenosis. Mitral stenosis is usually the result of rheumatic fever but may also be caused by tumors or calcification (Schakenbach, 1987). The normal mi-

tral valve area in adults is approximately 5 cm². When the valve orifice is reduced by stenosis to less than one-half its normal size, signs and symptoms of mitral stenosis ensue (Kenner et al., 1985). As stenosis develops, left atrial pressure rises, which serves to maintain blood flow and left ventricular filling. The left atrium dilates and eventually hypertrophies, often precipitating atrial fibrillation (Schakenbach, 1987). As the stenosis worsens, elevated left heart pressure is transmitted to the pulmonary vasculature. As pulmonary artery pressure rises, right ventricular afterload increases, causing a resultant increase in right ventricular end-diastolic pressure and ultimately an elevation in right atrial pressure. Pulmonary congestion leads to dyspnea, the most common presenting symptom of patients with mitral stenosis (Kenner et al., 1985; Schakenbach, 1987).

Generally, patients with mitral stenosis are asymptotic until the fourth decade of life, when the valve orifice has decreased to less than 2.5 cm² (Rappaport, 1975; Morgan et al., 1985) (Fig. 20–7). The left ventricular impulse may be normal or difficult to palpate unless the patient is in the left lateral position. The

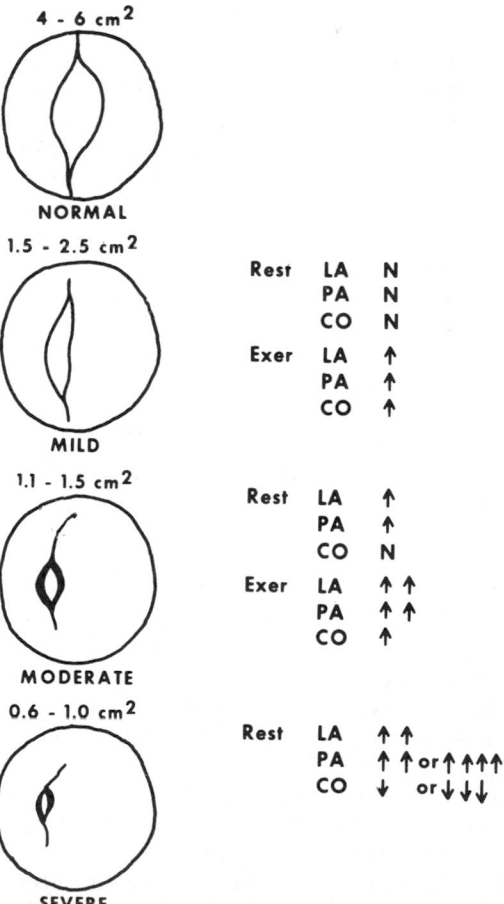

FIGURE 20–7. Diagrammatic representation of the hemodynamic changes that occur at various stages of severity of mitral stenosis. The valve area is listed above each stage. *Abbreviations:* ↓, decreased; ↑, increased; CO, cardiac output; Exer, exercise; LA, left atrial pressure; N, normal; PA, pulmonary arterial pressure. (From Rappaport, E. (1975). Natural history of aortic and mitral valve disease. *American College of Cardiology, 35,* 219–227.)

obstruction to flow through the mitral valve prevents detection of a presystolic impulse. In the presence of significant pulmonary hypertension and right ventricular hypertrophy, closure of the pulmonic valve can be palpated at the second intercostal space on the left sternal border. Frequently, a right ventricular heave can be observed and palpated at the left sternal border edge.

The classic heart sounds heard in patients with mitral stenosis are a pronounced first heart sound, an early diastolic opening snap, and an early mid-diastolic rumble. In the early stages of the disease, these abnormal heart sounds may often go unrecognized. Their detection depends upon valve mobility, blood flow, and cardiac rhythm. When atrial fibrillation is present, a presystolic murmur will be absent. Atrial fibrillation causes a decrease in left ventricular filling, an increase in heart rate, and stagnation of blood in the atrium. This condition predisposes to thrombus formation with the potential for subsequent pulmonary and systemic embolization (Morgan et al., 1985).

Indications for early surgical evaluation for mitral valve replacement are a prominent opening snap, a low probability of valve calcification, and a history that includes an episode of pulmonary edema or paroxysmal nocturnal dyspnea. In this patient population, an attempt is made to retain the native valve by performing either valvuloplasty (percutaneous or surgical) or an open commissurotomy (Kirklin and Barratt-Boyes, 1986). Emergent surgery may be indicated in patients who have undergone unsuccessful percutaneous valvuloplasty. For patients with previous commissurotomy or valvuloplasty, severe calcification, or concomitant mitral regurgitation, surgery is usually postponed until symptoms are more chronic and severe (NYHA functional Class III) (Kirklin and Barratt-Boyes, 1986). However, patients in NYHA functional Class IV who undergo operation have been demonstrated to have a 13% survival at 9 years after surgery (Chaffin and Dagget, 1978; Kirklin and Barratt-Boyes, 1986).

Mitral Regurgitation. Mitral regurgitation in its chronic form is usually the result of rheumatic disease in 25% to 40% of this patient population (Rappaport, 1975; Roberts, 1983). It may also be caused by mitral valve prolapse (in 6% to 10% of patients [Edwards, 1983]) or endocarditis (in 5% of patients [Roberts, 1983]). Less commonly, mitral regurgitation is caused by calcification, distortion of the annulus due to left ventricular dilation (Schakenbach, 1987), and, rarely, from congenital abnormalities or connective tissue disorders such as Marfan syndrome.

With mitral regurgitation the diseased mitral valve is incapable of full closure during systole. This causes regurgitant blood to flow from the left ventricle into the left atrium. Left ventricular stroke volume and cardiac output decrease as left atrial volume and pressure increase (Kenner et al., 1985). Over time, both the left atrium and the left ventricle dilate in response to the increased chamber volumes. As in mitral stenosis, the increased left atrial pressure associated with mitral regurgitation causes elevated pulmonary artery pressure and subsequent right heart failure (Kenner et al., 1985; Schakenbach, 1987).

Acute mitral regurgitation can develop after chest trauma or more commonly, in patients with coronary artery disease or myocardial infarction (McGoon and Brest, 1987; Schakenbach, 1987). Despite the cause, acute mitral regurgitation occurs suddenly, usually as a result of papillary muscle dysfunction or rupture, secondary to either ischemia or infarction (Stephenson et al., 1978; Schakenbach, 1987). Patients with acute mitral regurgitation have not developed the compensatory mechanisms of atrial and ventricular hypertrophy. With the sudden development of regurgitation, dramatic increases in left atrial pressure quickly lead to pulmonary congestion and biventricular failure. Emergent surgery is often indicated (Schakenbach, 1987). Coronary artery bypass grafting, valve reconstruction, or valve replacement may be performed depending upon the cause and extent of the lesion.

In chronic mitral regurgitation, symptoms often become worse slowly over time. The most common presenting symptoms in this patient population are fatigue and exhaustion caused by decreased cardiac output (Schakenbach, 1987). Upon inspection it is not uncommon for a parasternal systolic impulse to be observed. On palpation, the point of maximum intensity is displaced laterally and downward with a diffuse hyperactive impulse. An auscultatory hallmark in mitral regurgitation is a holosystolic murmur beginning with the first heart sound and extending through the second heart sound. The murmur is medium in pitch and blowing in intensity. It is best heard with the bell of the stethoscope. The second heart sound is usually normal but may be accentuated in the presence of pulmonary hypertension. Patients may have a third heart sound that corresponds with a high diastolic flow of ventricular filling.

Echocardiographic, cardiac catheterization, and radionuclide studies are performed to evaluate valvular function and chamber dimensions. This information, taken in conjunction with the patient's symptoms, is used to determine the need for and timing of surgical intervention. Patients are usually managed medically until they reach NYHA functional Class III or IV (Kirklin and Barratt-Boyes, 1986). However, the effects of acute left ventricular distention or chronic dilation and their reversibility after valve replacement generate concern (Braunwald, 1980; Ross, 1985). Morgan and colleagues (1985) recommend use of the following criteria for surgical intervention: (1) NYHA Class III or IV symptoms; (2) NYHA Class II symptoms if left ventricular diastolic dimensions are 6 cm or greater, regurgitant flow fraction is 40% or greater, or a 4+ mitral regurgitation with an ejection fraction of 60% or less is present.

Aortic Stenosis. Aortic stenosis can be caused by

rheumatic inflammation, idiopathic calcification, or congenital malformation (Kenner et al., 1985). The normal aortic valve area in adults measures 2.5 to 3.5 cm². In severe aortic stenosis this area is reduced to 0.5 to 0.7 cm² (Rappaport, 1975). During systole, the left ventricle must generate a significantly higher pressure to force blood through the stenotic valve. Pressure gradients of more than 50 mm Hg across the aortic valve are often necessary to maintain an adequate cardiac output (Khan and Gray, 1988). As a result of severe aortic stenosis, left ventricular systolic pressure is increased, causing the development of compensatory left ventricular hypertrophy. Myocardial oxygen demands are also increased due to increased left ventricular wall tension and muscle mass. Symptoms of angina may develop even in patients without coronary artery disease (Deverux and Reichek, 1980; Schakenbach, 1987). As the disease process progresses, left atrial pressure rises as the atrium attempts to empty into the stiff, hypertrophied left ventricle. During activity, the left ventricle may be unable to meet systemic cardiac output demands. If left ventricular preload is inadequate to "stretch" the noncompliant left ventricle, cardiac output and systemic blood pressure will fall, and dyspnea on exertion and syncope will result.

In acute aortic stenosis, patients present with severe low cardiac output, vasoconstriction, and intractable pulmonary edema. Assessment of the distal extremities reveals pale, cold, or cyanotic skin. The systolic blood pressure is normal or slightly elevated, and the diastolic pressure may be normal or slightly decreased.

Palpation of the carotid arteries may reveal a decrease in upstroke called *pulsus parvus* and a diminished pulse volume termed *pulsus tardus* (Khan and Gray, 1988). A palpable systolic thrill may be felt at the second right intercostal space on expiration with the patient sitting and leaning forward. The presence of this thrill has been reported to coincide with a 40-mm Hg gradient (Khan and Gray, 1988).

The murmur of aortic stenosis, which is a long systolic murmur heard best at the right sternal border at the second intercostal space, is often the first clinical sign of the disease process. As left ventricular hypertrophy worsens a fourth heart sound caused by left atrial contraction may be heard on auscultation at the apex.

Surgery is indicated in symptomatic patients when a pressure gradient of 50 mm Hg or more is present across the aortic valve. In patients with only minor symptomatology, surgery is usually not indicated unless the gradient across the valve is 75 mm Hg or more. Other determinants include a valve area measuring less than 0.8 cm², progressive left ventricular hypertrophy, syncope, or congestive heart failure, and a positive exercise tolerance test (Rappaport, 1978; Khan and Gray, 1988). Because many patients with aortic stenosis also have coronary artery disease, valve replacement is often undertaken with concomitant coronary artery bypass grafting (Khan and Gray, 1988).

Aortic Regurgitation. Aortic valvular regurgitant states may be acute, subacute, or chronic. The most common cause of acute aortic regurgitation is infective endocarditis involving a previously normal valve, an unrecognized bicuspid valve, or aortic dissection. Blunt chest trauma may lead to either acute or subacute regurgitation. In acute or subacute aortic regurgitation, there is a sudden volume overload on a relatively normal left ventricle. The ability of the left ventricle to compensate and distend acutely is diminished, causing an elevation in left ventricular end-diastolic pressure and volume. These elevations, accompanied by a normal or mildly elevated left atrial pressure, may cause the mitral valve to close prematurely. During ventricular systole, the left ventricle fails secondary to the acute increase in volume, further contributing to a decreased ejection fraction and a drop in systemic cardiac output.

Chronic aortic regurgitation is frequently the result of rheumatic heart disease (RHD). Other causes of chronic aortic regurgitation are syphilis, aortic calcification, aortic aneurysm, or senile dilation of the annulus (Schakenbach, 1987). Aortic regurgitation may also be caused by congenital malformations such as a bileaflet valve. In chronic aortic regurgitation, the previously stated volume and pressure changes occur over time, allowing for compensatory dilation of the left ventricle. As the left ventricular end-diastolic volume increases, the ejection of forward stroke volume increases based on Starling's law.

Patients with severe chronic aortic regurgitation may remain asymptomatic for long periods of time. Upon auscultation, the murmur of aortic regurgitation is heard as a systolic, high-pitched, decrescendo murmur. It is heard best at the lower left sternal border. Typically, the murmur is classified as blowing, and its duration rather than its quality is correlated with the severity of regurgitation. A third heart sound may also be heard as a result of rapid diastolic filling.

Physical assessment of the peripheral pulses, distal tissue perfusion, and blood pressure reveal classic findings associated with the disease process. In assessing the carotid pulses, the "water hammer" or Corrigan pulse may be noted. This is demonstrated by a rapid rise in upstroke followed by a quick collapse of the pulse wave. Visible pulsations may also be present in the carotid, subclavian, and brachial arteries and in the vessels of the fingers (Rappaport, 1975). Systolic hypertension associated with a diastolic pressure is often observed.

With acute aortic regurgitation, patients typically present with severe left ventricular failure and low cardiac output. They are tachycardic and acutely dyspneic. Assessment of the distal extremities reveals vasoconstriction with cold, pale, or cyanotic skin. The systolic blood pressure is normal or slightly elevated; the diastolic pressure may be normal or slightly decreased.

Because the disease process in chronic aortic regurgitation is often insidious, causing deterioration of left ventricular function prior to the onset of symptoms, surgical intervention is often not undertaken until moderate to severe symptoms of left ventricular failure are apparent (Kirklin and Barratt-Boyes, 1986; Hirschfield, 1986). Conversely, in patients with acute aortic regurgitation, surgical repair or replacement of the valve is usually indicated with the onset of symptoms because the compensatory mechanisms of hypertrophy and vasodilation are absent and the patient's condition is acutely compromised.

Valvular Reconstruction

To date, there remains no ideal substitute for the native human valve. All prostheses, whether mechanical or biologic, have inherent risks and may cause complications for the patient. Therefore, whenever possible it is better to retain and repair the native valve, negating or at least delaying valve replacement. Two major advantages of valve repair over replacement are (1) lowered mortality rate, and (2) decreased thromboembolic and anticoagulant-related complications (Pluth, 1987). In many patients with congenital or acquired valvular diseases, reparative or reconstructive surgery can be performed successfully (West and Weldon, 1978). Techniques commonly employed to repair diseased valves may include commissurotomy—splitting of fused leaflets; valvuloplasty—repair or reconstruction of the valve; and annuloplasty—repair or reconstruction of the ringlike base or annulus of the valve.

Mitral Valve. Mitral valve repairs are most successful if they can be performed fairly early in the course of the disease before the leaflets have been severely damaged by calcification or degeneration. Open commissurotomy, which involves incision of the left atrium and cardiopulmonary bypass, is indicated in patients with pure mitral stenosis, without associated regurgitation or calcification (Seifert, 1987). Closed commissurotomy, in which bypass is not necessary, is seldom performed. The rationale for this change is twofold: (1) In patients who prefer not to undergo an open heart procedure, percutaneous balloon valvuloplasty is usually attempted first, and (2) open commissurotomy offers the distinct advantage of being able to visualize the valve. If, after examining the valve or attempting commissurotomy, it is determined that a successful repair cannot be achieved, valve replacement can be performed as long as the valve leaflets are mobile and noncalcified (Pluth, 1987) (Fig. 20–8).

In patients with mitral regurgitation secondary to rheumatic disease, ruptured chordae tendineae, prolapse, coronary artery disease, endocarditis, or congenital malformation, surgical valvuloplasty procedures can be performed successfully (Spencer et al., 1985). Carpentier (1985), a French surgeon, has described reparative techniques for patching perforated leaflets, revising elongated or fused chordae tendineae, and resecting excessive or redundant leaflet tissue. Carpentier's techniques are employed throughout the world and have spurred further research in the area of reconstructive valvular surgery. When mitral regurgitation results from a widened

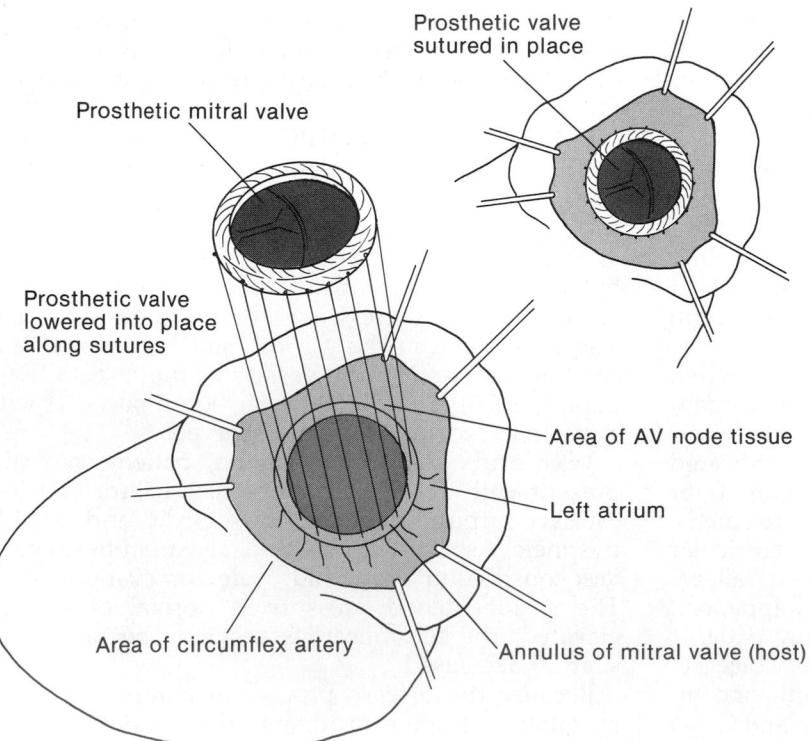

Prosthetic valve sutured in place

Prosthetic mitral valve

Prosthetic valve lowered into place along sutures

Area of AV node tissue

Left atrium

Area of circumflex artery

Annulus of mitral valve (host)

FIGURE 20–8. After excision of the diseased valve, the prosthetic valve is lowered into position along sutures placed in the host ring tissue and valve sewing ring.

annulus, annuloplasty can often be performed to reduce the size of the annulus and approximate the leaflets. This is accomplished by using either a prosthetic ring or a pursestring-type suture to draw the excess annular tissue together. Valvuloplasty or annuloplasty procedures are successful in approximately one-fourth of all patients with pure mitral regurgitation (Pluth, 1987). Severe destruction secondary to rheumatic or other infectious processes and extensive calcification are the limiting factors that most often preclude or contraindicate valvular reconstruction and indicate surgical repair (Spencer et al., 1985).

Aortic Valves. Aortic valve repairs have not been as successful as repair of the atrioventricular valves. The aortic valves are often heavily calcified, and the leaflets are more difficult to approximate (Carpentier, 1983; Seifert, 1987). In most cases, the condition of the valve determines the need for replacement (Fig. 20–9).

Types of Prosthetic Valves

Since the first successful valve replacements were performed in the early 1960s, many different varieties of valves have been developed and subsequently improved. The types of replacement valves available today are mechanical and tissue (biograft and homograft). The indications, advantages, and disadvantages of each type will be discussed in relation to the proposed properties of an ideal prosthetic valve (Table 20–3). These properties or characteristics are (1) adequate hydraulic performance, (2) durability, lasting the lifetime of the patient, (3) absence of thrombogenic tendencies, thus eliminating the need for anticoagulation and its resulting deleterious effects, (4) biocompatibility, absence of negative effects on blood cells or tissue, (5) ease of insertion, thus decreasing bypass time and related complications, and (6) silence, increasing patient comfort and satisfaction (Weiland, 1983; Campbell and Waldhausen, 1986; Bonchek, 1987).

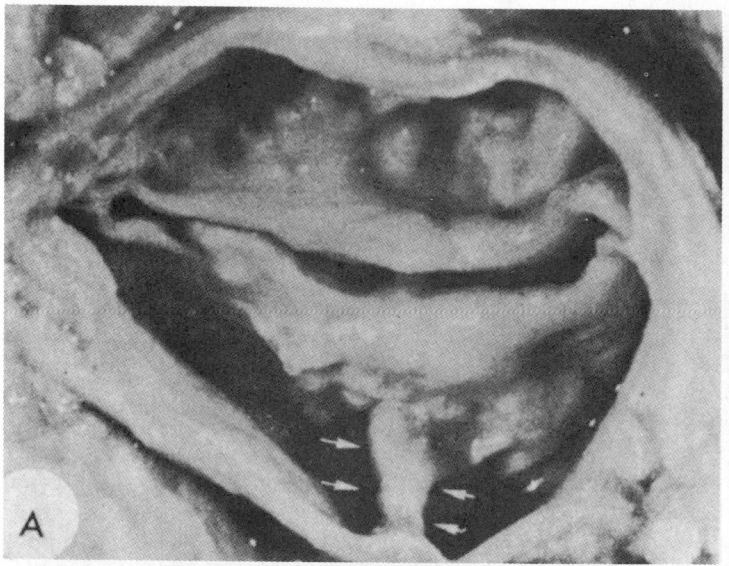
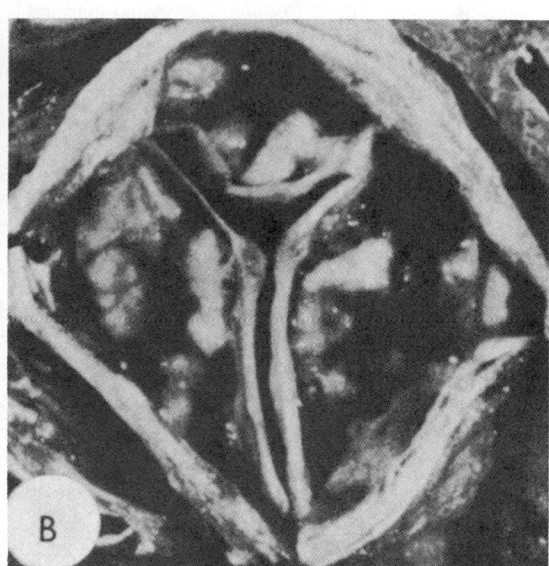
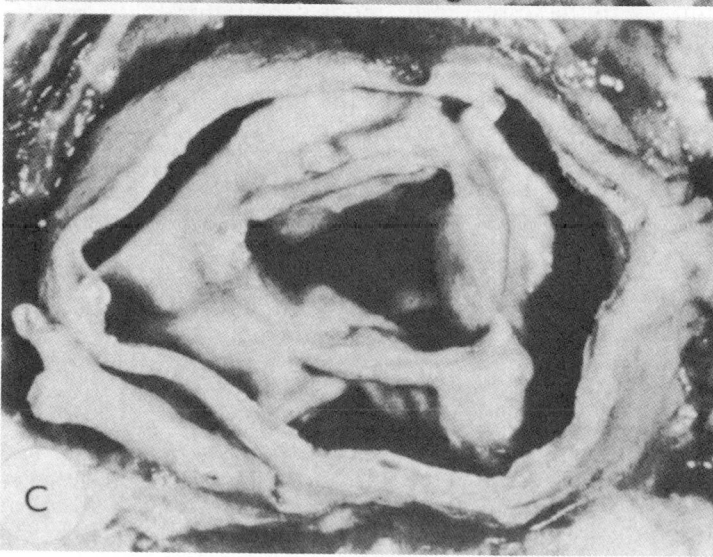

FIGURE 20–9. A, Calcified, stenotic, congenitally bicuspid aortic valve of a 59-year-old man. The cusps are situated anteriorly and posteriorly, with the commissures on the right and left. The valve has a raphe *(white arrows)* in the anterior cusp. Peak systolic gradient across the valve was 45 mm Hg, and the patient had complete heart block secondary to destruction of the atrioventricular bundle by calcium, which presumably had extended down from the aortic valvular cusps. B, Stenotic tricuspid aortic valve in an 81-year-old man. Aortic stenosis in the elderly is characterized by calcific deposits on the aortic surfaces of the cusps and typically no or little commissural fusion. C, Stenotic tricuspid aortic valve in a 55-year-old man. Each of the three commissures is fused, producing a triangular fixed central orifice that is both stenotic and incompetent. (From Roberts, W. C. (1973). Valvular, subvalvular and supravalvular aortic stenosis: Morphologic features. In J. E. Edwards (Ed.), *Clinical-pathologic correlations* No. 2 (pp. 100, 106, and 108). Philadelphia: F. A. Davis.)

TABLE 20–3. Comparison of Available Valve Prostheses to the Characteristics of the "Ideal Valve"

Characteristics of the "Ideal" Valve	Mechanical			Biologic		
	Caged-Ball (Starr-Edwards)	Single Tilting-Disc (Bjork-Shiley) (Omniscience) (Medtronic-Hall)	Bi-Leaflet Tilting-Disc (St. Jude) (Duramedics)	Porcine (Carpentier-Edwards) (Hancock-Vascor)	Bovine (Ionescu-Shiley)	Pulmonary Autografts and Aortic Homografts
Hydraulic performance	Good peripheral flow Sub-optimal in small sizes	Very good degree of laminar flow	Excellent near-laminar flow Best hemodynamics in small sizes	Very good laminar flow Higher gradients than mechanical in small sizes	Very good, especially in aortic position Laminar flow slightly better than porcine in small sizes	Excellent laminar flow
Durability	Excellent Abundant long-term experience	Very good	Very good	Limited to 10 years Accelerated tissue failure in patients >35 years of age	Limited to 10 years	Variable (10–20 years)
Non-thrombogenic	No To date, all mechanical prosthetic valves require long-term anticoagulation Prothrombin time should be 1.6–1.9 × control	No	No	Very low incidence of thromboembolism. Short-term anticoagulation		Yes Anticoagulation not required
Biocompatibility	Hemolytic anemia may result from destruction of RBCs	Minimal hemolytic tendencies		No hemolysis	No hemolysis	No hemolysis Minimal compatibility problems
Ease of insertion					Leaflets very fragile; may lead to more difficult insertion	Most difficult to obtain, size and insert
Silence	Yes	No	No	Yes	Yes	Yes

Mechanical Valves. Mechanical valve prostheses are composed of metal or synthetic materials and have either a ball or a disc that moves in response to pressure changes within the adjacent cardiac chambers or arteries (Fig. 20–10). For example, in the mitral position, when left atrial pressure supersedes that in the left ventricle, the ball or disc will move, thus allowing blood to flow from the left atrium into the ventricle. When the pressure in the left ventricle becomes greater than that in the atrium, the movable component of the valve will close, thus preventing regurgitation of blood into the atrium during subsequent ventricular ejection.

In 1960, Starr and Edwards developed and implanted the first caged-ball prosthetic mitral valve. Since that time, this valve has been updated and the mechanics further refined. Current versions of the Starr-Edwards caged-ball valve are used for both aortic, (model 1260) and mitral (model 6120) valve replacements. The major advantages of these valves are their durability and silence. Disadvantages include thrombogenic properties requiring long-term anticoagulation, and turbulence of peripheral blood flow around the ball with resultant decreases in both hydraulic performance and biocompatibility. Rates of thromboembolism for the Starr-Edwards ball-cage valve range from 2.5% to 3.5%/patient per year in the aortic position, and 3.5% to 6.3% for mitral

prostheses in anticoagulated patients (Edmunds, 1987). Of note also is that this type of valve has a fairly large profile and may cause some outflow obstruction in patients with a small left ventricle (mitral position) or small aortic root (aortic position) (Roberts, 1976).

Tilting disc valves such as the Bjork-Shiley valve emerged in the late 1960s. Initially, these prostheses consisted of a ring with two struts, which held the tilting disc. Early models had durability problems secondary to strut fracture and thrombosis of the disc (Bonchek, 1987). Current models of the Bjork-Shiley valve, such as the Monostrut, are constructed from a single piece of metal with no welded points or struts that can fracture. The disc is made of pyrolytic carbon, which is moisture resistant, non-traumatic to blood, and very durable (Levine et al., 1981). The Omniscience (Lillehel-Haster) and Medtronic-Hall (Hall-Kaster) valves are also tilting disc devices similar to the Bjork-Shiley. These valves are also constructed from single metal blocks and contain pyrolytic carbon discs. The opening angle of these disc-type valves ranges from 60 to 80 degrees (Bonchek, 1987; Stelzer and Elkins, 1989). In the open position, blood flows on either side of the disc. There is less turbulence and more laminar type flow with these devices.

Another type of tilting disc valve that has become

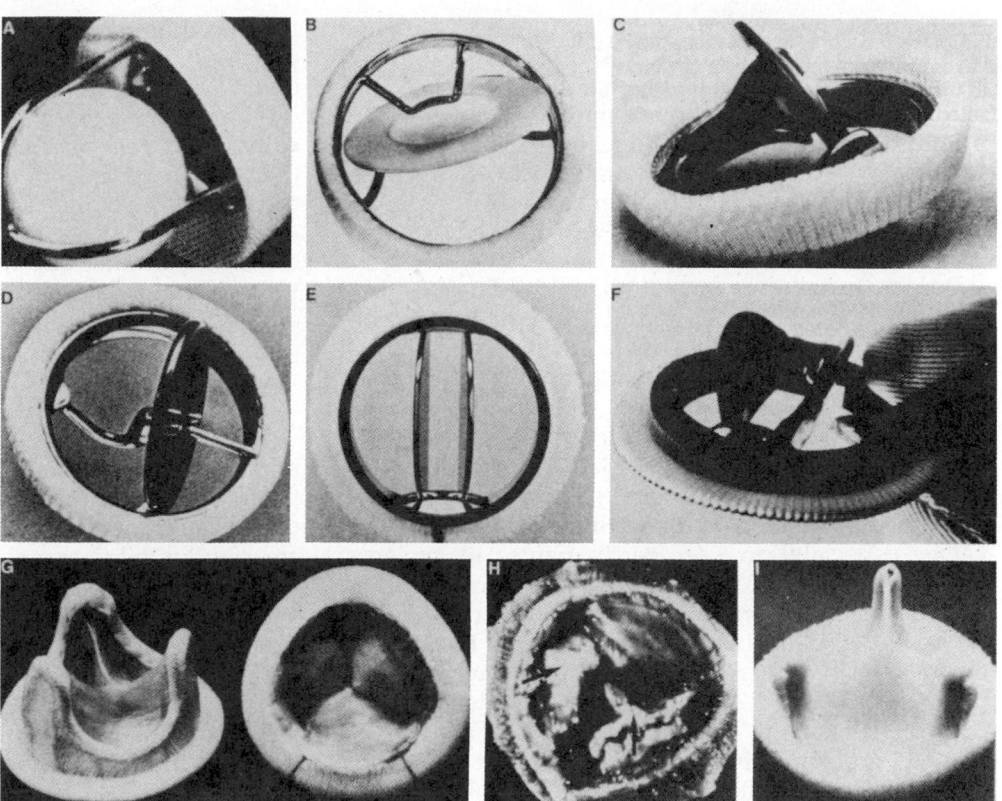

FIGURE 20–10. Prosthetic cardiac valves. *A,* Starr-Edwards caged ball valve with cloth sewing ring and bare struts. *B,* Bjork-Shiley tilting disc valve. *C,* Omniscience tilting disc valve. *D,* Medtronic-Hall tilting disc valve. *E,* St. Jude medical bileaflet valve as viewed end-on. Note the large size of the effective orifice area compared with the potential orifice area and the minimal obstruction of flow by the leaflets. *F,* Duromedics bileaflet valve. *G,* Carpentier-Edwards prosthetic valve. *H,* Porcine valve removed several years following implantation because of primary valve failure; arrows point to areas of calcification and destruction of leaflets. *I,* Ionescu-Shiley pericardial valve. (*A* from Starek, P. J. K., and *F,* from Clark, R. E. (1987). In *Heart valve replacement and reconstruction* (pp. 223–286). Chicago: Year Book Medical Publishers; *B* from Bjork, V.; *C* from Austin, E. H., III.; *E* from Crawford, F. A., Jr.; *G* and *H* from Magilligan, D. J., Jr.; and *I* from Crawford, F. A., Jr., In Crawford, F. A. (Ed.) (1987), *Cardiac surgery: Current heart valve prostheses* (Vol. 1, pp. 184, 204, 252, 270, 271, and 286). Philadelphia: Hanley and Belfus; *D* from Cobanoglu, A., and Brockman, S. K. (1986). *Valvular heart disease: Comprehensive evaluation and management. Cardiovascular Clinics,* 16, 404.)

very popular is the St. Jude Medical. This apparatus consists of a base ring with two semicircular discs or leaflets. The entire mechanism is made of pyrolytic carbon. With an 85-degree opening angle, this valve has the highest degree of laminar or central flow (Stelzer and Elkins, 1989).

The major advantages of the tilting disc valves are their durability and improved hydraulics as demonstrated by more direct and less peripheral, or turbulent flow. Disadvantages include audible sounds easily perceived by the patient and thrombogenic properties, necessitating anticoagulation. Thromboembolic rates for the disc valves vary in the literature and range from 0.7% to 3.7%/patient per year for aortic replacements, and 2.4% to 4.7%/patient per year for mitral prostheses in anticoagulated patients (Edmunds, 1987). Hemorrhage secondary to anticoagulation with valve replacement may occur in as many as 4.0% to 5.0% of patients per year (Edmunds, 1987).

Biologic Valves. Biologic or tissue valves are prostheses developed from either animal or human tissue. The most commonly used heterograft valves are the porcine, made from pig valves, and the bovine, made from calf pericardium. Human homograft cardiac valves, preserved from cadavers, are also being used in valve replacement surgery.

Heterografts. The two most widely used porcine valves are the Hancock/Vascor and the Carpentier-Edwards prostheses. These porcine valves and materials are preserved with glutaraldehyde, which enhances the formation of collagen bonds, increases the strength of the tissue, and decreases antigenicity (Bonchek, 1987; Siefert, 1987). Both the Hancock/Vascor valve and the Carpentier/Edwards valve are made from excised pig valves and are mounted on stents to support the valve leaflets. Both types of porcine heterografts are fairly nonthrombogenic, with embolic rates of 1% to 2%/patient per year for aortic valves, and 2% to 4%/patient per year for mitral replacements in nonanticoagulated patients (Bonchek, 1987; Edmunds, 1987). Patients receiving porcine valves are usually given either warfarin (Coumadin) or aspirin and dipyridamole for 6 weeks to 3 months postoperatively (Bonchek, 1987). Patients who have received mitral porcine valves and also have concomitant left atrial enlargement or atrial fibrillation may require long-term anticoagulation (Bonchek, 1987; Seifert, 1987).

Porcine prostheses are completely silent when implanted, mimicking the sounds of a native human valve. They do not cause hemolysis, and the blood flow is laminar in nature. Functionally, however, they tend to be stenotic with small valvular orifices, and they have higher valvular gradients than mechanical prostheses (Bjork, 1987). The major disadvantage of porcine heterografts is their limited durability secondary to primary tissue failure of the valve, especially in younger patients. In patients under the age of 35 years, the rate of calcification and tissue degeneration is very high. Mechanical valves are usually preferred for patients in this age group. In the over-30 age group, primary tissue failure of the valve occurs in approximately 15% to 25% of patients at 10 years. After 10 years, valve-related problems increase significantly (Bonchek, 1987; Stelzer and Elkins, 1989).

The Ionescu-Shiley bioprosthesis, which was developed in 1971, is a bovine heterograft made from calf pericardium (Crawford, 1987). The pericardial tissue is cut and molded into three leaflets and mounted on a Dacron-covered titanium stent. Like the porcine heterografts, these prostheses are also treated with glutaraldehyde (Stelzer and Elkins, 1989). On insertion, extra care must be taken to avoid trauma to the fragile leaflets (Bonchek, 1987). Although the hemodynamics of these valves seem significantly better, especially in the smaller sizes, the general characteristics are comparable to those of the porcine heterografts (Stelzer and Elkins, 1989).

Homografts. The first aortic valve homograft was inserted in 1962. Various types of sterilization and preservation procedures have been used to prepare cadaver valves. Fresh organ donor valves have also been transplanted, but availability of these is extremely limited. Currently, these homografts are obtained from organ donors, treated with antibiotic solutions, and cryopreserved at temperatures as low as 4° C (Stelzer and Elkins, 1989). Factors that affect homograft viability are the conditions existing during procurement and storage, techniques of sterilization, and age of the donor. Recipients of these grafts include patients with congenital, rheumatic, infectious, or degenerative processes involving the aortic valve or aortic root. Advantages of the aortic valve homograft include its excellent hemodynamics and virtual freedom from thromboembolic sequelae (Stelzer and Elkins, 1989). Statistics from Britain and New Zealand, where many of these grafts have been placed, show a patient survival rate of 65% at 10 years and 51.6% at 20 years (Pena et al., 1984; Matsuki et al., 1988).

Aortic homografts have also been used in Bentall procedures. These procedures, first described by Bentall in 1972, include excision and replacement of the aortic valve with the proximal aortic root, and subsequent reimplantation of the coronary arteries (Bentall and DeBono, 1968). Rather than using a prosthetic valve and a Dacron conduit, a homograft aortic valve and its root are used. Ross (1988) has described another use for the aortic homograft. His technique entails excision of the diseased aortic valve and the patient's pulmonic valve. The healthy, fresh, pulmonic valve is used as an autograft in the aortic valve position, and the aortic homograft is placed in the pulmonic valve position (Ross, 1988).

Advantages of using autografts and homografts include excellent hemodynamics, silence, virtual freedom from thromboembolic sequelae without the use of anticoagulants, blood compatibility, and increased durability compared with bovine and porcine heterographs. Their disadvantages, which have resulted in limited use of homograft aortic valve replacements in the United States, include scarce donor supply, sizing problems, increased expense related to limited availability and procurement and preservation problems; and difficult operative techniques involved in implantation (Stelzer and Elkins, 1989).

Prosthetic Valves: Selection Criteria

Although there are significant variations among the different types of mechanical and tissue valves, the long-term advantages and disadvantages are fairly evenly matched (Braunwald, 1988). Generally, mechanical prostheses demonstrate the best durability and are theoretically capable of lasting for the patient's lifetime. Their major disadvantage is thrombogenicity and the subsequent need for anticoagulation. Conversely, tissue valves are fairly nonthrombogenic and do not require long-term anticoagulation. The durability of these prostheses, however, is limited, especially in younger patients. In choosing the best prosthesis for a particular patient, the advantage of durability is weighed against the implications and risks associated with the need for long-term anticoagulation inherent in mechanical devices. In the bioprostheses, the advantage of low thrombogenicity is tempered by their short-term durability (Braunwald, 1988; Kirklin and Barratt-Boyes, 1986). It is important to discuss these advantages and disadvantages with the patient, who should be an active participant in the decision-making process.

In young and middle-aged adults, mechanical prostheses are usually preferred. Because of the long-term durability of these devices, patients generally will not need to undergo another operation to replace the prosthesis. If the patient and the members of the health care team decide on a mechanical valve, the specific type of device is chosen by the surgical team, taking into consideration the valve lesion, annular size, heart dimensions, and the surgeon's expertise and preference. Because all mechanical prostheses require continual anticoagulation, any medical or patient-specific situation that precludes use of long-term anticoagulation may, in many instances, be considered a contraindication to use of a mechanical valve. Such specific medical conditions include bleeding ulcer disease, cerebrovascular hemorrhage, and intended pregnancy in women of childbearing age. Patient-related factors that must be considered in valve selection include the patient's motivation to adhere to specific life-style changes, such as dietary restrictions, and strict medication follow-up regimens. Other considerations may be hazardous occupations or vocations, geography, availability of follow-up services, and psychosocial issues related to the audible sounds made by most mechanical prostheses (Siefert, 1987). After consideration of these medical and patient-related factors, biologic or tissue valves may be deemed more appropriate for specific patients in the young and middle-aged groups.

Patients over the age of 65 to 70 years, those with a life expectancy of less than 10 years, and those in whom anticoagulation is deemed undesirable or contraindicated usually receive a biologic prosthesis. Exceptions to these guidelines may include patients who for cultural or religious reasons do not want specific types of animal valves or who require anticoagulation for chronic atrial fibrillation or past thromboembolic episodes. In the latter group, the primary advantage of having a tissue valve is cancelled because the patient will need long-term anticoagulation for other medical conditions (Bonchek, 1987). Individuals with chronic renal failure or hypercalcemia in most instances should not receive a tissue heterograft because of the high probability of primary tissue failure within a few years (Braunwald, 1988; Kirklin and Barratt-Boyes, 1986).

In patients with isolated aortic valvular disease or those requiring Bentall-type procedures, aortic homografts and pulmonary autografts have been used successfully. These valves and conduits may be especially promising for young patients in whom anticoagulation is contraindicated. Unfortunately, because the donor supply of homografts is limited, only specific patient populations can be considered for this type of valve replacement (Stelzer and Elkins, 1989).

Long-term Results

Long-term results following valvular surgery are dependent upon patient, valve, and health care–related factors. Patient-related factors include preoperative left ventricular function, associated coronary artery disease, other medical problems such as diabetes, hypertension, renal insufficiency, and chronic obstructive pulmonary disease, and the patient's attitude and compliance with medication, diet, and follow-up regimens. Valve-related factors include complications associated with the type and size of the prosthesis implanted.

The predominant complications associated with mechanical valves are related to the relative adequacy or inadequacy of anticoagulation, thrombosis, thromboembolism, and hemorrhage (Stelzer and Elkins, 1989). In 1987, in a review of thrombotic and bleeding complications associated with prosthetic valves, Edmunds found that 30% to 50% of patients had prothrombin times outside the therapeutic range, either above or below (Edmunds, 1987). This researcher also found that 80% to 90% of all thromboembolic complications and 20% to 30% of all bleeding complications involved the central nervous system (Edmunds, 1987). Rare complications associated with mechanical valves include perivalvular leak, valve thrombosis, hemolysis, and mechanical failure.

Porcine and bovine bioprostheses are subject to higher rates of primary tissue failure after 5 to 10 years. All heterograft prostheses are inherently stenotic compared with the orifice of the normal native valve. "Prosthesis to patient mismatch" is an uncommon complication that can occur with either a mechanical or a biologic valve (Westaby, 1985). This phenomenon results when the orifice of the prosthetic valve is too small to meet the patient's requirements adequately, especially during exercise. Prosthesis to patient mismatch is suspected when a patient demonstrates worse hemodynamic function and symptoms after a technically satisfactory valve replacement (Westaby, 1985).

Foremost among health care–related factors that affect patient morbidity, mortality, and long-term results are the expertise of the medical and surgical teams. Additionally, the timing of surgery in relation to the course of the disease process, the quality and expertise of the care received throughout the postoperative period, and access to cardiac rehabilitation and patient teaching programs all have an impact on patient outcome (Rahimtoola, 1988).

In addition to these factors, intraoperative improvements in myocardial preservation, better postoperative management of left ventricular dysfunction employing the intra-aortic balloon, inotropic and vasodilator drug therapy, and revascularization for patients with concurrent coronary artery disease all have had a positive influence on hospital morbidity, mortality, and long-term survival (Winters and Samuels, 1986). Recent studies have demonstrated that mitral valve repair seems to be associated with a lower operative mortality, a decreased incidence of thromboembolism, improved left ventricular function, and better long-term survival than mitral valve replacement in patients with amenable lesions (Cohen et al., 1988; Rahimtoola, 1988).

PREOPERATIVE CARE

Initial Assessment. Comprehensive systematic assessment elicits vital information in the preliminary stages to prepare the patient for cardiovascular surgery. The initial assessment of the patient and family, focusing upon physiologic, psychological, psychosocial, and spiritual factors and concerns, will enable the critical care nurse to compile an extensive and informative data base. Upon completion, identification of actual and potential problems will assist the nurse in delineating factors that may affect the surgical outcome and in formulating an individualized plan of care. Sharing the plan and any other vital information among caregivers assists in maximizing continuity of care. Reducing fragmentation of care resulting from the shortened lengths of stay in acute care areas represents a continuous challenge to the health team. Thus, pertinent patient information must be relayed in a manner that includes nurses in the operating room, intensive care unit, and progressive care unit who will eventually be caring for the patient.

Diagnostic Studies. A series of preoperative routine laboratory studies are utilized in the assessment of physiologic function (Table 20–4). Modifications should be made on an individual basis, utilizing discretion to determine need for extensive testing in an attempt to promote cost efficiency.

Routine complete blood count (CBC), electrolytes, blood urea nitrogen (BUN), creatinine, prothrombien time (PT), partial thromboplastin time (PTT), and bleeding time are evaluated. Chest radiographs and electrocardiograms are done to establish baseline information. Urinalysis may be done to rule out urinary tract infection. In patients about to undergo valvular surgery, dental consultations are obtained to confirm the absence of any periodontal infection. These measures are enacted to reduce the risk of postoperative endocarditis.

Pulmonary function tests (PFTs) may be obtained to identify patients at high risk for respiratory complications or respiratory failure in the postoperative period. However, there is conflicting evidence about the relationship between preoperative pulmonary status and postoperative outcome. Some reports indicate that vital capacity and flow greater than 80% represents a low risk and that results that are less than 50% of the predicted value signify a high risk for postoperative pulmonary complications (Braunwald, 1988). Ingersoll (1991), however, demonstrated no correlation between diminished pulmonary function and the need for prolonged mechanical ventilation. Thus, the need for preoperative pulmonary function measurements remains questionable.

Cardiovascular performance and valvular function are evaluated through findings from the electrocardiogram, echocardiogram, cardiac catheterization, and magnetic resonance imaging. The echocardiogram provides valuable baseline data regarding chamber dimensions, wall excursion, valvular motion, thickening, calcification, and prolapse. Coronary angiography reveals details of the location, severity, and shape of coronary lesions. Close study of the coronary anatomy will assist the surgeon in devising and formulating an appropriate plan for revascularization. Valvular function is assessed through calculation of transvalvular pressure gradients and estimation of valve area. Ventriculography determines the left ventricular ejection fraction and the degree of mitral regurgitation, and aortography

---

TABLE 20–4. Common Preoperative Diagnostic Studies

Cardiac	Respiratory	Renal/Metabolic
Electrocardiogram	Arterial blood gases	Serum electrolytes
Exercise tolerance test	Chest roentgenogram	Blood urea nitrogen (BUN)
Cardiac echocardiogram	Pulmonary function tests*	Creatinine
Cardiac catheterization		Urine analysis
Magnetic resonance imaging		

Neurologic*	Vascular*	Miscellaneous
Carotid flow studies	Doppler flow profile	Blood bank specimen
Carotid angiography	Ankle brachial index	Type and crossmatch
		HIV screen
		Heparin sensitivity screen

Hepatic	Hematologic	
Bilirubin	Hematocrit	
Lactic dehydrogenase	White blood count	
SGOT; SGPT	Hemoglobin	
Total protein	Platelet count	
Albumin	Prothrombin time	
Lipid profile	Partial thromboplastin time	
	Bleeding time	
	Fibrinogen	

*If indicated by clinical findings or past medical history.

aids in evaluating regurgitant flow in patients with aortic regurgitation. Magnetic resonance imaging is gaining closer attention for use in patients with poor ventricular function or valvular disease to determine the presence of thrombus and the need for prophylactic intervention.

The presence of carotid atherosclerotic disease is significant for the patient about to undergo CABG or valve replacement. The use of angiography or duplex scanning is the most reliable method of detecting carotid disease. Studies have shown a significantly higher neurologic complication rate after CABG in patients with greater than 50% narrowing of carotid vessels. When indicated, carotid endarterectomy is often performed concomitantly with CABG to reduce the risk of ischemic induced neurologic injury (Hurst et al., 1986). Thus, the role of preoperative carotid screening serves as a valuable tool in identifying patients at risk for stroke following CABG (Faggioli et al., 1990).

Close examination of the coagulation profile is of paramount importance. Consumption of aspirin products, nonsteroidal anti-inflammatory agents, or warfarin alters bleeding time on studies, predisposing the patient to an increased risk of coagulopathy as a postoperative complication and potentially requiring transfusion. Type and crossmatch, autologous blood donations, and direct donor donations are currently used to ensure the presence of an adequate blood reserve prior to surgery.

Autologous blood donation is encouraged in many centers for patients undergoing elective surgery. It is estimated that only 5% of all eligible patients participate in the program, indicating a significant underutilization of this service (Toy et al., 1987). Predonation has been considered safe for patients with cardiovascular disease. Eligibility criteria include patients with chronic angina but precludes those with preinfarction angina. Use of autologous blood programs have helped to reduce the need for homologous transfusions as well as transmission of blood-borne diseases. Some centers have reported a 50% decrease in the need for homologous blood transfusion postoperatively. Approximately 73% to 75% of patients who predonated blood avoided homologous transfusions compared to 18% to 20% who did not donate (Britton et al., 1989). Most patients donate an average of one unit of blood per week. The American Association of Blood Banks has established guidelines for autologous blood donation (Table 20–5). Factors affecting donation are progression of angina, anemia, and development of new symptoms. Current investigations are now focusing on the use of synthetic growth hormones such as erythropoietin to stimulate red blood cell production, increasing the ability of patients to donate. In addition to red cell autologous transfusion, interest has also increased in the readministration of plasma and platelets during cardiopulmonary bypass to reduce bleeding risk and augment hemostasis (Boldt et al., 1990).

TABLE 20–5. General Guidelines for Predonation of Autologous Blood

1. No upper age limit
2. No more than 450 mL (or 12% of estimated blood volume, whichever is less) may be withdrawn per single donation
3. Saline solution used for isovolemic replacement
4. Minimum hemoglobin concentration = 11 g/dL
5. Minimum hemocrit = 0.34 or greater at time of donation
6. Maximum of one donation every 3 days
7. Oral iron supplementation recommended. Administration should begin 1 week prior to first donation and should be continued for several months following last donation. Dosage of ferrous sulfate, 325 mg three times a day

Adapted from Walker (1990). American Association of Blood Banks (AABB) Technical Manual. Arlington, VA: AABB Publishers, pp 433–448.

Medications. The value of obtaining a complete medication history cannot be overemphasized. Prior to surgery, the modification of certain medications is warranted to avert the development of perioperative complications. First and foremost, all aspirin and nonsteroidal anti-inflammatory products must be discontinued at least 7 to 10 days prior to surgery. Aspirin acts to inhibit thromboxane synthesis, thereby inhibiting platelet aggregation and vasoconstriction. This effect persists 5 to 7 days or for the life of the platelet. This action, in combination with the effects of cardiopulmonary bypass on platelet membranes, has been associated with an increased perioperative blood loss (Ferraris et al., 1988). Resultant bleeding increases the risk of cardiac tamponade, reoperation, and transfusion requirement. Other agents known to interfere with platelet function are ampicillin, carbenicillin, diphenhydramine, furosemide, gentamicin, ibuprofen, indomethacin, nitrofurantoin, papaverine, penicillin, phenothiazines, propranolol, sulfinpyrazone, and tricyclic amines (Bick, 1984). Recent reports have linked the intake of large amounts of omega-3 fatty acids to increased risk of bleeding times, especially in patients taking coumarin or aspirin (Leaf and Weber, 1988). Patients on warfarin are advised to refrain from consumption 5 days prior to surgery. Knowledge of the impact of these agents upon hemostasis will assist the nurse in identifying high-risk patients. Postoperative bleeding remains a risk in some cases when prothrombin times have returned to normal. Administration of vitamin K may be considered to ensure adequate reversal and hemostasis. If continuous anticoagulation is warranted, as is often the case in patients awaiting valvular surgery, heparin therapy is initiated upon admission and terminated 4 to 8 hours prior to anesthetic induction.

All antianginal agents such as beta-adrenergic blocking agents, calcium channel blockers, and nitrates are continued. With the increased emotional and physiologic stress experienced by patients preoperatively, continued administration of antianginal agents is warranted to prevent exacerbation of ischemic symptoms or myocardial damage. Propranolol has been found to be effective for controlling increased adrenergic stimulation, assisting in anesthetic induction, and reducing the incidence of perioperative ventricular dysrhythmias (Hurst et al., 1986). The use of propranolol has not been found to depress postoperative myocardial performance (Hurst et al., 1986).

Digoxin is usually withheld 1 to 2 days prior to surgery except in patients with atrial fibrillation with a poorly controlled ventricular response (Hurst et al., 1986). It has been found that serum digoxin levels tend to rise in these patients, a phenomenon that is poorly understood but is thought to be linked to the effects of cardiopulmonary bypass.

Additional medications administered include prophylactic antibiotics, most commonly a broad-spectrum cephalosporin. Many centers recently have added dipyridamole (100 mg three times a day) to the preoperative regimen. The role of antiplatelet therapy started early has shown to be effective in reducing the incidence of thrombosis and early vein graft occlusion (Goldman et al., 1988). Some centers also have focused on the administration of allopurinol preoperatively. Allopurinol acts to inhibit the formation of cytotoxic free radicals during myocardial ischemia and reperfusion. Johnson and colleagues (1991) found that allopurinol improved postoperative cardiac performance, demonstrated by a reduced need for inotropic support or mechanical support. The recommended dose is 200 to 400 mg (depending upon patient weight) administered once on the evening before the operation and once 4 hours prior to surgery.

Preoperative Teaching. The value of preoperative teaching cannot be overemphasized. Patients undergoing CABG have increased levels of emotional anxiety and stress (Pieper et al., 1985). Consequently, many patients experience an increase in frequency and severity of angina, potentially inducing untoward ischemia. The nursing literature now cites research validating the efficacy of preoperative preparation resulting in decreased anxiety, prevention of postoperative complications, and quicker recovery (Christophersen and Pfieffer, 1980; Lindeman and Stetzer, 1973). A variety of programs, both structured and unstructured, exist to provide the necessary information to prepare the patient for surgery (Sutcliffe and Ridder, 1984; Gross, 1988).

Most patients arrive the day before surgery. With increasing financial constraints, many institutions now admit patients on the day of surgery, creating the need to develop innovative teaching strategies for this population. However, traditionally, during the preoperative period the patient is seen by the anesthesiologist, the surgeon, and the chest physical therapist. The primary nurse plays a vital role in initiating the teaching process or helping the patient focus on key points. The provision of sensory and environmental information will help the patient to formulate more realistic expectations about the anticipated events during the postoperative period (Johnson, 1972). A tour of the surgical intensive care unit may be helpful. Also, a visit from the critical care nurse may offer the patient the increased security of becoming acquainted with his or her caregivers. The development of preoperative visits by critical care nurses has been effective in decreasing postoperative patient anxiety as well as providing advance information for the nurse to use in formulating an initial plan of care (Sutcliffe and Ridder, 1984; Gross, 1988).

Information is provided to patients about the course of events. Concepts about invasive monitoring, mechanical ventilation, respiratory care or therapy, pain management, and visiting hours are discussed and reinforced by the critical care nurse. Incorporating the family in the teaching process and encouraging them to ask questions and voice concerns is extremely important in assisting both patient and family through the recovery period.

INTRAOPERATIVE MANAGEMENT

Cardiopulmonary Bypass

The first successful use of extracorporal cardiopulmonary bypass (CPB) in humans was undertaken by Gibbson in 1954. Cardiopulmonary bypass is a method by which venous blood is diverted from the arrested heart's right atrium to pass through either a membrane or a bubble oxygenator. In the oxygenator, through the process of diffusion, carbon dioxide is given off and oxygen is bound to hemoglobin. Once arterialized, the blood is returned to the body through the aorta for systemic distribution (Edmunds and Stephenson, 1983; Blanche et al., 1990; Moores and Willford, 1989). The diversion of blood provides the surgeon with a bloodless immobilized heart muscle on which to work. Improvements in the delivery of hypothermia, myocardial protection, anesthesia, blood conservation, and surgical techniques all have contributed to the ever decreasing mortality associated with various types of cardiac operations.

Although CPB clearly has contributed greatly to the art and science of cardiac surgery, it is not without consequences. Nurses caring for these patients in the perioperative phase need to understand the operative events that affect common postoperative clinical problems. This section will review the components of the cardiopulmonary bypass machine, myocardial preservation, the systemic pathophysiologic responses associated with the conduct of CPB, common nursing problems, and the management of cardiac surgical patients.

Hemodilution. The CPB machine is usually primed with a crystalloid solution. A volume of 1800 to 2000 mL of fluid, or the equivalent of 20 mL/kg, is used, resulting in dilution of the serum hematocrit to the range of 20% to 25% (Edmunds and Stephenson, 1983; Milam, 1983; Blanche et al., 1990). Because of loss of pulsatile pressure while on CPB and hemodilution, some of the perfusate becomes translocated into the interstitial space (Milam, 1983). Albumin may be used in the priming solution to balance the changed oncotic pressures and maintain volume in the intravascular space. However, Marelli and associates (1989) conducted a randomized study on the efficacy of the use of albumin in the priming solution on clinical outcomes. These investigators found no significant difference in the group in which albumin was used.

Heparinization. After the chest is opened and prior to cannulation of the great vessels and cardiac chambers, heparin at 3 mg/kg is administered to prevent spontaneous clot formation as blood comes in contact with the approximately 40 feet of polyvinylchloride tubing associated with the CPB system (Milam, 1983; Blanche et al., 1990). A baseline activated clotting time (ACT) is measured prior to the first injection of heparin, which inhibits clotting factors V, IX, XI, XIIa, and thrombin (Blanche et al., 1990; Edmunds and Stephenson, 1983). While on CPB, the ACT is measured every 30 to 60 minutes and should be maintained between 350 and 500 seconds during both normothermic and hypothermic states with supplemental heparin (Gralee et al., 1990).

At completion of the cardiac operation, protamine sulfate is given in a dose of approximately 1.3 mg to each 1-mg dose of heparin given, including any used in the priming solution to reverse the clotting inhibition (Edmunds and Stephenson, 1983; Milam, 1983; Blanche et al., 1990). Protamine administration at the completion of CPB has been demonstrated to cause significant hemodynamic effects due to systemic vasodilation, hypotension, and myocardial dysfunction (Levy et al., 1989; Michaels and Barash, 1983). Right ventricular dysfunction caused by pulmonary vasoconstriction due to protamine has also been demonstrated (Lewenstein et al., 1983). Patients with a history of insulin-dependent diabetes using protamine zinc insulin or with allergies to seafood may also be at risk of developing anaphylaxis with protamine administration. Another population at risk is male patients who have had a vasectomy. In this group, it is reported that 1 year after the vasectomy, up to 55% of patients develop antibodies to human protamine produced by sperm (Samuel, 1977). Because protamine is derived from salmon gonadal tissue, vasectomized patients are at risk of having developed a sensitivity to the drug and therefore a potential anaphylactoid reaction (Levy et al., 1989). When a reaction is anticipated, pretreatment using steroids, diphenhydramine hydrochloride (Benadryl), and ranitidine (Zantac) is recommended. Blanche and associates (1990) recommend that protamine be administered after removal of the venous catheters but before removal of the arterial catheter because CPB may need to be reinitiated emergently.

Arterial Cannulation. Cannulation of the ascending aorta proximal to the innominate artery provides a route for returning the arterialized blood back to the patient after he has been heparinized. Care must be taken not to dislodge plaques during placement of the cannula, precipitating embolic events. In patients with conditions such as a severely calcified ascending aorta or with surgery involving the aortic arch or brachiocephalic vessels, or with initiation of emergency bypass, the femoral arteries can be used as an alternative route for cannulation. On rare occasions, the axillary artery is also used to initiate CPB (Edmunds and Stephenson, 1983; Blanche et al., 1990). However, cannulation of smaller arteries may increase the risk of embolic phenomena or ischemia to a limb. If alternate approaches are used, nurses need to survey the extremities involved closely for potential alterations in tissue perfusion. Additionally, patients need to be assessed for changes in baseline mental status.

Venous Cannulation. Systemic venous blood from the right atrium and inferior vena cava (IVC) and superior vena cava (SVC) is diverted from the heart, usually by one single right atrial catheter (Edmunds and Stephenson, 1983; Blanche et al., 1990). This catheter is usually placed through the lateral wall of the right atrial appendage (Blanche et al., 1990). A newer catheter is also available that utilizes the same placement position but has two extensions capable of cannulating both the IVC and SVC independently (Blanche et al., 1990). Venus return to the CPB machine occurs by gravity in the manner of a siphon and is completely dependent upon a closed system without air. Therefore, any procedure that has the potential to introduce air into the right side of the heart requires independent cannulation of the cavae. Patients requiring atriotomy, ventriculotomy (Blanche et al., 1990), or procedures involving the pulmonary arteries or repair of communications between the atria or ventricles require separate cannulation of the IVC and SVC. Once either cannulation method has been accomplished, venous blood returning to the right atria through the coronary sinus is stopped with the institution of aortic cross clamping and cardioplegic arrest (McKnight et al., 1985). Cannulation of either the arterial or the venous side of the heart can lead potentially to introduction of air or dislodgement of plaque, causing systemic embolization.

As the blood travels through the various components of the CPB machine, destruction of the blood cells can occur in the suction system, reservoirs, heat exchanger, or oxygenator. A review of these components and their normal function follows. The intent of this section is to demystify the operation of the CPB machine and to provide a basis for anticipating care.

Cardiotomy Suction System. Blood conserved from the operative field is removed and returned to the extracorporeal perfusion system by way of the cardiotomy suction system (Edmunds and Stephenson, 1983). This aspirate contains calcium, bits of sutures, fat, or fibrin, and foreign materials that are filtered through the CPB system to prevent systemic embolization. Delong and associates (1980) demonstrated that the intense blood–air contact made during suctioning has a major effect upon blood cell hemolysis in conjunction with use of the CPB oxygenator. Although blood conservation is the objective, some hemolysis does occur.

Venous Reservoirs. A venous reservoir is a conduit for deoxygenated blood and is a part of the CPB machine. It is usually positioned 30 cm below the right atrium to facilitate passive venous drainage before blood enters the oxygenator. In the bubble oxygenator system, venous blood enters the oxygenator directly and is arterialized (Edmunds and Stephenson, 1983; Blanche et al., 1990) (Figs. 20–11 and 20–12). These conduits also receive filtered blood from the operative field from the cardiotomy system.

Bubble Oxygenator. The bubble oxygenator is the most commonly used oxygenator because it is thought to have little hemolytic effect on the red blood cells (RBCs) (Milam, 1983). Oxygenation occurs when venous blood comes in contact with oxygenated bubbles. During this interface, oxygen diffuses from the bubbles and is absorbed by the RBCs of the venous blood while CO_2 diffuses in the opposite direction. Bubbles in the arterialized blood are removed by passing the blood over a large mesh or sponge surface area that is treated with an antifoam agent. The arterialized blood then enters a large settling chamber or reservoir in which heat exchange occurs (Edmunds and Stephenson, 1983; Blanche et al., 1990). Arterialized blood is then pumped into a chamber, where it is filtered again for potential

gaseous emboli prior to being returned to the aorta for systemic distribution.

Membrane Oxygenator. Venous blood passes through a separate heat exchanger before entering the membrane oxygenator. Once inside the oxygenator, blood never comes in direct contact with oxygen but instead covers a large semipermeable capillary-type membrane. Arterialization of the venous blood occurs by diffusion when CO_2 is given off by the RBCs and oxygen diffuses across the membrane from the oxygenator. A filter is not needed in this system because the arterialized blood is then returned directly to the patient after oxygenation.

The bubble oxygenator causes less damage to blood cells on CPB runs of 3 hours or less (Clark et al., 1979). When CPB runs are anticipated to be longer than 3 hours, the membrane oxygenator causes less damage to blood cells (Boonstra et al., 1986). In clinical use, the bubble oxygenator has the advantage of being easy to prime and assemble, simple to use, and relatively inexpensive.

Pumps. Both the roller pump and the centrifugal pump are used at present to conduct cardiac operations. Originally designed by Dr. DeBakey in 1934, the roller pump used today is virtually unchanged (DeBakey, 1934) (Fig. 20–13). It is simple to use, reliable, produces low blood trauma, and delivers accurate perfusion rates. Flow through the roller pump is delivered by the degree of partial occlusion applied to the CPB tubing by the roller. Pump output is proportional to the speed of rotation and the internal diameter of the compressible tubing (Edmunds and Stephenson, 1983). Flow rates of 1.6 to 2.2 liters/m² per minute in conjunction with hypothermia are thought to deliver adequate blood volume while on CPB without causing cerebral dysfunction (Edmunds and Stephenson, 1983). The roller

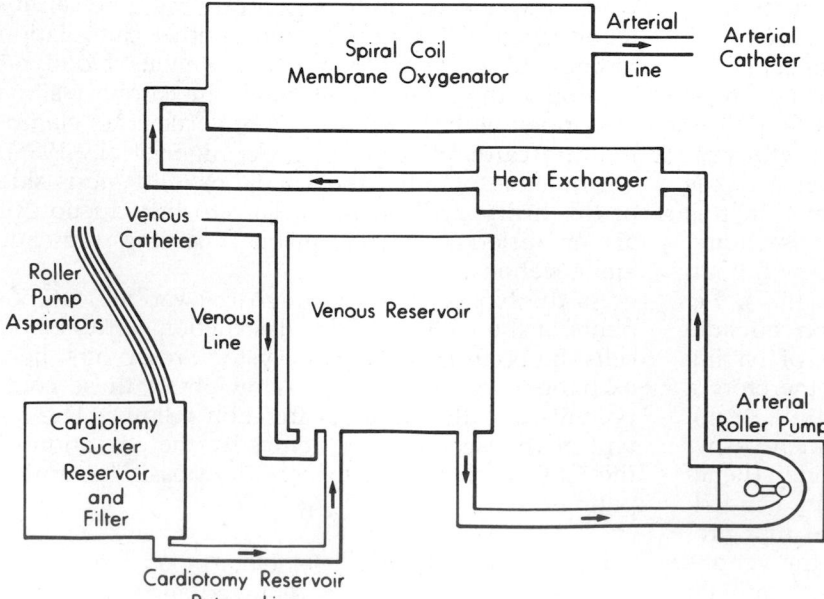

FIGURE 20–11. Diagram of a typical set-up for cardiopulmonary bypass using a spiral coil type membrane oxygenator. (From Edmunds, H., and Stephenson, L. (1983). Cardiopulmonary bypass for open heart surgery. In Geha, A., et al. (Eds.), *Thoracic and cardiovascular surgery* (4th ed., p. 1092). E. Norwalk, CT: Appleton-Century-Crofts.)

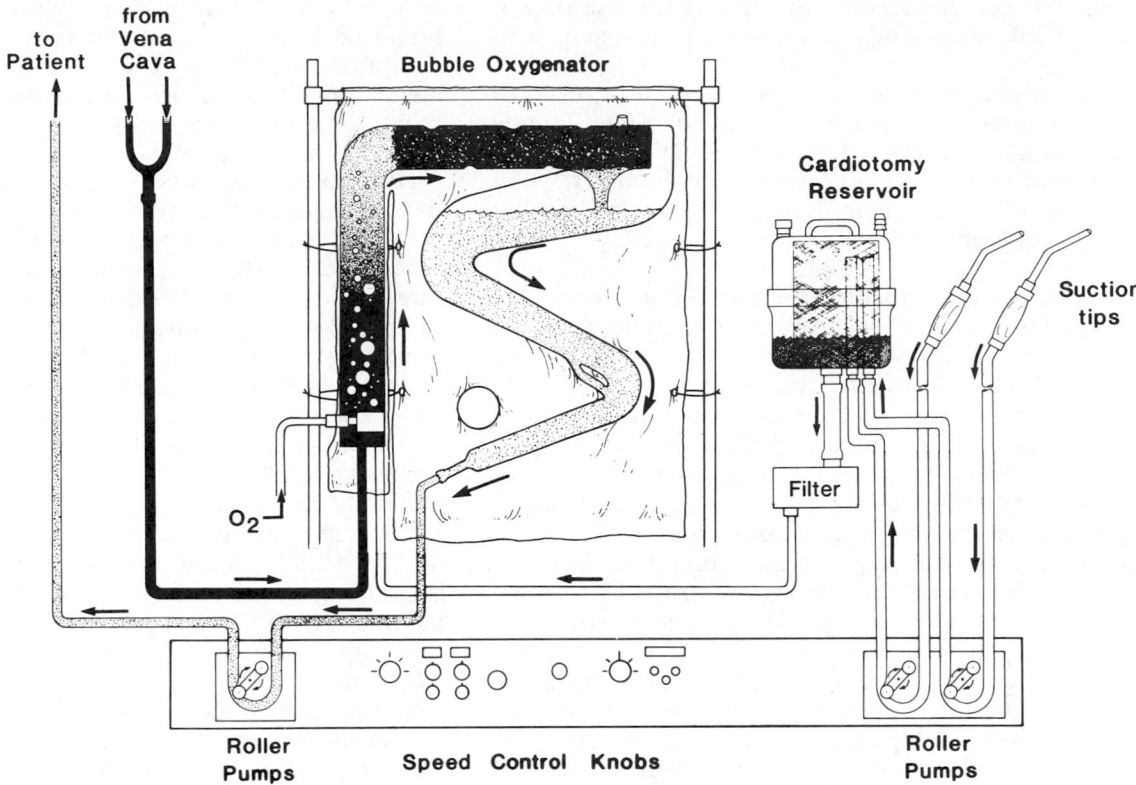

to Patient

from Vena Cava

Bubble Oxygenator

O_2

Cardiotomy Reservoir

Suction tips

Filter

Roller Pumps

Speed Control Knobs

Roller Pumps

FIGURE 20–12. Composite illustration of a cardiopulmonary bypass system utilizing a bubble oxygenator system. (From Milam, J. (1983). Blood transfusion in heart surgery. *Surgical Clinics of North America*, 65, 1127–1146.)

pump delivers continuous nonpulsatile blood flow to the tissue. Although adequate for CPB, this flow state contributes to the pathophysiologic systemic changes seen in the postoperative period.

Use of a pump that delivers pulsatile flows during CPB has been thought to be more physiologic. Very little clinical use of this pump has been documented (Reis et al., 1987; Moores et al., 1977; Niemmen et al., 1980; Singh et al., 1980). However, pulsatile flow

is thought to produce less metabolic acidosis, lower peripheral arterial resistance, improved cerebral perfusion, less hepatocellular injury, improved myocardial perfusion to the subendocardium, and expedient cooling and warming of body tissues (Ries et al., 1987). Study of the effects of pulsatile flows on the cooling and rewarming of tissues has not proved this approach to be beneficial (Singh et al., 1980; Niemmen et al., 1983). At present, clinical study has not

FIGURE 20–13. Diagram of a roller pump used in both the membrane and bubble oxygenator systems. (From Milam, J. (1983). *Surgical Clinics of North America*, 63 (5), 1127–1147.)

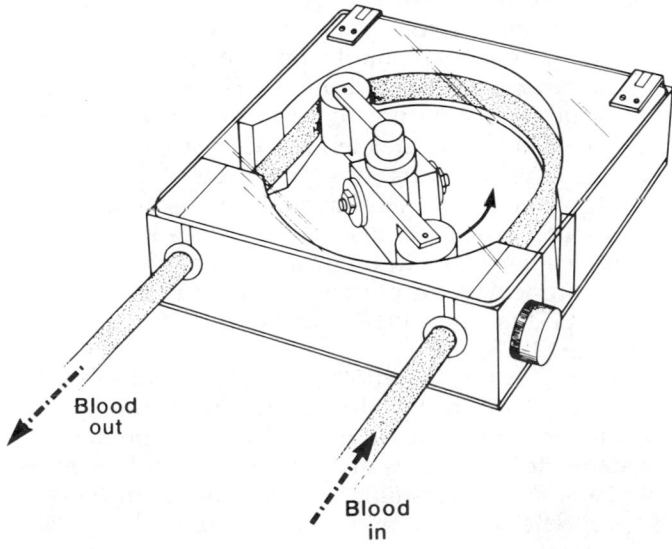

Blood out

Blood in

provided conclusive data to support the use of pulsatile CPB; more study is needed on the use of such pumps.

Centrifugal pumps move blood by an impeller or vortexing motion (Blanche et al., 1990). These pumps have been used for long-term cardiac-assist devices and appear to cause less trauma to blood. They are gaining more consideration in routine use during cardiac operation.

Hypothermia and Blood Flows. Hypothermia reduces the metabolic need for oxygen and provides an important margin of safety during cardiac surgery (Reitz, 1982). Biochemical reactions are described as a function of a 10°C change in temperature (Moores and Willford, 1989; Milam, 1983). It has been stated that for every 10°C increase in temperature, the metabolic rate increases by 50%. The converse occurs when the temperature decreases by 10°C. Likewise, moderate systemic hypothermia (temperatures of 25° to 32°C) has several advantages during CPB: lower perfusion flow requirements, less myocardial rewarming, less blood trauma, and protection of organs during brief hypothermia (Moores and Williford, 1989). Initially, surface-induced hypothermia was thought to be safer than core cooling through CPB (Haneda et al., 1982). However, use of the surface method prolonged cooling and was abandoned because of the need for prolonged rewarming time and increased metabolic acidosis. Also, its use was prohibitive in hemodynamically unstable patients (Cameron and Gardner, 1988).

During the hypothermic state, a left shift in the oxyhemoglobin dissociation curve occurs. This results in less unloading of oxygen from the hemoglobin molecule. However, as long as the tissue metabolic need for oxygen is decreased, a balance of oxygen supply and demand is maintained.

While on CPB perfusion flow rates take the place of the cardiac index and may range from 1.8 to 2.4 liters/minute per square meter during systemic hypothermia of 25°C (Cameron and Gardner, 1988; Blanche et al., 1990). Hickey and Hoor (1983) conducted a clinical trial that monitored oxygen consumption in a small population of patients undergoing coronary revascularization. Flow rates of 1.2 liters/minute/m^2 did not produce formation of detrimental acidosis or deleterious decreases in mixed venous oxygen saturations compared with flows of 2.2 liters/minute/m^2. The advantage of using low flow rates while on CPB is that they produce less venous return to the heart through noncoronary collaterals of the bronchial and pulmonary vessels because less blood perfuses through the body (Cameron and Gardner, 1988).

Optimal systemic hypothermia and perfusion flow rates are individualized. Patients with few or no collaterals benefit least from deeper hypothermia. Systemic temperatures of 28° to 30°C with flow rates of 2.2 to 2.4 liters/minute per square meter are appropriate. In patients with extensive collateralization, anticipated complex procedures, and or a compromised heart, the converse is true. Systemic temperatures of 20° to 25°C and flow rates of 1.6 liters/minute per square meter may be appropriate (Cameron and Gardner, 1988).

Heat Exchanger. Both oxygenator systems have heat exchanges that allow for the cooling and rewarming of body temperature. Body temperature is monitored closely using a nasopharyngeal temperature probe, which reflects brain temperature and is the most sensitive indicator of systemic temperature changes (Cameron and Gardner, 1988). Core temperature is usually monitored using a pulmonary artery catheter or rectal probe. Most cardiac surgeons at present use systemic hypothermia to depress the metabolic cellular rate, thereby decreasing tissue vulnerability to ischemia (Moores and Willford, 1988). Adult temperatures are usually decreased at a rate of 0.7° to 1.5°C/minute to achieve moderate systemic hypothermia ranging from 25° to 32°C (Edmunds and Stephenson, 1983; Cameron and Gardner, 1988). Rewarming occurs at a slower rate of 0.2° to 0.5°C/minute (Edmunds and Stephenson, 1983). Clinically, the rate of systemic rewarming is limited by perfusion flow rates in the extracorporeal circuit and temperature gradients between the heat exchanger, blood, and tissue (Cameron and Gardner, 1988). The temperature of blood generated by the heat exchanger should not exceed 40° to 42°C during rewarming because a risk of protein denaturation and hemolysis to blood cells occurs at 44°C (Edmunds and Stephenson, 1983; Cameron and Gardner, 1988; Blanche et al., 1990). Close monitoring of temperature gradient differences between the perfusate temperature and the nasopharyngeal temperature is maintained to ensure that the gradient remains between 6° and 8°C. Such a gradient is maintained during systemic cooling and rewarming because gases may be liberated from solution when cool blood perfuses warmed tissue or when cool blood is rewarmed (Blanche et al., 1990).

Myocardial Protection

This review of the technical aspects of the conduct of CPB is most helpful for nurses caring for cardiac surgical patients. The advent of the use of CPB has allowed surgeons to perform delicate cardiac operations while supporting the patient's systemic metabolic function. However, one of the most crucial aspects of the operation is myocardial preservation. This section will give nurses an understanding of the basic approaches to myocardial preservation as it affects ventricular functioning in the postoperative period. Such information, in conjunction with a knowledge of the conduct of CPB, will provide a foundation for anticipating nursing care for these patients.

Optimal subendocardial preservation during cardiac operations has a major impact on morbidity and mortality during the perioperative period. The initial techniques used to protect the subendocardium and provide the surgeon with a bloodless arrested heart were hypothermic intermittent ischemic arrest with aortic cross clamping (Olinger, 1988) and the induction of ventricular fibrillation (Buckberg, 1983). These techniques were attempts to decrease the oxygen debt during the period of myocardial anoxia. However, the former approach accentuated changes in anaerobic metabolism, causing increased intracellular acidosis, and altered cellular enzymatic functions (Kirklin and Barrat-Boyes, 1986). Further, the latter approach depleted ATP and high-energy phosphate stores within the myocardial cells (Buckberg, 1983; Cameron and Gardnar, 1988). Both approaches were associated with subendocardial injury and support the present use of a high-potassium cardioplegic solution to precipitate global myocardial arrest.

The key considerations in preventing subendocardial damage depend on decreasing myocardial energy demands during the ischemic period while salvaging enough energy stores to meet these demands. Care is also taken to prevent both iatrogenic injury due to excessive cold, excessive retraction on the organ, trauma, or potassium-induced fibrosis and damage caused by the reperfusion process (Silverman et al., 1988). Therefore, the goals of myocardial protection are prevention of cardiac muscle injury through induction of rapid electromechanical arrest, adequate hypothermia, buffering of the myocardial and systemic acidotic state, and prevention of intracellular edema (Silverman et al., 1988).

Cardinal to subendocardial protection is the provision of continuous, even myocardial hypothermia. Maintenance of hypothermic myocardial temperatures during aortic cross clamping depends upon maintaining the balance between heat escaping and heat entering the tissues (Rosenfeldt, 1988). Rosenfeld and colleagues (1988) studied the effects of noncoronary blood flow of pulmonary venous return to the left heart and inadequate systemic venous drainage to the CPB system on rewarming the hypothermic heart. These investigators demonstrated that bronchial venous return increased septal temperatures. Systemic and pulmonary venous return entering the cardiac chambers was found to be a significant heat source that precipitated early rewarming and ischemic injury to the myocardium. These data support the notion that such venous return may also cause injury to the conduction system through early rewarming.

To prevent these injuries from warmed venous blood entering the cardiac chambers, cold cardioplegia and topical cooling techniques are used. Typically, concern about the evenness of cooling the dense ventricular mass, specifically in the hypertrophied left ventricle, warrants the common practice of using adjunctive topical cooling with a cold cardioplegia infusion (Rosenfeldt and Watson, 1979; Blanche et al., 1990). Various methods of topical

cooling have been used. For example, recirculating solutions have been used in both open techniques, such as cold saline ice solution poured into the operative field (Edmunds and Stephenson, 1983; McKnight et al., 1985; Silverman et al., 1988), and closed techniques, such as cooling jackets (Bonchek and Olinger, 1981). Although the use of the cooling jacket theoretically has advantages, it has proved to be inadequate in maintaining uniform myocardial temperatures and interferes with surgical logistics (Rosenfeldt and Arnold, 1982). Whichever method is used, myocardial hypothermic temperatures between 12° and 20°C have been demonstrated to provide adequate protection in both hypertrophic and normal ventricular myocardium (Rosenfeldt, 1988; Blanche et al., 1990). Protection of the subendocardium (i.e., swift induction and maintenance of diastolic arrest), global myocardial hypothermia, and use of cardioplegia are attempts to minimize cell injury.

Investigation into the determinants of adequate myocardial protection has focused on ventricular preservation and recovery. However, early study has demonstrated that inadequate interatrial temperatures of 25° to 30°C result from the use of hypothermic antegrade cardioplegic techniques (Smith et al., 1983). Atrial activity secondary to early rewarming of the atrial septum has been suggested as an explanation for the high incidence of postoperative tachydysrhythmias (Tchervenkov et al., 1983; Ferguson et al., 1986) and conduction defects (Fergusson et al., 1987; Williams, 1988). Preliminary data on using warm blood cardioplegia via the retrograde method (Salerno et al., 1991) and the use of the right atrial method of cardioplegia delivery seem to offer decreased supraventricular dysrhythmias.

Upon aortic cross clamping, an intracellular ischemic period occurs just prior to the onset of rapid diastolic arrest. During this period, endogenous catecholamines are secreted that deplete intracellular high-energy stores while myocardial cells undergo a hyperfunctional and hypermetabolic state. In efforts to reduce these cellular demands quickly, high potassium crystalloid or blood cardioplegia is widely used in conjunction with systemic hypothermic cooling measures to minimize cellular ischemic injury.

Adequate delivery of cardioplegic solution is cardinal to the prevention of myocardial injury. Although the majority of surgeons presently utilize the antegrade or aortic root method, either retrograde or cardioplegic administration via the coronary sinus (Chitwood, 1988) or the right atrial delivery method (Fabiani et al., 1986) is beginning to demonstrate promise. Although popular, antegrade delivery of cardioplegic solutions does have the disadvantages of uneven distribution of the solution past the stenotic native coronaries (Lust, 1987) and a potential for right ventricular intraoperative injury secondary to its thin-walled muscled mass and anatomic position (Morris and Whechler, 1988). The retrograde method has been documented to promote better distribution of the cardioplegic solution (Fabiani et al., 1987). Use of the right atrial method has provided data supporting a lowered incidence of postoperative tachydysrhythmias through the maintenance of even atrial hypothermia and diastolic arrest. Its usage may increase as research involving atrial preservation continues.

Cold high-potassium crystalloid solution is the most common cardioplegic solution used to produce global cardiac hypothermic arrest. Cardiac arrest is achieved through perfusion of the high-potassium solution through the native coronary vessels, which ultimately perfuse the myocardial cells. This causes an elevation in the extracellular potassium level, which decreases the resting membrane potential and inactivates the sodium channels. As a result, the cardiac cell is inactive and remains in diastolic arrest (Guyton, 1988; Silverman et al., 1988). Optimal temperature range for the delivery of cold crystalloid cardioplegia is between 10° and 15°C (Buckberg, 1988; Rosenfeldt, 1988; Blanche et al., 1990). Both the delivery of cardioplegic solution and the continuous maintenance of adequate temperatures may be impeded by perfusion gradients in diseased vessels, ventricular position, and muscle mass differences.

As long as the extracellular potassium level remains high, diastolic arrest will prevail. However, noncoronary flow can lower extracellular potassium and precipitate electrical mechanical activity, causing ischemic damage created by an oxygen debt. Use of intermittent reinfusion of hyperkalemic cardioplegia every 20 to 30 minutes, through either an antegrade or a retrograde approach, is a common practice used to prevent this washout (Silverman et al., 1988).

The superiority of blood cardioplegia over crystalloid cardioplegia remains controversial. Sanguineous cold cardioplegia has the major advantages of oxygen-carrying capacity (Edmunds and Stephenson, 1983; Cameron and Gardner, 1988; Blanche et al., 1990), excellent buffering capacity supporting a normal pH (Bodenhamer et al., 1983), and oncotic properties (Kresh et al., 1987). However, cold blood cardioplegia demonstrates a leftward shift of the oxyhemoglobin dissociation curve when used in conjunction with hypothermia. This impedes unloading of oxygen to the tissues (Cameron and Gardner, 1988; Cusmano et al., 1988). These effects are counterbalanced by a decrease in cellular oxygen demand. Clinical studies show that optimal temperatures for the delivery of cold blood cardioplegia are 15° to 20°C (Singh et al., 1981; Femes et al., 1984).

An emerging practice in maintaining myocardial protection is the use of normothermia in conjunction with high-potassium, warm blood cardioplegia delivered retrograde through the coronary sinus. Avoidance of hypothermia has the advantages of not interfering with biochemical cellular functions, maintaining the normal oxyhemoglobin dissociation curve, and avoiding the clinical problems associated with reperfusion (Salerno et al., 1991). Further, normothermia and the continuous circulation of warm whole blood has the advantages of providing oxygen and needed substrates to the myocardial cells during diastolic arrest. Through using the retrograde method via the coronary sinus, warm blood cardioplegia is evenly distributed to both the right and left ventricles and the interventricular septum (Drinkwater et al., 1990; Salerno et al., 1991).

Salerno and associates (1991) reported the first clinical use of these methods in 113 consecutive patients who underwent both coronary bypass and valve surgery. In this series, 6% of patients experienced perioperative myocardial infarction, 7% required the use of inotropic support, and 96% spontaneously converted to normal sinus rhythm without the need for defibrillation. Although still inconclusive, these data appear to be encouraging and may well change the recovery pattern for cardiac surgical patients.

Left Ventricular Venting

Ventricular distention is an intraoperative condition characterized by increased diastolic volume, impaired endocardial blood flow, and decreased cardiac output (Buckberg, 1983). During the myocardial arrested state, ventricular distention can elevate aortic root pressures, wash out cardioplegic solution, precipitate early rewarming of the heart, and potentially initiate ventricular or atrial contractions causing ischemic damage (Guyton, 1988). Techniques used to avoid ventricular distention are either active or passive. Active techniques such as placing a catheter in the left ventricle, ascending aorta, or pulmonary veins (Guyton, 1988; Blanche et al., 1990) are no longer commonly practiced. These active interventions have not demonstrated a clear benefit over passive methods (Roberts et al., 1983). Additionally, the risk of introducing air into the systemic circulation is high (Guyton, 1988).

Passive techniques such as ventricular massage, creation of a stab wound in a pulmonary vein, or amputation of the tip of the left atrial appendage all allow air to escape from the heart and prevent ventricular distention (Guyton, 1988). However, the most commonly practiced maneuver is to elevate the operating room table and place the operating team on stools. This method increases suction to the right atrium, decreases the need for other approaches, and avoids cannulation of the heart (Guyton, 1988). Regardless of which passive method is used, once it has been decompressed, adequate ventricular function generally returns.

Operative Procedure

Initial entry into the chest wall is most commonly achieved through a median sternotomy. This approach provides optimal exposure and visualization of the myocardium and related structures. In addition, use of a median sternotomy incision affords less interruption in respiratory mechanics and reduced postoperative chest wall discomfort, which facilitate earlier mobilization and recovery.

The incision extends longitudinally between the suprasternal notch and the xiphoid process. Following the spread of soft tissue, a sternal saw is used to open the sternum. Lateral placement of retractors facilitates stabilization and separation of the chest wall. The pericardium is incised and tacked to obtain an unobstructed view of the epicardial surface (Fig. 20–14).

Dissection and mobilization of the internal mam-

mary artery from the chest wall is performed while the saphenous vein is harvested from the lower extremities and prepared for implantation. Once the aorta has been cross clamped, injection of cold, hyperkalemic cardioplegic solution into the aortic root or coronary ostia induces electromechanical diastolic arrest (Loop, 1983).

The sequencing of anastomotic construction is dictated by the urgency of the situation, the degree of disease, and the preference of the surgical team. Emergent situations resulting from acute coronary closure or occlusion induced during cardiac catheter-

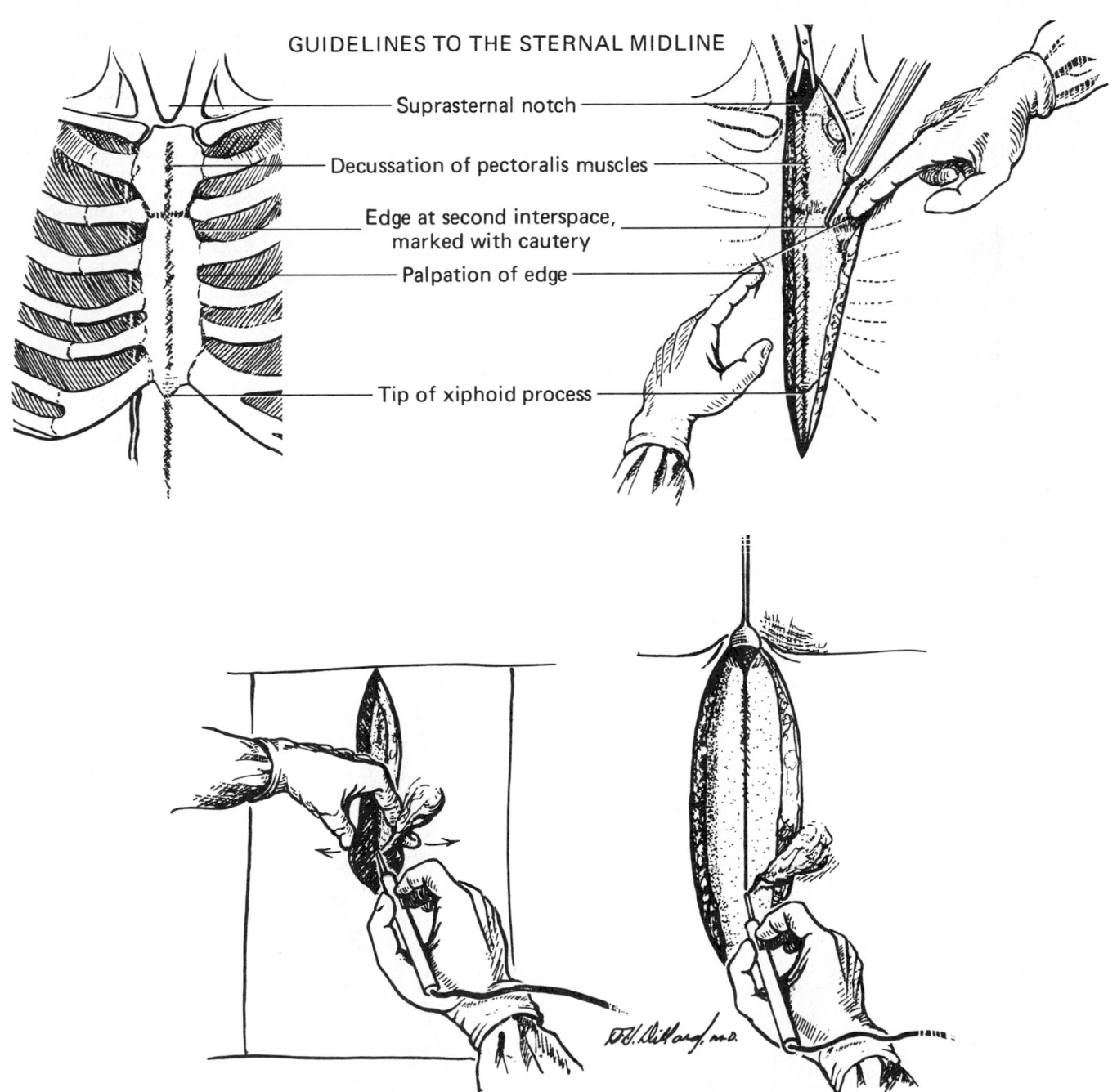

FIGURE 20–14. Median sternotomy incision. (From Dillard, D. H., and Miller, D. W. (1983). *Atlas of cardiac surgery* (p. 21). New York: Macmillan.)

ization or angioplasty procedures require prompt restoration of flow. To expedite the revascularization process, the saphenous vein may be used as the primary conduit. The relative ease in preparation and large graft flow add to the appeal of use of the saphenous vessel in the face of hemodynamic instability or evolving ischemia.

In general, the distal anastomoses to the posterior vasculature (circumflex and right coronary systems) can be performed first. Vessels to be bypassed on the anterior surface of the heart are exposed and incised. Selection of an anastomosis site requires a minimum size of 1 mm in diameter and a disease-free lumen. A vein graft end-to-side anastomosis is constructed to the most distal diagonal branch, and side-to-side anastomoses are made to bypass more proximal obstructions (Fig. 20–15). Finally, the internal mammary artery graft is attached to the LAD using an end-to-side technique. Every 20 to 30 minutes or after each distal anastomosis, infusion of cardioplegic solution distends the vein graft to enhance cardioplegic delivery and distribution to the myocardium in that region, contributing to tissue protection.

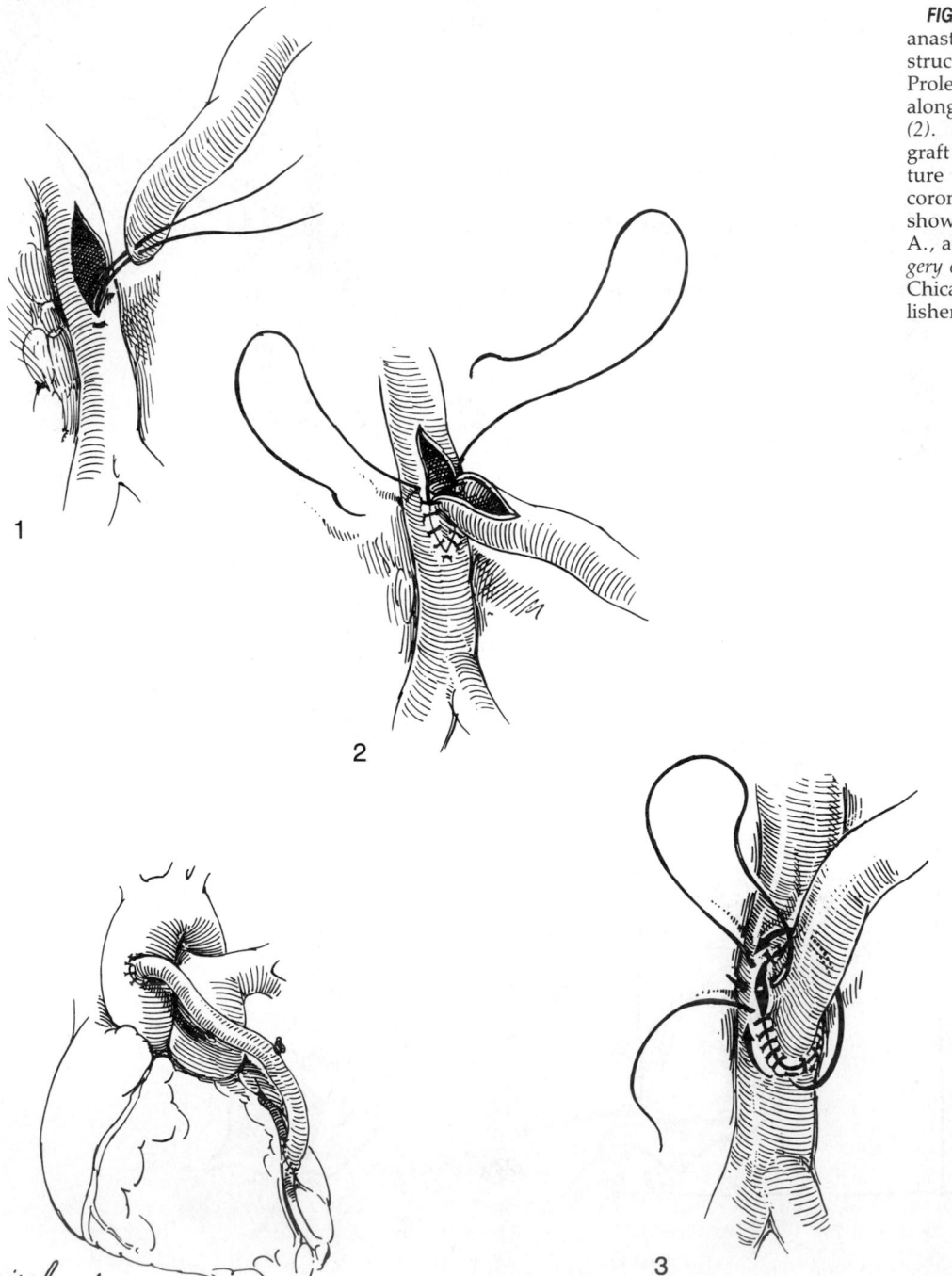

FIGURE 20–15. Saphenous vein anastomosis. Anastomotic construction starts distally *(1)* using Prolene sutures and continues along both edges of arteriotomy *(2)*. Cold cardioplegia de-airs graft prior to completion of suture line *(3)*. Completed aorto-coronary saphenous vein graft is shown *(4)*. (From Waldhausen, J. A., and Pierce, W. S. (1985). *Surgery of the chest* (5th Ed., p. 467). Chicago: Year Book Medical Publishers.)

Sequential grafting, most commonly used by surgeons, involves attachment of a single conduit to a coronary artery in one or more sites (Fig. 20–16). This technique facilitates the ease and speed of performing multiple bypass grafts, reducing the number of aortic manipulations. *Simple grafts* bypass a single lesion, usually beginning at the ascending aorta, with the distal attachment below the obstruction. A *skip graft* is used to bypass a coronary vessel that has both proximal and distal lesions such as is commonly seen in the LAD. *Y grafts* may be utilized when a conduit shaped like a Y is used to bypass two adjacent vessels (Fig. 20–17).

Construction of anastomoses may be performed with either continuous or interrupted sutures. Some evidence suggests that interrupted sutures provide a better anastomosis. Excellent results have been achieved, however, with both techniques. Optical magnification affords the surgeon excellent visualization of the coronary vasculature and minimizes the risk of technical error.

After completion of the distal anastomosis, the cross clamp is removed. Rewarming is performed gradually, initiated at a rate of 1°C/minute. At this time the vein grafts are directed up to the ascending aorta. Each vein is distended with cold cardioplegic solution each time it is fitted between anastomotic sites and finally again prior to aortic attachment. This helps to determine adequate graft length and tension. Evaluation and adjustment of each graft must be performed to ensure proper symmetry and angulation to prevent kinking or early graft closure. A special device (Goosen aortic punch) is used to punch out circular pieces of aorta for construction of each proximal graft.

Prior to separation from cardiopulmonary bypass, basal flow rates are measured within the coronary system. Target flow rates range from 40 to 80 mL/minute depending on the size of the recipient coronary artery and the particular conduit used. The use of transesophageal two-dimensional Doppler echocardiography (TEE) is gaining increasing popularity. Placement of an esophageal transducer provides continuous real-time color flow imaging. The information obtained allows rapid assessment of ventricular function and visualization of coronary graft flow. Clinical reports validate the efficacy of TEE in precise detection of undiagnosed lesions and prevention of postoperative myocardial ischemia due to poor graft construction or procedural defects (Currie, 1989).

Weaning from cardiopulmonary bypass is accomplished following evacuation of air from the grafts and chambers. The cannulas are removed following satisfactory recovery of cardiovascular and hemodynamic function. Atrial and ventricular pacing wires are implanted on the epicardial surface of the right ventricle and brought out to the skin through the chest wall. Pleural and mediastinal tubes are inserted to evacuate blood and drainage and prevent cardiac tamponade. Administration of protamine sulfate and desmopressin (DDAVP) aids in reversing the effects of heparin to minimize postoperative bleeding. The pericardium may be left open or partially closed and resutured; the sternum is then wired for closure. The skin is approximated with sutures or staples.

Following satisfactory hemodynamic recovery, the surgical team prepares the patient for transport to the surgical intensive care unit. Portable monitoring devices are applied to ensure maximum safety during transport. Upon arrival at the intensive care unit, the patient is carefully assessed and evaluated collaboratively by intensive care nursing and medical staff. After admission and stabilization, a report of intraoperative events is communicated among nursing and medical staff. Information exchanged at this time allows the nurse an opportunity to plan the patient's care and to anticipate the pathophysiologic response during the immediate postoperative period.

Systemic Pathophysiologic Changes Characteristic of Cardiopulmonary Bypass

Although the mortality with cardiac surgery is low, there are many pathophysiologic systemic responses to cardiopulmonary bypass as a result of hemodilution, heparinization, hypothermia, hemolysis, and nonpulsatile blood flow. The following section will review these sequelae in relation to common postoperative clinical problems as result of CPB. This information will provide cardiac surgical nurses with valuable data in anticipating and constructing nursing interventions for this patient population.

Fluid. Intravascular volume changes occur secondary to cardiopulmonary bypass. These changes are associated with a decreased serum protein level producing a lowering of osmotic pressure and an increase in capillary permeability mediated by complement activation. Plasma protein concentration is altered by hemodilution and trauma caused by blood coming into contact with the CPB tubing system. Increased capillary permeability to small proteins and water has been demonstrated experimentally to be caused by the release of serotonin from platelets, histamine from mast cells, and lysosomal enzymes from white cells (Buckberg, 1983). Additionally, elevation in C3 complement levels can pose particular organ problems such as gas exchange problems in the lung (Lavelle et al., 1984), increased myocardial cell permeability, and altered gastric motility (McKnight et al., 1985). These changes occur through increasing capillary permeability and interstitial water in these organs. Overall extravascular fluid volume may increase as much as 150 mL/kg. This increase in total body water appears to be proportional to the length of CPB (McKnight et al., 1985) and to increases in aldosterone and antidiuretic hormone (Roth et al., 1981). These changes often precip-

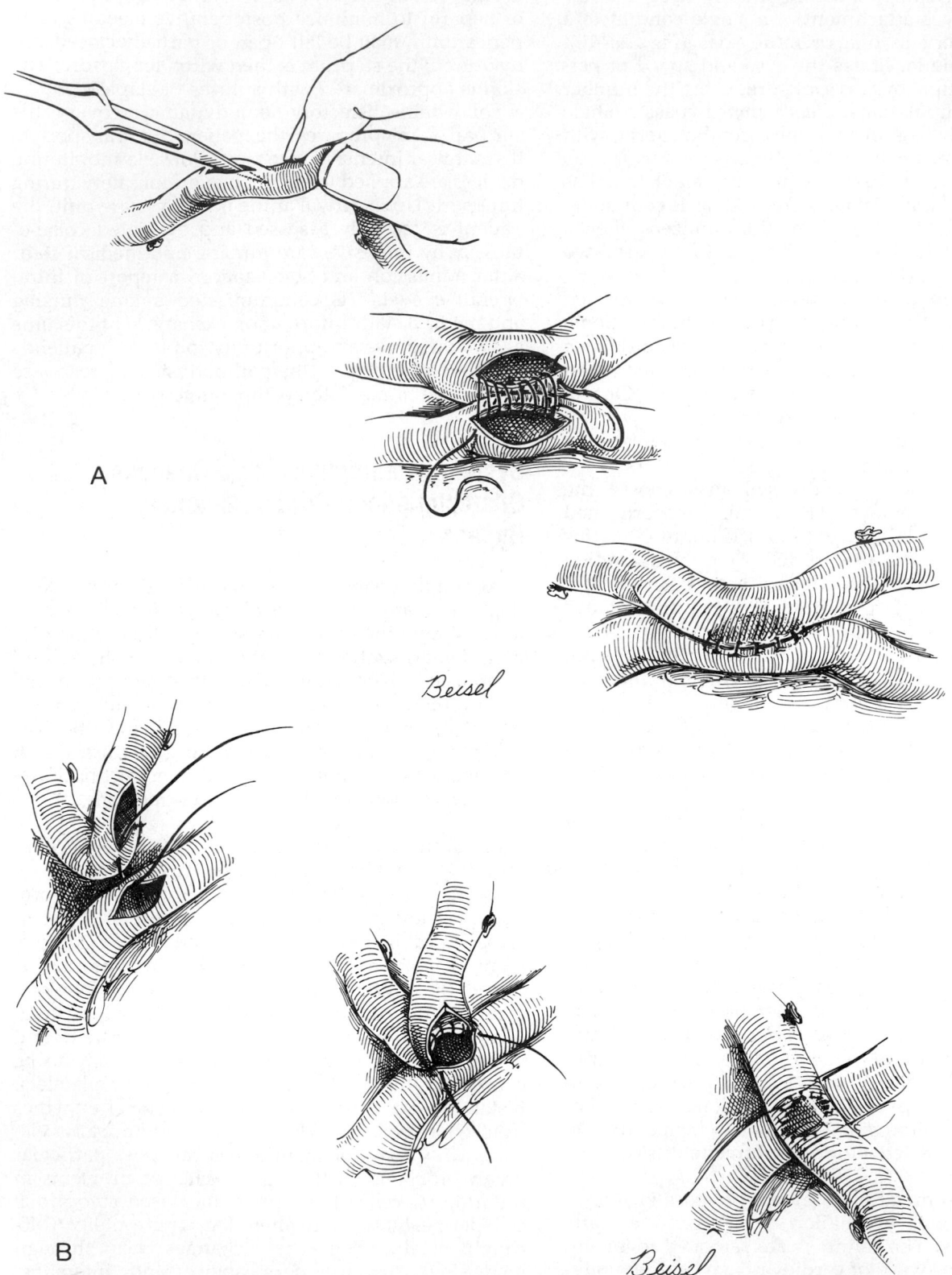

FIGURE 20–16. Sequential graft construction. *A*, Construction of parallel sequential anastomosis is frequently used to revascularize left anterior descending diagonal coronary artery. *B*, Perpendicular anastomosis is used when venotomy lies perpendicular to long axis of coronary artery. (From Waldhausen, J. A., and Pierce, W. S. (1985). *Surgery of the chest* (5th ed., p. 471). Chicago: Year Book Medical Publishers.)

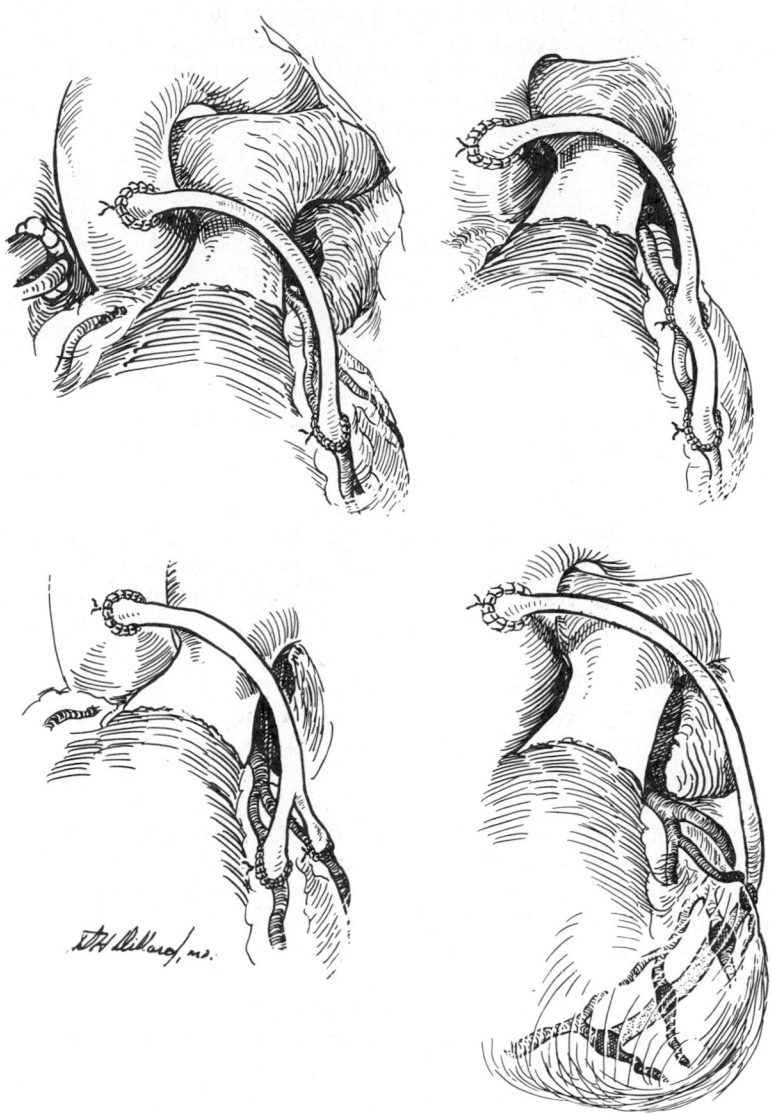

FIGURE 20–17. Types of bypass grafts. (From Dillard, D. H., and Miller, D. W. (1983). *Atlas of cardiac surgery* (Plate XXIX, p. 77). New York: Macmillan.)

itate the clinical problem of hypotension due to decreased intravascular volume.

Cardiac Changes. As a result of disruption of normal coronary perfusion, cardioplegia, uneven rewarming, and surgical manipulation, varying degrees of intracellular myocardial edema occur. These changes can contribute to potential injury of the conduction system, which may precipitate dysrhythmias, ventricular dysfunction, and perioperative ischemia or infarction. Additionally, alterations in hemodynamics caused by hypotension or hypertension are commonly observed.

During CPB, some degree of cardiac cellular edema occurs (Buckberg, 1983; Guyton, 1988; Williams, 1988). These changes may be caused by ischemia, changes in serum oncotic pressures, high cardioplegic perfusion pressures, or ventricular distention (Kirklin et al., 1986; Silverman et al., 1988). Restoration of coronary blood flow after global arrest often accentuates cardiac edema produced by ischemia.

Changes in cell membrane functions and serum oncotic pressures promote an increase in cell water volume upon reperfusion. Damage to the cell membrane has been attributed to cytoxic hydroxyl (OH) radicals (Silverman et al., 1988). The addition of mannitol to cardioplegic solutions has proved beneficial for reducing reperfusion injury because of its hyperosmolarity effects (Lucus et al., 1980). Experimental data seem to support the notion that mannitol may also have a scavenger effect, which eliminates the OH radical, thereby improving postischemic reperfusion injury and coronary blood flow (Magovern et al., 1984). Clinical studies conducted by Johnson and colleagues (1991) demonstrate promising outcomes using allopurinol preoperatively to decrease the effects of OH free radicals.

Dysrhythmias. Commonly, patients who undergo coronary artery bypass or valvular surgery are observed to have tachydysrhythmias, premature ventricular contractions (PVCs), and bradydysrhythmias

(Moore and Wilkoff, 1991). These dysrhythmias may range in severity from benign to life-threatening and are one of the most common complications encountered after cardiac operations. Many operative factors can contribute to the development of these dysrhythmias such as premature myocardial rewarming, electromechanical atrial activity during anoxic states (Smith et al., 1983; Fergusen and Smith, 1983; Magillian et al., 1985), hypoxemia, hypotension, increased sympathetic stimulation, fluid shifts (Estanfanous, 1981), metabolic imbalances (commonly due to digitalis and potassium), and irritation due to prosthetic valves (Moore and Wilkoff, 1991).

The incidence of supraventricular tachydysrhythmias is reported as 48% in coronary artery bypass patients (Caby et al., 1986) and as high as 83% in patients who undergo aortic valve replacement (Vecht et al., 1986; Hoie and Forfaug, 1980). Onset of dysrhythmias usually occurs on the third or fourth postoperative day with deleterious consequences stemming from their hemodynamic effects. The increased time spent in systole increases myocardial oxygen demand. However, the diastolic time is decreased, lending to reduced coronary flow, ventricular filling, and cardiac index. These imbalances set the stage for ischemia, ventricular dysfunction, or infarction.

Treatment, which may vary by institution and physician, is aimed toward control of the ventricular response relative to the individual patient. Once hypoxemia and metabolic derangements are ruled out, the most common pharmacologic medications used are digoxin, which remains controversial, verapamil and low-dose beta blockers. Class 1 antidysrhythmics such as procainamide or quinidine can be used to convert atrial fibrillation or atrial flutter to normal sinus rhythm. These drugs are helpful only after the ventricular rate is controlled in the absence of atrial enlargement (Moore and Wilkoff, 1991). Commonly, atrial overdrive pacing is effective in restoring atrial flutter to normal sinus rhythm (Figs. 20–18 and 20–19).

Ventricular dysrhythmias ranging from isolated PVCs to nonsustained ventricular tachycardias (VT) requiring treatment occur in 36% of postoperative patients (Moore and Wilkoff, 1991). Their occurrence is particularly high in the operating room during anesthesia, induction, cardiac cannulation for CPB, rewarming, and weaning from CPB. The hemodynamic consequences are related to the frequency and duration of the dysrhythmia as it relates to adequate perfusion pressures.

Once physiologic deficits are ruled out as the cause, lidocaine or bretylium may be used as a common first-line medication. In the case of polymorphic VT, usually a result of drug toxicity, magnesium sulfate is the drug of choice (Gray and Mandel, 1991). The presence of ventricular fibrillation is life-threatening and is treated with defibrillation and cardiopulmonary resuscitation as recommended by the American Heart Association.

Bradydysrhythmias caused by injury to the conduction system during CABG or valve surgery are common. In CABG patients 45% are reported to develop a new bundle branch block (BBB), with 4% developing a complete atrioventricular (AV) block. However, resolution of the new BBB prior to discharge has been reported to occur in 54% (Moore and Wilkoff, 1991). Development of new conduction defects after aortic valve replacement is reported to occur in 29% (Thompson et al., 1980).

These defects are commonly precipitated by oper-

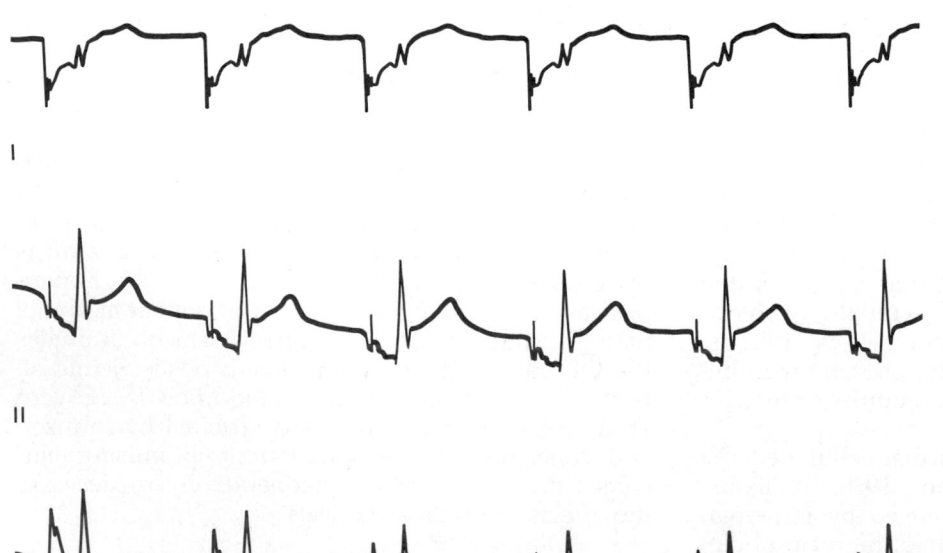

I

II

III

FIGURE 20–18. Atrial electrogram (AEG); the rhythm is normal sinus rhythm. The lead I recording is bipolar; note the very small ventricular complex. Leads II and III are unipolar; both the atrial and the ventricular complexes are easily seen. The atrial complex in lead III is significantly larger than that seen in lead II. This signifies that the atrial pacing wire attached to the left arm lead is farthest away from the ventricle and would be the best pacing wire to use for rapid atrial pacing.

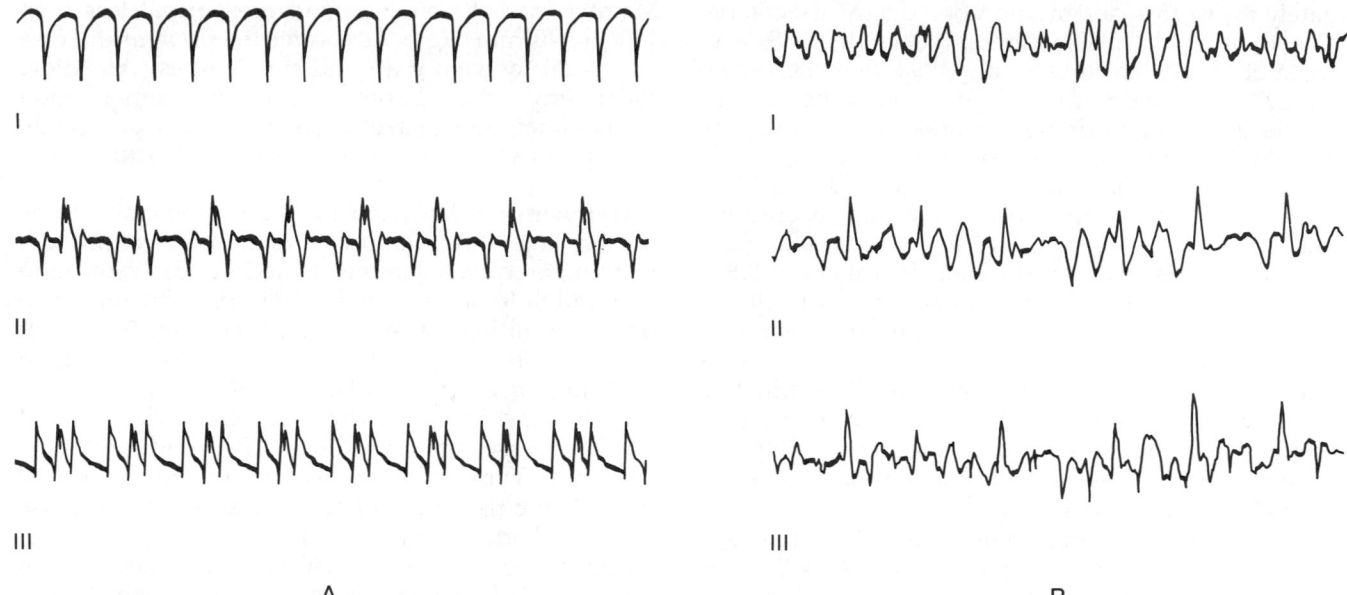

FIGURE 20–19. *A,* Atrial electrograms recorded during atrial flutter. Atrial rate is approximately 290 bpm; ventricular rate is 145 bpm. Lead I is bipolar; only the atrial activity is visible. Leads II and III are unipolar; both atrial and ventricular activity are seen. *B,* Atrial electrograms recorded during atrial fibrillation. Note the chaotic atrial activity seen in both the bipolar (lead I) and the unipolar (leads II and III) atrial electrograms.

ative events associated with hypothermia, potassium concentration of cardioplegia, number of coronaries bypassed, aortic cross clamp time, and time on CPB (Moore and Wilkoff, 1991; Gray and Mandel, 1991). The clinical significance of these defects will depend upon their hemodynamic outcome. The most common treatment is the use of temporary atrial or ventricular pacing until the normal intrinsic conduction pathways resume. In rhythm patterns in which loss of the atrial contribution to the cardiac output occurs, temporary AV sequential pacing is used.

Ventricular Dysfunction. Transient biventricular dysfunction to a varying degree occurs after CPB. Common contributors to this phenomenon are preexisting ventricular dysfunction, microemboli to the subendocardium, inadequate cardioplegic protection, premature or uneven rewarming, elevation in systemic and pulmonary vascular resistance, or ischemic ventricular injury. These causes are commonly thought to be associated with left ventricular (LV) dysfunction after CPB. However, increasing attention is being directed toward factors that specifically put the right ventricle (RV) at risk for dysfunction. In addition to the causes previously stated, RV dysfunction is caused by cold potassium cardioplegia (Christakis et al., 1985), right coronary artery air embolism, elevated pulmonary vascular resistance, and LV dysfunction (Hines and Barash, 1985; Coleman, 1989). Likewise, biventricular dysfunction can be caused by independent injury to the right or left ventricle, cardiac cellular edema, or loss of high-energy phosphates due to initiation of global arrest. Recovery of LV dysfunction may take up to 8 days (Pennington et al., 1985), whereas RV recovery may

be reversed in 3 to 5 days depending on the severity of injury and the absence of pulmonary hypertension (Hines and Barash, 1985). Although multifactorial, any or all of these factors can contribute to the development of low cardiac output states observed postoperatively. These patients often need fluid administration, mechanical assist devices, or inotropic support to maintain an acceptable cardiac index, urine output, and mentation level.

Cardiac Tamponade. Careful assessment for signs and symptoms of cardiac tamponade must not be overlooked as a cause of ventricular dysfunction. Cardiac tamponade results from accumulation of blood or fluid in the pericardial space, impairing ventricular diastolic filling, which eventually causes the equalization of all cardiac chamber pressures. A major factor in the development of tamponade is the rapidity with which fluid accumulates in the pericardial space. However, slow subtle bleeding into the mediastinum also can cause tamponade. Occluded mediastinal chest tubes secondary to clot formation in the anterior mediastinum may induce a precipitous fall in drainage output. Manifestations of hypotension, elevation and equalization of diastolic filling pressures, low cardiac output, a decrease in chest tube drainage, and a widening mediastinum on x-ray are the clinical sequelae of cardiac tamponade. Immediate recognition of this situation is imperative to ensure expeditious intervention, which most often requires reexploration.

Perioperative Myocardial Infarction. The incidence of perioperative myocardial infarction (MI) in patients after coronary revascularization is approximately 5% to 15% depending upon diagnostic criteria (Chartman et al., 1983; Guiteras Val et al., 1988; Van Lente et al., 1989; Force et al., 1990; Seitelberger et al., 1991). To date, there is no consensus on the criteria used to determine the presence of perioperative MI. However, the presence of a new Q wave on the electrocardiagram (Force et al., 1990) and the presence of a prolonged peak elevation in creatine kinase (CK)-MB isoenzyme 12 to 15 hours after surgery are criteria often used (Guiteras Val et al., 1983; Van Lente et al., 1989). Both of these primary criteria have been documented to provide false-negative and false-positive results. Given an index of clinical suspicion for the presence of a perioperative MI, the above criteria, taken in conjunction with myocardial scanning techniques or ventricular contractility assessment, provide additional data that help to determine the presence of a perioperative MI.

The single most important factor that has decreased the incidence of perioperative MI is the use of potassium cardioplegia. Conditions in which adequate myocardial preservation might not be achieved promote high-risk states. Patients at risk are those with a left main stenotic lesion greater than 50% with accompanying stenosis of the right coronary artery, prolonged aortic cross clamp and CPB time, multivessel bypass, and/or a concomitant valve replacement (Guiteras Val et al., 1983). In addition to these operative risks, patients who undergo surgery emergently, or have cardiomegaly or unstable angina, or are female are also at risk.

Postoperative consequences associated with a suspected perioperative infarction are significant ventricular irritability, low cardiac output, and poor hemodynamic response. The intra-aortic balloon pump and pharmacologic inotropic support are common treatment modalities used to support the failing ventricle(s) until recovery. Seitelberger and colleagues (1991) conducted a randomized study on the use of nifedipine in reducing the incidence of MI. These investigators demonstrated a reduction in myocardial infarction and necrosis with the use of this calcium channel agonist. Although these results are encouraging, larger clinical trials are needed.

Hypertension. Hypertension is most commonly seen in the immediate postoperative period as a result of peripheral arterial constriction and hypothermia (Connors and Avioli, 1981). Hypertension is rapidly alleviated following administration of sedatives and analgesics and initiation of the rewarming process. Efforts to control hypertension and reduce arterial blood pressure help to decrease left ventricular workload and wall tension while lessening myocardial oxygen demand. Intravenous nitroglycerin and sodium nitroprusside are effective vasodiliating agents used to lower systemic vascular resistance through preload and afterload reduction. Reduced arterial pressure allows more complete left ventricular emptying and ejection, facilitating a rise in stroke volume and a redistribution of coronary blood flow.

Maintenance of systolic blood pressure at less than 120 to 140 mm Hg is advocated to prevent adverse effects on the vein graft and suture lines (Wheatley, 1986; Gray, 1990). Excessive pressure exerted upon suture lines and anastomosis sites may precipitate serious consequences such as leakage or rupture.

Hypotension. Hypotension may be precipitated by hemorrhage, vasodilation, intravascular volume depletion, or catecholamine depletion. Early recognition and volume reexpansion will prevent complications resulting from prolonged episodes of hypotension such as tissue hypoperfusion, organ ischemia, or cardiovascular collapse. Severe volume deficits may induce early vein graft closure and myocardial ischemia and injury (Behrendt and Austen, 1981). Typically, volume replacement of colloidal fluids is the treatment of choice (rather than the use of crystalloid) to improve hypotension. In a two-group randomized trial, Ley and colleagues (1990) demonstrated reduced fluid replacement needs, improved hemodynamics, and shortened ICU stays in the patient group given replacement volume with colloid as compared with the crystalloid group.

Coronary Artery Spasm. Coronary artery vasospasm has been postulated as a cause of postoperative morbidity and mortality following CABG (Tanimoto et al., 1984). It occurs early in the postoperative period in approximately 0.8% of cases (Gurley et al., 1990; Maleki and Manley, 1989). Common manifestations have been identified as ST-segment elevations, hypotension, atrioventricular block, ventricular tachycardia, and cardiovascular collapse. Many centers routinely employ prophylactic use of intravenous nitroglycerin and nifedipine in the postoperative period to promote vasodilation and counteract the potential for perioperative MI or ischemia caused by spasm (Maleki and Manley, 1989).

Coronary artery spasm has been found to affect both normal coronaries, endarterectomized vessels, recipient bypassed vessels, and conduits such as the internal mammary artery or saphenous vein. The etiology of this syndrome is unknown; researchers propose that calcium infusion, increased catecholamine levels, or myocardial ischemia may be factors linked to the development of coronary artery vasospasm (Behrendt and Austen, 1981). Recognition is extremely difficult because angiographic confirmation may not be feasible. However, once it has been identified, treatment with intracoronary vasodilators has proved effective (Fischell et al., 1989).

Acute Valvular Rupture. In managing patients who have undergone valvular surgery, close monitoring of heart sounds and frequent analysis of hemodynamic waveforms are common nursing practices. Normally, tilting disc valves should be fairly silent on opening and produce a crisp sound on closure. Biologic valves mimic the sounds produced by normal native valves. Assessment for changes in heart sounds, such as loss of the crisp closing sound produced by the tilting disc or occurrence of new murmurs, should be included with hemodynamic assessment. Any unexplained changes in cardiac output, filling pressures, or changes in left atrial or pulmonary capillary wedge waveform support a suspicion of acute valve rupture (Fig. 20–20).

A left atrial line may be placed after mitral valve surgery has been performed to provide continuous monitoring of left atrial pressure and better hemodynamic assessment of mitral valve function. An increase in the amplitude of the *a* wave may indicate late or sticky valve opening; a heightened *v* wave may indicate regurgitation or perivalvular leak. Changes in the appearance of the left atrial waveform may also denote pressure changes or conduction disturbances (Fig. 20–21). Depending on the severity of hemodynamic consequences, these patients may require reoperation.

Hematologic Changes. At the time of sternotomy, bone marrow emboli are liberated into the blood and are thought to be the mediators of subclinical disseminated intravascular coagulation associated with a decrease in platelet count seen prior to initiation of CPB (Milam, 1983; Thayman, 1985). Once on CPB, blood is subject to turbulence causing hemolysis, pressure producing trauma to the cells, low flow states precipitating clumping of cells, and denaturing of blood cells as a result of contact with CPB tubing. Further damage to blood cells results from the direct interface of blood and oxygen in the bubble oxygenator or suctioning of the surgical field (Milam, 1983;

Heynan, 1985). In addition, blood coagulability is further hindered by heparinization, hemodilution, and hypothermia.

One of the most important contributions to the development of postoperative bleeding is platelet dysfunction. The definitive mechanism of injury to platelets as they travel through the oxygenator is unclear. However, there is evidence to support the development of cell membrane injury (Harker, 1986) and impaired platelet binding to fibrinogen (Musial et al., 1985) in conjunction with low levels of factor V or von Willebrand factor (Salzman et al., 1986; Czer et al., 1985). Additionally, the use of aspirin and antiplatelet medications contributes to the development of this dysfunction (Sethi et al., 1990). Common alterations in other blood indices observed after CPB are slight thrombocytopenia, elevation in fibrin degradation products, increases in factors VII and IX, and a decrease in factor V (Edmunds and Stephenson, 1983; Milam, 1983; Heynan, 1985). Decreased fibrinogen values while on CPB have also been documented; these values elevate immediately postoperatively and remain high for 24 to 48 hours (Moores and Willford, 1989). Thorough assessment of clotting factor activity, bleeding time, and platelet function will provide an appropriate treatment plan. Interventions commonly used are autologous platelet transfusions (Giordano et al., 1988), DDAVP (Salzman et al., 1986), and cryoprecipitate (Harker, 1986). Treatment should be directed towards repletion of the specific clotting factor(s) needed.

Postoperative mediastinal bleeding usually stems from a coagulation disturbance or vascular interrup-

Prosthesis type	Mitral Prosthesis	Acoustic Characteristics	Aortic Prosthesis	Acoustic Characteristics
Ball Valves	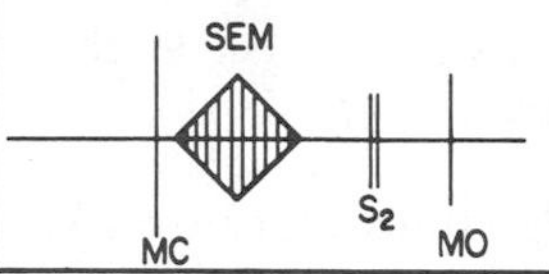 SEM / MC / S_2 / MO	1) A_2–MO interval 0.07–0.11 sec. 2) MO > MC 3) II–III / VI Systolic ejection murmur (SEM) 4) No diastolic murmur	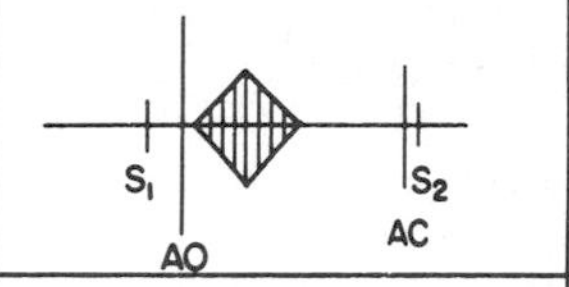 S_1 / AO / S_2 / AC	1) S_1–AO interval 0.07 sec. 2) AO > AC 3) II / VI harsh SEM 4) No diastolic murmur
Disc Valves	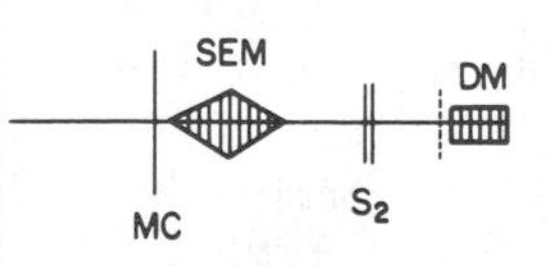 SEM / MC / S_2 / DM	1) A_2–MO interval 0.05–0.09 sec. 2) MO is rarely heard 3) II / VI SEM is usually heard 4) I–II / VI diastolic rumble is usually heard	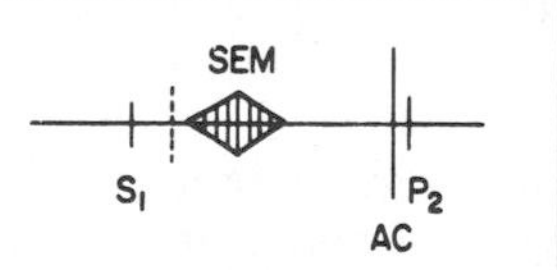 SEM / S_1 / P_2 / AC	1) S_1–AO interval 0.04 sec. 2) AO is uncommonly heard, AC is usually heard 3) II / VI SEM is usually heard 4) Occasional diastolic murmur
Porcine Valves	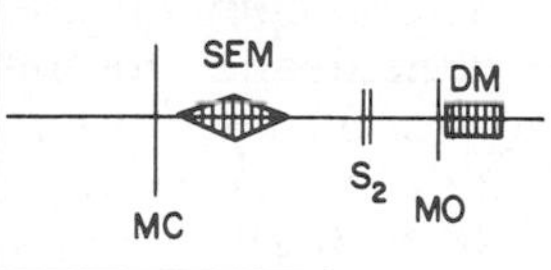 SEM / MC / S_2 / MO	1) A_2–MO interval 0.1 sec. 2) MO is audible 50% 3) I–II / VI apical SEM 50% 4) Diastolic rumble $\frac{1}{2}$ – $\frac{2}{3}$	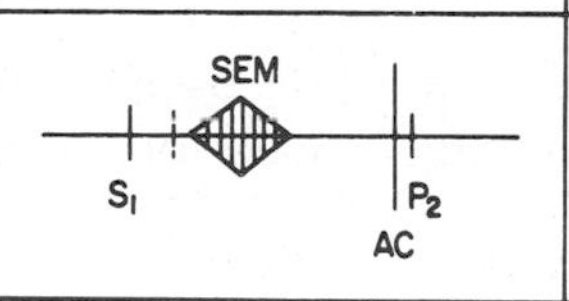 SEM / S_1 / P_2 / AC	1) S_1–AO interval 0.03–0.08 sec. 2) AO is uncommonly heard, AC is usually heard 3) II / VI SEM in most 4) No diastolic murmur
Bileaflet Valve (St. Jude)			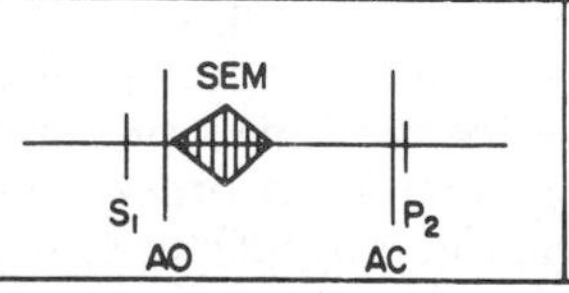 SEM / S_1 / AO / P_2 / AC	1) AO and AC commonly heard 2) A soft SEM is common

FIGURE 20–20. Summary of the acoustic characteristics of each valve prosthesis according to type and location. *Abbreviations*: SEM, systolic ejection murmur; DM, diastolic murmur; S_1, first heart sound; S_2, second heart sound; P_2, pulmonic second sound; A_2, aortic second sound; AO, aortic valve opening sound; AC, aortic valve closure sound; MO, mitral valve opening sound; MC, mitral valve closure sound. (From Smith, N., Raizada, V., and Abrams J. (1981). *Annals of Internal Medicine*, 95, 594–598.)

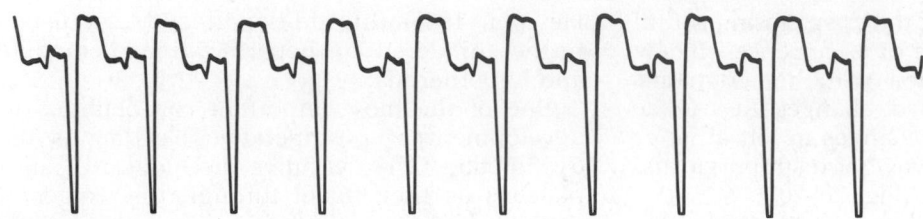

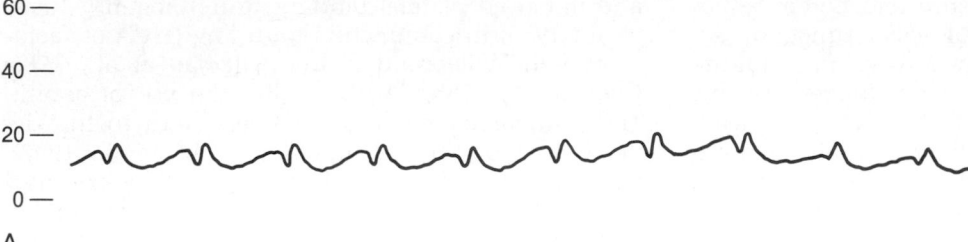

A

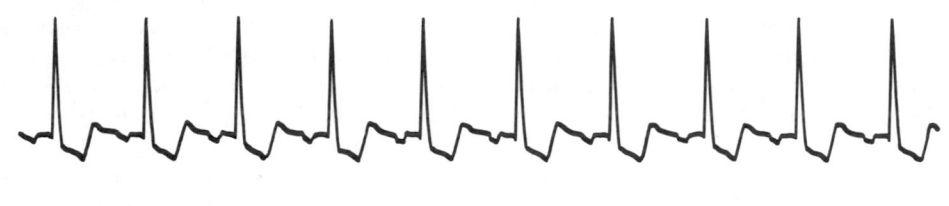

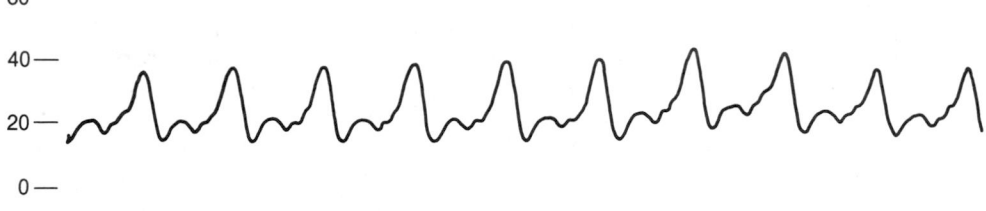

B

FIGURE 20–21. Left atrial pressure (LAP) recordings. *A*, Recording taken from a 66-year-old male after coronary artery bypass graft surgery. The patient is in sinus rhythm; LAP is approximately 15 mm Hg. *B*, Recording taken from a 56-year-old woman after mitral and aortic valve replacements. This patient is also in sinus rhythm. LAP is approximately 25 to 28 mm Hg. Note the large *v* wave associated with the higher LAP in this patient.

tion. Care is taken intraoperatively to avoid unnecessary dissection, although persistent bleeding may result despite precautions taken to achieve intraoperative hemostasis. Identification of the causative factors will determine the appropriate therapy. Coagulation abnormalities can result from incomplete heparin reversal, heparin rebound effect, thrombocytopenia, platelet dysfunction, depletion of clotting factors, or disseminated intravascular coagulation (Bojar, 1989).

In the absence of a hemostatic defect, bleeding most likely results from an anastomotic site, warranting return to the operating room for urgent surgical reexploration. Anastomotic bleeding usually occurs in the presence of diseased vessels. When grafts are sutured to thin-walled, poor-quality recipient vessels, excessive intraluminal pressure may cause rupture or tearing. Increased pressure may be a product of vasoconstriction or hypertension. Repair of the anastomosis may induce further compromise or damage to the vessel. Bleeding may also occur from side branches of the vein graft sites, areas of intracardiac cannulation, or acute disruption of su-

tures at the valve site. All such conditions require emergent reoperation.

Endocrine Changes. Controlled trauma of cardiopulmonary bypass, hypothermia, diversion of circulation from the heart and lung, hemodilution, and the loss of autonomic innervation contribute to changes in the endocrine system (Edmunds and Stephenson, 1983; Philibin, 1985; Reyes, 1985). As a result of these factors, epinephrine may be elevated to nine times normal and norepinephrine to two times normal in response to an empty heart (Reyes, 1985), and changes in glucose regulation have been demonstrated. Reyes found an elevation in endogenous catecholamines when CPB began and during weaning (Reyes, 1985). These elevations have been documented to persist up to 8 hours postoperatively (Landymore et al., 1979; Estanfanous, 1981). Such impressive elevations in these potent vasoconstrictors, in combination with hypovolemia and hypothermia, precipitates the common problem of hypertension.

Elevations in vasopressin levels have been demonstrated to be 20 times normal after cardiopulmonary bypass (Edmunds and Stephenson, 1983; Philibin, 1985). These extremely high circulating levels not only cause water retention and result in hyponatremia but also exert a potent vasoconstricting effect upon the vascular beds (Reyes, 1985). In conjunction with elevations in serum vasopressin levels, renin and angiotensin levels are also elevated, contributing to a 35% to 45% incidence of postoperative hypertension (Philibin, 1985; Estanfanous, 1981). Treatment focuses upon maintaining adequate intravascular volume, slow rewarming, and vasodilation therapy.

Changes in serum glucose patterns can be observed in all patients during CPB when exogenous glucose is not used in the priming solution (Kuntschen et al., 1985). During hypothermia, inhibition of both insulin secretion and hepatic glucose production occurs. Hypothermic patients have been found to have no insulin secretion or an elevated serum glucose response during CPB (Kuntschen et al., 1985). However, post CPB, after rewarming occurs, hyperglycemia and hyperinsulinemia (Kuntschen et al., 1985, 1986) with some insulin resistance have been observed in both diabetic and nondiabetic patients (Kuntschen et al., 1986). These data are helpful because hyperglycemia is commonly observed in all patients post CPB. However, diabetic patients may require insulin drips to gain control of the serum glucose.

Crystalloid prime solutions often contain metabolically active substrates that have been thought to modulate the hormonal and metabolite responses to CPB. McKnight and associates conducted a randomized control trial on the effects of four different crystalloid prime solutions. Patients were randomized to four groups and received prime solutions containing either glucose, lactate, glucose and lactate, or neither glucose nor lactate. Four hours postoperatively, no significant changes in endocrine or metabolic responses were found between the groups. However, in groups in which glucose or lactate was used in the prime, serum glucose and lactate levels were found to be elevated. These findings support the use of non-glucose or lactate additives to the prime solution (McKnight et al., 1985). Whatever solution is used, an increase in total body water results at completion of CPB.

Pulmonary Changes. The lungs remain deflated and underperfused during CPB. During this process there is a decrease in chest wall compliance with a resultant decrease in function residual capacity (FRC) (Bartlett, 1980). General anesthesia and muscle paralysis cause cephalad movement of the dependent portion of the diaphragm, which decreases static and dynamic spontaneous lung volume.

Following CPB, an increase in the alveolar-arterial oxygen difference with a resultant increase in intrapulmonary shunting occurs (Edmunds and Stephen-

son, 1983; Svennevig et al., 1984; Chulay et al., 1982). Further changes in the pneumocytes as a result of CPB lead to a loss of surfactant (Chulay et al., 1982), increased alveolar permeability secondary to C5a complement activation, swelling of endothelial cells, sequestering of leukocytes with release of lysosomal enzymes (Bartlett, 1980; Edmunds and Stephenson, 1983), and development of atelectasis secondary to intraoperative ventilation at high oxygen levels, which dilutes normal alveolar nitrogen and impairs clearance of secretions (Asada and Yamaguchi, 1981).

Left lower lobe atelectasis is the most common sequel of CPB with a reported incidence of 68% to 72% (Chulay et al., 1982) in cardiac surgical patients. Factors proposed to explain this phenomenon include the operative factors previously stated, the supine position in combination with an enlarged heart, which may interfere with left lower lobe expansion (Sheland et al., 1983), the presence of an endotracheal tube (Freedman and Goodman, 1982), and phrenic nerve damage (Benjamie et al., 1982; Curtis et al., 1989). Recovery is usually accompanied by return of normal diaphragmatic function. Other reports indicate that exposure to hypothermia interferes with surfactant production (Rouson et al., 1985). Interruption of lung surfactant may produce transient alveolar collapse, potentiating atelectasis. In the population of patients who undergo cauterization of the internal mammary artery, development of an ipsilateral pleural effusion further prevents alveolar expansion and predisposes patients to the development of atelectasis (Jansen and McFadden, 1986).

Diaphragmatic dysfunction secondary to phrenic nerve injury, particularly that involving the left hemidiaphragm, has been seen to persist for up to 48 to 72 hours or for up to 2 years postoperatively (Lewis, 1980; Asada and Yamaguchi, 1981; Luce, 1984; Dajee et al., 1988; Curtis et al., 1989). This reported variable recovery pattern is attributed to the severity (i.e., unilateral or bilateral) of involvement and the mechanism of injury to the phrenic nerve. Injury to the phrenic nerve may also result from the use of ice slush for myocardial cooling (Curtis et al., 1989), take-down of the IMA for CABG, and electrocautery (Abd et al., 1989). Whatever the cause, these patients are prone to develop atelectasis, may require prolonged mechanical ventilation, and are at risk for respiratory infection. Treatment focuses upon managing the airway, strengthening the ventilatory muscles, promoting adequate patient communication, and managing anxiety.

Preoperative variables that predispose patients to postoperative lung problems include chronic obstructive lung disease, poor lung compliance, decreased activity tolerance, advanced age, malnutrition, and a prior long hospitalization with pulmonary complications (Rich et al., 1988). Prevention and management of atelectasis is a primary nursing concern. Interventions such as early turning (Chulay et al., 1982), progressive increases in activity, and the use of incentive spirometry (Lewis, 1980) should be initiated in the ICU and continued throughout the patient's hospital stay.

Renal/Serum Electrolyte Changes. Cardiopulmonary bypass decreases overall blood flow distribution to the kidney, impairing autoregulation as a result of hemodilution and hypothermia (Utley et al., 1981). Additionally, hypotension, microemboli, and nonpulsatile CPB flow states contribute to development of a drop in glomerular filtration rate (GFR) to 50% to 60% of normal while the patient is on CPB, which usually normalizes by the second postoperative day (Kristensen, 1990). The reported incidence of renal dysfunction is 1.5% to 5% in the cardiac surgical patient population.

Acute tubular necrosis (ATN) as a result of these factors is not an uncommon clinical problem after cardiac surgery (Davis et al., 1982; Myers and Moran, 1986). Episodes of hypotension or the use of potent vasoconstrictor medications in the perioperative period may precipitate a sudden decrease in renal perfusion and output (Utley et al., 1981). This may be compounded by hypothermia, which contributes to a potential decrease in renal blood flow by increasing renal vascular resistance, resulting in a decrease in free water clearance, urine osmolarity, and a subsequent decrease in urine output (Davis et al., 1982; Edmunds and Stephenson, 1983). Hemolysis of red cells is a common problem of CPB and requires the kidney to clear the degraded byproducts such as hemoglobin. Free hemoglobin binds to plasma albumin producing methemalbumin, which is secreted in the kidney (Kristensen, 1990). As long as urine output is adequate, free hemoglobin will be excreted and will be of no consequence to the renal tubules. To differentiate between hemoglobinuria and hematuria by observation, hemoglobinuria does not precipitate and usually clears with adequate urine output within the first 1 to 2 hours following CPB (Edmunds and Stephenson, 1983).

As a result of these renal perfusion changes and the use of electolyte-based cardioplegic solutions and diuretics, common changes in serum electrolytes observed after CPB include hypokalemia, hyponatremia, and hypomagnesemia. These serum electrolytes should be monitored closely in conjunction with renal function indices and urine output and altered as needed.

Central Nervous System. Central nervous system problems resulting from CPB are most commonly caused by emboli or ischemia (Santillan et al., 1985). Perfusion pressures below 50 mm Hg, prolonged CPB runs, and advanced age can contribute to postoperative cerebral manifestations (Brewer et al., 1983; Rebeyka et al., 1987). CPB does not cause changes in cerebral blood flow (CBF) unless perfusion pressures drop below 50 mm Hg (Brewer et al., 1983). If the perfusion pressure decreases to less than 40 mm Hg, carbon dioxide levels can cause a decrease in CBF and precipitate an ischemic event (Brewer et al., 1983; (Johnson et al., 1987).

Cerebrovascular Accidents. Microemboli from the CPB machine or cardiotomy suction system or release of plaque from artery walls can cause stroke. Generally, neurologic sequelae due to air embolization elicit transient symptoms that resolve completely. However, neurovascular injury secondary to particulate matter results in less predictable recovery and prognosis. Reports of permanent deficits range from 2% to 10% (Faggioli et al., 1990; Glenn et al., 1990; Brewer et al., 1983). This incidence is increasing and is attributed to the advanced age of patients and the presence of carotid stenosis at the time of bypass. Faggioli and associates (1990) demonstrated that the risk of stroke is higher in patients older than 60 years who have carotid stenosis of 50% to 70%.

The mechanism of injury that produces stroke remains unclear. It is thought to be related to the duration of CPB, the presence of aortic arch disease, and sudden blood pressure changes during the postoperative period (Faggioli et al., 1990; Brener et al., 1987; Turnipseed et al., 1980).

Cognitive changes such as short-term memory loss, impaired visual motor ability, difficulty in problem-solving, and lack of ability to concentrate have been found to exist in the absence of stroke (Raymond et al., 1985; Townes et al., 1989). These deficits may persist up to 6 months post CPB (Townes et al., 1989). Such changes have implications for nurses in developing teaching strategies of patients, particularly those older than 60 years, in whom the pattern of resolution may not be predictable.

Peripheral Nerve Injury. Neuralgia and numbness are common symptoms in patients with saphenous vein grafts (Nair et al., 1988). Some patients experience sensory deficits around the ankle and leg such as pain and paresthesias. Injury to the saphenous nerve at the time of operation may result from surgical handling, trauma, or postoperative compression. Patients experience the most numbness during the first 48 hours. Numbness is attributed to a combination of surgical trauma and tissue inflammation.

Different methods of repairing the leg incision have been proposed to alleviate the problem. A single-layer technique of suture closure may result in improved protection of cutaneous sensation compared to subcuticular sutures (Angelini et al., 1984). The optimum technique of closure is directed toward minimizing pressure on the saphenous nerve as healing progresses (Angelini et al., 1984).

Upper extremity nerve injury has been reported in approximately 10% to 15% of patients undergoing CABG (Green, 1989). Development of this syndrome is not related to arm position, internal mammary artery dissection, or internal jugular vein catheterization. Attempts to explain the etiology focus upon compression of the brachial plexus caused by sternal retraction (Loop, 1989). Symptoms stem from the ulnar or median nerve region. This syndrome is transient, and complete resolution usually occurs in several weeks (Loop, 1989).

Immune System. Complement activation results from blood coming in contact with the tubing of the cardiopulmonary bypass machine (Hammerschmidt et al., 1981). Such activation causes release of PMNs from bone marrow. However, overall PMN levels are decreased during this hypothermic state because they are sequested along with lymphocytes in the lung (Quiroga et al., 1985), adhere to the surface of the CPB tubing (Hammerschmidt et al., 1981), and tend to aggregate in small vessels within the lung, leading to pulmonary dysfunction (Hammerschmidt et al., 1981; Lavelle et al., 1984; Quiroga et al., 1985).

Also observed at the beginning of CPB is an overall increase in WBC count, which continues until rewarming is complete. Upon rewarming, the serum PMN count is elevated with further uptake of these white cells in the lung (Quiroga et al., 1985). Significant elevation in the PMN count causes the development of perivascular edema in the endothelial cells of the pneumocytes, impairing gas exchange and increasing pulmonary A-a gradients (Edmunds and Stephenson, 1983; Lavalle et al., 1984; Quiroga et al., 1985).

T cells are likewise depressed following CPB. Roth and associates have demonstrated that the T cell–dependent lymphocyte response was significantly diminished after cardiac operation (Hisatomi et al., 1989; Roth et al., 1981). These levels were found to be diminished for the first week postoperatively. Such findings suggest a vulnerable period in which patients may be susceptible to bacterial and viral infections.

Infection. Sternal wound infections infrequently complicate the postoperative period. Approximately 1% to 5% of patients develop major wound infections involving the chest wall and mediastinum (Jeevanandam et al., 1990; Grossi et al., 1985). These patients are at extremely high risk with potentially fatal consequences.

Signs and symptoms of infection are usually manifested by the second postoperative week but can occur anywhere from 6 to 21 days following surgery. Diagnosis and confirmation of sternal wound infection is made following comprehensive examination and testing. Development of fever, leukocytosis, incisional pain, sternal instability, and wound drainage commonly describe the clinical picture. *Staphylococcus aureus* and *Staphylococcus epidermidis* are the common causative organisms (Grossi et al., 1985).

Bacterial invasion of the myocardium and surrounding structures due to mediastinitis can jeopardize the integrity of the coronary grafts and suture lines. Erosion caused by release of endotoxin may precipitate anastomotic instability and potential rup-

ture. The risk of graft occlusion in these patients arises from the potential formation of septic thrombi.

Factors related to the development of mediastinitis are advanced age (over 80 years), early chest reexploration, and prolonged low cardiac output (Behrendt and Austen, 1981). Some evidence exists linking the use of the IMA to an increased risk of sternal wound infection (Culliford et al., 1985). An increased incidence of infection has been documented with use of bilateral internal mammary artery grafts (Culliford et al., 1985). Multivariate analysis, however, indicates that factors such as age and diabetes have a greater impact than use of the IMA in determining the risk of infection (Cosgrove et al., 1988). Subsequent reports have failed to support a relationship between use of the internal mammary artery and mediastinitis (Cosgrove et al., 1988).

Leg wound infections occur in less than 1.0% of patients (Delaria et al., 1981). Necrosis or sloughing of wound edges may result from postoperative low cardiac output or poor skin perfusion. Edema along the incision contributes to suture tension and may interrupt the wound healing process. In patients with large hematomas, accumulation of serous fluid acts as a suitable medium for bacterial proliferation. It is recommended that infected hematomas be evacuated and drained to promote granulation. Certain wound closure techniques have also been associated with infection. Some authors note that use of subcuticular sutures facilitates improved wound healing compared to metal staples (Angelini et al., 1984).

POSTOPERATIVE MANAGEMENT OF CARDIAC SURGICAL PATIENTS

Nursing and medical staff collaborate on the management of the patient throughout the postoperative recovery phase. During the acute postoperative phase, patients are monitored continuously as systemic recovery from anesthesia occurs and body temperatures return to normal. The primary goals of management are to ensure the adequacy of the cardiac index and tissue perfusion and to monitor neurologic recovery. Systemic responses to the operative procedure and the cardiopulmonary pump run are monitored. Nursing and medical management of these patients is accomplished through monitoring of direct and derived hemodynamic parameters, clinical assessment, and laboratory tests.

The focus of management for these patients is continuous assessment and prompt intervention to maintain an adequate cardiac index to meet metabolic needs. Concurrently the critical care nurse assists the family in coping with the situational crisis of the illness, receiving communications about the patient's progress, and verbalizing their feelings. Common nursing diagnoses, operative correlations of the clinical problem, nursing interventions, and rationale for treatment are listed in the nursing care plan.

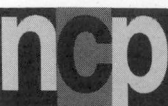 **nursing care plan**

1. Alteration in cardiac output related to:
Decreased contractility
Decreased preload
Increased afterload
Conduction defects
    Bradycardias
    Supraventricular tachydysrhythmias
Ventricular dysrhythmias
    Premature ventricular beats
    Ventricular tachycardia
    Ventricular fibrillation
Perioperative infarction
Cardiac tamponade

Outcome Criteria	*Nursing Interventions*
Patient will have an adequate cardiac output as evidenced by: Mean arterial pressure greater than 60 mm Hg BP within normal limits (WNL) for the patient Hemodynamic values within optimal prescribed parameters Adequate cardiac output and index Sa_{O_2} greater than 90% Sv_{O_2} greater than 70% Urine output greater than 30 ml/hour Adequate rewarming process after surgery and return to normothermia state Normal sinus rhythm with no conduction defects and ventricular dysrhythmias No occurrence of cardiac tamponade	Monitor cardiac direct and derived parameters—i.e., dysrhythmias, Sv_{O_2}, hypertension, hypotension, urine output, sensorium, and presence of distal tissue perfusion—within normal limits for the individual patient Anticipate interventions for abnormalities Anticipate volume replacement to maintain adequate tissue perfusion, using colloid or crystalloid solutions, or directed donor or autologous blood replacement Anticipate use of vasodilators to decrease SVR and prevent vascular interruption Rewarm slowly, monitoring temperature Monitor for signs of shivering because its presence can increase metabolic demands, O_2 consumption, and blood pressure and precipitate or accentuate a metabolic acidotic state and/or bleeding Initiate standby temporary pacing using mode appropriate to maintain adequate cardiac index Anticipate overdrive pacing or pharmacologic interventions Monitor serum arterial blood gases, K^+, MG^{++}, vital signs, and cardiac hemodynamics Anticipate use of antidysrhythmic medications Monitor creatine kinase levels with MB fraction, ECG, and clinical presentation for the presence of perioperative myocardial infarction Monitor cardiac hemodynamics for equalization of pressures, decrease or increase in chest tube drainage, widening mediastinum on chest x-ray, and decrease in blood pressure as high index of suspicion for cardiac tamponade Monitor distal pulses and capillary fill

2. Impaired gas exchange related to:
Atelectasis
Increased $A\text{-}a_{O_2}$
Decreased functional residual capacity
Changed breathing patterns
Impaired secretion clearance
Pain

Outcome Criteria	*Nursing Interventions*
Patient will have adequate gas exchange as evidenced by: Arterial blood gases WNL for the patient Clear breath sounds bilaterally Respiratory rate, depth, and rhythm WNL for the patient Sa_{O_2} greater than 90% Vital signs WNL for the patient Minimal amount of incisional pain	Monitor ABG values and ventilator settings and perform pulmonary examination; compare to baseline prior to making changes in setting In the presence of rhonchi or secretions, suction using preoxygenation, hyperinflation, suction, and rehyperinflation techniques. Patients should be preoxygenated to minimize pulmonary vasoconstriction Weigh patient when stable or following a day; anticipate a 3- to 5-kg weight gain Monitor SaO_2, FIO_2, and PEEP levels as appropriate Monitor muscle strength, static lung volumes, respiratory effort, mentation, hemodynamic parameters, heart rate, and anxiety level prior and during weaning process Monitor clinical readiness for weaning Post-weaning, instruct patient in use of incentive spirometry as an inspiratory maneuver to recruit collapsed alveoli. Encourage patient to cough only to remove secretions because coughing is an expiratory maneuver that predisposes to atelectasis Turn the patient every 2 hours to maximize V/Q matching and promote return of normal lung volumes Monitor hydration status because hydration impairs secretion clearance Encourage progressive activity/ambulation as condition allows Provide analgesia as needed Provide chest splint pillow Instruct patient in arm or leg exercises

3. Potential for bleeding related to:
Coagulopathy
Vascular interruption of suture lines

Outcome Criteria	*Nursing Interventions*

Patient will have normal bleeding times and no abnormal bleeding problems as evidenced by:
    PT, PTT, H/H, DIC panel, platelet count and bleeding WNL for the patient
    Chest tube will be patent and free of air leaks
    Chest tube drainage will be less than 50 ml/hour
	Monitor PT, PTT, H/H, DIC panel, platelet count, bleeding time for elevations in normal values per physician's order
	Anticipate transfusion with autologous platelets, autotransfusion, or repletion of specific clotting factors
	Monitor chest tube drainage and report increase of greater than 100 ml/2 hours or sudden decrease in chest tube drainage
	Anticipate the need for hematology consult
	Anticipate the use of positive end-expiratory pressures as a means of slowing the bleeding
	Maintain chest tube patency through 20 cm of negative pressure on pleural space and milk chest tubes as per orders
	Assess drainage system for presence of air leak, which may be normal in patients in whom the pleural space was opened

4. Potential for decreased cerebral tissue perfusion related to:
    Stroke
    Prolonged hypotension
    Anoxia secondary to cardiac arrest
    Confusion secondary to sensory overload, sleep deprivation

Outcome Criteria	*Nursing Interventions*

Patient will have adequate cerebral tissue perfusion as evidenced by:
    Mental status WNL for the patient
    Neurologic assessment will be WNL for the patient
    No periods of confusion or disorientation
	Monitor, assess, and document patient neurologic examination reponse as per unit protocol. Compare motor response of each extremity with the other on one-step and two-step commands
	Provide reorientation prn
	Correct hypoxic state
	Encourage family to speak and touch patient
	Decrease sensory overload
	Provide rest periods and adequate sleep during night hours

5. Ineffective family and patient coping related to:
    Situational crisis

Outcome Criteria	*Nursing Interventions*

Patient and family will have effective coping mechanisms as evidenced by:
    Knowledge of the surgical procedure and what will happen to the patient in the postoperative period
    Identification and use of support systems
    Demonstration of appropriate coping techniques
	Nurse introduces self to family members or significant others, preferably before receiving patient from operating room
	Conduct a family assessment to determine:
	    How well the family unit is coping and what are the usual coping patterns
	    Who will be involved in decision-making
	    Who is supporting the family
	    What the significance of religion may be in the coping process of the family
	    What institutional supports may be needed—the family should be informed of these resources
	Ensure that the family's needs are met and that language used is simple and clear
	Additionally, ensure that communications are delivered in a sensitive manner. Establish clear communication patterns with family
	Assist the family in determining a spokesperson for the purpose of receiving and disseminating information
	Encourage family to write questions and verbalize feelings and concerns
	Evaluate the family's ability to adapt to the crisis
	Initiate family conference with physician, nursing, and support services as needed
	Once the patient is able to verbalize, encourage him to express feelings about health status, discharge planning, or needed life-style changes
	Support patient through periods of anxiety about illness, feelings of "setbacks," or regressive behaviors that impede progress

SUMMARY

During the past decade, innovations in cardiac surgery have produced exciting and provocative information for the scientific community caring for these patients. Coronary artery bypass operations have increased during the last decade. In 1983, 188,000 procedures were performed compared to 353,000 operations in 1991. Simultaneously, PTCA procedures have also experienced tremendous growth. A reported 227,000 procedures were performed in 1988, and the number anticipated for the 1990s is more than 400,000 per year, which far exceeds the number of coronary artery bypass procedures (American Heart Association, 1991).

What are the implications for the future? What trends can be expected in the twenty-first century? With $7.7 billion currently being spent on PTCA, valve, and CABG procedures, the inherent socioeconomic ramifications are evident. Researchers are now focusing on risk factor stratification in an attempt to evaluate the outcomes associated with various modes of therapy. What factors can be derived to indicate or predict operative outcomes of coronary artery bypass surgery?

As angioplasty and valvuloplasty techniques become more sophisticated, the patient population selected for these procedures will change. Consequently, patients undergoing surgical revascularization will also be different, characterized by more advanced preexisting pathologic disease states compared to the population observed during the last decade.

Changes during past years in patients undergoing valvular procedures have included a diminishing incidence of rheumatic heart disease. Similarly, improvements in valvular bioprostheses, myocardial preservation, and management of left ventricular dysfunction have improved the mortality statistics of valvular surgery. Improvements in anticoagulation protocols are also occurring. The dominant clinical issue for patients with valvular disease continues to be maintaining the dynamic balance between adequate anticoagulation and the prevention of embolic phenomena. As clinical experience accumulates, specific criteria governing the optimal timing of valve replacement are expected to further decrease morbidity and mortality statistics in this population. It is to be hoped that, with ongoing research to better define the associated risks and outcomes, the 1990s will be marked by continued progress and treatment for patients suffering from coronary atherosclerosis and valvular diseases.

References

Abd, A., Braun, N., Baskin, M., et al. (1989). Diaphragmatic dysfunction after open heart surgery. Treatment with a rocking bed. *Annals of Internal Medicine*, 111, 881–886.

Abernathy, W. and Willis, P. (1973). Thromboembolic complications of rheumatic heart disease. *Cardiovascular Clinics*, 5, 131–175.

Alderman, E. L., Fisher, L. D., Litwin, P., et al. (1983). Results of coronary artery surgery in patients with poor left ventricular function (CASS). *Circulation*, 68(4), 785–795.

American Heart Association (1987). *Textbook of advanced cardiac life support*. Dallas: Author.

American Heart Association (1991). *1991 Heart and stroke facts*. Dallas: Author.

Anderson, K., Waaben, J., and Husum, B. (1985). Nonpulsatile cardiopulmonary bypass disrupts the flow metabolism couple in the brain. *Journal of Thoracic and Cardiovascular Surgery*, 90, 570–579.

Angelini, G. D., Butchart, E. G., Armistead, S. H., et al. (1984). Comparative study of leg wound skin closure in coronary artery bypass graft operations. *Thorax*, 39(12), 924–925.

Asada, S., and Yamaguchi, F. (1981). Fine structural changes in the lung following cardiopulmonary bypass: Its relationship to early postoperative course. *Chest*, 50(3), 478–486.

Bartlett, R. (1980). Pulmonary pathophysiology in surgical patients. *Surgical Clinics of North America*, 60(6), 1323–1338.

Baumann, F. G. (1981). Vein contraction and smooth muscle extensions as causes of endothelial damage during graft preparation. *Annals of Surgery*, 194, 199–210.

Behrendt, D., and Austen, G. (1981). *Patient care in cardiac surgery* (3rd ed.). Boston: Little, Brown.

Benjamine, J., Cascade, P., Rubenfire, N., et al. (1982). Left lower lobe atelectasis and consolidation following cardiac surgery. The effects of topical cooling on phremo nerve. *Radiology*, 142(1), 11–14.

Bentall, H., and DeBono, A. (1968). A technique for complete replacement of the ascending aorta. *Thorax*, 23, 338–339.

Bick, R. L. (1984). Alterations of hemostasis associated with surgery, cardiopulmonary bypass, and prosthetic devices. In O. D. Ratnoff, and C. D. Forbes (Eds), *Disorders of hemostasis*. New York: Grune & Stratton.

Bjork, W. O. (1987). The Bjork-Shiley tilting disc valve: Past, present and future. *Cardiac Surgery*, 1, 183–202.

Blanche, C., Matloff, J., and Mackay, D. (1990). Technical aspects of cardio-pulmonary bypass. In R. Gary and J. Matloff (Eds.), *Medical management of the cardiac surgical patient* (p. 55). Baltimore: Williams & Wilkins.

Bojar, R. M. (1989). *Manual of perioperative care in cardiac and thoracic surgery*. Boston: Blackwell Scientific Publications.

Boldt, J., Kling, D., Zickmann, B., et al. (1990). Acute preoperative plasmapheresis and established blood conservation techniques. *Annals of Thoracic Surgery*, 50, 62–68.

Bonchek, L. (1987). Basis for selecting a valve prosthesis. In D. McGoon and A. Brest (Eds.), *Cardiac surgery* (2nd ed.). Philadelphia: F. A. Davis.

Bonchek, L. and Olinger, G. (1981). An improved method of topical hypothermia. *Journal of Thoracic and Cardiovascular Surgery*, 82(6), 878–882.

Bonser, R., Dave, J., Davies, E., et al. (1990). Reduction of complement activation during bypass by prime manipulation. *Annals of Thoracic Surgery*, 49, 279–283.

Boonstra, P., Vermenlen, F., Levsink, J., et al. (1986). Hematologic advantages of a membrane oxygenater over a bubble oxygenater in long perfusions. *Annals of Thoracic Surgery*, 41(3), 297–300.

Braunwald, E. (1983). Effects of coronary artery bypass grafting on survival. *New England Journal of Medicine*, 309, 1181–1188.

Braunwald, E. (Ed.). (1988). *Heart disease: A textbook of cardiovascular medicine* (3rd ed). Philadelphia: W. B. Saunders.

Brenner, B., Brief, D., Alpet, J., et al. (1987). The risk of stroke in patients with asymptomatic carotid stenosis undergoing cardiac surgery: A followup study. *Journal of Vascular Surgery*, 5, 269–279.

Brewer, A., Furlan, A., and Hansen, E. (1983). Central nervous system complications of coronary artery bypass graft surgery: Prospective analysis of 421 patients. *Stroke*, 45(5), 682–687.

Britton, L. W., Eastlund, D. T., and Dziuban, S. W. (1989). Predonated autologous blood use in elective surgery. *Annals of Thoracic Surgery*, 47, 529–532.

Brockman, S. and Cobanoglu, A. (1986). How cold cardioplegia and other myocardial protective modalities changed valvular surgery. In W. Frankl and A. Brest (Eds.), *Valvular heart disease: Comprehensive evaluation and management* (p. 396). Philadelphia: F. A. Davis.

Buckberg, G. (1975). Ventricular fibrillation: Its effects on myocardial flow, distribution, and performance. *Annals of Thoracic Surgery*, 20(1), 76–81.

Califf, R. M., Harrell, F. E., Lee, K. L., et al. (1989). The evolution of medical and surgical therapy for coronary artery disease. *Journal of American Medicine*, 261(14), 2077–2086.

Camara, M. L., Aris, A., Padro, J. D., et al. (1988). Long term results of mitral valve surgery in patients with severe pulmonary hypertension. *Annals of Thoracic Surgery*, 45(2), 133–136.

Campbell, D. and Waldhausen, J. (1986). The basis of choice of heart valve prostheses: Fact or fancy. *Annals of Thoracic Surgery*, 42, 487–493.

Carpentier, A. (1983). Cardiac valve surgery: The French correction. *Journal of Thoracic and Cardiovascular Surgery*, 86, 323–337.

CASS principal investigators (1984). Myocardial infarction and mortality in the coronary artery surgery study (CASS) randomized trial. *New England Journal of Medicine*, 310(12), 750–758.

Caulfield, J. B., Leinbach, R. C., and Gold, H. K. (1976). The relationship of myocardial infarct size and prognosis. *Circulation*, 53(Suppl. 1), 141–145.

Chaffin, J. and Daggett, W. (1978). Mitral valve replacement. Nine year followup of risk and survival. *Annals of Thoracic Surgery*, 27(4), 312–319.

Chaikhouni, A., Crawford, F. A., Kochel, P. J., et al. (1986). Human internal mammary artery produces more prostacyclin than saphenous vein. *Journal of Thoracic Cardiovascular Surgery*, 92(1), 88–91.

Chaitman, B. R., Alderman, E. L., Sheffield, L. T., et al. (1983). Use of survival analysis to determine clinical significance of new Q waves after coronary artery bypass surgery. *Circulation*, 67, 302–310.

Chaitman, B. R., Fisher, L. D., Bourassa, M. G., et al. (1981). Effect of coronary bypass surgery on survival patterns in subsets of patients with left main coronary artery disease: (CASS). *American Journal of Cardiology*, 48:765–777.

Chesebro, J. H., Knatterud, G., Roberts, R., et al. (1987). Thrombolysis in myocardial infarction (TIMI) trial, phase I: A comparison between intravenous tissue plasminogen activator and intravenous streptokinase. *Circulation*, 76, 142–154.

Chitwood, W. (1988). Myocardial protection by retrograde cardioplegia. Coronary sinus and right atrial methods. *Cardiac Surgery: State of the Art Reviews*, 2(2), 197–218.

Christakis, G., Fremes, S., Weiser, R., et al. (1985). Right ventricular dysfunction following cold potassium cardioplegia. *Journal of Thoracic Cardiovascular Surgery*, 90(2), 243–250.

Christopherson, B., and Pfieffer, C. (1980). Varying the timing of information to alter preoperative anxiety and postoperative recovery in cardiac surgery patients. *Heart & Lung*, 9(5), 854–861.

Chulay, M., Brown, J., and Summer, W. (1982). Effect of postoperative immobilization after coronary artery bypass surgery. *Critical Care Medicine*, 10, 176–182.

Chunlay, M., Brown, J., and Summer, W. (1982). Effects of postoperative immobilization after coronary artery bypass surgery. *Critical Care Medicine*, 10(3), 176–179.

Clark, R., Beauchamp, R., and McGrath, R. (1979). Comparison of bubble and membrane oxygenators in short and long perfusions. *Journal of Thoracic Cardiovascular Surgery*, 78(5), 655–666.

Cohn, L. H., Kowalker, W., Bhatia, S., et al. (1988). Comparative morbidity of mitral valve repair versus replacement for mitral regurgitation with and without coronary artery disease. *Annals of Thoracic Surgery*, 45(3), 53.

Coleman, B. (1989). Nursing implications for pulmonary artery balloon counterpulsation: A treatment for right ventricular dysfunction after cardiac surgery. *Critical Care Nursing Clinics of North America*, 55, 373–379.

Connors, J. P., and Avioli, L. V. (1981). An update on cardiac surgery. *Heart & Lung*, 10, 323–330.

Coronary Artery Surgery Study (CASS) principal investigators and associates. (1983). A randomized trial of coronary artery bypass surgery: Survival data. *Circulation*, 68, 939–950.

Cosgrove, D. M., Lytle, B. W., Loop, F. D., et al. (1988). Does bilateral internal mammary artery grafting increase surgical risk? *Journal of Thoracic and Cardiovascular Surgery*, 95, 850–856.

Crawford, F. A. (1987). The Ionescu-Shiley pericardial xenograph. *Cardiac Surgery*, 1, 285–293.

Culliford, A. T., Cunningham, J. N., and Zeff, R. H. (1976). Sternal and costochondral infections following open heart surgery. *Journal of Thoracic and Cardiovascular Surgery*, 52, 714–726.

Currie, P. J. (1989). Transesophageal echocardiography. *Circulation*, 80(1), 215–217.

Curtis, J., Nawaraawong, W., Walls, J., et al. (1989). Elevated hemidiaphragm after cardiac operation: Incidence, prognosis, and relationship to the use of topical ice slush. *Annals of Thoracic Surgery*, 43, 764–768.

Cusmano, R., Ashe, K., Salerno, P., et al. (1988). Oxygenated solutions in myocardial preservation. *Cardiac Surgery: State of the Art Reviews*, 2(2), 167–180.

Czer, L. Bateman, T., Gray, R., et al. (1985). Prospective trial of DDAVP in treatment of severe platelet dysfunction and hemorrhage after cardiopulmonary bypass. *Circulation*, 72(Suppl. 3), 111–130.

Daily, P. O. (1989). Early and five year results for coronary artery bypass grafting. *Journal of Thoracic and Cardiovascular Surgery*, 97(1), 67–77.

Davidson, D. M. (1980). Long-term results of coronary artery bypass surgery for unstable angina: Incidence of mortality, myocardial infarction, and angina resumption. *Clinical Cardiology*, 3:297–306.

Davis, R., Lappas, D., and Kirklin, J. (1982). Acute oliguria after cardiopulmonary bypass: Renal functional improvement with low-dose dopamine infusion. *Critical Care Medicine*, 10, 852–856.

DeBakey, M. (1934). A single continuous flow blood transfusion instrument. *The New Orleans Medical Surgical Journal*, 87(1), 386–394.

DeLaria, G. A., Hunter, J. A., and Goldin, M. D. (1981). Leg wound complications associated with coronary revascularization. *Journal of Thoracic and Cardiovascular Surgery*, 81, 403–407.

Delong, J., Ten-Ovis, H., Sibinga, C., et al. (1980). Hematologic aspects of cardiotomy suction in cardiac operations. *Journal of Cardiovascular Surgery*, 79(2), 227–236.

Deverux, R., and Reicher, N. (1980). Left ventricular hypertrophy. *Cardiovascular Reviews*, 1(2), 55–67.

Dewer, M., Rusengarten, M., Sampson, C., et al. (1980). Is high potassium solution necessary for reinfusion in "multidose" cold cardioplegia? A randomized prospective study using computerized Holter system. *Annals of Thoracic Surgery*, 43(4), 409–415.

DiSesa, V. J. (1987). The rationale for selection of inotropic drugs in cardiac surgery. *Journal of Cardiac Surgery*, 2(3), 385–406.

Drinkwater, D. K., Laks, H., and Buckberg, G. (1990). A new simplified method of optimizing cardioplegia delivery without right heart isolation. *Journal of Thoracic and Cardiovascular Surgery*, 77, 56–64.

Edmunds, L. H. (1987). Thrombotic and bleeding complications of prosthetic heart valves. *Annals of Thoracic Surgery*, 44(3), 430–445.

Edmunds, H., and Stephenson, L. (1983). Cardiopulmonary bypass for open heart surgery. In A. Getta, W. Glen, G. Hammond, et al. (Eds.); *Thoracic and cardiovascular surgery* (4th ed., p. 1091). Norwalk, CT: Appleton-Century Crofts.

Edwards, J. (1983). Pathology of mitral incompetence. In M. Silvers (Ed.), *Cardiovascular pathology* (Vol. 1; pp. 575–598). New York: Churchill Livingstone.

Ellis, R., Mauroudis, C., Gardner, C., et al. (1980). Relationship between atrioventricular arrhythmias and the concentration of potassium ion in cardioplegia solution. *Journal of Thoracic Cardiovascular Surgery*, 80(4), 517–526.

Epstein, S. E., Palmeri, S. T., and Patterson, R. E. (1982). Evaluation of patients after acute myocardial infarction: Indications for cardiac catheterization and surgical intervention. *New England Journal of Medicine*, 307, 1487.

Estanfanous, F. (1981). Hypertensive episodes during and after open heart surgery. *Cleveland Clinic Quarterly*, 48(1), 139–141.

Eugene, J., Ott, R. A., Piters, K. M., et al. (1983). Operative risk factors associated with unstable angina pectoris. *Archives of Surgery*, 120, 279–282.

European Coronary Surgery Study Group. (1982). Long-term results of prospective randomized study of coronary artery bypass surgery in stable angina pectoris. *Lancet*, 2, 1173–1181.

Fabiani, J., Deloche, A., Swansen, J., et al. (1986). Retrograde cardioplegia through the right atrium. *Annals of Thoracic Surgery*, 41(1), 101–102.

Fabiani, J., Swansen, J., and Deloche, A. (1987). Right atrial cardioplegia. In A. Roberts (Ed.), *Myocardial protection in cardiac surgery,* (p. 505). New York: Marcel Dekker.

Faggioli, G. L., Curl, G. R., and Ricotta, J. J. (1990). The role of carotid screening before coronary artery bypass. *Journal of Vascular Surgery,* 12(6), 724–730.

Farmilo, R. W., Scott, D. J. A., Cole, S. E. A., et al. (1990). Role of duplex scanning in the selection of patients for carotid endarterectomy. *British Journal of Surgery,* 77, 388–390.

Favalaro, R. G. (1969). Saphenous vein graft in the surgical treatment of coronary artery disease: Operative technique. *Journal of Thoracic and Cardiovascular Surgery,* 58, 178–185.

Ferguson, T., Smith, P., and Buhrman, W. (1983). Studies of the physiology of the conduction system during hyperkalemic hypothermic cardioplegic arrest. *Surgery Forum,* 34(2), 302–318.

Ferguson, T., Smith, P., Damiano, R., et al. (1987). Electrical activity on the heart during hyperkalemic hypothermic cardioplegic arrest: Site of origin and relationship to specialized conduction tissue. *Annals of Thoracic Surgery,* 43(4), 373–379.

Ferguson, T., Smith, P., Lofland, G., et al. (1986). The effects of cardioplegic potassium concentration on myocardial temperature on electrical activity in the heart during elective cardioplegic arrest. *Journal of Thoracic and Cardiovascular Surgery,* 92(4), 755–765.

Ferraris, V. A., Ferraris, S. P., Lough, F. C., et al. (1988). Preoperative aspirin ingestion increases operative blood loss after coronary artery bypass grafting. *Annals of Thoracic Surgery,* 45, 71–74.

Fischell, T. T., McDonald, T., Grattan, M., et al. (1989). Occlusive coronary artery spasm as a cause of acute myocardial infarction after coronary artery bypass grafting. *New England Journal of Medicine,* 320, 400–401.

Fitzgibbon, G. M., Leach, A. J., Keon, W. J., et al. (1986). Coronary bypass conduit fate after operation. *Journal of Thoracic and Cardiovascular Surgery,* 91, 773–778.

Fletcher, G. F., Froelicher, V. F., Hartley, L. H., et al. (1990). Exercise Standards AHA Medical/Scientific Statement. *Circulation,* 82(6), 2286–2315.

Force, T., Hibberd, P., Weeks, G., et al. (1990). Perioperative myocardial infarction after coronary artery bypass surgery. *Circulation,* 82, 903–912.

Forker, A., McCallister, B., and Giuliani, E. (1970). Atypical presentations of patients with calcific aortic stenosis. *Journal of American Medical Association,* 212(8), 774–779.

Foster, E. D., and Kranc, M. (1989). Alternative conduits for aortocoronary bypass grafting. *Circulation,* 79(Suppl 1), 34–40.

Freedman, A., and Goodman, L. (1982). Suctioning the left bronchial tree in the intubated adult. *Critical Care Medicine,* 10(1), 43–45.

Fremes, S., Christakis, G., Weiser, R., et al. (1984). A clinical trial of blood and crystalloid cardioplegia. *Journal of Thoracic and Cardiovascular Surgery,* 104, 726–741.

Fremes, S. E., Weisel, R. D., Mickle, D. A., et al. (1985). A comparison of nitroglycerine and sodium nitroprusside: Treatment of postoperative hypertension. *Annals of Thoracic Surgery,* 39(1), 53–59.

Galvin, I., Mosleri, J., Paneth, M., et al. (1988). An analysis of isolated aortic valve surgery and combined procedures in patients over 70 years of age. *Journal of Cardiovascular Surgery,* (Torino) 29(5), 577–581.

Geltman, E. M. (1987). Coronary thrombolysis with intravenous streptokinase. In B. E. Sobel (Ed.), *Cardiology clinics: Thrombolysis and the heart* (Vol. 5, pp. 91–99). Philadelphia: W. B. Saunders.

Gersh, B. J., Califf, R. M., Loop, F. D., et al. (1989). Coronary bypass surgery in chronic stable angina. *Circulation,* 79(Suppl 1), 46–59.

Gibbson, J. (1954). Application of a mechanical heart and lung apparatus to cardiac surgery. *Minnesota Medicine,* 37, 171–178.

Glancy, D. L. (1980). Medical management of adults and older children undergoing cardiac operations. *Heart & Lung,* 2(2), 277–283.

Goldman, S., Copeland, J., Moritz, T., et al. (1988). Improvement in early saphenous vein graft patency after coronary artery bypass surgery with antiplatelet therapy: Results of a Veterans Administration Cooperative Study. *Circulation,* 77(6), 1324–1332.

Goran, S. F. (1989). Vascular complications of the patient undergoing intra-aortic balloon pumping. *Critical Care Clinics of North America,* 1(3), 459–467.

Gordon, M. (1989). *Manual of nursing diagnosis.* St. Louis: C.V. Mosby.

Gortner, S. R., Gillis, C. L., Paul, S. M., et al. (1989). Expected and realized benefits from cardiac surgery: An update. *Cardiovascular Nursing,* 25(4), 18–24.

Gravlee, G., Haddon, S., Rothberger, H., et al. (1990). Heparin dosing and monitoring for cardiopulmonary bypass. *Journal of Thoracic and Cardiovascular Surgery,* 99, 518–527.

Gravlee, G., Roy, R., Stump, D., et al. (1990). Regional cerebrovascular reactivity to carbon dioxide during cardiopulmonary bypass in patients with cerebrovascular disease. *Journal of Thoracic and Cardiovascular Surgery,* 99, 1022–1029.

Gray, R. (1990). Postoperative hypertension. In R. Gray and J. Matloff (Eds.) *Medical management of the cardiac surgical patient.* Baltimore: Williams & Wilkens.

Gray, R., and Mandel, W. (1991). Management of common postoperative arrhythmias. In R. Gray and J. Matloff (Eds.), *Medical management of the cardiac surgical patient* (p. 208). Baltimore: Williams & Wilkins.

Green, G. E. (1989). Use of internal thoracic artery for coronary artery grafting. *Circulation,* 79(6), Suppl. 1, 1-30–1-33.

Greene, A., Gray, L. A., Slater, A. D., et al. (1991). Emergency aortocoronary bypass after failed angioplasty. *Annals of Thoracic Surgery,* 51, 194–199.

Greenberg, B. H. and Murphy, E. (Eds.). (1987). *Valvular heart disease.* Littletown, MA: PSG Publishing.

Grondin, C. M., Campeau, L., Thornton, J. C., et al. (1989). Coronary artery bypass grafting with saphenous vein. *Circulation,* 79(Suppl 1), 24–29.

Gross, S. (1988). Effect of a preoperative education/orientation visit by a critical care nurse on patient anxiety. Unpublished manuscript.

Grossi, E. A., Culliford, A. T., and Krieger, K. H. (1985). A survey of 77 major infectious complications of median sternotomy: A review of 7949 consecutive operative procedures. *Annals of Thoracic Surgery,* 126, 214–221.

Guiteras, P., Pelletier, C., Hernandez, M., et al. (1983). Diagnostic criteria and prognosis of perioperative myocardial infarction following coronary bypass. *Journal of Thoracic and Cardiovascular Surgery,* 88, 878–886.

Gurley, J., Booth, D., and DeMaria, A. (1990). Circulatory collapse following coronary bypass surgery: Multivessel and graft spasm reversed in the catheterization laboratory by intracoronary papaverine. *American Heart Journal,* 119, 1194–1195.

Gutmann, M. C., Knapp, D. N., and Pollack, M. L. (1982). Coronary bypass patients and work status. *Circulation,* 66, 33–38.

Guyton, R. (1988). Myocardial protection as an integral part of overall operative strategy. *Cardiac Surgery: State of the Art Reviews,* 2(2), 279–289.

Guzman, L. (1981). Nursing management of the parenteral drug abuser with infective endocarditis. *Heart & Lung,* 10(2), 289–294.

Hamlet, M. (1989). Personal communication.

Hammermeister, K. E., Fisher, L., Kennedy, J. W., et al. (1978). Prediction of late survival in patients with mitral valve disease from clinical hemodynamic, and quantitative angiographic variables. *Circulation,* 57, 341–348.

Hammerschmidt, D., Irncek, D., Bowers, T., et al. (1981). Compliment activation and neutropenia occurring during cardiopulmonary bypass. *Journal of Thoracic and Cardiovascular Surgery,* 81(3), 370–377.

Haneda, K., Thomas, R., and Breasale, D. (1982). Whole body temperature gradients under surface perfusion and combined surface perfusion hypothermia. *Cryobiology,* 19(1), 119–128.

Harker, L. (1986). Bleeding after cardiopulmonary bypass. *New England Journal of Medicine,* 314, 446–448.

Heyman, S. (1985). Effects of cardiopulmonary bypass on coagulation. *Dimensions of Critical Care Nursing,* 4(2), 70–78.

Hickey, R., and Hoor, P. (1983). Whole body oxygen consumption during low flow hypothermic cardiopulmonary bypass. *Journal of Thoracic and Cardiovascular Surgery,* 86(6), 903–906.

Hines, R., and Barash, P. (1985). Right ventricular function in the perioperative period. *Mount Sinai Journal of Medicine*, 52(2), 529–537.

Hinohara, T., Simpson, J. B., Phillips, H. R., et al. (1988). Transluminal intracoronary reperfusion catheter: A device to maintain coronary perfusion between failed coronary angioplasty and emergency coronary bypass surgery. *Journal of American College of Cardiology*, 11, 977–982.

Hirshfeld, J. (1986). Role of laboratory diagnostic methods in evaluation and followup of patients with valvular heart disease: Relation to prognosis and outcome after valve replacement. In W. Frankl and A. N. Brest (Eds.), *Valvular heart disease: Comprehensive evaluation and management* (pp. 151–158). Philadelphia: F. A. Davis.

Hisatomi, K., Isomura, T., Kawara, T., et al. (1989). Changes in lymphocyte subsets mitogen responsiveness and interleukin-2 production after cardiac operations. *Journal of Thoracic and Cardiovascular Surgery*, 948, 580–591.

Hoie, J., and ForFang, K. (1980). Arrhythmias and conduction disturbances following aortic valve replacement. *Scandinavian Journal of Thoracic Cardiovascular Surgery*, 14, 177–183.

Horran, J. (1985) Protamine: A review of its toxicity. *Anesthesia Analog*, 64, 348–361.

Hurst, J. W., King, S. B., and Friesinger, G. C. (1986). *The heart*. New York: McGraw Hill.

Ingersoll, G. L., and Grippi, M. A. (1991). Preoperative pulmonary status and postoperative extubation outcome of patients undergoing elective cardiac surgery. *Heart & Lung*, 20(1), 137–143.

Isaacson, J., Walker, H., Hayes, S., et al. (1982). Post pump psychosis. *Critical Care Nurse*, 2(1), 14–16.

Jais, M., Chaitman, R., Dupras, G. K., et al. (1983). Diagnostic criteria and prognosis of perioperative myocardial infarction following coronary bypass. *Journal of Thoracic and Cardiovascular Surgery*, 86, 878–886.

Jansen, K. J., and McFadden, P. M. (1986). Postoperative nursing management in patients undergoing myocardial revascularization with the internal mammary artery bypass. *Heart & Lung*, 15(1), 48–54.

Jeevanandam, V., Smith, C., Rose, E., et al. (1990). Single stage management of sternal wound infections. *Journal of Thoracic and Cardiovascular Surgery*, 99, 256–263.

Johnson, J. E. (1972). Effects of structuring patients' expectations on their reactions to threatening events. *Nursing Research*, 21, 499–504.

Johnson, P., Messter, K., Ryding, E., et al. (1987). Cerebral blood flow and autoregulation during hypothermic cardiopulmonary bypass. *Annals of Thoracic Surgery*, 43(4), 386–390.

Johnson, W., Flemma, R. J., and Lepley, D. (1969). Extended treatment of severe coronary artery disease: A surgical approach. *Annals of Surgery*, 170, 460–467.

Johnson, W. D., Kayser, K. L., Brenowitz, J. B., et al. (1991). A randomized controlled trial of allopurinol in coronary bypass surgery. *American Heart Journal*, 121(1), 20–23.

Kaiser, G. C., Schaff, H. V., and Killip, T. (1989). Myocardial revascularization for unstable angina. *Circulation*, 79(6) Suppl 1, 60–67.

Kaiser, G. C., Davis, K. B., Fisher, L. D., et al. (1985). Survival following coronary artery bypass grafting in patients with severe angina pectoris (CASS) An observational study. *Journal of Thoracic and Cardiovascular Surgery*, 89(4), 513–522.

Karp, R. (1987). Infective endocarditis. In D. C. McGoon and A. N. Brest (Eds.), *Cardiac Surgery* (2nd ed., pp. 141–160). Philadelphia: F. A. Davis.

Kay, J. H. (1982). Emergency operation for complications of myocardial infarction. *Heart & Lung*, 11, 40–45.

Kennedy, J. W., Ivey, T. D., Misbach, G., et al. (1989). Coronary artery bypass graft surgery early after acute myocardial infarction. *Circulation*, 79(6) Suppl 1, 68–72.

Khan, S. and Gray, R. (1988). Recent development in aortic stenosis. *Comprehensive Therapy*, 14(4), 33–39.

Killip, T., Passamani, E., and Davis, K. (1985). Coronary artery surgery study (CASS) A randomized trial of coronary bypass surgery: Eight years follow-up and survival in patients with reduced ejection fraction. *Circulation*, 72(Suppl 5), 102–109.

Kirklin, J. W., Akins, C. W., Blackstone, E. H., et al. (1991).

Guidelines and indications for coronary artery bypass graft surgery. *Journal of American College of Cardiology*, 17(3), 543–589.

Kirklin, J. W., and Barratt-Boyes, B. G. (Eds.). (1986). *Cardiac surgery*. New York: John Wiley & Sons.

Kirklin, J. K., and Kirklin, J. W. (1981). Management of the cardiovascular subsystem after cardiac surgery. *Annals of Thoracic Surgery*, 32(3), 311–319.

Kirklin, J. W., Naftel, D. C., Blackstone, E. H., et al. (1989). Summary of a consensus concerning death and ischemic events after coronary artery bypass grafting. *Circulation*, 170, 81–91.

Kresh, J., Nastala, C., and Bianchi, P. (1987). The relative buffering power of blood cardioplegic solution. *Journal of Thoracic and Cardiovascular Surgery*, 93, 309–311.

Kristensen, C. (1990). Renal failure. In Gray, R., and Matloff, J. (Eds), *Management of cardiac surgical patients*. Baltimore: Williams & Wilkins.

Kruse, D. (1983). Postoperative hypothermia. *Focus on Critical Care*, 10(2), 48–50.

Kuntschen, F., Galletti, P., and Hahn, C. (1986). Glucose-Insulin interactions during cardiopulmonary bypass, hypothermia versus normothermia. *Journal of Thoracic and Cardiovascular Surgery*, 91(3), 451–459.

Kuntschen, F., Galletti, P., Hahn, C., et al. (1985). Alteration in insulin and glucose metabolism during cardiopulmonary bypass under normothermia. *Journal of Thoracic and Cardiovascular Surgery*, 89(1), 97–106.

Landymore, R., Murphy, D., and Kinley, C. (1979). Does pulsatile flow influence the incidence of postoperative hypertension? *Annals of Thoracic Surgery*, 28(1), 261–272.

Lavelle, J., Duigan, J., and Neligan, A. (1984). The effects of cardiopulmonary bypass on immune mechanisms of man. *Irish Journal of Medical Science*, 153(12), 431–436.

Leaf, A., and Weber, P. C. (1988). Cardiovascular effects of n-3 fatty acids. *New England Journal of Medicine*, 181, 549–557.

Leimgruber, P. P., Roubin, G. S., Hollman, J., et al. (1986). Rest enosis after successful angioplasty in patients with single vessel disease. *Circulation*, 73, 710–718.

Levine, F. H., Carter, J. E., Buckley, M. J., et al. (1981). Hemodynamic evaluation of Hancock and Carpentier-Edwards bioprostheses. *Circulation*, 64 (Suppl II), 192–195.

Levy, J., Schwieger, I., Zaidan, J., et al. (1989). Evaluation of patients at risk for protamine reactions. *Journal of Thoracic and Cardiovascular Surgery*, 948, 200–204.

Lewenstein, E., Johnsen, W., and Lappas, D. (1983). Catastrophic pulmonary vasoconstriction associated with reversal of heparin. *Anesthesiology*, 50(4), 470–473.

Lewis, R. (1980). Management of atelectasis and pneumonia. *Surgical Clinics of North America*, 60(6), 1391–1401.

Ley, J., Miller, K., Skov, P., et al. (1990). Crystalloid versus colloid fluid therapy after cardiac surgery. *Heart & Lung*, 19, 31–40.

Lindeman, C. A., and Stetzer, S. L. (1973). Effect of preoperative visits by operating room nurses. *Nursing Research*, 22(1), 4–16.

Livesey, S., Caine, N., Spiegelhalter, D. J., et al. Cardiac surgery for patients aged 65 years and older: A long term survival analysis. *British Heart Journal*, 60(6), 480–484.

Loop, F. D. (1983). Progress in surgical treatment of coronary atherosclerosis. Part 1. *Chest*, 84, 611.

Loop, F. D. (1983). Progress in surgical treatment of coronary atherosclerosis. Part 2. *Chest*, 84, 740.

Loop, F. D., Lytle, B. W., and Cosgrove, D. M. (1989). New arteries for old. *Circulation*, 79(Suppl 1), 40–45.

Loop, F., Lytle, B., Cosgrove, D., et al. (1990). Sternal wound complications after isolated coronary artery bypass grafting: Early and late mortality and morbidity, and cost of care. *Annals of Thoracic Surgery*, 49, 179–187.

Loop, F. D., Lytle, B. W., Cosgrove, D. M., et al. (1986). Influence of the internal mammary-artery-graft on 10 year survival and other cardiac events. *New England Journal of Medicine*, 314, 1–6.

Loop, F. D., Lytle, B. W., Gill, C. C., et al. (1983). Trends in selection of and results of coronary artery reoperations. *Annals of Thoracic Surgery*, 36, 380–388.

Luce, J. (1984). Clinical risk for postoperative pulmonary complications. *Respiratory Care*, 29(5), 484–495.

Luce, J. M., Tyler, M. L., and Pierson, D. J. (1984). *Intensive respiratory care*. Philadelphia: W. B. Saunders.

Lucus, S., Gardner, F., Flatherty, J., et al. Beneficial effects of mannitol administration during reperfusion after ischemic arrest. *Circulation*, 62(1), 1–34.

Lust, R. (1988). Physiologic influences of alterations in coronary anatomy on cardioplegia and reperfusion. *Cardiac Surgery: State of the Art Reviews*, 2(2), 351–382.

Lytle, B. W., Cosgrove, D. M., Stewart, R. W., et al. (1987). Right gastroepiploic artery: Alternative coronary bypass conduit. *Circulation*, 76, 351.

Lytle, B. W., Loop, F. D., Cosgrove, D. M., et al. (1987). Fifteen hundred coronary reoperations: Results and determinants of early and late survival. *Journal of Thoracic and Cardiovascular Surgery*, 205, 847–859.

Magilligan, D., Vij, D., Peper, W., et al. (1985). Failure of standard cardioplegic techniques to protect the conduction system. *Annals of Thoracic Surgery*, 39(5), 403–408.

Magovern, G., Bolling, S., Casale, A., et al. (1984). *Circulation*, Suppl. 70(1), 1–91.

Maleki, M., and Manley, J. (1989). Venospastic phenomena of saphenous vein bypass grafts. *British Heart Journal*, 62, 57–60.

Marelli, R., Paul, A., Samson, R., et al. (1989). Does the addition of albumin to the prime solution in cardiopulmonary bypass affect clinical outcome? *Journal of Thoracic and Cardiovascular Surgery*, 98, 757–766.

Massell, B., Ameccua, F., and Czohiczer, G., (1966). Prognosis of patients with pure predominant aortic regurgitation in the absence of surgery. *Circulation*, 34 (Suppl II), 164–170.

Matsuki, O., Robles, A., Gibbs, S., et al. (1988). Long-term performance of 555 aortic homographs in the aortic position. *Annals of Thoracic Surgery*, 46, 187–191.

McGoon, D., and Brest, A. (Eds.). (1987). *Cardiac surgery* (2nd ed., pp. 40–50). Philadelphia: F. A. Davis.

Michaels, I., and Barash, P. (1983). Hemodynamic changes during protamine administration. *Anesthesia Analog*, 60(1), 33–36.

Milam, J. (1983). Blood transfusions in heart surgery. *Surgical Clinics of North America*, 63(5), 1127–1147.

Mills, N. L., and Everson, C. T. (1989). Right gastroepiploic artery: A third arterial conduit for coronary artery bypass. *Annals of Thoracic Surgery*, 47, 706–711.

Mnami, K., Korner, M., Vyska, K., et al. (1990). Effects of pulsatile perfusion on plasma catecholemine levels and hemodynamics during and after cardiac operations with cardiopulmonary bypass. *Journal of Thoracic and Cardiovascular Surgery*, 99, 82–91.

Moore, S., and Wilkoff, B. (1991). Rhythm disturbances after cardiac surgery. *Seminars in Thoracic and Cardiovascular Surgery*, 3, 24–28.

Moores, W., Gago, O., Morris, J., et al. (1977). Serum and urinary amylase levels following pulsatile and continuous cardiopulmonary bypass. *Journal of Thoracic and Cardiovascular Surgery*, 74(1), 73–76.

Moores, W., and Willford, D. (1989). Modification of cardiopulmonary bypass to optimize myocardial protection. *Cardiac Surgery: State of the Art Reviews*, 2(2), 331–350.

Morel, D., Zapol, W., Thomas, S., et al. (1987) C5a and thromboxane generator associated with pulmonary vaso- and bronchoconstriction during protamine reversal. *Anesthesiology*, 66, 597–604.

Mori, T., Ivey, T., Itoh, T., et al. (1987). Effects of pulsatile on postishemic recovery of myocardial function after global hypothermic cardiac arrest. *Journal of Thoracic and Cardiovascular Surgery*, 93, 719–727.

Morgan, R., Davis, T. and Fraker, T. (1985). Current status of valve prostheses. *Surgical Clinics of North America*, 65(3), 699–722.

Morris, J., and Wechsler, A. (1988). Right ventricular performance and protection. *Cardiac Surgery: State of the Art Reviews*, 2(2), 303–329.

Murphy, D. A., Craver, J. M., Jones, E. L., et al. (1982). Surgical revascularization following unsuccessful percutaneous transluminal coronary angioplasty. *Journal of Thoracic and Cardiovascular Surgery*, 84, 342–348.

Musial, J., Neiwiarowski, S., Hershock, D., et al. (1985). Loss of fibrinogen receptors from the platelet surface during simulated extracorpeal circulation. *Journal of Laboratory and Clinical Medicine*, 105, 514–522.

Myers, B., and Moran, S. (1986). Hemodynamically mediated acute renal failure *New England Journal of Medicine*, 314, 97–105.

Myers, W. O., Schaff, H. V., Gersh, B. J., et al. (1989). Improved survival of surgically treated patients with triple vessel coronary artery disease and severe angina pectoris. (CASS). *Journal of Thoracic and Cardiovascular Surgery*, 97(4), 487–495.

McKnight, C., Elhot, M., Pearson, D., et al. (1985). The effects of four different crystalloid bypass pump priming fluids upon the metabolic response to cardiac operation. *Journal of Thoracic Cardiovascular Surgery*, 90(1), 90–97.

Nair, U. R., Griffiths, G., and Lawson, R. A. (1988). Postoperative neuralgia in the leg after saphenous vein coronary artery bypass graft. *Thorax*, 43(1), 41–43.

New York Heart Association Criteria Committee. (1964). *Diseases of the heart and blood vessels: Nomenclature and criteria for diagnosis* (6th ed., pp. 110–114). Boston: Little, Brown.

Niemmen, M., Philbin, D., Rosow, C., et al. (1983). Gradients and rewarming time during hypothermic cardiopulmonary bypass with and without pulsatile flow. *Annals of Thoracic Surgery*, 35(5), 488–493.

Norris, S. O. (1989). Managing postoperative mediastinitis. *Journal of Cardiovascular Nursing*, 3(3), 52–65.

O'Keefe, J. H., Hartzler, G. O., McConahay, D. R., et al. (1990). Procedural risk and long term effectiveness of multi-vessel coronary angioplasty 1980–1989. *Journal of American College of Cardiology*, 15, 205.

Olinger, G. (1988). Hypothermic intermittant ischemic arrest. *Cardiac Surgery: State of the Art Reviews*, 2(2), 155–165.

O'Rouke, M. F., Sammel, N., and Chang, V. P. (1979). Arterial counterpulsation in severe refractory heart failure complicating acute myocardial infarction. *British Heart Journal*, 41, 308–316.

O'Rourke, R., and Walsh, R. (1983). Recognition and treatment of acute aortic regurgitation. *Journal of Intensive Care Medicine*, 1(1), 33–46.

Pairolero, P. (1984). Management of recalcitrant median sternotomy wounds. *Journal of Thoracic and Cardiovascular Surgery*, 88, 357–365.

Parsonnet, V., Dean, D., and Bernstein, A. D. (1989). A method of uniform stratification of risk for evaluating the results of surgery in acquired adult heart disease. *Circulation*, 79(Suppl 1), 3–12.

Pennington, G., Merjavy, J. and Swartz, M. (1985). Important biventricular failure in patients with postoperative cardiogenic shock. *Annals of Thoracic Surgery*, 39(1), 16–28.

Penta, A., Qureshi, S., Radley-Smith, R., et al. (1984). Patient status 10 or more years after "fresh" homograph replacement of the aortic valve. *Circulation*, 70(Suppl 1), 182–186.

Philbin, D. (1985). Endocrine response to cardiopulmonary bypass. *The Mount Sinai Journal of Medicine*, 52(7), 508–510.

Phillips, R., and Skov, P. (1988). Rewarming and cardiac surgery: A review. *Heart & Lung*, 17(5), 511–520.

Phillips, S. J., Kongtahworn, C., Skinner, J. R., et al. (1983). Emergency coronary artery reperfusion: A choice therapy for evolving myocardial infarction. *Journal of Thoracic and Cardiovascular Surgery*, 86, 679–688.

Pieper, B., Lepczzyk, M., and Caldwell, M. (1985). Perceptions of the waiting period before coronary artery bypass grafting. *Heart & Lung*, 14(1), 40–44.

Pluth, J. R. (1987). Mitral valve reconstruction versus mitral replacement. In D. C. McGoon and A. N. Brest (Eds.), *Cardiac surgery* (2nd ed., pp. 127–140). Philadelphia: F. A. Davis.

Puig, R. B., Ciongolli, W., Cividanes, G. V. L., et al. (1990). Inferior epigastric artery as a free graft for myocardial revascularization. *Journal of Cardiovascular and Thoracic Surgery*, 99, 251–255.

Quiroga, M., Miyagishima, R., Haendschen, L., et al. (1985). The effects of body temperature on leukocytes kinetics during cardiopulmonary bypass. *Journal of Thoracic Cardiovascular Surgery*, 90(1), 91–96.

Rahimtoola, S. H. (1985). A perspective on the 3 large multicenter randomized clinical trials of CABG for chronic stable angina. *Circulation*, 72(Suppl V), 123–135.

Rahimtoola, S. H. (1988). Lessons learned about the determinants of the results of valve surgery. *Circulation*, 78(6), 1503–1507.

Randall, E. (1989). Recognizing cardiac tamponade. *Journal of Cardiovascular Nursing*, 252(3), 42–51.

Rankin, J. S., Newton, J. R., Jr., Califf, R. M., et al. (1984). Clinical characteristics and current management of medically refractory unstable angina. *Annals of Surgery*, 200(4), 457–464.

Rapport, E. (1975). Natural history of aortic and mitral valve disease. *American College of Cardiology*, 35, 221–227.

Raymond, M., Conklin, C., Schaeffer, J., et al. (1985). Coping with transient intellectual dysfunction after coronary bypass surgery. *Heart & Lung*, 13(5), 531–539.

Rebeyka, M., Coles, J., Wilson, G., et al. (1987). The effects of low flow cardiopulmonary bypass on cerebral function: An experimental and clinical study. *Annals of Thoracic Surgery*, 43(4), 391–396.

Reis, C., Evora, P., Ribeiro, P., et al. (1987). A simple mechanical system for pulsatile cardiopulmonary bypass. *Journal of Cardiovascular Surgery*, 28(1), 143–144.

Reitz, B. A. (1982). Uses of hypothermia in cardiovascular surgery. In A. K. Ream (Ed.), *Acute cardiovascular management: Anesthesia and intensive care*. Philadelphia: J. B. Lippincott.

Rentrop, K. P. (1985). Thrombolytic therapy in patients with acute myocardial infarction. *Circulation*, 71, 627–631.

Reves, J. (1985). Adrenergic response to cardiopulmonary bypass. *The Mount Sinai Journal of Medicine*, 52(7), 511–515.

Rich, M. W., Keller, A. J., Schechtman, K. B., et al. (1988). Morbidity and mortality of coronary bypass surgery in patients 75 years of age or older. *Annals of Thoracic Surgery*, 46, 638–644.

Roberts, A., Faro, R., Williams, L., et al. (1983). Relative efficacy of left ventricular venting techniques commonly used during coronary artery bypass graft surgery. *Annals of Thoracic Surgery*, 3694), 444–452.

Roberts, W. (1983). Morphologic features of the normal and abnormal mitral valve. *American Journal of Cardiology*, 51(7), 1005–1028.

Roberts, W. C. (1976). Choosing a substitute cardiac valve: Type, size, surgeon. *American Journal of Cardiology*, 38(5), 633–644.

Rodrigues, J. L., Weissman, C., Damask, M. C., et al. (1983). Morphine and postoperative rewarming in critically ill patients. *Circulation*, 68(6), 1238–1246.

Rosenfeldt, F. (1988). The theory and practice of cardiac cooling. *Cardiac Surgery: State of the Art Reviews*, 2(2), 219–240.

Rosenfeldt, F., and Arnold, M. (1982). Topical cooling by recirculation: Comparison of a closed system using a cooling pad with an open system using topical spray. *Annals of Thoracic Surgery*, 34(2), 138–145.

Rosenfeldt, F., and Watson, D. (1979). Interference with local myocardial cooling by heart gain during aortic cross clamping. *Annals of Thoracic Surgery*, 27(1), 13–16.

Ross, D. (1988). Pulmonary valve autotransplantation. Journal of *Cardiac Surgery*, 3(Suppl. 1), 313–319.

Ross, J. (1985). Afterload mismatch in aortic and mitral valve disease. Implications for surgical therapy. *Journal of American College of Cardiology*, 5(5), 811–826.

Roth, J., Golub, S., Cukingnan, R., et al. (1981). Cell mediated immunity is depressed following cardiopulmonary bypass. *Annals of Thoracic Surgery*, 31(4), 350–356.

Rousou, J. A., Parker, T., Engelman, R. M., et al. (1985). Phrenic nerve paresis associated with use of iced slush and the cooling jacket for topical hypothermia. *Journal of Thoracic and Cardiovascular Surgery*, 89(6), 921–925.

Sadler, P. D. (1981). Incidence, degree, and duration of postcardiotomy delirium. *Heart & Lung*, 10, 1084–1092.

Salerno, T., Houch, J., Barrozo, C., et al. (1991). Retrograde continuous warm blood cardioplegia. *Annals of Thoracic Surgery*, 51, 245–247.

Salzman, E., Weinstein, M., Weintraub, R., et al. (1986). Treatment with desmopressin acetate to reduce blood loss after cardiac surgery. *New England Journal of Medicine*, 314, 1402–1411.

Samuel, T. (1977). Antibodies reacting with salmon and human protamines in sera from infertile men from vasectomized men and monkeys. *Clinical Experimentation Immunology*, 21, 65–74.

Santillan, G., Chemnitius, M., and Bing, P. (1985). The effects of cardiopulmonary bypass on cerebral blood flow. *Brain Research*, 280, 1–9.

Sarabu, M. R., McClung, J. A., Fass, A., et al. (1987). Early

postoperative spasm in left internal mammary artery bypass grafts. *Annals of Thoracic Surgery*, 44, 199–200.

Schakenbach, L. (1987). Physiologic dynamics of acquired valvular disease. *Journal of Cardiovascular Nursing*, 1(3), 1–17.

Schneider, R. M., and Helfant, R. H. (1986). Timing of surgery in chronic mitral and aortic regurgitation. In W. Frankl and A. N. Brest (Eds.), *Valvular heart disease: Comprehensive evaluation and management* (pp. 361–371). Philadelphia: F. A. Davis.

Seifert, P. C. (1987). Surgery for acquired valvular heart disease. *Journal of Cardiovascular Nursing*, 1(3), 26–40.

Settelberger, R., Zwolfer, W., Huber, S., et al. (1991). Nifedipine reduces the incidence of myocardial and transient ischemia in patients undergoing coronary bypass grafting. *Circulation*, 83, 460–468.

Sethi, G., Copeland, J., Goldman, S., et al. (1990). Implications of preoperative administration of aspirin in patients undergoing coronary artery bypass grafting. Department of Veteran Affairs Coop Study on Antiplatelet Therapy. *Journal of American College of Cardiology*, 15, 15–20.

Sheland, J., Hirleman, M., and Hoang, A. (1983). Lobar collapse in the surgical intensive care unit. *British Journal of Radiology*, 247, 531–534.

Shultz, C., and Woodall, C. (1989). Using epicardial pacing electrodes. *Journal of Cardiovascular Nursing*, 3(3), 25–33.

Silverman, K. J., and Grossman, W. (1984). Angina pectoris: Natural history and strategies for evaluation and management. *New England Journal of Medicine*, 310(26), 1712–1717.

Silverman, N., Del Ndio, P., Kruken-Kamp, I., et al. (1988). Biological rationale for antegrade c cardioplegic solution. *Cardiac Surgery: State of the Art Reviews*, 2(2), 181–195.

Singh, R., Barratt-Boyes, B., and Morris, E. (1980). Does pulsatile flow improve perfusion during hypothermic cardiopulmonary bypass? *Journal of Thoracic and Cardiovascular Surgery*, 79(6), 827–832.

Singh, A., Farrugia, R., Teplitiz, C., et al. (1981). Electrolyte versus blood cardioplegia: Randomized clinical and myocardial intrastructural study. *Annals of Thoracic Surgery*, 33(3), 218–227.

Smith, N., Raizada, V. and Abrams, J. (1987). Ascultation of the normally functioning prosthetic valve. *Annals of Internal Medicine*, 95(5), 594–597.

Smith, P. K., Buhrman, W., Levett, J., et al. (1983). Supraventricular conduction abnormalities following cardiac operation. *Journal of Thoracic and Cardiovascular Surgery*, 85(1), 105–115.

Solem, J. O., Steen, S., Tengborn, L., et al. (1987). Mediastinal drainage blood: Potentialities for autotransfusion aftercardiac surgery. *Scandinavian Journal of Thoracic and Cardiovascular Surgery*, 21(2), 149–152.

Sones, F. M., and Shirey, E. K. (1962). Cine coronary arteriography. *Modern Concepts in Cardiovascular Diseases*, 31, 735–745.

Spenser, F. C., Colvin, S. B., Culliford, A. T., et al. (1985). Experiences with the Carpentier techniques of mitral valve reconstruction in 103 patients (1980–1985). *Journal of Thoracic and Cardiovascular Surgery*, 90, 341–350.

Stelzer, P., and Elkins, R. (1989). Homograph valves and conduits: Applications in cardiac surgery. *Current Problems in Surgery*, 259, 389–445.

Stephan, Y., Jebara, V. A., Fabiani, J., et al. (1990). The internal mammary vein: A new conduit of coronary artery bypass. (Editorial.) *Journal of Thoracic and Cardiovascular Surgery*, 99(1), 178.

Stephenson, L. W., MacVaugh, H., and Edmunds, L. H. (1978). Surgery using cardiopulmonary bypass in the elderly. *Circulation*, 58(2), 250–254.

Suma, H., Takeuchi, A., and Hirota, Y. (1989). Myocardial revascularization with combined arterial grafts utilizing the internal mammary and the gastroepiploic arteries. *Annals of Thoracic Surgery*, 47, 712–715.

Sutcliffe, S. A., and Ridder, M. E. (1984). Individualized preadmission teaching program. *Critical Care Nurse*, 4, 35–39.

Svennevig, L., Linberg, H., Geiran, O., et al. (1984). Should the lungs be ventilated during cardiopulmonary bypass? Clinical, hemodynamic, and metabolic changes in patients undergoing elective coronary artery surgery. *Annals of Thoracic Surgery*, 37(4), 295–300.

Takaro, T., Hultgren, H. N., Lipton, M. J., et al. (1976). The VA Cooperative randomized study of surgery for coronary arterial occlusive disease. II: Subgroup with significant left main lesion. *Circulation*, 54 (Suppl 3), 107–117.

Talley, J. D., Jones, E. L., Weintraub, W. S., et al. (1989). Coronary artery bypass surgery after failed elective percutaneous transluminal coronary angioplasty. *Circulation*, 79 (Suppl 1), 126–131.

Tanimoto, Y., Matuda, Y., and Kobayaski, Y. (1984). Coronary spasm as a cause of perioperative myocardial infarction. *Japanese Heart Journal*, 25, 275–281.

Tchervenkov, C., Wynands, J., and Symes, J. (1983). Persistent atrial activity during cardioplegic arrest: A possible factor in the etiology of postoperative supraventricular tachyarrhythmias. *Annals of Thoracic and Cardiovascular Surgery*, 36(4), 453–459.

Teoh, K. H., Christakis, G. T., Weisel, R. D., et al. (1987). Increased risk of urgent revascularization. *Journal of Thoracic and Cardiovascular Surgery*, 93, 291–299.

Thompson, R., Mitchell, A., Ahmed, M., et al. (1980). Conduction defects in aortic valve disease. *American Heart Journal*, 948, 3–10.

Thorpe, C. J. (1979). A nursing care plan—the adult cardiac surgery patient. *Heart & Lung*, 8(4), 690–698.

TIMI Study Group. (1989). Comparison of invasive and conservative strategies after treatment with intravenous tissue plasminogen activator in acute myocardial infarction. TIMI trial. Phase II. *New England Journal of Medicine*, 320, 618–627.

Townes, B., Bashein, G., Hornbein, T., et al. (1989). Neurobehavioral outcomes in cardiac operations. A prospective controlled study *Journal of Thoracic Cardiovascular Surgery*, 98, 774–782.

Toy, P., Strauss, R. G., and Stehling, L. C. (1987). Predeposited autologous blood for elective surgery. *New England Journal of Medicine*, 316, 517–520.

Tsai, T. P., Matloff, J. M., Gray, R. J., et al. (1986). Cardiac surgery in the octogenarian. *Journal of Thoracic and Cardiovascular Surgery*, 91(6), 924–928.

Turnipseed, W., Berkoff, H., and Belzer, F. (1980). Postoperative stroke in cardiovascular and peripheral vascular disease. *Annals of Surgery*, 192, 365–368.

Underhill, S. L., Woods, S. L., Sivarajan, E. S., et al. (1982). *Cardiac nursing*. Philadelphia: J. B. Lippincott.

Utley, J., Wachtel, C., and Cain, R. (1981). Effects of hypothermia, hemodilution, and pump oxygenation on organ water content, blood flow and oxygen delivery, and renal function. *Annals of Thoracic Surgery*, 31(2), 121–133.

VanLente, F., Martin, A., Ratliff, N., et al. (1989). The predictive value of serum enzymes for perioperative myocardial infarction after cardiac operation. *Journal of Thoracic and Cardiovascular Surgery*, 98, 704–710.

Vecht, R., Nicolaides, E., and Ireuke, J. (1986). Incidence and prevention of supraventricular tachydysrhythmias after coronary bypass surgery. *International Journal of Cardiology*, 13, 125–134.

Vineberg, A. M. (1946). Development of an anastamosis between coronary vessels and transplanted internal mammary artery. *Canadian Medical Association Journal*, 55, 117.

Waggoneer, P. C. (1981). Postoperative care of the patient undergoing cardiac valve replacement: A nursing perspectie. *Critical Care Quarterly*, December, 57–66.

Waldhausen, J. A., and Pierce, W. S. (Eds.). (1985). *Johnson's surgery of the chest* (5th ed. pp. 433–460). Chicago: Year Book.

Walker, R. H. (Ed.). (1990). *Autologous transfusion*. American Association of Blood Banks technical manual, pp. 433–448. Arlington, VA: American Association of Blood Banks.

Wechsler, A. S., and Junod, F. L. (1989). Coronary bypass grafting in patients with chronic congestive heart failure. *Circulation*, 79(6), 92–96.

Weiland, A. (1983). A review of cardiac valve prostheses and their selection. *Heart & Lung*, 12(2), 498–509.

Westaby, S. (1985). Unexpected failure to improve after valve replacement surgery. *Quarterly Journal of Medicine*, 55(217), 103–108.

Wheatley, D. J. (1986). *Surgery of coronary artery disease*. St. Louis: C. V. Mosby.

Williams, J. (1988). Effects of cardioplegia on arrhythmias and conduction. *Cardiac Surgery: State of the Art Reviews*, 2(2), 259–269.

Wingate, S. (1987). Rehabilitation of the patient with valvular heart disease. *Journal of Cardiovascular Nursing*, 1(3), 52–63.

Winters, W. L., and Samuels, D. A. (1986). Long term prognosis following valvular heart surgery. In W. Frankl and A. N. Brest (Eds.), *Valvular heart disease: Comprehensive evaluation and management* (pp. 437–501). Philadelphia: F. A. Davis.

Zeff, R. H., Kongtahworn, C., Iannone, L. A., et al. (1988). IMA vs. SVG to the left anterior descending coronary artery: Prospective randomized study with 10 year follow-up. *Annals of Thoracic Surgery*, 45(5), 533–536.

Zema, M. (1986). Left ventricular failure: Clinical recognition and management. *Hospital Medicine*, 5(1), 63–99.

21

Patients with Vascular Emergencies

Maria Beasley Dixon

Vascular emergencies encompass a wide range of arterial and venous problems, some of which may result in risk to an extremity, vital organ, or loss of life. Vascular emergencies, whether from trauma or secondary to peripheral vascular disease, offer major challenges to the critical care nurse.

Significant advances have been made in caring for patients with vascular emergencies. Delivery of optimal nursing care requires a thorough understanding of vascular anatomy, specific clinical manifestations, pathophysiology, current methods of diagnosis and treatment, and a high index of clinical suspicion for vascular abnormalities.

This chapter addresses selected vascular emergencies, current methods of diagnosis and treatment, and appropriate nursing diagnoses and related nursing care in the critical care setting. The topics chosen are limited to conditions that are limb- or life-threatening and that require immediate or emergent attention.

The nursing care plan provided at the end of the chapter represents a sample of the nursing diagnoses that would be appropriate for a vascular emergency or disease process accompanying a vascular emergency.

ABDOMINAL AORTIC ANEURYSM

An aneurysm is an irreversible dilatation of an artery secondary to a localized weakness of the arterial wall that may predispose the artery to thrombosis, distal embolization, or rupture (Spittell and Wallace, 1980; Haimovici, 1989).

Aneurysms are described and categorized by a variety of criteria including shape, location, and etiology. There are two types of true aneurysms:

fusiform and saccular. A fusiform aneurysm involves the entire circumference of the aorta and is the most common type of aortic aneurysm. A saccular aneurysm is an outpouching from the aorta that results from localized thinning and stretching (Spittell and Wallace, 1980; Haimovici, 1989; Roberts, 1981).

A false aneurysm or pseudoaneurysm occurs when the entire aortic wall is disrupted, resulting in communication of blood with the surrounding tissues, producing a pulsatile hematoma. False aneurysms may be classified as traumatic, anastomotic, degenerative, or mycotic (Fig. 21–1) (Ochsner, 1982).

Aortic dissection is frequently referred to in the literature as a dissecting aneurysm, although vascular experts discourage its categorization as an aneurysm. Due to its unique pathophysiology, aortic dissection will be discussed separately.

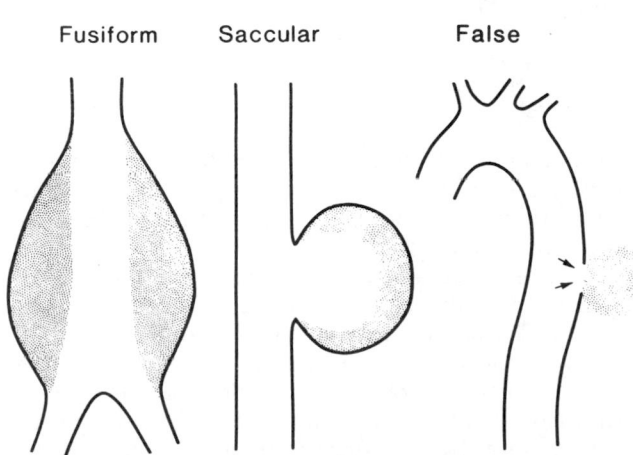

Fusiform   Saccular   False

FIGURE 21–1. Types of basic aneurysms. (From Dalsing, M., and Sawchuk, A. (1988). Surgery of the aorta. In V. Fahey (Ed.), *Vascular nursing* (p. 187). Philadelphia: W.B. Saunders.)

Aneurysms may involve the ascending aorta, the aortic arch, descending aorta, thoracoabdominal aorta, abdominal aorta, or a combination of these. Abdominal aortic aneurysms (AAA) are the most common type; they usually arise just below the renal arteries and frequently involve the iliac arteries at the bifurcation. Suprarenal aneurysms are usually seen in thoracoabdominal aneurysms.

Etiology

More than 95% of abdominal aneurysms are caused by atherosclerosis. Atherosclerosis is more extensive in individuals with hypertension. Other factors strongly associated with atherosclerosis are diabetes, cigarette smoking, hyperlipidemia, and heredity. Other causes may include infections, poststenotic dilatation, syphilis, arteritis, congenital abnormalities, and trauma (Spittell and Wallace, 1980; Haimovici, 1989; Roberts, 1981; Rob, 1987).

Pathophysiology

The infrarenal abdominal aorta is particularly prone to the formation of aneurysms and atherosclerotic occlusive disease. Atherosclerosis causes a weakening of the aortic wall due to destruction of the media, the middle layer containing elastic fibers. The gradual weakening of the media in combination with hemodynamic forces may cause thickening and compression of the vasa vasorum, which supplies nutrition to the aortic wall. The muscle fibers then become damaged and may be replaced with fibrous tissue and calcium deposits (Spittell and Wallace, 1980). As the aneurysm increases in diameter, wall tension increases also, allowing further enlargement.

As dilatation occurs, changes in laminar blood flow allow the formation of an intraluminal thrombus. In some cases, the thrombus may become dislodged and may produce distal thromboembolism, causing acute ischemia of vital organs or a distal extremity.

Clinical Presentation

Aortic aneurysms are most common in males between 50 and 70 years of age. Approximately one-half of patients with AAA are asymptomatic. Since aneurysmal changes of the abdominal aorta are only one of the effects of atherosclerosis, the patient may be referred to the vascular surgeon because of other vascular disease complaints. Often an aneurysm remains unnoticed by the patient and is detected on routine physical examination. On the basis of the history and physical examination, AAA are frequently described as symptomatic, symptomatic/expanding, or ruptured.

An asymptomatic AAA is usually discovered by a widened midline pulsation just proximal to the um-

bilicus. The pulsations are typically described as pushing the examiner's fingers apart. If the hand of the examiner can be placed between the upper aspect of the aneurysm and the xiphoid, the aneurysm probably originates below the renal arteries, as do 95% of all AAA (Hertzer, 1979).

A symptomatic AAA indicates expansion or impending rupture. Excruciating back pain is the cardinal symptom and may be accompanied by abdominal pain and tenderness on palpation. The back pain may also radiate to the lower back, groin, or legs. The pain may be due to stretching of the adventitia or pressure on the anterior spinal ligament (Haimovici, 1989; Hertzer, 1979).

Frank rupture of an AAA is a catastrophe, and immediate diagnosis and treatment are crucial. In spite of significant medical and surgical advances, the morbidity and mortality of a ruptured AAA still remain very high. The diagnosis of a ruptured AAA is based on the presence of a pulsatile mass or retroperitoneal hematoma, accompanied by excruciating abdominal or back pain. Evidence of hemorrhage may include severe hypotension, tachycardia, diaphoresis, pallor, and oliguria. Mottling of the abdomen or of the extremities and progressive loss of pulses may also be noted (Haimovici, 1989).

Laboratory Findings

Leakage of blood into the peritoneal space may be indicated by leukocytosis. The hematocrit is usually normal but may be decreased in the patient with a ruptured AAA and if massive fluid resuscitation is administered.

Diagnostic Findings

X-Rays. Routine anteroposterior and lateral roentgenograms of the abdomen may suggest the presence of an aortic aneurysm on the basis of calcifications outlining the aneurysm. Large aneurysms may appear as soft masses, displace other organs, or cause abnormal gas patterns. The estimated accuracy of routine radiography is approximately 88% (Rob, 1987; Hertzer, 1979).

Ultrasound. Ultrasound is a simple and safe technique for the diagnosis and measurement of an abdominal aortic aneurysm. It is a good way to follow the size of an abdominal aneurysm in patients who are being treated conservatively. Ultrasound has correlated well with measurements taken at the time of surgery and is considered a reliable diagnostic tool.

CT Scan. Computed tomography (CT) scan provides information similar to that of ultrasound but is considered more accurate than ultrasound. The CT scan may be more beneficial in documenting proximal extension of the aneurysm to the renal or iliac arteries (Rob, 1987; Hertzer, 1979).

Aortogram. Aortography is not performed routinely for the purpose of diagnosing abdominal aortic aneurysm. Aortography demonstrates only the blood flow in the lumen, which may be occupied by thrombus, and cannot estimate the total diameter of the aneurysm (Fig. 21–2). Except with aneurysm rupture, aortography is useful for evaluating the number and location of the renal arteries; for determining the presence of renal, inferior mesenteric, iliac, and distal artery disease or aneurysm; for confirming a suspicion of a thoracoabdominal aneurysm; and for determining whether the abdominal aortic aneurysm extends above the level of the renal arteries.

Management

Generally, the patient with an abdominal aortic aneurysm should undergo surgery. The risk of aneurysmal rupture balanced against the risk of elective operation supports resection. The mortality rate is usually less than 4% provided that the patient is a good operative risk. Untreated aortic aneurysms put the patient at high risk for potential rupture, infection, or embolization of thrombotic debris. (Crisler and Bahnson, 1972; Hertzer, 1979; Thompson et al., 1983).

The most important predictor of aneurysmal rupture is the size of the aneurysm. Rupture occurs when the aortic wall can no longer sustain the sheer stress. It is a known fact that larger aneurysms rupture more than smaller aneurysms, and patients with hypertension are at greater risk for rupture. An aneurysm of 4 cm has less than a 15% chance of rupture within 5 years, whereas an aneurysm of 8 cm has a 75% chance of rupture. The risk of rupture is more significant than the risk of operation when an aneurysm reaches 5 cm in diameter; therefore, surgery is recommended for aortic aneurysms greater than 5 cm. The risk of rupture for aneurysms less than 5 cm is small; however, an average growth rate of 0.4 cm/year determined by ultrasound is an indication for surgery (Rob, 1987; Thompson et al., 1983; McIntyre and Bernhard, 1987).

Elective operation for repair of an abdominal aortic aneurysm requires optimal preoperative evaluation of the cardiac, pulmonary, renal, and endocrine systems. A cardiology consultation should be obtained for all patients except in extreme emergencies. Pulmonary function studies may be indicated for patients with emphysema or a long smoking history. Patients with renal disease may have an elevated creatinine level following the aortogram and should be well hydrated prior to surgery. Diabetes should be well controlled.

Prophylactic antibiotics are generally given the night before or 1 to 2 hours prior to surgery. A mechanical bowel preparation is usually recommended. Electrocardiographic (ECG) monitoring, arterial pressure, pulmonary artery pressure, urinary catheter, and a nasogastric tube are used to ensure optimal fluid management during surgery.

OPERATIVE TECHNIQUE

Minimal dissection is desired to expose the aneurysm. After proximal and distal control has been obtained, the aneurysmal sac is opened, the intraluminal thrombus is removed, and bleeding lumbar arteries are oversewn. The aortic clamp can be placed below the renal arteries in 90% to 95% of cases. Clamping above the renal arteries (less than 60 minutes) is usually tolerated by the kidneys. If distal perfusion is necessary, partial aortic occlusion for placement of an end-to-side proximal anastomosis or the use of a shunt may allow adequate distal perfusion. The graft limbs are flushed with arterial blood to clear atherosclerotic debris and thrombus to prevent distal embolization. A preclotted, woven Dacron graft is sutured in place, and the remaining aneurysm wall is wrapped around the graft. If the iliac arteries are free from disease, a straight tube graft is used. In the presence of aneurysmal or aortoiliac occlusive disease, a bifurcated graft is placed to the segment with adequate open vessels (Fig. 21–3) (Rob, 1987; Thompson et al., 1983).

When rupture is impending, the chest may be opened to obtain proximal control of the aorta prior to resection of the aneurysm.

Ruptured aneurysms require emergent surgery.

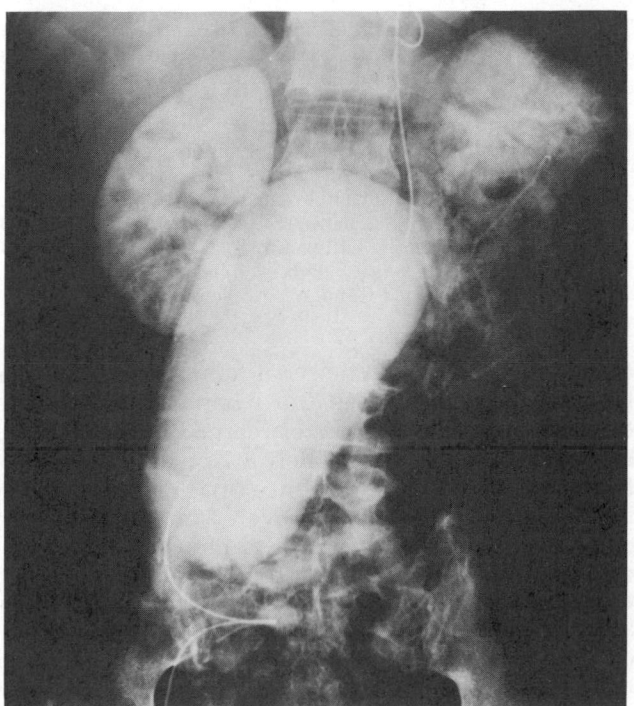

FIGURE 21–2. Angiographic demonstration of an abdominal aortic aneurysm. (Compliments of Larry-Stuart Deutsch, M.D., Chief Cardiac/Vascular/Interventional Radiology, University of California Irvine Medical Center.)

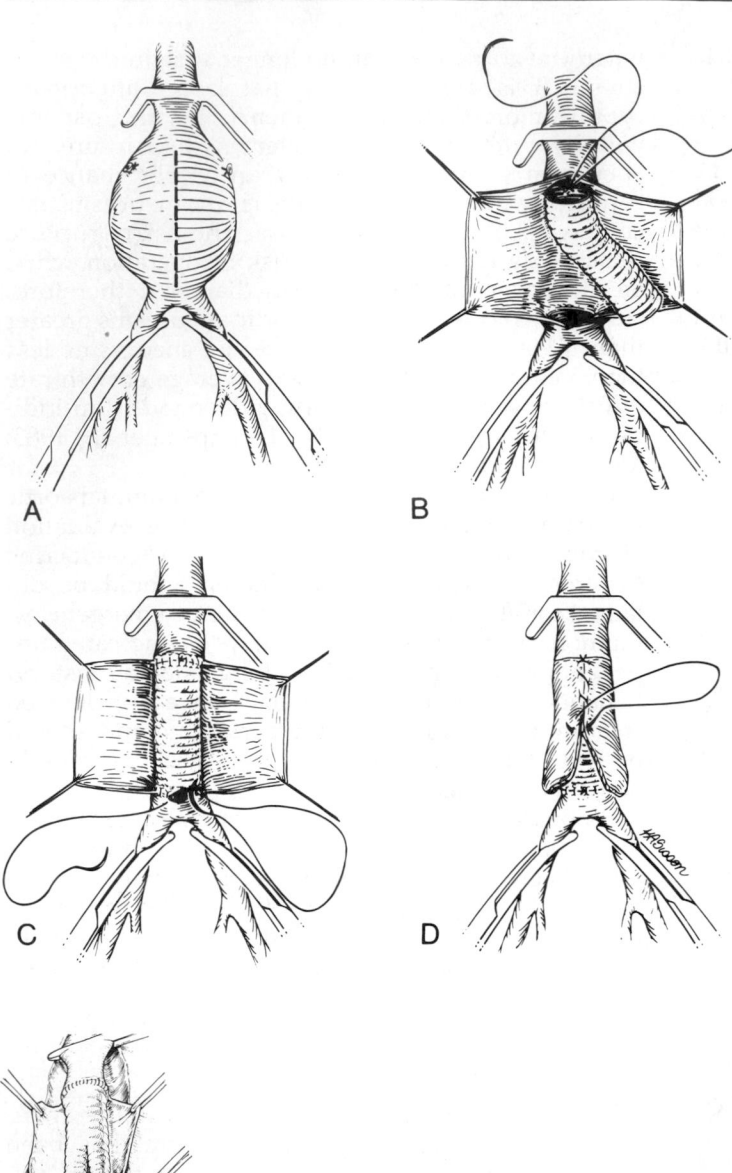

FIGURE 21–3. Repair of abdominal aortic aneurysm not involving the iliac arteries. *A,* Vascular control using clamps. *B,* Aneurysm is opened, and tube graft is inserted. *C,* Proximal and distal anastomosis. *D,* Posterior wall of aneurysm is wrapped around new graft. *E,* Repair of abdominal aortic aneurysm involving iliac arteries. (*A* to *D* from Yao, J., Flinn, W. R., and Bergan, J. (1984). Technique for repairing infrarenal abdominal aortic aneurysms. In L. M. Nyhus and R. J. Baker (Eds.), *Mastery of surgery* (pp. 1361–1365). Boston: Little, Brown; *E* from Haimovici, H. (1984). *Vascular surgery: Principles and techniques* (2nd ed., p. 702). Englewood Cliffs, NJ: Appleton & Lange.)

X-rays, CT scans, and blood tests are avoided to expedite treatment. The site of aneurysmal rupture depends on the location of the aneurysm, but aneurysms most commonly rupture into the retroperitoneum. The abdomen is opened and bleeding controlled by compressing the aorta against the vertebra. Once the aorta has been cross-clamped, the aneurysm is opened, and the preclotted Dacron graft is flushed, sutured in place, and wrapped by the remaining posterior aneurysm wall (Coselli and Crawford, 1989).

POSTOPERATIVE COMPLICATIONS

Acute Renal Failure. Renal failure can result from prolonged ischemia, inadequate hydration, and atheromatous emboli. Acute renal failure occurs in less than 1% of elective cases, but when clamping above the renal arteries lasts longer than 60 minutes, renal failure occurs in approximately 8% of patients (Crawford et al., 1989). The incidence of acute renal failure increases in patients with severe shock, prolonged cross-clamping, and massive transfusions. The decrease in renal perfusion combined with the presence of myoglobinuria may lead to intrinsic tubular damage, which is responsible for the acute renal shutdown. Renal failure is frequently irreversible, and hemodialysis may be required in the early postoperative stages. Decreasing the clamp time, operating time, and blood loss can significantly decrease the potential for tubular necrosis (Haimovici, 1989).

Renal failure is significantly less common in elective aneurysm repair.

Colon Ischemia. Ligation of the inferior mesenteric artery during aneurysm resection may result in ischemia of the descending and retrosigmoid colon (Haimovici, 1989). Manifestations include cyanotic discoloration of the colon, melena, diarrhea, abdominal pain, and leukocytosis.

Thromboembolism. Manipulation of the aneurysm during surgery can result in mobilization of intraluminal thrombus and distal embolization. Distal embolization can be prevented by initial distal clamping of the iliac arteries with minimal manipulation of the aneurysm. Distal embolization may result in renal failure or acute tissue ischemia of the lower extremities characterized by areas of discoloration or petechia-like lesions on the toes or bottom of the foot (blue toe syndrome or trash foot).

Spinal Cord Ischemia. Spinal cord ischemia associated with resection of the infrarenal aortic aneurysm is rare but may result from interruption of the spinal cord's arterial supply. Spinal cord ischemia may be temporary or permanent. Manifestations include sensory and motor deficits as well as rectal and urinary incontinence.

Myocardial Infarction. The major cause of death following aortic surgery is myocardial infarction. The need for preoperative coronary angiography is controversial. Indications for angiography should be based on preoperative risk factors and cardiac evaluation. Myocardial infarction, dysrhythmias, or congestive heart failure can occur concurrent with the operation or postoperatively. Diagnosis can be made with serial ECG tracings and elevation of the creative phosphokinase (CPK)-MB isoenzymes. Myocardial infarction may be difficult to manage postoperatively due to major fluid shifts and electrolyte disturbances.

Infection. Infection may occur in 1% to 2% of aortic procedures but carries a high mortality when a prosthetic graft is in place. Fevers, prolonged ileus, and leukocytosis may indicate a smoldering infection (Dalsing and Sawchuk, 1988).

PROGNOSIS

Abdominal aortic aneurysms left untreated have a 40% to 50% mortality in 1 year, 75% to 80% mortality at 5 years, and a 100% mortality at 10 years. Current operative mortality is 3% to 4%, with deaths usually related to associated cardiac and pulmonary disease (Thompson et al., 1983).

NURSING MANAGEMENT

Preoperative. Preoperative evaluation of the patient for elective aneurysm repair requires a thorough history and physical examination. Baseline data including risk factors, vital signs, peripheral pulses, breath sounds, and heart sounds should be documented.

Preparation for surgery involves a variety of tasks including completion of diagnostic tests and laboratory work and carrying out specific preoperative protocols. Four to eight units of blood should be available in the blood bank.

The high-risk patient may be admitted to the intensive care unit prior to surgery for insertion of a Swan-Ganz catheter for continuous monitoring of the pulmonary artery wedge pressure and cardiac output. Arterial line placement is also done to monitor blood pressure and to secure easy access for blood samples.

Most patients and families have a high level of anxiety about the impending surgery, lack of knowledge about the surgery, and hospital routine. Although preoperative time is shorter in most hospital settings, preoperative education should not be overlooked. Explanations of the equipment (endotracheal tube, ventilator, tubes, drains, monitors), routines, procedures, and visiting hours should be discussed. A tour of the intensive care unit should be offered when possible. Specific fears and concerns of the patient and family should be discussed and included in the care plan.

Postoperative. The main goal of postoperative care is to prevent complications. Patients with aortic rupture are at much higher risk for complications than those with elective surgery.

The patient is transferred to the surgical intensive care unit for continuous monitoring of urine output, arterial blood gases, and hemodynamics for the next 48 to 72 hours. Optimal fluid management may be obtained by monitoring cardiac output, pulmonary artery wedge pressure, and mixed venous oxygenation (Sv_{O_2}). Fluids are replaced to optimize cardiac output and renal function.

Meticulous attention should be paid to pulmonary toilet to prevent serious pulmonary complications. Mechanical ventilation is used for the first 24 to 48 hours. Early activity, suctioning, postural drainage, and chest percussion are important aspects of management.

Tissue perfusion should be evaluated hourly by using the six Ps: pulselessness, pain, paresthesia, paralysis, pallor, poikilothermia (cold). Distal pulses may be difficult to palpate initially, especially if the patient is hypothermic. It may be necessary to use Doppler echocardiography to assess blood flow to the extremities. Palpation of the femoral pulses should be readily apparent, and absence of these pulses indicates graft failure.

Doppler ankle pressures are useful in assessing the status of blood flow to the lower extremities. Postoperative pressures should be compared to baseline pressures. Any significant change in ankle pressure should be noted and the vascular status further evaluated by duplex scan imaging or angiography.

Capillary refill time should be assessed and documented as brisk (<3 seconds), delayed (>3 seconds), or absent. Warming the patient with overhead warmers, warmed blankets, and heat lights may be necessary. Blood transfusions should also be given through blood warmers.

The incidence of postoperative hemorrhage is approximately 1% to 4% and can result from the extensive retroperitoneal dissection and vascular anastomoses. Intra-abdominal bleeding may be suspected with increasing abdominal girth, decreasing urine output, pulmonary artery wedge pressure, and hematocrit. When significant bleeding occurs, immediate surgical exploration is necessary (Dalsing and Sawchuk, 1988).

Ischemic colitis occurs in approximately 2% of infrarenal aortic aneurysm repairs and has a 50% mortality. Signs and symptoms may include diarrhea, melena, abdominal tenderness, prolonged ileus, sepsis, fever, leukocytosis, metabolic acidosis, and shock. Any suspicion of ischemic bowel should be reported and requires a colonoscopic inspection of the bowel.

Care of the patient with repair of an abdominal aortic aneurysm requires an understanding of both the disease process and the needs of the patient. The nurse is in a unique position to provide the necessary education and support for the patient undergoing such a major operation. A sample nursing care plan that addresses the common needs of the individual with peripheral vascular disease or a vascular emergency will be found at the end of this chapter.

ACUTE AORTIC DISSECTION

Acute aortic dissection is a catastrophic event that is characterized by an intimal tear and separation of the medial layers by a column of blood creating a false lumen. Pulsatile flow in the false lumen may cause proximal or distal extension of the dissection, resulting in compression of the true lumen, occlusion of arterial branches, or rupture through the adventitia resulting in hemorrhage (Ergin et al., 1985; Saunders, 1979; Wheat, 1980; Roberts, 1981).

The term dissecting aneurysm was first used in 1761 by Morgagni, who described a hematoma separating the medial layer (Anagnostopoulos, 1975). Although the term is widely applied in the literature, the pathogenesis of acute aortic dissection differs from that of a true aneurysm.

Histology

The aorta consists of three basic layers. The inner layer, or intima, is composed primarily of endothelium and connective tissue. The media is the thick middle layer and is composed of elastin, collagen, and smooth muscle cells. The outer layer, the adventitia, is thin and is composed of connective tissue.

This layer serves to anchor the vessel to the surrounding structures, providing strength and stability to the aorta. The blood supply to the media flows through the vasa vasorum, a network of capillaries embedded in the adventitia.

Incidence

Approximately five to ten aortic dissections per million population occur each year in the United States, which is two to three times the incidence of a ruptured abdominal aortic aneurysm (Anagnostopoulos, 1975; Griffith and Todd, 1985). There is evidence that the incidence of aortic dissection is increasing, probably due to the increasing elderly population and increased clinical awareness of aortic dissection (Burchell, 1955).

Acute aortic dissection occurs two to three times more frequently in men between the ages of 50 and 70 than in women the same age. Below the age of 40, aortic dissection is rare except in those with a familial predisposition to it as in patients with Marfan syndrome (McKusick, 1955). As many as 50% of aortic dissections occurring in patients under the age of 40 may occur during pregnancy (Mandell et al., 1954). It is more common in blacks, perhaps as a result of the higher incidence of hypertension in that population (Saunders, 1979; Pate et al., 1976).

Etiology

CYSTIC MEDIAL NECROSIS

Medial degeneration, specifically Erdheim cystic medial necrosis, has been considered the primary basis for most acute aortic dissections. The lesion is characterized by focal accumulation of mucoid material in the media of the ascending aorta and aortic arch. A form of medial degeneration is seen in Marfan syndrome. Marfan syndrome is characterized by increased elasticity of the aortic wall secondary to a deficiency of connective tissue (Spittell and Wallace, 1980; Lie and Juergens, 1980).

Medial degeneration has also been linked to hypertension, injury to the vasa vasorum, loss of nutritional supply to the media, atherosclerosis, intimal thickening, injury to the intima from hemodynamic forces, and the normal aging process (Spittell and Wallace, 1980).

HYPERTENSION

The theory that hypertension is a major contributing factor to medial stress and aortic dissection is supported by the fact that approximately 70% of patients with aortic dissection have hypertension, and at autopsy, 90% of patients have left ventricular hypertrophy (Hirst et al., 1958). The combination of hypertension and the steepness of the pulse wave (dP/dT) is thought to injure the vasa vasorum, resulting in sclerosis and ischemia of the medial layer (Roberts, 1981; Spittell and Wallace, 1980; Lindsay, 1979).

PREGNANCY

During pregnancy the body produces hormones to relax smooth muscle and connective tissue for normal uterine expansion. A combination of these hormonal changes, increased blood volume, and hypertension may increase the risk of aortic dissection (Roberts, 1981; Glagov and Zarins, 1983).

AORTIC COARCTATION

Approximately 10% of untreated patients with aortic coarctation die from aortic dissection and hemopericardium. The dissection usually occurs in the proximal aorta and is thought to be associated with hypertension and a high frequency of congenital bicuspid aortic valve disease (Roberts, 1981; Burchell, 1955).

TRAUMA

Blunt trauma due to deceleration accidents is a well-recognized cause of aortic tears and dissection. The tear usually occurs just distal to the left subclavian artery at the aortic isthmus. It is here that the mobile aortic arch joins a relatively fixed thoracic aorta and is vulnerable to injury.

Iatrogenic dissections may result from direct arterial injury during angiography, cardiopulmonary bypass, intra-aortic balloon procedures, cardiac catheterization, or direct operative procedures. The tip of the catheter may be wedged into the media instead of the aortic lumen, resulting in dissection (Roberts, 1981).

Pathology

The distinctive underlying pathology of aortic dissection is medial degeneration, particularly Erdheim cystic medial necrosis associated with Marfan syndrome (Wheat, 1980).

Recent studies suggest that medial degeneration also occurs in the aging aorta. During systole the aortic wall expands and thins, temporarily squeezing the vasa vasorum. When hypertension is present, the aortic wall is exposed to additional hemodynamic stresses that can cause medial degeneration. This theory is supported by the fact that dissection occurs more frequently in the ascending aorta and arch, where hemodynamic stresses are greatest (Wheat, 1980).

Most aortic dissections are characterized by a transverse intimal tear. The tear is usually found just distal to the left subclavian artery. During the normal cardiac cycle, the ascending aorta and arch undergo a side-to-side motion or flexion. As a result of this continuous motion, the underlying degeneration in the media, and the force of blood ejected from the left ventricle, the ascending aorta is subjected to intimal tears (Wheat, 1980).

Most aortic dissections are characterized by a longitudinal separation of the media in a course parallel to that of the blood flow. As a hematoma develops, it separates the degenerated medial layer, producing an acute aortic dissection. The dissection may be propagated for varying distances throughout the aorta by a combination of the steepness of the pulse wave (dP/dT), the blood pressure, and the extent of the medial degeneration (Wheat, 1980; Roberts, 1981). The progressing dissection produces a false channel and may undermine the aortic valve leaflets, occlude branch vessels, or rupture through the adventitia, resulting in hemorrhage and death (Lindsay, 1979).

Classification

According to the classification model devised by DeBakey, dissections are characterized according to the originating tear and the extent of the dissection (Fig. 21–4). Type I dissections are characterized by a tear in the ascending aorta with subsequent dissection into the descending aorta. The intimal tear is frequently located just above the aortic valve and may involve the valve leaflets, resulting in aortic valve insufficiency. Approximately 60% of dissections are type I. Type II dissections occur in approximately 10% of cases, are limited to the ascending

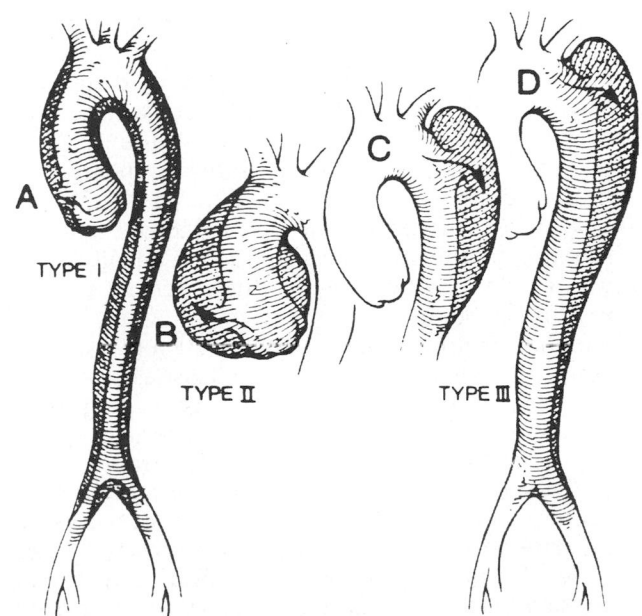

FIGURE 21–4. DeBakey's classification of aortic dissection types I, II, and III. (From page 28 of *The Journal of Cardiovascular Nursing*, Vol. 1, No. 2, February 1987.)

aorta, and are common in patients with Marfan syndrome. Type III dissections typically originate just distal to the left subclavian artery and may extend distally to the descending thoracic aorta and bifurcation. Type III dissections account for 20% to 30% of cases.

Recently, experts have classified dissections as proximal (DeBakey's types I and II) and distal (DeBakey's type III) because types I and II are treated similarly. Shumway has classified ascending dissections as class A and descending dissections as class B.

Clinical Presentation

The diagnosis of acute aortic dissection should be suspected in any patient who has severe back pain, anterior chest pain, epigastric pain, abrupt onset of a pulseless extremity, acute aortic valve insufficiency without known heart disease, and a history of hypertension or Marfan syndrome (Wheat, 1980; Griffith and Todd, 1985). Although diagnostic techniques have become more sophisticated, early diagnosis depends primarily on a high index of clinical suspicion and excellent assessment skills. The four main clinical manifestations of aortic dissection are pain, cardiovascular symptoms, neurologic symptoms, and gastrointestinal symptoms.

Pain is the classic symptom of aortic dissection and may be described as sharp, ripping, or tearing and is in synchrony with the heart beat. The onset of pain is usually sudden and typically begins in the anterior chest, epigastric area, shoulders, or back (Griffith and Todd, 1985; Cooke and Safford, 1986). The pain may migrate to the neck, back, or extremities as the dissection progresses. Typically, patients with pain localized to the anterior chest have proximal dissections. Radiation of the pain to the back, abdomen, or legs is highly suggestive of distal dissection (Spittell and Wallace, 1980; Cooke and Safford, 1986). Severe pain that occurs suddenly, subsides, and then recurs may indicate impending rupture or significant extension of the dissection. In rare instances, dissection can occur without pain. In these patients, the initial presentation is usually heart failure, aortic insufficiency, or pulse deficits (Cooke and Safford, 1986).

From a cardiovascular viewpoint, most patients present with diaphoresis and restlessness as if in shock, yet may have severe hypertension. Hypotension may occur if the aorta ruptures, which occurs more commonly with ascending dissections. The blood pressure may be unobtainable or significantly different in one or both arms as a result of occlusion of the true aortic lumen or arterial branches. Pulses may be absent or diminished in both upper and lower extremities or carotids, reflecting decreased tissue perfusion. Occasionally, duplication of pulses may be noted due to the difference in flow rates in the true and false channels.

Examination of the heart may reveal tachycardia, murmurs, or a pericardial friction rub if bleeding has occurred into the pericardial sac. Aortic insufficiency is seen in approximately half the patients with ascending dissections and is loudest at the right sternal border (Cooke and Safford, 1986). Dyspnea is usually due to failure from aortic insufficiency or cardiac tamponade. Conduction abnormalities and myocardial infarction may be noted secondary to dissection into the septum or coronary arteries (Griffith and Todd, 1985).

Neurological deficits are more common in patients with proximal dissections. Disturbances in the level of consciousness may occur secondary to hypotension or compromised subclavian or carotid arteries. Neurologic deficits, including stroke, ischemic peripheral neuropathy, and ischemic paralysis may occur secondary to compression or occlusion of spinal arteries.

Gastrointestinal symptoms such as acute abdominal pain, melena, hematemesis, nausea and vomiting may suggest mesenteric artery involvement (Lindsay, 1979).

Diagnostic

Laboratory Findings. Because there is no consistent pattern of abnormal laboratory findings, laboratory tests are of little help in the diagnosis of acute aortic dissection. If aortic rupture occurs, a decrease in the hemoglobin and hematocrit may be reflected with massive fluid resuscitation.

Electrocardiogram. The most common electrocardiographic abnormality is usually left ventricular hypertrophy. Ischemic patterns, dysrhythmias, and bundle branch blocks may also be seen but are not diagnostic.

Radiologic Findings. Abnormal findings on anteroposterior chest radiographs may include widened mediastinum, increase in the size of the aortic shadow, loss of the aortic knob, increased aortic diameter, deviation of the trachea to the right, and cardiac enlargement. A small percentage of patients with dissection may have a normal chest film; therefore, a normal film does not rule out the possibility of aortic dissection (Anagnostopoulos, 1979; Griffith and Todd, 1985; Cooke and Safford, 1986).

Computed Tomography. Computed tomography (CT) scan is a quick means of making the diagnosis of aortic dissection. When contrast medium is used, the CT scan is highly accurate and can clearly delineate the intimal tear and false channel within the aorta. It may also visualize collections of fluid in the pericardial, pleural, and mediastinal spaces. CT is used primarily as a screening tool to determine which patients should undergo aortography (Cooke and Safford, 1986).

Magnetic Resonance Imaging. Magnetic resonance imaging (MRI) offers the same advantages as CT but does not require the use of contrast agents for imaging. Stagnant blood, turbulent flow, atheromatous plaques, and thrombi produce signals of variable intensity and appear as shades of gray. Normal blood flow emits little or no signal and appears black. MRI can readily identify the site and extent of the intimal flap and the false channel. A disadvantage of MRI is that patients with vascular clips, pacemakers, or metal equipment cannot be scanned due to the magnetic forces involved (Cooke and Safford, 1986).

Aortography. Although aortography is an invasive technique that puts the patient at risk for renal compromise, it is still considered by many vascular surgeons the optimal diagnostic tool. Abnormal findings may include demonstration of a false lumen, splitting of the contrast column, evidence of intraluminal thrombus, increased thickness of the aortic wall, narrowing or occlusion of aortic branches, and alterations in flow patterns (Fig. 21–5) (Griffith and Todd, 1985; Lindsay, 1979).

Management

Immediate therapy for acute aortic dissection requires prompt lowering of the systolic blood pressure to 90/110 mm Hg to prevent extension of the dissection. Generally, patients are started on nitroprusside and a beta blocker such as propranolol. Nitroprusside is infused at a rate of 0.5 μg/kg per minute, titrated to achieve optimal blood pressure. Uncomplicated distal dissections may be successfully managed medically unless expansion of the aneurysm, compromise of aortic branches, or an increase in pain occurs.

SURGICAL TREATMENT

Proximal Dissection. Indications for surgical management include aortic valve insufficiency, impending rupture, progression of the dissection, symptoms of cerebral or coronary ischemia, pericardial tamponade, and failure to control the blood pressure with appropriate drug therapy (Wheat, 1980; Griffith and Todd, 1985; Spittell and Wallace, 1980).

Surgical treatment for ascending dissection is aimed at preventing aortic rupture and correcting the dissection and related complications. Cardiopulmonary bypass is required. The operative repair consists of resection of the aneurysmal portion and site of the tear, repair or replacement of the aortic valve if the aortic root is involved, and restoration of blood flow to major branches of the aorta. Replacement of the excised segment is done with prosthetic graft material (Fig. 21–6) (Anagnostopoulos, 1979; DeBakey et al., 1955; Cooke and Safford, 1986).

Descending Dissection. Indications for surgical intervention in type III/B distal dissection include continued progression of the dissection, hypertension, or pain despite adequate drug therapy, evidence of compromise or occlusion of major aortic

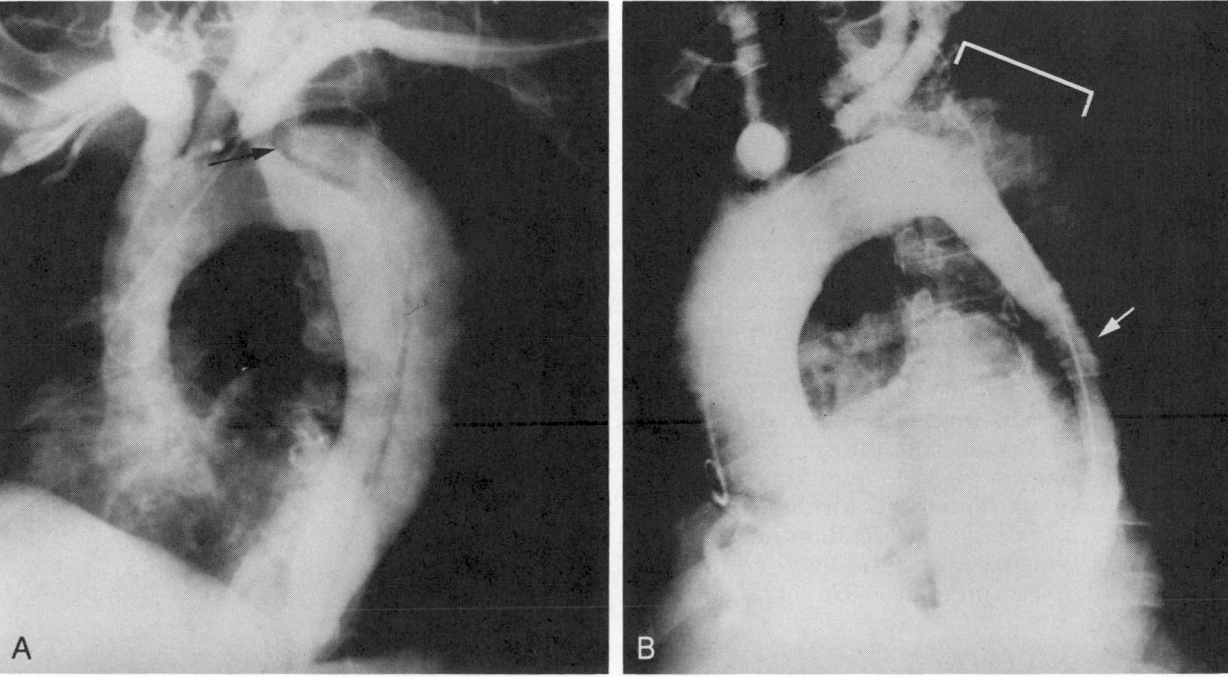

FIGURE 21–5. *A* and *B,* Angiographic demonstration of acute aortic dissection, type I. Note narrowed true lumen *(arrow in A)* and evidence of double lumen *(arrow in B)* in descending aorta. Evidence of clotted false lumen *(bracket in B)* just distal to the left subclavian artery. (Compliments of Larry-Stuart Deutsch, M.D., Chief Cardiac/Vascular/Interventional Radiology, University of California Irvine Medical Center.)

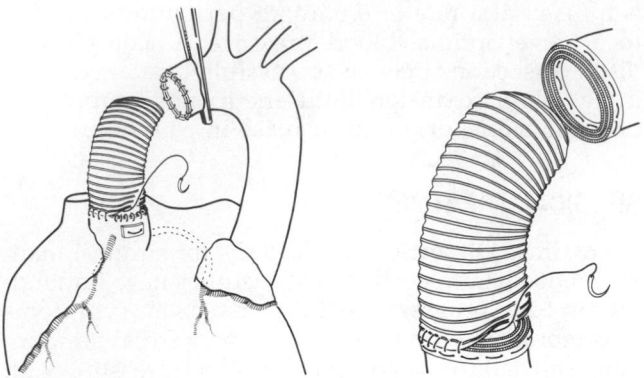

FIGURE 21–6. Repair of a type I dissection. (From Symbas, P. N. (1979). Treatment of thoracic aortic diseases. In J. Lindsay and J. W. Hurst (Eds.), *The aorta* (p. 380). New York: Grune & Stratton.)

branches such as the renal or mesenteric artery, impending rupture, and cardiac tamponade (Griffith and Todd, 1985; Cooke and Stafford, 1986).

Operative repair consists of resection of the dissection, obliteration of the false lumen, and graft replacement. A femorofemoral, atriofemoral, or ventriculofemoral bypass or shunt is used to maintain blood supply distally (Fig. 21–7) (DeBakey et al., 1982).

COMPLICATIONS

Major complications of acute aortic dissection such as rupture and hemorrhage are directly related to the extent of the dissection. Complications that carry the greatest threat to the patient include myocardial infarction, stroke, renal or visceral ischemia, and paraplegia (Griffith and Todd, 1985). Major causes of death include cardiac tamponade, cerebral ischemia, aortic rupture, and obstruction of major aortic branches (Pate et al., 1976).

PROGNOSIS

If left untreated, 50% of patients may die within 48 hours, 60% to 70% within 1 week, and 90% within 3 months (Wheat, 1980). It is imperative that patients receive prompt medical attention with emphasis on controlling the blood pressure.

Surgical mortality in acute ascending dissections is 10% to 20%, with long-term survival greater than 60%. Survival is essentially the same for descending dissections that are treated successfully with antihypertensive agents. Patients with descending dissections who do undergo an operation have a mortality rate of less than 10%, and the long-term survival is excellent (Applebaum et al., 1976).

NURSING MANAGEMENT

Acute Phase. The overall objective in the acute phase is to prevent extension of the dissection. Continuous monitoring of vital signs and titration of the

antihypertensive drips is important to achieve hemodynamic stability. An arterial line for continuous pressure monitoring is a must. Nitroprusside is titrated to keep the systolic blood pressure between 90 and 110 mm Hg yet still maintain adequate perfusion to the vital organs. Nitroprusside may cause an increased dP/dT and increased myocardial contractility by increasing adrenergic discharge. This negative effect can be treated successfully by administering a beta blocker such as propranolol. Fluid management can be optimized by taking frequent pulmonary artery measurements, including cardiac output and mixed venous oxygenation. Urine output should be measured hourly.

Pain can best be controlled by lowering the blood pressure and medicating the patient with morphine. Assessment of the type and location of the pain should be documented. An increase or recurrence of the pain may indicate progression of the dissection and should be reported immediately.

Physical and environmental stresses should be reduced to prevent unnecessary stimulation of the patient. Relaxation techniques such as deep breathing and imagery may be helpful. The combination of high-tech equipment, restricted visiting hours, and use of disposable gloves has significantly limited the patient's contact with human touch. A calm approach and a caring touch is important in developing patient trust and reducing anxiety. The emotional stress and anxiety of emergency hospitalization can be overwhelming for the patient and family. This can be compounded by a knowledge deficit related to hospital routines, potential surgery, financial burdens, and separation from loved ones. Appropriate resources should be utilized to assist the patient and family in identifying effective coping skills and supports.

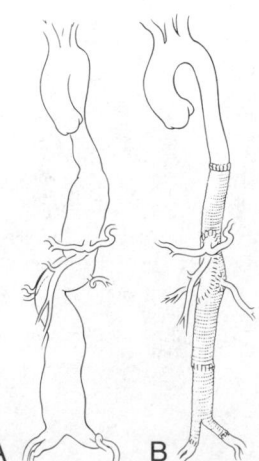

FIGURE 21–7. Illustrations of a degenerative aneurysm that involves the distal half of descending thoracic aorta and the entire abdominal aorta (type III). *A,* Drawing showing the location and extent of disease. *B,* Drawing showing graft in place and functioning. (Courtesy of Baylor College of Medicine, 1987.)

Postoperative Phase. Postoperative care requires continued control of blood pressure by continuous infusion of nitroprusside and beta blockers. Hemodynamic monitoring via an oximetric pulmonary artery catheter and arterial line is required. The potential for redissection and postoperative bleeding requires constant monitoring of the vital signs, hemodynamic trends, peripheral pulses, neurologic status, and level of pain. Aggressive pulmonary toilet should be done to avoid pulmonary complications. Close monitoring of the blood pressure is necessary during suctioning to avoid hypertension.

Incorporating the family into the plan of care must not be overlooked. Scheduled patient care conferences are helpful in bringing the family up-to-date on the patient's status and serve to enhance communication between members of the health care team. A multidisciplinary approach including the primary nurses, social worker, physician, and other caregivers is encouraged.

The surgical intensive care unit at the University of California, Irvine, for example, coordinates a weekly family support group that has been extremely successful. The group consists of families, staff nurses, clinical nurse specialists, social workers, and interpreters. General information is shared between families, specific questions and concerns are addressed, and short educational presentations are given.

Despite advances in the diagnosis and treatment of aortic dissection, its morbidity and mortality can still be devastating. Although diagnostic techniques have become more sophisticated, nurses should maintain a high index of clinical suspicion for aortic dissection as well as excellent physical assessment skills.

ACUTE ARTERIAL OCCLUSION

Acute arterial occlusion was first recognized in 1628 by William Harvey, and the first successful embolectomy was performed by Labey more than a century later. In the early 1940s, heparin was discovered, and anticoagulation became the focus of treatment. In 1963, the introduction of the Fogarty embolectomy balloon catheter made it possible to extract emboli and thrombi directly from arteries (Cranley et al., 1964; Fogarty et al., 1963). Significant tissue ischemia can result from acute arterial occlusion. Prompt diagnosis and treatment are critical to avoid limb loss, tissue or organ ischemia, or death.

Etiology

Acute arterial occlusion results either from embolism from the heart, an aneurysm, or ulcerative plaque, or from thrombosis of pre-existing occlusive disease or iatrogenic causes. A thorough history and assessment of the cardiovascular status is important in determining the etiology (Fig. 21–8).

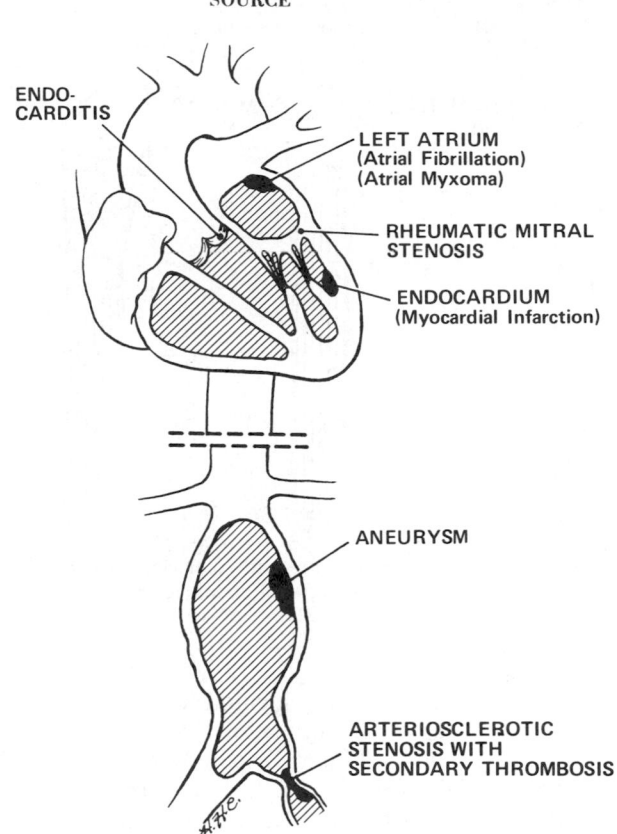

SOURCE

FIGURE 21–8. Emboli may originate from cardiac, aneurysmal, or atherosclerotic disease. (From Zimmerman, J. J., and Fogarty, T. J. (1986). Acute arterial occlusion. In W. S. Moore (Ed.), *Vascular surgery: A comprehensive review* (p. 694). New York: Grune & Stratton.)

EMBOLISM

Arterial embolism appears to be increasing as a result of the aging of the population, increased survival of cardiac patients, and the availability of invasive diagnostic procedures (Fairbairn et al., 1980).

Emboli can be divided into cardiac and noncardiac sources. The most common cause of acute aortic occlusion is emboli from cardiac sources. Four major causes of cardiac emboli are rheumatic mitral stenosis, atrial fibrillation, acute myocardial infarction, and coronary artery disease (Fairbairn et al., 1980).

Patients with mitral stenosis have an enlarged left atrium and stasis, predisposing to thrombus formation. With the decrease in rheumatic heart disease and successful valvular replacement surgery, coronary artery disease with atrial fibrillation has become the most common cause of embolism, accounting for 60% to 70% of cases (Cranley et al., 1964). Atrial fibrillation is present in 50% to 80% of patients with coronary artery disease and further predisposes the patient to atrial stasis and thrombosis formation (Connett et al., 1984).

Myocardial infarction with subsequent thrombus formation is a common precursor of cardiogenic emboli. The infarct is usually large and transmural,

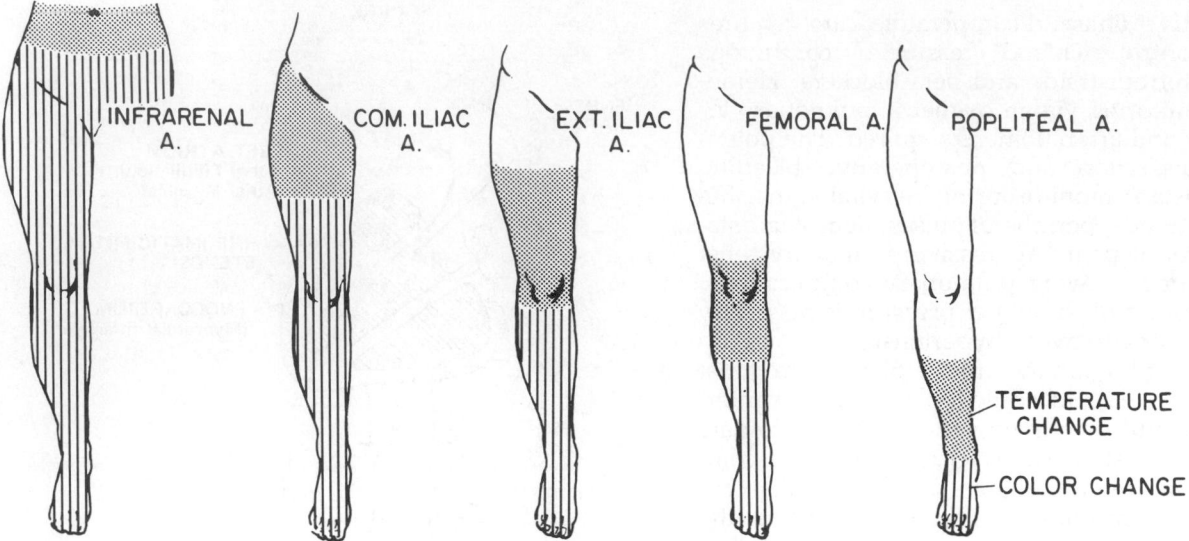

FIGURE 21–9. Level of temperature and color change with occlusion of different arteries. (From Smith, J., Holcroft, J., and Blaisdell, W. (1987). Acute arterial insufficiency. In S. Wilson, F. Veith, R. Hobson, and R. Williams (Eds.), *Vascular surgery: Principles and practice* (p. 327). New York: McGraw-Hill.)

and the thrombus is usually located in the apex. The left ventricle is also the source of emboli from ventricular aneurysms, dilated cardiomyopathy, and myocarditis (Fairbairn et al., 1980). Other cardiac sources include prosthetic heart valves, endocarditis, cardiac tumors, and poor ventricular function (Chin et al., 1986).

Noncardiac emboli may originate from proximal lesions such as an atherosclerotic plaque or aneurysm. Atheromatous plaques consisting of thrombus, fibrin, platelets, or cholesterol as well as mural thrombus within an aneurysm may fragment and dislodge distally, resulting in distal occlusions and ischemia.

Iatrogenic embolization is an unfortunate complication of invasive vascular procedures. Embolization of catheter tips, guidewires, and dislodged atherosclerotic debris can result in acute arterial occlusion (Fairbairn et al., 1980).

THROMBOSIS

More than half of all acute arterial occlusions are caused by arterial occlusive disease with subsequent thrombosis. Spontaneous thrombosis usually occurs in patients in whom a low flow state exists due to a narrowed atherosclerotic artery. Systemic conditions predisposing to arterial thrombosis include dehydration, congestive heart failure, fever, infection, thrombocytosis, disseminated intravascular coagulation, and polycythemia vera (Chin et al., 1986).

TRAUMA

Blunt and penetrating trauma may directly cause arterial injury and thrombosis. Blunt trauma can cause damage to the intima or dislodge pre-existing

plaque, resulting in embolus or thrombosis. Penetrating trauma may lead to thrombosis, intimal dissection, hematoma, or spasm (Juergens and Pluth, 1980). Bony fractures and dislocations may directly cause arterial laceration, transection, or contusion. Closed fractures in the extremities put the patient at risk for compartment syndrome due to bleeding or soft tissue swelling, leading to acute arterial occlusion.

Pathophysiology

Emboli of cardiac origin tend to obstruct large arteries at their bifurcations where the luminal diameter is decreased. Atheroemboli tend to occlude smaller vessels. The size of the obstructed vessel may help to determine the origin of the emboli. For example, an embolus that obstructed the common femoral artery is usually of cardiac origin; an embolus that causes local ischemia of a toe (blue toe syndrome) usually arises from the descending aorta or common iliac artery. Cardiac embolization accounts for most upper extremity, cerebral, and visceral ischemia (Smith et al., 1987).

The majority of peripheral emboli lodge in the lower extremities. Generally, the effects of the occlusion are proportional to the size of the vessel involved and the degree of collateral circulation present (Fig. 21–9) (Blaisdell et al., 1978).

Sudden occlusion of a severely stenotic vessel may produce only mild intermittent claudication because the pre-existing atherosclerotic disease has prompted the formation of a well-developed collateral circulation. Conversely, severe acute ischemia may result from an embolic event in a patient with marginal vascular status in whom the involved artery and collateral circulation are affected with chronic occlusive disease. Severe ischemia may also result from occlusion of a normal artery in the absence of collateral channels (Fig. 21–10) (Chin et al., 1986).

Once an embolus or thrombus occludes an artery, the vasculature distal to the obstruction goes into spasm for up to 8 hours. The clot propagates distally and proximally from the obstruction, blocking branch vessels and collaterals and worsening the ischemia (Fairbairn et al., 1980).

The extent of ischemic damage depends on the adequacy of the collateral circulation, blood viscosity, the oxygen-carrying capacity of the hemoglobin, the patient's underlying cardiovascular status, the extent of the clot propagation, and the promptness of diagnosis and treatment. Skeletal muscle and peripheral nerves can endure acute ischemia for 6 to 8 hours without permanent damage; skin can withstand severe ischemia for up to 24 hours (Blaisdell et al., 1978; Zimmerman and Fogarty, 1983).

Once muscle damage occurs, the muscle becomes paralyzed and acquires a firm, doughy consistency. Peripheral nerve damage results in loss of motor and sensory function. The skin appears blotchy, cold, cyanotic, or pale.

Reperfusion of the extremity poses a risk to the

DISTRIBUTION

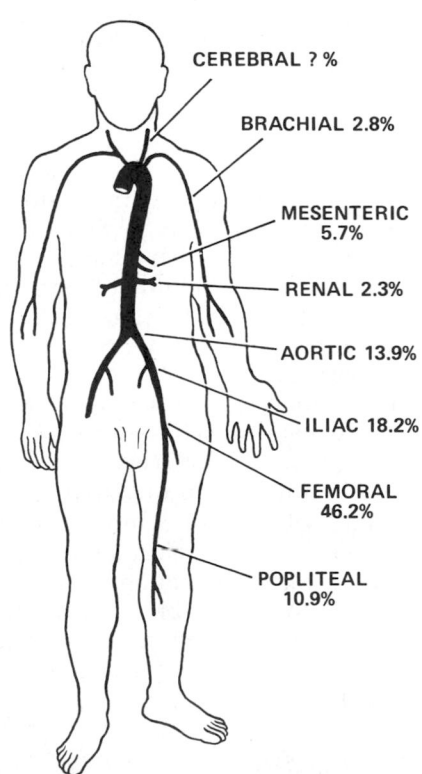

FIGURE 21–10. Emboli may obstruct various arteries but most frequently compromise flow to the extremities. (From Zimmerman, J. J., and Fogarty, T. J. (1986). Acute arterial occlusion. In W. S. Moore (Ed.), *Vascular surgery: A comprehensive review* (p. 864). New York: Grune & Stratton.)

systemic circulation and vital organs. Anaerobic metabolism produces unbuffered acid, injured cells release potassium and myoglobin, microemboli form in areas of stasis and acidosis, and platelet aggregation is enhanced (Karmody and Leather, 1984). When these toxins are released into the circulation, pulmonary, cardiac, renal, and neurologic embarrassment can result. The degree of insult depends on the degree of ischemia and necrosis, the length of the revascularization procedure, and the previous condition of the organs (Blaisdell et al., 1978).

Clinical Manifestations

A thorough history should include the type of symptoms and their duration. A history of prior cardiac disease, dysrhythmias, vascular disease, claudication, and smoking may help to differentiate between embolic and thrombotic occlusions. If there is no history of peripheral vascular disease, the acute ischemia is most likely to be of cardiac origin. A recent history of chest pain, myocardial infarction, atrial fibrillation, or murmurs is suggestive of cardiac embolus. Pain, paresthesia, pallor, pulselessness, paralysis, and poikilothermia (cold) are the classic signs and symptoms of acute arterial occlusion.

Acute pain is present in the majority of patients. The pain usually worsens with movement of the extremity. Muscle tenderness and rigidity are seen as tissue swelling worsens.

Paresthesia is an early sign of ischemia. It is important to distinguish the perception of light touch from that of pressure, pain, and temperature. The small nerve fibers responsible for soft touch are more sensitive to hypoxemia than the nerve fibers serving the latter functions. The patient may be able to detect a pinprick yet not perceive the touch from a cotton swab (Perry, 1980a).

Pallor results from decreased arterial blood flow and is an ominous sign of arterial occlusion when accompanied by pulselessness and paresthesia. Capillary refill is sluggish or absent. As ischemia worsens, pallor may be replaced by cyanosis or mottling.

Absence of peripheral pulses may be acute or chronic. The pulses are absent distal to the arterial occlusion. Pulses may be bounding proximal to the area of occlusion. Doppler arm and ankle pressures should be done to estimate the extent of ischemia.

Paralysis is a late symptom. It signifies significant neural and skeletal muscle ischemia and is frequently not reversible. Inability to dorsiflex and plantarflex the toes indicates significant ischemia. When the extremity becomes rigid or when the time of ischemia is longer than 6 to 8 hours, fasciotomy is usually necessary.

Temperature should be compared in both extremities using the back of the hand. An abrupt temperature change distal to the level of the obstruction is common.

Deep venous thrombosis (DVT) is most easily

confused with acute arterial occlusion. The normal or increased skin temperature, edema, distended veins, and normal pulses seen in DVT should help distinguish it from acute arterial occlusion. Swelling is not an early component of acute arterial occlusion but is classic in DVT (Fairbairn et al., 1980).

It is also important to evaluate the presence of visceral arterial emboli (cerebral, mesenteric, renal, coronary). Their presence adds to the complexity of the prognosis and may alter the priority of management (Haimovici, 1989).

Diagnostic Studies

Doppler pressures or imaging provides an accurate assessment of the acute aortic occlusion as well as a standard by which postoperative results can be measured.

Laboratory tests help evaluate hydration, oxygenation, renal function, cardiac function, and the degree of muscle damage. Prothrombin time, partial thromboplastin time, antithrombin III, platelet count, and hematocrit should be evaluated. Antithrombin III deficiency has been documented as a causative factor in arterial and graft thrombosis (Towne et al., 1981). Routine urinalysis may show protein or myoglobin. Creatinine phosphokinase isoenzymes help in evaluating the presence of muscle necrosis (Smith et al., 1987).

An *electrocardiogram* can identify the presence of dysrhythmias or a myocardial infarction and can help in judging the overall status of the heart.

Two-dimensional echocardiography identifies the heart chamber size and condition of the valves, estimates ejection fraction and wall motion, and occasionally identifies intracardiac thrombus or tumor (Wagner and Martin, 1973).

Ultrasound of the abdominal aorta or popliteal fossa may demonstrate the presence of an aneurysm or intraluminal clot.

Arteriography is not always indicated but provides useful information when it is done. A sharp cutoff of a normal artery is indicative of an embolus. Underlying atherosclerosis and aneurysmal disease may also be demonstrated (Fig. 21–11) (Smith et al., 1987).

Management

All patients with limb-threatening acute arterial occlusion should be given anticoagulation with heparin to prevent propagation of the clot. A bolus of 5000 to 10,000 units, followed by continuous infusion of 1000 units/hour should be started immediately. The guidelines of heparin administration are 100 to 200 units/kg per bolus, followed by 15 to 30 units/kg per minute in a constant infusion (Smith et al., 1987). Heparin should be administered regardless of whether surgical intervention is planned because it

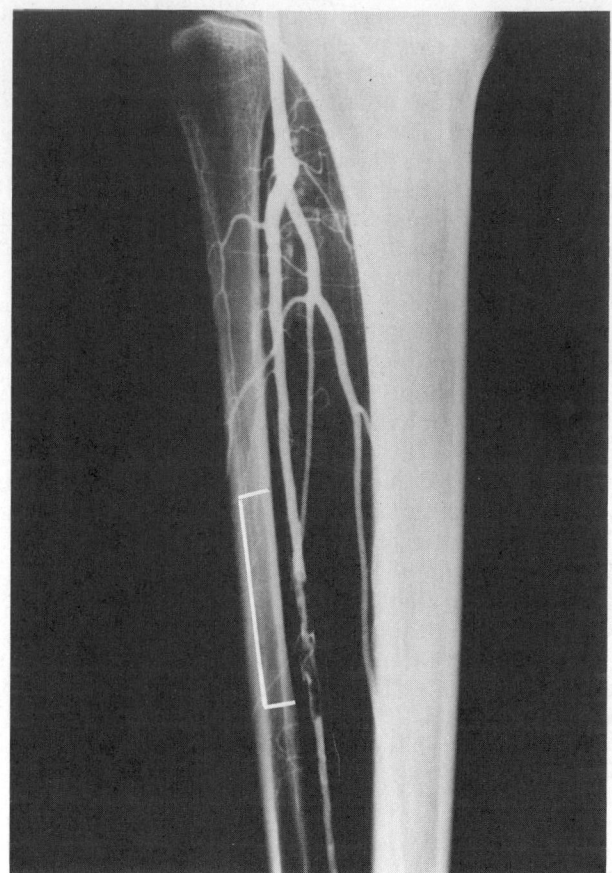

FIGURE 21–11. Angiographic demonstration of distal emboli to anterior tibial artery. Note intraluminal clot *(brackets).* (Compliments of Larry-Stuart Deutsch, M. D., Chief Cardiac/Vascular/Interventional Radiology, University of California Irvine Medical Center.)

can easily be reversed with protamine sulfate in the operating room (Fairbairn et al., 1980).

Once anticoagulation has been established, treatment of cardiac disorders should be initiated as soon as possible. Adequate hydration may help to restore perfusion. Appropriate pain management should be provided as necessary.

Fluid management can be optimized by monitoring the pulmonary wedge pressure and cardiac output. A Foley catheter should be placed and urine output maintained at 100 mL/hour. If myoglobinuria is present, alkalinization of the urine and diuresis may be advisable. Infusion of low-molecular-weight dextran may improve the microcirculation by (1) increasing blood volume, (2) improving blood flow and volume secondary to decreased blood viscosity, and (3) decreasing platelet adhesiveness (Chin et al., 1986; Nunnelee, 1988).

FIBRINOLYTIC THERAPY

Streptokinase is a nonenzymatic protein from group C beta-hemolytic streptococci that combines with plasminogen to form an active enzyme that converts plasminogen to plasmin. A low-dose, intra-arterial, selective infusion of 5000 to 10,000 IU/hour given over 12 to 48 hours effectively restores patency in occluded vessels. The arterial catheter is placed just proximal to the clot, thus avoiding systemic complications as much as possible. Thrombin time, fibrinogen levels, prothrombin time, partial thromboplastin time, platelet count, hematocrit, and fibrin split products should be monitored every 6 hours to allow early detection and treatment of bleeding complications associated with fibrinolytic therapy (Rush et al., 1982).

Urokinase is a protease harvested from human renal cells that directly converts plasminogen to plasmin. Low-dose urokinase at 20,000 IU/hour selectively has shown a high success rate in restoring vessel patency. Urokinase is much more expensive than streptokinase and therefore may be used less frequently (Smith et al., 1987).

Complications of fibrinolytic therapy can include intracranial hemorrhage, local hematoma, distal embolization, retroperitoneal hemorrhage, lysis of graft pseudointima, and mild allergic reaction (Smith et al., 1987; Rush et al., 1982).

SURGICAL PROCEDURE

The type of surgical procedure used to correct acute arterial occlusion varies with the location and underlying cause of the occlusion. When atherosclerotic occlusive disease or aneurysmal disease is suspected, a reconstructive procedure is indicated. The level of bypass grafting is chosen according to the location of the disease and thrombosis (Fairbairn et al., 1980). When arterial occlusion of the graft occurs, thrombectomy of the graft or a new bypass procedure may be necessary.

When acute ischemia is caused by an embolus, balloon embolectomy is the definitive surgical treatment. A Fogarty balloon catheter is inserted through an arteriotomy and is passed through the clot or embolus, the balloon is inflated slowly, and the catheter is withdrawn, dragging out the embolic material (Fairbairn et al., 1980; Smith et al., 1987). Embolectomy can be done under local anesthesia (Fig. 21–12). Complications of balloon embolectomy include arterial rupture, perforation, intimal injury, arterial dissection, and embolization. These complications can be readily visualized by obtaining an arteriogram after the embolus extraction.

Fasciotomy is often required following revascularization in patients with severe ischemia and edema lasting 6 to 8 hours. The fasciotomy is done to release pressure within the muscle compartments and preserve distal circulation. Subcutaneous vertical incisions are made in the involved compartments, releasing the pressure. The major complication of fasciotomy is infection.

NURSING MANAGEMENT

Proper treatment and protection of the ischemic limb are essential. The extremity should never be

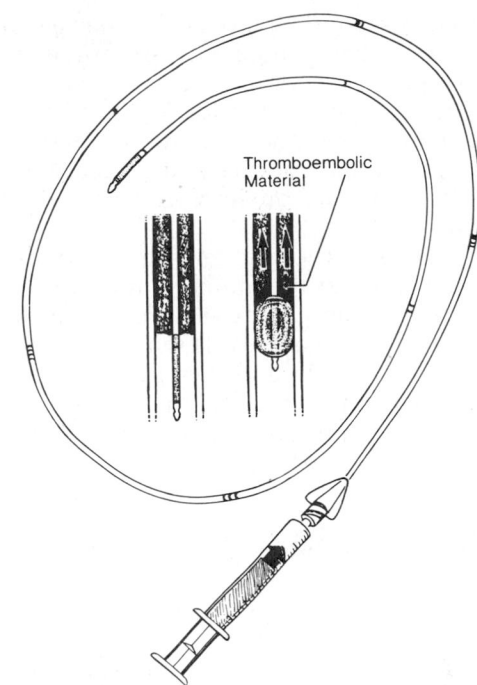

FIGURE 21–12. Demonstration of balloon embolectomy. (Balloon Embolectomy Catheter (Figure 3) from page 45 of *Critical Care Quarterly*, Vol. 8, No. 2, © September 1985.)

elevated because this only serves to diminish capillary perfusion and worsen the ischemia and pain. Decreased blood supply and decreased sensation put the extremity at risk for injury. Application of heat or chemical agents that will burn the skin should be avoided. Protection from mechanical trauma can be ensured with appropriate foot padding, use of an eggcrate mattress or specialized air bed, lambs wool placed between the toes, sheepskin, protective boot or bedcradle, avoidance of tape, and elevation of the heels off the bed. Absolutely no venipunctures or injections should be initiated on the ischemic extremity.

Hemorrhage is the major complication of anticoagulation or fibrinolytic therapy. Close observation of vital signs, IV or injection sites, and operative incisions is necessary. Coagulation values, hemoglobin, and hematocrit should be monitored frequently.

In preparation for surgery, appropriate laboratory tests should be done, including a complete blood count, prothrombin and partial thromboplastin times, potassium, platelet count, and blood type and cross-match. A Foley catheter as well as appropriate venous lines should be inserted. The use of a pulmonary artery catheter may be necessary to ensure optimal fluid management.

Hourly neurovascular checks should be done and any changes reported immediately. If recurrent embolus or thrombosis is suspected, the patient should be returned to the operating room immediately. Routine nursing care should be done to manage pain and prevent infection, pulmonary complications, and alteration in skin integrity.

Continuous emotional support of the patient and family must not be overlooked. Appropriate hospital resources such as clinical nurse specialists, social workers, and chaplains should be utilized as needed. Effective communication and mutual goal setting will enhance optimal patient care and decrease the sense of powerlessness and anxiety often experienced by the patient.

The management of acute arterial occlusion remains a challenge to the medical and nursing staffs. Early diagnosis and treatment are crucial for limb salvage. The critical care nurse who maintains excellent assessment skills and familiarity with proper treatment measures can greatly increase the success rate in treating acute arterial occlusion (see nursing care plan at end of chapter).

VASCULAR TRAUMA

More than 50 million injuries occur each year, and more than 100,000 victims die as a result of those injuries, making trauma the fourth leading cause of death in the United States (Perry, 1981). Many of these patients present with multiple trauma, but injuries to the major vessels are often the cause or major contributing factor in deaths. Patients who survive may suffer from residual disability, impaired function, or amputation (Perry, 1986). Successful management of vascular injuries depends on prompt evaluation, accurate diagnosis, and skillful management. Major advances in rapid transportation, including helicopter retrieval, and the use of highly trained paramedic and nursing personnel have resulted in the survival of many trauma victims.

Etiology

Penetrating trauma from knives and bullets is the most common cause of vascular injuries in urban areas (Jacobs and Jacobs, 1991; Perry, 1986; McCann and Makhoul, 1988). Other causes include multiple trauma from motor vehicle and motorcycle accidents, farm accidents, fractures, dislocations, lacerations, falls from great heights, crushing injuries, and iatrogenic injuries.

Mechanism of Injury

Most penetrating injuries are caused by stab or low-velocity bullet wounds, and damage is usually confined to the wound tract. High-velocity bullet wounds have a cavitation effect that may directly injure vessels, nerves, tissue, and bone. Vascular injuries may occur directly or secondarily to bone fractures. Such injuries may not be appreciated on initial inspection of the surface wound (Perry, 1985).

Motor vehicle accidents are also a cause of trauma and vascular injury. More than 1.6 million people have died on the nation's highways in the last century. Auto crashes alone result in more than 500,000 hospital admissions annually (McCann and Makhoul, 1988). Although seatbelts have proved to save lives, vascular injuries such as contusions, lacerations, and thrombosis of the abdominal aorta and the mesenteric, hepatic, subclavian, and carotid vessels have been reported (States et al., 1987).

Iatrogenic complications are not always avoidable, but many can be prevented. Intravenous infusions of hypertonic solutions may result in thrombophlebitis. Accidental intra-arterial infusions may cause arteriospasm and arteritis. Flushing air bubbles through an arterial line can result in necrosis and loss of the distal extremity and digits. Arterial puncture or cannulation for diagnostic studies or therapeutic procedures may cause local hematoma, thrombosis, dissections, and false aneurysms.

Pathophysiology

The usual pathogenesis of blunt trauma is intimal tear or contusion with associated thrombosis. Compression injuries are commonly seen in the femoral, popliteal, brachial, carotid, and renal arteries. Shearing and deceleration injuries may involve the thoracic, innominate, carotid, and subclavian arteries and may result in transection, dissection, thrombosis, aneurysm, or rupture. Penetrating arterial injury may result in hematoma, tamponade, dissection, transection, pseudoaneurysm formation, and arteriovenous fistula formation (Mattox, 1989).

Arterial insufficiency and organ ischemia may be a devastating result of arterial injury. Significant cerebral ischemia may result in permanent brain damage within 4 minutes; irreversible renal damage can occur within 1 hour; and skeletal muscle necrosis may occur within 6 hours or more. Compartment syndrome may result following revascularization of tissue that has been ischemic for 3 to 6 hours. This problem is commonly seen as a result of popliteal injury and crushing injuries to the lower leg. The compartments can be relieved by performing a fasciotomy (Mattox, 1989).

Clinical Manifestations

Injuries of large vessels are usually readily identified because of obvious hemorrhage, but deeper, less extensive wounds may not be as evident. Hemorrhage, hematoma, and pulse deficits are the cardinal signs of vascular injury. Specific presentations will be discussed under specific vascular injuries.

DIAGNOSTIC STUDIES

Doppler signals and measurement of distal arterial blood pressure are helpful in detecting vascular injury, but the specificity of these tests depend on the hemodynamics and the presence of pre-existing vascular disease. Extensive hemorrhage may be accompanied by a decrease in hemoglobin and hematocrit, especially with hemodilution from fluid resuscitation.

Routine x-rays may reveal retained bullets, bone fragments and fractures, and soft tissue damage.

The CT scan is effective in identifying injuries to the abdominal organs, hematomas, and displacement of other structures (Federle et al., 1982).

Magnetic resonance imaging provides a clear delineation of structures and can detect minor injuries.

The use of arteriography in the diagnosis of vascular injury remains controversial (McCann and Makhoul, 1988). In a stable patient, preoperative arteriography may be quite valuable in identifying vascular injury. Abnormalities may include an abrupt cutoff of a vessel, extravasation of contrast media, and evidence of an intraluminal clot. If the patient is unstable, or when firm indications for operation are present, arteriograms may not be necessary, and further evaluation is best performed in the operating room (Perry, 1986).

Management

Management of trauma patients requires a rapid yet thorough assessment. Measures of first priority are controlling obvious hemorrhage, establishing and maintaining an airway, and stabilizing the cervical spine if necessary. Once these vital precautions have been taken, a more generalized evaluation can be made.

Patients who arrive in severe hemorrhagic shock who are too unstable to be transferred to the operating room may need an operation performed in the emergency room to control the hemorrhage. An emergency thoracotomy may be necessary to treat the unstable patient with an injury to the aorta or major abdominal vascular structure. The patient should be taken to the operating room for more definitive repair as soon as possible (McCann and Makhoul, 1988).

Patients who have major hemorrhage but are in less distress should be resuscitated in the emergency room while preparations are being made for surgery. Large central catheters should be placed for rapid fluid and blood replacement. Blood and fluids should be infused through blood warmers to prevent hypothermia.

An arterial line and pulmonary artery catheter are helpful in monitoring, especially when the patient is hemodynamically unstable. The Allen test should be performed prior to inserting the arterial line to ensure a patent palmar arch.

MANAGEMENT OF SPECIFIC VASCULAR INJURIES

Aorta and Great Vessel Injury. Injury to the aorta and great vessels may be the result of penetrating or blunt trauma. Massive hemorrhage resulting in hypovolemia, shock, and death is associated with a high mortality if not rapidly treated. The presence of the Beck triad: hypotension, distant heart sounds, and elevated central venous pressure (CVP) are indicative of cardiac tamponade. However, the most reliable signs of cardiac tamponade in the traumatized patient are elevated CVP accompanied by hypotension and tachycardia. The presence of paradoxical pulse and narrow pulse pressure may also be noted (Markovchick, 1988).

The physical examination usually reveals marked hypotension, occasionally a difference in blood pressures in the extremities, pulse deficits, and an aortic murmur. A penetrating wound of the chest or abdomen is frequently the cause of aortic injury. Abdominal distention due to hemorrhage may be seen, although retroperitoneal bleeding may go undetected. Because these vessels cannot be readily examined, surgical exploration is indicated. It is important to remember that a patient with blunt trauma may present with little or no evidence of injury (Perry, 1986).

Radiographic signs of aortic injury include widened mediastinum, loss of the aortic knob, loss of sharpness of the aortic outline, deviation of the trachea and nasogastric tube to the right, depression of the left mainstem bronchus, and hematoma in the left apex. Foreign objects such as bullets may also be seen (Peyton and Wolfe, 1988).

If the patient's condition is not deteriorating, a CT scan or aortogram may be useful in identifying injury to the vessels as well as to organs and surrounding structures. Characteristics of an abnormal aortogram include extravasation of contrast medium, interruption of the aorta, intimal tears visualized as filling defects, and medial dissection (Peyton and Wolfe, 1988).

Hemodynamically unstable patients should be taken directly to the operating room. The nature of the vascular reconstruction depends on the nature of the injury. Small lacerations may be repaired by simple suturing. More extensive wounds may require extensive vessel repair, cardiopulmonary bypass, bypass grafting, as well as repair of surrounding tissues and organs (Perry, 1985).

Carotid Injury. Approximately 75% of carotid artery trauma is related to penetrating gunshot wounds, and 25% is due to stab wounds. The mechanism of injury and direction of penetration may be helpful in locating the site of carotid injury. Gunshot wounds frequently cause complete transection of the artery with significant tissue loss. Stab wounds may result in lacerations or perforations (Perry, 1985). Injuries associated with blunt trauma may present with no external evidence of injury. These injuries may remain undetected until neurologic symptoms develop resulting from thrombus formation (Perry, 1980b).

Physical examination may reveal evidence of local

trauma, frank bleeding, tracheal or esophageal trauma, crepitus, stridor, pulse deficits, neurologic deficits, hematoma, thrills, and bruits (Kelly, 1984).

Neck x-rays may reveal cervical spine injuries, soft tissue injuries, tracheal deviation, or foreign bodies. Chest x-rays are useful in detecting hemopneumothorax. Noninvasive oculopneumoplethysmography and Doppler scanning are helpful in documenting carotid occlusion.

The carotid arteriogram provides direct assessment of the location and extent of the arterial disruption as well as intraluminal thrombus. Patients who are unstable and hemorrhaging should be taken immediately to the operating room for exploration and repair (Kelly, 1984).

Initial therapy is directed at controlling the bleeding and maintaining cerebral perfusion. Maintenance of blood pressure and adequate oxygenation can help prevent cerebral infarction. An expanding hematoma may cause tracheal compression and respiratory compromise. Penetrating wounds that are not bleeding should not be probed in the emergency room because this may dislodge a thrombus or activate hemorrhage (McCann and Makhoul, 1988).

Carotid repair must be done using precise suture and graft techniques to avoid thromboembolic complications. Isolation and control of the artery both proximal and distal to the injury is obtained. The artery is flushed, any clot is removed, and the artery is then repaired. The various methods of carotid repair include lateral arteriorrhaphy with or without vein patch, end-to-end anastomosis, interposition vein graft, prosthetic graft, and ligation (McCann and Makhoul, 1988). Complications include embolus, stroke, bleeding, and death. Maintenance of adequate blood pressure and blood volume is extremely important preoperatively and postoperatively to preserve cerebral perfusion.

Patients with severe hemispheric neurologic deficits are at high risk for cerebral hemorrhage following attempts at revascularization. Most experts recommend treating these patients conservatively (Perry, 1986; Kelly, 1984).

Patients should be closely monitored in the intensive care unit for bleeding and neurologic problems. When occlusion from a thrombus or technical error occurs, rapid restoration of flow is often successful in preventing permanent neurologic deficits (Perry, 1986).

Injuries to Arteries of the Extremities. Vascular injuries to the upper extremity result primarily from gunshot wounds or stab wounds (Graham et al., 1980). Iatrogenic injuries may result from such procedures as venous access, percutaneous angiography, or cardiac catheterization. Although blunt trauma is an infrequent cause of upper extremity vascular injury, fractures and dislocations can potentially lacerate or compress adjacent vessels (Graham, 1984).

Femoral arteries are among the most frequently injured vessels. Large veins and vital nerves are located near the femoral arteries, and associated injuries are common. Most femoral injuries result from penetrating trauma from stab wounds and gunshot wounds, but they may be associated with femoral fractures (Perry, 1986).

Popliteal artery injuries are frequently associated with lower extremity injury. Although penetrating trauma may be more severe, blunt trauma may cause intimal disruption and thrombosis with no visible external injury. Blunt trauma is frequently seen in hyperextension or posterior dislocations of the knee (Perry, 1986; Davis, 1984). Failure to diagnosis popliteal injury can lead to severe tissue ischemia and limb loss.

The most important factors associated with successful management of vascular wounds of the extremities are the ischemic time and the extent of the associated injuries to bones, muscles, joints, and nerves (McCann and Makhoul, 1988). Most experts agree that muscle can tolerate approximately 6 to 12 hours of ischemia before necrosis and permanent nerve damage occur (Rush et al., 1985).

The recognition of vascular injury in the extremity is often difficult in the presence of multiple trauma and hypovolemia. Doppler assessment of the distal circulation may be helpful when pulses are difficult to palpate. A difference of 10 mm Hg between extremities is considered significant.

Arteriography is helpful in identifying the location and extent of the vascular injury. However, if arterial injury is obvious or if the patient is unstable, arteriography can be performed in the operating room (McCann and Makhoul, 1988; VanWay, 1984).

The type of vascular repair depends on the location

TABLE 21–1. General Indications for Fasciotomy

Vascular trauma
  Prolonged arterial ischemia
  Massive venous stasis
  Combined venous-arterial injury
  Popliteal arterial or venous injuries
  Arterial ligation or failed reconstruction
  Prolonged shock
  Massive tissue swelling
  Distal soft tissue injury
"Crush syndrome"
  Massive soft tissue injury
  External limb compression (drug overdose, constricting
    bandages)
Major extremity fractures
Limb reimplantation
Circumferential extremity burns
Stress-induced compartment syndromes (anterior compartment
  syndrome)
Wringer injuries
High-pressure tissue injections
Snake bite or other envenomation
Bleeding dyscrasia
Phlegmasia cerula dolens

Reprinted from Management of Vascular Trauma, by M. Kerstein (Ed.), p. 137, with permission of Aspen Publishers, Inc., © 1985.

and extent of the injury. The opposite extremity should be prepared in case a saphenous vein graft is required. Proximal and distal control is achieved before the hematoma is explored. Damaged tissue is resected, and an end-to-end anastomosis is completed. Once the necessary vascular repairs have been done, stabilization of fractures and other orthopedic repairs can be done.

Complications can include graft thrombosis, thromboembolism, bleeding, infection, and limb loss (Perry, 1986).

Fasciotomy should always be considered when the arterial supply has been disrupted for 3 hours or more and is recommended when ischemic time is greater than 6 hours (VanWay, 1984). Other indications for fasciotomy include crush injuries, closed distal extremity fractures, and swelling and tenseness of the extremity (Table 21–1) (Davis, 1984; VanWay, 1984).

Signs and symptoms diagnostic of compartment syndrome are swelling and tenderness of the compartment; pain greater than anticipated for the clini-

ncp nursing care plan

1. Impaired airway clearance, related to compromised energy state.
Validating data includes:

Dyspnea, shortness of breath
Altered respiratory pattern
Nasal flaring
Ineffective cough
Cyanosis
Diaphoresis

Inability to remove secretions
Absence of, or abnormal breath sounds
Fever
Compromised energy state
Presence of secretions

Outcome Criteria	*Nursing Interventions*
Patient's airway is patent Patient demonstrates knowledge/skill of activities designed to restore/promote/maintain effective airway clearance as indicated Patient verbalizes knowledge of pertinent follow-up resources as indicated	1.0 Assessment data 1.0.1 Assess ability to clear airway every 2 hours 1.0.2 Assess respiratory pattern every 2 hours 1.0.3 Assess for influencing risk factors: smoking, lung disease 2.0 Institute measures to restore/maintain airway clearance 2.0.1 Collaborate with physician in planning/implementing care 2.0.2 Monitor/report patient's response to treatment 2.0.3 Position patient for optimal airway clearance 2.0.4 Plan activities to provide rest periods 2.0.5 Assist patient in effective deep breathing and coughing every 4 hours as indicated/prn 2.0.6 Suction/turn prn 3.0 Instruct patient in measures to restore/promote/maintain airway patency as indicated 3.0.1 Instruct patient in specific measures: proper positioning, deep breathing/coughing, suction techniques, warning signs of ineffective airway clearance 3.0.2 Instruct patient in choices of pertinent follow-up resources 4.0 Initiate referral(s): CNS, respiratory as indicated 5.0 Evaluate status of patient in relation to outcome criteria

2. Anxiety related to impending surgery, knowledge deficit, or separation from home/family.

Patient is tense
Apprehension
Agitated
Impaired memory
Tearful
Shaky
Withdrawn
Increased activity
Distressed
Jittery
Sleep disturbance

GI disturbance
Forgetful
Inability to concentrate
Tachycardia
Tachypnea
Elevated BP
Flushing cool extremities
Diaphoresis
Impaired learning
Incongruent affect
Impulsive behaviors

Nursing Care Plan continued on following page

Outcome Criteria	Nursing Interventions

Patient verbalizes decreased feelings of uneasiness and demonstrates decreased anxiety as evidenced by positive changes in presenting data
 	
Patient demonstrates knowledge/skill of measures designed to decrease or eliminate anxiety as outlined
 	
Patient verbalizes knowledge of pertinent follow-up resources
	1.0 Assessment data
	1.0.1 Assess patient's level of anxiety
	1.0.2 Assess patient's past/present coping mechanisms
	1.0.3 Assess patient's knowledge/understanding of present situation
	2.0 Institute measures to manage anxiety
	2.0.1 Provide opportunities for verbalization of feelings
	2.0.2 Maintain quiet environment
	2.0.3 Assist patient with coping strategies:
	    Reality orientation
	    Family support
	    Positive reinforcement
	    Problem solving
	3.0 Instruct patient in measures to manage anxiety
	3.0.1 Instruct patient in specific measures:
	    Relaxation, imagery, soft music, preoperative teaching, identification of sources of anxiety, situations that trigger anxiety, effective coping strategies
	3.0.2 Instruct patient in choices of pertinent resources
	4.0 Initiate referral as indicated: CNS, social worker, psychological counseling
	5.0 Evaluate status of patient in relation to criteria

3. Altered cardiac output; decreased, related to alteration in preload/afterload, inotropic changes, alteration in rate, rhythm, conduction, structural changes.
    Validating data include:

Restlessness	Dysrhythmias
Confusion	Tachycardia
Changes in level of consciousness	Angina
Vertigo	Decreased urine output
Cool, clammy skin	Rales
Cyanosis	Angina
Decreased blood pressure	Edema
Narrowing of pulse pressure	Jugular vein distention
Increased CVP/PAP	Evidence of related factors

Outcome Criteria	Nursing Interventions

Patient demonstrates optimum cardiac output as evidenced by positive changes in presenting data
 	
Patient demonstrates knowledge/skill of activities designed to restore/promote/maintain optimum cardiac output
	1.0 Assessment data
	1.0.1 Assess BP, heart rate, respirations, mental status every hour; breath sounds, peripheral pulses, skin color/temperature every 4 hours or prn
	1.0.2 Assess for ECG changes every 4 hours and prn
	1.0.3 Assess hemodynamics as indicated:
	    PA, PAP, PCWP, CO, CI, PVR, SVR
	1.0.4 Assess for risk factors influencing cardiac output: cardiac disease, fluid status
	2.0 Institute measures to restore/promote/maintain optimum cardiac output
	2.0.1 Collaborate with physician in planning/implementing patient care
	2.0.2 Monitor/report patient's response to treatment
	2.0.3 Monitor input and output every hour and prn
	2.0.4 Weigh patient every day as indicated
	2.0.5 Monitor hemodynamic drips to optimize hemodynamic status as ordered
	3.0 Instruct patient in measures to restore/promote/maintain optimum cardiac output as indicated
	3.0.1 Instruct patient in specific measures:
	    Risk factors: diet, weight, activity
	    Medications: purpose, dosage, schedule, precautions, side effects
	    Warning signs requiring follow-up
	3.0.2 Instruct patient in choices of pertinent follow-up resources
	4.0 Initiate referrals as indicated
	4.0.1 CNS, dietary, social services
	5.0 Evaluate status of patient in relation to outcome criteria

4. Fluid volume deficit, related to excessive loss of fluid (hemorrhage, third spacing, drains).
    Validating data include:

Extremes of age/weight	Defining characteristics:
Excessive losses	Increased fluid output
Deviations affecting fluid balance	Urinary frequency
Medications	Thirst
	Altered intake

Outcome Criteria	Nursing Interventions
Patient maintains optimum fluid balance as evidenced by improved vital signs, laboratory values, intake and output Patient demonstrates knowledge/skill of activities designed to promote/maintain optimum fluid balance	1.0 Assessment data 1.0.1 Assess vital signs hourly, assess for orthostatic hypotension, skin turgor, mucous membranes every 4 hours 2.0 Institute measures to promote/maintain optimum fluid balance 2.0.1 Collaborate with physician in planning care 2.0.2 Monitor/report patient's response to treatment 2.0.3 Monitor intake and output 2.0.4 Weigh patient as indicated 2.0.5 Check wounds/dressings for excessive drainage 2.0.6 Monitor for laboratory values as indicated 3.0 Instruct patient in measures to promote/maintain optimum fluid balance 3.01 Instruct patient in: Fluid intake, medications, warning signs of fluid imbalance 2.0.2 Instruct patient in choices of pertinent follow-up resources 4.0 Initiate referrals as indicated: CNS, dietary 5.0 Evaluate status of patient in relation to outcome criteria

5. Pain related to tissue ischemia, operative procedure, aortic dissection/aneurysm.
Validating data include:

Complaints of severe pain/discomfort	Guarding
Fluctuation in vital signs	Grimacing
Pupil dilation	Alteration in muscle tone
Diaphoresis, flushed, pale skin	Irritability/restlessness
Tremors	Crying, moaning
Protective positioning	

Outcome Criteria	Nursing Interventions
Patient verbalizes/demonstrates increased comfort as evidenced by positive changes in presenting data Patient demonstrates knowledge/skill of activities designed to restore/promote/maintain comfort Patient verbalizes knowledge of pertinent follow-up resources as indicated	1.0 Assessment data 1.0.1 Assess patient's level of pain, type, location, duration 1.0.2 Assess for influencing factors affecting level of pain: anxiety, infection, noise 1.0.3 Assess patient's usual response to pain 2.0 Institute measures to restore/promote/maintain comfort 2.0.1 Maintain proper positioning/alignment 2.0.2 Provide backrubs, reassurance, rest, medication 2.0.3 Collaborate with physician in planning/implementing care 2.0.4 Monitor/report patient's response to treatment and medication 2.0.5 Plan activities to provide rest periods after therapies and pain medication 2.0.6 Institute music, quiet environment, relaxation techniques to augment pain control 3.0 Instruct patient in measures to restore/promote/maintain comfort 3.0.1 Instruct patient in specific measures: Relaxation techniques, imagery, splinting 3.0.2 Instruct patient in choices of pertinent resources 4.0 Initiate referral to CNS, social worker, pain management team as indicated 5.0 Evaluate status of patient in relation to outcome criteria

6. Potential for impaired skin integrity related to decreased tissue perfusion, poor nutritional status, infection, edema.
Validating data include:

    Poor tissue perfusion
    Bedrest

Outcome Criteria	Nursing Interventions
Patient's skin will remain intact Patient demonstrates knowledge/skill of activities designed to maintain skin integrity	1.0 Assessment data 1.0.1 Assess risk factors influencing skin integrity: tissue perfusion, age, nutritional status 1.0.2 Assess skin every shift and prn 2.0 Institute measures to promote/maintain skin integrity 2.0.1 Maintain optimum hygiene/skin care 2.0.2 Avoid tape/constricting garments 2.0.3 Institute pressure prevention devices prn: sheepskin, cradle, heel protectors, eggcrate mattress, air mattress 2.0.4 Maintain optimum nutritional status 3.0 Instruct patient in measures to maintain skin integrity 3.0.1 Instruct patient in specific measures: Foot care, appropriately fitting shoes/garments; avoid crossing legs; nutrition 4.0 Initiate referral(s): CNS, dietary consult as indicated 5.0 Evaluate status of patient in relation to outcome criteria

Nursing Care Plan continued on following page

7. Altered cerebral tissue perfusion related to interruption of arterial/venous flow, hypovolemia (embolization, aortic dissection, stroke, aneurysm rupture).
Validating data include:

Headache
Dizziness
Changes in level of consciousness
Confusion
Restlessness

Memory loss
Changes in motor/sensory signs
Changes in speech pattern
Tongue deviation

Outcome Criteria	*Nursing Interventions*
Patient demonstrates optimum neurologic functioning as evidenced by positive changes in presenting data or maintenance of baseline data Patient demonstrates knowledge of or skill in activities designed to restore/promote/maintain optimum neurologic status/function as outlined	1.0 Assessment data 1.0.1 Assess neurologic status: Glasgow Coma Scale every hour and prn 1.0.2 Assess vital signs every hour and prn 1.0.3 Assess intracranial pressure every hour and prn 1.0.4 Assess impact of related factors influencing cerebral tissue perfusion 2.0 Institute measures to restore/promote/maintain optimum cerebral tissue perfusion 2.0.1 Collaborate with physician in planning/implementing patient care 2.0.2 Monitor/report patient's response to treatment 2.0.3 Minimize patient stimulation 2.0.4 Maintain vital signs, position to ensure optimum cerebral tissue perfusion 3.0 Instruct patient in measures to restore/promote/maintain optimum cerebral tissue perfusion, as indicated 3.0.1 Instruct patient in specific measures: activity, medications, warning signs and symptoms: transient ischemic attacks, stroke 3.0.2 Instruct patient in choices of pertinent follow-up resources 4.0 Initiate referral(s): CNS, dietary, social worker as indicated 5.0 Evaluate status of patient in relation to outcome criteria

8. Altered gastrointestinal tissue perfusion related to interruption of arterial/venous flow (embolus, cross-clamping aorta, mesenteric ligation), hypovolemia.
Validating data include:

Severe and escalating abdominal pain
Pain after eating
Bowel sounds (hyper/hypo/absent)
Diarrhea/constipation
Fever
Distention

Nausea/vomiting
Melena
Hematemesis
Tachycardia
BP changes
Weight changes

Outcome Criteria	*Nursing Interventions*
Patient demonstrates optimum GI tissue perfusion as evidenced by positive changes in presenting data Patient demonstrates knowledge of or skill in activities designed to restore/promote/maintain optimum GI tissue perfusion	1.0 Assessment data 1.0.1 Assess bowel sounds, abdominal distention, abdominal pain, tenderness every 4 hours and prn 1.0.2 Assess pattern of nausea and vomiting as indicated 1.0.3 Monitor appetite, food/fluid intake as indicated 1.0.4 Assess stools for frequency, consistency, character, melena, as indicated 1.0.5 Assess for impact of related factors affecting GI perfusion 2.0 Institute measures to restore/promote/maintain optimum GI tissue perfusion 2.0.1 Collaborate with physician in planning/implementing patient care 2.0.2 Monitor/report patient's response to treatment 2.0.3 Monitor intake and output 3.0 Instruct patient in specific measures to restore/promote/maintain optimum GI tissue perfusion 3.0.1 Instruct patient in specific measures: diet, medications, warning signs/symptoms 4.0 Initiate referral(s): dietary, CNS as indicated 5.0 Evaluate status of patient in relation to outcome criteria

9. Alteration in renal tissue perfusion related to interruption of arterial/venous flow, impairment of microcirculation, hypovolemia, change in vascular resistance (hypotension, embolization, aortic dissection/aneurysm rupture).
Validating data include:

Pruritus
Anemia
Edema, generalized
Trend of increased body weight
Decreased urinary output

Level of consciousness: confused/lethargic
Shortness of breath
Abnormal lung sounds
Abnormal SMA: creatinine, electrolytes, magnesium, phosphorus, arterial blood gases, complete blood count

Outcome Criteria	Nursing Interventions
Patient demonstrates optimum renal tissue perfusion as evidenced by positive changes in presenting data Patient demonstrates knowledge of or skill in activities designed to restore/promote/maintain optimum fluid balance	1.0　Assessment data 1.0.1　Assess pulse, respirations, BP, lung sounds every 4 hours and prn 1.0.2　Assess skin integrity every 8 hours and prn 1.0.3　Assess impact of related factors influencing renal tissue perfusion: cardiac function, medications 2.0　Institute measures to restore/promote/maintain optimum renal tissue perfusion 2.0.1　Collaborate with physician in planning/implementing patient care: renal diet, fluid restriction, medications 2.0.2　Monitor/report patient's response to therapeutic regimen 2.0.3　Weigh patient every day as indicated 2.0.4　Monitor intake and output every 1–2 hours and prn; specific gravity every 4 hours 3.0　Instruct patient, if indicated, in measures to restore/promote/maintain optimum fluid balance/renal tissue perfusion 3.0.1　Instruct patient in specific measures: medications, diet, fluid intake, weight control 3.0.2　Instruct patient in choices of pertinent follow-up resources 4.0　Initiate referral(s): dietary, CNS, as indicated 5.0　Evaluate status of patient in relation to outcome criteria

10. Altered peripheral tissue perfusion related to interruption of arterial/venous flow, hypovolemia, impaired gas exchange (aneurysm rupture, peripheral vascular disease, embolization, compartment syndrome).
Validating data include:

Pain	Thick, brittle nails
Numbness/tingling	Claudication/rest pain
Coolness of extremities	Bruits
Pallor/cyanosis	Slow healing lesions
Decreased arterial pulses	Edema, peripheral
Shiny skin surfaces	Decreased motor/sensory function
Gangrene	

Outcome Criteria	Nursing Interventions
Patient demonstrates optimum peripheral tissue perfusion as evidenced by positive changes in presenting data Patient demonstrates knowledge of or skill in activities designed to restore/promote/maintain optimum peripheral tissue perfusion	1.0　Assessment data 1.0.1　Assess peripheral pulses, color, movement/sensation of extremity every 1–2 hours and prn 1.0.2　Assess impact of related factors influencing tissue perfusion: risk factors, BP, medications 2.0　Institute measures to restore/promote/maintain optimum tissue perfusion 2.0.1　Collaborate with physician in planning/implementing patient care 2.0.2　Monitor patient's response to treatment 2.0.3　Monitor anticoagulant laboratory data 2.0.4　Position extremity at level to best ensure optimum tissue perfusion 2.0.5　Implement ambulation/activity as needed 2.0.6　Determine appropriate pressure prevention: sheepskin, sequential pump stockings, special mattress (eggcrate), foot cradle 3.0　Instruct patient in measures to restore/promote/maintain optimum peripheral tissue perfusion 3.0.1　Instruct patient in specific measures: activity, medications, precautions, warning signs of decreased circulation 4.0　Initiate referral(s): CNS, dietary, social worker, as indicated 5.0　Evaluate status of patient in relation to outcome criteria

cal situation, pain not relieved by analgesics, pain on passive stretch of the compartment, and decreased motor and sensory function (Bess, 1984).

Postoperatively, the patient should be monitored in the intensive care unit. Hourly neurovascular checks should be done by assessing the pulses, color, temperature, sensory and motor function, and level of pain. If there is any question about the patency of the graft or the distal circulation, the surgeon should be notified immediately.

SUMMARY

Remarkable advancements in the diagnosis and treatment of vascular disease and emergencies have been made. Major advances in rapid transportation, including helicopter retrieval, and the use of specially trained paramedic personnel have resulted in successful management of many vascular emergencies. Effective management depends on a high index of clinical suspicion for certain injuries as well as a solid knowledge base of the vascular anatomy and physiology.

Nurses play a vital role in the initial assessment and management of vascular emergencies. Although vascular surgery is an emerging subspecialty of medical practice, the nursing profession as a whole has not recognized the requirements for nursing vascular problems in nursing curricula, continuing education programs, nursing research, or nursing literature.

Recognition of the unique needs of vascular patients and the need for education, research, and publications on vascular disease continue to be a challenge to the nursing profession. Vascular nurses throughout the country are dedicated to the advancement of peripheral vascular nursing and quality patient care by supporting basic and advanced education in vascular nursing, providing local and national education programs, developing standards of care for vascular problems, and encouraging clinical research.

Although this chapter has not been all-inclusive, it is hoped that the topics will enhance the reader's understanding of vascular emergencies, related nursing diagnoses, and the exciting challenges of caring for the patient with peripheral vascular problems.

References

Anagnostopoulos, C. E. (1975). *Acute aortic dissections.* Baltimore: University Park Press.

Applebaum, A., Karp, R. B., and Kirklin, J. W. (1976). Ascending versus descending aortic dissections. *Annals of Surgery, 183,* 296–300.

Bess, R. (1984). Fasciotomy. In E. Moore, B. Eiseman, and C. VanWay (Eds.), *Critical decisions in trauma* (pp. 530–537). St. Louis: C. V. Mosby.

Blaisdell, F. W., Steele, M., and Allen, R. E. (1978). Management of acute lower extremity arterial ischemia due to embolism and thrombosis. *Surgery, 84,* 822–834.

Burchell, H. (1955). Aortic dissection. *Circulation, 12,* 1068–1079.

Chawla, S. K., Najafi, H., Ing, T. S., et al. (1975). Acute renal failure complicating ruptured abdominal aortic aneurysm. *Archives of Surgery, 110,* 521.

Chin, A., Zimmerman, J., and Fogarty, T. (1986). Acute arterial occlusion. In W. Moore (Ed.), *Vascular surgery, a comprehensive review* (2nd ed., pp. 861–880). Orlando: Grune & Stratton.

Connett, M. C., Murray, D. H., and Denneker, W. W. (1984). Peripheral arterial embolus. *American Journal of Surgery, 148,* 14–19.

Cooke, J., and Safford, R. (1986). Progress in the diagnosis and management of aortic dissection. *Mayo Clinic Proceedings, 61,* 147–153.

Coselli, J. S., and Crawford, S. (1989). Thoracic aortic aneurysms. In H. Haimovici (Ed.), *Vascular emergencies* (pp. 591–611). Norwalk, CT: Appleton and Lange.

Cranley, J. J., Krause, R. J., Strasser, E. S., et al. (1964). Peripheral arterial embolism: Changing concepts. *Surgery, 55,* 57–64.

Crawford, E. S., Coselli, J. S., and Safi, H. J. (1989). Thoracoabdominal aortic aneurysm. In R. B. Rutherford (Ed.), *Vascular surgery* (3rd ed., pp. 927–942). Philadelphia: W. B. Saunders.

Crisler, C., and Bahnson, H. (1972). *Aneurysms of the aorta, current problems in surgery.* Chicago: Year Book.

Dalsing, M., and Sawchuk, A. (1988). Surgery of the aorta. In V. Fahey (Ed.), *Vascular nursing* (pp. 185–221). Philadelphia: W. B. Saunders.

Davis, J. (1984). Popliteal and tibial vascular trauma. In E. Moore, B. Eiseman, and C. VanWay (Eds.), *Critical decisions in trauma* (pp. 290–293). St. Louis: C. V. Mosby.

DeBakey, M., Cooley, D., and Creech, O., Jr. (1955). Surgical considerations of dissecting aneurysms of the aorta. *Annals of Surgery, 142,* 586–610.

DeBakey, M., McCollum, C., Crawford, S., et al. (1982). Dissecting aneurysms of the aorta. In J. Bergan, and J. Hao (Eds.), *Aneurysms: Diagnosis and treatment* (pp. 97–193). New York: Grune & Stratton.

Dixon, M. (1987). Acute aortic dissection. *Journal of Cardiovascular Nursing, 1* (2), 24–35.

Dragon, R., Saranchak, H., Lakin, P., et al. (1981). Blunt injuries to the carotid and vertebral arteries. *American Journal of Surgery, 141,* 497–500.

Ergin, A., Galla, J., Lansman, S., et al. (1985). Acute dissections of the aorta, current surgical treatment. *Surgical Clinics of North America, 65,* 721–741.

Fairbairn, J., Joyce, J., and Pairolero, P. (1980). Acute arterial occlusion of the extremities. In J. Juergens, J. Spittell, and J. Fairbairn (Eds.), *Peripheral vascular diseases* (pp. 381–401). Philadelphia: W. B. Saunders.

Federle, M. P., Richard, A. C., Jeffrey, R. B., et al. (1982). Computed tomography in blunt abdominal trauma. *Archives of Surgery, 117,* 645–650.

Fogarty, T. J., Cranley, J. J., Krause, R. J., et al. (1963). A method of extraction of arterial emboli and thrombi. *Surgical Gynecology and Obstetrics, 116,* 241–244.

Glagov, S., and Zarins, C. (1983). Pathology of aneurysm formation. In M. Kerstein, P. Moulder, and W. Webb (Eds.), *Aneurysms* (pp. 1–17). Baltimore: Williams & Wilkins.

Graham, J. M., Feliciano, D., Mattox, K., et al. (1980). Management of subclavian vascular injuries. *Journal of Trauma, 20,* 537–544.

Graham, J. M. (1984). Subclavian, axillary, and brachial artery injuries. In E. Moore, B. Eiseman, C. VanWay (Eds.), *Critical decisions in trauma* (pp. 282–285). St. Louis: C. V. Mosby.

Griffith, G., and Todd, E. (1985). Acute aortic dissection. *Southern Medical Journal, 78,* 1487–1493.

Haimovici, H. (1989). Abdominal aortic and iliac aneurysms. In H. Haimovici (Ed.), *Vascular emergencies* (pp. 622–649). Norwalk, CT: Appleton and Lange.

Haimovici, H. (1989). Arterial embolism of the lower extremity and technique of embolectomy. In H. Haimovici (Ed.), *Vascular emergencies* (pp. 330–353). Norwalk, CT: Appleton and Lange.

Hertzer, N. (1979). Abdominal aortic aneurysm: A guide to diagnosis and management. *Hospital Medicine,* March, 65–81.

Hirst, A. E., Johns, V., Jr., and Kime, S. W., Jr. (1958). Dissecting aneurysms of the aorta: A review of 505 cases. *Medicine, 37,* 217–279.

Jacobs, B. B., and Jacobs, L. M. (1991). Injury epidemiology. In E. E. Moore, K. L. Mattox, and D. V. Feliciano (Eds.), *Trauma* (2nd ed., pp. 15–36). Norwalk, CT: Appleton and Lange.

Juergens, J., and Pluth, J. (1980). Trauma and peripheral vascular disease. In J. Juergens, J. Spittell, and J. Fairbairn (Eds.), *Peripheral vascular diseases* (pp. 607–627). Philadelphia: W. B. Saunders.

Karmody, A. M., and Leather, R. P. (1984). Atherothrombotic microemboli of the lower limb. In R. B. Rutherford (Ed.), *Vascular surgery* (2nd ed., pp. 536–546). Philadelphia: W. B. Saunders.

Kelly, G. (1984). Carotid artery injuries. In E. Moore, B. Eiseman, and C. VanWay (Eds.), *Critical decisions in trauma* (pp. 278–281). St. Louis: C. V. Mosby.

Lie, J. T., and Juergens, J. (1980). Degenerative arterial diseases other than atherosclerosis. In J. Juergens, J. Spittell, and J. Fairbairn (Eds.), *Peripheral vascular diseases* (pp. 237–293). Philadelphia: W. B. Saunders.

Lindsay, J. (1979). Thoracic aneurysms. In J. Lindsay, *The Aorta* (pp. 121–130). New York: Grune & Stratton.

Mandell, W., Evans, E. W., and Walsford, R. C. (1954). Dissecting aortic aneurysms during pregnancy. *New England Journal of Medicine, 251,* 1059.

Markovchick, V. (1988). Acute pericardial tamponade. In P. Rosen, F. Baker, R. Barkin, et al. (Eds.), *Emergency medicine, concepts and clinical practice* (2nd ed., pp. 501–506). St. Louis: C. V. Mosby.

Mattox, K. L. (1989). Vascular trauma. In H. Haimovici (Ed.), *Vascular emergencies* (pp. 370–385). Norwalk, CT: Appleton and Lange.

McCann, R., and Makhoul, R. (1988). Peripheral vascular injuries. In J. Moylan (Ed.), *Trauma surgery* (pp. 333–359). Philadelphia: J. B. Lippincott.

McCarthy, W. J., and Williams, L. R. (1985). Femoral artery reconstruction. *Critical Care Quarterly, 11* (2), 39–50.

McIntyre, K., and Bernhard, V. (1987). Aortic aneurysms: Complications of aneurysms of the abdominal aorta and iliac arteries. In S. Wilson, F. Veith, R. Hobson, et al. (Eds.), *Vascular surgery: Principles and practice* (pp. 481–486). New York: McGraw-Hill.

McKusick, V. A. (1955). Cardiovascular aspects of Marfan's syndrome: A heritable disorder of connective tissue. *Circulation, 11,* 321.

Nunnelee, J. (1988). Medications used in vascular patients. In V. Fahey (Ed.), *Vascular nursing* (pp. 169–183). Philadelphia: W. B. Saunders.

Ochsner, J. (1982). Management of femoral pseudoaneurysms. *Surgical Clinics of North America,* 62 (3), 431–44.

Pate, J., Richardson, R., and Eastridge, C. (1976). Acute aortic dissections. *The American Surgeon,* 42, 395–404.

Perry, M. O. (1980a). Acute arterial insufficiency of the extremities. In R. B. Rutherford (Ed.), *Vascular surgery* (2nd ed., pp. 440–448). Philadelphia: W. B. Saunders.

Perry, M. O. (1980b). Carotid artery injuries caused by blunt trauma. *Annals of Surgery,* 192, 74–77.

Perry, M. O. (1981). *Management of acute vascular injuries.* Baltimore: Williams & Wilkins.

Perry, M. O. (1985). Vascular injuries. In T. Shires (Ed.), *Principles of trauma care* (3rd ed., pp. 177–196). New York: McGraw-Hill.

Perry, M. O. (1986). Vascular trauma. In W. Moore (Ed.), *Vascular surgery* (2nd ed., pp. 831–860). New York: Grune & Stratton.

Perry, M. O. (1987). Vascular injuries to the neck and thoracic outlet. In S. Wilson, F. Veith, R. Hobson, et al. (Eds.), *Vascular surgery: Principles and practice* (pp. 834–842). New York: McGraw-Hill.

Peyton, R., and Wolfe, W. (1988). Traumatic thoracic aneurysm. In J. Moylan (Ed.), *Trauma surgery* (pp. 183–196). Philadelphia: J. B. Lippincott.

Rob, C. (1987). Aortic aneurysm: Infrarenal, aortoiliac, and hypogastric. In S. Wilson, F. Veith, R. Hobson, et al. (Eds.), *Vascular surgery: Principles and practice* (pp. 475–480). New York: McGraw-Hill.

Roberts, W. (1981). Aortic dissection: Analogy, consequences and causes. *American Heart Journal,* 101, 195–215.

Roberts, W. (1982). Pathology of arterial aneurysms. In J. Bergan, and J. Yao, (Eds.), *Aneurysms, diagnosis and treatment* (pp. 17–43). New York: Grune & Stratton.

Rush, D., Adinolfi, M., and Haddad, R. (1985). Fasciotomy in vascular surgery. In M. Kerstein (Eds.), *Management of vascular trauma* (pp. 128–147). Baltimore: University Park Press.

Rush, D., Gewertz, B., Lu, T., et al. (1982). Selective infusion of streptokinase for arterial thrombosis. *Surgery,* 93, 828–833.

Saunders, J. (1979). Aortic dissection. In J. Bergan, and J. Yao (Eds.), *Surgery of the aorta and its body branches.* New York: Grune & Stratton.

Smith, J., Holcroft, J., and Blaisdell, W. (1987). Acute arterial insufficiency. In S. Wilson, F. Veith, R. Hobson, et al. (Eds.). *Vascular surgery: Principles and practice* (pp. 325–343). New York: McGraw-Hill.

Spittell, J., and Wallace, R. (1980). Aneurysms. In J. Juergens, J. Spittell, Jr., and J. Fairbairn, II (Eds.), *Peripheral vascular diseases* (pp. 415–439). Philadelphia: W. B. Saunders.

Spittell, J., and Wallace, R. (1980). Dissecting aneurysms of the aorta. In J. Juergens, J. Spittell, Jr., and J. Fairbairn, II (Eds.), *Peripheral vascular diseases* (pp. 403–413). Philadelphia: W. B. Saunders.

States, J., Huelke, D., Dance, M., et al. (1987). Fatal injuries caused by underarm shoulder belts. *Journal of Trauma,* 27, 740–749.

Thompson, J., Garrett, W., Patman, D., et al. (1983). Elective surgery for abdominal aortic aneurysms. In J. Bergan, and J. Yao (Eds.), *Aneurysms: Diagnosis and treatment* (pp. 287–300). New York: Grune & Stratton.

Towne, J. B., Bernhard, V. M., Hussey, C., et al. (1981). Antithombin III deficiency: A cause of unexplained thrombosis in vascular surgery. *Surgery,* 89, 735–742.

VanWay C., III (1984). Iliofemoral vascular injuries. In E. Moore, B. Eiseman, and C. VanWay (Eds.), *Critical decisions in trauma* (pp. 530–537). St. Louis: C. V. Mosby.

Wagner, R. B., and Martin, A. S. (1973). Peripheral atheroembolism: Confirmation of a clinical concept with a case report and review of the literature. *Surgery,* 73, 353–359.

Wheat, M. (1980). Acute dissecting aneurysms of the aorta, diagnosis and treatment. *American Heart Journal* 99, 373–386.

Zimmerman, J. J., and Fogarty, T. J. (1983). Acute arterial occlusion. In W. S. Moore (Ed.), *Vascular surgery: A comprehensive review.* New York: Grune & Stratton.

22

Patients with Hypertension

Rita M. Barden

Hypertension is a major health problem in the United States, afflicting over 58 million Americans of every age (American Heart Association, 1989). Hypertension is defined as a systolic pressure (SBP) greater or equal to 140 mm Hg or a diastolic pressure (DBP) of greater or equal to 90 mm Hg, or both (Joint National Committee on Detection, Evaluation and Treatment of High Blood Pressure, 1988). Hypertension is the major contributing factor in the development of cerebral vascular accidents, renal failure, and congestive heart failure. It is a significant risk factor associated with cardiovascular heart disease (Frohlich, 1989). Although the cause in most cases is unknown, the disease is easily detected and treated.

Largely through the efforts of the Joint National Committee on Detection, Evaluation and Treatment of High Blood Pressure and other national education programs, detection and treatment of high blood pressure has been successful. Aggressive treatment has resulted in a 50% reduction in deaths from strokes, a 35% reduction in deaths from myocardial infarction, and an overall reduction in deaths from cardiovascular disease by 8% (Frohlich, 1989). Research efforts are currently aimed at finding the cause or causes of primary hypertension and refining treatment regimens.

The National Joint Committee (1988) recommends that an individual's blood pressure be obtained at every exposure to the health care system. Mass public screenings for detection of high blood pressure are seldom necessary. The emphasis of the committee is on treatment of persons already identified as hypertensive in an effort to mitigate untoward vascular events and target organ damage. The critical care nurse is in a pivotal position to administer treatment and evaluate the hypertensive patient's clinical response to medical treatment. Nursing's emphasis on prevention of disease and education of patients makes the profession particularly well suited to address this major health issue.

This chapter will address the definition, prevalence, and classification of hypertension. A review of the homeostatic mechanisms that maintain normal blood pressure, the pathophysiology of the development of primary (essential) and secondary hypertension, and the medical and nursing treatment of this disease process are also included. Hypertensive crisis and the intensive nursing care required to manage this emergency effectively will be highlighted.

REGULATION OF ARTERIAL BLOOD PRESSURE

Blood pressure is determined by cardiac output (blood flow) and the resistance to flow or total peripheral resistance. Simply put, arterial pressure equals cardiac output times total peripheral resistance (Guyton, 1986). Total peripheral resistance is the sum of resistance in all vascular beds. Direct determinants of arterial pressure include cardiac output, aortic impedence, and vascular resistance. Figure 22–1 diagrams those factors affecting blood pressure regulation. Indirect determinants that maintain control of arterial pressure are the autonomic nervous system, hormonal regulation, the renin/angiotensin pressor system, and the volume of extracellular fluid (Dustan, 1986). Guyton (1986) divides these indirect determinants into rapid-acting systems and long-term control mechanisms. Rapid-acting systems are effective in seconds, whereas long-term control mechanisms may take minutes to hours to manifest their effects on arterial pressure.

Autonomic Nervous System

The autonomic nervous system's mechanisms for control of arterial pressure include the baroreceptor

BLOOD PRESSURE = CARDIAC OUTPUT × PERIPHERAL RESISTANCE

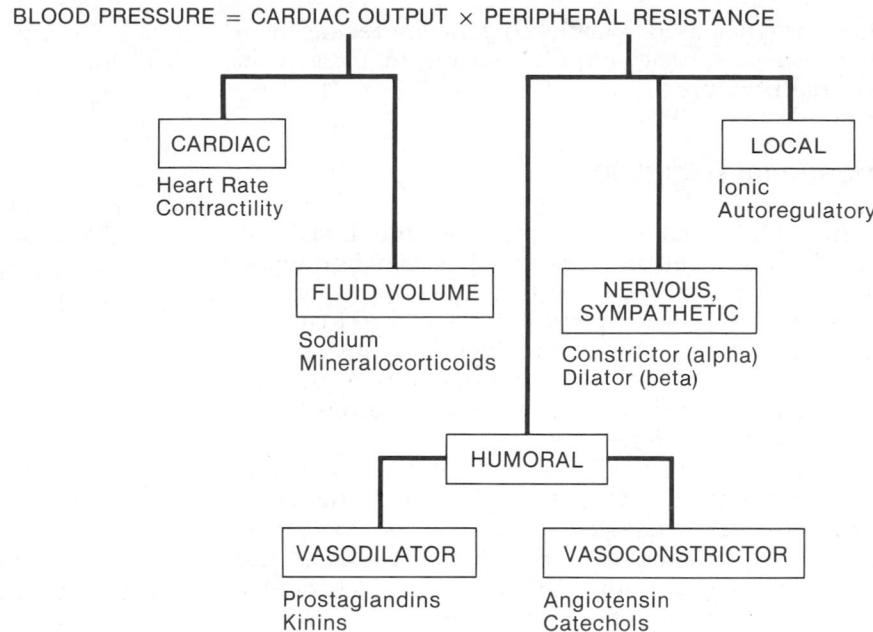

FIGURE 22-1. Factors affecting blood pressure. Some of the factors involved in the control of blood pressure = cardiac output times peripheral resistance. (From Kaplan, N. (1984). Systemic hypertension: Mechanisms and diagnosis. In E. Braunwald (Ed.). *Heart disease: A textbook of cardiovascular medicine* (2nd ed.). Philadelphia: W. B. Saunders.)

reflex, the chemoreceptor reflex, and the central nervous system ischemic mechanism. Baroreceptors are located in the walls of the large systemic arteries, most notably the internal carotid artery and the aortic arch. When these receptors are stimulated by stretching they send signals to the medullary area of the brain stem. These signals inhibit the vasoconstrictor center of the medulla and innervate the vagal center, causing vasodilatation of the peripheral vascular circuit. Stimulation of the vagus nerve also results in a decrease in heart rate and a decrease in the strength of myocardial contractions (Guyton, 1986). Arterial pressure declines secondary to a decrease in peripheral resistance and cardiac output. When arterial pressure is too low, the baroreceptor reflex system creates the opposite effect, resulting in a rise in blood pressure. The baroreceptor system reacts immediately to variations in arterial pressure, making it an effective mechanism for short-term control of blood pressure. However, this system adapts to the pressure it is exposed to within 1 to 2 days, making it an ineffective system for long-term arterial pressure control.

Changes in arterial pressure also stimulate chemoreceptors located in small bodies in the carotid artery and the aorta. These bodies are in close contact with the arterial pressure system via an artery that flows through the chemoreceptors. As arterial pressure declines, the chemoreceptors are stimulated because of a decrease in oxygen and the build-up of carbon dioxide and hydrogen. The chemoreceptors stimulate the vasomotor center, which creates a rise in arterial pressure (Guyton, 1986). These receptors respond to low arterial pressures only, not to normal arterial pressures.

Other reflexes located in the atria are stimulated

by excess fluid volume. These stretch receptors, when stimulated, cause reflex dilatation in afferent arterioles, most notably in the kidneys. As dilatation occurs, the glomerular capillary pressure rises, causing increased deposition of fluid into the tubules. As the atria stretch, they also stimulate the hypothalmus to decrease the excretion of antidiuretic hormone. This results in increased excretion of fluid into the urine. Loss of blood volume results in a decline in arterial pressure (Guyton, 1986).

As atrial pressure increases, the stretching of the sinoatrial node stimulates a 15% increase in heart rate. As the atria is stretched, the receptors of the Bainbridge reflex are also stimulated, resulting in an additional 40% to 60% increase in heart rate. This significant increase in heart rate is due to stimulation of the vagal and sympathetic nerves. This mechanism increases arterial pressure but does not serve to maintain arterial pressure within the normal range and may actually be detrimental to blood pressure control for brief periods (Guyton, 1986).

The central nervous system (CNS) ischemic response exerts powerful control over arterial pressure. As arterial pressure declines to below 60 mm Hg, the build-up of carbon dioxide and lactic acid stimulates the vasomotor center, resulting in innervation of the sympathetic nervous system. The sympathetic discharge results in an increase in heart rate and contractile force, causing arterial pressure to rise. The CNS ischemic response is activated in lethal situations of low arterial pressure (Guyton, 1986).

Stimulation of the sympathetic nervous system also results in venous constriction. This constriction decreases capacity in the veins, forcing blood into the heart. As the heart receives an increased blood volume, both the heart rate and the strength of contractions are increased. Venous constriction results in an increase in cardiac output, causing an increase in arterial pressure.

Hormonal Regulation

In addition to neural responses the body also regulates arterial pressure using certain hormones. Rapid hormonal responses include the release of epinephrine and norepinephrine into the circulation via stimulation of the sympathetic nervous system. These catecholamines increase heart rate and the force of contractions and exert a vasoconstrictive effect on both arteries and veins.

Another hormone involved in the regulation of arterial pressure is vasopressin. This hormone causes profound vasoconstriction and elevates blood pressure by increasing total peripheral resistance and vascular filling pressure (Guyton, 1986). Vasopressin is also known as antidiuretic hormone (ADH). The principal action of ADH is the reabsorption of water in the renal tubules. With the increase in vascular volume, the arterial pressure rises (Orten and Neuhaus, 1982).

Renin-Angiotensin System

Both vasopressin and the renin-angiotensin system are rapid-acting and are also long-term control mechanisms in the maintenance of arterial pressure. When the blood pressure is inadequate to maintain sufficient blood flow through the kidneys, the juxtaglomerular cells of the kidneys secrete renin. Renin secretion is also increased with sympathetic nervous system stimulation and oliguria (Dustan, 1986). Renin is converted in the bloodstream to angiotensin I, which is converted in the lungs to angiotensin II. Orten and Neuhaus (1982) write that "angiotensin I has only a slight effect on blood pressure, whereas angiotensin II is the most powerful pressor agent now known, having an activity 200 times greater than norepinephrine." Angiotensin II affects arterial pressure in several ways. It acts as a powerful vasoconstrictor of the arterial system and has a mild vasoconstrictive effect on the venous circulation as well. Angiotensin II inhibits the excretion of salt and water as regulated by the kidneys and stimulates the production of aldosterone, which further reduces the excretion of salt and water. This results in an increase in blood volume, creating an increase in arterial pressure (Kaplan, 1986). Aldosterone is not a pressor agent in itself; rather, it causes retention of sodium by the kidneys, which results in an excess accumulation of water. Figure 22–2 represents the renin-angiotensin-aldosterone mechanism. The renin-angiotensin system and the regulation of aldosterone are part of a feedback loop that can either increase or decrease blood volume in an effort to maintain normal arterial pressure.

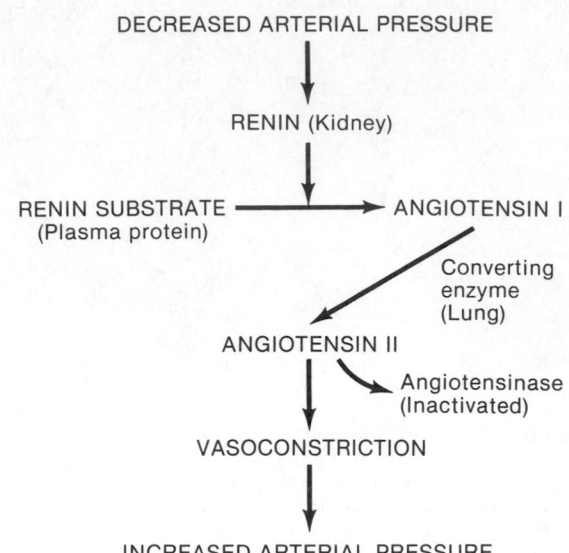

FIGURE 22–2. Renin-angiotensin mechanism. The renin-angiotensin vasoconstrictor mechanism for arterial pressure control. (From Guyton, A. C. (1986). *Textbook of Medical Physiology* (7th ed., p. 254). Philadelphia: W. B. Saunders.)

Extracellular Fluid Volume

The kidneys' ability to regulate the volume of extracellular fluid plays a major role in the maintenance of long-term arterial pressure control. With a rise in arterial pressure the kidneys are stimulated to excrete water and salt into the urine. This is called pressure diuresis and pressure natriuresis (Guyton, 1986; Dustan, 1986). This decrease in fluid volume causes a decline in the pumping action of the heart and diminishes cardiac output, resulting in a decline in arterial pressure. With a decline in arterial pressure the kidneys reabsorb water and sodium, thereby increasing extracellular fluid volume and blood volume. With an increase in blood volume, the cardiac output increases, and arterial pressure rises. This system is involved in the long-term regulation of blood pressure.

Ingestion of large quantities of water rarely result in a dramatic and sustained elevation in arterial pressure. Rather, the ingestion of salt results in the increase in vascular volume. As the amount of salt increases in the body, the osmolality in the plasma volume increases, stimulating the thirst center in the brain, resulting in increased consumption of water. This excess salt intake also stimulates secretion of antidiuretic hormone, which results in reabsorption of more water by the kidneys, all of which increase extracellular fluid volume. Fluid overload results in vasoconstriction resulting in increased peripheral resistance, which, if chronically elevated, will quickly lead to abnormal thickening of the vascular wall. This is believed to be one of the mechanisms associated with the development of hypertension.

The inherent ability of the vascular beds to increase or decrease blood flow depending on the metabolic needs of the tissues is called autoregulation. As blood flow in the vascular bed increases beyond demand, vasoconstriction occurs, decreasing the volume of blood in the vascular bed. When blood flow is diminished, the vessels dilate to increase the volume of blood required to meet the metabolic needs of the tissues adequately. As the vascular bed constricts and dilates, it influences resistance to flow, creating a fluctuation in arterial pressure (Kaplan, 1986; Guyton, 1986).

DEFINITION AND PREVALENCE OF HYPERTENSION

Hypertension is defined according to the criteria of the Joint National Committee (1988). Hypertension is defined as multiple averaged blood pressure readings in persons 18 years of age or older that are greater than or equal to 140/90 mm Hg or an isolated systolic blood pressure greater than or equal to 160 mm Hg or an isolated diastolic blood pressure greater than or equal to 90 mm Hg (Table 22–1).

The prevalence of hypertension has increased with the growth in our population. Some 58 to 60 million Americans have high blood pressure or are receiving antihypertensive therapy. Age significantly affects the percentage of hypertensive individuals, with some 50% of all diagnosed individuals falling in the over-65 age category. Isolated systolic hypertension is common in the elderly and is associated with an increased risk of cardiovascular events, predominantly stroke. Thirty-eight per cent of all hypertensive individuals are black, and 29% are white (Kaplan, 1986). Blacks continue to sustain increased morbidity and mortality from hypertension, most

TABLE 22–1. Classification of BP in Adults Aged 18 Years or Older*

BP Range, mm Hg	Category†
DBP	
<85	Normal BP
85–89	High-normal BP
90–104	Mild hypertension
105–114	Moderate hypertension
≥115	Severe hypertension
SBP, when DBP	
<90 mm Hg	
<140	Normal BP
140–159	Borderline isolated systolic hypertension
≥160	Isolated systolic hypertension

*Classification based on the average of two or more readings on two or more occasions. BP indicates blood pressure; DBP, diastolic blood pressure; and SBP, systolic blood pressure.

†A classification of borderline isolated systolic hypertension (SBP, 140 to 159 mm Hg) or isolated systolic hypertension (SBP, ≥160 mm Hg) takes precedence over high-normal BP (DBP, 85 to 89 mm Hg) when both occur in the same person. High-normal BP (DBP, 85 to 89 mm Hg) takes precedence over a classification of normal BP (SBP, <140 mm Hg) when both occur in the same person.

From the Joint National Committee (1988). The 1988 report of the joint national committee on detection, evaluation and treatment of high blood pressure. *Archives of Internal Medicine, 148,* 1023–1038.

commonly renal disease and strokes. Males suffer more cardiovascular morbidity and mortality than females with every degree of severity of hypertension (Kaplan, 1988a).

CLASSIFICATION OF HYPERTENSION

Classification of hypertension is based on cause and severity. Primary (also known as essential or idiopathic) hypertension accounts for 90% to 95% of all hypertension. The causes of primary hypertension are still unknown. Secondary hypertension has a distinct cause and accounts for 5% to 10% of all hypertensives (Kaplan, 1986; Joint National Committee, 1988; Dustan, 1986). There are numerous causes of secondary hypertension (Table 22–2). A third classification is hypertensive crisis, which is usually manifested by a diastolic blood pressure greater than 130 mm Hg, significant neurologic deficits, and a fundoscopic examination revealing retinal hemorrhages, exudate, or papilledema (Kaplan, 1986; Ram, 1984). Although this phenomenon is rare, it is life-threatening and must be promptly and aggressively treated.

Classification of hypertension according to severity is based on diastolic pressure and is labeled as follows (Kaplan, 1986):

Mild	90–104 mm Hg
Moderate	105–114 mm Hg
Severe	≥ 115 mm Hg

The risk of cardiovascular, renal, and neurologic morbidity and mortality increasing with the severity of hypertension is well documented (Hypertension Detection and Follow-up Program Cooperative Group, 1979; Multiple Risk Factor Intervention Trial Research Group, 1982; Veterans Administration Cooperative Study Group on Antihypertensive Agents, 1967, 1970).

PRIMARY (ESSENTIAL) HYPERTENSION

Several hypotheses have been postulated to explain primary hypertension. The factors that regulate normal arterial pressure, as previously discussed, have all been implicated in the development of hypertension. The dysfunction in these interrelated factors contributes to sustained elevated arterial pressure, indicating the multifactorial aspect of primary hypertension. Currently, there are several hypotheses postulated to explain primary hypertension. They are the autoregulatory, the renal-volume retention, and the sodium transport theories. There is much debate among clinicians about which theory most likely explains the development of primary hypertension. Kaplan (1988a, 1986) believes that blood pressure is the result of several complex mechanisms in the body, namely, cardiac output, vessel

TABLE 22–2. Types of Hypertension

I. *Systolic and diastolic hypertension*
  A. Primary, essential, or idiopathic
  B. Secondary
    1. Renal
      a. Renal parenchymal disease
        (1) Acute glomerulonephritis
        (2) Chronic nephritis
        (3) Polycystic disease
        (4) Connective tissue diseases
        (5) Diabetic nephropathy
        (6) Hydronephrosis
      b. Renovascular
      c. Renin-producing tumors
      d. Renoprival
      e. Primary sodium retention (Liddle's syndrome, Gordon's syndrome)
    2. Endocrine
      a. Acromegaly
      b. Hypothyroidism
      c. Hypercalcemia
      d. Hyperthyroidism
      e. Adrenal
        (1) Cortical
          (a) Cushing's syndrome
          (b) Primary aldosteronism
          (c) Congenital adrenal hyperplasia
        (2) Medullary: pheochromocytoma
      f. Extraadrenal chromaffin tumors
      g. Carcinoid
      h. Exogenous hormones
        (1) Estrogen
        (2) Glucocorticoids
        (3) Mineralocorticoids: licorice, carbenexolone
        (4) Sympathomimetics
        (5) Tyramine-containing foods and MAO inhibitors
    3. Coarctation of the aorta
    4. Pregnancy-induced hypertension
    5. Neurological disorders
      a. Increased intracranial pressure
        (1) Brain tumor
        (2) Encephalitis
        (3) Respiratory acidosis: lung or CNS disease
      b. Quadriplegia
      c. Acute porphyria
      d. Familial dysautonomia
      e. Lead poisoning
      f. Guillain-Barré syndrome
    6. Acute stress, including surgery
      a. Psychogenic hyperventilation
      b. Hypoglycemia
      c. Burns
      d. Pancreatitis
      e. Alcohol withdrawal
      f. Sickle cell crisis
      g. Postresuscitation
      h. Postoperative
    7. Increased intravascular volume
    8. Ethanol drugs and other substances
II. *Systolic hypertension*
  A. Increased cardiac output
    1. Aortic valvular regurgitation
    2. AV fistula, patent ductus
    3. Thyrotoxicosis
    4. Paget's disease of bone
    5. Beriberi
    6. Hyperkinetic circulation
  B. Rigidity of aorta

From Kaplan, N. (1988). In E. Braunwald (Ed.), *Heart disease* (3rd ed.). Philadelphia: W. B. Saunders.

diameter and resistance, and fluid volume. All of these factors are interrelated in the maintenance of arterial pressure control. All have been implicated in the development of chronic arterial pressure elevation.

The autoregulatory hypothesis explains the increase in arterial pressure as a direct result of an increase in cardiac output, presumably due to an increase in extracellular volume or increased stimulation of the sympathetic nervous system. This increase in cardiac output causes an elevation in arterial pressure. With this oversupply of blood and nutrients, the autoregulatory mechanism of the arterial vessels will begin vasoconstriction to bring supply and demand into balance. This chronic constriction leads to structural thickening of the vessel wall and the sequence of events discussed in the following section on vascular changes associated with hypertension. Even though cardiac output may fall to normal or low, the vessels remain structurally damaged, resulting in a chronic increase in peripheral resistance (Guyton, 1986).

The renal-volume retention hypothesis claims that, with normal elevation in arterial pressure, renal blood flow is increased. This increase in flow increases the glomerular filtration rate, enhancing the excretion of sodium and water into the urine, thus returning blood pressure to normal. This mechanism is called pressure natriuresis-diuresis. In hypertension, there appears to be an increase in renal efferent arteriolar constriction possibly due to overstimulation of catecholamines or increased sensitivity to these catecholamines. This arteriolar constriction results in an increased filtration fraction and peritubular oncotic pressure, which increases reabsorption of sodium and water. The kidneys become accustomed to higher arterial pressures, requiring markedly increased arterial pressures to begin excreting sodium and water. This is labeled the resetting of the pressure natriuresis curve (Kaplan, 1986; Guyton, 1986).

Alterations in sodium transport have recently been postulated as an explanation for primary hypertension. Due to a genetic defect, the kidneys are unable to excrete sodium in sufficient quantities, resulting in an increase in extracellular fluid. A natriuretic hormone secreted in response to this elevated volume decreases the activity of the intracellular sodium pump. The sodium-potassium ATPase pump is located on receptor sites of the semipermeable membrane and functions to maintain homeostatic balance between intra- and extracellular sodium, potassium, and calcium. This system malfunctions (presumably due to an inherited defect), increasing the amount of intracellular sodium. Sodium heightens contraction of the vascular tissues. Studies also indicate an increase in intracellular calcium, which results in increased vascular tone and reactivity. This increase in intracellular sodium and calcium leads to sustained peripheral resistance, the hemodynamic hallmark of hypertension (Kaplan, 1986). Figure 22–3 presents this hypothesis.

These various hypotheses explain the chemical and

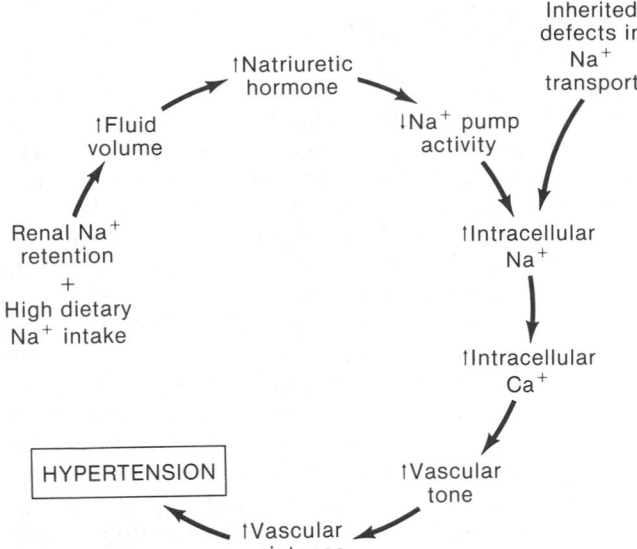

FIGURE 22–3. Sodium transport defect leading to hypertension. An overall scheme for a "sodium transport" defect for the pathogenesis of primary hypertension. The defect is shown to arise either from an acquired inhibitor of the sodium pump or from an inherited defect of sodium transport. (From Kaplan, N. (1986). *Clinical hypertension* (4th ed.) © 1986, The Williams & Wilkins Co., Baltimore.)

structural changes found in persons with hypertension, but factors such as heredity, obesity, cigarette smoking, diabetes, alcohol, and others have also been associated with the development of hypertension. Discussion of these factors follows.

Heredity

The role of heredity in the development of hypertension is accepted among scientists and practitioners. Hypertension aggregates in families, and individuals with hypertensive parents have twice the possibility of developing hypertension (Kaplan, 1986). What is not clearly understood is the exact contribution of heredity and the method of genetic transmission necessary for the development of hypertension. Without a clearer understanding of the causes of primary hypertension, the exact weight of heredity in hypertension may never be known.

The mode of inheritance of hypertension is also a mystery. It is postulated that hypertension may be due to a genetic defect in cellular transport of sodium, a defect in renal excretion of sodium, or an exaggerated sympathetic response to stress. Hypertension may be the result of one or all of these genetic abnormalities.

Factors Affecting Hypertension

A variety of factors are implicated in the acute or chronic elevation of blood pressure. These factors include cigarette smoking, caffeine, alcohol, obesity, diabetes, and stress.

Smoking. With acute inhalation of nicotine there is a rise in both systolic and diastolic blood pressures, probably due to the release of norepinephrine. Chronic smoking has not been found to contribute to the development of hypertension. There is no more likelihood of smokers developing hypertension than nonsmokers. However, because smoking has been found to increase the possibility of development of other cardiovascular diseases and has been linked to an increased death rate in hypertensives, abstinence is advocated (Kaplan, 1988a, 1986).

Caffeine. Caffeine does not appear to affect hypertension, although ingestion of this substance in individuals who do not normally ingest it has been found to elevate arterial blood pressure and renin and catecholamines levels. Chronic ingestion results in development of a tolerance, which results in normal secretion of renin and catecholamines as well a return to a normal blood pressure (Kaplan, 1986).

Alcohol. Alcohol has been associated with a rise in arterial pressure in persons consuming more than 2 to 3 ounces daily. Alcohol increases vascular tone, which results in vasoconstriction. Increasing amounts of alcohol appear to correlate with higher blood pressure levels. Therefore, an individual who consumes 6 to 7 ounces daily is likely to have higher blood pressure than an individual who consumes 4 to 5 ounces daily. A reduction in blood pressure and coronary mortality has been associated with modest (1/2 to 2 ounces daily) consumption of alcohol (Kaplan, 1986).

Obesity. There is a strong correlation between obesity and hypertension. There is a relationship between weight gain and the development of hypertension, especially in young adults and children. The association between obesity and the worsening of atherogenesis was noted in the Framingham Study (Kannel, 1976). Obesity creates an increase in blood volume, resulting in an increase in cardiac output.

Diabetes. Diabetes and hypertension commonly coexist. This relationship is not clearly understood, but the combination of disease processes results in a significant increase in cardiovascular morbidity and mortality (Assmann and Schulte, 1989). Poor glucose control causes arterial vessel damage and alteration in the glomerular basement membrane of the kidneys. Hypertension is likely to result from increased vascular tone and rigidity as well as an alteration in renal function (Kaplan, 1986).

Stress. Stress stimulates the sympathetic nervous system, resulting in increased cardiac output, vasoconstriction, and enhanced excretion of renin. Whether stress itself or an abnormality in the sympathetic nervous system results in hypertension is unknown. Hyperactivity of the sympathetic nervous system has been demonstrated in response to mental stress, physical activity, exposure to cold, and postural changes. This heightened sympathetic response is more acute in individuals with a genetic predisposition and documented hypertension (Kaplan, 1986).

SECONDARY HYPERTENSION

Although primary hypertension accounts for the majority of persons with hypertension, approximately 10% of all hypertensives have secondary hypertension, or hypertension with a known cause. After identifying the cause, the treatment may be tailored to eradicate hypertension. An extensive list of possible causes is found in Table 22–2.

Oral Contraceptives

Oral contraceptives containing estrogen are the most common cause of secondary hypertension (Kaplan, 1988a). Progestogen, contained in oral contraceptive preparations, has also been shown to increase blood pressure. Both estrogen and progestogen are dose dependent. With increasing amounts of each hormone, blood pressure levels elevate (Meade, 1988). The severity of hypertension is usually mild but does increase over time with oral contraceptive use. Hypertension is one of the major contributors to the increased incidence of cardiovascular mortality seen in women using oral contraceptives. Concomitant use of cigarettes and alcohol in excess of 10 ounces/week increases a woman's risk of cardiovascular mortality. Hypertension is probably caused by stimulation of the renin-angiotensin-aldosterone mechanism, creating volume expansion in oral contraceptive users. The structural and functional changes associated with contraceptive use include enhanced blood clot formation, increased coronary artery vascular tone, increased fibroblast deposition, and enhanced cellular replication in vessel walls (Stadel, 1981; Royal College of Practitioners Oral Contraception Study, 1981).

Renal Parenchymal Disease

Renal parenchymal disease resulting in hypertension is associated with chronic glomerulonephritis and acute oliguric renal failure. Both of these entities, if untreated, result in renal damage altering the renal-pressor system or inappropriate stimulation of the renin-angiotensin mechanisms (Linas and Schrier, 1981). Acquired infections or polycystic kidney disease can alter renal function as well. Renal parenchymal disease may account for 2% to 4% of the hypertensive population (Kaplan, 1988a).

Renovascular Disease

Another common cause of secondary hypertension is renovascular disease. Estimates indicate that about 2% of the hypertensive population has renovascular disease causing hypertension (Kaplan, 1986). This increase in systemic vascular resistance is due to stenosis caused by fibrous dysplasia or atherosclerosis of one or more of the renal arteries. This decrease in renal flow results in an overproduction and release of renin-angiotensin. Production of renin is also stimulated by the sympathetic nervous system, predominantly catecholamine release. Hypokalemia is a common finding of renovascular hypertension and is a result of the stimulation of aldosterone by angiotensin II. Aldosterone further elevates peripheral resistance by decreasing absorption of sodium, causing an increase in extracellular fluid (Linas and Schrier, 1981).

Primary Aldosteronism

Primary aldosteronism is caused by an adenoma on the adrenal gland or an adenomatous hyperplasia of the adrenal gland resulting in overproduction of aldosterone. This creates an excess of salt and water, which is the mechanism behind the development of hypertension with this disease. The percentage of hypertensives with this disease is estimated at less than 1%. This is the most common of the steroid-induced hypertensions. Other disease entities that alter steroid production and result in hypertension include Cushing's syndrome, adrenogenital syndrome, and 17- and 11-hydroxylase deficiencies (Dustan, 1986).

Pheochromocytoma

Pheochromocytoma, a tumor located in the adrenal glands, is a rare cause of hypertension. This tumor oversecretes catecholamine, causing an increase in peripheral resistance through vasoconstriction. This disease may cause fluctuations in blood pressure or may result in sustained hypertension. In addition to hypertension, the practitioner will see headache, sweating, palpitations, anxiety, and weight loss. Pheochromocytomas have a strong familial link. Stroke and myocardial infarction have been associated with rapid significant elevations in blood pressure in this disease process (Dustan, 1986; Kaplan, 1988a).

Coarctation of the Thoracic Aorta

This localized lesion develops in the thoracic portion of the aorta just below the ligamentum arteriosum. This constriction reduces the lumen of the aorta significantly or may result in complete obliteration (Kaplan, 1986; Dustan, 1986). The hallmark presentation of coarctation is an elevated arterial pressure in the upper extremities and low or absent pressures in the lower extremities. The mechanisms of hypertension are vasoconstriction and an increase in fluid volume secondary to alterations in renal function (Kaplan, 1986).

Pregnancy-Induced Hypertension

Pregnancy-induced hypertension (PIH) is an important cause of maternal morbidity and mortality and fetal mortality (Assche et al., 1989). PIH is the term used to include preeclampsia, toxemia, and chronic hypertension that is exacerbated by pregnancy. It may occur in previously normotensive women or may intensify in chronic hypertensive individuals (Koniak-Griffin and Dodgson, 1987). The definition of hypertension in PIH is a blood pressure greater than 140/90 mm Hg or a systolic increase of 30 mm Hg or a diastolic increase greater than 15 mm Hg from baseline readings. These measurements need to be obtained on two separate occasions at least 6 hours apart (Gant and Worley, 1980).

Signs of preeclampsia are hypertension, edema, and proteinuria after the twentieth week of gestation. Eclampsia is a severe manifestation of PIH and includes significant alterations in cerebral function resulting in grand mal seizures (Gant and Worley, 1980).

Another severe manifestation of pregnancy-induced hypertension is the HELLP syndrome. This acroynm stands for hemolysis, elevated liver function tests, and low platelets (Weinstein, 1982). Symptoms associated with this syndrome are malaise, nausea with or without emesis, epigastric pain, right upper quadrant tenderness on examination, and edema. Frequently these patients present with blood pressures greater than 160/110 mm Hg. Clinical signs include elevated levels of serum glutamic oxaloacetic transaminase (SGOT), serum glutamic pyruvic transaminase (SGPT), bilirubin, blood urea nitrogen (BUN), creatinine, and more than 2+ proteinuria. Disturbances in the hematologic profile include decreases in the hematocrit and platelet count and an abnormal peripheral blood smear (Weinstein, 1982). The HELLP syndrome may be superimposed on preeclampsia or eclampsia. Without rapid and aggressive treatment, infant and maternal mortality is high.

Hypertensive Crisis

Although hypertensive crisis is rare, its recognition and treatment must be rapid and aggressive. Most hypertensive crises occur in patients with any type of preexisting hypertension. Disease entities commonly associated with hypertensive crisis are essen-

tial hypertension, chronic renal disease, toxemia of pregnancy, renovascular hypertension, pheochromocytoma, acute glomerulonephritis, and certain medications (Rahn, 1989). The determinants of crisis are an elevated blood pressure (usually markedly so) and evidence of acute target organ damage. Ram (1984) categorized hypertensive crisis into emergencies and urgencies. Emergencies are defined as hypertension causing target organ damage such that prognosis will be poor unless the blood pressure is decreased within 1 hour. Urgencies are acute hypertensive episodes that pose a less immediate life threat but if sustained, will result in serious complications. Reduction of blood pressure should occur within several hours (Joint National Committee, 1988). Hypertensive emergencies include acute aortic dissection, pulmonary edema, hypertensive encephalopathy, pheochromocytoma crisis, intracranial hemorrhage, MAO inhibitors and tyramine interaction, and eclampsia (Gonzales and Ram, 1988). Hypertensive urgencies may include peri- and postoperative hypertension, severe hypertension in patients with kidney transplants, accelerated and malignant hypertension, hypertension associated with coronary artery disease, and uncontrolled hypertension in individuals requiring emergency surgery (Gonzales and Ram, 1988). Any hypertensive crisis classified as an urgency may rapidly develop into an emergency.

Accelerated hypertension is defined as significantly elevated blood pressure (DBP greater than 130 mm Hg) with hemorrhages and exudate (grade 3 on the Keith-Wagener scale, Table 22–3) on funduscopic examination (Ram, 1984; Kaplan, 1986). Malignant hypertension is defined as a marked elevation in blood pressure (DBP greater than 130 mm Hg) with a grade 4 Keith-Wagener funduscopic examination, which includes the findings of grade 3 and papilledema. Hypertensive crisis is more common in individuals who smoke or those with specific immune system abnormalities (Kaplan, 1986). Accelerated hypertension frequently precedes malignant hypertension and should be considered part of a continuum of hypertension. For that reason and also because of the similarities in signs and symptoms, they will be discussed together in this chapter.

TABLE 22–3. Keith-Wagener Scale for Funduscopic Examination

KW1 = Minimal arteriolar narrowing and irregularity.
KW2 = More marked narrowing and arteriovenous nicking. Implies arteriosclerotic as well as hypertensive changes.
KW3 = Flame-shaped or circular hemorrhages and fluffy "cotton wool" exudates.
KW4 = Any of the above plus papilledema, i.e., elevation of the optic disk, obliteration of the physiologic cup, or blurring of the disk margins. By definition, malignant hypertension is always associated with papilledema.

From Sokolow, M. (1985). In Krup, M., Chalton, M., and Werdegan, D. (Eds.), *Current medical diagnosis and treatment*. Los Altos, CA: Lange Medical Publications.

It is likely that significant elevations in blood pressure or involvement of other factors set off a cascade of events resulting in the bodily changes considered the hallmark of accelerated and malignant hypertension (Kaplan, 1986; Ram, 1984). Figure 22–4 outlines the structural and functional changes that occur in hypertensive crisis. The effects of elevated arterial pressure result in endothelial damage and platelet deposition. With this abnormality, myointimal proliferation occurs with fibrinoid necrosis found most notably in the interlobular arteries of the kidneys. This vascular damage may occur throughout the arterial system. Sections of the arterioles are constricted and dilated, creating a "sausage"-like pattern that likely enhances platelet deposition and the development of microangiopathic hemolytic anemia. There is an increase in secretion of renin, aldosterone, catecholamines, and vasopressin that sustains and potentially elevates the blood pressure, creating further vascular damage and tissue ischemia (Kaplan, 1986; Ram, 1984).

The clinical presentation of accelerated and malignant hypertension is a markedly elevated diastolic blood pressure, usually 130 to 140 mm Hg, with recent onset or progressive end-organ damage (Joint

National Committee, 1988). Headache is a frequent presenting symptom. Vision impairment may be present, especially if the funduscopic examination reveals papilledema. Urinalysis reveals gross or microscopic blood and is positive for protein and hyaline or red cell casts. Anemia is especially common in patients with renal insufficiency, as is an elevated blood urea nitrogen and creatinine. Hypokalemia is usually present due to hyperaldosteronism (Kaplan, 1986; Ram, 1984).

Hypertensive Encephalopathy

Due to aggressive detection and treatment of elevated arterial pressure, the occurrence of hypertensive encephalopathy is uncommon. Although any cause of a rapid elevation in blood pressure may precipitate this syndrome, it is more common as a complication of glomerulonephritis, eclampsia, and accelerated and malignant hypertension (Ram, 1984). As in eclampsia, the blood pressure need not be markedly elevated to produce the signs and symptoms of encephalopathy. An abrupt rise in a normotensive person may cause hypertensive encephalopathy, whereas a chronically hypertensive person may require markedly elevated pressures to develop this syndrome (Ram, 1984).

The mechanism of action in encephalopathy is thought to be significant vasodilatation overriding the autoregulatory response in the brain and the disruption in the permeability of the blood–brain barrier. Normally, as arterial blood pressure varies, the brain is able to maintain a constant cerebral blood flow by constricting or dilating the cerebral vessels—this is called autoregulation. As arterial pressure rises significantly, the autoregulatory mechanism is disrupted, and vasodilatation results. This causes a disruption in the permeability of the blood–brain barrier. Both of these physiologic abnormalities result in cerebral edema (Kaplan, 1986; Ram, 1984).

As cerebral edema worsens, the individual develops persistent headache and visual impairment ranging from blurred vision to transient blindness. Altered mental status is common and can present anywhere on the continuum from slight disorientation to coma. Seizures are more common in children but can occur in adults with encephalopathy. Nausea and vomiting may result as intracranial pressure increases.

EVALUATION OF HYPERTENSION

The Joint National Committee (1988) recommends that the diagnosis of hypertension not be made on the basis of only one measurement. Two readings should be obtained and averaged. The average of these readings should result in an SBP greater than or equal to 140 mm Hg or a DBP greater than or equal to 90 mm Hg. This elevation should be verified

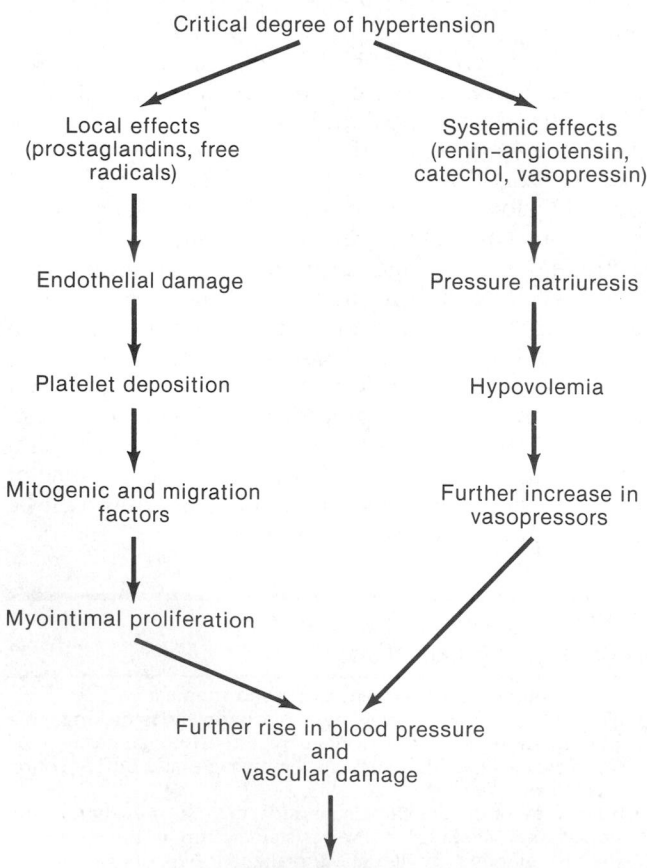

FIGURE 22–4. Malignant hypertension. A scheme for the initiation and progression of malignant hypertension. (From Kaplan, N. (1986). *Clinical hypertension* (4th ed.). © 1986, The Williams & Wilkins Co., Baltimore.)

a minimum of two additional times to make the diagnosis of hypertension.

Once the diagnosis has been made, evaluation and work-up need to address the issue of primary versus secondary hypertension, involvement of target organs, and determination of other cardiovascular risk factors (Joint National Committee, 1988; Kaplan, 1986; Hall et al., 1986).

A study done by Bulpitt and colleagues (1976) found that five symptoms appeared to be more prevalent in 99 hypertensives compared to 78 normotensive individuals. These symptoms were waking headaches, unsteadiness, blurred vision, depression, and nocturia. Additional questioning may reveal information regarding symptoms of asthma, fatigue, impotence, muscle cramps, hematuria, polyuria, and joint pain (Hall et al., 1986).

Assessment of additional cardiovascular risk factors is important. A thorough history to determine the occurrence of angina, previous myocardial infarction, transient ischemic attacks, stroke, claudication, family history, diabetes, and cigarette smoking is necessary.

Labile hypertension may be suggestive of pheochromocytoma, alcohol abuse, diet pills, or over-the-counter medications containing phenylpropanolamine. Stress stimulates the sympathetic nervous system and may create episodic hypertension. Encouraging the patient to discuss recent life events may determine the cause of labile hypertension.

Evaluation of Target Organ Damage

Physical examination, laboratory tests, and diagnostic procedures are performed to determine target organ damage and to search for clues that might yield a cause for hypertension. A thorough physical assessment provides the clinician with baseline health data as well. The target organs most affected by chronic hypertension are the heart, kidneys, and brain. Each of these systems will be reviewed to highlight the sequelae of uncontrolled hypertension.

CARDIOVASCULAR SYSTEM

The Framingham Study found that hypertension was the leading cause of heart failure (Kannel, 1976). Cardiac damage caused by hypertension is manifested as either coronary artery disease or left ventricular hypertrophy (Fig. 22–5).

Clinical signs including rales, jugular venous distention, ventricular gallop, edema, and an apical impulse diameter greater than 3 cm in the left lateral position indicate left ventricular hypertrophy. A cardiothoracic ratio greater than 0.5 on chest x-ray supports this diagnosis. An electrocardiogram (ECG) is valuable in determining evidence of left ventricular strain as well as for providing a baseline cardiac assessment. Although the chest x-ray and ECG can be of assistance, a more sensitive detector of early

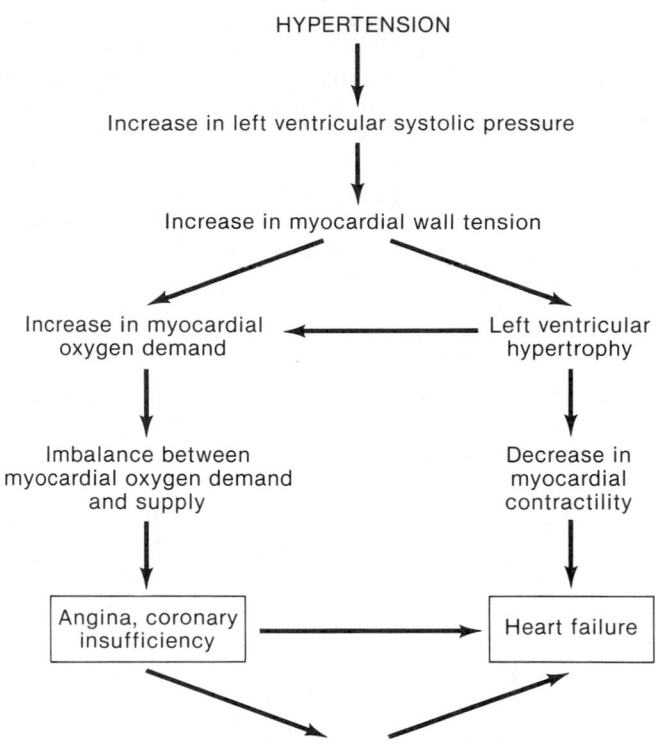

FIGURE 22–5. Effect of hypertension on myocardial function. (From Hollander, W. (1976). Role of hypertension in atherosclerosis and cardiovascular disease. *American Journal of Cardiology, 38,* 786.)

left ventricular hypertrophy is the echocardiogram (Savage et al., 1979). Left ventricular mass index, interventricular septal thickness, posterior wall thickness, and mean muscle mass can be determined from the echocardiogram and can provide the practitioner with valuable information about the effects of hypertension on the left ventricle (Kaplan, 1986).

Angina and myocardial infarction are twice as prevalent in hypertensives as in normotensive individuals. Angina may be related to a lack of adequate microcirculation for the increased muscle mass of left ventricular hypertrophy (Kaplan, 1986). Hypertension enhances the development of atherosclerosis. Myocardial infarction, recognized and unrecognized, is twice as common in individuals with hypertension. Frequently after a myocardial infarction the blood pressure normalizes and may elude detection. Kannel (1980) suggests performing frequent ECGs in hypertensive individuals to assist in earlier detection and prevention of myocardial damage.

RENAL SYSTEM

As many as one of six hypertensive individuals will develop renal failure (Kaplan, 1986). Renal effects include arteriosclerotic lesions, especially in the afferent and efferent tubules and glomerular capillary tufts. Structural and functional damage is common in hypertensive persons (Kaplan, 1986). The earliest signs of renal impairment are usually nocturia and albuminuria. Elevated uric acid is a common finding and is probably due to nephrosclerosis. In most hypertensives, renal impairment is slow and does not affect daily living, but in hypertensive individuals who develop accelerated or malignant hypertension, renal damage may progress rapidly and may result in death (Kaplan, 1986). Uncontrolled hypertension leads to progressive renal impairment, causing azotemia, uremia, and death.

CEREBRAL DAMAGE

Hypertensive hemorrhage, hypertensive encephalopathy, and lacunar infarction almost always occur in the presence of hypertension. Chronic arterial pressure elevation causes damage to the vessel wall, resulting in leakage of plasma into the wall and creating microaneurysms (Kaplan, 1986). This destruction occurs predominantly in the small resistance vessels in the brain. Occlusion of the larger vessels in the brain is the result of atherosclerosis and thrombosis. Hypertension is the dominant factor in the development of cerebral vascular accidents. Strokes are more prevalent in blacks and the elderly. Kannel and associates (1980) found that control of hypertension is necessary to prevent strokes in the eighth and ninth decades of life as well as in younger persons. Blacks have about a 50% higher mortality from hypertension than whites (Kaplan, 1986).

Structural and Functional Disturbances in Hypertension

Whether the cause is known or unknown the structural changes of hypertension are similar. Hypertension is a disease of resistance resulting in increased arterial wall rigidity. The changes in the arteries and arterioles are similar to the changes undergone by the vascular system with aging but are far more severe. As the tension in the arterial wall increases due to elevated arterial pressure, damage occurs to the vessel wall including medionecrosis, atherosclerosis, development of aneurysms, rupture, and hemorrhages (Kaplan, 1986). The chronic increase in arterial pressure results in more forceful pulsatile flow, which causes endothelial wall damage. This damage causes an increase in smooth muscle contraction and enhances the development of fibrosis and atherosclerosis. Areas of damage to the endothelial lining result in enhanced cell replication. Atherosclerosis is directly related to the rate and number of cell replications (Kaplan, 1986).

Specific arterial lesions associated with chronic elevation of arterial pressure have been identified. These lesions, which are more commonly found in hypertensives, include hyperplastic atherosclerosis, hyaline atherosclerosis, and miliary aneurysms. Hyperplastic atherosclerosis, or increased cell replication, results from vessel damage. This damage is manifested by deposition of fibroblasts, elastin fibers, and other damaging substances in the intima. The other layers of the vessel wall are affected, the adventitia becomes fibrotic, and the media is hypertrophied in hyperplastic atherosclerosis (Kaplan, 1986). The abnormal deposition of hyaline and the thickening of the basement membrane of the intima and media are the types of damage associated with hyaline atherosclerosis. Both forms of atherosclerosis result in a significant reduction in lumen size and elasticity of the vessel (Kaplan, 1986). Miliary aneurysms are usually found in the cerebral arterioles. Dilatation of the arteriole occurs just past an area of thickening or stenosis in the vessel wall. Miliary aneurysms are closely related to the increased incidence of cerebral vascular accidents found in hypertensive individuals (Kaplan, 1986).

The ischemia and infarction of target organs (kidneys, heart, and brain) probably result from thrombus formation over these arterial lesions. Medial layer damage in the aorta due to chronic arterial pressure elevation may result in development of aortic aneurysms and dissections, which are found more commonly in hypertensive individuals (Kaplan, 1986).

TREATMENT OF PRIMARY (ESSENTIAL) HYPERTENSION

The goal of treatment is lifelong maintenance of a blood pressure less than 140/90 mm Hg, no evidence of target organ damage, and little if any adverse effects from treatment (Joint National Committee, 1988). Treatment is dependent on the degree of severity of hypertension.

Non-pharmacologic Therapy

Mild hypertension (DBP 90 to 104 mm Hg) may respond to non-pharmacologic therapy. This includes weight reduction, sodium restriction, reduction of alcohol intake to less than 2 ounces daily, regular isotonic exercise, and relaxation to reduce stress (Kaplan, 1986; Joint National Committee, 1988; Wollam and Hall, 1986).

Pharmacologic Treatment

If non-drug therapy is unsuccessful in reducing the diastolic blood pressure, drug therapy is then indicated. Non-pharmacologic therapy needs to be maintained despite antihypertensive medications. The Joint National Committee in 1988 changed its recommendations regarding the step-care approach to management of hypertension. In previous reports (Joint National Committee, 1984), diuretics or beta blockers were recommended as the first step, whereas in the most recent report (1988), calcium antagonists and angiotensin-converting enzyme (ACE) inhibitors were added to the first step. These drugs may be used as monotherapy in the first step or in conjunction with other antihypertensive agents as the second step of therapy. Usually the physician starts with one drug given at the lowest possible dose (Fig. 22–6).

If the individual's blood pressure does not respond sufficiently, step two is then instituted. The physician will either increase the dose of the medication, substitute another medication, or add a second drug from a different class of antihypertensives. The third step involves substitution of a second drug or adding a third drug from a different class. If the individual's blood pressure remains elevated, the physician then adds a third or fourth drug. Further evaluation or referral may be necessary (Joint National Committee, 1988).

There are five classes of antihypertensive agents. See Table 22–4 for a list of antihypertensive drugs currently used in treatment (Joint National Committee, 1988). They are diuretics, adrenergic inhibitors, vasodilators, calcium antagonists, and angiotensin-converting enzyme inhibitors. Each class will be discussed in terms of their mechanisms of action and side effects. Table 22–5 lists the adverse effects of antihypertensive medications.

DIURETICS

Diuretics are the most commonly prescribed agents for the treatment of hypertension (Kaplan, 1986). They are considered the easiest, least expensive, and most effective treatment. They are very effective in reducing arterial pressure in black, elderly, and obese individuals. There are three main classes of diuretics: thiazides, loop diuretics, and potassium-sparing agents. Each has a different mode of action, varying degrees of potency, and specific side effects.

Thiazides. The thiazide diuretics act by inhibiting sodium and chloride reabsorption in the distal tubules. Plasma volume decreases, and cardiac output falls. There is a resultant decline in peripheral vascular resistance. In certain individuals a significant decline in plasma volume may result in excessive stimulation of renin and aldosterone, which may mitigate the decrease in arterial pressure.

Side effects of chronic thiazide therapy are most commonly hypokalemia and hypomagnesemia. The higher the dosage, the more dramatic the side effects, but even at lower doses there is a decrease in potassium and magnesium concentrations. Hollifield (1989) writes that "their undesirable metabolic consequences have been suspected of contributing to increases in cardiovascular morbidity and mortality." There is circumstantial evidence that thiazides increase the risk of malignant dysrhythmias and sudden cardiac death (Hollifield, 1989). Hypokalemia may be present in individuals before thiazide therapy is started, often due to primary aldosteronism. It is prudent to obtain a potassium level prior to instituting treatment. Hypomagnesemia is frequently not diagnosed because levels are not routinely obtained. The signs and symptoms of decreased magnesium are similar to those of hypokalemia. They may include nausea, weakness, neuromuscular irritability, tetany, mental changes, convulsions, stupor, and coma. Ventricular dysrhythmias may develop, especially in patients treated with digitalis. If treatment of the individual's hypokalemia does not suppress the dysrhythmias, hypomagnesemia should be suspected (Kaplan, 1986).

Elevated uric acid and calcium levels may occur in some individuals on chronic thiazide treatment. Hyperglycemia or worsening of diabetic control may occur in rare cases (Cressman and Gifford, 1989).

Of recent concern is the effect of thiazides on cholesterol levels. The Multiple Risk Factor Intervention Trial Research Group (1982) noted modest ele-

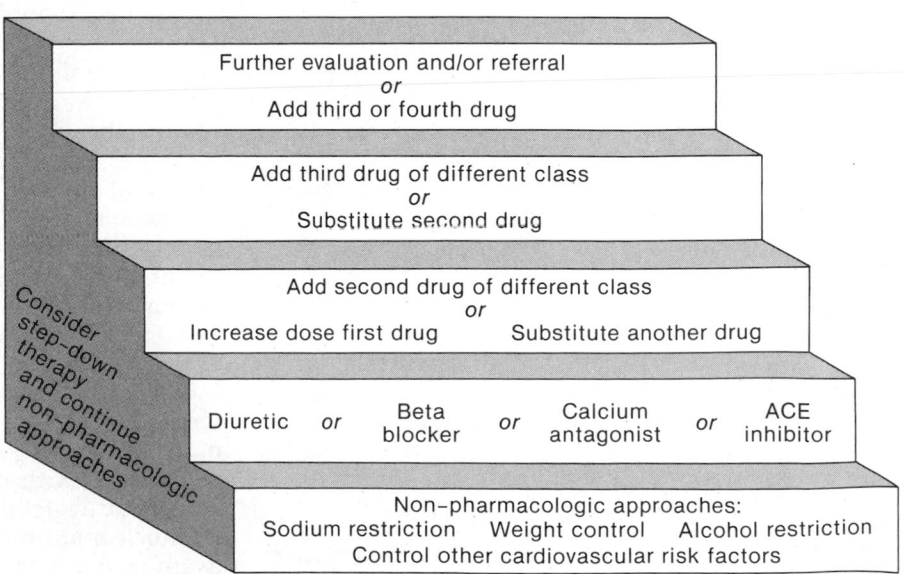

FIGURE 22–6. Step care approach to the treatment of hypertension. (From the Joint National Committee (1988). The 1988 report of the joint national committee on detection, evaluation and treatment of high blood pressure. *Archives of Internal Medicine,* 148, 1023–1038.)

Consider step-down therapy and continue non-pharmacologic approaches

Further evaluation and/or referral
or
Add third or fourth drug

Add third drug of different class
or
Substitute second drug

Add second drug of different class
or
Increase dose first drug   Substitute another drug

Diuretic   *or*   Beta blocker   *or*   Calcium antagonist   *or*   ACE inhibitor

Non–pharmacologic approaches:
Sodium restriction   Weight control   Alcohol restriction
Control other cardiovascular risk factors

TABLE 22-4. Antihypertensive Medications

Type of Drug	Usual Minimum	Usual Maximum
Diuretics		
Thiazides and related sulfonamide diuretics		
Bendroflumethiazide	2.5	5
Benzthiazide	12.5–25	50
Chlorothiazide	125–250	500
Chlorthalidone	12.5–25	50
Cyclothiazide	1	2
Hydrochlorothiazide	12.5–25	50
Hydroflumethiazide	12.5–25	50
Indapamide	2.5	5
Methyclothiazide	2.5	5
Metolazone	1.25	10
Polythiazide	2	4
Quinethazone	25	100
Trichlormethiazide	1–2	4
Loop diuretics†		
Bumetanide‡	0.5	5
Ethacrynic acid‡	25	100
Furosemide‡	20–40	320
Potassium-sparing agents		
Amiloride	5	10
Spironolactone	25	100
Triamterene	50	150
Adrenergic inhibitors		
β-Adrenergic blockers§		
Acebutolol	200	1200
Atenolol	25	150
Metoprolol	50	200
Nadolol	40	320
Penbutolol sulfate	20	80
Pindolol‡	10	60
Propranolol hydrochloride‡	40	320
Propranolol, long-acting	60	320
Timolol‡	20	80
Centrally acting α-blockers		
Clonidine‡	0.1	1.2
Clonidine TTS (Patch)‖	0.1	0.3
Guanabenz‡	4	64
Guanfacine hydrochloride	1	3
Methyldopa‡	250	2000
Peripheral-acting adrenergic antagonists		
Guanadrel sulfate‡	10	100
Guanethidine monosulfate	10	150
Rauwolfia alkaloids		
Rauwolfia (whole root)	50	100
Reserpine	0.1	0.25
α₁-Adrenergic blockers		
Prazosin hydrochloride‡	1–2	20
Terazosin hydrochloride	1–2	20
Combined α-β-adrenergic blocker:		
labetalol‡	200	1800
Vasodilators		
Hydralazine‡	50	300
Minoxidil‡	2.5	80
Angiotensin-converting enzyme inhibitors		
Captopril‡	25–50	300
Enalapril maleate	2.5–5	40
Lisinopril	5	40
Calcium antagonists		
Diltiazem hydrochloride¶	60	360
Nifedipine¶	30	180
Nitrendipine	5	40
Verapamil¶	120	480
Verapamil SR (long-acting)	120	480

*The dosage range may differ slightly from the recommended dosage in the *Physicians' Desk Reference* or package insert.

†Larger doses of loop diuretics may be required in patients with renal failure.

‡This drug is usually given in divided doses twice daily.

§Atenolol, metoprolol, and acebutolol are cardioselective; pindolol and acebutolol have partial agonist activity.

‖This drug is administered as a skin patch once weekly.

¶This drug is usually given in divided doses three or four times daily.

From the Joint National Committee. (1988). The 1988 report of the joint national committee on detection, evaluation and treatment of high blood pressure. *Archives of Internal Medicine*, 148, 1023–1038.

vations in patients' cholesterol and triglyceride levels and a reduction in their high-density lipoprotein (HDL) levels. Hulley and colleagues (1985), in their systolic hypertension study in the elderly, did not find a difference in cholesterol levels between the thiazide-treated group and the placebo-treated group. It appears that the elevation in cholesterol level may be transient, and with long-term thiazide use cholesterol may revert to prior treatment levels.

Loop Diuretics. The second group of diuretics is the loop diuretics. These agents are effective in controlling the abnormal sodium and water homeostasis of renal insufficiency or failure (Cressman and Gifford, 1989). They act by blocking the reabsorption of chloride in the loop of Henle, which interferes with sodium reabsorption. They are more potent and more rapid in onset than the thiazide agents (Kaplan, 1986). The side effects of the loop diuretics are similar to those seen with thiazide pharmaceuticals. Hypokalemia, hypomagnesemia, and elevated uric acid and calcium levels may result from chronic use of loop diuretics.

Potassium-Sparing Agents. The potassium-sparing agents block the excretion of potassium by varying mechanisms. Spironolactone is a popular steroidal compound that inhibits the excretion of aldosterone, diminishing reabsorption of sodium and water while sparing the excretion of potassium. The other potassium-sparing antihypertensive agents act on the distal tubules of the kidneys to enhance urinary excretion of sodium and decrease excretion of potassium (Govoni and Hayes, 1985). This group of antihypertensive medications does not have the same potency of blood pressure reduction as do thiazides and loop diuretics. Frequently, potassium-sparing agents are used in combination with other diuretics.

ADRENERGIC INHIBITORS

Adrenergic inhibitors used in the treatment of hypertension act on the sympathetic nervous system either centrally or peripherally on the alpha or beta receptors (Kaplan, 1986). The central alpha agonists act on the alpha receptors of the brain stem to decrease efferent sympathetic activity. This reduction in stimulation of the sympathetic nervous system results in a fall in cardiac output and a mild decrease in peripheral vascular resistance (Kaplan, 1986). Fluid retention is frequently noted with the decrease in arterial pressure and can be treated with a diuretic. See Table 22–4 for antihypertensive agents in this class.

Side effects include dry mouth, sedation, loss of mental alertness, impotence, fluid retention, and postural hypotension. Autoimmune side effects have been noted with chronic use of methyldopa. These include drug fever, positive Coombs' test, positive antinuclear antibody test, lupus-like syndrome, liver dysfunction, and hemolytic anemia (Kaplan, 1986).

TABLE 22–5. Adverse Drug Effects

Drugs	Selected Side Effects†	Precautions and Special Considerations
Diuretics‡		
Thiazides and related sulfonamide diuretics	Hypokalemia, hyperuricemia, glucose intolerance, hypercholesteremia, hypertriglyceridemia, sexual dysfunction, weakness	May be ineffective in renal failure; hypokalemia increases digitalis toxicity; may precipitate acute gout; may cause an increase in blood levels of lithium
Loop diuretics	Same as for thiazides	Effective in chronic renal failure; hypokalemia and hyperuricemia as above
Potassium-sparing agents	Hyperkalemia	Danger of hyperkalemia or renal failure in patients treated with ACE inhibitor or nonsteroidal anti-inflammatory drug; may increase blood levels of lithium
Spironolactone	Gynecomastia, mastodynia	Interferes with digoxin immunoassay
Triamterene		Danger of renal calculi
Amiloride		
Adrenergic inhibitors		
β-Adrenergic blockers§	Bronchospasm, peripheral arterial insufficiency, fatigue, insomnia, sexual dysfunction, exacerbation of congestive heart failure, masking of symptoms of hypoglycemia, hypertriglyceridemia, decreased HDL cholesterol (except for pindolol and acebutolol)	Should not be used in patients with asthma, COPD, congestive heart failure, heart block (>first-degree), and sick sinus syndrome; use with caution in insulin-treated diabetic patients and patients with peripheral vascular disease; should not be discontinued abruptly in patients with ischemic heart disease
Acebutolol		
Atenolol		
Metoprolol		
Nadolol		
Penbutolol sulfate		
Pindolol		
Propranolol hydrochloride		
Timolol		
Centrally acting adrenergic inhibitors		
Clonidine	Drowsiness, sedation, dry mouth, fatigue, sexual dysfunction	Rebound hypertension may occur with abrupt discontinuance, particularly with prior administration of high doses or with continuation of concomitant β-blocker therapy
Guanabenz	As above	As above
Guanfacine hydrochloride	As above	As above
Methyldopa	As above	May cause liver damage and Coombs-positive hemolytic anemia; use cautiously in elderly patients because of orthostatic hypotension; interferes with measurements of urinary catecholamine levels
Clonidine TTS (Patch)	As above; localized skin reaction to the patch	
Peripheral-acting adrenergic inhibitors		
Guanadrel sulfate	Diarrhea, sexual dysfunction, orthostatic hypotension	Use cautiously because of orthostatic hypotension
Guanethidine monosulfate	Same as for guanadrel	Same as for guanadrel
Rauwolfia alkaloids	Lethargy, nasal congestion, depression	Contraindicated in patients with history of mental depression; use with caution in patients with history of peptic ulcer
Reserpine	Same as for rauwolfia alkaloids	Same as for rauwolfia alkaloids
α₁-Adrenergic blockers		
Prazosin hydrochloride	"First-dose" syncope, orthostatic hypotension, weakness, palpitations	Use cautiously in elderly patients because of orthostatic hypotension
Terazosin hydrochloride	As above	As above

Table continued on following page

TABLE 22–5. Adverse Drug Effects Continued

Drugs	Selected Side Effects†	Precautions and Special Considerations
Adrenergic inhibitors *Continued*		
Combined α-β-adrenergic blocker: Labetalol§	Bronchospasm, peripheral vascular insufficiency, orthostatic hypotension	Should not be used in patients with asthma, COPD, congestive heart failure, heart block (>first-degree), and sick sinus syndrome; use with caution in insulin-treated diabetic patients and patients with peripheral vascular disease
Vasodilators	Headache, tachycardia, fluid retention	May precipitate angina pectoris in patients with coronary artery disease
Hydralazine	Positive antinuclear antibody test	Lupus syndrome may occur (rare at recommended doses)
Minoxidil	Hypertrichosis	May cause or aggravate pleural and pericardial effusions; may precipitate angina pectoris in patients with coronary artery disease
ACE Inhibitors	Rash, cough, angioneurotic edema, hyperkalemia, dysgeusia	Can cause reversible, acute, renal failure in patients with bilateral renal arterial stenosis or unilateral stenosis in a solitary kidney; proteinuria may occur (rare at recommended doses); hyperkalemia can develop, particularly in patients with renal insufficiency; rarely can induce neutropenia; hypotension has been observed with initiation of ACE inhibitors, especially in patients with high plasma renin activity or in those receiving diuretic therapy
Calcium antagonists	Edema, headache	Use with caution in patients with congestive heart failure; contraindicated in patients with second- or third-degree heart block
Verapamil	Constipation	May cause liver dysfunction
Diltiazem hydrochloride	Constipation	May cause liver dysfunction
Nifedipine	Tachycardia	
Nitrendipine	Tachycardia	

*Sexual dysfunction, particularly impotence in men, has been reported with the use of all antihypertensive agents. ACE indicates angiotensin-converting enzyme; HDL, high-density lipoprotein; and COPD, chronic obstructive pulmonary disease.

†The listing of side effects is not all-inclusive, and health practitioners are urged to refer to the package insert for a more detailed listing.

‡See Table 22–4 for a list of these drugs.

§Sudden withdrawal of these drugs may be hazardous in patients with heart disease. See Table 22–4 for a list of these drugs.

From the Joint National Committee (1988). The 1988 report of the joint national committee on detection, evaluation and treatment of high blood pressure. *Archives of Internal Medicine*, 148, 1023–1038.

Abrupt withdrawal from the central alpha agonists such as clonidine, methyldopa, and guanabenz may result in excessive catecholamine release and a sharp rise in blood pressure (rebound hypertension).

PERIPHERAL ADRENERGIC INHIBITORS

The peripheral adrenergic inhibitors act by inhibiting either the storage or the release of norepinephrine. When the sympathetic nervous system is stimulated, the norepinephrine response is significantly blunted, causing a decrease in peripheral vascular resistance. Side effects include drowsiness, depression (especially with reserpine), postural hypotension, fluid retention, and diarrhea.

Alpha-adrenergic receptor blockers act by inhibiting the alpha-1 and alpha-2 receptor sites. More efficacious antihypertensives in this group are the alpha-selective agents. Prazosin is an example of an alpha-1 selective drug that acts by blocking the post-synaptic receptors, thus decreasing the effect of norepinephrine on the neuron. This causes a decline in peripheral resistance, no change in cardiac output, and an increase in plasma volume (Kaplan, 1986). Side effects include drowsiness, fatigue, weakness, sexual dysfunction, and postural hypotension.

Beta-adrenergic receptor blockers are among the most popular agents for the treatment of hypertension. They are classified by their cardioselectivity, lipid solubility, and the presence of intrinsic sympathomimetic activity. Agents with beta-1 selectivity, such as atenolol and metoprolol, act to lower blood pressure by decreasing cardiac contractility and heart rate. The advantage of using a cardioselective drug lies in the reduced side effects of beta-2 blockade in the lungs, vascular system, and pancreas. In larger doses the cardioselective properties decline.

Nonselective beta blockers, such as propranolol, block beta-1 and beta-2 receptors. In addition to the effects of blockade of beta-1 receptors, the blockade of beta-2 receptors results in vasodilatation of the peripheral vascular system. Peripheral resistance may not decrease with blockade by nonselective agents because the alpha receptors, which cause vasoconstriction, are unopposed and may counterbalance the dilatation of the peripheral vascular system.

Drugs in this class that have intrinsic sympathomimetic activity are not as potent in reducing blood pressure. The chemical structure of these agents, such as pindolol, have only one rather than two sites of attachment to the receptor. This allows partial stimulation of the beta receptor. The more intrinsic sympathomimetic activity a drug has, the less reduction in blood pressure can be expected (Kaplan, 1986). Side effects, such as extreme bradycardia, bronchospasm, and decreased myocardial contractility resulting in heart failure, are also diminished.

Side effects of this class of antihypertensives include fatigue, bronchospasm, bradycardia, negative inotropy, peripheral vasospasm, impotence, insomnia, bad dreams, hallucinations, and depression.

Diabetics should be treated with these agents with care. Beta blockers blunt the hypoglycemic reaction and delay the elevation of blood sugar by blocking epinephrine from stimulating the release of glucagon. Type 2 diabetics are more prone to hyperglycemia with this group of antihypertensive agents, especially with concomitant use of diuretics. Beta blockers elevate serum triglycerides and lower HDL cholesterol. This effect is less with cardioselective drugs and may not occur with drugs with intrinsic sympathomimetic activity.

Labetalol is currently the only alpha and beta blocker available in the United States. This drug blocks beta-1 and beta-2 and alpha-1 receptor sites. It reduces blood pressure by reducing cardiac output and peripheral resistance. Symptomatic orthostatic hypotension is the most common side effect of labetalol. In rare instances, this drug has increased arterial pressure, especially in persons with pheochromocytoma or individuals taking other antihypertensives. There is no evidence that labetalol causes a rise in serum lipid levels.

VASODILATORS

Vasodilators are classified as either direct or indirect. Examples of indirect vasodilators are the calcium antagonists and the angiotensin-converting enzyme inhibitors. The fourth Joint National Committee

(1988) has added these agents to the first step of treatment because their efficacy has been established.

Direct vasodilators such as hydralazine and minoxidil act on the peripheral arterioles and relax the smooth muscle. They are extremely potent agents and do result in a reflex increase in cardiac output and heart rate. Minoxidil is longer acting and more potent than hydralazine and is very effective in the treatment of severe hypertension associated with renal insufficiency (Kaplan, 1986). Because of their propensity to increase cerebral blood flow, they should be avoided in patients with cerebral infarction.

Side effects of hydralazine include a lupus-like syndrome that may disappear with decreasing dosages or, in certain individuals may require discontinuation of the medication. Headaches, flushing, tachycardia, anorexia, nausea, vomiting, and diarrhea are also side effects of hydralazine. Minoxidil elicits hirsutism in approximately 80% of individuals on this medication. Generalized hair growth appears to be directly related to vasodilatation. The hair will disappear gradually after minoxidil is discontinued. Pericardial effusions have been noted in rare instances with drug administration (Kaplan, 1988b).

CALCIUM ANTAGONISTS

All four of the currently available calcium antagonists decrease arterial pressure by vasodilating the vascular bed. Intracellular calcium is essential for smooth muscle contraction. By blocking calcium uptake in the cells, the smooth muscle relaxes and dilates. Verapamil acts to decrease heart rate and cardiac contractility as well as dilate vascular smooth muscle. Nifedipine and nitrendipine act only on vascular smooth muscle to relax the arterioles (Frohlich, 1989). Nifedipine is short acting and may produce reflex cardiac stimulation by increasing heart rate and myocardial contractility. Nitrendipine is longer acting and appears to produce less cardiac stimulation. Verapamil, due to its negative inotropic effects, does not stimulate reflex cardiac symptoms. The pharmacologic response of diltiazem is between that of nifedipine and verapamil. It decreases the heart rate and conduction and produces mild cardiac stimulation (Frohlich, 1989).

Nifedipine and nitrendipine can cause headache, tachycardia, and palpitations as well as peripheral edema. Beta blockers can be used to decrease the reflex tachycardia seen with nifedipine and nitrendipine. Verapamil causes constipation, and its negative inotropic action necessitates caution when it is used in patients with cardiac failure. Calcium antagonists increase the serum levels of digoxin, theophylline, and phenytoin (Kaplan, 1986).

ANGIOTENSIN-CONVERTING ENZYME (ACE) INHIBITORS

These agents inhibit the enzyme that converts angiotensin I to angiotensin II. Angiotensin II is a potent vasoconstrictor. ACE inhibitors, by blocking conversion of angiotensin I to angiotensin II, result in vascular bed dilation and a reduction in blood pressure. Heart rate, cardiac output and fluid volume do not seem to be affected by these medications. Captopril, enalapril, and lisinopril are effective agents in patients with mild to severe hypertension. Their efficacy is enhanced by the concomitant use of diuretics. ACE inhibitors mitigate the hypokalemic effects of diuretics (Cressman and Gifford, 1989).

Side effects include marked hypotension, usually with the first dose, elevation in serum potassium levels, and worsening of renal insufficiency due to renal artery stenosis, probably secondary to decreased renal blood flow. Rare occurrences of proteinuria and leukopenia, especially in individuals with renal impairment, may result from ACE administration (Kaplan, 1986). Drug interactions in antihypertensive therapy are listed in Table 22–6.

MANAGEMENT OF SECONDARY HYPERTENSION

Despite pharmacologic treatment of hypertension with a combination of medications, if the blood pressure remains elevated, the search for secondary causes may prove fruitful. Medical and surgical interventions are discussed for each of the identified causes.

Oral Contraceptives

Decreasing the dose of estrogen and progestogen found in oral contraceptives may be effective in reducing blood pressure. Discontinuation of oral contraceptives may be necessary; results indicate a return of blood pressure to normal within 3 to 6 months (Kaplan, 1986). Recent studies indicate that oral contraceptives with low-dose estrogen can be prescribed in healthy, nonsmoking, premenopausal women between the ages of 35 and 44 (Mishell, 1988). Women over the age of 35 with hypertension or cardiovascular risk factors (obesity, cigarette smoking, or family history) should be encouraged to use alternative means of birth control (Kaplan, 1988b; Mishell, 1988). If this is not possible, antihypertensives can be effective in controlling hypertension. Close monitoring of blood pressure is necessary in this group of patients.

Renal Parenchymal Disease

Chronic renal disease is one of the most common causes of hypertension. Glomerulonephritis, pyelonephritis, polycystic disease, and diabetic nephropathy damage the kidneys, creating insufficiency and ultimately failure. Glomerulonephritis and pyelonephritis are becoming less common causes because

---

TABLE 22–6. Drug Interactions in Antihypertensive Therapy

Diuretics
 Diuretics can raise lithium blood levels by enhancing proximal tubular reabsorption of lithium.
 Nonsteroidal anti-inflammatory agents, including aspirin, may antagonize antihypertensive and natriuretic effectiveness of diuretics
 Angiotensin-converting enzyme (ACE) inhibitors magnify potassium-sparing effects of triamterene, amiloride, or spironolactone.
 ACE inhibitors blunt hypokalemia induced by thiazide diuretics.

Sympatholytic agents
 Guanethidine monosulfate and guanadrel sulfate: Ephedrine and amphetamine displace guanethidine and guanadrel from storage vesicles. Tricyclic antidepressants inhibit uptake of guanethidine and guanadrel into these vesicles. Cocaine may inhibit neuronal pump that actively transports guanethidine and guanadrel into nerve endings. These actions may reduce antihypertensive effects of guanethidine and guanadrel.
 Hypertension can occur with concomitant therapy with phenothiazines or sympathomimetic amines.
 Monoamine oxidase inhibitors may prevent degradation and metabolism of released norepinephrine produced by tyramine-containing foods and may thereby cause hypertension.
 Tricyclic antidepressant drugs may reduce effects of clonidine and guanabenz.

β-Blockers
 Cimetidine may reduce bioavailability of β-blockers metabolized primarily by the liver by inducing hepatic oxidative enzymes. Hydralazine, by reducing hepatic blood flow, may increase plasma concentration of β-blockers.
 Cholesterol-binding resins, ie, cholestyramine and colestipol, may reduce plasma levels of propranolol hydrochloride.
 β-Blockers may reduce plasma clearance of drugs metabolized by the liver (eg, lidocaine, chlorpromazine, coumarin).
 Combinations of calcium channel blockers and β-blockers may promote negative inotropic effects on the failing myocardium.
 Combinations of β-blockers and reserpine may cause marked bradycardia and syncope.

ACE inhibitors: Nonsteroidal anti-inflammatory drugs, including aspirin, may magnify potassium-retaining effects of ACE inhibitors.

Calcium antagonists
 Combinations of calcium antagonists with quinidine may induce hypotension, particularly in patients with idiopathic hypertrophic subaortic stenosis.
 Calcium antagonists may induce increases in plasma digoxin levels.
 Cimetidine may increase blood levels of nifedipine.

From the Joint National Committee (1988). The 1988 report of the joint national committee on detection, evaluation and treatment of high blood pressure. *Archives of Internal Medicine*, 148, 1023–1038.

---

early diagnosis and treatment are preventing their chronic occurrence. Hemodialysis or renal transplantation is the treatment for renal failure. Hypertension may or may not accompany renal failure. If present, antihypertensive medications are indicated to control the blood pressure. On occasion, severe refractory hypertension may necessitate a nephrectomy. The advent of potent agents such as minoxidil has decreased the need for surgical removal of the kidney or kidneys.

Renovascular Hypertension

Atherosclerosis, fibromuscular disease, and renal artery aneurysms are common causes of renovascular hypertension. Although medical management can control blood pressure, surgical procedures produce excellent long-term relief of hypertension and preservation of renal function in most patients (Lawrie et al., 1989). Common surgical procedures include Dacron grafting, endarterectomy, and angioplasty. Recurrence of hypertension requires reoperation or medical management. Fibromuscular disease appears to respond favorably to angioplasty, whereas atherosclerotic lesions respond well to grafting and endarterectomy. Angioplasty can only be performed on accessible vessels, and thus its use is limited. There is an approximate reocclusion rate of 20%, necessitating another angioplasty procedure. Lawrie and colleagues (1989), in a retrospective review of 916 patients with renovascular lesions, found that age significantly affected long-term prognosis. Diffuse atherosclerosis in the elderly may have affected their prognosis in that myocardial infarction was the most common cause of death in the age group older than 62. These physicians recommend conservative medical management of the elderly unless hypertension is refractory or renal impairment occurs.

Primary Aldosteronism

In those patients with bilateral hyperplasia, those who are unable or unwilling to undergo surgery, and those who remain hypertensive postoperatively, medical management is indicated (Kaplan, 1986). Spironolactone and amiloride are the agents of choice. Large doses of spironolactone, 300 to 400 mg daily, are used to initiate treatment. After adequate blood pressure control has been achieved, daily doses may be as low as 50 mg. Low-dose thiazides may be added to maintain adequate blood pressure control and to decrease the dose of spironolactone, thereby mitigating the side effects of both medications.

In individuals with solitary adenomas, surgical intervention is indicated. Preoperative management includes administration of spironolactone to assist in determining the hypertensive response postsurgery and to correct fluid and electrolyte deficits. Removal of the adenoma usually results in a return to normal of the fluids and electrolytes within 6 months. Hypertension may persist and can be medically managed. If bilateral hyperplasia is found during surgical exploration, surgical removal of the left adrenal is preferred. There are significant complications from bilateral adrenalectomies. The removal of only one adrenal gland may be a judicious course (Kaplan, 1986; Wells and Santen, 1986).

Pheochromocytoma

Pheochromocytoma results in excessive secretion of catecholamines. These tumors arise from chromaffin cells that may be found anywhere along the sympathetic system but are most commonly located in the adrenal gland. If missed, a pheochromocytoma may result in fatal hypertensive crisis during anesthesia, childbirth, or other stress (Kaplan, 1986).

Medical management is indicated if the patient is unable to have surgery or is in hypertensive crisis. Alpha-blocking agents such as dibenzyline or prazosin are effective in reducing the blood pressure. Beta blockers may be added only after adequate alpha blockade has been achieved. These agents blunt the tachycardia and dysrhythmias seen with excessive catecholamine excretion. Intravenous administration of phentolamine (an alpha-blocking agent) in 2- to 5-mg boluses every 5 minutes is effective in treatment of hypertensive crisis to achieve rapid control of the arterial pressure (Kaplan, 1986).

Surgical intervention is the preferred treatment for pheochromocytomas. There is a high mortality if blood pressure is not adequately controlled at the time of surgery. Preoperative treatment requires medication to control blood pressure and restore diminished blood volumes. Minimal mortality rates are associated with adequate preoperative treatment and vigorous intraoperative blood volume restoration.

Coarctation of the Thoracic Artery

Surgical correction of this damaged artery is the preferred treatment. The hypertension associated with coarctation can be treated with antihypertensive medications. Balloon angioplasty has been tried in limited numbers and appears to be effective but requires long-term follow-up to determine its efficacy (Marvin and Mahoney, 1985).

Pregnancy-Induced Hypertension

The most effective treatment is delivery of the fetus if maturity of the infant allows. Magnesium sulfate is administered to alleviate seizures, and an antihypertensive agent is given intravenously to control diastolic blood pressure greater than 110 mm Hg (Shannon, 1987; Weinstein, 1982). When the fetus is immature, the mother is placed on bedrest. If diastolic blood pressure remains greater than 105 mm Hg, antihypertensive medications are indicated. Hydralazine is the most common medication used, but nifedipine and labetalol have been tried with success. For further discussion see Chapter 63.

Hypertensive Crisis

Rapid and aggressive treatment of arterial pressure is indicated in patients in hypertensive crisis. A history and physical examination as well as laboratory tests are performed as quickly as possible before treatment is initiated. Admission to an intensive care unit and insertion of venous access and arterial invasive lines should be accomplished in a timely manner. Initiation of antihypertensive therapy is best accomplished using the intravenous route. Oral agents may be efficacious in hypertensive urgencies.

The decision about the type of medication to be administered depends on the clinical status of the patient. The most widely used and safest drug, if monitored closely, is nitroprusside. Intravenous nitroglycerin and diazoxide are also effective in reducing blood pressure immediately (see Table 22–7 for commonly used medications in hypertensive crisis). Caution is needed to avoid too rapid a reduction in blood pressure. Reduction of the diastolic blood pressure to around 110 mm Hg within the hour will prevent underperfusion of cerebral and coronary arteries. If the patient is in heart failure after reduction in blood pressure, a pulmonary artery catheter may be needed. Diuretics may be indicated if the patient is in heart failure or has fluid overload. As blood pressure declines, renal sodium reabsorption occurs and may necessitate the use of diuretics to maintain desired blood pressure levels. In individuals with markedly elevated arterial pressures and no evidence of acute target organ damage, blood pressure reduction can occur over several days.

NURSING IMPLICATIONS

Intensive care nurses monitor and provide intervention to numerous patients with all degrees of severity of hypertension. The nurse's relationship with the patient and family plays a vital role in assessing the patient's response to therapy, his understanding of the disease process, health beliefs, degree of compliance, and other psychological and social factors affecting adequate arterial pressure control. These data assist the nurse in developing a plan to address the educational needs of the patient and significant others.

As a pivotal member of the health care team, the nurse's initial and ongoing assessment of the patient's clinical status is essential to proper management of hypertension. Nurses also play a vital role in identifying hypertension in patients in whom it was previously undiagnosed. Physical examination includes assessment of heart sounds for an S_3 and/or S_4, which are present in heart failure, and determination of the width and location of the point of maximal impulse, which, if widened and displaced, indicates cardiac enlargement. Examination of the jugular veins for distention and evidence of peripheral and sacral edema further confirm the diagnosis of heart failure. Auscultation of the lungs every 4 hours to determine the absence or presence of rales is necessary to confirm heart failure and monitor therapy. A review of the patient's ECG for signs of left ventricular strain assists the nurse in directing the care provided.

A neurologic assessment is obtained during every shift and prn, if changes in mental status, development of gait disturbance, and/or rapid marked elevations in arterial pressure are noted. Scrupulous attention to fluid status with notations of intake and output and daily weights is important in managing hypertension due to the frequency of renal impair-

TABLE 22–7. Parenteral Drugs for Treatment of Hypertensive Emergencies

	Dose*	Reaction Time (min)	Adverse Reactions
Vasodilators			
Sodium nitroprusside	0.5–10 μg/kg/min as IV infusion	Instantaneous	Nausea, vomiting, muscle twitching, thiocyanate intoxication, methemoglobinemia
Nitroglycerin	5–100 μg/min as IV infusion	2–5	Headache, tachycardia, vomiting, methemoglobinemia
Diazoxide	50–150 mg/IV bolus, repeated, or 15–30 mg/min by IV infusion	1–2	Hypotension, tachycardia, aggravation of angina pectoris
Hydralazine	10–20 mg IV, 10–50 mg IM	10 20–30	Tachycardia, headache, vomiting, aggravation of angina pectoris
Adrenergic Inhibitors			
Phentolamine hydrochloride	5–15 mg IV	1–2	Tachycardia, orthostatic hypotension
Trimethaphan camsylate	1–4 mg/min as IV infusion	1–5	Paresis of bowel and bladder, orthostatic hypotension, blurred vision, dry mouth
Labetalol	20–80 mg IV bolus every 10 min, 2 mg/min IV infusion	5–10	Bronchoconstriction, heart block, orthostatic hypotension
Methyldopa	250–500 mg IV infusion	30–60	Drowsiness

*IV indicates intravenous; IM, intramuscular.
From the Joint National Committee, (1988). The 1988 report of the joint national committee on detection, evaluation and treatment of high blood pressure. *Archives of Internal Medicine*, 148, 1023–1038.

ment and fluid retention seen with vasodilators used to control arterial pressure.

Examination of the abdomen may reveal a bruit over the flank area indicating renal artery stenosis. Weak femoral and popliteal pulses combined with hypertension in the upper extremities may be indicative of coarctation of the thoracic aorta.

The physical examination, history, laboratory findings, and radiologic procedures such as echocardiography, aortography, renal artery arteriography, and renal ultrasound provide the nurse with sufficient data to develop a care plan to meet the needs of these patients. Nursing care plans used in the treatment of hypertension follow.

ncp nursing care plan

PRIMARY HYPERTENSION

1. Alteration in health maintenance

Outcome Criteria	Nursing Interventions
Blood pressure will remain less than 140/90 mm Hg	Monitor blood pressure periodically Administer antihypertensive medications Monitor intake and output Obtain daily weights Monitor electrolytes Administer potassium supplements Assist patient in identifying and modifying risk factors Encourage cessation of smoking Reinforce moderation in alcohol consumption: less than 2 ounces daily

2. Knowledge deficit of disease process and consequences of uncontrolled blood pressure

Outcome Criteria	Nursing Interventions
Patient/significant other will verbalize understanding of the disease process	Review blood pressure control mechanism Review name, dose, action, and side effects of antihypertensive medications Review signs and symptoms of inadequate blood pressure control, i.e., headache, nocturia, fatigue, weakness, and depression Obtain dietary consult to reinforce need for sodium restriction and weight reduction Reinforce importance of frequent blood pressure monitoring and teach home blood pressure monitoring if indicated

3. Noncompliance related to:

Knowledge deficit	Mental status
Financial status	Health belief system denial
Immobility	Negative consequence of the treatment regimen
Decreased energy levels	Negative perception of the treatment regimen

Outcome Criteria	Nursing Interventions
Patient will be able to verbalize rationale of treatment plan, desired blood pressure and weight, and consequences of nonadherence	Assess patient's ability to adhere to treatment plan: understanding, financial status, age, culture, and health status Review consequences of nonadherence to treatment plan Involve patient/significant other in treatment decisions Design program that is compatible with patient's life style

SECONDARY HYPERTENSION

1. Alteration in comfort related to:
Surgical or radiology procedure
Headache
Antihypertensive drug effect
Electrolyte disturbances

Nursing Care Plan continued on following page

Outcome Criteria	Nursing Interventions
Patient will state absence or decrease in pain	Assess pain location, duration, and intensity Administer analgesics Maintain quiet environment Limit activities Position patient for comfort Use ice packs, binders, pillows to ease discomfort Avoid constipation Reassure patient Explain treatment plan

2. Potential for infection related to:
   Surgery or invasive monitoring

Outcome Criteria	Nursing Interventions
Patient will remain free of infection as evidenced by normal temperature and white blood cell count, clean and dry incision or puncture sites	Obtain and monitor temperature Monitor WBC Clean incision site or puncture sites and inspect for evidence of infection Assess lungs every 4 hours Note respiratory pattern and amount color and odor of sputum if present Change intravenous sites and tubing every 72 hours Change body position every 2 hours Note clarity and odor of urine output; obtain specimen for culture and sensitivity Note risk factors that predispose patient to infection, i.e., steroids, malnutrition, immobility

3. Knowledge deficit

Outcome Criteria	Nursing Interventions
See preceding plan for primary hypertension	See preceding plan for primary hypertension

4. Noncompliance

Outcome Criteria	Nursing Interventions
See preceding plan for primary hypertension	See preceding plan for primary hypertension

HYPERTENSIVE CRISIS

1. Alteration in tissue perfusion related to:
   Overperfusion of target organs resulting in fluid excess

Outcome Criteria	Nursing Interventions
Blood pressure within normal range: goal is reduction of DBP to less than 110 mm Hg, then slower reduction to less than 90 mm Hg	Monitor arterial pressure via invasive pressure readings every 5 minutes Rapidly administer intravenous antihypertensive medication Observe for side effects or toxic effects of medication Monitor neurologic status Monitor input and output hourly Obtain daily weights

2. Alteration in thought process related to
   Hypertensive encephalopathy

Outcome Criteria	Nursing Interventions
Patient will resume pre-morbid mental status	Rapidly reduce DBP to 110 mm Hg Administer IV medications Monitor blood pressure every 5 minutes Assess neurologic status every 4 hours Orient patient frequently Explain all procedures and treatments to patient Maintain hygiene and skin integrity

3. Potential for injury related to
   Change in mental status

Outcome Criteria	Nursing Interventions
Patient will remain free of injury	Side rails up and bed in low position when unattended Padded side rails, bite block, and oral airway are at bedside in event of seizures Assist patient with all activities Frequently orient patient Restrain or position patient as indicated

4. Potential of fluid volume excess related to
Vasodilator therapy/heart failure
Cerebral edema

Outcome Criteria	Nursing Interventions
Patient will maintain normal fluid volume	Monitor intake and output Inspect patient for evidence of edema Administer diuretics to counterbalance vasodilator effects of sodium retention Restrict fluid and sodium Assess lungs every 4 hours and prn

5. Knowledge deficit

Outcome Criteria	Nursing Interventions
Note preceding plan on primary hypertension	

6. Noncompliance

Outcome Criteria	Nursing Interventions
Note preceding plan on primary hypertension	

SUMMARY

Critical care nurses are integral to the effective management of hypertension at all levels of severity. Understanding of the mechanism of blood pressure control and the pathophysiology of primary and secondary hypertension will assist the nurse to focus attention on the important aspects of the history and physical examination. The review of physical findings and laboratory and radiologic results in primary and secondary hypertension and hypertensive crisis provides the critical care nurse with the knowledge to manage hypertension effectively.

References

American Heart Association. (1989). *1989 Heart facts reference sheet.* Dallas, TX: American Heart Association.

Assche, F., Spitz, B., and Vansteelant, L. (1989). Severe systemic hypertension during pregnancy. *American Journal of Cardiology,* 63, 22–25c.

Assmann, G., and Schulte, H. (1989). Diabetes and hypertension in the elderly: Concomitant hyperlipidemia and coronary heart disease risk. *American Journal of Cardiology,* 63, 33–37H.

Brown, M., and Albright, J. (1989). Hypertension. In M. Kinney, D. Packa, and S. Dunbar (Eds.), *AACN's clinical reference for critical care nursing* (pp. 659–680). St Louis: C. V. Mosby.

Bulpitt, C. J., Dollery, C. T., and Carne, S. (1976). Change in symptoms of hypertensive patients after referral to hospital clinic. *British Heart Journal,* 38, 121–133.

Cressman, M., and Gifford, R. (1989). Pharmacologic management of hypertension: New guidelines based on latest studies. *Postgraduate Medicine,* 85, 259–268.

Dustan, H. (1986). Systemic arterial hypertension. In J. Hurst, R. Logue, C. Rackley, et al. (Eds.), *The heart* (6th ed., pp. 1038–1048). New York: McGraw-Hill.

Frohlich, E. (1989). Calcium antagonists for initial therapy of hypertension. *Heart & Lung,* 18, 370–376.

Gant, N. F., and Worley, R. J. (1980). *Hypertension in pregnancy: Concepts and management* (pp. 95–96). New York: Appleton-Century-Crofts.

Gonzalez, D., and Ram, V. (1988). New approaches for the treatment of hypertensive urgencies and emergencies. *Chest,* 93, 193–195.

Govoni, L., and Hayes, J. (1985). *Drugs and nursing implications.* Norwalk, CT: Appleton-Century-Crofts.

Guyton, A. (1986). Arterial pressure regulation: Parts 1 and 2. In *Textbook of medical physiology* (7th ed., pp. 244–271). Philadelphia: W. B. Saunders.

Hall, W., and Wollam, G. (1986). Treatment of systemic hypertension. In J. Hurst, R. Logue, C. Rackley, et al. (Eds.), *The heart* (6th ed., pp. 1071–1090). New York: McGraw-Hill.

Hall, W., Wollam, G., and Tuttle, E. (1986). Diagnostic evaluation of the patient with hypertension. In J. Hurst, R. Logue, C. Rackley, et al. (Eds.), *The heart* (6th ed., pp. 1048–1070). New York: McGraw-Hill.

Hollifield, J. (1989). Electrolyte disarray and cardiovascular disease. *American Journal of Cardiology,* 63, 21B–31B.

Hulley S., Furberg, C., Gurland, B., et al. (1985). Systolic hypertension in the Elderly Program (SHEP): Antihypertensive efficacy of chlorthalidone. *American Journal of Cardiology,* 56, 913–920.

Hypertension Detection and Follow-up Program Cooperative Group (1979). Reduction in mortality of persons with high blood pressure, including mild hypertension. *Journal of the American Medical Association,* 242, 2562–2573.

Joint National Committee. (1988). The 1988 report of the Joint National Committee on Detection, Evaluation and Treatment of

High Blood Pressure. *Archives of Internal Medicine,* 148, 1023–1038.

Joint National Committee. (1984). The 1984 report of the Joint National Committee on Detection, Evaluation and Treatment of High Blood Pressure. (No. 84-1088). Washington, DC: National Institute of Health Publications.

Kannel, W. (1976). Some lessons in cardiovascular epidemiology from Framingham. *American Journal of Cardiology,* 37, 269–282.

Kannel, W., Dawber, T., and McGee, D. (1980). Perspectives on systolic hypertension: The Framingham Study. *Circulation,* 61, 1179–1187.

Kaplan, N. (1986). *Clinical hypertension* (4th ed.). Baltimore: Williams & Wilkins.

Kaplan, N. (1988a). Systemic hypertension: Mechanism and diagnosis. In E. Braunwald (Ed.), *Heart disease,* (3rd ed., pp. 819–861). Philadelphia: W. B. Saunders.

Kaplan, N. (1988b). Systemic hypertension: Therapy. In E. Braunwald (Ed.), *Heart disease* (2nd ed., pp. 863–895). Philadelphia: W. B. Saunders.

Koniak-Griffin, D., and Dodgson, J. (1987). Severe pregnancy induced hypertension: Postpartum care of the critically ill patient. *Heart & Lung* 16, 661–669.

Lawrie, G. M., Morris, G. C., Glaser, D. H., et al. (1989). Renovascular reconstruction: Factors affecting long term prognosis in 919 patients followed up to 31 years. *The American Journal of Cardiology,* 63, 1085–1092.

Linas, S., and Schrier, R. (1981). The renin-angiotensin-aldosterone system and the etiology of hypertension in renal disease. In B. Brenner and F. Rector (Eds.), *The kidney* (pp. 2344–2379). Philadelphia: W. B. Saunders.

Marvin, W., and Mahoney, L. (1985). Balloon angioplasty of unoperated coarctation in young children. *Journal of the American College of Cardiology,* 5, 405.

Meade, T. (1988). Risks and mechanisms of cardiovascular events in users of oral contraceptive. *American Journal of Obstetrics/Gynecology,* 158, 1646–1652.

Mishell, D. (1988). Use of oral contraceptives in women of older reproductive age. *American Journal of Obstetrics/Gynecology,* 158, 1652–1657.

Multiple Risk Factor Intervention Trial Research Group. (1982). Multiple risk factor intervention trial: Risk factors changes and mortality results. *Journal of the American Medical Association,* 248, 1465–1477.

Orten, J., and Neuhaus, O. (1982). *Human biochemistry.* St. Louis: C. V. Mosby.

Rahn, K. (1989). How should we treat a hypertensive emergency? *American Journal of Cardiology,* 63 (Suppl.), 48–50c.

Ram, C. (1984). Hypertensive crisis. *Cardiology Clinics,* 2, 211–225.

Royal College of Practitioners, Oral Contraception Study. (1981). Further analyses of mortality in oral contraceptive users. *Lancet,* 1, 541.

Savage, D., Drayer, J., Henry, W., et al. (1979). Echocardiographic assessment of cardiac anatomy and function in hypertensive subjects. *Circulation,* 59, 623–632.

Shannon, D. (1987). HELLP Syndrome: A severe consequence of pregnancy induced hypertension. *Journal of Obstetrical and Gynecological Nursing,* Dec/Jan, 395.

Stadel, B. (1981). Oral contraceptives and cardiovascular disease. *New England Journal of Medicine,* 305, 672.

Tucker, S., Canobbio, M., Paquette, E., et al. (1988). *Patient care standards: Nursing process, diagnosis, and outcome.* St Louis: C. V. Mosby.

Veterans Administration Cooperative Study Group on Antihypertensive Agents (1967). Effects of treatment on morbidity in hypertension. Results in patients with diastolic blood pressure averaging 115 through 129 mm Hg. *Journal of the American Medical Association,* 202, 116–127.

Veterans Administration Cooperative Study Group on Antihypertensive Agents (1970). Effects of treatment on morbidity in hypertension. Results in patients with diastolic blood pressure averaging 90 through 114 mm Hg. *The Journal of the American Medical Association,* 213, 1143–1152.

Weinstein, L. (1982). Syndrome of hemolysis, elevated liver enzymes, and low platelet count: A severe consequence of hypertension in pregnancy. *American Journal of Obstetrics and Gynecology,* 142, 159–154.

Wells, S. A., Jr., and Santen, R. J. (1986). The pituitary and adrenal glands. In D. Sabiston (Ed.), *Textbook of surgery: The biological basis of modern surgical practice* (13th ed., pp. 639–696). Philadelphia: W. B. Saunders.

Wollam, G. L., and Hall, W. D. (1986). Treatment of systemic hypertension. In J. Hurst, R. Logue, C. Rackley, et al. (Eds.), *The Heart* (6th ed., pp. 1071–1090). New York: McGraw-Hill.

Pulmonary System

23

Respiratory Physiology*

Kathleen S. Stone

Respiration can be defined as two separate processes: *external respiration*, the process of gas exchange within the lungs, which includes the absorption of oxygen (O_2) and the elimination of carbon dioxide (CO_2), and *internal respiration*, the utilization of oxygen at the cellular level in the mitochondria in oxidative phosphorylation and the production of adenosine triphosphate (ATP) and CO_2.

The primary functions of the respiratory system are threefold: (1) regulation of the partial pressure of oxygen, (2) maintenance of the partial pressure of carbon dioxide at a constant, and (3) maintenance of the plasma hydrogen (H) ion concentration.

The components of the respiratory process include (1) pulmonary ventilation, which is the exchange of air between the external atmosphere and the alveoli, (2) the diffusion of oxygen and carbon dioxide between the alveoli and the blood, (3) transport of oxygen and carbon dioxide in the blood to and from the cells, and (4) control of ventilation. This chapter will focus on the anatomy of the respiratory tract and the four components of the respiratory process.

ANATOMY OF THE RESPIRATORY TRACT

The respiratory tract is composed of upper and lower passageways whose primary function is to conduct air in and out of the respiratory system. In contrast, the respiratory gas exchange portion of the respiratory system is the site where oxygen is exchanged from the alveolus into the blood and carbon dioxide from the blood into the alveolus.

Upper Respiratory Tract

Air can enter the respiratory system through either the nose or mouth, the nose serving as the normal route. The nasal cavity is irregularly shaped. It extends from the bony palate on the floor of the mouth upward to the base of the cranial cavity, which comprises the roof. The nose is divided into right and left nasal cavities by the nasal septum. The nostrils have a wide opening called the vestibule, which is lined with coarse hairs in the external nares that trap foreign substances such as dust. The roof of the nasal cavity contains the olfactory receptors for the sense of smell. The sense of smell is diminished by smoking or upper respiratory infections and is enhanced with hunger.

The nasal cavity contains three bony projections called the superior, middle, and inferior conchae. Under each conchae is an air space called a meatus. Air swirls around and under the conchae as it enters the nose, where it is warmed and humidified by the blood vessels in the surface epithelium covering the conchae.

The sinuses (frontal, paranasal, and sphenoidal), located in the face, are large air pockets lined with mucous membrane. Mucus from the sinuses drains into the nasal cavity. The sinuses add resonance to the voice and decrease the weight of the skull.

The posterior nasal opening is called the internal nares. Distal to the internal nares is the nasal pharynx, which contains the pharyngeal tonsils, or adenoids, composed of lymphoid tissue that is responsible for trapping bacteria and foreign particles. The oropharynx, surrounded by the palatine tonsils, serves as the common passageway for food and air. Distal to the oropharynx is the larynx (Fig. 23–1).

The larynx is the air passageway between the pharynx and the lungs. The epiglottis, a thin, leaf-shaped structure located immediately posterior to the root of the tongue, covers the entrance to the larynx. The larynx acts as a sphincter to prevent solids and liquids from passing into the bronchi and the lungs. Contained within the larynx are the vocal cords, which are composed of the true and false

---

*Please refer to glossary on p. 528.

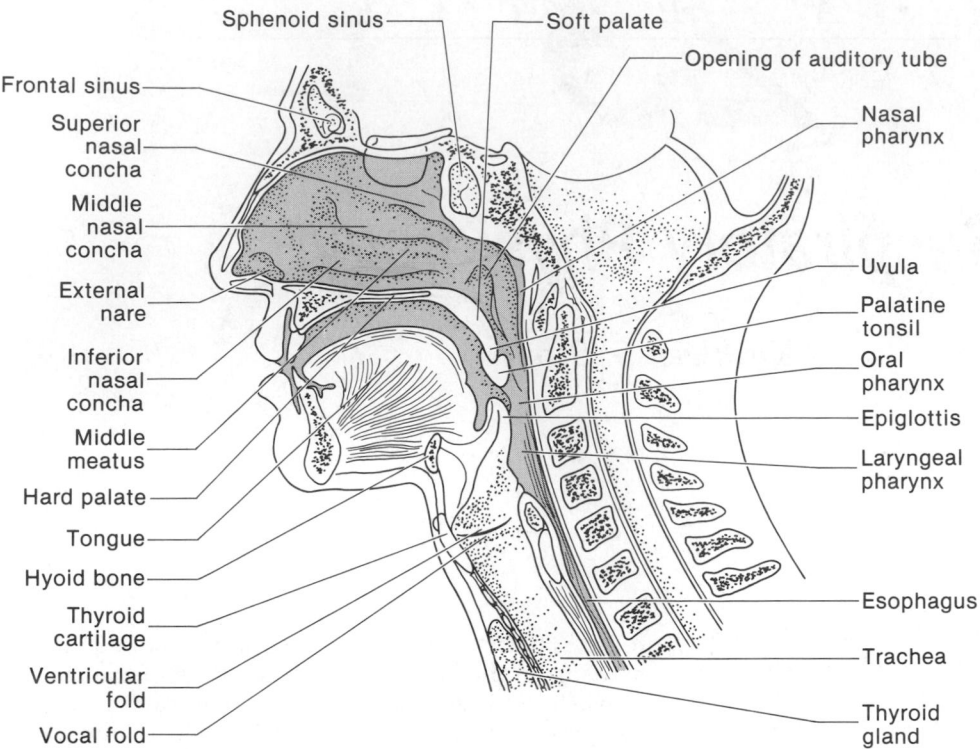

Sphenoid sinus — Soft palate
Frontal sinus —
— Opening of auditory tube
Superior nasal concha —
— Nasal pharynx
Middle nasal concha —
External nare —
— Uvula
— Palatine tonsil
Inferior nasal concha —
— Oral pharynx
Middle meatus —
— Epiglottis
Hard palate —
— Laryngeal pharynx
Tongue —
Hyoid bone —
Thyroid cartilage —
— Esophagus
Ventricular fold —
— Trachea
Vocal fold —
— Thyroid gland

FIGURE 23–1. Sagittal section of the human head, showing the right nasal cavity; superior, middle, and inferior conchae; sinuses, frontal and sphenoidal; and the pharyngeal and laryngeal portions of the respiratory system.

cords. The vocal cords are open with inspiration and closed during swallowing. During swallowing, the vocal cords assist in preventing the aspiration of food into the lungs. The vocal cords vibrate during the expiration of air, resulting in the production of sound. The vocal cords are innervated by the recurrent laryngeal nerve, which is a branch of the vagus nerve (cranial nerve X). Stimulation of the vocal cords during endotracheal intubation can cause stimulation of the vagus nerve, resulting in a decline in heart rate.

The major functions of the upper respiratory tract include (1) filtration of dust, dirt, foreign materials, and bacteria larger than 5 to 10 microns, and (2) humidification and warming of the air. Alteration of these functions is an important consideration when the upper respiratory tract is bypassed with an endotracheal tube or a tracheostomy.

Lower Respiratory Tract

The lower respiratory tract begins at the level of the trachea. The trachea in an adult is approximately 5 inches long and 1 inch in diameter. The trachea is continuous with the larynx above and terminates at the carina, the point of bifurcation into the right and left mainstem bronchi in the thoracic cavity. The trachea is composed of 16 to 20 regularly placed, horseshoe-shaped cartilaginous rings. The cartilaginous rings are incomplete posteriorly and have a musculomembranous sheath that lies anterior to the esophagus (Fig. 23–2).

The paired lungs occupy most of the space in the thoracic cavity. The right lung is composed of three lobes and the left lung of two lobes. Each lung receives a branch from the right and left mainstem bronchus respectively. The right bronchus is shorter and wider and has a more vertical position. This anatomic structure increases the risk of aspiration of food and foreign objects as well as the introduction of endotracheal tubes and suction catheters into the right bronchus. The right and left bronchi branch distally into numerous hollow tubes. Bronchi are differentiated into two categories. Bronchi not surrounded by lung tissue are called *extrapulmonary bronchi*, as opposed to bronchi that are surrounded by lung tissue, which are called *intrapulmonary bronchi*. Smooth muscle and irregularly shaped (ovals or crescents) cartilage plates maintain the patency of the intrapulmonary bronchi during lung inflation. With very distant branching the cartilage becomes less complete. The secondary bronchi give rise to innumerable smaller branches called bronchioli.

The bronchioli are distinguished from the bronchi by a lack of cartilage and a single layer of epithelium. The bronchioli give rise to between 50 and 80 terminal bronchioli in each lobule. The terminal bronchioli are the last purely conducting portion of the bronchial tree where no gas exchange occurs (Fig. 23–3).

Histology of the Conduction Portion of the Respiratory Tract

The innermost layer of the respiratory tract is composed of pseudostratified columnar ciliated epi-

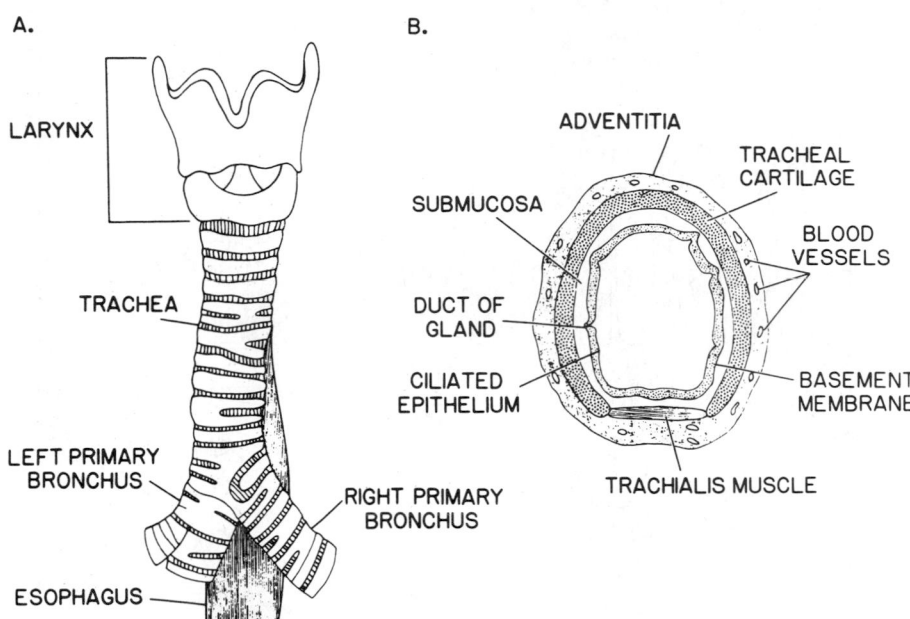

A.

LARYNX

TRACHEA

LEFT PRIMARY
BRONCHUS

RIGHT PRIMARY
BRONCHUS

ESOPHAGUS

B.

ADVENTITIA

SUBMUCOSA

TRACHEAL
CARTILAGE

BLOOD
VESSELS

DUCT OF
GLAND

CILIATED
EPITHELIUM

BASEMENT
MEMBRANE

TRACHIALIS MUSCLE

FIGURE 23–2. Gross anatomy of the trachea, from the ventral aspect *(A)* and cross section *(B)*. (From Jensen, D. (1980). *The principles of physiology* (2nd ed., p. 652). New York: Appleton-Century-Crofts.)

thelium. The cells are rectangular-shaped columns that are anchored in a basement membrane. The cells give the appearance of being stratified in layers but are not, because each cell is individually anchored in the basement membrane. Projecting out of each columnar cell are 15 to 200 cilia, which measure 7 microns in height. The name pseudostratified columnar ciliated epithelium is reflective of the visual appearance of this layer. Interspersed between the columnar cells are goblet cells, which produce mucus. Mucus is a protective mechanism that traps particulate matter such as dust, foreign material, and bacteria. The mucus is constantly propelled by the swaying cilia, which move at a rate of 16 times/second, to the pharynx, where it is either expectorated or swallowed and eliminated by the gastrointestinal tract. The epithelium lines the entire conducting respiratory passageway. The terminal bronchioli do not have mucus-secreting goblet cells nor cilia on the columnar cells. In the terminal bronchioli the epithelial cells are cuboidal in shape and flattened (Fig. 23–4).

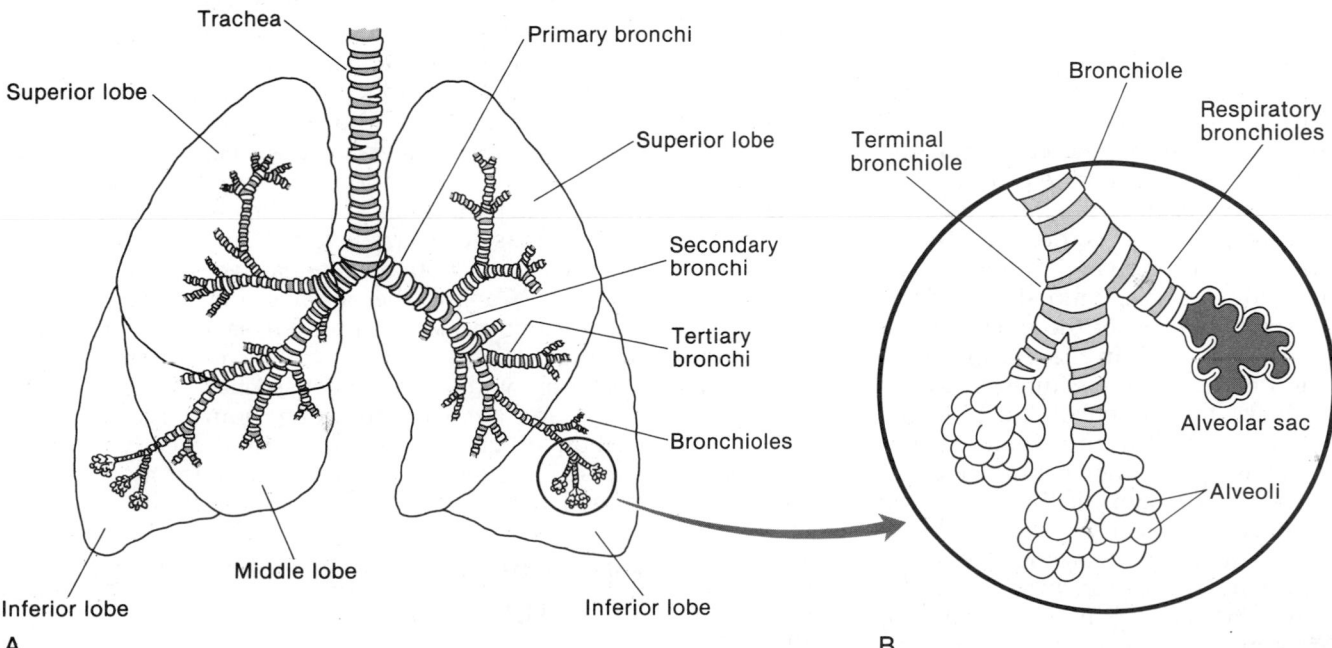

A

Trachea

Superior lobe

Primary bronchi

Superior lobe

Secondary
bronchi

Tertiary
bronchi

Bronchioles

Middle lobe

Inferior lobe

Inferior lobe

B

Bronchiole

Terminal
bronchiole

Respiratory
bronchioles

Alveolar sac

Alveoli

FIGURE 23–3. Gross anatomy of the lower respiratory tract, including the right lung composed of three lobes and the left lung of two lobes; the right and left mainstem bronchus; the extrapulmonary bronchi, intrapulmonary bronchi, bronchioli, and terminal bronchioli.

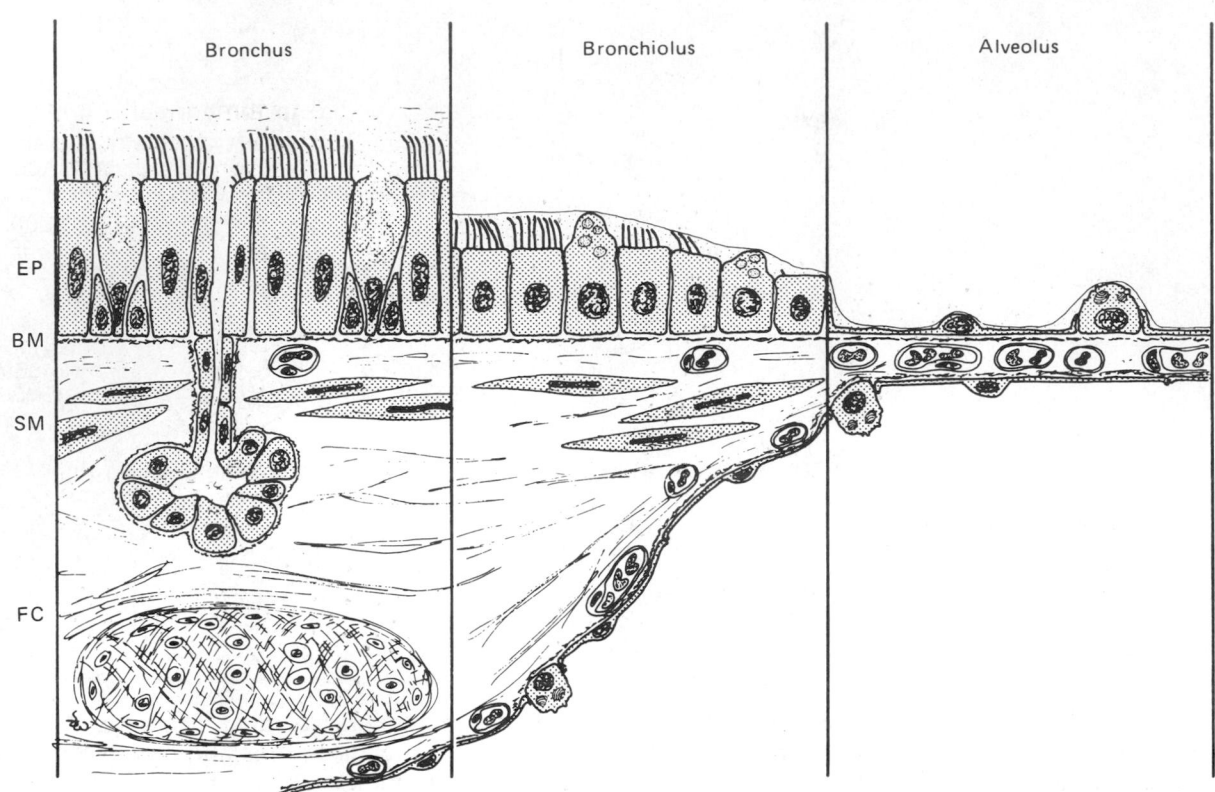

FIGURE 23–4. Change of airway wall structure at the three principal levels. The epithelial layer (*EP*) gradually becomes reduced from pseudostratified to cuboidal and then to squamous but retains its organization as a mosaic of lining and secretory cells. The smooth muscle layer (*SM*) disappears in the alveoli. The fibrous coat (*FC*) contains cartilage only in bronchi and gradually becomes thinner as the alveolus is approached. BM, basement membrane. (From Weibel, E. R., and Burri, P. H. (1973). *Funktionelle aspekte der lungenmorphologie.* In W. A. Fuchs and E. Voegeli (Eds.), *Aktuelle probleme der roentgendiagnostik* (Vol. 2, pp. 1–17). Berne: Huber Publishers.)

Immediately below the basement membrane is the membrane propria. The membrane propria has a different appearance depending on its location in the upper or lower respiratory tract. In the trachea, the membrane propria is composed of loose elastic fibers, whereas in the bronchi there are strong strips of elastic tissue. The membrane propria contains macrophages—phagocytic cells that engulf bacteria. In addition, the membrane propria is very vascular and assists in warming the inhaled atmospheric air.

Smooth muscle is located immediately under the membrane propria in portions of the upper and lower respiratory tracts. Smooth muscle is located in the posterior portion of the trachea and in the extrapulmonary bronchi. In the intrapulmonary bronchi, the smooth muscle constitutes a layer that completely encircles the lumen of the bronchi. There are two sets of spirally arranged smooth muscle fibers, one clockwise, the other counterclockwise. The state of muscle contraction of this smooth muscle layer can significantly affect the size of the bronchial lumen. Contraction and relaxation of the smooth muscle, especially in the bronchioli, can alter resistance to air flow. The smooth muscle fibers are innervated by the autonomic nervous system. Parasympathetic influence through vagal innervation results in bronchial constriction and mucus secretion. Sympathetic in-

nervation as well as stimulation of beta-2 adrenergic receptors due to increased circulating epinephrine levels cause bronchial relaxation. Mast cells situated beneath the epithelium near the blood vessels and smooth muscle release histamine in antigen-antibody reactions, causing bronchoconstriction.

The level of carbon dioxide in the respiratory gas in the bronchi influences the degree of muscular contraction. Increased levels of carbon dioxide cause bronchodilation, thus enhancing exhalation of the gas, whereas decreased levels of carbon dioxide cause bronchoconstriction and enhanced carbon dioxide retention. Cooling the airways due to inhaled cold atmospheric air, as during exercise, can trigger bronchoconstriction. There is a circadian rhythm in bronchial tone, with maximal constriction occurring commonly in the early morning hours and maximal dilation occurring commonly in the early evening hours. As a result, asthma attacks are more severe in the late night and early morning hours.

ANATOMY OF THE RESPIRATORY GAS EXCHANGE UNIT

The functional unit of the lung in which gas exchange occurs (external respiration) is called the primary lobule or the acinar. An acinar gas exchange unit is composed of (1) respiratory bronchioli, (2) alveolar ducts, (3) alveolar sacs, (4) alveoli (Fig. 23–5).

Bronchioli

The respiratory bronchioli are short tubular structures that have an internal diameter of approximately 0.5 mm. The respiratory bronchioli are continuous with the terminal bronchioli. The epithelial cells in the respiratory bronchioli are cuboidal in shape and lack cilia and interspersed goblet cells. The walls of the respiratory bronchioli consist of collagenous connective tissue, smooth muscle bundles, and sparse elastic fibers. Alveoli appear in the walls of the bronchioli, hence the name *respiratory bronchioli*.

Alveoli

The alveolar ducts are thin-walled tubular structures that give off numerous branches. The alveolar sacs contain two or more individual alveoli. The alveoli are thin-walled polyhedral sacs. The walls of the alveoli are really spaces in a huge mesh of spongelike elastic tissue fibers lined with a layer of epithelium, which is a single cell in thickness. Surrounding the walls of the alveoli are capillary networks for gas exchange between the respiratory system and the blood. In the normal adult there are approximately 300 million alveoli, thereby creating a tremendously large surface area for gas exchange (Fig. 23–6).

The alveolar capillary membranes have four layers.

1. Alveolar squamous epithelium
2. Basement membrane of elastic fibers and collagen
3. Basement membrane of the pulmonary capillary
4. Capillary endothelium

These four layers, which are 0.5 micron thick, form the morphologic interface between the alveoli and the capillary blood for the diffusion of oxygen from the alveoli and carbon dioxide from the blood. In the adult the total surface area of alveoli in contact with the capillaries is 70 m^2 (Fig. 23–7).

The alveoli are lined by two types of epithelial cells. Type I cells are flat cells and are the primary lining cells. Type II cells, or granular pneumocytes, are highly active metabolically and produce surfactant. Alveolar macrophages are present in the alveoli and are responsible for phagocytizing foreign particles and bacteria.

PULMONARY CIRCULATION

The pulmonary artery arises from the right ventricle and branches almost immediately into the right and left pulmonary arteries to join the bronchi in the mediastinum at the hilus of the lung (Fig. 23–8). The pulmonary arterial vessels transport deoxygenated venous blood to the lungs. The pulmonary circulation delivers the cardiac output from the right ventricle and distributes it as a very thin film of blood in the pulmonary capillaries to enhance gas exchange between the alveoli and the capillaries. The pulmonary vascular system is a network of highly distensible vessels with thin, incomplete smooth muscle in the tunica media layer resulting in a low resistance system. In a normal person the average systolic and diastolic pressures in the pulmonary artery are approximately 25 and 10 mm Hg respectively, with a mean pressure of 15 mm Hg. These pressures are much lower than those in the aorta, which reflects the lower pressures produced in the right ventricle during systole and the low resistance network. The mean diastolic pressure in the left atrium is 5 to 8 mm Hg, so the total pulmonary arteriovenous pressure gradient is approximately 10 mm Hg compared to about 90 mm Hg in the systemic circulation. The pressure fall from the pulmonary artery to the pulmonary capillaries is negligible, resulting in a mean hydrostatic pressure in the pulmonary capillaries of approximately 10 mm Hg. The oncotic pressure in the pulmonary capillaries is 25 mm Hg, resulting in an inward directed pressure gradient of 15 mm Hg,

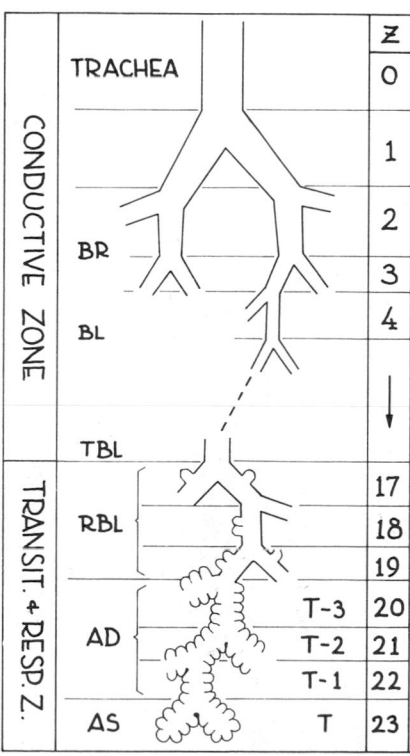

FIGURE 23–5. Airway branching in human lung by regularized dichotomy from trachea (generation z = 0) to alveolar ducts and sacs (generations 20 to 23). The first 16 generations are purely conducting: transitional airways lead into the respiratory zone made of alveoli. (From Weibel, E. R. (1963). *Morphometry of the human lung.* Heidelberg: Springer-Verlag.)

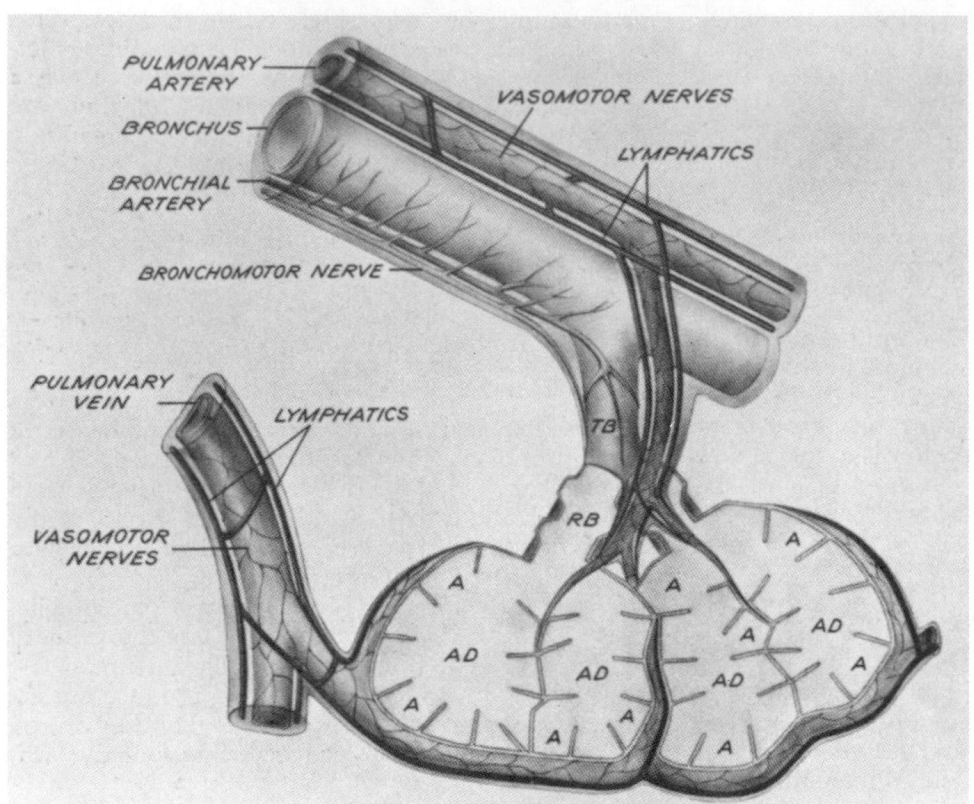

FIGURE 23–6. Structure of the lung. *Abbreviations:* A, anatomic alveolus; AD, alveolar duct; RB, respiratory bronchiole; TB, terminal bronchiole. (From Staub, N. C. (1970). The pathophysiology of pulmonary edema. *Human Pathology*, 1, 419.)

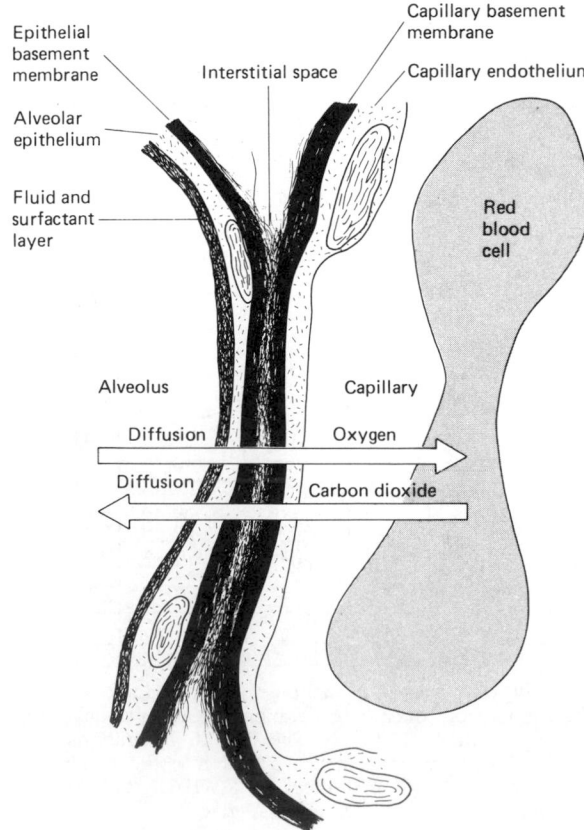

FIGURE 23–7. Ultrastructure of the respiratory membrane as shown in cross section. (From Guyton, A. C. (1991). *Textbook of medical physiology* (8th ed, p. 429). Philadelphia: W. B. Saunders.)

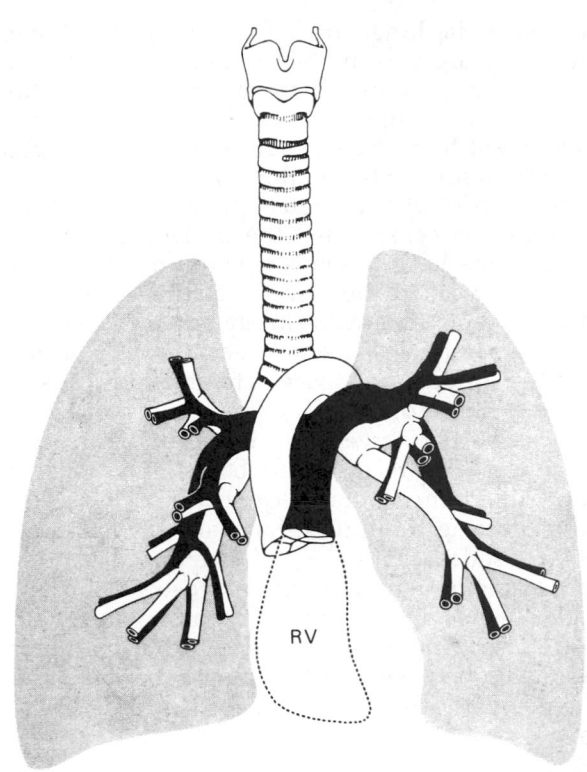

FIGURE 23–8. Main branches of pulmonary artery in relation to bronchi. RV, right ventricle. (Reproduced with permission from Fishman, A. P. (1980). *Assessment of pulmonary function* (p. 20). New York: McGraw-Hill.)

Despite this innervation and the reactivity to vasoactive agents, the overall regulation of pulmonary blood flow is passive, and local adjustments to ventilation and perfusion are determined by the local concentration of oxygen and H^+ ion. This local control will be addressed later in the chapter under ventilation-perfusion mismatch.

Because the pulmonary circulation receives all of the venous blood of the body before it is recycled, the lungs play an important metabolic role in regulating the level of vasoactive substances in the circulation. The surface area of the pulmonary capillary endothelium is large, and the cells have many projections and indentations that contain many enzyme-rich sites. Prostaglandins E and F types, serotonin, norepinephrine, and histamine are removed from the blood while passing through the lungs. Angiotensin I is converted to the powerful vasoconstrictor angiotensin II during passage through the lung.

The bronchi and lung tissue receive blood through the bronchial vessels that originates from the mid-thoracic aorta or from branches of the intercostal, internal mammary, or subclavian arteries. Two or three arteries accompany the bronchi to form a peribronchial plexus. Venous blood drains into the azygous and hemizygous systems. Venous blood from the small bronchi enter the pulmonary veins, thus adding deoxygenated blood to the overall oxygenated blood leaving the lungs.

which keeps the alveoli free of fluid. When pulmonary capillary pressure is increased above 25 mm Hg as in left ventricular failure, pulmonary congestion and edema result. The lymphatic channels, which end near the terminal bronchioli, drain fluid from the interstitial space and propel the fluid by active contraction of the smooth muscle in the wall of the lymphatics to the hilus of the lung (Fig. 23–9). Lymph flow from the lung is normally about 20 mL/minute and greatly increases in pulmonary edema. The four pulmonary veins that transport oxygenated blood course independent of the bronchial tree and are collected at the hilus to return the blood to the left atrium for distribution through the systemic circulation (Fig. 23–10).

The pulmonary blood vessels are innervated by the sparse sympathetic vasoconstrictor fibers and by the parasympathetic dilator fibers. The fetal pulmonary circulation responds to both parasympathetic and sympathetic stimulation. The pulmonary arterioles are constricted by such substances as norepinephrine, epinephrine, angiotensin II, thromboxanes, and prostaglandin F_{2alpha}. They are dilated by isoproterenol, acetylcholine, and prostaglandin I_2. In the body, both constrictor and dilator substances may be released simultaneously, resulting in a mixed response. The pulmonary venula are constricted by serotonin, histamine, and *Escherichia coli* endotoxin.

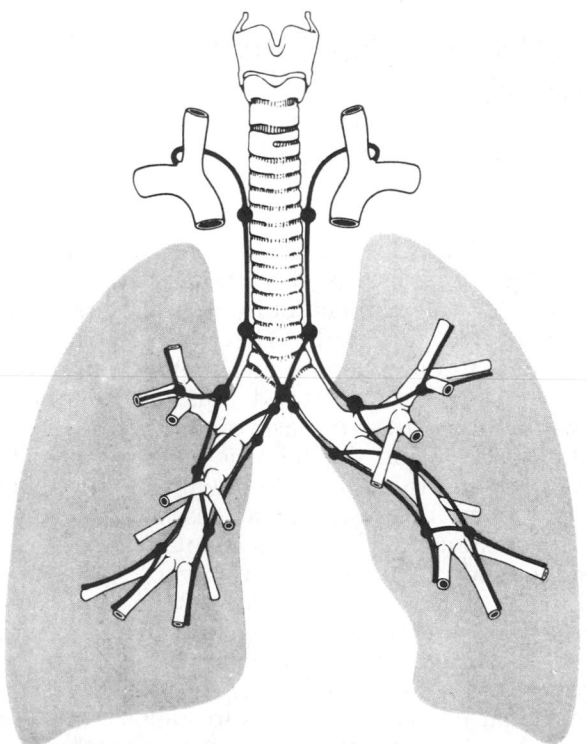

FIGURE 23–9. Schematic diagram of distribution of lymph nodes and main lymphatic channels along bronchial tree. (Reproduced with permission from Fishman, A. P. (1980). *Assessment of pulmonary function* (p. 50). New York: McGraw-Hill.)

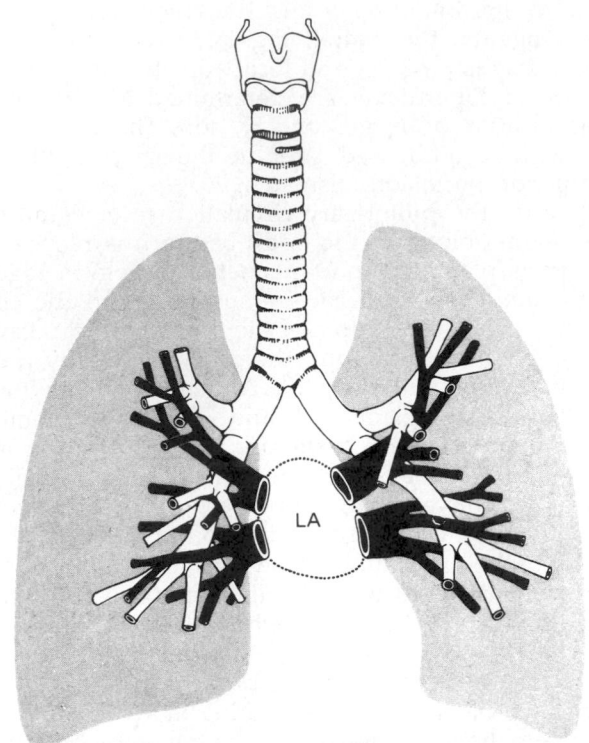

FIGURE 23–10. Two main stems of pulmonary vein penetrate into lung on each side. LA, left atrium. (Reproduced with permission from Fishman, A. P. (1980). *Assessment of pulmonary function* (p. 20). New York: McGraw-Hill.)

MECHANICS OF PULMONARY VENTILATION

Relationship of the Lungs to the Thoracic Cage

The lungs are located in a closed compartment called the thoracic cage. The thoracic cage is composed of the sternum anteriorly, the 12 pairs of ribs, and the spine posteriorly. The intercostal muscles, both internal and external, are located between the ribs. The large dome-shaped muscular diaphragm forms the floor of the thoracic cage (Fig. 23–11).

The space inside the thoracic cage is called the thoracic cavity. In addition to the lungs, the thoracic cavity houses the heart, great vessels, esophagus, and mediastinum. The lung is maintained in a stable position within the thoracic cavity by the root or hilus. The hilus is a depression in the lung where the airways and blood vessels enter the lung from the mediastinum. The pulmonary ligament, a long narrow band of attachment between the visceral and mediastinal pleura, also serves to stabilize the lung. When the lung retracts during a pneumothorax, it remains attached to the mediastinal wall of the thoracic cavity because of these attachments. When the lungs are expanded they fill the entire chest cavity to a total lung capacity of 5 to 6 liters.

Although the lungs are stable within the thoracic cavity, they are very mobile to allow for expansion during inspiration and retraction during expiration. The mobility of the lung is due to morphologic development from the mesoderm of a serosal space. The interior surface of the thoracic cavity is lined by a delicate sheet of squamous epithelial cells (serosal or mesothelial cells) called the parietal pleura. The surface of the lung tissue is covered by an identical serosal layer called the visceral pleura. The parietal and visceral pleura are so closely apposed that there is only a potential space between the two surfaces called the intrapleural space. The intrapleural space is filled with a thin film of fluid produced by the serosal cells that serves as a lubricant between the two layers. The relationship between the parietal pleura lining the thoracic cavity and the visceral pleura covering the lung tissue can be compared to two glass slides with a drop of water between them. The two pleural surfaces are as closely apposed as the glass slides, which slide easily along one another but are also adherent to one another. This intimate relationship between the two pleural surfaces is important for breathing, as described in the next section.

Inspiration and Expiration

The process of inspiration followed by expiration is called the respiratory cycle and is the result of pressure gradients. To understand the process of ventilation, it is important to understand the pressures that exist on the thorax and within the lungs at rest and during the respiratory cycle. The external pressure exerted on the thorax is atmospheric pressure, which is equal to 760 mm Hg. The alveoli, which are in direct communication with the atmosphere through the nose or mouth, are also at atmospheric pressure equal to 760 mm Hg. The pressure within the alveoli is termed intra-alveolar.

The pressure between the chest wall and the lungs is called intrapleural pressure and is −2.5 mm Hg subatmospheric, or 757.5 mm Hg. The intrapleural subatmospheric pressure results from the two opposing forces of deflation and inflation (Fig. 23–12).

The forces tending toward deflation in the lung are due to the elastic recoil of the lung tissue and the surface tension at the liquid–air interface. The lungs have a continual tendency to recoil or collapse because they are composed of elastic fibers that when stretched by inflation attempt to shorten. This process is similar to an elastic band, which, when stretched, will recoil upon the release of tension.

The second and most important force tending toward deflation of the lung is the surface tension of the fluid lining the alveoli. The surface tension is due to the intermolecular attraction between the water molecules at the surface of the liquid–air interface in the alveoli. The water molecules at the surface are pulled downward toward the water molecules

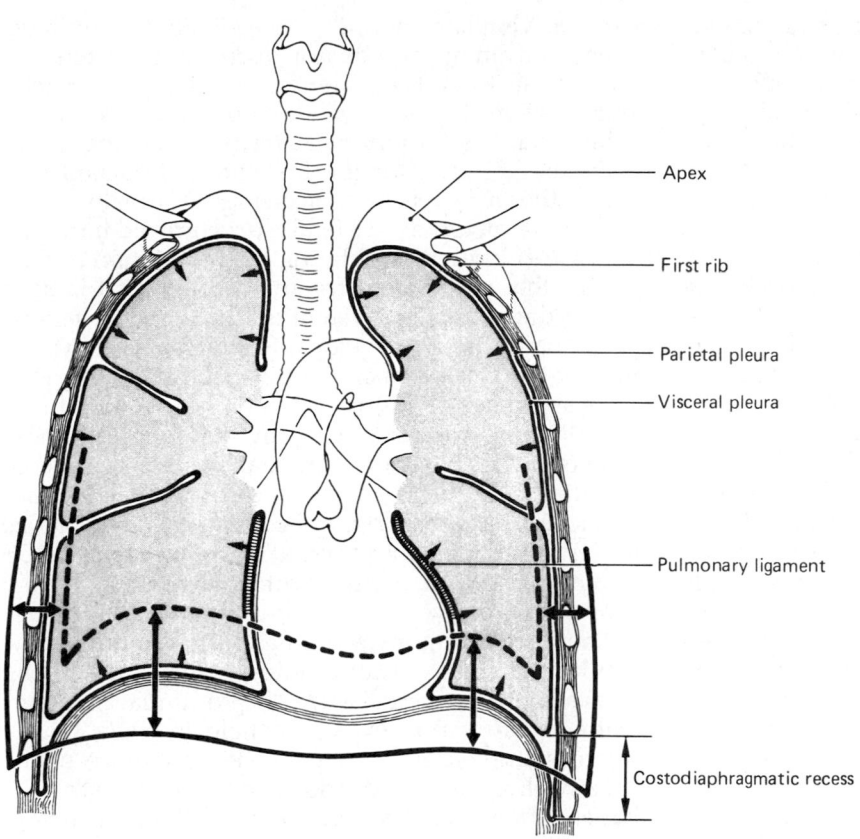

Apex

First rib

Parietal pleura

Visceral pleura

Pulmonary ligament

Costodiaphragmatic recess

FIGURE 23–11. Frontal section of the chest and lung, depicting the thoracic cage and the structures contained within the thoracic cavity. The single arrows indicate retractive force; the double arrows show the excursion of the lung bases and the periphery between deep inspiration and expiration. (Reproduced with permission from Fishman, A. P. (1980). *Assessment of pulmonary function* (p. 19). New York: McGraw-Hill.)

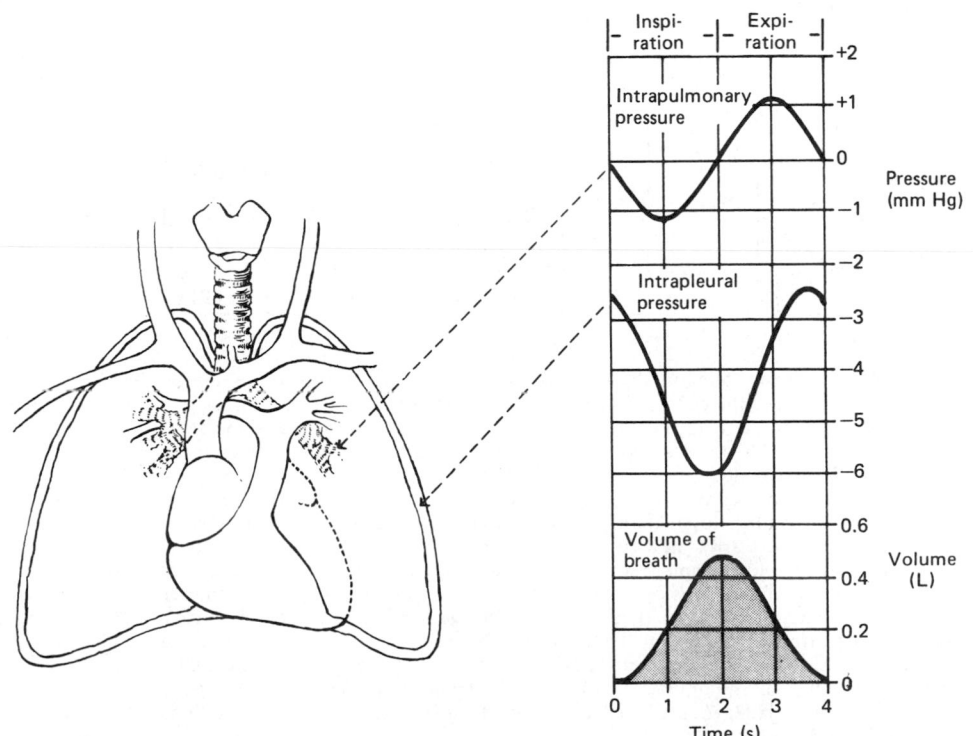

FIGURE 23–12. Changes in intrapleural (intrathoracic) and intrapulmonary pressure relative to atmospheric pressure during inspiration and expiration. (From Ganong, W. F. (1989). *Review of medical physiology* (14th ed.). Norwalk, CT: Appleton & Lange.)

below the surface due to the attraction of unlike charges on the water molecules. This intermolecular attraction results in a sheet of fluid lining the alveolar surface that is continually trying to collapse inward. About one–third of the elastic recoil of the lung and two–thirds of the surface tension account for the forces acting toward deflation in the lung (Fig. 23–13).

Surfactant, a lipoprotein substance secreted by the type II pneumocytes in the alveoli, is important in lowering the surface tension at the air–liquid interface, thereby decreasing the tendency of the alveoli to collapse. Surfactant is composed of dipalmitoylphosphatidylcholine (DPPC). DPPC molecule has a hydrophilic (water-loving) "head" and two parallel hydrophobic (water-fearing) fatty acid "tails." The surfactant molecules are oriented parallel at the air–liquid interface in the alveoli. The heads of the molecule are oriented toward the water in the alveoli, whereas the tails are oriented toward the air. The orientation of the surfactant molecule disrupts the intermolecular interaction between the surface water molecules, thereby decreasing the surface tension. The surfactant molecules are spread apart during inspiration as the alveolar size increases but move together during expiration, thus adjusting surface tension during breathing.

Surfactant is produced and replaced on a regular basis by type II cells. The importance of surfactant in reducing surface tension in the alveoli is exemplified by commonly seen derangements. Cigarette smoking decreases the amount of surfactant at the air–liquid interface in the alveoli. Fresh water drowning victims loose their surfactant, resulting in increased alveolar tension that necessitates high pressures to ventilate the individual. Patients who have been on a pump-oxygenator during cardiac surgery have a surfactant deficiency, resulting in patchy atelectasis in the immediate postoperative period.

Surfactant is important at birth, when the infant expands the lungs for the first time. Surfactant prevents the lungs from collapsing. Normally, near term, both maternal and fetal glucocorticoid hormone levels are elevated, facilitating the maturation of type II cells that produce surfactant. If the infant is born before the surfactant system is functional, a serious pulmonary disease develops, formerly called hyaline membrane disease and now termed respiratory distress syndrome (RDS) in the newborn. Without surfactant, the surface tension in the lungs of these infants is high, and there are many collapsed alveoli, resulting in atelectasis. The type II cells that produce surfactant have also been shown to increase in size under the influence of thyroid hormone, hence RDS is more severe in infants with low plasma thyroid levels.

The force acting toward inflation in the lung is the result of the chest wall tending to expand, pulling outward on the lung tissue. The continual tendency of the chest wall to expand is held in check by the intercostal muscles. When the circumference of the chest wall is measured prior to and after death, it is larger upon postmortem examination. At death, when the chest wall is no longer under the restraining influence of the intercostal muscles, the chest wall naturally expands. The opposing forces of deflation in the lungs and inflation of the chest wall create a vacuum between the visceral and parietal pleura, resulting in an intrapleural pressure that is subatmospheric (757.5 mm Hg).

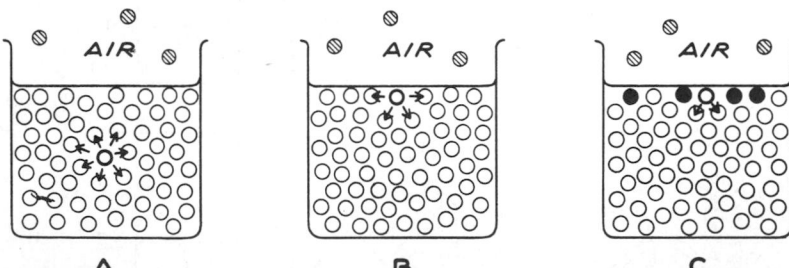

A **B** **C**

FIGURE 23–13. Surface tension. "In a liquid such as water at rest, the intermolecular forces acting on the molecule in *A* are equal in all directions; molecular forces pull it downward, to the left, to the right, and upward. However, the water molecule in *B*, at the water-air surface, does not experience equal attracting forces in all directions. *B* is attracted by water molecules directly beneath it, but there are relatively few molecules in the gas above it to exert an upward force. Therefore, more molecules pull it down than pull it up, and typical of surface molecules, it tends to dive downward. As a result of this imbalance of intermolecular forces, the surface shrinks to the smallest possible area. The resulting force in the surface is referred to as surface tension" (description from Comroe, 1965). In *C*, surface tension lowering substances (e.g., surfactant), denoted by the black circles, decrease the attraction between the surface water molecules and therefore lower the surface tension at the liquid-air interface. *Abbrevations:* Open circles, molecules of water; shaded circles, molecules of air; black circles, surface-active molecules. (From Comroe, J. H. (1965). *Physiology of respiration* (p. 106). Chicago: Year Book Medical Publishers.)

Inspiration

Inspiration is an active process that requires energy for the contraction of the inspiratory muscles to expand the thoracic cavity. The diaphragm is the most important muscle of inspiration. Neural innervation of the diaphragm occurs through the phrenic nerve, which exits from the spinal cord between the third and fourth cervical vertebrae. At rest between breaths, the diaphragm is bowed upward into the thoracic cavity to the level of the fourth intercostal space. With neural stimulation, the diaphragm contracts, moving downward and pushing on the abdominal contents while raising the rib margins upward and outward, thus increasing the transverse diameter of the thoracic cavity. The external intercostal muscles, which run obliquely downward and forward from rib to rib, contract to raise the ribs during inspiration and increase the anteroposterior (AP) diameter of the thoracic cavity.

In normal persons, the accessory muscles of inspiration assist only during high levels of ventilation by enlarging the upper part of the thoracic cavity. The scalene muscles in the neck elevate the first two ribs. The sternocleidomastoid elevates the sternum and enlarges slightly the AP diameter of the chest.

As the thoracic cavity expands, the parietal pleura that lines the thoracic cavity pulls outward on the visceral pleura that surrounds the lung tissue, causing the intrapleural pressure to become more subatmospheric (-6 mm Hg). There is a pressure gradient difference between the intra-alveolar air pressure and the intrapleural pressure that causes air to flow from the atmosphere into the alveoli. Air enters the lungs by bulk flow to the region of the terminal bronchioli and by gaseous diffusion to the alveolar spaces. The volume of air entering the lungs during a normal breath at rest is approximately 500 cc or 0.5 liter (see Fig. 23–12).

Expiration

Expiration is normally a passive process in the sense that no muscles contract. During expiration the diaphragm relaxes, the external intercostals relax, and the size of the thoracic cage decreases. The elastic tissue of the lungs recoil, pulling the chest back to the expiratory position, where the recoil pressure of the lungs and the chest wall balance. As the stretched lung tissue recoils, the alveolar air is compressed; the intra-alveolar pressure exceeds atmospheric pressure, and air flows from the alveoli to the atmosphere by bulk flow. Normally, passive expiration takes one-third longer than inspiration due to the increase in airway resistance during expiration.

Although normally passive, expiration can become active during high levels of ventilation or when resistance to air flow is increased. The accessory muscles of expiration include the internal intercostals and the abdominal muscles. With contraction, the internal intercostals, which run upward and backward between the ribs, cause the ribs to move inward, thus decreasing the anteroposterior diameter of the thoracic cage. The abdominal muscles compress the abdominal contents and raise the intra-abdominal pressure.

Relationships Between Pressure Gradients, Airway Resistance, and Compliance

The volume of air that flows in or out of the alveoli during breathing is directly proportional to the pressure gradient. During deep breathing, the accessory muscles of inspiration and expiration are called into play, resulting in greater negative pressure gradients during inspiration and greater positive pressure gradients during expiration. In addition, the flow of air into and out of the alveoli is inversely proportional to airway resistance. As airway resistance increases, as in patients with asthma, chronic obstructive pulmonary disease (COPD), or a tumor, the flow of air into the lungs decreases.

$$\text{Flow} = \frac{\text{Pressure gradient}}{\text{Resistance}}$$

A number of factors determine airway resistance including (1) the number of interactions between the flowing gas molecules, (2) the length of the airway, and (3) the airway radius. The airway radius is extremely important because resistance to air flow is inversely proportional to the fourth power of the airway radius.

$$\text{Resistance} = \frac{1}{r^4}$$

Airway resistance may be altered by physical, nervous, or chemical factors. During normal inspiration, simple expansion of the lungs acts as a physical factor that pulls on the airways and widens them, thereby decreasing airway resistance. Conversely, during expiration, when airway pressures are above atmospheric, airway resistance is increased, and expiration takes one-third longer than inspiration. As discussed earlier, nervous regulation of the bronchiolar smooth muscle through the autonomic nervous system can decrease (sympathetic) or increase (parasympathetic) airway resistance. The bronchiolar smooth muscle is also sensitive to chemicals such as histamine and low carbon dioxide levels, causing bronchoconstriction, whereas high levels of carbon dioxide cause bronchodilation. The radius of the airways can become severely decreased with certain disease processes. Asthma is characterized by severe bronchiolar smooth muscle constriction and plugging of the airways by secretions. Airway resistance may become great enough to impede air flow completely despite large pressure gradients. Due to physical factors, asthmatics have much less difficulty with inhaling than with exhaling, resulting in air trapping in the lungs.

Compliance refers to the stretchability, distensibility, or elasticity of the lungs and the thoracic structures. The lungs and thorax have elastic properties—that is, they return to their resting shape after deformation by an external force. When pressure changes are applied to these structures, the resulting volume changes are proportional to the applied force (pressure) within limits. As intrapleural pressure decreases or intra-alveolar pressure increases, lung volume increases proportionally according to the following formula:

$$\frac{\Delta V}{\Delta P}$$

in which V equals lung volume and P equals pressure. The compliance of the normal lungs and the thorax combined is 0.1 liters/centimeter of water pressure. That is, every time the alveolar pressure is increased by 1 cm of water the lung volume increases by 100 milliliters:

$$\frac{1}{\text{Total compliance}} = \frac{1}{C_L} = \frac{1}{C_T} = 0.1 \text{ liter/cm } H_2O$$

in which C equals compliance, L equals lungs, and T equals thorax.

The compliance of the lungs alone, when removed from the thoracic cage, is 0.2 liter/cm water. This highlights the fact that the lungs are twice as distensible as the thorax and that the muscles of inspiration must expend energy to expand the lungs and the thoracic cage. Lung compliance can be determined indirectly in man by measuring the pressure developed in an intraesophageal balloon during respiration with the glottis open. The pressure changes in the intraesophageal balloon reflect the intrapleural pressure changes. The pressure is recorded at the end of expiration and again while holding the breath after inspiring a known volume of air in increments of 50 to 100 mLs.

Lung compliance provides an indication of the elastic recoil of the lung tissue and the surface tension of the lung. Normally, lung compliance decreases with age. Lung compliance also decreases in disease processes such as pulmonary fibrosis and pulmonary edema. Decreased lung compliance is a hallmark sign in adult respiratory distress syndrome (ARDS) and RDS in the newborn and in oxygen toxicity. Deformities of the thoracic cage such as kyphosis, scoliosis, and muscular dystrophy can significantly reduce thoracic compliance. Thoracic compliance can also be reduced with obesity, trauma, and postoperative surgical splinting.

Work of Breathing

The work of inspiration can be divided into three components: (1) work required to expand the elastic forces of the lung, called compliance work; (2) work required to overcome the viscosity of the lung and thoracic cage, called tissue resistance work; and (3) work required to overcome the resistance to the flow of air into and out of the lungs, called airway resistance. During normal quiet breathing, the majority of the work is expended to overcome compliance, with tissue resistance and airway resistance requiring only a small percentage of the total work of breathing. In pulmonary disease, any or all of the components of the work of breathing may be increased. Expiration is normally passive due to elastic recoil of the lungs and the thoracic cage, thus requiring no work. In rapid breathing or when tissue resistance or airway resistance is increased, expiratory work becomes greater than inspiratory work. In order to perform work, the respiratory muscles require oxygen. Oxygen consumption by the respiratory muscles is an indirect measure of the work of breathing. The oxygen cost of breathing is assessed by determining the total oxygen consumption of the body at rest and at an increased level of ventilation. The oxygen cost of normal breathing is approximately 1 mL/liter of ventilation and comprises less than 3% to 5% of total body consumption. During rapid respiration, the oxygen requirement may increase 25-fold. In pulmonary disease, respiratory oxygen consumption increases markedly, resulting in respiratory muscle fatigue and overall skeletal muscle fatigue, which limits severely the amount of energy that can be exerted for other daily activities.

PULMONARY FUNCTION MEASUREMENTS

Spirometry is a simple method of measuring pulmonary function by recording the volume of air movement into and out of the lungs (Fig. 23–14). A spirometer consists of a drum inverted over a chamber of water, with the drum counterbalanced by a weight. The inverted drum is filled with air or oxygen, and a tube connects the mouth of the subject with the gas filled drum. The water in the chamber prevents the gas mixture from escaping from the inverted drum. When the subject breathes through the tubing, the inverted drum rises and falls with expiration and inspiration respectively while a recording (spirogram) is made simultaneously on a moving sheet of paper. Figure 23–15 illustrates a spirogram during different breathing conditions. The values have been divided into four volumes and four capacities. The values reported below are "average" values for a 70-kg man. The values are dependent on height, weight, sex, and age. The volumes and

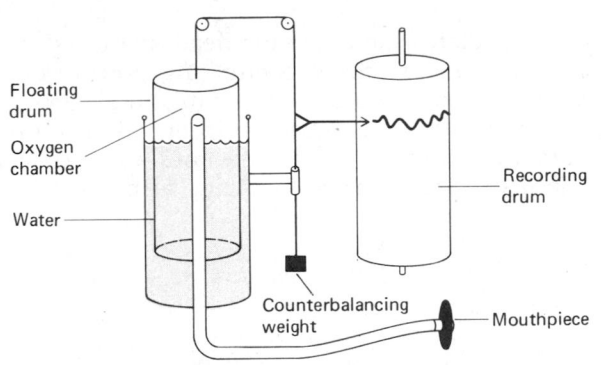

FIGURE 23–14. A spirometer. (From Guyton, A. C. (1991). *Textbook of medical physiology* (8th ed, p. 407). Philadelphia: W. B. Saunders.)

capacities are 20% to 25% lower in females. With increasing age, all of the values are lower.

Pulmonary Volumes

1. *Tidal volume* (V_T) is the volume of air entering or leaving the lungs during a single breath in the resting state (500 mL)
2. *Inspiratory reserve volume* (IRV) is the amount of air that can be inspired over and above resting tidal volume (3100 mL)

3. *Expiratory reserve volume* (ERV) is the air remaining in the lungs at the end of a normal expiration that can be exhaled by active contraction of expiratory muscles (1200 mL)
4. *Residual volume* (RV) is the amount of air remaining in the lungs after maximum expiration (1200 mL)

Pulmonary Capacities

1. *Vital capacity* (VC) is the sum of normal tidal volume, inspiratory reserve volume, and expiratory reserve volume (4800 mL)
2. *Inspiratory capacity* (IC) is the sum of inspiratory reserve volume and tidal volume (3600 mL)
3. *Functional capacity* (FC) is the sum of the expiratory reserve volume and the residual volume (2400 mL)
4. *Total lung capacity* (TLC) is the amount of air in the lungs after a maximum inspiration (6000 mL, the sum of all volumes)

Alterations in body position can affect pulmonary volumes and capacities. When a subject lies down, the values decrease because the abdominal contents exert pressure on the diaphragm and increased pulmonary blood volume decreases available space for

FIGURE 23–15. The lung volumes and capacities. The upper diagram illustrates the four principal lung volumes: RV, residual volume; ERV, expiratory reserve volume; TV, tidal volume; IRV, inspiratory reserve volume. The same shading is used in the lower part of the figure to indicate the same volumes. The four lung capacities are shown to the right of the figure. TLC, total lung capacity; VC, vital capacity; IC, inspiratory capacity; FRC, functional residual capacity. (From Jensen, D. (1980). *The principles of physiology* (2nd ed., p. 668). New York: Appleton-Century-Crofts.)

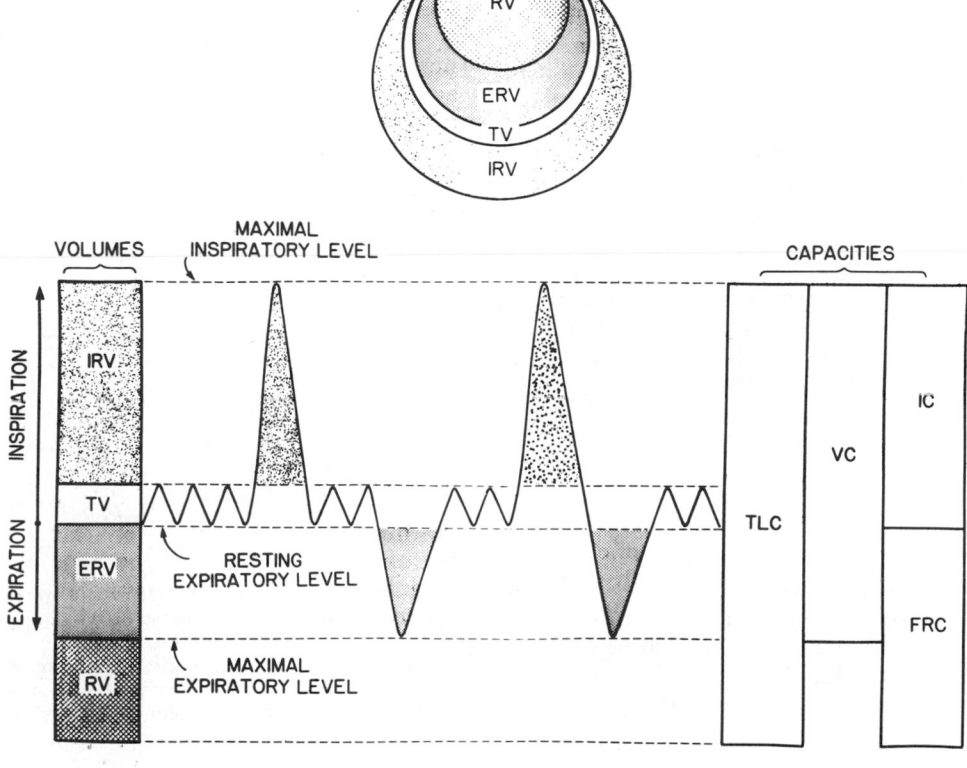

pulmonary air. This becomes important in patients with cardiac and pulmonary dysfunction.

Minute Ventilation and Maximum Voluntary Ventilation

Minute ventilation or volume (MV) is the volume of air moved in or out of the respiratory tract per minute in the resting state. This volume is equivalent to the product of tidal volume and respiratory rate. Therefore, if the tidal volume is 500 cc during the resting state and respiratory rate is 12 breaths/minute, the minute respiratory volume is 500 cc times 12 breaths/minute = 6000 cc/minute (or 6 liters/minute). During strenuous breathing, the tidal volume can equal vital capacity and the respiratory rate may reach as high as 50/minute, thereby markedly increasing minute ventilation. At extremely rapid respiratory rates, maintenance of tidal volume at much above one-half of vital capacity is limited by the work of breathing.

Maximum voluntary ventilation (MVV) is the total volume of air that can be moved into and out of the respiratory tract while breathing as rapidly and as deeply as possible for 12 seconds. This volume can be as high as 170 liters/minute for short intervals. Because the respiratory system has an enormous reserve, respiratory volume can increase up to 20- to 25-fold for short intervals.

Anatomic and Physiologic Dead Space

Air that enters the purely conducting portions of the respiratory tract including the nose, mouth, pharynx, larynx, trachea, bronchi, and bronchioli to the respiratory zone where gas exchange does not occur is called the anatomic dead space. The volume is difficult to determine but rough estimates based on age, sex, and tidal volumes indicate that in the adult anatomic dead space is equal to "ideal weight" in milliliters, or approximately 150 mL in a 70-kg man.

Alveolar dead space is a less well defined volume that consists of a variable number of alveoli whose perfusion is reduced or absent due to gravitational shifts in pulmonary blood flow in the normal person and to impaired blood flow in the diseased person.

Physiologic dead space is the sum of the anatomic and alveolar dead spaces; it is the functional dead space ventilation. In normal persons, the anatomic dead space is equivalent to the physiologic dead space.

Dead space ventilation (V_{DS}) is the amount of air that ventilates the physiologic dead space per minute, whereas alveolar ventilation (V_A) is the volume per minute that ventilates all perfused alveoli and is the difference between minute ventilation and dead space ventilation.

During a normal breath at rest, the tidal volume is equal to 500 cc. Approximately 150 cc of the total

500 cc ventilates the anatomic dead space, which is composed of the purely conducting portion of the respiratory tract. The alveolar ventilation is 350 cc of the total 500 cc. The relationship between the tidal volume, dead space ventilation, and alveolar ventilation is expressed in the following formula.

$$V_T = V_{DS} + V_A$$
$$500 \text{ cc} \quad 150 \text{ cc} \quad 350 \text{ cc}$$

V_T = Tidal volume
V_{DS} = Dead space ventilation
V_A = Alveolar ventilation

Single Breath Nitrogen Analysis

A new test has been developed to assess pulmonary function entitled the modified single breath nitrogen analysis (Fig. 23–16). The anatomic dead space can be measured by this technique. Starting from midinspiration, the subject takes as deep a breath of pure oxygen as possible and exhales steadily while the nitrogen content of the expired gas is continuously measured. When the subject inhales pure oxygen, it fills the conducting portion of the respiratory tract, or the anatomic dead space. Consequently, the initial gas that is exhaled (phase I) contains no nitrogen. The exhaled gas that follows is first a mixture of dead space and alveolar gas (phase II) and then the alveolar gas (phase III) alone. The dead space volume is the volume of gas expired from peak inspiration to the midportion of phase II. Phase III of the single breath nitrogen curve, the alveolar plateau, terminates at the closing volume (CV), where there is an abrupt increase in slope of phase IV to residual volume. The closing volume is the lung volume above residual volume where the airways begin to close off because of increasing positive transmural pressure during expiration. The modified single breath nitrogen test is currently being used in longitudinal studies of normal subjects and individuals with lung disease. The alveolar plateau increases

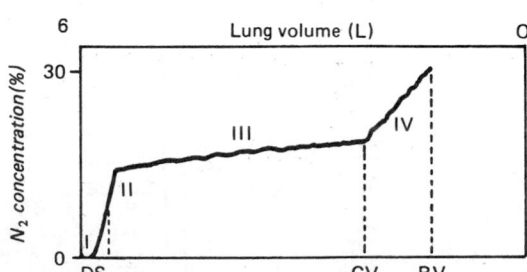

FIGURE 23–16. Single breath nitrogen curve. From mid-inspiration, the subject takes a deep breath of pure oxygen, then exhales steadily. The changes in the nitrogen concentration of expired gas during expiration are shown, with the various phases of the curve indicated by roman numerals. *Abbreviations:* DS, dead space; CV, closing volume; RV, residual volume. (Reprinted, by permission, from the New England Journal of Medicine, 293, 438, 1975.)

with age, and the closing volume increases in subjects exposed to pollutants and cigarette smoke. The closing volume is increased in subjects with premature airway closure as with emphysema.

Forced Expiratory Vital Capacity

Forced expiratory vital capacity is measured using a spirometer or a pneumotachograph. The subject inhales to total lung capacity and then exhales in a rapid forceful maximal expiration. Figure 23–17 illustrates a graph of volume versus time. Several measurements are commonly obtained from the volume-time presentation of the forced vital capacity including the volume exhaled in one second (FEV_1) and the volume exhaled in 3 seconds (FEV_3). These values can be expressed as a ratio of total forced vital capacity.

$$\frac{FEV_1}{\text{Forced vital capacity}}$$

Patients with airway obstruction show drastic changes in the appearance of the forced vital capacity tracing. There is a flattening of the slope of the curve at any given volume, indicating a reduced rate of air flow upon expiration. In addition, the duration of the forced expiratory maneuver is prolonged, and the cessation of air flow is delayed as indicated by a plateau at the bottom of the curve. The smaller the ratio of FEV_1 to forced vital capacity, the more difficult it is to exhale. Pre- and postexpiratory forced vital capacity tests are used to determine the effectiveness of bronchodilating drugs on patients with airway obstructive disease.

DIFFUSION OF RESPIRATORY GASES

The diffusion of oxygen from the alveoli to the pulmonary capillary blood and the diffusion of carbon dioxide from the blood to the alveolus is the result of the partial pressure gradients of the gases. The partial pressure of a gas is the desire of the gas to escape from the liquid state into the gaseous state. This phenomenon can be exemplified by a carbonated soft drink in an enclosed glass container. With the cap on, the gas is contained within the liquid state. When the cap is removed, the gas in the liquid begins to escape, as visualized by the bubbles escaping into the atmosphere from an area of higher partial pressure in the container to an area of lower partial pressure in the atmosphere. The respiratory gases are carried in the liquid portion of the plasma of the blood and on the hemoglobin molecule and exert a partial pressure. This partial pressure is the result of the individual gas molecules bombarding the walls of the blood vessels. The magnitude of the pressure is dependent upon the concentration of the gas and the temperature. At higher gas concentrations there will be a greater number of molecules colliding with the vessel wall. At higher temperatures the speed of the moving molecules will be greater and the number of collisions with the vessel wall will be greater. The exchange of oxygen from the alveoli and carbon dioxide from the blood is the result of partial pressure gradients. In order to understand the diffusion of respiratory gases from areas of higher concentration to areas of lower concentration the composition of atmospheric air must be considered.

Composition of Air

Atmospheric air is composed of the following gases in different percentages.

Nitrogen	78.6%
Oxygen	20.9%
Carbon dioxide	0.04%
Inert gases	0.92%
Water vapor	Variable

The total pressure of a mixture of gases is simply the sum of the individual pressures according to the Dalton law of partial pressures. With the atmospheric pressure at sea equal to 760 mm Hg, the individual partial pressures of the gases can be calculated by taking the percentage of each of the respiratory gases comprising the total pressure. The partial pressures (P) of the inspired atmospheric air is stated in the following formula.

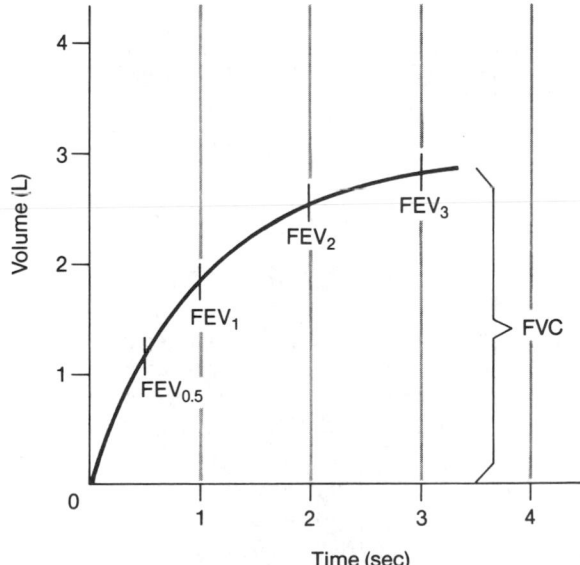

FIGURE 23–17. A spirogram of a forced vital capacity (FVC) maneuver with forced expiratory volume (FEV) labeled at various time intervals. The FEV at 1 second (FEV_1) is the most important measurement. (From Kersten, L. D. (1989). *Comprehensive respiratory nursing* (p. 375). Philadelphia: W. B. Saunders.)

$$\underset{\text{760 mm Hg}}{\text{Partial pressure atmospheric}} = \underset{158}{P_{O_2}} + \underset{0.3}{P_{CO_2}} + \underset{597}{P_{N_2}} + \underset{5}{P_{H_2O}}$$

The partial pressure of water vapor is dependent upon the temperature of the atmospheric air. At low temperatures, atmospheric air has very little water in vapor form. At high temperatures, as in the summer months, atmospheric air will have more water in vapor form, as indicated by the increased "humidity" of the air.

Oxygen is consumed by the body at the cellular level for the production of ATP in the process of oxidative phosphorylation, and carbon dioxide is produced as a byproduct. Therefore, oxygen and carbon dioxide are considered essential respiratory gases. Nitrogen is in high concentration in the atmospheric air, and although it is inert (devoid of active properties), it does serve a useful purpose. Nitrogen serves to dilute the concentration of oxygen, thereby protecting the alveolar cells from the effects of oxygen toxicity. In addition, nitrogen is not as soluble as oxygen and therefore does not diffuse as readily from the alveoli into the blood. Nitrogen stays in the alveoli, keeping them inflated and thereby reducing their tendency to collapse.

Factors Affecting Diffusion

The movement of gas molecules occurs by physical diffusion from a region of higher partial pressure to one of lower partial pressure. The rate of diffusion depends upon the following factors:

1. The difference in partial pressure between the two sides
2. The surface area for diffusion
3. The thickness of the tissue separating the two sides
4. The diffusibility of the gas

In the respiratory system, the difference in partial pressures lies in the partial pressure of oxygen and carbon dioxide in the alveoli versus the partial pressure in the blood. The total surface area available for diffusion is 70 m² due to the large number of alveoli and pulmonary capillaries surrounding the alveoli. The total surface area available for diffusion in the lungs is the size of a badminton court. In health, the alveolar capillary membrane thickness is 0.5 micron. The diffusibility of a gas is directly proportional to the solubility of the gas in the liquid and inversely proportional to the square root of the molecular weight and is expressed in the following formula:

$$\text{Diffusibility} = \frac{\alpha \text{ Solubility of the gas}}{\sqrt{\text{Molecular weight of the gas}}}$$

As a result of this relationship, carbon dioxide is 20 times more diffusible than oxygen. The reason for this difference in the two gases is that carbon dioxide is 24 times more soluble than oxygen. Using the formula, carbon dioxide is 24 times more soluble than oxygen, but its molecular weight is greater, resulting in carbon dioxide being 20 times more

diffusible than oxygen. Carbon dioxide moves 20 times as fast across the alveolar capillary membrane as oxygen. For this reason, the elimination of carbon dioxide is almost never limited by alterations in the diffusion component of the respiratory process. However, the diffusion of gases between the alveoli and the capillaries can be impaired in a number of disease processes. In emphysema, which is frequently related to cigarette smoking, alveolar capillary walls are broken down, resulting in fewer but larger alveoli and a reduction in the total surface area available for diffusion. Alveolar capillary membrane thickening, as in ARDS or RDS and pulmonary edema, increases the distance needed for the diffusion of gas molecules. The alveolar capillary walls may become denser and less permeable with inhaled substances such as beryllium.

The diffusion of oxygen from the alveoli and carbon dioxide from the pulmonary capillaries is depicted in Figure 23–18. As discussed earlier, the partial pressure of oxygen in the atmospheric air is 158 mm Hg and the partial pressure of carbon dioxide is 0.3 mm Hg. During inspiration, as atmospheric air is inhaled it becomes mixed with the air in the anatomic dead space and the gases contained in the alveoli. As a result, in the alveoli the partial pressure of oxygen is 100 mm Hg, and the partial pressure of carbon dioxide is 40 mm Hg. In addition, the partial pressure of the water vapor is increased because the temperature of the body is higher at 98°F than the atmosphere at 70°F.

As discussed earlier, the pulmonary arteries (right and left) are transporting deoxygenated blood from the right ventricle to the lungs. At the level of the pulmonary capillaries that surround the individual alveoli the partial pressure of oxygen in the venous

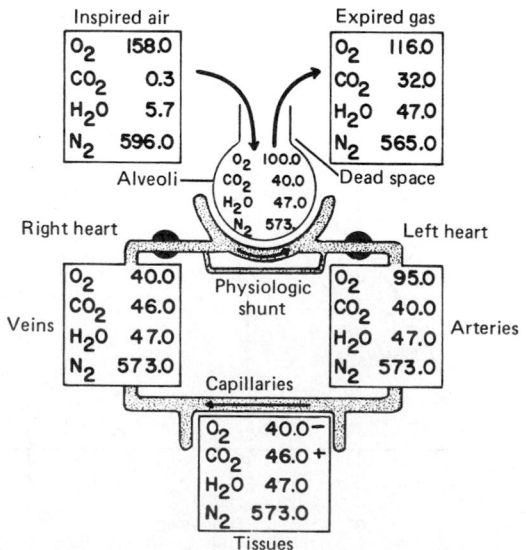

FIGURE 23–18. Partial pressures of gases (mm Hg) in the respiratory and cardiovascular system. (From Ganong, W. F. (1989). *Review of medical physiology* (14th ed.). Norwalk, CT: Appleton & Lange.)

blood is 40 mm Hg and the partial pressure of carbon dioxide is 46 mm Hg. Due to pressure gradient differences, oxygen moves from an area of higher partial pressure (100 mm Hg in the alveoli) into the capillaries at a lower partial pressure of 40 mm Hg. The partial pressure gradient (the difference between the two pressures) in the diffusion of oxygen from the alveoli to the capillaries is therefore 60 mm Hg. This large pressure gradient is advantageous to ensure adequate oxygenation of blood. The partial pressure of carbon dioxide in the pulmonary capillaries is 46 mm Hg, whereas the partial pressure of carbon dioxide in the alveoli is 40 mm Hg, resulting in a pressure gradient of 6 mm Hg that "drives" carbon dioxide into the alveoli. Although the pressure gradient for carbon dioxide is only 6 mm Hg, it is sufficient to provide adequate diffusion because carbon dioxide is 20 times more diffusible than oxygen.

The four pulmonary veins return oxygenated arterialized blood to the left atrium and left ventricle to be distributed to the cells of the body through the arterial system. At the tissue level, the partial pressure of oxygen is 40 mm Hg and the partial pressure of carbon dioxide is 46 mm Hg due to the utilization of oxygen and the production of carbon dioxide by the cells in oxidative phosphorylation. The pressure gradient for the diffusion of oxygen to the cells is 60 mm Hg, whereas the diffusion gradient for the movement of carbon dioxide from the cells to the capillaries is 6 mm Hg. The diffusion process results in a partial pressure of 40 mm Hg for oxygen and 46 mm Hg for carbon dioxide in the returning venous blood.

Venous blood returns from the lower portions of the body through the inferior vena cava and from the upper portions through the superior vena cava to the right atrium and right ventricle, exiting into the two pulmonary arteries, which carry the deoxygenated blood to the lung to reinitiate the entire process. Under normal circumstances the diffusion process is immediate and blood flow through the pulmonary capillaries is slow enough (a single red cell remains in the pulmonary capillary approximately 0.75 second) that equilibrium is easily achieved. With strenuous exercise, an increase in cardiac output results in a decrease in the time available for diffusion to 0.3 second, thereby challenging the respiratory system. High altitudes, where the atmospheric pressure is reduced, pose a respiratory challenge. At high altitudes, the partial pressure of atmospheric oxygen is less, thereby reducing the normal "driving" pressure gradients and compromising the diffusion process. As a result, physical activity is limited by the partial pressure of oxygen in the arterial blood.

Ventilation-Perfusion Ratio

Diffusion of the respiratory gases is optimal when both ventilation and blood flow are evenly matched.

However, even this ideal situation does not exist in the normal lung. At rest, pulmonary ventilation averages 5.1 liters/minute. Cardiac output averages 6.0 liters/minute, resulting in a ventilation-to-perfusion ratio (V_A/Q) of 0.85. The discrepancy between ventilation and perfusion is due to the difference in the distribution of pulmonary gases and pulmonary circulation due to gravity. In an upright subject at rest between breaths, the alveoli in the apex of the lung will be filled with air due to the fact that air rises. During inspiration more ventilation will be distributed to the base of the lung than to the apex. Similarly, perfusion of the lung is lowest in the apex and greatest in the base due to gravity. However, in the apex of the lung, ventilation is three times greater than perfusion. At the base of the lung, alveolar ventilation is less than pulmonary capillary blood flow, and the V_A/Q is 0.6. This results in an overall ventilation-to-perfusion ratio of 0.85. The range of V_A/Q throughout the normal lung is relatively narrow, so that differences in arterial blood gases in different regions of the lung are small.

However, in pulmonary diseases in which airway resistance is increased, pulmonary compliance is decreased, and blood vessel caliber is altered, ventilation-perfusion mismatches can occur, resulting in a decreased capacity for gas exchange. Normally, physiologic mechanisms attempt to reduce the degree of ventilation-perfusion mismatch. As discussed earlier, high carbon dioxide concentrations result in bronchodilation, whereas low concentrations result in bronchoconstriction, altering pulmonary ventilation. Pulmonary arteriolar smooth muscle is very sensitive to the partial pressure of oxygen in the alveoli. Increased alveolar oxygen results in vasodilation, whereas decreased alveolar oxygen results in vasoconstriction. This local control permits perfusion of well-ventilated alveoli and the "shunting" of blood away from poorly ventilated alveoli. Systemic hypoxia also causes the pulmonary arterioles to constrict, resulting in an increase in pulmonary arterial pressure and pulmonary hypertension. The pulmonary arteriolar smooth muscle is also sensitive to the concentration of H^+ ion, which is indirectly related to the concentration of carbon dioxide. When carbon dioxide combines with water, carbonic acid forms and rapidly breaks down into H^+ and HCO_3^-. An increased concentration of H^+ results in pulmonary vasoconstriction and the "shunting" of blood away from poorly ventilated alveoli with high alveolar carbon dioxide levels to better ventilated alveoli.

TRANSPORT OF RESPIRATORY GASES

The oxygen delivery system and the carbon dioxide elimination system in the body are composed of the lungs, heart and blood vessels, and the blood. The adequacy of the system is dependent upon the processes of ventilation, diffusion, perfusion, and the capacity of blood to carry the respiratory gases.

Oxygen Transport

Oxygen is transported in the blood in two forms: (1) physically dissolved in the liquid or plasma portion of the blood, and (2) chemically bound to hemoglobin. The amount of oxygen that is physically dissolved in blood is directly proportional to the partial arterial pressure of oxygen (Pa_{O_2}). However, as discussed earlier, oxygen is relatively insoluble in water, and thus only 0.30 cc of oxygen can be dissolved in 100 mL of blood. If the oxygen requirement of the body were to be met simply by the dissolved oxygen in the plasma, then the P_{O_2} would have to be 2000 mm Hg. The largest amount (98%) of oxygen is transported by hemoglobin, the bright red pigmented protein found in red blood cells. Oxygen binds rapidly (0.01 second) and reversibly with hemoglobin to form oxyhemoglobin (HbO_2). Hemoglobin that is not combined with oxygen is called reduced hemoglobin (Hb).

Hemoglobin is a protein made up of four subunits, each containing a heme moiety attached to a polypeptide chain. The four polypeptide chains comprise the globin portion of the hemoglobin molecule. Two of the subunits, alpha chains, have 140 amino acid residues, whereas the other two subunits, beta chains, have 146 amino acid residues. Individuals who have equal quantities of alpha and beta chains in their hemoglobin are said to have hemoglobin A. The heme moiety is a complex made up of a porphyrin and one atom of iron (Fe^{2+}). Each of the four iron atoms can bind reversibly with one O_2 molecule according to the following formulas:

$$Hb_4 \quad + \; O_2 \rightleftharpoons Hb_4O_2 \; (25\% \text{ saturated})$$
$$Hb_4O_2 + \; O_2 \rightleftharpoons Hb_4O_4 \; (50\% \text{ saturated})$$
$$Hb_4O_4 + \; O_2 \rightleftharpoons Hb_4O_6 \; (75\% \text{ saturated})$$
$$Hb_4O_6 + \; O_2 \rightleftharpoons Hb_4O_8 \; (100\% \text{ saturated})$$

The reactions of oxygen with heme are called oxygenation, not oxidation, because the iron remains in the ferrous (Fe^{2+}) state. Frequently, the reactions of oxygen with hemoglobin are abbreviated to $Hb + O_2 \rightleftharpoons HbO_2$ when in reality each molecule of hemoglobin can bind four molecules of O_2.

The structure of the hemoglobin molecule determines its affinity for oxygen by shifting the position of its four component polypeptide chains, fostering either O_2 uptake or O_2 delivery. The movement of the polypeptide chains results in a change in position of the heme moieties, which assume an R state (relaxed state), favoring O_2 binding, or a T state (tense state), decreasing O_2 binding. The transition from the R state to the T state is due to the breaking or forming of salt bridges between the polypeptide chains. When hemoglobin binds to oxygen the two beta chains move close together, and when oxygen is given up they move farther apart. The oxygen hemoglobin dissociation curve (Fig. 23–19), relating the percentage of oxygen saturation of hemoglobin to the P_{O_2}, is characteristically sigmoid-shaped due

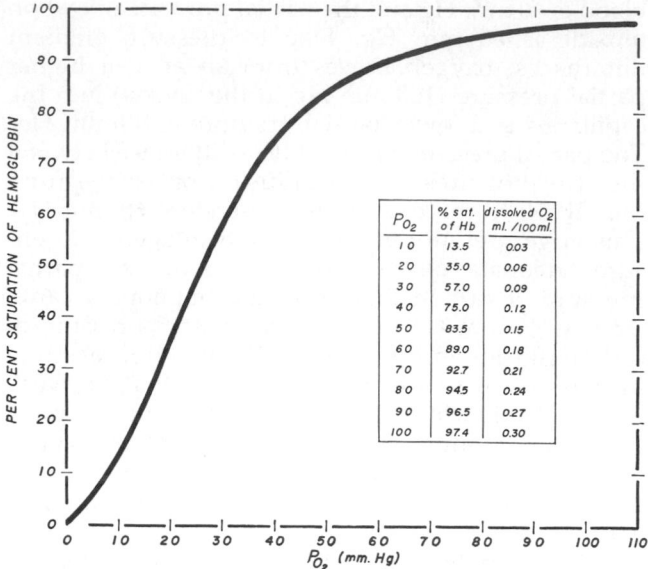

P_{O_2}	% sat. of Hb	dissolved O_2 ml. /100 ml.
10	13.5	0.03
20	35.0	0.06
30	57.0	0.09
40	75.0	0.12
50	83.5	0.15
60	89.0	0.18
70	92.7	0.21
80	94.5	0.24
90	96.5	0.27
100	97.4	0.30

FIGURE 23–19. Oxyhemoglobin dissociation curve at temperature 38° C, pH 7.40.

to the movement of the polypeptide chains of the hemoglobin molecule. The combination of oxygen (O_2) with the first heme increases the affinity of the second heme for O_2, which in turn increases the affinity of the third, and so on. Similarly, the release of O_2 by each of the four iron atoms enhances the release of O_2 molecules from the remaining iron atoms.

One gram of hemoglobin is capable of combining with 1.34 mL of oxygen and is called the oxygen capacity. At a normal hemoglobin concentration of 15 g/100 mL of blood, the blood is capable of carrying approximately 20 mL O_2/100 mL, or 20 volume percent.

$$\frac{15 \text{ g Hb}}{100 \text{ mL blood}} \times \frac{1.34 \text{ mL } O_2}{1 \text{ g Hb}} = 20.1 \text{ mL } O_2/100 \text{ mL blood}$$

Oxygen-carrying capacity of the blood is dependent upon the amount of hemoglobin in the blood. The actual amount of O_2 in combination with hemoglobin is less than the capacity. The actual amount of O_2 carried on the hemoglobin is called the oxygen content. The ratio of the O_2 content to the O_2 capacity is expressed as a percentage and is called the oxygen saturation (Sa_{O_2}).

$$\frac{\text{How much oxygen carried by hemoglobin (content)}}{\text{How much oxygen hemoglobin is capable of carrying (capacity)}}$$

$$Sa_{O_2} = 100 \times \frac{\text{Content}}{\text{Capacity}}$$

The oxygen content and oxygen saturation of blood increase progressively with increasing P_{O_2} as depicted in Figure 23–19. The upper flat region of the oxyhemoglobin dissociation curve indicates that the oxygen saturation and hence hemoglobin affinity are relatively constant (92.7% to 97.5%) over an approximate range of 70 to 110 P_{O_2}. Therefore, small changes in P_{O_2} produced by changes in alveolar ventilation ordinarily have little effect on oxygen saturation. However, changes in oxygen saturation are more pronounced in the lower P_{O_2} ranges below 55 mm Hg. Because of the steep slope of the oxyhemoglobin dissociation curve below 55 mm Hg P_{O_2}, large quantities of O_2 can be unloaded from the blood to the tissues with a relatively small decrease in blood P_{O_2}.

The amount of oxygen bound to hemoglobin is affected not only by the oxygen tension (P_{O_2}) but also by the partial pressure of carbon dioxide (P_{CO_2}), the pH, the temperature of the blood, and the concentration of 2,3-diphosphoglycerate (2,3-DPG). The HbO_2 dissociation curve is shifted to the right by an increase in carbon dioxide, a decrease in pH, an increase in temperature, or an increase in the concentration of 2,3-DPG (Fig. 23–20). Therefore, at any given partial pressure of O_2, hemoglobin is less saturated, and the delivery of oxygen from the blood to the tissues is enhanced. Increased tissue metabolism, as occurs with an increase in body temperature, results in increased CO_2 production and a local decrease in pH. The shift in the oxyhemoglobin dissociation curve to the right with increased CO_2, decreased pH, and increased temperature facilitates the unloading of O_2 from the hemoglobin to the blood to meet the increased metabolic needs of the cell.

2,3-DPG is very plentiful in red cells. It is formed in the erythrocyte by anaerobic glycolysis and has a half-life of 6 hours. It is a highly charged anion that binds to the beta chains of deoxygenated hemoglobin but not to those of oxyhemoglobin, thereby causing the release of oxygen.

$$HbO_2 + 2,3\text{-DPG} \rightleftharpoons Hb\text{-}2,3\text{-DPG} + O_2$$

2,3-DPG concentration in the red blood cells is decreased in patients with acidosis due to inhibition of red blood cell glycolysis. Thyroid hormone, growth hormone, androgens, exercise in the untrained athlete, high altitude, and chronic anemia increase the concentration of 2,3-DPG, thereby enhancing oxygen delivery to the tissues. In stored bank blood, 2,3-DPG levels fall, reducing the ability of the transfused blood to release O_2 to the tissues.

In contrast, the HbO_2 dissociation curve is shifted to the left with decreased carbon dioxide levels, increased pH, decreased temperature, or decreased 2,3-DPG, enhancing the affinity of hemoglobin for oxygen and improving oxygen saturation at lower P_{O_2} levels. However, the enhancement of hemoglobin's affinity for oxygen decreases the unloading of oxygen at the tissue level. This phenomenon should be kept in mind when caring for patients with hypothermia, which reduces cellular metabolism while simultaneously decreasing the availability of oxygen at the tissue level.

Carbon Dioxide Transport

Carbon dioxide is transported to the lungs in the plasma of blood and in the erythrocyte in three forms: (1) dissolved in the plasma or liquid portion of the erythrocyte, (2) as a carbamino compound combined with blood proteins and plasma proteins, and (3) as bicarbonate (HCO_3^-) ion. The volume of carbon dioxide dissolved in the blood depends on the partial pressure of CO_2, as with oxygen. Because carbon dioxide is 24 times more soluble than oxygen, more is transported in the dissolved form. A small fraction, about 20% of the total CO_2, is carried to the lungs in the blood as carbamino compounds formed by the reaction between CO_2 and the amino groups (NH_2 groups) of the proteins in both plasma and erythrocytes. The amino groups of hemoglobin, for example, react with carbon dioxide in the following manner:

$$Hb - NH_2 + CO_2 \rightleftharpoons Hb - NHCOO^- + H^+$$

As oxygen is given up to the tissues from Hb, CO_2 combines very rapidly with Hb. Deoxyhemoglobin is able to form carbamino compounds more readily than oxyhemoglobin, and consequently CO_2 transport in venous blood is achieved more readily than in arterial blood.

The carbon dioxide that diffuses into the plasma and the erythrocytes combines rapidly with water

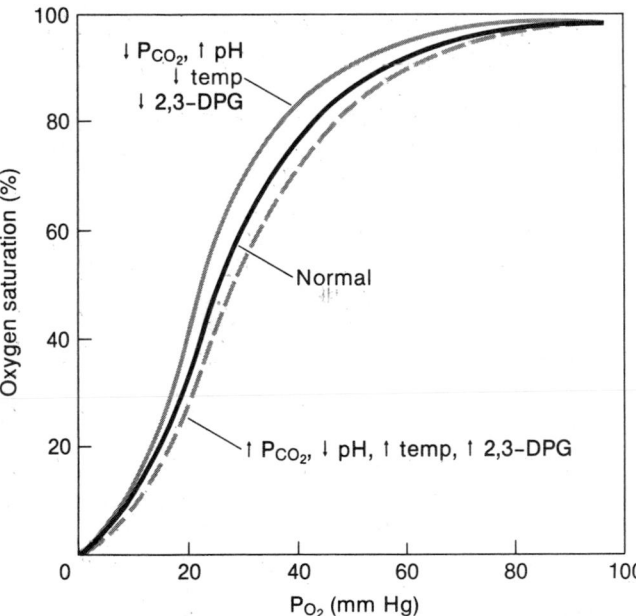

FIGURE 23–20. The effects of changes in P_{CO_2}, pH, temperature, and 2,3-diphosphoglycerate (2,3-DPG) on oxygen binding to hemoglobin. An increase in partial pressure of CO_2, decrease in pH, increase in temperature, or increase in 2,3-DPG produce a shift to the right of the hemoglobin oxygen dissociation curve. The hemoglobin oxygen dissociation curve is shifted to the left by a fall in carbon dioxide, increase in pH, decrease in temperature, or decrease in concentration of 2,3-DPG. (Modified from Berne, R. M., and Levy, M. N. (1988). *Physiology* (2nd ed., p. 610). St. Louis: C. V. Mosby.)

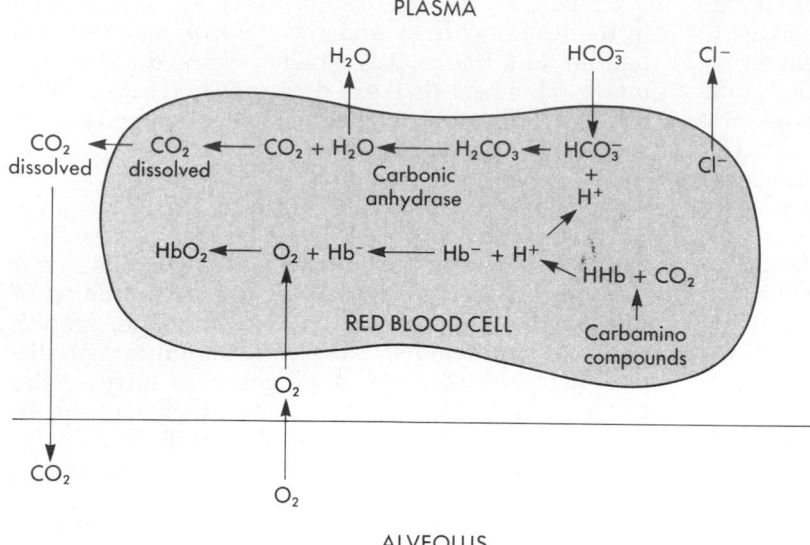

PLASMA

ALVEOLUS

FIGURE 23–21. Carbon dioxide transport in blood. (From Berne, R. M., and Levy, M. N. (1988). *Physiology* (2nd ed.). St. Louis: C. V. Mosby.)

(hydration reaction) in the presence of the enzymatic catalyst carbonic anhydrase to form carbonic acid (H_2CO_3). The H_2CO_3 dissociates rapidly to H^+ and HCO_3^- according to the formula depicted in Figure 23–21. The hydration reaction takes approximately 200 seconds and is rapidly reversed in the lungs to permit the diffusion of carbon dioxide into the alveoli. The H^- ion formed in the hydration reaction is buffered by deoxygenated hemoglobin, and the HCO_3^- enters the plasma. Because the HCO_3^- content rises 70% in the plasma as the blood passes through the tissue capillaries, electrochemical neutrality is maintained by Cl^- entering the red cells in exchange for HCO_3^-; this is called the chloride shift. The hydration reaction allows large amounts of carbon dioxide to be carried to the lungs in the form of HCO_3^-.

Arterial blood gases provide important information about the concentration of the respiratory gases in the arterial blood and about the effectiveness of ventilation, perfusion, and diffusion. The normal arterial blood gas values are as follows:

Pa_{O_2}	95–100 mmHg	⎫ Oxygenation
Sa_{O_2}	97%	⎬ status
pH	7.35–7.45	⎫
Pa_{CO_2}	38–42 mmHg	⎬ Acid-base status
HCO_3^-	23–25 milliequivalents/liter	⎭

Pa_{O_2} and the Sa_{O_2} provide information about the oxygenation status of the individual, whereas the pH, Pa_{CO_2}, and HCO_3^- reveal information about acid-base status. For the body to function optimally these values must remain within these narrow ranges. A complete discussion of acid-base balance is provided in Chapter 24.

CONTROL OF RESPIRATION

The respiratory system has fine controls to adjust the rate of alveolar ventilation to meet the demands of the body exactly and to maintain the partial pressures of oxygen and carbon dioxide and the pH of the blood at normal levels. Control of the respiratory system is achieved through both neural and chemical control.

Neural Control

The nervous system provides both voluntary control through the cerebral cortex via the corticospinal tracts to the respiratory muscles and automatic control through the medulla and pons of the brainstem. Normal resting respiration requires cyclical respiratory muscle excitation from the brain through the phrenic nerves to the diaphragm and from the spinal nerves to the external intercostals resulting in active contraction of the inspiratory muscles, thereby producing expansion of the thoracic cage and inspiration. The accessory muscles of inspiration, including the scalene and sternocleidomastoid muscles, are activated in stimulated respiration. Passive relaxation of the inspiratory muscles causes the thoracic cage and the lungs through their own weight to resume a resting state. The motor neurons to the expiratory muscles are inhibited, whereas the inspiratory muscles are stimulated through reciprocal innervation. When expiration must be facilitated, stimulation through the spinal nerves causes contraction of the internal intercostals and the abdominal muscles. An individual can voluntarily alter the rate and depth and pattern of breathing through mechanisms in the cerebral cortex.

Medullary and Pontine Neural Control

Rhythmic cyclical discharge of neurons located in the medulla oblongata produces automatic respiration. The precise anatomic and physiologic function of the respiratory medullary neurons is under investigation. Current research indicates that there are two groups of respiratory neurons in the medulla. The dorsal group of neurons is in or near the nucleus of the tractus solitarius and is the source of rhythmic drive to the contralateral phrenic motor neurons. The neurons in the dorsal group project to and drive the ventral group. The ventral group has two divisions: The cranial division is composed of neurons in the nucleus ambiguous that innervate the accessory muscles of respiration on the same side, and the caudal division is composed of neurons in the nucleus retroambigualis that provide inspiratory and expiratory input to the intercostal muscles (Fig. 23–22).

Although the rhythmic discharge of the neurons in the medullary respiratory center is spontaneous, research to date has failed to demonstrate actual pacemaker cells similar to those in the sinoatrial (SA) node in the heart, which drive respiration. Research has shown that the rhythmic discharge of the medullary neurons is modified by centers in the pons and by afferent information via the vagus nerve from stretch receptors (mechanoreceptors) in the lungs. Research studies examining the role of the pneumotaxic and apneustic centers in the pons have been performed in anesthetized animal models in which the brainstem was transected above the pons. When the brainstem is transected at this point, normal regular breathing occurs (point A in Fig. 23–23). When the pneumotaxic center is intact and the vagus nerve is cut, the depth of respiration is increased, indicating that the vagus nerve sends information from stretch receptors in the lung that provide information about the stretch of the lungs during inspiration. With the vagus intact, stretching of the lungs during inspiration reflexly inhibits the inspiratory drive, reinforcing the function of the pneumotaxic center in producing intermittent inspiratory neuron discharge. The pneumotaxic center causes stimula-

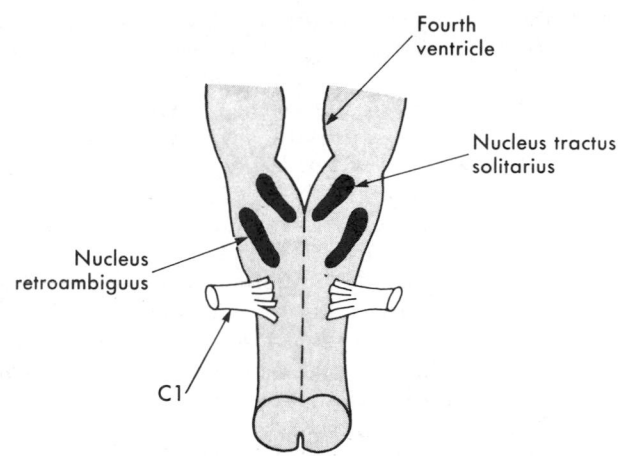

FIGURE 23–22. Neuronal group in the brainstem that controls respiration. (From Berne, R. M., and Levy, M. N. (1988). *Physiology* (2nd ed., p. 625). St. Louis: C. V. Mosby.)

tion of the expiratory neurons and simultaneously inhibits the inspiratory center, thus promoting regular cyclical respirations. Transection of the brainstem in the inferior portion of the pons (point B in Fig. 23–23) results in continuous inspiratory discharge with the vagus intact. When the vagi are cut, respiration in inspiration is arrested (called apneusis, hence the name apneustic center). When all pontine tissue is separated from the medulla (point C in Fig. 23–23) respirations are irregular and gasping, indicating that the medullary respiratory neurons may be capable of spontaneous rhythmic discharge. Complete transection of the brainstem below the medulla (point D in Fig. 23–23) stops all respirations.

Chemical Control

Central chemoreceptors are located in the medulla and account for 70% to 80% of the increase in

FIGURE 23–23. Respiratory patterns following complete transection of the brainstem at four levels: A, B, C, and D. (From Jensen, D. (1980). *The principles of physiology* (2nd ed., p. 674). New York: Appleton-Century-Crofts.)

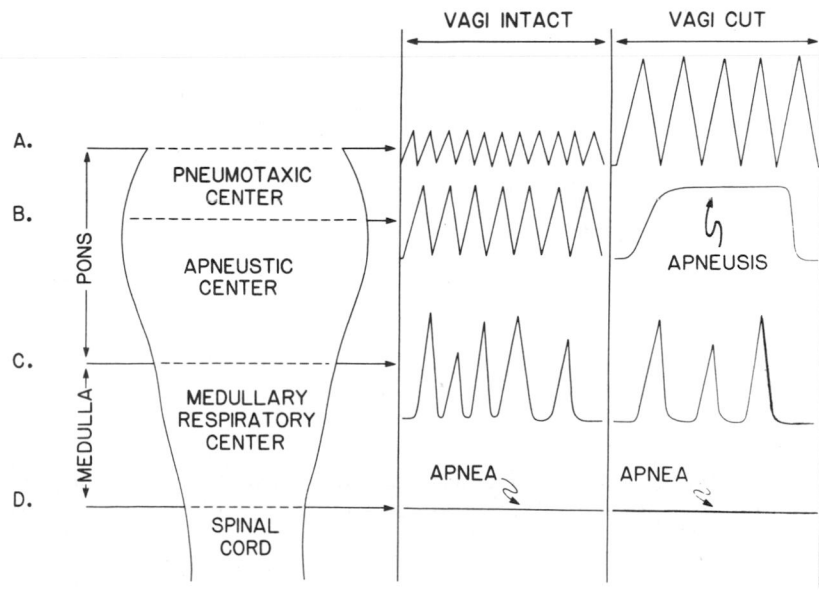

ventilation when carbon dioxide levels are elevated. The peripheral chemoreceptors, located in the carotid and aortic bodies, are responsible for 20% to 30%. The exact location of the central chemoreceptors is unknown, but it is hypothesized to be near the ventrolateral surface of the medulla. The medullary chemoreceptors monitor the H^+ ion concentration of the cerebrospinal fluid (CSF) and the brainstem interstitial fluid. Unfortunately, H^+ ion and HCO_3^- ions are unable to cross the blood–brain barrier and the blood–CSF barrier easily. On the other hand, carbon dioxide readily penetrates these barriers and immediately following hydration forms carbonic acid (H_2CO_3), which dissociates into H^+ ion and HCO_3^-. The H^+ ion concentration in brain interstitial fluid parallels the arterial P_{CO_2} and acts as the stimulus for increases in respiration. There is a linear relationship between the respiratory minute volume and the alveolar P_{CO_2} to an upper limit of 100 mm Hg Pa_{CO_2}. Accumulation of CO_2 in the body (called hypercapnia) depresses the central nervous system and the respiratory center and produces headache, confusion, and eventually coma.

The peripheral chemoreceptors include the carotid body near the bifurcation of the internal and external

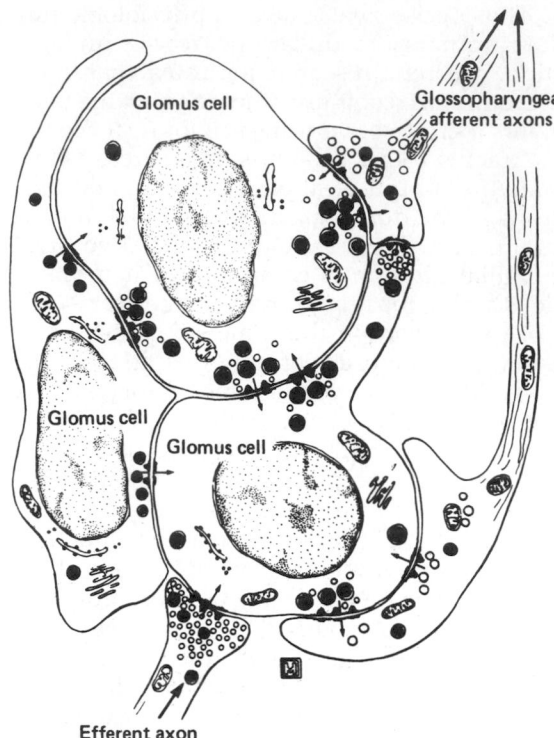

FIGURE 23–25. Organization of the carotid and aortic bodies. (Modified from McDonald, D. M., and Mitchell, R. A. (1975). The innervation of glomus cells, ganglion cells, and blood vessels in the rat carotid body. A quantitative ultrastructural study. *Journal of Neurocytology*, 4, 177. Chapman & Hall, London.)

carotid arteries and the aortic bodies near the arch of the aorta (Fig. 23–24). The carotid and aortic bodies are composed of islands of type I and type II cells surrounded by capillaries with large openings or fenestrations (Fig. 23–25). The carotid bodies receive a tremendous blood supply (0.04 mL/minute or 2000 mL/100 g of tissue per minute). The type I cells are surrounded by nerve endings from the glossopharyngeal nerve to the carotid bodies and from the vagi to the aortic bodies. Type I cells are sensitive to the concentration of the partial pressure of oxygen dis-

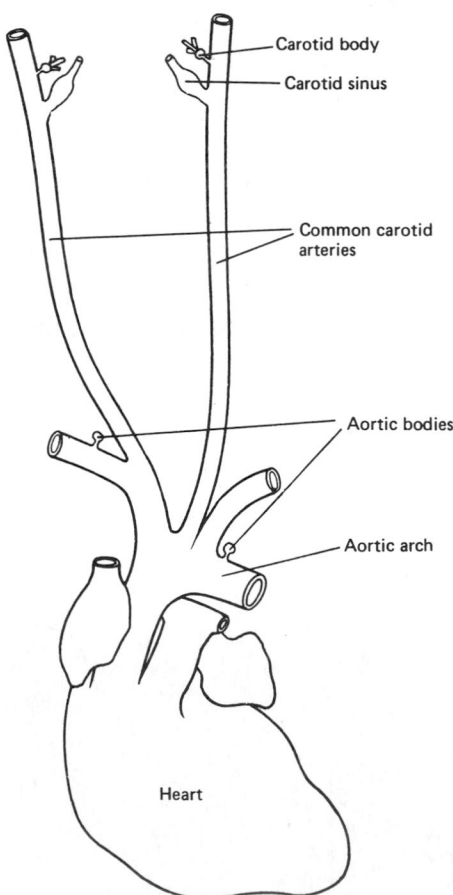

FIGURE 23–24. Location of the carotid and aortic bodies. (From Ganong, W. F. (1983). *Review of medical physiology* (11th ed.) Los Altos, CA: Lange Medical Publications.)

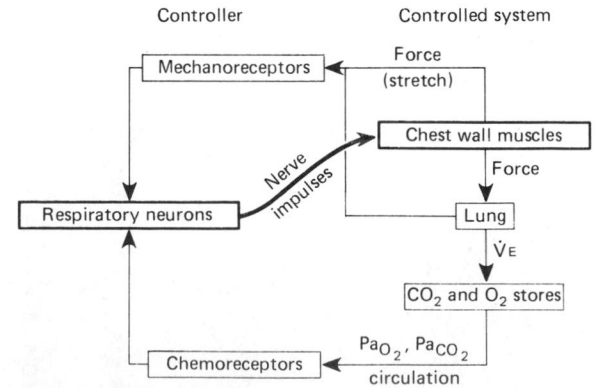

FIGURE 23–26. Control of the respiratory system. (Reproduced with permission from Fishman, A. P. (1980). *Assessment of pulmonary function.* New York: McGraw-Hill.)

solved in the liquid plasma of the blood. Afferent nerve fibers from the carotid and aortic bodies ascend to the medulla and cause an increase in ventilation when the Pa_{O_2} falls below 60 mm Hg, which is the point at which hemoglobin saturation declines. Because the receptors are sensitive to Pa_{O_2} dissolved in the plasma, they do not respond in patients with such conditions as anemia or carbon monoxide poisoning, which affect the concentration of Hb or the content of oxygen on the hemoglobin molecule. The carotid and aortic bodies are primarily stimulated by an elevated Pa_{CO_2} or an increased H^+ ion concentration and secondarily by a marked decrease in Pa_{O_2}. Chronic sustained hypoxia appears to depress the carotid and aortic chemoreceptor response to low Pa_{O_2}, and peripheral control is dependent upon the levels of Pa_{CO_2} and H^+ ion to increase ventilation.

SUMMARY

The relationship of the neural and chemical control of the respiratory system is summarized in Figure 23–26. Control of respiration is an intricate interplay between neural and chemical factors that serve to maintain the levels of Pa_{O_2}, Pa_{CO_2}, and pH at a constant level to promote the optimal functioning of the cells of the body.

References

Berne, R. M., and Levy, M. N. (1988). *Physiology* (2nd ed.). St. Louis: C. V. Mosby.

Comroe, J. H., Jr. (1965). *Physiology of respiration.* Chicago: Year Book.

Fishman, A. P. (1980). *Assessment of pulmonary function.* New York: McGraw-Hill.

Ganong, W. F. (1987). *Review of medical physiology* (13th ed.). Norwalk, CT: Appleton & Lange.

Guyton, A. C. (1991). *Textbook of medical physiology* (8th ed.). Philadelphia: W. B. Saunders.

Jensen, D. (1980). *The principles of physiology* (2nd ed.). New York: Appleton-Century-Crofts.

Kersten, L. D. (1989). *Comprehensive respiratory nursing.* Philadelphia: W. B. Saunders.

Luciano, D. S., Vander, A. J., and Sherman, J. H. (1978). *Human function and structure.* New York: McGraw-Hill.

Vander, A. J., Sherman, J. H., and Luciano, D. S. (1975). *Human physiology: The mechanisms of body function* (2nd ed.). New York: McGraw-Hill.

24

Acid-Base Physiology

Carol F. Baker

Man is an acid-producing system that continually forms acids by means of carbohydrate, fat, and glucose metabolism. The hydrogen ion concentration (H^+) of body fluids is represented by the symbol pH. For human life, the pH of extracellular fluids must be maintained within a fairly narrow range (7.35 to 7.45). Other fluids of the body such as urine undergo wide fluctuations in pH. Immediately on detecting a change from normal, feedback mechanisms are initiated to adjust for the altered state. Usually these compensatory mechanisms are successful in returning the blood pH to within the normal range. The body cells and organs, especially the brain and heart, are very susceptible to changes in pH and tolerate them poorly. The range of blood pH compatible with life is 6.8 to 8.0. Thus, the regulation of hydrogen ion concentration is one of the most important aspects of homeostasis or the steady state necessary to maintain health (Guyton, 1991).

Interestingly enough, the body tolerates acidosis better than alkalosis. The regulatory mechanisms are designed primarily to remove acid and restore base. Carbon dioxide is normally the most potent stimulus of the respiratory center. Increases in the partial pressure of carbon dioxide stimulate the respiratory center, causing increased ventilation. Carbon dioxide in water forms carbonic acid: $CO_2 + H_2O \rightarrow H_2CO_3$. With the increased loss of carbon dioxide, carbonic acid is reduced. One of the primary functions of the kidney tubules is to retain base and excrete organic and inorganic acids. This mechanism facilitates neutralization or removal of unwanted acid. Though regulatory mechanisms exist to correct alkalosis, they are less powerful and may take a longer period of time. The body tolerates this condition poorly, though it is less severe or life threatening.

KEY DEFINITIONS

In order to understand the regulation of acid-base balance, appropriate principles and terms need to be defined first (Appel and Chase, 1986; Goldberger, 1986; Guyton, 1991).

1. An *acid* is a molecule or ion that can release a hydrogen ion into a solution. Carbonic acid ionizes in water to form $H^+ + HCO_3^-$, and hydrochloric acid ionizes to $H^+ + Cl^-$. An acid can be a simple or complex ion. Some other acids in the body are acetic, uric, and lactic acids.

2. *Acidosis* is the state of excess addition of hydrogen ions or a loss of basic ions to solutions.

3. A *base* is a molecule or an ion that combines with hydrogen ions and removes them from a solution. Some examples of base in the body are bicarbonate, phosphate, proteins, and hemoglobin.

4. *Alkalosis* is the excess removal of hydrogen ions or the addition of basic ions to solutions. An alkali is the combination of one of the alkaline metals (sodium or potassium, for example) with a highly basic ion such as the hydroxyl ion (OH^-).

5. *Strong versus weak reaction:* A strong acid is one in which the hydrogen ion has a very strong tendency to dissociate and discharge its hydrogen ion into solution, such as hydrochloric acid (HCl). A weak acid releases hydrogen ions more slowly, such as carbonic acid (H_2CO_3). A strong base reacts powerfully with hydrogen ions to remove them rapidly from solution, such as the hydroxyl ion (OH^-). The bicarbonate ion (HCO_3^-) is a weak base but is the primary buffering system of the body.

6. *pH* is the symbol used to express the concentration of hydrogen ions in solutions. The actual hydrogen ion concentration in extracellular fluid

(ECF) is normally regulated at a constant value of approximately 4×10^{-8} mEq/liter. To alleviate cumbersome calculation, a logarithmic figure (pH) was derived for ease of expression. pH is related to actual hydrogen ion concentration by the following formula:

$$pH = 6.1 + \log HCO_3^-/H_2CO_3 + CO_2$$

A low pH (6.7 to 7.35 in ECF) corresponds to a high hydrogen ion concentration, acidosis. A high pH (7.45 to 7.9 in ECF) corresponds to alkalosis.

7. *Compensatory mechanisms* are the responses of the buffers, the respiratory or the renal systems, to alterations in the opposite system; that is, respiratory acidosis is compensated by the kidney's reabsorption of bicarbonate.

An *uncompensated* state is a single or complex acid-base disorder resulting in an abnormal pH and abnormal respiratory or renal signs.

A *compensated* state occurs when the pH returns to normal after an acid-base imbalance, but respiratory or renal signs may remain abnormal until the imbalance is corrected.

8. Measured *anions* are ions with a negative valence, such as bicarbonate (HCO_3^-) and chloride (Cl^-).

9. Measured *cations* are ions with a positive valence, such as sodium (Na^+), potassium (K^+), calcium (Ca^{2+}). The sum of measured cations is greater than the sum of measured anions due to the presence of unmeasured anions.

10. An *anion gap* describes the residual (R) of unmeasured anions, proteins, phosphates, sulfates, and organic acid, usually 16 mEq/liter.

SOURCES OF ACIDS AND BASES IN THE BODY

Large amounts of *carbon dioxide* are continuously formed from the metabolism of carbohydrates and fats. Some of the carbon dioxide combines with water to form carbonic acid ($CO_2 + H_2O = H_2CO_3$). The majority of the gas is eliminated through the lungs and is regulated by the rate and depth of pulmonary ventilation. *Fixed acids* consist of all other acids in the body, sulfuric, lactic, acetoacetic, and so on. The majority are formed as a result of protein metabolism. Hydrogen ions produced from the dissociation of fixed acids are excreted by the kidneys. The amount of fixed acids produced daily is much less than the amount of carbon dioxide (Muir, 1980).

Glucose Metabolism

The metabolism of glucose results eventually in the formation of carbon dioxide and water. Complete oxidation of one mole of glucose releases 686,000 calories of energy to form a total of 38 moles of ATP (Guyton, 1987). There are several steps in the process of the oxidation of glucose for energy:

1. Glycolysis is the splitting of the glucose molecule to form two molecules of pyruvic acid, 2 moles of ATP, and hydrogen atoms. The efficiency of energy in the formation of ATP is 43%, whereas 57% of the energy is lost as heat.

2. Pyruvic acid is converted into two molecules of acetyl coenzyme A (acetyl Co-A), carbon dioxide, and hydrogen atoms.

3. In the citric acid cycle (Krebs cycle), the acetyl portion of acetyl Co-A is degraded to carbon dioxide, hydrogen atoms, and coenzyme A. Two molecules of ATP are formed in the citric acid cycle for each molecule of glucose metabolized.

4. Oxidative phosphorylation is the process by which 95% of the ATP is formed during oxidation of the hydrogen atoms released in earlier mechanisms. The hydrogen atoms are changed into hydrogen ions (H^+) and electrons, these are used to change the dissolved oxygen into hydroxyl ions (OH^-), and finally the hydrogen and hydroxyl ions combine to form water. Tremendous quantities of energy are released to form ATP. The overall efficiency of energy transfer into ATP is 66%, whereas the remaining 34% becomes heat. End products of metabolism are carbon dioxide and water.

Anaerobic Glycolysis

When oxygen becomes unavailable or is insufficient to allow cellular oxidation of glucose, anaerobic glycolysis occurs. Anaerobic metabolism can be a life-saving process. When the buildup of pyruvic acid and hydrogen atoms becomes excessive, lactic acid is formed. It can diffuse into extracellular and intracellular fluids, allowing the conversion of ATP to continue and glycolysis to proceed much longer without oxygen. Large amounts of lactic acid are released from skeletal muscle during heavy exercise or during severe tissue hypoxia, such as with a myocardial infarction, causing metabolic acidosis. When oxygen is again available, lactic and pyruvic acids are oxidized in the liver and can be used in glucose reconversion or directly for energy. Heart muscle is especially capable of converting lactic to pyruvic acid and utilizing it for energy, especially during heavy exercise (Guyton, 1991).

Protein Metabolism

Protein metabolism results in the production of strong organic acids: sulfuric and phosphoric acids. There is a limit to the amount of protein that can be used in any cell. Once that limit has been reached, any additional amino acids in body fluids will be degraded in the liver and used for energy or stored as fat. The process of deamination of protein is the removal of amino groups from amino acids. This can occur by one of two processes. The first is transamination, or the transfer of amino groups to another substance, such as to glutamic acid, which then releases it in the form of ammonia. The ammonia is converted in the liver into urea and is excreted by the kidney. The second method of deamination is the oxidation of amino acids into pyruvic acid and glucose or into keto (fatty) acids with ketogenesis.

Fat Metabolism

Fat metabolism occurs with the degrading and oxidation of fatty acids in the cell, resulting in the production of acetyl Co-A. Acetyl Co-A enters the citric acid cycle and is converted into carbon dioxide and hydrogen ions in the liver. Excess accumulation of acetyl Co-A results in pairing to form acetoacetic acid. This is converted into large quantities of beta-hydroxybutyric acid and small amounts of acetone. During abnormal states such as starvation, diabetes mellitus, or a high fat diet, ketosis occurs. Ketosis is the production of ketone bodies, which are converted into beta-hydroxybutyric acid and acetone.

Diet and Medication

The diet can be a source of acid ranging from fruits containing citric, acetic, tannic, or ascorbic acids, to fat and especially protein. Heavy meat eaters tend to have an increased production of acid. The major source of alkali production in the body is the catabolism of dietary organic anions such as lactate, citrate, and isocitrate to carbon dioxide and water. They are present in all foods but are especially prevalent in fruits and vegetables. Other sources of base in the diet include milk products, which contain calcium. Vegetarians tend to have a net production of alkali (Guyton, 1987, 1991; Muir, 1980). Medications such as ammonium choride and aspirin are sources of acid. Antacids are a source of base.

pH OF NORMAL BODY FLUIDS

Although the range of pH in the extracellular fluid that is compatible with life approximates that of water and is narrow, the relative acid or alkaline characteristics of other body fluids vary considerably and are dependent on the particular organ's function. For instance, gastric fluid is highly acid, reflecting the large concentration of hydrochloric acid in the stomach. On the other hand, fluids containing pancreatic enzymes are basic. Urine has the widest range in pH, varying from highly acidic to highly basic depending on the pH of plasma. Normal values of pH of body fluids are shown in Table 24–1.

DEFENSE AGAINST CHANGES IN ACID-BASE BALANCE

To maintain a homeostatic balance and a normal pH, the body first buffers the acids produced by

TABLE 24–1. pH of Normal Body Fluids

Extracellular fluid	7.35–7.45
Cerebrospinal fluid	7.35–7.45
Intracellular fluid	6.9–7.2
Bile–gallbladder	5.0–6.0
Pancreatic	7.6–8.2
Urine	4.0–8.0
Gastric	1.0–2.0
Intestine	6.5–7.6
Bile–liver	7.4

metabolism and then removes excess H^+ from the body (Appel and Chase, 1986). Several regulatory systems are sequentially available to readjust for constant fluctations in acid-base balance. The chemical buffer system response is both intracellular and extracellular and occurs within seconds. This mechanism is temporary until the other regulatory mechansims go into effect. The respiratory system buffer response occurs in a few minutes to hours, and is primarily concerned with the excretion of carbon dioxide. The renal system buffer response occurs within hours to days and is the most powerful response. It removes excess acid or base from the body and restores or retains the bicarbonate buffer base.

The Buffer System

A chemical buffer is a substance that prevents rapid or great change in the pH of a solution when an acid or a base is added. A buffer system usually consists of a pair of compounds: a weak acid and its conjugate base. For example, when hydrochloric acid is added to water, the strong acid dissociates completely, releasing many hydrogen ions into solution and markedly lowering the pH of the solution. When sodium bicarbonate is added as a weak base, it dissociates in water. The hydrogen ions combine with bicarbonate, forming carbonic acid, a weak acid, and a salt, sodium chloride:

$$H^+ + Cl^- + Na^+ \ HCO_3^- \rightarrow H_2CO_3 + NaCl$$

The strong acid is replaced with a weak acid that dissociates only slightly. If a strong base such as sodium hydroxide were added to the system, carbonic acid would dissociate to release hydrogen ions, forming a weak base and water:

$$NaOH + H_2CO_3 = Na \ HCO_3 + H_2O$$

A buffer system works most efficiently when the concentrations of the weak acid and conjugate base are equal (Muir, 1980).

There are several major buffer systems in the body. Extracellular buffers include bicarbonate, proteins, plasma, and bone. The most important buffer of the extracellular fluid, especially the interstitial fluid, is the bicarbonate–carbonic acid system. However, bicarbonate cannot buffer carbonic acid because it would simply regenerate itself ($H_2CO_3 = H^+ + HCO_3^-$). The intracellular compartment may provide up to 50% of the total body buffering response by intracellular proteins, hemoglobin, phosphates, and other organic buffers (Appel and Chase, 1986).

The *bicarbonate buffer system* is a mixture of carbonic acid and sodium bicarbonate in solution, as seen in the formula above. The concentrations of carbonic acid and dissolved carbon dioxide form the total "carbonic acid pool" available for buffer action. Because the amount of carbonic acid in body fluids is small, the strength of the buffer pool is determined by the amount of dissolved or partial pressure of carbon dioxide P_{CO_2}.

Maximal buffering occurs when the ratio of available base (bicarbonate concentration) to the carbonic acid pool is 20 to 1. This ratio is measured in terms of the pH of the acid-containing solution. Different acids have various buffering capacities depending on their pK (the pH at which half the acid is undissociated). This ratio is called the Henderson-Hasselbach equation and is expressed as:

pH = pK (a constant of 6.1)
  + log[$BHCO_3$ bicarbonate]/[HA carbonic acid pool]

The buffer pair loses buffering capacity if either the base or carbonic acid is totally consumed. Even though considerable amount of base is required to buffer the acid, the strength of the system lies in the fact that each member is capable of being regulated independently by either the kidneys or the lungs. If there is a shift in the ratio, an imbalance occurs. An excess of base (30:1) or a deficit of acid (20:0.5) produces an alkalotic state and an increase in pH. On the other hand, an excess of acid (20:2) or a deficit of base (10:1) produces an acidotic state and a decrease in pH. A change in the bicarbonate buffer system will be reflected by changes in the other buffer systems in solution.

The *phosphate buffer system* is important in red blood cells and especially in the cells of kidney tubules, where it enables the kidneys to excrete hydrogen ions. The buffer system is composed primarily of a weak acid, sodium dihydrogen phosphate ($NaH_2PO_4 = Na^+ + H^+ + HPO_4^{2-}$) and its conjugate base, sodium monohydrogen phosphate (Na_2HPO_4). In the kidneys' intracellular fluid, high concentrations of the monohydrogen phosphate are available to combine with hydrogen ions, which are secreted into the urine and eliminated along with NaCl. On the other hand, if a strong base is introduced into the body, the dihydrogen phosphate can combine with it, forming a weak base and water (Goldberger, 1986).

The *protein buffer system* consists of a weak acid (H^+-protein) and a weak base (Na^+-protein) and is found in proteins in cells and in plasma. Carbon dioxide diffuses readily through the cell membranes, followed more slowly by bicarbonate and hydrogen ions. This diffusion causes the intracellular pH to change in proportion to changes in the extracellular fluid. However, the change occurs over several hours; it cannot respond to rapid changes in the extracellular fluid. Fixed acids produced inside the cells, such as sulfuric acid, are also initially buffered by proteins and phosphate before they enter the extracellular fluid. Proteins act as anions, carrying many negative charges in the alkaline pH of body fluids (Goldberger, 1986; Muir, 1980).

Hemoglobin of the red blood cells is a protein buffer that is very important in buffering carbon dioxide while it is being transported to the lungs for elimination. Carbon dioxide enters the blood as a byproduct of tissue metabolism. Some (5%) is immediately transformed into carbonic acid and carried in solution by the plasma. This process occurs slowly, and the remainder of the carbon dioxide diffuses into red blood cells. Twenty per cent of it reacts to form a carbamino compound with hemoglobin.

The enzyme *carbonic anhydrase* is a catalyst for the formation of carbonic acid from the remaining 75% of the carbon dioxide:

$$CO_2 + H_2O \rightarrow \text{carbonic anhydrase} \rightarrow H_2CO_3$$

This compound dissociates into $H^+ + HCO_3^-$ ions, the H^+ ion reacts with reduced deoxygenated hemoglobin ($H^+ + Hb^- \rightarrow HHb$), and the bicarbonate reacts with potassium in the red blood cells to form $KHCO_3$. Bicarbonate later diffuses into the plasma. To maintain electrical neutrality, chloride ions diffuse inside the red blood cells (the *chloride shift*) to form KCl. In the lungs, the opposite reaction occurs. The reduced hemoglobin is oxygenated ($HHbO_2$). Hydrogen ions are released from the hemoglobin and react with bicarbonate salts to form carbonic acid, which is converted to carbon dioxide by carbonic anhydrase (Fig. 24–1) (Goldberger, 1986). Chloride diffuses back

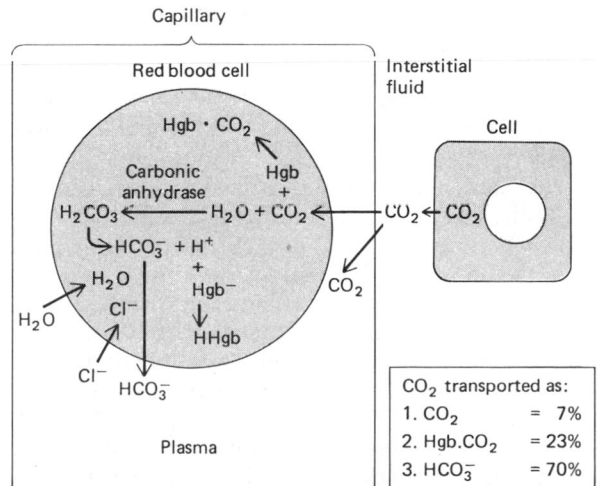

FIGURE 24–1. Mechanisms of carbon dioxide transport. (From Guyton, A. C. (1991). *Textbook of medical physiology.* Philadelphia: W. B. Saunders.)

into the plasma, and potassium reacts with bicarbonate:

$$HHbO_2 + KHCO_3 \rightarrow H_2CO_3 + KHbO_2$$

Carbonate in the bone can act as a cellular buffer when acid is present in the extracellular fluid. Hydrogen ions are absorbed to the crystal lattice of bone, and sodium is released into the ECF. This exchange provides a vast buffering capacity in patients with chronic conditions of H$^+$ retention such as chronic renal failure (Appel and Chase, 1986). Calcium is also released in exchange for the uptake of phosphorus by the bone. When alkaline substances are being buffered, more carbonate is deposited. In acid-base abnormalities, a large proportion of the buffering is carried out in bone: in respiratory alkalosis, 99%; in respiratory acidosis, 97%; in metabolic acidosis, 57%; and in metabolic alkalosis, 32% (Goldberger, 1986).

Respiratory Regulation of Acid-Base Balance

Because the ultimate goal of respiration is to maintain normal levels of carbon dioxide, hydrogen ions, and oxygen, changes in their concentrations are integral to respiratory regulation. Excess carbon dioxide and hydrogen ions have excitatory effects on the respiratory center, causing increased strength of both inspiratory and expiratory signals to the respiratory muscles. This ventilatory stimulus increases the elimination of carbon dioxide and carbonic acid from the plasma. It is thought that a chemosensitive area, receptive to changes in carbon dioxide and hydrogen ion concentrations, is located directly beneath the surface of the medulla near the entry of the glossopharyngeal and vagal nerves. The chemosensitive area then excites other portions of the respiratory center, especially the inspiratory center. Though it is believed that hydrogen ions are the only direct stimulus for this area, they are slow to cross the blood–brain barrier. Because carbon dioxide readily diffuses across all cell membranes, changes in this concentration have the most powerful effect on control of respiration, though the effect is indirect. Carbon dioxide reacts with water of the tissues to form carbonic acid. This then dissociates into hydrogen ions, which have a potent direct stimulatory effect, and bicarbonate (Guyton, 1991; Shapiro, et al., 1982).

Changes in metabolism affect the amount of carbon dioxide produced, whereas changes in pulmonary ventilation affect the rate of excretion of carbon dioxide, creating a cyclical feedback mechanism. Because the carbon dioxide concentration is directly related to the pH of tissue fluids, tissue fluid P_{CO_2} must be regulated exactly by the respiratory system. Its ability to stimulate ventilation is especially great in the *normal* P_{CO_2} and pH ranges: P_{CO_2} between 30 and 50 mm Hg and pH between 7.5 and 7.3. When venous blood reaches the pulmonary capillaries, the

P_{CO_2} is approximately 46 mm Hg. The P_{CO_2} in the alveoli is normally 40 mm Hg. This difference in partial pressure facilitates the diffusion of carbon dioxide from the plasma into the alveoli for elimination. Increasing the carbon dioxide concentration can result in an increase in ventilation up to 11-fold. This concentration is the primary chemical regulator of normal respiration. If the P_{CO_2} rises above 65 mm Hg, carbon dioxide acts as a depressant, and other stimulants to respiration must intervene.

Ventilatory rate also affects hydrogen ion concentration; an increase in ventilation causes the excretion of excess carbonic acid with a net increase in pH. On the other hand, hydrogen ion concentration also controls alveolar ventilatory rate by acting directly on the chemosensitive area of the respiratory center. Due to the blood–brain barrier, respiratory regulation is slower when it is dependent on a change in pH. Up to a fourfold increase in hyperventilation occurs when the pH drops to 7.2; however, hyperventilation stops when the pH reaches 7.0. Figure 24–2 (Guyton, 1991) demonstrates the effect on alveolar ventilation with increases in carbon dioxide and hydrogen ion concentrations.

The respiratory center is affected in varying degrees by the partial pressure of oxygen in the alveolar air. Normally, the respiratory system maintains an alveolar P_{O_2} that is much higher than that needed to saturate the hemoglobin. Ventilation can decrease to as low as one-half normal and the hemoglobin will still remain essentially saturated. Chemoreceptors, located outside the central nervous system in the carotid and aortic bodies of the carotid arteries and aorta, respectively, are sensitive to changes in oxygen concentration. Low blood P_{O_2} will not increase alveolar ventilation appreciably until the P_{O_2} is one-half normal. Hypoxia, a P_{O_2} between 60 and 30 mm Hg, will increase ventilation by 1.5 to 1.7 times, a much weaker effect than occurs with increased carbon dioxide and hydrogen ion concentrations. A reduced P_{O_2} becomes the primary stimulus to respiration only

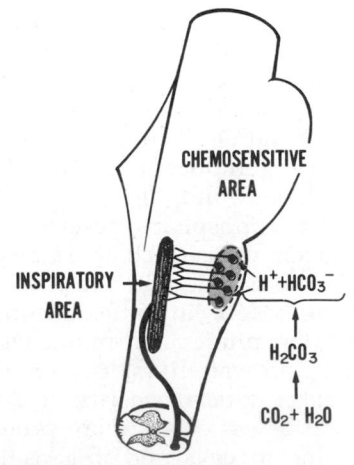

FIGURE 24–2. Stimulus of the respiratory center. (From Guyton, A. C. (1991). *Textbook of medical physiology*. Philadelphia: W. B. Saunders.)

URINE FILTRATE
IN TUBULE

KIDNEY TUBULE
CELLS

ECF

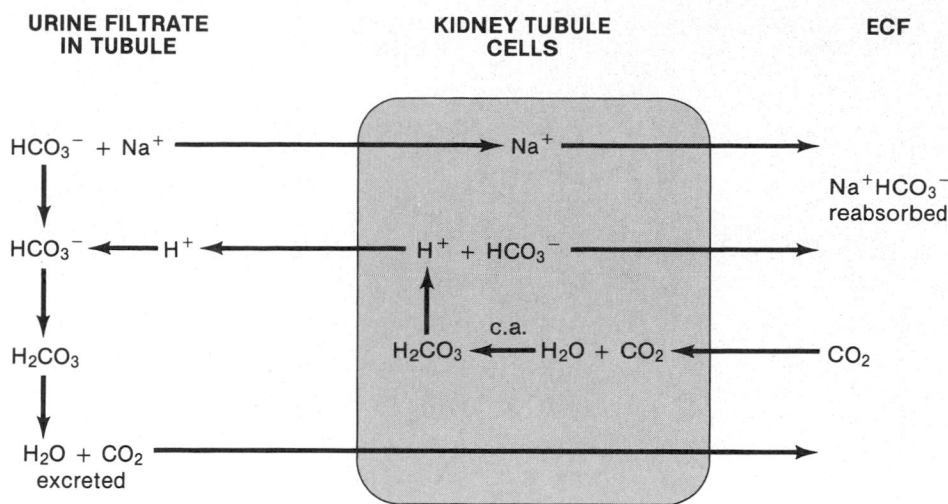

FIGURE 24–3. Renal regulation of hydrogen and bicarbonate ion concentration. *Abbreviations:* ECF, extracellular fluid; c.a., carbonic anhydrase.

in conditions of acute or chronic pulmonary disease when carbon dioxide and hydrogen ions cannot be excreted and their concentrations remain elevated.

Renal Regulation of Acid-Base Balance

Metabolic control and the restoration of acid-base balance are regulated by the kidneys. The kidneys control hydrogen ion concentration primarily by increasing or decreasing the bicarbonate concentration of the body fluids and secreting fixed acids. Although it may take 1 to 3 days for the kidney to restore acid-base balance, the mechanism provides for complete removal of excess acid or base unless the abnormality persists. The pH of the urine can vary from 4.4 to 8.0, depending on the need to conserve or excrete acid. Dietary intake has a major influence on urinary pH; a heavy protein intake will acidify the urine, whereas a vegetarian intake causes an alkaline urine. The usual urinary pH is 6.0, more acid than the 7.4 pH of blood because 50 to 80 mmol more acid than alkali is produced each day and excreted (Guyton, 1991).

BICARBONATE "REABSORPTION" AND HYDROGEN ION SECRETION

There are three major processes by which the kidneys excrete acid and retain bicarbonate. Sodium bicarbonate is filtered, and then Na^+ is reabsorbed into the proximal tubule. *Carbon dioxide* in the tubular cells combines with water, under the catalytic action of carbonic anhydrase, to form carbonic acid. This dissociates, and hydrogen ions are exchanged for sodium ions in the tubular fluid in a process called countertransport. A carrier protein combines with sodium and moves it along a concentration gradient to the interior of the cell. At the same time, hydrogen attaches to the same protein and is moved actively against a concentration gradient into the tubular lumen. As sodium crosses into the ECF, the lumen

is electronegative, and hydrogen ion secretion occurs (Fig. 24–3). In this way, hydrogen can be excreted even though acid already exists in the tubular fluid (Puschett and Piraino, 1985). About 84% of all hydrogen ion secretion occurs in the proximal tubules. The gradient is only three to four times the tubular concentration compared with a gradient of 900 times greater in the collecting ducts.

Under normal conditions, the amount of hydrogen ions secreted from the tubular cells is approximately the same as the amount of bicarbonate filtered into the tubular lumen by the glomerulus. They combine with each other to form carbon dioxide and water, thereby neutralizing each other. Usually there is an excess of acid to be excreted. However, if an alkalotic condition exists, increased bicarbonate would be filtered and fewer hydrogen ions secreted into the tubular lumen, with a net loss of bicarbonate and a return of the pH toward normal.

The normal process of restoring bicarbonate to the extracellular fluid occurs inside the tubular cell. When carbonic acid dissociates, it releases bicarbonate as well as hydrogen ions. These bicarbonate ions diffuse into the extracellular fluid in combination with sodium ions that were reabsorbed from the tubular fluid to form sodium bicarbonate.

Several other mechanisms exist to facilitate the removal of hydrogen ions through the kidney tubules. In the tubular filtrate, the *phosphate buffers* become more concentrated. Once filtered, they are relatively impermeable to reabsorption. Although weak in the plasma, they are powerful buffers in the filtrate in transporting a major portion of the hydrogen ions into the urine. As excess hydrogen ions are secreted into the filtrate in the distal tubule, they combine with Na_2HPO_4 to form NaH_2PO_4. The remaining sodium ions are reabsorbed into the extracellular fluid along with bicarbonate ions (Fig. 24–4). This allows excretion of a titratable acid with a pH of 4.5 (Appel and Chase, 1986; Guyton, 1991).

Another potent buffer in the tubular filtrate is composed of *ammonia* (NH_3) and the ammonium ion

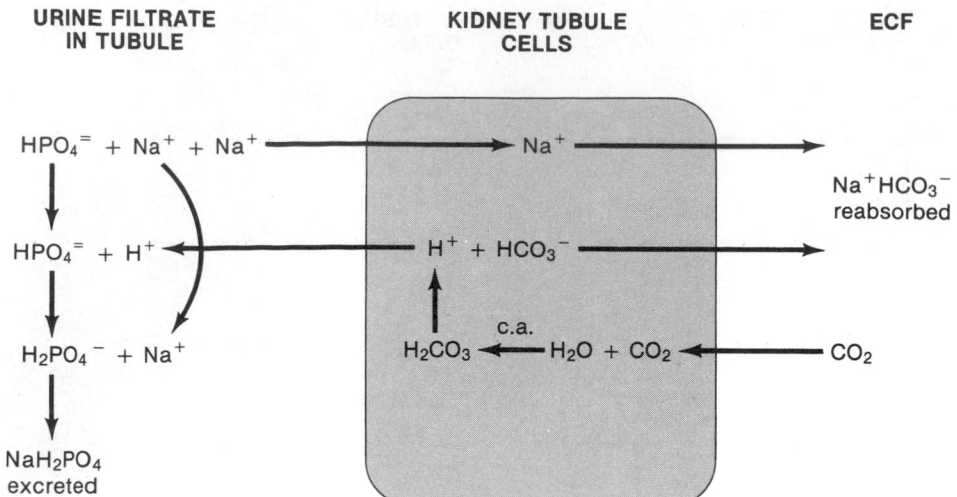

URINE FILTRATE IN TUBULE   KIDNEY TUBULE CELLS   ECF

FIGURE 24–4. Renal regulation of the phosphate buffer system.

(NH_4^+). The epithelial cells of the entire tubule except the thin segment of the loop of Henle continually synthesize ammonia, which diffuses into the tubules. This combines with hydrogen to form an ammonium ion (NH_4^+). The tubular cells are less permeable to NH_4^+, helping to excrete the hydrogen. The major anion of the filtrate is chloride. Much of it combines with the ammonium ion to form ammonium chloride, a weak acid that gives urine its characteristic odor. This process facilitates the removal of hydrogen, ammonium, and chloride ions, avoiding the formation of a strong acid, hydrochloric acid, and keeps the pH of the urine within acceptable limits. At the same time, a bicarbonate ion is reabsorbed into the extracellular fluid as a substitute for the chloride ion. The ammonia buffer system allows the tubules to secrete many times the number of hydrogen ions that would otherwise be possible and facilitates the retention of bicarbonate, thus enhancing the ability of the kidney to correct acidotic states (Fig. 24–5) (Guyton, 1991; Porth, 1986).

Potassium Exchange

A fourth process exists at the cellular level to compensate temporarily for an acidotic state. Normally, extracellular sodium is exchanged for intracellular potassium by means of the sodium pump. If other cations such as excess hydrogen or ammonium ions are present, these will compete with potassium. Hydrogen ions can be transported intracellularly in exchange for potassium. To maintain a fairly narrow range of extracellular potassium levels, excess amounts of the ion are excreted in the urine. This mechanism is another means by which the blood pH maintains its delicate balance.

The urine pH is not an indication of the total amount of acid excreted by the kidney. If the concentration of buffer is high, the amount of acid excreted will also be great, but the pH will be maintained above 4.5. Disruption of any of the cell transport mechanisms, NH_3 production, or aldosterone deficiency in the distal tubule will decrease maximal acid production (Appel and Chase, 1986).

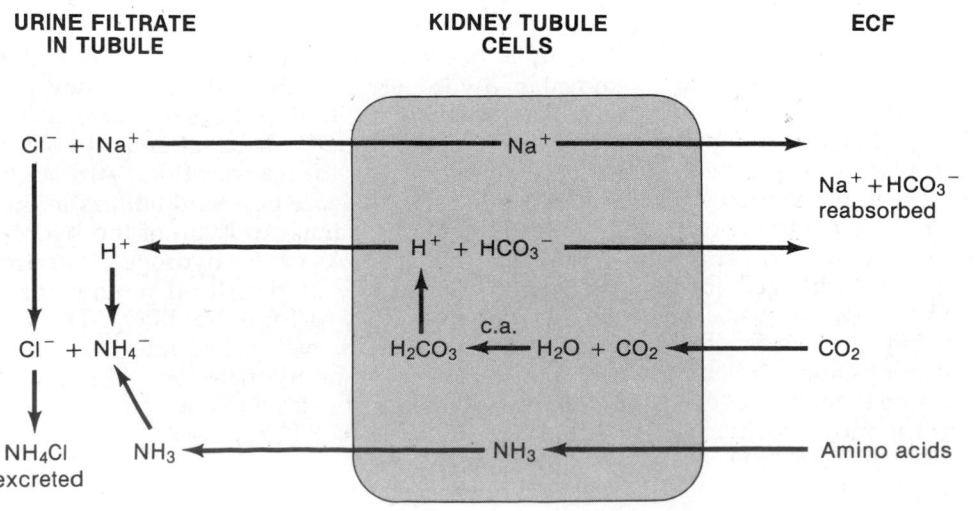

URINE FILTRATE IN TUBULE   KIDNEY TUBULE CELLS   ECF

FIGURE 24–5. Renal regulation of ammonia secretion.

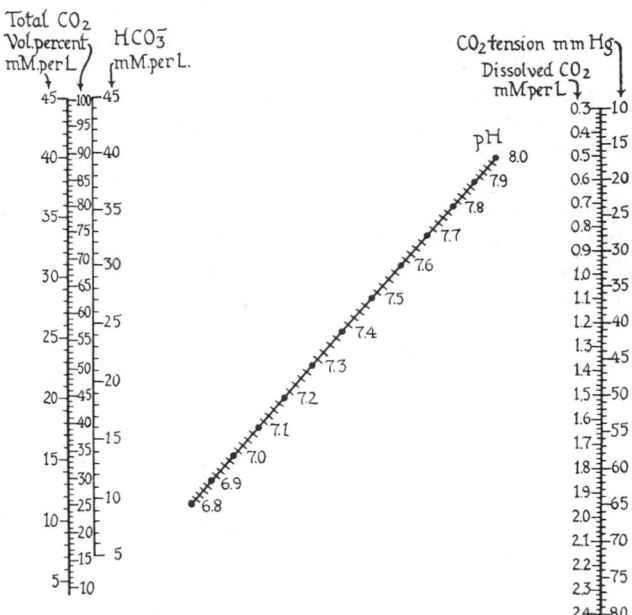

FIGURE 24–6. Nomogram to determine P_{CO_2} from pH and CO_2 content. (From McLean, F. C. (1938). *Physiological Review*, 18, 495.)

Compensation

When a single disorder of acid or base balance occurs, the concentration of acid or base is excessive and causes an abnormal blood pH. The unaffected pulmonary or renal system will adjust for the altered state. If there is an excess in hydrogen ion, pulmonary ventilation will be increased to remove carbon dioxide, and the kidney will remove excess acids and retain bicarbonate. If the hydrogen ion concentration is decreased, the pH will be returned toward normal by raising the carbon dioxide concentration or decreasing the bicarbonate concentration. *Compensation* exists when the pH is returned to normal by a change in the unaffected system, i.e., the kidneys retain more bicarbonate and secrete hydrogen ions to compensate for an increased P_{CO_2}. However, the P_{CO_2} and bicarbonate may not be within normal limits. Compensation requires normal function of the lungs and kidneys. Though the pH may return to normal, an abnormality in the secondary system may be created. A condition of respiratory acidosis will be compensated by an increase in plasma HCO_3^-. If the primary disease is corrected and the P_{CO_2} decreases, an elevated HCO_3^-, or metabolic alkalosis, will remain.

A *correction* occurs when the pH is returned to normal by alleviating the problem of the primary system, i.e., the P_{CO_2} is lowered by putting the patient on a mechanical ventilator and eliminating excess carbon dioxide. All parameters return to normal in a corrected state. *Overcompensation* occurs when one parameter (i.e., metabolic) continues to be abnormal after the primary imbalance has been corrected. If the primary abnormality in acid-base balance persists, the other system will not be able to adjust fully or compensate, and an *uncompensated*

state will exist. The specific mechanisms of compensation will be discussed with each alteration in acid-base balance (Guyton, 1991).

ASSESSMENT OF ACID-BASE BALANCE AND IMBALANCE

Laboratory Assessment

To describe the patient's state of acid-base balance, it is necessary to determine at least two of the three parameters: serum pH and bicarbonate concentration (often measured indirectly as CO_2 content). The third parameter, usually serum carbonic acid measured as P_{CO_2}, can then be calculated from a chart called a nomogram (Fig. 24–6) (McLean, 1938). The two known parameters are plotted on the chart, and a line is drawn between them. The point of intersection with the right column represents the carbonic acid concentration. This method was derived when arterial blood gases were less easily obtained and is currently useful in patients in whom arterial vascular access is lacking. More commonly, four parameters of acid-base balance are measured directly from the arterial blood gases. Normal values for blood gases are listed in Table 24–2 (Halperin and Goldstein, 1988; Hudak et al., 1986; Romanski, 1986).

Serum pH is obtained from an arterial (usually radial) sample that is not exposed to air. The usual sample for blood gas analysis is also obtained from an artery. Normal values for mixed venous blood are more variable and represent only the extremity from which the blood was drawn. However, these values are useful when arterial samples are unavailable. Respiratory parameters of oxygenation, the partial pressure of oxygen (P_{O_2}) and oxygen saturation (O_2 Sat), are also included in blood gas analysis, but their values do not directly affect blood pH. Indirectly, the respiratory response to insufficient oxygenation can result in hyperventilation and respiratory alkalosis.

The partial pressure of carbon dioxide (P_{CO_2}) is a measurement of the pressure or tension exerted by dissolved carbon dioxide in the blood. It is proportional to the P_{CO_2} in alveolar air. To maintain a normal P_{CO_2}, the rate and depth of ventilation vary "automatically" with changes in metabolism (Metheny, 1987).

There is a direct relationship between the degree

TABLE 24–2. Normal Blood Gas Values of Acid-Base Balance

Parameter	Arterial Blood	Mixed Venous Blood
pH	7.35–7.45 (7.4)	7.33–7.43 (7.38)
P_{CO_2}	35–45 mm Hg	
HCO_3	22–26 mEq/liter	24–28 mEq/liter
Base excess or	−2.5 to +2.5	0 to +4
plasma anion gap	10–15 mEq/liter	

of ventilation and the partial pressure of carbon dioxide in the blood. If the P_{CO_2} is too high, it is a result of inadequate ventilation and removal of carbon dioxide. This is called "hypoventilation." Increased concentrations of carbonic acid accumulate. If the condition persists, respiratory acidosis will develop. A P_{CO_2} that is lower than normal due to excessive ventilation (hyperventilation) causes a depletion of carbonic acid. Prolonging this condition causes the development of respiratory alkalosis. P_{CO_2} is more important than P_{O_2} in determining alveolar ventilation because factors other than ventilation affect levels of oxygenation.

Metabolic parameters of acid-base balance are determined from direct or indirect measurements of bicarbonate concentration or the degree of base excess or plasma anion gap. Serum bicarbonate and base excess or deficit can be measured directly from blood gas analysis. Plasma anion gap and CO_2 content are measured from venous blood (Corbett, 1987).

If arterial blood gases are not available, the concentration of bicarbonate can be determined by using an indirect measure from venous blood serum, the carbon dioxide content. The approximate bicarbonate ion concentration can be determined by subtracting 1 mEq/liter from the CO_2 content or using the formula

$$bicarbonate = CO_2 \text{ content} - (0.03 \times P_{CO_2})$$

The normal values are 24 to 30 mEq/liter (Goldberger, 1986; Metheny, 1987).

Base excess refers to the sum of the concentration of buffer anions in whole blood: available bicarbonate ions, plasma proteins, red blood cells, hemoglobin, and phosphates in plasma and hemoglobin. This determination is made to quantify the patient's total base excess or deficit so that clinical treatment of acid-base disturbances (especially metabolic disturbances) can be initiated. The total quantity of buffer anions is normally 45 to 50 mEq/liter, or twice that of bicarbonate. This measure gives a more complete picture of the nonrespiratory causes of acid-base imbalance. A negative value reflects a metabolic disturbance and a deficit of buffer base (metabolic acidosis). A positive value reflects a loss of metabolic acid or an excess of buffer base (metabolic alkalosis) (Corbett, 1987).

The anion gap is the sum of the unmeasured anions in serum: phosphate, sulfates, ketones, and lactic acid. Normally these anions are less than 16 mEq/liter of the total anion production. The anion gap can be determined by subtracting the sum of the measured anions (HCO_3^- and Cl^-) from the cation concentration (represented by Na^+) (Methany, 1987):

$$\text{Anion gap (AG)} = Na^+ - [Cl^- + HCO_3^-] = 12–15 \text{ mEq/liter}$$

Blood pH is a measure of the chemical balance in the body and is a ratio of acids to bases. Low pH numbers (<7.36) represent an acid state, whereas higher pH numbers (>7.44) indicate an alkaline state in the extracellular fluid. The sources of hydrogen ions are both gases and nonvolatile or fixed acids.

When attempting to interpret acid-base states, the following steps are needed: (1) First observe the arterial pH to determine whether an acidotic or an alkalotic state exists. (2) Look for the cause, which may be respiratory, metabolic, or both. Also look for the expected compensatory response. If it is respiratory, then the P_{CO_2} will be changed as follows:

Respiratory acidosis: Increase in P_{CO_2}, decrease in pH, no change or increase in base excess or HCO_3^-.

Respiratory alkalosis: Decrease in P_{CO_2}, increase in pH, no change or decrease in base excess or HCO_3^-.

If the cause is metabolic, then the base excess will be changed as follows:

Metabolic acidosis: negative base excess or HCO_3^-, decrease in pH, no change or decrease in P_{CO_2}.

Metabolic alkalosis: positive base excess or HCO_3^-, increase in pH, no change or increase in P_{CO_2} (Fig. 24–7).

Clinical Assessment

Clinical signs of acid-base imbalance appear as indications of compensatory mechanisms for various states. For example, metabolic acidosis, an accumulation of nonvolatile acids with a lowered blood pH, stimulates the respiratory center, resulting in the observed sign of hyperventilation. Respiratory acidosis, an accumulation of carbon dioxide, is compensated by the reabsorption of sodium bicarbonate from the kidney filtrate and the secretion of hydrogen ions or metabolic acids. The clinical sign is an acid urine with a strong odor of ammonia. Electrolyte and fluid abnormalities can also occur with acid-base imbalances. The specific clinical and laboratory signs will be discussed later under each respiratory or metabolic alteration.

Systematic Method of Assessing Acid-Base Balance and Imbalance

To assess acid-base disorders accurately, a systematic method needs to be used to evaluate laboratory values and clinical signs in the specific context of a clinical situation. Although the four basic alterations, respiratory and metabolic acidosis and respiratory and metabolic alkalosis, can occur independently, more frequently a combination of two or more can be observed. The disturbances may be antagonistic to or synergestic of each other. Factors to be considered in the assessment include the following (Holloway, 1984):

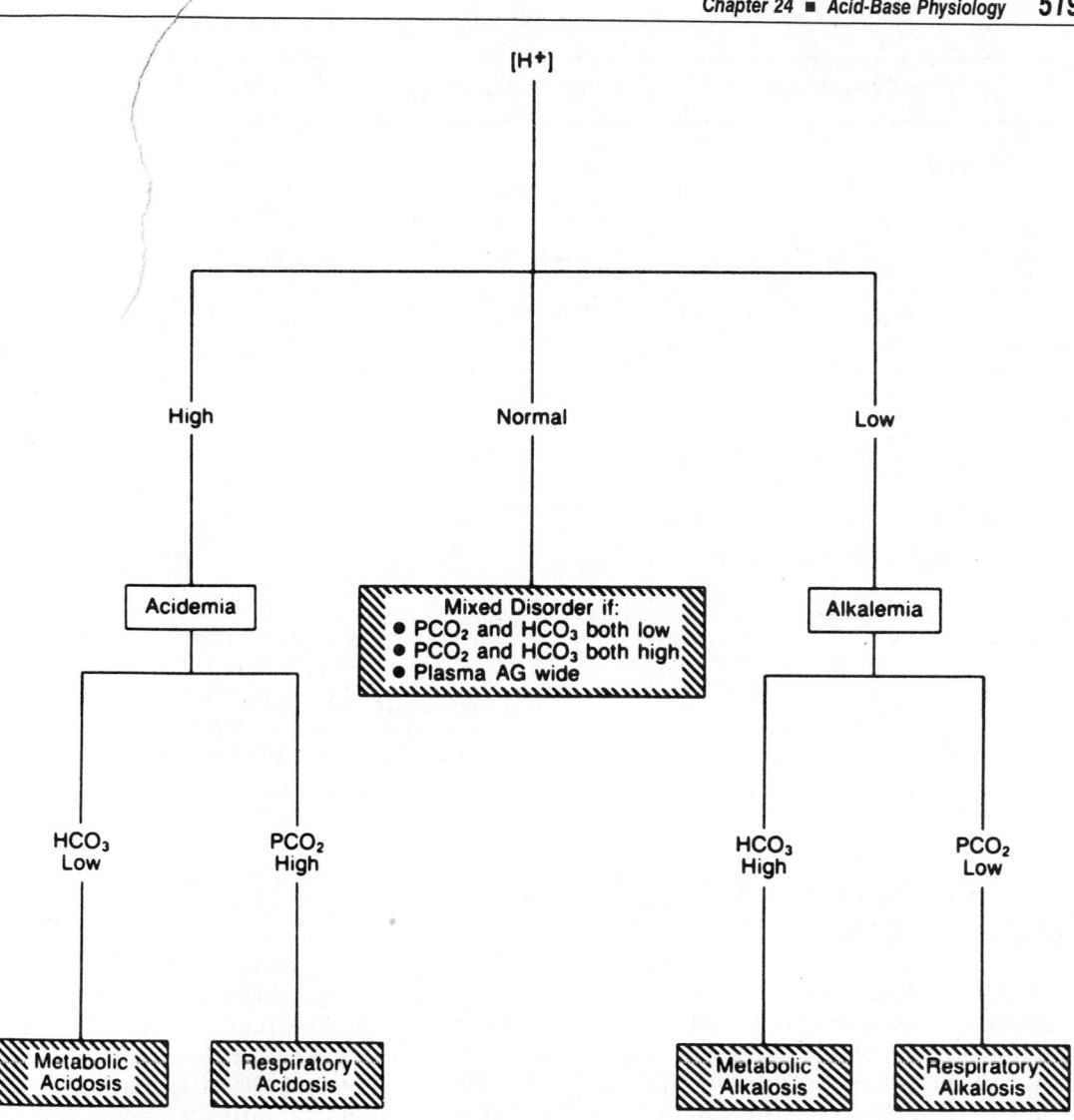

FIGURE 24–7. Systematic assessment of acid-base disorders. AG, anion gap. (From Halperin, M. L., and Goldstein, M. B. (1988). *Fluid, electrolyte, and acid-base emergencies*. Philadelphia: W. B. Saunders.)

1. Conditions in the patient's history predisposing to acid-base imbalance
   a. Respiratory: pneumonia, COPD, use of a ventilator, extreme anxiety
   b. Renal/metabolic: diabetes mellitus, kidney disease, starvation states (NPO), loss of gastrointestinal fluids, liver disease, hypoxic states, heart disease
2. Clinical signs and symptoms of acid-base imbalance
   a. Changes in cerebral status: confusion, coma (acidosis), dizziness, giddiness (alkalosis). Cerebral changes occur sooner with respiratory disorders than with metabolic states because carbon dioxide crosses the blood–brain barrier faster
   b. Changes in respiratory status (changes are more rapid if acute): hypo- or hyperventilation (rate and depth of pattern), restlessness or cyanosis (hypoxia), changes in pattern of respiration
   c. Changes in cardiovascular status: hypoxia or electrolyte imbalances (can lead to arrhythmias, angina, or shock); acute myocardial infarction (results in altered perfusion and lactic acidosis); acid-base imbalances (cause changes in the oxygen dissociation curve: Alkalosis causes a shift to the left with decreased dissociation of oxygen from hemoglobin and hypoxia; acidosis causes a shift to the right, allowing oxygen to be released more readily from hemoglobin. Acidosis also results in a decreased response to catecholamines, decreased myocardial contractility, and decreased peripheral vasoconstriction)
   d. Changes in renal status: electrolytes, urine characteristics (color or ammonia odor), urine output

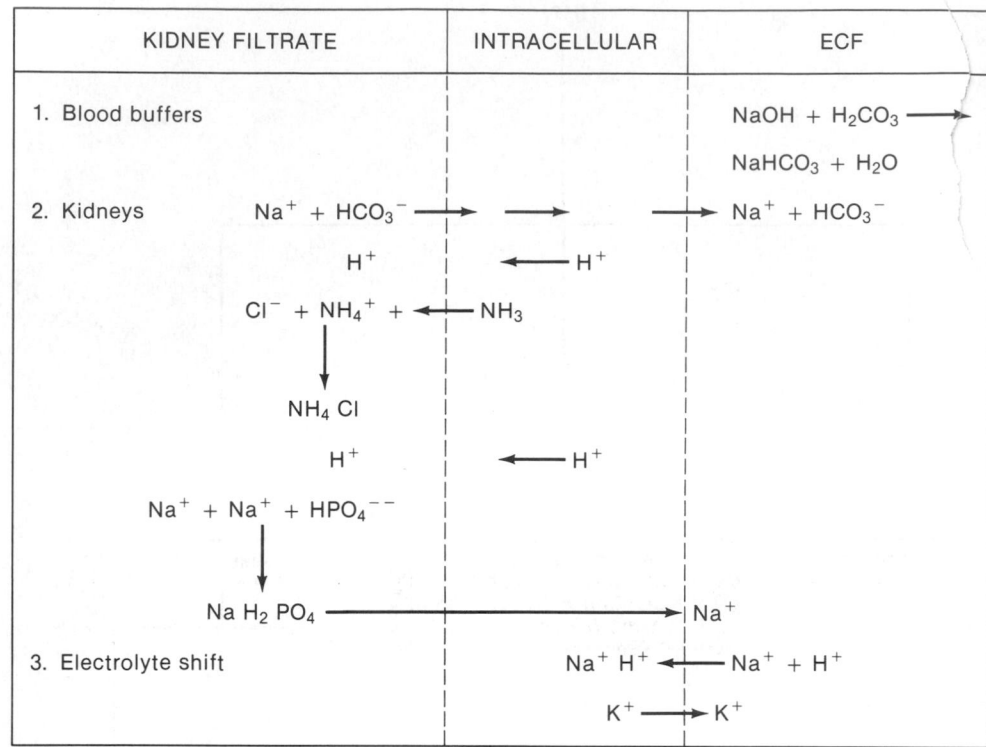

KIDNEY FILTRATE	INTRACELLULAR	ECF
1. Blood buffers		$NaOH + H_2CO_3 \longrightarrow$
		$NaHCO_3 + H_2O$
2. Kidneys $\quad Na^+ + HCO_3^- \longrightarrow \rightarrow$		$\rightarrow Na^+ + HCO_3^-$
H^+	$\longleftarrow H^+$	
$Cl^- + NH_4^+ + \longleftarrow NH_3$		
$\downarrow$		
NH_4Cl		
H^+	$\longleftarrow H^+$	
$Na^+ + Na^+ + HPO_4^{--}$		
$\downarrow$		
$Na\,H_2\,PO_4 \longrightarrow$		Na^+
3. Electrolyte shift	$Na^+ H^+ \longleftarrow Na^+ + H^+$	
	$K^+ \longrightarrow K^+$	

FIGURE 24–8. Compensatory mechanisms in respiratory acidosis.

Diagnostic Procedures and Laboratory Tests

Electrolyte Imbalances

Sodium. Hyponatremia, if associated with hypochloremia, may also be associated with *alkalosis* and a decreased potassium. Bicarbonate is reabsorbed with sodium instead of with chloride, and potassium is lost in exchange for sodium, which is conserved (Holloway, 1984).

Potassium. Hyperkalemia is associated with *acidosis*. Because an elevated potassium concentration can quickly be fatal due to its effect on cardiac muscle, an intracellular mechanism exists whereby potassium ions in the ECF can be exchanged for hydrogen ions in the intracellular fluid. The inverse is also true. The kidneys exchange hydrogen ions instead of potassium to retain sodium, resulting in increased potassium. *Alkalosis* is related to *hypokalemia*.

Calcium. The ionization of calcium in the ECF increases with acidosis and decreases with alkalosis. Acidosis can mask the muscular signs of true hypocalcemia. With overcorrection of the acidosis, symptoms of tetany, carpopedal spasms, paresthesias, or convulsions may occur.

Chloride. Chloride is primarily an extracellular ion. The concentration varies inversely with that of bicarbonate. A *chloride shift* occurs across the cellular membrane in exchange for bicarbonate during buffering. The renal reabsorption of chloride varies inversely with bicarbonate, and therefore a decreased chloride level is related to metabolic alkalosis and an increased chloride concentration to metabolic aci-

dosis. If a patient has lost considerable amounts of sodium and chloride, such as from gastrointestinal drainage or a low-salt diet without chloride replacement, metabolic alkalosis can develop.

Carbon Dioxide. Carbon dioxide content is normally 95% bicarbonate and 5% carbonic acid. The CO_2 content will rise (>30 mEq/liter) with a respiratory acidosis and a metabolic alkalosis due to an increased production of bicarbonate or carbonic acid. The CO_2 content will drop (<24 mEq/liter) with a metabolic acidosis or a respiratory alkalosis due to the depletion of bicarbonate or carbonic acid.

Anion Gap. The *anion gap* is the difference between the total unmeasured anions in the body (such as protein and phosphates) subtracted from the measured cations (such as sodium and potassium). Normally this is 10 to 15 mEq/liter. Plasma proteins usually constitute most of the anion gap. An increase in the anion gap occurs in metabolic acidosis with an increase in organic acids (starvation, ketoacidosis, lactic acidosis). With metabolic acidosis resulting from bicarbonate or chloride loss, the anion gap remains normal.

CLINICAL ALTERATIONS IN ACID-BASE BALANCE

Respiratory Acidosis

Respiratory acidosis is an accumulation of carbon dioxide and carbonic acid in the body as a result of hypoventilation, an increase in P_{CO_2} above 46 mm Hg, and a lowering of the pH below 7.34. Respiratory acidosis can result from breathing air with an abnormally high carbon dioxide content, as is done experimentally or during anesthesia administration. Respiratory acidosis more commonly occurs as a result of pulmonary, abdominal, or central nervous system alterations that interfere with respiration and the elimination of carbon dioxide (Kersten, 1989).

Respiratory acidosis may occur acutely or may develop chronically over a period of time. For a given increase in P_{CO_2}, there is a greater change in pH with an acute condition. In a chronic condition, a compensatory mechanism exists to increase retention of bicarbonate and enhance secretion of hydrogen and chloride ions by the kidneys. For each 10 mm Hg increase in P_{CO_2}, there is a rise in bicarbonate by 35 mEq/liter. However, this mechanism takes several days to compensate. Often, hypoxia occurs simultaneously with hypercarbia as a result of hypoventilation. The effect of hypoxia is much more life-threatening than that of hypercarbia. The limit to life from hypercarbia is not known.

The pathophysiology of respiratory acidosis is a result of alveolar hypoventilation. This may occur if the tidal volume or respiratory rate is decreased (rapid shallow breathing to compensate for metabolic alkalosis or CNS depression) or if there is obstruction of the diffusion or ventilation of carbon dioxide (Guyton, 1991).

Because retention of CO_2 interferes with the normal respiratory response to hypercarbia, the following compensatory mechanisms develop (Fig. 24-8): (1) the blood buffers react with carbonic acid to form more basic salts; (2) the kidneys increase the secretion and excretion of hydrogen ions, ammonium ions are formed and excreted, bicarbonate ions (along with sodium) are retained in exchange for chloride ions, and phosphate ions combine with hydrogen and are excreted; and (3) there is a shift in electrolytes: hydrogen and sodium ions move intracellularly, raising the blood pH, in exchange for which potassium enters the extracellular fluid, causing a tendency toward hyperkalemia. With these compensatory changes, the bicarbonate concentration and pH rise toward normal, producing a partially compensated respiratory acidosis.

Many patients may actually overcompensate. The pH may rise over 7.46 as serum bicarbonate increases, a positive base excess is achieved, and total body potassium decreases as it is excreted in urine. As the P_{CO_2} returns to normal, the lost chloride ions must be replaced before bicarbonate can return to normal. Until this occurs, a metabolic alkalosis exists. Excessive loss of potassium ions due to use of diuretics will also potentiate alkalosis (Goldberger, 1986).

The causes and signs of respiratory acidosis are listed in Table 24-3 according to acute or chronic conditions. Acute conditions are often the result of a temporary and sudden problem occurring in a previously normal respiratory system. Chronic condi-

TABLE 24-3. Respiratory Acidosis

Cause	Signs	Laboratory Findings
Acute Respiratory Acidosis		
Congestive heart failure and pulmonary edema	Palpitations Warm, flushed skin Ventricular fibrillation may be first sign in anesthetized patient Fullness in head Mental cloudiness, dizziness Muscular twitching Convulsions Decreased LOC May be respiratory signs: rales, wheezing	pH = 7.4 to 7.0 P_{CO_2} = 45–120 mm Hg CO_2 content = upper normal or above HCO_3 = normal or slightly elevated Base excess = upper normal Elevated serum K^+
Massive pulmonary embolism		
Severe pulmonary infections		
Bronchial obstruction, atelectasis		
Aspiration		
Pneumothorax, open chest wound		
Hypoventilation with mechanical ventilation		
Severe abdominal distention		
Trendelenburg positions		
Neuromuscular: Guillain-Barré syndrome		
CNS depression: Head trauma, oversedation, anesthesia, high cord injury		
Chronic Respiratory Acidosis		
Bronchiectasis Emphysema Pulmonary fibrosis Cystic fibrosis Pickwickian syndrome (obesity) Poliomyelitis Amyotrophic lateral sclerosis Myasthenia gravis Multiple sclerosis (advanced)	Hyperpnea (maybe), productive cough, thick-colored sputum Weakness Headache Stupor Irritability, poor judgment and coordination Symptoms of underlying disease: Dependent edema Weight gain Orthopnea Use of accessory muscles Pursed lip breathing	Changes in pH and CO_2 content are similar to above HCO_3 > 26 mEq/liter pH rises to or near normal Decreased Cl^-, increased Na^+ and K^+

tions usually result from prolonged disease states in which there is a gradual buildup in the carbon dioxide concentration. Pulmonary disorders include those in which gas exchange is limited by an abnormal alveolar-capillary membrane, airway obstruction, or inadequate lung tissue, such as emphysema, pulmonary edema, or bronchial obstruction. Neurologic disorders include problems with innervation of the lung (Guillain-Barré syndrome), or CNS depression (head injuries). Drugs that reduce respiratory drive, such as sedatives, analgesics, anesthesia, or alcohol, produce hypoventilation. Abdominal distention may interfere with lung expansion and reduce ventilation, as in pregnancy, obesity, or ascites (Flomenbaum, 1984; Hudak, 1986; Metheny, 1987).

Nursing Diagnoses and Interventions. Nursing diagnoses often associated with respiratory acidosis include the following:

1. Alteration in respiratory function: ineffective airway clearance and impaired gas exchange
2. Alteration in acid/base and electrolyte balance
3. Alteration in sensory-perceptual awareness

Implications for nursing interventions revolve around improving ventilation, allowing for rest and comfort, and correcting fluid and electrolyte imbalances.

Improving Ventilation

1. Expand respiratory capacity: Increase cough and deep breathing by use of unassisted blow bottles or incentive spirometry, postural drainage, or bronchodilators; humidify secretions mechanically and by encouraging fluid intake; use mechanical ventilation if the patient is in respiratory failure.
2. Treat documented infection with antibiotics.

Providing rest and comfort

1. Plan activities to allow for rest periods between treatment or care.
2. Provide a position of comfort and support with a backrest, overbed table, or pillows. The use of a chair with arm supports instead of reclining in bed allows the patient to bend his or her legs for better support and chest expansion.
3. Help alleviate anxiety of patient by teaching slow breathing exercises when condition is stable. Use comfort touch measures and relaxation tapes or music.
4. Maintain a cool, low-humidity environment to promote ease of breathing; adjust humidity level to comfort of patient.

Correcting Fluid and Electrolyte Imbalances

1. Diurectics are often necessary to treat edema.
2. If the acidosis and hyperkalemia are corrected, potassium chloride may be given to replace these electrolytes in both the intracellular and extracellular fluids, respectively.
3. If a metabolic alkalosis persists after the respiratory acidosis has been corrected (e.g., as with mechanical ventilation), administration of calcium gluconate may be indicated to prevent tetany.
4. Acidosis *may* be treated occasionally with bicarbonate administration.

Respiratory Alkalosis

Respiratory alkalosis results from stimulation of the respiratory center with a resulting decrease of P_{CO_2} in the alveolar air due to hyperventilation. There is an increase in tidal volume or depth of respiration and increased alveolar ventilation; however, respiratory rate may or may not be increased. When this situation occurs, a large amount of carbon dioxide is eliminated from the body, increasing the acid-base ratio and the pH.

Compensatory processes can occur to restore the pH to within normal limits. The kidney excretes less acid in the urine by suppressing hydrogen ion formation, ammonia production, and chloride excretion, and it conserves less bicarbonate. Potassium moves into the intracellular space in exchange for hydrogen and sodium ions, which move extracellularly.

Respiratory alkalosis is the least common type of acid-base disturbance. Some of the causes are psychogenic in origin, such as pain or anxiety. Other causes are central nervous system stimulation due to head injury or lesions, early salicylate poisoning, alcohol intoxication, paraldehyde ingestion, thyrotoxicosis, or fever. Cardiac or pulmonary causes often indicate an attempt to increase oxygenation during conditions of hypoxia such as congestive heart failure or pulmonary embolism. Patients receiving excessive mechanical ventilation or those with respiratory acidosis who have been treated with a tracheostomy experience a sudden increase in alveolar ventilation. Exercise and change to a higher altitude may precipitate temporary hyperventilation.

The most characteristic signs of respiratory alkalosis occur in the "hyperventilation syndrome" associated with anxiety. The patient may complain of lightheadedness or dizziness; circumoral paresthesias; numbness of fingers and toes; sweating, sometimes profusely; palpitations, dyspnea, and a feeling of panic; and muscle cramps or tetany, such as carpopedal spasm. Other sensations in the chest or abdomen may be present. The condition is usually temporary and self-limited.

Laboratory findings are a low P_{CO_2}, an elevated blood pH, and a normal or low bicarbonate concentration. The base excess may be negative in a chronic state. It may be difficult to diagnose a primary respiratory alkalosis; however, tetany does not occur with the compensatory hyperventilation associated with a primary metabolic acidosis. The causes, signs and laboratory findings of a respiratory alkalosis are listed in Table 24–4.

Nursing Diagnoses and Interventions. Nursing diagnoses often associated with respiratory alkalosis include the following:

1. Anxiety related to known or unknown factors
2. Alteration in respiratory function: ineffective breathing patterns
3. Alteration in fluid and electrolytes

TABLE 24–4. Respiratory Alkalosis

Cause	Signs	Laboratory Findings
Hyperventilation, extreme anxiety	Dizziness	pH > 7.45
Hypoxemia	Lightheadedness	P_{CO_2} < 35 mm Hg
Excessive mechanical ventilation	Numbness of fingers	Low CO_2 content, normal or low HCO_3^-
Hypermetabolic states: high fever, thyrotoxicosis	Tinnitus	Base excess normal in acute and low in chronic
	Palpitations	
	Sweating	Decreasing Ca^{2+} and K^+
	Feeling of panic	
	Muscle cramp	
Toxic stimulation of resp. center: CNS lesions, drug intoxication (early salicylate)	Tetany	
	Tightness of chest	
	Dry mouth	
	Blurred vision	
Pregnancy		
Gram-negative septicemia		

Implications for nursing interventions revolve around relieving anxiety, correcting hypoxia, and increasing the partial pressure of carbon dioxide.

Relieving Anxiety

1. Measures to relieve anxiety depend partly on the clinical state of the patient and the underlying psychological mechanisms of each person. A soothing but firm touch on the shoulders and a calm voice or asking the person to concentrate on when to breathe may greatly facilitate a decrease in ventilatory excursion.

2. If the cause of the hyperventilation is primarily anxiety, use of psychotherapeutic interventions or minor tranquilizers may be indicated.

Correcting Hypoxia

If the patient has an underlying disease of cardiac or pulmonary origin and has some degree of hypoxia, increasing the partial pressure of oxygen should relieve the hyperventilation and respiratory alkalosis. Oxygen therapy, diuretics, cardiotonic drugs, antibiotics, pulmonary hygiene, or mechanical ventilation may be indicated.

Increasing Partial Pressure of Carbon Dioxide

1. Teaching an anxious patient to breathe into a paper bag held closely around the nose and mouth or using rebreathing oxygen masks acts to retain carbon dioxide momentarily, which the patient then inhales.

2. Adjusting the settings on a mechanical ventilator to decrease tidal volume or rate and perhaps adjusting the pulmonary end-expiratory pressure (PEEP) will help restore a normal P_{CO_2}.

Metabolic Acidosis

Metabolic acidosis results either from an excess of inorganic or organic acids not being freely excreted by the kidney or from a loss of base from the body. As a result, the normal bicarbonate–carbonic acid ratio decreases, and the pH falls to less than 7.35. The decreased pH stimulates the respiratory center, and an increased depth and rate of respirations occur in an attempt to lower the carbonic acid concentration and restore the pH to a normal range.

As in respiratory acidosis, there is a shift of electrolytes, with hydrogen and sodium ions moving intracellularly in exchange for potassium. This creates a tendency toward hyperkalemia. Compensation by the pulmonary system is usually not complete. The renal mechanism involving sodium bicarbonate retention and acid excretion may occur depending on the cause and duration of the metabolic acidosis. The compensatory hyperventilation may persist after the acidotic state has been corrected, especially if sodium bicarbonate or lactate has been used.

Metabolic acidosis can result from a variety of conditions. An acid excess or an increase in the absolute amount of acid in the blood may occur with metabolic conditions that interfere with the normal catabolism of nutrients or with excess tissue breakdown. Accumulation of acid due to abnormal protein and fat metabolism occurs in diabetic acidosis and starvation. The unavailability of glucose for metabolism due to either lack of insulin or limited intake results in the mobilization of fats and protein to supply energy. Large amounts of nitrogenous wastes and ketones then accumulate in the blood, causing a metabolic acidosis. The body may be depleted of large amounts of sodium and potassium from a diuresis associated with hyperosmotic plasma.

Increased metabolic demands during surgical anesthesia, fever and infectious disease, and hyperthyroidism cause increased catabolism of all nutrients and acid accumulation. Anaerobic metabolism resulting from violent exercise, shock, acute myocardial infarction, sepsis, pancreatitis, and other conditions cause the accumulation of lactic and pyruvic acids. These conditions often occur acutely compared with diabetic or other metabolic conditions, which usually occur on a more chronic basis.

An excess of acids due to retention of those produced under normal conditions of metabolism occurs in renal disease and renal failure. The acidosis is related to several disturbances in renal function. Decreased glomerular filtration causes the retention of urea, creatinine, uric acid, and other nitrogenous products and organic acids. These react with serum bicarbonate, which is excreted as CO_2. Because the kidneys have a limited ability to reabsorb bicarbonate, the acid-base ratio falls, decreasing the pH. The tubules lose part of their ability to conserve water and secrete ammonia and sulfuric, phosphoric, and other inorganic acids. The net effect is a retention of metabolic acids and a decrease in base excess. Due to the chronic nature of renal disease, respiratory compensation usually does not occur until the bicarbonate concentration falls below 10 mEq/liter.

An acute metabolic acidosis can result from excessive intake of oral or parenteral acids, e.g., admin-

TABLE 24–5. Classification of Metabolic Acidosis According to Type

Elevated anion gap
  Chronic renal failure
  Lactic acidosis
  Diabetic ketoacidosis
  Starvation
  Ingestions and intoxications (methanol, late salicylate
    poisoning, ethylene glycol)
  Alcoholic ketolactic acidosis

Hyperchloremic metabolic acidosis
  Excessive gain of chloride (large quantities of normal saline,
    ammonium chloride)
  Renal tubular acidosis
  Administration of carbonic anhydrase inhibitors (Diamox)
  Extrarenal bicarbonate loss: diarrhea, ureterosigmoidostomy,
    or fistulas

(Data from Methany, 1987; Puschett and Piriano, 1985)

istration of intravenous fluids containing chloride ions such as hypertonic saline, when given in excessive amounts. The sodium is converted to sodium bicarbonate, and chloride is retained with hydrogen ions. Medications such as ammonium chloride, calcium chloride, or carbonic anhydrase inhibitors can result in metabolic acidosis, and their administration needs careful monitoring.

The more common cause is a drug overdose: salicylic acid, methanol, or ethylene glycol (antifreeze) poisoning. Methanol breaks down into formic acid; ethylene glycol breaks down into oxalic acid, which crystallizes in the kidney and causes acute renal failure. Salicylic acid poisoning causes two types of acid-base disturbance: a primary respiratory alkalosis and, within 8 hours, a primary metabolic acidosis. Salicylate disturbs carbohydrate metabolism and causes a depletion of liver glycogen, resulting in an accumulation of ketone bodies and lactic and pyruvic acids. When respiratory alkalosis develops, the renal compensatory mechanism causes an excretion of bicarbonate, producing a compensatory metabolic acidosis.

A fourth type of metabolic acidosis can result from excessive loss of alkaline body fluids such as intestinal secretions, as with severe diarrhea or a small bowel or biliary fistula. When diarrhea occurs, large amounts of bicarbonate are secreted into the intestinal tract and excreted, lowering the acid-base ratio and the pH. An excess accumulation of hydrogen ions in the serum also contributes to metabolic acidosis.

Two general types of metabolic acidosis can occur: (1) that with an excessive fixed acid accumulation or an increase in the unmeasured anion gap; or (2) that with a normal anion gap with a net loss of bicarbonate leading to its replacement in the ECF by chloride (hyperchloremic metabolic acidosis). Table 24–5 lists conditions causing each type of metabolic acidosis. Figure 24–9 compares the anion gap and electrolyte balance in different types of metabolic acidosis.

Signs of metabolic acidosis may not become readily apparent until the acidosis becomes more advanced. When the CO_2 content falls to 18 mEq/liter, the patient may complain of weakness, malaise, dull headache, nausea, vomiting, and abdominal pain. Kussmaul respirations, especially very deep respirations as opposed to a rapid rate, usually develop when the pH is 7.2 or lower. Vasodilation with a flushed face and a bounding pulse may be seen. Other signs depend on the underlying clinical process. Patients with diabetes and renal disease develop a fruity odor on the breath and may show signs of severe water and sodium loss due to diuresis.

The laboratory findings vary depending on whether or not compensation has occurred. If the condition is uncompensated, the pH is low and the P_{CO_2} is normal. The bicarbonate is low, and there is a base deficit. When compensation occurs, the pH rises slightly, and the P_{CO_2} falls due to hyperventilation. The serum bicarbonate level will vary depending on the underlying condition, but usually it remains low. Chloride and potassium levels are often elevated, the potassium producing electrocardiographic changes of a spiked T wave and prolonged QRS complex. A normal or low potassium value is a sign of total body fluid and potassium depletion. The causes and signs of metabolic acidosis are listed in Table 24–6 (Alexander, 1986; Methany, 1987).

Nursing Diagnoses and Interventions. Nursing diagnoses associated with metabolic acidosis are often related to the cause of the disorder or to clinical or laboratory signs. They may include the following:

1. Alteration in nutrition: more or less than body requirements

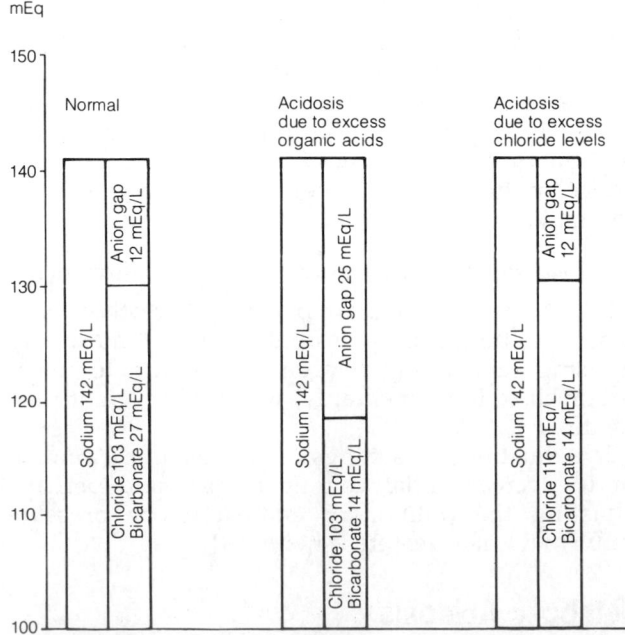

FIGURE 24–9. Comparisons of the anion gap in metabolic acidosis. (From Porth, C. M. (1986). *Pathophysiology.* Philadelphia: J. B. Lippincott.)

TABLE 24–6. Metabolic Acidosis

Cause	Signs	Laboratory Findings
Increase in acid retention or production: renal failure, ketoacidosis, acute MI, starvation, salicylate intoxication, anaerobic metabolism	Headache Confusion Kussmaul respirations Weakness Nausea Stupor	pH < 7.35 HCO_3^- < 22 mEq/liter P_{CO_2} < 35 mm Hg Negative base excess
Hyperchloremia: prolonged diarrhea, intestinal fistulas, ureterosigmoidostomy, renal tubular acidosis	Delirium Arrhythmias Warm, flushed skin	Increased K^+ Decreased Ca^{2+} in some

2. Alteration in electrolytes: potassium excess, sodium deficit

3. Alteration in acid-base: hydrogen ion excess or base deficit

4. Fluid volume excess or deficit: altered elimination

5. Alteration in cardiac output: decreased

6. Potential for injury related to alterations in sensory-perceptual awareness

Implications for nursing interventions revolve around stopping the metabolic disturbance, restoring the electrolytes that have been lost, preventing any further catabolism, and supporting respiration.

Stopping the Metabolic Process and Restoring Electrolytes

1. If the metabolic acidosis results from chloride excess, the chloride salt should be stopped immediately; the kidneys usually can eliminate the excess.

2. If the problem is diabetes, treating the patient with insulin and replacing the sodium, potassium, and water lost in diuresis should reverse the diabetic acidosis. Long-term treatment must be aimed at controlling the diabetes with a balanced dietary, medication, and activity program.

3. In patients with chronic renal failure, the acidosis cannot be reversed without dialysis. However, before they need dialysis, patients are often dehydrated. Replacing lost sodium and water will facilitate any remaining renal function. In patients with acute renal failure, water, sodium, and potassium need to be restricted until kidney function returns. Elevations of potassium need immediate treatment because they may be life-threatening.

4. In salicylate poisoning the patient may be supported by dialysis. Sodium bicarbonate may be given; however, it is dangerous because it may cause a metabolic alkalosis with a sodium overload.

5. Lactic acidosis can be treated with oxygen, rest, and medications to improve cardiac output and perfusion.

Preventing Catabolism

Preventing further catabolism is also necessary. Any additional stress such as invasive lines or wounds that would contribute to tissue trauma or breakdown should be avoided. Preventing the occurrence of or treating existing infection is a major factor in reducing metabolic need. Adequate intake of essential nutrients either orally or by means of total parenteral nutrition will facilitate maintenance of a positive nitrogen balance, reduce excess acid production, and help in building new tissue.

Supporting Respiration

Support respiration by maintaining a patent airway, using positioning to facilitate breathing, and giving oxygen or using mechanical ventilation as necessary. Because hyperventilation is the primary respiratory compensation, this mechanism should be supported while treatment is aimed at correcting the underlying problem. Replacement of fluids and electrolytes will help to rehydrate the patient and loosen respiratory secretions. Mechanical ventilation may be used when the blood pH is very low or when the patient is in respiratory failure.

Metabolic Alkalosis

Metabolic alkalosis results from an accumulation of excess base (bicarbonate) or a loss of hydrogen ions from the body. When hydrogen ions are lost, the bicarbonate–carbonic acid ratio increases, and the serum pH rises above 7.46. The kidneys try to compensate by excreting excess bicarbonate and retaining hydrogen ions. However, this process seldom fully corrects the serum pH because it is antagonistic to the normal regulatory mechanisms.

Metabolic alkalosis can occur in the following types of conditions: oral or parenteral intake of excessive base, such as sodium bicarbonate; loss of acid from the body through the gastrointestinal tract or in the urine; and electrolyte abnormalities such as loss of potassium, chloride, or calcium. The expected respiratory compensation of hypoventilation to retain carbon dioxide and elevate pH is not very efficient in correcting alkalosis. The P_{CO_2} will not exceed 60 mm Hg in patients with metabolic alkalosis, who are breathing room air, because a decreased oxygen saturation and hypoxia would result. The kidneys attempt to compensate by excreting large amounts of bicarbonate in the urine. In prolonged metabolic alkalosis, this renal compensatory mechanism is impaired often due to enhanced bicarbonate reabsorption, decreased filtration if the person is in renal failure, or a low serum potassium.

The pathophysiologic state of metabolic alkalosis is a result of excess concentrations of bicarbonate in the extracellular fluid. For instance, when excessive amounts of base, such as milk or absorbable alkali salts, are ingested, they combine with the hydrochloric acid of the gastric juice, the hydrogen ions are neutralized, and carbon dioxide is formed and eliminated, leaving excessive concentrations of bicarbonate and an elevated pH.

When hydrogen ions are lost from the gastrointestinal tract, as in vomiting, the base that has been absorbed cannot be neutralized, causing an alteration in the acid-base ratio and an increase in pH. Acids can also be lost through excessive use of diuretics. The ability of the distal tubules to reabsorb sodium and especially chloride ions is reduced with the use of diuretics. Along with the loss of these ions, potassium and ammonium ions are excreted. The excretion of each ammonium ion is associated with the loss of a hydrogen ion. When large amounts of salt and water are excreted as a result of diuretic use, the extracellular fluid becomes more concentrated around a constant amount of bicarbonate, resulting in a contraction alkalosis.

The reduction of potassium ions with gastrointestinal or renal fluid losses aggravates a metabolic alkalotic state. Potassium loss causes a metabolic alkalosis and vice versa. When potassium is lost from the intracellular fluid, sodium and hydrogen ions move into the cells, causing a decreased concentration of hydrogen in the extracellular fluid. A similar loss of potassium occurs in the renal tubular cells. Potassium is not available to combine with hydrogen ions, and they are lost in the urine, causing an increase in pH (Methany, 1987).

In addition to losses through the kidneys with diuretics or renal tubular acidosis, many other conditions of metabolic alkalosis are associated with the loss of potassium. Loss of potassium occurs through the gastrointestinal tract from vomiting, gastric suction, intestinal fistulas, or diarrhea. Gastric secretions contain approximately ten times the amount of potassium in the serum and twice the amount in the intestine. Cirrhosis of the liver and non–insulin-secreting tumors of the pancreas are associated with loss of potassium ions and metabolic alkalosis. Potassium is lost in malnourished or semistarved patients due to a very low intake despite continued urinary excretion. Hypersecretion of adrenal cortical hormones, as in Cushing syndrome or hyperaldosteronism, results in retention of sodium and the secretion of potassium. Certain antibiotics, such as sodium penicillin and amphotericin B, cause potassium loss through the kidneys.

Signs of metabolic alkalosis may be difficult to differentiate from the signs of the associated disease processes. After ingestion of large amounts of absorbable antacid medication over a long time, symptoms of anorexia, nausea, and painless vomiting may occur. Confusion and mental "unreliability" may develop, followed by drowsiness and coma. Another symptom is tetany. In alkalosis, more calcium is bound to protein, producing a low serum calcium concentration. Tetany does not occur in an acidotic state or with hypokalemia. Electrocardiographic changes can occur in alkalosis and hypokalemia. Sinus tachycardia may be apparent with a prolonged Q–T interval and the T wave approaching or merging with the P wave. The causes and signs of metabolic alkalosis are listed in Table 24–7.

Nursing Diagnoses and Interventions. Nursing

TABLE 24–7. Metabolic Alkalosis

Cause	Signs	Laboratory Findings
Acute loss of hydrogen ions: vomiting, nasogastric suction	Tingling of fingers and toes Dizziness Nausea Vomiting	pH > 7.45 HCO_3^- > 0.26 mEq/liter Positive base excess
Potassium or chloride loss: diuretics, corticosteroids, liver disease	Lethargy Coma Paralytic ileus Disorientation Convulsions	Pco_2 normal or high K^+ normal or low, Ca^{2+} low Urinary Cl^- low
Addition of base: excess use of bicarbonate, lactate administration in dialysis	Weakness Muscle cramps Tetany Depressed respirations Electrocardiographic changes	with vomiting, higher with K^+ loss

diagnoses often associated with metabolic alkalosis include the following:

1. Fluid volume deficit: gastrointestinal or renal
2. Alteration in electrolyte balance: potassium, calcium, chloride
3. Alteration in acid-base balance
4. Alteration in thought processes
5. Potential for injury related to neuromuscular irritability

Implication for nursing interventions revolve around restoring fluid and electrolyte balance and limiting alkaline intake.

Restoring Fluid and Electrolyte Balance

1. Restore fluid volume and electrolyte balance either orally or parenterally to correct the cause of the alkalosis. Observe for vomiting, diarrhea, or excess use of diuretics. Electrolytes such as chloride and potassium need to be replaced if diuretics are used or gastrointestinal fluid losses have occurred. Records of intake and output and laboratory results should be noted frequently.

2. Tetany can be corrected either by lowering the pH or raising the serum calcium. A low potassium should be treated only if a low serum calcium is increased at the same time. Correcting the alkalosis will allow the serum calcium to return to normal.

Limiting Alkaline Intake

1. Administration of alkaline antacids should be done cautiously to patients who have gastric ulcers or a metabolic acidosis.

2. Occasionally, acidifying agents, such as carbonic anhydrase inhibitors (Diamox), are used to treat alkalosis such as that produced from prolonged diuretic use. They should be used with caution.

SUMMARY

Many patients have more than one acid-base abnormality due to either multiple system involvement, normal compensatory mechanisms, or various therapies. An assessment of the underlying disease state, clinical signs, and laboratory values obtained from both arterial blood gases and venous serum is necessary to diagnose and use the appropriate interventions for acid-base alterations.

References

Adinaro, D. (1987). Liver failure and pancreatitis; Fluid and electrolyte concerns. *Nursing Clinics of North America*, 22(4):843–851.

Alexander, E. (1986). Metabolic acidosis: Recognition and etiologic diagnosis. *Hospital Practice*, 21(1):100E–100R.

Appel, G. B., and Chase, H. S. (1986). Diagnosis and treatment of acid-base disorders. In Askanazi, J., Starker, P. M., and Weissman, C. (Eds.), *Fluid and electrolyte management in critical care*. Boston: Butterworth.

Butts, D. (1987). Fluid and electrolyte disorders associated with diabetic ketoacidosis and hyperglycemic hyperosmolar nonketotic coma. *Nursing Clinics of North America*, 22(4):827–836.

Carpenito, L. J. (1987). *Handbook of nursing diagnosis* (2nd ed.). Philadelphia: J. B. Lippincott.

Chaffee, E. E., and Lytle, I. M. (1980). *Basic physiology and anatomy* (4th ed.). Philadelphia: J. B. Lippincott.

Chambers, J. K. (1987). Fluid and electrolyte problems in renal and urologic disorders. *Nursing Clinics of North America*, 22(4):815–825.

Corbett, J. V. (1987). *Laboratory tests and diagnostic procedures with nursing diagnoses* (2nd ed.). Norwalk, CT: Appleton & Lange.

Flomenbaum, N. (1984). Acid-base disturbances. *Emergency medicine* 16:59–89.

Goldberger, E. (1986). *A primer of water, electrolyte and acid-base syndromes* (7th ed.). Philadelphia: Lea & Febiger.

Guyton, A. C. (1991). *Textbook of medical physiology* (8th ed.). Philadelphia: W. B. Saunders.

Guyton, A. C. (1987). *Human physiology and mechanisms of disease* (4th ed.). Philadelphia: W. B. Saunders.

Halperin, M. L., and Goldstein, M. B. (1988). *Fluid, electrolyte, and acid-base emergencies*. Philadelphia: W. B. Saunders.

Holloway, N. M. (1984). *Nursing the critically ill adult* (2nd ed.). Menlo Park, CA: Addison-Wesley.

Hudak, C. M., Gallo, B. M., and Lohr, T. (1986). *Critical care nursing* (4th ed.). Philadelphia: J. B. Lippincott.

Kersten, L. D. (1989). *Comprehensive respiratory nursing. A decision-making approach*. Philadelphia: W. B. Saunders.

Mathewson, M., and Mathewson, R. E. (1987). Establishing acid-base balance. *Critical care nurse* 7(5), 77–80, 82–85.

McLean, F. C. (1938). *Physiological Review*, 18, 495.

Metheny, N. M. (1987). *Fluid and electrolyte balance*. Philadelphia: J. B. Lippincott.

Muir, B. L. (1980). *Pathophysiology*. New York: John Wiley & Sons.

Porth, C. M. (1986). *Pathophysiology* (2nd ed.). Philadelphia: J. B. Lippincott.

Price, S. A., and Wilson, L. M. (1987). *Pathophysiology* (3rd ed.). New York: McGraw-Hill.

Puschett, J. B., and Piraino, B. (1985). Disorders of acid-base balance. In *Disorders of fluid and electrolyte balance*. New York: Churchill Livingstone.

Romanski, S. D. (1986). Interpreting ABG's in four easy steps. *Nursing 86*, September, 27–32.

Shapiro, B. A., Harrison, R. A., and Walton, J. R. (1982). *Clinical application of blood gases* (3rd ed.). Chicago: Year Book.

Shires, G. T. (Ed.). (1988). *Fluids, electrolytes and acid base*. New York: Churchill Livingstone.

York, K. (1987). The lung and fluid-electrolyte and acid-base imbalances. *Nursing Clinics of North America* 22(4), 805–814.

25

Patients with Acute Respiratory Failure

Elizabeth A. Henneman

Glossary

PA_{O_2}	Partial pressure of alveolar oxygen
Pa_{O_2}	Partial pressure of arterial oxygen
$P\bar{v}_{O_2}$	Partial pressure of mixed venous oxygen
PA_{CO_2}	Partial pressure of alveolar carbon dioxide
Pa_{CO_2}	Partial pressure of arterial carbon dioxide
$F_{I_{O_2}}$	Fraction of inspired oxygen
$P_{I_{O_2}}$	Partial pressure of inspired oxygen
$\dot{V}_D$	Dead space
$\dot{V}_E$	Minute ventilation
$\dot{V}_A$	Alveolar ventilation
$\dot{V}/\dot{Q}$	Ventilation-perfusion ratio
A-a gradient	Alveolar-arterial gradient
$\dot{Q}_T$	Cardiac output
$\dot{Q}_S/\dot{Q}_T$	Shunt fraction
Ca_{O_2}	Oxygen content of arterial blood
$C(a-v)_{O_2}$	Arterial-venous oxygen content difference
$\dot{D}_{O_2}$	Oxygen delivery
$\dot{V}_{O_2}$	Oxygen utilization
$\dot{V}_{CO_2}$	Carbon dioxide production
Sa_{O_2}	Oxygen saturation of arterial blood
$S\bar{v}_{O_2}$	Oxygen saturation of mixed venous blood
$ETCO_2$	End-tidal carbon dioxide monitoring

Acute respiratory failure (ARF) is a medical emergency frequently encountered in the critical care setting. Critical care nurses must be able to identify patients at risk for developing ARF, recognize its signs and symptoms, and be able to provide appropriate life-saving intervention.

Respiratory failure occurs when the body is unable to meet its need for tissue oxygenation or carbon dioxide (CO_2) removal. Events leading to the development of ARF are varied and include primary lung dysfunction as well as extrinsic problems such as circulatory insufficiency (Luce, 1988). The diagnosis of ARF is made on the basis of arterial blood gas (ABG) results. A sudden deterioration in the partial pressure of arterial oxygen (Pa_{O_2}) to less than 50 mm Hg or in the partial pressure of carbon dioxide (Pa_{CO_2}) to greater than 50 mm Hg constitutes ARF (Petty, 1974). Blood gas values should serve only as a guide and must be used in conjunction with other data derived from the clinical assessment. Factors such as age and altitude affect ABGs even in healthy people. Patients with chronic obstructive pulmonary disease (COPD) may have ABGs outside the normal range. In these instances, changes from baseline and not absolute values should be considered.

An assessment of a patient's respiratory status depends on more than an evaluation of arterial blood gases. Arterial blood gases reflect only the adequacy of ventilation and the efficiency with which gas is exchanged across the pulmonary-capillary membrane. Ultimately, the purpose of respiration is to provide the tissues with oxygenated blood so that normal cellular processes may occur. This cannot happen unless well-oxygenated blood can be delivered to and utilized by the tissues. Oxygen delivery and utilization are dependent not only on pulmonary function but also on nonpulmonary factors such as cardiac output and hemoglobin levels. This chapter will review the pathophysiology, clinical assessment, and management of patients with ARF.

PATHOPHYSIOLOGY

The process of respiration involves four steps: (1) ventilation, (2) diffusion of gases across the pulmonary-capillary membrane (i.e., arterial oxygenation and CO_2 elimination), (3) oxygen delivery, and (4) oxygen utilization. A sudden impairment in one or more of these processes will result in acute respiratory failure (Fig. 25–1).

Acute Ventilatory Failure

Acute ventilatory failure (AVF) is a common cause of ARF in trauma patients, drug overdose victims, and patients with neurologic disorders. The result of acute ventilatory failure is alveolar ventilation ($\dot{V}_A$), which is inadequate for removing the CO_2 produced

by the body ($\dot{V}_{CO_2}$). Elevated CO_2 levels result from an inability to eliminate CO_2 or an increase in physiologic dead space ($\dot{V}_D$), or secondary to an increased production of CO_2 (Table 25–1). An inability to maintain an adequate minute ventilation ($\dot{V}_E$) to eliminate CO_2 is the most common cause of AVF. As minute ventilation falls, effective ventilation (i.e., alveolar ventilation) also falls, resulting in an increased Pa_{CO_2}.

$$Pa_{CO2} = \frac{\dot{V}_{CO_2}}{\dot{V}_A}$$

Decreased minute ventilation may occur secondary to mechanical obstruction (aspiration), decreased ventilatory drive (head trauma, drug overdose), or restrictive processes (muscle weakness).

Increased dead space, or wasted ventilation, will also contribute to ventilatory failure (Fig. 25–2). This occurs when areas of the lung are ventilated but not perfused. Poor perfusion inhibits the transfer of CO_2 from the pulmonary capillary into the alveoli, resulting in an increased Pa_{CO_2}. Increased dead space is seen with pulmonary embolism and other disorders that compromise the pulmonary vasculature, such as

FIGURE 25–1. Process of gas exchange leading to tissue oxygenation. An interruption at any point in the cycle will lead to acute respiratory failure.

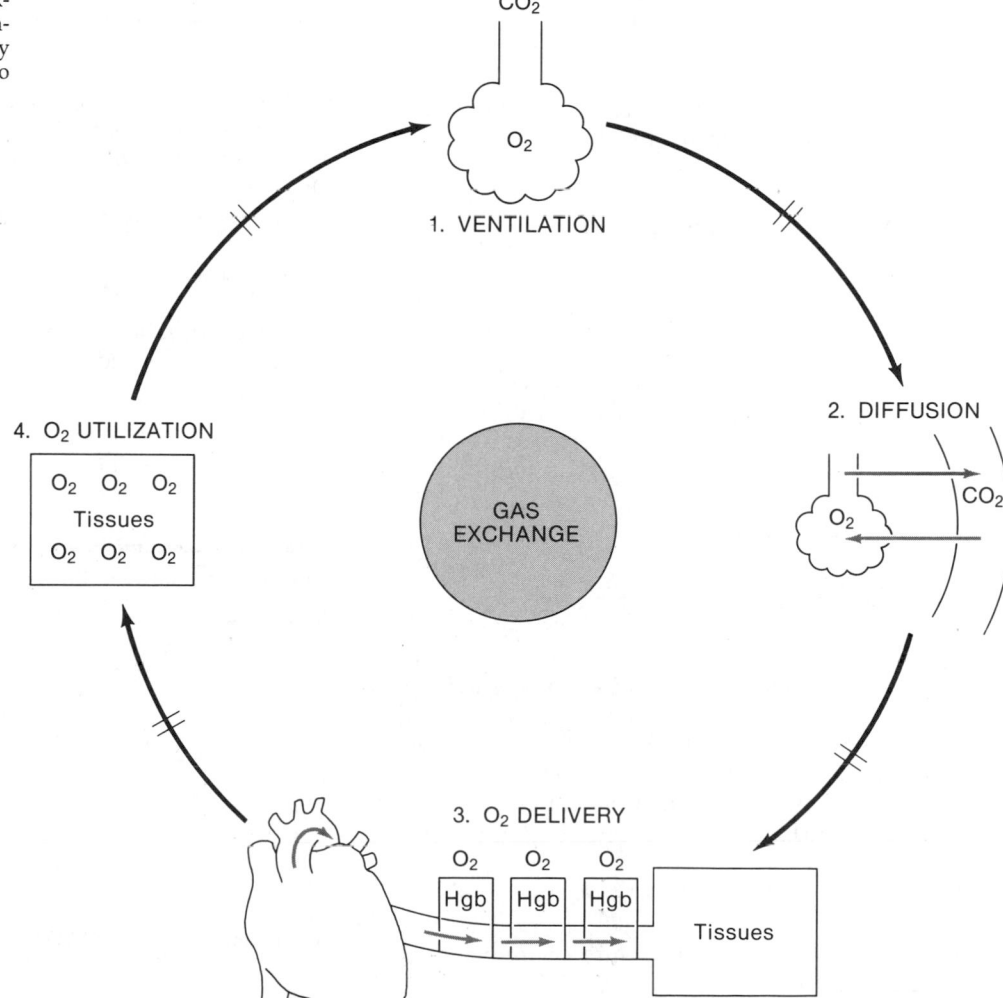

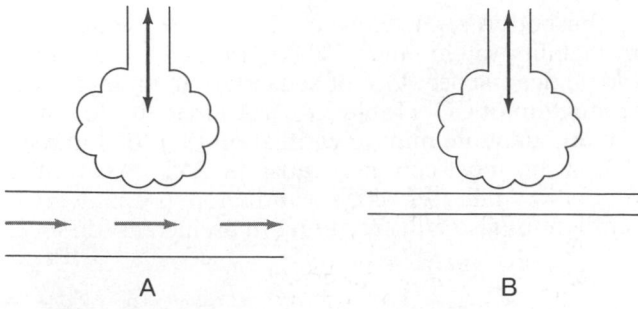

FIGURE 25–2. Relationship between ventilation and perfusion in normal (*A*) and dead space (*B*) units.

the adult respiratory distress syndrome (ARDS). In most cases, however, although CO_2 transfer is impaired, the measured Pa_{CO_2} will be normal or low because the patient has been stimulated to compensate by hyperventilating (Luce, 1988).

Although an increase in CO_2 production is rarely the primary cause of AVF, it may complicate the clinical course of a patient with underlying pulmonary dysfunction. Increases in CO_2 production occur with the administration of high carbohydrate loads or when metabolic activity is increased (e.g., with fever, exercise, seizures, or agitation).

AVF may occur with or without a concomitant decrease in oxygenation. Ventilatory failure without hypoxemia occurs when the patient's minute ventilation is affected but gas exchange in the lung is otherwise normal (e.g., after head trauma).

Failure of Arterial Oxygenation

A primary failure of arterial oxygenation is a common cause of ARF in critically ill patients (e.g., those with ARDS, pneumonia, or pulmonary edema). When the level of arterial oxygenation falls below normal, hypoxemia is present. There are five conditions that lead to impaired arterial oxygenation and hypoxemia: low inspired O_2, hypoventilation, diffusion abnormalities, ventilation-to-perfusion ($\dot{V}/\dot{Q}$) mismatching, and shunt (Table 25–2).

LOW PARTIAL PRESSURE OF INSPIRED OXYGEN

A low partial pressure of inspired oxygen (PI_{O_2}) is rarely a cause of impaired arterial oxygenation in the critical care setting. At high altitudes (as in Denver), where atmospheric pressure is less than at sea level, the PI_{O_2} will be lower despite equal concentrations of inspired oxygen (FI_{O_2}).

$$PI_{O_2} = FI_{O_2} \times (\text{atmospheric pressure} - 47)^*$$

Decreases in the partial pressure of inspired oxy-

---

*47 = Vapor pressure of water at 37° C.

TABLE 25–1. Causes of Acute Ventilatory Failure (AVF)

Decreased minute ventilation ($\dot{V}_E$)	Mechanical obstruction
	Upper airway
	Edema
	Hemorrhage
	Aspiration of solid object
	Lower airway
	Asthma
	Emphysema
	Chronic bronchitis
	Pulmonary edema
	Restrictive disorders
	Obesity
	Kyphoscoliosis
	Muscle weakness
	Neuromuscular defects
	Pneumonia
	Decreased ventilatory drive
	Drug poisonings
	Sedatives
	Head trauma
	Postoperative complications
Increased dead space ventilation ($\dot{V}_D$)	Pulmonary embolus
	ARDS
Increased CO_2 production ($\dot{V}_{CO_2}$)	Fever
	Seizures
	High carbohydrate loads
	Exercise

gen also occur during a fire, when combustion diminishes the availability of O_2 (Tyler, 1986). Purposeful or inadvertent discontinuation of delivered O_2 (FI_{O_2}) can also decrease the partial pressure of inspired oxygen, leading to hypoxemia.

HYPOVENTILATION

Hypoventilation results in an increased Pa_{CO_2} and therefore decreased PA_{O_2}, as evidenced by the following equation:

$$PA_{O_2} = FI_{O_2} \times (PB - 47) - \frac{Pa_{CO_2}}{0.8}$$

TABLE 25–2. Causes of Impaired Arterial Oxygenation

Low PI_{O_2}	High altitude
	Administration of low FI_{O_2}
Hypoventilation	Mechanical obstruction
	Restrictive disorders
	Decreased ventilatory drive
	Increased dead space ($\dot{V}_D$)
Ventilation-to-perfusion ($\dot{V}/\dot{Q}$) mismatch	Asthma
	COPD
	Atelectasis
	Congestive heart failure
	Pulmonary embolism
	Pulmonary edema
Intrapulmonary shunt ($\dot{Q}S/\dot{Q}T$)	ARDS (as above but more severe)
Diffusion defects	Pulmonary fibrosis

Only severe hypoventilation accompanied by significant increases in Pa_{CO_2} will have an impact on the PA_{O_2}. Hypoventilation as a singular problem, therefore, rarely produces hypoxemia.

DIFFUSION ABNORMALITIES

Another rare but potential cause of impaired oxygenation in the critically ill patient is diffusion defects. Optimal diffusion of gases into and out of the alveoli is dependent on the characteristics of the alveolar capillary membrane. Equilibrium between the alveoli and capillaries occurs so rapidly and efficiently that even severe diffusion defects rarely result in hypoxemia. Diffusion abnormalities occur in such conditions as interstitial fibrosis, sarcoidosis, asbestosis, and primary alveolar disease (Albert, 1988).

VENTILATION-PERFUSION ABNORMALITIES

The mismatching of ventilation to perfusion is the primary cause of impaired oxygenation and hypoxemia in the critically ill patient. Hypoxemia results when alveoli are underventilated relative to the amount of perfusion (i.e., blood flow) they receive (i.e., low $\dot{V}/\dot{Q}$) (Fig. 25–3). Unoxygenated blood passing by underventilated alveoli mixes with oxygenated blood and lowers the Pa_{O_2} (Kersten, 1989).

Decreased ventilation relative to perfusion is the mechanism of hypoxemia in such conditions as asthma, COPD, and pulmonary edema. Bronchospasm, mucus plugging, and atelectasis can also reduce ventilation of well-perfused alveoli, resulting in impaired arterial oxygenation.

SHUNT

The most severe form of low ventilation-perfusion mismatching is intrapulmonary shunt. Shunting occurs when alveoli are completely collapsed due to atelectasis or are filled with fluid or mucus (Fig. 25–3). Shunted blood returns to the systemic arteries without ever having come in contact with gas-exchanging areas of the lung.

Normal physiologic shunting comprises 3% to 5% of the cardiac output (5 mL/dL) and results from bronchial and thesbian veins emptying into the left side of the heart (Williams, 1985). The equation for

determining the ratio of shunted blood ($\dot{Q}_S$) to cardiac output ($\dot{Q}_T$) is:

$$\frac{\dot{Q}_S}{\dot{Q}_T} = \frac{Cc_{O_2} - Ca_{O_2}}{Cc_{O_2} - C\bar{v}_{O_2}}$$

where $Cc_{O_2} = O_2$ content of end capillary blood, $Ca_{O_2} = O_2$ content of arterial blood, and $C\bar{v}_{O_2} = O_2$ content of mixed venous blood.

Because the equation for calculating the shunt fraction is somewhat cumbersome, it can be estimated as follows: when breathing 100% O_2, each 20 mm Hg reduction in Pa_{O_2} (below 700 mm Hg) is equal to a 1% shunt. This rule holds true until the Pa_{O_2} falls below 150 mm Hg (severe shunt) (Zagelbaum and Pare, 1982).

Example: $Pa_{O_2} = 300$ mm Hg on 100% oxygen

Shunt = Approximately 20%

Shunting can occur with atelectasis, pneumonia, pulmonary edema, or ARDS and can be differentiated from low ventilation-perfusion abnormalities by administering 100% O_2 to the patient. Hypoxemia due to shunting will not respond to high FI_{O_2}, whereas hypoxemia due to low ventilation-perfusion problems will.

Failure of Oxygen Delivery

Patients with normal ventilation and oxygenation may still develop ARF if they are unable to deliver the well-oxygenated blood to the tissues where it is needed. Oxygen delivery is dependent on two variables, oxygen content (Ca_{O_2}) and cardiac output ($\dot{Q}_T$) (Fig. 25–4).

$$O_2 \text{ delivery} = Ca_{O_2} \times \dot{Q}_T$$

OXYGEN CONTENT

The majority of O_2 in the blood is bound to hemoglobin (97%); the rest is dissolved in the plasma. The oxygen content of the arterial blood is calculated by adding the amount of O_2 carried on the hemoglobin to the amount of dissolved O_2:

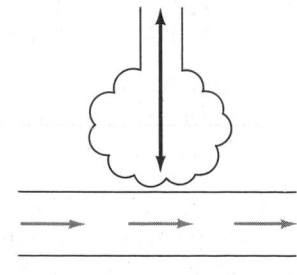
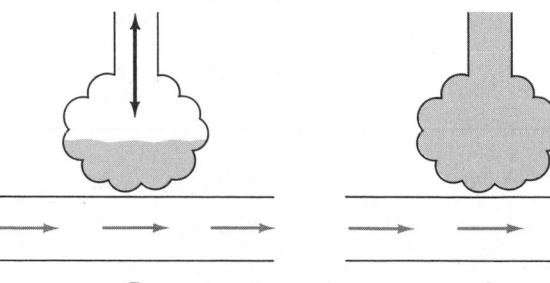

FIGURE 25–3. Normal (*A*), low $\dot{V}/\dot{Q}$–low ventilation/normal perfusion (*B*), and shunt–no ventilation/normal perfusion (*C*) units.

A

B

C

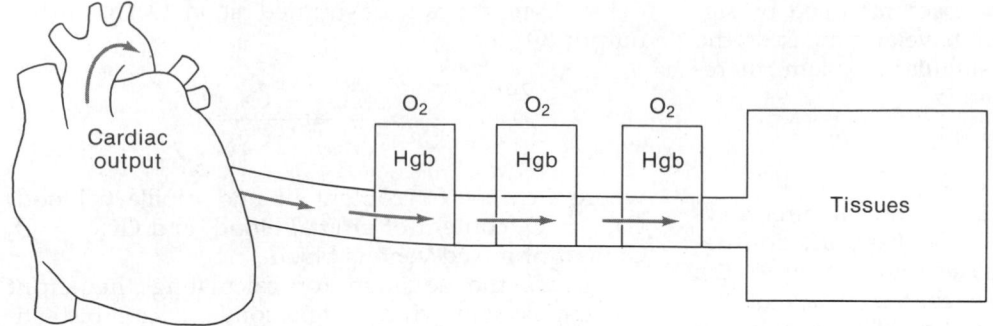

FIGURE 25–4. Components of oxygen delivery: cardiac output, hemoglobin (Hgb), and oxygen saturation.

$$Ca_{O_2} = O_2 \text{ saturation} \times \text{hemoglobin} \times 1.34 + (Pa_{O_2} \times 0.0031)$$

where 1.34 = the maximal amount of oxygen that can combine with one gram of hemoglobin. Oxygen saturation has a significant impact on the oxygen content of the arterial blood. Factors that influence the affinity of hemoglobin for O_2, such as temperature and metabolic factors, will influence O_2 saturation and enhance or impede O_2 delivery. Conditions that shift the oxyhemoglobin-dissociation curve to the right (e.g., acidosis, increased Pa_{CO_2}, fever, increased 2,3-diphosphoglycerate [2,3-DPG]) facilitate the dissociation of O_2 from hemoglobin and decrease the oxygen content of the arterial blood. Alkalosis, hypothermia, decreased Pa_{CO_2}, and decreased 2,3-DPG have the opposite effect, resulting in a greater affinity of hemoglobin for oxygen and higher O_2 saturations (shift to the left).

The amount of hemoglobin available to carry O_2 will also influence the oxygen content of the arterial blood. Anemia resulting either from blood loss, impaired red blood cell (RBC) production, or increased RBC destruction will decrease the O_2-carrying capacity of the blood.

CARDIAC OUTPUT

The cardiac output ($\dot{Q}_T$) also influences the amount of O_2 delivered to the tissues. An inadequate cardiac output results from disturbances in heart rate or stroke volume. Although cardiac output normally increases to compensate for a low oxygen content, this mechanism is often compromised in severely ill patients (Marini, 1988) (Table 25–3).

Failure of Oxygen Utilization

The final step in the process of respiration is the uptake and utilization of oxygen by the tissues. If this final step is impaired, ARF will result. When the tissues are unable to utilize oxygen, aerobic processes in the cell come to a halt. The result is a dramatic reduction in energy (adenosine triphosphate [ATP])-producing reactions and a compromise in cellular metabolic activity. The cells become dependent on anaerobic metabolism, and lactic acid accumulates.

The amount of O_2 utilized by the tissues is not related (under normal conditions) to the amount of O_2 delivered to it. Rather, the amount of O_2 utilized determines how much O_2 will be delivered. This process involves local autoregulatory mechanisms, which allow increased blood flow when O_2 requirements are high (Clemmer et al., 1988). However, studies suggest that when O_2 content reaches critically low levels, oxygen utilization becomes dependent on O_2 supply (Danek et al., 1980; Abraham et al., 1984).

The relationship between O_2 utilization and delivery is expressed by the Fick principle. Oxygen utilization is calculated by multiplying the cardiac output by the amount of O_2 extracted by the tissues (i.e., the arterial-venous O_2 content difference):

$$\dot{V}_{O_2} = \dot{Q}_T \times C(a\text{-}v)O_2$$

where $\dot{V}_{O_2}$ = O_2 utilization, $\dot{Q}_T$ = cardiac output, and $C(a\text{-}v)O_2$ = arterial-venous O_2 content difference.

A primary failure of O_2 utilization occurs in septic shock and cyanide poisoning. Patients in septic shock commonly exhibit signs of tissue hypoxia yet do not utilize available O_2, as evidenced by high mixed venous O_2 levels (i.e., oxygenation of the blood returning to the right side of the heart). It is presently unclear what mechanism is responsible for this impairment in O_2 uptake, although peripheral tissue

---

TABLE 25–3. Factors Leading to Failure of O_2 Delivery and Utilization

O_2 Delivery ($\dot{D}_{O_2}$)	
Decreased cardiac output	
Heart rate	Arrhythmias
Stroke volume	Hypovolemia
	High systemic vascular resistance (SVR)
	Myocardial infarction
	Cardiac tamponade
	Congestive heart failure
Decreased O_2 content of arterial blood (Ca_{O_2})	
Decreased hemoglobin	Anemia
Decreased O_2 saturation	Fever
	Acidosis
O_2 Utilization ($\dot{V}_{O_2}$)	Sepsis
	Cyanide poisoning

damage plays a role (Danek et al., 1980). Cyanide poisoning also results in a failure of O_2 utilization. When cyanide ions react with the enzyme cytochrome oxidase, a complex is formed that interferes with intracellular respiration. The result is a decreased utilization of oxygen, an increased amount of oxygenated blood returning to the heart (partial pressure of venous oxygen [$P\bar{v}_{O_2}$]), and a narrowing arterial-venous oxygen content difference.

CLINICAL ASSESSMENT

A comprehensive clinical evaluation of the patient with ARF includes a history, physical examination, laboratory studies, and diagnostic testing. Because ARF frequently presents as an emergency situation requiring immediate intervention, the clinical assessment is often limited. It is not uncommon to collect the majority of data after therapy has been initiated.

The patient history can be very useful in determining the etiology of ARF. If the patient is unable to provide information, data can be collected from family or other medical personnel. As much information as possible should be obtained about the details of the precipitating event (e.g., trauma, drug ingestion, flu, allergen exposure, and so on). The patient's past medical, family, occupational, and travel history may all provide useful data in reaching a diagnosis.

The chief complaint (e.g., cough, chest pain, dyspnea) may also be helpful in making a diagnosis and determining a plan of care. Unfortunately, because the signs and symptoms of ARF are nonspecific, laboratory and diagnostic testing are usually necessary to confirm a diagnosis.

The presence of cough, sputum production, chest pain, dyspnea, and mental status changes, alone or in combination, may be suggestive of respiratory failure. A cough productive of large amounts of sputum suggests chronic bronchitis or bronchiectasis. Purulent sputum points to an infectious process, and foul-smelling sputum indicates an anaerobic organism. Pink, frothy sputum is seen with pulmonary edema, whereas grossly bloody sputum occurs with pulmonary infarction or malignancy.

If the patient complains of chest pain, attempts must be made to ascertain if the discomfort is of pulmonary or cardiac origin. Pleuritic chest pain is acute, localized, and intermittent and is aggravated by breathing. This type of pain is associated with conditions such as pneumonia, pleurisy, and pulmonary infarction. Cardiac chest pain is more constant than pleuritic pain and is unaffected by respirations.

Dyspnea is a useful diagnostic finding when it is considered together with other clinical signs and symptoms. For example, dyspnea associated with cough and a history of allergen exposure is suggestive of asthma. Paroxysmal nocturnal dyspnea and orthopnea occur with left-sided heart failure. Dyspnea associated with stridor is consistent with upper airway obstruction. Transient episodes of dyspnea at rest may indicate a pulmonary embolism (Zagelbaum and Pare, 1982).

Complaints by the patient or family about mental status changes deserve particular attention. Alterations in level of consciousness (LOC) or mentation may be early signs of respiratory insufficiency.

Physical Examination

The clinical manifestations of ARF include those of the underlying disease as well as the signs and symptoms of hypoxemia or hypercapnia (Table 25–4). Respiratory failure may present in a dramatic fashion (e.g., tension pneumothorax, asthma, massive pulmonary embolism, aspiration) or so subtly that it goes unnoticed and is appreciated only by laboratory testing. Because the brain and heart have high O_2 requirements, they are particularly vulnerable to O_2 deprivation. As a result, the neurologic and cardiovascular systems deserve particular attention during the physical examination of a patient with ARF.

NEUROLOGIC SYSTEM

Headache, restlessness, and confusion are among the most common signs of ARF (Petty, 1974). Neurologic disturbances arise from both hypoxemia and hypercapnea. Altered LOC can range from a mild inability to concentrate to profound coma.

Central nervous system (CNS) disorders may also be the precipitating event in ARF. Respiratory center depression and hypoventilation result from a number of CNS insults, including head injury and sedative overdosage. Altered LOC may also precipitate ARF by predisposing the patient to aspiration.

CARDIOVASCULAR SYSTEM

Early cardiovascular changes associated with ARF represent the body's attempt to compensate for hypoxemia. These findings include tachycardia, mild hypertension, peripheral vasoconstriction, and increased cardiac output. However, if left to progress, ARF will result in cardiovascular collapse and inad-

TABLE 25–4. Clinical Manifestations of ARF

Low Pa_{O_2}	Increased Pa_{CO_2}
Hypoxemia	Hypercapnia
Restlessness	Headache
Confusion	Altered level of consciousness
Poor judgment	Coma
Coma	Cardiovascular collapse
Tachycardia	Arrhythmias
Hypertension (early)	Hypotension
Hypotension (late)	Poor peripheral perfusion
Cyanosis	
Dyspnea	
Tachypnea	

TABLE 25–5. Pulmonary Embolism

Predisposing Factors

History of deep vein thrombosis (DVT)
Immobilization (e.g., bedrest)
Postoperative patients
Right atrial thrombi (e.g., associated with atrial fibrillation)
Hypercoagulability
Trauma
Estrogen therapy
Pregnancy
Obesity

Pathophysiology

Clot lodges in pulmonary vasculature resulting in: (1) increased dead space ventilation ($\uparrow$ $\dot{V}/\dot{Q}$) + pulmonary hypertension $\rightarrow$ $\uparrow$ $\dot{V}_E$ (minute ventilation); (2) platelet aggregation, serotonin, and thromboxane $\rightarrow$ bronchoconstriction $\rightarrow$ alveolar hypofunction $\rightarrow$ atelectasis $\rightarrow$ $\downarrow$ $\dot{V}/\dot{Q}$ $\rightarrow$ hypoxemia

Clinical Presentation

Tachypnea
Tachycardia
Dyspnea
Apprehension
Pleuritic chest pain
Cough
Crackles
Fever
Wheezing
Hemoptysis
Pleural friction rub/pleural effusions

Diagnostic Tests

Laboratory tests
Arterial blood gases: Pa_{O_2} < 80 mm Hg; Pa_{CO_2} < 35 mm Hg; pH > 7.45
A-a gradient: increased
Mild leukocytosis
Elevated fibrin degradation products (FDP)

Electrocardiographic
Sinus tachycardia
Right axis deviation
Nonspecific T-wave changes
Right bundle branch block

Chest x-ray (rarely diagnostic)
Elevated hemidiaphragm
Atelectasis
Pulmonary infiltrates
Wedge-shaped density in periphery
Pleural effusions
Enlarged hilar pulmonary arteries

Ventilation/perfusion scans—see multiple segmental or lobar perfusion defects with normal ventilation

Angiography will show "cut off" of blood flow or filling defect

Medical Therapy

Goal: To stabilize cardiopulmonary function (i.e., maintain adequate oxygen delivery), prevent reembolization, and avoid pulmonary damage

1. Stabilize cardiopulmonary function (particularly for patients with hemodynamic compromise (i.e., in shock)
   a. Basic and advanced life support
   b. Ventilatory support/supplemental O_2
   c. Maintenance of cardiac output
      (1) Vasopressors
      (2) Fluids
2. Prevent reembolization with anticoagulation therapy to prevent new clots
   a. Heparin
      (1) Initial dose = 140–200 units/kg IVP
      (2) Maintenance dose = 25 units/kg IV per hour to keep PTT at 1.5 to 2.5 times control
   b. Sodium warfarin (Coumadin) = 5–10 mg/day to keep PT at 2.0 to 2.5 times control (long-term up to 12 months)
3. Avoid further pulmonary damage with thrombolytic therapy to dissolve embolus
   a. Indicated for patients with significant hemodynamic disturbances
   b. Streptokinase
      (1) Initial dose = 250,000 IU IV (over 30 minutes)
      (2) Maintenance dose = 100,000 IU/hour IV for 24–72 hours
   c. Urokinase
      (1) Initial dose = 4400 IU/kg IV (over 30 minutes)
      (2) Maintenance dose = 4400 IU/kg/hour IV for 12 hours
4. Surgical management—indicated for patients in whom medical management is contraindicated and for patients with recurrent pulmonary embolism despite adequate anticoagulation
   a. Femoral vein ligation
   b. Inferior vena cava ligation
   c. Intraluminal umbrella
   d. Pulmonary embolectomy (rare)

From Arabian, A. A. (1986). In S. V. Spagnolo and A. Medinger (Eds.), *Handbook of pulmonary emergencies* (pp. 193–204). New York: Plenum Publishing Corp.

equate perfusion, manifested by arrhythmias, ischemic pain, and hypotension.

PULMONARY SYSTEM

An in-depth evaluation of the pulmonary system is indicated for all patients with suspected or proved ARF. This comprehensive examination includes observation, palpation, percussion, and auscultation.

Skillful observation may provide useful diagnostic information about the presence and severity of ARF, although not in all cases. For example, patients who are hypercapnic may appear somnolent and not in any acute distress when in fact their Pa_{CO_2} levels are dangerously high. On the other hand, respiratory distress may be suspected in other groups of patients simply by noting their facial expressions (e.g., apprehension or fear in patients with asthma).

Careful attention must be paid during the physical examination to observation of the respiratory rate, pattern, and depth. Irregular or labored respirations may provide early clues to respiratory failure. Patients who are hypoxemic frequently present with tachypnea, whereas hypercapnic patients may have depressed respirations.

Observation of chest and abdominal movements may be useful in assessing ventilatory status. The use of accessory muscles (e.g., sternocleidomastoid) suggests air hunger, whereas the development of inward abdominal retraction indicates diaphragm fatigue, usually an ominous sign.

Palpating the trachea and chest wall is also a useful diagnostic tool in patients with ARF. Tracheal deviation and asymmetric chest wall movements occur in such conditions as pneumothorax and hydrothorax. Areas of abnormal density can be discovered by percussing the chest wall. Pneumothoraces are characterized by hyperresonance, whereas pneumonia and pleural effusions are associated with dullness.

Auscultation is used to identify the presence or absence of breath sounds and to identify obstruction or fluid in the airways or lungs. Breath sounds are diminished or absent when the alveoli are collapsed or underventilated, as in atelectasis or pneumothorax. Upper airway obstruction usually results in inspiratory wheezes (heard best over the trachea), and lower airway obstruction results in expiratory wheezes. When severe, these findings are audible without the aid of a stethoscope. Other adventitious breath sounds such as crackles occur when fluid is present in the airway or alveoli or when collapsed alveoli are opened during inspiration (e.g., in pulmonary edema). Rhonchi are indicative of large airway obstruction due either to mucus accumulation or stricture. A pleural friction rub, a harsh, grating sound, is suggestive of an inflammation of the pleura or a loss of pleural fluid (as with pulmonary emboli, infarction, or fractured ribs) (Williams, 1985). See Table 25–5 for specific findings associated with pulmonary embolism.

DIAGNOSTIC TESTS

Arterial Blood Gas Monitoring

Critically ill patients with ARF require monitoring of the adequacy of ventilation (Pa_{CO_2}), oxygenation of arterial blood (Pa_{O_2}), oxygen delivery (oxygen saturation, cardiac output, and hemoglobin), and oxygen utilization. Adequacy of ventilation can be monitored intermittently through arterial blood gas analysis of Pa_{CO_2}. The Pa_{CO_2} varies directly with alveolar ventilation and therefore can be used as an indicator of whether or not the patient is ventilating enough to meet his metabolic needs. A low Pa_{CO_2}, less than 35 mm Hg (hypocapnia), occurs in ARF either secondary to pain or anxiety or as a compensatory response to a metabolic acidosis or in an attempt to improve oxygenation. Hypercapnia (Pa_{CO_2} greater than 45 mm Hg) suggests that the patient is unable to ventilate adequately to meet his metabolic needs. Hypoventilation and resultant hypercapnia are dangerous in that they will lead to respiratory acidosis if left untreated.

The adequacy of ventilation can also be measured continuously with end-tidal CO_2 (ET_{CO_2}) monitoring. This noninvasive technique utilizes mass spectrometry or infrared spectroscopy to detect variations in expired CO_2. It may be used to trend CO_2 levels, particularly if continuous monitoring is indicated such as during weaning from mechanical ventilation.

Arterial blood gas monitoring also allows for intermittent evaluation of Pa_{O_2} and oxygen saturation (Sa_{O_2}). A Pa_{O_2} of less than 50 to 60 mm Hg or an Sa_{O_2} of less than 90% on room air (at sea level) is indicative of hypoxemia. A comprehensive evaluation of the cause and extent of hypoxemia requires the use of formulas such as the alveolar-arterial (A-a) gradient and shunt fraction. Calculation of the A-a gradient is useful in determining whether the hypoxemia is due to a problem with gas exchange in the lung or is secondary to an extrapulmonary event. A normal A-a gradient is 10 mm Hg on room air and 100 mm Hg on an F_{IO_2} of 1.0. If the A-a gradient is widened (greater than normal), the hypoxemia is due to a primary lung problem (e.g., diffusion defect, ventilation-perfusion mismatch, shunt); normal A-a gradients are seen with such extrapulmonary causes of hypoxemia as hypoventilation and low partial pressures of inspired oxygen.

$$\text{A-a gradient} = PA_{O_2} - Pa_{O_2}$$

$$PA_{O_2} = F_{IO_2} \times (PB - 47) - \frac{Pa_{CO_2}}{0.8}$$

Noninvasive oxygen monitoring that permits continuous evaluation of Sa_{O_2} is available. Although these oximeters (pulse or ear) can assess arterial oxygenation, they may be of limited value in certain situations (e.g., in patients who have hypothermia or vasoconstriction or are agitated).

Monitoring of oxygen delivery and utilization requires a pulmonary artery catheter to determine cardiac output and obtain mixed venous blood gas samples. The newest hemodynamic monitoring technology uses reflectance spectrophotometry to monitor continuously the saturation of mixed venous oxygen ($S\bar{v}_{O_2}$), which is an indicator of the balance between O_2 delivery and utilization.

Laboratory Tests

As previously mentioned, ABG analysis is critical in diagnosing ARF. In addition to ABGs, a complete blood count (CBC) and electrolytes should be routinely ordered for all patients with ARF, paying particular attention to hemoglobin, potassium, magnesium, phosphorus, and calcium. Patients in whom an infectious pulmonary process is suspected (e.g., a patient with COPD who is admitted with an acute exacerbation of the illness) should have a sputum specimen taken and sent for culture and sensitivity. More specific tests such as toxicology screens or thyroid function studies should be ordered if indicated by the patient's history or other clinical findings.

Chest X-ray

An evaluation of the anteroposterior (AP) and lateral chest x-ray (CXR) is valuable in substantiating the findings from the physical examination and determining the etiology of ARF. Possible CXR findings include areas of consolidation (e.g., pneumonia), hyperinflation (e.g., emphysema), pulmonary venous congestion, cardiomegaly (e.g., left heart failure), pleural effusion, collapsed lung (e.g., pneumothorax), fractured ribs, or flail chest.

Pulmonary Function Tests

Measurement of pulmonary function tests (PFTs) are useful in diagnosing obstructive airway disease and in evaluating the effectiveness of bronchodilator therapy. Patients with COPD typically have a reduction in expiratory volume during the first second of a forced exhalation (FEV_1) and a reduction in the ratio of FEV_1 to forced vital capacity (FEV_1/FVC). Asthmatics also have diminished flow rates but experience improvement after bronchodilator therapy. This difference in response of FEV_1 to bronchodilator therapy is used to distinguish reversible (e.g., asthma) from nonreversible (e.g., COPD) airway disease (Zagelbaum and Pare, 1982). Pulmonary function studies require an alert, cooperative patient and are often difficult to perform during a critical illness.

Miscellaneous Tests

A variety of other diagnostic tests are available to assist in the differential diagnosis of ARF, including bronchoscopy, ventilation-perfusion ($\dot{V}/\dot{Q}$) scans, and angiography. Bronchoscopy permits direct visualization of the tracheobronchial tree using a flexible fiberoptic scope. The bronchoscope can also be used to obtain specimens, either by suction or biopsy, to confirm or provide a diagnosis.

Pulmonary $\dot{V}/\dot{Q}$ scans and angiography are used in the evaluation of pulmonary embolism (PE). Although $\dot{V}/\dot{Q}$ scans are among the major diagnostic tests for PE, they lack specificity and can only suggest a low, intermediate, or high probability of PE. Pulmonary angiography is considered the "gold standard" diagnostic tool for PE but is associated with some risk (Chandler, 1979) (Table 25–5).

MANAGEMENT OF ACUTE RESPIRATORY FAILURE

Effective management of ARF requires the combined efforts of a skilled multidisciplinary team. Although each member of the team (nurse, physician, respiratory therapist) has specific functions, the goals of therapy are similar. The critical care nurse's role in management of ARF includes assessing and monitoring the patient, developing a plan of care, administering therapy, and evaluating the effectiveness of the plan. Interventions employed by the nurse include those prescribed by the physician as well as other independent therapies. Specific nursing goals and interventions for patients with ARF are addressed in the nursing care plan at the end of this chapter.

A primary goal in the management of ARF is treatment of the underlying condition that precipitated the acute event while supporting respiratory function at the same time. The specifics of patient management for the multitude of possible causes of ARF are beyond the scope of this chapter. (See Chapters 26, 27, and 28 for management of ARDS, pulmonary infection, and COPD.) The essentials of management of pulmonary embolism are addressed in Table 25–5 to serve as an example.

Regardless of the underlying cause, the principles of providing airway management, ventilatory support, and supplemental oxygenation are the same. The approach used ultimately depends on the mechanism of respiratory failure present in a particular patient (i.e., ventilatory failure, oxygenation failure, failure of O_2 delivery, or failure of O_2 utilization).

Managing Acute Ventilatory Failure

A patient with AVF requires immediate assessment and stabilization of the airway (basic cardiac life support). If the airway is obstructed, steps must be taken to ensure its patency. This may require repositioning the patient (chin-tilt) or removing foreign material (e.g., Heimlich maneuver, suctioning). Opening the patient's airway may be the only step necessary for treating AVF.

If the patient's minute ventilation is inadequate, experienced personnel should intubate the patient, allowing for artificial ventilation as well as airway protection. Types of artificial airways are listed in Table 25–6. (See Chapter 29 for a discussion of mechanical ventilators.) Once ventilatory support has been established, the priority of management is treatment of the underlying condition and interventions for complications.

Improving Arterial Oxygenation

A failure of arterial oxygenation may occur alone or in combination with AVF. As soon as the patient's

TABLE 25–6. Artificial Airways

Airway	Indications	Precautions	Potential Complications	Miscellaneous
Nasopharyngeal	Pharyngeal obstruction Secretion removal Mouth to nose ventilation		Trauma from insertion (bleeding)	Useful with facial or jaw fractures or when oral airways are inappropriate May be used in conscious or unconscious patients Humidification is necessary to maintain airway patency
Oropharyngeal	Pharyngeal obstruction Secretion removal Holds tongue anteriorly Mouth to mouth ventilation	Will cause gagging in conscious patients	Trauma from insertion Vomiting Aspiration	Improper insertion technique could push tongue back and occlude airway
Endotracheal	Establishes airway when nasopharyngeal or oropharyngeal airways are inadequate Allows for mechanical ventilation Secretion removal	Requires skilled personnel to insert	Improper placement (esophageal intubation) Mucosal damage Laryngeal or tracheal edema Vocal cord damage Tracheal stenosis (rare) Obstruction of tube Kinking of tube Cuff herniation Tracheoesophageal fistula Sinusitis	Has cuff to prevent aspiration Cuff should be maintained below capillary filling pressure of trachea (20 mm Hg) to avoid damage
Tracheostomy	Provides long-term airway management Allows for mechanical ventilation Secretion removal Bypasses upper airway obstruction Assists in prevention of aspiration		Complications associated with insertion (e.g., bleeding, infection, pneumothorax) Obstruction of tube Cuff herniation Tracheoesophageal fistula Dislodged tube Hemorrhage	Requires surgery
Cricoidthyroidotomy	Provides an immediate airway in extreme emergencies	Requires skilled personnel	Bleeding	Only a temporary measure to be used until a more stable airway is secured

airway and ventilation are supported, efforts are directed toward improving alveolar oxygenation. Hypoxemia is managed by maximizing ventilation, increasing the FI_{O_2}, decreasing ventilation-perfusion mismatching, and diminishing shunt.

IMPROVING VENTILATION

Any attempt to influence oxygenation will be futile if the patient does not have an adequate airway or effective alveolar ventilation (see previous section on management of AVF). In some patients (e.g., those with COPD or asthma) both ventilation and oxygenation can be optimized by relieving air flow obstruction through such interventions as bronchial hygiene or bronchodilators. In other instances, the need for artificial support may be averted through performing vigorous interventions aimed at improving airway patency (e.g., bronchodilators, bronchial hygiene).

INCREASING FI_{O_2}

Increasing the FI_{O_2} will improve the Pa_{O_2} when a low partial pressure of inspired oxygen, hypoventi-

lation, diffusion impairment, or ventilation-perfusion mismatch is the cause of hypoxemia. Only intrapulmonary shunting will not respond significantly to increased O_2 administration.

There are a variety of methods available for administration of O_2 therapy (Table 25–7). Because O_2 is a drug, it should be administered cautiously, with an awareness of the dosage being given and potential side effects.

Serious complications of O_2 therapy include suppression of hypoxic drive in patients with COPD, absorption atelectasis, and parenchymal damage. Prolonged periods of high Pa_{CO_2} with acidosis in patients with COPD reduce the sensitivity of the medulla to changes in cerebrospinal pH. The result is that hypoxia instead of hypercapnia becomes the stimulus to breathe. If high levels of O_2 are administered without ventilatory support, CNS depression, hypoventilation, and acidosis may occur (Mecca, 1986).

Alveoli are normally filled with a combination of gases, including CO_2, O_2, and nitrogen (N_2). Because N_2 is not absorbed into the pulmonary capillaries, it keeps the alveoli open. However, when 100% O_2 is

TABLE 25–7. O_2 Delivery Systems

System	Amount of O_2 Delivered	Advantages	Disadvantages	Miscellaneous
Nasal cannula	0.5 liter–5 liters/min (20%–40%)	Easy to apply Comfortable Patient able to eat	Variable amounts of O_2 delivered depending on patient's minute ventilation, O_2 flow rate, and the way patient breathes (mouth or nose) Causes mucosal drying at high flow rates (greater than 4 liters/minute)	Requires humidification at flow rates greater than 4 liters/minute
Simple face mask	40%–60%	Easy to apply	Variable amounts of O_2 delivered depending on patient's V_E, O_2 flow rates, and mask fit Must be removed to eat May cause skin irritation if applied too tightly Uncomfortable	May be used with a nebulizer to humidify inspired gas
Partial rebreathing mask	35%–60%	Allows for delivery of higher concentrations of O_2 than a simple mask Humidification of inspired gas is unnecessary	Increases in CO_2 may occur if O_2 reserve bag collapses, allowing the rebreathing of expired gases Uncomfortable	High flow rates are necessary to prevent the reserve bag from collapsing
Nonrebreathing mask	60%–100%	One-way valve prevents rebreathing of expired gases and allows for delivery of higher FI_{O_2} than with partial rebreather masks	Skin irritation Uncomfortable	Loose masks allow room air to enter during inspiration Requires high flow rates to prevent collapse of reservoir bag
Venturi mask	24%–50%	Maintains FI_{O_2} within a narrow range Allows for minimal rebreathing of CO_2 Humidification not necessary	Uncomfortable	Utilized in patients with COPD to avoid depression of hypoxic drive (or other patients with specific O_2 needs)
T-piece tracheal mask	21%–100%	Delivers variable amounts of humidified O_2 to intubated patients		May be used with oral or nasal endotracheal tubes, or tracheostomy tubes Requires heated nebulizer and large-bore tubing Requires high flow rates to prevent CO_2 accumulation in T-tube reservoir
Mechanical ventilation	21%–100%	Allows for high concentrations of O_2 in patients with concomitant ventilatory failure or in patients requiring constant high FI_{O_2}	Requires skilled personnel to operate	O_2 must be warmed and humidified High FI_{O_2} may be offset with PEEP

COPD, chronic obstructive pulmonary disease; PEEP, positive end-expiratory pressure.

delivered, N_2 is replaced by O_2, and the alveoli collapse when all their oxygen is absorbed before the next breath (i.e., absorption atelectasis).

O_2 toxicity may also result in damage to the lung parenchyma itself. If high levels of O_2 are administered for prolonged periods, pulmonary capillary damage can also occur, resulting in an ARDS-like picture of pulmonary edema (Mecca, 1986). The actual incidence of oxygen toxicity is difficult to determine because it occurs in the context of other lung injuries associated with the same histologic changes.

DECREASING $\dot{V}/\dot{Q}$ MISMATCH

Efforts directed toward improving the ratio of alveolar ventilation to perfusion may also improve hypoxemia. Low $\dot{V}/\dot{Q}$ is managed by decreasing airway obstruction (secretions, bronchospasm) or lung fluid (pneumonia, pulmonary edema). Bronchial hygiene and pharmacologic interventions (bronchodilators, diuretics) are utilized in the treatment of patients with low $\dot{V}/\dot{Q}$ ratios.

Bronchial Hygiene. Vigorous bronchial hygiene is

frequently the mainstay of therapy for ventilation-perfusion abnormalities; methods include chest physical therapy (CPT), effective coughing, and suctioning. Chest physical therapy is used to facilitate the transfer of mucus from the lower to the upper airways, where they can be removed by suctioning or coughing. Theoretically, CPT prevents the accumulation of secretions and aids in their removal, thereby improving oxygenation. However, there is little evidence that CPT as a singular modality improves Pa_{O_2} (Graham and Bradley, 1978). Studies do suggest that CPT improves mucus clearance and air flow in patients with copious secretions (e.g., cystic fibrosis, chronic bronchitis) (Feldman et al., 1979; May and Munt, 1979). Techniques of CPT (postural drainage, percussion, vibration) have been described in detail elsewhere (Dean, 1987). Typically, a combination of methods is employed to optimize removal of secretions.

Postural drainage utilizes gravity to assist in the drainage of secretions from localized areas of the lung. This technique is commonly used in conjunction with other methods to enhance their effectiveness. Percussion and vibration are used to loosen and dislodge mucus and assist in the movement of secretions into the bronchi and trachea.

Coughing and deep breathing may be employed singly or in combination with the techniques mentioned earlier as part of a bronchial hygiene regimen. It has been suggested that coughing is the most effective method of mobilizing and removing secretions (Oldenburg et al., 1979).

It is important that the clinician document the efficacy of CPT as well as the patient's tolerance of the procedure. Breath sounds, heart rate and rhythm, blood pressure, and O_2 saturation should be evaluated before and after CPT. The risk-benefit ratio of CPT must always be considered. For example, patients with a head injury and increased intracranial pressure may benefit from CPT and improved oxygenation but should not be placed in a head-down position. In this instance, a modification of traditional CPT is necessary (e.g., gentle vibration and deep breathing). The effect of CPT (and any intervention) on intracranial pressure should always be monitored closely.

Suctioning the trachea and mainstem bronchi is necessary when patients are unable to cough effectively and clear their secretions. This situation is typically seen in patients with decreased levels of consciousness and in those with weak muscular strength. Various techniques have been suggested to improve the efficacy of suctioning. One such technique is the instillation of normal saline into the endotracheal tube prior to suctioning. This method is believed to improve Pa_{O_2} by loosening secretions and opening the airway. Several studies have been conducted to examine the usefulness of this practice. In one study, investigators instilled technetium-tagged saline into tracheal tubes and found that all of the normal saline remained in the trachea or mainstem bronchi even after hyperinflation (Hanley et al., 1978). Instillation of normal saline has also been reported to be of questionable value in facilitating removal of secretions and to be ineffective in improving Pa_{O_2} (Bostick and Wendelgrass, 1987). Some clinicians theorize that the major benefit of saline is its propensity to elicit a cough (Demers and Saklad, 1973).

Pharmacologic Agents. Bronchospasm, either alone or in combination with increased secretions, can impair ventilation. A variety of bronchodilators are now available, including sympathomimetics and corticosteroids (Table 25–8). The advent of beta-2 selective agents has minimized the adverse side effects (e.g., tachycardias) once common with bronchodilator therapy.

Diuretics are indicated in the treatment of low ventilation-to-perfusion abnormalities secondary to pulmonary edema of cardiac or noncardiac origin (i.e., ARDS). Cardiogenic pulmonary edema is treated by improving left ventricular function (by optimizing preload, afterload, and contractility). Noncardiogenic pulmonary edema is not related to heart function and therefore will not respond to similar interventions. In both instances, however, diuresis may be useful in reducing intravascular hydrostatic pressure and excessive filtration of fluid into the alveoli (Albert, 1988).

Decreasing Shunt. Intrapulmonary shunting is the most extreme form of low V/Q mismatching. As a result, many of the techniques described in the previous section will also improve shunt. Administration of high F_{IO_2}s, however, will be futile in the patient with shunt.

Positive end-expiratory pressure (PEEP) in the ventilated patient, or continuous positive airway pressure (CPAP) in the spontaneously breathing patient is used in the treatment of severe shunt (i.e., hypoxemia refractory to the administration of greater than 60% O_2 for at least 30 minutes) (Demers and Irwin, 1983). Positive end-expiratory pressure opens collapsed alveoli, increases the lung's functional residual capacity, and improves compliance. When pulmonary edema is present, the application of PEEP converts areas of shunt to areas of low $\dot{V}/\dot{Q}$ by opening alveoli and allowing the edema to spread over a greater surface area. The result is improved transport of gases across the pulmonary capillary membrane, an increased responsiveness to O_2 therapy, and an improvement in Pa_{O_2}.

Potential complications of PEEP include pulmonary barotrauma and a reduction in cardiac output. Barotrauma, the presence of extra-alveolar air resulting from positive pressure ventilation, occurs in up to 25% of patients receiving PEEP. Barotrauma may be manifest as subcutaneous emphysema, pneumothorax, tension pneumothorax, pneumopericardium, pneumoperitoneum, interstitial emphysema, and, rarely, air embolism.

PEEP reduces cardiac output by impeding venous

TABLE 25–8. Pharmacologic Agents Commonly Utilized in Acute Respiratory Failure

Drug	Indications	Mechanism of Action	Dosage	Adverse Effects	Miscellaneous
Aminophylline	Bronchospasm	Inhibits phosphodiesterase, which catalyzes the degradation of cyclic AMP resulting in beta-adrenergic stimulation and bronchodilation	Loading dose (IV): 3–6 mg/kg over 30 minutes Continuous infusion (IV): 0.5–0.9 mg/kg per hour	CNS disturbances Arrhythmias GI disturbances Seizures	Serum blood levels should be used to guide dosages Therapeutic levels are between 5 and 20 mg/liter
Epinephrine	Bronchospasm	Alpha and beta agonist	0.3–0.5 mL of a 1/1000 solution SC every 20 to 30 minutes (may be repeated 3 times)	Cardiac stimulation: palpitations arrhythmias hypertension	Avoid use in patients with ischemic heart disease
Isoproterenol (Isuprel)	Bronchospasm	Nonselective beta agonist	0.3–0.5 mL of a 5% solution via nebulizer every 3 hours prn	As above	
Isoetharine (Bronkosol)	Bronchospasm	Selective beta-2 agonist	0.5 mL of a 1% solution via nebulizer every 4 hours prn	As above (less severe)	
Metaproterenol (Alupent/Metaprel)	Bronchospasm	Selective beta-2 agonist	0.5–1.0 mL of a 5% solution via nebulizer every 4 to 6 hours prn	As above	Longer duration of action than isoproterenol or isoetharine
Racemic epinephrine (Vaponephrin)	Laryngeal edema	Alpha and beta stimulation	0.25–0.5 mL of a 2.25% solution via nebulizer every 2 hours prn	Cardiac stimulation	
Corticosteroids	Bronchospasm	Anti-inflammatory	Dose dependent on type of corticosteroid administered	Gastric disturbances Hypokalemia Metabolic alkalosis	
Furosemide (Lasix)	Heart failure Pulmonary edema	Loop diuretic Decreases intravascular volume Increases venous capacitance	20–80 mg IV/po	Volume depletion Hypokalemia Hyponatremia Hypochloremic metabolic alkalosis Ototoxicity	
Antibiotics	Pulmonary infection		Varies	Hypersensitivity reactions Superinfections	Antibiotic therapy should be based on results of culture and sensitivity tests
Heparin	Pulmonary embolism Proved or suspected deep venous thrombosis	Inactivates clotting factors	Loading dose (IV): 140–200 units/kg Maintenance dose (continuous infusion): 20 units/kg per hour	Bleeding	Heparin dosages should be adjusted to maintain partial thromboplastin time at 1.5 to 2.5 times control
Streptokinase	Pulmonary embolism resulting in unstable cardiopulmonary status	Antithrombolytic	Initial dose (IV): 250,000 IU over 30 minutes Maintenance dose (IV): 100,000 IU/hr for 24–72 hr	Hemorrhage Allergic reactions Fever Hypotension Arrhythmias	Monitor thrombin time to maintain 2.5 times normal
Urokinase	Same as for streptokinase	Same as above	Initial dose (IV): 4400 IU/kg over 30 minutes Maintenance dose (IV): 4400 IU/kg/hr for 12 hours	Same as above	Same as above

Data from Brenner and Yanos, 1985; Zagelbaum and Pare, 1982.

return and possibly by impairing ventricular disten-sibility (Dorinsky and Whitcomb, 1983). Of note is that PEEP adversely affects patients with normal, compliant lungs more than those with abnormal lungs (e.g., those with ARDS) because the PEEP is dissipated across the stiff lungs more than normal lungs. As a result, patients on PEEP with noncom-pliant lungs experience less change in intrathoracic pressure, and therefore there is less impact on ve-nous return than in patients with normal lungs.

PEEP is generally applied in small increments (3 to 5 cm H_2O) while ABGs and hemodynamics are being monitored. The goal is to determine the "op-timal PEEP," i.e., the amount of PEEP that allows optimal oxygenation without compromising cardiac output. Monitoring O_2 delivery allows the best eval-uation of PEEP therapy because it includes the ben-eficial effect on oxygen content as well as the detri-mental effect on cardiac output. The level of PEEP at which O_2 delivery is maximized is the optimal PEEP.

Improving O_2 Delivery

Optimizing O_2 delivery requires interventions aimed at maximizing O_2 saturation, cardiac output, and hemoglobin. Oxygen saturation can be improved by optimizing Pa_{O_2} and by stabilizing blood pH and temperature so that shifts in the oxyhemoglobin dissociation curve (i.e., hemoglobin's affinity for O_2) do not occur.

Anemia also has an impact on O_2 delivery. Fortu-nately, the body will compensate for a fall in hemo-globin by increasing cardiac output. However, this ability to increase cardiac output in compensation for anemia is often compromised in critical illness. Treat-ment of anemia is essential to optimize O_2 delivery and may require blood transfusions. Iron replace-ment may also be used as an adjunctive therapy.

Without an adequate cardiac output, oxygenated blood is unable to reach the tissues. Optimizing cardiac output may necessitate altering heart rate or stroke volume. Abnormal heart rates or rhythms can impede ventricular filling and cardiac function. Treat-ment of arrhythmias requires normalizing oxygena-tion and electrolytes and possibly administering an-tiarrhythmics. Stroke volume can be improved by optimizing preload (left ventricular end-diastolic vol-ume), contractility, and afterload (systemic imped-ance to ventricular ejection). Preload is optimized by administering fluid or diuretic therapy and noting its effect on the pulmonary capillary wedge pressure (PCWP) and other variables (blood pressure, cardiac output, urine output).

Correction of acid-base and electrolyte imbalances is useful in ensuring optimal cardiac contractility. When necessary, inotropic agents (e.g., digitalis, catecholamines) may be used to improve ventricular performance.

Afterload reduction may be necessary when sys-temic vascular resistance (SVR) is impeding ventric-ular ejection. Nitroprusside is often the drug of choice, although other agents (e.g., hydralazine) may also be effective. The combination of an afterload reducer and a selective inotrope (e.g., dobutamine) may be beneficial in optimizing O_2 delivery (Miller et al., 1977).

Optimizing O_2 Utilization

Impaired utilization of O_2 is perhaps the least understood of all the mechanisms of ARF and as a result is difficult to manage. At least in certain situations, however, it has been shown that by im-proving O_2 delivery, O_2 utilization also improves. The current recommendation in patients with septic shock is to increase O_2 delivery until O_2 utilization no longer increases (i.e., supply independent) (Abra-ham et al., 1984; Danek et al., 1980).

Patients with cyanide poisoning also suffer from a primary failure of O_2 utilization but are more easily treated. Administration of sodium nitrate and so-dium thiosulfate allows cyanide to convert to thio-cyanate, a relatively nontoxic, excretable substance (Clemmer et al., 1988).

MANAGING COMPLICATIONS OF ACUTE RESPIRATORY FAILURE

Complications of ARF will arise if hypoxemia and hypercapnia are left untreated. Hypoxemia affects all bodily functions but particularly the central nervous and cardiovascular systems. Hypercapnia associated with respiratory acidosis also affects the CNS and may lead to cardiovascular collapse. Although re-medial steps may be helpful in managing the com-plications of ARF, the underlying condition must ultimately be resolved.

In addition to the complications of hypoxemia that have previously been addressed, acid-base disorders pose particular problems for the patient in respiratory failure. Not only do acid-base disorders interfere with normal cellular processes, they also aggravate other complications.

Acute respiratory acidosis occurs when the Pa_{CO_2} is allowed to rise suddenly without intervention. Treatment of respiratory acidosis involves facilitating the removal of CO_2 by improving alveolar ventilation.

Respiratory alkalosis results from hyperventilation, which may be a compensatory response to hypox-emia or may be iatrogenically induced through me-chanical ventilation. Therapy is directed at treating the cause of the hyperventilation; it is seldom nec-essary to treat the alkalosis itself.

For specific management, see the nursing care plan that follows.

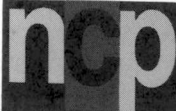 **nursing care plan**

1. **Impaired airway clearance related to:**
   Mechanical obstruction (foreign body, bronchospasm, edema)
   Neuromuscular impairment (Guillain-Barré syndrome, multiple sclerosis, myasthenia gravis, cerebrovascular accident, CNS depression)
   COPD
   Anesthesia
   Suppressed cough reflex
   Thick or large amounts of secretions

Outcome Criteria	*Nursing Interventions*

Patient will have a patent airway and optimal ventilatory capacity as evidenced by:
Clear breath sounds bilaterally
Respiratory rate, depth, and rhythm within normal limits (WNL) for the patient
Sa_{O_2} greater than 90%
Arterial blood gases WNL for the patient
Vital signs WNL for the patient
Mental status WNL for the patient
Pulmonary function tests WNL for the patient
	Monitor patient for signs or symptoms of ineffective airway clearance:
	  Weak, ineffective cough
	  Shortness of breath, dyspnea
	  Cyanosis
	  Use of accessory muscles
	  Presence of adventitious breath sounds (wheezes, crackles, rhonchi)
	  Alterations in level of consciousness
	  Tachycardia
	  Pa_{CO_2} greater than 50 mm Hg (or greater than normal for the patient)
	  O_2 saturation less than 90%
	Maintain patent airway
	  Be aware of patients at high risk for aspiration (e.g., patients emerging from anesthesia, elderly patients)
	  Take steps to prevent aspiration
	    Position patient upright or on side
	  Establish and maintain patent airway
	    Perform chin-lift (basic cardiac life support)
	    Remove foreign material (Heimlich maneuver or suction)
	    Suction prn
	      Assess need for suctioning
	        Increased respiratory rate
	        Tachycardia
	        Tachypnea
	        Dyspnea
	        Restlessness
	        Crackles, rhonchi
	        Coughing
	        Increased peak inspiratory pressure (PIP) on ventilator
	      Preoxygenate with 100% O_2 prior to suctioning
	      Utilize sterile technique
	      Suction intermittently for no greater than 10 seconds while withdrawing catheter
	      Monitor for arrhythmias
	      Monitor Sa_{O_2} and $S\bar{v}_{O_2}$
	      Document results of suctioning in nurses' notes
	  Provide humidification (aerosols) for patients with artificial airways
	  Turn and position patient every 2 hours as tolerated
	  Chest physical therapy every 2 to 4 hours and prn (when appropriate)
	  Administer bronchodilators as ordered (e.g., aminophylline); assist with placement and maintenance of artificial airways
	  Monitor for complications of artificial airways (see Table 25–6)
	Maintain adequate hydration
	  Monitor fluid status
	    Record intake and output
	    Perform daily weights
	    Assess skin turgor
	    Assess for edema
	    Assess characteristics of secretions
	  Administer oral and intravenous fluids (as ordered)
	  Maintain awareness of potential causes of fluid imbalance in the critically ill patient
	    Insensible losses amount to approximately 300 to 500 mL/day (increases with fever, vomiting, diarrhea)

2. Ineffective breathing pattern related to:

Anesthesia	Pain
Sedation	Anxiety, fear
Analgesia	Trauma
Fatigue	Drug overdose

Outcome Criteria	Nursing Interventions

Patient will demonstrate an effective breathing pattern as evidenced by:
Arterial blood gases WNL for the patient
Vital signs WNL for the patient
Mental status WNL for the patient
Respiratory rate, rhythm, and depth WNL for the patient
Minute ventilation WNL for the patient
	Monitor patient for signs and symptoms of ineffective breathing patterns
	  Abnormal respiratory patterns (e.g., hypoventilation, hyperventilation, apnea, bradypnea, tachypnea)
	  Splinted, guarded respirations
	  Decreased minute ventilation
	  Hypoxemia (Pa_{O_2} <50 mm Hg) on room air
	  Hypercapnia (Pa_{CO_2} >50 mm Hg)
	  pH <7.35 or >7.45
	
	Monitor patients at high risk for development of altered breathing patterns
	  Postoperative patients
	  Patients receiving sedatives or narcotics
	  Patients with pain or anxiety
	  Patients with CNS disorders
	  Patients with metabolic disorders (e.g., acid-base imbalances)
	Provide ventilatory support
	  Assist with obtaining spontaneous mechanics to determine need for artificial ventilatory assistance (e.g., tidal volume, respiratory rate)
	  Assist with monitoring or adjusting of ventilator settings to maintain appropriate level of assistance and minute ventilation
	  Monitor patient's response to artificial ventilation
	    Psychological response
	    Arterial blood gases
	    Effect on cardiovascular status
	  Assist in correction of the underlying disorder
	  Nursing interventions for decreasing pain or anxiety
	    Analgesics and sedatives
	    Comfort measures
	    Distraction (visitors, music)

3. Imparied gas exchange related to:
  V̇/Q̇ mismatch, diffusion defects, shunt

Outcome Criteria	Nursing Interventions

Patient will exhibit optimal gas exchange as evidenced by:
Arterial blood gases WNL for the patient
Vital signs WNL for the patient
Mental status WNL for the patient
	Monitor patient for signs or symptoms of altered gas exchange
	  Restlessness
	  Confusion
	  Headache
	  Somnolence
	  Dyspnea
	  Cyanosis
	  Pa_{O_2} less than 50 mm Hg on room air
	  Pa_{CO_2} greater than 50 mm Hg
	  Sa_{O_2} less than 90%
	  Accessory muscle use
	  Arrhythmias
	  Hypotension
	Maintain patent airway (see under Impaired airway clearance)
	Administer O_2 therapy as ordered (see Table 25–7)
	Maintain adequate hydration (see under Impaired airway clearance)
	Improve V̇/Q̇ mismatching and shunt
	  CPT
	  Suctioning
	  Increase functional residual capacity
	    Elevate head of bed
	    Administer positive end-expiratory pressure (PEEP)
	    Assist in determining "optimal PEEP" (see text)
	Optimize O_2 delivery (see text)
	  Maintain cardiac output WNL
	  Maintain hemoglobin WNL

Nursing Care Plan continued on following page

4. Altered tissue perfusion, cardiopulmonary, related to pulmonary embolism

Outcome Criteria	Nursing Interventions

Patient will have normal tissue perfusion (lung) as evidenced by:
  Arterial blood gases WNL for the patient
  Vital signs WNL for the patient
  Mental status WNL for the patient
	Monitor patient for signs or symptoms of altered tissue perfusion (lung)
	  Tachypnea
	  Dyspnea
	  Cyanosis
	  Tachycardia
	  Confusion
	  Anxiety
	  Feeling of impending doom
	  Cough
	  Hemoptysis
	  Pleuritic chest pain
	Maintain high degree of suspicion in patients with increased risk of PE
	  Immobility
	  Venous thrombosis
	  Pregnancy or childbirth
	  Postoperative patients
	Prevent development of thrombosis
	  Antithromboembolic stockings
	  Encourage mobility
	  Range of motion exercises
	  Heparin therapy as ordered
	Assist in resuscitation of patients with massive pulmonary embolism
	  Basic cardiac life support/advanced cardiac life support
	  Thrombolytic therapy (see Tables 25–5 and 25–7)
	Assist with diagnostic tests
	  V̇/Q̇ scans
	  Pulmonary angiography

5. Anxiety related to dyspnea secondary to ARF

Outcome Criteria	Nursing Interventions

Patient will demonstrate a decreased level of anxiety as evidenced by:
  Vital signs WNL
  Mental status WNL
  Subjective report by the patient of feeling less anxiety
	Monitor for signs and symptoms of increased anxiety
	  Tachycardia
	  Hypertension
	  Tachypnea
	  Restlessness/confusion
	Institute measures to relieve dyspnea
	  Improve oxygenation/ventilation
	  Administer pharmacologic agents as ordered (e.g., morphine)
	  Provide comfort measures
	  Allow for rest periods
	Institute measures to decrease anxiety of hospitalization
	  Explain procedures and administer care in an unhurried manner
	  Encourage family participation

SUMMARY

Successful management of the patient with acute respiratory failure requires the combined efforts of a skilled multidisciplinary team. The critical care nurse is responsible for the ongoing assessment and treatment of patients with this potentially life-threatening problem. An understanding of the pathophysiology of acute respiratory failure and current monitoring and treatment modalities provides the nurse with the knowledge base necessary for effective management of these patients.

References

Abraham, E., Bland, R. D., Cobo, J. C., et al. (1984). Sequential cardiorespiratory pattern associated with outcome in septic shock. *Chest*, 85, 75–80.

Adlkofer, R. M., and Powaser, M. M. (1978). The effect of endotracheal suctioning on arterial blood gases in patients after cardiac surgery. *Heart & Lung, 7*, 1011–1014.

Albert, R. K. (1988). Physiology and management of failure of arterial oxygenation. In R. J. Fallot (Ed.), *Cardiopulmonary critical care management* (pp. 37–59). New York: Churchill-Livingstone.

Arabian, A. A. (1986). Embolic pulmonary disease. In S. V. Spagnolo, and A. Medinger (Eds.), *Handbook of pulmonary emergencies* (pp. 193–204). New York: Plenum.

Bell, W. R. (1982). Pulmonary embolism: Progress and problems. *American Medical Journal, 72*, 181–183.

Bostick, J., and Wendelgrass, S. T. (1987). Normal saline instillation as part of the suctioning procedure. Effects on Pa$_{O_2}$ and amount of secretions. *Heart & Lung, 16*, 532–537.

Brenner, B. E., and Yanos, J. (1985). Asthma. In B. E. Brenner (Ed.), *Comprehensive management of respiratory emergencies* (pp. 315–339). Rockville, MD: Aspen.

Chandler, A. B. (1979). Pathogenesis of thrombosis. In S. Sheny (Ed.), *Thrombosis and thrombolysis* (2nd ed., pp. 37–57). Somerville, NJ: Hoechst-Rossel Pharmaceuticals.

Clemmer, A. B., Orme, J. F., and Thomas, F. O. (1988). Physiology and management of failure of oxygen transport and utilization. In R. J. Fallot (Ed.), *Cardiopulmonary critical care management* (pp. 61–87). New York: Churchill-Livingstone.

Danek, S. J., Lynch, J. P., Wey, J. G., et al. (1980). The dependence of oxygen uptake on oxygen delivery in the adult respiratory distress syndrome. *American Review of Respiratory Disease 122*, 387–395.

Dean, E. (1987). The ICU: Principles and practice of physical therapy. In D. L. Frownfelter (Ed.), *Chest physical therapy and pulmonary rehabilitation* (2nd ed., pp. 377–442). Chicago: Year Book.

Demers, R. R., and Irwin, R. S. (1983). Positive end-expiratory pressure. In J. M. Rippe (Ed.), *Manual of intensive care medicine* (pp. 142–145). Boston: Little, Brown.

Demers, R. R., and Saklad, M. (1973). Minimizing the harmful effects of mechanical aspiration. *Heart & Lung, 2*, 542–545.

Dorinsky, P. M., and Whitcomb, M. E. (1983). The effect of PEEP on cardiac output. *Chest, 82*, 210–216.

Duff, J. H., Groves, A. C., McLean, A. P., et al. (1969). Defective oxygen consumption in septic shock. *Surgery, Gynecology, and Obstetrics, 128*, 1051–1060.

Feldman, J., Traver, G. A., Taussig, L. M. (1979). Maximal expiratory flows after postural drainage. *American Review of Respiratory Disease, 119*, 239–245.

Fell, T., and Cheney, F. W. (1971). Prevention of hypoxia during endotracheal suctioning. *Annals of Surgery, 174*, 24–28.

Goodnough, J. K. (1985). The effects of oxygenation and hyperinflation on arterial O_2 tension after endotracheal suctioning. *Heart & Lung, 14*, 11–17.

Graham, W. G., and Bradley, D. A. (1978). Efficacy of chest physiotherapy and intermittent positive pressure breathing in the resolution of pneumonia. *New England Journal of Medicine, 229*, 624–627.

Hanley, M., Rudd, T., and Butler, J. (1978). What happens to intratracheal saline instillations? (Abstract). *American Review of Respiratory Disease, 117*, 124.

Kersten, L. O. (1989). *Comprehensive Respiratory Nursing* (pp. 68–69). Philadelphia: W. B. Saunders.

Luce, J. M. (1988). Pathophysiology and management of ventilatory failure. In R. J. Fallot (Ed.), *Cardiopulmonary critical care management* (pp. 11–35). New York: Churchill-Livingstone.

Marini, J. J. (1988). Hemodynamic assessment and management of patients with respiratory failure. In R. J. Fallot (Ed.), *Cardiopulmonary critical care management* (pp. 179–214). New York: Churchill-Livingstone.

May, D. B., and Munt, P. W. (1979). Physiologic effects of chest percussion and postural drainage in patients with stable chronic bronchitis. *Chest, 75*, 29–32.

Mecca, R. S. (1986). Complications of therapy. In R. Kirby, and R. W. Taylor (Eds.), *Respiratory failure* (pp. 583–601). Chicago: Year Book.

Miller, R. R., Awan, N. A., Joye, H. A., et al. (1977). Combined dopamine and nitroprusside therapy in congestive heart failure. *Circulation, 55*, 881–884.

Naigow, D., and Powaser, M. M. (1977). The effect of different endotracheal suctioning procedures on arterial blood gases in a controlled experimental model. *Heart & Lung, 6*, 808–816.

Oldenburg, F. A., Dolovich, M. B., Montgomery, J. M., et al. (1979). Effects of postural drainage, exercise, and cough in mucus clearance in chronic bronchitis. *American Review of Respiratory Disease, 120*, 739–745.

Petty, T. L. (1974). Acute respiratory failure. In T. L. Petty (Ed.), *Intensive and rehabilitative respiratory care* (pp. 1–13). Philadelphia: Lea & Febiger.

Rosen, M. A. (1985). Pulmonary embolism. In B. E. Brenner (Ed.), *Comprehensive management of respiratory emergencies* (pp. 273–288). Rockville, MD: Aspen Publications.

Shin, C., Fine, N., Fernandez, R., et al. (1969). Cardiac arrhythmias resulting from tracheal suctioning. *Annals of Internal Medicine, 71*, 1149–1153.

Tyler, M. L. (1986). Acute respiratory failure. In M. L. Patrick, S. L. Woods, R. F. Clover, et al. (Eds.), *Medical-surgical nursing* (pp. 449–457). Philadelphia: J. B. Lippincott.

Williams, S. M. (1985). The pulmonary system. In J. G. Alspach, and S. M. Williams (Eds.), *Core curriculum for critical care nursing* (pp. 1–100). Philadelphia: W. B. Saunders.

Zagelbaum, G. L., and Pare, J. A. (1982). *Manual of acute respiratory care* (pp. 19–50). Boston: Little, Brown.

26

Patients with Adult Respiratory Distress Syndrome

Elaine L. Enger

Adult respiratory distress syndrome (ARDS) is a severe form of acute respiratory failure that can occur in individuals with or without preexisting pulmonary disease as a consequence of acute lung injury (ALI). To date, there is no universally accepted definition of this syndrome. In its broadest usage, ARDS refers to the acute onset of pulmonary edema that is not due to cardiogenic factors but to increased permeability factors. Hence, the term noncardiogenic pulmonary edema has been used interchangeably with ARDS. More specifically, ARDS is a term used to encompass the pathophysiologic, clinical, and pathologic alterations that occur when there is a fundamental loss in alveolar-capillary (a-c) membrane integrity. Development of increased permeability resulting from damage to the microvascular endothelial barrier or the alveolar epithelium is common to all cases of ALI. Therefore, the patient will present with pulmonary edema with a high protein content. This, however, represents only the first pathologic response on a continuum of complex responses found in ARDS. Damage to the endothelial capillary membrane will result in an increased permeability interstitial edema. Damage to the alveolar barrier will result in alveolar flooding as well as a series of other gas exchange and metabolic derangements not necessarily encompassed by the term noncardiogenic pulmonary edema. Therefore, the terms are not necessarily synonymous.

In 1967, Ashbaugh and co-workers published a report describing the clinical characteristics of 12 patients who developed acute respiratory failure. These patients, admitted for such conditions as major trauma, pancreatitis, drug overdose, and viral pneumonia, all consequently developed respiratory failure during the course of their hospitalization. The authors noted that the clinical and physiologic characteristics of these patients' respiratory impairment were remarkably similar to those of neonates exhibiting infant respiratory distress syndrome. Therefore, the term adult respiratory distress syndrome was used to describe this respiratory impairment. The recognition that acute respiratory failure could occur as a consequence of nonpulmonary conditions was not new in 1967. Since World War II, the occurrence of severe pulmonary dysfunction had been noted in soldiers suffering from nonthoracic trauma. The terms wet lung, shock lung, and DaNang lung have been applied to the pulmonary edema associated with severe combat injury (Putterman, 1988). The contribution made by Ashbaugh and associates was grouping the acute respiratory failures that occurred in patients afflicted with a variety of underlying diseases into a single entity. In addition, the authors suggested that there might be a single pathogenic mechanism common to all of these cases despite the diversity of underlying disorders.

Since this report, the term ARDS has become firmly entrenched in medical terminology. There is general agreement that it is characterized by (1) a history compatible with the development of the syndrome, (2) bilateral diffuse infiltrates on the chest roentgenogram, (3) tachypnea, and (4) progressive hypoxemia despite increasing levels of inspired oxygen (Dalnogare, 1989). Although the precise incidence of ARDS is unknown, it is estimated to exceed 150,000 cases annually in the United States alone, making it one of the most common diagnoses in the critical care setting (Murray, 1977).

STRUCTURE OF THE ALVEOLAR-CAPILLARY MEMBRANE

Integral to the understanding of the pathogenesis of ARDS is the comprehension of normal alveolar-capillary membrane structure as well as fluid dynamics in the lung (Fig. 26–1).

The Microvascular Barrier: Capillary Endothelial Layer

The capillaries of the lung comprise the microvascular barrier and consist of primarily endothelial cells. The thin cytoplasmic projections of these cells overlap to form a continuous tube, facilitating maximal gas exchange with minimal tissue mass. At each of the areas of overlap are clefts that serve as communication channels between the pulmonary capillaries and the interstitial space. These clefts have been referred to as "loose junctions" because their width can be enhanced as a result of increases in vascular pressures or by toxic damage. It is across these junctions that water, lipid-insoluble molecules, and macromolecules may pass (Simionescu and Simionescu, 1984).

Interstitium and Lung Lymphatics

The interstitium is organized into two interconnecting compartments (Taylor and Parker, 1985). First is the perimicrovascular compartment, which comprises the alveolar wall interstitium. The second is the peribronchovascular compartment, which consists of the loose connective tissue spaces around the bronchi and blood vessels. The peribronchovascular interstitium is wider and more compliant than the perimicrovascular interstitium. This makes it more susceptible to liquid accumulation if the capacity of the lymph channels is exceeded. In addition, there

is a pressure gradient from the alveolar interstitium (which is exposed to alveolar pressure) to the peribronchovascular interstitium (which possesses a more negative pressure approximating pleural pressure). This pressure gradient encourages fluid drainage from areas of high to low pressure into the peribronchovascular interstitium in an effort to prevent fluid accumulation near the air–blood interface (Havill and Gee, 1984).

Lymphatic channels are not present in the perimicrovascular interstitium (Staub, 1974). They originate in the connective tissue of the peribronchovascular compartment. Under normal conditions, fluid and protein filtered into the interstitium are directed along lymphatic ducts and are pumped via thoracic ducts into the superior vena cava as rapidly as they accumulate. Therefore, the lymph channels serve as an indispensable means of draining extravasated fluid and proteins from the interstitium. Although no method for measuring lymph flow in humans exists, it has been estimated by Staub (1974, 1980) to average 20 mL/hr in the resting 70-kg individual. Drainage away from the alveolar wall also occurs by the filling of loose connective tissue spaces called cuffs of the peribronchovascular compartment. The capacity of these cuffs to fill with fluid increases as the lungs are inflated and the cuff pressures fall (Havill and Gee, 1984). These cuffs are then drained slowly into the surrounding blood vessels or down the prevailing pressure gradient to the openings of lymph channels in the mediastinum.

The Alveolar Barrier: Alveolar Epithelial Layer

The alveolar barrier consists of two types of epithelial cells. The type I cells are thin, flat cells that cover 95% of the surface area. They are extremely vulnerable to injury and possess limited regenerative capabilities. The remaining surface area of the alveolar barrier is covered by the more compact type II cells, which secrete surfactant, a regulatory product that decreases alveolar surface tension. These cells appear to be far less susceptible to injury and possess remarkable reparative abilities (Connors et al., 1981). Like the cells of the capillary endothelium, the alveolar epithelial cells abut and overlap. However, because the areas of overlap in the capillary endothelium are loose junctions, the alveolar epithelium must serve as the principal protector against alveolar fluid accumulation. To achieve this, alveolar epithelial cell clefts are obliterated by complete fusion of the membranes of the adjacent cells. The alveolar barrier, therefore, has a very low permeability, and much greater distending forces are required before any disruption or transport can occur. Therefore, these junctions have been referred to as "tight junctions." In addition, the interstitial pressure gradient favors the movement of fluid away from the alveolar wall so that it may be drained by the lymphatics. This

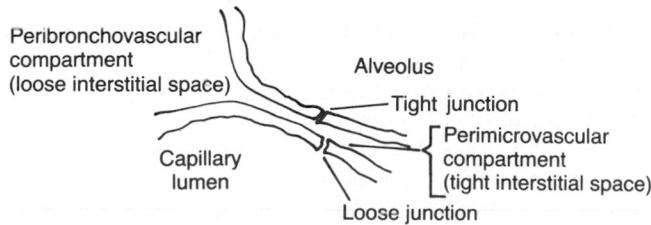

FIGURE 26–1. Schematic representation of the ultrastructure of the alveolar-capillary membrane (see text). (Adapted from Ingram, R.H., and Braunwald, E. (1988). Pulmonary edema: Cardiogenic and noncardiogenic. In E. Braunwald (Ed.), *Heart disease* (3rd ed., p. 544). Philadelphia: W. B. Saunders.)

explains why interstitial edema precedes alveolar edema. Even though fluid leaks into the interstitial tissues, it will not accumulate and lead to gas exchange abnormalities because it is efficiently removed by the lymphatics. Therefore, the alveoli will flood only if the rate of fluid filtration increases beyond the capacity of the lymphatics to drain it away and of the peribronchovascular cuffs to sequester it from the alveolar walls (Staub, 1983).

PHYSIOLOGIC BASIS OF FLUID MOVEMENT

Microvascular Barrier: Capillary-Interstitial Exchange

The lung is not a dry organ. In fact, it has one of the highest water contents of any organ. There is normally a continuous exchange of liquid, colloid, and solutes between the vascular bed and the interstitium due to the loose endothelial capillary junctions as well as to the balance of the driving filtration forces (Taylor, 1981). These driving forces, including both hydrostatic and osmotic pressures, have been referred to collectively as Starling forces because Ernest Starling first recognized that fluid flow out of a vessel was determined by a balance of these forces acting across a semipermeable membrane. A pathologic state will exist only when there is an increase in the net flux of liquids and colloids from the vascular into the interstitial space. The dynamic equilibrium between the capillary and interstitial forces that determines net transvascular fluid flux is mathematically described by the Starling equation (Staub, 1978). The equation is generally expressed as the balance between hydrostatic and osmotic forces (Connors et al., 1981) (Fig. 26–2).

Although the Starling equation appears quite complex, it can be simplified by summarizing that three major factors influence net transvascular fluid flux across the pulmonary capillary endothelium: hydrostatic pressure, colloidal osmotic pressure, and the integrity of the capillary endothelial membrane (Staub, 1978).

HYDROSTATIC PRESSURE

Transvascular hydrostatic pressure, or the difference between the microvascular and interstitial hydrostatic pressure, will influence the outward movement of fluid from the vasculature. In other words, hydrostatic pressure is considered a "push" pressure, and it is the primary force regulating fluid flux. If hydrostatic pressure is higher in the microvascular space (the capillary) than in the interstitial space, fluid will be pushed out of the capillary. Conversely, if interstitial hydrostatic pressure exceeds capillary hydrostatic pressure, fluid will be pushed out of the interstitial space. An indirect estimate of microvas-

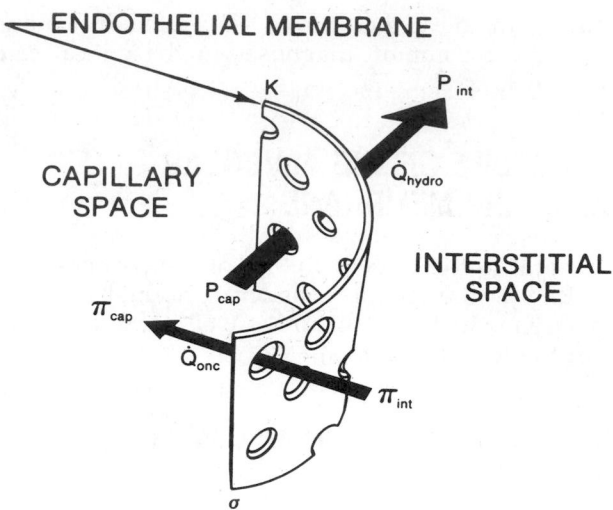

THE STARLING EQUATION
$$\dot{Q}_f = K(P_{cap} - P_{int}) - K\sigma(\pi_{cap} - \pi_{int})$$

FIGURE 26–2. Fluid filtration across the endothelial membrane into the interstitial space is the sum of the fluid filtration generated by the hydrostatic pressure gradient, which tends to push fluid into the interstitial space, and the filtration generated by the oncotic pressure gradient, which tends to pull fluid into the capillary. The final factor influencing fluid filtration is the inherent permeability of the membrane. The relationship of these factors is mathematically expressed by the Starling equation. (Adapted from Connors, A.F., McCaffrie, D.R., and Rogers, R.M. (1981). The adult respiratory distress syndrome. *Disease-a-Month*, 27, 1–75.)

cular hydrostatic pressure or pulmonary capillary pressure can be easily obtained from the pulmonary artery wedge pressure (PAWP) or left atrial pressure measurements. Interstitial hydrostatic pressure is very difficult to measure. It is assumed to be closely related to pleural pressure and thus is estimated to be subatmospheric (Staub, 1974). Consequently, under normal conditions hydrostatic pressure is higher in the intravascular space, and thus the net fluid flux as influenced by this pressure is from capillary to interstitium. In addition, because pulmonary blood flow is gravity dependent and is greater in the basilar regions, filtration of fluid into the interstitium will also be highest in the lung bases.

COLLOIDAL OSMOTIC PRESSURE

Transvascular colloidal osmotic pressure, or the difference between microvascular and interstitial osmotic forces, opposes transvascular hydrostatic pressure at fluid exchange sites. Because molecules smaller than plasma proteins pass unhindered across the microvascular barrier, colloidal osmotic forces are generated primarily by the plasma proteins and macromolecules. Colloidal osmotic (oncotic) pressure is considered a "pull" pressure. Fluid will be pulled or drawn toward the compartment where protein concentration is greatest. Plasma osmotic pressure is generally about 1.3 mOsm or 24 mm Hg (Nita et al.,

1981). Interstitial osmotic pressure is generated by extravasated proteins in the interstitial fluid. Although this pressure has not been measured directly, it has been calculated to be approximately 0.8 mOsm or 14.5 mm Hg (Erdmann et al., 1975). Consequently, under normal conditions the net fluid flux as influenced by colloidal osmotic pressure is from interstitium into capillary (Staub, 1974, 1980).

MICROVASCULAR BARRIER PERMEABILITY

The last factor influencing fluid flux is the inherent permeability of the microvascular barrier. This permeability is expressed in the Starling equation by two descriptors, the Kf and the σf. The Kf is a measure of how easily fluid crosses the barrier per unit of barrier filtering area. It therefore is the primary measure of permeability and is determined by the structure and function of the endothelial cells forming the barrier. Although it cannot be measured directly, it is believed that the Kf is normally quite low because fluid filtration is quite low relative to the large surface area of the lung (Staub, 1980). The σf is a measure of how effectively the barrier hinders the passage of solutes and thus also reflects capillary membrane permeability. It is an intrinsic property of the barrier. The σf of the microvascular barrier appears to be quite high, so the barrier is quite proficient at hindering the passage of solutes (Staub, 1980).

BALANCE OF FORCES: CAPILLARY-INTERSTITIAL FLUID EXCHANGE

In summary, three factors determine the flux of fluid across the microvascular barrier: hydrostatic pressure, colloidal osmotic pressure, and the inherent permeability or integrity of the capillary endothelial membrane. Under normal conditions, both hydrostatic pressure and osmotic pressure are higher in the intravascular space than in the interstitial space. Consequently, there is a relative balance of forces pushing fluid out of and pulling fluid into the capillary across a semipermeable membrane, the net flux being in an outward direction. This fluid flux, which constitutes approximately 20 mL/hr, can easily be drained by the lymphatics. A pathologic state will exist only when there is an increase in the net flux of extravasated fluid.

The Alveolar Barrier: Interstitial-Alveolar Exchange

As previously indicated, fluid and protein do not normally cross into the alveoli because the alveolar barrier possesses a low permeability. In addition, fluid is continuously drained away from the alveolar walls through the interstitium and removed by the lymphatics (Crandell, 1983).

GENERAL PATHOGENESIS OF PULMONARY EDEMA

Pathogenic Mechanisms

From the foregoing discussion of the alveolar-capillary membrane structure and the regulatory factors of fluid movement, three potential predisposing mechanisms of pulmonary edema can be identified (Bernard and Brigham, 1986). The first of these mechanisms is an imbalance of the Starling forces leading to an increase in fluid filtration into the interstitium that exceeds lymphatic capacity. This situation is generally referred to as an increased pressure edema. Increased microvascular hydrostatic pressure (PAWP) constitutes the most common alteration in Starling forces. Congestive heart failure resulting in increased pulmonary venous pressure is the most frequent clinical cause. For this reason, increased pressure edema is sometimes called cardiogenic pulmonary edema regardless of the fact that other Starling forces besides microvascular hydrostatic pressure may be contributing to the increased extravascular fluid flux.

The second mechanism is a primary lymphatic insufficiency that limits the rate of removal of extravascular fluid. This is the mechanism that is probably responsible for the edema that develops when lymphatics are disrupted following lung transplantation.

The third mechanism is fundamental damage to the alveolar-capillary membrane that increases the microvascular barrier's permeability to fluid and protein. This renders the normal Starling forces that limit fluid extravasation inoperative. This situation is referred to as increased permeability pulmonary edema, and it is the mechanism responsible for the development of pulmonary edema in ARDS. Normally, the capillary endothelial barrier deters most protein filtration. When this membrane is damaged, permeability to protein is greatly enhanced. On examination of the Starling equation, it is evident that with the loss of barrier integrity, the major determinant of fluid flux will be hydrostatic pressure. Because capillary hydrostatic pressure normally far exceeds interstitial hydrostatic pressure, capillary endothelial damage will result in increased water conductance into the interstitium. Lymphatic capability to pump excess filtrate away will be enhanced even at low capillary hydrostatic driving pressures (PAWP). The increased permeability pulmonary edema witnessed in ARDS, therefore, is identified by a concomitant increase in pulmonary lymph flow and lymph protein content (Sibbald et al., 1983).

Process and Sequence of Fluid Accumulation

Regardless of the specific mechanism involved, the sequence of fluid exchange and accumulation can be described in three separate stages, the last of which consists of two almost simultaneous substages (Fishman, 1980; Staub et al., 1967) (Fig. 26–3).

Stage I. During this stage, an increase in mass transfer of fluid and colloid from the capillaries occurs across the microvascular barrier to the interstitium. The capillary endothelial junctions may have been widened by an increase in filtrative forces or by toxic damage. However, no measurable increase in interstitial volume is seen because lymphatic outflow also increases. In addition, fluid and protein are pumped down the prevailing pressure gradient away from the alveolar walls into the loose perivascular tissue. As a result, development of pulmonary edema is limited.

Stage II. Stage II occurs when the amount of fluid filtered out of the capillary approaches and exceeds lymphatic drainage capacity. If the integrity of the microvascular barrier is maintained and there is no alteration in its permeability, the filtered fluid will be relatively free of protein. This will result in a dilution of interstitial protein, a decrease in the osmotic forces pulling fluid into the interstitium, and a maintenance of blood protein osmotic pull. All of these factors will help to deter further progression of edema. If, however, this safety mechanism does not sufficiently protect the interstitium or if the barrier is injured, liquid and colloid will begin to accumulate in the peribronchovascular interstitium. Increases in interstitial volume, however, will result in only small elevations of interstitial pressure until the interstitial volume is quite large. This mechanism serves as an attempt to keep the hydrostatic driving pressure across the alveolar barrier suitably low.

Stage III. In this stage, the volume limits of the loose interstitium have been exceeded. Therefore, fluid will begin to distend the less compliant perimicrovascular (alveolar wall) interstitium. As fluid fills the alveolar interstitium, several mechanisms come into play in an attempt to protect the alveoli from edema. The first protective mechanism is the alveolar epithelial membrane. The junctions of this membrane are quite tight and thus serve as excellent barriers to fluid flux. In addition, surfactant plays a role in keeping the alveoli dry by reducing surface tension at the air–liquid interface. If, however, the pressure developing in the alveolar wall interstitium is sufficient to disrupt the tight junctions of the alveolar epithelium, alveolar edema occurs in two substages. In the normal adult, the interstitial space can accommodate 200 to 300 mL of fluid before alveolar edema occurs (Staub et al., 1967).

Initially, fluid accumulates in the corners of the alveoli. This small fluid accumulation will, however, eventually alter the surface tension of the alveoli. As a result, alveolar size will be diminished, gas volume will be replaced by edema fluid, and alveolar flooding will ensue. During alveolar flooding, the alveoli are filled individually in an "all or none" fashion (Staub et al., 1967). The exact process by which alveolar flooding occurs remains unclear. However, it is believed that this flooding occurs when alveoli reach a critical configuration, at which point inflation pressures can no longer maintain the existing structure.

PREDISPOSING FACTORS FOR ARDS

Diffuse alveolar capillary membrane injury, the hallmark of ARDS, can result from a variety of direct mechanisms such as inhaled or blood-borne toxins as well as from indirect mechanisms such as the release of various intervening mediators or neuro-

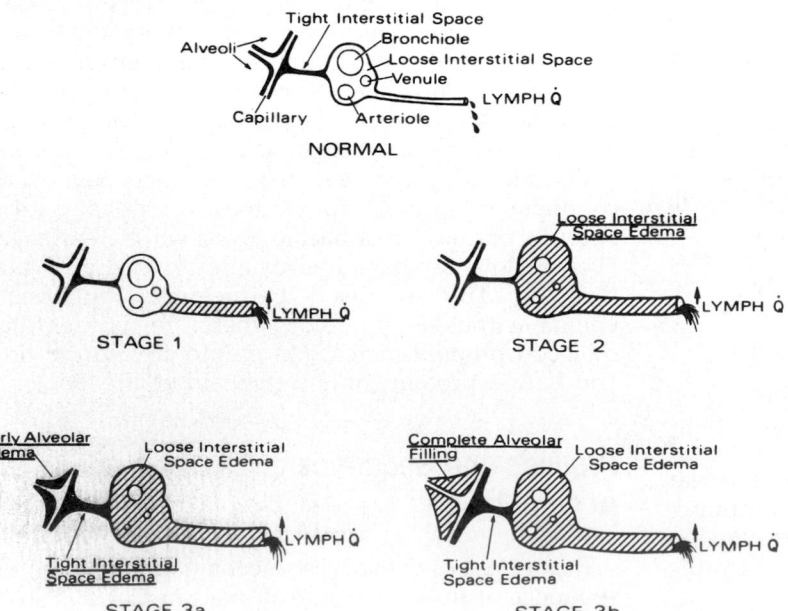

FIGURE 26–3. Schematic representation of the a-c membrane, loose interstitial space, and lymphatic system at the several stages of pulmonary edema. The new feature at each stage from normal to fully developed alveolar edema is underlined. (From Ingram, R.H., and Braunwald, E. (1988). Pulmonary edema: Cardiogenic and noncardiogenic. In E. Braunwald (Ed.), *Heart disease* (3rd ed., p. 547). Philadelphia: W. B. Saunders.)

humoral factors. Therefore, a large number of clinical predispositions have been described (Maunder, 1986). The most commonly cited predispositions are listed in Table 26–1. Recent epidemiologic studies suggest that the incidence of ARDS differs greatly among these predisposed groups.

The highest incidence appears to occur in patients with septic syndrome. This is described as a combination of leukocytosis or leukopenia, a known source of infection, fever or hypothermia, and hypotension regardless of whether blood cultures are positive for a gram-negative bacterial pathogen. More than one-third of these patients develop ARDS (Fowler et al., 1983; Pepe et al., 1982).

The second most common predisposition appears to be aspiration of gastric contents, which has an incidence of associated ARDS of approximately 30%. It has been suggested that aspiration of gastric contents that have a pH of less than 2.5 is particularly likely to lead to lung injury (Fowler et al., 1983; Pepe et al., 1982).

All types of shock have been associated with lung injury. Historically, shock was felt to be such an important predisposition for ARDS that the syndrome was termed "shock lung" by many investigators (Ayres, 1982; Shoemaker and Hauser, 1979). The relative importance of the various types of shock as a single risk factor is difficult to ascertain. Only 2% to 7% of patients presenting with hemorrhagic shock alone are reported to develop ARDS (Fowler et al., 1983). Because many of these patients have sustained trauma and have received multiple blood transfusions, it is difficult to implicate hemorrhagic shock as an isolated risk factor. Cardiogenic shock has also been described as a predisposing factor (Keren et al., 1980). However, it is difficult to differentiate increased pressure from increased permeability pulmonary edema in these cases.

The patient who has sustained multiple trauma is at high risk for ARDS. Fulton and Jones (1975) reported post-traumatic pulmonary insufficiency in 22% of patients with multiple trauma associated with pulmonary involvement and in 14% of patients with multiple trauma without primary chest involvement. ARDS has also been associated with head trauma as well as near drowning.

TABLE 26–1. Predisposing Factors for ARDS

Septicemia or septic syndrome
Aspiration of gastric contents
Shock syndrome
Nonpulmonary/pulmonary trauma
Drug overdose
Pneumonias
Oxygen toxicity
Hypertransfusion
Disseminated intravascular coagulation
Fat, amniotic fluid, thrombotic, or air embolism
Acute hemorrhagic pancreatitis
Cardiopulmonary bypass
Burns or smoke inhalation
Toxemia of pregnancy

Many drugs, when taken in excess, have been classified as predispositions to ARDS. These include narcotics, especially heroin, and barbiturates as well as aspirin, colchicine, and thiazides (Taylor and Duncan, 1983).

One of the mainstays in treatment of ARDS is also a potent lung toxin. High concentrations of oxygen may cause significant lung injury by facilitating the production of oxygen-free radicals (Jenkinson, 1982). Other inhalants such as smoke and nitrogen dioxide have also been linked with ARDS (Taylor and Duncan, 1983).

It is most important to note that the risk of developing ARDS has been reported to increase dramatically if more than one predisposing factor exists. In addition, it has been shown that the onset of ARDS usually occurs within 48 hours of the occurrence of a risk factor. Thus, patients who survive for 2 days after a risk factor event will usually not develop ARDS (Fowler et al., 1983; Pepe et al., 1982).

MECHANISMS AND MEDIATORS OF ACUTE LUNG INJURY: THE ROLE OF POLYMORPHONUCLEAR LEUKOCYTES

There are many potential mechanisms and mediators of lung injury in ARDS (Boxer et al., 1990) (Fig. 26–4). Which mediators are involved and their cells of origin remain unclear. Because information from humans is difficult to obtain and interpret, most of our knowledge about the mechanisms of ALI comes from experimental animal models. From these models it has been learned that many cells and cell interactions are likely to be involved in the pathogenesis of ARDS. These cells include alveolar macrophages, neutrophils, lymphocytes, platelets, and endothelial cells. Most research to date has focused on the role of the neutrophil or polymorphonuclear leukocyte (PMN) because these cells are capable of being activated by and producing most of the potential inflammatory and toxic products that have been linked to ALI. Therefore, rather than attempt to describe all the cells and mediators that have been implicated in the pathogenesis of ARDS, this review concentrates on the role of the PMN. The reader should be aware, however, that PMN-independent pathways undoubtedly exist (Rinaldo and Bogers, 1986).

Overview

Normally, the pulmonary circulation contains a large pool of marginated or inactive PMNs (Cooper et al., 1985). The premise is that a catastrophic clinical insult leads to the activation of these PMNs. This activation results in increased PMN adherence and entrapment in the lungs. In this aggregated, trapped state, PMNs generate and secrete toxic substances

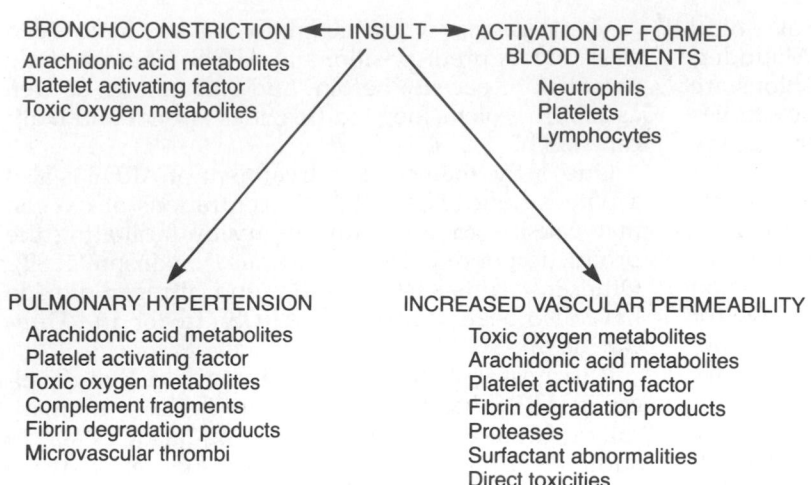

FIGURE 26–4. Potential mediators of the physiologic derangements in ARDS. (Adapted from Boxer, L.A., Axtell, R., and Suchard, S. (1990). The role of the neutrophil in inflammatory diseases of the lung. *Blood Cells*, 16, 25–42.)

and degradative enzymes that promote the physiologic derangements in ARDS. Many of these factors can directly injure the microvascular and alveolar barriers, promoting the development of pulmonary edema. They can also disrupt normal pulmonary blood flow and coagulation, thus leading to the onset of pulmonary hypertension. They can amplify the inflammatory response by attracting more neutrophils. Consequently, activated PMNs create a vicious self-perpetuating cycle that inevitably leads to severe lung injury (Putterman, 1988) (Fig. 26–5).

There is considerable experimental evidence that PMNs play a critical role in ARDS. If PMNs are instrumental, it would be expected that activation of leukocytes would be abnormal in patients with ARDS and that their number would be at least transiently diminished in the peripheral blood and increased in bronchoalveolar lavage samples as a consequence of lung sequestration. Indeed, these findings have been reported. Neutrophils obtained from pulmonary artery blood from critically ill patients with ARDS appear to be in a functionally and metabolically activated state compared to those from patients with-

out ARDS (Zimmerman et al., 1983). Increased numbers of neutrophils have been found by several investigators in the bronchoalveolar lavage of patients with ARDS. In healthy lungs, neutrophils constitute approximately 1% to 3% of the recovered cells. These studies, however, have reported that within 24 hours of the onset of ARDS, 68% to 82% of the lavaged cells were neutrophils; increased numbers of neutrophils were not present in the bronchoalveolar lavage obtained from intubated patients with non-ARDS respiratory failure (Christner et al., 1985; Parson et al., 1985; Weiland et al., 1986). In a prospective study of 40 patients at risk of developing ARDS, blood leukocyte counts were measured serially (Thommasen et al., 1984). Of the 10 patients who developed ARDS, eight demonstrated peripheral blood leukocyte counts that fell to extremely low levels. Only four of the remaining 30 patients without ARDS demonstrated a similar fall in number of circulating leukocytes. Thommasen and colleagues (1984) found a predictable relation between an acute fall in circulating neutrophils and the onset of ARDS in septic patients. In another study aimed at identi-

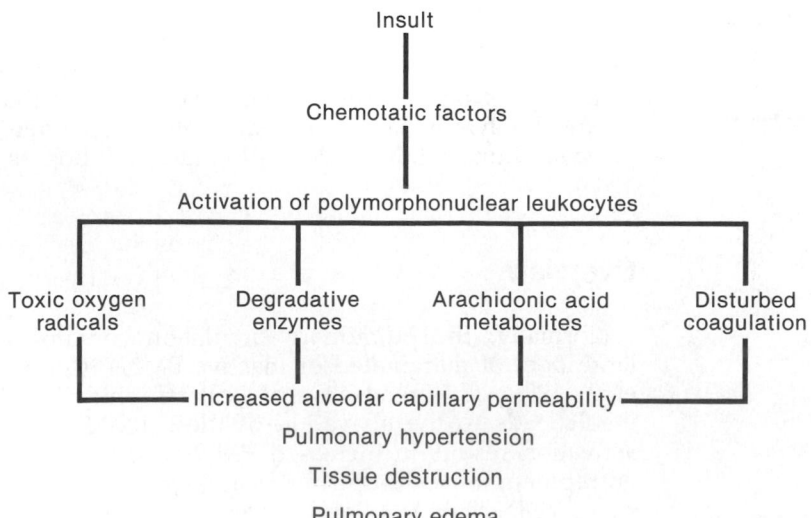

FIGURE 26–5. Flow chart showing the proposed mechanism of PMN activation promoting the physiologic derangements in ARDS.

fying the reason for this decrease in circulating leukocytes, patients who were injected with indium-labeled autologous neutrophils demonstrated an increased amount of radioactivity accumulating in the lung (Powe et al., 1982). It was inferred, therefore, that the decreased number of reported circulating leukocytes may well be a mark of the sequestration of leukocytes in the lungs.

Mechanism of PMN Activation

If PMN activation is critical to the onset of ARDS, what mediators are responsible for this activation? At least three inflammatory mediators have been postulated: complement, bacterial lipopolysaccharide (LPS), and tumor necrosis factor (TNF). Of these agents, the complement system has generated the most investigative interest. Sepsis and trauma are two clinical conditions commonly associated with ARDS in which complement activation is known to occur. The premise is that activation of the complement system results in the production of chemotaxins, especially C5a, which induce PMN activation (Goldstein, 1988). A prospective study of 61 patients at risk for ARDS reported an increase in C5a levels prior to ARDS onset in 31 of 33 patients developing ARDS; only 5 of the 28 patients not developing ARDS had similar elevations of C5a (Hammerschmidt et al., 1980). LPS has a number of proinflammatory direct effects. PMNs exposed to LPS have been reported to develop increased adhesiveness (Pohlman et al., 1986) and to release large amounts of toxins (Strieter et al., 1989). Again, because sepsis frequently precedes ARDS, these direct LPS effects may be important in initiating pulmonary injury. TNF is a potent cytokine that is released by macrophages. In vitro concentrations of TNF have been shown to cause PMN activation and to potentiate the release of toxic enzymes (Klebanoff et al., 1986). Administration of small amounts of TNF has been shown to cause increased permeability pulmonary edema in animals (Stephens et al., 1987).

Consequences of PMN Activation

Once activated, PMNs can damage the lung through several mechanisms: (1) release of toxic oxygen metabolites, (2) release of degradative enzymes, (3) release of arachidonic acid metabolites, and (4) activation of disturbed coagulation.

RELEASE OF TOXIC OXYGEN METABOLITES

Oxygen metabolites represent a group of molecules that are generated through the reduction of oxygen (Klebanoff, 1980). Activated PMNs possess an enzyme that catalyzes the reduction of oxygen by facilitating the addition of an electron to the oxygen molecule. When oxygen picks up this electron, it becomes a superoxide anion, a free radical (Babior et al., 1973). Oxygen-derived free radicals can participate in a variety of reactions with other molecules as well as with themselves. They can be further reduced to several toxic metabolites or can react with arachidonic acid to produce chemotactic factors that attract more PMNs to the site of injury. In general, the various molecules formed from superoxide are very reactive. The cell interior is protected by antioxidant enzymes that scavenge toxic oxygen metabolites. However, because normal extracellular defenses against oxygen-derived free radicals are not very potent, these compounds are not readily converted to nontoxic products outside cells. It has been shown that when antioxidant protective mechanisms are not present, reduced oxygen metabolites damage endothelial (Varani et al., 1985) and lung parenchymal cells (Martin et al., 1981) in vitro. Thus, oxygen-derived free radicals have the potential to cause considerable lung damage in humans.

RELEASE OF DEGRADATIVE ENZYMES

When PMNs are activated, granules in their cytoplasm are stimulated to release a variety of degradative enzymes (Ayars et al., 1984). The proteases that degrade elastin, collagen, and basement membranes have been studied the most intensively (Dalnogare, 1989). These proteases have been implicated as major factors contributing to the production of experimental acute lung injury and have been found in the bronchoalveolar lavage fluid from patients with ARDS (Lee et al., 1981).

RELEASE OF ARACHIDONIC ACID METABOLITES

Arachidonic acid (AA) is a fatty acid precursor present in all cell membranes that can be released whenever a cell membrane is hormonally, neurally, or mechanically activated. Released AA is then metabolized via two major pathways. The cyclooxygenase pathway produces several eicosanoids, sometimes generically termed prostaglandins, including prostaglandins D_2, E_2, $F_{2\alpha}$, thromboxane, and prostacyclin (Lefer, 1987). The lipooxygenase pathway produces leukotrienes. The biologic effects of these AA metabolites on vascular and airway smooth muscle as well as on formed blood elements such as platelets have made them attractive candidates for initiating or modulating some of the abnormalities witnessed in ARDS. The role of these metabolites has, therefore, been studied in various models (Brigham, 1985).

The prostaglandins have been shown to have potent effects on lung vascular function in sheep (Ogletree, 1982). Thromboxane, a potent vasoconstrictor and platelet aggregator, has been shown to be elevated in blood and lungs of sheep with endotoxin-induced ARDS (Brigham and Ogletree, 1981). In addition, it has been reported that the administration of cyclooxygenase inhibitors blunted the early increase in pulmonary artery pressure and lung lymph flow witnessed following endotoxin infusion into various animals (Brigham and Ogletree, 1981). Thromboxane has also been reported to increase the adhesiveness of PMNs in vitro (Spagnuolo et al., 1980), whereas the vasodilating prostaglandins (prostacyclin and PGE_2) have been shown to increase PMN influx into inflammatory sites (Issekutz and Movat, 1982).

Little information is known about the role of leukotrienes in ARDS. Certain leukotrienes cause long-lasting, intense bronchoconstriction in peripheral airways (Lewis and Austen, 1984). Morganroth and coworkers (1984) reported that a variety of inhibitors of leukotriene synthesis or action were found to inhibit hypoxic pulmonary vasoconstriction. Edema fluid concentrations of leukotrienes also were found to be higher in patients with ARDS than in patients with increased pressure pulmonary edema (Matthay et al., 1984).

ACTIVATION OF DISTURBED COAGULATION

Disturbed coagulation is common in ARDS and is hypothesized to be potentiated by PMN activation and the release of platelet-activating factor (Braquet and Hosford, 1989). Two-thirds of patients with ARDS have evidence of thrombocytopenia and increased platelet turnover rates with platelet deposition in the lungs (Schneider et al., 1980). Factor VIII antigen (which participates in platelet adherence to vessel walls) and fibrinogen degradation products (specifically D antigen) are increased in patients with ARDS (Boggis and Greene, 1983). Frank disseminated intravascular coagulation (DIC) was found in 23% of patients in one study (Bone et al., 1976). Histologically, platelet aggregates and fibrin-rich microthrombi are frequently observed (Stevens and Raffin, 1984). Angiographic examination of the pulmonary vasculature in patients with ARDS frequently demonstrates fibrin thrombi (Boggis and Greene, 1983). Pathophysiologically, platelet and fibrin thrombi may mechanically obstruct the vascular bed, release vasoactive substances, and promote increased permeability pulmonary edema (Stevens and Raffin, 1984). There has also been a recent emphasis on the possible role of fibronectin deficiency in ARDS. There appears to be a reticuloendothelial system suppression in most patients with ARDS due to decreased levels of fibronectin (Saba and Jaffe, 1980). Because the reticuloendothelial system plays a major role in the clearance of particulate debris from the circulation, its depression in ARDS patients may allow this debris to accumulate for long periods and amplify its injurious effects on the pulmonary membranes.

Summary

Although this review has emphasized that the PMN is fully capable of producing ARDS, a funda-

mental question that remains unanswered is whether pulmonary sequestration of PMNs is both necessary and sufficient for the development of ARDS. Further research on the role of PMN-dependent and -independent pathways in the pathogenesis of ARDS is required.

THE CLINICAL AND PATHOLOGIC PHASES OF ARDS

ARDS can be divided into four major clinical phases. The first three phases parallel the stages of edema formation described earlier, whereas the fourth phase specifically represents a structural response to the alteration in alveolar-capillary (a-c) membrane integrity (Modig, 1986; Putterman, 1988).

Latent Phase

During this phase, the primary disorder responsible for the development of ARDS dominates the clinical picture. Unless the underlying disorder is pulmonary in nature, no respiratory distress is apparent and the lungs are clear to auscultation. In fact, little evidence of dysfunction exists except for an increased lymphatic flow. However, it is during this period that the ultrastructural changes in the a-c membrane begin to occur. This phase may last from several hours to a few days.

Acute Interstitial Edema Phase

During this period, pathologic evidence of pulmonary capillary damage and the development of widened endothelial pores exists. The endothelial barrier thus offers less resistance to flow, and hydrostatic pressure is unopposed by osmotic pressure. As a consequence, protein-rich edema fluid rapidly leaks into the lung interstitium, swelling its gel and reducing its compressibility. Alveolar distensibility is reduced, vital capacity is impaired, and mild ventilation-perfusion (V/Q) mismatch is present. However, regardless of the diminished lung distensibility or compliance, the amount of air remaining in the lungs at the end of a normal expiration is not greatly affected. This volume, referred to as functional residual capacity (FRC), is normal because alveolar collapse is prevented by normal surfactant activity and airway closure mechanisms. Pulmonary vascular resistance may increase due to morphologic changes of the microvascular endothelium (Wang et al., 1985).

Clinically, the patient is often apprehensive, restless, and may complain of dyspnea. Tachypnea is present as a result of excitation of sensory nerve endings called J receptors in the alveolar wall by the interstitial fluid. Therefore, minute ventilation is substantially increased. Capillary hydrostatic driving pressure, measured by PAWP, is generally low to normal unless cardiovascular disease coexists. However, an increase in pulmonary artery pressures with a widening of the pulmonary artery end-diastolic and wedge pressure gradient often exists, reflecting the increase in pulmonary vascular resistance. Chest auscultation reveals few, if any, abnormalities. The chest roentgenogram may be normal or demonstrate increased interstitial markings if at least a 20% to 30% increase in extravascular lung water is present (Staub, 1981). These interstitial findings might include patchy peripheral clouding as well as poor definition of the vascular markings. Edema of the interlobular septa, which produces radiographic linear densities referred to as Kerley lines, is generally not present in increased permeability edema states. In addition, many of the other findings of increased pressure edema such as peribronchial cuffing, pleural effusions, and an enlarged vascular pedicle are often not seen (Staub, 1985). Arterial blood gas values reveal an acute respiratory alkalosis secondary to hyperventilation as well as moderate arterial hypoxemia. Another method of evaluating pulmonary gas exchange is through the alveolar-arterial oxygen tension gradient $[P(A-a)O_2]$, which measures the ability of oxygen to cross the a-c membrane. Normally the gradient is less than 15 to 20 mm Hg on room air, but it will be widened in these patients as a result of ventilation-perfusion mismatch.

Acute Intra-alveolar Edema Phase

During this phase, alveolar flooding occurs and, thus, many alveoli are completely filled with high-protein fluid. There is morphologic evidence that both type I and type II alveolar epithelial cells may be injured or their function altered (Barrett et al., 1979). Type I cells, comprising most of the alveolar surface, appear to be more seriously damaged. Injury to these cells diminishes the geometric stability of the alveoli, lung compliance, the efficacy of gas exchange, and the ability of the alveolar barrier to protect against fluid accumulation. Although type II cells, responsible for surfactant production, appear to be less susceptible to injury, evidence exists that the surface-active material recovered from the lungs of patients with ARDS is abnormal (Hallman et al., 1982). This implies that although surfactant is produced, what is available is functionally abnormal. This chemical alteration may be caused by interactions between surfactant and the plasma proteins in edema (Balis et al., 1971). Surfactant may, likewise, be inactivated by compression at low lung volumes (Massard et al., 1980) or by substances released by the injured lung (Tierney and Johnson, 1965). As a consequence, high surface tension promotes alveolar collapse, leading to severe decreases in lung compliance. Functional residual capacity is now markedly diminished, and the work of breathing is tremendously increased. Gas exchange is severely compro-

mised owing to the development of absolute intrapulmonary shunting as perfusion continues to flooded, airless alveoli. However, perfusion is also compromised due to hypoxemic-induced enhancement of pulmonary vascular resistance. This compensatory response is viewed as beneficial in that an attempt is made to reduce perfusion to airless alveoli. This may better preserve ventilation-perfusion matching and minimize the severity of intrapulmonary shunting. Unfortunately, vasoconstriction in gas exchange units that remain aerated will result in wasted or dead space ventilation and further intensify the V/Q inequality and hypoxemia (Dantzker et al., 1979).

Clinically, the patient is often agitated and markedly short of breath. Tachypnea persists now as a consequence of profound hypoxemia, and changes in mental acuity reflect the severity of respiratory distress. The patient may use the accessory muscles of inspiration to optimize ventilation in noncompliant lungs; thus, intercostal retractions are seen. Excessive work of breathing leads to respiratory muscle fatigue, and the associated increase in oxygen consumption is far too costly in the face of progressing hypoxemia. Even if the patient is being mechanically ventilated, peak inspiratory pressures required to deliver a given tidal volume progressively increase. Increases in pulmonary artery pressures associated with enhanced pulmonary vascular resistance persist, and these may precipitate the development of right heart failure, decreased left ventricular filling volumes, and a deleterious reduction in cardiac output. Auscultation of the chest generally reveals fine, diffuse crackles, but the distinctive fluid-derived crackles of increased pressure pulmonary edema are often notably absent. Breath sounds, however, are diminished reflecting altered air movement and atelectasis. The chest roentgenogram demonstrates a diffuse, bilateral, fluffy alveolar filling pattern referred to as white lung (Staub, 1985). Arterial blood gas values generally reveal acute respiratory alkalosis, severe arterial hypoxemia unresponsive to supplemental oxygen even at increased FI_{O_2} levels, and a markedly widened $P(A-a)O_2$. Because some gas exchange units will have adequate ventilation but limited perfusion whereas others will have adequate perfusion but no ventilation, a rise in physiologic deadspace (V_D/V_T) and an increase in shunt fraction (QS/QT), respectively, are also characteristic (Dantzker et al., 1979). V_D/V_T reflects alveoli that are underperfused and thus wasted ventilation. QS/QT reflects the percentage of blood flowing from the right to left heart that does not perfectly exchange with alveolar gas; as such, this is a particularly useful parameter to measure in these patients. Calculated shunts of between 20% and 30% reflect an intrapulmonary abnormality that requires intervention. Any calculated shunt that exceeds the 30% value is considered life-threatening because it is incompatible with maintaining oxygenation (Dalnogare, 1989).

TABLE 26–2. Differentiation of Cardiogenic and Increased Permeability Pulmonary Edema

	Cardiogenic Pulmonary Edema	Increased Permeability Pulmonary Edema
History	Acute cardiac event	Predisposing condition of ARDS (see Table 26–1)
Clinical examination	S_3/cardiomegaly	No gallop
	Jugular venous distention	No jugular venous distention
	Crackles (wet)	Crackles (dry)
Diagnostic data	Chest x-ray: Perihilar distribution	Chest x-ray: Peripheral distribution
	Pulmonary artery wedge pressure (PAWP) ≥ 18 mm Hg	Pulmonary artery wedge pressure (PAWP) < 18 mm Hg
	PAD* − PAWP gradient ≤ 5 mm Hg	PAD* − PAWP gradient > 5 mm Hg
	Intrapulmonary shunt: Small increase	Intrapulmonary shunt: Large increase
	Edema fluid/serum protein ratio < 0.6	Edema fluid/serum protein ratio > 0.7

*PAD = pulmonary diastolic pressure.

Subacute–Chronic Phase

If recovery or death does not occur, a subacute stage results following the development of interstitial and alveolar edema. Pathologic evidence shows that with the natural progression of acute lung injury, alveolar damage appears to be more severe than damage to the capillary endothelium (Barrett et al., 1979). Type I pneumocytes are destroyed, leaving a denuded basement membrane. Condensed aggregates of plasma protein, cellular debris, fibrin strands, and remnants of surfactant adhere to the denuded alveolar surface, forming characteristic hyaline membranes. Over the course of the next few days, fluid is reabsorbed from the air spaces. The alveolar septum thickens markedly and is infiltrated by proliferating fibroblasts, plasma cells, and leukocytes. Hyaline membranes begin to organize, and microatelectasis is seen. These membranes can be a formidable barrier to gas diffusion. In addition, as a result of the limited regenerative properties of type I pneumocytes, proliferation of type II cells occurs. Fibrogenesis may begin at this point. Alveoli may be obliterated, alveolar walls coalesced, and functional lung units lost, leading to end-stage pulmonary fibrosis within a matter of weeks (Bachofen and Weibel, 1982). However, even these very severe changes may be reversible with slow recovery toward normal lung function. Recovery is probably related to the severity of the initial damage to the architecture of the lungs and to the intensity of the fibrotic response. Death can result either from a complicating event or from unrelenting, progressive pulmonary failure.

Clinically, peak ventilator pressures increase progressively, and the chest roentgenogram shows evidence of interstitial fibrosis. As carbon dioxide normally diffuses with ease across the a-c membrane, an increase in arterial carbon dioxide tension (Pa_{CO_2}) represents a grave prognostic sign suggesting severe membrane damage. Elevated Pa_{CO_2} levels may also represent increased work of breathing, an increase in wasted ventilation, or muscle respiratory fatigue in patients not supported by mechanical ventilation (Estenne and Yernault, 1984).

THE CLINICAL DIAGNOSIS OF ARDS

Identifying ARDS in its early stage, increased permeability interstitial edema, is very difficult. Because its onset may be sudden or insidious, any patient presenting with a predisposing condition associated with ARDS should be viewed with a high index of suspicion. This is by far one of the most powerful diagnostic tools. Additional features that are reasonably reliable during this stage include (Dalnogare, 1989; Putterman, 1988):

1. FI_{O_2} of 0.35 or higher required to maintain an arterial P_{O_2} greater than 60 mm Hg
2. Chest radiograph compatible with increased permeability interstitial edema and without pneumonia infiltrates or atelectasis
3. An elevated minute ventilation (greater than 20 L/minute) associated with an acute respiratory alkalosis
4. Absence of COPD and increased pressure cardiogenic edema

The major differential diagnosis is increased pressure cardiogenic pulmonary edema (Sibbald et al., 1983) (Table 26–2). Pulmonary artery and wedge pressure measurements can facilitate this differentiation. In ARDS, the PAWP is generally normal, mild to moderate pulmonary hypertension is often present, and the pulmonary artery diastolic pressure (PAD)–PAWP gradient is often increased to greater than 5 mm Hg. Conversely, in cardiogenic pulmonary edema, the PAWP is increased, and pulmonary hypertension, when present, is secondary to pulmonary venous congestion. Therefore, no significant PAD–PAWP gradient exists. It is, however, important to note that pressures obtained from pulmonary artery catheterization may be misleading in patients who are on mechanical ventilators, in particular those receiving positive end-expiratory pressure (PEEP), because alveolar pressure may exceed capillary hydrostatic pressure in different regions of the lung (Lozman et al., 1974; Rajacich et al., 1989). If the pulmonary artery catheter is located in a vessel where alveolar pressure is greater than capillary hydrostatic pressure, capillary narrowing or collapse can occur, disrupting the continuous column of blood from the catheter tip to the left heart and jeopardizing the validity of the PAWP pressure (Enger, 1989) (Fig. 26–6). Confirmation of the position of the catheter tip in a vessel below the level of the left atrium (West lung zone III) by lateral roentgenogram will minimize this discrepancy because hydrostatic pressure should exceed alveolar pressure in this zone, and therefore PAWP should be reflective of the left atrial pressure (Enger, 1989).

Once the alveolar edema, gas exchange abnormalities, and metabolic derangements of ARDS ensue, the syndrome is more easily identified by the following parameters (Dalnogare, 1989; Putterman, 1988):

1. Refractory hypoxemia (arterial P_{O_2} less than 60 mm Hg at an $F_{I_{O_2}}$ of 0.5 or higher)
2. A markedly diminished static lung compliance (less than 50 mg/cm H_2O on mechanical ventilatory assistance)
3. A chest radiograph with diffuse bilateral parenchymal infiltrates
4. An increased shunt fraction (QS/QT)

An additional diagnostic technique that has been advocated for distinguishing between increased pressure and increased permeability alveolar edema is the edema fluid–plasma protein ratio (Fein et al., 1979). Calculation of this ratio requires the measurement of protein content in edema and plasma collected simultaneously from endotracheal suctioning and blood sampling. Because the microvascular barrier is functionally intact in increased pressure alveolar edema, plasma proteins will remain confined to the intravascular space, and edema fluid protein content will be low relative to plasma protein content with a ratio generally of less than 0.6. Conversely, with increased permeability alveolar edema, as the barrier is injured, the edema–plasma protein content ratio will be greater than 0.7 (Crandell, 1983; Fein et al., 1979).

MEDICAL TREATMENT

The medical treatment of ARDS is divided into three major areas of concentration: (1) reversing the underlying associated disorder; (2) blocking the specific mechanism of alveolar-capillary membrane injury; and (3) minimizing the pathologic consequences of acute lung injury through supportive measures. The first two areas address preventing the development of ARDS whereas the last area focuses on attempting to minimize the morbidity and mortality of ARDS once it occurs. Therapy aimed at reversing the underlying disorder will vary according to the specific precipitating cause. The common disorders associated with ARDS have been discussed earlier, and their therapy can be found in other areas of this text. Therefore, measures addressing only the second two areas of treatment priority will be highlighted here.

Blocking the Specific Mechanism of a-c Membrane Injury

Several agents have been investigated in both human and animal models to determine their efficacy in blocking cell damage and subsequent pulmonary dysfunction. Animal studies, however, cannot totally duplicate the physiologic conditions of human ARDS. In addition, human studies are difficult to design in which the lung injury is physiologically well defined, in which the time from insult to intervention can be established, and in which endpoints are clearly defined. Therefore, data from these studies are often inconclusive. Until the mechanisms and mediators of acute lung injury in ARDS have been clearly elucidated, all aspects of specific therapy will remain controversial. However, based on the previous discussion, it seems logical that pharmacologic therapy be directed at stabilizing PMNs and inactivating the toxic mediators they release including oxygen-derived free radicals, degradative proteases,

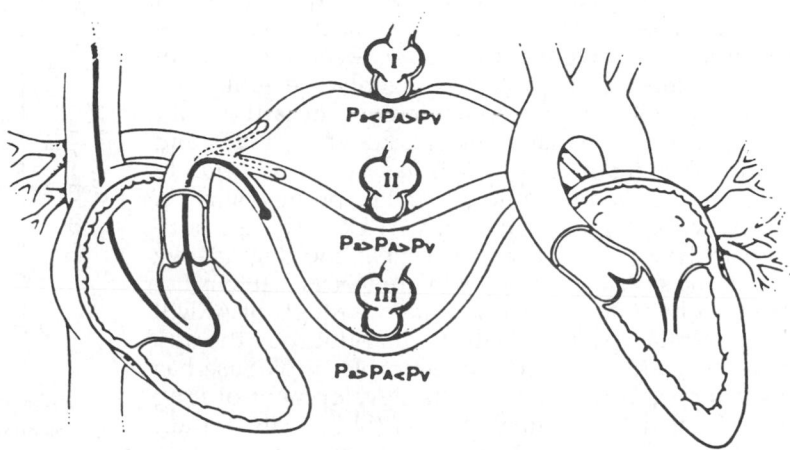

FIGURE 26–6. West lung zones. In lung zone III pulmonary arterial and venous pressures exceed alveolar pressure. PAWP reflects left atrial pressure only under lung zone III conditions, which allow for a continuous column of blood to exist from the tip of the pulmonary artery catheter to the left atrium. (From Enger, E.L. (1989). Pulmonary artery wedge pressure: When it's valid, when it's not. *Critical Care Nursing Clinics of North America,* 1, 603–618.)

and arachidonic acid metabolites (Raffin, 1987; Roberts, 1990).

Several beneficial effects have been postulated for the use of corticosteroids in ARDS. These include the ability of corticosteroids to inhibit the production of arachidonic acid metabolites, to impair PMN adherence, to stabilize lysosomal membranes, to prevent superoxide damage, and to decrease complement activation (Roberts, 1990). Sibbald and colleagues (1981) have demonstrated a reduced passage of radiolabeled albumin from serum to pulmonary edema fluid in patients with ARDS after methylprednisolone administration. However, Bernard and associates (1987) conducted a prospective, randomized, double-blind, placebo-controlled trial of high-dose methylprednisolone therapy in 99 ARDS patients with various underlying diseases and observed no statistical differences between groups in pulmonary shunting, oxygenation variables, chest radiograph severity, compliance, pulmonary artery pressures, infectious complications, or mortality. In addition, Bone and co-workers (1987) evaluated whether early methylprednisolone treatment would decrease the incidence or severity of ARDS in 304 patients with septic syndromes. They concluded that early corticosteroid therapy did not prevent the development of ARDS but actually impeded the reversal of ARDS and increased the mortality rate. Based on these and other trials, corticosteroid therapy for patients with ARDS cannot currently be recommended unless they present with shock secondary to or associated with adrenal insufficiency.

Although there are no agents other than corticosteroids that have been extensively evaluated in human lung injury, several classes of agents have been investigated in various animal models. Because the arachidonic acid metabolite thromboxane has been mechanistically implicated with ARDS, agents that inhibit its production including nonsteroidal anti-inflammatory agents such as indomethacin and ibuprofen (Begley et al., 1984) as well as thromboxane synthetase inhibitors (Said and Foda, 1989) have been examined. Two additional arachidonic acid metabolites with protective actions opposing thromboxane, prostacyclin (Perlman et al., 1986) and PGE_1 (Shoemaker and Appel, 1986), have been shown to inhibit hypoxic vasoconstriction and stabilize neutrophil membranes. Scavengers of oxygen-free radicals appear promising as protective agents. Several scavengers including N-acetylcysteine (Bernard et al., 1984), superoxide dismutase (Parker et al., 1983), and catalase (Milligan et al., 1985) have been reported to attenuate increased microvascular permeability in sheep with endotoxin-induced ARDS. Alpha-1 antitrypsin has been shown to combat the degradative effects of several proteases (Vered et al., 1985). Because pulmonary fibrosis is a major sequela of ARDS, the potential beneficial effects of antifibrotic therapy have been investigated. For example, urokinase has been reported to suppress the development of lung fibrosis in ARDS animal models (Shigematsu et al., 1980). Although preliminary communications on these investigational therapies have been promising, controlled human studies will determine which, if any, of these agents is effective. Until success is achieved, supportive intensive care will remain the focal point of therapy for ARDS.

Minimizing the Pathologic Consequences: Supportive Measures

Supportive measures are divided into three major objectives:

1. Minimizing edema formation
2. Maintaining tissue oxygenation while reducing exacerbating factors
3. Preventing and recognizing complications

MINIMIZING EDEMA FORMATION

With increased permeability pulmonary edema, the urgent problem is not that the driving pressure for edema formation is abnormally elevated but that the edema will form in great quantities even at low driving pressures (Fig. 26–7). Because of this fact, microvascular hydrostatic pressure (PAWP) is generally kept as low as possible to minimize fluid flux. Diuretics are often administered to achieve this outcome. However, diuresis often does not decrease lung water considerably. In fact, efforts to minimize fluid exudation may result in microvascular pressures inadequate to maintain effective blood flow to the tissues. It should be clear that the maintenance of cardiac output is of paramount importance because impairment of flow will have a profound effect on oxygen delivery to the tissues. Hence, fluid therapy may be required to maintain adequate cardiac performance even in the presence of wet lungs. This careful balancing of cardiopulmonary performance

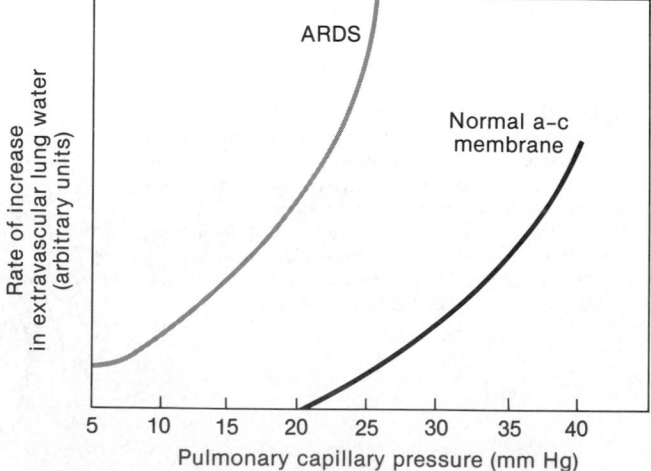

FIGURE 26–7. Schematic representation of the deleterious effects of essentially normal PAWP in combination with the loss of a–c membrane integrity in ARDS.

may be facilitated by invasive hemodynamic monitoring (Snider, 1990).

The choice of fluid to maintain vascular volume has received a great deal of attention. In patients with a low wedge pressure as well as a low hematocrit, packed red blood cells are effective not only in expanding intravascular volume but also in increasing the oxygen-carrying capacity of the blood. However, increased blood viscosity may intensify the workload of the right heart, which is already enhanced as a consequence of pulmonary hypertension. In patients with a normal hematocrit, both colloids and crystalloids have been advocated. Those favoring the use of colloid solutions argue that they are more effective for intravascular volume expansion than equal volumes of crystalloid solutions (Hauser et al., 1980). It is further argued that much of the crystalloid solution ends up in the pulmonary interstitium and alveoli, thus worsening gas exchange (Shoemaker et al., 1981). Large volume crystalloid infusion also lowers colloidal osmotic pressure (Haupt and Rackow, 1982). Proponents of crystalloid therapy suggest that since the barriers restricting colloid movement from the vascular space into the lungs do not function normally when the lungs have been injured, osmotic pressure differences favoring fluid movement into the vascular space cannot be established. Indeed, recent data from animal studies support that albumin readily crosses into the interstitium (Moss et al., 1981). This would mitigate against using albumin. Therefore, there appears to be no advantage to fluid resuscitation with expensive colloid solutions. In fact, they may even compound edema formation.

The goal of therapy is to maintain the lowest possible wedge pressure that is consistent with adequate cardiac output and perfusion to vital organs. If cardiac output is adequate, no wedge pressure is considered too low (Putterman, 1988). Vasodilator therapy may be beneficial because it will lower systemic afterload, which may improve cardiac output yet maintain low pulmonary vascular pressures. Blood pressure can then be supported as appropriate with inotropic agents. Vasodilators must be used cautiously, however, because they may increase intrapulmonary shunt in the later stages of ARDS by interfering with hypoxic vasoconstriction, which attempts to preserve ventilation-perfusion matching by decreasing perfusion to airless alveoli (Wood and Prewitt, 1981).

MAINTAINING TISSUE OXYGENATION

Tissue oxygen delivery (transport) is the product of arterial blood oxygen content (primarily determined by hemoglobin concentration and oxygen saturation of that hemoglobin) and cardiac output. Oxygen uptake (consumption) by the tissues is reflected by the product of the difference in oxygen content in arterial and venous blood and cardiac output. Oxygen uptake is determined by the metabolic re-

quirements of the tissues until oxygen delivery falls below these requirements, at which time oxygen uptake becomes dependent upon and varies directly with oxygen delivery. Normal oxygen delivery (1000 mL/minute) is greater than oxygen consumption (250 mL/minute). Therefore, the human body can experience a large fall in oxygen content, cardiac output, or both yet still supply sufficient oxygen to meet metabolic requirements (Snyder, 1987). However, some evidence exists that in ARDS, oxygen uptake is dependent upon oxygen delivery over a much greater range and, therefore, that oxygen uptake is extremely delivery dependent. As a result, maintaining oxygen delivery is of paramount importance in establishing adequate tissue oxygenation in ARDS patients (Dantzker, 1990; Karima and Burns, 1985). In addition, oxygen delivery must be maintained with a minimum $F_{I_{O_2}}$ because the lungs are already damaged, making them especially sensitive to the effects of alveolar hyperoxia and consequent oxygen-free radical production, as previously discussed. Fortunately, during the interstitial edema stage of ARDS, if adequate fluid balance and cardiovascular support have been achieved, the patient should be sufficiently oxygenated with $F_{I_{O_2}}$ concentrations below 0.50. In fact, the inability to achieve an arterial P_{O_2} of greater than 60 mm Hg with a maximum $F_{I_{O_2}}$ of 0.45 should be considered a warning signal of patient deterioration and the development of intra-alveolar edema. The appropriateness and timeliness of therapy directed at the early stage of ARDS will greatly determine whether the patient will progress into later, more severe stages. Hypotension, volume overload, and oxygen toxicity must be strictly avoided (Keogh et al., 1989).

Mechanical Ventilation. Patients with fully developed ARDS invariably require mechanical ventilation to minimize the work of breathing associated with their stiff, noncompliant lungs. When mechanical ventilation is initiated, tidal volumes of 10 to 15 mg/kg of body weight are generally employed to minimize atelectasis. Controversy persists with regard to which mode of ventilation is best suited for these patients. Advocates of the assist-control mode believe that it will better decrease the work of breathing. Advocates of the intermittent mandatory ventilation mode believe that it will diminish respiratory alkalemia, sparing the patient from difficulties in oxygen unloading at the tissues owing to increased pH-induced alterations in oxygen hemoglobin affinity (Keogh et al., 1989).

Several nontraditional ventilatory modes have been evaluated in the management of ARDS (Keogh et al., 1990; Toben and Levandowski, 1988). Inverse ratio ventilation represents a variation of conventional ventilation in which inspiratory to expiratory ratios greater than 1:1 are applied. The prolonged application of inspiratory-positive pressure may recruit collapsed alveoli, and the brief expiratory period, although adequate for carbon dioxide clearance, may retard expiration sufficiently to keep these alveoli above their closing volume. Another mode, airway pressure release ventilation, maintains lung volume and oxygenation by continuous positive airway pressure. Carbon dioxide clearance with this mode is achieved by the transient release of circuit pressure, allowing gas to exit and lung volume to fall. Continuous positive pressure is then reestablished, allowing fresh gas to enter into the system. The patient may breathe spontaneously throughout the respiratory cycle, and the need for conventional positive pressure breaths is eliminated. High-frequency jet ventilation utilizes high-pressure pulses of gas delivered at supranormal frequencies (60 to 600/minute) for a preset percentage of each inspiratory cycle. The clinical efficacy of these ventilatory modes and their ability to improve outcome in patients with ARDS remains to be established. The use of tidal volume preset ventilation, positive end-expiratory pressure (PEEP), and an inspiratory-expiratory ratio of less than 1:1 remains the mainstay of respiratory support in patients with ARDS.

Positive End-Expiratory Pressure. Although conventional mechanical ventilation can eliminate the high work of breathing in this disorder, it does not address the critical problem of impaired oxygen exchange. Keep in mind that no amount of oxygen administration can correct hypoxemia if this oxygen never reaches the alveoli because they are fluid filled. Therefore, the use of positive pressure ventilation with PEEP has a well-documented role in the management of refractory hypoxemia secondary to intrapulmonary shunting in ARDS (Dalnogare, 1989). PEEP is the artificial maintenance of positive (superatmospheric) pressure after passive exhalation is complete. This technique is termed continuous positive pressure ventilation (CPPV) when PEEP is added to intermittent positive pressure ventilation provided by a ventilator, whereas it is called continuous positive airway pressure (CPAP) when PEEP is applied to patients without ventilator assistance. Regardless of the technique used, the effect of PEEP on the lungs is an increase in functional residual capacity, which recruits or maintains open alveoli that are otherwise collapsed. This increase in lung volume, in return, improves pulmonary compliance, minimizes intrapulmonary shunting, and reduces the alveolar arterial oxygen tension difference (Shapiro et al., 1984). Accordingly, the beneficial use of PEEP generally improves oxygen delivery and allows reduction of the inspired oxygen concentration to levels less likely to produce oxygen toxicity and free radical production. Several additional effects of PEEP have been explored. It has been hypothesized that PEEP may alter surface tension by a yet unproven interaction with surfactant and thus reduce atelectasis. It has also been hypothesized that a relationship exists between PEEP and actual lung water (Shapiro et al., 1984). Despite initial reports, PEEP does not reliably decrease lung water. In fact, in some settings, it has

been reported to increase it, possibly by increased filtration through extra-alveolar vessels (Permutt, 1979). The question of whether PEEP may reduce the extent of ALI and therefore may be prophylactic if introduced early in patients at risk of developing ARDS has also arisen. Despite early encouraging data that this might be true, more recent controlled studies have not supported the prophylactic value of PEEP (Pepe et al., 1984).

Considerable controversy exists about how best to establish the optimum level of PEEP. Criteria that have been advocated to determine this optimal level include adjusting the PEEP to attain:

1. A P_{O_2} of approximately 60 mm Hg with an $F_{I_{O_2}}$ of 0.5 or less (Weisman et al., 1982)
2. The lowest intrapulmonary shunt percentage (Gallagher et al., 1978)
3. The greatest oxygen delivery (transport) (Suter et al., 1975)
4. The greatest measured lung compliance (Suter et al., 1975)
5. The point where mixed venous oxygen tension and/or saturation falls (Hurewitz and Bergofsky, 1981)

Despite differing emphasis in these approaches to establishing a PEEP level, there is no clear evidence that any one method has a distinct advantage in reducing morbidity or mortality. To better understand how to adjust this modality, its potential deleterious effects must be appreciated, the most significant of which are barotrauma (Balk and Bone, 1983) and a reduction in cardiac output (Weisman et al., 1982). Barotrauma involves the development of pneumomediastinum, pneumothorax, or subcutaneous emphysema. Decreased cardiac output results from a reduction in venous return as well as an increase in pulmonary vascular resistance. As right heart afterload increases, right ventricular emptying is impeded, shifting the intraventricular septum to the left, thus reducing left ventricular internal dimension and compliance (Weisman et al., 1982). Recall that arterial oxygen delivery is the product of arterial blood oxygen content and cardiac output. Any increase in oxygen content that results from the use of PEEP will not beneficially improve oxygen delivery if it is associated with a counterbalancing fall in cardiac output. Therefore, to determine the optimal level of PEEP, it is necessary to determine the level that provides combined optimal respiratory and cardiac function. This level should establish optimal tissue oxygenation (Putterman, 1988). Generally, PEEP is instituted in 3- to 5-cm H_2O increments until a predetermined measure of optimal tissue oxygenation is achieved. The efficacy of levels of PEEP in the range of 1 to 20 cm H_2O has been fairly thoroughly documented. Levels of PEEP in excess of 20 cm H_2O have also been studied, but efficacy remains to be shown (Brandstetter, 1986; Dalnogare, 1989). It has been suggested that excessive PEEP levels may compress alveolar vessels adjacent to well-ventilated alveoli, thus diverting more blood flow to poorly ventilated areas and increasing the shunting phenomenon (Shapiro et al., 1984).

Extracorporeal and Intravascular Gas Exchange. Several attempts to improve gas exchange by the use of extracorporeal membrane lungs have been made in patients with severe ARDS. Extracorporeal membrane oxygenation (ECMO) was first used in patients with ARDS in 1972 (Hill et al., 1972). With this technique, blood is usually taken from the inferior vena cava via the femoral vein, passed through a membrane oxygenator at high flow rates where it undergoes gas exchange, and then is returned to the circulation through the femoral artery. Results of a national multicenter collaborative study (Zapol et al., 1979) as well as several subsequent studies have not shown a significant decrease in mortality with the use of ECMO (Keogh et al., 1990). However, all patients in these studies have been severely ill prior to entry. More recently, a modified form of extracorporeal gas exchange termed extracorporeal carbon dioxide removal has been demonstrated to improve survival in patients with ARDS (Pesenti et al., 1988). With this technique, the lungs are still used for oxygenation and supplied with low-frequency positive pressure ventilation. However, carbon dioxide is removed through the membrane. This technique has several advantages. Because the removal of carbon dioxide requires a lower rate of blood flow through the extracorporeal circuit than that needed to achieve full oxygenation, it is possible to perform this procedure via a simple venovenous cannulation. In addition, barotrauma is minimized and lung movement reduced, thus providing better conditions for lung repair (Keogh et al., 1990).

Mortensen (1987) has pioneered the construction of an intravenous capillary membrane lung, the IVOX, which is designed to be placed percutaneously into the inferior vena cava. Gas exchange occurs by passive diffusion sufficient to supply 90% of the basal oxygen requirements of a resting adult.

The future role of these devices in the supportive treatment of patients with ARDS remains to be determined.

Nutritional Support. Patients with ARDS are at risk for developing protein–calorie malnutrition, which will further compromise the respiratory system and tissue oxygenation (Rochester and Esau, 1984). In undernourished patients, pulmonary defense mechanisms become impaired (Moriguchi et al., 1983), and an altered ventilatory response to hypoxemia is common (Weissmann et al., 1983). Surfactant function is also abnormal in the malnourished patient (Sahebjami et al., 1978), structural parenchymal changes have been documented (Sahebjami et al., 1978), and diaphragmatic mass may be dramatically decreased (Arora and Rochester, 1977). These responses can lead to markedly altered lung mechanics. Therefore, some form of nutritional ther-

apy that maintains a positive protein balance is imperative. Nutritional supplementation is not, however, without risk. If the carbohydrate load exceeds energy needs, lipogenesis and a greater production of carbon dioxide relative to oxygen consumption can predispose to hypercapnia. Therefore, judicious nutritional support must be provided (Majors, 1988).

PREVENTING AND RECOGNIZING COMPLICATIONS

The complications of ARDS can be divided into two broad categories, mechanical and medical complications (Pingleton, 1982). Because the majority of ARDS patients will be receiving mechanical ventilatory assistance, which entails control of the airway either by endotracheal intubation or tracheotomy, all of the mechanical complications associated with these procedures may be experienced (see Chaps. 29 and 30). In addition, because virtually every organ system can be involved with ARDS, whether from underlying disease processes, concomitant disease processes, or as a result of therapeutic interventions, a number of medical complications may occur as well (Table 26–3).

NURSING MANAGEMENT (PRIMARY NURSING DIAGNOSIS: IMPAIRED PULMONARY GAS EXCHANGE)

Throughout this chapter, it has been emphasized that maintenance of a sufficient, balanced amount of oxygen diffusion across the a-c membrane (ventilation) and intrinsic blood flow (perfusion) is essential to tissue oxygenation in ARDS patients. Therefore, the critical care nurse's responsibility is not only to implement and monitor the efficacy of the medical treatment plan but also to identify, implement, and

TABLE 26–3. Medical Complications of ARDS

Pulmonary	Infection
Pulmonary emboli	Sepsis
Pulmonary fibrosis	Nosocomial pneumonia
Oxygen toxicity	
Barotrauma	**Hematologic**
	Anemia
Renal	Thrombocytopenia
Renal failure	Disseminated intravascular
Fluid retention	coagulation
Cardiac	**Other**
Dysrhythmia	Hepatic
Hypotension	Endocrine
Low cardiac output	Neurologic
	Psychiatric
Gastrointestinal	Malnutrition
Hemorrhage	
Ileus	
Gastric distention	
Pneumoperitoneum	

evaluate nursing interventions targeted at addressing alterations in this pulmonary gas exchange process.

Causes and Manifestations

Several factors may potentially impair pulmonary gas exchange in ARDS patients (Roberts, 1990). Adequate ventilation may be threatened by bronchoconstriction, interstitial edema, decreased pulmonary compliance, intra-alveolar edema, and atelectasis. Manifestations that signal inadequate ventilation include tachypnea, decreased tidal volume, dyspnea, restlessness, tachycardia, and diminished or adventitious breath sounds. Optimal perfusion may be compromised by hypoxia-induced vasoconstriction, pulmonary microemboli, continuous positive pressure ventilation, and inadequate circulating blood volume secondary to diuresis. Warning signs of insufficient perfusion include tachycardia, arrhythmias, hypotension, decreased urine output, and a decreased level of consciousness.

Desired Outcomes

Collaborative and independent nursing interventions should be directed at attaining the following outcomes consistent with the goal of optimizing pulmonary gas exchange and thus tissue oxygenation (Dalnogare, 1989; Putterman, 1988; Roberts, 1990; Shapiro et al., 1984; Wood and Prewitt, 1981):

1. The lowest PAWP that will minimize the hydrostatic gradient for edema formation yet not compromise the adequacy of left ventricular filling and cardiac output
2. The lowest $F_{I_{O_2}}$ that will minimize toxic lung injury by oxygen-derived free radicals yet not compromise alveolar ventilation or arterial blood oxygen content
3. The lowest PEEP value that will minimize pressure-related barotrauma and cardiac output reduction yet not compromise alveolar expansion, FRC, and V/Q matching
4. The lowest intrapulmonary shunt percentage that will minimize refractory hypoxemia
5. The highest pulmonary compliance that will minimize the work of breathing
6. The highest arterial oxygen delivery that will optimize tissue oxygen utilization

Interventions

DECREASE THE METABOLIC REQUIREMENTS FOR OXYGEN

Anxiety, pain, and dyspnea notoriously increase basal metabolic rate, thus increasing inspired oxygen requirements (Snyder, 1987). Even in patients with good respiratory support, these factors often prevail.

Consequently, implementing strategies to control these factors is ultimately beneficial. It is important to ensure that the ventilator's circuit is properly set up and functioning. Sedation can also be used to control the discomfort of the endotracheal tube or other sources of pain as well as to calm the patient.

Fever is another factor that increases the demand for oxygen (Snyder, 1987). However, temperature must be regulated judiciously with cooling blankets and antipyretics because shivering, which increases oxygen consumption and masks sepsis, can be equally detrimental.

ENSURE OPTIMUM PATIENT POSITIONING

Patient positioning can be an important factor in optimizing gas exchange in that perfusion needs to be directed to areas of good ventilation to promote optimal matching. As such, patients with unilateral disease should be positioned with the "good lung" down to promote preferential dependent perfusion (Gottlieb, 1988). In patients with bilateral disease, which is commonly experienced with ARDS, the prone position has been advocated as practicality allows (Langer et al., 1988). Objective determination of the efficacy of various patient positions can probably best be achieved by measuring oxygen delivery or some other agreed upon gas exchange variable such as mixed venous oxygen saturation in each of the various positions. These measurements are best made 30 minutes following the position change to allow for stabilization.

MAINTAIN CONTINUOUS PEEP

In patients with ARDS supported by continuous positive pressure ventilation, removing the ventilator and PEEP for short time periods has been reported to decrease rapidly arterial oxygen tension as well as FRC (Enger, 1989; Weisman et al., 1982). An ideal tracheal suctioning or tubing change procedure, therefore, uses principles of preoxygenation, minimal suctioning time, postsuctioning hyperinflation to reverse atelectasis, and uninterrupted PEEP facilitated by an adaptor valve or a closed airway suctioning system (Roberts, 1990; Schumann and Parsons, 1985). Discontinuation of PEEP during measurements of PAWP has also been advocated because PEEP can introduce uncertainty in the validity of the values by inducing changes in left ventricular compliance and intrathoracic pressure. Alveolar pressure in patients on PEEP will equal the PEEP value, and, thus, in less dependent regions of the lung, it will be greater than capillary hydrostatic pressure. In these cases, the alveolar pressure will collapse the pulmonary capillary and the PAWP will reflect the alveolar pressure instead of left heart filling pressures (Enger, 1989). However, due to the fact that removing PEEP can induce serious gas exchange abnormalities as well as artificial hemodynamic changes, it is recommended that PAWP measurements be done with the patient on PEEP. PAWP is not generally affected by low levels of PEEP (less than 10 cm H₂O) (Lozman et al., 1974). As previously discussed, ensuring that the pulmonary artery catheter is positioned properly below the level of the left atrium will also maximize the accuracy of the values. At higher levels of PEEP, a mathematical adjustment of PAWP has been advocated (Enger, 1989; O'Quin and Marini, 1983).

IDENTIFY HEMOGLOBIN-RELATED ALTERATIONS IN OXYGEN DELIVERY

An important yet often overlooked threat to oxygen delivery and subsequent tissue oxygenation is anemia. The nurse, therefore, needs to monitor the patient's hemoglobin level closely. In addition, those factors that make it more difficult for hemoglobin to unload oxygen at the tissue level due to an increase in oxygen hemoglobin affinity should be detected and corrected. Conditions predisposing to this state (a leftward shift in the oxyhemoglobin dissociation curve) include hypophosphatemia, alkalemia, decreased Pa_{CO_2}, and decreased levels of 2,3-DPG that result from banked blood administration (Gottlieb, 1988).

ASSESS INTRAPULMONARY SHUNTING (QS/QT)

Intrapulmonary shunting refers to blood flowing from the right side of the heart to the left side of the heart that does not perfectly exchange with alveolar gas. Shunting has three potential components: (1) anatomic, (2) capillary, and (3) venous admixture. The first two of these are absolute shunting mechanisms in that blood reaches the left ventricle without having been exposed to the air-alveolar interface. Absolute shunt mechanisms are, therefore, refractory to oxygen therapy. No matter how much oxygen is available, blood volume that bypasses does not participate in oxygen exchange. Anatomic shunting includes blood flow leaving the right ventricle without passing through the pulmonary capillaries. Normally, this comprises 2% to 5% of the cardiac output. Pathologic anatomic shunting can result from intrapulmonary arteriovenous fistulas and right-to-left intracardiac shunts. Capillary shunting is a result of pulmonary capillary blood passing totally collapsed or airless alveoli. The third type of shunt mechanism is venous admixture, also referred to as the shunt effect. It is the result of perfusion in excess of ventilation, yet some ventilation still exists. This mechanism is responsive to oxygen therapy. In the later stages of ARDS, intrapulmonary shunting is primarily secondary to the absolute capillary mechanism. The percentage of intrapulmonary shunting can be quantified by calculating QS/QT in which QS is the shunted perfusion and QT is the total perfusion. Because pathologic anatomic shunting can easily be ruled out, QS/QT generally reflects the percentage of capillary and venous admixture shunting. If the parameter is abnormal or greater than 10%

when measured on an Fi_{O_2} of at least 0.5, it reflects primarily absolute capillary shunting (Gottlieb, 1988; Reischman, 1988). It then is a very valuable parameter to use to assess the severity of gas exchange abnormalities witnessed in ARDS.

Calculation of QS/QT requires simultaneously drawn arterial and mixed venous (pulmonary artery) blood samples. QS is determined by subtracting the arterial blood oxygen content (Ca_{O_2}), which represents the amount of oxygen content in pulmonary capillary blood immediately after it has passed the average alveolus, from the ideal end pulmonary capillary oxygen content (Cc_{O_2}). As such, any difference between ideal pulmonary capillary oxygen content and the actual oxygen content reflected by the systemic arterial sample is attributed to pulmonary shunting. QT is determined by subtracting mixed venous blood oxygen content (Cv_{O_2}), once again from ideal pulmonary capillary oxygen content. Dividing QS by QT will yield the shunt fraction, which may be multiplied by 100 to arrive at the percent shunt.

$$\frac{QS}{QT} = \frac{Cc_{O_2} - Ca_{O_2}}{Cc_{O_2} - Cv_{O_2}}$$

Ca_{O_2} is calculated by the following equation:

$$(Hgb \times 1.38 \times Sa_{O_2}) + (Pa_{O_2} \times 0.003)$$

Cv_{O_2} is calculated by the following equation:

$$(Hgb \times 1.38 \times Sv_{O_2}) + (Pv_{O_2} \times 0.003)$$

The calculation of Cc_{O_2} requires some explanation of underlying assumptions. The alveolar gas equation is used to calculate end-pulmonary capillary oxygen tension because ideally they should be the same. The patient's Fi_{O_2}, barometric pressure (P_B usually equals 760 mm Hg), and water vapor pressure ($P_{H_2O} = 47$ mm Hg) need to be known to determine the oxygen tension of inspired air. In addition, the patient's arterial carbon dioxide tension needs to be measured. These values are then inserted into the alveolar gas equation. The oxygen saturation of end capillary blood should be 100%. However, in order to eliminate any source of error induced by carboxyhemoglobin or other mechanisms, it is generally assumed to be 98%. Cc_{O_2} is then calculated by the following equation:

$$(Hgb \times 1.38 \times 0.98) + (PA_{O_2} \times 0.003)$$

$$\text{where } PA_{O_2} = Fi_{O_2}(P_B - P_{H_2O}) - (Pa_{CO_2})(1.25)$$

A shunt of less than 10% is considered normal. A shunt of 10% to 20% implies a noncritical pulmonary abnormality. A shunt of 20% to 30% is considered very serious. A shunt of 30% or greater may be life-threatening. It should be clear that calculating and trending this parameter can assist the practitioner in

TABLE 26-4. Outcome in Survivors of ARDS

Outcome Variable	Number of Patients	Normal (%)	Comments
Clinical status	84	83.3	7.1% mild DOE, 2.4% moderate DOE
Chest roentgenogram	81	80.2	7.4% hyperinflation, 11.1% interstitial changes
Lung volumes	122	72.1	5.7% hyperinflation, 22.1% restrictive (no improvement after 1 year in the few patients studied serially)
Expiratory flow	122	83.6	5.7% had reversible obstruction; the others had irreversible obstruction
Airway resistance	26	88.5	
Resting Pa_{O_2}	91	73.6	
Exercise Pa_{O_2}	65	52.3	3.1% developed an increased Pa_{O_2} with exercise
QS/QT	38	89.5	
DLCO	74	5.14	Those with abnormal values tended to return toward normal over time

Adapted from Alberts, W., Michael, M. D., Priest, G. R., et al. (1983). The outlook for survivors of ARDS. *Chest*, 84, 272–274.
Abbreviations: DOE, dyspnea on exertion; QS/QT, shunt fraction; DLCO, diffusing capacity for carbon monoxide, either single breath or steady state.

evaluating the efficacy of various interventions in improving gas exchange and V/Q equality in ARDS patients (Reischman, 1988).

MONITOR OXYGEN DELIVERY

In patients with ARDS, a simple cardiac output determination to evaluate whether the value falls within normal limits is not sufficient. Remember that high cardiac output values do not necessarily benefit the patient if, to attain them, PEEP values must be kept very low or PAWP values representing left ventricular filling pressures must be very high. Low PEEP values can compromise gas exchange by allowing alveolar units to recollapse. High PAWP values can increase the pressure gradient for edema development. Either situation will lead to a compromise in arterial blood oxygen content, and good perfusion to the tissues is wasted if the blood is not well oxygenated. Therefore, the clinician does not need to determine the normality of cardiac output but rather its adequacy in ensuring adequate oxygen delivery to the tissues (Snyder, 1987).

To calculate oxygen delivery, also referred to as transport, arterial blood oxygen content and cardiac output need to be determined. Cardiac output is measured using a pulmonary artery catheter via the thermodilution technique. Arterial blood oxygen content is measured by collecting an arterial sample for blood gas and hemoglobin determination.

$$\text{Oxygen delivery} = Ca_{O_2} \times CO \times 10$$

Recall that Ca_{O_2} is calculated by the following equation:

$$(Hgb \times 1.38 \times Sa_{O_2}) + (Pa_{O_2} \times 0.003)$$

An oxygen delivery of 1000 mL/minute is considered normal. Although achieving normal may be an unrealistic goal, calculating this parameter following

different interventions will assist the practitioner in determining the adequacy of cardiac output as well as which combination of therapies best facilitates tissue oxygenation.

MEASURE STATIC PULMONARY COMPLIANCE

Compliance is an expression of the elastic properties of the lung. It is the change in volume accomplished by a change in pressure. As such, it reflects the distensibility of the lung. When compliance is low, the lung is stiff, work of breathing is increased, and ineffective breathing patterns ensue (McCauley and Von Rueden, 1988). The calculation for measuring static compliance (C_{ST}) for patients on ventilatory assistance is:

$$C_{ST} = \frac{\text{Tidal volume } (V_T)}{\text{Plateau pressure} - \text{PEEP}}$$

All of these values are readily available in the ventilatory-assisted patient. A static compliance of greater than 50 mL/cm H_2O is generally considered acceptable. However, calculating C_{ST} at different tidal volume and PEEP levels can assist the practitioner in determining at what level compliance is optimum, work of breathing is reduced, and breathing patterns are most effective (McCauley and Von Rueden, 1988).

PROGNOSIS

The prognosis of ARDS is determined by the underlying cause, the extent of injury, the patient's response to therapy, and the development of multisystem organ failure, a dreaded and deadly complication of ARDS (Putterman, 1988). Mortality rates are reported to range from 50% to 90% (Fowler et al., 1983; Montgomery et al., 1985; Pepe et al., 1982; Seidenfeld et al., 1986). However, it is difficult to interpret these mortality rates because no definition of ARDS is uniformly accepted and applied as well as because milder forms of this syndrome probably go unrecognized.

ARDS is often a complication that occurs late in the natural course of other diseases. Although prognostic indicators have not been extensively studied, mortality directly correlates with the number and severity of the underlying disease or diseases (Fowler et al., 1983; Pepe et al., 1982). In addition, severe pulmonary hypertension and multisystem organ failure as a consequence of sepsis are apparently more predominant in nonsurvivors (Bell et al., 1983). Deaths as a result of respiratory failure are less common (Dalnogare, 1989). Patients with self-limited causes of ARDS such as those with air emboli, isolated trauma, or massive blood transfusions as well as those with milder degrees of edema also have a greater chance of survival (Lamy et al., 1976).

The outlook for patients who survive diffuse lung injury, even if severe, is favorable. Most recover completely or possess a residual reduction in diffusing capacity. Histologic abnormalities may also gradually regress. Alberts and colleagues (1983) summarized the findings in 21 publications providing prognostic information. The authors included only those publications that they agreed described ARDS based on its association with widely accepted etiologic and clinical descriptors. Their data are summarized in Table 26–4. As is evident, the outlook for those who do survive the acute event appears optimistic. On the other hand, the mortality rates for patients with severe ARDS are unlikely to improve until more is known specifically about how the lungs are injured and repaired. Therapy directed at these mechanisms as opposed to supportive therapy still needs to be identified so that it may be administered prophylactically or very shortly following the lung insult.

nursing care plan

1. Impaired pulmonary gas exchange

Outcome Criteria	Nursing Interventions
Pulmonary artery wedge pressure (PAWP) will be maintained at the lowest level that will minimize the hydrostatic gradient for edema formation and yet not compromise left ventricular filling Fi_{O_2} will be maintained at the lowest level that will minimize toxic lung injury yet not compromise alveolar ventilation or arterial blood oxygen content	Maintain oxygen delivery with a minimum Fi_{O_2} that is still adequate to maintain arterial oxygen content Decrease the metabolic requirements for oxygen 　Take nursing measures to decrease anxiety, pain, and shivering related to fever Ensure optimum patient positioning 　Utilize oxygen delivery measurement techniques to determine best position for patient 　Take measurement 30 minutes after the position change to allow for stabilization Maintain continuous positive end-expiratory pressure (PEEP) 　Utilize postsuctioning hyperinflation 　Utilize a closed airway suctioning system 　Take PAWP measurements without interrupting PEEP (a mathematical adjustment may be needed if the patient is on high levels of PEEP) Identify hemoglobin related alterations in oxygen delivery 　Closely monitor the patient's hemoglobin level 　Monitor for conditions that would shift the oxyhemoglobin curve to the left (hypophosphatemia, alkalemia, decreased CO_2); correct if possible Assess intrapulmonary shunting by measuring QS/QT (refer to text for calculation) Monitor oxygen delivery by determining cardiac output and arterial blood oxygen content (refer to text for calculation) Measure static pulmonary compliance (refer to text for calculation) Maintain adequate nutritional intake in order to maintain a positive protein balance without providing excessive carbohydrates

References

Alberts, W. M., Priest, G. R., and Moser, K. M. (1983). The outlook for survivors of ARDS. *Chest*, 84, 272–274.

Arora, N. S., and Rochester, D. F. (1977). Effect of general nutritional and muscular states on the human diaphragm. *American Review of Respiratory Disease*, 115, 84–87.

Ashbaugh, D. G., Bigelow, D. B., Pelty, T. L., et al. (1967). Acute respiratory distress in adults. *Lancet*, 2, 319–323.

Ayars, G. H., Altman, L. C., Rosen, H., et al. (1984). The injurious effects of neutrophils on pneumocytes in vitro. *American Review of Respiratory Disease*, 130, 964–973, 1984.

Ayres, S. M. (1982). Mechanisms and consequences of pulmonary edema: Cardiac lung, shock lung, and principles of ventilatory therapy in adult respiratory distress syndrome. *American Heart Journal*, 103, 97–102.

Babior, B. M., Kipnes, R. S., and Curnutte, J. T. (1973). Biological defense mechanisms: The production by leukocytes of superoxide, a potential bactericidal agent. *Journal of Clinical Investigation*, 52, 741–744.

Bachofen, M., and Weibel, E. R. (1982). Structural alterations of lung parenchyma in the adult respiratory distress syndrome. *Clinical Chest Medicine*, 3, 35–56.

Balis, J. U., Shelley, S. A., McCue, M. J., et al. (1971). Mechanism of damage to the lung surfactant system: Ultrastructure and quantification of normal and in vitro inactivated lung surfactant. *Experimental Molecular Pathology*, 14, 243–262.

Balk, R., and Bone, R. C. (1983). The adult respiratory distress syndrome. *Medical Clinics of North America*, 67, 685–699.

Barrett, C. R., Bell, A. L. L., and Ryan, S. F. (1979). Alveolar epithelial injury causing respiratory distress in dogs: Physiologic and electron-microscopic correlations. *Chest*, 75, 705–711.

Begley, C. J., Ogletree, M. L., Meyrick, B. O., et al. (1984). Modification of pulmonary responses to endotoxemia in awake sheep by steroid and nonsteroidal anti-inflammatory agents. *American Review of Respiratory Disease*, 130, 1140–1146.

Bell, R. C., Coalson, J., Smith, J., et al. (1983). Multiple organ system failure and infection in adult respiratory distress syndrome. *Annals of Internal Medicine*, 99, 293–298.

Bernard, G. R., and Brigham, K. L. (1986). Pulmonary edema: Pathophysiologic mechanisms and new approaches to therapy. *Chest*, 89, 594–600.

Bernard, G. R., Luce, J., Sprung, C., et al. (1987). High-dose corticosteroids in patients with the adult respiratory distress syndrome. *New England Journal of Medicine*, 317, 1565–1570.

Bernard, G. R., Lucht, W. D., Niedermeyer, M. E., et al. (1984). Effect of N-acetylcysteine on the pulmonary response to endotoxin in the awake sheep and upon in vitro granulocyte function. *Journal of Clinical Investigation*, 73, 1772–1784.

Boggis, C. R. M., and Greene, R. (1983). ARDS. *British Journal of Hospital Medicine*, 29, 167–174.

Bone, R. C., Fisher, C., Clemmer, T., et al. (1987). The Methylprednisolone Severe Sepsis Study Group: Early methylprednisolone treatment for septic syndrome and the adult respiratory distress syndrome. *Chest*, 92, 1032–1036.

Bone, R. C., Francis, P. G., and Pierce, A. K. (1976). Intravascular coagulation associated with the adult respiratory distress syndrome. *American Journal of Medicine*, 61, 585–589.

Boxer, L. A., Axtell, R., and Suchard, S. (1990). The role of the neutrophil in inflammatory diseases of the lung. *Blood Cells*, 16, 25–42.

Brandstetter, R. D. (1986). The adult respiratory distress syndrome—1986. *Heart & Lung*, 15, 155–164.

Braquet, P., and Hosford, D. (1989). The potential role of platelet-activating factor (PAF) in shock, sepsis and adult respiratory distress syndrome (ARDS). *Progress in Clinical and Biological Research*, 308, 425–439.

Brigham, K. L. (1985). Metabolites of arachidonic acid in experimental lung vascular injury. *Federation Proceedings*, 44, 43–45.

Brigham, K. L., and Ogletree, M. L. (1981). Effects of prostaglandins and related compounds on lung vascular permeability. *Bulletin of European Physiology*, 17, 703–722.

Christner, P., Fein, A., Goldberg, S., et al. (1985). Collagenase in the lower respiratory tract of patients with adult respiratory distress syndrome. *American Review of Respiratory Disease*, 131, 690–695.

Connors, A. F., McCaffree, D. R., and Rogers, R. M. (1981). The adult respiratory distress syndrome. *Disease-a-Month*, 27, 1–75.

Cooper, J. A., Bizios, R., and Malik, A. B. (1985). Pulmonary neutrophil kinetics in sheep: Effects of altered hemodynamics. *Journal of Applied Physiology*, 59, 1796–1801.

Crandell, E. D. (Ed.) (1983). Fluid balance across the alveolar epithelium. *American Review of Respiratory Disease*, 127(5), S1–S65.

Dalnogare, A. R. (1989). Southwestern Internal Medicine Conference: Adult respiratory distress syndrome. *American Journal of Medical Science*, 298, 413–430.

Dantzker, D. R. (1990). The role of oxygen supply dependence in the adult respiratory distress syndrome. *Critical Care Report*, 1, 260–265.

Dantzker, D. R., Brook, C. J., Dehart, P., et al. (1979). Ventilation-perfusion distributions in the adult respiratory distress syndrome. *American Review of Respiratory Disease*, 120, 1039–1052.

Enger, E. L. (1989). Pulmonary artery wedge pressure: When it's valid, when it's not. *Critical Care Nursing Clinics of North America*, 1, 603–618.

Erdmann, A. F., Vaughan, T. R., Brigham, K. L., et al. (1975). Effect of increased vascular pressure on lung fluid balance in unanesthetized sheep. *Circulation Research*, 37, 271–284.

Estenne, M., and Yernault, J. C. (1984). The mechanism of CO_2 retention in cardiac pulmonary edema. *Chest*, 86, 936–938.

Fein, A., Grossman, R. F., Jones, J. G., et al. (1979). The value of edema fluid protein measurements in patients with pulmonary edema. *American Journal of Medicine*, 67, 32–38.

Fishman, A. P. (1980). Pulmonary edema. In A. P. Fishman (Ed.), *Pulmonary diseases and disorders* (p. 733). New York: McGraw-Hill.

Fowler, A. A., Hamman, R., Good, J., et al. (1983). Adult respiratory distress syndrome: Risk with common predispositions. *Annals of Internal Medicine*, 98, 593–597.

Fulton, R. L., and Jones, C. E. (1975). The cause of post-traumatic pulmonary insufficiency in man. *Surgery, Gynecology and Obstetrics*, 140, 179–184.

Gallagher, T. J., Civetta, J. M., and Kirby, R. R. (1978). Terminology update: Optimum PEEP. *Critical Care Medicine*, 6, 323–326.

Goldstein, I. M. (1988). Complement: Biologically active products. In J. I. Gallin, I. M. Goldstein, and R. Snyderman (Eds.), *Inflammation* (pp. 55–74). New York: Raven Press.

Gottlieb, J. (1988). Breathing and gas exchange. In M. Kinney, D. Packa, and S. Dunbar (Eds.), *AACN's clinical reference for critical care nursing* (2nd ed.). New York: McGraw-Hill.

Hallman, M., Spragg, R., and Harrell, J. H. (1982). Evidence of lung surfactant abnormality in respiratory failure: Study of bronchoalveolar lavage phospholipids, surface activity, phospholipase activity and plasma myoinositol. *Journal of Clinical Investigation*, 70, 673–683.

Hammerschmidt, D. E., Weaver, J., Hudson, L., et al. (1980). Association of complement activation and elevated plasma C_{5A} with adult respiratory distress syndrome. *Lancet*, 1, 947–949.

Haupt, M. T., and Rackow, E. R. (1982). Colloid osmotic pressure and fluid resuscitation with hetastarch, albumin and saline solution. *Critical Care Medicine*, 10, 159–165.

Hauser, C. J., Shoemaker, W. C., and Turpin, I. (1980). Oxygen transport responses to colloid and crystalloid in critically ill surgical patients. *Surgery, Gynecology and Obstetrics*, 150, 811–816.

Havill, A. M., and Gee, M. H. (1984). Role of interstitium in clearance of alveolar fluid in normal and injured lungs. *Journal of Applied Physiology*, 57, 1–6.

Hill, J. D., O'Brien, T. G., and Muray, J. T. (1972). Prolonged extracorporeal oxygenation for acute post traumatic respiratory failure (shock lung syndrome). *New England Journal of Medicine*, 286, 629–634.

Hurewitz, A., and Bergofsky, E. H. (1981). Adult respiratory distress syndrome. *Medical Clinics of North America*, 65, 33–51.

Issekutz, A. C., and Movat, H. Z. (1982). The effect of vasodilator prostaglandins on polymorphonuclear leukocyte infiltration and vascular injury. *American Journal of Pathology*, 107, 300–309.

Jenkinson, S. G. (1982). Pulmonary oxygen toxicity. *Clinical Chest Medicine*, 3, 109–120.

Karima, N. K., and Burns, S. (1985). Regulation of tissue oxygen extraction is disturbed in adult respiratory distress syndrome. *American Review of Respiratory Disease*, 132, 109–114.

Keogh, B. F., Hunter, D. N., Morgan, C. J., et al. (1989). The management of adult respiratory distress syndrome (Part I). *British Journal of Hospital Medicine*, 42, 468–474.

Keogh, B. F., Hunter, D. N., Morgan, C. J., et al. (1990). The management of adult respiratory distress syndrome (Part II). *British Journal of Hospital Medicine*, 43, 26–30.

Keren, A., Klein, J., and Stern, S. (1980). Adult respiratory distress syndrome in the course of acute myocardial infarction. *Chest*, 77, 161–166.

Klebanoff, S. J. (1980). Oxygen metabolism and the toxic properties of phagocytes. *Annals of Internal Medicine*, 93, 480–489.

Klebanoff, S. J., Vadas, M., Harlan, J., et al. (1986). Stimulation of neutrophils by tumor necrotic factor. *Journal of Immunology*, 136, 4220–4225.

Lamy, M., Fallat, R., Koeniger, E., et al. (1976). Pathologic features and mechanisms of hypoxemia in adult respiratory distress syndrome. *American Review of Respiratory Disease*, 114, 267–284.

Langer, M., Mascheroni, D., Marcolin, R., et al. (1988). The prone position in ARDS patients. *Chest*, 94, 103–107.

Lee, C. T., Fein, A. M., Lippmann, M., et al. (1981). Elastolytic activity in pulmonary lavage fluid from patients with adult respiratory distress syndrome. *New England Journal of Medicine*, 304, 192–196.

Lefer, A. M. (1987). Physiologic and pathophysiologic role of cyclo-oxygenase metabolites of arachidonic acid in circulatory disease states. *Cardiovascular Clinics*, 18, 85–99.

Lewis, K. A., and Austen, K. F. (1984). The biologically active leukotrienes: Biosynthesis, metabolism, receptors, functions, and pharmacology. *Journal of Clinical Investigation*, 73, 889–897.

Lozman, J., Powers, S. R., Older, T., et al. (1974). Correlation of the pulmonary wedge and left atrial pressures: A study in the patient receiving positive end-expiratory pressure ventilation. *Archives of Surgery*, 109, 270–277.

Majors, M. (1988). Nutritional support of the mechanically ventilated patient. *Critical Care Nursing Quarterly*, 11, 50–61.

Martin, W. J., Gadek, J. E., Hunninghake, G. W., et al. (1981). Oxidant injury of lung parenchymal cells. *Journal of Clinical Investigation*, 68, 1277–1288.

Massaro, D., Thet, L. A., Massaro, G. D., et al. (1980). A hypothesis relating breathing pattern to some forms of the "adult respiratory distress syndrome." *American Journal of Medicine*, 69, 113–115.

Matthay, M. A., Eschenbacher, W. L., and Goetzl, E. J. (1984). Elevated concentrations of leukotriene D_4 in pulmonary edema fluid of patients with the adult respiratory distress syndrome. *Journal of Clinical Immunology*, 4, 479–483.

Maunder, R. J. (1986). Clinical predictors of the ARDS. *Clinical Chest Medicine*, 6, 413–426.

McCauley, M., and Von Rueden, K. (1988). Noninvasive monitoring of the mechanically ventilated patient. *Critical Care Nursing Quarterly*, 11, 36–49.

Milligan, S. A., Hoeffel, J. M., and Flick, M. R. (1985). Endotoxin induced acute lung injury in unanesthetized sheep is prevented by catalase. *American Review of Respiratory Disease*, 131, A422.

Modig, J. (1986). ARDS: Pathogenesis and treatment. *Acta Chirurgica Scandinavica*, 152, 241–249.

Montgomery, A. B., Stager, M. A., Carrico, C. J., et al. (1985). Causes of mortality in patients with the adult respiratory distress syndrome. *American Review of Respiratory Disease*, 132, 485–489.

Morganroth, M. L., Reeves, J. T., Murphy, K. C., et al. (1984). Leukotriene synthesis and receptor blockers block hypoxic pulmonary vasoconstriction. *Journal of Applied Physiology*, 56, 1340–1346.

Moriguchi, S., Sone, S., and Kishino, Y. (1983). Changes of alveolar macrophages in protein-deficient rats. *Journal of Nutrition*, 113, 40–46.

Mortenson, J. D. (1987). An intravenacaval blood gas exchange device: A preliminary report. *Transactions of the American Society of Artificial Internal Organs*, 33, 570–572.

Moss, G. S., Lowe, R. J., and Jilek, J. (1981). Colloid or crystalloid in the resuscitation of hemorrhagic shock: A controlled clinical trial. *Surgery*, 89, 434–440.

Murray, G. F. (1979). Mechanisms of acute respiratory failure. *American Review of Respiratory Disease*, 115, 1071–1078.

Nitta, S., Ohnuki, T., Ohkuda, K., et al. (1981). The corrected protein equation to estimate plasma colloid osmotic pressure and its development on a nomogram. *Tohoku Journal of Experimental Medicine*, 135, 43–49.

Ogletree, M. L. (1982). Pharmacology of prostaglandins in the pulmonary microcirculation. *Annals New York Academy Science*, 384, 191–205.

O'Quin, R., and Marini, J. J. (1983). Pulmonary artery occlusion pressure: Clinical physiology, measurement and interpretation. *American Review of Respiratory Disease*, 128, 319–326.

Parker, J. C., Martin, D. J., Rutili, G., et al. (1983). Prevention of free radical mediated vascular permeability increase in lung using superoxide dismutase. *Chest*, 83, S52–S53.

Parson, P. E., Fowler, A., Hyers, T., et al. (1985). Chemotatic activity in bronchoalveolar lavage fluid from patients with adult respiratory distress syndrome. *American Review of Respiratory Disease*, 132, 490–493.

Pepe, P. E., Hudson, L. D., and Carrico, C. J. (1984). Early application of PEEP in patients at risk for the adult respiratory distress syndrome. *New England Journal of Medicine*, 311, 281–288.

Pepe, P. E., Potkin, R., Holtman-Reus, D., et al. (1982). Clinical predictors of the adult respiratory distress syndrome. *American Journal of Surgery*, 144, 124–128.

Perlman, M. B., Lo, S. K., and Malik, A. B. (1986). Effect of prostacyclin on pulmonary vascular response to thrombin in awake sheep. *Journal of Applied Physiology*, 60, 546–553.

Permutt, S. (1979). Mechanical influences on water accumulation in the lungs. In A. P. Fishman and E. M. Renkin (Eds.), *Pulmonary edema* (p. 175). Bethesda, MD: American Physiological Society.

Pesenti, A., Gattinoni, L., and Kolobow, T. (1988). Extracorporeal circulation in adult respiratory failure. *Transactions of the American Society of Artificial Internal Organs*, 34, 43–47.

Pingleton, S. K. (1982). Complications associated with the adult respiratory distress syndrome. *Clinical Chest Medicine*, 5, 143–151.

Pohlman, T. H., Stanness, K., Beatty, P., et al. (1986). An endothelial cell surface factor induced in vitro by lipopolysaccharide, interleukin 1 and tumor necrosis factor-alpha increases neutrophil adherence by a CDW18-dependent mechanism. *Journal of Immunology*, 136, 4548–4553.

Powe, J. E., Short, A., and Sibbald, W. J. (1982). Pulmonary accumulation of polymorphonuclear leukocytes in the adult respiratory distress syndrome. *Critical Care Medicine*, 10, 712–718.

Putterman, C. (1988). Acute respiratory distress syndrome: Current concepts. *Resuscitation*, 16, 91–105.

Raffin, T. ARDS: Mechanisms and management. *Hospital Practice*, 22, 65–76; 78–80.

Rajacich, N., Burchard, K. W., and Hasan, F. M. (1989). Central venous pressure and pulmonary capillary wedge pressure as estimates of left atrial pressure: Effects of PEEP and catheter tip malposition. *Critical Care Medicine*, 17, 7–11.

Reischman, R. R. (1988). Impaired gas exchange related to intrapulmonary shunting. *Critical Care Nurse*, 8, 35–49.

Rinaldo, J. E., and Rogers, R. M. (1986). Acute respiratory distress syndrome. *New England Journal of Medicine*, 315, 578–580.

Roberts, S. L. (1990). High-permeability pulmonary edema: Nursing assessment, diagnosis and intervention. *Heart & Lung*, 19, 287–300.

Rochester, D. F., and Esau, S. A. (1984). Malnutrition and the respiratory system. *Chest*, 85, 411–416.

Saba, T. M., and Jaffe, E. (1980). Plasma fibrinectin: Its synthesis by vascular endothelial cells and role in cardiopulmonary integrity after trauma as related to reticuloendothelial function. *American Journal of Medicine*, 68, 577–594.

Sahebjami, H., Vassallo, C. L., and Wirman, J. A. (1978). Lung mechanics and ultrastructure in prolonged starvation. *American Review of Respiratory Disease*, 117, 77–82.

Said, S. I., and Foda, H. D. (1979). Pharmacologic modulation of lung injury. *American Review of Respiratory Disease*, 139, 1553–1564.

Schneider, R. C., Zapol, W. N., and Corvalb, A. H. (1980). Platelet consumption and sequestration in severe acute respiratory failure. *American Review of Respiratory Disease*, 122, 455–461.

Schumann, L., and Parsons, G. (1985). Tracheal suctioning and ventilator tubing changes in adult respiratory distress syndrome: Use of a positive-end expiratory pressure value. *Heart & Lung*, 14, 362–367.

Seidenfeld, J. J., Pohl, D. F., Bell, R. C., et al. (1986). Incidence, site and outcome of infections in patients with the adult respiratory distress syndrome. *American Review of Respiratory Disease*, 134, 12–16.

Shapiro, B. A., Cane, R. D., and Harrison, R. A. (1984). Positive end-expiratory pressure in adults with special reference to acute lung injury: A review of the literature and suggested clinical correlations. *Critical Care Medicine*, 12, 124–141.

Shigematsu, N., Matsuba, K., and Shirakusa, T. (1980). The preventative effect of urokinase on experimental bleomycin-induced interstitial pneumonia. *American Review of Respiratory Disease*, 121, 188.

Shoemaker, W. C., and Appel, P. L. (1986). Effect of prostaglandin E_1 in ARDS. *Surgery*, 99, 275–282.

Shoemaker, W. C., and Hauser, C. J. (1979). Critique of crystalloids versus colloid therapy in shock and shock lung. *Critical Care Medicine*, 7, 117–124.

Shoemaker, W. C., Schluchter, M., and Hopkins, J. A. (1981). Comparison of the relative effectiveness of colloids and crystalloids in emergency resuscitation. *American Journal of Surgery*, 142, 73–75.

Sibbald, W. J., Anderson, R. R., and Reid, B. (1981). Alveolocapillary permeability in human septic ARDS: Effect of high-dose corticosteroid therapy. *Chest*, 79, 133–138.

Sibbald, W. J., Cunningham, D. R., and Chin, D. N. (1983). Noncardiac or cardiac pulmonary edema? A practical approach to clinical differentiation in critically ill patients. *Chest*, 84, 453–462.

Simionescu, M., and Simionescu, N. (1984). Ultrastructure of the microvascular wall: Functional correlations. In E. M. Renkin, and C. C. Michel (Eds.), *Handbook of physiology* (Section 2), *the cardiovascular system* (Part 2), *microcirculation* (pp. 41–101). Bethesda, MD: American Physiological Society.

Snider, M. T. (1990). Adult respiratory distress syndrome in the trauma patient. *Critical Care Clinics*, 6, 103–110.

Snyder, J. V. (1987). Patterns of hemodynamic response. In J. V. Snyder, and M. R. Pinsky (Eds.), *Oxygen transport in the critically ill* (pp. 46–66). Chicago: Year Book.

Spagnuolo, P. J., Ellner, J. J., Hassid, A., et al. (1980). Thromboxane A$_2$ mediated augmented polymorphonuclear adhesiveness. *Journal of Clinical Investigation*, 66, 406–414.

Staub, N. C. (1974). Pulmonary edema. *Physiological Reviews*, 54, 678–811.

Staub, N. C. (1978). Lung fluid and solute exchange. In N. C. Staub (Ed.), *Lung water and solute exchange* (pp. 3–16). New York: Marcel Dekker.

Staub, N. C. (1980). The pathogenesis of pulmonary edema. *Progress in Cardiovascular Disease*, 23, 53–80.

Staub, N. C. (1981). Clinical measurement of lung water content. *Chest*, 79, 3–18.

Staub, N. C. (1983). Alveolar flooding and clearance. *American Review of Respiratory Disease*, 127(5), S44–S51.

Staub, N. C. (1985). Only the shadow knows. *American Journal of Roentgenology*, 144, 1086–1087.

Staub, N. C., Nagano, H., and Pearce, M. L. (1967). Pulmonary edema in dogs, especially the sequence of fluid accumulation in lungs. *Journal of Applied Physiology*, 22, 227–240.

Stephens, K. E., Ishizaka, A., Larrick, J., et al. (1987). Tumor necrosis factor causes increased pulmonary permeability and edema. *American Review of Respiratory Disease*, 137, 1364–1370.

Stevens, J. V., and Raffin, T. A. (1984). ARDS: Etiology and mechanisms. *Postgraduate Medical Journal*, 60, 505–513.

Strieter, R. M., Kunkel, S., Showell, H., et al. (1989). Endothelial cell gene expression of a neutrophil chemotactic factor by TNF-alpha, LPS and IL-1 beta. *Science*, 243, 1467–1469.

Suter, P. M., Failey, H. B., and Isenberg, M. D. (1975). Optimum end-expiratory pressure in patients with acute pulmonary failure. *New England Journal of Medicine*, 292, 284–289.

Taylor, A. E. (1981). Capillary fluid filtration: Starling forces and lymph flow. *Circulation Research*, 49, 557–575.

Taylor, A. E., and Parker, J. C. (1985). Pulmonary interstitial spaces and lymphatics. In A. P. Fishman, and A. B. Fisher (Eds.), *Handbook of physiology* (Section 3), *The respiratory system* (Vol. 1), *Circulation and nonrespiratory function* (pp. 167–230). Bethesda, MD: American Physiological Society.

Taylor, R. W., and Duncan, C. A. (1983). The adult respiratory distress syndrome. *Res Medica*, 1, 17–40.

Thommasen, H. V., Russell, J. A., and Boyko, W. J. (1984). Transient leukopenia associated with adult respiratory distress syndrome. *Lancet*, 1, 809–812.

Tierney, D. F., and Johnson, R. P. (1965). Altered surface tension of lung extracts and mechanics. *Journal of Applied Physiology*, 20, 1253–1260.

Toben, B., and Lewandowski, V. (1988). Nontraditional and new ventilatory techniques. *Critical Care Nursing Quarterly*, 11, 12–28.

Varani, J., Fligiel, S. E. G., Till, G. O., et al. (1985). Pulmonary endothelial cell killing by human neutrophils: Possible involvement of hydroxyl radical. *Laboratory Investigation*, 53, 656–663.

Vered, M., Dearing, R., and Janoff, A. (1985). A new elastase inhibitor from Streptococcus pneumoniae protects against acute lung injury induced by neutrophil granules. *American Review of Respiratory Disease*, 131, 131–133.

Wang, C. G., Hakim, T. S., Michel, R. P., et al. (1985). Segmental pulmonary vascular resistance in progressive hydrostatic and permeability edema. *Journal of Applied Physiology*, 59, 242–247.

Weiland, J. E., Davis, W., Holter, J., et al. (1986). Lung neutrophils in the adult respiratory distress syndrome. *American Review of Respiratory Disease*, 133, 218–225.

Weisman, I. M., Rinaldo, J. E., and Rogers, R. M. (1982). Positive end-expiratory pressure in adult respiratory failure. *New England Journal of Medicine*, 307, 1381–1384.

Weissmann, C., Askanazi, J., and Rosenbaum, S. (1983). Amino acids and respiration. *Annals of Internal Medicine*, 48, 41–46.

Wood, L. D. H., and Prewitt, R. M. (1981). Cardiovascular management in acute hypoxemic respiratory failure. *American Journal of Cardiology*, 47, 963–972.

Zapol, W. M., Snider, M. T., Hill, J. D., et al. (1979). Extracorporeal membrane oxygenation in severe acute respiratory failure: A randomized prospective trial. *Journal of the American Medical Association*, 242, 2193–2196.

Zimmerman, G., Renzetti, A., and Hill, A. (1983). Functional and metabolic activity of granulocytes from patients with ARDS: Evidence of activated neutrophils in the pulmonary circulation. *American Review of Respiratory Disease*, 127, 290–300.

27

Patients with Chronic Obstructive Pulmonary Disease

Diane Cooper

Chronic obstructive pulmonary disease (COPD) is a clinical term that generally refers to a group of chronic diseases that are associated with obstruction to air flow within the airways or the lung parenchyma. Although several terms are often used synonymously with the term COPD (chronic airflow obstruction [CAO], chronic obstructive lung disease [COLD], chronic airflow limitation [CAL]), COPD remains the most commonly used term. The diseases considered to belong under the umbrella of COPD are (1) chronic bronchitis, (2) emphysema, and (3) asthma. Cystic fibrosis and bronchiectasis are categorized as obstructive diseases also but are seen more frequently in the younger age group and will not be discussed in this chapter. Because asthma is felt to be a more reversible obstructive disease, it is now often addressed separately from chronic bronchitis and emphysema. The term ROAD (reversible obstructive airway disease) is sometimes used to describe the picture of asthma.

Whatever terms are used, the usual clinical findings for chronic obstructive diseases are:

1. Significant and progressive reduction in expiratory air flow as measured by the forced expiratory volume in 1 second (FEV_1) (Fig. 27–1)
2. Varying degrees of exertional dyspnea
3. Chronic cough and sputum production

"The bottom line becomes the degree of air flow obstruction (or limitation) as measured by FEV_1, the age of the patient when the abnormality is found, the degree of reversibility, and the rate of change of the FEV_1 over time" (Hodgkin and Petty, 1987).

Epidemiology

It is estimated that between 10% and 25% of adult Americans have some degree of chronic bronchitis, and deaths attributed to COPD run as high as 50,000/year in the United States alone (Weinberger, 1986).

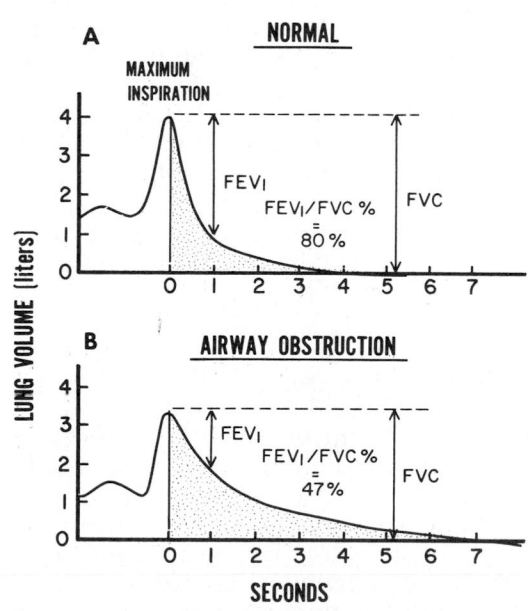

FIGURE 27–1. Recordings during a forced vital capacity maneuver. *A*, In the normal person. *B*, In the person with airway obstruction. (From Guyton, A. C. (1986). *Textbook of medical physiology* (7th ed., p. 477). Philadelphia: W. B. Saunders.) *Abbreviations:* FEV_1, forced expiratory volume in 1 second; FVC, forced vital capacity.

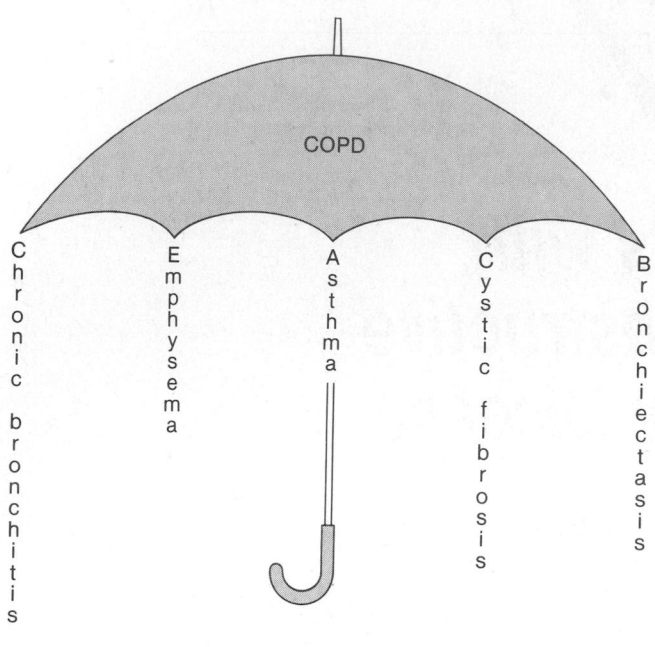

COPD is the fifth to sixth leading cause of death in the United States (Hodgkin and Petty, 1987; MacDonnell et al., 1987). The U.S. Social Security Administration reported that disability due to COPD is second only to heart disease in people over the age of 40 (MacDonnell et al., 1987).

The National Center for Health Statistics reported data from their National Health Interview Survey showing that at least 7.5 million Americans are diagnosed with chronic bronchitis, more than 2 million with emphysema, and approximately 6.5 million with some form of asthma (Hodgkin and Petty, 1987). The Tecumseh Community Health Survey of over 9000 men and women of all ages found that about 14% of adult males and 8% of adult females suffer from chronic bronchitis, obstructive airways disease, or both. In the same report, days of disability, as defined by activity restriction, averaged 12 days/year for those patients with chronic bronchitis, 68 days/ year for those with emphysema, and approximately 17 days/year for patients suffering from asthma (Hodgkin and Petty, 1987).

Distribution

A U.S. Department of Health Task Force Report (NIH Publication No. 81-2019) reported that the incidence, prevalence, and mortality rates for COPD, chronic bronchitis, and emphysema increase with age, are higher in males than females, and are higher in whites than in nonwhites. Morbidity and mortality are related to socioeconomic status—blue-color workers and those with fewer years of formal education having higher rates. COPD is also seen more frequently in offspring of affected parents as well as in affected siblings. Several studies indicate correlations between COPD and genetics and between COPD and the environment.

Although statistics of the numbers of people diagnosed, treated, or dying from COPD vary, it is agreed that health care costs from this group of diseases are rising and that the challenges to the health care team to deliver high-quality care in the most cost-efficient manner are also increasing. It is estimated that as many as 35% of intensive care unit admissions comprise patients with COPD in respiratory failure (MacDonnell et al., 1987). Critical care nurses have a major role in the coordination and delivery of care for these patients.

Etiology

On a scientific level, the etiology of COPD is unknown, but on a practical basis, several factors have been implicated in the pathogenesis of COPD, depending on the specific disease discussed. Tobacco, air pollution, occupational exposure, infection, and genetics all may play important roles in the development of diseases characterized by air flow obstruction. Clearly, the most important factor is the link between disease and the chronic inhalation of tobacco smoke.

It has been clearly established from data collected in longitudinal, cross-sectional, and case control studies that smokers have a higher death rate than nonsmokers. Pipe and cigar smokers have higher morbidity and mortality rates than nonsmokers but lower rates than cigarette smokers. It appears clear that cessation of smoking is beneficial, resulting in a decrease in symptoms, respiratory illnesses, and disease compared with smokers who continue to smoke. If permanent lung damage has occurred, lost function does not seem to return after smoking cessation. However, the age at which the patient stopped smoking, the amount of cigarette smoking that had already occurred, and the stage of the disease at time of smoking cessation do influence outcome.

It is important to realize that while cigarette smoking as a cause of COPD is established, not all smokers suffer the same effects in regard to frequency or severity of illness. The change in cigarette composition during recent years also plays a part in implicating smoking as a health hazard. Filtered cigarettes, cigarettes with lower tar and nicotine contents, and use of synthetic products all play a part in how cigarettes affect the pattern of COPD. There is an increasing amount of literature reporting the effects of involuntary exposure to smoking. Rates of respiratory symptoms and diseases are higher in nonsmoking wives of smoking husbands and in nonsmoking children of smoking parents. (Lefioe et al., 1984).

Certain occupations place a person at higher risk for developing COPD and, combined with cigarette smoking, increase the morbidity-mortality rates. Data from the United States, England, and Wales all list higher rates of COPD among coal miners, metal molders, workers manufacturing stone, glass, and clay products, those who work with cotton or grain dust, firefighters, and workers exposed to asbestos. Statistics indicate that exposure to asbestos, cotton dust, and crystalline silica is more harmful to smokers than nonsmokers (Higgens, 1984).

Episodes of severe air pollution have been associated with a sudden increase in morbidity and mortality, especially in persons with heart or lung disease. Although extremely high levels of pollution are rare, the effects on health of long-term exposure to low levels of pollution are being studied. Research is presently being done looking at such things as indoor pollutants versus outdoor pollutants (levels may be higher indoors and we tend to spend more time indoors) and changes in building and construction, in which the desire to conserve energy often reduces ventilation, which may affect indoor pollution. More research is also needed on the link between air pollution and cigarette smoking or occupation, active versus passive smoking, automobile emissions, and so on.

The role of infection in COPD as an etiologic factor is unproved, but some studies indicate that viral upper respiratory infections in children may predispose them to the development of COPD in adulthood. It is not clear whether viral infections change the progression of the disease. There is even less evidence that bacterial infections contribute to the progression of COPD.

Genetic factors indicating a link to the development of COPD are important considerations. Factors such as the alpha-1 protease inhibitor link seen in some emphysema patients (to be discussed in a later section), allergic conditions that are apparently passed on to offspring, as well as personal behaviors such as cigarette smoking should be considered when identifying risk factors for COPD. Whether or not these factors are inherited or acquired, more research based on methods that can be used in population-based epidemiologic studies needs to be carried out.

Other factors associated with COPD but generally not considered as important as those discussed include nutrition, leanness, alcohol consumption, and climate.

Although the term COPD refers to conditions in which a reduction in expiratory flow exists, the pathophysiologic basis for the reduced flow is different in the different diseases. The difference often provides the basis for the clinical diagnosis. The discussion that follows covers the specific diseases of chronic bronchitis and emphysema. Asthma, because of its potential reversibility, will be discussed separately. It should be remembered that although these diseases are treated separately here, it is not uncommon for patients to exhibit symptoms relating to all of them.

CHRONIC BRONCHITIS

The commonly accepted definition for chronic bronchitis relates to the symptomatology of chronic cough and sputum production. For epidemiologic purposes, chronic bronchitis is defined as a condition causing a chronic productive cough that is present for most days during at least three consecutive months for not less than two successive years. Other specific causes of the cough (i.e., tuberculosis or tumor) must be ruled out before a diagnosis of chronic bronchitis is made.

Etiology

Middle-aged males are most often afflicted, and cigarette smoking is the most important etiologic factor. The correlation between the amount of cigarette smoked and the duration of smoking with the severity of bronchitis has been established. The prevalence of chronic bronchitis increases as the lifetime cigarette consumption increases beyond approximately 8 pack years of exposure (calculated by the number of packs/day times the number of years smoked) (Tisi, 1983).

The etiologic role of other factors previously mentioned earlier in this chapter appears relatively unimportant in chronic bronchitis. Although not proved as an etiologic factor, the role of infection is significant in the exacerbation of symptoms and progression of the disease.

Pathophysiology

There is an increased production of mucus due to the enlargement of the bronchial mucous glands and an increase in the number of goblet cells. Other changes include inflammation of the bronchial and bronchiolar walls, loss of cilia, and the presence of mucous plugs. In later stages, changes associated with emphysema can be seen.

Physiologic changes are related to the narrowed airways. Chronic bronchitis is a disease of the central airways, and approximately 80% of the measurable airway resistance lies in these central airways. Normally, the airways narrow uniformly as they extend to the lung periphery, and their walls are smooth. Bronchography shows that in chronic bronchitis the degree of tapering is nonuniform, and airway wall surfaces and outpouchings are irregular. It is believed that these changes account for the increased airway resistance seen in bronchitis. Functionally, this resistance results in inspiratory and expiratory air flow obstruction, overinflation of the alveoli, and abnormal distribution of ventilation. In bronchitis, expiratory air flow is decreased because of the increased airway resistance. The narrowed airway leads to overinflation of the alveoli with increases in total lung capacity (TLC) and residual volume (RV) and a decrease in vital capacity (VC) (Fig. 27–2).

Clinical Manifestations

The signs and symptoms of chronic bronchitis vary greatly. For many, the cough and sputum production have been with them so long that they deny any symptoms. Often, too, the symptoms depend on the stage of the disease in which the patient presents.

The patient who has had only cough and sputum production for many years is considered to have simple (or uncomplicated) chronic bronchitis. Those who have no decrease in air flow or other serious complications other than the cough and mucus production have a good prognosis. In contrast, those with air flow reduction do have increased morbidity and mortality. It appears clear that the prognosis is related less to the symptoms than to the degree of air flow obstruction as measured by the forced expiratory volume in 1 second (FEV_1) and to the age at which these abnormal flow rates were first identified. The rate of change in flow rates also predicts prognosis, those patients who lose function rapidly dying sooner than those with a slower rate of decline. Most patients become symptomatic in their 40s and 50s

and become disabled from the disease in their late 50s and early 60s.

Some patients have a history of frequent chest colds and increased purulent sputum production with complaints of dyspnea, an indication of airway obstruction. The symptoms are usually insidious, with infections causing bouts of exacerbations. Although patients often adjust their life style to avoid dyspnea, the disease progresses so that it takes less and less exertion or activity to cause the dyspnea. In the later stages, patients may be dyspneic at rest with severe airway disease and may have severe derangements in ventilation-perfusion ratios and arterial blood gases, pulmonary hypertension, and cor pulmonale. The World Health Organization reports that the mortality rate from bronchitis in the United States per 100,000 deaths is 3.4 for men and 1.4 for women (Tisi, 1983).

In 1955 Dornhorst coined the phrase "blue bloater" to characterize chronic bronchitis patients and "pink puffer" to characterize those with emphysema (Table 27–1). Burrows and associates (1964) used the type B designation for bronchitics and type A for patients with emphysema. Robin and O'Neill (1963) called the emphysema patient the "fighter" and the bronchitic patient the "quitter." This distinction emphasizes that the bronchitic patient generally maintains low minute volumes and develops arterial hypoxemia and hypercapnia, whereas the emphysema patient "fights" by maintaining a larger minute ventilation and normal arterial blood gases.

The blue bloater may present as a stocky or obese male with both central and peripheral cyanosis. There is less barreling of the chest wall than is seen in persons with emphysema. There may be evidence of wheezing. Crackles (rales) may be present due to airway secretions and usually clear with coughing. This patient usually gives a history of smoking for years and experiencing chronic smoker's hack for as long as he can remember and multiple episodes of "bronchitis" over the years. A good history will uncover a pattern of decreasing activity over a period of many years.

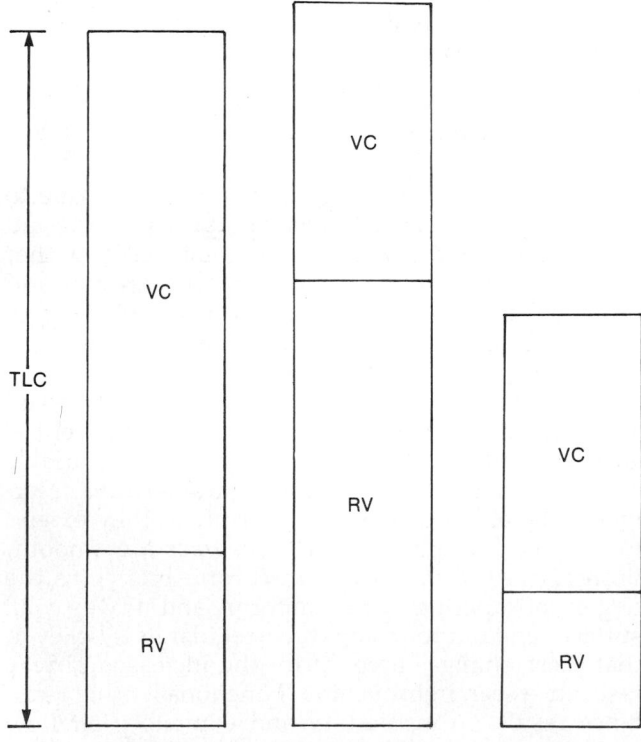

FIGURE 27–2. Diagram of lung volumes (TLC and subcompartments VC and RV) in normal individuals and in patients with obstructive and restrictive disease. See text for definitions. (From Weinberger, S. (1992). *Principles of pulmonary medicine* (2nd ed., p. 55). Philadelphia: W. B. Saunders.)

TABLE 27–1. Clinical Distinctions Between Type A and Type B Pathophysiology

Feature	Type A	Type B
Commonly used name	Pink puffer	Blue bloater
Disease association	Predominant emphysema	Predominant bronchitis
Major symptom	Dyspnea	Cough and sputum
Appearance	Thin, wasted, not cyanotic	Obese, cyanotic
P_{O_2}	↓	↓↓
P_{CO_2}	Normal or ↓	Normal or ↑
Elastic recoil of lung	↓	Normal
Diffusing capacity	↓	Normal
Hematocrit	Normal	Often ↑
Cor pulmonale	Infrequent	Common

From Weinberger, S. (1992). *Principles of pulmonary medicine* (2nd ed.). Philadelphia: W. B. Saunders.

Routine Laboratory Data

Usually the urinalysis and chemistry panels are normal. Patient with cor pulmonale may have polycythemia.

Radiographic Studies. Radiographs usually are normal in uncomplicated chronic bronchitis. If seen, abnormalities usually are due to concomitant changes resulting from emphysema (Fig. 27–3).

Pulmonary Function Tests. In the early stages and in uncomplicated chronic bronchitis, pulmonary function tests (PFTs) with spirometry are usually normal. Pulmonary function tests may also show an increased residual volume and mild reductions in vital capacity consistent with the degree of hyperinflation. Flow rates are reduced with indications of moderate increases in airway resistance. Some improvement occurs with bronchodilators, but values are still abnormal.

Electrocardiographic Findings. Although the electrocardiogram (ECG) is normal in uncomplicated chronic bronchitis, some typical changes are seen in the more severe stages of the disease. Once pulmonary hypertension, hypoxemia, and air flow obstruction are present, the ECG often shows:

1. P waves smaller in lead I but larger in leads II, III, and Avf
2. Shift of the P wave axis to the right
3. Reduced voltage due to the hyperinflation
4. Signs of right ventricular hypertrophy
5. Atrial or ventricular dysrhythmias, often managed by treating the underlying respiratory failure, acid-base imbalance, hypoxemia, or potassium abnormalities (Fig. 27–4)

Course and Prognosis

Most patients with chronic bronchitis experience chronic cough and sputum production for years but have little disability and a normal life span. Those who do develop increased airway obstruction and loss of pulmonary function and who have frequent infections will reach the stage of respiratory insufficiency and failure. The prognosis in these cases is much less favorable. Cessation of smoking and proper medical and nursing management are essential for possible prolongation of life and definitely for enhancing the quality of life.

EMPHYSEMA

In Greek, the word emphysema means "blown up," and in anatomic terms these patients have

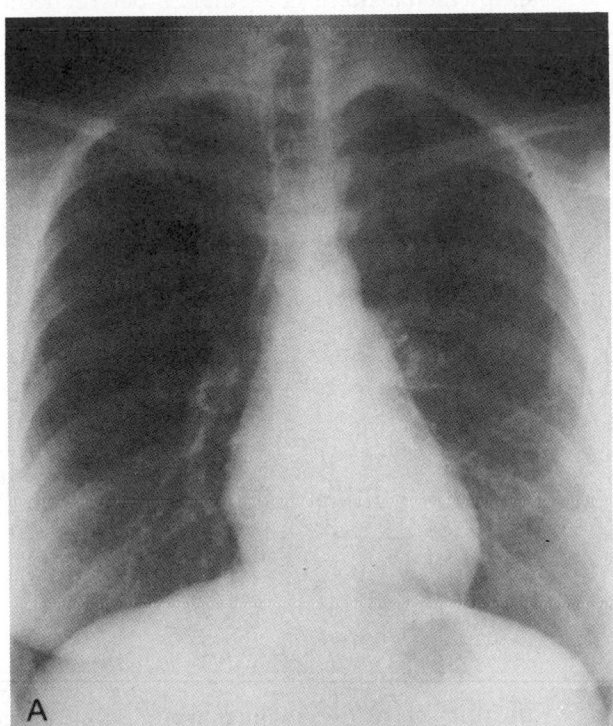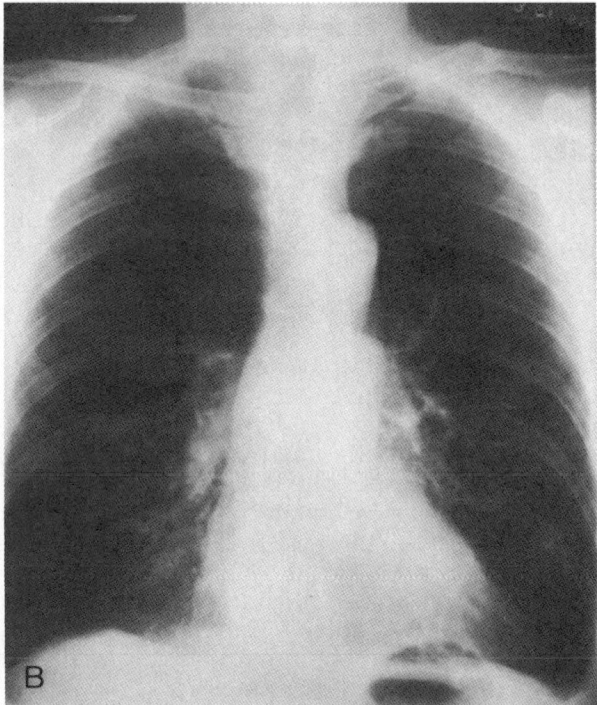

FIGURE 27–3. *A,* Normal chest roentgenogram. Posteroanterior view. *B,* Chest radiograph of a patient with severe chronic obstructive lung disease, showing the arterial deficiency pattern of emphysema. The lungs are hyperinflated, the diaphragms are low and flat and there is a paucity of vascular markings. (From Weinberger, S. (1992). *Principles of pulmonary medicine* (2nd ed., pp. 35, 102). Philadelphia: W. B. Saunders.)

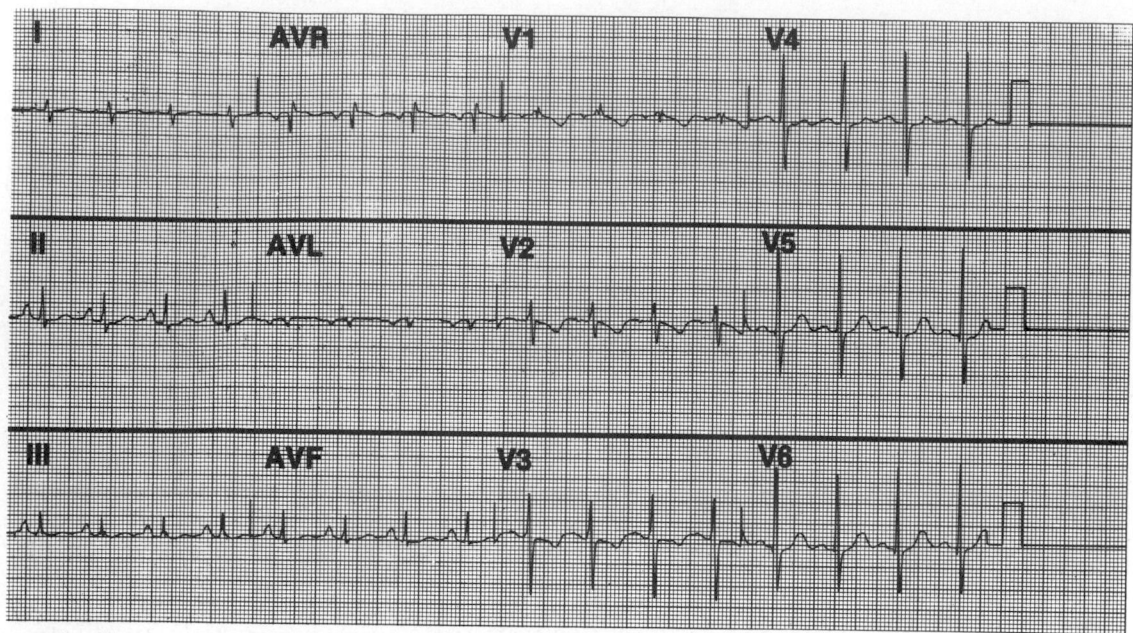

FIGURE 27-4. Pulmonary disease. A right axis together with prominent S waves in leads V_4 to V_6 and repolarization changes in leads V_1 to V_3 suggests right ventricular hypertrophy. An incomplete right bundle branch block is also present. The P waves are peaked in leads II, III, and aVF, indicative of right atrial enlargement. This group of findings is suggestive that this patient has pulmonary disease. (From Johnson, R., and Swartz, M. (1986). *A simplified approach to electrocardiography* (p. 106). Philadelphia: W. B. Saunders.)

abnormal permanent enlargement of the air spaces distal to the terminal bronchioles. This abnormality is accompanied by destruction of the alveolar walls and occurs without obvious fibrosis. Destruction is defined as "nonuniformity in the pattern of respiratory airspace enlargement so that the orderly appearance of the acinus and its components is disturbed and may be lost" (Snider, et al., 1985).

Etiology

Two primary etiologic factors are linked specifically with emphysema—cigarette smoking and genetic predisposition. This genetic factor is a deficiency in a serum protein, alpha-1 protease inhibitor (formerly called alpha-1 antitrypsin). This is a glycoprotein made in the liver that normally circulates in the blood. Patients with a decreased serum level of this protein are strongly predisposed to premature development of emphysema, as early as the third to fourth decade, especially if they also smoke.

Experimental production of emphysema in animal models indicates that enzymes that are capable of breaking down elastin (a complex structural protein found in alveolar walls) lead to the development of emphysema. The greater the elastolytic activity of the enzyme, the more pronounced the changes in the lung become.

Two types of cells seen in inflammatory responses in the lung are alveolar macrophages and polymorphonuclear leukocytes (PMNs). These two cells manufacture elastase, the enzyme capable of breaking down elastin. PMNs are believed to be the major source of elastase in the lung. In most people, there is an inhibitor of elastase in the lung—alpha-1 protease inhibitor. It is believed that in patients without emphysema there is a balance between the elastase and its inhibitor. When this balance is disturbed, either by an increase in elastase or a decrease in its inhibitor, damage to elastin and to the walls of the alveoli occurs (Fig. 27-5). The end result of this imbalance is the development of emphysema. This theory is thought to explain the small percentage of patients who develop the disease at an earlier age and, after testing, are found to have a deficiency in the inhibitor.

There are also reasons to believe that the balance between elastase and anti-elastase is disturbed by cigarette smoking. One reason is that smokers have an increased number of alveolar macrophages and PMNs, a source of elastase. Additionally, studies indicate that cigarette smoke oxidizes a critical amino acid residue of alpha-1 protease inhibitor, which then interferes with the activity of this protein (Weinberger, 1986).

Pathology

As just discussed, emphysema is characterized by destruction of the alveolar walls and enlargement of the air spaces distal to the terminal bronchioles. The terminal bronchioles are purely air-conducting structures, but distal to these are the increasingly more numerous alveoli. The portion of lung distal to the

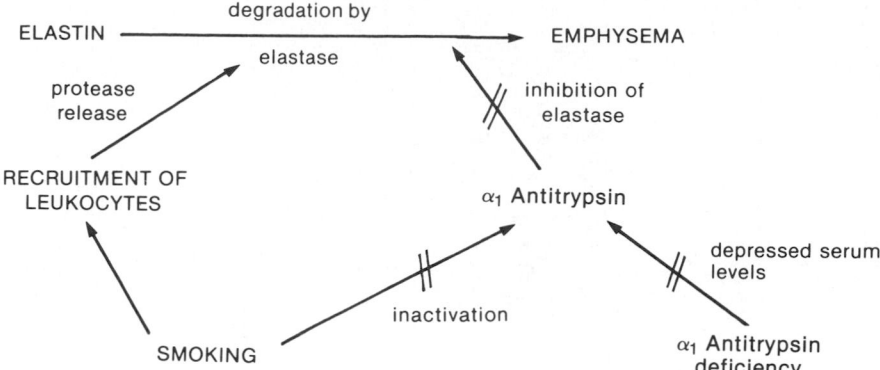

FIGURE 27–5. Schematic diagram of the hypothesized relationship between elastase and alpha 1 antitrypsin (α 1 PI), indicating how smoking and α 1 antitrypsin alter the balance, leading to degradation of elastin. (From Weinberger, S. (1992). *Principles of pulmonary medicine* (2nd ed.). Philadelphia: W. B. Saunders.)

terminal bronchioles is called the acinus. These are the functional units of the lung. There are about 25,000 of these acini in the lung, comprising approximately 300 million total alveoli.

The loss of airway support contributes to airway narrowing due to collapse of airways on expiration. This loss of alveolar wall and reduced elastic recoil also contribute to increased lung compliance, decreased driving pressure on expiration and subsequent hyperinflation, and increased residual volumes and total lung capacity. Additionally, there is a decrease in the surface area available for gas exchange, causing alterations in diffusing capacities and ventilation-perfusion abnormalities. These abnormalities lead to the hypoxia seen in emphysema. With the destruction of the elastic properties of the alveolar walls causing the decreased elastic recoil of the lungs, the increased intrathoracic pressure produced during expiration results in the collapse and premature closure of the airways. Because these changes affect chiefly flow rates on expiration, flow rates on inspiration are relatively normal unless obstructive bronchitis is also present. It should be emphasized that it is the destructive changes characteristic of emphysema that separate it from simple overdistention seen in the elderly, during asthma attacks, or with compensation of a remaining lung after a pneumonectomy.

Emphysema is often divided according to the site of pulmonary involvement (Fig. 27–6). In centrilobular (or centriacinar) emphysema, the lesion is located in the center of the lobule and is distinct from the periphery of the acinus. This form of disease most often involves the upper lung zones and is almost always associated with chronic bronchitis. This type is the most common form and is rarely seen in nonsmokers.

In panlobular (or panacinar) emphysema, less commonly seen, the entire acinus is involved. The normal architecture of the alveoli is lost. There is loss of septa with enlargement of the air spaces, leading to loss of pulmonary parenchyma. Although this form can occur anywhere in the lung, it is more often seen in the lower and anterior lungs. There is little association between this form and chronic bronchitis, it can occur in nonsmokers, and it is the type usually

seen in patients with the alpha-1 protease inhibitor deficiency. Some pathologists feel that centrilobular emphysema progresses into the panlobular form.

Clinical Manifestations

The signs and symptoms of pulmonary emphysema are insidious and variable. The main components of emphysema clinically are progressive expiratory flow obstruction and overinflation. Dyspnea, usually occurring only with exertion in the beginning, gradually increases in intensity. Some patients will experience very slow progression of their shortness of breath whereas others become markedly disabled more rapidly. The majority of patients adjust their activity levels to minimize the dyspnea. As the disease progresses, they find the symptoms occurring with less and less activity until, as previously mentioned, they are dyspneic at rest. The fact that some patients' dyspnea does not seem to correlate with the degree of pathology appears to be due to differences in sensitivity of the individual's respiratory centers or chemoreceptors. Like chronic bronchitis, the course of emphysema varies, with periods of exacerbations that are most often associated with infections.

Physical findings may be very mild or moderate. In the more advanced cases, enlargement of the anteroposterior diameter of the chest, dorsal kyphosis, elevated ribs, and wide costal angle produce the typical barreling effect. Besides the barrel chest, clinical characteristics include a thin physique with muscle wasting, an acyanotic, unproductive, minimal cough, and, in the later stages, signs of right heart failure. These patients may appear dyspneic, using the accessory muscles of respiration, and they may breathe through pursed lips with a prolonged expiration. As previously mentioned, they have been termed "pink puffers." On percussion, they are found to have increased resonance (hyperresonance) due to the increased lung volumes. Breath sounds are decreased and often difficult to hear because of the barrel chest. Heart sounds are also distant for the same reason. Expiratory wheezes may be present.

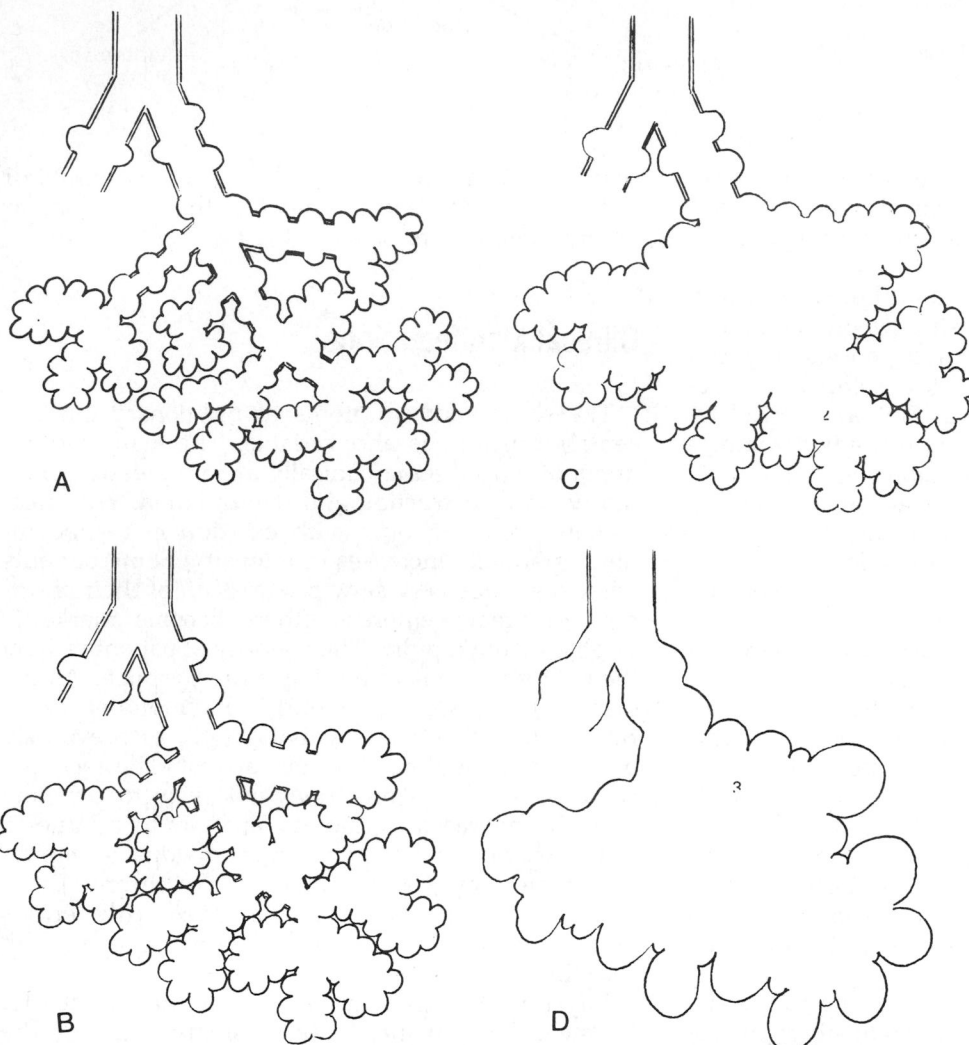

FIGURE 27–6. Comparison of the differences in the distal airways in *(A)* the normal patient, *(B)* simple hyperinflation, *(C)* centrilobular emphysema, and *(D)* panlobular emphysema. (Modified from Farzan, S., et al. (1992). *A concise handbook of respiratory diseases* (3rd ed., pp. 131–132). Norwalk, CT: Appleton & Lange.)

Respiratory excursion of the chest wall is normally decreased due to the hyperinflated state.

Routine Laboratory Data

In patients with pure emphysema, especially younger patients, the alpha-1 antiprotease phenotype should be determined. Other routine data are relatively unhelpful.

Electrocardiography. As discussed earlier under chronic bronchitis, changes seen on the ECG relate more to the stage and severity of the disease than to the type of disease.

Radiographic Changes. Again, x-ray changes seen in emphysema relate more to the severity and type of disease. Classic findings seen in the later stages of emphysema include flattening of the diaphragm, hyperlucency, decreased vascular markings, widening of the rib spaces, and increased anteroposterior diameter. All of these findings are related to the hyperinflation seen in emphysema. Careful interpretation of x-ray findings must rule out other reasons for the hyperinflation. The most common cause of hyperlucent lung fields is an overexposed x-ray film in a thin, elderly patient (Tisi, 1983). Bullous lesions seen on x-ray are unequivocal indications of emphysema.

Pulmonary Function Tests. Common findings on the most frequently run pulmonary function tests include:

1. Increased residual and functional residual volumes
2. Decreased vital capacity
3. Increased total lung capacity
4. Decreased diffusing capacity
5. Increased FEV_1 and maximal midexpiratory flow rate (MMFR)
6. Flow volume loop showing coved appearance (Fig. 27–7)

Both the FEV_1 and the MMFR are useful parameters in evaluating the severity and progression of the disease. Arterial blood gases may be normal in mild to moderate emphysema. In advanced cases, the most common abnormality is the decreased P_{O_2}. The P_{CO_2} may be normal or increased, especially in individuals with infections or other complications.

Course and Prognosis

Although the course varies from patient to patient, most will experience a fairly predictable decline in pulmonary function, with an average time between onset of disease and the stage of severe disability ranging from 20 to 25 years. The correlation between severity of air flow obstruction (as measured by FEV_1)

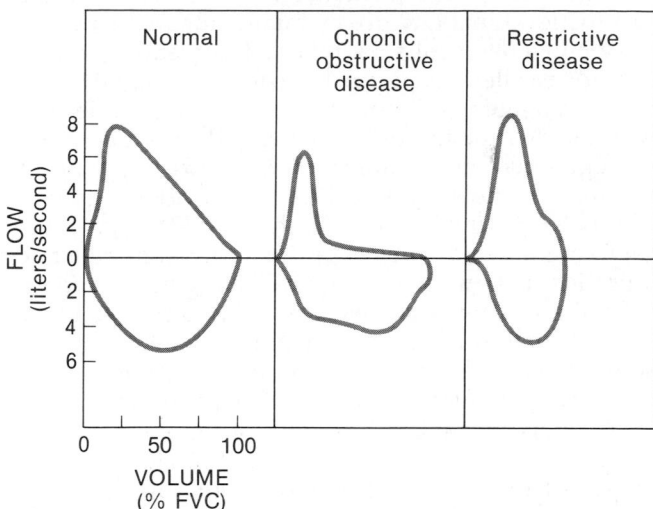

FIGURE 27–7. Illustration depicting flow-volume curves seen in *(A)* the normal patient, *(B)* the patient with COPD, and *(C)* the patient with restrictive disease. (Redrawn from Ayers, L., Whipp, B., and Ziment, I. (1978). *A guide to the interpretation of pulmonary function tests* (2nd ed.). New York: Roerig, a division of Pfizer Pharmaceuticals.)

and mortality is good. Few patients survive more than 5 years with an FEV_1 less than 750 mL (Farzan, 1985).

MANAGEMENT OF CHRONIC BRONCHITIS AND EMPHYSEMA

Smoking Cessation

Almost all books and articles that discuss management of these two diseases list smoking cessation as the single most important intervention to alter the progression of air flow obstruction. Both medical and nursing interventions must address this fact in a realistic, practical manner, realizing that avoidance of further insult to the lung should be one of the main objectives of management.

Techniques of behavioral modification, support groups, and use of nicotine-containing gum (Nicorette) may help to combat the addictiveness of nicotine. Research indicates that smokers with premature loss of pulmonary function who stopped smoking before the age of 50 had a rate of loss of ventilatory function that was comparable to the age-related loss seen in nonsmokers. Even those who stopped smoking at age 65 with advanced ventilatory impairment had a better survival than those who continued to smoke (Petty, 1986).

Sputum Mobilization

Good hydration with appropriate use of aerosol treatments may assist in mobilizing secretions in patients who have evidence of increased sputum production. Inability to maintain adequate pulmonary hygiene results in retained secretions, which are an excellent medium for bacterial growth. Postural drainage may improve, at least temporarily, the ventilatory function of the patient. Postural drainage is segmental lung drainage. It utilizes gravity to facilitate the flow of secretions from various segments of the lung to the bronchi, trachea, and throat, where they can more easily be expectorated. Percussion and vibration aid mechanically in dislodging secretions once the patient is in position. Vibration is administered over the affected area during exhalation. For some patients, however, postural drainage is difficult and can aggravate hypoxia. The condition of the patient, age, complications, and observation will determine the best position, degree of angle used, and length of the treatment period. Increasing dyspnea, labored respirations, and change in color or heart rate are some of the warning signs indicating that the treatments should be stopped. Oropharyngeal, tracheal, endotracheal, and transtracheal suctioning (depending on patient status) may be indicated.

Prevention of Infection

As stated earlier, the role of infection in exacerbating chronic bronchitis is evident, and both nursing and medical interventions should be focused on preventing infection. Adequate hydration, removal of secretions as mentioned previously, proper nutrition, avoidance of exposure to sudden changes in climate, and adherence to the prescribed antibiotic and physical therapy regimen are crucial. The Center for Disease Control recommends annual prophylaxis with multivalent influenza vaccine because it believes that these vaccines provide a substantial degree of protection. The influenza vaccine is usually given each fall if epidemics are predicted. In addition, it is highly recommended that patients with COPD also receive the pneumococcal vaccine. Although the effectiveness of the pneumococcal vaccine is still debatable, many experts recommend a one-time vaccination for their COPD patients.

Bronchodilators

Even if pulmonary function tests indicate only a small degree of reversibility of air flow obstruction (a 15% improvement over baseline is considered significant), treatment with bronchodilators may be able to prevent accelerated losses in lung function. This topic will be discussed in more detail following the asthma section of this chapter. It should be remembered that therapeutic blood levels of the theophylline compounds must be monitored closely in the patients with COPD because smokers tend to metabolize theophylline faster than nonsmokers, and patients with liver or cardiac disease metabolize theophyllines slower, so dosages must be individualized.

Pulmonary Rehabilitation

Proper education of patients and family is critical for the management of chronic disease. Their cooperation and compliance often depend on their understanding of their illness and treatment regime. Although this education can and should be done individually, pulmonary rehabilitation programs offer the opportunity to meet others with similar disabilities. Programs are generally organized to include instruction on reconditioning, breathing retraining, proper nutrition, psychosocial considerations, vocational counseling, energy conservation techniques, support for smoking cessation, and sexual counseling. Although it has not been established that these programs extend patients' life expectancy, it appears clear that they favorably affect the quality of life (Table 27–2).

PATIENTS IN THE INTENSIVE CARE UNIT

Clinical Presentation

A patient with COPD admitted to the intensive care unit (ICU) presents some special problems for those managing his care. These patients frequently present with a recent history of increasing dyspnea, increased cough, and fatigue. Family members may have noticed the recent onset of mental confusion or other changes in personality such as irritability or lethargy. Physical examination may reveal use of the accessory muscles to breathe, tachycardia, and tachypnea. The presence of hypoxia, abnormal breath sounds (crackles, wheezes, stridor) or consolidation (increased voice and whispered sounds and egophony), and cor pulmonale (increased neck vein distention, enlarged liver, edema) is additional indication of respiratory failure (see Chap. 25).

TABLE 27–2. Demonstrated Benefits of Pulmonary Rehabilitation

Reduction in respiratory symptoms.
Reversal of anxiety and depression and improved ego strength.
Enhanced ability to carry out activities of daily living.
Increased exercise ability.
Better quality of life.
Reduction in hospital days required.
Prolongation of life in selected patients, i.e., use of continuous oxygen in patients with severe hypoxemia.

From Hodgkin, J., and Petty, T. (1987). *Chronic obstructive pulmonary disease*. Philadelphia: W. B. Saunders.

Assessment Data

Upon admission to an ICU it is important to obtain an arterial blood gas sample for evaluation, sputum for analysis, a chest x-ray, blood for a complete blood count (CBC) and electrolyte evaluation, and an electrocardiogram. Much of the responsibility for obtaining these data rests with the critical care nurse. All this information will assist in determining the possible cause of the acute failure. Frequently, patients with underlying COPD present in the ICU because of infections, heart failure, pulmonary embolus, pneumothorax, bronchospastic episodes, gastrointestinal bleeding, or metabolic abnormalities. Sometimes these patients have changed the dosages of their medications without physician knowledge or have been unable to keep the medication regimen due to coughing, nausea, or vomiting. These patients sometimes change their oxygen dosage, which may also trigger an episode of acute respiratory failure. It is critical to teach these patients the importance of their medical regimens, and, again, it is often the nurse who is the "educator" of these patients.

Management

The primary goal of therapy for any patient admitted to the ICU in respiratory failure is to maintain adequate cellular respiration. Identifying and reversing the precipitating cause of the failure is critical. Although this is true for any patient in respiratory failure, even a relatively healthy person, it is even more important with patients with COPD. The parameters that are used to identify respiratory failure (Pa_{O_2} <60 mm Hg; Pa_{CO_2} >50 mm Hg) are frequently "normal" values in the patient with COPD. Clinically, the key to identification of acute or chronic respiratory failure is the pH. A pH in the severely acidotic range (<7.25) is often given as the marker for acute respiratory failure when it appears in conjunction with an elevated carbon dioxide level and a decreased oxygen level.

Oxygen Support. Supplemental oxygen is considered the mainstay of therapy. An adequate Pa_{O_2} improves tissue O_2 delivery and reverses the pulmonary hypertension that occurs in response to hypoxia. This in turn improves cardiac output because of the reduced afterload. The goal of therapy is to maintain the Pa_{O_2} between 55 and 65 mm Hg. In this range, saturation of hemoglobin is optimal without disruption of the "hypoxic drive" stimulus that is so critical for many of these patients. There are several ways to deliver this oxygen, ranging from Venturi masks, nasal cannulas, rebreathing masks, and mechanical ventilation (see Chap. 25).

Hemodynamic Monitoring. Because careful monitoring of these patients requires frequent blood gas sampling, many critically ill patients have indwelling catheters in place. Hemodynamic monitoring principles are the same in pulmonary patients as they are in any critically ill patient (see Chap. 10). There are, however, a few hemodynamic findings that may differ depending on the extent of pulmonary compromise. For instance, many of the patients admitted to the ICU with severe COPD have increased pulmonary vascular pressure. Measurements of pulmonary artery systolic and diastolic pressures and mean pulmonary artery pressures may be above normal. Changes in chest wall, pleural, and pulmonary compliance also may affect readings. In addition, a COPD patient with pulmonary hypertension also may have a pulmonary artery diastolic pressure that is 5 to 20 mm Hg higher than the pulmonary capillary wedge pressure (PCWP). Normally, these two readings are within 1 to 2 mm Hg of each other. This increased gradient between the two measurements is due to the increased pulmonary vascular resistance found in many of these patients.

The actual measurement technique used is another consideration in the pulmonary patient. As discussed in Chapter 10, equipment calibration is done prior to use, using an accurate and consistent right atrial reference point (the transducer is kept at the level of the right atrium). This reference point may change with a pulmonary patient, who may be very restless, agitated, or unable to cooperate and who changes position frequently due to dyspnea, coughing, hypoxia, and so on. Accuracy of measurement may also be altered by the phase of the respiratory cycle present at the time of measurement. Because the most accurate measurement occurs when intrathoracic pressures and airway pressures are stable, it is recommended that readings be taken at the end of expiration. If the patient is being mechanically ventilated, the positive pressures generated can create falsely elevated readings. There has been much debate about whether the patient should be taken off the ventilator during the actual reading. This is especially true if positive end-expiratory pressure (PEEP) is being used. Because the trends in readings are the important factor and because taking a patient on and off the ventilator may result in hypoxemia and sudden increases in venous return to the heart, it is generally recommended that the measurements be done while the patient remains on the ventilator. This also provides important information about the effects of the ventilator support system and establishes actual baseline readings.

Besides invasive monitoring techniques, oxygen saturation can be monitored by ear or by digital oximetry. This noninvasive monitoring technique has been found to have a high degree of accuracy, correlation, and speed compared with direct arterial O_2 saturation measurements as long as the saturation values are greater than 70% and the patient has an adequate cardiac output. If the patient has poor perfusion because of a decreased cardiac output or if the saturation is less than 65%, values may be inaccurate.

Removal of Secretions. Because of the critical condition of many COPD patients admitted to the ICU and because increased viscosity of sputum and inflammation of the airways are common in these patients, good hydration, frequent suctioning, and chest physiotherapy are often required.

Suctioning is not without hazards (dysrhythmias, laryngospasms, microatelectasis, hypoxemia), and many studies have been done to determine the best way for the nursing staff to maintain patent airways without causing these complications. Although a review of suctioning procedures is beyond the scope of this chapter, it appears that the most accepted recommendations for suctioning include hyperoxygenation with 100% oxygen and hyperinflation. When PEEP is used with mechanical ventilation, it is most important to maintain PEEP during oxygenation and suctioning if greater than 10 mm H_2O is used (Barnes and Kirchhoff, 1986). Drugs to thin secretions are sometimes used (e.g., glyceral quaiacolate) but may not be clinically helpful. Supplemental humidification with ultrasonic nebulization may be used to help liquify secretions, although this can be irritating to the airways of some patients, especially those prone to bronchospasm. Increasing fluid intake can also be effective, but because many of these patients are also on fluid restrictions due to heart or kidney involvement, careful individual assessment must be done.

Bronchodilator Therapy. Although the use of these drugs will be discussed later in this chapter in the section on asthma, bronchodilators can be of major benefit in the patient with chronic bronchitis or emphysema. Theophylline does relax the bronchial smooth muscle in the lung and has also been found to increase the hypoxic ventilatory drive and decrease the diaphragmatic fatigue seen in these patients. The usual goal with theophylline therapy is to maintain blood levels of 10 to 20 μg/mL, and, as mentioned previously, it must be remembered that these levels can vary in the critically ill because of changes in clearance rates.

Steroids. Although the use of steroids is discussed further in the asthma section, their use in COPD patients has been a source of dispute. It appears that, for some people with COPD who have a strong component of asthma, steroids may be helpful. Short courses of treatment appear to be relatively safe as long as the ICU nurse carefully monitors the patient for the major side effect of short-term therapy, hyperglycemia.

Steroids such as intravenous methylprednisolone for 1 to 2 days followed by oral prednisone may be ordered in increasingly lower doses until a maintenance dose is reached. Aerosol steroids have not been shown to be helpful in patients with COPD unless asthma is present. Close observation of improvement in condition is crucial; if there is no evidence of objective improvement, steroids should be discontinued.

Antibiotics. Because infections are a common precipitating cause of respiratory failure in patients with COPD, antibiotics are frequently ordered. Initial choice of the drug used is commonly based on Gram stain of the sputum; if necessary, it is changed if blood and sputum cultures suggest a more appropriate choice.

Treating the patient with an already compromised respiratory system for elevated temperatures is recommended, primarily because it is estimated that CO_2 production and O_2 consumption increase by as much as 10% for each degree Fahrenheit rise in temperature above normal (Chin and Pesce, 1983). This increase puts additional strain on the respiratory system.

Nutritional Support. There are some special considerations that should be emphasized when dealing with patients with COPD. Many of these patients show evidence of malnutrition not only because of decreased caloric intake due to nausea, vomiting, coughing, dyspnea, and fatigue, but also because of the increased metabolic demands brought on by the increased work of breathing and fever in some cases. Although the treatment regime may include an increase in calories, excess carbohydrates, when converted to fat, result in an increased production of carbon dioxide. This can result in a worsening of the respiratory failure. It is therefore recommended that less than one-third of the calories provided be made up of carbohydrates (MacDonnell et al., 1987).

Ventilatory Management. The use of intubation and mechanical ventilation in the critically ill patient does not cure the cause of the respiratory failure but does allow the patient to "rest" his respiratory muscles, allows easier access for suctioning, and can improve gas exchange. The problem with using mechanical ventilators for patients with COPD is that weaning from the ventilator is then often difficult (see Chap. 30). The decision to intervene with mechanical ventilation must be made in light of the expected outcome. These are difficult decisions because many of these patients are alert and awake, and it is clear that although their lives could be extended, it would mean being attached to a mechanical device for extraordinary intervals if not until death. These are decisions that must take into account the wishes of the patient first, with input from family and the medical management team.

ASTHMA

The Task Force on Respiratory Disease of the National Heart, Lung and Blood Institute reports that management of the asthma patient continues to be a challenge to the health profession despite the fact that newer drugs and better techniques for using them are available. Asthma remains a common cause of admission to hospitals and emergency rooms, and despite maximal drug therapy, some patients remain incapacitated and some die from this disease. Status asthmaticus occurs in 3% to 5% of asthmatics, and it is estimated that as many as 2000 patients die annually from asthma, with half of these deaths occurring outside the hospital (MacDonnell et al., 1987). Approximately 2.5% of the U.S. population is afflicted with asthma, 10 to 12 million people, with males affected twice as often as females. Asthma is a common respiratory disease that can begin at any age, though half the cases begin before the age of 10. There appears to be a genetic predisposition in some patients; more than one-third of patients have an immediate family member with asthma.

Asthma is characterized by increased airway responsiveness to a variety of stimuli and is manifested by widespread narrowing of the airways. This bronchoconstriction, which is induced by many different agents, does not occur in normal individuals.

Etiology

PRECIPITATING STIMULI

Some of the stimuli that can precipitate an attack of asthma include the following:

Allergens. Despite the widespread belief that asthma is an allergic disorder, allergy is only one of the etiologic factors. In children the role of allergy is more clear when development of an attack is associated with a specific substance. When a specific allergy is associated with the attack, asthma is often referred to as *extrinsic* or allergic. When the attack is seemingly unrelated to a specific allergen, though there may be a frequent association with a respiratory tract infection, this type of asthma is known as *intrinsic* (Kersten, 1989). It is not uncommon for children with severe asthma to have a strong history of allergic conditions such as hay fever or eczema and have more strongly positive skin tests and higher levels of immunoglobulin E (IgE) than children with milder asthma.

It is well documented that asthmatics have an increased responsiveness to certain chemical substances such as histamine and methacholine. There is also an increased reactivity to cold air, fumes, dust, and exercise.

Infection. As already indicated, there is a strong correlation between respiratory tract infections and the onset of an asthma attack, both intrinsic and extrinsic types. It does appear that in children the onset of asthma following infection has a better prognosis than asthma whose onset was more related to an allergy (Tisi, 1983).

Occupational History. Asthma related to an occupational inhalant can cause fixed airway obstruction after chronic exposure. Some of the irritants implicated in occupational asthma are listed in Table 27–3. It is possible that there are different mechanisms of response depending on the occupational irritant present in the environment, but circulating antibodies and elevated IgE levels in these patients often make it difficult to identify the direct effects of the irritant or to distinguish direct effects from reactions to these chemicals.

Exercise. Asthma attacks related to exercise are common in children and young adults. An attack that occurs after vigorous exercise is thought to be due to the cooling of the airways. Normally, inspired air is humidified and temperature regulated (37° C). This process occurs by heat exchange and evaporation of water from the airway mucus. Heat loss is proportional to minute ventilation, which, in vigorous exercise, is markedly increased. Heavy exercise in cold, dry air (e.g., ice skating) is much more likely to cause an attack than exercise in warm, humid air (e.g., indoor swimming).

Emotions. There is no evidence indicating a psychogenic basis for asthma, but sudden emotional reactions or stress reportedly reduce airway caliber in asthmatics. Hyperventilation resulting in hypocapnia may increase airway resistance by constricting the smooth muscles of the airways.

Nasal Polyps. Recurrent nasal polyps, asthma, and aspirin sensitivity is a well-recognized triad. There are some data that indicate a worse prognosis in these asthmatics compared with patients who do not have polyps. Approximately 10% of asthmatics belong in this category. These patients may also be hypersensitive to tartrazine, the yellow food coloring used in many products.

MECHANISMS PRODUCING ASTHMA

The classic mechanism producing asthma is a biochemical one (Fig. 27–8). Sensitized mast cells in the lungs have an antibody (IgE) fixed to their surface. When exposed to an allergen, the antigen-antibody

TABLE 27–3. Occupational Irritants Implicated in Asthma

Tobacco smoke
Ozone
Nickel
Platinum
Pigeon droppings (bird breeder's lung)
Moldy bark exposure (maple bark stripper's lung)
Moldy vegetable compost (farmer's lung/bagassosis)
Contaminated air conditioning systems
Polyurethane fumes
Sulfur dioxide
Formaldehyde
Cotton fiber (byssinosis)

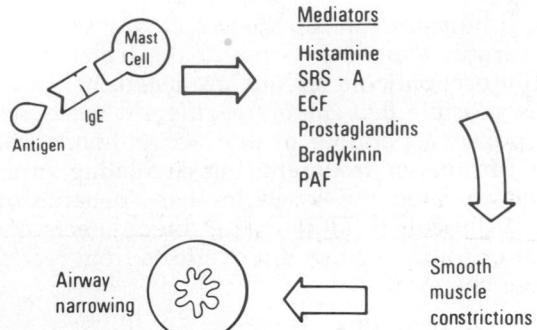

FIGURE 27–8. Biochemical mechanism for asthma. *Abbreviations:* SRS-A, slow-reacting substance of anaphylaxis; ECF, eosinophilic chemotactic factor; PAF, platelet-activating factor; IgE, immunoglobulin E. (From Tisi, G. (1983). *Pulmonary physiology in clinical medicine* (2nd ed., p. 169). © 1983, the Williams & Wilkins Co., Baltimore.)

reaction triggers the release of chemical mediators that are responsible for the bronchoconstriction seen in asthma. These mediators include:

1. Histamine: produces smooth muscle contraction, increased vascular permeability, and increased production of mucus
2. Slow-reacting substance of anaphylaxis (SRS-A): a sulfur-containing substance that produces long-lasting smooth muscle contraction
3. Eosinophilic chemotactic factor (ECF): a small peptide that attracts eosinophils
4. Other mediators: prostaglandin, bradykinin, and platelet-activating factor

Cyclic nucleotides modulate these mediators (Fig. 27–9). Increased levels of cyclic adenosine monophosphate (cAMP) inhibit their secretion, and decreased levels of cAMP facilitate mediator release. Increased levels of cAMP can occur when beta-adrenergics (catecholamines) stimulate the conversion of adenosine triphosphate (ATP) to cAMP or when the degradation of cAMP is prevented by the inhibition of phosphodiesterase (the enzyme that breaks cAMP down). There is also a decrease in cAMP when alpha-catecholamines stimulate phosphodiesterase to degrade cAMP. This cyclic nucleo-

BIOCHEMICAL MODULATION

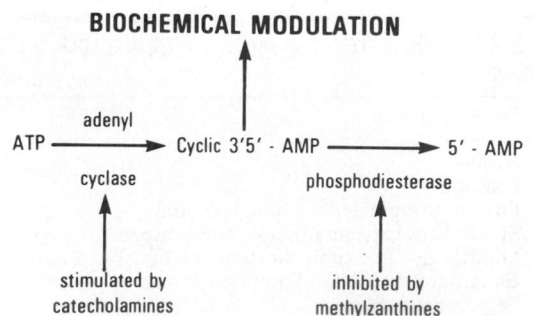

FIGURE 27–9. Modulation of cAMP levels (see text). (From Tisi, G. (1983). *Pulmonary physiology in clinical medicine* (2nd ed., p. 169). © 1983, the Williams & Wilkins Co., Baltimore.)

tide mechanism of action is the basis for many of the drugs used in the treatment of asthma.

There may also be a neurogenic mechanism responsible for asthma (Fig. 27–10). Studies indicate that antigen-antibody responses stimulate a vagally mediated reflex. Animal studies show that bronchoconstriction in animals could be inhibited by cooling and cutting the cervical vagi.

Pathophysiology

The pathologic changes seen in asthma include bronchospasm, airway edema, and hypersecretion of mucus. The bronchoconstriction that affects the central and peripheral airways initially leads to edema, cellular infiltration, and hypersecretion. Hypertrophy of the smooth muscle layer, thickening of the epithelial basement membrane, and infiltration of eosinophils within the bronchial wall are identified by microscopy. If the attack goes untreated, mucous plugging occurs. There are several end results of airway narrowing:

Flow Obstruction. The early stages of an asthmatic attack produce the clinical signs and symptoms related to smooth muscle contraction. The rhonchi result from the narrowed central airways (Caw), and the wheezing is a result of the narrowing of the peripheral airways (Paw). Due to the absence of cartilage in the Paw, these airways are particularly susceptible to airway narrowing and collapse. Inspiratory and expiratory flow rates are reduced because of this narrowing.

Hyperinflation. Quite early in an asthmatic attack, the residual volume and size of the chest cage increase in order to preserve the vital capacity (VC). As the limits to expansion of the chest wall are reached and as the residual volume increases, the VC begins to drop. The severity of the asthmatic attack can be correlated with the decrease of the VC (in severe overinflation the VC is less than 60% of predicted).

Ventilation-Perfusion Abnormalities. Because the narrowing of the Paw is nonuniform, ventilation to the lungs becomes unequal. In areas of the lung that are underventilated due to airway narrowing, increased secretions, and edema, the perfusion of blood exceeds ventilation, producing a low ventilation to perfusion ratio. It is this abnormality that causes arterial hypoxemia and a widened A-a gradient (AaD_{O_2}) during the early stages of an attack. As the attack continues, with increasing edema and secretions, ventilation of the affected units reaches zero, and this causes the right-to-left shunting that produces the progressive hypoxemia that gets harder and harder to treat.

Arterial Blood Gases. Arterial blood gases (ABGs)

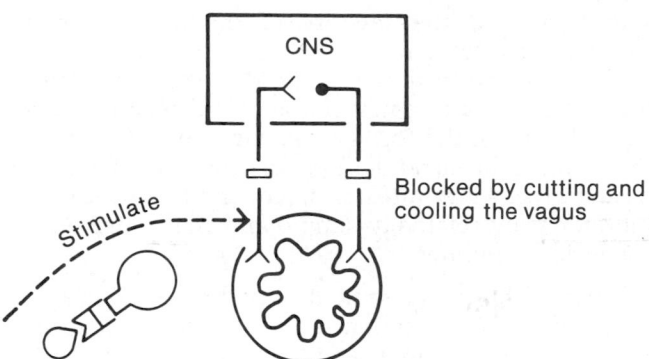

FIGURE 27–10. Neurogenic mechanism for asthma. (From Tisi, G. (1983). *Pulmonary physiology in clinical medicine* (2nd ed., p. 169). © 1983, the Williams & Wilkins Co., Baltimore.)

are a valuable way to evaluate the severity and duration of the attack. The anxiety that is common early in an attack results in an increased minute ventilation, resulting in hypocapnia along with the hypoxemia. As ventilation becomes more abnormal, the patient develops more severe hypoxemia, and as the severity of the attack worsens, arterial CO_2 increases. In the most severe cases, the patient is hypoxic and hypercapnic. In the stages of an attack showing progression of hypoxemia and increasing Pa_{CO_2}, the patient should be hospitalized, if he is not already, due to the higher mortality risk.

Clinical Manifestations

As in most diseases, the clinical signs and symptoms are often as varied as the type of patients that develop the disease. A combination of clinical findings and laboratory data assists the practitioner to select the appropriate therapies.

Vital Signs. A respiratory rate of more than 30 means that the adult patient is using a majority of his energy reserves to ventilate. Careful observation is needed to determine the cause of the increase. If not associated with a change in activity, increasing respiratory rates may be early indicators of impending trouble.

An elevated pulse rate above 130 is associated with increased work of breathing. It may be a result of a dropping P_{O_2}, an increasing CO_2, or both. Acidosis and some drugs can also increase pulse rates. It is crucial to evaluate whether the cardiac symptoms are caused by bronchospasm and airway obstruction (treatment may require an increase in bronchodilator medication or more aggressive pulmonary management) or whether the pulse increase is due to the drug therapy itself. In that case, a change or reduction in bronchodilator medication may be needed.

An elevated temperature indicates infection, and identification of the cause and proper treatment are required. The use of rectal thermometers may be necessary due to the patient's respiratory distress.

Large intrathoracic pressure shifts can cause hemodynamic changes due to alterations in left ventricular compliance. The reduced cardiac output results in a drop in blood pressure during inspiration. This is known as pulsus paradoxus if there is a drop in systolic blood pressure of 10 mm Hg or more on inspiration, and its presence is considered an indicator of the severity of the attack. A 20-mm Hg drop is a sign of a severe attack.

Work of Breathing. There is good correlation between the decrease in flow rates and the use of accessory muscles. The subjective response to an increase in the work of breathing is dyspnea. Central airway spasm or obstruction results in both dyspnea and accessory muscle use. It should be remembered, however, that symptoms may improve when the large airways are dilated even though the small airways remain severely impaired. Complaints of progressive muscle fatigue with a history of profound exhaustion, lack of sleep, and repeated coughing on mild effort correlate with a more severe attack.

Patient Presentation. A patient sitting upright, sweating, and very short of breath with personality changes, hoarseness, and a telegraphic (short choppy sentences) speech pattern indicates severe distress. The presence of any other major organ abnormality may be enough to cause a simple attack to become an acute one. Pneumonia, heart failure, tachydysrhythmias, or pulmonary emboli are just a few examples of potential factors that can worsen the situation.

The duration and pace of the attack may correlate with increased mortality. Patients who have prolonged subacute episodes with incomplete recovery despite therapy require extremely close monitoring.

It is particularly important to appreciate the circadian rhythms of asthmatic attacks. Many patients may be well during the day and symptomatic at night. This diurnal rhythm reflects the occurrence of a fall in lung function during the night (lowest at 3 A.M.) with a recovery to peak function 12 hours later. Sleep and cyclic variations in plasma epinephrine also play a part in this reduced function, and all these factors indicate the need to ensure that the therapy of these patients provides 24-hour coverage. It is recommended that measurement of peak air flow be done the last thing at night and the first thing in the morning prior to administration of medications so that the extent of the "morning dip" can be monitored (Clark, 1986).

Other factors that may indicate an impending asthma attack or deterioration are:

1. Increased dyspnea
2. Increased sleep disturbance with increased use of a bronchodilator during the night
3. Early morning chest tightness with increasingly less relief achieved from the medication
4. Increased frequency and severity of cough

5. Increased allergic state (atopy) with nasal hyperse-cretions and early morning sneezing bouts

Laboratory Data

Radiographic Findings. The findings on x-ray during an asthmatic attack reflect the hyperinflation from increased lung volumes. Hyperlucency of the affected lung fields is evident. If an infectious process is present, the chest x-ray may reveal areas of atelectasis, infiltration, or other densities.

Sputum Examination. The sputum examination provides information about the presence of infection and whether or not there are increased numbers of eosinophils (which are frequently present during an asthma attack).

Pulmonary Function Tests. As in most lung diseases, the findings on PFTs vary greatly, not only between patients but also in the same patient depending on the stage of the disease existing at the time of the test. Without a doubt, the most consistent changes seen on PFTs in patients with asthma are measured by expiratory flow studies. It is these studies that assist the health care team in evaluating the severity of the airway obstruction, the progression of the attack, and the response to treatment.

Between attacks, although some patients have normal pulmonary function, the majority show evidence of small airway obstruction. During the acute attack, common findings include:

1. Marked decrease in flow rates
2. Reduced forced vital capacity (FVC)
3. Increased residual volume (RV) and functional residual volume (FRV)
4. Ventilation-perfusion abnormalities

These findings are very similar to those noted in emphysema except that they usually respond to bronchodilators to a much greater extent than in COPD.

Arterial Blood Gases. Although ABGs have been discussed earlier in the section on asthma, it should be reemphasized that the common findings are mild to moderate hypoxemia and hypocapnia. Again, in the early stages the patient's anxiety and apprehension and the response to hypoxemia may be the cause of the increased respiratory rate. There is also some thought that neurogenic reflexes from irritant and stretch receptors may play a part in the increased minute volume (Farzan, 1985).

Management of Asthma

Management of the patient with asthma should take into account that:

1. There is not a strong correlation between the

symptoms and the severity of the disease or its response to treatment.

2. The return of flow rates to the patients' normal level rather than achievement of an asymptomatic state should be the focus of management. Obtaining the optimal bronchodilation for the patient should be the goal. Flow rates and bronchodilation can be monitored by relatively simple and inexpensive spirometric techniques.

Much of the management of asthma involves the cooperation of the patient and the family. Ensuring that both the patient and the family thoroughly understand the disease and the treatment regimen is a priority. In general, prevention of future attacks is the primary goal of treatment, and this includes (1) eliminating or avoiding allergens known to trigger the asthma attack, and (2) instituting drug therapy that is most effective in maximizing bronchodilation with a minimum of side effects (Table 27–4).

DRUG THERAPY

The fact that so many drugs are used in the management of asthma emphasizes how difficult it is to treat this disease. A drug that is very effective with one patient may have little effect on another. Most of the drugs that are used fall into one of the following categories:

Sympathomimetics
Theophylline compounds
Glucocorticoids
Cromolyns
Anticholinergics

Sympathomimetics. Used because of their ability to "mimic" the sympathetic nervous system, these drugs, also known as beta-adrenergics, have a direct bronchodilating effect on the airways and inhibit mast cell release of the mediators that cause bronchoconstriction. They may also have beneficial effects on mucociliary transport. These drugs vary in the selectivity of their effect on beta-2 receptors and in their duration of action. Although beta-agonist aerosol therapy has been the mainstay of treatment of acute asthma, current recommendations from the National Heart, Lung, and Blood Institute now say that for long-term control of asthma, it is more important to use anti-inflammatory agents. This is discussed later. The mode of delivery of sympathomimetics directly to the lungs via aerosol allows a reduced dosage with a subsequent reduction of side effects.

Metered dose inhalers (MDI), jet nebulizers, and intermittent positive-pressure breathing (IPPB) are the usual modes of delivery for these drugs. There are advantages and disadvantages to each of these systems. The IPPB system is not used anymore except for those few patients who may be psychologically dependent on the machine. This system offers no advantage and can cause pneumothorax in sus-

TABLE 27-4. Drug Therapy of Asthma

Drug	Examples	Possible Routes of Administration	Mechanism of Action
Bronchodilators Sympathomimetics	Epinephrine Isoproterenol Isoetharine Metaproterenol Terbutaline Albuterol Bitolterol	Inhaled, oral, parenteral (depending on particular drug)	↑ cAMP via stimulation of adenyl cyclase
Xanthines	Theophylline Aminophylline	Oral Oral, parenteral	? ↑ cAMP via inhibition of phosphodiesterase
Anticholinergics	Ipratropium	Inhaled	Blockade of cholinergic (bronchoconstrictor) effect on airways
Mast cell stabilizers Cromolyn		Inhaled	Inhibition of mediator release from mast cells; ? additional mechanisms
Anti-inflammatory drugs Corticosteroids		Oral, parenteral, inhaled	Decreased inflammatory response in airways; ? additional mechanisms

From Weinberger, S. (1992). *Principles of pulmonary medicine* (2nd ed.). Philadelphia: W. B. Saunders.

ceptible patients. Studies comparing MDI versus jet nebulization indicate no significant difference. The MDI system requires use of proper technique that a severely respiratory-compromised patient may not be able to accomplish. One particular advantage is that MDI can deliver a very small dose of the drug. The advantage of jet nebulizers is that patient cooperation is not required. If a continuous nebulizer system is used, the onset, peak, and duration of action depend on the drug used.

Although dosages vary, the usual dose of a beta-adrenergic agonist (e.g., albuterol) is 2 puffs four times a day via MDI; this dose can be increased to 4 to 6 puffs four times daily if necessary. Given over a 24-hour period, this dose is still less than the oral dose required. If a patient does not respond adequately to 4 to 6 puffs of albuterol or an equivalent drug given four times a day, it is unlikely that the addition of some other type of bronchodilater will be helpful.

Theophylline Compounds. These drugs are among the most commonly used agents for the treatment of asthma, aminophylline being the only one used intravenously. With careful monitoring of theophylline levels and the availability of slow-release oral preparations, theophylline preparations are often used for preventive therapy. The desired therapeutic level of 10 to 20 $\mu q/mL$ may, in some sensitive patients, cause toxic effects. Side effects to look for include nausea, vomiting, seizures, and supraventricular and ventricular dysrhythmias. When blood levels exceed 35 $\mu q/mL$, seizures and arrhythmias may occur. The fact that theophylline levels vary so greatly among patients, even with the same dosages, points to the need for close monitoring. Patients who have increased clearance of theophylline require increased dosages. These include cigarette smokers, patients with cystic fibrosis, marijuana users, and

patients on oral contraceptives. Some patients have decreased clearance of the drug. Conditions that tend to decrease clearance of these drugs and thus require decreased dosages include both young and old age (neonates and the elderly), patients with hepatic disorders, patients taking cimetidine, and those with cor pulmonale and other cardiac decompensation disorders (MacDonnell et al., 1987).

Corticosteroids. Although their exact mechanism of action in asthma is not known, it is believed that corticosteroids potentiate the effects of bronchodilators and reduce inflammation. Because inflammation is the predominant feature in asthma, an expert panel convened by the National Institutes of Health (1991) now recommends the use of anti-inflammatory drugs to reduce and prevent recurrence rather than reliance on drugs used to relieve bronchial constriction alone. With the availability of aerosol delivery and the subsequent decrease in dosage requirements, their use is considered safer and effective in severe asthmatics. Oral steroids are reserved for patients who do not respond to inhaled steroid therapy or for short courses during an acute attack. When used intravenously, steroids should be limited to use in life-threatening situations. Dosages and choice of steroid vary, but generally the sicker the patient, the higher the dosage. There is a delay of about 6 hours before clinical and laboratory evidence of improvement in air flow is seen with the use of intravenous prednisone or hydrocortisone (MacDonnell et al., 1987).

Sodium Cromoglycate (Cromolyn). Used most frequently in children, cromolyn is thought to be effective in asthma as a prophylactic agent. It has no role in an acute attack. Its effect lies in its ability to inhibit the release of histamine and other mediators from the mast cells. In adults, it may take 1 to 2 months to determine whether or not cromolyn is effective. Because of this potential delay in adequate therapy, use of inhaled steroids are recommended for adults instead.

Anticholinergics. Although anticholinergics do have a bronchodilating effect, their systemic side effects generally limit their use. Atropine is occasionally given in aerosol form in patients with intractable asthma when cholinergic stimulation is believed to play a role (Farzan, 1985).

VENTILATOR SUPPORT

Although the mainstay of the treatment of asthma is pharmaceutical, special attention must be paid to other aspects of patient care. The appearance of inadequate ventilation as evidenced by increasing fatigue, accessory muscle use, increasing Pa_{CO_2} arterial blood levels, obtundation, and refractory hypoxemia is clearly an indication of patient deterioration. These signs and symptoms indicate the need for intubation and mechanical ventilation. Intubation initially may irritate an already irritated airway; the use of topical lidocaine may prevent this and help to relax the tracheal smooth muscle.

The primary goal of ventilator management is to relieve hypoxemia with resultant stabilization of the cardiovascular and central nervous systems. Use of high levels of oxygen is not unusual initially, but $F_{I_{O_2}}$ levels should be carefully lowered following the crisis.

In some asthmatics increased secretions result in widespread mucous plugging, and some experts recommend segmental saline lavage through bronchoscopy. Evidence of infection should be managed with the appropriate antibiotics.

There may be a need to evaluate the patient for his ability to cope with this often frightening disease. In those who appear to have underlying emotional problems that may be partially responsible for triggering the attack, proper psychological counseling should be encouraged. With proper medical and nursing management, the majority of asthmatics should be able to lead normal lives.

Discussion of asthma would not be complete without including the problem of status asthmaticus. This condition is defined as "a severe asthmatic attack that does not respond to treatment with an adequate amount of commonly used bronchodilators . . . within a few hours" (Farzan, 1985). This life-threatening event can quickly lead to respiratory failure, and immediate hospitalization with institution of adequate hydration, intravenous aminophylline, large doses of intravenous corticosteroids, O_2 ther-

apy, and antibiotics if infection is present is necessary. If the patient's condition continues to deteriorate, intubation and ventilation are required (see Chap. 29).

Course and Prognosis

Approximately half of all patients with childhood asthma recover spontaneously. Beyond childhood, the incidence of spontaneous recovery lessens. When the onset of asthma occurs in later life, most patients will continue to suffer with asthma all their lives. Many adults will have progressively more frequent attacks, with respiratory infections assuming a more important role. The chronic airway obstruction may be mistaken for chronic bronchitis. The literature differs as to whether asthma may actually predispose the patient to emphysema-like pathologic symptoms.

NURSING DIAGNOSIS

The use of nursing diagnoses as a basis for planning nursing care for critically ill patients is still relatively new to some nurses. Although still in its infancy, the theoretical and research bases for the use of nursing diagnoses are progressing rapidly. The Seventh Conference on the Classification of Nursing Diagnoses (March, 1986) in conjunction with the North American Nursing Diagnoses Association (NANDA) approved a list of diagnoses that included three diagnoses with specific reference to problems frequently seen in patients with chronic obstructive pulmonary disease. These diagnoses are:

1. Ineffective airway clearance
2. Ineffective breathing pattern
3. Impaired gas exchange

In addition to these, Carpenito (1987) has suggested a new diagnostic category called potential alterations in respiratory function to describe patients whose entire respiratory system may be affected by their illness, and the cause of which cannot be attributed to one factor. For example, she states that "smoking, allergy, and immobility are examples of factors that affect the entire system and thus make it incorrect to say impaired gas exchange related to immobility, since immobility also affects airway clearance and breathing patterns" (Carpenito, 1987). She recommends that the nurse use one of the three accepted nursing diagnoses only when the nurse can, through her own interventions, affect the specific contributing factors (e.g., increased secretions, ineffective cough).

An example illustrating the use of one of these diagnoses is included in the nursing care plan.

ncp nursing care plan

1. Ineffective airway clearance related to:
Chronic air flow limitation
Ineffective cough

Outcome Criteria	Nursing Interventions

The patient will have increased air flow to both lungs and an effective cough as demonstrated by
1. Clear breath sounds
2. Objective improvement in vital signs, chest x-ray results, and pulmonary function flow rates
3. Effective cough techniques
	A. Assess for contributing factors
	  1. Thick secretions
	  2. Ineffective cough
	  3. Inadequate bronchodilator therapy
	  4. Presence of infection
	  5. Fatigue
	B. Reduce or eliminate the causes
	  1. Thick secretions
	    a. Administer humidifying agents as ordered
	    b. Perform/assist with percussion and postural drainage
	    c. Maintain adequate hydration, taking into account possible cardiac and renal contraindications
	    d. Encourage incentive breathing via incentive spirometer device
	    e. Administer bronchodilators as ordered
	    f. Observe for changes in amount, color, viscosity, and odor of sputum
	    g. Perform aseptic tracheal suctioning prn
	    h. Consider recommending therapeutic bronchoscopy if needed
	  2. Ineffective cough
	    a. Instruct patient on proper techniques of coughing and importance of proper coughing (therapeutic coughing)
	    b. Encourage frequent coughing following rest periods and after bronchodilator or humidifying treatments
	    c. Observe effects of coughing on vital signs
	    d. Maximize positioning for coughing and air flow
	    e. Ambulate patient as tolerated to facilitate expectoration
	  3. Inadequate bronchodilator therapy
	    a. Monitor subjective and objective responses to medication (cough, flow rates on spirometry, dyspnea, breath sounds, ABGs)
	    b. Consider timing medication to coincide with activities
	    c. Educate patient about medication regimen (drugs, dosages, side effects, reasons for being prescribed); assess for compliance
	    d. Consult with physician and/or pharmacist to evaluate effectiveness of prescribed regimen
	  4. Presence of infection
	    a. Identify usual cough, secretions to establish baseline
	    b. Monitor vital signs indicative of infection (respiratory rate, pulse, temperature)
	    c. Assess chest x-ray for indications of abnormalities
	    d. Send sputum specimen for culture and sensitivity as needed
	    e. Maintain medication regimen as ordered
	    f. Encourage incentive breathing and therapeutic coughing
	  5. Fatigue
	    a. Plan activities around frequent rest periods
	    b. Allow rest periods after coughing and prior to meals
	    c. Minimize causes of ineffective coughing (assess environmental irritants, e.g., allergens, smoking)
	    d. Provide periods of uninterrupted rest
	    e. Restrict visitors if necessary
	    f. Instruct patient on energy conservation measures

SUMMARY

The respiratory-compromised patient presents many challenges to the nursing profession. More than ever before, nurses must be knowledgeable, compassionate clinicians able to assess, diagnose, and plan interventions that will assist the patient to his maximum potential. This practitioner must also be able to evaluate the selected interventions and alter them when the established outcome criteria are not being met. In addition, the nurse must provide this care within a cost-conscious environment. This chapter has been intended to assist the nurse in meeting the needs of the patient, family, and facility caring for patients with chronic obstructive pulmonary disease.

References

Barnes, C., and Kirchoff, K. (1986). Minimizing hypoxemia due to endotracheal suctioning. *Heart & Lung*, 15(2), 164–176.

Burrows, B., Neden, A. V., Fletcher, C. M., et al. (1964). Clinical types of COLD in London and Chicago. *American Review of Respiratory Diseases*, 90, 14.

Carpenito, L. J. (1987). *Nursing diagnosis: application to clinical practice*. Philadelphia: J.B. Lippincott.

Chin, R., and Pesce, R. (1983). Practical aspects in management of respiratory failure in chronic obstructive pulmonary disease. *Critical Care Quarterly*, 6(2), 1–21.

Clark, T. (1986). Chronic asthma. In R. Cherniack (Ed.), *Current Therapy of Respiratory Disease* (Vol. 2, pp. 102–105). Philadelphia: B.C. Decker.

Dornhorst, A. C. (1955). Respiratory insufficiency. *Lancet*, 1, 1185.

Farzan, S. (1985). *A concise handbook of respiratory diseases*. Reston, VA: Reston Publishing Co.

Higgens, M. (1984). Epidemiology of COPD: State of the art. *Chest*, 85(6), 3s–8s.

Hodgkin, J., and Petty, T. (1987). *Chronic obstructive pulmonary disease: Current concepts*. Philadelphia: W.B. Saunders.

Kersten, L. D. (1989). *Comprehensive respiratory nursing*. Philadelphia: W.B. Saunders.

Lefioe, N. M., Ashley, M. J., Pederson, L. L., et al. (1984). The health risks of passive smoking. *Chest*, 1, 90–95.

MacDonnell, K., Fahey, P., and Segal, M. (1987). *Respiratory intensive care*. Boston: Little, Brown.

Petty, T. (1986). Chronic bronchitis. In R. Cherniack (Ed.), *Current therapy of respiratory disease* (Vol. 2, pp. 119–122). Philadelphia: B. C. Decker.

Robin, E. D., and O'Neill, R. P. (1963). The fighter versus the non-fighter. *Archives of Environmental Health*, 7, 125.

Snider, G. L., Kleinerman, J., Thurlbeck, W. M., et al. (1985). The definition of emphysema: *American Review of Respiratory Disease*, Report of a National Heart, Lung and Blood Institute, Division of Lung Disease Workshop, 132, 182–185.

Task Force Report on Epidemiology of Respiratory Diseases. (1980). NIH Publication No. 81-2019. Washington, D.C.: U.S. Dept. of Health and Human Services.

Tisi, G. (1983). *Pulmonary physiology in clinical medicine* (2nd ed.). Baltimore: Williams & Wilkins.

Weinberger, S. (1992). *Principles of pulmonary medicine*. (2nd ed.). Philadelphia: W.B. Saunders.

28

Patients with Pulmonary Infections

Catherine J. Ryan

The respiratory tree is kept free of infection by the normal airway defense mechanisms. These mechanisms include the cough reflex; ciliary activity; secretion of mucous lysosome, lactoferrin, and immunoglobulins; phagocytic cells; and the lung parenchyma containing the lymphatic system. Failure of one or more of the components of the pulmonary defense system may result in a pulmonary infection. Stratton (1986) has identified six possible mechanisms of infection of the lung: aspiration, colonization, inhalation, inoculation, direct spread from contiguous sites, and hematogenous spread.

INCIDENCE

It is estimated that 15% of hospital associated deaths are related to pulmonary infection (Gross et al., 1980). During the past decade dramatic changes have occurred in the types of patients with pulmonary infections requiring intensive care as well as in the infecting organisms. The significance of these phenomena is demonstrated in the changing population seen in hospitals today. Persons with cancer who are immunosuppressed are surviving to develop infections, organ transplantation is more common, cardiovascular surgical procedures are being performed more frequently, and persons have emerged with autoimmune deficiency syndrome. People with health problems not encountered in the past and who certainly would never have survived are now patients in our intensive care units. Additionally, the elderly population is growing at a dramatic rate. Serious respiratory infections are common in elderly patients and constitute the fourth leading cause of death in persons 65 years of age and older (Hawley, 1986).

PNEUMONIA

Pneumonia is an inflammation of the lung parenchyma caused by any one of a large number of etiologic factors. It is the fourth leading cause of death in the United States and the most common cause of death from infection (Finegold and Johnson, 1975). Nosocomial pneumonia represents 10 to 20% of all nosocomial infections (Simons and Wong, 1983) and may cause up to 60% of all deaths attributed to nosocomial infection (Gross et al., 1980). Each of the pneumonias has characteristic clinical findings. The critical care nurse can make a significant contribution to patient care and cost containment through prevention and early identification of patients with pneumonia.

In the literature, pneumonias have been categorized in a multitude of ways. Clinically, the presentation of pneumonia can be divided into two categories: bacterial pneumonias and atypical pneumonias. Classification of pneumonia into these two categories is important for selection of the appropriate method of treatment and for prediction of outcome. Tables 28–1 and 28–2 summarize the causative organisms for various types of pneumonia.

Pathophysiology

COMMON BACTERIAL PNEUMONIAS

Bacteria cause half of the cases of adult pneumonia. Bacterial pneumonia is most commonly seen in the elderly population and may be caused by a number of different organisms. Any anatomic or physiologic alteration in the tracheobronchial tree or in the defenses of the host increases the risk of infection to

TABLE 28–1. Etiology of Bacterial Pneumonias

Gram-Positive Cocci	Gram-Positive Rods
Streptococcus pneumoniae	Nocardia species
Staphylococcus aureus	Actinomyces species
Streptococcus pyogenes	Bacillus anthracis
Anaerobes: Peptococcus, Peptostreptococcus	

Gram-Negative Cocci	Gram-Negative Rods
Neisseria meningitidis	Haemophilus influenzae
	Klebsiella pneumoniae
	Pseudomonas aeruginosa
	Escherichia coli
	Acinetobacter species
	Serratia species
	Proteus species
	Enterobacter species
	Legionella species
	Anaerobes: Bacteroides species, Fusobacterium nucleatum

the lungs. Causative organisms may enter the lungs in a variety of ways. Many of the organisms that are capable of invading the lungs are components of the oro- or nasopharyngeal flora in states of health and disease (Austrian, 1986). The most common cause of pneumonia is aspiration of oropharyngeal or gastric secretions, including their flora, into the lower respiratory tract (Bjornson, 1987).

Streptococcus pneumoniae. Streptococcus pneumoniae (commonly referred to as pneumococcal pneumonia) is a major cause of community-acquired bacterial pneumonia (Gross and Levine, 1983). It is spread via inhalation of droplets or air-borne nuclei, or it may enter the pharynx from the skin through direct contact. Aspirated bacteria lodge in the upper airway and produce local edema with transudation into the alveoli. Transudation produces pulmonary congestion as well as an environment in which pneumococci may multiply. Adjacent capillaries become congested, and red cells as well as polymorphonuclear leukocytes appear in the alveoli (red hepatization). Later, polymorphonuclear leukocytes ingest the pneumococci and fibrin precipitates in the alveoli (gray hepatization). Finally, there is resolution with

TABLE 28–2. Etiology of Atypical Pneumonias

Viruses	Mycoplasma
Paramyxovirus	Mycoplasma pneumoniae
Respiratory syncytial virus	
Parainfluenza virus types 1, 2, 3, and 4	**Protozoa**
	Pneumocystis carinii
Influenza viruses A and B	Toxoplasma gondii
Adenovirus	
Rhinovirus	**Other**
Varicella-zoster virus	Strongyloides species
Herpes simplex virus	
Measles virus	
Coxsackie viruses A and B	
Echovirus	
Cytomegalovirus	

complete healing as macrophages clear the particulate debris, fibrin, and remaining bacteria (Lerner and Jankauskas, 1975). Mortality from this type of bacterial pneumonia is 10 to 20% overall and 50% in those who are debilitated (Rytel, 1983).

Staphylococcal Pneumonia. Staphylococcal pneumonia occurs most often as a secondary infection with or following influenza. It is frequently seen in infants and children under the age of 3 and in persons who are chronically ill. *Staphylococcus pneumoniae* usually enters the respiratory tract through inhalation of contaminated air or after aspiration of carrier staphylococci from the nasopharynx. It may also enter the lungs after bacteremia from a septic focus elsewhere in the body. There are two types of staphylococcal pneumonia, acute hemorrhagic and subacute.

Acute hemorrhagic staphylococcal pneumonia is most frequently seen in association with influenza. In this type, the bronchi and bronchioles are stripped of their mucosa, and their walls are infiltrated with polymorphonuclear leukocytes, histiocytes, and fibrin. Abscesses may form and rupture into the pleural space to form a fistula or pneumothorax. Empyemas are not an uncommon complication.

Subacute staphylococcal pneumonia causes the lungs to become heavy and engorged with a moderate amount of thin fluid present in the pleural cavity. The trachea and bronchi become filled with plugs of yellow-gray tenacious exudate. Abscesses that communicate with the bronchi and bronchioles may develop as a complication.

Gram-Negative Pneumonias. Gram-negative pneumonia, which carries the highest mortality (Hawley, 1986), is frequent in the elderly as well as the chronically ill populations. It is most often attributed to aspiration of oropharyngeal contents. Colonization of the lungs may result from the use of broad-spectrum antibiotics in patients with endotracheal tubes. The patient with gram-negative pneumonia may follow a chronic course with a slow response to treatment. Healing results in fibrosis of lung tissue and loss of functional lung volume. Destruction of lung tissue with abscess formation is a frequent complication (Biller, 1987).

NOSOCOMIAL PNEUMONIA

Nosocomial pneumonia is an infection of the lower respiratory tract involving the pulmonary parenchyma that develops in hospitalized patients (Stratton, 1986). Recent statistics reveal that nosocomial pneumonia is the second most frequent cause of hospital-acquired infection in the United States (Centers for Disease Control, 1986) and the leading cause of mortality directly related to nosocomial infection (Gross et al., 1980). Although nosocomial pneumonias may be caused by any bacterial, viral, or fungal organism, they are most frequently gram-negative bacterial bronchopneumonias (Pugliese and Lichtenberg, 1987). Celis and colleagues (1988) noted that hospital-acquired infection with *Pseudomonas aeruginosa* and *Enterobacter* species as well as other gram-negative bacilli, *Streptococcus faecalis*, *Staphylococcus aureus*, *Candida* species, *Aspergillus* species, and polymicrobial episodes of pneumonia carried a particularly high risk of mortality.

Critically ill patients are most likely to acquire nosocomial pneumonia due to their debilitated state, altered defenses, and frequent colonization of the upper airway with gram-negative bacilli. Many factors in the critical care environment contribute to the development of nosocomial pneumonia, including tracheal intubation, a depressed level of consciousness allowing for aspiration of oropharyngeal secretions, underlying chronic lung disease, thoracic or upper abdominal surgery, prior episodes of large-volume aspiration, advanced age, poor oral hygiene, and inhibition of the normal cough mechanism. Endotracheal intubation is the most commonly named risk factor for nosocomial pneumonia (Bjornson, 1987; Pugliese and Lichtenberg, 1987) because the endotracheal tube bypasses the upper airway and the host defense mechanisms of nasopharyngeal filtration and mucociliary clearance. These tubes and related respiratory procedures such as suctioning may also create mechanical irritation or injury to the mucosa, predisposing the lungs to inoculation and colonization with bacteria. Respiratory therapy equipment and the people who care for the equipment may also contaminate the respiratory tract. Widespread and inappropriate use of antibiotics has also been implicated as a predisposing factor in the development of nosocomial pneumonia. Antibiotics cause suppression of the normal upper airway flora, which may permit colonization with drug-resistant organisms.

ATYPICAL PNEUMONIAS

Viral Pneumonia. Viruses are a common cause of community-acquired pneumonia but may also cause pneumonia in patients who are already hospitalized. Paramyxoviruses are most common in younger populations, and influenza A or B virus is more common in adults (Belshe, 1986). Transmission occurs by inhalation of aerosolized virus. The virus enters the respiratory tract, attaches to columnar epithelial cells, and replicates in a cycle of 4 to 6 hours. Particles of the replicated virus are shed, causing illness to occur 18 to 72 hours after exposure to the virus. The severity of the illness correlates with the quantity of the virus shed and the number of ciliated columnar epithelial cells that are killed as a result of viral replication (Belshe, 1986). Severe forms of viral pneumonia are more common in pregnant women and persons with cardiovascular disease. It carries a high mortality because it progresses rapidly to a clinical picture of adult respiratory distress syndrome (ARDS).

The denuded airway is also more susceptible to colonization and infection by bacteria. The phenomenon of secondary bacterial infection in viral pneumonia is more commonly noted in patients with underlying chronic pulmonary disease and in the elderly population. Pneumococcus (*Streptococcus*) and *Staphylococcus aureus* are the secondary bacterial organisms most frequently isolated.

Mycoplasmal Pneumonia. Mycoplasmal pneumonia is the most common cause of atypical pneumonia and is the prototype of "walking pneumonia." It is more common in young adults than in children or the elderly. The disease is transmitted through droplets in the air and frequently spreads from one family member to another. Exactly how mycoplasmas cause local irritation of the pulmonary tissue is not clear (Pennington, 1981). Direct damage to the pulmonary tissue may not be as significant as the production of an antigen through the immune system. The clinical course of the disease is usually benign and self-limiting.

Pneumocystis carinii. *Pneumocystis carinii* pneumonia is an opportunistic infection in which the infecting organism is a protozoan. Until the discovery of acquired immune deficiency syndrome (AIDS) in 1981, the infection was noted primarily in severely immunosuppressed persons who were undergoing chemotherapy. Since that time it has become possibly one of the most well known and most commonly recognized opportunistic pulmonary infections, causing pneumonia at least once in 50% to 90% of all AIDS patients (Murray et al., 1987) and recurring in 30% to 50% of AIDS patients per year (Rankin et al., 1988). *Pneumocystis carinii* is primarily an alveolar process (Rankin et al., 1988). Studies suggest that this infection in the AIDS patient may be attributed to reactivation of a latent infection (Hughs, 1982; Meuwissen et al., 1977; Pifer et al., 1978). Persons with AIDS possess complex immunologic abnormalities that encompass all arms of the immune system (Rankin et al., 1988). Macrophages and monocytes are antigen-presenting cells that are required for optimal immune responses to invading pathogens. Studies suggest that the alveolar macrophage-monocyte system in patients with AIDS does not function normally and produces a local pulmonary immune deficit (Rankin et al., 1988), which allows the lungs to be infected with *Pneumocystis carinii*.

Clinical Presentation (Figs. 28–1 and 28–2)

The clinical presentation of the patient with pneumonia is varied because unique properties of the interaction between the host and the organism determine the presentation. Pneumonia may present with an acute or chronic onset and a productive or dry cough. The patient may be cyanotic or tachypneic. The chest film may reveal lobar consolidation

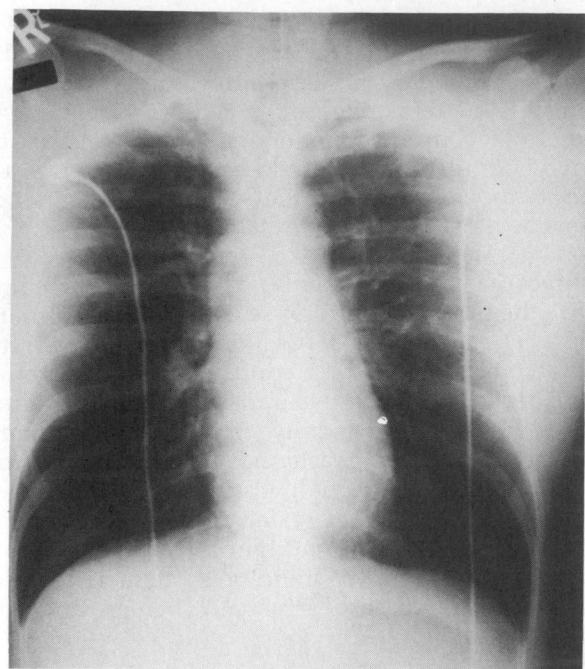

FIGURE 28–1. Chest x-ray of a female patient with bacterial pneumonia. There is a prominent infiltrate in the right base and atelectasis in the left upper lobe.

or scattered interstitial infiltrates, or it may be normal in appearance. Pneumonia generally requires a combination of clinical observations and microbiologic and radiographic findings to be diagnosed accurately. Signs and symptoms of infection may be absent in the immunocompromised patient.

PHYSICAL ASSESSMENT

Bacterial Pneumonia. The patient with pneumococcal pneumonia presents with a sudden onset of illness that includes shaking chills, fever of 102° to 105°F, and a cough that is initially dry but becomes productive of rusty sputum early and yellow green sputum later. Rusty sputum is due to a mixture of red blood cells and inflammatory cells in infected alveoli. The patient may be dyspneic, tachypneic, tachycardiac, cyanotic, and have pleuritic chest pain. Accompanying symptoms include malaise, weakness, headache, myalgia, and possibly cyanosis, depending on the degree of respiratory compromise. The elderly patient may also present with an altered mental state and dehydration. Complications involve dissemination of the bacteria into a site other than the lungs, causing meningitis, endocarditis, empyema, disseminated intravascular coagulation (DIC), lung abscess, and nephritis. Infection with *Haemophilus influenzae* may mimic pneumococcal pneumonia.

Chest examination in the patient with pneumococcal pneumonia will reveal consolidation that is manifested by dullness to percussion, increased tactile fremitus (palpable vibrations transmitted through the bronchopulmonary system to the chest wall when the patient speaks), bronchophony (voice sounds louder and clearer than usual because the higher pitched components are better transmitted through airless lung tissue), coarse inspiratory rales, egophony ("ee" to "ay" change because of altered filtration of sound), and whispered pectoriloquy (whispered sounds louder and more clearly heard than normal because of enhanced transmission through airless lung tissue), indicating that air is being replaced with exudate and crepitant rales. A friction rub may be present. Pneumococcal pneumonia takes some time to resolve, with consolidation in the lungs taking up to 6 weeks to clear completely.

Staphylococcal pneumonia has an insidious onset in chronically ill and elderly patients and an acute onset in infants. High fever with chills may last up to 1 week in severe cases despite the use of antibiotics. Cough with blood-streaked sputum production and tachypnea with cyanosis occur early in the course of the disease. Lung abscesses and pneumatoceles are not uncommon with this form of pneumonia (Smith and Hartz, 1986).

Gram-negative bacterial pneumonia has a highly variable clinical presentation depending on the underlying condition of the patient and the infecting organism. It may progress slowly or rapidly over a few days. Patients will have fever with cough that is productive of purulent sputum and pleuritic chest pain as with other bacterial pneumonias. Mortality is most often related to concomitant host disease rather than to the type of gram-negative infection.

Atypical Pneumonia. In contrast to bacterial pneumonia, only 50% of patients with viral pneumonia show clinical manifestations. Those that do have a gradual onset of symptoms and a milder course of illness. Headache is often the first symptom (Fuller,

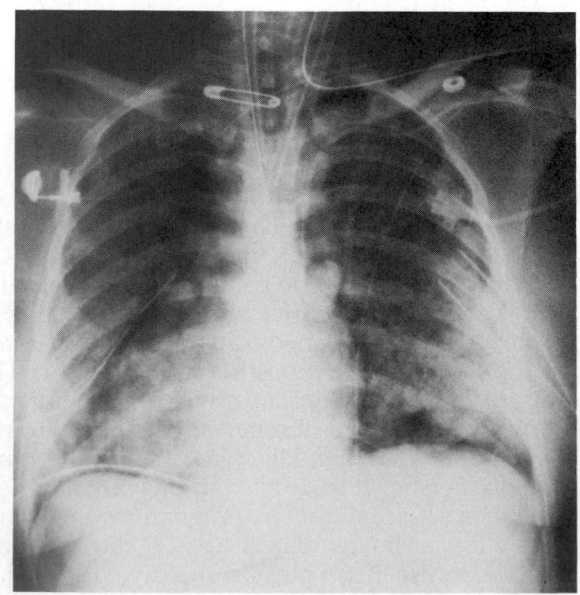

FIGURE 28–2. Chest x-ray of a female patient with viral pneumonia showing diffuse interstitial infiltrates bilaterally.

1986), which may be followed by rhinorrhea, dry cough, low-grade fever without chills, pharyngitis, and muscle pain. Myalgias are the hallmark of influenza A (Belshe, 1986). If sputum is present, it will be scanty and nonpurulent. Chest examination of the patient with viral pneumonia will reveal rales and rhonchi. In fulminating cases of viral pneumonia, however, the alveoli are filled with fibrin, fluid, red blood cells, and macrophages, causing profound hypoxemia that may respond poorly to oxygen administration.

Symptoms of mycoplasmal pneumonia appear gradually and are nonspecific, including fever without chills, nonproductive cough, headache, myalgia, arthralgia, and general malaise. Diffuse pleuritic chest pain on inspiration occurs rarely. Mycoplasmal pneumonia is frequently associated with pharyngitis and bullous myringitis.

Pneumocystis carinii presents with nonspecific chronic respiratory symptoms, which are usually present for some time before the patient seeks medical attention. The symptoms include a nonproductive cough, fever, and dyspnea (Murray et al., 1987). The patient with *Pneumocystis carinii* infection may have inspiratory crackles but frequently has normal breath sounds (Rankin et al., 1988). The patient may be tachypneic.

LABORATORY FINDINGS AND DIAGNOSTIC PROCEDURES

Sputum evaluation is a critical part of the evaluation of the patient with pneumonia. The nurse must be extremely careful when collecting the sputum sample to avoid collection of saliva because it may be colonized with many of the organisms that cause pneumonia and may be misleading. Early morning specimens are preferred because secretions that have pooled during the night can be mobilized. A sputum sample with more than 25 polymorphonuclear leukocytes and less than 10 buccal squamous epithelial cells per $100\times$ field is considered to be from the lower respiratory tract and to be diagnostic of pneumonia (Biller, 1987; Gleckman, 1983). If it is impossible to collect an acceptable specimen using traditional methods (cough or suction through an endotracheal or nasotracheal tube), the physician may elect to use more invasive means such as transtracheal aspiration (operating on the assumption that the lower airway is sterile), fiberoptic bronchoscopy, or open lung biopsy.

Bacterial Pneumonia. Initial therapy of the patient with bacterial pneumonia is determined by the Gram stain of the sputum and later verified by the culture. Arterial blood gases may be normal or show significant desaturation, depending on the extent of the pneumonia and the presence of other pulmonary pathology. Other laboratory tests helpful in diagnosis may include a complete blood count (CBC), blood cultures, and antigen assays of body fluids. The

white blood cell count is usually elevated (12,000 to 30,000/mL) but may be normal in debilitated persons (Rytel, 1983). If a significant pleural effusion is seen on the chest x-ray, thoracentesis is indicated to obtain a sample for culture of the pleural fluid (Biller, 1987).

The chest x-ray of the patient with pneumococcal pneumonia classically shows a dense infiltrate of one or more lobes or the pattern of bronchopneumonia (a "patchy" pattern) with no consolidation. This pattern may not be seen in the patient with underlying chronic obstructive pulmonary disease (COPD).

In the patient with gram-negative pneumonia, the chest x-ray shows interstitial infiltrates early in the course of the disease that may be unilateral or bilateral and rapidly progress to consolidation, a clinical picture that may be confused with congestive heart failure and atelectasis.

Atypical Pneumonia. Traditional laboratory tests will not reveal a diagnosis in patients with viral pneumonia. The total leukocyte count may rise, with neutrophilia and relative lymphopenia within the first 48 hours, but it will quickly return to normal (Belshe, 1986). Therefore, if the white blood cell count is performed early in the course of the disease, it will not be significantly elevated. Arterial blood gases usually show no arterial desaturation. Although viral pneumonia may be suspected clinically, the diagnosis can be confirmed only with serologic studies, which may take several days to complete. The chest x-ray of the patient with viral pneumonia will show scattered and diffuse interstitial infiltrates involving one or more lobes. Infiltrates are most common in the lower lobes and represent inflammation of pulmonary interstitial areas.

In mycoplasmal pneumonia the chest x-ray shows segmental areas of consolidation that are usually isolated in the lower lobes. The sputum Gram stain will not reveal a particular organism in mycoplasmal pneumonia. Definitive diagnosis is by sputum culture, which requires 5 days of incubation. The leukocyte count is normal or only mildly elevated. Serum cold agglutinins, which were previously used as a diagnostic tool for mycoplasmal pneumonia, are not specific because they may be elevated in adenovirus or influenza virus infections and other conditions. Complement fixation titers are now recommended; these often show a fourfold rise in titer between acute and convalescent specimens (Gross and Levine, 1983).

Pneumocystis **Pneumonia.** In the patient with AIDS, more than one organism is frequently involved in the pulmonary pathology, and thus the diagnosis of *Pneumocystis carinii* pneumonia may not be classic. Evaluation of a sputum specimen is the first procedure to be done; it may be diagnostic in as many as 70% of cases (Bigby et al., 1986; Pitchenik et al., 1986). Arterial oxygen tension may be normal or low when the patient is breathing room air. The amount of pulmonary involvement by *Pneumocystis carinii* is best evaluated through pulmonary function studies, which will show changes consistent with diffuse alveolar disease. These changes include decreases in total lung capacity (TLC) and vital capacity (VC), an increase in expiratory flow rates, and a decrease in single breath diffusing capacity for carbon monoxide (Hopewell and Luce, 1985; Murray et al., 1987).

Medical Management

Medical management of the patient with pneumonia is specific to the needs of the individual patient. In addition to providing appropriate antibiotic therapy, it includes providing respiratory and nutritional support, managing fluids and electrolytes, treating concomitant medical disorders, and managing pulmonary and extrapulmonary complications. Pulmonary treatment begins with providing humidified oxygen. Arterial blood gases must be evaluated and supplemental oxygen provided as necessary. Significant oxygen desaturation with a P_{O_2} of less than 60 mm Hg and a rising P_{CO_2} indicate that the patient may need to be intubated and provided with the respiratory support of a ventilator. Chest physical therapy is beneficial in mobilizing and promoting expectoration of secretions. Postural drainage is useful when there are large quantities of sputum (Smith and Hartz, 1986).

PHARMACOLOGIC TREATMENT

Table 28–3 summarizes the pharmacologic treatment commonly recommended for pneumonia. Pneumococcal pneumonia is one type of pneumonia that has a vaccine available. It is recommended prophylactically in high-risk groups, including the elderly and those with chronic lung disease, congestive heart failure, renal failure, alcoholism, cirrhosis, splenic dysfunction or splenectomy, Hodgkin's disease, myeloma, and other immunocompromised states. The vaccine should be given only once to adults to avoid significant adverse reactions. Influenza vaccines are also available.

Nursing Management

The previous discussion has demonstrated that nearly all patients admitted to the critical care unit who do not have a pulmonary infection have a potential to develop pneumonia. With this in mind, nursing management must be aimed first at preventing pneumonia. The nurse must be aware of the risk factors previously described and the susceptible patient population. When caring for patients in these populations careful attention must be paid to aseptic technique, including handwashing and handling of respiratory equipment, to prevent cross-contamination to susceptible patients. In addition, pulmonary hygiene measures of frequent turning, coughing, and

TABLE 28–3. Organisms Causing Pneumonia and Commonly Prescribed Treatments

Organism	Antibiotic
Streptococcus pneumoniae (Pneumococcus)	Penicillin Alternate: erythromycin, cephalosporin
Staphylococcus aureus	Nafcillin Alternate: vancomycin, cephalosporin
Haemophilus influenzae	Ampicillin Alternate: trimethoprim-sulfamethoxazole
Escherichia coli	Gentamicin Alternate: ampicillin, cephalosporin
Klebsiella pneumoniae	Gentamicin with cephalosporin Alternate: choramphenicol
Pseudomonas aeruginosa	Gentamicin and penicillin Alternate: gentamicin with cephalosporin
Mycoplasma pneumoniae	Erythromycin Alternate: tetracycline
Legionella	Erythromycin with or without rifampin
Pneumocystis carinii	Trimethoprim-sulfamethoxazole (TMP-SMX) with or without pentamidine

deep breathing exercises must be facilitated. Assessment of the airway protective mechanisms (cough, gag, and swallowing reflexes) is essential to identify patients who are at risk for aspiration of oral secretions as well as gastric contents. Positioning with the head of the bed elevated will decrease gastric reflux and facilitate swallowing. The supine position should be avoided. Careful and frequent assessment of temperature, pulse, respiratory rate, chest sounds, and chest x-ray along with observation of any sputum produced will assist the nurse in prompt identification of development of a pulmonary infection.

When a diagnosis of pneumonia has been made, the focus of nursing care will change to provision of appropriate therapy, maintenance of adequate oxygenation, and prevention of complications. Antibiotic therapy is the basis of medical therapy. The nurse is responsible for administering the appropriate therapy as well as monitoring the response to it.

Provision of respiratory support is essential in nursing a patient with a pulmonary infection. The additional pulmonary secretions produced have the potential to compromise the patency of the airway. Airway management techniques include assessment of the effectiveness of the cough, chest percussion and drainage for improved sputum clearance, and possibly nasotracheal or endotracheal suctioning for the patient who is unable to clear his own secretions. Provision of humidified oxygen liquifies the secretions and helps the patient mobilize secretions. Supplemental oxygen also helps to reverse hypoxemia and improves tissue oxygenation. The patient should also be placed in a comfortable position for breathing. Assessment techniques for evaluating the effectiveness of these measures include observing the respiratory rate and depth, use of accessory muscles for breathing, color and circulation, and evaluating the arterial blood gases. Tracheal intubation is necessary if the patient is unable to clear his own secretions or becomes hypoxemic despite the provision of supplemental oxygen.

The patient with a pulmonary infection may also have a poor oral intake and intravascular volume depletion related to increased insensible losses due to fever. Assessment of the patient's total volume status and provision of additional fluids are essential. If the patient is able to take oral fluids, the nurse should assess and provide the patient's fluid preferences. Most often, the febrile patient prefers cool fluids. Fruit juices provide the necessary fluids and help to replace electrolytes lost during diaphoresis. Intravenous fluid therapy is necessary if the patient is unable to ingest an adequate amount of oral fluids.

A number of nursing diagnoses may apply to the patient with pneumonia regardless of the cause. The nurse must choose which diagnoses apply when developing the patient care plan. The nursing care plan at the end of this chapter summarizes the potential nursing diagnoses and interventions needed for the patient with pneumonia.

LEGIONNAIRES' DISEASE

Pathophysiology

Legionnaires' disease is a type of gram-negative bacterial pneumonia that has an etiology and clinical course different from those of other gram-negative pneumonias. The bacterium termed *Legionella pneumophila* has four serologic groups (McKinney et al., 1979). It may present sporadically but is usually associated with an outbreak. Soil and water are the sources of the bacterium, and transmission is air borne with inhalation of the bacterium in contaminated soil, dust, or water. The incidence of legionnaires' disease typically is greatest in the summer and fall and is associated with specific buildings, geographic areas, and excavation (Kirby et al., 1980). The initial incubation period is 2 to 10 days (Kirby et al., 1980). Pathologically, legionnaires' disease resembles other forms of bacterial pneumonia. Intraalveolar exudation of polymorphonuclear leukocytes, macrophages, and fibrin occurs. Lysis of the inflammatory cells in association with large numbers of bacteria is unusual in bacterial pneumonia but is seen in *Legionella* pneumonia (Blackmon et al., 1978; Winn et al., 1978). Most victims are immunocompromised, but in patients with normal immunodefenses, *Legionella* infections are more likely to be acquired in the community by patients 50 years of age or older

who are heavy smokers or who have significant underlying disease (Wing, 1982).

Clinical Presentation

Legionella pneumophila infection may present as an asymptomatic seroconversion in which antibody titers and skin test become positive but symptoms of the disease never become manifest (Haley et al., 1979); as a mild, self-limiting, febrile illness characterized by headache, chills, and myalgia and unassociated with pneumonia; or as a severe, potentially fatal illness with progressive pneumonia that is known as legionnaires' disease. In the more serious cases of legionnaires' disease, the patient presents with anorexia, malaise, and weakness. Shaking chills with a high fever begin during the first 3 days of the illness and have a tendency to recur. A dry cough is present initially but then becomes productive of purulent and sometimes blood-tinged secretions. If chest pain is present it will be pleuritic. Watery diarrhea unassociated with blood, mucus, or abdominal cramping as well as nausea and vomiting may be present. In patients who die of legionnaires' disease, the cause of death is usually progressive respiratory insufficiency and hypotension (Kirby et al., 1980).

Examination of the chest is often normal at the onset of the illness. Rales will develop and may progress to consolidation as the disease progresses.

Laboratory Findings and Diagnostic Procedures

Traditional radiographic and laboratory findings are nonspecific. *Legionella* organisms are not identified on a sputum Gram stain. The CBC reveals a leukocytosis. Arterial blood gases reveal hypoxemia and hypocarbia commensurate with the amount of infiltrate on the chest x-ray. Hyponatremia is a common finding, as is elevated lactate dehydrogenase (LDH), alkaline phosphatase, aspartate aminotransferase (AST), and bilirubin. Antibody titers begin to rise by the third week (Kirby et al., 1980). Serologic testing with immunofluorescent antibody titers and direct fluorescent antibody stains are recommended for definitive diagnosis, but these results may take weeks. The initial chest x-ray typically reveals a unilobar, patchy alveolar infiltrate (Kirby et al., 1980), which rapidly progresses to consolidation (Dietrich et al., 1978; Fraser et al., 1977). Diagnosis is difficult because these patients may not produce sputum, and the organism does not grow in commonly used media (Wing et al., 1982). When diagnosis and treatment are delayed in the patient with *Legionella* infection, mortality becomes high. The principal diagnostic methods are open lung biopsy and retrospective serologic analysis and microbiologic techniques. Gleckman (1983) states that recovery of the organism from other organs, demonstration of the organism's presence in organs by means of immunofluorescence or special stains, and antigen detection in the urine may also be useful in the diagnosis of *Legionella pneumophila*.

Medical Management

The prognosis is related to the extent of underlying disease and timely initiation of appropriate therapy. These patients may be treated at home, and no special treatment is required unless the disease is severe and respiratory compromise is present. In these cases, medical management is similar to that used for patients with other forms of pneumonia, focusing on appropriate antibiotic therapy, maintenance of the airway and oxygenation, and prevention of complications.

Pharmacologic Treatment. Erythromycin 2 to 4 g/day given either intravenously or orally is the first line antibiotic therapy. Patients usually respond to this treatment within 2 to 3 days. If they fail to respond to erythromycin alone, oral rifampin 600 mg/day or double-strength sulfamethoxazole-trimethoprim may be added. Pharmacologic therapy is prolonged for 3 weeks because relapse is a problem if antibiotics are discontinued sooner (Kirby et al., 1980; Wing et al., 1982).

Nursing Management

The patient with *Legionella* infection is treated symptomatically in a manner similar to that of patients with other forms of pneumonia. The nursing diagnoses that may be chosen along with suggested nursing interventions are summarized in the nursing care plan at the end of this chapter.

TUBERCULOSIS

Pathophysiology

Tuberculosis is a serious pulmonary infection that is seen most frequently in large cities in areas of poverty and overcrowding (Wolinsky, 1983). It differs from the other bacterial pulmonary infections because it is a chronic condition. Modern treatment has resulted in lower mortality rates from tuberculosis. Persons with human immunodeficiency virus (HIV) appear to be at an increased risk for developing tuberculosis.

Tuberculosis is an infiltrative disease caused by the tubercle bacillus (*Mycobacterium tuberculosis*). It is spread by droplets emitted from persons infected with cavitary tuberculosis and is transmitted through the air and inhaled into the alveoli. In the alveoli the tubercle bacilli cause dilatation of the capillaries and moderate swelling of epithelial cells that contain phagocytized tubercle bacilli. The organism proliferates and spreads to the regional lymph nodes and within several weeks disseminates hematogenously. In most instances, cell-mediated immunity to the organism develops, halting further bacterial replication. This prevents clinical development of the disease at that time even though live tubercle bacilli remain in the body. The remaining bacilli may proliferate and cause clinical disease when cell-mediated immunity is weakened long after the initial infection. When cell-mediated immunity does not halt bacterial replication, the organism will infiltrate the alveolar structures. Although the process is not completely understood, a process of necrosis termed caseation that is characteristic of tuberculosis may occur (Wolinsky, 1983). Infiltration usually occurs in the upper zones of the lung tissues (Pierson, 1988), creating inflammation. The tubercular lesion in the lung may persist as a granuloma, progress through caseation to tissue necrosis, or heal as a scar (Wade, 1982). Often the hilar lymph nodes are involved in the infection.

Clinical Presentation

In the early stages the patient may be asymptomatic. As the disease progresses, malaise, fatigue, weight loss, night sweats, cough, and hemoptysis develop. Hemoptysis may occur in patients with active infection or in those with old, inactive disease (Pierson, 1988).

Laboratory Findings and Diagnostic Procedures

The chest x-ray is variable but classically shows cavitary upper lobe infiltrates (Pierson, 1988). Diagnosis requires demonstration of the organism in sputum or cultures of other body fluids. A presumptive diagnosis is made when acid-fast bacilli can be demonstrated with special stains of sputum or other body fluids. A tuberculin skin test will be positive in most cases.

Medical Management

All hospitalized patients with tuberculosis should be isolated in a private room. Masks should be used if the patient is coughing or sneezing. The patient may be taken out of isolation after 7 to 10 days of appropriate pharmacologic treatment. Special pulmonary treatments are usually not necessary. If, however, the patient develops respiratory compromise, medical management is the same as it would be for a patient with pneumonia.

Pharmacologic Treatment. Active tuberculosis is

treated with at least two antituberculin drugs because of the presence of small numbers of organisms that are naturally resistant to any individual drug (Pierson, 1988). Isoniazid and rifampin are the most potent agents used to treat tuberculosis, but streptomycin, ethambutol hydrochloride, pyrazinamide, ethionamide, cycloserine, *p*-aminosalicylic acid, kanamycin, or capreomycin may be chosen instead. Treatment is continued for several months because the organism is slow growing and has long periods of inactivity.

Nursing Management

Nursing management is primarily aimed at prevention of disease and identification of asymptomatic individuals. Most persons with positive skin reactions to standard tuberculin tests have been infected but may not have clinical symptoms. Nurses may be instrumental in facilitating care, including encouraging adherence to the prolonged medication regimen and compliance with follow-up chest x-rays.

In the majority of cases, the primary nursing diagnosis is a knowledge deficit, which is summarized in the nursing care plan at the end of this chapter. In patients with active tuberculosis, the nursing diagnoses and management are the same as they are in patients with pneumonia.

ASPIRATION PNEUMONITIS

Pathophysiology

Aspiration pneumonitis occurs in three different forms: acute aspiration pneumonitis, also known as septic pneumonitis or Mendelson syndrome, chronic aspiration pneumonia, and lipoid pneumonia.

Acute aspiration pneumonitis is caused by inhalation of large amounts of gastric contents into the lungs, primarily hydrochloric acid, resulting in severe and almost instantaneous chemical pneumonitis. The pneumonitis is characterized by epithelial degeneration of the bronchi, pulmonary edema, hemorrhage, isolated areas of atelectasis, and necrosis of type I alveolar cells (Modell and Boysen, 1989). After 24 to 36 hours, alveolar consolidation occurs, and the airways may begin mucosal sloughing. Hyaline membrane appears after 48 hours. By 72 hours, resolution has begun with regeneration of bronchial epithelium (Modell and Boysen, 1989).

Chronic aspiration pneumonia leads to localized consolidation of dependent portions of the lungs or bilaterally in the midzones due to repeated aspiration of small quantities of infected pharyngeal secretions. It is common in alcoholics, drug abusers, and obtunded patients.

Lipoid aspiration pneumonia is a result of aspiration of milk or oil-based substances. It often occurs in elderly persons with swallowing defects.

Clinical Presentation

Gastric acid aspiration causes aspiration pneumonitis with a rapid onset of dyspnea, bronchospasm, wheezing, fever, leukocytosis, and production of frothy, nonpurulent sputum. This stage usually occurs within 2 hours of aspiration. In acute gastric acid aspiration, the patient may become severely hypoxic with normal or low P_{CO_2}. Hypoxemia is thought to be caused by a reflex airway closure in response to aspiration of fluid (Modell and Boysen, 1989). The chest x-ray shows infiltrates in the dependent lung segments (Bjornson, 1987). The endotracheal secretions have an acid pH.

Localized consolidation of dependent portions of the lungs is characteristic of chronic aspiration pneumonia. If aspiration is allowed to continue, necrosis and abscess formation are common.

In lipoid aspiration the chest x-ray shows chronic consolidation that resembles carcinoma. These patients may not appear particularly toxic, and often the clinical appearance is very similar to that of the patient with a mild case of bacterial pneumonia.

Medical Management

As soon as possible after aspiration, the airway must be suctioned to remove any aspirated material and stimulate coughing. Arterial blood gases and shunt studies are used to assess the degree of respiratory embarrassment. If the patient is alert, continuous positive airway pressure with a mask may be attempted to restore adequate P_{O_2}. Intubation with a cuffed endotracheal tube is recommended to restore adequate oxygenation and to protect the airway from further aspiration in the patient who is not able to manage his own secretions. Mechanical positive end-expiratory pressure ventilation (PEEP) may be necessary to reverse arterial hypoxemia. Fluid therapy is necessary to replace intravascular volume that is lost to pulmonary edema (extravascular fluid).

Pharmacologic Treatment. Bronchodilators are used for patients who develop bronchospasm as a result of aspiration. Patients with aspiration do not always develop an infectious pneumonia that can be treated with antibiotics, and therefore antibiotics are withheld until a specific organism can be identified.

Nursing Management

Nursing management of aspiration pneumonitis is aimed primarily at prevention. The nurse must carefully evaluate the ability of each patient to swallow and manage his own secretions. Careful attention should be paid to patients in high-risk groups, including those with a decreased level of consciousness, persons receiving tube feedings, and persons with neuromuscular disorders. Prophylactic endotracheal intubation may be suggested for individuals in this high-risk group. Appropriate positioning during feeding and procedures is essential. Elevation of the head of the bed will decrease gastropharyngeal reflux. Parenteral nutrition, gastrostomy, or jejunostomy feedings should be considered for patients who aspirate tube feedings despite appropriate positioning. Should identification and prevention techniques fail and the patient develop aspiration pneumonitis, the nursing diagnoses and orders for pneumonia will apply.

PULMONARY ABSCESSES

Pathophysiology

Pulmonary abscesses are necrotic areas of lung parenchyma containing purulent material. Necrosis of lung tissue is due to bacterial infection. The most common causes of lung abscess are the bacteria that normally colonize the upper airways. Smith and Hartz (1986) noted that *Staphylococcus aureus* and *Klebsiella pneumoniae* are commonly isolated from abscesses. Other causative conditions may be aspiration pneumonitis, which predisposes to lung abscess, and septic pulmonary emboli.

Lung abscesses have been classified traditionally on the basis of clinical observation. Acute and chronic pulmonary abscesses are differentiated by the duration of symptoms when the patient presents for treatment. Symptoms lasting 4 to 6 weeks prior to presentation classify the syndrome as chronic (Bartlett, 1983). Primary lung abscesses are usually seen in patients prone to aspiration or in previously healthy persons. Secondary abscesses are a complication of a local lesion such as pulmonary malignancy or systemic disease.

Clinical Presentation

Lung abscesses usually develop slowly, with symptoms developing and worsening over several weeks. The patient often presents with nonspecific symptoms associated with a background of aspiration, such as a history of alcoholism, sedation, narcotic abuse, coma, or general anesthesia. All of these conditions cause altered levels of consciousness and suppression of the cough reflex, which normally clears the airways. Periodontal disease also increases the amount of bacterial flora in the mouth and is associated with increased risk of lung abscess. The patient is febrile but does not have chills. The patient will have pleuritic chest pain with dyspnea, weakness, malaise, anorexia, and weight loss. Cough is present with production of purulent or bloody sputum. Often the sputum has an extremely foul odor.

Laboratory Findings and Diagnostic Procedures

Laboratory procedures include collection and identification of a specimen that is diagnostic of the pathogen involved. Initially, the chest x-ray may show a pattern of pneumonitis. The findings vary depending on the evolutionary stage of the abscess. The diagnosis of lung abscess is made through identification of an abscess cavity on chest x-ray and determination of a causative organism in a sputum culture. Anaerobic lung abscesses are most frequently located in lung segments favored by gravitational flow, making body position at the time of bacterial entry into the lungs significant (Bartlett, 1983).

Medical Management

Medical management of a pulmonary abscess is directed at eliminating the source of the infection and providing antibiotic therapy specific to the organism. Postural drainage and chest physical therapy assist in draining the abscess cavity. Bronchoscopy is recommended for patients with an atypical presentation or who show a poor response to antibiotic therapy. If traditional medical management fails to produce improvement, a lobectomy may be performed (Bartlett, 1983).

Pharmacologic Treatment. Penicillin given orally or parenterally is the unanimously agreed upon agent of choice for lung abscesses involving anaerobic bacteria. Other studies show that tetracycline and clindamycin are effective in treatment of chronic pulmonary abscess. Aerobic abscesses are treated with agents selected by results of sensitivity testing. The agent of choice is continued for an extended period of 4 to 8 weeks or until the chest x-ray is either clear or shows only a small, stable lesion.

Nursing Management

The patient with a pulmonary abscess most likely has significant underlying disease and may also already have been treated for pneumonia. Nursing management is directed toward maintenance of a patent airway and prevention of tissue hypoxemia. Possible nursing diagnoses and interventions are outlined in the nursing care plan.

ncp nursing care plan

1. Activity intolerance related to:
Generalized weakness
Bedrest or immobility
Hypoxemia
Other

Outcome Criteria	Nursing Interventions

Develop activity/rest pattern consistent with physiologic limitations	Protect patient from injury
	Active/passive range of motion
	Assess response to activity:
	    Dangle
	    Stand
	    Chair
	    Walk
	Plan care with rest periods
	Assist with use of aids:
	    Cane
	    Walker
	    Wheelchair
	Encourage patient participation in planning activities
	Teach safety measures to prevent injury
	Increase activity level gradually

2. Ineffective airway clearance related to:
Decreased energy and weakness
Tracheobronchial infection secretions
Other
Impaired swallowing reflexes

Outcome Criteria	Nursing Interventions
Patient will maintain a patent airway	Assess breath sounds, respiratory rate, and circulation Position patient to promote airway clearance Teach coughing and deep breathing techniques; reinforce performance of techniques Assess cough and gag reflexes Provide oxygen and humidity Suction prn, preoxygenate with 100% oxygen Evaluate need for additional respiratory treatments Turn every 2 hours Maintain hydration Evaluate need for or recommend medications to promote expectoration of secretions

3. Altered body temperature related to:
Infection

Outcome Criteria	Nursing Interventions

Patient attains normothermia	Check temperature every 2 hours
	Monitor intake and output
	Assess level of consciousness
	Assess need for antipyretics
	    Administer as ordered, note response
	Assess need for cooling mattress
	Assess and document:
	    Breath sounds
	    Urine output
	    Chilling
	    Skin turgor
	Provide tepid baths
	Provide mouth care

Nursing Care Plan continued on following page

4. **Potential for infection related to:**
   Inadequate pulmonary defense mechanisms
   Impaired immunity
   Environmental exposure

Outcome Criteria	*Nursing Interventions*
Patient is free of signs and symptoms of infection Sputum culture is negative Patient is afebrile Vital signs and WBC are within normal limits	Monitor vital signs, temperature, and breath sounds frequently Monitor sputum for changes in color, consistency, amount, and odor Limit use of antipyretics, which may mask fever Promote/provide oral hygiene Monitor CBC/WBC Use good handwashing and aseptic technique Monitor and provide appropriate foods and fluids Teach signs and symptoms of infection and appropriate intervention

5. **Potential for fluid volume deficit related to:**
   Diaphoresis
   Fever

Outcome Criteria	*Nursing Interventions*
Patient maintains adequate fluid volume and electrolyte balance	Monitor intake and output Weigh daily Provide meticulous skin care and oral care Assess skin turgor and mucous membranes Monitor laboratory values Push fluids Dietary consult Provide humidified oxygen Administer IV therapy as ordered

6. **Impaired gas exchange related to:**
   Bronchopulmonary secretions
   Infection
   Other

Outcome Criteria	*Nursing Interventions*
Patent airway Adequate alveolar ventilation and perfusion Arterial blood gases within normal limits for patient Normal respiratory rate	Provide oxygen and humidity as ordered Encourage cough and deep breathing Position for pulmonary drainage Assess airway patency Suction prn, preoxygenate with 100% oxygen Assess respiratory rate, quality, and pattern Assess color and circulation Assess and monitor breath sounds for signs and symptoms of obstruction Maintain fluid balance Monitor arterial blood gases and chest x-ray Assess presence and strength of gag, cough, and swallow reflexes

7. **Knowledge deficit related to:**
   Lack of exposure
   Lack of recall
   Misinterpretation of learning
   Other

Outcome Criteria	*Nursing Interventions*

Patient verbalizes signs and symptoms of infection
Patient seeks appropriate medical intervention
Patient complies with treatment plan
	Provide information on
	  Treatment
	  Risk factors
	  Avoidance of recurrence
	Assess learning level
	Reinforce medical treatment plan
	Provide written instructions
	Teach signs and symptoms of pulmonary infection
	Teach appropriate intervention

SUMMARY

Pulmonary infections remain a significant problem in the critical care environment despite recent advances in pharmacologic treatment and advances in nursing care. In fact, advances in treatment, including ventilatory support equipment, immunosuppressive therapy, and widespread use of antibiotics have created new populations at risk for the development of pulmonary infections. As noted earlier, nurses can make a significant contribution to patient care and cost-containment through early identification of persons at risk, proper preventive measures, and aggressive management of persons with pulmonary infections.

References

Austrian, R. (1986). Pneumococcal pneumonia: Diagnostic, epidemiologic, therapeutic and prophylactic considerations. *Chest,* 90, 738–743.

Bartlett, J. G. (1983). Lung abscess. In G. L. Baum, and E. Wolinsky (Eds.), *Textbook of pulmonary diseases* (3rd ed., pp. 595–603). Boston: Little, Brown.

Belshe, R. B. (1986). Viral respiratory disease in the intensive care unit. *Heart & Lung,* 15, 222–226.

Bigby, T. D., Margolskee, D., Curtis, J. L., et al. (1986). The usefulness of induced sputum in the diagnosis of *Pneumocystis carinii* pneumonia in patients with the acquired immunodeficiency syndrome. *American Review of Respiratory Disease,* 133, 515–518.

Biller, P. L. (1987). Diagnosis and management of acute bronchitis and pneumonia in the ambulatory setting. *Nurse Practitioner,* 12(10), 12–28.

Bjornson, H. S. (1987). Diagnosis and treatment of bacterial pneumonia in the intensive care unit: An overview. *Respiratory Care,* 32, 773–780.

Blackmon, J. A., Hicklin, M. D., Chandler, F. W., et al. (1978). Legionnaire's disease: Pathological and historical aspects of a "new" disease. *Archives of Pathological Laboratory Medicine,* 102, 337.

Celis, R., Torres, A., Gatell, J. M., et al. (1988). Nosocomial pneumonia: A multivariate analysis of risk and prognosis. *Chest,* 93, 312–324.

Centers for Disease Control (1986). Nosocomial infection surveillance, 1984. *Surveillance summaries,* 35, 17–29.

Dietrich, P. A., Johnson, R. D., and Fairbank, J. T. (1978). The radiograph in Legionnaires' disease. *Radiology,* 127, 577.

Finegold, S. M., and Johnson, C. C. (1975). Lower respiratory tract infection. *American Journal of Medicine,* 79(73), 687–694.

Fraser, D. W., Tsai, T. F., and Orenstein, W. (1977). Legionnaires' disease: Description of an epidemic of pneumonia. *New England Journal of Medicine,* 297, 1189.

Fuller, E. (1986). What's different about atypical pneumonia? *Patient Care,* 12(19), 14–47.

Gleckman, R. A. (1983). Antibiotic treatment of community-acquired pneumonia. *Practical Cardiology,* 9(4), 129–136.

Gross, P. A., Neu, H. C., and van Antwerpen, C. (1980). Deaths from nosocomial infections: Experience in a university and community hospital. *American Journal of Medicine,* 68, 219–223.

Gross, P. A., and Levine, J. F. (1983). *Rouche handbook of differential diagnosis* (pp. 1–25). Nutley, NJ: Rouche Laboratories.

Haley, C. E., Cohen, M. L., and Halter, J. (1979). Nosocomial Legionnaires' disease: A continuing common-source epidemic at Wadsworth Medical Center. *Annals of Internal Medicine,* 90, 583.

Hawley, H. B. (1986). Pulmonary infections in critical care medicine: Challenges and dilemmas. *Heart & Lung,* 15, 221–222.

Hopewell, P. C., and Luce, J. M. (1985). Pulmonary involvement in the acquired immunodeficiency syndrome. *Chest,* 87, 104–112.

Hughs, W. (1982). Natural mode of acquisition for de novo infection with *Pneumocystis carinii. Journal of Infectious Disease,* 145, 842–848.

Kirby, B. D., Snyder, K. M., and Meyer, R. D. (1980). Legionnaires' disease: Report of sixty-five nosocomially acquired cases and review of the literature. *Medicine,* 59(3), 188–205.

Lerner, A. M., and Jankauskas, K. (1975). The classic bacterial pneumonias. *Disease-a-Month,* February, 3–46.

McKinney, R. M., Thacker, L., and Harris, P. P. (1979). Four serogroups of Legionnaires' disease bacteria by direct immunofluorescence. *Annals of Internal Medicine,* 90:621, 1979.

Meuwissen, J. H., Taber, I., and Leewenberg, A. D. (1977). Parasitologic and serologic observations of infection with *Pneumocystis* in humans. *Journal of Infectious Disease,* 136, 43–49.

Modell, J. H., and Boysen, P. G. (1989). Pulmonary aspiration of gastric contents. In W. C. Shoemaker, W. L. Thompson, and P. R. Holbrook (Eds.), *Textbook of critical care medicine* (pp. 272–275). Philadelphia: W. B. Saunders.

Mostow, S. R. (1986). Pneumonia complicated by bacteremias: Therapeutic options. *Hospital Practice,* 12(21), 105–113.

Murray, J. F., Garay, S. M., and Hopewell, P. C. (1987). Pulmonary complications of the acquired immunodeficiency syndrome: An update. *American Review of Respiratory Disease,* 135, 504–509.

Pennington, J. E. (1981). *Mycoplasmas and human disease: A brief review.* Chicago: Abbott Laboratories.

Pierson, D. J. (1988). Tuberculosis. In J. M. Luce, and D. J. Pierson (Eds.), *Critical care medicine* (pp. 193–196). Philadelphia: W. B. Saunders.

Pifer, L. L., Hughs, W. T., and Stagno, S. (1978). *Pneumocystis carinii* infection: Evidence for high prevalence in normal and immunosuppressed children. *Pediatrics,* 65, 35–41.

Pitchenik, A. E., Ganjei, P., Torress, A., et al. (1986). Sputum examination for the diagnosis of *Pneumocystis carinii* pneumonia in the acquired immunodeficiency syndrome. *American Review of Respiratory Disease,* 133, 226–229.

Pugliese, G., and Lichtenberg, D. A. (1987). Nosocomial bacterial pneumonia: An overview. *American Journal of Infection Control,* 15, 249–265.

Rankin, J. A., Collman, R., and Daniele, R. P. (1988). Acquired immune deficiency syndrome and the lung. *Chest,* 94, 155–164.

Rytel, M. W. (1983). Pneumococcal pneumonia: Diagnosis and management. *Journal of Respiratory Diseases,* 4(9), 80–87.

Simons, B. P., and Wong, E. S. (1983). CDC guidelines for the prevention and control of nosocomial infections: Guidelines for prevention of nosocomial pneumonia. *American Journal of Infection Control,* 11, 230–233.

Smith, J., and Hartz, R. S. (1986). Bacterial infections of the thorax. *Critical Care Quarterly,* 9(3), 41–49.

Stratton, C. W. (1986). Bacterial pneumonias: An overview with emphasis on pathogenesis, diagnosis and treatment. *Heart & Lung,* 15, 226–244.

Wade, J. F. (1982). *Comprehensive respiratory care: Physiology and techniques* (3rd ed.). St Louis: C. V. Mosby.

Wing, E. J., Schafer, F. J., and Pasculle, A. W. (1982). The use of tracheal and pulmonary aspiration to diagnose *Legionella micdadei* pneumonia. *Chest,* 82, 705–707.

Winn, W. C., Glavin, F. L., Perl, D. P., et al. (1978). The pathophysiology of Legionnaires' disease: Fourteen fatal cases from the 1977 outbreak in Vermont. *Archives of Pathological Laboratory Medicine,* 102, 344–350.

Wolinsky, E. (1983). Tuberculosis. In G. L. Baum, and E. Wolinsky (Eds.), *Textbook of pulmonary diseases* (3rd ed., pp. 507–525). Boston: Little, Brown.

29

Advances in Mechanical Ventilation

John Wright
Peter R. Doyle
Gary Yoshihara

Mechanical ventilators have been used for decades to support the respiratory function of patients with various degrees of respiratory distress or failure. Patients who have weak or absent spontaneous respirations usually require mechanical support to assist in ventilation and oxygenation. Patients with post-cardiac or respiratory arrest, neurologic disease or trauma, drug overdose or postoperative anesthesia are a few examples of patients who may require mechanical support until spontaneous respirations resume. Because the ventilator is an integral and vital piece of life support equipment in the intensive care unit, it is important for the practitioner to know the basic concepts and applications of mechanical ventilation. In this chapter we will review the indications for and concepts of conventional mechanical ventilation and introduce new modalities currently in clinical use.

HISTORICAL OVERVIEW

For centuries, medical pioneers have experimented with the idea of artificially mimicking the respiratory function of the lungs to maintain human life. Twenty-eight centuries ago, reference to supportive ventilation appeared in the Bible.

And he put his mouth upon his mouth. . . . and the flesh of the child became warm.

II KINGS 4:34

The Biblical story of Elisha, who restored the life of a young boy, recognized the principle that respiratory function could be supported artificially (Burton et al., 1984). In the centuries to follow, many experiments were conducted with animal and human subjects using a variety of mechanical devices to support ventilation. Paracelsus in the sixteenth century placed a tube in the mouth of a patient and used a fireplace bellows to inflate the lungs and assist his ventilation. Similar experiments continued through the seventeenth and eighteenth centuries. Late in the 1800s the first successful use of an endotracheal tube was reported.

Modern mechanical ventilation was a result of the popularity and technology of the iron lung (negative pressure ventilation) developed by Drinker and Shaw in 1929 (Burton et al., 1984; Shapiro et al., 1982). The iron lung, used primarily for polio victims, provided ventilatory support without the use of endotracheal intubation or tracheostomy.

World War II introduced several devices that were later adapted and developed for mechanical ventilation. Continuous positive pressure breathing to increase the altitude tolerance of pilots was used during World War II and was later adapted for use in intermittent positive pressure ventilation (IPPV) (Burton et al., 1984). Positive pressure ventilation gained support and acceptance during and after World War II because of the questionable effectiveness of the negative pressure ventilators. This acceptance is thought to mark the beginning of the modern era of respiratory care (Burton et al., 1984; Shapiro et al., 1982).

Early ventilators were pressure-cycled or volume-cycled. Pressure-cycled ventilators were designed to terminate gas flow to the patient when the preset pressure was reached. The problems of this design included large air leaks and the fact that changes in the patient's airway resistance or lung compliance would result in delivery of inconsistent tidal volumes.

Early volume ventilators were designed to terminate the mechanical breath once the set tidal volume was delivered. These early volume ventilators often lacked the capability to detect patient disconnection or volume loss due to a leak. Up to this time both pressure- and volume-cycled ventilators were used in conjunction with cuffless tracheostomy and endotracheal tubes. The dangers of aspiration of gastric contents and the need to deliver the precise volume and pressures for cycling the ventilator into exhalation led to the development of cuffed tracheal tubes.

Mechanical ventilators have come a long way since the days of the cumbersome iron lung. Ventilators today incorporate space-age technology to regulate and monitor all ventilatory parameters. The newer ventilators are capable of performing all ventilator functions. Time-, pressure-, or volume-cycled ventilation can be performed by a single ventilator just by flipping a switch. Most modern ventilators are the result of a modification of basic techniques and modalities rather than new ideas, with the exception of high-frequency ventilators.

GENERAL VENTILATORY CONCEPTS

Indications for Mechanical Ventilation

Many factors affect the decision to institute mechanical ventilation, not the least of which is the fact that this invasive procedure is not without potentially harmful effects. It must also be understood that no mode of mechanical ventilation can or will cure a disease process but merely supports the patient until resolution of the symptoms is accomplished.

Although no absolute reasons exist for the institution of mechanical ventilation, there are some common indications. Mechanical failure, or failure of the normal respiratory neuromuscular system, often requires the institution of mechanical ventilatory support. This may occur in patients with neuromuscular diseases such as myasthenia gravis, Guillain-Barré syndrome, and poliomyelitis. Respiratory paralysis, whether immediate or gradual, often necessitates ventilatory support to maintain adequate alveolar ventilation. Musculoskeletal abnormalities, such as chest wall trauma (flail chest), may impede the function of respiratory mechanics and thus require ventilatory support. Similarly, dysfunction of the neuromuscular system, either from trauma, infectious lesions, central disorders, or progressive central nervous system diseases, often requires ventilatory support. Each of the different disease processes has different ventilatory requirements; however, in many cases prolonged mechanical ventilatory support will result.

Abnormalities of pulmonary gas exchange account for the majority of patients requiring mechanical ventilatory support. Obstructive lung disease in the form of asthma, chronic bronchitis, or emphysema may result in gas exchange impairment necessitating ventilatory support to oxygenate and ventilate the patient adequately. These patients offer a unique challenge in that they often have abnormal arterial blood gas values as their normal baseline and must be maintained within these new "normal values." Furthermore, they are at greater risk for respiratory muscle fatigue secondary to diaphragmatic nonuse.

Finally, patients undergoing general anesthesia and post–cardiac arrest patients often require ventilatory support until they have recovered from the initial insult. In all cases a complete understanding of airway management, the use of mechanical ventilators, and the implications of each disease process is required to ensure a successful outcome.

Negative Pressure Ventilation

The Drinker and Shaw tank-type ventilator of 1929 was the first negative pressure ventilator to be widely used for mechanical ventilation (Burton et al., 1984). Better known as the iron lung, this device utilized negative pressure applied to the outside of the patient's chest to cause a drop in the intrapulmonary pressure and flow of ambient air into the patient's lungs. Upon termination of the breath, the negative pressure applied to the chest would drop to zero, and the elastic recoil of the chest and lungs would permit passive exhalation. A tight-fitting cylinder completely engulfed the patient up to the neck, allowing the negative pressure generated by a pump to be exerted on the patient's chest. Although neither a tracheostomy nor an endotracheal tube was needed to maintain a patent airway, patient discomfort and inaccessibility by health care providers made the Iron Lung a less favorable form of mechanical ventilation. Furthermore, significant negative pressure exerted on the abdomen occasionally resulted in venous blood pooling in the lower torso, resulting in a decrease in cardiac output. Further developments in design led to the production of the "cuirass" or shell unit. This device consisted of a shell and soft bladder combination that covered the patient's chest only.

Although these types of ventilators gave way to positive pressure devices (because of inability to control tidal volumes accurately, patient inaccessibility, and difficulty in maintaining a tight seal around the chest), a resurgence in their use for specific situations has recently been seen. Some patients with neuromuscular disorders, especially those with residual muscular function, may benefit from nocturnal use of this type of ventilator because it does not require a tracheostomy with its inherent problems. Furthermore, some patients find that even full-time home ventilation may be attained using a chest cuirass.

Positive Pressure Ventilation

Reference can be found as early as biblical times to the use of positive pressure for purposes of respiration or ventilation. In recent history advances in the design and function of positive pressure devices have led to mechanical ventilators. Although the earlier models terminated the delivered breath when a preset pressure was achieved, more recent models are volume cycled (the breath is terminated after a set volume has been delivered). In either case, positive pressure applied at the patient's airway (usually through an endotracheal or tracheostomy tube) causes the flow of gas into the lungs until the ventilator breath is terminated. Passive exhalation occurs as the airway pressure drops to zero, and elastic recoil of the chest then pushes the tidal volume out.

By and large, the positive pressure type of ventilator is used most often in the hospital setting. Due to improvements in the mechanical ventilators and advances in the design of endotracheal and tracheostomy tubes, positive pressure ventilators have become the mainstay of ventilatory support. Clinical uses of positive pressure devices include intermittent positive pressure breathing (IPPB) therapy as well as many modes of mechanical ventilation.

Effects of Positive Pressure

Pulmonary System. The effects of positive pressure on the pulmonary system are numerous and are often dependent upon the amount of positive pressure delivered and the patient's lung pathology. Beneficial effects usually occur in the form of reversal of atelectatic changes in the lung or regression of pulmonary congestion. With improvement in the resting volume (functional residual volume, FRC) of the lung, positive pressure may in some instances reduce pulmonary vascular resistance and improve arterial oxygenation. The work of breathing is often reduced, and cough effectiveness augmented.

Numerous forms of barotrauma may be the result of the deleterious effects of positive pressure on the lungs. These include pneumothorax, pneumomediastinum, pulmonary interstitial emphysema, bronchopulmonary dysplasia, and subcutaneous emphysema. Positive pressure can rupture alveoli, allowing movement of air into the interstitium, which can track into the pleural space (pneumothorax), into the pericardium (pneumopericardium), or into the mediastinum (pneumomediastinum). Tension pneumothorax (air in the thorax under pressure) or pneumopericardium can decrease venous blood return and reduce left ventricular function. This situation could be life-threatening, and emergent decompression of the air is indicated. (Although the presence of subcutaneous emphysema is not in itself dangerous, it may suggest concurrent barotrauma and warrants further investigation.)

The combination of elevated levels of inspired oxygen, the presence of an endotracheal tube, and positive pressure may over time result in a chronic form of respiratory distress syndrome in neonatal patients termed bronchopulmonary dysplasia. These patients often require long-term ventilatory and oxygen support until the pulmonary insult regresses.

Currently, many believe that the single most important contributory factor in the development of barotrauma is the production of sheer forces caused by high initial inspiratory flow rates into the patient's airways. This, together with a high mean airway pressure (MAP) and variances in lung compliance and airway resistance within the lung, leads to the complications of positive pressure collectively known as barotrauma. Thus, it may be that with the use of slower inspiratory flow rates and lower mean airway pressures the incidence of this type of pulmonary insult will be reduced.

Cardiovascular System. Although it has been believed that the reduction in venous blood return secondary to positive pressure in the thoracic space caused alterations in cardiac output, other factors may be involved. Ultrasound studies of postcardiac surgery patients undergoing positive pressure ventilation indicate that increased intrapulmonary pressures cause an apparent increase in pulmonary vascular resistance with an elevation of right ventricular pressures. This, in turn, shifts the ventricular septum into the left ventricular space, thus decreasing left ventricular filling and output. In either case, cardiac output may be impaired. The degree to which this occurs appears to depend upon the mean airway pressure, cardiac reserve and function, circulating blood volume, and lung compliance or airway resistance.

Renal System. Any form of circulatory embarrassment may result in hypoperfusion of the kidneys with an alteration in urinary output. Although this phenomenon has been noted during positive pressure ventilation, it may also be secondary to positive pressure effects on antidiuretic hormone (ADH) secretion. A reduction in venous drainage secondary to increased intrathoracic positive pressure could stimulate osmoreceptors in the hypothalamus to mediate secretion of ADH. This, in turn, will result in diminished urinary output. Judicious use of plasma expanders and diuretics and careful observation of renal function should allow patients to maintain adequate fluid homeostasis.

Classifications of Positive Pressure Ventilators

Commonly, ventilators are classified by their method of cycling from the inspiratory phase to the expiratory phase (changeover from inspiratory to expiratory phase). The term cycle will be used here to indicate a terminating event as opposed to an initiating event.

Volume-Cycled. Termination of the delivered breath is achieved when a set volume has left the ventilator. This is the most common form of ventilator cycling because it allows a more consistent delivery of volumes. As a safety device, many ventilators have a pressure pop-off, or limit, which prevents overpressurization of the pulmonary circuit on any given breath. Depending upon the type of pressure-regulating device in use, the breath may be terminated before the entire volume has been delivered to the patient. This, however, can be monitored with exhaled volume-measuring devices, available on most volume ventilators. These devices also serve to monitor for leaks in the patient circuit. Although changes in airway resistance or lung compliance could result in lost ventilation into the ventilator tubing (compressible volume loss), some newer ventilators automatically compensate for this.

Pressure-Cycled. The delivered volume is terminated when a preset pressure is reached. Although this system often avoids overpressurization of the pulmonary circuit (over what the operator has set), the delivered breaths are not as consistent in volume. The size of the tidal volume depends upon the patient's airway resistance and lung compliance and on the peak pressure that has been selected. Thus, changes in the patient's pulmonary status may result in delivery of grossly inadequate volumes. Furthermore, large leaks or patient disconnect may not allow the peak pressure to be reached, resulting in failure of the ventilator to cycle off. Often this type of ventilator does not have the capacity to deliver precisely controlled levels of inspired oxygen. Because of these inconsistencies, this type of ventilator is more commonly used for intermittent treatment modalities only (i.e., IPPB).

Time-Cycled. The delivered breath is terminated when a preset time has been reached. Often a pressure limit is also incorporated, so that the pressure limit is reached and the remainder of the inspiratory phase is in the form of an inspiratory pause. This type of ventilation became the mainstay of neonatal ventilation in the late 1960s and early 1970s and is currently the mode of choice for neonates and small infants in many medical centers.

Although this type of ventilator does not guarantee a set tidal volume, it does allow precise control of inspired fraction of oxygen and adequate humidification systems. It must also be noted that monitoring of tidal volumes in the neonatal population has been notoriously difficult, further justifying this type of ventilator.

Note: Some time-cycled ventilators occasionally utilize a constant flow of gas delivered to the patient while the exhalation valve is completely closed. Thus, the tidal volume is constant (tidal volume = flow ×

time). These types of devices are often used as transport ventilators or in emergency rooms as manual resuscitators (Elder Valve).

STANDARD MODES OF MECHANICAL VENTILATION

Control Mode Ventilation

When a patient is placed on a ventilator in the control mode, the ventilator initiates and controls both the volume delivered and the frequency of the breaths. The respiratory pattern, delivered by the ventilator, therefore has very regular intervals (Fig. 29–1A). When used strictly in the control mode, the ventilator will not respond (give a breath) if the patient attempts to initiate a ventilator breath. In between the machine breaths, the patient is unable to breathe spontaneously or initiate (trigger) a ventilator breath. The patient's ventilatory pattern may become asynchronous if the patient tries to breathe faster than the set rate. When the ventilator fails to give a breath on demand, the patient may become agitated and increase the work of breathing and may cause increases in carbon dioxide production and oxygen consumption.

The control mode can be used to override (control) a patient with a high respiratory rate. The patient can be deliberately hyperventilated by increasing the minute ventilation delivered by the ventilator. If the patient is not hypoxemic, the resulting hypocapnia often may remove the normal stimulus to breathe, allowing the ventilator to control all inspirations.

Other clinical uses of control mode ventilation (Burton et al., 1984) include patients with:

> Apnea
> Drug overdose
> Spinal cord injuries
> Central nervous system dysfunction
> Flail chest
> Paralysis from drugs
> Neuromuscular disease
> Back-up rate for the assist mode ventilation

With the advent of newer technologies for modes of ventilation, the use of the control mode as a sole form of ventilation is limited. The control mode combined with other modes of augmented ventilation is still widely used and will be discussed later.

Assist Mode

The assist mode of ventilation was developed during the early years of modern respiratory care. Initially, assist was designed for pressure-cycled ventilators, such as IPPB devices. The assist mode is a mode of ventilation in which the patient is able to

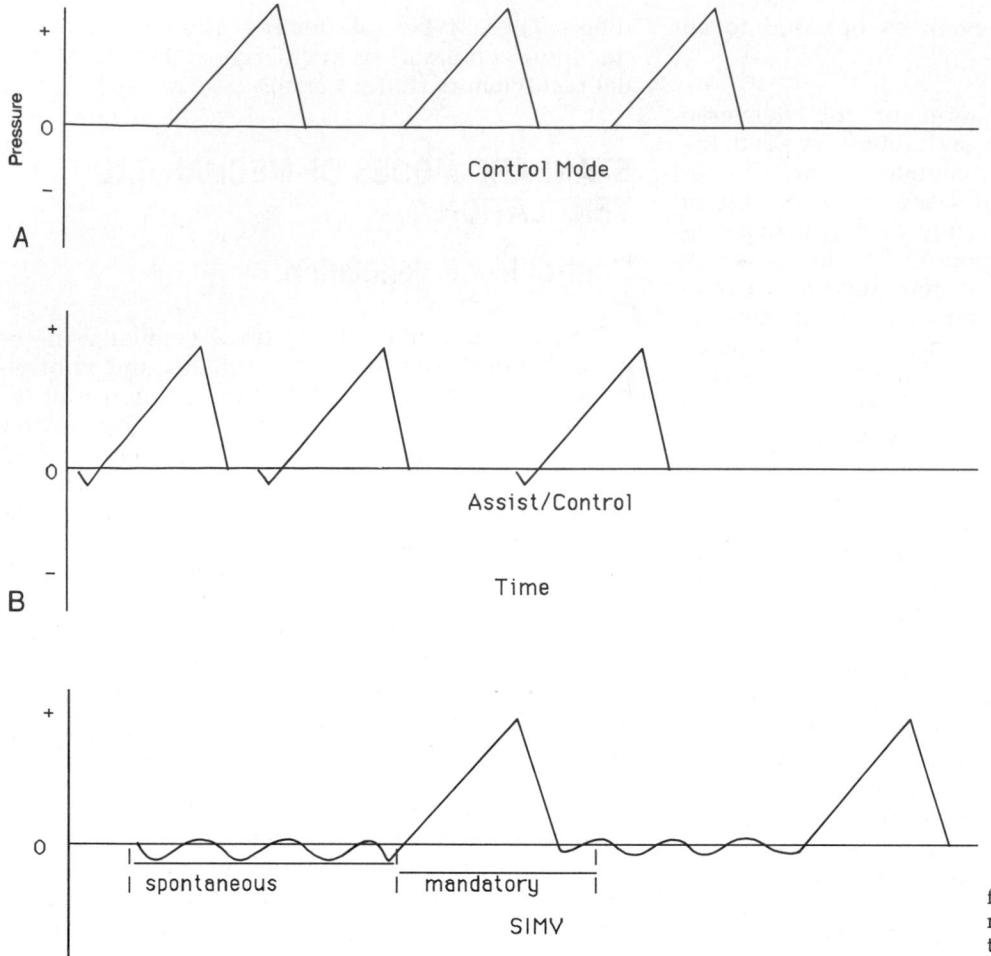

FIGURE 29–1. Pressure waveforms for conventional modes of mechanical ventilation. _A_, Control mode. _B_, Assist mode. _C_, Synchronized intermittent mandatory ventilation (SIMV).

initiate inspiration and to control the frequency of breathing. The major disadvantage of assist was the lack of a back-up rate if the patient became apneic. Because this mode requires the patient to cycle the ventilator on, ventilation may become inadequate if apnea occurs subsequently. The control mode was later incorporated with the assist mode (assist/control, A/C) to alleviate this problem.

Assist/Control Mode

This mode of ventilation is a combination of the assist and control modes. As in controlled ventilation, a tidal volume and rate are preset. However, on A/C, whenever the patient makes an inspiratory effort, the ventilator senses the effort and delivers the preset tidal volume. Therefore, the respiratory pattern may have irregular intervals (depending on the timing of patient efforts) (see Fig. 29–1B). If the patient fails to initiate inspiration, the ventilator automatically goes into the back-up mode (control mode) and delivers the preset rate and tidal volume until it senses an inspiratory effort. This back-up rate ensures a minimum minute ventilation in the event of apnea.

Clinical Uses of A/C. The A/C mode is indicated when the work of breathing must be reduced, for example, in patients who require a set back-up rate but also need an assisted breath on demand to reduce the work of breathing. Assist/control devices can be used in patients with the following conditions:

Neuromuscular diseases such as myasthenia gravis or Guillain-Barré syndrome
Postcardiac or respiratory arrest
Pulmonary edema
Adult respiratory distress syndrome (ARDS)
Anxiety or apprehension

There are two theoretical advantages of the A/C mode. First, the pH and Pa_{CO_2} may be more normal compared with the control mode, and the patient is therefore able to control his or her own respiratory rate and minute ventilation because he is not subjected to a fixed rate and volume (Burton et al., 1984). The second possible advantage is that cycling the ventilator into the inspiratory phase maintains normal ventilatory activity and therefore prevents atrophy of the respiratory muscles (Burton et al., 1984).

There are two potential disadvantages of the A/C

mode. The first is respiratory alkalosis. Because the ventilator will deliver the set tidal volume on demand, there is a potential for alveolar hyperventilation resulting in hypocapnia. The second possible disadvantage is that the patient may "stack" breaths (take several breaths in a row). This may lead to ineffective ventilation and asynchronous breathing.

Intermittent Mandatory Ventilation

Originally intermittent mandatory ventilation (IMV) was developed for weaning infants from the ventilator. Later this mode was found to be effective as a primary means of ventilating adult patients. This mode of ventilation evolved from combining the advantages of spontaneous breathing with those of conventional mechanical ventilation. In addition, not all patients require total support of ventilation and oxygenation. Many are capable of maintaining some (not all) of their spontaneous ventilations and may require additional respiratory support (Kirby, 1988).

Intermittent mandatory ventilation allows the patient to breathe spontaneously with the ventilator providing some mandatory breaths at a predetermined rate. Like the control mode, the ventilator delivers the mandatory breaths at a preset tidal volume and at a controlled rate. For spontaneous breathing the ventilator provides a gas source of oxygen of the same concentration, temperature, and humidity as is available to the patient for mandatory breathing. During the spontaneous phase of ventilation the patient determines the respiratory rate and tidal volume. Unfortunately, with this mode of ventilation, asynchronous breathing may be experienced. Because IMV has a controlled rate, the mandatory breath may be imposed on the patient's spontaneous inspiration or exhalation.

The advantages of IMV compared with the control and assist/control modes are:

1. The iatrogenic effects of mechanical ventilation are minimized (barotrauma, decreased cardiac output) because mean airway and intrapleural pressures are lower (Kirby, 1988; Shapiro et al., 1982).
2. Higher levels of pulmonary end-expiratory pressure (PEEP) can be used because mean intrapleural pressure is relatively lower (Burton et al., 1984).
3. There is less likelihood of hyperventilation (respiratory alkalemia) (Burton et al., 1984).
4. IMV can be used as a means of weaning the patient from mechanical ventilation because it provides a gradual transition from the control mode or the assist/control mode to spontaneous breathing. Decreasing the back-up rate will allow the patient to do more of the work of breathing.

The disadvantages of IMV include:

1. Asynchronous breathing. Mandatory breaths may be imposed on the patient's spontaneous inspiration or expiration, which may cause the patient to breathe asynchronously with the ventilator, become agitated, or receive abnormally large tidal volumes.
2. Apnea or hypoventilation. A patient on a low backup rate may become apneic, resulting in an inadequate level of ventilation.

Clinical uses for IMV include:

1. Use as a primary means of mechanical ventilation (as an alternative to the control mode or the assist/control mode).
2. Use in patients who have respiratory patterns that are asynchronous on the control mode.
3. Use in patients who hyperventilate (respiratory alkalosis on the assist/control mode.
4. Use in patients who require some respiratory support but are able to breathe spontaneously.
5. Use as a means of weaning patients from mechanical ventilation.

Synchronized Intermittent Mandatory Ventilation

Synchronized intermittent mandatory ventilation (SIMV) was developed to prevent the "stacking" effect. The mandatory breath delivered from the ventilator is synchronized with the beginning of the patient's spontaneous inspirations (if the patient is breathing spontaneously). Because of this additional feature, three types of breaths are possible on SIMV:

1. Mandatory mechanical ventilation breaths are delivered at the back-up rate if patient effort is absent.
2. If the patient makes a spontaneous inspiratory effort reasonably near the time of the next mandatory mechanical ventilation breath, the effort triggers that mandatory mechanical breath. Thus, the patient's effort is synchronized with the mandatory ventilation, preventing the stacking of mandatory and spontaneous breaths and providing a more comfortable form of mechanical ventilation (Fig. 29–1C).
3. If the patient makes a spontaneous inspiratory effort that is not within reasonable proximity to the time that the next mandatory mechanical ventilation breath is due, the patient generates an unassisted spontaneous breath.

The advantages of SIMV compared to the control mode or the assist/control mode are the same as those of IMV except that SIMV is probably more comfortable for the patient. The disadvantages of SIMV are also the same as those of IMV except that the spontaneous breaths on SIMV may be more difficult for pediatric or weak patients to trigger on ventilators with mechanical demand valves. The clinical uses are the same as those for IMV. In addition, SIMV is used whenever lack of synchronous breathing seems to affect the patient's ability to be weaned.

Positive End-Expiratory Pressure

Positive end-expiratory pressure (PEEP) is a mode of therapy that is used in conjunction with mechanical ventilation. At the end of exhalation (either mechanical or spontaneous) the patient's airway pressure is maintained above atmospheric. PEEP therapy can be effective when used in patients with a diffuse lung disease that results in an acute decrease in functional residual capacity (FRC), which is the volume of gas that remains in the lung at the end of a normal expiration. FRC is determined primarily by the elastic characteristics of the lung and chest wall. In many pulmonary diseases, FRC is reduced due to the collapse of the unstable alveoli. This reduction in lung volume decreases the surface area available for gas exchange and results in intrapulmonary shunting (unoxygenated blood returning to the left side of the heart). For this reason, if FRC is not restored, a high concentration of inspired oxygen may be required to maintain the arterial oxygen content of the blood in an acceptable range. Refractory hypoxemia due to intrapulmonary shunting secondary to a decreased FRC may be effectively treated with PEEP. Applying continuous positive pressure at the end of exhalation causes an increase in alveolar pressure and increases the alveolar volume (Craig et al., 1988). This increase in lung volume increases the surface area by reopening or stabilizing collapsed or unstable alveoli. This "splinting" or "propping open" of the alveoli with positive pressure may provide a better matching of ventilation to perfusion, thereby reducing the shunt effect. Therefore, lower concentrations of oxygen can be used to maintain an adequate Pa_{O_2}.

It has been reported that PEEP therapy is also effective in improving lung compliance (Craig et al., 1988; Shapiro et al., 1982). A decrease in compliance also increases the patient's work of breathing. When FRC and lung compliance are decreased, it takes more energy and volume to inflate the lung. By applying PEEP, the lung volume at the end of exhalation is increased. This decreases the work of breathing because the lung is already partially inflated, so less volume and energy are needed to inflate the lung. This concept is analogous to inflating a toy balloon. When inflating the balloon initially it takes a considerable amount of energy to overcome the elastic properties of the balloon. If the balloon is deflated completely, it takes just as much energy to reexpand it. If it is deflated only partially, less energy and less volume are needed to reinflate it.

In summary, when used to treat patients with a diffuse lung disease, PEEP should improve compliance, decrease dead space, and decrease the intrapulmonary shunt effect (Shapiro et al., 1982). The most significant benefit of the use of PEEP is that it enables the patient to maintain an adequate Pa_{O_2} at a lower concentration of oxygen, thereby reducing the risk of oxygen toxicity.

PEEP is not a benign mode of therapy and can lead to serious consequences. Elevated levels of PEEP may result in overdistention of the alveoli, with increased intrapleural pressures that may result in a decrease in cardiac output (due to a decrease in venous return), an increase in intrapulmonary shunting (overdistention of nondiseased areas may decrease blood flow to these areas), and a decrease in lung compliance (Shapiro et al., 1982) and barotrauma.

Continuous Positive Airway Pressure

Continuous positive airway pressure (CPAP) has the same physiologic characteristics as PEEP. The goal of CPAP therapy is to restore or maintain FRC in a patient who is intubated and on a ventilator but is able to breathe spontaneously. When placed on CPAP, the patient does all the work of breathing on his own without the aid of a mechanical back-up rate from the ventilator. This mode of therapy is primarily used to wean the patient from mechanical ventilation. A concise comparison of PEEP and CPAP is outlined in Table 29–1.

NEWER MODES OF MECHANICAL VENTILATION

Several unconventional modes of ventilation have recently become popular or at least have been the source of much controversy. Whenever a divergence from the customary clinical solution is considered, substantial capacity for debate usually exists. When the issue of implementing a nontraditional form of mechanical ventilation is deliberated, the question often asked is whether or not to risk straying from the norm in order to offer a different approach to treatment. The final decision, of course, depends on several factors, including the probability of success in treating the patient's condition with the current conventional modes of ventilation. For example, a recent review of patients with ARDS indicates that in the last decade the survival rate has changed

---

TABLE 29–1. Comparison of PEEP and CPAP

PEEP	CPAP
Patient is intubated	Patient is usually intubated (CPAP mask is available)
Used in conjunction with control, assist-control, and SIMV	Not used with other modes of ventilation
Back-up rate and tidal volume are provided	No back-up rate is set, all breathing is done spontaneously
Goal is to improve or maintain FRC	Goal is to improve FRC
	Used for weaning patients from mechanical ventilation

Abbreviations: PEEP, positive end-expiratory pressure; CPAP, continuous positive airway pressure; SIMV, synchronized intermittent mandatory ventilation; FRC, functional residual capacity.

insignificantly (Petty and Fowler, 1982). Therefore, a patient with ARDS who is failing on a conventional mode of ventilation may be a candidate for an unconventional mode of therapy.

This section will provide some basic information on these newer modes of ventilation, including indications and contraindications, applications, and monitoring. Knowledge of the material presented in this section by no means qualifies an individual to manage ventilators in these modes. Unless the clinician has acquired the appropriate knowledge and skills, managing one of the newer modes of ventilation may only increase the potential for harming the patient.

Pressure Control Ventilation (PCV)

A pressure-limited, time-cycled ventilator is used (i.e., Servo 900C or Puritan Bennett 7200a). The clinician sets a specific inspiratory pressure and inspiratory time. The ventilator delivers a flow of gas until the pressure is reached. The pressure is then maintained within the lung for the set inspiratory time. Like A/C, the patient is able to initiate a breath, and in the event of apnea a back-up rate will support the patient's respirations. But unlike A/C, with changes in airway resistance and lung compliance, the delivered tidal volumes may vary. Pressure control may be an alternative method of ventilating a patient who does not respond to conventional therapy. With PCV, the initial flow is high (peak flow is determined automatically). This rapid flow fills the ventilator circuit and the upper airways with gas. Therefore, flow reaches the small airways early in the inspiratory phase, allowing more time for gas distribution according to regional variations in compliance and resistance. The rapid introduction of gas into the airways may be uncomfortable for the patient and may require sedation and/or paralyzation. The tidal volume delivered to the patient is a result of the change in pressure from the baseline pressure to the set peak inspiratory pressure (PIP). Any ventilator changes that result in a change in the PIP or the baseline pressure (total end-expiratory) may cause a change in the tidal volume delivered. Pressure control can be used in conventional I/E ratios or inverse ratio ventiation (IRV). Pressure control ventilation is closely related to inverse ratio ventilation, which is described in detail below.

Inverse Ratio Ventilation

Inverse ratio ventilation (IRV) is an alternative method of providing ventilatory support to a group of patients with refractory hypoxemia. With conventional ventilation, the expiratory phase of the respiratory cycle is usually longer than the inspiratory phase. In IRV, the duration of inspiration exceeds that of expiration. The duration of the inspiratory phase can be reversed to up to 80% of the total cycle time (inspiratory-expiratory [I/E] ratio, 4:1), which results in a shortened expiratory time.

Physiology. Theoretically, a prolonged inspiratory time exposes the lung to a longer period of positive pressure, which may cause recruitment of unstable alveoli, thus improving gas exchange. It has been suggested that prolonged inspiration decreases dead space ventilation (V_D/V_T) and improves the matching of ventilation to perfusion (V/Q) in patients who have a decreased lung compliance. The mean airway pressure is usually higher in the IRV mode compared to conventional ventilation despite the lower peak pressures delivered to the patient's lungs. It is felt that either an increased mean airway pressure (MAP) or an increased total end-expiratory pressure (see below) is responsible for the increase in oxygenation. However, physiologically, it is not known exactly why IRV improves oxygenation and ventilation.

The significant effects of PEEP are thought to be associated with the increased FRC, which recruits collapsed or unstable alveoli for gas exchange (Cole et al., 1984). Like PEEP, IRV can also increase FRC because the shortened expiratory time may prevent full expiration. Because inspiration is prolonged and the expiratory phase is short, the lung is reinflated before expiratory flow from the previous breath ends (Fig. 29–2A and B). The incomplete exhalation causes a PEEP-like effect. This "air trapping" at the end of exhalation due to a short expiratory time is referred to as auto-PEEP. This PEEP-like effect causes the alveolar pressure to remain positive throughout the entire respiratory cycle. This constant pressure prevents the alveoli from collapsing at the end of exhalation.

Indications

1. Diffuse lung injury demonstrated by chest radiograph
2. Refractory hypoxemia on conventional mechanical volume ventilation requiring high concentrations of oxygen (>60%), high levels of PEEP, and high

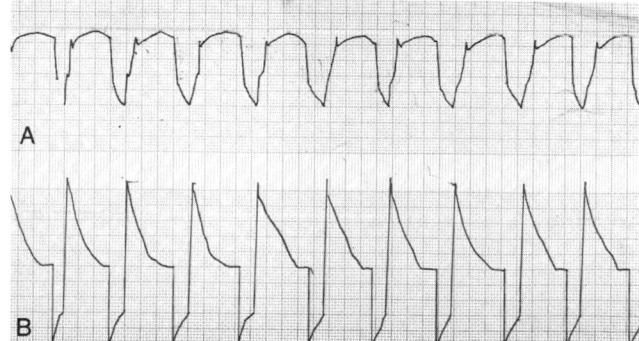

FIGURE 29–2. *A*, Pressure waveform on inverse ratio ventilation. *B*, Flow waveform on inverse ratio ventilation.

peak inspiratory pressures to deliver the set tidal volume
3. Hemodynamic stability

Contraindications

1. A nondiffuse lung disease process (e.g., lobar pneumonia)
2. Obstructive pulmonary disease
3. Presence of copious secretions

All of these contraindications may cause severe air trapping and thus may result in barotrauma or inadequate ventilation.

Applications. A pressure-limited, time-cycled ventilator in the pressure control mode is used when implementing IRV. The pressure control mode is used because it can obtain peak inspiratory pressure and maintain this level for the entire duration of the set inspiratory time. The prolonged exposure to positive pressure facilitates "splitting open" atelectatic alveoli (Gurevitch, 1988).
Conversion to IRV includes the following sequential steps:

1. PEEP should be optimized on conventional ventilation. In addition, the peak inspiratory pressure (PIP) and static pressure on the conventional ventilator settings should be noted.
2. The patient must undergo neuromuscular paralysis and/or sedation because prolonged inspiration with a pause is an unnatural way to breathe. This will prevent the patient from fighting the ventilator and allow the maximum benefit to be derived from IRV.
3. The patient should be placed on a ventilator that can provide the pressure control mode and on which the inspiratory time can be set (for example, the Siemens Servo 900C ventilator). The ventilator should have the capability of measuring auto-PEEP and mean airway pressures.
4. F_{IO_2} should be 100% because onset hypoxemia may occur when the mode of ventilation is changed.
5. The mode of ventilation is changed to pressure control and the preset inspiratory pressure level is adjusted to one-half to two-thirds the peak inspiratory pressure noted on the previous ventilatory mode (Gurevitch, 1988). This should yield a tidal volume that is slightly less than 10 mL/kg.
6. The percentage of inspiratory time is increased as the set PEEP is decreased to a level of 5 to 7 cm water in a fashion that maintains optimal oxygenation without cardiac compromise. This increase in inspiratory time usually increases the level of auto-PEEP and total end-expiratory pressure (set PEEP plus auto-PEEP).
7. Changes in the rate, inspiratory pressure level, and inspiratory time are used to adjust the level of auto-PEEP and optimize CO_2 and O_2 levels without compromising the cardiac system (e.g., decreased cardiac output). Any changes in these parameters

may affect the tidal volume delivered. These adjustments require previous experience or training.
8. Oxygenation is primarily regulated by the total end-expiratory pressure (TEEP). F_{IO_2} can also be adjusted to maintain the level of oxygenation.
9. Ventilation is dependent on ΔP (the change in pressure from TEEP to PIP) and must be monitored and maintained.

Monitoring. The following parameters should be monitored when a patient is on IRV:

1. Heart rate, blood pressure, cardiac output, and Sv_{O_2}
2. Hemodynamic measurements including those obtained from a pulmonary artery catheter
3. Noninvasive parameters—pulse oximetry and capnography
4. Arterial blood gases and mixed venous blood gases
5. Airway pressure and flow tracings
6. Mean airway pressure (MAP), auto-PEEP, total end-expiratory pressure, and all ventilator parameters

Adverse Effects. Although IRV reduces the peak airway pressures needed to ventilate and oxygenate the patient, it may increase the mean airway pressure. As the inspiratory phase is increased, the MAP may also increase, affecting venous return to the heart. This could result in a decreased cardiac output. For this reason, it is imperative to monitor closely the hemodynamic status of the patient on IRV.
In addition, as the ratios are reversed further (I/E ratio 4:1), the resulting increase in MAP will expose the lung to the possible hazard of barotrauma. Chest radiographs, breath sounds, chest rise, MAP and auto-PEEP levels, and all vital signs should also be closely monitored for any signs of barotrauma.

Summary. There is evidence that IRV may be beneficial when conventional means of mechanical ventilation have failed to correct refractory hypoxemia due to acute lung injuries. (Gurevitch et al., 1986; Gurevitch, 1988). The improvements in gas exchange make this mode of ventilation an appealing alternative to conventional ventilation. Sometimes it is not necessary to reverse the I/E ratios, but pressure control ventilation is used to better oxygenate and ventilate the patient at a lower peak inspiratory pressure.
IRV ventilation cannot be indiscriminately used on any patient. The patient must meet the IRV criteria (mentioned earlier), and trained personnel with the proper understanding, technique, and equipment must be used to obtain the maximum benefit from IRV safely.

Pressure Support Ventilation

Pressure support ventilation (PSV) is a mode of ventilation that provides augmentation of spontaneous breaths with selected levels of positive pressure. As the patient initiates a breath, the preselected inspiratory pressure is reached quickly, and a pressure plateau is sustained for as long as the patient continues to make an inspiratory effort or until a certain minimum peak flow level is reached (MacIntyre, 1988a). Unlike other modes of conventional ventilation, PSV requires the patient to make an inspiratory effort continuously in order for the ventilator to deliver the pressure support. Therefore, the ventilator aids in a portion of the work of breathing for spontaneous breathing. The level of pressure support will determine the ratio of work done by the ventilator versus the work done by the patient.

PSV is in some ways similar in concept to IPPB. When using IPPB, inspiratory flow and the pressure limit are preset. When the patient makes an inspiratory effort, the ventilator turns on. The breath is terminated as soon as the preset pressure is reached. However, there are significant differences between IPPB and PSV. The patient must also trigger the ventilator in PSV, but as the set pressure is reached, instead of the breath being terminated, the pressure plateaus for as long as the patient continues to make an inspiratory effort. Second, in PSV the patient is able to determine his own rate, tidal volume, and inspiratory flow on a breath-to-breath basis.

Physiology. The respiratory center in the central nervous system receives input from chemoreceptors (arterial blood gas tensions) and neural pathways that sense the mechanical work of breathing (mechanoreceptors). The respiratory rate, respiratory pattern, and tidal volume are the result of input from these chemoreceptors and mechanical receptors. From this input, the respiratory center can regulate gas exchange with the minimum amount of work (MacIntyre, 1988a). Any variation in the input can cause dyspnea. It is thought that pressure support may interact with the mechanical receptors and can achieve this balance in a more physiologic fashion in a spontaneously breathing patient (MacIntyre, 1988a). In addition, patient comfort is improved with PSV because the patient has control of the respiratory rate, tidal volume, and inspiratory flow.

Indications. The following clinical situations may indicate the possible utilization of PSV:

1. Patients who are difficult to wean from mechanical ventilation using conventional means (i.e., T-piece, SIMV, CPAP)
2. Anxious patients, because they will have control over the respiratory rate, tidal volume, and inspiratory flow
3. Patients who have a less than optimal artificial airway. Small diameter airways (endotracheal or tracheostomy tubes) will increase the work of breathing because the patient must overcome the resistance to flow. PSV may help overcome this resistance (Kacmarek, 1988)

4. Patients with chronic obstructive pulmonary disease (COPD) or any patient with evidence of ventilatory muscle weakness who is being maintained on a low SIMV rate (<4/minute) or has been on CPAP for 24 to 48 hours (Kacmarek, 1988)
5. Weak patients or those with COPD who have difficulty in maintaining ventilation while on continuous flow IMV at a low rate (<4/minute) or on CPAP (Kacmarek, 1988)
6. Patients who have problems "synchronizing" with other modes of mechanical ventilation

Contraindications. Apnea is a contraindication for PSV. When a patient is on pressure support only, he will not receive a back-up ventilatory support if he should become apneic. Also, patients who become fatigued easily may experience hypoventilation if they are placed on PSV only, or if they are placed on SIMV with PSV with a low back-up rate.

Applications. The patient must be switched to a ventilator that has the capability of providing pressure support. There are several ways in which to use PSV when weaning a patient. The first is to use low levels of PSV (2 to 10 cm H_2O) in conjunction with SIMV, the PSV being utilized during the spontaneous breaths. The low levels of PSV are used to overcome the resistance of the endotracheal tube, which may provide improved patient comfort and respiratory muscle function. The second is to use low levels of PSV for nonventilatory support (patients intubated for airway protection or for alveolar stabilization using CPAP) (MacIntyre, 1988a). PSV is used to help overcome the resistance of the endotracheal tube. The third is to use PSV alone (PSVmax). In this situation, the pressure level is set so that the measured tidal volume is approximately equal to that received during conventional ventilation (10 ml/kg of body weight) (MacIntyre, 1988a). It is thought that this will reduce the work of the muscles (MacIntyre, 1987). The level of PSV is gradually reduced, allowing the patient to do more of the work of breathing. The rationale for using PSV in such a way is to provide patient comfort and a more physiologic workload for the respiratory muscles.

If all other parameters are stable (blood pressure, heart rate, respiratory rate, and so on), the patient can be extubated if the PSV level has been reduced to 5 cm H_2O and all other weaning criteria are met (Kacmarek, 1988).

Monitoring. The patient should be monitored in the same manner as any patient being weaned from mechanical ventilation. Hemodynamic parameters that are monitored are heart rate, blood pressure, and cardiac output. The patient is also monitored for signs of fatigue. Fatigue may be clinically present as dyspnea, paradoxical abdominal movement, diaphoresis, increased respiratory rate and effort, or a decrease in tidal volume at the same PSV pressure level. Arterial blood gases (or pulse oximetry) are also followed.

High-Frequency Ventilation

High-frequency ventilation should be considered a term that includes any form of mechanical ventilation that functions at a frequency of at least four times the normal respiratory rate, that is, at least 60 breaths/minute (Froese and Bryan, 1987; Slutsky et al., 1981). In the last several years, this form of ventilation has generated both interest and controversy. The variety of reactions probably stems from the concerns engendered by setting ventilator parameters beyond the conventional range as well as by the challenges presented by questioning the traditional theory of ventilation.

For clinicians to work safely with high-frequency ventilation of any type, they must (1) have an understanding of concepts common to all types of high-frequency ventilation, (2) have a knowledge of the various types of high-frequency ventilation including the terminology used and the indications for each type, and (3) be able to determine which method is optimal for the particular clinical situation.

Applications of this new type of ventilatory therapy can be divided into two general classifications. The extracorporeal type administers high-frequency ventilation indirectly by means of a device (Gross et al., 1985; Harf et al., 1985; Ward et al., 1985) similar to the negative pressure ventilators described earlier in this chapter. The type of high-frequency ventilation more commonly used delivers inspired gases directly to the airways through an endotracheal tube. In this classification there are three subtypes: high-frequency positive pressure ventilation (HFPPV), high-frequency jet ventilation (HFJV), and high-frequency oscillation (HFO). Because this classification is utilized more often in the intensive care setting, our focus will be on it. These three subtypes are compared in Table 29–2.

Physiology. All forms of high-frequency ventilation use smaller than normal tidal volumes. As tidal volume is lowered, the airways and lungs are exposed to less peak inspiratory pressure. This lower airway pressure may decrease the potential for trauma to the pulmonary system, but, as the tidal volume and airway pressure diminish, often so does alveolar ventilation. To make up for this loss, the respiratory rate is increased. Therefore, a normal tidal volume delivered at a normal rate is replaced by a smaller tidal volume delivered at the appropriately chosen higher rate. However, according to the traditional theory of ventilation, if the delivered tidal volume is smaller than the dead space volume (the part of the respiratory tract not involved with gas exchange), logically, this mode should not be successful.

The traditional theory of ventilation and gas exchange centers around the principle that two distinct regions of the lung exist: the dead space region, where gas is carried predominantly by bulk flow, and the alveolar region, which is primarily the area of molecular diffusion (gas exchange). This view, however, does not explain how normal arterial blood gas values can be obtained during experiments with high-frequency ventilation in which the tidal volume is much smaller than the dead space volume (New modes, 1984).

Several studies offer data that might help to demystify this confusion. They indicate that, instead of two mechanisms of ventilation (i.e., bulk flow and molecular diffusion), gas transport may be the result of possibly six different mechanisms (Carlon et al., 1985; Fredberg et al., 1984; Hazelton and Scherer, 1980; Henderson et al., 1915; Lehr et al., 1985; Slutsky, 1981). As the respiratory rate and tidal volume are altered from the norm, the four nontraditional forms of gas transport may come into play at different points and to various degrees. In other words, it appears that, as the respiratory rate increases and the tidal volume decreases, the physiologic dead space diminishes to allow adequate ventilation, or the point at which bulk flow of gas terminates and molecular diffusion commences is repositioned to a location "higher" in the airways (toward the larger airways). Alterations such as this would allow gas to diffuse to the alveoli over a longer distance. This concept is known as augmented diffusion.

HIGH-FREQUENCY POSITIVE PRESSURE VENTILATION

Definition. In general, high-frequency positive pressure ventilation (HFPPV) is defined as positive pressure ventilation delivered at a rate of 60 to 100

TABLE 29–2. Comparison of High-Frequency Ventilation

	HFPPV	HFJV	HFO
Rate	60–100/minute	100–150/minute	100–3000/minute
Tidal volume	3–5 cc/kg	3–5 cc/kg	1–2 cc/kg
Applications	Air leaks pulmonary	Air leaks pulmonary Laryngeal surgery Bronchoscopy	Pulmonary interstitial emphysema PPHN

Abbreviations: HFPPV, high-frequency positive pressure ventilation; HFJV, high-frequency jet ventilation; HFO, high-frequency oscillatory ventilation; PPHN, persistent pulmonary hypertension of the newborn.

breaths per minute (bpm) with tidal volumes in the range of 3 to 5 mL/kg through a system that does not involve gas entrainment (Froese and Bryan, 1987; Sjostrand, 1980)—that is, draw in additional gas from an outside source. Slight variations from this definition depend on the properties of the ventilator being used and will be discussed later in this section.

Indications and Contraindications. HFPPV is primarily used in patients who have major pulmonary air leaks, such as a bronchopleural fistula or a tracheoesophageal fistula, with the intention of minimizing leakage through the fistula by lowering the peak inspiratory pressure. HFPPV has indeed been shown to achieve adequate ventilation and arterial oxygenation at lower inspiratory pressures and with less circulatory compromise than occurs with conventional ventilation (Bjerager et al., 1977). Because of these traits, HFPPV has also been shown to be effective in the treatment of pneumomediastinum and pneumothoraces (which are also pulmonary air leaks) in neonates (Wren, 1983).

When HFPPV is used to treat respiratory failure or ARDS, however, the results are mixed (Carlon et al., 1979; Wattwil et al., 1983), and it is recommended that other modes be considered first. Because the tidal volume in this mode is an unpredictable product of the preset inspiratory pressure, the inspiratory time percentage, and the back-pressure generated by the patient's respiratory system, patients with low lung compliance (stiff lungs) will probably not receive adequate ventilation from HFPPV.

Application. If a patient has the indications for HFPPV mentioned previously, the appropriate ventilator must be obtained. The ventilator must have the following characteristics: (1) the capability of achieving respiratory rates of 60 to 100 bpm, (2) an "inspiratory time percentage" parameter that can be adjusted to below 30% (the ability to adjust to greater than 30% is also very useful), and (3) the capability of functioning in a "pressure control" mode (Sjostrand, 1980). One example of a ventilator that meets this description is the Siemens-Elema Servo 900C.

Before connecting the patient to the ventilator, certain considerations must be taken into account. Ineffective ventilation should be minimized by using noncompliant tubing, and the humidification system must be verified to be functioning properly. It should be kept in mind that HFPPV is primarily used for major pulmonary air leaks. The cuff on the patient's endotracheal tube (or tracheostomy tube) should be deflated before the patient is connected to the ventilator, especially if the pathologic leak is minimal or intermittent. Placing a patient without a significant air leak on this mode can result in deleterious effects.

The initial ventilator settings may vary according to the functional limits of the type of ventilator being used. The respiratory rate should be set at about 90 bpm. Respiratory rates of less than 90 bpm may be clinically indicated as well as beneficial to the patient,

but 90 bpm has been observed to be efficacious in most cases (Bjerager et al., 1977; Froese and Bryan, 1987). Rates higher than 90 bpm may exceed the functional limits of some ventilators (indicated by an inability to maintain a reasonable tidal volume or flow) and should not be used in such situations.

The inspiratory time percentage parameter determines how much of the respiratory cycle will be devoted to inspiration. For example, if the inspiratory time percentage is set at 33% and the respiratory rate is set at 90 bpm, the time allowed for each respiration would be 0.66 second per breath (60 seconds/minute divided by 90 bpm), and the time dedicated to inspiration would be 33% of the 0.66 second (0.22 second). To provide a normal inspiratory-expiratory ratio (I/E ratio), the inspiratory time percentage should initially be set at 20% to 25%.

Once the patient has been connected to the ventilator this parameter should be adjusted to achieve an expired tidal volume of 3 to 5 mL/kg. The mode dial should be set to deliver "pressure control." This setting enables the ventilator to attain the preset pressure level (and therefore the tidal volume) quickly. The $F_{I_{O_2}}$ should be set to achieve adequate oxygenation (an O_2 saturation level of at least 90% or a Pa_{O_2} of at least 60 mm Hg). If the ventilator being used has an adjustable driving pressure, it must be maximized to ensure proper function in this mode.

Monitoring. When placing the patient on the ventilator, all hemodynamic parameters and airway pressures should be noted. Arterial blood gas values should be obtained shortly after initiating HFPPV to ensure adequate ventilation and oxygenation. Pulse oximeters are sufficient for monitoring oxygenation, but capnography is usually ineffective in this mode for monitoring ventilation. Before, during, and after any change in setting the ventilator parameters, airway pressures, hemodynamic parameters, and arterial blood gas values should be assessed.

Always keep in mind that HFPPV is delivered through a pressure ventilator, which means that tidal volumes may vary greatly and therefore need to be monitored closely. Decreased lung compliance due to pulmonary edema, fluid overload, and so on can cause a significant drop in tidal volume because of the back-pressure generated. Also, any obstruction of the tubing, such as from water condensation, or secretions of the airway, can grossly affect the value of the delivered tidal volume. Therefore, patients on HFPPV need to be routinely lavaged and suctioned as well as closely monitored for decreased lung compliance. If the tidal volume drops significantly, one should try to determine the cause quickly and act appropriately (i.e., rule out the simplest causes first, such as secretion build-up, water in the tubing, kinked tubing, circuit leak or disconnection). At this point, if the tidal volume remains significantly low, the preset inspiratory pressure should be increased to a level that seems clinically appropriate for the patient (at least 3 to 5 mL/kg). If this attempt is not effective, then the ventilator circuit should be disconnected from the endotracheal tube and the patient manually ventilated with a hand-bag resuscitator.

If the patient starts to retain too much CO_2 (Pa_{CO_2} > 45 mm Hg), the inspiratory time percentage should be increased by an increment of 5% to 15%. This will allow a longer period of inspiration and therefore a larger tidal volume, which will provide better ventilation. This is the optimal method for regulating ventilation in this mode.

Increasing the respiratory rate does not necessarily result in a decrease in the Pa_{CO_2} as it does in conventional ventilation. Delivering more breaths/minute will shorten the amount of time allowed for each breath to be delivered, resulting in an even smaller tidal volume and possibly a higher Pa_{CO_2}.

If the respiratory rate is not up to the desired initial setting (90 bpm), increasing the preset inspiratory pressure as well as the respiratory rate may provide an increase in the tidal volume as well as effective ventilation.

Adequate oxygenation may be maintained by the Fi_{O_2} alone, but another factor involved with determining oxygenation exists, namely, total end-expiratory pressure. Total end-expiratory pressure (the sum of set PEEP plus auto-PEEP, or TEEP) is the actual pressure remaining in the patient's lungs at the end of expiration. This value is not readily observed and therefore must be actively sought. It can be measured on the pressure manometer if the expiratory port is temporarily blocked at the end of expiration. TEEP increases oxygenation in the same way that traditional PEEP does, and, like traditional PEEP, it can cause cardiac compromise if the level is too high. In most cases, oxygenation should increase and decrease as the TEEP level increases and decreases. Attempts should be made to avoid inadvertent decreases in cardiac output by routinely monitoring TEEP. Because the TEEP level is a dynamic value, it can fluctuate with changes in lung compliance and other factors, indicating a need for routine monitoring.

Traditional PEEP can also be used to improve oxygenation in the usual fashion, but it does not eliminate the need to measure TEEP routinely. TEEP should be monitored at least every 2 hours and after every change in ventilator parameters.

Four ventilator parameters can influence the TEEP level: the respiratory rate, the preset inspiratory pressure, the preset PEEP level, and the inspiratory time percentage. An increase or decrease in any one of these factors may cause an increase or decrease, respectively, in the TEEP level. If some of these factors are increased and some are decreased, the resulting TEEP level will be unpredictable due to the possible cancellation effect of this action. The TEEP level must be measured to be determined.

Because HFPPV is used primarily in patients with major pulmonary air leaks, close monitoring of fistula leaks is usually indicated with this mode (for details,

see under Monitoring in the next section on high-frequency jet ventilation).

Adverse Effects. The major adverse effects seen with HFPPV are associated with hypoventilation. Special concern should always be given to airway management and the monitoring of lung compliance and tidal volume, with proper patient selection and effective monitoring, HFPPV can be a successful mode of ventilation.

HIGH-FREQUENCY JET VENTILATION

Definition. High-frequency jet ventilation (otherwise known as HFJV or jet ventilation) in essence comprises the intermittent delivery of high-pressure gas (usually 2 to 40 psi, which is about 140 to 2800 cm H_2O) through a small-bore injector cannula placed in the proximal end of the endotracheal tube. Additional gas is drawn in from an outside source (i.e., entrained). Respiratory rates can range from 60 bpm to more than 200 bpm, but rates of 100 to 150 bpm are commonly used for adults.

Indications and Contraindications. HFJV is primarily intended for use in the treatment of large pulmonary air leaks such as bronchopleural fistulas and tracheoesophageal fistulas and for bronchoscopic and laryngoscopic procedures. HFJV is similar to HFPPV in that the tidal volume is an unpredictable product of the preset inspiratory pressure, inspiratory time percentage, and the back-pressure generated by the patient's respiratory system (Froese and Bryan, 1987). Therefore, HFJV should not be used in patients with decreased lung compliance.

Because of the stronger driving pressure in jet ventilators, HFJV might be indicated in patients with large pulmonary air leaks when HFPPV ventilators cannot provide adequate tidal volumes.

Physiology. Several different gas transport mechanisms may come into play during HFJV. The traditional mechanisms (bulk flow and molecular diffusion) are considered to dominate (Beahrendtz, 1983), but other, less traditional mechanisms have been shown to occur (Korventranta et al., 1987). For more information, see under Physiology in the preceding section on high-frequency ventilation.

Unlike the HFPPV systems, in which the ventilator is used as the sole source of gas for the delivered tidal volume, HFJV systems deliver one portion of the tidal volume through the high-pressure jet injector cannula while another portion is being entrained or "sucked into" the system from an external source, usually a conventional ventilator. An exception to this is the neonatal jet ventilator (e.g., Bunnell).

Applications. The ventilator used for HFJV is different from the ventilator used to deliver HFPPV in many respects. Some of its unique features include the following: (1) driving pressures that can be adjusted from 15 to 40 psi (approximately 1000 to 2800 cm H_2O), and (2) an injector cannula that protrudes into the most proximal portion of the endotracheal tube. Some manufacturers that have developed jet ventilators include Bear Medical, Healthdyne, Bunnell, and Siemens.

Although the ability to deliver adequate humidification is not a drawback with most forms of mechanical ventilation, it is a persistent problem with most HFJV systems used on adult patients. Usually 60% of the delivered tidal volume originates from the jet injector cannula, which pulls in (entrains) the other 40% from another interlinked gas source, usually a conventional ventilator. Gas from the conventional ventilator is easily humidified, whereas gas from the jet ventilator is often completely dry.

To provide adequate humidification to the respiratory tract, a second source of humidification must be integrated into the system. This usually entails hooking up a drip system. An intravenous infusion pump connected to IV tubing can be attached to the appropriate port on the jet injector cannula. Through this set-up, sterile water is introduced at the gas outlet of the injector cannula so that the jet stream can nebulize the fluid (Bear Jet Manual, 1984). Clinical experience shows that water set at a drip rate of 1 mL/minute for every liter/minute of minute ventilation appears to be adequate (Hodel, personal communication).

To monitor airway pressures adequately, the pressure monitoring tubing should be advanced through its designated port on the injector cannula system to a point where it is at least 10 cm away from the tip of the injector cannula. If the tubing is any closer to the injector cannula, the subatmospheric pressure created by the jet stream will affect the pressure readings. When it is properly positioned, the pressure monitor tubing will display what is considered to be alveolar pressures (Bear Jet Manual, 1984).

A respiratory rate of 100 bpm and an inspiratory time percentage of 30% are often used as initial settings for HFJV. The FI_{O_2} is adjusted to achieve adequate oxygenation (O_2 saturation > 90% or Pa_{O_2} > 60 mm Hg). The driving pressure is adjusted to deliver the desired tidal volume (usually 1 to 4 mL/kg).

Monitoring. Managing a patient on HFJV is similar to the method described in the previous section on HFPPV. Because jet ventilators are a type of pressure ventilator, tidal volumes, as with HFPPV, can vary greatly with changes in lung compliance and secretion build-up. Therefore, tidal volumes need close monitoring, and any significant variations must be addressed and acted upon immediately (see under *Monitoring* in the previous section on high-frequency positive pressure ventilation).

When initiating HFJV, hemodynamic parameters, airway pressures, tidal volumes, and arterial blood gas levels must be monitored routinely as well as before, during, and after any change in the ventilator parameters.

Regulation of Pa_{CO_2} is done primarily by adjusting the driving pressure. Increasing the driving pressure should decrease the Pa_{CO_2} level and vice versa. Tidal volumes correlate directly with the driving pressure.

With respiratory rates of 100 bpm or more, it may be difficult to obtain increased ventilation with increased respiratory rates. As the respiratory rate increases, less time is available for each inspiration, and subsequently ventilation diminishes. Increased respiratory rates as well as increased levels of the inspiratory time percentage (greater than 30%) in this mode usually cause increased auto-PEEP with decreased ventilation.

Oxygenation, of course, can be regulated by the FI_{O_2} and PEEP in the traditional fashion. Also, TEEP levels can be regulated by adjusting the respiratory rate and the inspiratory time percentage. An increase or decrease in either parameter will cause an increase or decrease respectively in the level of TEEP. (For more information on TEEP, see under *Monitoring* in the earlier section on high-frequency positive pressure ventilation.)

Because HFJV is primarily used on patients with major pulmonary air leaks, leakage from the fistula should be monitored closely and routinely. A recent study (Roth et al., 1988) indicates that chest tube suction may influence the efficacy of a jet ventilator in the treatment of a bronchopleural fistula. Just as increasing levels of back-pressure (caused by decreased lung compliance, secretion build-up, and so on) can cause any pressure ventilator to deliver less tidal volume, chest tube suction levels may generate a "negative back-pressure." In other words, the suction system creates subatmospheric pressure in the region of the lung adjacent to the chest tube. Therefore, a pressure gradient may exist, flowing from the positive pressure of the ventilator toward the subatmospheric region adjacent to the chest tube. In this study, as suction was increased, the minute volume inspired (V_I) had to be increased to maintain an equivalent Pa_{CO_2} (Fig. 29–3). The need for an increase in V_I may have been due to an increase in leakage through the fistula, facilitated by the pressure gradient (Fig. 29–4). Therefore, routine observation of fistula leaks is necessary to monitor the effect of chest tube suction on jet ventilator function as well as to monitor the leak itself.

Adverse Effects. If water condensation or secretions obstruct the pressure monitor tubing, the ventilator may sense falsely high airway pressures. When pressures reach the driving pressure limit, the ventilator may stop functioning until the line is cleared. Such a situation may adversely affect the patient. Routine purging of the pressure-sensing line may prevent obstruction of the tubing.

Even if a secondary humidification system is implemented, inadequate humidification remains a concern. Thicker secretions are often one of the first clinical manifestations of poor humidification. As a consequence, routine suctioning with lavage is a

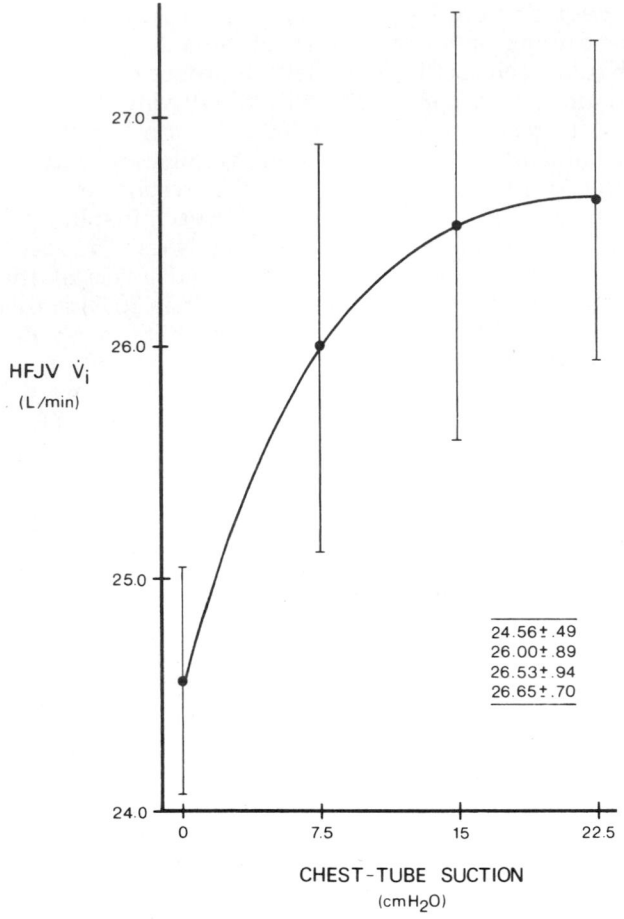

FIGURE 29–3. Relationship of chest tube suction to delivered minute ventilation delivered by high-frequency jet ventilation (HFJV). (From Roth, M. D., Wright, J. W., and Bellamy, P. E. (1988). Gas flow through a bronchopleural fistula. *Chest*, 93, 210, 213.

simple yet effective means of preventing the adverse effect of secretions obstructing the airway.

Because HFJV is delivered through a pressure ventilator, a common adverse effect of this mode is hypoventilation caused by a decrease in lung compliance or a build-up of airway secretions. This further emphasizes the need for routine suctioning with lavage.

HIGH-FREQUENCY OSCILLATORY VENTILATION

Definition. High-frequency oscillatory ventilation is the application of high-frequency (100 to 3000 cycles/minute) pulsations of gas in a sinusoidal wave pattern providing tidal volumes lower than normal physiologic dead space levels to support ventilation with significantly lower airway pressures.

Indications. Much additional research defining the indications for this type of ventilatory support is needed before specific recommendations can be made. However, recent studies have demonstrated improvement of gas exchange in patients suffering

from either IRDS or ARDS. It is believed that in these patients the high-frequency technique serves to apply a form of distending pressure (similar to CPAP) while effectively removing carbon dioxide (Froese and Bryan, 1987).

Other possible patient groups include those with pulmonary interstitial emphysema, persistent tracheoesophageal fistulas, and persistent pulmonary hypertension of the newborn (PPHN). The main goal, again, would be to allow adequate oxygenation and ventilation while lowering intrapulmonary pressures. Conclusive evidence for this result is still pending.

Contraindications. Due to the experimental nature of this mode of ventilation, specific contraindications have yet to be established. It does appear that obstructive lung disease has the greatest potential to produce inadvertent PEEP or overdistention. Thus, any patient in whom the expiratory phase of the

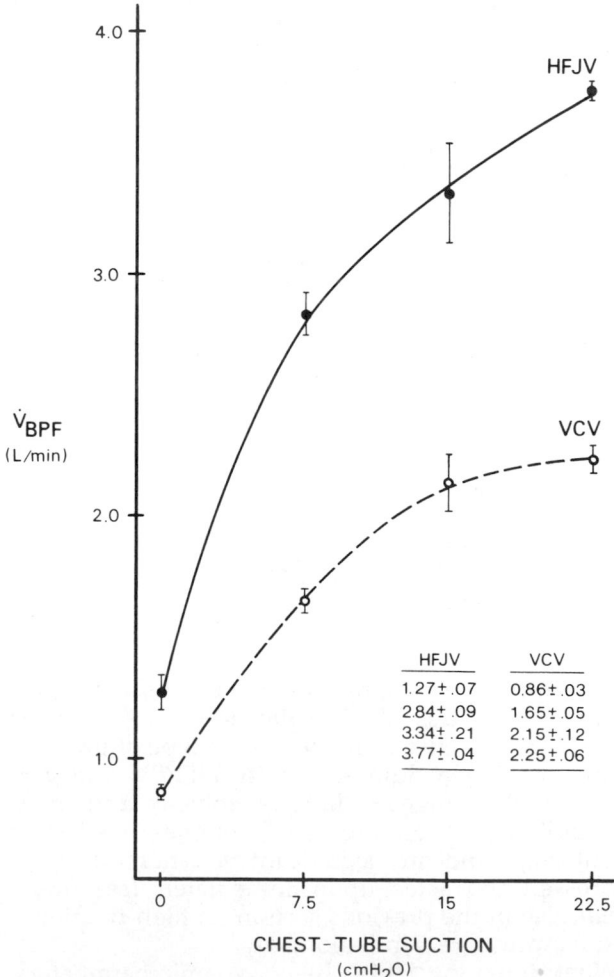

FIGURE 29–4. Flow rates through a bronchopleural fistula ($\dot{V}_{BPF}$) as a function of chest tube suctioning and ventilator type. VCV, volume-cycled ventilation. (From Roth, M. D., Wright, J. W., and Bellamy, P. E. (1988). Gas flow through a bronchopleural fistula. *Chest*, 93, 210, 213.)

breathing cycle is prolonged must be considered a poor candidate for this mode of ventilation.

Physiology. Contrary to past accepted respiratory physiologic beliefs, carbon dioxide can be effectively removed (ventilated) with tidal volumes less than those of the normal anatomic dead space. The mechanism for this phenomenon appears to be multifactorial and is not totally understood. Although bulk movement of gas still plays a role in gas exchange, other and possibly more dominant effects contribute. These include molecular diffusion (the normal movement of gas at and below the terminal bronchioles); the pendeluft effect (the movement of gas from areas of greater airway resistance or lower lung compliance to areas of lower airway resistance or higher lung compliance); cardiogenic mixing (in essence, the pounding of the heart adding to the normal gas mixing inside the lung); and velocity profiles (inspiratory gas characteristics that are unlike those of exhaled gas due to the presence of directional changes [bifurcations of the airway direction into the lung]) (Froese and Bryan, 1987).

Oxygenation appears to be improved by mechanisms that result in increased mean airway pressures. Specifically, PEEP-like effects are achieved, allowing for recruitment of collapsed alveoli, which in turn reduce the overall shunt fraction. Furthermore, animal research indicates that surfactant secretion is enhanced with high-frequency oscillatory ventilation, consequently providing improvement in alveolar stability (Nicholas, 1983).

Application. Oscillatory ventilators vary in design and function. Some require augmentation from another ventilator to assist with carbon dioxide removal or to supply bias flow. Others operate as a stand-alone ventilator. Still others actively suck out exhaled volumes. In any case, often a frequency of approximately 10 to 15 Hz (600 to 900 cycles/minute) is established. Peak inspiratory pressures and PEEP are adjusted to optimize gas exchange. Usually tidal volumes (amplitude) are adjusted to maximize ventilation, and then rate adjustments are made if needed. Exact tidal volume–frequency ratios have not yet been established. Weaning from high-frequency oscillation usually occurs by reducing tidal volumes (amplitude), with return to a conventional mode of ventilation. The patient is then further weaned from the conventional mode of ventilation.

Monitoring. Monitoring of these patients requires observation of those parameters often associated with other modes of ventilation. These include arterial blood gases, hemodynamic parameters, airway pressures, oximetry, and so on. In addition, the potential for gas trapping is high, and attempts to detect it are required. Detection can be achieved by measuring the differences between static and effective compliances. The use of an oscilloscope for monitoring the

high frequency rates and wave forms may be recommended.

Adverse Effects. Adverse effects include air trapping with overdistention of the lungs, carbon dioxide retention, hypoxemia, and a transient increase in the production of respiratory secretions. Any or all of these may constitute a hazard to the patient, and a change to another mode of ventilatory support may be indicated.

Differential Lung Ventilation

Definition. Differential lung ventilation is a method of ventilating each lung independently. In other words, the patient is mechanically ventilated by two ventilators, one for each lung. The parameters of each ventilator can therefore be different for each lung.

Indications and Contraindications. The primary indication for differential lung ventilation is unilateral lung disease that has failed conventional treatment. It may be advantageous during the course of unilateral lung disease to ventilate the more diseased lung in a manner dissimilar to the method used on the more normal lung. Differential lung ventilation has also been shown to be effective for the treatment of pediatric burn patients, for patients with acute diffuse lung disease or acute respiratory failure, and for patients undergoing surgery in the lateral posture (Beahrendtz, 1983). Differential lung ventilation should not be implemented when personnel are inadequately trained to work with this mode, or when the difficulty of performing bilateral intubations outweighs the benefits of using the mode.

Physiology. Although ventilations are mainly distributed toward the nondependent regions (upper lobes) of the lungs in both healthy subjects and patients with respiratory failure, perfusion, on the other hand, tends to be predominantly distributed toward the dependent lung regions (lower lobes). This physiologic mismatching may supplement the similar mismatching caused by the pulmonary disorder, creating further mismatching and eventually severe hypoxemia.

If PEEP is implemented in an attempt to improve oxygenation, it usually does so in a nonuniform manner. Because PEEP causes some alveoli to inflate (and some to overinflate), the pulmonary capillary beds are compressed, forcing the perfusion distribution even more toward the dependent regions of the lung. In this area, where perfusion dominates, the alveoli tend to expand less due to the swollen capillary beds, and thus airway closure is more extensive. Therefore, PEEP not only distributes itself away from a zone where it is needed, it also indirectly shifts perfusion and, subsequently, airway closure, toward the area that is lacking in airway distention pressure. PEEP is more readily accepted in the nondependent region, where perfusion is decreased and the alveoli are highly likely to be overdistended. This imbalance places the nondependent regions in jeopardy of barotrauma as PEEP levels are increased in an attempt to recruit not only pathologic alveoli but also those alveoli in the dependent region.

One can see, from this example of PEEP, that some pulmonary disorders will only add to the maldistribution problem. A possible solution is to attempt to segregate lung regions that are underexpanded from regions that are overdistended. Differential lung ventilation makes such a concept a possibility.

Application. The first step in implementing differential lung ventilation is to verify that the indications are appropriate: namely, the presence of unilateral lung disease. Although the criteria for qualification as unilateral lung disease may vary from vague to obvious (e.g., one traumatized lung), chest x-rays are always helpful.

One major step that must be taken before initiating differential lung ventilation is to institute the appropriate intubation process. Ventilation can be provided separately to each lung by (1) selectively intubating each mainstem bronchus, (2) selectively intubating one mainstem bronchus and then placing a second endotracheal tube in the trachea, or (3) utilizing a double-lumen endotracheal tube. When a double-lumen endotracheal tube is used, the distal end is inserted into a mainstem bronchus (usually the right mainstem because its angle of bifurcation allows easier intubation). One lung is ventilated from gas exiting this distal opening while the other lung is ventilated from gas exiting a port located just above the level of the carina. An inflatable cuff is located above each port to prevent cross-ventilation and airway leaks.

After intubation, two ventilators that can be electronically synchronized (such as the Siemens-Elema Servo 900C) may need to be obtained. Synchronization allows inspiration for the two ventilators, and thus the two lungs, to be exactly simultaneous. One ventilator (the master) controls the initiation of inspiration on the other (the slave).

The sum of the two delivered tidal volumes should be kept at 7 to 10 mL/kg (Beahrendtz, 1983). PEEP may be added to the more diseased (or traumatized) lung by methods to be mentioned later in this section.

Monitoring. The three general areas to be monitored are the various airway pressures, hemodynamic parameters, static compliance, and arterial blood gas values. Pulse oximeters are adequate for oxygenation monitoring. Capnography can be utilized to monitor end-tidal CO_2, provided a separate monitoring line (or system) is used for each ventilator.

Considering the need implied previously (in the physiology section) for more ventilation to the dependent region of the lung to offset its increased perfusion, airway closure, and atelectasis, the clinician might suspect that delivery of large tidal volumes to the more diseased (or traumatized) lung would be beneficial. However, studies indicate that use of the same size tidal volume for both lungs is optimal. With conventional ventilation, the one delivered tidal volume tends to migrate away from the atelectatic lung to the healthier, more compliant, lung. When equal tidal volumes are delivered during differential lung ventilation, the more diseased lung should receive more ventilation than it would have with conventional ventilation simply because a portion of the total volume is differentially selected to be delivered directly toward that lung, minimizing migration away from it (Beahrendtz, 1983). When a larger portion of the tidal volume is directed toward the more diseased lung, pulmonary vascular resistance increases, as does dead space volume, but cardiac output and Pa_{O_2} decrease (Beahrendtz, 1983). Needless to say, similar tidal volumes should be set on both ventilators.

During differential lung ventilation, the healthier lung will tend to have peak inspiratory pressures and mean airway pressures that may be lower than those received with conventional ventilation (Beahrendtz, 1983). The more diseased lung should have peak inspiratory pressures and mean airway pressures that are higher than those received with conventional ventilation (Beahrendtz, 1983) because this lung actually experiences more ventilation (and thus more positive pressure).

Improved ventilation of the diseased (or traumatized) lung probably results from a reduction in low V/Q regions. True shunt should be reduced, possibly due to the opening of atelectatic areas and closed airways. A slight decrease in cardiac output can be observed, possibly due to decreases in pulmonary vascular resistance and mean intrathoracic pressure. (Beahrendtz, 1983).

Adverse Effects. Differential lung ventilation can potentially increase risk to the patient if (1) inexperienced personnel perform it, (2) monitoring of airway pressures, hemodynamic parameters, arterial blood gas values, and static lung compliance is inadequate, (3) the endotracheal tube becomes dislodged or rotated, or (4) secretions are allowed to build up in the endotracheal tube or tubes, which have relatively small internal diameters and therefore are more prone to obstruction.

Extracorporeal Membrane Oxygenation (ECMO)

Definition. Extracorporeal membrane oxygenation (ECMO) is the implementation of a circuit and membrane lung to remove the majority of a patient's circulating blood volume for the purpose of oxygenation and ventilation, followed by return of the blood to the patient's circulation.

Indications. ECMO is the treatment of last resort for term infants who would otherwise die because of decreased lung function. The patient must meet certain criteria before institution of ECMO can be considered. The patient is usually a newborn weighing at least 2 kg who has been on mechanical ventilatory assist for no more than 7 days, has no intracranial hemorrhage or congenital heart disease but does have reversible lung disease and meets the respiratory failure index indicating a 80% to 100% predicted mortality. Often these patients suffer from either meconium aspiration syndrome (MAS), severe respiratory distress syndrome (IRDS), persistent pulmonary hypertension (PPHN), or sepsis. The common denominator in all of these patients is the presence of pulmonary hypertension.

Contraindications. Failure to meet the above stated criteria or lack of parental or guardian consent constitutes a contraindication for ECMO.

Physiology. Some newborn infants develop pulmonary hypertension secondary to any number of disease processes. As a result, significant right-to-left (cyanotic) shunting can occur, leaving the patient in a state of cyanosis and acidosis. This essentially is a persistence of fetal blood flow or circulation (commonly called persistent fetal circulation [PFC]). In a select group of these patients reduction of the pulmonary and cardiac blood flow for 5 to 7 days allows the pulmonary pressures to return to near normal while the heart and lungs are rested. This can be accomplished by draining approximately 75% of the cardiac output from the venous side of the patient and circulating it through a membrane oxygenator. This will permit artificial oxygenation and ventilation of the blood. Once this has been achieved the "arterialized" blood is returned to the aorta of the patient through a circulating pump where it can supply the body with the necessary oxygen and nutrients (Fig. 29–5).

Application. Once the decision has been made to institute ECMO, the patient is heparinized to prevent embolic events from occurring while on circulatory assist. The right jugular vein is cannulated to allow insertion of a venous catheter down into the right atrium. Similarly, an arterial catheter is inserted into the right carotid artery so that the tip is inside the aortic arch. Once attached to the ECMO pump circuit, venous blood can drain via gravity toward a circulating pump. From there it is pumped through a membrane oxygenator. Here oxygen and carbon dioxide can be exchanged by the same mechanisms that operate in the natural lung functions. By adjusting the flow of oxygen and carbon dioxide through the membrane lung, arterialization of the venous blood is achieved. The blood is rewarmed and then is returned to the patient through the arterial catheter located in the arch of the aorta. The blood then can enter the brain through the left carotid artery and

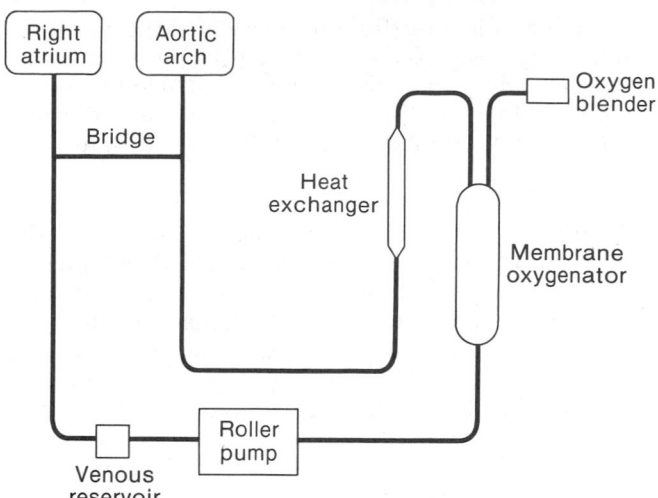

FIGURE 29–5. Extracorporeal membrane oxygenation (ECMO) circuit.

continue on through the rest of the body through the normal circulation. The lungs and heart are now able to "rest" and healing of the diseased lungs is promoted.

Weaning involves reducing the circulating blood flow so that the patient's lungs and heart begin to carry the bulk of the respiratory and circulatory flow. Once the patient has been weaned from the majority of the circulatory bypass, the patient is removed from the ECMO circuit. The right carotid artery and the jugular vein are ligated to prevent cranial embolisms. Note that prior to institution of ECMO these patients require high levels of inspired oxygen and ventilatory support. However, once on ECMO they can be rapidly weaned to very low ventilatory settings.

Monitoring. The bulk of the monitoring of these patients consists of close observation of the ECMO circuit, heparinization of the patient and circuit, adjustments in circulatory flows, stabilization of arterial blood gases, and observation of blood pressure. The greatest concern is the regulation of coagulation times. These patients are at greater risk of intracranial bleeding, and thus a combination of overanticoagulation and elevated intracranial blood pressure could be lethal. The need for adjustments of the sweep gases (gases that ventilate and oxygenate the membrane lung) and pump flows is determined by analyzing the results of arterial, postmembrane, and mixed venous blood gases. Routine CNS evaluations are performed to alert the clinician to any possibility of intracranial hemorrhage. Aseptic techniques are strictly adhered to when dealing with any part of the ECMO circuit. Airway care and pulmonary toilet are carried out as per ICU protocols, and full-time, one-to-one nursing care is mandatory. Blood products, especially platelets, are replenished as needed, and electrolyte balances are carefully maintained. Surprisingly, these patients, once on ECMO, become very stable from a cardiopulmonary standpoint. And, despite the loss of the right jugular vein and the right carotid artery, the outcome is usually quite favorable. In fact, these patients, with a predicted mortality of over 85%, have a 90% survival rate with the institution of ECMO.

Adverse Effects. By far the most serious complication occurring during ECMO is the development of an intracranial hemorrhage. Patients with this complication constitute the great majority of the 10% to 15% of patients who die during or soon after the institution of ECMO. Although sepsis is always a constant threat, it has a relatively low incidence (<1.5%). Other complications include bleeding, failure to be weaned from ECMO, and mechanical failure of the ECMO circuit or pump.

ROUTINE CARE OF PATIENTS ON MECHANICAL VENTILATION

Humanistic Approach

All patients have a resistance to being placed on mechanical ventilation. Often it is the primary means of life support for the patient. On other occasions, it is a very temporary measure. At all times, however, the clinician must recognize the fact that he is managing the care of the patient connected to the ventilator, not the ventilator itself. The needs of the patient should be addressed through frequent communication with the patient. The patient can best determine his own comfort and is the source of valuable feedback for the clinician.

Ventilator Checks and Humidification

The ventilator should be checked regularly for proper functioning, proper settings, appropriate alarm settings, and proper delivery of humidification. To maintain adequate humidification, the humidifier reservoir must be filled with water to the level indicating "full," and the water level should not be allowed to descend below the "refill" level. The heating device should be adjusted so that inspired gas is kept between 34° and 37°C. Higher airway temperatures (up to 39°C) are occasionally used on hypothermic patients. Warmer airway temperatures (approximately 37°C) usually facilitate the mobilization of tenacious secretions. The tenacity of secretions is a clinical manifestation that is often used to determine the efficacy of the current airway temperature setting. Higher airway temperatures will increase the ability of gas to hold water vapor. Therefore, condensation or "rain out" also increases as a result. Water should be drained as it accumulates in the tubing of the ventilator circuit. The water condensation problem is significantly minimized by using a heated-wire circuit. This system stabilizes the temperature, preventing condensation.

Suctioning

A significant mechanism clearing the patient's airways and the artificial airway is suctioning. Secretion build-up can increase airway pressure readings, diminish ventilation and oxygenation, limit the patient's comfort, and obstruct the airway. Lavaging the airway before suctioning is very effective in loosening tenacious secretions, thereby facilitating secretion removal (see also Chap. 30).

Assessment

Mechanical ventilation is a dynamic mode of therapy. The patient's status can change quickly. Breath sounds must be checked routinely for adverse clinical signs, adequacy of ventilation, and endotracheal tube position. Endotracheal tubes must be taped securely, and tracheostomy tubes should be cleaned routinely. Frequent monitoring of hemodynamic parameters, airway pressures, and arterial blood gas values are essential. Breath sounds are also essential in determining whether bronchodilators are called for or if mucolytics or increased humidification is needed for mucokinesis.

VENTILATOR TROUBLESHOOTING

The optimal response to problems with ventilators is, by far, calm and systematic action. On many occasions, the clinician may become overwhelmed by the copious amount of technologic equipment found in the intensive care unit setting and may respond irrationally to alarms or problems with the performance of the ventilator. To rectify the situation, he or she must quickly assess whether or not the patient is in immediate danger. If so, the clinician is responsible for ensuring that the fundamentals of ventilation and oxygenation have been implemented.

Whenever a problem occurs with a patient on mechanical ventilation, the basics of ventilation and oxygenation can be provided with a hand-bag resuscitator connected to an oxygen source and suctioning. If these two items are readily available at the bedside (and they must be), the clinician should have confidence that, if all else fails, he or she can maintain ventilation and oxygenation and manage the airway as well. Once the patient is out of danger and stabilized, the problem-solving process can begin. Using the systematic approach, the simplest problems and their potential solutions are sought first, and the more difficult problems and their solutions are then gradually considered.

A quick general surveillance of the immediate area is often the starting point. In other words, the clinician should look for the obvious, such as a disconnected ventilator circuit, crimped ventilator tubing, or a need for suctioning. If this process does not unveil the problem, then the alarm system must be checked. One should determine which alarm or alarms have been triggered and then search for possible causes (e.g., pressure limit alarm for obstruction, low tidal volume due to a loosely fitted section of tubing, and so on).

The systematic approach to the ventilator itself begins at the main gas outlet (where tubing is connected to a fitting protruding from the ventilator) and works toward the patient. If the patient is being ventilated by a hand-bag resuscitator, the tubing can be disconnected at this point, and a volume-measuring device such as a Wright's respirometer can be connected to the outlet port. If the volume measured is grossly different from the volume preset on the ventilator, the ventilator itself may be malfunctioning and must be replaced. If the volume measured approximates the preset volume, then the ventilator is probably not the source of the trouble.

The next step in the systematic check-out is the humidifier. It can be ruled out as a leak source by simply bypassing it. The volume is measured distally (toward the patient). If the volume measures less with the humidifier connected, then it is the source of a leak.

All of the ventilator circuit tubing should be checked for an airtight fit. Be sure to rule out an endotracheal tube cuff leak. If the circuit has an in-line nebulizer for aerosol treatments, it should be bypassed to rule it out as a leak source. As long as a hand-bag resuscitator is readily available, troubleshooting can be done without haste and without harm to the patient.

References

Beahrendtz, S. (1983). Differential ventilation and selective positive end-expiratory pressure; effects on patients during anesthesia and intensive care. *Opuscula Medica,* Suppl. LXI.

Bear Medical Company (1984). *Bear jet high frequency ventilator operator manual.* Riverside, CA.

Bjerager, K., Sjostrand, U., and Wattwil, M. (1977). Long-term treatment of two patients with respiratory insufficiency with IPPV/PEEP and HPPV/PEEP. *Acta Anaesthesiologica Scandinavica* Suppl. 64, 55.

Burton, B. G., Hodgkin, J. E., and Gee, G. N. (1984). *Respiratory care, a guide to clinical practice.* Philadelphia: J. B. Lippincott.

Carlon, G. C., Miodownik, S., and Ray, C., Jr. (1985). *High frequency jet ventilation: Technical evaluation and device characterization* (pp. 77–110). New York: Marcel Dekker.

Carlon, G. C., Klain, M., Kalla, R., et al. (1979). High frequency positive pressure ventilation-applications in acute respiratory failure (abstract). *Critical Care Medicine,* 7, 82.

Chatburn, R. (1984). New modes of ventilation: high frequency

ventilation: A report on a state of the art symposium; overview of HFV technology. *Respiratory Care,* 29, 8.

Cole, A. G. H., Weller, S. F., and Sykes, M. K. (1984). Inverse ratio ventilation compared with PEEP in adult respiratory failure. *Intensive Care Medicine,* 10, 227–232.

Craig, K., Pierson, D., and Carrico, J. (1988). The clinical application of positive end-expiratory pressure (PEEP) in the adult respiratory distress syndrome (ARDS). *Respiratory Care,* 30, 185–201.

Duncan, S. R., Rizk, N. W., and Rabbin, T. A. (1987). Inverse ratio ventilation. PEEP in disguise? (editorial). *Chest,* 390–392.

Fredberg, J. J., Keffe, D. H., Glass, G. M., et al. (1984). Alveolar pressure nonhomogeneity during small amplitude high-frequency oscillation. *Journal of Applied Physiology,* 57, 788–800.

Froese, A. B., and Bryan, A. L. (1987). State of art/high-frequency ventilation. *American Review of Respiratory Diseases,* 135, 1363–1374.

Gross, D., Zidulka, A., O'Brien, C., et al. (1985). Peripheral mucociliary clearance with high frequency chest wall compressions. *Journal of Applied Physiology,* 58, 1157–1163.

Gurevitch, M. J., Van Dyke, J., Young, E. et al. (1986). Improved oxygenation and lower peak airway pressure in severe adult respiratory distress syndrome; treatment with inverse ratio ventilation. *Chest,* 89, 211–213.

Gurevitch, M. J. (1988). Selection of the inspiratory, expiratory ratio. *Current respiratory care.* Philadelphia: B. C. Decker.

Harf, A., Zidulka, A., and Chang, H. K. (1985). N_2 washout during tidal breathing with superimposed high frequency chest wall oscillation. *American Review of Respiratory Disease,* 132, 250–253.

Hazelton, F. R., and Scherer, P. W. (1980). Bronchial bifurcations and respiratory mass transport. *Science,* 208, 69–71.

Henderson, Y., Chillingworth, F. P., and Whitney, J. L. (1915). The respiratory dead space. *American Journal of Physiology,* 38, 1–19.

Hodel, R. Clinical observations. Personal communication, 1986.

Kacmarek, P. R. (1988). The role of pressure support ventilation in reducing work of breathing. *Respiratory Care,* 33, 99–120.

Kirby, R. (1979). *Design of mechanical ventilators, neonatal pulmonary care.* Reading, MA: Addison-Wesley.

Kirby, R. (1988). *Modes of mechanical ventilation, current respiratory care.* Toronto, Philadelphia: B. C. Decker.

Korvenranta, H., Carlo, W. A., Goldthwait, D. A., et al. (1987). Carbon dioxide elimination during high frequency jet ventilation. *Journal of Pediatrics,* 111, 107–113.

Lehr, J. L., Butler, J. P., Westerman, P. A., et al. (1985). Photographic measurement of pleural surface motion during lung oscillation. *Journal of Applied Physiology,* 59, 623–633.

MacIntyre, N. R. (1986). Pressure support ventilation (editorial). *Respiratory Care,* 31, 189–190.

MacIntyre, N. R. (1987). Pressure support ventilation: Effects on ventilatory reflexes and ventilator muscle workloads. *Respiratory Care,* 32, 447–453.

MacIntyre, N. R. (1988a). Pressure support: Inspiratory assist. In R. M. Kacmarek and J. K. Stoller (Eds.), *Current Respiratory Care,* Toronto: B. C. Decker.

MacIntyre, N. R. (1988b). Weaning from mechanical ventilatory support: Volume-assisting intermittent breaths versus pressure-assisting every breath. *Respiratory Care,* 33, 121–125.

Maunder, R., Rice, C., Benson, M., et al. (1986). Managing positive end-expiratory pressure (PEEP): the Harborview approach. *Respiratory Care,* 31, 1059–1064.

McPherson, S. (1985). *Respiratory therapy equipment* (3rd ed.). St. Louis: C. V. Mosby.

Nicholas, T. E., and Barr, H. A. (1983). The release of surfactant in rat lung by periods of hyperventilation. *Respiratory Physiology,* 52, 69–83.

Petty, T. L., and Fowler, A. A. (1982). Another look at ARDS. *Chest,* 82, 98–104.

Roth, M. D., Wright, J. W., and Bellamy, P. E. (1988). Gas flow through a bronchopleural fistula. *Chest,* 93, 210–213.

Shapiro, B., Harrison, R., and Trout, C. (1982). *Clinical application of respiratory care* (2nd ed.). Chicago: Year Book.

Shelledy, D. C., and Mikles, S. P. (1988). Newer modes of mechanical ventilation, part I: Pressure support. *Respiratory Management,* 18, 21–28.

Sjostrand, O. (1980). High frequency positive pressure ventilation (HFPPV): A review. *Critical Care Medicine*, 8, 345–364.

Slutsky, A. S., Brown, R., Lehr, J., et al. (1981). High frequency ventilation: A promising new approach to mechanical ventilation. *Medical Instrument*, 15, 229–233.

Slutsky, A. S. (1981). Gas mixing by cardiogenic oscillations: A theoretical quantitative analysis. *Journal of Applied Physiology*, 51, 1287–1293.

Ward, H. E., Armemgol, J., and Jones, R. L. (1985). Ventilation by external high frequency oscillation in cats. *Journal of Applied Physiology*, 58(4), 1390.

Wattwil, L. M., Sjostrand, U. H., and Bog, U. R. (1983). Comparative studies of IPPV and HFPPV with PEEP in critical care patients. A critical evaluation. *Critical Care Medicine*, 11, 30–37.

Wren, W. S. (1983). High frequency positive pressure ventilation (HFPPV) in a newborn infant with ruptured lungs. *The British Journal of Anaesthesia*, 55, 575.

Chronic Ventilator-Dependent Patients

Donna J. Wilson

Critically ill patients requiring mechanical ventilation for longer than 2 weeks face several potential complications. The primary goals of care for these patients include preventing these complications and weaning the patient from dependence on chronic ventilation. Many challenges are faced by critical care nurses as they assist patients in reaching these goals. This chapter will focus on the care of the chronically ventilated patient, including causes of respiratory decompensation and airway management, and emphasizing weaning, including criteria used to assess weaning capability, weaning methods, airway management during weaning, and causes of failure to wean.

AIRWAY MANAGEMENT

Airway management is an essential part of nursing care of the ventilator-dependent patient. The artificial airway is either an oral or nasal endotracheal tube or a tracheostomy tube. A discussion of the advantages and disadvantages of each airway and the design of standard and specialized airway appliances follows.

Endotracheal Tubes

Endotracheal intubation or tracheostomy is performed to provide positive pressure ventilation, to protect the airway from aspiration, to remove tracheobronchial secretions, and to relieve airway obstruction. The three approaches that must be considered are oral endotracheal intubation, nasal endotracheal intubation, and tracheostomy. The advantages and disadvantages of each approach are summarized in Table 30–1 (Wilson, 1988). The type of tube selected is based on assessment of the patient, need for a long-term artificial airway and mechanical ventilation, patient tolerance, and the related advantages and disadvantages of each situation.

Oral endotracheal tubes are generally placed in emergency situations because of the ease of insertion. This tube can be larger in size and is shorter in length; therefore, access for suctioning and bronchoscopy is not limited. Patients tolerate the oral tube poorly because it stimulates the gag reflex, increases the production of saliva, and swallowing is more difficult compared with the nasal tube. Oral hygiene is often difficult to perform because of the taping necessary to hold the tube in place and the use of bite blocks or oral airways to prevent the patient from biting the tube, causing airway obstruction. Maintaining the proper position of the endotracheal tube as well as skin integrity is the responsibility of the nurse.

Nasal endotracheal tubes are better tolerated for extended periods of time and are far more comfortable for the conscious patient. Patients can swallow more easily and can communicate with lip motion. Nurses can perform mouth care more effectively. Stabilization of the nasal tube is easier, and thus self-extubation and migration of the tube into the mainstem bronchus is less likely. The disadvantages of a nasal tube include the size limitation due to the nasal passageway, tube kinking due to the acute curvature of the nasal route, and poor drainage of sinuses causing sinusitis. If a patient complains of an earache or if drainage is observed from the nose, sinusitis or otitis media should be suspected. At this time the nasal tube should be removed and replaced with an oral tube, or a tracheostomy should be considered.

TABLE 30–1. Advantages and Disadvantages of Various Airway Appliances

Type	Advantages	Disadvantages
Oral endotracheal tube	Easy to insert Large bore; work of breathing less Shorter length; easier to suction Less acute angle; less likely to kink	Requires laryngoscopy Easily dislodged Poorly tolerated by some patients Patients require more sedation Occluded by patient biting tube Oral hygiene difficult Patient has difficulty swallowing Unable to communicate Lip laceration Difficult to stabilize Inadvertent extubation common Laryngeal pathology

Nasal endotracheal tube	Easily secured
	Tolerated better by patient
	Insert blindly when neck motion or
	   visualization is limited
	Allow for oral hygiene
	Able to swallow
	Requires less sedation
	Communication; mouthing of words
		Skilled personnel for placement
		Nasal passageway limits size of tube
		Tube kinking due to curvature
		Inability to drain sinuses; sinusitis
		Obstruction of eustachian tube; otitis
		   media
		Nasal soft tissue injury
		Laryngeal pathology

Tracheostomy tube	Most comfortable
	Easiest to suction
	Communication; mouthing words,
	   talking or fenestrated tracheostomy
	   tubes
	Ability to swallow
	Reinsertion of trach tube relatively
	   easy with mature stoma
	No laryngeal injury
		Surgical procedure
		Complications postsurgery
		   Bleeding
		   Pneumothorax
		   Subcutaneous emphysema infection
		Posterior tracheal wall rupture during
		   insertion
		False passage in subcutaneous tissue
		Stenosis, stoma; cuff
		Granulation tissue formation
		Innominate artery erosion

From Wilson, D. J. Airway appliances and management. In: Kacmarek, R. M., and Stoller, J. K., eds. Current Respiratory Care. Toronto: B. C. Decker, 1988.

Tracheostomy Tubes

In the chronically mechanically ventilated patient a tracheostomy tube is preferred. Although there are no firm guidelines, it is common practice to place a tracheostomy tube 10–14 days following oral or nasal tracheal intubation if an airway appliance is deemed necessary for the foreseeable future (Whited, 1984; Heffner et al., 1986). The decision for tracheostomy must be individualized in any given situation.

Types of Tracheostomy Tubes. Tracheostomy tubes are available in a variety of designs, which differ according to the manufacturer. They differ in composition, type of neck flange, size, length, and cuff design. The most common material used to make cuff tracheostomy tubes is polyvinylchloride (PVC) (for example, those made by Portex, Inc., Concord, NH; or Shiley, Irving, CA). The tube size is printed on the neck flange. The tubes are sized according to the inner and outer diameters of the tube. The most common tube sizes are 7.0 mm and 8.0 mm inner diameter (ID) (i.e., a number 6 Shiley is a 7.0-mm ID tube). The lengths of tracheostomy tubes differ depending on the design and the manufacturer (Table 30–2). There is a relationship between the size and the length of the tubes—that is, the smaller the inner

diameter of the tube the shorter it is in length. There are extra-long tubes for the obese and patients with short "bull" necks (Fig. 30–1). The need for an extra-long tube is determined at the time of surgery or when there is difficulty in sealing a tube because of anatomic variation.

Tracheostomy tube cuffs are designed to be high volume and low pressure. These cuffs are soft, thin-walled, and compliant. The purpose of this design is to prevent tracheal injury. The large-volume diameter cuff conforms to the shape of the trachea, creating a seal with a low lateral tracheal wall pressure. The most common cuff inflation techniques are the minimal leak and the minimal occlusive techniques (Crabtree-Goodnough, 1988). The minimal leak technique is recommended to avoid excessive cuff pressure against the trachea while maintaining an adequate seal for positive pressure ventilation and airway protection. Cuff inflation is adjusted so that a small air leak is audible only at the end of the inspiratory phase with a positive pressure breath. In the minimal occlusive technique, the cuff is inflated so that there is no air leak on inspiration. In patients who cannot protect their airway it is advisable to use a minimal occlusive technique. After reinflation of the cuff, the pressure in the cuff should be measured. The cuff pressure should be maintained at a maxi-

TABLE 30–2. Tracheostomy Tube Size Chart

Size	Portex Standard (mm)	Portex Extra (mm)	Shiley Single Cannula (mm)	Shiley Double Cannula (mm)	Jackson* Stainless Steel (mm)
6.0 mm ID	67	—	67	—	69
7.0 mm ID (No. 6)	73	84	80	78	69
8.0 mm ID	78	95	89	—	69
8.5 mm ID (No. 8)	—	—	—	84	69
9.0 mm ID	84	106	99	—	69
10.0 mm ID (No. 10)	84	—	105	84	69

ID, interior diameter.
*Jackson No. 7 extra long = 85 mm.

mum level of 20 to 30 mm Hg to minimize the adverse effects of cuff pressure on blood flow to the tracheal mucosa. The perfusion pressure of tracheal tissue in a normotensive patient has been estimated at approximately 30 mm Hg. Ischemia results whenever the cuff tracheal pressure exceeds the perfusion pressure. The cuff should never be maintained at a volume higher than that necessary to just prevent a leak from occurring. Maintaining a cuff volume higher than this renders the patient vulnerable to a wide spectrum of tracheal damage. It should be emphasized again that the lowest possible cuff pressure and cuff volume should be maintained to prevent tracheal injury.

Specialized Airway Appliances

Inability to speak with an artificial airway is frustrating for the patient, family, and health care team. Patients and nurses are often anxious because of the difficulties with lip reading. A variety of appliances are available to promote communication. The talking tracheostomy tubes, fenestrated tracheostomy tubes, and cuffless tracheostomy tubes require functioning vocal cords to allow speech.

Talking Tracheostomy Tubes. Several manufacturers supply talking tracheostomy tubes. A talking tracheostomy tube allows speech with the cuff inflated, thus providing airway protection and the use of positive pressure ventilation (Safar and Grenvik, (1975) (Fig. 30–2). The tube has a single-lumen cannula with two external ports. There is a cuff inflation line and a talking port. The talking port is a small tube set into the curvature of the tube, terminating

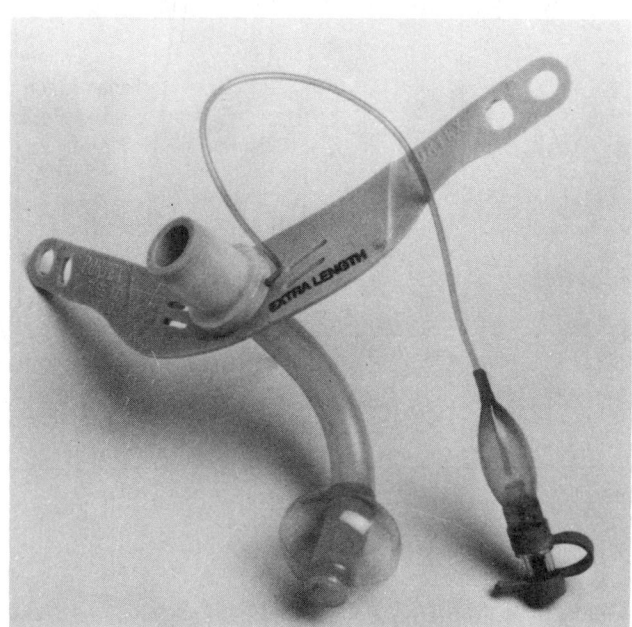

FIGURE 30–1. Extra long tracheostomy tube for the obese and for patients with short bull necks.

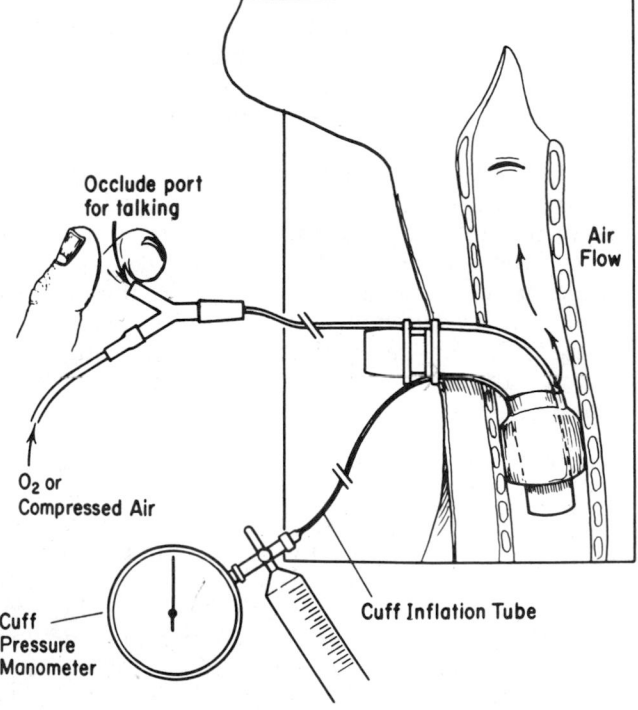

Occlude port for talking

O₂ or Compressed Air

Air Flow

Cuff Pressure Manometer

Cuff Inflation Tube

FIGURE 30–2. Talking tracheostomy tube.

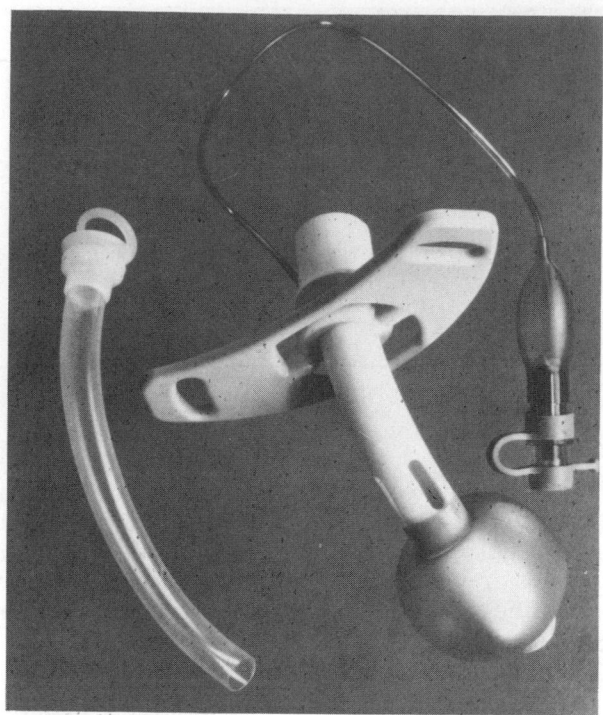

FIGURE 30–3. Cuffed fenestrated tracheostomy tube with disposable inner cannula (Portex, Concord, NH).

function are the methylene blue test and a modified barium swallow. The nurse can perform the methylene blue test at the bedside. Deep tracheal suction is performed, the cuff is deflated, and the patient is given 1 ounce of water or ice chips stained with methylene blue. When swallowing is completed, the cuff is inflated, deep tracheal suction is performed again. The sputum is evaluated for color. The test is considered negative if no dye appears in the aspirate, and positive if dye does appear in the aspirate. If the test is positive or if an accurate observation of swallowing is preferred, a modified barium swallow is done. The test is often performed by the Speech Pathology or the Radiology department.

The purpose of a fenestrated tracheostomy tube is to allow patients to breathe, speak, and cough normally, using the upper airway. The two manufacturers that provide fenestrated tracheostomy tubes are Portex and Shiley (Fig. 30–3). This type of tube is designed with a standard cuff, precut fenestration, inner cannula, and plug. The fenestration is a hole in the outer cannula of the tube that will direct air flow through the vocal cords for speaking (Fig. 30–4). A fenestrated tube must be positioned correctly within the lumen of the trachea. This position is determined by bedside measurement or by a lateral

just above the cuff. A flow of gas (compressed air or oxygen) is attached to the two-way connector of the external talking port. The open end of the two-way connector allows air flow to be regulated on or off via a thumb-controlled valve. The flow of gas exits above the cuff, forcing gas through the vocal cords and allowing vocalization. The flow of gas connected to the talking port ranges from 4 to 8 liters/minute. Some patients have a clear audible voice at 5 liters of flow, whereas others require a higher flow rate, and their voice may be a whisper. One reason for poor voice quality is partial obstruction of the talking port with mucus. This can be removed by instilling a 50% solution of Mucomyst and saline and then applying suction to the talking port. The two requirements for use of this tube are that the patient have intact oral motor function and that he be alert.

Another device used for speaking by the mechanically ventilated patient is the artificial larynx. This device is placed against the mandibular triangle; the vibration results in audible speech. This device does not require functioning vocal cords for speech.

Cuffed Fenestrated Tracheostomy Tubes. The cuffed fenestrated tracheostomy tube is utilized in patients who are actively weaning, can maintain spontaneous respirations for at least 2-hour intervals, and can provide airway protection from aspiration with the tracheostomy tube cuff deflated. This type of tube allows preservation of the tracheal air flow and normal glottic function. Before this tube is placed, the patient's ability to swallow must be evaluated. The two tests to evaluate swallowing

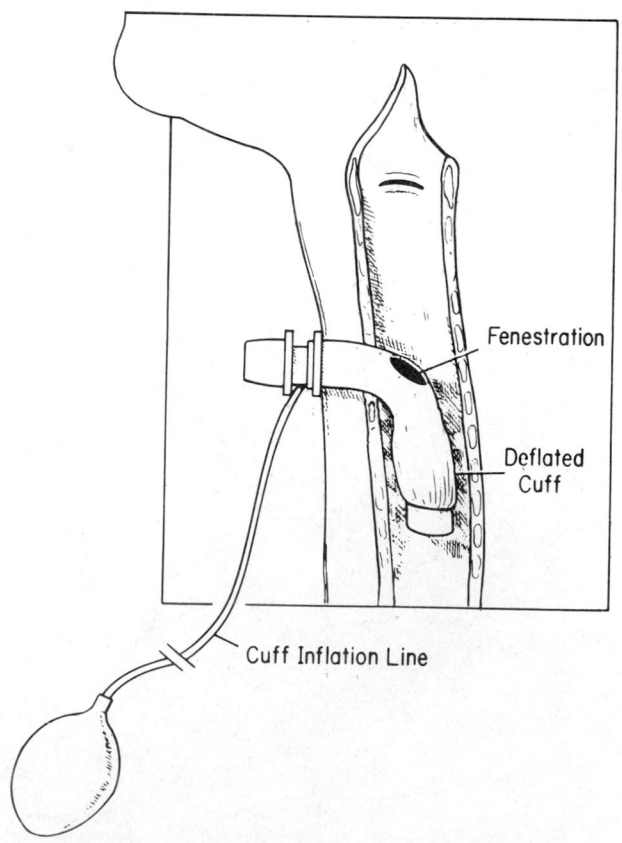

FIGURE 30–4. Proper positioning of a cuffed fenestrated tracheostomy tube in the trachea. The tube is plugged with the fenestration open and the cuff deflated to allow the patient to breathe and speak normally.

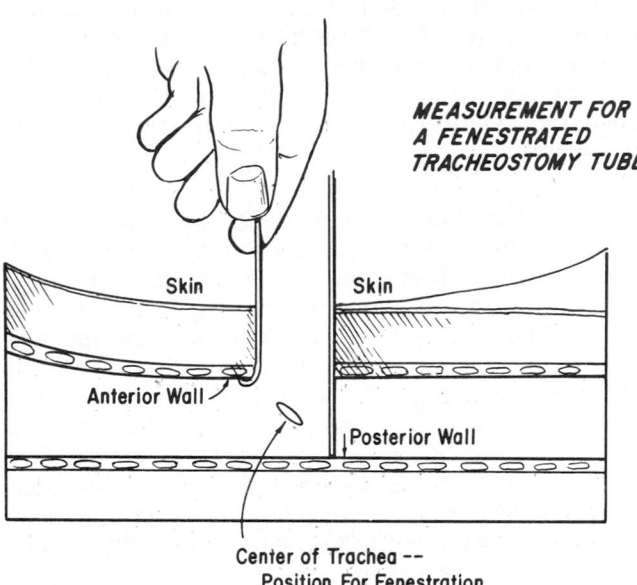

FIGURE 30-5. Bedside technique in measuring for fenestration.

neck x-ray. The bedside measurement is done with sterile pipe cleaners to determine the distance between the anterior and posterior tracheal walls and the skin (Fig. 30–5). The pipe cleaners are placed on the tracheostomy tube to determine whether the fenestration will be positioned correctly in the lumen of the trachea (Fig. 30–6) (Wilson, 1988). If the measured distance is larger than the precut tube, a tube must be custom designed for proper fit. If the fenestration is not placed in the proper position, there is a potential for the growth of granulation tissue occluding the fenestration, thus causing bleeding with each insertion and removal of the inner cannula. If proper placement is questionable, a flexible fiberoptic laryngoscope or bronchoscope can be used to inspect the tube (Snyder, 1983). Nurses should check the placement of the fenestration routinely by removing the inner cannula and examining it by direct vision, using a flashlight. If tissue is observed in the fenestration, the physician should be notified and the tube repositioned or replaced by a new tube to prevent further complications of tracheal injury.

When a cuff fenestrated tube is properly positioned, the patient can breathe, speak, and cough using normal glottic function. To allow use of the upper airway to breathe, the inner cannula must be removed, the cuff deflated, and the tube plugged. Mechanical ventilation and airway protection are secure when the plug is removed, the cuff inflated, and the inner cannula placed to occlude the fenestrations.

If a patient cannot tolerate the fenestrated tube being plugged, a one-way speaking valve may be useful. This can be useful for patients with vocal cord or tracheal pathology, neuromuscular disease, or chronic obstructive pulmonary disease (Passy,

1986). The valve is referred to as a Passy-Muir speaking valve. The valve fits on any tracheostomy tube with a 15-mm adapter. On inspiration the valve opens to allow air to enter through the tube and on expiration the valve closes, directing the air into the trachea and the upper airway to allow vocalization (Figs. 30–7 and 30–8).

Common Problems

Cuff Leak. The most common problem with an artificial airway is a cuff leak. This is evidenced by an audible leak from the patient's mouth or tracheostomy stoma with each positive pressure breath. The causes are faulty tube position, a crack or slow leak in the housing of the one-way inflation line valve, and cuff rupture. Evaluation of a cuff leak is performed before changing the tube. The tube is examined first. Any cause of pull or torque on the tube should be removed. The tracheostomy tube flange should be examined to ensure that it is flush with the patient's neck. The cuff pressure should be measured with the cuff deflated to compare it with the known values. The cuff should be reinflated, using minimal leak technique. When an air leak is present one should inspect the plastic housing of the one-way valve for cracks. Air leaks can be detected by placing the inflation line under water and observing any air bubbles with each positive pressure breath. If air bubbles are present, a hemostat is placed on the pilot balloon, and the tube should be changed within 24 hours. If the hemostat is placed on the small-bore tubing of the inflation line, it will collapse the small tubing and create difficulty in deflating the cuff prior to changing the tube. This procedure will not be helpful if the cuff is ruptured. In this situation the tube must be changed immediately.

Tracheal Stenosis. Tracheal stenosis develops in three main regions of the airway—subglottic area,

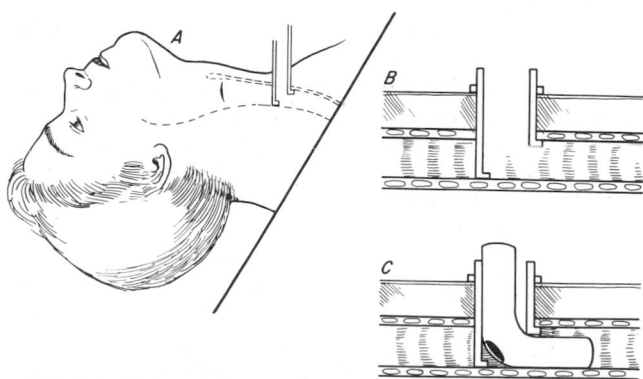

FIGURE 30-6. Measurement for fenestration. *A,* Hyperextend head for good visualization. *B,* Bedside measurements with sterile pipe cleaners determining anterior and posterior wall to skin measurement. *C,* Measurements determine location of fenestration on the tracheostomy tube.

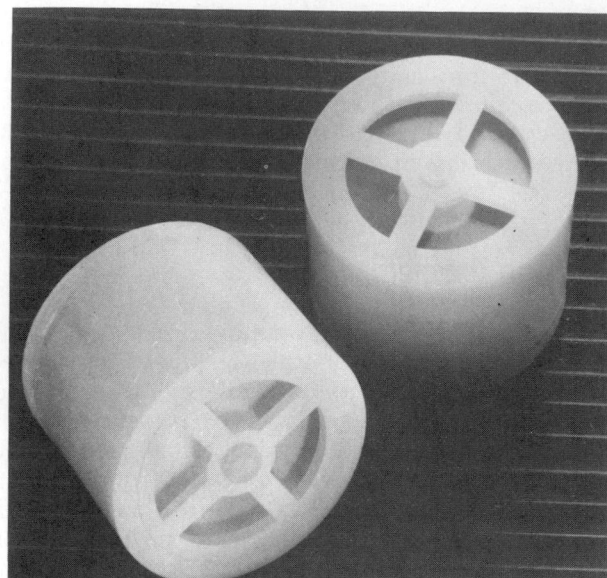

FIGURE 30–7. Passy-Muir speaking valve.

cuff site, and stoma site. Subglottic stenosis is rare but may develop if the tracheostomy is performed too high at the time of surgery, therefore causing damage to the cricoid cartilage (Heffner et al., 1986). Tracheal damage leading to stenosis at the cuff still occurs despite the use of high-volume, low-pressure cuffs. The cuff design will not ensure that low pressure is maintained if the cuff is overinflated. Cuff volumes and pressures that are larger than necessary can cause this stenosis-related, tube pressure necrosis (Grillo et al., 1971). The tracheal mucosa becomes inflamed, ulcerated, and necrotic, resulting in fragmentation of the cartilaginous rings when the cuff to tracheal wall pressure exceeds the capillary perfusion pressure. Excessive pressure destroys the tracheal architecture, causing scarring and narrowing of the tracheal lumen at the cuff site.

Tracheostomy can produce tracheal damage at the stoma site, resulting in stenosis. Factors that cause this process include faulty initial dimensions of the tracheal incision, use of an oversize tracheostomy tube, excessive movement of the tracheostomy tube within the stoma, and persistent stomal infection (Colice, 1987). Prevention of stomal injury begins at the time of surgery. Chronic inflammation and infection at the stoma site may lead to the formation of granulation tissue. Granulomas commonly form above and below the anterior tracheal stoma site. Stomal infection and inflammation should be prevented with local care and antibiotics, if necessary. A bacterial culture of the stoma area is obtained if purulent drainage occurs. If the area around the stoma is a large open wound with continuous purulent drainage and routine care with antibiotic ointment has been performed with no results, a wet-to-dry gauze dressing may be applied with half-strength povidone-iodine solution (Betadine) every 4 hours until the drainage has ceased. The skin around the stoma area should be examined closely for any irritation from the Betadine. If the area around the stoma is not infected, but irritation and redness are present, an occlusive dressing (stoma adhesive or Tegaderm) should be placed on the area to protect the skin.

Tracheomalacia. Tracheomalacia may develop at the cuff site, stoma site, or the area between the cuff and stoma site. It is thought to result from thinning of the tracheal wall due to incomplete erosion around the tracheal cartilage secondary to pressure necrosis or infection (Dane and King, 1975). Tracheomalacia should be suspected if the cuff volume required to create a seal increases progressively. The tracheostomy tube and cuff are examined on the chest x-ray. If the cuff diameter is 1.5 times the tracheal diameter, tracheomalacia can be suspected. As a result, a larger or longer tube may be required to change the position of the cuff in the airway.

When the patient is weaned from mechanical ventilation and tracheostenosis or tracheomalacia is suspected, an ear, nose, and throat (ENT) or thoracic surgery consult is suggested. The consulting physician will evaluate the need for surgical repair or

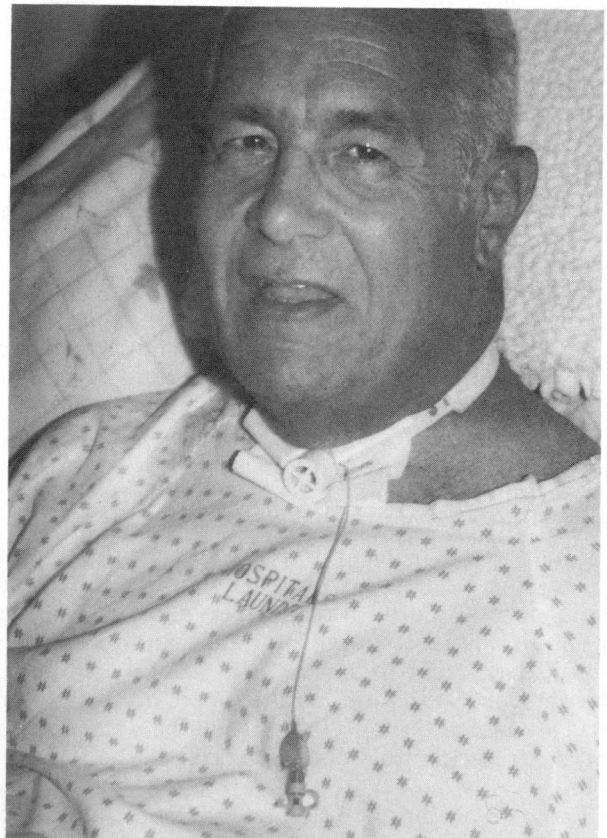

FIGURE 30–8. Patient with muscular dystrophy and COPD finds it easy to speak with the Passy-Muir speaking valve. The valve opens on inspiration and closes as the patient exhales, and the air is directed to the upper airway to allow clear speech.

stinting of the airway with a cuffless tracheostomy tube or T tube.

Suctioning

Nurses are required to suction the intubated patient to remove secretions that interfere with oxygenation and ventilation. Indications for deep tracheal suctioning are coarse rhonchi upon auscultation and a patient's inability to raise secretions.

Complications of Suctioning. Suctioning is performed frequently. Thus, nurses should be familiar with all aspects of the procedure, which is not a benign one. There are many documented complications that are life-threatening. The recognized complications are hypoxia, arrhythmias, discomfort, bronchospasm, and trauma. Thus, one must take precautions in patients with instability of the cardiovascular system, such as arrhythmias, recent myocardial infarction, or severe hypoxemia with respiratory failure. In these situations one must discuss the procedure with the clinical nurse specialist or physician who is familiar with the case. Remember, suctioning should be done only as often as necessary, not on a rigid time schedule.

Hypoxemia is a hazard of endotracheal suctioning because not only are secretions removed but also large amounts of gas are evacuated during the suctioning procedure. Patients should be observed for signs of hypoxemia. These signs are tachypnea, tachycardia, hypertension, diaphoresis, and restlessness. The patient is also at risk for cardiac arrhythmias due to systemic hypoxia. Suctioning may stimulate a vagal response, thus causing bradycardia and other life-threatening arrhythmias. Trauma can result from the repetition, vigor, duration, or amount of negative pressure applied during suctioning of the airway. Trauma is evident by the presence of bloody aspirates in the catheter. When blood is noted, stop the suctioning procedure and assess the situation. Another complication is bronchospasm, which may result from excessive coughing or the stimulation of a foreign body (catheter) in the airway. The techniques recommended to reduce the incidence of such complications include administering 100% oxygen before and after suctioning, limiting the duration of suctioning to 15 seconds or less, and limiting the amount of negative (suction) pressure applied (Demers and Saklad 1975; Fell and Cheney, 1971; Rindfleish and Tyler, 1983). Especially designed airway adapters are available to permit suctioning without disconnecting the patient from positive pressure ventilation. These have been shown to decrease the incidence of hypoxemia in postoperative, open heart, and trauma patients (Skelley et al., 1980; Brown et al., 1983). Similar recommendations have been made by other researchers (Jung and Newman, 1982). This idea suggests that a closed airway system decreases

the complications of hypoxia during suctioning. No study to date has demonstrated improved secretion clearance with a closed system. The closed system suction catheter (Trach Care catheter, Ballard Medical Products, Midvale, Utah) is designed for multiple use; also, suctioning is possible without disconnecting the patient from the positive pressure ventilator throughout the procedure. To date, little research has been published about the effectiveness of this catheter and its effect on the infection rate. One aspect of this new method (Trach Care catheter) is that because it is a closed system it is a more esthetically attractive and sanitary technique. It is not uncommon for a patient with a forceful cough to propel saline and secretions out of the tube, thus becoming a source of contamination to personnel. This method requires further study to determine whether it decreases nursing time for suctioning and thus creates a favorable cost-benefit ratio. As indicated previously, the complications associated with deep tracheal suctioning can be fatal. Thus, techniques must be instituted to minimize these complications as far as possible.

Suctioning Procedure. Suctioning is a very frightening experience for the patient; therefore, the nurse should fully explain and give verbal instructions to the patient throughout the procedure. Once the patient has been assessed, one can ready the equipment and begin the procedure, maintaining principles of asepsis.

Equipment includes a 100% manual resuscitator bag, oxygen wall outlet, suction regulator connected to a wall suction outlet and pharyngeal suction bottle, sterile suction catheter, sterile gloves, and sterile water. The suction regulator is turned on, maintaining negative pressure of 100 to 200 mm Hg. High negative pressure may cause mucosal trauma. The oxygen flowmeter should be set at 15 liters for the 100% manual resuscitator bag. The sterile water that will be used for clearing the suction tubing, sterile gloves, and catheter are opened. The patient is disconnected from the ventilator and preoxygenated with five hyperinflated breaths of 100% oxygen using the manual resuscitator bag (Chulay and Graeber, 1988). Sterile gloves are put on, and the catheter is removed from the package and connected to the suction tubing. If a cough is desired or secretions are thick, saline is instilled down the artificial airway. The catheter is gently inserted in the artificial airway as far as it will go, then withdrawn 1 to 2 cm, and suction is applied intermittently for a maximum of 15 seconds while the catheter is rotated between the thumb and index finger as it is removed. The patient is postoxygenated with five hyperinflated breaths. The procedure can be repeated or the patient returned to the mechanical ventilator or oxygen source system.

RESPIRATORY DECOMPENSATION
Clinical Signs and Symptoms

The primary role of the critical care nurse, in connection with ventilator failure, is to recognize the early signs of respiratory difficulty. Chest assessment should be done on mechanically ventilated patients, ideally every shift. At this time, abnormal findings or significant changes must be evaluated for cause and treated.

Physical signs in selected abnormalities of the lungs produce different findings. For example, in a patient with lobar pneumonia, the consolidated lung will be dull to percussion, breath sounds will be decreased or bronchial, and crackles will be present on inspiration. In a patient with asthma, the hyperinflated lung has a hyperresonant note with percussion, wheezes will be present, chest wall expansion is decreased, and use of accessory muscles will be increased. In patients with a pneumothorax, breath sounds are absent, percussion will be hyperresonant over the affected area, and the trachea may shift to the opposite side.

When the ventilator is checked, breath sounds should be evaluated and the overall appearance of the patient assessed. If the breath sounds are low-pitched, sonorous rhonchi, the patient may need deep tracheal suctioning; if the sounds are high-pitched wheezes a bronchodilator may be needed. The combination of physical and ventilator findings can confirm the cause of the abnormal findings. For example, causes of increases in peak airway pressure are secretions, obstruction of the artificial airway, kinking of the airway due to airway position, bronchospasm, lobar consolidation, pulmonary edema, patient "fighting" the ventilator, or a tension pneumothorax. The causes of a decrease in peak airway pressure are improvement in airway patency and lung function, artificial airway cuff leak, leak in the ventilator breathing circuit, or disconnection of the patient from the ventilator circuit.

An important part of the respiratory assessment is the evaluation of the patient's pattern of breathing. A discoordinated breathing pattern or excessive use of the accessory muscles indicates an increase in the patient's inspiratory work of breathing. The patient may not be coordinated with the ventilator, or respiratory muscle fatigue may be present. To decrease the patient's work of breathing, the mode of ventilation may be changed—for example, continuous positive airway pressure (CPAP) to intermittent mandatory ventilation (IMV); the sensitivity may be adjusted to the patient's efforts; the rate or tidal volume may be increased, or sedation of the patient may be instituted.

Causes of Respiratory Decompensation

Ventilator Malfunction. Mechanical ventilators are complex machines. A patient is dependent on this machine to provide adequate oxygenation and ventilation. A small change in the delivered tidal volume, respiratory rate, or flow rate can cause major physiologic changes in the patient. Ventilator malfunction can be a cause of morbidity in any ventilator-assisted patient (Feeley and Bancroft, 1982; Abramson et al., 1980). These malfunctions may be due to equipment failure or human error. Feeley and Bancroft reviewed 280 incident reports of equipment problems. Equipment failure resulted from disconnection or leaks in the breathing circuits, dysfunction of the exhalation valves, electrical problems, or failure of different components of the ventilator such as compressors, control switches, or alarms. Abramson and colleagues collected 57 incident reports during a period in the intensive care unit (ICU). Of these 57 incident reports of equipment malfunction, 34 were directly related to equipment problems and 23 were due to human error. Ventilator malfunctions due to human error included inappropriate assembly of the patient's breathing circuit, failure to set the correct rates, alarms turned off, power turned off during a procedure (e.g., during suctioning), and failure to turn the power source on. At present, dependable equipment is available with good alarm systems, but this does not replace careful monitoring by the critical care nurse. Therefore, standardization of procedures and education of all members of the health care team about equipment function can help to keep human error to a minimum. The responsibilities of the critical care nurse include becoming familiar with the different types of ventilators and their basic functions. See Chapter 29 for more information.

Pneumothorax. Pneumothorax is the collection of gas within the pleural cavity. This can cause respiratory decompensation in the ventilated patient. The most common causes of pneumothorax are chest trauma, placement of a central venous catheter, thoracentesis, chest tube placement, and, least often, barotrauma from mechanical ventilation (Cullen and Caldera, 1979; Pierson, 1982). Cullen and Caldera followed 200 ICU patients, of whom only 22 developed pneumothorax, pneumomediastinum, or subcutaneous emphysema. Only one patient had barotrauma related to mechanical ventilation. Other causes of pneumothorax were related to chest tube placement, chest trauma, thoracic surgical procedures, ruptured esophagus, central line placement, necrosis of the skin flap covering the remaining trachea following a reconstructive operation, and post-tracheostomy. In a study of 1700 ventilator patients by Pierson and colleagues (1986), only 39 (2%) had a significant bronchopleural air leak. The most common cause identified was chest trauma. The other causes identified did not result directly from mechanical ventilation. Patient populations at high risk for pneumothorax include those with severe underlying lung disease, necrotizing pneumonia, adult respiratory distress syndrome, and high airway pressures when on mechanical ventilation. Utilization of lower airway pressures, volumes, and flow rates may help to keep the incidence of this problem to a minimum.

If respiratory difficulty is evident, the patient should be disconnected from the ventilator and manually ventilated with 100% oxygen. Troubleshooting as to the cause of the respiratory difficulty can then be accomplished (Fig. 30–9). If the patient can be ventilated easily manually and respirations readily stabilize, a mechanical ventilator problem is suspected. An air leak in the system is suspected if the peak airway pressures are decreased compared to known values. Other patient complaints that can cause respiratory distress are difficulty in triggering the machine on inspiration, complaints of not receiving enough air or receiving too much air, or an inspiratory phase that is too long or too short. The

mechanical ventilator should be checked so that the sensitivity will *not* register a negative pressure of greater than 2.0 cm of water just prior to the beginning of inspiration. If the inspiratory phase is too long or too short, the flow rates should be checked and adjusted (flow rate is decreased if inspiration is too short; flow rate is increased if inspiration is too long). If the patient complains that it is difficult to exhale, the inspiratory-expiratory (I/E) ratio should be measured. To increase the expiratory time, the flow rate should be increased. Once the problem has been corrected, the patient can be safely placed back on the ventilator.

If increased resistance to manual ventilation is noted, the chest is examined for bilateral breath sounds and chest expansion. If either is abnormal, a pneumothorax can be suspected. Other signs of a

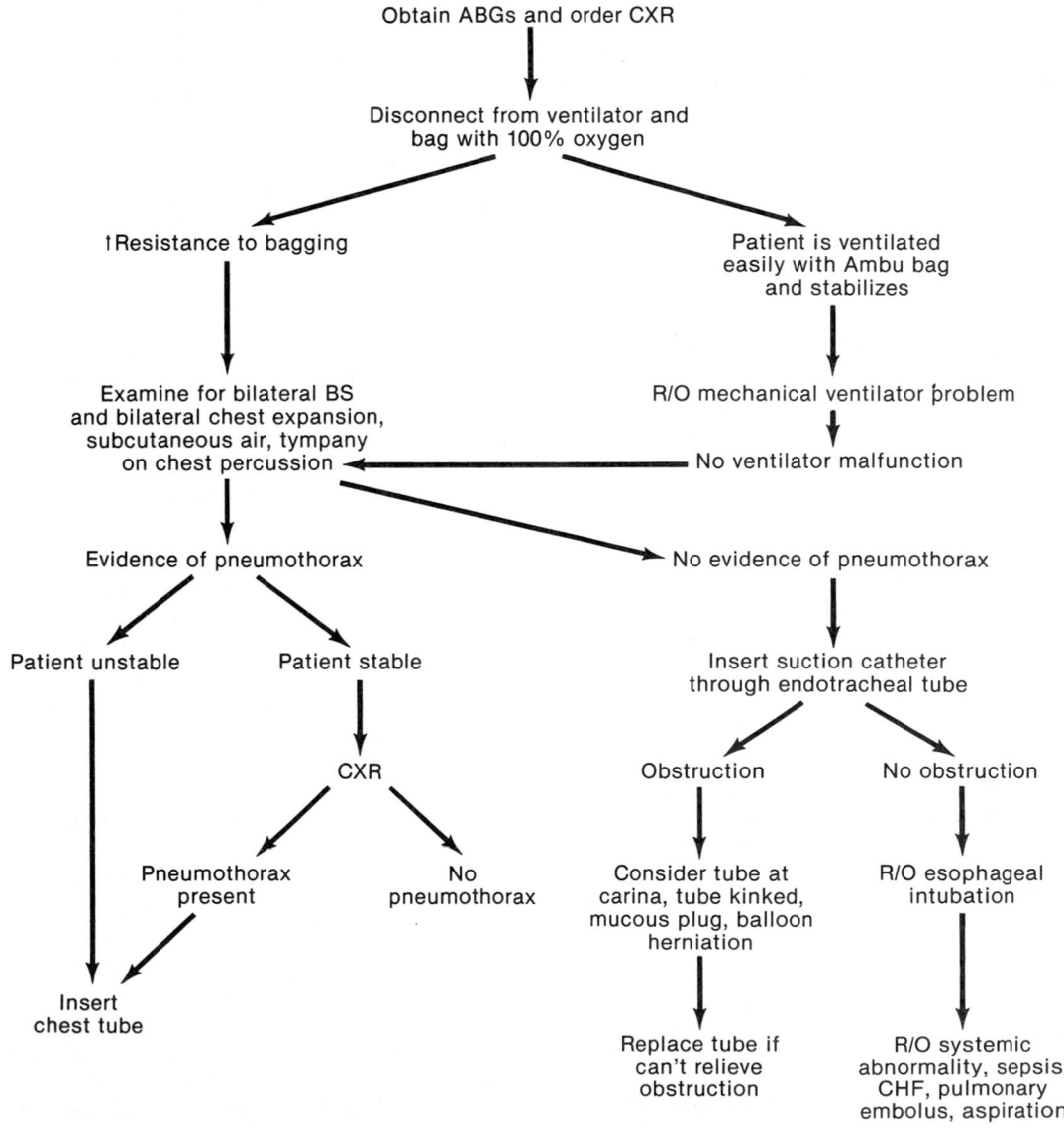

FIGURE 30–9. Approach to the patient who decompensates on a mechanical ventilator. *Abbreviations*: ABGs, arterial blood gases; CXR, chest x-ray; BS, breath sounds; R/O, rule out; CHF, congestive heart failure. (From Hotchkiss, R.S., and Wilson, R.S. (1983). *Surgical Clinics of North America, 63*, 417–438.)

pneumothorax include tympanic sounds on percussion, tracheal deviation, or subcutaneous emphysema. If a pneumothorax exists, cardiovascular instability will be present with hypoxemia and respiratory acidosis. If any of these signs are present, a chest x-ray should be obtained immediately. A chest tube will be placed if a significant pneumothorax is present.

Persistent Bronchopleural Air Leak. Persistent bronchopleural air leak with positive pressure ventilation can cause loss of the delivered tidal volume and loss of positive end-expiratory pressure (PEEP) through the chest tube; therefore, the patient's arterial blood gases are closely monitored for both oxygenation and acid-base abnormalities. The goal is to minimize the air leak by changing the ventilator pattern and maintaining adequate gas exchange. The ventilator pattern can be changed by using smaller tidal volumes and higher rates to maintain the same amount of ventilation. PEEP should be used at the lowest possible level and expiratory retard should not be used. If the patient's spontaneous respiratory pattern interferes with this goal, sedation should be used, and paralysis may be necessary.

These changes are made to try to lower the intrathoracic pressure and decrease the air leak. Other aggressive treatments have been reported in the literature such as high-frequency ventilation, ventilation of each lung separately using two mechanical ventilators through a double-lumen endotracheal tube, application of PEEP to the chest tube, and surgical repair (Sjostrand, 1980; Rafferty et al., 1980; Downs and Chapman, 1976). However, none of these methods have proved to be consistently successful.

If the mechanical ventilator is functioning properly and the chest x-ray shows no pneumothorax, other causes of respiratory decompensation that can cause an increase in peak airway pressure should be ruled out. The artificial airway could be obstructed or kinked. Deep tracheal suctioning is performed to eliminate any possibility of obstruction of the artificial airway.

Bronchospasm. If airway obstruction due to bronchospasm is suspected, treatment with a bronchodilating nebulizer is the fastest therapy. However, if no relief from the treatment is observed (decrease in respiratory rate, decrease in inspiratory work of breathing), other causes of bronchospasm that may be considered include the presence of secretions, collapse due to poorly supported airways, a foreign body in the airway, or airway pathology.

Patient or Ventilator Asynchrony. Another cause of respiratory distress is the patient breathing out of synchrony with the ventilator. When out of phase with the ventilator, the patient is often exhaling while the machine is delivering a breath. This causes an increase in the peak inspiratory pressure, which often exceeds the pressure limit set on the machine, thus triggering the pressure alarm. Increasing the delivered minute ventilation or increasing both the tidal volume and the respiratory rate may gain control of the patient's respirations. If the patient's respiratory status does not change after a bronchodilator nebulizer treatment and deep tracheal suctioning, sedation may be indicated.

If these causes for respiratory decompensation have been ruled out, systemic abnormalities should be suspected. These possibilities include sepsis, congestive heart failure, pulmonary embolus, and aspiration.

WEANING

Weaning from mechanical ventilation to spontaneous breathing is often a difficult process for both patient and staff. It is important to realize that weaning is a critical time, both psychologically and physiologically. This process may be long and frustrating for the patient, primary nurse, respiratory therapist, and physician, but consistency of care, patience, and persistence will make a difference.

Evaluation for Weaning

The ability to be weaned is governed by several factors including the patient's overall physical condition and psychological state (Morganroth et al., 1984; Nett et al., 1987). Weaning should be considered whenever the following conditions are met: The initial pulmonary pathology (e.g., pneumonia, low lung volumes, and abdominal distention) that necessitated intubation and mechanical ventilation should be resolving (Kirsten, 1989). Cardiovascular function should be stable with minimal or no need for vasopressors, a regular heart rate and rhythm, and a cardiac index of greater than 2. Fluid balance is especially important when weaning patients with limited cardiac function. Thus, daily weights and strict intake and output amounts should be measured. An increased metabolic demand secondary to fever, burns, and shivering will increase oxygen consumption and carbon dioxide production. Such conditions usually prevent successful weaning. The nutritional state should not be overlooked (Majors, 1988). While malnutrition exists, weaning is hindered due to weakness and abnormalities of pulmonary mechanics. Malnutrition is a leading cause of impaired respiratory muscle function, affecting both endurance and strength. If muscle wasting is present with deficits in nitrogen balance, albumin, phosphate, magnesium, and calcium levels, there will be significant atrophy and weakness of the respiratory muscles, resulting in poor ventilatory effort (Chernow, 1982; Askanazi et al., 1981; Dougherty, 1988).

Respiratory Parameters. A variety of respiratory parameters and tests are available to assess a patient's ability to be weaned from mechanical ventilation. This assessment can be divided into three aspects: (1) oxygenation, (2) ventilation, and (3) mechanical function (Fitzgerald and Huber, 1976; Sahn and Lakshminarayan, 1973). The arterial oxygen tension during mechanical ventilation should usually be greater than 70 mm Hg with an FI_{O_2} of 40% and the A-aD_{O_2} less than 300 mm Hg. The above condition should exist with a level of PEEP that is less than 10 cm H_2O. When PEEP is greater than 10 cm H_2O, weaning is usually contraindicated.

The next aspect to be assessed is the patient's ventilation requirement. Ventilation is a given amount of gas exchange required to eliminate carbon dioxide adequately. The necessary level of minute ventilation (tidal volume × respiratory rate) is determined by both carbon dioxide production and dead space ventilation. The dead space to tidal volume ratio (V_D/V_T) defines the percentage of the tidal volume that does not participate in CO_2 elimination and thus can be considered wasted ventilation. This dead space ratio is increased in diseases that affect the lung parenchyma and the distribution of gas flow (e.g., acute respiratory distress syndrome, pulmonary embolism, chronic obstructive pulmonary disease, and hypovolemia) (Marini, 1986). If V_D/V_T is 0.60 (i.e., 60% of tidal volume) or greater, the minute volume required to maintain adequate carbon dioxide elimination is frequently too great to permit total weaning (Skillman et al., 1971). Thus, it is not surprising that a useful estimate of weaning ability is the minute ventilation required during mechanical ventilation. Sahn and Lakshminarayan have shown that a minute ventilation of 10 liters/minute or less during mechanical ventilation usually indicates that a patient can be safely weaned.

There is an important relationship among V_D/V_T, minute ventilation, and carbon dioxide production. An increased V_D/V_T or increased CO_2 production will require increased minute ventilation. The CO_2 is elevated with fever, shivering, pain, sepsis, or overfeeding or a high-carbohydrate diet. Under such circumstances, weaning may be difficult to accomplish because of the potential need for an unusually high respiratory rate and large tidal volumes.

The patient's mechanical function may be assessed by measuring the vital capacity, inspiratory force, and the spontaneous respiratory rate. The vital capacity is the maximum volume of gas that can be exhaled following maximal inspiration. This serves as an index of ventilatory reserve. The vital capacity should usually be 10 to 15 mL/kg of actual body weight to institute weaning. Inspiratory force (the amount of negative pressure generated against an occluded airway) is a measurement of muscle strength. Weaning can be instituted when the inspiratory force is minus 20 cm H_2O. This measurement has an advantage in that it does not require patient cooperation and thus can be used in unresponsive or uncooperative patients. The vital capacity and the inspiratory force are the easiest parameters to follow at the bedside and are the two most important

indicators of weaning ability and progress in weaning. The respiratory rate should not exceed 35 breaths/minute because this commonly results in fatigue, CO_2 retention, and respiratory acidosis (Morganroth et al., 1984).

Psychological Readiness. Psychologically, the patient must be prepared to be weaned. The patient's anxiety stems from fear of ventilator malfunction, fear of suffocation, and loss of control. To reduce the patient's fear of ventilator failure, the nurse should explain the safety mechanisms of ventilator (e.g., alarms), keep the manual resuscitator in the patient's view, and give verbal reassurance that the ventilator is functioning properly. The respiratory therapist should announce to the patient when the ventilator is being checked and explain what changes are being made.

The fear of suffocation is breathlessness. This is often related to the weaning process. Monitoring oxygen saturation is suggested to reassure the patient that oxygen levels stay within a safe range.

Several aspects of treatment on a mechanical ventilator are anxiety-provoking and frustrating for the patient. One major component of this is the patient's impaired ability to communicate. A variety of communication modalities are available for the mechanically ventilated patient. These include eye signals, lip reading, palm writing, pen and paper, magic slate, alphabet board, flash cards, deflating tracheostomy cuff, talking tracheostomy tubes, and the use of computers. Encourage the patient to use the least frustrating mode. Remember that while weaning is recognized as a sign of improvement for some ventilated patients, for others with chronic respiratory disease it signals a return to ever increasing respiratory work.

An important aspect of successful weaning is the patient's trust in the staff responsible for his care. The staff should maintain a consistent approach to the patient throughout the weaning process. If there is disagreement among the medical and nursing teams and information presented to the patient is inconsistent, the patient becomes distrustful. Negative experiences with staff increase patient anxiety. Therefore, repeated explanations help minimize the occurrence of misinterpretation.

Methods of Weaning

Currently, there are two acceptable methods of weaning from mechanical ventilation—the conventional and the intermittent mandatory ventilation (IMV) techniques (Bendixen et al., 1965; Downs et al., 1973; Sporn and Morganroth, 1988).

Conventional Weaning. The conventional or Briggs (T piece) technique is an accepted and time-honored method. This technique is often modified by application of CPAP. The patient is disconnected from the ventilator for a specific period of time and allowed to breathe spontaneously using the Briggs (T piece) or CPAP system. CPAP may be used to improve the functional residual capacity and thus increase arterial oxygenation. Weaning is generally begun using short time intervals such as 5 to 10 minutes every hour. As the weaning time increases to 1 hour or more, the patient often requires a "rest" period with mechanical ventilation for 1 or more hours. Weaning should not be attempted during the night until the patient can maintain spontaneous ventilation through most of the day. By increasing each period of weaning time, respiratory muscle strength and endurance are increased to maintain spontaneous respiration. Thus, the monitoring of the patient's vital capacity and inspiratory force are of utmost value. The vital capacity represents the ventilatory reserve, and the inspiratory force represents the muscle strength. There is no technical measurement for endurance except the increasing time endured by the patient off the ventilator.

IMV Weaning. Intermittent mandatory ventilation (IMV) is a technique by which patients can breathe spontaneously and in addition receive mechanically ventilated breaths at specific preselected rates (Downs et al., 1973; Feeley and Hedley-Whyte, 1975). This weaning process is achieved by decreasing the number of mechanically ventilated breaths delivered. The patient then assumes a greater proportion of the total minute ventilation. Ventilators are equipped with a control that is sensitive enough to regulate the respiratory rate of the mechanical ventilator over a wide range of breaths ranging from 12 to a minimum of 1 breath every 2 to 3 minutes. Weaning is accomplished by instituting a gradual decrease in the frequency of ventilator breaths to rates as low as one breath/minute or one breath every 3 minutes with the Emerson ventilator.

The IMV method is popular for several reasons: (1) respiratory muscle tone is maintained to decrease muscle atrophy, (2) there is a reduction in the need for sedatives and narcotics, (3) there is possible improved distribution of ventilation with the combination of spontaneous and mechanical breaths, (4) weaning is initiated earlier in the course of disease, and (5) there is less cardiovascular disturbance and less time is needed for direct observation by nurses, therapists, or physicians (Luce et al., 1981). The IMV method is valid when patients are receiving four IMV breaths or more per minute, but at lower IMV rates (four or fewer breaths per minute), the patient requires close observation of vital signs and respiratory pattern. It is during this time that the patient assumes control over most of his total minute volume. It is at these lower IMV rates that patients tend to fail because of fatigue, increased work of breathing, or other factors including fever, atelectasis, or poor nutritional state. These problems often are evident when the patient controls the bulk of his own total minute ventilation. As this weaning process proceeds

with continued reductions in the number of mechanical breaths, arterial blood gases and spontaneous tidal volume (vital capacity, inspiratory force) should be measured and recorded every 2 to 4 hours. Any significant or adverse trend in vital signs should be noted. If no difficulty is observed, the IMV rate is decreased further until the patient can support his total minute ventilation. Most patients who require short-term mechanical ventilation following major surgery and anesthesia are suitable candidates for IMV techniques.

Modified Conventional IMV Weaning. Patients who are being mechanically ventilated for acute lung disease or an exacerbation of chronic obstructive pulmonary disease are often difficult to wean. Several factors may contribute to this finding such as poor nutritional state, poor spontaneous parameters due to muscle weakness and atrophy, or fear. If the primary cause of failure to wean is respiratory muscle dysfunction, an individualized weaning approach is suggested by combining aspects of conventional and IMV weaning techniques. This weaning process could be considered a modified conventional IMV wean. This method is designed like a training program with the goal of improving strength and then the endurance of respiratory muscle function. The resting IMV rate should arbitrarily provide 80% of the patient's minute ventilation. Incorporating techniques from the conventional wean, the weaning is done four times a day for 30 minutes to 1 hour on an IMV rate that is half the resting IMV rate. At the end of each day the patient is evaluated, and if the spontaneous parameters are normal for that patient and are not decreased, illustrating respiratory muscle dysfunction, the next day the weaning IMV rate is decreased again. Once the patient progresses to CPAP, the four 1-hour intervals are increased. The rest of the wean is accomplished in a fashion similar to a conventional wean.

Assessment During the Weaning Process

Regardless of the weaning technique employed, weaning time is increased by utilizing sound clinical judgment. First the proper position for optimal conditions for weaning must be assessed. The patient should be sitting or in a high Fowler's position whenever possible. Weaning should not be undertaken in the supine position except with individuals in the Stryker frame. Obese patients should be out of bed if at all possible. If in bed, the reverse Trendelenburg position helps to allow maximum chest expansion. Attention to airway secretions is vital. The patient should be suctioned prior to weaning if necessary and during weaning as needed.

As weaning begins, pulse, blood pressure, respiratory rate and spontaneous ventilatory parameters (tidal volume, vital capacity, and inspiratory force) should be measured and recorded. During the period of weaning it may be helpful for the nurse to place a hand on the patient's lateral chest wall and provide verbal instructions to inspire and expire at an appropriate rate. For the average patient, an inspiratory-expiratory ratio of 1:2 is desirable. For the patient with chronic obstructive pulmonary disease an inspiratory-expiratory ratio of 1:4 is acceptable. This instruction will help to facilitate a slow and regular breathing pattern.

Supervision during the weaning process is most important to help alleviate the patient's fears and provide emotional support. At the termination of the weaning period, the vital signs, arterial blood gases, and spontaneous parameters should again be measured and recorded. All of these parameters are needed to predict the length of time the patient can breathe spontaneously before stress, fatigue, hypoxemia, hypercapnia, or a major change in vital signs occurs. It is mandatory to stop weaning if the patient appears stressed. Stress may be demonstrated by a respiratory rate greater than 35/minute, a significant increase in heart rate (i.e., increased by 20 beats per minute from the resting heart rate), a dramatic increase in the blood pressure (systolic pressure increased 20% from the resting level), diaphoresis, air hunger, excessive use of accessory muscles or discoordinate breathing pattern. When a patient exhibits such stress, he or she should be manually ventilated with a self-inflating resuscitator bag for several minutes, and spontaneous parameters should not be checked at this time because this will stress him or her too much. Following the weaning period, mechanical ventilation is instituted at a rate and volume that will provide adequate rest. At the next scheduled weaning interval the patient should be reevaluated.

Causes of Failure to Wean

Failure to wean from mechanical ventilation never has a simple solution and often has multiple reasons. These include intrinsic pulmonary disease, poor nutritional state, respiratory muscle dysfunction or fatigue, cardiac disease, and sepsis (Norton and Neureuter, 1989).

The major causes of failure to wean due to pulmonary disease are extensive atelectasis, consolidation, edema, fibrosis and bronchospasm due to decreased recruitable air space and increased airway resistance. Therapy consists of positive end-expiratory pressure, use of bronchodilators, and chest physical therapy. Nursing interventions include auscultation of breath sounds every 2 hours; reporting the presence of adventitious breath sounds or absent breath sounds; monitoring the rate, rhythm, and depth of respirations; tracheobronchial suctioning; and monitoring arterial blood gases with each ventilator change or changes in patient clinical status. (Carroll, 1986; Daly and Allen, 1987).

Nutritional Status. A very important aspect of weaning is the patient's nutritional status. Nutrition must be considered during the acute phase of illness. It is well documented that starvation and protein loss cause breakdown of muscle mass for gluconeogenesis (Barrocas et al., 1983; Hyman et al., 1982). This results in a decrease in respiratory muscle function (intercostal, diaphragm, and abdominal), thus decreasing vital capacity and inspiratory force and causing failure to wean. Studies have indicated that 30% to 40% of adults with chronic obstructive pulmonary disease are undernourished based on body weight, anthropometric measures, and estimates of body fat and muscle mass (Wilson, 1985). Inability to maintain adequate nutritional status has been associated with compromises in pulmonary defense mechanisms, structure, and function (Rochester, 1984).

If the patient requires central intravenous hyperalimentation for nutritional support, the problems that can exist with high glucose diets must be appreciated (Sheldon and Baker, 1980). Askanazi and others (1981) have documented that high glucose loads result in lipogenesis rather than utilization as an energy source. Lipogenesis resulting from excess glucose will increase CO_2 production. This can be demonstrated by measuring the respiratory quotient (CO_2 production–oxygen consumption). The normal value is 0.8. When glucose is burned alone, the RQ is 1 or greater. When excess glucose is given, it is converted to fat; thus carbon dioxide is produced in excess of oxygen consumed. The excess carbon dioxide produced must be excreted by the lungs at an energy cost for additional respiratory work, increasing tidal volume and minute ventilation. Thus, in the compromised pulmonary patient with marginal reserve, this can be a cause of inability to wean. Therefore, there should be a balance between dietary intake of fats and carbohydrates. When the patient is able to switch to an enteral intake, parenteral nutrition should be withdrawn slowly while enteral nutrition is gradually advanced. Small feeding tubes are generally well tolerated for an enteral diet. These liquid diets are lactose-free and contain a balance of fat and carbohydrate calories. Most standard enteral feedings contain 30% to 35% fat and 50% carbohydrates.

Patient tolerance to tube feedings is essential for provision of adequate nutritional intake. The effects of intolerance to tube feedings can compound any existing deficiencies and defeat the effort to achieve adequate nourishment of the patient. Complications that are both critical and frequent in ventilator-dependent patients include aspiration pneumonia, gastric retention, diarrhea, abdominal distention, nausea, vomiting, hypophosphatemia, hypokalemia, and hypomagnesemia (Openbrier, 1985). These complications can be contributing factors that cause patients to fail weaning. The incorporation of fiber into the diet has been documented to help maintain normal bowel function and decrease the incidence of diarrhea and constipation caused by intolerance to low-residue feedings (Kelsay, 1978). Nursing interventions include auscultation of bowel sounds every 4 hours; monitoring the calorie count; and assessment of muscle mass, skin integrity, and wound healing.

Respiratory Muscle Weakness. The goal of mechanical ventilation should be to preserve and increase the functional capacity of the respiratory muscles; however, respiratory muscle weakness or fatigue is often the reason for failure to wean (Kim, 1984). This problem is often secondary to poor nutrition, asynchronous breathing pattern, abdominal distention, chest trauma, or phrenic palsy. When one or more of these problems is present, spontaneous respirations are not performed in a coordinated way. Discoordination of respiratory muscle activity can develop as a result of prolonged mechanical ventilation. A discoordinated breathing pattern is a sign of respiratory muscle dysfunction. This dysfunction results in a lack of synchronized function between the intercostal, diaphragmatic, and abdominal muscles during spontaneous respirations. The chest wall and abdomen appear to function with a rocking motion. On inspiration, the lower chest is pulled inward and the upper chest expands; then on expiration, the inward movement of the abdomen is interrupted by a bounce as the outward flow of air is suddenly expelled. This process may vary in severity, and these patients appear to be working much harder and moving less air and are unable to meet the demands of respiratory work. The cause is unknown, and there is no known treatment. Thus, therapy is continued use of ventilatory and nutritional support. Many clinicians have demonstrated that as the ability to breathe spontaneously improves, so does coordination of the breathing pattern. If a discoordinate breathing pattern is observed during weaning, patients generally tire easily because of the high respiratory rates and small tidal volumes. Ventilation of the lower lobes will be compromised. Thus, during weaning, it is helpful to institute diaphragmatic and lateral basal expansion breathing exercises with manual resistance to the chest wall and abdomen. These exercises emphasize the synchronized motion of the respiratory muscles to increase chest wall expansion, thus requiring less work to maintain ventilation. Frequently, respiratory muscle power will be slow to improve. Therefore, assessment of the patient's mechanical function (tidal volume, vital capacity, inspiratory force, minute ventilation) in the work of breathing will reveal trends in the strength and endurance of the respiratory muscles. No one criterion will determine whether the patient needs a rest, but the overall picture needs to be assessed.

Ventilator Design. Another reason for weaning difficulty may be that the ventilator is designed with a high gas flow or demand-valve system. Some demand-valve mechanical ventilators may require increased respiratory work because additional work is required to activate the valves or because the ventilator is unable to supply peak flow upon patient demand (Gibney et al., 1982). This produces an increase in the work of breathing resulting in tachypnea, dyspnea, and wide fluctuations in airway pressure during the respiratory cycle. When respiratory rates are 30/minute or more, the inspiratory effort required to open the demand valve can cause a decrease in compliance, tachypnea, and increased work of breathing. Thus, changing the ventilator to a high gas flow system or inspiratory pressure support can decrease the work required on inspiration, allowing the patient to breathe easier at a lower respiratory rate. The inspiratory pressure support is designed to maintain a constant preset positive airway pressure during spontaneous inspiration. The patient regulates the respiratory rate, tidal volume, and inspiratory time, and the work performed by the respiratory muscles is reduced (Kacmarek, 1989). Several researchers have demonstrated that inspiratory pressure support decreases the respiratory rate, increases the patient's spontaneous tidal volume, and decreases the use of accessory muscles (McIntyre, 1986; Brochard et al., 1989).

Cardiac Failure. Cardiac failure is another reason for failure to wean. Positive pressure ventilation increases intrathoracic pressure, which can be beneficial to a failing ventricle by decreasing the preload. In the weaning process, as the mean intrathoracic and airway pressure are reduced, the central intravascular volume is increased, causing an increase in preload. This may lead to cardiac ischemia or congestive heart failure (Hotchkiss and Wilson, 1983; Mathru et al., 1982). During the weaning process one should monitor the clinical indicators (central venous pressure, and pulmonary arterial, diastolic, and wedge blood pressures) of preload and afterload. If these parameters are increased, weaning should be stopped and the patient returned to positive pressure ventilation. Reevaluation of the weaning process is indicated, and diuretics, nitrates, or inotropic support may be necessary to accomplish a successful wean.

HOME CARE

Patients who are unweanable or need mechanical ventilation at night may be candidates for home care if the appropriate family or caregiver support systems are available. This process demands planning that involves the input of the family, nursing, respiratory therapy, physical therapy, dietary and social service, physicians, third-party payment providers, and appropriate representatives from community resources. The transition of a patient living in the intensive care unit to the home requires a change in thinking about health care that will be successful only if all involved understand and are committed to it. The patient and family must be motivated to learn all the procedures and must be willing to alter their life styles, roles, and responsibilities to accommodate a ventilator at home.

Nurses must have a complete understanding of the care of airway and ventilator to be able to teach the family and have them assume all responsibilities. The nurse acts as a resource and coordinator of all professionals and agencies involved. Due to the complex nature of this process, weekly conferences should be organized with everyone involved to discuss the progress of the discharge plans. This comprehensive plan of management includes education, bedside instruction, demonstration, organizing equipment and supplies, and provision of emotional support for the patient and family throughout the discharge process. This planning is time-consuming and requires the complete cooperation of workers in all disciplines for a successful outcome.

nursing care plan

1. Ineffective airway clearance related to:
Respiratory muscle weakness
Artificial airway

Defining Characteristics	Nursing Interventions
Cough	Auscultate lungs
Sputum production	Instruct patient on deep breathing exercises
Adventitious breath sounds	Assess cough
Altered chest expansion	Chest physical therapy treatment—percussion, vibration, and deep tracheal suctioning
Change in depth, rate, and rhythm of respirations	Monitor sputum production—color, amount, consistency
	Evaluate gag reflex
	Monitor spontaneous mechanics—tidal volume, vital capacity, and inspiratory force
	Monitor intake and output
	Out of bed to chair; ambulate with oxygen

2. Ineffective breathing pattern related to:
Respiratory muscle weakness
Discoordinate breathing pattern
Airway obstruction
Anxiety

Defining Characteristics	Nursing Interventions
Tachypnea	Perform chest assessment:
Decreased spontaneous tidal volume	Evaluate chest excursion
Tachycardia	Auscultate lungs
Expiratory abdominal muscle tensing	Monitor respiratory rate and rhythm
Recruitment of inspiratory scalene muscles	Provide verbal instruction to assist with a more effective breathing pattern
Nasal flaring	Reposition patient to provide for most effective chest expansion
Discoordinate breathing pattern	Stop wean and manually ventilate
Inability to perform vital capacity maneuver on command	Establish patency of airway
Increased $Paco_2$	Return to control ventilation or resting IMV rate
Decreased Pao_2	
Adventitious breath sounds	
Diaphoresis	
Altered level of consciousness	

Nursing Care Plan continued on following page

3. **Anxiety related to:**
   Environment
   Fear of ventilator failure
   Fear of suffocation
   Loss of control

Defining Characteristics	Nursing Interventions
Irritability	Fear of ventilator failure
Agitation	Frequent physical presence
Restlessness	Announce when ventilator is being checked
Muscle tension	Explain what is being checked or changed each time you do it
Headache	Explain safety mechanisms of ventilator, e.g., alarm systems, back-up equipment
Fatigue	Follow up with verbal reassurance, i.e., everything is working well
Increase in respiratory rate	Keep Ambu bag in patient's view
Inability to concentrate	Fear of suffocation
	Accept patient's feeling as valid and frightening
	When suctioning, pre- and postoxygenate and limit duration of suctioning to 10 to 15 seconds
	Remind patient of good skin color and pink nail beds, if present
	Remind patient of staff presence
	Loss of control
	Identify yourself and your role
	Establish a daily routine
	Give direct clear explanations
	Keep same nurse whenever possible
	Leave call bell, other communication devices within patient reach
	Develop ability to listen and discuss emotional issues with patient
	Give choice about timing or preparation for procedure if possible

4. **Impaired communication related to:**
   Artificial airway
   Impaired understanding
   Impaired interpersonal communication
   Language barrier

Defining Characteristics	Nursing Interventions
Presence of tracheostomy tube	Use plain, nontechnical language explaining mechanical ventilation and weaning
Inability to read or write	Focus on basic needs at present and during immediate future
Frustration	Repeat explanations often
Anger	Be alert to nonverbal clues
	Allow time for patient to respond to questions
	Observe carefully for all attempts to communicate
	Provide patient with paper and pencil, magic slate, alphabet board, flash cards, computer
	Place talking tracheostomy tube or cuffed fenestrated tracheostomy tube
	Deflate cuff on artificial airway
	Develop code of communication such as eye signals, head nodding, palm writing, or lip reading
	Use nonverbal communication, i.e., touch, facial expressions, voice tone

SUMMARY

Every step taken during management of the chronic ventilator patient must be directed toward relieving the patient of his dependency on the ventilator. The transition from artificial to spontaneous ventilation should be attempted when objective data indicate that lung function is adequate to permit this change. The need for careful monitoring of blood gas exchange and spontaneous parameters during the weaning process cannot be overemphasized. Regardless of the technique utilized, the critical care nurse needs to organize a plan of care that is individualized and to approach weaning as the first priority of the day. The nurse has the responsibility of coordinating all other services involved in the weaning process, involving ambulation, muscle training, communication, proper nutrition, and emotional support. Caring for the chronic ventilator patient is complex and demanding, both in the hospital and at home, but can be rewarding with a successful outcome.

References

Abramson, N. S., Wald, K. S., and Grenvik, A. N. A. (1980). Adverse occurrences in intensive care units. *Journal of the American Medical Association*, 244, 1582–1584.

Askanazi, J., Carpentier, Y. A., and Elwyn, D. H. (1980). Influence of total parenteral nutrition on utilization in injury and sepsis. *Annals of Surgery*, 191, 40–46.

Askanazi, J., Nordenstrom, J., and Rosenbaum, S. H. (1981). Nutrition for the patient with respiratory failure. Glucose vs. fat. *Anesthesiology*, 54, 373–377.

Barrocas, A., Tretola, R., and Alonso, A. (1983). Nutrition and the critically ill pulmonary patient. *Respiratory Care*, 28, 50–61.

Bendixen, H. H., Egbert, L. D., and Hedley-Whyte, J. (1965). *Respiratory Care*. St. Louis: C.V. Mosby.

Brochard, L., Harf, A., Lorino, H., et al. (1989). Inspiratory pressure support prevents diaphragmatic fatigue during weaning from mechanical ventilation. *American Review of Respiratory Disease*, 139, 513–521.

Brooks, C. G. (1983). The adult way to wean from mechanical ventilation. *Critical Care Nurse*, 3, 64–78.

Brown, D. R. G. (1984). Weaning patients from mechanical ventilation. *Intensive Care Medicine*, 10, 55.

Brown, S. F., Merrill, E. J., and Light, R. W. (1983). Prevention of suctioning related arterial oxygen desaturation. Comparison of off-ventilator and on-ventilator suctioning. *Chest*, 4, 621–627.

Carroll, P. F. (1986). Caring for ventilator patients. *Nursing '86*, 16, 34–40.

Chernow, B. (1982). Hypomagnesemia: Implications for the critical care specialist. *Critical Care Medicine*, 10, 193–196.

Chulay, M., and Graeber, G. (1988). Effectiveness of hyperinflation and hyperoxygenation for suctioning interventions. *Heart & Lung*, 17, 15–22.

Colice, G. L. (1987). Prolonged intubation versus tracheostomy in the adult. *Journal of Intensive Care Medicine*, 2, 85–107.

Crabtree-Goodnough, S. K. (1988). Reducing tracheal injury and aspiration. *Dimensions of Critical Care Nursing*, 7, 324–331.

Cullen, D. J., and Caldera, D. L. (1979). The incidence of ventilator-induced pulmonary barotrauma in critically ill patients. *Anesthesiology*, 50, 185–190.

Daly, B. J., and Allen, M. L. (1987). Nursing care of the mechanically ventilated patient. In M. L. Nochomovitz, and H. D. Montenegro (Eds.), *Ventilatory support in respiratory failure*. Mt. Kisco, N.Y.: Futura.

Dane, T. E. B., and King, E. G. (1975). A prospective study of complications after tracheostomy for assisted ventilation. *Chest*, 67, 398–404.

Davis, H., Letrak, S., and Miller, D. (1980). Prolonged mechanical assisted ventilation: Analysis of outcomes and changes. *Journal of the American Medical Association*, 243, 43–45.

Demers, R. R., and Saklad, M. (1975). Mechanical aspiration: A reappraisal of its hazards. *Respiratory Care*, 20, 661–666.

Dougherty, S. (1988). The malnourished respiratory patient. *Critical Care Nurse*, 8, 13–22.

Downs, J. B., and Chapman, R. L. (1976). Treatment of bronchopleural fistula during continuous positive pressure ventilation. *Chest*, 69, 363–366.

Downs, J. B., Klein, E. P., Desautels, D., et al. (1973). Intermittent mandatory ventilation: A new approach to weaning patients from ventilation. *Chest*, 64, 331–335.

Downs, J. B., Perkins, H. M., and Sutton, W. W. (1974). Successful weaning after five years of mechanical ventilation. *Anesthesiology*, 40, 602–603.

Feeley, T. W., and Bancroft, M. L. (1982). Problems with mechanical ventilators. *International Anesthesiology Clinics*, 20, 83–93.

Feeley, T. W., and Hedley-Whyte, J. (1975). Weaning from controlled ventilation and supplemental oxygen. Weaning from intermittent positive-pressure ventilation. *New England Journal of Medicine*, 292, 903–906.

Fell, T., and Cheney, F. W. (1971). Prevention of hypoxia during endotracheal suction. *Annals of Surgery*, 174, 24–28.

Fitzgerald, L. M., and Huber, G. L. (1976). Weaning the patient from mechanical ventilation. *Heart & Lung*, 5, 228–234.

Gibney, R. T. N., Wilson, R. S., and Pontoppidan, H. (1982). Comparison of work of breathing on high gas flow and demand valve continuous positive airway pressure systems. *Chest*, 82, 692–695.

Grillo, H. C., Cooper, J. D., Geffin, B., et al. (1971). A low-pressure cuff for tracheostomy tube to minimize tracheal injury: A comparative clinical trial. *Journal of Thoracic Cardiovascular Surgery*, 62, 898–907.

Heffner, J. E., Miller, K. S., and Sahn, S. A. (1986). Tracheostomy in the intensive care unit. Part 2: Complications. *Chest*, 90, 430–436.

Hess, D. (1983). Bedside monitoring of the patient on a ventilator. *Critical Care Quarterly*, 6, 23–31.

Hotchkiss, R. S., and Wilson, R. S. (1983). Mechanical ventilatory support. *Surgical Clinics of North America*, 63, 417–438.

Hyman, A. L., Rodriquiz, J., and Weissman, C. (1982). Nutritional support of the critically ill patient. *Seminars in Anesthesia*, 1, 354–361.

Jung, R. C., and Newmans, J. (1982). Minimizing hypoxia during endotracheal airway care. *Heart & Lung*, 11, 208–212.

Kacmarek, R. M. (1989). Inspiratory pressure support: Does it make a clinical difference? *Intensive Care Medicine*, 15, 337–339.

Kelsay, J. L. (1978). A review of research on effects of fiber intake on man. *American Journal of Clinical Nutrition*, 3, 142–159.

Kim, M. J. (1984). Respiratory muscle training: Implications for patient care. *Heart & Lung*, 13, 333–340.

Kirsten, L. D. (1989). *Comprehensive respiratory nursing*. Philadelphia: W.B. Saunders.

Landis, K., and Smith, S. (1983). The mechanically ventilated patient. A comprehensive nursing care plan. *Critical Care Quarterly*, 6, 43–52.

Luce, J., Pierson, D., and Hudson, L. (1981). Intermittent mandatory ventilation. *Chest*, 79, 678–685.

Majors, M. (1988). Nutritional support of the mechanically ventilated patient. *Critical Care Nursing Quarterly*, 11, 50–61.

Marini, J. J. (1986). The physiologic determinants of ventilator dependence. *Respiratory Care*, 31, 271–282.

Mathru, M., Rao, T. L. K., and Venus, B. (1982). Hemodynamic response to changes in ventilatory patterns in patients with normal and poor left ventricular reserve. *Critical Care Medicine*, 10, 432–426.

McIntyre, N. R. (1986). Respiratory function during pressure support ventilation. *Chest*, 89, 677–683.

Morganroth, M. L., Morganroth, J. L., Nett, L. M., et al. (1984). Criteria for weaning from prolonged mechanical ventilation. *Archives of Internal Medicine*, 144, 1012–1016.

Nett, L. M., Morganroth, M. L., and Petty, T. L. (1987). Weaning protocols that work; Weaning in specific clinical situations; Weaning the unweanable. *American Journal of Nursing*, 87, 1174–1184.

Norton, L. C., and Neureuter, A. (1989). Weaning the long-term ventilator-dependent patient: Common problems and management. *Critical Care Nurse*, 9, 42–52.

Openbrier, D. (1985). A delicate balance: Strategies for feeding ventilated patients. *American Journal of Nursing*, 3, 247–280.

Passy, V. (1986). Passy-Muir tracheostomy speaking valve. *Otolaryngology*, 95, 247–248.

Pierson, D. J., Horton, C. A., and Bates, P. W. (1986). Persistent bronchopleural air leak during mechanical ventilation. A review of 39 cases. *Chest*, 90, 321–323.

Pierson, D. J. (1982). Persistent bronchopleural air leak during mechanical ventilation: A review. *Respiratory Care*, 27, 408–416.

Rafferty, T. D., Palma, J., Motoyama, E. K., et al. (1980). Management of a bronchopleural fistula with differential lung ventilation and positive end-expiratory pressure. *Respiratory Care*, 25, 654–657.

Rindfleish, S. H., and Tyler, M. L. (1983). Duration of suctioning: An important variable. *Respiratory Care*, 28, 457–459.

Rochester, D. F. (1984). Malnutrition and the respiratory system. *Chest*, 85, 411–415.

Safar, P., and Grenvik, A. (1975). Speaking cuffed tracheostomy tube. *Critical Care Medicine*, 3, 23–26.

Sahn, S. A., and Lakshminarayan, S. (1973). Bedside criteria for discontinuation of mechanical ventilation. *Chest*, 63, 1002–1005.

Sheldon, G. F., and Baker, C. (1980). Complications of nutritional support. *Critical Care Medicine*, 9, 35–37.

Shepherd, K. E., Wilson, D. J., and Wilson, R. S. (in press). Use of modified IMV as an approach to weaning patients from prolonged mechanical ventilation.

Sjostrand, U. (1980). High frequency positive pressure ventilation (HFPPV): A review. *Critical Care Medicine*, 8, 345–364.

Skelley, B. F. H., Deeren, S. M., and Powaser, M. M. (1980). The effectiveness of two preoxygenation methods to prevent endotracheal suction-induced hypoxemia. *Heart & Lung*, 9, 316–323.

Skillman, J. J., Malhotra, I., Pallotta, J. A., et al. (1971). Determinants of weaning from controlled ventilation. *Surgical Forum*, 22, 198–200.

Snyder, G. M. (1983). Individualized placement of tracheostomy tube fenestration and in-situ examination with the fiberoptic laryngoscope. *Respiratory Care*, 28, 1294–1298.

Sporn, P. H. S., and Morganroth, M. L. (1988). Discontinuation of mechanical ventilation. *Clinics in Chest Medicine*, 9, 113–126.

Venus, B., Smith, R. A., and Mathru, M. (1987). National survey of methods and criteria used for weaning from mechanical ventilation. *Critical Care Medicine*, 15, 530–533.

Walsh, J. J., and Rho, D. S. (1985). A speaking endotracheal tube. *Anesthesiology*, 63, 703–705.

Whited, R. E. (1984). A prospective study of laryngotracheal sequela in long-term intubation. *Laryngoscope*, 94, 367–377.

Wilson, D. J. (1988). Airway appliances and management. In R. M. Kacmarek, and J. Stoller (Eds.), *Current respiratory care* (pp. 80–89). Philadelphia: B. C. Decker.

Wilson, D. J. (1985). State of the art: Nutrition and chronic lung disease. *American Review of Respiratory Disease*, 124, 376–381.

Woodward, C. G., and Kacmarek, R. M. (1983). Failure to wean an adult from mechanical ventilation. *Respiratory Care*, 28, 775–776.

Nervous System

C · H · A · P · T · E · R 31

Neurophysiology

Victor G. Campbell

The human nervous system is composed of two constituent cells: neurons and neuroglia. The neurons are the basic structural and functional units for conduction in the nervous system, and the neuroglia cells serve in a supportive capacity for the neurons.

NEUROGLIA CELLS

About 40% of the microscopic structures of the brain and spinal cord are composed of neuroglia cells (Fig. 31–1). The purpose of these cells is to protect, support, and nourish the neuron. There are four different types of neuroglia cells: (1) ependyma, (2) astrocyte, (3) oligodendroglia, and (4) microglia.

Ependyma. Ependymal cells are found throughout the epithelial lining of the cerebral ventricles, the choroid plexuses, and the central canal of the spinal cord. Ependymal cells assist in the production of cerebrospinal fluid.

Astrocyte. Astrocytes, or astroglia, are starlike in appearance because of the many processes that extend out from the cell body. The functions of the astrocytes include (1) maintenance of the chemical environment for the conduction of impulses; (2) information storage; (3) maintenance of the blood–brain barrier; (4) maintenance of the nutritional needs of the neuron; and (5) structural support for the neuronal cells.

Oligodendroglia. Oligodendroglia are cells that synthesize a lipid-protein complex that forms the myelin sheaths around the axons of neurons in the central nervous system. The functions of the myelin sheath include (1) insulation along the processes of the nerve; (2) holding the nerve fibers together; (3) promotion of ionic flow across the cell membrane of the nerves; and (4) transmission of nerve impulses

(this type of transmission is termed saltatory conduction). Although considered homologous to the Schwann cells of the peripheral nervous system, oligodendrogliocytes lack the neurilemma membrane. Therefore, when structures are damaged, they are replaced with astrocytes that eventually form scar tissue that can disrupt the surrounding tissue and impair neuronal transmission.

Microglia. The microglial cells are formed from the embryonic mesodermal cells that migrated along branches of blood vessels into the central nervous system (Jensen, 1980). Microglia are found throughout the central nervous system, primarily in the white matter. The main function of the normally stationary microglia cells is phagocytosis. During this process, the microglia become mobile in order to ingest and digest tissue debris.

THE NEURON

The neuron (Fig. 31–2) is the principal structural cell of the nervous system whose function is transmission of specific nervous stimuli. Neurons have the specialized properties of excitation and electrical-chemical conductivity.

The neuron is composed of a cell body, or perikaryon; an axon, or axis cylinder; and a number of short receptive fibers called dendrites. The axons carry information away from the nerve body and thus are termed *efferent* fibers. The dendrites carry information to the neuron and are therefore called *afferent* fibers.

Neurons are classified according to their structure as unipolar, bipolar, or multipolar (Fig. 31–3). *Unipolar* neurons have one process or pole that divides close to the body of the cell. One branch of this division, termed the *peripheral process,* carries afferent (sensory) impulses from the periphery to the cell body. Another branch, called the *central process,* car-

A.

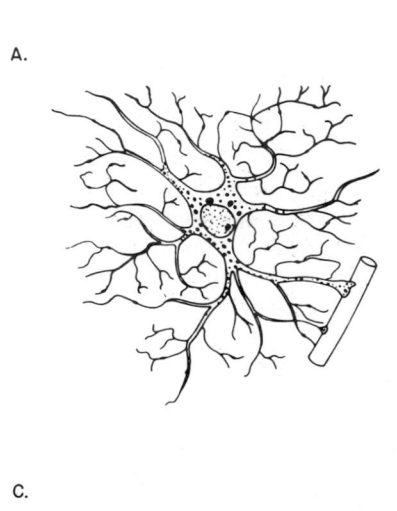

B.

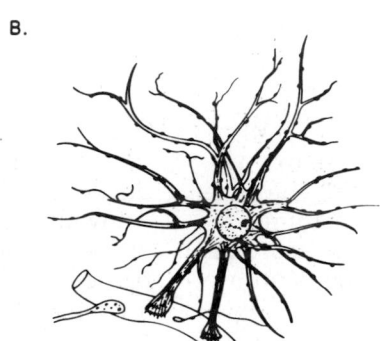

FIGURE 31–1. Neuroglia (interstitial) cells found in the central nervous system. Protoplasmic *(A)* and fibrous *(B)* astrocytes with end feet terminating on capillaries. Oligodendroglia *(C)* and *(D)* are shown. (From Jensen, D. (1980). *The principles of physiology* (2nd ed). New York: Appleton-Century-Crofts.)

C.

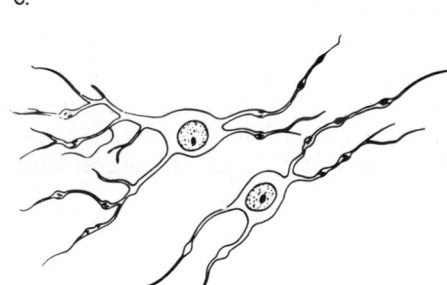

D.

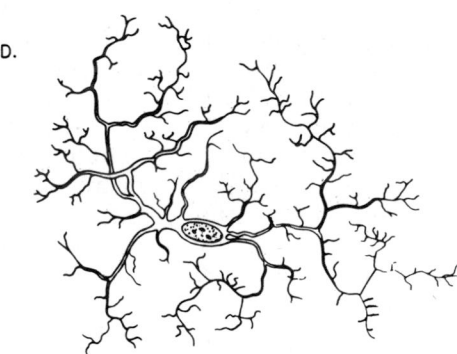

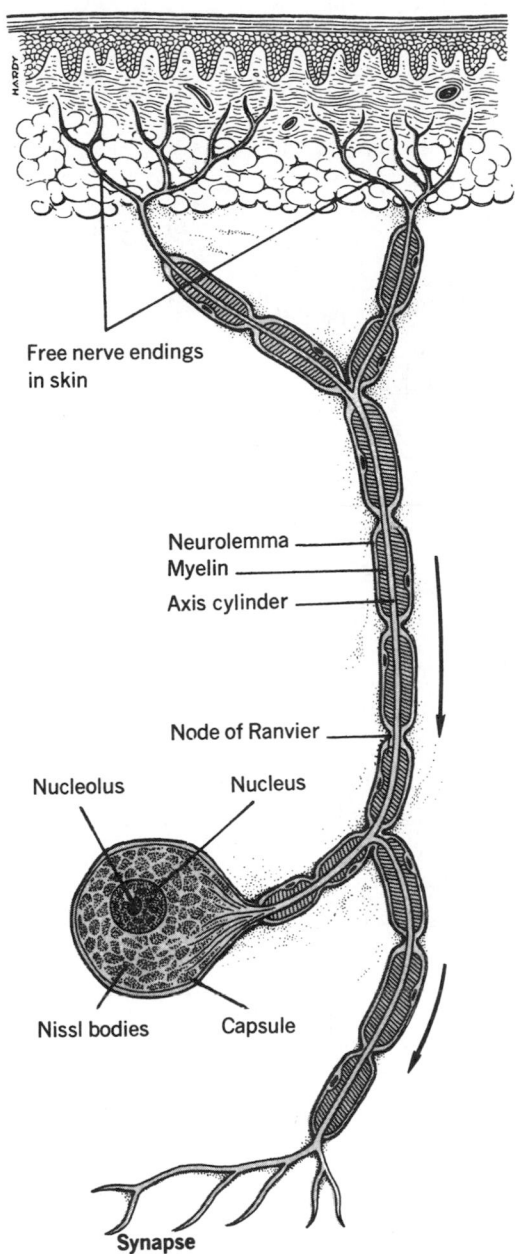

Free nerve endings
in skin

Neurolemma
Myelin
Axis cylinder

Node of Ranvier

Nucleolus   Nucleus

Nissl bodies   Capsule

Synapse

Unipolar neuron

FIGURE 31–2. Typical afferent (sensory) neuron. (From Chaffee, E. E., and Greisheimer, E. M. (1974). *Basic physiology and anatomy* (3rd ed., p. 164). Philadelphia, J.B. Lippincott.)

ries efferent (motor) impulses away from the cell body to the spinal cord and brainstem. *Bipolar* neurons have two processes consisting of one axon and one dendrite. Bipolar neurons are found only in spinal ganglia, the olfactory mucous membrane, and rod and cone cells of the retina. *Multipolar* neurons are found throughout the central nervous system, including all association (internuncial) and motor neurons. These neurons consist of a cell body, one long projection called the axon, and one or more shorter branches (dendrites).

Functionally, neurons are classified as afferent or efferent. Afferent neurons conduct sensory impulses from the peripheral nerve endings toward the cell body in the central nervous system. *Efferent* neurons transmit motor impulses away from the cell body via the axon to effector organs and tissues.

Cytologic Features. The neuron is composed of a cell body, or perikaryon, prosections called dendrites, and an axon (Fig. 31–4). In the cell body, which is located in the gray matter of the CNS, there is a centrally located *nucleus*. The nucleus is a large structure with a double membrane and contains deoxyribonucleic acid (DNA). Within the nucleus is a single prominent *nucleolus*, which contains ribonucleic acid (RNA). RNA is crucial for protein synthesis and serves as the messenger from the genes of the nucleus.

Surrounding the nucleus is the cellular cytoplasm, which contains numerous organelles including the Nissl bodies, mitochondria, the Golgi complex, neurofilaments, and microtubules. *Nissl bodies* are ordered masses of granular endoplasmic reticulum with ribosomes that function as the protein-synthesizing machinery of the cell. The *mitochondria* are rod-shaped structures that regulate the respiratory metabolism of the cell. Structurally, the mitochondria consist of outer and inner lipid bilayer-protein membranes. The *outer membrane* is smooth. The *inner membrane* forms a number of narrow folds that provide sites of attachment for oxidative enzymes. Between the narrow folds is an inner cavity called the mitochondrion *central cavity.* This cavity is filled with the dense *matrix granules,* which contain large numbers of dissolved enzymes that facilitate energy extraction from nutrients (Guyton, 1987). Mitochondria primarily function as the "powerhouse" of the cell. Specifically, the oxidative enzymes and the enzymes contained in the matrix granules act in a specific sequence to cause oxidation of nutrients. As a result of this oxidative process, water and carbon dioxide are formed, and the liberated energy is used to synthesize the high-energy compound adenosine triphosphate (ATP) from adenosine diphosphate (ADP) and inorganic phosphate. ATP then is transported from the cell to provide energy where it is needed for cellular functions (Guyton, 1987).

The *Golgi complex* is located in the cytoplasm and condenses and stores substances necessary for transmission of impulses. Throughout the cytoplasm as well as the processes of the axon and dendrites are the dense neurofilaments. Individual *neurofilaments* consist of structures called neurotubules or microtubules. Together, the neurotubules and microtubules make up the *neurofibril.* The neurofibril is involved in intracellular axoplasmic transport.

Neuronal Processes. Neuronal processes consist of the axon and the dendrites. The *axon,* or axis cylinder, is a long smooth projection that extends from

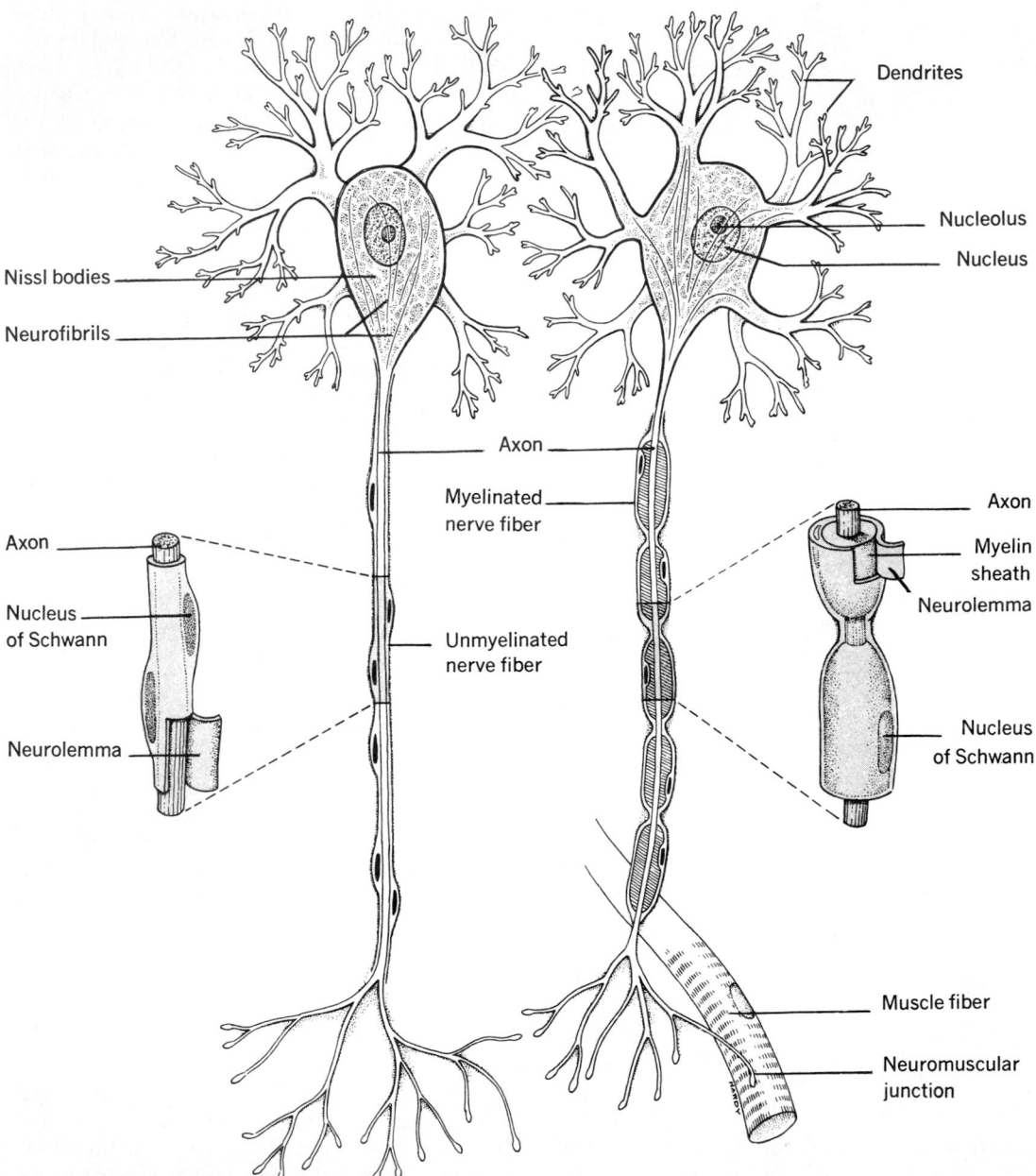

Dendrites

Nucleolus

Nucleus

Nissl bodies

Neurofibrils

Axon

Myelinated
nerve fiber

Axon

Axon

Myelin
sheath

Neurolemma

Nucleus
of Schwann

Neurolemma

Unmyelinated
nerve fiber

Nucleus
of Schwann

Muscle fiber

Neuromuscular
junction

FIGURE 31–3. Typical efferent (motor) neuron. (From Chaffee, E. E., and Greisheimer, E. M. (1974). *Basic physiology and anatomy* (3rd ed., p. 165). Philadelphia, J.B. Lippincott.)

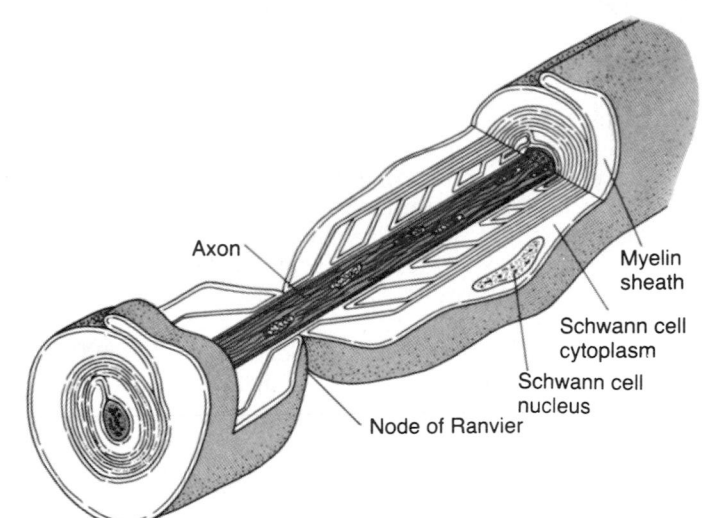

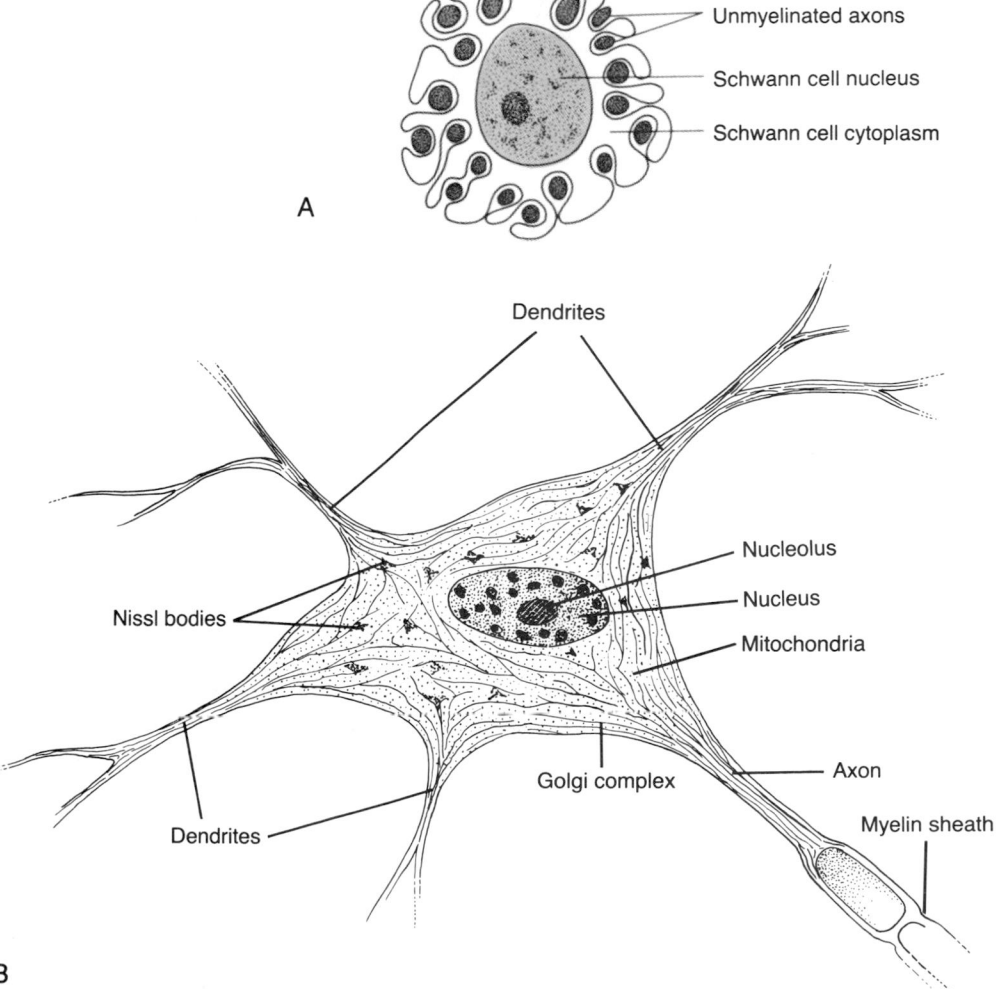

FIGURE 31–4. *A*, Cross-section of a myelinated neuron. *B*, Cell body of multipolar neuron. (*A* modified from Leeson, C. R., and Leeson, T. S. (1979). *Atlas of histology.* Philadelphia: W.B. Saunders; *In* Guyton, A. C. (1991). *Basic neuroscience.* (2nd ed., p. 78). Philadelphia: W. B. Saunders. *B* reproduced by permission from: Conway, B. L. *Pediatric neurologic nursing.* St. Louis, 1977, The C.V. Mosby Co.)

the cell body. Generally, the axon originates from the cell body at a point called the *axon hillock*. The axon carries efferent impulses away from the cell body and forms the white matter (myelinated) of the central nervous system. Surrounding the axon is the myelin, which protects and insulates the axonal structure. The terminal branches of the axon are called *terminal filaments* or axon telodendria. Short receptive processes called the *dendrites* extend from the cell body to the immediate surrounding areas. The dendrites are unmyelinated and lie in the gray matter of the central nervous system. The dendritic branches increase the surface area from which neuronal impulses may be picked up. The dendrites transmit afferent impulses to the cell body. Terminal endings of the dendrite, or dendritic spines, provide increased surface area for synaptic transmission of nerve impulses.

THE NERVE

The primary function of the neuron in the peripheral nervous system is the conduction of impulses to and from the central nervous system. This function of the neuron is accomplished by chainlike groupings of neuronal cell fibers into nerves.

The nerve component responsible for impulse conduction is the axon. Surrounding the axon is the discontinuous layer of the myelin sheath, which protects, insulates, and nourishes the axon (see Fig. 31–4). Periodic interruptions of the myelin sheath in the peripheral nervous system are called *nodes of Ranvier*. These nodes increase the speed of impulse conduction by allowing the nerve impulse to skip from node to node.

All the peripheral nerves are enveloped in a thin cytoplasmic membrane called the neurilemma. The *neurilemma* is formed by the Schwann cells and wraps segmentally around the myelin sheaths of myelinated nerves or the axons of unmyelinated nerves in the peripheral nervous system. The neurilemma protects and supports the vital nerve processes.

Surrounding the nerve are three layers of connective tissue (Fig. 31–5). The innermost *endoneurium* ensheathes the neurilemma cells. Next to the endoneurium is the *perineurium*, which surrounds bundles of nerve fibers (fascicles) with connective tissue. The outermost covering is the *epineurium*, which binds the groups of fascicle together.

As with the neuron, nerve fibers in the peripheral nervous system are classified according to their function. Afferent nerves receive sensory input. *Internuncial*, or association, nerves convey incoming stimuli to the various centers in the central nervous system. Efferent nerves transmit motor impulses to effector organs.

Impulse Conduction. Like other cells in the body, nerve fibers are charged, or polarized, in their resting state. In this state, the inside of the cell is charged negatively in relation to the outside. This difference in electrical polarity is the result of a high concentration of sodium (Na^+) outside the cell and a high concentration of potassium in the cell, causing unequal electrical charges across the cell membrane. The difference in electrical polarity is caused by the impermeability of the cell membrane to sodium and maintained by the sodium-potassium pump. The *sodium-potassium pump* is the mechanism by which sodium is pumped continuously out of the cell while potassium is being pumped into the cell.

When a chemical, mechanical, or electrical stimulus of threshold intensity (the amount of stimulus required to elicit tissue response) is applied, there is a rapid, marked change in the permeability of the cell membrane. This change in membrane permeability causes a rapid influx of sodium and a loss of intracellular potassium via diffusion. As the sodium rushes into the cell, the plasma membrane becomes charged positively in relation to the interstitial space, and an action potential *(depolarization)* results. The depolarization stimulus excites one local area of the cell membrane, which then excites adjacent areas of the cell membrane (conduction), until the whole membrane is stimulated at the same intensity. Consequently, the wave of depolarization is self-propagated along the entire length of the nerve process. Following depolarization, there is a reversal of ionic flow across the cell membrane. Specifically, sodium is pumped out as potassium is pumped back into the cell. This reversal in ionic flow *(repolarization)* restores the membrane polarization, and the membrane returns to its resting potential. To prevent repeated excitation, the neuron cannot be restimulated with another action potential during the entire phase of depolarization and during about one-third of the repolarization phase. This time interval is termed the *absolute refractory period*. Following the absolute refractory period is the *relative refractory period*. During this time interval, which lasts about one-quarter to one-half as long as the absolute refractory period, a stronger than normal stimulus can excite the nerve fiber. The relative refractory period is caused by (1) sodium channels that have not been reversed from inactivation, and (2) potassium channels that generally are wide open, producing hyperpolarization and making it more difficult to stimulate the nerve fiber (Guyton, 1987). The rate of transmission of the nerve impulse is dependent upon whether the nerve is myelinated. In heavily myelinated nerve fibers, the axon is exposed only at the nodes of Ranvier; therefore, the influx of sodium is possible only at these points. When depolarization occurs, there is a rapid influx of sodium ions (termed the sodium sink) at the node. The impulse then "skips" in a discontinuous manner to another node of Ranvier. This node-to-node transmission (termed *saltatory transmission*) results in a more rapid conduction of the action potential, increasing the velocity of impulse transmission and decreasing energy demands. In unmye-

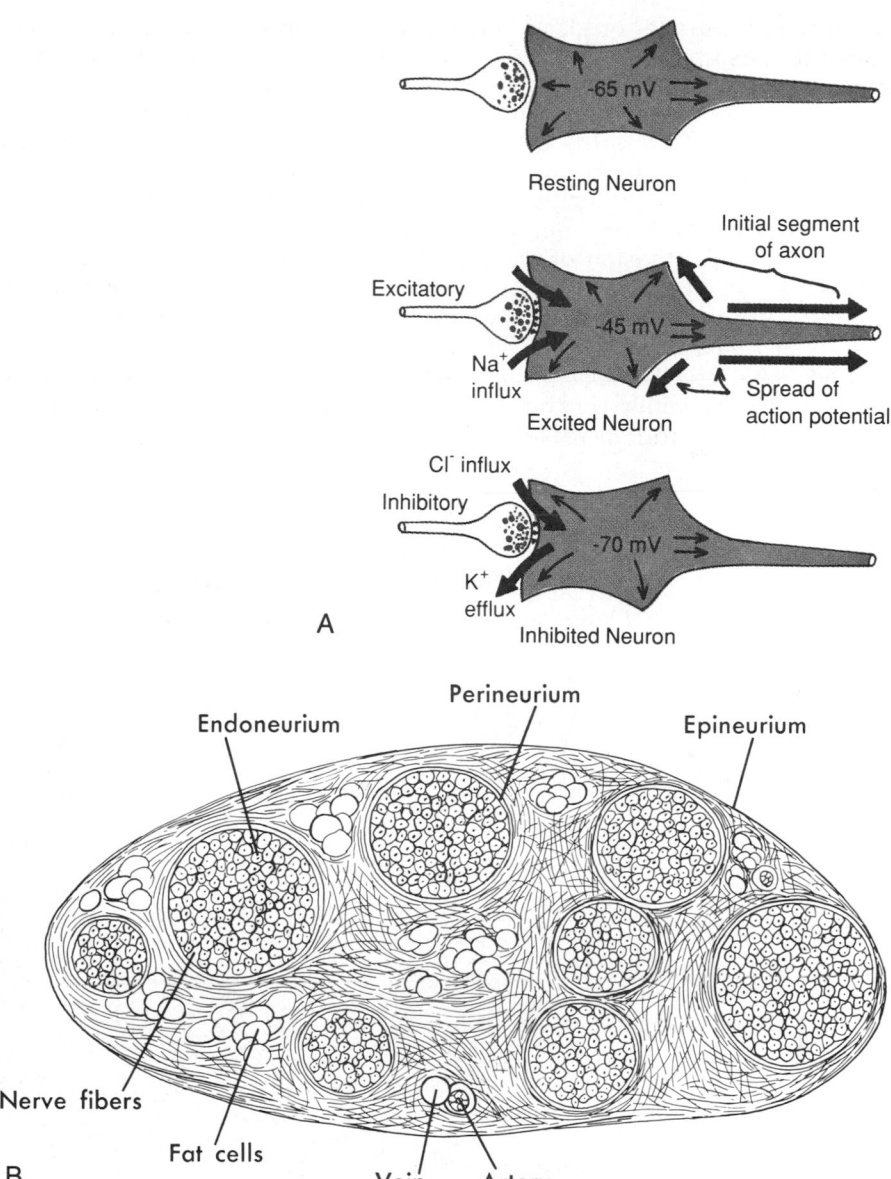

FIGURE 31–5. *A,* Examples of excitatory and inhibitory transmission. *B,* Transverse section of peripheral nerve trunk. (*A* From Guyton, A. C. (1991). *Basic neuroscience* (2nd ed., p. 95). Philadelphia: W. B. Saunders; *B,* reproduced by permission from: Conway, B. L. *Pediatric neurologic* nursing. St. Louis, 1977, The C. V. Mosby Co.)

linated nerves, the action potential must travel the entire length of the nerve fiber.

Synapse. Because neurons are physically distinct, impulses must travel via "signal transmission" from one neuron to another by way of gap junctions called synapses. Unlike impulse conduction, which is an electrical process, synaptic transmission is a chemical process that is accomplished by substances called *neurotransmitters.* Synaptic junctions between neurons are located in the gray matter. Anatomic structures of the synapse include the (1) presynaptic terminals, (2) synaptic cleft, and (3) postsynaptic membrane. *Presynaptic terminals,* also referred to as presynaptic knobs, store excitatory or inhibitory neurotransmitters in the synaptic vesicles. When the presynaptic terminals are stimulated by an impulse,

a specific type of neurotransmitter is released into the synaptic cleft. The synaptic cleft is a microscopic space between the terminals and receptor membranes. The release of the neurotransmitter stimulates specific receptor sites on the postsynaptic membrane (dendrite cell body area) of the next neuron in the pathway. Following synaptic transmission, the neurotransmitter is inactivated chemically or removed by reabsorption to prevent overstimulation of the postsynaptic membrane.

Neurotransmitters (see Fig. 31–5). Neurotransmitters are chemical substances that conduct impulses from nerve cells to target cells (Hickey, 1986). At least 30 neurotransmitters have now been identified. Each of these synaptic transmitters has a characteristic excitatory (facilitating) or inhibitory effect on the target nerve, muscle, or gland cell. *Excitatory* neurotransmitters stimulate the receptor sites on the postsynaptic membrane to enhance permeability to sodium, chloride, and potassium ions. The influx of the sodium ion lowers the cell membrane potential (depolarization) and forms an excitatory postsynaptic potential (EPSP). The principal excitatory neurotransmitter of the voluntary nervous system and the parasympathetic division of the autonomic nervous system is *acetylcholine* (ACh). In addition to acetylcholine, other central excitatory neurotransmitters include *dopamine, serotonin, norepinephrine, L-asparate,* and *glutamic acid. Inhibitory* neurotransmitters decrease the permeability of the postsynaptic receptor sites to sodium and increase their permeability to

potassium and chloride ions. The postsynaptic cell is hyperpolarized (membrane potential is raised) and forms an inhibitory postsynaptic potential (IPSP). Formation of an IPSP is called *direct inhibition*.

Another type of inhibitory action is caused by the stimulation of the excitatory presynaptic terminals by an inhibitory neuron. With presynaptic inhibition, there is a partial depolarization of the terminal fibrils and the excitatory presynaptic terminals, causing less excitatory neurotransmitters to be released from these endings. Consequently, the velocity of the action potential is reduced, and end-excitation of the neuron is decreased. Inhibitory neurotransmitters include *gamma-aminobutyric acid* (GABA) (presynaptic) and *glycine* (postsynaptic).

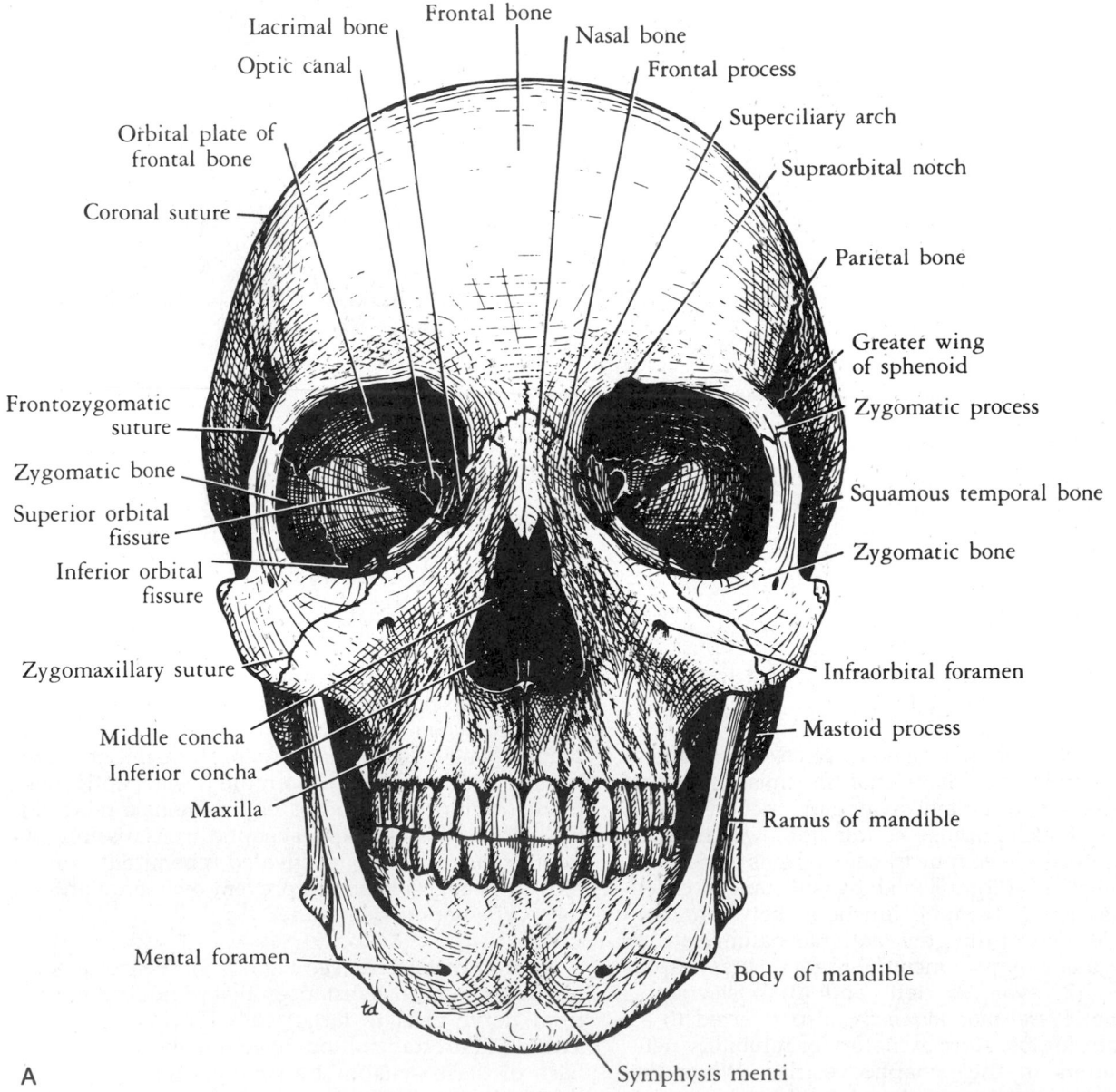

FIGURE 31–6. *A,* Anterior view of the skull. (From Textbook of Neurological Nursing, Pallet, P. J., and O'Brien, M. T., © 1985. Reprinted by permission of Scott, Foresman and Company.)

CENTRAL NERVOUS SYSTEM

Skull

The *skull* (Fig. 31–6) encloses and protects the vulnerable brain tissue. The two major anatomic divisions of the skull are the cranium and the facial bones. The cranial portion consists of eight irregularly shaped bones that are joined together by fixed joints or sutures. Internally, the cranial cavity is divided into three major areas—the anterior, middle, and posterior fossae. The *anterior fossa* contains the frontal lobes of the brain. The *middle fossa* contains the temporal, parietal, and occipital lobes. The *posterior fossa* contains the brainstem and the cerebellum. The opening at the base of the skull is called the *foramen magnum* and is the area in which the brain and spinal cord join.

The 14 facial bones are fused together as a unit to support the facial structures. The facial skull encloses the eye sockets, a portion of the nasal cavity, and the oral cavity.

Meninges

The brain is covered by three layers of connective tissue referred to collectively as the *cranial meninges* (Fig. 31–7). Each of the three meningeal layers is a continuous sheet of connective tissue that protects the vulnerable brain.

The outermost meningeal layer is the *dura mater* or "hard mother." The dura mater is a double-layered sheath that encloses the brain and separates the skull into various compartments by its folds and processes. The *falx cerebri* process is formed by a vertical fold at the midsagittal line and divides the two cerebral hemispheres. The *tentorium cerebelli* is a horizontal fold that separates the cerebral hemispheres from the brainstem and the cerebellum. Anatomically, structures that lie above the tentorium cerebelli are called *supratentorial*, whereas structures below this fold are termed *infratentorial*. The *falx cerebelli* is a dural process that divides the two cerebellar hemispheres.

The second meningeal layer is the *arachnoid*. The arachnoid has two thin layers of delicate and elastic

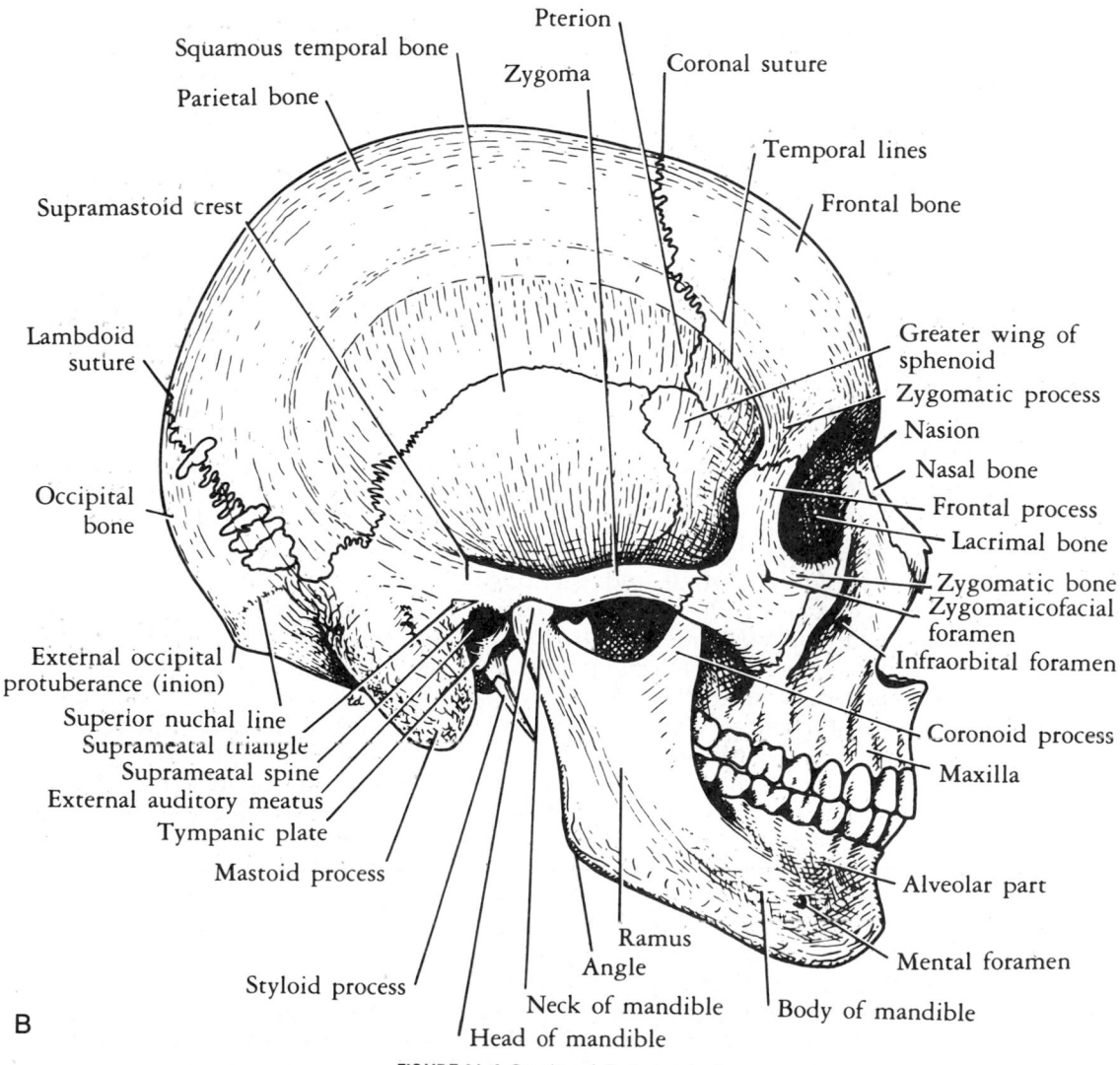

FIGURE 31–6 *Continued B*, Lateral view.

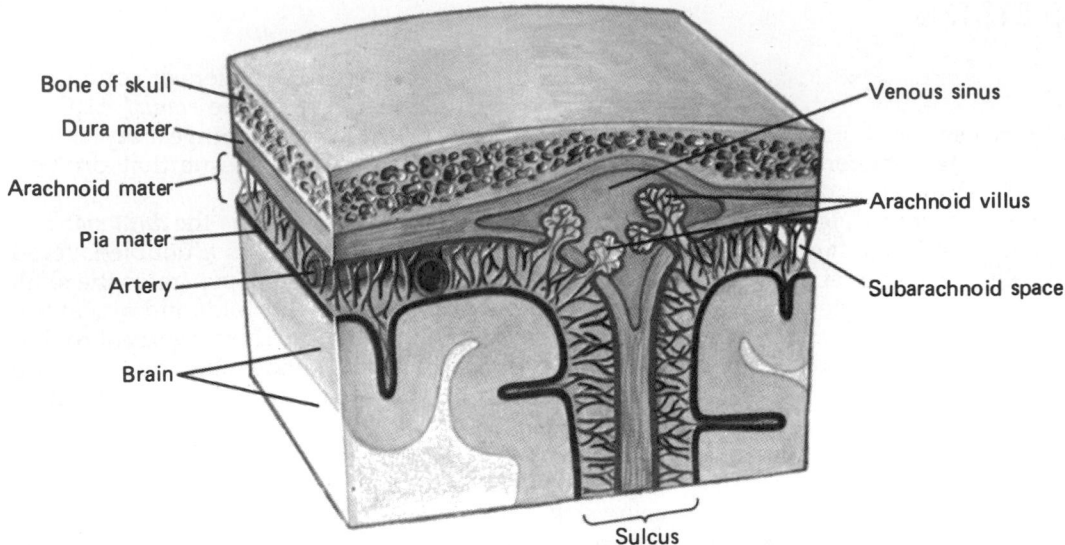

FIGURE 31–7. Schematic diagram illustrating the relationships among the meninges, their spaces, and the ventricles of the brain. Thickness of the pia mater has been exaggerated. (From Guyton, A. C. (1987). *Basic neuroscience*. Philadelphia: W. B. Saunders.)

membranes that create the cobweblike subarachnoid space. Located within the subarachnoid space are a number of cerebral vessels, and it is in this space that cerebrospinal fluid circulates around the brain. The cerebrospinal fluid is formed from three primary sources: the *choroid plexus*, located in portions of the lateral, third, and fourth cerebral ventricles; the *ependymal cells* that line the ventricles and meningeal blood vessels; and *cerebral* and *spinal blood vessels*.

The third and innermost meningeal layer is the meshlike *pia mater*. This vascular membrane is supplied with blood from the internal carotid and vertebral arteries and provides a large volume of blood to the brain.

Cerebral Circulation

The primary sources of the cerebral blood supply are the two pairs of internal carotid and vertebral arteries (Fig. 31–8). The pair of *internal carotid arteries* provide the brain with approximately 80% of the needed blood supply. These vessels originate from the right and left *common carotid arteries*, respectively, at about the level of the thyroid cartilage. The internal carotid artery enters the skull at the foramen lacerum. At approximately the level of the optic chiasm, the internal carotids give rise to the anterior and middle cerebral arteries. The *anterior cerebral artery* passes medially along the base of the brain anterior to the optic chiasm and then runs along the longitudinal fissure between the frontal lobes. The anterior cerebral artery primarily supplies the corpus callosum, medial portions of the frontal and parietal lobes, portions of the internal capsule, and the nuclei of the basal ganglia. The *middle cerebral artery* is the largest branch of the internal carotid artery and

supplies the lateral surfaces of the frontal, temporal, and parietal lobes. The middle cerebral artery is the primary source of blood to the precentral (motor) and postcentral (sensory) gyri (wrinkles or convolutions).

The remaining 20% of cerebral blood supply is delivered by the pair of vertebral arteries that originates from the right and left subclavian arteries and enters the skull through the foramen magnum in front of the spinal cord. The arteries run along the anterior surface of the medulla oblongata and unite at the level of the pons to form the *basilar artery*. The basilar artery lies in the median groove of the pons. Branches of the vertebral and basilar arteries provide blood to the brainstem and cerebellum. Within the midbrain, the basilar artery bifurcates into the two *posterior cerebral arteries* that supply inferior and medial portions of the temporal and occipital lobes, the vestibular organs, and the cochlear apparatus.

Circle of Willis. Located at the base of the brain is a small circle of arteries that surround the pituitary stalk and the optic chiasm. This ring of blood vessels, called the *circle of Willis*, is formed by communicating branches of the posterior and anterior cerebral arteries (Fig. 31–9). Specifically, the posterior and middle cerebral arteries are joined together by the two *posterior communicating arteries*. The two anterior arteries are connected by one *anterior communicating artery*. The circle of Willis is thought to be a protective mechanism by which cerebral circulation is maintained if blood flow from one of the four primary vessels is occluded or interrupted.

Venous Drainage. Cerebral venous drainage is accomplished by venous sinuses that are created by two layers of the dura mater. The major venous

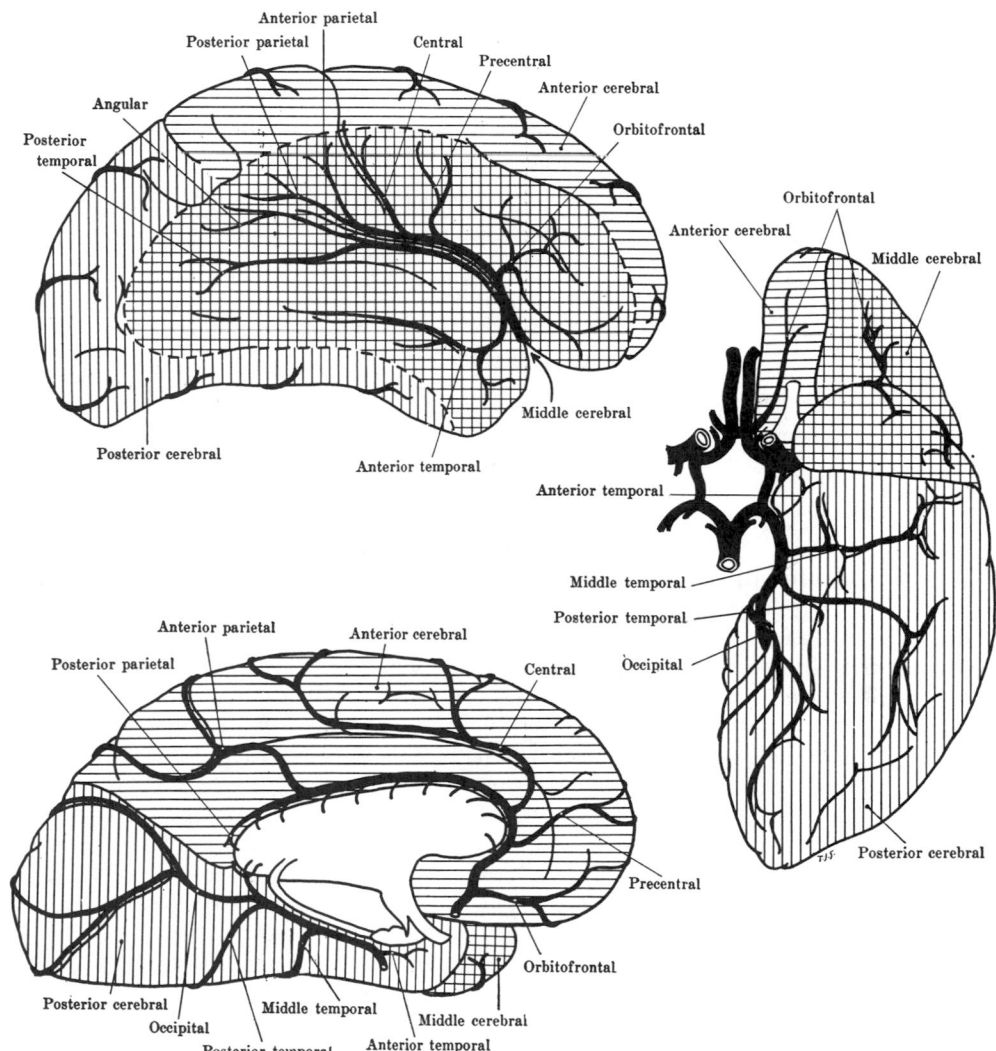

FIGURE 31–8. Diagram of areas of distribution of anterior, middle, and posterior cerebral arteries. (Reproduced by permission from: Mettler, F. A. *Neuroanatomy* (2nd ed.). St. Louis, 1948, The C.V. Mosby Co.)

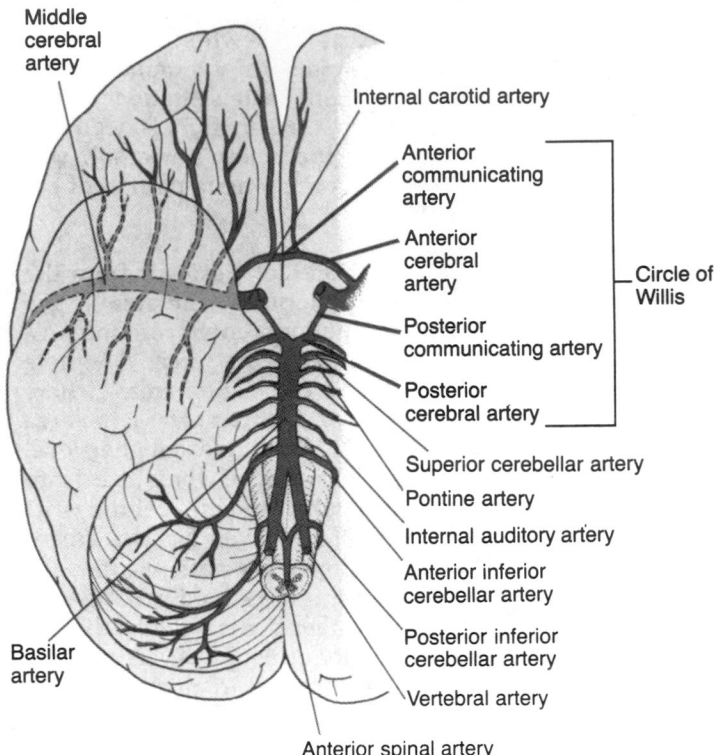

Middle
cerebral
artery

Internal carotid artery

Anterior
communicating
artery

Anterior
cerebral
artery

Posterior
communicating artery

Posterior
cerebral artery

Circle of
Willis

Superior cerebellar artery

Pontine artery

Internal auditory artery

Anterior inferior
cerebellar artery

Posterior inferior
cerebellar artery

Basilar
artery

Vertebral artery

Anterior spinal artery

FIGURE 31–9. Diagram of principal cerebral arteries and circle of Willis. (From Ignatavicius, D. D., and Bayne, M. V. (1991). *Medical-surgical nursing: A nursing process approach.* Philadelphia: W. B. Saunders.)

sinuses include the superior sagittal sinus, the inferior sagittal sinus, the straight sinus, the transverse sinuses, and the cavernous sinuses. The *superior sagittal sinus* arises at the frontal lobe and traverses the top of the falx cerebri. This sinus drains the cerebrospinal fluid and the superior cortical veins. The *inferior sagittal sinus* passes along the lower edge of the falx cerebri and drains the medial surface of the brain. The *straight sinus* runs between the superior and inferior sinuses and drains the vein of Galen. The *transverse sinuses* are continuations of the superior sagittal sinus and are found on each side of the skull. The transverse sinuses drain blood from the superior sagittal and straight sinuses into the internal jugular vein. The *cavernous sinuses* run along the sphenoid bone and drain the inferior surfaces of the brain.

Cerebral Blood Flow Regulation

Normal cerebral blood flow (CBF) is approximately 750 mL/minute and is maintained by a cerebral perfusion pressure (CPP) of approximately 85 mm Hg (Simon and Sayre, 1987). The cerebral vasculature, and thus CBF, is regulated by a number of mechanisms to maintain sufficient blood flow to meet the cerebral metabolic needs. These mechanisms include autoregulation, chemical control, and metabolic regulation.

Autoregulation is a mechanism that permits variation in cerebral perfusion pressure within certain

limits without significantly altering cerebral blood flow (Lindsay et al., 1986). Normally, CBF is maintained at a relatively constant level by vasoconstriction and vasodilation of the cerebral vessels. Specifically, an increase in cerebral perfusion pressure causes the vascular smooth muscles and the vessels to constrict. Similarly, a decrease in cerebral perfusion pressure produces a myogenic effect resulting in vasodilation. The autoregulatory mechanism fails when the CPP is less than 50 mm Hg or greater than 160 mm Hg. At these extreme pressures, CBF is dependent passively upon CPP (Lindsay et al., 1986). When the CPP falls below 50 mm Hg, an extremely powerful sympathetic reflex is initiated. This reflex is called the *Cushing response,* and when stimulated, it produces a rapid elevation in systemic blood pressure.

The Cushing response is an ischemic reflex that occurs when there is an increase in pressure within the cranial vault. Such an increase in pressure occurs when CSF pressure equals arterial pressures, thereby compressing cerebral vessels and cutting off the blood supply to the brain (Guyton, 1987). The purpose of this response is to maintain medullary perfusion, and it is mediated through the vagus nerve and the sympathetic system. When initiated, the Cushing response produces three significant changes in cardiorespiratory physiology. First, there is an increase in arterial pulse pressure that results from a rise in systolic blood pressure. With the increase in arterial pressure above that of the CSF, blood flow is reestablished to the ischemic area. Second, there is a decrease in heart rate. Third, there is a decrease in the respiratory rate (Simon and Sayre, 1987). The main goal in treating the Cushing response is to make a direct attempt to widen the cerebral perfusion pressure (Simon and Sayre, 1987).

Chemical control of cerebral blood flow is achieved through alterations in the carbon dioxide, hydrogen, and oxygen concentrations. Increased levels of carbon dioxide (i.e., hypercarbia) and increased hydrogen ion concentrations (i.e., lactic acidosis) result in vasodilatation and increased CBF. In contrast, an increased oxygen concentration or decreased carbon dioxide level (hypocarbia) produces vasoconstriction and lowers the CBF.

Metabolic regulation is another mechanism that significantly affects arteriolar diameter and CBF. During ischemia, large amounts of *adenosine* are released, producing a powerful vasodilatation effect. Adenosine levels have been shown to increase in response to falling cerebral perfusion pressures and increased cerebral metabolic rate of oxygen ($CMRO_2$) (Simon et al., 1987). $CMRO_2$ is the rate of cerebral oxygen utilization during metabolism.

A number of clinical factors can alter CBF significantly. The factors that can produce a decrease in CBF include hypocarbia, hypothermia, and barbiturates. Clinical factors that increase CBF include seizures, fever, narcotics, hypoxia, and anesthetic agents such as halothane (Simon et al., 1987).

Blood–Brain Barrier

The brain tissue is very sensitive to any changes in the concentration of ions. For the central nervous system to function normally, the brain's internal environment must be delicately balanced. This stable environment is accomplished by the blood–brain and blood–cerebrospinal fluid barriers. These barriers are physiologic mechanisms that protect the homeostatic balance of the brain tissue by selective capillary permeability. The *blood–brain barrier* consists of a dense network of astroglial membranes and capillary endothelial cells that form tight junctions around the cerebral capillaries (Hickey, 1986). These tight junctions affect capillary permeability, thus providing selective permeability of substances that cross the neuronal membrane. The *blood–cerebrospinal fluid barrier* is found in the choroid plexuses and also provides selective permeability of substances that gain entrance to the neuron (Hickey, 1986). Both the blood–brain and the blood–cerebrospinal fluid barriers are permeable to oxygen, carbon dioxide, water, and glucose. These barriers are somewhat permeable to circulating electrolytes such as Na^+, Cl^-, and K^+, but are impermeable to many drugs, fixed acids, and bases.

Cerebrospinal Fluid

Cerebrospinal fluid (CSF) is normally a clear, odorless, and colorless fluid that contains oxygen, carbon dioxide, glucose, electrolytes, small quantities of protein, and a few leukocytes. The purpose of the CSF is to protect and cushion the brain and spinal cord by acting as a shock absorber. In addition, the CSF participates in the nutrition and removal of metabolic wastes for the central nervous system.

CSF Formation. CSF is formed from three different sources. The primary source of CSF is the *choroid plexus,* which is a dense network of capillaries located in the lateral, third, and fourth ventricles (Fig. 31–10). The choroid plexus secretes approximately 500 to 750 mL of CSF daily; however, only 125 to 150 mL are present in the cerebral ventricular system at any given time. A smaller amount of CSF is formed by the *ependymal cells* that line the ventricles and meningeal blood vessels. The third source of CSF is the *blood vessels* of the brain and spinal cord (Hickey, 1986).

CSF Flow. After the CSF is secreted, it passes through the two foramina of Monro to the third ventricle. From the third ventricle, the CSF flows slowly through the aqueduct of Sylvius to the fourth ventricle. The CSF then passes through the medial foramen of Magendie and the paired lateral foramina of Luschke to the cisternal magnum. It then enters the subarachnoid space, where it slowly diffuses upward over the brain and fills the spinal cisterns.

CSF Absorption. Most of the CSF is reabsorbed slowly from the subarachnoid space by the arachnoid villi. The *arachnoid villi* are clusterlike projections from the subarachnoid space into the venous sinuses. The CSF flows through the arachnoid villi into the venous sinuses and is reabsorbed into the venous system.

Cerebral Structures

Brain. The brain (Fig. 31–11) constitutes approximately 2% of body weight, receives approximately 20% of the cardiac output, and requires about 20% of the body's oxygen utilization. The brain (encephalon) can be divided into the three anatomic areas—cerebrum (see p. 657), brainstem (see p. 659), and cerebellum (see p. 660).

Cerebrum. The cerebrum is the largest portion of the brain and consists of two cerebral hemispheres that are divided partially by the *great longitudinal fissure* (Fig. 31–12). The cerebral hemispheres are joined at the bottom of the great longitudinal fissure by a large tract of white commissural fibers, the *corpus callosum.* On the outside of the cerebrum are multiple layers of gray cells called the *cerebral cortex.* Internally, the cerebrum consists of a large number of myelinated nerve fibers and neuroglial cells collectively called the white matter. The major sulci (grooves) and fissures (deep grooves) of the cerebral cortex divide each hemisphere into four pairs of lobes that are named after the overlying cranial bones: frontal, parietal, temporal, and occipital (Fig. 31–12).

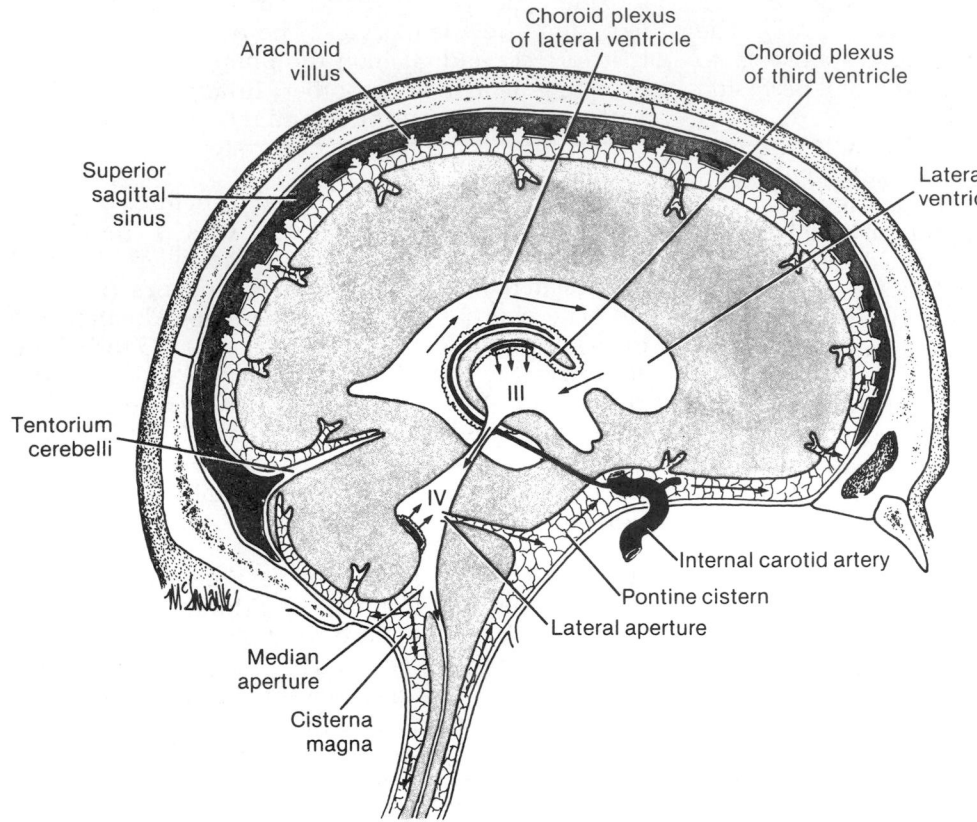

Arachnoid villus

Choroid plexus of lateral ventricle

Choroid plexus of third ventricle

Superior sagittal sinus

Lateral ventricle

Tentorium cerebelli

III

IV

Internal carotid artery

Pontine cistern

Lateral aperture

Median aperture

Cisterna magna

FIGURE 31–10. Path of circulation of cerebrospinal fluid from its formation in the ventricles to its absorption into the superior sagittal sinus. (Reproduced by permission from: Nolte, J. *The human brain* (2nd ed.). St. Louis, 1988, The C.V. Mosby Co. Redrawn from Hamilton W. J., ed.: *Textbook of human anatomy* (2nd ed.). St. Louis, 1976, The C.V. Mosby Co. By permission of Macmillan Press, London and Basingstoke.)

FIGURE 31–11. Sagittal section of the cerebrum. (Reproduced by permission from: Conway-Rutkowski, Barbara Lang: Carini and Owens' *Neurological and neurosurgical nursing,* ed. 8, St. Louis, 1982, The C.V. Mosby Co.)

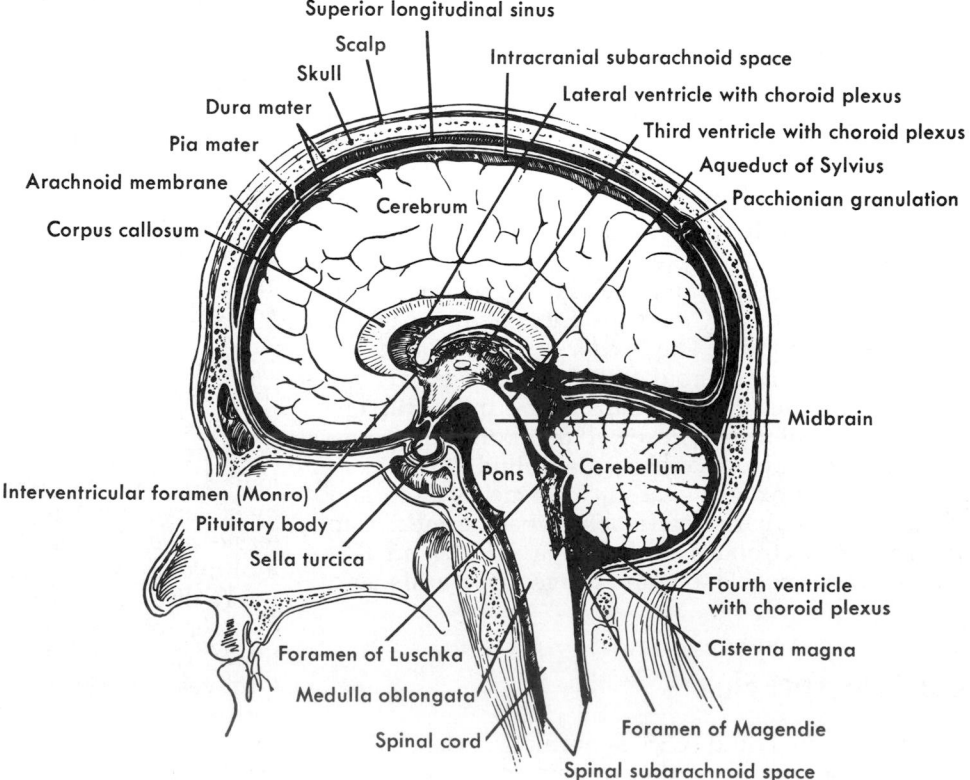

Superior longitudinal sinus

Scalp

Skull

Intracranial subarachnoid space

Dura mater

Lateral ventricle with choroid plexus

Pia mater

Third ventricle with choroid plexus

Arachnoid membrane

Aqueduct of Sylvius

Pacchionian granulation

Corpus callosum

Cerebrum

Midbrain

Pons

Cerebellum

Interventricular foramen (Monro)

Pituitary body

Sella turcica

Fourth ventricle with choroid plexus

Cisterna magna

Foramen of Luschka

Medulla oblongata

Spinal cord

Foramen of Magendie

Spinal subarachnoid space

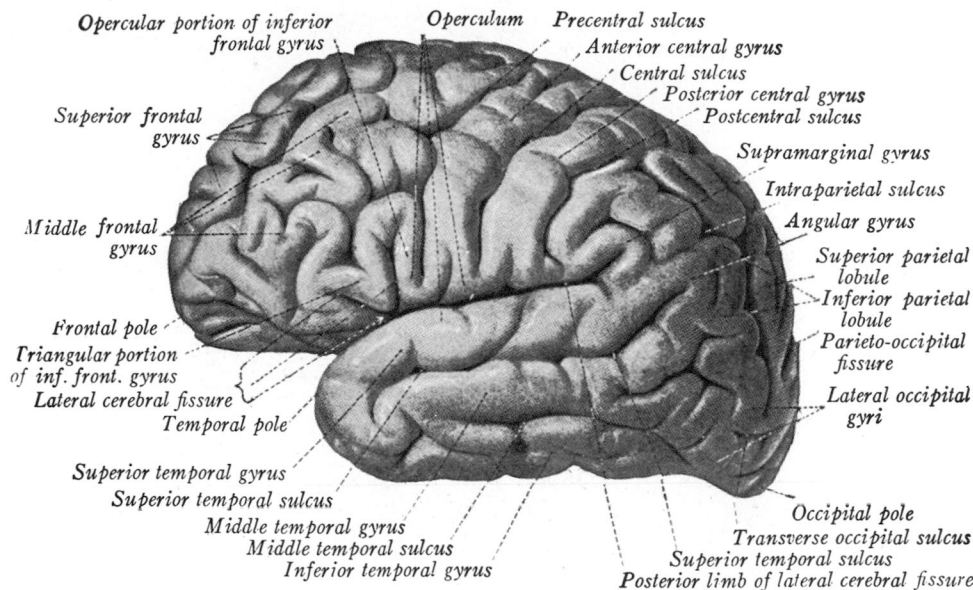

Opercular portion of inferior frontal gyrus
Operculum
Precentral sulcus
Anterior central gyrus
Central sulcus
Posterior central gyrus
Postcentral sulcus
Superior frontal gyrus
Supramarginal gyrus
Intraparietal sulcus
Middle frontal gyrus
Angular gyrus
Superior parietal lobule
Inferior parietal lobule
Frontal pole
Triangular portion of inf. front. gyrus
Lateral cerebral fissure
Temporal pole
Parieto-occipital fissure
Lateral occipital gyri
Superior temporal gyrus
Superior temporal sulcus
Middle temporal gyrus
Middle temporal sulcus
Inferior temporal gyrus
Occipital pole
Transverse occipital sulcus
Superior temporal sulcus
Posterior limb of lateral cerebral fissure

FIGURE 31–12. Lateral surface of the cerebrum. (From Ranson, S. W., and Clark, S. L. (1966). *The anatomy of the nervous system: Its development and function* (p. 55). Philadelphia: W.B. Saunders.)

Certain areas of the cerebral cortex have been identified as having specific functions. In 1909, Brodmann developed a cytoarchitectural map of 47 primary and association function areas of the human cerebral cortex (Fig. 31–13). Primary function areas include those in which movement or perception of movement occurs. Association function areas surround the primary function areas and provide a higher level of integration for sensory experiences.

Frontal Lobes. The frontal lobes are located in the anterior fossa, extending from the front of each cerebral hemisphere to the fissure of Rolando. The function of the frontal lobe is related primarily to motor activity, psychic activity, and higher intellectual activities. Along with the thalamus and hypothalamus, the frontal lobes also control autonomic functions such as respiration, blood pressure, and gastrointestinal activity. Located at the inferior frontal gyrus is Broca's area. *Broca's area* is an association area (areas 44 and 45) that is involved in the formulation of words. When this area is damaged or destroyed, the individual can no longer speak in sentences (expressive aphasia).

Parietal Lobes. The parietal lobes lie in the middle fossa in the area between the fissure of Rolando and the parieto-occipital fissure. The function of the parietal lobes is the processing of input to the primary sensory cortex. The primary sensory cortex is concerned with the gross aspects of sensation and sends input of its interpretation to the thalamus and other cortical structures (Hickey, 1986). The association areas of the parietal lobes are specific to shape, texture, size, and consistency of objects, comprehension of written words, and the ability to discriminate between two simultaneous skin contacts (Rudy, 1984).

Temporal Lobes. The temporal lobes are located in the middle fossa. They lie inferior to the fissure of

Sylvius and extend back to the parieto-occipital fissure. Primary functions of the temporal lobes are memory storage and hearing. Located in the temporal lobe is an auditory association area called *Wernicke's area.* If Wernicke's area is damaged or destroyed, the individual is unable to understand the meaning of spoken words (receptive asphasia).

Occipital Lobes. The occipital lobes lie in the middle fossa, just above the cerebellum and posterior to the parieto-occipital fissure. The occipital lobes contain the primary vision cortex and the visual association areas. Damage or destruction of the visual association areas will result in an ability to see objects clearly but an inability to recognize or identify those objects (visual agnosia).

Limbic Lobes. Anatomically, the limbic lobes are part of the temporal lobes; however, they do have a separate function. The limbic lobes are concerned with visceral activities, self-preservation, moods, and emotions. The limbic lobes also are referred to as the *rhinencephalon.*

Basal Ganglia. The basal ganglia are a group of gray nuclei that lie deep within each cerebral hemisphere. The basal ganglia provide a vital subcortical link between the cerebral cortex and the motor cortex (Schmidt, 1985). Paired structures of the basal ganglia include the caudate nucleus, the lenticular nucleus, the amygdaloid body, and the claustrum. Functions of the basal ganglia include the initiation and execution of fine motor movements.

Commissural Fibers. Commissural, or interhemispheric, fibers connect the cerebral hemispheres with each other and maintain higher sensory and motor functions of the cortex (Rudy, 1984). Commissural fibers consist of the *corpus callosum, commissure of the fornix, anterior commissure,* and the *habenular commis-*

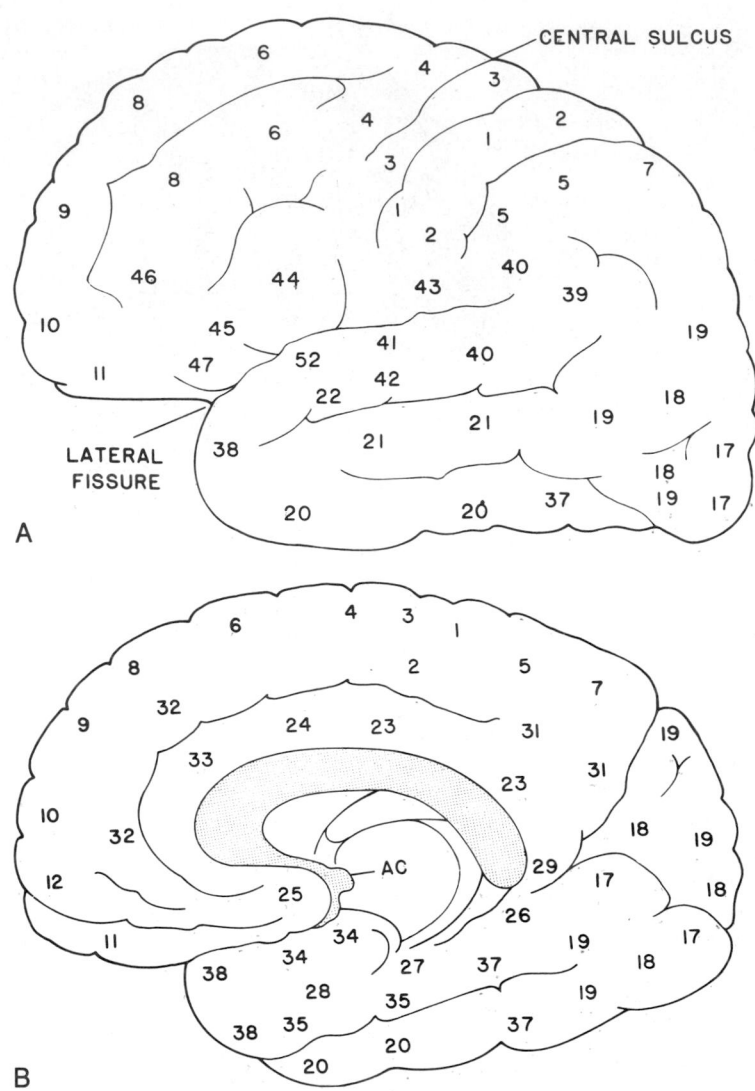

FIGURE 31–13. *A,* Lateral aspect of left cerebral hemisphere showing the cortical areas according to Brodmann. Area 8 = frontal eye movement, pupillary change area. Area 6 = premotor area (portion of extrapyramidal system). Area 4 (precentral gyrus) = primary motor area. Areas 3, 2, 1 (postcentral gyrus) = primary sensory areas. Areas 5, 6, 7 = secondary sensory association areas. Areas 39, 40 = association areas. Areas 18, 19 = visual association areas. Area 17 = primary visual cortex. Area 41 = primary auditory cortex. Area 42 = associative auditory cortex. Area 44 = motor speech area of Broca.

B, Medical aspect of left cerebral hemisphere showing the cortical areas according to Brodmann. Functions of specific areas are given in the legend to part A. AC = anterior commissure. Shaded area indicates the corpus callosum. (From Jensen, D. (1980). *The principles of physiology* (2nd ed., pp. 229–230). New York: Appleton-Century-Crofts.)

sure. The largest of these connective pathways is the corpus callosum, which connects every area of one cerebral hemisphere with the corresponding area in the other hemisphere. The connection of the two sides of the brain by the corpus callosum prevents interference between the two hemispheres and ensures coordinated and complementary motor responses and thoughts (Guyton, 1987).

Hemispheric Dominance. The term *hemispheric dominance* refers to the fact that the interpretative functions of the angular gyrus and the temporal lobe are developed more highly in one or the other of the cerebral hemispheres. At birth, both of these regions have almost the same capacity for development. However, Wernicke's area in the left hemisphere is as much as 50% larger in more than half of newborn

babies. Because the left side is larger, the temporal lobe in this hemisphere begins to be used to a greater extent than the right (Guyton, 1987). Since the rate of learning occurs much faster in the better developed hemisphere, there is a tendency to continue to direct attention to that hemisphere, resulting in hemispheric dominance. In approximately 90% to 95% of the population, the temporal lobe and the angular gyrus of the left cerebral hemisphere become dominant. In the remaining 10%, there is dual dominance, or, in rare cases, the right side becomes the dominant hemisphere (Guyton, 1987).

Diencephalon. The oval-shaped diencephalon (Fig. 31–14) is a major division of the cerebrum and consists of the epithalamus, thalamus, hypothala-

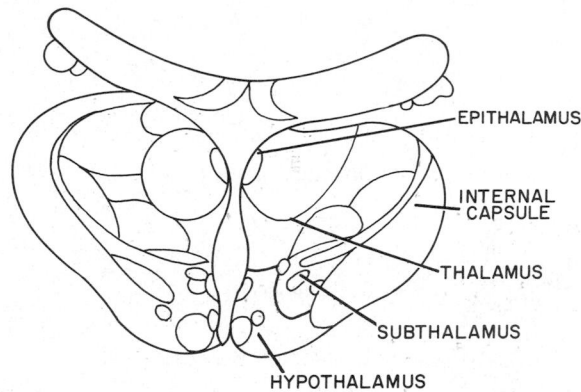

FIGURE 31–14. Diencephalon. Cross section of the brainstem at the diencephalic level. (From B. Curtis, et al.: *An introduction to the neurosciences.* Philadelphia: Lea & Febiger, 1977. Reprinted with permission.)

mus, and subthalamus. The internal capsule and pituitary gland (hypophysis) also are located in the area of the diencephalon.

Epithalamus. The epithalamus is located in the most dorsal area of the diencephalon and consists of the pineal body, habenula, habenular commissure, posterior commissure, and striae medullares. The most important structure in the epithalamus is the *pineal body*, which is believed to have a role in growth and sexual development. The epithalamus also is believed to have a role in the primitive reflex of getting food (Hickey, 1986).

Thalamus. The thalamus also is located in the dorsal portion of the diencephalon and is composed of two connected ovoid masses of gray matter located deep within each cerebral hemisphere. The thalamus essentially is the "main entrance" for all sensory input (except that from the olfactory system) to the cerebral cortex (Guyton, 1987). As such, the thalamus is involved intricately in several important functions including direction of attention to specific areas of one's mental environment, the sleep-wake cycle, and influence on voluntary movements and motor responses.

Hypothalamus. The hypothalamus is located under the thalamus, forming the floor and parts of the walls of the third cerebral ventricle. The hypothalamus functionally is the most important efferent pathway by which the limbic system controls many of the essential functions of the body (Guyton, 1987). These functions include:

1. Regulation of body temperature
2. Regulation of body water by controlling water excretion into the urine and creation of the thirst sensation
3. Control of appetite
4. Control of secretions of the pituitary gland such as corticotropin, thyrotropin, luteinizing hormone, and the follicle-stimulating hormone
5. Regulation of uterine contractility and expelling of breast milk
6. Cardiovascular regulation including increased

or decreased blood pressure, and increased or decreased heart rate
7. Subcortical regulation of somatic and visual activities of the autonomic nervous system
8. Influence on the sleep-wake cycle, motivation, learning, and sexual behavior

Subthalamus. The subthalamus is located between the tegmentum of the midbrain and the dorsal part of the thalamus. The functions of the subthalamus are related closely to those of the basal ganglia.

Pituitary Gland. The pituitary gland (or hypophysis) lies in the sella turcica at the base of the brain and is directly above the sphenoid air sinus and slightly anterior to the optic chiasm. The pituitary gland is connected to the hypothalamus by the *hypophyseal stalk*. Structurally, the gland is divided into two major lobes, the *anterior pituitary lobe* and the *posterior pituitary lobe*. The anterior lobe secretes seven major hormones: (1) growth hormone, (2) prolactin, (3) adrenocorticotropin, (4) thyroid-stimulating hormone, (5) follicle-stimulating hormone, (6) luteinizing hormone, and (7) melanin-stimulating hormone. The posterior pituitary lobe stores oxytocin and antidiuretic hormone (ADH).

Internal Capsule. Located deep in the region of the thalamus and hypothalamus is a dense mass of white matter called the internal capsule. This area is called a capsule because of the way the pyramidal and other tracts essentially encapsulate the thalamus as they pass between it and the basal ganglia (Schmidt, 1985). Damage to the structures of the internal capsule may result in the stroke syndrome due to the blockage of conduction in motor pathways.

Brainstem

The brainstem (Fig. 31–15) consists of the midbrain, pons, and medulla oblongata. Overall, the purpose of the brainstem is control of involuntary reflexes necessary for maintaining vital functions.

Midbrain. The midbrain, or mesencephalon, lies between the diencephalon and the pons. The top of the midbrain is made up of four rounded elevations called the *corpora quadrigeminal*. The superior pair of colliculi control eye tracking, whereas the posterior pair of colliculi have a role in the auditory system. Cranial nerves III (oculomotor) and IV (trochlear) emanate from the midbrain. The lower surface of the midbrain consists of two fiber bundles called the *crura cerebri*. These bundles are composed of the corticospinal, corticopontine, and corticobulbar tracts of the voluntary nervous system. The primary functions of the midbrain are the relay of stimuli between the cerebrum and the lower brain, and central control of auditory and visual reflexes.

Pons. The pons (metencephalon) lies between the midbrain and the medulla. The pons contains cranial nerve V (trigeminal), and three other cranial nerves

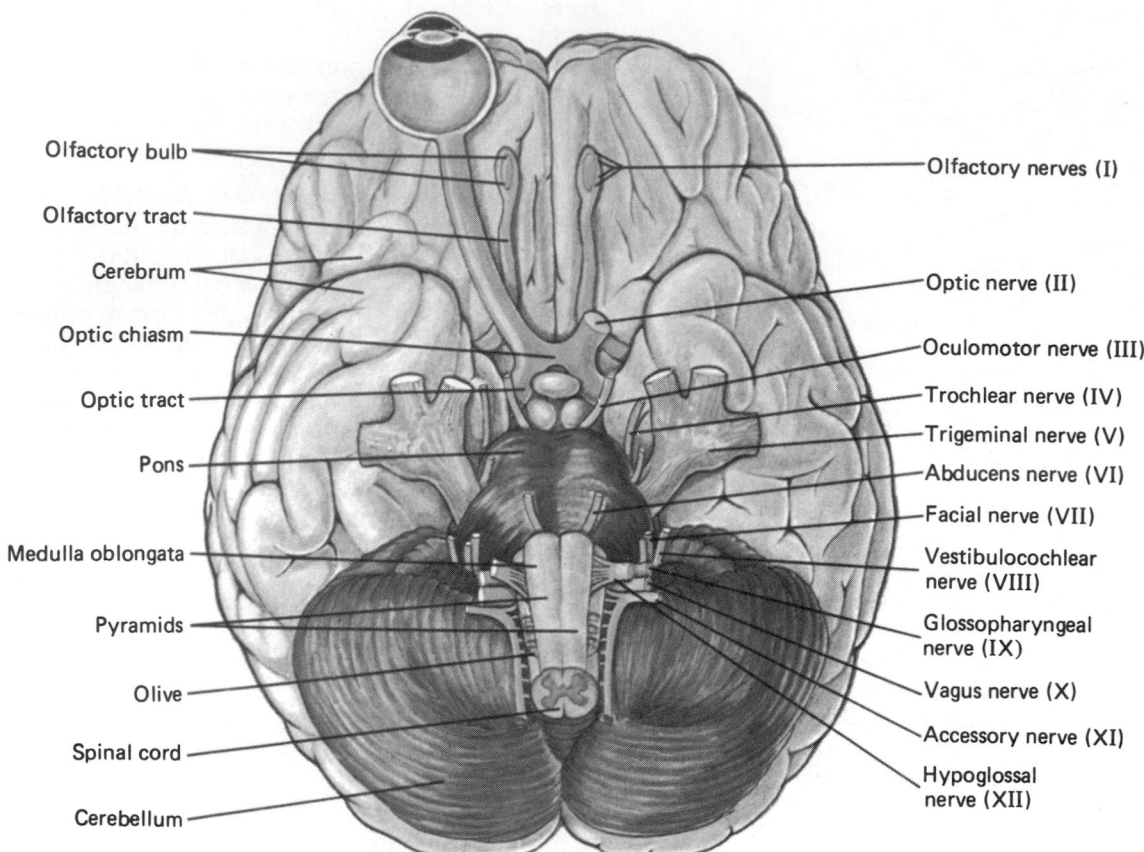

Olfactory bulb

Olfactory tract

Cerebrum

Optic chiasm

Optic tract

Pons

Medulla oblongata

Pyramids

Olive

Spinal cord

Cerebellum

Olfactory nerves (I)

Optic nerve (II)

Oculomotor nerve (III)

Trochlear nerve (IV)

Trigeminal nerve (V)

Abducens nerve (VI)

Facial nerve (VII)

Vestibulocochlear
nerve (VIII)

Glossopharyngeal
nerve (IX)

Vagus nerve (X)

Accessory nerve (XI)

Hypoglossal
nerve (XII)

FIGURE 31–15. Anterior brainstem showing the cranial nerves. (From Guyton, A. C. (1987). *Basic neuroscience.* Philadelphia: W. B. Saunders.)

(VI, abducens; VII, facial; and VIII, acoustic) originate at the pons–medulla junction. The white matter of the pons is made up of the corticobulbar and corticospinal tracts.

Medulla Oblongata. The medulla, or myelencephalon, is located directly under the pons and is continuous with the spinal cord at the foramen magnum. The medulla contains cranial nerves IX (glossopharyngeal), X (vagus), XI (spinal accessory), and XII (hypoglossal). The decussation (cross-over) of the pyramidal tract forms a ridge on either side of the median fissure in the medulla. Functionally, the medulla contains important involuntary reflex centers for breathing, sneezing, coughing, swallowing, salivating, vomiting, and vasoconstriction.

Cerebellum

The *cerebellum* (Fig. 31–16) is separated from the cerebrum by the tentorium cerebelli and is connected to the midbrain, medulla, and pons by three pairs of *cerebellar peduncles*. It consists of two lateral hemispheres and a middle section called the *vermis*. The outer covering is composed of a cortex of gray matter, and the inner medulla consists of white matter. Deep

within the white matter are four pairs of cerebellar nuclei: *dentate, emboliform, globose,* and *fastigial*. These nuclei receive input from the cerebellar cortex and all sensory afferent tracts to the cerebellum. The major function of the cerebellum is the monitoring and corrective adjustment of motor activities elicited by other parts of the brain (Guyton, 1987).

Reticular Formation

Located throughout the entire brainstem are diffuse areas of neurons that collectively are called the *reticular formation*. The majority of neurons in the reticular formation are excitatory and are known collectively as the *bulboreticular facilatory area*. Diffuse stimulation of this facilatory area produces a general or localized increase in muscle tone. A small area of the reticular formation in the lower medulla, the *bulboreticular inhibitory area*, decreases general muscle tone when stimulated (Guyton, 1987). Under normal circumstances, both the facilitory and inhibitory areas are activated, and therefore the spinal cord's motor functions are neither excited nor inhibited. However, in situations such as cerebral infarction, in which the inhibitory area is damaged or destroyed, facilitation becomes dominant with resultant muscle spasticity.

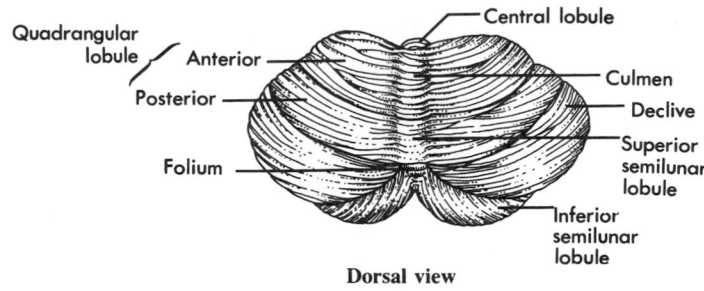

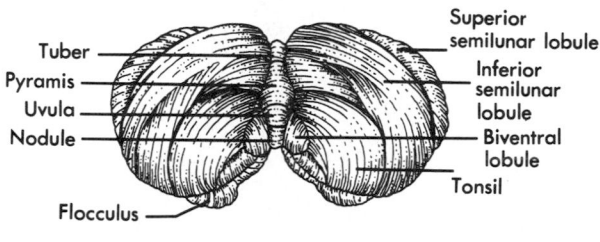

Ventral view

FIGURE 31–16. Cerebellum. (Reproduced by permission from: *Mosby's medical and nursing dictionary*, ed. 2, St. Louis, 1986, The C.V. Mosby Co.)

Another important function of the reticular formation is support of the body against gravity.

Reticular Activating System

Extending from the lower portion of the brainstem through the diencephalon and into the cerebral cortex are multiple diffuse sensory pathways that collectively are called the *reticular activating system* (RAS) (Fig. 31–17). Most of the RAS is excitatory and is involved in the processes of regulation of visceral functions; consciousness; temperature control; emotional states; learning; regulation of skeletal muscle activity and tone; and perception of sensory stimuli (Jensen, 1980). Stimulation of different areas of the RAS produces different effects on specific parts of the brain. For example, stimulation of the brainstem (mesencephalic) portion of the RAS provides intrinsic activation of the whole brain, whereas stimulation of the thalamic portion activates specific areas of the cerebral cortex.

Vertebral Column and Spinal Cord

The vertebral column consists of 33 vertebrae that are divided into five anatomic and functional areas: cervical, thoracic, lumbar, sacral, and coccygeal (Figs. 31–18 and 31–19). The vertebrae are joined together by multiple ligaments and cartilage pads called intervertebral discs.

The first two cervical vertebrae differ from the other cervical vertebrae. C1 is referred to as the *atlas* because it supports the skull and does not have a vertebral body or spinous process. C2, or the *axis*, also is modified in that it has a toothlike projection called the *odontoid process*, extending upward from

the vertebral body. The odontoid process is the point on which the atlas articulates (see Fig. 31–19).

Most vertebrae have similar anatomic characteristics (Fig. 31–20). The *vertebral body* supports weight bearing and is separated from other vertebral bodies by cartilage and fibrous tissue called *intervertebral discs*. The dorsal part of the vertebrae is the *vertebral arch* that is formed by two pedicles and two laminae. The posterior portion of the vertebrae is called the *spinous process*. In the middle of the vertebrae is the

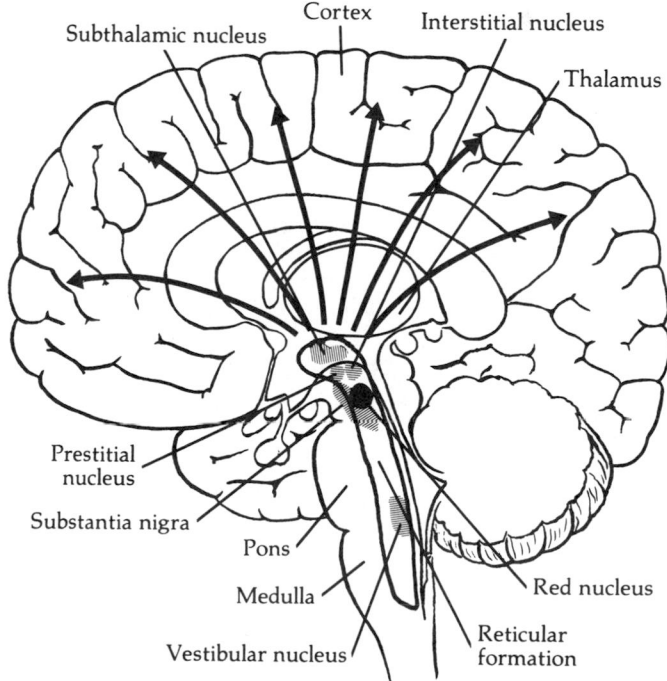

FIGURE 31–17. Reticular activating system. (Reproduced by permission from: Thompson, J. M., et al. *Mosby's manual of clinical nursing*, ed. 2, St. Louis, 1989, The C.V. Mosby Co.)

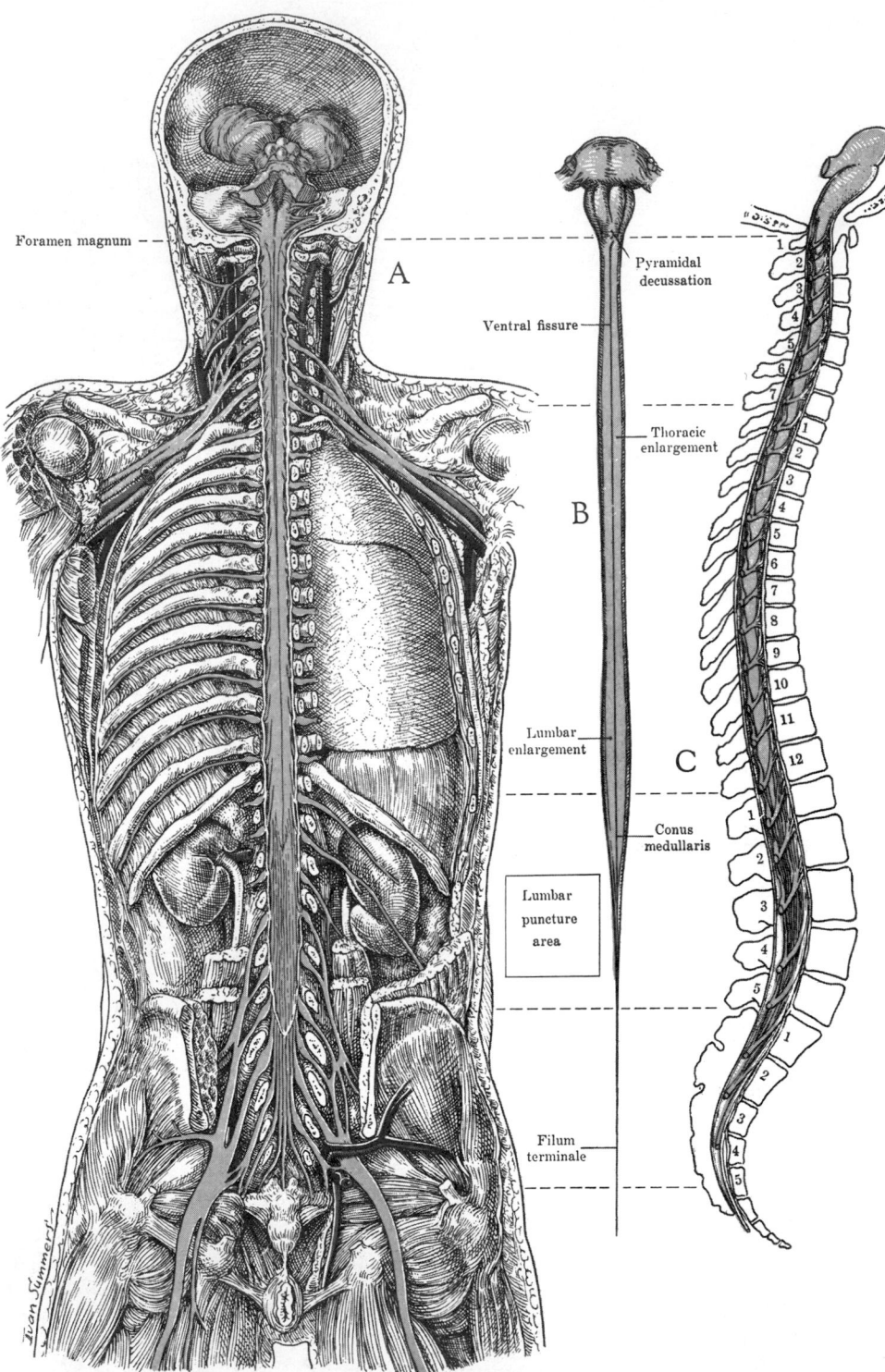

FIGURE 31–18. *A,* Posterior view of brainstem and spinal cord in situ with spinal nerves and plexuses. *B,* Anterior view of brainstem and spinal cord. *C,* Lateral view, showing relationship of spinal cord to vertebrae. (Reproduced by permission from: Mettler, F. A. *Neuroanatomy* (2nd ed.). St. Louis, 1948, The C.V. Mosby Co.)

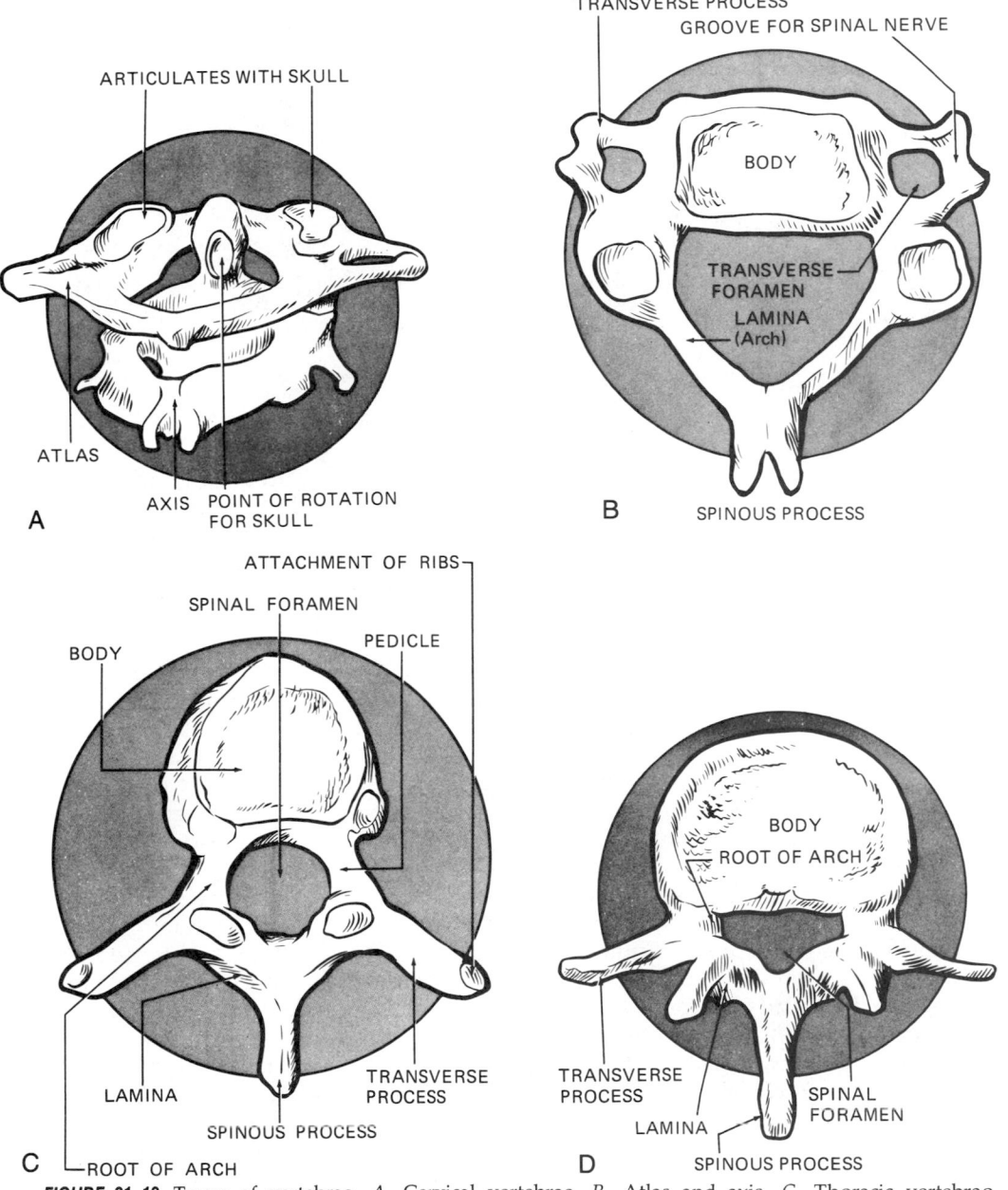

FIGURE 31–19. Types of vertebrae. *A*, Cervical vertebrae. *B*, Atlas and axis. *C*, Thoracic vertebrae. *D*, Lumbar vertebra. (From Snyder, M., and Jackle, M. (1981). *Neurologic problems: A critical care nursing focus.* Bowie, MD: Robert J. Brady.)

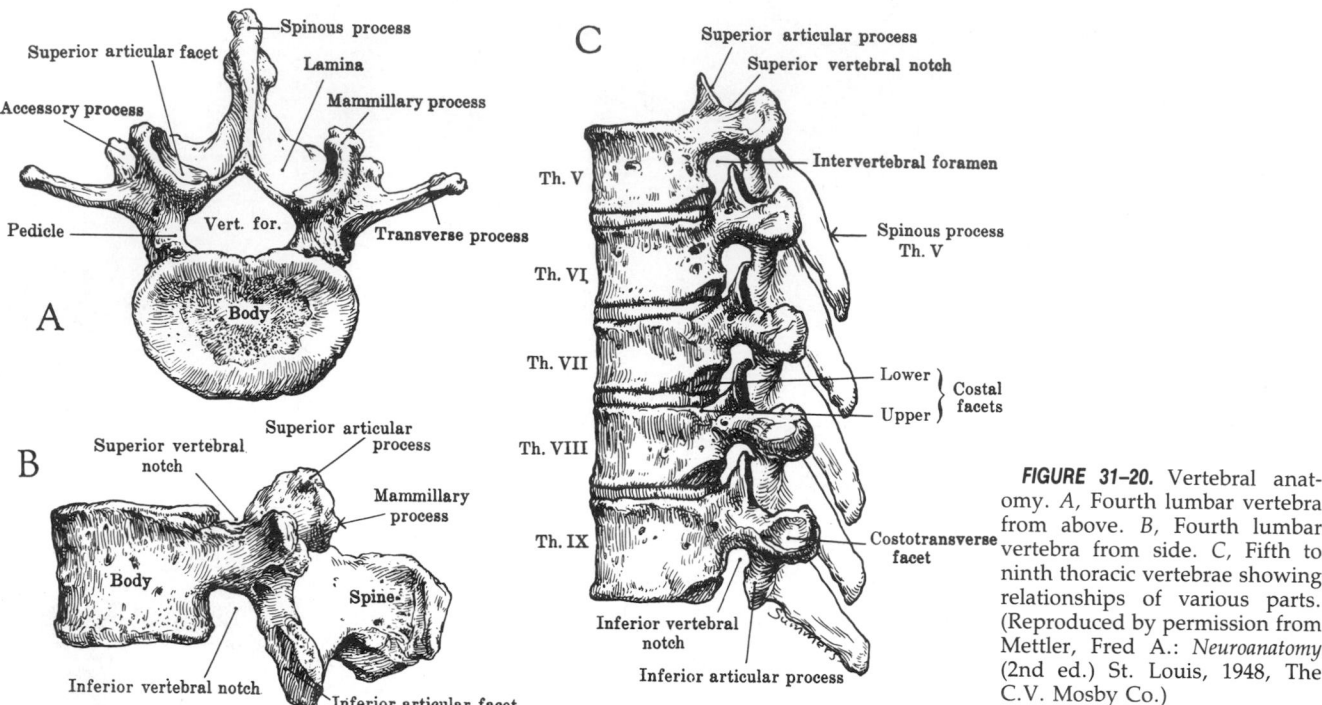

FIGURE 31–20. Vertebral anatomy. *A*, Fourth lumbar vertebra from above. *B*, Fourth lumbar vertebra from side. *C*, Fifth to ninth thoracic vertebrae showing relationships of various parts. (Reproduced by permission from Mettler, Fred A.: *Neuroanatomy* (2nd ed.) St. Louis, 1948, The C.V. Mosby Co.)

vertebral foramen. This foramen is the opening that contains the spinal cord and spinal meninges. A portion of the vertebral foramen, the *vertebral notch,* is the point at which the spinal nerves and blood vessels leave the spinal cord. Extending from either side of each vertebrae are the *transverse processes,* which provide sites for articulation of adjacent vertebrae and for attachment of ligaments and muscles. The *pedicle* is a bony connection between the body of the vertebrae and the transverse process.

Spinal Meninges. Like the brain, the spinal cord is surrounded by three meningeal coverings: dura mater, arachnoid, and pia mater. The spinal *dura mater* extends from the cranial dura to the second sacral vertebra, where it fuses with the filum terminale. The dura also covers the roots of the spinal nerves. The second spinal meningeal layer, the *arachnoid,* extends from the foramen magnum to the lower surfaces of the cauda equina and the filum terminale. The spinal arachnoid also covers the spinal nerve roots to the point where they exit the vertebral canal. Between the arachnoid and innermost meningeal layer is the *subarachnoid space,* which contains a delicate network of cells and cerebrospinal fluid. The third meningeal layer is the *pia mater.* The fibrous pia mater extends to the filum terminale, where it is attached by denticulate ligaments to the dura mater between the spinal nerve roots.

Spinal Vascular Supply. The primary supply of blood to the spinal cord is provided by the *vertebral artery* and small *spinal arteries* (Fig. 31–21). The spinal arteries enter the intervertebral foramina at successive vertebral levels and divide into a number of *anterior* and *posterior radicular arteries.*

Three longitudinal arteries, the *anterior* and two *posterior spinal arteries,* supply the entire spinal cord. The anterior spinal artery is formed by the fusion of two branches of the vertebral artery at the level of the foramen magnum. Small branches of the anterior spinal artery enter the gray and white matter of the spinal cord and join together in the anterior median fissure to form the anterior central artery. The two posterior spinal arteries have many tiny branches that enter the spinal cord and help to form the posterior central artery (Rudy, 1985).

There are a number of venous plexuses extending along the entire inside and outside of the vertebral canal. Outside the vertebral column, venous plexuses receive blood from the spinous processes, vertebral bodies, facets, laminae, and surrounding muscles. Inside the canal, venous plexuses located between the dura and vertebral surfaces receive blood from the spinal matter and nearby bony structures. A series of venous rings are formed from these venous plexuses at each vertebral level. Blood from the internal and external plexuses drains into the intervertebral veins that exit the canal through the intervertebral foramina.

Intradural veins of the spinal cord follow the general distribution pattern of the spinal arteries and form the *anterior* and *posterior radicular veins.* Blood from the radicular veins and the two venous plexuses at each vertebral level drain into the *intervertebral vein.*

Spinal Cord. The spinal cord (Fig. 31–22), which originates at the foramen magnum, is essentially a downward continuation of the medulla oblongata. In the lower thoracic region, the cord tapers into the cone-shaped *conus medullaris.* Extending below the

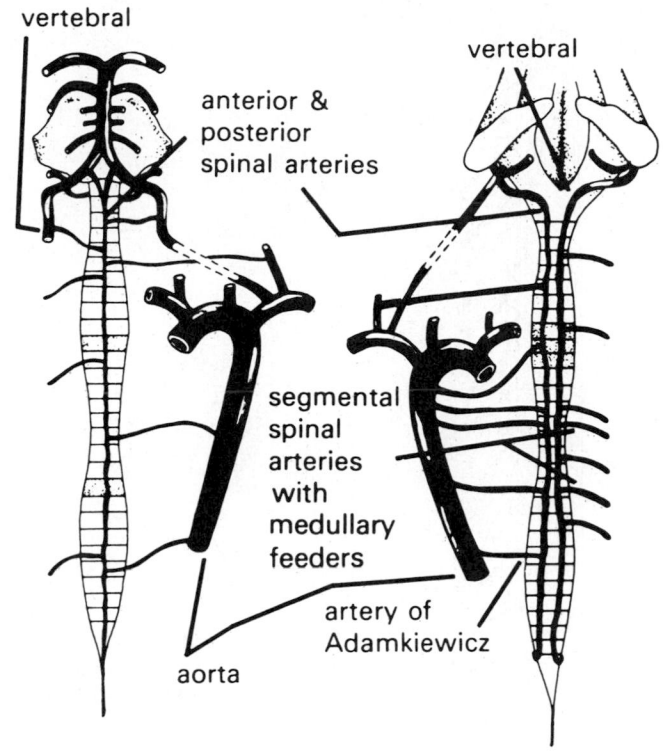

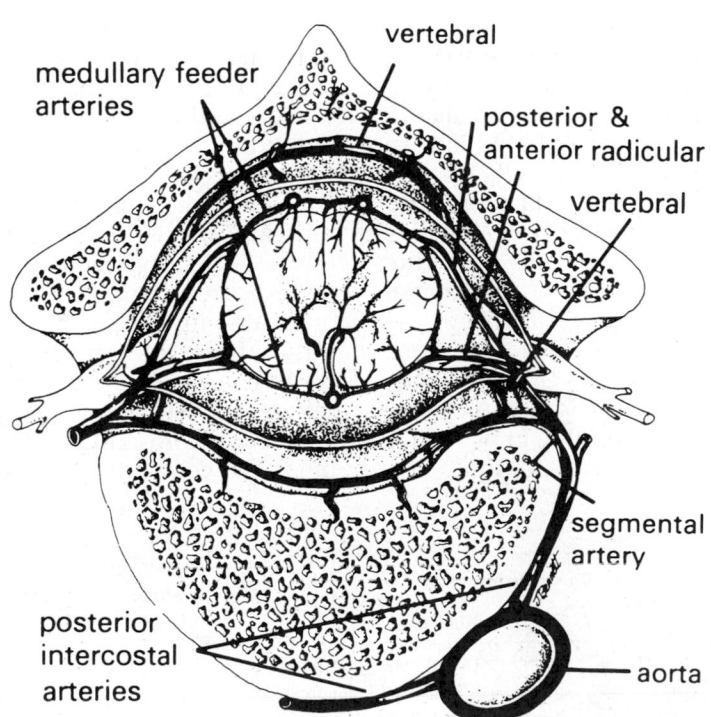

FIGURE 31–21. Vascular supply of the spinal cord. (From Romero-Sierra, C. (1986). Neuroanatomy: A conceptual approach. New York: Churchill Livingstone.)

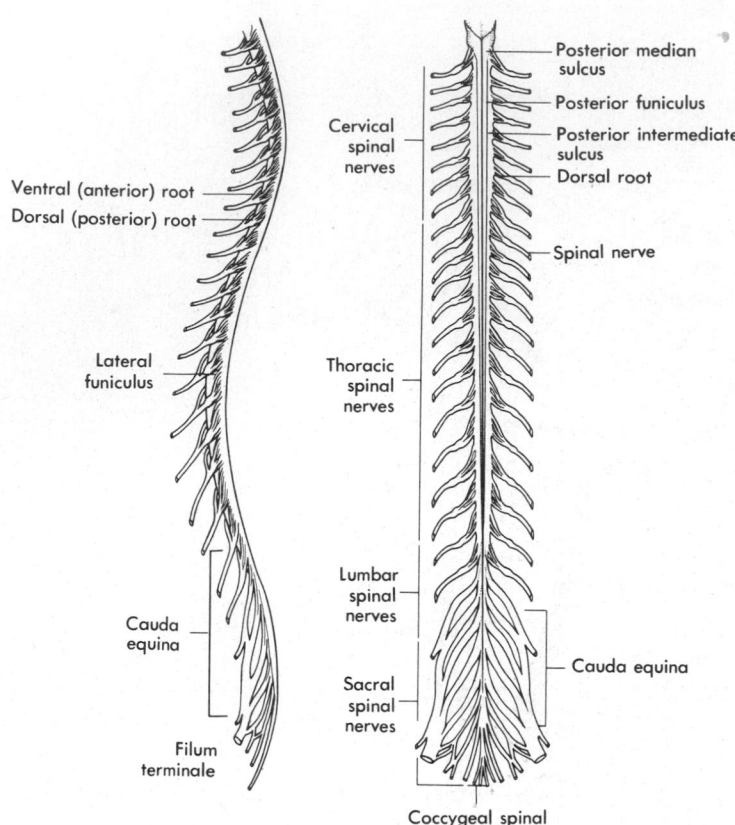

FIGURE 31–22. Two views of gross anatomy of the spinal cord. (Reproduced by permission from: *Mosby's medical and nursing dictionary,* ed. 2, St. Louis, 1986, The C.V. Mosby Co.)

conus medullaris is a thin prolongation, the *filum terminale,* which attaches the cord to the coccyx.

The spinal cord itself consists of gray (unmyelinated) and white (myelinated) microscopic matter (Fig. 31–23). The gray matter is concentrated into an internal core that can be divided functionally into the anterior horn, the intermediate zone and lateral horn, and the posterior horn. The *anterior horn* contains alpha and gamma motor cells. These cells constitute the final common motor pathway of the spinal nerves. The *intermediate zone* and *lateral horn* of the gray matter give rise to the preganglionic *sympathetic* fibers in T1 to L2 and L3. At the level of S2 to S4, cell bodies give rise to the preganglionic *parasympathetic* fibers. The *posterior horn* of the gray matter contains sensory cells from peripheral neurons.

The white matter of the spinal cord surrounds the gray matter, and is composed of ascending and descending spinal tracts that serve as pathways for sensory and motor impulses between the spinal cord and brain.

Neurons of the *ascending* pathways transmit sensory impulses from peripheral receptors (i.e., skin, muscles, and tendons) to the spinal cord and brain (Fig. 31–24). The sensory pathway is made up of a three-neuron chain. The cell body of the first neuron originates in the spinal ganglion and conducts impulses from the peripheral receptors to the spinal cord. The cell body of the second neuron occurs at different levels within the gray matter of the brain and spinal cord and conducts impulses to the thalamus. The cell body of the third neuron is located in

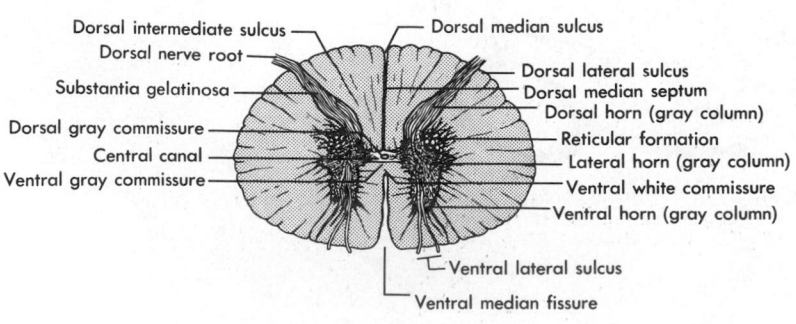

FIGURE 31–23. Cross section of the spinal cord. (Reproduced by permission from: *Mosby's medical and nursing dictionary,* St. Louis, 1983, The C.V. Mosby Co.)

CROSS-SECTION OF SPINAL CORD

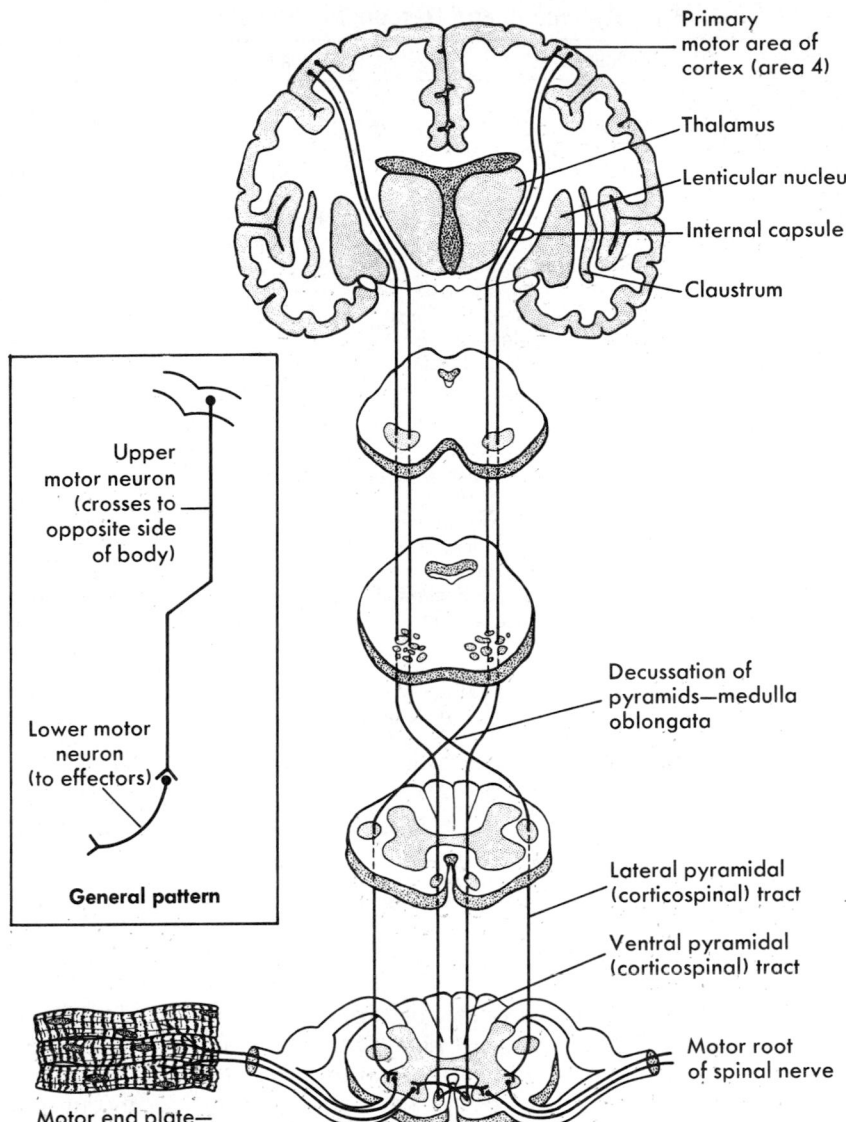

Primary motor area of cortex (area 4)

Thalamus

Lenticular nucleus

Internal capsule

Claustrum

Upper motor neuron (crosses to opposite side of body)

Lower motor neuron (to effectors)

General pattern

Decussation of pyramids—medulla oblongata

Lateral pyramidal (corticospinal) tract

Ventral pyramidal (corticospinal) tract

Motor root of spinal nerve

Motor end plate—skeletal muscle

FIGURE 31–24. Pyramidal tracts. Upper motor neurons cross to muscles on opposite side of body. Lateral pyramidal tracts cross high at decussation in medulla oblongata. Ventral tracts cross low. (Reproduced by permission from: Conway-Rutkowski, B. L. *Neurological and neurosurgical nursing* (8th ed.). St. Louis, 1982, The C.V. Mosby Co.)

the thalamus and conducts sensory impulses from the thalamus to the cerebral cortex. The major ascending pathways are summarized in Table 31–1.

Descending pathways consist of two primary types of neurons: upper motor neurons and lower motor neurons (Fig. 31–25). *Upper motor neurons*, which originate and terminate within the central nervous system, transmit impulses from the brain to the motor neurons in the anterior horn cell of the spinal cord and motor neurons in the cranial nerves. *Lower motor neurons* constitute the final common pathway and consist of motor neurons in the anterior spinal horn cell and motor nuclei of the cranial nerves. The major subdivisions of the descending tracts are the pyramidal and extrapyramidal pathways (Table 31–1).

Reflexes. The reflex arc (Fig. 31–26) is the basic unit that maintains the body's integrity by the automatic conduction of impulses from afferent (sensory) receptors to efferent (motor) neurons. The reflex arc

consists of the stimulation of a sensory nerve ending that conducts an impulse via sensory (afferent) neurons to the nuclei in the gray matter of the spinal cord. In the gray matter, the sensory neuron may synapse directly with lower motor neurons, or it may synapse with one or more association neurons, which transfer the impulse to the lower motor neuron. The impulse then is carried by the lower motor neurons, via the anterior spinal roots, to the neuroeffector junction. Stimulation of the neuroeffector junction elicits a response in the effector organ such as muscle contraction or glandular secretion (Campbell, 1985).

Peripheral Nervous System

Spinal Nerves. The 31 pairs of spinal nerves arising from different spinal cord segments are categorized as follows: 8 cervical; 12 thoracic; 5 lumbar; 5 sacral; and 1 coccygeal. Each spinal nerve is composed of

TABLE 31–1. Major Ascending and Descending Spinal Cord Tracts

Name	Function	Location	Origin*	Termination†
Ascending				
Lateral spinothalamic	Pain, temperature and crude touch opposite side	Lateral white columns	Posterior gray column opposite side	Thalamus
Ventral spinothalamic	Crude touch, pain, and temperature	Anterior white columns	Posterior gray column opposite side	Thalamus
Fasciculi gracilis and cuneatus	Discriminating touch and pressure sensations, including vibration, stereognosis, and two-point discrimination; also conscious kinesthesia	Posterior white columns	Spinal ganglia same side	Medulla
Spinocerebellar	Unconscious kinesthesia	Lateral white columns	Posterior gray column	Cerebellum
Descending				
Lateral corticospinal (or crossed pyramidal)	Voluntary movement, contraction of individual or small groups of muscles, particularly those moving hands, fingers, feet, and toes of opposite side	Lateral white columns	Motor areas of cerebral cortex (mainly areas 4 and 6) opposite side from tract location in cord	Intermediate or anterior gray columns
Ventral corticospinal (direct pyramidal)	Same as lateral corticospinal except mainly muscles of same side	Lateral white columns	Motor cortex but on same side as tract location in cord	Intermediate or anterior gray columns
Lateral reticulospinal	Mainly facilitory influence on motor neurons to skeletal muscles	Lateral white columns	Reticular formation, midbrain, pons, and medulla	Intermediate or anterior gray columns
Medial reticulospinal	Mainly inhibitory influence on motor neurons to skeletal muscles	Anterior white columns	Reticular formation, medulla mainly	Intermediate or anterior gray columns

*Location of cell bodies of neurons from which axons of tract arise.
†Structure in which axons of tracts terminate.
  Reproduced by permission from: Anthony, C. P., and Thibodeau, G. M. *Textbook of anatomy and physiology* (12th ed.). St. Louis, 1987, The C. V. Mosby Co.

an anterior (ventral) and a posterior (dorsal) root in the spinal cord. The *anterior root* lies within the gray matter of the spinal cord and carries motor (efferent) impulses from the cord to the muscles and glands. The *posterior root* is made up of sensory (afferent) fibers that conduct impulses from the body's sensory receptors to the spinal cord. As the anterior and posterior fibers exit the spinal cord, they pass side by side and exit the vertebral column through the intervertebral foramina. Once outside the vertebral column, the two sets of nerve fibers join together and form the *spinal nerve*. Some spinal nerves join together and form dense networks of nerve fibers called *plexuses*. Table 31–2 summarizes the spinal nerves, plexuses, and peripheral innervation.

Dermatomes. Each of the spinal nerves is distributed to a specific area of the body to receive superficial or cutaneous sensations. The specific body areas supplied by the spinal nerves are known as *dermatomes*. The many sensory fibers of the spinal nerves distributed to each of the dermatome regions provide many types of sensory reception including touch, kinesthetic sensation, vibration, heat and cold, and pain. Figures 31–27*A* and *B* illustrate the anterior and posterior distribution of dermatomes for cutaneous sensation.

Cranial Nerves. There are 12 pairs of cranial nerves (Table 31–3). The first two pairs of cranial nerves are not true peripheral nerves but are actually tracts of the central nervous system. The cranial nerves transmit impulses for sensation, voluntary control of muscles, and autonomic functions in the head, and are involved in transmitting impulses for the special senses of vision, hearing, smell, and taste. Table 31–3 summarizes the origin and functions of each of the cranial nerves.

Autonomic Nervous System

The autonomic nervous system (ANS) is considered to be a part of the peripheral nervous system because it is outside of the central nervous system. However, the function of the ANS is substantially different from that of the rest of the peripheral nervous system. More specifically, the ANS regulates the body's organs and internal environment in close conjunction with the endocrine system. The ANS has two major subdivisions: the sympathetic and parasympathetic systems. These subdivisions differ in (1) type of neurotransmitter released, (2) nerve fiber distribution, and (3) effector organ response (Campbell, 1985) (Fig. 31–28).

Text continued on page 673

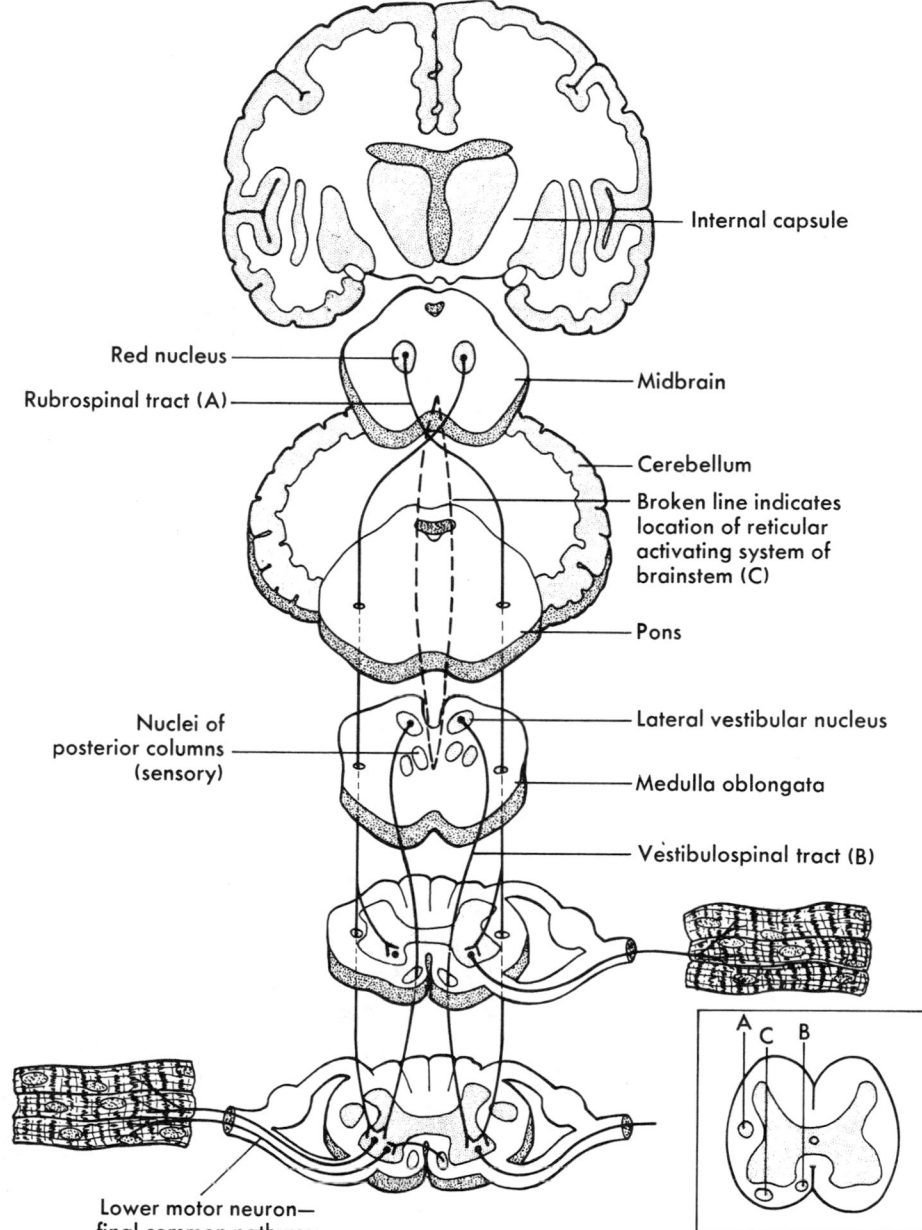

FIGURE 31–25. Extrapyramidal descending tracts. Upper motor neurons originate below level of cortex and converge on lower motor neurons (final common pathway) along with upper motor neurons of pyramidal tracts. *A,* Rubrospinal tract originates in the red nucleus of the midbrain, crosses immediately, and descends contralaterally in opposite cord. *B,* Vestibulospinal tract originates in vestibular nucleus of medulla oblongata and descends ipsilaterally. *C,* Reticulospinal tracts (medial and lateral) originate from reticular activating system of brainstem and descend in general area of *C.* (These are not so well organized as others are.) Interconnections between basal nuclei, midbrain, diencephalon, and cerebellum are extensive. (Reproduced by permission from: Conway-Rutkowski, B. L. *Neurological and neurosurgical nursing* (8th ed.). St. Louis, 1982, The C.V. Mosby Co.)

Internal capsule

Red nucleus

Rubrospinal tract (A)

Midbrain

Cerebellum

Broken line indicates location of reticular activating system of brainstem (C)

Pons

Nuclei of posterior columns (sensory)

Lateral vestibular nucleus

Medulla oblongata

Vestibulospinal tract (B)

Lower motor neuron— final common pathway

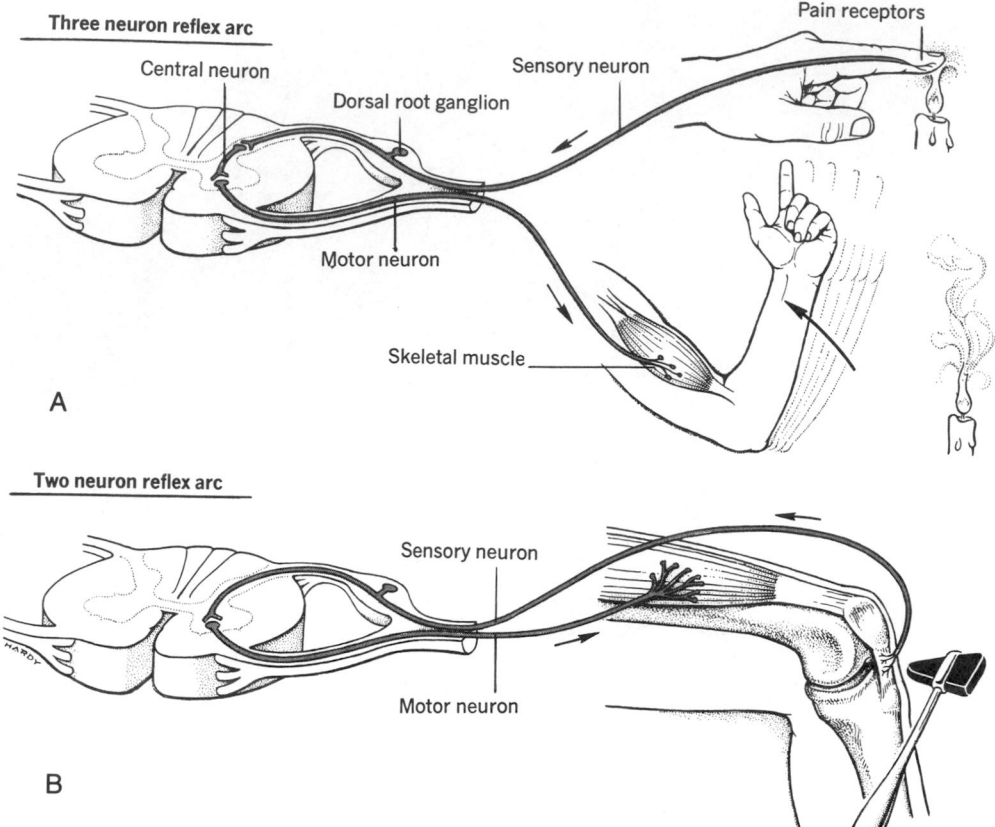

Three neuron reflex arc

Central neuron

Dorsal root ganglion

Sensory neuron

Pain receptors

Motor neuron

Skeletal muscle

A

Two neuron reflex arc

Sensory neuron

Motor neuron

B

FIGURE 31–26. Diagram of (A) flexor reflex and (B) stretch reflex. (From Chaffee, E. E., and Lytle, I. M. (1980). *Basic physiology and anatomy*. Philadelphia, J. B. Lippincott.)

FIGURE 31–27. Dermatomes. A, Anterior view. B, Posterior view. (From Snell, R. S. (1980). *Clinical neuroanatomy for medical students*. Boston: Little, Brown.)

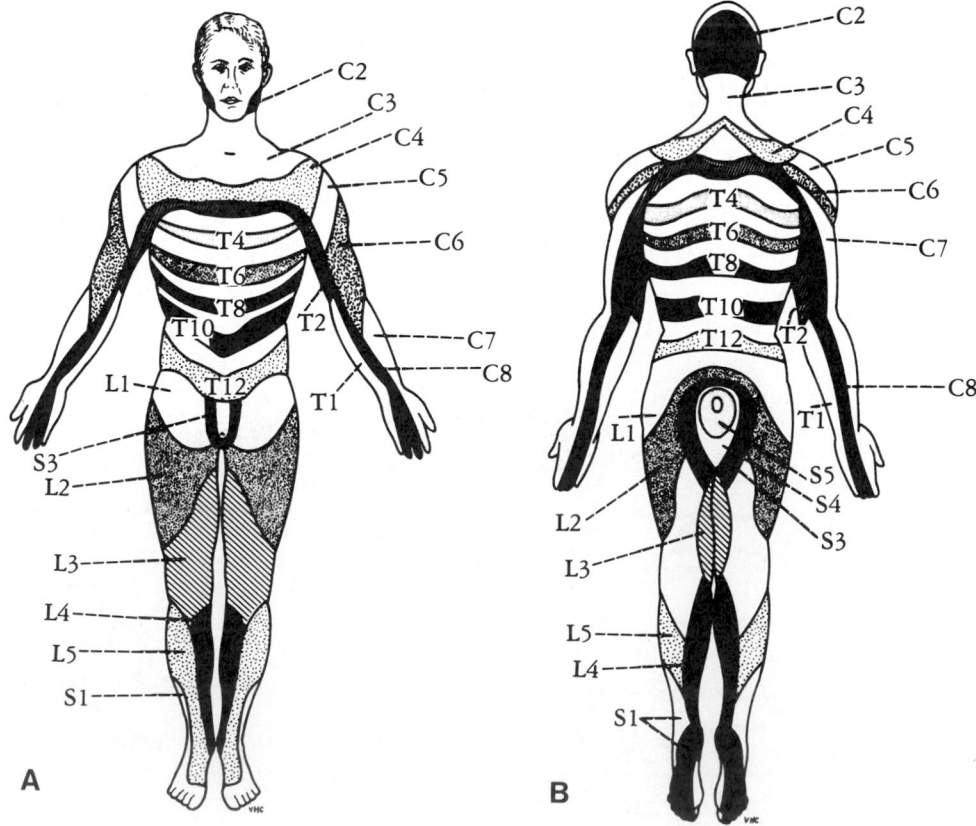

A

B

TABLE 31–2. Spinal Nerves, Plexuses, and Peripheral Innervation

Spinal Nerves	Plexuses Formed from Anterior Rami	Spinal Nerve Branches from Plexuses	Parts Supplied
Cervical 1 2 3 4	Cervical plexus	Lesser occipital Great auricular Cutaneous nerve of neck Anterior supraclavicular Middle supraclavicular Posterior supraclavicular Branches to numerous neck muscles	Sensory to back of head, front of neck, and upper part of shoulder, motor to numerous neck muscles
		Phrenic nerve	Diaphragm
		Suprascapular and dorsoscapular	Superficial muscles† of scapula
		Thoracic nerves, medial and lateral anterior	Pectoralis major and minor
		Long thoracic nerve	Serratus anterior
		Thoracodorsal	Latissimus dorsi
		Subscapular	Subscapular and teres major muscles
		Axillary (circumflex)	Deltoid and teres minor muscles and skin over deltoid
Cervical 5 6 7 8 **Thoracic (or Dorsal)** 1	Brachial plexus	Musculocutaneous	Muscle of front of arm (biceps brachii, coracobrachialis, and brachialis) and skin on outer side of forearm
		Ulnar	Flexor carpi ulnaris and part of flexor digitorum profundus; some of muscles of hand; sensory to medial side of hand, little finger, and medial half of fourth finger
2 3 4 5 6 7 8 9 10 11 12	No plexus formed; branches run directly to intercostal muscles and skin of thorax	Median	Rest of muscles of front of forearm and hand; sensory to skin of palmar surface of thumb, index, and middle fingers
		Radial	Triceps muscle and muscles of back of forearm; sensory to skin of back of forearm and hand
		Medial cutaneous	Sensory to inner surface of arm and forearm
		Phrenic (branches from cervical nerves before formation of plexus; most of its fibers from fourth cervical nerve)	Diaphragm
		Iliohypogastric } Sometimes fused Ilioinguinal	Sensory to anterior abdominal wall Sensory to anterior adominal wall and external genitalia; motor to muscles of abdominal wall
		Genitofemoral	Sensory to skin of external genitalia and inguinal region
Lumbar 1 2 3 4 5 **Sacral** 1 2 3 4 5 **Coccygeal** 1	Lumbosacral plexus	Lateral cutaneous of thigh	Sensory to outer side of thigh
		Femoral	Motor to quadriceps, sartorius, and iliacus muscles; sensory to front of thigh and to medial side of lower leg (saphenous nerve)
		Obturator	Motor to adductor muscles of thigh
		Tibial* (medial popliteal)	Motor to muscles of calf of leg; sensory to skin of calf of leg and sole of foot
		Common peroneal (lateral popliteal)	Motor to evertors and dorsiflexors of foot sensory to lateral surface of leg and dorsal surface of foot
		Nerves to hamstring muscles	Motor to muscles to back of thigh
		Gluteal nerves, superior and inferior	Motor to buttock muscles and tensor fasciae latae
		Posterior cutaneous nerve	Sensory to skin of buttocks, posterior surface of thigh, and leg
		Pudendal nerve	Motor to perineal muscles, sensory to skin of perineum

*Sensory fibers from the tibial and peroneal nerves unite to form the *medial cutaneous* (or *sural*) nerve that supplies the calf of the leg and the lateral surface of the foot. In the thigh, the tibial and common peroneal nerves are usually enclosed in a single sheath to form the *sciatic nerve,* the largest nerve in the body with its width of approximately ¾ of an inch. About two thirds of the way down the posterior part of the thigh, it divides into its component parts. Branches of the sciatic nerve extend into the hamstring muscles.

Reproduced by permission from: Anthony, C.P., and Thibodeau, G.M. *Textbook of anatomy and physiology* (12th ed.). St. Louis, 1987, The C.V. Mosby Co.

TABLE 31–3. The Cranial Nerves

Number	Name	Nerve Fiber Type(s)*	Origin; Primary Cell Body	Peripheral Termination(s)	Principal Function(s)
I	Olfactory	SVA	Rhinencephalon; olfactory epithelium	Olfactory epithelium	Olfaction
II	Optic	SSA	Diencephalon; retina, ganglionic layer	Bipolar retinal cells to rods and cones	Vision
III	Oculomotor	GSA, GSE, *GVE*	Superior collicular level; oculomotor nucleus, Edinger-Westphal nucleus	Superior, inferior, medial rectus, and levator palpebrae muscles. Pupillary constrictors and ciliary muscles of eyeball	Proprioceptive impulses; eye movements; accommodation reflex
IV	Trochlear	GSA, GSE	Superior cerebellar peduncle; trochlear nucleus	Superior oblique muscle	Proprioceptive impulses, eye movements
V	Trigeminal	GSA, SVE	Pons; masticator nucleus, semilunar ganglion, mesencephalic nucleus	Face, nose, mouth, jaw	Muscles of mastication; sensory to face, nose, mouth; proprioceptive to tooth sockets and jaw muscles
VI	Abducens	GSA, GSE	Pons; abducens nucleus	Lateral rectus	Eye movements
VII	Facial	GVA, SVA, SVE, *GVE*	Pons; facial nucleus, superior salivatory nucleus, geniculate ganglion	Glands of nose, lacrimal glands, palate; sublingual and submaxillary glands; anterior taste buds	Motor and sensory components to facial region, tongue
VIII	Vestibulocochlear: Cochlear division	SSA	Pons; spiral ganglion	Organ of Corti	Audition (hearing)
	Vestibular division	SSA	Pons; vestibular ganglion	Cristae of semicircular canals, maculae of saccule and utricle	Equilibrium
IX	Glossopharyngeal	SVA, GVA, SVE, *GVE*	Medulla; ambiguous nucleus, inferior salivatory nucleus, petrosal ganglion, superior ganglion	Superior constrictor, stylopharyngeus muscles; parotid glands, taste buds (vallate papillae), auditory tube	Motor to pharyngeal region; gustation (taste); motor to parotids; pain, tactile, thermal sensations from posterior tongue, tonsils, and eustachian tubes; regulates blood pressure
X	Vagus	GSA, GVA, SVA, *GVE*, SVE	Medulla; ambiguous nucleus, dorsal motor nucleus; nodose ganglion; jugular ganglion	Muscles of pharynx and larynx, viscera of thorax and abdomen; pinna of ear	Sensory and motor to thoracic and abdominal viscera, certain skeletal muscles of pharyngeal, laryngeal regions
XI	Spinal accessory	GSA, *GVE*, SVE	Medulla; accessory nucleus	Sternocleidomastoid and trapezius muscles; portions of laryngeal, pharyngeal muscles; heart (?)	Sensory and motor to muscles of larynx and pharynx; may form components of cardiac branches of vagus
XII	Hypoglossal	GSA, GSE	Medulla; hypoglossal nucleus	Tongue muscles	Sensory and motor to tongue muscles

Special afferent fibers are found only in the cranial nerves. SVA, special visceral afferent (sensory) fibers related only to nerves that subserve olfaction (1) and gustation (VII, IX, X). SSA, special somatic afferent (sensory) fibers that transmit impulses from the special sense organs, i.e., eye (II) and ear (VIII). SVE, special visceral efferent (motor) fibers of cranial nerves that innervate particular skeletal muscles derived embryologically from visceral (branchial) arch mesoderm. Some authors prefer the term "branchial motor fibers" to SVE when referring to the nerves that innervate the muscles derived from visceral arch mesoderm (e.g., the palatine, pharyngeal, laryngeal, and masticatory muscles as well as those of facial expression innervated by branches of cranial nerves V, VII, IX, X, and XI). GSA, general somatic afferent; GSE, general somatic afferent; GVA, general visceral afferent, *GVE*, general visceral efferent, GVE components of cranial nerves III, VII, IX, and X are in italics.
From Jensen, D. (1980). *The Principles of Physiology* (2nd ed.), Appleton-Century-Crofts.

The *sympathetic* system, also referred to as the thoracolumbar division of the ANS, is involved in maintaining the body's survival. Therefore, it is activated in situations that produce internal and external stress. Sympathetic stimulation results in a phenomenon called the flight-fight response that enables the body to respond to stressful situations. This response affects some of the body systems as follows:

1. Cardiovascular system—increased blood pressure and heart rate; peripheral vasoconstriction

2. Gastrointestinal system—decreased motility, contraction, and secretions; increased rectal sphincter tone; loss of appetite

3. Genitourinary system—relaxation of bladder muscles and contraction of the urinary sphincter

4. Eyes—pupillary dilation and slight elevation of the upper eyelid

The primary neurotransmitter of the sympathetic nervous system is norepinephrine, thus making the system an adrenergic one. Norepinephrine, or nor-

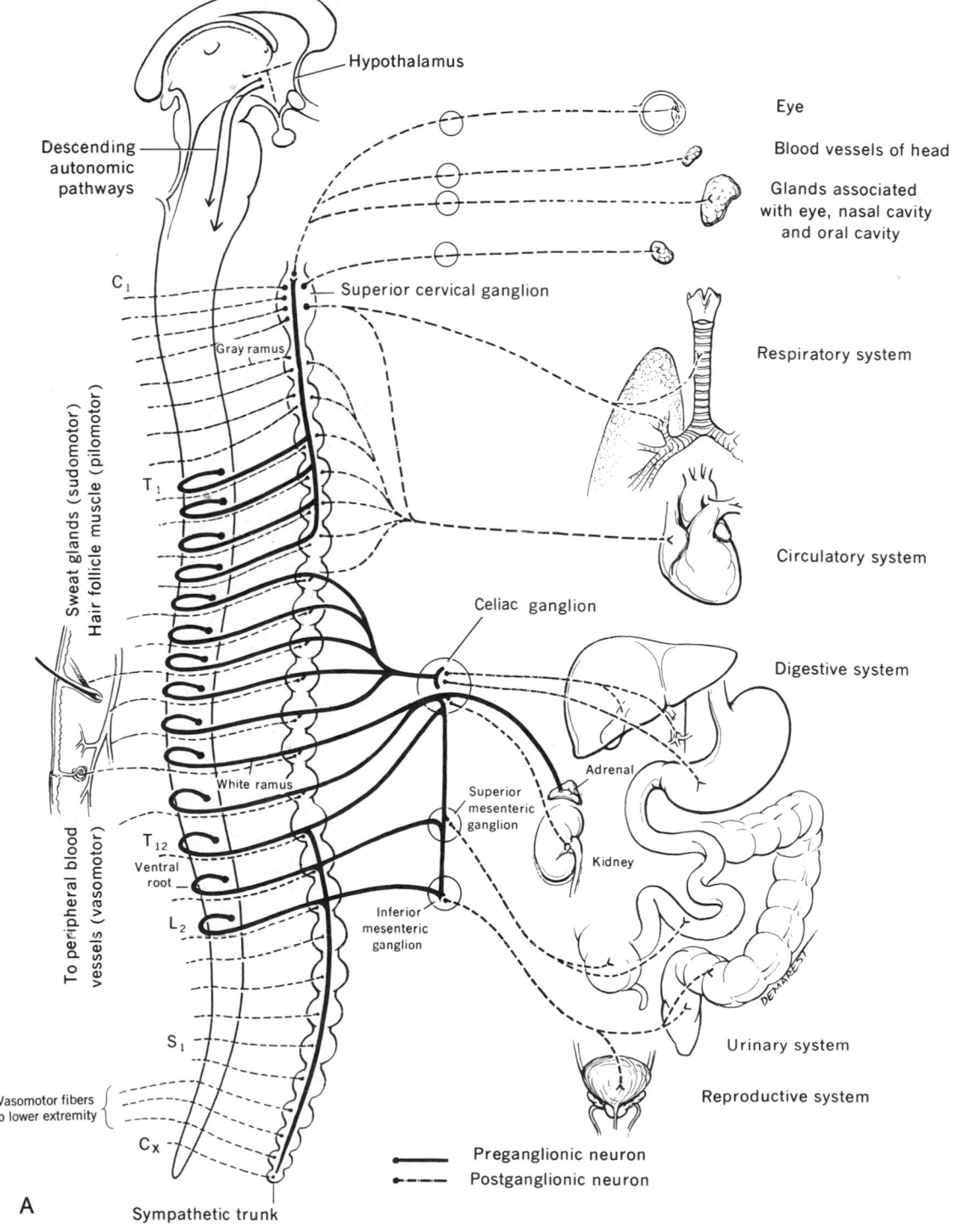

FIGURE 31–28. *A*, Sympathetic nervous system.

Illustration continued on following page

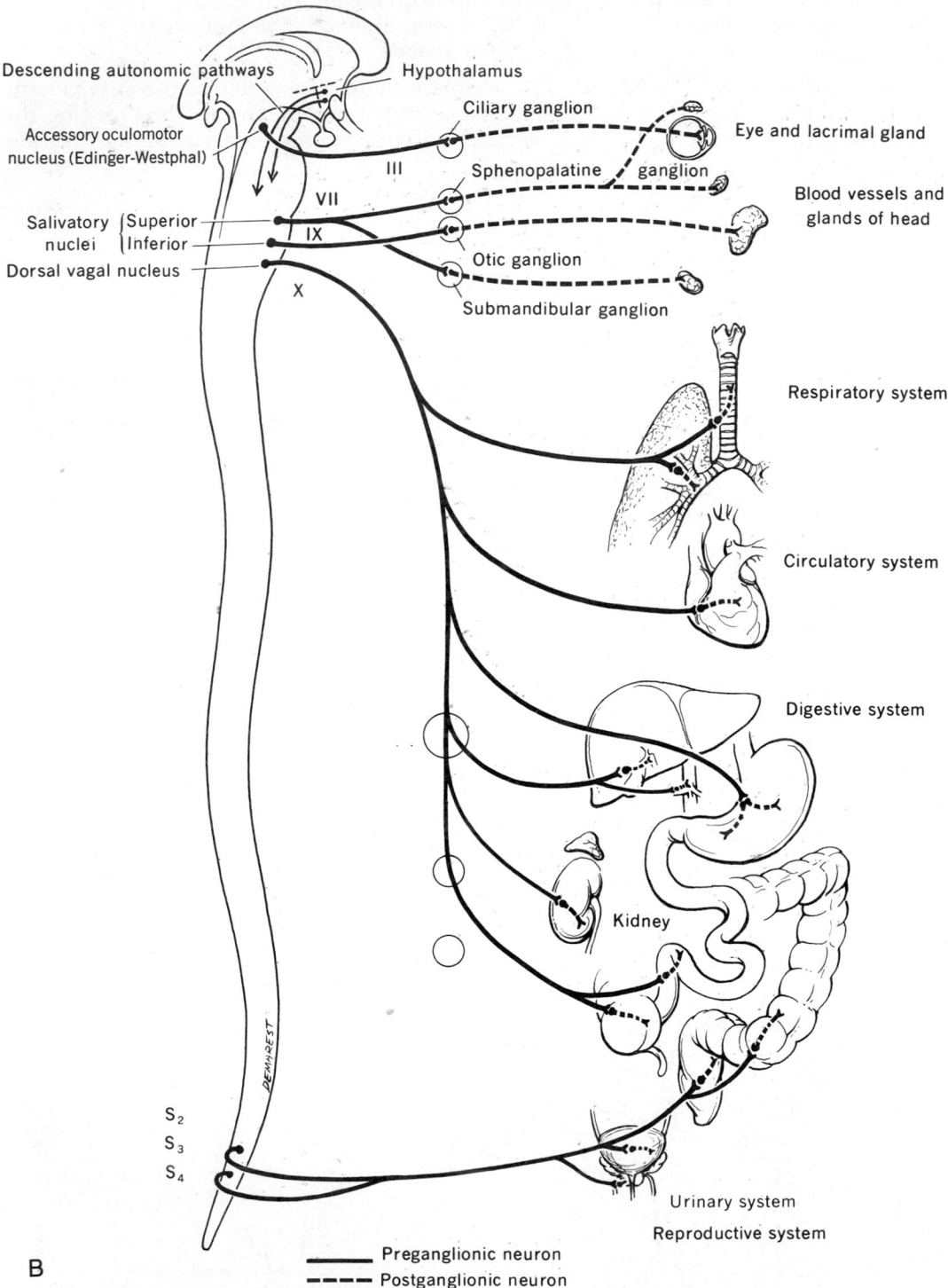

Descending autonomic pathways — Hypothalamus

Accessory oculomotor nucleus (Edinger-Westphal)

Ciliary ganglion

Eye and lacrimal gland

Sphenopalatine ganglion

III

VII

Salivatory {Superior nuclei {Inferior

IX

Dorsal vagal nucleus

X

Otic ganglion

Submandibular ganglion

Blood vessels and glands of head

Respiratory system

Circulatory system

Digestive system

Kidney

Urinary system

Reproductive system

S₂
S₃
S₄

B

——— Preganglionic neuron
- - - - Postganglionic neuron

Figure 31–28 *Continued B,* Parasympathetic nervous system. (From Adams, R. D., and Victor, M. (1977). *Principles of neurology.* New York: McGraw-Hill.)

adrenaline, is secreted by the postganglionic nerve terminals.

Structurally, the preganglionic neurons of the sympathetic system are found in the intermediolateral columns of all the thoracic and the upper two lumbar segments of the spinal cord. After exiting the spinal nerves, the preganglionic sympathetic axons enter, via a connection called the *white ramus*, a chain of ganglia that extends from the upper portion of the neck to the coccyx. This chain of ganglia is called the *sympathetic trunk, ganglionated cord*, or the *sympathetic chain*.

Most of the sympathetic fibers synapse with preganglionic neurons in the sympathetic trunk or pass up and down the trunk and synapse with postganglionic neurons in other ganglia of the chain. Some axons pass through the sympathetic trunk and synapse with a peripheral ganglion closer to the organ of innervation. Finally, some axons pass through the sympathetic trunk to the adrenal medulla and act as a preganglionic fiber along the entire path to the innervated organ, gland, or tissue.

Functionally, the *adrenal medulla* is an extension of the sympathetic nervous system. Sympathetic stimulation of the adrenal medulla results in the release of large amounts of epinephrine and norepinephrine. The discharge of adrenal sympathetic hormones produces almost the same response as direct sympathetic stimulation of the afferent organs; however, the effect lasts much longer. Generally, the organs or body tissues are stimulated simultaneously by the sympathetic fibers (direct stimulation) and by the adrenal medulla (indirect stimulation).

The *parasympathetic* division of the autonomic ner-

TABLE 31–4. Autonomic Effects on Various Organs of the Body

Organ	Effect of Sympathetic Stimulation	Effect of Parasympathetic Stimulation
Eye:	Dilated	Constricted
Pupil	Slight relaxation	Constricted
Ciliary muscle	Vasoconstriction and slight secretion	Stimulation of copious (except pancreas) secretion (containing many enzymes for enzyme-secreting glands)
Glands:		
Nasal		
Lacrimal		
Parotid		
Submandibular		
Gastric		
Pancreatic		
Sweat glands	Copious sweating (cholinergic)	None
Apocrine glands	Thick; odoriferous secretion	None
Heart:	Increased rate	Slowed rate
Muscle	Increased force of contraction	Decreased force of contraction (especially of atrium)
Coronaries	Dilated (β_2): constricted (α)	Dilated
Lungs:	Dilated	Constricted
Bronchi		
Blood vessels	Mildly constricted	? Dilated
Gut:	Decreased peristalsis and tone	Increased peristalsis and tone
Lumen		
Sphincter	Increased tone (most times)	Relaxed (most times)
Liver	Glucose released	Slight glycogen synthesis
Gallbladder and bile ducts	Relaxed	Contracted
Kidney	Decreased output and renin secretion	None
Bladder:	Relaxed (slight)	Excited
Detrusor		
Trigone	Excited	Relaxed
Penis	Ejaculation	Erection
Systemic arterioles:		
Abdominal	Constricted	None
Muscle	Constricted (adrenergic α) Dilated (adrenergic β_2) Dilated (cholinergic)	None
Skin	Constricted	None
Blood:		
Coagulation	Increased	None
Glucose	Increased	None
Basal metabolism	Increased up to 100%	None
Adrenal medullary secretion	Increased	None
Mental activity	Increased	None
Piloerector muscles	Excited	None
Skeletal muscle	Increased glycogenolysis Increased strength	None

From Guyton, A.C. (1986). *Textbook of Medical Physiology* (7th ed.). Philadelphia: W.B. Saunders.

vous system is involved primarily with vegetative activities that conserve and restore an individual's energy reserves. Such activities include decreased blood pressure, slower respiratory rate, decreased heart rate, and stimulation of the digestive system. The parasympathetic nervous system also is referred to as the *craniosacral system* because the preganglionic neurons exist from the brainstem through the cranial nerves and leave the spinal cord through the second, third, and fourth sacral spinal nerves. Parasympathetic fibers in the cranial and sacral spinal nerves synapse only with terminal ganglia in the effector organ; therefore, preganglionic fibers are long and postganglionic fibers are short. Both preganglionic and postganglionic fibers of the parasympathetic nervous system are called *cholinergic* because they secrete *acetylcholine*.

Autonomic Effects. Table 31–4 summarizes the autonomic effects on various organs. From this table, it is evident that both sympathetic and parasympathetic stimulation produce excitatory effects in some body organs and inhibitory effects in others. Also, as can be noted from the table, when sympathetic

stimulation excites a specific organ, parasympathetic stimulation usually inhibits that organ. However, most organs are dominated by one or the other system, so that the sympathetic and parasympathetic nervous systems do not oppose one another actively (Guyton, 1987).

References

Campbell, V. G. (1985). Neurologic system. In J. Thompson et al. (Eds.), *Clinical nursing*. St. Louis: C.V. Mosby.

Guyton, A. C. (1987). *Basic neuroscience: Anatomy and physiology*. Philadelphia: W. B. Saunders.

Hickey, J. (1986). *The clinical practice of neurological and neurosurgical nursing* (2nd ed.). Philadelphia: J.B. Lippincott.

Jensen, D. (1980). *The principles of physiology* (2nd ed.). New York: Appleton-Century-Crofts.

Lindsay, K. W., Bone, I., and Callander, R. (1986). *Neurology and neurosurgery illustrated*. London: Churchill Livingstone.

Rudy, E. B. (1984). *Advanced neurological and neurosurgical nursing*. St. Louis: C.V. Mosby.

Schmidt, R. F. (Ed.) (1985). *Fundamentals of neurophysiology*. New York: Springer-Verlag.

Simon, R. H., and Sayre, J. T. (1987). *Strategy in head injury management*. E. Norwalk, CT: Appleton and Lange.

32

Patients with Head Injury and Brain Dysfunction

Connie Walleck

The brain is a very sensitive organ and can be injured in many ways. When the brain is injured, physiologic, behavioral, cognitive, and psychological changes may occur. This chapter will review some major causes of brain injury, e.g., traumatic head injury, ischemic injury, metabolic disorders, and the effects of seizure on brain function. The pathophysiology of these events differs, but the medical and nursing interventions have the same goal: to protect the brain throughout the recovery process in order to restore the patient to his or her optimum level of functioning.

TRAUMATIC BRAIN INJURY

Over the years there has been a steady increase in the number of people who sustain traumatic head injuries. Each year approximately 5% of the population sustain a head injury serious enough to result in lost time from normal daily activities (Hickey, 1986; Rimel, 1982). Head injury is the leading cause of all trauma-related deaths, i.e., 70% of all fatal injuries involve the head (Rimel and Lundgren, 1986). Mortality from head injury alone is approximately 50%, with the majority of these deaths occurring before hospitalization.

The incidence of head injury is higher in males than in females (3:1) and higher in people 15 to 24 years of age. Most head-injured people are single and have a low median family income (Krause, 1987; Krause et al., 1984; Rimel and Lundgren, 1986).

The economic consequences of head injury are staggering. According to the National Head and Spinal Cord Survey (based on today's dollar), direct costs for diagnosis, treatment, and rehabilitation and the indirect costs to society from lost productivity total more than 5 billion dollars (Kalsbeck et al., 1980). This figure does not include such psychosocial and emotional issues as pain, suffering, effects on family and significant others, or the symbolic aspects of disability. Therefore, the total costs are probably enormous (Spielman, 1988).

Major causes of head injury are motor vehicle accidents, falls, and assaults. Vehicular accidents account for 48% of head-injured patients and occur most frequently in the 15- to 24-year-old age group (Rimel and Lundgren, 1986). Falls generally occur in the elderly and the under-15-year-old age group. The most significant contributing factor in all accidents is the use of alcohol (Rimel and Lundgren, 1986; Spielman, 1988).

Many preventive programs have been developed to ameliorate the death and disability associated with head injury. Failure to use safety restraint systems increases the risk of head injury in motor vehicle accidents. Most states have mandatory seat belt laws, but there is commonly a lack of compliance with the law. Advocates for passive restraints (e.g., air bags) feel that because compliance with seat belt usage will never be complete, mandatory passive restraints will ensure protection of people involved in motor vehicle accidents.

Motorcycle accidents account for many trauma victims. Laws mandating the use of helmets when riding a motorcycle have met with resistance from motorcyclists. The motorcyclists' lobby in most states has been effective in repealing or preventing the adoption of such laws.

Preventive programs designed to protect the trauma victim provide the means to decrease mortality and morbidity from head injury. Health care professionals involved in the care of trauma patients must become active in designing, implementing, and researching the effectiveness of preventive programs. These professionals then need to be active in sponsoring, supporting, and lobbying for legislation for mandatory safety equipment and more stringent safety requirements.

Types of Injury

Head injury is a generic term that refers to any injury of the scalp, skull (either the facial or cranial section), or brain. In this chapter, head injury will be divided into injuries of the head and injuries of the brain tissue. Injuries of the head include scalp lacerations and skull fractures. Traumatic brain injuries are those in which tissue disruption and injury occur. Tissue injuries include concussion, contusion, and laceration.

SCALP LACERATIONS

Scalp lacerations are among the most common head injuries (Nikas and Tolley, 1982). Because of the extensive vascularity of the scalp and poor contractility of these blood vessels, scalp injuries can result in significant blood loss, occasionally resulting in actual hypovolemia. Diagnosis of scalp injury is made by inspection. Skull radiographs, computed tomography (CT) scans, magnetic resonance imaging (MRI), and other diagnostic procedures may be ordered to rule out concurrent injury.

The bleeding of scalp lacerations is controlled by direct pressure, although sutures may be required for hemostasis with severe injuries. Careful inspection of the wound is important. Digital examination of the wound is conducted after infiltration with lidocaine and 1:1000 epinephrine for anesthesia and vasoconstriction (Hickey, 1986). Copious irrigation of the wound with normal saline cleanses the wound of dirt and debris. Severe lacerations require débridement of devitalized tissue.

SKULL FRACTURES

Skull fractures are categorized as linear, depressed, or basilar but may also be described as simple, comminuted, and compound. The type of fracture depends on the velocity, direction, and momentum of the object causing the injury (Hickey, 1986).

Linear skull fractures comprise about 80% of all skull fractures, half of which involve the temporoparietal area (Jennett and Teasdale, 1981). Generally, linear fractures are not displaced and require no treatment. If the fracture extends into the orbit or paranasal sinuses or crosses a major vascular channel (such as the sagittal sinus or middle meningeal artery), the patient should be admitted to the hospital for observation. Surgery may be necessary to correct these secondary injuries (Weiner and Eisenberg, 1985).

A depressed skull fracture is characterized by an inward depression of the outer table of the skull below the inner table of the adjacent bone (Jennett and Teasdale, 1981) (Fig. 32–1). Depressed skull fractures are classified as open, or compound, in the presence of a communicating scalp laceration. Most patients with depressed fractures caused by nonpenetrating injuries have symptoms associated with focal brain damage and therefore never, or briefly, lose consciousness. Half of the patients with compound fractures have a torn dura, which is associated with a higher incidence of prolonged post-traumatic amnesia and focal signs (Jennett and Teasdale, 1981).

When depressed skull fractures are open, surgical asepsis is used to care for the scalp laceration because of the obvious potential for infection. Surgery to elevate the depressed bone is accomplished within 24 hours with open fractures (Nikas, 1987).

Because of the risk of infection, fracture fragments are removed from grossly contaminated wounds. If these fragments cannot be replaced in the wound, a plate cranioplasty (with a plate made of acrylic or metal) may be needed. The cranioplasty may be delayed to prevent local infection. A course of antibiotics is recommended if removal of fragments is not possible or if more than 24 hours elapses before débridement (Nikas, 1987).

A basilar skull fracture involves the base of the skull, including the anterior, middle, or posterior fossa. Because these fractures are difficult to confirm with radiographs, diagnosis may be based on the clinical presentation of the patient.

The clinical signs of an anterior fossa basilar skull fracture include cerebrospinal fluid (CSF) rhinorrhea (Fig. 32–2) and bilateral periorbital ecchymosis (referred to as raccoon's eyes). CSF rhinorrhea occurs in 25% of patients with anterior basilar fractures, and in more than half of these the leak lasts for only 2 or 3 days, until the dura seals itself (Jennett and Teasdale, 1981). Anterior fossa fractures may be associated with other facial injuries.

Middle fossa basilar skull fracture results in ecchymosis over the mastoid bone, called Battle sign, and CSF otorrhea. The leaking fluid from the ear demonstrates a dural tear and a ruptured tympanic membrane. If the tympanic membrane remains intact, blood and CSF may be evident behind the membrane on otoscopic examination. CSF otorrhea is rare, but when it occurs, CSF flow is profuse (Jennett and Teasdale, 1981).

CONCUSSION

Concussion is a clinical diagnosis that involves transient neurogenic dysfunction caused by rapid acceleration-deceleration or by a sudden blow to the head. It is suspected that temporary alteration in function results from transient ischemia or neural depolarization after a sudden release of acetylcholine (Spielman, 1988).

Mild concussion is the most common brain injury. It is considered a minor injury generally not requiring

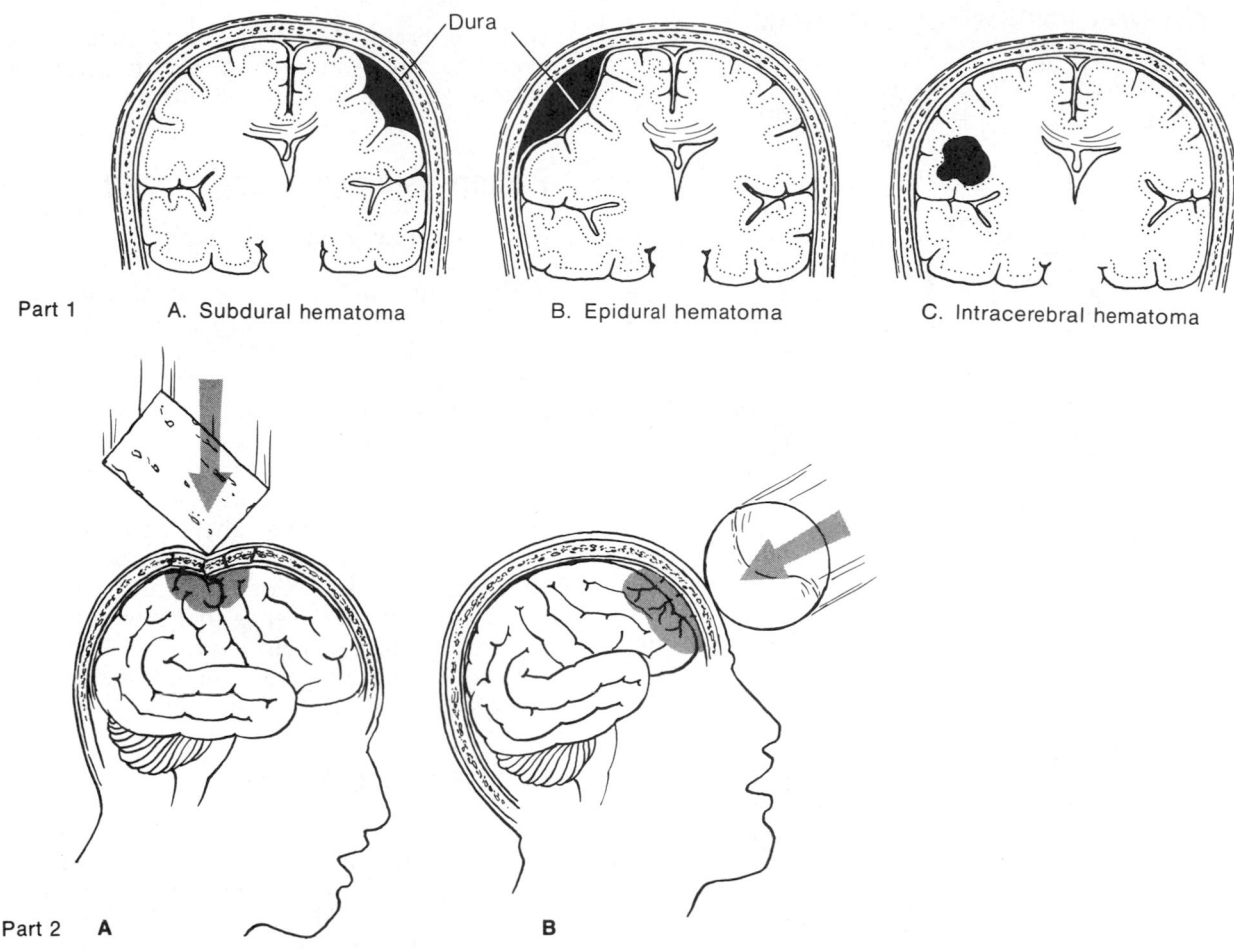

FIGURE 32–1. *Part 1, A* to *C,* Different types of hematoma. *Part 2,* Some mechanisms of head injury. Head injury results from penetration or impact. *A,* A direct injury (blow to the skull) may fracture the skull. Contusion and laceration of the brain may result from fractures. Depressed portions of the skull may compress or penetrate brain tissue. *B,* In the presence of skull fracture, a blow to the skull may cause the brain to move enough to tear some of the veins going through the cortical surface of the dura. Subsequently, subdural hematoma may develop. Note areas of cerebral contusion *(shaded).* In addition to the injuries depicted, secondary phenomena may result from the injury and cause additional brain dysfunction or damage. For example, ischemia, especially cerebral edema, may occur, elevating intracranial pressure. (From Luckmann, J., and Sorensen, K. C., (1987). *Medical-surgical nursing: A psychophysiologic approach* (3rd ed.). Philadelphia: W. B. Saunders.)

hospitalization. Symptoms include confusion, disorientation, and sometimes retrograde amnesia or post-traumatic amnesia. Symptoms generally only last a few minutes and are not related to permanent deficits. Preservation of consciousness is the distinguishing feature of mild concussion as opposed to classic concussion (Gennarelli, 1987). Classic concussion involves temporary loss of consciousness, retrograde amnesia, post-traumatic amnesia, and occasionally mild neurologic impairment. Unconsciousness usually lasts less than 5 minutes and no longer than 6 hours. The duration of post-traumatic amnesia is often a predictor of the severity of the injury (Spielman, 1988).

CONTUSION AND LACERATION

Contusions involve cortical bruising and laceration of vessels and brain tissues with subsequent tissue infarction and necrosis. These injuries usually in-

volve cortical and white matter petechial hemorrhages. The size and severity of the contusion and laceration vary depending on the area of contact between the striking object and the skull. The distinction between contusion and laceration is based on the degree of trauma, a laceration being more serious than a contusion.

The major sites of contusions and lacerations are the frontal and temporal lobes at the frontal poles, the orbital areas, the frontotemporal junction around the sylvian fissure, and the inferior and lateral surfaces of the temporal lobes (the temporal tips) (Hickey, 1986). The distribution of contusions in these particular areas is explained by the movement of the brain within the cranium and bony ridges on the inner plate of the cranium in these areas.

Assessment of the severity of contusion depends on the site and extent of brain injury. Isolated contusions do not generally produce immediate loss of consciousness but may subsequently if there is as-

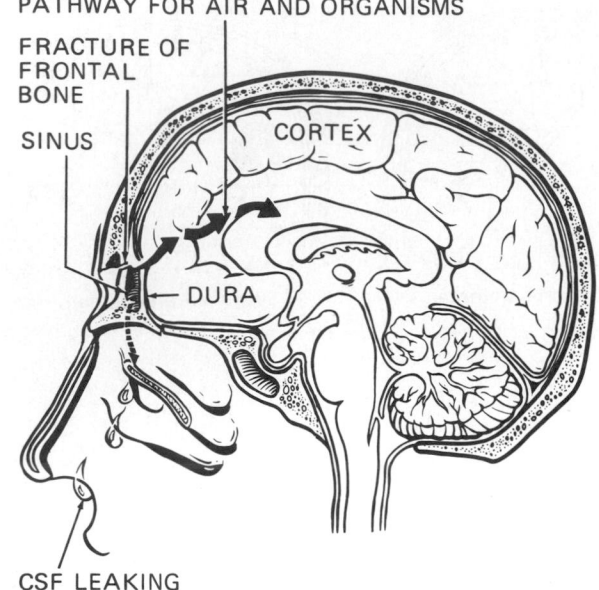

PATHWAY FOR AIR AND ORGANISMS

FRACTURE OF FRONTAL BONE

SINUS

CORTEX

DURA

CSF LEAKING

FIGURE 32–2. Frontal bone fracture with CSF leakage. (From Snyder, M., and Jackle, M. (1981). *Neurologic problems: A critical care focus.* Bowie, MD: Robert J. Brady.)

sociated ischemia. Coma is usually the result of concussion or diffuse injury. Frontal injuries result in personality, behavior, motor, and speech deficits. Temporal lobe contusions are closely monitored because of their proximity to the tentorium and midbrain, increasing the potential for herniation (Spielman, 1988).

PENETRATING INJURIES

Penetrating injury may be caused by missile injuries or impalement. Direct injury to the brain can result from penetration of the cranium. The wound created by a bullet depends on the size (caliber), shape, velocity, direction, and action within the intracranial space.

Wounds from missiles have been described as (1) tangential, when the missile produces a depressed skull fracture; (2) penetrating, when the missile enters but does not exit, resulting in metal, bone, hair, and skin fragments within the brain; and (3) through and through injuries, when the missile enters the cranium, traverses the cranial contents, and passes through an exit wound (Purvis, 1966).

The major effects of missile injuries are focal damage and generalized destruction of the brain from concussion, contusions, and lacerations of the brain. Necrosis of tissue and hemorrhage can occur. The amount of injury depends on the structures involved. There is an 80% mortality rate associated with through and through wounds (Hickey, 1986). Patients who are in deep coma on admission seldom survive. Forty-five per cent of the patients with missile injuries develop epilepsy within 5 years (Jennett and Teasdale, 1981).

Impalement injuries include piercing of the scalp,

skull, or brain. A foreign body that is protruding from the head should be left in place to control bleeding until it is removed during surgery.

Pathophysiology of Brain Injury

COUP-CONTRECOUP INJURIES

The brain has some movement within the skull, and this results in mass movement of the intracranial contents when the head incurs trauma (Fig. 32–3). An injury directly below the point of trauma can produce a coup injury, caused by the slapping effect of the brain hitting the skull. The contrecoup contusion, or laceration, occurs at the opposite pole of impact as the brain rebounds and strikes other parts of the skull. Wherever the impact occurs on the head, the resulting lesions are usually bilateral and symmetric. These lesions are most marked at the interfaces between tissues that have different physical properties, i.e., compliance or elasticity, such as between white and gray matter or brain and blood vessels (Jennett and Teasdale, 1981).

DIFFUSE AXONAL INJURY

Diffuse axonal injury (DAI) is the most severe form of brain injury and differs from concussion in degree rather than in kind of brain pathophysiology. This injury has also been called a shearing injury. The hallmark of DAI is immediate and prolonged coma (more than 6 hours). The coma is the result of severe, widespread damage to the white matter, essentially disconnecting the hemispheres from the brainstem's reticular activating system (RAS) by stretching and tearing the RAS fibers (Spielman, 1988). There is widespread neurologic dysfunction, diffuse white matter degeneration, and global cerebral edema.

DAI is classified as mild, moderate, or severe. Gennarelli and colleagues (1982) described mild injury as that restricted to the parasagittal white matter of the cerebral hemispheres; a moderate injury adds a focal injury in the corpus callosum; and a severe injury involves a large degree of axonal abnormality of the white matter of the cerebellum and upper brainstem. Because DAI involves microscopic changes, the severity of injury is not identified through radiographs but by the severity of symptoms and the duration of coma (Spielman, 1988).

The clinical findings of DAI include deep and prolonged coma, initial decortication (flexion) or decerebration (extension), increased intracranial pressure, hypertension, and an elevated temperature. The clinical course and outcome are dependent upon the severity of axonal injury. The patient may be comatose for up to 3 months and may never regain full consciousness. Major sequelae of severe DAI are deficits in cognition, memory, speech, motor function, and personality (Spielman, 1988). Mortality in severe DAI is around 51%, and only 15% of the

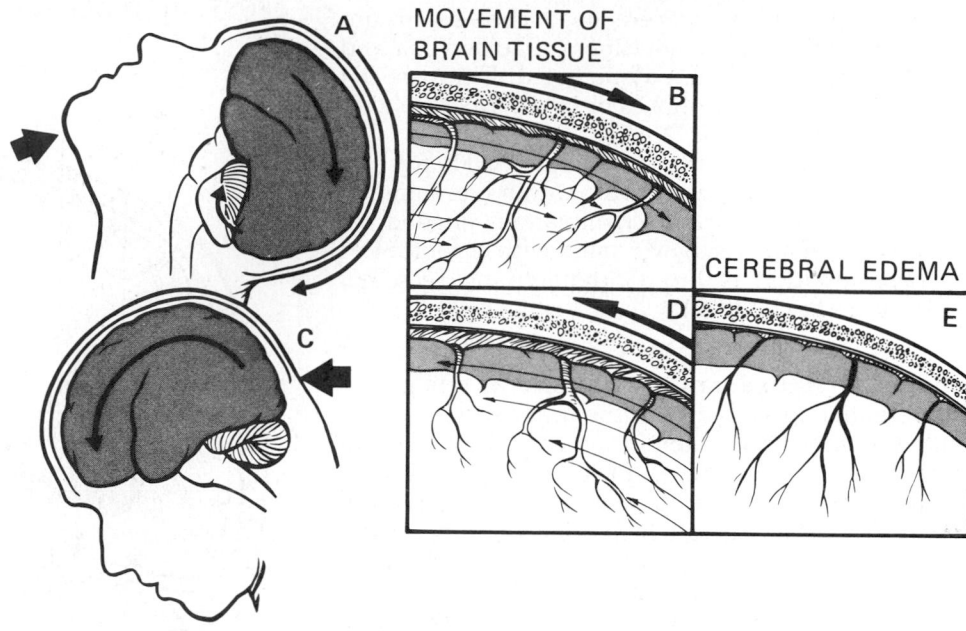

FIGURE 32–3. Acceleration-deceleration injury. *A* and *C*, Forceful extension and flexion of the neck. *B* and *D*, Movement of the brain within the skull. *E*, Cerebral edema. (From Snyder, M. and Jackle, M. (1981). *Neurologic problems: A critical care focus.* Bowie, MD: Robert J. Brady.)

A, C   Forceful extension and flexion of the neck

B, D   Movement of the brain within the skull

E   Cerebral edema

survivors have a good outcome (Gennarelli et al., 1982).

Complications of Brain Injury

POSTCONCUSSION SYNDROME

Concussion is considered a mild brain injury, but postinjury sequelae called postconcussion syndrome may be devastating for the patient. Major complaints with this syndrome include headache, dizziness, nervousness, irritability, fatigability, insomnia, poor concentration, poor memory, and changes in intelligence. Symptoms may be delayed several weeks to 2 years after the injury. Recognition of this syndrome has led to changes in follow-up for concussion patients. Patients whose symptoms persist have apparently sustained some organic injury and will have difficulty regaining their previous life style and level of function. Referral to a neuropsychologist for follow-up aids in early identification of the syndrome, facilitating the patient in adjusting to any disabilities.

HEMATOMA FORMATION

Subdural Hematoma. A subdural hematoma (SDH; see Fig. 32–1) refers to bleeding between the dura mater and the arachnoid layer of the meninges. This bleeding creates pressure on the brain. Bleeding into the subdural space is believed to result from

tearing of the bridging veins between the brain and the dura, bleeding from contused or lacerated brain tissue, or extension from an intracerebral hematoma. Ten to fifteen per cent of head-injured patients develop subdural hematomas.

Subdural hematomas have a poor prognosis because they are frequently not diagnosed rapidly enough after the injury. Mortality varies from 52% to 65% (Miller et al., 1981). Diagnosis is confirmed by CT scan, which demonstrates the typical half-moon–shaped area of increased density on the surface of the brain (Jennett and Teasdale, 1981).

Acute SDH occurs within 48 hours of injury and is associated with major cerebral trauma with contusion and laceration. Patients usually present with progressive and marked depression of consciousness, headache, drowsiness, agitation, and confusion. Pupillary and motor changes are present in many of these patients. Treatment consists of craniotomy (usually burr holes) with evacuation of the hematoma and coagulation of actively bleeding vessels. Patients are monitored in a critical care unit postoperatively.

Subacute SDH can develop 2 to 14 days following injury. Subacute SDH is strongly indicated by a failure to regain consciousness (Hickey, 1986).

Chronic SDH can occur up to several months following the initial injury. The pathogenesis of chronic SDH is not known. The hematoma tends to develop slowly, indicated by the same signs as a space-occupying lesion. Symptoms commonly include an increasingly severe headache, confusion, slow cerebration, and drowsiness. Papilledema and ipsilateral pupil dilation may be noted. Chronic SDH is more common in alcoholics or in older people with cerebral atrophy (Nikas, 1987).

Treatment of subacute or chronic SDH involves burr holes and evacuation. Some authors recommend craniectomy for recurrent accumulations of subdural fluid (Tyson et al., 1980). Mortality with chronic SDH has been reported as 0 to 5% (Jennett and Teasdale, 1981; Tyson et al., 1980).

Epidural (Extradural) Hematoma. Bleeding into the potential space between the inner surface of the skull and the dura mater forms an epidural hematoma (EDH) (see Fig. 32–1). Incidence of EDH is low, comprising only 5% of all severe head injuries and only 20% to 30% of all hematomas (Bruce et al., 1978). Epidural hematomas are associated with temporal or parietal skull fractures with involvement of a branch of the meningeal artery (Hirsh, 1980; Jennett and Teasdale, 1981). Fractures crossing a major venous channel, such as the sagittal or transverse sinus, lead to EDH of venous origin.

One-third of patients with EDH have the classic triad of symptoms, e.g., immediate loss of consciousness at the time of injury, a lucid interval lasting a few minutes to a few hours, then a lapse into unconsciousness again. Other symptoms include increasingly severe headache, seizures, vomiting, hemiparesis, and a fixed and dilated ipsilateral pupil (Hickey, 1986). Emergency surgery to evacuate the hematoma is done to prevent cerebral herniation (Fig. 32–4). Prognosis is good in patients with EDH who undergo surgical evacuation prior to the onset of neurologic decompensation (Langfitt, 1978). Eighty per cent of these patients show a rapid recovery with little neurologic deficit. Mortality rates of 8% are reported when surgery is done rapidly (Becker et al., 1977).

Intracerebral Hematoma. An intracerebral hematoma (ICH) is a well-defined blood clot within the brain tissue (see Fig. 32–1). Similar to contusion, the most frequent sites for ICH are the frontal and temporal lobes (Jameson and Yelland, 1972). ICH is uncommon, representing only 1.5 to 21% of intracranial mass lesions (Bowers and Marshall, 1980; Miller et al., 1981). Small, deep hematomas within the periventricular, medial, or paracentral area follow shear forces and indicate diffuse axonal injury (Gennarelli and Thibault, 1982). Intracerebral bleeding is found with lacerations following closed head injury but may also be found in patients with open or penetrating injury.

Signs and symptoms of ICH are similar to those of contusions, the course and outcome depending upon the size and location of the hematoma. ICH is complicated by progressive focal edema and mass effect, which result in neurologic deterioration. Deteriora-

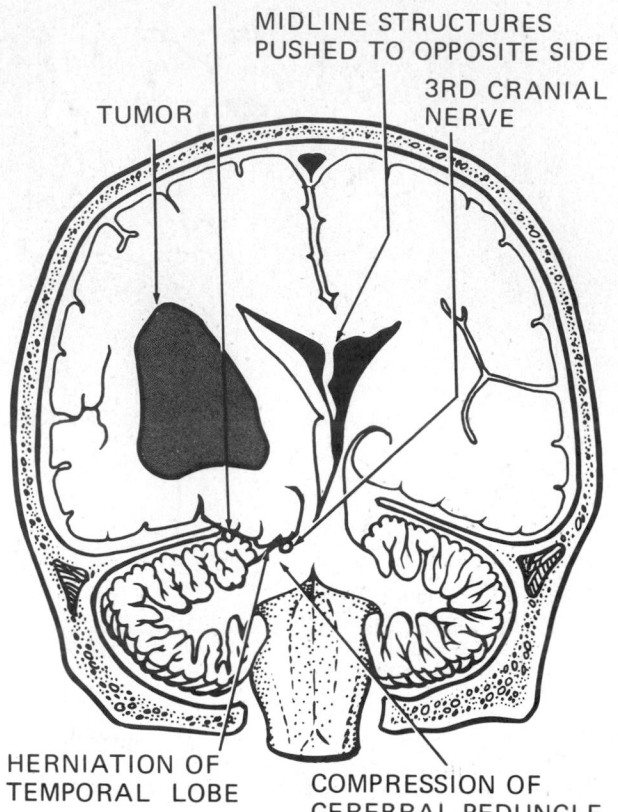

POSTERIOR CEREBRAL ARTERY

MIDLINE STRUCTURES PUSHED TO OPPOSITE SIDE

3RD CRANIAL NERVE

TUMOR

HERNIATION OF TEMPORAL LOBE

COMPRESSION OF CEREBRAL PEDUNCLE

FIGURE 32–4. Cerebral herniation. Lesions and/or edema in the supratentorial compartment tend to push the uncus of the temporal lobe through the tentorial notch. This is called uncal or tentorial herniation. The downward pressure of the uncus compresses the oculomotor nerve and the posterior cerebral artery. With increasing pressure, the midbrain is compressed against the opposite side of the tentorium. (From Snyder, M. and Jackle, M. (1981). *Neurologic problems: A critical care focus.* Bowie, MD: Robert J. Brady.)

tion may be immediate or may follow the injury by 7 to 10 days (Spielman, 1988).

Delayed hemorrhage following ICH is known as delayed traumatic intracerebral hemorrhage (DTICH). DTICH occurs in areas that were injured at the time of impact but appeared normal on the initial CT scan. Clot formation and deterioration occur within a few days of the original trauma (Cooper, 1985). DTICH is associated with a poor outcome and a high incidence of intracranial hypertension. Patients with disseminated intravascular coagulopathy, hypoxia, hypotension, or alcohol abuse have an increased incidence of DTICH (Cooper, 1985; Spielman, 1988).

CEREBRAL EDEMA/INCREASED INTRACRANIAL PRESSURE

Cerebral edema is a common complication of head injury that affects cerebral function, increases intracranial pressure, and may interfere with neural function in edematous brain tissues (Cooper, 1985). Klatzo (1967) was the first to classify brain edema

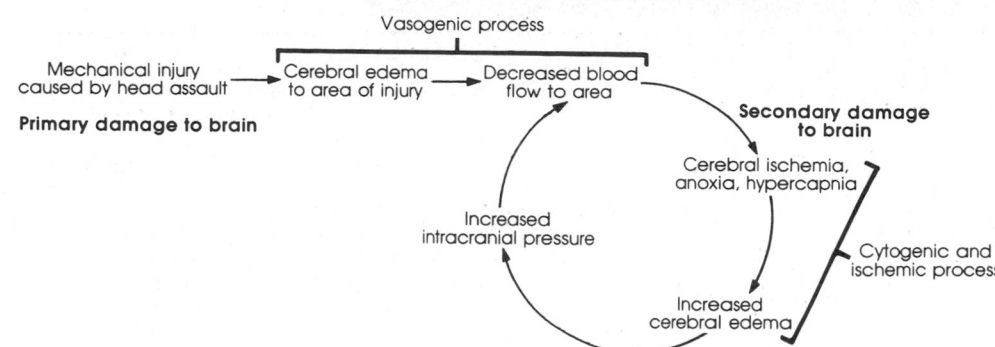

CEREBRAL EDEMA – INCREASED INTRACRANIAL PRESSURE

FIGURE 32–5. Mechanisms in cerebral edema from head trauma. (Reproduced by permission from: Rudy, E., *Advanced neurological and neurosurgical nursing*, St. Louis, 1984, The C. V. Mosby Company.)

into cytotoxic and vasogenic types. Cytotoxic edema results in cellular metabolism abnormalities that allow the accumulation of fluid that is rich in electrolytes but low in proteins (Klatzo, 1967). The relevance of cytotoxic edema for head injury is unclear (Cooper, 1985).

There appears to be a relationship between the type of cerebral injury and vasogenic edema (Fig. 32–5). Vasogenic edema results from a defect in cerebral capillaries that allows extravasation of plasma proteins and electrolytes into the extracellular cerebral tissues (Cooper, 1985). Edema spreads from the site of capillary injury into the white matter, diffusing into areas where capillaries remain intact.

Cerebral edema may be localized or diffuse. Diffuse cerebral edema of one or both hemispheres is common in traumatic brain injury. Cerebral edema exaggerates the amount and severity of any neurologic deficit that is present. The severity and extent of edema are related to the severity of the head injury. As the brain's compensatory mechanisms to accommodate additional brain mass fail, increases in intracranial pressure begin.

Intracranial hypertension is a major complication

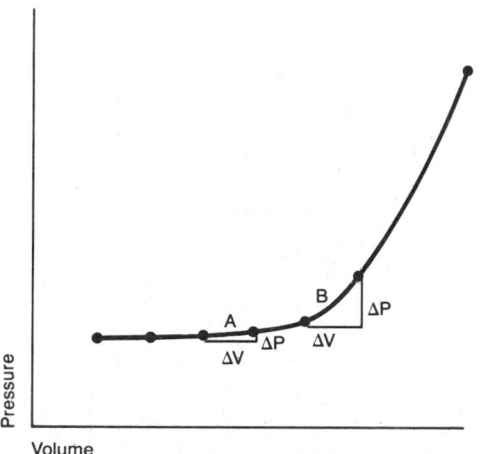

FIGURE 32–6. Pressure-volume curve. *A,* A change in volume (ΔV) causes only a small change in pressure (ΔP), and so elastance ($\Delta P/\Delta V$) is small. *B,* The elastance is high, and the same ΔV causes a much greater ΔP. (Reproduced from Bruce, D. A.: *The pathophysiology of increased intracranial pressure.* Kalamazoo, MI, The Upjohn Company, 1978, p. 19, with permission from the publisher.)

of head trauma and is the most frequent cause of death in head-injured patients (Walleck, 1990). The effects of cerebral edema and increased intracranial pressure (ICP) on cerebral tissues depend on their severity and duration. Compression of blood vessels results in ischemia and infarction of brain tissue.

Normal ICP reflects the intracranial volume within the rigid skull. Intracranial volume is composed of brain tissue (88%), cerebrospinal fluid (CSF, 8% to 9%), and blood within blood vessels (2% to 5%). Increased ICP results from an increase in the volume of one of these three constituents without a compensatory decrease in one of the other two. The chief compensatory mechanism is a reduction in CSF by increased resorption, displacement into the subarachnoid space, or decreased production of CSF. Vasoconstriction with reduced blood volume or shifts of brain tissue may also occur, but these are of time-limited assistance.

The concept of compliance also contributes to an understanding of increased ICP. Compliance is an index of the volume-pressure relationship within the skull. When compensatory mechanisms fail, compliance is minimal, and a small increase in volume causes autoregulation, which is influenced by a large increase in pressure (Fig. 32–6).

Autoregulation is the automatic change in the caliber of the cerebral blood vessels over a broad range of mean arterial blood pressures to ensure normal perfusion pressure. The brain regulates its blood flow by autoregulation, which is influenced by systemic changes in blood pressure, and metabolic factors. Primary control of ICP occurs through autoregulatory mechanisms. Head trauma interferes with maximum functioning of autoregulation. Most nursing and medical interventions to control increased ICP support these compensatory mechanisms.

Post-traumatic epilepsy is the most common sequela of brain trauma, occurring in 5% of patients with closed head injury and 50% of patients with open head injuries (Hickey, 1986). The interval between trauma and the onset of seizures varies greatly. Fifty per cent of patients develop seizures within 1 to 6 months of injury; by the end of 2 years 80% of the patients at risk will have had a seizure. Focal or tonic-clonic seizures are most common. Most seizures are amenable to anticonvulsant therapy.

TABLE 32–1. The Glasgow Coma Scale Response Chart

	Stimulus/Measure	Patient's Response	Score
Eye opening	Spontaneous	Opens eyes independently	4
	Speech	Opens eyes in response to loud command	3
	Pain	Opens eyes with painful stimulus	2
	Pain	Does not open eyes even with painful stimulus	1
Best motor response	Verbal command	Follows simple commands	6
	Pain	Pushes away the source of painful stimulus	5
	Pain	Pulls body part away from painful stimulus	4
	Pain	Flexes body inappropriately in response to pain	3
	Pain	Body becomes rigid in extended position in response to pain stimulus	2
	Pain	No motor response to deep pain (pressure on nailbeds or orbital arch)	1
Verbal response	Speech	Converses appropriately and is oriented to person, place, and time	5
	Speech	Confused or disoriented	4
	Speech	Speech is understandable but nonsensical	3
	Speech	Unintelligible speech	2
	Speech	Makes no sound	1

Adapted from Rimel, R. (1978). Emergency management of the patient with central nervous system trauma. *Journal of Neurosurgical Nursing*, 10(4), 185–188.

Because seizures tend to decrease in frequency over a period of years, it is estimated that 10% to 30% of these patients will eventually be seizure-free (Hickey, 1986).

Clinical Presentation

Assessment of the head trauma patient provides a dynamic overview of patient improvement or deterioration and guides diagnostic or therapeutic efforts. Complete physical assessment includes an assessment of the level of consciousness and brainstem reflexes (primarily pupillary responses). Laboratory data, radiologic procedures, imaging procedures, and neural monitoring techniques aid diagnosis and provide prognostic information.

Level of Consciousness. The level of consciousness is the most sensitive indicator of neurologic function. The Glasgow coma scale (GCS) is an internationally recognized tool for evaluating level of consciousness, both arousal and awareness (Table 32–1 and Fig. 32–7). The arousal component of consciousness depends on the function of the reticular activating system in the brainstem. Awareness is a measure of cortical activity. The three functions assessed with the GCS are eye opening, verbal response, and motor response. The scale ranges from 3 to 15, with a score derived by summing the three functions. A score of 13 to 15 indicates mild head injury; 9 to 12 signifies

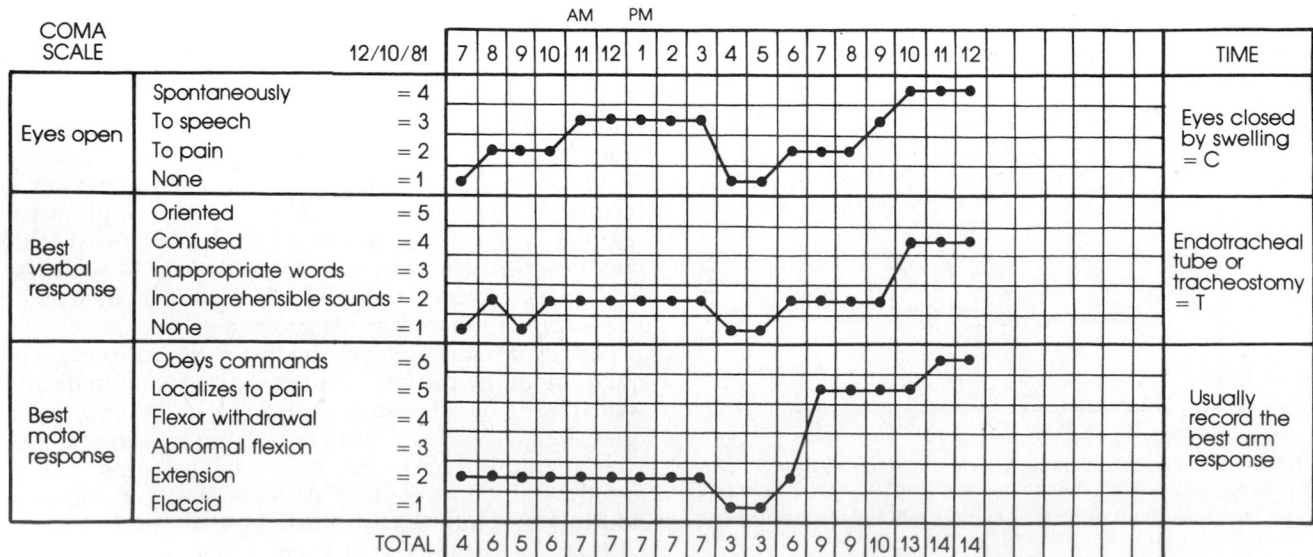

FIGURE 32–7. Glasgow coma scale for recording assessment of consciousness. (Reproduced by permission from Rudy, E., *Advanced neurological and neurosurgical nursing*, St. Louis, 1984, The C. V. Mosby Company.)

moderate head injury; and a score of 8 or less indicates severe head injury or coma. This scale aids clinicians in making meaningful comparisons between patients and in predicting head injury outcomes and mortality (Spielman, 1988). The lower the GCS score, the deeper the coma and the higher the mortality and morbidity.

Another useful head injury assessment scale is the Rancho Los Amigos scale (Table 32–2). This scale was designed by Chris Hagen, a speech and language pathologist (Hagen et al., 1979). The scale is based on standard evaluation criteria that provide a numerical reference for levels ranging from nonresponsiveness (level I) to purposeful and appropriate response (level VIII). This scale generalizes behavior via brainstem reflexes through high cortical activity and is useful in all phases of head injury care.

Pupillary Response. Pupils are normally equal in size, round, and react briskly to light. Changes in size or reaction time should be reported to the physician. If there is lateral transtentorial herniation from brain edema, mass lesion, or epidural or subdural hematoma, the ipsilateral pupil will become dilated and fixed because of pressure of brain matter on the oculomotor nerve (cranial nerve III). An oval-shaped pupil occurs with increased ICP and is associated with a poor prognosis (Marshall et al., 1983).

Other brainstem reflexes that can be assessed include corneal, gag, oculocephalic, and oculovestibular reflexes. The corneal reflex (cranial nerves V and VII), gag reflex (cranial nerves IX and X), and oculocephalic test, or doll's eye maneuver, are easily assessed at the bedside. The oculovestibular test involves instillation of ice water into the auditory canal and provides information on the function of cranial nerves III, VI, and VIII. Tests of these reflexes serve to assess the function of the brainstem. Absent reflexes indicate a poor prognosis.

Vital Signs. Vital signs are routinely monitored on all neurotrauma patients. Blood pressure and heart rate are assessed to ensure adequate perfusion of brain tissues. Cerebral blood flow depends on the cerebral perfusion pressure (CPP) and the diameter of the cerebrovascular bed. CPP is the difference between the mean arterial pressure (MAP) and the ICP. Normal CPP is 60 to 80 mm Hg (Miller, 1985). Alterations in CPP occur because of changes in the MAP, which reflects arterial pressure, or changes in ICP. CPP falls when there is arterial hypotension or increased ICP. As ICP rises and cerebral blood flow (CBF) falls, the systemic arterial blood pressure rises to maintain adequate cerebral perfusion. This is part of the Cushing reflex, e.g., increased systolic blood pressure, widened pulse pressure, and bradycardia. When autoregulation is lost following severe head injury, a rise in arterial pressure may be accompanied by a rise in ICP, leading to reduced CPP (Miller, 1985). A change in the blood pressure and heart rate without an accompanying change in the level of

consciousness indicates non-neurologic pathology. Classic Cushing reflex occurs late in the clinical course in patients whose condition is deteriorating.

Cardiac rate, rhythm, and conduction changes occur with a variety of intracranial injuries and may be neurogenic in origin. Dysrhythmias vary with the initial neurologic pathology. Progressive bradycardia, junctional escape rhythms, and idioventricular rhythms occur with cerebral hemorrhage and increased ICP. Atrial fibrillation and bundle branch blocks are more frequently seen with cerebral contusion. Acute subdural hematoma is associated with atrial and ventricular ectopy and conduction defects (Clifton et al., 1983; Staller, 1987).

ST- and T-wave changes follow cerebral ischemia resulting from severe head injury and increased ICP. Neurogenic T waves (inverted T waves with increased amplitude and duration) are associated with a variety of neurologic pathologies (Conner, 1969; Staller, 1987). The frequent, though inconsistent, electrocardiographic (ECG) changes associated with intracranial pathology require continuous cardiac monitoring of these patients in the critical care unit (Nikas, 1987).

Changes in respiratory pattern are associated with the level of intracranial injury or the degree of pressure exerted on the brainstem. Centers controlling the regulation of respirations are scattered throughout the cerebral hemispheres and brainstem, and each center is responsible for a unique respiratory pattern (Spielman, 1988). Changes in respiration assist in identifying the area of injury and indicate neurologic deterioration. The earliest and most common respiratory alteration is Cheyne-Stokes respirations, which result from hemispheric compression (Spielman, 1988). Although it is not essential that the nurse know the name of each respiratory pattern, it is vital to identify changes, recognize the potential neurologic origin of the changes, and be prepared to provide neurologic and ventilatory support (Plum and Posner, 1982).

Temperature monitoring is essential following head injury. Hyperthermia increases metabolic demand in already compromised cerebral tissues and may contribute to increased ICP. Fever indicates either infection or hypothalamic dysfunction. Body temperature fluctuations from hypothermia to hyperthermia occur frequently with these patients, requiring continuous temperature monitoring.

Intracranial Pressure Monitoring

Monitoring ICP allows aggressive management of patients with potential or actual increased ICP. Lundberg (1960) introduced ICP monitoring in 1960, employing direct cannulation of a ventricle with a catheter. Since Lundberg's work, several other monitoring methods have been introduced, including subdural, epidural, and intraparenchymal monitor-

TABLE 32–2. Rancho Los Amigos Hospital: Levels of Cognitive Functioning

I.	No response	Patient appears to be in a deep sleep and is completely unresponsive to any stimuli presented to him.
II.	Generalized response	Patient reacts inconsistently and nonpurposefully to stimuli in a nonspecific manner. Responses are limited in nature and are often the same regardless of stimulus presented. Responses may be physiologic changes, gross body movements, and/or vocalizations. Often the earliest response is to deep pain. Responses are likely to be delayed.
III.	Localized response	Patient reacts specifically but inconsistently to stimuli. Responses are directly related to the type of stimulus presented as in turning head toward a sound, focusing on an object presented. The patient may withdraw an extremity and/or vocalize when presented with a painful stimulus. He may follow simple commands in an inconsistent, delayed manner, such as closing his eyes, squeezing or extending an extremity. Once external stimuli are removed, he may lie quietly. He may also show a vague awareness of self and body by responding to discomfort by pulling at nasogastric tube or catheter or resisting restraints. He may show a bias toward responding to some persons (especially family, friends) but not to others.
IV.	Confused-agitated	Patient is in a heightened state of activity with severely decreased ability to process information. He is detached from the present and responds primarily to his own internal confusion. Behavior is frequently bizarre and nonpurposeful relative to his immediate environment. He may cry out or scream out of proportion to stimuli even after removal, may show aggressive behavior, attempt to remove restraints or tubes, or crawl out of bed in a purposeful manner. He does not, however, discriminate among persons or objects and is unable to cooperate directly with treatment efforts. Verbalization is frequently incoherent and/or inappropriate to the environment. Confabulation may be present; he may be euphoric or hostile. Thus gross attention to environment is very short, and selective attention is often nonexistent. Being unaware of present events, patient lacks short-term recall and may be reacting to past events. He is unable to perform self-care (feeding, dressing) without maximum assistance. If not disabled physically, he may perform motor activities as sitting, reaching, and ambulating, but as part of his agitated state and not as a purposeful act or on request necessarily.
V.	Confused-inappropriate-nonagitated	Patient appears alert and is able to respond to simple commands fairly consistently. However, with increased complexity of commands or lack of any external structure, responses are nonpurposeful, random, or at best, fragmented toward any desired goal. He may show agitated behavior, but not on an internal basis (as in level IV), but rather as a result of external stimuli, and usually out of proportion to the stimulus. He has gross attention to the environment but is highly distractible and lacks ability to focus attention to a specific task without frequent redirection back to it. With structure, he may be able to converse on a social-automatic level of short periods of time. Verbalization is often inappropriate; confabulation may be triggered by present events. His memory is severely impaired, with confusion of past and present in his reaction to ongoing activity. Patient lacks initiation of functional tasks and often shows inappropriate use of objects without external direction. He may be able to perform previously learned tasks when structured for him, but is unable to learn new information. He responds best to self, body, comfort, and often family members. The patient can usually perform self-care activities with assistance and may accomplish feeding with maximum supervision. Management on the ward is often a problem if the patient is physically mobile, as he may wander off either randomly or with vague intention of "going home."
VI.	Confused-appropriate	Patient shows goal-directed behavior but is dependent on external input for direction. Response to discomfort is appropriate, and he is able to tolerate unpleasant stimuli (as NG tube) when need is explained. He follows simple directions consistently and shows carry-over for tasks he has relearned (as self-care). He is at least supervised with old learning; maximally assisted for new learning with little or no carry-overs. Responses may be incorrect due to memory problems, but they are appropriate to the situation. They may be delayed to immediate situation and he shows decreased ability to process information with little or no anticipation or prediction of events. Past memories show more depth and detail than recent memory. The patient may show beginning immediate awareness of situation by realizing he does not know an answer. He no longer wanders and is inconsistently oriented to time and place. Selective attention to tasks may be impaired, especially with difficult tasks and in unstructured settings, but is now functional for common daily activities (30 minutes with structure). He may show a vague recognition of some staff, has increased awareness of self, family, and basic needs (as food), again in an appropriate manner as in contrast to level V.
VII.	Automatic-appropriate	Patient appears appropriate and oriented within hospital and home settings, goes through daily routine automatically, but frequently robotlike, with minimal to absent confusion, but has shallow recall of what he has been doing. He shows increased awareness of self, body, family, foods, people, and interaction in the environment. He has superficial awareness of, but lacks insight into his condition, decreased judgment and problem-solving, and lacks realistic planning for his future. He shows carry-over for new learning but at a decreased rate. He requires at least minimal supervision for learning and for safety purposes. He is independent in self-care skills for safety. With structure he is able to initiate tasks such as social or recreational activities in which he now has interest. His judgment remains impaired, such that he is unable to drive a car. Prevocational or avocational evaluation and counseling may be indicated.
VIII.	Purposeful-appropriate	Patient is alert and oriented, is able to recall and integrate past and recent events, and is aware of and responsive to his culture. He shows carry-over for new learning if acceptable to him and his life role, and needs no supervision once activities are learned. Within his physical capabilities, he is independent in home and community skills, including driving. Vocational rehabilitation, to determine ability to return as a contributor to society (perhaps in a new capacity), is indicated. He may continue to show a decreased ability, relative to premorbid abilities, in abstract reasoning, tolerance for stress, judgment in emergencies or unusual circumstances. His social, emotional, and intellectual capacities may continue to be at a decreased level for him, but functional in society.

From Hagen, C., Malkmus, D., Durham, P., et al. (1979). Rancho Los Amigos Hospital, Levels of Cognitive Functioning. Head Trauma Service, Rancho Los Amigos Medical Center, Downey, CA.

ing (see Chap. 13 for more information on ICP monitoring).

Overall, ICP monitoring allows early identification and rapid treatment of intracranial hypertension, a complication of head injury. Any head-injured patient with a Glasgow coma scale score of 8 or less is a candidate for ICP monitoring. Ability to monitor ICP allows critical evaluation of treatments used to prevent or control increased ICP. Because nursing activities have been implicated in elevating ICP, use of ICP monitoring allows assessment while performing these activities and facilitates nursing research into the best methods to use in caring for these patients.

Laboratory Studies

Initial laboratory data provide a baseline for comparison with future laboratory studies. Baseline data also indicate the patient's overall physiologic status.

Because hypoxemia and hypercarbia aggravate brain injury, arterial blood gases should be monitored every 6 hours during intensive care. A Pa_{O2} of 80 to 100 mm Hg is necessary to prevent hypoxia. A Pa_{CO2} of 35 to 45 mm Hg is normal, but with mandatory hyperventilation the Pa_{CO2} should be 27 to 33 mm Hg. A normal hemoglobin and hematocrit aid in ensuring adequate oxygen transport to the brain.

White blood cell counts with differential should be done daily to monitor for infection. Daily coagulation profiles assess for disseminated intravascular coagulation as a complication of neurologic injury. Early diagnosis of coagulopathy allows early diagnosis, reducing mortality and morbidity from this complication.

It is important to monitor serum sodium, potassium, glucose, and chloride levels. Because of their role in nervous system function, changes in sodium and glucose levels may complicate the clinical course of patients with head injury. Iatrogenic fluid and electrolyte imbalance must be monitored when dehydration or diuresis therapies are used. The serum osmolality should be closely monitored in these patients because diuretics and fluid restriction can cause dangerously high osmolality levels (>310 mOsm). Complications of diabetes insipidus (DI) and syndrome of inappropriate secretion of antidiuretic hormone (SIADH) can lead to hypo-osmolar and hyper-osmolar states. Assessment of blood serum osmolality, urine osmolality, urine specific gravity, and urine electrolytes (Na, K, and Cl) should be monitored as indices of fluid balance.

Diagnostic Procedures

SKULL FILMS

The skull x-ray is used to diagnose skull fractures in the emergency department. This is the most com-

mon neuroradiologic procedure used. These films also demonstrate facial fractures, especially orbital rim injuries.

COMPUTED TOMOGRAPHY

CT scanning has revolutionized the care of patients with head injury. CT scanning clearly identifies space-occupying lesions, contusions, and hemorrhagic or edematous areas in the brain. An accurate diagnosis can be made within minutes, allowing rapid initiation of therapy. CT scans have significantly reduced mortality and morbidity from epidural, subdural, and intracerebral hematoma.

MAGNETIC RESONANCE IMAGING

MRI promises to be an improvement over CT scanning. MRI is based on the interaction of protons, moved by radio waves, in a static magnetic field and provides excellent composites of the brain anatomy. No ionizing radiation or x-rays are associated with MRI. MRI surpasses CT scans in differentiating between gray and white matter and in detecting small hemorrhages in diffuse axonal injury (Spielman, 1988).

Because of technical problems, it is extremely difficult to use MRI in critically ill patients who are being mechanically ventilated with a ventilator that is not MRI-compatible or with ICP monitoring. These problems include the longer time needed for MRI versus CT scanning; the magnetic field of MRI will not function with ferrous-containing compounds in the imaging room; and the radio frequency generator disrupts function of hemodynamic monitoring devices, including ICP monitors. Efforts are underway to correct these problems to allow use of MRI in critically ill patients.

EVOKED POTENTIAL STUDIES

Evoked potential studies (EPS) have become valuable in locating lesions and in clarifying prognoses in head-injured patients. EPS reflect the brain's response to specific sensory stimulation (visual, auditory, or somatosensory). They can be performed at the bedside and are valuable in assessing and monitoring patients who would be considered untestable or are in a comatose state because of the influence of CNS depressants or barbiturate-induced coma.

CONTINUOUS CEREBRAL BLOOD FLOW STUDIES

A new technology introduced in the care of head-injured patients involves the continuous monitoring of cerebral circulation. Cerebral blood flow studies have been used in the past to define no-flow states in brain death. This technology involves the use of radiologically tagged xenon gas delivered by a computerized ventilator that monitors xenon uptake as a reflection of cerebral blood flow.

Although this technology is at present in limited use, it promises to be very helpful in determining the effect of brain injury on blood flow and monitoring the effects of treatment to improve blood flow in ischemic areas. Monitoring of cerebral blood flow may eventually replace ICP monitoring.

Assessment of the patient with brain injury involves the use of a variety of techniques to provide a comprehensive picture of the patient's neurologic status. Comparison of current and past assessment data identifies subtle changes in neurologic status, allowing appropriate intervention in the patient's care.

Medical Management

The goals of medical management of patients with closed head injury include creating a brain tissue environment conducive to recovery; avoiding hypoxia, hypercapnia, or hypotension; and preventing complications. Use of standard treatment protocols and early institution of therapy appropriate to the underlying pathology improve the potential for favorable outcomes.

OXYGENATION

The severely head-injured patient is intubated and placed on a ventilator to maintain the airway and prevent hypoxia and hypercapnia. High levels of supplemental oxygen should be provided to ensure adequate cerebral oxygenation (Nikas and Tolley, 1982). The goal of therapy is to achieve a Pa_{O_2} of 80 to 100 mm Hg.

Ability to maintain adequate oxygenation may be compromised by pulmonary pathology, e.g., pulmonary contusion, atelectasis, or pneumonia. Ventilation-perfusion abnormalities are found in many severely head-injured patients (Walleck, 1987). Meticulous pulmonary toilet is essential, including positioning, suctioning, and chest physiotherapy while attempts are made to maintain acceptable levels of ICP. Positive end-expiratory pressure (PEEP) may also be needed. PEEP prevents collapse of the alveoli at the end of expiration, improving gas exchange. In patients with normal pulmonary compliance, PEEP increases intrathoracic pressure, which may also increase ICP (Cepuzzo et al., 1977; Frost and Gildenberg, 1977). With pulmonary pathology, intrathoracic compliance is reduced, decreasing the impact on ICP (Frost and Gildenberg, 1977). Elevation of the head of the bed to 30 degrees reduces the effect of PEEP on ICP (Cepuzzo et al., 1977).

Evaluating the effectiveness of oxygen therapy includes monitoring arterial blood gases (ABGs), venous blood gases, oxygen extraction, and other cardiopulmonary parameters when available. Continuous assessment of tissue oxygenation is facilitated with pulse oximetry, intra-arterial electrodes, or transcutaneous or transconjunctival oxygen sensors. End-tidal CO_2 can also be monitored with a capnometer (Spielman, 1988).

HYPERVENTILATION

Hyperventilation has been part of most head injury protocols for the last two decades. Hyperventilation decreases the Pa_{CO_2} and therefore constricts cerebral blood vessels, decreasing cerebral blood volume, which in turn decreases ICP. Each millimeter of mercury decrease in Pa_{CO_2} results in a cerebral blood flow decrease of 2 to 3 mL/100 g of tissue per minute. This compromised blood flow can cause ischemia in injured brain tissues. Pa_{CO_2} levels of below 25 mm Hg should be avoided. Because of this potential for ischemia, many institutions are no longer using hyperventilation on a routine basis. In patients with severe head injury, the vasoreactivity of cerebral vessels may be reduced, which also limits the therapeutic effectiveness of hyperventilation. Although hyperventilation produces respiratory alkalosis, which combats brain tissue acidosis, this may also lower the seizure threshold (Bruce et al., 1978; Shapiro, 1975; Spielman, 1988). Monitoring Pa_{CO_2} is essential to ensure that it remains within 27 to 33 mm Hg.

GLUCOCORTICOSTEROIDS

Glucocorticosteroids have been used extensively to treat cerebral edema in patients with head injury. Most frequently used are dexamethasone and methylprednisolone. The usefulness of steroids in severe head injury is questionable—i.e., some researchers report positive effects, whereas others find no effect. Researchers who disclaim the effectiveness of steroids also feel that they may do harm by lowering resistance to infection and increasing the risk of gastrointestinal hemorrhage. Proponents of steroids feel that they reduce mortality from head injury as effectively as other therapeutic modalities.

It is speculated that steroids exert a stabilizing effect on the cell membrane. They may also improve neuronal function by improving cerebral blood flow and restoring autoregulation. Large doses and prolonged therapy are associated with complications including carbohydrate intolerance and hyperglycemia, immunosuppression, decreased resistance to infection, gastric ulceration, and water and sodium retention (Spielman, 1988).

DIURETIC THERAPY

Osmotically active agents have been used for over 50 years to treat cerebral edema. Hypertonic solutions remove cerebral tissue fluid via the vascular osmotic pressure gradient, reducing brain volume and lowering ICP. To be effective, the agent must remain within the intravascular compartment. If the blood–

brain barrier is disrupted, the therapy becomes more harmful than beneficial because the hypertonic solution could pass into the already edematous brain, increasing the edema in a rebound phenomenon.

Osmotherapeutic agents include mannitol, glycerol, and urea. Mannitol is most frequently used and has been found to be more effective than glycerol or pentobarbital in reducing ICP (Levin et al., 1979). Twenty per cent mannitol is given as an intravenous bolus or continuous infusion in dosages ranging from 0.5 to 2.0 g/kg of body weight. Optimal effect is acquired with rapid administration. Its rapid onset of action makes this the preferred drug for elevated ICP. Hyperosmolality and acute renal failure are complications of hyperosmotic therapy. Monitoring fluids, electrolytes, and serum osmolality is essential to avoid severe dehydration.

Recent research has demonstrated the potential usefulness of nonosmotic diuretics (furosemide and ethacrynic acid) in reducing ICP. Furosemide is a potent loop diuretic that is thought to reduce ICP by decreasing sodium transport within the brain, reducing systemic fluid volume and inhibiting CSF production (up to 70%) (Spielman, 1988; Walleck, 1990). Loop diuretics minimize the potential for electrolyte and osmolality disturbances (Bakay and Wood, 1985).

Fluid dehydration has also been advocated to control ICP. The patient with isolated head injury is not usually hypovolemic and thus does not require large-volume fluid replacement. Fluid replacement should be based on indicators of fluid and electrolyte balance and on serum osmolality. Osmolality in the head-injured person should be between 305 and 310 mOsm/liter (normal, 275 to 296 mOsm/liter. Osmolality greater than 310 mOsm/liter can be dangerous and indicates a need to reduce or eliminate diuretic therapy (Spielman, 1988).

CONTROLLING METABOLIC ACTIVITY OF THE BRAIN

The pharmacologic control of cerebral metabolism is well established as a means of preventing cerebral dysfunction and controlling ICP. High doses of barbiturates (pentobarbital or thiopental) have been successful in reducing elevated ICP and protecting against cerebral hypoxia and ischemia. High doses of barbiturates stabilize cell membranes and produce superimposed coma, which reduces cerebral metabolism and cerebral blood flow (Marshall et al., 1979; Platt and Schiff, 1984).

Barbiturate therapy requires close monitoring of the patient. Because the ability to assess the neurologic status is lost, it is vital to monitor ICP and cerebral perfusion pressures in these patients. Because large doses of barbiturates may cause hypotension, endangering cerebral blood flow, mean arterial pressure monitoring is mandatory. Vasopressors may be required to maintain an adequate cerebral perfusion pressure. Although barbiturates effectively reduce ICP, they have not been demonstrated to decrease mortality (Marshall et al., 1979; Spielman, 1988).

Narcotic sedation has been used as an alternative to barbiturate therapy to control agitation and ICP. Fentanyl, a short-acting narcotic, can be administered intravenously in doses of 1 to 5 mL. This agent may be used to blunt the effect of turning or suctioning. The advantage of narcotic therapy is the ability to reverse the effect with naloxone, allowing neurologic assessment. Morphine should be avoided because it dilates cerebral blood vessels and may raise the ICP.

Many agents are being investigated for use in head-injured patients and ICP management including alfaxalone, dimethyl sulfoxide, lidocaine, and phenytoin. These agents should be used only as part of approved clinical research protocols.

Alfaxalone is an intravenous steroid anesthetic that has properties similar to those of barbiturates. This agent combines the advantages of pentobarbital with the capability for rapid reversal and no systemic hypotension (Versari et al., 1980; Spielman, 1988).

Dimethyl sulfoxide (DMSO) has been used in experiments to treat cerebral stroke, acute brain injury, and spinal cord injury. DMSO is suspected to cause vasodilation, osmotic diuresis, decreased ICP, and decreased cellular oxygen consumption. A side effect, severe hypernatremia, has made this agent unacceptable for current use (Marshall et al., 1984).

Lidocaine is an anesthetic agent that suppresses neuronal activity and cerebral metabolism. This agent has been used to suppress the cough reflex and prevent arterial hypertension with endotracheal intubation. Lidocaine has been used prior to suctioning in doses of 50 to 100 mg given 2 minutes before the procedure to reduce sudden increases in ICP. This agent has not been shown to be effective in all subjects studied (Donegan and Bedford, 1980), making further study of its efficacy necessary.

Phenytoin is a widely used anticonvulsant similar to barbiturates that is known to decrease cerebral oxygen consumption. Clinical studies of this agent are required to test its effectiveness in the head-injured patient (Walleck, 1987).

CONTROLLING BRAIN ACIDOSIS

Based on the assumption that brain tissue and CSF acidosis follows brain injury and contributes to the injury, alkylating agents are being used experimentally in head-injured patients. Buffering agents used include tromethamine (THAM) and superoxidase dysmutane (SOD). Although clinical trials have just begun, results are promising (Becker, 1985).

SURGICAL MANAGEMENT

Recognition and rapid treatment of mass lesions are vital to improving outcomes in head-injured patients. A primary cause of death in patients who "talked and died" was delay in surgical intervention (Marshall et al., 1983; Rose et al., 1977). Causes of delay include failure to identify the rate and significance of neurologic deterioration and inappropriately relating deterioration to alcohol intoxication or other neurologic pathology. CT scanning has significantly reduced the misdiagnosis of mass lesions. Determination of the need for surgery is facilitated by assessment and CT scan findings.

Nursing Management

Nursing care of patients with traumatic head injury is guided by the severity of the injury and the medical plan of care. Nursing diagnoses involve actual and potential problems and focus on preventing secondary brain injury due to hypoxemia, hypercarbia, increased cerebral metabolism, and increased ICP in order to maximize functional outcome.

ALTERATION IN CEREBRAL TISSUE PERFUSION RELATED TO INJURY

Cerebral injury results in disrupted local blood supply, cerebral edema, and possible systemic cardiovascular instability, especially hypotension.

Expected Outcomes. Neurologic status improves or remains stable, ICP of the resting patient is less than 15 mm Hg, and cerebral perfusion pressure is more than 50 mm Hg.

Neurologic assessments focus on level of consciousness (using the Glasgow coma scale), pupillary reflexes, and motor function. Careful documentation of findings allows identification of subtle changes of deterioration over time.

ICP monitoring is essential in patients with severe head injury and may be accomplished through the intraventricular, subdural, subarachnoid, or epidural route. Accuracy of the system is important to ensure that interventions can be accomplished when indicated. ICP monitoring also reflects the impact of nursing care activities and therapy on ICP.

The head of the bed should be elevated 30 to 45 degrees to facilitate venous drainage of the head and decrease ICP. Head and body alignment should also be maintained.

POTENTIAL FOR INJURY DUE TO DECREASED INTRACRANIAL ADAPTIVE CAPACITY

Expected Outcomes. ICP remains at less than 15 mm Hg during nursing care activities or returns to baseline less than 15 mm Hg immediately, and cerebral perfusion pressure remains above 50 mm Hg.

Because routine care activities may increase ICP, patients with decreased adaptive capacity require use of interventions for positioning, suctioning, and hygiene that are based on research in this area.

Because activities have an accumulated effect on ICP, care activities should be spaced to allow inter-

vals of inactivity that permits the ICP to return to baseline. The patient's baseline should be assessed prior to any intervention to enable adequate evaluation of the effect of the intervention. If ICP is monitored, the cerebral perfusion pressure (CPP) should be calculated during all activities using the following formula:

$$MAP - ICP = CPP$$

Nursing care procedures may safely be performed as long as the CPP remains at or above 50 mm Hg.

Hyperoxygenation and hyperventilation before, during, and after suctioning blunt the effect of suctioning on ICP. Limiting suctioning to no more than 10 seconds at a time also limits elevation of ICP.

Controlling the cerebral metabolic rate (CMR) increases the adaptive capacity of the brain. A quiet environment with meaningful stimuli should be basic to the care of these patients. Barbiturate coma decreases $CMRO_2$ and protects the neuroglial cells but may also cause cardiovascular depression, requiring continuous monitoring and appropriate interventions for hypotension. Narcotic sedation appears to be more beneficial in controlling or decreasing cerebral metabolism.

INEFFECTIVE AIRWAY CLEARANCE DUE TO DECREASED LEVEL OF CONSCIOUSNESS AND POSSIBLE CRANIAL NERVE DYSFUNCTION

Expected Outcomes. Patent airway is maintained, there is no evidence of pulmonary complications, lungs are clear to auscultation, and ABGs remain within normal limits (with slight hyperoxemia and hypocarbia).

Respiratory parameters should be carefully monitored by taking vital signs including rate and pattern of respirations, airway pressures, breath sounds, and chest expansion. Gag and swallowing reflexes should be assessed as indicated.

The patient should be turned every 2 hours to facilitate mobilization of pulmonary secretions. If possible, chest physiotherapy also aids in removing secretions. Research by McQuillan (1986) demonstrated the safety of the Trendelenburg (head-down) position during chest physiotherapy in patients with closed head injury. Using the bedside monitor to record the MAP, mean intracranial pressure (MICP) and CPP (calculated) were measured throughout chest physiotherapy; an adequate CPP was demonstrated in the head-down position with improved general oxygenation following the therapy. Replications of this work are currently being done to validate the safety of this technique.

Viscosity of secretions should be monitored, and increased humidification of inspired air, added hydration, or mucolytic agents requested for patients with viscous secretions.

POTENTIAL ALTERED BODY TEMPERATURE DUE TO LOSS OF THERMOREGULATION OR INFECTION

Expected Outcome. Patient remains normothermic, or temperature elevations are rapidly identified and interventions begun before complications occur.

A rectal temperature probe allows continuous monitoring and identification of rapid temperature changes. Because of increased cerebral metabolism, temperature elevations should be avoided. Interventions to reduce temperature elevations need to be implemented quickly, including use of acetaminophen, tepid water baths, ice packs, or cooling blankets. Rapid cooling and prolonged use of hypothermia blankets should be avoided because of the potential for shivering, which increases cerebral metabolism and ICP. Shivering is avoided by reducing the temperature slowly and discontinuing use of hypothermia when the temperature reaches 100°F. Sometimes sedation with thorazine is required to control shivering (Spielman, 1988).

POTENTIAL FLUID VOLUME DEFICIT

Fluid volume deficits may be due to therapeutic osmotic diuresis or fluid restriction, or to complications of diabetes insipidus (DI) or syndrome of inappropriate secretion of antidiuretic hormone (SIADH).

Expected Outcome. Fluid and electrolyte balance is maintained.

Intake and output should be monitored hourly in these patients. Taking weights daily or biweekly assists in identifying the presence of fluid retention. Signs of DI that require notification of the physician include thirst, dehydration, diluted urine, diuresis, low specific gravity, decreased urine osmolality, elevated serum osmolality, and elevated serum sodium level. Patients with an altered level of consciousness are often unable to report their thirst and require astute observation by the nurse to recognize symptoms of DI. Therapy for DI involves replacement of free water and administration of aqueous vasopressin or vasopressin tannate in oil.

SIADH results in continuous resorption of water from the renal tubule causing a serum osmolality of less than 280 mOsm/kg of water and hyponatremia (<125 mEq/liter). SIADH leads to water intoxication and cerebral edema. Indicators that require notification of the physician include weight gain without obvious edema, neurologic deterioration, and increased urinary sodium. Treatment depends on severity but includes fluid restriction, furosemide, and, possibly, judicious use of hypertonic saline (3% sodium chloride).

Excess fluid loss may also result from "neurogenic sweats" during which 500 to 1000 mL of fluid may be lost. Calculation of fluid loss should include comment on the number of diaphoretic episodes.

POTENTIAL FOR INJURY DUE TO INCREASED CEREBRAL METABOLISM AND ICP DURING SEIZURES

Expected Outcome. Seizures do not occur, or, if they do, no injury results from the seizure.

Anticonvulsants are used to prevent and control seizures. Seizure precautions should be used with all patients with head injury, including keeping the bed in a low position, keeping side rails up and padded (as necessary), and keeping an airway at the bedside.

If a seizure occurs, the onset, characteristics, and duration of abnormal activity should be carefully documented. A patent airway should be maintained and supplemental oxygen provided. Objects that may injure the patient should be removed. Restraint of the patient during the seizure may result in injury and should be avoided.

POTENTIAL IMPAIRED SKIN INTEGRITY

Skin integrity may be impaired by immobility due to a decreased level of consciousness, enforced bed rest, or spasticity.

Expected Outcome. Skin remains dry, intact, and nonerythemic.

Because of decreased consciousness, these patients are especially prone to pressure necrosis. As long as the patient is able to respond to commands, he or she should be encouraged to change position frequently. Family members should be taught the importance of moving the patient and how to avoid shear forces during the process so that they can help the patient move appropriately. A turning schedule should be established and posted at the bedside to ensure that turning patterns are uniformly followed. Inspection, massage, and application of lotion to all bony prominences should be accomplished each time the patient is turned and positioned. Skin should be kept free from excess moisture but not allowed to become dry and scaly; bath oil is preferred to soap for bed baths. Plastic incontinent pads in direct contact with the patient's skin should be avoided because these trap moisture and heat and may macerate the skin.

Adjunctive devices cannot replace basic nursing interventions in preventing pressure necrosis, but they aid in preventing skin breakdown. Air mattresses and mechanical beds (kinetic tables, air-fluidized mattresses, circolectric beds, Stryker frames) may be useful depending on the patient's condition. Judicious use of heel and elbow pads may also be helpful.

POTENTIAL FOR INJURY FROM JOINT CONTRACTURES DUE TO MUSCLE WEAKNESS, HYPERTONICITY, OR IMMOBILITY

Expected Outcomes. Patient is able to use all extremities without residual loss of range of motion or complaints of pain or stiffness.

As long as the patient responds to commands, the patient and family should be instructed in the need for and how to perform range of motion exercises. An exercise program should be established in which all joints are moved through their full range of motion every 8 hours. Ideally, the exercise schedule is posted at the bedside to encourage patient and family participation.

Proper positioning is vital to maintain optimal joint function. The ideal joint position is neutral. Splints, orthoses, and adjunctive aids (antirotation boots) may be indicated to prevent or correct joint contracture.

INEFFECTIVE FAMILY COPING: COMPROMISED OR DISABLING

Family coping may be impeded by the overwhelming aspects of head injury to a family member.

Expected Outcome. Patient and family are able to cope effectively with the situation as shown by their positive adaptations to limitations.

Family members may experience fear, helplessness, and a loss of control. The family can be assisted in identifying tasks that they can perform (exercises, repositioning) that aid the patient's recovery. When the patient responds, encourage the family to listen to the patient's concerns and identify problem areas in which the staff can intervene. Encourage the family to talk about current events and reminisce about the patient's past to facilitate communication with the semicomatose or comatose patient. Incorporate the family's efforts into the care of the patient to the extent with which they are comfortable.

Extensive support services are available through the National Head Injury Foundation, Inc. This organization was established by the family of a severely head-injured child and has grown rapidly to become a national organization that emphasizes support for head-injured patients and their families as well as support for research in this area. For local chapters and support group information, families and patients may be referred to the National Head Injury Foundation, 333 Turnpike Road, Southborough, MA 01772; telephone (800) 444–6443. (See also Chap. 7, Psychosocial Needs of Families.)

POTENTIAL FOR INJURY BY DEEP VEIN THROMBOSIS DUE TO VENOSTASIS

Expected Outcome. Lower extremity circumference will be monitored daily, and increases of greater than 2 cm will be promptly reported; antithrombus regimen will be maintained.

Circumference of the lower extremities should be checked daily. Standard measurement sites are ensured by marking the positions on the legs with permanent markers. Measurements should be made at midcalf and midthigh on each leg.

When not contraindicated, a variety of methods may be used to prevent venostasis. Promotion of venous return is facilitated by range of motion exercises that should be done every 4 hours. Antiembolism hose or alternating pneumatic pressure devices on the legs aid venous return. Elevating the entire lower extremity 10 to 15 degrees prevents venostasis. Kinetic treatment beds, which rotate the patient for up to 20 hours a day, also promote venous return. Early mobilization is of benefit to these patients.

ALTERED THOUGHT PROCESSES DUE TO THE EFFECT OF BRAIN INJURY ON COGNITIVE PROCESSES

Expected Outcome. Patient will attain maximal cognitive function, and independent functioning will be encouraged.

Assessment of cognitive function aids in determining level of consciousness. The Rancho Los Amigos scale of cognitive function aids in this assessment (see Table 32–2) (Hagen et al., 1979). When scale scores of level I, II, or III are noted, the patient should receive low-level stimulation of all senses. Most stimulation of the patient is the natural outcome of nursing care, i.e., from turning and bathing. Soft conversational speech or music provides auditory stimuli. Taste is stimulated through oral hygiene or Popsicles. Pleasant smelling substances close to the patient stimulate the olfactory senses. To prevent confusion, stimulation of one sense at a time should be attempted (Spielman, 1988).

Additional nursing diagnoses for these patients may include self-care deficit, impaired verbal communication, and alteration in nutrition: less than body requirements. Holistic patient care will prevent secondary injury to the brain and avoid the many complications to which these patients are prone.

Medical and nursing management of the traumatic head-injured patient has changed dramatically in the past decade. Improved emergency medical care, improved CT scanning in diagnosis, and more aggressive treatment have combined to produce better patient outcomes.

ISCHEMIC BRAIN INJURY

Brain ischemia has many causes and may be focal or generalized. Focal ischemia may result from traumatic brain injury, cerebral vasospasm, or stroke, whereas generalized ischemia may be caused by asphyxiation, severe hypovolemia, or cardiorespiratory arrest. This section focuses on global ischemia as the cause of brain injury.

Pathophysiology of Ischemic Injury

METABOLIC CONSEQUENCES

Cessation of brain circulation results in depletion of oxygen and a loss of consciousness within about

10 seconds and in the depletion of glucose and adenosine triphosphate (ATP) within about 5 minutes (Safar, 1983). Without ATP the cellular sodium-potassium pump fails, leading to cerebral edema (cytotoxic edema). If ischemia continues, the blood–brain barrier is damaged, allowing vasogenic edema to increase the injury (Jordan, 1983). After 4 to 7 minutes of total ischemia, calcium enters the cell and mitochondria (Jordan, 1983; Safar, 1983). The occipital cortex, basal ganglia, and diencephalon are more susceptible to ischemic-anoxic damage than the frontal and temporal cortices (Nemoto, 1978).

REPERFUSION

Once cerebral perfusion is restored, reperfusion occurs nonhomogeneously throughout the brain. The nonuniformity of reperfusion probably results from varied degrees of vasospasm, increased local tissue pressures, capillary compression, and intravascular coagulation (Nemoto, 1978). Reperfusion may provoke secondary changes that evolve into microscopic infarctions (Safar, 1983). These microinfarctions probably result from transient vasoparalysis, hypoperfusion from blood cell sludging, catecholamine-stimulated hypermetabolism, tissue acidosis, free chemical radicals that damage cell membranes, or varying degrees of intra- or extracellular edema. These secondary changes may be exacerbated by noncerebral organ system failures.

NO-REFLOW PHENOMENON

In 1968, Ames and colleagues described a no-reflow phenomenon as causing continuing neuronal injury despite reestablished circulation (Jordan, 1983). Ames speculated that lack of perfusion resulted from increased blood viscosity in low- and no-flow states because of red blood cell aggregation. He theorized that during stasis of global ischemia, red blood cells aggregate in dependent areas, increasing blood viscosity. When circulation is reestablished, the vessels are unable to be reperfused, resulting in patchy areas of no flow (Fischer, 1974).

Clinical Presentation

Following global ischemia, the patient is usually comatose with a Glasgow coma scale score of less than 8. Duration of coma following resuscitation from global ischemia is the most reliable indicator of patient outcome (Epstein and Hamilton, 1983).

NEUROLOGIC ASSESSMENT

Neurologic assessment of the patient with ischemic brain injury is performed in the same way as that for traumatic brain injury (see p. 684). The following discussion focuses on predictors of outcomes that are based on assessment data.

LEVEL OF CONSCIOUSNESS

The coma following global ischemic injury implies bilateral diffuse dysfunction of the cerebral hemispheres or, less commonly, damage to the upper brainstem (Koehler and Michael, 1985). Although presentation in coma does not necessarily indicate a poor prognosis, coma lasting more than 2 days is associated with a poor neurologic outcome (Koehler and Michael, 1985; Safar, 1983). Motor unresponsiveness or flaccidity, assessed through the Glasgow coma scale, carries a poor prognosis (Snyder et al., 1977). Flexion and extension posturing are serious indicators but are not effective as predictors.

PUPIL CHANGES AND OTHER BRAINSTEM REFLEXES

Absence of pupillary light response and of oculocephalic (doll's eyes) and oculovestibular (caloric) reflexes at 6 and 12 hours after ischemic insult signifies a poor but not hopeless prognosis (Snyder et al., 1977). Pupil size and spontaneous eye movements are unreliable indicators of prognosis. Snyder and colleagues (1981) reported 100% mortality in patients with 3 or more reflex abnormalities or those without corneal or pupillary light reflexes 3 hours following global ischemic-anoxic injury from cardiac arrest.

VITAL SIGNS

Studies of the predictiveness of vital signs have been inconclusive. The presence or absence of spontaneous breathing shows promise as a predictor, but further study is needed.

INTRACRANIAL PRESSURE MONITORING

Although sudden ischemia results in a fluid shift causing cerebral edema, this may not raise ICP unless the insult is prolonged and severe (Safar, 1983). Monitoring ICP is not common following an ischemic insult, but most physicians assume that cerebral edema occurs and intervene to prevent elevated ICP.

LABORATORY FINDINGS

Examination of CSF provides important information about the degree of cellular injury. Concentrations of adenosine triphosphate and phosphocreatinine return to normal following brain injury even without functional recovery. Elevations of amino acids persist following injury, and the level of alanine increases in proportion to the duration of global ischemia (Debard, 1983).

The CSF creatine kinase level appears to be related to the amount of cellular injury and may eventually provide a means of assessing the potential for recovery. Measures of serum and CSF creatine kinase–BB fraction (CKBB) at 6 hours after cardiac arrest are related to neurologic outcome and survival (Longstreth et al., 1981). CSF CKBB levels of less than 2 units/liter are associated with a good recovery, whereas levels greater than 10 units/liter were associated with a poor outcome or death.

Diagnostic Procedures

A variety of procedures are used to diagnose ischemic injuries. Many of these diagnostic tests were discussed in greater detail in the previous section of this chapter on closed head injury (see p. 687). Only the specific utilization of these procedures for ischemic injuries will be described here.

After 72 hours, CT scans will identify cerebral edema and areas of infarction. CT scans also rule out other causes of coma, e.g., mass lesions.

Because MRI clearly demonstrates edema, it shows promise as a diagnostic tool in patients with ischemic injuries. MRI also demonstrates small areas of infarction earlier than CT scans. More experience with this tool is necessary to evaluate its effectiveness. The major problem with using MRI to follow global ischemia is that the patient often requires ventilatory support and no metal can be used in the area of the MRI because it creates a strong magnetic field.

Evoked potentials test neuronal pathway integrity and detect marginally functional neurons missed in neurologic assessment. Relationships between evoked potentials and patient prognosis have been identified (DeBard, 1983).

Electroencephalography (EEG) is most effective as a negative predictor, i.e., for identifying nonsurvivors. It is not effective in predicting survivors or disability (DeBard, 1983).

Monitoring of cerebral blood flow can determine areas of hyperemia and poor reperfusion following ischemic injury. With further research, this procedure may be shown to be effective in guiding treatment to maximize blood flow to ischemic areas.

Medical Management

Neurologic deficit may be intensified following a global ischemic insult by extracranial complications of hypoxemia, hypotension, hypercarbia, hyperthermia, or sepsis. Preventing these complications may ameliorate the neurologic deficit. Safar (1981) outlined the therapeutic goals that should be set following ischemic insult:

1. Control the MAP at between 90 and 100 mm Hg, maintaining systolic blood pressure at 100 mm Hg or higher.
2. Maintain Pa_{CO_2} at 25 to 35 mm Hg.
3. Provide for Pa_{O_2} at 100 mm Hg or more.
4. Keep arterial pH within a range of 7.3 to 7.6.
5. Decrease the cerebral metabolic rate for oxygen ($CMRO_2$) by immobilizing the patient with sedatives and paralytic agents.

6. Maintain the following blood value limits:
   a. Hematocrit, 30% to 40%
   b. Electrolytes, within normal limits
   c. Plasma colloidal osmotic pressure, 15 mm Hg or higher
   d. Albumin, 3 g/100 mL or above
   e. Serum osmolality, 280 to 315 mOsm/L
   f. Glucose, 100 to 300 mg/100 mL
7. Maintain normothermia or mild hypothermia for a short interval.
8. Monitor CNS status closely using the Glasgow coma scale, EEG, and CT scanning.

These are the immediate goals of therapy, and these procedures are maintained throughout the period of unresponsiveness (usually 2 to 7 days) (Safar, 1983).

OXYGENATION

The uninjured brain uses 20% of all consumed oxygen (3.5 cc/100 g tissue per minute). Mild hyperoxygenation ($Pa_{O_2} \geq 100$ mm Hg) should be provided immediately after an ischemic insult. Controlled ventilation with an FI_{O_2} of 1.0 ensures an adequate Pa_{O_2}, Pa_{CO_2}, and pH. Neuromuscular blockade may be needed to ensure controlled ventilation.

HYPERVENTILATION

Hyperventilation decreases Pa_{CO_2} and produces a constriction of cerebral blood vessels. Careful monitoring of hyperventilation and Pa_{CO_2} is important because a Pa_{CO_2} of less than 25 mm Hg may result in excessive vasoconstriction in reactive brain areas while also decreasing cardiac output (Jagger and Bobovsky, 1983).

GLUCOCORTICOSTEROIDS

Use of corticosteroids after an ischemic insult with coma is controversial (Safar, 1983). The potential benefits of steroids are discussed earlier in this chapter in the section on traumatic brain injury. There are no studies of the use of steroids following global ischemic injury. Following ischemic brain injury the use of steroids would be an adjunctive measure used as part of a combination of brain resuscitation measures (Safar, 1983).

DIURETIC THERAPY

Short-term, low-dose osmotherapy with mannitol may be used to control increased ICP. Although this therapy may be initially helpful with large doses of osmotic agents, rebound edema may occur, limiting its usefulness (Safar, 1983).

The use of dimethyl sulfoxide (DMSO) is currently being investigated to control ICP. DMSO is a water-soluble, organic industrial solvent. Low concentrations of DMSO have been used in clinical trials in patients with cerebral stroke, spinal cord injury, and acute brain injury. DMSO is suspected to cause cerebral vasodilation, osmotic diuresis, changes in prostaglandin actions, stabilization of mitochondria from tissue injury, decreased cellular oxygen consumption during anoxia, and decreased ICP. In humans this agent also acts as a potent diuretic.

The main side effects of DMSO are nausea, headache, ventricular toxicity demonstrated by dysrhythmias with prolonged use, respiratory stimulation, and hemolysis (Martin, 1983). Hemolysis appears to be related to use of high concentrations of DMSO. More research is needed on the use of this agent in global ischemic injury.

CEREBRAL METABOLIC CONTROL

Barbiturate coma (discussed earlier under traumatic brain injury, p. 689) reduces cerebral metabolism and suppresses seizure activity. Barbiturates may also block noxious stimuli through their anesthetic effects; scavenge-free chemical radicals resulting from ischemia alter metabolic pathways and suppress catecholamine hypermetabolism (Safar, 1983). Clinical trials show promising results with thiopental and pentobarbital. A recently published study reports research done in nine countries utilizing thiopental (30 mg/kg) as the barbiturate. This report noted that barbiturates do not exert a marked improvement on neurologic recovery after global ischemia. Because of the frequent cardiorespiratory side effects, the researchers did not recommend routine use of barbiturates after cardiac arrest (Abramson et al, 1985).

Phenytoin is being investigated for its action in controlling the cerebral metabolic rate by decreasing cerebral oxygen consumption ($CMRO_2$). Phenytoin promotes sodium efflux from neurons, stabilizing and protecting the neuron from hyperexcitability. Phenytoin may also enhance cerebral blood flow by promoting vasodilation after ischemia and may increase brain energy reserves (Martin, 1983). The loading dose is 7 mg/kg given intravenously, but dosage schedules for brain resuscitation have not been established. Administration of phenytoin should not exceed 50 mg/minute because of the associated potential for cardiac dysrhythmia, hypotension, or arrest.

MAINTAINING HOMEOSTASIS

Facilitating the patient's rapid return to homeostasis is assumed to be beneficial following ischemic injury. Initial therapy involves the ABCs of emergency care (airway, breathing, and circulation). Opening the airway and providing supplemental oxygen will reduce hypoxia and minimize further brain injury. Tracheal intubation and controlled ventilation are usually necessary.

Avoidance of hypotension or severe hypertension are essential; the usual goal is a normotension (MAP = 100 mm Hg). Safar (1983) has advocated the benefits of mild sustained hypertension (MAP ≤ 150 mm Hg) following the restoration of cerebral circulation. Severe hypertension increases cerebral blood volume and ICP, which may cause cerebral edema or hemorrhage and exacerbate the postischemic neurologic deficit.

Plain dextrose and water solutions should not be used for fluid replacement because they contribute to cerebral edema. Infusions of 5% to 10% dextrose in 0.25 to 0.5 normal saline solutions are preferred (Safar, 1983).

Normothermia or mild hypothermia should be maintained. Hypothermia reduces cerebral metabolism, but the actual mechanism of action following ischemic brain injury has yet to be documented. Complications of hypothermia include cardiac dysrhythmias, increased blood viscosity and reduced tissue blood flow, increased potential for infection, and stress ulcers (Safar, 1983). A study of the risks and benefits of hypothermia is needed to document the efficacy of this therapy.

OTHER INVESTIGATIONAL DRUGS

Calcium Channel Blockers. Safar has described the postischemic reperfusion phenomenon as a result of cerebral vasospasm, blood cell sludging, and clotting (1983). Calcium and sodium ions that accumulate within neurons may also contribute to destructive metabolic activity following cerebral ischemia. Calcium channel blockers may deter the increased blood viscosity and decrease vasospasm. For example, nifedipine counters elevated ionized calcium in cytosol and mitochondria, and flunarizine interferes with calcium ion entry into the plasma membrane (Raffsen and Davis, 1989). The future role of calcium channel blockers in patients with brain resuscitation is uncertain (Martin, 1983).

Lidocaine. Lidocaine's role in controlling increased ICP was discussed earlier (see p. 689). Lidocaine may also play a role as a calcium channel blocker, so that intravenous or endotracheal administration of lidocaine may eventually be used to treat ischemic injuries.

Other agents currently being studied are prostaglandin blocking agents, opiate blockers (naloxone), and brain-buffering agents (THAM). These agents may be useful in preventing or correcting the metabolic effects of global ischemia.

Nursing Management

Nursing care of survivors of global ischemic injury is challenging, as is the care of any comatose patient with an unknown prognosis. Recovery from global ischemic injury is determined not only by the course of the pathologic state but also by the intensity of the nursing care provided for the patient. In addition to the following nursing diagnoses, those discussed under traumatic brain injury are also applicable.

TOTAL SELF-CARE DEFICIT DUE TO UNCONSCIOUSNESS

Expected Outcome. The patient's basic care needs will be met until the patient is able to participate in self-care.

All basic care activities are provided based on the patient's tolerance. Care activities should be done at intervals to prevent the cumulative effects of these activities on ICP.

IMPAIRED VERBAL COMMUNICATION DUE TO COMA, INTUBATION, OR VARYING DEGREES OF UNCONSCIOUSNESS

Expected Outcome. Patient maintains optimal communication level for his or her physiologic state. Family members actively communicate with the patient.

An inability to communicate contributes to the overwhelming fear and frustration experienced by patients and families. The nurse needs to use imagination to help these patients communicate their needs as long as possible. Letter and picture boards may be used for selected patients. Although use of communication boards is tedious and time-consuming, they may be the only means of communication by the patient with others. It is important to spend time with the patient and family to teach them how to use the communication method adequately. The nurse should acknowledge the patient's frustration about the slowness of communication while encouraging patience. The family needs to be encouraged to continue to communicate with the patient, reminiscing about past experiences and discussing current events. If the patient has awareness, this will provide sensory stimulation while also allowing the family to feel capable of contributing to the care of the patient. (See also Chap. 6.)

ALTERATION IN NUTRITION: LESS THAN BODY REQUIREMENTS

Malnutrition may be due to immobility, decreased gastrointestinal mobility, dysphagia, anorexia, or depression.

Expected Outcome. Patient maintains ideal body weight.

Enteric or parenteral nutrition is necessary with comatose patients to accommodate the increased metabolism due to the stress of the injury. Patients who are receiving tube feedings should be assessed for excessive gastric residual (>50 mL in 2 hours for those on continuous feedings and >100 mL for those on every 4 hour feedings). Metoclopramide hydrochloride may be ordered to facilitate gastric emptying. Most institutions have established regimens for patients receiving total parenteral nutrition to ensure adequate hydration and nutrition while avoiding any iatrogenic influences of the therapy. Weights taken daily or every other day allow monitoring of nutritional status. Serum albumen and total lymphocyte counts also aid in determining the patient's nutritional status.

INEFFECTIVE FAMILY COPING: COMPROMISED OR DISABLING

Coping abilities may be ineffective due to the overwhelming aspects of the patient's illness on the family.

Expected Outcome. Patient, when appropriate, and family are able to cope effectively with the situation as shown by the absence of abnormal reactions.

Family members may also experience fear, helplessness, and a loss of control. The family can be helped to identify tasks that they can perform (range of motion exercises, sensory stimulation, repositioning) that aid the patient's recovery. Encourage the family to talk about current events and reminisce about the patient's past to distract the patient from the reality of the current situation and foster a sense of hope. The family should be allowed to participate in the care of the patient to the extent that they are comfortable. (See also Chap. 7.)

METABOLIC DISORDERS

Because the brain is sensitive to changes in homeostasis, disturbances in other body systems often affect brain function. Changes in consciousness are early indicators of most acute and subacute metabolic encephalopathies. Primary metabolic encephalopathies include Creutzfeldt-Jakob disease, Alzheimer syndrome, Huntington chorea, and Pick disease. Secondary encephalopathies, which are related to dysfunction of other organ systems, include pancreatic, liver, or kidney disease; toxic reactions to drugs or heavy metals; and hypoxia. This section focuses on secondary metabolic encephalopathies related to liver failure, hypoglycemia, renal failure, and toxic reactions.

Hepatic Encephalopathy

Severe liver disease eventually involves the central nervous system, usually with progressive mental, cerebellar, or extrapyramidal deterioration (Plum and Posner, 1982). The actual pathogenesis depends on the underlying hepatic disease. Although many toxic agents or deficiencies have been proposed as potential causes of hepatic coma, none has been clearly linked to this process.

Hypoglycemia

Hypoglycemia is a common cause of metabolic coma and is associated with great variation in the presenting findings (Plum and Posner, 1982). The major pathology of hypoglycemia involves the cerebral hemispheres, and the resulting encephalopathy presents in one of the following ways (Plum and Posner, 1982):

1. Delirium with mental changes varying from sleepy confusion to wild mania.
2. Coma with signs of multifocal brainstem dysfunction including central neurogenic hyperventilation, decerebration, and hypothermia with pupillary reaction preserved.
3. Strokelike findings with focal neurologic signs with or without coma and shifting neurologic deficits.
4. Single or multiple generalized convulsions and postictal coma.

Uremic Encephalopathy

Although no specific neurologic pathology has been identified, renal failure is associated with encephalopathy. The cause of symptoms is unknown, but symptoms are usually reversed following dialysis. Rapid onset of encephalopathy is associated with florid delirium, noisy agitation, delusions, and hallucinations. A slower onset is evidenced by dull confusion and inappropriate behavior that progresses to coma.

Toxic Reactions

Ingestion of large amounts of alcohol, barbiturates, sedatives, other drugs, poisons, and some heavy metals may result in encephalopathy. Toxic reactions may also follow absorption through the skin or inhalation. The mechanism of toxic reactions on the nervous system is unclear. With some drugs and alcohol there is a depression of central nervous system function, including the brainstem. Suggested mechanisms of action include interference with neurotransmitter synthesis or release, focal demyelination, axonal edema, or disruption of cellular biochemistry (Hickey, 1986).

Pathophysiology

The normal brain consumes 3.5 cc of oxygen/100 g tissue per minute; this is known as the cerebral metabolic rate for oxygen ($CMRO_2$) and represents 15% to 20% of the systemic oxygen consumed. $CMRO_2$ levels of 2.5 cc/100 g per minute are associated with changes in level of consciousness, and coma follows a $CMRO_2$ of 2.0 cc/100 g per minute. Normal cerebral blood flow is 50 to 60 mL/100 g per minute (Plum and Posner, 1982), and interferences in the rate of flow result in changes in consciousness.

Glucose is the main source of energy for the brain, but the brain is unable to store much glucose (only about 2 g). Each 100 g of brain tissue require 5.5 mg of glucose/minute. Lacking adequate glucose, the brain begins anaerobic metabolism, which results in lactic acidosis.

The severity of symptoms is related to the amount and areas of the brain affected. Symptoms are generally aggravated by the compensatory mechanisms of hyperpnea, hypoventilation, metabolic acidosis or alkalosis, or fluid shifts.

Clinical Presentation

Presenting signs are related to the etiology, depth of coma, complications associated with the primary illness, and treatment of the primary illness. Differential diagnosis of metabolic coma is difficult but is assisted by careful assessment of the level of consciousness, respirations, pupillary response, extraocular movements, motor function, and EEG evaluations.

Level of consciousness varies from mild drowsiness to total unresponsiveness. The pupillary response aids in distinguishing metabolic from structural disease. A preserved pupillary response to light in the presence of decerebrate rigidity or muscle flaccidity and respiratory depression suggests metabolic coma (Plum and Posner, 1982). The eyes in patients with metabolic coma usually rove randomly.

Motor changes may be either nonspecific in strength, tone, and reflexes accompanied by seizures, or they may involve adventitious movement with weakness, loss of tone, grasp reflexes, and prehensile sucking. Tremors may be present in patients with metabolic coma but are usually absent at rest. Asterixis is associated with metabolic coma and is characterized by sudden palmar or plantar flapping (liver flap), which can occur at rest or in response to dorsiflexion. Some patients develop multifocal myoclonus, which is a sudden nonrhythmic, nonpatterned gross twitching of all muscle groups.

Respiratory changes may include hyperventilation, hypoventilation, or Cheyne-Stokes respirations. Hypoventilation may indicate respiratory compensation characteristic of metabolic alkalosis or severe respiratory depression and acidosis.

EEG changes aid in diagnosing metabolic coma. They usually involve diffuse slowing with no focal change.

A complete history is vital because a past history of diabetes, liver disease, or renal pathology provides clues to changes in the level of consciousness. However, a history is often unobtainable, and neurologic assessment is difficult due to coma. Because hypoglycemia is the most frequent cause of metabolic coma, most patients are given a trial of 25 to 50 g of intravenous glucose in the emergency department.

Laboratory Findings

Laboratory findings aid in determining the primary cause of metabolic encephalopathy. Increases in serum ammonia aid in the diagnosis of hepatic encephalopathy. The CSF may also demonstrate bilirubin (Plum and Posner, 1982). In patients with hypoglycemia serum and CSF glucose levels (normally two-thirds of the serum glucose level) may be useful. Blood urea nitrogen and electrolyte levels do not reflect the presence of uremic encephalopathy. However, it is important to rule out water intoxication (serum osmolality <260 mOsm/liter and serum sodium <120 mEq/liter). A toxicology screen is helpful in assessing the presence of toxic etiologies of metabolic coma. Drug, alcohol, and heavy metal levels should be determined as indicated.

Diagnostic Procedures

LUMBAR PUNCTURE

CSF determinations aid in diagnosing the causes of coma. In addition to the changes in CSF mentioned earlier (see discussion of ischemic injuries, p. 692), uremia may cause an aseptic meningitis with increased lymphocytes and polymorphonuclear leukocytes in the CSF and increased CSF pressure (160 to 180 mm H$_2$O).

ELECTROENCEPHALOGRAPHY

EEG shows generalized diffuse slowing in patients with metabolic coma as opposed to focal changes in structural disease. Seizures often accompany metabolic coma, and EEG aids in diagnosing the seizure type.

COMPUTED TOMOGRAPHY

CT scanning can differentiate between structural and metabolic etiologies, but it cannot aid in determining the cause of metabolic encephalopathy.

Medical Management

Medical management begins with treatment of the primary cause of the metabolic encephalopathy while providing supportive care of the comatose patient. Most patients require intubation and ventilation for hypoventilation or hyperventilation. Arterial blood gases are assessed frequently to evaluate acid-base balance and oxygenation. Brain resuscitation measures (discussed earlier in the section on ischemic brain injury) should be initiated. Because cerebral edema may result from metabolic encephalopathy, management of increased ICP is critical (see earlier discussion in the section on traumatic brain injury).

Prognosis of these patients is good once the pri-
mary etiology has been treated. Hypoglycemia and uremic encephalopathy are usually reversed quickly through administration of glucose or dialysis.

Nursing Management

Care of patients with metabolic coma is complex, and the nurse must be aware of the underlying medical illness as well as the neurologic dysfunction. Nursing goals involve preventing further injury while the primary medical condition is being treated. The nursing diagnoses discussed for the patient with traumatic brain injury are also appropriate for the care of these patients.

SEIZURES

Epilepsy is a Greek word meaning "to be seized by a force from without." Epilepsy is a chronic seizure disorder of the cerebral tissues characterized by recurrent paroxysmal episodes of disturbed skeletal motor function, sensation, autonomic visceral function, behavior, or consciousness (Hickey, 1986).

Seizures are a symptom of central nervous system irritability characterized by abnormal neuronal discharge. Epilepsy is a syndrome rather than a disease because seizures are often a manifestation of a disease.

Classification of Seizures

Attempts to classify seizures began with Hippocrates, and since then classification schemes have been based on symptomatology, electrophysiology, anatomic origin, etiology, or response to therapy (Hickey, 1986). Two currently used classifications are partial (focal) and generalized (unlocalized) seizures.

Partial seizures affect certain areas of the brain, the signs and symptoms being dependent on the area involved. Consciousness is usually present as long as the seizure involves only one hemisphere. If midline structures such as the thalamus, hypothalamus, or midbrain are involved, unconsciousness results.

Both cerebral hemispheres and connections with subcortical nuclei are involved in generalized seizures, and consciousness is always impaired. Some generalized seizures begin as focal or parietal seizures and progress to the generalized form.

Since 1969, the International Classification of Epileptic Seizures by Gastaut has been used (Table 32–3). This classification system is based on the nature of the onset of seizures.

Most seizures are thought to be caused by a few abnormally hyperactive or hypersensitive neurons, which form an epileptogenic focus. These neurons are physiologically and chemically abnormal and are always hyperactive compared to normal neurons

TABLE 32–3. International Classification of Epileptic Seizures

I. Partial seizures (seizures beginning locally)
  A. Partial seizures with elementary symptomatology (generally without impairment of consciousness)
    1. With motor symptoms (includes Jacksonian seizures)
    2. With special sensory or somatosensory symptoms
    3. With autonomic symptoms
    4. Compound forms
  B. Partial seizures with complex symptomatology (generally with impairment of consciousness) (temporal lobe or psychomotor seizures)
    1. With impairment of consciousness only
    2. With cognitive symptomatology
    3. With affective symptomatology
    4. With "psychosensory" symptomatology
    5. With "psychomotor" symptomatology (automatisms)
    6. Compound forms
  C. Partial seizures secondarily generalized

II. Generalized seizures (bilaterally symmetrical and without local onset)
  A. Absences (petit mal)
  B. Bilateral massive epileptic myoclonus
  C. Infantile spasms
  D. Clonic seizures
  E. Tonic seizures
  F. Tonic-clonic seizures
  G. Atonic seizures
  H. Akinetic seizures

III. Unilateral seizures (or predominantly)

IV. Unclassified epileptic seizures (due to incomplete data)

From Gastaut, H. (1970). Clinical and electroencephalographical classification of epileptic seizures. *Epilepsia,* 11, 102–113.

(Hickey, 1986). The epileptogenic focus is autonomous and emits an excessive number of paroxysmal discharges.

It is unclear what cellular mechanism initiates a seizure, but it has been postulated that an autonomous discharge may be enhanced or minimized by neurotransmitter substances on the postsynaptic membrane. After neuronal stimulation, depolarization occurs followed by a period of hyperpolarization that probably results from an inhibitory postsynaptic potential. Hyperpolarization is replaced by depolarization, which then increases in amplitude, causing the cell to "fire" (depolarize) repeatedly, allowing sustained depolarization and seizure activity.

Cessation of seizure activity is associated with membrane hyperpolarization, thought to be the result of electrical potential generated by the sodium pump. On an EEG this result is evidenced by high-voltage spikes and waves that gradually decrease in size and frequency. Focal cells cease firing, suppressing in turn the abnormal firing of the surface cells.

The period following a seizure is called the postictal period; it is characterized by confusion, headache, lethargy, or a deep sleep. There may also be temporary paresis, aphasia, or hemianopsia (Hickey, 1986).

Cerebral blood flow during a seizure is increased dramatically to approximately 250% of normal to meet the metabolic demands; cerebral oxygen consumption is also increased. Increased cerebral blood flow meets demand as long as hypoxemia, hypoglycemia, and cardiac irregularities do not occur. In these situations the brain may require more energy than it can produce with the limited oxygen or glucose available. Cellular exhaustion and destruction occur in these situations.

Clinical Presentation

Because seizures are associated with numerous primary diseases, it is important to rule out any underlying causes. Diagnosis is based on the history and on the physical and neurologic assessments. Questions about seizure activity should include those relating to age at onset, progression of the seizure, loss of consciousness, subjective and objective details, frequency and length of the seizure, any associated prodrome or aura, and resulting injuries (Hickey, 1986). The status of the patient in the postictal phase should also be documented.

Diagnostic Data

Baseline laboratory data should include complete blood count, urinalysis, serum chemistries (especially glucose, urea, sodium, and potassium), and liver enzymes. If indicated, a toxicology screen may sometimes be helpful.

The most useful diagnostic tool is the EEG. EEGs not only aid in diagnosing the type of seizure but may also isolate the epileptogenic focus through its abnormal neuronal activity. Certain EEG waveform abnormalities are associated with specific seizure disorders. Absence (petit mal) seizures classically have a 3-second spike wave complex seen on all leads. High-voltage spikes are seen with tonic-clonic seizures. Temporal lobe, psychomotor, or complex partial seizures are illustrated by spike complexes over the involved temporal lobe; these complexes may be square-topped and occur at a rate of four to six per second. Other waves include theta and delta waves. Theta waves may be normal whereas delta waves are associated with necrotic brain tissue resulting from infarction, tumor, or abscess. Because EEG is frequently normal between seizure events, video EEGs and 24-hour EEGs are more commonly used.

Lumbar puncture may reveal CSF with an increased cell count indicating infection as the source of the seizures. CSF pressure exceeding 180 mm H_2O may indicate a tumor or other source of elevated ICP as the cause of the seizure.

Computed tomography is frequently used to rule out sources of seizures such as tumor, aneurysm, stroke, and cerebral edema. Normal CT scans rule out these potential causes of the seizure. When available, magnetic resonance imaging is becoming the diagnostic tool of choice over CT.

Medical Management

The first principle of therapy is to treat the underlying cause of the seizure when an underlying cause can be identified. When no primary cause is known, the goal of therapy is to control the seizures.

Seventy-five per cent of patients with seizures are controlled with medication (Hickey, 1986). It is important to remember that drugs control but do not cure the seizures. Some drugs are more effective than others for specific seizures. Once the seizure type has been identified, the drug of choice is prescribed and dosage regulated until a therapeutic level is achieved. If control is not achieved, then the initial drug is tapered as the alternative drugs are instituted. Some patients require combination therapy, e.g., phenytoin and phenobarbital. Sometimes a second drug is used to decrease the dosage of the initial drug to avoid toxicity. Of the many anticonvulsant drugs available, some appear to be better at controlling specific seizures than others (see Table 32–4). Patients on long-term drug therapy should be closely monitored for toxicity. Serum levels should be periodically assessed to ensure that adequate therapeutic levels are maintained.

TABLE 32–4. Drugs Used for Management of Seizures

Medication	Seizure Type
Phenytoin (Dilantin) Phenobarbital (Luminal) Primidone (Mysoline) Mephenytoin (Mesantoin)	Tonic-clonic (generalized) and focal sensory
Phenytoin (Dilantin) Phenobarbital (Luminal) Primidone (Mysoline) Carbamazepine (Tegretol) Mephenytoin (Mesantoin) Phenacemide (Phenurone)	Partial seizures with complex symptomatology (temporal lobe or psychomotor seizures)
Ethosuximide (Zarontin) Trimehadione (Tridione) Methsuximide (Celontin) Valproic acid (Depakane) Paramethadione (Paradione) Phensuximide (Milontin)	Generalized—absences (petit mal seizures)
Nitrazepam (Mogadon)	Generalized—myoclonus, akinetic seizures
Prednisone Corticotropin (ACTH)	Generalized—infantile spasms
Diazepam (Valium) Paraldehyde Thiopental Lorazepam	Status epilepticus

Surgical Intervention

Patients who fail to respond to drug therapy may be candidates for surgical ablation of the epileptogenic focus. Only 5% of epileptic patients fit this category (Hickey, 1986). Patients with loss of quality of life and a unilateral focus in an area that will not result in major neurologic deficit after surgery are considered for operative intervention (Norman, 1981). The procedure is done under local anesthesia to allow interaction with the patient and to permit EEG and cortical stimulation during the procedure. Once the epileptogenic focus has been identified and removed and the EEG no longer demonstrates abnormal activity, the patient is completely anesthetized to allow closure of the incision. The patient is managed in the same way as any postcraniotomy patient. Following postoperative recovery, anticonvulsants are slowly tapered as long as no seizure activity is encountered. Periodic EEG is done to monitor for recurrence. Drug tapering is done slowly over a period of 2 years; if no seizure activity occurs, the drug is discontinued.

Status Epilepticus

Status epilepticus is a medical emergency defined as recurrent, generalized seizures that occur at a frequency that does not allow the patient to regain consciousness between tonic-clonic activity. Metabolic exhaustion eventually occurs because of lack of sufficient oxygen and glucose to meet the metabolic demands of the brain. About 10% of all epileptics develop this condition. Concurrent impaired respirations compound the problem because they contribute to hypoxemia.

The goals of therapy are to control the seizures and restore normal cerebral metabolism. Establishing and maintaining an airway while providing supplemental oxygen are essential for these patients. An intravenous line should be used to replace fluids and provide medications. Valium and lorazepam are the drugs of choice; other drugs that may be used include phenobarbital, amobarbital, and phenytoin. As long as the seizure continues, a search should be made for a primary cause to allow treatment of the initiating etiology. Brain damage or death may result from status epilepticus, so control of the seizure activity is mandatory.

Nursing Management

Nursing management of patients with seizures focuses on preventing the complications of seizures and avoiding injury during seizures. Teaching the patient and family about seizures and anticonvulsant therapy begins in the intensive care unit. The following nursing diagnoses are aimed at the patient with status epilepticus and tonic-clonic seizure activity.

Impaired Gas Exchange

Due to Obstructed Airway or Changes in Respiratory Status During a Seizure

Expected Outcome. The patient's airway will remain patent, and the patient will demonstrate normal gas exchange.

An airway should be kept at the bedside of seizure-prone patients to aid in maintaining an open airway during seizures. Oxygen should also be available for administration during the seizure. Frequent assessment of respirations during and after the seizure should be performed. ABGs should be drawn in the postictal period to determine the patient's oxygen and carbon dioxide levels.

Aspiration is a common complication of tonic-clonic seizures and status epilepticus. Following a seizure, auscultation is important to note areas of decreased or absent breath sounds, which should then be reported to the physician. If aspiration is suspected, aggressive pulmonary toilet, including chest physiotherapy, should be begun promptly.

Potential for Injury

Due to Trauma Incurred During the Seizure

Expected Outcome. Patient is protected from injury.

During tonic-clonic movements the patient's side rails should be up and padded. Objects that may injure the patient should be removed from the immediate area. Loosen any tight clothing, especially around the neck. Do not restrain the patient's movements during the seizure, but ensure a clear area in the patient's immediate vicinity; ensure that restraints are removed from the previously restrained patient.

If the patient is aware of a pre-ictal aura, instruct the patient to lie down when this occurs to prevent injury from falling.

Knowledge Deficit

Related to Medication Therapy

Expected Outcome. Patient or family member is able to verbalize understanding of the rationale for therapy, name of the medication, dosage, schedule, precautions, and commonly encountered side effects.

When the patient or family is assessed as being ready to learn, he or they should be instructed about the need for medication to control seizures, including the need for continuous therapy to ensure adequate blood levels and periodic laboratory testing. The patient is taught the name, schedule, dosage, precautions, and potential side effects for the prescribed medication. A handout is provided that reviews this information so that the patient can refer to it at home (these are available from the American Association of Hospital Pharmacists). Ensure that the patient knows what to do if a dose is missed and that he has a phone number to call for any questions that arise. If the patient is taking other medications concurrently, ensure that there are no drug interactions or additional precautions of which the patient should be aware. Instruct the patient to check all new prescription and nonprescription drugs with a neurologist prior to taking them.

Noncompliance with Therapy

Due to Nonacceptance of the Diagnosis or Embarrassment

Expected Outcome. Patient verbalizes understanding of the need to adhere to therapy, and anticonvulsant serum levels are within therapeutic range.

Instruct the patient about the seizure process and the role of the medication in controlling, not curing, the seizure disorder. The need for continued follow-up by the physician should be stressed. Patient education begins in the intensive care unit and is continually reinforced until discharge.

Anxiety

Related to the Unpredictability of Seizure Activity

Expected Outcome. The patient is able to discuss the source of anxiety, and there is no evidence of uncontrolled anxiety.

The patient's verbal and nonverbal cues should be assessed for increased anxiety. Attempt to aid the patient in identifying the source of anxiety. Discuss with the patient means used in the past to cope and attempt to integrate one of these coping behaviors to control the current anxiety. Clarify information and correct misconceptions. Identify new stress reduction techniques for the patient. If necessary, contact a clinical specialist in psychiatric nursing for assistance. (See also Chap. 6.)

Disturbances in Self-Concept

Changes in Self-Esteem Related to the Diagnosis of Seizures

Expected Outcome. The patient maintains self-esteem.

Assess the patient's self-concept. Spend time with the patient, using touch to support the patient's self-concept and self-esteem. Allow the patient to participate in his care and give him as much control as possible in planning his own care. This is an essential aspect of care that will require increasing emphasis and expansion as the patient recovers, especially after transfer from the intensive care unit. However, intensive care nurses need to keep in mind this important aspect of the patient's care.

Patients and families may also be referred to the Epilepsy Foundation of America, 4351 Garden City Drive, Suite 406, Landover, MD 20785; telephone (800) 332-1000.

ncp nursing care plan

TRAUMATIC BRAIN INJURY

1. Altered cerebral tissue perfusion related to:
Cerebral injury

Outcome Criteria	Nursing Interventions
Neurologic status improves or remains stable. Intracranial pressure of resting patients is less than 15 mm Hg. Cerebral perfusion pressure is greater than 50 mm Hg.	Carefully assess neurologic status focusing on level of consciousness (using Glasgow coma scale), pupillary reflexes, and motor function. Document findings. Monitor intracranial pressure. Elevate the head of the bed 30 to 45 degrees and maintain head and body in alignment.

2. Potential injury related to:
Decreased intracranial adaptive capacity

Outcome Criteria	Nursing Interventions
Intracranial pressure remains less than 15 mm Hg during nursing care activities or returns to baseline immediately. Cerebral perfusion pressure remains greater than 50 mm Hg.	Space care activities to allow intervals of inactivity, allowing intracranial pressure to return to baseline. Assess baseline intracranial pressure prior to any intervention. Perform nursing care activities only if cerebral perfusion pressure remains greater than 50 mm Hg. Hyperoxygenate and hyperventilate before, during, and after tracheal suctioning. Limit suctioning to no more than 10 seconds at a time. Maintain a quiet environment with meaningful stimuli.

3. Ineffective airway clearance related to:
Decreased level of consciousness
Possible cranial nerve dysfunction

Outcome Criteria	Nursing Interventions
Patent airway is maintained. Patient is free of pulmonary complications. Lungs are clear to auscultation. Arterial blood gas values remain within normal limits.	Carefully monitor respiratory parameters by taking vital signs, including rate and pattern of ventilation, airway pressures, breath sounds, and chest expansion. Assess gag and swallowing reflexes. Turn patient every 2 hours to mobilize secretions. Perform chest physiotherapy as needed. Monitor viscosity of secretions and increase humidification by adding hydration and/or administer mucolytic agents as necessary.

4. Potential altered body temperature related to:
Loss of thermoregulation
Infection

Outcome Criteria	Nursing Interventions
Patient remains normothermic. If fever occurs, temperature elevations are rapidly identified and interventions begun before complications occur.	Monitor temperature continuously. Avoid temperature elevations and reduce elevations quickly, using acetaminophen, tepid water baths, ice packs, or cooling blankets. Avoid rapid cooling and prolonged use of cooling blankets. Control shivering using chlorpromazine (Thorazine) as needed.

5. Potential fluid volume deficit related to:
Therapeutic osmotic diuresis or fluid restriction
Complications of diabetes insipidus or syndrome of inappropriate secretion of antidiuretic hormone

Outcome Criteria	Nursing Interventions

Fluid and electrolyte balance is maintained.	Monitor intake and output hourly.
	Weigh patient daily or biweekly.
	Notify physician of symptoms of diabetes insipidus:
	   Thirst
	   Dehydration
	   Dilute urine
	   Diuresis
	   Low urine specific gravity
	   Decreased urine osmolality
	   Elevated serum osmolality
	   Elevated serum sodium
	Notify physician of symptoms of syndrome of inappropriate secretion of antidiuretic hormone:
	   Weight gain without obvious edema
	   Neurologic deterioration
	   Increased serum sodium
	Include the number of diaphoretic episodes in the calculation of fluid loss.

6. Potential impaired skin integrity related to:
Decreased level of consciousness
Enforced bedrest
Spasticity

Outcome Criteria	Nursing Interventions
Skin remains dry, intact, and nonerythemic.	If responsive, encourage patient to change position frequently. Establish and post a turning schedule. Teach family members the importance of moving the patient and how to avoid shear forces. Inspect, massage, and apply lotion to all bony prominences with each turn and repositioning. Keep skin free from excess moisture but prevent dry, scaly skin. Avoid plastic incontinence pads in direct contact with patient's skin. Use adjunctive devices such as air mattresses, mechanical beds, and heel and elbow protectors.

7. Potential injury: joint contractures related to:
Muscle weakness
Hypotonicity
Immobility

Outcome Criteria	Nursing Interventions
Patient is able to use all extremities without residual loss of range of motion. Patient experiences no joint pain or stiffness.	Instruct patient and family in the need for and how to perform range of motion exercises. Establish and post an exercise program in which all joints are moved through their full range of motion at least once every 8 hours. Maintain proper positioning—ideally in the neutral position. Use splints, orthoses, and antirotation boots as needed.

8. Ineffective family coping: compromised or disabling related to:
Patient's head injury

Outcome Criteria	Nursing Interventions
Patient and family members are able to cope effectively as shown by their positive adaptation to patient limitations.	Assist family members in identifying tasks that they can perform that aid in the patient's recovery. Encourage family members to listen to the patient's concerns and identify problem areas in which the staff can intervene. Encourage family members to talk about current events and reminisce about the patient's past if the patient is semicomatose or comatose. Incorporate the family's efforts into the patient's care to the extent that they are comfortable. Encourage family members to participate in support groups such as those sponsored by the National Head Injury Foundation, Inc.

9. Potential injury: deep vein thrombosis related to:
Venostasis
Immobility

Nursing Care Plan continued on following page

Outcome Criteria	Nursing Interventions
Lower extremity circumference will be monitored daily. Increases of greater than 2 cm in leg circumference are promptly reported. Antithrombus regimen is maintained.	Check the circumference of lower legs daily using standard, marked measuring sites at mid-calf and mid-thigh. Provide range of motion exercises every 4 hours to lower extremities. Use antiembolism hose or alternating pneumatic pressure devices. Elevate entire lower extremity 10 to 15 degrees. Consider use of a kinetic treatment bed. As soon as possible, assist with mobilization.

10. Altered thought processes related to:
   Effects of brain injury

Outcome Criteria	Nursing Interventions
Patient will attain maximal cognitive function. Independent functioning is encouraged.	Assess cognitive function using the Rancho Los Amigos scale. Provide low-level stimulation for patients at level I, II, and III. In addition to natural stimulation from nursing care (bathing, turning, etc.), provide sensory stimulation as follows: Auditory: soft conversational speech or music Taste: oral hygiene or Popsicles Olfactory: pleasant smelling substances Stimulate one sense at a time to prevent confusion.

PATIENTS WITH SEIZURES

1. Impaired gas exchange related to:
   Changes in ventilation during seizure
   Obstructed airway

Outcome Criteria	Nursing Interventions
Airway remains patent. Normal ventilation and gas exchange.	Keep an airway at the bedside to aid in maintaining an open airway. Ensure that oxygen, flowmeter, and mask are readily available. Frequently assess ventilation during and following seizures. Obtain arterial blood gases in the postictal period. Auscultate breath sounds following seizures to detect if aspiration occurred. If aspiration is suspected, begin aggressive pulmonary toilet immediately, including chest physiotherapy.

2. Potential injury related to:
   Trauma incurred during seizure

Outcome Criteria	Nursing Interventions
Patient does not sustain injury.	Keep side rails up and padded during tonic-clonic movements. Remove objects that might cause injury. Loosen any tight-fitting clothing, especially around the neck. Clear area immediately around the patient. Do not restrain patient movement. Remove restraints from patient if previously restrained. Instruct patient to lie down if aware of a preictal aura when it occurs.

3. Knowledge deficit related to:
   Medication therapy

Outcome Criteria	Nursing Interventions
Patient or a family member is able to verbalize an understanding of the medication therapy, including rationale, names of medications, their dose, schedule, precautions, and commonly encountered side effects.	After assessment indicates readiness, instruct patient or family member about the need for medications to control seizures, including the need for continuous and consistent therapy to ensure adequate blood levels and periodic laboratory testing. Teach patient (or family member) the names of the medication, the doses, schedule, precautions, and potential side effects. Provide a printed review of the medications for the patient (or family) to refer to at home. Ensure that the patient (or family member) knows what to do if a dose is missed. Ensure that the patient (or family member) has a phone number to call for answering any questions. If the patient is taking other medications, ensure that there are no drug interactions or additional precautions that require the patient's awareness. Instruct patient (or family member) to check all new prescriptions and nonprescription drugs with a neurologist prior to taking them.

4. **Noncompliance with therapy related to:**
   Nonacceptance of the diagnosis of seizure disorder
   Embarrassment

Outcome Criteria	Nursing Interventions
Patient verbalizes understanding of the need to adhere to therapy. Anticonvulsant serum levels are within the therapeutic range.	Instruct patient about the seizure process and the role of medications in controlling, not curing, the seizure disorder. Stress the need for continued follow-up by the physician.

5. **Anxiety related to:**
   Unpredictability of seizure disorder

Outcome Criteria	Nursing Interventions
Patient is able to discuss the source of anxiety. There is no evidence of uncontrolled anxiety.	Assess patient's verbal and nonverbal cues for increased anxiety. Attempt to aid the patient in indentifying the source of anxiety. Discuss with the patient means used in the past to cope and attempt to integrate one of these coping behaviors to control the current anxiety. Clarify information and correct misconceptions. Identify new stress reduction techniques for the patient. Contact a psychiatric clinical nurse specialist for assistance if necessary.

6. **Disturbance in self-concept related to:**
   Diagnosis of seizure disorder

Outcome Criteria	Nursing Interventions
Patient maintains self-esteem.	Assess the patient's self-concept. Spend time with the patient, using touch to support the patient's self-concept and self-esteem. Allow the patient to participate in his care and give as much control as possible in planning his own care. Refer patients and families to the Epilepsy Foundation of America as necessary.

PATIENTS WITH ISCHEMIC BRAIN INJURY

1. **Total self-care deficit related to:**
   Unconsciousness

Outcome Criteria	Nursing Interventions
Basic care needs are met until the patient is able to participate in self-care.	Provide all basic care activities based on the patient's ability to tolerate. Provide care activities at intervals to prevent cumulative effects on intracranial pressure.

2. **Impaired verbal communication related to:**
   Varying degrees of consciousness, including coma
   Intubation

Outcome Criteria	Nursing Interventions
Patients maintain optimal communication level for their physiologic states. Family members actively communicate with the patients.	Use alternate means of communication such as letter and picture boards. Spend time with the patient and family to teach them how to use the chosen communication method accurately. Acknowledge the patient's frustration about the slowness of communication while encouraging patience. Encourage family members to continue to communicate with the patient, reminiscing about past experiences and discussing current events.

3. **Altered nutrition: less than body requirements related to:**
   Immobility
   Decreased gastrointestinal motility
   Dysphagia
   Anorexia
   Depression

Nursing Care Plan continued on following page

Outcome Criteria	Nursing Interventions
Patient maintains ideal body weight. Plasma protein levels are normal.	Provide enteral or parenteral nutrition. For patients receiving enteral nutrition, assess for excessive gastric residual volumes. Administer metoclopramide as needed to facilitate gastric emptying. Monitor weight daily or every other day. Monitor serum albumin and total lymphocyte count weekly.

4. Ineffective family coping: compromised or disabling related to:
Overwhelming aspects of the patient's illness

Outcome Criteria	Nursing Interventions
Patient and family members cope effectively as evidenced by the absence of abnormal reactions.	Help family members identify tasks that they can perform that aid the patient's recovery. Encourage family members to talk to the patients about current events and reminisce about the past. Allow family members to participate in the care of patients to the extent that they feel comfortable.

SUMMARY

Brain injury has serious consequences for the patient. Whether the injury is traumatic, ischemic, or metabolic, these patients require vigilant and continuous nursing care. Accurate and knowledgeable assessment is important to identify the neurologic status and the subtle changes that may occur. Nursing care is aimed at meeting the physical, cognitive, and personal needs of these patients and can be a challenge for the nurse. This chapter has provided an overview of the major causes of brain injury and the current methods of medical and nursing care. This knowledge will aid the nurse in accepting the challenges of caring for these patients.

References

Abramson, N. S., Safar, P., Detre, K., et al. (1985). Randomized clinical study of thiopental loading in comatose survivors of cardiac arrest. *New England Journal of Medicine*, 314, 1982–83.

Ames, A., Wright, R. L., Kowanda, M., et al. (1968). Cerebral Ischemia II. The no reflow phenomenon. *American Journal of Pathology*, 52, 437.

Bakay, R. A. E., and Wood, J. H. (1985). Pathophysiology of cerebrospinal fluid. In D. P. Becker, and J. T. Povlishock (Eds.), *Central nervous system trauma status report 1985* (pp. 89–137). Bethesda, MD: National Institutes of Health/National Institutes of Neurological Disorders and Stroke.

Becker, D. P. (1985). Brain acidosis in head injury: A clinical trial. In D. P. Becker, and J. T. Povlishock (Eds.), *Central nervous system trauma status report 1985* (pp. 229– 242). Bethesda, MD: National Institutes of Health/National Institutes of Neurological Disorders and Stroke.

Becker, D. P., Miller, J. D., and Ward, D. (1977). The outcome from severe head injury with early diagnosis and intensive management. *Journal of Neurosurgery*, 47(3), 491–502.

Bowers, S. A., and Marshall, L. F. (1980). Outcome in 200 consecutive cases of severe head injury treated in San Diego County: A prospective study. *Neurosurgery*, 6(2), 237–242.

Bruce, D., Gennarelli, T., and Langfitt, T. (1978). Resuscitation from coma due to head injury. *Critical Care Medicine*, 6(4), 254–266.

Cepuzzo, M. L. J., Weiss, M. G., and Petersons, V. (1977). Effect of positive end-expiratory pressure ventilation on intracranial pressure in man. *Journal of Neurosurgery*, 46(2), 227–238.

Chapman, P. H. (1983). Infection with intracranial pressuring monitoring devices. In A. H. Ropper, S. K. Kennedy, and N. T. Zervas (Eds.), *Neurological and neurosurgical intensive care* (pp. 39–49). Baltimore: University Park Press.

Clifton, G. I., Robertson, G. S., and Kyper, K. (1983). Cardiovascular responses to severe head injury. *Journal of Neurosurgery*, 59(4), 447–454.

Conner, R. (1969). Myocardial damage secondary to brain lesions. *American Heart Journal*, 78(2), 145–148.

Cooper, P. R. (1985). Delayed brain injury: Secondary insults. In D. P. Becker, and J. T. Povlishock (Eds.), *Central nervous system trauma status report 1985* (pp. 217–228). Bethesda, MD: National Institutes of Health/National Institutes of Neurological Disorders and Stroke.

DeBard, M. L. (1983). Predictors in brain resuscitation. *Critical Care Quarterly*, 5(4), 91–98.

Donegan, M., and Bedford, R. (1980). Intravenously administered lidocaine prevents intracranial hypertension during endotracheal suctioning. *Anesthesiology*, 52(6), 516–518.

Epstein, F., and Hamilton, G. (1983). Initial approach to the brain injured patient. *Critical Care Quarterly*, 5(4), 13–29.

Fischer, E. G. (1974). Impaired perfusion following cerebrovascular stasis. *Archives of Neurology*, 33(1), 91–92.

Frost, E. A. M., and Gildenberg, P. L. (1977). Effect of positive end-expiratory pressure on intracranial pressure and compliance in brain injured patients. *Journal of Neurosurgery*, 46(2), 227–238.

Gennarelli, T. A. (1987). Cerebral concussion and diffuse brain injuries. In P. Cooper (Ed.), *Head injury* (2nd ed., pp. 108–123). Baltimore: Williams & Wilkins.

Gennarelli, T. A., Spielman, G. M., and Langfitt, T. W. (1982). Influence of the type of intracranial lesion on outcome from severe head injury. A multicenter study using a new classification system. *Journal of Neurosurgery*, 56(1), 26–32.

Gennarelli, T. A., and Thibault, L. (1982). Biomechanics of acute subdural hematoma. *Journal of Trauma*, 22(7), 680–685.

Hagen C., Malkmus, D., and Dunham, P. (1979). *Comprehensive physical management*. (pp. 87–88). Downey, CA: Professional Staff Association of Rancho Los Amigos Hospital.

Hickey, J. V. (1986). *The clinical practice of neurological and neurosurgical nursing* (2nd ed.). Philadelphia: J. B. Lippincott.

Hirsh, L. F. (1980). Chronic epidural hematomas. *Neurosurgery*, 6(4), 508–512.

Jagger, J. A., and Bobovsky, J. (1983). Nonpharmacologic therapeutic modalities. *Critical Care Quarterly*, 5(4), 31–41.

Jameson, K. G., and Yelland, J. D. N. (1972). Traumatic intracranial hematoma: Report of 63 surgically treated cases. *Journal of Neurosurgery*, 37(4), 528–532.

Jennett B., and Teasdale, G. (1981). *Management of head injuries*. Philadelphia: F. A. Davis.

Jordan, R. C. (1983). Pathophysiology of brain injury. *Critical Care Quarterly*, 5(4), 1–11.

Kalsbeck, W. D., McLaurin, R. L., and Harris, B. S. H., III (1980).

The national head and spinal cord injury survey: Major findings. *Journal of Neurosurgery*, 53(1), 19–31.

Klatzo, I. (1967). Neuropathological aspects of brain edema. *Journal of Neuropathophysiology and Experimental Neurology*, 20(1), 1–14.

Koehler, R. C., and Michael, J. R. (1985). Cardiopulmonary resuscitation, brain blood flow and neurologic recovery. In M. C. Rogers, and R. J. Fraystman (Eds.), *Critical care clinics: Neurologic intensive care*, 1(2), 195–204.

Krause, J. F. (1987). Epidemiology of head injury. In P. Cooper (Ed.), *Head injury* (2nd. ed., pp. 1–19). Baltimore: Williams & Wilkins.

Krause, J. F., Black, M. A., and Hessol, N. (1984). The incidence of acute brain injury and serious impairment in a defined population. *American Journal of Epidemiology*, 119(1), 186–201.

Langfitt, T. W. (1978). Measuring the outcome from head injury. *Journal of Neurosurgery*, 48(5), 673–678.

Levin, A., Duff, T., and Javid, M. (1979). Treatment of increased intracranial pressure: A comparison of different hyperosmotic agents and the use of thiopental. *Neurosurgery*, 5(5), 570–575.

Longstreth, W. T., Jr., Clayson, K. J., and Sume, S. M. (1981). Cerebrospinal fluid and serum creatine kinase BB activity after out-of-hospital cardiac arrest. *Neurology*, 31(3), 455–458.

Lundberg, N. (1960). Continuous recording and control of the ventricular-fluid pressure in neurosurgical practice. *Acta Psychiatrica Scandinavia*, 36 (Suppl. 149), 581–590.

Marshall, L. F., Barbar, D., and Toole, B. M. (1983). The oval pupil: Clinical significance and relationship to intracranial hypertension. *Journal of Neurosurgery*, 58(5), 566–568.

Marshall, L. F., Camp, P., and Bowers, S. (1984). Dimethylsulfoxide for the treatment of intracranial hypertension: A preliminary trial. *Neurosurgery*, 14(5), 659–663.

Marshall, L. F., Smith, R. W., and Shapero, H. M. (1979). The outcome with aggressive treatment in severe head injuries I: The significance of intracranial pressure monitoring. *Journal of Neurosurgery*, 50(1), 20–25.

Marshall, L. F., Toole, B. M., and Bowers, S. A. (1983). The national traumatic coma databank: II. Patients who talk and deteriorate: Implications for treatment. *Journal of Neurosurgery*, 59(2), 285–288.

Martin, M. L. (1983). Pharmacologic therapeutic modalities: Phenytoin, dimethyl sulfoxide, and calcium channel blockers. *Critical Care Quarterly*, 5(4), 72–81.

McQuillan, K. A. (1986). *The effects of the Trendelenburg position for postural drainage on cerebrovascular status in head injured patients.* Unpublished Master's thesis. Baltimore: University of Maryland, School of Nursing.

Miller, J. D. (1985). Head injury and brain ischemia—Implications for therapy. *British Journal of Anaesthesiology*, 57(1), 120–129.

Miller, J. D., Butterworth, J. F., Gudeman, S. K., et al. (1981). Further experience in the management of severe head injury. *Journal of Neurosurgery*, 54(3), 289–299.

Nemoto, E. M. (1978). Pathogenesis of cerebral ischemia-anoxia. *Critical Care Medicine*, 6(4), 203–214.

Nikas, D. L. (1987). Critical aspects of head trauma. *Critical Care Nursing Quarterly*, 10(1), 19–44.

Nikas, D. L., and Tolley, M. (1982). Acute head injury. In D. L. Nikas (Ed.), *The critically ill neurosurgical patient* (pp. 89–106). New York: Churchill Livingstone.

Norman, S. E. (1981). Surgical treatment of epilepsy. *American Journal of Nursing*, 81(5), 994–997.

Platt, J. H., and Schiff, S. J. (1984). High dose barbiturate therapy in neurosurgery and intensive care. *Neurosurgery*, 15(3), 427–444.

Plum, F., and Posner, J. B. (1982). *The diagnosis of stupor and coma* (3rd ed.). Philadelphia: F. A. Davis.

Purvis, J. (1966). Craniocerebral injuries due to missile and fragments. In W. Caveness, and A. E. Walker (Eds.), *Head injury* (pp. 133–141), Philadelphia: J. B. Lippincott.

Raffsen, M. L., and Davis, W. R. (1989). Cerebral function and preservation during cardiac arrest. *Critical Care Medicine*, 17(3), 283–292.

Rimel, R. W. (1982). Head injury: A challenging future for neurological nursing. *Journal of Neurosurgical Nursing*, 14(5), 207–209.

Rimel, R., and Lundgren, J. (1986). The head injured patient. In J. Lundgren (Ed.), *Acute neuroscience nursing: Concepts and care* (pp. 130–146). Boston: Jones and Barlett.

Rose, J., Valtonen, S., and Jennett, B. (1977). Avoidable factors contributing to death after head injury. *British Medical Journal*, 2(5), 615–623.

Safar, P. (1981). Dynamics of brain resuscitation after ischemic anoxia. *Hospital Practice*, (2), 67–72.

Safar, P. (1983). Brain resuscitation. In G. Tinker, and M. Rapin (Eds.), *Care of the critically ill patient* (pp. 751–763). Philadelphia: F. A. Davis.

Safar, P. (1988). Resuscitation from clinical death. *Critical Care Medicine*, 16(10), 923–941.

Shapiro, H. M. (1975). Intracranial hypertension: Therapeutic and anesthetic considerations. *Anesthesiology*, 43(3), 445–467.

Snyder, B. D., Gumnit, R. J., and Leppik, I. E. (1981). Neurologic prognosis after cardiopulmonary arrest. IV. Brainstem reflexes. *Neurology*, 31(9), 1092–1097.

Snyder, B. D., Ramirez-Lassepas, M., and Lippert, D. M. (1977). Neurologic status and prognosis after cardiopulmonary arrest. I. A retrospective study. *Neurology*, 27(7), 807–811.

Spielman, G. M. (1988). Central nervous system I: Head injuries. In V. D. Cardona, P. D. Hurn, P. J. B. Mason, et al. (Eds.), *Trauma nursing: From resuscitation through rehabilitation* (pp. 365–418). Philadelphia: W. B. Saunders.

Staller, A. G. (1987). Systemic effects of severe head trauma. *Critical Care Quarterly*, 10(1), 58–68.

Tyson, G., Strachan, W. E., and Newman, P. (1980). The role of craniectomy in the treatment of chronic subdural hematomas. *Journal of Neurosurgery*, 52(7), 776–781.

Versari, P., Vecci, C., and Arosio, M. (1980). Effects of althesin on intracranial hypertension in patients with severe head injury. In R. Shulman, A. Marmarrou, and J. Miller (Eds.), *Intracranial pressure* (pp. 610–613). New York: Springer-Verlag.

Walleck, C. A. (1987). Intracranial hypertension: Interventions and outcomes. *Critical Care Nursing Quarterly*, 10(1), 45–57.

Walleck, C. A. (1990). Acute head injury. In K. VonRueden, and C. A. Walleck (Eds.), *Critical care case studies*. Rockville, MD: Aspen.

Weiner, R. L., and Eisenberg, H. M. (1985). Radiologic evaluation of head injury: Key concepts. *Trauma Quarterly*, 2(1), 26–39.

33

Patients with Cerebral Vascular Disorders

Christina M. Whitney-Rainbolt

Cerebrovascular disease, or stroke, is a general term referring to an interruption in blood flow to or hemorrhage in an area of the brain, as shown by transient or permanent neurologic deficit. Since 1900 there have been significant advances in the understanding of the risk factors, etiology, and pathophysiology of stroke. Knowledge of cerebral structure and vascular anatomy, refinements in microneurosurgery, new and more accurate imaging techniques, and improved understanding of pharmacotherapy have enhanced our ability to treat stroke patients successfully. However, stroke continues to be a major cause of disability and is the third leading cause of death in the United States. In 1988, health care costs for stroke were estimated at $12.9 billion, including costs of health care providers, hospital and extended care use, medications, and loss of productivity (American Heart Association, 1988).

Stroke devastates the family and patient. Nearly half of the patients admitted for an acute neurologic condition have had a stroke. Nurses play a critical role in the care of these patients, making it imperative for them to understand thoroughly the etiology, risk factors, medical and surgical therapies, and nursing management of cerebrovascular disease. In addition to the preceding topics, this chapter will provide a brief overview of the cerebrovascular system (see also Chap. 31).

CEREBROVASCULAR SYSTEM

The cerebrovascular system is composed of extracranial and intracranial arteriovenous components. The extracranial arterial supply stems from the external carotid artery (ECA) and its main branches, the superficial temporal, posterior auricular, and occipital arteries. The occipital artery supplies the scalp and facial and neck muscles, whereas its terminal branches, through the cranial foramina, supply the meninges of the posterior fossa and dura mater. The supraorbital and supratrochlear branches of the ophthalmic artery, which arises from the internal carotid artery (ICA), supply the skin, muscles, and pericranium of the forehead (Sheldon, 1981).

The central nervous system receives 15% to 20% of the total cardiac output via the ICAs and vertebral arteries (Millikan et al., 1987). The ICA enters the skull through the foramen lacerum. The anterior and middle cerebral arteries and the terminal branches of the ICA and their subdivisions supply the cerebral hemispheres. Vertebral arteries, entering the skull through the foramen magnum, join to form the basilar artery, which branches terminally into the posterior cerebral artery. The vertebral-basilar system supplies the brainstem, cerebellum, and rostral portion of the midbrain.

Both superficial and internal cerebral venous systems drain through the dural sinuses, large collecting channels, which eventually empty into the internal jugular vein.

Collateral Circulation

The collateral vessel circulation may compensate for lost blood supply from an occluded primary vessel. Collateral circulation develops when there is a gradual decrease in cerebral blood flow through one of the primary arteries, provided that there has not been a prior occlusion of the collateral vessel. The three major collateral circulations are the extracranial, extracranial-intracranial, and intracranial anastomoses. The ECA is the main source of the extracranial collateral supply. The extracranial-intracranial anastomosis of the ECA and ICA occurs in the orbit. Also, cervical arteries may interconnect with the vertebral arteries (Millikan et al., 1987). The most important intracranial collateral channel is the circle of Willis (Fig. 33–1). The circle of Willis connects the anterior (carotid system) and posterior (vertebral-basilar system) circulations at the base of the brain. The anterior communicating artery allows collateral flow between the ICAs, and the posterior communicating artery connects the anterior and posterior circulations. There are many idiosyncratic variations of the circle of Willis that may affect the amount of collateral circulation provided. The leptomeningeal arteries, formed from the terminal branches of the anterior, middle, and posterior cerebral arteries, may provide intracranial collateral blood flow over the surface of the brain (Millikan et al., 1987).

Cerebral Blood Flow

Cerebral blood flow (CBF) is the blood flow (in mL) to a given amount of brain (100 g) per minute (Millikan et al., 1987). In a healthy adult the average CBF is 50 to 55 mL/100 g brain per minute. Blood flow to various areas of the brain are related to the activity of the area (Lassen et al., 1978), but cerebral autoregulation ensures constant CBF. The exact mechanism of cerebral autoregulation is incompletely understood (Strandgaard and Paulson, 1984), but by regulating the diameter of arterioles, CBF remains constant despite fluctuations in systemic blood pressure. Therefore, hypertension results in cerebral vasoconstriction, decreasing blood flow, whereas hypotension causes vasodilation and increased cerebral blood flow. When autoregulation fails, CBF is dependent on changes in systemic blood pressure. Situations associated with these changes are summarized

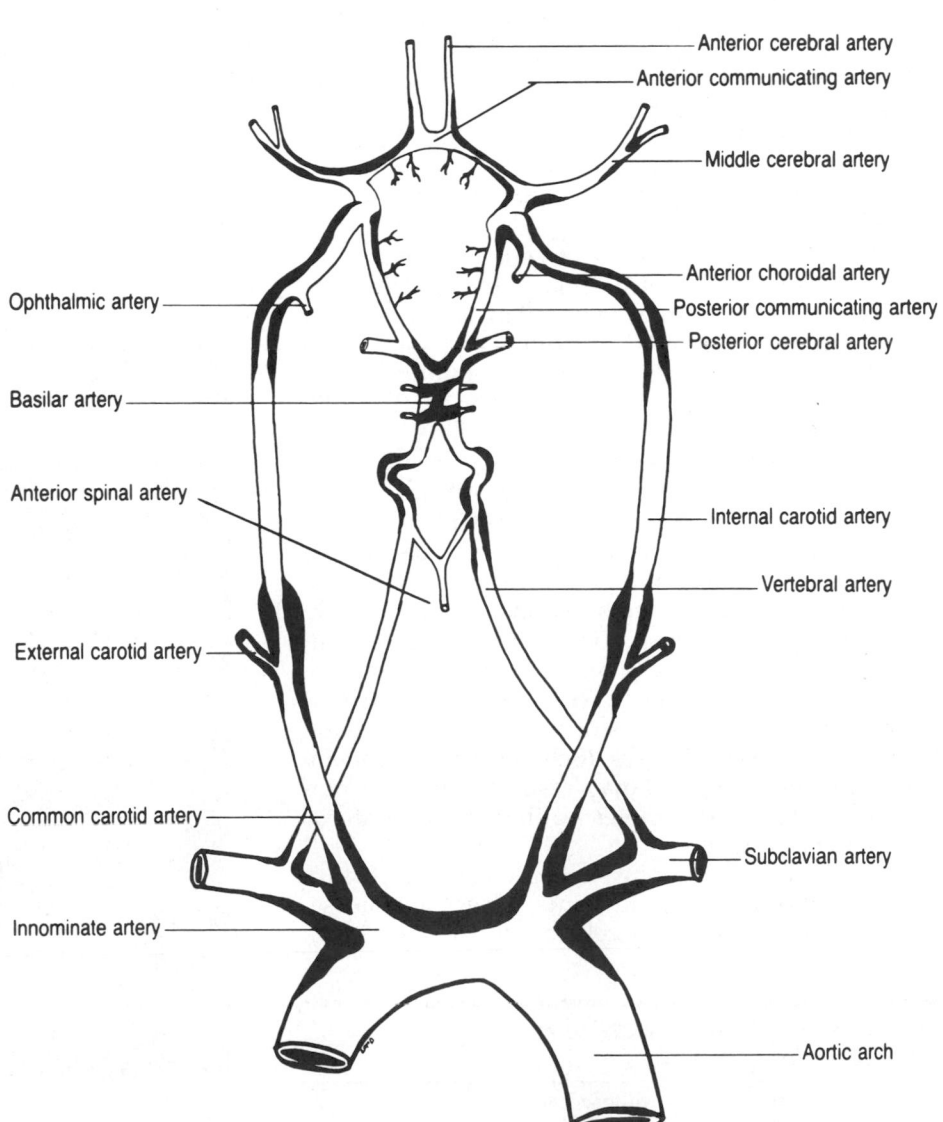

FIGURE 33–1. Diagram showing the carotid and vertebral arteries, their major branches, and the circle of Willis. The diagram also shows the common sites of atherosclerosis in extracranial and intracranial cerebral arteries, which are darkened. (From Millikan, C. H., McDowell, F., and Easton, J. D. (1987). *Stroke* (p. 41). Philadelphia: Lea & Febiger.)

in Table 33–1 (Millikan et al., 1987). The caliber of the resistance vessels is maximal at 40 mm Hg, so that autoregulation fails because no further decrease of resistance is possible, and blood flow becomes a function of pressure. Above 160 mm Hg the converse is true. Additional factors that alter CBF are listed in Table 33–2.

NONHEMORRHAGIC STROKE

Pathophysiology

Nonhemorrhagic, or ischemic, stroke results from significant reduction or obstruction of arterial or venous blood flow to or from an area of the brain. The size of the infarct is related to the vessel(s) involved, the length of time of critical reduction in CBF, and the availability of collateral circulation. Central nervous system function is affected when CBF is 20 mL/100 g brain per minute for 15 to 30 minutes (Millikan et al., 1987). With this rate of CBF, the amplitude of electrocortical activity on the electroencephalogram (EEG) as well as the amplitude of the evoked cortical responses decreases (Millikan et al., 1987). Changes in intracellular water and electrolyte concentration occur because the sodium-potassium pump is disrupted when the CBF is less than 10 to 15 mL/100 g brain per minute. Below this threshold cytotoxic (intracellular) edema immediately occurs (Schuier and Hossman, 1980). Cytotoxic edema results from an accumulation of extracellular potassium and intracellular sodium and calcium. A CBF of below 10 mL/100 g brain per minute results in irreversible cellular damage (Millikan et al., 1987). Also, lack of oxygen stimulates anaerobic glycolysis, leading to high lactic acid levels that contribute to permanent cellular damage (Raichle, 1983).

Collateral circulation may maintain CBF at 10 to 20 mL/100 g brain per minute, allowing normal cellular metabolism, avoiding permanent damage, and permitting partial or complete functional recovery. Without adequate perfusion, vasogenic (extracellular) edema resulting from cellular destruction and disruption of the blood–brain barrier occurs. Vasogenic edema occurs within hours of the original insult and peaks within 2 to 4 days (Schuier and Hossman, 1980). Extensive edema may result in shifts of portions of the brain, sometimes leading to transtentorial herniation and death.

Cerebral infarction occurs when an area of brain is deprived of oxygen and nutrients, especially glucose, long enough to produce cellular death (Fig. 33–2).

TABLE 33–1. Potential Causes of Failure of Cerebral Autoregulation

Acute cerebral lesion, either focal or global
Low perfusion pressure (below 40–60 mm Hg)
High perfusion pressure (greater than 160 mm Hg)

TABLE 33–2. Factors Influencing Cerebral Blood Flow (CBF)

Increase in CBF (Vasodilation)	Decrease in CBF (Vasoconstriction)
Increased arterial P_{CO_2}	Decreased arterial P_{CO_2}
Decreased arterial P_{O_2}	Increased arterial P_{O_2}
Decreased blood viscosity	Increased blood viscosity
Hyperthermia	Hypothermia
Increased cerebral metabolism	Increased intracranial pressure
	Drugs
	Anesthetics
	Barbiturates

This may result from thrombotic, embolic, or inflammatory processes.

Thrombosis

Thrombosis is a local obstruction of one or more vessels and is the most common cause of cerebral infarction. Thrombotic stroke most often results from atherosclerosis. In the Framingham study, 60% of all strokes were secondary to atherothrombotic brain infarction (Wolf et al., 1983). Factors that stimulate atheromatous plaque formation are poorly understood. From birth, the intima of the arterial wall begins to thicken. Smooth muscle cells, collagen, elastic fibers (elastin), and glycosaminoglycans con-

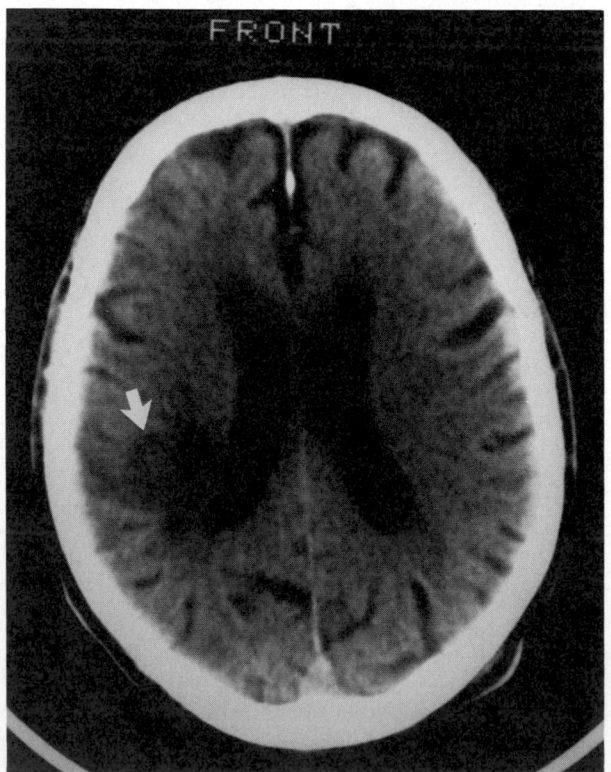

FIGURE 33–2. Axial CT scan of the head demonstrating a hypodense wedge-shaped area (*arrow*) in the right posterior hemisphere consistent with an ischemic infarct.

tribute to this thickening (Garcia and Geer, 1985). These components may act to trap elements of the plasma, including lipids, which form the core of the atheromatous plaque. Lipids, especially cholesterol, are released into the extracellular spaces, prompting an inflammatory response. Lipids are surrounded by collagen, smooth muscle cells, and fibrous tissue, all of which make up the plaque. Plaques vary in size, involving part or the entire circumference of the arterial wall. Over time, fibrous plaques may thicken, resulting in stenosis of the arterial lumen and restriction in CBF (Millikan et al., 1987). Extension of fibrous plaque is often related to mural thrombus formation. Also, hemorrhage into plaque, connective tissue synthesis, and lipid accumulation are thought to promote plaque enlargement (Garcia and Geer, 1985).

Atherosclerotic changes predominate in large arteries at points of bifurcation (Baker and Iannone, 1961). The process tends to begin in the aorta and then involve the coronary arteries; by the third decade of life there is evidence of atherosclerotic changes in the cerebral vessels (Moosey, 1959). Common loci of atherosclerosis in intra- and extracranial vascular systems are shown in Figure 33–1. Location, degree, rate of occlusion, and collateral supply influence the clinical response to a vascular lesion. Gradual narrowing of the arterial lumen allows development of collateral circulation, which may then become the primary blood supply of the area formerly supplied by the thrombosed vessel.

Cerebral venous thrombosis, though uncommon, may also cause ischemic brain disease. Most commonly involved are the dural sinuses and their tributary veins. Meningitis, local infection (e.g., sinusitis, otitis media, peritonsillar abscess), head injury, Behçet's disease, oral contraceptive use, and pregnancy may precipitate venous thrombosis, but the cause may also be idiopathic (Bousser et al., 1985).

Embolism

Ischemic stroke from embolism results from material formed proximally in the vascular tree that travels through the vascular system, lodging in a cerebral vessel and occluding distal blood flow. Although emboli may occur in any vessel, they are most commonly found in the distribution of the middle cerebral artery (Lhermitte, et al., 1970). Onset of symptoms is usually sudden, with maximal deficit at the onset, but a fluctuating course does not rule out the possibility of an embolus. Nineteen per cent of the Michael Reese Stroke Registry patients with embolic stroke presented with fluctuating, stepwise, or steady progression of a neurologic deficit (Caplan et al., 1983). Neurologic deficit may quickly resolve following break-up of an embolus or lysis of an associated thrombus (Furlan, 1985). Cardiac disease is the most common source of embolic stroke. Chronic atrial fibrillation, with or without valvular

disease, is the most common cause of cardioembolic stroke (Furlan, 1985; Hart et al., 1983; Sage and Van Uitert, 1983; Wolf et al., 1978). Young healthy adults (<45 years) with no other explanation of their cerebrovascular symptoms should be investigated for mitral valve prolapse as a possible cause of cerebroembolism (Jackson et al., 1984). The risk of emboli following myocardial infarction is greatest in the first 2 to 4 weeks (Komad et al., 1984; Millikan et al., 1987). Cardiac conditions associated with embolic stroke are listed in Table 33–3.

Other sources of embolic stroke include fat emboli following trauma or long bone fracture, tumor emboli, and atherosclerotic emboli (Thomas and Ayyer, 1972; Sandok et al., 1980; Soloway and Aronson, 1964).

Thromboembolism

Sometimes it is difficult to determine clinically whether a cerebral infarct results from emboli, thrombus, or a combination of the two. Thrombus of a vessel can lead to embolism of distal arteries. Nonatherosclerotic thromboembolic disease may result from hematologic disorders, migraine, use of illicit drugs, fibromuscular dysplasia, or moyamoya disease.

Hematologic Disorders. CBF is reduced when blood viscosity and platelet aggregability are increased. Decreased CBF may lead to ischemic stroke. Elevated hematocrit and fibrinogen indicate increased blood viscosity (Grotta et al., 1982). This occurs in disorders such as polycythemia, thrombocytosis, and sickle cell anemia. Less commonly, ischemic stroke has also been associated with serum lupus anticoagulant and disseminated intravascular coagulation (Levine and Welch, 1988; Reagan and Okazaki, 1974). Oral contraceptives may also cause hypercoagulability that results in thromboembolic stroke (Stadel, 1981).

Migraine. Strokes secondary to migraine, although rare, have been reported (Broderick and Swanson, 1987; Bogousslavsky et al., 1988). At greatest risk are patients with migraines associated with hemianopsia, ophthalmoplegia, or hemiparesis (migraine with

TABLE 33–3. Cardiac Sources of Cerebral Embolism

Atrial fibrillation
Rheumatic heart disease
Mitral valve prolapse
Myocardial infarction
Infectious endocarditis
Nonbacterial thrombotic endocarditis
Atrial myxoma
Mitral annulus calcification
Cardiomyopathy
Coronary artery disease
Prosthetic heart valve

aura) (Bogousslavsky et al., 1988; Broderick and Swanson, 1987; Featherstone, 1986). Migraine patients without aura appear to have the same risk of stroke as people without migraine (Featherstone, 1986). The pathogenesis of migraine and its role in stroke are poorly understood, although the clinical picture of stroke in migraine reflects a thromboembolic process (Featherstone, 1986).

Drug Abuse. Neurologic sequelae of drug abuse are difficult to study because multiple substances are often used and the subjects are unreliable (Caplan et al., 1982). Reviews of the literature in this area report cerebral infarction related to the intravenous use of heroin, Talwin, and pyribenzamine (Ts and blues); methylphenidate (Ritalin); intranasal, intramuscular, or inhaled cocaine and crack; or oral ingestion of lysergic acid diethylamine (LSD) (Caplan et al., 1982; Levine and Welch, 1988). The mechanism of infarction is probably multifactorial, including embolism from endocarditis, injection of foreign matter, or an immune-mediated response altering the cerebral vessels (Caplan et al., 1982).

Fibromuscular Dysplasias. This idiopathic nonatheromatous vascular process affects the systemic arteries, especially renal, carotid, and intracerebral vessels. Cerebral ischemia may result from either stenosis or emboli (Paulson et al., 1978).

Moyamoya. This rare, idiopathic cerebrovascular abnormality is characterized by acquired stenosis of the carotid arteries resulting in the development of extensive collateral circulation at the base of the brain (Millikan et al., 1987). Focal cerebral ischemia is a common manifestation of moyamoya.

Inflammation

Vasculitis, inflammation, and necrosis of blood vessels may result in ischemic cerebrovascular disease. Rarely, central nervous system (CNS) vasculitis presents as an intracranial hemorrhage (Biller et al., 1987). CNS vasculitis occurs in isolation, with peripheral vasculitides, or secondary to infection, toxins, neoplasia, or collagen vascular disease (Moore and Cupps, 1983). Isolated cerebral angiitis may involve any size artery or vein, but small vessel disease is always present. Untreated, this disease is fatal, usually as a result of recurrent cerebral infarctions. Cerebral vessel involvement may be associated with polyarteritis nodosa, Wegener granulomatosis, Behçet disease, systemic lupus erythematosus, lymphomatoid granulomatosis, hypersensitivity vasculitis, and giant cell arteritis (temporal arteritis and Takayasu arteritis) (Moore and Cupps, 1983). Secondary causes of cerebral vasculitis include bacterial, syphilitic, tubercular, herpetic, and fungal meningitis and drug abuse, especially with amphetamines and phenylpropanolamine (an amphetamine analog found in many over-the-counter nasal decongestants, diet pills, and stimulants) (Caplan and Stein, 1986; Fallis and Fisher, 1985; Stafford et al., 1975). Sarcoidosis also produces cerebral vasculitis, most often affecting the veins, manifested by ophthalmologic, cranial nerve, cortical, and cerebellar involvement (Caplan and Stein, 1986; Caplan et al., 1983).

Epidemiology

The incidence of stroke and stroke mortality have decreased for both sexes, blacks, whites, and all age groups, although the phenomenon is more pronounced in the elderly (Whisnant, 1974; Garraway et al., 1979; Gillum, 1988). These improvements may reflect better understanding and control of risk factors, especially hypertension.

Age, gender, race, and family history influence the incidence of stroke, but these factors cannot be altered. The incidence of stroke dramatically increases over the age of 55, with a twofold increase each decade (Robins and Baum, 1981). Blacks have a greater incidence of stroke and stroke mortality than whites, with black women having the highest rate (Gillum, 1988; Gross et al., 1984). Men have a higher incidence than women (Robins and Baum, 1981; Garraway et al., 1979). There is evidence that family history plays a role in the development of cerebrovascular disease (Gifford, 1966; Heydan et al., 1969). This can partially be attributed to known familial occurrence of several stroke risk factors, such as hypertension and diabetes mellitus.

Risk Factors

Hypertension. Hypertension (≥160/95 mm Hg) is the greatest risk factor for ischemic stroke. The degree of risk is directly related to the magnitude of blood pressure (Kannel et al., 1970). The Framingham study indicated that isolated systolic hypertension (systolic ≥160 mm Hg, diastolic <95 mm Hg) is significantly related to the risk of stroke, especially in the elderly (Kannel et al., 1981). Diastolic pressures were not demonstrated to be a better indicator of risk for stroke. Labile hypertension was found to be significantly related to stroke and should not be ignored. It was recommended that the diagnosis of hypertension be based on the *average* of serial blood pressure readings taken on different days (Kannel et al., 1980).

Cardiac Disease. People with cardiac disease, regardless of blood pressure, have more than twice the risk of stroke found in people with normal cardiac function (Wolf et al., 1983). Cardiac disease is also associated with increased morbidity among stroke survivors (Sacco et al., 1982). People who have had a transient ischemic attack are at high risk of mortality from myocardial infarction (Toole et al., 1978).

Transient Ischemic Attacks (TIAs). A recent TIA increases the risk of stroke. In the Rochester, Minnesota population study, 21% of the patients had a stroke within a month of suffering a TIA, and 51% within a year (Whisnant, 1974). Although TIAs are a significant risk factor, only 10% to 25% of strokes are preceded by a TIA (Whisnant, 1974; Mohr et al., 1978).

Previous Stroke. Cumulative recurrence rates vary among studies, but a previous stroke increases the risk of subsequent strokes (Meissner et al., 1988; Sacco et al., 1982). In the Framingham study, concomitant hypertension and cardiac disease increased the potential for recurrent stroke (Sacco et al., 1982). However, the Rochester study showed that management of hypertension following stroke did not decrease the recurrence rate (Meissner et al., 1988).

Diabetes. Adult diabetics, women more so than men, have an increased risk of atherothrombotic brain infarcts (Wolf et al., 1983). However, no evidence suggests that tighter control of serum glucose either decreases the incidence or improves the outcome of strokes (Helgason, 1988). There is some evidence that hyperglycemia at the time of ischemia increases the risk of infarction and that this is associated with poorer outcomes (Helgason, 1988).

Hyperlipidemia. Although elevated serum lipids (total and low-density lipoprotein-cholesterol) have been closely associated with coronary artery disease, the same relationship has not been consistently found with cerebrovascular atherosclerosis (Wolf et al., 1983; Tell et al., 1988). The Framingham study demonstrated a significant association between elevated serum cholesterol and atherosclerotic brain infarction only in men under the age of 55 (Kannel et al., 1974).

Blood Viscosity. Blood viscosity is largely determined by serum fibrinogen concentration and hematocrit. An increase in either component leads to increased blood viscosity, resulting in decreased CBF (Grotta et al., 1982). CBF is significantly lower when the hematocrit is in the upper limits of normal (47% to 53%). Hematocrit in the upper limits of normal has also been associated with an increased incidence of cerebral infarction (Tohgi et al., 1978). Thomas and colleagues, (1977) demonstrated that reducing the hematocrit by phlebotomy increased the CBF by 50%.

Asymptomatic Carotid Bruit. Carotid bruits often indicate advanced atherosclerosis and are associated with increased stroke risk. In the asymptomatic individual, however, a carotid bruit is a nonlocalizing sign. Data from the Framingham study showed that less than half of the strokes in people with an asymptomatic carotid bruit occurred in the distribution of the corresponding carotid artery (Wolf et al., 1981).

Oral Contraceptives. Oral contraceptives stimulate platelet aggregability and increase prothrombin-converting factor (factor III) activity (Stadel, 1981). It is believed that these characteristics lead to an increased risk of stroke (thromboembolic and hemorrhagic) and myocardial infarction among users of oral contraceptives. The risk of stroke among oral contraceptive users is greatest in women who also smoke cigarettes, are over 35 years of age, and have other risk factors, particularly hypertension. With the introduction of a low-estrogen and progesterone pill, the risk of stroke has decreased (Stadel, 1981).

There are many factors that by themselves may not increase the risk of atherothrombotic infarction but, when combined with other factors, may become significant. Some of these factors include obesity, cigarette smoking, and use of alcohol. Outcomes of the Framingham study delineate five characteristics that, when found together, identify 10% of the population that will have at least a third of all strokes. The profile characteristics include systolic hypertension, left ventricular hypertrophy on electrocardiography, hyperlipidemia (cholesterol), cigarette smoking, and glucose intolerance (Wolf et al., 1983).

Clinical Manifestations

Transient Ischemic Attacks. TIAs are vascular events that result in temporary, focal neurologic dysfunction. Characteristic TIAs are of rapid onset, reaching maximal dysfunction within 5 minutes (often in less than 1 minute) with resolution occurring within 2 to 15 minutes (Millikan et al., 1987). Symptoms rarely persist for 24 hours, but if they do and there is resolution within 21 days, the event is referred to as a reversible ischemic neurologic deficit (RIND) (Millikan et al., 1987). In either case, the patient is without permanent neurologic deficit.

TIAs result from a variety of conditions. Arterial obstruction from thrombus or embolus, arterial inflammation, and hematologic or coagulation abnormalities may reduce CBF to a point that allows transient focal ischemia. Cardiac or atherosclerotic plaque emboli are considered the most common source of TIAs (Barnett, 1979; Millikan et al., 1987). Lysis of emboli from intravascular enzymes or emboli that are small enough to pass through the affected vessel may account for the transient nature of focal abnormalities (Millikan et al., 1987).

The significance of hypotension induced by positional change, cerebral arteriography, or medications in chronically hypertensive patients as a mechanism for producing TIAs has been debated. Ruff and associates (1981) found that rapid lowering of blood pressure in hypertensive patients with hemodynamically significant carotid artery stenosis (greater than 85%) put the patient at risk for a TIA. Others have found no relationship (Kendall and Marshall, 1963). Nevertheless, nurses must be particularly attuned to monitoring postural blood pressure changes and assessing these patients for any transient focal neurologic signs.

Most TIAs are not witnessed by health care workers, making a careful history essential for diagnosis. TIA symptoms may be classified by localization to areas supplied by the carotid or vertebrobasilar systems; however, at times the distinction can be difficult. Common signs and symptoms of TIAs in both distributions are listed in Table 33–4. The most common symptoms associated with the carotid system are contralateral weakness and ipsilateral amaurosis fugax (painless, unilateral blindness). Amaurosis fugax indicates retinal ischemia and is usually the result of atherosclerotic plaque emboli from the ipsilateral ICA. Many patients describe this transient blindness as if a "shade were pulled down over the eye." Others describe a central scotoma that spreads to involve part or all of the visual field within seconds. Each episode is usually brief (<10 minutes), and often normal vision returns but generally more slowly than the visual defect began (Marshall and Meadows, 1968).

Vertigo and binocular visual complaints are most frequently associated with vertebrobasilar TIAs. Nausea and vomiting may accompany these findings. Less commonly, drop attacks and transient global amnesia (TGA) occur. A drop attack is an unprecipitated loss of strength in both legs, causing the patient to fall. The attack is so sudden that the patient is unable to break the fall. The patient remains conscious, and, usually by the time he lands on the ground, his strength has returned (Brust et al., 1979; Kubala and Millikan, 1964). TGA is an episode of memory loss which persists minutes to hours. The patient is oriented to self but confused about the environment, has retrograde amnesia, and conversation is vague. The episode gradually resolves with the patient returning to normal except for amnesia for the event. TGA, unless associated with risk factors or other symptoms of cerebral ischemia, is unlikely to recur or lead to stroke (Jensen and Olivarius, 1981; Shuping et al., 1980).

It is important to note that TIAs within the carotid system produce contralateral motor or sensory symptoms, whereas those of the vertebrobasilar system result in alternating or bilateral motor or sensory deficits. TIAs usually present as a constellation of symptoms as opposed to an isolated abnormality. For example, recurrent vertigo in the absence of other symptoms is probably not secondary to ischemia (Barnett, 1979; Millikan et al., 1987). The nurse should be aware that a TIA signals impaired cerebral circulation. Episodes that increase in frequency over a short period of time, "crescendo" TIAs, indicate the need for immediate medical intervention.

Progressing Stroke. Progression of stroke is a temporal phenomenon defined as the continued worsening of a neurologic deficit or the progressive development of new neurologic signs. Stroke may evolve steadily or in a stuttering fashion over minutes to days. Britton and Roden (1985) found that 43% of the patients admitted for stroke experienced an extension of their neurologic deficits, half of which occurred in the first 24 hours. Progression can result from cerebral edema, recurrent emboli, or failure of collateral blood supply. Complications such as pulmonary embolus, hypotension, and systemic infection may also contribute to a worsening neurologic status.

It is frequently the nurse who first notes deterioration of the patient's neurologic status, especially changes in the level of consciousness. Because this is a critical finding, it should be reported immediately. Repeated neurologic and cardiac assessments, comparing the findings to those of previous examinations, are essential. This information aids the physician in isolating the cause, allowing selection of appropriate diagnostic procedures and rapid institution of medical and surgical interventions to attempt to prevent further progression. Ischemia within the carotid artery distribution is unlikely to progress after 18 to 24 hours of *stable* neurologic status. However, progression of ischemia within the vertebrobasilar system may occur up to after 72 hours of neurologic stability (Millikan and McDowell, 1981).

Completed Stroke. A completed stroke is defined as a prolonged neurologic deficit, lasting more than 21 days, and is basically stable (Millikan et al., 1987). A completed stroke indicates infarction as opposed to ischemia. However, a completed stroke does not preclude the potential for gradual improvement. The term completed stroke does not reflect the cause or degree of associated neurologic dysfunction. Prognosis is dependent upon the size and location of the infarct and the availability of collateral circulation.

Lacunar infarcts are small deep "holes" that often result from occlusion of small arteries in the basal ganglia, thalamus, internal capsule, or brainstem (Mohr, 1982). Small vessel disease secondary to hy-

---

TABLE 33–4. Common Symptoms of Transient Ischemic Attacks

Carotid System	Vertebrobasilar System
Amaurosis fugax	Vertigo
Homonymous hemianopsia	Bilateral homonymous hemianopsia; diplopia
Unilateral weakness of one or both limbs	Weakness that may be bilateral or may alternate during subsequent TIAs*
Unilateral numbness or paresthesias	Numbness or paresthesias of any or all limbs
Aphasia	Dysarthria
dysarthria	Dysphagia
	Ataxia
	Perioral numbness

*TIAs, transient ischemic attacks.

pertension is the most likely cause. Lacunar infarcts may result in "pure sensory" or "pure motor" strokes, or dysarthria–clumsy hand syndrome (Fisher, 1982; Fisher and Curry, 1965). Prognosis is generally good for these patients.

Diagnosis

Diagnosis begins with a detailed history, including a family history. Activity and time of onset, first noticed symptom, and progression or resolution of symptoms are essential information. Some patients present with seizures or status epilepticus. Most commonly, focal motor seizures with or without generalization are noted (Cocito et al., 1982; Lesser et al., 1985). Risk factors should be identified, including history of hypertension, cardiac disease, diabetes mellitus, and TIAs. Questions should be very specific, that is, "Have you ever lost vision in one eye which lasted only a few minutes?" (Millikan et al., 1987). When the patient is dysarthric, aphasic, or confused, the history should be taken from family or friends.

Physical assessment focuses on vital signs, cardiac status, and assessment of skin. Hypertension, hypotension, atrial fibrillation, evidence of congestive heart failure, and coagulopathy (petechiae, ecchymosis) should be noted (Millikan et al., 1987). Laboratory studies should include a complete blood count, erythrocyte sedimentation rate, and platelet count; serum electrolytes, glucose, and calcium; coagulation studies; VDRL test; and urinalysis. Serum and urinary toxicology screens should be done for suspected substance abuse. Chest radiographs are also done. Electrocardiography and echocardiography are obtained on all patients with suspected embolic stroke or known cardiac abnormalities.

Neurologic assessment emphasizes the level of consciousness, mental status, cranial nerve function, and motor and sensory function. Frequent neurologic assessments should be carefully documented on a flow sheet. Fundoscopic examination and auscultation for subclavian, carotid, and orbital bruits are also useful. Specialized testing procedures used in assessing ischemia and infarction are discussed below.

Computed Axial Tomography (CT Scan). CT scan of the head is appropriate for most patients with transient or progressive neurologic symptoms. Intracerebral or subarachnoid blood appears as a hyperdensity when compared to normal brain. In contrast, a nonhemorrhagic (bland) infarct and cerebral edema are hypodense. Often a bland infarct will not be evident on CT for several days after the insult. CT is also valuable in uncovering previously unsuspected pathology, such as a structural lesion (tumor, abscess) or subdural hematoma, rather than stroke as an explanation for the patient's condition. In an emergency situation a contrast-enhanced study is not always necessary. Contrast agents should be avoided in patients with renal disease, congestive heart failure, or a known allergy to the contrast medium, although the latter is quite rare.

Cerebral Angiography. Angiography is performed by the direct intra-arterial injection of a radiopaque contrast medium into either the carotid or vertebral artery (or both), thus providing visualization of the vascular tree. The catheter is usually inserted through the femoral artery, passed to the aortic arch, and then passed to the carotid or vertebral artery. Angiography is done to delineate extracranial or intracranial occlusive vascular disease (such as that from atherosclerosis or vasculitis) and to guide subsequent treatment, medical or surgical. The major complication, though rare, of angiography is the onset of or progression of neurologic deficit. There is also a very small potential for allergic reaction to the contrast agent.

Magnetic Resonance Imaging. Magnetic resonance imaging (MRI) is more sensitive in detecting early changes in cellular water content, allowing new infarcts to be identified within hours (Brant-Zawadzki, 1988). MRI also enhances visualization of the cerebellum and brainstem, permitting better identification of vertebrobasilar infarcts. With multiple infarcts it is not possible to distinguish the age of infarcts without previous comparison scans (Brant-Zawadzki, 1988). MRI is contraindicated for patients with cardiac pacemakers or intracranial aneurysm clips because of the high magnetic fields generated (Brant-Zawadzki, 1988).

Digital Subtraction Angiography. Digital subtraction angiography (DSA) may be done intravenously (IV) or, preferably, intra-arterially (IA). IV-DSA is accomplished by means of systemic venous injection of contrast media. IA-DSA is done in the same way as cerebral angiography, but it requires less contrast medium, allows electronic subtraction of the overlying bony structures, and takes less time (Millikan et al., 1987).

Magnetic Resonance Angiography. Magnetic resonance angiography (MRA) is a new, rapid, noninvasive procedure that promises to define extracranial carotid artery disease as well as invasive IA-DSA (Masaryk et al., 1989). This procedure, with a short increase in examination time, can also image the brain parenchyma. The disadvantages of MRA are its sensitivity to patient movement and positioning (Masaryk et al., 1989).

Ultrasonography. Ultrasound noninvasively detects stenosis of the extracranial carotid arteries through Doppler or B-mode scanners. The Doppler provides a static image, whereas B-mode produces real-time images of the pulsating artery. A duplex scanner combines both of these techniques into a single instrument. The quality of the image is very dependent upon the technician and on patient cooperation. This device is unable to distinguish between severe stenosis and complete occlusion (Millikan et al., 1987). Ultrasound results should be confirmed by angiography before considering surgical correction.

Positron Emission Tomography. Position emission tomography (PET), a radionuclide scanning technique, allows study of cerebral metabolism. Injection of a positron-emitting radioisotope will provide information about regional cerebral blood flow (rCBF) and regional cerebral oxygen and glucose use. PET is still in the developmental stage and is not universally available. PET studies of ischemic cerebrovascular disease have provided information about metabolic and perfusion changes following ischemia and infarction, and have identified metabolic characteristics associated with transient neurologic dysfunction (Powers and Raichle, 1985).

Single Photon Emission Computed Tomography. Single photon emission computed tomography (SPECT) also studies rCBF, using an intravenous ^{123}I-labeled amine that crosses the blood–brain barrier and is then visualized in a format similar to that of a CT scan. SPECT can identify abnormal cerebral perfusion within hours of infarction, when the CT scan may still be normal (Brott et al., 1986).

Lumbar Puncture. Since the advent of CT scanning and MRI, the lumbar puncture (LP) has become less crucial in diagnosing ischemic stroke patients. However, patients with unexplained ischemic infarction may require LP for examination of the cerebrospinal fluid (CSF) for evidence of meningitis or vasculitis. LP is always contraindicated with clinical evidence of increased ICP.

Medical Management

The goals of treatment of patients with acute cerebral ischemic events are to prevent associated complications and further neurologic insult. Interventions are initiated in an attempt to restore normal perfusion to the injured area and prevent increased intracranial pressure secondary to cerebral edema, cautiously manage blood pressure, and identify and correct contributing systemic processes (e.g., cardiac disease, pneumonia, and pulmonary embolism). Treatment of cardiac and pulmonary conditions is discussed in Chapters 16, 17, 22, and 25, and the reader is referred to these chapters for specific details on treatment. Besides transtentorial herniation, the most common causes of death in the initial 35 days following stroke are pneumonia, cardiac disease, and pulmonary embolism (Bounds et al., 1981). Therefore, identification and treatment of these conditions are imperative.

MEDICAL TREATMENT

Platelet antiaggregants, anticoagulation, calcium channel blockers, hemodilution, and thrombolytic therapy are used to treat ischemic stroke. Inflammatory cerebrovascular disease is treated with corticosteroids and cyclophosphamide.

Platelet Antiaggregants. Agents that inhibit platelet aggregability, or adhesiveness, include dipyridamole (Persantine), sulfinpyrazone (Anturane), acetylsalicylcic acid (ASA), and ticlopidine. ASA is more effective for men than women in reducing the incidence of stroke after TIA or atherothrombotic stroke. Side effects of this therapy include gastrointestinal upset or bleeding. Although the optimum dosage has not been determined, as little as 40 mg (1/2 a baby aspirin) daily will inhibit platelet aggregation in vitro. Dipyridamole and sulfinpyrazone, by themselves or with ASA, are no better than ASA alone in preventing cerebral infarction (Bousser et al., 1983; American-Canadian Study Group, 1985; Weksler et al., 1985). Platelet antiaggregants are associated with less severe or disabling strokes (Grotta et al., 1985). Results of a large multicenter trial of ticlopidine, a newer platelet antiaggregant in the prevention of nonfatal stroke in patients with a history of TIA, RIND, or minor stroke demonstrated that ticlopidine was somewhat more effective in men and women than ASA. The risk of side effects from ticlopidine (diarrhea, skin rash, severe neutropenia), however, was greater than that from ASA (Hass et al., 1989).

Anticoagulation. Anticoagulants are used to prevent recurrent emboli and further formation of thrombus. Use of anticoagulation in an acute ischemic event is controversial. Anticoagulation is considered a treatment option in the treatment of "crescendo" or multiple TIAs and in progressive, acute partial or cardioembolic stroke (Miller and Hart, 1988). This therapy is not indicated in a patient with a completed infarction.

Before beginning anticoagulation CT or MRI is done to rule out hemorrhagic stroke and allow careful consideration of the risks and benefits for the patient. Lumbar puncture done within an hour of the advent of anticoagulation therapy increases the risk of a spinal hematoma (Ruff and Dougherty, 1981). Contraindications for anticoagulant therapy include hemorrhagic lesions (e.g., gastric ulcer), poorly controlled hypertension, high risk for falls (e.g., ataxia, vertigo), and an inability to adhere to specific instructions (e.g., cognitive impairment or dementia).

Therapy usually begins with a bolus of intravenous heparin (5000 to 10,000 units) followed by a continuous infusion of heparinized solution. Dose adjustments are made to maintain the activated partial thromboplastin time (APTT) within 1.5 to 2.5 times the control (normal, 35 to 40 seconds; therapeutic, 60 to 100 seconds) (Miller and Hart, 1988). A potential risk of anticoagulation is the transformation of an ischemic lesion into a hemorrhagic infarct or an intracerebral bleed. Hypertension and excessive anticoagulation are significantly associated with an increased risk of a fatal intracerebral bleed (Ruff and Dougherty, 1981). Anecdotal reports indicate a need to delay heparinization for 5 to 7 days and avoid bolus administration in patients with large embolic infarcts (Cerebral Embolism Study Group, 1984).

Patients on long-term anticoagulation will be converted to the oral medication warfarin (Coumadin). Dosage is adjusted to maintain a prothrombin time (PT) of 1.5 times normal. Heparin is continued until the PT is within the therapeutic range; hence, there is an overlap of treatment of about 4 days.

Patients beginning anticoagulation therapy need careful neurologic monitoring for intracerebral hemorrhage. Increasing neurologic deficit should be rapidly reported to the physician. Laboratory values, APTT and PT, should be monitored to ensure that therapeutic levels are met and not exceeded.

Patients and family members should be instructed in the rationale for anticoagulation therapy and taught the need to report evidence of petechiae, epistaxis, ecchymosis, hematuria, melena, hematemesis, hemoptysis, bleeding gums, or wounds that continue to bleed.

Co-administration of drugs known to alter the effect of anticoagulation therapy should be avoided, including salicylates, intravenous nitroglycerin, carbamazepine, and phenytoin. The reader is referred to *Drug Interaction Facts* (1988) or a similar handbook for a complete listing of potential interactions.

Calcium Channel Blockers. Cerebral ischemia results in an influx of calcium into the cell that may contribute to cellular death. Administration of nimodipine, a calcium channel blocker that crosses the blood–brain barrier, may modify this process. Nimodipine has improved outcomes and reduced mortality in patients with acute completed atherothrombotic infarcts, especially men, and those with moderate to severe neurologic deficits at onset of symptoms (Gelmers et al., 1988).

Hemodilution. A relationship between increased blood viscosity and decreased CBF has been identified. Hemodilution is used to decrease the hematocrit and increase CBF to ischemic but potentially viable tissue surrounding the infarct, called the ischemic penumbra. If the ischemic area is reperfused, the completed infarct may be smaller, improving patient outcome. Hemodilution is accomplished through phlebotomy and volume replacement (isovolemic hemodilution), administration of a plasma volume expander such as low molecular weight dextran (hypervolemic hemodilution), or a combination of both methods (Grotta, 1987). Strand and colleagues (1984) demonstrated that hemodilution through plebotomy and dextran in the acute phase of ischemic stroke improved patient outcome, whereas others have found no beneficial effect (Scandinavian Stroke Study Group, 1987). This treatment should not be considered for patients with impaired cardiac function, low hematocrit on admission, or evidence of cerebral edema. Further studies are needed to determine the effectiveness of hemodilution and, if found to be effective, to develop a protocol to ensure safe implementation.

Thrombolytic Therapy. Thrombolytic therapy may be useful in the treatment of cerebral vessels occluded by thrombus or emboli (Del Zoppo et al., 1986). In the past, unacceptable complications such as hemorrhagic transformation of the infarct have precluded clinical use of this therapy. However, development of intravenous tissue plasminogen activator (t-PA), which has less effect on systemic fibrinogen and clotting factors and tends to have a more specific action against fibrin of fresh thrombi, has renewed interest in this therapy (Sherry, 1985). Bleeding complications, however, are still evident, and controlled studies are needed to document the safety and efficacy of this therapy.

Hypertension. CBF remains constant as long as the autoregulation mechanism is intact. Cerebral edema or ischemia may impair autoregulation, and CBF then becomes dependent upon systemic blood pressure. Therefore, lowering the blood pressure in these circumstances may significantly reduce CBF, resulting in clinical deterioration. Most stroke patients are hypertensive on admission, but spontaneous reduction in blood pressure occurs gradually during the next 10 days (Wallace and Levy, 1981). Antihypertensive therapy is discouraged during this period except when there is hypertensive encephalopathy, a diastolic pressure of 130 mm Hg or more, or compromised vital organs (e.g., heart or kidney) (Lavin, 1986; Strandgaard, 1983). Hypertensive therapy should be done cautiously, using short-acting agents that can be precisely adjusted and promptly withdrawn.

Central Nervous System Vasculitis. Cyclophosphamide and prednisone are the agents of choice for isolated CNS vasculitis (Moore, 1989). If cerebral angiitis is due to an infectious process such as bacterial meningitis or neurosyphilis, specific antibiotic therapy is needed.

SURGICAL TREATMENT

Some patients with extracranial vascular disease are candidates for surgery. The goals of surgery are to prevent recurrent TIAs or stroke.

Carotid Endarterectomy. Carotid endarterectomy is the most common surgical procedure used for extracranial artery disease. Atherosclerotic occlusive disease usually occurs at the carotid bifurcation, an area easily accessible for surgical intervention (Fig. 33–3). During endarterectomy the vessels are tem-

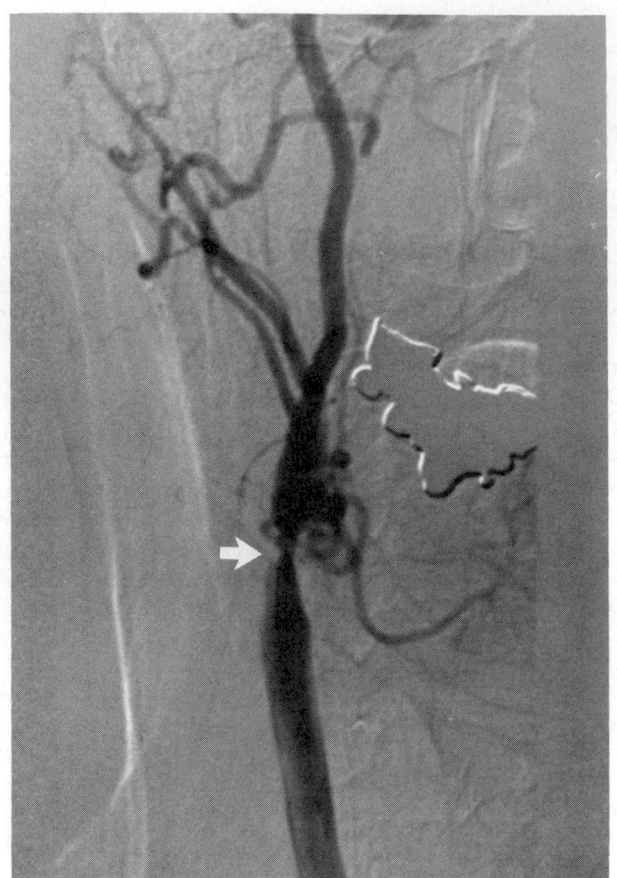

FIGURE 33–3. Intra-arterial digital subtraction angiogram demonstrating stenosis *(arrow)* of the right carotid artery at the bifurcation.

porarily clamped and opened, and the atheroma and associated thrombus are excised, leaving a smoother luminal surface. Intraoperative electroencephalography is frequently done to ensure adequate intraoperative perfusion and assess the need for surgical shunting. There is controversy, however, about when and for whom endarterectomy is indicated. The potential surgical mortality and morbidity must be carefully weighed against the risk of stroke. The potential for surgical complications increases in patients with major medical, neurologic, or angiographically defined risk factors (Sundt et al., 1987b). Medical risk factors include cardiopulmonary disease, severe hypertension, obesity, advanced peripheral vascular occlusive disease, and age over 70 years. Neurologic risk factors include crescendo TIAs, progressive neurologic deficit, deficit resolving within 24 hours of surgery, cerebral infarct less than 7 days old, and generalized cerebral ischemia. Occlusion of the contralateral ICA, a large plaque in the operative vessel, or a large plaque protruding from an ulcerative lesion are some angiographically defined risk factors (Sundt et al., 1987b).

Potential neurologic complications of surgery are stroke, TIAs, or cranial nerve injury. Ischemic stroke may result from perioperative embolization, postop-

erative ICA occlusion, or hyperperfusion syndromes due to significantly increased CBF during surgery. Intracerebral hemorrhage is an uncommon but devastating complication and may result from hyperperfusion. Cranial nerve injury, particularly to the hypoglossal, recurrent or superior laryngeal branches of the vagus, and facial nerves may occur (Sundt et al., 1987a) (Fig. 33–4). Postoperative assessments should include evaluation of tongue movement, quality and tone of voice, ability to swallow, and facial symmetry. Non-neurologic complications include wound infection, hematoma, carotid artery hemorrhage, and fluctuations in blood pressure. Transient dysfunction of carotid sinus baroreceptors is the suspected cause of postoperative hypotension and hypertension. Hypotension is managed with volume replacement and Trendelenburg positioning because the patient usually fails to respond to vasopressors. Hypertension is dealt with by intravenous nitroglycerin or nitroprusside (Sundt et al., 1987a).

Overall, mortality from carotid endarterectomy is approximately 1.3% (Sundt et al., 1987a). Obviously, the more medically and neurologically unstable a patient is, the greater the risk of surgery. The expertise and experience of the surgical team are critical factors in ensuring a favorable outcome.

Extracranial-Intracranial (EC-IC) Arterial Bypass. An international randomized study investigated the benefit of EC-IC arterial bypass in patients with symptomatic atherosclerotic disease. Bypass of the superficial temporal or occipital artery to the middle cerebral artery failed to decrease stroke recurrence and stroke mortality (EC-IC Bypass Stroke Group, 1985). Therefore, this procedure does not appear to be warranted for these patients.

HEMORRHAGIC STROKE

Hemorrhagic stroke results from bleeding into the subarachnoid space or brain parenchyma and accounts for approximately 14% of all cerebral infarctions (Wolf et al., 1983).

Subarachnoid Hemorrhage

Subarachnoid hemorrhage (SAH) results from a cerebral vessel that has "leaked" or "ruptured," allowing blood to flow into the subarachnoid space (Fig. 33–5*A* and *B*). This provokes several responses that alter regional CBF. Loss of cerebral autoregulation, decreased cerebral perfusion pressure, increased intracranial pressure, and arterial vasospasm combine to reduce CBF. Consequently, cerebral ischemia and infarction are frequent and devastating complications of SAH. The most common cause of SAH is a ruptured cerebral aneurysm. Less commonly, arteriovenous malformations, head injury, or blood dyscrasias result in SAH.

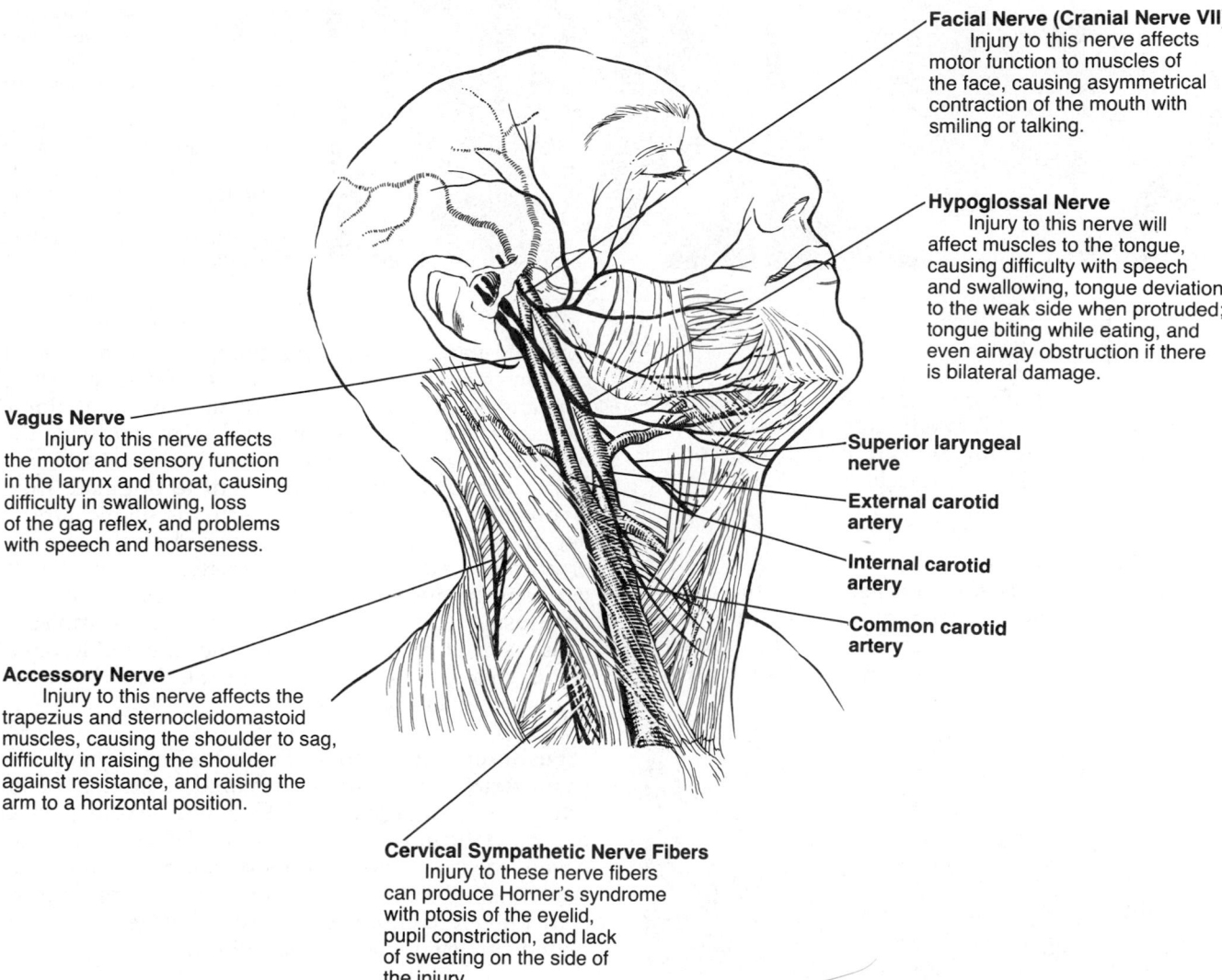

Facial Nerve (Cranial Nerve VII)
Injury to this nerve affects motor function to muscles of the face, causing asymmetrical contraction of the mouth with smiling or talking.

Hypoglossal Nerve
Injury to this nerve will affect muscles to the tongue, causing difficulty with speech and swallowing, tongue deviation to the weak side when protruded; tongue biting while eating, and even airway obstruction if there is bilateral damage.

Superior laryngeal nerve

External carotid artery

Internal carotid artery

Common carotid artery

Vagus Nerve
Injury to this nerve affects the motor and sensory function in the larynx and throat, causing difficulty in swallowing, loss of the gag reflex, and problems with speech and hoarseness.

Accessory Nerve
Injury to this nerve affects the trapezius and sternocleidomastoid muscles, causing the shoulder to sag, difficulty in raising the shoulder against resistance, and raising the arm to a horizontal position.

Cervical Sympathetic Nerve Fibers
Injury to these nerve fibers can produce Horner's syndrome with ptosis of the eyelid, pupil constriction, and lack of sweating on the side of the injury.

FIGURE 33–4. Cranial nerves exposed to trauma during carotid endarterectomy.

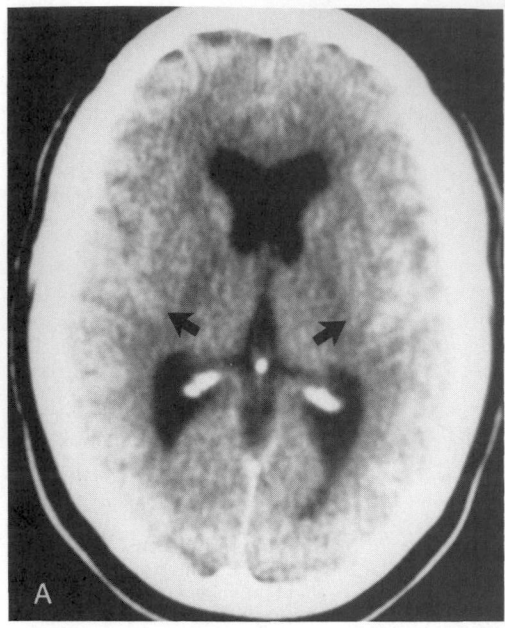 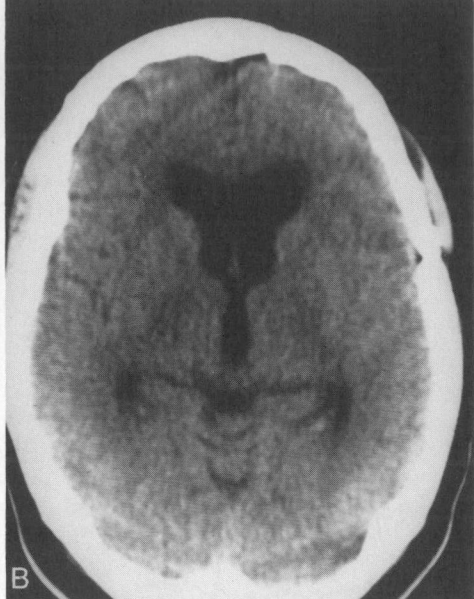

FIGURE 33–5. *A,* Axial CT scan of the head demonstrating hyperdensity around the cortical convexity, particularly in the area of the sylvian fissures *(arrows)* secondary to recent subarachnoid hemorrhage. Hyperdense areas in the posterior horns of the lateral ventricles and the third ventricle represents normal calcification of choroid plexus. *B,* Axial CT scan of the same patient as in *A* 3 1/2 months later. Note resolution of the subarachnoid blood. (The cut is lower than that in *A,* explaining the absence of calcification.)

ANEURYSMS

Aneurysms are formed from a weakness in the arterial wall and result in an outpouching or ballooning appearance. Aneurysms are classified according to their configuration as saccular, fusiform, or dissecting.

Saccular Aneurysms. Saccular, or berry, aneurysms are most common and usually form at places of arterial bifurcation, especially in the anterior cerebral circulation of the circle of Willis. Saccular aneurysms often have a narrow neck that extends

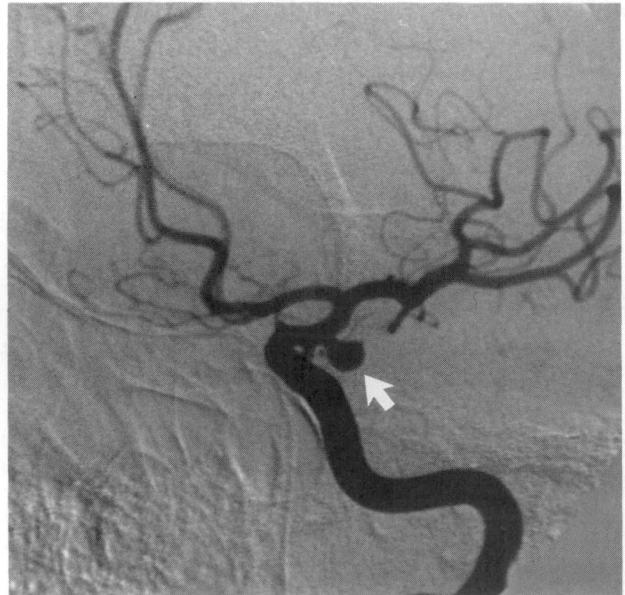

FIGURE 33–6. Cerebral arteriogram demonstrating a saccular aneurysm *(arrow)* of the left internal carotid artery at the origin of the posterior communicating artery.

from the parent vessel and expands into a broader portion or dome, giving them a saclike or berrylike appearance (Fig. 33–6). Size of the neck and dome varies. Although either portion may rupture, the dome is the more common site of hemorrhage.

Saccular aneurysms are thought to originate from a congenital defect of the muscularis of the artery, degenerative changes in the internal elastic lamina, or a combination of both processes that gradually weakens the arterial wall (Mohr et al., 1986a). Rarely, aneurysms form from infectious emboli (mycotic aneurysm), trauma, or neoplastic emboli. Mycotic aneurysms are usually found in the distal branches of major cerebral vessels.

Fusiform Aneurysms. Fusiform aneurysms are characterized by a spindle-shaped dilatation of an artery, with tapering at either end. Weir (1987a) described fusiform aneurysms as "shaped like deformed cigars." These are more commonly found in the vertebrobasilar artery and cause symptoms of cranial nerve compression, cerebral ischemia, or impaired CSF circulation (Weir, 1987a).

Dissecting Aneurysms. Dissecting aneurysms, often the result of trauma, form from a tear in the endothelium that creates a false channel. These rarely cause SAH because they usually occur extracranially.

Clinical Manifestations

Aneurysms rupture when the stress on the arterial wall exceeds the wall's strength. This may occur when there is an increase in intra-aneurysmal pressure, increased aneurysmal radius, or decreased arterial wall thickness (Ferguson, 1972). This could explain why aneurysms are more likely to rupture during hypertensive episodes, strenuous activity, straining to defecate (Valsalva maneuver), heavy lifting, or sexual intercourse. Spontaneous rupture, however, may occur at any time, even during nonstrenuous activity or sleep. Mortality rates after the initial hemorrhage are 27% to 43% at 1 week and 50% at 1 month (Weir, 1987a). Many patients die before reaching the hospital.

Characteristic symptoms of a SAH include sudden explosive headache, with or without loss of consciousness, and subsequent nuchal rigidity. The headache peaks in severity within seconds. The pain may initially be localized in the area of the bleed, but soon becomes holocephalic. Nausea, vomiting, neck pain, and stiffness are commonly associated with the headache. Frequently, there is loss of consciousness lasting minutes to hours; some patients never regain consciousness. Others may manifest only altered consciousness, e.g., lethargy, and altered mentation, including confusion or disorientation. Additional symptoms may include partial or generalized seizures, photophobia, diplopia, and vertigo. Seizure is most likely to occur at the onset of hemorrhage or with a rebleed (Hart et al., 1981). With extension of the hemorrhage intracerebrally or compression of adjacent brain by hematoma, the patient may exhibit focal neurologic signs such as hemiparesis or aphasia.

Prior to rupture, many patients (48%) have a warning leak (sentinel hemorrhage) or evidence of aneurysmal enlargement (Okawara, 1973). A warning leak may be enough to cause a headache with nausea, vomiting, and neck pain. Patients usually describe the headache as different from their typical headache. However, many times these symptoms do not prompt the patient to seek health care, or they are misdiagnosed. Cranial nerve palsies, particularly of the oculomotor and abducens nerves, visual field defects, and pain in, behind, or around the eye may indicate aneurysmal enlargement (Mohr et al., 1986b). The striking morbidity and mortality associated with SAH may be reduced through early recognition of these warning signs and rapid institution of definitive therapy before severe SAH occurs.

DELAYED NEUROLOGIC COMPLICATIONS

Major causes of delayed morbidity and mortality following SAH are symptomatic cerebral vasospasm, rebleeding, and delayed hydrocephalus. The onset of these complications is heralded by a change in the findings of the neurologic examination. The importance of consistent and frequent assessment and documentation of the patient's neurologic status by nurses and physicians cannot be overemphasized.

Vasospasm. Symptomatic cerebral vasospasm (abnormal narrowing of an artery) occurs in about 30% of patients with SAH following rupture of a saccular aneurysm (Fisher et al., 1977). The incidence in patients with arteriovenous malformation (AVM) is less because AVMs occur less frequently and rarely rupture into large basal cisterns.

Onset of cerebral vasospasm averages 4 to 14 days (range 3 to 21 days) following the initial hemorrhage (Mohr et al., 1986b). The size and location of SAH can be correlated with the occurrence, severity, and location of vasospasm (Kistler et al., 1983).

Cerebral artery vasospasm can lead to ischemia or infarction, the clinical findings varying with the specific arteries involved. Many patients with vasospasm exhibit altered mental status or consciousness. Signs of severe vasospasm of the anterior cerebral area include urinary incontinence, whispered voice, speaking with eyes closed, pursing lips, grasp reflex, and abulia (impaired ability to initiate spontaneous action) (Kistler et al., 1983). Ischemia of the middle cerebral artery's distribution may produce monoparesis, hemiparesis, facial weakness, anosognosia (nondominant hemispheric lesion), and dysphasia (dominant hemispheric lesion) (Kistler et al., 1983). Homonymous hemianopsia is often seen with posterior cerebral artery ischemia.

Rehemorrhage. Aneurysms are most likely to rebleed within the first 2 weeks after the initial hemorrhage, especially in the first 24 hours (Kassell and Torner, 1983). This fact significantly affects decisions about the timing of surgical interventions.

Hydrocephalus. Interruption or impairment of CSF flow due to blood in the subarachnoid space or intraventricular spaces can lead to hydrocephalus. Hydrocephalus is caused by impaired reabsorption of CSF. Communicating hydrocephalus usually occurs 4 to 20 days after aneurysmal rupture, although it may occur at any time. Patients may be completely asymptomatic, requiring no intervention, or they may exhibit marked deterioration of level of consciousness over a few hours, requiring emergency drainage of CSF (Mohr et al., 1986b).

Intracerebral Hemorrhage

Intracerebral hemorrhage (ICH) results from bleeding into the brain parenchyma (Fig. 33–7A and B). Although the most common source is small penetrating arterioles or capillaries, AVM and aneurysms may also cause ICH. ICH usually develops gradually, over minutes to hours, due to the low pressure of arterioles and capillaries. By comparison, SAH causes a rapid (within seconds) increase in intracranial pressure secondary to rupture of an aneurysm under systemic arterial pressure.

Most ICHs occur in the cerebral hemispheres, particularly within the putamen, thalamus, and lobar regions. A smaller percentage occur in the cerebellum and pons (Kase and Mohr, 1986). Hypertension is the usual cause, with vascular malformations the most common nonhypertensive cause. Oral anticoagulant therapy, cerebral amyloid angiopathy, and intracranial tumors may also result in ICH. Drug abuse may lead to both SAH and ICH.

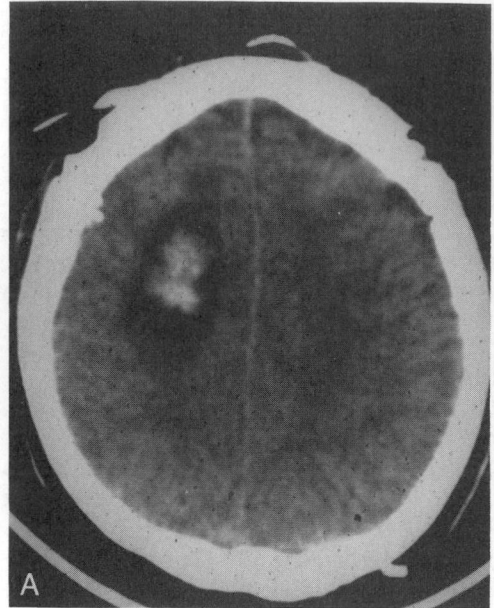 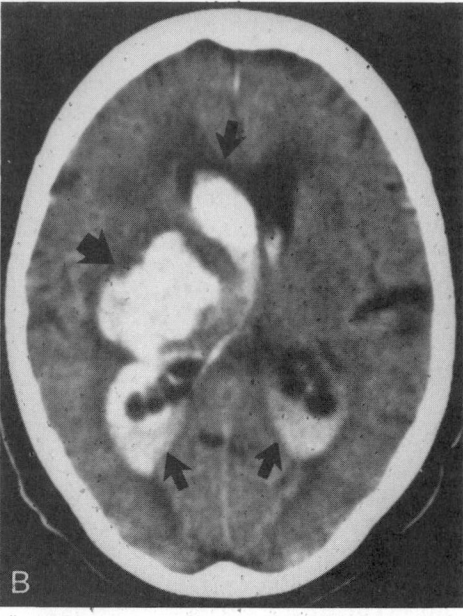

FIGURE 33–7. *A*, Axial CT scan of the head demonstrating a hyperdense lesion surrounded by a hypodense area in the right hemisphere. This is an intracerebral hematoma with surrounding edema. *B*, Axial CT scan of the head demonstrating a right hemispheric basal ganglian intracerebral hematoma *(wide arrow)* with intraventricular extension *(narrow arrows)*.

HYPERTENSIVE HEMORRHAGE

Chronic hypertension causes degenerative changes in cerebral vessels and the formation of microaneurysms (Charcot-Bouchard aneurysms). Blood pressure does not need to be in a critical range for this to occur; moderate hypertension for many years or a few years of severe hypertension produce the same changes (Furlan et al., 1979). ICH occurs when one or more affected vessels rupture. Many ICH patients are hypertensive on admission, the hypertension being either an acute process secondary to increased intracranial pressure or a chronic process, which is the primary cause of ICH. Therefore, a blood pressure history should be obtained for all patients admitted for ICH.

VASCULAR MALFORMATIONS

There are a number of cerebral vascular malformations besides aneurysms. McCormick's (1966) classification of vascular malformations includes venous angiomas, cavernous angiomas, capillary telangiectasis, varix, and arteriovenous malformations.

Venous Angiomas. Venous angiomas are formed by a group of anomalous veins, usually located deep within the white matter. These angiomas may serve to drain areas lacking normal venous drainage (Mohr et al., 1986b; Senegor et al., 1983). These rarely hemorrhage but may be associated with seizures and headaches (Mohr et al., 1986b).

Cavernous Angiomas. Cavernous angiomas are space-occupying lesions composed of large vascular cavernous channels most commonly found in the cerebral hemispheres. A large part of the malformation may be thrombosed. Unlike tumors, cavernous angiomas replace, instead of displace, normal brain

and therefore do not create a significant masslike effect. These lesions are associated with headache, seizures, and occasionally hemorrhage (Mohr et al., 1986b; McCormick, 1966).

Capillary Telangiectasis. This is a small group of thin-walled capillaries often found in the brainstem, cerebellum, or diencephalon. These rarely hemorrhage (Mohr et al., 1986b; McCormick, 1966).

Varix. A varix is a large, dilated vein or veins, usually found in the parenchyma or leptomeninges. Occasionally multiple veins are involved. These malformations have been associated with hemorrhage (McCormick, 1966).

Arteriovenous Malformation. AVM, the most common nonaneurysmal vascular anomaly, is composed of a tangle of abnormal arteries and veins larger than capillaries (Fig. 33–8). These are congenital or, less commonly, familial lesions. The normal capillary bed is absent, and blood flow, following the path of least resistance, creates an arteriovenous (A-V) fistula. Vessels supplying the lesion, feeding vessels, may be one or more of the major cerebral arteries and their branches. Venous drainage occurs through superficial and deep veins. Because of absent arteriolar and capillary resistance, blood flow increases and leads to increased venous pressure. Over time, as blood supply demand increases, arterial and venous dilation occurs. These veins transport oxygenated blood (i.e., little oxygen is extracted in the A-V fistula) called non-nutritive flow. In addition, blood shunted through the fistula may cause hypoperfusion of the surrounding brain, called cerebral steal. Cerebral vessels dilate in response to chronic hypoperfusion, and when maximal dilation is reached autoregulation may be lost. As a result, chronic

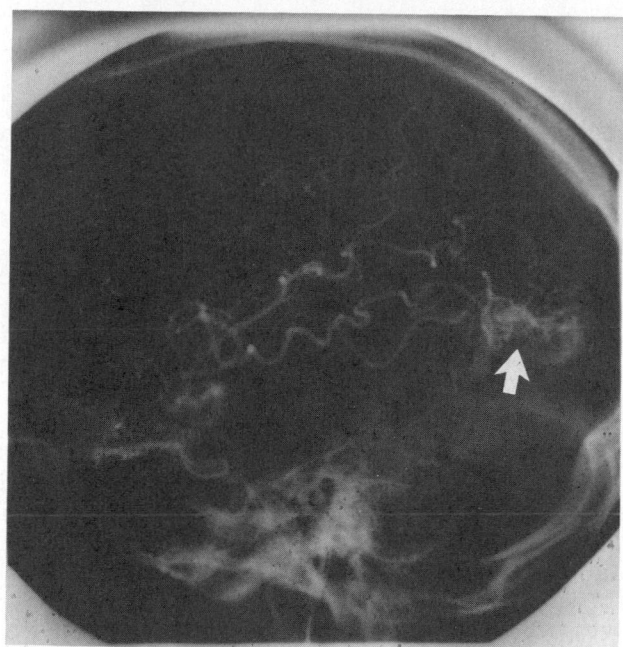

FIGURE 33–8. Cerebral arteriogram demonstrating left posterior temporal and occipital arteriovenous malformation *(arrow)* supplied by branches of the middle cerebral artery.

hypoperfusion can lead to ischemic changes in the surrounding brain and possible focal neurologic deficits (Mohr et al., 1986b).

CLINICAL MANIFESTATIONS

AVMs range in size from very small, cryptic lesions to lesions involving more than one lobe. AVMs enlarge with age and may not become symptomatic until the second or third decade of life. Early manifestations are usually hemorrhage or seizure (Fults and Kelly, 1984). Other findings include headache, progressive neurologic deficit, and, occasionally, bruits.

Hemorrhage. Approximately 50% of patients with AVM present with hemorrhage (Fults and Kelly, 1984). AVMs are most likely to cause ICH, but the hemorrhage can extend into the subarachnoid or intraventricular space. Although it is usually the smaller AVM that bleed, larger lesions may also hemorrhage.

About 10% to 15% of AVMs show evidence of previous hemorrhage when they are operated on (Mohr et al., 1986b). These hemorrhages often were asymptomatic or produced only minor symptoms. Unlike aneurysms, AVMs tend not to rebleed within a short time. The rate of rebleeding after the initial hemorrhage is difficult to determine with certainty. Fults and Kelly (1984) reported rebleeding rates of 17.9% during the first year, 3% per year after 5 years, and 2% per year after 10 years. However, Graf and colleagues (1983) estimated rebleeding at 6% during the first year and 2% per year thereafter.

Seizures. Prior small hemorrhages, chronic ischemia due to cerebral steal, cerebral cortex hemorrhage, and scarring all contribute to seizures (Berger et al., 1988). Seizures are often focal and correspond to the site of hematoma but may secondarily generalize or may be primarily generalized. Patients who present with a seizure unassociated with hemorrhage have a more favorable prognosis than those presenting with seizures with hemorrhage (Fults and Kelly, 1984).

Headache. Although headaches are very common in the general population, recurrent headaches may be a premonitory sign of AVM. Sentinel headaches may resemble atypical migraine. Headaches at the onset of ICH are often associated with vomiting (Gorelick et al., 1986).

Progressive Neurologic Deficit. The size and location of the hemorrhage determine the extent of the neurologic deficit. Ischemia or direct compression of adjacent brain may result in focal neurologic deficits in the absence of any episode of bleeding.

Bruit. Depending on the size and location of the AVM, a bruit may be heard over the eyes or skull. The patient may describe hearing a murmur within his or her head.

ANTICOAGULANT THERAPY

Bleeding associated with anticoagulation occurs infrequently, but people who take oral anticoagulants, often to prevent stroke, have a tenfold risk of ICH (Wintzen et al., 1984). Hemorrhages may occur without systemic bleeding, tend to be larger than those due to hypertension, and are associated with a higher mortality rate (62%) (Kase et al., 1985). Onset of focal neurologic deficit is often insidious, developing over hours to days. Increased risk of ICH is associated with excessively prolonged prothrombin time (>1.5 times normal). Other risk factors include hypertension, age, and duration of therapy (Kase et al., 1985).

CEREBRAL AMYLOID ANGIOPATHY

Cerebral amyloid angiopathy (CAA) is associated with amyloid deposits in the walls of small vessels in the cerebral cortex but not with systemic amyloidosis. Amyloid plaques may be found in patients with Alzheimer disease, senile dementia of the Alzheimer type, and Down syndrome (Vinters, 1987). CAA usually presents in normotensive people over 65 years of age with multiple or recurrent intracerebral hemorrhages, possibly due to vessel wall weakening. Most commonly, lobar hemorrhages occur, occasionally extending into the subarachnoid space. Hemorrhage in the basal ganglia, brainstem, or cerebellum is rare (Gilles et al., 1984; Vinters, 1987).

INTRACRANIAL TUMORS

An uncommon cause of ICH is bleeding into an intracranial tumor. Malignant tumors such as glioblastoma multiforme and metastatic lesions are most likely to hemorrhage because of their rich vasculature and neoplastic characteristics. In addition, some tumors invade and disrupt the vessel walls (Kase and Mohr, 1986).

DRUG ABUSE

Cocaine, amphetamine, pseudoephedrine, and ephedrine abuse have been temporally associated with ICH and SAH (Delaney and Estes, 1980; Loizou et al., 1982; Wojak and Flamm, 1987; Wooten et al., 1983). Bleeding from aneurysms and vascular malformations has been documented shortly after use of cocaine. Cocaine use has been shown to result in transient blood pressure increases that may precipitate the hemorrhage (Wojak and Flamm, 1987; Levine and Welch, 1988). Phenylpropanolamine, even used within dosage guidelines, has been associated with ICH (Fallis and Fisher, 1985; Glick et al., 1987; Kase et al., 1987). Even though ICH following drug abuse is uncommon, it is prudent to obtain a drug history, including use of illicit and over-the-counter medications, especially from young and otherwise healthy patients who present with ICH.

Epidemiology

A population study in Rochester, Minnesota, done between 1945 and 1974 showed decreasing rates of ICH, but not as striking as the decrease in ischemic stroke. No clear trend for SAH was identified (Garraway et al., 1979). The average age at onset for ICH increased from 65 to 71 years (Furlan et al., 1979), perhaps reflecting better control of hypertension, a major risk factor for ICH.

Prevalence of ruptured aneurysm increases with age, peaking in the fifth to sixth decades, after which the frequency declines. Aneurysms rarely are found in children (Weir, 1987a). Intracranial aneurysms are slightly more common in women after the sixth decade, possibly reflecting the longer life span of women (Weir, 1987a). Aneurysms are found in all races, but there are some geographic variations that are difficult to interpret because they may represent varied levels of health care rather than prevalence (Weir, 1987a).

The rate of primary ICH increases with age. Men have a higher rate of spontaneous ICH in all age groups (Furlan et al., 1979). The increased incidence among blacks may reflect a higher incidence of hypertension in this population (Gross et al., 1984; Brott et al., 1986).

Risk Factors

A variety of factors have been associated with hemorrhagic cerebrovascular disease. The most common are described below.

Hypertension. As in ischemic cerebrovascular disease, hypertension is considered a major risk factor for both ICH and SAH (Brott et al., 1986; Longstreth et al., 1985; Stemmerman et al., 1984). Conditions transiently elevating blood pressure produce an additive effect, such as cigarette smoking, alcohol consumption, and use of stimulants.

Oral Contraceptives. Current or past use of oral contraceptives increases a woman's risk of SAH, especially if the current oral contraceptive user is over 35 years of age and smokes cigarettes (Donaldson, 1986; Longstreth et al., 1985; Petitti et al., 1979). This increased risk associated with oral contraceptives may result from hormones that act directly on the arterial wall, weakening it and promoting formation or rupture of cerebral aneurysms (Petitti et al., 1979).

Pregnancy. Pregnancy increases the risk of both ischemic and hemorrhagic stroke. Although ischemic strokes related to pregnancy are rarely fatal, 5% to 10% of all maternal deaths result from ruptured aneurysms or AVMs (Donaldson, 1986). Aneurysms are most likely to bleed in the third trimester, whereas AVMs are more likely to bleed in the second trimester or during labor. Rebleeding from an aneurysm may occur during childbirth or in the postpartum period. AVMs rarely rebleed postpartum (Donaldson, 1986). Development of pregnancy-related hypertension is another complicating factor.

Cigarette Smoking. Cigarette smoking is a risk factor for hemorrhagic stroke (Petitti et al., 1979). Women who smoke more than a pack a day have twice the risk of hemorrhagic stroke as nonsmokers (Collaborative Group for the Study of Stroke in Young Women, 1975). Increased risk has also been identified for men (Abbott et al., 1986). The risk of hemorrhagic stroke is significantly reduced with cessation of smoking.

Diagnosis

The history, neurologic examination, and baseline laboratory work are similar to those described for ischemic cerebrovascular disease. Clinical presentation is often very suggestive of ICH. Due to the high morbidity and mortality associated with ICH, rapid and accurate diagnosis is important to allow appropriate medical and nursing management. CT scans, MRI, cerebral angiography, transcranial Doppler examination, and lumbar puncture are used for diagnosis.

Computed Tomography. Noncontrast CT scans done emergently upon suspicion of hemorrhage are excellent in detecting and determining the extent of acute bleeds (Mohr et al., 1986a). Although a very small volume SAH may be missed, the majority will be detected. CT scans may also identify hydrocephalus, if present. Contrast CT scans may locate and determine the size of an aneurysm or AVM, but this is not a definitive procedure for this condition; it must be confirmed with angiography.

Magnetic Resonance Imaging. The appearance of blood on MRI and CT scans changes with time. In the first 24 hours after an SAH, MRI detects an abnormal signal but cannot specify that it is blood, making the CT scan the preferred method during the first 24 hours (Brant-Zawadzki, 1988). The MRI is preferred in the subacute phase because hemorrhage may appear isodense on CT scan. Intracerebral hemorrhage and its relationship to the surrounding brain are readily visualized on MRI. MRI is more effective in identifying small ("cryptic") vascular lesions. MRI angiography may become the best noninvasive method of detection of intracranial AVMs and aneurysms in the future (Ross, 1988).

Cerebral Angiography. Depiction of the vascular anatomy and location of AVMs, aneurysms, and the degree of vasospasm are possible with cerebral angiography. Thrombosed vessels, vessels obliterated by hemorrhage, or very small malformations may not be visualized. Angiography is definitive for AVMs and aneurysms and is required prior to surgery.

Transcranial Doppler. Transcranial Doppler (TCD) is a noninvasive ultrasound procedure used to diagnose and monitor vasospasm in the middle and anterior cerebral arteries. Vasospasm in other cerebral arteries is difficult to detect with this method (DeWitt and Wechsler, 1988). TCD can detect increased blood velocity secondary to a narrowed vessel lumen that may precede symptomatic vasospasm by hours to days (DeWitt and Wechsler, 1988).

Lumbar Puncture. Lumbar puncture (LP) should be done to aid diagnosis if the CT scan is negative for SAH, intraventricular hemorrhage, mass, or obstructive hydrocephalus. The cerebrospinal fluid in SAH either contains frank blood that does not clear as the fluid is collected or fluid that is xanthochromic (deep yellow) due to the presence of blood breakdown products. Further examination of the CSF will reveal increased opening pressure, elevated protein, normal glucose, and a pleocytosis (Caplan and Stein, 1986).

Medical Management of the Patient with Acute Intracranial Hemorrhage

Treatment of acute intracerebral hemorrhage is aimed at preventing further hemorrhage, maintaining adequate cerebral perfusion pressure, and preventing neurologic sequelae. These goals are usually accomplished using combined medical and surgical interventions.

MEDICAL TREATMENT

Many of the signs and symptoms of ICH are due to increased intracranial pressure. Management of increased ICP is discussed in detail in Chapter 32.

To reduce the risk of rebleeding, patients are placed in a quiet, dimly lit room on complete bed rest. If tolerated, the head of the bed is elevated 30 degrees to aid venous drainage. Stool softeners are given to reduce straining during bowel movements. Mild, short-acting sedatives may be used with caution to aid restlessness and anxiety. Sedatives may mask subtle changes in the level of consciousness, thus interfering with accurate neurologic assessment. Platelet antiaggregants, such as ASA, are contraindicated. Anticonvulsants may be prescribed if the patient has had a seizure or as prophylaxis. Corticosteroids have not been shown to be useful in reducing cerebral edema associated with hemorrhage (Mohr et al., 1986; Poungvarin et al., 1987).

As in ischemic stroke, it is essential to obtain careful control of hypertension. Palliative measures for pain and anxiety may reduce blood pressure. If needed, short-acting antihypertensive medications may be used. It is essential to monitor the neurologic status and blood pressure closely. Mild hypotension may result in clinical deterioration.

Medical treatment of these patients is geared toward preventing rebleeding or treating syptomatic cerebral vasospasm. Several treatment modalities will be discussed in more detail.

Antifibrinolytics. Antifibrinolytic agents, aminocaproic acid (Amicar) or tranexamic acid (Cyklokapron), may be used to try to prevent rebleeding from a ruptured intracranial aneurysm. These drugs prevent the lysis of thrombus within and on the surface of an aneurysm. This thrombus may support the wall of the aneurysm, reducing the potential for rebleeding (Adams, 1987). The suggested dosage of aminocaproic acid is 5 g given in an IV bolus followed by a continuous infusion of 24 to 36 g/day for 10 to 14 days, unless surgery is attempted. Antifibrinolytic agents considerably reduce the 14-day rebleeding rate but do not significantly alter the overall mortality rate (Kassell et al., 1984) because these agents are associated with a greater incidence of hydrocephalus and ischemic complications (Kassell et al., 1984). Therefore, use of these drugs in patients with SAH is controversial (Adams, 1987; Weir, 1987b).

Calcium Channel Blockers. The mechanism for vasospasm is thought to be related to the presence of blood and blood products within the CSF, which stimulate arterial narrowing. Calcium channel blockers, which inhibit vascular smooth muscle contraction by blocking the influx of extracellular calcium, are thought to prevent or reverse vasospasm (Greenberg, 1987). Two agents currently under investigation for this use are nimodipine and nicardipine. Both of these agents have been associated with reduced severity of cerebral vasospasm and improved patient outcomes (Aver, 1984; Flamm et al., 1988; Petruk et al., 1988). Hypotension, a serious potential complication of calcium channel blockers, usually responds to increased intravascular fluid and rarely necessitates discontinuation of the drug (Flamm et al., 1988; Petruk et al., 1988).

Intravascular Volume Expansion. The most common treatment for symptomatic cerebral vasospasm is to increase cerebral perfusion pressure through plasma volume expansion. Vasopressors may be used to increase mean arterial pressure following surgery on an aneurysm. Because autoregulation is lost during vasospasm, an increase in systemic arterial pressure increases CBF. To be effective, this therapy must restore adequate CBF before infarction occurs.

Intravascular volume expansion is accomplished by administering fluid to create a positive fluid balance. The central venous pressure (CVP) is maintained at 10 to 12 mm Hg, and the pulmonary artery wedge pressure is kept at 15 to 20 mm Hg (Awad et al., 1987; Kassell et al., 1982). Kassell and associates (1982) used albumin or plasma fractionate along with packed cells or whole blood to maintain a hematocrit of 40%. Others advocate hypervolemic hemodilution, reducing the hematocrit to 33% to 38% (Awad et al., 1987). Crystalloid solutions are used to maintain normal serum electrolytes.

Blood pressure is kept at the minimal level necessary to maintain neurologic function. For patients awaiting surgery, the maximum systolic pressure is 160 mm Hg. When the aneurysm has been obliterated, the maximum systolic pressure is 240 mm Hg (Kassell et al., 1982). When necessary, a vasopressor (such as dopamine) may be administered to maintain optimum blood pressure.

Risks associated with intravascular volume expansion include aneurysmal rebleeding, pulmonary edema, myocardial infarction, dilutional hyponatremia, hemothorax, and coagulopathy (Kassell et al., 1982). Intensive monitoring of CVP, pulmonary artery wedge pressure, cardiac function, arterial blood gases, and serum and urinary electrolytes is mandatory.

SURGICAL TREATMENT

Operative treatment of saccular aneurysms involves placing a metal clip across the base of the lesion where it rises from the parent vessel. Definitive treatment of AVM is complete excision, when possible. Optimal timing for surgery (early versus delayed) is controversial. Prognosis and treatment decisions are often based on the size and location of the lesion as well as the clinical status of the patient on admission.

Surgery during the first 48 hours (early) eliminates the risk of aneurysmal rebleeding and may reduce vasospasm by removing the subarachnoid clot. Surgery performed 10 to 14 days after the initial hemorrhage allows resolution of cerebral edema and reduces postoperative vasospasm (Mohr et al., 1986b). The Hunt and Hess (1968) classification of intracranial aneurysms is frequently used to aid these decisions (Table 33–5). The current trend is to operate on grade I and grade II lesions as soon as diagnostic studies are complete.

The decision to intervene surgically to remove an AVM that has hemorrhaged is based on similar criteria. An unruptured AVM that presents with a seizure or headache may be managed appropriately without surgery. Because of their size or location, some AVMs are not amenable to surgical intervention. Embolization, Bragg-Peak proton beam therapy, or stereotactic radiosurgery may be used in these situations.

Embolization. Embolization obliterates inoperable vascular malformations, including some aneurysms. This procedure may precede surgical intervention in an attempt to reduce the size of the lesion. Superselective catheterization and angiography are used to deliver the embolizing material (e.g., particles [radiopaque Silastic spheres], detachable balloons, or liquid adhesive). Best results have been obtained with balloons or adhesive. Transient or permanent neurologic deficits may follow embolization. Some complications are specific to the technique, such as gluing the balloon in place, rupture of the balloon in a small feeder artery, or occlusion of normal arteries (Vinuela and Fox, 1986).

Bragg-Peak Proton Beam Therapy. In this procedure stereotactic neurosurgery is used to guide pro-

TABLE 33–5. Classification of Patients with Intracranial Aneurysms According to Surgical Risk

Category*	Criteria
Grade I	Asymptomatic, or minimal headache and slight nuchal rigidity.
Grade II	Moderate to severe headache, nuchal rigidity, no neurological deficit other than cranial nerve palsy.
Grade III	Drowsiness, confusion, or mild focal deficit.
Grade IV	Stupor, moderate to severe hemiparesis, possibly early decerebrate rigidity and vegetative disturbances.
Grade V	Deep coma, decerebrate rigidity, moribund appearance.

*From Hunt, W. E., and Hess, R. M. (1968). *Journal of Neurosurgery*, 28(1), 14.

ton beam radiation to the AVM. Within 1 to 2 years of treatment, the walls of small vessels thicken and reduce the lumen, causing associated arteries and veins to return gradually to near normal in size. Although this is a low-risk procedure, it is not widely available because of the elaborate equipment needed (Kjellberg et al., 1983).

Stereotactic Radiosurgery. In this procedure gamma radiation is focused stereotactically on an intracranial target. Although individual beams deliver very small doses of gamma radiation, the intersecting focus of all beams receives a large dose of energy that is capable of obliterating a vascular malformation. This procedure is most effective for smaller AVMs of which the entire nidus can be irradiated. The mechanism of occlusion is uncertain, but proliferation of endothelial lining and thrombosis are thought to contribute (Steiner, 1986).

The major drawback to radiosurgery is the length of time that elapses before results are seen. Hemodynamic changes, such as decreased flow rate, may be noted within 3 months, but complete obliteration may take from 6 to 22 months (Steiner, 1986). Angiographic evidence of obliteration has been identified in 85% of the patients who have undergone radiosurgery. Potential complications include delayed radiation necrosis or rebleeding, but the risk of rebleeding is the same as that noted in the natural history of an AVM (Steiner, 1986). Currently, this procedure is available in only a few centers due to the expense and type of equipment, but this situation is expected to change in the near future.

NURSING CARE OF THE PATIENT WITH AN ACUTE CEREBROVASCULAR EVENT

Optimal care of the patient with a stroke is provided through an interdisciplinary approach that utilizes the primary nurse, physician, social worker, dietitian, and physical, occupational, and speech therapists. Nursing care of the patient with a stroke should focus on stabilization in the acute phase, prevention of complications, psychological needs, rehabilitation, and discharge planning (Hickey, 1986). The quality of the care given during the earlier stages has a significant impact on the overall outcome and rehabilitation potential. Monitoring the neurologic, hemodynamic, and respiratory status throughout the patient's care is essential. Specific nursing care is guided by the patient's actual neurologic deficit. Monitoring activities, selective nursing diagnoses, and interventions are outlined below.

Monitoring Activities

Neurologic Status. The patient's neurologic condition can change rapidly and subtly. Hourly assess-

ments of the level of consciousness, mental status, cranial nerves, and general motor and sensory function should be carefully documented until the patient is stable. Decreased level of consciousness is often the first indicator of progression of the stroke. Any deterioration must be promptly reported to the physician.

Hemodynamic Status. Cardiovascular monitoring for arrhythmias (particularly atrial fibrillation), congestive heart failure, and variations in blood pressure is important. Blood pressure should be assessed prior to and after administration of antihypertensive agents. If there is a significant change from previous blood pressure readings or in the patient's condition, the nurse should notify the physician before giving the medication. A precipitous drop or rise in blood pressure may be associated with clinical decline. Fluid balance (intake and output), serum and urinary electrolytes, and osmolality should be closely monitored. A CVP line or arterial line is frequently used to monitor hemodynamic status. Specific guidelines for maintenance of the CVP and pulmonary artery wedge pressure during intravascular volume expansion were discussed earlier in this chapter.

Pulmonary Status. Recovery may be impeded by respiratory problems, such as hypostatic pneumonia, aspiration, or pulmonary embolism. To prevent or promptly treat these conditions, the respiratory status should be frequently monitored. Auscultation of breath sounds, observation of respiratory rate and pattern, and monitoring reports of arterial blood gases and chest x-rays should be included in the nurse's assessment.

Aggressive pulmonary toilet such as coughing and deep breathing, intermittent positive pressure breathing, chest physiotherapy, and suctioning is needed to maintain a patent airway and remove secretions. However, vigorous coughing, suctioning, and chest physiotherapy must be avoided in patients with intracranial hemorrhage or signs of increased intracranial pressure. Repositioning of the patient every 1 to 2 hours will also facilitate mobilization of secretions.

Patients with dysphagia should be carefully assessed prior to beginning oral feedings. It is important to note that the gag reflex is *not* a reliable indicator of the patient's swallowing ability (Horner, et al., 1988). Nurses must assess palatal function and the swallowing reflex. A small amount of water or soft food is given and the swallowing process observed. Speech therapists can be consulted for a formal swallowing evaluation. Dysphonia is present more often in patients who aspirate (Horner et al., 1988) and should prompt the nurse to assess carefully the patient's ability to swallow.

Minidose heparin may be ordered to decrease the risk of pulmonary embolism in patients who have suffered a nonhemorrhagic stroke and are not otherwise receiving anticoagulants. Antiembolic stockings are used for similar purposes.

Nursing Diagnoses

Alteration in Cerebral Tissue Perfusion Related to Increased Intracranial Pressure or Vasospasm. Cerebral injury results in disrupted local blood supply, edema, and possible systemic cardiovascular instability.

Expected Outcome. Neurologic status improves or remains stable.

Neurologic assessments focus on the level of consciousness using the Glasgow Coma Scale if appropriate (see Chap. 32), pupillary reflexes, and motor function. Careful documentation allows identification of subtle changes or deterioration over time.

The position and activity level best tolerated by the patient need to be determined. Postural changes, even changes achieved just by elevating the head of the bed, may produce clinical worsening. This can occur in the absence of orthostatic hypotension (Caplan and Sergay, 1976). In other patients it is desirable to elevate the head of the bed to reduce intracranial pressure and promote venous drainage.

Hyperoxygenation and hyperventilation before and after suctioning blunt the effect of suctioning on ICP. Limiting suctioning to no more than 10 seconds at a time also restricts elevation of ICP.

Ineffective Airway Clearance Due to Decreased Level of Consciousness and Decreased Neuromuscular Function

Expected Outcome. A patent airway is maintained, there is no evidence of pulmonary complications, lungs are clear to auscultation, ABGs remain within normal limits, and the patient is afebrile.

Respiratory parameters should be carefully monitored with vital signs, including rate and pattern of respirations, airway pressures, breath sounds, and chest expansion. Gag and swallowing reflexes should be assessed as indicated.

Patients should be turned every 2 hours to facilitate mobilization of pulmonary secretions.

Viscosity of secretions should be monitored, and increased humidification of inspired air, added hydration, or mucolytic agents requested for patients with viscous secretions.

Potential Impaired Skin Integrity Due to Sensory and Motor Deficits Following a Cerebrovascular Event

Expected Outcome. Skin remains dry, intact, and nonerythemic. A turning schedule is posted and continuously followed.

Because of paresis and decreased mobility, these patients are especially prone to pressure necrosis. Patients who are able to respond to commands should be encouraged to change position frequently. Family members should be taught the importance of helping patients move and how to avoid shear forces when helping them move. A turning schedule should be established and posted at the bedside to ensure that turning patterns are uniformly followed. Inspection, massage, and application of lotion to all bony prominences (including the back of the head) and the ears should be accomplished each time the patient is turned and positioned. Skin should be kept free of excess moisture but not allowed to become dry and scaly; bath oil is preferred to soap for bed baths. Avoid use of plastic incontinent pads in direct contact with the patient's skin because these trap moisture and heat and may macerate the skin.

Adjunctive devices cannot replace basic nursing interventions in preventing pressure necrosis, but they do help. Air mattresses and mechanical beds (kinetic tables, air fluidized mattresses, circolectric beds) may be useful depending on the patient's condition. Judicious use of heel and elbow pads may also be helpful.

Postoperative craniotomy patients will require sterile wound care to prevent infections. The nurse should also position the patient so that pressure is not applied to the incision site.

Impaired Physical Mobility Due to Muscle Weakness, Paresis, or Immobility

Expected Outcome. Patient is able to use all extremities without residual loss of range of motion or complaints of pain or stiffness.

Patients who respond to commands and family members should be instructed in the need for and how to perform range of motion exercises. An exercise program should be established that places all joints through their full range of motion every 8 hours. Joints with partial or complete function should also be placed through range of motion. Instructing the patient and family in the need for range of motion increases the potential for prevention of contractures. Ideally, the exercise schedule is posted at the bedside to encourage patient and family participation.

Proper positioning is vital to maintain optimal joint function. The ideal joint position is neutral. Splints, orthoses, and adjunctive aids (antirotation boots, antidrop foot splints, trochanter rolls, high-top tennis shoes, and wrist splints) may be indicated to prevent or correct joint contracture.

Paretic upper extremities are prone to injury, especially freezing or dislocation of the shoulder. Patients with nondominant (usually right-sided) cerebral hemispheric infarcts may completely neglect or deny their hemiplegic side or may be unable to recognize that their arm is caught between the bed and side rail. Special care needs to be taken to protect this extremity from injury on bedrails, hanging from the bedside, or out of a wheelchair. Sling and swathe restraints may be obtained from physical therapy to aid in supporting the extremity, decreasing the potential for injury.

Ineffective Family Coping: Compromised or Disabling Due to Overwhelming Aspects of Cerebrovascular Event on Family

Expected Outcome. Patient and family are able to cope effectively with the situation as shown by the absence of abnormal reactions.

Patients may experience loss of self-image and a sense of powerlessness, and the family and patient need assistance in adjusting to this change. Behavior and personality changes may be related to the area of infarct. Patients with left hemispheric infarcts are more likely to exhibit signs of depression. These patients are often aphasic, creating difficulty in evaluating the presence of depression. Antidepressants can often be effective in this group of patients (Caplan and Stein, 1986). Inappropriate cheerfulness may be associated with right hemispheric infarcts (Robinson et al., 1984). Emotional lability, loss of social inhibitions, and impulsiveness are behaviors found in some stroke patients. The nurse must inform the family and patient about the probable source of these reactions and aid the patient and family in developing individualized interventions to meet these problems.

Family members may experience fear, helplessness, and loss of control. Aid the family in identifying tasks that they can perform (exercises, repositioning) that aid the patient's recovery. Encourage the family to listen to the patient's concerns and to identify problem areas in which staff may intervene. Encourage the family to talk about current events and reminisce about the patient's past to facilitate communication with aphasic patients. Incorporate the family in the care of the patient as far as they feel comfortable in so doing. (See also Chap. 7.)

Impaired Verbal Communication Due to Dysarthria, Aphasia, or Altered Mental Status

Expected Outcome. Patient maintains optimal communication level for his physiologic state. Family members actively communicate with the patient.

The nurse should begin by assessing the patient's fluency, clarity, and content of speech, comprehension, and memory (Blanco, 1982; Ozuna, 1985). An inability to communicate may contribute to the fear and frustration experienced by patients and families. The nurse needs to use imagination to aid these patients in communicating their needs. Letter and picture boards may be useful. Although use of the communication boards is tedious and time-consuming, it may allow the patient his only means of communicating with others.

It is important to spend time with the patient and family teaching them how to use the communication method adequately. The nurse should acknowledge the patient's frustration about the slowness of communication while encouraging patience. (See also Chap. 6.)

Alteration in Nutrition: Less Than Bodily Requirements. Malnutrition may be due to immobility, decreased gastrointestinal mobility, dysphagia, anorexia, or depression.

Expected Outcome. Patient maintains ideal body weight and, when plausible, actively participates in the diet regimen.

The threat of aspiration can complicate the patient's ability to maintain adequate nutrition. Careful assessment of pharyngeal function is mandatory as a baseline in nutrition interventions. Patients with mild dysphagia may be able to ingest semisolid to solid foods while sitting upright. Liquids tend to be aspirated more easily. Enteric or parenteral nutrition are necessary with moderate to severe dysphagia. Patients on tube feedings should be assessed for excessive gastric residual (>50 mL in 2 hours for continuous feedings and >100 mL for every-4-hour feedings). Metoclopramide hydrochloride may be ordered to facilitate gastric emptying. If the patient is able to begin eating solid foods, calorie counts may be used periodically to ensure adequate caloric intake. If necessary, the patient should be aided in choosing foods that are nutritious. Encouraging the family to bring in home-cooked foods may be useful for some patients. Taking weights daily or every other day allows monitoring of nutritional status.

Total Incontinence Due to Patient's Lack of Awareness or Inability to Reach Commode or to Express a Need to Void

Expected Outcome. A bladder-emptying regimen should be established that allows maintenance of continence and prevents complications of urinary tract infection or urinary retention.

Stroke patients with frontal lobe involvement are particularly prone to urinary incontinence. Clean intermittent catheterization programs should be established for these patients, emptying the bladder every 4 to 6 hours, until urologic assessments of the potential for bladder control are accomplished. Use of a urinary output flow sheet aids in ensuring that appropriate intervals are maintained between bladder catheterizations.

Constipation and fecal impaction, frequent complications of immobility, must be prevented to the extent possible. The Valsalva maneuver, manual disimpaction, and the use of enemas all increase intracranial pressure and should be avoided during the most acute phase of the stroke.

Partial Self-Care Deficit Due to Partial Loss of Motor Function

Expected Outcome. Patient participates maximally in self-care, the degree of participation being based on the physiologic capabilities, and the patient demonstrates feelings of self-worth and exercises some degree of control.

Patients with cerebrovascular events experience a temporary, total loss of physical ability to perform some activities of daily living. The patient is initially dependent on others for most self-care. Dependence lowers a person's sense of control and self-worth and may lead to depression. Giving the patient as much control as possible is essential. Include the patient in planning of care and goal setting; provide instruction to allow the patient to make knowledgeable decisions. (See also Chap. 6.) Consult with physical therapists as soon as the patient's condition has stabilized.

Potential for Injury Due to Cognitive, Visual, or Motor Deficits Resulting from Cerebrovascular Event

Expected Outcome. Patients and families will verbalize their understanding of the necessary safety precautions. Safety precautions will be adhered to, and the patient will not receive any injuries.

Basic safety interventions include keeping bedrails raised, keeping the bed in its lowest position, ensuring proper lighting (including night lighting), keeping the call light within reach and ensuring that the patient understands how to use it and is capable of using it, and removing hazardous objects and unnecessary clutter from the patient's immediate area. When an identified seizure disorder is present, seizure precautions should be maintained (see Chap. 32).

Patients with anosognosia may deny their disability and may not recognize their paretic extremity. Because of this denial, these patients are prone to fall when getting out of bed (Booth, 1982). Soft restraints may be required to protect these patients, especially those with concurrent cognitive dysfunction.

The patient with a visual field deficit (such as homonymous hemianopsia) should be positioned in the room so that all activity occurs in his or her unaffected visual field. The patient's telephone, television, meal tray, and so on should all be placed within the normal visual field. The nurse should instruct other caregivers, family members, and visitors to announce their presence in the room and approach the patient from his or her unaffected side. The nurse should also instruct the patient and family to be aware of the safety hazards to the patient and provide instruction in measures to protect the patient.

Knowledge Deficit of Therapy and of How Much the Patient and Family Are Expected to Participate in Care

Expected Outcome. Patients and their family members verbalize understanding of their role in the rehabilitation of the patient and actively participate in care.

The patient's ability to comprehend and remember will influence how the nurse approaches this problem. Family should be included in all teaching sessions, which should be scheduled to allow family participation. Patients and family should be encouraged to participate in care whenever possible. Information about the illness, medications, intensive care therapy regimen, preventive measures, risk factors, and available community resources should be shared with the patient and family. The importance of adhering to the medication regimen (such as antihypertensive therapy), modification of risk factors, and follow-up care are stressed.

Impaired Home Maintenance Management Due to Lack of Understanding of the Goals of and Resources Available for Rehabilitation

Expected Outcome. The patient and family become active members of the rehabilitation team and are able to make realistic and knowledgeable choices about patient's care after hospitalization.

Discharge planning begins early in the hospitalization and requires involvement of the patient, family, and multiple health care disciplines. Both family members and the patient should be active members of the team. Realistic goals should be established and available resources assessed. Early in the hospitalization decisions on referral to a rehabilitation hospital, extended care facility, or home health agency will be made. Involving the patient and family in the patient's care, especially preventive and rehabilitative aspects, allows them to understand realistically the potential placement of the patient.

ncp nursing care plan

1. Altered cerebral tissue perfusion related to:
Increased intracranial pressure
Vasospasm

Outcome Criteria	Nursing Interventions
Neurologic status improves or remains stable.	Assess neurologic status, focusing on level of consciousness, and carefully document the findings. Determine the position and activity level best tolerated by the patient. Hyperoxygenate and hyperinflate lungs before and after suctioning. Limit suctioning to no more than two passes of 10 seconds each.

2. Ineffective airway clearance related to:
  Decreased level of consciousness
  Decreased neuromuscular function

Outcome Criteria	Nursing Interventions
Patient airway is maintained.
There is no evidence of pulmonary complications.
Lungs are clear to auscultation.
Arterial blood gases are within normal limits.
Patient is afebrile.	Carefully monitor vital signs, including ventilatory rate and pattern, airway pressures, breath sounds, and chest expansion.
Assess gag and swallowing reflexes as indicated.
Monitor viscosity of secretions and increase humidification of inspired air, add hydration or mucolytic agents as needed.
Turn patient every 2 hours to facilitate mobilization of secretions.

3. Potential impaired skin integrity related to:
  Sensory deficits following cerebrovascular event
  Motor deficits following cerebrovascular event

Outcome Criteria	Nursing Interventions
Skin remains dry, intact, and nonerythemic.
A turning schedule is posted and followed.	If responsive to commands, encourage patient to change positions frequently.
Teach family members the importance of helping patients move and how to avoid shear forces.
Establish and post a turning schedule.
Inspect, apply lotion, and massage all bony prominences (including the head and ears) each time the patient is turned and positioned.
Keep skin free of excess moisture, but prevent the skin from becoming dry and scaly.
Use bath oil rather than soap for bathing.
Avoid using plastic incontinence pads in direct contact with skin to avoid skin maceration.
Use adjunctive devices (such as air mattresses, mechanical beds, and heel and elbow protectors) to help prevent pressure necrosis.
Follow sterile procedures for wound care.
Position patient to avoid pressure on incisions.

4. Impaired physical mobility related to:
  Muscle weakness
  Paresis
  Immobility

Outcome Criteria	Nursing Interventions
Patient is able to use all extremities without residual loss of range of motion or complaints of stiffness or pain.	Instruct patient and family members in the need for and how to perform range of motion exercises.
Establish and post an exercise program that places all joints through their full range of motion every 8 hours (including joints with partial function).
If possible, position patient in neutral position and use splints, orthoses, and adjunctive aids to prevent or correct contractures.
Protect patient's hemiplegic side from injury on bedrail or from hanging from bedside or wheelchair.

5. Ineffective family coping: compromised or disabling related to:
  Overwhelming aspects of cerebrovascular event

Outcome Criteria	Nursing Interventions
Patient and family members are able to cope effectively with the situation as shown by the absence of abnormal reactions.	Inform the patient and family of the probable pathologic source of depression, cheerfulness, and emotional lability. Help develop individualized interventions for these problems.
Help family members identify tasks that they can perform that aid in the patient's recovery.
Encourage family members to listen to the patient's concerns and to identify areas in which the staff may intervene.
Encourage family members to talk about current events and to reminisce about the patient's past to facilitate communication with aphasic patients.
Incorporate family members into patient care as far as they feel comfortable.

6. Impaired verbal communication related to:
  Dysarthria
  Aphasia
  Altered mental state

Nursing Care Plan continued on following page

Outcome Criteria	Nursing Interventions
Patient maintains optimal communication level for his physiologic state. Family members actively communicate with the patient.	Assess the patient's fluency, clarity, and content of speech, comprehension, and memory. Help the patient communicate his needs by using adjuncts such as word or picture boards. Spend time with patient and family members, teaching them how to use communication aids. Acknowledge the patient's frustration about the slowness of communication while encouraging patience.

7. Altered nutrition: less than body requirements related to:
   Immobility
   Decreased gastrointestinal motility
   Dysphagia
   Anorexia
   Depression

Outcome Criteria	Nursing Interventions
Patient maintains target body weight. Patient actively participates in the diet program.	Carefully assess pharyngeal function. Assess patient's receiving tube feedings for excessive gastric residual volume. Administer metoclopramide to facilitate gastric emptying as needed. If the patient is eating, perform calorie counts periodically. Help the patient to choose foods that are nutritious, high in protein and vitamins. Encourage family members to bring home-cooked foods. Monitor weight daily or every other day.

8. Total incontinence related to:
   Lack of awareness
   Inability to reach commode
   Inability to express need to void

Outcome Criteria	Nursing Interventions
Continence. No urinary tract infections. No bladder distention.	Establish an intermittent bladder catheterization program, every 4 to 6 hours, until urologic assessment of the potential for bladder control is completed. Use a urinary output flow sheet. Prevent constipation and fecal impaction to the extent possible. Avoid the Valsalva maneuver, manual disimpaction, and the use of enemas during the acute phase of stroke.

9. Partial self-care deficit related to:
   Partial loss of motor function

Outcome Criteria	Nursing Interventions
Patient participates maximally in self-care. Patient demonstrates feeling of self-worth. Patient exercises some degree of control.	Give patient as much control as possible. Include patient in goal setting and care planning. Provide instruction to allow patient to make knowledgeable decisions. Consult physical and occupational therapists as soon as the patient's condition stabilizes.

10. Potential injury related to:
   Cognitive deficits
   Visual deficits
   Motor deficits

Outcome Criteria	Nursing Interventions
Patient and family members verbalize their understanding of necessary safety precautions. Safety precautions are enforced. Patient does not sustain injury.	Implement basic safety procedures: keep bedrails raised, keep bed in lowest position, keep call light within reach and ensure patient understands its use, provide adequate lighting, remove hazardous objects and unnecessary clutter. Maintain seizure precautions when a seizure disorder has been identified. Use soft restraints in patients with anosognosia, especially patients with concurrent cognitive dysfunction. Position patients with visual field deficits so that all activity occurs within his or her unaffected field of vision. Place patient's telephone, television, and bedside table within the patient's visual field. Instruct caregivers, family members, and visitors to announce their presence in the room and to approach the patient from his or her unaffected side. Instruct the patient and family members to be aware of safety hazards and provide instruction in measures to protect the patient.

11. Knowledge deficit related to:
   Therapy
   Expectations of patient and family to participate in care

Outcome Criteria	Nursing Interventions
Patient and family members verbalize an understanding of their roles in rehabilitation. Patient and family members actively participate in care.	Include family members in all teaching sessions, scheduling them to allow family participation. Encourage patient and family members to participate in care whenever possible. Share information about the illness, medications, and intensive care therapy regimen, preventive measures, risk factors, and the availability of community resources. Stress the importance of adhering to the established medication regimen, modification of risk factors, and follow-up care.

12. Impaired home maintenance management related to:
   Lack of understanding of the goals of the resources available for rehabilitation

Outcome Criteria	Nursing Interventions
Patient and family are active members of the rehabilitation team. Patient and family are able to make knowledgeable choices about patient's care after hospitalization.	Begin discharge planning early in hospitalization. Involve patient, family members, and other care providers. Establish realistic goals and assess available resources. Involve patient and family members in patient's care, especially in preventive and rehabilitative aspects.

References

Abbott, R. D., Yin, Y., Reed, D. M., et al. (1986). Risk of stroke in male cigarette smokers. *New England Journal of Medicine, 315,* 717–720.

Adams, H. P. (1987). Antifibrinolytics in aneurysmal subarachnoid hemorrhage: Do they have a role? Maybe. *Archives of Neurology, 44,* 114–115.

American Heart Association. (1988). *1988 Stroke facts.* Dallas.

American-Canadian Co-Operative Study Group. (1985). Persantine aspirin trial in cerebral ischemia. Part II: Endpoint results. *Stroke, 16,* 406–415.

Aver, L. M. (1984). Acute operation and preventive nimodipine improve outcome in patients with ruptured cerebral aneurysms. *Neurosurgery, 15,* 57–66.

Awad, I. A., Carter, P., Spetzler, R. F., et al. (1987). Clinical vasospasm after subarachnoid hemorrhage: Response to hypervolemic hemodilution and arterial hypertension. *Stroke, 18,* 365–372.

Baker, A. B., and Ionnone, A. (1961). Cerebrovascular disease VII. A study of etiologic mechanisms. *Neurology, 11,* 23–31.

Barnett, H. J. M. (1979). The pathophysiology of transient cerebral ischemic attacks therapy with platelet antiaggregants. *Medical Clinics of North America, 63,* 649–679.

Barnett, H. J. M., Jones, M. W., Boughner, D. R., et al. (1976). Cerebral ischemic events associated with prolapsing mitral valve. *Archives of Neurology, 33,* 777–782.

Beck, D. W., Adams, H. P., Flamm, E. S., et al. (1988). Combination of aminocaproic acid and nicardipine in treatment of aneurysmal subarachnoid hemorrhage. *Stroke, 19,* 63–67.

Berger, A. R., Lipton, R. B., Lesser, M. L., et al. (1988). Early seizures following intracerebral hemorrhage: Implications for therapy. *Neurology, 38,* 1363–1365.

Biller, J., Loftus, C. M., Moore, S. A., et al. (1987). Isolated central nervous system angiitis first presenting as spontaneous intracranial hemorrhage. *Neurosurgery, 20,* 310–315.

Blanco, K. M. (1982). The aphasic patient. *Journal of Neurosurgical Nursing, 14,* 34–37.

Bogousslavsky, J., Regli, F., Van Melle, G., et al. (1988). Migraine stroke. *Neurology, 38,* 223–227.

Booth, K. (1982). The neglect syndrome. *Journal of Neurosurgical Nursing, 14,* 38–43.

Bounds, J. V., Wiebers, D. O., Whisnant, J. P., et al. (1981). Mechanisms and timing of deaths from cerebral infarction. *Stroke, 12,* 474–477.

Bousser, M., Chiras, J., Bories, J., et al. (1985). Cerebral venous thrombosis—a review of 38 cases. *Stroke, 16,* 199–213.

Bousser, M. G., Eschwege, E., Haguenau, M., et al. (1983). "AICLA" controlled trial of aspirin and dipyridamole in the secondary prevention of athero-thrombotic cerebral ischemia. *Stroke, 14,* 5–14.

Brant-Zawadzki, N. (1988). MR imaging of the brain. *Radiology, 166,* 1–10.

Britton, M., and Roden, A. (1985). Progression of stroke after arrival at hospital. *Stroke, 16,* 629–632.

Broderick, J. P., and Swanson, J. W. (1987). Migraine-related strokes. *Archives of Neurology, 44,* 868–871.

Brott, T. G., Gelfand, M. J., Williams, C. C., et al. (1986). Frequency and patterns of abnormality detected by iodine-123 amine emission CT after cerebral infarction. *Radiology, 158,* 729–734.

Brott, T., Thalinger, K., and Hertzberg, V. (1986). Hypertension as a risk factor for spontaneous intracerebral hemorrhage. *Stroke, 17,* 1078–1083.

Brust, J. C., Plank, C. R., Healton, E. B., et al. (1979). The pathology of drop attacks: A case report. *Neurology* (Minneapolis), 29 (6), 786–790.

Canadian Cooperative Study Group. (1978). A randomized trial of aspirin and sulfinpyrazone in threatened stroke. *New England Journal of Medicine, 299,* 53–59.

Caplan, L., Corbett, J., Goodwin, J., et al. (1983). Neuro-ophthalmologic signs in the angiitic form of neurosarcoidosis. *Neurology, 33,* 1130–1135.

Caplan, L. R., Hier, D. B., and Banks, G. (1982). Current concepts of cerebrovascular disease—stroke: Stroke and drug abuse. *Stroke, 13,* 869–872.

Caplan, L. R., Hier, D. B., and D'Cruz, I. (1983). Cerebral embolism in the Michael Reese Stroke Registry. *Stroke, 14,* 530–536.

Caplan, L. R., and Sergay, S. (1976). Positional cerebral ischaemia. *Journal of Neurology, Neurosurgery, and Psychiatry, 39,* 385–391.

Caplan, L. R., and Stein, R. W. (1986). *Stroke: A clinical approach.* Boston: Butterworths.

Cerebral Embolism Study Group (1984). Immediate anticoagulation of embolic stroke: Brain hemorrhage and management options. *Stroke, 15,* 779–789.

Cocito, L., Favale, E., and Reni, L. (1982). Epileptic seizures in cerebral arterial occlusive disease. *Stroke, 13,* 189–195.

Collaborative Group for the Study of Stroke in Young Women (1975). Oral contraceptive and stroke in young women: Associated risk factors. *Journal of the American Medical Association*, 231, 718–722.

Delaney, P., and Estes, M. (1980). Intracranial hemorrhage with amphetamine abuse. *Neurology*, 30, 1125–1128.

Del Zoppo, G. J., Zeumer, H., and Harker, L. A. (1986). Thrombolytic therapy in stroke: Possibilities and hazards. *Stroke*, 17, 595–607.

DeWitt, L. D., and Wechsler, L. R. (1988). Transcranial Doppler. *Stroke*, 19, 915–921.

Donaldson, J. O. (1986). Cerebrovascular disease: Pregnancy, puerperium, and the Pill. *Neurology and Neurosurgery Update Series*, 6, 2–8.

EC/IC Bypass Study Group. (1985). Failure of extracranial-intracranial arterial bypass to reduce the risk of ischemic stroke. *New England Journal of Medicine*, 313, 1191–1200.

Edmunds, L. H. (1982). Thromboembolic complications of current cardiac valvular prostheses. *Annals of Thoracic Surgery*, 34, 96–106.

Fallis, R. J., and Fisher, M. (1985). Cerebral vasculitis and hemorrhage associated with phenylpropanolamine. *Neurology*, 35, 405–407.

Featherstone, H. J. (1986). Clinical features of stroke in migraine: A review. *Headache*, 26, 128–133.

Ferguson, G. G. (1972). Physical factors in the initiation, growth, and rupture of human intracranial saccular aneurysms. *Journal of Neurosurgery*, 37, 666–677.

Fisher, C. M. (1982). Pure sensory stroke and allied conditions. *Stroke*, 13, 434–447.

Fisher, C. M. and Curry, H. B. (1965). Pure motor hemiplegia of vascular origin. *Archives of Neurology*, 13, 30–44.

Flamm, E. S., Adams, H. P., Beck, D. W., et al. (1988). Dose-escalation study of intravenous nicardipine in patients with aneurysmal subarachnoid hemorrhage. *Journal of Neurosurgery*, 68, 393–400.

Fults, D., and Kelly, D. L. (1984). Natural history of arteriovenous malformations of the brain: A clinical study. *Neurosurgery*, 15, 658–662.

Furlan, A. J. (1985). Cardiac disease and stroke. In F. McDowell and L. R. Caplan (Eds.), *Cerebrovascular survey report for the National Institute of Neurological and Communicative Disorders and Stroke* (pp. 97–107). Bethesda: National Institute of Health.

Furlan, A. J., Whisnant, J. P., and Elveback, L. R. (1979). The decreasing incidence of primary intracerebral hemorrhage: A population study. *Annals of Neurology*, 5, 367–373.

Garcia, J. H., and Geer, J. C. (1985). Carotid artery atherosclerotic disease pathology and detection. In F. McDowell and L. R. Caplan (Eds.), *Cerebrovascular survey report for the National Institute of Neurological and Communicative Disorders and Stroke* (pp. 35–45). Bethesda: National Institutes of Health.

Garraway, W. M., Whisnant, J. M., Furlan, A. J., et al. (1979). The declining incidence of stroke. *New England Journal of Medicine*, 300, 449–452.

Gelmers, H. J., Gorter, K., de Weerdt, C. J., et al. (1988). A controlled trial of nimodipine in acute ischemic stroke. *New England Journal of Medicine*, 318, 203–207.

Gent, M., Blakely, J. A., Easton, J. D., et al. (1988). The Canadian American ticlopidine study (CATS) in thromboembolic stroke. Design, organization, and baseline results. *Stroke*, 19 (10), 1203–1210.

Gifford, A. J. (1966). An epidemiological study of cerebrovascular disease. *American Journal of Public Health*, 56, 452–461.

Gilles, C., Brucher, J. M., Khoubesserian, P., et al. (1984). Cerebral amyloid angiopathy as a cause of multiple intracerebral hemorrhages. *Neurology*, 34, 730–735.

Gillum, R. F. (1988). Stroke in blacks. *Stroke*, 19, 1–9.

Glick, R., Hoying, J., Cerullo, L., et al. (1987). Phenylpropanolamine: An over-the-counter drug causing central nervous system vasculitis and intracerebral hemorrhage. *Neurosurgery*, 20, 969–974.

Gorelick, P. B., Hier, D. B., Caplan, L. R., et al. (1986). Headache in acute cerebrovascular disease. *Neurology*, 36, 1445–1450.

Graf, C. J., Perret, G. E., and Torner, J. C. (1983). Bleeding from cerebral arteriovenous malformations as part of their natural history. *Journal of Neurosurgery*, 58, 331–337.

Greenberg, D. A. (1987). Calcium channels and calcium channel antagonists. *Annals of Neurology*, 21, 317–330.

Greenlee, J. E., and Mandell, G. L. (1973). Neurological manifestations of infective endocarditis: A review. *Stroke*, 4, 958–963.

Gross, C. R., Kase, C. S., Mohr, J. P., et al. (1984). Stroke in south Alabama: Incidence and diagnostic features—a population based study. *Stroke*, 15, 249–255.

Grotta, J. C. (1987). Current status of hemodilution in acute cerebral ischemia (editorial). *Stroke*, 18, 689–690.

Grotta, J., Ackerman, R., Correia, J., et al. (1982). Whole blood parameters and cerebral blood flow. *Stroke*, 13, 296–301.

Grotta, J. C., Lemak, N. A., Gary, H., et al. (1985). Does platelet antiaggregant therapy lessen the severity of stroke? *Neurology*, 35, 632–636.

Hart, R. G., Byer, H. A., Slaughter, J. R., et al. (1981). Occurrence and implications of seizures in subarachnoid hemorrhage due to ruptured intracranial aneurysms. *Neurosurgery*, 8, 417–421.

Hart, R. G., Coull, B. M., and Hart, D. (1983). Early recurrent embolism associated with nonvalvular atrial fibrillation: A retrospective study. *Stroke*, 14, 688–693.

Hass, W. K., Easton, J. D., Adams, H. P., et al., for the Ticlopidine Aspirin Stroke Study Group (1989). A randomized trial comparing ticlopidine hydrochloride with aspirin for the prevention of stroke in high-risk patients. *New England Journal of Medicine*, 321, 501–507.

Helgason, C. M. (1988). Blood glucose and stroke. *Stroke*, 19, 937–941.

Heyden, S., Heyman, A., and Camplong, L. (1969). Mortality patterns among parents of patients with atherosclerotic cerebrovascular disease. *Journal of Chronic Disease*, 22, 105–110.

Hickey, J. V. (1986). *The clinical practice of neurological and neurosurgical nursing* (2nd ed.). Philadelphia: J. B. Lippincott.

Horner, J., Massey, E. W., Riski, J. E., et al. (1988). Aspiration following stroke: Clinical correlates and outcome. *Neurology*, 38, 1359–1362.

Hunt, W. E., and Hess, R. M. (1968). Surgical risk as related to time of intervention in the repair of intracranial aneurysms. *Journal of Neurosurgery*, 28, 14–20.

Jackson, A. C., Boughner, B. R., and Barnett, H. J. M. (1984). Mitral valve prolapse and cerebral ischemic events in young patients. *Neurology*, 34, 784–787.

Jensen, T. S., and de-Fine-Olivarius, B. (1981). Transient global amnesia—its clinical and pathophysiological basis and prognosis. *Acta Neurologica Scandinavia*, 63 (4), 220–230.

Kannel, W. B., Gordon, T., and Dawber, T. R. (1974). Role of lipids in the development of brain infarction: The Framingham study. *Stroke*, 5, 679–685.

Kannel, W. B., Sorlie, P., and Gordon, T. (1980). Labile hypertension: A faulty concept? The Framingham study. *Circulation*, 61, 1183–1187.

Kannel, W. B., Wolf, P. A., McGee, D. L., et al. (1981). Systolic blood pressure, arterial rigidity, and risk of stroke: The Framingham study. *Journal of the American Medical Association*, 245, 1225–1229.

Kannel, W. B., Wolf, P. A., and Verter, J. (1983). Manifestations of coronary disease predisposing to stroke: The Framingham study. *Journal of the American Medical Association*, 250, 2942–2946.

Kannel, W. B., Wolf, P. A., Verter, J., et al. (1970). Epidemiologic assessment of the role of blood pressure in stroke: The Framingham study. *Journal of the American Medical Association*, 214, 301–310.

Kase, C. S., Foster, T. E., Reed, J. E., et al. (1987). Intracerebral hemorrhage and phenylpropanolamine use. *Neurology*, 37, 399–404.

Kase, C. S., and Mohr, J. P. (1986). General features of intracerebral hemorrhage. In H. J. M. Barnett, J. P. Hohr, B. M. Stein, et al. (Eds.), *Stroke: pathophysiology, diagnosis, and management* (Vol. 1, pp. 497–523). New York: Churchill Livingstone.

Kase, C. S., Robinson, K., Stein, R. W., et al. (1985). Anticoagulant-related intracerebral hemorrhage. *Neurology*, 35, 943–948.

Kassell, N. F., Peerless, S. J., Durward, O. J., et al. (1982). Treatment of ischemic deficits from vasospasm with intravascular volume expansion and induced arterial hypertension. *Neurosurgery*, 11, 337–343.

Kassell, N. F., and Torner, J. C. (1983). Aneurysmal rebleeding: A preliminary report from the cooperative aneurysm study. *Neurosurgery*, 13, 479–481.

Kassell, N. F., Torner, J. C., and Adams, H. P. (1984). Antifibrinolytic therapy in the acute period following aneurysmal subarachnoid hemorrhage: Preliminary observations from the Cooperative Aneurysm Study. *Journal of Neurosurgery*, 61, 225–230.

Kendall, R. E., and Marshall, J. (1963). Role of hypotension in the genesis of transient focal cerebral ischemic attacks. *British Medical Journal*, 2, 344–348.

Kistler, J. P., Crowell, R. M., Davis, K. R., et al. (1983). The relation of cerebral vasospasm to the extent and location of subarachnoid blood visualized by CT scan: A prospective study. *Neurology*, 33, 424–436.

Kjellberg, R. N., Hanamura, T., Davis, K. R., et al. (1983). Bragg-peak proton-beam therapy for arteriovenous malformations of the brain. *New England Journal of Medicine*, 309, 269–274.

Komrad, M. S., Coffey, C. E., Coffey, K. S., et al. (1984). Myocardial infarction and stroke. *Neurology*, 34, 1403–1409.

Kubala, M. J., and Millikan, C. H. (1964). Diagnosis, pathogenesis, and treatment of "drop attacks." *Archives of Neurology*, 11, 107–113.

Lassen, N. A., Ingvar, D. H., and Skinhoj, E. (1978). Brain function and blood flow. *Scientific American*, 239, 62–71.

Lavin, P. (1986). Management of hypertension in patients with acute stroke. *Archives of Internal Medicine*, 146, 66–68.

Lesser, R. P., Luders, H., Dinner, D. S., et al. (1985). Epileptic seizures due to thrombotic and embolic cerebrovascular disease in older patients. *Epilepsia*, 26, 622–630.

Levine, S. R., and Welch, K. M. A. (1987). Cerebrovascular ischemia associated with lupus anticoagulant. *Stroke*, 18, 257–263.

Levine, S. R., and Welch, K. M. A. (1988). Cocaine and stroke. *Stroke*, 19, 779–783.

Lhermitte, F., Gautier, J., and Derouesné, C. (1970). Nature of occlusions of the middle cerebral artery. *Neurology* (Minneap.), 20, 82–88.

Loizou, L. A., Hamilton, J. G., and Tsementzis, S. A. (1982). Intracranial hemorrhage in association with pseudoephedrine overdose (letter to the editor). *Journal of Neurology, Neurosurgery, and Psychiatry*, 45, 471–475.

Longstreth, W. T., Koepsell, T. D., Yerby, M. S., et al. (1985). Risk factors for subarachnoid hemorrhage. *Stroke*, 16, 377–385.

Marshall, J., and Meadows, S. (1968). The natural history of amaurosis fugax. *Brain*, 91, 419–434.

Masaryk, T. J., Modic, M. T., Ruggieri, P., et al. (1989). Three dimensional (volume) gradient echo imaging of the carotid bifurcation: Preliminary clinical experience. *Radiology*, 171 (3), 801–806.

McCormick, W. F. (1966). The pathology of vascular ("arteriovenous") malformations. *Journal of Neurosurgery*, 24, 807–816.

Meissner, I., Whisnant, J. P., and Garraway, W. M. (1988). Hypertension management and stroke recurrence in a community (Rochester, Minnesota, 1950–1979). *Stroke*, 19, 459–463.

Miller, V. T., and Hart, R. G. (1988). Heparin anticoagulation in acute brain ischemia. *Stroke*, 19, 403–406.

Millikan, C. H., McDowell, F., and Easton, J. D. (1987). *Stroke*. Philadelphia: Lea & Febiger.

Moore, P. M. (1989). Diagnosis and management of isolated angiitis of the central nervous system. *Neurology*, 39, 167–173.

Mohr, J. P. (1982). Asymptomatic carotid artery disease (editorial). *Stroke*, 13 (4), 431–433.

Mohr, J. P., Caplan, J. W., Melski, J. W., et al. (1978). The Harvard Cooperative Stroke Registry: A prospective registry. *Neurology*, 28, 754–762.

Mohr, J. P., Kistler, J. P., Zambramski, J. M., et al. (1986a). Intracranial aneurysms. In H. J. M. Barnett, J. P. Mohr, B. M. Stein, et al. (Eds.), *Stroke pathophysiology, diagnosis, and management* (Vol. 1, pp. 643–677). New York: Churchill Livingstone.

Mohr, J. P., Tatemichi, T. K., Nichols, F. C., et al. (1986b). Vascular malformations of the brain: Clinical considerations. In H. J. M. Barnett, J. P. Mohr, B. M. Stein, et al. (Eds.), *Stroke pathophysiology, diagnosis, and management* (Vol. 1, pp. 679–705). New York: Churchill Livingstone.

Moore, P. M., and Cupps, T. R. (1983). Neurological complications of vasculitis. *Annals of Neurology*, 14, 155–167.

Moosey, J. (1959). Development of cerebral atherosclerosis in various age groups. *Neurology*, 9, 569–574.

Okawara, S. (1973). Warning signs prior to rupture of an intracranial aneurysm. *Journal of Neurosurgery*, 38, 475–580.

Ozuna, J. (1985). Alterations in mentation: Nursing assessment and intravention. *Journal of Neurosurgical Nursing*, 17, 66–70.

Paulson, G. W., Boesel, C. P., and Evans, W. E. (1978). Fibromuscular dysplasia. *Archives of Neurology*, 35, 287–290.

Petitti, D. B., Wingerd, J., Pellegrin, F., et al. (1979). Risk of vascular disease in women smoking, oral contraceptives, non-contraceptive estrogens, and other factors. *Journal of the American Medical Association*, 242, 1150–1154.

Petruk, K. C., West, M., Mohr, G., et al. (1988). Nimodipine treatment in poor-grade aneurysm patients. *Journal of Neurosurgery*, 68, 505–517.

Poungvarin, N., Bhoopat, W., Viriyavejakul, A., et al. (1987). Effects of dexamethasone in primary supratentorial intracerebral hemorrhage. *New England Journal of Medicine*, 316, 1229–1233.

Powers, W. J., and Raichle, M. E. (1985). Positron emission tomography and its application to the study of cerebrovascular disease in man. *Stroke*, 16, 361–376.

Raichle, M. E. (1983). The pathophysiology of brain ischemia. *Annals of Neurology*, 13, 2–10.

Reagan, T. J., and Okazaki, H. (1974). The thrombotic syndrome associated with carcinoma. *Archives of Neurology*, 31, 390–395.

Robins, M., and Baum, H. M. (1981). Incidence. *Stroke*, 12 (Suppl. 1), I-45–I-55.

Robinson, R. G., Kubos, K. L., Starr, L. B., et al. (1984). Mood disorders in stroke patients. *Brain*, 107, 81–93.

Ross, J. S. (1988). MR angiography furnishes detailed vascular images. *Diagnostic Imaging*, 10, 96–103.

Ruff, R. L., and Dougherty, J. H. (1981). Evaluation of acute cerebral ischemia for anticoagulant therapy: Computed tomography or lumbar puncture. *Neurology*, 31, 736–740.

Ruff, R. L., Talman, W. T., and Petito, F. (1981). Transient ischemic attacks associated with hypotension in hypertensive patients with carotid artery stenosis. *Stroke*, 12, 353–355.

Sacco, R. L., Wolf, P. A., Kannel, W. B., et al. (1982). Survival and recurrence following stroke: The Framingham study. *Stroke*, 13, 290–295.

Sage, J. I., and Van Uitert, R. L. (1983). Risk of recurrent stroke in patients with atrial fibrillation and non-valvular heart disease. *Stroke*, 14, 537–540.

Sandok, B. A., von Estorff, I., and Guiliani, E. R. (1980). CNS embolism due to atrial myxoma. *Archives of Neurology*, 37, 485–488.

Scandinavian Stroke Study Group (1987). Multicenter trial of hemodilution in acute ischemic stroke I. Results in the total patient population. *Stroke*, 18, 691–699.

Schuier, F. J., and Hossman, K. A. (1980). Experimental brain infarcts in cats II. Ischemic brain edema. *Stroke*, 11, 593–601.

Senegor, M., Dohrmann, G. J., and Wollmann, R. L. (1883). Venous angiomas of the posterior fossa should be considered as anomalous venous drainage. *Surgical Neurology*, 19, 26–32.

Sheldon, J. J. (1981). Blood vessels of the scalp and brain. *Clinical Symposia*, 33, 3–36.

Sherry, S. (1985). Tissue plasminogen activator (t-PA) Will it fulfill its promise? *New England Journal of Medicine*, 313, 1014–1017.

Shuping, J. R., Rollinson, R. D., and Toole, J. F. (1980). Transient global amnesia. *Annals of Neurology*, 7, 281–285.

Soloway, H. B., and Aronson, S. M. (1964). Atheromatous emboli to central nervous system. *Archives of Neurology*, 11, 657–667.

Stadel, B. V. (1981). Oral contraceptives and cardiovascular disease (Pt. 2). *New England Journal of Medicine*, 305, 672–677.

Stafford, C. R., Bogdanoff, B. M., Green, L., et al. (1975). Mononeuropathy multiplex as a complication of amphetamine angiitis. *Neurology*, 25, 570–572.

Steiner, L. (1986). Radiosurgery in cerebral arteriovenous malformations. In E. Flamm and J. Fein (Eds.), *Textbook of cerebrovascular surgery* (pp. 1161–1215). New York: Springer-Verlag.

Stemmermann, G. N., Hayashi, T., Resch, J. A., et al. (1984). Risk factors related to ischemic and hemorrhagic cerebrovascular disease at autopsy: The Honolulu heart study. *Stroke*, 15, 23–28.

Strand, T., Aspuland, K., Eriksson, S., et al. (1984). A randomized controlled trial of hemodilution therapy in acute ischemic stroke. *Stroke*, 15, 980–989.

Strandgaard, S. (1983). Cerebral blood flow in hypertension. *Acta Medica Scandinavica Supplements, 678,* 11–25.

Strandgaard, S., and Paulson, O. B. (1984). Cerebral autoregulation. *Stroke, 15,* 413–416.

Sundt, T. M., Piepgras, D. G., Ebersold, M. J., et al. (1987a). Postoperative evaluation and management of complications with illustrative cases. In T. M. Sundt (Ed.), *Occlusive cerebrovascular disease: diagnosis and surgical management* (pp. 243–260). Philadelphia: W. B. Saunders.

Sundt, T. M., Piepgras, D. G., Ebersold, M. J., et al. (1987b). Risk factors and operative results. In T. M. Sundt (Ed.), *Occlusive cerebrovascular disease: diagnosis and surgical management* (pp. 226–231). Philadelphia: W. B. Saunders.

Szekely, P. (1964). Systemic embolism and anticoagulant prophylaxis in rheumatic heart disease. *British Medical Journal, 1,* 1209–1212.

Tell, G. S., Crouse, J. R., and Furberg, C. D. (1988). Relation between blood lipids, lipoproteins, and cerebrovascular atherosclerosis. A review. *Stroke, 19,* 423–430.

Thomas, D. J., du Boulay, G. H., Marshall, J., et al. (1977). Effect of haematocrit on cerebral blood-flow in man. *Lancet, 2,* 941–943.

Thomas, J. E., and Ayyer, D. R. (1972). Systemic fat embolism. *Archives of Neurology, 26,* 517–523.

Toole, J. F., Yuson, C. P., Janeway, R., et al. (1978). Transient ischemic attacks: A prospective study of 225 patients. *Neurology, 28,* 746–753.

Tohgi, H., Yamanouchi, H., Murakami, M., et al. (1978). Importance of the hematocrit as a risk factor in cerebral infarction. *Stroke, 9,* 369–374.

Vinters, H. V. (1987). Cerebral amyloid angiopathy: A critical review. *Stroke, 18,* 311–324.

Vinuela, F., and Fox, A. J. (1986). Interventional neuroradiology. In H. J. M. Barnett, J. P., Mohr, B. M. Stein, et al. (Eds.), *Stroke pathophysiology, diagnosis, and management* (Vol. 1, pp. 1173–1189). New York: Churchill Livingstone.

Wallace, J. D., and Levy, L. L. (1981). Blood pressure after stroke. *Journal of the American Medical Association, 246,* 2177–2180.

Weir, B. (1987a). *Aneurysms affecting the nervous system.* Baltimore: Williams & Wilkins.

Weir, B. (1987b). Antifibrinolytics in subarachnoid hemorrhage: Do they have a role? No. *Archives of Neurology, 44,* 116–118.

Weksler, B. B., Kent, J. L., Rudolph, D., et al. (1985). Effects of low dose aspirin on platelet function in patients with recent cerebral ischemia. *Stroke, 16,* 5–9.

Whisnant, J. P. (1974). Epidemiology of stroke: Emphasis on transient cerebral ischemic attacks and hypertension. *Stroke, 5,* 68–70.

Wintzen, A. R., de Jonge, H., Loeliger, E. A., et al. (1984). The risk of intracerebral hemorrhage during oral anticoagulant treatment: A population study. *Annals of Neurology, 16,* 553–558.

Wojak, J. C., and Flamm, E. S. (1987). Intracranial hemorrhage and cocaine use. *Stroke, 18,* 712–715.

Wolf, P. A., Dawber, T. R., Thomas, H. E., et al. (1978). Epidemiologic assessment of chronic atrial fibrillation and risk of stroke: The Framingham study. *Neurology, 28,* 973–977.

Wolf, P. A., Kannel, W. B., Sorlie, P., et al. (1981). Asymptomatic carotid bruit and risk of stroke: The Framingham study. *Journal of the American Medical Association, 245,* 1442–1445.

Wolf, P. A., Kannel, W. B., and Verter, J. (1983). Current status of risk factors for stroke. *Neurologic Clinics, 1,* 317–343.

Wooten, M. R., Khangure, M. S., and Murphy, M. J. (1983). Intracerebral hemorrhage and vasculitis related to ephedrine abuse. *Annals of Neurology, 13,* 337–340.

Brain Death

Ellen B. Rudy

To most people the term "death" is a clear-cut pronouncement. Death occurs when a person stops breathing and the heart stops beating. These criteria, cessation of function of the heart and lungs, continue to be synonymous with death. Biomedical advances, however, have provided us with the means to ventilate the lungs mechanically and ways to restart the heart and maintain circulation. Such advances in medical technology, coupled with pharmacologic support that can maintain physiologic function in patients well beyond any potential for recovery, have created the need to reexamine the definition of death.

Along with recognition of the inadequacy of the common law definition of death have come improvements in the area of organ transplantation. Early activities in the transplantation of solid organs, including the kidney, heart, liver, and pancreas, were limited due to surgical techniques, inadequate tissue typing, and subsequent rejection by organ recipients. This picture changed dramatically in the 1960s with perfection of transplant surgery and major advances in the field of immunology that allowed improved tissue typing. An even greater boost to organ transplantation occurred with the discovery of cyclosporin and its antirejection properties. These advances have led to organ transplantation as an accepted treatment modality, not just an experimental procedure (see Chap. 52). The need for healthy, viable organs can be met only by cadaveric sources, focusing attention on the necessity to declare a person dead as soon as irreversible brain damage can be established. The object, of course, is to hasten the process of recognizing death early enough to allow transplantable organs to be adequately perfused and kept healthy in order to increase the potential for successful transplantation.

Biomedical advances that allowed irreversibly brain damaged individuals to maintain cardiopulmonary function coupled with an increasing need for viable organs for transplantation resulted in recognition of the concept of brain death. *Brain death is the irreversible loss of all brain function.* This means loss of the higher centers of the cerebral hemispheres, which are involved in cognitive functioning, and loss of the lower centers of the brainstem, which control many involuntary functions, including respiratory and circulatory activities.

It should be clearly understood that brain death does not introduce a second type of death or a second means of determining death. Death is viewed as a single phenomenon that can be accurately demonstrated either by the traditional means of irreversible cessation of function of the heart and lungs or by irreversible loss of all functions of the entire brain (President's Commission, 1983). The President's Commission for the Study of Ethical Problems in Medicine and Biomedical and Behavioral Research, in its report *Defining Death* (President's Commission, 1981), took special note of the confusion that the term "brain death" has created in the literature by means of public discussions and legislative activity. The Commission advised that terminology such as "brain-based standard of death" be used rather than brain death. Their point was that the term brain death can refer either to "cessation of brain function" or to "the death of a person based on cessation of brain function." Such usage may indeed be confusing, particularly to the lay public. Brain death, however, has become a part of accepted medical and legal terminology. It seems unlikely that the term will be changed, and efforts will continue to be made to inform the public that brain death is not a second type of death apart from cardiac and respiratory death.

The three most common causes of brain death are (1) direct head trauma, such as occurs with motor vehicle accidents and gunshot wounds, (2) massive, spontaneous hemorrhage into the brain, and (3) lack of blood flow to the brain secondary to cardiac arrest or severe systemic hypotension (Cranford and Smith, 1979). In each of these cases, brain death occurs when the brain has inadequate cerebral perfusion to maintain cell integrity. This interruption of blood flow may be the result of inadequate systemic blood pressure (such as occurs with cardiac arrest) or the consequence of increased intracranial pressure that exceeds the cerebral perfusion pressure necessary to deliver blood to the brain cells. When the cerebral circulation is interrupted, all brain functions will cease within a matter of minutes to hours. The relationship between cerebral circulation and brain functioning is essential to the understanding of the clinical tests used to determine brain death and to an appreciation of the certainty of the prognosis in these cases.

Two developments have occurred that directly affect clinical practice and the application of brain death in critical care. First is the development of the legal, or statutory, criteria, to determine brain death, and the second is the development of clinical criteria to determine brain death.

STATUTORY RECOGNITION OF BRAIN DEATH

A variety of lawsuits concerning the determination of death for organ procurement and transplantation and for inheritance and criminal purposes first prompted the medical community to seek legal recognition of brain death. Such recognition has occurred through enactment of state statutes that include brain death along with general death. Not surprisingly, such laws, beginning in 1970 with the Kansas state law, were not uniform in wording or application.

Work began in the later 1970s by the American Medical Association, the American Bar Association, and the National Conference of Commissioners on Uniform State Laws to develop a uniform definition to be used in state statutes. The President's Commission for the Study of Ethical Problems in Medicine and Biomedical and Behavioral Research worked with those organizations and eventually endorsed the Uniform Determination of Death Act to replace earlier proposals. The definition in this act reads:

An individual who has sustained either (1) irreversible cessation of circulatory and respiratory functions, or (2) irreversible cessation of all functions of the entire brain, including the brain stem, is dead. A determination of death shall be made in accordance with accepted medical standards.

The President's Commission recommended adoption of this statute in all jurisdictions in the United States. By the end of 1991, most states gave legal recognition to brain death. As an aid to the implementation of the proposed statute, the President's Commission published *Guidelines for the Determination of Death* (Table 34–1). These guidelines were developed by a group of more than 50 medical and scientific consultants representing a wide range of medical specialties (President's Commission, 1983).

As noted in the statute on brain death, determination of brain death, or cessation of all brain func-

TABLE 34–1. Criteria for the Determination of Death

A. An individual with irreversible cessation of circulatory and respiratory functions is dead.
  1. Cessation is recognized by an appropriate clinical examination.
  2. Irreversibility is recognized by persistent cessation of functions during an appropriate period of observation and/or trial of therapy.
B. An individual with irreversible cessation of the entire brain, including the brainstem, is dead.
  1. Cessation is recognized when evaluation discloses finding of both:
  Absence of cerebral functions, and
  Absence of brainstem functions.
  2. Irreversibility is recognized when evaluation discloses *all* of the following:
  The cause of coma is established and is sufficient to account for the loss of brain functions; and
  The possibility of recovery of any brain functions is excluded.

From Medical Consultants on the Diagnosis of Death to the President's Commission for the Study of Ethical Problems in Medicine and Biomedical and Behavioral Research (1981). Report: Guidelines for the determination of death. *Journal of the American Medical Association,* 246 (19), 2184–2186. Copyright 1981 American Medical Association.

tions, must be made "in accordance with accepted medical standards." Such a phrase allows for altering of clinical criteria to determine brain function as medical technology improves and measurements become more precise. Recognizing the continuing advancements being made in biomedical technology, such leeway only makes sense to members of the health care profession. The lack, however, of any *one* test for brain death leaves questions in the mind of the public as to the validity of the tests used and again leads people to ask, "Is a person who is brain dead really dead?"

CRITERIA FOR DETERMINING BRAIN DEATH

Many different combinations of clinical criteria have been proposed for determining brain death. The earliest and most frequently cited are those developed by an Ad Hoc Committee of the Harvard Medical School in 1968 (Beecher, 1968), referred to as the "Harvard criteria." However, these criteria have been reported to be unnecessarily restrictive (Walker, 1983), and, as the lay and medical communities have become more confident in the use of brain death as a terminal diagnosis, the original criteria have been modified.

The criteria used to determine death based on irreversible cessation of all brain function provided by the President's Commission (see Table 34–1) require documentation of three items:

1. Cerebral and brainstem functions are absent.
2. The condition of the patient is irreversible. This necessitates that the condition has a known cause and that the possibility of recovery has been excluded.

3. Cessation of all brain functions has persisted for an appropriate period of observation or trial of therapy.

Absence of Cerebral and Brainstem Functions

Assessment of the function of the entire brain requires testing the functions of both the cerebral cortex and the brainstem. When possible, laboratory tests are used to confirm the clinical diagnosis. At one time the electroencephalogram (EEG) was considered important in the diagnosis of brain death. However, because an isoelectric EEG only measures the electrical activity of the cerebral hemispheres and not the physiologic function of the brainstem, it does not confirm the diagnosis of brain death. Furthermore, physical, electrical, and ventilator artifacts and variability in reading the EEG contribute to difficulties with interpretation. For these reasons, an isoelectric EEG is not considered mandatory for the diagnosis of brain death. The most widely used laboratory tests include cerebral blood flow studies by radioisotope cerebral angiography or CT scanning with contrast media.

Laboratory tests used to confirm brain function usually include only the most commonly available and clinically accepted tests. Laboratory testing is the most likely area of change as advances in medical technology allow more precise information. One example is the positron emission tomography (PET) scanner, which already has the capacity to measure not only cerebral circulation but also cerebral metabolism. Some writers believe that cerebral metabolism is the ultimate test of cerebral function. Results of a PET scan would certainly be a more definitive test of cerebral function than that presently used. However, the cost and limited availability of a PET scan prohibited its consideration as a "standard" medical practice for the establishment of brain death.

To establish the absence of cerebral and brainstem functions, tests of cerebral cortex function and tests of brainstem function are used as described in the following sections.

TESTS OF CEREBRAL CORTEX FUNCTIONING
(Rudy, 1984)

Cerebral or cognitive functioning is determined by responses to stimuli, such as light, sound, motion, or pain. Absence of cortical functioning is determined by a lack of verbal response, lack of spontaneous or coordinated eye movements, and absence of muscle flexion or extension (decorticate and decerebrate activity) in response to any of the foregoing stimuli. Complex spinal cord reflexes may be preserved in brain dead persons and must be differentiated from true decerebrate and decorticate posturing (Powner and Grenvik, 1979).

Documentation of the absence of cerebral circula-

tion through four-vessel (carotid and vertebral vessels) intracranial angiography in the normothermic patient is considered a definitive test of cerebral death. This test, however, involves considerable practical difficulties and some risks to the patient. For these reasons, tests assessing only the cerebral hemisphere circulation are usually employed. Tests of cerebral blood flow include radioisotope angiography, echo cerebrovascular pulsations, CT scans with contrast media, and regional cerebral blood flow studies.

TESTS OF BRAINSTEM FUNCTION

Brainstem function is determined by testing the cranial nerves whose nuclei are within the brainstem and the presence or absence of spontaneous respirations. The usual tests of brainstem function are as follows:

Pupillary Light Reflex. With an intact optic nerve (cranial nerve II) and oculomotor nerve (cranial nerve III), a light will stimulate the parasympathetic fibers to the iris, causing pupillary constriction. Absence of pupillary response to light indicates nonfunction of cranial nerves II and III. Pupils need not be equal or necessarily dilated but must be nonreactive to light to meet the criteria.

Pupillary response will be absent after administration of scopolamine, atropine, opiates, neuromuscular blocking agents, or glutamine. It may also be absent following eye trauma or eye disease. In the presence of either medication that interferes with pupillary response or eye trauma or disease, tests of the pupillary reflex will be omitted. Testing this reflex is not considered mandatory to the determination of brain death.

Oculovestibular Reflex. The patient is positioned with the head elevated 30 degrees, and the ear is inspected with an ophthalmoscope to ensure that the tympanic membrane is intact. Ice water is slowly introduced through a 30-mL syringe into the patient's ear canal. In the person with an intact brainstem, stimulation conducted from the vestibular portion of the acoustic nerve (cranial nerve VIII) via the pons and the abducens nerve (cranial nerve VI) to the midbrain and the oculomotor nerve (cranial nerve III) will result in a horizontal nystagmus, slow movement toward the irrigated ear and rapid movement away. In the absence of brainstem function, ice water will produce no eye movement.

Vagus Nerve Function. The tenth cranial nerve, the vagus nerve, with its parasympathetic fibers, acts to slow the heart. Thus, atropine, a parasympathetic inhibitor, given intravenously, inhibits the action of the vagus nerve, causing an increase in pulse rate when the vagus nerve is functioning and the cardiac muscle is capable of responding. Vagus nerve function is tested by administering 0.1 mg of atropine

740 Section 6 ■ Nervous System

intravenously. The pulse rate is expected to increase by 5 beats per minute if the vagus nerve is functioning.

Brainstem Auditory Evoked Response. Some physicians believe that one of the last portions of the brainstem to remain intact is the acoustic nerve (cranial nerve VIII). This nerve is tested by using the brainstem auditory evoked response (BAER) technique. An electrode is placed deep within the ear canal, and surface electrodes on the mastoid bone record the electrical evoked responses. Following administration of stimuli, evoked responses appear as electrical sequelae on a computer-averaged EEG. The presence of a response reflects activation of the eighth cranial nerve and auditory regions of the brainstem and cerebral cortex by sound stimuli. Absence of a BAER indicates severe, widespread CNS dysfunction consistent with brain death. Although the BAER is not widely used at present, there is evidence that the use of such electrophysiologic measurements may soon become more widespread.

Other Cranial Nerve Functions. Although the functions of other cranial nerves are often checked in determining brainstem responses in comatose patients, these are less often used to determine brain death. The *corneal reflex* is elicited by brushing the cornea of the eye lightly with a wisp of cotton. The normal response is an involuntary blink of the eye, indicating intact trigeminal (V) and facial (VII) cranial nerves. The corneal reflex may be absent due to facial muscle weakness or paralysis, and these possibilities should be ruled out before considering this reflex a reliable clinical test. The *gag reflex* may be elicited by touching the back of the throat or tongue, indicating intact glossopharyngeal (cranial nerve IX) and vagus (cranial nerve X) nerves. Assessment of this reflex is not practical in a patient who is intubated or has a tracheostomy tube in place.

Irreversible Condition of the Person

In essence, this criterion requires the physician to establish as nearly as possible the cause of the comatose state and rule out any conditions that may be treated and reversible. Although much attention has been focused on the pros and cons of the clinical tests used, most difficulties with determining brain death have occurred because inadequate attention has been paid to reversible complicating conditions.

When the cause of the patient's condition is well established and loss of brain function is not unexpected, there is little problem. Difficulties may occur when the cause of the comatose state is not known or is complicated by drugs, metabolic abnormalities, hypothermia, or shock. In order to document adequately the irreversibility of the loss of brain function, the possibility of complicating conditions must be investigated and treated.

DRUG OR METABOLIC INTOXICATION

When the cause of the coma is unknown or when drugs are suspected, comprehensive drug toxicology screening is required. A variety of sedative and anesthetic drugs produce clinical symptoms that mimic brain death including electrocerebral silence or an isoelectric EEG. Drugs most commonly producing brain dysfunction at toxic levels include barbiturates, benzodiazepines (Valium), meprobamate (Equanil, Miltown), methaqualone (Quaalude), and trichloroethylene. When toxic serum levels of a drug are present, death may not be declared until the drug is metabolized or until testing demonstrates absent cerebral circulation.

Another category of drugs that may cause complete muscle paralysis and areflexia is the neuromuscular blocking agents such as succinylcholine, pancuronium, or similar agents. Because these drugs can also cause deathlike symptoms, patients with prolonged paralysis with these drugs need to be tested for pseudocholinesterase deficiency by low-dose atropine stimulation, electromyography, or peripheral nerve stimulation. If there is any question about the possibility of a drug-induced coma, additional testing or extended observation is required (Medical Consultants, 1981).

Illnesses that cause severe metabolic abnormalities can produce prolonged deep coma, including hepatic coma with encephalopathy, hyperosmolar coma, and severe uremia. It seems unlikely that these metabolic abnormalities would go untreated, but efforts should be made to correct them before brain function is tested. Again, an isoelectric EEG or absence of cerebral circulation would be definitive test results.

HYPOTHERMIA

People are considered hypothermic when their core body temperature is below the physiologically normal limits (less than 35.6°C) (Elder, 1984). However, for purposes of establishing brain death, the core body temperature must be above 32.2°C (90°F) for the criteria to apply. Hypothermic victims may appear dead by all clinical signs, but successful resuscitation has been reported following a core body temperature of 28°C and below (DeRouboix, 1980; Pickering et al., 1977). Thus, the dictum, "No one is dead until he is warm and dead" (Reuler, 1978). With increased experience and success in treating severely hypothermic patients, brain death is usually not considered until rewarming procedures have been initiated. Hypothermia coupled with drug or alcohol intoxication can produce cerebral dysfunction that mimics brain death at temperature levels above the proposed 32.2°C, making careful diagnosis and toxicology screening essential prerequisites for the diagnosis of brain death.

SHOCK

A state of shock with its accompanying low levels of blood pressure can reduce cerebral circulation to the point where clinical tests can be inaccurate, making a determination of brain death unreliable. This is particularly true in patients with shock with coexisting multiple injuries. Early evidence of the combined effects of multiple injuries with shock came from battlefield determinations of death in soldiers later shown to be in a state of severe shock closely resembling death. In a clinical setting, patients should be treated appropriately for shock before any examination for brain death takes place.

Cessation of All Brain Functions Persisting for an Appropriate Period of Observation or Trial of Therapy

Once the cessation of all brain functions has been established by clinical criteria, the length of time required for observation or for further trials of therapy varies and is a matter of clinical judgment by the physician. Thus the term "appropriate" will depend on the clinical situation. The report to the President's Commission suggests the following observation guidelines (Medical Consultants, 1981).

Six Hours. Once clinical criteria for brain death have been documented and confirmed by appropriate clinical testing and the patient has no complicating conditions (e.g., drug intoxication, hypothermia, young age, shock), an observation period of 6 hours with no change in brain function is considered adequate for determination of brain death.

Twelve Hours. In the absence of confirmatory tests (e.g., electrocardiogram, cerebral blood flow, etc.) but when an irreversible condition is well established, a period of at least 12 hours of observation is recommended.

Twenty-four Hours. In cases of anoxic brain damage when the extent of damage may be more difficult to ascertain, 24 hours of observation with no evidence of brain function is suggested. This period of observation may be reduced if cerebral blood flow studies or an EEG support the loss of brain function.

MANAGEMENT OF PATIENTS WHO MEET BRAIN DEATH CRITERIA

There is evidence from clinical reports that in patients who are supported on mechanical ventilation, cardiac arrest usually occurs within 72 hours of brain death (Ibe, 1971; Jorgensen, 1973; Kimura et al., 1968; Korein, 1978). However, in a recent reported case a pregnant female who was declared brain dead following a craniotomy was kept on mechanical ventilation 53 days until her baby could be delivered by Caesarean section (*Akron Becon Journal*, 1986). Another publication reported a patient

with documented brain death following a cardiorespiratory arrest who was kept on mechanical ventilatory support for 68 days before removal from ventilatory support and electrocardiac silence occurred (Parisi et al., 1982). Because of the long duration of external support and attendant circumstances, these two cases are unusual. For the most part, once brain death has been determined, there are few circumstances when intensive care therapy is still indicated. Exceptions include cases in which the brain-dead patient is a pregnant woman with a viable fetus, or when the family (or patient) has agreed to organ donation and organ retrieval is scheduled.

Pregnant Female. In the case of a brain-dead woman who is pregnant with a viable fetus, there is already evidence that a live birth may occur if the fetus can be maintained through ventilatory and circulatory support to the mother (Dillon et al., 1982). Such circumstances are rare, and the birth can be successful only if the fetus is at least in the second trimester of development at the time of maternal death.

Organ Donor. With improved surgical technology and a more complete understanding of the immune system and tissue typing, organ transplantation has progressed from an experimental procedure to a recognized therapeutic modality. Publicity and increased long-term survival have resulted in a need for solid organs and tissues (cornea, skin, bones) that has far outstripped the supply. The only source of solid organs such as the pancreas, liver, or heart is brain-dead patients. In many states, statutes have been passed requiring the family of every patient who dies in an acute care setting and meets eligibility criteria for organ donation to be offered the opportunity to donate the patient's organs (see Chap. 52). If the family agrees to organ donation, the brain-dead patient must be kept on life-support therapy until organ procurement takes place. This is obviously necessary to keep the organ perfused and viable for subsequent transplantation.

Family Wishes. If one believes legally, morally, and ethically that brain death is no different from death that occurs when the heart and lungs stop functioning, there is little reason to maintain patients on intensive therapy after a determination of brain death has been made. In fact, termination of further medical intervention is ethically justifiable when that treatment is no longer deemed useful (Lucas et al., 1987). That is, there is no moral obligation to perform useless or futile therapy, and in the presence of a declaration of brain death, further therapy would be useless. The reality of clinical circumstances, however, sometimes dictates otherwise. In a survey of neurologists and neurosurgeons on the subject of brain death, they were asked what they would do if a patient met the brain death criteria but the family wanted the life support to be continued. A total of

76% said they would continue ventilatory support. There was variability in exactly what that meant, and responses ranged from declaring the patient dead but continuing support, not declaring the patient dead and continuing support, and declaring the patient dead and stopping support regardless of the family's wishes (Black and Zervas, 1984). Many respondents spoke of working with the family to help them accept the patient's death. This type of situation is mentioned to emphasize that family members may require additional time and help to understand that a beating heart and moving lungs are possible even when a person is dead.

PROBLEMS IN DETERMINING BRAIN DEATH

The established criteria for determining brain death and accepted clinical tests have been presented. There remain, however, practical problems in the performance and interpretation of test results.

Motor Response to Stimuli

Decerebrate or decorticate muscle activity is inconsistent with brain death criteria. Spinal reflexes, however, can occasionally produce complex integrated movement of muscle groups, and such movement may be difficult to ascribe to spinal reflexes on clinical evidence alone. If there is any doubt about the origin of muscle activity, cerebral blood flow studies should be done to confirm the absence of perfusion to the brain.

Electroencephalogram

In some places an isoelectric EEG may be required as part of brain death testing. Spontaneous muscle fasciculations may produce EEG tracing artifacts, making interpretation difficult. In such cases, drugs may be used to produce neuromuscular paralysis during the EEG recording. Clinical examination for cerebral and brainstem responses cannot be performed until the drug effects have worn off or a neuromuscular stimulator counteracts the initial drug effect. As mentioned earlier in the chapter, most physicians no longer require an EEG to determine brain death.

Spontaneous Respirations

Testing for the absence of spontaneous respirations is difficult because of the potential for producing further deterioration in the patient's status while he or she is apneic. The first problem is hypoxia, which can occur while the patient is disconnected from the ventilator. This problem is usually handled by preoxygenating the patient with 100% oxygen for several breaths before disconnecting him from ventilatory support, or providing passive oxygen through a catheter down the endotracheal tube during the disconnect time. Some patients require a hypoxic stimulus to initiate spontaneous breathing, so they must be allowed to become hypoxic to rule out spontaneous respirations. Blood gas determinations are required to validate the P_{CO_2} level.

For most patients, increased carbon dioxide is considered the strongest stimulus for spontaneous respirations. Because many ventilator-dependent patients, particularly head-injured patients, are maintained in a hypocarbic state, the respiratory rate should be decreased prior to testing, and P_{CO_2} levels should be allowed to rise to near normal values (40 to 50 mm Hg) before testing for spontaneous respirations is performed. This test is not considered valid unless the P_{CO_2} is at least 45 mm Hg, providing an adequate stimulus for spontaneous respiratory effort. In patients with increased intracranial pressure, increases in P_{CO_2} result in cerebral vasodilatation and subsequent increases in intracranial pressure. This sequence of events obviously has the potential to compromise brain function further. Therefore, tests of spontaneous respirations in patients with increased intracranial pressure should be reserved until all other criteria have been met.

Cerebral Blood Flow

Cerebral blood flow is the test that is probably considered the most definitive test for brain death. However, cerebral blood flow angiography requires visualization of all four vessels supplying the brain. This test is invasive, requires complicated radiologic techniques, and is often impractical for routine use in critically ill patients.

Indirect methods to determine cerebral blood flow include radioisotopic techniques, echoencephalography to demonstrate loss of the midline intracranial pulsations, and cerebral Doppler echoencephalography (Korein et al., 1975; Schwartz et al., 1983). Although not as definitive as four-vessel contrast cerebral angiography, these tests support other clinical determinations of brain death and are useful when clinical criteria are inconclusive or impractical.

BRAIN DEATH IN CHILDREN

Little information is available on the application of brain death criteria in pediatric patients. The President's Commission warns physicians to "be particularly cautious in applying neurological criteria to determine death in children younger than 5 years" (Medical Consultants, 1981). This warning, however, offers little in the way of explicit information about which clinical tests are to be used or which applications are to be changed in determining brain death. Some authors claim that the brains of infants and children have increased resistance to hypoxic damage and may recover substantial function even after exhibiting unresponsiveness on neurologic examination for long periods of time compared to adults (Green and Lauber, 1972; Pasternak and Volpe, 1979; Rowland et al., 1984). Keeping in mind the potential immaturity of the nervous system in children, the use of cerebral blood flow studies is recommended as a more accurate assessment of irreversible neurologic loss in these patients (Ashwal and Schneider, 1979; Schwartz et al., 1983).

Two additional factors are noteworthy with comatose children. First, many of these children may be hypothermic at the time of testing. Hypothermia occurs commonly in the critically ill child and may mimic brain death in the slowing of responses; it should be assessed and corrected before brain death criteria are examined. Second, barbiturates and muscle relaxants are frequently used to treat increased intracranial pressure in children. These medications make neurologized testing suspect, and therefore a serum barbiturate level is recommended before testing for brain death.

SUMMARY

The recognition and diagnosis of death by brain function criteria is an inevitable step in the evolution of twentieth century medical care. The increasing capacity to maintain man's physiologic functions through mechanical and medical means makes the concept of brain death increasingly necessary.

Ability to transplant human organs with increased success highlights the demand for viable organs from cadaveric sources. The statutes and the Uniform Determination of Death Act have paved the way for acceptance of brain death within the health care professions. The clinical criteria used to establish brain death require clear evidence of irreversible loss of both cortical and brainstem activity.

References

Ashwal, S., and Schneider, S., (1979). Failure of electroencephalography to diagnose brain death in comatose children. *Annals of Neurology*, 6, 512–517.

Baby girl born to woman legally dead seven and one-half weeks. (1986, July). *Akron Beacon Journal*, p. A12.

Beecher, H. K. A. (1968). Definition of irreversible coma. Report of the Ad Hoc Committee of the Harvard Medical School to examine the definition of brain death. *Journal of the American Medical Association*, 205, 337–340.

Benesch, K. (1989). Legal aspects of brain death certification and withdrawal of life support. In W. C. Shoemaker, W. L. Thompson, and P. R. Holbrook (Eds.), *Textbook of critical care* (2nd ed., pp. 973–980). Philadelphia: W. B. Saunders.

Black, P. L., and Zervas, N. T. (1984). Declaration of brain death in neurosurgical neurological practice. *Journal of Neurosurgery*, 15(2), 170–174.

Black's law dictionary (4th ed.) (1951). St. Paul: West Publishing.

Cranford, R. E., and Smith, H. L. (1979). Some critical distinctions between brain death and the persistent vegetative state. *Ethics in Science and Medicine*, 6, 199–209.

DeRouboix, J. A. M. (1980). Successful resuscitation in severe accidental hypothermia—a case report. *South Africa Medical Journal*, 57, 374–376.

Dillon, W. P., Lee, R. V., Tronolone, M. J., et al. (1982). Life support and maternal death during pregnancy. *Journal of the American Medical Association*, 248(9), 1089–1091.

Elder, D. T. (1989). Accidental hypothermia. In W. C. Shoemaker, W. L. Thompson, and P. R. Holbrook (Eds.), *Textbook of critical care* (2nd ed., pp. 85–93). Philadelphia: W. B. Saunders.

Green, J. B., and Lauber, A. (1972). Return of EEG activity after electrocerebral silence: Two case reports. *Journal of Neurosurgery and Psychiatry*, 35, 103–107.

Grenvik, A. (1984). Brain death and permanently lost consciousness. In W. C. Shoemaker, W. L. Thompson, and P. R. Holbrook (Eds.), *Textbook of critical care* (pp. 968–973). Philadelphia: W. B. Saunders.

Ibe, K. (1971). Clinical and pathophysiological aspects of the intravital brain death. *Electroencephalography and Clinical Neurophysiology*, 30, 272.

Jastremski, M., Downer, D., Snyder, J., et al. (1978). Problems in brain death determination. *Forensic Science*, 11, 201–212.

Jorgensen, E. O. (1973). Spinal man after brain death. *Acta Neurochirurgica*, 28, 259–273.

Kipmura, J., Gerber, H. W., and McCormick, W. F. (1968). The isolectric electroencephalogram. *Archives of Internal Medicine*, 121, 511–517.

Korein, J. (1978). The problem of brain death: Development and history. *Annals of New York Academy of Science*, 315, 1–5.

Korein, J., Braunstein, D., Kricheff, I., et al. (1975). Radioisotopic bolus technique as a test to detect circulatory deficit associated with cerebral death. *Circulation*, 51, 924–939.

Lucas, B. A., Clark, D. B., Belak, A., Jr., et al. (1987). Brain death in a murder victim: A medicolegal dilemma. *Hospital practice*, April 15, 251–276.

Medical Consultants on the Diagnosis of Death to the President's Commission for the Study of Ethical Problems in Medicine and Biomedical and Behavioral Research. (1981). Report: Guidelines for the determination of death. *Journal of the American Medical Association*, 246(19), 2184–2186.

Parisi, J. E., Kim, R. C., Collins, G. H., et al. (1982). Brain death with prolonged somatic survival. *New England Journal of Medicine*, 306, 14–20.

Pasternak, J. F., and Volpe, J. J. (1979). Full recovery from prolonged brainstem failure following intraventricular hemorrhage. *Journal of Pediatrics*, 95(6), 1046–1049.

Pickering, B. G., Bristow, G. K., and Craig, D. B. (1977). Case history number 97; case rewarming by peritoneal irrigation in accidental hypothermia with cardiac arrest. *Anesthesia and Analgesia*, 56, 574–577.

Powner, D. J., and Grenvik, A. (1979). Triage in patient care: From expected recovery to brain death. *Heart & Lung*, 8(6), 1103–1108.

President's Commission for the Study of Ethical Problems in Medical and Biomedical and Behavioral Research. (1981). *Defining death*. Washington, D. C.: U.S. Government Printing Office.

President's Commission for the Study of Ethical Problems in Medicine and Biomedical and Behavioral Research. (1983). *Summing up*. Washington, D. C.: U.S. Government Printing Office.

Reuler, J. B. (1978). Hypothermia. Pathophysiology, clinical settings and management. *Annals of Internal Medicine*, 89, 519–527.

Rowland, T., Donnelly, J. H., Jackson, A. H., et al. (1984). Brain death criteria. In Reply to Letters to the Editor. *American Journal of Diseases in Children*, 138, 102.

Rudy, E. B. (1984). *Advanced neurologic and neurosurgical nursing*, (pp. 255–261). St. Louis: C. V. Mosby.

Schwartz, J. A., Baxter, J., Brill, D., et al. (1983). Radionuclide cerebral imaging confirming brain death. *Journal of the American Medical Association*, 249, 246–247.

Walker, E. A. (1983). Current concepts of brain death. *Journal of Neurosurgical Nursing*, 15(5), 261–264.

35

Patients with Spinal Cord Injury

Connie Walleck

Anyone is at risk for a spinal cord injury (SCI). SCI with loss of motor and sensory function is one of the most catastrophic medical conditions possible (Krause, 1985). These injuries not only change the life style of the victim but also affect family, friends, the community, and society. SCI can result in permanent paralysis and total loss of sensation below the level of the injury. The ability to breathe may be diminished or destroyed. Bowel, bladder, and sexual function may also be affected. Significant psychologic, social, and economic ramifications are also related to SCI.

Care of SCI patients is complex and demanding. The critical care nurse must have a thorough understanding of the effects of SCI to be able to provide comprehensive care of the patient and avoid the associated complications.

EPIDEMIOLOGY

Although the incidence of SCI is low, 40.1/1 million people, it is considered a high-cost disability (Krause, 1985). Each year there are about 12,000 new paraplegics and quadriplegics in the United States as a result of SCI (Albin and White, 1987). About 40% of patients with SCI die before reaching the hospital or during the initial hospitalization. First-year hospital costs for patients with acute cervical SCI range from $35,000 to $70,000. Lifetime costs (all costs, including list income) for a quadriplegic are estimated to reach up to $750,000 and for a paraplegic, $225,000 (Young and Northrup, 1981). Total costs for care of all victims of SCI is estimated to be $2.4 billion a year (Hickey, 1986).

SCI occurs most frequently in younger people, with 80% of patients under the age of 40 years and 50% between 15 and 25 years. The "typical" SCI victim is a young male (82% males versus 18% females) injured in a motor vehicle accident. Most SCI patients (57%) possess a high school education and were either working or full-time students when they were injured (Young and Northrup, 1981).

Motor vehicle accidents account for 46% of cases of SCI, followed by falls (16%) and sports injuries (16%) (Young and Northrup, 1981). Penetrating wounds are responsible for 12% of all SCIs, most of these occurring in children (Leader, 1976).

Mortality and morbidity of SCI patients have dramatically changed during the past 60 years. During World War I, the life expectancy for a SCI victim was 6 to 12 months. During the past decade, improvements in acute care and treatment of complications have allowed these patients a near normal life expectancy. Factors affecting survival include the level at which the injury occurred, the extent of paralysis, associated injuries, age when injured, and survival for the first 3 months following injury. Ten per cent of those who survive the initial resuscitation die within 3 months due to cardiopulmonary complications.

"Prevention" refers to programs aimed at lowering the incidence of SCI. Because most SCI victims are young (15 to 25 years old), prevention programs are focused toward the middle and high school populations. In these groups there is a sense of invulnerability and peer pressure for risk-taking behaviors, especially among males. Males are also encouraged to be more exploratory during the preteenage and early teenage years. Public education about the consequences of drug and alcohol abuse when driving or during other high-risk activities can be effective in reducing SCIs. Prevention programs should include information about law enforcement of driving within the speed limits, drinking and driving, and use of passenger restraints. An aggressive public education program in Florida focuses on preventing SCI from diving accidents. The program, *Feet First, First Time,* focuses on preventing young people from diving head first into shallow water. In the first year following the program there was a 50% decrease in SCI in Florida (Green et al., 1985).

Today's challenge is to motivate the general public to use safety measures and minimize high-risk situations. Public education and media support are essential to disseminate the information needed to avoid this type of preventable trauma.

TYPES OF SPINAL CORD INJURY

SCI is classified by level, degree (complete or incomplete), and mechanism of injury. Vertebral injuries are also defined according to their contribution to SCI.

Spinal levels include cervical, thoracic, and lumbar. Cervical and lumbar injuries occur most commonly because these areas have the greatest flexibility and movement. A cervical injury may result in paralysis of all four extremities, called quadriplegia or, less frequently, tetraplegia. Injuries of the thoracic and lumbar areas leave the patient paraplegic. Table 35–1 provides a list of some levels of injury and the expected functional ability following rehabilitation.

Degree of involvement may be complete or incomplete (partial). Complete SCI results in initial flaccid paralysis and total loss of motor and sensory function below the level of the injury. Losses result from irreversible spinal cord damage. Incomplete cord injury (partial transection) results in a mixed loss of motor and sensory function because some spinal cord tracts remain intact. The degree of loss depends on the level of injury and the specific nerve tract damaged.

Central cord syndrome is an example of partial transection. This syndrome usually follows a hyperextension injury in a person with cervical spondylosis (degeneration or ankylosis of the spine from osteoarthritis) or stenosis (narrowing of the spinal canal) (Chilton and Dagi, 1985). Central cord syndrome is characterized by microscopic hemorrhage and edema in the central gray matter of the cord (Fig. 35–1). Motor weakness of the upper extremities occurs, but it is greater in the upper extremities. There is varying sensory and bladder dysfunction. Recovery depends on the number of undamaged spinal cord tracts and on resolution of the edema (Walleck, 1987).

Another partial injury is anterior cord injury, which is characterized by acute compression of the anterior portion of the spinal cord. Compression may impair blood flow through the anterior spinal artery, which supplies the anterior two-thirds to three-quarters of the spinal cord (Ducker et al, 1971). This syndrome may follow a flexion injury but is also associated with a herniated intervertebral disc or thrombosis of the anterior spinal artery. Signs of this injury include immediate motor loss, hypoesthesia (decreased sensation), or loss of sensation for pain and temperature below the level of injury. Since posterior cord function is preserved, the sensations

TABLE 35–1. Levels of Injury and Expected Functional Ability

Level	Normal Activity	Functional Expectation
C4	Head control Mouth control Shoulder/scapular elevation Diaphragm movement	Use of a mouthstick for turning pages, typing or writing Control of electric wheelchair ADL dependent
C5	Shoulder flexion Elbow flexion Increased scapular function	Feeds self with special adaptive devices Able to move wheelchair for short distances, does better with electric wheelchair Assists a little in self-care
C6	Good elbow flexion Wrist extension Shoulder rotation and abduction	Independent in feeding and some grooming with adaptive devices Weak hand grasp Can roll over in bed Uses regular wheelchair Can drive a car with hand controls Can assist in transfer
C7	Elbow extension Strong wrist extension Good shoulder movement	Transfers independently to chair Independent in most ADLs Excellent bed mobility
T1	Normal hand strength Normal upper extremity strength	Bed and wheelchair independent Performs self catheterization Wheelchair independent

ADL, activities of daily living.

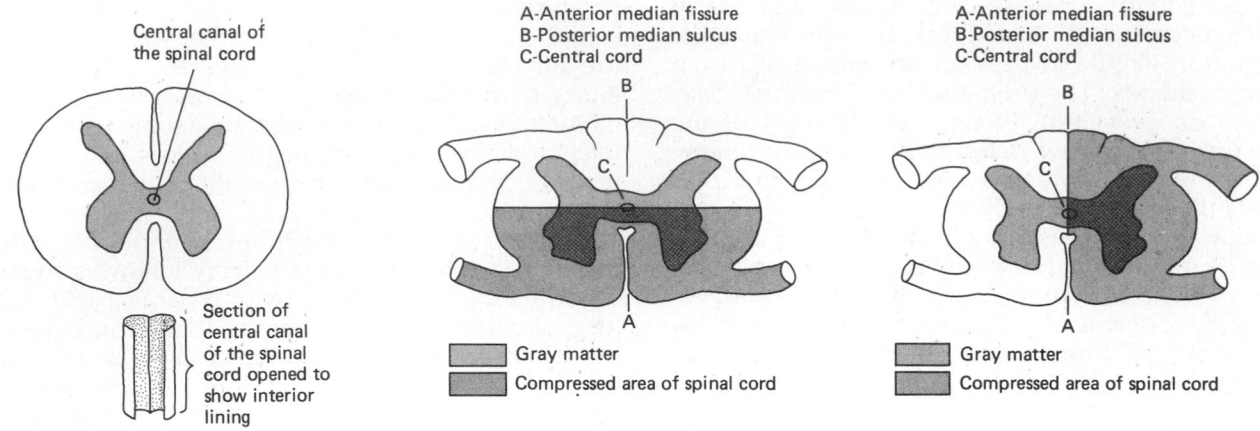

Central canal of the spinal cord

Section of central canal of the spinal cord opened to show interior lining

A-Anterior median fissure
B-Posterior median sulcus
C-Central cord

Gray matter
Compressed area of spinal cord

A-Anterior median fissure
B-Posterior median sulcus
C-Central cord

Gray matter
Compressed area of spinal cord

A. Central cord syndrome   B. Anterior cord syndrome   C. Brown-Sequard syndrome

FIGURE 35—1. Three syndromes associated with incomplete cord lesions. (Reproduced by permission from: Lewis, S. M., and Collier, I. C. (Eds). *Medical surgical nursing: Assessment and management of clinical problems* (p. 1602). New York: 1982, McGraw-Hill Book Co.; copyrighted by The C. V. Mosby Co., St. Louis).

of touch, position (proprioception), and vibration remain intact. If the syndrome is caused by compression of the anterior cord from bony fragments, surgical decompression is necessary.

Brown-Sequard syndrome, or hemisection of the cord (Fig. 35–1), results in ipsilateral motor loss and contralateral loss of pain and temperature sensation due to spinothalamic tract involvement. Penetrating injuries may cause pure Brown-Sequard syndrome, whereas blunt trauma may result in a more asymmetrical loss (Chilton and Dagi, 1985). The motorsensory dysfunction seen in this syndrome can be understood by knowing that the corticospinal tracts and posterior columns decussate (cross) in the medulla, but the spinothalamic fibers cross the spinal cord within one or two spinal segments before ascending to the thalamus.

Other incomplete injuries cause varying degrees of motorsensory dysfunction, sometimes sparing specific functions.

SCI results from compression, contusion, or transection of the spinal cord. The major mechanisms of injury are flexion, flexion-rotation, hyperextension, and compression (axial loading) (Figs. 35–2 and 35–3). Flexion injury with tearing of the posterior ligaments and dislocation is the most unstable injury. This injury is often associated with severe neurologic deficits. Hyperextension injury is the most common mechanism of cord injury.

Vertebral injuries can be classified as simple, compression, and comminuted, or as teardrop fracture, dislocation, subluxation (partial dislocation), and fracture-dislocation (Riggins and Kraus, 1983). Simple fractures usually involve the spinous or transverse processes and are seldom associated with neurologic deficits.

In a wedge or compression fracture the vertebral body is compressed due to hyperflexion injury. Neural compression may or may not occur. This fracture is common in elderly women with osteoporosis. Several successive fractured vertebral bodies may produce the clinical picture known as "dowager's back," in which the woman's spine is hunched forward.

The burst fracture, or comminuted fracture, results in a shattering of the vertebral body. This fracture is associated with a compression injury and often results in serious SCI.

Dislocation is defined as one vertebra overriding another with unilateral or bilateral facet joint dislocation. The dislocation results from torn or stretched ligaments that allow excessive vertebral movement. Subluxation is a partial or incomplete dislocation. Ligamentous injury and SCI may also be present following subluxation.

Fractures may be stable or unstable. Stability is maintained if all of the anterior ligaments and posterior ligaments, plus one additional structure (such as the lamina or spinous process), remain intact (Carol and Ducker, 1987). Even though an injury may be described as acutely unstable, delayed stability can occur following fracture healing. If severe ligamentous damage has occurred, fractures may remain chronically unstable unless they are internally fixed with spinal fusion or internal fixation devices.

PATHOPHYSIOLOGY OF SPINAL CORD INJURY

SCI is multiphasic, involving morphologic damage to the spinal cord, hemorrhage, vascular damage, structural changes in the gray and white matter, and subsequent biochemical responses to trauma (Gilbert, 1987).

The hemodynamic changes that occur following SCI are a major factor in the resulting damage to the spinal cord. Autoregulation is lost during the acute phase of injury, profoundly decreasing blood flow

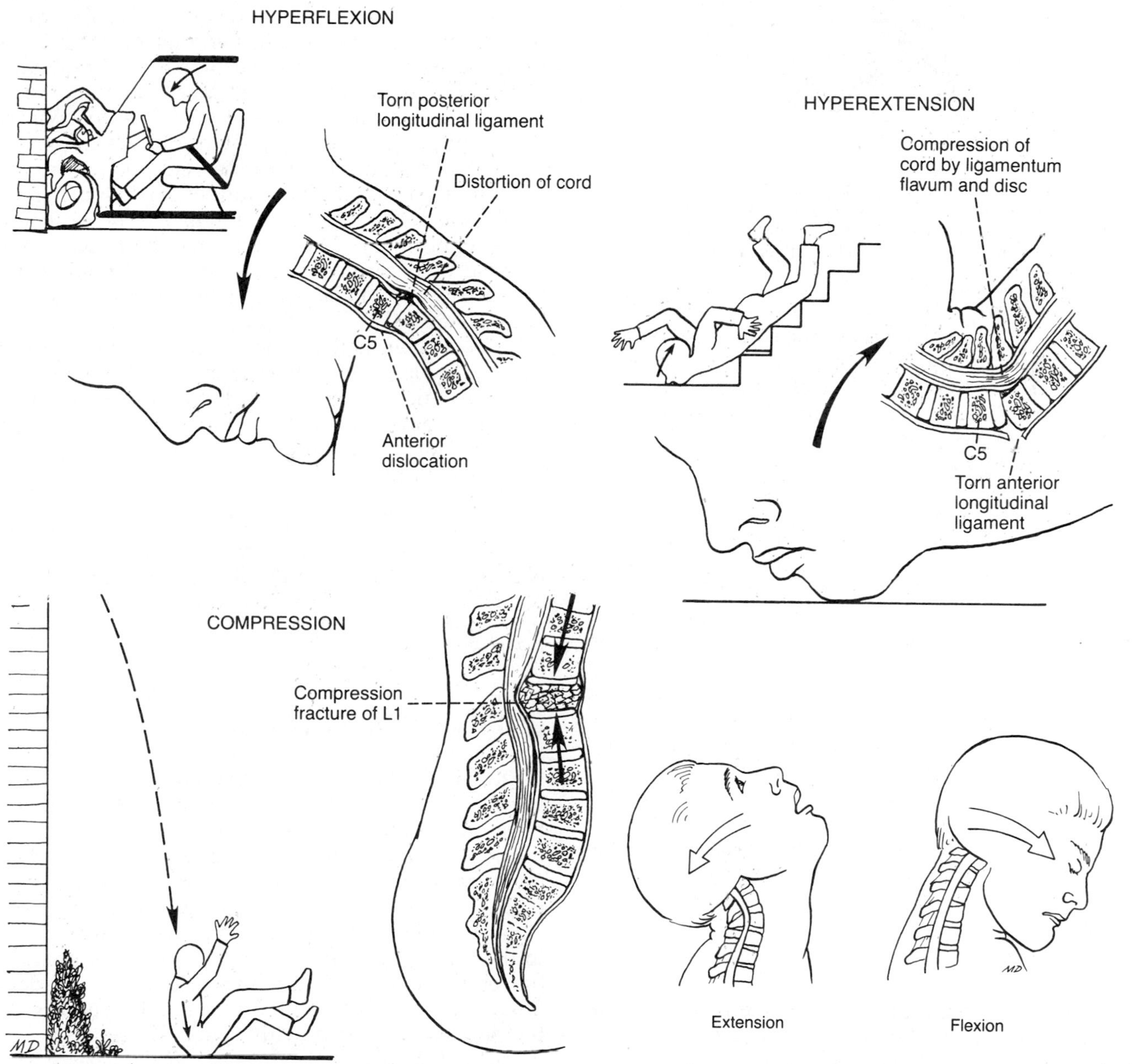

FIGURE 35—2. Closed spinal injury mechanisms. Many situations produce these consequences. This figure shows examples only. (From Luckmann, J., and Sorensen, K. C. (1987). *Medical-surgical nursing: A psychophysiologic approach* (3rd ed., pp. 427–428). Philadelphia: W. B. Saunders.)

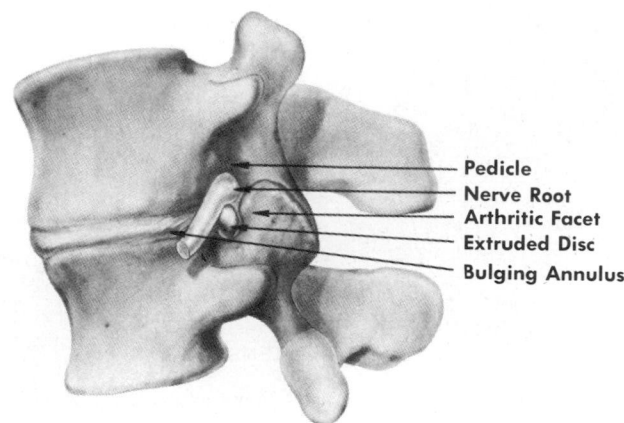

FIGURE 35—3. Normal vertebra. Note the comparatively protected position of the spinal cord relative to the transverse and spinous processes. (From Rothman, R. H., and Simeone, F. A. (Eds.) (1975). *The spine: Volume II* (p. 450). Philadelphia: W. B. Saunders.)

and causing ischemic injury to the cord. Concomitant with changes in blood flow are changes in the tissue oxygen tension that ultimately affect metabolic function. As blood flow is compromised, free radicals are released from ischemic areas, increasing the damage in the area of the original injury by means of increased ischemia, vasospasm, and hypoxia. The optimum time for intervention to limit or reverse these destructive processes is within 4 hours of injury, and preferably within 60 to 90 minutes (Senter and Venes, 1979).

In addition to morphologic and histologic changes, the injured spinal cord may also suffer concussion or contusion. Concussion, due to severe shaking of the cord, may cause temporary loss of function lasting 24 to 48 hours. No identifiable neuropathologic changes are usually present (Hickey, 1986). Contusion of the spinal cord is a bruising that includes bleeding, subsequent edema, and possible necrosis from the edematous compression. The neurologic involvement depends on the severity of the contusion and necrosis (Hickey, 1986).

Spinal Shock

Bony compression of the spinal cord can result in spinal shock, a temporary suspension of function and reflexes below the level of injury. Following acute injury, input from higher brain centers is abruptly lost. Symptoms of spinal shock occur below the level of injury and include flaccid paralysis of all skeletal muscles; loss of all spinal reflexes; loss of pain, proprioception, and other sensations; bowel and bladder dysfunction; and loss of thermoregulation and the ability to perspire.

Spinal shock may last days, weeks, or months. Generally it subsides within 7 to 10 days. It may be prolonged by infection or other complications (Guttman, 1976). A return of reflexes indicates the end of spinal shock. As spinal shock dissipates, spasticity of involved muscles begins (Nikas, 1988).

Neurogenic Shock

Neurogenic shock occurs following cervical and upper thoracic cord injury. This form of shock is the result of the loss of brainstem and higher center control of the sympathetic nervous system. Input from the brainstem contributes to basic reflex control of vital signs through cardiac accelerator and vasoconstrictive reflexes (Tyson, 1979). Loss of sympathetic outflow results in hypotension due to peripheral vasodilation, bradycardia (secondary to an overriding parasympathetic influence), loss of cardiac accelerator reflex, and loss of ability to sweat below the level of injury. The patient may be hypothermic because of disrupted transmission of impulses between the hypothalamus and the sympathetic nervous system.

In identifying neurogenic shock, it is important to rule out hypovolemic shock, which may worsen the hypotension. An active search for sources of hemorrhage must be done to ensure proper treatment. Hypotension in patients with neurogenic shock reflects displacement of fluid volume into the vasodilated periphery, not a true lack of fluid volume. Overhydration of these patients will not correct low blood pressure and may lead to pulmonary edema or congestive heart failure. The goal of therapy is to combat the cause of lost circulatory volume. The use of vasopressor agents will be discussed later under medical management.

CLINICAL PRESENTATION

Most patients with acute SCI are in spinal shock. They have lost all motorsensory and reflex function below the level of injury. Even when transection is incomplete, the patient may appear to have a complete transection. Once spinal cord shock resolves, upper motor neuron (UMN) signs appear. UMN signs include increased muscle tone, flexor spasms in the lower extremities, spasticity of trunk muscles, bowel and bladder incontinence, and increased reflexes. Recovery of voluntary motor function is not temporally associated with spinal shock resolution (Geisler, 1988).

Neurologic Assessment

Assessment of patients with SCI begins at the scene of the accident. It is critical to note the actual time of onset of loss of motorsensory function. Since treatment within 60 to 90 minutes is thought to limit or reverse neurologic deficits, noting the time of onset can guide the aggressiveness of therapy (Geisler, 1988).

Assessment focuses on motorsensory function and includes voluntary motor ability, proprioception, and pain. Motor function is assessed by requesting the patient to move all major muscle groups, beginning with the deltoids and biceps (C_5 innervation). Muscle groups are assessed by asking the patient to flex, extend, abduct, and adduct each extremity. If the patient is able to move against gravity, resistance is applied by the examiner, and the patient is asked to repeat the movement. A five-point motor scoring system is used to grade muscle function: 5 = normal movement, 3 = movement against gravity, 0 = total paralysis (Fig. 35–4).

Superficial and deep reflexes are also assessed (see Chap. 31). Although reflex testing does not provide specific information about motor function ability, it aids in identifying spinal shock and differentiates between partial and complete lesions (Nikas, 1988).

Sensory assessment includes evaluation of proprioception (position sense), temperature, and pain. Proprioception is assessed by asking the patient to close both eyes and identify whether the thumb or great toe is moved toward or away from the head (i.e., up or down). Spinothalamic tracts convey pain and temperature sensations. Pain sensation is tested with a pin. The patient closes both eyes, and the face is lightly touched with the pin to determine the patient's ability to differentiate sharp from dull. The pin is then touched to various places on the patient's body, progressing distally, to determine if and where sensation has been lost. Bilateral testing is necessary to rule out sensory sparing. Care must be taken not to break the skin while testing. Light touch is similarly tested using a wisp of cotton.

Initially, motorsensory function is assessed along with the vital signs to determine whether changes have occurred. Once the patient is stable, daily testing is sufficient. Careful documentation in the patient's record is important to detect neurologic deterioration.

Monitoring of vital signs, including cardiac rhythm, is important during the critical care phase. With the loss of sympathetic outflow, hypotension and bradycardia can occur. An arterial line, pulmonary artery catheter, and electrocardiographic monitoring aid in the assessment of these patients during the spinal and neurogenic shock phases (Carol and Ducker, 1987; Dunham and Cowley, 1986). Monitoring temperature carefully is important because hypothermia can result from peripheral vasodilation and loss of thermoregulation.

In addition to hypotension from decreased systemic vascular resistance (SVR), the cardiac preload is decreased. Cardiac output (CO) drops, and tissue perfusion decreases. A pulmonary artery catheter monitors SVR, CO, and pulmonary capillary occlusion pressure (PCOP).

Heart rate is closely monitored for bradycardia. Atropine should be available at the bedside in case the pulse drops below 40 beats/minute. Left ventricular function is also depressed. Beta endorphins released as a result of SCI have been implicated in exacerbating poor ventricular performance (Faden et al., 1980). Left ventricular dysfunction can lead to cardiac dysrhythmias.

Respiratory insufficiency is a serious threat following SCI. Some degree of respiratory insufficiency should be suspected in all quadriplegics and most paraplegics until this is disproved (Carter, 1979). Insufficiency may result from airway obstruction, intercostal or diaphragmatic muscle paralysis, or associated thoracic or tracheal trauma or aspiration.

Respiratory assessment is critical because respiratory failure is the leading cause of death for quadriplegics. Arterial blood gases, chest assessment, vital capacity, and chest radiographs are used to determine the patient's respiratory status. It may be normal for long-term quadriplegics to have a chronically low Pa_{O_2} (60 to 70 mm Hg) and an abnormally high Pa_{CO_2} (45 to 60 mm Hg), but during the immediate postinjury phase a much higher Pa_{O_2} is needed (Green et al., 1985). Hypoxemia can compromise injured neurons and exacerbate neurologic damage. A Pa_{O_2} of at least 80 mm Hg coupled with normalization of the Pa_{CO_2} is recommended.

Assessment of respiratory rate and pattern should be done hourly. Measurements of tidal volume, minute ventilation, and vital capacity should be included in the respiratory assessment.

Patients with injury at the C4 level or above require intubation and ventilation because of loss of phrenic innervation. Injuries involving C5 or lower may potentially involve respiratory compromise, requiring frequent respiratory assessment.

Laboratory Findings

Laboratory studies include baseline blood studies (serum electrolytes, glucose, hemoglobin, hematocrit, blood gases, and enzymes), urinalysis, and other studies as indicated, including a toxicology screen. This laboratory work provides a baseline for future blood work. If a pulmonary artery catheter is in place, mixed venous blood gases should be monitored.

Diagnostic Procedures

A cervical spine radiograph is obtained right after admission to the hospital. Thoracic and lumbar x-rays should also be taken. These x-rays add to information obtained from subsequent neuroradiologic tests (myelogram, tomograms, computed tomography [CT scans], and magnetic resonance imaging [MRI]) and facilitate therapeutic decisions.

The x-ray process must be accomplished with the patient in neutral position to prevent further spinal cord injury. Immobilization of the spinal column is important to prevent additional trauma. All seven cervical vertebrae must be seen to the top of T1 on anteroposterior and lateral films. It may be necessary

UNIVERSITY OF MARYLAND
MIEMSS — UMMS
SPINAL CORD INJURY FLOW SHEET

Muscle Strength

5 Normal
4 Active movement through range of motion
      against resistance
3 Active movement through range of motion
      against gravity
2 Active movement through range of motion with
      gravity eliminated
1 Palpable or visible contraction
0 Total paralysis
U Unable to test strength of extremity

Rectal Tone, Proprioception, Diaphragm

P–Present   A–Absent   U–Untestable

Medication   Sensation

Sedation-S   N–Normal
Paralytic-PL   ABN–Abnormal
Tranquilizer-T   A–Absent
Pain-P   U–Untestable

MOTOR LEVEL   *Circled entry means to refer to nurse's note*

Level of bony/ligamentous injury	
Anatomical Classification	
Date	
Time	
Medications	
*Diaphragm (P/A)	C4
Deltoid (raise arms) (R/L)	C5
*Biceps (elbow flexion) (R/L)	C5,6
Wrist Extensors (R/L)	C6
*Triceps (elbow extension) (R/L)	C7
*Flexor Digitorum Profundus (finger flexion) (R/L)	C8
Hand Intrinsics (finger abduction) (R/L)	T1
*Iliopsoas (hip flexion) (R/L)	L2
Quadriceps (knee flexion) (R/L)	L3
Tibialis Anterior (dorsiflex foot) (R/L)	L4
Extensor Hallucis Longus (great toe extenstion) (R/L)	L5
*Gastrocnemius (ankle plantar flexion) (R/L)	S1
Function	Level
Proprioception (finger) (R/L)	
Proprioception (toe) (R/L)	
Rectal Tone (P/A)	
INITIALS	
INITIALS/SIGNATURE	

A

FIGURE 35—4. *A* and *B,* Spinal cord injury flow sheet. (*Tested each time.) (Reproduced with permission from University of Maryland; MIEMSS–UMMS.)

SENSATION

DATE															
TIME															
C_2 (R/L)															
C_3 (R/L)															
C_4 (R/L)															
*C_5 (R/L)															
C_6 (thumb and forefinger) (R/L)															
C_7 (middle finger) (R/L)															
C_8 (ring and little finger) (R/L)															
T_1 (R/L)															
T_2 (R/L)															
T_3 (R/L)															
*T_4 (nipple) (R/L)															
T_5 (R/L)															
T_6 (R/L)															
T_7 (R/L)															
T_8 (R/L)															
T_9 (R/L)															
*T_{10} (umbilicus) (R/L)															
T_{11} (R/L)															
T_{12} (R/L)															
L_1 (R/L)															
L_2 (R/L)															
L_3 (R/L)															
L_4 (R/L)															
L_5 (R/L)															
S_1															
S_2															
$S_{3,4,5}$ (sacral sparing)															
Sensory Function															
INITIALS															

B

FIGURE 35–4 Continued

to depress the shoulders to visualize C7. A swimmer's view (one arm up and the other at the patient's side, with the x-ray taken through the axilla) may facilitate visualization. Views of the odontoid process (the dens of C2) may require films taken through the open mouth (Fig. 35–5).

If a major neurologic deficit is noted, a myelogram is done to determine any potential sources of pressure on the spinal cord. After reduction, a puncture at the C1–C2 level is made, and radiopaque dye (iophendylate, metrizamide, or iohexal) is instilled with the patient in the supine position (Carol et al., 1980). A CT scan may also be performed with the myelogram.

CT scans define and delineate bony injury and cord compression. The CT image is extremely helpful in visualizing spinal areas not seen on plain x-ray. Indications for CT scan with myelography include (Dunham and Cowley, 1986):

1. Neurologic deficit in the presence of normal x-rays at the level of the deficit
2. Thoracic spine injury with deficit to allow differentiation of injury of the conus medullaris from a cauda equina injury
3. After reduction of the spinal column in patients with a neurologic deficit to ensure adequate bony reduction and cord decompression
4. In preoperative patients if bone is suspected within the spinal canal

Magnetic resonance imaging is a new diagnostic procedure used to determine the extent of SCI. It is difficult to perform MRI on critically ill patients because no metal can contact the patient during the scan. However, newer MRI-compatible devices are being developed. MRI is useful for detecting soft tissue involvement, i.e., spinal cord contusion and edema.

Another diagnostic tool used in SCI is the somatosensory evoked potential (SEP). Evoked responses may establish a prognosis because they reflect neural pathway function. Although SEPs reflect only sensory function, findings in patients with acute cord injury show a high but incomplete correlation with motor function as well (Grundy and Friedman, 1987). In SEP a peripheral nerve in an arm or leg below the level of injury is stimulated, and the responses of the cord and cerebral cortex are recorded with electrodes. In patients with complete injury, SEPs are absent because no transmissions can pass the site of injury. In patients with an incomplete injury an altered response is noted. Early persistence and progressive normalization of evoked potentials generally precede clinical improvement (Green et al., 1985).

MEDICAL MANAGEMENT

The medical management of a patient with SCI begins at the scene of the accident. All trauma patients should be treated as if they had SCI until proved otherwise. A thorough assessment at the scene uses the priorities of airway, breathing, and circulation. The goals of treatment are immobilization of the spinal column, stabilization of all systems, ventilatory support, oxygen supplementation, and rapid transportation for emergency care.

Traditionally, fluid replacement is begun in the field using two large-bore (14- to 16-gauge) intravenous lines to treat hypovolemic shock. Dextrose 5% and lactated Ringer's solution is the usual fluid of choice for the initial resuscitation. However, this form of fluid replacement is inappropriate for patients with SCI because their hypotension arises from systemic vasodilation following neurogenic shock. Cautious fluid management is necessary until hemorrhagic shock is ruled out.

Upon admission to the emergency department, a

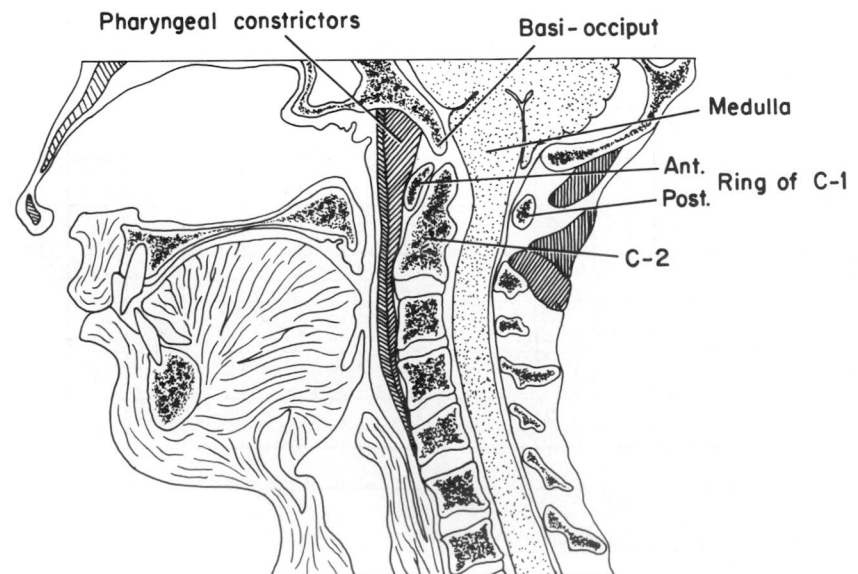

Pharyngeal constrictors
Basi-occiput
Medulla
Ant. Ring of C-1
Post.
C-2

FIGURE 35–5. Sagittal section through the base of the skull and upper cervical spine. Note the ring of C1 surrounding the dens of C2; also note the close relationship of the medulla to the basiocciput and upper cervical vertebrae. (From Rothman, R. H., and Simeone, F. A. (Eds.) (1975). *The spine: Volume I* (p. 103). Philadelphia: W. B. Saunders.)

report of prehospital management and a history of the injury are rapidly obtained. Immobilization with a spinal board is maintained until after spinal x-rays are completed and cleared. The priorities of care are to prevent further injury and reestablish physiologic homeostasis, i.e., normalize vital signs and blood gases and establish spinal alignment (Green et al., 1987).

Skeletal cervical traction is useful in patients with upper level SCI to realign the spinal column and relieve the spinal cord pressure from the displaced bony fragments. Biomechanical knowledge and experience are necessary for optimal application and to prevent complications (Geisler, 1988).

Patients must be evaluated individually for the amount of instability and damage they have sustained to determine the amount of traction needed. A variety of devices may be used for skeletal traction of cervical vertebrae (Fig. 35–6). At least 10 pounds of traction are initially applied. Weight is applied based on the 5-pound per interspace formula (for example, a C5–C6 injury would require between 25 and 30 pounds of traction). Serial x-rays are taken to determine the effect of the traction. Traction weights may be increased to as high as twice the initial weight (Greene et al., 1987). If this amount of traction is unable to reduce bony fragment displacement and neurologic deficit persists, muscle relaxants or paralytic agents may aid in reduction. If these agents are used, the patient will be intubated and placed on a ventilator. Open reduction, with or without internal fixation, may be needed. Aggressive reestablishment of spinal alignment is essential for physiologic homeostasis.

The decision to operate on patients with SCI depends on the type of injury and the patient's overall hemodynamic status. Once emergency department stabilization has been accomplished, decisions about immediate or delayed surgery or conservative therapy can be made.

In patients with SCI with a flexion or flexion-compression cervical fracture, closed cervical reduction is usually successful. If there are no associated fractures (i.e., unilateral or bilateral locked facet joints), traction is maintained until posterior cervical wire fixation or bony fusion can be performed in the operating room.

Patients with severe ligamentous injuries, compression unrelieved by traction, or a burst fracture require rapid surgical intervention. An anterior corpectomy (removal of the vertebral body) and fusion are performed. Progressive neurologic deficit from edema or intrathecal hemorrhage may require emergency decompression laminectomy (Fig. 35–7). Early surgery may preserve, improve, or restore spinal cord function (Hickey, 1986).

Thoracic and upper lumbar injuries may require surgical intervention utilizing a variety of methods to stabilize the injury. Autograft or allograft bone may be used to perform spinal fusion. A variety of internal fixation devices may be used to stabilize the

spine, including Harrington or Luque rods, Dwyer instrumentation, methylmethacrylate, and surgical wire (Fig. 35–8).

Once the airway, breathing, and circulation are stable, the patient should be started on a high dose of methylprednisolone. A bolus of 30 mg/kg is administered, followed by a 23-hour infusion of 5.4 mg/kg per hour. This treatment must be started within 8 hours of the injury to be effective (Brackman et al., 1990). The patient with a neurologic deficit is usually transferred to the critical care unit. The hemodynamic and pulmonary status of the patient is of major concern. The goal of care is to prevent life-threatening complications while maximizing function of all body systems. A holistic approach to care throughout the acute phase is needed because every system of the body is affected by SCI.

The intensive care of these patients has changed dramatically in the last decade due to the realization that hypotension and bradycardia are the result of neurogenic shock. Hypotension is not the result of circulatory volume deficit but is secondary to vasodilation from lack of sympathetic outflow. The use of inotropic drugs rather than fluid resuscitation is the treatment of choice. Dopamine hydrochloride (3 to 5 mg/kg per minute) may be supplemented with dobutamine hydrochloride in low doses to maintain mean arterial blood pressures of 80 to 90 mm Hg with an increased cardiac output (1 to 1.5 times normal) (Geisler, 1988). Augmentation of cardiovascular dynamics is maintained for 72 hours to counteract the effects of neurogenic shock and enhance spinal cord perfusion to promote neurologic recovery. Gilbert (1987) states that dobutamine rather than dopamine is preferred for the hemodynamic push because it does not increase pulmonary vascular resistance, which could contribute to pulmonary capillary extravasation and pulmonary edema.

Cardiovascular System

Bradycardia in patients with SCI complicates increased vascular capacitance and decreased circulatory volumes (Nikas, 1988). Pulse rates may be as low as 40 beats/minute. Slow heart rates are usually tolerated by patients with adequate volume replacement and an adequate cardiac index. Atropine sulfate may be used when hemodynamic changes accompany the low heart rate. Suctioning or turning that causes a vasovagal response with a heart rate of below 40 beats/minute should be treated with atropine sulfate.

Although not directly related to cardiovascular function, the sympathectomy resulting from SCI may result in loss of thermoregulation. Hypothermia and poikilothermia are frequently seen in patients with spinal shock. Poikilothermia occurs when the patient's temperature rises and falls in response to the environmental temperature (Nikas, 1982). Normo-

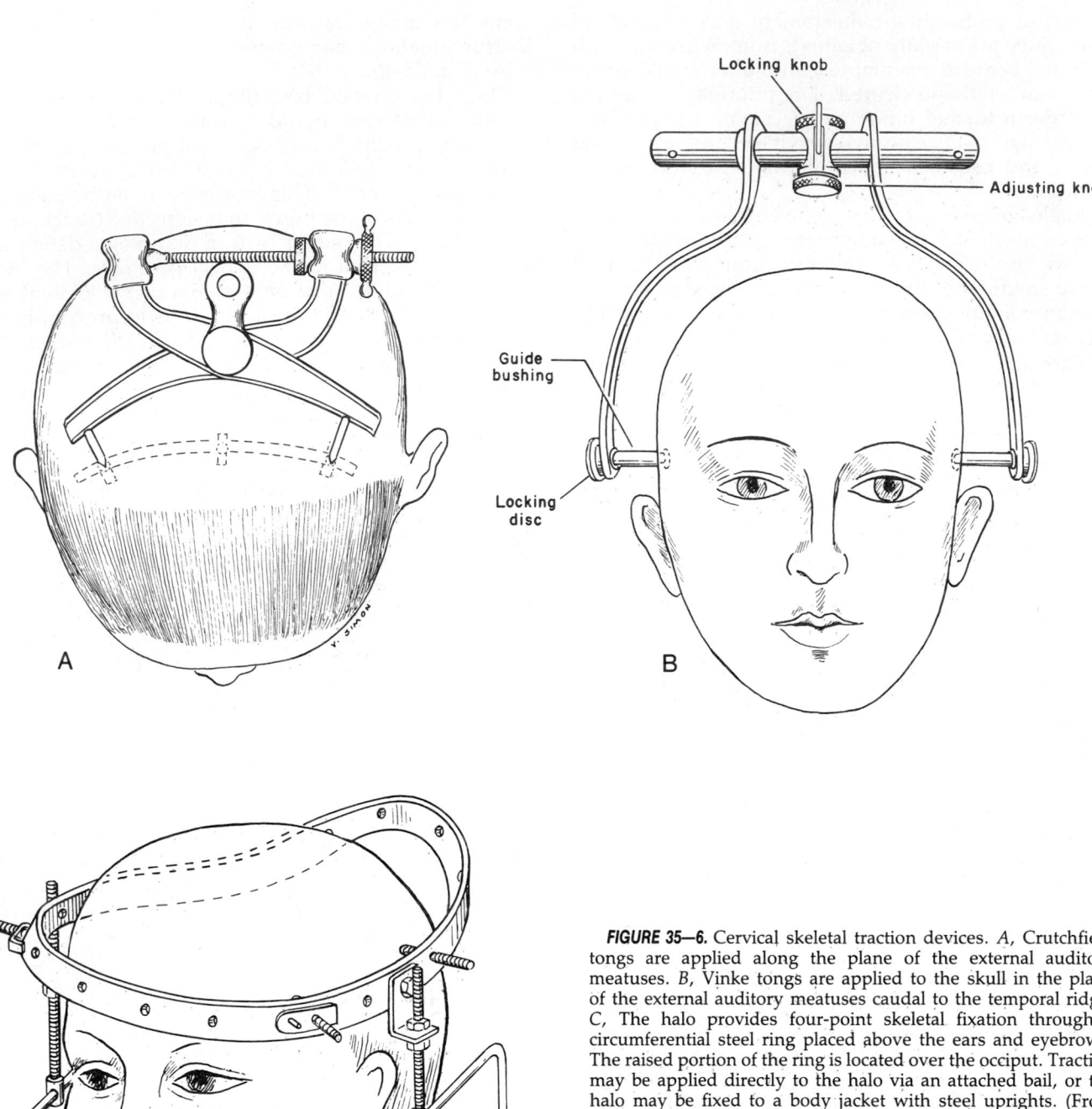

FIGURE 35—6. Cervical skeletal traction devices. *A*, Crutchfield tongs are applied along the plane of the external auditory meatuses. *B*, Vinke tongs are applied to the skull in the plane of the external auditory meatuses caudal to the temporal ridge. *C*, The halo provides four-point skeletal fixation through a circumferential steel ring placed above the ears and eyebrows. The raised portion of the ring is located over the occiput. Traction may be applied directly to the halo via an attached bail, or the halo may be fixed to a body jacket with steel uprights. (From Rothman, R. H., and Simeone, F. A. (Eds.) (1975). *The spine: Volume I.* (pp. 89, 91, and 92). Philadelphia: W. B. Saunders.)

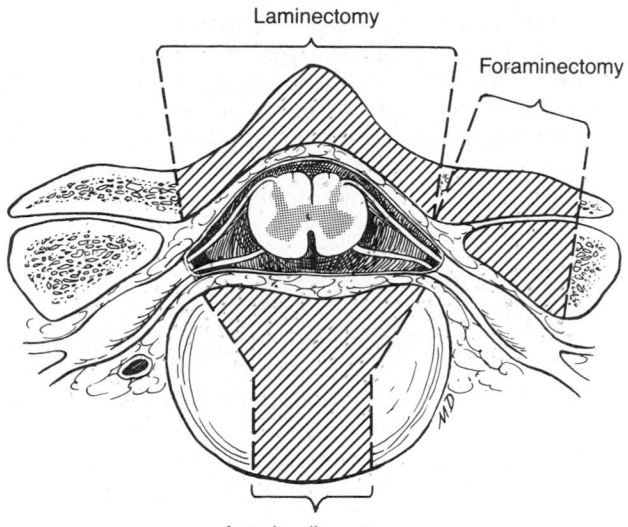

FIGURE 35—7. Operative approaches to the spinal cord. (From Luckmann, J., and Sorensen, K. C. (1987). *Medical-surgical nursing: A psychophysiologic approach* (3rd ed., p. 537). Philadelphia: W. B. Saunders.)

thermia should be maintained. If the patient is hypothermic, warming intravenous fluids and the use of warming lamps and blankets can elevate the patient's temperature. Hyperthermia may result in serious metabolic strain. Cooling may be encouraged by removing excess clothing, altering the environmental temperature, or using a cooling blanket.

The peripheral vascular system is also affected in patients with SCI. Decreased blood flow increases the risk of venous thrombosis in the legs and pelvis.

Venous stasis, intimal damage, and hypercoagulability are reported to exist in all patients with SCI (McCagg, 1986). Prevention of deep vein thrombosis (DVT) is a goal throughout hospitalization. Diagnosis of DVT is difficult because its signs and symptoms are unreliable. Daily calf and thigh measurements are recommended. Definitive diagnostic studies are indicated if an increase of 2 cm or more in circumference occurs (McCagg, 1986).

There is no agreement on the most effective way to prevent DVT. Elastic hose, pneumatic calf compression devices, elevation, and kinetic therapy have all been utilized (Becker et al., 1987; Green et al., 1982; Green et al., 1983). Prophylactic anticoagulation has been advocated as a form of definitive therapy (Hull et al., 1982). Anticoagulation may be avoided because of its potential for complications involving hemorrhage, especially in multiple trauma patients or preoperative or postoperative patients. Low-dose heparin (5000 to 7000 units every 12 hours) is recommended in high-risk patients, e.g., those with long bone fractures, the elderly, or the obese (Nikas, 1988). (See Chap. DD for care of the patient with diagnosed DVT.)

Respiratory System

Altered respiratory function is a major problem for patients with high thoracic or cervical SCI. Injuries at or above C4 result in ventilator dependency because of the inability to breathe spontaneously due to lost phrenic nerve function and paralysis of intercostal muscles. Edema or hemorrhage can result in compression of the spinal cord in patients with

FIGURE 35—8. Posterior interspinous fusion. *A,* Holes are drilled in the outer cortex of the spinous process adjacent to the lamina. *B,* The drill holes are connected with a towel clip. *C,* Wires are passed through the holes and adjacent vertebrae and are twisted in place. *D,* One additional wire is passed, to surround all of the vertebrae involved in the area of intended fusion. *E,* Corticocancellous strips of bone graft are laid down about the posterior elements in the area of intended fusion. (From Rothman, R. H., and Simone, F. A. (Eds.) (1975). *The spine: Volume I.* (p. 128). Philadelphia: W. B. Saunders.)

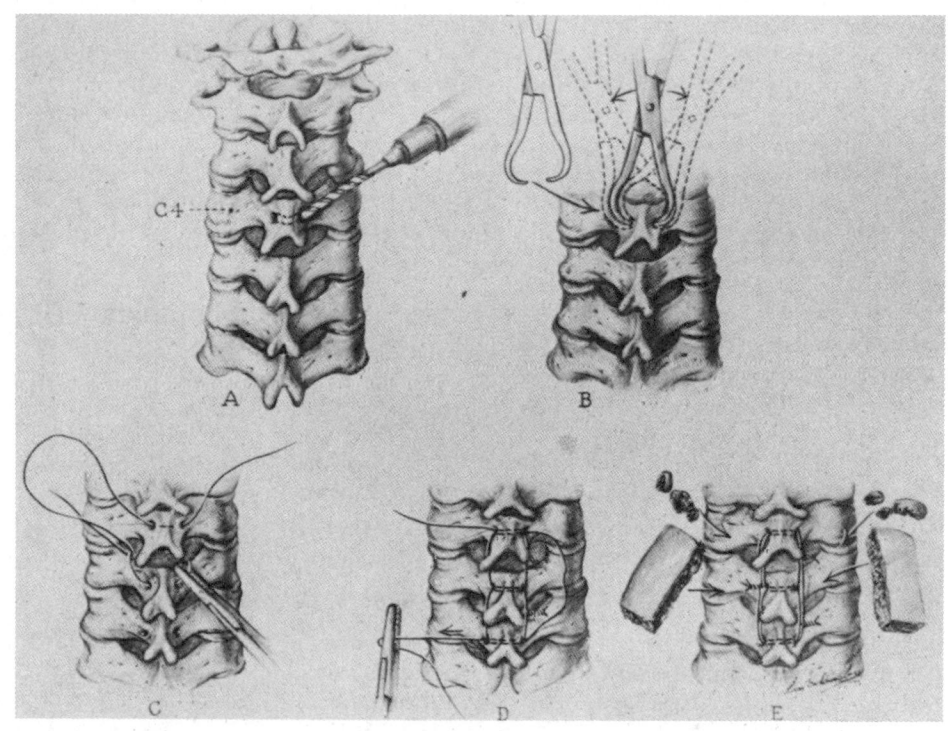

injuries below the level of C4, thus interfering with respirations. Prophylactic intubation (nasoendotracheal) is utilized in quadriplegics (Geisler and Salcman, 1987; Green et al., 1985). Paralysis of the abdominal and intercostal muscles aggravates the respiratory insufficiency, leading to ineffective cough and retention of secretions. Respiratory management of these patients must be aggressive, routinely utilizing chest physiotherapy every 4 hours. Ventilatory support is used to maintain normal blood gases.

Aspiration and pneumonia are common complications in patients with SCI. Aspiration may occur at the time of injury in water or diving accidents, or vomitus may be aspirated in motor vehicle accidents. Pneumonia usually occurs within the first few weeks of hospitalization resulting from hypostasis of secretions due to immobility. Pulmonary edema may follow aspiration or pneumonia but is most commonly due to fluid overload during resuscitation. Pulmonary emboli occur in about 13% of these patients and are seen in the first few weeks after injury (Gilbert, 1987).

Physical assessment of the chest, including observation, inspection, palpation, percussion, and auscultation, should be done with the vital signs for the initial 72 hours. Chest expansion and abdominal movement should be observed to determine whether accessory muscles are being used for respirations. Bedside pulmonary function studies can determine respiratory function and the need for ventilatory support. Tidal volume, inspiratory and expiratory reserve volumes, residual volume, total lung capacity, functional residual capacity, and vital capacity are assessed. Serial blood gas analysis aids in determining the need for ventilatory support. Pulse oximetry may also be used for continuous monitoring of Sa_{O_2}. Daily chest radiographs rule out the presence of pulmonary complications or allow early treatment of complications.

As mentioned earlier, all body systems are affected by SCI. Identification of cardiovascular and pulmonary complications is a high priority in critical care of these patients because they may be life-threatening. However, care of patients with SCI also includes identifying and managing complications of the gastrointestinal, urinary, musculoskeletal, and integumentary systems.

Gastrointestinal System

Gastrointestinal complications following SCI include gastric dilatation, paralytic ileus, and stress ulcers. A nasogastric, or sump, tube is placed while the patient is in the emergency department to decompress the stomach. Patients are usually started on intravenous hyperalimentation within 24 to 48 hours. When peristalsis returns, nasogastric feedings are begun, emphasizing calories, protein, and high fiber.

Stress ulcers occur in 10% to 20% of patients with SCI (Nikas, 1988). These are thought to be related to

vagal stimulation of gastric acid during spinal shock. Frequent testing of gastric pH and intravenous H_2 receptor blocking agents (ranitidine, cimetidine, fomatidine), or antacids are used to prevent gastrointestinal hemorrhage. Monitoring for melena and hematochezia is done for all patients with SCI, including hematests of all stools.

Urinary System

Areflexia caused by spinal shock leads to urinary retention. An indwelling catheter is placed on admission. The catheter is maintained until the hemodynamic push is stopped. Once hemodynamic stability is attained, scheduled intermittent catheterizations should be initiated (McCagg, 1986).

Musculoskeletal System

Management of musculoskeletal problems in the intensive care period is a priority. Primary concerns include ensuring stability of the spine and managing the consequences of immobility. Maintaining the mobility of the paralyzed joints while maintaining spinal stability is the key to care of these patients. A variety of devices may be used to maintain spinal stability besides traction and surgery. These include halo-pelvic external fixators (Fig. 35–9), hyperextension body casts, Minerva jacket casts, and many forms of orthoses.

Integumentary System

Prevention of skin breakdown is another important consideration in the intensive care unit, as it is throughout the patient's lifetime. Pressure necrosis can prolong spinal shock, complicate spasticity, delay rehabilitation, and lead to life-threatening systemic infection (Nikas, 1988). Frequent turning and use of Rotorest treatment tables (Fig. 35–10) and other specialty beds, such as low air loss types, can be helpful in preventing pressure necrosis and skin breakdown.

Experimental Drug Therapy

Naloxone Hydrochloride. Animal experiments with SCI demonstrate that endogenous opioids are released following spinal cord trauma. These opioids contribute to secondary ischemic injury by reducing microcirculatory blood flow, among other effects (Faden et al., 1982a; Faden et al., 1981). Naloxone hydrochloride, an endogenous opioid antagonist, has shown promising results in animal studies on SCI. Naloxone-treated animals subjected to SCI demonstrated nearly normal motor function 6 weeks following injury, whereas control animals remained quadriparetic (Faden et al., 1981). Naloxone treatment was

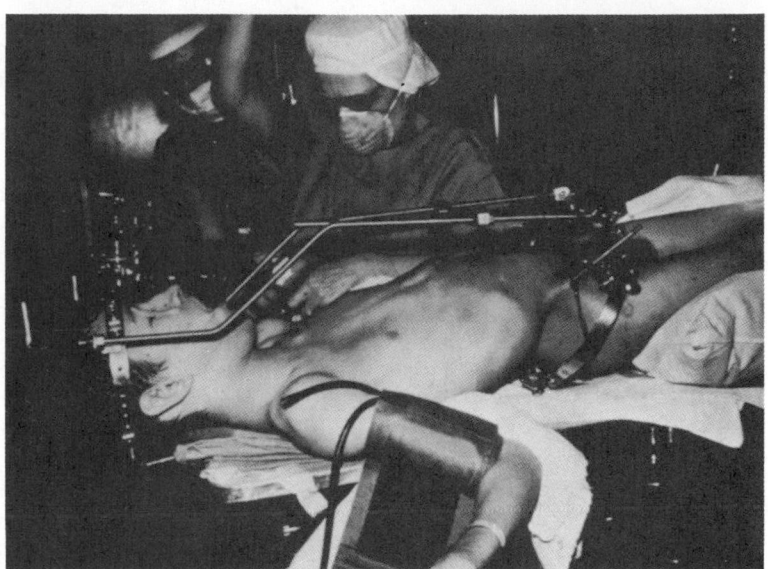

FIGURE 35—9. Halo-pelvic external fixator. (From Rothman, R. H., and Simeone, F. A. (Eds.) (1975). *The spine: Volume I* (p. 304). Philadelphia: W. B. Saunders.)

also associated with significant recovery of somatosensory evoked potentials even when treatment was delayed 4 hours after injury (Faden et al., 1982b; Young et al., 1981). Naloxone is now under investigation in 11 United States medical centers (Flamm et al., 1985). One major problem identified with naloxone therapy in humans is that it blocks the uptake of exogenous opioids such as narcotic analgesics. This limitation in the use of naloxone has lead to investigations of other endogenous opioid antagonists.

Thyrotropin-Releasing Hormone (TRH). This drug is a partial physiologic antagonist of endogenous opioids that does not interfere with narcotic analgesics. Beneficial effects of TRH on neurologic recovery are better than those produced with naloxone in experimental animals (Faden et al., 1981). In addi-

tion, TRH blocks the release of leukotrienes and other substances believed to be involved in secondary ischemic injury and improves spinal cord blood flow better than naloxone (Faden et al., 1981; Geisler, 1988). The beneficial effect of TRH was larger the sooner the drug was administered, although TRH was shown to be effective in treatment of SCI even when the initial dose was given 24 hours after injury (Faden et al., 1984). Several clinical trials are now being conducted.

Other Experimental Therapies

Hypothermia of the injured cord has also been studied. A small pad through which cooled saline solution is circulated is positioned surgically on the epidural layer of the newly injured spinal cord for 3 to 4 hours. Or fluid may be directly perfused through a C1–C2 stick and a lumbar drain. The temperature of the coolant is 6°C in most research protocols. The purpose of the procedure is to produce local vasoconstriction, decrease edema formation, and reduce intrinsic destructive processes (Hickey, 1986). Hypothermia in humans with SCI has improved neurologic function in some patients (Hansebout et al., 1984). This therapy requires further study to demonstrate its efficacy. One major problem with this therapy is the potential for infection from prolonged exposure of the spinal cord.

Hyperbaric oxygen therapy is a medical treatment in which the entire body is placed in a chamber under increased atmospheric pressure, and the patient breathes pure oxygen (Hickey, 1986). This treatment has been tried in patients with SCI in the belief that it may reduce ischemia and subsequent cord destruction by improving oxygen diffusion. Studies show conflicting results with this therapy (DeJesus-Greenberg, 1980; Gamache et al., 1981). Further study is needed to document the benefit of this therapy.

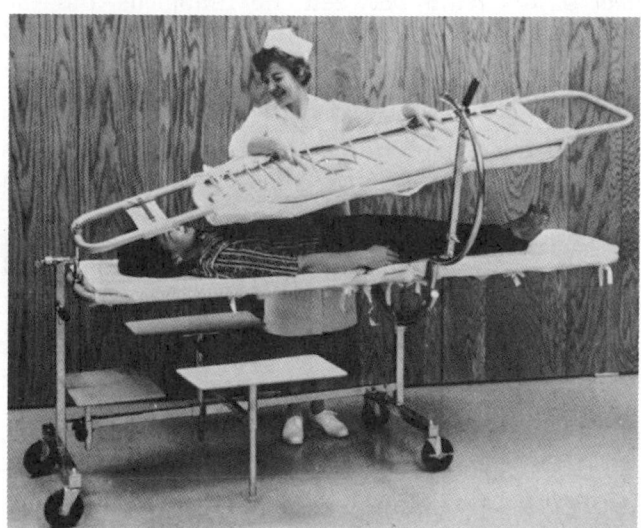

FIGURE 35—10. Stryker frame. (Reproduced with permission from: Lewis, S. M., and Collier, I. C. (Eds.), *Medical surgical nursing: Assessment and management of clinical problems.* New York, 1987, McGraw-Hill Book Co.; copyrighted by the C.V. Mosby Company, St. Louis.)

NURSING MANAGEMENT

The care of patients with acute SCI is complex because of the effect of this injury on all body systems. During the critical care phase the priorities of nursing care focus on the appearance of changes in major organ systems. The goals of nursing care are to prevent complications and prepare the patient for rehabilitation.

Altered Tissue Perfusion: Spinal Cord

Spinal cord tissue perfusion is altered due to inflammatory responses following injury, sympathetic blockade, and changes in intrathecal oxygen tension.

Expected Outcome. Blood pressure and Pa_{O_2} remain within normal limits for these patients; high cardiac output is maintained (1 to 1.5 times normal); urinary output exceeds 30 mL/hour.

Careful monitoring of all hemodynamic parameters is essential. Titration of vasopressor agents to maintain optimal hemodynamic status is often accomplished by the critical care nurse. Special attention should be paid to fluid and electrolyte balance, and careful monitoring of intake and output is essential. Fluid replacement should be judiciously accomplished to maintain adequate blood volume without risking pulmonary edema.

The patient's mental status should be closely monitored as a reflection of cerebral perfusion. Supplemental oxygen therapy should be provided during the first 24 hours and as indicated thereafter. Maintenance of normothermia during neurogenic shock prevents increased metabolic demand from hyperthermia. Vital signs should be monitored every 4 hours or more often as needed.

Ineffective Breathing Patterns

Breathing patterns may be altered due to upper level SCI (C4 and above) and because of possible loss of innervation of the intercostals and diaphragm. In patients with lesions above T1 the diaphragm is the only muscle of respiration. Gastric dilatation and paralytic ileus may also limit respiratory excursion. When only the diaphragm is active, fatigue may also contribute to ineffective breathing patterns.

Expected Outcome. Ventilation will be adequate as demonstrated by normal arterial blood gases, absence of respiratory distress, absence of pulmonary complications, absence of fever, and lungs that are clear to auscultation.

Physical assessment of the chest, including observation, inspection, palpation, percussion, and auscultation, should be done along with the vital signs during the first 72 hours following injury. Any changes from baseline respiratory function should be noted and reported, particularly the depth and pattern of respirations. As the injured spinal cord becomes edematous, respiratory arrest due to impaired innervation can occur in any patient with a cervical fracture. Serial vital capacity measurements are the most accurate method of predicting mechanical pulmonary failure. When serial vital capacity measurements demonstrate progressive decline, elective intubation and mechanical ventilation are required. Arterial blood gases or pulse oximetry are carefully monitored to detect impaired oxygenation and to guide the type of ventilatory support used. Initially, the Pa_{O_2} should be maintained at or above 80 mm Hg because systemic hypoxemia may exacerbate the SCI. Supplemental oxygen should be provided for the first 24 hours and as needed. The Pa_{CO_2} must be monitored carefully because quadriplegic patients retain CO_2 when they hypoventilate. Daily chest x-rays are done to rule out pulmonary complications and to allow early treatment of complications.

Assessment of the abdomen is important because abdominal distention interferes with respiratory excursion. An abdominal binder may be helpful in providing external support.

Ineffective Airway Clearance

Airway clearance may be impaired due to flaccid paralysis of the abdominal and intercostal muscles, which reduces the strength of the patient's cough (Richmond, 1985).

Expected Outcome. Patients will participate in assisted cough and will not show indications of retained secretions—that is, they are afebrile, the Pa_{CO_2} is within normal limits, and the sputum is clear and is present in normal amounts.

The "quad-assist" cough augments the abdominal muscles during the expiratory phase of a cough. As in the Heimlich maneuver, the nurse places a fist or heel of the hand between the umbilicus and the xiphoid process and presses downward and upward when the patient coughs. The patient is instructed to take a deep, slow breath and repeat it three times; then, instead of exhaling, the patient coughs on the last breath as the nurse assists. Performing this intervention hourly effectively assists patients in clearing respiratory secretions. Standard nursing interventions of turning (with mechanical beds) and ensuring adequate hydration aid in mobilizing and liquefying respiratory secretions. Patients and family members need to be instructed in the need for frequent pulmonary hygiene, drinking fluids, and turning to mobilize secretions.

Aggressive chest physiotherapy is needed to mobilize and clear secretions to prevent atelectasis. Care must be taken when the patient is in the head-down position for chest physiotherapy because of the risk of severe bradycardia resulting from vagal stimulation. Close monitoring of vital signs during and following therapy is necessary. Patients who are able to do so should be encouraged to use incentive spirometry hourly.

If the patient has an endotracheal tube or tracheostomy, suctioning will clear secretions. Care is needed when suctioning because of the vasovagal response, resulting in severe bradycardia.

Impaired Physical Mobility

Mobility is altered due to total loss of motor function below the level of injury during spinal shock. Flaccid paralysis progresses to spastic paralysis following spinal shock. If the patient is not paralyzed, immobility may be necessary to prevent SCI.

Expected Outcome. Further injury to the spinal cord does not occur, and range of motion of all joints is maintained.

Continuing assessment of motor function is critical during the acute phase. In-depth muscle testing should be performed every 4 hours. All major muscle groups should be graded for strength on a 5-point scale, i.e., 0 equals no movement and 5 equals movement against full resistance. Decreased motor function may accompany swelling at the injury site, loss of vertebral alignment, or intrathecal hematoma formation. Consistent documentation is important to identify trends of dysfunction. Significant changes should be promptly reported to the physician.

Immobilization is usually maintained with tongs (see Fig. 35–6). As with other bony injuries, observing the principles of traction is essential, including providing the ordered amount of weight and ensuring that the weights hang free. Maintenance of spinal stability is facilitated with mechanical beds. Two commonly used beds are Stryker frames (Fig. 35–10), which turn from supine to prone, and kinetic therapy beds (Fig. 35–11), which constantly rotate in a 60- to 60-degree arc. Turning or rotation in these beds should not begin until bony alignment is documented by x-ray and the issue is discussed with the physician.

The halo-pelvic external fixator (see Fig. 35–9) may be used to maintain vertebral stability. This fixator is a static traction device that permits increased patient mobility. A metal halo ring is secured to the outer table of the skull. Metal struts attach the halo to a metal pelvic ring, which is secured to the bony pelvis with Steinmann pins. Depending on the stability of the fracture, the halo may eventually be attached to a body cast or sheepskin-lined plastic vest for cervical immobilization.

Passive range of motion exercises should be done every 4 hours to prevent contractures. Poor positioning contributes to contracture formation. Joints should be positioned in the neutral position whenever possible. Adjunctive devices, antirotation boots, antidrop foot splints, trochanter rolls, high-top tennis shoes, and wrist splints are useful in maintaining the correct position. Joints with partial or complete function should also be placed through range of motion. Instructing the patient and family in the need for

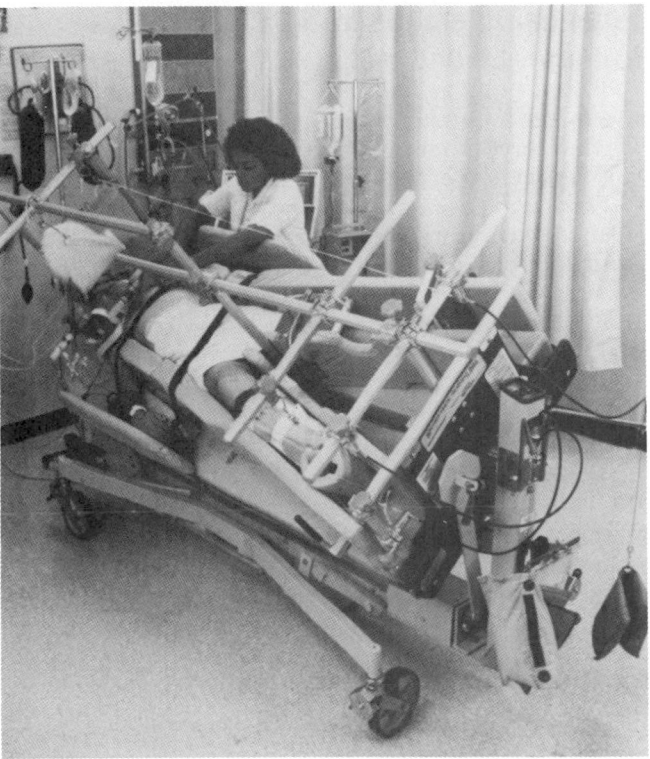

FIGURE 35—11. Kinetic therapy treatment table. (Reproduced by permission from Lewis, S. M., and Collier, I. C. (Eds.). *Medical surgical nursing: Assessment and management of clinical problems*, (p. 1607) New York (1987) McGraw-Hill Book Co.; copyrighted by The C. V. Mosby Co., St. Louis.)

range of motion exercises increases the potential for prevention of contractures of nonparalyzed areas.

Potential for Injury: Deep Vein Thrombosis Due to Venostasis

Expected Outcome. Lower extremity circumference will be monitored daily, and increases of more than 2 cm will be promptly reported; antithrombus regimen will be maintained.

Circumference of the lower extremities should be checked daily. Standard measurement sites are ensured by marking the positions on the legs with permanent markers. Measures should be made at midcalf and midthigh on each leg.

Promoting venous return is facilitated by range of motion exercises, which should be done every 4 hours. Antiembolism hose or alternating pneumatic pressure devices on the legs aid venous return. Elevating the entire lower extremity 10 to 15 degrees prevents venostasis. Kinetic treatment beds, which rotate the patient for up to 20 hours a day, also promote circulation in the patient with SCI (Green et al., 1983). Mobilization from bed to chair is still the best mechanism for decreasing the cardiovascular sequelae of immobility.

Potential Alteration in Skin Integrity Due to Paralysis and Immobility

Expected Outcome. Skin will remain dry, intact, and nonerythemic. Patient and family will verbalize understanding of the need for frequent repositioning.

Thorough assessment of the skin should be accomplished each time the patient is turned and positioned. A turning and positioning schedule should be established and posted at the bedside to ensure that all personnel maintain the same turning routine. Turning should be done every 2 hours unless it is contraindicated. Use of special mattresses and gel pads may add to the effectiveness of traditional nursing interventions but do not replace them.

Massage of bony prominences and application of moisturizing lotions should be done whenever the patient is turned. Preventing skin maceration from excessive moisture is essential. The patient and family should be instructed in the need for frequent repositioning and turning to prevent pressure necrosis.

Anxiety Due to Insecurity About Care and Long-Term Prognosis Following SCI

Expected Outcome. The patient does not demonstrate immobilizing anxiety and is able to verbalize concerns freely to caregivers.

Fear, uncertainty, and anxiety are the predominant emotions in the intensive care unit. The psychoemotional trauma of SCI can be overwhelming. Sudden paralysis does not permit any patient preparation. Fear revolves around the injury and life and death issues. Anxiety may stem from the intensive care environment, lack of familiarity with care providers, feelings of total dependence, helplessness, and an unknown future (Walleck, 1988). Anxiety is intensified by sensory deprivation and an inability to communicate if the patient is intubated.

It is important for all care providers to realize the patient's devastation. Dependence on the nursing staff for basic needs as well as for all therapies requires that a trusting relationship be established between the patient and the staff. Use of verbal communication, touch, eye contact, and patience are reassuring to the patient.

Encouraging self-care within the patient's abilities will decrease feelings of complete dependence. When possible, incorporating the patient and family in goal setting and decision making increases the patient's sense of autonomy.

The patient should be informed by the physician about the degree of injury, the diagnosis, and the prognosis as soon as possible after the injury. The family or significant others should be part of these discussions. This information will not ease the patient's fears but does allow him or her to begin to grasp the reality of the situation and thus begin to deal with fear (Green et al., 1985).

Patients who are able to talk should be encouraged to verbalize their fears. The nurse should be a receptive listener, making time for the patient to be able to verbalize concerns. The patient's self-worth should be reinforced by making time to spend talking with the patient. (See also Chap. 6.)

Ineffective Thermoregulation

Thermoregulation may be altered due to loss of hypothalamic control of the sympathetic nervous system in patients with SCI above the level T6.

Expected Outcome. Patients with poikilothermia will receive careful monitoring, and normothermia will be maintained.

Rectal temperature should be monitored every 4 hours during the first 72 hours following injury. Palpation of skin surfaces to note areas of warmth, coolness, and moisture augments temperature monitoring.

The nurse should be alert to environmental temperatures, adding blankets when it is cool and removing bed clothes when it is warm. Drafts should be eliminated when possible. Tepid baths should be used first in trying to reduce a fever. Care must be exercised with hypothermia blankets because these may result in a precipitous drop in the patient's temperature.

Constipation Due to Changes in Neural Function and Immobility Following SCI

Expected Outcomes. The patient will maintain his normal bowel habits or pass a formed stool every other day without straining.

The location and degree of SCI determines the degree of alteration in bowel elimination. Bowel sounds generally return within 2 days of injury, but elimination may not return. Patient with cervical or thoracic SCI lose the ability to feel the urge to defecate, but reflex defecation activity may remain intact in patients with nonsacral injuries. Sacral cord injuries may destroy the defecation reflex and anal sphincter tone, resulting in fecal retention and oozing of stool through a flaccid anal sphincter.

A bowel regimen is begun when peristalsis returns. The patient is given a pysllium hydrophilic mucilloid and stool softener daily. Every other day at the same time of day, the patient is given a cup of warm fluid to drink to stimulate the gastrocolic or duodenocolic reflex. If this is unsuccessful, a glycerine suppository is inserted, and digital stimulation of the internal anal sphincter provided. If this is unsuccessful, a laxative or bisacodyl suppository may be required. Use of the bowel regimen makes it possible to establish bowel continence. Avoid the use of enemas, which will dilate the rectum and sigmoid colon. Digital disimpaction may occasionally be necessary. Caution should be exercised when the anus is stimulated because it may create autonomic dysreflexia.

Potential for Injury

Autonomic dysreflexia may occur due to an uninhibited response of the sympathetic nervous system resulting from lack of higher level control in paraplegic and quadriplegic patients with upper level injury (above T6) (Fig. 35–12).

Expected Outcome. Assessments of autonomic dysreflexia are rapidly identified and treated before complications occur.

Autonomic dysreflexia may result from a variety of stimuli including an overdistended bladder, infection, skin stimulation, pressure necrosis, pain, sudden changes in environmental temperature, and, most commonly, a full rectum (Mason, 1981). Assessments of autonomic dysreflexia include a sudden onset of severe headache, hypertension, bradycardia, tachycardia, diaphoresis, and flushing above the level of injury, pallor and coolness below the level of injury, nasal stuffiness, and unusual apprehension. Hypertension may be so severe that it results in cerebral hemorrhage or myocardial infarction (Hickey, 1986). This is most likely to occur in the first year following injury, but it can occur anytime after spinal shock subsides. Patients and families need to be taught that this problem can occur, how to identify it, and the need for rapid intervention.

Once identified, these patients should have the head elevated to a sitting position and the blood pressure and pulse closely monitored. The physician should be promptly notified. If possible, the source should be identified and removed—i.e., check for a distended bladder and perform intermittent catheterization; check the indwelling catheter for kinks or plugs. Ganglionic blocking agents may be required to disrupt the hyper-reflexic state. Hydralazine hydrochloride, 20 mg, may be ordered and should be given slowly to avoid abrupt hypotension. Diazoxide may also be used. If this situation occurs during a bowel movement a local anesthetic should be applied to the anal canal to reduce further stimuli (Zejdlik, 1983).

Alterations in Urinary Elimination

Urinary elimination may be altered by the disruption of normal neurologic bladder innervation by the SCI. Areflexia resulting from spinal cord shock causes urinary retention. Sacral reflexes normally causing bladder contraction and detrusor muscle opening are lost (McCagg, 1986).

Expected Outcome. Urinary output will be maintained at 30 mL/hour when an indwelling catheter is in place; there are no findings of urinary tract infection on assessment.

When the patient with SCI is on vasopressor therapy an indwelling catheter is used. This catheter is removed as soon as possible because it contributes to bladder atonicity, making later reflex emptying more difficult.

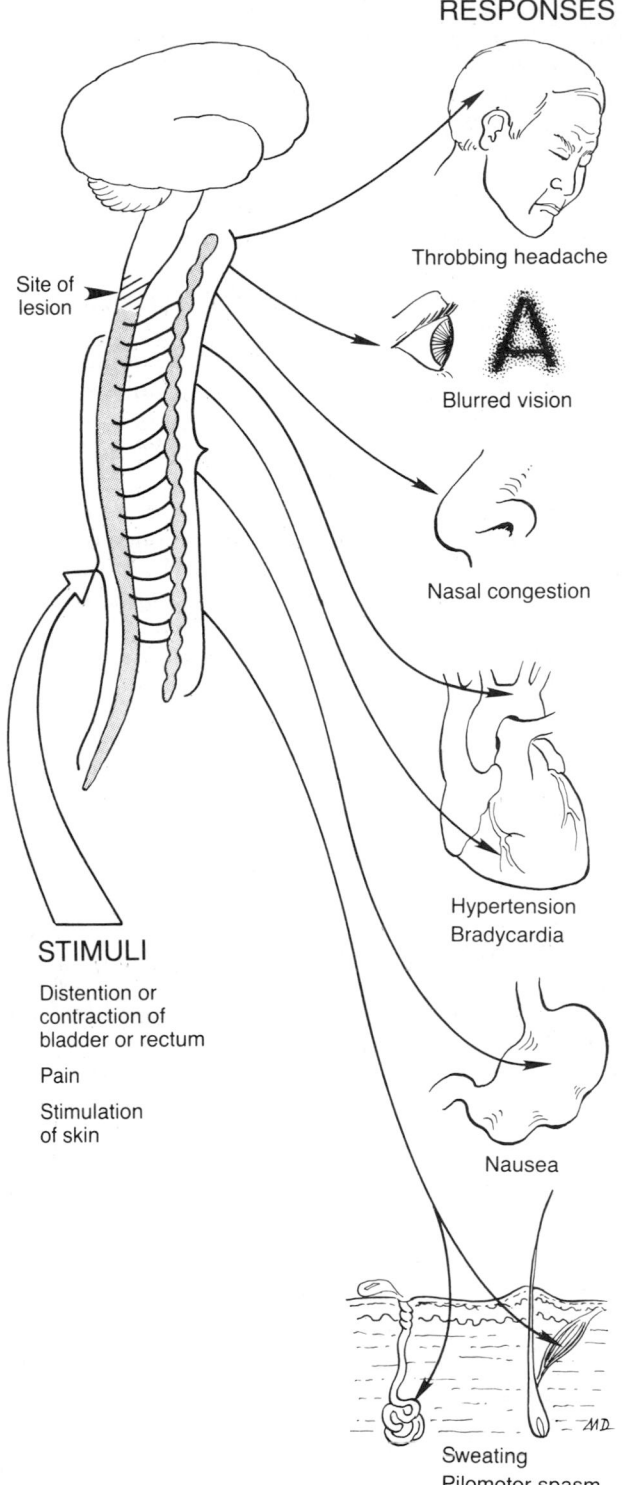

RESPONSES

Throbbing headache

Blurred vision

Nasal congestion

Hypertension
Bradycardia

Nausea

Sweating
Pilomotor spasm

Site of lesion

STIMULI

Distention or contraction of bladder or rectum

Pain

Stimulation of skin

FIGURE 35–12. Causes of hyperreflexia and assessment findings. (From Luckmann, J., and Sorensen, K. C. (1987). *Medical-surgical nursing: A psychophysiologic approach* (3rd ed. p. 434). Philadelphia: W. B. Saunders.)

Intermittent catheterization should be started as quickly as possible. Criteria for such a program include negative urine culture; patient tolerance of fluid restriction to 1800 to 2200 mL/24 hours; no use of diuretics. The goal of the program is to stimulate reflex emptying of the full bladder. The need for catheterizations is based on the amount of urine obtained from each catheterization, usually done every 4 hours. Frequency of catheterizations decreases as the bladder gains automaticity. After resolution of spinal cord shock, the patient may void spontaneously between catheterizations.

Self-Care Deficit: Partial Due to Partial Loss of Motor Function

Expected Outcome. Patients will participate maximally in self-care, the degree of participation being based on his or her physiologic capabilities. The patient will demonstrate feelings of self-worth and exercise some degree of control over his care.

Patients with SCI experience a temporary but total loss of physical ability to perform some activities of daily living. The patient is initially dependent on others for most self-care. This dependence decreases self-worth, interferes with role performance, and increases feelings of helplessness, powerlessness, and humiliation (Walleck, 1988). Giving the patient as much control as possible over his life is essential. Include the patient in planning of care and goal setting; provide instruction that will allow the patient to make knowledgeable decisions. Contracting with the patient and establishing behavior modification programs may be useful in setting limits for some patients (see also Chap. 6).

These patients are often depressed because of their forced dependency. Be honest and consistent about describing the patient's condition, and share realistic goals for the patient's future. Individualize the patient's care to meet the patient's needs. Beginning to teach patients to manage their disability in the ICU aids adaptation.

Sexual Dysfunction Due to Disruption of Normal Sexuality

Expected Outcome. Patient verbalizes understanding of potential for sexual functioning and demonstrates satisfactory adjustment.

Although sexuality may not be a high-priority issue in the care of ICU patients, it may be of great concern to the patient. Sexuality is a complex physical and emotional response. During the critical care phase, the nurse should be aware that the patient may be worried about sexual function. Sexual counseling is usually delayed until the intermediate phase of care. Create a climate of openness; answer any questions honestly. The degree of sexual function varies with the level of injury and the sex of the patient. Although the capability for orgasm is frequently lost, the ability to bear children remains for most women. For men, orgasm is lost and the ability to reproduce is severely limited, but the capability to engage in sexual intercourse may remain. Reassure the patient that sexual counseling will be available later.

ncp nursing care plan

1. Altered tissue perfusion related to:
Inflammatory responses following injury
Sympathetic blockade
Changes in intrathecal oxygen tension

Outcome Criteria	Nursing Interventions
Patient's blood pressure and Pa_{O_2} will remain at baseline. Patient will maintain high cardiac output (1 to 1.5 times normal) Urinary output will exceed 30 mL/hour	Monitor hemodynamic parameters. Titrate vasopressors to maintain optimal hemodynamic responses. Monitor fluid and electrolyte balance with careful monitoring of intake and output. Replace fluids judiciously to maintain adequate blood volume without pulmonary edema. Monitor mental status closely. Provide supplemental oxygen therapy during the first 24 hours and as needed thereafter. Monitor vital signs every 4 hours. Maintain normothermia.

2. Ineffective breathing pattern:
Injuries resulting in possible loss of innervation of the diaphragm and intercostals
Gastric dilation
Paralytic ileus
Fatigue

Outcome Criteria	Nursing Interventions
Adequate ventilation as evidenced by normal arterial blood gas analysis. Absence of respiratory distress and fever. Lung sounds clear on auscultation.	Physical assessment of the chest with each vital sign check during the first 72 hours. Note and report changes from baseline in the depth or pattern of ventilation. Measure serial vital capacities to determine the need for intubation and mechanical ventilation. Monitor arterial blood gas analyses and provide supplemental oxygen as needed to keep the Pa_{O_2} 80 mm Hg. Daily chest radiograph. Assess abdomen for distention and apply abdominal binder as needed.

3. Ineffective airway clearance related to:
    Flaccid paralysis of abdominal and intercostal muscles

Outcome Criteria	Nursing Interventions
Patient will participate in assisted cough. Patient will remain afebrile. Pa_{CO_2} will remain at baseline Sputum will remain clear and minimal in amount.	"Quad-assist" coughs hourly and as needed. Frequent turning and adequate hydration to mobilize secretions. Aggressive chest physiotherapy while closely monitoring vital signs. Incentive spirometry hourly, if spontaneously breathing. If present, suction artificial airways (endotracheal tube or tracheostomy tube) as needed.

4. Impaired Physical Mobility
    Loss of motor function below the level of injury

Outcome Criteria	Nursing Interventions
No further injury to the spinal cord. Range of motion of all joints is maintained.	Perform in-depth muscle testing every 4 hours. Consistently document motor function assessment and report significant changes to the physician. Ensure proper functioning of immobilization devices. Provide passive range of motion exercises every 4 hours and explain their importance to family members. Position joints in neutral position when possible to prevent contractures.

5. Potential for injury: deep vein thrombosis
    Venostasis

Outcome Criteria	Nursing Interventions
No increase in lower extremity circumference >2 cm. No complications of thromboembolism (e.g., pulmonary embolism).	Measure lower extremity circumference daily. Perform range of motion excercises every 4 hours. Apply antiembolism hose or alternating pneumatic pressure devices on legs. Elevate lower extremities 10 to 15 degrees. Mobilize patient from bed to chair when possible.

6. Potential altered skin integrity related to:
    Paralysis
    Immobility

Outcome Criteria	Nursing Interventions
Skin remains dry, intact, and nonerythemic. Patient and family will verbalize understanding of the need for frequent repositioning.	Thoroughly assess skin with each turning or repositioning. Establish and post a turning/positioning schedule. Turn every 2 hours unless contraindicated. Massage bony prominences and apply lotion with each turn. Avoid excessive moisture to prevent skin maceration.

7. Anxiety
    Uncertainty about care and long-term prognosis

Outcome Criteria	Nursing Interventions
Patient does not demonstrate immobilizing anxiety. Patient verbalizes concerns freely to caregivers.	Establish a trust relationship with patient using verbal communication, touch, eye contact, and patience. Encourage self-care within the patient's ability. Incorporate patient and family members in setting goals and making decisions when possible. Ensure that the physician informs the patients and significant others of the degree of injury, the diagnosis, and the prognosis as soon as possible after the injury. Encourage patient to verbalize fears and concerns. Take time to spend talking and actively listening to the patient.

8. Ineffective thermoregulation
    Loss of hypothalamic control of the sympathetic nervous system in patients with injuries above T6

Outcome Criteria	Nursing Interventions
Patients with poikilothermy will receive careful monitoring. Normothermia is maintained.	Monitor rectal temperature every 4 hours during the first 72 hours after injury. Palpate skin surfaces to note areas of warmth, coolness, and moisture. Monitor environmental temperatures, adding blankets when cool and removing bedding when warm. Eliminate drafts. Use tepid baths first when trying to reduce a fever. Use hypothermia units carefully to avoid precipitous drops in patient's temperature.

Nursing Care Plan continued on following page

9. Constipation related to:
    Changes in neural function
    Immobility

Outcome Criteria	Nursing Interventions
Patient will pass a formed stool every other day without straining.	Begin a bowel regimen when peristalsis returns. Administer psyllium hydrophilic mucilloid and stool softener daily. Administer a cup of warm fluid every other day at the same time of day to stimulate the gastrocolic or duodenocolic reflex. If necessary, administer a glycerin suppository and provide digital stimulation of the internal anal sphincter. If necessary, administer a laxative or bisacodyl suppository.

10. Potential for injury
    Dysreflexia

Outcome Criteria	Nursing Interventions
Symptoms of autonomic dysreflexia are rapidly identified and treated before any complications occur.	Monitor patient for sudden onset of severe headache, hypertension, bradycardia, tachycardia, diaphoresis and flushing above the level of injury, pallor and coolness below the level of injury, nasal stuffiness, and unusual apprehension. Once identified, elevate the head of the bed to the sitting position and monitor blood pressure closely. Notify the physician. Identify and remove the stimulus, if possible. Consider administering ganglionic blocking agents to disrupt the hyper-reflexic state. Administer antihypertensive medications (hydralazine hydrochloride, 20 mg; or diazoxide) slowly to avoid abrupt hypotension. If autonomic dysreflexia occurs during a bowel movement, administer a local anesthetic to the anal area. Teach patient and family members about autonomic dysreflexia, how to identify it, and the need for rapid intervention.

11. Altered urinary elimination related to:
    Disruption of nervous system innervation of the bladder

Outcome Criteria	Nursing Interventions
Urinary output will be at least 30 mL/hour while indwelling catheter is in place. No urinary tract infection.	Remove indwelling catheter as soon as possible. Begin intermittent catheterization every 4 hours. Decrease frequency of catheterization as the bladder gains automaticity.

12. Partial self-care deficit
    Partial loss of motor function

Outcome Criteria	Nursing Interventions
Patient will participate in self-care to the maximum of his or her physiologic capability. Patient will demonstrate feelings of self-worth and exercise some degree of control over his/her care.	Give patient as much control as possible over his/her life. Include the patient in care planning and goal setting. Teach the patient what is necessary to make knowledgeable decisions. Consider contracting or establishing behavior modification programs in setting limits. Be honest and consistent about describing the patient's condition. Share realistic goals for the patient's future. Individualize care to meet the patient's needs.

13. Sexual dysfunction related to:
    Disruption of normal sexuality

Outcome Criteria	Nursing Interventions
Patient verbalizes understanding of the potential for sexual functioning. Patient demonstrates satisfactory adjustment.	Be aware that the patient may be worried about sexual function. Create a climate of openness. Answer questions honestly. Reassure the patient that sexual counselling will be available later.

SUMMARY

Care of the patient with SCI has changed dramatically during the past decade. ICU care is complex, and these patients demand aggressive medical and nursing management. These patients represent a unique challenge to the critical care nurse. Every body system is affected by the injury and must be addressed in planning care. Continued research is aimed at reversing the pathophysiology seen at injury in the hope of improving the quality of life for these patients. The care provided by the critical care nurse will allow survivors of SCI to achieve maximal return to functional well-being.

References

Albin, M. S., and White, R. J. (1987). Epidemiology, physiopathology, and experimental therapeutics of acute spinal cord injury. *Critical Care Clinics*, 3, 441–452.

Becker, D. M., Gonzalez, M., and Gentilli, A. (1987). Prevention of deep vein thrombosis in patients with acute spinal cord injuries: Use of rotating treatment tables. *Neurosurgery*, 20, 675–677.

Braakman, R., and Penning L. (1976). Injuries of the cervical spine. In P. J. Venken and E. W. Bruyn (Eds.), *Injuries of the cervical spine and spinal cord: Part I*. New York: American Elsevier.

Brackman, M. B., Shepard, M. J., Collins, W. F., et al. (1990). A randomized controlled trial of methylprednisolone or naloxone in the treatment of acute spinal cord injury. *New England Journal of Medicine*, 322(20), 1405–1411.

Carol, M. P., and Ducker, T. B. (1987). Spinal cord injury and spinal shock syndrome. In J. H. Siegel (Ed.), *Trauma emergency surgery and critical care* (pp. 947–981). New York: Churchill Livingstone.

Carol, M. P., Ducker, T. B., and Brynes, D. P. (1980). Minimyelogram in cervical spinal cord trauma. *Neurosurgery*, 1 (2), 218–222.

Carter, E. R. (1979). Medical management of pulmonary complications of spinal cord injury. *Advances in Neurology*, 22, 267–268.

Chilton, J., and Dagi, T. F. (1985). Acute cervical spinal cord injury. *American Journal of Emergency Medicine* 3 (4), 340–351.

DeJesus-Greenberg, D. A. (1980). Acute spinal cord injury—hyperbaric oxygen therapy: A new adjunct in management. *Journal of Neurosurgical Nursing* 12 (3), 155–160.

Ducker, T B., and Kindt, G. W. (1971). The effect of trauma on the vasomotor control of spinal cord blood flow. *Current Topics in Surgical Research*, 3 (1), 163–181.

Dunham, C. M., and Cowley, R. A. (1986). *Shock trauma/critical care handbook*. Rockville, MD: Aspen.

Faden, A. I., Hallenbeck, J. M., and Brown, C. Q. (1982a). Treatment of experimental stroke. Comparison of naloxone and thyrotropin releasing hormone. *Neurology* 43, 1083–1087.

Faden, A. I., Jacobs, T. P., and Holaday, J. W. (1980). A possible pathophysiologic role for endorphins in spinal injury (abstract). *Federal Proceedings*, 39, 760–766.

Faden, A. I., Jacobs , T. P., and Holaday, J. W. (1981). Opiate antagonist improves neurologic recovery after spinal injury. *Science*, 211, 493–494.

Faden, A. I., Jacobs, T. P., and Holaday, J. W. (1982b). Comparison of early and late naloxone treatment in experimental spinal injury. *Neurology* 32, 677–681.

Faden, A. I., Jacobs, T. F., and Smith, M. T. (1984). Thyrotropin releasing hormone in experimental spinal injury: Dose response and late treatment. *Neurology*, 34, 1280–1284.

Flamm, E. S., Young, W., and Collins, W. F. (1985). Phase I trial of naloxone treatment in acute spinal cord injury. *Journal of Neurosurgery*, 63 (4), 390–397.

Gamache, F. W., Myers, R. A. M., Ducker, T. B., and Cowley, R. A. (1981). The clinical application of hyperbaric oxygen therapy in spinal cord injury. A preliminary report. *Surgical Neurology*, 15 (1), 85–87.

Geisler, F. H. (1988). Acute management of cervical spinal cord injury. *Trauma Quarterly*, 4 (3), 1–22.

Geisler, F. H., and Salcman, M. (1987). Respiratory system: Physiology, pathophysiology and management. In F. P. Wirth and P. A. Ratcheson (Eds.), *Neurological critical care* (pp. 1–50). Baltimore: Williams & Wilkins.

Gilbert, J. (1987). Critical care management of the patient with acute spinal cord injury. *Critical Care Clinics*, 549–567.

Green, B. A., Eismont, F. J, and O'Heir, J. T. (1987). Spinal cord injury—a systems approach: Prevention, emergency medical services, and emergency room management. *Critical Care Clinics*, 471–493.

Green, B. A., Green, K. L., and Klose, K. J. (1983). Kinetic therapy for spinal cord injury. *Spine*, 8 (7), 722–728.

Green, B. A., Klose, K. J., and Goldberg, M. I. (1985). Clinical and research considerations in spinal cord injury. In D. P. Becker and J. Povlishock (Eds.), *Central nervous system trauma status report 1985* (pp. 341–368). Bethesda, MD: National Institute of Neurologic and Communicative Disorders and Stroke/National Institute of Health.

Green, D., Rossi, E. C., and Yao, J. S. T. (1982). Deep vein thrombosis in spinal cord injury: Effect of prophylaxis with calf compression, aspirin, and dipyridamole. *Paraplegia*, 20, 227–234.

Grundy, B. L., and Friedman, W. (1987). Electrophysiological evaluation of the patient with acute spinal cord injury. *Critical Care Clinics*, 3, 519–548.

Guttman, L. (1976). *Spinal cord injuries: Comprehensive management and research*. Oxford, England: Blackwell.

Hansebout, R. R., Tanner, J. A., and Romero-Sierra, C. (1984). Current status of spinal cord cooling in the treatment of acute spinal cord injury. *Spine*, 9, 508–511.

Hickey, J. V. (1986). *The clinical practice of neurological and neurosurgical nursing* (2nd ed.). Philadelphia: J. B. Lippincott.

Hull, R., Hirsh, J., and Jay, R. (1982). Different intensities of oral anticoagulant therapy in the treatment of proximal vein thrombosis. *New England Journal of Medicine*, 307, 1076–1081.

Krause, J. F. (1985). Epidemiological aspects of acute spinal cord injury: A review of incidence, prevalence, causes and outcomes. In D. P. Becker and J. Povlishock (Eds.), *Central nervous system trauma status report 1985* (pp. 314–332). Bethesda, MD: National Institute of Neurologic and Communicative Disorders and Stroke/National Institute of Health.

Leader, W. (1976). *Statistical reports for traumatic spinal cord injury (1975–1976)*. Tallahassee: Florida Central Registry for Severely Disabled.

McCagg, C. (1986). Postoperative management and acute rehabilitation of patients with spinal cord injuries. *Orthopedic Clinics of North America*, 17, 171–182.

Mason, R. (1981). Autonomic dysreflexia: A nursing challenge. *Rehabilitation Nursing*, 6(1), 11–15.

Nikas, D. L. (1982). Acute spinal cord injuries: Care and complications. In D. L. Nikas (Ed.), *The critically ill neurosurgical patient* (pp. 107–124). New York: Churchill Livingstone.

Nikas, D. L. (1988). Pathophysiology and nursing interventions in acute spinal cord injury. *Trauma Quarterly*, 4 (3), 23–44

Richmond, T. (1985). The patient with a cervical cord injury. *Focus on Critical Care*, 12 (2), 23–33.

Riggins, R., and Kraus, J. (1983). The risk of neurological damage with fractures of the vertebrae. *Trauma*, 23 (5), 459–465.

Senter, H. J., and Venes, J. L. (1979). Loss of autoregulation and posttraumatic ischemia following experimental spinal cord trauma. *Journal of Neurosurgery*, 50 (2), 198–206.

Tyson, G. W. (1979). Acute care of the spinal cord injured patient. *Critical Care Quarterly*, 2, 45–60.

Walleck, C. A. (1987). Nursing role in management of peripheral nerve and spinal cord problems. In S. M. Lewis and I. C. Collier (Eds.), *Medical surgical nursing: Assessment and management of clinical problems* (pp. 1591–1621). New York: McGraw-Hill.

Walleck, C. A. (1988). Central nervous system II. Spinal cord injury. In V. D. Cardona, P. D. Hurn, P. J. Mason, et al. (Eds.). *Trauma nursing: From resuscitation through rehabilitation*, (pp. 419–448). Philadelphia: W. B. Saunders.

Yashon, D. (1986). *Spinal injury* (2nd ed.). Norwalk, CT: Appleton-Century-Crofts.

Young, J. S., and Northrup, N. E. (1981). *Statistical information pertaining to some of the most commonly asked questions about spinal cord injury*. Phoenix: National Spinal Cord Injury Data Center.

Young, J. S., Burns, P. E., Bowen, A. M., and McCutchen, R. (1982). *Spinal cord injury statistics*. Phoenix: Good Samaritan Medical Center.

Young, W., Flamm E. S., and Demopoulos, H. B. (1981). Naloxone ameliorates posttraumatic ischemia in experimental spinal contusion. *Journal of Neurosurgery*, 55 (2), 209–219.

Zejdlik, C. P. (1983). *Management of spinal cord injury*. Monterey, CA: Wadsworth Health Sciences Division.

36

Patients with Guillain-Barré Syndrome

Kathryn Sabo Thompson

The disorder known as Guillain-Barré syndrome (GBS) is a rare peripheral nervous system disease that may become a frustrating nightmare for the patient's family, and the nurses caring for the patient. GBS is characterized by an acute, ascending, symmetrical weakness that can progress to total paralysis of the extremities, trunk, respiratory musculature, and face. The incidence ranges from 0.6 to 1.9/100,000 population per year (Schonberger et al., 1981). The syndrome occurs in all seasons throughout the world; it affects both sexes and all age groups. GBS gained notoriety during the 1976 Swine flu immunization program when an increased incidence was noted and linked to an immune response to the vaccine (Retailiau et al., 1980). This syndrome was first described in 1859 by Jean Landry and again in 1916 by George Guillain, Jean Barré, and Andry Strohl (Guillain et al., 1916; Landry, 1859).

ETIOLOGY

The cause of GBS is unknown, but it has been classified as an acute demyelinating, inflammatory polyradiculopathy. The myelin sheath that surrounds the axon of the neuron is segmentally destroyed, making nerve impulse conduction impossible. Focal segmental demyelination is associated with infiltration of the endoneurial and perivascular areas by lymphocytes and monocytes (Pleasure and Schotland, 1984). Lesions may appear on cranial nerves, spinal nerve roots, and peripheral nerves. At first the myelin sheath breaks down and the axon remains intact (Figs. 36–1 and 36–2). As lymphocytes and monocytes invade the neuron, the axon may become damaged, resulting in muscle denervation and atrophy. Regeneration and recovery of the axon and myelin sheath depend on the amount of destruction incurred. Complete clinical recovery may take years, and permanent neurologic damage may result when there is extensive demyelination and axonal destruction.

Triggering Events

Although the etiology of GBS is unknown, a variety of preceding or triggering events are associated with its pathophysiology. Triggering events usually occur within 30 days of the onset of symptoms, and the pathophysiology is suspected to involve a delayed hypersensitivity reaction to the trigger. Some evidence suggests that GBS is caused by an immunologically mediated peripheral nerve injury (Korn-Lubetzki and Abramsky, 1986). It has also been suggested that immunosuppressive states, i.e., pregnancy or immunosuppressive therapy for malignant neoplasms or following organ transplantation, can trigger GBS (Cameron et al., 1958; Klingon, 1965). Viral infections, especially cytomegalovirus and the swine influenza virus, have also been associated with GBS (Kaplan et al., 1983; Schonberger et al., 1979).

It is suspected that both cellular and humoral components of the immune system are involved in the pathophysiology of GBS because there is frequently a preceding acute respiratory or gastrointestinal illness. The illness is thought to activate the cell-mediated immune system by sensitizing T lymphocytes to the person's own myelin sheath, initiating its destruction. Research has also suggested that B lymphocytes may respond to some antigens (the trigger) by producing a demyelinating antibody that activates myelin destruction (see also Chap. 54).

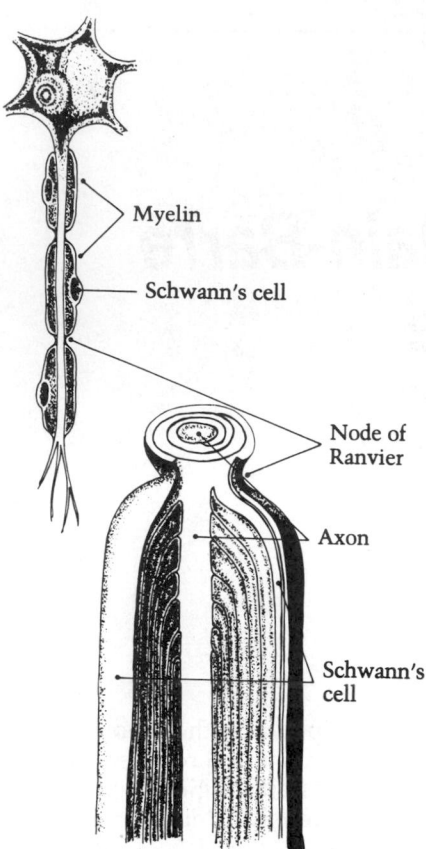

FIGURE 36-1. Microscopic enlargement of the anatomic components of the normal peripheral nerve. (From *Critical Care Nursing: Body-mind-spirit* by Cornelia Vanderstaay Kenner, Cathie E. Guzzetta, and Barbara Montgomery Dorsey. Copyright © 1985 by Cornelia Vanderstaay Kenner, Cathie E. Guzzetta, and Barbara Montgomery Dorsey. Reprinted by permission of Scott, Foresman and Company.)

Course of the Disease

Once the destruction of the myelin sheath has begun, the patient begins to experience muscle weakness, which may progress to flaccid paralysis. The disease course is variable but can be divided into three distinct phases: progression, plateau, and recovery. During the *progression phase*, muscle weakness and paralysis increase in severity; this phase may last from a few hours to 4 weeks. *Plateau phase* occurs when the patient does not develop further weakness or paralysis. The *recovery phase* usually begins 2 to 4 weeks after the plateau and is characterized by a slow return of muscular strength. Prognosis for complete recovery is generally excellent (Loffel et al., 1977). The rate and degree of an individual's recovery cannot be predicted. The slow recovery, which may be as long as 6 months to 2 years, can be very frustrating for the patient, family, and caregivers. There have been rare patients with residual disabilities, ranging from paresthesia to sensory ataxia, and resulting in major changes in activity level and life style (Sobue et al., 1983).

CLINICAL PRESENTATION

Although variable, the onset of symptoms is usually sudden, involving pain, muscle weakness, and autonomic dysfunction.

Pain

Pain is a major finding on assessment and varies from mild to extremely severe. Painful sensations can be categorized into paresthesias, muscular aches and cramps, and hyperesthesias. Paresthesias can include numb, prickly, tingling, and burning sensations, especially in the stocking and glove dermatomes. Perception of joint position (proprioception) and vibratory and temperature sensations may diminish. Hyperesthesia may cause the light touch of a hand or bed sheet to be perceived as severe pain.

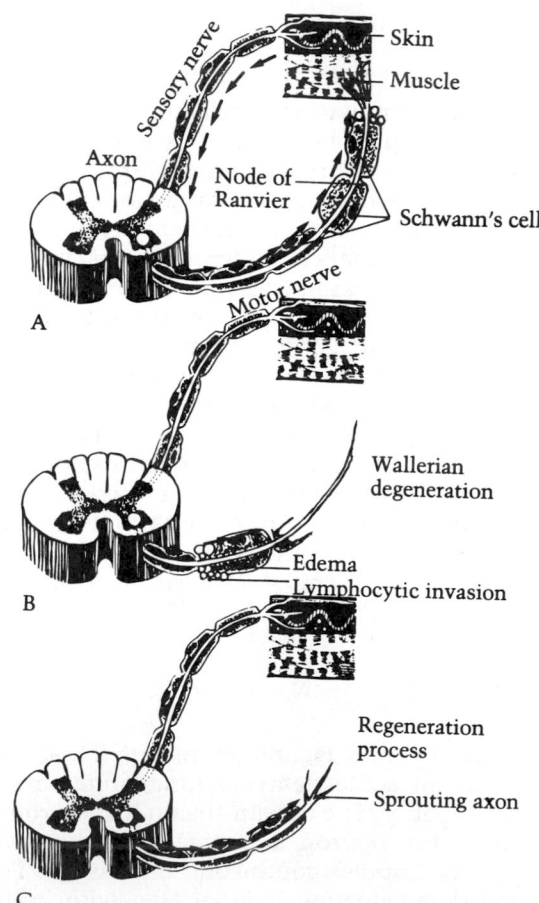

FIGURE 36-2. Cross section of the spinal cord illustrating the pathologic changes with Guillain-Barré syndrome. *A,* Anatomy of a motor and sensory peripheral nerve; the innervation of a muscle fiber with the sensory receptors is displayed. *B,* Response of a neuron to injury, with wallerian degeneration. *C,* Regeneration with the sprouting axon. (From *Critical Care Nursing: Body-mind-spirit* by Cornelia Vanderstaay Kenner, Cathie E. Guzzetta, and Barbara Montgomery Dorsey. Copyright © 1985 by Cornelia Vanderstaay Kenner, Cathie E. Guzzetta, and Barbara Montgomery Dorsey. Reprinted by permission of Scott, Foresman and Company.)

Ropper and Shahani (1984) reported that the patient's pain is usually worse at night and occurs most frequently in the buttocks, quadriceps, and hamstrings and less frequently in the calves, shins, shoulders, and lower back. It is unclear what causes the pain associated with GBS.

Muscular Weakness

Progressive muscular weakness usually develops rapidly. Muscle weakness begins distally and progresses in an ascending manner with relatively symmetrical muscle involvement. Severity of muscle involvement varies from weakness of the legs to total paralysis of all extremities, the trunk, face, and areas innervated by the bulbar (cranial) nerves. Bulbar nerve involvement can result in weakness or paralysis of the respiratory musculature, necessitating admission to the intensive care unit and ventilatory support.

Cranial nerve involvement can result in facial muscle weakness, dysphagia, and inability to talk or blink. The patient may be paralyzed but remains fully conscious and able to hear. Once the disease process begins to subside, pain and muscle weakness decrease, descending from head to toes.

Autonomic Dysfunction

Autonomic dysfunction is critically important in caring for the GBS patient. GBS may impair autonomic function due to lesions on the afferent limb of the baroreflex arc, interrupting homeostatic reflexes. Lesions may also involve the postganglionic sympathetic fibers of the spinal nerves. Autonomic disturbances are commonly seen in GBS patients with severe muscle involvement and respiratory muscle paralysis (Greenland and Griggs, 1980; Lichenfeld, 1971). The most dangerous autonomic dysfunctions include orthostatic hypotension, hypertension, abnormal vagal responses (bradycardia, heart block, asystole), and the syndrome of inappropriate antidiuretic hormone. Other autonomic dysfunctions include bowel and bladder dysfunction, facial flushing, and diaphoresis. The severity of autonomic disturbances varies and is a major cause of mortality (Traux, 1982); there is a 5% mortality rate associated with all of the complications of GBS. The literature describing the duration of autonomic dysfunction is inadequate, making it difficult to determine the length of time necessary for these patients to remain monitored in an intensive care unit.

Clinical Variants

GBS has several regional and functional variations reflecting the area of peripheral nerve demyelination (Ropper, 1986).

Ascending GBS. GBS most commonly presents with muscular weakness and pain in the legs, which progresses upward to the trunk, arms, or cranial nerves. In severe cases the patient presents with flaccid quadriplegia involving both spinal and cranial nerves. Deep tendon reflexes are diminished or absent. Life-threatening events associated with ascending GBS include respiratory muscle paralysis and autonomic dysfunction.

Pure Motor GBS. This variant is similar to ascending GBS except that the patient retains normal sensory function. Quadriparesis may occur but without muscular pain.

Descending GBS. A less common variation of GBS involves weakness beginning with the cranial nerves and progressing downward to the respiratory muscles, trunk, and extremities. Hyporeflexia or areflexia is absent. This type of disease may involve the facial, glossopharyngeal, and vagus nerves as manifested by facial paralysis, ophthalmoplegia, dysphagia, and cardiac dysrhythmias.

Miller-Fisher Syndrome (Fisher Variant). This variation of GBS is extremely rare and may also be called encephalomyeloradiculopathy. Prominent features include ophthalmoplegia, ataxia, and areflexia. This form is distinguished from descending GBS by the weakness of eye movement, limb and gait ataxia, minimum or no muscular weakness, and normal sensory function.

Chronic Idiopathic Polyneuritis (Chronic or Relapsing GBS). This rare process shares features with GBS. Chronic idiopathic polyneuritis is similar in the presentation of peripheral nerve demyelination, areflexia, muscular weakness, and pain. Unlike GBS, weakness in patients with chronic idiopathic polyneuritis develops slowly over 6 to 12 months, and muscular strength may take 2 years or longer to return. In some cases, there are cyclical episodes of progressive weakness and return of muscle strength. Evidence suggests that cell-mediated immunity plays a significant role in the pathogenesis of chronic idiopathic polyneuritis, thus linking it to GBS (Korn-Lubetzki and Abramsky, 1986).

Diagnostic Considerations

Diagnostic criteria for GBS were established in 1978 by the National Institute of Neurological and Communicative Disorders and Stroke (1978). Criteria include clinical assessments and laboratory and electrodiagnostic data. Illnesses such as spinal cord compression, acute intermittent porphyria, poliomyelitis, botulism, and diphtheria must be ruled out before GBS can be definitively diagnosed. Serial lumbar punctures are performed to identify elevations in cerebrospinal fluid (CSF) protein, which occur during the first week of symptoms. There is usually no increase in mononuclear leukocytes within the CSF. In most cases, electromyographic studies are abnormal, ruling out muscle disease as a cause of the patient's symptoms (Table 36–1).

MEDICAL MANAGEMENT

Initial medical management for GBS includes diagnosis, symptom management, and interventions to prevent major complications (such as infection and deep vein thrombosis). Therapeutic plasmapheresis (TP) has been used within 2 weeks of the onset of symptoms and has been associated with decreased length of stay and reduced need for mechanical ventilation (Consensus Conference, 1986). TP removes antibodies and other immunologically active substances that have been implicated in GBS (Fig. 36–3).

TABLE 36–1. Diagnostic Requirements for Guillain-Barré Syndrome

Required for Diagnosis
Progressive motor weakness of more than one limb
Definite hyporeflexia or areflexia

Strongly Supports Diagnosis
Cerebrospinal fluid protein elevated after 1 week of symptoms
Progression of motor weakness develops rapidly over days to 4 weeks
Motor weakness plateaus within 2 to 4 weeks
Relative symmetry of motor weakness
Mild sensory symptoms
Cranial nerve involvement
Recovery begins 2 to 4 weeks after plateau is reached
Autonomic dysfunction
Absence of fever
Abnormal electrodiagnostics (usually)

Possible Variants
Fever at onset
Severe sensory loss with pain
Progression beyond 4 weeks
Major permanent residual deficits
Transient bladder paralysis
Central nervous system involvement

Required to Rule Out Diagnosis
No evidence of:
  Porphyria
  Lead intoxication
  Polio
  Botulism
  No history of hexacarbon abuse
  Symptoms not purely sensory
  Organophosphates
  Tick paralysis
  Diphtheria infection
  Toxic neuropathy

Adapted from National Institute of Neurologic and Communicative Disorders and Stroke. (1978). Criteria for diagnosis of Guillain-Barré syndrome. *Annals of Neurology,* 3 (6), 565–566.

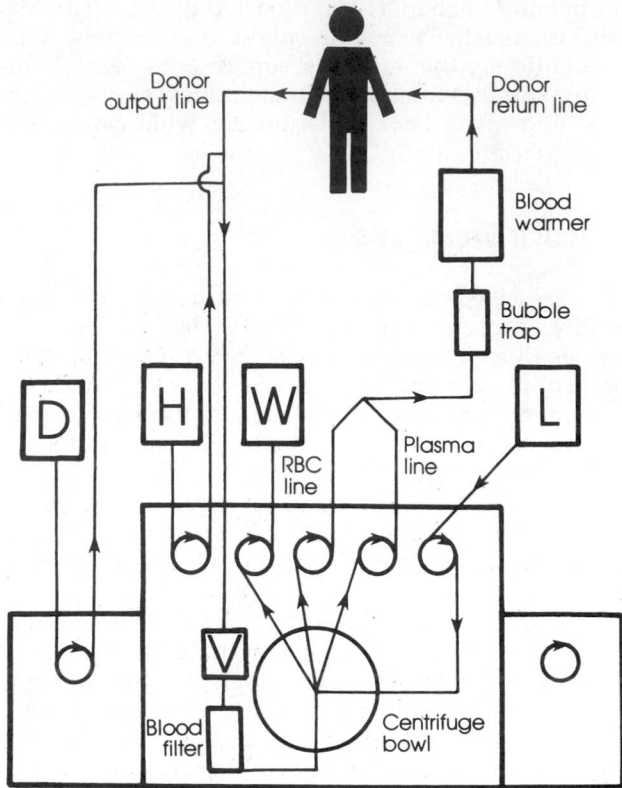

O	Peristaltic pumps
D	Red cell sedimenting agent (e.g., dextran, HES)
H	Heparin coagulant
W	Leukocyte collection
L	Saline lubrication for centrifuge bowl
V	Venous collapse sensor

FIGURE 36–3. Plasmapheresis. Diagrammatic representation of leukapheresis procedure using a continuous flow cell separator. (Reproduced by permission from: Rudy, E. B. *Advanced neurological and neurosurgical nursing* (p. 311). St. Louis, 1984, The C.V. Mosby Co.)

COLLABORATIVE MANAGEMENT

Treatments for respiratory support and autonomic monitoring are collaborative efforts between physicians and nurses. The nurse's role in collaborative care is to monitor the patient for progressive symptoms while also assessing the individual's response to therapy.

During the progressive phase, careful evaluation of muscular strength is done every 8 hours to determine further deterioration of clinical status. The Medical Research Council (MRC) scale provides a consistent, quantitative method for evaluating muscle group function (Griswold et al., 1984) (Table 36–2).

TABLE 36–2. Medical Research Council Scale

0 = No contraction
1 = Flicker or trace contraction
2 = Active movement with gravity eliminated
3 = Active movement against gravity
4 = Active movement against gravity and resistance
5 = Normal power

Adapted from Griswold, K., McKenna, M., and Ropper, A. (1984). An approach to care of patients with Guillain-Barré syndrome. *Heart & Lung,* 13 (1), 69.

RESPIRATORY MUSCLE DYSFUNCTION MANAGEMENT

During the progressive phase, the patient is monitored in an intensive care unit for potentially fatal respiratory muscle paralysis and autonomic dysfunction. It is critical to assess the trends of muscle weakness to anticipate acute respiratory dysfunction. It is useful to assess maximum inspiratory pressure and vital capacity every 2 to 4 hours (Ringel and Carroll, 1980). Testing the gag, cough, and swallow reflexes is mandatory to monitor pharyngeal function.

The danger of atelectasis, aspiration, and hypostatic pneumonia is great for patients with respiratory and pharyngeal muscle weakness. Pleuritic-type chest pain and dyspnea are insidious signs of respiratory tract infection in these patients. It is important to institute meticulous pulmonary toilet every 2 hours to mobilize secretions (Tanner, 1980).

Intubation and mechanical ventilation are recommended when the following clinical signs are noted:

1. Vital capacity is 1 liter or less or 30% or less of predicted value for the patient.
2. Negative inspiratory force is 20 cm H_2O or less.
3. Pharyngeal paralysis and inability to clear oral secretions are present.

Tracheostomy is indicated when the duration of intubation exceeds 10 days, unless there is rapid improvement and the potential for unassisted ventilation (Ropper and Kehne, 1985).

Weaning from mechanical ventilation begins once respiratory muscle strength returns, as evidenced by a vital capacity exceeding 30% of the predicted value for that patient and a negative inspiratory force of 20 cm H_2O or greater. Successful weaning of a patient with respiratory muscle weakness involves training of the respiratory muscles. It is not helpful to push these patients to fatigue during weaning trials. Several methods of weaning have been successful in patients with GBS. The eventual success of weaning involves not only the physical and mental readiness of the patient but also the skill of the caregiver. Depending on individual preference, either assist-control with intermittent T-piece trials or intermittent mandatory ventilation can be used for weaning. Assist-control ventilation provides patients with a preset tidal volume and respiratory rate. If the patient triggers the ventilator above the preset rate, the machine will deliver a preset tidal volume. During the weaning process, the patient is disconnected from the ventilator and provided with oxygen through a T-piece circuit. The patient is placed on the T-piece for 5 minutes, three times a day. The length of time off the ventilator is gradually increased, depending on the patient's tolerance. Close monitoring of the respiratory rate, level of consciousness, and work of breathing is essential. This method of weaning should include periods of rest when patients are on assisted ventilation and exercise as they are weaned intermittently.

Synchronized intermittent mandatory ventilation (SIMV) allows the patient to ventilate spontaneously from a demand valve opened by a patient-created pressure gradient. SIMV provides the patient with a preset rate and tidal volume but allows spontaneous breathing. If patients breathe more frequently than the preset rate, they will generate their own tidal volume. Weaning on intermittent mandatory ventilation (IMV) is accomplished by successively decreasing the preset rate, allowing more patient control of ventilation. IMV weaning requires continuous monitoring with preset mechanical alarms. Pressure support may be added to the SIMV mode to provide synchronous pressurization of the ventilator circuit during inspiration to decrease the work of breathing associated with opening the demand valve (MacIntyre, 1986). The pressure support mode reduces the work of breathing of patients on ventilatory support, making it a useful technique for weaning patients experiencing respiratory muscle dysfunction.

MANAGEMENT OF AUTONOMIC DYSFUNCTION

Cardiac monitoring is mandatory for GBS patients with respiratory muscle dysfunction and severe motor weakness because of the high incidence of autonomic dysfunction in these patients. Treatment of autonomic dysfunction is preventive and symptomatic.

Orthostatic hypotension may be avoided by maintaining positive pressure ventilation and slowly elevating the head while closely monitoring the blood pressure. Elevation of the head of the bed 30 degrees at night enhances renin secretion, resulting in sodium retention and increased blood volume, which may reduce orthostatic hypotension (Bannister, 1983; McLeod and Tuck, 1987). Severe or sustained hypertension should be treated with carefully titrated or short-acting antihypertensive agents. Vagal episodes are avoided by limiting the length of time of tracheal suctioning. Pacemakers may be necessary in patients with severe vagal episodes.

Bladder dysfunction is usually seen in patients with respiratory muscle failure and severe motor weakness (Traux, 1982). Urinary retention is treated with intermittent catheterization. Continuous catheterization is indicated for patients with severe, prolonged muscle weakness. Catheters are discontinued when the patient regains motor function of the trunk muscles. Often, intermittent catheterization is required for several days following continuous catheterization until the patient regains bladder tone.

Another autonomic dysfunction that occurs with GBS patients is hyponatremia and the syndrome of inappropriate secretion of antidiuretic hormone (SIADH). It is important to monitor serum sodium and osmolality in these patients. Treatment of SIADH involves crystalloid fluid restriction. (See also Chap. 42.)

NURSING DIAGNOSIS AND MANAGEMENT

Recovery from GBS is determined not only by the course of the disease but also by the intensity of the nursing care provided for the patient. The plan of care frequently changes due to the unpredictable nature of the disease and requires a high degree of resourcefulness by the nurse.

Potential for Aspiration Due to Dysphagia

Expected Outcome. The patient will demonstrate effective coughing and will be able to handle oral secretions without evidence of aspiration.

The threat of respiratory muscle failure and aspiration is of immediate concern in the progressive phase of GBS and requires intense monitoring, usually in a critical care unit. Inability to clear secretions because of paresis and an ineffective cough due to diaphragmatic paralysis are indications for intubation.

It is crucial that physical assessment include hourly monitoring of the patient's ability to gag, cough effectively, and clear secretions. An increase in oral secretions may signify that the patient is experiencing dysphagia.

Maintaining the head of the bed at 60 to 90 degrees if the patient is not hypotensive may facilitate a patent airway. The patient should be coached to cough forcefully every 2 hours.

Evidence of aspiration includes agitation, abnormal breath sounds, dyspnea, tachycardia, tachypnea, and abnormal arterial blood gases. Elective intubation should be done at the first sign of dysphagia with or without respiratory distress to prevent aspiration and its complications.

The nurse should explain to the patient and family why the patient's cough and swallow are being evaluated so frequently. The patient should be instructed to notify the nurse if he is experiencing increased difficulty in swallowing and coughing.

Alteration in Comfort: Pain, Due to Paresthesia, Hypesthesia, and Muscle Cramps

Expected Outcome. The patient states that he has no pain or the pain is controlled, and he does not demonstrate any evidence of uncontrolled pain.

Pain is one of the most difficult and frustrating symptoms to treat in GBS patients. The patient with uncontrolled pain may demonstrate varying degrees of anxiety, depression, hopelessness, hostility, and anger. Uncontrolled pain may be interpreted by the patient as a progression of disease, preventing him from participating in rehabilitation.

It is important on physical assessment to ask the patient to describe thoroughly the location, quality, and intensity of the pain. Information should also be elicited about what increases or relieves the pain. Sometimes it is possible to reduce the patient's pain by repositioning an extremity or removing a bed sheet or using a foot cradle. Pain may be so severe that it requires narcotic analgesics. Recording the assessment of pain and the treatment given on a flow sheet helps to track and communicate treatment success.

Pain can overwhelm the patient. Developing rapport with the patient allows the patient to relate his fears and demonstrates belief in his pain. Interventions to manage pain can include passive range of motion exercises, massage, distraction, ice, heat, cutaneous stimulation, oil of wintergreen, and transcutaneous electrical nerve stimulation (TENS). Analgesics used for these patients range from the nonsteroidal anti-inflammatory drugs (NSAIDs) to narcotic analgesics. Pain control needs to be individualized, considering the patient's response to pain and the phase of illness. For instance, if the patient is being weaned from the ventilator or is not intubated, an attempt should be made to use the least amount of narcotic analgesic possible because these drugs depress respirations. In the progressive phase, when the patient is intubated, narcotic analgesics may be very appropriate.

Impaired Verbal Communication Due to Intubation or Progressive Paralysis

Expected Outcome. Patient maintains optimal communication level for his physiologic state.

An inability to communicate contributes to the overwhelming fear and frustration experienced by the GBS patient and the family. Development of communication tools for these patients has been unsatisfactory to date. The nurse needs to use imagination to help these patients communicate their needs. One successful method, if the patient has little or no facial muscle weakness, is lip reading. It is important to encourage the patient to exaggerate lip movements, articulate key words, and go slowly.

This is a skill requiring patience on the part of both nurse and patient. When successful, patients express enormous relief and appreciation to nurses who can establish communication by means of lip reading.

If the patient has facial paralysis, lip reading is difficult or impossible. Letter and picture boards may be used (Easton, 1988). Diplopia may occur due to eye muscle involvement, making it difficult for the patient to see the communication board clearly. An eye patch covering one eye may help. Although use of the communication boards is tedious and time consuming, it may allow the patient his only means of communicating with others.

A "talk trach" may be useful for patients who have a tracheostomy but do not have vocal cord paralysis. The talk trach has air vents below the vocal cords. When the air port of the talk trach is connected to 4 to 6 liters of air flow, it is possible for the patient to speak. Problems with the talk trach include plugging of the air vents with secretions and gastric distention due to air leaking into the esophagus.

Other communication methods include the electronic artificial larynx and Morse code. Whichever method is used, it is important to spend time with the patient and family teaching them how to use the method adequately. The nurse should acknowledge the patient's frustration about the slowness of communication while encouraging patience. The patient and family should be reminded that verbal communication will return when the patient is extubated. Humor is frequently useful in promoting a positive attitude while using a variety communication methods.

Inability to communicate verbally means that the nurse must establish some means of allowing the patient to signal for help. Sometimes patients who cannot call out can still "click" with their tongue to gain attention. Clicking is useful when the nurse is in close proximity to the patient. Some very anxious patients may seem to click excessively. The nurse should investigate whether the patient has an actual physical need or is expressing anxiety indirectly and should deal with the situation accordingly.

There are pressure-sensitive call devices that require minimal pressure to be activated. The nurse may place the call device near the part of the patient that has the greatest remaining strength, e.g., the hand or the head. A "Sip-n-Puff" call system works well if the patient cannot use a pressure-sensitive plate. The ability to use a call device allows the patient to retain a sense of some control over the situation. Just one episode of being unable to summon help may cause severe anxiety or mistrust or even result in death if the ventilator-dependent patient becomes dislodged from the ventilator.

Potential Impaired Skin Integrity Due to Immobility from Paralysis

Expected Outcome. Skin remains dry, intact, and nonerythemic. A turning schedule is posted and continuously followed.

Because these patients may become completely paralyzed, they are especially prone to pressure necrosis. As long as possible in the progressive and recovery phases, the patient should be encouraged to change position frequently. Family members should be taught the importance of moving the patient and how to avoid shear forces when moving so that they can help the person move appropriately. A turning schedule should be established and posted at the bedside to ensure that turning patterns are followed uniformly. Inspection, massage, and application of lotion of all bony prominences should be accomplished each time the patient is turned and positioned. Skin should be kept free of excess moisture but not allowed to become dry and scaly; bath oil is preferred to soap for bed baths. Avoid use of plastic incontinent pads in direct contact with the patient's skin because these trap moisture and heat and may macerate the skin.

Adjunctive devices cannot replace basic nursing interventions in the prevention of skin breakdown. Air mattresses and mechanical beds (kinetic tables, air fluidized mattresses, Stryker frames) may be useful depending on the patient's condition. Judicious use of heel and elbow pads may also be helpful. When helping the patient into a chair, a gel pad such as the air flotation cushion may decrease excessive pressure.

Potential for Injury from Joint Contractures Due to Muscle Weakness or Paralysis

Expected Outcome. Patient will recover complete use of all extremities without residual loss of range of motion or complaints of pain or stiffness.

During the progressive and recovery phases the patient and family should be instructed in the need for and how to perform range of motion exercises for paralysed and weakened extremities. An exercise program should be established that places all joints through their full range of motion each 8 hours. Ideally, the exercise schedule is posted at the bedside to encourage patient and family participation.

Proper positioning is vital to maintain optimal joint function. The ideal joint position is neutral. Splints, orthoses, and adjunctive aids (antirotation boots) may be indicated to prevent or correct joint contracture.

Isometric and isotonic exercises of uninvolved or partially involved muscle groups should accompany range of motion exercises. Too frequent or vigorous exercise should be avoided because it may contribute to the demyelination process (Ross et al., 1979). Traction weight systems may be set up on the bed to allow the patient to perform isotonic exercises when confined to bed. Exercise goals set mutually with the patient and family should be posted at the bedside. Attained goals should be celebrated with effusive positive reinforcement and reward.

Potential Activity Intolerance Due to Orthostatic Hypotension from Associated Autonomic Dysfunction

Expected Outcome. Patient will tolerate getting out of bed without complaint of lightheadedness or occurrences of hypotension.

The judgment of when to get the patient out of bed to a chair varies with each individual. Autonomic nervous system stability and trunk muscle strength should be considered. Patients with unstable autonomic nervous system function should have their blood pressure taken and cardiac monitoring performed whenever the patient's head is elevated. If the patient has little or no upper body strength, it is difficult and painful for him or her to sit in a chair. Patients transferred into a cardiac chair should have adequate torso strength to maintain their position in the chair.

Elastic support stockings and elastic wraps applied to the upper legs may provide adequate compression to decrease venous pooling and decrease orthostasis. Slowly elevating the head of the bed over a period of several hours may aid in overcoming orthostasis in the patient who has been on prolonged bed rest. Tilt tables may also be necessary for some patients.

Alteration in Nutrition: Inability to Meet Bodily Requirements

Malnutrition may be due to immobility, decreased gastrointestinal mobility, dysphagia, anorexia, or depression.

Expected Outcome. Patient maintains his ideal body weight and actively participates in the diet regimen.

Because the threat of aspiration can complicate the patient's ability to maintain adequate nutrition, careful assessment of pharyngeal function is mandatory as a baseline in nutritional interventions. In patients with mild dysphagia it may be possible to provide semisolid to solid foods while the patient sits upright. Liquids tend to be more easily aspirated. Enteric or parenteral nutrition is necessary with patients who have moderate to severe dysphagia. Patients on tube feedings should be assessed for excessive gastric residual (>50 mL in 2 hours for continuous feedings and >100 mL for every 4 hour feedings). Metoclopramide hydrochloride may be ordered to facilitate gastric emptying. When the patient is again able to begin solid foods, calorie counts may be periodically used to ensure adequate caloric intake. If necessary, the patient should be aided in choosing foods that are nutritious. Encouraging the family to bring in home-cooked foods may be useful for some patients. Weights taken daily or every other day allow monitoring of nutritional status. Serum albumin and total lymphocyte counts also aid in determining nutritional status.

Fear

Fear may be due to lack of understanding of the disease process and prognosis, pain, inability to communicate, loss of control, and thoughts of dying.

Expected Outcome. Patients state that they are comfortable with their situation and do not demonstrate uncontrolled fear.

Fear is experienced by most if not all GBS patients. The experience of GBS may seem like a nightmare. Fearful feelings may be exacerbated by caregivers' inability to provide a precise estimate of the rate and degree of recovery. It is imperative that the critical care nurse keep the patient and family informed. Information provided varies from details about ICU routines to supplemental information about the disease and its therapy. Whenever possible, sensory information, from the patient's perspective, should be provided, especially for painful or uncomfortable procedures. It is important to spend time with the patient and family to identify misconceptions or distorted perceptions.

The GBS Society has published a booklet for patients and families that provides information about the disease and resources for financial, rehabilitative, and social support (Steinberg, 1984). The booklet is available from The Guillain-Barré Syndrome Support Group, P.O. Box 262, Wynnewood, PA 19096. It is sometimes helpful to direct families to the nearest GBS support group to share feelings, hope, and practical information on coping strategies. The National GBS Support Group Office (telephone [215] 649–7837) can direct patients and families to the nearest chapter.

Fear may be exacerbated by a lack of sleep. ICU syndrome has also been associated with a lack of sleep. This syndrome is described as a gradual loss of ability to perceive reality in response to restraints, sensory overload, sensory monotony, and sleep deprivation. Patients with GBS are prone to ICU syndrome because of changes in their ability to perceive the environment, chronic pain, sleep deprivation, and a feeling of being trapped within their own body. It is important to combat this complication because it can prolong hospitalization.

The patient's sleep routine should be monitored and hypnotics administered, if necessary, to promote rest. A day–night routine should be established and maintained for the patient. Allow the patient optimal control in establishing the daily schedule. A posted schedule of activities aids staff and family in maintaining the schedule for the patient.

Visits of former patients with GBS are helpful because they allow the patient to gain insight into the situation. They also provide a role model of the recovered patient and visible evidence of recovery for the patient. The timing of such a visit is crucial and may be best arranged during the plateau or recovery phase after the patient has experience the illness and gained a sense of ownership of it. (See also Chap. 6.)

Ineffective Family Coping: Compromised or Disabling Due to the Overwhelming Aspects of GBS on the Family

Expected Outcome. Patient and family are able to cope effectively with the situation as shown by the absence of abnormal reactions.

Family members may also experience fear, helplessness, and a loss of control. Aid the family in identifying tasks that they can perform (exercises, repositioning) that aid the patient's recovery. Encourage the family to listen to the patient's concerns and to identify problem areas in which the staff can intervene. Encourage the family to talk about current events and reminisce about the patient's past to distract the patient from the reality of the current situation and foster a sense of hope. Incorporate the family as much as possible in the care of the patient to the extent that they feel comfortable. (see also Chap. 7).

ncp nursing care plan

1. Potential aspiration related to:
Dysphagia

Outcome Criteria	Nursing Interventions
Patient will demonstrate effective cough. Patient does not aspirate oral excretions.	Monitor ability to gag, cough effectively, and clear secretions hourly. Maintain head of the bed at 60 to 90 degrees, if not hypotensive. Encourage coughing every 2 hours. Facilitate tracheal intubation at the first sign of dysphagia with or without respiratory distress. Explain to patient and family why coughing and swallowing are evaluated so frequently. Instruct patient to notify nurse if any increased difficulty in swallowing or coughing is experienced.

2. Altered comfort: pain related to:
Paresthesia
Hyperesthesia
Muscle cramps

Outcome Criteria	Nursing Interventions
Patient reports that he or she is pain free, or that pain is controlled. No objective evidence of uncontrolled pain (tachycardia, hypertension, facial grimacing).	Ask patient to thoroughly describe the location, quality, and intensity of pain, as well as what increases or relieves the pain. Attempt to manage the pain by repositioning the extremity, removing a bed sheet, using a foot cradle, passive range of motion exercises, massage, distraction, ice, heat, cutaneous stimulation, oil of wintergreen, or transcutaneous electrical nerve stimulation (TENS). Consider analgesics based on individual patient's responses to other interventions, ranging from non-steroidal anti-inflammatory agents to narcotics. Develop rapport with patient that allows fears and concerns to be relayed while demonstrating a belief in the patient's pain experience. Record the pain assessment, treatment, and patient's response on a flow sheet to track and communicate successful interventions.

Nursing Care Plan continued on following page

3. Impaired verbal communication related to:
   Tracheal intubation
   Progressive paralysis

Outcome Criteria	Nursing Interventions
Patient maintains optimal communication level for his or her physiologic state.	To facilitate lip reading, encourage patient to exaggerate lip movements, articulate key words, and speak slowly. Use letter, word, and picture boards if lip reading is difficult or impossible. Consider an eye patch on one eye if seeing the communication board is difficult due to diplopia. Consider a "talking tracheostomy tube," an electronic artificial larynx, or Morse code and teach patient and family how to use them. Acknowledge patient's frustration about the slowness of communication while encouraging patience. Remind patient and family that verbal communication will return when the patient's strength returns and extubation occurs. Consider the use of humor to promote a positive attitude while using a variety of communication methods. Establish some means for the patient to call for help.

4. Potential impaired skin integrity related to:
   Immobility due to paralysis
   Paresthesia

Outcome Criteria	Nursing Interventions
Skin remains dry, intact, and nonerythemic. A turning schedule is posted and followed continuously.	Encourage frequent position changes during the progressive and recovery phases. Teach family members the importance of how to avoid shear forces when moving. Establish and post a turning schedule. Inspect, apply lotion to, and massage all bony prominences with each turn. Keep skin free of excess moisture. Use bath oil with bed bathing rather than soap. Avoid using plastic incontinent pads in direct contact with patient's skin. Consider adjunctive devices to augment basic nursing interventions, such as air mattresses, low airloss beds, heel and elbow protectors, and gel pads.

5. Potential for injury: joint contractures related to:
   Muscle weakness
   Paralysis

Outcome Criteria	Nursing Interventions
Patient recovers complete use of all extremities without residual loss of range of motion or complaints of pain or soreness.	Instruct patient and family in the need for and how to perform range of motion exercises for paralyzed and weakened extremities. Establish an exercise program that places all joints through their full range of motion every 8 hours. Post exercise schedule and encourage patient and family participation. Position joints in neutral position if possible, using splints, orthoses, and other adjunctive aids as needed to prevent or correct joint contracture. Include isometric and isotonic exercises of uninvolved or partially involved muscle groups, using traction weight systems if necessary. Avoid too frequent or vigorous exercise. Set exercise goals with patient and family. Post at bedside. Celebrate attained goals with positive reinforcement and reward.

6. Potential activity intolerance related to:
   Orthostatic hypotension
   Autonomic dysreflexia

Outcome Criteria	Nursing Interventions
Patient will tolerate getting out of bed without complaint of lightheadedness or occurrence of hypotension.	Consider autonomic nervous system stability and trunk muscle strength before getting patient out of bed to a chair. Monitor heart rate, cardiac rhythm, and blood pressure whenever the patient's head is elevated if autonomic nervous system function is unstable. Apply elastic wraps or support stockings to legs (including thighs) to decrease venous pooling of blood and orthostasis. Elevate the head of the bed over a period of hours or use a tilt table.

7. Altered nutrition: less than body requirements related to:
Immobility
Decreased gastrointestinal motility
Dysphagia
Anorexia
Depression

Outcome Criteria	*Nursing Interventions*
Patients maintains ideal body weight. Patient actively participates in diet regimen.	Assess swallowing prior to nutritional interventions. For a patient with mild dysphagia, provide semisolid foods to patient sitting upright. For patients receiving enteral feedings, check gastric residual volume every 2 hours for those receiving continuous feeding or prior to each bolus feeding. Consider using metoclopramide hydrochloride (10 mg PO, IV, or IM four times per day given 30 minutes before meals and at bedtime) to facilitate gastric emptying. When patient is able to begin solid foods, obtain periodic calorie counts and help patient choose nutritious foods. Encourage family members to bring favorite home-cooked foods. Obtain weight at least every other day. Monitor serum albumin level and total lymphocyte count.

8. Fear related to:
Lack of understanding of the disease process and prognosis
Pain
Inability to communicate
Loss of control
Thoughts of dying

Outcome Criteria	*Nursing Interventions*
Patient states that he or she is comfortable. Patient does not demonstrate uncontrolled fear.	Keep patient and family informed about all aspects of situation, ranging from details about ICU routines to supplemental information about the disease and its therapy. Provide sensory information, from the patient's perspective, especially for painful or uncomfortable procedures. Spend time with patient and family to identify misconceptions or distorted perceptions. Consider referring families to the nearest Guillain-Barré support group. Monitor patient's sleep routine and consider the use of hypnotics to promote rest if necessary. Establish and post a day-night routine and allow patient maximal control in establishing the day routine. Consider planning a visit from former Guillain-Barré patients during the plateau or recovery phase.

9. Ineffective family coping: compromised or disabling related to:
Overwhelming aspects of Guillain-Barré syndrome

Outcome Criteria	*Nursing Interventions*
Patient and family are able to cope effectively with the situation as shown by the absence of abnormal reactions.	Help family members identify tasks that they can perform that aid the patient's recovery. Encourage family members to listen to the patient's concerns and to identify problem areas in which the staff can intervene. Encourage family members to talk about current events and reminisce about the patient's past. Incorporate the family into the patient's care wherever possible.

SUMMARY

Guillain-Barré syndrome is a debilitating neuromuscular disorder characterized by sensory, motor, and autonomic dysfunction. Nursing care is directed toward supportive care of these patients as they progress through the progressive, plateau, and recovery phases of the illness. Successful recovery of these patients is highly dependent upon the nurse's ability to prevent complications and support recovery.

References

Arnason, B. (1975). Inflammatory polyradiculoneuropathies. In P. Dyck, P. Thomas, and E. Lambert (Eds.), *Peripheral neuropathy* (Vol. II 5 pp. 1110–1148). Philadelphia: W. B. Saunders Co.

Bannister, R. (1983) (Ed.). *Autonomic failure.* Oxford: Oxford University Press.

Cameron, D., Howel, D. and Hutchinson, J. (1958). Acute peripheral neuropathy in Hodgkin's disease. Report of fatal case with histologic features of allergic neuritis. *Neurology,* 8, 575–577.

Consensus Conference (1986). The utility of therapeutic phasmaspheresis for neurological disorders. *Journal of the American Medical Association.* 256 (10), 1333–1336.

Easton, J. (1988). Alternative communication for patients in intensive care. *Intensive Care Nursing*, 4, 47–55.

Gracey, D., McMichan, J., Divertie, M., and Howard, F. (1982). Respiratory failure in Guillain-Barré syndrome. *Mayo Clinic Proceedings*, 57, 742–746.

Greenland, P., and Griggs, R. (1980). Arrhythmic complications in the Guillain-Barré syndrome. *Archives of Internal Medicine*, 140, 1053.

Griswold, K., McKenna, M., and Ropper, A. (1984). An approach to care of patients with Guillain-Barré syndrome. *Heart & Lung*, 13 (1), 66–72.

Guillain, G., Barré, J., and Strohl, A. (1916). Sur un syndrome de radiculonervite avec hyperalbuminose du liquide encephalorachidien sans reaction cellaire. *Bull Soc Med Hop*, 40, 1462.

Kaplan, J., Greenspan, J., Bomgaars, M., et al. (1983). Simultaneous outbreaks of Guillain-Barré syndrome and Bell's palsy in Hawaii in 1981. *Journal of the Medical Association*, 250, 2635–2640.

Klingon, G. (1965). The Guillain-Barré syndrome associated with cancer. *Cancer*, 18, 157–163.

Korn-Lubetzki, I., and Abramsky, O. (1986). Acute and chronic demyelinating inflammatory polyradiculoneuropathy. Association with autoimmune diseases and lymphocyte response to human neuritogenic protein. *Archives of Neurology*, 43, (6), 604–608.

Landry, O. (1859). Note sur la paralysic ascendante aigul. *Gaz Rebd Med Chir*, 6, 472–486.

Lichtenfeld, P. (1971). Autonomic dysfunction in the Guillain-Barré syndrome. *American Journal of Medicine*, 50, 772.

Loffel, N., Rossi, L., Mumenthaler, M., et al. (1977). The Landry-Guillain-Barré syndrome. *Journal of the Neurological Sciences*, 33, 71–79.

McLeod, J., and Tuck, R. (1987). Disorders of the autonomic nervous system: Part 2. Investigation and treatment. *Annals of Neurology*, 21 (6), 519–529.

National Institute of Neurologic and Communicative Disorders and Stroke (1978). Criteria for diagnosis of Guillain-Barré syndrome. *Annals of Neurology*, 3, (6), 565–566.

Pleasure, D., and Schotland, D. (1984). *Acquired neuropathies*. In L. Rowland (Ed.), *Merrit's textbook of neurology* (p. 484). Philadelphia: Lea & Febinger.

Retailiau, H., Curtis, A., Storre, G., et al., (1980). Illness after influenza vaccination reported through a nationwide surveillance system, 1976–1977. *American Journal of Epidemiology*, 111, 270–278.

Ringel, S., and Carroll, J. (1980). Respiratory complications of neuromuscular disease. In W. Weiner (Ed.), *Respiratory dysfunction in neurologic disease* (p. 122). New York: Futura.

Ropper, A. (1986). Unusual clinical variants and signs in Guillain-Barré syndrome. *Archives of Neurology*, 43, 1150–1152.

Ropper, A., and Shahani, B. (1984). Pain in Guillain-Barré. *Archives of Neurology*, 41, 511–514.

Ropper, A., and Kehne, S. (1985). Guillain-Barré syndrome: Management of respiratory failure. *Archives of Neurology*, 43, 1150–1152.

Ross, A. J., Herr, B. E., Norwood, M. L., et al. (1979). Neuromuscular diagnostic procedures. *Nursing Clinics of North America*, 14, 107–156.

Schonberger, L., Bregman, D., Sullivan-Bolyai, J., et al. (1979). Guillain-Barré syndrome following vaccination in the national influenza immunization program, United States, 1976–1977. *American Journal of Epidemiology*, 118, 105–123.

Schonberger, L., Hurwitz, E., Katona, P., et al. (1981). Guillain-Barré syndrome. Its epidemiology and associations with influenze vaccination. *Annals of Neurology*, 9, 31–38.

Sobue, G., Senda, Y., Matsuoka, Y., et al. (1983). Sensory ataxia. A residual disability of Guillain-Barré syndrome. *Archives of Neurology*, 40, 86–69.

Steinberg, J. (1984). *Guillain-Barré syndrome. An overview for the lay person*. Wynnewood, PA: Guillain-Barré Support Group.

Tanner, C. (1980). Respiratory dysfunction and peripheral neuropathy. In W. Weiner (Ed.), *Respiratory dysfunction in neurologic disease* (p. 95). New York: Futura.

Traux, B. (1982). Autonomic disturbances in the Guillain-Barré syndrome. *Seminars in Neurology*, 4, (4), 462–468

Patients with Craniotomies

June Romeo

There are several types of cranial lesions, including aneurysms, intracranial hemorrhage, trauma, abscess, metastatic disease, and neoplasms, that require various forms of craniotomy. Because several of these conditions are addressed in other chapters, this chapter will focus on craniotomies for neoplastic disease.

Intracranial lesions are often synonymous with a bleak prognosis. The neurologic symptoms associated with intracranial lesions depend upon the size of the lesion, its location, and the degree of invasiveness. Intracranial lesions commonly destroy the structures they invade, displace surrounding tissues, and cause increased intracranial pressure. Craniotomy is the treatment of choice for tumors and other masses in the brain. The future for patients who undergo craniotomies has improved because of advances in microsurgery, neuroanesthesia, pharmacology, diagnostic procedures, and postoperative management. In spite of these advances, intracranial neoplasms are often fatal even with surgical removal of the tumor mass.

CAUSES OF BRAIN TUMORS

The etiology of brain tumors remains enigmatic. Meticulous analysis of past medical records has offered no clue as to why a tumor begins to grow in the brain. Among the many causative agents suggested have been head injury, exposure to toxins, infection, and a variety of diseases; however, none of these agents has been associated with conclusive evidence. Some evidence indicates that certain viruses and radiation may contribute to development of neoplasms, but these are the exception rather than the rule (Bauman and Zumwalt, 1989).

PATHOPHYSIOLOGY OF BRAIN TUMORS

Symptoms of brain tumor growth are governed by the principles of physics and physiology. The Monro-Kellie hypothesis is based on the fact that the skull is a rigid container with a finite volume occupied by brain tissue, blood, and cerebrospinal fluid (Klatzo, 1967). These three elements fill the cranial vault to near capacity, and this capacity is a constant. Any increase in one of the three elements must be accompanied by compensatory reduction in one or both of the others. A tumor growing in the brain eventually exerts pressure on the surrounding tissues. To compensate for this pressure the brain must shift cerebrospinal fluid from the subarachnoid space surrounding the brain to the subarachnoid space surrounding the spinal cord. Vasoconstriction may also be necessary to reduce blood flow. These mechanisms are illustrated in the following equations:

Normal intracranial pressure:

$$V_{total} = V_{blood} + V_{CSF} + V_{brain}$$

Increased intracranial pressure due to other mass:

$$V_{total} = V_{blood} + V_{CSF} + V_{brain} + V_{other}$$

where V equals volume. V_{total} is the constant and remains the same no matter how much additional volume V_{other} assumes. Compensatory mechanisms that accommodate changes among these elements are discussed in Chapter 32. In the case of a growing tumor, these compensatory mechanisms eventually fail, allowing intracranial pressure to increase. If not relieved, intracranial pressure will eventually force the extrusion of the brain through the path of least resistance, usually through tentorial or cerebellar herniation. Such herniation will ultimately lead to death (Arsenault, 1985; Barnett et al., 1988; Chan, 1984; Youmans, 1982).

Space-occupying lesions cause signs and symptoms through compression, obstruction, and invasion, all three of which result in pressure. Signs and symptoms are the consequence of invasion of or pressure on brain tissue or of obstruction to the flow of blood or cerebrospinal fluid (CSF).

The first compensation for a space-occupying lesion is a reduction in the volume of CSF in the ventricles and subarachnoid space. Some of the CSF is displaced into the subarachnoid space of the spinal cord via the foramen magnum. As the neoplasm continues to grow, this means of compensation becomes inadequate, and CSF begins to flow through the optic foramina into the perioptic subarachnoid space. Increasing pressure in the perioptic space impairs axonal transport and venous drainage from the optic nerve and retina, resulting in *papilledema.*

The venous drainage of tissue compressed by the neoplasm is also impaired, leading to an increase in capillary pressure, especially in the cerebral white matter. Microvascular transudative factors, such as proteases, may be released by neoplastic tissue, disrupting the blood-brain barrier. These proteases are postulated to activate plasminogen, which breaks down fibrin and other proteins. As these proteins accumulate in the extravascular space within the cerebral white matter, they increase the colloidal osmotic pressure of these tissues, drawing fluid from the blood into the tissue in the form of edema. This is thought to be the source of localized edema around a neoplasm in the brain (Bleehan, 1986; Youmans, 1982).

TYPES OF BRAIN TUMORS

Tumors of the brain are classified according to the type of cell involved (Adams and Victor, 1985; Gerke, 1980; Zimmerman, 1969; Zulch, 1986). Primary tumors of the central nervous system are thought to arise from adult transformation of two embryologic tissues, nerve and glial cells. For instance, a normal astrocyte becomes transformed into a neoplastic cell, and its subsequent cells become more and more dedifferentiated as the degree of malignancy increases. Types of tumors are listed in Table 37–1.

Gliomas

Glioblastoma Multiforme. The most common primary neoplasm of brain is the glioblastoma multiforme. Glioblastoma multiforme accounts for 25% of all intracranial neoplasms, approximately 55% of all gliomal tumors, and 90% of cerebral hemispheric gliomas. This neoplasm is also found in the brain stem, cerebellum, or spinal cord. Peak incidence is

TABLE 37–1. Types of Intracranial Tumor and Percentage of Total*

Tumor	Percentage of Total
Gliomas	
Glioblastoma multiforme	20
Astrocytoma	10
Ependymoma	6
Medulloblastoma	4
Oligodendrocytoma	5
Meningioma	15
Pituitary adenoma	7
Neurinoma (schwannoma)	7
Metastatic carcinoma	6
Craniopharyngioma	4
Angioma	4
Sarcoma	4
Unclassified (mostly gliomas)	5
Miscellaneous (pinealoma, chordoma, granuloma)	3
Total	100

*Types derived from the combined series of Zulch, Cushing, and Olivecrona involving 15,000 cases.
From Adams, R. D., and Victor, M. (1985), *Principles of neurology.* New York: McGraw-Hill.

middle age, usually after 35 years, and men are affected twice as often as women. The tumor most commonly occupies the cerebral white matter. This virulently malignant, fast-growing, rapidly invasive neoplasm often spreads from one hemisphere to the other through the corpus callosum. The neoplasm is composed of several cell types, is very vascular, hemorrhages easily, and contains necrotic areas (Frankel and German, 1969; Walker and Posner, 1984, Youmans, 1982). These neoplasms may also be classified as grade 4 astrocytomas (see later discussion).

Findings on early assessment include diffuse cerebral symptoms and seizures (present in 30% to 40% of patients). Within a few weeks or months symptoms are localized to a more specific location with specific symptoms depending on the area of the neoplasm. In most patients symptoms are present for 3 to 6 months before a diagnosis is established. Ten per cent of these patients present with mental changes. In a few patients the onset of symptoms is sudden, and this is most commonly attributed to hemorrhage or rapid expansion of a cyst within the tumor. In these patients a lumbar puncture reveals blood in the CSF.

The prognosis of patients with glioblastoma multiforme is poor. Fewer than 20% survive 1 year past the onset of symptoms, and less than 10% survive 2 or more years. Median survival following surgical resection (without chemotherapy or radiotherapy) is 14 weeks. Radiotherapy may extend the median survival to 12 to 14 months (Walker and Posner, 1984; Youmans, 1982). Chemotherapy has shown little benefit. Death usually results from cerebral edema, increased intracranial pressure, and tentorial herniation.

Current therapy is ineffective in controlling the progression of glioblastoma multiforme. Because of the invasive quality of the neoplasm, the neoplasm is only partially resectable. Surgery through craniotomy is often necessary for diagnosis, to improve the quality of life, or to prevent impending transtentorial herniation. Stereotaxic procedures provide the least invasive method of confirmatory biopsy. Although there appears to be a trend away from surgical intervention, neither radiotherapy nor chemotherapy has improved the prognosis of these patients (Frankel and German, 1969; Harper and Stewart-Wynne, 1978; Shapiro, 1982; Youmans, 1982).

Astrocytoma. Astrocytoma is a relatively common primary brain neoplasm that can occur in both adults and children, with more benign forms found in children. Although this neoplasm may be found anywhere in the central nervous system, it occurs most frequently in the cerebral white matter, cerebellum, hypothalamus, optic nerve, optic chiasm, and pons. This infiltrative neoplasm tends to form large cavities or cysts. However, some of these neoplasms are noncavitating and are almost indistinguishable from normal white matter.

Most patients with astrocytomas present with a seizure, and up to 75% of these patients continue to have seizures throughout the course of their illness. People between 20 and 60 years old who experience onset of focal seizures should be investigated for potential astrocytoma. Temporal lobe astrocytomas may have subtle symptoms that precede seizures; this subtlety makes diagnosis difficult. Symptoms such as slight changes in mood and personality suggestive of schizophrenia may precede or follow the onset of seizures. Symptoms of frontal lobe astrocytomas may include slight arm drift, a mild limp, brisk tendon reflexes, or slight changes in language and sensation. These symptoms may be present for several years before diagnosis is made (Adams and Victor, 1985; Youmans, 1982).

The treatment of choice for astrocytoma is excisional craniotomy. The survival rate averages 5 years for cerebral astrocytoma and 9 years for cerebellar astrocytomas. These neoplasms are graded according to the degree of malignancy; I is the least malignant, and IV is the most malignant and is synonymous with glioblastoma multiforme. A newer system of classification being introduced in the literature consists of astrocytoma low grade, anaplastic astrocytoma, and glioblastoma multiforme.

Oligodendroglioma. Oligodendroglioma is a third form of glioma derived from oligodendrocytes, the myelin-producing brain cells. Although this neoplasm occurs throughout the life span, it is most common in the fourth and fifth decades. This infrequently found neoplasm represents 5% to 7% of all gliomas. Oligodendrogliomas are most commonly found deep in the white matter of the temporal lobes with little or no localized edema. Less commonly,

the neoplasm is found intraventricularly and most infrequently in the third ventricle, brain stem, cerebellum, or spinal cord. Oligodendrogliomas may metastasize to the ventriculosubarchanoid space.

Oligodendrogliomas are slow-growing tumors, the interval between the first symptom and surgical intervention ranging from 28 to 70 months. About 70% of these patients have seizures, and seizures are the most common presenting symptoms. Surgical excision through a craniotomy has allowed survival rates of 5 years. These tumors recur in about half of the patients within several months of surgery (Bailey, 1929; Walker and Posner, 1984; Weir and Elvidge 1968; Youmans, 1982).

Ependymoma. Ependymoma represents 5% of all gliomas and is more complex and variable than the other gliomas. This neoplasm occurs most commonly in the fourth ventricle within the brain and in the lumbosacral area of the spinal cord, especially the conus and filum terminale. This neoplasm tends to form canals and to radiate around blood vessels. About 40% of infratentorial ependymomas occur in the first decade of life, some within the first year. Supratentorial ependymomas occur throughout life. Symptomology depends on the location of the tumor. Seizures occur in about 35% of these patients. Fourth ventricle signs are common in patients with infratentorial ependymomas, e.g., headache, nuchal rigidity, and vomiting. Only about half of the patients survive for 1 year after surgical resection. Prognosis is highly dependent upon the degree of anaplasia, but less than 15% of these patients survive 10 years. Radiation following surgical resection has improved survival rates (Adams and Victor, 1985; Fokes and Earle, 1969; Youmans, 1982).

Medulloblastoma. Medulloblastoma is a rapidly growing embryonic tumor that arises from the cerebellar vermis and roof of the fourth ventricle in children and in the cerebellum in adults. This neoplasm frequently fills the fourth ventricle and invades its floor. Metastasis may occur to the meninges of the cisterna magna and spinal cord. Medulloblastoma occurs mainly in males between the ages of 4 and 8 years. Symptoms commonly precede diagnosis by 5 months.

Medulloblastomas have a distinct clinical picture. The child becomes listless, complains of morning headache, and vomits repeatedly. Although gastrointestinal disease is commonly suspected, dizziness, nystagmus, stumbling gait, falls, squinting, and papilledema soon follow. The child's head tends to tilt back and away from the side of the tumor when cerebellar herniation is present.

Medulloblastomas are highly sensitive to radiation. Although initial therapy with chemotherapy has not been shown to be effective, it has increased remission rates in some patients. Two-thirds of these patients survive 5 years following surgical excision, radiation of the entire neuraxis, and chemotherapy (Bleehan, 1986; Youmans, 1982).

Meningiomas

Meningiomas are benign growths that arise from the arachnoid or dura mater and comprise 15% of all primary brain tumors. This neoplasm occurs most commonly in the seventh decade in women. People who have had radiation therapy of the cranium or scalp are more prone to development of meningiomas (Bleehan, 1986; Cushing and Eisenhardt, 1962; Youmans, 1982).

Meningiomas most commonly occur on the parasagittal surface of the frontal or parietal lobes, the lesser wings of the sphenoid, olfactory grooves, tuberculum sellae, superior surface of the cerebellum, cerebellopontine angle, or spinal canal. Meningiomas commonly invade the overlying cranial bones and may manifest as an exostosis of the skull (Bellur et al. 1979; Bleehan, 1986; Youmans, 1982).

Small meningiomas are often found on autopsy of asymptomatic middle-aged and elderly people. Focal seizures are the most common presenting symptom. Parasagittal frontoparietal meningiomas may be manifest by a slowly progressive spastic weakness of the lower extremity. Other symptoms depend on the location of the neoplasm. Signs and symptoms may precede diagnosis by as long as 15 years. In neoplasms that are easily accessible, surgical excision often provides a permanent cure. Incomplete resection commonly results in recurrence. Rarely, meningiomas are malignant and invasive. Radiation following surgery has proved beneficial for inaccessible or malignant meningiomas (Berkshire and Watson-Evans, 1989; Chan and Thompson, 1984).

Cerebellopontine Angle Neoplasms

Lesions of the cerebellopontine angle may include acoustic neuromas (most common), meningiomas, cholesteatomas, metastatic tumor, cerebellar tumors, and neurinomas. Vascular lesions, angiomas and aneurysms, may also involve the basilar area. Because of its frequency, acoustic neuroma will be the focus of attention in this discussion (Davis et al., 1977; Youmans, 1982).

Neuromas may occur in any of the cranial or spinal nerves but most frequently affect the acoustic nerve. Neuromas occur from early adulthood and affect men and women equally. Unilateral neuromas are most common, but bilateral neuromas are found, particularly in families with a history of von Recklinghausen disease (neurofibromatosis) (Youmans, 1982).

This neoplasm arises from the Schwann cells within the auditory meatus on the vestibular portion of the eighth cranial nerve. As it grows, the neoplasm may compress the fifth and seventh cranial nerves at the cerebellopontine angle. If the tumor extends superiorly it may compress the third cranial nerve, whereas inferior extension will compress the ninth or tenth cranial nerve. This benign, encapsulated neoplasm may become cystic and degenerate into a malignant lesion (Davis et al., 1977). Recurrence is common unless it is completely excised. Symptoms usually appear in a specific order: decreased hearing, deafness, tinnitus, vertigo, and pressure in the ear that progresses to facial pain, facial muscular weakness, nystagmus, and ataxia. Hearing loss will be permanent unless surgical intervention is accomplished early (Salcman, 1985). Large tumors may compress the pons, medulla, and fourth ventricle, resulting in symptoms of increased intracranial pressure from disrupted flow of cerebrospinal fluid (Harner and Laws, 1983; Martuza and Ojemann, 1982; Youmans, 1982).

The goal of medical therapy is complete excision of the neoplasm. Surgery usually is undertaken in several stages through a transmeatal or posterior fossa craniotomy. Six months after the initial excision, reanastomosis of the hypoglossal and facial nerves may be accomplished to regain facial muscle tone. In general, the prognosis for longevity is good for these patients (Martuza and Ojeman, 1982; Youmans, 1982).

Pituitary Tumors

Tumors of the pituitary comprise 7% to 10% of all primary intracranial tumors. Tumors arise from one of the three basic cell forms comprising the pituitary gland, e.g., basophil, eosinophil, or chromophobe.

Adenomas are the most frequent neoplasm affecting the pituitary area. These adenomas may be categorized clinically into one of two groups. The first group is characterized only by indications of a space-occupying lesion without apparent endocrine or pituitary dysfunction. The second group exhibits endocrine hyperactivity, usually through clinical indications of Cushing's syndrome or acromegaly (Drayer et al., 1979; Youmans, 1982).

Growth of pituitary neoplasms is characterized by four distinct phases. The first phase involves growth of the neoplasm, stretching the diaphragma sella (the dural covering of the sella) and causing bitemporal headaches. In the second phase continued neoplastic growth results in pressure on the pituitary gland that eventually results in its destruction and a panhypopituitary syndrome (see Fig. 37–1). Panhypopituitary syndrome results in hypothyroidism, hypogonadism, and hypoadrenalism. Loss of libido is the first finding on assessment in males, whereas in women amenorrhea precedes decreased sex drive. In phase three the continued enlargement of the neoplasm results in pressure on the medial fibers of the optic chiasm causing bitemporal visual field defects. In the final phase the neoplasm invades the third ventricle, where it eventually blocks the passage of cerebrospinal fluid. Findings on assessment during the fourth

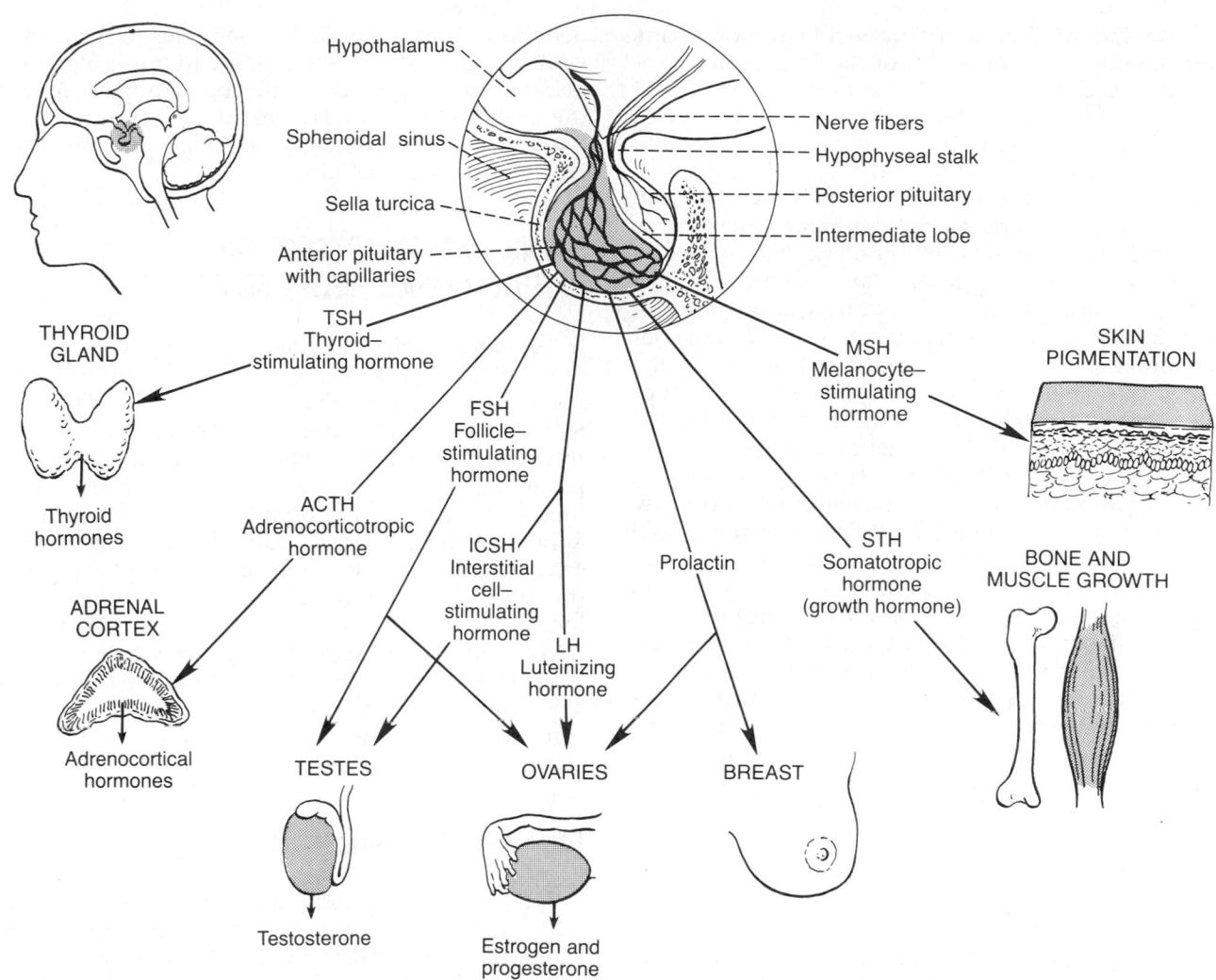

FIGURE 37–1. The anterior pituitary gland and its effects on the body. (Adapted from *Taber's Cyclopedic Medical Dictionary* (15th ed., p. 1306). Philadelphia: F. A. Davis, 1985. In Luckmann, J., and Sorensen, K. C. (1987). *Medical-surgical nursing: A psychophysiologic approach* (3rd ed., p. 1470). Philadelphia: W.B. Saunders.)

phase include headaches, motor and sensory dysfunction, and altered mentation. If the neoplasm continues to grow, the patient eventually experiences hypothalamic dysfunction, altered sleep patterns, and coma. Diagnosis of pituitary tumors is usually accomplished prior to erosion of the sella and optical nerve compression (phase three) (Cogan, 1974; Drayer et al., 1979).

Neoplasms arising from the anterior pituitary are commonly associated with changes in vision and symptoms associated with involvement of the sella turcica. Tumors of the pituitary increase in incidence with each decade. Endocrine abnormalities and visual disorders (especially bitemporal hemianopsia) are among the presenting findings for pituitary neoplasms. Although additional findings are rare, they may include seizures, rhinorrhea, and diabetes insipidus. Approximately 70% of pituitary neoplasms secrete prolactin, 15% secrete growth hormone, and a few secrete ACTH. Two major hormone-secretion syndromes are described below (Youmans, 1982).

Amenorrhea-Galactorrhea Syndrome. The classic

patient with this syndrome is a woman of childbearing age taking birth control pills who finds that her menses are not reestablished after cessation of the birth control pills. Galactorrhea may also be present. In general, longer periods of amenorrhea are associated with larger neoplasms. Serum prolactin is increased in patients with this neoplasm, in contrast to idiopathic galactorrhea, in which serum prolactin levels are normal. Men with prolactin-secreting pituitary neoplasms usually present with headache, impotence, and visual disturbances (Hebert and Breeding, 1979, Youmans, 1982).

Acromegaly. Acromegaly is due to excessive production of growth hormone after puberty. Oversecretion of growth hormone prior to puberty produces gigantism. Acromegaly produces findings of enlarged hands and feet, thickening and protrusion of the brow and jaw, and thickening and broadening of the lips and nose. These changes occur gradually over a period of years (Bleehan, 1986; Drayer et al., 1979).

If the growth hormone–producing tumor occurs after puberty, the epiphyses of the long bones have already fused with the shaft, and the person cannot grow taller. The soft tissues, however, do respond to this increase in growth hormone and continue to grow. This accounts for the thickening in the bones as well as the enlargements described earlier. Many other soft tissue organs may become enlarged as well, including the tongue, liver, and kidneys.

Neoplasms of the pituitary are usually removed through a transsphenoidal hypophysectomy (Fig. 37–2) or frontal craniotomy, proton beam therapy, or chemotherapy with bromocriptine. Because of the limited availability of proton beam therapy, this option is not often used. Bromocriptine therapy has not fulfilled the promise it demonstrated in early clinical trials (Youmans, 1982). Surgical excision through a frontal craniotomy is associated with high morbidity because it requires deep manipulation of the frontal lobes to accomplish the resection of the pituitary gland. The trans-sphenoidal approach has proved to be a simple procedure with fewer complications and a shorter hospital stay. Recent advances in microsurgery allow the surgeon to gain access to the sella via the nasal passages and sphenoid sinus. Because there is much less manipulation of neural tissues, the transsphenoidal approach is the procedure of choice when feasible (Salcman, 1985).

Other Neoplasms

Additional cranial neoplasms include teratomas, craniopharyngiomas and metastatic tumors. With the exception of metastases these are rare. The symptoms are dependent on the location of the neoplasm. The usual treatment of choice is surgical excision, but radiation and chemotherapy may be used when neoplasms have identified sensitivities to these interventions. Sometimes, especially with multiple metastases and poor quality of life, no treatment may be the preferred option. Treatments are chosen on the basis of accessibility, type of neoplasm, life expectancy, and quality of life.

SIGNS AND SYMPTOMS OF INTRACRANIAL NEOPLASMS

As stated earlier, space-occupying lesions cause their signs and symptoms through three mechanisms: compression, obstruction, and invasion, with increased pressure being the common product of all three. Symptoms vary with the location of the neoplasm and aid in identifying the location of the tumor, making it important for the nurse to be familiar with the cranial anatomy and neurophysiology. Knowing the location of the neoplasm allows the nurse to monitor the patient for appropriate indicators of tumor extension, associated complications, and response to therapy. Because some of these changes may be subtle, the more knowledgeable the nurse, the greater the chance for more comprehensive care of the patient in the intensive care unit.

Frontal Lobe Symptoms

Symptoms associated with pressure on the frontal lobe include changes in mentation and subtle changes in personality or mood. These may be reported by the patient's family as increased irritability, loss of inhibition, or inappropriate behavior (such as exhibitionism). In general, the patient is unaware that the behavior is inappropriate. These behaviors

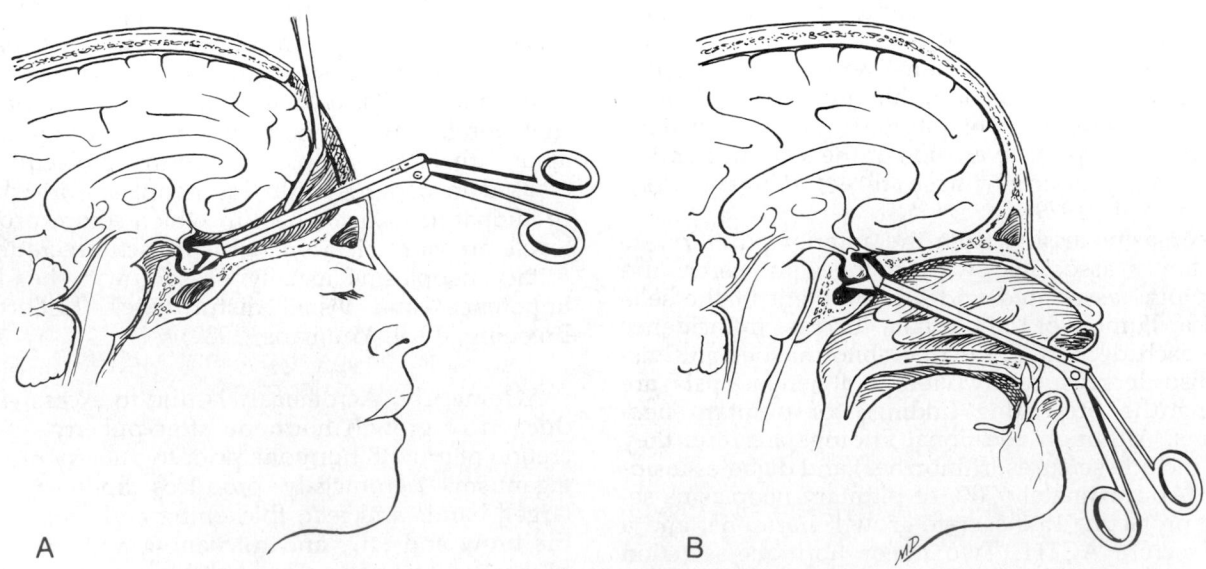

FIGURE 37–2. Pituitary surgery approaches. *A,* Transcranial. *B,* Trans-sphenoidal. (From Luckmann, J., and Sorensen, K. C. (1987). *Medical-surgical nursing: A psychophysiologic approach* (3rd ed., p. 528). Philadelphia: W.B. Saunders.)

may result from pressure on the inhibitory control center in the frontal lobe. The pressure may result from tumor growth, hemorrhage, or postoperative edema. If the behavior is associated with postoperative edema, resolution of the edema may result in return of normal behavior.

Pressure on the motor cortex results in motor deficits varying from weakness to severe and debilitating paralysis. Deficits may involve part or all of any of the extremities. Spasticity, flaccidity, and seizure activity may occur. Symptoms usually occur on the contralateral side of the neoplasm.

Involvement of Broca's motor speech center in the dominant hemisphere may result in aphasia. Aphasia may be partial or complete depending on the degree of pressure or neoplastic involvement.

Intellectual abilities may also be affected, including the ability to calculate, abstract, and make judgments. Apathy, dementia, and, more rarely, catatonia may also occur with temporal lobe neoplasms (Barnett et al., 1988; Hannegan, 1989).

Parietal Lobe Symptoms

Neoplasms of the parietal lobe may affect sensory stimulus processing. Abnormal testing response for extinction (loss of feeling to sensory stimulation) is often noted with parietal lobe involvement. Contralateral sensory paresthesias are common: tingling, numbness, burning, or anesthesia. Astereognosis (inability to recognize objects by feeling them) and loss of ability to localize stimuli may be noted. Since Broca's center extends into the parietal lobe of the dominant hemisphere, subtle difficulties with speech, reading, and writing may also be found. As with most neoplasms, seizure activity may occur (Chan and Thompson, 1984; Youmans, 1982).

Temporal Lobe Symptoms

Auditory disturbances are common findings with temporal lobe neoplasms, including tinnitus, auditory hallucinations, and distortion of sound. Visual hallucinations and feelings of deja vu may also occur with temporal lobe lesions. Psychomotor seizures with olfactory or auditory hallucinations, lip-smacking, chewing, or swallowing movements may be experienced by these patients. Other findings include unprovoked aggression and periods of amnesia (Adams and Victor, 1985; Youmans, 1982).

Occipital Lobe Symptoms

Defects in the visual field and other visual disturbances are the predominating findings for lesions involving the occipital lobe. Homonymous hemianopsia is the most common visual defect. Headaches may occasionally be identified as a complaint by patients.

Cerebellar Symptoms

The cerebellum is composed principally of ipsilateral pathways and functions that coordinate reflex and voluntary muscle activity. Symptoms of neoplasms involving the cerebellar area generally affect an entire limb and are manifested by poor coordination, unsteady gait, inability to maintain gait or posture, ataxia, tremor associated with fine motor function, and dysdiadochokinesia (inability to arrest one motor function and substitute it with a diametrically opposite motor impulse). Reflex function may be disturbed and tendon reflexes are prolonged. Nystagmus or ataxia of the eye muscles occurs as well as dysarthria causing slurred speech, jerky articulation, and explosive verbalizations.

Acute lesions of the cerebellum result in sudden, severe onset of symptoms and signs. Recovery may be complete, suggesting compensation by other areas of the central nervous system. Chronic lesions result in less severe symptoms than those of acute lesions, probably because of compensatory function.

The most common neoplasm of the vermis (midline cerebellum) is a medulloblastoma, which results in symptoms associated with the vestibular system. Muscle incoordination involves the head and trunk (instead of the extremities); the patient tends to fall backward or forward and has difficulty maintaining the head in an upright position (Bleehan, 1986).

It is important to note that cerebellar lesions do not result in paralysis or paresthesias. Although muscle hypotonia and incoordination are present, the disorder is not limited to specific muscle groups; rather, an entire extremity or entire half of the body is affected. Muscular contractions may be weak, and the patient is easily fatigued. This distinction aids in identifying the location of the lesion, and thus it is important to document associated symptoms carefully in the patient's record (Adams and Victor, 1985; Spritz, 1986; Youmans, 1982).

NEUROSURGICAL OPERATIVE PROCEDURES

Neurosurgical operative procedures may be grouped into the major classifications of craniotomy, transsphenoid procedures, laser surgery, and stereotaxic procedures (Ropper and Kennedy, 1988).

Craniotomy

Craniotomy for intracranial neoplasms and other lesions begins with an incision through the scalp, underlying muscle, and periosteum. This tissue is dissected away from the underlying skull in the form of a flap, and hemostasis is usually obtained with metal or plastic clips along the edge of the flap. The skull is usually entered first with large drill holes, called burr holes (Fig. 37–3). Burr holes alone may be used when the object of the craniotomy is to evacuate a hematoma, control superficial hemorrhage, perform a biopsy, drain an abscess, or place an intraventricular shunt. Burr holes may be made so that the bone is not replaced, in which case they are usually only 1 to 2 cm in diameter. Or larger burr holes may be made with the intention of replacing the bone, holding it in place with wire or heavy silk sutures at the end of the procedure. Larger burr holes may measure from 2 to 6 cm in diameter.

More extensive craniotomies are accomplished by making several burr holes (Fig. 37–4). These burr holes may be extended with a rongeur, or the bone between a series of drill holes may be separated from the remainder of the skull with a reciprocating saw or hand-held Gigli blade (a wire saw). The incised skull may be left attached to the overlying periosteum and muscle in a large craniotomy.

If the craniotomy is performed for a skull fracture, osteomyelitis, or neoplastic involvement of the skull, a craniectomy (removal of part of the cranium) may be necessary. Depending on the size of the bone removed, a cranioplasty may be performed. Cranioplasty involves replacement of excised bone with synthetic material (metal or plastic implants) or transplants of cadaver bone.

Once the craniotomy is performed, the underlying dura is carefully incised to allow access to the underlying brain. After the surgery is complete, the

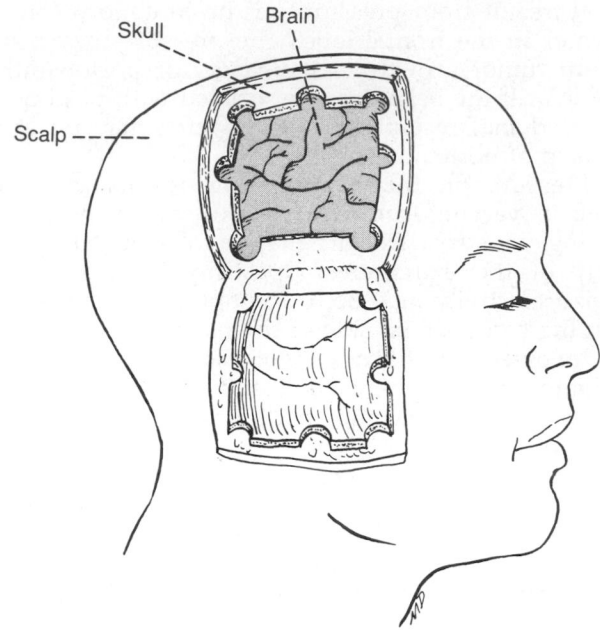

FIGURE 37–4. Craniotomy with osteoplastic bone flap. (From Luckmann, J., and Sorensen, K. C. (1987). *Medical-surgical nursing: A psychophysiologic approach* (3rd ed., p. 528). Philadelphia: W.B. Saunders.)

dura is sutured closed, and the cranial bone is replaced and held in place with sutures passing through small holes drilled in the surrounding bone and the flap. The periosteum and muscle are sutured in place, and the skin is either sutured or stapled closed. Depending on the type of surgery, drains may be left in place. Drains may be open (Penrose) or closed drainage systems with a plastic reservoir. Anatomic placement of the drains varies—i.e., they may be intracranial or extracranial. All drains should receive special care to prevent displacement or contamination.

Craniotomies are classified according to where they are made, i.e., frontal, temporal, parietal, occipital, or combinations of these (temporoparietal). Craniotomies may also be described as supratentorial (above the tentorium) or infratentorial (below the tentorium). Supratentorial craniotomies allow access to the cerebral hemispheres or midbrain, whereas infratentorial craniotomies provide an avenue to the cerebellum, medulla, or pons. Infratentorial procedures are most commonly accomplished via a suboccipital or posterior fossa approach (Fig. 37–5).

Some neurosurgical procedures, especially infratentorial approaches, are done with the patient in the barber chair position, i.e., sitting (Fig. 37–6). Because the head is higher than the heart and negative pressure is produced in the dural venous sinuses, these patients are at risk for air embolism. A central venous pressure (CVP) catheter may be inserted preoperatively to aspirate any air that enters during surgery. If air enters the venous system, it is rapidly carried to the heart where it produces a characteristic millwheel murmur. Treatment involves

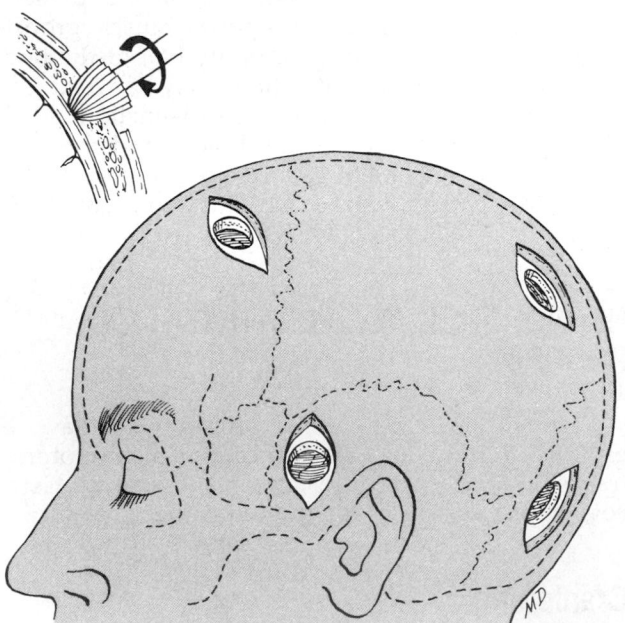

FIGURE 37–3. Placement of burr holes in the skull. (From Luckmann, J., and Sorensen, K. C. (1987). *Medical-surgical nursing: A psychophysiologic approach* (3rd ed., p. 510). Philadelphia: W.B. Saunders.)

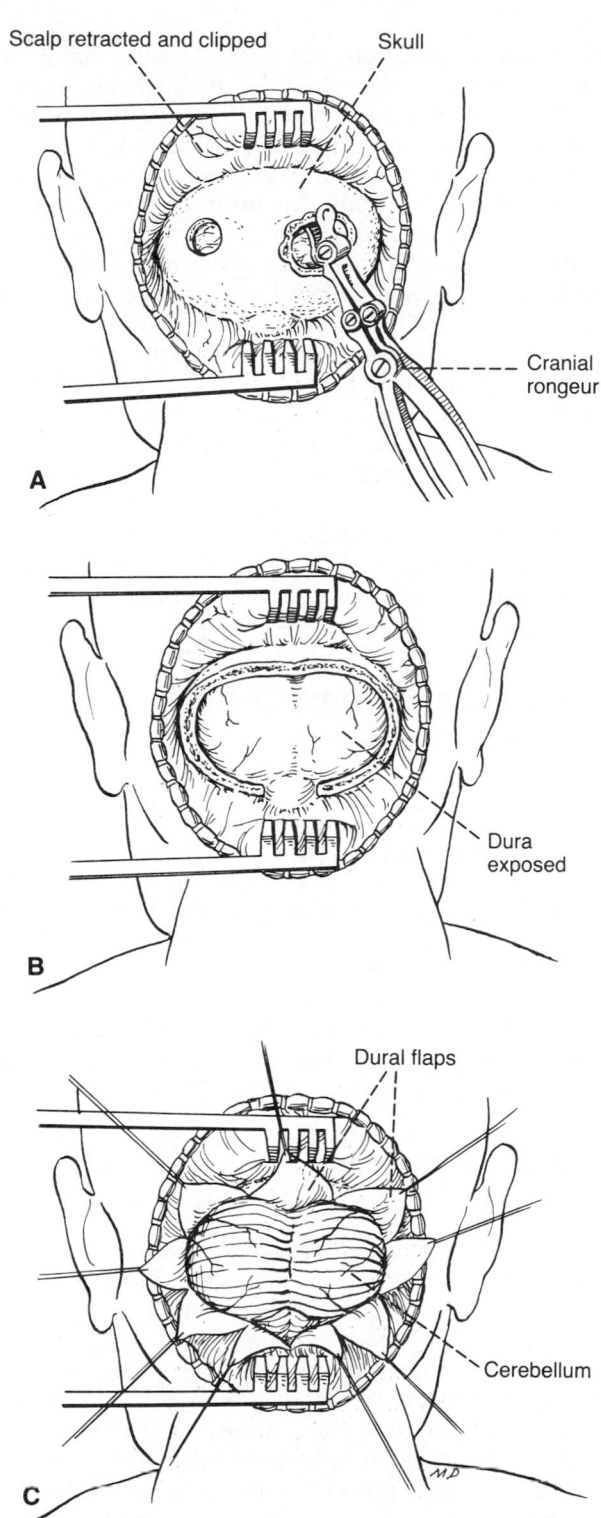

FIGURE 37–5. *A* to *C*, Suboccipital craniotomy. (From Luckmann, J., and Sorensen, K. C. (1987). *Medical-surgical nursing: A psychophysiologic approach* (3rd ed., p. 529). Philadelphia: W.B. Saunders.)

identifying and closing the source of the air leak and aspirating the air from the right atrium through the CVP catheter (Youmans, 1982).

Knowing the location of the craniotomy allows the nurse to determine the general area of the lesion,

which allows anticipation of possible deficits, complications, and the type of care needed by the patient postoperatively (Shapiro, 1982; Youmans, 1982).

Trans-sphenoidal Procedures

The trans-sphenoidal approach is used mainly to gain access to the pituitary gland. Transsphenoidal surgery may be used to resect pituitary adenomas, control metastatic bone pain via hypophysectomy, or aid in the removal of craniopharyngiomas. The incision is made through the upper gum and extended into both sides of the nasal septum (Fig. 37–1). Posterior dissection leads to the floor of the sphenoid sinus. Removal of the floor of this sinus allows access to the sella turcica, which is entered, and then the dura is entered. Specially created microinstruments are used by means of a microscope to perform the surgery. Closure involves harvesting a small muscle graft from the anterior thigh to patch the dura. The gum is sutured closed and the nasal septum is packed with petrolatum gauze. The donor site on the thigh is dressed with a dry sterile pressure dressing (Harris and Park, 1976; Youmans, 1982).

Stereotaxic Surgery

Stereotaxis involves the use of three-dimensional coordinates derived from the use of special frames. Use of stereotaxis allows precise targeting of a lesion for biopsy or resection deep within the brain with minimal trauma to surrounding and overlying brain. Once the frame has been placed on the patient, the three-dimensional coordinates (X, Y, and Z) for the target area are identified in relation to the frame. The target area has been pinpointed with a computed tomography (CT) scan. Using the referents of the frame, the neurosurgeon guides an electrode or

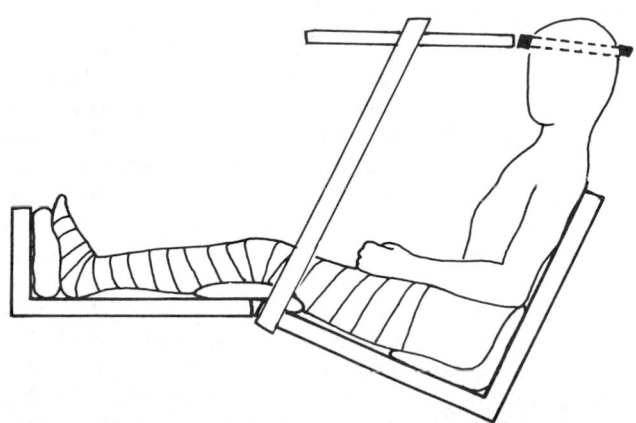

FIGURE 37–6. Sitting position. (Reproduced by permission from: Kneedler, J. A., and Dodge, G. H. *Perioperative patient care: The nursing perspective* (2nd ed., p. 472). Boston, 1987, Blackwell Scientific Publications; copyrighted by The C.V. Mosby Co., St. Louis.)

microinstrument to the target tissue. Positioning is verified by x-ray or, preferably, CT scan. Once the correct position is ensured, the surgeon performs the procedure.

Stereotaxic surgery has been used for resection or biopsy of small subcortical neoplasms deep within the brain, and it is promoted for use in aspirating intracranial hematomas, abscesses, and cystic lesions; for controlling chronic pain through placement of electrodes; for placing radiotherapeutic agents in the area of a neoplasm; and for treating extrapyramidal symptoms with ablative procedures (Ropper and Kennedy, 1988; Youmans, 1982).

Laser Surgery

In laser surgery a source of light energy intensely amplified into a narrow beam of monochromatic light is used to focus precisely on a specific tissue. As the tissue absorbs the light it is transformed into thermal energy, which vaporizes the tissue and provides hemostasis. The laser allows the neurosurgeon to use microsurgical techniques to identify and apply the laser to tissues requiring resection with minimal disruption of surrounding tissues. Thus, laser surgery allows the neurosurgeon to perform surgery on previously inaccessible areas of the brain and spinal cord (Salcman, 1985; Youmans, 1982).

NURSING CARE OF THE POSTOPERATIVE CRANIOTOMY PATIENT

The outcome in patients undergoing craniotomy is highly dependent on the nursing care provided, especially in the intensive care unit (Arsenault, 1985; Hebert and Breeding, 1979; Ropper and Kennedy, 1988). The following nursing diagnoses are helpful for the nurse caring for patients after a craniotomy.

Ineffective Airway Clearance

Poor airway clearance may be due to altered consciousness or neurologic deficit. The important thing is that the patient maintain a patent airway throughout the convalescent period to prevent hypoxic insult to the brain. Breath sounds should be auscultated hourly and more frequently if needed. Abnormalities such as wheezing, rhonchi, rales, and any decreased sounds should be noted. Any changes, either increases or decreases, should also be noted, as should dyspnea or cyanosis.

The conscious patient should be instructed in deep breathing and encouraged to change position at least hourly. Coughing should be avoided in the early postoperative period and in any patient who continues to be at risk for or demonstrates elevated intracranial pressure. Alignment of the head and neck promotes venous flow. Elevating the head of the bed to between 30 and 40 degrees facilitates respirations and decreases intracranial pressure (note: this meas-

ure is not appropriate for patients who have had posterior fossa surgery). The unconscious patient should not be placed supine but turned regularly on each side to facilitate drainage of secretions. When in the side-lying position, the head must be kept in alignment with the body. Suctioning should be done when necessary, keeping in mind that suctioning greatly increases intracranial pressure. The patient should be hyperoxygenated before and after each suctioning period, and actual suctioning time should be limited to 10 seconds. The patient must be assessed very carefully for signs of increased intracranial pressure during and after suctioning. If signs occur, the nurse should immediately hyperventilate the patient until the pressure returns to baseline. Sound nursing judgment is required for the decision to suction a patient who is at risk for increased intracranial pressure. Blood gas values must be monitored, and hypoxemia and hypercapnia reported to the physician.

Impaired Gas Exchange Due to Hypercapnia

The expected outcome of care is maintenance of the patient's arterial oxygen and carbon dioxide levels within normal limits; any changes are to be reported immediately. Tidal volumes must be monitored also when the patient is being mechanically ventilated. Before and after suctioning the patient should be hyperinflated with 100% oxygen. Unless contraindicated, the head of the bed should be kept elevated. Supplemental oxygen therapy is often part of preventive care for this nursing diagnosis.

Cognitive Impairment

Cognitive impairment may be due to neurologic impairment or deficit. The degree of impairment should be identified and the safety of the patient ensured until the patient regains the ability to care for himself. It is most important for the nurse to explain consistently what is going to be done and what is being done to the patient, even if the patient appears unconscious. Often the patient is able to hear but cannot respond or communicate. Repeat the information frequently and expect a shorter attention span as well as problems with retention of information. Maintain the patient's dignity at all times and call patients by name, not by demeaning terms such as "honey" and "sweetheart." Instruct the patient in rehabilitation activities and continually promote patient involvement in care as well as encouraging family involvement. Assess patient safety needs and ensure that safety measures are routinely instituted—side rails up, frequent observation, minimal restraint required to prevent injury.

Altered Cerebral Tissue Perfusion

Tissue perfusion may be altered by increased intracranial pressure from cerebral edema, cerebral hypoxia, hypercarbia, cerebral vasospasm, or intracranial hemorrhage. The hoped-for outcome is that intracranial pressure does not increase and remains within normal values (0 to 15 mm Hg). The patient will not manifest any symptoms of increasing intracranial pressure such as changes in level of consciousness (as subtle as irritability or as obvious as lethargy), any pupillary changes, changes in motor or sensory ability, headache, or nausea. Vital sign changes, it must be remembered, are *late* changes and generally signify extreme pressure. By the time bradycardia or widening pulse pressure is seen, it is too late for successful intervention. Because of the subtlety of many of the changes signifying alterations in cerebral perfusion, frequent and thorough assessments are of the utmost importance. Assessments at least hourly are conducted during the first 36 hours postoperatively. Abnormal findings in the assessment include restlessness, confusion, irritability, decreasing level of consciousness, motor or sensory deficits, headache, changes in pupil size, shape, or response, changes in vital signs, and any comments from family that indicate that the patient is " not himself." Abnormal findings should be reported promptly to the physician.

Nursing interventions include spacing activities to allow for adequate rest and maintaining the head of the bed at an elevation of 30 to 45 degrees unless contraindicated (as in patients with posterior fossa surgery). Strict fluid intake and output records must be kept, and fluid intake should be restricted when ordered. Adequate oxygenation must be maintained and suctioning performed only when absolutely necessary. Hyperventilate as necessary for increasing ICP. Prevention or control of events known to elevate ICP will greatly reduce the occurrence of increased ICP. These actions include the Valsalva maneuver, pain, hypercapnia, and talking about the patient at the bedside (especially when he or she appears unconscious). Careful observation of the ICP monitor and correlation of these findings with the patient's physical status is required, as is detection of trends rather than separate notations of ICP. If the pressure remains within normal limits but the trend has been from 3 mm Hg to 11 mm Hg during the shift, a rise in ICP is indicated and physician notification is required.

Self-Care Deficit Due to Neurologic Impairment or Deficit

The nurse must ensure that the patient's basic needs are met until the patient regains the ability for self-care. Assessment of deficits and impairment is accomplished early in the postoperative period, and interventions are developed specifically to aid the patient and family in correcting or compensating for these deficits. Assistance is provided as necessary until the patient is able to care for himself. Families are incorporated into the care of the patient with the caveat that they realize the importance of not "doing for" but rather assisting the patient to do for himself. Set realistic goals for the patient and reevaluate them as necessary. Do not talk down to the patient; treat patients with respect and call them by name.

Potential for Physical Injury

Cognitive or neurologic impairment or deficit may lead to injury. The desired outcome is that the patient does not incur physical injury while hospitalized. To ensure this, the nurse must regularly assess the safety needs of the patient, updating them as necessary. Side rails should always be kept up, and the bed should be in its low position. If restraints are indicated, they should be used judiciously and this should be documented. Patient and family should be instructed in appropriate safety measures and the rationale for their use.

Alteration in Comfort: Headache Due to Surgery

During the first 24 hours postoperatively it is expected that the patient will experience pain. Medication should be given at regular intervals during this time period. When the patient is fully recovered from the anesthesia, pain status should be frequently assessed. In less than fully conscious patients, signs such as restlessness, movement of hands toward the incision site, and grimacing should be taken as signs of pain. Analgesics are administered as needed. Generally, these will include codeine, aspirin, or Tylenol because these do not mask neurologic signs. Morphine may be given early in the postoperative period, but care must be taken because, like most pain medications, it will mask signs of neurologic deterioration.

Potential for Fluid Loss or Retention

Fluid status may change due to diabetes insipidus (DI), especially following pituitary surgery, or to the syndrome of inappropriate secretion of antidiuretic hormone (SIADH). Meticulous intake and output measurements are made and documented to anticipate or correct any fluid deficit, thereby maintaining normal fluid balance. Serum and urinary osmolality must be monitored and alterations reported promptly to the physician. Daily weights and determination of urine specific gravity will assist in determining any fluid imbalance; however, other signs or symptoms may occur first, such as increased or decreased urine output, poor skin turgor, and changes in osmolality. Replace or restrict fluid as directed by the physician.

Potential for Electrolyte Imbalance Due to Fluid Loss or Effects of Surgery

Of particular importance is sodium balance because of the release of arterial natriuretic factor during neurosurgery. Serum and urinary reports must be monitored and abnormalities and trends reported to the physician. The patient also must be monitored for indicators of electrolyte imbalance. Meticulous intake and output records must be kept and replacement therapy performed as indicated.

Alteration in Self-Image Due to Shaving Hair

Of great importance, especially to women patients, is waking up to find their hair gone. Most women are not permitted to wear a wig for several weeks following surgery to decrease the risk of infection to the incision. Loose scarves should be offered to the patient, and time should be set aside to assist her in using them becomingly. Offering light hand mirrors for use in applying make-up may also assist the patient in feeling more self-confident about her looks. Allowing time for the patient to talk about her looks and her apprehensions about returning to the "outside" while without hair is important in the nursing care of the craniotomy patient. The patient should not be made to feel that her hair is of no importance but instead helped to realize that her feminine image is manifested in other ways as well.

Alteration in Nutrition

Nutrition may be altered due to increased needs following surgery or altered level of consciousness. Adequate nutrition may be maintained as demonstrated by normal serum protein and lymphocyte counts. These counts should be monitored and alterations reported to the physician. The patient's nutritional intake should be monitored and documented. A nutrition consultation may be requested early in the postoperative period for semiconscious and unconscious patients who are unable to maintain their own nutritional needs. If intake is questionable, calorie counts may be performed.

Constipation

Constipation may exist due to altered diet, the effect of medications, and inadequate fluid intake. It is desirable for the patient to maintain the normal bowel elimination pattern without straining (straining will increase intracranial pressure). Determine the patient's preoperative bowel elimination pattern and monitor the patient for peristalsis and frequency of bowel movements. Provide the patient with a psyllium hydrophilic mucilloid and a stool softener daily. For patients (if conscious) who are unable to establish a regular elimination pattern, provide a cup of warm fluid to drink to stimulate gastrocolic or duodenocolic reflexes every other day at the same time of day. If this is unsuccessful or if the patient is semiconscious or unconscious, a glycerine suppository is inserted and digital stimulation of the internal anal sphincter is provided. If this is also unsuccessful, a laxative or bisacodyl suppository may be required. Use of a bowel regimen makes it possible to establish bowel continence. Avoid the use of enemas, which dilate the rectum and sigmoid colon. Digital disimpaction may occasionally be necessary.

See also Chapter 33 for discussion of the following nursing diagnoses:

Potential for injury: from joint contractures due to muscle weakness, paresis, or immobility

Potential for impaired skin integrity: due to sensory and motor deficit following cerebrovascular insult

Ineffective family coping: compromised or disabling due to the overwhelming aspects of cerebrovascular events on the family

Impaired verbal communications: due to dysarthria, aphasia, or altered mental status

Total incontinence: due to loss of cerebral control due to cerebrovascular events

Partial self-care deficit: due to partial loss of motor function

Knowledge deficit: of the therapy and how much the patient and family are expected to participate in care

The outcome of therapy following craniotomy depends in large part on the nursing care provided postoperatively. Appropriate assessments and interventions minimize neurologic deficits, reduce potential complications, and maximize the potential for an uneventful recovery. The critical care nurse needs to monitor carefully and identify the subtle signs of increasing intracranial pressure, changing levels of consciousness, and indicators of deterioration. Changes in vital signs are generally late indications of problems and emphasize the need for critical care nurses to identify the early physical signs of deterioration.

The nurse must rely on a knowledge of neuroanatomy and physiology, clinical signs and symptoms, and nursing interventions to care appropriately for these patients. Because of the lack of specific monitors for these functions, the postoperative craniotomy patient presents a special challenge for the critical care nurse. It is the nurse who identifies trends, correlates monitor readings with physical findings, and intervenes to prevent complications or progression toward an uneventful recovery.

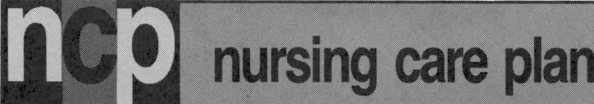 nursing care plan

1. Ineffective airway clearance related to:
Altered consciousness or neurologic deficit

Outcome Criteria	Nursing Interventions
Patent airway is maintained.	Auscultate breath sounds hourly or more frequently as needed and note any abnormality or changes. Instruct conscious patients to deep breathe and change position at least hourly. Caution patient against coughing. Maintain alignment of head and neck. Elevate the head of the bed to between 30 and 40 degrees, except for patients with posterior fossa surgery. Turn unconscious patients side to side and avoid supine positions to facilitate drainage or secretions. Suction only when needed and provide hyperoxygenation before and after each suctioning period. Limit actual suction time to 10 seconds and carefully monitor for signs of increased intracranial pressure during and after suctioning. If signs of increased intracranial pressure occur, hyperventilate patient until intracranial pressure returns to baseline. Monitor blood gas values and report hypoxemia or hypercapnia to the physician.

2. Impaired gas exchange related to:
Hypercapnia

Outcome Criteria	Nursing Interventions
Patient's arterial oxygen and carbon dioxide levels are maintained within normal limits.	Monitor arterial oxygen and carbon dioxide levels and report any changes immediately. If mechanically ventilated, monitor tidal volume. Provide hyperinflation with 100% oxygen before and after suctioning. Keep the head of the bed elevated unless contraindicated.

3. Cognitive impairment related to:
Neurologic impairment or deficit

Outcome Criteria	Nursing Interventions
The degree of impairment will be identified. The patient's safety will be ensured until he is able to care for himself.	Consistently explain current and future interventions, even if patient appears to be unconscious. Repeat information frequently and expect shorter attention span and problems with retention of information. Maintain patient's dignity at all times. Use patient's name and avoid demeaning terms such as "Honey" and "Sweetheart." Instruct patient in rehabilitation activities Continually promote patient and family involvement in care. Assess patient safety needs and ensure that safety measures are routinely instituted, such as side rails up, frequent observation, minimal restraints.

4. Altered cerebral tissue perfusion related to:
Increased intracranial pressure Cerebral vasospasm
Cerebral edema Intracranial hemorrhage
Cerebral hypoxia Paresthesia
Hypercapnia

Outcome Criteria	Nursing Interventions
Cerebral perfusion pressure at least 50 mm Hg. Intracranial pressure remains within normal range (less than 15 mm Hg).	Conduct assessments for increased intracranial pressure at least hourly for the first 36 hours postoperatively and report any abnormal findings or changes to the physician promptly. Space activities to allow for adequate rest. Maintain the head of the bed at 30 to 45 degrees unless contraindicated. Maintain strict fluid intake and output records. Restrict fluid intake. Maintain adequate oxygenation and suction only when needed. Hyperventilate as needed for increasing intracranial pressure. Prevent or control events known to increase intracranial pressure, such as Valsalva maneuver, pain, hypercapnia, and talking about the patient at the bedside. Carefully observe the ICP monitor to detect trends rather than separate notations.

Nursing Care Plan continued on following page

5. Self-care deficit related to:
Neurologic impairment or deficit

Outcome Criteria	Nursing Interventions
Patient's basic needs are met until patient regains ability for self-care.	Assess deficits and impairment early in the postoperative period. Develop interventions to aid patient and family in correcting or compensating for deficits. Post exercise schedule and encourage patient and family participation. Provide assistance as needed until the patient is able to care for himself. Incorporate family members into patient's care and point out need to help patient do for himself rather than "doing for" the patient. Set realistic goals and reevaluate as necessary. Treat patients with respect, using their names. Avoid "talking down" to patients.

6. Potential physical injury related to:
Cognitive impairment
Neurologic impairment or deficit

Outcome Criteria	Nursing Interventions
Patient does not incur physical injury while hospitalized.	Regularly assess the safety needs of the patient, updating interventions as necessary. Keep side rails up and the bed in low position. Use restraints judiciously. If used, document their use. Instruct patient and family members about appropriate safety measures and the rationale for their use.

7. Altered comfort: headache related to:
Surgery

Outcome Criteria	Nursing Interventions
Pain's frequency and intensity will decrease.	Provide analgesic at regular intervals during the first 24 hours postoperatively. Frequently assess patient's pain when he or she is fully recovered from anesthesia. In patients who are not fully conscious, consider restlessness, movement of hands toward the incision, and grimacing to be signs of pain. Administer codeine, aspirin, or acetaminophen as needed. Reserve morphine for the early postoperative period.

8. Potential electrolyte imbalance related to:
Fluid loss
Effects of surgery

Outcome Criteria	Nursing Interventions
Electrolytes will be maintained within normal limits.	Monitor serum and urinary electrolyte values. Report trends and abnormalities to the physician. Monitor signs of electrolyte imbalance. Maintain meticulous intake and output records and perform replacement therapy as indicated.

9. Altered self-image related to:
Shaving of hair

Outcome Criteria	Nursing Interventions
Patient will verbalize feelings and apprehensions regarding self-image.	Allow time for patient to talk about his looks and returning to the "outside." Offer loose scarves or caps and assist in their placement. Offer light hand mirror for use in applying make-up. Avoid minimizing the importance of hair, but help patients realize other ways that their image is maintained.

10. Altered nutrition related to:
Increased needs following surgery
Altered level of consciousness.

Outcome Criteria	Nursing Interventions
Adequate nutrition will be maintained as demonstrated by normal serum albumin level and total lymphocyte count.	Monitor serum albumin level and total lymphocyte count. Report alterations to the physician. Monitor and document patient's nutritional intake. Consider a nutrition consultation early in the postoperative period for semiconscious and unconscious patients. Perform calorie counts if intake is questionable.

11. Constipation related to:
Altered diet
Immobility
Medications
Decrease fluid intake

Outcome Criteria	Nursing Interventions
Patient will maintain normal bowel elimination pattern without straining.	Determine the patient's preoperative bowel elimination pattern. Assess for peristalsis and frequency of bowel movements. Provide psyllium hydrophilic mucilloid and stool softener daily. For conscious patients unable to establish a regular elimination pattern, provide a cup of warm fluid every other day at the same time of day. Administer a glycerin suppository and provide digital stimulation of the internal anal sphincter if necessary. Administer laxative or bisacodyl suppository if necessary. Avoid the use of enemas.

References

Adams, R. D., and Victor, M. (1985). *Principles of neurology.* New York: McGraw-Hill.

Arsenault, L. (1985). Selected postoperative complications of cranial surgery. *Journal of Neurosurgical Nursing,* 17 (3), 155–163.

Bailey, P., and Bucy, P.C. (1929). Oligodendrogliomas of the brain. *Journal of Pathologic Bacteriology,* 32, 735.

Bailey , P., and Cushing, H. (1926). *A classification of tumors of the glioma group on a histogenetic basis with a correlated study of prognosis.* Philadelphia: J.B. Lippincott.

Barnett, G., Ropper, A., and Romeo, J. H. (1988). Intracranial pressure and outcome in adult encephalitis. *Journal of Neurosurgery,* 68(4), 585.

Bauman, C. K., and Zumwalt, C. B. (1989). Intracranial neoplasms: An overview. *AORN Journal,* 50(2), 240–255.

Bellur, S. N., Chandra, V., and McDonald, L. W. (1979). Association of meningiomas with extraneural primary malignancy. *Neurology,* 29; 1165.

Berkshire, J., and Watson-Evans, H. (1989). Meningioma: A nursing perspective. *Journal of Neuroscience Nursing,* 21(2), 96–103.

Bleehan, N. (1986). *Tumors of the brain.* New York: Springer-Verlag, 1986.

Chan, R. C., and Thompson, G. B. (1984). Morbidity, morality, and quality of life following surgery for intracranial meningiomas. *Journal of Neurosurgery,* 60, 52–60.

Cogan, D. G. (1974). Tumors of the optic nerve. In P. J. Vinken, and G.W. Bruyn (Eds.), *Handbook of clinical neurology* (Vol. 17). Amsterdam, North-Holland.

Cushing, H., and Eisenhardt, L. (1962). *Meningiomas.* New York: Hafner.

Davis, K. R., Parker, S. W., and New, P. F. J. (1977). Computed tomography of acoustic neuroma. *Radiology,* 124, 81.

Drayer, B., Kattah, J., Rosenbaum, A., et al. (1979). Diagnostic approaches to pituitary adenomas. *Neurology,* 29, 161.

Fokes, E. C., Jr., and Earle, K. N. (1969). Ependymomas: Clinical and pathological aspects. *Journal of Neurosurgery,* 30, 585.

Frankel, S. A., and German, W. J. (1969). Glioblastoma multiforme: A review of 219 cases with regard to natural history, pathology, diagnostic methods and history. *Journal of Neurosurgery,* 30, 585.

Gerke, M. (1980). Identifying brain tumors. *Journal of Neurosurgical Nursing,* 12(2), 103–205.

Hannegan, L. (1989). Transient cognitive changes after craniotomy. *Journal of Neuroscience Nursing,* 21(3), 165–170.

Harner, S. G., and Laws, E. R. (1983). Clinical findings in patients with acoustic neurinoma. *Mayo Clinic Proceedings,* 58, 721.

Harris, L., and Park, E. (1976). Transsphenoidal approach to pituitary adenomas. *AORN Journal,* 23(6), 989.

Harper, C. G., and Stewart-Wynne, E. G. (1978). Malignant gliomas in adults. *Archives of Neurology,* 35, 731.

Hebert, P., and Breeding, P. (1979). Self-care after hypophysectomy. *Journal of Neurosurgical Nursing,* 11(2), 118.

Klatzo, I. (1967). Neuropathological aspects of brain edema. *Journal of Neuropathology and Expimental Neurology,* 26, 1.

Martuza, R. L., and Ojemann, R. G. (1982). Bilateral acoustic neuromas: Clinical aspects, pathogenesis and treatment. *Neurosurgery,* 10, 1.

Ropper, A. H., and Kennedy, S. F.(1988). *Neurological and neurosurgical intensive care* (2nd ed.) Rockville, MD: Aspen.

Salcman, M. (1985). The morbidity and mortality of brain tumors: A perspective on recent advances in therapy. *Neurologic Clinics,* 3 (2), 229–257.

Shapiro, W. R. (1982). Treatment of neuroectodermal brain tumors. *Annals of Neurology,* 12, 231.

Spritz, D. W. (1986). Brain tumor basics. *Critical Care Nurse,* 6(5), 94–96.

Walker, R. W., and Posner, J. B. (1984). Central nervous system neoplasms. In S.H. Appel (Ed.), *Current neurology,* (Vol. 5), New York: Wiley.

Weir, B., and Elvidge, A. R. (1968). Oligodendrogliomas: An analysis of 63 cases. *Journal of Neurosurgery,* 29, 500.

Youmans, J. R. (1982). *Neurological surgery* (3rd ed., Vols. 4 and 5). Philadelphia: W. B. Saunders.

Zimmerman, H. M. (1969). Brain tumors: Their incidence and classification in man and their experimental production. *Annals of the New York Academy of Science,* 159, 337.

Zulch, K. J. (1986). *Brain tumors: Their biology and pathology.* New York: Springer-Verlag.

38

Patients with Pain

Geraldine M. Goosen
Virginia A. Rahr

Pain management in the critically ill patient is a continuous challenge to the critical care nurse due to the complexity and diversity of patients in the critical care unit. Additionally, pain management is complicated by the fact that the nurse frequently causes discomfort yet is responsible for assessing and managing the pain of discomfort. Ability to address this perplexing issue requires a clear understanding of pain mechanisms as well as a knowledge of current, safe, and effective management modalities. The following chapter provides comprehensive information requisite for the critical care nurse to minister therapeutically and successfully to the pain management needs of the critically ill patient.

HISTORICAL EVENTS OF PAIN IN THE CRITICALLY ILL

Chronology of Key Contributions to the Concept of Pain

Recognition and descriptions of pain are as old as humanity. Reference to pain is evidenced in ancient writings, artworks, songs, and poetry and in Biblical writings that included terms such as "travail" and "suffering," which were associated with sickness and plagues, as well as responses such as "weeping" and "wailing" of individuals. Treatments included the use of herbs, concoctions, mandragora root, opium, and distraction. Cousins and Phillips (1986) provide a comprehensive listing of international resources of events relating to and contributions to the concept of pain from 1564 to the beginning of critical care medicine in 1950. It is important to note that the quantity of the literature devoted to some aspect of pain cannot be equated with the amount of suffering experienced by humans over time. In the past decade

the focus on pain research has provided the critical care nurse with exciting new information derived from the discovery of opiate receptors, extensive pharmacokinetic and pharmacodynamic studies of narcotics and their actions, the development of sensitive analytic techniques and mathematical knowledge, the development of new drugs and combinations of drugs, and novel methods of administration such as intraspinal narcotic therapy (Bonica, 1987). In spite of these advances, the search continues for effective ways to provide individual comfort in the safest possible manner, paying particular attention to individual needs.

Some ambiguities associated with pain assessment and management are reflected in the varied and broad definitions of pain. For example, Liebeskind (1977) stated that "Pain means many different things, and the variables which correlate with, inhibit or enhance one kind of pain, and the neural mechanisms which underlie it, may not be associated with or influence other kinds" (p. 41). Mersky (1975) defined pain as "an unpleasant experience which we primarily associate with tissue damage or describe in terms of tissue damage or hurt" (p. 6).

Although Meinhart and McCaffery (1983) agree with the need for a working definition and understanding of terms associated with pain, their major premise is that the individual experiencing pain is the true authority. Therefore, the authors follow an operational definition of pain. "Pain is whatever the experiencing person says it is, existing whenever he or she says it does" (p. 11).

The International Association for the Study of Pain defines pain as "an unpleasant sensory and emotional experience associated with actual or potential tissue damage, or described in terms of such damage" (Mersky, 1979). Pain is the most common symptom reported with disease or injury and the most aversive stimulus noted for altering behavior. Pain is viewed as a protective mechanism because individuals will withdraw from or avoid the source of pain, which may cause additional tissue damage, and is frequently the symptom that directs the individual to seek assistance for an illness or disease process. In general, pain is regarded as a signal of tissue injury, although injury can occur without pain, and pain can occur in the absence of injury or remain after healing or cure has occurred (Muir, 1988).

Cultural Factors Associated with Pain

Pain is a highly personal and variable experience that is influenced by cultural learning, by the meaning of the situation, and by attention and other cognitive activities (Sternbach and Tursky, 1965). Melzack (1973) considers pain a complex, perceptual, and affective experience determined by the unique past history of the individual, by the meaning of the stimulus to him, by his "state of mind" at the moment, and by the sensory nerve patterns evoked by physical stimulation.

Individual response to pain is believed to be due to a *sensation threshold*, which is defined as the lowest stimulus value at which sensation is first reported; *pain tolerance level* which is the point at which the subject refuses to tolerate further pain and withdraws from the stimulus; and *pain response*, which includes attitudes, emotions, attentiveness to painful sensations, and behaviors in which these orientations are displayed (Hardy, et al., 1952; Sternbach and Tursky, 1965).

Initial attempts to relate cultural aspects such as religion, ethnicity, race, age, and sex to pain were reported in the 1950s. Cultural components known to influence response to pain include occupation, socioeconomic status, family relationships, whether curative or palliative treatment is sought, to whom the pain is reported, and what types of pain require attention (Hardy, et al., 1952; Zborowski, 1952; Meinhart and McCaffery, 1983).

Cultural traditions dictate to members of a given society not only whether they should expect and tolerate pain but also the correct response to the pain experience. The rules may vary with sex, age, and social status, but because people in a society usually comply with the cultural rules, it is important to have a working knowledge of these rules when caring for the patient. The best source of information is the patient or the family. The American family is typically a supportive unit that becomes particularly concerned during a family member's illness or injury. This is evident by observation of the numbers of family members and friends in intensive care unit waiting rooms. Although there may be some cultural variations, in general, regardless of cultural affiliation, family members surround the suffering individual. Family members are especially attentive to the patient experiencing pain and focus on that aspect of illness. Pain is a recognizable and more familiar

symptom of the illness that family members can discuss and about which they can seek information. Because of the family's ongoing involvement with the patient's painful experience, these individuals can serve as a resource for information about the patient's previous pain response and coping ability. Family members or friends can serve as supports to the patient during extreme pain episodes. The ability of family members to support the patient during pain episodes may well correlate with the amount of teaching and interaction that develops between them and the critical care nurse (Edwards et al., 1985).

Cognitive activities associated with cultural values, anxiety, attention, and suggestion have a profound effect on the pain experience. There is evidence that the sensory input is localized, identified in terms of its physical properties, and evaluated in terms of past experience with the sensation (Sternbach, 1978). It is generally understood that cognitive processes are of critical importance in determining the nature of the pain experience. Individuals experiencing pain tend to interpret the source and personal meaning of the pain in terms of the immediate environment, their past history, and the future implications of any injury or disease.

In summary, the influence of cultural values on the response to and expression of pain is well established in the literature (Zola, 1966; Koopman et al., 1984; Lipton and Marbach, 1984), yet in actual practice, there is little evidence that cultural factors are included in diagnostic and therapeutic activities (Good and Good, 1980; Bates, 1987). Attention to individual cultural facets by the critical care nurse when assessing and managing pain can only enhance the management outcome. The ability of the nurse to recognize and suppress prejudice toward and stereotyping of different cultural beliefs and behavior is reflected in planning and caring for the critically ill patient without evidence of judgmental principles.

Psychological Factors Associated with Pain

Psychological factors such as affect, anxiety, anger, guilt, and depression are believed to alter the perception and response to acute pain. From documented reports, research findings, and experience, there is much evidence that psychological factors may cause pain, can frequently augment its severity, and may also serve to diminish or abolish pain in the presence of extensive physical trauma.

Even though discussion continues in regard to somatogenic pain and psychogenic pain, most references acknowledge that pain is a combination of mental and physical events. Psychogenic pain is usually defined as a discrepancy between the physical findings and the amount of pain reported or pain behavior observed (Sternbach, 1978). Support for the occurrence of psychogenic pain is presented in studies that show positive findings of hysterical neuroses or conversion hysteria, the state resulting from unconscious emotional conflicts originating in the past and hypochondriac pain, neuroses characterized by a preoccupation with the body and a constant fear of disease or malfunction of the body.

Psychological or cortical processes of attention, past experience with pain, and the meaning of the situation may exert considerable influence on the perception of painful stimuli. Pavlov's experiments with dogs, later applied to humans, support the concept that the meaning of the stimulus acquired during earlier conditioning modulates the sensory input before it activates brain processes that underlie perception and response. Attention to the stimulation also contributes to the intensity of pain experienced. This is evident in people engaged in sports or battle who may be seriously injured but do not perceive the injury until later or not at all (Beecher, 1959). The environment may serve as a distraction; conversely, if the person's attention is focused on a potentially painful experience, that individual will tend to perceive pain more intensely than he would under normal conditions (Hall and Strider, 1954).

Clinical experience and research yield inconclusive and sometimes contradictory results about the effects of anxiety upon pain and whether identified anxiety is wholly associated with pain or with other factors such as culture and socioeconomic status (Barak and Weisenberg, 1988). Although there are exceptions, increasing anxiety about pain increases the perceived intensity of pain, whereas reduction in anxiety decreases the perception of pain. Paradoxically, in some instances pain decreased while anxiety related to a specific situation temporarily increased (Sternbach, 1978). Modification of anxiety associated with the pain experience is considered an important theoretical basis for pain relief measures. Therefore, it is important to note the suspected interplay between anxiety and pain relief, especially when mild to moderate anxiety is associated with an episode of acute pain. During the anticipation of pain, relief for the impending pain may be enhanced if the patient has knowledge of the existing or anticipated pain, experiences a moderate amount of anxiety, and can channel the anxiety into methods of coping with pain. When a pain sensation is felt, reduction of anxiety tends to decrease the perceived intensity of the sensation or increase the tolerance for pain (Janis, 1958). The nurse's ability to promote pain relief could be enhanced by awareness that a moderate level of anxiety should be derived from the patient's knowledge of what may actually occur and only a minimal amount of anxiety should be derived from the threat of the unknown or a threat to self-concept. Studies have documented preoperative anxiety as a predictor of postoperative pain (Parbook et al., 1973; Scott et al., 1983).

Some degree of sadness and anger often accompany acute pain. Patients may express unhappiness or perhaps anger due to the illness or pain. They may be angry with themselves for doing something foolish or careless that led to the pain, or angry with the physician or nurse for failure to take steps that the patient believes could have prevented pain. Anger and sadness consume physical and mental energy. Theoretically, relief from anger and sadness will enable the patient to experience less pain, to handle pain more efficiently, and to increase tolerance to pain.

The functionally impaired, acutely ill patient is often saddened or depressed by his condition. In this instance, depression is a product of the pain problem. Anxiety that accompanies acute pain eventually becomes less prominent and is replaced by reactive depression. This depression has many possible characteristics, such as sleep and appetite disturbances, decreased physical and social activity, forgetfulness, mental dullness, irritability, and suicidal thoughts (Sternbach, 1974).

Intensive Care Unit Techniques Contributing to the Pain Experience

Within the organization of the modern hospital there is a political arena with certain ground rules and expectations. The body of the patient is viewed as the battleground against disease in which many activities, including pain, occur. Physicians and nurses make most of the rules that prevail in this interactional context. There are specific routines and work rhythms to which the staff adhere and to which the patient must conform and adapt. In a series of interviews with intensive care unit (ICU) patients 1 week following discharge, the common complaints noted were pain, sleeplessness, physiotherapy, noise, handling, and movement. More than 50% of the patients claimed to remember little about the ICU, but of those who did, pain, lights, noise, boredom, and nursing procedures were of greatest concern (Puntillo, 1988). The combination of fear, pain, anxiety, sleep deprivation, unpleasant physical surroundings, absence of day and night cycles, and other physical and psychological patient problems can cause a severe paranoid confusional decompensation that can magnify mildly painful procedures (Jones et al., 1979; Cousins and Phillips, 1986).

The ICU is viewed as a specialized area that is very different from other wards and units. The environment is usually efficiently organized and reflects ample staff, highly technical equipment, numerous and powerful drugs, critically ill patients (many close to death), continuous monitoring of vital signs, and perpetual activity. Many times the bustle of activity is directed toward insertion of wires or intravenous lines to monitor or support the body during a life-threatening insult. In addition, managing and maintaining these lines and devices causes discomfort and pressure that is usually perceived as pain by the patient. Restraining or limiting arm motion may be necessary to keep a delirious patient from removing vital tubes. This adds to the frustration, anxiety, and fear associated with painful stimuli. In this predominantly technical environment the nurse must continue to remember that the patient is a recipient of procedures and techniques that can be painful.

Critically ill patients commonly have two major sources of pain—the illness, injury, or treatment that brought them to the ICU, and the iatrogenic treatment that occurs while they are residents in the ICU. When nurses and physicians recognize various procedures and techniques as painful, they can prepare the patient with accurate information in addition to pain relief measures. Analgesia should be given one-half hour before any painful procedure. Additionally, the patient should be instructed in pain control strategies such as the relaxation response, imagery, and distraction.

The mechanically ventilated patient presents an extra management challenge in decreasing pain and anxiety. Many times the fear and discomfort associated with ventilation and suctioning are perceived as pain and can be adequately managed with relaxants such as diazepam (Cousins and Phillips, 1986). The interaction of unfamiliar technical devices, sounds, and lights, compounded by decreased ambient temperature and invasive procedures, create an alien environment and experience for ICU patients and can produce a significant stress response. As noted earlier, the relationship between pain and stress is somewhat unclear, but clinical observations while managing ICU patients indicate that administration of muscle relaxants and tranquilizers to diminish stress in addition to analgesics will enhance the response obtained from the use of analgesics alone (Puntillo, 1988).

Pain Syndromes Common to the Critically Ill

Most clinicians differentiate between acute pain and chronic pain. *Acute pain* is related to a known or well-defined cause, follows a predictable course, and is self-limiting and correctable. When healing is completed, the pain usually disappears. Acute pain has a rapid onset, varies in length, and includes phasic and tonic components. The phasic component is of short duration and occurs at the onset of pain. Patients tend to withdraw actively from the pain source during the phasic component. The tonic component varies in length and continues until healing has occurred. Reaction to pain results in response patterns that are usually protective in nature and help to restore the individual's natural equilibrium. Reflex muscle spasm and automatic splinting at a fracture site, and avoidance of foods that would increase the pain of a stomach ulcer are examples of response to acute pain. In clinical situations, acute pain generally represents either a symptom of a disease condition or a temporary aspect of treatment. In both cases, patients and health care professionals expect to have pain alleviated (Craig, 1984).

Chronic pain may begin as acute pain with the tonic component lasting far beyond the healing time. Some pain clinicians and researchers believe that chronic pain is the result of inadequately or poorly managed acute pain. Chronic pain may also begin as a low level input and continue for extended periods of time despite intervention. It is believed that chronic pain may incorporate neural mechanisms that are more complex than acute pain and involve adjacent body areas (Melzack and Dennis, 1978). Chronic pain becomes a constant companion, even when intermittent. Individuals with chronic pain may be admitted to the ICU for acute problems, requiring the nurse to consider the presence of both acute and chronic pain.

Two additional terms that are appearing more frequently in the literature are *intractable* and *deafferentation*. Intractable pain is viewed as unmanageable or untreatable pain. The goal is to change intractable pain to tractable pain so that it can be treated. Deafferentation refers to discomfort arising in any part of the body where the flow of afferent nervous impulses has been partially or completely interrupted (Tasker, 1984). This term is frequently used synonymously with *phantom limb pain*. Different types of pain distribution are expressed by patients; these may include reflex, dystrophy, or perverse reaction to stimuli. Patients who undergo amputation of a body part commonly experience a phantom sensation reflecting the presence of the body part at varying times postoperatively. For some individuals, the sensation may be distorted or painful. Formation of neuromas and a central mechanism may be instrumental in causing distorted sensations.

Phantom sensations may also occur with mastectomies, cosmetic surgery of the nose and other parts of the body, tooth extraction, amputation of the tongue, penis, or scrotum, and enucleation. Children who have a congenital amputation or are undergoing an amputation before the age of 6 usually do not experience phantom sensations, possibly due to the general instability of the mnemonic process of the brain, causing the phantom limb to be forgotten rapidly, or the presence of an immature body image at the time of amputation (Jensen and Rasmussen, 1984).

Additional studies have been done on phantom sensations in parts of the body that are surgically removed. Preoperative pain commonly involves concentrated areas of sensory nerves such as the palm, knuckles, tips of the fingers, thumb, instep of the foot, heels, and toes. Postoperatively, these areas are frequent sites of phantom pain. Because an estimated 450,000 amputees are now living in the United States, phantom pain should be viewed as a major clinical problem (Stein and Warfield, 1982).

Pain syndromes, described according to their general location in the body, may be superficial or cutaneous, deep visceral, deep somatic, ischemic, referred, or radiating. Patients may experience one, all, or any combination of these pain syndromes while in the ICU. *Superficial pain* usually refers to pain in the skin and mucous membranes and is described as sharp, pricking, or burning. *Deep pain* is divided into splanchnic and deep somatic, with splanchnic pain referring to the viscera, and deep somatic pain involving structures other than the viscera. *Ischemic pain* results from inadequate tissue oxygenation and occurs when metabolic substances or end products of cell degeneration accumulate in the tissues and come in contact with nerve endings (Phillips and Cousins, 1986). *Referred pain* is present in an area that is removed or distant from the point of origin (Fig. 38–1), and *radiating pain* reflects extension from the site of origin (Procacci and Zoppi, 1984). Further description regarding pathways and fibers involved in these pain syndromes will be discussed in relation to pathophysiology.

The interaction among complex illness, body response, and treatment variables in ICU patients has the potential to excite all known pain receptors—mechanical, thermal, and chemical. Mechanosensitive pain receptors are excited by excessive mechanical stress or damage to the tissues. Thermosensitive pain receptors react to extremes of heat or cold, and chemosensitive receptors are excited by bradykinin, serotonin, histamine, potassium ions, acids, prostaglandins, acetylcholine, and proteolytic enzymes. Cell damage can result from direct trauma or when the blood supply is interrupted to an area, resulting in accumulation of lactic acid from altered metabolism. Muscle spasm and pressure associated with clinical syndromes, medications, and immobility

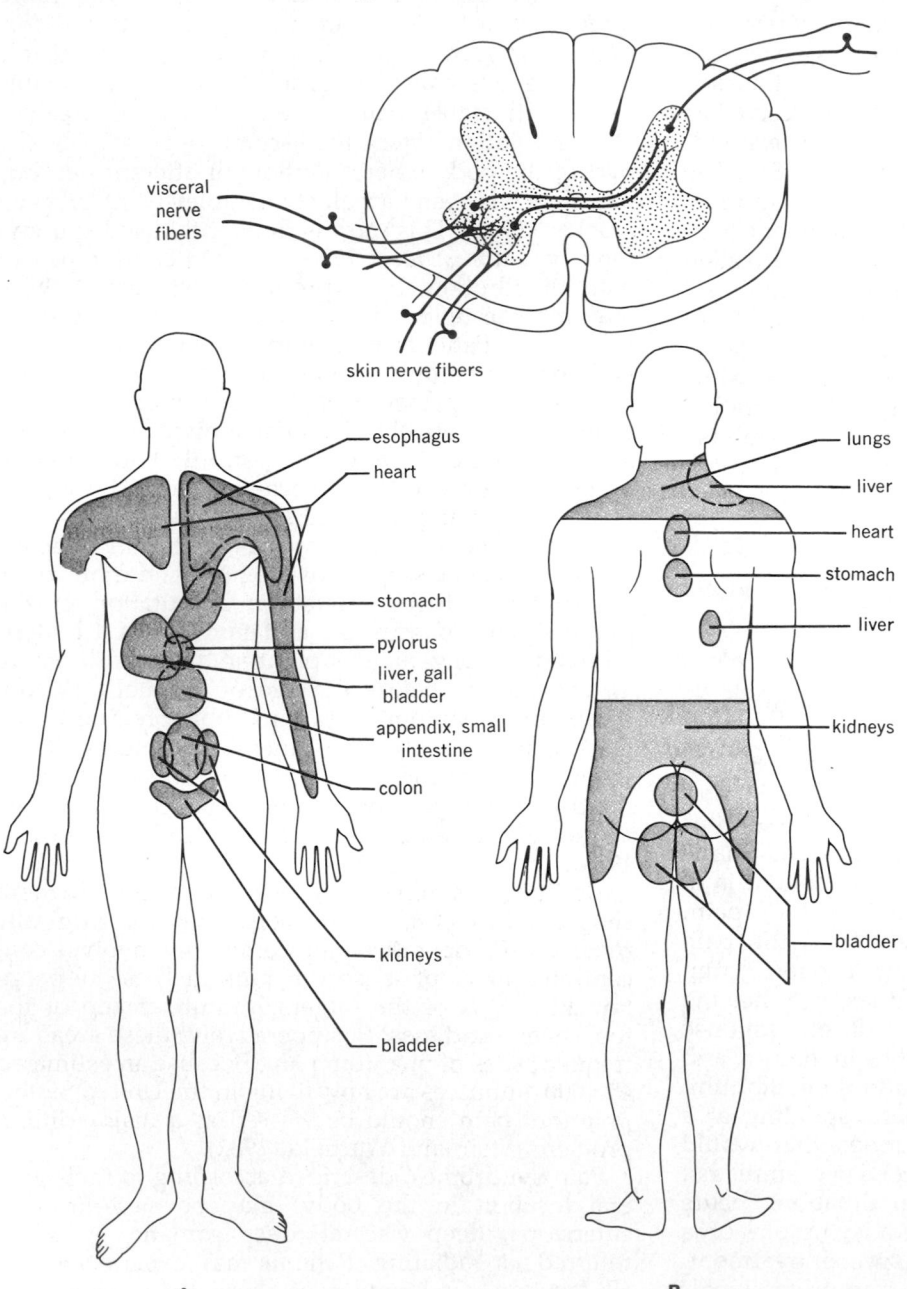

FIGURE 38–1. *A* and *B,* Referred pain. (From Silverstein, A. (1983). *Human anatomy and physiology* (2nd ed., p. 300). New York: John Wiley & Sons.)

stimulate mechanosensitive pain receptors and account for much of the discomfort experienced by the critically ill patient (Cousins and Phillips, 1986).

Cost and Dehumanization of Pain

Pain is more than a hurt and sometimes can become a way of life. The reaction to pain, which is extremely complex, is the determining factor in the outcome of pain. The toll of pain in terms of cost, utilization of energy, human suffering, and unhappiness is remarkable and totally undeterminable. In addition, the effect of pain on other body systems is a major concern for the critically ill patient. In the United States alone, pain affects between 60 and 70 million individuals. Lost wages, medical and other costs incurred for pain relief, disability compensation benefits, and court judgments cost approximately $70 billion in 1981 (Bonica, 1987). Therefore, critically ill patients who have suffered much pain may have some carryover to everyday life. Attitudes toward pain may affect job situations, personal relationships, and future development and creativity as well as feelings about health, illness, and treatment.

THEORIES OF PAIN

The concept of "theory based practice" is not foreign to modern critical care nurses nor to the area of pain assessment and management. Even though there is no consensus about which theories are most useful, existing theories provide guidance for clinical practice. Each theorist individually addresses cultural, affective, physiological, and/or psychological parameters. Currently, the emphasis is on underlying theories, reflecting a holistic construct. Melzack (1975) identified four guidelines that could serve to evaluate the merit of past and future theories. His view was that any new theory of pain must be able to account for four factors:

1. The high degree of physiological specification of receptor fiber units and of pathways in the central nervous system (CNS).
2. The role of temporal and spatial patterning in the transmission of information in the nervous system.
3. The influence of psychological processes on pain perception and response.
4. The clinical phenomena of spatial and temporal summation, spread of pain, and persistence of pain after healing (p. 153).

Although these guidelines were proposed nearly 15 years ago, they remain applicable today.

Affect Theory of Pain

The affect theory dates back to Aristotle and considers pain an emotion that colors all sensory events.

Aristotle described as painful both listening to badly played music and bereavement. Sherrington (1900) proposed that affective tone is an attribute of all sensation; skin pain is an example of an attribute of sensation. Titchener (1909) added the view that pain and unpleasantness were on a continuum. Even though he believed that a continuum of feeling was different from one of sensation, he did not explain the link between affect, unpleasantness, and pain (Melzack, 1973).

Specificity Theory

Specificity theory, the first reflection of a physiologic basis for pain, is the traditional theory still utilized in some medical and graduate schools (Bates, 1987). In general, it proposes that pain is a specific sensation that is proportional to the extent of tissue damage. The theory, first presented by Descartes in 1644, implies a fixed transmission system running straight through from a mosaic of somatic pain receptors to a pain center in the brain (Sternbach, 1978).

Von Frey extended the physiologic component of the specificity theory by using existing information from Muller, Helmholtz, and Volkmann to identify four types of sensory input: touch, cold, warmth, and pain. Von Frey further linked newly identified tissue types with the four types of sensations. Consequently, Meissner corpuscles are identified as touch receptors, Krause end-bulbs are cold receptors, Ruffini end-organs are warmth receptors, and Pacinian corpuscles detect pressure (Melzack, 1973). The sensorial end-organ is an apparatus by which an afferent nerve fiber is rendered amenable to some particular physical agent and simultaneously less amenable to other excitants.

A refinement of the original specificity theory was necessary when two different types and sizes of nerve fibers, the A delta epsilon fibers and the C fibers, were discovered to be involved in pain transmission. Each pathway is responsible for a different pain sensation. The A delta epsilon system, termed the epicritic pain pathway, is responsible for a sharp, pricking type of pain, carried via the lateral spinothalamic tract. The slower C fibers carry a burning type of pain called protopathic, which becomes more severe when stimulation of this pathway, due to summation, remains repetitive. This pathway is believed to be carried on the ventral spinothalamic tract. With this elaboration of neuroanatomy and physiology, neurosurgeons could become more precise in applying techniques of pain alleviation such as nerve blocks, tractotomies, sympathectomies, posterior rhizotomies, and cordotomies (Melzack, 1973).

Pattern Theory

As evidence mounted to refute the specificity theory, several new theories, presented by Goldschnei-

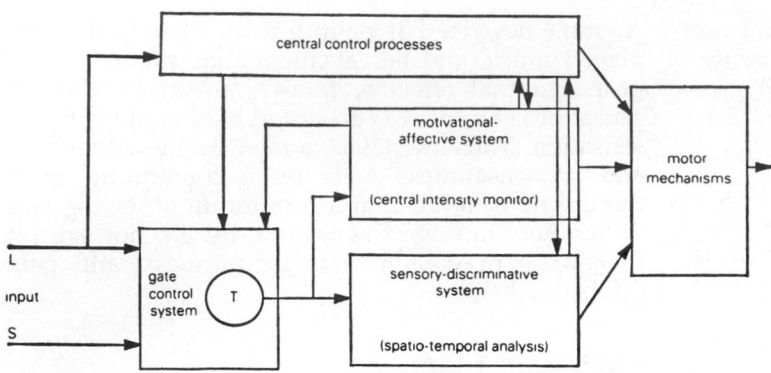

FIGURE 38–2. Conceptual model of gate control theory. (From Melzack, R., and Casey, K. L. (1988). In D. Kenshele (Ed.), *The skin senses.* Courtesy of Charles C Thomas, Publisher, Springfield, Illinois.)

der, Nafe, Livingston, and Noordenbos, were grouped into a pattern theory. Through studies of patients with syphilis, Goldschneider proposed that stimulus intensity and central summation are the critical determinants of pain. Pain sensation becomes cumulative, and the response increases as time increases. Goldschneider believed that the large cutaneous fibers comprise a specific touch system, whereas the smaller fibers converge on dorsal horn cells in the spinal cord that summate their input and transmit the pattern to the brain. Pain results when the total input goes beyond a certain level due to excessive stimulation or pathologic conditions (Melzack, 1973). The peripheral pattern component simply implies that excessive peripheral stimulation produces nerve impulses that are interpreted centrally as pain (Nafe, 1934). The sensory interaction theory, derived from Goldschneider's original beliefs, further proposes that a rapidly conducting firing system inhibits synaptic transmission from a more slowly conducting system.

Livingston (1943) proposed that intense pathologic stimulation of the body sets up reverberating circuits in spinal pools that can be triggered by normally non-noxious inputs and generate abnormal volleys that are interpreted centrally as pain. This theory is credited with explaining such central phenomena as causalgia and phantom pain because a central pat-

terning of impulse flow creates a "painful memory" for the patient. Amputation of a limb or healing of a peripheral nerve injury does not withdraw the peripheral stimulus. Instead, a fixed pattern is locked in the central structures, that cannot be modified because no normal sensory input from the original source is possible.

Noordenbos (1959) made an important contribution to concepts of sensory interaction. He viewed the small fibers as carriers of the nerve impulse pattern that produces pain and the large fibers as those that inhibit transmission. A shift in ratio of large to small fibers with an increase in small fibers would result in excessive pain.

The composite pattern theory holds that there are no specific pain pathways or nerve endings, and the sensation of pain does not depend on one pathway or two but on the total central projection system. Pain perception is related to the intensity of the stimulus and the summation of all impulses, so that when a hypersynchronization of impulse volleys occurs all at once, the individual interprets this sensation as pain (Melzack, 1975).

Gate Control Theory

The gate control theory utilizes and extends the principles presented in the pattern theory (Figs. 38–2 and 38–3). Pain perception is believed to be the result of both central and peripheral inputs that act upon a "gate" that controls transmission of impulses to the pain centers of the thalamus and cerebral cortex. Peripheral input occurs from the two types of fibers described in the pattern theory, large and small fibers. Large fibers are the rapidly conducting A-alpha and A-beta fibers, which inhibit transmission of impulses through the central transmission (T) cells in the dorsal horn (close the gate). To close the gate to pain, A fiber input must predominate, and this can be achieved by introducing touch, pressure, or thermal stimuli. These peripheral impulses are always subject to modification by emotion, experience (memory), and other cortical functions. Large diam-

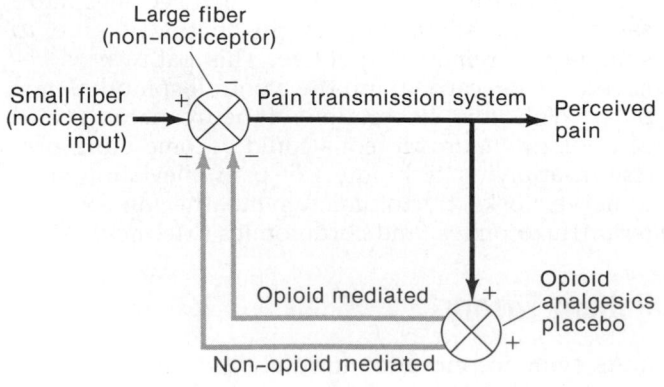

FIGURE 38–3. Pain modulation system(s).

eter fibers transmit impulses by way of the dorsal column of the spinal cord to a central control site in the brain; the central control triggers selective cognitive processes that then influence the gate-control mechanism by way of descending fibers.

Small-diameter, slowly conducting fibers are A-delta and C fibers, which facilitate transmission of impulses to the T cells, leading to perception of pain (open the gate). The gate is located in a portion of the dorsal column of the spinal cord at each segmental level called the substantia gelatinosa (SG). When the gate is open, impulses are transmitted to an action system in the brain. To open this gate to pain perception, a predominance of C fiber input must prevail. When the amount of information that passes through the gate exceeds a critical level, neural areas such as the brain stem reticular formation, thalamus, hypothalamus, limbic system, and cerebral cortex are activated; these are responsible for pain experience and response (Melzack and Wall, 1965).

The substantia gelatinosa seems to be the key in this theory because it receives axion terminals from many of the large- and small-diameter afferent fibers. The dendrites of cells in deeper laminae project into the gelatinosa. The SG consists of a highly specialized, closed system of cells throughout the length of the spinal cord. Melzack and Wall (1965) proposed that it acts as a spinal gating mechanism by modulating the conduction of nerve impulses from peripheral fibers to transmission cells in the spinal cord.

Melzack and Wall (1965, 1970) suggested that sensory fibers transmit patterned information about pressure, temperature, and chemical changes at the skin, depending on the specialized properties of each receptor fiber unit. These temporal and spatial patterns of nerve impulses have two effects at the dorsal horns: They excite the spinal cord T cells that transmit the information to the brain, and they activate the SG, which modulates or "gates" the amount of information projected to the brain by the T cells.

There are two ways in which the cells of the substantia gelatinosa can act as a gating mechanism that influences the transmission of impulses from afferent fiber terminals to spinal cord cells (Melzack and Wall, 1970). They can act directly on the presynaptic axon terminals, thereby blocking the impulses in the terminals or decreasing the amount of transmitter substance they release, or they can act postsynaptically on the spinal transmission cells by increasing or decreasing their level of excitability to arriving nerve impulses. Melzack and Wall (1965) proposed that the effect is primarily presynaptic. Hongo and colleagues (1968) supported the idea that modulating effects are exerted postsynaptically on the spinal transmission cells.

The reticular formation exerts a powerful inhibitory control over information projected by the gate control system. This central control system acts very rapidly in identifying, evaluating, and selectively modifying the sensory input and also clearly interacts with the action system when the output of the T cells exceeds a certain critical level, (Melzack, 1973). When the

output reaches or exceeds a critical level, the T cell output is transmitted to the reticular and cortical projection subsystems. Activation of the reticular structure underlies the motivational drive of unpleasant effects that triggers the organism into action toward escape or attack. Selection and modulation of sensory input through the cortical projection subsystem provide sensory discriminative information about the location, magnitude, and spatiotemporal characteristics of the noxious stimulus.

Behaviorist Theory

Because the behaviorist theory has greater meaning for chronic pain, only the key points that are pertinent to pain in the critically ill patient will be included here. Lazarus (1977) stated, "of course, nearly everyone will agree that the only way we can know anything about another person is through his behavior" (p. 553). It is through pain behavior that pain is recognized and interpreted by clinicians. Behaviors may include verbal descriptors, splinting, increase in heart rate, limping, rubbing a body part, sweaty palms, grimacing, or other overt expression. Behaviors have meaning both for the person demonstrating them and for the observer.

Skinner introduced two terms that are seen in literature related to pain: respondent and operant. *Respondents* are actions that occur in response to antecedent stimuli. The stimulus may be internal, external or reflexive in nature. A typical respondent may include glandular or smooth muscle action. *Operants* are actions of the organism that are overt or visible/audible and thereby have an effect on or with the environment. An operant is usually followed by reinforcement that will influence future behavior (Fordyce, 1978).

Endogenous Opiate Theory

Discovery of endogenous opiates in 1965 provided new knowledge about and clarification of existing pain theories. Viewed as neurophysiologic, biochemical substances associated with pain, endogenous opiates became the target of numerous research activities. Clarification of their role as neurotransmitters, neuromodulators, or neuroregulators is based on the knowledge that stimulation of known pain pathways produces analgesia. Enkephalins, small peptide molecules, and beta-endorphin, a large peptide involving long sequences of amino acids, are responsive to pain sensation and adaptation. According to this discovery, the body manufactures opiate-like substances to provide pain relief at specific receptor sites in the CNS. These substances are similar in effect to morphine and react at receptor sites to inactivate pain sensations. Enkephalins are found in the caudate nucleus, the periaqueductal gray matter, the anterior hypothalamus, and the substantia gelatinosa. Because of their relatively simple structure, enkephalins have a rapid-acting effect that terminates in about 2 minutes. Enkephalins appear to be neurotransmitters because they are found in the medial and intralaminar nuclei of the thalamus and in other areas of the brain involved with nociception. Enkephalins have an inhibitory effect on neurons that transmit impulses concerned with nociception. They also inhibit the release of substance P and other neuroregulators (Hokfelt et al., 1980).

Beta-endorphin is found in the pituitary gland, hypothalamus, and amygdala and has an effect of 4 hours or longer. A larger pain or stress stimulus is needed to generate the beta-endorphin response than the enkephalin response (Bloom et al., 1978; Terenius, 1981; Woods et al., 1982). Beta-endorphin and adrenocorticotropic hormone (ACTH) are synthesized together as one large molecule that is subsequently cleaved to produce the two substances. It has been postulated that the interaction between ACTH and beta-endorphin has a modulatory role that cannot function if exogenous opiates are chronically given (Jacquet, 1979). Both of these substances are released in response to stress. These substances, like morphine, can become addictive. As endogenous substances, however, the result of addiction may be expressed as the behavior of seeking specific stress- or pain-generating conditions. The example cited most often is the exercise fanatic who chooses to exercise for very long periods on a daily basis. It may be true that people with chronic or intractable pain are "addicted" to their pain through the beta-endorphin mechanism. Thus, although the role of these substances is pain alleviation, the interpretation chosen by such patients is the inappropriate one of seeking continued pain (Carr et al., 1981).

This summary of common pain theories is given in an attempt to explain the complex nature of pain and to increase our understanding of how pain occurs. Each approach is unique and lends insight into this phenomenal, complicated body response that is experienced by virtually everyone during his or her lifetime. It is evident from the brief data presented that the gate control theory is more sophisticated than the other theories because it attempts to incorporate bio-psycho-social components in addition to providing some explanation for variations in pain management. However, it is important to note that controversy exists about the value of the gate control theory because the activity proposed in the gating process has not been clearly identified. Discovery and acquisition of new knowledge about endogenous opiates continue to support the gate control theory and further explain some of the relationships within it. Current research and literature on pain commonly reflect the use of the gate control theory as a theoretical framework because it is the most comprehensive description of the pain process available. Knowledge of the available theories is requisite for each clinician. Following careful analysis of each theory, selection of one theory to guide and direct the clinical assessment, management, and evaluation of the pain experience will assist the critical care nurse to provide the best possible care to patients.

PATHOPHYSIOLOGY OF PAIN

Continued acquisition of new knowledge and insights into the neuroendocrine system allow greater understanding of the mechanism and pathophysiology of pain. Comprehension of nociception, pain receptors, pain pathways, pain centers, and biochemical mediators of pain will provide the critical care nurse with the background information required to assess and manage the specific type of pain experienced by each patient.

Relationship of Nociception to Perceived Pain

Nociceptors are widely branching, unencapsulated, free nerve endings that are found in varying amounts in all body tissues and respond to chemical, mechanical, and thermal stimulation. Areas of high nociceptor concentration include subcutaneous tissue, periosteum, deep fascia, ligaments, joint capsules, and the cornea; few are found in muscle and hardly any in bone and cartilage (DiGregorio et al., 1986; Chapman, 1988). Pain is produced when strong noxious stimuli such as heat, extreme cold, and mechanical injury excite these receptors. At weaker intensities, these stimuli may produce other somatic sensations, e.g., warmth, cold, and pressure. In skin and deep tissue, nociceptors typically react to burns, the severe pressure of crush, and cutting, whereas those in the viscera tolerate such stimuli but respond instead to stretch or distention (Chapman, 1988). The process of pain perception that depends on the transmission of electrical impulses from the site of tissue injury in the periphery to higher centers in the brain is termed nociception.

Primary afferent neuronal fibers transport impulses from nociceptors into the CNS and are classified into three groups based on their cross-sectional area and speed of conduction: A fibers are the largest and most rapid conducting, C fibers are the smallest and the slowest conducting, and B fibers are in between. A fibers include rapidly conducting myelinated A-alpha and A-beta plus the smaller, more slowly conducting A-delta fibers. The A-alpha and A-beta fibers innervate sensitive (low threshold) mechanoreceptors that are involved with proprioception and sensations of touch and light pressure. A-delta fibers are surrounded only by a thin myelin sheath and transmit impulses at a rate of 6 to 30 milliseconds. They are distributed primarily to the skin and mucous membranes. About 10% to 25% of A-delta fibers respond to a strong stimulus, producing a fast, sharp,

Posterior (dorsal)

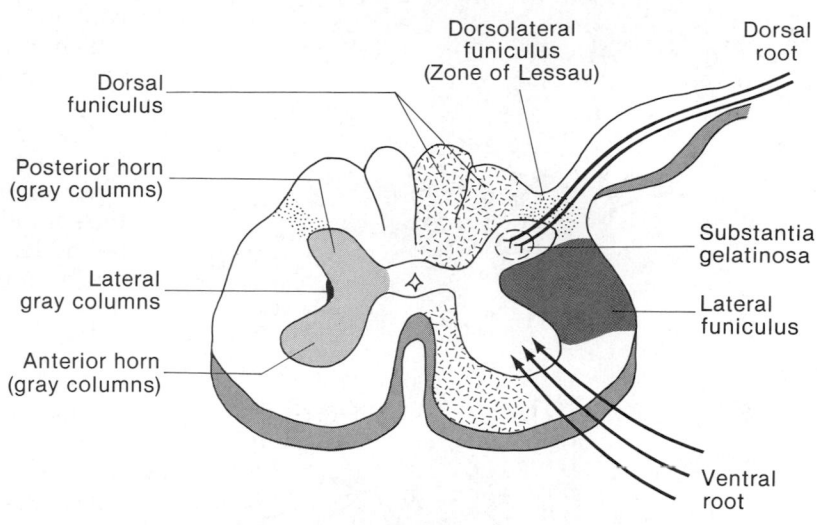

FIGURE 38–4. Cross section of spinal cord.

easily localized pain. These fibers may also respond to a cooling sensation (Guyton, 1991).

C fibers are the smallest fibers and, like some A-delta fibers, may respond to more than one type of stimulus (polymodal). About 50% to 70% of C fibers transmit pain impulses. These neurons are unmyelinated, conduct more slowly (0.5 to 2 milliseconds), and are responsible for duller, more prolonged pain (Guyton, 1991). This longer-lasting pain is associated with somatic and autonomic reflexes, usually sympathetic in nature (i.e., cardiac acceleration, peripheral vasoconstriction, pupillary dilatation, and sweating).

Both A-delta and C fibers innervate nociceptors and are involved with pain sensation, but they can also respond to innocuous stimuli such as warmth. A-delta and C fibers have high thresholds to mechanical and thermal stimuli. Unlike most types of receptors, which become less responsive when subjected to continued stimulation, nociceptors remain sensitive (nociceptors do not adapt to prolonged stimulation). Therefore, following trauma, pain persists. In fact, repetitive stimulation of nociceptors may lower the receptor threshold, causing increased sensitivity to noxious stimuli (hyperalgesia) (Muir, 1988).

Nociceptive units are now classified as high threshold mechanoreceptor units (HTMs), polymodal nociceptor units (PMNs), and multireceptive neurons, or wide dynamic range cells (WDR). HTM units are believed to be composed mostly of A-delta fibers, responding to strong pressure applied to a discrete point spread over an area of skin that can exceed 1 cm^2. There is a slow adaptation response to pressure. PMN units are predominantly C fibers that are excited by a range of irritant chemicals and have a slowly adapting response to firm pressure. Response to heat will accelerate with increasing skin temperature (Lynn, 1984). The role of WDR cells is unclear, but they are believed to respond to both noxious and non-noxious cutaneous or visceral stimuli. Activity in the dorsal horn suggests that these cells may provide more precise information about the noxious stimulus such as intensity, location, and quality (Zimmerman, 1984).

Physiologic Parameters of Pain

Primary (first-order) peripheral afferent neurons transmit impulses to the central nervous system, entering the spinal cord at various lamina levels in the dorsal roots, and forming cell bodies in the dorsal root ganglia (Fig. 38–4). The nerves bifurcate, and two processes extend from the cell body, one peripheral process terminating distally in a body tissue receptor and the central process terminating in the brain or spinal cord. This latter primary afferent neuron may terminate in the marginal layer (lamina I), substantia gelatinosa (lamina II and III), lamina V, and, to a smaller extent, lamina IV (Jacox, 1977). At this point, the message is transmitted to secondary neurons, most of which cross the midline and enter the lateral spinothalamic tract. Some ipsilateral tracts also exist. The dorsal horn acts as the site through which descending pathways modulate pain (Fig. 38–5) (Christensen and Perl, 1970; DiGregorio et al., 1986).

Transmission Pathways

Ascending and descending pathways have been identified in the literature and play a role in pain transmission. The naming and activity of these pathways vary from reference to reference, as does their

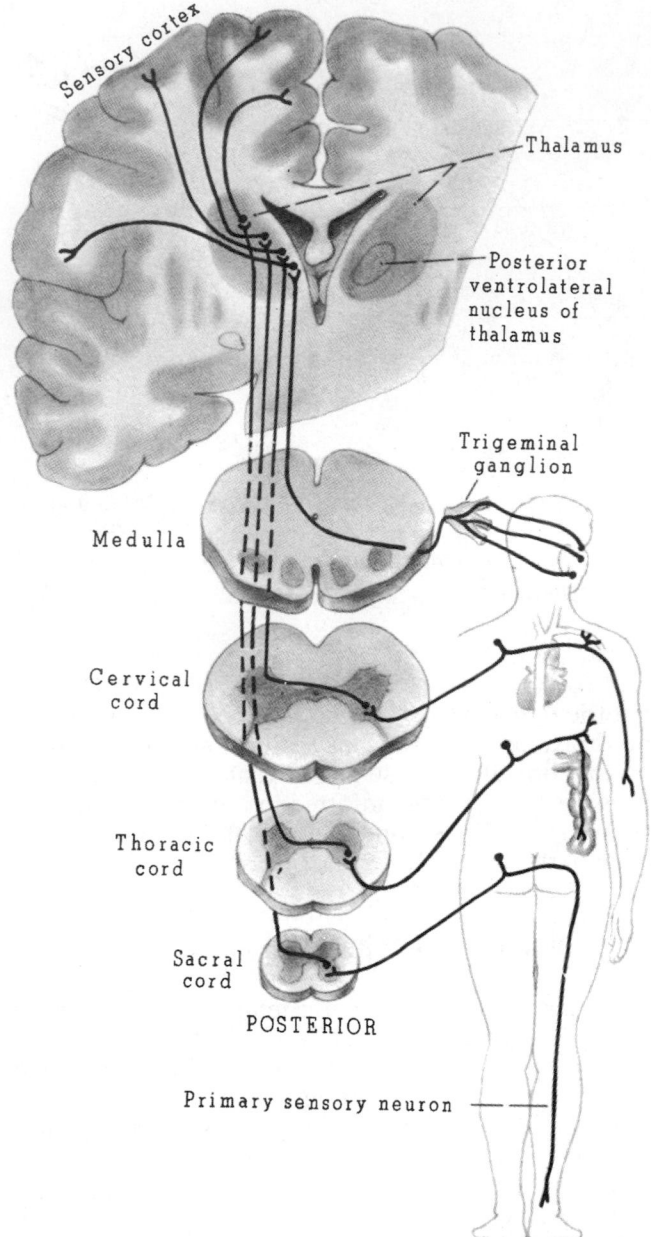

Sensory cortex

Thalamus

Posterior ventrolateral nucleus of thalamus

Trigeminal ganglion

Medulla

Cervical cord

Thoracic cord

Sacral cord

POSTERIOR

Primary sensory neuron

FIGURE 38–5. Central nervous system—spinothalamic tract. (From Jacob, S.W., Francone, C.A., and Lossow, W.J. (1978). *Structure and function in man* (p. 287). Philadelphia: W.B. Saunders.)

stated value to nociceptive transmission. The following five systems are believed to be important in the pain experience: the tract of Lissauer, the lemniscal-dorsal column system, the spinothalamic tract, the spinoreticular multisynaptic system, and the spinomesencephalic system. Of the five systems, the first two are controversial, and the last three are usually identified as the major pathways involved in pain transmission (see Fig. 38–5).

The tract of Lissauer is a bundle of fine dendrites from marginal cells that enter the dorsolateral horn and project the transmission of noxious stimuli ventrally into the substantia gelatinosa (lamina II) as part of the pain transmission process. The tract of Lissauer contains axons from substantia gelatinosa cells, which connect to the nucleus of the fifth cranial nerve in the brainstem; from this nucleus, fibers project to the thalamus.

The spinothalamic tract is generally regraded as the most important pathway for signaling the existence of painful stimuli in humans. As neurons of the spinothalamic tract traverse the spinal cord, fibers are added at each segment. Spinothalamic neurons can be subdivided into four categories:

1. The neospinothalamic tract terminates in the ventrolateral and posterior thalamus. From these thalamic nuclei, fibers project to the primary somatosensory area of the cerebral cortex and may be responsible for short, well-localized pain sensations.

2. The paleospinothalamic tract terminates in the medial thalamus but synapses with other neurons that connect to the reticular formation, midbrain, periaqueductal gray, limbic system, and hypothalamus. These connections may help to regulate respiration, endocrine function, and the cardiovascular system as well as modulate descending inhibitory neurons.

3. The lateral spinothalamic tracts have branches passing to the reticular nuclei of the brainstem. Impulses transmitted through the lateral spinothalamic tracts are thought to be responsible for spatial and temporal discriminative aspects of pain and touch sensations.

4. The ventral spinothalamic tracts have fibers that project to the brainstem reticular activating system and then to the medial and intralaminar thalamic nuclei. It is presumed that most impulses transmitted by spinothalamic cells cross over (decussate) at the anterolateral section of the spinal cord dorsal horn at the same level where they synapse.

The main thalamic nuclei receiving spinothalamic terminals include the ventral posterior lateral nucleus and the central lateral nucleus of the intralaminar complex. The ventral posterior lateral nucleus is somatotypically organized, that is, the neurons are organized in such a way that specific body surface areas can be easily identified and stimulated. Thus, a sensation on the finger can be transmitted to a specific area in the spinal cord and ascends to a particular area within the ventral posterior lateral nucleus of the thalamus, where the stimulus is perceived and a response is initiated. The termination zone of the spinothalamic tract in the ventral posterior lateral nucleus is in a region that overlaps with the termination zone of the dorsal column nuclei. Information derived from activity in spinothalamic neurons is thought to be forwarded to somatosensory cortices.

The spinoreticular multisynaptic system is likely to play a major role in pain mechanisms. The system has relatively short A-delta and C fibers with many synapses, allowing this pathway to transmit impulses more slowly. The most direct input to the reticular formation from the spinal cord is by way of the spinoreticular tract. Fibers from the spinoreticular system connect with the brainstem reticular activating system and then with the medial and intralaminar nuclei of the thalamus. From these thalamic nuclei, fibers project diffusely to the cerebral cortex, limbic system (including connections to the hypothalamus), and basal ganglia. Impulses passing through the medial and intralaminar nuclei of the thalamus are thought to take part in responses concerned with aversive motivation and other nondiscriminative aspects of pain. The reticular formation is likely to trigger arousal and to contribute to neural activity underlying the motivational-affective aspects of pain as well as somatic and autonomic motor reflexes. It is not clear whether relatively discrete sensory information transmitted by some spinoreticular neurons to the reticular formation is preserved in the postsynaptic responses of reticular formation neurons or if these responses are made less discriminative by convergent inputs from other neurons. In any event, reticular formation neurons are commonly responsive to noxious stimuli. The locations of the cells of origin of the spinoreticular tract in the human are unknown (Muir, 1988).

Higher Brain Centers

The pain tracts described earlier enter the reticular formation of the medulla, pons, and mesencephalon prior to activating neurons capable of transmitting the impulses to the thalamus, hypothalamus, and other cerebral or cortical areas of the brain. The thalamus is the lowest level of the brain where pain reaches consciousness but localization is poor. Pain information is disseminated from the thalamus to both cerebral hemispheres. Fibers from the thalamus terminate in the postcentral gyrus (somesthetic area) of the parietal lobe, which appears to be involved in discrimination of pain attributes such as localization and intensity. Other fibers terminate in the frontal lobe, which stimulates afferent fibers to the limbic system. This pathway appears to regulate the emotional or unpleasant aspects of pain. The response of the limbic system may determine how individuals respond to a noxious stimulus, adding the behavioral or subjective nature of pain. This may explain why different people respond differently to the same stimulus or why an individual responds differently at different times.

Biochemical Mediators of Pain

The previously described anatomic aspects of pain are only a small portion of the activity that takes place in the body in response to nociception. Neuroregulators such as neurotransmitters, neuromodulators, and neuroinhibitors play a vital role in the overall picture of pain. New information about these substances is discovered daily, and controversial issues about them are evident when the literature is scrutinized.

Many neuroregulators have been discovered. However, the exact role of each one and how it interacts with the others are not yet known. Several known neuroregulators influence pain perception and response. Some neuroregulators facilitate the activity of neurons involved in transmitting impulses for nociception. Other neuroregulators have an inhibitory effect, whereas others may produce an analgesic state. Neuroregulators such as monoamines (norepinephrine, epinephrine, dopamine, and serotonin), acetylcholine, amino acids (gamma-aminobutyric acid [GABA], glycine, and glutamine), substance P, prostaglandins, peptides (pituitary peptides, bradykinin, and peptides from other tissues), potassium chloride, and the endogenous opioids are substances that may act at different levels of the pain pathway as either neurotransmitters or neuromodulators (Willis, 1985; Guyton, 1991). Nociceptors are believed not to be directly stimulated by noxious stimuli. Rather, a noxious stimulus produces tissue injury, resulting in the release of chemical mediators that activate nociceptors. The activated nociceptors generate nerve impulses perceived as pain.

A neurotransmitter is synthesized within the presynaptic neuron and released into the synaptic cleft when an action potential reaches the end of the axon. The neurotransmitter then travels across the synaptic cleft to activate or inhibit other neurons in the pain transmission chain. The neurotransmitter binds with receptors on the membrane of the postsynaptic neuron, altering membrane excitability. Excess neurotransmitter is inactivated by enzymatic cleavage or by being actively taken up again by the presynaptic neuron (Fig. 38–6). Pain modulation reflects the basic activity of presynaptic, synaptic, and postsynaptic events that expedite the processes of facilitation, excitation, adaptation, summation, and inhibition (Guyton, 1991).

Neuromodulators alter the activity of neurons without the aid of a direct transfer of a signal through a synapse. They may influence the metabolism or receptor binding of a neurotransmitter at a synapse, or they may act directly on a large number of neurons at some distance from their release site.

Serotonin, found in various parts of the brain and spinal cord, is released from the ends of nerve fibers that descend from the brain and terminate in the dorsal horns of the spinal cord. It appears to inhibit neurons that transmit nociceptive signals (Muir, 1988).

Acetylcholine and amino acids such as aspartate and glutamate and some peptides are involved in higher brain centers. Gamma-aminobutyric acid may have an important role in the spinal regulation of pain. Histamine and bradykinin participate in peripheral mechanisms at the nociceptors.

Norepinephrine, also found in parts of the brain and spinal cord, appears to have different actions depending on the site. In the brain, norepinephrine

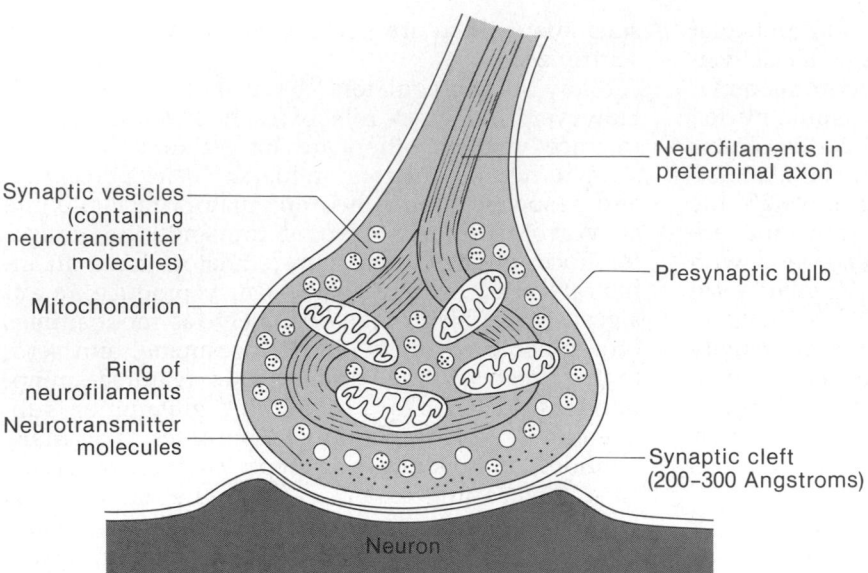

Synaptic vesicles (containing neurotransmitter molecules)

Mitochondrion

Ring of neurofilaments

Neurotransmitter molecules

Neurofilaments in preterminal axon

Presynaptic bulb

Synaptic cleft (200–300 Angstroms)

Neuron

FIGURE 38–6. The synapse.

seems to have an excitatory effect on neurons involved with nociception, whereas in the spinal cord it has an inhibitory effect. Catecholamines such as norepinephrine can exacerbate the pain of causalgia when applied locally by modulating polymodal nociceptors on C fibers.

Dopamine is located in the brain, with only insignificant amounts found in the spinal cord. This neurotransmitter appears to have an inhibitory effect on nociception.

Substance P has been identified as both a neurotransmitter at polymodal nociceptors and a neuromodulator because it facilitates transmission of nociceptive input. Substance P has also been shown to have analgesic effects on both physiologic and pathologic pain. This wide variation in activity is believed to be related to the amount of the substance that is present. The peptide is synthesized in cell bodies in dorsal root ganglia following stimulation of C fibers. It is released into peripheral tissues, cerebrospinal fluid, and inflammatory transudate. Particularly high concentrations of the peptide are found in the substantia gelatinosa of the dorsal gray horn and in parts of the brain associated both with processing nociceptive input and with the relay of information from the primary afferent fibers to secondary fibers (Terenius, 1978).

Prostaglandins (PGs) sensitize nociceptors to pain and modulate bradykinin activity at polymodal nociceptors, thus playing an important role as mediators in pain and the inflammatory process. PGs may be formed directly by the initial pain stimulus, whether thermal, chemical, or mechanical, and by the action of the peripheral pain mediators histamine, bradykinin, and substance P on the membranes of surrounding tissues. They sensitize nociceptors of C fibers by lowering the threshold of response to these stimuli. PGs are not stored free in tissues but are synthesized as a result of trauma or alteration in the cell membranes. PGs exert their physiologic or pathologic effects and are then rapidly biotransformed to inactive products. Prostaglandins are derived from arachidonic acid, which is present in all cell membranes (DiGregorio et al., 1986).

Leukotrienes, also derivatives of arachidonic acid, are not stored in tissue but with the appropriate stimuli are rapidly synthesized and released from leukocytes and are biotransformed to inactive products. These agents are important mediators of inflammation and allergic reactions by means of a synergistic action with other mediators such as histamine (DiGregorio et al., 1986).

Endogenous Analgesic Mechanisms

During the past decade it has been discovered that the brain contains a very important natural system for regulating pain including at least three groups of endogenous opioid peptides: enkephalins, dynorphins, and beta-endorphins. The findings that electrical stimulation of select loci in the brain elicit analgesia that can last for several hours and that endogenous substances modulate synaptic transmission in specific areas of the brain were key discoveries fostering ongoing studies.

Further study has more clearly explained the role of these opioids in direct transmission of painful stimuli. In the higher brain centers this role is believed to be more complicated. Endogenous opioid peptide neurons enhance the activity of descending inhibitory neurons to the spinal cord from the periaqueductal gray and rostral medulla, presumably by blocking inhibitory interneurons in higher centers. Inputs to these enkephalin-containing neurons may come from ascending substance P–containing neurons or from beta-endorphin–containing neurons from the pituitary or the hypothalamus.

Enkephalins are a pair of pentapeptides, identical in structure except for the C-terminal amino acid, which is methionine in one (met-enkephalin) and leucine in the other (leu-enkephalin). Enkephalins are viewed as neurotransmitters because they have been located in synaptosomal fractions and are rapidly inactivated by peptidases. Enkephalins are localized in areas associated with pain modulation including periaqueductal gray of the midbrain, raphe magnus, substantia gelatinosa, and marginal layer. The proposed mechanism of enkephalin-induced analgesia is inhibition of transmission of nociception, principally at the spinal cord; modulation of synaptic transmission; reduction of calcium transport across the membrane, thus inhibiting the release of substance P; and alteration of projection neurons of the spinothalamic tract.

The exact role of dynorphins in the regulation of pain is still unclear. Dynorphins and related substances are formed by the cleavage of a large polypeptide precursor, prodynorphin. The location and function of dynorphins overlap with those of enkephalin with some differences. Both groups of compounds are found in the periaqueductal grey, but dynorphins are located more ventrally, and there are more enkephalin-containing neurons in the medulla. Enkephalins and dynorphins appear to coexist in some dorsal horn neurons. Like the enkephalins, dynorphin-containing neurons have a close correlation with opioid receptors in the brain. It has been proposed that dynorphins might act by influencing projection neurons of the marginal layer of the spinal cord, secondarily affecting the descending inhibitory pathway.

Beta-endorphin, derived from pro-opiomelanocortin, a common precursor peptide of adrenocorticotropic hormone (ACTH) and melanocyte-stimulating hormone, is synthesized in the pars intermedia and pars distalis of the pituitary and in the basal hypothalamus. In response to painful stimuli of stress, beta-endorphin is released into the bloodstream from the pituitary or from pro-opiomelanocortin–containing neurons that terminate principally in the periaqueductal gray, where it may enhance the activity of the descending inhibitory system. Beta-endorphins have a more prolonged activity than met-enkephalin. The co-release of ACTH and beta-endorphin by hypothalamic neurons may also reach the cord via the cerebrospinal fluid, thus influencing spinal nociceptors directly. Pituitary endorphins may be involved in varying the threshold to pain and therefore, are important in pain control. In addition to analgesia, beta-endorphin mimics many of the other effects of morphine including tolerance and physical dependence, euphoria, respiratory depression, constipation, and hormonal and behavioral effects (Smith and Simon, 1981; Huhman, 1982; Akil et al., 1976; Fields and Basbaum, 1984; Muir, 1988).

Physiologic Responses to Pain

Even though there does not appear to be a direct or invariable relationship between a given stimulus and the perception and response to pain, certain factors appear to affect the pain response with some consistency. These factors include the integrity of the central nervous system, level of consciousness, training and previous experience in pain control, attention, distraction, fatigue, and anxiety (Jacox, 1979). The first and simplest response to a painful, external noxious stimulus is a flexor-withdrawal reflex, which is mediated at the spinal cord level. Internal sources of pain elicit reflex contraction of muscles over the affected area. This contraction or tension process can arise in either voluntary or involuntary muscles and increases the pain experience.

Activation of the sympathetic nervous system produces most of the recognizable responses to pain. Catecholamine release from the adrenal medulla evokes the fight or flight response, which is characterized by an increase in heart rate, an increase in blood pressure, a resulting increase in cardiac output, an increase in respiratory rate and depth, an increase in strength of muscle contractions, and vasoconstriction, which increases peripheral resistance. Blood is rapidly shifted from parts of the body that are considered nonvital or unnecessary in the fight or flight syndrome. Vessels of the skin and the abdominal viscera constrict, resulting in pallor and decreased gastric motility and digestive gland secretion. Muscle tension rises, and energy stores are mobilized to supply blood glucose. With the passage of time and marked intensity of pain, the parasympathetic response or rebound may occur, precipitating a fall in respiration rate, pulse rate, and blood pressure (Goosen and Bush, 1979).

Commonly observed behaviors of a person in pain include restlessness, perspiration, muscle tension, limping, splinting, rubbing the site, goose flesh, writhing, pacing, or fist clenching. Additional responses may include lip biting, teeth clenching, and facial expressions such as frowning or wrinkling the brow. Some individuals may withdraw from others and remain quiet, whereas others become noisy and strike out at those around them. The North American Nursing Diagnosis Association Taxonomy of Approved Diagnoses (Hurley, 1986) lists the following physical responses as defining characteristics for pain:

1. Guarding, protective behavior
2. Distracting behavior such as crying, moaning, pacing, or restlessness
3. Facial mask of pain, in which eyes lack luster, have a beaten look with fixed or scattered eye movements, or facial grimacing
4. Altered muscle tone that may range from rigid to listless
5. Presence of autonomic responses not seen in

chronic pain such as diaphoresis, vital sign changes, dilatation of pupils, and changes in respiration

Psychosocial reactions to pain are deeply influenced by the same factors that affect pain tolerance, including past experiences with pain. A verbally competent person may be able to describe accurately the location, duration, and intensity of the pain as well as the ability or willingness to tolerate it. A change in the tone of voice may be as revealing as the words spoken. Previous personal and family experiences with certain diseases, such as cancer, can significantly affect the degree of fear, anxiety, and depression associated with pain and consequently the individual's reaction. Vocalizations include responses such as crying, groaning, grunting, and gasping. Their frequency, loudness, and duration can assume greater significance in young children and the elderly who are either too young or too confused to be verbally competent.

Pain that persists or is repetitive results in adaptation of response, with observable reductions in sympathetic signs and symptoms. Pain receptors, however, show little if any adaptation. Reactions to long-term pain tend to be centrally mediated. With time, physiologic and psychological coping mechanisms evolve, but these behavioral responses do not necessarily indicate pain relief. The person may merely be too fatigued to respond.

Occasionally, pain is associated with neurogenic shock resulting from inhibition of the medullary vasomotor center with decreased vasomotor tone. This mechanism is not well understood but may be associated with circulatory collapse. Pain is believed to relate to other neurologic activities such as sleep. During rapid eye movement (REM) or dream sleep, the electroencephalogram (EEG) records increased brain activity. Certain disorders in which pain predominates, such as angina and ulcer, appear to be exacerbated during this stage of sleep (Phillips and Cousins, 1986).

Adverse Physiologic Effects of Pain

It is believed that continued acute pain begins to produce harmful physiologic effects in addition to the usual signs and symptoms associated with pain. Conversely, there are clinicians who are hesitant to treat abdominal pain or head injuries because relief of acute pain may alter or delay an accurate diagnosis. Although these concerns are well-founded, individuals should be assessed as rapidly as possible, and pain relief should be provided as soon as it is safe to do so.

Common respiratory problems caused by acute pain are associated with splinting that results from chest or abdominal pain and the patient's reluctance or inability to cough. Failure to cough, especially in individuals with chronic lung problems or after anesthesia, may result in retention of secretions with lung consolidation and possible atelectasis with resulting hypercapnia and hypoxemia. Physiologic splinting can result in a decreased tidal volume, vital capacity, functional residual capacity, and alveolar ventilation. Cardiovascular problems associated with acute pain may include an exaggeration of sympathetic indicators commonly associated with the pain response. Increased cardiac work load results from the tachycardia, increased peripheral resistance, hypertension, and increased myocardial oxygen consumption that result from pain. Ischemia of heart muscle and other tissue such as brain tissue may result. Muscle spasm in the area associated with acute pain sets up a cycle of increased discomfort and increased sympathetic activity frequently causes increased intestinal secretions and decreases intestinal motility, ultimately resulting in ileus with gastric stasis and dilation of the bowel. Skeletal muscle and bone immobilization may cause venous stasis and platelet aggregation that predispose to deep vein thrombosis and pulmonary embolism (Cousins and Phillips, 1986).

ASSESSMENT OF PAIN

Assessment of pain in the critically ill individual is challenging because of the patient's complex condition, altered interpretation of other stressful factors, and difficulty with communication. Nevertheless, comprehensive assessment is essential to determine the severity of pain and the proper method of management. The findings must be completely documented in the patient's record. Incomplete or absent documentation leads to the assumption that the nurse has treated pain without prior assessment (Puntillo, 1988).

Pain is not reliably quantifiable. Establishing reliability is problematic because pain varies over time, is confounded by memory, is unique to individuals, and includes sensory, affective, and evaluative components (Reading, 1984). A number of assessment scales are available to aid in determining the severity of pain. The success of any process of pain assessment is dependent upon consistent use and the ability to make modifications to meet the clinical needs of the patient (Huskisson, 1974).

Factors believed to alter the assessment of pain include individual patient characteristics (McCaffery, 1979); health professionals' attitudes (Baer et al., 1983); age, sex, education, and experience of health care workers (McCaffery, 1979; Amnad et al., 1982); and the patient's age and sex (Mather and Mackie, 1983). Children, men (Davitz et al., 1976), and postoperative patients (Cohen, 1980) present controversial assessment problems that are evident in the literature on pain and in clinical practice. Some nurses ignore patients' verbal or nonverbal complaints of pain, thereby undertreating a problem that should be well managed, especially during acute episodes.

Reading (1984) identified four objectives in clinical pain measurement:

1. Diagnostic, in that establishing a diagnosis and thereby selecting the appropriate treatment may depend on an accurate assessment of the precise characteristics of the pain.

2. Monitoring of fluctuations in pain levels during the course of treatment and thereby reducing reliance on the patient's making retrospective comparisons, which may be fraught with bias.

3. Evaluation of treatment efficacy, so that therapies having specific effects can be distinguished from the nonspecific or placebo effects, well documented in pain (Beecher, 1972).

4. Reliable monitoring of the pain over time, which permits controlling factors to be identified (p. 195).

Evaluation of pain begins by determining whether or not the pain exists. Critically ill patients may not be able to verbalize pain perception, making this task difficult. An understanding of a patient's past and current pathophysiology provides insight into the presence of pain and some initial expectations about the severity of pain (Johnson P., 1977). Once the existence of pain has been identified, the patient's subjective reports of pain must be evaluated. Information should be elicited about location, quality, pattern, intensity, verbal and nonverbal observations, symptoms associated with pain, aggravating or triggering factors, and duration. Differentiation between sensory and affective dimensions of pain is important and can be determined by means of patient interview (Gracely and Dubner, 1981; Gaston-Johansson, 1984; Gaston-Johansson and Asklund-Gustafsson, 1985). A few examples of rating scales and questionnaires are discussed in this chapter. Critical care nurses are responsible for selecting a feasible method for assessing patients in their setting.

Verbal reports of pain present the following potential problems: subject response bias or falsification, a response not proportional to the actual severity of the noxious stimuli, discordance with other indices, and reactive effect in sensitizing the patient to the pain (Reading, 1984). However, the advantages of subjective data far outweigh these difficulties. Because pain is a personal experience, the patient should be seen as the authority on what is experienced.

Pain location can be relatively easy to determine in the alert patient by asking the patient to point to the area or verbally describe the location. This information can be recorded in the nurses' notes or on an anatomic drawing. Pain assessment involves observing, measuring, and recording physiologic and behavioral indicators that are perceived as pain related. The challenge facing the critical care nurse is to differentiate these indicators from the patient's overall condition. The individual's perception of pain and the meaning that pain holds for him must also be investigated. This aspect is best assessed by more than one person, such as the patient's team of health care providers.

The final aspect of evaluation is the determination of the adaptive mechanisms that are used to cope with pain. Five typical methods of coping are used when an individual faces any disaster: (1) denial, (2) group affiliation, (3) information gathering, (4) religion, and (5) optimism. The nurse can help foster any coping mechanisms the patient identifies as successful. Maladaptive mechanisms that are indicative of failure to cope include social isolation, extreme anxiety with exacerbation of pain, and passive dependency.

Pain intensity is frequently evaluated based on the sensory component of pain alone. Patient statements may aid in gauging the severity and qualitative nature of pain, utilizing rankings of numbers or word descriptors. Words have different meanings for different people and even for the same person at different times because there is no universal anchorage. Thus, these scales are not reliable over time (Tursky, 1976).

Visual, verbal, and numerical rating scales are commonly used in clinical practice and pain research. Numerical scales can be used as visual or verbal responses. They are easily implemented by asking the patient to identify the amount of discomfort perceived on a scale of 0 to 10, with 0 reflecting no pain and 10 reflecting the worst pain the patient has ever experienced. Even with this simple and commonly used rating, it is expected that the patient will not reliably differentiate and correctly place value on the numbers (Shapiro, 1975). Determination of the patient's ability to discriminate between levels of pain is an important precursor to use of this method.

The visual analog scale of pain quantitation is similar to a numerical scale because the patient subjectively quantifies one aspect of the pain experience, usually its intensity (Fig. 38–7). These scales rate pain on a certain point scale with anchor words such as none, slight, moderate, and severe, which require evaluation by the patient, provided that he or she is able to perform such cognitive distinctions. Instead of choosing a number, the subject is asked to mark a point on a line. The line is divided into ten equal spaces and the interval that contains the subject's mark is then given a value of 1 to 10. Again, this approach requires patient discriminative response and memory.

The most widely used method of qualitative and quantitative measurement of pain is the McGill-Melzack Pain Questionnaire (MPQ), a multidimensional scale that assesses sensory, affective, and evaluative elements of the pain experience (Fig. 38–8). Descriptive words in these three categories are chosen to identify subjective pain. Words used to describe pain reflect not only the sensory-discriminative aspect but also motivational-affective and cognitive-evaluative dimensions. Pain has an unpleasant, negative-affective quality that distinguishes it from sensory experiences such as sight or hearing.

The two major measures obtained with the MPQ are the pain rating index rank (PRI) based on numerical values assigned to the chosen words and the

A. SIMPLE DESCRIPTIVE SCALE

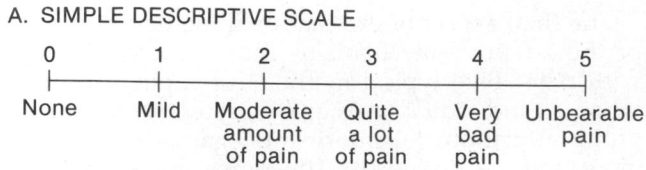

B. MELZACK'S SCALE

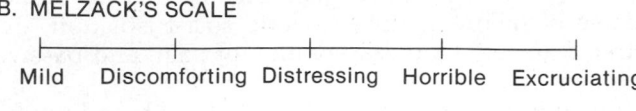

C. 0-100 NUMERIC SCALE

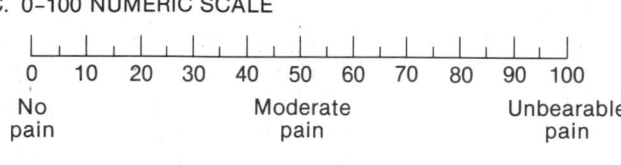

D. VISUAL ANALOGUE SCALE OR
GRAPHIC RATING METHOD

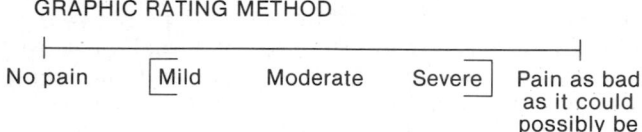

FIGURE 38–7. *A* to *D*, Examples of pain scales—visual analog scales. (Redrawn from Melzack, R. (1975). *Pain*, 1, 277.)

number of words chosen (NWC) (Melzack, 1975). Although difficult to administer and grade in the clinical setting due to its length and complexity, the questionnaire has demonstrated characteristic response patterns for different pain syndromes such as cancer pain, lower back pain, and arthritis. The exact role of the MPQ in the evaluation of acute pain syndromes is still being actively investigated, but in its present form it is unsuitable for frequent assessments of pain in the critically ill patient.

The Stewart Pain-Color Scale presents the patient with an array of yellow, orange, red, and black colors. Patients are asked where they would place their pain on the color chart. Research has indicated that patients with no pain select the left or yellow side of the scale, patients with moderate pain select the red or orange, middle range part of the scale, and patients with severe pain indicate the black or right side of the scale. The scale is easy to use by patients who are not color blind and may be especially useful for critically ill patients who are too ill to conceptualize numbers (Stewart, 1977).

Another method of pain analysis is the estimation of magnitude, a measurement technique adapted from psychophysics (Haber and Hershenson, 1980). Because all objects and events serve as potentially perceivable stimuli by the sensory apparatus, a measurable response results from a perceived stimulus. The purpose of the magnitude estimation technique is to form a ratio scale, mapping the magnitude of a sensory response in relation to the magnitude of a physical stimulus such as pain for each individual subject. An individual is asked to estimate the apparent strength or intensity of his sensory responses relative to a set of stimuli and reflect the magnitude of this intensity in some physical manner. The expression of this magnitude may be captured by an instrument such as a hand dynamometer. Tursky and colleagues (1982) used this principle to develop a pain perception profile that has been used successfully and reliably in a laboratory setting. A further application in the clinical setting has been reported for estimating the parameters of dyspnea (Nield et al., 1989).

Development of an instrument for assessment of pain has been reported and refined by Gaston-Johansson and Asklund-Gustafsson (1985). They found that the words "pain," "ache," and "hurt" commonly referred to painlike experiences in the English and Swedish languages. In addition, "these concepts were shown to differ in intensity and to be associated with particular sensory and affective word descriptors" (p. 541). Sensory (s) and affective (a) descriptors representing the concept of pain were listed as cutting (s), tearing (s), killing (a), and torturing (a). Words representing ache were grinding (s), gnawing (s), irritating (a), and troublesome (a). Hurt was represented by pricking (s), pinching (s), fearful (a), and unhappy (a) (Gaston-Johansson, 1984). These words were used to study the discriminating power of descriptors in nurses, nursing students, and patients. Comparison was made with a visual analog scale and the MPQ. It was found that all subject groups agreed on the difference in intensity among the words pain, ache, and hurt, encouraging further development of this descriptive measurement tool. The use of fewer descriptors might make this a more useful clinical assessment tool. Descriptors for pain, ache, and hurt can be given a numerical value, providing a basis for managing sensory and affective aspects of pain (Gaston-Johansson and Asklund-Gustafsson, 1985).

Assessment issues that require extra consideration by the critical care nurse when narcotic analgesics are used include size of the individual, age, and sex. The key to proper pain management is an individualized narcotic dosage based on the patient's needs.

Weight. Because of significant differences in body weight, obese patients are likely to require more narcotic than emaciated patients.

Elderly. The elderly may receive inappropriate dosages because of metabolic changes associated with aging. Use of the lowest drug strength initially, with subsequent titration upward, may prevent untoward side effects. Alterations in absorption, distribution, metabolism, and excretion can contribute to drug sensitivity (Greenblat et al., 1982). Decreased renal function and decreased cardiac output may result in drug concentration at a particular site of action (Cohen, 1986; Weinberg, 1988). Abrupt hos-

Patient's name _____ Age _____

Hospital No. _____

Clinical category (e.g., cardiac, neurological, etc.):

_____

Diagnosis: _____

_____

_____

Analgesic (if already administered):

1. Type _____

2. Dosage _____

3. Time given in relation to this test _____

Patient's intelligence: Circle number that represents best estimate.

1 (low)   2   3   4   5 (high)

****

This questionnaire has been designed to tell us more about your pain. Four major questions we ask are:

1. Where is your pain?
2. What does it feel like?
3. How does it change with time?
4. How strong is it?

It is important that you tell us how your pain feels now. Please follow the instructions at the beginning of each part.

Part 1. Where Is Your Pain?

Please mark, on the drawings, the areas where you feel pain. Put E if external, or I if internal, near the areas which you mark. Put EI if both external and internal.

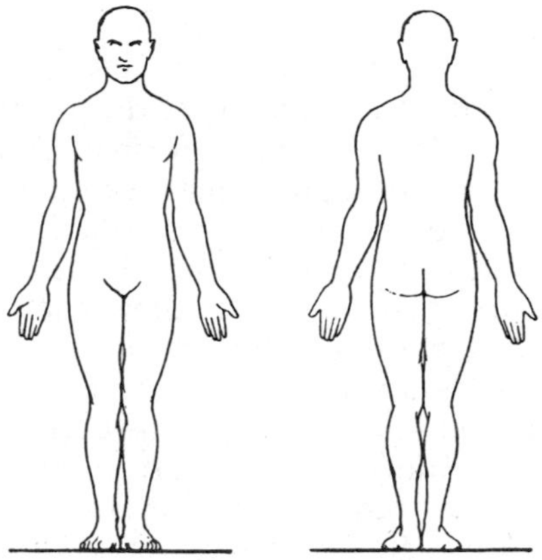

Part 2. What Does Your Pain Feel Like?

Some of the words below describe your present pain. Circle ONLY those words that best describe it. Leave out any category that is not suitable. Use only a single word in each appropriate category—the one that applies best.

1	2	3	4	5
Flickering	Jumping	Pricking	Sharp	Pinching
Quivering	Flashing	Boring	Cutting	Pressing
Pulsing	Shooting	Drilling	Lacerating	Gnawing
Throbbing		Stabbing		Cramping
Beating		Lancinating		Crushing

6	7	8	9	10
Tugging	Hot	Tingling	Dull	Tender
Pulling	Burning	Itchy	Sore	Taut
Wrenching	Scalding	Smarting	Hurting	Rasping
	Searing	Stinging	Aching	Splitting
			Heavy	

11	12	13	14	15
Tiring	Sickening	Fearful	Punishing	Wretched
Exhausting	Suffocating	Frightful	Gruelling	Blinding
		Terrifying	Cruel	
			Vicious	
			Killing	

16	17	18	19	20
Annoying	Spreading	Tight	Cool	Nagging
Troublesome	Radiating	Numb	Cold	Nauseating
Miserable	Penetrating	Drawing	Freezing	Agonizing
Intense	Piercing	Squeezing		Dreadful
Unbearable		Tearing		Torturing

Part 3. How Does Your Pain Change With Time?

1. Which word or words would you use to describe the pattern of your pain?

1	2	3
Continuous	Rhythmic	Brief
Steady	Periodic	Momentary
Constant	Intermittent	Transient

2. What kind of things relieve your pain?

_____

_____

_____

3. What kind of things increase your pain?

_____

_____

_____

Part 4. How Strong is Your Pain?

People agree that the following 5 words represent pain of increasing intensity. They are:

1   2   3   4   5

Mild Discomforting Distressing Horrible Excruciating

To answer each question below, write the number of the most appropriate word in the space beside the question.

1. Which word describes your pain right now? ____
2. Which word describes it at its worst? ____
3. Which word describes it when it is the least? ____
4. Which word describes the worst toothache you ever had? ____
5. Which word describes the worst headache you ever had? ____
6. Which word describes the worst stomach ache you ever had? ____

FIGURE 38–8. Pain assessment form. (From Melzack, R. (1975). *Pain*, 1, 277.)

pitalization may result in disorientation, decreased exercise, loss of control over one's life, inability to express pain, or regression. Depression and fear of death may also cause special problems. These problems must be considered particularly when dealing with pain in the elderly. Careful, frequent assessment of the elderly patient by the critical care nurse may prevent development or progression of complications resulting from overmedication. Inability or failure of elderly patients to complain of pain contributes to the erroneous notion that elderly patients do not perceive pain as readily as young adults.

Children. Literature on the pain experience in children is meager, controversial, and lacking in systematic research. Several investigators have reported that, contrary to a widely held belief, children can and often do suffer considerable pain. Children with an inaccurate understanding of what is happening may develop fantasies of mutilation, become extremely anxious, and doubt their ability to cope. Realistic reassurance can promote a sense of control and increase coping ability (Savedra et al., 1982; National Institutes of Health Consensus Development Conference, 1987; Porth, 1986).

Gender. The issue of pain assessment and management related to gender has been addressed intermittently in the literature during the past three decades. Most of the information provided merely compares male and female samples during statistical analysis on general issues centered around emotion, attitude, and/or behavior. Some of this information was addressed briefly in the section on cultural issues at the beginning of this chapter, but additional details are necessary to provide the critical care nurse with background data that can be used during assessment and planning of pain management. These previous references can be augmented by more recent studies that look carefully at gender and the stress response. Although little reference is made directly to pain in these studies, application of data related to the stress response is an appropriate transfer of information. The fact that pain-induced stress results in sympathetic nervous system activation is well documented by evidence of increases in heart rate, blood pressure, peripheral and vascular resistance, cardiac output, and cardiac work (Thoren, 1974). Hormone response to the stress of pain, surgery, or trauma is similar and depends on the magnitude and duration of the insult (Thoren, 1974; Traynor and Hall, 1981).

Gender-differentiated neuroendocrine (cortisol, epinephrine, norepinephrine, beta-endorphin, and beta-lipotropin) and cardiovascular stress response are two key areas that have value for the critical care nurse. Pain and stress promote the pituitary release of ACTH into the bloodstream, stimulating secretion of glucocorticoids (cortisol) from the cortex of the adrenal gland. The adrenal medulla is directly innervated by the sympathetic nervous system, which serves as a stimulus for release of the catecholamines—epinephrine and norepinephrine. About 80% of the adrenal secretion of catecholamines consists of epinephrine (Asterita, 1985). Research findings consistently indicate that in response to standard laboratory stressors women show a less pronounced elevation in urinary excretion of epinephrine than do men (Johansson and Post, 1974; Frankenhaeuser et al., 1976). The same relationship has been observed among 12-year-olds, indicating that the difference is related to gender rather than to age (Johansson, 1972). None of the investigations has revealed a corresponding sex difference in the urinary excretion of norepinephrine, which is consistent with observations that norepinephrine responds most to physical stress whereas epinephrine is more reactive to psychological stressors (Dimsdale and Moss, 1980; Ward et al., 1983).

Compared with women, men show exaggerated reactions to stress in some but not all of the variables measured. It has been consistently observed that both plasma and urinary excretions of epinephrine rise appreciably more in men than in women during exposure to achievement-oriented laboratory tasks or stressors. Other neuroendocrine reactions either do not differ between men and women (norepinephrine) or show no consistent pattern related to gender (cortisol). The few studies of the influences of the reproductive hormones on catecholamine or cortisol responses to laboratory stressors reveal no consistent effects of menstrual phase or, in postmenopausal women, of replacement therapy with an estrogen-progestin compound (Plante and Denvey, 1984).

In regard to cardiovascular reactivity, there is some inconsistent evidence that men exhibit larger systolic blood pressure responses and smaller heart rate reactions to psychological stressors than do women. Among ovariectomized women, systolic blood pressure responses to laboratory stressors are reduced following administration of an estrogen or estrogen-progestin compound. An attenuated systolic blood pressure response to stressors has also been found to accompany the use of oral contraceptives. These findings as well as a recent observation that heart rate and systolic blood pressure responses of postmenopausal women were greater than those seen in premenopausal controls suggest that the female reproductive hormones are associated with a reduced cardiovascular response (Polefrone and Manuck, 1987).

The influence of gender on beta-endorphin and beta-lipotropin levels has also been explored, with more recent studies reporting that women have higher levels than men (Furuhashi et al., 1984). Previous reports were varied. Findings in a study by Viswanathan and colleagues (1987) supported many previous reports that exercise induces increases in plasma beta-endorphins and beta-lipotropin. These investigators further found that eumenorrheic and amenorrheic women increased plasma levels at the end of the exercise period, whereas men did not significantly increase levels until exhaustion was reached.

The existence of gender-related differences in pain response is supported in a study of newborn infants, in whom sex differences were apparent in speed of response, with boys showing a shorter time to cry and to display facial action following heel-lance. The presence of variation in facial action was interpreted as an indication that the biologic and behavioral context of pain events affects behavioral expression even at this very early developmental stage before the opportunity for learned response patterns has occurred (Grunau and Craig, 1987).

MANAGEMENT OF PAIN

Pain management is a complex issue, and methods used to control or decrease pain range from simple, noninvasive relaxation techniques to invasive surgical procedures. Nurses are the key persons respon-

TABLE 38–1. Selected Narcotic Compounds

Classification	Generic Name	Common Trade Name
Agonists		
Phenanthrene derivatives		
	Morphine	
	Codeine	
	Hydromorphone	Dilaudid
	Oxymorphone	Numorphan
	Oxycodone	
Morphinan derivative		
	Levorphanol	Levo-Dromoran
Phenylpiperdine derivatives		
	Meperidine	Demerol
	Fentanyl	Sublimaze
Diphenylheptane derivatives		
	Methadone	Dolophine
	Propoxyphene	Darvon
Antagonists		
	Naloxone	Narcan
	Naltrexone	Trexan
Mixed Agonist-Antagonists		
	Buprenorphine	Buprenex
	Butorphanol	Stadol
	Nalbuphine	Nubain
	Pentazocine	Talwin

sible for pain alleviation and implementation of dependent, interdependent, and independent actions. The principles of pain management most appropriate for use by critical care nurses are presented here, emphasizing recent successful and innovative techniques. Pharmacologic and nonpharmacologic methods of management are included along with their physiologic effects. Ethical and legal issues related to pain management are also addressed.

Pharmacologic Management of Pain

Critical care nurses play a key role in the pharmacologic management of pain. Not only do nurses administer most drugs used for pain management, they also evaluate the desired and untoward effects of these drugs and identify life-threatening situations. Pharmacologic management of pain includes use of narcotic analgesia, non-narcotic analgesia, and anesthetic agents. Methods of administration and observed responses to these agents are within the domain of nursing.

NARCOTIC ANALGESIA

Narcotic analgesics include the naturally occurring opium alkaloids and their synthetic and semisynthetic derivatives. Because these drugs possess pharmacologic effects similar to the effects of opium, they are frequently called opioid analgesics. For this discussion, the narcotic analgesic agents will be divided into narcotic agonists, narcotic antagonists, and agents with mixed agonist and antagonist activity

(DiGregorio et al., 1986). Table 38–1 classifies the narcotic agents by generic and common trade names.

Narcotic Agonists. Narcotic agonists are frequently used in critical care and include the derivatives listed in Table 38–1. Morphine is the oldest known drug of this class and remains the prototype and the standard of comparison for all other narcotic analgesic compounds (Table 38–2).

The discovery of the endogenous opioids and their activity in the body has enhanced our understanding of exogenous opioids such as morphine. Studies support the hypothesis that specific opioid receptors exist to facilitate the action of endogenous opioids and mediate the action of narcotic drugs. Four receptor types have been identified as the sites of action for endogenous and exogenous opioidlike substances, including μ (mu), κ (kappa), δ (delta), and Σ (sigma). Experimentation suggests that the mu receptor is associated with supraspinal analgesia, respiratory depression, euphoria, and physical dependence; the kappa receptor is believed to mediate spinal analgesia, miosis, and sedation, and the sigma receptor appears to be involved with dysphoria, psychotomimetic effects, and respiratory stimulation. The delta receptors may influence affective behavior. Agonistic narcotics act as analgesics by binding to and activating both mu and kappa receptors in the brain and spinal cord. The agonist opioid drugs have an affinity for these receptors and can stimulate the receptors to produce an effect. Therefore, they mimic the activity of the endogenous opioid peptides. Despite the fact that all of the narcotic agonists stimulate both the mu and kappa receptors, differences in

TABLE 38–2. Potency Comparisons of Selected Narcotic Analgesics*

Drug	Equianalgesic Doses (mg)	
	IM	PO
Narcotic Agonists		
Morphine	10	60
Codeine	120	200
Fentanyl	0.1	−†
Hydromorphone	1.5	7.5
Levorphanol	2	4
Meperidine	75	300
Methadone	10	20
Oxycodone	15	30
Oxymorphone	1	6
Propoxyphene	−†	130
Narcotic Agonist-Antagonists		
Buprenorphine	0.3	−†
Butorphanol	2	−†
Nalbuphine	10	−†
Pentazocine	30	150

*The data in this table are based upon morphine, 10 mg, administered intramuscularly and represent the general consensus of medical opinion. Variability will occur among patients; therefore, these values should be used only as a guide for comparison.
†Not used by this route.

TABLE 38–3. Pharmacokinetic Data of Narcotic Analgesics

Drug	Onset of Effect* (Minutes)	Peak Effects* (Minutes)
Narcotic Agonists		
Morphine	30	30–60
Codeine	30	45–90
Fentanyl	10	20–30*
Hydromorphone	30	30–90
Levorphanol	30	60–90
Meperidine	15	30–60
Methadone	15	60–120
Oxycodone	—†	—†
Oxymorphone	10	30–90
Propoxyphene‡	30	60–90
Narcotic Agonist-Antagonists		
Buprenorphine	15	45–60
Butorphanol	10	30–60
Nalbuphine	15	45–60
Pentazocine	15	30–60

*Based on intramuscular administration.
†No data available.
‡Based on oral administration.

amounts needed to induce analgesia among the compounds are great (DiGregorio et al., 1986).

Agonist opioids are readily absorbed by the body after subcutaneous or intramuscular injection. However, hepatic first-pass biotransformation reduces the amount available to the entire body, and therefore the bioavailability of most of these drugs when administered orally is less than 60%. In general, the amount of drug needed for an effective oral dose is greater than the amount needed for a parenteral dose, resulting in a low parenteral-oral dose ratio. This varies, however, among patients and depends on the particular compound. The intravenous route is the preferred method of administration in critically ill individuals because life-support systems and altered consciousness alter accessibility to the oral route. In addition, the subcutaneous and intramuscular routes are frequently impaired by poor circulation.

Following intravenous injection of an agonist opioid, onset of analgesic effect occurs within 10 to 30 minutes and peak effect occurs between 20 and 120 minutes (Table 38–3). Most analgesics are biotransformed to inactive conjugates in the liver; however, approximately 10% of codeine, the 3-methyl derivative of morphine, is demethylated to morphine prior to inactivation. More than 90% of the administered dose of drug is excreted in the urine as inactive metabolites; the remainder appears in the feces through biliary excretion, mainly as the more lipid-soluble parent drug. The plasma half-life of these narcotics is generally 4 hours or less, with the exception of levorphanol, methadone, and propoxyphene (Table 38–4) (Jaffe and Martin, 1980; Twycross, 1984; DiGregorio et al., 1986). Additional information about each of the narcotics can be obtained from the drug reference literature.

Adverse Actions of Agonists. Although opioid agonists predominantly abolish pain, these drugs have profound pharmacologic activity throughout the body. In addition to the effects on the central nervous system, activity of the peripheral systems and organs may also be altered. Central nervous system effects of opioids include analgesia, drowsiness, alteration in mood, lethargy, inability to concentrate, apathy, and mental clouding. These symptoms occur both in pain-free individuals and in patients experiencing pain. Opioids relieve pain without a loss of consciousness, and patients retain sensations such as touch, vision, and hearing. Euphoria may be experienced in 10% to 20% of patients, especially as pain is alleviated; however, dysphoric reactions may also occur.

Narcotic agonists act directly on the brain stem respiratory centers, reducing the respiratory rate, minute volume, and tidal exchange and producing irregular and periodic breathing patterns. These effects are observable at therapeutic doses of the opioids and increase as the dose is raised. Death from narcotic overdose is almost always the result of respiratory depression and arrest.

Narcotic analgesics often cause constipation, nausea, and vomiting. Nausea and vomiting are frequently perceived as allergic responses to morphine and other narcotics. This possibility should be carefully evaluated by the critical care nurse, who should determine the patient's untoward response through careful history taking or skin testing. Both peripheral and central actions of these drugs cause constipation by decreasing the propulsive peristaltic motility of the small intestine (the duodenum is affected more than the ileum), enhancing the action of the gastrointestinal sphincter muscles, and reducing digestive secretions along the entire alimentary canal. Delay in movement of bowel contents leads to fecal dehy-

TABLE 38–4. Pharmacokinetic Data of Narcotic Analgesics

Drug	Duration of Effect (Hours)	Plasma Half-Life (Hours)
Narcotic Agonists		
Morphone	3–7	2–3
Codeine	4–6	3–4
Fentanyl	1–2	3–4
Hydromorphone	4–5	2–4
Levorphanol	4–8	10–12
Meperidine	2–4	3–4
Methadone	4–6	21–25
Oxycodone	4–5	—*
Oxymorphone	3–6	—*
Propoxyphene	4–6	6–12
Narcotic Agonist-Antagonists		
Buprenorphine	4–6	2–3
Butorphanol	3–4	2–4
Nalbuphine	3–6	4–6
Pentazocrine	2–3	2–3

*No data available.

dration, further reducing intestinal passage. Decreased perception of normal rectal sensory stimuli can also contribute to constipation.

Direct stimulation of the chemoreceptor trigger zone in the area postrema of the medulla causes nausea and emesis. A vestibular component is believed to be involved because there is a high incidence of nausea and vomiting when patients are ambulatory. This side effect rarely occurs in bedridden individuals.

Most narcotic agonists constrict the pupil through stimulation of the nuclei of the oculomotor nerve. This is a useful diagnostic sign of narcotic use or abuse. Tolerance generally does not develop to opioid-induced miosis.

Most agonists alter the cough reflex, and critical care nurses should be aware that even mild depression of the medullary-pontine (tussive) cough center may modify the triggering effect of mucus. Potential dependence and respiratory depression severely limit the antitussive benefit of some narcotics. The therapeutic effects of codeine and hydromorphone as cough suppressants, with their high antitussive activity and lower liability to dependence, make them more suitable for analgesia but less suitable if the patient needs to retain an ability to clear mucus from the respiratory tract.

Arteriolar vasodilatation and reduced peripheral resistance may occur with therapeutic doses of narcotics. While the patient is supine, these effects are usually insignificant, but orthostatic hypotension and fainting may occur in ambulatory patients. Most opioid analgesics promote histamine release from mast cells, enhancing the hypotensive effect of these compounds. In normal individuals, cardiac function is not significantly altered; however, in patients with coronary artery disease or myocardial infarction, a decrease in oxygen consumption, left ventricular end-diastolic pressure, and cardiac function may occur.

With the exception of vascular muscle, most smooth muscle, including the bronchioles, gallbladder, bile duct, sphincter of Oddi, and urinary bladder, is contracted by morphinelike drugs. Urinary retention is a common side effect. Morphine or its derivatives are contraindicated in patients experiencing pain from biliary stones unless atropine is administered concurrently to decrease smooth muscle contraction. Bronchiolar smooth muscle contraction is rarely significant.

Release of histamine from mast cells is partially responsible for the cutaneous vasodilation, pruritus, and sweating that accompany agonist narcotics. Although annoying, these symptoms are usually tolerated as long as pain relief occurs.

The issue of physical and psychological dependence raised by chronic use of narcotics should be a minor consideration in the ICU. Typically, the goal in an acutely ill individual is to abolish pain and to maintain comfort.

Tolerance occurs when the same dose elicits a decreased effect following repeated administration, or when increasingly greater doses are required to achieve the effect observed with the initial dose even after physiologic improvement. Careful consideration must be given to changing the dosage as evidence of tolerance is observed or if the patient has a history of chronic pain that has been managed by narcotics. Tolerance and physical dependence are dose- and time-dependent. Two to three weeks of therapeutic doses may lead to physical or psychological dependence. The critical care nurse should observe for signs of physical withdrawal such as autonomic hyperactivity, including diarrhea, vomiting, lacrimation, rhinorrhea, chills, and fever. Patients may also suffer abdominal cramps, pain, and tremors. Observation and documentation of these indicators should be reported to the physician and a collaborative plan devised to prevent further dependence or reverse existing dependence (Jaffe and Martin, 1980; Mather and Phillips, 1986; DiGregorio et al., 1986).

Narcotic Antagonists. Narcotic antagonists, naloxone and naltrexone, are competitive antagonists of agonist narcotics and mixed agonist-antagonist compounds. These drugs compete for opioid receptor sites and prevent or reverse activation of receptors by other opiate agents. These agents do not produce analgesia, respiratory depression, pupillary constriction, or physical dependence. Antagonists are used frequently in critical care to reverse the adverse effects of an agonist overdose.

Naloxone has a plasma half-life of about an hour in adults and 3 hours in neonates. Onset of action occurs within 2 minutes of administration of an IV dose; IM administration has a slightly longer onset. Because an individual response to naloxone is anticipated, it is necessary to titrate naloxone by giving small doses and observing any subsequent changes in the patient's appearance, behavior, and verbal response. The drug and its inactive metabolites are excreted in the urine. Oral administration of naloxone is ineffective due to its rapid biotransformation by hepatic conjugation; parenteral administration is required. Naltrexone may be given orally and has a duration of 24 to 72 hours.

Mixed Agonist-Antagonists. Mixed agonist-antagonists, butorphanol tartrate (Stadol) and nalbuphine (Nubain), are potent analgesics with opioid receptor selectivity. They cause some of the agonist agents' side effects; however, they are believed to cause less respiratory depression and less dependence due to antagonist properties. Signs of narcotic agonist dependence withdrawal result when mixed agonist-antagonists are given.

NON-NARCOTIC ANALGESIA

Numerous non-narcotic analgesic drugs have analgesic properties or potentiate narcotic analgesics. Non-narcotic analgesics are structurally dissimilar organic acids that fit into the subcategories of analgesic, antipyretic, and anti-inflammatory activity. Non-narcotics act peripherally, and their anti-inflammatory activity results from biochemical changes. These drugs are frequently referred to as nonsteroidal anti-inflammatory agents (NSAIDs). In the ICU these drugs are rarely used for anti-inflammatory action, but some are used as antipyretics. Because aspirin and acetaminophen are the two agents most commonly used, and acetaminophen lacks some of the side effects of aspirin, only major problems associated with aspirin in combination with other drugs will be addressed.

Epigastric distress progressing to gastric or intestinal ulceration and subsequent bleeding may be associated with the use of aspirin. The degree of involvement is usually dose-dependent. Gastric distress results from prostaglandin inhibition, which normally decreases stomach acid secretion and promotes secretion of cytoprotective intestinal mucus. There is also an increase in the mean bleeding time due to inhibited thromboxane A_2 formation in thrombocytes and reduced platelet aggregation. This effect persists for the life of the platelet. Bleeding time will be doubled for 4 to 7 days following administration of 650 mg of aspirin. All other non-narcotic analgesics, except acetaminophen, also inhibit platelet aggregation; however, the effect is "reversible" and is usually quantitatively less and shorter than that observed with aspirin. Increased bleeding time is exacerbated in patients with underlying hematologic defects and in those taking anticoagulants. Use of any NSAID should be approached with caution because of this potential problem. In small doses, other side effects from non-narcotic analgesics are minimal (Huskisson, 1974).

ANALGESIC ADJUVANT THERAPY

Adjuvant therapy offers a valuable addition to the available treatment modalities in critical care. This group of drugs can be divided into different pharmacologic categories including central nervous system stimulants, antidepressants, antispastic agents, skeletal muscle relaxants, antipsychotics, antihistamines, anxiolytics, and anticonvulsants. Mechanism of analgesic action of these agents is frequently conjectural, and critical proof of analgesic efficacy is often lacking. However, there are clinical situations in which adjuvant therapy may provide substantial analgesic benefit. It is interesting to note that as our understanding of pain transmission mechanisms improves, some observations of adjuvant drug therapy effectiveness have been validated.

Stimulant and antidepressant drugs are not widely used in various pain syndrome treatments due to fear of drug dependence and potential side effects involving CNS stimulation. However, these drugs have been extremely effective in patients with excessive narcotic analgesic sedation or illness-related depression. Caffeine and dextroamphetamine are the most popular drugs in this category. Oral dextro-

amphetamine given at a dose of 5 to 10 mg in the morning is especially useful for combating daytime sedation resulting from narcotic analgesics. A combination of morphine and dextroamphetamine has been found twice as effective for analgesia as morphine alone. Caffeine, a constituent of both over-the-counter and prescription medications, is an effective analgesic adjuvant at doses of at least 65 mg. When combined with various non-narcotic analgesics such as aspirin or acetaminophen, caffeine increases the analgesic activity of these agents. Tricyclic antidepressants such as amitriptyline, imipramine, and nortriptyline are commonly used to treat depression associated with chronic pain such as neuralgia or migraine headaches.

Skeletal muscle relaxants include antispastic and centrally acting agents. Primary antispastic agents are diazepam and baclofen, which act in the spinal cord, and dantrolene, which acts directly on skeletal muscle. These drugs reduce muscle spasticity, leading to reduced pain. Centrally acting skeletal muscle relaxants include carisporodol, chlorephenesin, chlorzoxazone, cyclobenzaprine, methocarbamol, and orphenadrine. The choice of agent depends upon the condition being treated, the presence of associated illnesses, and potential drug interactions. These drugs are frequently used in combination with other drugs and treatment regimens to obtain the best therapeutic effect.

Antipsychotics and antianxiety agents (anxiolytics) are used for their ability to alter the patient's behavioral status. Examples of antipsychotics are methotrimeprazine and haloperidol. In addition to its antipsychotic activity, methotrimeprazine also appears to produce analgesia directly through a nonopioid receptor system. It is useful in patients with tolerance to narcotic analgesics or who respond to them with respiratory depression or when both antipsychotic and analgesic effects are needed. In the anxiolytic group, benzodiazepine, like diazepam, is most popular. These agents reduce other symptoms, such as anxiety, that are often associated with pain. Tranquilizers may modify the undesirable side effects of narcotics such as nausea and vomiting. Minor tranquilizers are more specific for the treatment of anxiety and safer than phenothiazines.

The major *antihistamine* used as an adjuvant in pain therapy is hydroxyzine, given in doses of 50 to 100 mg intramuscularly with a narcotic analgesic. Promethazine may be used in a similar manner. Some clinicians believe that the sedative effect of antihistamine enhances the sedative activity of the narcotic and is the major benefit of this combination.

Anticonvulsant drugs have been demonstrated to be effective for certain types of neurologic pain such as phantom limb pain. Anticonvulsants most often prescribed include carbamazepine, phenytoin, and clonazepam. When these drugs are used baseline blood studies must be performed at regular intervals to determine the blood levels of the drug and to check for the presence of blood dyscrasias. Physicians and nurses should be thoroughly familiar with the pharmacologic properties of these agents.

ANESTHETIC AGENTS

Most anesthetic agents provide anesthesia and are generally considered poor analgesics except when the patient is semiconscious or unconscious. Clinical experience and research have demonstrated that anesthetic agents are useful because of their CNS depression properties. These agents include halothane (Fluothane), enflurane (Ethrane), and isoflurane (Forane). In contrast, inhaled anesthetics such as nitrous oxide and methoxyflurane (Penthrane) are potent analgesics at subanesthetic concentrations and are used for pain control in dental and obstetric procedures. They have also been extremely useful for intermittent, severe pain when routine analgesics are not adequate, such as during burn dressing changes or orthopedic procedures. When the critical care nurse is not satisfied with the adequacy of the analgesic agents used or believes they are unsafe in the doses required, the possible use of anesthetic agents should be pursued in consultation with the anesthesiologist.

Use of local anesthetics such as cainal agents is common in critical care to produce limited analgesia close to the site of administration. Frequently used agents include procaine (Novocain), lidocaine (Xylocaine), and bupivacaine (Marcaine). Benzocaine is a topical compound used for irritated areas of the skin or mucous membranes. These drugs prevent conduction and generation of nerve impulses, a process that is reversed when the drug concentration diminishes. Although all neurons in contact with these drugs are affected, the small-diameter fibers such as those that transmit pain (the A-delta and C fibers) are most susceptible (Bonica, 1987; DiGregorio et al., 1986; Mather and Cousins, 1986).

METHODS OF ADMINISTRATION

Much concern has been expressed by nurses about the adequacy of pain management, especially for postoperative pain, because pain relief continues to pose a significant problem in everyday clinical practice. Despite advances in anesthesia and analgesia, relief of postoperative pain has not changed drastically and remains inadequate (Nordberg, 1984; Donovan, 1983). Nordberg (1984) states that parenteral administration of narcotics persists as the major approach to postoperative pain relief, not because it offers optimal pain relief but because of its simplicity of administration. In a study by Donovan (1983) involving 200 general surgery patients, 31% reported insufficient postoperative pain relief. Sixty-three per cent of these dissatisfied patients stated that pain relief could have been more frequent. Donovan believes that medical and nursing staff are reluctant to depart from traditional routines to relieve pain. However, investigations in the last decade have increased

our understanding of the pharmacodynamics of narcotics and have opened new doors for pain treatment.

Continous and intermittent intravenous administration of narcotic analgesics has recently become popular. The continous method is most useful for terminally ill cancer patients unable to take oral medications. Morphine is most commonly used. In nontolerant patients of average weight with acute pain, the usual doses of morphine and meperidine are 3 mg/hr and 20 mg/hr, respectively. Some patients with severe acute pain may require higher doses. However, increasing the infusion rate more than once a day should be done with extreme caution because a new peak narcotic plasma level will not be attained for 12 to 24 hours after a rate change. Therefore, any adjustment in dose should be closely monitored for delayed respiratory depression 12 to 24 hours later. Frequent assessment of vital signs is mandatory during this period, and naloxone should be available for the immediate reversal of narcotic-induced toxicity. Patients with advanced cancer or terminal cancer-related pain can become rapidly tolerant. Because the major therapeutic goal for these patients is pain relief, they may require hourly analgesic doses that are substantially higher than those required for management of acute pain.

Patient-Controlled Analgesia (PCA). PCA is a recent innovative approach to pain management that allows self-administration of intravenous analgesia. A PCA device consists of an infusion pump and a timing unit that the patient triggers by depressing a thumb button. The device delivers analgesia, usually morphine, in a preset bolus amount through an indwelling catheter. The timing unit prevents overdosage by interposing an "inactivation period" between patient-initiated doses. A specified total dose is regulated over a period of time, usually 24 hours. Data regarding dosage and time of administration are recorded and are retrievable by the nurse at any time (Barkas and Duafala, 1988). Advantages of PCA include increased patient comfort, satisfaction of individualized needs, reduction of lag time from pain onset to drug administration, elimination of dependency on the nurse, decrease in tissue trauma from frequent parenteral injections, reduction in amount of analgesic used, early postoperative ambulation, increase in forced vital capacity and peak expiratory flow in postoperative patients, and enhanced bowel recovery following trauma or surgery (Bennett and Griffen, 1983; Atwell et al., 1984; Eisenach et al., 1988). A comparative study by Kleiman and associates (1988) reported no significant difference between PCA and regularly scheduled intramuscular injections in patients with severe postoperative pain. Subjectively, both patients and nurses liked the PCA, and observations of earlier and more comfortable ambulation were reported. The most frequently identified disadvantage to the pump is expense. Use of PCA should be selective, depending on patient alertness and ability to comprehend the function and purpose of the machine. Caution should be exercised in patients with incident pain and neuropathic pain syndromes, depressed and delirious patients, and patients with a history of drug or alcohol abuse (Barkas and Duafala, 1988).

Epidural Narcotics. Epidural narcotics alleviate visceral and somatic pain by direct application into the spinal epidural space. This new technique is gaining increasing popularity in clinical practice because opiates provide long-acting analgesia while avoiding many negative side effects, such as the central depressant effects associated with parenteral pain control. This form of analgesia allows increased mobility and improved respiratory dynamics, theoretically preventing further postoperative complications (Leib and Hurtig, 1985). Yeager and colleagues (1987) studied the effect of epidural anesthesia and postoperative analgesia on postoperative morbidity in high-risk surgery patients. Compared to the control group, patients receiving epidural anesthesia and analgesia had fewer respiratory, cardiovascular, and major infectious complications. Urinary cortisol excretion, a marker of the stress response, was also significantly diminished in this group. Finally, hospital costs were significantly reduced for these patients due to decreased postoperative morbidity.

Depending on hospital policy, nurses may administer epidural narcotics or monitor patients receiving epidural narcotics. Frequently, these patients are monitored in critical care units because close, continual nursing observation is a requirement for adequate epidural pain management (Leib and Hurtig, 1985). Therefore, critical care nurses need to be knowledgeable about epidural physiology, use of epidural narcotics, and implications for nursing care.

The epidural space, a potential space between the spinal dura mater and the vertebral canal, contains loose connective tissue, fat, and a plexus of veins and functions to cushion the spinal cord (Stewart, 1986) (Fig. 38–9). Discovery of endogenous narcotic-like peptides, called endorphins and enkephalins, and opiate receptors in the dorsal horn region of the spinal cord has improved our understanding of pain and epidural narcotic function (Parish and Thompson, 1987; Leib and Hurtig, 1985). Endorphins and enkephalins, released from interneurons, act like neurotransmitters by binding with opiate receptors on the surface of neurons at the neuronal synapses. Administration of narcotics presumably mimics the action of endogenous peptides. Epidural analgesia occurs when opioids, such as morphine, are placed in the epidural space, enabling the drug to cross the duralarachnoid layer passively and diffuse into the spinal fluid and then into the dorsal horn of the spinal cord to bind the opiate receptors located strategically along pain pathways (Parish and Thompson, 1987; Nordberg, 1984).

The analgesic effect of epidural narcotics depends upon diffusion to the opiate receptors in the dorsal

root horn. The rate of diffusion appears to be related to lipid solubility, molecular weight and volume of the drug, and specific receptor affinities (Leib and Hurtig, 1985). For example, 2 to 10 mg of epidural morphine, which is more water-soluble than lipid-soluble, slowly diffuses through the lipid neural sheath and exhibits a long latency period. This, combined with strong receptor affinity, contributes to its high analgesic potency and long duration of action. Fentanyl, in contrast, is highly lipid-soluble, diffuses rapidly, and immediately binds receptors. Therefore, it has a rapid onset and a short duration of action (Leib and Hurtig, 1985). Although several narcotics have been used, morphine sulfate remains the standard by which all epidural narcotics are measured. Meperidine, methadone, and beta-endorphin are all effective epidural analgesics. Drugs containing stabilizing agents, preservatives, and trioxidants or neurolytic agents such as phenol or alcohol are not recommended because of their potential for neurotoxicity.

Studies have supported the spinal epidural approach over the parenteral route for control of pain after thoracic, abdominal, orthopedic, vascular, urologic, and gynecologic surgery (Nordberg, 1984; Bromage et al., 1980; Yeager et al., 1987). Similar or smaller dose requirements of epidural morphine compared to those needed for systemic administration have been frequently reported (Nordberg, 1984; Martin et al., 1982). Onset of analgesia, however, has been reported to be slower than that observed with intramuscular morphine, with adequate analgesia frequently not obtained until 45 to 60 minutes after administration (Nordberg, 1984; Bromage et al., 1980).

The epidural catheter is placed by a trained anesthesiologist or anesthetist, the site of insertion usually being at the level closest to the segments innervated by the pain focus (Nordberg, 1984; Bromage et al., 1980; Leib and Hurtig, 1985) (see Fig. 38–3). Usually, the catheter is left in place for 48 hours. However, the time may vary depending on patient needs and agency policy (Stewart, 1986). Complications associated with epidural narcotics are attributable either to the technique of administration or to drug action and side effects (Leib and Hurtig, 1985). Side effects associated with epidural narcotics are well documented in the literature and include urine retention, nausea, vomiting, pruritus, and respiratory depression. Although the overall incidence is low, respiratory depression is the most untoward complication associated with spinal narcotics because it has been reported to occur many hours after administration of spinal opiates and to outlast a single reversing dose of naloxone (Nordberg, 1984). The itching caused by morphine is thought to be due to direct histamine release from tissue mast cells. However, antihistamines seldom completely block this type of pruritus and sometimes provide little relief (Bernstein and Swift, 1979). Sensations of both itch and pain are transmitted to the dorsal horns of the spinal cord and are probably integrated at a

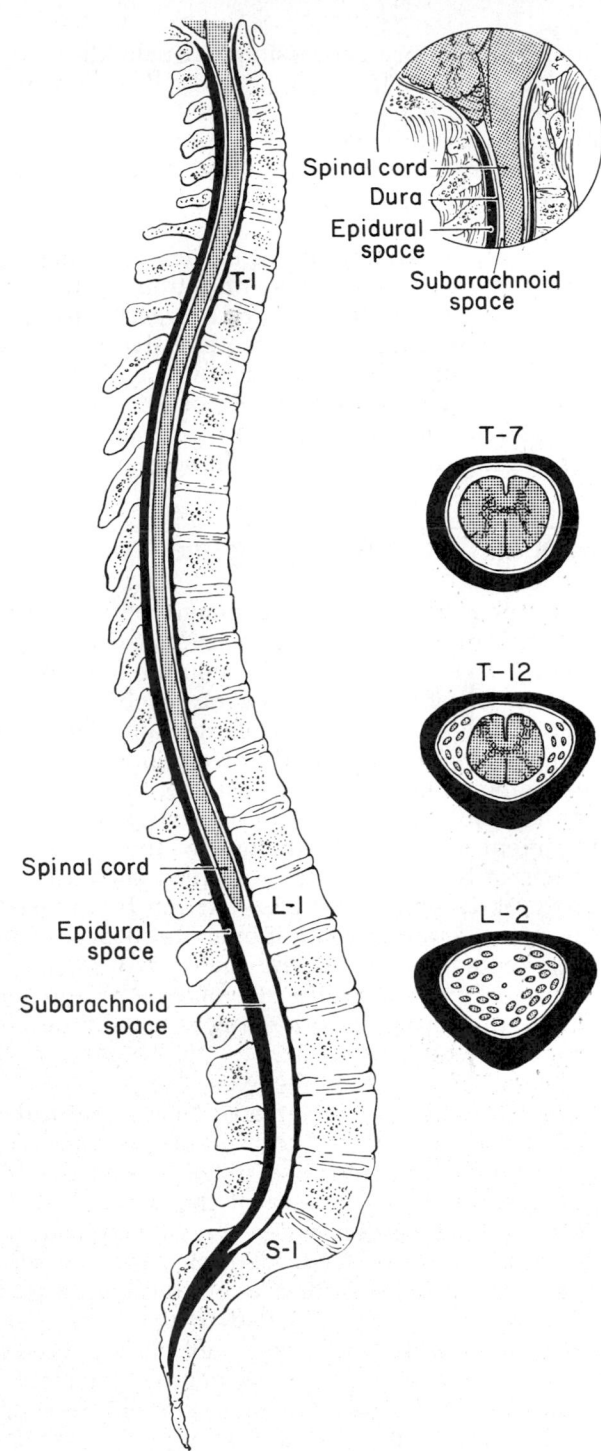

FIGURE 38–9. Epidural space. *Left*, Sagittal section of spinal column. *Inset*, Enlarged view of upper cervical region showing that the epidural space does not extend beyond the foramen magnum where the dura attaches to the entire circumference of the foramen. *Right*, Cross sectional view of various levels of vertebral column. Note the difference in shape of the epidural space in the midthoracic and midlumbar region. (From Bonica, J.J. (1967). *Principles and practice of obstetric analgesia and anesthesia* (p. 622). Philadelphia: F.A. Davis.

common site at each spinal segment (Summerfield, 1980). Therefore, a second theory suggests that, given the close link between pain and itching, the itching produced by morphine might also result from its binding to opiate receptors. It is believed that by blocking the encephalon and endorphin opiate receptors in the CNS, naloxone, an opiate antagonist, can relieve the itching associated with epidural morphine (Bernstein and Swift, 1979). A few reports suggest that the side effects induced by epidural narcotics may be reversed with small doses of naloxone with-

out reversing the analgesic effect (Leib and Hurtig, 1985). The incidence, duration, and rationale for the occurrence of these adverse effects remain controversial because many studies have revealed conflicting results.

Intrathecal Narcotics. Intrathecal narcotics are similar to epidural narcotics and are administered through a catheter placed in a selected area of the spinal cord. Respiratory depression and coma can be produced by rostral spread of the narcotic into the brain. Respiratory depression is usually delayed and can occur up to 12 hours after the dose. Morphine, meperidine, fentanyl, methadone, and beta-endorphins are also used effectively through the intrathecal routes. For acute pain, the dose of morphine varies from 0.2 to 2 mg/hour.

Inhalation Analgesia. Inhalation analgesia is achieved through the use of nitrous oxide, other inhalant-type anesthetics, and oxygen. Mixtures of nitrous oxide and oxygen are effective for management of minor and severe acute pain. Entonox is a commercially prepared mixture of 50% nitrous oxide and 50% oxygen that has been used successfully for performing dressing changes in burn patients.

Nonpharmacologic Management of Pain

Nonpharmacologic management of pain can be initiated independently by the critical care nurse. Numerous studies are available in the literature supporting the efficacy of techniques such as relaxation in reducing or even controlling pain. These techniques have been reported to work independently or in combination with analgesic agents. A major advantage of the use of nonpharmacologic management is patient safety and reduction of the possible side effects of body response to a given chemical. Some of the independent actions that can be initiated by the nurse require no additional instruction or training; however, to use the skills and instruments associated with relaxation techniques reliably, some degree of assistance or training is usually necessary to enhance outcomes.

Transcutaneous Electrical Nerve Stimulation (TENS). The use of electrical stimulation for analgesia and prevention of atrophy dates back to the 1800s; however, wide acceptance of the principle did not occur until the 1960s, when the gate control theory of pain was introduced. Clinical use of knowledge about dorsal column stimulation to decrease pain by Melzack and Wall (1965) led to the application of electrical stimulation to almost all parts of the body. Thus, the intent of peripheral nerve stimulation is to utilize large myelinated primary afferent nerve fibers (A fibers) to inhibit the transmission of activity in the small, unmyelinated primary afferent fibers (C fibers), inactivating local inhibitory circuits within the dorsal horn of the spinal cord and ultimately diminishing nociceptive transmission through the spinal cord (Wolff, 1985).

Research about the release of endogenous opiates from the appropriate neuronal tracts led to the discovery that electrical stimulation of neurons in specific areas of the CNS could elicit analgesia for several hours. These findings supported the premise that TENS units are effective because electrical nerve stimulation excites large mechanoreceptors in the periphery that subsequently stimulate the activity of enkephalins in the dorsal horn of the spinal cord, resulting in analgesia. This hypothesis is supported by findings reporting the ability of naloxone to reverse the effects of both acupuncture and TENS (Mayer et al., 1977).

Four electrical stimulation techniques can be employed to produce analgesia, including TENS, using surface electrodes applied to the skin; peripheral nerve stimulation through subcutaneously implanted electrodes; peripheral nerve stimulation using electrodes implanted directly on the nerve; and antidromic activation of primary afferent collaterals by the stimulation of the dorsal columns either directly or through the dura (Wolff, 1985).

The pulse generator used for electrical stimulation is a simple device and should be familiar to nurses. Trial and error is employed in regard to the sites used for the electrodes as well as the frequency used for stimulation. Stimulation should be adjusted to a strength that causes pain and then lowered until the patient's comfort level is obtained. Differences in the frequency used are influenced by individual variations as well as the origins of the pain. The usual frequency used is 50 to 100 pulsations per second. Electrodes should be tried at one site for 12 to 24 hours for a fair evaluation of a decrease in pain. Low-frequency stimulation or trains of stimulation have been associated with modification of acute pain.

For treatment of pain related to surgical incisions, electrodes are commonly placed 1 to 2 inches from the wound. Postoperative electrical stimulation appears to reduce the incidence of complications following abdominal procedures, to stimulate gastrointestinal tract function following surgery, and to reduce the amount of time spent by the patient in intensive care. Atelectasis is almost entirely eliminated, and the incidence of ileus is markedly reduced.

Complications or adverse effects of TENS may include skin irritation from the adhesives used to secure the electrodes or, rarely, from the electrodes themselves. Neovascularization has occurred in some individuals when the same site is used repeatedly for electrode placement. Vascularization promptly subsides when the positions are varied.

Acute pain can be successfully diminished by TENS in more than 60% of all patients. TENS has been reported to be moderately successful in male patients with sickle cell pain (Wang et al., 1988), dental operations (Hochman, 1988), and prostatectomy or penile prosthetic surgery (Merrill, 1989). TENS did not provide significant analgesic relief in patients with labor pains (Thomas et al., 1988), cholecystectomy (Reuss et al., 1988), acute postoperative pain (McCallum et al., 1988), and inguinal herniorrhaphy (Smedley et al., 1988).

Several issues emerge from the literature that may be advantageous for consideration by critical care nurses. TENS therapy alone is not appropriate for acute pain management. It should be considered part of a larger pain management program in combination with the use of other modalities. Use of TENS in patients with chronic pain syndromes appears to be successful. Finally, several studies report that electrical stimulation improves circulation and may be beneficial in patients with ischemic pain (Omura, 1987; Jivegard et al., 1987).

Acupuncture and Acupressure. Acupuncture, an ancient Chinese practice, through many beliefs and applications has become a common form of pain management in the Western world. The procedure involves inserting fine needles through specific points in the skin and twirling them for some time at a slow rate. The needles can be removed when relief is obtained or left in place for varying periods of time. Continued analgesia can be achieved by hooking the needles to a battery-driven stimulator to maintain the activity of the needle or needles. It is believed that acupuncture needles stimulate large afferent fibers that cause the release of endorphins and enkephalins. Ongoing research supports the belief that pain relief achieved by acupuncture is a result of CNS involvement and not simply a placebo effect (Melzack, 1975; Mayer et al., 1977). The use of TENS at auricular acupuncture points has provided a significant level of pain relief from induced pain (Noling et al., 1988).

Acupressure is a technique whereby pressure instead of needle insertion is applied to the designated points on identified meridians of the body. Use of electrical stimulation, heat, and a variety of intense sensory techniques indicates that acupressure is not a magical procedure but only one of many ways of producing analgesia by an intense sensory input that might be labeled "hyperstimulation analgesia." The use of these noninvasive techniques provides opportunities for paramedical personnel to employ them after learning the appropriate points on the body. Clearly, the points can be easily learned and applied by the critical care nurse to assist in pain management.

Relaxation Techniques. Various skills, techniques and rituals have been developed over many centuries for individuals who wish to achieve some level of relaxation and are willing to learn and practice the routine until a specified goal is achieved. These techniques incorporate autogenic training to reach relaxation through the use of commonly known approaches such as progressive relaxation, imagery, meditation, hypnosis, biofeedback, zen, and yoga. Autogenic training was developed in the 1920s in Germany by Johannes H. Schultz, who believed that voluntary and predictable control of the body could be attained by programming it to develop heavy and warm extremities, a warm abdomen, a calm and regular heartbeat, relaxed respiration, and a cool forehead. Actually, then, autogenic training is sensory biofeedback. Prior to that, Emil Coué, a French pharmacist, used a simple general approach composed of attunement through autosuggestion and repetition of the phrase, "Every day, in every way, I am getting better and better." Autogenic training

has been helpful for many individuals. Following this, Jacobsen (1978) introduced progressive relaxation. Many somatic conditions were improved through the routine use of relaxation. The benefits of relaxation techniques used by patients with acute and chronic conditions, including pain, are reflected in the literature (Benson et al., 1975; Tan, 1982; Snyder, 1984; Lawlis et al., 1985). Graffam and Johnson (1987) compared the use of imagery and progressive muscle relaxation by adult oncology patients and found both strategies equally effective in reducing pain and distress. Most patients, however, expressed a preference for using progressive muscle relaxation.

In 1959, Maharishi Mahesh Yogi introduced transcendental meditation (TM) to the western world. TM involves passive, dispassionate relaxation. This type of relaxation was more commonly used by cults, resulting in distaste for the technique by the general public.

Biofeedback, introduced in the early 1960s, gave the greatest boost to autogenic training. Like autogenics, biofeedback is based on the assumption that if patients can be taught to control an internal state, they can modify pain or any illness that is psychosomatic in nature. Biofeedback provides individuals with an opportunity to observe progress in their ability to manage body activities such as skin temperature, heartbeat, breathing, blood pressure, and, most importantly, pain. Patients learn to control their autonomic nervous system, which regulates the internal organs. The literature is filled with research and knowledge about the application, implementation, and benefits of biofeedback. Recent summaries and analyses of the literature, however, reflect the fact that the major current application of biofeedback is in patients with chronic pain (Turner and Chapman, 1982; Kewman and Roberts, 1983; Roberts, 1987). A study by Jacobs (1987) reflects an estimated medical cost-offset of $7 million when biofeedback was used by adult males as a method of managing stress, pain, vocational rehabilitation, and coping skills.

Biofeedback training involves the use of a machine such as a heart monitor, blood pressure machine, electromyography (EMG) machine, or thermometer that can be observed and a teaching device such as audiotapes that can be used to teach a progressive or consistent program. There are various types of biofeedback training: brainwave or ALPHA training teaches the patient to control brain wave output; temperature biofeedback instruction teaches the patient to raise or lower the skin temperature of a portion of the body; EMG training teaches how to relax certain muscle groups; and finally, the patient can be taught how to control a particular function of the body such as heart rate, blood pressure, or breathing. Many other types of biofeedback training are now being developed or proposed for control of almost any physiologic activity. The training is done with an electronic machine that is calibrated to pick up extremely small physiologic, electrical, or chemical changes as they take place. These minute changes are converted to either visual or auditory signals that can be recognized by the patient, providing immediate feedback.

Repeated use of the relaxation approach and the biofeedback machine allows patients to control (self-regulate) the particular function of the body being monitored. Patients become aware of the subtle changes in their conscious feelings (subjective response) that occur when the biofeedback machine reflects the desirable physical change. Continued monitoring and awareness of subjective feelings will eventually cancel the need for a feedback machine.

In the critical care setting the devices or machines already attached to the patient provide feedback on patients' ability to control certain functions such as heart rate. However, it is the nurse's skill and knowledge that makes it possible to teach the biofeedback technique to patients who are critically ill and are currently in a location that differs from the quiet and solitude of their own home.

Hypnosis. Hypnosis, a trancelike, altered state of consciousness, has been used in many different settings to manage acute and chronic pain and stress. A trance state may include a temporary suspension of critical judgment, a capacity for congruent ideas, and rapid assimilation of internal or external data (Spiegel and Spiegel, 1978). Like other non-narcotic methods of pain management, hypnosis is the target of myths and misconceptions by both patients and nurses. The major misconception is that hypnosis is caused by a force or person outside the patient. Hypnotic states can occur spontaneously through self-induction without the formal ceremony of induction (Crasilneck and Hall, 1975) and with minimal intervention from the nursing or medical staff. Hypnotic states may occur spontaneously in patients who focus on a symptom or on pain. Many critically ill or traumatized patients are already in a trancelike state, which can be enhanced by support and direction from the nurse. This trancelike state may explain the positive response to pain management in patients who have been severely traumatized, such as burn patients (Schafer, 1975). Clinical studies also support the premise that patients can direct their attention following injury or acute illness (Edmonston, 1981; Zahourek, 1982; Wain and Amer, 1986). One important observation is that the trance state is not altered by the injection of naloxone. This fact is believed to indicate that hypnosis reflects a higher level of consciousness that may not be mediated through endogenous opiates. It appears that spontaneous hypnosis-like states may be an outstanding adjunctive procedure of great use for the critical care nurse.

Additional Techniques for Managing Pain

Other approaches may be implemented to manage or decrease pain perception including music and other forms of distraction, cognitive dissonance, body massage, and ice application. Music has been especially beneficial due to its calming benefits.

ETHICAL ISSUES IN PAIN MANAGEMENT

Ethics may be defined as a body of principles relating to right or good conduct. Ethical principles relating to nurses' assessment and management of pain and suffering have not been clearly delineated. Lisson (1987) identified the balancing of therapeutic relief with toxic side effects as an ethical dilemma that is complicated by the failure of nurses to recognize pain control as a crucial ethical issue. Additionally, the presence of certain myths, attitudes, and behaviors in clinical practice results in restrictive, insensitive, and inappropriate rationing of pain relief (Copp, 1985).

In general, the nurse's role is usually described as the provision care, comfort, compassion, and protection for patients and their families. A compassionate, caring, and comforting approach to the pain and suffering experienced by patients who are critically ill should clearly be a high-priority goal for the critical care nurse. In addition, the mental and emotional suffering of the family and significant others must be addressed. Factors that may prevent attainment of this goal are numerous; only a few will be mentioned here. The necessary focus on technology in critical care settings can de-emphasize the importance of simple comfort measures. One example is the elderly patient who is cold but is not given a blanket because it would make it more difficult to monitor the many lines and tubes attached to the patient. Assessment of coldness and intervention for this discomfort may be overlooked because life-saving or life-sustaining measures take precedence. Hospital environments, especially critical care settings, may amplify the suffering caused by anxiety, loneliness, fear, confusion, anger, and possibly despair. Families as well as patients are likely to experience these feelings. Simple comfort measures such as a calm and reassuring voice, touching the patient in a manner that recognizes the person's importance as a human being, and allowing the expression of feelings are often overlooked in a setting that requires complicated technology and frequent decision making. However, these caring and comforting measures may be the efforts best remembered gratefully by patients' families who have lost their loved ones despite the best efforts of the health care team.

In the process of delivering nursing care to critically ill patients, not only is much pain and suffering left unrecognized or untreated, but also additional pain, discomfort, and suffering are necessary parts of many medical and nursing procedures. Critically ill patients are often unable to respond verbally; therefore, the nurse must be particularly vigilant in protecting these patients. The challenge for nurses is how to mitigate the pain, discomfort, and suffering as much as possible while providing the necessary high-tech care.

Jameton (1984) states that nurses, because of their close work with patients on a daily basis, may become "specialists in suffering." In critical care areas this special ability may take a back seat to technologic skills such as interpretation of data provided by the many monitoring devices. Jameton suggests that because caring skills are labor-intensive and the results are less tangible than technologically oriented work, the tendency may be to provide more rewards and respect to those with more technologically oriented skills.

Critical care nursing is particularly challenging because it requires the nurse to be highly competent in the knowledge and skills associated with sophisticated life-sustaining equipment, yet also to provide as much comfort as possible. The ethical issues involved in critical care pain management remain to be fully addressed. Nurses in intensive care should examine their care protocols to determine the best way to provide a consistent humanistic and research-based approach to assessing and managing pain and suffering of critically ill patients.

NURSING DIAGNOSES RELATED TO PAIN

This chapter has focused on pain and its relationship to other factors impinging on the care of the critically ill patient. As such, the entire chapter may be said to address the nursing diagnosis of alteration in comfort, pain. The remainder of this section addresses this specific nursing diagnosis.

The use of nursing diagnoses helps to define and give direction to care that is uniquely nursing. The critical care nurse is in a key position to affect the quality of life of critically ill patients who are experiencing pain, discomfort, and suffering. An example illustrating the difference in using a nursing diagnosis versus a medical diagnosis for the same patient is the following: Instead of identifying the patient's problem as myocardial infarction or multiple trauma, which are medical diagnoses, the nurse assesses the effects of the disease on functional status experienced by the patient. The nurse cannot directly intervene for the problem of myocardial infarction but can intervene for the nursing diagnosis of pain, or alteration in comfort, related to myocardial ischemia. The desired patient outcome is a decrease in pain or discomfort. The nurse simultaneously implements interventions to relieve pain and to decrease myocardial ischemia, such as administering analgesics and oxygen and taking appropriate measures to decrease the patient's fear and anxiety.

Pain, discomfort, or suffering, no matter what the specific etiology (myocardial infarction, multiple trauma) is likely to produce other changes in the patient's functional status and may result in one or more of the following nursing diagnoses:

Sleep pattern disturbance

Sensory-perceptual alterations

Altered thought process

Anxiety

Fear

Hopelessness

Powerlessness

Altered role performance

Impaired social interaction

Ineffective individual coping

Ineffective family coping

The preceding nursing diagnoses are more likely to be experienced by patients who perceive that their pain, discomfort, or suffering is not being addressed or managed adequately. They may blame themselves for not being able to decrease this problem, especially if their health care providers have made unsuccessful attempts to alleviate the pain. A change in the rate and rhythm of the heart is one of many physiologic alterations that can be produced by the stress of pain. Alleviation or decrease in pain, discomfort, and suffering in the critically ill patient, then, is an important priority. Management of these nursing diagnoses related to alterations in comfort, with outcomes and interventions focused on increasing comfort, is likely to affect the patient's overall well-being to a greater extent than we may anticipate.

References

Akil, H., Mayer, D., and Liebeskind, J. (1976). Antagonism of stimulation produced analgesia by naloxone, a narcotic antagonist. *Science*, 191, 961–962.

Amnad, R. E., Perry, S., and Genovese, V. (1982). Nonprocedural pain as perceived by burn patient and nurse. Reported at American Burn Association, 14th Annual Meeting, Boston.

Asterita, M. F. (1985). *The physiology of stress.* New York: Human Sciences Press.

Atwell, J. R., Flanigan, R. C., Bennett, R. L., et al. (1984). The efficacy of patient-controlled analgesia in patients recovering from flank incisions. *Journal of Urology,* 132, 701–703.

Baer, E., Davitz, L. J., and Lieb, R. (1983). Inferences of physical pain and psychological distress. 1. In relation to verbal and nonverbal patient communication. *Nursing Research,* 79, 32–35.

Barak, E., and Weisenberg, M. (1988). Anxiety and attitudes toward pain as a function of ethnic grouping and socioeconomic status. *Clinical Journal of Pain,* 3, 189–196.

Barkas, G, and Duafala, M. E. (1988). Advances in cancer pain management: A review of patient-controlled analgesia. *Journal of Pain and Symptom Management,* 3, 150–160.

Bates, M. S. (1987). Ethnicity and pain: A biocultural model. *Social Science Medicine,* 24 (1), 47–50.

Beecher, H. K. (1959). *Measurement of subjective responses.* New York: Oxford University Press.

Beecher, H. K. (1972). The placebo effect as a nonspecific force surrounding disease and the treatment of disease. In R. Jongen, W.D. Keidel, A. Herz, et al. (Eds.), *Pain: Basic principles, pharmacology and therapy.* Stuttgart: Thieme.

Bennett, R. L., and Griffen, W. O. (1983). Patient controlled analgesia. *Contemporary Surgery*, 22, 75–79.

Benson, H., Greenwood, A. B., and Klemchuk, A. B. (1975). The relaxation response: Psychophysiologic aspects and clinical applications. *International Journal of Psychiatry in Medicine*, 6, 87–98.

Bernstein, J. E., and Swift, R. (1979). Relief of intractable pruritus with naloxone. *Archives of Dermatology*, 115, 1366–1367.

Bloom, F. E., Rossier, J., Battenberg, E. L. F., et al. (1978). B-endorphin: Cellular localization, electrophysiological and behavioral effects. In E. Costa and M. Trabucchi (Eds.), *The endorphins. Advances in biochemical psychopharmacology* (pp. 18, 89). New York: Raven Press.

Bonica, J. J. (1983). The importance of education and training in pain diagnosis and therapy: The role of continuing education courses. In R. Rizzi, and M. Visentin (Eds.), *Pain therapy* (pp. 1-10). Amsterdam: Elsevier Biomedical Press.

Bonica, J. J. (1987). Importance of effective pain control. *Acta Anaesthesiology Scandinavica*, Supplement 85, 1–16.

Bromage, P. R., Camporesi, E., and Chestnut, D. (1980). Epidural narcotics for postoperative analgesia. *Anesthesia and Analgesia*, 59, 473–480.

Carr, D. B., Bullen, B. A., Skrinar, G. S., et al. (1981). Physical conditioning facilitates the exercise-induced secretion of beta-endorphins and beta-lipotropin in women. *New England Journal of Medicine*, 305, 560–563.

Chapman, R. C. (1988). Pain related to cancer treatment. *Journal of Pain and Symptom Management*, 3 (4), 188–193.

Christensen, B. N., and Perl, E. R. (1970). Spinal neurons specifically excited by noxious or thermal stimuli: Marginal zone of the dorsal horn. *Journal of Neurophysiology*, 33, 293–307.

Cohen, F. L. (1980). Postsurgical pain relief: Patients' status and nurses' medication choices. *Pain*, 9, 265–274.

Cohen, J. L. (1986). Pharmacokinetic changes in aging. *American Journal of Medicine*, 80 (Suppl.), 31–38.

Copp, L. A. (1985). *Recent advances in nursing: Perspectives on pain.* New York: Churchill Livingstone.

Cousins, M. J., and Phillips, G. D. (1986). *Acute pain management.* New York: Churchill Livingstone.

Craig, K. D. (1984). Emotional aspects of pain. In P. D. Wall, and R. Melzack (Eds.), *Textbook of pain*. New York: Churchill Livingstone.

Crasilneck H. B., and Hall, J. A. (1975). *Clinical hypnosis.* New York: Grune & Stratton.

Davitz, L. J., Sameshina, Y., and Davitz, J. (1976). Suffering as viewed in six different cultures. *American Journal of Nursing*, 76, 1296–1297.

DiGregorio, G. J., Barbieri, E. J., Sterling, G. H., et al. (1986). *Handbook of pain management.* West Chester, PA, Medical Surveillance.

Dimsdale, J. E., and Moss, J. (1980). Plasma catecholamines in stress and exercise. *Journal of the American Medical Association*, 243, 340–342.

Donovan, B. D. (1983). Patient attitudes to postoperative pain relief. *Anesthesia Intensive Care*, 11 (2), 125–129.

Duranti, R., Pantaleo, T., and Bellini, F. (1988). Increase in muscular pain threshold following low frequency–high intensity peripheral conditioning stimulation in humans. *Brain Research*, 452 (1–2), 66–72.

Edmonston, W. E. (1981). *Hypnosis and relaxation.* New York: J. Wiley & Sons.

Edwards, P. W., Zeichner, A., Kuczmierczyk, A. R., et al. (1985). Familial pain models: The relationship between family history of pain and current pain experience. *Pain*, 21, 379–384.

Eisenach, J. C., Grice, S. C., and Dewan, D. M. (1988). Patient-controlled analgesia following cesarean section: A comparison with epidural and intramuscular narcotics. *Anesthesiology*, 68, 444–448.

Fields, H. L., and Basbaum, A. L. (1984). Endogenous pain control mechanisms. In P. D. Wall, and R. Melzack (Eds.), *Textbook of pain*. New York: Churchill Livingstone.

Fordyce, W. E. (1978). Learning processes in pain. In P. A. Sternbach (Ed.), *The psychology of pain* (p. 200). New York: Raven Press.

Frankenhaeuser, M., Dunne, E., and Lundberg, U. (1976). Sex differences in sympathetic-adrenal medullary reactions induced by different stressors. *Psycho-pharmacology*, 47, 1–5.

Furuhashi, N., Takahashi, T., Kono, H., et al. (1984). Sex difference in human peripheral plasma beta-endorphin and beta-lipotropin levels. *Gynecological and Obstetrical Investigation*, 17, 145–148.

Gaston-Johanssen, F. (1984). Pain assessment: Intensity and quality of the words pain, ache and hurt. *Pain*, 20, 69–76.

Gaston-Johanssen, F., and Asklund-Gustafsson, M. (1985). A baseline study for the development of an instrument for the assessment of pain. *Journal of Advanced Nursing*, 10, 539–546.

Good, B. J., and Good, M. D. (1980). The meaning of symptoms: A cultural hermeneutic model for clinical practice. In L. Eisenberg and A. Kleinman (Eds.), *Relevance of social science for medicine* (pp. 165–196). Dordrecht: Reidel.

Goosen, G. M., and Bush, H. (1979). Adaptation: A feedback process. *Advances in Nursing Science*, 1 (4), 51–66.

Gracely, R. H., and Dubner, R. (1981). Pain assessment in human—a reply to Hall. *Pain*, 11, 109–120.

Graffam, S., and Johnson, A. (1987). A comparison of two relaxation strategies for the relief of pain and its distress. *Journal of Pain and Symptom Management*, 2, 229–231.

Greenblat, D. ,., Sellers, E. M., and Shader, R. I. (1982). Drug disposition in old age. *New England Journal of Medicine*, 306, 1081–1088.

Grunau, K. D., and Craig, R. V. (1987). Pain expression in neonates, facial action and cry. *Pain*, 28 (3), 395–410.

Guyton, A. (1991). *Textbook of medical physiology* (8th ed.). Philadelphia: W. B. Saunders.

Haber, R. N., and Hershenson, N. (1980). *The psychology of visual perception* (2nd ed.). New York: Holt, Rinehart, and Winston.

Hall, K. R., and Strider, E. (1954). The varying response to pain in psychiatric disorders: A study in abnormal psychology. *British Journal of Medical Psychology*, 27, 48.

Hardy, J. D., Wolff, H. G., and Goodell, H. (1952). *Pain sensations and reactions*. Baltimore: Williams & Wilkins.

Hochman, R. (1988). Neurotransmitter modulator (TENS) for control of dental operative pain. *Journal of the American Dental Association*, 116 (2), 208–212.

Hokfelt, T., Johansson, O., Jungdahl, A., et al. (1980). Peptidergic neurones. *Nature*, 284, 515–521.

Hongo, T., Jankowska, E., and Lundberg, A. (1968). Post-synaptic excitation and inhibition from primary afferents in neurones of the spinocervical tract. *Journal of Physiology*, 199, 569–592.

Huhman, M. (1982). Endogenous opiates and pain. *Advances in Nursing Science*, 4 (4), 62–71.

Hurley, M. E. (Ed.) (1986). *Classification of nursing diagnosis: Proceedings of the sixth national conference*. St. Louis: C.V. Mosby.

Huskisson, E. C. (1974). Treatment of rheumatoid arthritis with fenoprofen: Comparison with aspirin. *British Medical Journal*, 1, 176–180.

Jacobs, D. F. (1987). Cost-effectiveness of specialized psychological programs for reducing hospital stays and outpatient visits. *Journal of Clinical Psychology*, 43 (11), 729–735.

Jacobsen, E. (1978). *You must relax.* New York: McGraw-Hill.

Jacox, A. K. (1977). *Pain: A source book for nurses and other health professionals*. Boston: Little, Brown.

Jacox, A. K. (1979). Assessing pain. *American Journal of Nursing*, 79 (5), 895–900.

Jacquet, Y. F. (1979). B-Endorphin and ACTH—Opiate peptides with coordinated roles in the regulation of behaviour? *Trends in Neurosciences* 2, 140–143.

Jaffe, J. H., and Martin W. R. (1980). Opioid analgesics and antagonists. In A. G. Gilman, L. S. Goodman, and A. Gilman (Eds.), *The pharmacological basis of therapeutics* (6th ed., p. 494). New York: Macmillan.

Jameton, A. (1984). *Nursing practice: The ethical issues.* Englewood Cliffs, N.J: Prentice-Hall.

Janis, I. L. (1958). *Psychological stress.* New York: Wiley.

Jensen, T. S., and Rasmussen, P. (1984). Amputation. In P. D. Wall and R. Melzack (Eds.), *Textbook of pain* (pp. 402–412). New York: Churchill Livingstone.

Jivegard, L., Augustinsson, L. E., Carlsson, C. A., et al. (1987). Long-term results by epidural spinal electrical stimulation (ESES) in patients with inoperable severe lower limb ischaemia. *European Journal of Vascular Surgery*, 1 (5), 345–349.

Johansson, G. (1972). Sex differences in the catecholamine output of children. *Acta Physiologica Scandinavica*, 85, 569–572.

Johansson, G., and Post, B. (1974). Catecholamine output of males and females over a one-year period. *Acta Physiologica Scandinavica*, 92, 557–565.

Johnson M. (1977). Assessment of clinical pain. In A. K. Jacox (Ed.), *Pain: A source book for nurses and other health professionals* (pp. 139–166). Boston: Little, Brown.

Johnson, P. (1977). The long, hard dying of Joe Rodriguez. *American Journal of Nursing*, 77, 54–57.

Jones, J., Hoggart, B., and Withey, J. (1979). What the patients say: A study of reactions to an intensive care unit. *Intensive Care Medicine*, 5, 89–94.

Kewman, D. G., and Roberts, A. H. (1983). An alternative perspective on biofeedback efficacy studies: A reply to Stiener and Dince. *Biofeedback and Self-Regulation*, 8, 487–503.

Kleiman, R. L., Lipman, A. G., Hare, B. D., et al. (1988). A comparison of morphine administered by patient-controlled analgesia and regularly scheduled intramuscular injection in severe, postoperative pain. *Journal of Pain and Symptom Management*, 3 (1), 15–22.

Koopman, S., Eisenthal, S., and Stoeckle, J. (1984). Ethnicity in the reported pain, emotional distress and requests of medical patients. *Social Science Medicine*, 18, 487–490.

Lawlis, G. G., Selby, D., Minnant, D., et al. (1985). Reduction of postoperative pain parameters by presurgical relaxation instructions for spinal pain patients. *Spine*, 10, 649–651.

Lazarus, R. (1977). Cognitive and coping process in emotion. In A. Monat, and R. Lazarus (Eds.), *Stress and coping: An anthology*. New York: Columbia University Press.

Leib, R. A., and Hurtig, J. B. (1985). Epidural and intrathecal narcotics for pain management. *Heart & Lung*, 14 (2), 164–174.

Liebeskind, J. (1977). Psychological mechanisms of pain. *Annual Review of Psychology*, 28, 41–60.

Lipton, J. A., and Marbach, J. J. (1984). Ethnicity and the pain experience. *Social Science Medicine*, 19, 1279–1298.

Lisson, E. L. (1987). Ethical issues related to pain control. *Nursing Clinics of North America*, 22 (3), 649–659.

Livingston, W. K. (1943). *Pain mechanisms: A physiologic interpretation of causalgia and its related states*. New York: Macmillan.

Lynn, B. (1984). The detection of injury and tissue damage. In P. D. Wall and R. Melzack (Eds.), *Textbook of pain* (pp. 19–31). New York: Churchill Livingstone.

Martin, R., Salbaing, J., and Blaise, G. (1982). Epidural morphine for postoperative pain relief: A dose-response curve. *Anesthesiology*, 56 (6), 423–426.

Mather, L. E., and Cousins, M. J. (1986). Local anesthetics: Principles of use. In M. J. Cousins and G. D. Phillips (Eds.), *Acute pain management*. New York: Churchill Livingstone.

Mather, L. E., and Mackie, J. (1983). The incidence of postoperative pain in children. *Pain*, 15, 271.

Mather, L. E., and Phillips, G. D. (1986). Opioids and adjuvants: Principles of use. In M. J. Cousins and G. D. Phillips (Eds.), *Acute pain management* (pp. 77–101). New York: Churchill Livingstone.

Mayer, D. J., Price, D. D., and Rafii, A. (1977). Antagonism of acupuncture analgesia in man by the narcotic antagonist naloxone. *Brain Research*, 121, 368–372.

McCaffery, M. (1979). *Nursing management of the patient with pain* (2nd ed.). Philadelphia: J. B. Lippincott.

McCallum, M. I., Glynn, C. J., Moore, R. A., et al. (1988). Transcutaneous electrical nerve stimulation in the management of acute postoperative pain. *British Journal of Anesthetics*, 61 (3), 308–312.

Meinhart, N. T., and McCaffery, M. (1983). *Pain: A nursing approach to assessment and analysis*. Norwalk, CT: Appleton-Century-Crofts.

Melzack, R. (1973). *The puzzle of pain*. New York: Basic Books.

Melzack, R. (1975). The McGill pain questionnaire: Major properties and scoring methods. *Pain*, 1, 277–299.

Melzack, R., and Dennis, S. G. (1978). Neurophysiological foundations of pain. In R. A. Steinbach (Ed.), *The psychology of pain*. New York: Raven Press.

Melzack, R., and Wall, P. D. (1965). Pain mechanisms: A new theory. *Science*, 150, 971–973.

Melzack, R., and Wall, P. D. (1970). Evolution of pain theories. *International Anesthesiology Clinics*, 8, 3–34.

Merrill, D. C. (1989). Clinical evaluation of fasTENS, an inexpensive, disposable transcutaneous electrical nerve stimulator designed specifically for postoperative electroanalgesia. *Urology*, 33 (1), 27–30.

Mersky, H. (1975). Pain, learning and memory. *Journal of Psychosomatic Research*, 19, 319–324.

Mersky, H. (1979). IASP Subcommittee on Taxonomy: Pain terms: A list with definitions and notes on usage. *Pain*, 6, 249.

Muir, B. L. (1988). *Pathophysiology: An introduction to the mechanisms of disease*. New York: John Wiley & Sons.

Nafe, J. P. (1934). The pressure, pain and temperature senses. In C. Murchison (Ed.), *Handbook of general experimental psychology*. Worcester: Clark University Press.

Nield, M., Kim, M. J., and Patel, M. (1989). Use of magnitude estimation for estimating the parameters of dyspnea. *Nursing Research*, 38 (2), 77–80.

NIH Consensus Development Conference. (1987). The integrated approach to the management of pain. *Journal of Pain and Symptom Management*, 2 (1), 35–44.

Noling, L. B., Clelland, M. A., Jackson, J. R., et al. (1988). Effect of transcutaneous electrical nerve stimulation at auricular points on experimental cutaneous pain threshold. *Physiological Therapeutics*, 68 (3), 328–332.

Noordenbos, W. (1959). *Pain*. Amsterdam: Elsevier.

Nordberg, G. (1984). Pharmacokinetic aspects of spinal morphine analgesia. *Acta Anaesthesiologica Scandinavica*, 28, 7–38.

Omura, Y. (1987). Basic electrical parameters for safe and effective electro-therapeutics [electro-acupuncture, TES, TENMS (or TEMS), TENS and electro-magnetic field stimulation with or without drug field] for pain, neuromuscular skeletal problems, and circulatory disturbances. *Acupuncture Electrotherapy Research*, 12 (1), 53–70.

Parish, K., and Thompson, G. (1987). Epidural "port-a-cath": An analgesic find. *Australian Nurses Journal*, 17 (3), 44–47.

Phillips, G. D., and Cousins, M. J. (1986). Neurological mechanisms of pain and the relationship of pain, anxiety and sleep. In M. J. Cousins, and G. D. Phillips (Eds.), *Acute pain management* (pp. 32–35). New York: Churchill Livingstone.

Plante, T. G., and Denvey, D. R. (1984). Stress responsivity among dysmenorrheic women at different phases of their menstrual cycle: More ado about nothing. *Behavior Research and Therapy*, 22, 2491–2580.

Polefrone, J. M., and Manuck, S. B. (1987). Gender differences in cardiovascular and neuroendocrine response to stressors. In R. C. Barnett, L. Biener, and G. K. Baruch (Eds.), *Gender and stress* (pp. 45–55). New York: Free Press.

Porth, C. M. (1986). *Pathophysiology: Concepts of altered health states*. Philadelphia: J. B. Lippincott.

Procacci, P., and Zoppi, M. (1984). Heart pain. In P. D. Wall, and R. Melzack (Eds.), *Textbook of pain*. New York: Churchill Livingstone.

Puntillo, K. A. (1988). The phenomenon of pain and critical care nursing. *Heart & Lung*, 17 (3), 262–271.

Reading, A. E. (1984). The McGill pain questionnaire: An appraisal. In R. Melzack (Ed.), *Pain measurement and assessment* (pp. 55–61). New York: Raven Press.

Reuss, R., Cronen, P., and Abplanalp, L. (1988). Transcutaneous electrical nerve stimulation for pain control after cholecystectomy: Lack of expected benefits. *Southern Medical Journal*, 81 (11), 1361–1363.

Roberts, A. H. (1987). Literature update: Biofeedback and chronic pain. *Journal of pain and symptom management*, 3 (3), 169–171.

Savedra, M., Gibbons, P., Tesler, M., et al. (1982). How do children describe pain? A tentative assessment. *Pain*, 14, 95–104.

Schafer, D. W. (1975). Hypnosis use on a burn unit. *International Journal of Clinical and Experimental Hypnosis*, 23 (1), 1–14.

Scott, L. E., Clum G. A., and Peoples, J. B. (1983). Preoperative predictors of postoperative pain. *Pain*, 15, 283–286.

Shapiro, M. B. (1975). The single-variable approach to assessing the intensity of the feeling of depression. *European Journal of Behavior Analysis and Modification*, 1, 62-75.

Sherrington, C. S. (1900). Cutaneous sensations. In E. A. Schafer (Ed.), *Textbook of physiology* (pp. 19–20). Edinburgh: Pentland.

Smedley, F., Taube, M., and Wastell, C. (1988). Transcutaneous electrical nerve stimulation for pain relief following inguinal hernia repair: A controlled trial. *European Surgical Research*, 20 (4), 233–237.

Smith, J. R., and Simon, E. J. (1981). Endorphins, opiate receptors, and their evolving biology. *Pathobiology Annual*, 11, 87–126.

Snyder, M. (1984). Progressive relaxation as a nursing intervention: An analysis. *Advances in Nursing Science*, 2, 47–53.

Spiegel, H., and Spiegel, D. (1978). *Trance and treatment: Clinical uses of hypnosis*. New York: Basic Books.

Stein, J. M., and Warfield, C. A. (1982). The pain clinics: Phantom limb pain. *Hospital Practice*, 17, 166–167.

Sternbach, R. A. (1974). *Pain patients: Traits and treatments*. New York: Academic Press.

Sternbach, R. A. (1978). *The psychology of pain*. New York: Raven Press.

Sternbach, R., and Tursky, B. (1965). Ethnic differences among housewives in psychophysical and skin potential responses to electric shock. *Psychophysiology*, 1, 241–246.

Stewart, M. L. (1977). Measurement of clinical pain. In A. K. Jacox (Ed.), *Pain: A source book for nurses and other health professionals*. Boston: Little, Brown.

Stewart, S. M. (1986). Controlling pain with epidural narcotics: Nursing implications. *Critical Care Nurse*, 6 (3), 50–56.

Summerfield, J. A. (1980). Naloxone modulates the perception of itch in man. *British Journal of Clinical Pharmacology*, 10, 180–183.

Tan, S. (1982). Cognitive and cognitive-behavioral methods for pain control: A selective review. *Pain*, 12, 201–208.

Tasker, R. R. (1984). Deafferentation. In P. D. Wall, and R. Melzack (Eds.), *Textbook of pain* (pp. 119–132). New York: Churchill Livingstone.

Terenius, L. (1978). Endogenous peptides and analgesia. *Annual Review of Pharmacologic Toxicology*, 18, 189–192.

Terenius, L. (1981). Endorphins and pain. *Frontiers of Hormone Research*, 8, 162–177.

Thomas, I. L., Tyle, V., Webster, J., et al. (1988). An evaluation of transcutaneous electrical nerve stimulation for pain relief in labour. *Australia and New Zealand Journal of Obstetrics and Gynecology*, 28 (3), 182–189.

Thoren, L. (1974). General metabolic response to trauma including pain influence. *Acta Anaesthesiologica Scandinavica*, 55 (Suppl.), 9–14.

Titchener, E. B. (1909). *A textbook of physiology*. Philadelphia: Macmillan.

Traynor, C., and Hall, G. M. (1981). Endocrine and metabolic changes during surgery: Anaesthetic implications. *British Journal of Anaesthesia*, 53, 153–158.

Turner, J. A., and Chapman, C. R. (1982). Psychological interventions for chronic pain: A critical review. I. Relaxation training and biofeedback. *Pain*, 12, 1–21.

Tursky, B. (1976). The development of a pain perception profile: A psychophysical approach. In W. Weisenbert, and B. Tursky (Eds.), *Pain: New perspectives in therapy and research*. New York: Plenum.

Tursky, B., Jamner, L. D., and Friedman, R. (1982). The pain perception profile: A psychophysical approach to the assessment of pain report. *Behavior Therapy*, 13 (4), 376–394.

Twycross, R. G. (1984). Narcotics. In P. D. Wall, and R. Melzack (Eds.), *Textbook of pain* (pp. 514–526). New York: Churchill Livingstone.

Viswanathan, M., Van Dijk, J. P., Graham, R. E., et al. (1987). Exercise and cold-induced changes in plasma β-endorphin and β-lipotropin in men and women. *American Physiological Society*, 27, 622–626.

Wain, H. J., and Amer, D. G. (1986). Emergency room use of hypnosis. *General Hospital Psychiatry*, 8, 19–22.

Wang, W. C., George, S. L., and Williams, J. A. (1988). Transcutaneous electrical nerve stimulation treatment of sickle cell pain crises. *Acta Haematologica*, 80 (2), 99–102.

Ward, M. M., Mefford, I. N., Parker, S. D., et al. (1983). Epinephrine and norepinephrine responses in continuously collected human plasma to a series of stressors. *Psychosomatic Medicine*, 45, 471–486.

Weinberg, A. D. (1988). The etiology, evaluation and treatment of head and facial pain in the elderly. *Journal of Pain and Symptom Management*, 3 (1), 29–38.

Willis, W. D. (1985). *The pain system*. New York: Karger.

Wolff, B. B. (1985). Ethnocultural factors influencing pain and illness behavior. *Clinical Journal of Pain*, 1, 23–30.

Woods, J.H., Young, A. M., and Herling, S. (1982). Classification of narcotics on the basis of their reinforcing, discriminative, and antagonist effects in rhesus monkeys. *Federation Proceedings*, 41, 221–227.

Yeager, M. P., Glass, D. D., Neff, R. K., et al. (1987). Epidural anesthesia and analgesia in high-risk surgical patients. *Anesthesiology*, 66, 729–736.

Zahourek, K. P. (1982a). Hypnosis in nursing practice—emphasis on the "problem patient" who has pain. Part I. *Journal of Psychosocial Nursing Mental Health Service*, 20, 21–24.

Zahourek, K. P. (1982b). Hypnosis in nursing practice—emphasis on the "problem patient" who has pain. Part II. *Journal of Psychosocial Nursing Mental Health Service*, 20, 21–24.

Zborowski, M. (1952). Cultural components in response to pain. *Journal of Social Issues*, 8 (40), 16–24.

Zimmerman, M. (1984). Neurobiological concepts of pain, its assessment and therapy. In E. Bromm (Ed.), *Pain measurement in man* (pp. 15–35). Amsterdam: Elsevier Science Publications.

Zola, I. K. (1966). Culture and symptoms: An analysis of patients presenting complaints. *American Sociological Review*, 31, 615–630.

Renal System

39

Renal Physiology

Patricia Peschman

The human kidney is a complex organ that performs several major functions essential for survival (Table 39–1). The primary role of the kidney is to maintain the composition and volume of the extracellular fluid, thereby ensuring a constant environment in which normal cellular function can take place. The kidney accomplishes this fine-tuning by removing the waste products of metabolism while conserving substances needed by the body.

The kidney performs several additional functions. It participates in the regulation of blood pressure through the renin-angiotensin-aldosterone system. It contributes to acid-base balance by removing hydrogen ions and conserving bicarbonate. The kidney produces erythropoietin, which promotes red blood cell synthesis. Additionally, the kidney plays a role in the metabolism of vitamin D to its active form.

This chapter addresses the anatomic structures and physiologic principles underlying these functions of the human kidney. A clear understanding of normal renal function is helpful when studying the pathophysiology, symptomatology, and management of renal dysfunction. It will also assist the nurse with problem solving when confronted with concerns about a patient's renal function in the critical care setting.

RENAL ANATOMY

Gross Anatomy

The kidneys are paired, reddish-brown, bean-shaped organs. They are retroperitoneal organs whose posterior surfaces are adjacent to the muscles of the posterior abdominal wall. The kidneys lie on either side of the abdominal aorta, inferior vena cava, and lumbar spine between the twelfth thoracic and third lumbar vertebrae. The right kidney usually sits slightly lower than the left beneath the large right lobe of the liver.

Adult kidneys measure 10 to 12 cm in length and 5 to 6 cm in width (Zamboni, 1989). The weight of each kidney ranges between 125 and 170 grams in adult males and 115 and 155 grams in adult females (Tisher and Madsen, 1986). Determination of kidney size by ultrasound may be useful clinically in the differential diagnosis of renal failure. Small kidneys are suggestive of many forms of chronic renal disease. Large kidneys may be indicative of obstruction or polycystic kidney disease. Abdominal palpation is not always helpful in measuring kidney size because the kidneys are usually not palpable.

The kidneys move up and down within the abdominal cavity in association with respiration. This movement is clinically important during the performance of a kidney biopsy. The cooperation of the patient in holding the breath during the biopsy is essential to prevent complications.

The outside of each kidney is protected by a tough white fibrous coat known as the renal capsule. Additional protection is offered by a mass of perinephric fat that surrounds each kidney. An adrenal gland lies above each kidney within the perinephric fat. The renal fascia and surrounding organs help to hold the kidneys in place. On the medial aspect of each kidney there is a central indentation known as the hilum. The renal arteries and nerves enter and the renal veins, lymphatics, and ureters exit the kidney at the hilum.

Internal Structure

When the kidney is cut longitudinally and opened, three distinct sections become apparent: cortex, medulla, and renal sinus (Fig. 39–1). The outer three-quarters of an inch is known as the cortex. The cortex is pale in color and has a granular appearance. Most

TABLE 39–1. Functions of the Kidney

Maintenance of extracellular fluid volume and concentration
Regulation of blood pressure
Regulation of acid-base balance
Production of erythropoietin
Metabolism of vitamin D

parts of the nephrons, the primary functional units of the kidney, lie in the cortex.

The middle section, the medulla, is darker in color and has a striated appearance. The medulla is composed of 8 to 18 wedge-shaped structures known as pyramids. Within the pyramids a segment of the nephrons and the collecting ducts descend deep into the kidney, resulting in the striated appearance. Between the pyramids, blood vessels and nerves run to and from the cortex in areas known as the columns of Bertin. The apex of each pyramid forms a nipple-like projection known as the papilla, as seen in Figure 39–2. The collecting ducts end in the papillae, perforating their surfaces, allowing urine to flow out of the medulla.

The final section of the kidney is the renal sinus. The renal sinus is a cavity that is almost completely filled with blood vessels and structures formed by the expanded upper end of the ureter. Prior to entering the kidney, the ureter dilates to form the renal pelvis. The renal pelvis branches into two or three major divisions known as the major calices. Each major calyx branches further to form several minor calices. The upper part of each minor calyx cups itself around one to three papillae, collecting the urine that drains through the papillae from the collecting ducts.

Microscopic Structure

The primary functional unit of the kidney is the nephron, a long, tubular structure composed of several distinct parts. Each kidney contains approximately one million nephrons. Each nephron is capable of performing all of the kidney's necessary functions.

The kidney contains two types of nephrons, cortical and juxtamedullary, distinguished by their structure and location in the cortex (Fig. 39–3). Cortical nephrons have glomeruli that lie in the outer region of the cortex. These nephrons have relatively

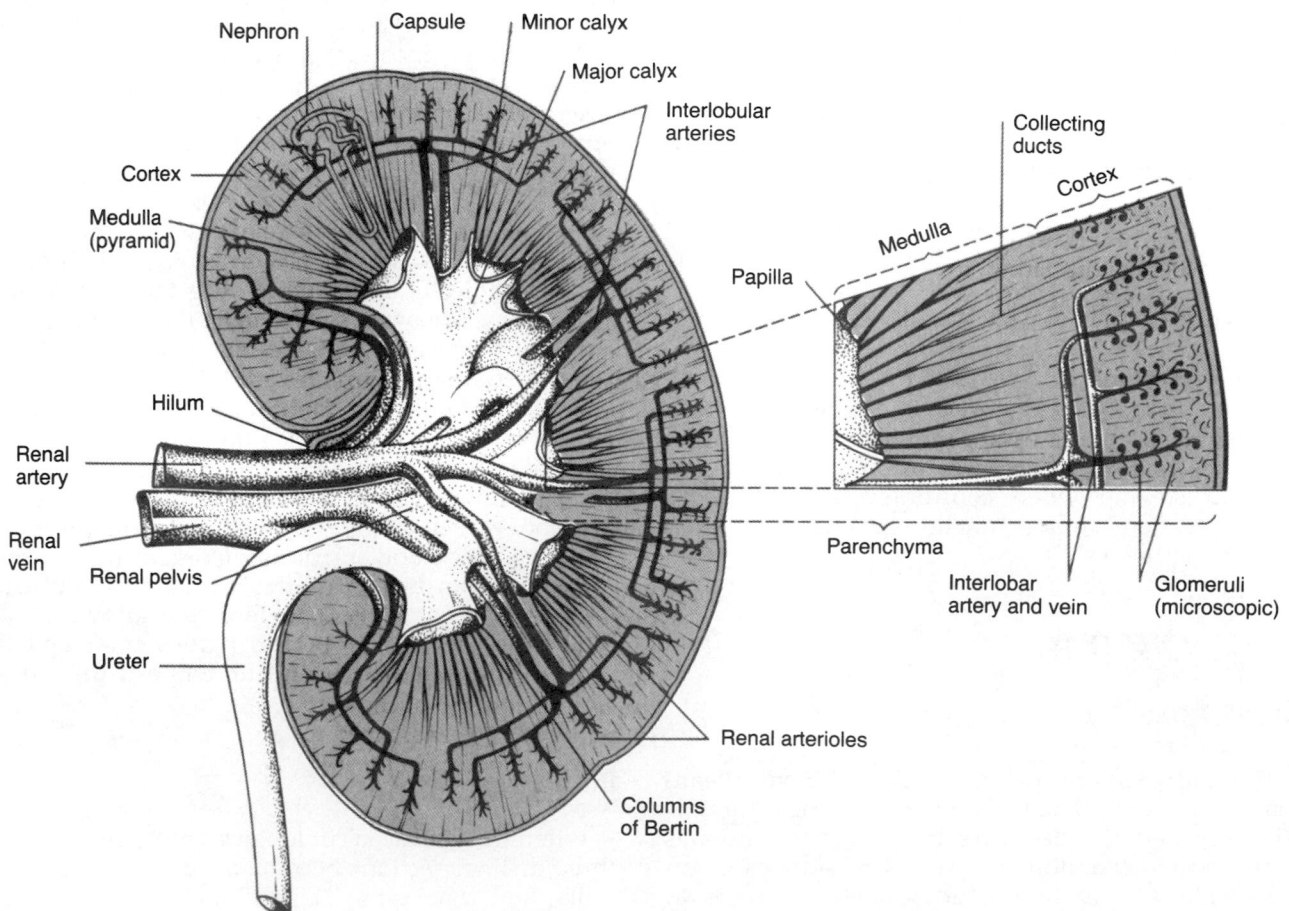

FIGURE 39–1. Major structures of the kidney. (From Ignatavicius, D. D., and Bayne, M. V. (Eds.). (1991). *Medical-surgical nursing: A nursing process approach* (p. 1801). Philadelphia: W. B. Saunders.)

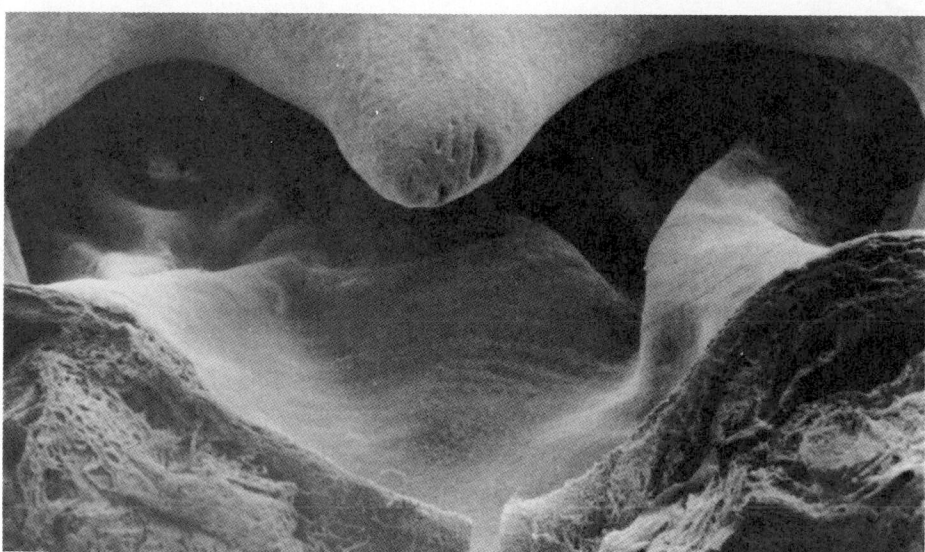

FIGURE 39—2. Scanning electron micrograph of papilla from a rat, illustrating the area cribrosa formed by the slit-like openings where the ducts of Bellini terminate. The renal pelvis surrounds the papilla. (From Tisher, C. C., and Madsen, K. M. (1986). In B. M. Brenner and F. C. Rector, (Eds.), *The kidney* (3rd ed., p. 5). Philadelphia: W. B. Saunders).

short loops of Henle that extend only a short distance into the outer medulla. Juxtamedullary nephrons have glomeruli situated in the inner region of the cortex, near the outer zone of the medulla. Juxtamedullary nephrons have long loops of Henle that penetrate deeply into the medulla. The structure of the juxtaglomerular nephrons is important to the kidney's ability to concentrate the urine.

Each nephron is composed of three major parts: the renal corpuscle, the renal tubules, and the collecting duct (Fig. 39–4). The renal corpuscle, consisting of the glomerulus and Bowman's capsule, is responsible for the formation of ultrafiltrate from the

blood. The renal tubules are responsible for the processes of reabsorption and secretion, which alter the volume and composition of the ultrafiltrate to form the final urine product. The collecting duct, which receives tubular fluid from many nephrons, transports the fluid from the cortex to the minor calyx.

Renal Corpuscle. Renal corpuscles are located in the cortex and columns of Bertin between the pyramids. As mentioned previously, they are composed of the glomerulus and Bowman's capsule (Fig. 39–5). The glomerulus is a complex anastomosing tuft

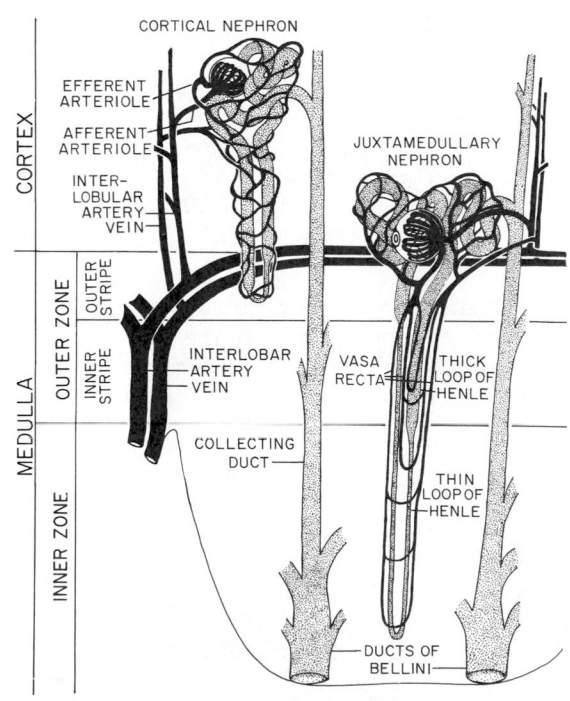

FIGURE 39—3. Differences between a cortical and a juxtamedullary nephron. (From Pitts, R. F. (1974). *Physiology of the kidney and body fluids* (3rd ed.). Chicago: Year Book Medical Publishers.)

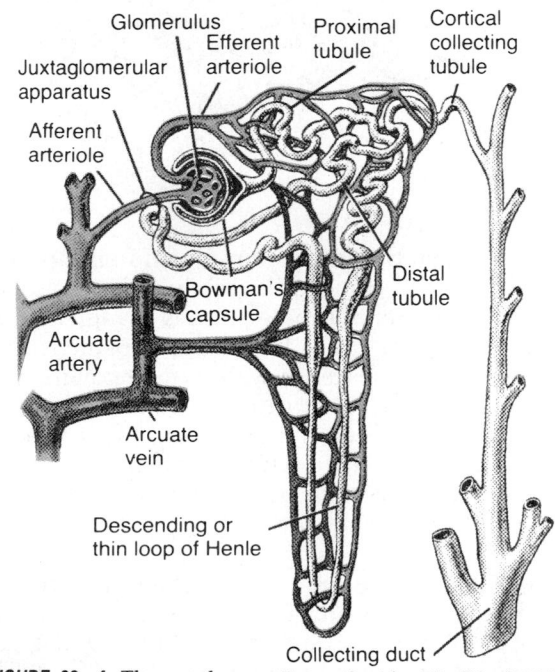

FIGURE 39—4. The nephron. (From Smith, H. W. (1951). *The kidney: Structure and functions in health and disease.* New York: Oxford University Press.)

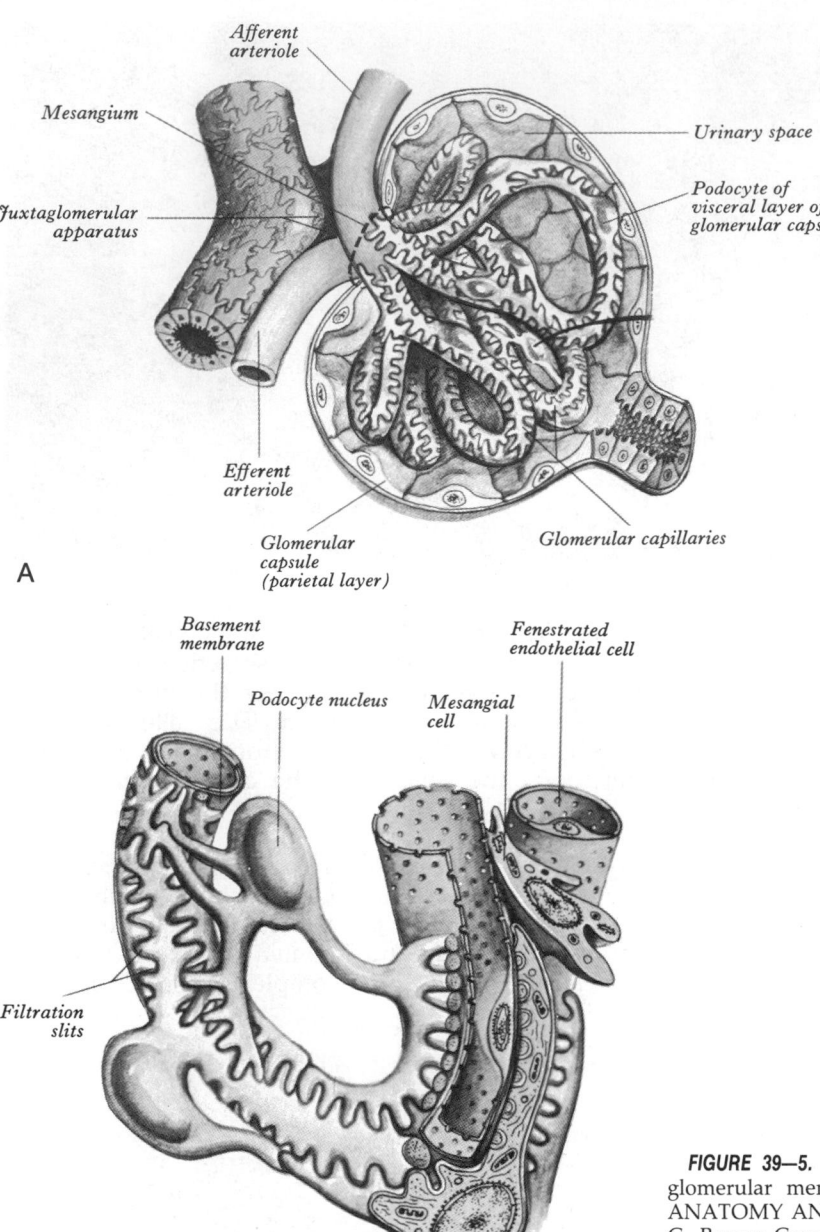

A

B

of capillaries that branches from the afferent arteriole (Zamboni, 1989). Bowman's capsule is the blind initial end of the renal tubules that is invaginated by the glomerular capillaries. Bowman's capsule is composed of an inner (visceral) wall, which covers most sides of the glomerular capillaries, and an outer (parietal) wall. Between the outer and inner walls of Bowman's capsule is an open area, the urinary space, which is continuous with the lumen of the proximal convoluted tubule (Williams et al., 1989).

Glomerular Membrane. The glomerular capillary membrane is composed of three distinct layers: the capillary endothelium, the basement membrane, and the epithelial cells or podocytes (see Fig. 39–5). The first layer, the endothelium, lines the lumen of the glomerular capillary. The endothelial cells are perfo-

rated by regularly spaced pores. The second layer, the glomerular basement membrane, is a filamentous support structure composed of the merged basement membranes of the glomerular endothelium and epi-

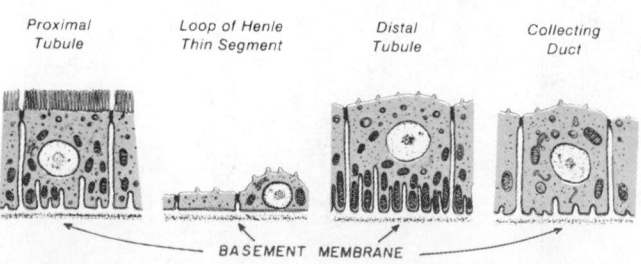

thelium (Zamboni, 1989). The glomerular basement membrane contains negatively charged molecules (Tisher and Madsen, 1986). The third layer of the glomerular membrane is actually the visceral epithelial wall of Bowman's capsule. The tightly interwoven epithelial cells that cover the outside of the glomerular capillaries are known as podocytes. Extending from the body of the podocytes are numerous projections or primary processes. These processes branch further to form foot processes, which wrap around the glomerular capillary loops, contacting the basement membrane (Tisher and Madsen, 1986). Adjacent foot processes do not arise from the same podocyte but interdigitate with foot processes from other epithelial cells (Zamboni, 1989). A thin diaphragm, the slit diaphragm, covers the narrow gap between adjacent foot processes.

Renal Tubules and Collecting Ducts. The ultrafiltrate formed in the renal corpuscle leaves Bowman's capsule and begins its journey through the tubular system of the nephron. Figure 39–6 illustrates the distinct anatomic structures of the three sections of the tubule: the proximal tubule, the loop of Henle, and the distal tubule and collecting duct.

Proximal Tubule. The proximal tubule lies entirely in the cortex. The initial part is convoluted, that is, looped or folded, whereas the later portion is straight. The proximal tubule is formed from a single layer of cuboidal epithelial cells. These cells are characterized by a dense brush border of microvilli on their luminal surface, multiple mitochondria, and relatively open junctions between adjoining cells. These cellular characteristics are responsible for the proximal tubule's ability to rapidly reabsorb and secrete various substances. Approximately 65% of the filtered sodium and water are reabsorbed in the proximal tubule (Vander, 1985).

Loop of Henle. The straight portion of the proximal tubule turns toward the medulla and tapers to become the thin descending limb of the loop of Henle. At the base of the loop, the tubule makes a hairpin turn, and the ascending limb of the loop of Henle begins. The tubule widens again to form the thick segment of the ascending limb. In juxtamedullary nephrons, the thin segment of the loop of Henle descends deep into the medulla and continues around the turn to form the initial one-third to one-half of the ascending limb. In cortical nephrons the thin segment is shorter and ends shortly before or after the hairpin turn. The result is that all or nearly all of the ascending limb is thick (Tisher and Madsen, 1986). The loop of Henle is made up entirely of cuboidal epithelial cells except for the thin ascending segment of the juxtamedullary nephrons. The thin ascending segment of juxtamedullary nephrons is composed of squamous epithelial cells.

Distal Tubule. The distal tubule may itself be divided into three distinct sections: the straight portion, the macula densa, and the convoluted portion (Zamboni, 1989). The thick ascending limb of the loop of Henle comprises the straight portion of the distal tubule. It extends from the outer medulla into the cortex to the point where it comes to lie between the afferent and efferent arterioles entering and exiting the glomerulus. Cells of the distal tubule lying between the afferent and efferent arterioles are known as the macula densa. These cells are distinguished by their taller height and more compact relationship. The macula densa is part of the juxtaglomerular apparatus, which will be discussed later in the chapter. The convoluted portion of the distal tubule extends from the macula densa to the collecting duct (Zamboni, 1989). Both the straight and convoluted portions of the distal tubule are made up of cuboidal epithelial cells with sparse microvilli on their luminal surface.

In some nephrons, fluid exiting the distal tubule enters a short, straight connecting tubule prior to entering a collecting duct. Many nephrons eventually connect to a single collecting duct. Small collecting ducts join together to form progressively larger collecting ducts as they progress downward through the medulla. The collecting duct is divided into three sections: the cortical collecting duct, the medullary collecting duct, and the papillary collecting duct or ducts of Bellini. The cells of the collecting duct begin as flat cuboidal epithelium in the cortical section enlarging to taller columnar epithelium in the ducts of Bellini. These cells have few microvilli and mitochondria indicating that little metabolic activity occurs in this area. The ducts of Bellini finally empty into the minor calices through the surface of the papillae.

Renal Vascular System

The kidneys are very vascular organs, receiving about 20% of the cardiac output under resting conditions (Brenner et al., 1986). As shown in Figure 39–1, the renal vascular structure closely follows the pattern of the various parts of the nephrons, an indication of the close link between structure and function.

Renal Arteries, Arterioles, and Capillary System. Arterial blood is supplied to the kidneys by the renal arteries, which branch directly off the abdominal aorta. Most individuals have only one renal artery supplying each kidney. Approximately 30% of individuals have one or more accessory renal arteries that branch off the aorta and supply a portion of the renal parenchyma (Williams et al., 1989).

The renal artery branches into approximately five segmental arteries, which divide the kidney into vascular segments (Williams et al., 1989). The segmental arteries then branch to form the lobar arteries, one of which supplies each pyramid. The lobar arteries divide into two or three interlobar arteries, which ascend toward the cortex on either side of the pyramid in the renal columns (Williams et al., 1989).

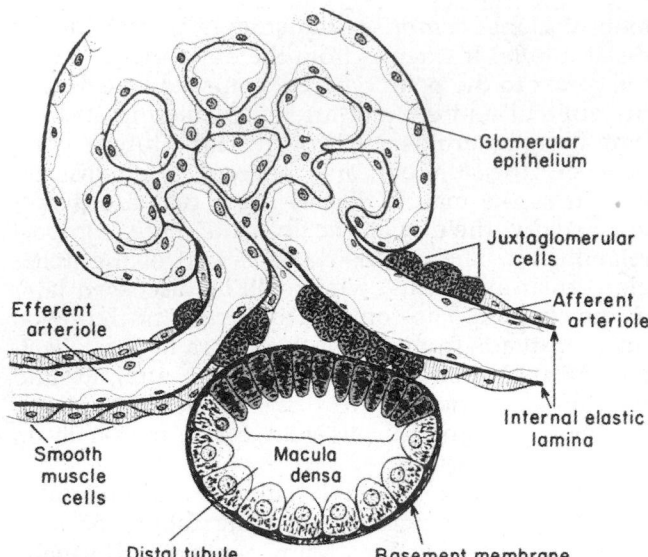

FIGURE 39—7. Structure of the juxtaglomerular apparatus. (From Guyton, A. C. (1991). *Textbook of medical physiology* (8th ed., p. 411). Philadelphia: W. B. Saunders).

At the point where the cortex and medulla meet, the interlobar arteries turn at right angles to form the arcuate arteries, which course along the tops of the pyramids. The arcuate arteries have multiple branches known as the interlobular arteries, which ascend at right angles from the arcuate artery into the cortex.

The vascular structure of the kidney has several unique features that distinguish it from vascular beds in other areas of the body (see Fig. 39–3). The afferent arteriole branches off the interlobular artery to supply blood to the glomerular capillaries. Blood leaving the glomerulus does not enter a vein but instead enters a second arteriole, the efferent arteriole. The kidneys are unique in having two separate capillary beds separated from each other by the efferent arteriole. The efferent arterioles leaving the glomeruli of cortical nephrons branch into a network of peritubular capillaries that surround the proximal and distal convoluted tubules. The efferent arterioles from the juxtamedullary nephrons form a very different capillary network known as the vasa recta (Brenner et al., 1986). The vasa recta is a complex of long, straight capillary loops connected by side branches at various levels that run parallel to the ascending and descending loop of Henle. The vasa recta play an important role in maintaining the concentrated interstitial fluid found within the medulla.

Juxtaglomerular Apparatus. The juxtaglomerular apparatus is a specialized anatomical structure made up of the macula densa and the juxtaglomerular cells (Fig. 39–7). As discussed previously, the macula densa is the part of the distal tubule that lies in close proximity to the afferent and efferent arterioles as they enter and exit the glomerulus. The cells of the arterioles in this region, particularly those of the afferent arteriole, are different from normal smooth muscle cells and are known as juxtaglomerular cells (Zamboni, 1989). The enzyme renin is produced and stored in the juxtaglomerular cells. The function of the juxtaglomerular apparatus will be discussed in the section on renal blood flow and blood pressure regulation.

Renal Veins. Blood drains from the peritubular capillaries and vasa recta into the interlobular veins, beginning the venous system in the kidneys. The veins of the kidney retrace the pattern formed by the renal arteries. Blood flows from the interlobular veins into the arcuate veins and then to the interlobar veins, ultimately forming the renal vein, which empties into the inferior vena cava.

RENAL HEMODYNAMICS

Renal Blood Flow and Distribution

Renal function is largely dependent upon maintenance of a normal rate and distribution of renal blood flow (RBF) and normal pressures within the renal vascular circuit. Although the function of the renal vasculature has many similarities to vasculature in other parts of the body, there are some special features and regulatory mechanisms that help to maintain normal renal hemodynamics.

The renal fraction—the part of the cardiac output that passes through the kidneys—averages around 20% or approximately 1000 to 1200 mL/minute (Navar et al., 1989). Blood flow is not distributed evenly throughout the kidney. Eighty-five to ninety per cent of renal blood flow is distributed to the cortex under normal circumstances (Brenner et al., 1986). The remaining blood circulates through the medulla. Only 1 to 2% of total renal blood flow passes through the vasa recta surrounding the loop of Henle, resulting in very sluggish flow through the vasa recta. The slow blood flow through the vasa recta is an important characteristic in the kidney's ability to form a concentrated urine.

Determinants of Renal Blood Flow

Pressure Gradients. Blood flow through any vessel is determined by the pressure gradient and the vascular resistance. The pressure gradient, or the difference in pressure between the two ends of a blood vessel, is the force that pushes blood through the vessel. Blood flow is opposed by the resistance offered by the walls of the blood vessel. The smaller the diameter of the vessel, the higher the resistance and the slower the blood flow through the vessel.

Normally, the diameter of the arterioles is the major determinant of resistance within an organ. This is true in the kidney, where mean arterial

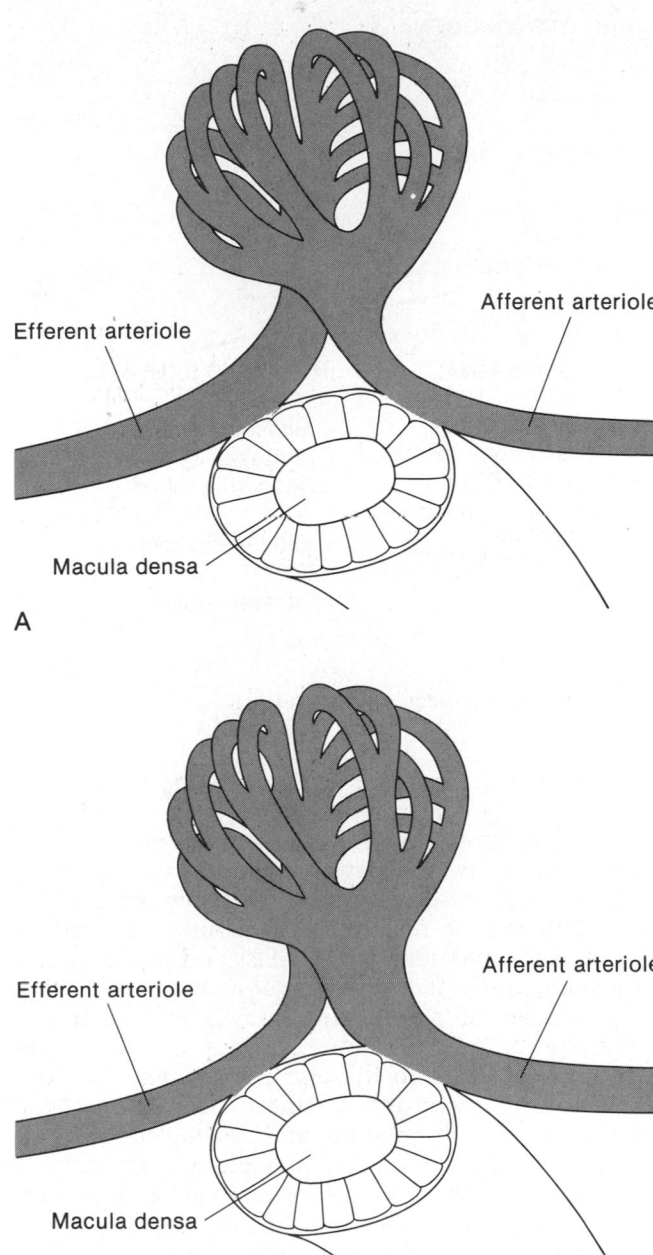

FIGURE 39—8. *A*, Response of afferent arteriole to increased intraglomerular pressure. *B*, Response of afferent and efferent arterioles to decreased intraglomerular pressure.

pressure does not fall significantly until the afferent arteriole is reached.

The mean arterial pressure inside the arcuate artery averages 100 mm Hg. The mean glomerular capillary pressure is estimated to be 55 to 60 mm Hg (Navar et al., 1989). These figures are estimates from animal studies because direct measurements in human kidneys are not available. Glomerular capillary pressure is much higher than in other capillaries throughout the body, where it is believed that mean-capillary pressure averages 17 mm Hg (Guyton, 1991). Changes in the diameter of the afferent and efferent arterioles determine resistance to renal blood flow

and intraglomerular pressure. The afferent arteriole controls blood flow into the glomerulus, whereas the efferent arteriole offers resistance to blood flow out of the glomerulus. Blood pressure drops significantly across the efferent arteriole, averaging 13 mm Hg in the peritubular capillaries and 8 mm Hg in the renal veins. The low pressure in the peritubular capillaries promotes reabsorption of fluid from the tubules back into the circulatory system (Guyton, 1991).

Autoregulation. Autoregulation refers to the kidney's ability to maintain a relatively constant RBF and intraglomerular pressure despite changes in mean arterial pressure between the range of 80 and 180 mm Hg (Vander, 1985). Autoregulation is extremely important in the fine tuning of renal regulation of the extracellular fluid. If autoregulation were not present, fluctuations in arterial blood pressure, such as normally occur with changes in activity level, would result in changes in RBF and the intraglomerular pressure. Consequently, the glomerular filtration rate (GFR) would also fluctuate widely. Because even small changes in the GFR can produce significant changes in the volume and content of the urine, the volume and composition of the extracellular fluid would ultimately be altered.

As discussed previously, blood flow through a vessel is determined by the pressure gradient and vascular resistance. It follows that the only way that RBF can remain constant despite changes in arterial pressure is through changes in the vascular resistance. In the kidney the predominant location of changes in vascular resistance is the afferent arteriole (Navar et al., 1989). The efferent arteriole also participates in autoregulation but to a lesser extent. (Brenner et al., 1986). Increases in the mean arterial pressure result in constriction of the afferent arteriole, which prevents the increased arterial pressure from raising the intraglomerular presure (Fig. 39–8*A*). A fall in blood pressure within the range of 80 to 180 mm Hg results in dilatation of the afferent arteriole (Fig. 39–8*B*). As the diameter of the afferent arteriole increases, more blood is allowed to flow into the glomerulus. The increased glomerular blood flow will increase intraglomerular pressure if efferent arteriolar resistance remains constant. Efferent arteriolar resistance may increase as the arterial blood pressure falls below 100 mm Hg, helping to maintain the intraglomerular pressure (Brenner et al., 1986).

The exact mechanism by which renal autoregulation occurs is not known. There are two theories of its operation—the myogenic theory and the macula densa theory (Navar et al., 1989). The myogenic theory suggests that changes in the diameter of the arteriole are an intrinsic response to changes in vascular wall tension (Brenner et al., 1986). A rise in arterial pressure would cause the walls of the afferent arteriole to stretch, triggering a subsequent contraction of the smooth muscle cells of the arteriole. The opposite would occur with a decrease in arterial pressure. Decreased stretch in the afferent arteriolar

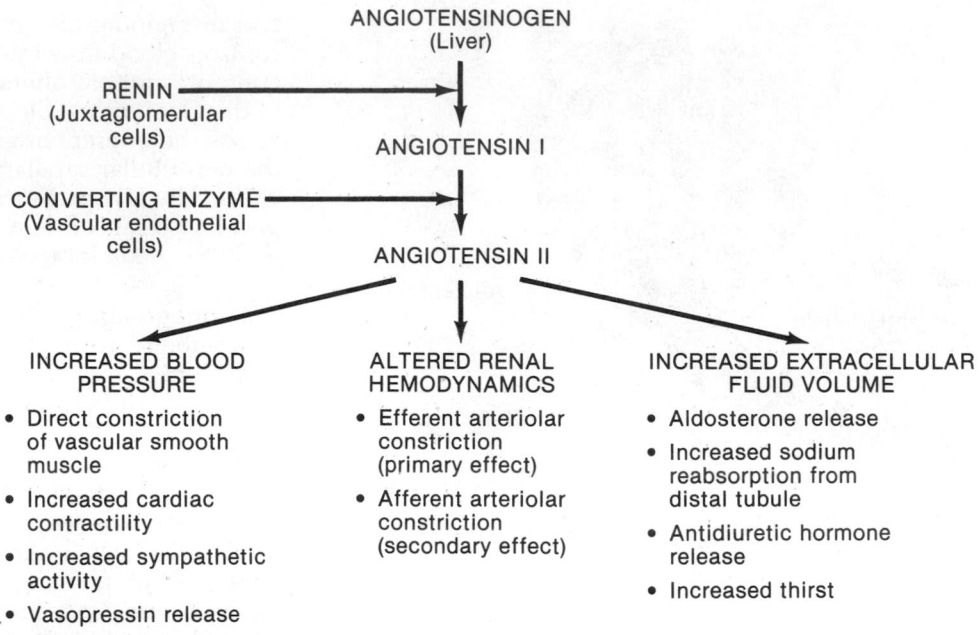

STIMULI FOR RENIN RELEASE

1. Baroreceptors in the afferent arteriole
2. Sympathetic nervous system
3. Increased NaCl at the macula densa
4. Prostaglandins

ANGIOTENSINOGEN
(Liver)

RENIN
(Juxtaglomerular cells)

ANGIOTENSIN I

CONVERTING ENZYME
(Vascular endothelial cells)

ANGIOTENSIN II

INCREASED BLOOD PRESSURE

- Direct constriction of vascular smooth muscle
- Increased cardiac contractility
- Increased sympathetic activity
- Vasopressin release
- Catecholamine release

ALTERED RENAL HEMODYNAMICS

- Efferent arteriolar constriction (primary effect)
- Afferent arteriolar constriction (secondary effect)

INCREASED EXTRACELLULAR FLUID VOLUME

- Aldosterone release
- Increased sodium reabsorption from distal tubule
- Antidiuretic hormone release
- Increased thirst

FIGURE 39—9. The renin-angiotensin-aldosterone system.

wall would cause the arteriole to dilate, thereby allowing increased blood flow into the glomerulus and maintaining intraglomerular pressure.

The macula densa theory is somewhat more complex. According to this theory, the macula densa participates in the autoregulation of RBF through the tubuloglomerular feedback mechanism (Navar et al., 1989). Tubuloglomerular feedback is believed to operate in the following way. As arterial pressure increases, intraglomerular pressure also increases, resulting in an increase in the GFR. An increase in the GFR increases the rate of fluid flow through the tubules, preventing them from reabsorbing normal amounts of water and sodium from the filtrate. The cells of the macula densa in the distal tubule sense the increase in fluid flow past them, probably by detecting the increase in the sodium concentration, and respond by releasing a vasoconstrictor substance. The vasoconstrictor substance constricts the afferent arteriole, thereby decreasing the intraglomerular pressure and the GFR. Tubular fluid flow is thereby returned toward normal. A fall in arterial pressure would have the opposite effect, resulting in inhibition of release of the vasoconstrictor substance, thus allowing afferent arteriolar dilation.

A number of other substances are being studied to determine whether they play a role in autoregulation of RBF. These substances, which include prostaglandins, kinins, angiotensin II, and adenosine, are known to affect RBF (Brenner et al., 1986). Their exact role in the kidney's response to changes in arterial blood pressure remains to be determined.

Renin-Angiotensin-Aldosterone System. Another important mechanism that affects RBF and the GFR is the renin-angiotensin-aldosterone system, which

is illustrated in Figure 39–9. The primary function of the renin-angiotensin-aldosterone system is to increase blood pressure and intravascular volume. Activation of this complex system produces a multitude of physiologic effects. Within the kidney these physiologic alterations result simultaneously in a reduction of RBF, maintenance of GFR, and conservation of sodium and water (Ingelfinger et al., 1989).

A number of stimuli are known to trigger the release of renin by the kidney. These stimuli include perfusion pressure in the afferent arteriole, sodium chloride delivery to the macula densa, sympathetic nervous system stimulation, and prostaglandins (Ballermann et al., 1986). The juxtaglomerular cells of the afferent arteriole are believed to act as a baroreceptor. When the pressure in these cells falls below the usual mean arterial pressure of 90 to 100 mm Hg, a direct stimulus for renin release results (Ingelfinger et al., 1989). Changes in tubular sodium chloride concentration, sensed by the macula densa, also result in renin release. Various studies have demonstrated renin release from the juxtaglomerular cells following both increases and decreases in distal tubular sodium chloride concentration (Ballermann et al., 1986). Additionally, stimulation of renal sympathetic nerves and the presence of prostaglandins have also been shown to be direct stimuli for renin release.

As previously discussed, the juxtaglomerular cells, located primarily in the afferent arteriole, contain many granules that are the site of renin storage. When these cells are stimulated, renin is released into the bloodstream, where it acts on the plasma protein angiotensinogen, splitting off part of the molecule to form angiotensin I. Angiotensin I is then rapidly split to form angiotensin II by a converting enzyme found in vascular endothelial cells throughout the body, particularly in the lung. The formation of angiotensin II then produces a variety of actions, including increased peripheral vascular resistance, altered renal hemodynamics, increased reabsorption of sodium and water by the kidneys, and increased thirst.

The renin-angiotensin-aldosterone system participates in the adjustment of vascular resistance in response to changes in arterial pressure that occur with changes in position and activity level. This system is particularly important in maintaining blood pressure in critically ill patients who experience extracellular fluid volume depletion (Ballermann et al., 1986). Angiotensin II increases blood pressure in several ways. It is a potent vasoconstrictor, directly stimulating contraction of vascular smooth muscle cells. Angiotensin II also directly increases cardiac contractility. Indirectly, angiotensin II increases blood pressure by acting on the central nervous system to stimulate increased sympathetic activity and vasopressin release. Angiotensin II also increases catecholamine release from peripheral nerve endings and from the adrenal medulla.

In the kidney, angiotensin II produces a fall in RBF and GFR. However, researchers have observed that the GFR does not fall as much as would be predicted by the fall in RBF. This observation led to the conclusion that the primary effect of angiotensin II in the nephron is constriction of the efferent arteriole (Ingelfinger et al., 1989). Constriction of the efferent arteriole raises the intraglomerular pressure. As a result, a greater proportion of the plasma filters across the glomerulus into the tubules, thereby maintaining the GFR.

Other physiological effects resulting from angiotensin II result in an increased extracellular fluid volume. Angiotensin II stimulates aldosterone release from the adrenal cortex. Aldosterone acts on the collecting duct in the nephron, stimulating increased sodium reabsorption. Angiotensin II also acts directly to increase sodium reabsorption by the distal tubule (Ballermann et al., 1986). Angiotensin II is also believed to stimulate antidiuretic hormone (ADH) release from the posterior pituitary, though the exact mechanism is not completely understood (Ballermann et al., 1986). As will be discussed later, ADH increases water reabsorption by the distal tubule and collecting duct of the nephron. Finally, angiotensin II increases the sensation of thirst, which should result in increased fluid intake.

Sympathetic Nervous System. The sympathetic nervous system is the third system that has an effect on RBF. The kidney is richly innervated with sympathetic fibers. Nerve fiber endings have been found in the afferent and efferent arterioles and in all sections of the tubules. Their presence implies that the sympathetic nervous system has a role in alteration of blood flow and reabsorptive processes (Pelayo and Quan, 1989). Under resting conditions the influence of the sympathetic nervous system on renal

function is thought to be minor. At low levels of stimulation, the sympathetic nervous system increases sodium reabsorption within the proximal tubule. At moderate levels of sympathetic nervous system stimulation, both the afferent and efferent arterioles constrict. This results in a decrease in both RBF and GFR, although RBF is impaired more (Navar et al., 1989). With higher levels of sympathetic nervous system stimulation, such as might occur with severe hypotension, afferent arteriolar constriction predominates. RBF may be reduced sufficiently to cause cessation of glomerular filtration. If RBF is reduced for a prolonged period of time, renal ischemia and acute renal failure may result.

Local Hormones. Prostaglandin and bradykinin are two hormones produced by the kidney and other tissues. They are considered local hormones because they are synthesized in the same location in which they exert their effect and they are rapidly inactivated. Prostaglandin production is promoted by the presence of angiotensin II, bradykinin, ADH, sympathetic stimulation, and renal ischemia (Garella and Matarese, 1989). Bradykinin release is stimulated by angiotensin II, aldosterone, prostaglandins, and ADH (Carretero and Scicli, 1989). Both prostaglandin and bradykinin cause vasodilation in the kidney. They are believed to help modulate the vasoconstricting effects resulting from angiotensin II and sympathetic stimulation, thereby helping to preserve renal blood flow. Nonsteroidal antiinflammatory agents, such as aspirin and ibuprofen, act by inhibiting prostaglandin formation. In individuals with renal insufficiency, these agents may decrease RBF enough to cause severe renal ischemia.

Extrinsic Vasoactive Substances. RBF may also be altered by a variety of vasoactive drugs administered to patients. Dopamine hydrochloride, epinephrine, and norepinephrine are three common examples of drugs that affect RBF. In low doses of 2 to 5 μg/kg per minute, dopamine acts primarily on the dopaminergic receptors in the renal artery, resulting in dilation of the artery. Low doses of dopamine are frequently utilized as a means of protecting renal function by improving RBF when blood flow to the kidneys has been impaired. In higher doses greater than 10 μg/kg per minute, dopamine may itself impair renal blood flow by causing constriction of the renal artery. Epinephrine and norepinephrine both result in renal artery constriction. Urine output is monitored as an index of RBF during administration of these drugs.

PHYSIOLOGIC FUNCTIONS PERFORMED BY THE KIDNEY
Formation of Urine

The kidney performs its primary function, regulation of the volume and composition of the extracellular fluid, through the processes involved in the formation of urine: glomerular filtration, reabsorption, and secretion. Urine formation begins with glomerular filtration, the movement of fluid across the glomerular membrane as a consequence of pressure gradients. The composition of the resulting filtrate is then altered by the processes of reabsorption and secretion. The process of reabsorption returns filtered substances to the blood. Secretion results in the movement of solutes from the blood into the tubules. The end result of all these processes is the excretion of waste products and excess water as urine and the selective adjustment of the composition and volume of the extracellular fluid. This section will discuss the specific processes involved in the formation of urine and will introduce the concept of clearance.

Glomerular Filtration. Glomerular filtration is similar to filtration of fluid from capillaries in other parts of the body. The rate at which fluid filters out of any capillary is determined by the net filtration pressure and the permeability of the capillary membrane. In nonrenal capillary systems, pressure dynamics result in a net pressure that pushes fluid into the interstitial space at the arterial end of the capillary. In the glomerulus there is also a net pressure moving fluid out of the capillaries into Bowman's capsule. The major difference between the glomerulus and other capillaries is the permeability of the capillary membrane. In comparison to other capillaries, the glomerular membrane is significantly more permeable, allowing a much greater amount of fluid to move out of the capillary for each mm Hg difference in pressure (Vander, 1985).

Net Filtration Pressure. The net filtration pressure for any capillary is determined by the opposing values of hydrostatic and colloid osmotic pressures across the capillary wall. Hydrostatic pressure refers to the pressure exerted by a fluid, for example, the pressure exerted by the blood in a capillary. Colloid osmotic pressure refers to the pressure that develops across a semipermeable membrane when large molecules, such as protein, are unable to cross the membrane. The net pressure responsible for glomerular filtration is the sum of the hydrostatic and colloid osmotic pressures in the glomerular capillary and Bowman's capsule (Fig. 39–10).

Glomerular capillary hydrostatic pressure and the colloid osmotic pressure of the fluid in Bowman's capsule promote filtration. Under usual circumstances, the glomerular membrane allows only a small amount of protein to filter out of the blood into Bowman's capsule. Therefore, the colloid osmotic pressure of the fluid in Bowman's capsule is too small to have any significant impact on filtration. For this reason, glomerular capillary hydrostatic pressure will be the only force promoting filtration considered in this discussion. Glomerular filtration is opposed by the colloid osmotic pressure of the blood in the

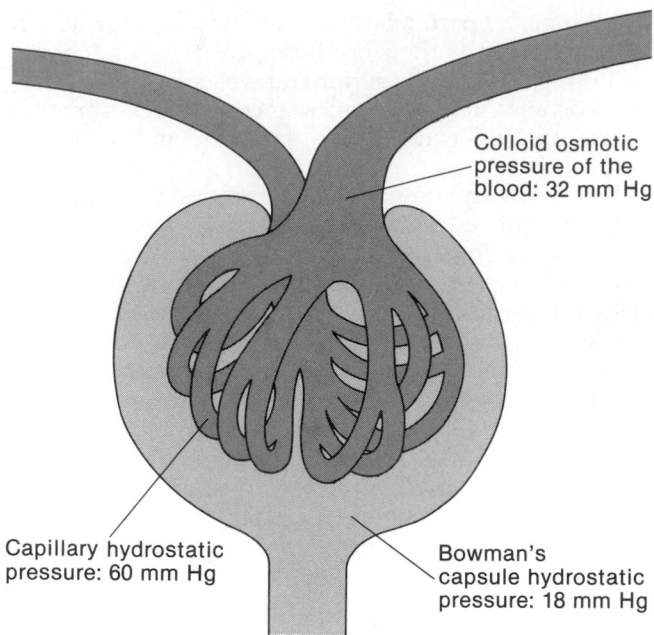

NET FILTRATION PRESSURE
60 − 32 − 18 = 10 mm Hg

FIGURE 39—10. Average pressures involved in filtration from the glomerular capillaries.

glomerular capillary and by the hydrostatic pressure exerted by the fluid inside Bowman's capsule.

The hydrostatic pressure exerted by the blood against the walls of the glomerular capillary has not been measured in humans. It has, however, been calculated to be around 55 to 60 mm Hg (Navar et al., 1989). As discussed previously, many factors have the potential to increase or decrease this pressure. The autoregulatory mechanisms within the kidney normally help to maintain intraglomerular hydrostatic pressure at a relatively constant level.

The normal colloid osmotic pressure of the blood averages 28 mm Hg. As plasma water leaves the glomerular capillary to filter into Bowman's capsule, the concentration of the proteins that are left behind increases. The resulting colloid osmotic pressure is approximately 36 mm Hg. An average colloid osmotic pressure in the glomerular capillaries would then be 32 mm Hg (Guyton, 1991). The osmotic pull exerted by the plasma proteins tends to hold fluid in the vascular space, opposing filtration in the glomerulus. This osmotic pressure is also important for the reabsorption of fluid back into the peritubular capillaries. Any factor that decreases the plasma protein concentration results in an increase in filtration. A decrease in filtration occurs with an elevation in the plasma protein concentration.

The fluid that filters into Bowman's capsule creates a hydrostatic pressure of its own that is believed to average around 18 mm Hg (Guyton, 1991). This is a pressure against which fluid leaving the glomerulus must flow, and thus it opposes filtration. Under normal conditions the hydrostatic pressure of the blood in the glomerulus is much higher than the pressure in Bowman's capsule, and fluid filters easily into the tubules. However, if the flow of urine through the urinary tract becomes obstructed, the pressure inside Bowman's capsule may begin to rise. This may result in a decrease in or even cessation of glomerular filtration.

Calculation of the difference between the forces promoting and the forces opposing filtration results in determination of the net filtration pressure. Utilizing the average pressures that have been discussed, the net filtration pressure in the glomerulus is calculated to be 10 mm Hg.

Glomerular Capillary Permeability and Composition of the Glomerular Ultrafiltrate. The glomerular capillary membrane is very permeable in comparison to most other capillary membranes (Vander, 1985). This permeability is the result of the large number of tiny perforations in the various layers of the membrane. Water and solutes of small molecular size filter freely across the glomerular membrane. The size of the perforations in the glomerular membrane, especially in the basement membrane layer, restrict the filtration of large molecules such as protein. As a result, the glomerular ultrafiltrate that enters Bowman's capsule has a composition that is almost identical to that of plasma except that it is protein free.

Filtration Fraction and Glomerular Filtration Rate. The renal filtration fraction is a term that refers to the portion of the plasma entering the glomerular capillaries that filters out of the capillary into Bowman's capsule. The renal filtration fraction is much higher than the filtration fraction in other capillaries. The filtration fraction in the glomerulus is approximately 20%, compared with 0.5% in most other capillaries (Guyton, 1991). The total amount of plasma flowing through the kidneys is around 650 mL/minute. If 20% of this amount were to filter across the glomerular membrane into Bowman's capsule, the GFR would be calculated at 130 mL/minute. Actual measurements in man have determined that the average amount of glomerular filtrate formed by both kidneys is 125 mL/minute or 180 liters/day.

The GFR can be altered by factors that affect the net filtration pressure or the permeability of the glomerular membrane. Disease processes that decrease the permeability of the glomerular membrane, e.g., acute or chronic glomerulonephritis or diabetes, decrease the amount of fluid that is able to filter across the membrane at a given filtration pressure. In patients with chronic renal disease, the GFR usually decreases slowly over a relatively long period of time. In most chronic renal diseases the nephrons are not all affected at the same time. Some nephrons cease to function while others remain intact. The nephrons that remain functional increase their GFR to compensate for the filtration capacity lost from diseased nephrons. It is not entirely clear how the intact nephrons are able to increase their GFR, but

this mechanism functions so efficiently that little alteration in the composition of the extracellular fluid occurs until 50% to 66% of the nephrons have ceased to function (Guyton, 1991).

Tubular Reabsorption. The process of glomerular filtration results in approximately 180 liters of ultrafiltrate entering the renal tubules every day. This huge volume of ultrafiltrate is equal to more than four times the volume of total body water. A carefully controlled process governing the reabsorption of water and solutes is essential to prevent significant alterations in the volume and composition of the extracellular fluid. Ordinarily, the renal tubules reabsorb 99% of the water and sodium from the 180 liters that filter into the tubules, resulting in the production of 1 to 2 liters of urine each day. Other substances that can be utilized by the body, such as glucose and amino acids, are also returned to the blood by the process of reabsorption. Some metabolic waste products, such as urea and uric acid, are partially reabsorbed. The majority of these wastes, however, are lost in the urine.

Substances reabsorbed by the nephrons move from the tubular lumen and pass through either the junctions between the tubular cells or the tubular cells themselves to enter the interstitial fluid. From the interstitial fluid, water and solutes readily enter the peritubular capillaries, which are extremely permeable and which together reabsorb about four times as much as all other capillaries in the entire body (Guyton, 1991). The majority of reabsorbed solutes must pass through the tubular cells, crossing both the luminal membrane (separating the tubular lumen from the interior of the cell) and the basolateral membrane (separating the interior of the cell from the interstitial fluid) in the process. A description of diffusion, osmosis, and active transport—the transport mechanisms utilized in reabsorption—follows.

Diffusion. The term diffusion refers to the movement of molecules or ions from an area of higher concentration to an area of lower concentration via the random motion of the molecule or ion (Fig. 39–11A). For diffusion to occur, there must be a concentration or electrical gradient across the cell membrane, and the membrane must be permeable to the substance. If the membrane is permeable, net movement of the substance from the area of higher concentration to the area of lower concentration will occur until equilibration is achieved. In the nephron, negatively charged ions are most frequently reabsorbed passively due to the electrical gradient created by sodium reabsorption. As sodium and water are transported out of the tubular lumen, the concentration of solutes that are left behind increases. This sets up a concentration and often an electrical gradient for these solutes between the tubular lumen and the interstitial fluid surrounding the tubular cell. If the tubular membrane is permeable to them, solutes will move down their concentration or electrical gradient and will be reabsorbed.

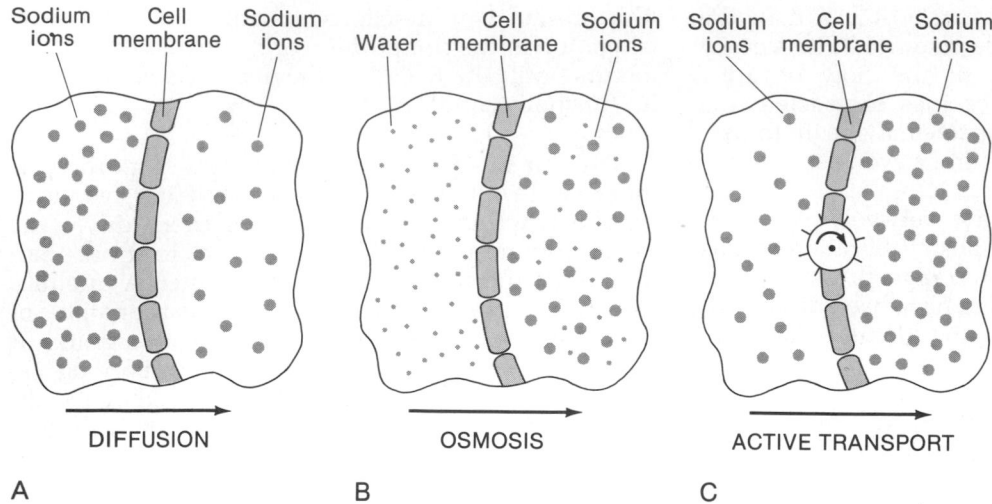

FIGURE 39—11. Movement of molecules across cell membranes. A, movement of sodium ions by diffusion. B, movement of water by osmosis. C, movement of sodium ions by active transport.

Some solutes that are not lipid soluble are able to cross the tubular membrane only if a specific carrier molecule is available to help them across—a process known as facilitated diffusion. The carrier molecule combines with the solute at the outside surface of the cell membrane. The carrier molecule transports the solute across the lipid inside of the membrane and releases it on the other side. In this type of system, the rate of diffusion is limited by the amount of carrier molecule available and the rate at which the chemical reaction can take place.

Osmosis. The movement of water from an area of higher water concentration to an area of lower concentration is referred to as osmosis (Fig. 39–11*B*). In the nephron, osmosis occurs when sodium molecules are transported out of the tubular lumen, decreasing the concentration of solutes in the lumen and increasing the concentration of solutes in the interstitial fluid. Concurrently, the concentration of water in the lumen increases and the concentration of water in the interstitial fluid decreases. If the tubular membrane is permeable, water will move from the lumen to the area of increased solute concentration in the interstitium to equalize the concentrations. Water in the interstitium then rapidly diffuses into the peritubular capillaries due to the movement of sodium and the osmotic pull created by the high concentration of plasma proteins in the blood leaving the glomerulus.

Active Transport. The term active transport refers to a cellular transport mechanism that moves a substance against its concentration or electrical gradient, requiring the expenditure of cellular energy (Fig. 39–11*C*). The majority of substances that are reabsorbed leave the tubular lumen through active transport. Sodium is an example of a molecule that is actively transported.

Each actively reabsorbed solute requires a specific carrier system. These systems operate like the mechanism described for facilitated diffusion except that energy is expended in the process. The rate at which reabsorption of the solute can occur is limited by the amount of carrier available and the time it takes for the completion of the chemical reaction between the carrier and the solute. As a result, each actively reabsorbed solute has a transport maximum—the maximum rate it can be transported across the tubular membrane. If the concentration of the solute in the tubular fluid is greater than the amount of the solute that can be actively reabsorbed, some of the solute in the tubular fluid will not be reabsorbed but will be excreted in the urine. Glucose is a substance that exhibits this property. When the serum glucose is within normal limits, about 125 mg of glucose filters into the tubules each minute and is reabsorbed by its carrier system. As the amount of glucose entering the tubules rises above 200 mg/minute, some of the glucose is not reabsorbed and begins to appear in the urine. The point at which it begins to appear in the urine is known as the threshold. The maximum amount of glucose that can be reabsorbed by the tubules is 325 mg/minute. The amount of glucose entering the tubules must increase above 400 mg/minute before the carrier system will begin to operate at that capacity (Guyton, 1991).

Disease processes within the tubular cell can increase or decrease the transport maximum of various substances. One example is gout, in which an increase in the tubular transport maximum for uric acid contributes to a rise in plasma and interstitial fluid levels (Duling, 1988). Eventually this elevated level leads to precipitation of uric acid in the joints and other tissues.

Factors Regulating Reabsorption. Under normal circumstances, the amount of a substance that is reabsorbed is dependent upon body needs and is regulated by changes in the concentration of the substance and by body hormones. When the concentration of a substance is decreased in the plasma, the amount of that substance that filters into the tubule will also be decreased. If the substance is normally reabsorbed by active transport, a fall in its concentration in the tubular fluid results in fewer molecules of the substance competing for the available carrier molecules in the cell membrane. As a result, the percentage of the substance reabsorbed from the tubular fluid will increase with a consequent decrease in the amount lost into the urine. The opposite occurs with an increase in the plasma concentration of a substance. More of the substance is filtered into the tubules, and there are more molecules of the substance competing for the available carrier molecules in the tubular cell membranes. A smaller percentage is reabsorbed and more is excreted in the urine.

Hormones also play a role in regulation of tubular reabsorption. A good example of this is aldosterone. As described previously, aldosterone release is one of the end results of stimulation of the renin-angiotensin-aldosterone system. Aldosterone stimulates the distal convoluted tubule to increase sodium reabsorption, which increases the intravascular volume and RBF. These adjustments of tubular reabsorption occur continuously to maintain a stable composition of the extracellular fluid.

Tubular Secretion. The process of tubular secretion transports substances from blood in the peritubular capillaries into the tubular lumen, adding substances to the urine that either are not filtered or are filtered in small amounts. In general, secreted substances are electrolytes present in excess amounts in the extracellular fluid, metabolic wastes, and chemicals or drugs. Examples of substances secreted by the nephron are hydrogen ion, potassium, creatinine, ammonia, thiamine, histamine, and penicillin. Secretion occurs by diffusion and active transport, though active transport plays a larger role.

The amount of a substance secreted is regulated by body needs and hormones. Tubular handling of potassium illustrates this well. A significant amount of the filtered potassium is reabsorbed in the proximal tubule, leaving a low concentration of potassium in the fluid that enters the distal tubule. As a result, a diffusion gradient is set up between the peritubular capillary blood and the distal tubular fluid, resulting in passive secretion of potassium. The higher the potassium content in the plasma, the wider the gradient and the greater the amount of potassium that is secreted. In addition, potassium is also secreted through a sodium-potassium pump in the cells of the distal tubule. This pump operates under the influence of aldosterone. A high plasma potassium concentration is a direct stimulus for aldosterone release from the adrenal cortex.

The terms net absorption and net secretion are used to discuss how a specific substance is handled by the nephron. Generally, one process takes precedence; however, a molecule or ion may be only reabsorbed, only secreted, or reabsorbed and secreted, or it may not undergo either process.

Clearance. Clearance is defined as the volume of plasma that can be completely cleared of a substance in one minute. It can be calculated for any substance by utilizing the following formula:

$$\text{Clearance (mL/minute)} = \frac{UV \times UC}{PC}$$

where UV = the volume of urine in mL/minute,
UC = the concentration of the substance in the urine, and
PC = the concentration of the substance in the plasma.

Most substances are not completely cleared from the plasma in one pass through the nephron. Instead, a percentage of the substance is actually removed from a given volume of plasma. The concept of clearance is helpful in comparing how much of one particular substance is removed by the kidney relative to another substance.

The clearance of creatinine and inulin is utilized as a measure of GFR. These molecules are unique in that they are freely filtered across the glomerulus and are not reabsorbed. Inulin is an exogenous polysaccharide that must be given intravenously to the patient for a clearance to be determined. Inulin is not secreted by the tubules, so the amount of inulin that enters the tubules is the same as the amount excreted in the urine. For this reason, the clearance of inulin is equal to the GFR.

To spare the patient the invasive administration of inulin, most practitioners utilize the creatinine clearance to measure GFR. Creatinine is an endogenous waste product released from muscle tissue. A tiny amount of creatinine is secreted into the tubules from the peritubular capillary blood. The creatinine clearance, therefore, slightly overestimates the GFR. The difference is so slight that in the clinical setting it is considered insignificant.

Transport of Specific Substances Throughout the Nephron

The processes of glomerular filtration, reabsorption, and secretion result in precise regulation of waste removal and conservation of water and other substances required for normal body functioning. This section will describe how each section of the nephron specifically regulates key substances to accomplish this task.

Proximal Tubule. The proximal convoluted tubule is structurally designed for reabsorption. Its cells have a large surface area and a large number of mitochondria to supply cellular energy. About two-thirds of the glomerular filtrate is normally reabsorbed in this first section of the tubules. Of particular importance is the reabsorption of electrolytes, water, and substances of nutritional value. Secretion of a few metabolic end-products also occurs in the proximal tubule.

Reabsorption of Electrolytes. Approximately 65% of the filtered sodium is actively reabsorbed in the proximal tubule. Figure 39–12 illustrates the processes involved in sodium reabsorption. Sodium moves by facilitated diffusion from the tubular fluid in the lumen of the proximal tubule, across the luminal membrane and into the cytoplasm of the proximal tubule epithelial cell. Sodium movement occurs as a result of an electrochemical gradient for sodium. The inside of the proximal tubule epithelial cell is negatively charged in relation to the luminal fluid, and the concentration of sodium inside the cell is low. This electrochemical gradient for sodium movement into the cell is maintained by an active transport mechanism or "sodium pump" within the basolateral membrane of the proximal tubule epithelial cell. The sodium pump moves sodium from the interior of the cell into the interstitial fluid. As the concentration of sodium in the interstitial fluid increases, sodium moves by simple diffusion into the blood in the peritubular capillaries.

The reabsorption of several other substances is closely linked to the reabsorption of sodium in the proximal tubule. As large amounts of the positively charged sodium ions leave the tubular lumen, negatively charged ions must also leave in order to maintain electroneutrality. For example, bicarbonate ions are passively reabsorbed with the sodium ions in the first part of the proximal tubule. Chloride is the preferred ion to accompany diffusion of sodium in the latter portion of the proximal tubule. Sodium is the most abundant ion reabsorbed, and its movement creates a large osmotic gradient resulting in the reabsorption of water. The reabsorption of other solutes also contributes to the osmotic gradient for water.

Potassium reabsorption in the proximal tubule involves both active transport and diffusion. The concentration of potassium in the lumen of the proximal tubule is around 5 mEq/liter. The potassium concentration inside the tubular cells is about 140 mEq/liter. This large concentration gradient acts against passive reabsorption. The reabsorption of sodium, however, causes the inside of the tubular cell to become very negative, setting up an electrical gradient for potassium diffusion. In addition, an active transport mechanism is present to assist in moving potassium into the cell against its concentration gradient. Potassium is able to move passively down its concentration gradient from the inside of the cell into the peritubular capillary blood. Ultimately, 65% of the filtered potasssium is reabsorbed from the proximal tubule.

Less is known about how the nephron handles calcium and phosphate. A large amount of the filtered calcium is actively reabsorbed from the proximal tubule. Phosphate is also actively reabsorbed under the principles of tubular transport maximum. If the serum phosphate level is low, virtually all filtered phosphate is reabsorbed. As serum phosphorus rises, increasing amounts of phosphate fail to be reabsorbed and are excreted in the urine. The tubular transport maximum for phosphate is under the influence of parathyroid hormone. The presence of this hormone decreases the transport maximum for phosphate, resulting in increased excretion into the urine.

Reabsorption of Nutrients. A number of substances are so important for maintenance of nutritional balance in the body that little, if any, of these substances are allowed to leave the proximal tubule. Glucose, amino acids, proteins, vitamins, and acetoacetate ions are all actively reabsorbed (Guyton, 1991). Glucose reabsorption operates by a transport maximum system as previously described. Protein molecules are too large to cross the cell membrane by the usual means and thus are transported into the cell by the process of pinocytosis. First, the protein molecule attaches itself to the cell wall of the tubular epithelial cell. The cell wall then forms a pocket around the protein molecule, which eventually is pinched off into the interior of the cell. Once inside the cell, the protein molecules are broken down into their component amino acids, which are then reabsorbed by diffusion.

Reabsorption and Secretion of Waste Products. Substances that are considered to be body wastes are either secreted, not reabsorbed, or only partially reabsorbed by the proximal tubule. For example, creatinine is not reabsorbed at all, and only 50% of filtered urea is reabsorbed. Reabsorption of waste substances is regulated by the permeability of the tubular membrane. Hydrogen ion is secreted by the proximal tubule. This process will be discussed in detail later when the kidney's role in maintenance of acid-base balance is addressed.

Effect of Diuretics on the Proximal Tubule. Osmotic diuretics, such as mannitol, exert their effect primarily in the proximal tubule because this is where most of the water is reabsorbed. Mannitol is a monosaccharide that is freely filtered at the glomerulus and is not reabsorbed by the tubules. The presence of

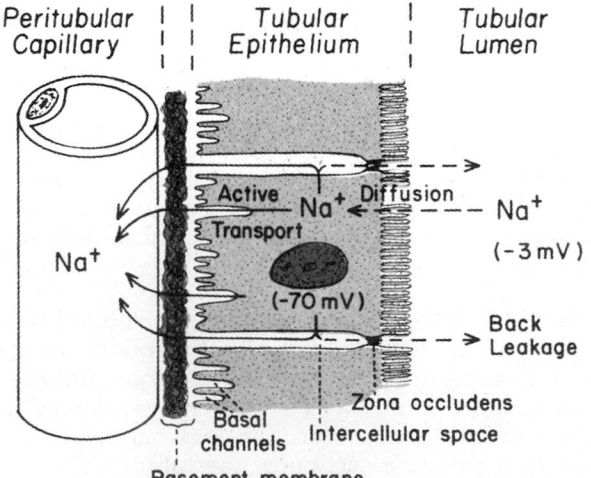

FIGURE 39–12. Mechanism for reabsorption of sodium from the tubular lumen into the peritubular capillary. (From Guyton, A. C. (1991). *Textbook of medical physiology* (8th ed., p. 400). Philadelphia: W. B. Saunders).

mannitol in the proximal tubule contributes to an osmotic gradient, decreasing the amount of water reabsorbed. The water, held in the tubules by the mannitol, passes into the more distal portions of the tubules and is excreted, thus increasing the urine volume.

Loop of Henle. The loop of Henle is also involved in the reabsorption of substances from the tubular fluid. Its configuration, cell structures, and management of sodium and water reabsorption are designed to cause a buildup of solutes within the interstitial fluid of the medulla, decreasing the solute concentration of the fluid moving into the distal tubule. This function is essential to the kidney's ability to control the volume and concentration of the urine.

The amount of sodium and water reabsorbed varies greatly from section to section of the loop of Henle. In the descending portion of the thin segment the membrane is highly permeable to water and moderately permeable to sodium and other ions. Movement of sodium and water in this portion of the loop occurs primarily by diffusion. The cell membrane in the ascending portion of the thin segment is much less permeable to water but remains permeable to solutes. Finally, in the thick portion of the ascending limb sodium is actively transported out of the tubular lumen into the interstitial fluid. The membrane here is almost completely impermeable to water. Because water cannot move along with sodium and other solutes, the fluid leaving the loop is quite diluted.

Potassium is reabsorbed from the loop of Henle. Potassium is actively transported from the thick portion of the ascending limb. Approximately 25% of the filtered potassium is reabsorbed from the loop, allowing only about 10% of the original tubular load of potassium to enter the distal tubule.

Furosemide and bumetanide belong to a class of diuretics known as the "loop diuretics." Their site of action is the thick segment of the ascending limb of the loop of Henle. These diuretics work by blocking sodium reabsorption. As a result, the sodium concentration of the fluid leaving the loop increases. The increased sodium content holds water in the distal tubule and collecting duct, increasing the volume of urine excreted.

Distal Tubule. Fine-tuning of the final urine product occurs in the distal tubule. The concentration of sodium, potassium, calcium, urea, and other substances continues to be altered by reabsorption and secretion. Whereas the fluid leaving the proximal tubule is isotonic at 300 mOsm/liter, the fluid leaving the distal tubule may vary between 100 and 300 mOsm/liter, depending upon the permeability of the tubule to water.

Reabsorption of Electrolytes. Sodium is actively reabsorbed throughout the length of the distal tubule. The transport process here is similar to that in the proximal tubule. A major difference is that the transport mechanism for sodium in the distal tubule

is under the influence of aldosterone. When aldosterone is present in large amounts, virtually all of the sodium entering the distal tubule is reabsorbed. The final urine normally contains less than 1% of the filtered sodium. If aldosterone is not present, a much smaller amount of sodium will be reabsorbed, resulting in the loss of large amounts into the urine. The exact mechanism by which aldosterone alters the sodium transport process is not known. It is believed that aldosterone either increases the amount of available carrier protein or increases the concentration of a particular enzyme, thus increasing the rate of sodium reabsorption (Guyton, 1991).

Another difference between the proximal tubule and the distal tubule is that sodium reabsorption in the distal tubule is coupled with potassium secretion. Potassium diffuses into the distal tubular cell down an electrical gradient and then diffuses into the tubular lumen down a concentration gradient. Control of potassium secretion is influenced by aldosterone, the plasma potassium concentration, and the amount of sodium which enters the distal tubule. The presence of aldosterone increases potassium secretion by increasing the electrical gradient for potassium diffusion. Potassium secretion is also increased by an elevation of the plasma potassium concentration above normal. The higher plasma potassium concentration creates a wider concentration gradient between the peritubular fluid and the tubular lumen, thus increasing diffusion. Finally, if the amount of sodium entering the distal tubule increases, as occurs following administration of a loop diuretic, sodium reabsorption and potassium secretion also increase.

An active transport mechanism for potassium reabsorption exists in the distal tubule, and this mechanism is capable of reabsorbing all of the remaining potassium. As a result, excretion of excess potassium is dependent upon the mechanisms that regulate potassium secretion.

Only about 10% of the filtered calcium reaches the distal tubule. When the plasma calcium concentration is within normal limits, little calcium reabsorption occurs in the distal tubule, and calcium is lost into the urine. If the plasma calcium concentration is low, most of the calcium will be reabsorbed from the distal tubule under the influence of parathyroid hormone. A low plasma calcium concentration is the stimulus for parathyroid hormone release. This hormone stimulates calcium reabsorption from the bone as well as from the distal tubule, leading to correction of the low plasma calcium concentration.

Water Reabsorption. Water reabsorption from the distal tubule is dependent upon the presence of ADH. ADH is produced in the supraoptic and paraventricular nuclei of the hypothalamus and is released from the posterior pituitary (Vander, 1985). There are two primary stimuli for ADH production and release. The first is a fall in blood pressure which is sensed by the baroreceptors, particularly in the left atrium. The second stimulus is an increase in serum osmolality, sensed by the osmoreceptors located in the hypothalamus and liver. ADH production and release is inhibited by an increase in blood pressure, a decrease in serum osmolality, or the presence of alcohol (Vander, 1985).

When ADH is absent, the distal tubular cell membranes are impermeable to water. Water remains in the distal tubule, so the fluid entering the collecting duct will be dilute. In the presence of ADH, the distal tubular cell membrane becomes more permeable to water. ADH is thought to cause pores within the cell wall to open, allowing water to move with sodium, because sodium is actively reabsorbed. Movement of water equalizes the concentration gradients between the tubular lumen and the peritubular capillary blood.

Secretion of Waste Products. Wastes and substances foreign to the body are secreted by the distal tubule and are not reabsorbed from the tubular fluid. As water is reabsorbed from the distal tubule, the concentration of these substances in the tubular fluid increases.

Connecting Tubule and Collecting Duct. The collecting duct epithelium functions like the distal tubule in the handling of sodium, potassium, water, and wastes. Sodium is actively reabsorbed under the influence of aldosterone. Potassium continues to be secreted, although potassium reabsorption may occur if potassium intake is reduced. It is in the collecting duct that the final volume and concentration of urine are determined. Water reabsorption is dependent upon the presence of ADH. As the collecting duct descends through the increasingly more concentrated interstitial fluid of the medulla, large amounts of water may move out of the collecting duct when ADH is present. ADH also makes the membrane of the collecting duct more permeable to urea, allowing urea to diffuse into the interstitial fluid of the medulla along with water.

Impact of Tubular Damage on Composition of the Extracellular Fluid. Disease processes, such as acute tubular necrosis, affect the tubules of the nephron. Consequently, there is a potential to create significant imbalances in the composition of the extracellular fluid. Tubular damage may impair the kidney's ability to reabsorb electrolytes, amino acids, and vitamins and to secrete body wastes. As a result, the plasma concentrations of these substances become altered and may eventually impair cellular function in organ systems and tissues.

Regulation of Urine Concentration and Volume

The various mechanisms for controlling urine volumes and concentration have already been described. When fluid intake increases and the extracellular fluid becomes more diluted, the kidney must be able to excrete the excess water without depleting sodium

or other solutes. Conversely, when fluid intake is limited, the kidneys must be able to rid the body of waste products while conserving water. Under ordinary circumstances, the kidney manages this by matching urine output closely to fluid intake minus fluid loss from other sources and by varying urine concentration within a range of 70 to 1400 mOsm/liter (Guyton, 1991). This section will discuss the integration of the various mechanisms controlling urine volume and concentration. Clinical problems that affect this important renal function will also be addressed.

Anatomic and Physiologic Features Contributing to Control of Urine Concentration and Volume. As previously described in the section on renal anatomy in this chapter, the loops of Henle in the juxtamedullary nephrons are structurally quite different from those of cortical nephrons. The specialized structures of the juxtamedullary nephrons are critical to the kidney's ability to concentrate the urine. The loops of Henle, distal convoluted tubules, and collecting ducts also play essential roles in the handling of sodium, water, and urea. A summary of water and solute handling is presented in Table 39–2. Table 39–3 outlines the differences between the fluid that filters into the tubules and the fluid that is ultimately excreted as urine.

Countercurrent Mechanism. The term countercurrent mechanism refers to the interaction of the specialized anatomic and physiologic features of the loops of Henle in juxtamedullary nephrons that result in the development of an interstitial fluid that becomes increasingly more concentrated with movement from the outer to the innermost regions of the medulla. An understanding of this mechanism's function in forming a concentrated interstitial fluid is fundamental to understanding how the kidney concentrates urine.

The process begins with entry of fluid from the proximal tubule into the loop of Henle as seen in Figure 39–13. At this point, the tubular fluid has a concentration of 300 mOsm/liter, the same as plasma. The thick segment of the ascending limb of the loop

TABLE 39–2. Water and Solute Handling by the Nephron

Loop of Henle	
Descending limb	Very permeable to water and solutes
Thin segment of the ascending limb	Permeable to sodium and chloride Low water permeability
Thick segment of the ascending limb	Active reabsorption of sodium Impermeable to water and urea
Distal Convoluted Tubule	Active reabsorption of sodium Permeable to water when antidiuretic hormone (ADH) is present Impermeable to urea
Collecting duct	Active reabsorption of sodium Permeable to water and urea when ADH is present

TABLE 39–3. Relative Concentrations of Substances in the Glomerular Filtrate and in the Urine

	Glomerular Filtrate (125 mL/min)		Urine (1 mL/min)		Conc. Urine/Conc. Plasma (Plasma clearance/per min)
	Quantity/min	Concentration	Quantity/min	Concentration	
Na$^+$	17.7 mEq	142 mEq/L	0.128 mEq	128 mEq/L	0.9
K$^+$	0.63	5	0.06	60	12
Ca^{2+}	0.5	4	0.0048	4.8	1.2
Mg^{2+}	0.38	3	0.015	15	5.0
Cl$^-$	12.9	103	0.134	134	1.3
HCO$_3^-$	3.5	28	0.014	14	0.5
H$_2$PO$_4^-$	0.25				
HPO$_4$2 −		2	0.05	50	25
SO$_4^{2-}$	0.09	0.7	0.033	33	47
Glucose	125 mg	100 mg/dl	0 mg	0 mg/dl	0.0
Urea	33	26	18.2	1820	70
Uric acid	3.8	3	0.42	42	14
Creatinine	1.4	1.1	1.96	196	140
Inulin	—	—	—	—	125
Diodrast	—	—	—	—	560
PAH	—	—	—	—	585

From Guyton, A. C. (1991). *Textbook of medical physiology* (8th ed., p. 407). Philadelphia: W. B. Saunders.

of Henle actively transports sodium from the tubular lumen into the interstitial fluid. Because the ascending limb is impermeable to water, water cannot follow the sodium into the interstitial fluid.

Consequently, the concentration of the interstitial fluid increases. As a concentration gradient develops between the fluid in the descending limb and the interstitial fluid, water begins to move out of the descending limb and solute diffuses into the descending limb until an equilibrium is reached. As a result, the fluid within the descending limb becomes more concentrated.

Sodium and urea also help to raise the concentra-

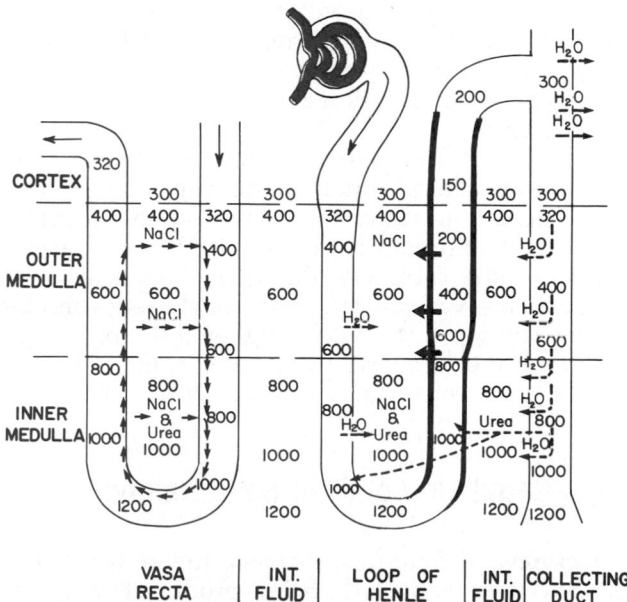

FIGURE 39–13. The countercurrent mechanism for concentrating the urine. (Numerical values are in milliosmoles per liter). (From Guyton, A. C. (1991). *Textbook of medical physiology* (8th ed., p. 415). Philadelphia: W. B. Saunders).

tion of the interstitial fluid as they are reabsorbed from the collecting duct. The addition of these solutes to the interstitial fluid pulls additional water out of the descending limb, further concentrating the fluid in this part of the tubule. The tubular fluid flows down toward the tip of the loop of Henle carrying the solutes with it. As the fluid rounds the bend and enters the ascending limb, the transport mechanisms there remove sodium, adding it to the solute accumulating in the interstitial fluid. Solute is constantly being added to the interstitial fluid by the ascending limb and the collecting duct. Therefore, solute becomes concentrated in the interstitial fluid of the medulla. The concentration becomes highest in the deepest regions of the medulla as solute is carried there by the loops of Henle and vasa recta, potentially reaching a concentration of about 1400 mOsm/liter.

The tubules of the loop of Henle have the capacity to maintain a concentration difference of up to 200 mOsm/liter between the fluid in the ascending and descending limbs. Thus, the distal segment of the ascending limb can reduce the concentration of the tubular fluid to as little as 100 mOsm/liter.

Excretion of a Diluted Urine. When the extracellular fluid becomes hypotonic, secretion of ADH is inhibited. Without ADH, the distal tubules and collecting ducts of the kidney become impermeable to water. Because sodium continues to be removed from the fluid and water cannot follow it, the diluted fluid entering the distal tubule becomes even more diluted as it passes onward, through the collecting duct. The concentration may decrease from 100 mOsm/liter at the start of the distal tubule down to 70 mOsm/liter in the collecting duct. The end result is the excretion of a large volume of diluted urine.

Excretion of a Concentrated Urine. When body fluids become hypertonic, the normal kidney conserves water. At the same time, the kidney must be able to excrete the end-products of metabolism. Increased osmolality of the extracellular fluid stimulates ADH secretion. The presence of ADH increases the permeability of the distal tubule and collecting duct to water. Water can leave the relatively diluted fluid inside the collecting duct to move into the concentrated interstitial fluid of the medulla. If a very large amount of ADH is present, the urine concentration may equilibrate with the concentration of the interstitial fluid, potentially reaching 1400 mOsm/liter. The end result is the excretion of a small volume of very concentrated urine.

The amount of ADH secreted determines the permeability of the collecting duct to water, the amount of water reabsorbed from the collecting duct, and therefore the final volume and concentration of the urine. If the urine is maximally concentrated to 1400 mOsm/liter, a urine volume of at least 400 mL is required to excrete the waste solutes produced in a 24-hour period (Vander, 1985). If the urine volume is less than 400 mL/24 hours, or if the urine volume is low and the urine cannot be maximally concentrated, waste products will begin to accumulate in the blood.

Physiologic Changes Affecting Urine Volumes.
Even small changes in the GFR can have a significant impact on urine volume. Changes in blood pressure, colloid osmotic pressure, or the level of sympathetic nervous system stimulation also have the potential to alter the amount of urine produced.

The impact of changes in blood pressure on the GFR has been previously discussed in the section on autoregulation. Briefly, an increase in blood pressure increases the pressure inside the glomerular capillary, pushing more fluid across the glomerular membrane into the tubules. The tubules are unable to reabsorb all of the additional tubular fluid, and urine output therefore increases. With a fall in blood pressure, the GFR falls. The corresponding fall in the rate and volume of tubular flow allows the tubules to reabsorb a proportionally greater amount of the tubular fluid than normal, and urine output decreases. The mechanism for autoregulation of the GFR helps to minimize the effects of changes in blood pressure. However, some change in the volume of urine produced will occur, particularly when blood pressure rises or falls outside of the range in which autoregulation is effective.

Changes in the colloid osmotic pressure affect glomerular filtration and the forces promoting tubular reabsorption. A rise in the colloid osmotic pressure decreases glomerular filtration by exerting an increased osmotic force that holds fluid in the vascular space. As the blood passes on into the peritubular capillaries, the higher colloid osmotic pressure attracts increased amounts of fluid out of the tubules, thus increasing tubular reabsorption and decreasing urine output. Conversely, a fall in the colloid osmotic pressure increases the GFR, decreases tubular reabsorption, and increases urine output.

Changes in the level of sympathetic nervous system stimulation may also affect GFR and urine output. Increased sympathetic stimulation causes increased constriction of the afferent arteriole. The resulting fall in blood flow decreases intraglomerular pressure and glomerular filtration. With less fluid filtering into the tubules, a higher percentage of tubular fluid is reabsorbed, and urine output decreases.

Clinical Problems Affecting Urine Concentration and Volume. Disease states or drug therapy utilized to treat illness may alter urine volume and concentration. A common example is diabetes mellitus. As blood glucose levels rise, the amount of glucose being filtered also increases. When the tubular load of glucose exceeds the transport maximum, some glucose fails to be reabsorbed and passes into the urine. The increase in urinary glucose molecules creates an increased osmotic pull, holding water in the tubule and increasing urine output.

Diabetes insipidus can also affect the volume and concentration of the urine. Diabetes insipidus is caused by either the insufficient production of ADH or the kidney's lack of ability to respond to ADH. In either case the distal tubule and collecting duct remain relatively impermeable to water, resulting in significant loss of water as urine. Conversely, when excessive amounts of ADH are present, water is maximally reabsorbed from the distal tubule and collecting duct, and a small volume of concentrated urine is excreted. This may occur in a condition known as the syndrome of inappropriate antidiuretic hormone secretion (SIADH). Administration of exogenous ADH (vasopressin) for therapeutic reasons may also result in excessive concentration of urine.

Acute or chronic renal failure impairs the kidney's ability to regulate urine volume and concentration. Both forms of renal failure result in a fall in GFR. Many disease processes also damage the tubules, impairing tubular function and the ability to concentrate the urine.

The use of diuretics to treat fluid overload results in a common clinical situation affecting urine volume and concentation. Administration of any of the major categories of diuretics results in an increased excretion of sodium. Table 39–4 describes the mechanisms by which the various categories of diuretics inhibit sodium reabsorption. With a higher sodium concentration in the tubules, water will remain in the tubules, and urine output will increase.

Renal Regulation of Acid-Base Balance

Overview of Acid-Base Balance Regulation. Acid substances are constantly being produced as a consequence of cellular metabolism. These acids must be removed from the body if a stable pH is to be maintained. Two physiologic mechanisms are in

TABLE 39–4. Mechanism of Action of the Major Classes of Diuretics

Class of Diuretic	Representative Drugs	Mechanism of Action
Loop diuretics	Furosemide (Lasix) Bumetanide (Bumex) Ethacrynic acid (Edecrin)	Inhibits sodium reabsorption in the thick segment of the loop of Henle
Thiazide diuretics and thiazidelike diuretics	Hydrochlorothiazide (Hydrodiuril, Esidrix) Metolazone (Diulo, Zaroxolyn)	Inhibit sodium reabsorption in the proximal and early distal tubules
Osmotic diuretics	Mannitol (Osmitrol)	Increase osmolality of the tubular fluid leading to decreased reabsorption of sodium and water
Potassium-sparing diuretics	Spironolactone (Aldactone) Triamterene (Dyazide, Dyrenium, Maxzide)	Aldosterone antagonist Blocks the sodium-potassium exchange mechanism in the distal tubule
Carbonic anhydrase inhibitors	Acetazolamide (Diamox)	Blocks the action of carbonic anhydrase in the proximal tubule preventing bicarbonate and sodium reabsorption

place to accomplish this: pulmonary excretion and renal excretion.

Cellular metabolism produces large amounts of carbon dioxide (CO_2). Carbon dioxide leads to the production of acid when it combines with water in the following reaction:

$$CO_2 + H_2O \rightleftarrows \underset{\text{(carbonic acid)}}{H_2CO_3} \rightleftarrows \underset{\text{(hydrogen ion)}}{H^+} + \underset{\text{(bicarbonate)}}{HCO_3^-}$$

This reaction is reversed as blood passes through the lungs. Carbon dioxide is excreted through the lungs, so that normally there is no net gain of hydrogen ion (Vander, 1985).

Cellular metabolism also results in the production of acid substances not amenable to pulmonary excretion known as "fixed acids." Examples of fixed acids are sulfuric, phosphoric, and lactic acids. These substances release a hydrogen ion as they dissociate. Fixed acids can be excreted only by the kidneys

(Cogan and Rector, 1986). The kidneys have two functions in regulating acid-base balance. First, hydrogen ions are secreted by the epithelial cells of the kidney tubules and excreted in the urine. Second, the kidneys help to maintain a normal bicarbonate concentration by reabsorbing filtered bicarbonate ions and forming bicarbonate inside the epithelial cells of the tubules (Vander, 1985).

Bicarbonate functions as a major buffering mechanism in the body. Bicarbonate combines with H^+ to prevent acidosis through the following reaction:

$$HCO_3^- + H^+ \rightleftarrows H_2CO_3 \rightleftarrows CO_2 + H_2O$$

The CO_2 produced by this reaction is either excreted through the lungs or utilized to form a bicarbonate ion inside the epithelial cells of the kidney tubules. This latter mechanism will be described later.

Regeneration of Bicarbonate by the Tubular Epithelial Cells. The processes responsible for renal secretion of hydrogen ion and conservation of bicarbonate are complex and intertwined. These processes are illustrated in Figure 39–14. Hydrogen ion secretion and regeneration of bicarbonate ion begin with the buildup of carbon dioxide inside the tubular epithelial cell. Carbon dioxide is either formed by the cell's own metabolic processes or diffuses into the cell from the tubular lumen or peritubular capillary blood. As the carbon dioxide concentration rises, the rate of hydrogen ion secretion and bicarbonate formation also increase.

Inside the cell, carbon dioxide combines with water to form carbonic acid under the influence of the enzyme carbonic anhydrase. Carbonic acid then dissociates into a hydrogen ion and a bicarbonate ion. The hydrogen ions are secreted into the tubular lumen. The bicarbonate ions combine with sodium and diffuse out of the cell into the extracellular fluid. In this way, bicarbonate ions, which were used

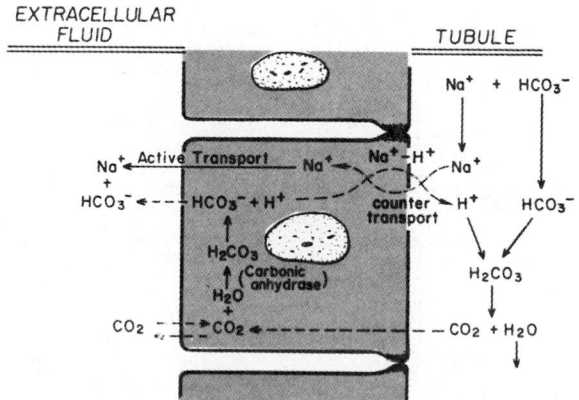

FIGURE 39–14. Chemical reactions for (1) hydrogen ion secretion, (2) sodium ion absorption in exchange for a hydrogen ion, (3) combination of hydrogen ions with bicarbonate ions in the tubules. (From Guyton, A. C. (1991). *Textbook of medical physiology* (8th ed., p. 444). Philadelphia: W. B. Saunders).

somewhere in the body to buffer hydrogen ions, are reformed and replenished in the extracellular fluid.

Hydrogen Ion Secretion. Secretion of hydrogen ion occurs primarily in the proximal tubule and to a smaller extent in the thick segment of the ascending limb of the loop of Henle, the distal tubule, and the collecting duct. Hydrogen ion secretion is linked to the reabsorption of sodium. Sodium combines with the carrier protein in the cell wall and is carried from the lumen of the tubule into the interior of the epithelial cell. Simultaneously, hydrogen ion from the inside of the cell combines with the other side of the carrier protein. As sodium diffuses into the cell, the carrier protein rotates, carrying the hydrogen ion from the inside of the cell and releasing it into the tubular lumen. The energy provided to the carrier protein by sodium diffusion allows the tubules to move hydrogen ion against its concentration gradient. Secretion may continue until the pH reaches approximately 6.8 in the proximal tubule, 6.0 to 6.5 in the ascending limb of the loop of Henle and the distal tubule, and 4.5 in the collecting duct (Guyton, 1991).

Reabsorption of Filtered Bicarbonate. Inside of the tubular lumen much of the secreted hydrogen ion again combines with bicarbonate. A small but significant amount of hydrogen ion combines with other tubular buffers. The bicarbonate ion in the tubular fluid originates from filtration of sodium bicarbonate from the glomerular capillary blood. As sodium is actively reabsorbed from the tubular fluid, bicarbonate is left behind. If bicarbonate did not combine with hydrogen ion, it would be lost into the urine because the epithelial cells of the tubules are generally not permeable to it. The combination of bicarbonate and hydrogen ion forms carbonic acid, which quickly dissociates into carbon dioxide and water under the influence of carbonic anhydrase. The carbon dioxide diffuses rapidly out of the tubule into the epithelial cell. From there, carbon dioxide may diffuse into the blood in the peritubular capillaries to be transported to the lungs. Carbon dioxide may also remain in the epithelial cell to combine with water, ultimately resulting in the reformation of a bicarbonate ion. In essence, this process results in the reabsorption of bicarbonate ions even though they cannot be reabsorbed directly across the tubular membrane. Approximately 80% of the filtered bicarbonate is reabsorbed from the proximal tubule.

Tubular Buffers. The number of hydrogen ions secreted into the tubular lumen is greater than the number of bicarbonate ions being filtered. This leaves an excess of hydrogen ions in the tubular fluid. Because there are limits on how far the tubular fluid pH may fall, only a small portion of the daily hydrogen ion production would be excreted in the urine if it were not for the presence of the tubular buffering systems. One method of removing a free hydrogen ion from the tubular fluid is to combine it with a weak acid. The two primary tubular buffers, phosphate and ammonia, combine with free hydrogen ions, allowing excretion of large amounts of hydrogen ion while minimizing the fall in urine pH.

Acid phosphates (H_3PO_4), by-products of cellular metabolism, are buffered by bicarbonate in the extracellular fluid as illustrated below:

$$(2\ NaHCO_3) + (H_3PO_4) \rightarrow Na_2HPO_4 + 2\ CO_2 + 2\ H_2O$$

This process produces two carbon dioxide molecules and Na_2HPO_4, which is then filtered. The concentration of Na_2HPO_4 in the tubular fluid increases because the tubular membrane is relatively impermeable to it. It remains in the tubular lumen as water is reabsorbed. Within the tubule Na_2HPO_4 combines with hydrogen ion in the following reaction:

$$Na_2HPO_4 + H^+ \rightarrow NaH_2PO_4 + Na^+$$

In this way, a free hydrogen ion is picked up to be excreted and a sodium ion is returned to the extracellular fluid (Fig. 39–15).

The other major tubular buffer is the ammonia buffer system. Ammonia (NH_3) is formed within the tubular cells of all portions of the tubules except the thin segment of the loop of Henle. It is produced by the metabolism of amino acids, particularly glutamine. Ammonia diffuses easily into the tubular lumen, where it combines with a free hydrogen ion to form ammonium (NH_4^+) (Fig. 39–16). Because the tubular membrane is much less permeable to ammonium than to ammonia, ammonium ion is trapped within the tubular lumen. Ammonium then combines with chloride or another negative ion and is excreted.

Renal Response to Acid-Base Imbalance. When acids and bases are in balance in the body, the ratio of the amount of hydrogen ion to the amount of bicarbonate remains constant. In a state of acidosis

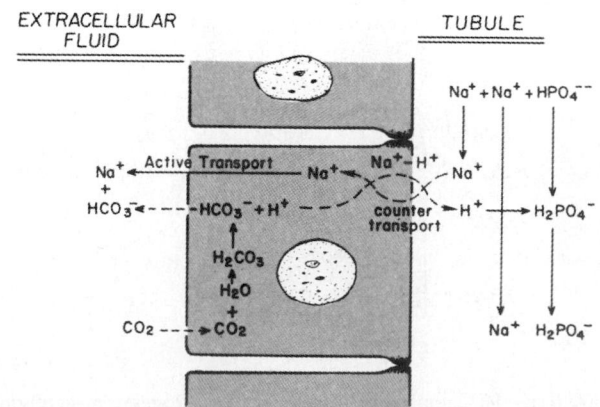

FIGURE 39–15. Chemical reactions in the tubules involving hydrogen ions, bicarbonate ions, sodium ions, and the phosphate buffer system. (From Guyton, A. C. (1991). *Textbook of medical physiology* (8th ed., p. 446). Philadelphia: W. B. Saunders).

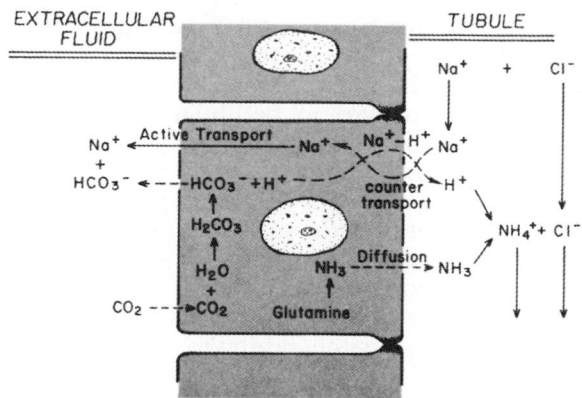

FIGURE 39—16. Secretion of ammonia by the tubular epithelial cells and reaction of the ammonia with hydrogen ions in the tubules. (From Guyton, A. C. (1991). *Textbook of medical physiology* (8th ed., p. 447). Philadelphia: W. B. Saunders).

hydrogen ion is increased in proportion to bicarbonate. In response to acidosis, the kidneys increase their secretion of hydrogen ion. Increased hydrogen ion secretion by the tubules helps to restore acid-base balance by (1) ensuring reabsorption of all filtered bicarbonate ions, (2) adding large amounts of bicarbonate to the blood via the process of bicarbonate regeneration, and (3) increasing excretion of hydrogen ion.

In a state of alkalosis, the ratio of bicarbonate to hydrogen ion increases. The kidney responds to alkalosis by decreasing hydrogen ion secretion. As a result, insufficient hydrogen ions are available to combine with filtered bicarbonate for reabsorption. Bicarbonate is lost into the urine, and the proportion of bicarbonate to hydrogen ion is brought back into range.

Clinical Problems Resulting in Altered Renal Handling of Hydrogen and Bicarbonate Ions. The normal renal processes for maintenance of acid-base balance may be impaired by either a defect in the tubular epithelial cells or by some other factor that impairs their ability to conserve bicarbonate and secrete hydrogen ion. Both metabolic acidosis and alkalosis may be the result of alterations in renal handling of hydrogen or bicarbonate ions. Examples of conditions leading to metabolic acidosis include proximal and distal renal tubular acidosis, renal failure, and carbonic anhydrase inhibition. Conditions known to cause metabolic alkalosis include administration of most diuretics and hyper-reninemic hyperaldosteronemia.

Proximal renal tubular acidosis is a defect of the epithelial cells that impairs bicarbonate recovery from the tubular fluid. The problem may be a defect in the carrier protein located on the luminal surface of the epithelial cell that transports sodium and hydrogen ion. It may also be caused by impaired carbonic anhydrase supply or function. In either case, bicarbonate cannot be reabsorbed and is lost in the urine. Because 80% of bicarbonate reabsorption normally occurs in the proximal tubule, this loss of bicarbonate eventually leads to acidosis. In addition, serum chloride levels rise as chloride is reabsorbed with sodium instead of bicarbonate.

In distal renal tubular acidosis the deficit is an inability to move hydrogen ion into the tubular lumen against its concentration gradient. This prevents net excretion of hydrogen ion as well as reabsorption of the small amount of bicarbonate that enters the distal tubule. Both of these factors contribute to the development of acidosis. Hypokalemia is also associated with distal renal tubular acidosis as increased amounts of potassium are secreted by the distal tubule to maintain electroneutrality in the face of decreased hydrogen ion secretion.

Metabolic acidosis is often a component of renal failure. The major defect in renal failure is an inability to produce adequate amounts of ammonia. Without ammonia available as a buffer, the amount of hydrogen ion that can be secreted is significantly reduced. The decreased GFR associated with renal failure also contributes to acidosis because a smaller amount of fixed acids can be filtered and excreted.

The administration of carbonic anhydrase inhibitors is another clinical situation that may promote the development of metabolic acidosis. Acetazolamide is a commonly used carbonic anhydrase inhibitor. This drug inhibits carbonic anhydrase on the luminal surface of the epithelial cells in the proximal tubule. As a result, carbonic acid formed in the tubular lumen cannot dissociate into carbon dioxide and water, and the indirect mechanism for the reabsorption of filtered bicarbonate cannot occur.

Administration of diuretics may lead to the onset of metabolic alkalosis. Osmotic, thiazide, and loop diuretics all promote increased flow of fluid and decreased sodium reabsorption. Consequently, the sodium load arriving at the distal tubule is greatly increased. As the distal tubule attempts to reabsorb this large amount of positive sodium ions, hydrogen ion is secreted into the tubules in large amounts to maintain electroneutrality. This increase in hydrogen ion loss eventually leads to metabolic alkalosis.

Alkalosis may also result from conditions that cause increased renin secretion such as renal artery stenosis. Renin initiates a series of reactions that culminate in angiotensin II formation. Angiotensin II then triggers secretion of aldosterone, which directly stimulates the distal tubule and collecting duct to secrete increased amounts of hydrogen ion (Vander, 1985).

Hormonal Function of the Kidney

Though it is not considered an endocrine organ, the kidney does participate in the formation of erythropoietin and in the metabolism of vitamin D, two systemic hormones. Although these functions are not necessary for survival, the kidney is essentially the only place in the body where they occur. Loss of these hormone functions may lead to significant problems for the individual.

Erythropoietin is believed to be produced by the epithelial cells of the proximal tubule and endothelial cells of the peritubular capillaries. Up to 90% of the erythropoietin produced in the body is contributed by the kidney. The stimulus for erythropoietin production and release is tissue hypoxia. Erythropoietin acts on the bone marrow to accelerate the production and release of red blood cells. Maximal erythropoietin production can increase red blood cell production up to 50 times the normal rate (Guyton, 1991). When erythropoietin production is diminished, few red blood cells are formed. Erythropoietin deficiency is one of the principal causes of the anemia seen in renal failure.

The kidney performs an important step in the formation of an active metabolite of vitamin D. It is this active metabolite that acts as a hormone within the body. Under normal circumstances, humans have two sources of inactive vitamin D: vitamin D_3, which is formed by the skin following exposure to ultraviolet light, and vitamin D_2, which is absorbed from ingested food. Both forms have identical biologic activity and are known together as vitamin D. Both forms of the vitamin are stored in the liver, where the initial conversion to 25-hydroxycholecalciferol (25-OHD_3) takes place. This substance is then converted by the mitochondria of the proximal tubular cells to 1,25-dihydroxycholecalciferol (1,25-$(OH)_2D_3$), known as calcitriol. Calcitriol is the active metabolite of vitamin D. Calcitriol stimulates calcium and phosphorus absorption from the gastrointestinal tract and is of critical importance to mineralization of newly formed bone. Individuals whose kidneys are unable to participate in vitamin D metabolism are at risk for hypocalcemia, secondary hyperparathyroidism, and osteomalacia.

SUMMARY

This chapter reviews the anatomic structure and major physiologic functions of the kidney as well as the close relationship between structure and function in this organ. The kidney's primary function is to maintain stability in the composition and volume of the extracellular fluid. This is accomplished through complex processes that culminate in the formation of urine. Each step—glomerular filtration, tubular reabsorption and secretion, concentration and dilution of the tubular fluid, and regulation of acids and bases—plays an important and necessary role in forming urine. The resulting urine is a fluid that eliminates precise amounts of water, waste, and excess electrolytes. Loss of the ability to form urine, which is responsive to changes in bodily needs, is usually incompatible with life. Replacement of this function by dialysis or renal transplantation is necessary for survival. The kidney is also the primary site of erythropoietin production and the final step in vitamin D metabolism. Although these two functions are not necessary for survival, they are required for maintenance of well-being. Integration of these complex functions allows the kidney to play a significant role in maintaining a relatively constant extracellular environment in which cells throughout the body can function normally.

References

Ballerman, B. J., Levenson, D. J., and Brenner, B. M. (1986). Renin, angiotensin, kinins, prostaglandins, and leukotrienes. In B. M. Brenner and F. C. Rector (Eds.), *The kidney* (3rd ed., pp. 281–340). Philadelphia: W. B. Saunders.

Brenner, B. M., Zatz, R., and Ichikawa, I. (1986). The renal circulations. In B. M. Brenner and F. C. Rector (Eds.), *The kidney* (3rd ed. pp. 93–123). Philadelphia: W. B. Saunders.

Carretero, O. A., and Scicli, A. G. (1989). Kallikrein-kinin system. In S. G. Massry, and R. J. Glassock (Eds.), *Textbook of nephrology* (2nd ed., pp. 185–191). Baltimore: Williams & Wilkins.

Cogan, M. G., and Rector, F. C. (1986). Acid-base disorders. In B. M. Brenner and F. C. Rector (Eds.), *The kidney* (3rd ed., pp. 457–517). Philadelphia: W. B. Saunders.

Duling, B. R. (1988). The kidney. In R. M. Berne and M. N. Levy (Eds.), *Physiology*. St. Louis: C. V. Mosby.

Garella, S., and Matarese, R. A. (1989). Renal effects of prostaglandins and clinical adverse effects of nonsteroidal anti-inflammatory agents. *Medicine*, 63(3): 165–181.

Guyton, A. C. (1991). *Textbook of medical physiology* (8th ed.). Philadelphia: W. B. Saunders.

Ingelfinger, J. R., Pratt, R. E., and Dzau, V. J. (1989), Renin-angiotensin system. In S. G. Massry, and R. J. Glassock. (Eds.), *Textbook of nephrology* (2nd ed., pp. 180–185). Baltimore: Williams & Wilkins.

Navar, L. G., Carmines, P. K., and Paul, R. V. (1989). Renal circulation. In S. G. Massry, and R. J. Glassock (Eds.), *Textbook of nephrology* (2nd ed., pp. 43–53). Baltimore: Williams & Wilkins.

Pelayo, J. C., and Quan, A. H. (1989). Neurogenic control of renal function. In S. G. Massry, and R. J. Glassock (Eds.), *Textbook of nephrology* (2nd ed., pp. 65–69). Baltimore: Williams & Wilkins.

Tisher, C. C., and Madsen, K. M. (1986). Anatomy of the kidney. In B. M. Brenner, and F. C. Rector (Eds.), *The kidney* (3rd ed., pp. 3–60). Philadelphia: W. B. Saunders.

Vander, A. J. (1985). *Real physiology* (3rd ed.). New York: McGraw-Hill.

Williams, P. L., Warwick, R., Dyson, M., et al. (1989). *Gray's anatomy* (37th ed.). London: Churchill Livingstone.

Zamboni, L. (1989). Anatomy of the kidney, bladder and urethra. Part I. Morphology and embryology. In S. G. Massry, and R. J. Glassock (Eds.), *Textbook of nephrology* (2nd ed., pp. 3–28). Baltimore: Williams & Wilkins.

40

Patients with Fluid and Electrolyte Disturbances

Marcia L. Keen

The kidney provides a myriad of important functions necessary for the maintenance of the body's internal environment. Among these functions is regulation of the physicochemical milieu, which supports cellular processes. This chapter deals with problems of fluid volume and composition associated with disease states or trauma frequently seen in the critical care setting. For a detailed discussion of renal regulation of electrolytes, the reader is referred to Chapter 39.

BODY FLUID COMPARTMENTS

Approximately 55% to 60% of the body is composed of water. This solution is crucial to the maintenance of life because essential solutes are dissolved or suspended in this medium. The total body water (TBW) is distributed in several discrete compartments or volumes. The intracellular (IC) fluid volume is the largest compartment, comprising 67% of TBW. IC fluid accounts for approximately 40% of body weight. The extracellular (EC) fluid volume is composed of several small compartments, including interstitial fluid (IS) and plasma volume (PV). The vascular volume also contains erythrocytes, which contain a portion of the IC fluid volume. The combined EC fluid makes up approximately 20% of body weight. The smallest compartment is the transcellular volume, which consists of fluid found in the peritoneum and pleural cavities, gastrointestinal tract, joints, and cerebrospinal fluid. The body water compartments and proportional sizes are shown in Table 40–1. Adult males tend to have a TBW of approximately 60% because of a somewhat larger proportion of muscle mass. Adipose tissue contains less water.

Thus, the average adult female has a TBW equal to about 50% of body weight, reflecting the gender predisposition to increased body fat. Infants and children up to the age of puberty also have higher values for TBW.

Intracellular water is separated from EC fluid by cell membranes. The plasma volume is confined to the vascular space by capillary membranes. These membranes selectively permit passage of solutes between compartments through a variety of active and passive mechanisms. The cell membranes are freely permeable to water. Thus, body water is distributed in the various anatomic compartments to achieve osmotic equilibrium throughout the total body water.

The cation and anion composition of the respective compartments is shown in Figure 40–1. Sodium salts are the primary osmotically active constituent of the EC fluid. The concentration of sodium in the interstitial subcompartment of EC fluid will be somewhat lower than the plasma concentration due to the effect of the Donnan equilibrium (Guyton, 1991). Since plasma proteins are negatively charged ions, a larger

TABLE 40–1. Body Compartment Volumes

Plasma volume (liters)	= 4.5% body weight (kg)
Interstitial fluid volume (liters)	= 13% body weight (kg)
Extracellular fluid volume (liters)	= 17.5% body weight (kg)
Intracellular fluid volume (liters)	= 33% body weight (kg)

Total body water (TBW) (liters)
Males, thin females, chronically ill patients—normal hydration:
  TBW = 55% to 60% body weight (kg)
Obese patients, normal females—normal hydration:
  TBW = 47% to 52% body weight (kg)

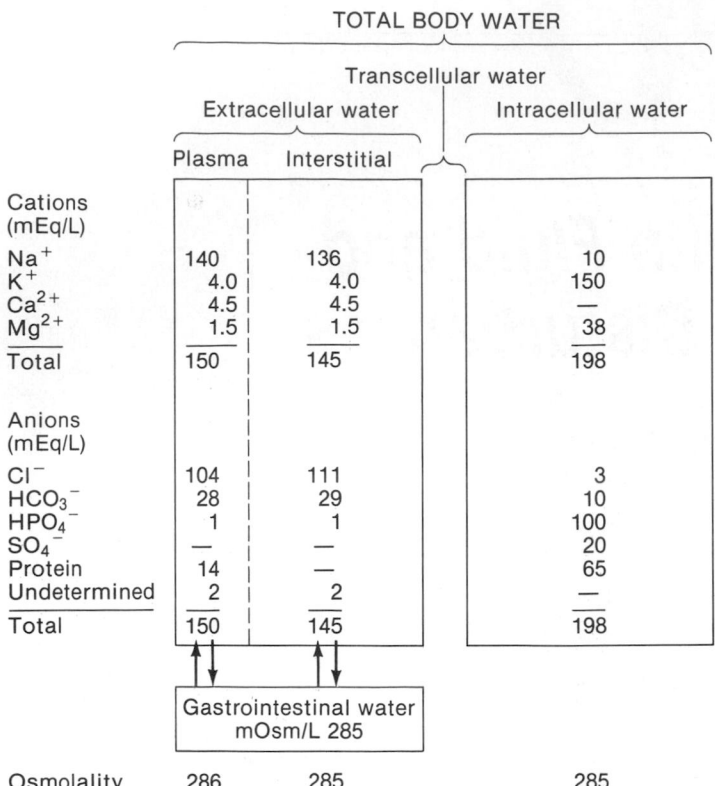

FIGURE 40–1. Body water composition.

TOTAL BODY WATER

Transcellular water

Extracellular water | Intracellular water

Plasma   Interstitial

	Plasma	Interstitial		Intracellular
Cations (mEq/L)				
Na^+	140	136		10
K^+	4.0	4.0		150
Ca^{2+}	4.5	4.5		—
Mg^{2+}	1.5	1.5		38
Total	150	145		198
Anions (mEq/L)				
Cl^-	104	111		3
HCO_3^-	28	29		10
HPO_4^-	1	1		100
SO_4^-	—	—		20
Protein	14	—		65
Undetermined	2	2		—
Total	150	145		198

Gastrointestinal water
mOsm/L 285

Osmolality	286	285	285

number of positively charged ions are required to achieve electrochemical balance. Concentrations of sodium (Na) and chloride (Cl) may differ in these two subcompartments because of the associated difference in protein concentrations.

The major electrolyte of the IC fluid is potassium (K). K is actively retained within the compartment by energy-consuming Na-K pumps found in the cell walls. These pumps remove Na from cells in exchange for K from the EC fluid. In this way, Na remains in EC fluid while K is confined to IC fluid. Other low-molecular-weight solutes (such as urea and glucose) can be considered freely diffusible between IC fluid and EC fluid. Other electrolytes, such as magnesium, are also osmotically active but exert a much smaller effective osmotic pressure in both the IC and EC compartments.

As described in Chapter 39, the normal physiologic regulation of water and sodium metabolism is primarily directed toward the preservation of three separate but related parameters of body water: (1) osmolality of total body water; (2) extracellular water volume; and (3) intracellular water volume. An integrated neuro-endocrine-renal system responds to significant alterations in volume or osmolality with the intent of restoring composition and volume toward normal.

Exchange of Water Between Plasma and Interstitial Volumes

Water exchange between the plasma (PV) and interstitial (IS) volumes is dependent on three important pressure relationships. One is the hydraulic or hydrostatic pressure in the capillary. This pressure gradient normally tends to move water out of the capillary into the interstitial space. Opposing that outward flow of water is the capillary oncotic pressure exerted by plasma proteins. About 65% to 70% of this plasma protein oncotic pressure in plasma is due to albumin, with the rest provided by globulins (Guyton, 1991). The third pressure results from a slow albumin leak in the capillary wall, which accounts for a low concentration of protein in the IS fluid. The protein in the IS fluid exerts an oncotic pressure, which tends to pull water into the interstitial compartment. Under normal conditions of hydration, the net result is that most of the fluid leaving the PV at the afferent end of the capillary is reabsorbed. However, there is a net filtration pressure that allows a small amount of fluid and solutes to remain in the IS fluid. This small volume eventually is returned to the circulation through the lymphatic system.

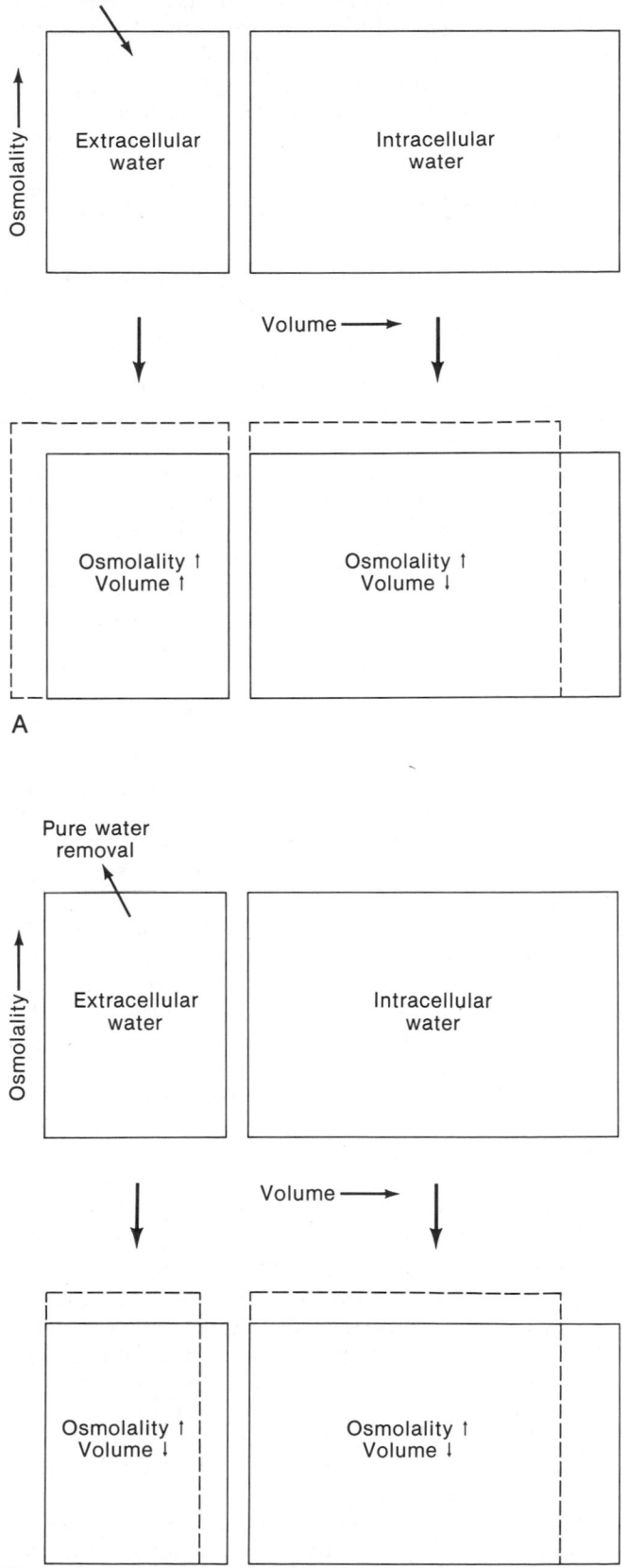

FIGURE 40-2. *A*, Effect of sodium addition on compartment osmolality and volumes. *B*, Effect of pure water removal on compartment osmolality and volumes.

Effective Arterial Volume

The mechanisms controlling the circulation and its regulation have been comprehensively discussed in previous chapters. The theoretical concept of effective arterial volume (EAV) associated with circulation and tissue perfusion has important implications for fluid and electrolyte control in health and illness. The EAV is essentially the degree of fullness of the arterial vascular tree relative to its capacity. This volume is a balance between peripheral resistance and cardiac output. Normally, if cardiac output falls, there is a compensatory increase in peripheral resistance. However, there may be situations in which the arterial vascular capacity is abnormally increased such that cardiac output cannot compensate completely. In this situation, EAV will decrease, and there will be renal conservation of sodium and water to augment volume. Major effectors for controlling EAV include the sympathetic nervous system as well as the renin-angiotensin II response.

The regulation of Na is closely associated with maintenance of the EAV. In general, EAV varies as the extracellular volume varies, and both of these volumes vary with total body sodium. In some instances, EAV may not reflect extracellular volume or, more specifically, plasma volume. Pathologic sequestration of extracellular water in the interstitium because of decreased plasma oncotic pressure will produce an expanded interstitial volume but a depleted plasma volume. If cardiac output falls, EAV will be decreased. The kidney will attempt to alleviate this situation by conserving Na. Water will also be retained but may be sequestered in the already expanded interstitial space. This situation produces a decreased EAV and plasma volume but a greatly expanded interstitial volume and extracellular volume.

Cation-Anion Balance

As illustrated in Figure 40-1, the sum of the plasma cations (150 mEq/liter) is balanced by the sum of the plasma anions (150 mEq/liter). Electroneutrality of the plasma is always maintained. Under normal circumstances, any increase or decrease in cation concentration will result in a similar increase or decrease in anion concentration.

Sodium and potassium are the major measured plasma cations, and chloride is the major measured anion. The other major plasma anion is bicarbonate, which can be estimated as $CO_2 - 1$ (Goldberger, 1986). The remainder of anions are phosphates, sulfates, proteins, and organic acid ions. These anions are not measured but may have clinical significance in certain disease states.

Anion Gap. Measurement of the anion gap is a simple method of describing the concentration of unmeasured plasma anions. In calculating the anion gap, the sum of the measured anions is subtracted from the sum of the measured cations:

$$\text{Anion gap} = (Na + K) - (HCO_3 + Cl)$$

The resulting "gap" represents the unmeasured anions present in the plasma. Normally, the anion gap is 8 to 16 mEq/liter.

As described in Table 40–2, the anion gap may be increased or decreased in disease states that alter the unmeasured anions or unmeasured cations. Fluid volume disorders will also affect the anion gap by elevating or lowering plasma Na. Metabolic acidosis is the most common cause of an increased anion gap in critically ill patients. The most frequent cause of decreased anion gap is hypoalbuminemia.

Calculation of the anion gap is clinically useful in differentiating between possible etiologies of metabolic acidosis. For example, the anion gap in patients with diabetic ketoacidosis is frequently greater than 22 mEq/liter. On the other hand, patients with metabolic acidosis resulting from excessive intestinal fluid losses will have a near normal anion gap.

FLUID VOLUME AND OSMOLALITY

Distribution of body water follows osmotic pressure relationships within the EC and IC compartments. The terms osmolality and osmolarity often are used interchangeably although they are different. Osmolality is expressed as the number of osmoles per *kilogram* (kg) of *water*, whereas osmolarity refers to the number of osmoles per *liter* of *solution*. With dilute solutions, such as EC or IC fluids, the difference is negligible, and osmolality is the more common term employed. Extracellular volume is determined by the total number of osmoles in the extracellular compartment. Therefore, extracellular volume regulation is accomplished through the regulation of extracellular osmoles. The intracellular volume generally is not manipulated directly but will

change as a consequence of alterations in extracellular volume and osmolality. Because extracellular osmolality is equal to intracellular osmolality, the respective volumes will be dictated by the requirements of osmotic equilibrium. In a state of fluid and solute balance:

Osmolality TBW = osmolality EC fluid = osmolality IC fluid

Tonicity refers to the osmolality of a solution relative to another. If one solution has a higher osmolality than another, it is described as being hypertonic relative to the second solution. Solutions of the same osmolality are isotonic. A solution with a lower osmolality than a second solution is described as hypotonic.

Since Na^+ and K^+ salts are the major osmotically active solutes anatomically confined to the EC fluid and IC fluid, respectively, they are the only solutes that exert an osmotic effect in each compartment. The passive movement of water across cell membranes by osmosis dictates that the osmolar concentration of Na in EC fluid must be equal to the osmolar concentration of K in IC fluid in order to maintain osmotic equilibrium.

If sodium is added to extracellular water, water will flow from the intracellular to the extracellular compartment to regain osmotic equilibrium between them, as shown in Figure 40–2A. The outcome will be that osmolality will be increased in both compartments, with the extracellular volume expanded at the cost of a reduced intracellular volume. On the other hand, if pure water is removed from the extracellular compartment, the loss will be proportionally distributed between the two compartments. The result will be an increase in osmolality and a decrease in volume in both compartments as shown in Figure 40–2B.

Sodium salts are the primary osmoles in extracellular water, and therefore regulation of the extracellular volume involves regulation of Na retention or excretion by the kidney. The principle is that if Na is retained or excreted, water will follow. Normally, EC volume is controlled through maintenance of the balance of Na intake and renal excretion.

This discussion of volume regulation emphasizes the principle premise of EC volume and osmolality regulation: EC volume is managed through the renal regulation of Na salts, whereas EC osmolality is regulated through thirst and renal handling of water. These two regulatory processes are closely associated, so that changes in one parameter may affect changes in the other.

The afferent and efferent mechanisms of renal Na excretion as well as their respective actions are shown in Table 40–3. No single afferent mechanism dominates this regulatory process. It is worth repeating that the body will protect volume at the expense of osmolality.

TABLE 40–2. Mechanisms Affecting the Anion Gap

Increased Anion Gap (>16 mEq/liter)	Decreased Anion Gap (<8 mEq/liter)
Increased unmeasured anion	Decreased unmeasured anion
Lactic acidosis	Hypoalbuminemia
Ketoacidosis	
Hyperosmolar coma	
Na penicillin	
Phosphate administration	
Sulfate administration	
Decreased unmeasured cation	Increased unmeasured cation
Hypocalcemia	Hypercalcemia
Hypomagnesemia	Hypermagnesemia
	IgG (multiple myeloma)
Water loss	Water excess
Hypernatremia	Hyponatremia
Metabolic alkalosis	

TABLE 40–3. Regulation of Renal Sodium Excretion

Mechanism	Action
Afferent	
Baroreceptors	Modifies peripheral and renal
Aorta and carotid sinus	vascular resistance
Juxtaglomerular apparatus	Produces renin/angiotensin II
	Direct renal effect
	Aldosterone
	Na transport in kidney
Low pressure volume receptors	Prostaglandin production
	ADH secretion
Atrial natriuretic peptide	Vasodilation
	Natriuresis and diuresis
	Reduces plasma renin,
	aldosterone, ADH
	concentrations
Efferent	
Kidney	
Proximal tubule	Regulates Na excretion/
Loop of Henle	conservation
Collecting tubule	
Prostaglandins	Renal hemodynamics
	Na excretion/conservation

Volume Disorders

Volume disorders tend to be classified as either depletion (contraction) or expansion derangements. This refers to both EC and IC compartments, although direct measurement of these states is restricted to the EC compartment, specifically the vascular volume.

VOLUME DEPLETION

Volume depletion is a relatively common disturbance in critically ill patients, occurring when fluid losses exceed intake. The fluid loss must occur acutely and must be of significant magnitude to produce volume depletion. Otherwise, the normal mechanisms for conservation of volume would compensate for the decreased TBW. If left uncorrected, hypovolemia can lead to a variety of serious secondary effects such as shock, myocardial ischemia, acute tubular necrosis, and, depending upon the composition of the fluid lost, electrolyte disorders and acid-base disturbances. The severity of symptomatic volume depletion reflects the proportion of volume lost from the EC compartment. An isotonic volume loss of 10% of body weight is considered serious, whereas a loss of 15% may be lethal.

The composition of the fluid lost will have a significant effect on TBW composition after volume depletion. A categorical approach to volume depletion is shown in Table 40–4, and the designation reflects the osmolality of the TBW following acute depletion. The losses come directly from the EC fluid. However, as discussed earlier, compartment volumes are dictated by osmotic equilibrium requirements, so that there may well be a secondary effect on IC volume. These categories and their effects on com-

partment volumes and osmolality are shown in Figure 40–3. All disorders will be associated with some depletion of EC volume and thus hypovolemia. However, laboratory and clinical findings associated with each of these volume disturbances will vary. The variability of the composition of these fluids can produce a spectrum of metabolic disturbances when fluid is lost from the body in excessive amounts. Gastrointestinal losses, depending on their origin and composition, may also induce acid-base disturbances. Vomiting and diarrhea will be associated with significant acid loss, with metabolic alkalosis as a possible consequence. Conversely, intestinal, biliary, and pancreatic fluids are alkaline, and large losses of these fluids may be associated with metabolic acidosis. With severe volume depletion, the kidney will conserve $NaHCO_3$ even though acid-base status is normal because of the need for Na and thus volume. As a result, a contraction alkalosis may be present. Chloride and potassium disorders can also occur in conjunction with volume depletion.

The laboratory findings common to extracellular volume contraction states are shown in Table 40–4.

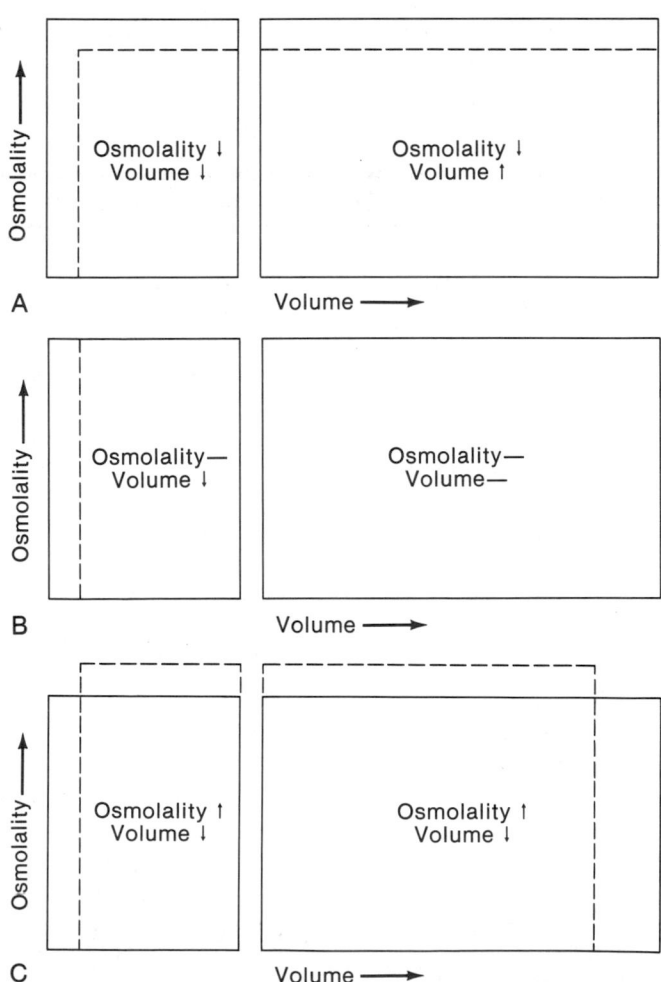

FIGURE 40–3. Osmolality and volume changes in depletion status. *A*, Hypotonic contraction. *B*, Isotonic contraction. *C*, Hypertonic contraction.

Urinary Na values reflect the appropriate renal response to volume contraction states. Under the influence of aldosterone, the renal tubules reabsorb Na in response to volume contraction, thereby decreasing the amount of Na lost in the urine. Water is also reabsorbed, which increases the osmolality of the urine. Some urinary Na values may be misleading in that inappropriate renal Na excretion is seen in patients with salt-wasting renal disease, osmotic diuresis, and following diuretic administration. All these disorders force Na excretion. In renal failure, urinary osmolality (uOsm) may be less than 350 mOsm/kg because of the renal concentrating defect associated with renal disease (Valtin, 1987).

Normal blood urea nitrogen (BUN) and creatinine ratios should be approximately 10:1. This value may be elevated in hypovolemia because of decreased glomerular filtration.

Plasma sodium (PNa) will be variably affected depending on the type of volume depletion. In iso-osmotic losses, PNa will probably be unchanged. However, volume depletion will stimulate thirst and ADH secretion, so that dilutional hyponatremia may be observed with isotonic contraction. Hypo-osmotic contraction, when solute loss exceeds water loss, will generally exhibit a decreased PNa. In hyperosmotic contraction, water is lost in excess of solute and thus may be reflected in hypernatremia.

Potassium may be increased or decreased depending on the etiology of volume loss. Acidosis is associated with increased serum K concentrations due to electroneutrality requirements as hydrogen ion (H^+) moves from the EC into the IC compartment.

Plasma protein and hematocrit values are frequently elevated when hypovolemia is present, reflecting hemoconcentration. These laboratory findings should be evaluated relative to baseline values.

Management of Volume Depletion. Both the volume and composition of replacement solutions will depend on the composition and estimated volume deficit. For replacement of a pure water deficit of a hyperosmotic contraction without significant solute loss, fluid replacement can be estimated as follows:

$$\text{Amount of water required (liters)} = \text{weight loss (kg)}$$

Fluid replacement can be given as 5% dextrose in water if only free water is desired, or isotonically if serum Na is normal (Carroll and Oh, 1989).

For many critically ill patients, both water and sodium are needed to correct volume depletion. For hypo-osmotic contraction, isotonic or hypertonic saline solutions are used. The solution chosen depends on the degree of Na deficit and on volume considerations. Normal saline (0.9%) contains approxi-

TABLE 40–4. Categorization and Laboratory Values in Extracellular Volume Depletion

| | Laboratory Values | | | | | |
| | Urine | | Blood | | | |
Etiology	Sodium	Osmolality	Sodium	BUN/Creatinine Ratio	Plasma Protein	Hematocrit
Iso-osmotic Solute and water lost in equal proportion Gastrointestinal losses Hemorrhage Third spacing Burns	Decreased	Increased	Unchanged	Increased	Increased	Increased
Hypo-osmotic Solute loss greater than water loss Aldosterone deficiency Diuretic therapy with water replacement Increased insensible loss with water replacement Salt-wasting renal disease Osmotic diuresis	Increased	Decreased	Decreased	Increased	Increased	Increased
Hyper-osmotic Water loss greater than solute loss No water or access to water Increased insensible loss with no replacement Untreated diabetes insipidus	Increased	Increased	Increased	Increased	Increased	Increased

mately 155 mEq/liter of sodium, whereas hypertonic saline contains approximately 515 mEq/liter. The amount of sodium replacement needed can be estimated by the following formula:

$$Na \text{ required (mEq)} = [(\text{normal PNa} - \text{current PNa}) \times \text{TBW (liters)}] + [(\text{normal PNa}) \times \text{weight loss (liters)}]$$

The amount of water replacement in liters is equal to the weight loss in kilograms.

Depending upon the value obtained from this equation, the clinician could prescribe an isotonic solution if renal function is adequate and no significant heart disease is present, or a mix of isotonic and hypertonic solutions. It is also important to consider potassium stores as well as acid-base status when choosing the appropriate solutions for restoring volume.

The rate of fluid replacement will be a function of the current or continuing deficit and the type of solution being used. The risk of volume overload from rapid administration of isotonic or hypertonic solutions must be minimized. Rapid addition of Na to EC fluid can produce a rapid influx of water into the vascular space, overwhelming marginal cardiac function in the critically ill patient.

Fluid Volume Deficit. Extracellular fluid volume depletion or contraction is frequently seen in critically ill patients. The goals of nursing care are to identify any fluid volume deficit and restore and support the patient's fluid balance.

Clinical manifestations of EC volume depletion may vary depending upon the type of volume contraction present. Therefore, it is important for the critical care nurse to carefully assess all aspects of the patient's fluid volume status. Patients with significant volume depletion frequently complain of thirst and dry mouth. Unfortunately, the intubated or comatose patient loses this ability, so early volume depletion may go unnoticed. Reduced skin turgor has long been purported to be a hallmark of volume depletion. However, normal skin turgor does not rule out a hypovolemic state. In fact, changes in skin turgor may not appear until late in the volume depletion process. Assessments of the patient's tongue and mucous membranes provide a more reliable indication of the volume status (Metheny, 1987).

Urine output is a sensitive indicator of fluid volume status. Hourly urine volumes are measured, and downward trends are noted and reported. Bedside serial specific gravity measurements may be indicative of the increasing urinary concentration seen in hypovolemia. Accurate daily weights provide the most valuable estimate of TBW loss. Weight loss, as determined by daily weights, is utilized by the physician in calculating fluid replacement (Whittaker, 1985).

Hemodynamic parameters provide objective measures of volume depletion. Documentation of hypotension should always be considered relative to base-line blood pressure reference values. Tachycardia is frequently present. Postural hypotension may be observed along with dizziness or syncope on assuming a sitting or erect position.

Central venous pressure (CVP) can be a useful parameter in the assessment of volume status, even without sophisticated monitoring technology. Visual inspection of the external jugular vein just above the clavicle with the patient supine and the neck muscles relaxed can provide useful information. If the external jugular is flat when the patient is supine, the patient is volume depleted. If the fluid wave can be seen in the external jugular vein when the patient is upright, the CVP is approximately 10 cm of water. Assessment of the CVP and jugular distention is valid in the absence of right or left heart failure. Left ventricular filling pressures, as measured by pulmonary capillary wedge pressure, and cardiac output will fall below baseline in patients with hypovolemia.

Although notoriously inaccurate, intake and output records may provide a useful estimate of the balance between fluid lost and fluid gained. The nurse carefully monitors the patient's intake and output for trends indicative of excessive fluid loss or inadequate fluid replacement.

If the patient is at risk of volume depletion, the nurse ensures the availability of intravenous lines. Prescribed infusions are carefully monitored, and the patient's response is closely observed and evaluated.

VOLUME EXPANSION

The kidney normally responds to an increase in Na intake by a compensatory increase in renal Na excretion. This process blunts the change in extracellular volume that might be associated with the

TABLE 40–5. Extracellular Volume Expansion

Primary Renal Salt Retention

Cause	Abnormal kidney function
Features	Extracellular and effective arterial volume increased
Associated findings	Hypertension
	Reduced sympathetic nervous system activity
	Decreased levels of renin, ADH, aldosterone

Secondary Renal Salt Retention

Cause	Kidney responds to decreased extracellular volume stimuli
Features	Extracellular volume increased
	Effective arterial volume decreased
Associated findings	Low blood pressure
	Increased sympathetic nervous system activity
	Increased levels of renin, ADH, aldosterone

increased Na intake. In some pathophysiologic states, this remarkable balance breaks down, with the immediate consequence of retention of ingested or infused Na and water. If uncorrected, the increase in vascular volume as well as an associated increase in capillary permeability to water leads to accumulation of fluid in the interstitial space and the formation of edema.

The fundamental problem in volume expansion states is that Na and water are not being excreted. There are two possible reasons why Na is retained. One is that abnormal kidney function may lead to inappropriately diminished Na excretion in the presence of increased Na intake. The other is that the kidney is responding appropriately to erroneous stimuli indicating that EC volume is contracted. This response is the mechanism that results in the Na and water retention observed in congestive heart failure. The classification and clinical features of extracellular volume expansion are described in Table 40–5.

The interstitial volume is about 75% of that in the EC compartment. As described earlier, movement of fluid into the interstitial space in the capillary bed is influenced by opposing capillary and oncotic pressures. Changes in the hydrostatic pressure before or after the capillary will influence the movement of fluid out of the capillary (Guyton, 1991). Precapillary constriction reduces hydrostatic pressure within the capillary and thus reduces water flux. In contrast, postcapillary vasoconstriction produces increased pressure within the capillary and thus increases water movement into the interstitial space. In hypoalbuminemic states, plasma oncotic pressure is decreased, which also favors movement of fluid out of the capillary. If capillary permeability to plasma protein is increased, migration of these proteins into the interstitium will also encourage water to move (Guyton, 1991).

In normal circumstances, once plasma fluid has entered the interstitial space it eventually returns to the vascular space through the lymphatic system. In clinical conditions in which lymph drainage is obstructed, the normal route of interstitial water return is lost. If lymph obstruction remains uncorrected, edema will result.

Edema may not be evident until interstitial volume is 30% greater than normal (Guyton, 1991). Obviously, if this process is localized, a smaller volume will produce demonstrable edema. Pitting edema is usually not seen until 3 to 4 liters have entered the interstitium from the plasma (Carroll and Oh, 1989). When a significant amount of fluid has left the vascular space, the plasma volume becomes decreased and the kidney begins to conserve Na and water to restore volume even though the total EC volume is expanded.

In summary, edema occurs through the three primary mechanisms described earlier: (1) increased hydrostatic pressure in the capillary. (2) decreased plasma oncotic pressure, and (3) lymph system obstruction. With the first two mechanisms, the vascular volume decreases and compensatory renal conservation of Na and water occurs. This renal maneuver attempts to restore the vascular volume to normal despite the accumulation of fluid in the interstitial space and the EC volume expands. This edema-producing mechanism is seen in disease states such as congestive heart failure, cirrhosis, and nephrotic syndrome.

Prostaglandins play a role in Na and water excretion and retention. Prostaglandins are fatty acid compounds whose production by the kidney depends on the availability of arachadonic acids and phospholipase. Prostaglandins are elevated in volume depletion states and decreased in volume expansion conditions, indicating a counter role in the primary processes of volume regulation. High levels of prostaglandins inhibit Na reabsorption in the kidney and thus counteract the direct effects of the renin-angiotensin II system in volume depletion.

Some drugs commonly used in the critical care environment, including peripheral vasodilators and some calcium channel blockers, also increase Na retention by the kidney. Nonsteroidal anti-inflammatory (NSAID) agents may encourage Na retention through their blocking action on prostaglandin synthesis. Estrogens and some synthetic mineralocorticoids also induce primary renal Na retention. The consequence of all these mechanisms of Na and water conservation is an expanded plasma volume and possible edema formation.

Physical findings associated with edema states generally reflect the underlying etiology of the disorder and thus the preferential location of edema formation.

Laboratory findings are not always specific to the underlying pathology. However, all these edema-forming disorders will be reflected in a decreased UNa, and, in some situations such as nephrotic syndrome, proteinuria may be pronounced. Primary renal Na retention may also produce proteinuria. Elevated blood urea nitrogen and serum creatinine values may be indicative of renal disease. Reduced serum protein values, specifically albumin, are seen in cirrhosis and nephrotic syndrome. Serum Na values are variable depending on the disorder and the degree of plasma volume expansion.

Management of Volume Expansion. Pulmonary edema is a life-threatening event and must be treated promptly. Other edematous states require remedial action but are not considered imminently lethal. In fact, in some situations a measured approach to volume correction will avoid secondary complications resulting from treatment.

The goal of treatment should be to resolve the underlying pathology and correct volume status to the degree consistent with adequate tissue perfusion. The objective is to mobilize the expanded interstitial fluid volume without causing a significant reduction in plasma volume, particularly in patients with edema states in which decreased EAV exists. Further reduction in this hemodynamic parameter may potentially decrease cardiac function and tissue perfusion, thereby preventing further volume correction. Diuretics are generally useful in the treatment of edema states. However, volume depletion caused by the overuse of diuretics may induce an increase in renin, aldosterone, and ADH production, all of which will act to conserve Na and water (Kaloyanides, 1980). An intravenous infusion of low-dose dopamine (<5 μg/kg) is frequently used to increase renal blood flow and enhance Na and water excretion.

Mobilization of interstitial fluid into the vascular volume occurs initially through the mechanism of decreased plasma volume through diuretic action, which decreases capillary hydrostatic pressure. The structure of the interstitial space is such that, normally, the pressure in that compartment is actually below zero. Therefore, there is a point beyond which interstitial fluid will not move, even if the volume is somewhat expanded. Patients with severe generalized edema may experience more rapid mobilization of fluid. Patients with hepatic disease and ascites will tend to have a slower rate of interstitial volume reduction because of the more localized deposition. Forced excretion of water through the use of diuretics may exceed the rate at which ascitic fluid can replace the plasma volume. In this situation, symptoms of volume depletion may be observed. These patients are also more prone to other electrolyte disorders when diuretics are used. To minimize this, an aldosterone-antagonist diuretic is generally utilized.

Sodium restriction, with or without concurrent administration of diuretics, is often applied successfully in edematous patients because it indirectly diminishes further water retention. In patients with chronic heart failure, the long-term use of diuretics combined with a low-sodium diet may prevent subsequent edema formation.

Fluid Volume Excess. A number of disease states may cause fluid volume expansion in critically ill patients. Nursing care is directed toward early recognition and prevention of fluid volume excess, monitoring, and evaluation of the patient's response to mobilization of fluid.

Nursing assessment of the patient with fluid volume overload includes identification of edema and the patient's response to changes in TBW. The patient's hemodynamic response to fluid volume overload is carefully monitored. Depending upon the underlying cause of volume overload, the patient's blood pressure may be elevated or decreased. If plasma volume is increased, the central venous pressure (CVP), and pulmonary capillary wedge pressure (PCWP) will be elevated. The jugular veins are assessed for distention.

The rate and quality of respirations are assessed. The presence of tachypnea may be indicative of evolving pulmonary edema. The lungs are auscultated for the presence of rales.

In performing a head-to-toe assessment, the nurse observes and documents the presence, location, and severity of peripheral edema. In patients at risk of sequestering fluid in the abdomen, abdominal girth is measured, and the presence or absence of a fluid wave is noted. Skin areas that may be gravitational sites for edema should be evaluated. In patients on bed best, edema collects along the flanks, lateral chest, lateral abdominal wall, lateral buttocks, and posteromedial thighs. It appears later in the presacral area.

The patient is weighed daily, and changes in body weight are noted and calculated in terms of liters of fluid retained. When fluid restriction is prescribed, the nurse educates the patient and family about the rationale for the restriction. The fluid allotment is appropriately distributed across the 24-hour period to facilitate patient comfort. Fluid administration is individualized to meet the patient's specific needs. Intake and output records assist the nurse to ration fluids appropriately.

The critical care nurse administers the prescribed diuretics and monitors the patient's response. The adequacy of diuresis is assessed. The nurse monitors the patient's serum electrolytes and anticipates the development of hypokalemia following diuretic administration.

Impaired Skin Integrity. Skin care is an important aspect of nursing care of the volume-overloaded patient. The skin in edematous areas is assessed frequently. Careful attention is paid to relieving pressure areas (Metheny, 1987).

Osmolality Disorders

Plasma osmolality (pOsm) is maintained within narrow limits (280 to 300 mOsm/liter) by body mechanisms that act to conserve or excrete water. This important physiologic parameter is regulated by several integrated neurohormonal-renal mechanisms. The vascular volume is monitored by osmoreceptors and, because it is a subcompartment of the EC volume, is a surrogate for EC osmolality. Changes in the osmolality of the EC compartment have implications for water shifts between the EC and IC compartments.

Thirst is an important mechanism in maintaining plasma osmolality. The thirst mechanism may be brought into play by nonosmotic factors such as hypovolemia (isotonic depletion) or decreased cardiac output. The body will defend volume at the expense of osmolality, which may lead to a situation in which activated drinking occurs in the presence of normal or reduced plasma osmolality. Angiotensin II is thought to be a potent dipsogen, and therefore, clinical events that increase renin production may also increase thirst (Arieff and Schmidt, 1980). To restore plasma osmolality, thirst must be accompanied by the ability of the individual to obtain water. Critically ill patients may lose either or both their ability to recognize the thirst sensation and their ability to obtain water.

ADH is a second mechanism involved in the regulation of pOsm. Its synthesis and release are stimulated when extracellular osmolality is increased. This response is marked even when the increase in osmolality is only a 1% to 2% deviation from baseline (Robertson et al., 1976). In addition to its effect on the renal collecting duct's permeability to water, ADH also plays a role in modulating peripheral vascular resistance and thus blood pressure. When extracellular fluid volume is lost, ADH and aldosterone secretion is increased regardless of the serum sodium concentration. These hormones encourage the conservation of Na and water. ADH release may also be stimulated by baroreceptor-perceived reduction in plasma volume as well as pain, stress, and drugs such as narcotics, nicotine, and tricyclic antidepressants. Factors stimulating or inhibiting ADH secretion are described in Table 40–6. Thus, as with thirst and drinking, these stimuli and the accompanying change in ADH secretion can cause a change in water excretion that is not indicated by osmolality alone. The action of ADH on the kidney results in the excretion of a small volume of concentrated urine. Enhanced aldosterone secretion results in renal conservation of available sodium. This provides an additional impetus for water conservation and thus volume repletion. Derangements in these important control mechanisms may produce serious perturbations in osmolality.

Osmolality of body water is closely correlated with serum sodium concentration because Na is the most abundant EC ion. Plasma osmolality can be reasonably estimated by the following formula:

$$\text{Plasma osmolality} = 2(\text{plasma Na}) + \text{BUN}/2.8 + \text{glucose}/18$$

where Na is mEq/liter, BUN is mg/dL, and glucose is mg/dL. Because Na is the major osmotically active ion, in the absence of hyperglycemia or renal insufficiency plasma osmolality can be reliably estimated using the following formula:

$$2(\text{Plasma Na[mEq/liter]})$$

It is helpful to utilize the calculated plasma osmolality to explain the effect of various disease states on osmolality. The following examples illustrate the normal calculated pOsm, hyperosmolality caused by hyperglycemia and hypernatremia, and hypo-osmolality caused by hyponatremia.

$$\text{Normal: } 2(140) + 12/2.8 + 100/18 = 290 \text{ mOsm/kg}$$

$$\text{Hyponatremia: } 2(130) + 12/2.8 + 100/18 = 270 \text{ mOsm/kg}$$

$$\text{Hyperglycemia: } 2(140) + 12/2.8 + 450/18 = 309 \text{ mOsm/kg}$$

$$\text{Hypernatremia: } 2(152) + 12/2.8 + 100/18 = 314 \text{ mOsm/kg}$$

The normal physiologic range for pOsm is 280 to 300 mOsm/kg H_2O. It should be noted that changes in the serum levels of urea and glucose do have an effect on the calculated pOsm. However, as demonstrated in the examples of calculated pOsm above, small changes in serum sodium concentration have the most significant effect on plasma osmolality. Further discussion of osmolality in this chapter will focus on problems with osmolality associated with hyponatremia or hypernatremia.

HYPONATREMIA

Hyponatremia or hypo-osmolality results from increased water loading or retention relative to plasma Na levels. The result is a decreased concentration of EC Na ions (<135 mEq/liter). The predominant change occurs in water content, not solute concentration. In this situation, thirst is inactivated, and inhibition of ADH occurs. The outcome of these responses is excretion of a large volume of dilute urine. In situations in which EC volume is severely compromised, the body will override these homeostatic functions in order to defend volume.

It has been suggested that hyponatremia is the most common electrolyte disorder seen in hospitalized patients (Dixon and Berl, 1984). Body fluid losses are usually isotonic or slightly hypotonic. Hyponatremia occurs when the patient drinks or is given hypo-osmotic solutions as a replacement for losses. To maintain a hypo-osmotic state, there also must be a decreased ability to excrete dilute urine because of diminished reabsorption of Na or increased reabsorption of water in the kidney. The clinical mechanisms associated with this disorder are shown in Table 40–7. In the critical care setting, hyponatremia is often associated with hypovolemic states in patients with congestive heart failure. It frequently results from diuretic therapy.

Isotonic or pseudohyponatremia is seen in patients with hyperproteinemia or hyperlipidemia. In these cases, the exaggerated protein or lipid fraction interferes with accurate measurement of plasma sodium. With many of the newer techniques used for biochemical analyses of electrolytes, the total sample is small enough to be artificially altered by this abnormally elevated plasma fraction. Consequently, the "measured" Na value will be erroneous because of the greater portion of the sample occupied by the

TABLE 40–6. Factors Affecting ADH Secretion

Factor	Effect on ADH Secretion
Hypovolemia	Increased
Low output cardiac failure	Increased
Hyperosmolality/hypernatremia	Increased
Narcotics	Increased
Nicotine	Increased
Tricyclic antidepressants	Increased
Pain	Increased
Stress	Increased
Hypo-osmolality/hyponatremia	Decreased
Hypervolemia	Decreased
Excess ADH	Decreased

TABLE 40–7. Mechanisms Contributing to Hyponatremia

Mechanism	Effect
Reduced sodium intake	Impairs formation of dilute urine
Excessive free water intake (5% dextrose/water)	
Primary ADH excess (syndrome of inappropriate antidiuretic hormone [SIADH])	Produces water retention, Na excretion
Mixed disorders:	
Nonosmotic ADH release	Produces water retention, Na excretion
Decreased urinary Na excretion	

protein or lipid. This represents an artifact and is not a true hyponatremic state.

Hypertonic hyponatremia, as shown in Figure 40–4, is the result of hyperglycemia or the administration of mannitol. In both situations, the EC compartment tonicity is elevated. In patients with hyperglycemia, glucose does not enter the cells because of the lack of insulin or insulin resistance. Therefore, glucose becomes an osmotically active substance. Mannitol also becomes an effective osmotic agent because it is confined to the EC compartment. Increased EC tonicity leads to a flow of water from the IC to the EC compartment and dilution of plasma Na. The net result of this osmotic activity is an expanded EC compartment and a contracted IC compartment.

The type of water and Na disorders that may produce isotonic hyponatremia are also described in Figure 40–4. These categories reflect the variable combination of Na and water disorders. Extracellular volume depletion may be caused by renal or extrarenal losses. Urinary Na (UNa) will vary depending upon the etiology. With diuretic excess or mineralocorticoid deficiency, Na will be inappropriately lost by the kidney. With an extrarenal etiology, Na will be conserved through normal homeostatic mechanisms.

The center section of Figure 40–4 depicts the consequences of an excess of TBW on EC volume. One of the causes of this clinical state is the syndrome of inappropriate antidiuretic hormone (SIADH). Hyponatremia occurs because of sustained production or release of ADH or ADH-like substances. This results in retention of water and volume expansion. Volume expansion induces natriuresis, so demonstrable edema is uncommon. Causes of SIADH are shown in Table 40–8. The differential diagnosis between hyponatremia caused by SIADH and a modest decrease in serum Na is that in the latter, Na is conserved so that UNa should be less than 10 to 15 mEq/liter. In contrast, in SIADH, the UNa will be high because of natriuresis (Valtin, 1987).

In the hyponatremic state associated with excess total body sodium and a larger excess of TBW, excess water will be distributed between EC and IC spaces proportional to their respective original compartment sizes. EC volume will be expanded such that edema is present. Further delineation of the problem may

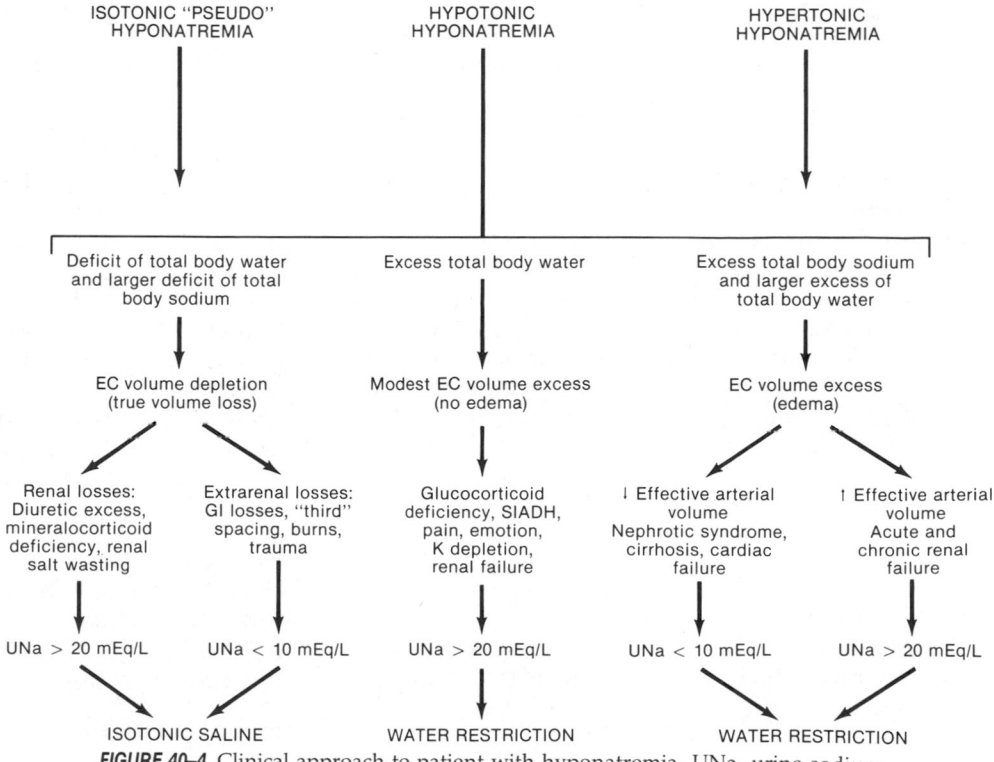

FIGURE 40–4. Clinical approach to patient with hyponatremia. UNa, urine sodium.

TABLE 40–8. Causes of Syndrome of Inappropriate Antidiuretic Hormone (SIADH)

CNS Disorders
Tumors
Infections
Head trauma
Hemorrhagic events

Tumor Production of ADH
Bronchogenic oat cell carcinoma
Hodgkin's disease
Cancer of pancreas
Cancer of prostate

Pulmonary Conditions (Nonmalignant)
Tuberculosis
Chronic obstructive pulmonary disease
Pneumococcal and viral pneumonia

Drugs
Carbamazepine (Tegretol)
Morphine
Oxytocin
Thiazide diuretics
Nicotine
Isoproterenol (Isuprel)

Miscellaneous
Positive pressure ventilation
Mitral commissurotomy

indicate the presence of decreased EAV, as seen in clinical entities such as cardiac failure, cirrhosis, or nephrotic syndrome. On the other hand, increased EAV may be present as a consequence of acute or chronic renal failure. Examination of UNa in these two situations will show opposite results. In patients with decreased EAV, the body is attempting to restore volume through renal conservation of Na, and urine Na will be very low. In patients with acute or chronic renal failure, the impaired renal mechanisms result in high urinary Na levels.

The hallmark of hyponatremia is that both pOsm and plasma Na are reduced. Symptoms associated with this disorder are dependent on the age and sex of the patient as well as the severity and rate of reduction in pOsm and Na. The primary symptoms are neurologic in origin and reflect the decreased Posm that leads to IC volume expansion in the brain cells. The relative plasma Na concentrations and associated symptoms are described in Table 40–9. Symptoms related to hyponatremia tend to be more severe in young women (<50 years of age). In some elderly patients, slow salt depletion may occur as a consequence of chronic diuretic therapy and pure water ingestion, leading to a long-term depletion of brain solute. These patients may be less symptomatic until plasma Na reaches significantly lower levels. Mortality seems to be correlated with symptomatic hyponatremia, which should be considered a medical emergency.

Management of Hyponatremia. Treatment of hy-

ponatremia (hypo-osmolality) depends on the level of plasma Na as well as the total body fluid volume and Na status. In edema-forming states, water restriction may be the only therapy required. If hyponatremia is the result of diuretic therapy, the diuretic should be discontinued. Administration of normal amounts of sodium and potassium usually permit a rapid return toward normal osmolality following diuresis.

Symptomatic hypo-osmolality must be treated expeditiously to prevent seizures and death. If plasma Na is less than 120 mEq/liter and the patient is symptomatic, hypertonic saline solutions of 3% or 5% may be administered intravenously. Hypertonic solutions are given at a rate that allows the serum Na to increase approximately 2 mEq/liter per hour (Arieff and Schmidt, 1980). When plasma Na reaches 120 to 125 mEq/liter, hypertonic saline infusion is discontinued and water restriction is implemented. Frequent monitoring of plasma Na is required to monitor serum Na reduction.

If the EAV is expanded, as in patients with SIADH, the infused sodium will be quickly excreted. To counteract natriuresis, intravenous furosemide may be administered during hypertonic infusion (Carroll and Oh, 1989). This will induce salt and water diuresis. In hyponatremic patients, some or most of the sodium will be retained while excess EC water will be excreted.

Stable, nonsymptomatic patients with SIADH may need only water restriction to restore fluid volume to normal. If water restriction alone is insufficient, an ADH-antagonizing medication, such as demeclocycline, may be administered (Dixon and Berl, 1984).

Potential for Injury. The patient with hyponatremia may experience alterations in central nervous system function, including coma and seizures. Early detection of decreased plasma Na and prevention of patient injury are important nursing goals.

Early hyponatremia is characterized by lethargy and malaise, followed by the development of nausea and vomiting. The nurse carefully assesses the patient's level of consciousness and level of response. The bedside environment is structured to prevent injury to the lethargic or somnulent patient. Suction or other equipment should be available to maintain airway patency in the vomiting patient.

Acute water-loading results in more severe CNS manifestations than a slowly developing hyponatremia. Following acute water ingestion, the nurse closely monitors the patient's plasma Na levels. The

TABLE 40–9. Clinical Manifestations of Acute Hyponatremia

PNa 125 mEq/liter	Nausea, malaise, muscle cramps
PNa 110–120 mEq/liter	Headache, dizziness, lethargy, obtundation
PNa < 110 mEq/liter	Seizures, coma, respiratory arrest

need for administration of hypertonic saline solutions should be anticipated. Seizure precautions are initiated because the patient is at high risk of convulsions.

HYPERNATREMIA

Hyperosmolality of the extracellular water is commonly the result of hypernatremia (Na>145 mEq/liter). The etiology of hypernatremia is either increased water loss in proportion to solute loss or solute gain in excess of water gain. The most common reasons for clinically significant hypernatremia include three pathogenic mechanisms: (1) impaired thirst or decreased access to water, (2) solute or osmotic diuresis, and (3) excessive renal or extrarenal losses of water. Generally, hypernatremia cannot occur in the presence of a normal thirst mechanism and an ability or opportunity to satisfy that sensation. However, the critically ill patient is at risk of developing hypernatremia due to impaired recognition of thirst and an inability to obtain or drink water.

The type of volume disorders resulting in hypernatremia are shown in Figure 40–5. These categories reflect the tonicity of fluid lost or gained by the patient relative to EC osmolality. As can be seen, the volume and tonicity changes will affect urinary sodium losses as well as total body sodium in different ways.

In the first classification of hypernatremia, shown on the left in Figure 40–5, the water loss is in excess of sodium loss. The possible renal causes include osmotic diuresis in association with uncorrected hyperglycemia and glucosuria, or administration of osmotic agents such as mannitol. Urinary sodium is inappropriately high because of the forced excretion. As a consequence, total body Na is low (Carroll and Oh, 1989).

Extrarenal mechanisms of hypernatremia include gastrointestinal losses or excessive loss of Na through the skin. In this situation, urinary sodium is low because the kidney is attempting to restore volume through the conservation of Na.

The second classification of hypernatremia located in the center of Figure 40–5 consists of clinical states in which pure water is lost. Total body sodium remains normal. Renal losses include central diabetes insipidus (CDI) in which ADH synthesis or release is diminished or absent. As a result, water is lost, and extracellular volume is decreased. Increased pOsm triggers the osmoreceptors. Because of the central abnormality, there is no attendant ADH secretory response. In critical care, this pathology is seen frequently in neurosurgery patients. It may be the consequence of head trauma, particularly basilar skull fractures, or ischemia due to cerebrovascular events.

Another mechanism by which free water is lost is nephrogenic diabetes insipidus (NDI). NDI is a condition in which the kidney, specifically the collecting duct, does not respond to ADH and thus does not

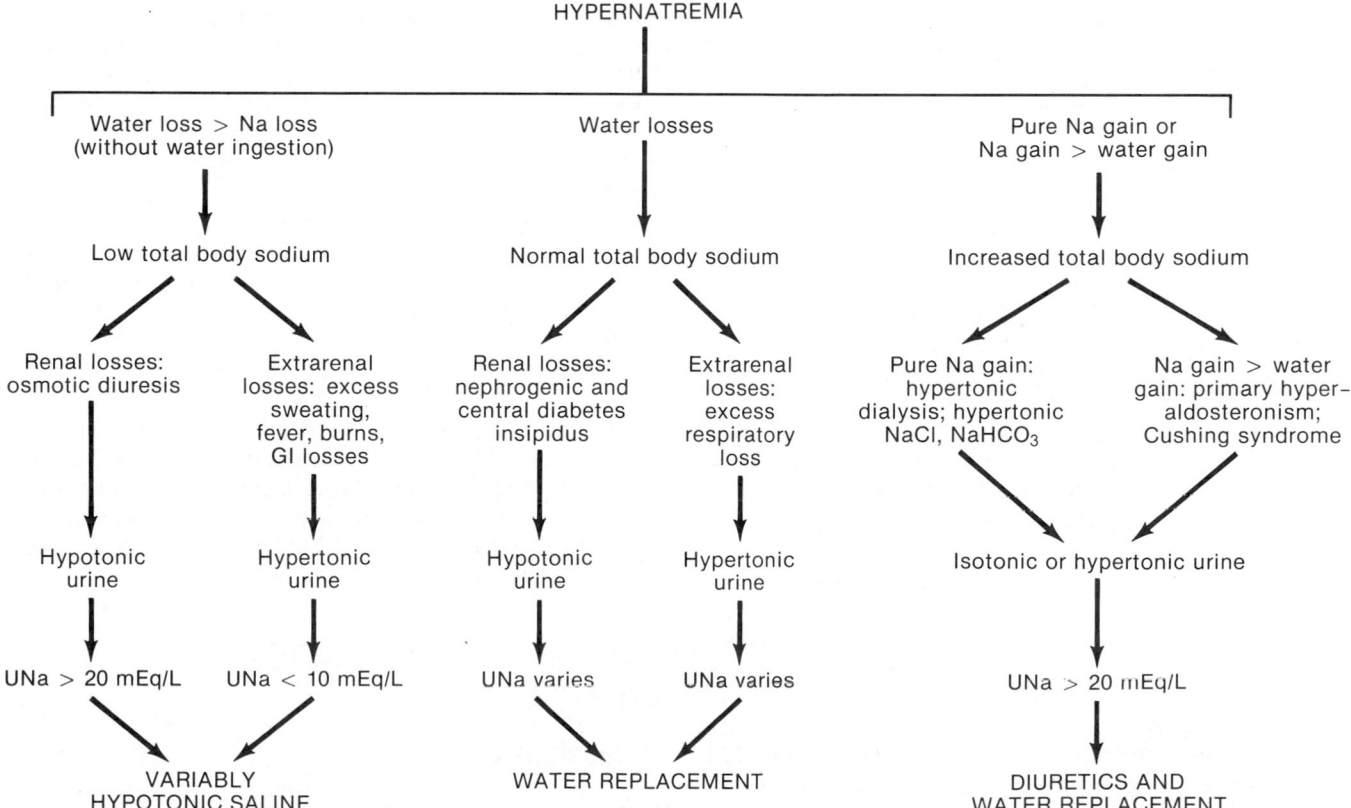

FIGURE 40–5. Clinical approach to patient with hypernatremia. UNa, urine sodium.

reabsorb water (Kleeman, 1984). Acquired NDI, which is the more common form, is characterized by the kidney's ability to concentrate urine to the level of plasma but not higher. Consequently, urine volumes are lower, on the order of 3 to 5 liters/day, compared to the larger urine volumes commonly seen with CDI. The causes of NDI include renal disease, in which medullary damage occurs or the number of functional nephrons is significantly reduced. Several mechanisms may adversely alter the medullary interstitial hypertonicity and thus the urinary concentrating process. Among these are severe prolonged protein deprivation or restriction, which decreases urea concentration in the renal interstitium. Significant sodium restriction may also be a contributing factor.

Clinical manifestations of disorders in which pure water is lost include polyuria and thirst. In some CDI states in which hypothalamic involvement includes the thirst center, the problem will be further complicated by a lack of the compensatory thirst mechanism. Urinary osmolality will be decreased as a consequence of the large excreted water volume and the pOsm will be elevated.

The third category of causes of hypernatremia is divided into those uncommon disorders in which there is pure Na gain and those in which the Na gain is larger than the water gain. Total body sodium stores are increased. Pure Na gain can occur through iatrogenic administration of hypertonic dialysis, $NaHCO_3$, or NaCl to a patient. This latter category represents a medical emergency in that the sudden change in EC osmolality induces the serious side effects of rapid expansion of EC volume (Kleeman, 1984). This may induce pulmonary edema in susceptible individuals. Serious central nervous system complications may arise from the rapid shift of water from the IC to the EC compartment in the brain. In the subgroup of Na gain larger than water gain, primary hyperaldosteronism leads to unregulated reabsorption of Na in excess of water by the kidney. This leads to a modestly elevated PNa. In either subgroup, UNa will be more than 20 mEq/liter as the kidney tries to respond to the body load of Na.

Symptoms associated with hypernatremia are related to the rate at which the plasma osmolality increases as well as the degree of increase. The clinical manifestations described in Table 40–10 reflect the central nervous system intracellular dehydration that occurs with increased pOsm.

Management of Hypernatremia. Treatment of hypernatremia is designed to address the specific deficits identified. Very rapid correction of hypernatremia can produce cerebral edema, seizures, and death because of rapid intracellular movement of water. The general approach is to decrease pOsm by 1 to 2 mOsm/kg H_2O per hour (Kleeman, 1984). Plasma Na should be lowered no more than 2 mEq/hour (Rose, 1984). Frequent serial plasma Na measurements will be necessary to guide fluid administration.

TABLE 40–10. Clinical Manifestations of Hypernatremia

Early Stage
Thirst/polydipsia
Restlessness/irritability
Confusion/somnolence

Second Stage
Ataxia
Muscle weakness/twitching

Late Stage
Focal or grand mal seizures

The type of solution used for volume replacement will depend on the etiology of the derangement. When hypernatremia exists in concert with water excess, diuretics may play a useful role in restoring plasma osmolality and returning volume toward normal.

Potential for Injury. Central nervous system alterations may become manifest from the elevated plasma Na or from cerebral edema resulting from too rapid a reduction in plasma Na. Nursing care is directed toward ensuring a gradual reduction in plasma Na and protecting the patient from possible injury.

The hypernatremic patient is assessed for signs of CNS irritability. The patient may appear confused and restless. The nurse assesses the patient's level of consciousness frequently and evaluates for change. As plasma Na decreases, the patient's neurologic status should improve (Metheny, 1987). The nurse provides a quiet, calm environment to decrease further stimulation. If the patient is restless and thrashing in bed, protective measures such as placement of bedrail padding are instituted. In patients with significant hypernatremia, seizure precautions are appropriate.

The nurse carefully reviews serial plasma Na measurements and evaluates the patient's response to the hypotonic infusion. The infusion is closely monitored to avoid overhydration and too rapid a reduction in sodium.

Osmolality disorders are frequently the consequence of a number of chronic disease processes. Therefore, the chronically ill patient is at risk for recurring episodes of hyponatremia or hypernatremia. Teaching the patient and family members about the causes and early signs of these osmolality disorders may result in earlier medical attention and may prevent the need for hospitalization.

ELECTROLYTE REGULATION AND BALANCE

Potassium

Potassium is an important electrolyte that serves two major physiologic purposes. One is a regulatory role in cell growth and metabolic processes. In the absence of appropriate K balance, cellular functions are impaired. The second important physiologic role of K is in the development of the resting membrane potential in neuromuscular tissue. This resting membrane potential is created by the difference between IC and EC potassium concentrations. The resting membrane potential is important for successful initiation of the action potential in nerve and muscle, including cardiac muscle. If EC potassium is elevated (hyperkalemia), the potential difference between EC and IC is less. The result is a decrease in the resting membrane potential, and the cell becomes more excitable. In the presence of low extracellular K (hypokalemia), the cell membrane is hyperpolarized and is less sensitive to excitation. These pathologic conditions will be discussed in detail in subsequent sections.

The normal plasma concentration of K is 3.5 to 5.0 mEq/liter. Potassium homeostasis is achieved through maintaining a balance among (1) K intake; (2) K distribution between the IC and EC compartments; and (3) renal management of filtered K. As described previously, K is the major intracellular cation and is preferentially confined to the IC compartment by the energy-consuming Na-K-ATPase pumps located in the cell membrane. The effectiveness of these pumps is demonstrated by the disparity normally maintained between the IC and EC potassium concentrations, as shown in Figure 40–1. Total body K stores in a normal adult are approximately 3000 to 4000 mEq. In normal steady-state conditions, K excretion occurs primarily through the kidney. Some K is lost through the gastrointestinal tract and in sweat. Thus, there is an obligatory K excretion regardless of K stores or the plasma concentration. The renal mechanism for EC potassium regulation requires several hours to become effective. Consequently, the more immediate regulation of K occurs endogenously through the mechanisms associated with IC and EC potassium distribution.

The mechanisms that influence the distribution of potassium in IC and EC compartments include the presence of Na-K-ATPase, insulin, exercise, and adrenergic nervous activity. In normal circumstances, plasma K concentration is precisely regulated because a small change in plasma concentration could be fatal. The IC concentration acts as a storage or supply depot for the EC compartment depending on the plasma K concentration.

The availability of Na-K-ATPase is an important requirement because the Na-K pump is responsible for the IC and EC distribution of potassium. If the pump is not functioning adequately, the distribution of Na and K will not be maintained in the EC and IC compartments, respectively. Any derangement in pump function has important implications for the fate of K added through the diet. Rapid addition of a large amount of K into a small EC volume would cause plasma K to rise to potentially lethal levels. Thus, the major body mechanism for handling a dietary load of K is rapid incorporation of this elec-

trolyte into cells via the Na-K pumps (Carroll and Oh, 1989). This immediate redistribution allows time for the remainder of the K load to be renally excreted. Plasma K concentration may directly affect the Na-K-ATPase pumps as well as aldosterone secretion.

Insulin is an important cofactor governing movement of K intracellularly, particularly into the liver and skeletal muscle. This explains the useful role played by insulin in conjunction with glucose in the treatment of hyperkalemia. Basal insulin levels also appear to enhance the movement of K into cells because suppression of the basal plasma insulin level will lead to an increase in plasma K concentration (Smith et al., 1985).

Exercise causes the release of K from cells, which, by means of a vasodilatory action, increases blood flow to exercising muscle. This process facilitates nutrient supply and waste removal from the working muscle. Once exercise stops, K rapidly moves back into cells. The restoration of K to the cellular compartment requires a process that involves the beta-adrenergic system. This mechanism of K distribution can be blunted by beta antagonists such as propranolol (Smith et al., 1985). Consequently, severe prolonged exercise in patients taking beta blockers may induce a potentially dangerous hyperkalemia.

Plasma K concentration is itself an influence on K distribution in the body. Plasma K concentration reflects total body stores of K, and variations in plasma concentration are correlated with changes in body stores. Exceptions to this clinical observation include significant changes in blood pH, plasma osmolality, and the rate of cell catabolism in the body. Under these circumstances, a change in plasma K concentration may instead reflect a redistribution of K between the EC and IC compartments.

Metabolic acidosis leads to an extracellular shift of K. This occurs because the body's attempt to buffer the acid load promotes the movement of hydrogen ion into the IC compartment. This reciprocal shift of K cations into the EC satisfies the requirements of electroneutrality. The effect of alkalosis on K distribution is not as striking, probably because of the decreased magnitude of hydrogen ion movement in patients with this condition. Respiratory acid-base disturbances do not lead to equally significant swings in plasma K concentrations because of the acid source CO_2 (Androgue and Madias, 1981).

Tissue catabolism will also affect EC potassium concentration. With cell breakdown, K will be liberated into the EC compartment. This situation commonly occurs in patients with surgery or trauma. In patients with normal renal function, the effect on plasma K concentration will be minimal. However, in critically ill patients with acute renal dysfunction, plasma K levels may rise rapidly due to tissue catabolism.

Potassium excretion is managed primarily by the kidney, most of it in the distal nephron by means of secretion and reabsorption. Thus, renal excretion is the important mechanism for varying K excretion as a function of K intake. The specific processes associated with K secretion or reabsorption in the nephron are discussed in Chapter 39.

Aldosterone, synthesized in the zona glomerulosa of the adrenal cortex, plays a powerful role in K homeostasis. When a K load is introduced into the body, aldosterone secretion is stimulated. Aldosterone increases excretion of K by the kidney while conserving the other major cation, Na. Conversely, under appropriate circumstances, decreased aldosterone availability minimizes urinary loss of K.

HYPOKALEMIA

A serum potassium value of less than 3.5 mEq/liter is classified as hypokalemia. The causes of hypokalemia are shown in Table 40–11. Decreased dietary intake is rarely the cause of hypokalemia because urinary losses can be minimized in the presence of a low K intake. Pica involving clay consumption may contribute to hypokalemia because this substance actually binds K and iron in the gut.

Increased gastrointestinal losses through the mechanisms of vomiting, nasogastric suction, or diarrhea are common causes of hypokalemia (Stein, 1988). Because the concentration of K in gastrointestinal secretions is relatively low, this loss alone cannot explain the significant degree of hypokalemia seen in these patients. The process by which hypokalemia is induced in this setting is associated with the metabolic alkalosis and volume depletion that accompanies severe vomiting or prolonged gastric drainage. An increase in pH of 0.1 will decrease plasma K concentration approximately 0.4 mEq/liter (Androgue and Madias, 1981; Carroll and Oh, 1989). In the presence of volume and acid-base disturbances, the renal dumping of bicarbonate coupled with high aldosterone levels leads to renal excretion of K and preservation of Na. Metabolic alkalosis favors movement of K into the IC compartment. Fecal loss of K can be sizable with significant diarrhea and can be responsible for K depletion.

Increased entry of K into the IC compartment may be the result of increased pH, insulin, or beta-adrenergic activity. Any situation in which there is an increase in supply or availability of insulin or catecholamines will promote intracellular movement of K.

Critically ill patients receiving dialysis treatments may become hypokalemic as a result of this therapy. Dialysis utilizing a low potassium bath may produce K depletion because of inappropriate removal of K during the treatment. Hypokalemia may be worsened by the correction of metabolic acidosis that occurs during dialysis. This will encourage K movement into cells and a further decrease in serum K.

The more common reasons for hypokalemia involve problems in renal regulation of K. As described earlier, the distal nephron plays the major role in regulating K balance. Hypokalemia may occur in the presence of mineralocorticoid excess, an increase in the tubular lumen fluid flow to the distal nephron, or a decrease in the reabsorption of K in the presence of a nonreabsorbable anion. If urinary K values are 10 mEq/day or more in conjunction with hypokalemia, renal K wasting is probably present (Levey and Harrington, 1984).

Hypokalemia is a common sequela of mineralocorticoid excess. This condition causes increased reabsorption of Na by the kidney and secretion of K and hydrogen ion. However, in order for K wasting to occur in the kidney, there must be adequate tubular fluid volume delivered to the distal nephron. Thus, in situations in which effective arterial volume is diminished, serum K values may be relatively normal. Depletion of EC volume stimulates aldosterone secretion but decreases the fluid volume delivered to the distal nephron as a result of the volume restoration effort by the kidney. Extracellular volume expansion produces the opposite effects.

An excess of mineralocorticoid conserves Na, an effort that, if successful, leads to EC volume expansion and hypertension. As a consequence of the increased volume, the fluid volume delivered to the distal nephron is increased and K wasting may occur. Causes of mineralocorticoid excess include hyperaldosteronism as a consequence of adrenal tumor or hyperplasia. Cushing's disease, in which there is bilateral hyperplasia, produces hypokalemia through glucocorticoid excess. Administration of corticosteroids for treatment of other disease processes may also result in hypokalemia.

Another common mechanism that leads to renal K wasting and hypokalemia is initiated by those states in which there is an increase in the fluid volume

---

TABLE 40–11. Etiology and Clinical Manifestations of Hypokalemia

Etiology	Clinical Findings
Extrarenal	**Neuromuscular**
Decreased K intake	Weakness
Increased gastrointestinal losses	Paralysis
Increased K entry into cells	
Increased pH	**Cardiac**
Increased insulin	ST depression
Increased beta-adrenergic	Decreased amplitude
activity	T wave inversion
Dialysis	Increased U wave (>1 mm)
	Prolongation of Q–T interval
Renal	Decreased amplitude of P
Mineralocorticoid excess	wave
Hyperaldosteronism	Prolonged P–R interval
Cushing's syndrome	Widened QRS complex
Hyperreninemia	
Increased Na delivery to distal	**Renal**
nephron	Increased urinary K
Diuretics	(concentration defect)
Osmotic diuresis	Na retention
Bartter syndrome	
Salt-wasting nephropathies	
Nonreabsorbable anions	
Penicillins	
Ketoacids	
HCO_3 (metabolic alkalosis)	

delivered to the distal nephron. This disorder is commonly seen in critically ill patients following the administration of diuretics that inhibit proximal Na reabsorption and force water excretion. In this situation, Na reabsorption in the proximal tubule is diminished, resulting in a higher volume of fluid delivered to the distal segment. Consequently, there is an increase in K excretion by the kidney. Chronic use of diuretics can cause EC depletion, which stimulates aldosterone secretion and thus K secretion by the kidney. An osmotic diuresis will also produce hypokalemia in essentially the same way. Hypomagnesemia may produce hypokalemia. This condition will be manifested by elevated aldosterone and renin blood levels but without hypertension.

The physiologic manifestations of hypokalemia are shown in Table 40–11. The severity of the manifestations tends to be correlated with the degree of hypokalemia, and these signs generally do not appear until serum K values are below 3.0 mEq/liter. A decrease in EC potassium concentration relative to the IC concentration causes hyperpolarization across the cell membrane and reduces the excitability of the cells. The resting membrane potential is below the normal level; thus the cell requires a larger stimulus to reach the threshold value and cause depolarization. The cell then requires a longer time to repolarize to baseline value. These facts have important clinical implications for nerve and muscle function.

One of the important clinical manifestations of hypokalemia is muscle weakness. Progression to muscle paralysis occurs when the plasma K is less than 2.5 mEq/liter (Carroll and Oh, 1989). Muscle dysfunction may first be evident in the lower extremities. With increasing severity, the trunk and upper extremities become involved, and respiratory failure may occur.

Cardiac arrhythmias induced by hypokalemia are varied and include premature contractions, both atrial and ventricular, tachyarrhythmias, and sinus bradycardia. Serious arrhythmias are usually not seen until plasma K is less than 3 mEq/liter. However, digitalis therapy may make the individual patient susceptible to serious arrhythmias at a higher plasma K value. The electrocardiographic (ECG) changes commonly seen in hypokalemia are all reversible with K repletion.

Severe muscle dysfunction may also lead to rhabdomyolysis and acute renal failure in patients with severe hypokalemia. This phenomenon appears to be the result of cellular ischemia caused by the lack of available K (Knochel and Schlein, 1972). As described earlier, the release of K from intracellular stores promotes vasodilation in the local area of an exercising muscle. If K depletion exists, this transcellular movement of K does not occur. Since there is no increase in blood flow to the area, ischemia necrosis of muscle cells, with release of cellular contents, may occur.

Hypokalemia may have a significant effect on renal function. Polyuria may be associated with low plasma K values. This may be a sequela of impaired urinary concentrating ability associated with K depletion. However, urine osmolality generally stays above 300 mOsm/kg with K depletion. Potassium depletion may lead to renal retention of Na, resulting in edema formation if Na intake is high.

Management of Hypokalemia. Treatment of hypokalemia includes identification and correction of the underlying cause as well as the electrolyte disorder. The underlying cause of hypokalemia may be discernible from a history of extrarenal losses or the extensive use of diuretics in the critically ill patient. Urinary K values may not be specific for renal wasting in the presence of either very low or very high urine volumes. Volume depletion may occur in association with significant extrarenal losses and diuretic usage. Hypovolemia may further cloud the issue with activation of the normal renal response of Na conservation and K secretion. In contrast, primary mineralocorticoid excess is more often associated with volume expansion. The presence of acid-base disturbances may be an important clue to the etiology of the observed hypokalemia. For example, hypokalemia and metabolic alkalosis may indicate excessive diuretic usage or upper gastrointestinal losses.

There is no good correlation between the plasma K concentration and the total K deficit. As noted above, the actual plasma K concentration at which signs and symptoms appear is variable. Symptomatic patients need to be treated promptly. The goal is K repletion to diminish the signs and symptoms of hypokalemia but not necessarily to completely restore body K stores immediately. Rapid administration of K supplements may induce a hyperkalemic state, which will be discussed in a later section. If the hypokalemia is not acute, oral K supplements may be appropriate. Oral replacement avoids K rebound because there is time for renal regulation to contribute to restoration of K balance. In hypokalemia associated with primary hyperaldosteronism, oral K replacement may not be adequate to replace losses because K will continue to be lost through the kidney. Intravenous K supplementation should be administered at an infusion rate of 10 to 20 mEq/hour unless paralysis or potentially fatal arrhythmias are present. When hypokalemia is severe or when serious ECG abnormalities are evident, intravenous K may need to be administered more rapidly, at a rate of up to 80 to 100 mEq/hour (Lunger, 1988). Under these circumstances, the ECG must be monitored closely to prevent *hyper*kalemic changes. Because of the insulin effect on K distribution, glucose solutions, which would stimulate endogenous insulin production, are not usually the solutions of choice for administration of K replacement in patients with severe hypokalemia (Metheny, 1987).

Alteration in Cardiac Output. In hypokalemia, the contractility of the cardiac muscle is impaired. The nurse assesses the patient for signs and symptoms of decreased cardiac output and the development of congestive heart failure. The effect of digitalis is enhanced in hypokalemia, placing the patient at risk of digitalis toxicity. The critical care nurse monitors the patient's serum K level and confers with the physician regarding withholding or reducing the dosage of digitalis. The ECG is observed for changes indicative of hypokalemia. Particular attention is paid to the patient's ECG during intravenous K repletion (Lunger, 1988). Emergency resuscitation equipment is kept readily available in case cardiac arrest occurs.

Potential for Injury. The patient with hypokalemia is at risk for injury from several sources. Muscle weakness is a common manifestation of hypokalemia. The patient may not have the strength to perform activities such as transferring himself from bed to chair. The nurse assesses the patient's muscle strength and provides appropriate support and assistance as necessary.

Maintenance of adequate intravenous access is vital in the treatment of K disorders. As with intravenous administration of any drug, K repletion carries some risk to the patient. Rapid repletion of K in a peripheral vein may cause localized pain and irritation of the vein. Therefore, if a peripheral site is used, it may be preferable to infuse lower K concentrations through two sites. Ideally, high K concentrations should be administered through a large-bore central line.

HYPERKALEMIA

Hyperkalemia is defined as a plasma K level of greater than 5.5 mEq/liter, although the level at which hyperkalemic complications occur may vary depending on the steady-state value for a given patient. Adaptation may occur when K intake is gradually increased to very high levels or may be a protective mechanism associated with chronic renal failure. This process blunts the effects of an acute increase in K load. In the case of chronic renal failure, the remaining functioning nephrons are capable of increasing their individual excretion of K and avoiding significant hyperkalemia until renal function approaches zero. There can be situations in which serum K as measured in the blood specimen is erroneously elevated. Hemolysis associated with venipuncture or specimen collection will artificially increase measured serum K values. Spuriously high plasma K values may also be seen in the patient with thrombocytosis or leukocytosis (Bronson et al., 1966; Katz and Defronzo, 1984).

Hyperkalemia can be the result of increased oral or intravenous intake of K, although this is uncommon in the presence of normal renal function. As discussed earlier, the body first defends against wide swings in EC potassium concentration by rapidly shifting K between the body compartments to reestablish appropriate concentrations in each compartment. The secondary regulatory mechanism involving the kidney can then restore true K balance during the course of 6 to 8 hours. Therefore, sustained hyperkalemia is almost always the result of impaired renal K regulation mechanisms. However, there may be instances, either because of the rate of K administration or the size of the patient (infants), in which potentially fatal serum K levels can be reached even with normal renal function.

The most common causes of true hyperkalemia are shown in Table 40–12. These causes are frequently the inverse of those described in the section on hypokalemia. Metabolic acidosis is a frequent cause of hyperkalemia in critically ill patients. With the intracellular movement of hydrogen ions, K moves out of the cells, thus increasing the EC potassium concentration. Hyperkalemia in patients with diabetic ketoacidosis is partially a consequence of the lack of insulin and thus the inability to move K intracellularly quickly. Hyperglycemia is also responsible for significant movement of K out of cells. The increased EC osmolality accompanying hyperglycemia pulls water out of cells, bringing K with it.

Beta blockers may play an indirect role in the production of hyperkalemia by preventing the movement of K into cells. This is usually expressed as a modest elevation in serum K. However, when there is a significant addition of K to the EC compartment, the normally rapid redistribution of K is attenuated. As discussed earlier, this may produce a dangerous situation when vigorous exercise is performed (Coester et al., 1973; Schultz and Nissenson, 1980).

Tissue catabolism, either through traumatic injury or surgery, may liberate large amounts of K into the EC compartment. This is further exacerbated by renal failure, which often occurs as a sequela to these insults.

Digitalis can also be responsible for the development of hyperkalemia. Large doses of digitalis preparations significantly inhibit the Na-K-ATPase pump, which is instrumental in transporting K into cells. Typical therapeutic doses of digitalis may cause an inconsequential increase in serum K values. However, in patients in which the renal regulatory mechanism is compromised or absent, hyperkalemia may be a serious complication of digitalis administration.

TABLE 40–12. Etiology and Clinical Manifestations of Hyperkalemia

Etiology	Clinical Findings
Extrarenal	***Neuromuscular***
Metabolic acidosis	Paresthesias
Decreased insulin availability/ hyperglycemia	Paralysis—distal moving to proximal
Beta blockers	
Exercise	***Cardiac***
Tissue catabolism	Peaked T wave
Digitalis overdose	Widened QRS complex
	Widened P–R interval
Renal	Disappearance of P wave
Mineralocorticoid deficiency	Appearance of sine wave
Renal failure	
Decreased effective arterial volume	

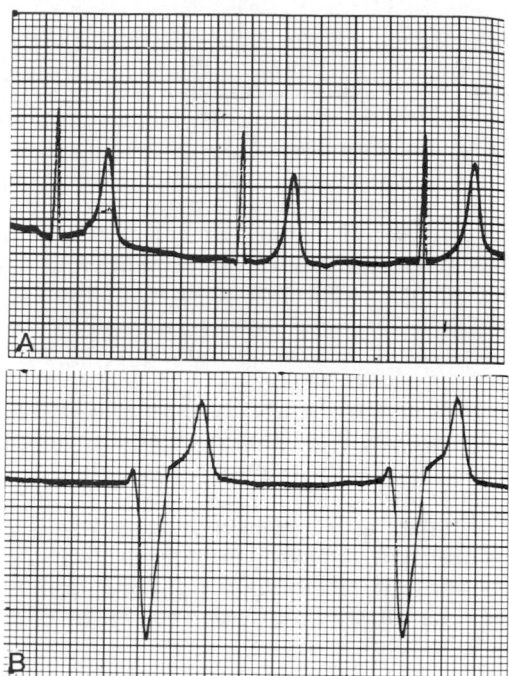

FIGURE 40–6. *A* and *B,* Characteristic electrocardiographic changes during hyperkalemia.

Persistent hyperkalemia may be indicative of an impairment of the mechanisms that regulate K excretion. Mineralocorticoid deficiency may result from either the production of aldosterone or the diminished effect of the hormone on the kidney (DeFronzo, 1980). Hypoaldosteronism can result from the administration of nonsteroidal anti-inflammatory drugs (NSAIDs), K-sparing diuretics, or any condition that affects the adrenal synthesis of the hormone.

Renal insufficiency or failure frequently leads to hyperkalemia because of a direct reduction in nephron excretory ability. Hyperkalemia may also result from the secondary problem of decreased flow of water and Na through the distal tubule. Hyperkalemia occurs more frequently in oliguric acute renal failure than in patients with nonoliguric renal failure.

Decreased EAV leads to diminished delivery of water and electrolytes to the distal nephron. As described earlier, this will reduce K secretion at this site. Any clinical condition that produces a reduced EAV will encourage K retention by the kidney and the possibility of hyperkalemia. In patients with chronic congestive heart failure, the addition of digitalis preparations and the imposition of renal insufficiency may result in significant hyperkalemia.

Clinical manifestations of hyperkalemia are described in Table 40–12. Because of the increase in EC potassium concentration, the cell transmembrane resting potential is reduced (becomes less negative). Thus, the resting potential is closer to the threshold value relative to the normal state. There is a corresponding increase in the velocity of repolarization and a decreased rate of diastolic depolarization (Carroll and Oh, 1989).

The most striking example of this phenomenon is seen in cardiac muscle, where significant conduction abnormalities may be seen in the ECG. The shortened Q–T interval and tall T waves demonstrate the rapid repolarization effects. The serum K at which these changes occur is variable. Figure 40–6 illustrates the cardiac effects of hyperkalemia.

The neuromuscular manifestations may be less common but are frequently the initial patient complaint. Paresthesias of the extremities may be present. Flaccid paralysis of the distal extremities with proximal progression may also be evident. Neuromuscular involvement tends to remain localized to the extremities.

Management of Hyperkalemia. Management of the hyperkalemic patient is directed toward treatment of the underlying etiology as well as the signs and symptoms of hyperkalemia. Electrocardiographic changes warrant prompt treatment to avoid progression of cardiac toxicity to ventricular fibrillation and cardiac arrest. The absolute value at which treatment must be initiated will vary, and management should be instituted based on ECG and physical findings. Hyperkalemia in the presence of ECG abnormalities or muscular weakness should be treated immediately.

There are a number of approaches that can be used to reduce EC potassium concentration effectively. Treatment is directed toward removal of K from the body or effective redistribution of K into the IC compartment. The therapeutic techniques most often used are shown in Table 40–13.

Calcium acts to antagonize the cell membrane effects of hyperkalemia directly by resetting the interval between the resting and the threshold potential. In cardiac muscle, this reverses the conduction defect observed with hyperkalemia. Acute infusion of calcium increases sodium flux through the sodium channels in muscle tissue, which also enhances conduction of the impulse. The action of calcium infusion is rapid, the effect being seen in 1 to 3 minutes. The action is sustained for up to 60 minutes (Smith et al., 1985). Continuous ECG monitoring must be done during acute calcium infusion. Administration of repeat doses of this agent will depend on the ECG changes produced with the first dose. Calcium may potentiate the digitalis effect. In this situation, calcium should be diluted in 5% dextrose and water and the infusion rate reduced to an appropriate level to avoid toxic effects (Rose, 1984).

TABLE 40–13. Therapy for Hyperkalemia

Membrane Antagonism	Removal of K
Calcium	Diuretics
Hypertonic Na	Exchange resin
	Dialysis
Redistribution of K	
Insulin and glucose	
Bicarbonate	

Hypertonic sodium chloride administration in a hyponatremic patient may be effective in correcting the cardiac conduction defect. This agent acts by increasing the number of Na channels in the muscle cells, which helps to conduct the electrical impulse once the threshold potential has been reached. The effectiveness of this technique with normal serum Na is less obvious.

Rapid redistribution of K from the extracellular to the intracellular compartment is effective in reducing the toxic effects of hyperkalemia. Insulin in association with a glucose infusion is used for this purpose. Insulin is effective in moving K intracellularly, and glucose prevents hypoglycemia resulting from the additional exogenous insulin. This combination is administered over 30 minutes and should be effective for 4 to 6 hours (Rose, 1984).

Sodium bicarbonate is effective in rapidly redeploying K even in the absence of acidemia. The renal tubule will also increase K secretion in the presence of an increase in blood pH. Sodium bicarbonate can be administered as a 50-mEq bolus dose over 5 to 10 minutes. This agent has a rapid onset (5 to 10 minutes) and will be effective for up to 2 hours (Rose, 1984). If volume expansion is present, the addition of this Na load may increase the risk of congestive heart failure or fluid volume overload.

The maneuvers described above will not reduce total body K. They serve as temporary measures that allow the physician and nurse time to consider ways in which K can be effectively removed from the body. If kidney function is adequate, diuretics such as furosemide will be useful in delivering increased water and Na flow to the distal tubule, thus enhancing K secretion by the kidney. More frequently, hyperkalemia is associated with renal impairment. In this case, extrarenal removal of K may be warranted. Hemodialysis with a zero K dialysate rapidly removes K from the body. However, this treatment requires a vascular access device, dialysis equipment, and skilled personnel, all of which may be difficult to obtain in an emergency situation. If time permits, however, this is the most efficient method of reducing serum K rapidly. Using standard operating parameters, approximately 40 mEq of potassium can be removed in the first hour of dialysis. Peritoneal dialysis can also be used to lower serum K, although this therapeutic technique will be much slower than hemodialysis.

Exchange resins, such as kayexalate, are also effective in removing K from the body. The resin exchanges a sodium ion for K and calcium in the gastrointestinal tract. It can be given either as an oral preparation or by retention enema to accomplish K removal. It is usually given with sorbitol to enhance K loss via the bowel. A 25-g dose will remove approximately 12.5 to 25 mEq of K. This method of K removal is slower and requires 1 to 2 hours before onset of action. In general, 50 g of kayexalate will lower serum K by approximately 0.5 to 1.0 mEq/liter (Smith et al., 1985). The additional Na from the resin, approximately 3 mEq/1 mEq K exchanged, may be contraindicated in patients with serious cardiac disease.

Alteration in Cardiac Output. Nursing care of a patient in hyperkalemic crisis is directed toward supporting and monitoring the patient's cardiac status while administering therapies designed to reduce the plasma K level. Hyperkalemia has no significant effect on cardiac contractility but can cause alterations in cardiac output owing to abnormalities in rhythm and conduction. Careful, ongoing evaluation of ECG monitoring in the hyperkalemic patient before and during treatment is an important nursing responsibility.

The critical care nurse observes the ECG for peaked T waves, shortened Q–T interval, and prolonged P–R interval. Following administration of prescribed medications and fluids, serial plasma K measurements are taken and monitored. Response is evaluated by observing the patient for resolution of the ECG changes. If bicarbonate, glucose, and insulin are used, the nurse anticipates the return of hyperkalemia in several hours.

The nurse maintains adequate intravenous access and monitors medication infusions carefully. Several of the drugs used to treat hyperkalemia are incompatible. Calcium and bicarbonate solutions should not be placed in the same intravenous line because calcium salts will precipitate out of solution. At least two intravenous lines should be maintained for emergency drug therapy in the hyperkalemic patient (Metheny, 1987).

Calcium

Calcium (Ca), phosphate (P), and magnesium (Mg) have important roles in bone structure, neuromuscular transmission, and regulation of many enzyme systems. These three electrolytes are maintained in balance by a careful coupling of intestinal absorption and renal excretion. Calcium and Mg are divalent cations that are also secreted by the intestine in digestive fluids.

Calcium plays an important role in the following body functions:

Bone structure

Neuromuscular transmission

Secretions of exocrine and endocrine glands

Cardiac action potential

Regulation of many enzyme systems

Blood clotting and activation of the complement system

Calcium is believed to bind with proteins in cellular sodium channels, thereby closing the Na channels in the cell membrane after depolarization has occurred. This allows the cell membrane to repolarize and return to its resting membrane potential (Guyton, 1991). When a stimulus of sufficient magnitude occurs, calcium ions are displaced, Na enters the cell, and depolarization begins. This process is of particular importance in tissues requiring repetitive rhythmic discharge such as the heart. Calcium is an essential participant in cardiac conduction and contractility.

Calcium is also vital to the secretory activity of many endocrine and exocrine glandular cells through the process of stimulus-secretion coupling. Moreover, Ca is a regulator of various enzyme activities within cells. It is essential to many cyclic AMP–mediated responses.

Calcium plays a number of roles in blood coagulation. It is essential in the formation of prothrombin activator. Calcium also interacts with fibrin-stabilizing factor (Factor XIII) to convert the fibrin strands into a stable clot.

Because of its significant contribution to these important functions, Ca concentration is maintained within narrow limits in both the IC and EC compartments. The normal plasma Ca level is 9 to 10.5 mg/dL (4.5 to 5.25 mEq/liter). Calcium exists in the plasma as two separate fractions—40% of plasma Ca is protein bound, primarily to albumin, and 50% exists as an ionized or active fraction. The remainder of total plasma Ca is complexed with other ions such as citrate or phosphate. There is a difference between total serum calcium and the ionized Ca concentration. Direct measurement of the ionized or active fraction of Ca is not routinely performed because of technical difficulties. However, the ionized Ca fraction is an important parameter because this is the free Ca that is physiologically relevant.

The level of plasma proteins also plays a role in determining total serum Ca. Any state associated with increased albumin will increase total calcium. Hypoalbuminemia produces the opposite effect. Protein binding of Ca is reversible and may be affected by blood pH and parathyroid hormone.

Regulation of Ca is multifactorial. Intestinal absorption of Ca is under the influence of vitamin D–1,25. Renal excretion of Ca is influenced by both parathyroid hormone (PTH) and serum Ca levels. Bone deposition and resorption are regulated by vitamin D, PTH, and serum phosphorus levels.

Under normal conditions, constant bone formation and resorption lead to little net change in serum calcium. However, when either the intake or excretion pathways are disturbed, bone acts as a reservoir to stabilize serum Ca levels. PTH in concert with vitamin D–1,25 can change the rate of bone resorption. High levels of PTH increase the liberation of Ca from the skeleton. Alterations in the bioavailability of either PTH or vitamin D–1,25 subsequently affect the utilization of bone as a source of Ca.

The renal regulation of calcium balance is accomplished through reabsorption in the proximal tubule. Final regulation of renal Ca excretion occurs in the distal nephron under the influence of PTH. There is a direct relationship between PTH and Ca reabsorp-

tion. As serum PTH levels increase, renal Ca reabsorption increases. It should be noted that clinical disorders that affect Na transport tend to affect Ca transport in a similar direction. Metabolic acidosis promotes Ca excretion by the kidney, whereas alkalosis leads to Ca conservation. Diuretics also influence Ca excretion depending on the site of action. Furosemide, ethacrynic acid, and osmotic diuretics inhibit Na reabsorption and thus force excretion of both Na and Ca. Thiazide diuretics result in decreased Ca renal excretion.

HYPOCALCEMIA

Hypocalcemia is defined as a plasma Ca level of less than 9 mg/dL (4.5 mEq/liter). The primary causes of hypocalcemia are shown in Table 40–14. In many of these states, there is a defect in either PTH or vitamin D–1,25. The normal synergistic relationship between PTH and vitamin D cannot compensate for this defect. As described earlier, low serum albumin affects the fraction of Ca bound to protein, thus lowering the total serum Ca. However, this state may have little clinical effect if the biologically important ionized fraction is normal.

Hypoparathyroidism is one of the common causes of hypocalcemia (Mawer et al., 1976). Hypoparathyroidism may be the result of trauma or of surgical removal or injury to the parathyroid gland during neck or thyroid surgery. Idiopathic hypoparathyroidism may occur at any time in life but is most common

TABLE 40–14. Etiology and Clinical Manifestations of Hypocalcemia

Etiology	Clinical Findings
Hypoalbuminemia	Neuromuscular
	Tetany
Parathyroid dysfunction	Seizures
Hypoparathyroidism	Muscle cramps
Surgical excision	Weakness
Idiopathic	
Pseudohypoparathyroidism	Cardiovascular
	Hypotension
Hypomagnesemia	Electrocardiographic
	changes
Vitamin D abnormalities	Shortened Q–T interval
Malnutrition/malabsorption	
Liver disease with decreased	Neurologic or cognitive
production of 25(OH) D	Cognitive impairment
Drugs—increased metabolism	Affective disorders
of 25(OH) D	
Nephrotic syndrome—increased	
loss of 25(OH) D	
Renal failure—decreased	
production of	
1,25-vitamin D	
Excessive removal of calcium	
Hyperphosphatemia	
Acute pancreatitis	
Rapid bone formation	
Massive transfusion of	
citrated blood	

in childhood or adolescence. True hypoparathyroidism is manifested by low PTH levels. Pseudohypoparathyroidism, in contrast, is characterized by normal circulating PTH levels and an inadequate tissue response to the hormone. In critically ill patients, hypocalcemia is frequently associated with hypomagnesemia. Hypomagnesemia is most often caused by inadequate magnesium content in total parenteral nutrition (TPN), although it can also result from prolonged diarrhea or renal Mg wasting. Hypomagnesemia is generally thought to be responsible for depressing PTH secretion. It may also decrease the responsiveness of bone to PTH action.

As described earlier, vitamin D–1,25 enhances absorption of dietary Ca as well as the effect of PTH on bone. Abnormalities in the chain of vitamin D metabolism and its transformation to the active form can affect these important processes and produce hypocalcemia. Vitamin D abnormalities include inadequate intake of this vitamin. Although this cause is uncommon in the general population, it must be considered in critically ill patients who may be NPO or on clear liquid diets for long periods of time. In addition, clinical states such as partial gastrectomy, pancreatitis, and intestinal resection may be associated with malabsorption, which also contributes to a vitamin D–1,25 deficiency. Also common in critically ill patients are vitamin D abnormalities resulting from disturbances in conversion of the vitamin to its intermediate and active forms. Liver dysfunction may impair conversion of vitamin D to the intermediate form because of a lack of bile salts. Anticonvulsant drugs, such as phenobarbital and phenytoin, may increase metabolism of the intermediate form to inactive metabolites, which then cannot undergo renal conversion to the active form. Nephrotic syndrome may cause increased excretion of the intermediate form. Acute or chronic renal failure renders the kidney incapable of converting the intermediate form to the biologically active vitamin D–1,25. Renal failure is accompanied by metabolic acidosis, which also may adversely affect the metabolism of vitamin D. The consequence of these pathologic states is decreased intestinal absorption of Ca and altered bone deposition and resorption, leading to hypocalcemia.

Abnormalities in phosphate excretion can also result in hypocalcemia. Excessive removal of Ca from the serum may be the consequence of hyperphosphatemia. Mechanisms in this situation may include impaired conversion of vitamin D–1,25, extravascular calcification resulting from the phosphate-calcium complexes, and reduced bone resorption. These mechanisms occur most often in the presence of an acute rise in serum phosphorus. Acute hyperphosphatemia may occur following acute ingestion of phosphate or administration of multiple phosphate enemas. Acute phosphatemia also occurs in rhabdomyolysis, when damaged muscle cells release intracellular phosphate ions into the blood.

Hypocalcemia is seen in conjunction with acute pancreatitis, although the exact mechanism is not known. It is believed that Ca ions combine with fatty acids, released from areas of lipolysis and fat necrosis, to form soaps (Parfitt and Kleerkoper, 1980; Greenberger, 1986). Elevated levels of glucagon may also play a role. The reduction in total serum Ca occurs at the expense of the ionized fraction. Severe hypocalcemia (<7 mg/dL) in patients with acute pancreatitis is not common and is associated with a poor prognosis (Agus and Goldfarb, 1985).

Rapid bone formation can also produce hypocalcemia. This condition may appear after correction of hyperparathyroidism, thyrotoxicosis, or nutritional rickets. In these situations, Ca is rapidly restored to the bone to replace that resorbed during the pathologic state.

Binding of Ca by citrate can cause hypocalcemia in critically ill patients who have received massive blood transfusions. This is a particular problem in patients with liver dysfunction because liver disease causes decreased metabolism of citrate.

The physiologic manifestations of hypocalcemia are shown in Table 40–14. The most common manifestations are expressed as neuromuscular irritability. Characteristic clinical findings include stiffness, muscle spasms, and cramps. These findings are seen most often in the hand, with carpopedal spasm. More serious complications of laryngeal stridor and respiratory muscle spasm may compromise respiratory effort.

Tetany is described as intermittent tonic spasms. Tetany can occur at variable levels of serum calcium deficiency, depending on coexisting conditions such as alkalosis and hypomagnesemia. However, this neuromuscular manifestation usually occurs when serum Ca is below 7 to 7.5 mg/dL. Tetany may be elicited by tapping over the facial nerve to produce twitching (Chvostek sign) or by prolonged blood pressure cuff inflation (>3 minutes) to elicit carpopedal spasm (Trousseau sign). These diagnostic signs may not be present in all hypocalcemic patients. Seizures of any magnitude may be an early sign of disordered serum Ca. Muscle cramps occur as a consequence of the tetany.

Cardiovascular manifestations of hypocalcemia include hypotension and decreased myocardial contractility. Electrocardiographic changes include a characteristic increase in the Q–T interval, which reflects a delay in ventricular repolarization. In contrast to hypokalemia, hypocalcemia usually does not cause ST depression. If hyperkalemia is present, which is frequently the case in critically ill patients with acute renal failure, the T waves may be peaked.

Cognitive and affective disorders may accompany hypocalcemia. Anxiety, lethargy, depression, confusion, and overt psychosis may be seen. These acute changes can be reversed with Ca replacement. Mental retardation may be a sequela of chronic hypocalcemia in children.

Management of Hypocalcemia. The correction of hypocalcemia includes fluid management as well as administration of Ca-containing medications. A complete evaluation to elicit the underlying cause of the disorder is also required and will help to guide treatment. A history of neck surgery, anticonvulsant therapy, or familial occurrence of hypoparathyroidism is valuable in helping to determine the etiology. In addition, laboratory assessment of serum albumin, magnesium, and phosphate levels is useful in the diagnostic process. Each 1 g/dL reduction in serum albumin produces a decrement of approximately 0.7 mg/dL in total serum Ca concentration. Hypomagnesemia (<0.8 mEq/liter) may prove to be the cause of hypocalcemia (Agus and Goldfarb, 1985). Serum phosphate may provide additional information, although its concentration is dependent on PTH levels in the absence of renal failure.

Severe acute hypocalcemia may present with serious cardiac and neuromuscular complications that require prompt and aggressive therapy with intravenous calcium. Solutions available for use include calcium gluconate and calcium chloride. Calcium gluconate is preferred because calcium chloride is known to produce thrombophlebitis and tissue necrosis should it infiltrate into the extravascular space (Agus and Goldfarb, 1985). It should be noted that standard preparations of calcium chloride contain four times as much calcium as an equal volume of calcium gluconate. The rate of calcium infusion should not exceed 50 mg/minute. A total dose of 2 grams should not be exceeded without a repeat measurement of the serum Ca level. Continued correction of serum Ca requires slow calcium infusion and careful monitoring of serum Ca levels.

Magnesium repletion may also be required to treat hypocalcemia. The presence of renal failure is a contraindication to magnesium administration unless severe hypomagnesemia exists.

If onset of hypocalcemia is slower, such as that occurring following parathyroid surgery, acute intravenous administration of Ca may still be necessary. However, if the patient is able to take oral medications, further Ca restoration may be accomplished with oral agents in combination with phosphorus restriction. If vitamin D deficiency is the underlying cause of hypocalcemia, vitamin D supplementation may be useful.

Potential for Injury. Acute symptomatic hypocalcemia is a medical emergency requiring immediate nursing attention. In addition to assisting the physician in monitoring and correcting the serum Ca deficit, nursing care is directed toward preventing patient injury due to seizures or airway obstruction.

Because hypocalcemia increases the irritability of the central nervous system, the hypocalcemic patient is at risk of developing seizures. The critical care nurse assesses the patient for signs and symptoms of neuromuscular irritability. Specific assessments include patient complaints of numbness or tingling in the digits, muscle cramps, and the presence of the Chvostek or Trousseau signs. In addition, the nurse observes the patient for changes in mentation, mood, and memory. If hypocalcemia is severe or if the patient demonstrates neuromuscular irritability, seizure precautions are instituted.

In addition to the risk of injury from the disease process itself, the hypocalcemic patient is also at risk of injury from therapy with intravenous medications. Calcium solutions are not compatible with bicarbonate-containing fluids. When mixed, precipitation of Ca salts will occur. Ca infusions should be accompanied by careful ECG monitoring. During the infusion, the nurse closely monitors the patient for the onset of ventricular irritability or heart block. If either of these cardiac changes occurs, the infusion should be immediately stopped.

Impaired Breathing Pattern. Among the life-threatening consequences of severe hypocalcemia are laryngospasm, airway obstruction, and respiratory arrest. The critical care nurse carefully assesses the patient's airway status for evidence of spasm or obstruction. The patient is observed for restlessness, tachypnea, and subtle arterial blood gas changes. These early signs are followed by inspiratory stridor, hoarseness, and decreased air movement. The nurse prepares for the possibility of airway obstruction by assembling emergency airway equipment and preparing for possible intubation.

HYPERCALCEMIA

Hypercalcemia can be classified as mild (<12 mg/dL), moderate (12 to 15 mg/dL), or severe (>15 mg/dL). The causes of hypercalcemia are listed in Table 40–15 and can be categorized as either increased gut absorption or increased bone resorption.

TABLE 40–15. Etiology and Clinical Manifestations of Hypercalcemia

Etiology	Clinical Findings
Malignancy	Cardiovascular
Breast	Positive inotropic effects
Lung	Increased myocardial
Multiple myeloma	contractility
Lymphoma	Decreased heart rate
Renal	Shortened systolic time
	interval
Granulomatous disorders	Shortened ventricular
	ejection time
Endocrine disorders	Conduction abnormalities
Primary	Shortened Q–T interval
hyperparathyroidism	Widened T wave
Thyrotoxicosis	Metastatic calcifications in
Acromegaly	cardiovascular system
	Gastrointestinal
Immobilization	Anorexia
	Nausea, vomiting
Milk-alkali syndrome	Constipation
Excess vitamin D	Renal
Thiazide diuretic	Acute renal insufficiency
administration	Nephrolithiasis
Renal failure	Metastatic calcifications
	Neurologic
	Confusion
	Stupor
	Coma

The two most common causes of hypercalcemia are malignancy and hyperparathyroidism. The incidence in each category may differ as a function of age, with malignancy a more common cause in the older patient. Bony metastatic lesions are thought to be responsible for most cases of malignancy-related hypercalcemia. The major types of primary malignancy associated with bony metastases and hypercalcemia are breast and lung cancer, multiple myeloma, lymphoma, and renal cell carcinoma. Granulomatous disorders such as sarcoidosis, tuberculosis, histoplasmosis, and coccidioidomycosis can also produce hypercalcemia.

Primary hyperparathyroidism is a major cause of hypercalcemia. The pathogenesis of this disorder remains unknown, although many patients have a past history of head and neck radiation. Primary hyperparathyroidism may also occur in conjunction with a more generalized syndrome of tumors in various endocrine organs (Rosai et al., 1972). Hypercalcemia may occasionally occur in the presence of endocrine disturbances such as hyperthyroidism, acromegaly, and adrenal insufficiency. Prolonged immobilization, particularly following severe trauma with multiple fractures or spinal cord injury with paralysis, may lead to an increase in bone resorption. This heavy load of Ca exceeds the kidney's regulatory capacity, resulting in hypercalcemia.

Patients with a markedly increased intake of Ca through milk products and antacids for ulcer therapy may exhibit hypercalcemia. Preexisting renal failure is a necessary prerequisite for this mechanism to produce hypercalcemia. The role of alkalosis due to ingested antacids may also be a cofactor because it promotes renal reabsorption of Ca. Vitamin D intoxication will lead to increased intestinal absorption of calcium as well as bone resorption, and hypercalcemia may be a consequence.

Administration of thiazide diuretics may be associated with hypercalcemia. This is usually expressed as a transient elevation in serum Ca, which reflects volume contraction and increased plasma protein as a result of hemoconcentration. If these drugs are used in patients with coexisting disease processes, which tend to increase serum Ca values, significant hypercalcemia may result.

Recovery of renal function via transplantation has been associated with hypercalcemia, probably because the prolonged hypocalcemia that occurs during chronic renal failure often leads to secondary hyperparathyroidism. With successful renal transplantation, it takes a variable period of time for the body to reset PTH secretion.

Hypercalcemia is also seen during the diuretic phase of acute renal failure. The exact mechanism is not known but may be correlated with the extent and severity of muscle damage associated with rhabdomyolysis (Grossman et al., 1974).

Acute hypercalcemic crisis may produce acute renal failure and a markedly depressed sensorium, a situation that represents a medical emergency. In general, hypercalcemia causes decreased neuromuscular excitability or muscle hypotonicity. The various clinical manifestations associated with hypercalcemia are shown in Table 40–15. The cardiac changes are the most specific indicator of hypercalcemia; both contractility and conduction changes are observed. Shortening of the Q–T interval is considered the most characteristic sign of hypercalcemia; however, it is not present in all hypercalcemic patients. In hypercalcemic crisis, the S and T waves merge. Other dysrhythmias associated with hypercalcemia include varying degrees of heart block and cardiac arrest (Parfitt and Kleerkoper, 1980). Hypercalcemia also increases the patient's susceptibility to digitalis toxicity.

Renal tubular nephropathy is a relatively common occurrence and is related to the degree of serum calcium elevation. Calcification of cellular debris within the renal tubules leads to tubular obstruction and renal failure. This renal damage is frequently reversed when therapy is initiated. Renal stone formation may occur in patients with chronic hypercalcemic states such as hyperparathyroidism.

Widespread soft tissue calcification can be a serious complication of chronic hypercalcemia. Calcifications are more common in the presence of hyperphosphatemia and chronic renal failure.

Management of Hypercalcemia. A serum Ca level of greater than 15 mg/dL combined with stupor or coma represents a hypercalcemic crisis and requires prompt treatment. Management efforts are directed toward determining the underlying cause of the hypercalcemia and instituting therapy to lower the serum calcium level. Diagnostic efforts to identify hyperparathyroidism include measurement of immunoreactive PTH levels. The presence of an elevated PTH level tends to support hyperparathyroidism as the cause. A history of neoplastic disease is an important clue to the presence of malignancy-associated hypercalcemia.

In moderate or severe hypercalcemia, prompt reduction of serum Ca is essential. The most important factor in treating hypercalcemia is to ensure adequate hydration (Carroll and Oh, 1989). Most patients with severe hypercalcemia are dehydrated as a result of increased urine volume and sodium diuresis. Rapid volume expansion with intravenous (IV) fluids and concomitant use of loop diuretics such as furosemide will augment urinary excretion of Ca. If renal function is good, 6 to 12 liters of IV fluid can be administered over 24 hours. Usually 0.9% or 0.45% sodium chloride is infused because this solution promotes excretion of both Na and Ca. Dextrose 5% may be used if the patient is hypernatremic or has congestive heart failure. Intravenous administration of furosemide every 4 to 6 hours will prevent fluid volume overload (Carroll and Oh, 1989). If diuresis is sustained over a long interval, Mg replacement may be necessary.

Reduction of bone resorption can be achieved through administration of pharmaceutical agents.

Administration of glucocorticoids has been useful in decreasing bone resorption and may also decrease gut absorption of Ca. Mithramycin is a cytotoxic antibiotic that inhibits bone resorption. It has a rapid onset (6 to 12 hours), and its action may be sustained for several days. If therapy is limited in duration, few side effects are seen. With prolonged administration, thrombocytopenia, platelet dysfunction, and nephrotoxicity are seen (Ahr et al., 1978). Calcitonin is also effective in suppressing bone resorption and may act faster than mithramycin. However, the effectiveness may not be as consistent, and drug resistance may occur with continued use (Au, 1975). Side effects of calcitonin are rare, and this may be the agent of choice when renal insufficiency, thrombocytopenia, or congestive heart failure is present.

Intravenous administration of phosphate causes Ca complex formation, which is a rapid method of lowering serum Ca. Unfortunately, this method is associated with significant risk. The complex of Ca and phosphate that is formed is usually deposited at extravascular sites and can result in renal failure or sudden death. Oral phosphate is generally considered a safer approach in patients who are not hyperphosphatemic.

Hemodialysis with a dialysate low in Ca is the most efficient way to correct serum Ca, particularly in patients with renal insufficiency. Severe hypercalcemia from hyperparathyroidism can usually be alleviated by surgery.

Mild hypercalcemia may not require major intervention, such as volume expansion with diuretics or agents inhibiting bone resorption. Alleviation of the underlying process may restore serum Ca to normal or near-normal values without aggressive intervention.

Altered Urinary Elimination and Potential Fluid Volume Excess. Severe hypercalcemia (serum Ca levels of greater than 15 mg/dL accompanied by neurologic or cardiac complications) requires prompt and aggressive treatment. The critical care nurse collaborates in lowering the serum Ca level by administering prescribed fluids and medications. The goals of nursing care include preventing calcium-induced renal insufficiency while maintaining optimal fluid balance.

The primary treatment for severe hypercalcemia is to enhance renal excretion of Ca by administering large volumes of intravenous fluid along with diuretics. The critical care nurse facilitates fluid administration by ensuring that intravenous access is adequate. At least two large-bore IV lines are necessary because fluid administration may need to be as high as 500 mL/hour. Urine volumes are assessed hourly, and careful intake and output records are maintained. The BUN and serum creatinine are monitored for elevations indicating renal tubular damage.

While promoting Ca excretion, the critical care nurse must also assess the patient's cardiovascular response to the large fluid load. The patient's hemodynamic parameters, including CVP, PCWP, blood pressure, heart rate, and cardiac output, are monitored frequently for evidence of impending congestive heart failure. The jugular veins are observed for distention, and the lungs are auscultated for the development of rales or crackles.

Alteration in Cardiac Output. Hypertension is one cardiovascular change that the nurse should anticipate in hypercalcemia. Elevated blood pressure may be partially the result of renal insufficiency; however, it is also seen in patients with normal renal function. It is thought that calcium increases peripheral resistance as well as exerting a positive inotropic effect on the cardiac muscle (Kleerkoper et al., 1978).

Hypercalcemia is also associated with a number of cardiac dysrhythmias that can adversely affect cardiac output. The critical care nurse carefully monitors the patient's electrocardiogram. The P–R, QRS, and Q–T intervals are measured and evaluated for change. If heart block does occur, the nurse evaluates the patient's response by assessing the available hemodynamic parameters as well as the patient's level of consciousness.

Hypercalcemia potentiates the effect of digitalis. The digitalized patient must be carefully observed for signs of digitalis toxicity.

Cardiac standstill may occur at serum Ca levels of greater than 17 mg/dL. The nurse anticipates this emergency by keeping resuscitation equipment and medications readily available.

Phosphate

Phosphorus is one of the principal IC anions and in the body is found as organic and inorganic phosphate salts, the latter form occurring in small amounts in EC water and blood. Normal serum phosphate values range from 2.5 to 4.5 mg/dL, whereas the IC concentration may be as much as 300 mg/dL.

Phosphate plays a number of important roles in the body. It is a structural element of bone. In fact, approximately 85% of total body P is found in bone. Phosphate is the major intracellular anion and plays a role in the metabolism of lipids, carbohydrates, and proteins. As a component of ATP, P is essential to oxidative phosphorylation, the main energy source of muscle tissue. It is also a critical component of 2,3-diphosphoglycerate (2,3-DPG), and is therefore involved in oxygen delivery to peripheral tissues. Phosphate is also a participant in one of the major renal buffering mechanisms controlling acid-base balance in the body.

Phosphate balance is maintained by dietary intake and by urinary and gastrointestinal losses. Protein is a significant source of phosphorus, particularly dairy products. There is little direct regulation of gastrointestinal absorption, so the major influence on body P content is the kidney. Renal excretion of P is influenced by the plasma P concentration and by PTH. Under normal circumstances, as plasma P rises, renal excretion increases. PTH also increases phosphate excretion by the kidney and is accepted as the major factor controlling renal excretion of P. PTH as well as vitamin D–1,25 shifts P from bone to EC water as a consequence of calcium homeostatic mechanisms (Carroll and Oh, 1989). Because the EC concentration is so small, a shift of phosphate across the cell membrane can have a significant effect on EC concentration. Acid-base disturbances also affect the transcellular distribution of P.

HYPOPHOSPHATEMIA

Hypophosphatemia can occur as a consequence of the events described in Table 40–16. Serum P concentrations of less than 1.0 mg/dL are classified as profound hypophosphatemia. Reduced intake alone is rarely the reason for hypophosphatemia of this magnitude because renal excretion can compensate for low intake. Phosphate-binding antacids, e.g., aluminum hydroxide, bind with P in the gut to decrease absorption and force elimination through the gastrointestinal tract. Vitamin D–1,25 deficiency results in decreased gastrointestinal absorption of P and causes some renal tubular dysfunction, which impairs P reabsorption. In addition, lack of vitamin D retards movement of P from bone to the EC. Malabsorption due to gastrointestinal disease may produce hypophosphatemia. This clinical problem causes a decrease in both vitamin D and Ca absorption and leads to secondary hyperparathyroidism, which in turn leads to increased renal excretion of phosphate.

Increased renal excretion of phosphate can be the consequence of either intrarenal or extrarenal mechanisms. Fanconi syndrome and vitamin D-resistant rickets are intrinsic renal disorders that produce tubular transport abnormalities. Extrarenal factors that promote renal wasting of P include hyperparathyroidism, glucosuria, some diuretics, and acute expansion of EC volume. Hyperparathyroidism, either primary or secondary, causes a decrease in renal tubular reabsorption of P. Glucosuria (e.g., in diabetic ketoacidosis) produces an osmotic diuresis that also limits P reabsorption in the kidney. Acute EC volume expansion increases urine flow through the renal tubules, thereby decreasing P reabsorption. Factors that may promote a redistribution of P from the EC to the IC include respiratory alkalosis, glucose infusion, and insulin administration. Hypophosphatemia associated with acute alkalosis is the result of rapid movement of H^+ from the intracellular space. The cellular response is to increase glycolysis, which results in a shift of P from the EC into the IC (Parfitt and Kleerekoper, 1980). Critically ill patients who are at risk of developing hypophosphatemia from acute alkalosis include those with heat stroke, acute salicylate poisoning, alcohol withdrawal, and thyrotoxicosis (Metheny, 1987).

Administration of intravenous glucose may be the most common cause of hypophosphatemia in hospitalized patients (Betro and Pain, 1972). Administration of glucose, along with endogenous or exogenous insulin, facilitates the transport of both glucose and P into skeletal muscle and liver cells. This response may be particularly severe in the malnourished alcoholic patient. Another common cause of hypophosphatemia in critical care patients is the administration of hyperalimentation (TPN) without an adequate P content (Metheny, 1987).

Phosphate is an ubiquitous electrolyte; a deficiency in serum or body stores is reflected in multisystem abnormalities. The two primary mechanisms through which cellular processes are disturbed by hypophosphatemia are (1) impairment of cellular synthesis of ATP, and (2) decreased amount of red cell 2,3-DPG, which adversely affects oxygen release in the tissues. Thus, energy for cell functions and processes is reduced. The primary manifestations of hypophosphatemia are shown in Table 40–16 and reflect the disordered cellular functions that result from hypophosphatemia. Signs and symptoms are usually not present unless severe hypophosphatemia is present (<1.5 mg/dL). The muscular abnormality, associated with ATP depletion, may be severe enough to compromise respiratory effort. Myocardial function may also be affected, as manifested by decreased stroke volume and possible development of congestive cardiomyopathy.

A variety of hematologic derangements may occur as a result of hypophosphatemia and may cause significant problems in critically ill patients. Decreased 2,3-DPG levels may result in reduced oxygen delivery to peripheral tissues. Tissue anoxia is manifested by pain and a buildup of lactic acid. Low ATP levels in the erythrocytes leads to RBC fragility and

TABLE 40–16. Etiology and Clinical Manifestations of Hypophosphatemia

Etiology	Clinical Findings
Decreased P intake	Neurologic
Anorexia, starvation	Confusion
Vomiting	Irritability
	Obtundation
Decreased gastrointestinal	Seizures
absorption	Coma
Phosphate-binding antacids	
Vitamin D deficiency	Musculoskeletal
Malabsorption syndromes	Myopathy
Diarrhea	Weakness
	Bone pain
Increased renal P excretion	Bone resorption
Hyperparathyroidism	
Osmotic diuresis (drug-induced	Hematopoietic
or diabetic ketoacidosis)	Hemolysis
Metabolic acidosis	Platelet dysfunction
	Impaired resistance to
Transcellular redistribution	infection
Acute respiratory alkalosis	
Glucose infusion	
Insulin administration	
Total parenteral nutrition without	
phosphate	
Rapid anabolism	

hemolytic anemia. Impaired leukocyte function places the patient at increased risk of infection.

Bone resorption and development of bone disease are associated with total body phosphate depletion. With erosion of the skeleton, Ca and Mg will also be released, resulting in increased Ca and Mg excretion by the kidney.

Management of Hypophosphatemia. Management of hypophosphatemia includes identification of the etiology and repletion of P stores. If possible, the underlying cause of hypophosphatemia should be identified and corrected. Urinary P concentration may be helpful in determining the cause. A high urinary P concentration in the presence of low serum P levels indicates an intrinsic renal disturbance or elevated PTH secretion. If urinary losses are in accord with the measured serum P, then problems with gastrointestinal absorption or EC distribution are the likely cause. Phosphate administration may not be necessary if the underlying problem is corrected.

The presence of severe neurologic or muscle disturbances necessitates P supplementation. As with hypocalcemia, IV administration of P may lead to soft tissue deposition of calcium-phosphate complexes. Oral administration is less likely to lead to untoward effects. However, IV administration of P may be the only route available in the critically ill patient. Intravenous P must be diluted and administered slowly. Careful monitoring of the patient as well as serial serum P measurements is necessary. Regardless of the route of administration, P repletion is usually continued only until the serum P reaches 2.5 to 3.0 mg/dL. Rapid elevation of the serum P level can result in hypocalcemia.

Impaired Breathing Pattern. When caring for the hypophosphatemic patient, the critical care nurse must keep in mind that the pathologic manifestations result from decreased levels of ATP and 2,3-DPG. Particular attention must be paid to problems associated with muscle weakness and those related to diminished peripheral tissue oxygenation.

Weakness of the muscles of respiration is a particular nursing concern in the hypophosphatemic patient. The nurse assesses the patient for changes in muscle strength. Hand-grasp strength can be tested to determine general muscle strength. More specifically, changes in the patient's speech may be indicative of muscle weakness (Metheny, 1987). Particular attention is paid to assessment of muscle strength in patients with chronic obstructive pulmonary disease (COPD) who utilize accessory breathing muscles. The nurse should carefully monitor the rate and quality of respirations in these patients. Changes in the patient's sensorium are evaluated in light of the potential for hypoventilation. Arterial blood gases are monitored for a rising $PaCO_2$.

The hypophosphatemic patient may lack sufficient respiratory muscle strength to be weaned from mechanical ventilation. Repletion of the serum P and careful evaluation of respiratory muscle function should be done prior to weaning and extubation.

Decreased Peripheral Tissue Perfusion. The decrease in 2,3-DPG results in peripheral tissue anoxia. This condition is manifested by muscle weakness, fatigue, and pain. The skin and muscles may be very tender to the touch. The patient may complain of extreme fatigue and muscle pain resulting from such nursing care activities as turning, range of motion exercises, and transferring from bed to chair.

Nursing goals are to reduce the oxygen requirements of peripheral tissues and promote the patient's comfort. The patient's physical activity is reduced to the level of the essential. Adequate rest periods are scheduled. Comfort measures, including patient positioning and analgesics, are administered. These interventions may need to continue for several days following serum P repletion because the clinical manifestations of severe hypophosphatemia do not immediately resolve.

HYPERPHOSPHATEMIA

Hyperphosphatemia (P> 4.5 mg/dL) represents a breakdown in the normal regulatory process, either through an acute increase in EC phosphate concentration or as a consequence of renal dysfunction. The causes of hyperphosphatemia are listed in Table 40–17. Oral intake of P is unlikely to produce elevation of the serum P because the kidney quickly responds by decreasing P reabsorption. The chronic use of phosphate-containing laxatives or administration of phosphate enemas in a susceptible individual may produce hyperphosphatemia. Severely injured patients may be at risk of hyperphosphatemia. Rhabdomyolysis liberates a large amount of P into the EC fluid, and if renal failure is present, marked serum P elevation may occur. Cytotoxic drugs, which are used to treat leukemia, may cause hyperphosphatemia as a result of cell lysis. These clinical situations reflect a shift of P from the IC to the EC compartment rather than an increase in total P load. Acidosis also encourages a transcellular shift of P. Phosphate ions are released from the cell as a result of tissue hypoxia and ATP degradation (O'Connor et al., 1977).

TABLE 40–17. Etiology and Clinical Manifestations of Hyperphosphatemia

Etiology	Clinical Findings
Increased P load	Neuromuscular
Phosphate enemas	Tetany
Oral phosphate	Seizures
supplementation	Muscle cramps
Rhabdomyolysis	Weakness
Cytotoxic drugs	
	Cardiovascular
Decreased P excretion	Hypotension
Hypoparathyroidism	Shortened Q–T interval
Renal insufficiency	
	Neurologic/cognitive
	Cognitive impairment
	Affective disorders

Decreased renal excretion of P is most often the result of hypoparathyroidism. This hormonal disorder is characterized by elevated serum P, hypocalcemia, and chronic tetany. PTH levels are usually depressed but may be elevated if tissue resistance to the hormone is present. Hypoparathyroidism may occur following neck surgery, most commonly for removal of the parathyroid glands or the thyroid.

Renal insufficiency leads to reduced renal excretion of P. In chronic renal failure, hyperphosphatemia tends to occur after 75% of renal function has been lost. Patients with acute renal failure may have more severe episodes of hyperphosphatemia, possibly related to the cause of the acute renal failure, e.g., rhabdomyolysis, in concert with decreased renal excretion. Fortunately, hyperphosphatemia quickly resolves once renal function returns.

The clinical manifestations of hyperphosphatemia are related to the hypocalcemia that frequently accompanies this disorder. Signs and symptoms are more likely to occur when the increase in serum P occurs rapidly. Soft tissue calcifications occur when the Ca × P product exceeds 70 (Brautbar, 1984). Calcium-phosphate complex deposition most commonly occurs in the aorta, kidneys, lungs, conjunctiva, and skin. Such deposits may produce other clinical complications such as hypoxia and renal failure.

Management of Hyperphosphatemia. Treatment of hyperphosphatemia is directed toward correction of the underlying pathophysiologic mechanisms and removal of P from the circulation. Phosphate can be removed by dietary restriction of P intake, and the use of phosphate binders to bind intestinal P. In the critically ill patient these methods may not be appropriate. Acute dialysis is often the best method of lowering serum P levels in the critically ill patient.

Careful and judicious monitoring of serum P during the treatment of *hypo*phosphatemia can help to avoid *hyper*phosphatemia. Maintaining adequate urine volumes through the use of IV fluids and diuretics is helpful in preventing hyperphosphatemia in patients at risk.

Impaired Tissue Integrity. Because serum P and Ca have a reciprocal relationship, hyperphosphatemia is often associated with hypocalcemia. For this reason, the nursing assessments and interventions described for the hypocalcemic patient are also appropriate for the patient with elevated serum P. The critical care nurse is concerned with assessing soft tissue calcification and maintaining tissue integrity.

Pruritus is frequently associated with Ca-P deposition in the skin. This may represent a significant problem in the already compromised integument of the critically ill patient. Uncontrolled patient scratching may lead to skin breakdown and infection. The nurse observes for signs of scratching and inspects the skin for areas of breakdown.

A variety of skin care protocols are available to promote patient comfort and protect skin integrity.

The patient's fingernails should be clipped short. If pruitus is particularly severe, sedation may be helpful.

Magnesium

Magnesium is an abundant intracellular cation, although the normal serum concentration is only 1.5 to 2.5 mEq/liter (1.6 to 2.2 mg/dL). Sixty of per cent total body Mg is found in the bone, which serves as a source for exchange with the plasma. Fifty-five to sixty per cent of the plasma Mg is in the ionized form, which is the physiologically active fraction. Seventeen per cent is complexed with other compounds such as citrate, phosphate, and bicarbonate. The remaining 25% is protein bound, primarily to albumin. This fraction varies directly with plasma protein concentration.

Magnesium is an important element of bone structure. It also functions as a cofactor in cellular enzyme systems. Magnesium has a direct effect on the neuromuscular junction and therefore plays a role in neuromuscular irritability and muscle contraction.

Magnesium is found in many foods, vegetables and cereals being the primary dietary source. The major site of gastrointestinal absorption is the small intestine. A number of factors influence intestinal absorption, including availability of Na and water, lactose, and, most importantly, Mg concentration in the body. There appears to be an inverse relationship between Mg absorption and the amount of Mg ingested (Levine et al., 1980). Magnesium absorption in the gut is at least partially stimulated by vitamin D and PTH (Carroll and Oh, 1989).

Gastrointestinal loss of Mg cannot be reduced to zero in the face of low intake, nor is there a protective mechanism to decrease gastrointestinal absorption with very large Mg loads. The kidney is responsible for blunting low Mg intake by decreasing renal Mg losses. Despite renal conservation, hypomagnesemia may occur as a result of continued gastrointestinal loss.

The kidney is quite effective in increasing renal excretion of Mg when serum Mg is elevated. Renal excretion of Mg is primarily regulated by the plasma Mg level. Renal regulation is also partially under the control of PTH, vitamin D, and thyrocalcitonin. The action of these hormones on Mg excretion appears to be a consequence of their role in calcium regulation. Any clinical disorder that increases urine volume results in increased renal excretion of Mg.

HYPOMAGNESEMIA

A serum Mg concentration of less than 1.6 mg/dL is classified as hypomagnesemia, although the serum level is not always a good indicator of total body Mg. Significant symptoms usually are apparent at serum Mg levels of less than 1.0 mg/dL.

The primary causes of hypomagnesemia are shown

in Table 40–18 and are classified into three categories: (1) decreased intake/absorption, (2) increased renal losses, and (3) redistribution into the IC compartment. Diminished intake is a common cause of hypomagnesemia in critically ill patients. Prolonged periods of use of magnesium-poor parenteral nutrition (TPN) may lead to Mg depletion. Malabsorptive states including diarrhea can interfere with gastrointestinal absorption of Mg. Large amounts of gastric or biliary fluid losses postoperatively have been demonstrated to result in hypomagnesemia (Vallee et al., 1960). Chronic ingestion of large amounts of alcohol also produces hypomagnesemia. Poor nutrition is the major cause of hypomagnesemia in alcoholic patients. Chronic alcohol intake also results in impaired gastrointestinal absorption of Mg and increased renal excretion (McCollister et al., 1960; Metheny, 1987).

Increased renal loss of Mg is a frequent cause of hypomagnesemia. Renal losses of Mg may be induced by a variety of pharmacologic and pathologic states. Loop or thiazide diuretics inhibit reabsorption of Mg, and continued use of these agents risks total body Mg depletion. Digitalis preparations also reduce renal Mg reabsorption, placing the patient at risk of hypomagnesemia-related digitalis toxicity (Iseri et al., 1975). Administration of carbenicillin and gentamicin may lead to hypomagnesemia, although the exact mechanism is unknown (Patel and Savage, 1979).

TABLE 40–18. Etiology and Clinical Manifestations of Hypomagnesemia

Etiology	Clinical Findings
Decreased intake/reabsorption	Neuromuscular
Protein-calorie malnutrition	Vertigo
Prolonged NPO status	Ataxia
Mg-free parenteral nutrition	Nystagmus
Malabsorption	Athetoid and choreiform
Diarrhea	movements
	Muscle tremors
Increased renal Mg Losses	Weakness
Pharmacologic agents	Hyperreflexia
Alcohol	Tetany with Chvostek sign
Diuretics	Muscle cramps
Cardiac glycosides	Seizures
Aminoglycosides	
Cisplatin	Cardiac
Diuretic phase of acute renal	Tachycardia
failure	Increased Q–T interval
Metabolic disturbances	Decreased S–T segment
Diabetic ketoacidosis	
Hypercalcemia	
Metabolic disturbances	
Hyperparathyroidism	
Hyperaldosteronism	
Redistribution to intracellular compartment	
Recovery from severe bone disease	
Acute hemorrhagic pancreatitis	
Recovery from protein-calorie malnutrition	

Excessive urinary loss of Mg can occur in patients with metabolic disturbances such as diabetic ketoacidosis (DKA). In DKA the accompanying osmotic diuresis contributes to the loss of Mg. The diuretic phase of recovery from acute renal failure can also produce renal Mg wasting.

Hormonal disturbances may produce hypomagnesemia. These disorders include hyperaldosteronism and hyperparathyroidism. Hyperparathyroidism is associated with hypercalcemia, which also increases renal Mg losses.

Redistribution of Mg to the IC compartment is seen with rapid restoration of bone following treatment of hyperparathyroidism. Acute hemorrhagic pancreatitis may lead to Mg deposition in tissue and may produce hypomagnesemia. During the recovery period of protein-calorie malnutrition, hypomagnesemia occurs as a result of rapid incorporation of Mg into regenerating cells. In critical care, this is commonly seen in the alcoholic patient (Metheny, 1987).

Clinical manifestations of hypomagnesemia are primarily observed in the neuromuscular and cardiac systems. These signs and symptoms are described in Table 40–18. The clinical picture may be complicated by the presence of other abnormalities such as renal potassium-wasting, producing hypokalemia. Hypocalcemia results from the impaired PTH secretion or action present in hypomagnesemia.

Management of Hypomagnesemia. The severity of the signs and symptoms will guide the treatment of hypomagnesemia. Treatment will include correction of the underlying disorder as well as Mg repletion. The presence of renal impairment influences management strategies because Mg repletion must be done with great caution in patients with renal insufficiency. Mild hypomagnesemia is treated by oral Mg replacement or by increasing the Mg content of parenteral nutrition infusions. Severe symptomatic hypomagnesemia requires parenteral administration of Mg. Dosage of intravenous Mg will depend on the severity of symptoms. In the presence of convulsions, a bolus loading dose of 500 mg is administered. An infusion of up to 3 mEq/kg of body weight is then administered over a 4-hour period. Less severe hypomagnesemia is treated with 0.5 to 1.25 mEq/kg body weight (Carroll and Oh, 1989). These suggested dosages should be administered only to patients with normal renal function. If renal insufficiency exists, the dose must be decreased. The patient's serum Mg concentration must be measured frequently to prevent hypermagenesemia. In hypomagnesemia associated with chronic states such as malabsorption, continued Mg supplementation may be necessary.

The clinical manifestations of hypomagnesemia are very similar to those of hypocalcemia. Major problems include irritability of the central nervous system with possible development of seizures, and the potential for laryngospasm and airway obstruction. Appropriate nursing assessments and interventions are discussed under hypocalcemia.

Potential for Injury. Up to this point, the discussion has centered around administration of parenteral Mg to hypomagnesemic patients. The critical care nurse may also be called upon to care for a critically ill obstetric patient receiving parenteral Mg as treatment for preeclampsia. For specifics regarding the care of the obstetric patient, the reader is referred to Chapter 63. Regardless of purpose, the goal of nursing care is to prevent complications during Mg infusion.

Parenteral Mg preparations are available in several concentrations ranging from 10% to 50% solutions. Before administering a loading dose or infusion, the critical care nurse must carefully check the concentration and dosage against the physician's prescription (Metheny, 1987).

Pertinent nursing assessments during Mg infusion include deep tendon reflexes, urine output, blood pressure, respirations, and level of consciousness. Deep tendon reflexes are checked at least hourly during Mg infusion. Patellar reflexes are the most commonly assessed; however, antecubital reflexes can also be used. Reflexes are usually reported on a scale of 1+ to 4+. The nurse observes for a trend toward diminishing reflexes. If deep tendon reflexes are absent, the Mg infusion must be stopped and the physician notified.

Because magnesium is excreted by the kidneys, urinary output is an important nursing assessment. Ideally, urine output should remain at or above 0.5 mL/kg body weight per hour. If urine output falls below this level, deep tendon reflexes must be assessed more frequently.

Blood pressure, pulse, respirations, and level of consciousness are checked at least hourly during Mg infusion. A sudden, significant fall in blood pressure or a decrease in respiratory rate is a sign of magnesium toxicity.

Any sudden or sustained change in deep tendon reflexes, urine output, or vital signs should alert the nurse to the development of Mg toxicity. The infusion must be stopped, and the nurse should prepare for the possible need for emergency resuscitation.

HYPERMAGNESEMIA

Significant hypermagnesemia (>5 mg/dl) rarely occurs in patients with normal renal function. Even in patients with chronic renal insufficiency, the kidney responds by increasing the efficiency of the remaining nephrons, thereby maintaining serum Mg at normal or near-normal levels. The causes of hypermagnesemia are listed in Table 40–19. Salt depletion, volume contraction, and mineralocorticoid deficiency all lead to increased Mg retention by the kidney despite normal body Mg. Significant reduction in thyroid function has also been shown to reduce Mg excretion by the kidney.

Magnesium salts that are administered to treat hypomagnesemia or preeclampsia/eclampsia can increase serum Mg acutely. Injudicious use of magne-

TABLE 40–19. Etiology and Clinical Manifestations of Hypermagnesemia

Etiology	Clinical Findings
Decreased renal excretion	Neuromuscular
Acute/chronic renal failure	Muscle weakness
Salt depletion	Hyporeflexia
Volume depletion	
Mineralocorticoid deficiency	Cardiovascular
Hypothyroidism	Increased P–R interval
	Increased QRS complex
Increased exogenous Mg load	Increased Q–T interval
Magnesium salts in diet or	Complete heart block
parenteral nutrition	Cardiac arrest
Magnesium-containing antacids	Hypotension
or laxatives	
Magnesium-containing enemas	
High magnesium dialysate	
Increased endogenous Mg load	
Burns	
Traumatic soft tissue injury	
Rhabdomyolysis	

sium containing laxatives and antacids may provide a sizable intake of Mg; these agents are particularly problematic in patients with diminished renal function. Hypermagnesemia may also result from liberation of Mg from the muscle cells. Clinical examples of the latter include rhabdomyolysis following crush injuries or soft tissue trauma and severe burns. When renal function is normal, the increase in serum Mg should be transient. Unfortunately, many of these severely injured patients also develop acute renal failure and are then unable to excrete the high Mg load.

Significant hypermagnesemia is associated with a variety of signs and symptoms, as listed in Table 40–19. Nonspecific nausea and vomiting may be the earliest symptoms of hypermagnesemia. Muscle weakness is also an early symptom. At serum Mg levels of 3 to 5 mg/dL, peripheral vasodilation occurs. This may result in significant hypotension. Hyporeflexia in deep tendons may be seen when serum Mg approaches 7 mg/dL. Respiratory paralysis occurs when the serum Mg exceeds 8 mg/dL. Intracardiac conduction defects are varied and will adversely affect cardiac output. Usually the ECG changes of prolonged P–R and QRS intervals are not seen until the serum magnesium level is above 15 mEq/liter (Zuspan and Zuspan, 1981).

Management of Hypermagnesemia. In patients with normal renal function, withdrawal of the exogenous source of Mg may be sufficient to lower serum Mg to near-normal levels. In patients with renal failure, hemodialysis or peritoneal dialysis is the most effective way to remove excess Mg from the body.

Patients with severe neuromuscular or cardiac symptoms may require additional support until serum Mg is corrected. Intravenous administration of Ca is the emergency treatment for hypermagnesemia in the presence of life-threatening symptoms. A dose of 10 mL of 10% calcium gluconate is administered slowly over a few minutes. Glucose and insulin can also be administered to facilitate the temporary intracellular movement of Mg (Au and Lee, 1984). Forced diuresis with large volumes of intravenous saline solutions can also be used in patients with normal renal function.

Decreased Tissue Perfusion. The critically ill patient with hypermagnesemia is at risk for several life-threatening complications. The goals of nursing care include early recognition and response to the development of neuromuscular complications.

Peripheral vasodilation occurs at Mg levels of more than 3 mg/dL, resulting in hypotension and decreased tissue perfusion. The nurse assesses the blood pressure and heart rate for change. The level of consciousness and urine output are monitored, and these measurements are used to evaluate the patient's response to blood pressure changes. Symptomatic patients may be placed in the head-down position to facilitate blood flow to the core. Volume expansion with intravenous fluids may be helpful in stabilizing the blood pressure.

Impaired Breathing Pattern. Paralysis of respiratory muscles followed by respiratory arrest is a life-threatening complication in patients with hypermagnesemia. Pertinent nursing assessments include monitoring muscle strength and respiratory status. Deep tendon reflexes, grasp strength, and head lift are all measures of muscle strength that can be utilized to assess the extent of neuromuscular depression. Respiratory rate, quality, and depth must be carefully monitored for minute changes. Continuous pulse oximetry monitoring, end-tidal carbon dioxide measurements, and arterial blood gas analysis may all be used to detect diminishing ventilation. In addition to ongoing assessment, the nurse prepares for the possibility of emergency intubation and ventilation.

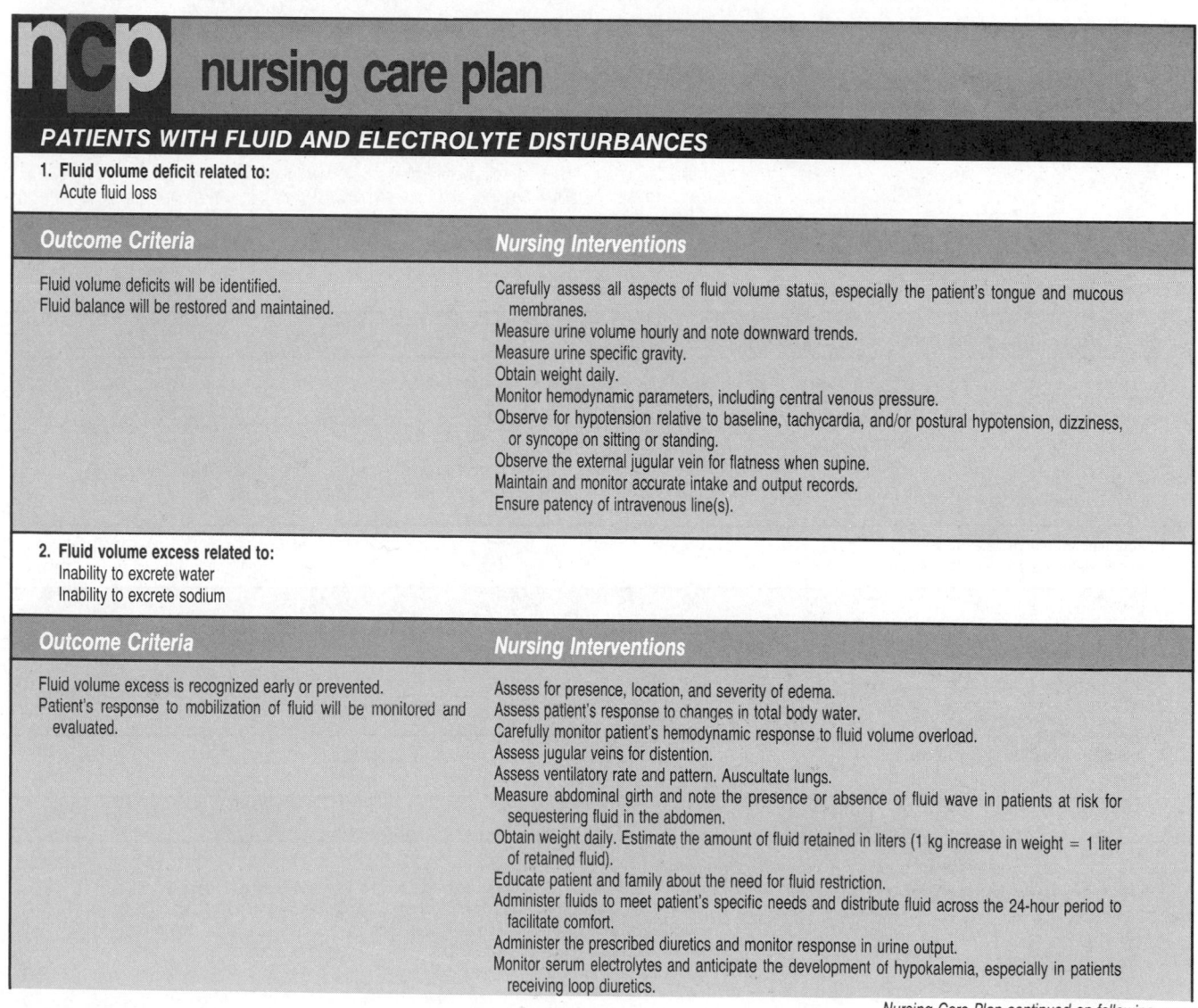

ncp nursing care plan

PATIENTS WITH FLUID AND ELECTROLYTE DISTURBANCES

1. Fluid volume deficit related to:
Acute fluid loss

Outcome Criteria	Nursing Interventions
Fluid volume deficits will be identified. Fluid balance will be restored and maintained.	Carefully assess all aspects of fluid volume status, especially the patient's tongue and mucous membranes. Measure urine volume hourly and note downward trends. Measure urine specific gravity. Obtain weight daily. Monitor hemodynamic parameters, including central venous pressure. Observe for hypotension relative to baseline, tachycardia, and/or postural hypotension, dizziness, or syncope on sitting or standing. Observe the external jugular vein for flatness when supine. Maintain and monitor accurate intake and output records. Ensure patency of intravenous line(s).

2. Fluid volume excess related to:
Inability to excrete water
Inability to excrete sodium

Outcome Criteria	Nursing Interventions
Fluid volume excess is recognized early or prevented. Patient's response to mobilization of fluid will be monitored and evaluated.	Assess for presence, location, and severity of edema. Assess patient's response to changes in total body water. Carefully monitor patient's hemodynamic response to fluid volume overload. Assess jugular veins for distention. Assess ventilatory rate and pattern. Auscultate lungs. Measure abdominal girth and note the presence or absence of fluid wave in patients at risk for sequestering fluid in the abdomen. Obtain weight daily. Estimate the amount of fluid retained in liters (1 kg increase in weight = 1 liter of retained fluid). Educate patient and family about the need for fluid restriction. Administer fluids to meet patient's specific needs and distribute fluid across the 24-hour period to facilitate comfort. Administer the prescribed diuretics and monitor response in urine output. Monitor serum electrolytes and anticipate the development of hypokalemia, especially in patients receiving loop diuretics.

Nursing Care Plan continued on following page

3. Impaired skin integrity related to:
   Fluid overload

Outcome Criteria	Nursing Interventions
Skin will remain intact.	Frequently assess skin in edematous areas. Relieve pressure areas as needed.

4. Potential for injury related to:
   Central nervous system alterations due to hyponatremia

Outcome Criteria	Nursing Interventions
Decreased plasma sodium will be detected early. Injury will be prevented.	Carefully assess patient's level of consciousness and level of response. Structure the bedside environment to prevent injury to the lethargic or somnolent patient. Ensure suction or other equipment is available to maintain a patent airway in the vomiting patient. Closely monitor the patient's sodium levels following acute water ingestion. Anticipate the need for administration of hypertonic saline solutions. Initiate seizure precautions.

5. Potential for injury related to:
   Central nervous system alterations secondary to hypernatremia

Outcome Criteria	Nursing Interventions
Patient will have a gradual reduction of plasma sodium. Patient injury will be prevented.	Assess for signs of CNS irritability. Assess for patient's level of consciousness frequently. Provide a quiet, calm environment. Institute protective measures, such as bedrail padding, if patient is restless and thrashing. Institute seizure precautions in patients with significant hypernatremia. Carefully review serial plasma sodium measurements and evaluate the patient's response to the hypotonic infusion. Monitor the infusion closely to avoid overhydration and too rapid a reduction in sodium. Teach patient and family members about the causes and early signs of hyponatremia and hypernatremia.

6. Alteration in cardiac output related to:
   Impaired cardiac muscle secondary to hypokalemia

Outcome Criteria	Nursing Interventions
Patient will not experience a decrease in cardiac output.	Assess patient for signs and symptoms of decreased cardiac output and the development of congestive heart failure. Monitor serum K levels and confer with the physician regarding withholding or reducing the dose of digitalis. Observe the ECG for changes indicative of hypokalemia, particularly during intravenous K repletion. Keep emergency resuscitation equipment readily available in case cardiac arrest occurs.

7. Potential for injury related to:
   Muscle weakness and vascular irritation

Outcome Criteria	Nursing Interventions
Patient will be free from injury.	Assess patient's muscle strength and provide appropriate support during activities such as transfers. If a peripheral site is used for intravenous K repletion, infuse lower concentrations through two sites.

8. Alteration in cardiac output related to:
   Dysrhythmias secondary to hyperkalemia

Outcome Criteria	Nursing Interventions
Patient's cardiac status will be monitored and supported. Therapies designed to reduce plasma K levels will be administered.	Carefully monitor ECG before and during treatment. Observe ECG for peaked T waves, shortened Q–T intervals, and prolonged P–R interval. Obtain plasma K measurements following administration of prescribed medications and fluids. Anticipate the return of hyperkalemia in several hours if bicarbonate, glucose, and insulin are used. Maintain adequate intravenous access and monitor medication infusions carefully. Maintain at least two intravenous lines for emergency drug therapy.

9. Potential for injury related to:
Seizures or airway obstruction secondary to hypocalcemia

Outcome Criteria	Nursing Interventions
Injury will be prevented.	Assess the patient for signs and symptoms of neuromuscular irritability, including complaints of numbness or tingling in the digits, muscle cramps, and the presence of Chvostek or Trousseau signs. Observe the patient for changes in mentation, mood, and memory. Institute seizure precautions if hypocalcemia is severe or if patient demonstrates neuromuscular irritability. Carefully monitor ECG for the onset of ventricular irritability or heart block and stop infusion immediately if either are present.

10. Impaired breathing pattern related to:
Laryngospasm, airway obstruction, and respiratory arrest secondary to hypocalcemia

Outcome Criteria	Nursing Interventions
Life-threatening airway emergencies will be prevented.	Carefully assess patient's airway status for evidence of spasm or obstruction. Observe patient for restlessness, tachypnea, and subtle arterial blood gas changes. Observe for later signs of inspiratory stridor, hoarseness, and decreased air movement. Prepare for the possibility of airway obstruction by assembling emergency airway equipment and prepare for possible intubation.

11. Altered urinary elimination and potential fluid volume excess related to:
Hypercalcemia

Outcome Criteria	Nursing Interventions
Calcium-induced renal insufficiency will be prevented. Optimal fluid balance will be maintained.	Ensure at least two large-bore IV lines are maintained. Assess urine volumes hourly and maintain careful intake and output records. Monitor the BUN and serum creatinine for elevations. Assess patient's response to the large fluid load. Frequently monitor patient's hemodynamic parameters for evidence of impending CHF. Observe for jugular vein distention and auscultate lungs for rales or crackles.

12. Alteration in cardiac output related to:
Hypertension, dysrhythmias, and/or arrest secondary to hypercalcemia

Outcome Criteria	Nursing Interventions
Patient's blood pressure will remain within baseline levels. Patient will experience no significant dysrhythmias. Cardiac arrest will be prevented.	Carefully monitor the patient's ECG for P–R, QRS, and Q–T changes. If heart block occurs, evaluate the patient's response by assessing the available hemodynamic parameters as well as the patient's level of consciousness. Carefully observe the digitalized patient for signs of digitalis toxicity. Anticipate the possibility of cardiac standstill by having resuscitation equipment and medications readily available.

13. Impaired breathing pattern related to:
Weakened respiratory muscles and diminished peripheral tissue oxygenation secondary to hypophosphatemia

Outcome Criteria	Nursing Interventions
Patient will not experience hypoxemic episodes. Oxygen requirements of peripheral tissues will be reduced. Patient will experience optimal comfort.	Assess for changes in muscle strength, including changes in speech. In patients with COPD, pay particular attention to changes in muscle strength and note the rate and quality of respirations. Monitor for changes in the patient's sensorium. Monitor arterial blood gases for a rising Pa_{CO_2}. Replace serum P and carefully evaluate respiratory muscle function prior to weaning and extubation. Reduce patient's physical activities to only those that are essential. Provide adequate periods of rest. Provide comfort measures, including positioning and the administration of analgesics for several days following serum P repletion.

Nursing Care Plan continued on following page

14. Impaired tissue integrity related to:
Hyperphosphatemia

Outcome Criteria	Nursing Interventions
Patient's skin will remain intact.	Assess soft tissue calcification. Observe for signs for scratching and inspect skin for areas of breakdown. Implement a skin care protocol to promote patient comfort and protect skin integrity. Clip patient's fingernails. Consider sedation if pruritus is particularly severe.

15. Potential for injury related to:
Hypomagnesemia

Outcome Criteria	Nursing Interventions
Complications during magnesium infusion will be prevented.	Carefully check the concentration and dosage of magnesium prior to administering the loading dose or infusion. Assess deep tendon reflexes at least hourly during infusion and monitor for a trend toward diminishing reflexes. Stop the infusion and notify the physician if deep tendon reflexes are absent. Monitor urine output, blood pressure, respirations, and level of consciousness during infusion and stop infusion for any sudden or sustained change.

16. Decreased tissue perfusion related to:
Hypermagnesemia

Outcome Criteria	Nursing Interventions
Neuromuscular complications will be prevented.	Assess the blood pressure and heart rate. Monitor level of consciousness and urine output. Place symptomatic patients in head-down position to facilitate blood flow. Consider volume expansion with intravenous fluids to stabilize blood pressure.

17. Impaired breathing pattern related to:
Paralysis of respiratory muscles secondary to hypermagnesemia

Outcome Criteria	Nursing Interventions
Respiratory complications will be prevented.	Monitor muscle strength, including deep tendon reflexes, grasp strength, and head lift. Monitor respiratory rate, quality, and depth for minute changes. Consider the use of pulse oximetry, end-tidal CO_2 measurements, and ABGs in detecting diminishing ventilation. Prepare for the possibility of emergency intubation and ventilation.

SUMMARY

Volume, osmolality, and electrolyte disorders are common complications of critical illness or injury. The critically ill patient may manifest one or several of these alterations in the course of his or her illness. The critical care nurse, along with the physician, is responsible for monitoring the patient's fluid volume and electrolyte status. Careful nursing assessment may uncover early manifestations of imbalance. This chapter has presented the etiology, clinical presentation, and management of the common fluid, osmolality, and electrolyte disorders. Appropriate nursing diagnoses and nursing care strategies have been identified.

References

Agus, Z. S., and Goldfarb, S. (1985). Calcium metabolism: Normal and abnormal. In A.I., Arieff and A.D. DeFronzo (Eds.), *Fluid, electrolye and acid-base disorders.* New York: Churchill Livingstone.

Ahr, D. J., Scialla, S. J., and Kimball, D. B., Jr. (1978). Acquired platelet dysfunction following mithramycin. *Cancer*, 41, 448–454.

Androgue, H. J., and Madias, N. E. (1981). Changes in plasma potassium concentration during acute acid-base disturbances. *American Journal of Medicine*, 71, 456a–467.

Arieff, A. I., and Schmidt, R. W. (1980). Fluid and electrolyte disorders and the central nervous system. In M.H. Maxwell, and C.R. Kleeman (Eds.), *Clinical disorders of fluid and electrolyte metabolism.* New York: McGraw-Hill.

Au, W. Y. W. (1975). Calcitonin treatment of hypercalcemia due to parathyroid carcinoma: Synergistic effect of prednisone on long-term treatment of hypercalcemia. *Archives of Internal Medicine*, 135, 1594–1597.

Aw, T. C., and Lee, D. B. (1984). Hypomagnesemia and hypermagnesemia. In R. J. Glassock (Ed.), *Current therapy in nephrology and hypertension 1984–1985.* Philadelphia: B.C. Decker.

Betro, W. R., and Pain, R. W. (1972). Hypophosphatemia in a hospital population. *British Medical Journal*, 1, 273–276.

Brautbar, N. (1984). Hypophosphatemia and hyperphosphatemia. In R. J. Glassock (Ed.), *Current therapy in nephrology and hypertension 1984–1985.* Philadelphia: B.C. Decker.

Bronson, W. R., DeVita, V. T., Carbone, P. P., et al. (1966). Pseudohyperkalemia due to release of potassium from white blood cells during clotting. *New England Journal of Medicine*, 274, 369–375.

Burnell, J. M. (1956). The effects in humans of extracellular pH changes on the relationships between serum potassium concentration and intracellular potassium. *Journal of Clinical Investigation*, 35, 935.

Carroll, H. J. and Oh, M. S. (1989). *Water, electrolyte and acid-base metabolism: Diagnosis and management* (2nd ed.). Philadelphia: J.B. Lippincott.

Coester, N., Ellioitt, J. C., and Luft, Y. C. (1973). Plasma electrolytes, pH and ECG during and after exhaustive exercise. *Journal of Applied Physiology*, 34, 677–682.

DeFronzo, R. A. (1980). Hyperkalemia in hyporeninemic hypoaldosteronism. *Kidney International*, 17, 118–134.

Dixon, B. S., and Berl, T. (1984). Hyponatremia. In R. J. Glassock (Ed.), *Current therapy in nephrology and hypertension 1984–1985*. Philadelphia: B.C. Decker.

Goldberger, E. (1986). *A primer of water, electrolytes and acid-base syndromes* (7th ed.). Philadelphia: Lea & Febiger.

Greenberger, N. (1986). *Gastrointestinal disorders*. Chicago: Year Book Medical Publishers.

Grossman, R. A., Hamilton, R. W., Morse, B. M., et al. (1974). Nontraumatic rhabdomyolysis and acute renal failure. *New England Journal of Medicine*, 291, 807–811.

Guyton, A. C. (1991). *Textbook of medical physiology* (8th ed.). Philadelphia: W.B. Saunders.

Iseri, L. T., Freed, J., and Barnes, A. R. (1975). Magnesium deficiency and cardiac disorders. *American Journal of Medicine*, 58 837–846.

Kaloyanides, G. J. (1980). Pathogenesis and treatment of edema with special reference to the use of diuretics. In M.H. Maxwell, and C.R. Kleeman (Eds.), *Clinical disorders of fluid and electrolyte metabolism*. New York: McGraw-Hill.

Katz, L. D., and DeFronzo, R. A. (1984). Hyperkalemia. In R. J. Glassock (Ed.), *Current therapy in nephrology and hypertension 1984–1985*. Philadelphia: B.C. Decker.

Kleeman, C. R. (1984). Hypernatremic and hyperosmolar syndromes. In R.J. Glassock (Ed.), *Current therapy in nephrology and hypertension 1984–1985*. Philadelphia: B.C. Decker.

Kleerkoper, M., Roa, D. S., and Frame, B. (1978). Hypercalcemia, hyperparathyroidism and hypertension. *Cardiovascular Medicine*, 3, 1283–1295.

Knochel, J. P., and Schlein, E.M. (1972). On the mechanism of rhabdomyolysis in potassium depletion. *Journal of Clinical Investigation*, 51, 1750.

Levey, A. S., and Harrington, J.T. (1984). Hypokalemia. In R. J. Glassock (Ed.), *Current therapy in nephrology and hypertension 1984–1985*. Philadelphia: B.C. Decker.

Levine, B. S., Brantbar, N., Walling, M.W., et al. (1980). Effects of vitamin D and diet magnesium on magnesium metabolism. *American Journal of Physiology*. 239, 515–523.

Lunger, D. G. (1988). Potassium supplementation: How and why? *Focus on Critical Care*, 15, 56.

Mawer, E. B., Backhouse, J., Davies, M., et al. (1976). Metabolic fate of administered 1,25-dihydroxycholecalciferol in controls and patients with hypoparathyroidism. *Lancet*, 1, 1203–1206.

McCollister, R. J., Flink, E. B., and Doe, R. P. (1960). Magnesium balance studies in chronic alcoholism. *Journal of Laboratory and Clinical Medicine*, 55, 998–1104.

Metheny, N. (1987). Fluid and electrolyte balance. Philadelphia: J. B. Lippincott.

O'Connor, L. R., Klein, K. L., and Bethune, J. E. (1977). Hyperphosphatemia in lactic acidosis. *New England Journal of Medicine*, 2997, 707–709.

Parfitt, A. M., and Kleerkoper, M. (1980). Clinical disorders of calcium, phosphorus, and magnesium metabolism. In M.H. Maxwell and O.R. Kleeman (Eds.), *Clinical disorders of fluid and electrolyte metabolism*(pp. 947–1152). New York: McGraw-Hill.

Patel, R., and Savage, A. (1979). Symptomatic hypomagnesemia associated with gentamicin therapy. *Nephron*, 23, 50–52.

Reineck, H. J., and Stein, J. H. (1980). Regulation of sodium balance. In M. H. Maxwell and C.R. Kleeman (Eds.), *Clinical disorders of fluid and electrolyte metabolism*. New York: McGraw-Hill.

Robertson, G. L., Shelton, R. L., and Athar, S. (1976). The osmoregulation of vasopressin. *Kidney International*, 10, 613–620.

Rosai, J., Higa, E., and Davie, J. (1972). Mediastinal endocrine neoplasms in patients with multiple endocrine adenomatosis. *Cancer*, 29, 1975–1083.

Rose, B. (1984). Clinical physiology of acid-base and electrolyte disorders (2nd ed.). New York: McGraw-Hill.

Rubini, M. (1961). Water excretion in potassium deficient man. *Journal of Clinical Investigation*, 40, 2215–2224.

Schultze, R.G., and Nissenson, A. R. (1980). Potassium: physiology and pathophysiology. In M.H Maxwell, and C.R. Kleeman (Eds.), *Clinical disorders of fluid and electrolyte metabolism*. New York: McGraw-Hill.

Smith, J. D., Bia, M. J., and DeFronzo, R. A. (1985). Clinical disorders of potassium metabolism., In A.J. Arieff, and R.A. Defronzo (Eds.), *Fluid electrolyte and acid-base disorders*. New York: Churchill Livingstone.

Stein, J. H. (1988). Hypokalemia—common and uncommon causes. *Hospital Practice*, March 30, 55–70.

Vallee, B. L., Wacker, W. E. C, and Ulmer, D. D. (1975). The magnesium deficiency tetany syndrome in man. *New England Journal of Medicine*, 262, 155–161.

Valtin, H. (1987). *Renal dysfunction: Mechanisms involved in fluid and solute imbalance*. Boston: Little, Brown.

Whittaker, A. A. (1985). Acute renal dysfunction: Assessment of patients at risk. *Focus on Critical Care*, 12, 12–17.

Zuspan, F. P., and Zuspan, K. H. (1981). Strategies for controlling eclampsia. *Conptemporary OB/GYN*, 18(1), 135–144.

41

Patients with
Acute Renal Failure

Alice A. Whittaker

Acute renal failure is a serious sequela of critical illness and traumatic injury. It is estimated that as many as 5% of patients hospitalized for medical or surgical problems experience some decrease in renal function (Hou et al., 1983). Despite advances in prevention, diagnosis, and medical treatment, the mortality associated with acute renal failure remains high. Overall mortality rates in patients with acute loss of renal function approach 40% to 50%. In surgical and traumatically injured patients, mortality may be as high as 60% to 70% (Schrier, 1981: Hou, 1985; Jacobsen et al., 1990).

Loss of renal function has a potentially negative impact on all body systems. This chapter will focus on the clinical challenge presented by the critically ill patient with oliguric acute renal failure.

PATHOPHYSIOLOGY OF ACUTE RENAL FAILURE

Acute renal failure (ARF) can be defined as a sudden decrease in renal function manifested by rapid accumulation of waste metabolites in the patient's body. In the majority of cases, the patient becomes oliguric. Oliguria exists when the urine flow is less than the volume required to excrete the body's metabolic waste load. In the adult patient, this obligatory urine volume is approximately 400 mL/24 hours.

Oliguria is considered the classic finding in ARF, but the syndrome also manifests in a more benign nonoliguric form (Meyers, 1977). Although patients with nonoliguric renal failure pass normal amounts of urine, they demonstrate the renal pathology and metabolic changes seen in oliguric failure.

Etiology

Acute renal failure is a syndrome of multiple etiologies. The various etiologies can be classified into three major categories: prerenal, postrenal, and renal.

Prerenal Causes. Prerenal causes of ARF are characterized by diminished renal perfusion resulting from a reduction in the volume of blood reaching the kidney. As listed in Table 41-1, the most common causes of renal hypoperfusion are related to an absolute loss of extracellular fluid volume or a redistribution of extracellular fluid from the cardiovascular system into other body compartments. Prerenal oliguria may also be caused by a reduction in the effective circulatory volume resulting from impaired cardiac function.

The kidneys react to the prerenal hypoperfusion state by increasing tubular reabsorption of sodium and water and by selective vasoconstriction of the glomerular arterioles. These are normal regulatory mechanisms designed to increase blood volume and improve renal perfusion. The urine volume falls and the patient becomes oliguric.

Renal function remains intact in prerenal states. Oliguria can be reversed if the underlying hypoperfusion disorder is corrected, and normal blood flow is restored to the kidneys before ischemic damage occurs.

Postrenal Causes. Disease states that interrupt or obstruct the outflow of urine from the body are the causes of postrenal ARF. Table 41-2 lists the major obstructive and traumatic processes seen in critically ill patients.

TABLE 41–1. Prerenal Causes of Acute Renal Failure

Cause	Clinical Example
Absolute Extracellular Volume Reduction	
Hemorrhage	Traumatic injury, postoperative bleeding, gastrointestinal bleeding
Gastrointestinal loss	Diarrhea, vomiting, gastrointestinal drainage tubes
Urinary loss	Excessive diuretics, diabetes insipidus, diabetic ketoacidosis
Skin loss	Burns, excessive sweating
Extracellular Volume Redistribution	
Third spacing	Bowel obstruction, peritonitis, pancreatitis, soft tissue injury
Vasodilatory states	Sepsis, anaphylaxis, vasodilating medications
Decreased Effective Circulatory Volume	
Decreased cardiac output	Congestive heart failure, cardiomyopathy, pericarditis, cardiac tamponade, pulmonary embolism, cardiogenic shock

TABLE 41–3. Renal Causes of Acute Renal Failure

Cause	Clinical Example
Glomerular	
Primary	Poststreptococcal glomerulonephritis
Secondary to systemic disease	Systemic lupus erythematosus, vasculitis, endocarditis
	Malignant hypertension
Tubulointerstitial	
Ischemic	Uncorrected prerenal hypoperfusion
	Alpha-adrenergic drug administration
	Renal artery thrombosis
Nephrotoxic	
Drugs or chemicals	Antibiotics: aminoglycosides, cephalosporins, penicillins, tetracyclines, amphotericin
	Heavy metals
	Organic solvents
	Pesticides, fungicides
	Cisplatin
Endogenous toxins	Hemoglobinuria
	Myoglobinuria
	Hypercalcemia

Impairment of renal function in postrenal ARF occurs as the intratubular pressure increases proximal to the obstruction. Glomerular filtration ceases as the pressure in Bowman's capsule becomes equal to the hydrostatic pressure in the glomerular capillaries. High intratubular pressure damages the tubular cells, resulting in impaired transport and concentration mechanisms (Papper, 1978; Finn, 1990). If the postrenal disorder is rapidly corrected, renal function can be preserved. Prolonged postrenal obstruction results in permanent damage to the nephrons.

Renal Causes. A variety of diseases and injuries intrinsic to the actual kidney tissue may lead to the development of ARF. As listed in Table 41–3, damage to the renal parenchyma may be related to abnormalities of the glomerulus, tubules or interstitium.

TABLE 41–2. Postrenal Causes of Acute Renal Failure

Cause	Clinical Example
Obstruction	
Ureteral	Calculi, crystals
	Retroperitoneal tumor
	Blood clot
Bladder	Prostatic hypertrophy, carcinoma
	Tumor
	Neurogenic, functional
	Stone, blood clot
Urethral	Stricture, stenosis
Traumatic Interruption	Severed ureter
	Bladder tear

Tubular damage, referred to as acute tubular necrosis (ATN), is the most frequently encountered form of ARF seen in critically ill patients (Corwin, 1986).

Both ischemic and toxic insults impair nephron function; however, renal cellular ischemia is the most common cause of ATN. In many patients, renal ischemia is preceded by severe, uncorrected prerenal hypoperfusion. Prolonged administration of alpha-adrenergic drugs, resulting in intense renal vasoconstriction, is another frequent cause of renal ischemia in critically ill patients.

Loss of nephron function may occur following exposure to a number of nephrotoxic chemicals and drugs. Damage to the renal tubules is a frequent sequela to accidental or intentional ingestion of organic solvents, such as carbon tetrachloride or ethylene glycol. Critically ill patients often receive a number of potentially nephrotoxic antibiotics. Aminoglycoside antibiotics are particularly nephrotoxic when administered to patients with fluid volume and electrolyte disorders. Approximately 10% to 15% of patients receiving aminoglycoside antibiotics will develop some degree of renal dysfunction (Tolkoff-Rubin et al., 1984).

Among the endogenous nephrotoxins, hemoglobin and myoglobin are implicated as causes of ATN accompanying critical illness. Hemoglobinuria, resulting from hemolytic transfusion reaction or another hemolytic process, may result in renal tubular injury. Following intravascular hemolysis, hemoglobin is released into the circulating plasma and exerts a toxic effect on the renal tubular epithelium. Myoglobin is a respiratory pigment present in muscle cells. When muscle injury occurs, myoglobin is released into the blood and filtered by the glomeruli, resulting in myoglobinuria. Rhabdomyolysis, with accompanying myoglobinuria, is a frequent cause of ARF in traumatically injured patients.

Pathogenesis of Acute Tubular Necrosis

Several theories have been proposed to explain the diminished glomerular filtration rate (GFR) that occurs in patients with ATN. As shown in Figure 41–1, either tubular factors or vascular factors contribute to the reduction in GFR. Different modes of injury may preferentially affect either the tubules or the renal vasculature.

Tubular Factors. The renal tubules are damaged by ischemic and nephrotoxic insults in two distinct patterns. Ischemic damage is characterized by *tubulorrhexic lesions*, which are scattered throughout the proximal tubule as well as portions of the distal tubule. Lesions are not evenly distributed among all nephrons. This type of necrosis results in destruction of both the tubular cells and the underlying tubular basement membrane (Oliver et al., 1951; Olsen and Solez, 1987). Tubular fluid leaks into the renal interstitium, causing additional inflammation. Disruption of the basement membrane results in delayed healing and regeneration of the tubular epithelium. In contrast to the patchy loss of tubular cells seen in ischemic injury, *nephrotoxic lesions* are evenly distributed throughout the proximal tubules of all nephrons. Necrosis of the tubular epithelial cells occurs throughout most of the proximal tubule; however, the basement membrane remains intact.

Proximal tubular dilatation and the presence of intraluminal casts and cellular debris are common findings in ATN. Studies in animal models have demonstrated blockage of 90% of the proximal tubules following experimentally induced renal ischemia (Donohoe et al., 1978). Desquamated microvilli fill the proximal tubule in the first hours following ischemic injury. Later these cellular debris combine with Tamm-Horsfall protein to form tubular casts, which further obstruct the tubules and the loop of Henle (Hoyer and Seiler, 1979 Bayati et al., 1990). The tubules remain obstructed until the casts are dissolved by proteolytic enzymes or flushed out by increased glomerular filtrate flow.

Disruption of the integrity of the tubular epithelium permits glomerular filtrate to leak back into the peritubular circulation. This backleak of filtrate is thought to result in interstitial edema and tubular collapse. The role of backleak in decreased GFR is controversial. Research measuring the fractional clearance of dextran/inulin has demonstrated the presence of tubular backleak (Myers et al., 1980). However, no evidence of backleak has been found in other experimental models of acute renal failure (Burke et al., 1980). Severe reductions in GFR may occur long before evidence of tubular disruption is present. It appears that backleak is not the major contributing factor in the decreased GFR seen in ATN.

A number of studies have demonstrated significant increases in intratubular pressure accompanying tubular obstruction in ATN (Tanner and Steinhausen, 1976). Others have been unable to establish a consistent correlation between increased intratubular pressures and decreased GFR (Mason et al., 1977). It is likely that variations in glomerular vasoconstriction and backleak of glomerular ultrafiltrate influence the rise of intratubular pressure in the obstructed nephron.

Vascular Factors. There is increasing support in the literature for the vascular theory of the pathogenesis of ATN. During the initial phase of ATN, renal blood flow (RBF) decreases by more than 50% (Kashgarian et al., 1976). In addition, there is a significant rise in renal vascular resistance. The reduction in RBF is preferential. Blood flow to the renal cortex is sharply decreased while perfusion to the medulla is maintained. The mechanisms responsible for these

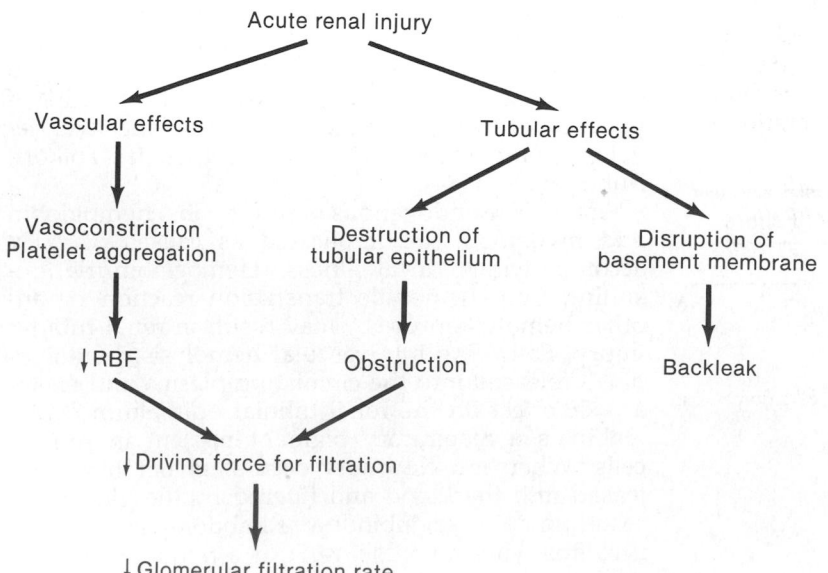

FIGURE 41–1. Schematic representation of the mechanisms theorized to initiate and maintain the reduction in glomerular filtration rate (GFR) in acute renal failure (ARF). (Adapted from Brenner, B. M., and Rector, F. L. (Eds.) (1988). *Acute renal failure* (2nd ed.). Philadelphia: W. B. Saunders.)

changes in the renal vasculature are not well understood. There is evidence to indicate that damaged endothelial cells swell, reducing the diameter of the renal arterioles. RBF falls as the arteriolar diameter diminishes (Flores et al., 1972). Increased peritubular capillary permeability results in a massive extravasation of plasma, leading to an elevated intracapillary hematocrit (Bayati et al., 1990a). Aggregation of red blood cells in the peritubular capillaries of the outer medulla has been shown to cause congestion and possible intravascular coagulation (Mason et al., 1984; Bayati et al., 1990a). Impaired tubular reabsorption of sodium chloride is thought to activate the renin-angiotensin system, resulting in afferent arteriolar constriction (Shapira et al., 1976). Abnormal glomerular permeability to proteins is another suggested mechanism explaining the decrease in GFR (Solez and Finckh, 1984).

Each of these proposed vascular mechanisms can be demonstrated in the early stages of acute renal failure. However, none can be shown to be totally responsible for maintaining the suppressed GFR beyond the initial phase. Most likely, sustained decreased GFR is a result of both tubular and vascular factors. The relative contribution of each factor varies with the mode of injury and individual patient characteristics.

Metabolic and Biochemical Disturbances

The physiologic disturbances seen in ARF are a result of the kidney's decreased ability to form and excrete urine. As the blood level of metabolic wastes and toxins rises, a variety of metabolic and biochemical derangements occur. As shown in Table 41–4,

---

TABLE 41–4. Physiologic Disturbances in Acute Renal Failure

Protein Metabolism
Increased protein degradation
Decreased protein synthesis

Acid-Base Balance
Metabolic acidosis

Carbohydrate Metabolism
Insulin resistance
Hyperglycemia
Decreased ATP production

Fluid/Electrolyte Balance
Fluid volume overload
Hyponatremia
Hyperkalemia
Hypocalcemia/hyperphosphatemia

Hematologic Function
Anemia
Platelet dysfunction
Leukopenia

---

these disturbances range from mild to life-threatening and involve all of the body systems.

Catabolism. Two terms are commonly used to describe the physiologic disturbances seen in ARF. The abnormal retention of nitrogenous waste products such as urea, creatinine, uric acid, and amino acids is known as *azotemia*. *Uremia* refers to the symptoms of the clinical illness caused by renal failure.

In ARF, the intensity of azotemia and the uremic syndrome is closely correlated with the patient's rate of catabolism. ARF is characterized by an increased rate of cellular decomposition (Knochel, 1988). The breakdown of cells releases intracellular products and their metabolites into the circulatory system. When renal excretion is suppressed, the blood level of these metabolites rises rapidly, and the patient becomes azotemic. In mildly catabolic patients, the blood urea nitrogen (BUN) increases approximately 10 to 20 mg/100 mL per day. When severe catabolism is present, the BUN may rise as much as 40 to 50 mg/100 mL per day (Cameron and Ogg, 1967).

The explanation for the high rate of catabolism in ARF is not well understood. Patients who are stressed by critical illness or traumatic injury demonstrate elevations of circulating catecholamines, cortisol, and glucagon. It is theorized that these hormones play an important role in stimulating catabolism. In addition to protein degradation, protein synthesis is also suppressed in ARF.

Acid-Base Imbalance. Under normal conditions, the kidney regulates acid-base balance by excreting hydrogen ion and selectively reabsorbing bicarbonate. When acute renal damage has occurred, organic and inorganic acids are retained, leading to metabolic acidosis. In catabolism, disintegrated cells release a number of organic acids and sulfate- and phosphate-containing acids into the circulation, thereby greatly increasing acid production. This is evidenced by a rapid fall in plasma bicarbonate levels of 15 to 20 mEq/24 hours.

The presence of uremia intensifies the harmful effects of metabolic acidosis in critically ill patients. Metabolic acidosis further stimulates protein degradation (May et al., 1986). Carbohydrate metabolism is impaired, and energy production is reduced (Relman, 1972).

Altered Carbohydrate Metabolism. Patients with ARF are unable to metabolize glucose normally. Hyperglycemia occurs during fasting, and there is a delay in the fall of blood glucose following a glucose challenge (Reaven et al., 1974). Insulin response to high blood glucose levels in acutely uremic patients is greater than that in normal patients, indicating that the defect in insulin activity is not impaired secretion. Rather, glucose intolerance is apparently a result of an inappropriate response of target tissue to insulin (Giordano et al., 1987). Peripheral muscle tissue is thought to be the site of insulin resistance in patients with acute uremia.

Electrolyte Disturbances. Acute loss of renal function results in a variety of fluid and electrolyte disturbances.

Sodium. Hyponatremia is the most common sodium disturbance observed in patients with ARF and is usually attributed to dilution. The serum sodium may become diluted by three mechanisms. First, administration of free water, such as 5% dextrose and water (D_5W) or oral water, may exceed the kidney's ability to excrete it. Second, metabolic water production in patients with ARF may be increased up to 160% over normal (Bluemle et al., 1951). In catabolic patients, additional water is released as body tissues are destroyed.

Disturbances in ion transport across the cellular membrane also contribute to hyponatremia in ARF. As cellular injury occurs, intracellular potassium is exchanged for sodium. Failure of the sodium-potassium pump results in increased intracellular osmolality and inward movement of water. Cell volume increases, and cellular transmembrane potential is depressed.

Potassium. Hyperkalemia is common and is often severe in patients with oliguric ARF. Intracellular potassium concentration is approximately 155 mEq/liter. When cellular injury occurs, potassium is released into the extracellular fluid and the serum potassium rises.

Hyperkalemia is aggravated by hyperglycemia and metabolic acidosis, both of which are commonly present in oliguric patients. It is theorized that the intracellular accumulation of hydrogen ions displaces potassium ions into the extracellular fluid (Knochel, 1985). Lowering of the intracellular pH decreases the rate of glycolysis, leading to reduction of energy needed to run the sodium-potassium pump (Relman, 1972).

Calcium-Phosphate. Calcium and phosphate derangements are expected in patients with ARF. Because phosphate ions are normally excreted in the urine, serum phosphate levels climb as renal function decreases. In hypercatabolic patients, phosphate levels rise rapidly as phosphate is released from injured tissue. Hyperphosphatemia is aggravated by metabolic acidosis. Acute acidosis interferes with intracellular glycolysis and causes hydrolysis of sugar-phosphates. The resulting free inorganic phosphate ions are released into the extracellular fluid (Knochel, 1977).

As hyperphosphatemia develops, phosphate ions interact with calcium ions to form calcium-phosphate salts. These salts are deposited in body tissues. Deposition of calcium salts leads to a fall in serum calcium levels (Andreucci, 1984). Synthesis of vitamin D is also suppressed in patients with ARF. Low levels of vitamin D decrease calcium mobilization from bone and have a negative effect on intestinal calcium absorption (Llach et al., 1981).

Hematologic Abnormalities. Several alterations in hematologic function are commonly seen in ARF.

Anemia. Anemia may develop rapidly in patients with ARF. Often these patients have sustained significant blood loss due to injury or surgery. The rapid onset of severe azotemia results in hemolysis of red blood cells. Uremic hemolysis is believed to be the major cause of anemia in the early phase of ARF (Steinman and Lazarus, 1988). As the course of acute uremia progresses, anemia is sustained by a decrease in erythropoiesis. Diminished erythropoiesis may be caused by a fall in erythropoietin-stimulating factor or by the action of an erythropoietin inhibitor (Radtke et al., 1979, 1981).

Hemostasis. Thrombocytopenia, platelet dysfunction, and abnormal prothrombin consumption are clotting abnormalities common to acutely uremic patients. Because these abnormalities are associated with other underlying disease processes in critically ill patients, it is difficult to specify the exact role of renal failure in inducing or augmenting them. It is known that the bleeding tendency is well correlated with the degree of renal dysfunction (Larrain and Adleson, 1956).

Leukopenia. Almost invariably, patients with ARF demonstrate immunologic abnormalities. Leukocytosis of neutrophils, lymphopenia, abnormal chemotaxis, and impaired inflammatory response are common findings (Goldblum and Reed, 1980; Clark et al., 1972). Infection with septicemia is the most common cause of death in acutely uremic patients.

CLINICAL PRESENTATION

Acute oliguria may be attributed to a number of causes, including prerenal, postrenal, and intrinsic renal factors. Because of the critical impact of ARF and the fact that treatment depends upon the underlying problem, it is essential that an accurate etiologic diagnosis be made.

Laboratory Analysis

Table 41–5 presents a comparison of the common laboratory findings observed in prerenal and postrenal disease and ATN. Although many of the blood and urine findings appear similar, the correct etiologic diagnosis can usually be made based on laboratory tests, patient history, and physical examination.

Urine from the prerenal kidney shows marked sodium and water reabsorption. Urine volume is low and highly concentrated and contains a minimal amount of sodium. The BUN to serum creatinine ratio is elevated because an increased amount of urea is reabsorbed into the peritubular vascular circulation.

Urine chemistry results in early postrenal oliguria are very similar to those seen in prerenal states.

TABLE 41–5. Comparison of Laboratory Findings in Prerenal, Postrenal, and Intrinsic Renal Acute Oliguric States

Value	Prerenal	Postrenal	Intrinsic Renal (ATN)
Urine volume	Decreased	May alternate between anuria and polyuria	Anuria <100 mL/24 hr Oliguria 100–400 mL/24 hr Nonoliguria >400 mL/24 hr
Urine osmolality	Increased (>500 mOsm)	Isotonic (≤350 mOsm)	Isotonic (≤350 mOsm)
Urine specific gravity	Increased (>1.020)	Fixed (1.008–1.012)	Fixed (1.008–1.012)
Urine sodium	<20 mEq/liter	>40 mEq/liter	>40 mEq/liter
Fractional excretion of sodium (FE$_{Na}$)*	<1%	>1%	>1%
Renal failure index†	<1%	>1%	>1%
Urine pH	<6.0	>6.0	>6.0
Urine protein	Minimal	Minimal	Increased
Urine sediment	Normal, few casts	Normal, histiocytes and crystals	Granular casts, tubular epithelial cells
Urine/plasma creatinine ratio	>40	<20	<20
BUN:serum creatinine	>20:1	10–15:1	10–15:1

*Fractional excretion of sodium = U/P sodium ÷ U/P creatinine × 100.
†Renal failure index = U sodium ÷ U/P creatinine.

Adapted from M. Brezis, S. Rosen, and F. H. Epstein. (1991). Acute renal failure. In B. M. Brenner and F. C. Rector (Eds.), *The Kidney* (4th ed., pp. 993–1061). Philadelphia: W. B. Saunders.

However, after several hours of bilateral obstruction, the concentration of the urine decreases, and the excretion of sodium rises. Urine volume may remain high, even in the presence of severe partial obstruction. The BUN and serum creatinine are both elevated.

Patients with ATN are usually oliguric; however, anuria may also occur. In nephrotoxic ATN, urine volumes may remain relatively normal. Damaged nephrons do not adequately process the glomerular filtrate. The resulting urine is high in sodium with a concentration close to that of plasma. Serum creatinine levels increase by 1 to 2 mg/dL per day in noncatabolic patients with ATN. The BUN to serum creatinine ratio remains 10 to 15:1 because the BUN and creatinine rise proportionately.

Diagnostic Studies

Occasionally the patient with acute oliguria has inconclusive laboratory and physical findings. In these cases, a number of diagnostic studies may be performed to determine the cause of renal failure.

Radiologic Studies. Intravenous urography (IVU) may provide useful information about renal perfusion and patency of the renal collection system in the patient with ARF. Following rapid injection of a radiocontrast agent, serial films (nephrograms) of the renal tubules and collecting system are taken. Normally, the contrast agent enters the tubules by glomerular filtration within a few minutes following injection and is rapidly cleared from the kidneys. Severe reduction in renal perfusion and glomerular filtration, as seen in ATN, produces characteristic changes in the nephrogram. Uptake of the contrast agent is usually delayed, and achievement of normal density may be delayed or prolonged (Cattell et al.,

1973). IVU is most reliably used to rule out urinary tract obstruction. The procedure is not without risk. Injection of an iodinated, hyperosmolar contrast medium may result in hypersensitivity reactions and has been observed to worsen congestive heart failure. Development of nephrotoxic ATN following exposure to radiocontrast agents is well documented and is especially problematic in diabetic patients and patients with severe renal hypoperfusion (VanZee et al., 1978; Whalley et al., 1987).

Ultrasonography. Renal ultrasonography is a safe and highly reliable technique used to rule out urinary tract obstruction in the acutely oliguric patient (Green and King, 1976). Dilatation of the renal calices and collecting ducts can be detected by ultrasonography within the first 24 to 36 hours following acute obstruction. In addition, intrarenal and ureteral calculi can be identified using renal ultrasonography (Edell and Zengel, 1978).

Renal Biopsy. Biopsy of the renal tissue may be useful in the diagnosis of acute glomerular disease, when cortical necrosis is the cause of ATN, and when ATN is suspected but no known cause can be found for it (D'Amico and Colasanti, 1987). Because of the risks involved in tissue biopsy and the usefulness of other diagnostic tests, renal biopsy is not indicated in the majority of patients with acute oliguria.

Physical Findings

The patient with ARF presents with alterations in urine output and increasing azotemia. As ARF progresses, all body and organ systems demonstrate abnormalities. Table 41–6 lists the physical findings

TABLE 41–6. Physical Findings in Acute Oliguric Renal Failure

Cardiovascular
Hypertension
Congestive heart failure
Arrhythmias
Pericarditis

Pulmonary
Pulmonary edema
Hypoxemia

Neurologic
Lethargy
Disorientation
Seizures
Coma

Gastrointestinal
Increased gastrointestinal hormones
Increased gastric ammonia
Gastritis/peptic ulcers
Gastrointestinal hemorrhage

Integument
Edema
Pallor
Hair loss

commonly observed in patients with acute oliguric failure.

Cardiovascular Abnormalities. Patients with ARF show several cardiovascular abnormalities. Hypertension is a common finding, resulting from fluid volume overload and increased peripheral resistance. Cardiac output may be elevated as the patient becomes progressively anemic. Fluid volume overload frequently results in congestive heart failure. Impaired contractility, secondary to metabolic acidosis, also decreases cardiac function in the acutely uremic patient. Physical findings include peripheral edema, pulmonary edema, elevated central venous pressure (CVP), and increased jugular venous distention.

Changes in the patient's electrocardiogram (ECG) demonstrate the electrolyte disturbances accompanying ARF. ECG changes are generally noted when the serum potassium level exceeds 5.5 mEq/liter. The typical progression of ECG abnormalities seen in a patient with ARF with hyperkalemia is presented in Figure 41–2.

Pericarditis is an infrequent complication of acute uremia. The patient with uremic pericarditis usually does not complain of significant chest pain. A pericardial friction rub may be the initial clinical finding.

Pulmonary Abnormalities. Pulmonary edema is a frequent complication of ARF, occurring in patients with congestive heart failure as well as in those with normal cardiac function. Studies have demonstrated increased pulmonary capillary permeability in acutely uremic patients (Rackow et al., 1978). Plasma proteins leak into the alveolae, resulting in impaired gas diffusion. Arterial blood gas analysis demonstrates

hypoxemia. Physical findings include tachypnea and tachycardia. The patient may complain of shortness of breath.

Neurologic Abnormalities. Neurologic disorders may be caused by the underlying disease process as well as by acute uremia. When the onset of ARF is rapid, neurologic abnormalities are the earliest and most common symptoms. At the onset of acute uremia, the patient complains of fatigue and may

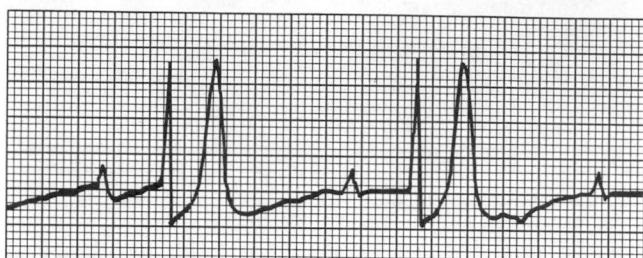

A

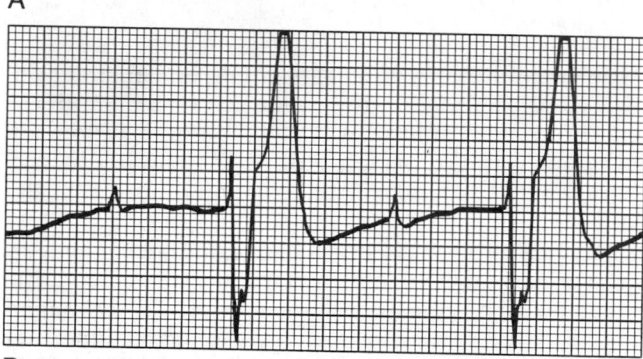

B

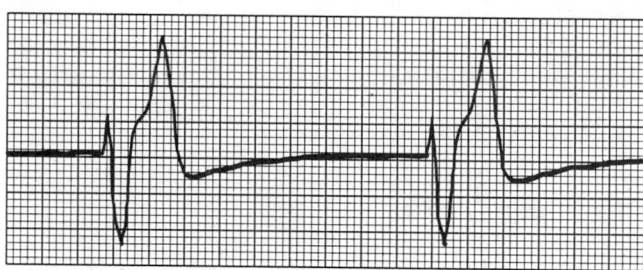

C

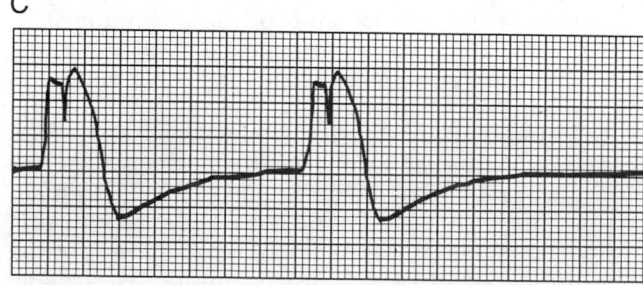

D

FIGURE 41–2. Electrocardiographic changes in hyperkalemia. *A,* Peaked T waves and AV block are evident at serum potassium levels of 5.5–6.5 mEq/liter. *B,* As the serum potassium concentration reaches 7.0–7.5 mEq/liter, the QRS interval widens and AV nodal conduction is further slowed. *C,* Atrial standstill occurs at serum potassium levels of 8.0–9.0 mEq/liter. *D,* As the serum potassium level exceeds 9.0 mEq/liter, the QRS and T wave merge. Conduction through the His bundle and Purkinje system is further delayed, leading to ventricular fibrillation or asystole.

appear lethargic or somnolent. As the oliguric phase progresses, the patient may reveal irritability, twitching, disorientation, and possibly psychosis. In advanced uremia, tonic-clonic seizure activity may occur, and the patient will eventually become comatose.

Gastrointestinal Abnormalities. The kidney plays a major role in the inactivation and removal of gastrointestinal hormones from the blood. When renal function is suppressed, plasma gastrin levels rise. In addition, the gastric ammonia level rises as a result of the increased BUN level. Patients complain of loss of appetite and nausea. Vomiting is a common occurrence. When gastritis or peptic ulcers develop, the patient may complain of abdominal pain. Gastrointestinal hemorrhage is manifested by occult blood in the stool or by frank upper intestinal bleeding.

Integument. Generalized subcutaneous edema is present in the patient with fluid volume overload. As anemia develops, the skin and mucous membranes become pale. Hair loss and abnormal nail growth may also be observed.

Clinical Course of ATN

The clinical course of ATN can be divided into three phases: an oliguric phase, a diuretic phase, and a recovery phase. Patients with nonoliguric ATN progress through a similar course.

The oliguric phase may last a few hours or several months. The average duration of oliguria is 10 to 14 days. In general, a prolonged oliguric phase is associated with a longer and less complete renal recovery. It is during the oliguric phase that the BUN and serum creatinine rise rapidly and the complications of uremia are most severe.

Following the onset of the diuretic phase, urine production begins to rise. In most cases, urine output increases incrementally over a period of days and weeks. A small number of patients have a profuse diuresis. The urine produced during the diuretic phase is not well concentrated. It contains less urea and creatinine than is produced by daily metabolic processes. Once urine output has exceeded 1 liter for several days, the BUN and serum creatinine levels will begin to fall. Uremic complications continue to be a threat during the diuretic phase.

The BUN and serum creatinine return to normal levels in the recovery phase. The biochemical and metabolic derangements of acute uremia resolve. Although renal function appears normal, defects in filtration and concentration remain for months to years following the renal injury (Levine et al., 1972).

MEDICAL MANAGEMENT

Because there is no "cure" for ARF once nephron damage has occurred, medical management focuses first on prevention and then on the complications arising from the various physiologic alterations accompanying uremia. Table 41–7 summarizes the medical management of the patient with acute oliguric renal failure.

Prevention

The most frequent cause of ARF is decreased renal perfusion leading to ischemia. Therefore, the efforts of medical management have been directed toward maintaining glomerular filtration and urine flow. Preventive management has focused on two areas: fluid challenge and pharmacologic support.

Fluid Challenge. A number of clinicians advocate the use of fluid challenge when acute oliguria occurs. If the patient is in a hypovolemic prerenal state, administration of fluid should improve renal perfusion, and the kidney will respond by increasing urine output. Unfortunately, patients with postrenal disease or ATN may also respond to fluid challenge by increasing urine output (Rudnick et al., 1988). In these patients, the additional fluid contributes to worsened hydronephrosis and may result in increased fluid volume overload. For these reasons, many clinicians reserve fluid challenge for patients whose hemodynamic and physical findings demonstrate hypovolemia.

Diuretic Challenge. In the oliguric patient with fluid volume overload, administration of a diuretic challenge is preferred to a fluid challenge. Diuretics must be used with caution in the presence of prerenal

---

TABLE 41–7. Medical Management of Acute Oliguric Renal Failure

Prevention
Fluid challenge
Diuretic challenge
  Mannitol
  Furosemide
Vasodilators
  Dopamine
  Calcium channel blockers

Fluid Management
Fluid restriction
Daily serum sodium monitoring

Management of Hyperkalemia
Potassium restriction
Intravenous insulin/glucose/bicarbonate
Ion exchange resin
Dialysis

Nutritional Management
Minimal carbohydrate requirement 100 g
Minimal protein requirement 20–30 g

Medication Management
Peak/trough serum drug levels

azotemia because they may contribute to further fluid volume depletion. In addition to their diagnostic value, diuretics are thought to offer protection against ARF. These protective mechanisms include increasing renal blood flow, increasing tubular urine flow, and decreasing nephron cellular energy requirements (Brezis et al., 1984). Both osmotic and loop diuretics have been utilized to treat ARF in the clinical setting.

Mannitol, an osmotic diuretic, is theorized to prevent tubular obstruction by increasing tubular urine flow. Increased flow washes out the solutes in the tubules, resulting in decreased tubular cast formation. Mannitol may also decrease endothelial cell swelling, thereby reducing renal vasoconstriction (Flores et al., 1972). Administration of mannitol has been shown to reduce the frequency of ATN development in patients receiving nephrotoxic agents (Zager, 1983).

Loop diuretics such as furosemide also have been observed to cause renal vasodilation and to increase tubular urine flow. A number of clinicians have used furosemide to convert oliguric ARF to a nonoliguric state (Schrier, 1981). It is theorized that treatment with loop diuretics reduces the total number of tubules blocked by Tamm-Horsfall casts (Bayati et al., 1990b). Because loop diuretics do not cause shifts of interstitial fluid into the intravascular space, they are safer than mannitol for use in patients with acute volume overload.

Vasodilators. Because renal vasoconstriction is a consistent finding in ARF, a number of clinicians have advocated the use of vasodilating agents to increase renal blood flow. Infusion of dopamine, a beta-receptor agonist, has been demonstrated to decrease the severity of azotemia in ARF. A number of studies confirm that the combination of dopamine and furosemide is particularly effective in converting oliguric to nonoliguric ARF (Linder, 1983; Graziani et al., 1984; Finn, 1990). Other studies suggest that infusion of calcium channel blockers may offer protection against renal ischemia. Administration of calcium channel blocking agents is thought to prevent the intracellular calcium overload observed in ischemic ARF (Burke et al., 1984; Schrier and Burke, 1988; Jacobsen et al., 1990).

Fluid Management

The patient with oliguric ARF will rapidly become fluid volume overloaded unless water intake is restricted. The prescribed fluid restriction will take into account the patient's daily urine output and the daily insensible fluid loss, which is approximately 500 mL. For example, if the patient produces 300 mL of urine in 24 hours, the daily fluid restriction would be 800 mL. Infusion of hypotonic intravenous fluids is discouraged because it may lead to hyponatremia. Daily serum sodium measurements will assist in maintaining water and solute balance.

Many critically ill patients sequester fluid in the extravascular compartments. This "third spacing" may significantly increase the patient's fluid volume requirements. Therefore, the physician must rely on the central venous pressure or the pulmonary capillary wedge pressure (PCWP) to guide fluid administration (Hou and Cohen, 1985). As the patient begins to produce increased amounts of urine, fluid requirements will need to be adjusted to prevent underhydration and hypovolemia.

Management of Hyperkalemia

Hyperkalemia is a common complication of oliguria ARF and is particularly problematic in patients with severe catabolism. Restriction of potassium intake may be all that is necessary to control serum potassium elevations of less than 6.0 mEq/liter (Schrier, 1981).

Hyperkalemia of greater than 6.0 mEq/liter must be actively treated, even in the absence of ECG changes. Initial therapy includes intravenous administration of insulin, glucose, and bicarbonate. This is a temporary measure that causes extracellular potassium ions to shift into the intracellular space. Because potassium is not actually removed from the body, hyperkalemia will recur within a few hours. Ion exchange resin (Kayexalate) may be effective in controlling serum potassium in noncatabolic patients. Potassium is exchanged across the gastrointestinal mucosa and is removed from the body in the feces. Kayexalate is of limited benefit in patients who do not have bowel function; dialysis therapy will be required to control extreme hyperkalemia in such patients.

Nutritional Management

Optimal caloric and protein intake is of critical importance in the treatment of ARF. The goals of nutritional management are to minimize endogenous catabolism and to prevent malnutrition (Schrier, 1981; Hou and Cohen, 1985). Adequate caloric intake is essential to prevent protein catabolism. At least 100 g of carbohydrates are necessary to supply energy requirements. Administration of hypertonic glucose solutions frequently results in hyperglycemia; therefore, insulin should be given to maintain normal blood glucose levels. Fat is an essential nutrient and is useful in providing a concentrated source of calories for the fluid restricted patient (Mitch and Wilmore, 1988).

Sufficient protein intake is necessary for wound healing to occur. In mildly catabolic patients, 20 to 30 g of protein are usually necessary to maintain neutral nitrogen balance (Mitch and Wilmore, 1988). Administration of additional essential and nonessential amino acids will be required in the more catabolic patient.

Medication Management

The dosage of drugs excreted by the kidneys must be adjusted to prevent toxicity in patients with ARF. Peak and trough serum drug levels are closely monitored. High serum trough levels appear to correlate best with nephrotoxicity and rising serum creatinine (Bernstein and Erk, 1990). Formulas for drug dosages based on the serum creatinine level may be useful once the serum creatinine reaches a steady state (Bennett, 1986).

NURSING MANAGEMENT

The patient with ARF presents with a number of complex nursing management problems. Nursing care requirements are multidimensional and include both preventive and supportive measures.

Potential for Injury

Renal injury may be caused by either ischemic insult or nephrotoxic exposure, and therefore it is essential for the nurse to assess the patient's clinical status to identify and correct factors that contribute to renal damage.

Because the most common cause of ARF in critically ill patients is prolonged renal ischemia, careful attention is paid to signs and symptoms that suggest impending renal hypoperfusion (Whittaker, 1985). Assessment of extracellular fluid volume loss includes careful consideration of all sources of fluid loss and fluid intake. Intake and output records provide useful information about fluid balance trends. Progressive loss of body weight is a very reliable indicator of fluid volume loss. If the patient is experiencing fluid shifts between body compartments (third spacing), body weight may not demonstrate significant change. Nursing assessment focuses on urinary output trends and hemodynamic findings. It is crucial that the nurse obtain a baseline urine output and monitor for a downward trend. Periodic bedside specific gravity measurements may be used to detect changes in urine concentration resulting from extracellular fluid volume depletion. Hemodynamic assessment reveals a falling PCWP and CVP. Tachycardia may be present. The blood pressure may show orthostatic changes.

If nursing assessment indicates that the patient is at risk of renal hypoperfusion, nursing interventions are implemented to restore and support circulating volume. The nurse investigates the sources of fluid loss and evaluates the appropriateness of the prescribed fluid replacement regimen. Significant changes or imbalances are reported to the physician.

Changes in fluid therapy are monitored for efficacy. Prescribed diuretics or renal vasodilators are administered and carefully evaluated for their effect on renal function.

Nursing assessment of patient exposure to toxic drugs or chemicals is a valuable aid in preventing nephrotoxic injury. A thorough nursing history may reveal evidence of toxin ingestion. In addition, the nurse possesses knowledge of numerous drugs, chemical agents, and endogenous substances known to cause renal damage. Identification of an ingested substance and knowledge of its toxic effects helps the nurse to plan appropriate interventions to prevent or minimize nephrotoxic injury.

The nephrotoxic effect of exogenous and endogenous agents is accentuated by hypovolemia. Maintenance of adequate fluid volume status before and during nephrotoxic exposure is essential. Prescribed diuretics may be given on a schedule to increase urine flow during antibiotic administration. Hypokalemia increases the potential for aminoglycoside toxicity (Molitoris and Schrier, 1984). Therefore, the serum potassium must be closely monitored when aminoglycoside antibiotics are administered. The nurse arranges for collection of peak and trough serum drug levels and monitors for rising trough levels.

Potential for Fluid Volume Excess

The patient with oliguric ARF requires close monitoring for fluid volume overload. Serial daily weights provide a reliable estimate of the patient's fluid status. An increase in weight of 1 kg is approximately equal to a fluid volume increase of 1 liter. Physical findings that provide evidence of volume overload include peripheral edema, pulmonary rales, and increased jugular venous distention. The patient may become hypertensive as a result of increased cardiac output. The CVP and PCWP will increase above baseline.

The patient's daily fluid requirements are prescribed by the physician. Since the daily restriction may frequently be less than 1000 mL, creative nursing strategies will be needed to stretch the allotment over the 24-hour period. Oral and intravenous fluid allotments must be appropriately divided among shifts. When possible, vasoactive infusions are mixed double strength to increase the amount of discretionary fluid available. Intake and output records can be utilized to guide the distribution of allowed fluids.

Management of thirst in the conscious patient who is able to take oral fluids is a particular challenge. The nurse explains the reasons for fluid restriction to the patient and family members. The patient may be very uncomfortable, and family members will feel pressured to provide extra fluids. Therefore, frequent explanations and support by the nurse will be necessary. Nursing actions to minimize thirst include providing periodic sips of water and ice chips. Some patients feel that chewing gum or hard sour candy is helpful. Others may prefer to have a cold wet gauze sponge available to suck on. Frequent, meticulous mouth care is essential to control thirst and maintain the integrity of the oral mucosa.

A large number of critically ill patients will need vasoactive drug infusions and total parenteral nutrition in volumes greatly in excess of their calculated daily fluid restriction. These patients will require dialysis therapy to prevent fluid volume overload.

Alteration in Cardiac Output: Decreased

Hyperkalemia is the most serious complication of oliguric ARF. Unless treatment is initiated, the patient will develop life-threatening cardiac dysrhythmias within a few days following the onset of oliguria. The nurse collaborates with the physician and clinical dietitian in evaluating sources of potassium intake and facilitating potassium removal from the body. The patient is placed on a low potassium diet, and potassium is removed from intravenous fluids. Medications containing potassium salts should be discontinued. The serum potassium is monitored at least daily. More frequent measurements will be required if the potassium is rising rapidly. The patient's ECG is monitored for the presence of peaked T waves, widened QRS complexes, and development of heart block or other rhythm disturbance.

Hyperkalemia can be treated by several methods. If glucose/insulin/bicarbonate is administered, the nurse must carefully monitor the patient to note its effects. Hyperkalemia will recur within several hours as potassium shifts back into the extracellular space. Kayexalate can be given by rectum or by the oral route. If given as an enema, Kayexalate is effective only if it is retained for at least 30 to 60 minutes. Oral administration is more effective because it allows the resin to remain in contact with the gastrointestinal mucosa for a longer period of time. Kayexalate can be very constipating when it is mixed with water. Therefore, it should be mixed with an osmotic agent such as sorbitol. Sorbitol produces an osmotic diarrhea that further increases potassium excretion.

Potential for Infection

Patients with ARF are at increased risk of infection because of leukopenia and impaired inflammatory response. Nursing actions to prevent infection emphasize careful technique and minimal manipulation of lines and catheters. Frequent pulmonary care will be required to prevent pooling of secretions in the lungs. The patient's body temperature curve is closely monitored, and elevations are reported. Blood, sputum, urine, and wound drainage are cultured. A white blood count (WBC) with microscopic differential is obtained on a daily basis.

Potential for Decreased Red Blood Cell Volume

The clotting abnormalities associated with ARF place the patient at increased risk of hemorrhage. In addition, synthesis of new red blood cells is depressed. Because of the potential for development of severe anemia, nursing actions are directed toward assessment for bleeding and minimizing blood loss. Daily hemoglobin and hematocrit levels are monitored for significant downward trends. Observations of the patient include noting the presence of bruising, petechiae, and hematoma formation. Urine, stool, and nasogastric drainage are tested for occult blood. Nursing measures to decrease blood loss include minimizing the number of times blood samples are drawn and ensuring that only minimal amounts of blood are collected for each specimen. Careful attention is paid to avoiding tissue trauma during tracheal suctioning and insertion of nasogastric tubes.

Alteration in Nutrition: Less Than Body Requirements

Management of the acutely oliguric patient's nutritional status is a challenge. A high caloric diet with adequate amounts of protein is essential for wound healing and prevention of infection. If the patient is able to eat, the nurse will assist the dietitian in obtaining a dietary history. The patient and family will need a thorough explanation of the dietary restrictions. The patient may be anorexic and have periods of nausea and vomiting. Nursing measures to maintain adequate intake include providing small meals or snacks at frequent intervals and performing mouth care often. If necessary, prescribed antiemetics are administered.

When total parenteral nutrition is utilized for nutritional management, the nurse carefully monitors the infusion and evaluates the patient's response to the fluid load. The serum glucose is routinely monitored, and an insulin prescription is obtained to correct hyperglycemia.

DIALYSIS THERAPY IN ACUTE RENAL FAILURE

Dialysis is a process in which waste materials in the blood are filtered through a semipermeable membrane and removed from the body. In ARF, the indications for dialysis therapy include fluid overload, rapidly progressing azotemia, hyperkalemia, and metabolic acidosis. Current clinical practice suggests that dialysis should be initiated early and at frequent intervals (Jameson and Weigmann, 1990). Early, aggressive dialysis minimizes fluctuations in serum chemistries and may decrease uremic complications.

Three dialysis methods are available for use in patients with ARF: hemodialysis, peritoneal dialysis, and continuous ultrafiltration. The advantages and disadvantages of each method are summarized in Table 41–8.

Hemodialysis

Hemodialysis is a highly efficient method of removing water and solutes from the body. The patient's blood is passed across a semipermeable membrane contained in a dialysis hemofilter. Dialysate fluid, containing prescribed concentrations of electrolytes, passes on the outside of the membrane. Water, electrolytes, and nitrogenous waste products diffuse freely across the membrane, but plasma proteins and blood cells are too large to pass through the membrane. The patient's electrolyte balance can be regulated by varying the ion concentration of the dialysate bath. For example, hyperkalemia is treated by using a low potassium concentration in the dialysate.

Water is removed during hemodialysis by means of ultrafiltration. Ultrafiltration depends on the presence of a pressure gradient across the semipermeable membrane. The hydrostatic pressure that produces this transmembrane pressure gradient has both positive and negative components (Gutch and Stoner, 1983). Positive hydrostatic pressure is applied to the blood compartment and acts to push water from the blood. Negative hydrostatic pressure is applied to the dialysate compartment and creates a vacuum that pulls water from the blood compartment. At any given transmembrane pressure, the amount of fluid

removed by ultrafiltration can be predicted. If the patient requires a higher rate of fluid removal, the ultrafiltration rate can be increased by increasing either the positive pressure on the blood side or the negative pressure on the fluid side.

Indications for Hemodialysis. The greatest advantage offered by hemodialysis to the patient with ARF is efficiency. The patient's fluid and electrolyte abnormalities can be corrected by an average of 4 hours of treatment every other day. Hemodialysis is particularly beneficial for patients with fluid volume overload and rapidly rising BUN and potassium levels. In extremely catabolic patients, daily hemodialysis treatments may be required to control azotemia and hyperkalemia.

Although hemodialysis is the dialysis therapy used most frequently in patients with ARF, it is not always well tolerated by critically ill patients. Cardiovascular instability is a common problem in patients undergoing acute hemodialysis. The rapid fluid shifts frequently result in severe hypotension. Other untoward cardiovascular effects include cardiac dysrhythmias, shortness of breath, and chest pain. Hemodialysis may be contraindicated in patients with severe brain injury. The rapid solute removal promotes movement of water across the blood–brain barrier, resulting in increased cerebral edema (Molitoris and Schrier, 1984).

Nursing Management of Acute Hemodialysis. Although critical care nurses do not routinely perform hemodialysis, the nursing care they provide between treatments is vital to the success of the dialysis

TABLE 41–8. Comparison of Hemodialysis, Peritoneal Dialysis, and Continuous Ultrafiltration

	Hemodialysis	Peritoneal Dialysis	Continuous Ultrafiltration
Efficiency	Highly efficient, rapid removal of water and solutes	Slow, inefficient removal of solutes	Continuous slow removal of water and solutes
Time requirements	Average 4 hours per treatment, usually 3–4 times/week	Continuous hourly exchanges	Continuous hourly exchanges
Access	Vascular access required: arterial or venous	Peritoneal catheter required. Cannot be used when peritoneal space is disrupted	Arterial and venous access required
Equipment	Complex: Dialysis machine Hemofilter Dialysate	Manual system can be easily performed at bedside	Manual system moderately complex: Blood tubing Hemofilter Dialysate (CAVHD) Infusion pump
Anticoagulation	Systemic or regional heparinization required	Little or no heparinization required	Heparinization of hemofilter/tubing required. Minimal systemic heparinization
Complications	Dialysis disequilibrium syndrome: Bleeding Cardiovascular instability Worsened cerebral edema	Peritonitis Protein loss (up to 500 mg/liter of dialysate)	Blood loss Hemofilter clotting Potential dehydration

Adapted from Holloway, N. M. (1988). *Nursing the critically ill adult* (3rd ed., p. 383). Menlo Park, CA: Addison-Wesley Publishing Co.

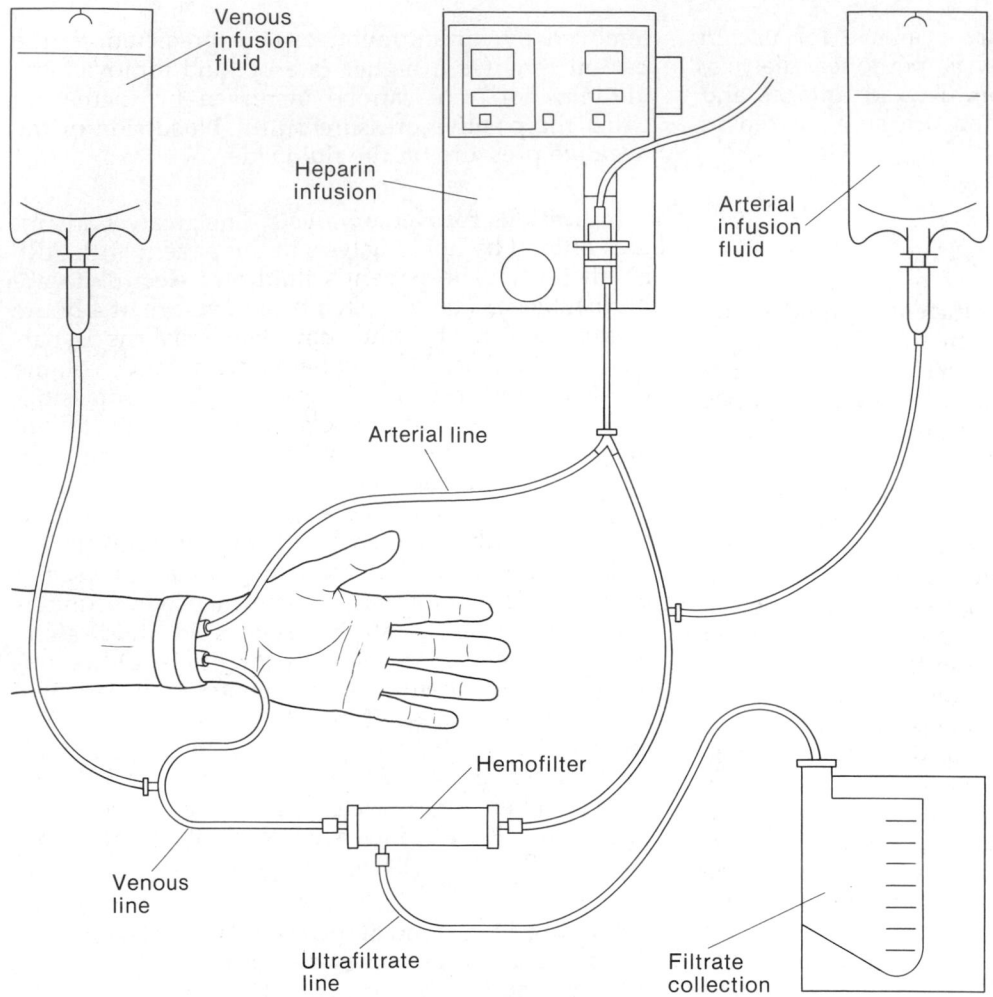

FIGURE 41–3. Continuous ultrafiltration system.

regimen. Nursing management of the patient undergoing acute hemodialysis is guided by the nursing diagnoses previously discussed in this chapter. In addition, special nursing consideration is given to maintaining the integrity of the patient's vascular access site. As seen in the nursing care plan for acute hemodialysis, nursing assessments and interventions are directed toward keeping the access patent and infection free.

Peritoneal Dialysis

Peritoneal dialysis is a renal replacement therapy that utilizes the peritoneum as the dialyzing semipermeable membrane. Sterile dialysate is instilled into the peritoneal cavity. Water, electrolytes, and metabolic wastes diffuse across the peritoneum from the blood in the peritoneal capillary network. These products are removed from the body when the dialysate is drained out of the peritoneal cavity. Diffusion of electrolytes, such as potassium, can be achieved by instilling dialysate that has a concentration lower

than that of plasma. Water removal is enhanced by using a more hypertonic dextrose solution.

Peritoneal dialysis is a slow, continuous therapy. Initially, hourly exchanges may be required to control fluid and electrolyte abnormalities in the patient with ARF. After the BUN has been controlled, exchanges may be done less frequently. Exchanges of 2000 mL performed every 3 hours achieve approximately the same solute clearance as 4-hour hemodialysis treatments performed every other day (Maher, 1990).

Indications for Peritoneal Dialysis. Since peritoneal dialysis does not cause rapid shifts in fluid and electrolyte balance, it does not contribute to cardiovascular instability. Critically ill patients with low mean arterial blood pressures and those with cardiac dysrhythmias can be effectively dialyzed. Solutes are removed slowly over a period of hours to days. Since the blood solute level does not fluctuate rapidly, peritoneal dialysis can safely be used in patients with cerebral edema. Anticoagulation is not required, so peritoneal dialysis may be indicated for patients with bleeding tendencies.

The major disadvantage of peritoneal dialysis is

that solute removal is relatively inefficient. Even hourly exchanges may not be sufficient to control the extreme elevations in BUN and potassium seen in hypercatabolic patients. In addition, significant amounts of plasma proteins and amino acids may be lost through peritoneal drainage. Protein losses of up to 0.5 g/liter further compromise the nutritional status of the catabolic patient. Peritoneal dialysis can be used only in patients with intact peritoneal membranes. The procedure is contraindicated in most patients with abdominal trauma and following surgery that disrupts the peritoneal space.

Nursing Management. The critical care nurse is responsible for performing and monitoring the peritoneal dialysis procedure. Careful assessment of the patient's fluid volume status is performed on an ongoing basis. Specific attention is paid to intake and output records and to changes in the patient's body weight. Strict aseptic technique is utilized during exchanges and in performing care of the catheter exit site.

In addition to fluid management and infection control, the nurse observes the patient for potential complications associated with peritoneal dialysis. The most common complications are pain, drainage problems, and development of peritonitis. Pertinent nursing assessments and interventions are outlined in the nursing care plan for acute peritoneal dialysis.

Continuous Ultrafiltration

Continuous ultrafiltration (CU) is an extracorporeal blood treatment used to control both fluid and solute balance in patients with ARF. The therapy does not require the use of hemodialysis machinery but relies instead on the patient's own arterial blood pressure to power the system. As shown in Figure 41–3, the ultrafiltration system is composed of arterial and venous tubing, the hemofilter, and an ultrafiltrate collection receptacle.

The success of CU is dependent upon maintenance of blood flow through the hemofilter. Both arterial and venous vascular access are required. Blood flows of up to 200 mL/minute can be obtained using an external arteriovenous shunt or percutaneous femoral catheters. In most patients, a mean arterial blood pressure of 60 mm Hg is required to maintain adequate blood flow.

During CU, water, electrolytes, and other solutes are removed as the patient's blood passes over semipermeable membranes contained in a hemofilter. The resulting ultrafiltrate is a protein-free fluid with a solute and electrolyte concentration similar to that of plasma. The plasma proteins and cellular components of the blood remain in the hemofilter circuit and return to the venous circulation. Mass transfer of water and solutes across a semipermeable membrane is a result of convection and diffusion. In CU, the convective forces applied across the hemofilter

membrane depend primarily on the patient's arterial blood pressure. The higher the blood pressure, the greater the hydrostatic pressure within the hemofilter. Diffusion is a process in which solutes are passively transferred across a membrane. Passive transfer of solutes is dependent upon the presence of a concentration gradient across the membrane. In CU therapy, a concentration gradient can be established by infusing dialysate fluid into the nonblood side of the hemofilter.

Indications for Continuous Ultrafiltration. Removal of plasma water and electrolytes by CU is a gradual process that closely resembles the kidney's normal function. Because it is gradual, rapid fluctuations in fluid and electrolyte status do not occur. Therefore, CU therapy is indicated for ARF patients with cardiovascular instability, abdominal wounds, or cerebral edema (Nahman and Middendorf, 1990). There are three distinct variations of CU in current clinical use. As summarized in Table 41–9, each of these treatment variations is designed to meet the renal replacement needs of a specific group of patients.

Slow Continuous Ultrafiltration. Slow continuous ultrafiltration (SCUF) is a CU therapy in which small amounts of plasma water and solutes are slowly removed from the patient. In most patients, fluid removal occurs at rates of 150 to 300 mL/hour. The therapeutic goal of SCUF is to control fluid balance and prevent fluid volume overload (Swan and Paganini, 1986). Because only small amounts of solutes are removed, SCUF is unsuitable as the primary dialysis therapy for patients with azotemia or significant electrolyte abnormalities. SCUF is highly effective in controlling fluid volume overload in patients with severe congestive heart failure who do not respond to diuretic therapy. Fluid removal by ultrafiltration can achieve significant preload reduction in these patients. SCUF can also be used as an adjunct to hemodialysis in patients with ARF who require large volumes of maintenance intravenous fluids. The patient is placed on SCUF between hemodialysis treatments to prevent hypervolemia and decrease the need for additional hemodialysis treatments.

Continuous Arteriovenous Hemofiltration. Continuous arteriovenous hemofiltration (CAVH) is a renal replacement therapy in which large amounts of plasma water and solutes are removed on a continuous basis. Fluid removal rates may range from 400 to 800 mL/hour. Because CAVH removes large volumes of plasma water, significant amounts of plasma electrolytes and solutes are also removed. Control of fluid volume and electrolyte balance is achieved through large-volume fluid exchanges. Hourly ultrafiltrate loss is replaced by prescribed amounts of a sterile intravenous electrolyte solution. CAVH provides a mechanism of diluting the patient's plasma by selective replacement of solutes. Therefore, CAVH can be utilized as the primary dialysis therapy for

TABLE 41-9. Clinical Application of Continuous Ultrafiltration Therapy

	Slow Continuous Ultrafiltration (SCUF)	Continuous Arteriovenous Hemofiltration (CAVH)	Continuous Arteriovenous Hemofiltration Dialysis (CAVHD)
Therapeutic goal	Prevention of hypervolemia	Control of fluid and solute balance	Control of fluid and solute balance
Indications	Volume overload in CHF. Adjunct to hemodialysis	Noncatabolic patients with oliguric ARF	Catabolic or noncatabolic patients with oliguric ARF
Rate of fluid removal	<300 mL/hour	400–800 mL/hour	Approximately 100 mL/hour
Efficiency of solute removal	Minimal solute removed	Solute control achieved dilution with large volume exchanges	Steady-state plasma, urea, and creatinine levels by 24–48 hours
Mechanism of solute removal	Convection resulting from hydrostatic pressure exerted by the arterial blood pressure	Convection	Primary—diffusion of solutes from blood into dialysate; Secondary—convection
Fluid replacement requirements	Fluid requirements usually met by maintenance intravenous infusions	Up to 20 liters/24 hours of prescribed intravenous fluids	Fluid requirements usually met by maintenance intravenous infusions

Abbreviations: ARF, acute renal failure.

ARF patients with mild to moderate azotemia and electrolyte disturbances (Olbricht, 1986).

Continuous Arteriovenous Hemodialysis. Continuous arteriovenous hemodialysis (CAVH) combines the convective transport of CAVH with diffusion dialysis. Sterile dialysate fluid is infused into the ultrafiltration compartment of the hemofilter shown in Figure 41–4. The dialysate flows countercurrent to the blood flow, which increases diffusion of solutes from the blood to the ultrafiltration compartment. Solute removal in CAVH is much greater than that in CAVH. Therefore, CAVHD can be effectively utilized as the primary dialysis therapy in a wide variety of critically ill patients, including ARF patients with severe azotemia and electrolyte imbalance. Plasma urea and creatinine levels reach a steady state after 24 to 48 hours of CAVHD treatment (Geronemus, 1986). Electrolyte abnormalities and acid-base disturbances are also well controlled.

Nursing Management. The major nursing goal in continuous ultrafiltration therapy is optimization of the patient's fluid volume status (Whitman, 1986). The large amount of fluid removed by ultrafiltration places the patient at risk of fluid volume depletion. Maintenance of the patency of the ultrafiltration system and prevention of blood loss are additional nursing goals. Nursing interventions to support these goals are described in the nursing care plan for continuous ultrafiltration therapy.

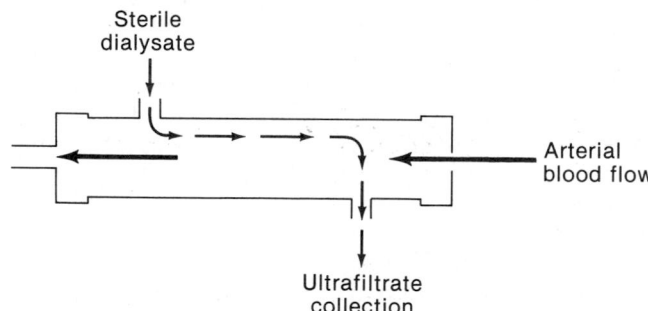

FIGURE 41–4. Continuous arteriovenous hemodialysis.

ncp nursing care plan

CONTINUOUS ULTRAFILTRATION THERAPY

Outcome Criteria		Nursing Interventions

1. Potential fluid volume deficit	Fluid volume balance remains optimal	1. Monitor and regulate ultrafiltration rate hourly
		  a. Use screw clamp on ultrafiltrate line to increase or decrease rate
		  b. Keep collection bag at same distance below hemofilter
		2. Monitor blood pressure hourly
		  a. Administer fluids or vasopressors to maintain mean arterial pressure at or above 60 mm Hg
		3. Monitor heart rate, CVP, PCWP for changes indicating hypovolemia

Outcome Criteria		Nursing Interventions

2. Alteration in hemofilter perfusion	Hemofilter and tubing remain patent	1. Assess hemofilter and blood tubing hourly
		  a. Blood in the hemofilter should appear bright red
		  b. Observe for darkening of blood, streaks, or separation of cells from plasma
		2. If clotting occurs, flush hemofilter with heparinized saline as prescribed
		3. Draw blood from venous port every 4 hours for clotting studies (PTT/ACT)
		4. Adust heparin infusion to maintain the PTT/ACT within the precribed range
		5. Secure tubing to prevent stasis from kinking or compression of tubing
		6. Maintain blood pressure above 60 mm Hg to prevent stasis of blood in hemofilter

Outcome Criteria		Nursing Interventions
3. Potential for injury	No blood loss from ultrafiltration system	1. Securely bridge-tape all blood tubing connections 2. Position hemofilter/blood lines to prevent accidental disconnection 3. Test ultrafiltrate for blood every 4 hours 4. Replace hemofilter if blood is present in ultrafiltrate

Outcome Criteria		Nursing Interventions
4. Potential for infection	Patient remains infection free	1. Utilize aseptic technique when entering the system to draw blood 2. Observe catheter exit sites for redness, drainage 3. Perform daily exit site care

Abbreviations: CVP, central venous pressure; PCWP, pulmonary capillary wedge pressure; PTT, partial thromboplastin time; ACT, activated clotting time.

ACUTE HEMODIALYSIS

Outcome Criteria		Nursing Interventions

1. Decreased perfusion through vascular access	Vascular access remains patent	*External Arteriovenous Shunt*
		1. Palpate:
		  The external cannula should feel warm. A "thrill" should be felt near the tip of the cannula
		2. Asculate:
		  A buzzing sound should be audible when the stethoscope bell is placed over the shunt
		3. Observe:
		  The column of blood in the cannula should appear a uniform red color
		4. Protect:
		  Elevate extremity on pillow for 48 to 72 hours. Avoid constrictions above access, e.g., BP cuff, tourniquets
		
		Subclavian Catheter
		1. Instill heparin into catheter following dialysis treatment
		2. Restrict use of catheter to hemodialysis treatments only. Do not infuse blood, fluids, or medications through it
		3. Secure catheter to prevent kinking or pulling
		
		Femoral Vein Catheter
		1. Keep leg straight while catheter is in place
		2. Restrict hip flexion to prevent kinking

Nursing Care Plan continued on following page

Outcome Criteria		Nursing Interventions
2. Potential for injury	No bleeding from vascular access	*Extrnal Arteriovenous Shunt* 1. Secure cannula limbs by bridge-taping and securely wrapping extremity 2. Minimize stress/pulling at the cannula exit sites 3. Keep a set of cannula clamps available at all times. If cannulas separate, clamp both immediately *Subclavian Catheter* 1. Secure catheter to prevent it from catching on bed linen 2. If patient is confused, restrain hands to prevent catheter dislodgement *Femoral Vein Catheter* 1. Immobilize patient during treatment to prevent displacement of catheter 2. Following removal of catheter, apply pressure to site for at least 10 minutes, then apply a tight dressing

Outcome Criteria		Nursing Interventions
3. Potential for infection	Access remains free of infection	*External Arteriovenous Shunt* 1. Clean and redress cannula exit sites daily 2. Use aseptic technique when drawing blood from shunt 3. Minimize manipulation of shunt *Subclavian Catheter* 1. Maintain a sterile, occlusive transparent dressing over exit site between treatments 2. Examine entry site for inflammation, swelling, tenderness, and discharge *Femoral Vein Catheter* 1. Catheters are usually removed following treatment 2. If catheter is left in place, provide meticulous site care

ACUTE PERITONEAL DIALYSIS

Outcome Criteria		Nursing Interventions
1. Alteration in comfort: Pain	Patient's pain is controlled	1. Warm dialysate to body temperature 2. Slow infusion rate to tolerable level 3. Administer pain medication as prescribed

Outcome Criteria		Nursing Interventions
2. Potential for fluid excess	Adequate fluid is removed	1. Maintain accurate records of dialysate infusion and drainage 2. Weigh daily at the end of the drain cycle 3. Change patient's position to facilitate drainage 4. Notify physician of significant fluid retention over two cycles

Outcome Criteria		Nursing Interventions
3. Potential for infection	Catheter exit site remains free of infection. Patient does not develop peritonitis	1. Assess exit site for signs of redness, drainage, leakage 2. Perform daily exit site care 3. Monitor patient's temperature curve 4. Assess drainage from each exchange: Report cloudiness, color change Send drainage for daily culture

SUMMARY

Acute renal failure is a serious complication of critical illness in which renal function is severely compromised. Acute renal failure may be due to renal hypoperfusion, obstruction of the urinary tract, or acute tubular necrosis resulting from renal ischemia or exposure to toxic agents. Oliguria is the most common manifestation and may persist from days to months. Goals of therapy include control of fluid and solute balance, adequate nutrition, and preven- tion of infection. Most patients with ARF recover near-normal renal function, although some deficits in tubular function may remain for months to years following the renal injury.

References

Andreucci, V. E. (1984). Myoglobinuria and acute renal failure. In V. E. Andreucci (Ed.), *Acute renal failure. Pathophysiology, prevention and treatment* (pp. 250–255). Boston: Martinus Nijhoff.

Bayati, A., Nygren, K., Kallskog, O., et al. (1990a). The long-term outcome of post-ischaemic acute renal failure II. A histopathological study of the untreated kidney. *AcTA Physiologica Scandinavia*, 138, 35–47.

Bayati, A., Nygren, K., Kallskog, O., et al. (1990b). The effect of loop diuretics on the long-term outcome of post-ischaemic acute renal failure in the rat. *AcTA Physiologica Scandinavia*, 139, 271–279.

Bennett, W. M. (1986). Update on drugs in renal failure. In J. P. Greenfeld, M. H. Maxwell, J. F. Back, et al. (Eds.), *Advances in nephrology* (Vol. 15, pp. 287–299). Chicago: Year Book.

Bernstein, J. M. and Erk, S. D. (1990). Choice of antibiotics, pharmacokinetics, and dose adjustments in acute renal failure. *Medical Clinics of North America*, 74, 1059–1076.

Bluemle, L. W., Potter, H. P., Elkinton, J. R. (1951). Changes in body composition in ARF. *Journal of Clinical Investigation*, 35, 1094–1099.

Brezis, M., Rosen, S., Silva, P., et al. (1984). Renal ischemia: A new perspective. *Kidney International*, 26, 375–383.

Burke, T. J., Arnold, P. E., Gordon, J. A., et al. (1984). Protective effect of intrarenal calcium membrane blockers before or after renal ischemia. *Journal of Clinical Investigation*, 74, 1830–1841.

Burke, T. J., Cronin, R. E., Duchin, K. L., et al. (1980). Ischemia and tubule obstruction during acute renal failure in dogs: Mannitol in protection. *American Journal of Physiology*, 238, 305–314.

Cameron, J. J., and Ogg, C. (1967). Peritoneal dialysis in hypercatabolic acute renal failure. *Lancet*, 1, 1188–1191.

Cattell, W. R., McIntosh, C. S., Moseley, I. F., et al. (1973). Excretion urography in acute renal failure. *British Medical Journal*, 2, 275–279.

Clark, R. A., Hamory, B. H., Ford, G. H., et al. (1972). Chemotaxis in acute renal failure. *Journal of Infectious Diseases*, 126, 460–465.

Corwin, H. L., and Bonventre, J. V. (1986). Acute renal failure. *Medical Clinics of North America*, 70, 1037–1054.

D'Amico, G., and Colasanti, G. (1987). The role of renal biopsy in acute renal failure. In A. Americo, P. Coratelli, V. M. Campese, et al. (Eds.), *Acute renal failure: Clinical and experimental*, (pp. 35–39). New York: Plenum.

Donohoe, J. F., Venkatachalam, M. A., Bernard, D. B., et al. (1978). Tubular leakage and obstruction after renal ischemia. Structural-functional correlations. *Kidney International*, 13, 208–222.

Edell, S., and Zengel, H. (1978). Ultrasonic evaluation of renal calculi. *American Journal of Roentgenology*, 130, 261–263.

Finn, W. F. (1990). Diagnosis and management of acute tubular necrosis. *Medical Clinics of North America*, 74, 373–380.

Flores, J., DiBona, D. R., Beck, C. H., et al. (1972). The role of cell swelling in ischemic renal damage and the protective effect of hypertonic solute. *Journal of Clinical Investigation*, 51, 118–125.

Geronemus, R. (1986). Continuous arteriovenous hemodialysis—Clinical experience. In E. Paginini (Ed.), *Acute continuous renal replacement therapy* (pp. 247–254). Boston: Martinus Nijhoff.

Giordano, C., Castellano, P., Pluvio, M., et al. (1987). Glucose metabolism. In A. Americo, P. Coratelli, V. M. Campese, et al. (Eds.), *Acute renal failure: Clinical and experimental* (pp. 105–111). New York: Plenum.

Goldblum, S. E., and Reed, W. P. (1980). Host defenses and immunologic alterations associated with chronic hemodialysis. *Annals of Internal Medicine*, 93, 597–613.

Graziani, G., Cantaluppi, S., Casati, S., et al. (1984). Dopamine and furosemide in oliguric acute renal failure. *Nephron*, 37, 39–42.

Green, W. M., and King D. L. (1976). Diagnostic ultrasound of the urinary tract. *Journal of Clinical Ultrasound*, 4, 55–59.

Gutch, C. F., and Stoner, M. H. (1983). *Review of hemodialysis for nurses and dialysis personnel* (4th ed., pp. 31–44). St. Louis: C.V. Mosby.

Hou, S. H., Bushinsky, D., Wish, J., et al. (1983). Hospital-acquired renal insufficiency: A prospective study. *American Journal of Medicine*, 74, 243–248.

Hou, S. H., and Cohen, J. J. (1985). Diagnosis and management of acute renal failure. *Acute Care*, 11, 59–84.

Hoyer, J., and Seiler, M. W. (1979). Pathophysiology of Tamm-Horsfall protein. *Kidney International*, 16, 279–289.

Jacobsen, W. K., Cole, D. J., Stewart, S. C., et al. (1990). Effect of calcium entry blocker nitrendipine on renal function after renal vascular occlusion. *Critical Care Medicine*, 18, 1403–1407.

Jameson, M. D., and Wiegmann, T. B. (1990). Principles, uses, and complications of hemodialysis. *Medical Clinics of North America*, 74, 945–960.

Kashgarian, M., Siegel, N. J., Ries, A. L., et al. (1976). Hemodynamic aspects in development and recovery phases of experimental post-ischemic acute renal failure. *Kidney International*, 10, 160–168.

Knochel, J. P. (1988). Biochemical, electrolyte, and acid-base disturbances in acute renal failure. In B. M. Brenner, and J. M. Lazarus (Eds.), *Acute renal failure*, (2nd ed., pp. 677–703). New York: Churchill Livingstone.

Knochel, J. P. (1985). Potassium gradients and neuromuscular excitability. In D. N. Seldin, G. Giebisch (Eds.), *The kidney: Physiology and pathology* (pp. 1207–1221). New York: Raven Press.

Knochel, J. P. (1977). The pathophysiology and clinical characteristics of severe hypophosphatemia. *Archives of Internal Medicine*, 137, 203–220.

Larrain, C., and Adleson, E. (1956). Hemostatic defect of uremia: Clinical investigation of three patients with acute post-traumatic renal insufficiency. *Blood*, 11, 1059.

Levine, M. L., Simon, N. M., Herdson, P. B., et al. (1972). Acute renal failure followed by protracted slowly resolving chronic uremia. *Journal of Chronic Disease*, 25, 645–649.

Linder, A. (1983). Synergism of dopamine and furosemide in diuretic-resistant, oliguric acute renal failure. *Nephron*, 33, 121–126.

Llach, F., Felsenfeld, A. J., and Haussler, M. R. (1981). Pathophysiology of altered calcium metabolism in rhabdomyolysis-induced acute renal failure. *New England Journal of Medicine*, 305(3), 117–122.

Maher, J. F. (1990). Physiology of the peritoneum. *Medical Clinics of North America*, 74, 985–996.

Mason, J., Olbricht, C., Takabarake, T., et al. (1977). The early phase of experimental acute renal failure, I. Intratubular pressure and obstruction. *Pflugers Archive*, 370, 155–163.

Mason, J., Torhorst, J., and Welsch, J. (1984). Role of the medullary perfusion defect in the pathogenesis of ischemic renal failure. *Kidney International*, 26, 283–286.

May, R. C., Kelly, R. A., and Mitch, W. E. (1986). Metabolic acidosis stimulates protein degradation in rat muscle by a glucocorticoid-dependent mechanism. *Journal of Clinical Investigation*, 77, 614–621.

Meyers, C., Roxe, D. M., and Hano, J. E. (1977). The clinical course of nonoliguric acute renal failure. *Cardiovascular Medicine*, 2, 669–672.

Mitch, W. E., and Wilmore, D. W. (1988). Nutritional considerations in the treatment of acute renal failure. In B. M. Brenner and J. M. Lazarus (Eds.), *Acute renal failure* (2nd ed., pp. 743–765). New York: Churchill Livingstone.

Molitoris, B. A., and Schrier, R. W. (1984). Prevention of acute renal failure. In R. J. Glassock (Ed.), *Current therapy in nephrology and hypertension 1984–1985* (pp. 231–235). Philadelphia: B. C. Decker.

Myers, B. D., Carrie, B. J., Yee, R. R., et al. (1980). Pathophysiology of hemodynamically mediated acute renal failure in man. *Kidney International*, 18, 495–502.

Nahman, N. S., and Middendorf, D. F. (1990). Continuous arteriovenous hemofiltration. *Medical Clinics of North America*, 74, 975–984.

Olbricht, C. (1986). Continuous arteriovenous hemofiltration—The control of azotemia in acute renal failure. In E. Paginini (Ed.), *Acute continuous renal replacement therapy* (pp. 123–142). Boston: Martinus Nijhoff.

Oliver, J., MacDowell, M., and Tracy, A. (1951). The pathogenesis of acute renal failure associated with traumatic and toxic injury: Renal ischemia, nephrotoxic damage and the ischemic episode. *Journal of Clinical Investigation*, 30, 1307–1440.

Olsen, S., and Solez, K. (1987). Acute renal failure in man: Pathogenesis in light of new morphological data. *Clinical Nephrology*, 27(6), 271–277.

Papper, S. (1978). *Clinical nephrology* (2nd ed., pp. 285–299). Boston: Little, Brown.

Rackow, E. C., Fein, I. A., Spring, C., et al. (1978). Uremic pulmonary edema. *American Journal of Medicine*, 64, 1084–1088.

Radtke, H. W., Claussner, A., Erbes, P. M., et al. (1979). Serum erythropoietin concentration in chronic renal failure: Relationship to degree of anemia and excretory function. *Blood, 54*, 877–884.

Radtke, H. W., Rege, A. B., LaMarche, M. B., et al. (1981). Identification of spermine as an inhibitor of erythropoiesis in patients with chronic renal failure. *Journal of Clinical Investigation, 67*, 1623–1629.

Reaven, G. M., Wisinger, J. R., and Swenson, R. S. (1974). Insulin and glucose metabolism in renal insufficiency. *Kidney International, 6*, 63–69.

Relman, A. S. (1972). Metabolic consequences of acid-base disorders. *Kidney International, 1*, 347–359.

Rudnick, M. R., Bastl, C. P., Elfinbein, I. B., et al. (1988). The differential diagnosis of acute renal failure. In B. M. Brenner and J. M. Lazarus (Eds.), *Acute renal failure* (2nd ed., pp. 177–232). New York: Churchill Livingstone.

Schrier, R. W. (1981). Acute renal failure: Pathogenesis, diagnosis, and management. *Hospital Practice, 16*, 93–112.

Schrier, R. W., and Burke, T. J. (1988). Calcium-channel blockers in experimental and human acute renal failure. In F. J. P. Grunfeld, M. H. Maxwell, J. F. Back, et al. (Eds.), *Advances in nephrology* (Vol. 17, pp. 287–299). Chicago: Year Book.

Shapira, J., Iaina, A., Eliahou, H. E., et al. (1976). High renin activity accompanying antiotensin II inhibition in rats with ischemic renal failure. *Israel Journal of Medical Sciences, 12*, 124–130.

Solez, K., and Finckh, E. S. (1984). Is there a correlation between morphologic and functional changes in human acute renal failure? In K. Solez, and A. Whelton (Eds.), *Acute renal failure: Correlations between morphology and function* (pp. 3–12). New York: Marcel Dekker.

Steinman, T. I., and Lazarus, J. M. (1988). Organ-system involvement in acute renal failure. In B. M. Brenner, and J. M. Lazarus (Eds.), *Acute renal failure* (2nd ed., pp. 705–742). New York: Churchill Livingstone.

Swan, S., and Paganini, E. (1986). The practical aspects of slow continuous ultrafiltration (SCUF) and continuous arteriovenous hemofiltration (CAVH). In E. Paginini (Ed.), *Acute continuous renal replacement therapy* (pp. 51–78). Boston: Martinus Nijhoff.

Tanner, G. A., and Steinhausen, M. (1976). Tubular obstruction in ischemia-induced acute renal failure in the rat. *Kidney International, 10*, 565–573.

Tolkoff-Rubin, N. E., McCluskey, R. T., Bhan, A. K., et al. (1984). Renal damage due to aminoglycoside administration in the Lewis rat. In K. Solez, and A. Whelton (Eds.), *Acute renal failure. Correlations between morphology and function* (pp. 249–260). New York: Marcel Dekker.

VanZee, B. O., Hoy, W. E., Talley, T. E., et al. (1978). Renal injury associated with intravenous pyelography in nondiabetic and diabetic patients. *Annals of Internal Medicine, 89*, 51–54.

Whalley, D. W., Ibels, L. S., Eckstein, R. P., et al. (1987). Acute tubular necrosis complicating bilateral retrograde pyelography. *Australian and New Zealand Journal of Medicine, 17*(5), 536–538.

Whitman, G. (1986). Hemofiltration and ultrafiltration: Nursing concerns. In E. Paginini (Ed.), *Acute continuous renal replacement therapy* (pp. 91–111). Boston: Martinus Nijhoff.

Whittaker, A. (1985). Acute renal dysfunction: Assessment of patients at risk. *Focus on Critical Care, 12*, 12–17.

Zager, R. (1983). Glomerular filtration rate and brush border debris excretion after mercuric chloride and ischemic acute renal failure: Mannitol versus furosemide diuresis. *Nephron, 33*, 196–201.

42

Patients with End-Stage Renal Disease

Sylvia Yarian

When the patient with chronic renal failure is admitted to a critical care unit, a critical illness or injury is superimposed on the existing renal pathophysiology. The critical care nurse may care for a number of patients along the continuum of renal failure, including those with mild renal insufficiency, those approaching end stage, and those who are already long-term dialysis patients. An understanding of chronic renal failure is the foundation on which development of nursing diagnoses and appropriate nursing interventions are based. The focus of this chapter is on the patient with end-stage renal disease (ESRD). However, the assessments and interventions presented are applicable to any patient with chronic renal disease.

HISTORICAL PERSPECTIVE ON ESRD AND DIALYSIS

End-stage renal disease was considered a uniformly fatal disease prior to the development of hemodialysis and transplantation. Before the 1960s, the patient with ESRD could be offered only conservative medical management of diet and fluids. Although hemodialysis and peritoneal dialysis were available, they could be used only in the acute care setting. Chronic hemodialysis first became a reality in 1960 when Scribner and Quinton developed an all-Teflon arteriovenous shunt—the first permanent access to the circulatory system. This shunt heralded the means of obtaining easy, repeated access to the circulation and the start of long-term therapy (Scribner and Babb, 1986). Technologic advances have continued over the past three decades and include improved access to the circulation, improved catheters for peritoneal dialysis, sophisticated equipment for dialysis therapies, efficient dialyzers, and advanced immunosuppressive therapy for transplantation. Morbidity and mortality rates have been reduced despite a marked rise in the mean age of patients on dialysis as well as an increased percentage of patients with multi-organ diseases.

In the beginning, selection committees decided who would be suitable candidates for hemodialysis. Selection was based upon criteria that included the person's potential contribution to society, rehabilitation potential, age, availability of space in a hemodialysis program, and ability to pay. When hemodialysis became more widely available, these committees were discontinued.

In 1972, the End Stage Renal Disease Program was enacted through federal legislation. This provided funding, under Medicare, to cover nearly the entire U.S. population with this catastrophic illness. During the first year of funding in 1973, 10,000 patients enrolled.

By the end of 1987, there were approximately 98,000 patients on dialysis (83,000 on hemodialysis and 15,000 on peritoneal dialysis). Nearly 9000 kidney transplants were performed, and an additional 12,000 patients were awaiting transplantation (National News, 1988). For 1989, the government's financial obligation to the ESRD program was approximately $3 billion.

Each renal replacement therapy has its complications. Cardiovascular complications account for approximately 50% of deaths in the ESRD population, and infections cause around 15% (ESRD Network 3, 1987). Infection is the most common cause of death of patients with ESRD in critical care units.

PATHOPHYSIOLOGY OF ESRD

A variety of mechanisms are responsible for kidney injury that ultimately progresses to ESRD. These include abnormal immunologic processes, coagulation disorders, vascular disorders, infection, and biochemical and metabolic disturbances. Several of these mechanisms may occur concurrently to cause advancing renal disease.

The typical clinical course of chronic renal failure culminating in ESRD is slow, progressive, and irreversible. The process may take from a few months to many years to become clinically evident. Clinical signs and symptoms may not occur until the glomerular filtration rate (GFR) is decreased by approximately 80%.

Etiology

Determination of the etiology of ESRD is often difficult. There is pathologic and histologic variability in the renal diseases as well as in their rate of progression. However, each results in a similar presentation of chemical and physiologic abnormalities. The hallmark of chronic renal disease is an irreversible, progressive decrease in GFR over a period of months to years. On x-ray, the kidneys generally appear small due to cortical thinning and eventual glomerular sclerosis, resulting in tubule loss, interstitial fibroses, and marked vascular disease (Coe, 1986). These changes result in a loss of the kidney's ability to excrete wastes and regulate the body's internal environment. The excretory failure can be treated with dialysis. The loss of biochemical and metabolic regulation leads to disturbances such as anemia and renal osteodystrophy.

The classification of disease states that progress to ESRD is variable and is constantly evolving. For ease of discussion only, the most commonly seen disorders will be summarized. Collectively, glomerular disease, polycystic kidney disease, hypertensive nephropathy, and diabetic nephropathy account for approximately 75% of all cases that progress to ESRD. A more extensive review of a particular disease can be found in any text specific to kidney disease.

Glomerular Disease. Glomerular diseases are one of the most frequent causes of ESRD. They result either from an immune process involving the glomerulus or as part of a systemic disorder that also involves other organ systems. The immune mechanism may be one of two types. Antibodies can react with a structural portion of the glomerulus, e.g., the glomerular basement membrane. More commonly, antibodies react with soluble antigen to form circulating immune complexes that are deposited in the glomerulus.

Chronic glomerulonephritis refers to an insidious, progressive functional impairment accompanied by varying degrees of proteinuria, hematuria, and hypertension. Progression of the disease to end stage occurs over a period ranging from 5 to 10 years or more, and the initiating problem is often impossible to determine (Glassock et al., 1986). Contributing to the progression of renal failure are an elevation of systemic blood pressure as well as increased flow and elevated glomerular pressures in the intact nephrons (Skorecki et al., 1986). Once these adaptive hemodynamic events are set into motion in the glomerular circulation, progression of renal failure occurs even when the initiating factor is no longer present. Blood pressure control and dietary protein restriction may slow the process.

In general, the glomerular diseases produce three different types of urinary sediment that may serve as clues to diagnosis and treatment. Nephrotic patterns are characterized by heavy proteinuria and lipiduria. The presence of hematuria is variable. Because the basement membrane is damaged, there is increased permeability but no inflammatory changes.

Nephritic patterns are characterized by red and white cells and a variable degree of proteinuria. There are frequent granular casts. Focal or diffuse involvement may occur, with diffuse glomerular disease resulting in more severe abnormalities.

Chronic patterns are characterized by less proteinuria and hematuria and by the presence of broad waxy casts and granular casts. The acute inflammatory changes are replaced by scarring. The decrease in GFR accounts for the presence of a less abnormal urinalysis.

Glomerular diseases account for 23% of the cases of ESRD that are treated by dialysis (ESRD Profile Tables, 1988). Research into methods of slowing the progression of these diseases focuses on dietary protein control and, especially, blood pressure control.

Polycystic Kidney Disease. Autosomal dominant polycystic kidney disease (ADPKD), which is generally classified as a tubulointerstitial disease, is a genetic kidney disorder that is responsible for approximately 10% of all cases of ESRD. It is characterized by the formation of multiple cysts of varying sizes that can develop anywhere in the nephron, but most often affect the proximal and collecting tubules. These cysts progressively enlarge and compress the adjacent nephrons. Renal function becomes compromised by the fourth to fifth decade of life (Grantham, 1988).

Cyst formation may also occur in other organs such as the liver, pancreas, and spleen. In 10% of these patients, the cerebral arteries may develop structural weaknesses leading to aneurysm formation and eventual intracerebral bleeding (Rose and Black, 1989).

Blood pressure is elevated in the majority of patients with ADPKD prior to the onset of renal failure. It is thought that compression of the intrarenal arteries by the cysts promotes renin secretion. Hypertension puts these patients at added risk for cerebral aneurysm rupture. Episodic gross hematuria, flank pain, vague abdominal discomfort due to bleeding into the cysts, and urinary tract infections are common features. The kidneys are generally palpable once the cysts have increased in size and number. Despite ESRD, a near normal hematocrit is generally the rule. This may be due to abnormal erythropoietin production by the cysts (Grantham, 1988). Patients with large polycystic kidneys may require nephrectomy prior to renal transplantation.

Hypertensive Nephropathy. Hypertension in conjunction with heart and renal disease accounts for nearly 25% of all ESRD cases (ESRD Profile Tables, 1988). The association between increasingly severe hypertension and the development of cardiovascular, cerebrovascular, and nephrovascular disease is well established. Systemic hypertension has adverse effects on the kidney and may initiate the development of renal disease or accelerate loss of function in the already diseased kidney (Baldwin and Newgarten, 1987).

The pathophysiology of the hypertension of chronic renal failure that progresses to ESRD is multifactorial. Sodium balance, hemodynamic factors, and the complex relationship between the renin-angiotensin system and the autonomic nervous system all play a role. These mechanisms have been covered in detail in Chapters 39 and 40 of this text.

Diabetic Nephropathy. Diabetic nephropathy is the single most important disorder leading to renal failure in the United States. It accounts for at least 25% of all cases of ESRD. An estimated 45% to 50% of insulin-dependent diabetics will develop nephropathy between 10 and 30 years following the onset of diabetes (Hostetter, 1986; Schmitz et al., 1985). Most often, this disease is the result of progressive glomerulosclerosis. For the diabetic who has reached ESRD, the major determinant of survival is related to the degree of cardiovascular disease that is present. These patients are also two- to threefold more likely than the nondiabetic patient treated by hemodialysis to succumb to infection (Keane and Maddy, 1989).

A poor outcome is predicted for diabetics with proteinuria of greater than 3 g/24 hours. The interval from the appearance of persistent proteinuria in the diabetic to established renal failure averages about 5 years. Studies have suggested that aggressive insulin therapy when subclinical albumin excretion occurs, plus effective hypertensive therapy, can slow the rate of decline of the GFR. In addition, the albumin excretion is decreased, thereby delaying progression to ESRD (Aubria et al., 1987; Morgensen, 1987).

Diabetics tolerate uremic symptoms less well than nondiabetics with ESRD. The uremic abnormalities associated with glucose intolerance and impaired insulin metabolism are even more complex in diabetics. The associated changes in diet, appetite, and physical activity complicate the clinical picture. For these reasons, renal replacement therapy is usually initiated at an earlier time in these patients, depending on the clinical symptoms.

Progression of Chronic Renal Failure

The usual clinical course of chronic renal failure is a slow progressive and irreversible process. Renal deterioration may take place over months to years until clinical symptoms become evident, and the patient reaches end stage. It is hypothesized that the kidney is able to maintain homeostasis in spite of a significant loss of functional nephrons because of its compensatory mechanisms. Bricker's intact nephron hypothesis suggests that nephrons, which are unaffected by the disease process, are essentially intact and increase their filtration rates (Brenner et al., 1986). This enables them to control solute and water excretion far along the course of the disease (Glassock et al., 1986). The compensatory hyperfiltration that occurs in the intact nephrons is able to maintain the GFR despite the disease activity until renal deterioration is quite severe. It has been proposed that the elevation in glomerular capillary hydrostatic pressure, which maintains the GFR, is the very mechanism that results in progressive glomerular damage (Fine, 1987).

The progression of chronic renal failure occurs in three stages. Each stage reflects an increasing loss of nephrons (Richard, 1987). The first stage, diminished renal reserve, reflects a 50% loss of nephron function. During this stage the patient is asymptomatic with serum creatinine levels within the high normal range. It is important to understand that serum creatinine concentrations above the normal range are highly significant in terms of the magnitude of nephron loss. Serum creatinine concentration doubles with a 50% loss of nephron function. Thus, a rise from 0.6 mg/dL to 1.2 mg/dL is significant even though this level is still within the normal range.

The second stage, renal insufficiency, reflects a nephron loss of 75% to 80%. Due to the decreased GFR and reduced clearance of solutes, the patient exhibits mild azotemia (elevated levels of plasma urea and creatinine), impaired ability to concentrate urine, and anemia. Conservative management with diet, fluid control, and medications may be adequate to control uremic symptoms. Chronic renal insufficiency, once established, tends to progress to the last stage, i.e., end-stage renal disease. Progression is influenced by the severity of hypertension, dietary protein intake, infection, nephrotoxic drugs, and other metabolic disturbances.

ESRD represents the final stage in which there is a 90% nephron loss. Homeostasis can no longer be maintained, and all body systems are affected. An accumulation of uremic waste products, fluid and electrolyte abnormalities, and disordered regulatory and hormonal functions are a few of the multiple chemical and physiologic changes that occur.

The patient with ESRD requires renal replacement therapy to maintain life. The options available include conservative management, home- or center-based hemodialysis, peritoneal dialysis, hemofiltration, and cadaver or living related donor renal transplantation (Prowant and Binkley, 1987). The patient's right to make choices regarding the options includes the right to refuse all therapy. The mortality rate for this last group is 100%.

CLINICAL MANAGEMENT

The systemic consequences of renal failure are evident to the nurse caring for the patient with ESRD. Admission of these patients into the critical care unit may involve a number of acute problems such as congestive heart failure, pulmonary edema, hyperkalemia, sepsis, and gastrointestinal bleeding. A review of systems for the patient with ESRD will be presented along with a discussion of medical management and specific nursing care. Because the majority of these patients are maintained by dialysis therapy, specific problems relating to this group will be emphasized.

Dialysis cannot replace the metabolic and endocrine functions of the kidney. Improvements occur in the function of some organ systems, but reversal of all the adaptive and maladaptive changes does not occur. Successful renal transplantation resolves many of the organ system problems. However, immunosuppression therapy brings with it a new set of systemic consequences, as described in Chapter 52.

Cardiovascular System

Cardiovascular complications account for approximately 50% of the mortality that occurs in the ESRD population. Table 42–1 summarizes the most common cardiovascular complications seen in patients with renal failure. For patients on hemodialysis, the mortality rate due to myocardial infarction and cerebrovascular disease is three times that of nonuremic, age-matched controls (Hakim and Lazarus, 1986).

TABLE 42–1. Factors Contributing to Myocardial Dysfunction in End-Stage Renal Disease (ESRD)

Atherosclerosis
Hypertension
Electrolyte abnormalities
Hypervolemia
Myocardial calcifications
Anemia
Arteriovenous fistula or graft
Autonomic neuropathy
Acetate in dialysate (vasodilatory effect)
Other systemic diseases (e.g., diabetes)

There are numerous potential factors in the development of atherosclerosis and subsequent myocardial damage and malfunction.

Hyperlipidemia has a role in vascular atherosclerosis and occurs in 50% of the dialysis population. Type IV hyperlipidemia is the most prevalent, with increases in total triglycerides and very low density lipoproteins, decreases in high-density lipoproteins, and normal total cholesterol levels (Golper, 1986). This pattern is associated with an increased incidence of ischemic coronary artery heart disease. Abnormal lipid metabolism may be related to an increased production of lipoproteins by the liver and impaired catabolism of low-density lipoproteins (Jacobson and McNatt, 1986). Other factors that contribute to hyperlipidemia are the ingestion of prescribed high-carbohydrate, high-fat diets and the decreased exercise patterns seen in patients with ESRD due to the effects of anemia. There have been improvements in hematocrit, triglyceride levels, and high-density lipoprotein levels in patients undergoing exercise programs (Kjellstrand, 1985). In peritoneal dialysis, hyperlipidemia can be aggravated by the continuous transperitoneal glucose absorption that occurs during dialysis exchanges.

Hypertension. Seventy to ninety per cent of patients with severe renal insufficiency are hypertensive. In the majority of these patients, hypertension can be controlled by a combination of dietary sodium and fluid restriction and sodium and water removal (ultrafiltration) during dialysis. This therapy reflects an expanded extracellular fluid volume.

Approximately 30% of patients require antihypertensive therapy for optimal blood pressure control (White and Rubin, 1983). Antihypertensive therapy is commonly instituted prior to the time of ESRD because there is evidence that reduction of systemic blood pressure slows the progression of renal failure (Baldwin and Neugarten, 1987).

If hypertension persists despite adequate volume control, elevated renin and angiotensin levels may be the cause. Prior to the development of effective antihypertensive medication regimens, bilateral nephrectomy was the most common method of treating renin-related hypertension. Now, medications such as captopril or propranolol are often used. If there is also a neurogenic cause of the hypertension, agents commonly used include prazosin or methyldopa and clonidine. To enhance the effects of these drugs and to minimize their side effects, a vasodilator may be added. For example, the antihypertensive regimen might include hydralazine used concomitantly with propranolol. Minoxidil, a very potent vasodilator, has been successfully used in conjunction with propranolol or captopril to eradicate the need for bilateral nephrectomy almost entirely (White and Rubin, 1983).

Hypertension in the renal transplant patient often occurs initially in response to high doses of prednisone. Resolution occurs after the dose has been tapered. Additionally, transplant renal artery stenosis may be the etiology of continued or worsening hypertension later in the course of transplantation (Strom and Tilney, 1986).

Alteration in Cardiac Output: Hypertension. Normally, hypertension in the patient with ESRD is managed in the outpatient setting with dialysis and antihypertensive medications. In some patients, however, severe hypertension is accompanied by cardiac or central nervous system manifestations (e.g., chest pain, pulmonary edema, syncope, visual disturbances) that require admission to the critical care unit.

Nursing assessment of the hypertensive patient with ESRD includes a careful history of the patient's antihypertensive medication regimen and his or her adherence to that regimen. The nurse obtains a description of the accompanying cardiac or CNS manifestations and observes the patient for further occurrences. The patient's usual blood pressure readings are obtained from the physician or dialysis nurse. Prescribed antihypertensive medications are administered, and their effect on blood pressure is carefully monitored.

The nurse assesses the patient's understanding and compliance with the prescribed medication and the fluid and diet regimen (Lancaster, 1987). A dietitian is consulted to provide appropriate diet instruction for the patient and family members. The critical care nurse reviews the patient's antihypertensive medications and teaches the patient the purpose, dosage, and effects of each drug. The pathophysiologic complications of noncompliance are identified, and adherence to the regimen is encouraged.

Hypotension. It is important to recognize hypotension as a less frequent but clinically significant problem for the patient with ESRD. There is impairment of patient rehabilitation if hypotension occurs between dialysis treatments. If the blood pressure falls during dialysis, fluid removal becomes impossible and congestion and cardiac compromise result.

The etiology of the hypotension seen in ESRD varies. It may be caused by a variety of pharmacologic agents. Anemia and intrinsic heart disease may aggravate hypotension. Pericardial effusion may precipitate hypotension during dialysis. In addition, the incidence of autonomic dysfunction is reported to be as high as 50% in dialysis patients (Henrich, 1986). Altered sympathetic tone in uremia may decrease conpensatory responses to hypotension. Acetate, which is commonly used in dialysis baths, has been implicated as a contributor to peripheral vasodilation during dialysis.

Alteration in Cardiac Output: Hypotension. The critical care nurse monitors the patient's blood pressure between dialysis treatments, noting and reporting significant hypotension. It is common practice to withhold antihypertensive medications for 6 hours prior to hemodialysis; however, this practice must be individualized for each patient. The critical care nurse should discuss the appropriateness of withholding antihypertensive drugs with the patient's physician and dialysis nurse.

Congestive Heart Failure. Congestive heart failure secondary to fluid volume overload is often a result of the dialysis patient's noncompliance with dietary restrictions. Prevention of heart failure requires sodium and fluid restrictions between dialysis treatments, control of hypertension with adequate fluid removal during dialysis, and adequate antihypertensive drug therapy (Schoenfeld, 1985b). The increased cardiac output due to the anemia seen in most patients with ESRD, in addition to large arteriovenous (AV) shunts or grafts, contributes to the development of heart failure. If vascular access is occluded to restrict blood flow through it and cardiac output improves, it may be necessary to decrease blood flow through the access surgically. If congestive heart failure persists despite correction of these factors, it may be necessary to digitalize the patient. Digoxin is commonly administered to patients on dialysis in its usual dosage every other day (Seffart, 1985).

Fluid Volume Excess. Fluid volume excess is a common cause of congestive heart failure in these patients. Nursing care of the patient with ESRD with volume overload is directed toward returning fluid balance to normal and teaching the patient how to prevent future recurrences (American Nephrology Nurses Association, 1988). If possible, the critical care nurse should obtain the patient's baseline weight from the physician or dialysis nurse. The degree of fluid volume overload can be estimated by comparing the baseline weight with the patient's admission weight. The patient is assessed for evidence of peripheral or dependent edema. Neck veins are observed for distention. The lungs are auscultated for the presence of rales.

Pertinent nursing interventions include maintaining the prescribed fluid restrictions. The anuric patient with ESRD is often restricted to 500 to 1000 mL/day. If the patient requires multiple vasoactive infusions, this restriction will be rapidly exceeded. Mixing the infusion in double or quadruple strength will give the nurse a larger amount of discretionary fluid. Serial daily weights are compared to the patient's baseline weight.

The nurse assesses the patient's understanding of the prescribed fluid regimen and encourages adherence.

Pericarditis. Pericarditis was once considered the hallmark of ESRD prior to the availability and early initiation of dialysis. Today it does not often occur after dialysis therapy is begun. The etiology is unknown, but it is often associated with inadequate dialysis, surgical procedures, and acute catabolic illness (Schoenfeld, 1985b). It is believed that the initiating factor in uremic pericarditis is a serositis exacerbated by the bleeding disorders frequently seen in the uremic patient. Myocardial contractions may perpetuate continued trauma to the inflamed pericardial surfaces. Myocarditis can occur with an increased risk of acute and chronic complications. If the patient is hemodynamically stable, intensive hemodialysis with minimal anticoagulation may lead to a resolution of the problem.

A major concern is the development of pericardial effusion. Echocardiography is used to monitor and assess the quantity of fluid in the pericardial sac; it can detect small collections of pericardial fluid. When the effusion is large or expands rapidly, the patient must be monitored for signs of impending cardiac tamponade. If there is early clinical evidence of cardiac compromise, right heart catheterization may be performed. Chest x-ray will reveal a rapid change in heart size and shape with normal-appearing lungs (Delano, 1983). Pericardiocentesis, pericardial window, or a total pericardectomy may be necessary if the situation does not resolve (Mako et al., 1986; Lancaster, 1987). Increased dialysis with careful management of anticoagulation is critical. Some clinicians advocate utilizing peritoneal dialysis during episodes of pericarditis to eliminate the need for anticoagulation.

Alteration in Cardiac Output: Pericarditis. The presenting signs of pericarditis in the patient on dialysis include the triad of fever, pain, and pericardial friction rub. The critical care nurse assesses the patient for the development of chest pain. The patient's temperature is monitored for low grade elevation. The chest is auscultated for the presence of a pericardial friction rub. The pulse and blood pressure are monitored for development of pulsus paradoxus of greater than 10 mm Hg. The ECG may show ST segment elevation with an upward concavity, a depressed PR segment, and low QRS voltage (Lancaster, 1987). Following diagnosis of pericarditis, the nurse prepares the patient for intensive dialysis. Equipment for pericardiocentesis is kept available.

Dysrhythmias. In the ESRD patient, dysrhythmias may be precipitated by multiple factors. These include pericarditis, atherosclerotic heart disease, conduction system calcifications, calcific or congestive cardiomyopathy, acute volume changes, electrolyte disorders, anemia, and congestive heart failure. Premature atrial contractions and premature ventricular contractions are the most frequently noted dysrhythmias. Atrial fibrillation and ventricular tachycardia may also occur.

Dialysis-related dysrhythmias are usually transient and remain unrecognized. During hemodialysis, there may be an increase in myocardial oxygen consumption due to the effects of acetate in the dialysate bath. Limited delivery of oxygen occurs due to the anemia and possible hypotension in individuals with coronary artery stenosis. Many dysrhythmias are related to these episodes of hypotension during dialysis treatment. Hypotension can often be avoided by administering antihypertensives, tricyclic antidepressants, or tranquilizers after the dialysis treatment.

Dysrhythmias associated with hypokalemia can be a result of intracellular movement of potassium due to glucose administration or to the metabolic alkalosis that may develop from the acetate or bicarbonate buffer used in the dialysis bath. Hypokalemia and hypomagnesemia may precipitate digitalis toxicity with associated dysrhythmias. Thus, it is usual to use a 3-mEq/liter potassium bath in the patient on hemodialysis therapy, who is also taking digoxin, to avoid this occurrence.

Dysrhythmias related to hyperkalemia can be life-threatening. Hyperkalemia usually results from noncompliance with dietary restrictions. Traumatically injured ESRD patients are also at high risk for development of hyperkalemia due to release of intracellular potassium from injured tissue.

Alteration in Cardiac Output: Hyperkalemia. The goals of nursing care for the hyperkalemic patient with ESRD are to prevent injury, reduce the serum potassium level, and assist the patient to prevent recurrences. Serial serum potassium levels are closely monitored. Serum potassium measurements will be required more frequently if acidosis is also present. The nurse closely monitors the electrocardiogram for peaked T waves, depressed ST segments, and widened QRS complexes.

The nurse prepares for emergency treatment of hyperkalemia. Intravenous insulin, glucose, and bicarbonate may be given as a temporary measure to reduce serum potassium. If the serum potassium level is not imminently life-threatening, ion exchange resins can be given as a retention enema. Emergency hemodialysis may be necessary to lower life-threatening hyperkalemia.

The nurse assesses the events leading to the hyperkalemic episode. If noncompliance with the dietary regimen is the cause, the nurse assesses the patient's level of understanding, provides the necessary patient instruction, and encourages the patient to adhere to the prescribed diet. Hyperkalemia can result from administration of blood transfusions. When possible, blood should be transfused during hemodialysis so that the excess potassium can be removed.

Vascular Access. Adequate access to the circulation is the single most important factor in the delivery of adequate hemodialysis therapy. Thrombosis, stenosis, and infections of the vascular access site account for a significant number of hospitalizations for the hemodialysis patient. Improved peritoneal catheters have made long-term peritoneal dialysis therapy possible. Peritonitis accounts for most hospitalizations in this group.

The arteriovenous shunt that connects the distal radial artery to a forearm vein is infrequently seen in patients on chronic dialysis therapy, due to the high incidence of clotting and infection. The use of these shunts has also decreased in patients with acute renal failure since the introduction of improved, long-term, dual-lumen subclavian catheters that are capable of delivering an adequate rate of blood flow.

An internal arteriovenous fistula is the vascular access route usually used in patients with ESRD. These can be composed of either a native vein or a prosthetic graft, e.g., polytetrafluoroethylene (PTFE) or bovine artery. As illustrated in Figure 42–1, the native vein fistula commonly involves the anastomosis of the cephalic vein to the radial artery (Brescia-Cimino fistula). Anastomosis of the basilic vein to the ulnar artery is also utilized. Approximately 4 to 6 weeks after the anastomosis is created, the venous walls hypertrophy, making repeated venipuncture for dialysis possible (Krupski et al., 1985).

Because patients with ESRD are often diabetic or elderly, and have inadequate or arteriosclerotic vessels, it may be impossible to create a native vein fistula. In these patients, placement of a prosthetic graft is necessary. The graft material is implanted subcutaneously to serve as a conduit between an artery and a vein. The superficial implant is made to facilitate easy needle placement. The forearm is the preferred site. Upper arm or thigh grafts can be done, but they increase the chance of high output failure due to the increased blood flow rates in these larger vessels (Golding, 1986). These large proximal grafts have been implicated in intractable pulmonary edema, which usually occurs in combination with fluid overload and myocardial dysfunction. Other complications of internally created fistulae include thrombosis, stenosis, steal syndrome, aneurysms, and localized and systemic infections.

Percutaneous cannulation of the subclavian or femoral vein provides temporary access to the bloodstream for hemodialysis. Percutaneous catheters are utilized when long-term access fails or when acute rejection occurs following renal transplantation.

If peripheral vascular disease is so severe that vascular access becomes a chronic problem, then peritoneal dialysis may be used. The mechanics of peritoneal dialysis are discussed in Chapter 41.

Alteration in Peripheral Tissue Perfusion. Maintenance of a patent and infection-free vascular access device is the goal of nursing care. The nurse monitors the color, temperature, and sensation of the extremity. A cool, pale, or cyanotic extremity may indicate vascular occlusion and should be reported. The patency of the access route is assessed by palpating for the thrill and auscultating for the bruit.

Temporary subclavian or femoral dialysis catheters are not ordinarily used for administration of intravenous fluids or medications. The critical care nurse should consult the dialysis nurse about how much heparin has been instilled in the catheter following dialysis and whether the catheter should be accessed for nondialysis purposes.

Particular care must be taken to prevent infection in femoral catheters that are left in place following dialysis. Because of their location, femoral catheters are easily contaminated by urine and fecal material. Frequent sterile dressing changes may be required.

Pulmonary System

There is a wide spectrum of pulmonary disease in the patient with renal failure. Abnormalities include asymptomatic changes in pulmonary capillary permeability, pulmonary edema, uremic pneumonitis, pleural effusion, and infectious pulmonary calcifications. Pulmonary edema is the most common problem in the patient with ESRD who is being treated by dialysis. In these patients pulmonary edema is primarily caused by fluid overload with subsequent left ventricular failure. There may also be increased pulmonary capillary permeability in the uremic patient; this would account for the development of pulmonary edema in the presence of low to normal pulmonary artery pressures (Mujais et al., 1986).

Uremic pneumonitis is an extreme form of pulmonary edema. Interstitial fibrosis occurs as a result of fibrin deposits with associated infiltrates of monocytes and lymphocytes.

Pleural effusions were seen more frequently when the initiation of dialysis therapy was delayed, usually in association with pericarditis. When pleural effusions occur, resolution typically results after thoracentesis and initiation of adequate dialysis therapy.

Pulmonary infections may occur more frequently in the ESRD patient due to decreased activity of pulmonary macrophages (Lancaster, 1986). The immunocompromised state that exists in patients with renal failure makes them more susceptible to a wide variety of infections (Jacobson and McNatt, 1986).

As a consequence of calcium and phosphorus imbalances, pulmonary calcifications can lead to impaired pulmonary function. Dyspnea, arterial hypoxemia, and decreased lung volume may result. Partial resolution may occur following good control of calcium and phosphorus concentrations through dietary restrictions, adherence to a phosphate binder regi-

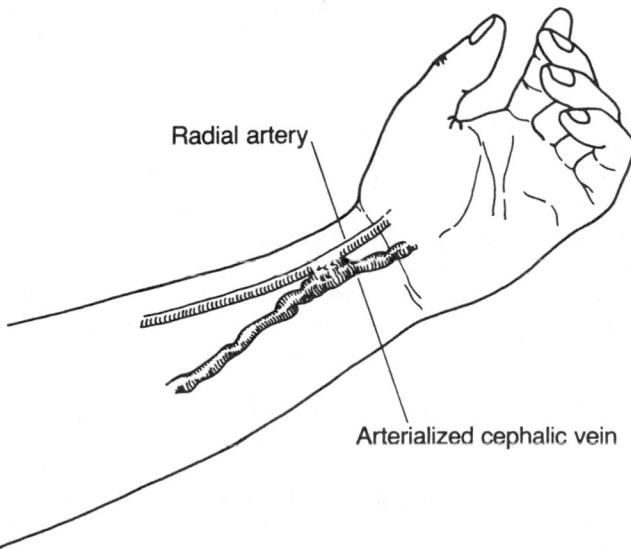

FIGURE 42–1. The native arteriovenous fistula. (Courtesy of Alice A. Whittaker.)

Radial artery

Arterialized cephalic vein

men, and subtotal parathyroidectomy if appropriate (Mujais et al., 1986). Pulmonary calcifications also tend to resolve following renal transplantation.

Impaired Gas Exchange. Maintenance of adequate ventilation and prevention of nosocomial pneumonia are major challenges for the nurse caring for the critically ill patient with ESRD. Breath sounds are frequently auscultated for the presence of rales, wheezes, and rubs. The respiratory pattern is assessed for tachypnea and the amount of breathing work required. The patient's subjective complaint of dyspnea is carefully assessed. Baseline data are compared with ongoing assessments to monitor increasing respiratory dysfunction.

Aggressive pulmonary toilet, including coughing, suctioning, percussion/postural drainage, turning, deep breathing, and incentive spirometry, is performed frequently. The patient's sputum is monitored for changes in amount and consistency.

Gastrointestinal System

Gastrointestinal disturbances are often the most disturbing problems experienced by the patient with ESRD prior to the initiation of renal replacement therapy.

Anorexia and Nutritional Disorders. Anorexia, nausea, and vomiting, especially in the morning, are common complaints associated with uremia. As a consequence, malnutrition may occur if renal replacement therapy is not instituted early enough. Nutritional status may be further compromised if the patient has a catabolic illness. Diabetic patients may experience gastroparesis and nephrotic albumin losses, placing them at higher nutritional risk. In addition, prolonged dietary protein restrictions prescribed to delay the initiation of renal replacement therapy may also result in a suboptimal nutritional status. Even when dialysis therapy is initiated, morbidity and mortality depend on an adequate state of nutrition, with protein intake levels in an acceptable range of 0.8 to 1.4 g/kg per day (Gotch and Sargent, 1985).

Albumin should not be lost during hemodialysis treatments. However, it is predicted that 9 to 10 g/day may be lost in patients on continuous ambulatory peritoneal dialysis (CAPD) and 12 to 15 g/treatment in patients undergoing intermittent peritoneal dialysis (IPD). These losses are increased during episodes of peritonitis. Thus, a protein intake of 1.5 g/kg per day is the recommended amount for patients on peritoneal dialysis (Schoenfeld, 1985a). Estimates of protein deficiency are best evaluated by obtaining serum transferrin levels. However, if iron stores are depleted, transferrin levels may be increased.

Nutrition Less Than Body Requirements. The goal of nutritional therapy for the patient with ESRD is provision of a diet adequate for repletion and main-

tenance of desirable body weight. Acceptable plasma levels of urea, sodium, potassium, magnesium, calcium, phosphorus, and albumin also must be maintained. Nutritional adjustments are necessary throughout the course of renal deterioration. During the stress of a critical illness or injury, further modifications become necessary depending upon individual requirements, rate of catabolism, and any changes made in renal replacement therapy.

For the nonstressed patient on hemodialysis, kinetic modeling is useful for individualizing the dialysis treatment and nutrition plan by determining the patient's protein catabolic rate. The typical recommendation is 1 g of protein per kilogram of ideal body weight, 2 to 3 g of sodium, 40 to 50 mEq of potassium, and 1200 mg of phosphorus per day. Calcium supplements are given if needed when phosphorus levels are controlled. Water-soluble vitamins are supplemented. Supplemental iron is given if stores are inadequate.

Dietary recommendations for the patient on peritoneal dialysis are similar to those for patients receiving hemodialysis. Protein losses are generally greater with peritoneal dialysis. Thus, recommended protein intake is usually 1.2 to 1.5 g/kg per day under normal circumstances. Protein loss is increased in the presence of peritonitis; therefore, dietary protein intake must also be increased. Critically ill patients also have increased protein requirements. It is important for the nurse to encourage the patient to eat a sufficient amount of protein.

Potassium restrictions are generally much more liberal for the patient on peritoneal dialysis. Dietary potassium prescriptions range from 75 to 90 mEq/day for patients on IPD to 3 to 4 g/kg per day for patients on CAPD or continuous cyclic peritoneal dialysis (CCPD). Fluid restrictions for patients on hemodialysis and IPD are generally limited to the sum of the urine output plus 500 to 1000 mL/day. For patients on CAPD and CCPD, there are generally no fluid restrictions due to the ease of controlling fluid loss through the dialysate glucose concentration (Hoffart, 1987).

In the renal transplant patient, dietary restrictions are based upon the level of function of the transplanted kidney. In addition, the adverse effects of corticosteroids must be considered when developing a diet prescription. Some of the more common dietary problems encountered include sodium and water retention with concomitant increased potassium excretion. The patient may be placed on sodium and fluid restrictions and given potassium supplements. Transplant patients frequently have an increased appetite, which results in excessive weight gain. At the same time, there is an elevated rate of protein catabolism. Many patients have varying degrees of glucose intolerance, and some develop steroid-induced diabetes mellitus. These problems will necessitate caloric restrictions and close serum glucose monitoring.

If the critically ill patient with ESRD is able to eat, it is important for the nurse to assess the patient's oral mucosa. Stomatitis is a common problem in these patients (Lancaster, 1987). Patients may complain of a dry mouth and an unpleasant taste in the mouth. Frequent mouth care will enhance the patient's ability and desire to eat.

Many critically ill patients with ESRD require total parenteral nutrition (TPN) to meet their nutritional needs. The prescription for TPN will follow the general dietary prescriptions previously described. Potassium and sodium are prescribed according to the patient's serum levels. Phosphate salts are usually not utilized because of the lack of renal phosphate excretion. Because magnesium excretion is also impaired, magnesium is given in TPN only if serum levels are low.

The patient's fluid balance and ability to handle the TPN fluid load will determine the amount of protein administered in the TPN. In general, if the patient requires fluid restrictions, the amount of amino acids is decreased, and a higher (70%) dextrose concentration is utilized. The nurse carefully assesses the patient's response to the TPN fluid load, specifically noting the presence of any signs of increasing congestive heart failure or pulmonary edema. The patient's serum glucose concentration is closely monitored and treated with the prescribed insulin dosage.

If the patient is catabolic, a higher TPN protein concentration is required to facilitate tissue or wound healing. These patients are at high risk of fluid volume overload and must be monitored closely. Daily hemodialysis or continuous peritoneal dialysis may be used to prevent fluid volume overload. An alternative method of fluid management is continuous ultrafiltration, described in Chapter 41.

Gastrointestinal Disorders. The most frequent disorders occurring in the patient with ESRD include gastritis, gastric and duodenal ulcers with bleeding in the upper gastrointestinal tract, diverticulosis, colonic perforation, and obstruction in the lower gastrointestinal tract. Ulcerations can occur at any point in the gastrointestinal tract. It is thought that urea conversion to ammonia influences the pathologic changes seen in the gastrointestinal mucosa.

The increased incidence of gastrointestinal blood loss is probably related to a number of factors. The platelet dysfunction seen in renal failure and the chronic heparinization used for hemodialysis are two contributing factors. In the renal transplant patient, the incidence of gastrointestinal bleeding and perforation is increased because of the use of steroid medications.

There is a higher incidence of diverticulosis and colonic perforation in the ESRD population, probably because of the chronic constipation experienced in this group due to ingestion of phosphate binders. Patients with polycystic kidney disease have an 80% incidence of diverticulosis, so these patients are particularly at risk when they reach ESRD (Hakim and Lazarus, 1986).

Alteration in Bowel Elimination: Constipation. Maintenance of the patient's normal bowel elimination pattern is an important nursing goal for the critically ill patient with ESRD (American Nephrology Nurses Association, 1988). A detailed history of the patient's bowel patterns and laxative use guides the nursing plan. The patient is assessed for abdominal distention, abdominal discomfort, presence of bowel sounds, and frequency of bowel movements. A prescription for the patient's usual laxative or stool softener should be obtained and administered on a regular basis. When the patient is able to tolerate an oral diet, the nurse encourages high fiber/high bulk foods.

Hematopoietic System

Chronic renal failure results in a number of changes in the hematopoietic system, placing the patient at increased risk of bleeding and infection.

Anemia. A common but not universal consequence of chronic renal failure is anemia. Anemia becomes evident when renal function falls below 50% and becomes progressively worse as kidney function deteriorates. By the time renal replacement therapy becomes necessary, the hematocrit is typically between 15% and 30% (Eschbach and Adamson, 1985).

The cause of anemia is primarily related to the decreased secretion of erythropoietin by the kidney. Although the exact secretory site of this substance in the kidney is unknown, it is presumed to be damaged with progression of renal failure. Consequently, erythropoietin levels are inadequate to stimulate the erythroid precursors in the bone marrow to maintain red blood cell production.

A variety of other factors contribute to the anemia of ESRD. RBC survival rates are decreased due to uremic toxins. External blood losses due to platelet dysfunction as well as those relating to the hemodialysis procedure itself may worsen the anemia. Aluminum has been shown to interfere with iron uptake in the RBC. Aluminum toxicity is evident in some ESRD patients and is associated with ingestion of aluminum hydroxide phosphate binders. Folic acid, a water-soluble vitamin vital to normal RBC production, is lost during dialysis. Hyperparathyroidism has been implicated in worsening anemia as an inhibitor of erythropoiesis, either as a result of osteosclerosis and marrow fibrosis or possibly due to parathyroid hormone itself (Rose and Black, 1989).

Apart from successful renal transplantation, complete reversal of anemia has not been possible. Good control of uremia with dialysis results in some increase in the hematocrit. Present methods of management include minimizing the chronic blood loss related to hemodialysis and laboratory sampling. Specific pharmacologic treatments include iron supplementation when a deficiency exists, vitamin B complex and folic acid supplements to replace those removed during dialysis, and weekly administration of androgen derivatives to stimulate renal and extra-renal production of erythropoietin (Vaziri, 1986). Routine blood transfusions are discouraged to avoid depression of the individual bone marrow production of RBCs, thereby causing transfusion dependency. The potential for transmission of hepatitis B, non-A, non-B hepatitis, and HIV virus is also an important consideration. Despite these precautions, an estimated 15% of patients, especially those with severe cardiac and pulmonary disorders, become symptomatic and require periodic blood transfusions (Paganini, 1988).

Future treatment for anemia will include recombinant human erythropoietin (rHuEPO). This compound was used successfully in Europe. Clinical trials with dialysis patients have been completed in the United States, and FDA approval was granted in 1989.

Activity Intolerance. Nursing care of the patient with ESRD is directed toward minimizing blood loss, thereby maintaining the patient's hematocrit at an adequate level. The patient's hematocrit and hemoglobin are monitored for downward trends. The nurse minimizes the number and amount of blood samples drawn from the patient. Iron, folate, and blood transfusions are administered as prescribed.

Platelets. There is a qualitative defect of platelet adhesiveness in the renal failure patient. Platelet factor III, necessary for conversion of prothrombin to thrombin, is also abnormal. Although there is some improvement with dialysis therapy, these defects do account for some of the increased bleeding tendencies associated with ESRD.

Potential for Bleeding. The critical care nurse anticipates the complication of bleeding in the patient with ESRD. Nursing care is directed toward early detection and prevention of bleeding. Stool, vomitus, and nasogastric aspirate are checked for occult blood. Antacids are administered as prescribed. Manipulation of the nasogastric tube is minimized. Tracheal suctioning is performed carefully to avoid tissue trauma.

Line insertion sites are assessed for bleeding. Manual pressure is applied to the fistula site until hemostasis is achieved following hemodialysis treatment.

Lymphocytes. Infection remains a major cause of morbidity in patients with ESRD. Although the WBC is normal, the patient's susceptibility to infection is increased. An immunosuppressed state in which the absolute numbers of T-cells and helper T-cells are reduced exists in the dialysis patient (Hakim and Lazarus, 1986).

A transient leukocytosis occurs at the beginning of hemodialysis, especially when a cuprophane or cellulose dialyzer membrane is used. The complement activation induced by these membranes results in neutrophil aggregation and sequestration in the lungs. In the critically ill patient, this process should

also be recognized as a possible cause of hypoxemia. More biocompatible membranes, which should eliminate this problem, are now available.

Potential for Infection. The critically ill patient with ESRD is at high risk for development of infection. Nursing care is directed toward prevention and early detection of infection processes. Nursing assessment includes monitoring of the patient's temperature curve and WBC count and observing for changes in odor, color, or consistency of drainage and secretions. Meticulous care is taken with line insertion and line maintenance. Vigorous pulmonary toilet is initiated to minimize pooling of pulmonary secretions. Wounds are carefully inspected for evidence of inflammation and infection.

Neurologic System

The nervous system is one of the earliest systems to show clinical signs and symptoms of advancing renal failure. These signs include impaired mentation, sleep disturbances, lethargy, gait abnormalities, and asterixis. If these are left untreated, the final result will be seizures and coma (Jacobson and McNatt, 1986; Lancaster, 1987). Peripheral neuropathy and electroencephalographic (EEG) abnormalities improve with dialysis but show even more improvement after renal transplantation.

Uremic Encephalopathy. Metabolic encephalopathy is thought to result from a combination of electrolyte disturbances, acidosis, and an accumulation of middle molecules. The symptoms of metabolic encephalopathy range from mild changes in concentration to deteriorating levels of consciousness including obtundation, stupor, and coma. The psychological stresses imposed by dealing with some of the early symptoms may result in depression and sometimes even psychotic episodes (Schoenfeld, 1985b). Dialysis dementia (dialysis encephalopathy) is a progressive neurologic disorder associated with high levels of aluminum in the gray matter of the brain. It was recognized in the early 1970s in hemodialysis patients who had been dialyzed for several years. The aluminum source was thought to be the water used to make the dialysate solution. Oral ingestion of aluminum hydroxide phosphate binders has also been implicated. The presenting symptoms include stuttering, dysphasia, personality changes, and impaired memory. Myoclonic jerking and focal or grand mal seizures may also be seen. Death usually occurs within 12 months of the onset of symptoms (Hakim and Lazarus, 1986). High aluminum levels in the dialysate are rarely seen with the improved water treatment systems currently used for hemodialysis. Chelation and removal of body aluminum have been successfully accomplished by administering deferoxamine. The chelation product is then made available for removal during dialysis (Abreo, 1988).

Alterations in Thought Processes. The patient with

ESRD is at high risk for alterations in mentation, not only as a complication of uremia but also due to the many electrolyte and metabolic disturbances that accompany critical illness. It is important that the critical care nurse obtain a baseline assessment of the patient's cognitive functioning on admission. This baseline assessment may be obtained by talking with the patient or from family members if the patient is unable to communicate. Information is obtained about the patient's orientation to person, place, and time, length of attention span, sleep disturbance, fatigue, increasing somnolence, irritability, and signs of depression. The patient's ability to understand requests or instruction is assessed. This information is then used to guide communication with the patient and, when appropriate, to develop a patient education plan. The effects of medication and treatment on the patient's mentation are observed and reported.

Peripheral Neuropathy. Uremic neuropathy cannot be distinguished from other types of neuropathy. Decreased motor and sensory nerve conduction is thought to be due to demyelination and axonal degeneration of the large distal nerve fibers. Sensory symptoms usually involve the lower extremities.

The "restless leg syndrome" is a sensory neuropathy that occurs at night. It is characterized by numbness, burning, and pain in the feet and lower legs that is often relieved by continuous leg movement. Motor abnormalities may develop if dialysis or transplantation does not occur. Slowing of motor nerve conduction velocity may result in muscle atrophy with irreversible damage.

Alteration in Comfort. Nursing goals for the patient with ESRD with peripheral neuropathy include providing comfort measures and encouraging ambulation. Assessment findings may include numbness or burning in the feet, restless leg movements, decreased muscle strength, cramps, paresthesias, and decreased deep tendon reflexes. Nursing measures that promote patient comfort include avoiding unexpected touching of the feet and keeping heavy bed linens off the feet. If there is sensory loss, the nurse teaches the patient how to inspect the feet visually for signs of injury. The nurse encourages and assists the patient with ambulation and collaborates with the physical therapist in developing an exercise program for the patient in the critical care unit.

Skeletal System

The term renal osteodystrophy encompasses a broad range of bone diseases that develop in 50% to 80% of patients with chronic renal failure (Teitebaum, 1985). The disorders include osteitis fibrosa, vitamin D–deficient osteomalacia, aluminum-induced osteomalacia, osteosclerosis, and combinations of these.

Hyperphosphatemia develops in the patient with ESRD because the kidney is no longer able to excrete phosphate ions. Phosphates are also poorly dialyzable. Because calcium and phosphorus function on a reciprocal basis, when the phosphorus rises, the calcium falls. The failed kidney is no longer able to convert vitamin D to its active form, 1,25-dihydroxy-vitamin D_3. This further disrupts calcium homeostasis because the vitamin D–activated metabolite is necessary to facilitate dietary calcium absorption from the gastrointestinal tract. Hypocalcemia triggers excessive secretion of parathyroid hormone (PTH) in an attempt to maintain normal calcium ion concentration. Secondary hyperparathyroidism often results as part of the trade-off for calcium and phosphorus balance. Unfortunately, parathyroid hormone causes an increase in the activity of osteoclasts, resulting in bone dissolution to maintain plasma calcium levels. The metabolic acidosis accompanying renal failure further promotes bone demineralization (Lancaster, 1987).

Because of the progressive nature of bone disease associated with renal failure, management of serum calcium, phosphorus, and PTH levels is critical. Therapy may include a combination of phosphate-binding medications, active vitamin D supplements, calcium supplements, and, if indicated, a subtotal parathyroidectomy (Lancaster, 1987).

Treatment of renal osteodystrophy must begin with control of serum phosphorus prior to instituting calcium and vitamin D therapy. If calcium levels are raised when serum phosphorus levels are elevated, a high calcium-phosphorus product will result, leading to metastatic calcification of soft tissues. Dietary phosphorus restriction and the use of aluminum hydroxide to bind the phosphate in the gut are the most common approaches. As discussed previously, use of aluminum hydroxide complicates existing bone disorders. A nonaluminum binder is currently not available. Calcium carbonate can be used as an alternative if the calcium-phosphorus (Ca × P) product is below 60 and can be controlled.

Alteration in Comfort. Although renal osteodystrophy is considered a chronic problem in patients with ESRD, it is important to direct nursing care in the critical care unit preventing immobility and maintaining acceptable calcium and phosphorus levels. The patient is assessed for muscular weakness, gait changes, and the presence of joint pain or deep bone pain. A history of any pathologic fractures is noted. The nurse encourages and assists the patient with ambulation or exercises to maintain mobility.

Baseline serum calcium and phosphorus levels are obtained. The patient is monitored for development of hypocalcemia. Phosphate-binding antacids are administered as prescribed.

Integument. Pruritus is reported to occur in as many as 86% of patients with renal failure (Mujais et al., 1986). The cause is unknown, but it is thought to be correlated with a variety of factors. Atrophy of the oil-secreting sebaceous glands and the sweat glands contribute to dry skin with resulting pruritus. Also implicated are urochrome deposits in the skin as well as disturbances in calcium and phosphorus metabolism, which may lead to deposition of calcium phosphate crystals in the cutaneous layer. The skin can become excoriated and infected secondary to scratching. If edema is present, the situation worsens. Widespread ecchymosis and purpura is associated with capillary fragility and the clotting abnormalities seen in the uremic state.

The yellow or gray-bronze skin coloration seen in the patient with ESRD is caused by the retained urochromes and pigmented metabolites normally excreted by the kidneys. The underlying pallor is attributed to anemia (Lancaster, 1987).

Wound healing is delayed in the patient with ESRD. This is even further magnified in the patient with chronic renal failure who has malnutrition secondary to uremia. In this situation, protein wasting with associated hypoalbuminemia may be evident by thin, brittle fingernails with pale, paired bands in the nail beds (Muerchke's lines).

Impaired Skin Integrity. An important goal of nursing care for the critically ill patient with ESRD is maintenance of intact, infection-free skin. The patient's skin is assessed for dryness, signs of infection, inflammation, excoriation, edema, and ecchymosis. Superfatted or lanolin-based soaps are used for bathing. Emollients are applied to relieve itching. The patient is turned frequently to prevent development of pressure areas. If prolonged immobility is expected, therapeutic mattresses or beds should be utilized to prevent skin breakdown.

Psychosocial Factors

Chronic renal failure and maintenance dialysis impose a number of stressors on the patient and family. The patient may feel that he has lost control of his life and is now controlled by the weekly schedule of dialysis. The presence of a fistula or peritoneal catheter, along with the outward changes that accompany ESRD, may lead to an alteration in body image. The patient may grieve for the loss of body functions, such as the loss of kidney or urinary function or the decrease in sexual and reproductive function (Finkelstein and Finkelstein, 1986). Critical illness or injury adds additional stress to the patient and family system.

Ineffective Coping. Nursing care of the critically ill patient with ESRD is directed toward assisting the patient and family to understand and adapt to the changes imposed by the critical illness. The patient and family are assessed for signs of depression, anger, withdrawal, and dependent behaviors. The nurse is alert for evidence of noncompliance or nonparticipation in therapy.

Nursing interventions that facilitate coping by the patient and family include providing an environment that is as quiet and nonstressful as possible. The patient and family are encouraged to express their feelings about the illness and treatment. The nurse assists them to identify their strengths and coping abilities. Information is provided in response to the patient and family's readiness and ability to learn. The nurse encourages the patient and family to set realistic goals and offers positive reinforcement toward meeting those goals.

On occasion, the critically ill patient and family members may decide to withdraw from dialysis treatment. When this occurs, the critical care nurse must recognize and honor the patient's right to choose his own treatment option—including the option of no treatment. In this case the nurse provides emotional support and comfort measures to ease the discomfort of advancing uremia and impending death.

RENAL REPLACEMENT THERAPY

There is no magic number with regard to creatinine clearance that determines when a patient must begin dialysis or receive a kidney transplant. Initiation of renal replacement therapy depends on the signs and symptoms displayed by the patient. However, as a rough index, considering that ESRD reflects a 90% nephron loss, we can predict that the patient may require dialysis or transplantation when the GFR is 10% of normal or less. For clinical purposes, the creatinine clearance closely approximates the GFR. Serial measurements of GFR show a linear decline with time prior to initiation of dialysis therapy. GFR may be maintained at varying levels after initiation of dialysis. In the majority of patients who are on dialysis, GFR falls substantially after 6 months to 1 year. The presence of any residual renal function is important in determining the optimal pharmacologic management and dialysis prescription (Gotch and Sargent, 1985).

Laboratory findings in patients with ESRD vary. Table 42-2 presents a range of acceptable values for patients on hemodialysis. These values differ somewhat for patients utilizing peritoneal dialysis, with variations for continuous compared to intermittent therapy.

Pharmacologic Management

The effects of renal failure on the absorption, distribution, metabolism, and excretion of drugs present a challenge to both the physician in modifying the dosage and the nurse in monitoring the effects of the medication. The kidney, by means of glomerular filtration and tubular secretion, is responsible for excreting at least part of most drugs. Drugs that are effectively bound to plasma protein are poorly filtered. Conversely, drugs that are not protein bound are cleared from the blood at a rate approximately equal to the creatinine clearance. The most obvious influence of renal failure on the pharmaco-

TABLE 42–2. Laboratory Values for ESRD Patients

	Adult Normal Value	Acceptable Predialysis Range for Dialysis Patients	Usual Causes of Abnormal Values	Important Considerations
Na^+	135–145 mEq/liter	135–145 mEq/liter	High: excessive Na intake; dehydration Low: dilution due to excessive water intake	Indicator of body hydration
K^+	3.5–5.5 mEq/liter	3.0–6.0 mEq/liter	High: excessive K intake; trauma; significant infection; respiratory/metabolic acidosis; rapid transfusion of stored bank blood	High levels can cause cardiac dysrhythmias Hyperkalemia must be considered in acute muscle weakness
			Low: vomiting, diarrhea; excessive diuretic administration	Hypokalemia can potentiate digitalis toxicity
CO_2	25–28 mEq/liter	15–18 mEq/liter	Metabolic acidosis	Dialysate bath to correct acidosis: Acetate (39–41 mEq/liter) or Bicarbonate (36–39 mEq/liter)
Ca^{2+}	8.5–10.5 mg/dL (4.5–5.5 mEq/liter)	8.5–10.5 mg/dL	High: secondary hyperparathyroidism; vitamin D metabolite overdose	Maintain calcium in upper normal range to minimize PTH stimulation
			Low: excessive phosphorus intake; noncompliance with phosphate binders	
PO_4	3.0–4.5 mg/dL	3.0–5.0 mg/dL	High: excessive dietary intake; PO_4 in TPN	Calcium-phosphorus product (Ca × PO_4) should be below 50. At 70, soft tissue calcification will occur
			Low: phosphate binder overdose	
Alkaline phosphatase	30–130 IU/liter	30–130 IU/liter	High: bone disease; liver disease	
Mg^+	1.5–2.5 mEq/liter	1.5–2.5 mEq/liter	High: ingestion of exogenous Mg (e.g., antacids, laxatives); Mg in TPN	Hypermagnesemia suppresses neuromuscular transmission
Blood urea nitrogen (BUN)	10–20 mg/dL	80–100 mg/dL	High: excessive protein ingestion; GI bleeding; catabolic state; inadequate dialysis Low: inadequate protein intake	Protein requirements may be increased in critically ill patients
Creatinine	0.6–1.3 mg/dL	6–25 mg/dL	High: inadequate dialysis; increasing muscle mass	Not influenced by diet or metabolic state
Albumin	3.5–5.0 g/dL	3.5–5.0 g/dL	Low: inadequate nutrition	Low plasma oncotic pressure can result in edema formation
Glucose	70–115 mg/dL	70–115 mg/dL	High: diabetes mellitus; persistent uremia Low: excess insulin administration	Uremia is associated with glucose intolerance and insulin resistance
Hematocrit	Male 40–54% Female 37–47%	20–30%	High: dehydration; polycystic disease Low: bleeding; anephric	Recent change in Hct is more important than the absolute value Transfuse only if symptomatic

Abbreviations: TPN, total parenteral nutrition; PTH, parathyroid hormone.

TABLE 42–3. Medications Commonly Prescribed for ESRD Patients

Drug	Purpose	Special Considerations
Propranolol Hydralazine Methyldopa Clonidine Metoprolol Minoxidil Prazosin	Antihypertensive	Dose is usually held until after dialysis to prevent hypotension resulting from fluid removal during hemodialysis
Acetaminophen	Analgesic	Aspirin is generally not prescribed due to increased risk of gastrointestinal bleeding
Sodium bicarbonate	Treatment of metabolic acidosis	Sodium can enhance fluid retention
Aluminum hydroxide Aluminum carbonate Calcium carbonate	Phosphorus binders	Must be taken with meals in order to bind with dietary phosphorus Can cause constipation Calcium-phosphorus product must be carefully monitored when calcium carbonate is used
Digoxin	Management of chronic congestive heart failure	Digitalis toxicity can develop when hypokalemia results from low potassium concentration in the dialysate bath
Furosemide Metolazone	Diuretic	Diuretics may be administered to ESRD patients with some residual renal function Administration schedule may need to be adjusted to avoid hypotension during dialysis
Folic acid	Required for red blood cell synthesis	Water soluble; lost during dialysis
Vitamin B complex Vitamin C	Replacement vitamins	Give after dialysis
Ferrous sulfate Ferrous fumarate	Iron repletion	Do not administer with antacids or when absorption is decreased
Iron dextran	Iron repletion	IV administration generally given during dialysis Test dose is critical to avoid severe allergic response
Activated vitamin D	Management of hypocalcemia May reduce elevated PTH levels Necessary for dietary calcium absorption from gastrointestinal tract	Monitor serum calcium levels during administration Fat-soluble so drug is not lost in dialysis
Nandrolone decanoate Testosterone enanthate	Anabolic steroid given to increase production of red blood cells	Given intramuscularly once each week
Deferoxamine	Chelates aluminum for removal during dialysis	IV or intraperitoneal administration Iron is also chelated; monitor serum ferritin levels

Abbreviations: PTH, parathyroid hormone.

kinetics of drug activity involves the distribution and excretion of drugs.

Abnormal distribution of drugs is related to volume excess and the decreased protein binding that occurs in uremia. It is hypothesized that in uremic patients retained molecules compete with drugs. This process can result in higher plasma concentrations of some drugs, or it may be associated with an enhanced pharmacologic effect at normal plasma concentrations (Anderson et al., 1981).

Renal failure prolongs the half-life of drugs. There is a gradual increase in half-life until the creatinine clearance falls below 30 mL/minute. As creatinine clearance falls below this level, the half-life of drugs increases rapidly (Baer, 1987). The extent of drug accumulation and the associated risk of toxicity will be more pronounced unless the usual dose or the dosage interval is modified. When dialysis is used,

the intermittent or continuous elimination of drugs through the dialyzer or peritoneal membrane must also be taken into consideration.

As previously discussed, patients with ESRD have other associated medical problems for which a variety of different drugs are routinely prescribed. Such patients will need additional medications when hospitalized for acute problems. A review of drugs commonly used by these patients is presented in Table 42–3. The purpose and special considerations for each drug are included. Additionally, Table 42–4 lists frequently used drugs with information on their dialyzability. This information can be used as a general reference in determining the optimal scheduling of medication administration. It is also useful in clinically assessing suboptimal therapy resulting from significant removal of a drug by means of hemodialysis or peritoneal dialysis. It must be kept

TABLE 42–4. Guidelines for Drug Administration in Renal Failure

Drug (Molecular Wt)	Plasma Protein Binding (%)	Volume of Distribution	Clearance in Dialysis	Dosage in ESRD with GFR < 10 ml/minute
Amikacin (782)	None	0.2–0.3 liters/kg BW	Some removal via PD and CAPD	Replacement dose required after HD
			Moderate clearance with HD	20% to 30% of usual dose every 12 hours
Amoxicillin (365)	15–25	0.24–0.42 liters/kg BW	Some removal through HD and PD but less than other antibiotics	HD: usual dose every 12–24 hours
				Replace with 30% of usual dose after HD treatment
				CAPD: usual dose every 15 hours
Amphotericin B (924)	90	4 liters/kg BW (very large)	No significant removal through HD and PD	Usual dose every 24–36 hours
Ampicillin (349)	8–20	0.17–0.30 liter/kg BW	Significant removal through HD and PD	HD: usual dose every 12 hours or 50% usual dose every 8–12 hours
				Give 50% of usual dose after dialysis
				CAPD: 75% of usual dose every 8 hours
Azathioprine (277)	30	Total body water	Moderately dialyzable	Usual dose in dialysis
Bretylium (237)	NA	Large	Moderately dialyzable	Reduced dosage with titration based on clinical effect
Captopril (217)	20–30	0.7 liter/kg BW	Significant removal through HD and PD	HD: 30% of usual dose
				Give 50% of usual dose after HD
				CAPD: 30% to 50% of usual dose (use BP as guide)
Cefamandole (463)	67–80	0.13 liter/kg BW	Moderate removal in HD Some removal in PD	50% of usual dose every 9–12 hours
Cephalexin (348)	15	0.18–0.38 liter/kg BW	Significant removal with HD and PD	HD: usual dose every 12–18 hours
				Give 50% of usual dose after HD
				CAPD: usual dose every 6–12 hours
Cimetidine (252)	20	0.8 liter/kg BW	Significant removal with HD and PD	75% of usual dose
				Give 50% of usual dose after HD
Clindamycin (461)	60–95	Very large	Insignificant removal with HD and PD	Usual oral dose
				Dialysis IV dose reduced to 50%
Clonidine (267)	40–50	3 liters/kg	Some removal with HD and PD	Usual dosage (use BP as guide)
Cloxacillin (476)	85–95	0.15–0.20 liter/kg BW	Insignificant removal with HD and PD	Usual dosage
Cortisone (361)	90%	NA	Not dialyzable	Usual dosage
Cyclosporine	High	3.5 liters/kg BW	Poorly dialyzed	
Diazepam (285)	94–98	Very large	Some removal with HD and PD	Usual dosage
Digitoxin (765)	90–97 decreased in uremia	0.6 liter/kg BW	Negligible removal in HD and PD	Adapt to individual needs, usually 0.1 mg/day
Digoxin (781)	25–35 (normal) 15–20 (ESRD)	5–12 liters/kg BW	Negligible removal in HD and PD	Usual dosage adapted to individual needs
				10%–25% of usual dose daily or usual dose every other day
Erythromycin (734)	70–75	0.57 liter/kg BW	Insignificant removal in HD Small removal in PD	Usual dosage
5-Fluorocytosine (129)	<10	0.6 liter/kg BW	Significant removal in HD and PD	HD and CAPD: usual dose every 24 hours
				Give 75% of usual dose after HD
Gentamicin (477)	2–25	0.20–0.25 liter/kg BW	Significant removal in HD Some removal through PD and CAPD	HD: 25% of usual dose every 24 hours
				Give 50% of loading dose after HD
				CAPD: 50% of usual dose every 24 hours
Heparin (6000–20,000)	Extensive	NA	Probably poorly dialyzed	Dosage titrated to partial thromboplastin time (PTT)
Insulin (6000)	1–10	0.6 liter/kg BW	No removal in HD or PD	HD: increase dosage interval
				CAPD: add to dialysate for intraperitoneal absorption
Lidocaine (234)	46–71	1.3 liters/kg BW	Not dialyzed	Usual dose
Meperidine (217)	58–64	3.7–4.2 liters/kg BW	Some removal through HD and PD	Usual dose
				Active metabolite accumulates in renal failure

Table continued on following page

TABLE 42–4. Guidelines for Drug Administration in Renal Failure *Continued*

Drug (Molecular Wt)	Plasma Protein Binding (%)	Volume of Distribution	Clearance in Dialysis	Dosage in ESRD with GFR < 10 ml/minute
Methyldopa (238)	<20	0.3 liter/kg BW	Some removal through HD and PD	Usual dose every 9–18 hours (use BP as guide)
Minoxidil (212)	None	3 liters/kg BW	Probably poorly dialyzed	Usual dose (use BP as guide)
Morphine (669)	35	0.66–1.5 liter/kg BW	Some removal through HD and PD	Usual dose
Nifedipine (346)	92–98	NA	Probably poorly dialyzed	Usual dose
Nitroprusside (252)	NA	NA	Metabolites are readily dialyzed	Usual dose (use BP as guide)
Penicillin G (334)	40–50	0.3–0.42 liter/kg BW	Some removal in HD and PD	HD: 50% of usual dose every 12 hours Give 75% of usual dose after HD CAPD: 75% of usual dose every 12 hours
Phenobarbital (232)	40–60	0.7–1.0 liter/kg BW	Significant removal in HD and PD	Usual dose every 12–24 hours
Prazosin (382)	97	0.6 liter/kg BW	Not dialyzable	Usual dose (use BP as guide)
Procainamide (272)	15–20	1.7–2.2 liters/kg BW	Substantial removal in HD and PD	Usual dose (use BP as guide)
Propranolol (259)	90–96	2.5–5 liters/kg BW	No removal in HD and PD	Usual dose; however, active metabolites may accumulate
Quinidine (324)	70–90	1.3–5.2 liters/kg BW	Very little removal with HD and PD	Usual dose
Theophylline (180)	25%	0.5 liter/kg BW	Significant removal in HD and PD	Usual dose
Tobramycin (468)	10–20	0.2–0.25 liter/kg BW	Substantial removal in HD and PD	HD: 20% to 30% of usual dose at normal intervals or usual dose every 24–48 hours Give 50% to 75% of usual dose after HD
Vancomycin (1800)	<10	0.47 liter/kg BW	Removal in HD unproved Significant removal in PD	HD: usual dose every 10 days PD: IV load of 1.0 g and 500 mg IV twice weekly
Verapamil (455)	87–93	Large	Probably poorly dialyzed	Usual dose

Abbreviations: GFR, glomerular filtration rate; BW, body weight; BP, blood pressure; HD, hemodialysis; PD, peritoneal dialysis; CAPD, continuous ambulatory peritoneal dialysis; NA, not available.

in mind that the new synthetic biocompatible membranes will increase the elimination rates of many drugs. However, limited data exist for the new membranes at this time.

As a general rule, lipid-soluble compounds are not readily dialyzable. Water-soluble drugs are more readily removed from the body. Drugs that are highly protein bound and those with high molecular weights are not dialyzable because the drug protein complexes are too large to cross the dialysis membrane effectively. Drugs with large volumes of distribution are not substantially dialyzed because the majority of the drug remains in tissue storage sites rather than in the blood compartment (Alexander and Gambertoglio, 1985).

Dialysis Therapy

The basic principles and complications of hemodialysis and peritoneal dialysis have been covered previously in Chapter 41. For the patient with ESRD, the goal of maintenance dialysis is to allow the individual to achieve the optimal level of functioning.

The patient receiving chronic hemodialysis therapy usually requires treatments lasting from 2 to 4 hours three times a week. Residual renal function, urea kinetic modeling, dialyzer capabilities, patient response, and ongoing clinical assessment by the nephrology team are used as parameters in determining the dialysis prescription for the individual patient. It is common for dialysis requirements to change during periods of acute illness or injury. The critically ill patient may require more frequent dialysis treatments due to administration of large amounts of total parenteral nutrition. More frequent dialysis will also be required when catabolism is increased following traumatic injury. As discussed earlier, maintenance of vascular access is critical to successful hemodialysis therapy.

Several treatment options are available to the patient with ESRD selecting chronic peritoneal dialysis. Intermittent peritoneal dialysis requires treatments of 10 to 14 hours each three to four times a week, or 8 to 12 hours nightly. No solution is left to dwell in the peritoneal cavity between dialysis treatments. Continuous cyclic peritoneal dialysis requires three to four overnight cycles, of 2 to 3 hours each. Solution is left in the peritoneal cavity for the 14 to 15 hours between dialyses. Continuous ambulatory peritoneal dialysis takes place 24 hours a day, 7 days a week, and usually involves four exchanges each day. Daytime exchanges last 4 to 6 hours, with a longer overnight exchange (Prowant and Binkley, 1987). The method chosen is determined by individual patient desires, physical and medical condition of the patient, and availability of these options for the patient. When a chronic peritoneal dialysis patient is admitted to the critical care unit, every possible means should be used to continue the usual dialysis routine. In some cases, as when the patient must undergo major abdominal surgery, peritoneal dialysis may be contraindicated. In these cases, a temporary vascular access is inserted, and the patient is hemodialyzed.

Renal Transplantation

The goal of renal transplantation for the patient with ESRD is achievement of an optimal level of function and reversal of many of the systemic consequences of renal failure. As with other types of therapy, long-term follow-up and teaching are crucial to the success of the transplanted kidney. The immunosuppressed transplant patient is at high risk of developing infection. In addition, these patients may have many problems associated with long-term steroid administration. General information related to medical management of the transplant patient is covered elsewhere in this text.

nCp nursing care plan

1. Alteration in cardiac output in hypertension related to:
Hypervolemia secondary to ESRD

Outcome Criteria	Nursing Interventions
Patient's blood pressure will remain within baseline levels.	Perform a careful history of the patient's antihypertensive medication regimen and his or her adherence to that regimen. Obtain a description of the accompanying cardiac or CNS manifestations and observe the patient for further occurrences. Obtain the patient's baseline blood pressure readings. Administer prescribed antihypertensive medications and carefully monitor their effect on blood pressure. Assess the patient's understanding and compliance with the prescribed medication, fluid, and diet regimen. Consult a dietitian to provide appropriate diet instruction for the patient and family. Review the patient's antihypertensive medications and teach the purpose, dosage, and effects of each drug. Identify the explain the pathophysiologic complications of noncompliance and encourage adherence to the regimen.

2. Alteration in cardiac output: hypotension related to:
Hypovlemia secondary to dialysis

Outcome Criteria	Nursing Interventions
Patient's blood pressure will remain within baseline levels.	Monitor the patient's blood pressure between dialysis treatments, noting and reporting significant hypotension. Discuss the appropriateness of withholding antihypertensive drugs with the patient's physician and dialysis nurse.

3. Fluid volume excess related to:
Hypervolemia

Outcome Criteria	Nursing Interventions
Patient's fluid balance will remain at or return to baseline levels. Patient will describe how to prevent future occurrences.	Obtain the patient's baseline weight. Assess the patient for evidence of peripheral or dependent edema. Observe neck veins for distention. Auscultate lungs for presence of rales. Maintain the prescribed fluid restrictions. Mix vasoactive infusions in double or quadruple strength. Obtain daily weights. Assess the patient's understanding of the prescribed fluid regimen and encourage adherence.

Nursing Care Plan continued on following page

4. Alteration in cardiac output: pericarditis related to:
Inadequate dialysis, surgical procedures, and acute catabolic illness

Outcome Criteria	Nursing Interventions
Pericarditis will be prevented or quickly detected.	Assess the patient for fever, chest pain, and pericardial friction rub. Monitor the pulse and blood pressure for the development of pulsus paradoxus of greater than 10 mm Hg. After diagnosis of pericarditis, prepare patient for intensive dialysis and keep equipment for pericardiocentesis available.

5. Alteration in cardiac output: hyperkalemia related to:
Diagnosis of ESRD

Outcome Criteria	Nursing Interventions
Injury related to hyperkalemia will be prevented. Serum potassium levels will be reduced. Reoccurrences of hyperkalemia will be prevented.	Closely monitor serum potassium levels. Measure serum potassium more frequently if acidosis is present. Monitor the ECG for peaked T waves, depressed ST segments, and wide QRS complexes. Have IV insulin, glucose, and bicarbonate available as well as a retention enema for the emergency treatment of hyperkalemia. Assess the events leading to the hyperkalemic episode. If noncompliance with the dietary regimen is the cause, assess the patient's level of understanding, provide necessary instruction, and encourage the patient to adhere to the prescribed diet. When possible, transfuse blood during hemodialysis so that excess potassium can be removed.

6. Alteration in peripheral perfusion related to:
Frequent vascular access secondary to dialysis

Outcome Criteria	Nursing Interventions
A patent and infection-free vascular access device will be maintained.	Monitor color, temperature, and sensation of the related extremity. Assess the patency of the access site by palpating for a thrill and auscultating for a bruit. Consult the dialysis nurse about how much heparin has been instilled in the catheter following dialysis and whether the catheter should be accessed for nondialysis purposes. Maintain a sterile and dry dressing at the catheter site. Assess femoral catheters more frequently because of ease of contamination by urine and fecal material.

7. Impaired gas exchange related to:
Fluid overload, increased capillary permeability, decreased activity of pulmonary macrophages, and increased susceptibility to infection

Outcome Criteria	Nursing Interventions
Adequate ventilation will be maintained. Nosocomial pneumonia will be prevented.	Frequently auscultate breath sounds. Assess for tachypnea and for the degree of respiratory effort. Compare baseline data with ongoing assessments to monitor for increasing respiratory dysfunction. Perform frequent and aggressive respiratory toilet, including coughing, deep breathing, suctioning, percussion/postural drainage, turning, and incentive spirometry. Monitor patient's sputum for changes in amount and consistency.

8. **Alteration in nutrition, less than body requirements related to:**
   Anorexia, nausea, vomiting, catabolic illness, prolonged dietary protein restrictions

Outcome Criteria	Nursing Interventions

Patient will receive diet adequate for repletion.
Patient will maintain desirable body weight.
Acceptable plasma levels of urea, sodium, potassium, magnesium, phosphorus, and albumin will be maintained.
	For non-stressed patients on hemodialysis:
	  Use kinetic modeling for individualizing the dialysis treatment and nutrition plan by determining the patient's protein catabolic rate.
	  Replace protein, sodium, potassium, and phosphorus based on recommendations per kg of ideal body weight (1 g of protein/kg of ideal body weight for protein, 2 to 3 g of sodium, 40 to 50 mEq of potassium, and 1200 mg of phosphorus per day).
	  Administer calcium supplements if needed and phosphorus levels are controlled.
	  Supplement diet with water-soluble vitamins and supplemental iron if stores are inadequate.
	For patients on peritoneal dialysis:
	  Encourage patient to eat sufficient amounts of protein, since protein losses are greater with peritoneal dialysis and peritonitis.
	  Consider that recommended protein intake is 0.2 to 0.5 g/kg per day greater than with patients on hemodialysis.
	  Ensure that patient complies with potassium restriction of 3 to 4 g/kg per day for patients on continuous peritoneal dialysis or 75 to 90 mEq/day for patients on intermittent peritoneal dialysis.
	  Ensure that fluids are restricted to urine output plus 500 to 1000 ml/day if on hemodialysis or intermittent peritoneal dialysis.
	For renal transplant patients:
	  Maintain dietary restrictions based upon the level of function of the transplanted kidney.
	  Consider the adverse effects of corticosteroids when developing a diet prescription.
	  Maintain caloric restrictions and closely monitor serum glucose levels.
	If patient is able to eat, assess his or her oral mucosa and provide frequent oral hygiene.
	If patient is on total parenteral nutrition (TPN), carefully assess the patient's response to the TPN fluid level, noting the presence of any signs of increasing congestive heart failure or pulmonary volume.
	Closely monitor catabolic patients for fluid volume overload.

9. **Alteration in bowel elimination: constipation related to:**
   Ingestion of phosphate binders

Outcome Criteria	Nursing Interventions
Patient's normal bowel elimination pattern will be maintained.	Obtain a detailed history of the patient's bowel patterns and laxative use. Assess patient for abdominal distention, abdominal discomfort, presence of bowel sounds, and frequency of bowel movements. Obtain and administer the patient's usual laxative or stool softener. Encourage a diet high in fiber and bulk.

10. **Activity intolerance related to:**
    Anemia secondary to decreased secretion of erythropoietin

Outcome Criteria	Nursing Interventions
Patient will experience minimal blood loss to maintain a hematocrit at an adequate level.	Monitor patient's hematocrit and hemoglobin for downward trends. Minimize the number and amount of blood samples drawn. Administer iron, folate, and blood transfusions as prescribed.

Nursing Care Plan continued on following page

11. Potential for bleeding related to:
Qualitative defect of platelet adhesiveness

Outcome Criteria	Nursing Interventions
Bleeding will be prevented or detected early.	Monitor stool, vomitus, and nasogastric aspirate for occult blood. Administer antacids as prescribed. Minimize manipulation of the nasogastric tube. Perform tracheal suctioning to avoid tissue trauma. Assess line insertion sites for bleeding. Apply manual pressure to fistula site until hemostasis is achieved following hemodialysis.

12. Potential for infection related to:
Immunosuppression

Outcome Criteria	Nursing Interventions
Patient will be free of infection and initial infectious process will be quickly identified.	Monitor the patient's temperature curve and WBC count. Observe for changes in odor, color, or consistency of drainage and secretions. Ensure meticulous care during line insertion and line maintenance. Initiate vigorous pulmonary toilet. Carefully inspect wounds for evidence of inflammation and infection.

13. Alterations in thought processes related to:
Uremia and electrolyte and metabolic disturbances

Outcome Criteria	Nursing Interventions
Patient will maintain optimum level of orientation and cognitive function.	Obtain a baseline assessment of the patient's cognitive functioning on admission, including orientation to person, place, and time; length of attention span; sleep disturbance; fatigue; increasing somnolence; irritability; and signs of depression. Assess the patient's ability to understand requests or instructions. Use assessment information to guide communication with the patient and, when appropriate, to develop a patient education plan. Observe and document the effects of medication and treatment on the patient's mentation.

14. Alteration in comfort related to:
Uremic neuropathy and renal osteodystrophy

Outcome Criteria	Nursing Interventions
Comfort measures will be provided. Patient will ambulate with increasing frequency. Immobility will be prevented. Calcium and phosphorus levels will be maintained at acceptable levels.	Assess for numbness or burning in the feet, restless leg movements, decreased muscle strength, cramps, paresthesias, and decreased deep tendon reflexes. Avoid unexpected touching of the feet, and keep heavy bed linens off the feet. Teach patient how to inspect the feet visually for signs of injury. Encourage and assist with ambulation and collaborate with the physical therapist in developing an exercise program for the patient. Assess for muscular weakness, gait changes, and the presence of joint pain or deep bone pain. Note history of pathologic fractures. Obtain baseline serum calcium and phosphorus levels and monitor for development of hypocalcemia. Administer phosphate-binding antacids as prescribed.

15. Impaired skin integrity related to:
Pruritus, delayed wound healing

Outcome Criteria	Nursing Interventions
Patient will have intact skin without infection.	Assess patient's skin for signs of infection, inflammation, excoriation, edema, and ecchymosis. Use superfatted or lanolin-based soaps for bathing. Apply emollients to relieve itching. Turn patient frequently to prevent pressure ulcers. Utilize therapeutic mattresses or beds is prolonged immobility is expected.

16. Ineffective coping related to:
Multiple stressors of chronic renal failure

Outcome Criteria	Nursing Interventions
Patient and family will demonstrate understanding and adaptation to the changes imposed by the critical illness.	Assess patient and family for signs of depression, anger, withdrawal, and dependent behaviors. Observe for evidence of noncompliance or nonparticipation in therapy. Encourage expression of feelings and discussion of concerns and frustrations. Consider referral to local support group via The National Kidney Foundation.

SUMMARY

Since the early 1970s, the dialysis and renal transplant population has steadily increased. Advances in renal replacement therapy have resulted in longer life expectancy for these patients. In fact, according to Dr. Belding H. Scribner, "A patient with end-stage renal failure who is in the 20 to 50 year age range and is otherwise well who starts renal replacement therapy in the 1980s should have a nearly normal life expectancy" (Maher, 1989, p. vii).

Although chronic renal failure and ESRD are not considered critical illnesses, the pathophysiology of renal disease frequently results in a need for hospitalization in a critical care unit. The medical and nursing management of these patients is complex, involving aspects of both the acute problem and the chronic disease process.

Physical and emotional support for the individual who has reached ESRD involves a collaborative effort by nurses, physicians, social workers, dietitians, family, and clergy. It may be the critical care nurse who provides the patient with the initial information about the diverse treatment options available to him. In many cases, hospitalization may be due to the patient's noncompliance with fluid or dietary restrictions. In such cases, ongoing patient education about the renal disease process and its relationship to the patient's critical illness is a vital nursing function.

References

Abreo, K. (1988). Use of deferoxamine in the treatment of aluminum overload in dialysis patients. *Seminars in Dialysis*, 1(1):55–61.

Alexander, D. P., and Gambertoglio, J. G. (1985). Drug overdose and pharmacologic considerations in dialysis. In M. G. Cogan, and M. R. Garovoy (Eds.), *Introduction to dialysis* (pp. 261–292). New York: Churchill Livingstone.

American Nephrology Nurses Association (ANNA) (1986). *Scope of practice for nephrology nursing*. Pitman, NJ: ANNA.

American Nephrology Nurses Association (ANNA) (1988). *Standards of clinical practice for nephrology nursing*. Pitman, NJ: ANNA.

Anderson, R. J., Bennett, W. M., Gambertoglio, J. G., et al. (1981). Fate of drugs in renal failure. In B. M. Brenner, and F. C. Rector (Eds.), *The Kidney* (2nd ed., pp. 2659–2708). Philadelphia: W.B. Saunders.

Aubria, J., Hojman, L., Chine, M., et al. (1987). Hypertension and nephrotoxicity in the rate of decline in kidney function in diabetic nephropathy. *Clinical Nephrology*, 27(1), 15–20.

Baer, C. L. (1987). The pharamacologic aspects of renal failure. In L. E. Lancaster (Ed.), *Core curriculum for nephrology nursing* (pp. 157–183). Pitman, NJ: American Nephrology Nurses Association (ANNA).

Baldwin, D. S. and Neugarten, J. (1987), Hypertension and renal diseases. *American Journal of Kidney Diseases*, 10(3), 186–191.

Brenner, B. M., Dworken, L., and Ichikawa, I. (1986). Glomerular ultrafiltration. In B. M. Brenner, and F. C. Rector (Eds.), *The kidney* (3rd ed., pp. 124–144). Philadelphia: W. B. Saunders.

Bukart, J. M., Hamilton, R. W., and Buchalew, V. M. (1989). Prevention of renal failure. In J. F. Maher (Ed.), *Replacement of renal function by dialysis* (3rd ed., pp. 1119–1132). Boston: Kluwer Academic Publishers.

Coe, F. L. (1986). Clinical and laboratory assessment of the patient with renal disease. In B. M. Brenner, and F. C. Rector (Eds.), *The kidney* (3rd ed., pp. 703–734). Philadelphia: W. B. Saunders.

Delano, B. G. (1983). Regular dialysis treatment. In W. Drukker, P. Parsons, and J. Maher (Eds.), *Replacement of renal function by dialysis* (pp. 391–409). Boston: Martinus Nijhoff.

Dzau, V. J. (1987). Renal and circulatory mechanisms in congestive heart failure. *Kidney International*, 31, 1402–1415.

Eddins, B. A. (1984). A review of the pathophysiologic basis of end-stage renal disease. *Journal of Nephrology Nursing*, 1(2), 85–94.

End-Stage Renal Disease Network 3. (1987). *Medical information systems 1987 data report*. Northern California–Nevada.

End-Stage Renal Disease Profile Tables—1986. (1988), *Contemporary dialysis and nephrology*, 9(5), 46–48.

Eschbach, J. W. and Adamson, J. W. (1985). Anemia of end stage renal disease (ESRD). *Kidney International*, 28, 1.

Eschbach, J. W. and Adamson, J. W. (1988). Recombinant human erythropoietin: Implications for nephrology. *American Journal of Kidney Diseases*, 11, 203.

Fine, L. G. (1987). The uremic syndrome: Adaptive mechanisms and therapy. *Hospital Practice*, 22(9), 63–73.

Finkelstein, S. H. and Finklestein, F. O. (1986). Sexual dysfunction in chronic renal failure. In A. R. Nissenson, and R. N. Fine (Eds.), *Dialysis therapy* (pp. 174–177). St. Louis: C. V. Mosby.

Glassock, R. J., Adler, S. G., Ward, H. J., et al. (1986). Primary glomerular diseases. In B. M. Brenner, and F. C. Rector (Eds.), *The kidney* (3rd ed., pp. 929–1013). Philadelphia: W. B. Saunders.

Golding, A. L. (1986). Complications of vascular access for chronic hemodialysis. In A. R. Nissenson and R. N. Fine (Eds.), *Dialysis therapy* (pp. 9–13), St. Louis: C. V. Mosby.

Golper, T. A. (1986). Management of hyperlipidemia in chronic dialysis patients. In A. R. Nissenson, and R. N. Fine (Eds.), *Dialysis therapy* (pp. 170–171). St. Louis: C. V. Mosby.

Gotch, F. A. and J. A. Sargent (1985). A mechanistic analysis of the national cooperative dialysis study (NCDS). *Kidney International*, 28, 526–534.

Grantham, J. J. (1988). The pathogenesis of renal cyst formation. In A. Davison (Ed.), *Nephrology*, Vol. II: *Proceedings of the Tenth International Congress of Nephrology* (pp. 11–19). Philadelphia: W. B. Saunders.

Hakim, R. M. and Lazarus, J. M. (1986). Medical aspects of hemodialysis. In B. M. Brenner and F. C. Rector (Eds.), *The kidney* (3rd ed, pp. 1791–1844). Philadelphia: W.B. Saunders.

Henrich, W. L. (1986), Hemodynamic instability during hemodialysis. *Kidney International*, 30, 605–612.

Hoffart, N. (1987). Nutrition in renal failure, dialysis and transplantation. In L. Lancaster (Ed.), *Core curriculum for nephrology nursing* (pp. 135–155). Pitman, NJ: American Nephrology Nurses Association (ANNA).

Hostetter, T. H. (1986). Diabetic nephropathy. In B. M. Brenner, and F. C. Rector (Eds.), *The kidney* (3rd ed. pp. 1372–1402). Philadelphia: W.B. Saunders.

Jacobson, P. M. and McNatt, G. E. (1986). Holistic nursing of the client with end stage renal disease. In C. J. Richard (Ed.), *Comprehensive nephrology nursing* (pp. 225–249). Boston: Little, Brown.

Keane, W. F. and Maddy, M. F. (1989). Host defenses and infectious complications in maintenance hemodialysis patients. In J. F. Maher (Ed.), *Replacement of renal function by dialysis* (pp. 865–880). Boston: Kluwer Academic Publishers.

Kjellstrand, C. M. (1985). Indicators for cardiovascular catastrophe in diabetic patients with renal failure. In N. Cummings and S. Klahr (Eds.), *Chronic renal disease* (pp. 277–283), New York: Plenum.

Klahr, S. (1988). The progression of renal disease. *New England Journal of Medicine*, 318(25): 1657–1666.

Krupski, W. C., Bruks, M. D., Webb, R. L., et al. (1985). Access for dialysis. In M. G. Cogan, and M. R. Garovoy (Eds.), *Introduction to dialysis* (pp.41–71). New York: Churchill Livingstone.

Lack, F., and Corburn, J. (1989). Renal osteodystrophy and maintenance dialysis. In J. F. Maher (Ed.), *Replacement of renal function by dialysis* (pp. 911–952). Boston: Kluwer Academic Publishers.

Lancaster, L. E. (1987). Manifestations of renal failure. In L. E.

Lancaster (Ed.), *Core curriculum for nephrology nursing* (pp. 75–104). Pitman, NJ: American Nephrology Nurses Association (ANNA).

Maher, J. F. (1989a). Pharmacological considerations for renal failure and dialysis. In J. F. Maher (Ed.), *Replacement of renal function by dialysis* (pp. 953–1111). Boston: Kluwer Academic Publishers.

Maher, J. F. (Ed.). (1989b). Foreword. *Replacement of renal function by dialysis*. Boston: Kluwer Academic Publishers.

Mako, J, Lengyel, M, Nagy, L, et al. (1986). Surgical window formation in the pericardium in uremic pericardial effusion. *Dialysis and Transplantation*, 15(8), 458–471.

Morgensen, C. E. (1987). Microalbuminuria as a predictor of clinical diabetic nephropathy. *Kidney International*, 31, 673.

Mujais, S. K., Sabatini, S., and Kurtzman, N. A. (1986). Pathophysiology of the uremic syndrome. In B. M. Brenner, and F. C. Rector (Eds.), *The kidney* (3rd ed., pp. 1587–1630). Philadelphia: W. B. Saunders.

McClusky, R. T. (1987). Immunopathogenic mechanisms in renal disease. *American Journal of Kidney Disease*, 10(3), 172–180.

National News. (1988). New facility and patient treatment statistics. *Nephrology News & Issues*, 2(10), 9.

Paganini, E. (1988). The treatment of anemia in dialysis patients: Present and future potentials of erythropoietin therapy. *Nephrology News & Issues*, 2(10), 36–40.

Prowant, B. F., and Binkley, L. S. (1987). Concepts and principles of peritoneal dialysis. In L. Lancaster (Ed.), *Core curriculum for nephrology nursing* (pp. 241–278). Pitman, NJ: American Nephrology Nurses Association (ANNA).

Richard, C. J. (1987). Causes of renal failure. In L. Lancaster (Ed.), *Core curriculum for nephrology nursing* (pp. 53–73). Pitman, NJ: American Nephrology Nurses Association (ANNA).

Rose, B. D., and Black, R. M. (1989). Chronic renal failure. In R. D. Rose, and R. M. Black (Eds.), *Manual of clinical problems in nephrology* (pp. 347–398). Boston: Little, Brown.

Ross, E. H., and Nissenson, A. R. (1988). Dialysis-associated hypoxemia: Insight into pathophysiology and prevention. *Seminars in Dialysis*, 1(1), 33–39.

Rutsky, E. A. (1986). Arrhythmias in patients on hemodialysis. In A. R. Nissenson, and R. N. Fine (Eds.), *Dialysis therapy* (pp. 90–91). St. Louis: C. V. Mosby.

Schmitz, O., Hansen, H. E., Orshon, H., et al. (1985). End-stage renal failure in diabetic nephropathy: Pathophysiology and treatment. *Blood Perfusion*, 3, 120–139.

Schoenfeld, P. (1985a). Care of the patient on peritoneal dialysis. In M. G. Cogan, and M. R. Garovoy (Eds.), *Introduction to dialysis* (pp. 145–196). New York: Churchill Livingstone.

Schoenfeld, P. (1985b). Care of the patient between dialysis. In M. G. Cogan, and M. R. Garovoy (Eds.), *Introduction to dialysis* (pp. 197–259). New York: Churchill Livingstone.

Scribner, B. H. and Babb, A. L. (1986). Chronic hemodialysis in Seattle: 1960–1966. *Dialysis and Transplantation*, 15(1), 33–45.

Seffart, G. (1985). Drugs in renal failure: Dosing guidelines for frequently used drugs in end-stage renal disease and dialysis patients. *Blood Purification*, 3, 140–168.

Skorecki, K. L., Nadler, S. P., Badr, K. F., et al. (1986). Renal and systemic manifestations of glomerular disease, In B. M. Brenner, and F. C. Rector (Eds.), *The kidney* (3rd ed., pp. 891–928). Philadelphia: W.B. Saunders.

Spital, A. and Sterns, R. H. (1988). Potassium homeostasis in dialysis patients. *Seminars in Dialysis*, 1(1), 14–20.

Sreepada Rao, T. K. (1989). Dialysis in the acquired immunodeficiency syndrome. In J. F. Maher (Ed.), *Replacement of renal function by dialysis* (pp. 704–910). Boston: Kluwer Academic Publishers.

Strom, T. B. and Tilney, N. L. (1986). Renal transplantation: Clinical aspects. In B. M. Brenner, and F. C. Rector (Eds.), *The kidney* (3rd ed., pp. 1941–1976). Philadelphia: W. B. Saunders.

Teitebaum, S. (1985). The pathology of the renal bone lesion. In N. B. Cummings, and S. Klahr (Eds.), *Chronic renal disease: Causes, complications and treatment* (pp. 127–138). New York: Plenum Medical Book Co.

Thompson, C. (1988). The spectrum of renal cystic disease. *Hospital Practice*, 23, 165–175.

Vaziri, N. D. (1986). Anemia in ESRD patients. In A. R. Nissenson, and R. N. Fine (Eds.), *Dialysis therapy* (pp. 158–161). St. Louis: C. V. Mosby.

White, R. P., and Rubin, A. L. (1983). Blood pressure control in chronic dialysis patients. In W. Drukker, P. Parsons, and J. Maher (Eds.), *Replacement of renal function by dialysis* (pp. 575–587). Boston: Martinus Nijhoff.

Gastrointestinal System

43

Gastrointestinal Physiology

Margaret Heitkemper
Una E. Westfall

The gastrointestinal (GI) tract is responsible for the digestion and absorption of nutrients. The accomplishment of this task requires appropriate and timely movement of nutrients through the GI tract (motility), the presence of specific enzymes to break down nutrients (digestion), and transport mechanisms to move nutrients from the GI tract lumen to the vascular system (absorption). The term GI system denotes the entire system responsible for these functions, whereas GI tract refers only to those organs that connect the mouth with the anus (Fig. 43–1). The anatomic parts of the GI tract include the mouth, esophagus, stomach, small intestine, and large intestine. The small intestine is further divided anatomically into duodenum, jejunum, and ileum, the duodenum being closest to the stomach. The large intestine is divided into the cecum, ascending colon, transverse colon, descending colon, sigmoid colon, and rectum. Accessory organs of the GI system include the liver, pancreas, and gallbladder. Each of these organs plays an important role in digestion of nutrients.

ANATOMY OF THE GUT WALL

Beginning in the esophagus and extending to the rectum, the GI tract is composed of multiple tissue layers.

Mucosa. The innermost layer that is exposed to dietary nutrients is the mucosa. The thickness and function of the mucosa vary according to the anatomic segment examined. The mucosal layer is composed of epithelial cells. These epithelial cells are connected by tight junctions, which produce an effective barrier against the entry of large molecular substances and bacteria. In addition, the mucosa contains goblet cells that produce and secrete mucus. In the stomach, the anatomic arrangement of epithelial cells as well as the production of mucus and the relatively rapid regeneration of cells provide what is known as the gastric mucosal barrier. However, some substances, such as salicylates and alcohol, are able to penetrate this barrier and thus are absorbed in the stomach. It is the disruption of this anatomic and physiologic barrier that is thought to play a role in ulcer development.

Submucosa. Beneath the mucosa is a nerve plexus known as the submucosal plexus (Fig. 43–2).

Serosa. Next is the first of two smooth muscle layers comprising the gut wall. The innermost muscle layer is the circular muscle, and the next is the longitudinal muscle. Both are so named because of their muscle fiber orientation. Combined, these muscle layers form what is called the serosa. Between the two muscle layers is another nerve plexus known as the *myenteric plexus*.

The anatomic arrangement of the gut wall including the nerve and muscle layers persists throughout the length of the GI tract. However, in the stomach there is an additional muscle layer known as the muscularis mucosa, which is located between the mucosa and the circular muscle layer.

NEURAL INNERVATION

Extrinsic

Functions of the GI system are influenced by neural as well as hormonal factors.

Autonomic Nervous System. The autonomic nervous system (ANS) exerts multiple effects. Table 43–

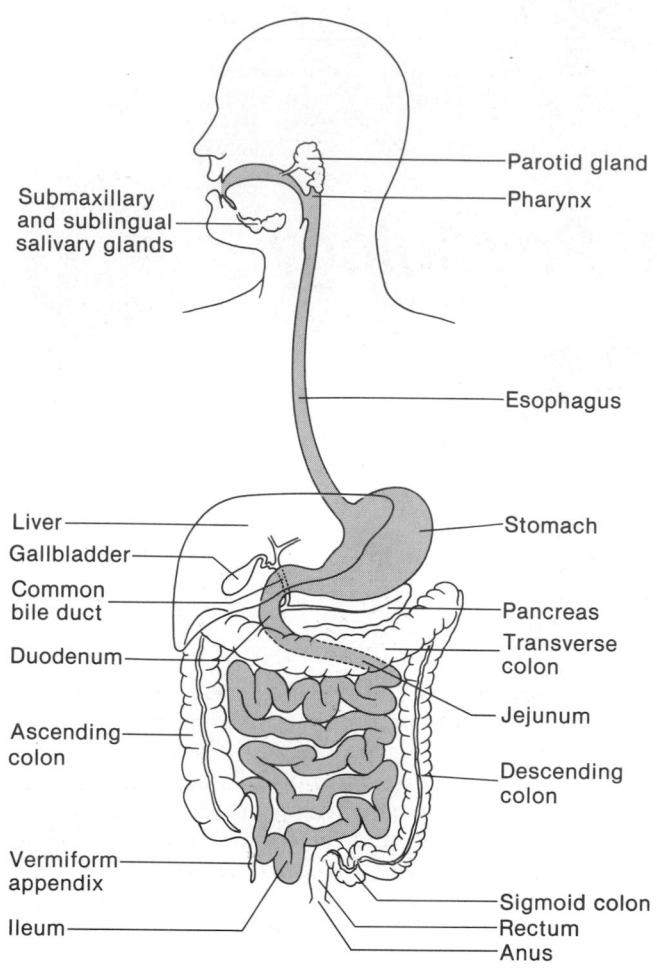

FIGURE 43–1. Digestive tract of the human being.

Labels (clockwise): Parotid gland, Pharynx, Submaxillary and sublingual salivary glands, Esophagus, Stomach, Pancreas, Transverse colon, Jejunum, Descending colon, Sigmoid colon, Rectum, Anus, Ileum, Vermiform appendix, Ascending colon, Duodenum, Common bile duct, Gallbladder, Liver

tract receives fibers from the vagus nerve; the distal GI tract receives fibers from the sacral division of the parasympathetic nervous system. As stated above, these fibers synapse on the enteric nervous system neurons, which are located between the muscle layers of the gut wall. In addition, these nerve bundles contain afferent (sensory) fibers whose receptors are located within GI tissues. The afferent nerve fibers relay information to the spinal cord and brain about such sensations as pain and distention.

Sympathetic Nervous System. The GI tract is also innervated by fibers from the sympathetic nervous system. Preganglionic fibers synapse upon leaving the spinal cord in ganglia located adjacent to the vertebral column. Long postganglionic fibers then travel to the GI tract organs to synapse on blood vessels and neurons located within the gut wall as well as some secretory cells.

Sympathetic and parasympathetic preganglionic fibers as well as postganglionic parasympathetic neurons release acetylcholine as their neurotransmitter, whereas postganglionic sympathetic fibers release norepinephrine. In general, parasympathetic cholinergic fibers (through vagal efferent fibers) are stimulatory to GI secretion and propulsive activity, in contrast to sympathetic nervous system input, which inhibits GI motor and secretory activity and produces contraction of GI sphincters and blood vessels. Clinical consequences include gastric stasis, adynamic or paralytic ileus, or colonic ileus. Parasympathetic and sympathetic fibers also innervate the gallbladder and pancreas.

Intrinsic

Extrinsic preganglionic parasympathetic and postganglionic sympathetic fibers synapse on neurons of the myenteric and submucosal plexi. The submucosal and myenteric nerve networks combined are referred to as the enteric nervous system of the gut. These

1 summarizes some of the common effects of the ANS on the GI system.

Parasympathetic Nervous System. The GI tract is innervated by preganglionic fibers of the parasympathetic nervous system (Fig. 43–3). The upper GI

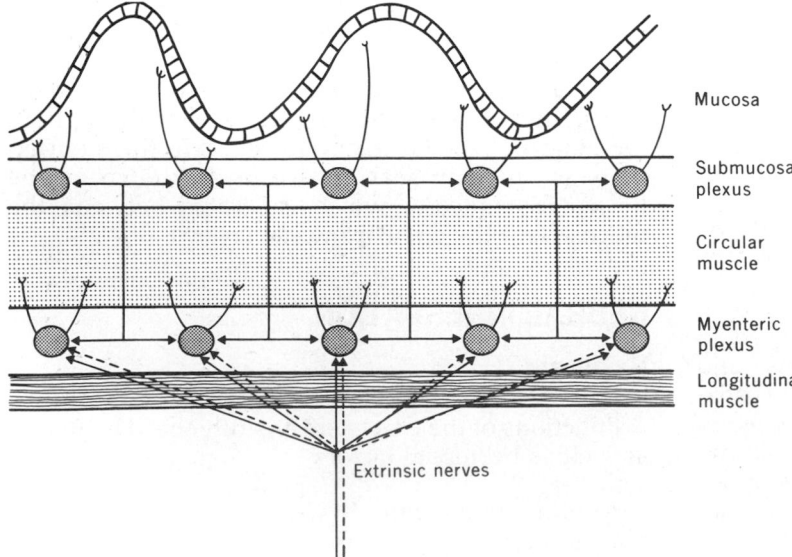

Labels: Mucosa, Submucosal plexus, Circular muscle, Myenteric plexus, Longitudinal muscle, Extrinsic nerves

FIGURE 43–2. The two main plexuses of the enteric nervous system, myenteric and submucosal, contain numerous cell bodies and processes. Neurons communicate with other neurons in the same plexus and with those in the other plexus. Additionally, plexus neurons communicate with both sympathetic and parasympathetic branches of the extrinsic nerves in the autonomic nervous system. Plexus neurons receive input from receptors located in the mucosa and muscle layers and supply efferent innervation to those same layers. Thus, the enteric nervous system can act autonomously to regulate integrated behavior of the gastrointestinal tract. (Reproduced by permission from: Johnson, L. *Gastrointestinal physiology* (3rd ed., p. 17). St. Louis, 1985, The C.V. Mosby Co.)

TABLE 43–1. Responses of Selected Effector Organs to Autonomic Nerve Impulses

Effector Organs	Receptor Type	Adrenergic Impulses: Responses	Cholinergic Impulses: Responses
Stomach			
Motility and tone	Alpha-2; beta-2	Decrease (usually)*+	Increase+ + +
Sphincters	Alpha	Contraction (usually)+	Relaxation (usually)+
Secretion		Inhibition (?)	Stimulation+ + +
Intestine			
Motility and tone	Alpha-1, beta-1; beta-2	Decrease*+	Increase+ + +
Sphincters	Alpha	Contraction (usually)+	Relaxation (usually)+
Secretion		Inhibition (?)	Stimulation+ +
Gallbladder and Ducts	Beta-2	Relaxation+	Contraction+
Liver	Alpha; beta-2	Glycogenolysis and gluconeogenesis†+ + +	Glycogen synthesis+
Pancreas			
Acini	Alpha	Decreased secretion+	Secretion+ +
Islets (B cells)	Alpha-2	Decreased secretion+ + +	—
	Beta-2	Increased secretion+	—
Fat Cells	Alpha; beta-1	Lipolysis†+ + +	—
Salivary Glands	Alpha-1	Potassium and water secretion+	Potassium and water secretion+ + +
	Beta	Amylase secretion+	
Nasopharyngeal Glands		—	Secretion+ +

*It has been proposed that adrenergic fibers terminate at inhibitory B receptors on smooth muscle fibers, and at inhibitory a receptors on parasympathetic cholinergic (excitory) ganglion cells of Auerbach's (myenteric) plexus.

†Gives estimated importance of ANS control for selected responses by organ. There is significant variation among species in the type of receptor that mediates certain metabolic responses; a and B responses have not been determined in man.

Adapted from Gilman, A. G., Goodman, L. S., Rall, R. W., et al. (1985). Goodman and Gilman's the pharmacologic basis of therapeutics (7th ed., pp. 72–73). New York: Macmillan, © 1985.

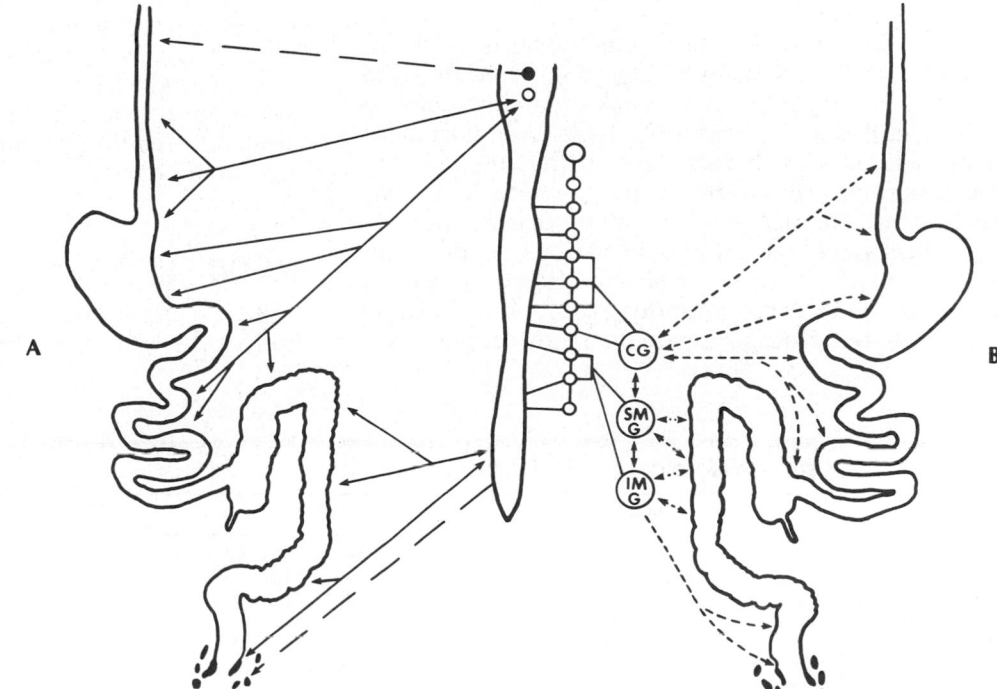

FIGURE 43–3. Extrinsic branches of the autonomic nervous system. *A,* Parasympathetic. Dashed lines indicate the cholinergic innervation of striated muscle in the esophagus and external anal sphincter. Solid lines indicate the afferent and preganglionic efferent innervation of the rest of the gastrointestinal tract. *B,* Sympathetic. Solid lines denote the afferent and preganglionic efferent connections between the spinal cord and the prevertebral ganglia (celiac, CG; superior mesenteric, SMG; inferior mesenteric, IMG). Dashed lines indicate afferent and postganglionic efferent innervation. (Reproduced by permission from: Johnson, L. *Gastrointestinal physiology* (3rd ed., p. 16). St. Louis, 1985, The C.V. Mosby Co.)

enteric neurons innervate target cells including smooth muscle cells, secretory cells, and absorptive cells. In addition, enteric neuron plexi communicate with each other throughout the length of the gut and contribute to intrinsic coordination. Enteric nerves generate propulsive activities (e.g., peristalsis, segmental contractions) and coordinate activities of the GI sphincters. Disturbances of these enteric neurons in a given segment of GI tract are related to lack of motility or movement. This is seen most dramatically in congenital megacolon (Hirschsprung disease), in which a segment of distal colon lacks enteric neurons. As a result, there is lack of movement of intestinal contents through this region, leading to distention of the region preceding the aganglionic segment.

HORMONAL CONTROL

Hormones that influence GI function include those produced by specialized cells within the GI tract as well as those synthesized by other endocrine organs (Fig. 43–4). In general, the GI tract is considered the largest endocrine organ in the body. Protein and peptide hormones produced by GI tissue are secreted into the portal venous circulation, pass through the liver and heart, and return to the GI tract to modulate activities such as motility, secretion, and absorption. Gastrointestinal hormones (e.g., gastrin) as well as other hormones (e.g., cortisol) may be involved in the normal maturation of GI tissues. There is some overlap in the function of gut hormones in that two or more hormones may produce similar effects in relation to motility, acid secretion, or fluid and electrolyte secretion.

The first hormone "discovered" was secretin in 1902. In 1905 gastrin was described, and in 1928 cholecystokinin (CCK) was named for its ability to cause gallbladder contraction. These three hormones were isolated and characterized in the 1960s. In the late 1960s, gastric inhibitory polypeptide (GIP) was isolated and characterized. A variety of other peptide hormones have been found in various segments of the gut; however, their physiologic functions remain to be clarified. These peptides (Table 43–2) include motilin, enteroglucagon, pancreatic polypeptide, va-

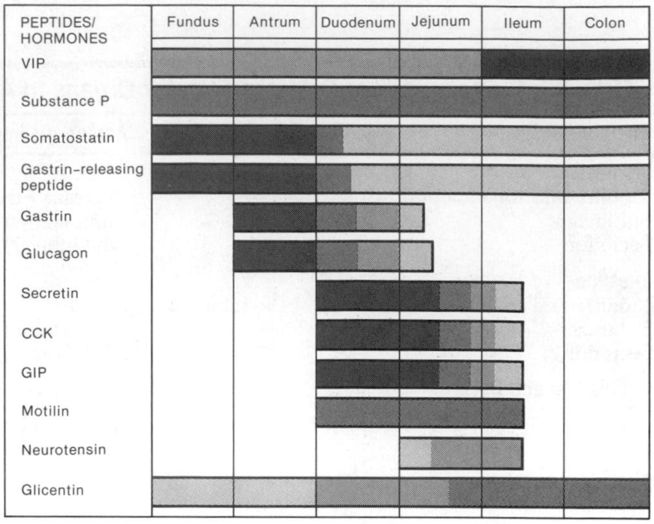

FIGURE 43–4. Distribution of gastrointestinal peptides along the gastrointestinal tract. The shading of each bar is proportionate to the concentration of the peptide in the mucosa.

soactive intestinal polypeptide, gastrin-releasing peptide, and enkephalins.

Table 43–3 lists the better known GI hormones and their actions. Gastrin, which is secreted by cells located in the gastric antrum and duodenum, stimulates release of hydrochloric acid. Serum levels of gastrin can be measured by radioimmunoassay, which may be performed in patients with Zollinger-Ellison (Z-E) syndrome, in which tumor cells produce gastrin. Cholecystokinin has the widest range of action. CCK is secreted by intestinal cells in response to the presence of fat and protein breakdown products and is a stimulant of pancreatic enzyme secretion and gallbladder smooth muscle contraction. Secretin, which is produced and secreted by the small intestine in response to the presence of acid, is known to stimulate secretion of pancreatic juice with a high bicarbonate content. These hormones also influence GI motility.

BLOOD SUPPLY

Of the various body organ systems, the GI system receives the largest percentage of the cardiac output.

TABLE 43–2. Candidate Hormones and Neurocrines

Peptide	Source	Action	Hormone/Neurocrine
Enkephalin	Gut mucosa and muscle	Smooth muscle tone	Neurocrine
Enteroglucagon	Intestinal mucosa	Glycogenolysis	Candidate hormone
Gastrin-releasing peptide or bombesin	Gastric mucosa	Gastric release	Neurocrine
Motilin	Duodenal mucosa	Gastric motility Intestinal motility	Candidate hormone
Pancreatic polypeptide	Pancreas	Pancreatic HCO_3 Enzyme secretion	Candidate hormone
Vasoactive intestinal polypeptide	Gut mucosa and muscle	Relaxation of gut and circular smooth muscle	Neurocrine

TABLE 43–3. Gastrointestinal Hormone Actions

Action	Gastrin	Cholecystokinin	Secretin	Gastrointestinal Peptide
		Hormone		
Acid secretion	S*	S	I*	I*
Gastric emptying	I	I*	I	I
Pancreatic HCO_3 secretion	S	S*	S*	0
Pancreatic enzyme secretion	S	S*	S	0
Bile HCO_3^- secretion	S	S	S*	0
Gallbladder contraction	S	S*	S	—
Gastric motility	S	S	I	I
Intestinal motility	S	S	S	S*
Insulin release	S	S	S	—
Mucosal growth	S*	S	I	—
Pancreatic growth	S	S*	S*	—

Abbreviations: S, stimulates; I, inhibits; 0, no effect; —, not yet tested
*Important physiologic response to endogenous hormone level following normal stimulus.
Reproduced by permission from Johnson, L. Gastrointestinal physiology (3rd ed., p. 8). St. Louis, 1985, The C. V. Mosby Co.

Approximately one-third of the cardiac output supplies these tissues. Blood supply to organs within the abdomen is referred to as the splanchnic circulation (Fig. 43–5). The stomach, small and large intestines, pancreas, and gallbladder are supplied by the superior and inferior mesenteric and celiac arteries, whereas the liver receives part of its blood supply from the hepatic artery. Circulation in the GI system is unique in that venous blood draining the GI tract empties into the portal vein, which then perfuses the liver. The portal vein supplies approximately 70% to 75% of blood flow to the liver. Because such a large percentage of cardiac output perfuses the tissues of the GI tract, the GI tract is a major source from which blood flow can be diverted to more vital organs during times of need, such as during exercise or hemorrhage.

At the tissue level, there is an overlap in perfusion

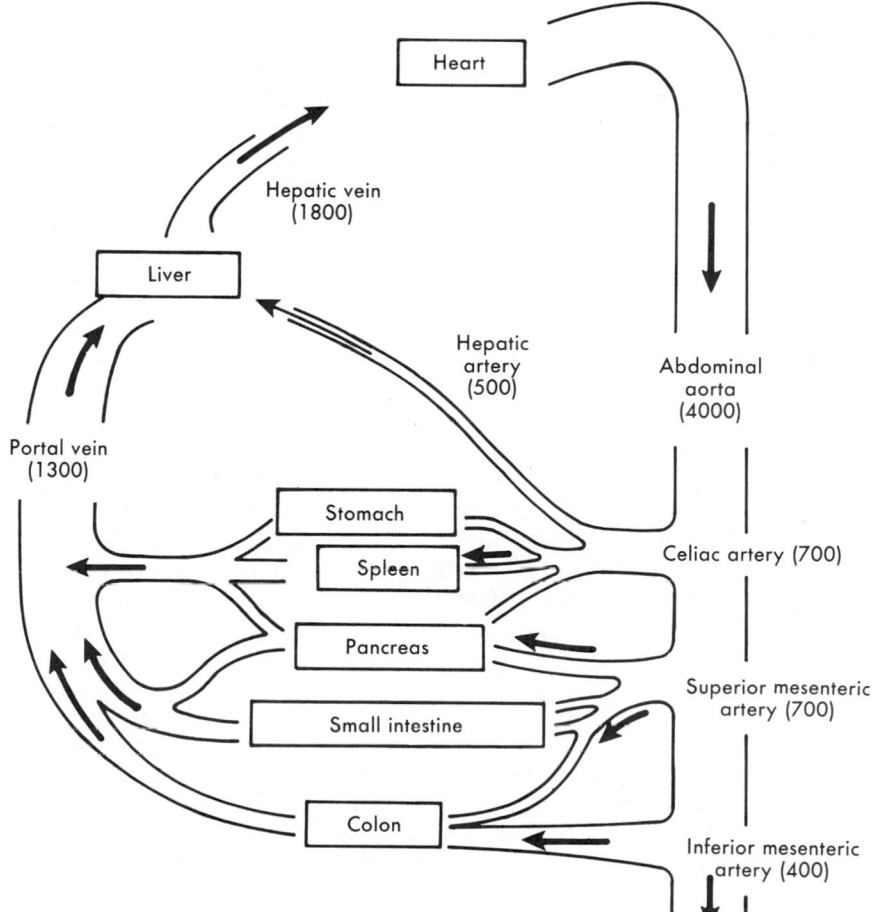

FIGURE 43–5. Blood flows and distributions within the major splanchnic vessels (ml/minute). (Reproduced by permission from: Johnson, L. *Gastrointestinal physiology* (3rd ed., p. 141). St. Louis, 1985, The C.V. Mosby Co.)

that ensures to some degree that occlusion of one artery due to, for example, thrombus or embolus will not completely deny the mucosa its blood supply. However, prolonged occlusion of a major artery supplying the GI tract can produce ischemic changes of the mucosal lining and ultimately necrosis. Non-occlusive intestinal ischemia or hemorrhagic necrosis of the gut is an example of potentially fatal damage produced by a prolonged reduction in intestinal blood supply. In the presence of a systemic problem such as congestive heart failure or a peripheral problem such as arteriosclerosis, there could be a reduction in the blood supply to the GI tract. As a result, necrosis of intestinal villi occurs, which can ultimately destroy the GI tract's barrier to harmful toxins and bacteria normally present in the intestinal lumen. These bacteria then enter the blood supply and can produce septic shock and, depending upon the severity, death of the patient. This process is referred to as bacterial translocation.

In the trauma patient with hemorrhagic shock in whom prolonged hypotension occurs, there is an increased risk of bacterial translocation. Animal studies have demonstrated that shock produces bacterial (e.g., *Escherichia coli*, *Enterococcus*) translocation. Histologic examination reveals that shock produces gut mucosal injury, which then promotes the movement of bacteria (Deitch and Berg, 1987). Poor nutrition has also been shown to alter the composition and amount of the intestinal flora. It has been suggested that malnutrition or lack of intestinal chyme may promote intestinal overgrowth and potentiate bacterial translocation. In addition, malnutrition impairs the body's immune function and thus may alter the body's ability to defend itself against these organisms. Studies done in severely burned children and adults demonstrated that enteral protein intake is associated with reduced mortality and reduced evidence of the septic state (Alexander et al., 1980; Antonacci et al., 1984).

MAJOR FUNCTIONS OF THE GI TRACT

Anatomic structures of the GI tract will be discussed as they pertain to the three main functions of the gut: motility, digestion, and absorption. In order to accomplish these functions, the segments of the GI tract secrete fluids that are important for lubrication, digestion, and absorption. Secretions will be presented as they pertain to these functions.

Motility

The term motility denotes the timely movement of nutrients through the GI tract. Under normal circumstances, nutrients move through the GI tract at a rate that allows the digestive enzymes to break down nutrients and that allows absorption to occur. Increased motility can result in decreased time for

digestion and absorption of nutrients, which can be manifested in whole body changes as well as in GI symptoms such as diarrhea.

Mouth. Normally, food and fluid enter the GI tract through the mouth. Here food is mechanically broken down into smaller pieces in a process known as mastication. Muscle activity involved in mastication is controlled in part by the fifth cranial nerve, the trigeminal nerve. During this process, food is mixed with saliva, which facilitates its transit to the back of the throat and down the esophagus. In addition, saliva facilitates exposure of taste receptors located along the tongue to the chemical properties of food. Approximately 1 to 2 liters of saliva are secreted each day. Three pairs of salivary glands located within the oral cavity are responsible for saliva production.

Swallowing is a complex function that requires an intact nervous system. Once food has been voluntarily moved to the back of the throat, it stimulates afferent nerve endings that travel by way of the vagus, glossopharyngeal, and trigeminal nerves to the brainstem to initiate the swallowing response. Neural fibers from the brainstem (i.e., pons, medulla) travel in the trigeminal, hypoglossal, and vagus nerves to innervate muscles of the mouth and throat. During swallowing, the jaw shuts, and the soft palate is elevated. The nasopharynx and the oropharynx close to prevent oral contents from moving upward into the nose or downward into the respiratory tract. Because of this, breathing ceases during swallowing. As a result of a pressure difference between the mouth and the esophagus, the bolus moves into the esophagus. Patients with neurologic damage, often related to a cerebrovascular accident, and those who have had resection of the oral cavity related to malignancy commonly experience swallowing difficulties.

Esophagus. The esophagus is a cylindrical tube that connects the mouth to the stomach (Fig. 43–6). It lies behind the trachea within the chest cavity and terminates at the level of the diaphragm. The upper third of the esophagus is striated muscle similar to skeletal muscle. The middle third is a transition area composed of a mixture of smooth and striated muscle. The lower third is similar to the remainder of the GI tract—that is, it has two layers of smooth muscle, the inner layer being circular and the next layer longitudinal.

There is no anatomic sphincter separating the distal end of the esophagus from the stomach. However, there is an area of high pressure called the lower esophageal sphincter (LES). This high-pressure zone is responsible for preventing the gastric contents from entering the esophagus. Without this physiologic sphincter, the risk of acidic gastric contents moving into the esophagus (regurgitation) when an individual is in a supine position is much greater. A number of clinical conditions can decrease the competency of the LES. Examples include pathologic

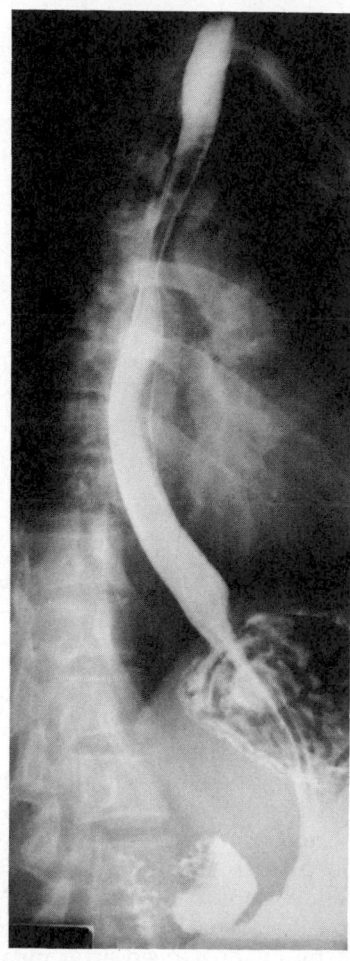

FIGURE 43–6. X-ray film of the entire barium-filled esophagus, showing the course of this organ through the mediastinum from hypopharynx to stomach. Note the three indentations produced by the aorta, left main stem bronchus, and left atrium.

states such as a hiatal hernia; pregnancy, with a concomitant elevation in serum progesterone level, which is thought to decrease LES pressure; and cigarette smoking, which reduces LES pressure. In addition, dietary substances can also influence LES pressure. The presence of protein in the stomach elevates the closing pressure; fat diminishes the closing pressure.

Movement of a food bolus from the mouth down the esophagus is promoted by a pressure gradient. In addition, contraction of the esophageal wall (peristalsis) behind the bolus promotes movement. When an individual swallows, the LES relaxes, allowing the bolus to enter the stomach. In the clinical condition known as achalasia the lower esophagus fails to relax or a spasm of the muscle prevents passage of the bolus into the stomach. Due to distention of the lower portion of the esophagus by the bolus, this condition is frequently painful. Patients often describe a sensation of pain that radiates down both arms. In patients with achalasia, symptoms frequently occur after eating.

Stomach. Anatomically, the stomach is divided into three parts—the fundus, body, and antrum. The distal portion of the antrum is known as the pylorus. The pylorus is a thick band of muscle that separates the stomach from the upper small intestine and thus acts like a physiologic sphincter. The stomach, like the lower esophagus, has longitudinal and circular muscle layers as well as two nerve layers. When food or liquids are ingested, the stomach acts like a reservoir that empties food into the small intestine at the optimum rate for digestion and absorption. This rate is normally dependent upon the characteristics of the diet. That is, foods that have a high osmolarity, such as "rich" foods with a high fat content, tend to empty more slowly than calorically less dense foods. In addition, the volume of liquid or food consumed can also modulate the rate of gastric emptying.

Motility of the stomach serves two purposes: (1) to promote movement of chyme (food mixed with GI secretions) through the pylorus, and (2) to mix and grind food, allowing exposure of food to gastric secretions. Stomach motor activity is controlled in part by extrinsic neural fibers and hormones as well as by intrinsic nerve fibers that respond to distention of the stomach wall. Vagotomy delays the rate at which the stomach empties solids and increases the rate at which liquids leave the stomach. The delayed emptying of solids is attributable to a decrease in antral peristalsis. In addition, the rate of gastric emptying is influenced by chyme characteristics such as fat content, acidity, and osmolarity. The caloric concentration, or nutrient density, of a solution is believed to play a major role in gastric emptying. When the calorie count of a fluid rises, the rate of gastric emptying declines (Murray, 1987). Temporal differences in gastric emptying rates have also been reported (Goo et al., 1987). Particularly for solid meals, more rapid emptying occurs with the morning meal rather than the evening one. Figure 43–7 summarizes other common factors influencing gastric emptying.

With the ingestion of a meal or liquid, the fundus and body of the stomach relax. This inhibition of stomach tone was termed "receptive relaxation" by Cannon and Lieb (1911). This response, which is initiated by swallowing, can be abolished by vagotomy and thus is mediated by extrinsic nerve fibers.

Vomiting. Vomiting is the forceful expulsion of gastric or intestinal contents up through the esophagus and out of the mouth. Frequently, vomiting is preceded by a variety of physiologic changes including increased salivation, sweating, tachycardia, retching, bradycardia, tachypnea, and nausea. The act of vomiting is a complex physiologic function that involves coordination of the GI organs and respiratory system. During vomiting there is relaxation of the upper stomach and esophagus and increased pressure in the duodenum due to contraction of the abdominal wall against these relaxed organs. This promotes the movement of chyme out of the small intestine and into the stomach. Contractile activity of the antrum then facilitates movement of chyme to the upper stomach and into the esophagus.

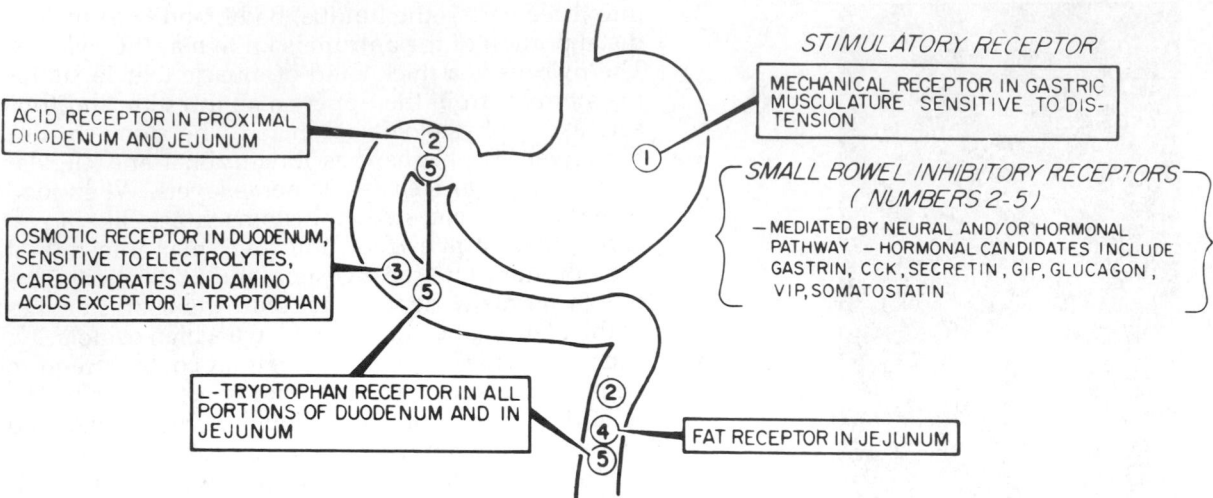

FIGURE 43–7. Physiology of gastric emptying. Various factors that influence gastric emptying are depicted. Location of mechanical and osmotic receptor (*1* and *3*) as determined by human studies. Other receptors localized by studies in dogs. *Abbreviations:* CCK, cholecystokinin; GIP, gastric inhibitory polypeptide; VIP, vasoactive intestinal polypeptide. (Reprinted with permission from Physiology and pathophysiology of gastric emptying in humans, by H. Minami and R. McCallum. GASTROENTEROLOGY, 86 (6), p. 1594. Copyright 1984 by the American Gastroenterological Association.)

During vomiting respiration ceases, and the chyme moves past the pharyngoesophageal sphincter and out of the mouth.

The mechanics of vomiting are controlled by an area in the brainstem frequently referred to as the vomiting or emetic center (Fig. 43–8). Electrical stimulation of this area in animals results in projectile vomiting without retching. This center receives input from its blood supply and from a variety of peripheral organs. Chemicals carried in the blood can activate the chemoreceptor trigger zone of the vomiting center, as can afferent fibers that are activated by noxious stimuli such as severe pain or injury to abdominal structures such as the kidney or bladder. Increases in intracranial pressure or stimulation of the vestibular system can also activate the vomiting center. Vomiting can also be induced psychogenically by the thought of unpleasant or noxious experiences. Conditions associated with nausea or vomiting, or both, in critically ill patients and potential adverse outcomes are shown in Table 43–4.

Drug therapy for the management of nausea and vomiting acts either peripherally to reduce peripheral input or centrally to decrease afferent nerve impulses in brain pathways. Peripherally acting drugs include topical anesthetics and antacids. Centrally acting antiemetics include antihistamines, phenothiazines, and anticholinergics. Drugs such as metoclopramide (Reglan) have a central effect on the chemoreceptor trigger zone and also increase gastric motility, which may decrease gastric distention and thus afferent stimulation.

Small Intestine. Most digestion and absorption activities occur in the small intestine (i.e., duodenum, jejunum, ileum). Motility of the small intestine is classified as either peristaltic (moving in one direc-

tion) or segmental (moving back and forth within an area). The primary purpose of segmentation is to promote the mixing of chyme with digestive enzymes and to allow greater exposure of chyme to the mucosa for digestion and absorption. However, such movement can also propel chyme in a caudal direction. Normal passage of chyme takes 3 to 5 hours from the pylorus to the ileocecal valve. Such movement in the small intestine is enhanced after meals.

Small intestinal motility is controlled by neural and hormonal inputs. Pathologic conditions, such as electrolyte imbalance (particularly hypokalemia) and pharmacologic agents can also influence small intestinal motility. A common condition associated with

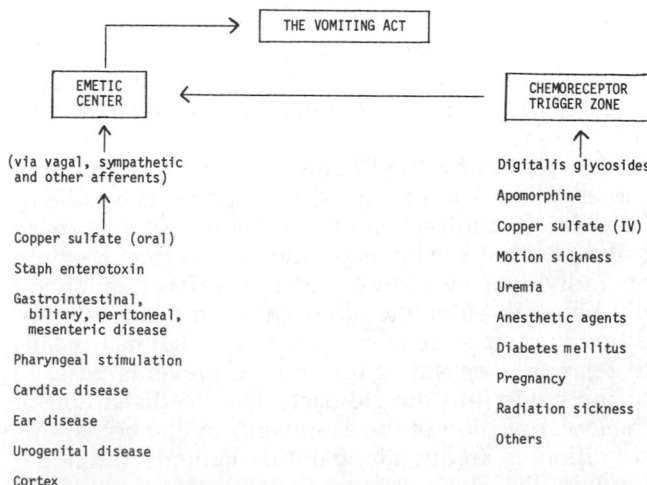

FIGURE 43–8. Diagram of proposed pathways in the act of vomiting. (From Greenberger, N. (1981). *Gastrointestinal disorders: A pathophysiologic approach* (2nd ed., p. 113). Chicago: Year Book Medical Publishers.)

TABLE 43–4. Selected Clinical Conditions Leading to and Adverse Consequences of Nausea and Vomiting

Common Conditions in Critically Ill Patients Associated with Nausea and Vomiting
Cholecystitis
Drug toxicity
Gastrointestinal obstruction
Hepatitis
Infection, including sepsis
Intracranial lesion
Increased intracranial pressure
Myocardial infarction, acute
Pancreatitis
Peritonitis

Selected Adverse Consequences
Acid-base imbalances
Aspiration pneumonia
Electrolyte imbalances
Esophageal rupture
Fluid depletion
Mallory-Weiss syndrome (nonperforating gastric mucosal tear at or near gastroesophageal junction)

altered small intestinal motility is paralytic ileus, which is often associated with abdominal surgery. In this condition manipulation of the intestinal tissue results in release of neurochemicals, which are thought to inhibit contraction of the intestine temporarily. This condition is most persistent in the left colon and is generally self-limiting (lasting until the third to fourth postoperative day); its resolution is evident by the presence of bowel sounds upon auscultation.

The distal portion of the small intestine is separated from the large intestine by the ileocecal junction. This is an important anatomic sphincter, which can control the rate of movement from the small intestine to the large intestine and prevents movement of colonic contents back into the small intestine. Flora of the colon contain bacteria, which, if allowed to move into the small intestine, can produce malabsorption and diarrhea. At the junction of the ileum and cecum there is a blind tube approximately the size of a little finger known as the vermiform appendix. This structure has no known purpose in humans; however, problems encountered with this structure include inflammation (appendicitis) and rupture.

Large Intestine. The colon is similar to the small intestine in regard to motor activity. Segmentation in an adult colon is called haustral formation. Haustral formation allows greater exposure of the colonic mucosa to the luminal contents. Multihaustral formation can propel the contents through the colon.

Expulsion of feces out of the rectal colon is under voluntary control. In the rectum there is an internal and an external sphincter. Under normal conditions the internal sphincter, which is not voluntarily controlled, is contracted. The external sphincter is composed of striated muscle and is under voluntary control. Distention of the rectum results in an urge

to defecate. As the pressure in the rectum increases, the internal and external sphincters relax, allowing the fecal material to pass. Delays in colonic transit can result in constipation, whereas excessively rapid transit can produce diarrhea.

Constipation. Constipation refers to delayed expulsion of the fecal contents. Because there is wide variation in what constitutes normal bowel function, constipation is generally denoted as a decrease in the individual's usual number of bowel movements or the passage of hard, dry stool or pellets. Constipation, which frequently is accompanied by abdominal discomfort and distention, is common in hospital patients, who experience marked changes in dietary and fluid intake and activity level.

Diarrhea. Diarrhea refers to the passage of frequent liquid or semiliquid stools. Diarrhea is the result of increased fluid secretion or decreased fluid absorption in the small intestine or colon. Secretagogues such as bacterial endotoxins (e.g., cholera enterotoxin) stimulate colonic fluid and electrolyte secretion through cyclic AMP activation. The ingestion of lactose by lactase-deficient individuals results in an increase in fecal water loss due to increased secretion of fluid in the small intestine and decreased net absorption in the colon.

Diarrhea as a symptom accompanies a number of pathophysiologic conditions. In immunocompromised patients, whose immune systems are impaired as a result of exogenous immunosuppressive therapy or acquired immune deficiency disease, diarrhea may result from the presence of viruses such as cytomegalovirus. This virus is a herpes virus, which is widely observed in people across all age ranges from newborns to adults. In healthy individuals its presence does not create problems. Like other herpes viruses, it is a lifelong infection that is usually latent (Dieterich, 1987). However, when T-cell–mediated immunity decreases, as in the immunosuppressed patient, this virus is activated. Such a virus creates lesions related to acute and chronic inflammation throughout the length of the GI tract and liver, and the patient may experience symptoms of abdominal pain, diarrhea, hematemesis, distention, and even perforation.

Digestion

As noted earlier, the bulk of digestion and absorption occurs in the small intestine. However, some minor digestive processes occur in the upper GI tract. In the mouth, amylase, which is secreted into salivary secretions, is the only digestive enzyme present. Amylase begins the breakdown of starch. The enzyme is inactivated by the acidity of the stomach and thus does not contribute substantially to carbohydrate digestion. No digestion or absorption occurs in the esophagus. Table 43–5 lists the volume, content, and major regulators of secretions throughout the GI system.

TABLE 43–5. Gastrointestinal Secretions

Site	Volume (day)	Content	Major Regulator
Oral cavity	1–2 liters	Mucus Water Electrolytes and amylase Immunoglobulins	Neural
Esophagus	300–800 mL	Mucus	Neural
Stomach	2 liters	Mucus Hydrochloric acid Water, electrolytes Intrinsic factor Pepsinogen	Neural Hormonal
Liver (bile)	500 mL–1 liter	Bile salts Water, electrolytes Bilirubin	Hormonal
Pancreas	1200–1800 mL	Water Electrolytes Enzymes	Hormonal Neural
Small intestine	3–4 liters	Water Electrolytes Mucus Brush border enzymes	Neural
Large intestine	Variable	Mucus	Neural

Stomach. In the stomach there are several secretions that contribute to digestion. Hydrochloric (HCl) acid is secreted by the parietal (oxyntic) cells, which are located primarily in the stomach body and fundus (Fig. 43–9). Under basal conditions, the intragastric pH is acidic (pH 2 to 4), and the rate of HCl acid secretion is approximately 2 to 3 mEq/hr. Stimulation of HCl acid secretion by a number of known stimulants can increase this rate 10-fold. Those factors known to stimulate HCl acid secretion include vagal stimulation, hormonal stimulation (e.g., gastrin), and chemical properties of the chyme. The antral hormone gastrin and the cholinergic neurotransmitter acetylcholine both directly stimulate the release of HCl acid by parietal cells. Diagnostic tests used to determine the ability of the stomach to secrete acid under "stimulated" conditions utilize pentagastrin, a synthetic form of the hormone gastrin. Because acetylcholine also stimulates release of gastrin, acetylcholine both directly and indirectly stimulates HCl acid secretion. Histamine, which is present throughout the GI tract, is also a stimulant of HCl acid secretion. Current drug therapies for peptic ulcer disease utilize histamine (H_2) receptor blockers (e.g., cimetidine, ranitidine) to decrease acid secretion. There appears to be some age-related decrease in gastric acid secretion; however, this decrease is much greater in patients with chronic atrophic gastritis.

The acid environment of the stomach promotes the conversion of pepsinogen, a proteolytic enzyme secreted by gastric chief cells, to pepsin. Pepsin begins the initial breakdown of proteins; however, it does not appear to be essential for normal protein breakdown and absorption.

A necessary protein secreted only by the stomach's parietal cells is intrinsic factor. Intrinsic factor binds to vitamin B_{12} and is essential for transport and absorption of this vitamin in the terminal ileum. Vitamin B_{12} is critical for formation of red blood cells; thus, surgical removal or atrophy of cells that secrete intrinsic factor can result in anemia. Similarly, resection of the terminal ileum, where absorption occurs, can also result in anemia.

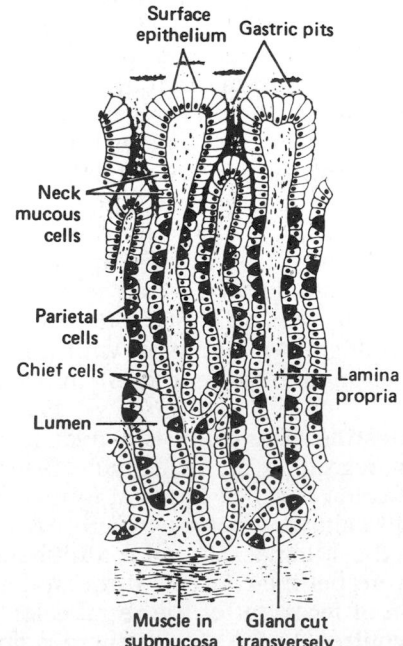

FIGURE 43–9. Diagram of glands in the mucosa of the body of the human stomach. (From Ganong, W. (1987). *Review of medical physiology* (13th ed., p. 409). Norwalk, CT: Appleton and Lange; adapted from Bell, G. H., Davidson, N. and Scarborough, G. (1965). *Textbook of physiology and biochemistry* (6th ed.). Edinburgh: Churchill Livingstone.)

In addition to HCl acid and pepsinogen, the stomach secretes fluid that is rich in electrolytes including sodium and potassium. Loss of these fluids through vomiting or gastric suction places the individual at risk for fluid and electrolyte imbalances as well as acid-base disturbances.

Though not actively contributing to digestion, mucus is secreted by the surface cells located in the body and fundus of the stomach. This mucus coats the organ mucosa and is believed to contribute to the gastric mucosal barrier. This barrier protects the gastric mucosa from autodigestion by gastric secretions, HCl acid, and pepsin.

In addition to the parietal, chief, and neck mucous cells, endocrine cells are interspersed among the gastric epithelial cells. The most abundant of these are the gastrin-producing cells in the gastric antrum.

Gastrin, a peptide hormone, is produced by specialized cells in the gastric and duodenal mucosa and is released by neural stimulation as well as by chemical properties of the diet and distention of the stomach wall. Tumors in patients with Zollinger-Ellison syndrome contain and release gastrin and thus are designated gastrinomas. The stomach also contains enterochromaffin cells, which release serotonin.

Small Intestine. Digestion of foodstuffs occurs primarily in the small intestine. The anatomic arrangement of the small intestine facilitates the digestive and absorptive processes that occur there. The small intestine is lined with villi and microvilli, which greatly increase the surface area (Fig. 43–10).

The functional unit of the small intestinal mucosal layer is the villus. Villi are composed of an inner core

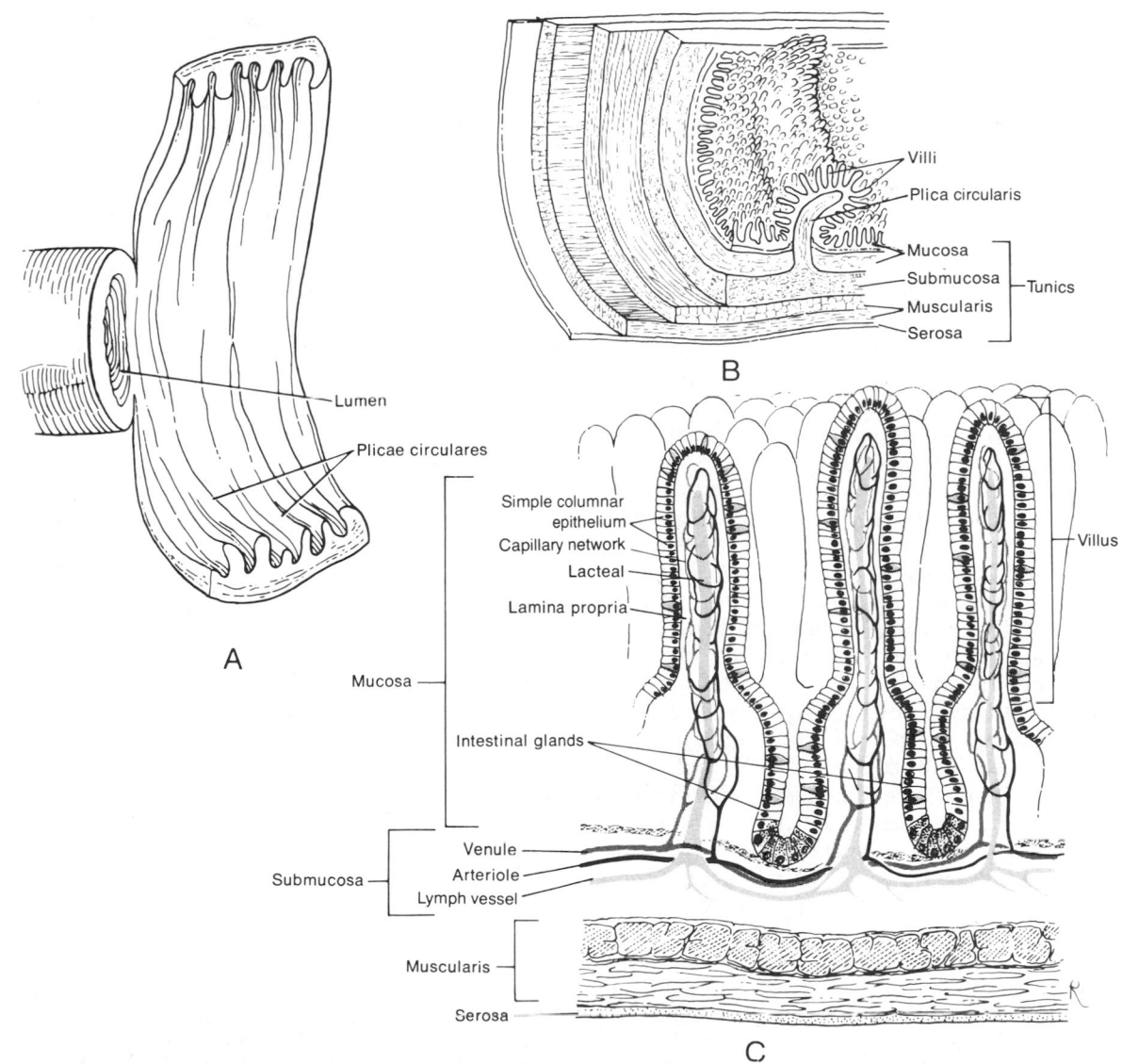

FIGURE 43–10. Small intestine. *A.* Section of small intestine cut open to expose plicae circulation. *B.* Villa in relation to the tunics of the small intestine. *C.* Enlarged aspect of several villa of the small intestine. (Figure from PRINCIPLES OF ANATOMY AND PHYSIOLOGY by G.J. Tortora and N.P. Anagnostokos. Copyright © 1981 by G.J. Tortora and N.P. Anagnostokos. Reprinted by permission of Harper & Row, Publishers, Inc.)

of lymph and capillary vessels surrounded by epithelial cells (i.e., enterocytes) and goblet cells. On each of the epithelial cells there are tiny projections known as microvilli. These tiny projections are referred to as the brush border and contain enzymes that are responsible for final breakdown of disaccharides and peptides. One characteristic of these epithelial cells is their relatively fast turnover rate. Cells migrate up from the crypts during a period of 5 to 7 days to replace cells that are sloughed off during the normal turnover process. This rapid turnover of epithelial cells makes intestinal epithelial cells particularly sensitive to regional radiation or systemic chemotherapy, which interrupts cell division. This feature allows rapid repair of the mucosa following injury.

The mucosa also contains goblet cells, which secrete mucus. The function of this mucus is not precisely known. However, it may play a protective role.

In the small intestine, digestion of proteins, fats, and carbohydrates begins with degradation of these food elements by pancreatic enzymes that are secreted into the duodenum. Additional enzymes located along the mucosal brush border complete the digestive processing of proteins and carbohydrates.

Protein. As stated earlier, protein digestion to a very limited extent begins in the stomach with pepsin. However, most protein digestion occurs after chyme has entered the small intestine. Proteolytic enzymes are synthesized in the pancreas and are secreted in an inactive form into the duodenum through the pancreatic duct. This duct often joins with the common bile duct to empty through the greater duodenal papilla. Once in the small intestine, enterokinase, an enzyme secreted into the small intestinal lumen, cleaves these enzymes to their active forms. This is a protective process that prevents proteolytic and lipolytic enzymes from destroying or autodigesting pancreatic or surrounding tissues outside the GI tract. Acute pancreatitis or inflammation of the pancreas results from premature activation of these enzymes within the pancreas.

Within the small intestinal lumen, pancreatic proteolytic enzymes break down proteins to peptides. Final digestion of peptide fragments to their constituent amino acid components is accomplished by proteolytic enzymes (i.e., peptidases) located on the microvilli brush border.

Carbohydrate. Digestion of carbohydrates is minimally influenced by salivary amylase. Stomach HCl acid causes some hydrolysis of starches and simple sugars. In the small intestine, carbohydrates are exposed to pancreatic amylase, which breaks down starches to their constituent disaccharides. There is also an enteric amylase. However, this amylase does not contribute significantly to the breakdown of starches. Because carbohydrates are absorbed in the form of monosaccharides, further digestion is required. Along the brush border of the intestinal mucosa there are disaccharidases, which cleave di-

saccharides to their constituent monosaccharide forms. Problems with carbohydrate maldigestion can result in abdominal discomfort, diarrhea, and possible malabsorption when the disaccharide is ingested. Such problems generally are secondary to lack of or insufficient brush border disaccharidase. A common example of this problem is lactase deficiency. Lactase is the enzyme that catabolizes the disaccharide lactose to glucose and galactose. Without this enzyme, undigested lactose remains in the lumen and enters the colon, where fermentation by intestinal bacteria occurs. This results in carbon dioxide production with subsequent distention and abdominal discomfort. Undigested lactose can also act as an osmotic agent, leading to decreased fluid absorption and increased fluid loss in the feces. Normally, in adults approximately 7 to 8 liters of water are absorbed by the small intestine each day.

Fat. Compared with proteins and carbohydrates, digestion of fats is somewhat more complicated (Fig. 43–11). The most common fats in the diet are neutral fats called triglycerides. Triglycerides are composed of glycerol and fatty acids. In the small intestine dietary fats are emulsified by bile salts. Bile salts are synthesized in the liver, stored in the gallbladder, and secreted into the small intestine as the gallbladder contracts. The bile salts emulsify fat, allowing pancreatic lipase to further break down the fat molecules into monoglycerides and fatty acids. These breakdown products are surrounded by a water-soluble barrier (i.e., micelle) and transported to the absorptive surface. After fat products enter the epi-

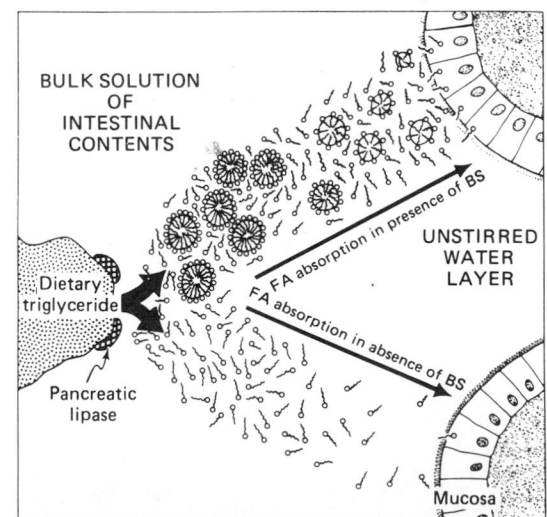

FIGURE 43–11. Lipid digestion and passage to intestinal mucosa. Fatty acids *(FA)* are liberated by the action of pancreatic lipase on dietary triglycerides and, in the presences of bile salts *(BS)*, form micelles (the circular structures), which diffuse through the unstirred water layer to the mucosal surface. (From Ganong, W. (1987). *Review of medical physiology* (13th ed., p. 396). Norwalk, CT: Appleton and Lange; Thomson, A.B.R. (1978). Intestinal absorption of lipids. Influence of the unstirred water layer and bile acid micelle. In J.M. Dietschy, A.M. Gotto, Jr., and J.A. Ontko (Eds.), Disturbances in lipid and lipoprotein metabolism. American Physiological Society.)

thelial cells, bile salts diffuse back into the lumen and either are reused for micelle formation or are reabsorbed in the ileum and returned to the liver.

The processes of digestion are completed within the small intestine. No digestion occurs in the colon.

Absorption

Absorption of dietary constituents occurs primarily in the small intestine. However, absorption of some substances such as ethanol and aspirin can occur in the stomach as well as in the small intestine.

As stated earlier, carbohydrates are absorbed in the form of monosaccharides, and proteins are absorbed in the form of amino acids. Multiple mechanisms including active and passive transport and facilitated diffusion contribute to absorption of nutrients. These substances then move into the blood supply. On the other hand, fats that are absorbed in the form of fatty acids and glycerol are reconstituted into triglycerides, cholesterol, and phospholipids to form what are known as chylomicrons. These chylomicrons are absorbed into the lymphatic system, and from there they enter the venous system. Figure 43–12 illustrates the expected absorptive locations for digested nutrients. In addition to nutrients, the small intestine also absorbs fluid and electrolytes arising from the diet or from gastric and intestinal secretions. Refer to Table 43–5 for expected adult daily fluid volumes secreted throughout the GI system.

No dietary absorption occurs in the colon. However, the colon is capable of absorbing certain drugs, as evidenced by the use of rectal suppositories. In addition, the large intestine is involved in the absorption of fluid and electrolytes. Of the 1500 mL of fluid delivered to the large intestine each day, only 100 to 200 mL is excreted in the feces. However, this fluid and electrolyte absorptive function is not vital to life. Nonetheless, for individuals who have had part or all of the large bowel removed, fluid and electrolyte imbalances are a major concern, particularly during the initial period following surgery and during times of illness when there is reduced intake or increased output of fluids.

PHYSIOLOGIC ADAPTATION TO PATHOLOGY

The body is resourceful in adjusting to changes. Surgical resection of parts of the GI tract can result in a number of problems including diarrhea and malabsorption, leading to the ultimate outcome of malnutrition. The severity and duration of these problems are related to both the location of the tissue removed and the amount of tissue resected. An example of the former is surgical removal of the terminal ileum for a disease such as Crohn's disease (inflammatory bowel disease). Because of tissue loss in this area, which is necessary for bile salt and vitamin B_{12} absorption, the patient may have problems related to fat malabsorption and anemia. Resection or loss of large sections of the intestine decreases the amount of absorptive surface area available for nutrient absorption. However, following resection the tissue remaining generally adapts to compensate for this loss of tissue. Therefore, symptoms of malabsorption are likely to decrease with time as adaptive changes occur in the remaining tissue.

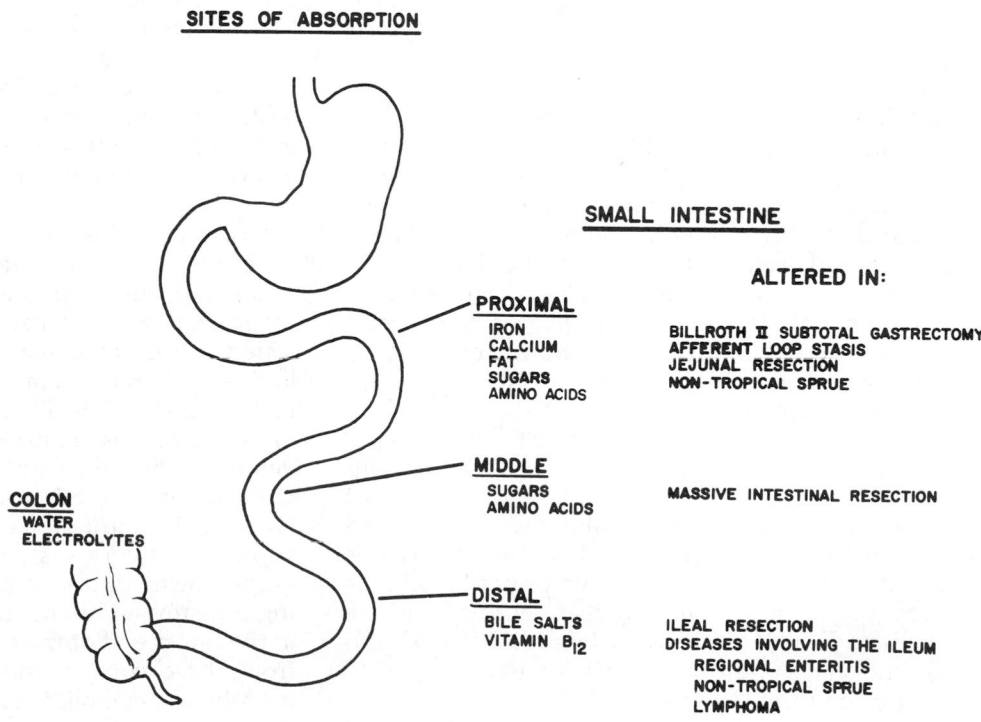

FIGURE 43–12. Sites of absorption of major nutrients across the small intestinal and colonic mucosa. (From Greenberger, N. (1981). *Gastrointestinal disorders: A pathophysiologic approach.* (2nd ed., p. 128). Chicago: Year Book Medical Publishers.)

SITES OF ABSORPTION

SMALL INTESTINE

ALTERED IN:

PROXIMAL
IRON
CALCIUM
FAT
SUGARS
AMINO ACIDS

BILLROTH II SUBTOTAL GASTRECTOMY
AFFERENT LOOP STASIS
JEJUNAL RESECTION
NON-TROPICAL SPRUE

MIDDLE
SUGARS
AMINO ACIDS

MASSIVE INTESTINAL RESECTION

DISTAL
BILE SALTS
VITAMIN B_{12}

ILEAL RESECTION
DISEASES INVOLVING THE ILEUM
REGIONAL ENTERITIS
NON-TROPICAL SPRUE
LYMPHOMA

COLON
WATER
ELECTROLYTES

Nutritional therapies such as total parenteral nutrition and tube feedings have also been associated with structural changes in the gut. Animal studies have demonstrated that colon length is reduced in response to parenteral feeding. Mucosal atrophy has been associated with both prolonged use of liquid diets and total parenteral nutrition. The impact of these structural changes on segmental function such as motility, digestion, and absorption is not known, however.

ACCESSORY GI ORGANS

Liver

The liver is an important and essential organ that performs multiple and complex functions. In an adult the liver weighs approximately 1500 g, making it the largest organ in the body. It is located primarily in the upper right quadrant of the abdomen and is divided into four lobes. These lobes are further subdivided into lobules. The liver has a rich blood supply that receives blood from both the hepatic artery and the portal vein, which drains the structures of the GI tract. Oxygen saturation of blood from the portal vein approaches 85%. This amount of oxygen is enough to meet about 30% to 35% of the oxygen requirements of the liver. Capillaries surrounding the hepatocytes are known as sinusoids. The sinusoids are lined with phagocytic cells known as Kupffer cells. In addition, the liver contains bile ducts called canaliculi that secret bile salts produced by the hepatocytes.

Multiple functions of the liver include (1) bile formation, (2) drug and hormone metabolism, (3) substrate metabolism, (4) protein synthesis including proteins important in blood coagulation, (5) detoxification of noxious substances, and (6) phagocytosis by means of the liver Kupffer cells.

Bile Formation. As noted in the earlier description of fat digestion and absorption, bile salts emulsify fats to allow their absorption along with fat-soluble vitamins. This action facilitates fat breakdown. Bile salts are then reabsorbed in the terminal portion of the ileum and transported back to the liver, where they can be reutilized. Bile fluid also contains electrolytes, phospholipids, and cholesterol. Bile travels to the gallbladder through the common hepatic duct, where it is stored and concentrated until needed for digestion. Approximately 500 to 1000 mL of bile is produced by the liver each day. Of this volume, approximately 96% to 97% is water, and the remainder comprises bile salts and bile pigments. The most common bile pigment is bilirubin, which is a red blood cell breakdown product. Because the liver is involved in the normal breakdown of red blood cells by way of the reticuloendothelial cells, bile is the mechanism for the excretion of bilirubin (Fig. 43–13). Under normal conditions, the liver handles 200 to 300 mg of bilirubin per day.

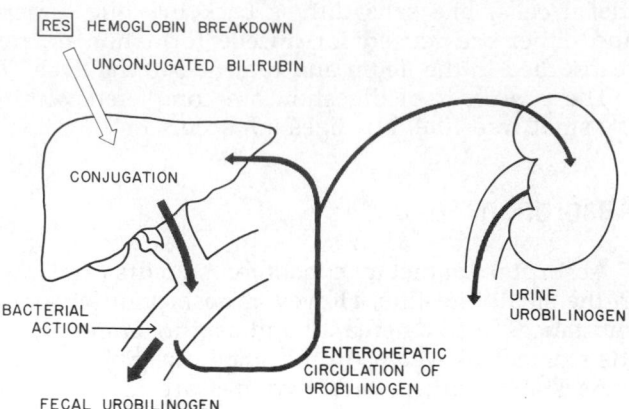

FIGURE 43–13. Schematic diagram illustrating the major steps in the normal metabolism of bilirubin. (From Greenberger, N. (1981). *Gastrointestinal disorders: A pathophysiologic approach* (2nd ed. p. 284). Chicago: Year Book Medical Publishers.)

Excess accumulation of bilirubin in the blood results in jaundice. There are several types of jaundice, including hemolytic (prehepatic). Hemolytic jaundice results from increased red blood cell destruction (e.g., sickle cell anemia, blood incompatibilities, and some lymphomas). In this situation, the ability of the liver to handle bilirubin is overwhelmed. This bilirubin is unconjugated and thus is lipid-soluble. Viral hepatitis is the most common cause of hepatocellular jaundice. Both cirrhosis and liver cancer can also decrease the liver's ability to excrete bilirubin. Due to hepatocellular failure, problems occur with bilirubin uptake, conjugation, or excretion. In this situation, serum levels of conjugated and perhaps unconjugated bilirubin increase. Because conjugated bilirubin is water-soluble, it can be excreted in the urine, and thus urine levels of bilirubin are elevated. Obstructive jaundice is generally due to gallbladder disease, such as that due to gallstones. Blockage of the common bile duct results in increased pressure within the bile ducts, resulting in movement of bile into tissues and blood. In this type of jaundice, blood levels of conjugated bilirubin increase.

Drug and Hormone Metabolism. Most medications and hormones such as testosterone, estrogen, and progesterone are metabolized at least in part by the liver. Enzymes located in hepatocytes are responsible for this catabolism. Morphine, an opioid alkaloid, is only one example of a commonly used drug metabolized in the liver and to a lesser extent, the intestinal mucosa (United States Pharmacopeial Convention, 1991). In therapeutic doses, morphine decreases both secretion and motility throughout the GI tract. In addition, it can precipitate contractions within the biliary system, including the sphincter of Oddi. These contractions may lead to spasm, increasing pressure within the biliary ducts, and constriction at the lower end of the common bile duct. Symptoms from these consequences may be sustained when morphine metabolism is prolonged. In patients with hepatic failure, the ability of the body to metabolize and excrete drugs as well as hormones is compromised. In addition, normal aging processes will result in decreased function of enzymes involved in drug metabolism, e.g., mixed function oxidases.

Substrate Metabolism. Because the liver is perfused by the portal vein, it is the first organ to be exposed to dietary substrates. As such, it plays an important role in the disposal of nutrients. In the liver monosaccharides are converted to glycogen (glycogenesis), which is the form in which a limited supply of unused glucose is stored. Because most cells of the body prefer glucose for energy, this glycogen can be broken down during periods of need. The liver can also convert amino acids and fats to glucose (gluconeogenesis).

Protein Synthesis. The liver is responsible for the synthesis of a variety of plasma proteins such as albumin, prothrombin, fibrinogen, and factors V, VII, VIII, and X. As part of the host response to injury or stress, the liver synthesizes acute phase proteins. These acute phase proteins include C-reactive protein, ceruloplasmin, heptoglobin, alpha-1 antitrypsin, alpha-1 acid glycoprotein, and fibrinogen. The synthesis of these proteins utilizes amino acids, which are obtained from catabolism of skeletal mus-

cle and mobilization of amino acids to the liver. As a result, liver synthesis of other proteins such as albumin and prealbumin probably decreases. The mediator of this acute phase response is interleukin-1, which is released from phagocytic cells, e.g., macrophages.

Gallbladder

The gallbladder is a saclike structure that lies beneath the right lobe of the liver (Fig. 43–14). The gallbladder holds approximately 30 mL of bile. Its primary function is to store and concentrate bile once it has been delivered from the liver. The gallbladder is connected to the duodenum via the common bile duct. Bile salts are delivered into the duodenum when nutrients are ingested. The flow of bile into the duodenum is controlled by contraction of the gallbladder and relaxation of the sphincter of Oddi, which is located at the junction of the common bile duct and the duodenum. The sphincter normally remains closed between meals and during fasting. Contraction of the gallbladder is mediated by hormonal and neural signals initiated by the presence of food.

The most common clinical problem associated with the gallbladder is cholecystitis (gallbladder inflam-

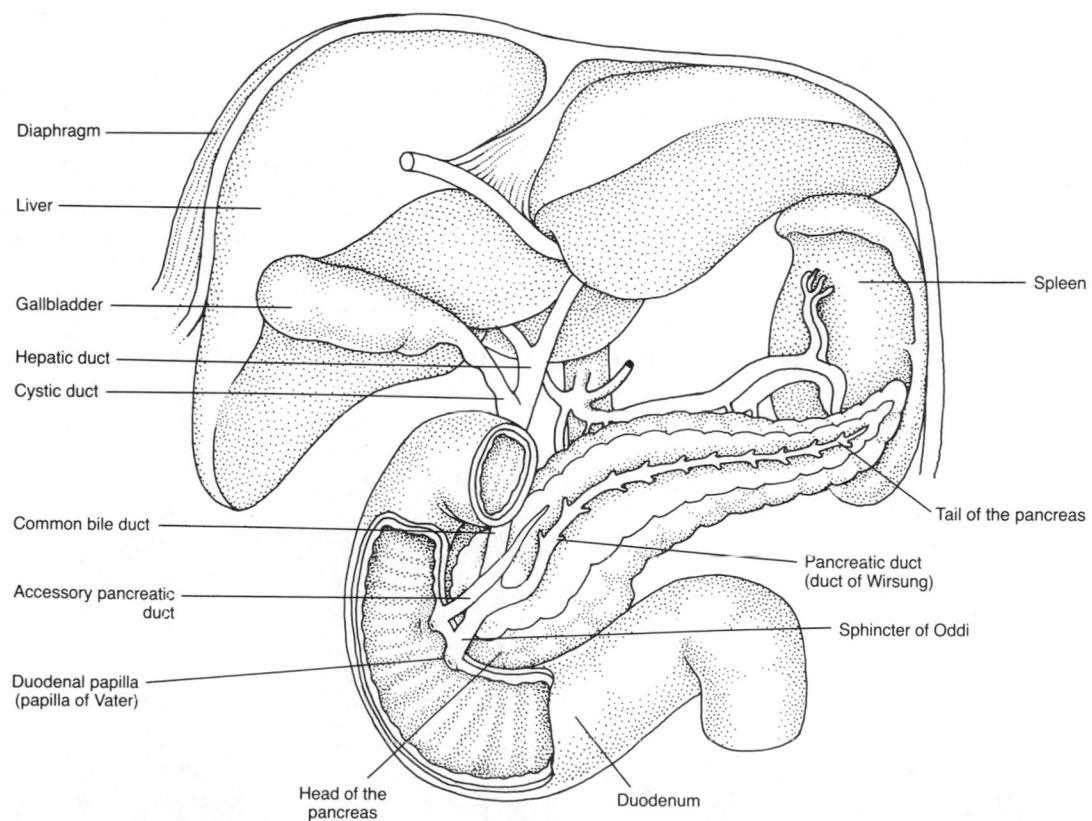

FIGURE 43–14. The gallbladder and its connections to the liver and intestine. (Adapted from Ignatavicius, D.D., and Bayne, M.V. (Eds.) (1991). *Medical-surgical nursing: A nursing process approach* (p. 1223). Philadelphia: W. B. Saunders.)

mation), which is frequently secondary to cholelithiasis (gallstones). Gallbladder stones are frequently composed of cholesterol and occur most commonly in middle-aged women. In addition to cholecystitis, gallstones can occlude the common bile duct and produce posthepatic jaundice or acute pancreatitis. In the patient with major trauma, surgery, or sepsis, cholecystitis can also occur, generally sometime after the initial injury. Although the etiology is unknown, it may be due to ischemia, bacterial invasion of the nonfunctioning gallbladder, or bile stasis.

Pancreas

The pancreas is a long slender organ located behind the spleen and duodenum. It is anatomically divided into head, body, and tail (see Fig. 43–14). The pancreas has both endocrine and exocrine (e.g., production of digestive enzymes) functions. Hormones are produced in specialized cells (e.g., alpha, beta, and delta cells) located in what is known as the islets of Langerhans. These specialized cells comprise only about 1% of the total pancreatic cells. The beta cells produce insulin, alpha cells glucagon, and delta cells somatostatin (Taborsky, 1989). The hormones are secreted into the rich organ blood supply and influence multiple tissues. Digestive enzymes produced by the clusters of exocrine cells known as acini are secreted into a central duct that runs the length of the pancreas. This duct then often connects to the common bile duct before it enters the duodenum.

The digestive enzymes are secreted in a small volume of fluid. Cells that line the ducts actively secrete bicarbonate into the duct lumen, producing a physiologically basic solution. This secretion of alkaline fluid into the intestine acts to buffer the acidic chyme entering the duodenum. The acinar cells are innervated by the vagus nerve, and thus their activity is also influenced by neural input.

In response to acute illness and hypotension, pancreatic ischemia can occur. This ischemia is thought to contribute to the release of cardiotoxic factors (e.g.,

myocardial depressant factor), which can lead to further complications of the critical illness. In addition, pancreatic ischemia can result in acute pancreatitis.

References

Alexander, J. W., MacMillan, B. G., Stinnet, J. D., et al. (1980). Beneficial effects of aggressive protein feeding in severely burned children. *Annals of Surgery, 192*, 505–517.

Antonacci, A., Cowles, S., and Reaves, L. (1984). The role of nutrition in immunologic function. *Infec. Surgery, 3*, 590–593.

Beisel, W. R. (1986). Sepsis and metabolism. In R. A. Little and K. N. Frayn (Eds.), *The scientific basis for the care of the critically ill*. London: Manchester University Press.

Buchan, A. (1989). Digestion and absorption. In H. Patton, A. Fuchs, B. Hille, et al. (Eds.), *Textbook of physiology* (21st ed., Vol. 2, pp. 1438–1460). Philadelphia: W. B. Saunders.

Cannon, W. B., and Lieb, C. W. (1911). The receptive relaxation of the stomach. *The American Journal of Physiology, 29* (2), 267–273.

Deitch, E. A., and Berg, R. D. (1987). Endotoxin but not malnutrition promotes bacterial translocation of the gut flora in burned mice. *Journal of Trauma, 27*, 161–166.

Dieterich, D. T. (1987). Cytomegalovirus: A new gastrointestinal pathogen in immunocompromised patients. *American Journal of Gastroenterology, 82*, 764–765.

Goo, R. H., Moore, J. G., Greenberg, E., et al. (1987). Circadian variation in gastric emptying of meals in humans. *Gastroenterology, 93*, 515–518.

Haglund, U. (1986). Gastro-intestinal, hepatic and renal complications of shock and trauma. In R. A. Little, and K. N. Frayn (Eds.), *The scientific basis for the care of the critically ill*. London: Manchester University Press.

Hinnat, K., Rotterdam, H. Z., Bell, E. T., et al. (1987). Cytomegalovirus infection of the alimentary tract: A clinicopathological correlation. *American Journal of Gastroenterology, 81*, 944–950.

Iwaski, T. (1987). Alimentary tract lesions in cytomegalovirus infection. *Acta Pathologica Japan, 37*, 549–565.

Murray, R. (1987). The effects of consuming carbohydrate-electrolyte beverages on gastric emptying and fluid absorption during and following exercise. *Sports Medicine, 4*, 322–351.

Taborsky, G. (1989). The endocrine pancreas: Control of secretions. In H. Patton, A. Fuchs, B. Hille, et al. (Eds.), *Textbook of Physiology* (1st ed. Vol. 2, pp. 1522–1543). Philadelphia: W. B. Saunders.

United States Pharmacopeial Convention (1991) USPDI: *Drug information for the health care professional* (Vol. IB 11th ed.). Rockville, MD: USP.

44

Patients with Gastrointestinal Bleeding

DeAnn M. Englert
Susan D. Ruppert

Throughout most of the gastrointestinal (GI) tract, the lumen of the gut is separated from the capillary blood supply only by a layer of epithelial cells. Any degree of injury to the epithelium may therefore cause bleeding. Blood loss can range in severity from chronic, intermittent, or nearly inconsequential bleeding to sudden massive hemorrhage that may be life-threatening or fatal.

Acute upper gastrointestinal bleeding is a common health problem that affects more than one-quarter of a million people annually in the United States (Elashoff and Grossman, 1980). Despite a number of recent advancements in diagnosis and treatment, the overall mortality rate associated with GI bleeding has remained 10% for the past 20 years (Kang and Piper, 1980). The majority of patients with moderate to severe upper GI bleeding, regardless of whether they are clinically stable at the time of initial presentation, are admitted to the critical care unit for observation, evaluation, and treatment. Many patients cease bleeding spontaneously. For those who do not, treatment is usually invasive and not always effective. Mortality is often disproportionately high in these individuals. Patients with esophageal varices and

peptic ulcer disease must be carefully monitored because they have a propensity for future hemorrhagic episodes. Fortunately, there is a lower mortality rate among patients with lower GI bleeding because of basic and improved diagnostic techniques such as guaiac testing, arteriography, and colonoscopy. In either event, the patient with acute GI hemorrhage represents an urgent and challenging opportunity for the critical care nurse.

PATHOPHYSIOLOGY

General

Because copious blood loss rarely occurs in the midjejunal or ileal segments of the bowel, GI bleeding is generally classified as either upper or lower in origin. Upper GI bleeding, defined as a loss of blood from the gastrointestinal system at a site above the ligament of Treitz at the duodenojejunal junction, accounts for 85% of all gastrointestinal bleeding episodes (Severance, 1986). Bleeding from a source below the ligament of Treitz is classified as lower GI bleeding.

The patient's presenting clinical signs may differentiate between an upper and a lower source of GI bleeding (Table 44–1). Upper GI bleeding is associated with hematemesis (vomiting of blood) or melena (passage of black tarry stools), or both, whereas lower GI bleeding results in hematochezia (passage of bright red blood from the rectum). If bleeding is rapid and massive from an upper GI source, both hematemesis and hematochezia will certainly occur. Concomitantly, patients with substantial blood loss

---

TABLE 44–1. Clinical Differentiation of Gastrointestinal Bleeding

Presenting sign	Upper GI Bleeding *Hematemesis or melena*	Lower GI Bleeding *Hematochezia*
Nasogastric aspirate	Positive for blood	Negative for blood
Bowel sounds	Hyperactive	Normal
Blood urea nitrogen	Elevated	Normal

will have clinical evidence of hypovolemic hemorrhagic shock.

Blood in the GI tract below the level of the duodenum rarely enters the stomach. Thus, the patient who is vomiting blood or coffee-ground material is usually bleeding from a site in the upper GI tract somewhere above the ligament of Treitz. The nature of the vomited blood can vary from bright red to coffee-ground color. Red blood, with or without clots, indicates a more recent or ongoing hemorrhage. Coffee-ground material may be present when blood that has accumulated in the stomach for a longer period of time is converted to acid hematin in the presence of gastric hydrochloric acid. Hematemesis may occur when as little as 100 mL of blood has been lost.

In passing through the gastrointestinal tract, blood becomes progressively darker and eventually black. The change in color depends upon the bleeding site, amount, rapidity of bleeding, and intestinal transit time. A transit time of 8 hours is typically required for melena to appear. The patient will describe the bowel movement as a "black" stool that is somewhat "sticky" with a characteristic foul odor. Melena is usually seen when there is prolonged bleeding from the upper gastrointestinal tract. As little as 50 to 100 mL of blood injected into the stomach can produce a melanotic stool. However, 400 to 500 mL is the usual amount necessary to produce melena consistently.

Following an acute episode of blood loss of 1 liter, melena will persist for 1 to 3 days. Although the patient's stools may then return to a normal color, occult blood may be guaiac positive for up to 12 days thereafter. Even when detected only by occult blood in the stool, gastrointestinal bleeding always represents a potentially serious symptom that must be investigated further.

Hemorrhagic Shock

Hemorrhagic or hypovolemic shock occurs when there is an acute loss of 15% to 20% of the circulatory blood volume (Porth, 1988). The clinical findings seen in patients with hypovolemic shock have been correlated with the magnitude of the volume deficit (Table 44–2).

There are four stages of hypovolemic shock as blood loss increases (Porth, 1988). Initially, the circulatory blood volume is decreased but not enough to cause serious effects. During the second phase, compensatory mechanisms work to maintain blood pressure and tissue perfusion at a level sufficient to prevent cell damage. Unfavorable clinical changes become evident during the third or progressive stage. The blood pressure begins to fall, blood flow to the heart and brain is impaired, capillary permeability is increased, fluid begins to leave the capillaries, blood flow becomes sluggish, and body cells and their enzyme systems are injured. The fourth and final

TABLE 44–2. Correlation of Clinical Findings and the Magnitude of Volume Deficit in Hemorrhagic Shock

Severity of Shock	Clinical Findings	Estimated Blood Loss (mL)
None	None	500*
Mild	Minimal tachycardia (<110 bpm) Slight decrease in BP Cool hands and feet	750–1250
Moderate	Tachycardia (100–120 bpm) Decrease in pulse pressure Systolic pressure (90–100 mm Hg) Restlessness Pallor Diaphoresis Oliguria	1250–1750
Severe	Tachycardia (≥120 bpm) Systolic pressure (<90 mm Hg) Mental stupor Extreme pallor Cold extremities Anuria	2500

*Based on blood volume of 7% in a 70-kg male of medium build.
Adapted from Weil, M., and Shubin, H. (1967). *Diagnosis and treatment of shock* (p. 118). Baltimore: Williams & Wilkins.

stage is irreversible. In this stage, death is imminent even though blood volume may have been temporarily restored and vital signs stabilized. Although the factors that determine recovery from severe shock have not been clearly identified, it appears that they may be related to blood flow at the level of the microcirculation. A summary of compensatory mechanisms active in hypovolemic shock is shown in Figure 44–1.

Sudden loss of blood volume (hemorrhage) decreases venous return to the heart and thereby lowers cardiac output. Thirty to sixty seconds after bleeding begins, the arterial baroreceptors note the decrease in blood pressure and signal a sympathetic response (Ross and Covell, 1985). The compensatory changes in heart rate, cardiac contractility, and vascular tone that develop in shock are mediated through the sympathetic nervous system. During the early stages, vasoconstriction causes a reduction in the size of the vascular compartment and an increase in peripheral vascular resistance. As blood loss increases, release of epinephrine and norepinephrine causes the alpha receptors in the skin, liver, lungs, intestines, and kidneys to constrict and the beta receptors in the striated muscle, heart, and brain to dilate. This reaction, a vascular response to decreased cardiac output and decreased right atrial pressure, shunts blood toward the cerebral and cardiopulmonary system. As vasoconstriction becomes more intense, heart rate and cardiac contractility increase. Decreased blood flow to the kidneys can then result in medullary tube

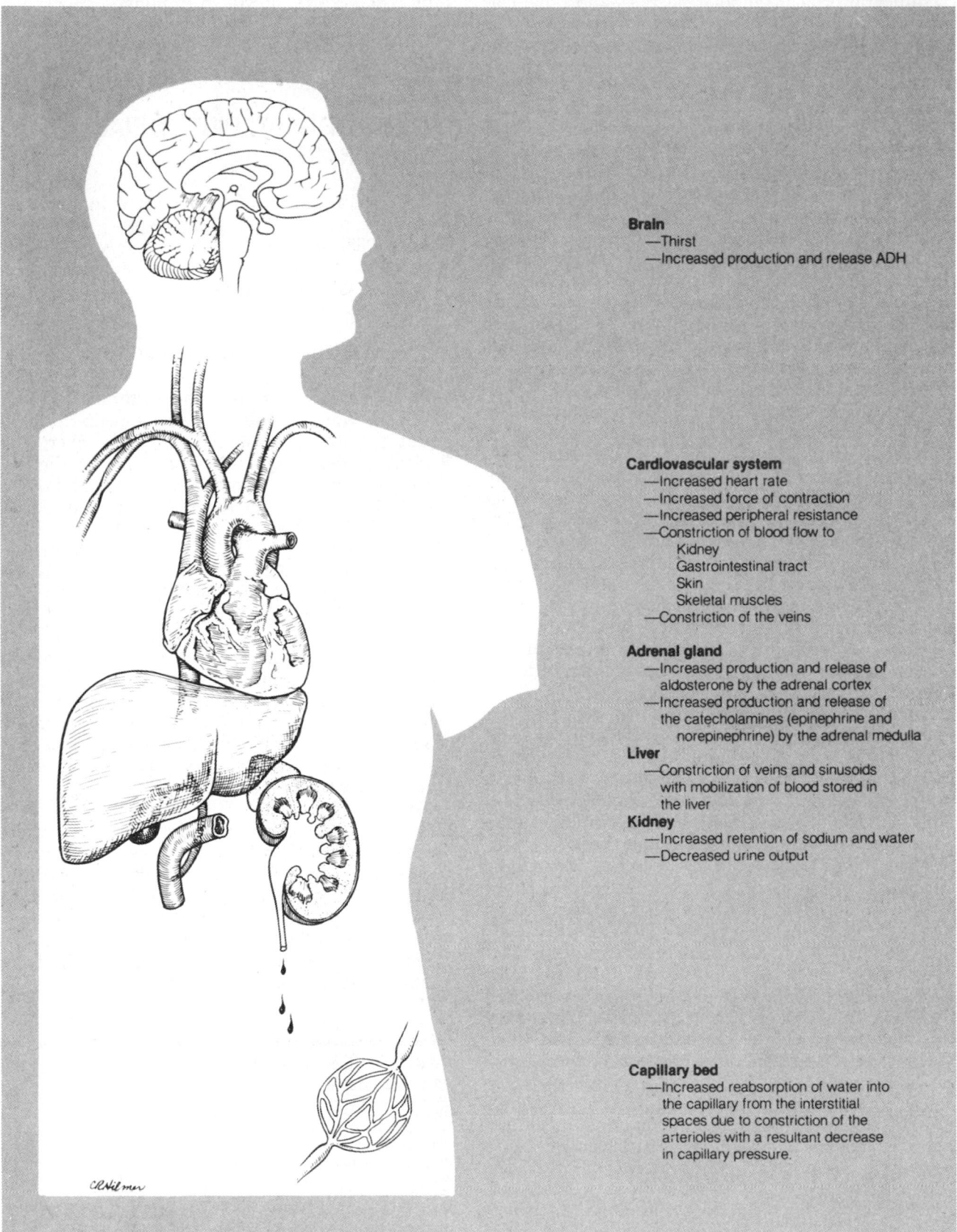

Brain
—Thirst
—Increased production and release ADH

Cardiovascular system
—Increased heart rate
—Increased force of contraction
—Increased peripheral resistance
—Constriction of blood flow to
    Kidney
    Gastrointestinal tract
    Skin
    Skeletal muscles
—Constriction of the veins

Adrenal gland
—Increased production and release of
    aldosterone by the adrenal cortex
—Increased production and release of
    the catecholamines (epinephrine and
        norepinephrine) by the adrenal medulla

Liver
—Constriction of veins and sinusoids
    with mobilization of blood stored in
    the liver

Kidney
—Increased retention of sodium and water
—Decreased urine output

Capillary bed
—Increased reabsorption of water into
    the capillary from the interstitial
    spaces due to constriction of the
    arterioles with a resultant decrease
    in capillary pressure.

FIGURE 44–1. Compensatory mechanisms in hypovolemic shock. (From Porth, C. (1990). *Pathophysiology: Concepts of altered health states* (3rd ed., p. 392). Philadelphia: J. B. Lippincott.)

dysfunction or acute tubular necrosis and renal failure. The organs of the GI tract can be equally affected, resulting in ischemia of the gut, liver, and pancreas.

Compensatory mechanisms to replace fluid lost from the vascular compartment also exist (Stephens, 1980). During shock, the decline in capillary pressure causes water to be drawn into the vascular compartment from the interstitial spaces. Maintenance of vascular volume is further enhanced by renal mechanisms that conserve fluid. As renal blood flow decreases during vasoconstriction, there is a decrease in the glomerular filtration rate and an increase in the reabsorption of sodium and water due to activation of the renin-angiotensin-aldosterone mechanism. The decrease in blood volume also stimulates the centers in the hypothalamus that regulate antidiuretic hormone release (ADH) and thirst.

The decreased tissue perfusion associated with vasoconstriction also causes cellular dysfunction. The body cells attempt to extract oxygen from the available blood until this mechanism is no longer adequate. As cellular hypoxia becomes manifest, metabolism of glucose changes from an aerobic to an anaerobic process (Robbins and Cotran, 1989). Energy production is decreased, and large quantities of lactic acid are produced. The depressed blood flow to the kidneys and liver impairs the ability of these systems to break down lactic acid or remove it from the bloodstream. The patient hyperventilates to exhale the waste products, but pulmonary circulation is also depressed. A profound metabolic acidosis develops as lactic acid accumulates.

During hypovolemic shock, the hematopoietic system produces an increase in white blood cells and platelets (Barsan and Baker, 1988). As the bone marrow is stimulated, red blood cell production and peripheral reticulocytosis result. Correction of abnormal hemoglobin can then occur naturally over a period of weeks following the hemorrhage.

When blood loss continues, cerebral blood flow becomes compromised. The patient may be confused at first, and these mental changes can progress to a loss of consciousness and brain damage. In patients with severe hypotension, there is decreased coronary perfusion while the shift of body fluids from the extravascular areas into the vascular space continues (Robbins and Cotran, 1989). Coronary blood flow insufficiency is detected by the presence of flattened T waves and ST-segment depression in the electrocardiogram.

Gastrointestinal hypoxia leads to decreased GI tract motility, venous congestion, edema, and small focal hemorrhages in the gut. Normal bacterial flora begin to release endotoxins in the absence of peristalsis. When circulation is decreased, normal colonic bacteria decompose and release ammonia. Metabolic wastes accumulate, and there is clumping and sludging of red blood cells in the microcirculation. This culminates in widespread microinfarctions, a condition known as disseminated intravascular coagulop-

athy (DIC) (Porth, 1988). In prolonged shock, when all of the patient's clotting factors have been expended, there is a strong tendency for the patient to bleed even more.

CAUSES OF GASTROINTESTINAL HEMORRHAGE

The major causes of GI bleeding in the United States are summarized in Table 44–3 (Barsan and Baker, 1988; Bitterman, 1988). These various pathophysiologic conditions can be divided into upper GI and lower GI disturbances.

Upper Gastrointestinal Bleeding

Duodenal ulcers are responsible for 25% to 40% of all GI bleeding episodes, whereas gastric ulcers account for 10% to 15% (Barsan and Baker, 1988). Therefore, peptic ulcer disease is by far the major cause of upper GI hemorrhage (Silverstein et al., 1981). Duodenitis has been the cause of bleeding in 5% to 10% of patients, and the incidence of hemorrhage from esophageal varices ranges from 6% to 18% (Barsan and Baker, 1988). Mallory-Weiss tears and esophagitis are seen in 1% to 10% of patients with upper GI bleeding (Barsan and Baker, 1988).

Peptic Ulcer Disease. An ulcer is defined as a loss of substance on a mucous surface causing a gradual disintegration and necrosis of the tissues extending below the musculous mucosae into the submucosa (Miller and Keane, 1987). Peptic ulcers can occur in any area of the gastrointestinal tract that is exposed to acid-pepsin secretions (Fig. 44–2).

At least one out of every 10 persons has or will develop peptic ulcer disease (Schiller, 1988). Men are affected three to four times as frequently as women. Duodenal ulcers are five to ten times more common than gastric ulcers. Duodenal ulcers occur at any age and are frequently seen in young adults, whereas gastric ulcers affect the older age group, peak incidence occurring in the sixth to seventh decades (Patras and Walsh, 1985). Interestingly, duodenal

TABLE 44–3. Major Causes of GI Hemorrhage in United States

Upper GI	Lower GI
Duodenal ulcer	Carcinoma of left colon
Erosive gastritis	Diverticular disease
Gastric ulcer	Inflammatory bowel disease
Esophageal varices	Polyps
Mallory-Weiss tears	Carcinoma of right colon
Esophagitis	Angiodysplasia of right colon
Duodenitis	

Adapted from Rosen, P. (1988). *Emergency medicine* (Vol. 2, pp. 1423, 1490). St. Louis: C. V. Mosby.

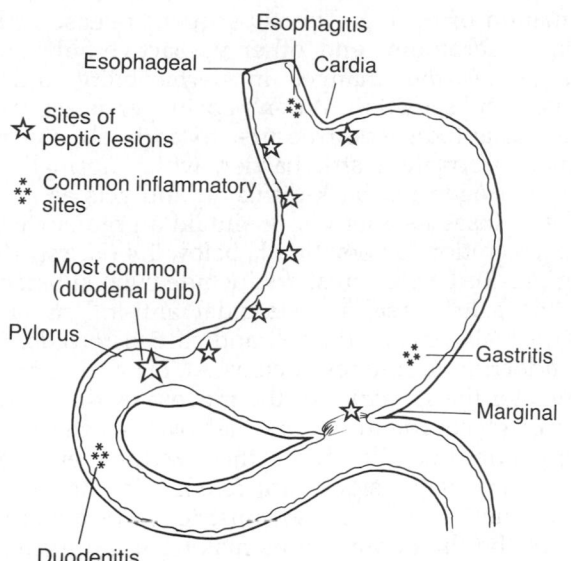

FIGURE 44–2. Upper gastrointestinal tract ulcer and inflammation sites.

ulcers seem to have a seasonal trend, with a higher incidence of recurrence in the spring and fall.

In general, it can be said that peptic ulcer formation reflects either an imbalance between acid and pepsin production or an inability of the affected mucosal layer to resist the destructive action of these digestive agents (Porth, 1988). Evidence suggests that hydrochloric acid may be the causative agent in duodenal ulcers, whereas decreased tissue resistance has a greater role in the genesis of gastric ulcers. Patients with gastric ulcers are known to have low hydrochloric acid secretion and a normal gastric emptying time. On the other hand, patients with duodenal ulcers have high gastric acid secretion, a low pH in the duodenum, and an abnormal gastric emptying time. Patients with duodenal ulcers may have an increased vagal drive or a greater mass of parietal cells than is normally present. More often than not, a number of factors contribute to the development of a peptic ulcer.

Hydrochloric acid is influenced by a number of factors, including neural and hormonal stimulation. The hormone gastrin, which is produced in the antrum of the stomach, is a potent stimulus for the production of hydrochloric acid. Increased levels of gastric acid have also been attributed to (1) increased acid or pepsin-producing cells in the stomach, (2) increased sensitivity of the parietal cells to food and other stimuli such as alcohol and caffeine, (3) excessive vagal stimulation, and (4) impaired inhibition of gastric secretions as food passes into the intestine. The intractable peptic ulcers associated with Zollinger-Ellison syndrome are caused by a gastrin-secreting tumor of the pancreas.

The defenses of the mucosal surface are dependent on an adequate blood flow and an intact mucosal barrier. Any disruption of the mucosal barrier there-

fore reduces these defenses and renders the mucosal surface more susceptible to injury.

It has been suggested that a basic abnormality in persons with gastric peptic ulcers is an increased permeability of the epithelial layer of the stomach to hydrogen ions. Bile is known to disrupt the mucosal barrier, and reflux of bile from the intestine into the stomach has been implicated in the pathogenesis of peptic ulcer disease.

The duodenum, acting as a passageway for digestive enzymes and acid-laden chyme, is a common site of peptic ulcers. Brunner's glands, which are located between the pylorus and the site where bile and pancreatic enzymes enter the duodenum, produce copious amounts of viscid mucus, which serve to protect this area. Because the activity of these glands is inhibited by sympathetic stimulation, this may explain why anxiety and stress contribute to the development of duodenal ulcers.

Certain drugs may contribute to the development of GI ulceration, but the exact mechanisms for this are not clearly understood. Table 44–4 identifies some of these offending pharmacologic agents and the proposed action of injury that can lead to GI bleeding. Anti-inflammatory agents such as indomethacin decrease mucosal resistance, are potentially ulcerogenic, and are contraindicated in patients with active or past ulcer disease. Reserpine and caffeine stimulate acid production (Robert and Kauffman, 1989). Phenylbutazone impairs epithelial cell metabolism and makes these cells more susceptible to injury. Antimetabolites and other chemotherapeutic agents damage the nuclei and cytoplasm of both normal and neoplastic cells, inhibiting mitosis and mucosal regeneration. Alcohol stimulates acid production and produces gastric mucosal hemorrhages.

Stress Ulcers. "Stress ulcer" is a nonspecific term that has been attached to a variety of gastric lesions and commonly refers to antral and duodenal ulcers. Changes in the mucosa can range from small petechial hemorrhages to deep ulceration with perfora-

TABLE 44–4. Pharmacologic Agents Associated with GI Bleeding

Possible Mechanism of Injury	Drugs
Acid stimulation	Reserpine, caffeine
Decreased mucosal blood flow	Vasopressors
Hydrogen back-diffusion	Aspirin, alcohol, bile salts, cinchopen, indomethacin, phenylbutazone, corticosteroids
Decreased mucus secretion	Corticosteroids, phenylbutazone
Decreased cell renewal	Antineoplastic agents, corticosteroids, phenylbutazone

tion. Endoscopic examinations have demonstrated that up to 100% of critical care patients develop gastric erosions within a few hours of admission to the unit (Gottlieb et al., 1986).

The development of stress ulcers has been associated with such conditions as sepsis, shock, renal failure, hepatic failure, major trauma, adult respiratory distress syndrome (ARDS), major operative procedures, and respiratory management using mechanical ventilation. In addition, burns and brain injury have been linked to ulcerative lesions. Curling's ulcers occur in patients who have sustained burns to 35% or more of the total body surface. This type of ulcer is thought to result from local ischemia. Decreased blood flow impairs mucus secretion and tends to make the mucosal surface less resistant to the damaging effects of hydrochloric acid. Cushing's ulcer is a special type of stress ulcer that is associated with severe brain injury including both brain tumors and lesions and head trauma. It occurs when the vagus nerve is overstimulated by way of the central nervous system. Cushing's ulcers are usually deep and can occur anywhere along the GI tract.

The clinical diagnosis of stress ulcers may be difficult because more than 25% of patients are asymptomatic (Hurst, 1988). The onset of hemorrhage occurs typically between 2 and 10 days after the original insult. Once stress ulceration has produced significant hemorrhage, mortality usually exceeds 50% (Bowen, 1984).

Although the pathogenesis of stress ulcers is not completely understood, several mechanisms have been implicated. These mechanisms include mucosal barrier breakdown, lowered intramural pH, decreased mucosal blood flow, increased acid secretion, decreased epithelial regeneration, and alteration in prostaglandin synthesis. The gastric mucosal barrier impedes the back-diffusion of hydrogen ions from the lumen into the interstitium. With barrier disruption, tissue damage results from the increase in permeability of the gastric mucosa to luminal hydrogen ions. Hydrogen ion back-diffusion leads to the

formation of edema. The subsequent release of histamine, serotonin, and other vasoactive substances exaggerates the changes in permeability and increases acid secretion. When pepsinogen is activated, mucosal autodigestion occurs. In addition, the mucous-bicarbonate gastric barrier, which normally delays hydrogen ion back-diffusion and acts as a neutralizer, loses its ability to maintain a gradient when hypersecretion lowers the pH below 1.4 (Hurst, 1988) (Fig. 44–3). Barrier breakers include such substances as bile salts, urea, nonsteroidal anti-inflammatory agents, salicylates, ethanol, and corticosteroids.

Endocrine hormones such as ACTH and cortisone may alter the structure of the mucosa or the production of glycoprotein mucus that overlies the gastric epithelium. In addition, it is theorized that emotional stress may play a significant role in ulcer formation. Sympathetic stimuli cause constriction of blood vessels in the duodenum, thus making it more susceptible to trauma due to gastric acid and pepsin. Activation of the adrenal cortex during the stress state may impair mucous production and stimulate gastric secretion. There is also a reduction in epithelial restoration and cellular proliferation during stress.

Another causative factor implicated in stress ulcer formation is an alteration in the synthesis of prostaglandins E and I (PGE and PGI) in the stomach. A deficiency in these prostaglandins results in a thinner mucous layer. Nonsteroidal anti-inflammatory agents are a causative factor because they block the synthesis of PGE and PGI.

Management of stress ulcers is aimed at prevention by decreasing the underlying risk factors, identifying patients at high risk early, and decreasing the hydrogen ion concentration in the stomach. Treatment of existing stress ulcers is basically the same as that used for other forms of ulcer disease.

Gastritis. Acute erosive or hemorrhagic gastritis is a transient irritation of the gastric mucosa that generally appears regional or patchy in nature. Mucosal destruction, however, does not extend beyond the

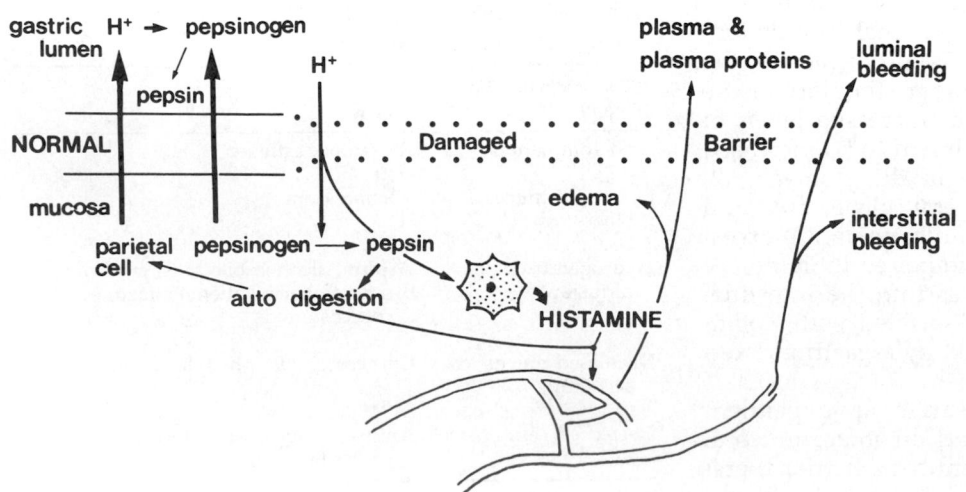

FIGURE 44–3. Pathophysiology of stress ulceration. (From Konopad, E. and Noseworthy, T. (1988). Stress ulceration: A serious complication in critically ill patients. *Heart & Lung,* 17 (4), 339–346.)

muscularis mucosae (MacDonald and Rubin, 1987). The mucosa may be red and friable, or it may appear normal. Multiple bleeding lesions may be distributed throughout the gastric mucosa or may be localized to the fundus, body, or antrum of the stomach. Pathologic changes may include vascular congestion, edema, acute inflammatory cell infiltration, and degenerative changes in the epithelium (MacDonald and Rubin, 1987). The surface epithelium becomes depleted of mucus, and blood extravasates into the lamina propria (MacDonald and Rubin, 1987).

The seriousness of acute hemorrhagic gastritis cannot be overemphasized. Its onset may be precipitated by a single mucosal insult, which may be chemical, thermal, mechanical, bacterial, or viral in nature. Spontaneous remission may occur when the offending agent is removed. An acute fulminating form of gastritis has been reported in patients with acquired immunodeficiency syndrome (AIDS) who have cytomegalovirus (CMV) or opportunistic infections (Haeney, 1989). There is empirical evidence suggesting that alcohol, salicylates, iodine, digitalis, chemotherapeutic agents, and chlortetracycline cause gastritis (Fall, 1986). Indomethacin, phenylbutazone, cinchopin, caffeine, ferrous salts, ammonium chloride, and steroids are potentially caustic to the gastric mucosa. Reserpine in large doses stimulates gastric secretion by accentuating the vagal release of gastrin. Uremia, shock, cirrhosis, severe stress, portal hypertension, and lesions of the central nervous system have been associated with erosive gastritis. Finally, certain foods such as tea, coffee, mustard, paprika, and cloves have the potential to precipitate a bleeding episode when an ulcer is present. Foods high in roughage and those at extreme temperatures may also be irritating to the mucosa.

The signs and symptoms of acute gastritis may vary according to the local irritant. For example, gastritis caused by infectious organisms such as the *Staphylococcus* species usually has an abrupt and violent onset with gastric distress and vomiting about 5 hours after the ingestion of a contaminated food source. Often, patients with aspirin-related gastritis are totally unaware of their condition or may complain only of heartburn. Gastritis associated with excessive alcohol consumption is a different situation. In these patients, transient gastric distress may lead to vomiting and, in more severe cases, to bleeding and hematemesis. Acute gastritis may be a self-limiting disorder, and complete regeneration and healing can occur within several days. It also can lead to major life-threatening situations.

Chronic gastritis, a separate entity from acute gastritis, is characterized by progressive and irreversible atrophy of the glandular epithelium of the stomach (Fall, 1986). The pepsin-producing chief cells and the acid-producing parietal cells of the epithelial layer are atrophied in patients with chronic gastritis. There appear to be two forms of chronic gastritis (Eastwood, 1983). The more common form, referred to as simple atrophic gastritis, is seen in elderly persons

and those who drink or smoke heavily. Atrophic gastritis predisposes to gastric ulcer, pernicious anemia, and cancer of the stomach. The second form of the disorder, autoimmune atrophic gastritis, is thought to be caused by autoantibodies that destroy the gastric mucosal cells. Acid and pepsin secretion are thereby impaired. This retention of acid production in a mucosal surface that has impaired defenses predisposes the patient to peptic ulcer formation.

Esophageal Varices. A detailed description of the pathophysiology of bleeding esophageal varices is covered in Chapter 45.

Mallory-Weiss Tears. A Mallory-Weiss (MW) tear is defined as a longitudinal laceration in the cardioesophageal region (Peterson, 1989). This disorder may be related to prolonged retching and vomiting. It is sometimes seen in patients with anorexia nervosa. In other patients, increased abdominal pressure caused by severe coughing, straining, convulsions, trauma, or childbirth has been implicated. Frequently, MW tears occur in alcoholics. They are also associated with a hiatal hernia. About 49% of the tears are located just below the gastroesophageal junction, whereas other tears may be found around the cardioesophageal junction and the esophagus (Spiro, 1983). The condition generally occurs suddenly and requires immediate treatment. Mallory-Weiss tears are responsible for about 10% of massive episodes of GI bleeding (Spiro, 1983).

Lower Gastrointestinal Bleeding

Hemorrhage from the lower intestine is relatively rare and does not usually necessitate admission into the critical care unit unless there is massive bleeding. Approximately 10% of rectal bleeds are classified as severe, which means that blood loss is substantial enough for the patient to require a transfusion (Bitterman, 1988). The most common source of bright red blood from the rectum is an anal lesion such as hemorrhoids or a fissure. In elderly patients, carcinoma of the colon is the most common cause of lower gastrointestinal bleeding, and diverticulosis is the most frequent cause of massive blood loss (Bitterman, 1988). Inflammatory colitis commonly occurs in young adults, and juvenile polyps are the most common cause of lower GI bleeding in children.

Diverticulosis. Diverticular disease, the most common cause of massive rectal bleeding, affects about 60% of persons over age 60 (Bitterman, 1988). It is thought that a lack of sufficient fiber content in the diet, a decrease in physical activity, poor bowel habits in which the urge to defecate is neglected, and the effects of aging are contributing factors to development of the disease. Diverticulosis is a condition in which herniation of the mucosal layer of the colon occurs through the muscularis layer (Porth, 1988).

Most diverticuli occur in the sigmoid colon. In the large intestine, the longitudinal muscle does not form a continuous layer but consists of three separate bands called the taeniae coli. It is between these muscles, in the area where the blood vessels pierce the circular muscle layer to carry blood to the mucosa, that diverticuli develop.

An increase in intraluminal pressure provides the force creating these herniations. The greater pressure is thought to be related to the volume of the colonic contents. The more scanty the contents, the more vigorous the contractions, and the greater the pressure. When forceful contractions continue for a period of time, both the circular and longitudinal muscle layers hypertrophy. Sometimes the haustra may become so thick that they are approximated during contractions, causing a marked increase in the pressure within the isolated segment. According to the laws of physics, the pressure within a tube increases as its diameter decreases. The sigmoid colon, which was mentioned earlier as the segment most vulnerable to the development of diverticulosis, is the segment of the colon with the narrowest diameter.

Vascular Anomalies. Figure 44–4 outlines the normal arterial and venous blood supply to the organs of the alimentary tract. Vascular malformations, known as angiodysplasia, are an important cause of lower GI bleeding. Although they most often produce chronic or recurrent bleeding, these vascular malformations are responsible for 10% of cases of massive, recurrent lower GI bleeding (Peterson, 1989). Angiodysplasia of the cecum and right colon is found primarily in patients older than 50 years with a history of hypertension (Bitterman, 1988).

Colorectal Cancer. Colorectal cancer is the second most frequent cause of fatal malignancy in the United States today (Kafonek et al., 1988). Almost all cancers of the colon and rectum are carcinomas. Although the cause of cancer of the colon and rectum is unknown, its incidence increases with age, as evidenced by the fact that 95% of persons who develop this type of malignancy are over age 50 (Porth, 1988). Its incidence is increased in persons with a family history of cancer, in persons with ulcerative colitis, and in those with familial polyposis of the colon.

Neoplasms do not often produce exsanguinating hemorrhage but tend to present with chronic, occult bleeding or with intermittent bouts of acute, self-limited bleeding (Peterson, 1989). Usually cancer of the colon and rectum is present for a long period of time before it produces symptoms. Bleeding is a highly significant early symptom and usually prompts the patient to seek medical attention. Commercially prepared tests for detecting occult blood in the stool and colonoscopy are used to diagnose lower GI bleeding caused by cancer. The only recognized treatment for cancer of the colon and rectum is surgical removal of the tumor mass.

Ulcerative Colitis. Ulcerative colitis is a nonspecific inflammatory condition of the colon affecting primarily the mucosa, although it can extend into the submucosal layer (Glickman, 1987). The disease is relapsing and usually follows a course of remissions and exacerbations. The cause of ulcerative colitis is largely unknown, but some evidence suggests a hereditary predisposition (Glickman, 1987). Psychogenic factors may also contribute to its onset and severity.

The inflammatory process tends to be confluent and continuous, causing pinpoint mucosal hemorrhages to appear. These bleeding sites may suppurate and develop into crypt abscesses. Although the ulcerations are usually superficial, they can extend to become large, denuded areas. Bloody diarrhea is always present during the fulminating form of the disease. Major complications of this disease include massive hemorrhage, perforation of the colon, and toxic megacolon (dilatation and hypertrophy of the colon).

Other Lesions. Hemorrhoids are probably the most common cause of lower GI bleeds, but with these usually only small amounts of bright red blood are present on the outside of formed stools (Peterson, 1989). In children, juvenile polyps are the most common cause of bleeding and can be eradicated easily using polypectomy through the sigmoidoscope or colonoscope (Bitterman, 1988).

CLINICAL ASSESSMENT

History

It is often difficult or even impossible to elicit a complete nursing history in critically ill patients with upper GI hemorrhage. When the patient is incapable of providing this important information, the nurse may consult with family members or close friends who have some knowledge of the health history. Not only is the nursing history helpful in ascertaining the origin of the hemorrhage, but also it provides a data base with which to monitor the patient's progress, reactions, and complications throughout hospitalization.

When patients seek medical attention for GI bleeding, research has shown that as many as 20% of them are in fact not really bleeding (Barsan and Baker, 1988). Emesis with red discoloration is often misinterpreted as "bloody" vomiting. Ingestion of beets, iron, charcoal, and bismuth-containing preparations gives the stool a dark red color or tarry appearance that is erroneously thought to be blood. Nosebleeds and hemorrhage secondary to recent oropharyngeal trauma have also been mistaken for GI bleeding.

Demographic data such as age, sex, and ethnic origin can be pertinent in patients with gastrointes-

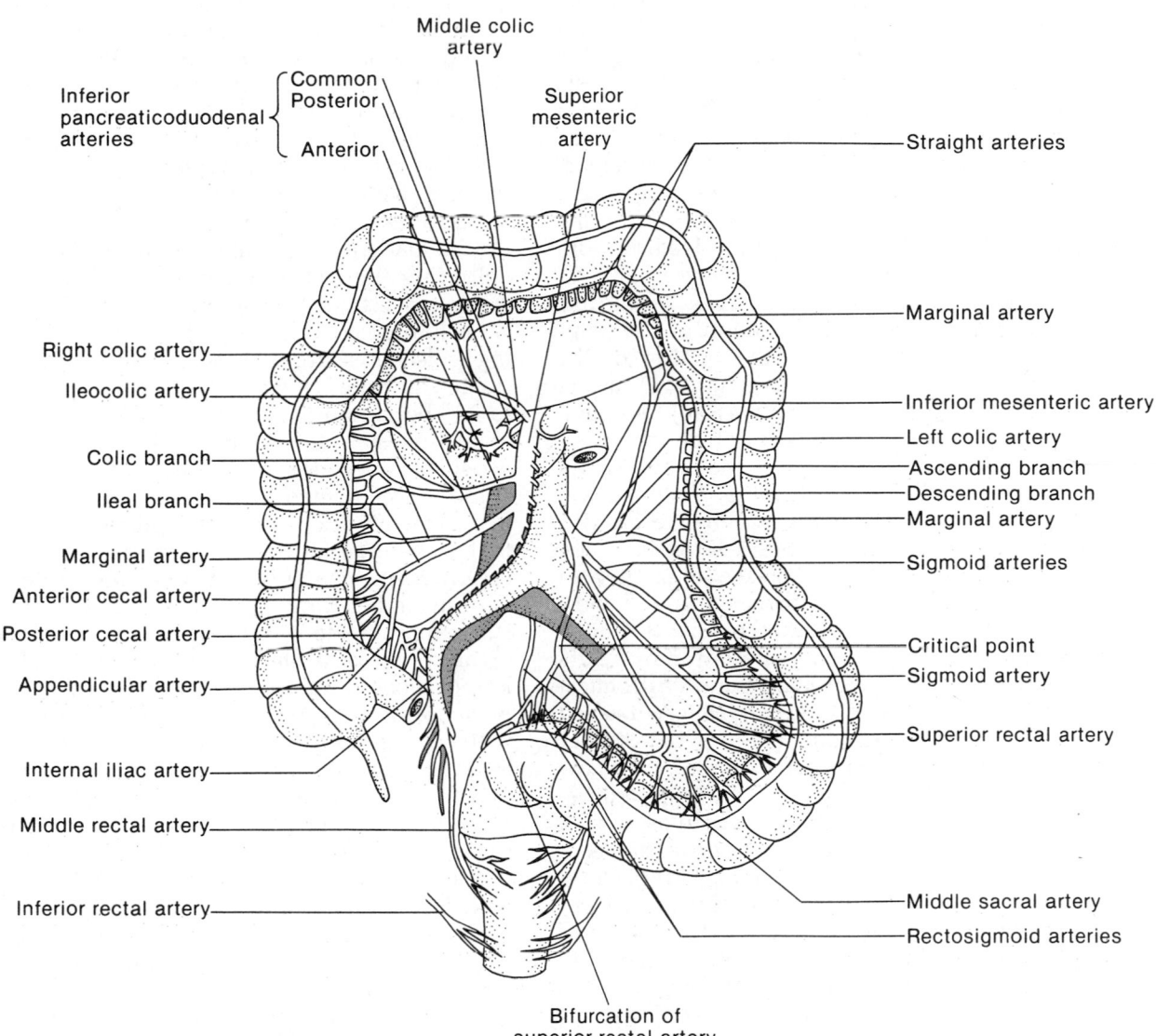

FIGURE 44–4. Arterial and venous blood supplies to primary and accessory organs of the alimentary canal.

tinal bleeds. For example, the incidence of gastric ulcers is twice as common in men as in women until menopause (Knauer and Silverman, 1989). More than 50% of all bleeding patients are older than 60 years (Quigley, 1989). Ulcerative colitis has a high incidence among the Jewish population (Glickman, 1987).

The presence of pain with GI bleeding is diagnostic and should be thoroughly investigated during the nursing history. Pain is often suggestive of mucosal lesions associated with peptic ulcer, esophagitis, and gastritis. A history of gradually increasing epigastric pain that resolves with the onset of bleeding suggests a duodenal ulcer. Blood in the stomach acts as a buffer for gastric acid, and the pain resolves in much the same way as it does with the ingestion of antacids. Up to 60% of patients with erosive gastritis have epigastric distress (Barsan and Baker, 1988). On the other hand, Mallory-Weiss tears and bleeding from esophageal varices are almost always painless. Whenever possible, the critical care nurse should ask the patient to describe (1) the location of the pain, (2) its radiation or extent, (3) the quality of the discomfort, (4) its quantity or frequency, (5) factors that alleviate or aggravate the distress, (6) its timing and patterns, and (7) the setting in which it occurs.

A careful history of the patient's medications and alcohol intake can be of great value. For instance, there is a high association between erosive gastritis and aspirin or alcohol intake. Besides predisposing to gastritis, alcohol causes an increase in gastric acid production. Alcohol-induced cirrhosis is the most common cause of esophageal varices in the United States. Also, alcohol ingestion is present in over 70% of patients with Mallory-Weiss tears and gastrointestinal bleeding (Barsan and Baker, 1988). A detailed history concerning ingestion of over-the-counter (OTC) drugs may be beneficial in identifying how much aspirin the patient has actually ingested because many of these preparations contain aspirin.

A history of vomiting preceding the onset of bleeding is present in at least 50% of patients with Mallory-Weiss tears (Barsan and Baker, 1988). Chronic weight loss is reported in patients with malignancy and mesenteric vascular insufficiency. A previous history of dysphagia suggests esophageal carcinoma or reflux esophagitis as a possible bleeding site. Questions should be geared to screen for a history of bleeding disorders and blood dyscrasias. A history of previous gastrointestinal bleeding is helpful but can also be misleading. Forty per cent of hemorrhaging patients who have a known lesion in the upper gastrointestinal tract, for example, are actually bleeding from a different site (Barsan and Baker, 1988). Twenty per cent of patients with peptic ulcer disease bleed from a site distant from the site of the ulcer (Barsan and Baker, 1988).

Physical Examination

An extensive physical examination is not always possible in patients with massive upper GI bleeding,

nor should it ever take precedence over the immediate treatment of shock. Clinical manifestations of GI bleeding are dependent upon volume of blood loss, rate of bleeding, associated diseases, and extent of cardiovascular compensation. Unless anemia is present prior to the onset of bleeding, loss of less than 500 mL of blood is not usually associated with signs or symptoms (Bogoch, 1985).

The vital signs are crucial in evaluating the patient's clinical condition at the time of the initial examination. Body temperature in patients with hematemesis and melena is often elevated. At least 80% of patients with upper GI hemorrhage have a temperature in the 37.5° to 38.5° C (100° to 102° F) range for at least 1 to 2 days (Barsan and Baker, 1988). The presence of hypothermia is ominous in patients with GI hemorrhage and suggests severe shock. Pulse and blood pressure are key indices in the evaluation of the patient's hemodynamic status. Following the trend in pulse pressure, which indirectly reflects stroke volume, is one of the simplest ways to predict or diagnose hypovolemia. A narrowing pulse pressure is seen in an advancing shock state. The patient's pulse may be increased from 100 to 120 beats/minute, even when blood pressure remains normal. Of course, the pulse may be an unreliable indicator in certain cases, especially in persons accustomed to vigorous sports and in those taking medications, such as digitalis or propranolol, that prevent an increase in heart rate.

Orthostatic changes in blood pressure can be diagnostic in bleeding patients. A diastolic blood pressure drop of 10 to 20 mm Hg and a pulse increase of greater than 20 beats/minute indicate a 25% to 50% loss of blood volume (Barsan and Baker, 1988). The presence of a "normal" blood pressure in a patient with other signs of clinical shock does not necessarily indicate a stable hemodynamic status. The patient may experience tachycardia, a thready peripheral pulse, and an increased respiratory rate in response to lactic acidosis.

The skin should always be examined in patients with upper GI hemorrhage. The skin may be pale, cool, and clammy with or without peripheral cyanosis. These changes, which indicate the presence of shock, represent a sympathetic response to hypovolemia (Barsan and Baker, 1988). Petechial and purpuric lesions may signal blood dyscrasias as the cause of bleeding. In patients with cirrhotic liver disease, the nurse may discover ecchymoses, spider angiomas, palmar erythema, and jaundice while inspecting the skin.

An abdominal examination is also relevant in bleeding patients. The size of the liver and spleen are assessed by palpation, even though the spleen cannot be palpated until it is at least two to three times its normal size. Splenomegaly suggests the presence of portal hypertension. Hepatomegaly may be found in patients with malignancy and those with Laennec's cirrhosis or acute hepatitis. The patient with gastritis or peptic ulcer disease may experience epigastric pain during palpation.

Bowel sounds are auscultated during the physical examination. Bowel sounds are typically hyperactive in patients with upper GI bleeding, whereas hypoactive or normal bowel sounds are more commonly heard in patients with lower GI bleeding (Peterson, 1989). Blood is a potent cathartic that stimulates peristalsis. Decreased or absent bowel sounds in a patient with upper GI bleeding raise the question of whether there is a perforated bowel or intestinal ileus.

Diagnostic Procedures

Laboratory. A complete blood count is obtained immediately in all patients with acute upper GI hemorrhage, and the hematocrit and hemoglobin are monitored serially to follow the clinical course of the bleeding and the extent of blood loss. In patients with chronic blood losses, the initial values may be low and do not accurately reflect an acute blood loss in the differential diagnosis. This information must be considered in order to avoid erroneous interpretations during subsequent laboratory studies.

After an acute episode of GI hemorrhage, 12 to 72 hours may elapse before the hematocrit reflects the true extent of the blood loss (Peterson, 1989). A normal hematocrit in a patient with active GI bleeding does not imply that the blood loss is not extensive. On the contrary, a normal or high hematocrit in the presence of severe hemorrhage suggests that the blood loss has occurred too rapidly to allow for equilibrium of the hematocrit by dilution. A low hematocrit, on the contrary, suggests that the blood loss has occurred at a much slower rate, allowing some equilibrium to occur, or that an acute bleeding episode has been superimposed on a chronic bleed-

ing condition. Table 44–5 summarizes the pertinent changes in laboratory values that may occur during GI hemorrhage. The patient's blood values are carefully considered along with the history, physical examination, and other diagnostic findings.

Nasogastric Intubation. Passing a nasogastric (NG) tube to obtain gastric aspirate will confirm active bleeding in the upper GI system. NG intubation is indicated in patients with melena or hematochezia and in those reporting bloody emesis. If no blood is present in the aspirated contents, it can be assumed that there is no active bleeding from the distal duodenum. If no blood is present initially, the NG tube is left in place to empty the stomach and aspirate bilious material. Some clinicians do not use NG intubation when esophageal varices are suspected because irritation from the tube may precipitate bleeding episodes.

Endoscopy. Endoscopy is considered the diagnostic test of choice in the majority of patients with persistent bleeding. This study can detect 90% to 95% of bleeding lesions in the upper GI system (Hurst, 1988). For upper GI endoscopy, a flexible tube is passed through the mouth into the stomach and duodenum to allow complete examination of the mucosal lining. Proctosigmoidoscopy allows visualization of the distal sigmoid colon, the rectum, and the anal canal. If a flexible sigmoidoscope is used, the descending colon can also be seen. Colonoscopy is performed to examine the lining of the large intestine, using a flexible endoscope inserted anally. Endoscopic procedures enable the gastroenterologist performing the procedure to remove tissue specimens for microscopic examination or control localized bleeding (see Chap. 45).

TABLE 44–5. Changes in Laboratory Indices During GI Hemorrhage

Laboratory Index	Change	Comment
Hematocrit	↑ or ↓	Results can be misleading (see text)
White blood cell count	↑ Up to 40,000 cells/mm³	Cause of leukocytosis is unknown. WBC usually returns within normal range 24 to 48 hours after bleeding stops
Platelet count	↑ sometimes within 1 hour after bleeding begins	Thrombocytosis may be absent in patients with bone marrow suppression or cirrhosis
Reticulocyte count	↑	Reticulocytosis is found within 24 hours after bleeding begins and may persist for 14 days after bleeding stops
Mean corpuscular volume (MCV)	↓ or within normal limits	Decreased levels suggest chronic bleeding
Hypochromic microcytic red blood cells	↓ or absent	Presence indicates chronic blood loss
Blood urea nitrogen	↑ as high as 80 mg/dL in patients who otherwise have normal renal function	Usually begins to fall 12 hours after bleeding stops
Sodium	Within normal limits or ↑ in dehydration	Low levels may indicate hemodilution or chronic blood loss

Guaiac Testing. The presence of occult blood should be confirmed in patients without melena or hematochezia whenever GI blood loss is suspected. Because some medications and food products may simulate melena, the stool should always be tested for the presence of blood. False-positive results using Hemoccult slides occur in 1% to 2% of patients, usually those who are taking vitamin C (Adrien and Mailhot, 1986).

Electrocardiography. An electrocardiogram is necessary in all patients older than 40 with GI bleeding and in younger patients when hemorrhagic shock is suspected (Barsan and Baker, 1988). In shock states, low voltage is usually present because of decreased central vascular volume. Although ischemic changes in the anterolateral precordial leads are common in patients with hypovolemic shock, these usually resolve spontaneously after adequate fluid resuscitation. Persistence of an ischemic state 24 to 36 hours after the bleeding episode suggests myocardial infarction. Of course, patients who have had abnormal electrocardiographic results prior to the hemorrhage must be carefully evaluated according to their previous history. In general, the incidence of myocardial infarction with upper GI bleeding is 1% to 2% (Barsan and Baker, 1988). Most of these myocardial infarctions, which may be subendocardial or transmural, are "silent" and are not manifested in the usual manner by substernal pain.

Chest and Abdominal Films. Chest radiographs and supine and upright abdominal films may be obtained to rule out perforation, masses, bowel obstruction, and signs of mesenteric vascular ischemia. If a central venous catheter has been placed for fluid replacement, the anteroposterior chest x-ray will enable the physician to confirm placement of the tip of the cannula in a central location. These large-bore catheters are placed in critically ill patients with profound blood loss when the patient's survival may depend on the rapidity of fluid replacement.

Arteriography. When GI bleeding is so brisk that it is impossible to perform endoscopy, selective mesenteric arteriography will localize the site of bleeding in 75% of patients (Peterson, 1989). Blood loss must be 0.5 to 0.6 mL/minute for this procedure to be useful as a diagnostic tool. If the rate of bleeding is less, or if the patient is bleeding from a venous lesion, results of arteriography will be negative. During the procedure, bleeding can be stopped temporarily by infusing vasopressin intra-arterially to cause short-term vasoconstriction.

Barium Radiographs (Upper GI Series and Barium Enema). Barium radiographs are not usually the diagnostic procedure of choice, especially in patients with acute active bleeding, due to the patient's vomiting and unstable condition. Double contrast barium x-rays are more diagnostic than single contrast x-rays for determining the bleeding site; however, both are less accurate than endoscopy and will detect only

80% to 85% of bleeding sites (Peterson, 1989). Furthermore, the ability to visualize the lesion on radiographs does not necessarily confirm that it is bleeding. When barium studies are done, endoscopy has to be postponed temporarily because the presence of barium precludes accurate endoscopic results.

TREATMENT OF GASTROINTESTINAL BLEEDING

The goals for immediate treatment of GI bleeding include (1) stabilizing the patient's condition, (2) identifying the source of the bleeding, (3) stopping the bleeding, and (4) initiating treatment to prevent further bleeding. Of patients with acute upper GI bleeding, 85% will stop bleeding spontaneously (Grendell, 1988). However, 25% will rebleed during the hospitalization, and 10% will die (Hurst, 1988). Accurate assessment and vigorous treatment are required until the patient has been successfully stabilized.

Fluid Replacement

Depending on the magnitude of blood loss, the primary nursing objective is volume replacement. One or more large-bore intravenous devices are started, and crystalloid solutions such as normal saline and Ringer's lactate are infused to replace volume during the initial phase of fluid resuscitation. A central venous pressure (CVP) cannula or pulmonary artery catheter may be placed to achieve rapid fluid replacement and closer hemodynamic monitoring. Blood samples are obtained for complete blood count, clotting studies, type and crossmatch, blood urea nitrogen, serum electrolytes, creatinine, and blood glucose levels. An arterial line may be placed to monitor blood pressure and arterial blood gases.

Blood products may be necessary depending on the estimated amount of blood loss. Estimated losses of 20% or more necessitate replacement with blood in order to restore oxygen transport (Hurst, 1988). Replacement is accomplished with the use of packed red blood cells (PRBC) milliliter for milliliter of estimated blood loss and crystalloid solutions used in a 3:1 ratio (Hurst, 1988). Albumin or plasmanate may also be used as volume expanders. Fresh frozen plasma will be necessary in patients who have been transfused with 5 or more units to replace clotting factors (Bogoch, 1985). Massive transfusion with 10 or more units necessitates administration of platelets (Peterson, 1989). Hematocrit and hemoglobin are monitored at least every 2 to 4 hours initially. With hydration, each unit of PRBCs increases the hematocrit by approximately 4% and the hemoglobin by 1 g.

The patient must be carefully monitored for complications during massive transfusion therapy (Table 44–6). Hyperkalemia may be present if the aging red blood cells release potassium in the banked blood.

TABLE 44–6. Complications of Massive Blood Transfusions

Complication	Mechanism
Hyperkalemia	Due to release of potassium from breakdown of aging RBCs in stored blood
Hypocalcemia	Due to binding of ionized calcium in stored blood with the preservative citrate-phosphate-dextrose
Hypothermia	Due to rapid administration of large amounts of cold blood
Circulatory overload	Due to infusion of large fluid volumes
Metabolic acidosis	Due to acidity that gradually occurs in stored blood
Decreased tissue oxygenation	Due to a decrease in 2,3-diphosphoglycerate (DPG) in stored blood, which results in a left shift on the oxyhemoglobin dissociation curve (impaired oxygen transfer at tissue level)
Infections	Due to risk of exposure to hepatitis, AIDS, and other infections despite increased processing precautions
Coagulopathies	Due to a decrease in clotting components because packed RBC infusions do not contain plasma or platelets
Disseminated intravascular coagulation	Due to release of a thromboplastin-like substance from red blood cells during hemolysis and the antigen-antibody complex as seen in transfusion reactions
Febrile transfusion reactions	Due to formation of antileukocyte antibodies (Abs) after previous transfusions
Adult respiratory distress syndrome	Thought to be due to aggregation of microemboli in the pulmonary system from transfusions

Hypocalcemia results when ionized calcium in the banked blood binds to the citrate derivative used as a preservative and anticoagulant. Preservatives in large amounts can also decrease the oxygen-carrying capacity of the blood. Supplemental oxygen is used, and oxygen saturations are monitored until the patient is stabilized. Microaggregate filters may be used for blood administration.

During high-volume fluid replacement therapy, the critical care nurse observes the patient carefully for signs and symptoms of fluid overload. Hemodynamic indices are monitored as well as physical signs and symptoms such as dyspnea, neck vein distention, and rales. An indwelling urinary catheter is inserted, and hourly urine outputs are measured as an index of volume replacement and renal perfusion.

Nasogastric Intubation or Lavage

As mentioned earlier, a large-bore nasogastric tube is inserted to obtain a gastric specimen for occult blood testing and to clear the stomach for endoscopic examination. After confirmation of upper GI bleeding, the tube remains indwelling to evacuate blood from the stomach. An Ewald tube in which additional side holes have been cut is sometimes used to remove large clots. It is very important to remove as much clot and intragastric material as possible because emptying the stomach allows its walls to collapse, contributing to hemostasis and helping to prevent vomiting and aspiration.

Lavaging the stomach with iced saline has long been used to stop upper GI bleeding. However, the efficacy of this practice has never been firmly established (Tobin, 1989). Some evidence suggests that iced saline may actually damage the stomach's mucosa and promote bleeding (Dworkin, 1989). The use of vasoconstrictors in lavage fluid has also not been proved to be effective. Either room temperature saline or tap water may be used for lavage. Lavage is done to cleanse the stomach for endoscopy and provide an indication of the rapidity of bleeding. Procedurally, 500 to 1000 mL of fluid is instilled and then removed by gravity drainage or gentle suction. As much as 10 liters may be necessary for optimal results.

The duration of nasogastric intubation varies according to the patient's condition. After the patient's condition is stabilized, the tube can be used for instilling antacids and for obtaining gastric aspirate for pH testing. Newer nasogastric tubes are now available that contain a disposable electrode for continuous pH monitoring. When the use of the tube becomes unimportant, it should be removed. Besides being uncomfortable, prolonged nasogastric intubation may predispose the patient to gastroesophageal reflux and esophagitis.

Pharmacologic Therapy

Histamine Receptor Antagonists. Histamine (H_2) receptor antagonists (cimetidine, ranitidine, famotidine, nizatidine) competitively inhibit the action of histamine on the H_2 receptors of parietal cells, thus reducing gastric acid output and concentration. Some studies indicate that histamine antagonists may be effective for the treatment of stress ulcers and GI bleeding when hemorrhage is not caused by the erosion of major blood vessels (Quigley, 1989). However, H_2 receptor antagonists have not been shown to be more effective in controlling gastric pH than antacids (Hurst, 1988).

Side effects of H_2 receptor antagonists include confusion, lethargy, seizures, hypotension, hepatotoxicity, thrombocytopenia, gynecomastia, and male impotence. Ranitidine has been shown to be twice as effective as cimetidine but is more likely to produce the above side effects. The usual intravenous or oral dose of cimetidine is 300 mg four times daily. Ranitidine can be given at a dosage of 150 mg twice daily to obtain the same effect. Because antacids may interfere with the oral absorption of ranitidine, administration of the drug and antacids should be separated by 1 hour. Nizatidine can be given at a dosage of 300 mg at bedtime or 150 mg twice daily. Maintenance dosage is 150 mg at bedtime. Famotidine 40 mg orally at bedtime is recommended for use in patients with an active duodenal ulcer or pathologic hypersecretory conditions.

Antacids. Antacids are the most common pharmacologic agents used to treat upper GI bleeding (Table 44–7). Antacids are inorganic salts that dissolve in gastric acid secretions, releasing anions that partially neutralize gastric hydrochloric acid. The clinical use of antacids is based on their ability to increase the pH of gastric acid secretions.

There are four major classifications of antacids. They are, in decreasing order of their ability to neutralize gastric acids, calcium carbonate, sodium bicarbonate, magnesium hydroxide, and aluminum hydroxide. Although aluminum hydroxide antacids usually do not raise the gastric pH above 5, magnesium hydroxide can increase the gastric pH above 9 (Thompson and Mahachai, 1985). Although antacids do not usually neutralize all gastric acids, increasing the gastric pH from 1.3 to 2.3 neutralizes 90%, and raising the pH to 3.3 neutralizes 99%. Consequently, the amount of gastric acid back-diffusing through the gastric mucosa and reaching the duodenum is decreased.

Although generally uncommon, some side effects are associated with the chronic use of antacids. All antacids promote some degree of metabolic alkalosis. Due to the high prevalence of this, as well as its high sodium content, sodium bicarbonate is not commonly used for its antacid effect. Calcium carbonate is not usually prescribed because it may produce hypercalcemia and impair renal function. Aluminum-containing antacids are known to cause constipation, whereas magnesium-containing antacids may produce diarrhea. To avoid these undesirable colonic effects and to balance the neutralizing effects, many commercially prepared antacids are combinations of aluminum and magnesium compounds. Aluminum-containing antacids may occasionally contribute to phosphate depletion. Magnesium-containing antacids may cause hypermagnesemia, but this is rare and occurs primarily in patients with impaired renal function. Amphogel, composed only of aluminum hydroxide, can be used for patients in renal failure to help control hyperphosphatemia.

In the management of patients with GI bleeding, antacids may be administered every 1 to 4 hours to maintain the gastric pH above 3.5 (McEvoy, 1988). Suspensions are generally preferable to tablets because they have a superior buffering ability (McEvoy, 1988). In some patients, treatment may require the use of both H_2 receptor antagonists and antacids for adequate results. Doses of H_2 antagonists and antacids should be staggered to allow for maximum absorption when both are administered orally.

Sucralfate. Sucralfate, an ionic, sulfated disaccharide, is an inhibitor of pepsin and an antiulcer agent (McEvoy, 1988). The exact mechanism of its pharmacologic action is unclear, but the therapeutic effects of the drug are the results of local rather than systemic activity. It does not appreciably affect gastric acid output or concentration.

The negatively charged sucralfate molecule binds to positively charged molecules such as leukocytes, mucosal debris, and fibrinogen in gastric and duodenal ulcer craters. This provides a protective barrier

TABLE 44–7. Composition of Commonly Used Antacids (mg/30 mL)

Name	Aluminum Hydroxide	Magnesium Hydroxide	Other	Sodium	Acid Neutralizing Capacity (mEq/30 mL)	GI Effects
ALternaGEL	3600	—	—	<15	96	Constipation
Amphogel	1920	—	—	<13.8	60	Constipation
Gelusil	1200	1200	Simethicone (150 mg)	4.2	72	Constipation or diarrhea
Maalox	1200	1200	—	8.4	79.8	Constipation or diarrhea
Maalox TC	3600	1800	—	4.8	163.2	Constipation or mild diarrhea
Mylanta	1200	1200	Simethicone (120 mg)	4.1	76.2	Constipation or diarrhea
Mylanta II	2400	2400	Simethicone (180 mg)	7.8	152.4	Constipation or diarrhea
Riopan	—	—	Magaldrate (3240 mg)	0.6	90	Mild constipation or diarrhea
Basaljel	—	—	Aluminum carbonate (2400 mg, equivalent to ALOH)	17.4	72	Constipation

against hydrogen ions and pepsin. The drug has a greater affinity for the ulcer site than for normal GI mucosa, although binding to normal mucosa does occur. Sucralfate also binds to acute gastric erosions produced by alcohol or other gastric irritating drugs such as aspirin.

The usual dose is 1 g four to five times daily by mouth. The most common side effect is constipation. A gastric pH of 3 to 4 is necessary for sucralfate to be effective (Hurst, 1988).

Recent studies have advocated the use of sucralfate rather than antacids and H₂ receptor antagonists in mechanically ventilated patients because those agents appear to raise the gastric pH and allow growth of microorganisms (Driks et al., 1987; Tryba, 1987). This is thought to increase the risk of nosocomial pneumonia or bacteremia. More controlled studies are needed before definitive conclusions can be drawn.

Prostaglandins. Prostaglandin (PG) therapy is a relatively new treatment for ulcer disease (Hurst, 1988). The E series of prostaglandins acts by suppressing parietal cell activity and curtailing gastric acid secretion. These agents also are considered cytoprotective in that they potentiate the effects of gastric mucus and bicarbonate. Further studies are needed to substantiate their effectiveness as prophylactic therapy. Side effects are mainly GI in nature and include nausea, vomiting, diarrhea, and abdominal cramping. This therapy is strictly contraindicated in pregnant patients because it can cause spontaneous abortion. Misoprostal, a synthetic prostaglandin E₁ analogue, is given at a dosage of 200 μg four times a day by mouth. Because this drug is available only in an oral form it is not used during acute bleeding episodes.

Vasopressin Infusion. Systemic infusion of vasopressin (Pitressin) has been shown to be effective in the treatment of massive GI hemorrhage. Vasopressin acts by constricting the arteries and contracting the bowel wall. Thus, mucosal blood flow is reduced, and thrombus formation can occur.

Vasopressin is a polypeptide hormone secreted by the hypothalamus and stored in the posterior pituitary gland of mammals. Exogenous vasopressin elicits all the pharmacologic responses usually produced by endogenous vasopressin (antidiuretic hormone). The primary physiologic role of vasopressin is to maintain serum osmolality within a normal range and to conserve up to 90% of the water that might otherwise be excreted in the urine. In larger doses, the hormone causes vasoconstriction, particularly of capillaries and of small arterioles, resulting in decreased blood flow to the splanchnic, coronary, GI, pancreatic, skin, and muscular systems (Peterson, 1989). When injected into the celiac or superior mesenteric artery, vasopressin constricts the gastroduodenal, left gastric, superior mesenteric, and

splenic arteries. In the intestinal tract, vasopressin increases peristaltic activity, particularly in the large bowel. Vasopressin also causes an increase in GI sphincter pressure and a decrease in gastric secretion but has no effect on gastric acid concentration.

Vasopressin may be given by regional perfusion using an angiographically placed arterial catheter or by systemic venous infusion (Table 44–8). The usual dosage is 0.2 to 0.4 units/minute given through an infusion pump. The intravenous route of administration is usually the first choice because intra-arterial infusion has not been shown to be more efficacious (Peterson, 1989). However, some patients who do not respond to the intravenous route may respond positively to an intra-arterial infusion. The use of vasopressin in such situations is a temporary measure for controlling bleeding because there is no clinical evidence that its use substantially improves the overall survival rate.

Because vasopressin can have major cardiovascular complications, its use may be contraindicated in patients with preexisting cardiovascular disease. Vasopressin reduces coronary blood flow, thus leading to such complications as angina, dysrhythmias, hypertension, and myocardial infarction. Other side effects include fluid retention, water intoxication, oliguria, pulmonary edema, confusion, headache, nausea and vomiting, and peripheral or intestinal ischemia. Extravasation of vasopressin can result in subcutaneous tissue sloughing. Nursing assessment of patients on vasopressin therapy should include monitoring of the electrocardiogram (ECG), vital signs, lung sounds, level of consciousness, intake and output, and daily weights. Any symptoms of chest pain or abdominal pain should be reported to the physician immediately. IV catheter insertion sites should be inspected frequently for signs of infiltration.

Studies have shown that combining vasodilator therapy (such as nitroprusside or nitroglycerin with vasopressin) reduces the detrimental cardiac effects of vasopressin by reducing cardiac oxygen demand and increasing coronary blood flow (Gelman and Ernst, 1978; Gimson et al., 1986). These agents may actually augment the effect of vasopressin in controlling bleeding from esophageal varices because they reduce portal venous resistance. More clinical studies are needed to establish definitive protocols for the use of vasopressin and vasodilators in combination.

TABLE 44–8. Selective Vasoactive Infusion Therapy

Bleeding Source	Vessel Used
Esophageal	Superior mesenteric artery or left gastric artery
Gastric	Left gastric artery
Duodenal	Gastroduodenal artery
Large bowel (right half)	Inferior mesenteric artery
Large bowel (left half)	Superior mesenteric artery

Other. Omeprazole is the newest pharmacologic agent being used in the treatment of ulcer disease (Mahachai, 1985). It has also been shown to be effective in treating Zollinger-Ellison syndrome and may indeed become the medical therapy of choice in these patients. Omeprazole is thought to bond to the proton pump of the parietal cell, acting as a hydrogen-potassium pump inhibitor. This results in inhibition of acid secretion regardless of the source of stimulation (acetylcholine, gastrin, or histamine). This drug is administered after bleeding is controlled. The regime is short-term, for a period of up to 8 weeks. The oral form should be given on an empty stomach. Side effects include dizziness, weakness, headache, fatigue, nausea, diarrhea, numbness of the extremities, and transient elevations of hepatic enzymes.

Medical Procedures

Endoscopic Electrocoagulation. In a variety of upper GI lesions, electrocoagulation can be accomplished through the use of a bipolar (BICAP) probe (Hurst, 1988). This form of therapy uses an electric current that flows between two electrodes in close proximity to each other to induce coagulation of bleeding lesions. Coagulation can also be achieved with the use of a heater probe. In this method direct heat is used to seal the vessel thermally (Fig. 44–5). Both types of therapy can be done using endoscopy. With the portability of this form of therapy and lower cost than laser therapy, endoscopic coagulation is becoming an accepted and popular form of treatment.

Transcatheter Embolization. An angiographic modality may be used if vasopressin is unsuccessful in controlling bleeding lesions in patients who are con-sidered to be poor surgical candidates (Hurst, 1988). Once the bleeding artery has been identified through angiography, embolic material is injected through the catheter selectively into the bleeding artery. The material proximally occludes the artery. Substances such as Gelfoam, cyanoacrylate glue, coils, autologous clots, and polyvinyl alcohol have been used for embolization. The choice of material depends on the desired length of action of embolization. Complications include tissue ischemia or infarction if collateral circulation is inadequate.

Photocoagulation. The use of lasers for coagulation of bleeding sources has gained in popularity as a treatment modality (Hurst, 1988). The neodymium: yttrium-aluminum-garnet (Nd:YAG) laser can be used to treat bleeding esophageal varices, Mallory-Weiss tears, ulcers, and gastric erosions. Results are similar to those achieved with endoscopic electrocoagulation. However, it is a more expensive form of therapy and may require endotracheal intubation and general anesthesia.

Sclerotherapy. A detailed description of this form of therapy is covered in Chapter 45.

Surgical Procedures for Upper Gastrointestinal Bleeding

Although the majority of lesions that cause upper GI bleeding are treated primarily medically, there are several indications for surgical treatment (Knauer and Silverman, 1989). Surgery is indicated (1) if healing is not accomplished with medical treatment, (2) if ulcer recurrence is a problem, (3) when malignancy is suspected, or (4) if complications such as perforation, obstructive pyloric stenosis, or intractable hemorrhage occur.

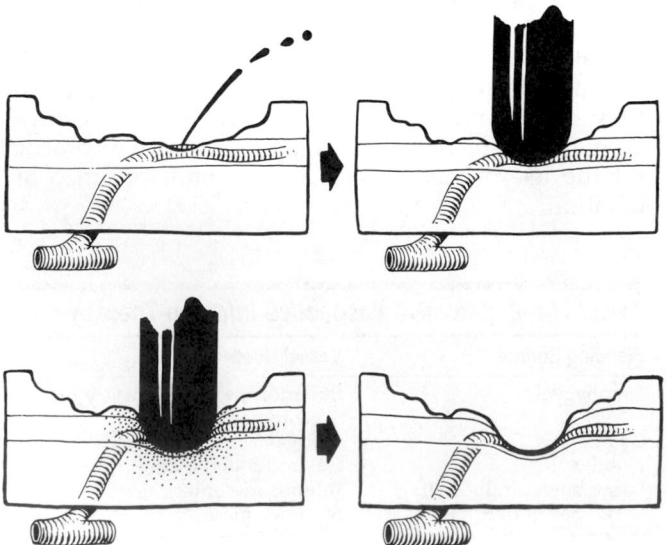

FIGURE 44–5. Heater probe therapy being used to seal vessel thermally. (Adapted from Johnston, J. H. (1985). *Endoscopy Review,* 2, 23; in Chung, R., *Therapeutic endoscopy in gastrointestinal surgery* (p. 23). New York: Churchill Livingstone, 1987.)

Types of Surgical Procedures. A gastric oversew may be indicated as treatment for a subcardial gastric ulcer. This procedure, which is usually considered palliative, involves suture ligation of the bleeding vessel and closure of the ulcer crater. Ulcer excision or gastric resection is preferred to prevent the possibility of rebleeding or the development of malignancy.

To decrease stomach acid production, two surgical approaches are used. The approaches involve (1) severing the nerves that stimulate cellular acid production, and (2) removing the acid-production section of the stomach. A vagotomy to eliminate the stimulus to gastric cells is accomplished by severing the vagus nerve to the stomach. Several types of vagotomy are possible (Table 44–9). Because the vagus nerve also stimulates motility, this procedure necessitates a gastroenterostomy or pyloroplasty to provide for gastric emptying. This is not necessary with the highly selective vagotomy (HSV), because motility is preserved.

Surgical treatment for gastric ulcer also includes gastric resection as a means of removing the acid-secreting parietal cells or gastric acid–secreting cells in the antrum of the stomach (Fig. 44–6). Resection is accomplished with either a Billroth I or Billroth II procedure. In the Billroth I procedure, the distal portion of the stomach is removed with an anastomosis of the proximal portion to the duodenum (gastroduodenostomy). The Billroth II procedure involves removal of the lower portion of the stomach with anastomosis to the jejunum (gastrojejunostomy). The duodenal stump is closed. The Billroth II procedure is more frequently performed as a treatment for duodenal ulcer because the incidence of ulcer recurrence is lower than that after the Billroth I. However, postoperative sequelae occur more frequently after the Billroth II (Table 44–10).

A total gastrectomy with anastomosis of the esophagus to the jejunum (esophagojejunostomy) is a radical procedure reserved for intractable ulcer disease such as that seen with Zollinger-Ellison syndrome (Fig. 44–7). Multiple ulcers of the stomach and duodenum occur in this syndrome as a result of hypersecretion of gastric acid caused by a pancreatic non–islet cell gastrinoma. Although the success of medical regimes is improving, the only definitive treatment is removal of all gastric acid–secreting tissue.

Implications for Care. Immediate postoperative nursing care is aimed at providing the routine care needed for an abdominal surgery patient, assessing for immediate postoperative complications, and providing support as the patient adapts to the changes in the gastrointestinal system.

The patient who undergoes emergency gastric surgery is at risk for development of numerous complications (Table 44–11). Due to the extent of the anastomosis, the potential for postoperative hemorrhage is significant. Other causes of hemorrhage may be intraluminal or extraluminal in nature (Table 44–12). The mortality rate for patients with postoperative bleeding is as high as 57% (Haring and Berger, 1988). Postoperatively, the patient will have a nasogastric tube, which should not be manipulated or irrigated unless specifically ordered. Normally, the patient may lose up to 300 mL of bloody drainage within the first 24 hours (Haring and Berger, 1988). There is less drainage after a total gastrectomy because there is no reservoir to collect the drainage. Excessive drainage or failure of the tube to drain should be reported immediately. A clogged tube may lead to gastric distention and increased pressure at the site of the anastomosis. An anastomotic leak usually occurs between the first and the eighth postoperative days. The result may be peritonitis, cellulitis, or abscess formation. Signs and symptoms include sudden severe pain, high fever, chills, tachycardia, abdominal rigidity, absent bowel sounds, tachypnea, and leukocytosis. Relaparotomy usually is necessary.

Afferent loop syndrome is a complication associated with the Billroth II. In this syndrome, pancreatic secretions and bile fill the afferent loop of the duodenal stump due to obstruction or stenosis of the afferent loop. As the afferent loop becomes dis-

TABLE 44–9. Types of Vagotomies

Name	Effect	Comments
Truncal vagotomy (TV)	Denervates stomach, upper abdominal organs, and intestine as far as left flexure of colon	Most widespread method used; used as treatment for duodenal ulcer as well as recurrent ulcers and marginal jejunal ulcers
Selective gastric vagotomy (SGV)	Denervates stomach only; weakens motility of the antrum	Used for treatment of duodenal ulcer or pyloric/prepyloric ulcer
Proximal gastric vagotomy (PVG) or	Denervates only proximal acid-producing portion of stomach; innervation and motility of antrum undisturbed	Decreased incidence of "dumping" and diarrhea; used as treatment of duodenal ulcer.
Selective proximal vagotomy (SPV, also known as highly selective vagotomy [HSV] and parietal cell vagotomy [PCV])		Need for drainage anastomosis eliminated

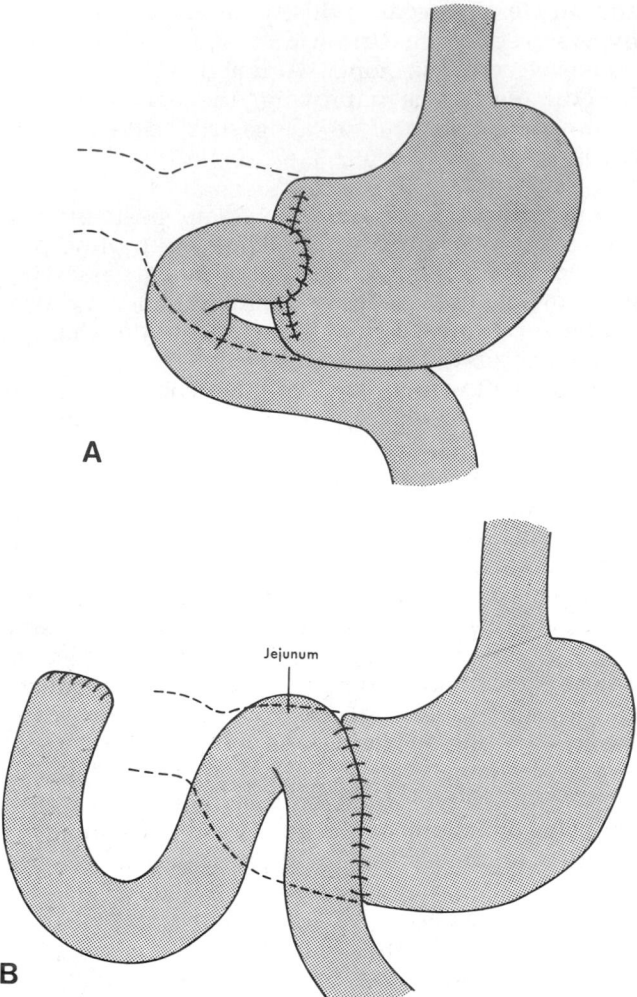

A

B

Jejunum

FIGURE 44–6. *Top,* Billroth I procedure (gastroduodenostomy). Removal of distal portion of stomach with anastomosis to duodenum. Dotted lines show portion removed. *Bottom,* Billroth II procedure (gastrojejunostomy). Removal of lower portion of stomach with anastomosis to jejunum. Dotted lines show portion removed. A duodenal stump remains and is closed. (From Given, Barbara A., and Simmons, Sandra J. (1984). *Gastroenterology in clinical nursing* (4th ed., pp. 274 and 275). St. Louis: C. V. Mosby.)

tended, there is pressure, pain, and gastric backflow. Typically, the patient experiences vomiting of bilious material after feedings.

After gastric surgery the patient is likely to develop nutritional problems. Removal of the proximal portion or all of the stomach results in loss of intrinsic factor, which is necessary for absorption of vitamin

TABLE 44–10. Pathologic Sequelae Following Gastrojejunostomy

Dumping syndrome
Diarrhea
Weight loss
Steatorrhea
Iron deficiency
Calcium metabolism disturbances

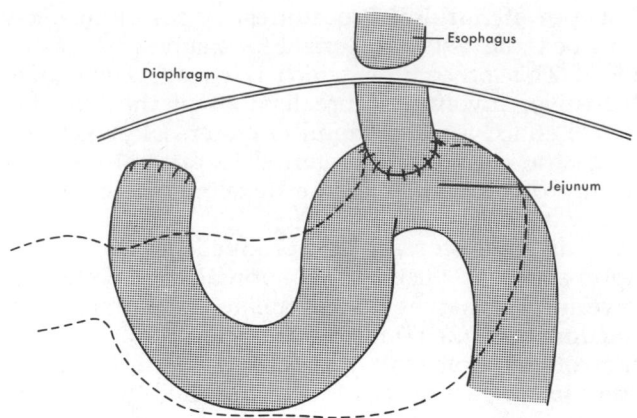

FIGURE 44–7. Total gastrectomy with anastomosis of esophagus to jejunum (esophagojejunostomy). Dotted lines show portion removed. (From Given, Barbara A., and Simmons, Sandra J. (1984). *Gastroenterology in clinical nursing* (4th ed., p. 288). St. Louis: C. V. Mosby.)

B_{12}. In addition, deficiencies in iron, folic acid, calcium, and vitamin D may occur. Malabsorption of nutrients can occur due to decreased pancreatic secretions and bile. The dumping syndrome is a postprandial problem that often occurs after gastric resection. Rapid passage of a hypertonic bolus of food into the jejunum results in an osmotic shift of fluid into the bowel. Symptoms include abdominal distention, vertigo, palpitations, sweating, and diarrhea. Late manifestations including sweating, vertigo, hunger, and headache may occur 1 to 3 hours after eating. The pathogenesis of these systemic symptoms is excessive carbohydrate absorption, which triggers an excessive release of insulin. Patient teaching includes instructing the patient to eat small, frequent meals, avoid high-carbohydrate foods, restrict fluids with meals, and rest after meals.

Surgical Procedures for Lower Gastrointestinal Bleeding

With adequate medical therapy, most lower GI bleeding stops spontaneously. However, surgical

TABLE 44–11. Postoperative Complications

Wound infection
Dehiscence/evisceration
Hemorrhage
Peritonitis
Pancreatitis
Anastomotic leak
Duodenal stump leak
Afferent loop syndrome
Stomach wall necrosis
Anastomotic loop necrosis
Postoperative enteritis or necrosis
Subphrenic/subhepatic abscesses
Postoperative jaundice
Gastric retention

TABLE 44–12. Causes of Hemorrhage Following Gastric Surgery

Extraluminal	Intraluminal
Slipped arterial ligatures	Intraluminal
Unligated vessels	Missed ulcers
Liver lacerations	Stress ulcers/erosions
Pancreatic injuries	Mucosal injuries
Coagulation disturbances	Loose anastomotic sutures
	Suture dehiscence
	Coagulation disorder

treatment is indicated when complications such as uncontrolled hemorrhage, perforation, or obstruction occurs. Extent of surgical resection depends on the source of the problem (Table 44–13).

Implications for Care. Removal of any part of the intestinal tract has an effect on the normal digestive, absorption, and elimination functions. Although operations involving segmental resection with reanastomosis affect these functions only minimally, major resections involving removal of large sections or all of the large intestine with creation of an ostomy produce significant changes for the patient. Removal of the entire colon as treatment for ulcerative colitis necessitates the creation of an ileostomy. Because of the loss of the large bowel for fluid reabsorption, drainage through the ileostomy is very liquid and unformed. With the conventional ileostomy, an appliance must be worn at all times. Skin protection is important because the drainage contains digestive enzymes that cause extreme excoriation of the skin. The area surrounding the stoma should be kept clean and dry. Protective barriers such as karaya gum and Stomahesive (Squibb) provide skin protection from the corrosive drainage. Appliances must be applied snugly around the stoma.

TABLE 44–13. Common Surgical Treatment of Lower Gastrointestinal Bleeding*

Condition	Surgical Procedure Used
Ulcerative colitis	Total colectomy with creation of an ileostomy
Diverticulitis	Ligation and removal of sac(s) Segmental resection Temporary colostomy may be necessary
Colorectal cancer	Colon resection (right hemicolectomy, transverse colon resection, left hemicolectomy, abdominal-perineal resection) Colostomy may be necessary
Hemorrhoids	Hemorrhoidectomy

*Surgical procedures may vary based on patient's condition and physician preference.

Two alternative surgical approaches are also used in creating an ileostomy (Fig. 44–8). These approaches give the patient more control over elimination. The continent Kock pouch involves creation of a pouch from the terminal ileum that is sutured to the abdominal wall. A nipple valve is constructed as an outlet. The pouch reservoir retains the feces until the patient drains it with a catheter. This must be done several times a day. No appliance is necessary unless the valve becomes incompetent. The other approach involves construction of an ileal pouch–anal anastomosis. Because the anal sphincter is intact, the patient retains voluntary control of elimination.

Resection of the colon may necessitate the creation of a temporary or permanent colostomy. A temporary colostomy is done if the goal is to divert the fecal flow from an inflamed area to allow healing. Because fluid absorption occurs in the large intestine, the stool eliminated from the colostomy is more formed than that eliminated from an ileostomy. The stool becomes more formed when the colostomy is nearer the terminal portion of the colon. An appliance is not always necessary depending on the location of the colostomy and the preferences of the patient. Some patients are able to control elimination through daily irrigations. Skin protection from drainage is necessary to prevent skin excoriation and breakdown.

Postoperative concerns during the critical care phase include assessment of the stoma for signs of ischemia such as cyanosis or necrosis, abdominal assessment for distention, and observation of patient status for signs and symptoms of fluid and electrolyte imbalances. Function of the ostomy including the color, amount, and consistency should be noted. Temperature and white blood cell count should be monitored for signs of infection. As patient recovery progresses, patient and family teaching about the ostomy and its care is necessary. Referral to the nurse enterostomal therapist and local support groups will help the patient deal physically and psychologically with the change in body image and function.

If an abdominal-perineal reaction is done, the patient will have a perineal wound in addition to a colostomy and abdominal incision. Frequent dressing changes are necessary because drainage is usually profuse in the first 24 to 48 hours. Wound irrigations and packings are usually done to debride the wound and stimulate granulation. Profuse bleeding or purulent drainage should be reported immediately. The patient should be positioned to avoid pressure on the perineal wound. Postoperative complications include hemorrhage, wound infection, dehiscence, peritonitis, obstruction, and pneumonia.

Although patients with lower GI bleeding are not seen as frequently in critical care units as those with an upper GI bleed, their care provides unique challenges for the critical care nurse. Astute assessment

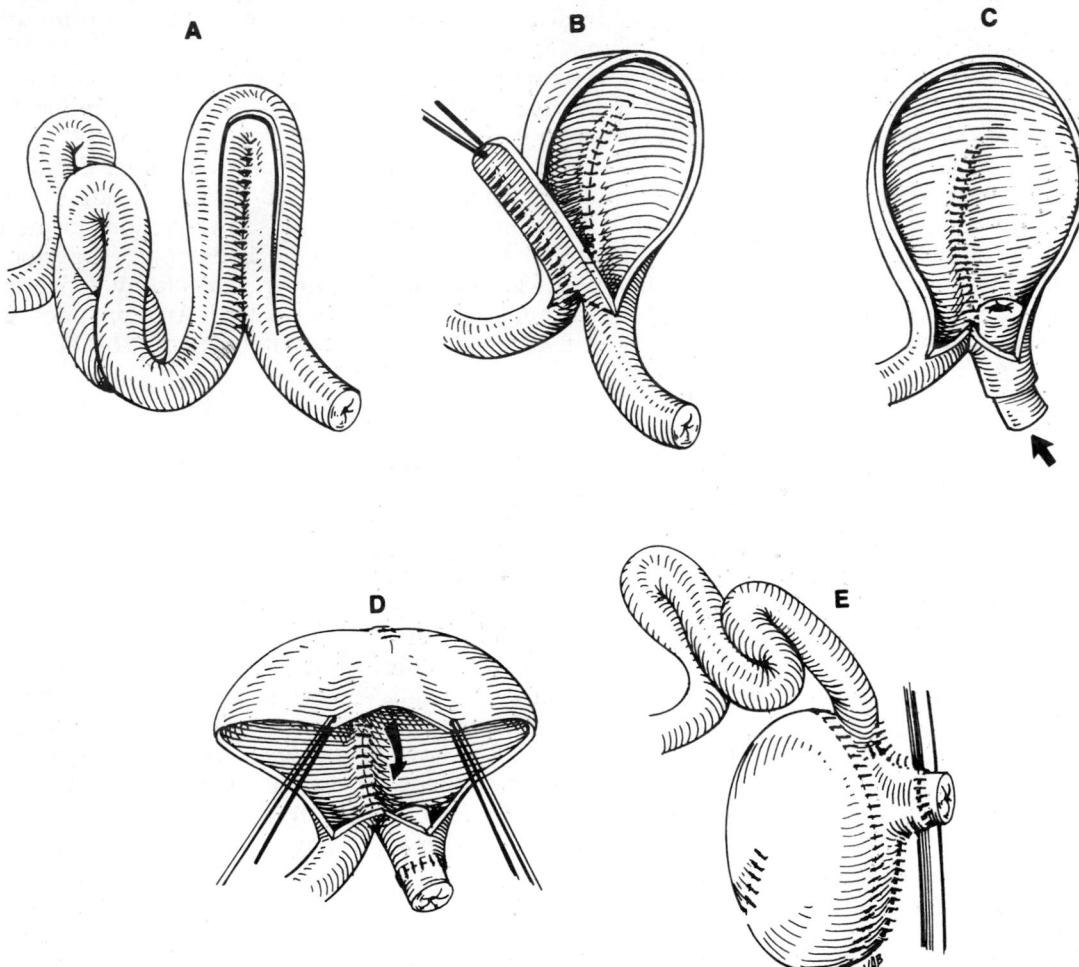

FIGURE 44–8. Continent Kock pouch. *A,* Loop of bowel sewn together. *B,* Removal of anterior portion. *C,* Nipple valve made by pushing bowel back on itself. *D,* Pouch formation. *E,* End brought through stoma. (From Long, B., and Phipps, W. (1989). *Medical-surgical nursing: A nursing process approach* (p. 1099). St. Louis, C. V. Mosby.)

and systemic support can result in stabilization. If surgical intervention becomes necessary, nursing care is aimed at preventing postoperative complications, implementing patient teaching, and providing emotional support in dealing with alterations in body image, body function, and life style.

NURSING DIAGNOSES AND INTERVENTIONS

The patient with acute GI bleeding presents a challenge to the critical care nurse. Nursing management includes close assessment and monitoring of the patient to establish and support a stable condition. An understanding of treatment modalities and their effects and side effects is essential. Special

TABLE 44–14. Primary Nursing Diagnoses for the Patient Following Gastric Surgery

Alteration in comfort related to	Incision
Impaired gas exchange related to	Anesthesia effects Location of incision Aspiration of gastric material
Altered nutrition: less than body requirements related to	Loss of intrinsic factor for vitamin B_{12} absorption Reduced absorption of calcium and vitamin D Reduction in pancreatic juices and bile (in Billroth II and gastrectomy) Iron deficiency (in duodenal bypass procedures) Increased metabolic need
Diarrhea related to	Dumping syndrome
Potential for infection related to	Organism invading wound Hematoma formation Decreased local blood flow Malnutrition
Potential fluid volume deficit related to	Operative fluid losses Postoperative bleeding Nasogastric losses Diarrhea (dumping syndrome) Inadequate intake
Knowledge deficit related to	Wound care Dietary needs or restrictions Possible complications or treatments
Anxiety related to	Body function changes Dietary needs or restrictions Life-style changes Body image changes

TABLE 44–15. Primary Nursing Diagnoses for the Patient Following Intestinal Surgery

Alteration in comfort related to	Incision/wound Surgical manipulation
Impaired gas exchange related to	Anesthesia effects Location of incision Postoperative pain
Diarrhea related to	Loss of route for fluid absorption
Altered nutrition: less than body requirements related to	Electrolyte losses (Na, K, Ca) Loss of fat and protein digestion (in small intestine resection) Decreased fat-soluble vitamin (A, D, E, K) absorption Increased metabolic need
Body image disturbance related to	Change in elimination route (ileostomy or colostomy)
Potential fluid volume deficit related to	Operative fluid losses Nasogastric losses Diarrhea Decreased fluid absorption Inadequate intake
Anxiety related to	Altered body functions Life-style changes Real or perceived alterations in sexual function Loss of control
Potential for infection related to	Decreased wound healing (poststeroid treatment) Disruption of bowel with spread of flora
Potential for impaired skin integrity	Surgical incision or resection Fistula formation Drainage from ostomy Decreased wound healing
Knowledge deficit related to	Wound care Ostomy care or ostomy products Dietary needs or restrictions Possible complications Need for local support groups (i.e., ostomy, cancer)

consideration should be given to providing emotional support to the patient and family, because this crisis can be extremely anxiety producing.

The following nursing care plan presents the basic nursing diagnoses and interventions for a patient experiencing GI bleeding. Due to the variety of possible etiologies, it is important to individualize care plans for each patient. Table 44–14 addresses the primary nursing diagnoses for the patient who has had gastric surgery, and Table 44–15 includes nursing diagnoses for the patient who has undergone intestinal surgery.

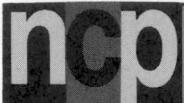 **nursing care plan**

1. Actual fluid volume deficit related to:
Decreased circulatory volume
Active blood losses
Losses from vomiting, diarrhea, and nasogastric tube

Outcome Criteria	Nursing Interventions
Vital signs stable Hemodynamic parameters within normal range for patient Urine output at least 30 mL/hour	*(Note:* Frequency of measurements depends on present clinical condition) 1. Monitor intake and output every hour. 2. Monitor vital signs including orthostatic vital signs. Be alert for a systolic decrease of 10 mm Hg or more and an increase in pulse of 10 bpm or more, which reflects a volume depletion of 15% to 20%. 3. Monitor level of consciousness for signs of confusion or decreased awareness. 4. Monitor hemodynamic parameters (CVP, pulmonary arterial pressure, systemic venous resistance, pulmonary capillary wedge pressure, cardiac output). 5. Monitor CBC, electrolytes, clotting studies, BUN, and creatinine. 6. Administer crystalloid solutions as ordered. Observe patient for signs and symptoms of fluid overload such as pulmonary congestion, distended neck veins, elevated CVP. 7. Weigh daily. A change in weight of 1 kg reflects a fluid loss or retention of 1 liter. 8. Administer blood products as ordered. Observe for signs and symptoms of transfusion reactions or other complications (Table 44–6). 9. Assess mucous membranes and skin turgor for hydration. 10. Provide frequent oral hygiene and skin care.

2. Altered tissue perfusion related to:
Decreased oxygen transport
Increased oxygen tissue demand
Metabolic acidosis
Vasoconstriction

Outcome Criteria	Nursing Interventions
Vital signs stable Warm, dry skin; rapid capillary refill Urine output at least 30 mL/hour Arterial blood gases within normal range for patient Hemoglobin and hematocrit within normal range for patient S_vO_2 60–80	1. Monitor hematocrit and hemoglobin every 2 to 4 hours until stable. Hypovolemia may cause false elevations in the values. 2. Monitor arterial blood gases. Be alert for P_{O_2} less than 80 and O_2 saturation below 90%. (Oximetry may also be used for assessing O_2 saturation.) 3. Monitor urine output every hour. 4. Monitor ECG for ischemic changes and dysrhythmias. 5. Monitor respiratory status for signs of distress. 6. Assess skin for color, temperature, dryness, pulses, and capillary refill. 7. Assess for alterations in level of consciousness. 8. Administer oxygen as ordered. 9. Reduce tissue oxygen demands through bedrest and comfort measures; reduce fever if present. Monitor S_vO_2 for changes. 10. Place patient in Fowler's or semi-Fowler's position to support perfusion to organ systems. 11. Position patient to maintain a patent airway. 12. Position patient to prevent aspiration.

3. Potential for injury related to:
Development of stress ulcers
Failure to control bleeding source
Nasogastric intubation
Altered levels of consciousness

Outcome Criteria	Nursing Interventions
Gastric pH maintained at over 3.5 No evidence of bleeding Minimal discomfort from nasogastric intubation Full level of consciousness exhibited	1. Perform gastric lavage until returned fluid is clear with saline or tap water as indicated for active bleeding. Notify physician if active bleeding occurs. 2. Test gastric aspirate every 1 to 4 hours as indicated for occult blood and pH. Administer antacids as ordered to maintain gastric pH above 3.5. (*Note:* pH indicator paper that tests below 4.5 must be used.) Irrigate and clamp nasogastric tube for 30 minutes after administration. 3. Administer H_2 receptor antagonists to maintain adequate blood levels of drug. If given orally with antacids, stagger administration by at least 1 hour. 4. Stagger administration of sucralfate and antacids so that there is at least a 30-minute interval between their administration times. 5. Maintain nasogastric suction at low level to avoid further trauma to gastric mucosa. 6. Maintain tube placement and patency; observe for abdominal distention. 7. Retape nasogastric tube every shift to avoid erosion of the nares. 8. Provide frequent oral hygiene. Avoid the use of lemon and glycerine swabs, which can be drying to the mucosa. 9. Measure and record gastric drainage every shift. Describe color and consistency. (*Note:* For personal protection wear gloves when handling any body fluid and during exposure to bloody substances.) 10. Monitor serum electrolytes. 11. Test all stools for occult blood. Record stool frequency, color, and consistency. 12. Auscultate bowel sounds every 4 to 8 hours. Hyperactive bowel sounds may indicate the presence of blood in the intestines, whereas absence of bowel sounds may indicate an ileus perforation, or peritonitis. 13. Provide safety measures such as side rails and soft restraints, if necessary, to protect the patient if changes in mentation occur.

4. Anxiety related to:
   Fear of death
   Sight of blood
   Procedures/treatments
   Anemia

Outcome Criteria	Nursing Interventions
Verbalizes feelings Expresses (verbally or nonverbally) feeling of relaxation	(*Note:* Include family members in interventions to decrease their feelings of anxiety and helplessness.) 1. Explain all procedures and equipment. 2. Encourage patient to verbalize fears and concerns, and address these accordingly. 3. Assess nonverbal behavior for inconsistencies with verbal expressions. 4. Use touch as a fear-allaying technique. 5. Focus on positive treatment outcomes when reached (i.e., increase in hematocrit and hemoglobin values, lack of present bleeding, stable vital signs.) 6. Allow patient an opportunity to make choices about his care. 7. Keep family informed about patient's condition and positive treatment outcomes as reached. Assist patient and family in setting realistic goals. Arrange for chaplain intervention or other support sources if warranted. 8. Allow family to participate in care as much as possible and as condition allows. 9. In the case of unsuccessful treatment outcomes, provide emotional support to patient and family in reaching difficult decisions and accepting the inevitable outcome.

5. Knowledge deficit related to:
   Contributing factors (i.e., diet, medications, smoking, alcohol, life style)
   Treatment regimen

Outcome Criteria	Nursing Interventions
Verbalizes understanding of causes of bleeding and effect of contributing factors on condition Uses stress management techniques	1. Assess understanding of cause of present condition (if known). Consult with physician for patient teaching plan concerning etiology. 2. When patient is ready, institute teaching concerning the purpose, dose, schedule, and side effects of medications (i.e., antacids, H_2 receptor antagonists). 3. Review the signs and symptoms of recurrent bleeding (i.e., pain, tarry stools, bloody or coffee-ground emesis) upon which medical attention should be sought. 4. Assess risk factors (i.e., smoking, alcohol use) that contribute to delayed healing and gastric irritation. Institute teaching accordingly. 5. Discuss dietary changes if necessary (i.e., restrictions on coffee, chocolate, hot and spicy foods, high roughage, and milk products, which may contibute to mucosal irritation, acid secretion, or varices irritation). 6. Discuss life-style modifications to reduce stress and instruct the patient about stress management techniques (i.e., deep breathing exercises, physical exercise, imagery). Refer to counseling groups if warranted. 7. Discuss the effects of medications such as aspirin and nonsteroidal anti-inflammatory agents on the gastrointestinal system. Educate the patient and family about reading labels on over-the-counter drugs for such ingredients.

SUMMARY

Most patients who require admission to the critical care unit are bleeding from an upper GI source, and one out of ten of these will die (Hurst, 1988). Gastrointestinal bleeding is caused by a myriad of primary disease processes. Clinical management of the patient with GI hemorrhage depends upon the site, extent, and rate of bleeding. The foremost consideration is the necessity to maintain adequate intravascular volume and circulatory stability. After this has been established, the second treatment priority is to control the source of bleeding.

The critical care nurse can significantly affect the patient's clinical progress. Nursing assessment must be astute and accurate. Because the acuity level of the patient is often labile, it is frequently necessary to update the nursing care plan. Prognosis will depend upon the pathophysiology, but outcome is often positive because most patients cease bleeding spontaneously before medical or surgical intervention is required.

References

Adrien, L. M., and Mailhot, C. B. (1986). Fecal occult blood test. In *Diagnostics* (2nd ed., pp. 804–806). Springhouse, PA: Springhouse Corporation.

Altman, D. F. (1987). Drugs used in gastrointestinal diseases. In B. G. Katzung (Ed.), *Basic and clinical pharmacology* (3rd ed., pp. 781–787). Norwalk, CT: Appleton & Lange.

Barsan, W. G., and Baker, P. B. (1988). Upper gastrointestinal tract disorders. In P. Rosen, E. J. Baker, R. M. Barkin, et al. (Eds.), *Emergency medicine: Concepts and clinical practice* (Vol. 2, pp. 1403–1432). St. Louis: C.V. Mosby.

Bitterman, R. A. (1988). General disorders of the large intestine. In P. Rosen, F. J. Baker, R. M. Barkin, et al. (Eds.), *Emergency medicine: Concepts and clinical practice* (Vol. 2, pp. 1479–1493). St. Louis: C.V. Mosby.

Bogoch, A. (1985). Bleeding. In J. E. Berk (Ed.), *Bockus gastroenterology* (4th ed., Vol. 1, pp. 65–110). Philadelphia: W. B. Saunders.

Bowen, J. C. (1984). Surgical therapy in stress ulcerations. *Scandinavian Journal of Gastroenterology*, 19 (Suppl. 105), 97–99.

Driks, M. R., Craven, D. E., Celli, B. R., et al. (1987). Nosocomial pneumonia in intubated patients given sucralfate as compared with antacids or histamine type 2 blockers. *New England Journal of Medicine*, 317 (22), 1376–1382.

Dworken, H. J. (1989). Gastrointestinal hemorrhage. In W. C. Shoemaker, S. Ayres, A. Grenvik, et al. (Eds.), *Textbook of critical care medicine* (2nd ed., pp. 697–703). Philadelphia: W. B. Saunders.

Eastwood, G. L. (1983). Gastritis and other gastric diseases. In J. S. Trier and J. H. Stein (Eds.), *Internal medicine* (pp. 104–107). Boston: Little, Brown.

Elashoff, J. D., and Grossman, M. I. (1980). Trends in hospital admissions and death rates for peptic ulcer in the United States from 1970 to 1978. *Gastroenterology*, 78 (2), 280–285.

Fall, D. J. (1986). Gastrointestinal disorders: Stomach and duodenum. In S. A. Price and L. M. Wilson (Eds.), *Pathophysiology: Clinical concepts of disease processes* (3rd ed., pp. 242–258). New York: McGraw-Hill.

Gelman, S., and Ernst, E. (1978). Nitroprusside prevents adverse hemodynamic effects of vasopressin. *Archives of Surgery*, 113, 1465–1471.

Gimson, A., Westaby, D., Hegarty, J., et al. (1986). A randomized trial of vasopressin and vasopressin plus nitroglycerin in the control of acute variceal hemorrhage. *Hepatology*, 6, 406–409.

Glickman, R. M. (1987). Inflammatory bowel disease: Ulcerative colitis and Crohn's disease. In E. Braunwald, K. J. Isselbacher, R. G. Petersdorf, et al. (Eds.), *Harrison's principles of internal medicine* (11th ed., pp. 1277–1290). New York: McGraw-Hill.

Gottlieb, J., Menaske, P., and Cruz, E. (1986). Gastrointestinal complications in critically ill patients: The intensitivist's overview. *American Journal of Gastroenterology*, 81 (4), 227–238.

Grendell, J. H. (1988). Upper gastrointestinal bleeding. In J. M. Luce and D. J. Pierson (Eds.), *Critical care medicine* (pp. 385–388). Philadelphia: W. B. Saunders.

Haeney, M. (1989). Gastrointestinal disease in the immunocompromised host. In L. A. Turnberg (Ed.), *Clinical gastroenterology* (pp. 317–355). Boston: Blackwell Scientific Publications.

Haring, R., and Berger, G. (1988). Postoperative complications and postoperative care. In H. D. Becker, C. Herforth, W. Lierse, et al. (Eds.), *Surgery of the stomach: Indications, methods, complications* (pp. 331–366). New York: Springer-Verlag.

Hurst, J. (1988). Gastrointestinal bleeding. In J. Civetta, R. Taylor, and R. Kirby (Eds.), *Critical care* (pp. 1271–1281). Philadelphia: J. B. Lippincott.

Kafonek, D. R., Herlong F., Giardiello, F. M., et al. (1988). Gastrointestinal bleeding. In A. M. Harvey, R. J. Johns, V. A. McKusick, et al. (Eds.), *The principles and practices of medicine* (26th ed., pp. 805–812). Norwalk, CT: Appleton & Lange.

Kang, J. Y., and Piper, D. W. (1980). Improvement in mortality rates in bleeding peptic ulcer disease. *Medical Journal of Australia*, 1 (5), 213–215.

Knauer, C. M., and Silverman, S. (1989). Alimentary tract and liver. In S. A. Schroeder, M. A. Krypp, L. M. Tierney, et al. (Eds.), *Current medical diagnosis and treatment* (pp. 343–428). Norwalk, CT: Appleton & Lange.

MacDonald, W. C., and Rubin, C. E. (1987). Gastric tumors, gastritis, and other gastric diseases. In E. Braunwald, K. J. Isselbacher, R. G. Petersdorf, et al. (Eds.), *Harrison's principles of internal medicine* (11th ed., pp. 1253–1260). New York: McGraw-Hill.

McEvoy, G. K. (Ed.) (1988). *Drug information 1988* (pp. 1606–1612). Bethesda: American Society of Hospital Pharmacists.

Miller, B. F., and Keane, C. B. (1987). *Encyclopedia and dictionary of medicine, nursing and allied health* (4th ed.). Philadelphia: W. B. Saunders.

Patras, A. Z., and Walsh, M. (1985). Intervening in upper GI inflammation. In *Gastrointestinal disorders* (pp. 88–99). Springhouse, PA: Springhouse Corporation.

Peterson, W. L. (1989). Gastrointestinal bleeding. In M. H. Sleisenger and J. S. Fordtran (Eds.), *Gastrointestinal disease: Pathophysiology, diagnosis, management* (4th ed., pp. 397–427). Philadelphia: W. B. Saunders.

Porth, C. M. (Ed.) (1990). *Pathophysiology: Concepts of altered health states* (3rd ed., pp. 697–718). Philadelphia: J. B. Lippincott.

Quigley, E. M. (1989). Acute upper gastrointestinal hemorrhage. In L. A. Turnberg (Ed.), *Clinical gastroenterology* (pp. 54–86). Boston: Blackwell Scientific Publications.

Robbins, S. L., and Cotran, R. S. (1989). Fluid and hemodynamic derangements—shock. In R. S. Cotran, V. Kumar, and S. L. Robbins (Eds.), *Robbins pathologic basis of disease* (4th ed., pp. 138–140). Philadelphia: W. B. Saunders.

Robbins, S. L., and Kumar, V. (1987). The gastrointestinal tract. In *Basic pathology* (4th ed., pp. 506–563). Philadephia: W. B. Saunders.

Robert, A., and Kauffman, G. L. (1989). Stress ulcers, erosions, and gastric mucosal injury. In M. H. Sleisenger and J. S. Fordtran (Eds.), *Gastrointestinal disease: Pathophysiology, diagnosis, management* (4th ed., pp. 772–792). Philadelphia: W. B. Saunders.

Ross, J., and Covell, J. W. (1985). Heart failure, hypertrophy, and other abnormal circulatory states. In J. B. West (Ed.), *Best and Taylor's physiological basis of practice* (11th ed., pp. 307–308). Baltimore: Williams & Wilkins.

Schiller, L. R. (1988). Epidemiology, clinical manifestations, and diagnosis. In J. B. Wyngaarden and L. H. Smith (Eds.), *Cecil textbook of medicine* (Vol. 1, pp. 684–688). Philadelphia: W. B. Saunders.

Severance, S. R. (1986). Gastrointestinal bleeding. In D. A. Zschoche (Ed.), *Mosby's comprehensive review of medicine* (3rd ed., pp. 540–552). St. Louis: C. V. Mosby.

Silverstein, F. E., Gilbert, D. A., Tedesco, F. J., et al. (1981). The National ASGE survey on upper gastrointestinal bleeding study design and baseline data. *Gastrointestinal Endoscopy*, 27 (1), 73–79.

Spiro, H. M. (1983). *Clinical gastroenterology* (3rd ed., pp. 88–128). New York: Macmillan.

Stephens, G. J. (1980). Disorders of water and solute balance. In *Pathophysiology for health practitioners* (pp. 21–27). New York: Macmillan.

Thompson, A. B., and Mahachai, V. (1985). Medical management of uncomplicated peptic ulcer disease. In J. E. Berk (Ed.), *Bockus gastroenterology* (4th ed., Vol. 2, pp. 1116–1154). Philadelphia: W. B. Saunders.

Tobin, M. J. (1989). *Essentials of critical care medicine* (pp. 409–419). New York: Churchill Livingstone.

Tryba, M. (1987). Risk of acute stress bleeding and nosocomial pneumonia in ventilated intensive care unit patients: Sucrafate versus antacids. *American Journal of Medicine*, 83 (Suppl. 3B), 117–124.

Patients with Liver Dysfunction

Susan L. Smith

ANATOMY OF THE LIVER AND HEPATOBILIARY SYSTEM

The Liver

The liver is the largest solid organ in the body, weighing about 1.5 kg in the adult. It is located mostly in the right upper quadrant (RUQ) but extends across the midline into the left upper quadrant (LUQ). In the RUQ the superior aspect of the liver lies at about the level of the fifth rib or, more simply stated, at the level of the nipples (Fig. 45–1). The inferior aspect does not extend more than 1 to 2 cm below the right costal margin in normal conditions.

The liver can be anatomically divided into two main lobes, right and left (Fig. 45–2*A*). The imaginary line that separates the two lobes runs from the fossa of the inferior vena cava (IVC) above to the notch of the gallbladder below. The right lobe can be further divided into anterior and posterior segments (Fig. 45–2*B* and *C*), which can be further divided into superior and inferior subsegments. The left lobe can likewise be divided into medial and lateral segments and further subdivided into superior and inferior subsegments.

The right and left lobes are divided anteriorly by the falciform ligament, inferiorly by the ligamentum teres, and posteriorly by the ligamentum venosum (the remnant of the embryonic venous shunt between the umbilical and caval vessels). However, this division does not correspond to the intrahepatic branching and distribution of blood vessels and bile ducts. Although the right lobe appears to be much larger than the left, they are actually almost equal in size.

The liver is attached to the anterior abdominal wall and the inferior surface of the diaphragm by the coronary, triangular, falciform, and round ligaments. The anterior and posterior coronary ligaments secure the liver to the diaphragm. The right and left triangular ligaments are formed by leaves of the coronary ligaments. The anterior coronary ligament forms a fold over the superior surface of the liver, dividing the medial and lateral segments of the left lobe. This fold is the falciform ligament. The round ligament (ligamentum teres) emerges between the two layers of the falciform ligament. At the porta hepatis, the visceral peritoneum of the liver forms the lesser omentum, which extends as the gastrohepatic ligament to the lesser curvature of the stomach.

The porta hepatis or hilum is a fissure on the inferior surface of the right lobe. The portal vein and

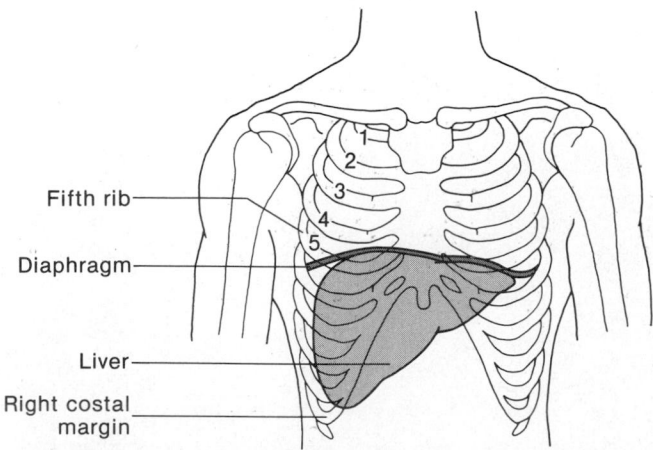

FIGURE 45–1. Anatomic location of the liver. The upper border normally lies at the level of the fourth intercostal space or fifth rib, and the lower border does not normally extend more than 1 to 2 cm below the right costal margin.

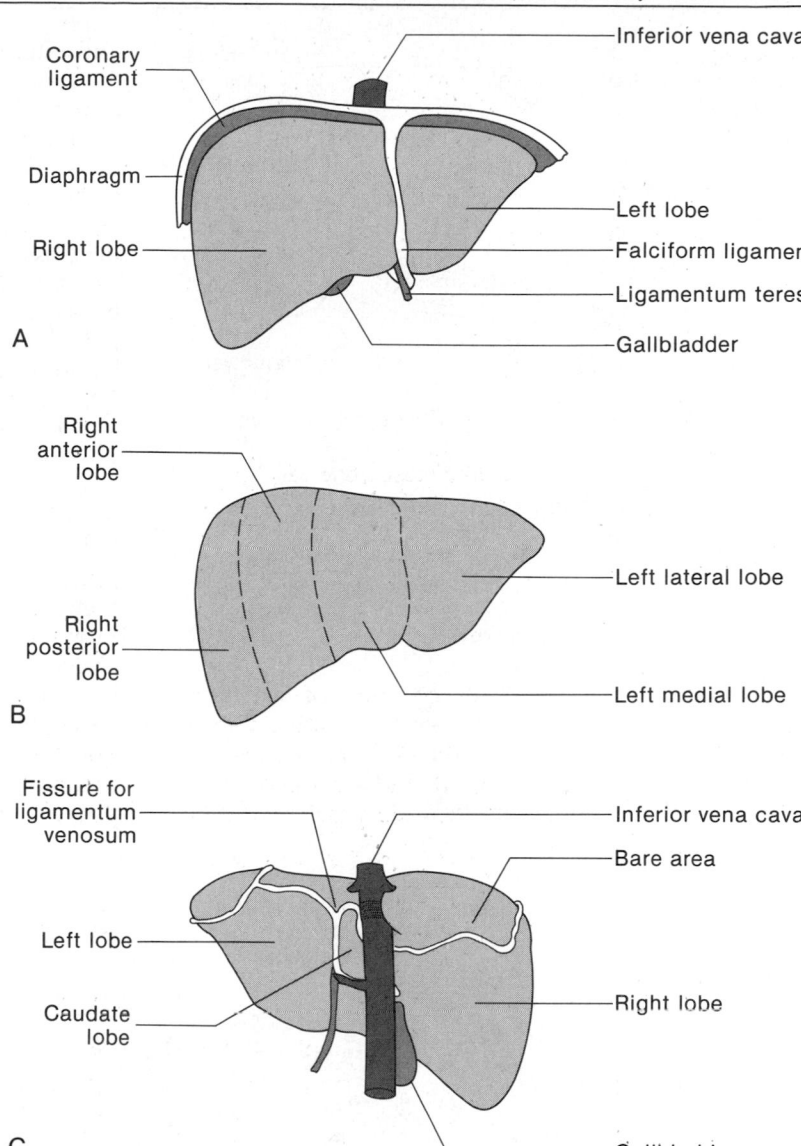

FIGURE 45–2. *A,* Anterior view of the liver. *B,* Segments of the liver, anterior view. *C,* Posterior view of the liver.

hepatic artery enter the liver through the porta hepatis, and the common bile duct exits the liver at the porta hepatis.

Portal Circulation

The liver is a highly vascular organ that holds about 600 mL of blood at any given time. However, the venous capacitance of the liver is great, allowing for expansion of its blood volume to approximately 1 liter in conditions such as hypervolemia or right heart failure. Approximately 25% of the cardiac output flows through the liver before it is returned by the IVC to the right atrium.

The liver has an unusual vascular system in that both a vein and an artery supply blood to the liver. The larger portal vein is formed behind the pancreas

by the confluence of the superior mesenteric and the splenic veins (Fig. 45–3). The portal vein delivers about two-thirds of the liver's blood supply. The superior mesenteric vein and the portal vein drain the splanchnic circulation; portal venous blood therefore is rich in nutrients and insulin. The smaller hepatic artery branches off the aorta at the celiac axis and divides into the right and left hepatic arteries just before it enters the liver adjacent to the portal vein. It delivers about one-third of the liver's blood supply and is the liver's chief source of oxygen.

Glisson's capsule is an innervated membrane that covers the liver and lies beneath the visceral peritoneum. This capsule converges at and enters the liver at the porta hepatis. Inside the porta hepatis this membrane branches to form the division tracts for the portal vein and the hepatic artery. Within the liver the portal vein and hepatic artery divide and form thousands of branches to the right and left

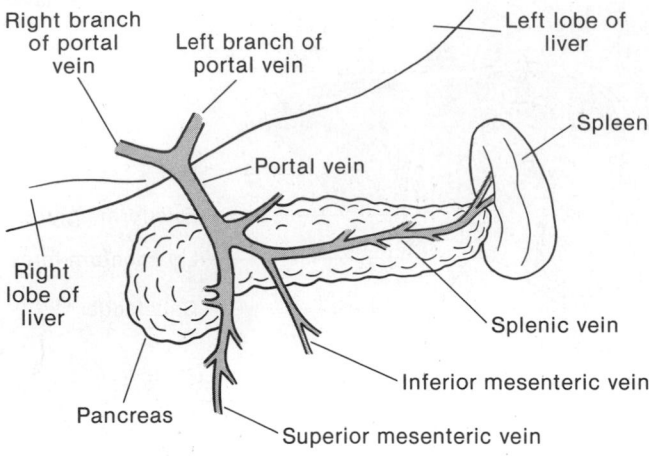

FIGURE 45–3. Portal venous circulation.

and efferent (hepatic venule) blood supply (Fig. 45–4). Small parallel branches of the portal vein and hepatic artery, called venules and arterioles, respectively, perfuse the lobules. Blood from these vessels flows through structures called sinusoids before it empties into tributaries of the hepatic veins and is carried from the liver. Sinusoidal blood is a mixture of blood from the portal venous and hepatic arterial systems. Exchange of oxygen, nutrients, and waste between blood and hepatocytes occurs in the sinusoids. Normally, two or three hepatic veins drain blood from the liver into the IVC. Together with small bile ducts that *exit* the lobules, portal venules and hepatic arterioles make up what are referred to as *portal triads*. Portal triads lie at the center of each lobule, and hepatic venules lie at the periphery of each lobule.

The walls of hepatic sinusoids contain highly phagocytic cells called *Kupffer cells*. Kupffer cells are members of the mononuclear phagocytic system. They function to remove particulate matter (denatured protein, lysosomal enzymes, foreign particles, bacteria, yeasts, viruses, and endotoxin) from the vascular system by removing it from the portal blood. The *space of Disse* is a tissue space located between the hepatocytes and sinusoidal cells. Hepatic lymphatics are located in periportal connective tissue

lobes. Portal and arterial inflow vessels unite at the level of the hepatic sinusoids.

Normal hepatic structure consists of functional units called simple hepatic acini or lobules. Lobules are composed of small cords of hepatocytes supported by a reticulin framework and arranged around their afferent (portal venule and hepatic arteriole)

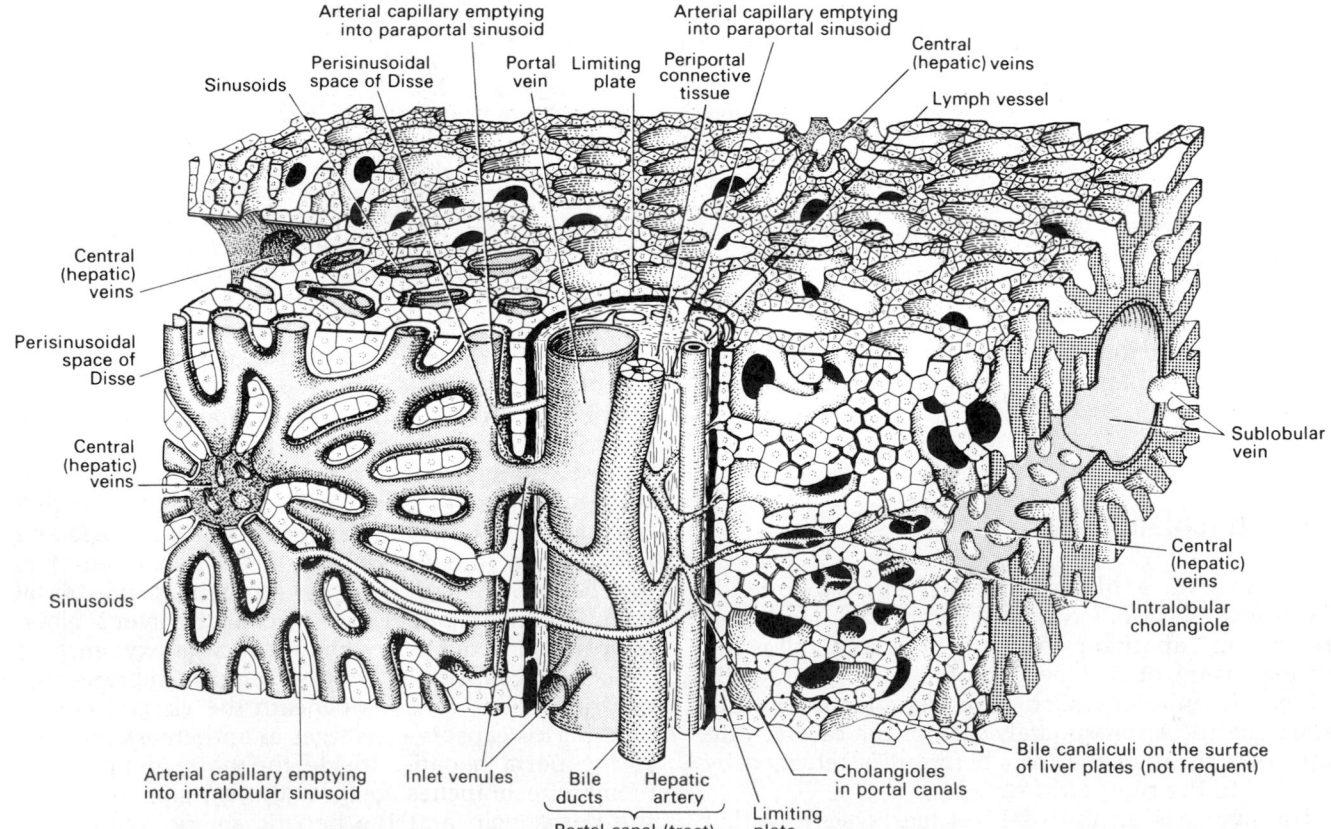

FIGURE 45–4. Synopsis of the structure of the normal human liver. (From Sherlock S. (1985). *Diseases of the liver and biliary system* (7th ed., p. 7). London: Blackwell Scientific Publications.)

and are lined with endothelial cells that allow uptake of hepatic interstitial fluid. When sinusoidal pressure increases, lymph production in the space of Disse increases, contributing to ascites formation when hepatic outflow obstruction occurs. To summarize, blood enters the liver by the portal vein and hepatic artery, is filtered free of foreign matter through hepatic sinusoids, and empties into the central veins. The central veins drain into two or three large hepatic veins that empty into the IVC.

Excretory System of the Liver

A major function of the liver is the production and secretion of bile. The bile excretory system begins as tiny bile canaliculi that emerge from hepatocytes and drain into terminal bile ductules. Terminal ductules branch into larger and larger ducts, until eventually large right and left hepatic ducts are formed (Fig. 45–5). The right and left hepatic bile ducts join to form the common hepatic duct. The common bile duct is then formed by the confluence of the common hepatic duct and the cystic duct from the gallbladder. The common bile duct enters the duodenum at the ampulla of Vater. The terminal end of the common bile duct is the sphincter of Oddi.

The gallbladder is a small, pear-shaped organ that lies under the surface of the right lobe of the liver. The function of the gallbladder is to store and concentrate bile. Although the liver produces about 1 liter of bile/day, the capacity of the gallbladder for bile is only about 50 mL. When chyme enters the duodenum from the stomach, the hormone cholecystokinin is secreted from the duodenum, causing the gallbladder to contract and the sphincter of Oddi to relax so that bile can flow into the intestine to participate in digestion and metabolism of fats.

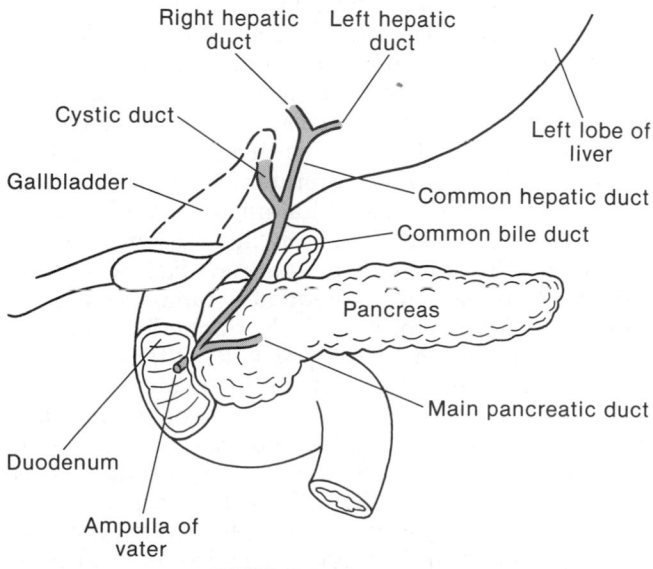

FIGURE 45–5. Biliary tract.

PHYSIOLOGY OF THE LIVER AND HEPATOBILIARY SYSTEM

Liver Function

The chemical versatility of the liver allows it to perform more than 400 separate functions (Sherlock, 1985). However, liver function can be summarized to include the synthesis of bile acids and excretion of bilirubin, carbohydrate metabolism, synthesis and release of plasma proteins, amino acid metabolism, conversion of ammonia to a less toxic substance, lipid metabolism, storage of fat-soluble vitamins and iron, detoxification of drugs, inactivation of hormones, control of procoagulants and removal of products of coagulation, and phagocytosis of foreign antigen.

BILE PRODUCTION AND BILIRUBIN METABOLISM

Bile acids, which largely consist of bile salts, are synthesized only by the liver as derivatives of cholesterol synthesis. Bile acids are conjugated in the liver with glycine or taurine to form bile salts. Bile salts are then excreted by active transport mechanisms into bile canaliculi and carried to the small intestine, where they are used to solubilize cholesterol in bile, emulsify and absorb fat, assist the pancreas with lipolysis, and secrete gastrointestinal hormones. In the ileum bile salts are reabsorbed and are eventually circulated through the liver by portal venous blood, where they are reconjugated and reexcreted. Bile salt deficiency results in cholelithiasis (the formation of gallstones) and the malabsorption of fats.

Cholestasis, or the failure of normal amounts of bile to reach the duodenum, can result from inhibition of bile flow anywhere from the conjugating site in the hepatocytes to the duodenum. Cholestasis results in the accumulation of bile in the hepatocytes and bile ducts and is manifested clinically by elevation of serum bile acid levels and differing degrees of jaundice. Prolonged cholestasis leads to biliary cirrhosis (Galambos, 1979). Bilirubin is the chief bile pigment and is the end product of heme released during the metabolism of hemoglobin, myoglobin, and respiratory enzymes. Approximately 80% of bilirubin is formed in the reticuloendothelial cells of the liver, and 20% is formed in the bone marrow. Approximately 6 g of hemoglobin is metabolized to approximately 30 mg of bilirubin each day. Bilirubin formed in the liver and bone marrow is called *unconjugated* bilirubin. Unconjugated bilirubin is lipid-soluble and is tightly bound in the plasma to albumin. In this form it is extracted by the liver and *conjugated* to a water-soluble form so that it can be excreted.

Normal serum bilirubin level is 0.2 to 0.9 mg/dL. Serum bilirubin can be measured as *total* bilirubin, *indirect* (unconjugated) bilirubin, or *direct* (conjugated) bilirubin. The normal indirect bilirubin level is 0.1 to 0.5 mg/dL, and the normal direct bilirubin level is 0.1 to 0.4 mg/dL. Therefore, the total bilirubin level is about 0.2 to 0.9 mg/dL. Indirect bilirubin is elevated in conditions such as hepatocellular necrosis and hemolysis, whereas direct bilirubin is elevated during cholestasis.

Jaundice, the most visibly apparent manifestation of altered bilirubin metabolism, can be obstructive, hepatocellular, or hemolytic in etiology. *Obstructive jaundice* occurs most commonly from biliary duct stones but also from cancer of the head of the pancreas, duodenum, or hepatocellular ducts and from metastatic or granulomatous intrahepatic lesions. Obstructive jaundice is associated with an increase in serum levels of enzymes (alkaline phosphatase [ALP] is the most commonly measured one) that are released when the bile duct epithelium is damaged. Intrahepatic biliary duct obstruction, e.g., primary biliary cirrhosis, produces higher elevations in ALP than extrahepatic obstruction (Widmann, 1987). ALP is elevated in growing children and during pregnancy and is therefore not diagnostic in these conditions. In these situations biliary duct obstruction can be diagnosed by measuring other enzymes such as 5'-nucleotidase, leucine aminopeptidase, and gamma-glutamyl transpeptidase (GGT). In obstructive jaundice the direct bilirubin is also increased, the serum glutamic oxaloacetic transaminase (SGOT) and serum glutamic pyruvic transaminase (SGPT) are normal or slightly elevated, and the prothrombin time (PT) is increased due to vitamin K malabsorption. *Hepatocellular jaundice* results from acute destruction of hepatocytes and is associated with such conditions as acute viral hepatitis and acute toxic or ischemic liver injury. The enzymes most commonly associated with hepatocellular jaundice are the aminotransferases. Hepatocellular jaundice is associated with an increase in the SGOT and SGPT. Both indirect and direct bilirubin are elevated, ALP is normal, and PT is normal or slightly elevated. If hepatocellular damage is extensive, the PT will be extremely elevated. *Hemolytic jaundice* occurs when the heme load in the circulation is increased to such a level that the liver cannot metabolize it. Conditions causing hemolytic jaundice are hemolysis of a large volume of red blood cells such as occurs with massive blood transfusion or a hemolytic transfusion reaction (mismatched ABO type). Hemolytic jaundice is associated with an increased indirect bilirubin and normal SGOT, SGPT, ALP, and PT.

CARBOHYDRATE METABOLISM

A major function of the liver is to maintain normal serum glucose for energy metabolism. Three mechanisms are responsible: *glycogenesis, glycogenolysis,* and *gluconeogenesis.* Carbohydrates in the diet are converted to simple sugars that can be metabolized by the liver for energy substrate. Excess carbohydrates can be converted to glycogen and stored in the liver for metabolic reserve. This process is called glycogenesis. Approximately 900 kcal are stored in the liver as glycogen in the adult (Keithley, 1985). A much larger reserve of glycogen is stored in skeletal muscle. When glucose is needed but unavailable, the first response by the liver is to convert stored glycogen to glucose. This process is called glycogenolysis. If glycogen reserves are depleted, the liver has the ability to manufacture glucose from noncarbohydrate sources, namely, fat (glycerol and fatty acids) and protein (amino acids). This catabolic process is called gluconeogenesis.

PROTEIN METABOLISM

Protein metabolism by the liver involves both the synthesis of plasma proteins from available amino acids and amino acid metabolism. With the exception of gamma globulins and immunoglobulins, all plasma proteins are manufactured by the liver (Galambos, 1979). Plasma proteins include albumin, clotting factors, transferrin, haptoglobin, ceruloplasmin, alpha-1-antitrypsin, the C_3 component of complement, and alpha-fetoprotein. The most sensitive indices of severity of liver disease are serum albumin and the vitamin K–dependent clotting factors.

Albumin is a low-molecular-weight protein responsible for about 60% to 70% of the serum colloid osmotic pressure. Approximately 10 g of albumin is produced by the normal liver each day; production drops to about 4 g daily in the cirrhotic patient (Galambos, 1979). Because the half-life of serum albumin is about 22 days, a decreased serum albumin level will not be apparent in patients with acute liver dysfunction unless there is predisposing malnutrition. Serum albumin levels will not normally decrease from liver dysfunction that lasts less than 3 weeks. Prealbumin, a precursor of albumin, has a much shorter half-life than albumin. Decreased plasma protein production is therefore more quickly identified by measuring serum prealbumin levels.

It is thought that liver cells probably synthesize and secrete all proteins necessary for coagulation (Galambos, 1979). Hepatic synthesis of clotting factors II, VII, IX, and X is dependent on hepatocellular function and vitamin K. Vitamin K is lipid-soluble and therefore is dependent on the presence of bile salts in the intestine for absorption. Failure of bile salt secretion leads to inadequate vitamin K absorption and deficiency of vitamin K–dependent clotting factors. Sterilization of the gut with antibiotics also inhibits the synthesis of vitamin K to some degree.

The most commonly used tests of coagulation are the PT and the partial thromboplastin time (PTT). Deficiencies in vitamin K–dependent clotting factors prolong the PT and PTT. The PT and PTT are therefore extremely sensitive indices of liver function. A PT greater than 3 seconds over the control time and a PTT greater than 10 seconds over the control time are significant. Prolongation indicates a deficiency of clotting factors, which may be a sign of acute or chronic liver dysfunction.

Metabolism of amino acids in the diet and from senescent tissue occurs either through the process of deamination (removal of an NH_2) or through the process of conversion of amino acids to ammonia and conversion of ammonia to urea. Deamination must occur before amino acids in the diet can be utilized for energy, tissue growth, or healing. Ammonia, as a byproduct of protein metabolism, can be formed as a result of deamination, from degradation of protein by gut flora, or from metabolism of blood in the gut secondary to upper gastrointestinal (GI) bleeding. Hepatocellular dysfunction leads to elevated serum ammonia levels, which are associated with hepatic encephalopathy. However, there is evidence that ammonia is not the only toxic compound responsible for this condition (Breen and Schenker, 1972; Schenker et al., 1974; Maddrey and Weber, 1975; Galambos, 1979; Jacques, 1985).

LIPID METABOLISM

The liver is the principal site of lipid synthesis and degradation. Cholesterol, phospholipids, and lipoproteins are formed in the liver, and excess carbohydrates are converted by the liver to triglycerides, which are then stored in adipose tissue. When needed for energy production, triglycerides are metabolized to glycerol and fatty acids. Fatty acids are split into acetyl CoA, which is used in the Krebs cycle in the liver mitochondria for energy production. Phospholipids are necessary for cellular wall integrity and many chemical cellular reactions. Lipoproteins are necessary for lipid transport.

The liver also acts as a storage depot for fat. There are fat-storing cells in the sinusoidal walls in the space of Disse. These cells store triglycerides and the fat-soluble vitamins A, D, E, and K. The healthy human adult has about a 2 years' supply of vitamin A and about a 6 months' supply of vitamin D stored in the liver (Sherlock, 1985).

Patients with cholestatic syndromes and acute viral hepatitis have elevated serum triglyceride levels (Sherlock, 1985). Triglyceride levels in the cirrhotic patient are normal unless the patient is malnourished, in which case they are decreased.

DRUG AND HORMONE METABOLISM

Another metabolic function of the liver is the metabolism of a wide variety of drugs commonly administered to critically ill patients such as bronchodilators, antibiotics, corticosteroids, and histamine blockers. Hepatic clearance of drugs depends on the presence of drug-metabolizing enzymes, hepatocyte integrity, liver blood flow, and the plasma protein–binding affinity of the particular drug. Chronic ingestion of the same drug initially increases metabolism of that drug and therefore shortens the drug's half-life (Galambos, 1979). However, with time and with

hepatocellular damage and hepatic dysfunction, drug metabolism may be significantly impaired. Many drugs, including alcohol, are potentially toxic to the liver (Table 45–1). Toxic agents are converted in the endoplasmic reticulum of the hepatocyte to water-soluble substances that can be excreted either in the urine or in the bile.

The adrenal response to stress or alterations in fluid volume status is to secrete glucocorticoids (cortisol) and mineralocorticoids (aldosterone). The liver plays an important role in inactivating these and other hormones when they are no longer needed to maintain homeostasis. Antidiuretic hormone is also cleared by the liver.

VASCULAR CLEARANCE FUNCTION

As mentioned earlier, Kupffer cells within the liver sinusoids function as tissue macrophages for the clearance of potentially pathogenic microorganisms. Patients with cirrhosis have a predisposition to bac-

TABLE 45–1. Potentially Hepatotoxic Drugs

Acetaminophen (Tylenol)
Allopurinol (Zyloprim)
Amiodarone
Azathioprine (Imuran)
Carbamazepine (Tegretol)
Chlorambucil (Leukeran)
Chlordiazepoxide (Librium)
Chlorpromazine (Thorazine)
Chlorpropamide (Diabinese)
Cyclosporine (Sandimmune)
Desacetylmethylcolchicine (Cocemid)
Diazepam (Valium)
Phenytoin (Dilantin)
Erythromycin estolate (Ilosone)
Estrogen, natural and synthetic
Ferrous sulfate
Halothane
Imipramine (Tofranil)
Indomethacin (Indocin)
Isoniazid (INH, Nydrazid)
Ketoconazole (miconazole)
Meprobamate (Equanil)
Methotrexate (Mexate)
Methyldopa (Aldomet)
Monoamine oxidase (MAO) inhibitors
Nicotinic acid
Nitrofurantoin (Furadantin, Macrodantin)
Oxacillioxymetholone (Anadrol, Adroyd)
Penicillin
Phenazopyridine (Pyridium)
Phenobarbital
Phenylbutazone (Butazolidin)
Probenecid (Benemid)
Prochlorperazine (Compazine)
Propoxyphene (Darvon)
Propylthiouracil
Salicylates (aspirin)
Sulfonamides
Tetracycline (Achromycin, Sumycin)
Thiouracil
Tolbutamide (Orinase)
Trimethobenzamide (Tigan)
Tripelennamine (Pyribenzamine)

terial infections due to shunting and decreased clearance of bacteria by the liver. Procoagulants, or activated clotting factors, and byproducts of coagulation are also cleared by these cells in the liver.

ASSESSMENT OF LIVER FUNCTION

Liver function, liver dysfunction, and effects of liver disease can be assessed or evaluated in various ways. The effects of liver disease on other organ systems can be assessed by laboratory techniques and physical examination. The degree of liver dysfunction is routinely assessed by standard laboratory tests, and true liver function is assessed by using sophisticated quantitative studies.

Physical Assessment

The four components of physical assessment—inspection, auscultation, percussion, and palpation—can be employed to elicit significant physical findings in the patient with suspected or known liver disease. These findings, however, are not evident until the disease is far advanced.

Inspection. Typical physical findings in the patient with advanced liver disease are described in Table 45–2.

Auscultation. Auscultation should be performed before percussion or palpation of the abdomen to prevent the creation of artifactual sounds that could be misinterpreted during auscultation. The patient with advanced liver disease has a hyperdynamic cardiovascular system. There are several reasons for this. First, the vascular space increases as a result of extensive collateral vessel development, and vascular volume is not necessarily increased adequately to fill this space. Therefore, cardiac output, as part of the oxygen transport system, accelerates to meet tissue oxygen requirements. Second, anemia due to malnutrition, splenomegaly, and coagulopathy is common in the patient with advanced liver disease. Cardiac output accelerates for the same reason in

---

TABLE 45–2. Table of Physical Findings in Liver Disease

Finding	Rationale	Finding	Rationale
Jaundice	Yellowish discoloration of skin, sclera, and secretions. Due to alteration in bilirubin metabolism. If the problem is "prehepatic," such as hemolysis, the light-skinned patient will manifest mild jaundice and appear mildly yellow. If the problem is "hepatic," such as acute hepatocellular necrosis, the light-skinned patient will appear deep yellow or orange. If the problem is cholestasis, jaundice will become manifest insidiously, and the light-skinned patient will appear greenish.	Clubbing of fingers	Thought to be due to extensive peripheral collateral vessel formation and alteration in hormone metabolism.
		Hyperpigmentation	Diffuse muddy-gray hypermelanosis more prominent in sun-exposed areas. Due to chronic cholestasis.
		Easy bruising	Due to insufficient coagulation factors and thrombocytopenia; seen especially on the legs.
Spider nevi (Fig. 45–6)	Cutaneous angiomas commonly seen on the anterior thorax, shoulders, neck, and face, and rarely on the posterior thorax. They are part of the arteriovenous (AV) collateral system that develops as a result of portal hypertension. A central arteriole feeds each clump of dilated blood vessels and will blanch when suppressed. The tiny vessels are quickly refilled as pressure is released. This is one feature distinguishing spider nevi from petechial hemorrhages.	Dry skin and scratch marks	Due to chronic cholestasis and formation of bile crystals in skin. Pruritus is most common skin symptom. It often precedes onset of jaundice and clears as liver insufficiency progresses except in patients with cholestatic liver disease.
		Brittle hair, hair loss	Body hair is thinned or lost; nails become white and flat with white striations. Due to increased levels of circulating estrogen and zinc deficiency.
Caput medusae	Dilated abdominal veins radiating from the umbilicus. Part of the AV collateral vessel system that develops as a result of portal hypertension.	Hypogonadism, feminization in males	Manifested by testicular atrophy, impotence, decreased beard and pubic hair, female escutcheon, and gynecomastia. Exact etiology is unclear, but chronic alcohol abuse thought to be a significant factor (Van Thiel et al., 1974).
Striae	"Stretch marks" prominent on inner aspect of arms, lower abdomen, thighs, and buttocks seen in both males and females. Due to increased levels of circulating cortisol.	Peripheral edema	Due to hypoalbuminemia.
Palmar erythema	Palmar surfaces of hands appear bright red. Thought to be due to (1) diffuse formation of AV collaterals in hands, and (2) increased levels of circulating estrogen.	Xanthomas	Flat round lesions on eyelids, extensor surfaces of palms, creases of hands, and sometimes on the trunk, face, and extremities. Due to hyperlipidemia and seen commonly in patients with primary biliary cirrhosis.

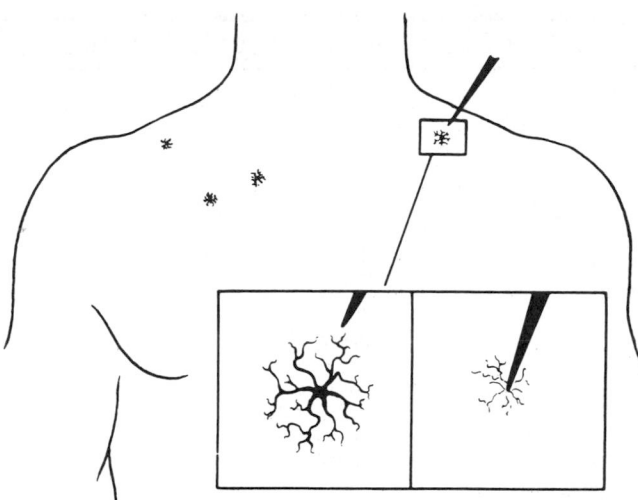

FIGURE 45–6. Cutaneous angiomas, or spider nevi. Notice blanching produced by pressure on central arteriole. (From Prior, John A., Silberstein, Jack S., and Stang, John M.: *Physical diagnosis: The history and examination of the patient*, ed. 6, St. Louis, 1981, The C. V. Mosby Co.)

this condition to increase oxygen transport. Third, gastrointestinal peptides responsible for vasodilation are normally cleared from the circulation by the liver (Galambos, 1979; Sherlock, 1985). In advanced liver disease they remain in the systemic circulation and cause a compensatory increase in cardiac output. An auscultatory abdominal finding associated with the hyperdynamic circulatory system in advanced liver disease is the *venous hum*. A venous hum is usually heard on auscultation of the abdomen over the upper aspect of the liver. This sound is a murmur that is continuous throughout the cardiac cycle and is associated with rapid flow through collateral portacaval vessels.

Percussion. Although advances in radiographic and angiographic technology are more frequently employed, percussion is sometimes useful for determining liver size, splenic enlargement, and the presence of ascites. Liver size can be estimated by percussing from the right clavicle straight down the right midclavicular line (MCL) (see Fig. 45–7). Over lung tissue the percussion tone will be resonant. At about the level of the fifth intercostal space the percussion tone becomes dull; this marks the upper edge of the liver. The percussion tone over the bowel is normally tympanic. Percussing upward from the level of the umbilicus, again at the MCL, over tympanic bowel until a dull percussion tone is heard locates the lower edge of the liver. The distance between the upper and lower edges of the liver at the midclavicular line, as determined by percussion, is normally about 12 cm (Fig. 45–7). The liver enlarges in acute inflammatory states such as alcoholic and viral hepatitis and in the early stages of chronic liver disease. In most advanced forms of disease, such as chronic active hepatitis, the liver atrophies. Atrophy

of the liver also occurs rapidly in acute hepatic necrosis.

The spleen cannot normally be percussed. However, in conditions in which the spleen is grossly enlarged, it may be percussed at the left midclavicular line but very low in the abdomen. Dull percussion tones may be heard over the intercostal spaces and below the left costal margin.

Although ascites may be obvious on inspection, smaller collections of peritoneal fluid that are not visible can sometimes be detected by percussion.

Palpation. Palpation is more easily performed than percussion. This technique is most useful for assessing liver size but can be used to assess the spleen as well. Palpation of the liver is always performed at the patient's right side by supporting the right flank area with the left hand and sliding the fingertips of the right hand under the right costal margin using firm pressure. The fingertips are advanced as the patient inhales deeply. The liver edge moves 1 to 3 cm downward during inspiration. Position of the fingertips is held steady as the patient exhales and inhales again. As the patient inhales, exhales, and inhales, the smooth edge of the liver may be felt moving past the fingertips. The liver is more easily palpated in thin individuals than in obese individuals. Liver palpation is deep palpation and is therefore slightly uncomfortable in most individuals if it is done correctly.

Normally, the liver cannot be palpated more than 1 to 2 cm below the right costal margin. However, there is one pathologic condition in which the liver may be palpated far below the right costal margin when it is not enlarged. This occurs in the patient with advanced chronic obstructive pulmonary disease (COPD) when the diaphragm becomes flattened and immobile. The flattened diaphragm pushes the liver farther down into the right abdominal quadrant. Percussion of liver size is useful when caring for the patient with COPD because cor pulmonale, which accompanies advanced COPD, causes hepatic congestion and enlargement.

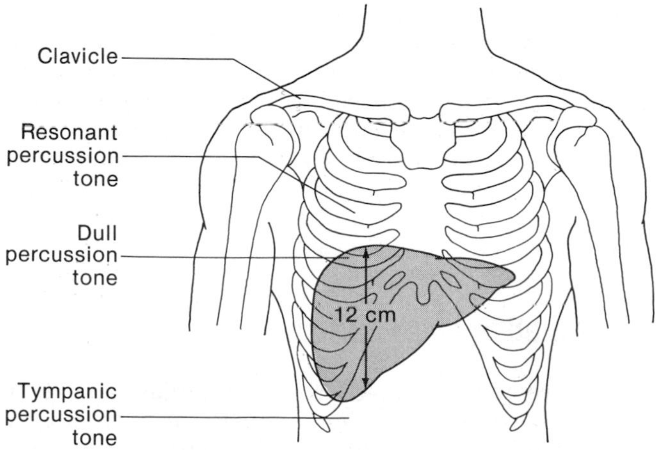

Clavicle

Resonant percussion tone

Dull percussion tone

12 cm

Tympanic percussion tone

FIGURE 45–7. Percussion to determine liver size.

The spleen cannot be palpated in normal conditions. To be palpated, it must be enlarged to at least twice its normal size, which often occurs in advanced liver disease. Palpation of the spleen is gentle because the spleen is a more superficial organ than the liver. As with percussion, palpation of the spleen should be done low in the abdomen to locate this organ. A word of caution about palpation of the enlarged spleen: If it is enlarged enough to be palpated, that in itself is an absolute contraindication to palpating it. The reason is that the risk of rupture is very high.

Standard Laboratory Assessment

Liver function is the capacity of the liver to perform specific tasks or functions. The conventional tests of bilirubin, albumin, PT, and liver enzymes, although referred to as "liver function" tests, do not actually assess liver function. Instead, these tests provide information about liver "dysfunction" and, to some extent, the specific type of liver injury.

The serum bilirubin value indicates the efficiency of the hepatic uptake and excretory system and the rate of production of bilirubin. Serum bilirubin, albumin, and PT were discussed in a previous section.

Liver enzymes are released during cellular injury and stop being released as injured hepatocytes heal. If hepatocellular injury is severe enough to cause massive necrosis, serum enzyme levels will be initially extremely high and then decline because there are no more enzymes to be released. Liver enzymes can be classified into two major types: *aminotransaminases* and *phosphatases*.

Liver aminotransaminases include SGOT and serum SGPT. SGOT is also referred to as aspartate aminotransferase (AST), and SGPT is also called alanine aminotransferase (ALT). SGOT is released into the circulation when cells of the heart, skeletal muscle, kidney, or liver are injured. Therefore, an increased SGOT level is not specific to hepatocellular injury. SGPT is released in the same conditions but in much larger quantities from injured liver cells and is considered a more specific liver cell enzyme. However, in liver disease, elevations in SGOT and SGPT are most often parallel.

The phosphatases include ALP and GGT. Although serum phosphatase levels increase with hepatocellular damage, these increases are more specific to bile duct injury or cholestasis. GGT is more likely to be elevated during biliary obstruction than during hepatocellular damage, and GGT is elevated in alcoholics. Normal serum transaminase and phosphatase values are listed in Table 45–3.

Quantitative Liver Function

As previously stated, the traditional laboratory methods for assessing liver function can be grossly misleading. Acute hepatocellular damage can produce significant changes in serum values of bilirubin,

TABLE 45–3. Normal Values for Hepatic Function Tests

Test	Normal Value
Bilirubin (total)	1.0 mg/dL
Indirect	0.5 mg/dL
Direct	0.5 mg/dL
Urobilinogen (urine)	0.2–3.0 mg/24 hours
Urinary bilirubin	0
SGOT (AST)	40.0 units
SGPT (ALT)	45.0 units
ALP	1.5 U/dL (Bodansky)
	4.0–13.0 U/dL (King-Armstrong)
	0.8–2.3 U/mL (Bessey-Lowry)
	15.0–35.0 U/mL (Shinowara-Jones-Rinehart)
GGT	5–55 U/liters
Prothrombin time	Greater than 3 seconds over control
Fibrinogen	200–400 mg/dL
Albumin	3.5–5.0 g/dL
Ammonia	11–35 Umol/liter
Cholesterol	100–250 mg/dL

Abbreviations: SGOT, serum glutamic oxaloacetic transaminase; AST, aspartate aminotransferase; SGPT, serum glutamic pyruvic transaminase; ALT, alanine aminotransferase; ALP, alkaline phosphatase; GGT, gamma-glutamyl transpeptidase.

liver enzymes, and PT. However, as acute damage resolves, these values can return to normal. Conversely, these values may be practically normal in the patient who has far advanced liver disease and little functional capacity of the liver. It is clear that reliance on the patient's physical appearance and the laboratory evaluation can result in errors in diagnosis, prognosis, and treatment for the patient with liver dysfunction and disease.

Liver function can be quantified by assessing the metabolic and clearance functions of the liver, which are dependent on functional liver cell mass and blood flow. Some of the more useful quantitative tests are the galactose elimination capacity (GEC), antipyrine metabolism and clearance, galactose clearance, and protein load.

The GEC measures the functional hepatocyte mass by calculating the maximal removal rate of galactose, which is exclusively and rapidly converted to glucose in the liver. In this test a known quantity of galactose is administered intravenously (IV), and several blood samples are taken over a given time span. Assays of these samples are plotted on a semilogarithmic plasma concentration curve over time. The maximal rate of galactose removal is calculated from the slope of this curve. Normal GEC is 500 mg/minute or 33 mg/kg per minute (Henderson and Warren, 1986). The antipyrine clearance test measures mixed function oxidase reactions in the liver (Henderson and Warren, 1986). Antipyrine is a drug similar to aspirin that is completely absorbed in the GI tract and metabolized by the liver. It is excreted in the saliva. In this test a known quantity of antipyrine is administered orally, and saliva samples are analyzed during the following 24 to 48 hours. The galactose clearance is used to evaluate hepatocyte function and is an index of "nutritive" liver blood flow. In this test a 5% solution of galactose is administered IV, and several blood samples are taken over time. Assays of these samples are plotted on a standard plasma concentration versus time curve, and galactose clearance is calculated using a steady-state equation. Normal galactose clearance is between 1100 and 1600 mL/minute (Henderson and Warren, 1986). The protein load test measures amino acid and ammonia tolerance. A known quantity of an oral protein solution is administered. Baseline fasting levels of serum and urine amino acids and ammonia are subtracted from the levels determined after administration of the protein load. A plasma response curve is plotted to evaluate the liver's ability to metabolize protein, and the patient's clinical tolerance is assessed. The danger in this test is that some patients will become encephalopathic after administration of the protein load. Although some quantitative studies of liver function are more invasive than assessment techniques, the precision of the results is highly beneficial when determining optimal treatment options for the patient with liver disease.

ACUTE FULMINANT HEPATIC FAILURE

Acute fulminant failure of the liver is discussed as a separate entity because the causes, manifestations, clinical course, and prognosis are very different from those characteristic of chronic hepatic disease and failure. Acute fulminant hepatic failure or necrosis is defined as the clinical and biochemical presence of liver disease in someone whose liver function was normal prior to the development of signs and symptoms. Hepatic encephalopathy generally develops within less than 8 weeks after the onset of clinical signs (Willson, 1977; Bonnice, 1985). A similar syndrome, subacute hepatic failure, becomes manifest after 8 weeks but usually by the twentieth week after exposure to the hepatotoxin. This condition is characterized by a sudden onset of altered mental status, progressive jaundice, coagulopathy, hepatorenal syndrome, respiratory alkalosis, fetor hepaticus, hepatic encephalopathy, and cerebral edema.

Prognosis for the patient with acute or subacute fulminant hepatic necrosis is very poor. With the exception of hepatic failure from acetaminophen toxicity, the outcome is almost always fatal within a few days. The overall mortality rate is between 75% and 95% (Bonnice, 1985). The neurologic complications of cerebral edema account for the majority of deaths. The depth of encephalopathy is an important index of the severity of hepatic necrosis, and the age of the patient plays a role in survival. Death is almost a certain outcome for the patient who descends to a grade IV hepatic coma.

Etiology

The most common causes of acute fulminant hepatic necrosis are acute viral hepatitis, acetaminophen toxicity, and fulminant Wilson's disease (Iwat-

suki et al., 1985). Other causes include mushroom poisoning, acute Budd-Chiari syndrome, anesthetic agents, acute fatty liver of pregnancy, and industrial toxins. Viral hepatitis accounts for about 80% and drug toxicity for about 15% of cases (Willson, 1977). Hepatitis A; hepatitis B; hepatitis C; and hepatitis non-A, non-B, non-C viruses can cause acute hepatocellular necrosis, the hepatitis B virus being the most common causative agent. In all types of viral hepatitis this condition is rare.

A major function of the liver is drug metabolism, especially of drugs taken or administered through the oral route. Because only lipid-soluble drugs can be absorbed by intestinal membranes, it is necessary for the liver to convert these lipid-soluble compounds to water-soluble compounds that can be excreted by the kidneys. The most common pharmacologic agents associated with acute hepatocellular necrosis are the anesthetic halothane and acetaminophen.

Halothane toxicity is rare and is more common in the patient who has been previously exposed to halothane or who has preexisting liver dysfunction. Halothane is metabolized to trifluoroacetic acid, bromine, and chloride, which are potentially hepatotoxic substances. These substances are stored in the adipose tissue, so halothane toxicity is more common in obese patients. Halothane toxicity usually becomes manifest with a fever on about the seventh day after exposure, accompanied by malaise, RUQ pain, nonspecific GI symptoms, and jaundice.

Currently, there are over 200 preparations that contain acetaminophen. The sudden ingestion of 10 or more g of acetaminophen, usually taken as a suicide attempt, can induce acute hepatocellular necrosis. Alcohol ingestion, which often accompanies purposeful acetaminophen overdose, enhances acetaminophen toxicity. Chronic ingestion of at least 3 g can also lead to hepatic necrosis (Leoni, 1985). Two metabolic pathways are involved in the detoxification of acetaminophen: conjugation and the cytochrome P450 mixed function oxidase pathway. Approximately 97% of acetaminophen is metabolized through conjugation, and about 2% to 3% is metabolized by the P450 pathway when therapeutic doses are taken (Russo and Pratter, 1985). The process of conjugation produces an unidentified, potentially hepatotoxic compound that combines with hepatic glutathione to form the nontoxic compound mercapturate, which is excreted in the urine. When excessive amounts of acetaminophen are ingested, the conjugation pathway becomes saturated, the P450 pathway becomes the primary metabolic system, and increased amounts of the potentially hepatotoxic metabolite are produced. As hepatic glutathione becomes depleted, this metabolite combines with hepatocellular proteins and causes necrosis.

The half-life of therapeutic doses of acetaminophen is approximately 2½ hours. This time period increases to at least 4 hours when larger than therapeutic doses are ingested, and to more than 12 hours if hepatic necrosis occurs. The serum acetaminophen level is a good prognostic indicator for the probability of hepatic necrosis, but blood should not be drawn until at least 4 hours after ingestion because absorption is slowed with large quantities.

During the first 24 hours after ingestion of a toxic dose the patient may experience nonspecific symptoms such as anorexia, malaise, nausea, vomiting, diaphoresis, and dehydration. If hepatic necrosis develops, the first signs and symptoms will become manifest after 24 to 48 hours. They are RUQ pain, increased serum transaminase and bilirubin levels, prolonged PT, and oliguria. On about the third or fourth day after acute ingestion of a toxic dose the individual becomes hypoglycemic and jaundiced, coagulopathy worsens, and encephalopathy develops. Severe renal and myocardial dysfunction can occur. Renal dysfunction is thought to be due to dehydration and possibly renal toxicity, and myocardial necrosis can also occur as a toxic side effect of acetaminophen.

Because no specific signs of hepatic dysfunction occur until approximately 24 to 48 hours after ingestion, it may seem that admission of the patient with an acetaminophen overdose to an intensive care unit (ICU) is unnecessary. On the contrary, these patients can become very ill over a short period of time. Nursing responsibilities include careful monitoring of the cardiovascular, renal, gastrointestinal, hematologic, and neurologic systems for the signs and symptoms already discussed.

The goal of initial management is to prevent continued drug absorption. Interventions include evacuating the stomach and adsorbing acetaminophen with activated charcoal. However, charcoal will also adsorb another therapeutic drug used to treat acetaminophen overdose, N-acetyl-L-cysteine. Treatment with N-acetyl-L-cysteine (Mucomist, Parvolex), which is a glutathione precursor, can prevent severe liver damage if it is administered within 8 hours of the acetaminophen overdose (Leoni, 1985). Considerable psychosocial support is necessary for the patient who has taken an intentional overdose, a psychiatric consultation is indicated.

Other causes of acute hepatic failure include toxic mushroom poisoning (*Amanita phalloides*, *A. verna*, and *A. virosa*; *Galerina autumnaas*, *G. marginata*, and *G. venenata*; and *Gyromitra* sp.) (Gould and Pratter, 1985), industrial toxins such as carbon tetrachloride, pesticides such as DDT, herbicides such as paraquat, infectious organisms such as *Aspergillus*, abdominal sepsis, hepatic artery thrombosis, shock, acute fatty liver of pregnancy, massive blastic infiltration of the liver such as occurs with acute leukemia and lymphoreticular malignancies, and Reye syndrome (Willson, 1977; Mar, 1982; Bonnice, 1985; Frank and Cummins, 1987).

Clinical Presentation

The critical role played by the liver in the body is evidenced by the changes that occur with liver fail-ure. Although the causes may vary, the clinical presentation is fairly uniform and predictable. There is a prodromal period of vague symptoms followed by rapidly progressive liver and multisystem failure. Frequently, progression from a fully alert and productive state to encephalopathic coma occurs in a period of only a few days.

Subtle mental status changes are often the first sign of acute liver failure. As massive necrosis of the liver occurs, the patient may progress through all stages of hepatic encephalopathy to deep coma. Cerebral dysfunction is attributed to three factors: (1) decreased synthesis of glucose required by the brain for metabolism; (2) faulty detoxification of nitrogenous byproducts of protein metabolism; and (3) replacement of normal neurotransmitters by "false" neurotransmitters that induce sedation (Galambos, 1979). Increased levels of free ammonia stimulate the respiratory center, causing hyperventilation and respiratory alkalosis. The electroencephalogram (EEG) shows generalized slowing and nonspecific changes consistent with metabolic encephalopathy (Galambos, 1979; Aring, 1982; Jacques, 1985). Development of papillary edema is an ominous sign indicative of cerebral edema. Grade III and IV hepatic coma are associated with complications such as renal failure, GI hemorrhage, bacteremia, and sepsis. The mortality rate is between 75% and 90% for patients who reach grade IV hepatic coma (Bonnice, 1985).

On physical examination the patient's liver is found to be enlarged during the inflammatory phase but becomes progressively smaller with massive necrosis. Rapid reduction in liver size, increasing bilirubin concentration with severe jaundice, severely prolonged PT with hemorrhagic complications, and hypoglycemia are prognostic of impending death. The hemodynamic changes seen in patients with acute fulminant hepatic failure are similar to those associated with septic shock—a decrease in systemic vascular resistance with a compensatory increase in cardiac output (Iwatsuki et al., 1985). And indeed, the necrotic liver serves as a septic focus.

Laboratory findings are remarkable. Serum transaminase levels are markedly elevated early in the course of disease as high as 20,000 U/mL but fall toward the normal range as the liver mass becomes necrotic. Therefore, a decrease in serum transaminase levels is not always a sign of improvement. In addition to signaling that the necrotic process has been arrested, this finding may also indicate that complete necrosis of the liver has occurred. The serum bilirubin is elevated, and coagulation times are significantly prolonged. Serum ammonia levels are elevated, but values do not correlate well with the degree of encephalopathy. The patient may be profoundly hypoglycemic. Serum albumin levels remain normal unless the patient is already malnourished.

As the liver dies, multisystem shock and failure ensue. The clinical syndromes of circulatory collapse secondary to hypovolemia and sepsis, acute respiratory failure, acute renal failure, disseminated coagulopathy, and increased intracranial hypertension become manifest. Acute hemorrhagic pancreatitis occurs in about 30% of patients (Willson, 1977). More than 50% of patients develop severe GI bleeding (Willson, 1977).

CASE HISTORY

G.H., a 23-year-old black male, presented to the emergency department of a large community hospital with a 3-week history of nausea, vomiting, anorexia, and malaise. His liver was tender and palpable at 7 cm below the right costal margin. He was jaundiced with a serum bilirubin of 19.1 mg/dL. His SGOT and SGPT were 16,000 U/mL and 19,000 U/mL, respectively. His PT and PTT were 18.2 and 40.1 seconds, respectively. He was alert and oriented.

Within several hours G.H. became lethargic and less attentive to the environment. At this time he was transferred to a university medical center to be considered a candidate for emergent liver transplantation. At the time of admission to the university medical center the patient was difficult to arouse. His respirations were 36/minute and shallow. He was prophylactically intubated as his level of encephalopathy deepened.

A computed tomographic (CT) scan of his head showed no diffuse swelling with normal ventricles, but when an intracranial pressure monitoring device was inserted, his intracranial pressure (ICP) was found to be 40 mm Hg. His cerebral perfusion pressure (CPP) was 70 mm Hg. Mannitol was used intermittently to decrease his ICP to between 20 and 25 mm Hg, and he was mechanically hyperventilated to a $P_{A_{CO_2}}$ of 30 mm Hg.

A meeting with his family yielded conflicting information regarding his social behavior. Some family members insisted that he was a "drug addict," whereas those closer to him denied this. He was employed, and it was learned that there had been no problems with his recent or past work performance. As it became clear that his condition was not going to improve, the decision was made to perform transplantation.

He was registered with the local organ procurement agency as the most urgent status outlined by the United Network on Organ Sharing (UNOS) because he was not expected to live more than 48 hours. Approximately 12 hours later a liver that matched his in size and blood type was donated. While the procurement team was recovering the liver, despite medical therapy G.H.'s blood pressure decreased, and his ICP increased until his CPP was 12 mm Hg. Shortly thereafter the brainstem herniated, and G.H. was pronounced brain dead.

Interventions

Survival depends on the capability of hepatocellular regeneration or preservation of organ systems until hepatic regeneration occurs or until definitive treatment such as liver transplantation can be employed. The need for intensive care and multisystem support is obvious. However, in spite of the fact that neurologic complications account for 67% of deaths (Bonnice, 1985), prompt and appropriate interventions to decrease cerebral edema are often overlooked.

The patient with acute fulminant hepatic failure is critically ill. The severity of the situation and the rapidity of deterioration must be recognized early by the health care team, and a protocol for managing this patient population should be in place to avoid unnecessary delays in diagnosis and interventions. Endotracheal intubation should be done before the patient loses consciousness to prevent pulmonary aspiration. A nasogastric (NG) tube is also necessary to allow gastric decompression, administer antacids, and serve as an alert to upper GI bleeding, a common complication of fulminant hepatic failure. Replacement of clotting factors with fresh frozen plasma is necessary to treat coagulopathy. Placement of any invasive catheters or other devices should be done before coagulopathy becomes so severe that these procedures are prohibited. Hemofiltration may be necessary for stabilization of fluid, electrolyte, and acid-base imbalances if acute renal failure and oliguria occur. It is important to avoid overhydration because it can increase cerebral edema.

The goals of treatment of the patient with hepatic encephalopathy are to remove the precipitating factors of encephalopathy, decrease intracranial pressure, and preserve cerebral integrity. Prophylactic insertion of an ICP monitoring device is useful for managing intracranial hypertension. However, neurosurgeons are frequently reluctant to perform this procedure because of the risks associated with coagulopathy.

Stimuli that increase ICP should be avoided: Physical and verbal stimulation should be kept to a minimum, and the lights should be dimmed. Increases in intra-abdominal and intrathoracic pressure should be prevented. Cerebral edema can be treated in the traditional manner with mannitol.

Parenteral amino acids are avoided, and the GI tract should be evacuated to minimize interactions between nitrogenous substances and enteric bacterial flora that produce ammonia. Colonic irrigation with tap water enemas until there is a clear return is one effective method. Lactulose enemas can also be used, and the gut can be sterilized with nonabsorbable antibiotics such as neomycin. Other methods of removing toxins from the body have also been used with varying degrees of success. In general, modalities such as exchange blood transfusions, plasmapheresis, hemodialysis, and charcoal hemoperfusion have not been very successful (Bonnice, 1985; O'Grady et al., 1988).

Although the efficacy of liver transplantation for the patient in acute fulminant hepatic failure has not yet been established, it is the only therapeutic option for someone with an irreversibly necrotic liver. Limited experience at a few centers has shown that some patients can be saved with liver transplantation (Iwatsuki et al., 1985; Buckels, 1987; Stieber et al., 1988). At the University of Pittsburgh the survival rate after acute or subacute fulminant hepatic failure has increased from less than 20% to 55% (Stieber et al., 1988). The efforts discussed earlier aimed at preserving cerebral integrity seem to be key factors in the survival of these patients. Patients who reach grade IV hepatic coma, however, are not likely to survive liver transplantation. This is an area in which much clinical research is needed.

The patient in acute fulminant hepatic failure presents not only physiologic but also intense psychosocial challenges to the critical care nurse. Family members often cannot comprehend how someone can be well one day or week and dying the next. Explaining the link between a failing liver and unconsciousness is difficult at best. Preparing a family for organ transplantation is a process that is optimally done over days or weeks. In this situation, there is no time to assess important psychosocial factors vital to the long-term success of transplantation or to provide preoperative education. If the patient is not a candidate for liver transplantation, then, in most cases, the critical care team and family will have to cope with the death of the patient.

Nursing Diagnoses for the Patient with Acute Fulminant Hepatic Failure

Altered nutrition: Less than body requirements
Potential for infection
Altered body temperature: Hypothermia,
    hyperthermia
Ineffective thermoregulation
Altered bowel elimination: Diarrhea
Altered urinary elimination: Total incontinence
Altered tissue perfusion: Renal, cerebral,
    cardiopulmonary, gastrointestinal, peripheral
Fluid volume excess
Impaired gas exchange
Ineffective airway clearance
Ineffective breathing pattern
Potential for injury: Suffocating, trauma
Impaired skin integrity, potential
Impaired tissue integrity, oral mucous membranes
Impaired communication, verbal
Altered role performance
Altered family processes
Ineffective coping, family: Compromised, disabled
Impaired physical mobility
Self-care deficit: Feeding, bathing/hygiene, toileting
Powerlessness
Altered thought processes
Anticipatory grieving, dysfunctional

HEPATITIS

The different types of hepatitis are clinically similar in many respects but differ with regard to epidemiology, serologic markers, prophylaxis, and prognosis. Causes of hepatitis include viral, drug-related, and autoimmune disease processes. There are at least

seven viruses responsible: hepatitis A, B, C, D, and E viruses; cytomegalovirus; and Epstein-Barr virus. In addition, it is presumed that hepatitis non-A, non-B, non-C (NANBNC) viruses exist. This chapter will specifically address viral hepatitis—hepatitis A (HAV), hepatitis B (HBV) and hepatitis C (HCV).

Hepatitis is defined as an acute inflammation of the entire liver, characterized by centrilobular necrosis and infiltration of the portal tracts by leukocytes (Galambos, 1979). Approximately 500,000 new cases of viral hepatitis are diagnosed in the United States each year (Gurevich, 1983). The incidence in the general public is less than 5%, but the incidence in health care workers is about 30% (Gurevich, 1983).

Those at high risk in the population at large include those with lepromatous leprosy, homosexuals, intravenous drug abusers, those institutionalized with Down syndrome, hemophiliacs, those of ethnic origin from a country with a high carrier rate, those receiving blood transfusions in underdeveloped countries, and neonates of carrier mothers (Jackson, 1980; Gurevich, 1983). Health care personnel who are particularly at risk are surgeons, hemodialysis personnel, those caring for transplant or oncology patients, those caring for patients with GI bleeding, burn unit personnel, laboratory personnel, and dentists.

The basic pathophysiology of hepatitis A, B, C, and NANBNC is the same. Again, the lesion is one of acute inflammation of the entire liver. Hepatitis can present as an acute process, an acute fulminant process, or a chronic process. Acute hepatitis can become manifest clinically anywhere along a spectrum ranging from an anicteric, nearly asymptomatic episode to acute fulminant hepatic necrosis. Nearly 50% of those contracting acute hepatitis are asymptomatic (Gurevich, 1983).

In symptomatic cases of acute nonfulminant hepatitis an icteric attack occurs that includes a prodromal period of a few days to several weeks. During this time the patient feels "flulike" with RUQ tenderness and experiences a lack of desire to smoke cigarettes or drink alcohol. Serum transaminase levels are elevated at this time. The urine then becomes dark and the feces colorless; this is followed by jaundice and an elevated serum bilirubin. At this time symptoms begin to decrease. After a few weeks the patient usually recovers without sequelae other than persistent fatigue. A list of serologic markers used to diagnose hepatitis is shown in Table 45–4.

There are three types of chronic sequelae of acute hepatitis: the asymptomatic carrier state, chronic persistent hepatitis, and chronic active hepatitis. A carrier state occurs when the infected individual is unable to clear the antigen from the serum. Immunosuppressed individuals such as organ transplant recipients, oncology patients, and those with chronic renal failure are at high risk of becoming chronic carriers. The common etiologic factor in this group of patients is an ineffective cellular immune response (Galambos, 1979). When the virus is HBV, the hep-

TABLE 45–4. Hepatitis Serology Nomenclature

HAV	Hepatitis A virus (enterovirus); detectable in stool prior to disease
Anti-HAV	Antibody to HAV; detectable at onset of disease prior to jaundice; confers lifelong immunity
IgM	Detectable at 4 to 6 weeks after exposure
IgG	Detectable at 8 to 12 weeks after exposure
HBV	Hepatitis B virus (DNA virus)
HBsAg	Hepatitis B surface antigen; detectable within 30 days of exposure and persists up to 3 months after jaundice unless a carrier state develops (in which case it will persist longer); indicates that disease is infectious
HBcAg	Hepatitis B core antigen; *not* detectable in serum, only detectable in liver cells
HBeAg	Hepatitis B "e" antigen; indicates high titer of HBV and increased infectiousness (ongoing viral replication); appears at 4 to 12 weeks after exposure
Anti-HBs	Antibody to HBsAg; appears 1 to 2 months after HBsAg disappears from serum or in person who has had Heptavax or immune globulin vaccination
Anti-HBc	Antibody to HBcAg; appears at 6 to 14 weeks after exposure in the "window phase" (after HBsAg disappears but before Anti-HBs appears); indicates low infectiousness
Anti-HBe	Antibody to HBeAg; possibly indicates dormant infection
Anti-HCV	Antibody to HCV
Anti-HDV	Antibody to HDV (hepatitis delta virus)

Criteria for diagnosing hepatitis B:
HBsAg positive *or*
Anti-HBsAg *or*
Anti-HBcAg

atitis B surface antigen (HBsAg) and the antibody-to-surface antigen (anti-HBsAg) are found in the serum. The chronic carrier suffers no liver damage but can transmit the virus to others. There are approximately 200 million carriers in the world (Sherlock, 1985). In the United States about 5% to 10% of the population and 1% of health care workers are carriers (Gurevich, 1983). Carrier states develop after HBV, HCV, and NANBNC infections but not after HAV infections. A chronic persistent state develops in about 5% to 10% of those who contract acute hepatitis B, hepatitis C, or hepatitis NANBNC. With chronic persistent hepatitis there are no signs or symptoms, and liver damage is limited.

In chronic active hepatitis (CAH) liver damage is progressive. A weak cellular immune response is ineffective in clearing the virus. Continued viral replication in the liver leads to progressive hepatocellular necrosis. Chronic active hepatitis is more likely to occur in the individual who has had a mild or asymptomatic case of acute HBV, HCV, or NANBNC infection (Gurevich, 1983; Sherlock, 1985; Seef and Koff, 1986). The most important sequela of CAH is primary hepatocellular carcinoma (Seef and Koff, 1986). Cirrhosis can develop after a severe case of acute hepatitis, in which case it is called postnecrotic cirrhosis, and it can develop as the end stage of CAH (Galambos, 1979).

Hepatitis A

The HAV is an enterovirus similar to the polio virus. Hepatitis A ("infectious hepatitis") accounts for approximately 20% to 25% of all hepatitis cases worldwide (Sherlock, 1985). About 20,000 people with hepatitis A are hospitalized in the United States each year (Gurevich, 1983).

The mode of transmission is the fecal-oral route. The virus is found in the stool from about 2 weeks before until 1 week after the onset of jaundice. The incubation period is from 2 to 6 weeks. As the stool becomes negative for HAV, serum antibody (anti-HAV) appears and is detectable for years. Therefore, the virus is transmissible before it is apparent that the disease exists. Serum IgM anti-HAV suggests recent infection, and serum IgG anti-HAV confers immunity to HAV.

Hepatitis A is more common in children than adults because of the route of transmission. Those at highest risk for hepatitis A are those of lower socioeconomic status living in crowded conditions, those confined to crowded psychiatric wards, and those living in or traveling to areas with contaminated food and water sources.

Although asymptomatic cases of acute hepatitis can occur, clinical presentation usually involves an acute onset of signs and symptoms including malaise, jaundice, and diarrhea. Often this condition is mistaken for gastroenteritis. Hepatitis A is more severe in adults than in children, but recovery in almost all cases is complete without sequelae. Chronic states do not develop after an acute HAV infection.

Hepatitis B

Hepatitis B infection ("serum hepatitis") is a serious health problem in the United States and worldwide. Approximately 200,000 new cases of hepatitis B are diagnosed in the United States each year (Gurevich, 1983). Of those, approximately 10,000 patients are hospitalized, and 20,000 become carriers (Gurevich, 1983).

Carriers are the major source of disease transmission. The major vector is blood and body fluids of infected individuals. The virus is known to be transmitted through whole blood, semen, and saliva. Other body fluids (urine, tears, wound drainage, bile, peritoneal and synovial fluid) of infected individuals contain the HBsAg but not the complete virus, so it is not clear whether these fluids are vectors as well (Seef and Koff, 1986; Hoofnagle and Schafer, 1986).

Hepatitis B disease transmission patterns have changed in the last decade. Previously, male homosexuals were the highest risk group, but currently, intravenous (IV) drug users and heterosexuals with multiple sexual partners are at highest risk (Alter et al., 1990a).

The HBV is a DNA virus originally referred to as the Dane particle that belongs to the class of viruses called hepadnaviruses. The HBV has an outer component of surface antigen (HBsAg or "Australia antigen") and an inner component called the hepatitis B core antigen (HBcAg). HBV is not highly virulent (likely to produce severe illness), but it is highly infective (easily transmissible). It is estimated that 300,000 new cases occur each year, with approximately 18,000 occurring in health care workers (Department of Labor, 1987).

The incubation period for HBV is 6 to 26 weeks. In the initial stage of the infection the HBsAg is found in the serum for 4 to 12 weeks. This is the replicating phase when the virus enters the liver cells, replicates, and produces complete virions (Dane particles) and excess surface antigen (HBsAg and HBeAg), which are components of the viral capsid. During this time the infection is very contagious. Then a period of time occurs called the "window" phase between the disappearance of antigen (HBsAg) from the serum and the appearance of antibody (anti-HBsAg). During this time the only serologic marker present is the anti-HBcAg. This is why it is important that a complete hepatitis serology panel be done in the individual with suspected hepatitis infection. Failure to look for the anti-HBcAg can lead to a false assumption that the patient does not have or has not had HBV infection. The window phase lasts for 2 to 12 weeks. Eventually (after 2 to 10 months) anti-HBsAg will appear in the serum.

As stated previously, an acute hepatitis B infection can be entirely asymptomatic. Subclinical disease is frequent, as suggested by the high incidence of anti-HBsAg found in those with no knowledge or history of infection. In symptomatic cases the onset of signs and symptoms is insidious. A prodromal period of flulike symptoms of fatigue, nausea, taste changes, and anorexia occurs approximately 2 weeks prior to the onset of jaundice and dark urine. Complete recovery can take as long as several months.

Hepatitis B is associated with serum sickness or immune complex disease. Fever, malaise, liver tenderness, arthralgias, and rashes are common. Less common are arthropathies such as rheumatoid arthritis or polyarteritis, and necrotizing vasculitis. Elevated serum transaminase and bilirubin levels accompany this phase.

Delta Hepatitis

Delta hepatitis is always associated with a coexistent HBV infection. Delta virus and HBV may coinfect, or delta virus hepatitis may be superimposed on the HBV carrier state. The mode of transmission is similar to that of HBV. Diagnosis is made by identification of the viral antigen in the serum or liver, or by detection of IgM antibody to delta virus.

Hepatitis C

The major cause of what was previously referred to as non-A, non-B (NANB) hepatitis has been identified (Cuthbert, 1990). A newly developed enzyme immunoassay allows for the identification of a serologic marker (antibody) to the hepatitis C virus (HCV). HCV is a single-stranded linear RNA virus similar to flavivirus. Infection with HCV is diagnosed by the presence of anti-HCV antibodies in 90% of patients with chronic NANB hepatitis. HCV has also been implicated in autoimmune liver disease, CAH in patients with alcoholic cirrhosis, and hepatocellular carcinoma (Cuthbert, 1990). Intravenous drug users are at highest risk, and others at risk include heterosexuals with multiple sexual partners or an infected partner, health care personnel exposed to blood and blood products, hemophiliacs, and chronic hemodialysis patients (Alter et al., 1990b).

Hepatitis E

Hepatitis E virus is also called enterically transmitted NANB hepatitis, epidemic NANB hepatitis, and fecal-oral NANB hepatitis, but should not be confused with HBV e antigen. The epidemiologic and clinical courses are similar to those of HAV infection, except that the incidence and prevalence are highest in young adult males.

Caring for the Patient with Hepatitis

The patient presenting with acute hepatitis should be questioned about specific risk factors and close personal contacts so that follow-up with those who are potentially infected can be done. Treatment of acute hepatitis has very little effect on outcome. The patient needs to rest until symptoms disappear, the liver is no longer tender, and the serum bilirubin has decreased to within normal range. A low-fat, high-carbohydrate diet is most palatable for these patients but does not necessarily play a role in recovery. Corticosteroids do not favorably alter the course of acute hepatitis; in fact, they have been found to enhance viral replication (Perillo, 1986). However, many patients with hepatitis, especially chronic active hepatitis, are treated with corticosteroids to slow the progression of disease and to palliate symptoms. This fact must be taken into consideration when caring for these patients to prevent acute steroid withdrawal.

The major implication for nurses caring for the patient with suspected or known acute viral hepatitis is protection of self, co-workers, and other patients from the highly contagious virus. Exposure to blood and possibly other body fluids is the risk, not the patient himself. Strict observation of universal precautions or maintenance of body substance isolation procedures is crucial. A common practice of critical care nurses is recapping contaminated needles. The benefits of this practice in terms of convenience and time saved do not outweigh its extreme risk. The Centers for Disease Control has recommended not recapping needles since 1975 (Centers for Disease Control, 1988).

Nursing Diagnoses for the Patient with Hepatitis

Altered nutrition: Less than body requirements
Potential for infection
Altered bowel elimination: Diarrhea
Social isolation
Altered role performance
Altered family processes
Altered patterns of sexuality
Ineffective coping: Individual
Ineffective coping, family: Compromised
Impaired physical mobility
Disturbance in self-concept: Body image, self-esteem

ALCOHOLIC LIVER DISEASE

Alcohol is the most abused drug in the United States (Malin, 1981), affecting more than 9 million Americans (Hubmayer et al., 1985). No other habit or culturally determined behavior creates more problems than does alcohol (Olsen, 1985). Although the association between alcohol and cirrhosis was recognized as early as 1793 (Galambos, 1978), the problem continues to affect the young and old, females and males, and knows no social barriers. Approximately 15% of alcoholics develop cirrhosis (Moore and Gerstein, 1985). Alcohol plays a major role in the four most common causes of death in men between 20 to 40 years old: suicide, homicide, accidents, and cirrhosis (Olsen, 1985). One-half of fire-related deaths, automobile fatalities, shootings, and drownings; two-thirds of beatings; and three-fourths of stabbings are alcohol-related (Deluca, 1981).

Alcoholic hepatitis is a precirrhotic lesion that progresses to cirrhosis in about one-third of cases (Galambos, 1979). Approximately 50% to 80% of all cases of cirrhosis are caused by alcohol abuse. Alcoholic cirrhosis usually, but not always, develops after many years of persistent alcohol consumption. Daily consumption of more than 60 g of alcohol for a period of at least 5 years is a prerequisite for 80% of those who develop alcoholic cirrhosis (Galambos, 1979). The type of alcohol is not relevant. The widely held belief that chronic consumption of beer or wine is less harmful (or not harmful at all) than chronic consumption of distilled liquor is a fallacy. Women suffer irreversible hepatocellular injury more quickly than men, and the mortality rate is greater in women with alcoholic cirrhosis (Galambos, 1979).

Alcohol has a direct toxic effect on liver cells. Ethanol is oxidized in the liver to acetaldehyde, which is oxidized to acetate. Acetaldehyde disrupts cell membranes, resulting in water retention, swelling, hepatomegaly, and eventually permanent hepatocellular damage. Acetate is oxidized to free fatty acids, which accumulate in the liver (fatty infiltration of the liver). However, the major injury to the liver occurs through the nutritional defects that develop. Alcohol replaces fatty acids as fuel, leading to fatty infiltration of the liver and alterations in nutritional absorption.

Chronic effects of alcoholism on other body systems must be taken into consideration when caring for the patient with alcoholic liver disease. Cardiovascular effects include hypertension, hyperlipidemia, atherosclerosis, and cardiomyopathy. Patients with alcoholic liver disease may have a significant cigarette smoking history and may have COPD. In addition, chronic bronchitis, tuberculosis, and aspiration pneumonia are common. Gastrointestinal effects include peptic ulcer disease, gastritis, reflux esophagitis, and pancreatitis. Malnutrition is associated with hypoalbuminemia, hypomagnesemia, hypocalcemia, hypophosphatemia, and vitamin K deficiency. Megaloblastic anemia secondary to folate deficiency is common.

Cirrhosis

Cirrhosis is the fourth leading cause of death in the United States in adults over the age of 40 and the third leading cause of death in men between the ages of 40 and 55 (Galambos, 1979). Cirrhosis is a chronic and usually slowly progressive disease involving diffuse formation of connective tissue (fibrosis) and nodular regeneration following hepatic parenchymal necrosis and inflammation. The pathophysiologic mechanism can be greatly simplified into three major events: hepatocellular injury, nodular regeneration, and loss of the original lobular architecture.

Causes of hepatocellular injury and necrosis are many: ischemia, toxemia, and viremia. Persistent necrosis stimulates hepatocellular regeneration, which involves the laying down of increased amounts of connective tissue, particularly collagen, by portal fibroblasts. Regenerating hepatocytes and fibrous connective tissue form nodules that distort the normal hepatic lobular and acinar structure. The septa connecting the hepatocytes become fibrous as well, creating increased resistance to venous flow through the septa and across the liver.

The major consequences of the resultant reconstruction of the normal hepatic parenchyma are (1) obstruction of normal portal venous flow and diversion of this blood past functional liver tissue through intrahepatic and perihepatic collateral vessels; (2) formation of basement membranes in the space of Disse; and (3) impedance of metabolic exchange leading to loss of functional capacity of the liver. The most common causes of cirrhosis are listed in Table 45–5.

Portal Hypertension

Portal hypertension is defined as increased hydrostatic pressure within the portal venous system. Specifically, portal hypertension is defined as a portal venous pressure of greater than 5 to 10 mm Hg. There is very little or no pressure drop across the sinusoid because blood flows from the portal venous system to the hepatic veins. Therefore, if hepatic

TABLE 45–5. Etiology of Chronic Liver Disease

Cirrhosis
    Laennec's cirrhosis (alcoholic cirrhosis)
    Postnecrotic cirrhosis* (acute viral hepatitis, shock, drug
      toxicity)
    Cardiac cirrhosis (congestive cirrhosis)
    Cryptogenic cirrhosis (unknown etiology)

Cholestatic disease
    Primary biliary cirrhosis
    Secondary biliary cirrhosis
    Primary sclerosing cholangitis

Metabolic liver disease
    Intestinal (jejunoileal) bypass surgery
    Malnutrition
    Diabetes mellitus

Inborn errors of liver metabolism (genetic disorders)
    Glycogen storage disease (type I, IV)
    Alpha-1 antitrypsin deficiency (Pi^{zz} phenotype)
    Wilson's disease
    Hemochromatosis
    Tyrosinemia
    Galactosemia
    Hereditary fructose intolerance
    Thalassemia
    Cystic fibrosis
    Hepatic porphyrias
    Hepatic amyloidosis
    Familial hypercholesterolemia
    Mucopolysaccharidoses

*Theoretically, all cirrhosis is postnecrotic cirrhosis, but for purposes of clarification of etiology, these distinctions have been made.

venous outflow is blocked, 100% of the increase in pressure is transmitted back to the sinusoids and portal venous system. Normal pressures in the sinusoids and hepatic venous system are slightly lower than portal venous pressure, thus creating the pressure gradient necessary for blood flow through the liver and into the IVC.

Portal hypertension can be classified according to the site of obstruction as *presinusoidal*, *sinusoidal*, and *postsinusoidal*. Portal hypertension resulting from cirrhosis is considered sinusoidal in nature. In the United States, cirrhosis is the most common cause of portal hypertension. Presinusoidal implies that the site of obstruction is before the sinusoids. Causes of presinusoidal portal hypertension include extrahepatic portal vein thrombosis, tumors, schistosomiasis, congenital hepatic fibrosis, and primary biliary cirrhosis. The term postsinusoidal implies that the site of obstruction is past the sinusoids. Causes of postsinusoidal portal hypertension include the Budd-Chiari syndrome (hepatic vein thrombosis) and other veno-occlusive diseases.

Portal venous flow is normally "hepatopedal" or toward the liver. Portal flow can be assessed by visualizing contrast medium in the portal venous branches during the venous phase of superior mesenteric artery arteriography. As cirrhosis develops, resistance to flow increases, resulting in dilation of portal veins proximal to the site of obstruction and increased portal venous pressure. Dilation of the portal veins initially helps to maintain portal blood flow. But eventually portal flow is impeded, and reversal of flow may occur, in which case it is said to be "hepatofugal," or away from the liver. Portal flow is classified according to arteriographic studies from grade I to grade IV, with grade I defined as good hepatopedal flow with contrast medium visible to the periphery of the liver, and grade IV defined as nonvisualization of the portal vein and reversal of flow documented on wedged hepatic venography.

Collateral Vessel Formation

Another consequence of increased resistance to portal venous flow is the development of collateral vessels that bypass the obstruction as a compensatory mechanism to maintain venous return to the right heart. These vessels are called portacaval vessels because they develop between the portal venous system and the caval system (inferior or superior vena cava) (Fig. 45–8).

Portasystemic collateral circulation develops at several sites, particularly within the peritoneal, retroperitoneal, and thoracic cavities. An arteriogram of the patient with severe portal hypertension shows hundreds of collateral vessels that use the abdominal wall, duodenum, stomach, and esophagus as "bridges" to the systemic circulation. Collateral branches can also form in the rectum and may be visible as large hemorrhoidal vessels. For this reason,

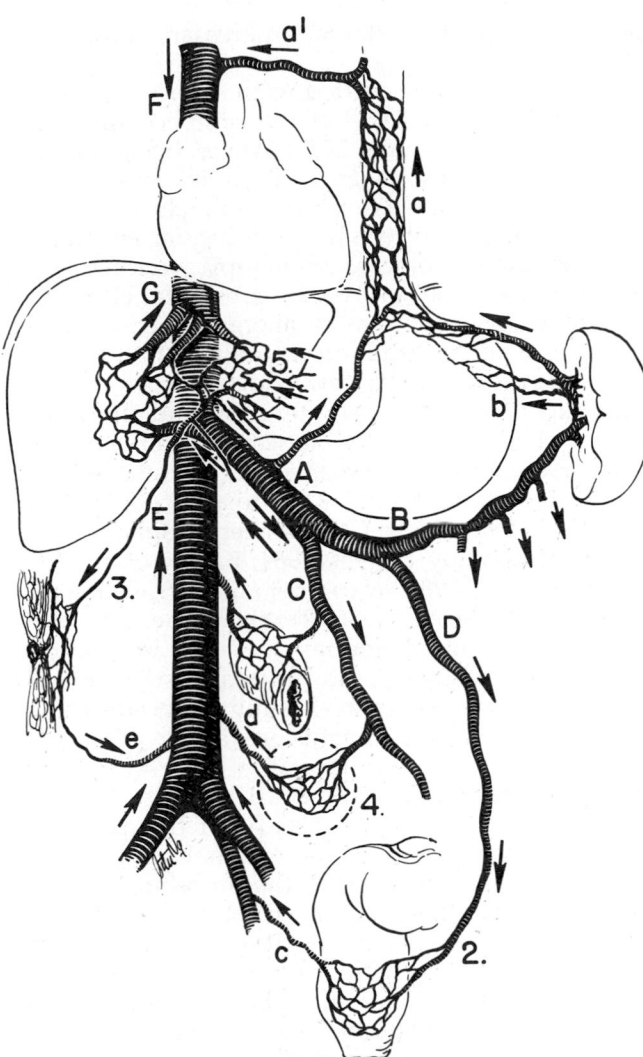

FIGURE 45–8. Collateral circulation. *1*, coronary vein; *2*, superior hemorrhoidal veins; *3*, paraumbilical veins; *4*, veins of Retzius; *5*, veins of Sappey; *A*, portal vein; *B*, splenic vein; *C*, superior mesenteric vein; *D*, inferior mesenteric vein; *E*, inferior vena cava; *F*, superior vena cava; *G*, hepatic veins; *a*, esophageal veins; *a¹*, azygos system; *b*, vasa brevia; *c*, middle and inferior hemorrhoidal veins; *d*, intestinal; *e*, epigastric veins. (From Schwartz, S. I. (1964). *Surgical diseases of the liver.* Reproduced with permission of McGraw-Hill, Inc.)

insertion of anything into the rectum such as a thermometer or rectal tube should be done with great caution.

The collateral vessels of greatest clinical significance are the gastric and esophageal vessels called varices. Varices are dilated, convoluted veins with very little elastic tissue in their walls. Therefore, they are vulnerable to spontaneous rupture and hemorrhage. The risk of variceal bleeding, however, does not correlate with the degree of portal hypertension (Henderson and Warren, 1988). About 50% of deaths in cirrhotics are due to variceal hemorrhage (Rector, 1986). If an individual is admitted to the hospital for bleeding varices, there is a good chance that rebleeding will occur during that admission, and if not during that admission, within 1 year (Benhamou, 1982).

A crucial first component in the management of the patient with upper GI bleeding suspected to be due to gastric or esophageal varices is diagnostic endoscopy. Fifty per cent of patients with varices will experience upper GI bleeding from other causes such as gastritis, peptic ulcer disease, or Mallory-Weiss tears (Clark et al., 1980). Potentially fatal complications of GI bleeding such as exsanguination, aspiration pneumonia, adult respiratory distress syndrome, hepatic encephalopathy, and acute renal failure can occur (Carrithers and Fairman, 1989). The differential diagnosis is important because the treatment for these conditions varies widely and must be timely for patient survival.

INTERVENTIONS FOR BLEEDING VARICES

Endoscopy
A responsibility of the nurse caring for the patient requiring endoscopy is to reassure the patient that the procedure is necessary and safe. Explanations that the procedure will cause some gagging may help the patient to be more cooperative. Gastric lavage with a large-bore (Ewald) tube may be necessary prior to endoscopy to allow adequate visualization. Approximately 5 minutes before the procedure the patient is sedated, usually with diazepam, midazolam, or meperidine. Care is taken not to oversedate the uncooperative patient.

Endoscopy is performed with an instrument called a fiberoptic endoscope or gastroscope. This instrument has a fiberoptic light source that permits an undistorted view of the entire upper GI tract. It is equipped with multiple channels for water, air, and the passage of instruments such as needles, forceps, and lasers. The patient is placed in the left lateral recumbent position. After a rubber mouthpiece is inserted to protect the patient's teeth and facilitate passage of the endoscope, the endoscope is gently advanced, first through the cricopharynx into the esophagus, and then down into the stomach and duodenum. Complications of diagnostic endoscopy include aspiration of gastric contents into the lungs, perforation of a viscus, and rupture of stable varices.

Endoscopic Injection Sclerotherapy
Endoscopic injection sclerotherapy, or injection of a "sclerosing" or coagulating substance into varices to stop or decrease the risk of bleeding, was first used in 1939 (Sivak, 1982) in a 16-year-old girl who was hemorrhaging from varices after a splenectomy (Sivak, 1982). Sclerotherapy was abandoned as a treatment for varices with the advent of surgical portacaval shunt procedures (Terblanche et al., 1979). But, as history often repeats itself, sclerotherapy has made a recent revival as a first-line treatment option for varices and is currently considered the safest method of treating acute variceal bleeding (Warren et al., 1986).

Sclerotherapy, in combination with intravenous vasopressin (Pitressin) is the mainstay of treatment for acute variceal bleeding today and has an 85% to

90% control rate (Henderson and Warren, 1988). Sclerotherapy is usually indicated for the individual who has had at least one variceal hemorrhage, but it is performed prophylactically in some patients. Control of hemorrhage with sclerotherapy is attempted before balloon tamponade. Several prospective, randomized trials have shown no difference in long-term survival between patients treated with sclerotherapy and those who have distal splenorenal shunts (Alwmark et al., 1982; Copenhagen Esophageal Varices Sclerotherapy Project, 1984; Korula et al., 1985; Westaby et al., 1985; Warren et al., 1986; Cello et al., 1986; Larson et al., 1986). Although the rebleeding rate is significantly lower in the shunt group (Warren et al., 1986; Rikkers et al., 1987; Teres et al., 1987), sclerotherapy with surgical back-up in case of failure of the procedure achieves a better quality of life and long-term survival than distal splenorenal shunt alone (Warren et al., 1986).

Sclerotherapy is performed using a modified fiberoptic endoscope with an injection port through which a flexible cable injector is inserted. The injector is equipped with a needle for injection at one end and a Luer-lok attachment for the syringe filled with the sclerosing agent at the other end. The actual injection technique requires two people who simultaneously visualize the varix, one placing the needle in the varix and the other injecting the sclerosing agent. Injection can be "paravariceal" or "intravariceal." Paravariceal injection is done into the tissue surrounding the varix. This induces formation of fibrous tissue around the varix and obliterates bleeding. Intravariceal injection is done directly into the lumen of the varix, which causes thrombus formation in the vein and obliterates bleeding. The number of injections required is dependent on the number of varices and the patient's response to sclerotherapy. Usually, regular injection sessions are required every 2 to 3 months to prevent and control bleeding. During each session as many as 10 to 20 injections may be made. The sclerosing agent used most commonly in the United States is a 5% solution of sodium morrhuate. Other sclerosants used include ethanolamine oleate and sodium tetradecylsulfate. No studies on humans have shown any one sclerosing agent to be superior (Sivak, 1982).

Sclerotherapy can be performed during acute variceal bleeding or, preferably, when the patient is stable. It may be performed in the patient's hospital room, or general anesthesia may be required to protect the airway and keep the patient still to prevent complications. On the other hand, general anesthesia may be contraindicated in the patient with decompensated liver disease. During the procedure the patient is placed on his or her left side with the head of the bed elevated 30 degrees to prevent aspiration. The confused or agitated patient who cannot tolerate general anesthesia may require neuromuscular paralysis to facilitate a complication-free procedure. In this situation, of course, mechanical ventilation will be necessary. Close monitoring of the patient's respiratory status is necessary during and after sclerotherapy.

The mortality rate related to the procedure is less than 1% (Waye, 1987), but the complication rate is 10% to 15% (Bradford, 1983; Waye, 1987). Complications include esophageal ulceration and mucosal sloughing, usually associated with chronic sclerotherapy, perforation of the esophagus, esophageal stenosis after chronic sclerotherapy, variceal bleeding, venous embolism, fever, substernal chest pain due to esophageal spasm, allergic reaction to the sclerosant, and aspiration pneumonia.

The success of sclerotherapy depends on the technical expertise of the sclerotherapists and on whether or not obliteration of the varices is complete (Cello et al., 1986). In several prospective, randomized trials rebleeding occurred in 23% to 75% of patients (Alwmark et al., 1982; Copenhagen Esophageal Varices Sclerotherapy Project, 1984; Korula et al., 1985; Westaby et al., 1985; Warren et al., 1986; Cello et al., 1986; Larson et al., 1986; Terblanche et al., 1981). Short-term results comparing operative time, number of blood transfusions, and hospital costs favor sclerotherapy over portacaval shunt procedures, although more blood transfusions are required after sclerotherapy and the mortality rates of the two groups do not differ (Cello et al., 1986).

It cannot be overemphasized that this procedure is potentially hazardous to health care personnel performing or assisting with the procedure. Patients requiring sclerotherapy, either because of their disease or because of the need for frequent blood transfusions, are at high risk for transmitting hepatitis. Universal precautions or body substance isolation procedures, including the wearing of protective eye covering, is recommended.

Intravenous Vasopressin (Pitressin)

Intravenous Pitressin was first introduced as a treatment for bleeding varices in 1956 (Kehne et al., 1986), but it was not until 1968 that it was applied clinically (Nussbaum et al., 1968). Pitressin is a vasoconstrictor of precapillary arterioles of the gut. It contracts smooth muscle in the arterioles and thus decreases blood flow to the gut. The result is decreased portal flow and pressure.

Pitressin infusion is indicated when sclerotherapy is contraindicated or fails to control an acute bleeding episode. It is indicated before balloon tamponade because it is associated with fewer complications (Rector, 1986). Although Pitressin can be administered intra-arterially, the intravenous route is just as effective and is associated with fewer complications. Pitressin is effective in controlling hemorrhage in 50% of cases, but rebleeding is likely to occur (Getzen et al., 1978; Rector, 1986).

A reasonable protocol for IV administration of Pitressin is a loading dose of 20 U in 50 mL of 5% dextrose given over 30 minutes followed by a maintenance infusion of 0.1 to 0.5 U/minute. The safe maximal infusion rate is 0.9 U/minute (Rector, 1986).

Discontinuation of the infusion should be done by tapering it slowly over at least 24 hours.

Administration of Pitressin is not a benign action. Intravenous Pitressin is associated with several important side effects: coronary vasoconstriction, cardiac arrhythmias, myocardial ischemia, decreased heart rate, decreased cardiac output, systemic hypertension, abdominal cramps, and a hypermotile bowel. Continuous ECG monitoring is necessary to detect ST segment changes associated with myocardial ischemia. Intravenous nitroglycerin may be useful or necessary during Pitressin infusion to prevent myocardial ischemia.

Because Pitressin is a synthetic antidiuretic hormone, another side effect is salt and water retention. Water intoxication and hyponatremia can occur. Pitressin is also a potent vasoconstrictor that causes tissue necrosis and sloughing when it infiltrates into the subcutaneous tissue. Tissue damage due to inadvertent Pitressin infiltration is frequently of such a magnitude that skin grafting is required. For this reason, administration through a central venous access is recommended.

Propranolol

Propranolol has been used with variable results for the treatment of variceal bleeding. The proposed benefit of propranolol is that it decreases heart rate, cardiac output, and hepatic venous pressure through beta receptor blockade (Lebrec et al., 1980). Other studies, however, do not support these findings (Lebrec et al., 1980; Colman et al., 1985). The dose response is extremely variable; patients require between 40 and 280 mg/day for results (Colman et al., 1985; Fleig et al., 1987).

Balloon Tamponade

From the 1930s until the late 1950s balloon tamponade was a standard treatment for bleeding varices even though the potentially lethal complications of this mode of therapy were recognized (Conn, 1958; Conn et al., 1981). Indeed, today, Hanna and colleagues (1981) describe the Sengstaken-Blakemore tube as "an ingenious device capable of taking as well as saving lives."

Balloon tamponade of bleeding varices is accomplished most frequently with a device called a Sengstaken-Blakemore tube. This tube is a triple-lumen, red rubber catheter with inflatable gastric and esophageal balloons attached (Fig. 45–9A). The proximal end of the catheter branches into three clearly marked ports, each representing a separate lumen. One port is used for inflation of the gastric balloon, one is used for inflation of the esophageal balloon, and the third is used for gastric aspiration and suction.

Prior to insertion, the tube is lubricated, the patient's posterior pharynx is sprayed with a topical anesthetic, and the head of the bed is elevated 30 to 45 degrees. The necessity for insertion of the tube and the insertion procedure are explained to the patient. Patient cooperation is necessary for smooth and uneventful insertion of the tube. Unfortunately, patients requiring this intervention are often in crisis due to upper GI hemorrhage, or they are encephalopathic. The patient is instructed to swallow as the tube is passed through a nostril and into the esophagus. Although the tube has two balloons, gastric balloon tamponade is attempted first; if this is successful, the esophageal balloon remains deflated. When the 50-cm mark on the tube is even with the patient's nostril the gastric balloon is partially inflated with 50 mL of air while the area over the epigastrium is auscultated for the sound of air insufflation. A chest x-ray is then taken to verify placement of the gastric balloon below the gastroesophageal (GE) junction before it is fully inflated. Failure to verify correct balloon placement could result in full inflation of the balloon within the esophagus with resultant esophageal rupture, mediastinitis, and death.

When balloon placement below the GE junction is verified, it is filled with 300 to 500 mL of air, and the gastric balloon port is double-clamped with rubber-shod clamps. The result is a tamponading effect on the bleeding varices located in the proximal gastric and GE junction mucosa. The gastric aspiration port is connected to low, intermittent suction. Initially, the stomach may need to be lavaged until the return fluid is clear to prevent clotting of the gastric aspiration lumen and to monitor control of bleeding.

Secretions can pool in the esophagus above the inflated balloon, increasing the risk of pulmonary aspiration. For this reason, an NG tube is inserted just to the level of the GE junction and connected to low, intermittent suction.

Traditionally, traction has been applied at the proximal end of the tube to ensure that the gastric balloon is placed tight against the cardia of the stomach and the GE junction. Methods employed to maintain traction include pulling the tube taut and attaching it to the face bar of a football helmet or baseball catcher's mask, or attaching orthopedic traction to the proximal end of the tube. Regardless of the method used, this intervention is uncomfortable for the patient and family, and the psychosocial implications can be significant. The nursing literature is void of studies comparing outcomes of patients in whom traction is applied with those in whom it is not. However, Teres found that this practice is not necessary, that adequate tension of the balloon can be maintained without traction, and that application of traction is associated with more patient discomfort and complications (Teres et al., 1978). In spite of these findings, the use of traction remains a common practice.

If bleeding cannot be controlled using gastric balloon tamponade alone, the esophageal balloon is also inflated to 25 to 40 mm Hg using a mercury manometer, and the esophageal lumen is double-clamped with rubber-shod clamps. Pressure in the esophageal balloon should be checked every 30 to 60 minutes. Continual monitoring of gastric secretions for blood is necessary to determine whether hemostasis is

1. Lumen to gastric balloon
2. Gastric aspiration lumen
3. Lumen to esophageal balloon

1. Esophageal aspiration lumen
2. Gastric aspiration lumen
3. Lumen to gastric balloon

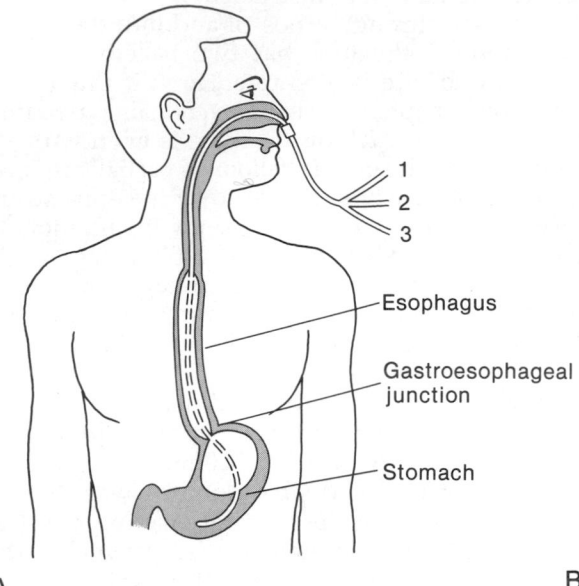

Esophagus

Gastroesophageal
junction

Stomach

A

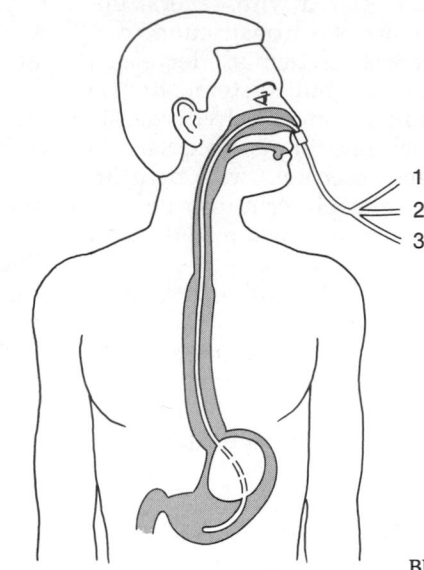

B

FIGURE 45–9. *A,* Sengstaken-Blakemore tube. *B,* Linton-Nachlas tube.

attained. If not, the pressure in the esophageal balloon can be increased to 45 mm Hg, and the gastric balloon can be inflated to hold up to 400 mL of air. However, at these high pressure levels ulceration of the mucosa will occur in only a few hours. Therefore, esophageal balloon pressure should be maintained at the lowest pressure that will control bleeding, and it should be continued only as long as necessary.

Balloon tamponade achieves primary hemostasis in 70% to 80% of cases, but results are rarely permanent (Rector, 1986). Balloon tamponade is not meant to be employed as a long-term therapy. Esophageal balloon pressure should not be maintained for longer than 72 hours and should be discontinued in less than 72 hours if possible. When hemostasis is attained, the tube is left in place and the balloons are deflated 12 to 24 hours prior to removal.

The major complications of balloon tamponade are (1) rupture or deflation of the balloon(s) and subsequent upper airway obstruction, (2) pulmonary aspiration, and (3) rupture of the esophagus. Scissors should be kept visible at the bedside at all times to be used in case the balloons migrate proximally and occlude the upper airway. In this life-threatening situation the lumens are immediately cut to facilitate prompt removal of the tube. Application of suction above the most proximally inflated balloon will help prevent pulmonary aspiration. Esophageal rupture is manifested by a sudden onset of upper abdominal or back pain and a sudden decrease in blood pressure. Necrosis of the affected nare can occur if it is not protected from constant pressure from the tube. Just as after nasotracheal intubation with an endotracheal tube, nasoesophageal intubation can lead to a life-threatening sinusitis. The onset of fever associated with purulent and foul-smelling nasal and nasopharyngeal drainage are signs of sinusitis. Novis found that the in-hospital mortality rate was 60% when the Sengstaken-Blakemore tube was used as the only mode of therapy (Sivak, 1982).

Other tubes are commercially available and are used for the same purpose as the Sengstaken-Blakemore tube. The Linton-Nachlas tube (Fig. 45–9B) is also a triple-lumen tube, but has only one large gastric balloon. The gastric balloon can be inflated with up to 800 mL of air. The two remaining lumens are for gastric and esophageal aspiration, a distinct advantage over the Sengstaken-Blakemore tube. The Linton-Nachlas tube is used to control bleeding from gastric varices. Because the tube does not have an esophageal balloon, varices in the middle and proximal esophagus cannot be tamponaded with this tube. The Minnesota tube is a quadruple-lumen tube. It has the advantages of both the Sengstaken-Blakemore tube and the Linton-Nachlas tube: gastric and esophageal aspiration capabilities, and both gastric and esophageal balloons.

Summary of Medical Treatment Considerations for the Patient with Bleeding Varices

Medical therapy is employed as a first-line treatment for bleeding varices. Patients who continue to bleed acutely in spite of sclerotherapy are first administered Pitressin. If Pitressin fails to stop the bleeding, angiography is indicated. An emergent portacaval shunt, although not desirable, may be necessary to control acute variceal bleeding before other forms of medical intervention are tried. The Sengstaken-Blakemore tube may be necessary to maintain hemostasis in the patient who bleeds rapidly and profusely and who does not respond to Pitressin. Emergent portacaval shunts are required more often in this group of patients.

The patient who is bleeding from varices is at risk for hypotension and decreased tissue perfusion. The nurse should routinely assess the patient for end-organ effects of decreased tissue perfusion such as oliguria, signs of myocardial ischemia, altered mentation, adult respiratory distress syndrome (ARDS), and ileus. The goal of treating hemorrhage is prevention of end-organ ischemia and associated complications. The patient's cardiac history is very important. The patient with a compromised cardiac reserve is at high risk for acute myocardial infarction (MI).

Volume resuscitation with packed red blood cells, fresh frozen plasma for clotting factors, and crystalloids is a priority intervention. However, the potential harm of maintaining adequate plasma volume for organ perfusion is the risk of increasing portal pressure and thus the chances of variceal bleeding. Placement of a pulmonary artery catheter is necessary to ensure optimal fluid resuscitation and management. Supplemental oxygen is also indicated.

The patient with upper GI bleeding from varices requires vigorous mouth care for both infection control and aesthetic reasons. This patient will also be passing melanotic stools, which may be frequent enough to cause breakdown of the perianal tissue. Attention to skin and mucous membrane care is important in this high-risk patient.

CASE HISTORY

B.G., a 67-year-old white man weighing 70 kg, was admitted emergently at 9:00 P.M. to the surgical ICU for acute upper GI bleeding, presumed to be from gastroesophageal varices. He had a 4-day history of intermittent hematemesis for which he had been treated medically at another hospital. On admission he was pale, diaphoretic, and slightly confused. He had had 20 mL of urine output over the previous 2 hours, and his lungs were clear. His BP was 110/80, HR 135/minute, and in lead II of the ECG there was a 2 mm ST depression. His hemoglobin and hematrocrit were 7.3 g/dL and 19.1%, respectively. Thirty minutes after admission he vomited approximately 750 mL of bright red blood. His HR increased to 150/minute and the BP decreased to 80/60.

Rapid transfusion of 2 units of packed red blood cells was begun, and a right subclavian pulmonary artery catheter was inserted. Initial hemodynamic readings were CVP, 2 mm Hg, PA, 18/10 mm Hg, PCWP, 8 mm Hg, CO, 9.5 liters/minute, and SVR, 600 dynes/sec per cm⁵. Endoscopy revealed that he was bleeding from a large gastric varix.

One hour later he was more confused, there had been no further urine output, and his lungs were congested. His hemodynamic readings were CVP, 15 mm Hg, PA, 40/25, PCWP, 25 mm Hg, CO, 3.0 liters/minute, and SVR, 1900 dynes/second per cm⁵. A 12-lead ECG confirmed a massive anterior MI. Despite oxygen, inotropic support, and judicious blood replacement he developed cardiogenic shock and died at 5:30 A.M. the next day.

Nursing Diagnoses for the Patient with Bleeding Varices

Altered nutrition: Less than body requirements
Potential for infection
Altered bowel elimination: Diarrhea
Altered tissue perfusion: Renal, cerebral, cardiopulmonary, gastrointestinal, peripheral
Actual fluid volume deficit
Altered cardiac output: Decreased
Impaired gas exchange
Ineffective airway clearance
Potential for injury: Suffocating
Potential for impaired skin integrity
Impaired tissue integrity: Oral mucous membranes
Altered family processes
Ineffective coping, individual
Ineffective coping, family: Compromised
Impaired physical mobility
Self-care deficit: Feeding, bathing/hygiene, toileting
Disturbance in self-concept: Body image, self-esteem
Altered thought processes

ASCITES

Ascites is an abnormal accumulation of fluid in the peritoneal cavity. Although there are many causes of ascites (malnutrition, severe congestive heart failure, nephrotic syndrome, pancreatitis, and neoplastic disease, to name a few), the most common cause of ascites in cirrhotics is the cirrhosis itself. Ascitic fluid of cirrhosis is normally clear with a yellow tinge. If the patient is deeply jaundiced the fluid will be a deeper shade of yellow. Ascites is a late sign in the continuum of cirrhosis; in other words, its presence indicates advanced disease. The patient who develops ascites has only a 40% chance of being alive after 2 years (Sherlock, 1979).

Another form of ascites, "chylous" ascites, is rare in patients with cirrhosis (Schumann, 1983). The most common cause of chylous ascites is malignant disease that results in occlusion and rupture of intestinal lymphatics with leakage of fluid rich in triglycerides into the peritoneal cavity. The triglyceride level of chylous ascites is greater than the plasma level. Chylous ascites also occurs in some patients after distal splenorenal shunt surgery when intestinal lymphatics are transected during the procedure.

There are two theories of ascites formation (Lautt and Greenway, 1987). The first is called the *underfilling theory*. According to this theory, the triad of portal hypertension, decreased colloid osmotic pressure, and increased hepatic lymph transudation results in retention of sodium and water and accumulation of ascites. Because there is no pressure gradient from the sinusoids to the hepatic veins, 100% of the increase in pressure due to blockage of venous outflow is transmitted back to the sinusoids and the portal system, resulting in increased lymph production. Hepatic lymph is returned to the systemic circulation by the large thoracic duct. Normal thoracic duct flow is about 800 to 1000 mL/day, but this can increase to 20 liters/day in patients with severe portal hypertension (Cattau et al., 1982). Hepatic flow increases by about 60% for every milliliter of mercury increase in intrahepatic venous pressure (Cattau et al., 1982). Fluid weeping from the hepatic vasculature and the splanchnic bed increases thoracic duct flow. Ascites develops when maximal thoracic duct flow is exceeded. There is a net movement of fluid into the peritoneal cavity, resulting in a reduced "effective" plasma volume.

The second theory is called the *overflow theory*. In this theory it is postulated that the diseased liver releases substances that cause renal vasoconstriction and excessive tubular reabsorption of sodium. Expansion of blood volume results in increased hepatic lymph formation. In other words, retained sodium and water are the initiating factors.

Ascites results in plasma volume contraction and stimulation of neuroendocrine compensatory responses of epinephrine, renin-angiotensin, and antidiuretic hormone release. Consequently, renal blood flow is decreased, and urinary sodium is retained.

Several important problems and complications are associated with ascites. From a pathophysiologic perspective the most important are the predisposition to renal failure and variceal bleeding. The most obvious are the related physical disfigurement and physical dysfunction. Not only are the body and the body image changed, ascites also interferes with erect posture and balance and adds to muscle fatigue in the already malnourished and fatigued individual. Minor complications include incisional, inguinal, and femoral hernias. Premature satiety interferes with nutritional intake at a time when nutrient metabolism is compromised. Reflux esophagitis can exacerbate esophageal varices and predispose the individual to esophageal ulceration.

An elevated diaphragm displaces the heart, causing increased right heart filling pressures and jugular venous distention. Right heart filling pressures may be falsely normal or elevated when the patient is hypovolemic and are almost always falsely elevated in the supine position. An important factor to be considered when assessing hemodynamic parameters is the position of the patient. Depending on the extent of accumulation of ascites, the patient may not be able to tolerate the supine position. This is another reason why it is important to measure heart pressures in the upright position that is best tolerated by the patient. The patient's baseline pressures with an elevated diaphragm are established and used for comparison with changing trends. These pressures will of course change if ascitic fluid is drained, necessitating reestablishment of baseline pressures. Other parameters such as urine output may be more

useful in assessing volume status and tissue perfusion.

Pleural effusions occur in 5% to 10% of patients with ascites (Carrithers and Fairman, 1989). Fluid transgresses upward through the transdiaphragmatic lymphatics and through tiny ruptures of the diaphragm that occur secondary to increased intra-abdominal pressure created by the ascites. End-stage patients may require regular thoracenteses to control reaccumulating pleural effusions. Atelectasis and pleural effusions increase the risk of infection in these already immunocompromised individuals.

Infection of ascitic fluid is common. Peritonitis develops in approximately 8% of cirrhotic patients with ascites (Gregory et al., 1977), and is more common in those with decompensated cirrhosis. Spontaneous bacterial peritonitis is diagnosed when the polymorphonuclear granulocyte count of the ascitic fluid is greater than 250/mm^3 and culture of ascitic fluid is positive. Associated signs and symptoms include localized abdominal pain, fever, leukocytosis, and increased serum bilirubin and creatinine. The development of spontaneous bacterial peritonitis is often the cause of a sudden deterioration in the patient's condition. Frequently, such a patient is admitted to the ICU in a "septic" state.

Ascitic fluid in the immunocompetent individual contains humoral substances that are active against gram-negative organisms. Gram-positive organisms are more often the cause of peritonitis than gram-negative organisms (Sherlock, 1985). However, in the cirrhotic patient both gram-positive and gram-negative organisms cause peritonitis and lead to seeding of infection in other organs, particularly the lungs. Treatment consists of broad-spectrum antibiotics.

Interventions for Ascites

The treatment regimen for ascites in general consists of diuresis and fluid and salt restriction (Frakes, 1980; Perez and Schiff, 1988). Paracentesis may be necessary to prevent pulmonary compromise and immobility.

Sodium Restriction. Sodium restrictions of from 0.5 to 2.0 g/day may be prescribed. These diets are not generally palatable and can be expensive. Therefore, patient compliance is not likely to be good, especially if the patient is not hospitalized. If the patient is hospitalized, restriction to a low-sodium diet may lead to significant decreases in food intake and further catabolism. Care must also be taken to identify sources of sodium intake such as sodium-rich antacids and antibiotics and drugs that can interfere with renal sodium excretion such as nonsteroidal anti-inflammatory agents and beta blockers.

Diuretics. Diuresis must be accomplished at a safe rate to avoid precipitating hypovolemia, prerenal azotemia, and encephalopathy. According to Sherlock (1985), it may be better to have a patient who is "wet and wise instead of one who is dry and demented." Therefore, replacement of effective plasma volume with plasma should accompany induced diuresis, and the serum creatinine, creatinine clearance, and blood urea nitrogen (BUN) are monitored closely.

The maximal rate of ascites reabsorption is 700 to 900 mL/day (Galambos, 1979). Therefore, diuresis of amounts greater than this results in removal of fluid from spaces other than the peritoneal cavity. This is relatively safe in the patient who also has peripheral edema but can be very hazardous in the patient who does not, resulting in renal failure.

The aim of diuretic therapy is to inhibit renal sodium conservation mechanisms. Potassium-sparing diuretics such as the aldosterone antagonist spironolactone (Aldactone) and triamterene are used for initial control. The onset of action of spironolactone occurs in 2 to 3 days, whereas the effects of triamterene can be seen in a few hours. A side effect of long-term use of spironolactone in men is gynecomastia. Serum potassium levels are monitored regularly in patients taking spironolactone because hyperkalemia is another side effect. Potassium-wasting or loop diuretics, namely, furosemide, may be necessary. In more severe cases, a combination of intravenous plasma, furosemide, and mannitol may be employed. Bedrest, up to 18 hours a day, is prescribed by some physicians because this initiates diuresis (Galambos, 1979). Compliance with this prescription is also difficult to control in the nonhospitalized patient.

Hyponatremia can occur after urinary excretion of sodium in the already sodium-restricted patient. Overhydration can also exacerbate this condition, leading to a state of water intoxication. Unless the serum sodium level is less than 130 mEq/liter, it is usually not treated. Treatment may consist of restriction of water intake and osmotic diuresis with mannitol to increase free water clearance. Hypokalemia can also occur after administration of loop diuretics or from secondary hyperaldosteronism, which develops as a compensatory response to decreased effective plasma volume.

Paracentesis. Paracentesis may be indicated for removal of ascites when it is interfering with breathing, eating, and activities of daily living. It is also indicated when ascites is resistant (responds to intravenous therapy but reaccumulates) or refractory (does not respond to other therapies). Repeated paracenteses for the removal of large amounts of fluid are frequently necessary in combination with administration of diuretics and salt-poor albumin. The patient's hemodynamic response to removal of large fluid volumes must be monitored closely. With release of pressure on the IVC, venous return and cardiac output generally improve, resulting in increased diuresis. Also, ventilatory status and appetite improve.

A protocol for sterile insertion of a peritoneal drain and for sterile management of the catheter and drainage system must be developed to prevent peritonitis. Abdominal assessment for peritoneal signs indicative of acute abdomen or peritonitis is an ongoing nursing responsibility.

Peritinoneovenous Shunting. The LeVeen valve (Fig. 45–10) for peritinoneovenous shunting was described by LeVeen in 1974 as a procedure for "continual reinfusion of ascitic fluid into the circulation via a pressure-activated valve inserted into the peritoneum and connected to a larger interthoracic vein through subcutaneous tubing" (Schumann, 1983). In the past, and even to some extent today, this device was considered another treatment option for patients with intractable ascites.

The LeVeen valve is contraindicated in patients who are encephalopathic, have had recent abdominal surgery, or have congestive heart failure, dissemi-

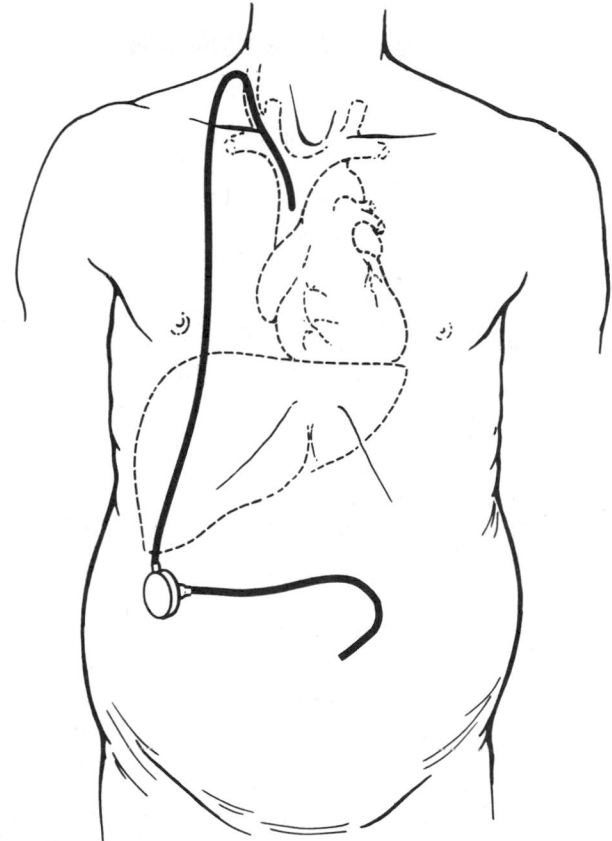

FIGURE 45–10. Placement of the peritoneovenous shunt. The collecting cannula lies within the peritoneal cavity, the valve is positioned extraperitoneally, and the outflow tubing extends from the valve through the subcutaneous tissue on the chest wall to an entrance point in the internal jugular vein. This tip is advanced to the superior vena cava within 1 to 2 cm of the right atrium, or within the right atrium. (From Schumann, D. (1983). *Heart & Lung*, 12, 248–255.)

nated intravascular coagulopathy, or severe decompensated liver disease (Galambos, 1979). One reason for the decrease in the initial popularity of the LeVeen valve is the high associated operative mortality (13%) (Sherlock, 1985). Infection is the major fatal complication. Plugging of the valve with proteinaceous material also occurs, rendering it ineffective and in need of being replaced. Less than 50% of LeVeen valves remain patent for 1 year (Sherlock, 1985). For these reasons, the LeVeen valve is a therapeutic option for only a select few patients with intractable ascites.

A functional LeVeen shunt will lead to the following changes in the patient's condition: hemodilution, diuresis and urinary loss of potassium, weight loss, decreased abdominal girth, and more comfortable respirations. Mobilization of ascitic fluid into the systemic circulation can lead to acute volume overload, congestive heart failure, and pulmonary edema. Excessive diuresis can trigger the hepatorenal syndrome. Patients receiving LeVeen shunts frequently require intensive care to provide close observation of and treatment for these problems.

Nursing Diagnoses for the Patient with Ascites

Altered nutrition: Less than body requirements
Potential for infection
Altered tissue perfusion: Renal
Fluid volume deficit: Actual
Impaired gas exchange
Ineffective breathing pattern
Potential for impaired skin integrity
Impaired social interaction
Altered role performance
Ineffective coping, individual
Noncompliance to diet and medical regimen
Impaired physical mobility
Sleep pattern disturbance
Disturbance in self-concept: Body image, self-esteem, personal identity

HEPATORENAL SYNDROME

Hepatorenal syndrome is defined as progressive acute renal failure in the patient with advanced liver disease, most commonly alcoholic liver disease, when the etiology of the renal failure cannot be explained by other causes (Clive, 1985; Carrithers and Fairman, 1989). This diagnosis is made on clinical grounds in the patient with manifestations of liver disease or is based on biopsy findings. Causes other than liver disease of acute renal failure in the patient with liver disease such as metabolic, toxic, and septic causes must be ruled out before the diagnosis of hepatorenal syndrome can be made. Hepatorenal syndrome is a "functional" disorder of the kidneys characterized by renal hypoperfusion that develops

as a result of decreased effective plasma volume. Vasoconstrictive mechanisms such as the release of endotoxins (Hollenberg, 1983), activation of the renin-angiotensin system (Zipser et al., 1983), thromboxanes (Zipser et al., 1979), and prostaglandins (LeVeen et al., 1976) have been implicated as precipitating factors of hepatorenal syndrome. The production of vasoconstrictive substances is increased while production of vasodilatory substances is decreased, favoring renal hypertension. The hepatorenal syndrome can be induced by excessive diuresis or diarrhea, hemorrhage, infection, or administration of nephrotoxic or nonsteroidal anti-inflammatory drugs to the patient with decompensated liver disease.

Sodium reabsorptive and urinary concentrating ability of the kidneys remains intact during hepatorenal syndrome. Therefore, the condition is reversible, as demonstrated by the fact that kidneys from patients with hepatorenal syndrome have been successfully transplanted (Finn, 1988).

The differential diagnosis for hepatorenal syndrome includes prerenal azotemia and acute tubular necrosis. Prerenal azotemia can be ruled out by the fluid challenge test. The patient with prerenal azotemia will respond to a fluid challenge by increasing urine output; the patient with hepatorenal syndrome will not. A fluid challenge is not recommended when the patient has pulmonary or venous congestion. If the patient has extreme ascites, rapid volume expansion increases the risk of variceal bleeding. In patients with acute tubular necrosis urine sodium concentration is greater than 40 mEq/liter, and in those with hepatorenal syndrome it is less than 10 mEq/liter (Frakes, 1980).

Hepatorenal syndrome is manifested by progressive oliguria in the presence of normovolemia, azotemia with anorexia, weakness, nausea, vomiting, increased thirst, highly concentrated urine that is free of sodium, and elevated serum creatinine and BUN. Even though the patient's cardiovascular system is hyperdynamic, renal blood flow is diverted away from the renal cortex. Because of this the patient's ability to excrete free water is decreased. As with any patient in renal failure, the patient with hepatorenal syndrome must be closely monitored for electrolyte imbalances (hyperkalemia, hyponatremia), hypervolemia with pulmonary edema, pleural effusions, and sepsis. In patients with decompensated cirrhosis the serum creatinine is not the most reliable index of renal function. Creatinine clearance is a better index. Therefore, 24-hour urine collections are commonly done on a regular basis to manage this problem.

Patient survival depends on reversing the initiating factors such as restoring effective plasma volume to optimal levels and restoring some degree of liver function. Dialysis may be employed as a life-saving measure while initiating factors are being reversed in the patient who has the potential for long-term survival, or as a bridge to transplantation if the patient is a candidate for liver transplantation.

Care of the patient in hepatorenal syndrome is complex because so many other problems coexist. Efforts at multisystem stabilization are ongoing. Finding the right balance between fluid volume deficit and overload can be difficult. The patient in acute renal failure is at high risk of acquiring an infection; the most frequent cause of death resulting from acute renal failure is sepsis (Cascino et al., 1978). Therefore, diligent observation of infection control measures is a vital component of the overall plan of care for this patient. Correction of etiologic factors is a primary goal, with protection of renal perfusion during diuresis and dialysis a secondary goal.

Nursing Diagnoses for the Patient with Hepatorenal Syndrome

Altered nutrition: Less than body requirements
Potential for infection
Altered pattern of urinary elimination:
    Urinary retention
Altered tissue perfusion: Renal
Fluid volume excess
Potential for fluid volume deficit
Impaired gas exchange
Ineffective breathing pattern
Potential for impaired skin integrity
Impaired physical mobility
Altered thought processes

HEPATIC ENCEPHALOPATHY

The brain of the individual with advanced liver disease is particularly sensitive to insults that do not affect the brain of the normal individual. Hepatic encephalopathy is defined as neuropsychiatric dysfunction resulting from liver disease and failure. In general, hepatic encephalopathy is characterized by a deterioration in intellectual function, personal behavior, and level of consciousness. Hepatic encephalopathy may occur spontaneously, or it may be precipitated by several important factors, to be discussed later.

The patient who develops hepatic encephalopathy has an altered circulation pathway through which toxic substances in the portal blood enter the systemic circulation and reach the brain without first being metabolized by the liver. This altered pathway consists of intrahepatic and perihepatic collateral vessels that develop because of portal hypertension. The result is that brain cells are poisoned by these toxic substances, which are usually intestinal in nature and which are not metabolized by the liver (Breen and Schenker, 1972; Schenker et al., 1974; Maddrey and Weber, 1975).

Development of spontaneous hepatic encephalopathy indicates that at least 50% of the liver's ability to synthesize urea has been lost (Galambos, 1979).

Spontaneous hepatic encephalopathy usually occurs in patients who are deeply jaundiced with ascites and heralds the end stage of advanced liver disease. Not surprisingly, the prognosis for the patient with precipitated encephalopathy is better than that for the patient with spontaneous encephalopathy.

Ammonia is postulated to be the key toxic stimulus to hepatic encephalopathy. Ammonia uptake normally occurs in the brain, liver, and skeletal muscle. Changes in brain, liver, and skeletal muscle metabolism contribute to increased serum ammonia accumulation. Cirrhosis is associated with muscle wasting and portasystemic shunting, both of which interfere with hepatic uptake of ammonia. Decreased hepatic uptake of ammonia increases the uptake of ammonia by the brain. Ammonia concentrations in the cerebrospinal fluid and blood increase in hepatic encephalopathy, and interventions that decrease serum ammonia concentrations improve encephalopathy. However, there is an inconsistent correlation between ammonia levels and the degree of neurologic impairment. For this reason, it is thought that other factors must also be responsible.

The patient who develops hepatic encephalopathy is thought to have increased cerebral sensitivity and possibly a deficiency of an essential factor required for normal brain metabolism, resulting in decreased energy utilization by the brain (Galambos, 1979). Mercaptans, which are derived from bacterial metabolism of toxic methionine, are normally removed by the liver. The patient in a state of hepatic encephalopathy, however, excretes mercaptans through pulmonary respiration, which produces the characteristic fruity, odorous breath called fetor hepaticus. The presence of fetor hepaticus is used by some clinicians as a criterion for diagnosing hepatic encephalopathy. Hypovolemia decreases hepatic perfusion and cerebral blood flow and decreases clearance of ammonia. Diuretics that induce a hypokalemic alkalosis with an increased extracellular fluid pH promote diffusion of ammonia from blood into tissues such as the brain.

Failure of deamination functions and altered ammonia metabolism by the diseased liver result in increased levels of aromatic amino acids and decreased levels of branched chain amino acids in the CNS (Bouletreau et al., 1979). Aromatic amino acids have an inhibitory effect on normal neurotransmitters favoring sedation, and branched chain amino acids have arousal properties favoring wakefulness. Tryptophan, the most toxic of the aromatic amino acids, is converted to serotonin, which produces sedation.

Accumulated systemic ammonia may impair normal synaptic transmission. Normal neurotransmitter synthesis is controlled by brain concentrations of precursor amino acids. Under normal conditions phenylalanine is converted by hydroxylation to tyrosine, which is further hydroxylated to dopa for the synthesis of the neurotransmitters dopamine and norepinephrine. In hepatic encephalopathy it is postulated that (1) phenylalanine is hydroxylated to phenyl ethylamine, which is further hydroxylated to phenyl ethanolamine, and (2) tyrosine is hydroxylated to tyramine, which is further hydroxylated to octopamine (Kaplan, 1987). Phenyl ethanolamine and octopamine are "false" neurotransmitters that replace norepinephrine at synaptic junctions, altering cerebral metabolism and favoring sedation.

Common precipitants of hepatic encephalopathy in the cirrhotic patient include hypoxia, infection, electrolyte abnormalities, increased amounts of ammonia in the diet, certain drugs (sedatives, alcohol, anesthetics), GI bleeding, hypovolemia, altered renal function, and surgically created portacaval shunts (Breen and Schenker, 1972; Galambos, 1979; Sherlock, 1985). It is important not to lose sight of the cause of encephalopathy when caring for a patient with advanced liver disease in whom encephalopathy has been precipitated by iatrogenic measures. Appropriate interventions to correct the underlying problem will usually reverse this type of encephalopathy.

The most common precipitant of hepatic encephalopathy in the cirrhotic patient is vigorous diuresis followed by azotemia (Galambos, 1979; Sherlock, 1985). Diuretics can precipitate encephalopathy by increasing ammonia production in either of two ways. First, prerenal azotemia secondary to reduced circulating plasma volume and decreased renal perfusion provides substrate for ammonia production. Renal tubular acidosis impairs hydrogen ion and ammonia transport in the urine, resulting in increased serum ammonia. Second, hypokalemia and metabolic alkalosis that occur as a result of hyperaldosteronism and as a side effect of administration of potassium-wasting diuretics, particularly the thiazides, increase renal production of ammonia. The higher the pH, the more freely ammonia penetrates the blood–brain barrier. Therefore, invasive and noninvasive measurements of plasma volume, as well as serum potassium and ammonia levels, are followed closely in the cirrhotic patient treated with diuretics.

Infection is often found to be the cause of unexplained hepatic encephalopathy. Remember that the patient with advanced liver disease is inherently immunosuppressed and has other risk factors related to the potential for infection such as ascites, malnutrition, and the frequent necessity for hospitalization. Fever increases the metabolic rate of tissues, which in turn increases the rate of amino acid metabolism and ammonia production. Fever can also contribute to decreased extracellular fluid and plasma volume. Detection of septicemia based on hemodynamic assessment of the critically ill patient with advanced liver disease is difficult because the classic signs of septicemia, increased cardiac output, and decreased SVR are normal findings in this patient. Exaggerated changes from the patient's baseline do occur and can be used in this assessment.

GI bleeding places an increased protein load on the GI tract, leading to increased amino acid and ammonia levels. An increased demand for hepatic detoxification occurs at a time when hepatic perfusion is decreased. Hemorrhage that is significant

enough to decrease renal perfusion also increases BUN and provides additional substrate for intestinal ammonia production.

An individual with hepatic encephalopathy may be entirely asymptomatic in the very early stages. The clinical manifestations of hepatic encephalopathy may fall anywhere on a continuum from completely asymptomatic to deep coma. Hepatic encephalopathy can be classified clinically into four grades. Table 45–6 outlines the clinical signs and defining characteristics of these stages.

In grade I hepatic encephalopathy, sometimes referred to as the prodromal stage, early signs include decreased intellectual capacity and mild alterations in level of consciousness. Because of the vague nature of these signs, early diagnosis is difficult. Later signs of grade I hepatic encephalopathy include loss of memory, confusion, and insomnia. It is important not to treat the insomnia of the individual with encephalopathy, even in this early stage, with sedatives or hypnotics. To do so would exacerbate the condition. Methods for assessing early encephalopathy include testing the ability of the patient to subtract by ones from 20 and adding or subtracting serial sevens, testing for apraxia by serial comparison of the patient's signature and the patient's attempts to draw a well-known object such as a star or house, and the Reitan trailmaking test. In this test the patient is asked to connect successively numbered dots with a line. The time it takes the patient to do this mental exercise is compared to a normal standard. As the degree of encephalopathy increases, the patient's ability to perform these simple tasks deteriorates.

In grade II hepatic encephalopathy speech becomes slower and slurred, and spontaneous movement decreases. The patient becomes intermittently confused, agitated, and drowsy. Asterixis, the characteristic "flapping" tremor of advanced liver disease, can be elicited in this stage. Asterixis is a condition in which the patient cannot maintain a fixed position or posture. To test for this response, ask the patient to hold his or her arms straight out at right angles to the body for 10 seconds. A loss of posture of the extremities is recovered by a flapping motion. To elicit this response, the patient must be able to cooperate. Asterixis can also be elicited by dorsiflexing the patient's wrist and watching for the characteristic downward flapping motion of the hand. The patient may also have a positive Babinski reflex, seizures, or myoclonic twitching. Myoclonic twitching must be differentiated from status epilepticus to avoid treatment with phenobarbital. Phenobarbital would exacerbate the condition.

In grade III hepatic encephalopathy severe bilateral forebrain involvement occurs, manifested by somnolence, stupor, decortication, and decerebration. The patient will respond to noxious stimuli. In grade IV hepatic encephalopathy the patient cannot be awakened and is said to be in a deep coma. Cerebral edema can be diagnosed in about 50% of cases (Sherlock, 1985).

The electroencephalogram (EEG) is useful in di-

TABLE 45–6. Clinical Assessment of Hepatic Encephalopathy

	Grade I	Grade II	Grade III	Grade IV
Level of consciousness	Awake	Decreased, but opens eyes spontaneously	Patient sleeps, but is arousable to verbal and painful stimuli; does not open eyes spontaneously	Comatose; no response to pain
Orientation	Total orientation with progression to confusion; then disorientation to time and place	Disoriented to time and place; severe confusion	Complete disorientation when aroused	Comatose
Intellectual functions	Mental clouding; slowness in answering questions; impaired handwriting; subtle changes in intellectual function, psychometric test scores decrease	Amnesia for past events; psychometric test scores decrease	Inability to make computations	Comatose
Behavior	Forgetful, restless, irritable, untidy, apathetic, disobedient	Decreased inhibitions, lethargic	Bizarre behavior (rage)	Comatose
Mood	Euphoria, depression, crying	Apathetic, paranoid	Apathy increases	Comatose
Neuromuscular	Muscular incoordination, tremors, yawning, insomnia	Hypoactive reflexes, asterixis, ataxia, slurred speech	Cannot cooperate; nystagmus and Babinski sign; clonus, decortication, decerebration, rigidity, seizures	Seizures; rigidity decreases to flaccidity; dilated pupils
Electroencephalography	Mild to moderate abnormalities	Moderate to severe abnormalities	Severe abnormalities	Severe abnormalities

agnosing hepatic encephalopathy and in differentiating metabolic encephalopathy from other conditions that can alter the level of consciousness. The EEG changes of hepatic encephalopathy are those of high-voltage slow waves in the delta range. In the early stages of encephalopathy changes occur in the frontal lobe. As encephalopathy progresses, the posterior lobes are affected as well, and by grade IV changes are evident in the entire brain. Although the majority of patients who suffer hepatic encephalopathy recover completely, the condition can lead to permanent neurologic damage and even death, especially if it progresses to grade IV.

Laboratory assessment of hepatic encephalopathy is nonspecific. As previously stated, serum ammonia levels do not necessarily correlate with the grade of encephalopathy (Galambos, 1979). Again, many precipitating factors may be reflected in analysis of fluid and electrolyte and acid-base status.

Treatment of hepatic encephalopathy involves searching for and treating all possible precipitants. Treatment of the encephalopathy of acute fulminant hepatic failure as discussed earlier is very different from the treatment of encephalopathy that develops with end-stage liver disease. The following discus-

sion relates to interventions for encephalopathy of chronic liver disease.

Dietary protein may be decreased or deleted altogether. Sufficient calories and carbohydrates are important because, according to Galambos (1979), a "low calorie diet in a cirrhotic is a high protein diet" due to catabolism and endogenous protein production. Most patients can tolerate at least small amounts of protein. Galambos (1979) recommends a 1200-calorie diet with 3 to 6 g of essential amino acids and a high carbohydrate content. Excessive amounts of fats, which delay gastric emptying, and glucose, which is hyperosmolar and can exacerbate nausea, are avoided.

Blood in the gut of the cirrhotic can significantly contribute to the ammonia load. Catharsis, or vigorous cleansing of the gut, is one method of removing bacteria that produce ammonia, ammonia itself, and blood. Any ongoing bleeding, of course, must be stopped. Interventions are aimed at interfering with the colonic production and absorption of ammonia. Neomycin and lactulose are the most commonly used pharmacologic agents for this purpose.

Neomycin is a nonabsorbable antibiotic that is effective against ureolytic gram-negative organisms.

It also induces regular bowel movements and is gentler in this respect than lactulose. Neomycin is administered in amounts of up to 4 to 6 g/day in divided doses. An important responsibility of the nurse caring for the patient receiving neomycin is monitoring for signs of nephrotoxicity and ototoxicity. Because of these undesirable side effects, neomycin is not intended for long-term use. It is used as a short-term treatment to return patients to a compensated state with regard to dietary intake and ammonia metabolism.

Lactulose is a saline laxative that is converted in the gut to lactic acid and acetic acid. One effect of lactulose is that ammonia in the gut remains in the ionized form and hence cannot cross the gut membranes into the systemic circulation. Another effect is a decrease in fecal pH (5.0), which inhibits growth of ammonia-forming bacteria. Lowering fecal pH creates a gradient of 2.4 between the extracellular fluid pH (7.4) and fecal pH (5.0). This promotes diffusion of ammonia from the systemic circulation into the acidified bowel contents and produces diarrhea. The amount of lactulose administered must be sufficient to decrease the fecal pH to create this gradient. Thirty milliliters of lactulose syrup every 6 to 8 hours or a 20% retention enema solution will usually accomplish this goal. Side effects of lactulose include abdominal cramps and gas. Protection of the perianal area with barrier cream may be necessary depending on the length of treatment and the amount of diarrhea produced. Caution is needed to prevent trauma to hemorrhoidal vessels when inserting rectal tubes for administration of an enema.

Evacuation of blood from the gut of the patient with a GI hemorrhage can also be accomplished with phosphorus or magnesium purgatives or with plain tap water. Although these interventions are time-consuming, the results are worth it. Equally important in the hemorrhaging patient, of course, is the replacement of lost circulating volume. Compensatory mechanisms for hypovolemia exacerbate the condition by decreasing hepatic and renal perfusion.

If encephalopathy is precipitated by diuretic therapy, these drugs should be discontinued. Alterations in plasma volume and electrolyte and acid-base balance should be promptly corrected. Potassium supplements are indicated if loop diuretics have been used. In intractable cases of hepatic encephalopathy, colon resection may be indicated to remove the major source of ammonia production.

A primary nursing responsibility in care of the encephalopathic patient is protection of the patient from self-harm to whatever degree this is necessary. It is fruitless to try to reason with or expect compliance with normally accepted behavior in an encephalopathic patient. Entering this vicious cycle will only lead to frustration and may further agitate the patient. Family members or friends often need emotional support to cope with observing the sometimes bizarre behavior changes in the encephalopathic patient. Particularly upsetting can be failure of the patient to recognize a significant other.

Nursing Diagnoses for the Patient with Hepatic Encephalopathy

Altered nutrition: Less than body requirements
Altered bowel elimination: Diarrhea
Altered tissue perfusion, cerebral
Potential fluid volume deficit
Ineffective airway clearance
Ineffective breathing pattern
Potential for injury: Suffocating, trauma
Potential for impaired skin integrity
Impaired verbal communication
Altered role performance
Altered family processes
Ineffective coping, individual
Ineffective coping, family: Compromised
Impaired physical mobility
Sleep pattern disturbance
Self-care deficit: Feeding, bathing/hygiene, toileting
Disturbance in self-concept: Body image, self-esteem, personal identity
Sensory/perceptual alterations: Visual, auditory
Altered thought processes

SPLENOMEGALY

Splenic enlargement occurs as a direct consequence of portal hypertension. In fact, splenic enlargement is the single most important diagnostic sign of portal hypertension (Sherlock, 1985). However, the exact size of the spleen does not necessarily correlate with the degree of portal hypertension. Unless the spleen is quite enlarged, noninvasive diagnosis of splenic enlargement is difficult. Because the spleen must enlarge to two to three times its normal size before it can be palpated, the diagnosis of splenic enlargement is usually made radiologically or angiographically. In contrast to palpation of the liver, the enlarged spleen must be palpated gently to prevent injury and rupture.

The most prominent finding associated with an enlarged spleen is pancytopenia: leukopenia, anemia, and thrombocytopenia. Therefore, frequent laboratory monitoring of these parameters is needed, especially before invasive procedures are performed. Invasive procedures may be precluded until platelets and clotting factors can be replaced. In extreme cases, the patient may complain of left-sided "spleen" pain and may unconsciously physically protect his or her left side.

METABOLIC BONE DISEASE

Bone disease is a metabolic complication of liver disease, especially chronic cholestasis and alcoholism (Stone, 1977; Mills et al., 1981; Cuthbert et al., 1984; Michison et al., 1988). The mechanism of bone disease associated with cholestatic liver disease is impaired calcium absorption and vitamin D deficiency.

Vitamin D_2 (ergo-calciferol) is absorbed in the gut, and vitamin D_3 (cholecalciferol) is synthesized in the skin. Both are transported in the serum by a vitamin D–binding globulin that is synthesized in the liver, and both are hydroxylated in the liver. The main defect is a lack of vitamin D substrate, either from lack of exposure to the sun or from malnutrition. Intraluminal (duodenal) bile acids necessary for vitamin D absorption are decreased or absent in patients with cholestatic disease, and because calcium will not be absorbed in the absence of vitamin D absorption, calcium malabsorption occurs. The parathyroid glands stimulate calcium resorption from bones in response to this perceived hypocalcemia. In alcoholic liver disease a defect in this process does contribute to bone disease, but other factors such as malnutrition and hypogonadism are thought to play a role (Stone, 1977). In the acutely ill or chronically debilitated patient, immobility and lack of weight-bearing exacerbates this condition.

The bone diseases that complicate life for these patients are osteopenia, osteomalacia, and osteoporosis. Osteomalacia is a reduction in mineralization of the bone. The bones are weakened, kyphosis occurs, and pseudofractures are common. Bone pain is a frequent complaint. Dental problems arise as the lamina dura around the teeth disappears and the teeth fall out. The oral cavity can become a source of infection and sepsis, and loss of teeth can contribute to poor dietary intake. A thorough dental or oral surgery consultation is often indicated. Osteoporosis is decreased bone density of normally mineralized bone associated with increased porosity and softening of the bone. Osteoporosis is more important clinically than osteomalacia because it is not usually diagnosed in this patient population until spontaneous fractures occur. Although the efficacy of various treatment modalities for metabolic bone disease has not been proved, the most common treatments for this problem include calcium supplementation, vitamin D or vitamin D metabolite supplementation, and estrogen therapy.

CASE HISTORY

J.C. is a 47-year-old white woman with a diagnosis of sclerosing cholangitis. She was unaware of her liver disease until she underwent general anesthesia and exploratory laparotomy for diagnosis and treatment of a gynecologic problem. During the laparotomy her liver was noted to be normal in size but nodular and greenish in color. About 10 days after the surgery she became extremely jaundiced and ill. Her liver enzymes and bilirubin level were significantly elevated. Because she appeared to be in acute fulminant hepatic failure she was referred to a large university medical center for evaluation for possible liver transplantation. The acute liver failure did begin to resolve, but it was decided to complete the evaluation.

Early one morning near the end of the evaluation period while getting out of bed to use the bathroom she experienced excruciating lower back pain and could not continue to the bathroom. Spinal x-rays showed a spontaneous fracture of L1 and L2 vertebrae. Her recovery was uneventful, but based on the results of quantitative liver function tests, liver transplantation in the near future was recommended. While waiting for a compatible donor, J.C. suffered a spontaneous fracture of the left calcaneous, causing her to fall and subsequently fracture the right ulna. Five days later she received her liver transplant. It is expected that she will continue to have metabolic bone problems in the early phase after transplantation due to the effect of high-dose steroids on calcium metabolism.

SURGICAL TREATMENT OF PORTAL HYPERTENSION

Patients with portal hypertension sufficient to cause variceal bleeding face a 30% risk of death with each bleeding episode. A variety of medical treatments for control of variceal bleeding have been described, but none has been successful in prevention of recurrent bleeding. Surgical procedures, however, have been perfected that do accomplish this goal.

In 1877 Nickolai Eck demonstrated the feasibility of portacaval anastomosis in a dog, and in 1903 Vidal performed the first portacaval shunt in a human (Henderson, 1988). This early patient suffered some of the same problems associated with portacaval shunts today, including encephalopathy. This procedure, therefore, fell out of favor within the surgical community for a time but was repopularized in 1945 by Whipple, who showed that portacaval shunts could be used effectively to treat portal hypertension (Henderson, 1988).

Evaluation of the Patient with Portal Hypertension

Evaluation of the patient with portal hypertension includes analysis of clinical, hematologic, biochemical, endoscopic, histologic, radiologic, and quantitative liver function data. Many of these parameters have been discussed. *Clinical* data include the patient's presenting symptoms and the presence of cutaneous stigmata suggestive of advanced liver disease. *Hematologic* data include the coagulation status of the patient and evidence of pancytopenia secondary to hypersplenism. *Biochemical* data include the standard laboratory tests associated with liver disease, as well as hepatitis serology, nutritional status, and fluid and electrolyte status. All patients evaluated for portal hypertension undergo upper GI endoscopic examination to either identify the exact site of bleeding or define the extent of collateral vessel development in the esophagus, stomach, and duodenum.

Percutaneous liver biopsy is performed in some patients to determine the exact nature and extent of disease. The most widely used method is needle biopsy without x-ray visualization using an intercostal transthoracic approach. While the patient is in a supine position under local anesthesia, a small aspiration needle is inserted through the eighth or ninth intercostal space at the midaxillary line. The patient is asked to take a deep breath and hold it. At this time the liver is lower in the abdominal cavity, and the biopsy needle is quickly inserted and withdrawn. This procedure is repeated two or three times to obtain adequate pathologic specimens. A safer method for performing percutaneous biopsy is to perform it under computed tomographic guidance.

Regardless of the method used, this procedure is not without complications. The major complication is hemorrhage, which can be significant enough to cause shock. A branch of the portal vein or hepatic artery within the liver, or an intercostal artery, can be lacerated. Because a branch of the hepatic artery and portal vein lie in juxtaposition to a bile ductule (the portal triad), injury of either vessel through the bile ductule can cause hemobilia, or bleeding into the bile ductule. If the patient has a T-tube, this will be immediately evident as frank bleeding or blood-stained bile in the drainage bag. This is abnormal and should be brought to a physician's attention promptly. Intraperitoneal hemorrhage from a lacerated liver vessel or tumor can occur. Significant hemorrhage will become manifest by a slowly decreasing hematocrit and compensatory cardiovascular signs such as increasing heart rate and decreasing pulse pressure. Other complications include laceration of a dilated bile duct, peritonitis, and pneumothorax.

Nursing responsibilities to the patient who has had a liver biopsy include close monitoring of vital signs and physical assessment parameters for signs of vascular or pulmonary compromise. Postbiopsy protocols vary from institution to institution, but generally the patient is required to be on bedrest lying on his or her right side for 6 to 8 hours.

Radiologic evaluation of the patient with portal hypertension can be extensive. CT scanning is used to measure liver and spleen size (normally 1100 to 1500 cm³ and 150 to 250 cm³, respectively) and to detect the presence of lesions within the liver. Hepatoma is associated with some types of advanced liver disease, particularly chronic active hepatitis B.

Angiography (portography) is used to visualize portal venous anatomy and sometimes to determine portal pressure. Splenoportography during venous phase imaging of the SMA and splenic artery allows visualization of the portal vein, splenic vein, and collateral vessels. Retrograde catheterization of the hepatic vein using the balloon occlusion method allows measurement of the wedged and free hepatic vein pressures in much the same way as wedged and free pulmonary artery pressures are measured with a pulmonary artery catheter. The hepatic vein pressure gradient (hepatic vein wedged pressure minus the free hepatic vein pressure) correlates well with and is used to calculate the portal venous pressure. Doppler ultrasound can be used to assess patency and flow velocities of the portal and superior mesenteric veins and the hepatic artery.

Child's Classification

The Child's classification of liver disease (Table 45–7) was developed to categorize patients according to surgical risk, based on the clinical parameters of ascites, encephalopathy, nutritional status, and the laboratory findings of bilirubin, albumin, and PT (Jackson et al., 1971). Patients are classified into one of three categories: A, B, or C. The Child's class A patient has no detectable stigmata of liver disease and normal hepatic reserve, and is a good surgical candidate. The Child's class B patient has visible stigmata, limited hepatic function, and an increased risk of surgical mortality. The Child's class C patient has minimal to no hepatic reserve, is in and out of hepatic failure, and is at high risk for surgical mortality.

Anesthesia and the Patient with Liver Disease

The patient requiring surgery for treatment of portal hypertension is at particular risk. The overall condition of the patient, as outlined by Child's classification, is an important preoperative predictor of outcome. Anesthetic agents decrease hepatic blood flow, so there is a potential for hepatic hypoxia. In

---

TABLE 45–7. Clinical and Laboratory Classification of Hepatic Function

Class	A	B	C
Functional impairment	Minimal	Moderate	Severe
Serum bilirubin (mg/dl)	<2.0	2.0 to 3.0	>3.0
Serum albumin (gm/dl)	>3.5	3.0 to 3.5	<3.0
Ascites	None	Easily controlled	Poorly controlled
Neurologic disorders	None	Minimal	Moderate to severe
Nutrition	Excellent	Good	Poor, wasted
Operative mortality	<1%	10%	>50%

Adapted from Tables 1–4 and 1–5 in Child, C. G., III (1967). *The liver and portal hypertension.* Philadelphia: W. B. Saunders; in Stone, H. H. (1977), *Surgical Clinics of North America,* 57, 409–419.

this situation, drug delivery to the liver is decreased and drug effects are enhanced, especially drugs with high hepatic extraction ratios such as lidocaine and propranolol. The presence of ascites places the patient at increased anesthetic risk for at least three reasons. First, it is unusual for significant ascites to exist without at least some degree of atelectasis and pleural effusion. Second, the patient with ascites in a supine position is more likely to vomit. Third, ascites increases the distribution and disposition of IV drugs. The onset of drug action is delayed, but the duration of action is prolonged. Actively bleeding varices also pose anesthetic risks, namely, pulmonary aspiration and hypovolemia. A Sengstaken-Blakemore tube left in place may also be vomited into the airway during induction of anesthesia.

The alcoholic patient undergoing surgery for portal hypertension presents special problems. These patients are often systemically debilitated with poor cardiac and pulmonary status. They frequently go to surgery emergently to stop acute life-threatening hemorrhage. The amount of anesthesia required may be increased, but again the duration of action will be prolonged, potentially affecting postoperative recovery. Alcoholic patients undergoing surgery, elective or emergent, may have minor withdrawal signs within 6 to 8 hours after anesthetics are metabolized. These signs include tremors, irritability, and insomnia. More severe signs of alcohol withdrawal usually occur after 48 to 72 hours and include disorientation, hallucinations, diaphoresis, hyperpyrexia, tachycardia, hypertension, and seizures. This is truly a medical emergency. Treatment involves prompt sedation, thiamine replacement, and electrolyte balance.

Shunt Surgery

Shunt surgery is one of several treatment options for the patient with bleeding varices, including pharmacotherapy, endoscopic sclerotherapy, and liver transplantation. The rationale for choosing one of these therapies is based on the patient's risk of continued bleeding and the risk of acute liver failure (Henderson et al., 1990).

Shunt surgery for decompression of varices falls into two main categories: nonselective and selective. In nonselective shunt surgery all of the portal blood flow can or does enter the systemic circulation without first circulating through the liver. In other words, total portal blood flow is diverted around the liver. In selective shunts portal venous flow through the liver is preserved. Regardless of the type of shunt performed, it must be remembered that these procedures are not curative but palliative in nature. Shunt surgery for portal hypertension is performed for one reason and that is to prevent death from variceal bleeding. Eventually the patient will succumb to liver failure. Shunts are not performed prophylactically for variceal bleeding because of the

morbidity associated with shunts compared with sclerotherapy.

NONSELECTIVE SHUNTS

Nonselective or "total" shunts accomplish total portal decompression. Total shunts fall into two categories: (1) end-to-side shunts, and (2) side-to-side shunts.

End-to-Side Portacaval Shunt. The end-to-side portacaval shunt (Fig. 45–11A) divides the portal vein at its bifurcation before it enters the liver at the porta hepatis; this access of the portal vein to the liver is then tied off. The proximal segment of the transected portal vein is then anastomosed to the side of the infrahepatic IVC, hence the term "portacaval" shunt (from the portal venous system to the caval system, bypassing or shunting around the liver). Portal venous flow now empties into the IVC instead of the liver, and venous return to the right heart is ensured. Therefore, resistance to flow is decreased, varices are decompressed, and bleeding is prevented. Although the splanchnic bed is decompressed, the liver is not. Pressure can no longer back up through the portal vein and collaterals (varices), and this is the mechanism that prevents variceal bleeding.

Side-to-Side Portacaval Shunts. There are several versions of side-to-side portacaval shunts, including portacaval, mesocaval, central splenorenal, mesorenal, portorenal, and the Clatworthy cavomesenteric shunt. In the side-to-side portacaval, mesocaval, and mesorenal shunt (Fig. 45–11B), the portal vein is left intact and serves as the hepatic outflow tract. Therefore, the liver and splanchnic bed are decompressed. Not only is variceal bleeding prevented, but development of postoperative ascites is inhibited. Long-term patency of side-to-side portacaval shunts is better if the shunt is short and direct. In the longer, curved shunts (mesocaval, mesorenal, and central splenorenal), the risk of thrombosis is greater (Henderson and Warren, 1988). The preferred procedure, should a total shunt be necessary, is the short portacaval H-graft anastomosis (Henderson and Warren, 1988). In this procedure a short synthetic graft (14- to 18-mm Gore-Tex) is placed between the portal vein and the IVC. This procedure is relatively easy to perform and affords the same benefits as the side-to-side portacaval shunt.

The cost of total loss of portal blood flow is eventual deterioration of the patient from hepatic failure and encephalopathy. Although these procedures are still used in emergent situations to control acute variceal bleeding or when sclerotherapy fails in someone who is not for anatomic reasons a candidate for a selective shunt, use of nonselective shunts has for the most part been abandoned because several investigators have found that survival is not prolonged with total portacaval shunts (Resnick et al., 1974; Rueff et al., 1976; Reynolds et al., 1981; Millikan et

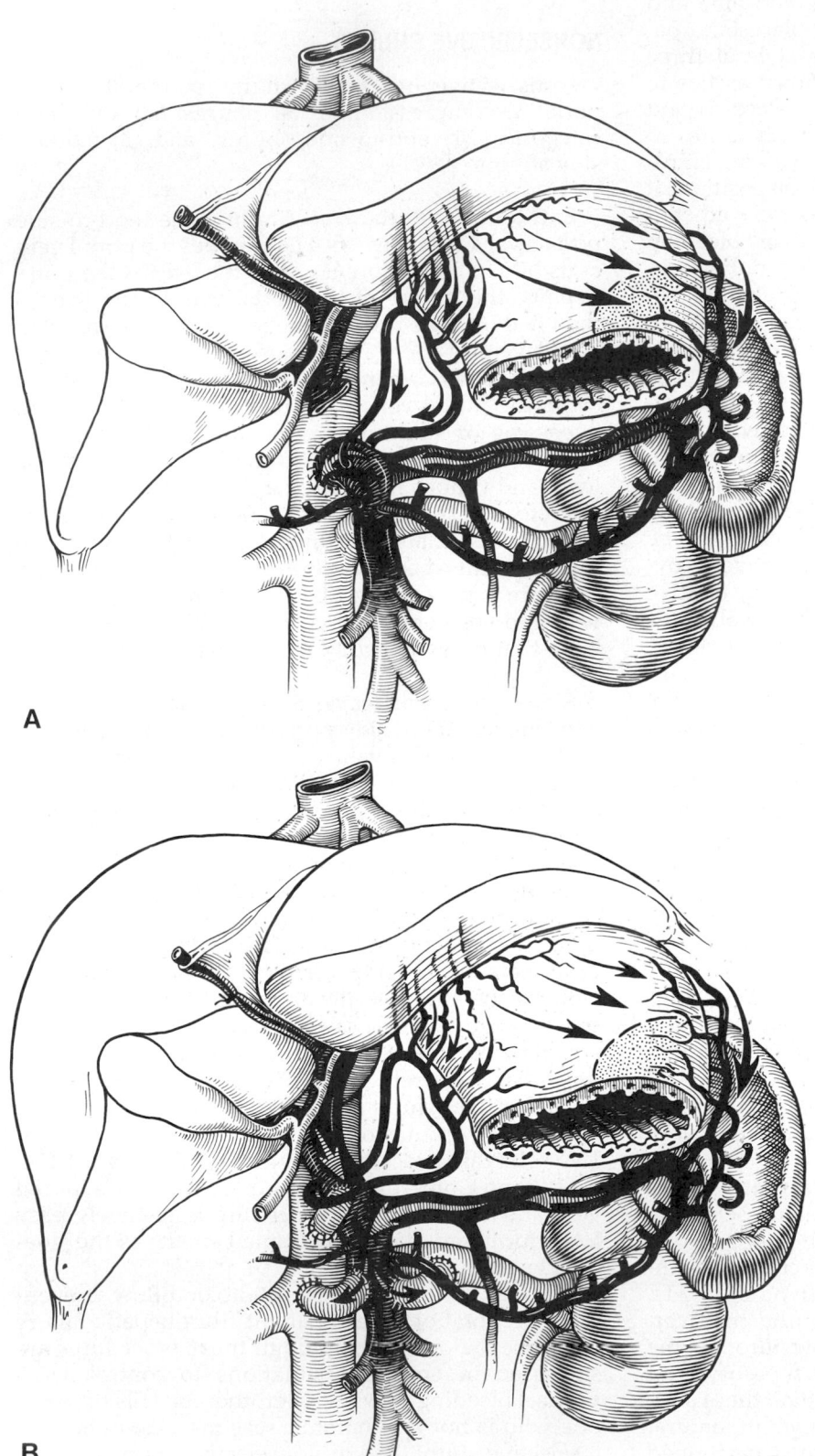

A

B

FIGURE 45–11. *A*, Schematic representation of an end-to-side portacaval shunt. Division of the portal vein at its bifurcation irrevocably interrupts portal flow. The splanchnic bed venous hypertension is relieved, but the hepatic sinusoidal hypertension is maintained. *B*, Three examples of side-to-side total portal systemic shunts: portacaval, mesocaval, and mesorenal interposition grafts. The same physiologic effects are achieved with side-to-side portacaval, central splenorenal, and Clatworthy shunts: venous hypertension is lowered in both the liver and the splanchnic bed. The portal vein now serves as a hepatic outflow tract. (From Henderson, J. M., and Warren, W. D. (1988). Portal hypertension. *Current Problems in Surgery*, 25, 151–223.)

al., 1985). If possible, a selective shunt is the procedure of choice.

SELECTIVE SHUNTS

The distal splenorenal shunt (DSRS) is a low pressure, high flow shunt that reduces esophagogastric and splenic variceal pressure and thereby controls bleeding. The DSRS maintains the portal hypertension necessary to sustain portal flow through the high resistance cirrhotic liver and provides a low pressure decompression pathway for varices through the splenorenal anastomosis. The DSRS is reserved for patients who still have hepatopedal or prograde portal flow. There would be no advantage in performing this shunt, which is in general technically more challenging, in someone with retrograde portal flow.

Suitability of a patient for a DSRS is also dependent on the status of portal and systemic venous anatomy, as anomalies of these structures may make the surgery technically more difficult, and the extent of liver disease. The ideal candidate for a DSRS has stable liver disease with good hepatocellular reserve.

The goals for a DSRS are (1) selective reduction of pressure and volume of flow through gastroesophageal varices, (2) maintenance of portal venous perfusion of the liver, and (3) maintenance of venous hypertension in the splanchnic bed (Warren et al., 1967).

In this procedure (Fig. 45–12) the splenic vein is detached from the portal vein and anastomosed to the left renal vein. Portal flow is not diverted, but varices are decompressed through the short gastric veins, spleen, and splenic vein to the left renal vein, which empties into the IVC. The advantages of the DSRS are prevention of bleeding and preservation of whatever portal flow the patient had prior to surgery. Ascites after DSRS is common due to the maintenance of portal hypertension, but it is manageable with diuretic therapy and dietary sodium restrictions. Hepatic encephalopathy is not a problem after successful DSRS.

Six controlled randomized trials have compared the results of DSRS to those achieved with portacaval shunts (Conn, 1958; Reichle et al., 1979; Fischer et al., 1981; Rikkers et al., 1978; Harley et al., 1986; Langer et al., 1987). The DSRS was not found to be superior in improving long-term survival, but, for reasons already stated, the patient's quality of life was better after DSRS.

SPLENOPANCREATIC DISCONNECTION

The survival pattern after DSRS is different between alcoholics and nonalcoholics. Survival after DSRS is better in nonalcoholic patients than in alcoholic patients (Van Thiel et al., 1974; Zeppa et al., 1978; Henderson et al., 1983; Warren et al., 1986). The metabolic response of the nonalcoholic patient after DSRS differs from that of the alcoholic patient after DSRS. In nonalcoholic patients portal perfusion, liver blood flow, and cardiac output do not change postoperatively. However, in alcoholics approxi-

FIGURE 45–12. The distal splenorenal shunt decompresses gastroesophageal varices through the short gastric veins, spleen, and the splenic vein to the left renal vein. Portal hypertension and prograde portal flow are maintained in the superior mesenteric and portal veins. (From Henderson, J. M., and Warren, W. D. (1988). Portal hypertension. *Current Problems in Surgery, 25, 151–223.)*

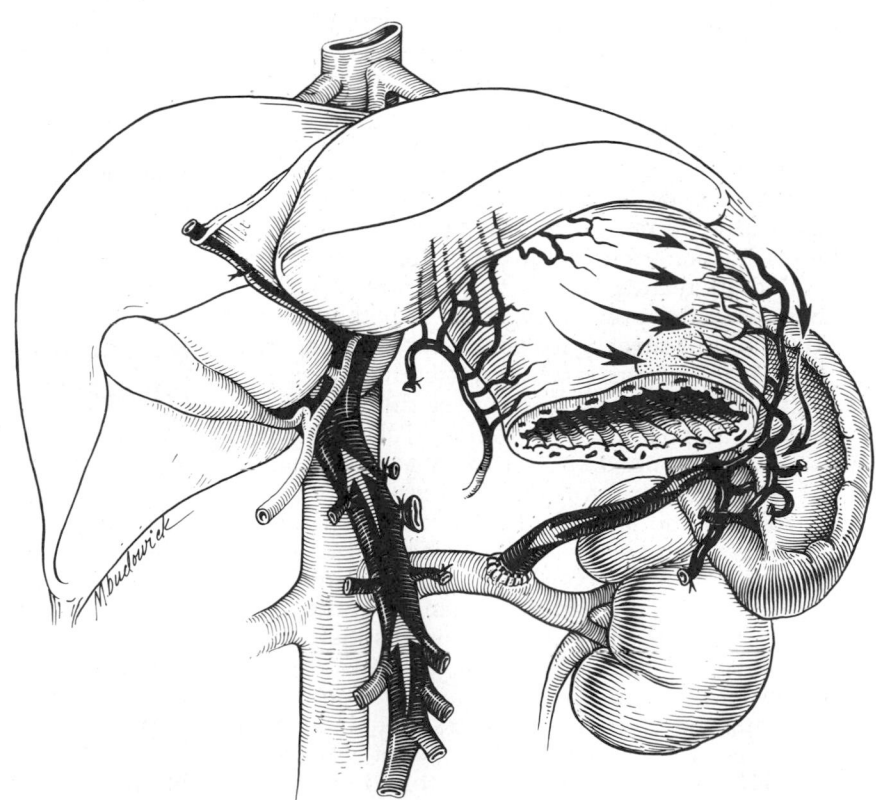

mately 50% of portal perfusion is lost through a siphon effect created by pancreatic and colonic collaterals. This loss in portal perfusion is compensated for by an increase in cardiac output and hepatic arterial flow, but vital nutrients and insulin are lost from the enterohepatic circulation.

A surgical intervention to prevent this problem and improve portal perfusion is the splenopancreatic disconnection. In this procedure the splenic vein is completely dissected out of (or disconnected from) its normal route of passage through the pancreas. This disconnection prevents siphoning of portal venous flow through the pancreas, and the metabolic response to DSRS is similar in alcoholics and nonalcoholics.

DEVASCULARIZATION PROCEDURES

Occasionally both selective and nonselective shunts are contraindicated or unsuccessful in the patient with portal hypertension and bleeding varices. In such cases a surgical devascularization procedure to remove collateral bleeding sources may be performed. These procedures include splenectomy, esophageal transection, and gastric and esophageal devascularization. Regardless of the procedure performed, portal hypertension and hepatic perfusion are maintained, but the rebleeding rate approaches 50% (Henderson and Warren, 1988).

CARING FOR THE POSTOPERATIVE SHUNT PATIENT

Shunt surgery for complications of portal hypertension may be done electively or emergently. Certainly the precipitating factors and the condition of the patient just prior to surgery have an important bearing on postoperative recovery. Based on Child's classification alone, the sicker the patient before surgery, the greater is the anticipated morbidity and mortality directly related to any surgical procedure. Problems encountered in the immediate postoperative period are related directly to the underlying liver disease. As stated previously, there is nothing curative about shunt surgery for portal hypertension. All of the complications and manifestations, except bleeding varices, of preexisting liver disease will be present in the postoperative period. Taking the patient's past and immediate history into consideration when planning care for this patient is therefore important. Additionally, the full impact of intraoperative events, such as severe hemorrhage and hemodynamic instability, is often not realized until the postoperative phase when the patient is in the ICU.

There is a potential for large interstitial (third space) fluid loss due to the physiologic response to stress and the dissection of abdominal lymphatics. The aldosterone response to stress and interstitial fluid loss is exaggerated in the patient with liver disease. Hemodynamic assessment for adequate circulating plasma volume based on right and left heart pressures, mean arterial pressure, and urine output is routine. Crystalloid replacement is accomplished with 5% dextrose in the DSRS patient. Saline solutions are avoided to help prevent ascites, which is generally not apparent until about 2 weeks after surgery. Fresh frozen plasma may be indicated for replacement of clotting factors and osmotic proteins depending on the patient's condition. Optimal blood pressure control is necessary to protect the integrity of the graft from hypertension and prevent thrombosis secondary to hypotension. Just as before surgery, the patient's circulation is hyperdynamic. The "normal" cardiac output for this patient is relatively high, in the range of 10 to 15 liters/minute. A functional systolic ejection murmur is a common and normal finding. Commonly, the CVP and PCWP are low due to increased venous capacitance and rapid movement of vascular volume into interstitial spaces.

Gastric decompression with an NG tube is necessary until ileus resolves. Abdominal assessment is important to monitor for (1) gastric and abdominal distention due to failure of the NG tube to decompress the gut, (2) ascites formation, and (3) intra-abdominal bleeding. The abdominal incision is a large "rooftop" incision below the right and left costal margins, the apex of the roof being below the xiphoid process. This wound is assessed for progression of healing and evidence of infection.

Because of the likelihood of compromised pulmonary status before surgery, mechanical ventilation is sometimes necessary for as long as several days after surgery. Mechanical ventilation combined with a large abdominal incision increases the potential for atelectasis and pneumonia. Pulmonary hygiene and meticulous attention to aseptic technique are most important in these patients, who have compromised immune defenses.

Finally, assessment for rebleeding and of liver compared with the patient's baseline indicators are important because shunt thrombosis may occur. Shunt thrombosis is the primary cause of rebleeding after a DSRS (Henderson et al., 1990).

Nursing Diagnoses for the Patient After Portacaval or Distal Splenorenal Shunt Surgery

Altered nutrition: Less than body requirements
Potential for infection
Altered bowel elimination: Constipation
Fluid volume excess
Potential fluid volume deficit
Impaired gas exchange
Ineffective breathing pattern
Potential for injury: Trauma
Impaired skin integrity: Actual
Impaired physical mobility
Sleep pattern disturbance

Self-care deficit: Feeding, bathing/hygiene, toileting
Disturbance in self-concept: Body image
Knowledge deficit related to surgical procedure and
  expected outcome
Altered thought processes
Altered comfort: Pain

SOCIAL ASPECTS OF LIVER DISEASE

There is a social stigma attached to "liver" disease. It is true that the majority of liver disease in the United States is alcohol related, and it is this fact that leads the average American to assume that anyone with liver disease must be a drinker. A common frustration and complaint of patients with nonalcoholic liver disease is that they have to defend themselves repeatedly, even to those close to them, against this stigma. Another feeling expressed by those with nonalcoholic liver disease is "Why me? I've never even had a drink!"

Ascites creates special problems. Aside from the physical restraints and discomfort associated with ascites, the patient suffers from an alteration in body image due to the changes and disfigurement that occur. Women with ascites are frequently asked by strangers, "When is the baby due?" This is distressing to some, especially young girls or women in their 50s and older. Men with ascites are assumed to have "beer bellies." Regardless of sex, their clothes no longer fit, and there may not be funds to purchase new ones.

The cost of liver disease, like that of any other chronic progressive disease, is high. As advanced liver disease begins to take its toll on bodily functions and robs its host of energy and motivation, gainful employment and providing for oneself or a family is no longer possible. Roles and family dynamics change. The burden of responsibility on the spouse, child, or parent of the patient with end-stage liver disease is heavy. Even the most productive members of society are forced to accept financial support from others or apply for disability payments. Too often insurance coverage is lost after many years of payments, just when it is needed most. Homes and other worldly possessions are sold to provide living and medical expenses. In the final years, patients with chronic liver disease bounce in and out of hospitals for palliative management of ascites, encephalopathy, and infections. The cost of medical treatment during these final years averages $25,000 per year.

nursing care plan

The Patient with Bleeding Varices
1. Fluid volume deficit related to:
  Upper gastrointestinal hemorrhage

Outcome Criteria	Nursing Interventions
The patient will maintain effective circulating plasma volume and adequate hemoglobin level for adequate tissue perfusion and oxygenation.	1. Monitor frequently for physical assessment, and hemodynamic and laboratory indicators (e.g., hemoglobin, hematocrit, BUN) of fluid volume to assess for hypovolemia and responses to therapy. 2. Monitor laboratory indicators (e.g., PT, PTT, fibrinogin, platelets, DD dimers) of coagulation status. 3. Monitor laboratory indicators (e.g., arterial blood gases) of pulmonary gas exchange. 4. Monitor laboratory indicators (e.g., serum transaminases, phosphatases, bilirubin, and ammonia) of liver function. 5. Monitor signs of insidious (e.g., melena) or acute (e.g., hematemesis) variceal bleeding. 6. Maintain adequate venous access for large volume fluid administration. 7. Keep patient NPO. 8. Ensure that suction apparatus is functional at bedside. 9. Prepare patient for gastroesophageal endoscopy (GED); sedate patient as ordered and turn to left lateral decubitus position; perform gastric lavage as ordered. 10. Prepare patient (as for GED) for endoscopic injection sclerotherapy. 11. Administer intravenous (IV) crystalloids and fresh frozen plasma for volume expansion and replacement of clotting factors. 12. Administer vasopressin (Pitressin) through a central venous catheter as ordered; monitor for chest pain and ST segment depression on ECG; administer IV nitroglycerin as ordered; monitor for abdominal cramps, decreased urine output, and dilutional hyponatremia. 13. Prepare patient for insertion of Sengstaken-Blakemore (SB), Linton, or Minnesota tube as ordered; for SB tube, insert nasogastric (NG) tube above esophageal balloon and maintain constant suction; maintain constant suction to gastric aspiration port; keep scissors at bedside to cut tube if it dislodges into airway; release balloon pressure regularly and frequently to prevent esophageal or gastric mucosal necrosis; monitor for nare pressure injury; provide frequent oral care. 14. Administer beta-adrenergic blocking agents as ordered. 15. Prepare patient for surgery (e.g., portacaval or distal splenorenal shunt) if indicated.

Nursing Care Plan continued on following page

2. Knowledge deficit related to: Cause and treatment of variceal bleeding	
Outcome Criteria	**Nursing Interventions**
The patient will verbalize understanding of the disease process responsible for variceal bleeding and the nature of interventions.	1. Provide explanation of variceal bleeding and why it occurred; relate to patient's type of liver disease. 2. Explain current and potential treatment options for variceal bleeding; include nature of options, potential, and goals. 3. When appropriate, explain any life-style or behavior changes that are recommended to decrease risk of rebleeding.

SUMMARY

Caring for the critically ill patient with liver dysfunction or liver disease challenges the nurse to understand the complex and vital role the liver plays in health and disease. The patient with acute fulminant hepatic failure generally demands prompt assessment and appropriate referral to a liver transplant center, as medical treatment is not effective in this life-threatening condition. The patient with cirrhosis may become critically ill for a variety of reasons that are most often related to the end effects of portal hypertension. The prognosis for many patients with cirrhosis has improved with the successes that have been achieved in the field of liver transplantation. Therefore, caring for the patient with end-stage liver disease is no longer a palliative process in most cases, which further emphasizes the need for critical care nurses to understand the nature of the pathophysiologic processes of and interventions for these patients.

References

Alter, M. J., Hadler, S. C., Margolis, H. S., et al. (1990a). The changing epidemiology of hepatitis B in the United States. *Journal of the American Medical Association*, 263, 1218–1222.

Alter, M. J., Hadler, S. C., Judson, F. N., et al. (1990b). Risk factors for acute non-A, non-B hepatitis in the United States and association with hepatitis C virus infection. *Journal of the American Medical Association*, 264, 2231–2235.

Alwmark, A., Bengmark, S., Borjesson, B., et al. (1982). Emergency and long-term transesophageal sclerotherapy of bleeding esophageal varices: A prospective study of 50 consecutive cases. *Scandinavian Journal of Gastroenterology*, 17, 409–412.

Aring, C. D. (1982). Metabolic encephalopathy: Neurologic and psychiatric considerations. *Heart & Lung*, 11, 516–521.

Benhamou, J. D. (1982). Risk factors of gastrointestinal bleeding in alcoholic cirrhosis. In D. Westaby, B. R. D. Macdougall, and R. Williams (Eds.), *Variceal bleeding* (pp. 5–15). Bath, U.K.: Pittman Press.

Bonnice, C. A. (1985). Fulminant hepatic failure. In J. M. Rippe, R. S. Irwin, J. S. Alpert, et al. (Eds.), *Intensive care medicine* (pp. 747–754). Boston: Little, Brown.

Bouletreau, P., Delafosse, B., Auboyer, C., et al. (1979). Role of branched chain amino acids in cirrhotic encephalopathy. In *Postgraduate course: XIth international meeting of anesthesiology and resuscitation* (pp. 239–254). Paris.

Bradford, K. S. (1983). Injection sclerotherapy in the management of bleeding esophageal varices. *Critical Care Nurse*, March/April, 36–40.

Breen, K. J., and Schenker, S. (1972). Hepatic coma: Present concepts of pathogenesis and therapy. In H. Popper, and F. Schaffner (Eds.), *Progress in liver disease* (Vol. 4). New York: Grune & Stratton.

Buckels, J. A. C. (1987). Liver transplantation in acute fulminant hepatic failure. *Transplantation Proceedings*, 19, 4365–4366.

Carrithers, R. L., and Fairman, R. P. (1989). Critical care of patients with severe liver disease. In W. C. Shoemaker, C. Ayers, A. Grenvik, et al. (Eds.), *Textbook of critical care* (2nd ed.). St. Louis: C. V. Mosby.

Cascino, A., Cangiano, C., Calcaterra, V., et al. (1978). Plasma amino acid imbalance in patients with liver disease. *American Journal of Digestive Diseases*, 23, 591–598.

Cattau, E. L., Benjamin, S. B., and Knuff, T. E. (1982). The accuracy of the physical exam in the diagnosis of suspected ascites. *Journal of the American Medical Association*, 247, 1164–1169.

Cello, J. P., Grendall, J. H., Crass, R. A., et al. (1986). Endoscopic sclerotherapy versus portacaval shunt in patients with severe cirrhosis and acute variceal hemorrhage. *New England Journal of Medicine*, 316, 11–15.

Centers for Disease Control. (1988). Update: Universal precautions for prevention and transmission of human immunodeficiency virus, hepatitis B virus, and other bloodborne pathogens in health-care settings. *Morbidity and Mortality Weekly Report*, 37, 377–387.

Clark, A. W., Westaby, D., Silk, D. B. A., et al. (1980). Prospective controlled trial of injection sclerotherapy with cirrhosis and recent variceal hemorrhage. *Lancet*, 2, 552–554.

Clive, D. M. (1985). Renal dysfunction in the patient with liver disease. In J. M. Rippe, R. S. Irwin, J. S. Alpert, et al. (Eds.), *Intensive care medicine* (pp. 755–757). Boston: Little, Brown.

Colman, J., Magnot, P., and Dudley, F. (1985). The effect of acute and chronic propranolol on portal venous pressure (Abstract). *Gastroenterology*, 86, 1315.

Conn, H. O. (1958). Hazards attending the use of esophageal tamponade. *New England Journal of Medicine*, 259, 701–707.

Conn, H. O., Resnick, R. F., Grace, N. D., et al. (1981). Distal splenorenal shunt versus portacaval shunt: Current status of a controlled trial. *Hepatology*, 1, 151–160.

Copenhagen Esophageal Varices Sclerotherapy Project. (1984). Sclerotherapy after first variceal hemorrhage in cirrhosis: A randomized multicenter trial. *New England Journal of Medicine*, 311, 594–600.

Cuthbert, J. (1990). Southwestern internal medicine conference: Hepatitis C. *American Journal of the Medical Sciences*, 299, 346–355.

Cuthbert, J. A., Pak, C. Y. C., Zerwekh, J. E., et al. (1984). Bone disease in primary biliary cirrhosis: Increased bone resorption and turnover in the absence of osteoporosis or osteomalacia. *Hepatology*, 4, 1–8.

Deluca, E. D. (1981). *Fourth Special Report to the United States Congress on Alcohol and Health*. Washington, D.C.: U.S. Government Printing Office.

Department of Labor, Occupational Health and Safety Administration. (1987). Occupational exposure to hepatitis B virus and human immunodeficiency virus: Advance notice of proposed rulemaking. *Federal Register*, 52, 45438–45441.

Finn, F. (1988). Recovery from acute renal failure. In B. M. Brenner, and J. M. Lazarus (Eds.), *Acute renal failure* (2nd ed.). New York: Churchill Livingstone.

Fischer, J. E., Bower, R. H., Atamian, S., et al. (1981). Comparison of distal and proximal splenorenal shunts. A randomized prospective trial. *Annals of Surgery*, 194, 531–544.

Fleig, W. E., Stange, E. F., Hunecke, R., et al. (1987). Prevention of recurrent rebleeding in cirrhosis with recent variceal hemorrhage: Prospective randomized comparison of propranolol and sclerotherapy. *Hepatology*, 7, 355–361.

Frakes, J. (1980). Physiologic considerations in the medical management of ascites. *Archives of Internal Medicine*, 140, 620–621.

Frank, I. C., and Cummins, L. (1987). Amanita poisoning treated with endoscopic biliary diversion. *Journal of Emergency Nursing*, 13, 132–136.

Galambos, J. T. (Ed.). (1979). *Cirrhosis. Major problems in internal medicine* (Vol. 17). Philadelphia: W. B. Saunders.

Getzen, L. C., Brink, R. R., and Wolfman, E. F. (1978). Survival following infusion of pitressin into the superior mesenteric artery to control bleeding esophageal varices in cirrhotic patients. *Annals of Surgery*, 187, 337–342.

Gould, B. E., and Pratter, M. R. (1985). Mushroom poisoning. In J. M. Rippe, R. S. Irwin, J. S. Alpert, et al. (Eds.), *Intensive care medicine* (pp. 962–965). Boston: Little, Brown.

Gregory, P., Broekelschen, P., Hill, M., et al. (1977). Complications of diuresis in the alcoholic patient with ascites: A controlled trial. *Gastroenterology*, 73, 534–538.

Gurevich, I. (1983). Viral hepatitis. *American Journal of Nursing*, April, 571–586.

Harley, H. A. J., Morgan, T., Redeker, A. G., et al. (1986). Results of a randomized trial of end-to-side portacaval shunt and distal splenorenal shunt in alcoholic liver disease and variceal bleeding. *Gastroenterology*, 91, 802–809.

Henderson, J. M., Millikan, W. J., and Galloway, J. R. (1990). The Emory perspective of the distal splenorenal shunt in 1990. *The American Journal of Surgery*, 160, 54–58.

Henderson, J. M., Millikan, W. J., Wright-Bacon, L., et al. (1983). Hemodynamic differences between alcoholic and nonalcoholic cirrhotics following distal splenorenal shunt—Effect on survival? *Annals of Surgery*, 198, 325–334.

Henderson, J. M., and Warren, W. D. (1986). A method of measuring quantitative hepatic function and hemodynamics in cirrhosis: The changes following distal splenorenal shunt. *Japanese Journal of Surgery*, 16, 158–168.

Henderson, J. M., and Warren, W. D. (1988). Portal hypertension. *Current Problems in Surgery*, 25, 151–223.

Hollenberg, N. K. (1983). Renin, angiotensin and the kidney: Assessment by pharmacological interruption of the renin-angiotensin system. In M. Epstein (Ed.), *The kidney in liver disease* (2nd ed., pp. 395–411). New York: Elsevier.

Hoofnagle, J. H., and Schafer, D. F. (1986). Serologic markers of hepatitis B infection. *Seminars in Liver Disease*, 6, 1–10.

Iwatsuki, S., Esquivel, C. O., Gordon, R. D., et al. (1985). Liver transplantation for fulminant hepatic failure. *Seminars in Liver Disease*, 5, 325–328.

Jackson, F. C., Perrin, E. B., Felix, R., et al. (1971). A clinical investigation of the portacaval shunt: Analysis of the therapeutic option. *Annals of Surgery*, 174, 672–701.

Jackson, M. M. (1980). Viral hepatitis. *Nursing Clinics of North America*, 15, 729–746.

Jacques, E. A. (1985). Hepatic encephalopathy. In J. M. Rippe, R. S. Irwin, J. S. Alpert, et al. (Eds.), *Intensive care medicine* (pp. 755–757). Boston: Little, Brown.

Kaplan, F. S. (1987). Osteoporosis. Pathophysiology and prevention. *Clinical Symposia*, 39 (1), 1–32.

Kehne, J. H., Hughes, F. A., and Gompertz, M. L. (1956). The use of surgical pituitrin in control of esophageal varix bleeding: Experimental study and report of two cases. *Surgery*, 39, 917–925.

Keithley, K. J. (1985). Nutritional assessment of the patient undergoing surgery. *Heart & Lung*, 14, 449–454.

Korula, J., Balart, L. P., Radvan, G., et al. (1985). A prospective, randomized controlled trial of chronic esophageal variceal sclerotherapy. *Hepatology*, 5, 584–589.

Langer, B., Taylor, B. R., Mackenzie, D. R., et al. (1987). Further report of a prospective randomized trial comparing distal splenorenal shunt with end-to-side portacaval shunt. *Gastroenterology*, 88, 424–429.

Larson, A. W., Cohen, H., Zweiban, B., et al. (1986). Acute esophageal variceal sclerotherapy: Results of a prospective, randomized controlled trial. *Journal of the American Medical Association*, 255, 497–500.

Lautt, W. W., and Greenway, C. V. (1987). Conceptual review of the hepatic vascular bed. *Hepatology*, 7, 952–963.

LeVeen, H. H., Wapnick, S., Grosberg, S., et al. (1976). Further experience with peritoneo-venous shunt for ascites. *Annals of Surgery*, 184, 574–581.

Lebrec, D., Nouel, O., Corbic, M., et al. (1980). Propranolol, a medical treatment for portal hypertension? *Lancet*, 2, 180–182.

Leoni, M. P. (1985). Management of acetaminophen overdose. *Critical Care Nurse*, 5, 44–47.

Maddrey, W. C., and Weber, F. J. (1975). Chronic hepatic encephalopathy. *Medical Clinics of North America*, 59, 937–944.

Malin, H. (1981). *An epidemiologic perspective on alcohol use and abuse in the United States.* Rockville, MD: National Institute of Alcohol Abuse and Alcoholism.

Mar, D. D. (1982). Drug-induced hepatotoxicity. *American Journal of Nursing*, January, 124–126.

Millikan, W. J., Warren, W. D., Henderson, J. M., et al. (1985). The Emory prospective randomized trial: Selective versus nonselective shunt to control variceal bleeding. Ten-year followup. *Annals of Surgery*, 201, 712–722.

Mills, P. R., Birnie, P. R., Quigley, B. E. M. M., et al. (1981). A prospective survey of radiologic bone and joint changes in primary biliary cirrhosis. *Clinical Radiology*, 3, 297–302.

Mitchison, H. C., Malcolm, A. J., Bassendine, M. F., et al. (1988). Metabolic bone disease in primary biliary cirrhosis at presentation. *Gastroenterology*, 94, 463–470.

Moore, M., and Gerstein, D. R. (1985). *Alcoholism and public policy: Beyond the shadow of Prohibition.* Washington, DC: National Academy Press.

Nussbaum, M., Baum, S., Kuroda, K., et al. (1968). Control of portal hypertension by selective mesenteric arterial drug infusion. *Archives of Surgery*, 97, 1005–1113.

O'Grady, J. G., Gimson, A. E. S., O'Brien, R. D., et al. (1988). Controlled trials of charcoal hemoperfusion and prognostic factors in fulminant hepatic failure (Part 1). *Gastroenterology*, 94, 1186–1192.

Olsen, S., and Gerstein, D. R. (1985). *Alcohol in America. Taking action to prevent abuse.* Washington, DC: National Academy Press.

Perez, G., and Schiff, E. R. (1988). The hepatorenal syndrome. In T. J. Gallagher, and W. C. Shoemaker (Eds.), *Critical care. State of the art.* (Vol. 9). Fullerton, CA: The Society of Critical Care Medicine.

Perillo, R. P. (1986). Corticosteroid therapy for chronic active hepatitis: Is a little too much? *Hepatology*, 6, 1416–1418.

Rector, W. G. (1986). Drug therapy for portal hypertension. *Annals of Internal Medicine*, 105, 96–107.

Reichle, F. A., Fahmy, W. E., and Golsorkhi, M. (1979). Prospective comparison clinical trial with distal splenorenal and mesocaval shunts. *American Journal of Surgery*, 137, 13–21.

Resnick, R. H., Iber, F. L., Ishihara, A. M., et al. (1974). A controlled study of the therapeutic portacaval shunt. *Gastroenterology*, 67, 843–857.

Reynolds, T. B., Donovan, A. J., Mikkelsen, W. P., et al. (1981). Results of a 12-year randomized trial of portacaval shunts in patients with alcoholic liver disease and bleeding varices. *Gastroenterology*, 80, 1005–1011.

Rikkers, L. F., Rudman, D., Galambos, J. T., et al. (1978). A randomized controlled trial of the distal splenorenal shunt. *Annals of Surgery*, 188, 271–282.

Rikkers, L. F., Burnett, D. A., Volentine, G. D., et al. (1987). Shunt surgery versus endoscopic sclerotherapy for long term treatment of variceal bleeding: Early results of a randomized trial. *Annals of Surgery*, 206, 261–271.

Rueff, B., Degos, F., Prandi, D., et al. (1976). A controlled study of the therapeutic portacaval shunt in alcoholic cirrhosis. *Lancet*, 1, 655–659.

Russo, J. M., and Pratter, M. R. (1985). Acetaminophen and phenacetin overdose. In J. M. Rippe, R. S. Irwin, J. S. Alpert, et al. (Eds.), *Intensive care medicine* (pp. 947–950). Boston: Little, Brown.

Schenker, S., Breen, K. J., and Hoyumpa, A. (1974). Hepatic encephalopathy: Current status. *Gastroenterology*, 66, 121–151.

Schumann, D. (1983). Correction of ascites with arteriovenous shunting: A study of clinical management. *Heart & Lung*, 12, 248–256.

Seef, L. B., and Koff, R. S. (1986). Evolving concepts of the clinical and serologic consequences of hepatitis B virus infection. *Seminars in Liver Disease*, 6, 11–22.

Sherlock, S. (1985). *Diseases of the liver and biliary system* (7th ed.). London: Blackwell Scientific Publications.

Sivak, M. V. (1982). Therapeutic endoscopy of the esophagus. *Surgical Clinics of North America*, 62, 807–820.

Stieber, A. C., Ambrosino, G., Van Thiel, D., et al. (1988). Orthotopic liver transplantation for fulminant and subacute hepatic failure. *Gastroenterology Clinics of North America*, 17, 157–165.

Stone, H. H. (1977). Preoperative and postoperative care. *Surgical Clinics of North America*, 57, 409–419.

Terblanche, J., Northover, J. M. A., Bornman, P., et al. (1979). A prospective controlled trial of sclerotherapy in the long-term management of patients after esophageal variceal bleeding. *Surgery, Gynecology & Obstetrics*, 148, 323–333.

Teres, J., Cecelia, A., Bordas, J., et al. (1978). Esophageal tamponade for bleeding varices. Controlled trial between the Sengstaken-Blakemore tube and the Linton-Nachlas tube. *Gastroenterology*, 75, 566–569.

Teres, J., Bordas, J. M., Bravo, D., et al. (1987). Sclerotherapy versus distal splenorenal shunt in the elective treatment of variceal hemorrhage: A randomized controlled trial. *Hepatology*, 7, 430–436.

Van Thiel, D. H., Lester, R., and Sheras, R. J. (1974). Hypogonadism in alcoholic liver disease: Evidence for a double effect. *Gastroenterology*, 67, 1188–1199.

Warren, W. D., Millikan, W. J., Henderson, J. M., et al. (1986). Splenopancreatic disconnection. Improved selectivity of distal splenorenal shunt. *Annals of Surgery*, 204, 346–355.

Warren, W. D., Zeppa, R., and Foman, J. S. (1967). Selective transplenic decompression of gastroesophageal varices by distal splenorenal shunt. *Annals of Surgery*, 166, 437–442.

Waye, J. D. (1987). Expanding uses of therapeutic endoscopy. *Hospital Practice*, August 15, 143–158.

Westaby, D., Macdongall, B. R. D., and Millikan, W. J. (1985). Improved survival following injection sclerotherapy for esophageal varices: Final analysis of a controlled trial. *Hepatology*, 5, 827–830.

Widmann, F. K. (Ed.). (1987). *Clinical interpretation of laboratory tests* (9th ed.). Philadelphia: F. A. Davis.

Willson, R. A. (1977). Acute hepatic failure. *Hospital Medicine*, October, 8–23.

Zeppa, R., Hensley, G. T., and Levi, J. U. (1978). Factors influencing survival after distal splenorenal shunt. *Annals of Surgery*, 187, 510–542.

Zipser, R. D., Hoefs, J. C., Speckart, P. F., et al. (1979). Prostaglandins: Modulators of renal function and pressor resistance in chronic liver disease. *Journal of Clinical Endocrinology and Metabolism*, 48, 895–890.

Zipser, R. D., Radvan, G. H., Kronberg, K. J., et al. (1983). Urinary thromboxane B_2 and prostaglandin E_2 in the hepatorenal syndrome: Evidence for increased vasoconstrictor and decreased vasodilator factors. *Gastroenterology*, 84, 697–703.

Patients with Acute Pancreatitis

Kathryn Hennessy

Pancreatitis is an inflammation of the pancreas that may be acute or chronic. The intensity of the disease may vary from mild edema to a partial or generalized pancreatic necrosis. The manifestations of acute pancreatitis disappear when the causative factors are eliminated. Chronic pancreatitis is a degenerative process that causes pathologic structural and functional changes in the absence of a causative agent. Although most patients presenting with acute pancreatitis recover rapidly, the disease can run a fulminant and fatal course in 10% of all patients (Sabesin, 1987).

PATHOPHYSIOLOGY (Figs. 46–1 and 46–2)

Acute pancreatitis is an autodigestive disease resulting from the "premature activation of zymogens to active enzymes within the pancreas" (Soergel, 1983). The events that trigger the sequence of enzyme activation and subsequent autodigestion of the pancrease remain unknown. Acute pancreatitis can be divided into two stages. The mild stage, acute edematous pancreatitis, is characterized by interstitial edema with exudation of small numbers of polymorphonuclear leukocytes. Exocrine, endocrine, and ductular cells are not damaged. Progression of the disease process leads to hemorrhagic or necrotizing pancreatitis, which is characterized by coagulation necrosis of the gland and the surrounding fatty tissue. The factors that promote this disease progression are unknown (Soergel, 1983).

Theories of the Pathophysiologic Events of Pancreatic Autodigestion

Six theories have been proposed to explain the process of enzyme activation and autodigestion that overcomes the body's protective mechanisms:

1. One theory is that some agents act as direct cellular toxins or in some way alter the metabolic and secretory processes of the acinar cells (Sabesin, 1987).
2. The bile reflux or common channel theory proposes that a stone may obstruct the flow of bile, allowing it to flow through a common channel into the pancreatic duct (Soergel, 1989).
3. The duodenal reflux theory is that duodenal contents containing activated enzymes enter the pancreatic duct, causing inflammation (Soergel, 1989).
4. Another possibility, called ductal hypertension, is that distal obstruction of the biliary ductal system causes pancreatic outflow obstruction and continued secretion of pancreatic enzymes into the occluded areas. This leads to ductal hypertension, resulting in pancreatitis (Sabesin, 1987).
5. The theory of intracellular protease activation refers to the process of crinophagy, in which lysosomes and zymogen granules are fused, and these, when extruded across the acinar cell wall, lead to the delivery of digestive and lysosomal enzymes to the interstitial and peripancreatic fatty tissue. The lysosome hydrolases include cathepsin B, which can activate trypsinogen, and trypsin will then activate other protease precursors. The normal pancreatic

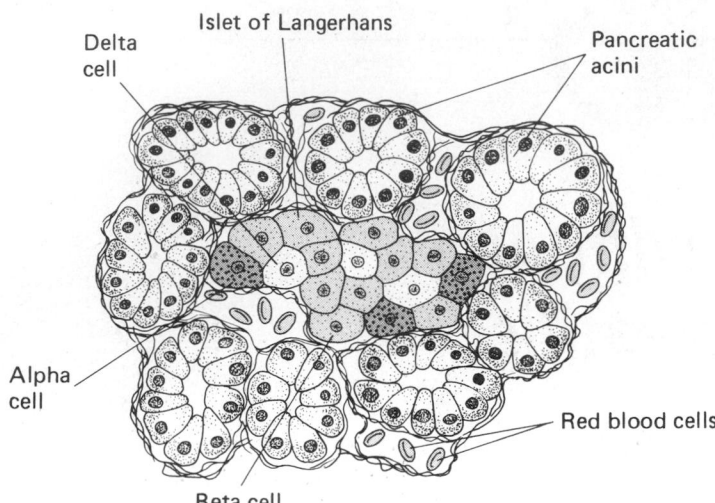

Delta cell
Islet of Langerhans
Pancreatic acini
Alpha cell
Red blood cells
Beta cell

FIGURE 46–1. Physiologic anatomy of the pancreas. (From Guyton, A. C. (1986). *Textbook of medical physiology* (7th ed., p. 923). Philadelphia: W. B. Saunders.)

trypsin inhibitor protein is inactive at the acidic pH that exists in lysosomes (Soergel, 1989).

6. The use of alcohol has been implicated in the development of chronic pancreatitis and is said to promote duct obstruction through precipitation of pancreatic secretory proteins (Grendell, 1983). Whether this mechanism can initiate acute pancreatitis remains unknown (Table 46–1).

ENZYME ACTIVATION

The process of enzyme activation, regardless of etiology, is the basis of the disease process (Fig. 46–3). Initial damage to the acinar cells causes a cycle of local inflammation and necrosis as well as systemic complications (Table 46–2).

Trypsinogen, a pancreatic enzyme, may undergo spontaneous activation to trypsin in the presence of an alkaline pH. This release of trypsin can convert kallikrein, a vasoactive substance, to bradykinin, which produces effects on the vascular system such as capillary permeability, vasodilation, and hypotension. The release of these vasoactive substances may be a major pathogenetic mechanism in the production of shock and the cardiovascular complications

of acute pancreatitis. Trypsin also produces abnormalities in blood coagulation and thrombotic tendencies. Trypsin can convert prothrombin to thrombin, leading to the formation of clots and the conversion of plasminogen to plasmin, a fibrinolytic enzyme, which leads to clot lysis.

Phospholipase A and elastase, other pancreatic enzymes, have been proposed as the primary enzymes responsible for autodigestion. Phospholipase A, in the presence of bile that has refluxed into the pancreas, causes severe pancreatic parenchymal and adipose tissue necrosis and fluid accumulation. It is believed that this release of phospholipase is instrumental in producing the pulmonary abnormalities characteristic of acute pancreatitis, especially that of adult respiratory distress syndrome (ARDS). Pulmonary surfactant, a phospholipid, may be decreased in the presence of circulating phospholipases. Elastase dissolves the elastic fibers of the blood vessels and is responsible for the hemorrhage seen in patients with necrotizing pancreatitis. Local venous thrombosis, splenic or portal vein thrombosis, and rare instances of disseminated intravascular coagulation result from the activation of elastase.

Fat necrosis in the pancreas occurs as a result of the digestion of lipid by lipase and the precipitation

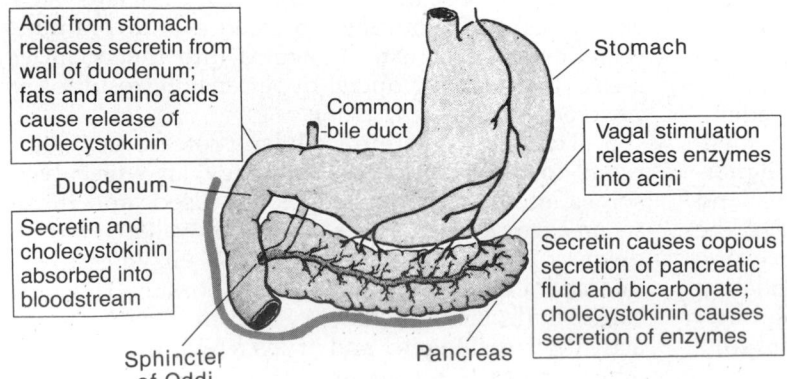

Acid from stomach releases secretin from wall of duodenum; fats and amino acids cause release of cholecystokinin

Common bile duct

Stomach

Vagal stimulation releases enzymes into acini

Duodenum

Secretin and cholecystokinin absorbed into bloodstream

Secretin causes copious secretion of pancreatic fluid and bicarbonate; cholecystokinin causes secretion of enzymes

Sphincter of Oddi

Pancreas

FIGURE 46–2. Regulation of pancreatic secretions. (From Guyton, A. C. (1986). *Textbook of medical physiology* (7th ed., p. 781). Philadelphia: W. B. Saunders.)

TABLE 46–1. Possible Effects of Alcohol on Pancreas

Increased secretion of pancreatic enzymes with decreased water and bicarbonate output

Formation of protein plugs in pancreatic ducts that may cause partial outlet obstruction (increased concentration of protein and volume of pancreatic secretions)

Increased tone of sphincter of Oddi with increased pressure in biliary tract and pancreas

Increased reflux of duodenal contents into pancreas. Alcohol bile more toxic than pure bile

Direct toxic effect on acinar cells

Data from Creutzfeldt and Lankisch, 1985.

of insoluble calcium and magnesium salts. The formation of calcium soaps causes a sequestration of calcium, thus leading to hypocalcemia.

PRECIPITATING CAUSES

Acute pancreatitis can have a variety of causes, but the most common are biliary tract stone disease and alcohol abuse. These account for at least 80% of cases (Sabesin, 1987). Other causes are listed in Table 46–3.

TABLE 46–2. Complications of Acute Pancreatitis

Systemic
Cardiovascular: Hypotension, nonspecific ST-T segment changes, pericardial effusion
Pulmonary: Pleural effusion, adult respiratory distress syndrome, atelectasis
Renal: Acute renal failure
Gastrointestinal: Gastritis, peptic ulcer disease
Hematologic: Disseminated intravascular coagulation, involvement of adjacent organs
Metabolic: Hypocalcemia, hyperglycemia, hypertriglyceridemia
Central nervous system: Psychosis
Pancreatic
Phlegmon: Solid mass of inflamed pancreas with patchy areas of necrosis
Pseudocyst: Collection of tissue, fluid, debris, enzymes, and blood
Abscess: Secondary infection of necrotic pancreatic or peripancreatic tissue
Ascites: Due to disruption of main pancreatic duct
Other
Fat necrosis: Subcutaneous, bone

CLINICAL PRESENTATION

Abdominal pain can be very severe in patients presenting with acute pancreatitis. The pain is usu-

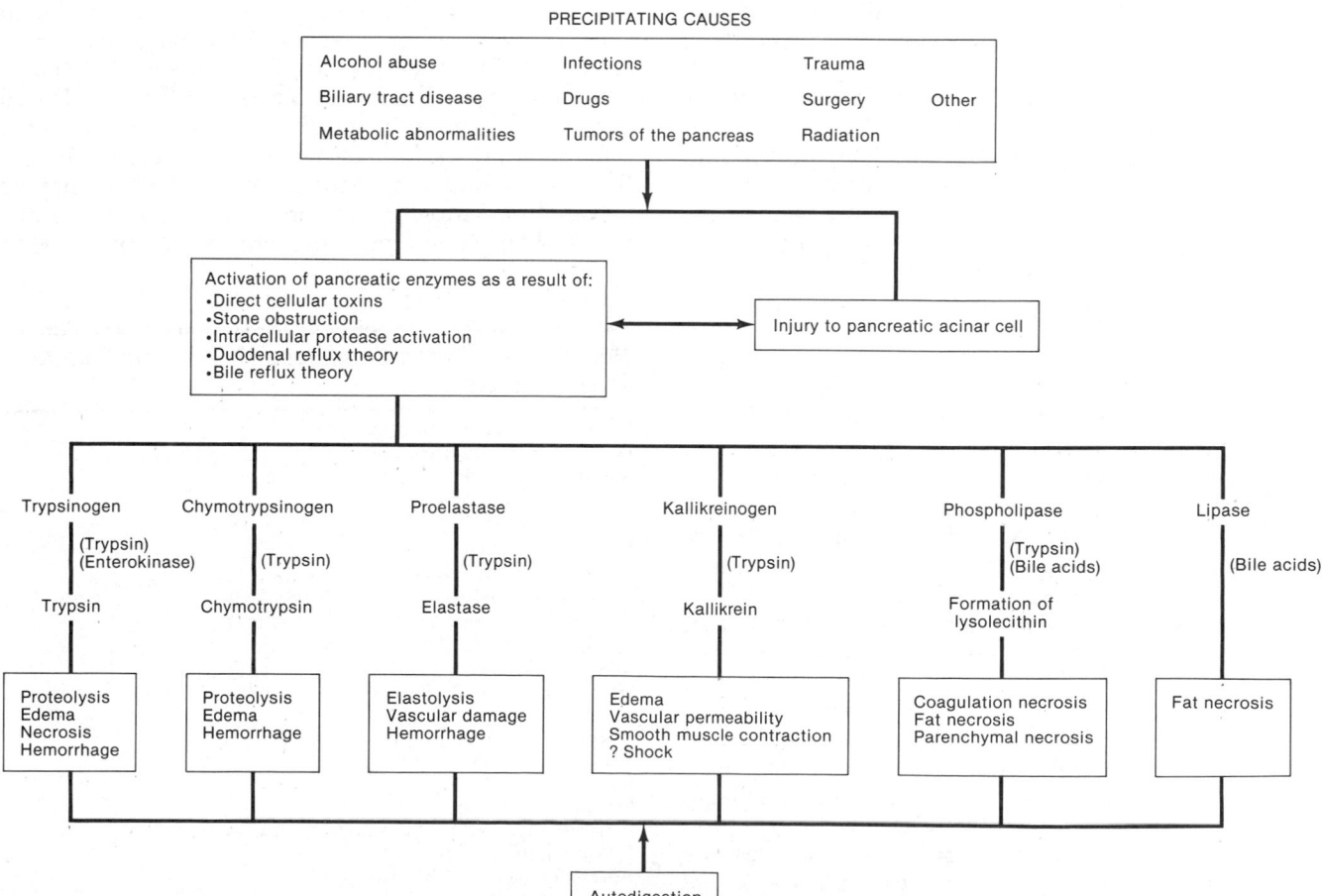

FIGURE 46–3. The activation of pancreatic enzymes in acute pancreatitis. (Adapted from Creutzfeldt, W., and Schmidt, H. (1970). *Scandinavian Journal of Gastroenterology,* 6, 47, by permission of Scandinavian University Press.)

TABLE 46–3. Precipitating Causes of Acute Pancreatitis

Biliary tract disease
Alcohol abuse
Duodenal disease, peptic ulcer
Drugs—thiazide diuretics, furosemide, estrogens, azathioprine,
    asparaginase, methyldopa, sulfonamides, pentamide,
    procainamide, tetracycline, mercaptopurine, excessive
    vitamin D
Pancreatic tumors
Severe hypertriglyceridemia (type I, IV, V)
Trauma, surgery, radiation injury
Pregnancy—third trimester
Hereditary pancreatitis (pancreas divisium)
Infectious agents (viral, bacterial)
Hypercalcemia
Vascular insufficiency
Idiopathic—no cause known (possibly pancreas divisium)

ally located in the epigastric region but may be present in the left upper quadrant radiating to the back. It may increase gradually for several hours before reaching maximum intensity, or it may begin suddenly after a large meal. This sudden onset of pain may mimic an acute vascular condition or a gastrointestinal disorder. Once the pain begins, it persists without diminishing for hours and even days. Abdominal pain that fluctuates in intensity or ceases for periods of time is generally not related to pancreatitis but is more often a result of biliary tract disease.

Nausea, vomiting, and retching occur frequently in patients with acute pancreatitis. Abdominal pain persists even after episodes of vomiting and is considered a hallmark sign of acute pancreatitis.

Fever is common in patients with acute pancreatitis but can be a result of other infectious processes. If the temperature is greater than 102°F it is probably related to peritonitis, cholecystitis, or perhaps an intra-abdominal abscess.

Jaundice occurs in 15% to 50% of patients with acute pancreatitis (Sabesin, 1987). Mild elevations in liver enzymes may also be present and reflect pancreatic edema. Hyperbilirubinemia greater than 3 mg/dL may be present (Thompson et al., 1986).

Changes in the circulatory system such as tachycardia, hypovolemia, and hypotension may be present and may progress to circulatory shock and coma in the late stages of the disease.

Patients with severe disease have symptoms that reflect the late stages of pancreatitis. These patients may have pleural effusion and infiltrates, pleuritic pain, diaphragmatic irritation with referred shoulder pain, and possibly respiratory compromise and ARDS. Abdominal rigidity, masses, and ascites may be present as a result of fat necrosis, hemorrhage, pseudocyst, or abscess. A bluish-brown discoloration of the flank, Grey Turner sign, signifies the presence of hemorrhagic pancreatitis and the retroperitoneal dissection of blood into that area. Cullen sign is a bluish-brown discoloration in the periumbilical area and indicates blood in that region. Renal function

may also be altered as a result of the combined effect of hypovolemia, shock, and mild disseminated intravascular coagulation. Oliguria is usually associated with acute tubular necrosis.

Although the clinical appearance of acute pancreatitis has a wide range of symptoms, most patients present with epigastric pain unrelieved by nausea and vomiting and with guarding of the upper abdomen area. A careful interview should elicit precipitating causes such as alcohol ingestion or biliary tract disease and possibly a history of similar attacks during the preceding years.

DIAGNOSTIC STUDIES

A variety of laboratory and diagnostic tests are ordered in an attempt to confirm the diagnosis of acute pancreatitis.

Laboratory Tests

Amylase. Amylase is the digestive enzyme released from the pancreas into the duodenum to assist in the digestion of carbohydrates. The serum amylase level is a widely used, sensitive test for the diagnosis of acute pancreatitis, but it is in no way a specific or exclusive test. Other illnesses can increase the serum amylase level as well (Table 46–4) (Banks, 1985).

Serum amylase is metabolized rapidly and cleared by the kidney, and in the absence of continued inflammation, a transient elevation occurs. In patients with mild pancreatitis, serum amylase may be elevated for 24 to 48 hours and then return to normal levels. The patient may present for treatment after

TABLE 46–4. Disease Conditions That Elevate Serum Amylase Levels

Biliary colic—biliary tract disease
Perforated peptic ulcer
Mesenteric infarct
Salivary gland dysfunction
Renal insufficiency
Macroamylasemia
Tumors of lung and ovary
Diabetic ketoacidosis
Pregnancy
Prostatic disease
Cerebral trauma
Gynecologic disorders—ruptured ectopic pregnancy or ovarian cyst
Pneumonia
Acquired bisalbuminemia
Burns and traumatic shock
Chronic alcoholism
Pancreatic carcinoma, pseudocyst, abscess, ascites
Intestinal obstruction
Aortic aneurysm with dissection
Peritonitis
Acute appendicitis

Data from Banks, 1985; Sabesin, 1987.

the initial elevation has returned to normal, making a diagnosis of pancreatitis difficult using this laboratory value. Serum amylase levels remain elevated longer in those conditions previously mentioned (Table 46–4). Serum amylase may be falsely low in patients with hypertriglyceridemia (Sabesin, 1987).

Serum amylase isoenzymes have been used to improve the diagnostic specificity of increased amylase levels (Banks, 1985). There are two types of serum amylase isoenzymes, pancreatic type (p type) and salivary type (s type). In patients with acute pancreatitis, p-type isoenzymes are elevated, and in those with salivary gland dysfunction and tumors, s-type isoenzymes are increased. Elevations in p-type isoenzymes also occur in patients with other intra-abdominal conditions such as perforated ulcer or mesenteric infarction (Banks, 1985).

Measurement of urinary amylase excretion may be a more sensitive indicator of acute pancreatitis than serum amylase. When serum amylase is elevated, an increased urinary amylase level also occurs. In patients with acute pancreatitis the urinary amylase rises just before the serum amylase, although this correlation does not always occur. Elevated urinary amylase levels may persist for 7 to 10 days after serum amylase levels have returned to normal. Therefore, urinary amylase is a useful diagnostic tool in patients with mild or resolving pancreatitis (Bell and Go, 1985).

An increase in the amylase-creatinine clearance ratio of greater than or equal to 5% has been proposed as a diagnostic tool in acute pancreatitis (Sabesin, 1987). However, it appears that the serum amylase level must be elevated, and even with this elevation, the clearance ratio can be nonspecific and is affected by other conditions. With the increasing use of isoenzyme measurements, the amylase-creatinine ratio is losing favor as a specific diagnostic test (Sabesin, 1987).

Serum Lipase. Serum lipase concentrations are increased in patients with acute pancreatitis and usually remain elevated longer than serum amylase. However, serum lipase, like amylase, can be elevated in patients with other serious abdominal illnesses such as those listed in Table 46–4. Normal serum lipase levels can rule out some nonpancreatic conditions such as macroamylasemia, tumors, pelvic inflammatory disease, and salivary dysfunction. Hyperlipidemia may also interfere with serum lipase results (Banks, 1985).

Trypsin. Trypsin is found exclusively in the pancreas. It does not circulate in free form and is measured by radioimmunoassay (RIA), which measures the presence of alpha-1 globulin, a trypsin inhibitor. Trypsin RIA levels tend to parallel the degree and duration of serum amylase levels. There is no correlation between the degree of elevation and the severity, complications, or prognosis of acute pancreatitis. Trypsin RIA levels may also be elevated in patients with pancreatic carcinoma (Bell and Go, 1985).

Nonspecific Laboratory Tests. Other nonspecific laboratory tests are used to evaluate the extent of acute pancreatitis (Table 46–5). Although these test results do not identify pancreatitis as the cause of the process, they help to identify the complications of the process.

Procedures

Radiographs and Barium Studies. Radiographs of the chest and abdomen may be the first diagnostic studies done when the patient presents with acute abdominal pain. These x-rays are taken with the patient in the recumbent and upright positions to exclude the presence of free air in the abdominal cavity, which suggests a perforated hollow viscus. Some findings that point to acute pancreatitis as the cause include regional or localized ileus, sentinel loop (distended small intestinal loop near the pancreas), presence of pancreatic pseudocyst, blurring of the renal outline and left psoas margin, elevation of the diaphragm, pleural effusion, pericardial effusion, atelectasis, and pulmonary edema (Baltaxe, 1985). Pancreatic calculi may also be seen on x-ray.

Contrast studies for patients with acute pancreatitis have been largely replaced by ultrasound and computed tomography because they provide such limited information. Barium studies are helpful only when the head of the pancreas is inflamed. Contrast studies will demonstrate pancreatic enlargement, widening of the duodenal c-loop, and enlargement of papilla of Vater. The stomach may also be displaced by a pseudocyst (Baltaxe, 1985).

Ultrasound. Ultrasound imaging of the pancreas can be very accurate in the thin person. It shows enlargement or abnormal texture of the pancreas, gallstones, enlargement or distention of the common bile duct, pancreatic mass, pseudocyst, or accumulation of fluid in the abdominal cavity. It can also be used to localize a cyst for percutaneous drainage. Limitations on the use of ultrasound occur in obese patients and in patients with excessive bowel gas because the loops of bowel obscure the imaging process. Because ultrasound is available in most hospitals, this procedure plays an important part in diagnosing acute pancreatitis.

Computed Tomography. Computed tomographic (CT) scanning provides better imaging of the pancreas and abdominal cavity compared with that provided by ultrasound. Unlike ultrasound, imaging of the pancreas shows up well on CT scans surrounded by adipose tissue. Although textural changes caused by edema cannot be identified as on ultrasound, enlargement of the gland can be identified. Enlargement of the gland is the most frequent CT finding in

TABLE 46–5. Nonspecific Laboratory Tests Used to Evaluate Acute Pancreatitis

Diagnostic Test	Test Result	Cause
White blood count	Moderately elevated	Infectious process
Serum glucose	Transient mild elevation in glucose in initial attacks	Excess glucagan released from alpha cells of islets of Langerhans in pancreas
	Hyperglycemia greater than 200 mg/dL	Widespread pancreatic necrosis
Serum calcium	Hypocalcemia 2 to 3 days after onset of disease	Possibly related to hypoalbuminemia; deposition and sequestration of ionized calcium in fat necrosis
	Calcium levels less than 8 mg/dL indicate poor prognosis	Inadequate parathyroid hormone release and end-organ refractoriness to parathyroid hormone
Hematocrit	Elevated on admission	Hemoconcentration is a result of extensive fluid sequestration
	Continuing or declining hematocrit after fluid restoration	Bleeding site rare in acute pancreatitis
Serum albumin	Hypoalbuminemia	Fluid restoration
Arterial P_{O_2}	Decreased arterial P_{O_2}	Development of ARDS; pulmonary edema caused by increased permeability of the alveolar-capillary membrane
Serum lipids	Hyperlipidemia—serum triglyceride levels increased; serum cholesterol normal or moderately elevated	Serum triglycerides elevated in alcohol-induced pancreatitis; lipemic serum is due to the cause of acute pancreatitis (hyperlipidemia I, IV, V)
Serum C-reactive protein	Markedly elevated	Predicts progression of disease to severe, necrotizing pancreatitis (95% accuracy)
Liver enzymes	AST, SGOT elevated ALT, SGPT, alkaline phosphatase elevated	Biliary tract disease
Serum bilirubin	Slight increase	Compression of common bile duct
Serum methemalbumin	Present	Breakdown of hemoglobin in and around pancreas, followed by hematin entering plasma and combining with albumin
BUN (blood urea nitrogen)	Elevated	Significant hemoconcentration as a result of fluid sequestration
Serum magnesium	Decreased	Found in patients who abuse alcohol. May contribute to hypocalcemia
Electrocardiography	ST-T segment alteration (depression or elevation) Inversion of T waves Extended T-wave negativity Arrhythmias	May be due to 1. Cardiac damage due to shock 2. Electrolyte imbalance 3. Effect of severe pain on coronary circulation 4. Influence of circulating pancreatic trypsin 5. Vagal influences on cardiac function arising from stimuli from inflamed pancreas

Data from Ammann, 1985; Bell and Go, 1985; Soergel, 1989.

patients with acute pancreatitis (Neff and Ferrucci, 1984) (Figs. 46–4, 46–6, and 46–7).* The development of a pancreatic phlegmon, a diffuse inflammation with induration of peripancreatic tissues, is the second most common finding in patients with acute pancreatitis on CT scan (Fig. 46–5). Overall, ultrasound and CT scans can detect at an early stage such complications of pancreatitis as phlegmon, pseudocyst, and abscess and can also monitor the treatment response of these complications and of overall pancreatitis. Percutaneous needle aspiration and drainage can be guided with the aid of these imaging procedures. Finally, these noninvasive procedures provide insight into the acute disease process.

---

*The author would like to acknowledge the valuable assistance of Michael Powalish, Supervisor of CT Scan, Alexian Brothers Medical Center, Elk Grove Village, IL. Without his enthusiasm and expertise, these CT scan photographs would not have been possible.

Magnetic Resonance Imaging. The development of magnetic resonance imaging (MRI) is the most promising diagnostic technique of this decade (Baltaxe, 1985). With the use of contrast media, it may prove useful in the diagnosis of acute pancreatitis. At present, inflamed pancreatic tissue is difficult to differentiate from viable pancreatic tissue, and MRI currently has no advantage over CT scan as the procedure of choice in diagnosing acute pancreatitis.

PROGNOSTIC ASSESSMENT

Patients with acute pancreatitis present with a wide spectrum of clinical conditions. Steady, dull, or boring pain located in the epigastric area is the hallmark symptom of acute pancreatitis. This pain may be accompanied by nausea, vomiting, fever, or jaundice and by cardiovascular, respiratory, or renal compli-

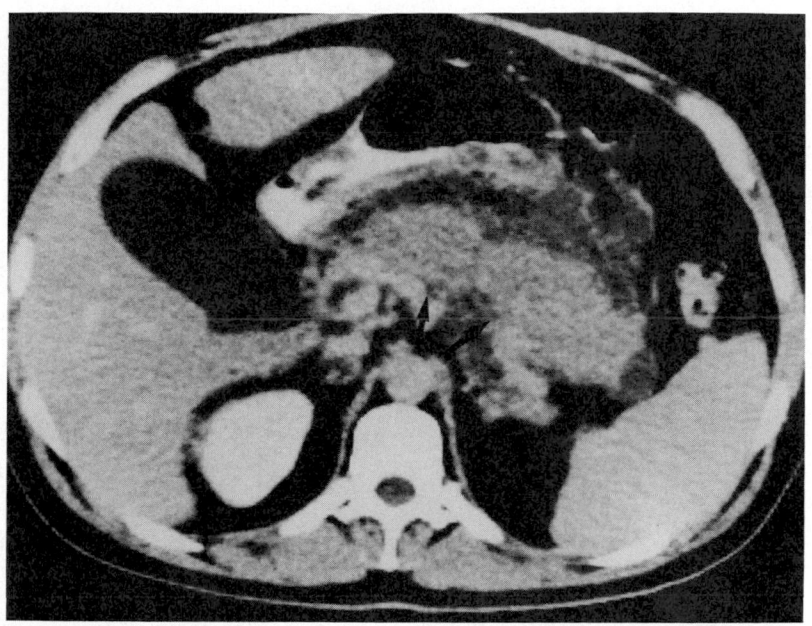

FIGURE 46–4. Computed tomographic (CT) scan showing marked enlargement of the pancreas with severe peripancreatic inflammatory changes extending into the mesenteric fat anteriorly *(arrows)*.

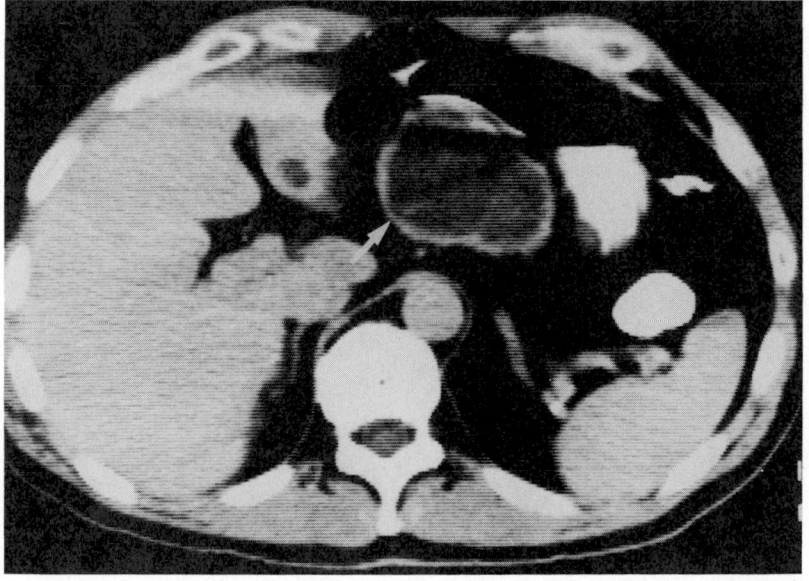

FIGURE 46–5. CT scan showing an 8 × 6 cm sized well demarcated space occupying process in the projection of the body of the pancreas *(arrow)*. This mass appears to be solid in nature.

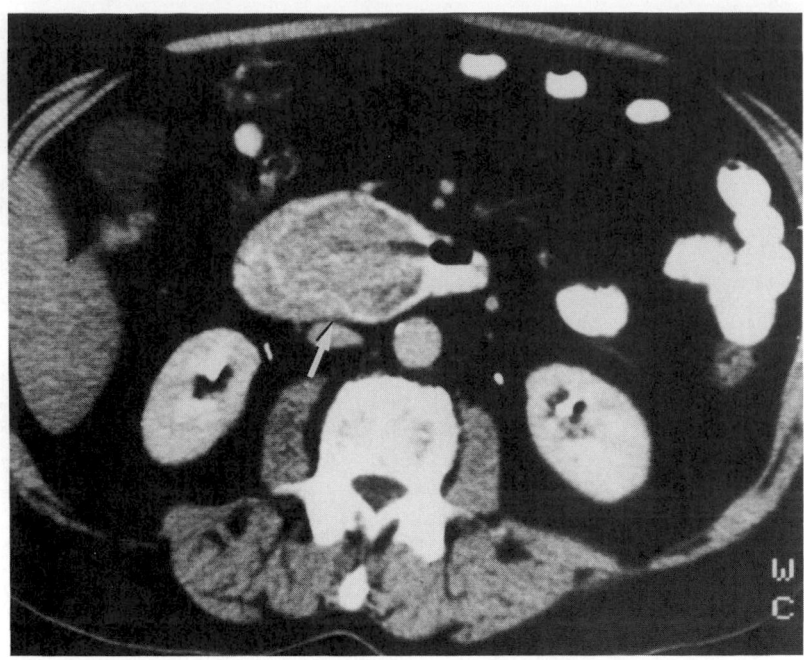

FIGURE 46–6. CT scan showing a 7 × 5 cm sized well encapsulated, solid type of mass involving the head of the pancreas, which could be consistent with malignant neoplasm *(arrow)*. Dilatation of the biliary duct and gallbladder is seen. This could be due to obstruction of the distal common duct, where there is a mass.

FIGURE 46–7. CT scan showing a 3.5 cm sized lobulated lucent space occupying process in the head of the pancreas with suggestion of neoplasm *(arrow)*. Diffuse enlargement of the pancreas is noted. The pancreatic duct and common bile duct are dilated.

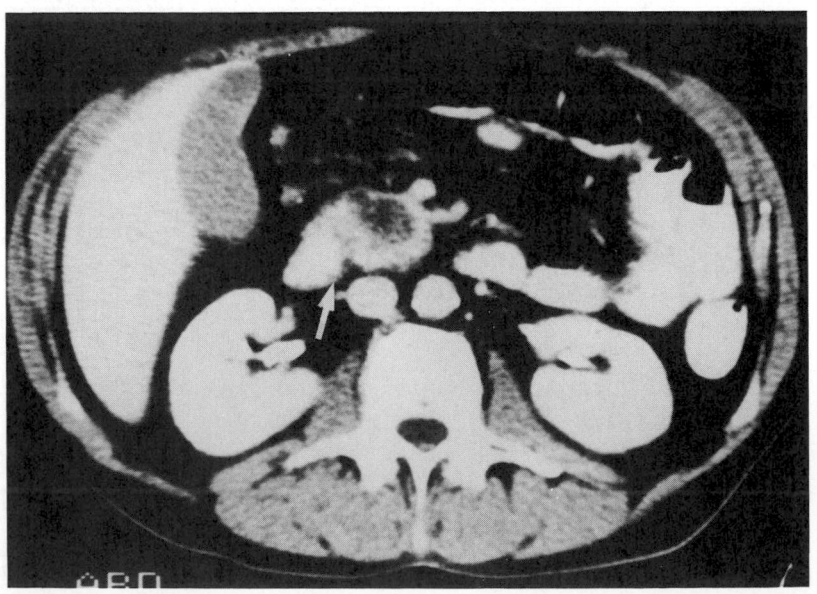

cations. The outcome is often unpredictable at the onset of the disease (Williamson, 1984). The overall mortality is 10%, and it exceeds 50% in patients with acute hemorrhagic pancreatitis (Sabesin, 1987). The need to predict outcome at the time of admission is invaluable in determining the type and aggressiveness of treatment and also for providing a comparison between the results of prospective studies (Williamson, 1984). It is for these reasons that researchers have attempted to establish criteria that assess prognosis early in the course of acute pancreatitis.

Ranson's Prognostic Signs. Of the many protocols that have been developed, the most widely accepted is the list of 11 prognostic signs devised by Ranson, which are determined within the first 48 hours of the hospital stay (Ranson, 1979). This scale has a 96% accuracy rate in predicting the severity and outcome of the disease in patients with acute pancreatitis (Table 46–6). In Ranson's study, mortality as a result of acute pancreatitis can also be predicted (Table 46–7).

Williamson's Factors. Other researchers have looked at single prognostic factors to predict disease severity and outcome (Williamson, 1984). The presence of methemalbumin in the blood, hypoxemia, early hypocalcemia, fluid sequestration, and blood in ascitic fluid have been evaluated for their usefulness in predicting severity of disease. Williamson (1984) used a combination of four factors: hypotension (blood pressure less than 100 mm Hg), hypocalcemia, hypoxemia, and the presence of "toxic broth" (dark fluid obtained from abdominal paracentesis). The presence of any one of these criteria indicated a severe attack with an overall diagnostic accuracy rate of 84%. Either of these sets of prognostic signs can be used to identify those patients who will require intensive care and management.

MEDICAL AND NURSING MANAGEMENT

In 85% to 90% of patients with acute pancreatitis, the disease is self-limiting and will subside within 3 to 7 days after treatment is initiated (Greenberger et al., 1987). Treatment of the patient with acute pancreatitis is aimed at stopping the progression of damage to the pancreas and preventing and treating the local complications. Because specific therapeutic agents for the prevention and treatment of pancreatitis have not been identified, medical interventions are symptomatic and supportive in nature.

Supportive Treatment

In keeping with the overall goals of nursing management, several key areas of treatment have been identified. They include provision of

TABLE 46–6. Ranson's Prognostic Signs Used to Predict Severity and Outcome in Patients with Acute Pancreatitis

Upon admission to hospital:
Age greater than 55 years
Blood glucose greater than 200 mg/dL (no history of diabetes)
WBC greater than 16,000 mm³
Serum aspartate transaminase greater than 250 units/liter
During first 48 hours of hospitalization:
Decrease in hematocrit greater than 10%
Serum calcium less than 8 mg/dL
Arterial P_{O_2} less than 60 mm Hg
Increase in BUN of greater than 5 mg/dL
Base deficit of greater than 4 mEq/liter
Fluid sequestration greater than 6 liters

From Ranson, J. H. C. (1979). *Current Problems in Surgery,* 16 (11), 1–84.

1. Intravenous fluids and colloids to maintain normal intravascular volume and restore electrolyte balance.

2. Nasogastric suction to decrease gastrin release from the stomach and prevent gastric contents from entering the duodenum.

3. Elimination of oral intake.

4. Analgesics for pain control.

5. Respiratory support.

The following sections will address these key areas as they relate to the management of acute pancreatitis.

Fluid Replacement. In patients with acute pancreatitis large quantities of fluid collect in the retroperitoneal spaces and occasionally within the peritoneal cavity itself. As a result of this third spacing, patients often experience some degree of dehydration. Fluid replacement is a high priority in preventing systemic hypotension. Hypovolemia and shock are major causes of death early in the disease process. Intravenous fluids, especially high-volume electrolyte and colloid solutions, need to be given to replenish losses. An accurate flow sheet of intake and output should be maintained so that all losses can be replaced with an equal amount of intravenous solution. Patients who are significantly dehydrated should receive isotonic solutions such as Ringer's lactate to replace plasma volume. Leese and colleagues (1987) conducted a study that suggested that fresh frozen plasma be used as a specific therapy for

TABLE 46–7. Using Ranson's Prognostic Signs to Predict Mortality in Patients with Acute Pancreatitis

Presence of Ranson's Prognostic Signs	Mortality Rates (%)
One to two signs	1
Three to four signs	15
Five to six signs	40
Seven signs or more	100

From Banks, P. A. (1985). *Annals of Internal Medicine,* 103, 91–97.

acute pancreatitis because it would replenish the naturally occurring antiprotease system. The results, however, showed no significant difference in terms of clinical outcome between the control group who received colloids and the experimental group. Regardless of the type of fluid used for replacement, fluid restoration helps to prevent the development of acute renal failure as well as to maintain perfusion of the pancreas and possibly diminish the severity of the pancreatitis. A urinary Foley catheter is inserted to monitor the adequacy of renal perfusion by measuring urinary output hourly. Central venous catheters are also helpful in monitoring the hydration status in these patients. Adequate volume resuscitation is indicated when the patient has a stable blood pressure, a stable pulse, and adequate left and right ventricular filling pressures (Crist and Cameron, 1987). Other indications of successful fluid replacement are a urinary output of 30 to 50 mL/hour and the presence of warm extremities indicating an adequate peripheral circulation.

For patients who fail to respond to intravascular fluid replacement, a pulmonary artery catheter needs to be inserted and intravenous fluids administered until the pulmonary artery wedge pressure reaches 15 mm Hg. If hypotension persists, medications to support circulation are administered. The preferred drug is dopamine, which should be started at a dose of 3 to 5 μg/kg per minute (Burch, 1988). Adjustments of the dopamine dosage can be made according to hemodynamic parameters and urinary output. Patients with severe hemorrhagic pancreatitis may require 6 to 8 liters of fluid or more during the initial 24 hours. They may require packed red blood cells or, rarely, whole blood. Albumin has also been shown to be effective in restoring intravascular volume in patients with marked hypoalbuminemia (Crist and Cameron, 1987). Renal failure may occur as a result of hypovolemia and shock and is prerenal in nature.

Electrolyte Replacement. Along with fluid replacement, electrolyte replacement is extremely important in preventing the complications of acute pancreatitis. The monitoring and replacement of calcium is of particular significance in the early stage of the disease because hypocalcemia reflects a graver prognosis. Hypocalcemia is generally related to a decrease in albumin. Calcium replacement is reserved for patients with clinical signs of hypocalcemia such as a positive Chvostek or Trousseau sign or a decreased ionized calcium level. Low calcium levels are related to disease severity, and it is believed that calcium and magnesium are sequestered in the area of pancreatic necrosis (Shearson and Finlayson, 1982).

Hypomagnesium may be present alone or in combination with a decreased serum calcium level; it requires parenteral administration of magnesium sulfate. Correction of the magnesium level may be necessary before the calcium level can be restored.

Potassium levels must also be followed carefully because hyperkalemia and acidosis may result from excess tissue destruction. Hypokalemia may result from vomiting, nasogastric suction, or loss of potassium into an atonic bowel lumen (Burrell and Burrell, 1982).

Another metabolic complication in patients with severe disease is hyperglycemia, which is a result of extensive damage to the pancreas. Regular insulin, on a sliding scale, should be given cautiously because glucagon levels are elevated only transiently in patients with acute pancreatitis. Serum glucose should be monitored frequently.

Minimizing Pancreatic Secretions

Nasogastric Suction. Nasogastric (NG) suction has been considered part of standard therapy for patients with acute pancreatitis for years (Crist and Cameron, 1987). Theoretically, nasogastric suction should indirectly suppress pancreatic exocrine secretion by preventing acid-induced release of secretin from the duodenum, thereby resting the pancreas (Crist and Cameron, 1987). However, clinical studies have not demonstrated that the use of nasogastric suction alters the course of acute pancreatitis. Therefore, because NG suction has no specific therapeutic effect, it should be reserved for patients with ileus, persistent vomiting, or gastric distention or those with a decreased level of consciousness to prevent pulmonary aspiration.

Oral Intake. Oral intake should be eliminated in patients with acute pancreatitis and should not be resumed until after abdominal pain, tenderness, and ileus have resolved and serum amylase levels have returned to normal or near normal (Banks, 1985). Resumption of oral intake prior to this time may lead to recurrence of abdominal pain and continued inflammation of the pancreas and may increase the risk of pancreatic abscess formation (Crist and Cameron, 1987). In patients with mild to moderate disease, oral fluids can usually be resumed in 3 to 6 days and a regular diet by day 5 to 7 (Greenberger et al., 1987).

Nutritional Support. Intravenous nutritional support is indicated for patients who develop complications or who have pancreatic pseudocyst or abscesses. Levine (1981) proposes that patients who meet four of the criteria established by Ranson are candidates for total parenteral nutrition (TPN). TPN is also beneficial if the patient will require surgery during hospitalization. The goal of nutritional support is to provide adequate amounts of calories and protein to meet the patient's increased metabolic demands and to promote anabolism without stimulating the pancreas. Both essential and nonessential amino acids with dextrose can be used to provide the necessary amounts of calories and protein. Supplemental vitamins and minerals, especially calcium, are also indicated in patients with acute pancreatitis (Boudeman et al., 1985). Insulin may be necessary if the patient has extensive pancreatic damage. The addition of lipids to the parenteral nutrition regimen is still somewhat controversial. Silberman concluded that patients with underlying hyperlipidemia and those with elevations of serum cholesterol and triglycerides without hyperlipidemia should not be given lipids (Rombeau and Caldwell, 1986). In patients without these abnormalities, lipids can be given safely and effectively (Rombeau and Caldwell, 1986).

TPN should be continued until the symptoms abate. Once the acute phase has resolved, patients may be fed orally. Pancreatic enzyme replacement may be needed. In summary, although TPN cannot change the pathophysiology of acute pancreatitis, by promoting bowel rest it can reduce the length of time needed for recovery, decrease complications, and prevent malnutrition. The usefulness of elemental diets in pancreatitis is still being evaluated (Levine, 1981).

Drug Therapy. Anticholinergic drugs such as atropine have been used as therapy for patients with acute pancreatitis, their purpose being to decrease the stimulation of the pancreas. However, there have been no controlled trials demonstrating the effectiveness of anticholinergics (Greenberger et al., 1987). Because the use of anticholinergics may decrease urine output and cause bowel hypomobility, tachycardia, increased need for fluid replacement, and signs of toxicity, it is difficult to determine whether the side effects are medication-related or are signs of worsening pancreatitis.

The use of histamine (H_2) receptor antagonists such as cimetidine or ranitidine (Zantac) has also not been shown to be effective in reducing pancreatic secretions as an indirect result of the decrease in gastric acid. Although pancreatic secretions are not affected, these drugs may be useful in preventing stress ulcers in the critically ill patient.

Pain Control. Pain control is essential in the management of the patient with acute pancreatitis. The abdominal pain is constant and severe and can persist for several days; analgesics are needed to control it. However, the analgesics that cause spasm of the sphincter of Oddi such as morphine have been routinely avoided; meperidine is administered instead (Banks, 1985). Because the quantity and quality of the pain are hallmark signs of pancreatitis, assessment should be carefully completed and maintained on an ongoing basis. The use of a pain rating scale can provide qualitative and quantitative assessment (Table 46–8). Frequent administration, at least every 2 to 3 hours, of the analgesic should control acute pain. Patient-controlled analgesia (PCA) may be more effective in relieving the patient's pain because it allows self-administration of the analgesic as needed. When the pain is severe and is unrelieved by analgesics, sympathetic, splanchnic, or epidural block may be necessary. The benefit of epidural block is

---

TABLE 46–8. Pain Rating Scale: McGill-Melzack Present Pain Intensity

0—No pain
1—Mild pain
2—Discomforting
3—Distressing
4—Horrible
5—Excruciating

Data from Meissner, J. E. (1980). *Nursing 80*, 10(1), 50.

---

that it interrupts the sensory pathways of both visceral and cerebrospinal afferent fibers. Also, an epidural catheter can remain in place for more frequent use (Ammann, 1985).

Respiratory Support. Respiratory complications are well recognized in patients with acute pancreatitis. Pleural effusion, atelectasis, pneumonia, and acute respiratory insufficiency (arterial hypoxemia) have been documented in a significant number of patients (Crist and Cameron, 1987). Ranson (1979) found early arterial hypoxemia in patients with mild to moderate disease in the absence of clinical or radiologic findings. It has been recommended that arterial blood gases be measured every 12 hours for the first 3 to 5 days in all patients with acute pancreatitis (Crist and Cameron, 1987). If arterial hypoxemia is found, oxygen should be administered. In mild to moderate disease the hypoxemia should resolve as the pancreatic inflammation subsides (Crist and Cameron, 1987). Two possible causative agents in the development of acute respiratory insufficiency may be the presence of circulating phospholipase, which may destroy pulmonary surfactant, or the free fatty acids produced by lipolysis of triglycerides in pulmonary capillaries. To date, there is no clinical evidence supporting either of these two theories (Crist and Cameron, 1987).

Treatment of respiratory insufficiency is primarily supportive. Frequent turning and vigorous pulmonary hygiene will reduce the risk of atelectasis. Supplemental oxygen should be used to maintain an adequate Pa_{O_2}. Careful monitoring of the amounts of intravenous fluid administered is necessary to prevent fluid overload.

Respiratory failure is common in patients with severe pancreatitis and is indistinguishable from ARDS (Burch, 1988). For patients with arterial hypoxemia who have persistent tachypnea and a falling P_{O_2}, endotracheal intubation and mechanical ventilation may be required. Positive end-expiratory pressure (PEEP) may be helpful in maintaining an adequate P_{O_2} in patients who require high fractional inspiratory oxygen concentrations (Fi_{O_2} greater than 50%). Weaning from mechanical ventilation may begin when patients show improvements in P_{O_2}, lung compliance, tidal volume, and vital capacity (Burch, 1988).

Peritoneal Lavage. Peritoneal lavage was first suggested as treatment for acute pancreatitis in 1965. Its efficacy is attributed to the removal of toxic substances such as vasoactive kinins, phospholipase A, trypsinogen, and prostaglandinlike histamine that are present in the peritoneal fluid. These substances are thought to cause many of the adverse systemic effects characteristic of pancreatitis such as decreased blood pressure, increased vascular permeability, and respiratory failure. By removing these substances before they can be absorbed, many of the early systemic complications can be eliminated (Banks, 1985). Many clinical experiences have been reported with conflicting results. It appears that peritoneal lavage may influence the early clinical course of acute pancreatitis but does not prevent the late formation of abscess or reduce the overall mortality of the disease. Consequently, peritoneal lavage is used for patients who have failed to respond to intensive supportive care during the first 24 to 48 hours of hospitalization. The response to peritoneal lavage is usually immediate and dramatic (Crist and Cameron, 1987).

The technique of peritoneal lavage requires the placement of a dialysis catheter either percutaneously or through a small incision. The catheter is secured and covered with an occlusive dressing. Ranson recommends the use of isotonic peritoneal solution with 20 g dextrose, 100 USP units of heparin, 250 mg ampicillin, and 8 mEq potassium to each 2 liters of dialysate. This solution is infused over 15 minutes and allowed to dwell for 30 minutes and is then drained by gravity. This cycle is repeated hourly for at least 48 hours depending on the clinical status of the patient (Crist and Cameron, 1987).

Respiratory compromise may result due to restricted diaphragmatic movement. Blood glucose levels need to be monitored and insulin administered as needed because the dextrose will be absorbed transperitoneally (Crist and Cameron, 1987).

Antibiotics. Finally, even the use of antibiotics is controversial in the management of patients with acute pancreatitis. There have been no clinical trials that have shown prophylactic antibiotics to be effective in patients with mild to moderate disease (Greenberger et al., 1987). Although there is a high incidence of infection in these patients, antibiotic use does not prevent the formation or extension of pseudocysts or abscesses (Sabesin, 1987). Thus antibiotics are used simply for the treatment of established infection and not as a preventive measure. Carr and associates (1987) identified patients with acute pancreatitis who had documented or suspected intra-abdominal sepsis and administered gentamicin to these patients. Their findings showed that a 25% increase in dose was necessary to achieve peak serum gentamicin concentrations. It is believed that body fluid sequestration and the increase in total body fluid caused the increased dosing requirements for gentamicin.

Experimental Agents. Steinberg and Schlesselman (1987) reviewed 13 studies of human acute pancreatitis and 25 studies involving experimentally induced pancreatitis in animals. These studies evaluated the use of aprotinin, glucagon, 5-fluorouracil, somatostatin, and peritoneal lavage as possible therapeutic agents in the treatment of acute pancreatitis. Although 81% of the animal studies showed a positive outcome, only 7.7% of the human studies showed a positive outcome on survival. These reviewers concluded that experimentally induced pancreatitis in animals does not compare to the pathophysiology of human pancreatitis, and therefore, animals may not be effective in the testing of therapeutic agents for use in humans. It is their belief that these negative studies have influenced the lack of development of therapeutic agents for acute pancreatitis. Glucagon, 5-fluorouracil, and somatostatin may prove beneficial with the development of studies based on large sample sizes and prolonged therapeutic regimes (Steinberg and Schlesselman, 1987).

Surgical Management

Although patients with acute pancreatitis generally do not require surgery, there are four categories of conditions necessitating surgical intervention (Martin et al., 1984). They are (1) uncertain diagnosis, (2) deterioration of patient's clinical condition, (3) presence of cholelithiasis, and (4) suspicion of intra-abdominal infection. The first three categories are indications for immediate surgery because they usually occur within the first 24 to 48 hours after admission. Late surgical intervention is usually reserved for patients with complications of intra-abdominal infection.

When acute pancreatitis cannot be differentiated from other intra-abdominal emergencies, exploratory surgery may be necessary. During diagnostic surgery, the pancreas should be inspected for edema, necrosis, and hemorrhage. Peritoneal fluid can be obtained for culture and for amylase and lipase determinations. Cholelithiasis should also be ruled out. It remains controversial whether to drain the pancreas or place lavage catheters. Pancreatic resection or débridement is debatable, and little evidence suggests that pancreatic resection is indicated if there is no secondary infection (Crist and Cameron, 1987).

The most controversial indication for surgical intervention is severe hemorrhagic pancreatitis in patients who fail to respond to conventional supportive management. Both pancreatic drainage and resection have been proposed for this group of patients. Pancreatic resection has ranged from local débridement of necrotic tissue to total pancreatectomy. However, there is a lack of clinical data supporting these approaches. Crist and Cameron (1987) suggest that patients whose condition continues to deteriorate with supportive care should be managed with nonoperative peritoneal lavage. Operative exploration should then be reserved for these patients and should be limited to local débridement of nonviable tissue and the placement of drainage catheters.

It is generally a well-accepted practice to operate on patients with gallstone pancreatitis to reduce the risk of recurrent attacks. Because there is little evidence to suggest that immediate surgical intervention is required, most surgeons provide initial supportive care followed by biliary surgery during the same hospitalization (Crist and Cameron, 1987). A cholecystectomy and operative cholangiogram are usually performed to remove gallstones in the gallbladder and common bile duct (Shearson and Finlayson, 1982).

The final indication for surgical intervention is the presence of abdominal infection. A pancreatic abscess is a life-threatening complication of acute pancreatitis, and without surgical intervention it has a mortality of 100% (Crist and Cameron, 1987). Pancreatic abscess formation involves the secondary infection of necrotic pancreatic and peripancreatic tissues. The most common causative agents include *Escherichia coli, Klebsiella, Proteus, Enterobacter, Pseudomonas,* and *Enterococcus.* Most abscesses are polymicrobial and may be single or multiple (Crist and Cameron, 1987). They usually form between the first and fourth weeks of hospitalization and present with abdominal pain, distention, tenderness, fever, leukocytosis, tachycardia, and hypotension. A palpable mass may be present (Soergel, 1989). Persistent elevations of amylase, bilirubin, and alkaline phosphatase levels are present in 50% of patients with abscesses. Antibiotics, such as piperacillin and gentamicin, are given prior to surgical drainage (Soergel, 1989). Surgical débridement is followed by percutaneous catheter drainage and lavage of the infected area. Postoperative complications are common and include chest infections, fistula, upper gastrointestinal bleeding, intestinal obstruction, and perforation (Shearson and Finlayson, 1982). Reoperation is necessary in about 25% of patients as a result of further abscess formation, acute bleeding, and involvement of the adjacent organs (Soergel, 1989).

Pseudocysts are collections of tissue, fluid, debris, enzymes, and blood within the pancreas (Greenberger et al., 1987). They develop over a period of 1 to 4 weeks after the onset of acute pancreatitis. About 30% of patients with pseudocysts present with an abdominal mass (Soergel, 1989). Other signs and symptoms may include abdominal pain, nausea, vomiting, jaundice, and weight loss (Shearson and Finlayson, 1982). Because pseudocysts cause a variety of complications such as bleeding and obstruction, early surgical drainage is indicated if these cysts continue to enlarge or if they persist for greater than 6 to 8 weeks without resolution.

An external pancreatic fistula may develop following drainage of either a pancreatic abscess or a pseudocyst. Fluids, electrolytes, and pancreatic juice are lost through the fistula opening. These losses may lead to dehydration and electrolyte imbalance. The abdominal wall can become infected and irritated from the pancreatic enzymes. Meticulous skin care is necessary to prevent skin breakdown and infection. Pancreatic fistulas usually heal in 6 months with adequate nutritional and electrolyte maintenance.

NURSING MANAGEMENT OF THE PATIENT WITH ACUTE PANCREATITIS

The patient with acute pancreatitis presents a challenge to nursing care because no specific treatment is available. Nursing management of the patient is supportive, and the emphasis is on symptom relief, pancreatic "rest," and the detection and treatment of complications. Special consideration is placed on reducing the patient's anxiety during the acute phase of the disease and providing health education on causative agents, medications, and dietary modifications in the chronic phase.

The following care plan has been developed using nursing diagnoses and highlighting pertinent information included in the preceding discussion on management of the patient with acute pancreatitis.

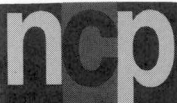 **nursing care plan**

---

1. Altered comfort: Pain, related to:
Obstruction of pancreatic duct
Diminished blood supply

Outcome Criteria	Nursing Interventions
Pain remains at tolerable level Vital signs stable	1. Assess patient's pain using pain-rating scale. Utilize pain rating to evaluate response to pain management interventions. 2. Instruct patient to tell nurse when pain is present so that interventions can be initiated prior to the onset of severe pain. 3. Provide analgesics as ordered and prior to activity or diagnostic procedures. Avoid use of morphine because it stimulates spasm of biliary and pancreatic ducts, resulting in increased pain. Remember to draw blood to determine amylase levels prior to giving first dose of analgesic to avoid false elevations in amylase. 4. Assist patient to assume a comfortable position to decrease pain. Knee-chest or fetal position may provide relief in patients with mild pain. 5. Maintain bedrest and limit activities to reduce metabolic stress. 6. Administer humidified oxygen to avoid hypoxemia and help to decrease respiratory efforts. 7. Administer sedatives as ordered. 8. Eliminate oral intake and maintain nasogastric suction, if ordered, to decrease nausea and vomiting, thereby improving patient comfort. 9. Provide alternative methods of pain control, i.e., back massage, guided imagery, relaxation techniques.

---

2. Fluid volume deficit: Actual, causing hemodynamic instability; related to:
Fluid, plasma, albumin, and blood losses into peritoneum and retroperitoneal space
Dehydration due to nausea and vomiting
Fever

Outcome Criteria	Nursing Interventions
Hemodynamic stability (blood pressure, pulse, central venous pressure, pulmonary arterial pressure (PAP), adequate peripheral circulation, urine output within normal limits) Absence of fever Absence of bleeding; stable hematocrit and hemoglobin	1. Monitor and record intake and output every hour. 2. Monitor and record central venous pressure, pulmonary arterial pressure. 3. Weigh patient daily. 4. Assess peripheral circulation and level of consciousness. 5. Monitor laboratory values for abnormal hemoglobin and hematocrit, electrolyte imbalance (calcium, magnesium, potassium), and BUN and creatinine. 6. Monitor for signs of bleeding (hemorrhagic pancreatitis: Cullen sign, Grey Turner sign, increased abdominal girth). 7. Monitor for signs of hypocalcemia: Chvostek sign, Trousseau sign. 8. Monitor vital signs and blood pressure every hour. 9. Monitor for signs of cardiac failure such as dyspnea, chest pain, edema. 10. Provide IV fluids and blood products. Monitor for signs of fluid overload, such as shortness of breath, edema, abnormal breath sounds (crackles).

---

3. Potential for tissue injury related to:
Pancreatic inflammation
Peritonitis
Formation of pseudocysts
Formation of abscesses, bleeding
Formation of fistulas

Outcome Criteria	*Nursing Interventions*
Absence or resolution of peritonitis Absence of fever Absence of pseudocyst Absence of abscesses	1. Administer antibiotics as ordered if causative organism(s) have been identified. Preventive antibiotics are not indicated. 2. Monitor vital signs, especially increases in temperature, and monitor for increase in white blood count. 3. Observe for signs of pseudocyst: upper abdominal pain, mass, tenderness, fever, deterioration, or no improvement in condition. 4. Observe for signs of abscess: abdominal pain, distention, and tenderness; fever, leukocytosis, tachycardia, hypotension. 5. Assess for paralytic ileus: adynamic bowel, fluid accumulation. Ascultate bowel sounds every shift. 6. Observe for respiratory distress resulting from ascites, abdominal mass; check breath sounds, presence of cough, sputum production, shallow breathing, elevated diaphragm, fluid accumulation. 7. Monitor arterial blood gases for early signs of hypoxemia. 8. Provide skin care for draining fistulas. Use skin barrier to protect skin from pancreatic enzymes. Monitor fistula output. 9. Prepare patient for surgery if an abscess forms.

4. Alteration in nutrition and metabolic status: Related to:
Pancreatic dysfunction with altered production of digestive enzymes, insulin, and glucagon
Decrease or absence of oral intake
Alcoholism
Abnormal metabolism

Outcome Criteria	*Nursing Interventions*

Normal nutritional status
Weight gain or maintenance
Positive nitrogen balance
	1. Eliminate oral intake during acute phase of illness.
	2. Assess nutritional status and general apperance for
	  a. Poor skin turgor
	  b. Lethargy
	  c. Anorexia
	  d. Dry, flaky, discolored skin
	  e. Sunken eyeballs
	  f. Decreased muscle mass and decreased muscular control
	  g. Tremors, twitching
	3. Monitor
	  a. Serum amylase
	  b. Urine amylase
	  c. Lipase
	  d. Glucose
	4. Provide nutritional support as ordered
	  a. Peripheral nutritional solutions
	  b. Total parenteral nutrition
	  c. Jejunal feedings
	5. Monitor laboratory results to prevent complications of nutritional support
	  a. Electrolyte imbalances
	  b. Hyperglycemia
	  c. Hyperosmolar hyperglycemic nonketosis
	6. Provide oral care every 4 to 8 hours.
	7. Monitor nasogastric output.
	8. Maintain ongoing assessment of nutritional status and therapy including
	  a. Daily weights
	  b. Intake and output
	  c. Nutritional laboratory data (albumin, transferrin, total lymphocyte count)
	  d. Nitrogen balance
	  e. Altered mental status
	  f. Skin turgor
	  g. Muscle atrophy, weakness
	9. Monitor fistula drainage and record output every shift.

5. Impaired gas exchange related to:
Inflammatory process and aggressive fluid therapy
Respiratory distress syndrome
Atelectasis
Microemboli
Pain
Pleural effusion

Nursing Care Plan continued on following page

Outcome Criteria	Nursing Interventions
Effective breathing patterns with adequate ventilation and oxygenation ($P_{A_{O_2}}$ and $P_{A_{CO_2}}$ within normal limits) Absence of atelectasis Absence or resolution of pleural effusion, pulmonary edema, microemboli	1. Administer analgesics to relieve pain and allow adequate ventilation. 2. Provide chest physiotherapy and reposition every 1 to 2 hours to prevent atelectasis. 3. Provide oxygen therapy as ordered to prevent hypoxemia. 4. Monitor daily chest x-rays for presence of atelectasis, effusion, edema, and microemboli (review coagulation studies if microemboli are present). 5. Perform respiratory assessments every 1 to 2 hours and note presence of tachypnea, dyspnea, wheezing. Identify presence of adventitious breath sounds and absence of normal breath sounds. 6. Suction whenever necessary and record amount, consistency, and color of secretions. 7. Monitor arterial blood gas results for hypoxemia, hypercapnia, or acidosis.

6. Anxiety (patient or family) related to:
Insufficient knowledge of disease process, treatment, diagnostic procedures

Outcome Criteria	Nursing Interventions
Reduction in patient's or family's anxiety with information about disease process, treatment, and diagnostic procedures Patient and family participate in care planning process	1. Assess patient's or family's reasons for and level of anxiety. 2. Provide information to patient and family about disease process, treatment(s), and diagnostic procedures. 3. Include patient and family in care planning process. 4. Evaluate reduction in patient's or family's anxiety.

SUMMARY

The patient with acute pancreatitis presents a challenge to critical care nurses to recognize and initiate supportive and life-saving interventions. The patient's recovery from this devastating disease is due in part to the knowledge and expert clinical skills of the critical care nurse.

References

Ammann, R. (1985). Acute pancreatitis: Clinical aspects and medical and surgical management. In J. E. Berk (Ed.), *Bockus gastroenterology* (4th ed., pp. 3993–4008). Philadelphia: W. B. Saunders.

Baltaxe, H. A. (1985). Diagnostic imaging of the pancreas. *Annals of Internal Medicine*, 103, 90–91.

Banks, P. A. (1985). Clinical manifestations and treatment of pancreatitis. *Annals of Internal Medicine*, 103, 91–97.

Batra, S. K. (1987). Pancreatitis. In F. H. Messerk (Ed.), *Current clinical practice* (pp. 428–430). Philadelphia: W. B. Saunders.

Bell, J. S., and Go, U. L. W. (1985). Laboratory diagnosis of pancreatic disease. In J. E. Berk (Ed.), *Bockus gastroenterology* (4th ed., pp. 3877–3892). Philadelphia: W. B. Saunders.

Boudeman, K. A., Cherlock, P. A., and Rowley, S. G. (1985). Pancreatic disease—Special feeding problems. *Nutritional Support Services*, 5 (11), 22–27.

Browder, W., Sherwood, E., Williams, D., et al. (1986). Protective effect of glucan-enhanced macrophage function in experimental pancreatitis. *American Journal of Surgery*, 153, 25–32.

Burch, J. M., (1988). Acute pancreatitis. In R. E. Rakel (Ed.), *Conn's current therapy, 1988* (pp. 438–442). Philadelphia: W. B. Saunders.

Burrell, L. O., and Burrell, Z. L., Jr. (1982). *Critical care* (pp. 319–324). St. Louis: C. V. Mosby.

Carr, M. R., Dick, S. P., Bordley, J. D., et al. (1987). Gentamicin dosing requirements in patients with acute pancreatitis. *Surgery*, 103 (5), 533–537.

Creutzfeldt, W., and Lankisch, P. G. (1985). Acute pancreatitis: Etiology and pathogenesis. In J. E. Berk (Ed.), *Bockus gastroenterology* (4th ed., pp. 3971–3992). Philadelphia: W. B. Saunders.

Crist, D. W., and Cameron, J. L. (1987). The current management of acute pancreatitis. *Advances in Surgery*, 20, 69–123.

Freeny, P. C., Lewis, G. P., Traverso, L. W., et al. (1988). Infected pancreatic fluid collections: Percutaneous catheter drainage. *Radiology*, 167 (2), 435–441.

Greenberger, N. J. (1986). *Gastrointestinal disorders* (3rd ed., p. 250). Chicago: Year Book Medical Publishers.

Greenberger, N. J., Joskes, P. P., Isselbacher, K. J. (1987). Diseases of the pancreas. In E. Braunwald, K. J. Isselbacker, R. G. Petersdorf, et al. (Eds.), *Harrison's principles of internal medicine* (pp. 1372–1380). New York: McGraw-Hill.

Grendell, J. H., and Cello, J. P. (1989). Chronic pancreatitis. In M. H. Sleisenger, and J. S. Fordtran (Eds.), *Gastrointestinal disease: Pathophysiology, diagnosis, management* (4th ed., p. 1844). Philadelphia: W. B. Saunders.

Imrie, C. W., Buist, L. J., and Shearer, M. G. (1988). Importance of cause in the outcome of pancreatic pseudocysts. *American Journal of Surgery*, 156, 159–162.

Jain, J. A., and Amato-Vealey, E. (1989). Acute pancreatitis: A gastrointestinal emergency. *Critical Care Nurse*, 8 (5) 47–64.

Johanson, B. C., Wells, S. J., Hoffmeister, D., et al. (1988). *Standards for critical care* (pp. 374–378). St. Louis: C. V. Mosby.

Leese, J., Holliday, M., Heath, D., et al. (1987). Multicentre clinical trial of low volume fresh frozen plasma therapy in acute pancreatitis. *British Journal of Surgery*, 74, 907–911.

Levine, G. M. (1981). Nutritional support in gastrointestinal disease. *Surgical Clinics of North America*, 61(3), 701–708.

Levitt, M. D. (1988). Pancreatitis. J. B. Wyngaarden and L. H. Smith (Eds.), *Cecil textbook of medicine* (18th ed., pp. 774–780). Philadelphia: W. B. Saunders.

Martin, J. K., Jr., Vanheerden, J. A., and Bess, M. A. (1984). Surgical management of acute pancreatitis. *Mayo Clinic Proceedings*, 59, 259–267.

Meissner, J. E. (1980). McGill-Melzach Pain Questionnaire. *Nursing 80*, 10(1), 50–51.

Neff, C. C., and Ferrucci, J. T. (1984). Pancreatitis. *Surgical Clinics of North America*, 64 (1), 23–36.

Ranson, J. H. C. (1979). Acute pancreatitis. *Current Problems in Surgery*, 16 (11), 1–84.

Rombeau, J. L., and Caldwell, M. D. (1986). *Parenteral nutrition* (pp. 338, 380–408, 437–444, 602–614). Philadelphia: W. B. Saunders.

Sabesin, S. (1987). Countering the dangers of acute pancreatitis. *Emergency Medicine*, 19 (17), 71–96.

Saunders, C. E., and Gentile, D. A. (1986). Treatment of mild exacerbations of recurrent alcoholic pancreatitis in an emergency department observation unit. *Southern Medical Journal*, 81(3), 317–320.

Sax, H. C., Warner, B. W., Talamini, M. A., et al. (1986). Early total parenteral nutrition in acute pancreatitis: Lack of beneficial effects. *American Journal of Surgery*, 153, 117–124.

Shearson, D. J. C., and Finlayson, N. D. C. (1982). *Diseases of the gastrointestinal tract and liver* (pp. 783–785). Edinburgh: Churchill Livingstone.

Soergel, K. H. (1989). Acute pancreatitis. In M. H. Sleisenger, and J. S. Fordtran (Eds.), *Gastrointestinal disease: Pathophysiology, diagnosis, management* (4th ed., pp. 1814–1842). Philadelphia: W. B. Saunders.

Steer, M. L., Meldolesi, J., and Figarella, C. (1984). Pancreatitis: The role of lysosomes. *Digestive Diseases and Sciences*, 29 (10), 934–938.

Steinberg, W. M., and Schlesselman, S. E. (1987). Treatment of acute pancreatitis: Comparison of animal and human studies. *Gastroenterology*, 93 (6), 1420–1427.

Thompson, J. M., McFarland, G. K., Hirsh, J. E., et al. (1986). *Clinical nursing* (pp. 1261–1265). St. Louis: C. V. Mosby.

Williamson, R. C. N. (1984). Early assessment of severity in acute pancreatitis. *Gut*, 25, 1331–1339.

Endocrine System

47

Patients with Disorders of Glucose Metabolism

Kathy Kigerl

Diabetes mellitus is a group of metabolic disorders characterized by a relative or absolute deficiency in insulin resulting in a glucose intolerance. The two main types of diabetes are type I, or insulin-dependent diabetes mellitus, and type II, or noninsulin-dependent diabetes mellitus. Diabetic ketoacidosis (DKA) and hyperglycemic hyperosmolar nonketotic coma (HHNC) are two of the most common acute complications of diabetes that may necessitate admission to the intensive care unit. Both complications may result in death if not treated promptly.

DIABETIC KETOACIDOSIS

Diabetic ketoacidosis is a metabolic disorder characterized by hyperglycemia with a blood sugar level exceeding 300 mg/dL and ketonemia and acidosis with a pH reduced to less than 7.30 and a serum bicarbonate less than 15 mEq/liter (Sperling, 1984). It occurs primarily in patients with type I diabetes mellitus and has a mortality of 5% to 17% (Krane, 1987). DKA can be precipitated by infection, stress, trauma, or an imbalance between the intake of food and the amount of exogenous insulin received. The National Diabetes Data group (1985) reports that 20% to 30% of patients with newly diagnosed cases of diabetes present with diabetic ketoacidosis.

Pathophysiology

Insulin and Counterregulatory Hormones. To understand the pathophysiology of DKA, one must first understand the role of insulin in the body. Insulin is an anabolic hormone produced by the pancreatic beta cells in the islets of Langerhans. Insulin permits glucose to be transported into the cells throughout the body, especially in the muscle, fat, and liver, to be used as an energy source. It facilitates the storage of glucose as glycogen in the liver, the storage of amino acids as proteins in the muscles, and the storage of free fatty acids as triglycerides in the fat. The nerve tissue, intestinal mucosa, liver cells, kidney tubules, and the formed blood elements are the only cells that do not depend on insulin to transport extracellular glucose across the cell membrane. Hepatic breakdown of glucose is also inhibited in the presence of insulin.

Insufficient levels of circulating insulin result in cellular starvation. This causes a catabolic process in which glycogen from the liver, proteins, and fats are broken down to glucose in an effort to provide an energy source for the cells. The speed of this catabolic process is determined by the counterregulatory hormones that are stimulated by stress.

Cortisol, glucagon, growth hormone, and epinephrine are the four hormones that oppose the action of insulin. In their presence insulin requirements increase. Cortisol and glucagon stimulate the breakdown of glycogen to glucose. Growth hormone assists with the breakdown of proteins to amino acids. Epinephrine increases blood glucose by inhibiting glucose uptake by the muscles and also activates protein breakdown. These hormones, in their effort to provide glucose to the cells, compound the problem of hyperglycemia in DKA.

Insulin Deficiency. Insulin deficiency is the major endocrine abnormality responsible for the metabolic changes of DKA. This deficiency allows unrestricted production of glucose without peripheral utilization of the glucose by the body. This results in a marked hyperglycemia leading to glycosuria and osmotic diuresis and ketosis.

Hyperglycemia. As plasma glucose concentrations rise, the renal threshold for glucose reabsorption by the proximal tubules of the kidneys is exceeded. This causes an osmotic diuresis in which water and glucose are excreted from the body in the urine. Large amounts of water can be lost by the body in this way, resulting in dehydration. The body attempts to compensate for this pathologic condition by stimulating the thirst center in the brain to increase fluid intake (polydipsia). The kidneys are also stimulated to secrete renin, which facilitates the conversion of renin substrate to angiotensin-I. Angiotensin-I is converted to angiotensin-II by angiotensin-converting enzyme in the lungs, stimulating the adrenal glands to secrete aldosterone. This hormone assists the kidneys in reabsorbing additional sodium and water to reduce fluid loss. Antidiuretic hormone is also secreted from the posterior pituitary gland in an effort to reduce free water loss.

This marked hyperglycemia also causes a change in the osmotic gradient at the cellular level. The presence of excess glucose throughout the extracellular free water results in a movement of water from the intracellular to the extracellular compartment. This occurrence may mask the clinical severity of the body's dehydration.

The body is unable to compensate for this ongoing water loss indefinitely. This loss can be between 100 and 150 mL/kg body weight depending on the severity and the duration of the illness (Krane, 1987). Severe dehydration, hypovolemia, and eventually a reduced glomerular filtration rate occur. This reduction in glomerular filtration rate limits the body's attempt to secrete glucose, augments hyperglycemia, and exacerbates hypertonicity and cellular dehydration. Nausea and vomiting, hemoconcentration, hypotension, and vascular collapse may ensue if the patient with DKA is not treated.

Ketosis. During this period of increasing hyperglycemia and cell starvation, the counterregulatory hormones are activated. Glucagon stimulates glycogen, which is stored in the liver to be released into the bloodstream in a process called glycogenolysis.

When the glycogen stores are exhausted, gluconeogenesis begins. Gluconeogenesis is the process by which fats and proteins are converted to glucose in the liver. Triglycerides from fat deposits are broken down to fatty acids and glycerol. The free fatty acids are transported to the liver and converted to keto-acids, acetoacetate, and beta-hydrobutyric acid. These acids are metabolized in the liver faster than the rate of gluconeogenesis. As a result, the excess acids are converted to ketones and transported to the peripheral circulation where they accumulate and eventually result in ketonemia. These ketone bodies dissociate to yield hydrogen ions that interfere with the normal serum pH and produce a metabolic acidosis.

The body attempts to buffer this acidosis with bicarbonate. Bicarbonate reserves in the body, however, are depleted by the osmotic diureses. As the

blood pH drops to approximately 7.20, the respiratory center attempts to remove the excess carbonic acid from the body by ''blowing off'' carbon dioxide. This results in an increase in the rate and depth of respirations known as Kussmaul breathing. Acetones, which are formed from the acetoacetate, are also blown off during respirations, giving the breath a characteristic fruity or sweet odor.

Kussmaul breathing causes a hypocapnia to occur, which reduces cerebral vasoconstriction and cerebral blood flow. As this respiratory compensatory mechanism fails to maintain the acid-base balance, carbon dioxide passes freely through the blood-brain barrier. The reduced cerebral blood flow and the accumulation of carbon dioxide reduce the central nervous system pH and lead to decreasing levels of consciousness.

Electrolyte Imbalances. Patients in DKA can present with a myriad of electrolyte imbalances resulting from the marked hyperglycemia. Potassium moves from the intracellular to the extracellular compartment with free water during the change in the osmotic gradient. This phenomenon may give the illusion that the patient has a high serum potassium value. If the patient has experienced a large amount of osmotic diuresis or vomiting, large amounts of potassium can be passively lost, resulting in hypokalemia.

Sodium and phosphate are also transported into the extracellular compartment. An initial low sodium value may be obtained due to a dilutional effect in the blood. Aldosterone activity also causes retention of sodium and may produce an abnormally high serum value if large amounts of this hormone have been secreted in an effort to control free water loss. Phosphate may be lost passively in the urine. This occurrence may be masked by the shift of the electrolyte to the extracellular space. When treatment for DKA is initiated, the electrolytes will shift back into the intracellular space as the body tissues are rehydrated.

Clinical Presentation

The patient with DKA has a history of lethargy, polyuria, polydipsia, and polyphagia often accompanied by weight loss. Various signs of dehydration such as loss of skin turgor, sunken eyeballs, flushed dry skin, and a weak thready pulse may be seen. The patient may complain of abdominal pain and may be nauseated or vomiting. Kussmaul respirations and a fruity odor to the breath due to ketosis may be present.

Laboratory tests show an elevated serum glucose and decreased serum bicarbonate and blood pH. Ketonuria and glycosuria are present. The total white blood cell count may be elevated with a marked shift to the left. This may be due to a predisposing infection or to the catecholamine activity. Blood urea nitrogen (BUN), creatinine, hematocrit, and hemoglobin values are usually elevated due to dehydration. Arterial oxygen levels may be lowered if the respiratory status is compromised.

The patient may present with an altered level of consciousness due to the high osmolality. This will usually resolve with fluid and insulin replacement therapy.

Medical Management

The three goals of managing DKA are (1) improve the circulatory volume and tissue perfusion, (2) decrease blood glucose levels, and (3) correct electrolyte imbalances. Table 47–1 delineates the medical management of these patients.

Intravenous fluids are required to improve circulatory blood volume and tissue perfusion. Fluids are given initially as a bolus of an isotonic solution (0.9 normal saline or lactated Ringer's). Hyperosmolality is a factor for these patients due to the marked hyperglycemia. An isotonic solution will allow a gradual decline in osmolality, which is desirable. Too rapid a decline is a proposed variable in cerebral edema. A hypotonic solution (0.45 normal saline) is used after the initial bolus to compensate for the loss of sodium by the body in the urine. This volume expansion reduces hemoconcentration, improves hemodynamics, improves glomerular filtration rate, and lowers the serum glucose in the blood. A 5% dextrose solution is added to the infusate when the blood sugar reaches 200 to 300 mg/dL. A 10% solution may be added when the blood sugar reaches 150 mg/dL to prevent hypoglycemia.

Insulin therapy to lower the blood glucose level is given by a continuous low-dose infusion method after an initial bolus of fast-acting insulin has been given. This method is simple and effective and results in a lower incidence of hypoglycemia and hypokalemia (Kitabchi and Murphy, 1988). It allows a steady cellular metabolic response without fluctuations in the blood sugar that had occurred from the intermittent injections of insulin that were used previously. This low-dose infusion method allows a linear decline in the serum glucose with an average drop of 75 to 100 mg/dL per hour.

Electrolytes are added to the IV fluids after the initial bolus has been given and when renal function has been assessed as adequate. Potassium supplements are begun early in therapy, and serum levels are monitored frequently. This supplement should be given as half potassium chloride and half potassium phosphate. This treatment avoids delivery of an excess of chloride to the patient and prevents hypocalcemia.

The use of bicarbonate replacement in the treatment of patients with DKA is controversial. Bicarbonate concentrations in the blood are depleted because extracellular bicarbonate is the body's first buffer against metabolic acidosis. Proponents of its

TABLE 47–1. Medical Management of Diabetic Ketoacidosis

IV Fluids

First Hour	200 to 1000 mL/hour of 0.9 normal saline depending on the degree of dehydration
Second and subsequent hours	200 to 1000 mL/hour of 0.45 normal saline depending on the degree of dehydration
Within the first 12 hours	Add 5% dextrose to the IV fluid when serum glucose reaches 200 to 300 mg/dL
	Add 10% dextrose to the IV fluid when serum glucose reaches 150 mg/dL (Kitabchi and Murphy, 1988)

Insulin

Initial	IV bolus of 0.1 units/kg of fast-acting insulin
First and subsequent hours	IV continuous infusion of 0.1 units/kg per hour of fast-acting insulin. When serum glucose falls to 150 mg/dL, reduce insulin to 0.05 units/kg per hour (Sperling, 1984)

Electrolytes

First hour	If initial serum K^+ is greater than 3.5 mEq/liter give 40 mEq/liter in the IV maintenance fluid, one-half as KCl, one-half as KPO_4
Second and subsequent hours	If urine output is adequate with serum K^+ of less than 5.5 mEq/liter, give 20 to 30 mEq/liter of IV fluid (Kitabchi and Murphy, 1988)

Laboratory Tests

Initial	Serum glucose, pH, bicarbonate, electrolytes, calcium, phosphate, serum osmolality, complete blood count, BUN, creatinine, arterial blood gases, blood culture, urine culture
Subsequent	Hourly monitoring of blood glucose electrolytes and HCO_2 every 3 hours

Monitoring

	Hourly vital signs, neurologic checks, intake and output
	Central venous pressure monitoring or pulmonary artery pressure may be necessary for patients with a compromised respiratory status
	Continuous electrocardiographic monitoring needed to evaluate abnormalities with K^+ balance

Ancillary measures

	Plasma expanders may be necessary for persistent hypotension
	Antibiotic and oxygen therapy as needed

use recommend that it be used only in patients with severe acidosis (pH less than 7.10). The use of bicarbonate to correct acidosis above a pH of 7.1 may result in a paradoxical CNS acidosis and cause severe hypokalemia if too rapid a correction occurs.

When a patient's serum glucose is less than 250 mg/dL, the pH is greater than 7.30, the serum bicarbonate is greater than 15 mEq/liter, and the patient is able to take food by mouth, conversion to subcutaneous insulin may be initiated. Two-thirds of the previous day's total dose is given as an intermediate-acting insulin, and the remaining one-third is given as a short-acting insulin. The patient receives two-thirds of his total subcutaneous dose prior to the morning meal and one-third of the total dose before the evening meal. Blood glucose monitoring should continue before meals and at bedtime to assess glycemic control.

Nursing Management and Nursing Diagnoses

A complete nursing assessment will provide the needed data to contribute to the development of the nursing care plan. Four primary diagnoses can be utilized for implementing nursing care for the patient with DKA and HHNC. The nursing care plan lists these nursing diagnoses, expected outcomes, and nursing interventions for this type of patient. These interventions are generalized for all patients with DKA. Individualization of these interventions will be necessary as determined by the nursing assessment.

NURSING DIAGNOSIS I: FLUID VOLUME DEFICIT RELATED TO OSMOTIC DIURESIS INDUCED BY HYPERGLYCEMIA

During fluid replacement therapy the patient must be closely monitored. Vital signs, intake and outputs, central venous pressure, and pulmonary artery wedge pressures must be recorded to prevent unrecognized shock, overhydration, or worsening dehydration. The patient must also be observed for signs and symptoms of cardiovascular overload, pulmonary edema, or inadequate central perfusion during fluid volume restoration. Laboratory values must be assessed to monitor the progression of the patient's hydration status and to make the necessary changes. Oral hygiene and skin care should be maintained for the patient's comfort and to prevent skin breakdown.

NURSING DIAGNOSIS 2: ALTERATION IN NUTRITION: LESS THAN BODY REQUIREMENTS RELATED TO INSULIN DEFICIENCY

Nursing interventions for this diagnosis are aimed at providing close observation of the patient's serum glucose level and at maintaining the insulin infusion at a rate that allows for a drop of serum glucose of 75 to 100 mg/dL per hour. Hourly glucose values are needed to assess the status of the hyperglycemia. Bedside glucose monitoring and laboratory tests can provide this information. IV insulin should be delivered in a separate line to allow for immediate changes in dosage as the patient's condition warrants. Standard solutions of insulin infusions vary from insti-

tution to institution. A convenient mix is 100 units of fast-acting insulin in 500 mL of normal saline. This concentration delivers 0.2 units of insulin with every milliliter of fluid given. Flushing of the intravenous line prior to administration with 50 to 100 mL of the insulin solution is recommended to limit the amount of insulin that is absorbed by the IV tubing.

The patient must be monitored for signs of hypoglycemia and hyperglycemia. The physician will need to be notified when serum glucose levels reach between 200 and 300 mg/dL and again at 150 mg/dL to order the necessary dextrose to be added to the hydration line.

NURSING DIAGNOSIS 3: SENSORY PERCEPTUAL ALTERATIONS RELATED TO INCREASED PLASMA OSMOLALITY AND ELECTROLYTE IMBALANCES

These interventions are directed toward evaluating the patient's neurologic status and monitoring him or her for physical signs of electrolyte imbalances. Laboratory values for potassium, chloride, phosphorus, and calcium will be drawn frequently, and the results need to be monitored so that the needed changes in electrolyte supplements can be made.

NURSING DIAGNOSIS 4: KNOWLEDGE DEFICIT RELATED TO THE PRECIPITATING EVENTS, SIGNS AND SYMPTOMS AND PREVENTION OF DKA OR HHNC

A nursing assessment of the patient's knowledge of the events leading to his hospitalization needs to be made. The patient needs to be able to verbalize the factors of diabetes that predispose to these emergency situations. The patient needs to be educated about the early signs and symptoms of hyperglycemia, how to manage diabetes when he is ill, and when to call the physician based on blood glucose or urine ketone readings. This education can be incorporated into the patient's daily care when his condition has stabilized.

HYPERGLYCEMIC HYPEROSMOLAR NONKETOTIC COMA

Hyperglycemic hyperosmolar nonketotic coma (HHNC) is a metabolic disorder characterized by hyperglycemia with a blood sugar of greater than 600 mg/dL, serum osmolality greater than 330 mOsm/kg, absent or minimal serum ketones, an arterial pH higher than 7.30, serum bicarbonate greater than 20 mEq/liter, and moderate to severe mental obtundation. It most commonly occurs in the elderly and type II or noninsulin-dependent diabetics. It is differentiated from DKA by the absence of significant ketosis or acidosis. The most common cause of HHNC is undiagnosed type II diabetes accompanied by a delay in seeking medical treatment after an associated illness. Other predisposing factors include stress, infections, steroid or diuretic usage, dialysis, or hyperalimentation. Mortality has been reported to be as high as 60% to 70% if the condition is not recognized and treated quickly (Kitabchi and Murphy, 1988).

Pathophysiology

Unlike the type I diabetic, the type II diabetic has a "relative" deficiency in insulin production. These patients may control their diabetes with diet management or oral hyperglycemic agents.

The patient with HHNC experiences the effects of marked hyperglycemia in the same way as a patient with DKA. Blood glucose levels are considerably higher and result in a more severe osmotic diuresis. This results in increased intracellular and extracellular dehydration and a higher serum osmolality.

The reason for the absence of ketosis in HHNC is not well understood. Several theories have been proposed to explain this occurrence. One prevalent theory is that the patient with HHNC has enough beta cell function to produce the needed insulin to inhibit fatty acid mobilization and the formation of ketones but not enough insulin to prevent hyperglycemia. Another theory is that the patient with HHNC may lack a substrate for hepatic ketogenesis. The hyperosmolar state may itself inhibit protein breakdown. Hyperosmolarity depresses pancreatic insulin secretion, inhibits adipose tissue lipolysis, and impairs the central nervous system's control of growth hormone and cortisol response.

These patients present with the same electrolyte imbalances as do those with DKA. Due to the higher serum osmolality, these patients have an altered sensorium. They may experience grand mal seizures, positive Babinski reflexes, nystagmus, or other neurologic deficits.

Medical Management

Medical management for these patients is very similar to that for patients with DKA (Table 47–2). Intravenous hydration is given as a bolus and then as a continuous infusion of 0.45% normal saline. Normal saline is given only if the patient is hypotensive due to the high serum osmolality. Half of the water deficit is given in the first 12 hours as 0.45 normal saline. The remainder is given during the next 24 hours as 5% dextrose, 5% dextrose and 0.45% normal saline, or 5% dextrose and 0.9% normal saline. Insulin is given as an initial IV bolus of 0.15 units/kg followed by a continuous infusion of 5 to 7 units/hour (Kitabchi and Murphy, 1988). Plasma glucose is maintained at 300 mg/dL for the first 24 hours. Since most patients in HHNC have some endogenous insulin available, the insulin requirements needed to

TABLE 47–2. Medical Management of HHNC

IV Fluids	
Hours 1 to 12	0.9 normal saline may be used if the serum sodium is less than 130 mEq/liter or if the plasma osmolarity is less than 330 mOsm/liter.
	0.45 normal saline is used if serum sodium is above 145 mEq/liter
	May require 8 to 12 liters of fluid over a 24-hour period; replace half of the water deficit in the first 12 hours
	When the blood glucose reaches 250 to 300 mg/dL add 5% dextrose to the infusate to prevent brisk lowering of serum osmolarity
Insulin	
Initial	IV bolus of 0.15 units/kg of fast-acting insulin
Subsequent hours	5 to 7 units/hour of continuous fast-acting insulin (Kitabchi and Murphy, 1988)
Electrolytes	
Initial	Same as for DKA
Laboratory Tests	Same as for DKA
Monitoring	Same as for DKA
Ancillary measures	Same as for DKA

correct hyperglycemia are usually less than those in DKA. Electrolytes, laboratory studies, and ancillary measures are the same as those used for patients with DKA. Due to the fact that these patients are usually older and have preexisting illnesses, their response to the treatment must be carefully monitored. The type II diabetic who has recovered from HHNC may require small amounts of subcutaneous insulin daily or may be able to control the diabetes with diet or oral medications.

Nursing Management and Nursing Diagnoses

The nursing diagnoses described for the patient with DKA are also appropriate for the patient with HHNC (see the Nursing Care Plan at the end of this chapter). It is necessary to educate the family as well as the patient about this disease because the patient may not be able to identify the subtle changes in mental status that often are the early indicators of HHNC.

PANCREAS TRANSPLANTS

DKA is only one of the emergent situations faced by the diabetic. Diabetes mellitus predisposes the patient to many serious long-term complications such as diabetic retinopathy, neuropathy, end-stage renal disease, and premature atherosclerosis. It is estimated that diabetes will shorten a patient's life expectancy to two-thirds that of a nondiabetic (National

Diabetes Advisory Board, 1985). Researchers believe that establishing a constant euglycemic state would prevent or stop the progression of these complications.

Pancreas transplants have been performed since 1966 in an attempt to provide this continuous euglycemic state for diabetics. Between December 1966 and March 1988, 1394 pancreas transplants were reported to the International Pancreas Transplant Registry. The overall 1-year graft and survival rates since 1982 have been 46% and 82%, respectively (Sutherland and colleagues, 1989).

Pancreas transplants had previously been performed only in patients who had already received a kidney transplant and were receiving immunosuppressive therapy. Since 1980 many centers have begun transplanting nonuremic, nonkidney transplant diabetic patients whose developing diabetic complications are more serious than the potential side effects of the antirejection therapy.

The diabetic who is a candidate for a pancreas transplant must go through an extensive pretransplant evaluation. Base-line studies to measure serum glucose, insulin, and C-peptide levels as well as pancreatic hormone levels are required. Nerve function studies, an ophthalmic examination, and a renal evaluation are performed. A psychiatric examination is done to ensure that the patient has a thorough understanding of the magnitude of the operation and the potential complications including lifetime follow-up.

Procedure

Cadaver or living related donors are used for this procedure. Whole pancreas or segmental grafts are used, and many double grafts including a kidney are performed. Islet transplants have been attempted but have produced poor results. The most important technical problem in pancreas transplants is the need to provide drainage of the exocrine secretions of the transplanted organ. The exocrine function of the patient's own pancreas remains intact, so the exocrine functions of the graft need to be controlled to prevent destruction of the body tissues. Between 1983 and 1988 the three most common techniques used to solve this problem included occlusion of the pancreatic duct with a synthetic polymer, anastomosis of the duct to the bowel, and anastomosis of the duct to the bladder. The 1-year graft survival rates for these techniques were 47%, 45%, and 51% respectively (Sutherland and colleagues, 1989).

Postoperative Care

The postoperative care of the patient with a pancreas transplant includes observing the patient for potential complications. The most common complications with this procedure include rejection, infec-

tion, venous thrombosis, technical problems with duct anastomoses, and the potential recurrence of diabetes.

The patient's vital signs should be monitored closely, as should central venous pressure, intake and output, and nasogastric drainage. A triple-lumen catheter may be used for total parenteral nutrition and for drawing blood samples. Laboratory studies include a complete blood count, electrolyte measurements, and coagulation profiles every 6 hours. Plasma glucose levels are monitored every 6 hours for 5 days. Daily laboratory work includes electrolytes, complete blood count, hemoglobin, and serum and urine amylase measurements. Blood samples for insulin, glucagon, and human C-peptide levels are done three to four times per week. Pancreatic scans and ultrasound examinations are performed on the first day and then once a week until discharge (Mittal and Tolego-Pereyra, 1986). The patient may require some exogenous insulin for 1 to 2 days postoperatively.

The patient will receive immunosuppressive and antirejection drugs. Immunosuppressive regimens that include both cyclosporine and asathioprine have been associated with higher graft survival rates than those that have included only one of these drugs (Sutherland and associates, 1989).

BLOOD GLUCOSE MONITORING

Bedside blood glucose monitoring has become one of the keystones in the care of the diabetic patient. It can assist the nurse in the intensive care setting to monitor a patient's serum glucose level quickly utilizing only one drop of blood, a reagent strip, and a reflectance meter. This technique has replaced urine tests for glucose due to the body's inconstant renal threshold. Any changes in a patient's diabetic control can affect the glomerular filtration rate and tubular glucose reabsorption in the kidneys, thus affecting the blood glucose concentration at which urine glucose excretion normally occurs.

Accuracy

The accuracy of bedside glucose monitoring by staff nurses has been shown to be between 83% and 96% when the procedure is correctly performed (Godine and associates, 1988; Kruger and associates, 1988). Strips read by a reflectance meter that gauges the reagent strip's colorimetric reaction provide greater accuracy than visually read strips.

Equipment and Technique

A variety of reagent strips and reflectance meters are available on the market. A small finger puncture is made on the lateral aspect of the finger pad midway on the distal interphalangeal joint. A drop of blood is placed on the strip's reagent pad for a specific period of time. The blood is then wiped or blotted well from the strip, and the strip is inserted into the reflectance meter. After another short period of time the meter provides a digital readout of the glucose level.

Some common errors during performance of this procedure include covering the reagent pad with an inadequate amount of blood or smearing the blood over the pad in an effort to cover it. These errors may give falsely low readings. Inaccurate timing of the blood as well as inadequate removal of the excess blood from the strip after the first waiting period may also affect the results. Reagent strips and reflectance meters need to be kept in good condition. Strips must be kept dry and away from light. The calibration of reflectance meters must be checked by using either a test strip or a standard aqueous solution. Meters need to be calibrated as per the manufacturer's specifications.

Recent developments in reflectance meters include a memory option in many models that store up to 350 readings. Some models also offer the option of a computer interface for recording and graphing the monitored data.

ncp nursing care plan

DIABETIC KETOACIDOSIS

1. Fluid volume deficit actual, related to:
Osmotic diuresis induced by hyperglycemia
Inadequate oral intake
Vomiting

Outcome Criteria	Nursing Interventions

Urine output greater than 30 mL/hour
Central venous pressure 7 to 12 cm H$_2$O
Vital signs within the patient's normal range
Moist mucous membranes and good skin turgor
Laboratory data returning to normal (BUN 10 to 15 mg/dL; HCT: men 40% to 54%, Na 132 to 140 mEq/liter, plasma osmolality 280 to 300 mOsm/liter)
	Assess vital signs hourly
	Maintain hourly intake and output
	Assess and document hydration status:
	  Skin turgor
	  Mucous membranes
	Monitor CVP hourly
	Administer IV fluid replacement as prescribed
	Obtain laboratory samples as ordered
	Observe for cardiovascular overload and pulmonary edema:
	  Jugular venous distention
	  Auscultated S$_3$ heart sound
	  Increasing CVP or PAWP
	  Increasing pulse rate
	  Dyspnea
	  Breath sounds for crackles
	Monitor for inadequate central perfusion:
	  Decreased urine output
	  Lowered BP elevated heart rate
	  Decreased CVP
	Provide oral hygiene and facilitate skin integrity every 2 hours

2. Alteration in nutrition; less than body requirements, related to:
Insulin deficiency
Effects of counterregulatory hormones
Impaired secretion of glucose by the kidneys due to decreased GFR

Outcome Criteria	Nursing Interventions

Blood glucose less than 300 mg/dL
No ketones present in serum or urine
	Monitor insulin infusion as ordered for correct rate and line patency
	Monitor serum glucose hourly
	Monitor urine for ketones every 2 to 4 hours
	Assess and document for signs and symptoms of hyperglycemia
	  Increased thirst
	  Polyuria
	  Drowsiness
	  Flushed dry skin

Nursing Care Plan continued on following page

3. Sensory perceptual alterations related to:
Plasma osmolality
Electrolyte imbalances

Outcome Criteria	Nursing Interventions

Pupils equal and reactive to light
Moves all extremities
Ventilatory rate regular and pattern normal
	Assess and document neurologic status
	  Level of consciousness
	  Pupil size, equality, and reaction to light
	  Response to verbal and tactile stimuli
	Monitor electrolyte values as ordered
	Assess for symptoms of K^+ imbalance
	  ECG displaying peaked T waves, flattened P waves, and widened QRS complex indicates
	    possible hyperkalemia
	  Depressed T waves and ST segments and prominent U wave indicates possible hypokalemia
	  Dysrhythmias
	Assess for symptoms of Na imbalance
	  Agitation, restlessness, or convulsions may indicate hypernatremia
	  Weakness, confusion, lethargy, or stupor may indicate hyponatremia

4. Knowledge deficit concerning precipitating events, signs and symptoms and prevention of DKA

Outcome Criteria	Nursing Interventions
Patient will be able to verbalize events leading to hyperglycemia Patient will be able to state signs and symptoms of DKA Patient will able to verbalize how to manage diabetes during an illness and when to notify the physician based on blood glucose values and urine ketone testing	Patient will be able to list stress, infection, trauma as precipitating events Early signs of polyuria, polydipsia, glycosuria, ketonuria, and elevated blood glucose will be verbalized Patient can relate sick day management of diabetes, and when to notify the physician based on home testing

References

Godine, J., Hurxthal, K., and Nathan, D. (1986). Bedside capillary glucose monitoring by staff nurses in a general hospital. *American Journal of Medicine*, 80(5), 803–806.

Kitabchi, A., and Murphy, M. (1988). Diabetic ketoacidosis and hyperosmolar hyperglycemic nonketotic coma. *Medical Clinics of North America*, 72(6), 1545–1563.

Krane, E. (1987). Diabetic ketoacidosis. *Pediatric Clinics of North America*, 35(4), 935–960.

Kruger, D., Horst, M., and Whitehouse, F. (1988). Bedside capillary blood glucose measurement in surgical intensive care units using a reflectance meter (summary). *Diabetes*, 37 (Suppl. 1), 26A.

Mattal, V., and Toledo-Pereyra, L. (1986). Pancreatic transplantation. *AORN Journal*, 42(3), 620–629.

National Diabetes Advisory Board. (1985). *Diabetes: A major public health problem* (annual report). Washington, D.C.: Author.

Sperling, M. (1984). Diabetic ketoacidosis. *Pediatric Clinics of North America*, 31(3), 591–607.

Sutherland, D., Moudry, K., and Fryd, D. (1989). Results of pancreas transplant registry. *Diabetes*, 38 (Suppl. 1), 46–54.

48

Patients with Disorders of the Thyroid and Neurohypophysis

Danni Brown

Cellular metabolism largely depends on and is regulated by the nervous system and the endocrine system. Therefore, alterations in hormonal function, regardless of the cause, commonly result in systemic manifestations. This chapter will discuss disorders of the pituitary, thyroid, and adrenal glands. Emphasis will be placed on primary diseases of these endocrine glands rather than on changes in hormonal function as a result of other system failure (i.e., renal failure). Acute alterations that are commonly encountered in the critical care patient population will be highlighted.

DISORDERS OF THE NEUROHYPOPHYSIS

Diabetes Insipidus

PATHOPHYSIOLOGY

The neurohypophysis, or posterior pituitary, stores two major hormones, arginine vasopressin (AVP), also known as antidiuretic hormone (ADH), and oxytocin. These hormones are actually synthesized in the hypothalamus and move by axonal transport into the neurohypophysis. They are then secreted from the pituitary into the systemic blood circulation following appropriate stimulation. Oxytocin regulates uterine contractions at parturition and milk release after parturition (Hadley, 1983). Alterations in oxytocin levels will not be discussed in this chapter.

Arginine vasopressin is one of several hormones that regulate the conservation of water to maintain fluid osmolality and systemic blood pressure and volume. It works on receptors in the distal renal

tubules. Stimulation of these receptors causes the reabsorption of water and subsequent concentration of urine. Diabetes insipidus (DI) is the condition that results from the absolute or relative lack of arginine vasopressin, the results of which cause excessive amounts of dilute urine output. This condition can be either neurogenic or nephrogenic (Blevins and Wand, 1992).

Neurogenic, or central, DI is the result of a defect in either the synthesis or secretion of AVP in the hypothalamus or pituitary, respectively. Some causes of this reduction in hormone include defective osmolreceptors, decreased numbers of secretory cells in the hypothalamus, impaired transport or release of AVP, and production of antibodies to the hormone (Rice, 1983).

The most common cause of an abnormal reduction in circulating AVP is a tumor of the hypothalamus or pituitary (Ingbar, 1987). These tumors may be either primary, such as chromophobe adenomas and craniopharyngiomas, or metastatic, most commonly from breast cancer (Rice, 1983).

The second most common cause of neurogenic DI is trauma. Trauma can be either accidental or iatrogenic from a surgical procedure. Severe head injury with resultant basilar skull fractures is the most common accidental cause of DI (Smith, 1981). Surgical procedures for tumor removal or aneurysm repair also often result in central DI (Smith, 1981). Traumatic DI is often transient in nature. Determining factors include the area of the lesion and the amount of destruction produced. Lesions of the hypothalamus and of the axonal tract above the median eminence produce permanent DI. However, lesions below the median eminence, even total removal of the pituitary gland, result only in temporary cessation of circulating hormone.

Certain medications also may have a central effect, decreasing the amount of circulating hormone. Some of these drugs are ethanol, reserpine, morphine sulfate, chlorpromazine, and phenytoin (Germon, 1987). Discontinuing the drug usually corrects the condition.

Local ischemia to the hypothalamus or the pituitary can cause neurogenic DI. This ischemia can be the result of decreased blood supply due to hemorrhage, thrombus formation, or severe hypotension.

Other causes of DI include central nervous system infections such as encephalitis, meningitis, tuberculosis, and syphilis. Granulomatous diseases, sarcoidosis and eosinophilic granuloma, also may cause central DI (Rice, 1983).

Nephrogenic diabetes insipidus results when the kidneys do not respond appropriately to the hormone. The renal tubules are resistant to AVP and therefore do not reabsorb water. Any renal disease in the advanced stages may cause nephrogenic DI. Examples of the more common causes include polycystic kidney disease, medullary cystic disease, and pyelonephritis. It may also occur following renal transplantation (Rice, 1983).

Other causes of nephrogenic DI include dietary factors, medications, pregnancy, and electrolyte imbalance. A rare familial form may also be seen; it is an X-linked recessive or autosomal dominant disease that is seen in male infants (Germon, 1987).

Nephrogenic DI is usually less severe than central DI. Fluid loss averages only 3 liters a day. An intact thirst mechanism will allow an individual to maintain an adequate fluid balance.

CLINICAL PRESENTATION

Regardless of the cause, patients with diabetes insipidus have abnormal water loss. Urine output can be as high as 16 to 17 liters/day. The patient with an intact thirst mechanism who is able to obtain enough water will prevent severe dehydration simply by drinking sufficient quantities. The hospitalized patient, however, may not have access to sufficient amounts of water, either because of physical limitations (i.e., too weak or too ill) or environmental limitations (i.e., too little water left at the bedside).

The patient with DI presents with polyuria and polydipsia. Profound weight loss is usually present. If fluid intake is insufficient, dehydration will occur. The patient will be hypotensive and have poor skin turgor and dried mucous membranes. In an attempt to conserve fluid, there will be decreased amounts of saliva and sweat.

Laboratory findings will include a high serum osmolarity (above 300 mOsm/liter) and hypernatremia (above 150 mmol/liter). Urine studies show an osmolarity under 200 mOsm/liter and a specific gravity of less than 1.005.

The diagnosis of diabetes insipidus is based on these laboratory findings and on diagnostic tests, such as the dehydration test and the hypertonic saline infusion test. The dehydration test is used most often. It provides adequate stimulation for AVP release and therefore readily identifies an abnormal state. During the test the patient is fluid restricted. Urine output, osmolality, and specific gravity are recorded. The patient with DI will continue to void dilute urine despite the fluid restriction. The patient should be watched closely due to the risk of severe dehydration resulting from the lack of fluid intake.

The diagnosis of neurogenic DI or nephrogenic DI can be made by administering an exogenous form of the hormone, commonly aqueous vasopressin. If the urine osmolality shows a moderate to marked increase (greater than 9%), neurogenic DI is diagnosed. Nephrogenic DI will show little to no response to the exogenous hormone because abnormal endogenous hormone production is not the cause of the disorder.

The hypertonic saline infusion also provides a stimulus for AVP release, i.e., a hyperosmolar state. If the infusion of hypertonic saline does not increase the urine concentration, then DI is confirmed. Other laboratory findings include an assay of the serum hormone level both before and after the infusion.

MEDICAL MANAGEMENT

Medical management of diabetes insipidus depends in part upon the etiology. Adequate fluid replacement and maintenance are essential regardless of the cause. Neurogenic DI is treated with hormone replacement. Aqueous vasopressin may be administered through either the subcutaneous or the intramuscular route. Its used with patients who have experienced an acute onset of DI, commonly following accidental trauma or surgery. Return of normal neurohypophyseal function can be recognized more easily due to the short duration of aqueous vasopressin. This prevents fluid overload and water intoxication in patients receiving intravenous fluids. Other longer acting forms of AVP are also available. Several nonhormonal agents are also available for clients who have some AVP production. These agents increase AVP release or potentiate its actions on the renal tubules.

Nephrogenic DI is more difficult to treat. The only drugs of clinical value are diuretics, most commonly the thiazide diuretics. These drugs produce sodium depletion, which leads to a fall in the glomerular filtration rate. This in turn causes an increase in fluid reabsorption from the proximal section of the nephron. Because less sodium reaches the ascending loop of Henle, the ability to dilute the urine is reduced (Ingbar, 1987). The patient with nephrogenic DI must restrict his or her sodium intake.

NURSING MANAGEMENT

Nursing management of patients with diabetes insipidus is aimed at preventing complications during the acute phase and providing patient education for long-term control. In the critical care setting the emphasis is on the former. However, the critical care nurse must remember that the disorder may persist for weeks to months or may even be permanent, and therefore patient and family teaching should be started as soon as possible. The nursing care plan provides nursing diagnoses and interventions that are applicable to the patient with diabetes insipidus.

Syndrome of Inappropriate Antidiuretic Hormone

PATHOPHYSIOLOGY

The opposite of diabetes insipidus, the syndrome of inappropriate antidiuretic hormone (SIADH), is the result of excessive amounts of circulating arginine vasopressin. There is a breakdown in the normal negative feedback system regulating the release and inhibition of the hormone. Circulating AVP acts directly on the renal tubules, causing reabsorption of water inconsistent with the body's needs. This leads to water overload and dilutional hyponatremia.

There are multiple causes of SIADH. Tumor tissue, commonly oat cell carcinoma, can produce AVP and release it independent of normal stimuli (Mundy, 1987). Nontumorous lung diseases also can cause SIADH either by independent synthesis and secretion of AVP or by altering left atrial filling pressures, thereby altering the stimulus for AVP release from the pituitary. Disorders of the central nervous system can affect the neurohypophysis, thereby increasing AVP release. These disorders include head trauma with skull fractures, cerebral vascular accidents, CNS infections, and Guillain-Barré syndrome (Ingbar, 1987). Certain medications increase the secretion of AVP from the pituitary. These include chlorpropamide, the antineoplastic drugs vincristine and vinblastine, general anesthetics, and tricyclic antidepressants (Ingbar, 1987).

CLINICAL PRESENTATION

Patients with SIADH produce a small amount of very concentrated urine. The symptoms are a result of the increased water retention. If the symptoms are not recognized and treated, they may progress to water intoxication. The symptoms are weight gain, anorexia, weakness, nausea, vomiting, diarrhea, confusion, aberrant respirations, hypothermia, and coma (Johndrow and Thornton, 1985).

Laboratory findings for the client with SIADH are a serum sodium level of less than 130 mmol/liter and a serum osmolality of less than 275 mOsm/liter. Other laboratory values, such as blood urea nitrogen (BUN), creatinine, hematocrit, and albumin may also be decreased. Hypokalemia is rare in SIADH. Urine sodium is usually greater than 20 mmol/liter. The diagnosis of SIADH is suspected in any patient with the above laboratory findings. Care should be taken to exclude other causes of hyponatremia. If SIADH is suspected and no cause can be identified, a malignancy should be strongly considered. SIADH may occur before a lesion can be detected by chest x-ray (Ingbar, 1987).

Also helpful in the diagnosis is a water load test. To prevent any serious side effects from the fluid load, the patient must have a sodium level greater than 125 mmol/liter and must not display any symptoms consistent with hyponatremia prior to administration of the test. The patient is then given an oral fluid load (usually 20 mL/kg body weight). Urine is collected over the next 5 to 6 hours. Patients with SIADH will excrete less than 40% of the water load in this period of time. Normal individuals will excrete 80%.

MEDICAL MANAGEMENT

Medical management of SIADH is largely dependent upon the etiology. Treatment is biphasic, the fluid overload being treated first and the underlying cause afterward. At present there are no drugs that successfully inhibit the secretion of AVP from either the pituitary or a tumor. Treatment therefore consists of restricting fluid intake. If the condition is mild to moderate a fluid restriction of 800 to 1000 mL/24 hours is usually sufficient to increase the serum sodium concentration. If the client has any signs of more severe water intoxication such as mental confusion, seizures, or coma more expedient correction of the hyponatremia must be implemented. The treatment of choice for the acute phase is infusion of 3% hypertonic saline solution and intermittent doses of furosemide. Although this will be only a temporary measure to increase the serum sodium, it will prevent the deleterious effects of severe hyponatremia, and the diuresis from the furosemide will help prevent pulmonary edema that might otherwise occur as a result of the fluid overload.

Long-term management of SIADH includes strict water restriction. There are also certain drugs that interfere with the actions of AVP at the nephron. These can be used to limit the effect of the hormone on water reabsorption and prevent fluid overload and hyponatremia. The most commonly used drug is demeclocycline. Other pharmacologic agents that have been used, but with less success, in the treatment of SIADH are lithium and phenytoin.

NURSING MANAGEMENT

The nursing management of patients with SIADH is aimed at preventing or limiting the complications of fluid overload and hyponatremia, and educating the patient long-term management. Nursing diagnoses applicable to the client with SIADH are given in the nursing care plan.

THYROID DISORDERS

The thyroid gland is directly regulated by the anterior piuitary gland and indirectly by the hypothalamus. The hypothalamus secretes thyrotropin-releasing hormone (TRH). This hormone travels through the hypophyseal portal system to the anterior pituitary. In response to TRH, the anterior pituitary secretes thyroid-stimulating hormone (TSH). This hormone is secreted into the general circulation and has as its target tissue the thyroid gland. This is called the hypothalamic-pituitary-thyroid axis.

The thyroid gland in response to TSH secretes thyroxine (tetraiodothyronine or T_4) and triiodothyronine (T_3). Synthesis of both hormones within the thyroid gland is dependent upon sufficient quantities of iodine. Both hormones are bound to carrier proteins in the bloodstream. The largest amount of circulating hormone is T_4. This hormone is also relatively physiologically inactive. In the peripheral tissue, however, T_4 is converted to T_3 by the enzymatic removal of an iodine atom from the T_4 outer ring. Unbound T_3 has considerable effect on cellular metabolism. Thyroid hormones affect tissue growth and maturation, energy expenditure, and vitamin and hormone degradation (Ingbar, 1987).

Secretion of the thyroid hormones is under negative feedback control. High serum levels of circulating hormones (T_3 and T_4) decrease the pituitary's response to TRH. Thyroid-releasing hormone is secreted in response to sleep, cold temperatures, and nonspecific stress.

Alteration in hormone levels results in widespread systemic dysfunction. Abnormal levels of thyroid hormones can result from either dysfunction of an organ in the physiologic axis or from other severe illness, physical trauma, or stress (Ingbar, 1987). The latter conditions result in a condition referred to as sick euthyroid syndrome (SES).

There are several variants of SES. The concentration of T_4 may be normal with a decreased concentration of T_3. This is a result of a decrease or peripheral conversion of T_4 to T_3. The total T_3 concentration is dependent upon the severity of the illness. This variant of SES can be separated from intrinsic hypothyroidism by the presence of normal T_4 and TSH levels.

A second variant of SES involves a low T_4 concentration and occurs in severely ill individuals. Triiodothyronine levels are also low. The low T_4 levels may be a result of hyposecretion of TSH. Low T_4 SES hypothyroidism can be differentiated from pituitary hypothyroidism by rT_3 levels. (rT_3 is produced by removal of an iodine atom from the inner ring of T_4. It is physiologically inactive.) rT_3 concentrations are increased in SES and decreased in pituitary hypothyroidism (Ingbar, 1987).

Hypothyroidism can be induced in critically ill individuals by other mechanisms. A drug commonly used in critically ill individuals, dopamine, is known to induce hypothyroidism. Dopamine inhibits TSH release from the pituitary gland.

Patients with nontoxic goiters (thyroid gland enlargement) can also become hypothyroid. Nontoxic goiters are the result of an imbalance between the supply of hormone produced and the demand by the body's needs. To provide for the supply required the thyroid enlarges. Lack of iodine, a necessary element in the production of thyroid hormones, can lead to a goitrous state. In most individuals enlargement of the gland allows the production of sufficient hormone to maintain normal metabolic functioning. Some individuals, however, are unable to meet the body's demands despite the glandular enlargement. They become both goitrous and hypothyroid. The addition of iodine to table salt has effectively decreased the incidence of endemic goiters.

Simple goiters can cause problems solely as a result of their size. The trachea and the esophogus can be compressed and displaced. Obstruction of either structure can occur if the goiter is large enough. Large retrosternal goiters can cause superior mediastinal obstruction.

Treatment of simple goiters is aimed at reducing the size and therefore the obstructing nature of the goiter. Exogenous hormone therapy is used to suppress the secretion of TSH from the pituitary. If the cause of the enlargement can be determined, treatment can be aimed more specifically. If iodine deficiency has resulted in the goitrous state, supplemental iodine should be used to treat the condition rather than hormone therapy.

Sodium L-thyroxine (levothyroxine) is the drug most commonly used to treat simple goiters. The dose usually starts at 100 μg/24 hours and is increased up to 200 μg/24 hours. Adequate suppression can be determined by measuring the radioactive iodine uptake (RAIU). Suppression of the thyroid gland is successful if the uptake of radioactive iodine (^{131}I or ^{123}I) is less than 5%.

Surgical intervention is used to treat simple goiters only if the goiter is causing severe obstruction and other medical means to reduce its size have failed. If a subtotal thyroidectomy is done, levothyroxine should be used (150 μg/24 hours) to prevent the recurence of the goiter from hyperplasia of the remaining tissue.

Hypothyroidism

PATHOPHYSIOLOGY

Hypothyroidism, regardless of the cause, is the condition that results when the levels of circulating T_3 and T_4 are inadequate. A variety of causes, both structural and functional, affect hormonal synthesis. Primary disease of the thyroid itself accounts for approximately 95% of hypothyroid conditions. The remaining 5% of cases arise from secondary (pituitary) and tertiary (hypothalamic) causes.

Failure of the thyroid gland to synthesize and secrete sufficient amounts of hormone (primary disease) can arise from several causes. These include congenital defects, surgical removal of the gland or radioiodine ablation, and dysfunction as a result of radiation for another condition such as lymphoma. Thyroid dysfunction can also be idiopathic.

Primary thyroid failure results in high levels of circulating TSH. Low to absent levels of T_3 and T_4 do not provide the negative feedback that is inhibitory to TSH production. The high levels of TSH stimulate tissue enlargement and the formation of a goiter. In the United States the most common cause of goitrous hypothyroidism is Hashimoto's disease, which is the result of defective organic binding of iodide and abnormal secretion of iodoproteins (Ingbar, 1987).

Cretinism is a hypothyroid state seen in infancy. If left untreated it will result in both physical and mental developmental handicaps. Most infants in the United States today are tested for thyroid function before leaving the hospital and between 7 and 10 days of age. Early detection and proper treatment with hormone replacement prevent any disability.

CLINICAL PRESENTATION

Early symptoms of hypothyroidism are nonspecific. They may include lethargy, constipation, and weight gain. Hair and skin may become dry. Ob-structive sleep apnea may also occur. The range of symptoms associated with hypothyroidism is found in Table 48–1. If left untreated, severe hypothyroidism may develop.

Severe hypothyroidism in adults can lead to accumulation of mucopolysaccharides in tissue. Lack of thyroid hormones also causes fluid retention and electrolyte imbalance. The excess fluid leaks into the tissue due to increased capillary permeability and the osmotic pull of the mucopolysaccharides. This results in nonpitting edema in the eyelids, periorbital tissue, hands, and feet. This condition is collectively called myxedema. This state can be treated and, more appropriately, prevented by early detection and prompt treatment of hypothyroidism.

MEDICAL MANAGEMENT

Hypothyroidism in the critically ill is treated with a synthetic thyroid preparation, levothyroxine, because of its uniform potency. Thyroid replacement is gradual. Initially, the daily dose of levothyroxine may start at 50 μg for 2 weeks, followed by 100 μg for 2 weeks, and then 150 μg. The daily dose of levothyroxine is usually given orally or by nasogastric tube. In patients with myxedema coma or in patients unable to absorb the drug from the gastrointestinal tract, it may be given intravenously. The maintenance dose varies with individuals. Some require

---

TABLE 48–1. *Clinical Manifestations of Hypothyroidism*

Cardiovascular	**Respiratory**
Cardiomegaly	Hypoventilation
Pericardial effusions	Impaired ventilatory response to hypoxia and hypercarbia
Decreased beta-adrenergic receptors	Pleural effusions
Impaired contractility	Edema and thickening of vocal cords
Decreased intravascular volume	Airway obstruction (i.e., enlarged tongue)
Hypotension	Muscle discoordination
Peripheral edema	Decreased diffusing lung capacity for carbon monoxide, vital capacity
Defect in baroreceptor responses	
Increased sensitivity to digitalis	**Neurologic**
Electrocardiography: sinus bradycardia; low voltage QRS complexes, prolonged PR and QT intervals, flattening of T waves	Obtundation, coma
	Slowed mentation
Renal	Dementia
Decreased renal blood flow and glomerular filtration rate	Psychosis
Urinary retention	Seizures
	Slowed relaxation of deep tendon reflexes
Gastrointestinal	Decreased hearing
Ascites	Vertigo
Ileus	Peripheral neuropathy
Atonic bowel	Abnormal EEG
Constipation	Elevated CSF protein
Miscellaneous	**Muscular**
Cold intolerance	Myopathy
Periorbital edema	Aches and pains
Hypothermia	Cramps
Arthralgias	
Joint effusions	**Hematologic**
Pseudogout	Anemia
Decreased drug metabolism	Coagulopathy
Hypercholesterolemia	Capillary fragility
Hypoglycemia	
Hyperuricemia	**Skin**
Hyponatremia	Cool, dry skin
Elevated creatine kinase, lactate dehydrogenase, SGOT, aldolase	Dry, coarse hair, brittle fingernails
Decreased cortisol response to stress	Nonpitting edema
	Alopecia

From Shoemaker, W. C., Ayres, S. M., Grennik, A., et al. (1989). Society of Critical Care Medicine: Textbook of critical care (2nd ed.). Philadelphia, W. B. Saunders Co.

TABLE 48–2. Clinical Features of Hyperthyroidism

Signs	Symptoms
Thyroid enlargement	Nervousness, anxiety
Thyroid bruit	Diaphoresis
Ophthalmopathy	Emotional lability
Lid retraction	Heat intolerance
Lid lag	Palpitations
Hyperkinesis	Dyspnea
Tremor	Fatigue and weakness
Hyperactive reflexes	Weight loss
Tachycardia	Increased appetite
Atrial fibrillation	Eye complaints (e.g., irritation,
Hot and moist skin	pain, diplopia)
Thin and fine hair	Hyperdefecation
Onycholysis	Personality change
Hyperpigmentation and/or vitiligo	Impaired concentration and
Impaired renal concentrating	cognitive function
ability	Insomnia
Muscle weakness	Difficulty swallowing
Hoarseness	
Gynecomastia	
Amenorrhea, oligomenorrhea	
Congestive cardiomyopathy	

Laboratory Tests:
Elevated total and free T_4
Elevated total and free T_3
Elevated RT_3U
Elevated (Graves' disease), normal and low (thyroiditis) RAIU
No response of TSH to TRH
Low creatinine phosphokinase, cholesterol, and triglycerides

RT_3U = T_3 resin uptake; RAIU = radioiodine uptake; TSH = thyrotropin; TRH = thyrotropin releasing hormone.
From Shoemaker, W. C., Ayres, S. M., Grennik, A., et al. (1989). Society of Critical Care Medicine: *Textbook of critical care* (2nd ed.), Philadelphia, W. B. Saunders Co.

doses as low as 50 μg/24 hours whereas others require as much as 400 μg (Gilman and colleagues, 1990).

NURSING MANAGEMENT

Nursing diagnoses for the patient with hypothyroidism are:

Activity intolerance
Alteration in bowel elimination; constipation
Fluid volume deficit
Knowledge deficit
Altered nutrition; more than body requirements
Disturbance in self-concept; body image
Ineffective thermoregulation
Altered thought processes

Hyperthyroidism

PATHOPHYSIOLOGY

Multiple etiologies can produce the clinical state of excessive circulating thyroid hormone. All produce essentially the same clinical picture. Treatment, however, varies depending on the cause.

The most common cause of hyperthyroidism is Graves' disease. It is an autoimmune disorder sometimes referred to as diffuse toxic goiter. The thyroid gland is enlarged and highly vascular. The follicles

are both hyperplastic and hypertrophic. Excessive TSH is not the cause of enlargement of the gland. Abnormal immunoglobulins that have TSH-like properties are found in the plasma of individuals with Graves' disease. These immunoglobulins are termed thyroid-stimulating immunoglobulins (TSI). The first immunoglobulin discovered had a much longer physiologic effect than TSH and it was named long-acting thyroid stimulator (LATS). TSI bind to the thyroid membrane, activate adenylate cyclase, increase the accumulation of iodide within the follicle, and induce glandular hyperplasia. The high circulating hormone levels that result inhibit TSH secretion from the pituitary gland.

Much less common than Graves' disease, hyperthyroidism can result from a toxic nodular goiter in a hyperfunctioning state. Adenoma of the thyroid gland may secrete thyroid hormones inappropriate to stimuli and may cause hyperthyroidism. Rare causes include thyroiditis, metastatic thyroid carcinoma, and overtreatment for hypothyroidism.

Secondary causes of hyperthyroidism are related to disorders of the pituitary or hypothalamus. Inappropriate secretion of thyrotropin (IST) results in excessive amounts of TSH with respect to the clinical picture. This elevation can result from a TSH-secreting tumor or resistance to thyroid hormone, thereby eliminating the negative feedback component (Faglia and colleagues, 1987).

Thyrotoxic crisis, or thyroid storm, is a complication of hyperthyroidism. Although it is seen rarely, it is associated with a high mortality. The exact etiology is unknown. Several factors are thought to contribute to the development of this complication. They include an abrupt release of thyroid hormones or an increased sensitivity of peripheral receptors to the circulating hormones (Evangelisti and Thorpe, 1983).

CLINICAL PRESENTATION

The clinical presentation of the client with hyperthyroidism is quite variable. The thyroid gland is

TABLE 48–3. Treatment of Hyperthyroidism

Antithyroid therapy
  Drugs
    Propylthiouracil 100–400 mg q 6 h
    Methimazole 20–40 mg q day
    Iodide
    Lithium 300 mg q 8 h
  Radioactive iodine (RAI)
  Thyroidectomy
Agents inhibiting T_4 to T_3 peripheral conversion
  Propylthiouracil
  Glucocorticoids
  Propranolol 40–60 mg q 6 h
  Ipodate (Oragrafin) 1 g q day
Agents ameliorating symptoms
  Propranolol 40–60 mg q 6 h
  Reserpine 1.0–2.5 mg/day
  Guanethidine 50–150 mg/day

From Shoemaker, W. C., Ayres, S. M., Grennik, A., et al. (1989). Society of Critical Care Medicine: *Textbook of critical care* (2nd ed.). Philadelphia, W. B. Saunders.

palpable in approximately 95% of the cases. A bruit can usually be heard over the superior thyroidal arteries. Other signs and symptoms include excess sweating, heat intolerance, tachycardia, tremor, nervousness, and excitability. Wasting of the skeletal muscles often occurs and results in a proximal myopathy. The muscle wasting may be severe even when the client has only mild to moderate hyperthyroidism. The cardiovascular findings—sinus tachycardia, systolic flow murmurs, and atrial fibrillation—develop in severe cases of long duration and are more common in the elderly. Chest pain may occur with myocardial infarction in 4% to 10% of patients with thyrotoxicosis. Patients in thyroid storm present with exaggerated symptoms of hyperthyroidism. There is a rapid rise in temperature, quickly reaching up to and in excess of 41°C (Table 48–2).

LABORATORY FINDINGS

Diagnosis of advanced hyperthyroidism typically is not difficult and is based on the clinical findings. However, the insidious onset often delays diagnosis well into the disease course. Thyroid function tests are diagnostic in most cases. If the T_4 and free T_4 index are borderline or normal, plasma T_3 should be measured. In approximatley 5% of patients with hyperthyroidism T_3 alone will be elevated.

MEDICAL MANAGEMENT

Medical management of the critically ill patient with hyperthyroidism involves three strategies. The first is to suppress the thyroid hormones, the second is to inhibit conversion of T_4 to T_3, and the third is to ameliorate the patient's symptoms (Table 48–3). Definitive therapy aimed at decreasing the overproduction of thyroid hormone often involves radioactive iodine or surgery.

NURSING MANAGEMENT

Nurses must monitor these patients carefully for signs of thyroid storm. Fever, tachycardia, hypertension, and myocardial ischemia can all be life-threatening. It is important to watch for these symptoms and to the patient's response to drug therapy such as propranolol.

nursing care plan

1. Actual fluid volume deficit

Outcome Criteria	Nursing Interventions

Maintenance of a euvolemic state as measured by
  A stable body weight
  A stable blood pressure
  A urine output appropriate to fluid intake
  A serum sodium level of 135 to 145 mmol/liter
  A serum osmolality of 285 to 295 mOsm/liter
	Record intake and output at least every hour. Maintain a cumulative total body balance for the duration of the acute phase. This will provide ongoing information about the patient's fluid balance. Simply doing 24-hour totals may allow subtle fluid deficits to accumulate over days, producing marked dehydration. A Foley catheter may be necessary to record accurate output figures as well as allowing the patient to rest.
	Adjust fluid intake to match urine output plus 10%. This will provide sufficient fluid to offset urine loss and other fluid losses from the skin and respiratory tract. If the patient is febrile or tachypneic, he will require greater fluid intake.
	Check urine specific gravity at least every hour until medical management is initiated or until the urine specific gravity is above 1.006. Then check at least every 2 to 4 hours for the duration of the acute phase. Consult with the physician if urine specific gravity does not increase after medical therapy or drops below 1.005.
	Weigh the patient at least daily. Weight is another indicator of fluid level. (Note: One liter of fluid equals one kilogram.)
	Monitor serum sodium and osmolality levels. Consult with physician if sodium is greater than 150 mmol/liter, serum osmolality is greater than 295 mOsm/liter, or the patient shows signs or symptoms of a hypernatremic hyperosmolar state. These symptoms include confusion, stupor, seizures, and muscle fasciculations.
	Check vital signs, including postural signs if client is able, every hour. Tachycardia and hypotension are indicators of a dehydrated state.

2. Knowledge deficit

Outcome Criteria	Nursing Interventions
Patient is prepared to care for himself at discharge. He must have adequate information about the disease process, drug administration, and the signs and symptoms of inadequate control.	As soon as the patient is able to comprehend the information, explain the disease process in terms he can understand. Watch for verbal cues that he understands the information. Have the patient start to administer his own medication if he will be taking it when he goes home. If possible, teach a significant other how to administer the medication also. Explain the signs of hormonal imbalance to the patient. Excessive urine output, particularly nocturia, should alert the client to notify his physician.

Nursing Care Plan continued on following page

3. Fluid volume excess	
Outcome Criteria	*Nursing Interventions*

Maintenance of a euvolemic state as measured by
  A stable body weight
  A stable blood pressure
  No evidence of edema
  Clear bilateral breath sounds
  Urine output appropriate to fluid intake
  A serum sodium level of 135 to 145 mmol/liter
  A serum osmolality of 285 to 295 mOsm/liter
	Record intake and output at least every hour. Maintain a cumulative total body balance for the duration of the acute phase. This will provide ongoing information about the patient's fluid status. Weigh the patient daily. Weight is an excellent indicator of fluid balance. Consult with the physician if the patient gains any weight.

References

Blevins, L. S., and Wand, G. S. (1992). Diabetes insipidus. *Critical Care Medicine, 20,* 69–79.

Evangelisti, J., and Thorpe, J. (1983). Thyroid storm—a nursing crisis. *Heart & Lung,* 12(2), 184–193.

Faber, J., Kirkegaard, C., Rasmussen, B., et al. (1987). Pituitary-thyroid axis in critical illness. *Journal of Clinical Endocrinology and Metabolism,* 65, 315–320.

Faglia, G., Beck-Peccoz, P., Piscitelli, G., et al. (1987). Inappropriate secretion of thyrotropin by the pituitary. *Hormone Research,* 26, 79–99.

Germon, K. (1987). Fluid and electrolyte problems associated with diabetes insipidus and syndrome of inappropriate antidiuretic hormone. *Nursing Clinics of North America.* 22(4), 785–796.

Gilman, A. G., Rall, T. W., Nies, A. S. et al. (1990). *The pharmacological basis of therapeutics* (8th ed.). New York: Pergamon Press.

Gregerman, R. (1980). The thyroid gland. In A. Harvey, R. Jones, V. McKusick, et al. (Eds.), *The principles and practice of medicine* (12th ed., pp. 868–892). New York: Appleton-Century-Crofts.

Hadley, M. E. (1983). *Endocrinology.* Englewood Cliffs, NJ: Prentice Hall.

Ingbar, S. (1987). Diseases of the thyroid. In E. Braunwald, K. Isselbacher, R. Petersdorf, et al. (Eds.), *Harrison's principles of internal medicine* (11th ed., pp. 1732–1752). New York: McGraw-Hill.

Johndrow, P., and Thornton, S. (1985). Syndrome of inappropriate antidiuretic hormone: A growing concern. *Focus on Critical Care,* 12(5), 29–34.

Kohrle, J., Brabant, G., and Hesch, R.-D. (1987). Metabolism of the thyroid hormones. *Hormone Research,* 26, 58–78.

Mundy, G. (1987). Ectopic hormonal syndromes in neoplastic disease. *Hospital Practice,* April 15, 179–194.

Rice, V. (1983). Problems of water regulation: Diabetes insipidus and syndromes of inappropriate anti-diuretic hormone. *Critical Care Nurse,* 3(1), 63–82.

Smith, J. (1981). Nursing management of diabetes insipidus. *Journal of Neurosurgical Nursing,* 13(6), 313–317.

Streeten, D., Moses, A., and Miller, M. (1987). Disorders of the neurohypophysis. In E. Braunwald, K. Isselbacher, R. Petersdorf, et al. (Eds.), *Harrison's principles of internal medicine* (pp. 1722–1732). New York: McGraw-Hill.

10

Hematologic System

49

Hematologic Physiology

Diane K. Dressler

Critical care nurses are confronted daily with clinical problems related to cellular respiration, immunity, and hemostasis. All these functions depend directly on blood. The nursing care of patients with hematologic disorders is challenging. It requires knowledge of the anatomy of the hematologic system (much of which continually moves around), the physiology of the blood elements, the effects of deficiencies of blood elements, and the processes of hemostasis and thrombosis. The purpose of this chapter is to present the anatomy and physiology of the hematologic system with an emphasis on blood coagulation.

THE COMPOSITION OF BLOOD

Blood is a mixture of living cells and plasma. The major functions of blood include the transportation of oxygen and food products, the removal of carbon dioxide and metabolic wastes, the transport of hormones from endocrine glands, and the protection of the body from infection. In addition, the flow of blood plays a role in the regulation of body temperature.

The average adult has 5 to 6 liters of blood in the intravascular compartment. Fifty-five per cent of this is in the form of plasma, and 45% is solid suspended cellular components. The solid suspended cellular component portion is commonly referred to as the hematocrit. Table 49–1 outlines the more specific composition of plasma and cellular components. The red blood cells are by far the most numerous of the cellular components. It is important to note that the red blood cells (RBCs) and platelets remain in the intravascular compartment. Most white blood cells (WBCs) are extravascular, and the blood serves mainly as a transport system for these cells (Clements, 1981).

All blood cells originate from primordial cells in the bone marrow, as shown in Figure 49–1. The marrow is considered to be one of the largest organs in the body. It produces 2.5 billion RBCs, 2.5 billion platelets, and 1 billion WBCs daily (Williams et al., 1983). The bone marrow is stimulated to differentiate cells into RBCs, platelets, and specific types of WBCs according to physiologic requirements. As the cells mature, they proceed through developmental stages before being released from the bone marrow and becoming fully functional. These stages will be described in more detail as the specific cell types are discussed.

Red Blood Cells

Normal red blood cells have a unique structure that facilitates the transport of oxygen from the lungs to the tissues. They are shaped like biconcave discs, allowing greater flexibility as they pass through tiny capillaries. Their biconcave structure also increases the surface area for absorption of oxygen.

TABLE 49–1. Composition of Blood

Plasma (55%)	Cellular Components (45%)
Water (92%)	Red blood cells (erythrocytes): 5 million/mm³
Protein (7%)	
Albumin	White blood cells (leukocytes): 5,000– 10,000/mm³
Other plasma proteins	Granulocytes
Immunoglobulins	Neutrophils (60–70%)
Fibrinogen	Eosinophils (1–3%)
Prothrombin	Basophils (.05–1%)
Other (1%)	Monocytes (macrophages) (4–8%)
Metabolites	Lymphocytes (20–40%)
Respiratory gases	B-cells
Enzymes	T-cells
Hormones	Platelets (thrombocytes): 150,000– 400,000/mm³
Clotting factors	

PRIMITIVE CELLS   MATURE CELLS

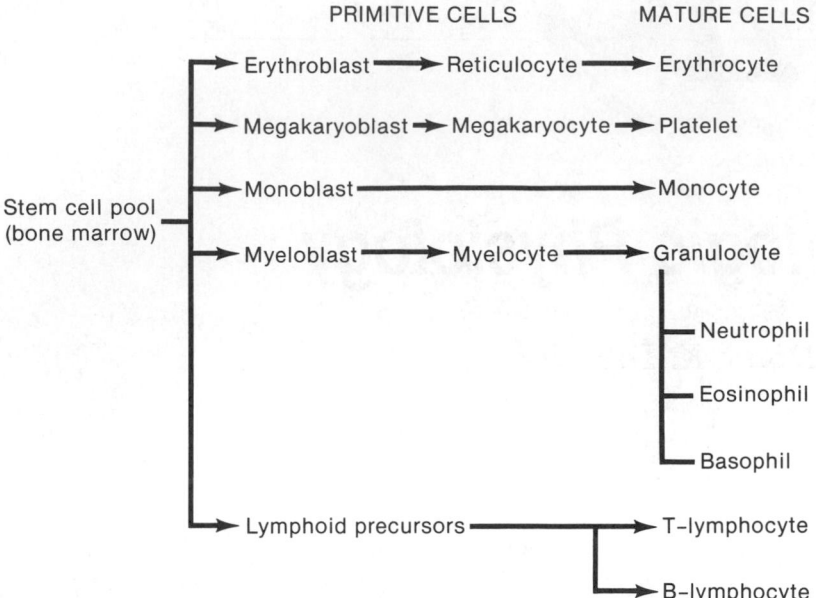

FIGURE 49–1. The production of cellular components.

The production of RBCs is regulated by tissue oxygenation. Under conditions of hemorrhage, hypoxia, and anemia, the bone marrow is stimulated to produce more RBCs. As the cells are formed, they begin to synthesize hemoglobin during the primitive stages. The cytoplasm eventually fills with hemoglobin, the cell nucleus becomes extremely small, and the cells are released into the circulation as reticulocytes. The number of reticulocytes can be measured to assess the rate of erythrocyte production. The reticulocytes mature in a few days into functional erythrocytes.

The process of erythropoiesis, or red blood cell production, is controlled by a feedback mechanism involving a circulating hormone, erythropoietin. Cellular hypoxia leads to an increased production of erythropoietin by the kidney, which produces 95% of this hormone. Erythropoietin then circulates to the bone marrow, where it causes stem cells to differentiate into erythrocytes. In addition, when severe hypoxia is present, more erythropoietin is produced, and the rate of production increases. When the kidneys are nonfunctional, anemia results because the other sites of erythropoietin production (possibly the liver and macrophages) can produce only a fraction of the needed amount (Guyton, 1991). Until recently, transfusion therapy was the only treatment option available for these individuals, but the development of genetically engineered recombinant human erythropoietin promises to change this situation.

Specific nutrients are necessary for RBC production. Vitamin B_{12} is essential for all tissue growth and is especially important for tissues that are rapidly proliferating. Lack of vitamin B_{12} inhibits the rate of RBC production and leads to the formation of abnormal RBCs. This maturational failure can be caused by inadequate intake of vitamin B_{12} or failure to absorb it (pernicious anemia). Folic acid, like vitamin B_{12}, is also a necessary nutrient for RBC production. Iron absorbed from the small intestine is formed into a substance called transferrin, which allows the iron to circulate to the parts of the body where it is needed. Excess iron is stored in the liver in the form of ferritin. When the plasma iron level falls, iron is transported to the bone marrow, where transferrin molecules bind with erythroblasts. Transferrin moves into the cells, where mitochondria synthesize heme from iron and porphyrin. The heme molecule then combines with a long polypeptide chain to form hemoglobin. The most important feature of this molecule is its ability to combine with oxygen in a bond that is easily reversible, allowing the oxygen to be readily released into the tissues (Guyton, 1991).

Red blood cells live an average of 120 days. When the cells become old and fragile, they rupture or are taken up by the red pulp of the spleen. The iron from the used cells is transported by macrophages into the blood, where it can be carried as transferrin back to the liver to be stored or to the bone marrow to be used in more hemoglobin production. The porphyrin portion of the hemoglobin molecule is converted by the macrophages into bilirubin, which is eventually secreted by the liver as bile (Guyton, 1991).

White Blood Cells

Six types of WBCs are found in peripheral blood and are known to participate in either nonspecific or specific immune responses. The granulocytes, also called polymorphonuclear leukocytes, are named for their granular appearance and for the fact that mature cells have multiple nuclei. These cells have the ability to engulf and digest invading organisms through the process of phagocytosis. The three types of granulocytes include neutrophils, eosinophils, and basophils. The monocytes and lymphocytes, which include plasma cells, comprise the nongranulocytic leukocytes. A seventh type of leukocyte found in the bone marrow, the megakaryocyte, produces platelets.

The production of WBCs takes place in the bone marrow. Production of sufficient numbers of WBCs depends on adequate nutrition. Both amino acids and B vitamins are used in production of WBCs. It is thought that specific hormones stimulate immature granulocytes to increase the rate of production. The bone marrow is thought to contain approximately 30 granulocytes for each granulocyte found in the peripheral blood. Since the life span of many of these cells is short, the granulocyte pool can be quickly depleted during an acute infection, especially if the body does not have the resources to increase production (Clements, 1981).

WBCs play a major role in the body's defense against infection. Granulocytes are the most numerous type of WBC and have a relatively short life span. Neutrophils, the most abundant type of granulocyte, play a major role in the destruction of microorganisms, particularly bacteria. A much smaller number of eosinophils are found in the blood. These cells seem to have less phagocytic activity than neutrophils. Eosinophils are found in high concentrations during parasitic infections and during allergic reactions (Jett and Lancaster, 1983). Even fewer basophils are found in peripheral blood. They are associated with the inflammatory response and are known to release both histamine and heparin (Jett and Lancaster, 1983).

The monocytes are the largest cells found in the peripheral blood and are a unique type of WBC. In both blood and tissues they recognize and phagocytize foreign organisms and particles. After transport through the blood, monocytes can travel to the tissues, where they are transformed into much larger cells called tissue macrophages. Both circulating and fixed macrophages are extremely phagocytic and serve to filter unwanted particles and organisms from the blood and body fluids (Jett and Lancaster, 1983).

In addition to the nonspecific inflammatory response initiated by neutrophils and macrophages, a sophisticated immune response can develop, enabling the body to mount a defense against specific invading organisms, toxins, or cells. This response is carried out by the lymphocytes. There are two major types of specific immunity. Humoral immunity, mediated by B-lymphocytes, involves the production of specific antibodies. Cellular immunity, mediated by T-lymphocytes, involves the production of small sensitized lymphocytes that can bind to and destroy invaders (Bellanti, 1985). For more detailed information about WBC function and the immune system, see Chapter 51.

Platelets

Platelets are the smallest and most fragile of the cellular components of the blood. They normally circulate as flattened discs (Williams et al., 1983). They originate as small particles that bud from large megakaryocytes. Platelets contain granules that in turn contain substances that directly affect the coagulation process. The granules contain actin and myosin molecules, which can cause platelet aggregation. They also contain enzyme systems capable of forming adenosine triphosphate (ATP) and adenosine diphosphate (ADP), enzymes that synthesize prostaglandins, and a growth factor that facilitates the repair of damaged vessels. The platelet cell membranes contain glycoproteins that cause the platelets to adhere to damaged cells. The membranes also contain phospholipids, which can activate the intrinsic pathway of blood coagulation (Guyton, 1991).

Platelets play several roles in the hemostatic process. They nurture the vascular endothelium, increasing its structural integrity. Without this nurturing by adequate numbers of platelets, petechiae develop easily. Platelets are able to plug small tears in capillaries physically. When a blood vessel is severed, platelets aggregate and release mediators that cause vascular constriction and initiate clot formation (Hirsh and Brain, 1983).

Platelet production is under the control of a hormone called thrombopoietin. The site of synthesis of this hormone is unknown, but production of the hormone is stimulated by thrombocytopenia. Thrombopoietin increases the number of megakaryocytes formed and appears to speed their maturation and the release of platelets.

After the platelets are released, they circulate as cytoplasmic discs. Approximately 80% of the body's platelets circulate while the rest are stored in the spleen. Normal length of platelet survival is 8 to 10 days, but this time period is influenced by many factors, including the need for hemostasis.

THE NORMAL HEMOSTATIC MECHANISM

The purpose of the hemostatic mechanism is to prevent blood loss from normal vessels and to stop bleeding from injured vessels. Normally blood circulates through smooth endothelial-lined vessels without platelet aggregation, coagulation, or hemorrhage (Colman et al., 1991). Injury to the blood vessel is what usually triggers the hemostatic process. Effective hemostasis is accomplished through the harmonious interplay among three factors: the blood vessel wall, the platelets, and the plasma coagulation factors. The precise mechanisms governing hemostasis are somewhat complex, but it is essential to understand these basic processes to understand coagulopathies.

Physical Events in Blood Clotting

There are several mechanisms that assist in achieving hemostasis following injury to a blood vessel. As shown in Figure 49–2, these mechanisms include vascular constriction, platelet plugging, clot formation, and fibrinolysis plus wound healing.

Vascular Constriction. When a blood vessel is injured, it constricts to slow the flow of blood. This constriction is thought to result from nervous reflexes in the vessel walls and local myogenic contraction of the vessel. It is also thought that platelets release a powerful vasoconstrictor, thromboxane A_2, at the injury site. Later, this effect is reversed when the vessel walls, under the influence of the procoagulant thrombin, release a powerful vasodilator called prostacyclin (PGI_2) (Hirsh and Brain, 1983). The greater the trauma, the greater the vascular spasm that occurs. This process can last from minutes to hours while the subsequent processes of platelet plugging and actual clot formation are under way (Guyton, 1991).

Platelet Plugging. Following an injury, the platelets change their form from discs to spheres (Colman et al., 1991). They become sticky and immediately begin to adhere to the damaged endothelium. They then release ADP and thromboxane A_2. These substances act on nearby platelets to activate them, resulting in their adhesion to the original platelets. The platelet adhesion process requires the presence of von Willebrand factor VIII and normal receptor sites for this substance.

Contact with tissue collagen on the damaged endothelium is the signal that sparks the platelet release reaction. The chemical mediators act quickly to promote platelet aggregation, and an unstable platelet plug may form over the injured site within seconds (Hirsh and Brain, 1983). If the tear in the vessel is very small, it may be sealed by a platelet plug. This process is particularly important in sealing ruptured capillaries. The larger vessels that are damaged in more severe injuries are not sealed with platelet plugging. Here the aggregated platelets provide a surface on which blood coagulation can occur. Once a fibrin clot forms, the platelet plug is strengthened.

Blood Clot Formation. A blood clot will begin to form within minutes after a vessel is damaged. The clot develops even faster if the trauma has been severe. Activating substances are released from platelets as described previously. Other activating substances are released from the vessel wall and from the plasma proteins. These substances activate the extrinsic and intrinsic blood coagulation pathways to initiate clotting. Fibrin strands appear over the injured site and eventually form a mesh that traps red blood cells. The fibrin clot should form within 3 to 6 minutes (the normal bleeding time) unless the opening in the vessel is very large. After about 30 minutes to an hour, serum is expressed from the clot, and it retracts. This further closes the vessel and stabilizes the clot (Guyton, 1991).

Fibrinolysis. Fibrinolysis is the process that eventually dissolves the clot. The fibrin is digested by enzymes from the plasma fibrinolytic system. Leukocytes also move in to phagocytize the debris by a process known as cellular fibrinolysis. Dissolution of the clot prepares the way for formation of fibrous scar tissue and wound healing.

The Biochemical Steps in Clot Formation

The process of blood clotting occurs as a series of steps that result in the formation of fibrin, the main substance of a clot. The physical events in blood clotting are controlled by biochemical reactions occurring between the procoagulant proteins and enzymes present in blood. There are four essential steps in clot formation:

1. Initiation of the extrinsic or intrinsic pathway.
2. Formation of prothrombin activator.
3. Conversion of prothrombin to thrombin.
4. Conversion of fibrinogen to fibrin.

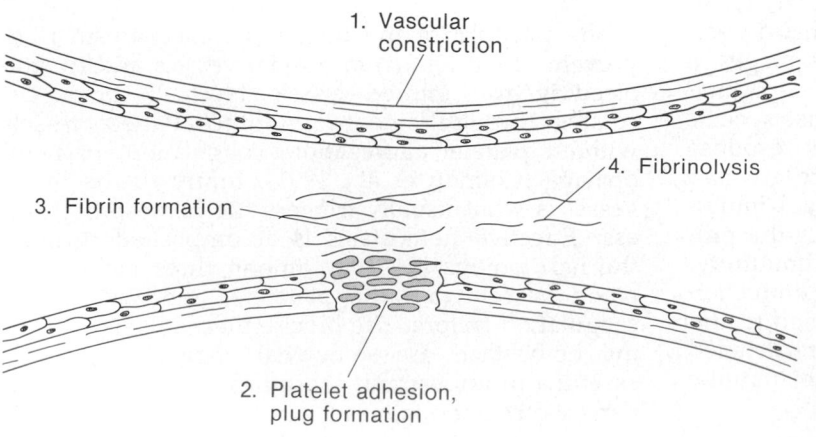

1. Vascular constriction

4. Fibrinolysis

3. Fibrin formation

2. Platelet adhesion, plug formation

FIGURE 49–2. Physical events in blood clotting.

TABLE 49–2. Plasma Coagulation Factors

Factor I	Fibrinogen
Factor II	Prothrombin
Factor III	Tissue thromboplastin
Factor IV	Calcium
Factor V	Proaccelerin
Factor VII	Proconvertin, serum prothrombin conversion accelerator
Factor VIII	Antihemophilic factor (AHF)
Factor IX	Plasma thromboplastin component (Christmas factor)
Factor X	Stuart-Prower factor
Factor XI	Plasma thromboplastin antecedent
Factor XII	Hageman factor
Factor XIII	Fibrin-stabilizing factor

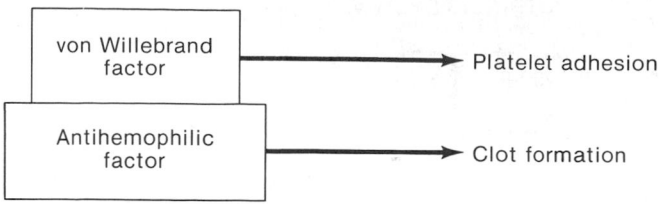

FIGURE 49–3. The factor VIII molecule.

Each of these important steps will be discussed in greater detail subsequently.

The Plasma Coagulation Factors. All steps in the coagulation process involve interaction among the plasma coagulation factors. These factors, listed in Table 49–2, play a role in the initiation and completion of the clotting process. The first four factors—fibrinogen, prothrombin, tissue thromboplastin, and calcium—are usually referred to by their common names. The other factors are most frequently referred to by their designated roman numeral. No factor VI is listed because this substance was found to be an activated form of factor V and was taken off the list.

Most coagulation factors are produced in the liver, many in conjunction with vitamin K. Many of the factors are basically inactive forms of proteolytic enzymes. When activated, these enzymes cause the cascading reactions that result in clotting.

A few factors require a closer look. Factor VIII, the antihemophilic factor, actually has two components. Each component has its own function and genetic control. First, there is the coagulant protein known as antihemophilic factor, which has a role in the intrinsic pathway. People who lack this factor have hemophilia A. The other portion of factor VIII is a large polymeric protein known as von Willebrand factor, as illustrated in Figure 49–3. This component

is necessary for normal platelet adhesion to collagen in a damaged vessel wall.

Factor XII is unique in that it functions not only in coagulation but also in interaction with other related processes that occur during an injury. As seen in Figure 49–4, surface activation of factor XII also activates the kinin system and the fibrinolytic system. In this way, factor XII links the initiation of clotting with the subsequent activation of the inflammatory process and fibrinolysis during the contact phase of coagulation (Hirsh and Brain, 1983).

The clotting process is initiated through two basic mechanisms termed the extrinsic and intrinsic pathways. Both pathways have the same endpoint, the activation of factor X, which becomes what is called prothrombin activator.

The Extrinsic Pathway. The extrinsic pathway is associated with trauma to body tissues. When an injury occurs, blood comes in contact with the damaged tissues, which release tissue thromboplastin. As seen in Figure 49–5, this substance, along with factor VII and calcium, forms activated factor X. The activated factor X then interacts with platelet phospholipids and factor V to produce the prothrombin activator complex. This complex is then able to split prothrombin to thrombin within seconds.

The extrinsic pathway is a much faster pathway than the intrinsic pathway. The addition of tissue thromboplastin enables clotting to begin without some of the early time-consuming steps involved in the intrinsic system (Colman et al., 1991).

The Intrinsic Pathway. The intrinsic pathway is thought to be the more important coagulation path-

FIGURE 49–4. The activation of factor XII links a number of homeostatic reactions. It promotes blood coagulation through activation of factor XI, inflammation through kinins, fibrinolysis through plasmin, and subsequent complement activation.

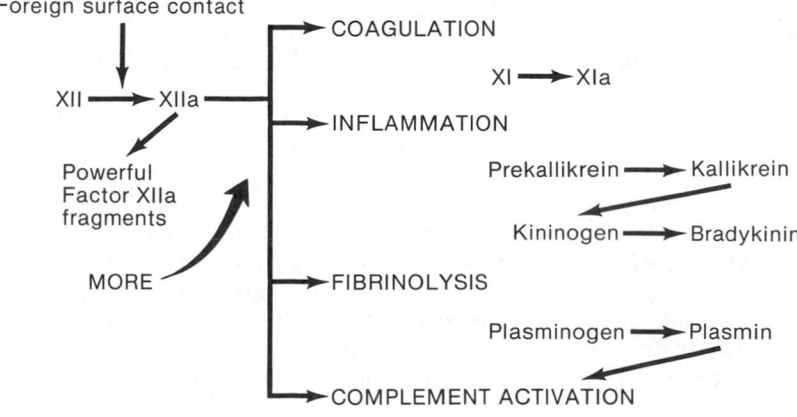

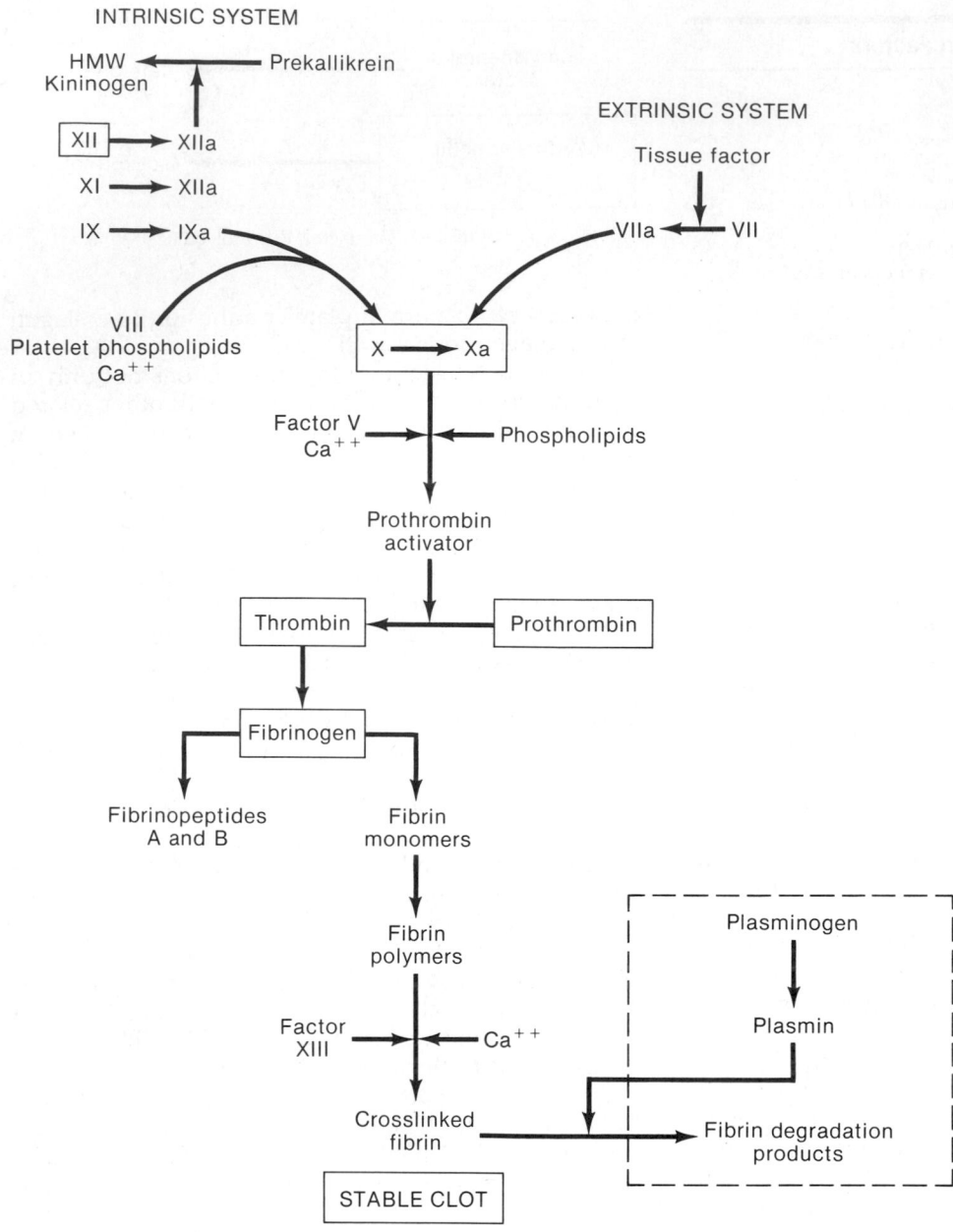

INTRINSIC SYSTEM

HMW ← Prekallikrein
Kininogen

EXTRINSIC SYSTEM

Tissue factor

XII → XIIa

XI → XIIa

IX → IXa

VIIa ← VII

VIII
Platelet phospholipids
Ca^{++}

X → Xa

Factor V
Ca^{++} → ← Phospholipids

Prothrombin
activator

Thrombin ← Prothrombin

Fibrinogen

Fibrinopeptides
A and B

Fibrin
monomers

Fibrin
polymers

Plasminogen

Plasmin

Factor
XIII → ← Ca^{++}

Crosslinked
fibrin → Fibrin degradation
products

STABLE CLOT

FIGURE 49–5. The coagulation process. HMW, high molecular weight.

way compared with the extrinsic pathway (Colman et al., 1991). All factors necessary to activate this pathway are already present in the intravascular compartment. The intrinsic pathway is activated when blood comes in contact with a foreign surface, such as a damaged vessel, or when the blood itself is traumatized (Guyton, 1991).

The intrinsic pathway has been called the *coagulation cascade*. It involves a series of reactions through which each inactive precursor is converted in turn into an active enzyme, which then goes on to convert another precursor. When a blood vessel is damaged and the subendothelium is exposed, the "contact" phase of coagulation begins. As shown in Figure 49–5, activated factor XII subsequently activates factor XI. This factor in turn activates factor IX. Factor IX then acts with factor VIII and the phospholipids

released from traumatized platelets to activate factor X. A deficiency of any of these factors interferes with this process and prevents adequate initiation of the intrinsic pathway. It should also be noted that calcium ions are necessary for many steps in this process.

After factor X is activated, a common final pathway is utilized in which prothrombin activator goes on to begin the actual formation of a clot. In most situations involving damage to blood vessels, clotting is initiated through both the extrinsic and intrinsic pathways. Tissue thromboplastin released from damaged tissues initiates the extrinsic pathway. Exposure of the damaged endothelium initiates the intrinsic pathway. The clot is then formed through the final common pathway.

Clot Formation. Following the activation of factor

X and formation of the prothrombin activator complex, fibrin strands begin to form within seconds. The production of fibrin depends on a rapid series of reactions through which prothrombin is cleaved to thrombin, a powerful procoagulant. The presence of thrombin accelerates clotting by stimulating the intrinsic pathway. It is thought that the extrinsic pathway may yield only small amounts of thrombin and fibrin. Adequate clot formation depends largely on activation and continued stimulation of the intrinsic pathway. Thrombin stimulates platelets to release ADP and continue to aggregate, and also stimulates the production of PGI$_2$ and is thus responsible for vessel relaxation following the formation of the clot (Colman et al., 1991). Figure 49–6 illustrates the complex role played by thrombin in hemostasis.

The reactions described so far take place on the surface of platelets and involve platelet phospholipids, as shown in Figure 49–7. Specific glycoproteins in the platelet membrane act as receptors for coagulants such as activated factor X. After the thrombin is formed, it detaches from the platelet surface and goes on to cleave fibrinogen enzymatically into fibrinopeptides and fibrin monomers, an unstable form of fibrin. The fibrin monomers spontaneously become polymers and develop into fibrin threads, which become the basis for the clot. Fibrin-stabilizing factor (factor XIII) is present in the plasma and can also be released from platelets. Fibrin-stabilizing factor converts the fibrin strands by cross-linking them into a strong fibrin mesh. This mesh then traps cellular components of the blood and becomes the stable clot (Guyton, 1991).

The clot retraction that follows is yet another reaction that depends on platelets. Platelets attach to the fibrin threads, where they release fibrin stabilizing factor and the contractile proteins actin and myosin. These substances cause both the platelets themselves and the clot to retract. Contraction of the edges of the injured vessel further stops the loss of blood.

The Fibrinolytic System. The fibrinolytic system provides the mechanism through which clots are eventually dissolved. This promotes the clearing of clot material from tissues and blood vessels. The fibrinolytic process is particularly important in small

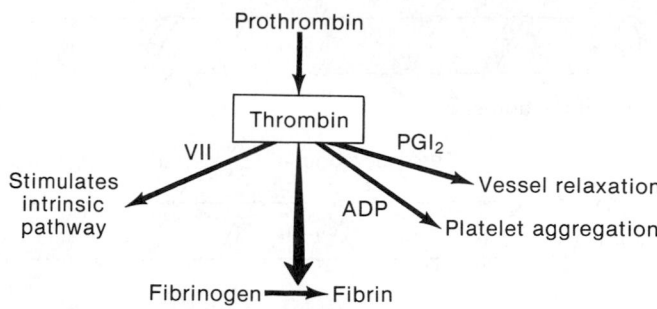

FIGURE 49–6. The role of thrombin in hemostasis. VII, factor VII; PGI$_2$, prostaglandin I$_2$; ADP, adenosine diphosphate.

peripheral vessels, which can easily become occluded by microclots (Guyton, 1991).

Both plasma fibrinolysis and cellular fibrinolysis are important in accomplishing the process of clot dissolution. The plasma fibrinolytic system can physically break apart the fibrin clot, as shown in Figure 49–5. When a clot forms, a certain amount of plasminogen becomes part of the clot along with other plasma proteins. Both tissues and blood contain factors that can activate plasminogen to become plasmin, the substance capable of chemically lysing clots. These factors include a substance released from the vascular endothelium called tissue plasminogen activator (t-PA). Genetically engineered t-PA is used clinically as thrombolytic therapy. Plasmin is also thought to be activated by thrombin, activated factor XII, and lysosomal enzymes from damaged tissues (Colman et al., 1991).

Plasmin is an active proteolytic enzyme that has the ability to hydrolyse fibrin and dissolve clots. The lysis of fibrin by plasmin takes place on the surface of the clot because both plasminogen and the activator substances are located there. This reaction results in the formation of fibrin degradation products (FDP), also called fibrin split products (Colman et al., 1991). The fibrinolytic system's activity is ultimately limited by an inhibitor, alpha-2 antiplasmin. This substance rapidly inactivates plasmin in the circulation, preventing uncontrolled fibrinolysis. If this inhibitor of fibrinolysis is exhausted, as it might be during fibrinolytic therapy, continuous fibrinolysis can occur.

FIGURE 49–7. Coagulation on the platelet surface.

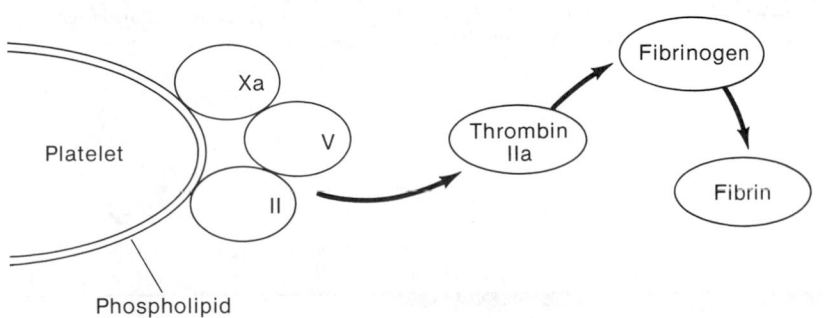

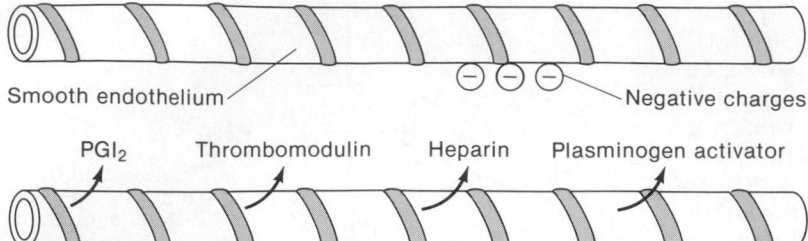

FIGURE 49–8. Anticoagulant characteristics of the vascular endothelium.

Cellular fibrinolysis has recently been found to make a significant contribution to clot destruction. Leukocytes release proteolytic enzymes that break down fibrin.

Hemostasis ultimately results in the fibrinolytic breakdown of fibrin, relaxation of the blood vessel, and healing. As a result of these processes, the vessel is usually returned to its normal state.

Control of Hemostasis

The hemostatic process is controlled by a number of mechanisms that prevent uncontrolled activity and help to ensure that clots form only where they are needed. The blood contains at least 40 substances that influence clotting. The procoagulant substances promote clotting, whereas the anticoagulant substances inhibit it. In the normal situation, the anticoagulants predominate, and the blood does not clot.

Some properties of the vascular endothelium also discourage clotting in normal blood vessels. As shown in Figure 49–8, endothelial cells are negatively charged and tend to repel the negatively charged platelets. Endothelial cells also synthesize prostaglandin I_2 (PGI$_2$), an inhibitor of platelet aggregation, and other substances that inhibit thrombin. Thrombomodulin is a substance released by the vascular endothelium that inhibits clotting. It inactivates thrombin and interacts with another natural anticoagulant, protein C, to inhibit other activated clotting factors (Colman et al., 1991).

Other naturally occurring coagulation inhibitors circulate in the blood. One of the most important is antithrombin III. The role of antithrombin III is removal of the powerful procoagulant thrombin from the circulation. Excess thrombin that is not used in the clotting process is inactivated by antithrombin III so that excessive clotting does not occur (Guyton, 1991).

Heparin is another naturally occurring substance that interferes with blood clotting. It is produced by a number of different cells, particularly the mast cells located near the capillaries. These cells and basophils secrete small amounts of heparin, which is thought to help prevent clots in the capillaries, particularly those of the lungs and liver. Heparin acts by combining with antithrombin III to remove thrombin from the circulation, thereby preventing clot formation (Guyton, 1991).

SUMMARY

The complex system of checks and balances related to hemostasis enables the body to control bleeding rapidly. Inappropriate clot formation away from the site of injury is prevented, and clots are broken down when they are no longer needed. Alterations in any part of this ongoing process can lead to clinically significant problems involving either hemorrhage or thrombosis.

References

Bellanti, J. A. (1985). *Immunology* (2nd ed.). Philadelphia: W. B. Saunders.

Clements, M. J. (1981). Functional hematology. In S. Ellerbe (Ed.), *Fluid and blood component therapy in the critically ill and injured* (pp. 21–32) New York: Churchill Livingstone.

Colman, R. W., Hirsh, J., Marder, V. J., et al. (1991). *Hemostasis and thrombosis: Basic principles and clinical practice* (2nd ed.). Philadelphia: J. B. Lippincott.

Guyton, A. C. (1991). *Human physiology and mechanisms of disease* (8th ed.). Philadelphia: W. B. Saunders.

Hirsh, J., and Brain, E. A. (1983). *Hemostasis and thrombosis* (2nd ed.). New York: Churchill Livingstone.

Jett, M. F., and Lancaster, L. E. (1983). The inflammatory-immune response: The body's defense against invasion. *Critical Care Nurse*, 3 (5), 64–84.

Williams, W. J., Beutler, E., Ersley, A. J., et al. (1983). *Hematology* (3rd ed.). New York: McGraw-Hill.

50

Patients with Coagulopathies

Diane K. Dressler

Few clinical problems are more challenging to the critical care nurse than hemorrhage. With advances in hematologic screening tests, it might be expected that bleeding problems would be predictable and preventable. However, most coagulopathies are difficult to predict. Even exhaustive screening for clotting abnormalities may not correlate with a patient's clinical course.

Nurses play a key role in the recognition and management of patients in a coagulation crisis. Because of this, it is essential for nurses to understand the complexities of both the clinical and laboratory manifestations of coagulation disorders. Acquired coagulation disorders rather than the inherited disorders are seen most commonly in critical care and in general clinical practice (Hirsh and Brain, 1983). This chapter will present the bleeding disorders associated with disseminated intravascular coagulation (DIC), vitamin K deficiency, liver insufficiency, renal insufficiency, excessive anticoagulation, primary fibrinolysis, and thrombocytopenia.

DISSEMINATED INTRAVASCULAR COAGULATION

The syndrome of DIC is known by many names—diffuse intravascular coagulation, defibrination syndrome, consumption coagulopathy, and intravascular coagulation–fibrinolysis syndrome (Wintrobe et al., 1981). This syndrome is a unique disorder of coagulation in which both hemorrhage and thrombosis, conditions that are usually diametrically opposed, occur simultaneously. DIC always occurs as a secondary process or a complication of another disease process. The syndrome has both acute and chronic forms. In critical care the acute form is seen most often and is usually considered a medical emergency (Hirsh and Brain, 1983). The chronic form of DIC is associated with certain chronic disease states, particularly oncologic disorders.

Pathophysiology

The pathophysiology of DIC is somewhat complicated and not yet completely understood (Wintrobe et al., 1981). The major pathophysiologic feature is the formation of fibrin in the bloodstream and the deposition of fibrin in the microcirculation. This excessive and inappropriate fibrin formation depletes the blood of essential clotting components, which is why DIC is referred to as a "consumption coagulopathy." As illustrated in Figure 50–1, microclots form where they are not needed. The blood becomes so depleted of coagulation factors that a stable clot cannot form at a site of injury. The ultimate result of this process is determined by the balance between the rate of fibrin formation and the rate of its clearance from the circulation. In general, clotting components are often used up faster than the liver and bone marrow can replace them.

The intravascular clotting of DIC is different from the physiologic clotting that occurs in response to an injury. In DIC clots form within the blood in response to a thrombogenic stimulus that has overwhelmed the normal inhibitors of coagulation. Multiple microclots develop and subsequently embolize into the microcirculation, where they can cause ischemia of organs and tissues (Colman et al., 1991). As shown in Figure 50–2, the process of DIC begins as a thrombotic problem and eventually becomes manifest clinically as a bleeding problem. The vascular occlusion, hemorrhage, and shock that result from this process produce profound alterations in the function of many organ systems.

The bleeding manifestations of DIC are perpetuated by the activation of the fibrinolytic system. In

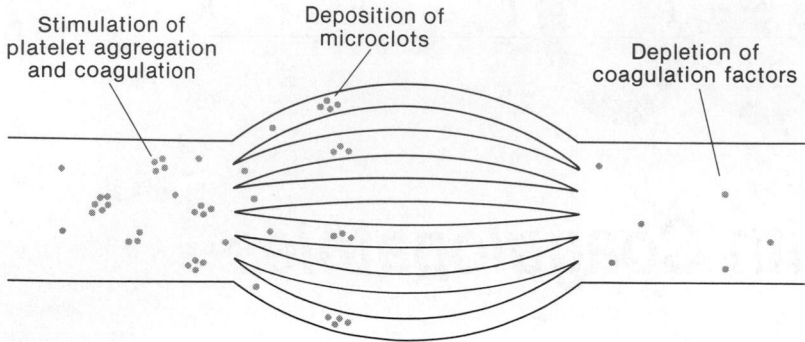

FIGURE 50–1. The process of disseminated intravascular coagulation (DIC).

DIC, plasminogen activators are released from the vascular endothelium following fibrin deposition and may also be released from platelets and leukocytes (Wintrobe et al., 1981). The plasminogen activators activate fibrinolysis, the physiologic process that breaks up fibrin clots and eventually reopens blood vessels. In DIC the fibrinolysis is often extensive and results in the release of large amounts of fibrin degradation products or fibrin split products. When fibrin degradation products (FDPs) are released, they exert an anticoagulant effect that results in more bleeding (Hirsh and Brain, 1983). The FDPs act like antithrombins, which prevent the formation of normal fibrin and impair platelet function. The presence of large amounts of FDPs in the circulation is thought to be a major factor in the hemorrhagic features of DIC (Wintrobe et al., 1981).

The syndrome of DIC was first described in the 1950s in connection with obstetric disorders. However, it may have been described around 1900 as "temporary hemophilia" (Colman et al., 1991). It was identified as a specific disorder of coagulation in the 1960s. The DIC syndrome is associated with many disease processes and can occur as a complication of a variety of disorders ranging from shock to snake-bite. As shown in Table 50–1, many disorders commonly seen in critical care can be complicated by DIC (Newland, 1985; Mersky, 1982). Chronic DIC is associated with disseminated cancer, giant hemangiomas, aneurysms, and intrauterine fetal death (Wintrobe et al., 1981). Shock states and sepsis are the most common precipitators of DIC in critically ill patients. It is thought that a clinical situation that includes hypoxia, hypotension, acidosis, and liver dysfunction may predispose the patient to DIC.

There is little information about the incidence of DIC because much of the literature is in the form of case reports. The overall incidence may be as common as 1 in 1000 hospital admissions (Wintrobe et al., 1981). Because DIC is not always manifested clinically, it may remain unrecognized in some patients.

Factors Triggering DIC

To initiate the DIC process, physiologic changes that are capable of altering the normal blood coagulation sequence must be present. So many disease processes are associated with the syndrome that most

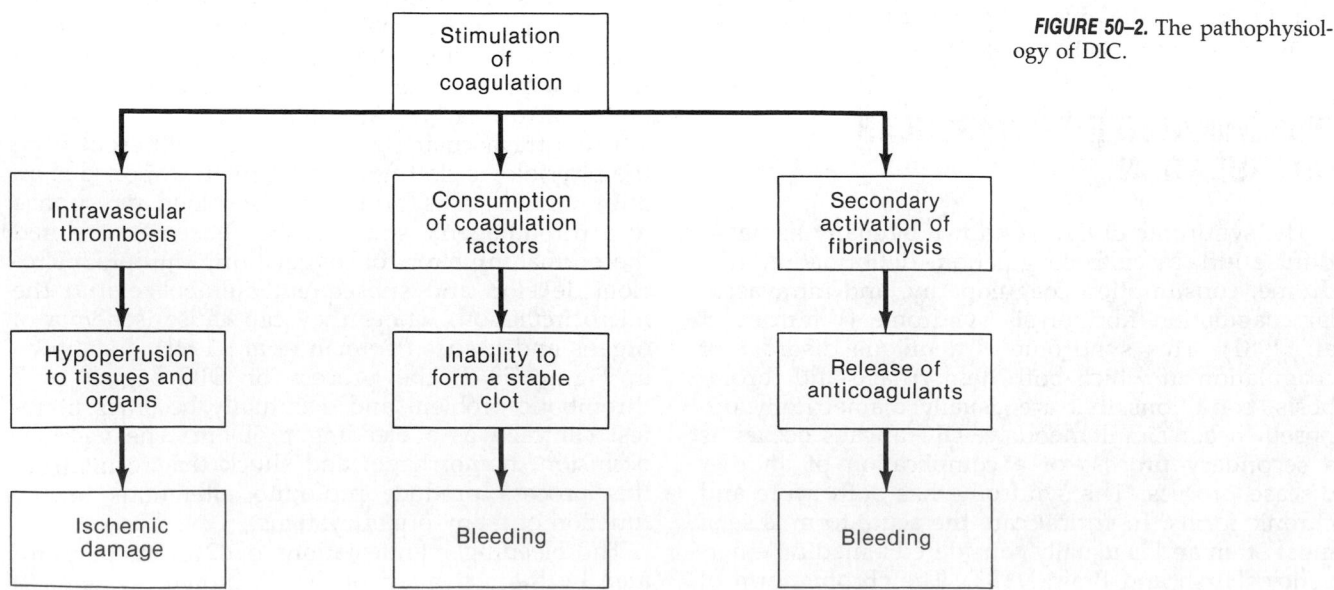

FIGURE 50–2. The pathophysiology of DIC.

TABLE 50–1. Clinical Conditions Associated with Disseminated Intravascular Coagulation (DIC)

Category	Associated Conditions
Septic processes	Bacterial infections (gram-negative most common), viral, rickettsial, protozoal, and mycotic infections
Shock states	Traumatic, septic, hemorrhagic, and cardiogenic shock
Obstetric complications	Abruptio placentae, amniotic fluid embolism, intrauterine fetal death, saline or urea-induced abortion, toxemia
Extensive trauma	Traumatic injury, severe burns, extensive surgical procedures, extracorporeal circulation, head injury
Neoplastic disorders	Acute and chronic leukemia, solid tumors of the prostate, pancreas, breast, lung, ovary, colon, and stomach
Immunologic disorders	Allograft rejection, incompatible blood transfusion, immune complex disease, anaphylactic drug reaction
Intravascular disorders	Dissecting aneurysm, giant hemangioma, vasculitis, pulmonary embolism
Miscellaneous	Venomous snake bite, heat stroke, liver failure, diabetic acidosis

authors feel that the many types of DIC do not have a common pathogenesis or even a final common pathway (Mersky, 1982). As shown in Figure 50–3, three of the processes associated with the triggering of DIC include tissue factors, factors that produce platelet aggregation, and factors that damage the blood vessel endothelium (Hirsh and Brain, 1983).

Tissue Factors. The addition of procoagulant tissue factors to the blood can be an initiating factor in DIC. When tissue damage occurs, tissue thromboplastin is released into the circulation, activating factor VII and the extrinsic coagulation pathway. This release of thromboplastic material is associated with massive trauma, obstetric complications, and tissue breakdown due to various neoplasms (Mayberry and Forte, 1985). When DIC is associated with trauma, major surgical procedures, or extensive burns, it is thought that thromboplastic substances released from the damaged tissues initiate DIC (Wintrobe et al., 1981). In patients with obstetric complications such as amniotic fluid embolism, abruptio placentae, or intrauterine fetal death, thromboplastic substances enter the maternal circulation and activate the coagulation process. In patients with neoplasms, tissue fragments and tumor microemboli may enter the circulation and act like thromboplastins. There is also evidence that some tumor cells release substances that can activate factor X directly (Greenberg et al., 1985).

Platelet Aggregation. Platelet aggregation is an early and necessary step in physiologic clotting. However, it is thought that extensive stimulation of platelet aggregation may lead to the inappropriate clotting seen in DIC. Septic processes may be associated with platelet aggregation. As endotoxin is released from the infectious organisms, the endothelium of the blood vessel walls and red blood cells may be injured. The injury may stimulate contact activation and platelet aggregation. The eventual result is excessive platelet aggregation and deposition of fibrin in the microcirculation.

The generalized Shwartzman reaction is an important experimental model of DIC (Mersky, 1982). Endotoxin injected into animal models results in fibrin formation in the glomerular capillaries with subsequent renal tubular necrosis. Changes in blood coagulation parameters are similar to those seen in patients with DIC. It is thought that the endotoxin

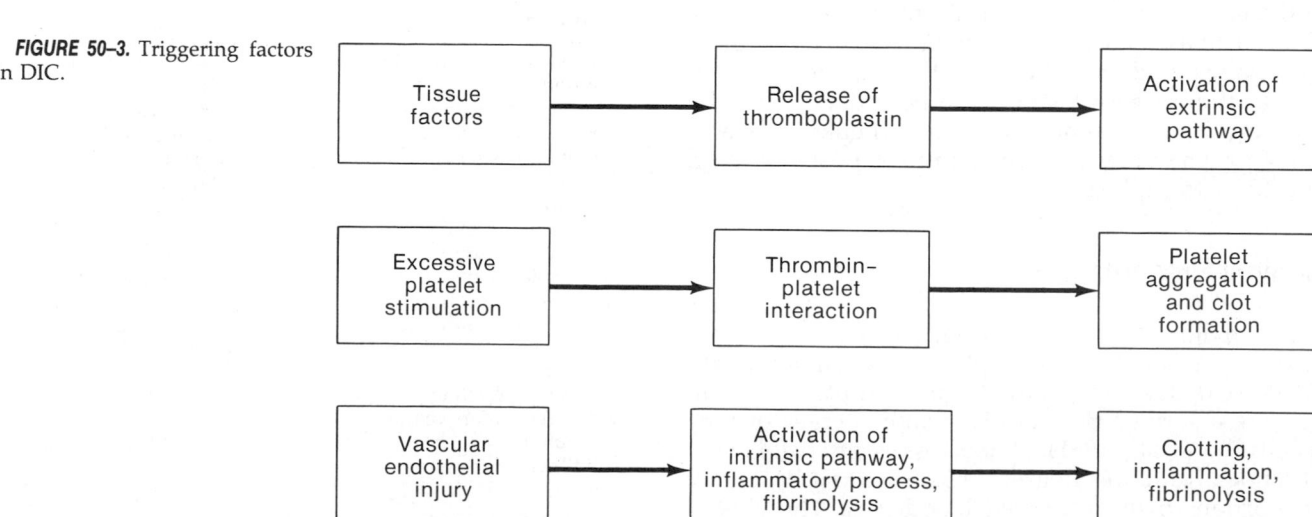

FIGURE 50–3. Triggering factors in DIC.

damages the platelets themselves as well as the endothelium, although it is unclear whether platelet injury is the cause or the result of the coagulopathy (Colman et al., 1991).

Vascular Endothelial Injury. In addition to the vascular damage done by endotoxins, the vascular endothelium may be injured during shock, acidosis, and hypoxia. This damage may directly activate the intrinsic pathway as collagen is exposed and mediators are released (Colman et al., 1991). Damage to the vascular endothelium initiates a number of interactive processes (Hirsh and Brain, 1983). Hypoperfusion, acidosis, and hypoxemia are known to initiate hypercoagulability and platelet aggregation. In addition, the inflammatory process is triggered, causing increased capillary permeability and chemotaxis of white blood cells. The WBCs may further damage the vascular endothelium as they migrate through the blood vessel walls. Monocytes in particular may play a major role in perpetuating the DIC process (Wintrobe et al., 1981). Hypoxia contributes to this process by causing a rise in chemotaxic substances.

Shock is thought to play an important role in the pathophysiologic process. Widespread endothelial damage is known to be extensive in the presence of hypoperfusion. The process of DIC is also enhanced by stasis, which inhibits the inflow of inhibitors of coagulation and impairs clearance of activated factors by the reticuloendothelial system (Colman et al., 1991). Because of this, all forms of shock can both precipitate and perpetuate DIC.

Although the specific initiating processes may vary, the pathophysiologic result is the same. Excessive production of activated coagulation factors overwhelms the normal inhibitors of coagulation, triggering DIC. In addition to the clotting and inflammation characteristic of DIC, the fibrinolytic process is initiated in an attempt to reopen the microcirculation. FDPs then perpetuate the vicious circle by contributing to the bleeding diathesis.

Three physiologic mechanisms aid recovery from this complex and destructive disorder. Reticuloendothelial cells in the liver and other organs phagocytize activated coagulation factors and remove them from the circulation. The fibrin that has been deposited in the microcirculation can be broken down by fibrinolysis, reopening the vessels. Leukocytes also assist in removing microcirculatory deposits of fibrin and fibrin complexes.

Clinical Presentation

The major clinical manifestation of acute DIC is bleeding, often from multiple sites (Colman et al., 1991). The bleeding may begin abruptly and can become a serious problem in a short period of time (Wintrobe et al., 1981). Blood loss is often followed by shock, and the degree of shock may be out of proportion to the observed blood loss. The clinical

signs of DIC are outlined in Table 50–2. There may be oozing of blood from incisions, injury sites, and puncture sites (Williams et al., 1983). Sites that were previously observed to be dry and healing may begin to bleed as fibrinolysis begins to dissolve clots. Petechiae or purpura may be observed as well as expanding hematomas. Bleeding from apparently healthy mucous membranes may occur.

In some patients a major hemorrhagic event is the first sign of DIC. Bleeding may begin in the gastrointestinal tract, genitourinary tract, or central nervous system. In surgical patients, postoperative hemorrhage may be precipitated.

The deposition of fibrin in the microcirculation can produce hypoperfusion and ischemic damage to tissues and organs. An unusual type of skin discoloration called acral cyanosis may develop on the patient's lips, nose, ears, fingers, and toes (Wintrobe et al., 1981). This type of cyanosis is characterized by gray to purple discoloration of the skin with sharp irregular lines of demarcation from normal areas. It results from the obstruction of the microcirculation and in some instances can lead to tissue necrosis.

Ischemia of major organs can occur as a result of DIC. Acute tubular necrosis (ATN) is the most common example of this process, as fibrin begins to block the glomerular capillaries (Colman et al., 1991). Respiratory insufficiency may develop as the alveolar capillaries are affected. Diarrhea and abdominal pain may indicate involvement of the gastrointestinal tract. Confusion and seizure activity may indicate that the central nervous system is affected. The circulatory and hypovolemic shock that occur in addition to vessel thrombosis further contribute to organ ischemia.

The clinical signs of DIC vary considerably depending on the initiating process, the extent of tissue and organ damage, and the severity of bleeding. In general, signs of DIC result from bleeding and from

TABLE 50–2. Clinical Features in DIC

Hemorrhagic	Thrombotic
Obvious cutaneous bleeding	Cutaneous ischemia
Incisions	Acral cyanosis
Mucous membranes	Tissue necrosis
Recent trauma sites	Gastrointestinal tract
Old trauma sites	Diarrhea
Petechiae	Abdominal pain
Purpura	Genitourinary/renal
Hematoma formation	Oliguria
Gastrointestinal tract	Anuria
Active bleeding	↑ BUN and creatinine
Genitourinary/renal	Central nervous system
Active bleeding	Convulsions
Hematuria	Coma
ulmonary	
Interstitial bleeding	
Adult respiratory distress syndrome	
Central nervous system	
Fatal hemorrhage	

microcirculatory occlusion. However, in the subacute form of DIC, thrombosis may dominate the clinical picture. Occasionally, patients in whom DIC is suspected may have no obvious signs or symptoms, and DIC is detected only by abnormal laboratory results.

Laboratory Findings

Acquired disorders of blood coagulation such as DIC are associated with multiple abnormalities in the clotting scheme. There is no one diagnostic test for DIC. When this disorder is suspected, a complete coagulation panel should be obtained. Key laboratory tests that screen for DIC include the prothrombin time (PT), the activated partial thromboplastin time (APTT), the thrombin time (TT), fibrinogen level, platelet count, and the presence of FDPs (Wintrobe et al., 1981).

The PT, APTT, and TT are general screening tests of coagulation. As seen in Table 50–3, they test the intrinsic, extrinsic, and common pathways of coagulation and may all be prolonged in a patient with DIC (Williams et al., 1983). The fibrinogen level is usually low in patients with DIC. The level may drop precipitously as fibrinogen is consumed in the formation of fibrin. Thrombocytopenia is an early and consistent indicator of DIC (Colman et al., 1991). The platelet count usually falls to less than 50,000/mm³ and may be depressed out of proportion to other coagulation abnormalities. It is thought that platelets may be readily consumed as they adhere to damaged surfaces (Wintrobe et al., 1981).

Measurement of the FDPs assesses the rate of fibrinolysis that is occurring. FDPs are frequently elevated to over 100 μg/mL in patients with DIC, indicating excessive fibrinolysis. Other tests for fibrinolysis may be done as well. The plasminogen level may be assessed; decreased plasminogen indicates that plasminogen has been converted to plasmin, and fibrinolysis is taking place (Colman et al., 1991). The euglobulin clot lysis time may be measured and

is shortened when excessive fibrinolysis is taking place.

There are other coagulation panel results that may indicate DIC. Factors V and VIII may be depleted. The peripheral blood is examined for schistocytes, which are distorted and fragmented red blood cells. The red cells become physically damaged when they try to pass through the fibrin strands that obstruct the microcirculation (Newland, 1985). A test for fibrin monomers, an unstable form of fibrin, such as the protamine sulfate test may be performed. This test is indicative of abnormal fibrin formation, and a positive result is a strong indicator of DIC. Severe depletion of antithrombin III usually occurs in DIC and can be revealed through an antithrombin III assay (Wintrobe et al., 1981).

Some physiologic and pathophysiologic states may change a patient's baseline coagulation panel. In patients with hepatic insufficiency the liver is often unable to synthesize normal levels of prothrombin, fibrinogen, and other factors. Certain stress states such as pregnancy, neoplasms, and infection can increase the levels of fibrinogen and factor VIII (Colman et al., 1991). When coagulation parameters are monitored, serial tests are usually done to detect trends in clotting times and factor levels. Trends are the most important assessment parameters because often the patient's baseline values are unknown.

Even after analysis of multiple coagulation panel results, laboratory diagnosis of DIC can be difficult. At times a definite laboratory diagnosis of DIC cannot be made. A hematologist may be consulted to assist in the interpretation of coagulation parameters and to discuss treatment options.

Medical Management

The DIC syndrome usually is a complication of a serious underlying disorder, and the original problem must be considered in the treatment plan. Treatment of DIC is challenging because three hematologic

TABLE 50–3. Coagulation Tests for DIC

Test	What Is Measured	Normal Result	Result in DIC
Prothrombin time	Extrinsic and common pathways	12 seconds	Prolonged
Activated partial thromboplastin time	Intrinsic and common pathways	≤33 seconds	Prolonged
Thrombin time	Rate of conversion of fibrinogen to fibrin	25–45 seconds	Prolonged
Fibrinogen level	Amount of fibrinogen available to form fibrin	170–410 mg/dL	Usually low, fibrinogen consumed
Platelet count	Platelets available for clot formation	150,000–400,000/mm³	Low, platelets consumed
Fibrin degradation products	Action of plasmin on fibrin or fibrinogen	<10 μg/mL	Often >100 μg/mL
RBC morphology	Look for abnormal RBCs	Normal RBCs	Schistocytes present
Plasminogen	Amount available to become plasmin	75–125%	Low due to excessive fibrinolysis
Protamine sulfate test	Presence of normal fibrin strands	Monomers negative	Monomers (unstable fibrin) positive
Antithrombin III assay	Amount available to inactivate thrombin	75–125%	Low

abnormalities—thrombosis, hemorrhage, and fibrinolysis—may be occurring simultaneously. The major treatment options for DIC are outlined in Figure 50–4.

Most sources agree that reversal of the DIC syndrome depends first on prompt treatment of the underlying disorder (Hirsh and Brain, 1983; Mayberry and Forte, 1985; Wintrobe et al., 1981). For example, if the syndrome was precipitated by gram-negative sepsis, appropriate intravenous antibiotic therapy is begun immediately. Nonspecific supportive therapy is also very important in preventing further deterioration in the patient's condition. Ventilatory assistance may be necessary to ensure adequate oxygenation. Circulatory support with fluid replacement and inotropic drugs are often needed until hemodynamic factors are stabilized. When acute tubular necrosis complicates the situation, hemodialysis may eventually be necessary. The circulatory shock that accompanies the DIC syndrome contributes to the degree of shock and acidosis. Because DIC is perpetuated by these pathophysiologic alterations, every attempt is made to reverse them. Aggressive treatment of the underlying disorder and appropriate supportive treatment will halt the DIC process in some patients.

Anticoagulant Therapy. Anticoagulant therapy may be used in the treatment of DIC. Heparin therapy is used occasionally in patients with acute DIC. More commonly, heparin is utilized in the subacute form of DIC because it seems to be most effective when major thrombosis is part of the clinical picture (Mayberry and Forte, 1985). Heparin activates the antithrombin III system. It interrupts the intravascular generation of thrombin, preventing further deposition of fibrin in the microcirculation (Franco, 1981). When heparin is used, the antithrombin III level is measured first. Fresh frozen plasma may be administered to increase the plasma antithrombin III level (Greenberg et al., 1983). Therapeutic or low doses of heparin may be given, and the patient is carefully monitored for response to the drug. Laboratory control of heparin therapy is difficult due to the multiple alterations in coagulation parameters already present. Administration of heparin to a patient with actual or potential bleeding seems paradoxical, and this is probably the only time heparin may be given to a bleeding patient (Williams et al., 1983). It may be contraindicated in some patients such as those with bleeding from the central nervous system, gastrointestinal tract, or recent surgery (Greenberg et al., 1985).

Other pharmacologic agents may be used in the treatment of DIC. Platelet inhibitors such as dipyridamole and aspirin are being investigated for use in DIC (Franco, 1981). Antifibrinolytic agents such as epsilon-aminocaproic acid (Amicar) may be avoided because of potential complication of fatal thromboembolism associated with their use (Mersky, 1982). When antifibrinolytic agents are used, heparin is administered first (Colman et al., 1991). Thrombolytic agents such as streptokinase have been tried experimentally with varying results (Wintrobe et al., 1981).

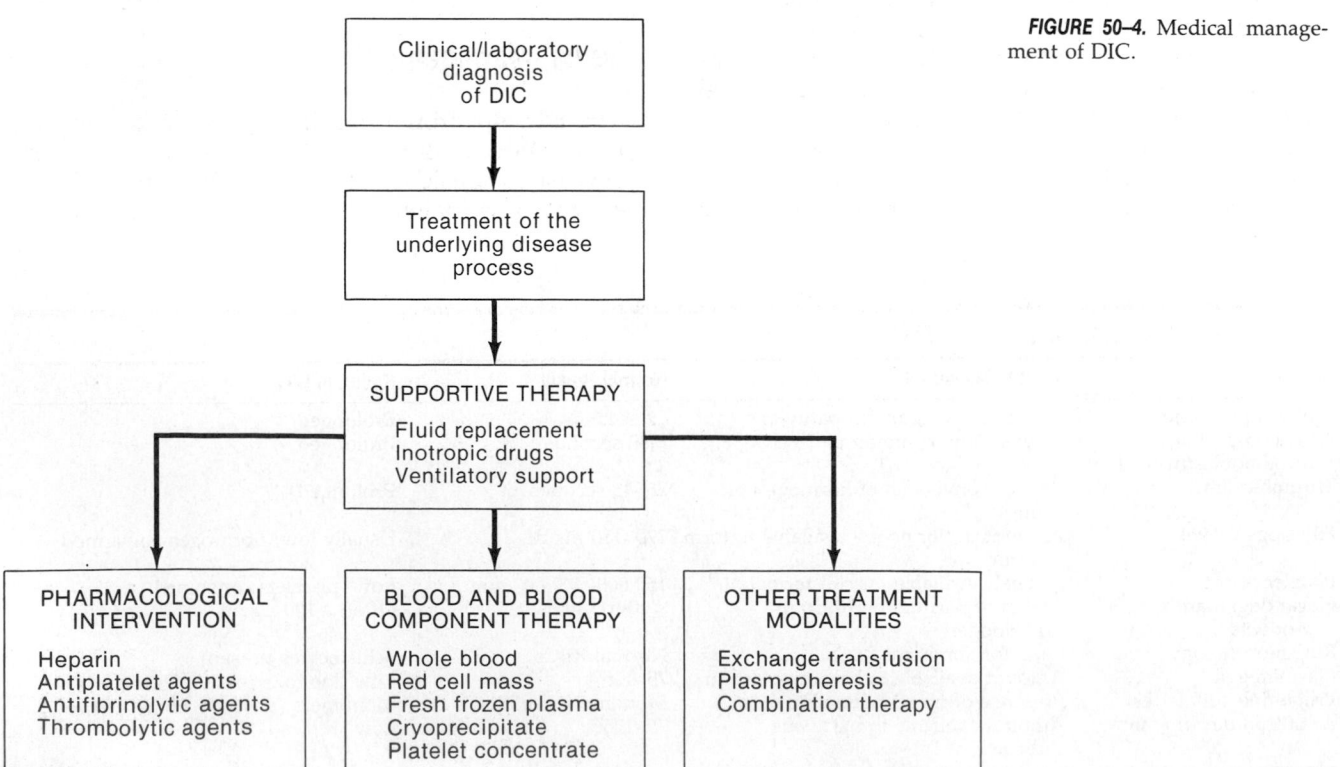

FIGURE 50–4. Medical management of DIC.

Blood Component Therapy. The value of whole blood and blood component therapy in DIC is somewhat controversial. Some sources caution that administration of components may be adding "fuel to the fire" because more fibrinogen and platelets are available for further clotting (Wintrobe et al., 1981). However, in patients who develop a bleeding diathesis due to DIC, it is usually necessary to replace the losses. In clinical practice, the greater the blood loss, the more blood and blood components will be given to replace lost volume and restore hemostasis and oxygen-carrying capacity (Mersky, 1982). Most commonly, red cell mass, whole blood, fresh frozen plasma, platelet concentrate, and cryoprecipitate are given. Fresh frozen plasma restores factor V, prothrombin, and other essential clotting factors. Fibrinogen and factor VIII can be replaced with cryoprecipitate. Whole blood and blood components do not contain active platelets, so platelet concentrate may be given to replace these (Greenberg et al., 1985).

Other Therapeutic Measures. As in all situations involving hypovolemic shock, intravenous fluid resuscitation is necessary to restore depleted intracellular and extracellular fluid volume. Lactated Ringer's solution, normal saline, and plasma protein fraction (albumin) are titrated to maintain adequate blood pressure, central venous pressure, pulmonary capillary wedge pressure, and urine output.

Other therapeutic measures may include exchange transfusions and plasmapheresis. It is thought that exchanging the patient's plasma removes fibrin degradation products and supplies fresh clotting components. Often a combination of therapies may be used such as heparin and blood transfusion. Research on these and other therapeutic measures for DIC continues.

Even with prompt and aggressive treatment, it may take hours to days to control the bleeding (Colman et al., 1991). Mortality from DIC is estimated to range from 54% to 68% (Greenberg et al., 1985; Rooney and Haviley, 1985). Mortality increases with the patient's age, the number of clinical manifestations present, and the severity of alterations in the coagulation parameters.

OTHER ACQUIRED COAGULATION DISORDERS

In addition to DIC, other acquired coagulation problems are commonly seen in critical care. The basic pathophysiology, clinical features, laboratory features, and medical management of the more common disorders will be described next.

Vitamin K Deficiency

Vitamin K is normally obtained from food, especially green leafy vegetables. It is also synthesized by microbiologic flora in the normal gastrointestinal tract. As shown in Figure 50–5, vitamin K is absorbed by the gastrointestinal tract in the presence of bile salts and pancreatic lipases (Hirsh and Brain, 1983). It is required for the hepatic synthesis of prothrombin (factor II) and factors VII, IX, and X. A deficiency of vitamin K is uncommon in healthy people but can result from inadequate intake in critically ill and chronically ill patients. Patients receiving total parenteral nutrition are at risk because this vitamin is not metabolized when it is administered through a central venous line (Colman et al., 1991); it must be administered separately.

Other patients may have inadequate absorption of the vitamin due to fat malabsorption or a lack of bile

FIGURE 50–5. Production of coagulation factors by the liver.

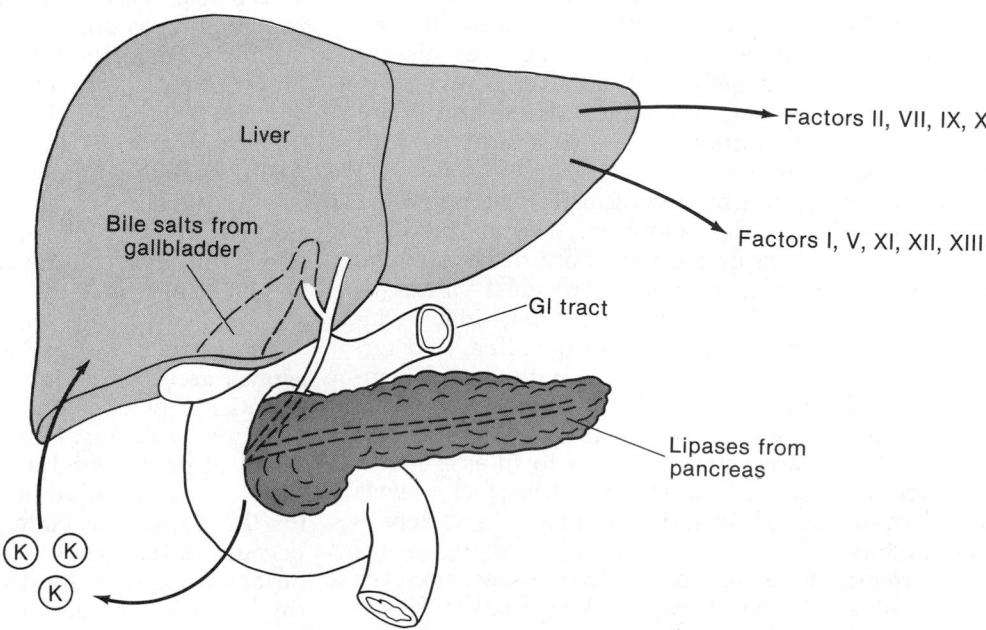

Liver

Bile salts from gallbladder

GI tract

Factors II, VII, IX, X

Factors I, V, XI, XII, XIII

Lipases from pancreas

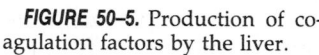

salts, as might occur in patients with biliary obstruction or pancreatic disease. Antibiotic therapy, especially therapy with broad-spectrum antibiotics, may interfere with the synthesis of vitamin K by intestinal flora. The amount of vitamin K available for production of coagulation factors may be significantly decreased.

Clinical features of vitamin K deficiency include cutaneous ecchymosis, epistaxis, gastrointestinal bleeding, and the potential for postoperative hemorrhage. There are no specific laboratory tests diagnostic of vitamin K deficiency. In most instances, the prothrombin time is prolonged. The patient's history is important in making the diagnosis.

Treatment of vitamin K deficiency generally involves administration of vitamin K preparations. Attempts are also made to correct the cause of the disorder. Transfusion therapy may be appropriate if severe hemorrhage and factor deficiencies develop.

In addition to acquired vitamin K deficiency, the syndrome is commonly present in newborn babies (Hirsh and Brain, 1983). During the first few days of life, the liver may be unable to synthesize vitamin K–dependent clotting factors, and intestinal flora are not yet present to synthesize the vitamin. This syndrome, called hemorrhagic disease of the newborn, is generally treated with prophylactic administration of vitamin K at birth.

Liver Disease

Alterations in liver function often result in coagulation abnormalities. As shown in Figure 50–5, the liver synthesizes almost all coagulation factors (except factor VIII), including fibrinogen, factor V, and the vitamin K–dependent factors (Colman et al., 1991). Liver problems such as cirrhosis and hepatic failure limit the production of these coagulation factors, resulting directly in clotting deficiencies. In addition, thrombocytopenia may complicate the situation because patients with chronic liver disease and portal hypertension may have congestive splenomegaly and pooling of platelets (Hirsh and Brain, 1983). Increased fibrinolysis is also associated with hepatic insufficiency.

Easy bruising is a mild clinical feature associated with these deficiencies. However, serious bleeding may follow trauma or surgery. Local lesions in the gastrointestinal tract such as esophageal varices or peptic ulcer can also lead to severe bleeding. Portacaval shunt surgery, fulminating hepatitis, and terminal liver disease are associated with severe hemorrhage (Colman et al., 1991).

The prothrombin time is usually prolonged when liver problems are severe enough to interfere with production of coagulation factors. Other factor levels are often depressed, including the vitamin K–dependent factors.

Treatment of bleeding due to liver disease involves treatment of the underlying problem. Vitamin K may

be administered. Transfusion with whole blood and blood components is often necessary and may be helpful but is only a temporary measure unless there is hope for recovery of hepatic function.

Bleeding Due to Anticoagulation Therapy

Clinical indications for the use of anticoagulants include actual or potential thromboembolism. This suppression of the normal coagulation process always carries with it the risk of bleeding, either spontaneous or provoked. Spontaneous bleeding most often occurs in the form of ecchymoses, gastrointestinal bleeding, hematuria, and retroperitoneal hemorrhage. Bleeding may also be precipitated during trauma from surgery or invasive procedures. Patients at increased risk of bleeding complications from anticoagulant therapy include those who have had recent surgery and those with a history of gastrointestinal bleeding.

Warfarin. Warfarin, because of its predictable action and duration of effect, is the oral anticoagulant most commonly used (Walsh, 1983). It is thought to compete with vitamin K–dependent factors, including the pivotal factor prothrombin. The prothrombin time is monitored in patients receiving warfarin; the usual therapeutic goal is to achieve a prothrombin time of 1½ to 2 times the control value. Antiplatelet agents are often given concurrently, so that the prothrombin time does not need to be prolonged beyond 1½ times the control, decreasing the incidence of bleeding. The effects of warfarin can be reversed by stopping the drug. More rapid reversal can be achieved by administering vitamin K and fresh frozen plasma.

Heparin. Heparin, the most commonly used intravenous anticoagulant, acts by combining with antithrombin III to inhibit thrombin and other factors, preventing clot formation (Deykin, 1982). The modes of heparin therapy include full-dose intravenous therapy and low-dose subcutaneous heparin. The APTT is most commonly monitored in patients receiving heparin. Therapeutic levels are usually considered to be 1½ to 2½ times the control value (Goodwin, 1985). Intravenous protamine sulfate can be given to reverse the effects of heparin.

Antiplatelet Drugs. Antiplatelet drugs such as aspirin are used commonly in patients with cardiovascular problems and have been associated with bleeding problems. Aspirin affects the platelet synthesis of prostaglandin and thus interferes with the platelet release reaction, inhibiting platelet function for the life of the platelet (Hirsh and Brain, 1983). Because of this, aspirin ingestion will have an effect on blood platelets for 4 to 7 days. In most patients, this effect will prolong the bleeding time only slightly. However, defects in hemostasis are magnified in patients who have taken aspirin. Ingestion of a single aspirin tablet can potentially lengthen the bleeding time to 30 minutes (from a normal of 5 to 8 minutes) and can induce hemorrhage in patients who are prone to coagulation problems. The drug 1-deamino-8-D-arginine vasopressin (DDAVP) may be used to promote hemostasis in patients who have ingested aspirin (Colman et al., 1991).

Renal Failure

The coagulation derangements that accompany renal failure can result in serious clinical problems. The bleeding tendency in these patients is thought to be caused mainly by a qualitative platelet defect (Colman et al., 1991). The metabolic imbalances that result from uremia have an adverse effect on platelet function.

Treatment of the renal failure itself, such as with dialysis and a low-protein diet, often improves coagulation abnormalities because the problem is proportional to the blood urea nitrogen (BUN). Blood and blood component therapy are frequently used, especially because these patients are anemic due to the lack of erythropoietin. The drug DDAVP has been used to improve platelet function temporarily in patients with renal failure.

Primary Fibrinolysis

Primary pathologic fibrinolysis is an acute and severe bleeding disorder that can resemble DIC. However, it must be distinguished from DIC because the treatment differs. As shown in Figure 50–6, excessive fibrinolysis results when tissue plasminogen activator (t-PA) is suddenly released into the blood (Hirsh and Brain, 1983). This syndrome can be induced by cardiothoracic surgery, metastatic cancer of the prostate, injury to the genitourinary tract, or other extensive trauma. Following the release of plasminogen activator, newly formed clots are broken down, and recently injured blood vessels resume bleeding. The disorder is most severe when it occurs in conjunction with hepatic insufficiency because in this condition there is insufficient production of alpha-2 antiplasmin, the naturally occurring substance

that inactivates plasmin and controls fibrinolysis. A fibrinolytic state may also be produced intentionally with administration of fibrinolytic agents such as streptokinase, urokinase, and recombinant t-PA. Bleeding resulting from excessive fibrinolysis may be a complication of the drug therapy.

The major clinical feature of primary fibrinolysis is post-traumatic or postoperative bleeding. In addition to bleeding from injury sites, internal bleeding from ulcerations in the gastrointestinal tract may occur.

Coagulation parameters pertinent to fibrinolysis are abnormal. The level of FDPs is elevated, the euglobulin clot lysis time short, and the plasminogen level decreased. Factors such as platelets may not be depleted as they are in DIC. Differential diagnosis can be difficult because fibrinolysis occurs as a secondary process in DIC.

The usual treatment for primary fibrinolysis is administration of an inhibitor of fibrinolysis such as epsilon-aminocaproic acid (Amicar). Following a series of intravenous doses of this drug, bleeding will usually cease (Colman et al., 1991). The drug is usually contraindicated in DIC because of the risk of major thrombosis following its administration in these patients (Wintrobe et al., 1981).

Thrombocytopenia

Platelets play a role in many places in the coagulation process, from plugging small tears in capillaries to providing phospholipids for clot formation and retraction. An inadequate number of platelets inhibit the coagulation process and can lead to both minor and major bleeding problems.

Thrombocytopenia can occur as a result of decreased production, increased destruction, or pooling of platelets in the spleen (Hirsh and Brain, 1983). Decreased production of platelets in the bone marrow is associated with leukemia, various anemias, and uremia. This is also a well-recognized side effect of cancer chemotherapy and radiation therapy. Increased destruction of platelets can occur in patients with severe infectious processes, diseases of the liver and spleen, and autoimmune disease. Reduced platelet survival is also associated with cardiopulmonary bypass and the intra-aortic balloon pump. Pooling of platelets in the spleen is associated with disorders that produce splenomegaly.

FIGURE 50–6. Primary fibrinolysis. FDP, fibrin degradation products.

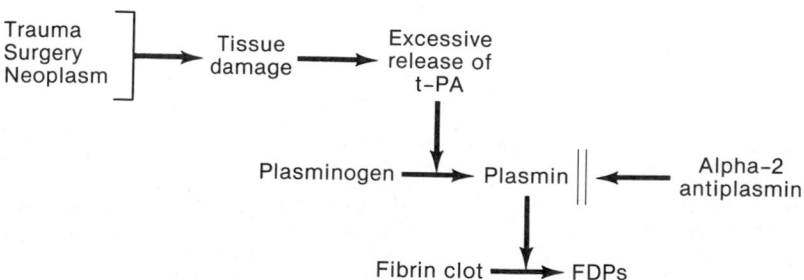

A platelet count of under 150,000 is diagnostic of thrombocytopenia. The clinical features of thrombocytopenia may include petechiae, bleeding from mucous membranes, and actual hemorrhage. However, bleeding due to thrombocytopenia is difficult to predict. Some patients with a severely low platelet count may not bleed, whereas others with moderately depressed counts may experience major bleeding. As shown in Table 50–4, spontaneous bleeding usually does not occur until the platelet count falls below 50,000 (Guyton, 1991). As the platelet count falls, the risk of bleeding increases, and at below 10,000 there is considerable risk of spontaneous central nervous system or gastrointestinal hemorrhage (Hirsh and Brain, 1983).

When possible, thrombocytopenia is treated by treating the underlying cause. For example, if it is thought to be a side effect of a drug, the drug is stopped. Platelet transfusions are indicated in patients at risk of spontaneous or provoked bleeding.

It must also be recognized that there are qualitative disorders of platelet function. The number of platelets present in the blood may not always predict their hemostatic capability, especially in patients who have received platelet-inhibiting drugs. When platelet dysfunction is suspected, platelet concentrate may be administered to provide active platelets. The drug DDAVP may be given to increase the plasma level of von Willebrand factor and improve hemostasis in conditions associated with defective platelet function (Salzman et al., 1986).

Another type of thrombocytopenia that is not associated with bleeding is seen in conjunction with heparin administration. Heparin can cause two types of thrombocytopenia (Deykin, 1982; Herring and Shelburne, 1984). There may be a transient fall in the platelet count with an initial loading dose of heparin due to the direct action of heparin on platelets. In addition, a second and more serious reaction can occur, involving a delayed but precipitous fall in the platelet count following the administration of full- or low-dose heparin. The mechanism is thought to involve the production of antiplatelet antibodies that induce clotting. This syndrome of heparin-induced thrombocytopenia is associated with recurrent venous and arterial thrombosis. Major thrombotic events such as stroke, myocardial infarction, pulmonary emboli, and thrombotic occlusion of major vessels may occur (King and Kelton, 1984). The documented incidence of this syndrome in patients receiving heparin is as high as 10%. Because of this risk, it is recommended that platelet counts be mon-

itored before and during heparin administration. Laboratory testing for heparin antibodies may also be appropriate in certain patients who have received heparin on numerous occasions. When the syndrome is suspected, heparin must be discontinued, including even small amounts used in hemodynamic monitoring lines.

NURSING MANAGEMENT OF THE PATIENT WITH COAGULOPATHY

In addition to medical diagnosis and treatment, specific nursing interventions are necessary to treat existing problems and prevent potential problems during a coagulation crisis. An understanding of the pathophysiology of bleeding disorders plus their clinical recognition and medical management suggests the following nursing diagnoses, expected outcomes of nursing care, and strategies needed to achieve the outcomes (Dressler, 1987, 1989).

Potential for Fluid (Blood) Volume Deficit

In patients with coagulopathy, essential clotting components are often depleted, and fibrinolysis may be activated, predisposing the patient to potential hemorrhage and severe volume depletion. The expected outcomes of nursing care include early recognition of overt and covert bleeding and early control of bleeding.

The critical care nurse plays a key role in the recognition of a bleeding problem. All incisions, puncture sites, and skin lesions are observed for signs of bleeding (Caplan, 1984). Because the mucous membranes bleed easily, it is important to watch for epistaxis and bleeding from the gums after mouth care is given. Expanding hematomas and swollen extremities need to be measured and monitored because bleeding into the muscles and compartments can occur insidiously. Abdominal girth should be assessed at intervals when peritoneal bleeding is suspected.

Exit sites of tubes and catheters are inspected periodically (Kirchner and Reheis, 1982). Surgical drainage containers need to be checked for increased drainage. Tracheal secretions are observed for evidence of pulmonary hemorrhage. It is particularly important to watch for bleeding from more than one source. Bleeding from multiple sites is often a sign of a coagulation problem and must be reported. Early identification of bleeding and initiation of treatment can minimize blood loss.

In critically ill patients, bleeding can lead to shock within a short period of time. Vital signs are evaluated for evidence of hypotension, labile blood pressure, low central venous pressure (CVP) or low pulmonary capillary wedge pressure (PCWP), tachy-

TABLE 50–4. Bleeding from Thrombocytopenia

Platelet Count	Effect on Hemostasis
150,000–400,000/mm³	No abnormal bleeding
50,000–150,000/mm³	Abnormal bleeding with trauma
10,000–50,000/mm³	Spontaneous bleeding possible
<10,000/mm³	Severe spontaneous bleeding common

cardia, and weak thready pulse. These signs may be indicative of occult bleeding. Extremities are inspected for evidence of poor perfusion such as coldness, delayed capillary refill, weak or absent peripheral pulses, and cyanosis. Urine output is assessed frequently because oliguria may result from hypotension, decreased blood volume, or thrombi in the renal vasculature (Mayberry and Forte, 1985).

Urine, stools, and nasogastric drainage are tested for occult blood. X-rays are checked for unexpected fluid collection. Changes in the level of consciousness are carefully evaluated because cerebral anoxia can occur as a result of hypovolemia, hypoxemia, and emboli. Patient reports of headache, joint pain, or abdominal pain are carefully assessed.

When a coagulation problem is suspected, laboratory data are monitored for a drop in hemoglobin and hematocrit and for changes in coagulation parameters. A flow sheet or computerized report that displays trends in laboratory data may be helpful in detecting problems, such as a falling platelet count. Changes in the laboratory data may be evident before clinical bleeding occurs, and likewise, improvement in coagulation parameters may be evident before bleeding decreases.

When a bleeding problem is identified, nursing care is directed toward minimizing the loss of blood. The patient is placed on bedrest, and oxygen therapy is adjusted to meet specific needs. The amount and character of the bleeding are reported to the physician. Care is taken not to disturb any clots during dressing changes because patients with coagulopathy may be unable to form new clots. Local measures such as pressure and cold compresses may be used to control bleeding from skin sites. Topical hemostatic agents may be prescribed. Bleeding from the gastrointestinal tract, genitourinary tract, or respiratory tract may require specific medical intervention.

Actual Fluid (Blood) Volume Deficit

In patients with a coagulopathy, a large amount of blood may be lost within a short period of time. Expected outcomes of nursing care include prevention of acute anemia, acute anoxia, and hypovolemic circulatory failure.

The patient with a coagulopathy must be continuously monitored for signs and symptoms of hypovolemic shock. These signs, plus any overt or covert signs of bleeding, must be reported to the physician. Fluid volume replacement is initiated to replace extracellular and intracellular volume and restore adequate blood pressure and cardiac filling pressures.

It is important to be aware of all drug actions and interactions related to coagulation. For example, aspirin or other anticoagulants should not be given unintentionally to a patient with a coagulopathy (Rooney and Haviley, 1985). When anticoagulant medication such as heparin is ordered for patients with DIC, the patient must be closely monitored for increased bleeding or other untoward effects. Laboratory values such as APTT are checked periodically but are often difficult to interpret due to multiple abnormalities. Because of this, clinical assessment of the patient is particularly important.

When active hemorrhage occurs, whole blood and blood components need to be administered to ensure maximum effectiveness. Table 50–5 outlines the blood components used most often to treat coagulopathies. Whole blood may be used in patients with acute hemorrhagic shock (Tannenbaum, 1983). It restores blood volume and oxygen-carrying capacity. Red cell mass is used more commonly. Each unit of red cell mass has the same oxygen-carrying capacity as whole blood but less volume and less serum containing the undesirable amounts of potassium, glucose, ammonia, and anticoagulant.

TABLE 50–5. Blood and Blood Components

Component	Contents	Indication	Shelf Life	Comments
Whole blood cells	Red cells, plasma, all components	Acute active hemorrhagic, hypovolemic shock	35 days	Restores blood volume and oxygen-carrying capacity
Red cell mass	Red cells, little plasma, WBCs, or platelets	Anemia, hypovolemic shock	Same as whole blood	Same oxygen-carrying capacity as whole blood; less volume, less plasma decreases reactions
Fresh frozen plasma	Plasma with most coagulation factors, no platelets	Many coagulation disorders, factor deficiencies	12 months frozen, 2 hours thawed	Give as soon as thawed
Cryoprecipitate	Factors I and VIII	DIC, hemophilia, von Willebrand factor deficiency	12 months frozen, 4 hours thawed	Give as soon as thawed
Platelet concentrate	Platelets, few WBCs and some plasma	Bleeding due to thrombocytopenia	5 days	No refrigeration; multiple units given together. Each unit should raise count by 5000 to 10,000
Albumin, plasma protein fraction	Heat-treated fraction of pooled plasma	Volume or colloid deficiency	3 to 5 years	Use as volume expander while blood is cross-matched

Fresh frozen plasma contains most active coagulation factors except platelets. It is used for patients with specific factor deficiencies, such as a low level of factor V. Fresh frozen plasma may also be administered when the specific deficiency is unknown because it contains so many essential components. This particular component should be infused as soon as it is thawed because some of the coagulation factors become inactive with time (Tannenbaum, 1983).

Cryoprecipitate is also commonly prescribed to treat patients with coagulation disorders such as DIC. It contains fibrinogen and factor VIII. Infusion of multiple units is required to replace depleted factors. Cryoprecipitate should also be infused as soon as possible after thawing (Massorli and Piercy, 1984).

Platelet concentrate is frequently given for bleeding due to thrombocytopenia or qualitative platelet disorders. Multiple donor units are given to attempt to raise the platelet count above 40,000 and prevent spontaneous bleeding (Mersky, 1982).

Patients with a coagulopathy frequently undergo massive blood transfusion. They must be closely monitored for adverse reactions related to the infusion of blood and blood components. Table 50–6 outlines the adverse reactions that may be observed.

During massive transfusion it is particularly important to measure hemodynamic parameters, including CVP and PCWP, before, during, and after the infusion of each unit of blood or blood component. Replacing the patient's blood loss is important to prevent shock, yet volume overload can easily become a complication of transfusion therapy. The appearance of dyspnea, rales, and pulmonary congestion may indicate fluid volume overload.

Hypothermia can result from rapid infusion of cold blood and blood components, leading to chills, decreased body temperature, and ventricular dysrhythmias. These symptoms are especially prevalent when the blood is infused through a central venous line (Smith, 1984). It may be necessary to use a blood warmer when infusing multiple units.

Hyperkalemia can result from the infusion of multiple units of blood as potassium diffuses from the intracellular space into the extracellular fluid in stored blood, increasing the serum potassium level in the plasma. When large volumes of blood are infused, the electrocardiogram should be continuously monitored for changes indicative of hyperkalemia, such as peaked T waves, widening QRS complexes, and bradycardia.

Citrate intoxication and hypocalcemia may also result from the infusion of large amounts of stored blood. The anticoagulant that prevents blood from clotting in the blood bag is citrate. Citrate acts by precipitating the serum calcium. Because calcium is necessary for blood coagulation, the blood does not clot. Infusion of large amounts of citrate can potentially precipitate the patient's serum calcium. This further decreases the ability of the blood to clot and may result in signs of hypocalcemic tetany. Because of these potential problems, the physician may prescribe intravenous calcium chloride to be administered in patients undergoing multiple blood transfusions.

Massive transfusion syndrome, a severe depletion of coagulation components, can occur as blood is lost and replaced with stored blood. When blood is stored, platelets and coagulation factors are inactivated over hours to days. Following transfusion, the patient's blood becomes diluted and deficient in active coagulation factors (Hirsh and Brain, 1983). This problem is magnified in patients who are unable to produce new coagulation factors, such as those with liver disease. Because of the potential for this problem in patients undergoing massive transfusion, periodic coagulation panels are analyzed to determine the need for specific component replacement.

In addition to the complications associated with massive transfusion, other reactions to the transfusion of blood and blood components may occur. The most common reaction is a febrile response caused by the reaction to donor platelets, lymphocytes, and granulocytes (Smith, 1984). Fever, chills, and tachycardia may be observed during or following transfusion, and the transfusion may need to be stopped. Patients known to have a history of this type of reaction can be premedicated with an antipyretic such as acetaminophen.

Hypersensitivity reactions can occur when a patient is hypersensitive to transfused allergens. These reactions may be mild or serious. Urticaria and wheezing occur most commonly, but an anaphylactic reaction is possible. The transfusion is stopped when a hypersensitivity reaction occurs, and the patient is given an antihistamine. For severe reactions, steroids or vasopressors may be necessary. Allergy-prone patients may be premedicated with an antihistamine such as diphenhydramine hydrochloride.

With current blood banking standards and typing and crossmatching techniques, hemolytic reactions due to incompatible blood are extremely rare. However, it is always necessary to follow policies related to checking patient and blood identification. Patients are observed closely for signs of hemolytic reaction such as chest tightness, chills, low back pain, he-

TABLE 50–6. Transfusion Reactions

Complications of massive transfusion
  Fluid overload
  Hypothermia
  Hyperkalemia
  Citrate intoxication, hypocalcemia
  Massive transfusion syndrome
Febrile reaction
Hypersensitivity reaction
Hemolytic reaction
Bacterial reaction
Late reactions
  Hepatitis
  Cytomegalovirus
  HIV infection

moglobinuria, and shock. Bacterial contamination is also rare. Nevertheless, blood should be examined prior to administration for unusual color, separation, or gas bubbles. Clinical manifestations of diseases transmitted by transfusion such as hepatitis, cytomegalovirus, and other organisms do not appear for many weeks. Patients who have received multiple transfusions of components containing pooled plasma are at greatest risk.

For some bleeding patients, autotransfusion of shed blood may be an option. Autotransfusion of mediastinal blood is used in many centers during and following cardiac surgery. The growing availability of autotransfusion systems and the concern about disease transmission from homologous blood have resulted in an increase in the use of autotransfusion. The advantages of autotransfusion include high oxygen-carrying capacity due to high levels of 2,3-diphosphoglycerate, normal pH, and normal temperature. Shed blood contains near-normal clotting factors but a lower hematocrit. It is relatively inexpensive, and there is no risk of disease transmission (Tector et al., 1985). An option for the future may be the use of artificial blood.

Potential for Injury

Because of the patient's potential for bleeding, trauma and hemorrhage can occur with routine critical care procedures. Prevention of vascular and tissue trauma is a crucial expected outcome of nursing care.

Bleeding precautions need to be instituted immediately when a patient develops a coagulopathy (Rooney and Haviley, 1985). Needle sticks must be avoided to minimize the risk of bleeding and hematoma formation. Indwelling arterial and venous lines are used whenever possible to draw blood and to administer medications. If needle sticks are necessary, a small-gauge needle should be used, and pressure should be applied to the site for 5 to 10 minutes with periodic inspection of the site later (Kirchner and Reheis, 1982).

All staff members must be alerted to the patient's potential for bleeding when invasive procedures are planned. Invasive and surgical procedures may need to be postponed in patients with a coagulopathy until hemostasis is restored. The risk of inserting hemodynamic monitoring lines may be too great during periods of active bleeding.

Other measures can be taken to prevent trauma in these high-risk patients. Patients need to be bathed and turned with enough assistance to prevent trauma. Side rails and sharp objects in the environment need to be padded if the patient is restless. Gentle skin care can be carried out with a mild lotion to minimize skin trauma. Only electric razors should be used for shaving. The teeth should be brushed gently using a foam toothbrush or swab. Frequent mouth care prevents drying and cracking of the oral mucosa, which bleeds easily in patients with coagulation disorders. In patients who are able to take food and fluids orally, liquids and soft foods are tolerated best because there may be irritated or ischemic areas within the oral cavity.

It may be necessary to avoid using a blood pressure cuff because the pressure of the inflated cuff can cause petechiae and ecchymotic skin lesions. Rectal temperature taking and suppositories are also avoided to prevent trauma to the mucous membranes.

If oral or tracheal suctioning is necessary, very low suction is used to prevent trauma to the trachea (Caplan, 1984). Continuous humidity is provided to the respiratory tract to minimize drying and bleeding of mucous membranes.

Alteration in Comfort

Painful hematomas can result from bleeding into the tissues. Ischemic tissue pain can result from the deposition of fibrin in the peripheral circulation. Fear and anxiety in patients experiencing hemorrhage or thrombosis can increase the perception of pain and block the effectiveness of usual coping behaviors. Expected outcomes of nursing care include the verbalization of increased comfort and demonstration of a relaxed posture and facial expression.

Patients who are ill with a coagulopathy may be unable to communicate that they are having pain. It may be necessary to observe them for physiologic indicators of discomfort, such as diaphoresis, pallor, tachycardia, and tachypnea. The skin and extremities need to be carefully assessed for the presence of joint or muscle pain, which indicate bleeding into these tissues.

Intervention for pain is difficult because these patients are often hypovolemic and easily become hypotensive following administration of intravenous analgesics. It may be necessary to give small doses of medication and monitor the blood pressure frequently. In addition to analgesic medication, all other comfort measures need to be provided. These patients may benefit from the use of a flotation mattress. Periodic repositioning with pillows or soft bath blankets will also enhance comfort.

Patients with DIC or other coagulopathies can easily become exhausted because of the need for continuous care. This can further increase their degree of stress and discomfort. Allowing rest periods of 30 minutes after activities such as turning, bathing, or x-rays can help to prevent exhaustion.

Isolation from the patient's family tends to increase as the complexity of care increases. Short visits by the family can help to minimize the distress experienced by the bleeding patient and promote relaxation and comfort. Providing reassurance to a patient and family during events as distressing as hemorrhage is always difficult. The situation can be particularly distressing because the coagulopathy is often a complication of another life-threatening disorder such as sepsis, extensive trauma, or malignancy. It may be helpful to list all the measures being used to control the bleeding such as transfusion of blood components and medications. It can also be helpful to point out any signs of improvement that may not be obvious, such as a rising platelet count. Providing honest information and emotional support can help the patient and family set realistic short-term goals and enhance their coping abilities during what is obviously a complex situation.

PREVENTION OF COAGULOPATHIES

Prevention of bleeding problems is a combined medical and nursing responsibility. The following strategies can be helpful in minimizing bleeding problems.

A careful patient history related to bleeding should be obtained prior to performing invasive procedures or surgery. A history of repeated bleeding problems such as epistaxis, bleeding following dental procedures, and bleeding following labor and delivery can be a reliable predictor of postoperative problems. A careful history should also include the family history related to spontaneous bleeding or bleeding following trauma (Schafer, 1984).

Each patient's medication history is very important, especially that related to the times anticoagulants were started and stopped. With the increasing number of drugs that affect coagulation in common use, it has become an important role of nurses to assist in the identification of patients at risk of bleeding (Goodwin, 1985). Nurses may also be involved in coordinating regimens prescribed by different physicians who are unaware of the patient's cumulative medication profile. For example, in a patient who develops complete heart block and is scheduled for insertion of a permanent pacemaker, the cardiologist may be unaware that warfarin has been prescribed by another physician.

Table 50–7 lists some of the drugs commonly used in critically ill patients that have a known effect on coagulation. It should be recognized that many drugs can potentially cause thrombocytopenia. Other drugs may not affect coagulation by themselves but may potentiate the effect of anticoagulants through drug interactions.

During physical examination, patients should be assessed for evidence of hematologic abnormalities. The skin is inspected for petechiae, easy bruising, and jaundice. The abdomen is palpated for hepatosplenomegaly.

TABLE 50–7. Drugs with Anticoagulant Effects

Major anticoagulants
  Heparin
  Warfarin
  Dicumarol
Thrombolytic agents
  Streptokinase
  Urokinase
  Tissue plasminogen activator
Nonsteroidal anti-inflammatory agents
  Aspirin
  Indomethacin
  Naproxen
  Ibuprofen
  Phenylbutazone
Corticosteroids
Platelet-inhibiting agents
  Dipyridamole
  Sulfinpyrazone
  Clofibrate
  Dextran
  Aspirin
Antibiotics
  Carbenicillin
  Ampicillin
  Penicillin
  Chloramphenicol
Ethanol

Prior to invasive and surgical procedures, laboratory work is done to assess liver and kidney function. Coagulation parameters are measured when indicated depending on the patient's history and the nature of the proposed procedure. However, it is recognized that laboratory values may not always accurately predict the potential for bleeding.

Certain clinical situations are associated with bleeding problems, especially in surgical patients. Patients undergoing reoperations have more bleeding complications due to adhesions from the initial surgery. The length of the operation can also influence the potential for bleeding. Extensive and prolonged procedures lead to the loss of more blood and blood components. Operations requiring the use of cardiopulmonary bypass are associated with a greater risk of bleeding because of the trauma to platelets and other factors. In addition, the potential for bleeding may be greater in surgery involving the heart and lungs because the entire cardiac output passes through these organs and they are constantly in motion.

Patients themselves can be involved in the prevention of coagulation problems. Teaching patients about the anticoagulant effects of their medications can begin in the critical care unit and continue throughout the recovery period.

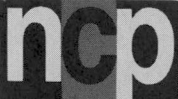 nursing care plan

1. Potential for fluid (blood) volume deficit related to:
Depleted clotting components and activated fibrinolysis

Outcome Criteria	Nursing Interventions
Early recognition and control of bleeding.	Observe all incisions, puncture sites, and skin lesions for signs of bleeding. Watch for epistaxis and bleeding from gums after mouth care is given. Measure expanding hematomas and swollen extremities and closely monitor. Assess abdominal girth periodically when peritoneal bleeding is suspected. Inspect exit sites of tubes and catheters periodically. Check surgical drains for increased drainage. Observe tracheal secretions for evidence of pulmonary hemorrhage. Watch for bleeding from multiple sites. Evaluate vital signs for evidence of hypotension; labile blood pressure; low CVP or low PCWP; tachycardia; and weak, thready pulse. Inspect extremities for evidence of poor perfusion. Assess urine output frequently. Test urine, stools, and vasogastric drainage for occult blood. Check x-rays for unexpected fluid collection. Carefully evaluate changes in the level of consciousness and carefully assess reports of headache, joint pain, or abdominal pain. Monitor patient's hemoglobin, hematocrit, and coagulation parameters. When bleeding is identified, place patient on bedrest and administer oxygen therapy to meet specific needs. Monitor and report the amount and character of bleeding. Change dressings carefully so that clots are not disturbed. Consider cold compresses and pressure to control bleeding from skin sites. Administer topical hemostatic agents as prescribed.

2. Actual fluid (blood) volume deficit related to:
Overt hemorrhage

Outcome Criteria	Nursing Interventions
Prevention of acute anemia, anoxia, and hypovolemic circulatory failure.	Continuously monitor for signs and symptoms of hypovolemic shock plus any overt or covert signs of bleeding and report findings. Initiate fluid volume replacement. Be aware of all drug actions and interactions related to coagulation. Closely monitor patients with DIC, when heparin is ordered, for increased bleeding or other untoward effects. Check laboratory values, such as APTT, periodically and evaluate considering the clinical assessment of the patient. Administer whole blood and blood components when active hemorrhage occurs. Infuse fresh frozen plasma and cryoprecipitate as soon as it is thawed. Monitor patients receiving transfusions for adverse reactions to related infusions. Measure hemodynamic parameters before, during, and after each infusion. Assess for dyspnea, rales, and pulmonary congestion. Consider using a blood warmer when infusing multiple units of cold blood. Continuously monitor ECG for changes indicative of hyperkalemia. Administer calcium chloride as ordered to prevent hypercalcemia secondary to citrate intoxication. Periodically analyze coagulation panels in patients undergoing massive transfusions. Consider premedication with acetaminophen in patients with a history of transfusion reactions. When a hypersensitivity reaction occurs, stop the infusion and administer an antihistamine, steroids, or vasopressors as prescribed. Examine blood prior to administration for unusual color, separation, or gas bubbles.

Nursing Care Plan continued on following page

3. Potential for injury related to:
Coagulopathy

Outcome Criteria	Nursing Interventions
Prevention of vascular and tissue trauma.	Institute bleeding precautions immediately. Avoid needle sticks. Utilize indwelling arterial and venous lines to draw blood and administer medications. If needle sticks are necessary, use a small-gauge needle and apply pressure to the site for 5 to 10 minutes with periodic inspection of the site later. Alert the staff to the patient's potential for bleeding when invasive procedures are planned. Consider postponing invasive and surgical procedures. Bathe and turn with enough assistance to prevent trauma. Pad side rails and sharp objects in the environment if the patient is restless. Provide skin care gently. Use only electric razors for shaving. Brush teeth using a foam toothbrush or swab. Provide frequent mouth care to prevent drying and cracking. Provide liquids and soft foods. Avoid using a blood pressure cuff and avoid rectal temperatures and suppositories. Use very low suction if oral or tracheal suctioning is necessary. Provide continuous humidity.

4. Alteration in comfort related to:
Painful hematomas, ischemic tissue pain, fear, and anxiety

Outcome Criteria	Nursing Interventions
Patient will verbalize increase in comfort. Patient will demonstrate a relaxed posture and facial expression.	Observe for physiologic indicators of discomfort such as diaphoresis, pallor, tachycardia, and tachypnea. Carefully assess the skin and extremities for presence of joint or muscle pain. Consider giving small doses of medication for pain and monitor blood pressure frequently. Consider the use of a flotation mattress. Periodically reposition patient with pillows or soft bath blankets. Allow rest periods of 30 minutes after activities of turning, bathing, or x-rays. Allow short visits by the family to minimize distress. Provide reassurance to patient and family by listing all measures being used to control bleeding and pointing out signs of improvement. Provide honest information and emotional support.

SUMMARY

Few patients challenge the critical care nurse as do those with coagulopathies. Nursing management of the patient with a coagulation disorder includes careful assessment of the patient's clinical status and identification of bleeding risk factors. Special nursing interventions are directed toward prevention of bleeding. The nurse collaborates with the physician in treating coagulation problems through the use of anticoagulant medications and blood component therapy.

References

Caplan, M. (1984). Disseminated intravascular coagulation: A multisystem problem. *Dimensions of Critical Care Nursing*, 3 (5), 76–83.

Colman, R. W., Hirsh, J., Marder, V. J., et al. (1991). *Hemostasis and thrombosis: Basic principles and clinical practice* (2nd ed.). Philadelphia: J. B. Lippincott.

Deykin, D. (1982). Current status of anticoagulant therapy. *American Journal of Medicine*, 72 (4), 659–664.

Dressler, D. K. (1987). Disseminated intravascular coagulation (DIC). In M. F. Moorhouse, A. C. Geissler, and M. E. Donges (Eds.), *Critical care plans* (pp. 319–328). Philadelphia: F. A. Davis.

Dressler, D. K. (1989). Disseminated intravascular coagulation (DIC). In K. T. VonRueden and C. A. Walleck (Eds.), *Case studies in critical care*. Rockville, MD: Aspen Publishers.

Franco, L. M. (1981). Acute disseminated intravascular coagulation. *Critical Care Update*, 8 (1), 17–20.

Goodwin, S. A. (1985). Drug-induced coagulation. *Critical Care Quarterly*, 7 (4), 1–18.

Greenberg, H. J., Vogel, J. M., and Sanders, M. (1985). Disseminated intravascular coagulopathy. *Physician Assistant*, 9 (2), 106–112.

Guyton, A. C. (1991). *Human physiology and mechanisms of disease* (8th ed.). Philadelphia: W. B. Saunders.

Herring, W. B., and Shelburne, P. F. (1984). Heparin-induced thrombosis. *North Carolina Medical Journal*, 45 (3), 159–162.

Hirsh, J., and Brain, E. A. (1983). *Hemostasis and thrombosis* (2nd ed.). New York: Churchill Livingstone.

King, D. J., and Kelton, J. G. (1984). Heparin-associated thrombocytopenia. *Annals of Internal Medicine*, 100 (4), 535–540.

Kirchner, C. W., and Reheis, C. E. (1982). Two serious complications of neoplasia: Sepsis and disseminated intravascular coagulation. *Nursing Clinics of North America*, 17 (4), 595–606.

Massorli, S. T., and Piercy, S. (1984). A lifesaving guide to blood products. *RN*, 47 (9), 32–37.

Mayberry, L. J., and Forte, A. B. (1985). Pregnancy-related disseminated intravascular coagulation (DIC). *Maternal Child Nursing*, 10 (3), 168–173.

Mersky, C. (1982). DIC: Identification and management. *Hospital Practice*, 17 (12), 83–94.

Newland, J. R. (1985). Coagulation and the tests for DIC. *Consultant*, 25 (3), 112–120.

Rooney, A., and Haviley, C. (1985). Nursing management of disseminated intravascular coagulation. *Oncology Nursing Forum*, 12 (1), 15–22.

Salzman, E. W., Weinstein, M. J., Weintraub, R. M., et al. (1986). Treatment with desmopressin acetate to reduce blood loss after cardiac surgery. *New England Journal of Medicine*, 314 (22), 1402–1406.

Schafer, A. I. (1984). Bleeding disorders: Finding the cause. *Hospital Practice*, 19 (11), 88K–88HH.

Smith, L. (1984). Reactions to blood transfusions. *American Journal of Nursing*, 84 (9), 1096–1101.

Tannenbaum, S. (1983). Blood—which component and why? *Physician Assistant*, 7 (11), 133–141.

Tector, A. J., Dressler, D. K., and Glassner-Davis, R. M. (1985). A new method of autotransfusing blood drained after cardiac surgery. *Annals of Thoracic Surgery*, 40 (3), 305–307.

Walsh, P. N. (1983). Oral anticoagulant therapy. *Hospital Practice*, 18 (1), 101–120.

Williams, W. J., Beutler, E., Erslev, A. J., et al. (1983). *Hematology* (3rd ed.). New York: McGraw-Hill.

Wintrobe, M. M., Lee, G. R., and Boggs, D. R. (1981). *Clinical hematology* (8th ed.). Philadelphia: Lea & Febiger.

Immune System

51

Physiologic Response to Infection

Mary Cusella Seller
Donna C. Owen

Advances in science and technology have led to the development of complex and high-risk therapeutic medical interventions. Interventions such as organ transplantation and ablative cytotoxic chemotherapy directly affect immune function. Patients receiving these aggressive therapies more and more frequently require nursing support in critical care settings. Esperson (1986) suggests that all patients exposed to a critical care environment may have lowered immunologic defenses. Thus, a working knowledge of the parts of the immune system and their interaction is essential. Knowing how the immune system works will allow nurses to increase the natural defenses of patients in the critical care setting. This chapter introduces readers to the science of immunology and highlights aspects of immune function most relevant to the critical care setting.

The term *immune* derives from the Latin word *immunis*, which means free from taxes or free from burden. Classically, immunity referred to resistance of the host to reinfection by a given pathogen. A more contemporary definition focuses on the physiologic mechanisms involved in immunity. Immunity enables the body to recognize certain microbes as foreign and to metabolize, neutralize, or eliminate them with or without injury to its own tissues (Stites et al., 1987). Note that the immune response is a physiologic reaction to the introduction into the body of foreign material regardless of whether it is harmful or not.

BASIC CONCEPTS OF IMMUNOLOGY

Three basic concepts describing the fundamental aspects of immune function are presented prior to a more complete discussion of immune function. Antigens are the primary stimulants of all immune responses. The major histocompatibility complex provides the basis for discerning foreign substances from our own molecules. Antibody is the key product of immune cell stimulation by antigen. These three concepts lay the foundation for a more complex discussion of the interaction between antigen and antibody in distinguishing self from nonself, which is the hallmark of all immune response.

Antigens and Antigenicity

Antigen is any substance that, when introduced parenterally into an animal, elicits an immune response specifically directed at the inducing substance (Barrett, 1988). Immunogen is a term used to clarify the fact that antigens foster both antibody production and activation of specific immune cell responses. Now the terms antigen and immunogen are used interchangeably. Before describing antigens further, it is necessary to define antibody briefly. Antibodies are proteins produced by specific immune cells. These proteins bind specifically to antigen.

Several characteristics of antigen foster stimulation of an immune response. Both the molecular shape and size of antigen are important. Antigen triggers an immune response only after immune cells recognize the specific shape of parts of the antigen molecule. A better immune response occurs as the molecular weight of a substance increases. The larger the antigen, the stronger the immune response. With bigger antigens, more parts of the molecule (antigenic determinants) stimulate production of specific antibody. Antigenic determinants are important in stimulating the production of many different antibodies during one immune response. Increased complexity of an antigen's molecular structure also enhances the stimulating properties of the antigen. The more "foreign" a substance is considered by the body, the more antigenic the substance is. Solubility and availability of a substance for degradation by cellular mechanisms enhance the antigenic property of that substance (Barrett, 1988). Table 51–1 lists the physical and chemical properties associated with antigenicity.

Mitogens, substances that induce mitosis, mimic antigens. Mitogens, like antigens, induce the activation of immune cells and the production of antibodies (Barrett, 1988). However, the mechanisms by which mitogens and antigens produce an immune response are different. Both mitogens and antigens are used experimentally to assess the function of the immune system.

The Major Histocompatibility Complex

Histocompatibility antigens, or self antigens, are a specific set of antigens with unique properties. Histocompatibility antigens are found on all cells in the body that have a nucleus. Histocompatibility antigens are those molecules that characterize each individual as unique. These antigens are inherited from one's parents. Parents and offspring may have some of the same histocompatibility antigens but not *all* of them.

The major histocompatibility complex (MHC) is an intricate set of genes that directs the production of histocompatibility antigens and other antigens involved in the elicitation of an immune response. The MHC is on chromosome 6 in humans (Fig. 51–1). Based on differences in tissue distribution, antigen structure, and antigenic function, three distinct classes of genes reside on the MHC. Class I genes code for histocompatibility antigens located on all nucleated cells. Class I histocompatibility antigens identify nucleated cells as targets for destruction (Bach and Sachs, 1987). Class II genes code for proteins of lymphocyte cell membranes. Macrophages, B-lymphocytes, and activated T-lymphocytes

TABLE 51–1. Properties Associated with Antigenicity

Characteristics	Property that Enhances Response
Size	Large molecule
Complexity	Very complex structures
Stability	Fixed structural configuration
Degradability	Timing of degradation process allows for interaction of antigen and processing cells
Foreignness	Greatest molecular difference from self antigen

express class II gene products. Class III antigens code for two complement proteins, C4 and factor B (Stites et al., 1987).

In humans, human lymphocyte antigens (HLA) are produced by the MHC. The MHC and HLA play a particularly significant role in organ transplantation (Bach and Sachs, 1987). The ability to match the HLA types of two individuals is important in determining the intensity of the potential rejection by the recipient of the donor's tissue graft (see Chaps. 52 and 53).

Antibodies

In developing methods of vaccination, Pasteur recognized the protective nature of serum. Antibody was the part of serum thought to confer immunologic protection (Tizard, 1984). Antibodies refer to a vast array of proteins produced by B-lymphoctyes following stimulation by antigen. The major function of antibody is to bind a specific antigen and remove that antigen from the body (Jeske and Capra, 1984). In a specific response to a specific antigen a single antibody is produced. Thus, for each antigen there is a matching antibody. There are hundreds of thousands of potential antigens, and there are an equal number of antibodies. Each of these antibodies has slightly different characteristics and specificities.

The many individual types of antibodies are grouped into five different immunoglobulin (Ig) classes: IgG, IgM, IgA, IgE, and IgD. Table 51–2 describes some physical and biologic properties of the five major immunoglobulin classes.

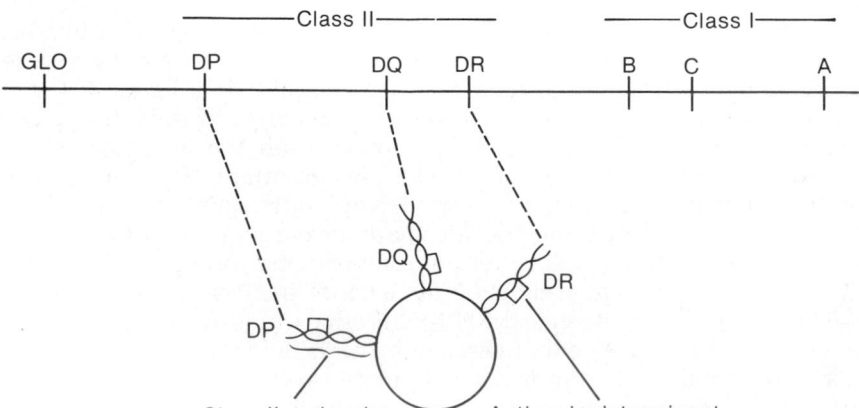

FIGURE 51–1. Schematic representation of major histocompatibility complex located on short arm of chromosome 6. The DP, DQ, and DR loci encode for class II molecules; the A, B, and C loci encode for class I molecules. The products of the MHC, DP, DQ, and DR genes are randomly expressed on cells, e.g., macrophages, B-cells, and some activated T-cells. These class II molecules express antigenic determinants that are detected by antibodies. (From Lockey, R., and Bukantz, S. (Eds.) (1987). *Fundamentals of immunology and allergy* (p. 70). Philadelphia: W. B. Saunders.)

TABLE 51-2. Classification of Immunoglobulins

Class	Mean Survival		Biologic Function
	Per Cent of Total	Half-life (Days)	
IgG	75	23	Fix complement Cross placenta Active against many blood-borne infectious organisms (e.g., bacteria, viruses, parasites, and some fungi) Primary antibody of the secondary antibody response
IgA	15	6	Secretory antibody Activates complement through alternate properdin pathway
IgM	10	5	Fix complement Primary antibody of the primary antibody response
IgD	1	2.8	Unknown but proposed as lymphocyte surface receptor
IgE	0.002	1.5	Reaginic antibody (allergy) Homocytotropic antibody

Adapted from Bernier, G. M. (1985). In J. A. Bellanti (Ed.), *Immunology III* (p. 91). Philadelphia: W. B. Saunders.

IgG, the most abundant of the immunoglobulins, makes up about 75% of the total concentration of immunoglobulins in the serum. Vascular and extravascular spaces contain high concentrations of IgG. IgG has a relatively long half-life (23 days), can cross the placenta, and can activate complement. This class of immunoglobulin provides immunity against many blood-borne infectious agents such as bacteria, viruses, parasites, and some fungi. Receptors for IgG exist on many immune cells including monocytes, polymorphonuclear leukocytes, accessory cells in spleen and liver, and some lymphocytes.

IgA provides immunity through the external secretory system. Through this system, IgA moves across mucous membranes within body secretions. Fifteen per cent of the total serum concentration of immunoglobulins consists of IgA, making it the second most abundant immunoglobulin. The lymphoid tissues lining the gastrointestinal, respiratory, and genitourinary tracts secrete IgA. Saliva and tears contain large amounts of IgA. IgA combines with a protein that confers IgA protection with proteolytic enzymes found in these lymphoid tissues. IgA does not cross the placenta; however, it gives immunity to the newborn by virtue of its high concentration in colostrum. Lymphocytes, polymorphonuclear cells, and monocytes have receptors for IgA.

IgM accounts for 10% of the total serum concentration of immunoglobulins. IgM is the largest immunoglobulin. It is confined almost entirely to the intravascular space because of its large size. IgM molecules have the ability to fix complement and are highly efficient agglutinators of particulate antigens such as red blood cells and bacteria. Both of these properties make IgM an important participant in host defense. IgM antibodies are the first class of antibody synthesized after primary stimulation by antigen. The level of IgM antibodies peaks within days and declines more rapidly than does the level of IgG antibodies.

IgD accounts for only 1% of the total serum concentration of immunoglobulins; its specific biologic role as a humoral antibody is unclear. This immunoglobulin class is found on the surface of lymphocytes much more frequently than in serum. IgD is expressed on neonatal lymphocytes more often than on adult lymphocytes. Both of these findings suggest that IgD serves as a specific surface receptor in the initiation of the immune response. Penicillin hypersensitivity is another instance of IgD participation in the immune response.

IgE is present in only trace amounts in the serum. It has the ability to attach to human skin and to start an allergic reaction. Also called the reaginic antibody, IgE functions to mediate the severe anaphylactic type of hypersensitivities. Like IgA, IgE is produced chiefly in the linings of the respiratory and intestinal tracts. Both IgA and IgE are part of the external secretory system of antibody (Barrett, 1988).

THE BASIC FUNCTIONS OF THE IMMUNE SYSTEM

The basic function of the immune system is to detect and eliminate from the body any substance recognized as foreign or nonself. Typically, each encounter of the body with a foreign substance activates an immune response. When analyzed individually, immunologic responses serve three functions—defense, homeostasis, and surveillance (Bellanti, 1985).

Defense

Response to infection is one defense function commonly attributed to the immune system. The defense action of the immune system has important consequences not only for the invading organism but also for normal human tissue. When immune system components or interactions between components are hyperactive, allergy or hypersensitivity may occur (Kirkpatrick, 1987). Conversely, when these elements are hypoactive, increased susceptibility to repeated infections may occur. The immune deficiency disorders are examples of repeated infections in the presence of a hypoactive immune system (Church and Schlegel, 1985).

Homeostasis

By maintaining homeostasis, the immune system preserves the internal environment. Cellular components of the body continually grow, mature, die, and are replaced. In this process of orderly senescence, antigens defining the cells as self become altered. The immune system is thus able to mount a response against normal cells that are no longer functioning competently. Specialized immunocompetent cells serve as scavengers that degrade and remove damaged or dead cells from the body. Other immunocompetent cells serve to control and regulate the homeostatic function of the immune system. The regulation of homeostasis is an important normal immunologic function. Failure of the regulation of homeostatic mechanisms often results in autoimmune disease (Barrett, 1988).

Surveillance

Controversy surrounds the surveillance function of the immune system. The *immune surveillance theory*, first posited by Thomas (1959) and later changed by Burnet (1967), suggests that T-lymphocytes of the immune system serve to detect and remove the abnormal cells that constantly arise within the body. These abnormal cells arise through spontaneous neoplastic transformation or induction by certain viruses and chemicals. Failure of this surveillance mechanism is thought to play a causal role in the development of malignant disease. Evidence supporting or refuting this theory is equivocal. Supporting evidence includes (1) the increased incidence of cancer in the elderly, (2) failure of rejection of tumor transplant by genetically thymectomized mice, and (3) a 300-fold increased incidence of cancer in individuals on long-term immunosuppressive therapy (Groenwald et al., 1988). Contradictory evidence suggests that the proposed mechanism of immune surveillance is too simplistic (Mitchell and Bertram, 1985). More recently, non–T-lymphocytes (natural killer cells) have been reported to have the primary role in surveillance rather than T-lymphocytes (Herberman and Gorelik, 1989). A further change in the immune surveillance theory suggests that the target of surveillance is the immunogen or stimulus of the immune response (Groenwald et al., 1988).

TISSUES OF THE IMMUNE SYSTEM

Lymphoid or immune tissues are the special tissues that participate in the development of competent immune cells. These tissues, as shown in Figure 51–2, are located throughout the entire body and are subdivided into central and peripheral lymphoid tissues. Differentiation of lymphoid stem cells into lymphocytes that can react with antigen takes place in the central lymphoid tissues. The central lymphoid system has three major subdivisions: (1) the bone marrow, (2) the thymus, and (3) a component whose identity is known with certainty only in birds (the bursa of Fabricius). The peripheral lymphoid tissues are found in areas in which the lymphocytes can later react with antigen (Barrett, 1988). The peripheral lymphoid system includes lymph nodes, spleen, tonsils, bronchus-associated lymphoid tissue, Peyer patches, appendix, and other gut-associated lymphoid tissue. Many patches of lymphoid tissue are scattered throughout tissues that initially confront antigens from the external environment. Characteristics of primary and secondary lymphoid organs are compared in Table 51–3.

TABLE 51–3. Comparison of Primary and Secondary Lymphoid Organs

	Primary Lymphoid Organ	Secondary Lymphoid Organ
Origin	Ectoendodermal junction	Mesoderm
Time of development	Early in embryonic life	Later in fetal life
Persistence	Involutes after puberty	Persists through adult life
Effect of removal	Loss of lymphocytes	No effect or only minor consequences
Response to antigen	Unresponsive	Fully reactive
Examples	Thymus; (bursa)	Spleen; lymph nodes

Table from IMMUNOLOGY: AN INTRODUCTION, by Ian R. Tizard, copyright © 1984 by Saunders College Publishing, reprinted by permission of the publisher.

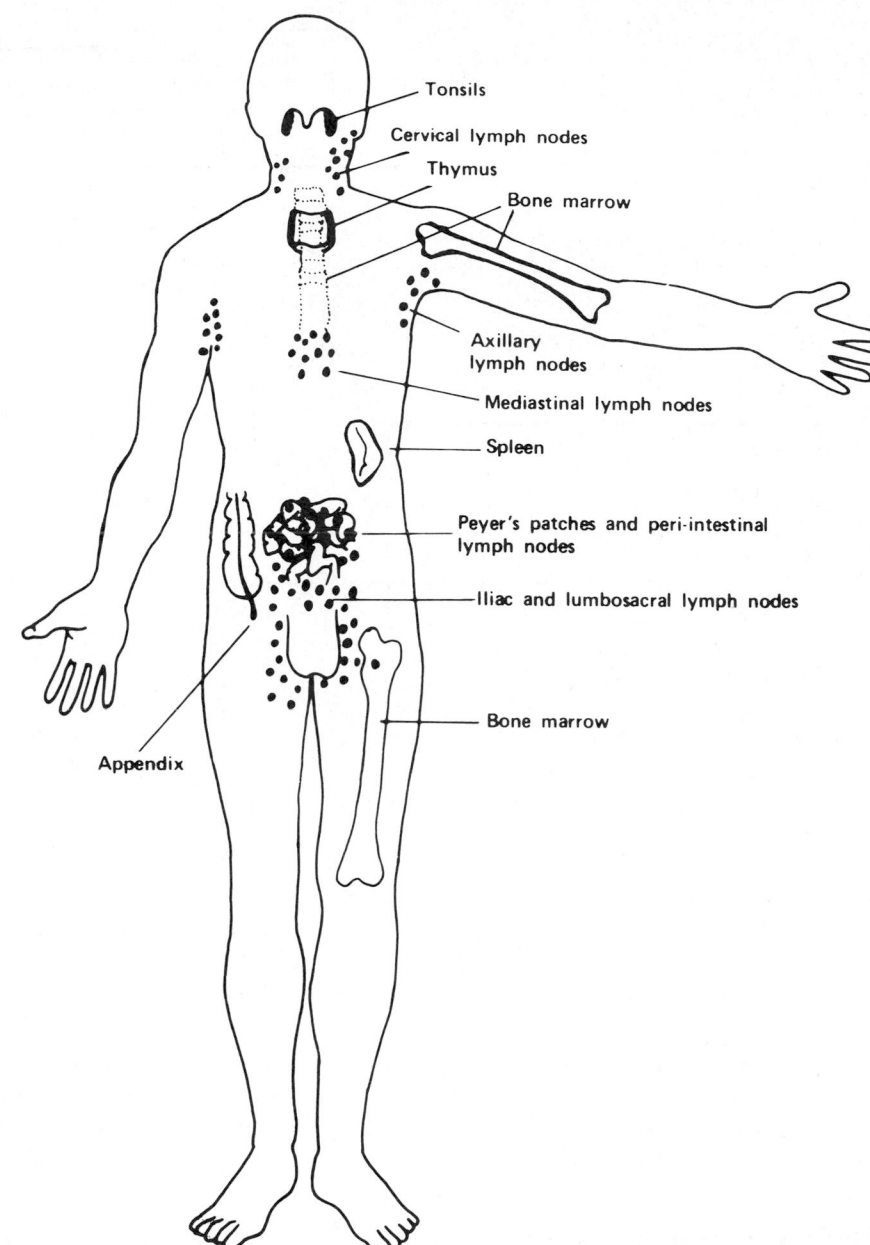

Tonsils

Cervical lymph nodes

Thymus

Bone marrow

Axillary
lymph nodes

Mediastinal lymph nodes

Spleen

Peyer's patches and peri-intestinal
lymph nodes

Iliac and lumbosacral lymph nodes

Bone marrow

Appendix

FIGURE 51–2. Diagrammatic representation
of the distribution of lymphoid tissues in
humans. (Reprinted from Virella, G. J. M.,
Fudenberg, H., and Patrick, C. (Eds.)
(1986). *Introduction to medical immunology*
(p. 13). By courtesy of Marcel Dekker, Inc.)

The Central Lymphoid Organs

Bone Marrow. Cells of the immune system originate, mature, and move from the bone marrow into the circulatory system. Erythrocytes, platelets, granulocytes, monocytes, and lymphocytes arise from a primitive undifferentiated stem cell. Figure 51–3 shows the development of the cells of the bone marrow. The granulocytic, monocytic, and lymphocytic cell lines are effector cells of the immune system (Barrett, 1988).

Thymus. The thymus consists of a bilobed sack of epithelial cells surrounding an interior core of lymphocytes. Structurally, each lobe of the thymus divides into an exterior cortex and an interior medulla.

Lymphocytes coalesce primarily in the cortex of the thymus. These thymic lymphocytes are morphologically indistinguishable from lymphocytes in other tissues. Thymic lymphocytes are, however, antigenically isolatable by Thy 1, a surface marker antigen, and are called T-lymphocytes (Barrett, 1988).

Bursa of Fabricius. The bursa of Fabricius is a lymphoid organ located in the gut of fowl. The bursa serves as the site of B-cell maturation in birds. Within the bursa there are three main types of cells: macrophages, B-lymphocytes, and plasma cells. Mammals do not have a bursa but do have B-lymphocytes. Much research effort has gone into attempts to identify a bursal equivalent in man. Despite these efforts, no one tissue has been fully supported empirically.

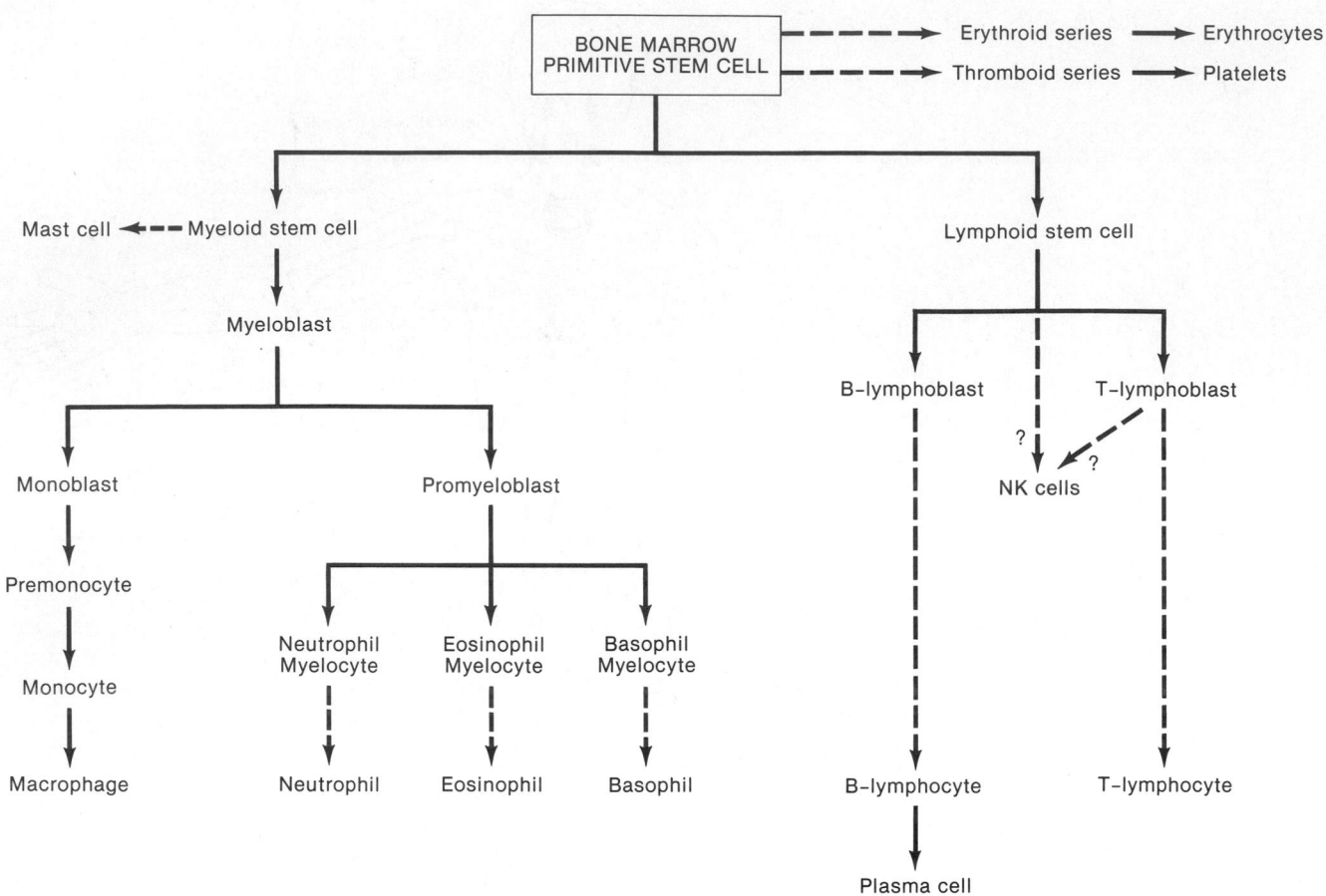

FIGURE 51–3. Differentiation of primitive stem cell in the bone marrow.

One potential tissue is gut-associated lymphoid tissue (GALT). B-lymphocyte activity is impaired with the removal of GALT in the early development of experimental animals (Barrett, 1988).

The Peripheral Lymphoid Organs

The spleen and lymph nodes are the two major peripheral lymphoid organs. Lymphocytes leave the central lymphoid organs, enter the circulatory system and peripheral lymphoid organs, and reenter the thymus. The tonsils, appendix, Peyer patches, and other lymphoid tissues play a lesser role in immune response (Barrett, 1988). Many other lymphoid tissues are scattered throughout the body. All of these tissues are capable of trapping antigen and are sites of immune response.

The spleen is physically divided into two sections—one as a storage site for erythrocytes and the second as the site of immunologic response. The spleen acts as a filter for antigen from the blood. The spleen also sequesters scavenger cells called macrophages and is a site of B-lymphocyte activation in response to antigen stimulation. Lymph nodes trap antigen in the lymph and provide maximal exposure

of antigen to antigen-sensitive cells. Antigen-sensitive cells in lymph nodes include lymphocytes, macrophages, and other accessory cells.

CELLS OF THE IMMUNE SYSTEM

One of the most interesting features of the immune system is the great diversity of white blood cells involved in the events comprising the immune response. Four categories of white blood cells involved in the immune response are (1) macrophages and antigen-processing and antigen-presenting cells (accessory cells), (2) granulocytic phagocytes, (3) B-lymphocytes, and (4) T-lymphocytes. The lymphocytes are primary participants in the recognition of nonself elements. Other white blood cells, including monocytes and granulocytes, help lymphocytes in either the early or late stages of the immune response. In the early stages, accessory cells present antigen in such a way that lymphocytes can recognize the antigen as nonself. In the later stages of an immune response macrophages and granulocytes ingest and digest nonself elements set for destruction (Barrett, 1988; Roitt et al., 1985).

Antigen-Presenting and Antigen-Processing Cells

The term accessory cells refers collectively to monocytes, macrophages, and many other antigen-presenting and antigen-processing cells. Accessory cells include cells that either participate in the initiation of an immune response or help the lymphocytes with their effector or inflammatory functions. Two broad groups of accessory cells are antigen-presenting cells and granulocytic phagocytes. Mononuclear phagocytes (monocytes and macrophages) and dendritic cells are nonlymphocytic antigen-presenting cells. These cells aid in the presentation of antigen to lymphocytes. A common characteristic of these cells is their ability to participate in the induction of the immune response. Macrophages also are active participants in the elimination of dead or damaged cells through phagocytosis.

Mononuclear Phagocytes. Mononuclear phagocytes arise from a single stem cell in the bone marrow and consist of a series of cells that develop from premonocyte to monocyte to macrophage. In the bone marrow, premonocytes undergo proliferation and move to the blood as monocytes after a period of maturation. After about 1 to 2 days in the blood, monocytes migrate to the main tissue site of their action. Monocytes become fixed in these tissues, where they differentiate into macrophages (Unanue, 1989).

Under normal conditions neither macrophages nor monocytes divide. Proteins secreted by T-lymphocytes, fibroblasts, macrophages, and epithelial cells stimulate monocytes to mature. Colony-stimulating factors (CSFs) start the differentiation of the premonocyte to monocyte and monocyte to macrophage. Colony-stimulating factors increase in amount during infection and during strong immune response (Unanue, 1989). Table 51–4 lists the actions of some CSFs involved in mediating the activity of mononuclear phagocytes.

Monocytes represent 3% of the circulating white blood cells in the adult, or about 300 cells/mL^3 of blood. Both monocytes and macrophages process and then present antigen to T-cells and B-cells. Processing of antigen requires internalization of antigens by the monocyte or macrophage. The exact biochemical events that take place within antigen-presenting cells remain unclear. Internalization and biochemical processing result in cell surface expression of antigen fragments (Unanue, 1989).

Most monocytes and macrophages express class II MHC molecules. Chemical mediators influence the amount of MHC protein found on the accessory cell membrane. These chemical mediators include both enhancers (gamma-interferon) and suppressors (prostaglandins) of monocyte/macrophage participation in the immune response. The expression of MHC on monocytes enhances the ability of the monocyte to present antigen fragments to lymphocytes and thus strengthens the lymphocyte response to antigen. Interleukin-1, a lymphokine secreted by monocytes, also enhances antigen presentation by monocytes (Unanue, 1989).

Macrophages are found in all tissues, often surrounding the blood vessels, near the epithelium. At times macrophages attach to vascular endothelial cells (Unanue, 1989). Macrophages serve at least three distinct functions in host defense: (1) secretion of biologically active molecules, (2) removal of excess antigen, and (3) antigen presentation. The secretory products of macrophages include prostaglandin E$_2$, leukotrienes, interleukin-1, tumor necrosis factor, interferon, growth factors, complement proteins, and enzymes (Table 51–5). Interleukin-1, tumor necrosis factor (TNF), and alpha- and beta-interferon are par-

TABLE 51–4. Colony-Stimulating Factors Involved in Differentiation of Monocytes

Colony-Stimulating Factors	Secreted By	Action
Multi-CSF (interleukin-3)	T-lymphocytes	Stimulates growth of granulocytes, mast cells, and lymphocytes
M-CSF	Macrophages	Stimulates differentiation of premonocyte to monocyte to macrophage. Increases longevity of mature macrophages
GM-CSF	Granulocytes Macrophages	In vitro administration of GM-CSF increases circulation of neutrophils, eosinophils, and macrophages
G-CSF	Granulocytes	Stimulates differentiation of myeloid precursor cell to granulocytes and monocytes

Compiled from Ihle, J. N., and Weinstein, Y. (1985). Interleukin 3 (pp. 291–324). In J. D. Watson and J. Marbrook (Eds.). *Recognition and Regulation in Cell-Mediated Immunity*. New York: Marcel Dekker.
Young, D., Lowe, L., and Clark, S. (1990). Comparison of the effects of IL-3, granulocyte-macrophage colony-stimulating factor, and macrophage colony-stimulating factor in supporting monocyte differentiation in culture.
Gillis, S., (1989). T-cell-derived lymphokines. In W. Paul (Ed.). *Fundamental Immunology* (2nd ed, pp 621–638). New York: Raven Press.
Roitt, I. (1991). *Essential Immunology* (7th ed). Boston: Blackwell Scientific Publications.
Guilbent, L. J. (1985). Mononuclear phagocyte progenitors and growth factors. In R. vanFurth (Ed.). *Mononuclear Phagocytes: Characteristics, Physiology, and Function* (pp. 233–241). Boston: Martinus Nijhoff Publishers.

ticularly important in the promotion of host defense (Unanue, 1989).

Tissue macrophages have specific names according to their anatomic location. Histiocytes are found in connective tissue, Kupffer cells in liver, alveolar macrophages in lung, and microglial cells in the neural system (Werb, 1987). Both free and fixed macrophages reside in the spleen, lymph nodes, and other organs. Blood monocytes have a half-life of only a few hours. However, tissue macrophages have a long lifespan, possibly extending for many months or years. Macrophages participating in inflammatory lesions have short lifespans because they die or fuse with other macrophages.

Dendritic Cells. Dendritic accessory cells reside primarily in the epithelium, lymphatics, spleen, and lymphoid organs. Morphologically distinct from mononuclear phagocytes, dendritic accessory cells express characteristically high levels of class II MHC molecules. Dendritic accessory cells are believed to be important in presenting antigens that have been introduced into the body through skin or other epithelial tissues. Details of the exact mechanism of antigen presentation by accessory cells have not yet been clarified (Unanue, 1989).

Of all the accessory cells, the follicular dendritic cells are the least understood. Follicular dendritic accessory cells are found in lymph nodes. These accessory cells participate with B-lymphocytes in antigen trapping within the follicles. These follicular dendritic cells have, however, been studied by indirect immunologic techniques only and have not been isolated or cultured. Thus, their exact nature, origin, and role in antigen trapping or in presentation of antigen to lymphocytes are not known.

Granulocytic Phagocytes

Most granulocytes have large lobular nuclei, leading to the name polymorphonuclear (PMN) leukocytes. Three varieties of circulating granulocytes exist—neutrophils, basophils, and eosinophils. Of the 5000 to 10,000 white blood cells in each cubic milliliter of blood, about 60% to 70% are neutrophils, 1% to 3% are eosinophils, and only 0.5% to 1% are basophils.

Neutrophils. Neutrophils go through a five-stage maturing process beginning with the myeloblast, myelocyte, metamyelocyte, and nonfilamented neutrophil and ending with the mature neutrophil. Neutrophils contain large cytoplasmic granules that produce enzymes with bactericidal activity (Patrick et al., 1986). During cell maturation the granules become more concentrated in the center of the cell. This readies the cell edges for movement to the sites of injury. At the metamyelocyte stage, complement and immunoglobulin G receptor are expressed on the cell surface. These surface antigens are important

TABLE 51–5. Some Secretory Products of Macrophages

Factors synthesized and secreted continuously	Lysozyme Complement components C2, C3, C4, C5 Fibronectin
Factors released during phagocytosis	Plasminogen activators Procoagulants Collagenase Elastase Lysosomal proteases Leukotrienes Thromboxanes Thromboplastin
Regulatory factors released during immune responses	Interferon Interleukin-1 Lymphocyte-activating factors Prostaglandins E_1 and E_2 Cyclic AMP

Table from IMMUNOLOGY: AN INTRODUCTION, by Ian R. Tizard, copyright © 1984 by Saunders College Publishing, reprinted by permission of the publisher.

facilitators of bacterial ingestion and cell motility. Only fully mature neutrophils are able to respond maximally to foreign particles (Densen and Mandell, 1987).

Neutrophils can migrate in response to chemical stimuli. Chemotactic factors also enhance the adhesiveness of neutrophils to endothelial cells, thus providing a mechanical means for motion (Werb, 1987). Chemotactic factors attract neutrophils to areas where antigen is present. Neutrophils engulf and destroy foreign substances such as bacteria and represent an important primary line of defense. Pus forms from neutrophils that die during the inflammatory process and their debris (Patrick et al., 1986).

Neutrophils synthesize and store in granules chemicals that are destructive to bacteria and cause injury in the surrounding tissue. Neutrophil degranulation has been implicated as a source of local tissue injury in adult respiratory distress syndrome and pulmonary emphysema (Densen and Mandell, 1987). Neutrophil secretory products include leukotrienes (slow-reactive-substance of anaphylaxis), vasoactive kinins, and toxic oxide metabolites such as hydrogen peroxide and myeloperoxidase (Bellanti and Kadlec, 1985).

Eosinophils. Eosinophils share many features with neutrophils in that both are removed from the body at the tissue site and do not return to the circulation. Like neutrophils, eosinophils contain many granules. Eosinophils concentrate at the mucosal surfaces of the respiratory and gastrointestinal tracts. Eosinophils do engage in phagocytosis; however, they are less efficient in the phagocytic process than neutrophils. Eosinophils concentrate in tissues during allergic reactions and parasitic infections, yet their specific role is unknown. Major roles postulated include destruction of some parasites, ingestion of immune complexes, and limitation of inflammatory reactions (Tizard, 1984).

Eosinophilia occurs in diseases involving increased levels of IgE, such as allergic gastroenteropathy and IgE-mediated anaphylaxis (Goust, 1986). Eosinophils are chemically attracted to sites of IgE concentration. These cells carry certain enzymes that neutralize chemicals responsible for anaphylaxis; however, the overall effect of eosinophilic degranulation is cell destruction. Eosinophils cause inflammation, bronchospasm, and tissue damage by releasing potent chemical mediators.

Some cytotoxic proteins within the eosinophilic granules include major basic protein, eosinophilic peroxidase, eosinophilic cationic proteins, eosinophil-derived neurotoxin, and a variety of enzymes (Gleich and Butterfield, 1987). These cytotoxic proteins not only exert a direct cytolytic effect on the microorganism, but some proteins also elicit the support of other cells. For example, eosinophilic peroxidase binds to another granulocyte, the mast cell, and triggers mast cell degranulation and later destruction of the microorganism.

Basophils. Basophils play an important role in cutaneous hypersensitivity reactions but show little phagocytic action. Basophils contain many cytoplasmic granules containing histamine and heparin, two chemical mediators involved in immunologic reactions. Structurally, the basophil is very delicate and is susceptible to easy rupture and release of granule contents into blood and tissues. Both the anticoagulant properties of heparin and the vasoactivity of histamine increase the severity of IgE-dependent allergies (Barrett, 1988).

Basophils contain a variety of vasoactive substances, such as histamine and serotonin. The mediators released from basophils cause a variety of biologic activities. The biologic actions of these mediators include increased vascular permeability, contraction of smooth muscle, and enhancement of the inflammatory response (Barrett, 1988).

Mast Cells. Mast cells arise in the bone marrow from a myeloid stem cell. Found at the point of antigen entry into the body, mast cells are called the sentinels of the immune system. Mast cells reside primarily in cutaneous and mucosal surfaces (Austen, 1983). They are the only immunologically active cells that can immediately recognize nonself antigens without presensitization in the blood or lymph systems. Mast cells function as effectors of immediate hypersensitivity or allergic reactions.

Mast cells concentrate most of the body's IgE on their cell membranes. Complexing of antigen and surface-expressed IgE triggers degranulation of the mast cell and alters the cell membrane. Degranulation releases histamines and other mediators into the extracellular environment. Changes in the cell membrane lead to arachidonic acid metabolism and the secretion of prostaglandin D_2 and leukotrienes, potent mediators of immediate hypersensitivity responses (Austen and Fisher, 1987).

Lymphoid Cells

The lymphoid cells of the immune system differ from other cells in their ability to react specifically with antigen and to produce specific cell products. Lymphoid cells include B- and T-lymphocytes, plasma cells, and large granular lymphocytes. The most well defined population of large granular lymphocytes is natural killer cells.

Lymphocyte is a morphologic term that describes a population of cells with many different immune functions. About 30% of the total white blood cell count is lymphocytes. One subset of lymphocytes (T-lymphocytes) participates in the primary recognition of antigen. Structurally similar but functionally different, B-lymphocytes produce circulating antibody.

Both B- and T-lymphocytes arise from a single lymphoid stem cell. As shown in Figure 51–4, the process of maturation differentiates B-cells from T-cells. Morphologic separation of T- and B-lymphocytes by visual inspection through blood smears is not possible. These lymphocytes can, however, be separated by function and cell surface markers (antigens). Some distinguishing functional and antigenic features of T- and B-lymphocytes are listed in Table 51–6.

B-Lymphocytes. B-lymphocytes are those cells that contain completely formed chains of immunoglobulin. These immunoglobulin molecules, expressed only on the cell surface of the B-lymphocyte, allow in vitro identification of B-cells (Kincade and Gimble, 1989). Immunoglobulin serves as a unique surface marker for B-lymphocytes. There are, however, many other proteins expressed on the cell membrane of the B-lymphocyte. The function of many of these surface markers remains unknown (Kincade and Gimble, 1989). One functionally important surface marker expressed on B-lymphocytes is MHC class II antigens. The MHC binds antigen fragments to the B-cell surface and helps B-cells interact with other immune cells (Kincade and Gimble, 1989).

Immunoglobulins are one of the few surface marker proteins made only by B-cells. The proteins expressed on the cell surface of B-cells change according to the stages of B-cell maturity. A certain number of receptors and glycoproteins are required for proper immune function; however, there can be great diversity in how and when these molecules are acquired (Kincade and Gimble, 1989).

In the resting state, B-lymphocytes have not been exposed to antigenic stimuli. On stimulation, many biochemical changes take place in the resting B-cell. These changes result in an increase in cell size and in the cellular structures responsible for protein synthesis (Kincade and Gimble, 1989). B-lymphocytes undergo a distinct developmental process. Early identifiable pre-B-cells, which express incomplete immunoglobulin molecules, go through intermediate stages of development and activation. Final differentiation of B-lymphocytes leads to plasma cell for-

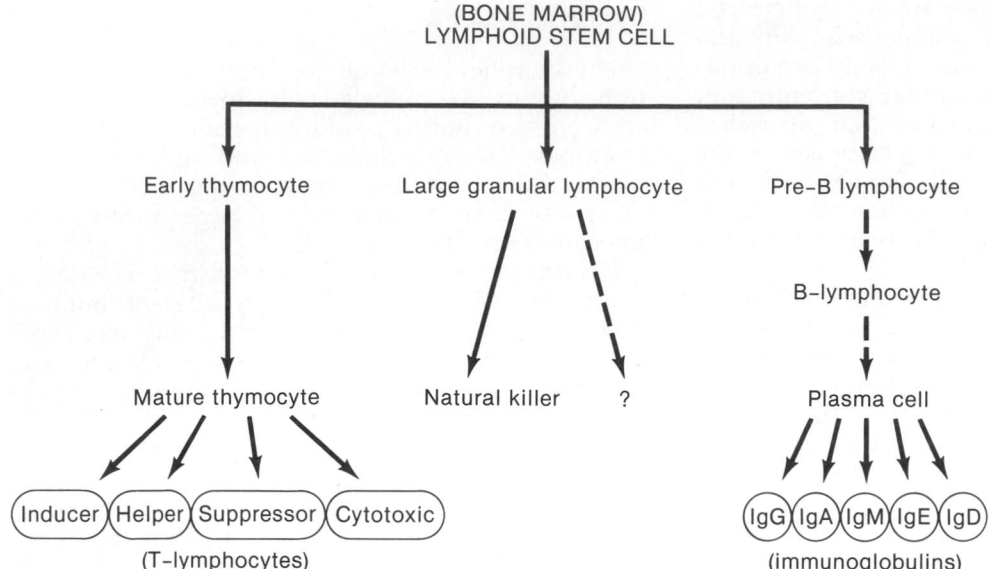

FIGURE 51–4. Maturation process of lymphocytes.

mation. Plasma cells are the major secretors of antibody (Kincade and Gimble, 1989). Thousands of antibody molecules can be released by a single plasma cell. The plasma cell does not usually divide and has a lifespan of approximately 4 days (Stobo, 1987).

One of the most mystifying aspects of B-lymphocyte function has been the generation of an endless variety of immunoglobulins. Two complementary and antigen-independent processes that create this diversity have been identified. First, the specific genes (variable region genes) in pre-B-lymphocytes undergo a series of orderly rearrangements. Each rearrangement creates a new type of B-cell clone. The second process is polyclonal proliferation. Almost 1 million clones of B-cells, never exposed to antigen and each with a different antigen specificity,

bring about the wide variety of antibodies (Cooper, 1987).

Activation of the B-lymphocyte requires extensive short-range communication between antigen, B-cells, and other immune cells. Communication occurs through a host of lymphokines. B-cells have receptors for interleukin, interferon, growth factors, and transferrin. Note that these lymphokines act in concert to enhance and counteract each other. The concentration of these lymphokines varies considerably throughout a specific immune response. Expression of class II molecules is greatly increased when resting B-cells are activated, thus enchancing antigen presentation.

T-Lymphocytes. From 65% to 80% of all lymphocytes in the blood are of the T-type. These cells,

TABLE 51–6. Relative Comparison of T- and B-Lymphocytes

Characteristic	T-Lymphocytes	B-Lymphocytes
Immune mechanism	Cell-mediated immunity	Humoral immunity
Site of precursor origin	Thymus	Bursal equivalent (fetal liver, bone marrow, gastrointestinal tract)
Distribution in tissue	High in thoracic duct (90%), blood (80%), lymph (75%)	High in bone marrow (>75%), gut-associated lymphoid tissue (70%)
Functions	Protection against most viruses, fungi, and slow-acting bacteria via macrostimulation and complement activation Mediation of cutaneous delayed hypersensitivity reactions Rejection of foreign grafts Regulation of the immune response Immunologic surveillance	Differentiation into plasma cells that secrete antibody Mediation of immediate phage hypersensitivity reaction (allergy) Protection against pyogenic infections and toxic reactions
Cell product	Lymphokines	Immunoglobulins
Surface markers	T antigen	Surface immunoglobulin
Immune tolerance	Occurs early and persists immunity	Less sensitive than T-cells

which have a longer lifespan than B-cells, are the major recirculating cell in the lymph nodes. The T-cell receptor (TcR) is perhaps the most critical surface marker protein on the cell membrane of the T-lymphocyte. The amino acid and DNA sequence of the receptor is known, revealing a pentameric T3–Ti antigen receptor complex (Royer and Reinherz, 1987). Identification of the T-cell receptor has allowed definitive isolation of T-lymphocytes. The T-cell receptor functions as an identity marker and allows the T-lymphocyte to interact with antigen, other cells, and specific antibodies.

There are several types of functionally distinct T-cells. Helper T-lymphocytes aid the triggering of the immune response. These cells help B-cells in the synthesis of immunoglobulins to T-cell–dependent antigens. These antigens are more complex than antigens that activate B-cells directly. Suppressor T-lymphocytes hold back immune responses. These cells restrict antibody production by B-cells. Cytotoxic T-lymphocytes can kill other cells recognized as non-self, for example, tumor cells and transplanted tissues.

In addition to the three functional groups of T-cells just described, T-lymphocytes are grouped by distinct proteins expressed on the cell membrane. At least four different taxonomies are used in the literature to identify these T-lymphocyte surface markers (Sprent, 1989). These taxonomic structures include a system developed in mice (Lyt), two human T-lymphocyte models (T_1, T_H), and a universal nomenclature proposed by the World Health Organization (CD). The T-lymphocyte subsets identified by any one taxonomic system only partially correspond with the functional categories of inducer, helper, suppressor, and cytotoxic T-lymphocytes.

The monoclonal antibodies specific for CD4+ and CD8+ have identified two T-lymphocyte subsets that are functionally distinct. Mature T-cells express CD4+ or CD8+ but rarely both. The ratio of CD4+ to CD8+ varies considerably with disease but is usually 2:1. The functional role of the CD8+ subset is restricted by class I MHC antigens. CD4+ functional activity is restricted by class II MHC antigens. This means that T-lymphocytes that are CD4+ bind to class II MHC molecules, and T-lymphocytes that are CD8+ bind to class I molecules. Because class I antigens are present on nearly all cells, CD8+ cells interact with virtually every cell in the body. Class II antigens are expressed only on immune cells, and therefore CD4+ cells interact primarily with B-cells and macrophages. One must keep in mind that MHC molecules help lymphocytes interact with antigens, thus strengthening the immune response.

Following the initial identification of these two T-lymphocyte subsets, CD8+ cells were mistakenly identified as suppressor cells (Ts), and CD4+ cells were identified as helper cells (Th). CD4+ cells consist primarily of helper T-lymphocytes and to a lesser extent cytotoxic T-lymphocytes. CD8+ cells consist of both cytotoxic and suppressor lymphocytes (Royer and Reinherz, 1987).

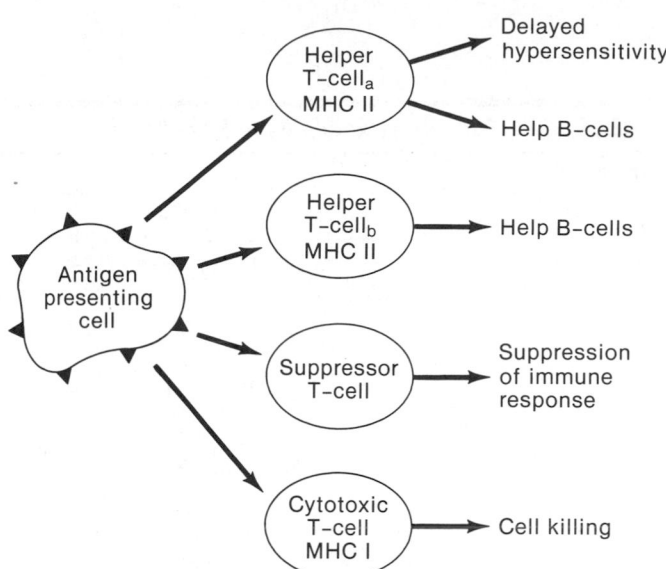

FIGURE 51–5. Major functions of T-lymphocytes. MHC, major histocompatibility complex. T-cell$_a$, subclass associated with delayed hypersensitivity; T-cell$_b$, subclass associated with modulation of B-cell response.

The major functions of the T-lymphocytes include mediation of cytolytic reactions, regulation of delayed hypersensitivity reactions, and overall regulation of immune responses (Fig. 51–5). The regulatory function of T-cells can be either positive or negative. The subpopulations of T-cells act in a variety of ways to enhance or suppress the immune response. Cytotoxic T-lymphocytes provide protection against most viral, fungal, and slow-acting bacterial infections and against some tumor cells. Delayed hypersensitivity is a localized immune reaction to a previously encountered antigen. Activation of T-lymphocytes requires the carefully orchestrated interaction of the TcR, the lymphokine interleukin-2 (IL-2), and the receptor for IL-2 (Royer and Reinherz, 1987).

Activation of T cells is triggered by the interaction of immunogen, the TcR, and MHC antigens and leads to the surface expression of IL-2 receptors. Activated T lymphocytes synthesize and secrete IL-2, which becomes bound to IL-2 receptors on T-lymphocytes (Royer and Reinherz, 1987). Once a critical number of IL-2 receptors have been bound, DNA synthesis and T-cell proliferation occur. Activation responses are maximized in the presence of interleukin-1, a lymphokine secreted by macrophages. Activated T-cells release soluble lymphokines that influence growth and differentiation of other cells (Sprent, 1989).

These lymphokines are not dependent upon the specific antigen-inducing activation response nor on the MHC antigens expressed by macrophages. The lymphokines produced through lymphocyte activation amplify the immune reaction (Dinarello and Mier, 1987). The same lymphokines are also produced by lymphocytes and macrophages. These lymphokines are able to stimulate or inhibit a variety of functions in T- and B-lymphocytes and macrophages.

TABLE 51–7. Functional Activities of Lymphokines

Abbreviation	Names	Functions
IL-1	Interleukin-1 Lymphocyte-activating factor Endogenous pyrogen	Potentiation of T- and B-cell responses Elevation of body temperature Osteoclast activation and bone resorption Induction of fibroblast proliferation
IL-2	Interleukin-2 T-cell growth factor	Stimulation of T-cell growth Costimulation of B-cell differentiation
IL-3	Interleukin-3 Mast-cell growth factor Multicolony-stimulating factor	Stimulation of mast-cell growth Multipotential hematopoietic cell growth
IL-4	Interleukin-4 B-cell stimulatory factor 1 B-cell growth factor T-cell growth factor 2 Mast-cell growth factor 2 IgE-IgG$_1$ enhancing factor	Costimulation of B-cell proliferation Stimulation of limited T-cell growth Synergy with IL-3 in mast-cell growth Enhancement of IgE and IgG$_1$ production Ia expression on B-cells and macrophages Enhanced proliferation of hematopoietic progenitors
IL-5	Interleukin-5 T-cell replacing factor B-cell growth factor 2 IgA-enhancing factor Eosinophil differentiation factor	Stimulation of in vitro antibody responses Costimulation of B-cell growth Enhancement of IgA production Stimulation of eosinophil differentiation
IFNγ	Interferon-γ	Inhibition of viral replication Induction of Ia expression on macrophages Activation of macrophages for killing Inhibition of all activities of IL-4 on B-cells Enhancement of IgG$_{2a}$ synthesis by B-cells
TNF	Tumor necrosis factor Cachectin	Cytotoxic factor Induction of "wasting disease" Activation of granulocytes and eosinophils Osteoclast activation and bone resorption Stimulation of fibroblast proliferation Chemotaxis of granulocytes and phagocytes
LT	Lymphotoxin Tumor necrosis factor-β	Cytotoxic factor Activation of granulocytes and eosinophils Osteoclast activation and bone resorption Stimulation of fibroblast proliferation Chemotaxis of granulocytes and phagocytes
GM-CSF	Granulocyte-macrophage colony-stimulating factor	Stimulation of growth of mixed colonies (granulocytes and macrophages) from progenitor cells
ppENK	Preproenkephalin	Opioid peptide Stimulation of natural killer cells

From Feldman, M., Lamb, J., and Owen, M. (1989). *T cells* (p. 181). New York: John Wiley & Sons.

Table 51–7 lists the functional activities of lymphokines involved in lymphocyte activation.

Natural Killer Cells. Large granular lymphocytes make up almost 3% of the peripheral blood cells. These lymphocytes share some T-lymphocyte, B-lymphocyte, and macrophage surface antigens but are clearly a distinct subpopulation of lymphocytes (Trincheri and Perussia, 1984). Several different cell lines are included under this term. Natural killer (NK) cells are the cells most frequently described (Barrett, 1988).

Natural killer cells participate as effector cells in immune reactions and do not require prior sensitization to exhibit cytotoxicity. Natural killer cells act directly as cytotoxic cells and also produce cytotoxicity by combining with antibody-coated target cells (termed the antibody-dependent cellular cytotoxic [ADCC] reaction). MHC class I or II proteins do not restrict NK cytotoxicity (Bolhuis, 1989). In their resting state NK cells exhibit maximal killing potential.

The cytotoxic mechanisms of NK cells are not fully understood. The lytic action of agents such as perforins offers one possible mechanism (Anegon et al., 1988). Lymphokines also increase the cell-killing ability of NK cells. Lymphokines released by NK cells include interferon, tumor necrosis factor, and growth factor. Release of lymphokines is triggered by NK cell interaction with IL-2 or target cells (Anegon et al., 1988). Target cells for NK cells include foreign host tissue as in allografts, some viruses, and neoplastic cells (Nakamura, 1989). In vitro exposure to IL-2 has been used to induce the production of lymphokine-activated killer cells (LAK cells). The therapeutic efficacy of concurrent administration of LAK cells and IL-2 is now undergoing clinical evaluation in the treatment of malignant disease. In vivo LAK cell counterparts have not been isolated, however (Lefor et al., 1989).

The immunoregulatory function of NK cells is under extensive exploration. Lymphokines produced by T- and B-lymphocytes influence NK cell function. Some NK cells also exert immunoregulatory effects upon T- and B-lymphocytes. The exact mechanisms underlying the immunoregulatory role of NK cells have yet to be defined (Kumagai et al., 1989; Tilden and Clement, 1989).

The cells and tissues of the immune system have been reviewed. Some of the interactions between different cell types have been briefly described. In the next sections, the interactions among immune system components will be described more fully in the context of how the immune system protects body integrity.

NONSPECIFIC IMMUNITY

Nonspecific immunity (innate immunity) refers to the type of natural resistance each individual characteristically exhibits. Innate immunity varies widely between species and to a lesser extent between individuals (Barrett, 1988). Each exposure to a foreign substance activates nonspecific immune responses. These responses are the body's first line of defense (Roitt et al., 1985). Although selective in differentiating self from nonself, innate immunity is not dependent upon specific antigenic recognition.

In comparison, specific immune responses (or acquired immune responses) depend upon exposure to a foreign substance and later recognition of and reaction to the substance (memory) (Barrett, 1988). When foreign agents penetrate the innate immune defenses of the body, the acquired immune system specifically recognizes and selectively eliminates them.

Natural Resistance: External Defense System

Nonspecific immunity enables the individual to resist the penetration of foreign substances, fosters the inhibition or destruction of agents invading tissues, and promotes the elimination of toxic wastes (Graziano and Bell, 1985). The first resistive forces met by an invading organism are those outside the physiologic milieu of the body and therefore are categorized as the external defense system (Table 51–8). These forces do not represent a coordinated system and indeed function independently of one another. Nevertheless, they are effective against a variety of potential pathogens.

Anatomic Barriers. The first line of defense encountered by most potential pathogens are the skin and mucous membranes. These tissues act in nonspecific immunity by providing a physical barrier to invasion. The skin is the more resistant barrier be-

TABLE 51–8. External Defense System

Respiratory System
Mucus
Cilia
Macrophages
Antiviral and antimicrobial secretions

Gastrointestinal System
Acid pH in stomach
Normal flora

Integumentary System
Anatomic barrier
Antimicrobial secretions

Genitourinary System
Flow rate of urine
Acid pH of urine
Lysozyme
Vaginal lactic acid

Eyes
Tears have physical cleansing action
Lysozyme

cause of its thick outer layer. However, the skin is more than a mere anatomic barrier. The antimicrobial functions of the skin are an important defense mechanism and are discussed more fully in the next section (Adams, 1985). Breaks in skin integrity increase the risk of infection. The skin should be kept relatively dry because in the presence of continuous moisture, skin tends to break down. On the other hand, if the skin is too dry, lubrication should be provided to maintain its integrity. Appropriate skin care of the hospitalized patient will maintain this important defense barrier.

The mucous membranes are structurally more susceptible to penetration than the skin. However, mucosal tissues are protected by several antimicrobial activities. The mucous secretions themselves tend to trap and inactivate organisms. The mucous membranes of the respiratory tract not only act as a trapping mechanism but, together with the action of the ciliated epithelial cells, sweep away foreign microbes (Janson-Bjerklie, 1983). In addition, alveolar macrophages patrol the surface of the mucous membranes. The major function of these cells is the phagocytic destruction of inhaled objects. Tobacco smoke decreases the viability of these macrophages, thus putting smokers at increased risk for respiratory problems (Barrett, 1988).

Lymphoid tissues line the gastrointestinal, respiratory, and genitourinary tracts. IgA and secretory component, found in the secretions from these tissues, increase the protective capacity of lymphoid tissues. IgA also provides antibacterial and antiviral properties to mucosal membranes (Barrett, 1988).

Microbial Barriers. There are many microorganisms that colonize the skin and mucosal surfaces. Both internally and externally, a normal flora develops. This flora acts to suppress overgrowth and later infection by pathogenic organisms. The importance of the normal flora of the intestine is often demonstrated in patients receiving long-term antibacterial therapy with a broad-spectrum antibiotic. After about 1 week of therapy, patients may complain of increased flatulence. Stool cultures frequently reveal an increase in number of the yeast *Candida albicans*. This organism is part of the normal intestinal flora and is resistant to antibacterial antibiotics. When antibiotics remove the normal bacterial flora, the yeast thrives and overpopulates the bowel. Continued drug therapy may cause candidiasis of the intestine, in which erosion of the mucous membranes may occur. By this means, the yeast can enter the body and produce a disseminated candidiasis. Normal flora also protect other regions of the body such as the nasopharynx and the vagina.

Physiologic Barriers. Secretions of the stomach, skin, and female genitourinary system provide a physiologic barrier against antigens. Hydrogen chloride is secreted in the stomach. Lactic acid and saturated and unsaturated fatty acids are secreted in sweat and on the skin. Lactic acid is secreted in the female genitourinary system. Lysozyme and mucus of the upper respiratory tract and lung are also physiologic barriers (Barrett, 1988).

The gastric juice is an unfavorable environment for many pathogenic organisms, which are destroyed in the stomach following ingestion. The lactic acid in sweat and the unsaturated fatty acids in the exogenous secretions from the sebaceous glands are potent antibacterial agents. The saturated fatty acids in these secretions are fungistatic.

Normal urine flow clears bacteria from the urinary tract, preventing infection. Inside the mature female reproductive tract, cells synthesize and store glycogen. As the cells die, the glycogen degrades to lactic acid, creating a bacteriostatic environment in the vagina (Adam, 1985; Bellanti and Kadlec, 1985).

Ciliary action in the respiratory tract is another important physiologic mechanism of resistance. Cilia constantly sweep mucus upward toward the throat. This movement allows organisms trapped in the mucus to be swallowed, exposing them to the potent bactericidal actions of the gastric juices (Adam, 1985; Bellanti and Kadlec, 1985).

The tendency to weep when objects enter the eye is an effective cleansing action and protects the mucosal surfaces of the eye. In the absence of weeping, the action of the enzyme lysozyme is far more important. Lysozyme has the ability to split the bacterial cell wall, causing destruction of the cell. This enzyme is present in high concentration in tears and to a lesser extent in nasal mucus, urine, and plasma and within phagocytic cells. Gram-negative bacteria are highly resistant to lysozyme, but gram-positive microorganisms are not (Adam, 1985; Bellanti and Kadlec, 1985).

Natural Resistance: Internal Defense Systems

Phagocytosis. When a foreign substance or antigen enters the body, a chain of events called the phagocytic response is set in motion. The primary role of phagocytosis is to localize an antigen, destroy it or inactivate it, and process it for handling by other parts of the immune system. Phagocytosis is a multiphasic act requiring the following steps: recognition of the material to be ingested, movement toward the object (chemotaxis), attachment, ingestion, and subsequent intracellular digestion by several antimicrobial mechanisms (Fig. 51–6). Very little phagocytosis occurs in the blood because the movement of the blood tends to hold cells apart. Phagocytosis is best accomplished on surfaces and is described as a surface phenomenon (Barrett, 1988).

First, phagocytes are drawn to the area of antigen invasion by a process called chemotaxis. A chemical is released by the antigen itself or by the tissue it has injured. This chemical, the chemotactic factor, stim-

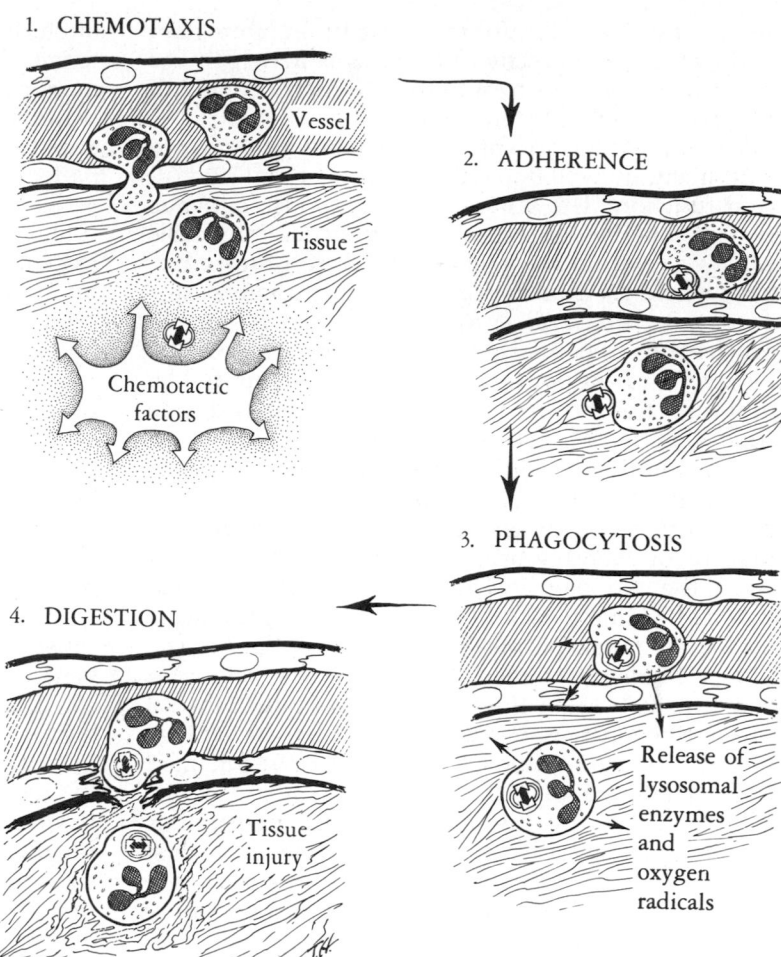

1. CHEMOTAXIS

Vessel

Tissue

Chemotactic factors

2. ADHERENCE

3. PHAGOCYTOSIS

Release of lysosomal enzymes and oxygen radicals

4. DIGESTION

Tissue injury

FIGURE 51–6. Sequence of reactions leading to tissue injury associated with neutrophil influx. Note that in addition to chemotaxis, adherence, phagocytosis, and digestion processes that normally result in particle inactivation, there may also be release of neutrophilic granule content (lysosomal enzymes) that results in tissue injury. (From Henson, P. M. (1985). In J. A. Bellanti (Ed.), *Immunology III* (p. 255). Philadelphia: W. B. Saunders.)

ulates the body's initial efforts to search and destroy. The next step in the sequence is phagocytosis, the process by which a particle is ingested by a phagocytic cell. This process has two steps: the attachment phase and the ingestion phase. During the attachment phase, firm contact occurs between the cell and the particle (Densen and Mandell, 1987). Such contact is largely dependent upon the surface properties of the particle. Many bacteria are unencapsulated and are rapidly taken up by phagocytes and destroyed. Encapsulated strains such as the pneumococcus, however, are poorly ingested and hence are not destroyed.

Molecular factors that promote attachment of phagocytes to the objects they will engulf are called opsonins (Densen and Mandell, 1987). Virtually any substance that improves phagocytosis is an opsonin. The best opsonin is antibody against the cell targeted for ingestion. If it is coated with antibody, its surface charge is unable to repel the phagocytic cell. These phagocytic cells tend to carry immunoglobulins of the IgM and IgG class on their surfaces. When an antigen contacts its specific antibody on the phagocytic surface, it is held there by the serologic reaction that takes place. This activity enables phagocytosis to occur. Immunoglobulins are opsonins and share

this property with other blood proteins (Barrett, 1988).

The ingestion process is the next step of phagocytosis and includes engulfment of the particle. The phagocyte extends its cell membrane to form a vacuole, which surrounds and encloses the antigen. The membrane enclosing the antigen pinches off from the cell surface. Finally, the antigen is internalized and digested by lysosomal enzymes contained within the phagocyte (Densen and Mandell, 1987).

The fate of the ingested antigen depends upon its interaction with the phagocyte. Usually antigen is completely destroyed; however, antigen fragments can stay within the phagocyte. Occasionally, both the antigen and the phagocyte die. The necrotic debris that results becomes purulent matter or pus. Another outcome of the interaction between the antigen and the phagocyte is survival of the antigen. If the phagocyte lives, it may spread disease as it travels through the body carrying a live organism. With death of the phagocyte, release of antigen may trigger specific immunologic defense mechanisms.

Inflammation. Inflammation is a complex series of events that occurs when the body is injured (Ward, 1985). There is a tendency to consider the inflammatory response harmful to the body. Inflammation is, however, a protective mechanism in which the body tries either to return to the pre-injury condition or to repair itself after injury.

The clinical signs of inflammation are well known. They include swelling, redness, heat, pain, and altered function. The inflammatory response depends on both intact blood vessels and the circulating cells and fluids within these channels. According to histologic criteria, three states of inflammation exist—acute, subacute, and chronic. The acute inflammatory response begins by the dilatation of blood vessels and the outpouring of leukocytes and fluids. Clinically, this results in redness (erythema) due to blood vessel dilatation, swelling (edema) due to escape of fluids into soft tissues, and firmness (induration) due to accumulation of fluids and cells. The result of these processes leads to a loss of the normal capacity of blood vessels to keep fluids and cells within the vasculature. The release of certain factors, such as histamine, from tissue mast cells may make the vessel more permeable to plasma fluids. The acute inflammatory response reflects the effects of mediators acting on the blood vessels rather than a nonspecific injury to the vessel. The mediators cause selective release of fluids and cells from the inflamed tissues (Gallin, 1989).

Within 30 to 60 minutes of injury, neutrophils appear, representing the first line of defense against invading microorganisms. As discussed earlier, the prime function of neutrophils is to ingest and destroy pathogens. If the acute inflammatory response progresses, mononuclear cells (including monocytes and lymphocytes) appear within 4 to 5 hours. Monocytes also phagocytose pathogens, whereas lymphocytes respond to foreign agents by specific humoral and cell-mediated phenomena that will be discussed later (Ward, 1985).

Although the inflammatory response is protective, if it becomes aberrant, serious consequences may occur. For example, the outpouring of too much fluid from the vasculature into the brain may cause a serious rise in intracranial pressure. Accumulation of fluid due to inflammation in the pleural or pericardial cavities may compromise organ function in these areas. In addition, the arrival of excessive numbers of neutrophils and the subsequent release of their enzymatic contents may result in serious structural damage (e.g., vasculitis, nephritis) (Ward, 1985).

The subacute inflammatory response is a somewhat delayed phase of the acute inflammatory response and is characterized by the accumulation of lymphocytes and monocytes and the formation of granulation tissue. For example, 1 to 3 days following a skin laceration, a dramatic proliferation of endothelial cells and fibroblasts occurs. Within 5 days a bridge of connective tissue has formed across a previously open and exposed area (Ward, 1985).

If the inflammatory response is not completely successful in restoring the injured tissue to its original state or if repair of tissue is not accomplished, a state of chronic inflammation may ensure. This is characterized by the continued presence of lymphocytes, monocytes, and plasma cells. Persistence of foreign material that mobilizes immunologic reactions may also cause chronic inflammation. For example, in patients with viral hepatitis, replicating virus may persist within the liver (Ward, 1985).

Depending upon the severity of the inflammatory response, a variety of systemic effects may occur. Many microorganisms and certain white blood cells produce pyrogenic materials, which act on the hypothalamus to increase temperature (McCarron, 1986; Norwood, 1988). Although there is a tendency to consider fever as harmful to the body, it has several beneficial effects. An elevation in body temperature of only a few degrees results in inhibition or death of a variety of microorganisms. Pneumococci are killed by temperatures as low as 40°C. It has been suggested that one of the reasons why fever may be beneficial during viral infections is that it leads to lysosomal breakdown. Perforation of lysosomes causes autodestruction of the infected cell and prevents viral replication (Cunha, 1985; Cunha et al., 1984). Release of interferons by T-cells and fibroblasts during inflammation also inhibits viral replication. Temperature increases of only 2° to 3° F are necessary to increase the production of antiviral interferons. It has frequently been observed that patients who are unable to mount a febrile response or who have subnormal temperatures have a poorer prognosis than those who mount a normal febrile response (Cunha et al., 1984).

Another systemic effect of inflammation may be an increased production of white blood cells (WBCs). A serum WBC level of greater than 10,000/mm^3 is called leukocytosis. Extreme elevations of WBCs may indicate a lymphoproliferative disease such as leukemia. Low-grade WBC elevations can occur with cell injury due to myocardial infarction and bone fracture or with other events such as digestion, exercise, and increased stress. Total elevation of the WBC count is, therefore, a nonspecific phenomenon (Gurevich, 1985).

The WBC differential count provides more specific information. In this test, 100 or more white cells in the peripheral blood are classified according to the two major types of leukocytes—granulocytes (neutrophils, eosinophils, and basophils), and nongranulocytes (lymphocytes and monocytes). The percentage of each is also determined. The differential count is the relative number of each type of white cell in the blood. The absolute number of each type of white cell is obtained by multiplying the percentage value of each type by the total WBC count. When the total number of immature neutrophils (blasts, bands, or stabs) is increased in the differential count, it is termed a "shift to the left" because cell maturation is visualized from the left side to the right side with less mature cells on the left (Gurevich, 1985).

Prolonged bacterial infections tend to cause a shift to the left. In such infections mature cells are killed by bacterial action and are replaced by immature white cells. In an attempt to replace the mature neutrophils, the bone marrow releases cells prematurely. The release of immature cells results in an increased number of circulating neutrophils, but these immature neutrophils are poor participants in phagocytosis (Gurevich, 1985). Overwhelming infection may result from an imbalance in the proportion of immature to mature neutrophils. Careful attention to the results of WBC differential counts is essential in critically ill patients. A "shift to the right" signifies the presence of mature neutrophils with more nuclear segments than normal. Commonly, this occurs with hepatic disease and pernicious anemia. A "degenerative shift" indicates an increased number of band cells and a low WBC count and reflects bone marrow depression. A "regenerative shift" occurs with bone marrow stimulation. Stimulation of the bone marrow causes increased numbers of band cells, metamyelocytes, myelocytes, and a high WBC count. This situation frequently occurs with pneumonia and appendicitis (Gurevich, 1985).

The hallmark of leukopenia is a decreased serum white blood cell count of less than 4500 cells/mm³. Leukopenia commonly occurs in viral infections, typhoid fever, or toxic reactions that depress the bone marrow. Viral and tuberculous infections usually produce an increase in mature lymphocytes (Gurevich, 1985).

An increased erythrocyte sedimentation rate may occur as another systemic effect of inflammation. The technique for determining the sedimentation rate requires the addition of an anticoagulant to blood in a test tube. The red blood cells settle to the bottom more rapidly than normal in patients with an elevated sedimentation rate. An increase in the sedimentation rate occurs during the acute inflammatory stage of infection, coinciding with an increase in the protein fibrinogen, which is essential for the healing process.

It is vital for the nurse to understand the physiologic changes that occur during the inflammatory process. One can then better understand the many defense mechanisms that may be operating during different disease states.

The Complement System. One of the most complex and powerful results of antigen-antibody binding is the activation of complement. Discovery of complement within serum occurred in the nineteenth century. The bactericidal activity of fresh serum required not only antibody but also a nonspecific component that enchanced antibody activity (Barrett, 1989). That nonspecific component was later identified as complement.

Recent research has shown a broad role for complement as a participant in inflammation, immune tissue injury, and modulation of the immune response. Elevated levels of activated complement are associated with pulmonary injury in adult respiratory distress syndrome (Langlois et al., 1989). There are

at least 20 complement proteins and fragments that circulate in the plasma in an inactive form. Activation of complement proteins results from splitting the inactive protein into two parts. The larger part attaches to target cells and bacteria. The smaller part is released into the fluid around the cell. Most small complement fragments have biologic activity and interact with other proteins in the complement sequence (Frank and Fries, 1989). Table 51–9 describes some of the major complement proteins.

The role of biologically active byproducts of complement activation assumes great importance in the immune response. First, the coating of bacteria or other immune complexes with components of complements aids ingestion of the bacteria by phagocytic cells. The cooperation of complement and immune complexes demonstrates the opsonic function of complement. Second, several of the products of complement proteins serve as chemotactic factors that attract phagocytes to the site of the reaction (inflammatory function of complement). When certain complement proteins are activated, other complement fragments are released. Some complement fragments act to release histamine from mast cells and are chemoattractants for polymorphonuclear leukocytes. Histamine increases vascular permeability and enhances smooth muscle contraction. The result is very

TABLE 51–9. Some Proteins of the Complement Cascade

Protein		Concentration in Serum (mg/ml)	Biologic Function
C1	q	80	Binds to Ag-Ab complexes
	r	34	Subunit of C1
	s	30	Enzymatic activity cleaves C4 and C2
C4		350	C4a anaphylatoxin C4b viral neutralization
C2		15	
C3		1200	C3a anaphylatoxin, immunoregulatory
			C3b key component of alternative pathway; major opsonin in serum
			C3e fragment induces leukocytosis
C5		75	C5a anaphylatoxin; principal chemotactic factor in serum; induces neutrophil attachment to endothelium
			C5b initiates membrane attack
C6		70	Participates with C5b in formation of membrane attack complex (MAC) that lyses cells
C7		60	
C8		80	
C9		60	
Factor B		225	Bb causes macrophage spreading on surfaces
Factor D		1	
Properdin		25	Stabilizes alternative pathway convertase

From Lockey, R., and Bukantz, S. (1987). *Fundamentals of immunology and allergy* (p. 42). Philadelphia: W. B. Saunders.

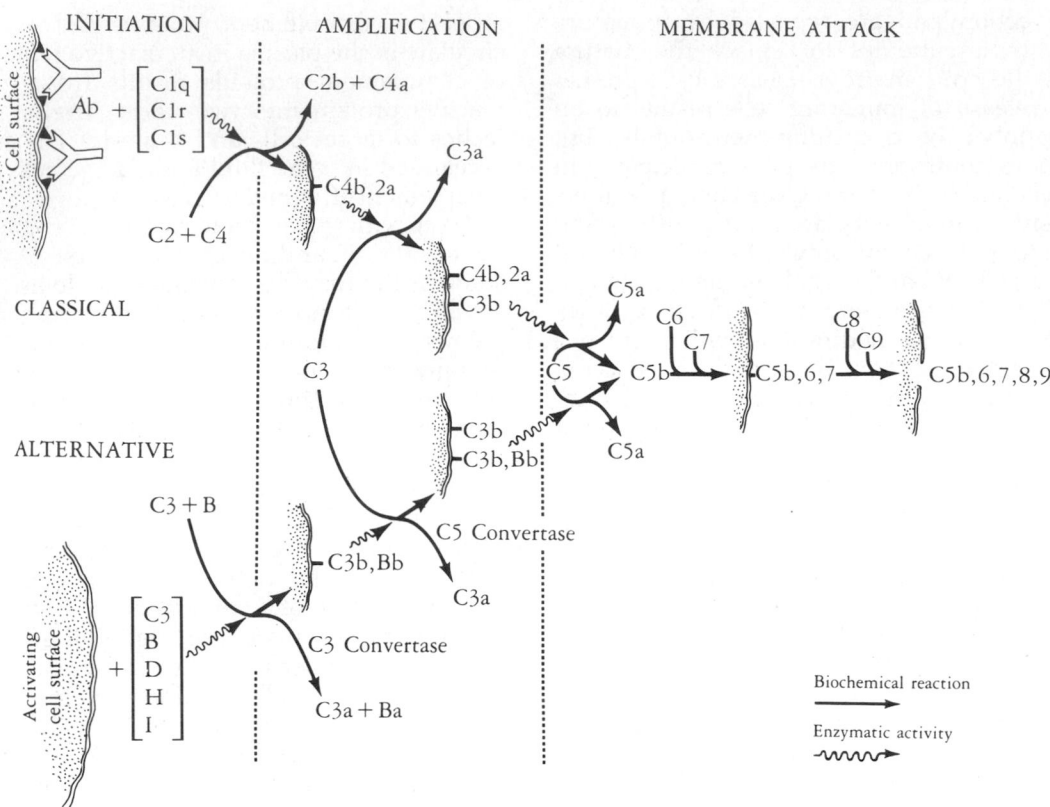

INITIATION   AMPLIFICATION   MEMBRANE ATTACK

FIGURE 51–7. Schematic representation of the two pathways of complement activation. (From Kimkel, S. L., et al. (1985). In J. A. Bellanti (Ed.), *Immunology III* (p. 107). Philadelphia: W. B. Saunders.)

similar to that seen in the classic anaphylactic reaction. Third, the late-acting proteins of the complement cascade form the complex that attacks and causes the death of target cells. The cytotoxic activity of complement is directed against viruses, bacteria, fungi, parasites, virus-infected cells, and tumor cells (Barrett, 1989).

Several cell types synthesize complement proteins. Two of the most important cell types are the liver hepatocyte and mononuclear phagocytic cells. Activation of complement proteins results in a rapid cascade of protein degradation. Degraded complement protein fragments activate the later steps in the cascade. These proteins are activated by two independent pathways termed the classic pathway and the alternative pathway (Fig. 51–7).

Activation of the classic complement pathway, C1 through C9, starts with complexing of antigen of antibody. Antibody and complement proteins circulate in the blood and lymph. Antibody undergoes a conformational change upon interaction with antigen. This requisite change in antibody structure allows interaction between antibody and complement. It is the antibody conformational change that is the basis for specific activation of the classic complement pathway (Barrett, 1988; Cooper, 1987). Table 51–10 lists the activators of the classic pathway.

Another group of activators of the complement system includes many types of aggregated proteins,

bacterial and other microbial membranes, and various cell walls (Table 51–11). These components activate the complement sequence through the alternative pathway (also known as the properdin pathway). This pathway is an alternative to the classic pathway in that this system begins the complement sequence at C3. The alternative pathway does not absolutely require antibody, C1, C4, or C2 for activation (Cooper, 1987).

Parts of bacterial membranes from gram-negative bacteria and the walls of certain gram-positive organisms are some of the most powerful activators of the alternative pathway. Consider, for example, an in-

---

TABLE 51–10. Activators of the Classic Pathway

Immunoglobulins
IgG (human subclasses 1, 2, and 3)
IgM

Nonimmunoglobulin Activators
Bacterial lipopolysaccharide (lipid A portion)
C-reactive protein bound to pneumococci
Retroviruses
Heart mitochondrial membranes
Polyanions (e.g., polynucleotides)
Urate crystals

From Kunkel, S. L., et al. (1985). In J. A. Bellanti (Ed.), *Immunology III* (p. 108). Philadelphia: W. B. Saunders.

TABLE 51–11. Activators of the Alternative Pathway

Polysaccharides (e.g., inulin)
Yeast cell walls (zymosan)
Bacterial cell wall components (lipopolysaccharide, peptidoglycan)
Influenza and other viruses
Schistosoma and other parasites
Cryptococci and other fungi
Certain tumor cells
Cobra venom factor
Nephritic factor (autoantibody that stabilizes C3b, Bb)
X-ray contrast media
Dialysis membranes

From Kunkel, S. L., et al.: In J. A. Bellanti (Ed.), *Immunology III* (p. 110). Philadelphia: W. B. Saunders.

fection with a gram-negative organism. Because we have low levels of antibody to most bacteria, some limited classic pathway activation occurs in response to such an infection. In the presence of large numbers of bacteria, low levels of specific antibody are absorbed from the serum by the antigenic complexes. This allows uncoated bacteria to escape the classic pathway. Prior to production of specific antibody, the alternative pathway components (C3b, factor B, factor D, and properdin) are spontaneously deposited on the bacteria, thus beginning the alternative complement sequence. Most bacteria, fungi, and viruses activate the alternative pathway to some degree (Barrett, 1988; Cooper, 1987). Hence, activation of this pathway is extremely important during the early phase of infection when specific antibody is limited. After the formation of antibodies, the classic and alternative pathways work in tandem.

SPECIFIC IMMUNITY

There are three general characteristics of the specific immune response that distinguish it from nonspecific responses: (1) specificity, (2) heterogeneity, and (3) memory. Specificity is the precise selectivity by which the products of the immune response react solely with the antigen that started the response. Heterogeneity refers to the variety of cell types and cell products that can respond to a single antigen but do so through many different mechanisms. Some of these cells also give rise to a wide variety of antibodies (immunoglobulins). Memory, the third hallmark of the immune response, refers to the fact that once the immune system has been exposed to an antigen, future encounters with that antigen will produce an even more vigorous and accelerated response.

Primary and Secondary Immune Response

Upon initial exposure to an antigen, antibody production and distribution are delayed. Antibody reaches detectable levels in the blood 3 to 4 days after the injection of foreign erythrocytes, 5 to 7 days after exposure to soluble proteins, and 10 to 14 days after exposure to bacterial cells (Barrett, 1988). During these delays, antigen is recognized by the B-lymphocyte. Antigen recognition causes the B-cell to divide and differentiate into a plasma cell. The plasma cell secretes antibody specific to the antigen. In this primary antibody response, the first antibody class synthesized is usually IgM. Later, IgG antibodies will predominate over IgM antibodies. The ratio between IgM and IgG antibodies is a useful index for discriminating between recent and past infections, particularly in viral infections.

Antibody does not reach a high level or persist without a second dose of antigen. The combination of antibody with antigen decreases detectable antibody in the blood. Within 1 to 2 days a rapid rise in the level of antibody occurs that can be from 10 to 50 times higher than the primary response. The persistent high level of antibody characterizes this secondary response. Antibody levels decline slowly over a period of months. Once an individual has responded to an antigen, the immune system retains a memory of that antigen. It is the G globulin that carries the memory of exposure. IgG remains in the bloodstream for long periods. Later exposure of IgG to the same antigen stimulates B-lymphocyte memory cells. Even after an interval of months or years, the immune system may mount a secondary response. Such a response is possible because presensitized antibody-secreting cells are mobilized within 1 to 2 days (Barrett, 1988).

A common example of an immunizing antibody response occurs in people with hepatitis A virus infection. It is during the acute phase that specific hepatitis A IgM is detectable. Once IgG titers become elevated, IgM disappears, and the patient enters the recovery phase. Levels of IgG remain detectable for life, a reminder of past infection and immunity. After a second encounter with the hepatitis A virus, IgG titers rise rapidly. The rapid presence of antibody precludes viral takeover and prevents a repeat infection. Vaccinations against the common childhood illnesses produce a similar immune response.

There are some diseases, however, in which the presence of IgM or IgG antibody provides neither protection nor immunity (Barrett, 1988). Herpes virus reinfection and reactivation can occur even in the presence of antibody. Recurrences are often less severe than the initial infection because the rapid IgG response shortens their duration to some extent.

Acquired Immunity

Specific host resistance can be acquired. Acquired immunity develops as a result of exposure to a specific pathogen. Unlike phagocytosis, which is a nonspecific response to an antigen, acquired immune defense is responsible for very specific responses.

Acquired immunity occurs following infection with pathogens or passively.

Active Immunity. Naturally acquired active immunity occurs following overt or subclinical infection. During the illness, the individual receives an antigenic stimulus that begins production of antibody against the specific pathogen involved. Upon reinfection by the same or an antigenically related pathogen, the antibodies are ready to help defend the body. This naturally acquired defense system lasts for months or years.

Exposure to an antigen (immunogen) by vaccination produces artificially acquired active immunity. Some infections, such as diphtheria, whooping cough, smallpox, and mumps, usually induce a lifetime immunity. Others, such as the common cold, influenza, and pneumococcal pneumonia, induce immunity for a shorter time, sometimes for only a few weeks. The organisms producing these diseases undergo frequent mutations, resulting in a constant supply of new strains. Acquisition of immunity to one strain does not prevent infection by another strain of the same organism. Regardless of the type of infection, active immunity appears only after a specified lapse of time after exposure to the antigen (Barrett, 1988). Like naturally acquired immunity, artificially induced immunity endures for years.

Passive Immunity. Natural and artificial methods are also used to confer passive immunity. In humans, the classic example of naturally acquired passive immunity is the passage of maternal antibody across the placenta during the latter part of pregnancy. IgG alone is transferred from mother to fetus. IgM, IgE, IgD, and IgA do not cross the placental barrier. During breastfeeding, colostrum contains IgA and IgM. Ingestion of colostrum provides passive immunity to infants during the early days postpartum.

Artificially introduced passive immunity develops in one individual following injection of antibodies produced by another individual. Pooled human immunoglobulin (gamma globulin) is a source of antibody used to confer passive immunity. Given during the incubation period of measles infection or infectious hepatitis, pooled human immunoglobulin modifies the intensity of disease symptomatology.

Because passive immunity acquired naturally or artificially involves the transfer of preformed antibodies, its onset of action is immediate. Nonetheless, because there may be no stimulus for continued production, its effect is usually of short duration (Barrett, 1988).

Specific Mechanisms of Immune Response

Specific immunologic defense mechanisms recognize antigens as nonself, as do nonspecific immune mechanisms. They are also capable of more precise immunologic reactions and respond in a matter unique to each antigen's composition. There are two mechanisms that mediate specific immune responses—humoral immunity and cell-mediated immunity. Antibody production by lymphoid tissues is the focal point of humoral immunity. Cell-mediated immunity focuses on specifically sensitized lymphocytes.

Humoral Immunity. It is now accepted that the triggering of a humoral response to antigens requires the cooperation of B-cells, macrophages, and T-cells. For participation in a humoral response, B-cells require more than one signal prior to activation. Macrophages and helper T-cells aid B-lymphocyte activation. The precise mechanism by which B-cell activation occurs is unknown (Fig. 51–8). Many pieces of the puzzle are, however, emerging. Both specific subsets of cells and cell products called lymphokines influence humoral immunity.

The first step involves antigen processing by the macrophage. During antigen processing, the macrophage releases interleukin-1, a lymphokine that fosters differentiation of inducer T-cells. This subset of T-cells releases a second lymphokine, interleukin-2. This second lymphokine promotes the maturation of helper T-lymphocytes.

Cell-Mediated Immunity. The primary component of cellular immunity is the T-lymphocyte. A basic misconception formerly held about cell-mediated immune was that T-lymphocytes acted independently of antibody. A variety of cell types, antibody, humoral substances, and combinations of these constitute most cell-mediated immune responses.

Like antigen–antibody reactions, cell-mediated immune reactions are divided into primary, secondary, and tertiary stages. After initial processing by the phagocytes, antigens travel to the regional lymph node that drains the area invaded by antigens. The primary stage of the cell-mediated reaction begins when the T-lymphocyte binds antigen with an antigen receptor on its surface. During the secondary stage, a variety of morphologic and biochemical changes occur that include DNA, RNA, or protein synthesis. The tertiary stage consists of the generation of helper, suppressor, cytotoxic, and memory T-cells. In the tertiary stage the T-cells that release the mediators of cell-mediated immunity emerge.

It is the tertiary stage that is the most complex. Initially, macrophages activate the small number of helper T-cells that have receptors for the antigen. In response to contact with the antigen, helper T-cells release lymphokines. Some of these lymphokines activate macrophages and recruit other lymphocytes and monocytes-macrophages to participate in the reaction. Activated macrophages produce monokines. Monokines are secretory products of monocytes or macrophages. Monokines and lymphokines often are the same chemical but are secreted by different cell types.

Some monokines, such as interleukin-1, are nec-

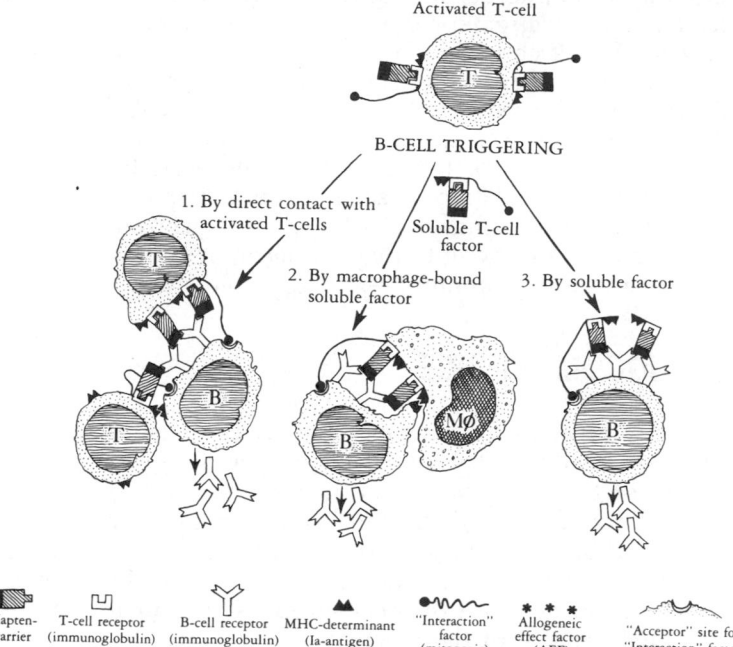

FIGURE 51–8. B-cells may be activated and triggered to grow and produce antibody in three ways: (1) by direct contact with antigen-bearing activated T-cells; (2) by macrophage-bound soluble factors; or (3) by soluble antigen specific T-cell factors. (Adapted from Herscowitz, H. B. (1985). In J. A. Bellanti (Ed.), *Immunology III* (p. 148). Philadelphia: W.B. Saunders.)

essary for T-cell activation (Fig. 51–9). The release of interleukin-1 by macrophages expands the activation of a single T-cell by antigen to activation of many T-cells. IL-1 is released locally into tissue and into blood and activates all T-lymphocytes within its reach. Therefore, a reaction that initially involves a small number of sensitized cells is amplified. Now the immune response includes many T-cells that were not directly sensitized by antigen.

Like the humoral immune response, the cell-mediated immune response results in the formation of long-lived, memory T-lymphocytes. Due to the production of memory cells, later exposure to the same antigen will evoke a more rapid and intense cell-mediated immune response.

Cell-mediated immunity includes those manifestations of the specific immune response expressed by a variety of cells and cell products. As opposed to humoral antigen–antibody reactions, cell-mediated reactions have a delayed onset and require activated lymphocytes or their products to elicit a response. This mechanism is instrumental when dealing with antigens that are cell bound or in other ways inaccessible to the antibody response.

Regulation of the Immune Response

Regulation of immune responses is a complex and intricate process. Many different subpopulations of

FIGURE 51–9. Schematic representation of the cellular events involved in T-cell activation. Mo, macrophage; T_H, helper T-cell. (From Herscowitz, H. B. (1985). In J. A. Bellanti (Ed.), *Immunology III* (p. 146). Philadelphia: W. B. Saunders.)

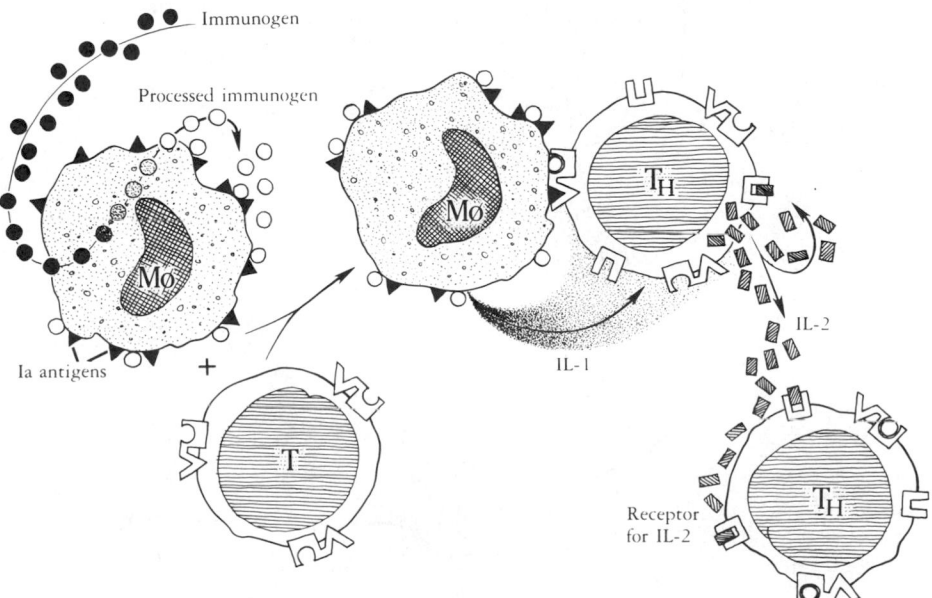

regulatory cells interact among themselves and with effector cells to augment or suppress the immune response. Research to date has largely been directed toward identification and characterization of individual subpopulations of regulatory cells, effector cells, and their secretory products. Understanding how each cell type and mediator interact to provide careful and controlled regulation of each immune response is the true challenge. Figure 51–10 depicts the current understanding of the interplay between immunocompetent cells and immunoregulatory mediators.

IMMUNOCOMPETENCE

The word *immunocompetence* is used by lay persons and many health professionals to describe the effectiveness of the immune system in warding off disease. Although this definition oversimplifies the meaning of immunocompetence, it serves as a common interdisciplinary starting point. The key to the multiple interpretations of this concept is our inherent understanding of the mechanism by which disease can or should be warded off. For example, in medicine immunocompetence describes the ability of humans to respond to a particular infectious or

tumorigenic challenge (Wyngaarden and Smith, 1988). In contrast, the lay literature implies that a state of immunocompetence will prevent an individual from succumbing to disease. For example, to the layman, the immunocompetent individual is perceived to be less likely to get a cold than the immunocompromised individual. This view of immune functioning is not supported by empirical evidence.

In nursing, the meaning of immunocompetence has been derived from an exploration of human responses in disorders that suppress immune function. Examples include cancer, acquired immunodeficiency syndrome, genetic immune system defects, and the effects of therapeutic modalities that assault the immune system. Specific pharmacologic agents and radiation therapy also compromise immune function. Halliburton (1986) describes an immunocompetent person as a host that responds adequately to an antigenic stimulus. An adequate response maintains bodily integrity. She further states that immunocompetence is a human response that is within the nature and scope of nursing practice.

Nurses in critical care settings need to take advantage of what is known about the immune system and the effects of the environment upon immunocompetence. We are only beginning to realize that

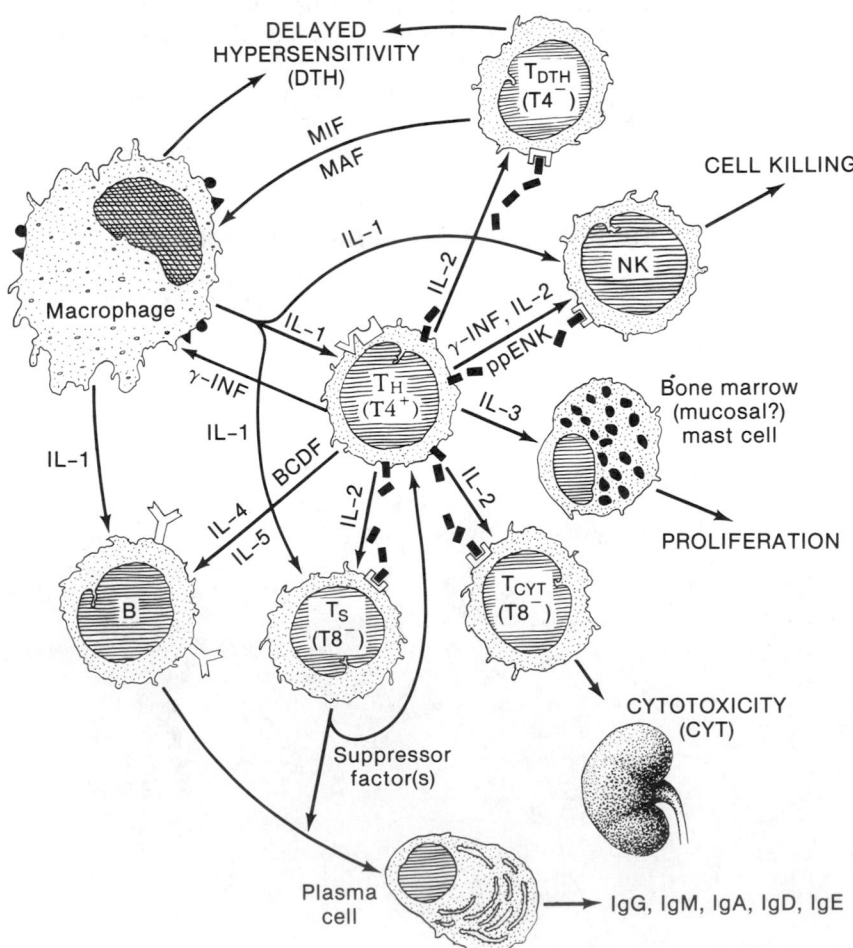

FIGURE 51–10. Cellular events that make up the tertiary stage of cell-mediated immunity in the human, illustrating the central role of the T-cell in the immunoregulatory network. γ-INF, interferon-gamma; IL-1, interleukin-1; IL-2, interleukin-2; IL-3, interleukin-3; IL-4, interleukin-4; IL-5, interleukin-5; MIF, migratory inhibitory factor; MAF, macrophage activating factor; CSF, colony stimulating factor; BCDF, B-cell differentiating factor; ppENK, preproenkephalin. (Adapted from Bellanti, J. A., and Rocklin, R. E. (1985). In J. A. Bellanti (Ed.), *Immunology III* (p. 181). Philadelphia: W. B. Saunders.)

the immune system can be artificially controlled. In vitro enhancement of immune function is a burgeoning area of research. Knowledge of potential threats to immunocompetence will help critical care nurses protect patients from or ameliorate the effects of immunosuppressive agents.

Threats to Immunocompetence

There are many factors that modify immune function. External and internal defense forces do not function at the same level of efficiency in all individuals. Individuals requiring intensive medical and surgical treatment are exposed to additional immunosuppressive conditions. Age, hormonal balance, nutrition, surgery, trauma, and psychologic distress influence both specific and nonspecific immunity.

Age. Age influences immunity, and infectious diseases are more severe at the extremes of life. In the very young, immaturity of the immune system leads to poor antigen recognition or antibody production. In the elderly, there is evidence that a hypofunctional state of the immune system occurs.

Diminished responsiveness to externally administered antigens and increased responsiveness to internal antigens are the immunologic changes associated with aging (Effros, 1984). Functional changes at the cellular level occur in both T- and B-lymphocytes (Gillis et al., 1981; Whisler et al., 1985). Immune responses of elderly subjects vary greatly from individual to individual, even in the absence of disease. Responses range from those that are no different from responses in the young adult to responses that are significantly diminished. The most overt change is that of thymic involution (atrophy of the thymus). This change leads to decreased ability of immune cells to discriminate between self and nonself. Thymic involution also causes diminished T-cell proliferation responses to mitogens, self antigens, and conventional antigens. There is conflicting evidence on whether the numbers and proportion of B-cells change in old age. There is, however, general agreement that serum immunoglobulin does show age-related changes (Effros, 1984). The defects in humoral immunity associated with old age are related to defective T-cell collaboration, defective monocyte function, and regulation of B-cell responses.

Changes in immune function occur gradually and are not precipitated by achieving a certain chronologic age. A greater proportion of the very old (>85 years) do, however, exhibit diminished immune function than younger adults. Therefore, although the aging process does influence immune function, the effects are subtle in nature and appear to be most influential at the extreme age ranges (Whisler et al., 1985).

Hormones. Changes in the levels of many hormones modulate immune function. These changes occur in response to nonpathogenic stimuli and in many disease states. Insulin deficiency affects the integrity of cell membranes, making diabetics more susceptible to infectious agents. Thus, diabetics are more susceptible to staphylococcal, streptococcal, and several fungal diseases. There is also an increased susceptibility to infection in both hypoadrenal and hypothyroid states.

Nutrition. Nutrition plays a major role in maintaining the functional capacity of the immune system (Gross and Newberne, 1980). Some clinical studies of cancer and obesity conclude that an imbalance in nutrient intake correlates with decreased immune function (Brookes and Clifford, 1981; Chandra, 1980). Severe, prolonged protein-calorie malnutrition profoundly alters cell-mediated immunity (Chandra, 1980). Severe malnutrition has less effect on humoral immunity and phagocytic function (Stiehm, 1980).

Dietary factors other than protein and calories such as vitamins and minerals (Lahita et al., 1984) also contribute to these alterations. Insufficient intake of vitamin A, pyridoxine, biotin, folic acid components, zinc, and iron alter immune function (Halliburton, 1986).

Altered cellular immune function occurs in association with gross obesity. Chandra (1981) reported that the altered cellular immunity seen with obesity correlated with subclinical deficiencies of zinc and iron. Additionally, high caloric intake, particularly fat-related calorie intake, can affect immune function. Excess cholesterol, saturated fatty acid, and polyunsaturated fatty acid decrease immune function (Beisel, 1981).

Surgery and Anesthesia. Surgical intervention and anesthesia lead to impaired immune function (Browder and Williams, 1988). A transient severe lymphopenia occurs in the immediate postoperative period. Complete return of normal immune function may take 10 days to 2 weeks (Lundy and Ford, 1983). The complement system is activated in certain types of operations, particularly abdominal and cardiovascular surgery (Watkins and Salo, 1982). Anesthesia partially inhibits T-cell function and reduces phagocytosis. Length of exposure to anesthetic agents and degree of surgical trauma affect both the quality and the quantity of these immune changes (Halliburton, 1986).

Trauma. Burn injury suppresses all aspects of immune function (Moran and Munste, 1987). The exact mechanisms of the pervasive immunosuppressive effect of thermal injury are not well understood. There is a decrease in the regulation of the immune response, with a marked decrease in IL-2 production. Nonspecific immune response is also diminished. Most of these responses are seen in patients about 4 to 5 days after injury (Antonacci, 1986). Because of the many possible contributing factors such as age and infection, it is difficult to discern what causes the persistence of immune dysfunction.

Blunt injury is primarily associated with alterations in nonspecific immune responses. Neutrophil migration to the site of inflammation is impaired. The degree of dysfunction is related to the magnitude of the injury. Immune dysfunction occurs almost immediately after injury and is most intense in the first 24 hours. Although immune dysfunction is of short duration, this time period is associated with a higher rate of infection and septicemia (Meakins, 1987).

Therapeutic Agents. A wide variety of drugs used to treat many clinical diseases display immunosuppressive activity. The most common therapeutic immunosuppressive agents are corticosteroids, azathioprine, cyclophosphamide, actinomycin, mercaptopurine, and antithymocyte globulin. Many of these agents were first developed to treat cancer. These drugs are now used to treat overactive immune responses in autoimmune diseases including rheumatoid arthritis, multiple sclerosis, and inflammatory bowel disease (Halliburton, 1986).

The use of corticosteroids is pervasive in the critical care setting. Treatment with corticosteroids reduces the inflammatory response, depresses phagocytosis, alters the functional ability of T-lymphocytes, and inhibits immunoglobulin synthesis (Smith, 1986). Corticosteroids thus increase susceptibility to bacterial infection (e.g., staphylococcal infection) as well as to certain viral diseases (e.g., varicella) (Sheagren and Young, 1987).

Psychological Distress. Studies of the psychological influence on immune function have explored the relationship of acute stressors to a variety of humoral and cellular indicators of immune function. Studies have also measured immune function during events considered by investigators to be distressing. More recently, research has focused on the relationship between emotional distress and immune function in the context of distressing situations (Rabin et al., 1989).

Emotionally distressing experiences influence many parameters of immune function, including cellular and humoral responses. Most recent studies have focused upon examination of cellular immune function, perhaps due to the relative insulation of this response to transient external stimuli. Transient external stimuli such as engaging in conversation are reported to affect humoral immune function. For example, salivary IgA levels are particularly sensitive to events that represent a change in the environment. Changes in IgA levels do not solely reflect responses to specific distressing situations (Stone et al., 1987). On the other hand, measures of cellular immune function change in response to intense and focused emotional distress.

Suppression of in vitro T- and B-lymphocyte proliferation in response to antigenic and mitogenic stimulation occurs in persons experiencing loss. Immunosuppression occurs in bereaved spouses (Bartrop et al., 1977), spouses of persons admitted to critical care units with life-threatening diseases (Schleifer et al., 1983), unemployed women (Arnetz et al., 1987), and separated and divorced women (Kiecolt-Glaser et al., 1987a). Immunosuppression has also been reported in students when they take major examinations (Halvorsen and Vassend, 1987; Kiecolt-Glaser, et al., 1984, 1986). Research is only beginning in patients with acute medical problems.

Augmentation of Immune Function

Although popular interest in stimulation or boosting of the immune system is high, little research has been done in this arena. Three main avenues of exploration are (1) therapeutic agents, (2) nutrition, and (3) psychological stimulation. To date, most research in these areas has focused on the ability to modulate single cells or mediators of specific immunologic responses reliably. Dietary supplementation with arginine increases in vitro lymphocyte proliferation (Daly et al., 1990). Pavlovian conditioning techniques are used to enhance lymphocyte proliferation in vitro. Importantly, the clinical or in vivo effect of these reported modulators has not been determined nor have the mechanisms of effect been clearly elucidated. Thus, the area of immune function augmentation is ripe for further research (Rabin et al., 1989).

SUMMARY

The manifestations of the immune response may be viewed as the capacity of the host to recognize and dispose of foreign substances. Once an antigen has been introduced, the body will attempt to eliminate it by phagocytosis. During this first encounter, there is no preexisting antibody to facilitate engulfment. Disposal of the antigen is determined by the efficiency of the phagocytic process. If phagocytosis is successful, the organism is eliminated, and disease symptoms are not seen or are minimal. The specific immune response may be induced to stimulate activity of cells capable of either producing antibody or inducing cell-mediated events. Future encounters with the same organism will result in a more rapid and intense response. Regulation of the immune system is now recognized to be orchestrated by a host of chemical mediators interacting with many different types of cells.

Immunocompetence depends not only on the state of health of an individual but also on biologic and environmental factors. Surgery, trauma, nutrition, and many therapeutic drugs pose a particular threat to the immune function of critically ill patients. Phagocytosis or cellular immune responses may be unsuccessful if the immune system is suppressed by medication or a state of poor health. Impairment of the immune system can lead to active disease or even death.

Competency of both nonspecific and specific immune responses is critical to the body's management of infections. The course of many diseases is determined by the efficiency of the immune response. Antigen must be successfully recognized and removed. This requires not only lymphocyte and macrophage involvement but also a granulocytic response. Production of antibody, synthesis and secretion of mediators, and many other chemicials including complement further enhance the effectiveness of the immune response. Effective immune system component responses are not enough to achieve an immunocompetent state; the timing and coordination of individual component responses must be carefully regulated as well.

There is much yet to be learned about the immune system. It is essential that all parts of the system work together to maintain health, including the primitive responses of phagocytosis and inflammation, which can dispose of most foreign substances. In the case of pathogens that escape these responses, the specific immune response leads to release of products that facilitate or enhance these primitive responses. The outcome of this encounter of the host with a pathogen can be either beneficial or harmful depending upon the efficiency of the immune system.

References

Adams, A. (1985). External barriers to infection. *Nursing Clinics of North America, 20,* 145–149.

Anegon, I., Cuturi, M., Trinchieri, G., et al. (1988). Interaction of Fc receptor (CD16) with ligands induces transcription of IL-2 receptor (CD25) and lymphokine genes and expression of their products in human natural killer cells. *Journal of Experimental Medicine, 167,* 452–472.

Antonacci, A. C. (1986). Immune dsyfunction and immunomodulation following trauma. In J. I. Gallin and A. S. Fauci (Eds.), *Advances in host defense mechanism* (Vol. 6, pp. 81–109). New York: Raven Press.

Arnetz, B., Wasserman, J., Petrini, B., et al. (1987). Immune function in unemployed women. *Psychosomatic Medicine, 49,* 3–12.

Austen, K. F., and Fisher, D. (1987). The biology of the mast cell (pp. 177–192). In R. Lockey, and S. Bukantz (Eds.), *Fundamentals of immunology and allergy.* Philadelphia: W. B. Saunders.

Austen, K. F. (1983). Tissue mast cells in immediate hypersensitivity. In F. Dixon and D. Fisher (Eds.), *The biology of immunologic disease* (pp. 223–233). Sunderland, MA: Sinauer Associates.

Bach, F., and Sachs, D. (1987). Transplantation immunology. *New England Journal of Medicine, 317,* 489–492.

Barber, J. (1986). Immunologic responses to trauma. *Critical Care Quarterly, 9,* 57–67.

Barrett, J. (1988). *Textbook of immunology* (5th ed.). St. Louis: C. V. Mosby.

Bartrop, R., Luckhurst, E., Lazarus, L., et al. (1977). Depressed lymphocyte function after bereavement. *Lancet, 1,* 834–836.

Beisel, W. (1981). Impact of infectious disease upon fat metabolism and immune function. *Cancer Research, 41,* 3797–3798.

Bellanti, J. A. (1985). *Immunology III.* Philadelphia: W. B. Saunders.

Bellanti, J. A., and Kadlec, J. (1985). Introduction to immunology. In J. A. Bellanti (Ed.), *Immunology III* (pp. 1–15). Philadelphia: W. B. Saunders.

Bierer, B., Sleckman, B., Ratnofsky, S., et al. (1989). The biologic roles of CD2, CD4, and CD8 in T-cell activation. *Annual Review of Immunology, 7,* 579–599.

Bolhuis, R. (1989). T-cell responses to cancer. In M. Feldman, J. Lamb, and M. Owen (Eds.), *T cells* (pp. 347–364). New York: John Wiley & Sons.

Brookes, G. B., and Clifford, P. (1981). Nutritional status and general immune competence in patients with head and neck cancer. *Journal of The Royal Society of Medicine, 74* (2), 32–39.

Browder, W. and Williams, D. (1988). Immunosuppression and surgery. *Journal of the National Medical Association, 80* (5), 531–536.

Burdette, S., and Schwartz, R. (1987). Idiotypes and idiotypic networks. *New England Journal of Medicine, 317,* 219–224.

Burnet, F. M. (1967). Immunologic aspects of malignant disease. *Lancet, 1,* 1171–1174.

Chandra, R. K. (1980). Cell-mediated immunity in nutritional imbalance. *Federation Proceedings, 39* (13), 3088–3092.

Chandra, R. (1981). Immune response in overnutrition. *Cancer Research, 41,* 3795–3796.

Church, J., and Schlegel, R. (1985). Immune deficiency disorders. In J. A. Bellanti (Ed.), *Immunology III* (pp. 471–507). Philadelphia: W. B. Saunders.

Claman, H. (1987). The biology of the immune response. In R. Lockey, and S. Bukantz (Eds.), *Fundamentals of immunology and allergy* (pp. 7–38). Philadelphia: W. B. Saunders.

Cooper, N. (1987). The complement system. In D. Stites, J. Stobo, and J. V. Wells (Eds.), *Basic and clinical immunology* (6th ed., pp. 114–127). Norwalk, CT: Appleton & Lange.

Cooper, M. (1987). B lymphocytes: Normal development and function. *New England Journal of Medicine, 317,* 1452–1456.

Corman, L. (1985). The relationship between nutrition, infection, and immunity. *Medical Clinics of North America, 69,* 519–529.

Cunha, B. (1985). Significance of fever in the compromised host. *Nursing Clinics of North America, 20,* 163–169.

Cunha, B., Digamon-Beltran, M., and Gobbo, P. (1984). Implications of fever in the critical care setting. *Heart & Lung, 13,* 460–465.

Daly, J., Reynolds, J., Sigal, R., et al. (1990). Effect of dietary protein and amino acids on immune function. *Critical Care Medicine, 18* (Suppl.), 86–93.

Densen, P., and Mandell, G. L. (1987). Phagocytosis. In R. Lockey, and S. Bukantz (Eds.), *Fundamentals of immunology and allergy* (pp. 51–64). Philadelphia: W. B. Saunders.

Dinarello, C. A., and Mier, J. W. (1987). Lymphokines. *New England Journal of Medicine, 317* (15), 940–945.

Dion, L. D., and Blalock, J. E. (1988). Neuroendocrine properties of the immune system. In T. P. Bridge (Ed.), *Psychological, neuropsychiatric and substance abuse aspects of AIDS* (pp. 15–20). New York: Raven Press.

Effros, R. (1984). Aging and immunity. In E. L. Cooper (Ed.), *Stress, immunity, and aging* (pp. 277–290). New York: Marcel Dekker.

Esperson, S. (1986). Nursing support of host defenses. *Critical Care Quarterly, 9,* 51–56.

Frank, M., and Fries, L. (1989). Complement. In W. Paul (Ed.), *Fundamental immunology* (pp. 679–701). New York: Raven Press.

Gallin, J. (1989). Inflammation. In W. Paul (Ed.), *Fundamental immunology* (pp. 721–733). New York: Raven Press.

Gillis, S., Kozak, R., Durante, M., et al. (1981). Immunological studies of aging. *Journal of Clinical Investigation, 67,* 937–942.

Glaser, R., Rice, J., Speicher, C., et al. (1986). Stress depresses interferon production by leukocytes concomitant with a decrease in natural killer cell activity. *Behavioral Neuroscience, 100,* 675–678.

Gleich, G., and Butterfield, J. (1987). Eosinophilia. In Lockey, R. and Bukantz, S. (Eds.), *Fundamentals of immunology and allergy* (pp. 217–234). Philadelphia: W. B. Saunders.

Goust, J. (1986). Immediate hypersensitivity. In G. Virella, J. Goust, H. H. Fundenberg, et al. (Eds.), *Introduction to medical immunology* (pp. 317–332). New York: Marcel Dekker.

Graziano, F., and Bell, C. (1985). The normal immune response and what can go wrong. *Medical Clinics of North America, 69,* 439–451.

Groenwald, S. (1980). Physiology of the immune system. *Heart & Lung, 9,* 645–650.

Groenwald, S. (Ed.) (1987). *Cancer nursing: Principles and practice.* Boston: Jones and Bartlett.

Groenwald, S., Fisher, S., and McCalla, J. (1988). Biological response modifiers. In S. Groenwald (Ed.), *Cancer nursing: Principles and practice* (pp. 385–404). Boston: Jones and Bartlett.

Gross, R., and Newberne, P. (1980). Role of nutrition in immunologic function. *Physiology Review*, 60, 188–302.

Gurevich, I. (1985). The competent internal immune system. *Nursing Clinics of North America*, 20, 151–161.

Halliburton, P. (1986). Impaired immunocompetence. In V. Carrieri, A. Lindsey, and C. West. (Eds.), *Pathophysiological phenomena in nursing*. Philadelphia: W. B. Saunders.

Halvorsen, R., and Vassend, O. (1987). Effects of examination stress on some cellular immunity functions. *Journal of Psychosomatic Research*, 31, 693–701.

Herberman, R., and Gorelik, E. (1989). Role of the natural immune system in control of primary tumors and metastasis. In C. Reynolds and R. Wiltrout (Eds.), *Functions of the natural immune system* (pp. 3–37). New York: Plenum Press.

Jackson, A. (1985). Antigens and immunogenicity. In J. A. Bellanti (Ed.), *Immunology III* (pp. 79–88). Philadelphia: W. B. Saunders.

Janson-Bjerklie, S. (1983). Defense mechanisms: Protecting the healthy lung. *Heart & Lung*, 12, 643–649.

Jeske, D., and Capra, J. D. (1984). Immunoglobulins: Structure and function. In W. Paul (Ed.), *Fundamental immunology* (pp. 131–166). New York: Raven Press.

Kiecolt-Glaser, J., Garner, W., Speicher, C., et al. (1984). Psychosocial modifiers of immunocompetence in medical students. *Psychosomatic Medicine*, 46, 7–14.

Kiecolt-Glaser, J., Fisher, L., Ogrocki, P., et al. (1987a). Marital quality, marital disruption, and immune function. *Psychosomatic Medicine*, 49, 13–34.

Kiecolt-Glaser, J., Glaser, R., Shuttleworth, E., et al. (1987b). Chronic stress and immunity in family caregivers of Alzheimer's disease victims. *Psychosomatic Medicine*, 49, 523–535.

Kiecolt-Glaser, J., Glaser, R., Strain, E., et al. (1986). Modulation of cellular immunity in medical students. *Journal of Behavioral Medicine*, 9, 5–21.

Kincade, P., and Gimble J. (1989). B Lymphocytes. In W. Paul (Ed.), *Fundamental immunology* (pp. 41–67). New York: Raven Press.

Kirkpatrick, C. H. (1987). Mechanisms of allergic injury. In Lockey, R., and Bukantz, S. (Eds.), *Fundamentals of immunology and allergy* (pp. 153–176). Philadelphia: W. B. Saunders.

Kumagai, K., Suzuki, S., and Suzuki, R. (1989). Role of the natural immune system in the antibody response: Regulatory effects of NK cells. In C. Reynolds and R. Wiltrout (Eds.), *Functions of the natural immune system* (pp. 213–227). New York: Plenum Press.

Lahita, R., Levy, J., Weksler, J., et al. (1984). Effects of sex hormones, nutrition and aging on the immune response. In D. Stites, J. Stobo, H. Fundenberg, et al. (Eds.), *Basic and clinical immunology* (5th ed., pp. 288–311). Los Altos, CA: Lange Medical.

Langlois, P. F., Gawryl, M. S., Zeller, J., et al. (1989). Accentuated complement activation in patient plasma during the adult respiratory distress syndrome: A potential mechanism for pulmonary inflammation. *Heart & Lung*, (1), 71-84.

Lefor, A., Mule, J., and Rosenberg, S. (1989). Lymphokine-activated killer cells: Biology and therapeutic efficacy. In C. Reynolds and R. Wiltrout (Eds.), *Functions of the natural immune system* (pp. 39–56). New York: Plenum Press.

Lind, M. (1980). The immunologic assessment: A nursing focus. *Heart & Lung*, 9, 658-661.

Lundy, J., and Ford, C. (1983). Surgery, trauma, and immune suppression: Evolving the mechanism. *Annals of Surgery*, 197, 434-438.

Malech, H., and Gallin, J. (1987). Neutrophils in human disease. *New England Journal of Medicine*, 317, 687–694.

McCarron, K. (1986). Fever—the cardinal vital sign. *Critical Care Quarterly*, 9, 15–18.

Mitchell, M., and Bertram, J. (1985). Immunology and biomodulation of cancer. In P. Calabresi, P. Schein, and S. Rosenberg (Eds.), *Medical Oncology*. New York: Macmillan.

Moran, K., and Munster, A. M. (1987). Alterations of the host defense mechanism in burn patients. *Surgical Clinics of North America*, 67, 47–56.

Nakamura, I. (1989). Involvement of natural effector cells in bone marrow transplantation and hybrid resistance. In C. Reynolds

and R. Wiltrout (Eds.), *Functions of the natural immune system* (pp. 321–339). New York: Plenum Press.

Norwood, S. (1988). An approach to the febrile ICU patient. In J. Civetta, R. Taylor, et al. (Eds.), *Critical care*. Philadelphia: J. B. Lippincott.

Patrick, C., Goust, J., and Virella, G. (1986). Tissues and cells in the immune response. In G. Virella, J. Goust, H. H. Fundenberg, et al. (Eds.), *Introduction to medical immunology* (pp. 7–24). New York: Marcel Dekker.

Perussia, B., Ramoni, C., Anegon, I., et al. (1987). Preferential proliferation of natural killer cells among peripheral blood mononuclear cells cocultured with B lymphoblastoid cell lines. *Natural Immunity and Cell Growth Regulation*, 6, 171–188.

Rabin, B., Cohen, S., Ganguli, R., et al. (1989). Bidirectional interaction between the central nervous system and the immune system. *Critical Reviews in Immunology*, 9, 279–312.

Rana, A., and Luskin, A. (1980). Immunosuppression, autoimmunity, and hypersensitivity. *Heart & Lung*, 9, 651–657.

Ristuccia, P. (1985). Microbiologic aspects of infection in the compromised host. *Nursing Clinics of North America*, 20, 171–179.

Roitt, I. M., Brostoff, J., and Male, D. K. (1985). *Immunology*. St. Louis: C. V. Mosby.

Royer, H., and Reinherz, E. (1987). T lymphocytes, ontogeny, function, and relevance to clinical disorders. *New England Journal of Medicine*, 317, 1136–1142.

Schleifer, S., Keller, S., Camerino, M., et al. (1983). Suppression of lymphocyte stimulation following bereavement. *Journal of the American Medical Association*, 250, 374–377.

Serafin, W., and Austen, K. F. (1987). Mediators of immediate hypersensitivity reactions. *New England Journal of Medicine*, 317, 30–34.

Shaver, J. (1982). The basic mechanisms of fever: Considerations for therapy. *Nurse Practitioner*, 7 (9), 15–19.

Sheagren, J., and Young, M. (1987). Glucocorticoids. In J. Parrillo and H. Masur (Eds.), *The critically ill immunosuppressed patient* (pp. 245–263). Rockville, MD: Aspen.

Siskind, G. (1983). Immunologic tolerance. In W. Paul (Ed.), *Fundamental immunology* (pp. 537-559). New York: Raven Press.

Smith, S. (1986). Immunosuppressive drugs used in clinical practice. *Critical Care Quarterly*, 9, 19–24.

Sprent, J. (1989). T lymphocytes and the thymus. In W. Paul (Ed.), *Fundamental immunology* (pp. 69–93) New York: Raven Press.

Stiehm, E. (1980). Humoral immunity in malnutrition. *Federal Proceedings*, 39, 3093–3097.

Stites, D., Stobo, J., and Wells, J. V. (Eds.) (1987). *Basic and clinical immunology* (6th ed.). Norwalk, CT: Appleton & Lange.

Stobo, J. (1987). Lymphocytes: T cells. In D. Stites, J. Stobo, and J. V. Wells (Eds.), *Basic and clinical immunology* (6th ed., pp. 65–72). Norwalk, CT: Appleton & Lange.

Stone, A., Cox, D., Valdimarsdottir, H., et al. (1987). Secretory IgA as a measure of immunocompetence. *Journal of Human Stress*, 6 (2), 136–140.

Thomas, L. (1959). *Cellular and humoral aspects of the hypersensitive states*. New York: Harper & Row.

Tilden, A., and Clement, L. (1989). Role of natural effector cells in the regulation of cell-mediated immune responses. In C. Reynolds and R. Wiltrout (Eds.), *Functions of the natural immune system* (pp. 229–247). New York: Plenum Press.

Tizard, I. (1984). *Immunology: An introduction*. Philadelphia: Saunders College Publishing.

Trinchieri, G., and Perussia, B. (1984). Human natural killer cells: Biologic and pathologic aspects. *Laboratory Investigation*, 50, 489–513.

Unanue, E. (1989). Macrophages, antigen-presenting cells, and the phenomena of antigen handling and presentation. In W. Paul (Ed.), *Fundamental immunology* (2nd ed., pp. 95–115). New York: Raven Press.

Virella, G. (1986). Diagnostic evaluation of phagocyte function. In G. Virella, J. Goust, H. H. Fundenberg, et al. (Eds.), *Introduction to medical immunology* (pp. 283–298). New York: Marcel Dekker.

Ward, P. (1985). Inflammation. In J. A. Bellanti (Ed.), *Immunology III* (pp. 208–217). Philadelphia: W. B. Saunders.

Watkins, J., and Salo, M. (Eds.) (1982). *Trauma, stress, and immunity in anaesthesia and surgery*. Boston: Butterworth Scientific.

Weigle, W. (1983). Immunologic tolerance and immunopathology. In F. Dixon and D. Fisher (Eds.), *The biology of immunologic disease* (pp. 107–116). Sunderland, MA: Sinauer Associates.

Werb, Z. (1987). Phagocytic cells: Chemotaxis and effector functions of macrophages and granulocytes. In D. Stites, J. Stobo, and J. V. Wells (Eds.), *Basic and clinical immunology* (6th ed., pp. 96–113). Norwalk, CT: Appleton & Lange.

Whisler, R., Newhouse, Y., Ennist, D., et al. (1985). Human B-lymphocyte colony responses: Suboptimal colony responsiveness in aged humans associated with defective function of B cells and monocytes. *Cellular Immunology, 94,* 133–146.

Wyngaarden, J. B., and Smith, L. H., Jr. (Eds.). *Cecil textbook of medicine* (18th ed.). Philadelphia: W. B. Saunders.

Organ Donation

Marilyn Rossman Bartucci

OVERVIEW OF TRANSPLANTATION

The art and science of transplantation have developed a great deal since the first kidney transplant was performed in 1954. The advances made in surgical techniques, tissue typing and matching, understanding the immune system, preventing and treating rejection with powerful and effective immunosuppressive drugs, and improved organ procurement and preservation techniques have brought a dramatic increase in the demand for organs and tissues for transplantation. In 1988 there were 36,900 cornea transplants, 9123 kidney transplants, 1647 heart transplants, 1680 liver transplants, 243 pancreas transplants, 74 heart/lung transplants, and 31 lung transplants performed in the United States (Eye Bank Association of America, 1988; *UNOS Update*, 1989). More than 200,000 orthopedic surgical procedures required donated bone grafts (American Council on Transplantation, 1988). Transplantation has offered new life to individuals dying of heart, liver, and lung failure and an improved quality of life for individuals with kidney failure, diabetes, blindness, and bone diseases. Implementation of an efficient national computerized system has made it possible to distribute organs equitably to patients with the greatest need who have the greatest chance of a successful outcome. Conservative medical management of patients with end-stage kidney, liver, or heart disease is costly. Although transplant procedures are expensive, the current success rates have made transplantation a cost-effective treatment option when compared with traditional medical management. For example, a patient undergoing chronic hemodialysis costs the federal government, through Medicare, about $40,000/year. The cost of a kidney transplant is approximately $40,000 for the first year and $5000/year for follow-up care. If the transplant functions for 5 years (the actual rate approaches 75%), the cost is $60,000 as opposed to $200,000 for 5-year chronic hemodialysis. Likewise, patients with end-

stage heart or liver disease have multiple, extended, and costly intensive care unit admissions for conservative management of the disease before death occurs as the final outcome. Table 52–1 shows the estimated cost of each transplant procedure and the current success rates. Other financial factors that increase the cost effectiveness of transplantation are the potential earning power of the transplant recipient and the discontinuation of disability benefits previously required. In short, transplantation is a therapy that can restore dignity and quality to the lives of patients and families dealing with end-stage organ disease and provide the potential for patients to become productive members of society again.

SHORTAGE OF DONOR ORGANS

During the last 5 years the number of patients awaiting organs and tissues for transplantation has grown exponentially because the advances made in transplantation have made it possible to transplant both a larger number and a larger variety of organs

TABLE 52–1. Organ Transplant Success Rates and Average Costs

	Success Rate (%)	Average Cost ($)
Kidney		
Cadaver	85–90	40,000
Living—related	95	40,000
Heart	80–85	90,000–100,000
Heart/Lung	68–70	130,000–200,000
Liver	70	100,000
Pancreas	60	30,000–40,000
Kidney/pancreas	80	70,000

Success rates are reported by the percentage of functioning grafts after one year since the greatest number of organs fail within the first year from rejection, technical problems, or other complications.

and tissues. Currently, there are over 18,000 individuals awaiting vital organs for transplantation (kidney, heart, liver, heart/lung, pancreas) in the United States (*UNOS Update*, 1989). Many individuals die while waiting because of the large gap that exists between the small available supply and the great demand for organs. The shortage of organs does not result from a lack of suitable donors as documented by the Centers for Disease Control (CDC). A study undertaken by the CDC revealed that only 15% of the 20,000 persons who die each year who meet donor eligibility criteria actually become organ donors (Kolata, 1983). Another study attributed the shortage to a failure to identify suitable donors, obtain consent from the next of kin, and procure the organs rather than to a lack of suitable donors (Bart et al., 1981).

Some of the difficulties in initiating the organ procurement process are related to the definition and declaration of death. In the past, both the medical and lay public agreed that the absence of a heart beat and respirations were acceptable criteria for a declaration of death. However, the advances in life-support technology that have enabled health care professionals to maintain respiration and circulation in individuals whose brain function is minimal or absent have also created uncertainty about death. Although the Uniform Definition of Death Act adopted by the President's Commission for the Study of Ethical Problems in Medicine and Biomedical and Behavioral Research (1981) includes the cessation of all function of the entire brain as a criterion for death, many health care professionals continue to feel uncertainty about implementing these criteria. People are strongly conditioned to view a breathing body with a beating heart as alive even when those functions continue only as a result of life-support systems.

METHODS OF OBTAINING CONSENT

Various methods have been tried in an effort to keep pace with the growing demand for organs and tissues for transplantation. Public education and media coverage of transplant success stories were implemented to raise the consciousness of the general public about the need for donated organs and the success rates achieved through transplantation. In 1968 the Uniform Anatomical Gift Act was passed, legalizing donor cards and the right of next-of-kin to consent to organ/tissue donation. In the past, health care providers relied on *voluntarism*, through which the next-of-kin initiated the offer to donate their loved one's organs or tissues after death. In the United States, voluntarism was ineffective even though it was encouraged by the passage of the Uniform Anatomical Gift Act. In Europe an attempt was made to increase organ/tissue donation by the passage of *presumed consent* laws. These laws gave physicians authority to simply remove needed organs or tissues from cadavers unless the individual carried a card prohibiting such donations or the next-of-kin

objected. These laws, however, did not succeed in narrowing the gap between the need for and the availability of organs or tissues for transplantation.

In an attempt to overcome the reluctance of health care professionals to ask grieving families for organ/tissue donation, all 50 states in the United States have now passed *required request* laws. These laws mandate that all families be given the opportunity to donate the organs or tissues of a loved one who has died if the deceased meets eligibility criteria. The premise of the law is that all families have the right to decide about donation. If this decision-making opportunity is not provided by health care professionals, then these professionals are, in a sense, making the decision for the family *against* donation. A policy of required request can lead hospital personnel to consider the need for transplantable organs or tissues routinely. It can ensure that the burden of decision concerning donation is equitably allocated among all families whose relatives might serve as donors. This policy may standardize the process of routine inquiry about organ/tissue donation in such a way that it lessens the psychological burden on both health care professionals and family members at a time of great stress and emotional upheaval. It removes the chance that a family may not be offered this option to donate while preserving their right to refuse consent, because voluntary choice remains the ethical foundation on which organ/tissue donation rests (Caplan, 1984).

The federal government has required all hospitals to establish organ/tissue procurement protocols to obtain Medicare reimbursement for patient care. Some states have made a similar requirement for Medicaid reimbursement. Government legislation is certainly one mechanism for increasing the likelihood that families of dying patients will be asked for organ/tissue donation, but the chronic shortage of organs and tissues cannot be alleviated solely by the passage of required request laws. Experience with this legislation has shown as much as a 300% increase in the number of tissue donors but no significant increase in the number of organ donors. This result does not necessarily mean that required request laws have been ineffective in increasing the number of organ donors. Changes in other public health policies are in a state of flux and may have clouded the issue. For example, in some states laws about drunk driving have been enacted and strictly enforced. In others, the age for legally purchasing alcohol has been raised. Still other states have enacted mandatory seat belt laws, lowered speed limits, and improved their ability to transport accident victims quickly to tertiary care centers through air transport. The fact that organ donation has remained constant despite the significant decrease in traffic fatalities provides some evidence that the laws have had a small positive impact on the organ supply.

Since required request laws were implemented, some states have reported a greater percentage of families saying "no" to the request. Part of the difficulty in evaluating this claim lies in the incomplete, inconsistent data collected prior to implementation of the laws compared to the more complete data currently collected. Certificates on every death are now required. These certificates include information about whether or not the deceased met donor eligibility criteria and the family's response to the request for an anatomical gift. Second, health care professionals formerly relied on voluntarism or carefully evaluated families, making the request only of families they were certain would respond favorably. A careful selection process was utilized prior to required request. Now, all potential donor families are offered the opportunity to make an anatomical gift. Another criticism is that there has not been enough preparation of health care professionals on how to identify potential donors and approach grieving families to implement the law effectively. If required request is to have a positive impact on the supply of organs and tissues for transplantation, health care providers must acquire the necessary knowledge to identify potential donors and the skills to enable them to communicate sensitively and effectively with grieving families. In addition, education of the public must continue emphasizing the need for individuals to discuss their wishes regarding organ/tissue donation with loved ones before a tragedy occurs. The public's attitude toward organ donation and the ability of the medical community to influence that attitude will have a profound effect on the future availability of organs and tissues for transplantation. (See also Chapter 35.)

ROLE OF NURSING IN DONATION PROCESS

The most recent Gallup poll conducted by the Batelle Human Affairs Research Center and the Gallup Organization (1987) showed that 99% of the general public is knowledgeable about transplantation and that 84% have received information about organ/tissue donation. Although many families have discussed their wishes in regard to organ/tissue donation, in an emergency situation the surviving loved one cannot be expected to initiate the idea of donation.

Nurses are frequently the first health care professionals to identify a potential organ donor and make the appropriate referral to the local Organ Procurement Organization. The ongoing physical assessment and hemodynamic monitoring provided by critical care nurses help direct care to maintain all transplantable organs and tissues in optimal condition. In addition, they provide both the factual information and the emotional support necessary for the next-of-kin to arrive at a decision about organ/tissue donation. Nurses are in the best position to provide compassionate support because they usually have a close relationship with the family and are well prepared both educationally and often through experience to help the family through their crisis. Research

by Morton and Leonard (1979) showed that the families' positive attitudes about organ donation and transplantation were strengthened by their donation experience in the hospital. Donor families' attitudes toward the health care team were closely related to the amount of time spent with them. The nursing staff was complimented without exception by all of the families interviewed.

DONOR FAMILY SUPPORT

Dealing with the Family's Reaction to Sudden Illness and Death

In our society people expect to live until the seventh or eighth decade. The death of a younger family member, which is common in the organ donation situation, in which the mean age of the donor is 26 years, is outside the natural order of life events. When a sudden illness or accident and death occur earlier in an individual's life span, the family is not psychologically prepared for the death. Shock and disbelief interfere with the family's ability to accept the fact of death. Caregivers can help by providing emotional support to families and by gently and sensitively assisting them to recognize the gravity of the loved one's condition.

Providing information to the family about the progress of their loved one consistently, simply, and repeatedly is the way caregivers can gradually assist the family to understand, assimilate, and accept the gravity of the situation. The critical care nurse is in the best position to assess constantly and evaluate the accuracy of the family's perception of the loved one's condition by asking questions like "What did the doctor tell you?" Any misconceptions should be corrected immediately. It may be helpful to convey to the family the recognition that it must be very hard for them to understand all that is happening to their loved one and to offer to call the physician to return and further clarify information about the clinical condition. It is very effective to provide explanations repeatedly because when anxiety is high, perceptions are narrowed. With narrowed perceptions, family members may hear only a small portion of what they are told in each interaction. In most instances of sudden illness, the family is looking for information that supports the hope that their loved one will survive, and therefore they may listen to information selectively.

Hope is a multidimensional, dynamic life force characterized by a confident yet uncertain expectation of achieving some future good. To the hoping person, the future good is realistically possible and personally significant (Dufault and Martocchio, 1985). Although it is important to be honest and straightforward with the family about the clinical situation, it is important not to destroy hope. The hope that families cling to can be therapeutic because it gives strength and energy at a time when sickness, pain, and fear are threatening to take over. It is important to remember that the family's hope for recovery can evolve into hope for their loved one's release from suffering and hope for meeting the person again in the afterlife.

Anxious family members often seek opinions from many staff members. Because nurses are most accessible to families at all hours, they are often the target for such requests for information. It is therefore critical that a nurse hears what the physician tells the family so that the information can be consistently reinforced during subsequent interactions with other caregivers.

Providing Emotional Support to Family Members

It is helpful if the family is permitted to visit their loved one as often as they wish. This is a good opportunity for the nursing staff to build trust and rapport. These interactions provide the foundation for the initial task of grieving, which is the recognition of the loss by the family when the patient dies. Conveying interest and concern about the patient as a unique individual by asking the family to tell about the patient during these interactions can strengthen the nurse-family relationship. The nurse must understand that the family may need to recount the circumstances leading up to the sudden illness or accident over and over again. It is important that the family be allowed to work through this situation with the help of an empathic listener.

The intensive care unit is a busy place, and extended conversations are not always possible. In such instances, simply personalize the care as much as possible to build rapport. The caregiver can engage the family in talking about the patient while providing care in the room. The family may feel less helpless in this crisis situation if they are able to provide simple comfort measures for their family member, such as wiping the face, applying skin lotion, combing hair, and shaving.

A family's response to a crisis is variable. It is influenced by the specific circumstances of the illness or accident, the relationship to the loved one, and sociocultural factors. Often rage or anger is expressed initially, particularly if the family feels responsible for the illness. Angry reactions are often directed at staff because there is no other target. Listening attentively and with empathy is the most effective intervention. It is important to remember to avoid becoming defensive because this will only provide fuel for their anger. (See also Chapter 7.)

Donor Identification and Referral

One of the biggest obstacles to organ donation in the past has been a failure to identify potential donors early in the process. Nurses must be knowledgeable about potential donor eligibility criteria and be able to activate the resources necessary to evaluate the situation. Early awareness can prevent the unfortunate circumstance of families being approached unnecessarily or not being approached at all. It is imperative that the local organ procurement agency be contacted to determine suitability for organ/tissue donation and to initiate appropriate donor management.

Eligibility criteria are different for organ and tissue donors. Cadaver organ donors (donors of heart, lung, liver, kidney, and pancreas) are previously healthy individuals who have suffered irreversible brain injury of a known cause. The most common causes of injury are cerebral trauma from motor vehicle accidents or gunshot wounds, intracerebral or subarachnoid hemorrhage, primary brain tumor, and anoxic brain damage resulting from drug overdose or cardiac arrest. The brain-dead donor must have effective cardiovascular function and must be supported on a ventilator to preserve organ viability. The age range of most suitable donors is newborn to 65 years of age. The age of the donor, however, is generally less important than the quality of organ function. The donor must be free of extracranial malignancies, sepsis, and communicable diseases including hepatitis, syphilis, tuberculosis, and human immunodeficiency virus (HIV). The organ donor eligibility criteria and necessary laboratory tests are listed in Tables 52–2 and 52–3. The specific criteria used may vary from transplant center to transplant

TABLE 52–2. Organ Donor Eligibility Criteria

	Heart	Heart/Lung	Lung
Age	Center-specific	Center-specific	1–50 years
Cardiac arrest, resuscitated	Center-specific	Center-specific	Possibly OK
Blood type	Yes	Yes	Yes
Laboratory Studies			
Hematology Chemistry	CBC with differential, platelets, PT/PTT Electrolytes, osmolality, arterial blood gases		
	CPK-MB	CPK-MB	N/A
Culture	Blood	Blood Sputum	Blood Sputum
Procedures			
Chest x-ray	Yes, within last 6 hours	Yes, within last 6 hours	Yes, within last 4 hours
12-lead electrocardiogram	Yes, within last 6 hours	Yes, within last 6 hours	Yes
Central venous pressure	Yes	Yes	Yes
Arterial line	Yes	Yes	Yes
Miscellaneous	Weight Height	Weight Height	Weight Height Chest circumference, left main stem bronchus measurement

From LifeBanc Donor Criteria Card 1990, LifeBanc, Cleveland, OH.

TABLE 52–3. Organ Donor Eligibility Criteria

	Kidney	Liver	Pancreas
Age	2–65 years	Center-specific	10 months–50 years
Cardiac arrest, resuscitated	OK	Possibly OK	Possibly OK
Blood type	Yes	Yes	Yes
Laboratory Studies			
Hematology	Complete blood count with differential, platelets, prothrombin time/partial thromboplastin time		
Chemistry	Electrolytes, arterial blood gases, osmolality		
	Blood urea nitrogen Creatinine Urinalysis	Liver Profile	Amylase Fasting blood glucose
Culture	Blood Sputum Urine	Blood	Blood
Procedures			
Chest x-ray	Yes	Yes	Yes
12-lead electrocardiogram	Yes	Yes	Yes
Central venous pressure	Yes	Yes	Yes
Arterial line	Yes	Yes	Yes
Miscellaneous		Height Weight Abdominal girth	

From LifeBanc Donor Criteria Card, LifeBanc, Cleveland, OH.

center. Always contact the local organ procurement agency for more information. These agencies have health care professionals on 24-hour call to answer questions, evaluate potential donors, make recommendations about proper donor management, and help provide information to potential donor families about the organ donation process.

Unlike organ donors, tissue donors (donors of eyes, bone, skin, heart valves) need not have a beating heart. Death may be pronounced and tissue recovered hours after the heart has stopped beating. Again, it is imperative to determine whether the donor meets eligibility criteria as specified by the local organ procurement agency. The general tissue donor eligibility criteria are listed in Table 52–4.

Treatment of the patient changes to management of the donor when brain death is determined, declared, and documented in the medical record and the legal next-of-kin has provided consent for organ donation (spouse, adult son or daughter, either parent, adult brother or sister, guardian of deceased at the time of death, or any person authorized to dispose of the body).

The Asking Process

A common question that arises in the minds of caregivers about organ/tissue donation is related to religious beliefs. Though the answers vary from denomination to denomination and from individual to individual within each denomination, research by the American Council on Transplantation (1987) found that the major religious groups in the United States support donation and transplantation. Many groups, such as Roman Catholics, Amish, Moslems, and Jews, view organ donation as an act of charity, fraternal love, and self-sacrifice. Other religions, such as the Buddhists, Christian Scientists, Hindus, Jehovah's Witnesses, and various Protestant groups, express the belief that donation is a matter of individual conscience. Gypsies are the only group opposing donation. Their opposition is associated with the belief that for 1 year after a person dies, the soul retraces its steps. It is believed that all of the body parts must be intact because the soul maintains a physical shape.

Timing is critical to sensitive and effective requests for organ/tissue donation. Only after the physician conveys the hopelessness of the clincial situation and the family has had time to assimilate this information can the donation process be initiated. The success of the request is related primarily to how the caregiver deals with a family during this sensitive period. The family should be approached, not to acquire organs, but to show compassion and offer assistance and support during their bereavement. The request for donation must be handled only as part of the natural support provided to a family at the time of their loved one's death. It is the death that is the most important event, not the organ/tissue donation. Research by Morton and Leonard (1979) showed that some family members were dissatisfied with the manner in which they were approached. Some found the person who approached them blunt and callous, especially if they had not understood the donor's hopeless prognosis until donation was requested. Nevertheless, most families were pleased that they

TABLE 52–4. Tissue Donor Eligibility Criteria

	Bone	Skin	Eye	Heart Valve	Middle Ear	Saphenous Vein
Age	15–65 years	12–75 years	2–75 years	Newborn to 60 years	6–80 years	5–55 years
Cardiac arrest resuscitated	N/A	N/A	N/A	No	N/A	N/A
Malignancy	No	No	Yes	No	N/A	N/A
Culture	Blood	Blood	N/A	Blood	N/A	N/A

From LifeBanc Donor Criteria Card 1990, LifeBanc, Cleveland, OH.

were offered the opportunity to donate their loved one's organs or tissues.

Once the next-of-kin have been informed of their family member's death by the physician, the physician, nurse, procurement coordinator, or hospital designee can offer the family the opportunity to donate organs or tissues. The discussion should take place in a comfortable, private area, conducive to the family's expression of grief. The approach to the family should be planned after they have had time to assimilate the news that their loved one's brain is dead. It is very effective and conveys sensitivity to begin the conversation with an extension of sympathy. Allowing time for the family to express their feelings at this time further conveys the sympathy of the caregivers. It is important then to elicit the family's understanding of the loved one's condition and to re-explain, if necessary, why the patient is considered dead. The caregiver can say something like, "Tell me what you understand about your son's condition." If the family does not understand what has occurred, it may be necessary to bring the physician back to explain the clinical situation. Likewise, if the family needs more time to absorb the idea that their loved one is dead, the interaction is stopped and the caregiver returns after a specified interval. At this point, the caregiver might say, "I can see the news of your son's death is still very overwhelming. I will leave you alone together for awhile . . . . I will return in 20 minutes."

Making the Request

If trust and rapport with family members have been established successfully, a conversation about donation can be a major step toward recognition of the loss. The subject can be introduced with a simple question such as, "Did your son ever mention the desire to donate his organs or tissues at the time of death?" The first sentence is the most difficult to get out, but once the subject has been introduced, the caregiver can follow the family's cues. Then pause to allow the family to think about and respond to the question. If the family asks questions, answer and explore any concerns they express.

A decision to donate is personal and voluntary. It is important for families to recognize the request as just another option to consider and a personal decision. It is often the first time families feel in control after the tragic death of a loved one. The caregiver should not feel like a failure as an asker if the family refuses. The refusal can mean many things, ranging from an informed decision to an expression of anger and anguish over the loss, to concern about what body parts are needed in the afterlife. Families have the right to say no. So, how is a negative response handled? Simply, the caregiver can thank the family for considering organ/tissue donation and then close

the conversation by saying, "Would you like to see your son one more time?"

If the family seems positive about donation or needs more information or time, continue to discuss their questions. Nurses cannot be expected to be able to answer every question a family asks. They can consult a procurement coordinator. The coordinator will explain the donation procedure to the family in more detail, including the fact that life supports are continued until the organs are removed in the operating room, as well as answering any other questions. In addition, the coordinator may handle communication with the coroner or funeral director about the donor's burial, when appropriate.

Questions frequently asked by the family concern pain experienced by the donor, payment, disfigurement, funeral delays, and confidentiality. A brief explanation of brain death again can allay family fears about their loved one experiencing pain during the organ/tissue procurement surgery. With regard to payment, once an organ or tissue donor has been identified, the procurement agency pays all costs associated with the care of the donor and organ/tissue procurement. These costs include additional laboratory tests, operating room costs, and intravenous fluids and medications required to maintain viable organs or tissues for transplantation. Families are often concerned about whether or not donation interferes with an open casket funeral. Assurance can be given that the donor will appear normal, and donation does not preclude an open casket. Funeral delays usually do not occur unless procurement teams are coming from various parts of the country. It can take up to 18 hours in some instances, but family members are kept informed of the delays. If delays are causing additional stress for the family, a decision may be made to proceed with the donation of those organs or tissues for which procurement teams are immediately available. After procurement, the body is released to the funeral home. If it is logistically possible, the family should be offered the opportunity to see their loved one after the heart has stopped beating. This can ease the transition from the hospital to the funeral home and again reinforce the family's recognition of the loss. This viewing can take place in the recovery room, the intensive care unit, or the morgue. Most families, however, leave the hospital when the deceased is taken to surgery. Often a telephone call informing them that the procurement has been completed is all the communication the family desires. This can be accomplished by the organ procurement coordinator, who is present in the operating room. Gifts of organs or tissues are confidential. No one who receives a transplant is told the identity of the donor. Likewise, donor families are only told the age and sex of the various recipients and how they are doing after transplantation. The organ procurement agency provides this information in a letter within a few weeks after the donation.

DONOR MANAGEMENT

Prior to a declaration of brain death, therapeutic modalities are employed to maximize neurologic recovery. Ventilation and fluid therapy are altered to reduce intracranial pressure. Systemic blood pressure is supported with vasopressors to maintain adequate cerebral perfusion pressure. When brain death has been declared, therapy changes to optimize organ function. At this point, the management of the donor becomes the responsibility of the organ procurement team.

The goals of donor management are to maintain organ perfusion and organ oxygenation. Organ perfusion is a function of intravascular volume, vascular resistance, and cardiac function. Failure to maintain and balance these three components will result in impaired tissue perfusion, cellular dysfunction, organ deterioration, and organ death. Organ donors usually have conditions such as thoracic injuries, shock, pneumonia, atelectasis, and other clinical problems that may result in diminished oxygenation and ventilation. Delivery of oxygen is essential to the maintenance of viable organ function. The nursing care plan at the end of the chapter outlines the nursing diagnoses, interventions, and expected outcomes for organ donor management.

BEREAVEMENT

Teaching family members about what to expect during the grieving process can help prepare them for the next few months. Bereaved families need others for continued comfort and support, such as extended family, friends, and clergy. Grief needs to be shared. It is important to tell families that the mourning process varies from person to person, but for most people healing occurs without complications with time. A variety of thoughts, feelings, behaviors, and physical sensations may be experienced by the family. It is important for family members to understand that these are a normal part of healthy grieving. (See also Chapter 7.)

Family Reactions to Donation

Health care professionals often fear that asking grieving families for organ/tissue donation will have negative consequences or that it will add to the family's grief. However, studies have shown that the strongest advocates of organ/tissue donation are donor families because they view donation as the highest form of charity, believing that they are giving the ultimate gift, life, to another person (Morton and Leonard, 1979; Bartucci and Seller, 1986; Christopherson and Lunde, 1971; Goldsmith and Montefusco, 1985; Bartucci, 1987).

In addition to the gift-giving aspect of donation, families have reported that the grief experienced due to an abrupt and tragic loss of a loved one was lessened when they knew that other people were leading new lives because of donation. The donation of vital organs was reported to be a meaningful part of the normal grief process (Morton and Leonard, 1979; Bartucci and Seller, 1986; Christopherson and Lunde, 1971; Goldsmith and Montefusco, 1985; Bartucci, 1987; Fulton et al., 1980; Gideon, 1981). Furthermore, it was found that families maintain very favorable attitudes over time because they view donation as the one positive aspect of death, seeing it as a chance for their loved one to achieve a type of immortality by living on in another human being through transplantation (Fulton et al., 1980; Bartucci and Seller, 1986; Bartucci, 1987).

In a recent study of families who donated the organs of loved ones, Bartucci (1987) found that 85% identified organ donation as something positive during their time of grief. Ninety-one per cent had no regrets about the decision to donate their loved one's organs. The three respondents who regretted the donation identified some problem with the procurement process, but later they reported extremely positive feelings about the recipients of their loved one's organs. One wife stated, "You'll never know how good (for the first time) I felt knowing that part of my husband was helping a little boy to live a normal life." The two most common reasons cited in the decision to donate were: (1) Their loved one would have wanted to help someone, and (2) organ donation seemed to be a way of deriving something positive from the loss.

The majority of donor families studied had good feelings about their donation experience because they were able to help someone else. It comforted them to know that the death of their loved one was not in vain, and the donation itself gave some meaning to the sudden, untimely death of a previously healthy person. If health care professionals consider the perspective of donor families, they may be less fearful about offering this life-giving, life-sustaining opportunity. Donation can be a vehicle for beginning the resolution of grief and an opportunity for the donor family to turn a tragic death into a heroic gesture. The following describes a mother's organ donation experience.

Jeffrey's Story

Peggy Rickard Bishop

During the Christmas season of 1982, my three-year-old son Jeffrey died of an intracerebral hemorrhage. There had been no indication that anything was wrong with Jeffrey. The day had been a very ordinary day in his life. He played with his two older brothers and exhibited normal three-year-old behavior. Several times that day he went to a corner of the living room, patted the floor, and announced to the family that was where he wanted the Christmas tree.

Because Jeffrey had a long nap and was quite cheerful, he stayed up to play with his brothers. At 11:00 P.M., after his prayers and good night kisses, he went to bed with his favorite stuffed animal and a Christmas book. I heard him talking and singing in his bed shortly before I heard a cry I had never heard before. I found Jeffrey holding the left side of his head, rolling back and forth in his crib. I carried him to the living room and as he lay on the couch, he began to vomit.

The rescue squad was called and by the time the paramedics arrived, Jeffrey was unconscious. He was transported to the local community hospital. Within minutes after arrival, he had a respiratory arrest and was placed on a respirator. After three hours, Jeffrey was transferred to a university-affiliated children's hospital where a CAT scan revealed a massive hemorrhage in his brain. At 4:00 A.M., I learned my son was brain dead, that nothing could make him well again. I was stunned and could not believe what was happening. I soon became aware Jeffrey's condition was deteriorating. His body was being artificially warmed, his blood pressure maintained with medications, and his heart beat and respirations dependent upon a machine.

I offered to donate any of Jeffrey's organs for transplant. The physician was very surprised when I brought up the subject of organ donation. A transplant coordinator from the local Organ Procurement Agency arrived at 12:00 noon and began preparations for the removal of Jeffrey's kidneys, eyes, and liver. My only stipulation to the donation was the organs be sent not only as gifts of life, but with the message they were also gifts of love.

During the course of the day, Jeffrey's brothers, grandparents, and a few close friends came to the hospital to spend time with him and give each other much needed support. It was an extremely painful experience to explain to Jay and Michael that their little brother, who had been running around the house hours before, was now being kept alive by a machine. My own pain of trying to cope with the loss was only heightened by experiencing their pain.

The atmosphere in the Intensive Care Unit was one of extreme caring. I was provided with a rocking chair in which I could sit and hold Jeffrey. I was given time to cuddle him, talk to him, and say a very special goodbye to my youngest child. When I requested hand and foot prints, the nurses found ink pads and I got my prints. I was also given a pair of scissors to cut a lock of his hair.

The Director of the Intensive Care Unit gave the family much consideration during that day and the following weeks. He spent time explaining what most likely caused Jeffrey's death, what kind of medical care was being provided, and the procedure for donating his organs. He took special time with Jay and Michael, explaining what had happened to Jeffrey and answering their many questions in terms they could understand.

At 4:00 P.M., eighteen hours after Jeffrey became ill, he was taken to surgery for the removal of his kidneys, eyes, and liver. As he left for the operating room, the family prepared to leave for home. I had Jeffrey's hand and foot prints, a lock of his hair, and the belief he had received the best possible care available. I spoke with the Director of the Intensive Care Unit and asked him to take care of Jeffrey for me. I left behind his favorite blue blanket that went everywhere with him and asked the doctor to cover Jeffrey with it following surgery. The doctor assured me he would be cared for as the little boy he was and my wish would be carried out.

Many people have made the comment that the decision to donate Jeffrey's organs must have been difficult. For me, it was a decision bringing comfort, not additional pain. Facing the death of my son was nearly unbearable, but because I had previously thought about organ donation, the decision was much easier. When I was twelve, a friend and I made our own non-legal wills donating our organs to their respective organ banks. It was at this time I first became aware of such medical advances as transplantation. While visiting my parents a few months after Jeffrey's death, I found the copy of the "pretend" will. It was so ironic to relate its contents to the events that had transpired in my life.

Another seed relating to organ donation was planted when I was taking a Medical Terminology class just six months before Jeffrey's death. After a serious class discussion about transplant, I continued to give the idea of organ donation much thought, and expressed the wish to donate my organs by signing the back of my driver's license. Although I decided to donate my organs, I had not allowed myself to consider what I would do if one of my sons was to die. For several weeks after the class the subject of organ donation was in my thoughts. I finally made up my mind, I would donate my child's organs if faced with the decision, so very unaware that within six months I would carry out that decision.

My purpose in sharing this experience is to convey to others that even in this dark tragedy new hope and new life can result. I view Jeffrey as a very precious gift, just as I view Jay and Michael, and through organ donation Jeffrey was again a gift, to five other people and their families.

From Bartucci, M. R., and Bishop, P. R. (1987). The meaning of organ donation to donor families. *ANNA Journal*, 14 (7), 369–372, 410. © 1987, *ANNA Journal*, official journal of the American Nephrology Nurses' Association. Reprinted with permission. Reprints of article available only from *ANNA Journal*; North Woodbury Road/Box 56; Pitman, NJ 08071.

PSYCHOSOCIAL IMPLICATIONS FOR NURSES

There are many sources of stress for nurses involved in the organ donation/procurement process. One major stressor is the declaration of brain death and the issues surrounding the termination of treatment. There is a great deal of uncertainty and ambivalence about the determination of brain death because there are no absolute rules. A physician makes the diagnosis based on state law, hospital policy, and the criteria currently accepted by experts in the neurosurgical and neurologic professions. The haunting question of whether or not one can ever be certain there is no potential for recovery remains. Even nurses who understand and accept the concept of brain death may find it difficult to ignore the signs of life they see. In addition, ambivalent feelings may be exacerbated by interactions with family members who are clinging to the hope for recovery and are less intellectually and emotionally prepared to accept the finality of death despite so much apparent life (Youngner et al., 1985). Nurses are forced to examine their own concerns about the meaning of a declaration of death made on brain death criteria because they must be able to answer the family's questions and respond to their concerns or misperceptions.

Other stressors include questions of professional competence because of the inability of the health care team to save the life of this previously healthy individual. Additionally, there are feelings of conflict and dissonance because the intensive care unit and operating room suddenly become the places where one life is given to save another through transplantation. The conflict occurs because the donor's welfare no longer provides the rationale for aggressive management, treatment, and surgery. This violation of the general belief that human beings should be treated as ends in themselves, rather than as means to other ends, creates the dissonance.

Further conflict arises because these nurses are also responsible for other critically ill patients in the intensive care unit. Caring for the organ donor requires intense hemodynamic monitoring and careful management to preserve organ viability for transplantation. Legitimate concerns arise about donor management detracting from the care of living patients.

Responsibility for donor management is stressful in itself. A study of intensive care unit nurses' perceptions of cadaver organ procurement revealed that nurses are fearful of making a mistake in the nursing management of a potential donor, thus jeopardizing the donor's ability to donate (Sophie et al., 1983).

Implementing interventions and strategies to help nurses deal with the psychosocial and stress factors surrounding the care of donors can help to alleviate the stresses or teach nurses to deal with the stresses in a healthy, constructive manner. The most critical intervention is professional education. A program should be designed to help nurses evaluate their personal feelings about their own mortality and their beliefs about the benefits of organ donation and transplantation. In addition, there should be discussion about what constitutes brain death, how the determination is made, and what the implications are for making such a declaration. Becoming informed about the documented benefits of organ donation to donor families can help the nurse view donation in a positive way. Learning and practicing the words to say when making a request for organ/tissue donation can lessen the fear of approaching a grieving family.

Development of a detailed orientation program for new staff prior to involving them in organ procurement is critical. The new staff member must be adequately prepared emotionally as well as technically to deal with donor management and supportive care of family members. A preceptorship or buddy system can be beneficial because it provides not only good role models for teaching new staff how to handle their personal feelings but also opportunities for practicing appropriate behaviors. Mutual support benefits not only the new staff member but also the more experienced nurse. It is helpful to use established guidelines and procedures to prepare the new caregiver to function with confidence and to gain the ability to deal with the most common complications that may occur. All caregivers may not be able to participate in organ donation/procurement for a variety of reasons and should not be required to do so.

Many organ donation/procurement procedures occur in hospitals not involved in transplantation. The process becomes very one-sided because the nurses involved in the care of the cadaver donor do not have the chance to benefit from caring for the recipients and seeing the fruits of their labor. One way to accomplish this is to request and share feedback from the organ procurement agency about the recipients of the organs they helped to procure. It is also valuable to provide special recognition for all who participated.

A mechanism for providing support to staff is vital for encouraging positive coping behaviors. It is imperative for staff members to receive the message that emotional upset is legitimate. There must be a forum for discussing these feelings on a regular basis or after each donor experience. If problems occur with the approach to a family or in management of a donor, it is constructive to review what might have been done differently so that all staff can learn what needs to be changed for the next time.

In summary, participation in donor care is emotionally draining because of the support and comfort needed by the grieving family. It is time-consuming and requires intense monitoring and expert application of physical and psychosocial assessment skills. In addition, it requires the nurse to be in touch with his or her personal feelings about death in general, brain death specifically, and beliefs about organ/tissue donation and transplantation. (See also Chapter 8.)

TRANSPLANTATION

Once the transplantable organs have been surgically removed, they are preserved in a sterile, iced electrolyte solution and transported to the respective transplant center. Heart, liver, heart/lung, and pancreas recipients are identified prior to the procurement procedure because of the short time these organs can maintain their viability after recovery. Kidney recipients are usually identified after procurement because kidneys can maintain viability for as long as 72 hours before they must be transplanted.

All potential organ recipients are entered into the national computer system through the United Network for Organ Sharing (UNOS). A point system has been instituted to allow equitable distribution of this scarce resource. Blood type compatibility between donor and recipient is mandatory. For potential kidney recipients there are five factors. First, priority is given to the potential recipient with the best antigen match. The reason is that recognition of the transplanted organ as nonself depends on the presence of major histocompatibility complex (MHC) antigens on the surface of the cells in the transplant. A small number of recipient T-lymphocytes are able, through their receptors, to interact with the MHC antigens on the transplant, triggering the immune response. To the extent that the antigens on the transplant are the same as those of the recipient, a less vigorous immune response may result. Second, consideration is given to how long the individual has been waiting compared to other potential recipients in the same locale. Priority is also given to potential recipients who have preformed antibodies to MHC antigens because the presence of these antibodies can limit the number of kidneys for which the potential recipient would be eligible. Priority is also given to potential recipients who are medical emergencies. There are a few circumstances that qualify a renal patient as an emergency for transplantation; one of the most common is the inability to maintain arteriovenous access for hemodialysis. The final criterion has to do with logistic factors based on the ease and rapidity with which the transplant can be performed.

Similar criteria are used for extrarenal organ recipients with the addition of degree of medical urgency and size. Because heart, liver, and heart/lung transplants are life-saving operations, the potential recipient who is most critically ill receives priority.

Immunosuppression After Transplantation

Regardless of the type of organ transplanted, immunosuppression is critical to graft survival. The goal of therapy is to prevent the body from recognizing the transplanted organ as foreign while preserving the body's ability to mount an immune response to infection. Greater potency and specificity and less toxicity have been the objectives in developing immunosuppressive therapies. Several drugs are currently used in a variety of combinations, which are individualized by each transplant center. The major drugs used in transplantation are listed in Table 52–5 as well as the immune system effect, dosage and administration, and adverse reactions.

TABLE 52–5. Immunosuppressives Used in Transplantation

1. Antilymphocytic Globulin (ALG)

Immune system effect
 Antibody destruction of transplant recipient's T-cells resulting in decreased population of T-cells
Dosage and administration
 Dosage based on mg/kg of body weight
 Administered intravenously through central venous line (usually subclavian) over 4–6 hours
 Used prophylactically for 5–12 days after transplantation and can also be used to treat acute rejection episodes
Adverse reactions
 Allergic reactions including fever, chills, rash, joint pain, back pain, dyspnea, tachycardia, and hypotension
 Serum sickness
 Thrombophlebitis or thrombosis
 Thrombocytopenia
 Latent viral infections (cytomegalovirus, herpes)

2. Azathioprine (Imuran)

Immune system effect
 Competes with enzymes required for cell nucleic acid synthesis and inhibits replication in rapidly dividing cells resulting in decreased immunoblast
  ability to clone daughter T- and B-cells
Dosage and administration
 Dosage based on mg/kg of body weight
 Administered orally once daily, usually in the evening
 Dosage may be adjusted downward if white blood cell count drops below 5000
Adverse reactions
 Hepatotoxicity manifested by elevated liver function test results and jaundice
 Anemia
 Alopecia
 Leukopenia
 Increased susceptibility to infection
 Increased potential to develop cancer

3. Corticosteroids (Prednisone)

Immune system effect
 Inhibits interleukin-1 secretion resulting in decreased replication and development of killer T-cells
Dosage and administration
 Dosage based on mg/kg of body weight
 Administered orally once daily
 Dosage tapered over first 6 months after transplantation
Adverse reactions
 Body image changes including increased weight, moon face, buffalo hump, pot belly, acne
 Delayed wound healing
 Increased susceptibility to infection
 Ulcer formation (duodenal or gastric)
 Cataracts
 Insulin-dependent diabetes, either temporary (dose-related) or permanent
 Aseptic necrosis (primarily of femoral head)
 Increased susceptibility to skin cancer
 Pancreatitis
 Mood swings
 Sodium and water retention
 Increased skin fragility
 Hyperlipidemia
 Night sweats

4. Cyclosporine

Immune system effect
 Reduces ability of accessory cells to produce interleukins, resulting in decreased replication of helper and killer T-cells
Dosage and administration
 Dosage based on mg/kg of body weight
 Administered once or twice daily in chocolate milk or juice in a minimum 1:10 dilution
 Must be given in glass container because drug adheres to plastic and is adsorbed in styrofoam
 Dosage tapered based on 12- or 24-hour trough blood levels and standard tapering schedule
Adverse reactions
 Hepatotoxicity manifested by elevated liver function test results and jaundice
 Nephrotoxicity (often mimicking rejection)
 Lethal fungal infections
 Lymphomas
 Hypertension
 Fine hand tremors
 Hyperkalemia

5. Orthoclone OKT3

Immune system effect
 A monoclonal antibody to the T3 antigen of human T-cells, which functions as an immunosuppressant
 Blocks both killing by cytotoxic human T-cells and the generation of other T-cell functions
Dosage and administration
 One dose of 5 mg given daily for 10 days
 Administered intravenously over 30–60 seconds
 First three doses administered in the hospital and remainder can be administered in the outpatient setting
Adverse reactions
 First and second doses:

Pyrexia	Nausea
Chills	Vomiting
Tremor	Diarrhea
Dyspnea	Headache
Chest pain	Photophobia
Wheezing	

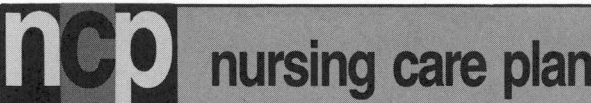 **nursing care plan**

ORGAN DONOR MANAGEMENT

1. Decreased cardiac output related to:
Central nervous system dysfunction (loss of vasomotor control)
Hypovolemia

Outcome Criteria	Nursing Interventions
Normal cardiac output as evidenced by systolic blood pressure greater than 100 mm Hg, heart rate within normal limits, and central venous pressure greater than 10 cm H_2O or 7 mm Hg	1. Monitor hourly heart rate and blood pressure 2. Maintain continuous electrocardiographic monitoring 3. Monitor hourly central venous or pulmonary artery pressures 4. Monitor hourly fluid intake and output 5. Administer intravenous fluids as ordered 6. Administer vasopressors as ordered and monitor for untoward effects 7. Obtain serum cardiac enzymes as ordered

2. Impaired tissue perfusion related to:
Central nervous system dysfunction
Hypovolemia

Outcome Criteria	Nursing Interventions
Adequate tissue perfusion as evidenced by systolic blood pressure, greater than 100 mm Hg, central venous pressure greater than 10 cm H_2O or 7 mm Hg, urine output greter than 2 to 3 mL/kg per hour, good quality periphral pulses, absence of cyanosis, and normal blood pH, urea nitrogen, and creatinine	1. Monitor hourly heart rate, blood pressure, central venous pressure, or pulmonary artery pressure 2. Monitor quality of peripheral pulses 3. Monitor skin temperature and color 4. Check capillary refilling in fingertips 5. Observe nailbeds and lips for cyanosis 6. Obtain arterial blood gases as indicated 7. Monitor hourly urine output 8. Obtain serum electrolytes, blood urea nitrogen, and creatinine 9. Administer vasopressors as ordered and document changes in blood pressure and urine output after administration

3. Impaired gas exchange related to:
Central nervous system dysfunction (loss of respiratory mechanics)
Neurogenic pulmonary edema
Aspiration pneumonia

Outcome Criteria	Nursing Interventions
Adequate gas exchange as evidenced by Pa_{O_2} between 80 and 120 mm Hg, oxyhemoglobin saturation above 90%, Pa_{CO_2} between 35 and 45 mm Hg, IMV rate between 8 and 14 breaths per minute, tidal volume 12 to 15 mL/kg, pH 7.35 to 7.45, hemoglobin 12% to 18% to maximize content of oxygen in arterial blood Adequate ventilation as evidenced by normal breath sounds bilaterally on auscultation and equal bilateral chest wall movement with respiration	1. Monitor mechanical ventilation 2. Maintain patent airway with sterile suctioning to remove tracheobronchial secretions 3. Auscultate breath sounds bilaterally 4. Obtain arterial blood gases every 4 to 6 hours and after ventilator changes 5. Observe tracheobronchial secretions for amount, color, consistency, and odor 6. Culture tracheobronchial secretions as indicated 7. Turn every 2 hours and administer chest physiotherapy 8. Chest x-ray as indicated

4. Potential fluid volume deficit related to:
Diabetes insipidus

Outcome Criteria	Nursing Interventions
Adequate fluid and electrolyte balance as evidenced by stable vital signs, appropriate urine output, stable weight, and normal serum and urine electrolytes	1. Monitor hourly intake and output 2. Monitor hourly heart rate, blood pressure, central venous pressure, or pulmonary artery pressure 3. Administer intravenous maintenance and replacement fluids 4. Daily weights 5. Monitor urine specific gravity every 2 hours 6. Administer aqueous vasopressin as ordered and document changes in urine output after administration 7. Monitor serum and urine electrolytes every 4 hours 8. Obtain urine and serum osmolality

Nursing Care Plan continued on following page

5. Potential for impaired temperature control related to:
Central nervous system dysfunction (damage to hypothalamus)

Outcome Criteria	Nursing Interventions
Adequate temperature control as evidenced by normal body temperature, 97° to 100°F	1. Monitor body temperature for hyperthermia or hypothermia 2. Restore normal body temperature with the use of heating/cooling blankets as indicated 3. Warm intravenous fluids before administration if hypothermia is present

6. Potential for infection related to:
Presence of indwelling catheters and an endotracheal tube

Outcome Criteria	Nursing Interventions
Absence of infection as evidenced by clear urine, WBC count within normal limits, absence of fever, absence of purulent secretions and purulent wound drainage	1. Careful handwashing 2. Obtain complete blood count with differential 3. Maintain aseptic care of indwelling Foley catheter, observing urine for cloudiness, sediment, and odor 4. Maintain sterile suction technique to remove tracheobronchial secretions observing amount, color, odor, and consistency 5. Turn and reposition every 2 hours and administer chest physiotherapy to prevent pneumonia 6. Monitor wounds, incisions, and puncture sites for erythema and drainage 7. Culture tracheobronchial secretions, urine, and blood 8. Administer antibiotics as ordered 9. Keep skin clean and dry

7. Potential skin impairment related to:
Immobility

Outcome Criteria	Nursing Interventions
Absence of skin impairment as evidenced by good skin turgor and no areas of redness or breakdown	1. Keep skin clean and dry 2. Turn and reposition every 2 hours; establish and post a turning schedule at the bedside 3. Assess for redness and skin breakdown, especially over bony prominences and areas prone to pressure 4. Apply lotion to dry skin 5. Maintain hydration to ensure good skin turgor 6. Apply heel protectors 7. Use sheepskin, air mattress, water mattress, or Flexicare bed

8. Grieving related to:
Imminent death or death of a loved one

Outcome Criteria	Nursing Interventions
Completion of the first task of grieving as evidenced by the family's ability to discuss feelings about loss of a loved one. Knowledge and understanding of the normal grief process as evidenced by family's ability to identify thoughts, feelings, behaviors, and physical sensations they experience as a result of their loss. Support system(s) in place as evidenced by the presence of other family members, friends, clergy, or counselor to help the family begin to work through their grief.	1. Provide information about loved one's progress consistently, simply, and repeatedly 2. Assess and evaluate accuracy of family's perceptions of loved one's condition 3. Support family's hope 4. Listen attentively and with empathy to accounts of circumstances leading up to sudden illness 5. Encourage family to talk about loved one 6. Allow family to visit any time and participate in care if they so desire 7. Participate in making request for organ/tissue donation once death has been pronounced and support family's decision 8. Explain variety of thoughts, feelings, behaviors, and physical sensations family may experience as normal part of healthy grieving 9. Evaluate support systems, i.e., other family members, friends, clergy 10. Refer for bereavement therapy if appropriate

Adapted from Goldsmith, J., and Montefusco, C. (1985). Nursing care of the potential organ donor. *Critical Care Nurse*, 5 (6), 22–29.

SUMMARY

Tremendous progress has been made in transplantation in the last ten years, with 1-year graft survivals reaching 90% and 5-year survivals averaging 70%. With the increasing success rates, more and more patients suffering from end-stage organ disease are opting for transplantation. Although more than 14,000 organ transplants are performed annually, the national waiting list continues to grow. There are currently almost 18,000 patients awaiting organs for transplantation. These people and their families are in limbo, walking a tightrope of hope and despair. Many patients will die before an organ becomes available.

The challenge of the 1990s is to prevent the organ supply and demand problem from escalating. The future of organ transplantation rests partially in the hands of critical care nurses. They have the ability to identify and refer potential donors and possess the necessary expert physical assessment and hemodynamic monitoring skills to help direct care toward maintaining organ and tissue viability. Critical care nurses are caring and empathic and have the skills to communicate with families in crisis. They have developed the ability to assess and evaluate the accuracy of the family's perception of a loved one's condition and therefore can identify when a family is ready to hear about the option of donation. They are able to provide both the factual information and the emotional support necessary to allow the next-of-kin to arrive at a decision about donation, and they have the support of their colleagues through this often emotionally draining experience.

References

American Council on Transplantation (1987). *Religious views of organ/tissue donation*. News release, National Organ and Tissue Donation Awareness Week Promotional Kit. Alexandria, VA.

American Council on Transplantation (1988). Organ transplants in 1988 showed dramatic increase in most categories. *Newsline*, Alexandria, VA.

Bart, K., et al. (1981). Increasing the supply of cadaveric kidneys for transplantation. *Transplantation*, 31 (5), 383–387.

Bartucci, M. R. (1987). Organ donation: A study of the donor family perspective. *Journal of Neuroscience Nursing*, 19 (6), 305–309.

Bartucci, M. R., and Bishop, P. R. (1987). The meaning of organ donation to donor families. *ANNA Journal*, 14 (7), 369–371; 410.

Bartucci, M. R., and Seller, M. C. (1986). Donor family responses to kidney recipient letters of thanks. *Transplantation Proceedings*, 18 (3), 401–405.

Caplan, A. L. (1984). Ethical and policy issues in the procurement of cadaver organs for transplantation. *New England Journal of Medicine*, 311 (15), 981–983.

Christopherson, L., and Lunde, D. (1971). Heart transplant donors and their families. *Seminars in Psychiatry*, 3 (1), 26–35.

Dufault, K., and Martocchio, B. (1985). Hope: Its spheres and dimensions. *Nursing Clinics of North America*, 20, 379–391.

Eye Bank Association of America (1988). *Eye bank statistics*. Washington, DC.

Fulton, J., Fulton, R., and Simmons, R. (1980). *The gift of life*. Spring Lake, MI: Books of Value.

Gideon, M. (1981). Kidney donation: Care of the cadaver donor's family. *Journal of Neurosurgical Nursing*, 13 (5), 238–251.

Goldsmith, J., and Montefusco, C. (1985). Nursing care of the potential organ donor. *Critical Care Nurse*, 5 (6), 22–29.

Kolata, G. (1983). Organ shortage clouds new transplant era: Organs are used from only one in ten potential donors; some say legislation is needed to make more organs available. *Science*, 221, 32–33.

LifeBanc (1987). *Organ and tissue donor eligibility criteria* (unpublished). Cleveland, OH.

Morton, J., and Leonard, D. (1979). Cadaver nephrectomy: An operation on the donor's family. *British Medical Journal*, 1, 239–241.

President's Commission for the Study of Ethical Problems in Medicine and Biomedical and Behavioral Research (1981). *Defining death: Medical, legal, and ethical issues in the determination of death*. Washington, DC: U.S. Government Printing Office.

Sophie, L. R., Salloway, J. C., Sorock, G., et al. (1983). Intensive care nurses' perceptions of cadaver organ procurement. *Heart & Lung*, 12 (3), 261–267.

United Network for Organ Sharing (UNOS) Update (1989). UNOS releases 1988 transplantation statistics (Vol. 5), p. 1. United Network For Sharing, Richmond, VA.

Youngner, S., Allen, M., Bartlett, T., et al. (1985). Psychosocial and ethical implications of organ retrieval. *New England Journal of Medicine*, 313 (5), 321–324.

53

Immunocompromised Patients

Jan L. Hawthorne

In recent years the treatment of cancer has become progressively more aggressive with the use of immunotherapies and high-dose chemotherapy. Although the success of these treatments is encouraging, the intensity of treatment has created new challenges for nurses caring for these patients. The nurse must be knowledgeable about these therapies to be able to provide the intensive support needed by patients and their families.

Immunotherapy, chemotherapy, and the resultant granulocytopenia can combine with the systemic effects of cancer to compromise the immune system of the patient. The immunocompromised patient has an increased risk of life-threatening infection (Oniboni, 1985; Reheis, 1985; Ristuccia, 1985). It is vital that the immunocompromised patient be protected from sources of infection, and in this area nurses play a significant role.

Leukocytes (white blood cells [WBCs]) act primarily to protect the host from invading foreign bodies. WBCs may be classified as nongranular (or mononuclears) and granular. Nongranular leukocytes include lymphocytes and monocytes. Granulocytes may be subclassified, based on their staining properties, as neutrophils, basophils, or eosinophils. Granulocytes are primarily responsible for combating infection. The total WBC count is usually 4.7 to 11.4 thousand cells/mm³. Of this total, 27% to 39% (1700 to 3400) are usually nongranulocytes and 61% to 73% (3000 to 7000) are usually granulocytes (Corbett, 1987). If the granulocyte count is below 3000 cells/mm³ the condition is termed granulocytopenia. Because granulocytes are primarily responsible for combating infection, granulocytopenia significantly increases the patient's risk of acquiring an infection. When neutropenia (less than 1000 cells/mm³) occurs, patients should be hospitalized. Neutropenic patients are placed in a protective environment to prevent infection while neutrophil counts return to normal (Smith, 1986a).

Granulocytopenia and neutropenia can be either the direct result of chemotherapy or immunotherapy or the systemic effect of cancer (Table 53–1). Cancer may develop from or metastasize to the bone marrow. Because the hematopoietic tissues of the marrow are responsible for the production of blood cells, bone marrow cancer will directly affect the production of WBCs. The altered nutrition and metabolism of cancer patients also have a direct effect on the production of these cells. Chemotherapeutic and immunotherapeutic agents attack rapidly dividing cells, including granulocytes. Therefore, the therapy itself frequently depresses granulocyte counts. Whatever the actual cause, the result of granulocytopenia is an exaggerated risk of infection.

NURSING ASSESSMENT

Granulocytopenia is associated with more frequent and severe infections and increased difficulty in diagnosing the infection (Becker, 1981; Oniboni, 1987; Reheis, 1985; Ristuccia, 1985). In patients with a decreased inflammatory response, infections may develop and spread rapidly. The nurse must be alert for subtle signs of infection (e.g., exudate, edema, erythema, tenderness, localized warmth, fever, regional adenopathy) because these signs will be attenuated due to the inadequate numbers of granulocytes. In patients with granulocytopenia the only signs of infection may be fever, erythema, and pain (Becker, 1981; Oniboni, 1985; Reheis, 1985).

Fever is the most important indicator of infection in the granulocytopenic patient (McCarron, 1986;

TABLE 53-1. Causes of Neutropenia

Bacterial—typhoid paratyphoid
Viral—influenza, measles, infectious hepatitis, infectious mononucleosis, chickenpox, rubella, yellow fever
Rickettsia—rickettsial pox, typhus, Rocky Mountain spotted fever
Protzoal—malaria, kala-azar

Overwhelming Infections (Especially in Debilitated Patients Such as Alcoholics or Malnourished Individuals)
Miliary tuberculosis
Pneumococcal pneumonia
Gram-negative bacteremia

Physical Agents—Chemicals and Drugs
Chemical and physical agents that always produce marrow hypoplasia and aplasia if given in sufficient dose
    Ionizing radiation
    Benzene
    Alkylating agents (nitrogen mustards, busulfan, chlorambucil, cyclophosphamide)
    Urethane
    Antimetabolites (methotrexate, 6-mercaptopurine, 5-fluorocytosine)
    Periwinkle alkaloids (vinblastine, vincristine)
    Antibiotics (daunomycin, Adriamycin)
Chemicals and drugs that occasionally cause neutropenia
    Analgesics (aminopyrine, salicylates)
    Anticonvulsants (Dilantin)
    Antithyroid drugs (propylthiouracil, methimazole)
    Anti-inflammatory drugs (phenylbutazone)
    Antimicrobial agents (Chloramphenicol, penicillins, sulfonamides)
    Tranquilizers (meprobamate)
    Phenothiazine (chlorpromazine, promazine)
    Cardiac antiarrhythmic drugs (lidocaine, quinidine, procainamide, phenytoin)

Hematologic and Other Conditions
Those due to decreased or ineffective production
    Anemias (pernicious, aplastic, chronic hyperchromic)
    Leukemia
Those due to increased utilization, destruction, or sequestration
    Cirrhosis of the liver with splenomegaly
    Lupus erythematosus
    Felty's syndrome
    Gaucher's disease
    Hemodialysis

Cachexia and Debilitated States
Alcoholism (folate deficiency)
Vitamin B_{12} deficiency
Copper deficiency

Anaphylactoid Shock and in Early Stages of Reaction to Foreign Protein

Hereditary, Congenital, or Familial and Miscellaneous Disorders
Cyclic neutropenia
Chronic idiopathic neutropenia
Infantile genetic agranulocytosis
Primary splenic neutropenia

Wintrobe, M.M., et al. (1981). *Clinical hematology* (8th ed.). Philadelphia: Lea & Febiger.

Oniboni, 1985). In these patients vital signs should be monitored at least every 4 hours (Becker, 1981). Temperatures above 38° C should be reported to the physician and assessments begun to attempt to identify the source of infection (Reheis, 1985).

The most frequent source of infection is through breaks in the skin (Oniboni, 1985; Reheis, 1985; Smith, 1986a), especially those made by venipuncture and intravenous catheters (Becker, 1981; Reheis, 1985). These sites should be inspected daily for indications of infection; if noted, the physician should be notified (Becker, 1981). Povidone iodine ointment should be applied to the site but not until all necessary cultures are obtained. To decrease the potential for infection, meticulous care should be taken with the routine changing of peripheral intra-venous catheters every 48 hours and intravenous tubing every 24 hours (Becker, 1981).

In addition to the obvious invasive sources that interrupt skin integrity, the entire body, including the oral mucosa, should be frequently inspected. Pressure necrosis is a frequent source of infection in immunocompromised patients. Side effects of chemotherapy combined with poor nutrition due to accompanying anorexia leave these patients at risk for breakdown of the oral mucosa. Frequent diarrheal stools, another side effect of chemotherapy, increase the patient's risk of perianal abscess, anal fissures, and excoriation. These areas should be assessed at least daily and more frequently as indicated by the individual's clinical condition (Reheis, 1985). Thorough abdominal assessments should be performed, including a search for distention, listening for bowel sounds in each quadrant, and feeling for abdominal wall firmness. Instruct the patient to report promptly abdominal pain, tenderness, feelings of fullness, nausea, and vomiting.

The respiratory tract is also at risk for infection in patients with granulocytopenia. Complaints of chest pain, discomfort, dyspnea, or shortness of breath require close follow-up. Breath sounds should be auscultated at least every 8 hours. It is possible for a chest radiograph to demonstrate pulmonary infiltrates without clinical findings of decreased or absent breath sounds, rales, or consolidation. In addition to noting patient complaints and performing chest assessment, the nurse should monitor the patient for changes in the amount and quality of sputum, the rate and rhythm of respirations, and fever.

Because of the granulocytopenic patient's increased risk of life-threatening infection, it is vital that the nurse monitor these patients vigilantly and rapidly report untoward findings.

MEDICAL TREATMENT

In the granulocytopenic patient a medical work-up is begun when infection is first suspected in an attempt to identify the source of infection rapidly (Fig. 53–1). This work-up should include cultures of the nasopharynx, urine, blood, sputum, perianal area, and any draining wounds (Oniboni, 1985; Reheis, 1985). The urine should also be examined for bacterial sediment. Chest radiographs should be taken to identify pulmonary infiltrates, pneumonia, and atelectasis.

After cultures are taken, broad-spectrum antibiotic therapy is promptly initiated in granulocytopenic patients to prevent rapid and life-threatening spread of infection (Oniboni, 1985; Reheis, 1985). Untreated infection in these patients has a 48-hour mortality rate of 18% to 40% (Reheis, 1985). Infection-related morbidity increases proportionately with delayed antibiotic therapy.

Granulocyte transfusions have been suggested for

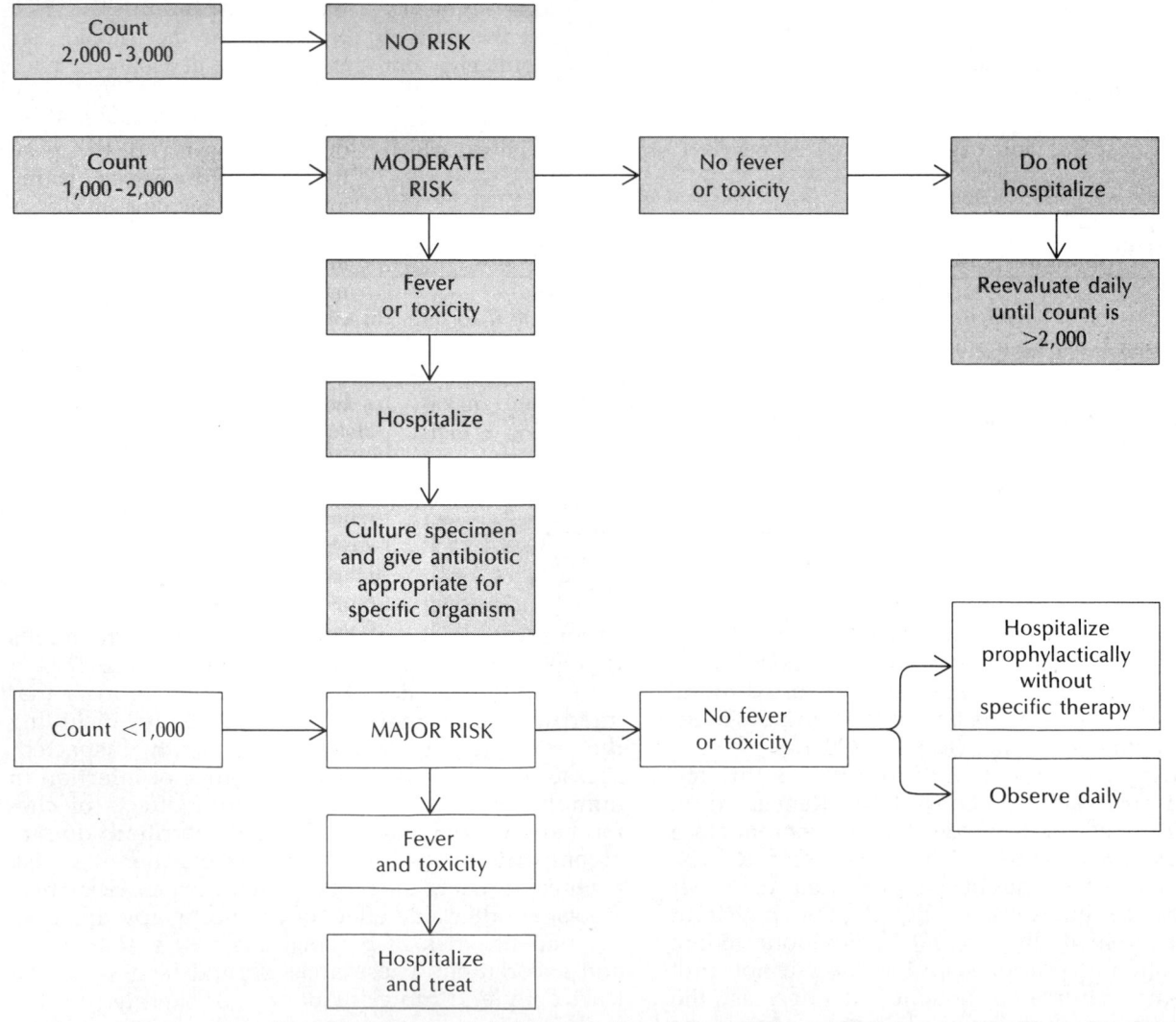

FIGURE 53–1. Managing chemotherapy-induced leukopenia (granulocytopenia): a selective approach. (Reproduced with permission from Lokich, J. J. (1976). Managing chemotherapy-induced bone marrow suppression in cancer. *Hospital Practice,* 11 (8), 61–67.)

patients with infections that do not respond to antibiotic therapy (Oniboni, 1985; Reheis, 1985). However, the expense and risks of these transfusions may outweigh the benefits. Risks of granulocyte transfusion include viral infection, acute hypersensitivity reaction, and sensitization to human leukocyte antigens (HLA) (Oniboni, 1985; Reheis, 1985). One research study has shown that use of granulocyte transfusions was no more effective than appropriate antibiotic therapy (Winston et al., 1982).

NURSING DIAGNOSIS AND MANAGEMENT

The following nursing diagnoses along with the expected outcomes and proposed interventions are those that are most frequently used with the immunocompromised patient.

Potential for Infection

Infection may arise because of the immunocompromised status.

Expected Outcomes. No signs or symptoms of infection will be noted, or, if identified, they will receive rapid intervention and not become life-threatening. Patient will verbalize understanding of indicators and symptoms that should be reported to caregivers.

Nursing Interventions. As already noted, a priority in granulocytopenic patients is monitoring for infection. Vital signs should be routinely monitored every 4 hours, and elevated temperature, the cardinal indicator of infection, should be reported immediately. Decreased blood pressure may precede bacterial sepsis, and tachypnea may indicate pneumonia or atelectasis.

The patient should be encouraged to perform oral hygiene every 4 hours. Supplemental oral hygiene with normal saline or bicarbonate solution and sponge sticks should be initiated in patients with oral lesions. Half-strength hydrogen peroxide solution aids in débriding significant oral lesions.

Similar ulcerations can occur throughout the gastrointestinal tract, and these may be monitored by performing Hematests on stools. Patients with diarrhea may be afforded some protection of the perianal area through the application of petroleum jelly or A + D ointment to irritated skin.

Soap with hexachlorophene should be used in the axillary and perineal areas to decrease colonization of these areas. However, excessive use of such soaps may result in dry skin, which is prone to cracking, thus allowing bacterial invasion. Bath oil should be used to bathe the rest of the body when bed baths are necessary.

Careful handwashing is important in any intensive care situation, but it is absolutely mandatory with these patients. Effective handwashing alone has proved effective in reducing infectious episodes (Armstrong, 1984; Garner and Simmons, 1983). The need for careful handwashing by caregivers cannot be overemphasized with the immunocompromised patient.

Granulocytopenic patients should be placed in a protective environment. Inform the patient and family why this is necessary and what it entails. The degree and form of isolation varies from institution to institution. The protective environment can be as simple as a private room, meticulous handwashing, and the omission of plants and flowers from the patient's environment or as complex as the use of near-sterile environments with laminar flow rooms, high energy particulate area (HEPA) filtration, and use of a sterile diet (Crane et al., 1980; Daly, 1983; Foon and Gale, 1982; Nauta, 1979) (Figs. 53–2, 53–3, and 53–4). Although protective isolation protects these patients from infection, it may produce nega-

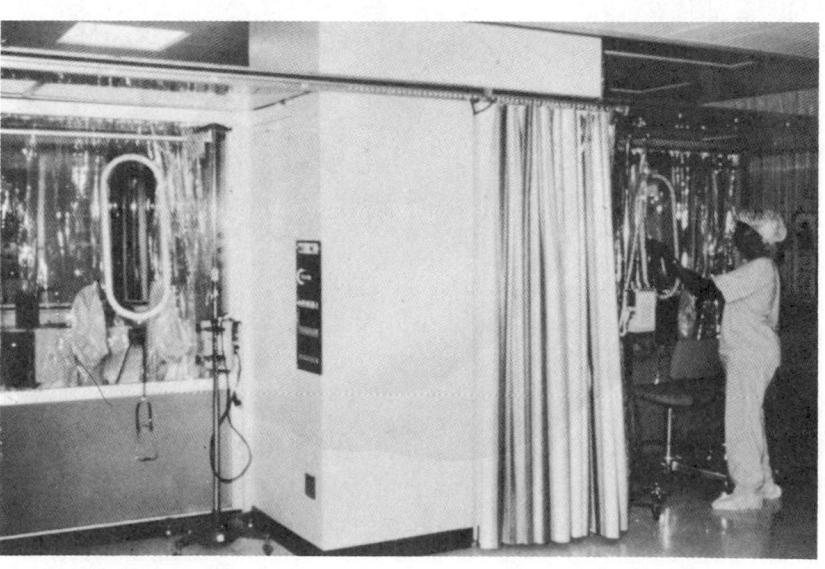

FIGURE 53–2. The Harper Hospital protective environment unit. (From Crane, L. R., Emmer, D. R., and Grguras, A. (1980). Prevention of infection on the oncology unit. *Nursing Clinics of North America*, 15 (4), 843–856.)

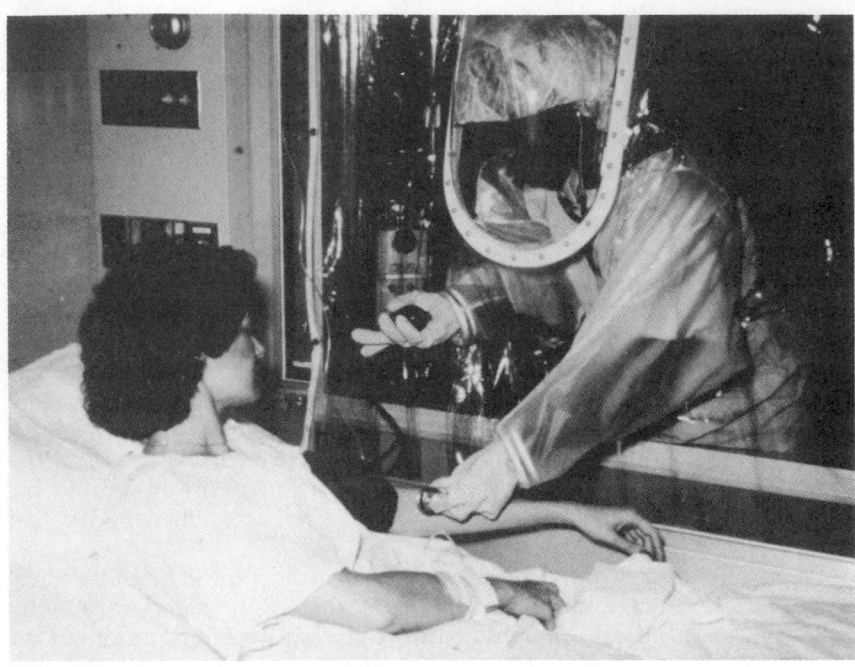

FIGURE 53–3. Clear, sliding plastic barriers allow the nurse to perform many necessary procedures without entering the laminar flow room. (From Crane, L. R., Emmer, D. R., and Grguras, A. (1980). Prevention of infection on the oncology unit. *Nursing Clinics of North America*, 15 (4), 843–856.)

tive psychological effects including depression, anxiety, and, in extreme cases, even psychosis.

Ineffective Individual Coping

Poor coping abilities may result from social and physical separation enforced by protective isolation measures.

Expected Outcomes. The patient appears to cope with physical and social isolation and does not demonstrate any impaired adjustment.

Nursing Interventions. The nurse, patient, and family should work together to identify problems related to isolation and alternative activities that the patient can use as distractions during the length of confinement. Sources of distraction include television, computer games, puzzles, music, and similar activities in which the patient has an interest. To decrease isolation, family and friends should be encouraged to spread visits throughout the day. In-person visits should be interspersed with telephone calls from family and friends. Hospital volunteers, social workers, housekeeping staff, and clergy should be encouraged to visit outside the confines of the

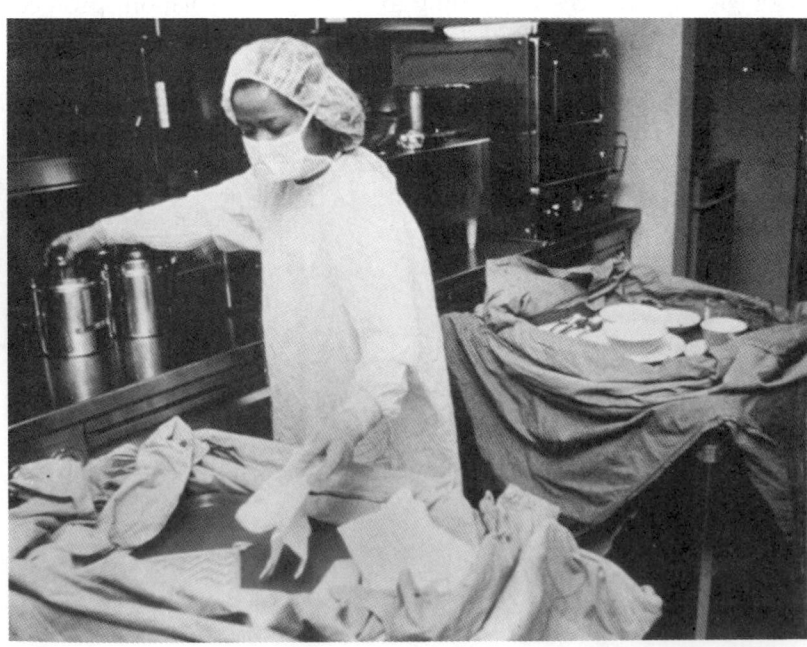

FIGURE 53–4. Bacteria, particularly *Pseudomonas aeruginosa*, can be transmitted by hospital food. (From Crane, L. R., Emmer, D. R., and Grguras, A. (1980). Prevention of infection on the oncology unit. *Nursing Clinics of North America*, 15 (4), 843–856.)

isolation. When problems in adjustment occur, a psychiatric nurse clinician may be consulted. (See also Chapters 6 and 7.)

Alterations in Nutrition

The patient may be malnourished due to altered gustatory sense, nausea, vomiting, and excessive diarrhea resulting from chemotherapy.

Expected Outcomes. Patient maintains adequate nutrition as demonstrated through maintenance of body weight and total protein and serum albumin levels within normal limits. The patient and family verbalize their understanding of food sources appropriate to the needs of the patient. The patient takes in adequate amounts of calories through meals and between-meal snacks.

Nursing Interventions. The nurse, patient, and family should identify nutritious foods that the patient enjoys, and these should be provided to the patient whenever possible. Encouraging smaller and more frequent meals (six per day) may avoid bloating, nausea, and diarrhea, which can cause the patient to become discouraged. The availability of a continuous supply of high-protein snacks ensures that the patient always has something to eat when he wants it. Warm foods and fluids should be served warm and cold foods and fluids cold, or at the temperature preferred by the patient. Instruct the patient and family about the need for high-protein foods that allow adequate tissue repair following chemotherapy. Instruct the family about sources of high-protein foods including meats, poultry, fish, eggs, milk, cheese, yogurt, legumes, and nuts.

Monitor the patient's dietary intake closely. Perform daily weights and monitor appropriate laboratory values. Initiate a dietary consultation and calorie counts in patients at risk.

Impaired Skin Integrity

Skin integrity may be impaired due to side effects of chemotherapy, intravenous therapy, and other invasive procedures.

Expected Outcomes. Skin integrity will be maintained. Areas where skin breakdown occurs will be promptly reported and therapy initiated immediately.

Nursing Interventions. Strict surgical asepsis should be used for care of intravenous catheters. Scheduled dressing and luminal cap changes should be maintained. Routine care of invasive catheters should be maintained without fail.

The patient and family should be instructed about

the need for frequent positional changes, at least every 2 hours. Areas prone to pressure should be inspected and massaged and lotion applied every 2 hours. A turning schedule should be established and posted at the bedside to ensure uniformity in turning by all caregivers. Skin should be kept free of excessive moisture but not allowed to become dry and scaly; bath oil is preferred to soap for bed baths. Avoid direct contact of the patient's skin with plastic incontinent pads because these may trap moisture and heat, macerating the skin.

Adjunctive devices cannot replace basic nursing measures to prevent pressure necrosis, but they can help. Air mattresses, heel protectors, elbow pads, sheep skins, and similar devices should be considered for immobile patients.

BONE MARROW TRANSPLANTATION

Bone marrow transplantation is a specialized treatment for certain neoplastic and hematologic diseases that places the patient at particular risk through its disruption of the entire immune system. Transplantation is an aggressive treatment with inherent risks, but the incidence of risks has decreased with refinements in techniques. As a mode of therapy, its increased use makes it highly likely that a nurse may be involved in referring a patient for bone marrow transplantation or caring for a patient who has had a bone marrow transplant.

Types of Bone Marrow Transplantation

Autologous transplantation involves the patient's own tissues (Fig. 53–5). The patient's bone marrow is harvested and frozen and then can be reconstituted for later use. This form of transplantation is used for patients who have had a relapse or have a high potential for relapse on standard therapy. When relapse occurs, patients may receive potentially lethal high-dose chemotherapy alone or in combination with total body irradiation in an attempt to halt the progression of the disease. An autologous transplant rescues patients imperiled by high doses of chemotherapy (Stewart and Thomas, 1985).

Allogeneic bone marrow transplantation involves bone marrow harvested from human leukocyte antigen (HLA)-compatible or HLA-identical donors. The patient's sibling is frequently used as a donor. This type of transplantation has been most successful in patients with acute or chronic leukemia.

Syngeneic bone marrow transplantation uses bone marrow from a genetically identical twin donor. It reduces the potential for tumor contamination, which can occur with autologous transplantation, or for incompatibility, which can occur with allogeneic transplantation (Table 53–2).

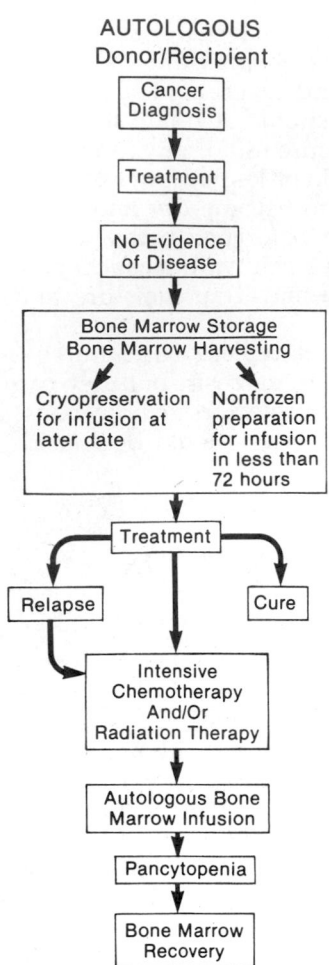

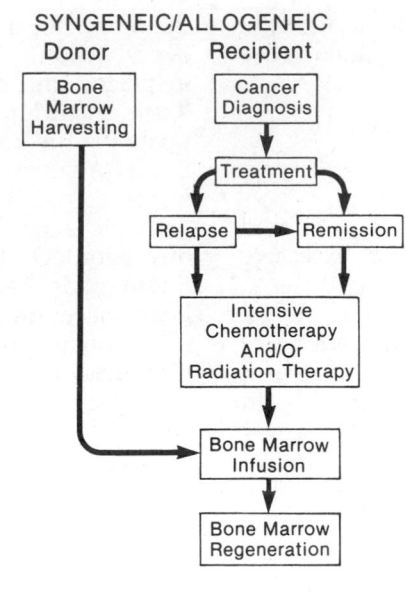

FIGURE 53–5. A comparison of autologous, syngeneic, and allogeneic treatment regimens. (From Cogliano-Shutta, N. A. and Broda, E. J. (1985). Bone marrow transplantation: An overview and comparison of autologous, syngeneic, and allogeneic treatment modalities. *Nursing Clinics of North America*, 20 (1), 49–66.)

Bone Marrow Harvesting

Patients who undergo bone marrow transplantation require intense medical and nursing care. An interdisciplinary, collaborative effort is necessary to be able to meet the multiple needs of these patients and provide high quality care.

A bone marrow transplant begins with the harvesting of bone marrow from a donor to obtain viable stem cells. Stem cells are immature hematopoietic cells that differentiate as they mature to form erythrocytes, granulocytes, lymphocytes, and platelets. Bone marrow harvesting is a relatively short procedure (30 to 45 minutes) done under general anesthesia in an operating room. The marrow is obtained by multiple aspirations from the posterior iliac crest. The goal is to extract 10 mL of marrow/kg body weight (i.e., an 80-kg man would donate approximately 800 mL of marrow) (Cogliano-Shutta and Broda, 1985; McGlave, 1985; Stewart and Thomas, 1985). The number of stem cells obtained is more important than the amount of marrow. The number of nucleated marrow cells required for consistent hematopoietic reconstitution is 0.5×10^8 cells/kg.

Processing bone marrow begins in the operating room, where the marrow is immediately mixed with preservative-free heparin in culture media. The marrow is then filtered to remove large particles. Allogeneic and syngeneic transplants are infused within 3 hours. Autologous transplants are treated with a cryoprotective agent, dimethylsulfoxide (DMSO), to prevent lysis of stem cells and stored in liquid nitrogen at $-40°$ to $-50°$ C. When needed, the autologous transplant marrow is reconstituted in sterile isotonic normal saline and warmed to body temperature before being infused intravenously.

After harvesting, pressure dressings are applied to aspiration sites. The donor returns to his or her room following recovery in the postanesthesia recovery room. Hematocrit and hemoglobin levels are monitored carefully for the first 24 hours to assess the need for blood replacement. Dressings are closely monitored for bleeding. This procedure is painful and requires careful management of postoperative pain with narcotic analgesics.

Recipients of marrow transplants require intensive supportive therapy including antibiotic therapy, parenteral nutrition, multiple blood products, and hydration. Because of the long-term intravenous therapy required for these patients, an indwelling central venous line is usually placed, most commonly a Hickman or Broviac catheter. The catheter is placed

TABLE 53–2. Comparison and Contrast of Side Effects and Nursing Interventions in Autologous, Syngeneic, and Allogeneic Transplantation

Transplantation Procedure	Complication	Pathophysiology	Time of Presentation	Signs and Symptoms	Nursing Intervention	Comments
Autologous, syngeneic, autologous	Discolored urine (red)	Excretion of phenol used in culture media	Time of infusion to 24 hr post-infusion	First void discolored	Note color changes, alleviate possible anxiety	Urine will gradually clear. Seen primarily with autologous
	Fever	Infusion of pyrogens and TBI	Evening of the bone marrow infusion	Elevated temperature	Frequent vital signs, acetaminophen	
	Veno-occlusive disease	Hepatic central vein fibrosis	One to three weeks post-transplant	Hepatomegaly, ascites	Abdominal girth measurements, fluid management	About half of cases are progressive
	Acute graft-versus-host disease	Donor T cells react to host	5 to 70 days	Skin: Erythema, maculopapular eruption, bullae, desquamation	Mild rash: Lubricate skin with oil-based lotions, such as Alpha Keri; antihistamine and steroid creams may be helpful. Frank desquamation: Use sterile technique, sterile sheets, débride skin twice daily; cover major areas with normal saline/ Betadine- impregnated gauze, and antimicrobial creams	Note: Rash in syngeneic BMT must have GVHD ruled out. Also note temporal change in medications
				Liver: Elevations of liver enzymes, bilirubin	Observe for jaundice, bleeding; check liver enzymes, coagulation	
				GI: Diarrhea to greater than 2 L/day	Meticulous intake and output; weights twice daily; good rectal care including sitz baths	
Autologous, syngeneic, autologous	Chronic graft-versus-host disease	Primary immunologic	Greater than 100 days post-transplant	Increased skin pigmentation/ thickening, contractures, conjunctivitis, photosensitivity	Physical therapy, sunscreens, Alpha Keri lotion, sunglasses	
	Infections: Bacterial, fungal, viral	Loss of immune function	Primarily during aplasia or GVHD	Fever, chills, malaise, rise in pulse, fall in blood pressure	Prevention: Assure compliance with oral prophylactic antibiotics, maintain protective isolation. With possible infection: Monitor vital signs carefully, fever/sepsis evaluation, anticipate use of broad-spectrum antibiotics with blood level determinations of drug; remember perirectal area as possible site of infection in these patients. Meticulous catheter care is of prime importance	
	Common preparative regimen toxicities					Note: Increased severity of toxicities is secondary to higher doses
	Cystitis	Cytoxan metabolites in bladder TBI	Shortly after administration; may be delayed	Hematuria, pain	Hydration before, during, and after drug administration; forced voiding every 2 hr for 24 hr after drug is given; careful intake and output	Drug may cause fluid retention so intake and output is critical

Table continued on following page

TABLE 53–2. *Comparison and Contrast of Side Effects and Nursing Interventions in Autologous, Syngeneic, and Allogeneic Transplantation* Continued

Transplantation Procedure	Complication	Pathophysiology	Time of Presentation	Signs and Symptoms	Nursing Intervention	Comments
Autologous	Garlic smell, unpleasant taste	Excretion of DMSO by lungs	Time of infusion to 36 hr post-infusion	Decreased appetite, garlic odor	Give patient hard candy, room deodorizer, peppermint oil	
	Transient hemoglobinuria	Release of hemoglobin during lysis after thawing	Within 48 hr after infusion	Positive Hemastix	Hematest all urine, monitor results for 48 hr	
	Potential for infusion of tumor cell	Related to the harvest of unsuspected tumor cell and subsequent infusion after ablative therapy	After transplant	Tumor recurrence	Plan therapy as feasible	
Primarily allogeneic	Interstitial pneumonitis	Multifactorial including virus (CMV) and pneumocystis	Most commonly in the first 4 months, especially at end of second month	Fall in FVC, fall in P_{O_2} dyspnea	Monitor for compromise of pulmonary function by daily FVC, careful fluid balance in patients with interstitial pneumonitis	Thirty to forty per cent of patients develop interstitial pneumonitis; half have no demonstrated etiologic agent; mortality is high
	Graft rejection	Not well understood	Either no engraftment or transient engraftment	No rise in blood counts or rise followed by fall	Continued protection as severely immuno-compromised patient; continued colonization surveys and observation for infection; minimize invasive procedures; bleeding precautions; continued irradiated blood product support	
Primarily allogeneic	Chronic graft-versus-host disease	Primarily immunologic	Greater than 100 days post-transplant	Liver: Jaundice coagulopathy	Enzyme replacement; early recognition	
				Gut: Malabsorption, chronic diarrhea	Diet manipulation; antidiarrheal medications	
				Musculoskeletal: Arthritis	Encourage increased ROM; physiotherapy	
				Pulmonary insufficiency; SOB, DOE, cough	Encourage increased activity to preserve function	
				Immunopathy: Opportunistic infection	Teach importance of good hygiene and environment protection; observe for signs of any infectious disease—systemic, superficial or fungal	
Syngeneic	Skin rash	Etiology unclear, question mild GVHD	One week	Variable in character and distribution, maculopapular, erythematous pruritic	Lubricate skin with oil-based lotion; may require antihistamines and steroid creams	
Autologous, syngeneic, autologous	Anxiety, depression	Isolation, concerns of complications	Any time during and after transplant	Emotional reactions	Encourage verbalization, reinforce reasonable expectations, activity, family involvement	
	Respiratory distress	Transient pulmonary hypertension secondary to infusion of cell particles from cell lysis, volume overload	During bone marrow infusion	Tachycardia, hypertension, anxiety, cyanosis	Monitor vital signs, oxygen, and drugs as ordered; monitor intake and output weights	

TABLE 53–2. Comparison and Contrast of Side Effects and Nursing Interventions in Autologous, Syngeneic, and Allogeneic Transplantation Continued

Transplantation Procedure	Complication	Pathophysiology	Time of Presentation	Signs and Symptoms	Nursing Intervention	Comments
Autologous, syngeneic, autologous	Cardiomyopathy	Associated with high dose Cytoxam	Shortly after administration	Decreased ECG voltage; decreased cardiac function by any of several laboratory tests; signs/symptoms of congestive heart failure	Baseline ECG with follow-up tracings; observation for clinical evidence of congestive heart failure	
	Mucositis	Multifactorial: Radiation, virus, drug	5 days onward	Intiially small oral lesions progressing to full oral cavity, peri-oral involvement	Meticulous oral care with frequent normal saline rinses; antimicrobial rinses may be of use if lesions progress	Emphasis is on prevention; new antiviral drugs are of significant help
	Marrow depression	Direct toxicity of preparative regimen	5 to 7 days after therapy	Depression in all counts of all three cell lines	See failure to engraft	
	"Capillary leak"	Probably direct toxicity of preparative regimen	3 to 5 days	Decreased FVC, decreased P_{O2}	Weigh twice daily, careful intake and output	

Abbreviations: TBI, total body irradiation; GVHD, graft versus host disease; BMT, bone marrow transplantation; CMV, cytomegalovirus; FVC, forced vital capacity; ROM, range of motion; DOE, dyspnea on exertion; SOB, shortness of breath; ECG, electrocardiography.

From Cogliano-Shutta, N. A., and Broda, E. J. (1985). Bone marrow transplantation: An overview and comparison of autologous, syngeneic, and allogeneic treatment modalities. *Nursing Clinics of North America*, 20 (1), 49–66.

when the patient is in the operating room in the external cephalic or internal jugular vein. Placement is done under local or general anesthesia. Fluoroscopy is used to ensure proper positioning of the proximal tip of the catheter. Two small incisions are needed, one to secure the access port of the catheter to the thoracic wall and one to enter the chosen vein (DeVita, 1985). Each device has a Dacron cuff that allows ingrowth of fibroelastic tissue, anchoring the device to the thorax and decreasing potential migration of bacteria along the outer surface of the device. During recovery, the nurse must carefully monitor the patient for hemorrhage (external bleeding or hematoma) from the site of vascular entry.

Autologous Transplantation

To be considered for autologous transplantation, the patient must meet the following criteria (Cogliano-Shutta and Broda, 1985):

1. Bone marrow must be free of detectable tumor.
2. The patient must be able to tolerate anesthesia and bone harvesting.
3. The patient's disease is expected to respond to increased chemotherapy using agents with myelosuppression as the main dose-limiting toxic factor.
4. The patient must be able to tolerate prolonged myelosuppression resulting in a WBC count of less than 1000 cells/mm^3 and a granulocyte count of less than 500 cells/mm^3 for 2 to 3 weeks.

The bone marrow transplant patient may be asked to choose between low-dose therapy with fewer life-threatening side effects and a low chance of cure,

and higher dose therapy plus bone marrow transplant with more life-threatening complications but a higher rate of cure. Reports in the literature suggest that high-dose chemotherapy and autologous bone marrow transplantation prolong survival in patients with some malignant conditions (Cogliano-Shutta and Broda, 1985). Patients with relapsed solid tumors that are resistant to conventional therapy who received high-dose chemotherapy and bone marrow transplantation had a 30% complete response rate with 16% in remission for at least 15 months following therapy (Deisseroth et al., 1982). Patients with acute leukemia who were treated with autologous bone transplants harvested during remission had response rates equal to those seen in patients who received syngeneic transplants. Autologous transplants were also effective for long-term survival of patients with non-Hodgkin's lymphoma. However, tumor cell contamination may result in recurrence, the rate of recurrence varying with the malignant condition (Cogliano-Shutta and Broda, 1985). The effectiveness of the transplant procedure is predicated on the ability of the preceding chemotherapy to eradicate malignant cells.

POST-TRANSPLANTATION/ENGRAFTMENT PERIOD

The induction phase (i.e., the period before transplantation) varies with the underlying disease and the treatment protocol. Patients typically receive high-dose chemotherapy alone or with radiation therapy. After the treatment regimen is complete, the bone marrow is transfused intravenously, allowing the stem cells to repopulate the recipient's depleted marrow. Following transplantation it takes several weeks for the transplanted marrow to engraft (i.e., to replace the patient's existing marrow as it is slowly destroyed). During this period the patient's blood cell counts drop precipitously, leaving the patient profoundly granulocytopenic.

Many complications may arise and require prompt nursing intervention. Platelet transfusions are required when the platelet count falls below 20,000 cells/mm^3. If the hematocrit falls below 30% and hemoglobin levels below 10 g/100 mL, the patient may require transfusion of packed red cells. Blood products for these patients are usually irradiated to inactivate immunologically competent cells and avoid possible graft-versus-host reactions.

The bone marrow begins to regenerate about 14 days following transplantation. For recipients of autologous transplants it may take up to 4 weeks for the granulocytes to recover to 500 cells/mm^3. It may take up to 6 weeks for platelets to reach 50,000 cells/mm^3. Autologous bone marrow recovery rates are slower than those with allogeneic and syngeneic transplants because of the myelosuppressive therapy needed prior to harvesting and the effect of freezing and storage on the bone marrow.

NURSING DIAGNOSIS AND MANAGEMENT

Gustatory Sensory Alterations. These changes are due to side effects from the preservative DMSO used to freeze the bone marrow for autologous transplantation.

Expected Outcomes. Patient states that he can tolerate the altered sensation and does not develop nausea or vomiting.

Side Effects. Side effects of autologous transplantation include a garlic breath odor and an unpleasant taste that results from the excretion of DMSO by the lungs. The patient should be informed of this side effect before the transplantation procedure to reduce anxiety when it occurs. Patients with sensitivity to taste may become nauseated and vomit. These side effects last up to 36 hours and may be diminished by sucking on hard candy or drinking sweet beverages. Some patients may require antiemetics to control nausea and vomiting.

Altered Patterns in Urinary Elimination. Urination is altered due to the presence of phenol dye in the transplant culture media and to lysis of erythrocytes during reconstitution.

Expected Outcomes. Patient verbalizes understanding of the reason why urine becomes red after autologous transplantation.

Nursing Interventions. Following autologous transplantation, the patient's urine usually becomes dark red, gradually lightening to an amber color within 24 hours. The patient should be informed about this change prior to the transplant to reduce anxiety. Clearing of this discoloration is facilitated by forcing

fluids. The patient should be instructed about the need for increased fluid intake and his or her fluid preferences determined. The patient's intake and output should be closely monitored to ensure adequate output. Patients should be informed about the need to monitor urinary output.

Potential for Altered Body Temperature. Temperature is increased due to pyrogens released from white blood cells injured during reconstitution.

Expected Outcomes. Patient verbalizes understanding of expected temperature elevations; elevations above 38° C will be rapidly identified and reported.

Nursing Interventions. Patients and families should be informed about the potential for post-transplant fever and told to inform caregivers if the patient feels warm. Vital signs should be monitored every 4 hours for the first day after transplantation. Temperatures exceeding 38° C should be reported to the physician. Acetaminophen may be required as an antipyretic.

Fear. Fear may be due to the known potential for infusion of malignant cells with the transplanted bone marrow.

Expected Outcomes. Patients freely verbalize their concerns and do not demonstrate uncontrolled fear.

Nursing Interventions. The patient and family should be allowed and encouraged to verbalize their concerns about recurrence of malignancy. The nurse can remind the family that precautions are taken at the time of the harvest to avoid malignancy (e.g., by means of chemotherapy and/or radiation therapy). Patients and family experiencing uncontrolled fear may require referral to psychiatric nurse clinicians for assistance. (See also Chapters 6 and 7.)

Allogeneic Transplantation

Allogeneic bone marrow transplantation is the treatment of choice for the first remission of acute myelogenous leukemia (AML) and for other hematologic malignancies that are refractory to standard therapy. Data from major transplant centers show the following survival rates with allogeneic transplantation for leukemia (Champlin and Gale, 1983; Stewart and Thomas, 1985): acute myelogenous leukemia, 60%; acute lymphoblastic leukemia, 40%; chronic myelogenous leukemia, 65%; aplastic anemia, 60%.

Although rates varied with the stage of each disease, these results indicate a potential benefit in the use of allogeneic bone marrow transplantation. Variations may have been due to the nature of each disease process or the resistance of the individual patient to the induction therapy.

Human Leukocyte Antigen (HLA) Typing. Allogeneic bone marrow transplantation is preceded by HLA typing to determine the compatibility of the donor and recipient. A blood specimen is used to perform HLA typing. There is a one in four chance of a sibling being HLA-compatible with the recipient.

Genes encoding the HLA antigens are found on chromosome 6. One set of genes is inherited from each parent. Each set of HLA genes has components labeled A, B, C, DP, DQ, DR, MB, MT, and Te, each of which has numerous subcategories. HLA-A and HLA-B antigens are identified serologically. Because of the large number of combinations of the five major antigens and the subgroups, it is unlikely for a close HLA match to be found outside of the family.

Preparation of the Recipient. Induction therapy for an allogeneic bone marrow transplant usually includes high-dose chemotherapy and total body irradiation (TBI). The goal of these therapies is to eradicate malignant cells and suppress host immune function to prevent rejection of the allogeneic bone marrow.

High-dose intravenous cyclophosphamide (50 μmol/kg per day) for 2 days followed by a high dose of TBI (1000 rad) in divided doses or a single dose is an example of an induction therapy (Cogliano-Shutta and Broda, 1985; DeVita, 1985; McGlave, 1985; Stewart and Thomas, 1985). TBI has proved effective because of its immunosuppressive effects and its ability to penetrate tumor growth areas (CNS and testicles) that are inaccessible to chemotherapy.

Complications of Therapy. The first complications encountered are usually related to the induction therapy, e.g., immunosuppression and gastrointestinal side effects. There are also complications unique to allogeneic transplantation (see Table 53–2).

Graft-versus-host disease (GVHD) is unique to allogeneic bone marrow transplantation because of the potential for reaction of the donor's marrow to the recipient. Once infused, the immunologically competent donor T-cells may recognize the recipient's tissue as foreign (Cogliano-Shutta and Broda, 1985; McGlave, 1985; Stewart and Thomas, 1985). Organs most commonly affected by this reaction are the skin, liver, and gastrointestinal tract. Clinical findings include erythema and sloughing of skin, elevated liver transaminases, jaundice, diarrhea, and fluid and electrolyte imbalances. The severity of GVHD for any one of the target organ systems may be graded on a scale of one to four, with four being most severe.

Graft-versus-host disease has been divided into acute and chronic forms. Acute GVHD occurs within the first 100 days following transplantation (Cogliano-Shutta and Broda, 1985; McGlave, 1985). GVHD persisting after 100 days is labeled chronic GVHD. Chronic GVHD results in changes similar to those seen in collagen vascular diseases, including joint contractures, skin thickening, and dry eyes and mouth. Although not immediately life-threatening, chronic GVHD has a high long-term mortality rate if it remains untreated (Cogliano-Shutta and Broda, 1985).

Approximately 60% of all patients with allogeneic transplants develop some degree of GVHD. Of this group, 30% to 50% will succumb to complications of GVHD. Prevention of GVHD includes use of prophylactic methotrexate or cyclosporine following transplantation. Severe GVHD may be treated with high doses of steroids or antithymocyte globulin (Cogliano-Shutta and Broda, 1985; Doney and Weiden, 1981).

Long-Term Complications of Allogeneic Transplantation. Most long-term complications of allogeneic transplantation are the result of high-dose chemotherapy, TBI, or chronic GVHD or are related to the original disease (Table 53–3). As allogeneic transplantation becomes more successful in controlling disease outcomes, the care of these patients becomes more challenging for nurses.

Cataracts that occur following allogeneic transplantation are thought to result from TBI or long-term steroid therapy for GVHD (Corcoran-Buchsel, 1986). Fifty per cent of patients who receive single-dose TBI experience cataracts compared to 20% of those who receive in TBI in divided doses. Age has not been identified as a risk factor for the development of cataracts. The average length of time for cataract formation is 3 years following transplantation (range 1 to 5.5 years). Cataract formation is usually bilateral. The treatment of choice is intraocular lens replacement (Corcoran-Buchsel, 1986). The nurse should instruct the patient and family about the potential for this complication and encourage yearly eye examinations.

Because patients with allogeneic transplantation have an immature immune response, they are at risk for numerous opportunistic infections for the first year after transplantation. About half of these patients develop herpes zoster–varicella infections in the first year (Atkinson and Meyers, 1980). Patients with chronic GVHD or mismatched transplants are at greater risk for development of herpes zoster infections because of the profound immunosuppression that occurs following the transplant. Chronic GVHD patients remain at high risk for developing bacterial pneumonia, septicemia, and sinusitis because of their immature immune response (Witherspoon and Storb, 1981).

Most transplant recipients experience some degree of gonadal dysfunction because of the high-dose chemotherapy or TBI. The incidence of gonadal dysfunction and sterility is related to the patient's age at the time of transplantation and the total dose and length of chemotherapy (Ruccione and Fergusson, 1984). When high-dose chemotherapy is used alone, especially cyclophosphamide, patients of either sex who are prepubertal will have normal sexual development. However, the long-term prognosis for postpubertal patients is uncertain. Menses and luteiniz-

TABLE 53–3. Possible Late Effects of Bone Marrow Transplantation Caused by High-Dose Chemotherapy and/or Irradiation in Conditioning Regimens

Late Effect	Incidence Rate	Time Post-BMT	Signs and Symptoms	Nursing Management	Diagnostic Tools	Medical Treatment
Late infectious complications Bacterial, viral, fungal infections with or without chronic graft-versus-host disease (GVHD)	>50%	100–365 days	Fever, wheezing, rales, postnasal drip, signs of infection	Preventive teaching Mask-wearing until 6 months post-BMT Good hand-washing techniques Avoid infectious persons (measles, chickenpox, mumps) Avoid school/work until 6 months post-BMT Avoid hot tubs, public swimming pools until 6–9 months post-BMT Limit number of sexual partners Avoid live virus vaccines	Positive blood culture for bacteria, fungus, virus Abnormal chest x-ray studies, pulmonary function tests (PFT) Pulmonary infiltrates Open lung biopsy Changes in CBC	Appropriate antibiotic support
Varicella zoster virus without chronic GVHD with chronic GVHD	<50% >75%	100–365 days	Lesions, pain, malaise, tenderness, neurological manifestation	Relieve pruritus with calamine lotion Cool compresses Prevent secondary infection	Positive herpes zoster varicella (HZV) cultures	Strict isolation until lesions are crusting IV acyclovir, 10 mg/kg/dose, q8h × 7 days
Pulmonary complications Interstitial pneumonia Cytomegalovirus *Pneumocystis carinii*	70%	100–400 days	Fever, sepsis, hypotension, lethargy, cough	Anticipatory preventive teaching Routine vital signs Chest auscultation and percusion (A&P) Monitor PFT, arterial blood gases (ABG)	Chest x-ray studies, CBC, ABG, PFT Positive cultures for bacterial, fungal, and viral microorganisms Bronchoscopy IgA, IgG levels	
Restrictive disease	5%		May be asymptomatic or Cough	Anticipatory teaching of pulmonary toilet Routine vital signs Chest A&P	Total lung capacity, diffusion capacity	Respiratory therapy Bronchodilation
Obstructive disease	11%		Decreased ability to perform daily living activities due to pulmonary insufficiency	Monitor PFT and ABG		

From Corcoran-Buchsel, P. (1986). Long-term complications of allogeneic bone marrow transplantation: Nursing implications. *The Oncology Nursing Forum*, 13 (6), 61–70.

ing hormone (LH) and follicle-stimulating hormone (FSH) levels in postpubertal women may return to normal, but early menopause and elevations of both LH and FSH have been noted. Outcomes for postpubertal men include the possibility of a return to normal gonadotropin levels and low-to-normal sperm counts, or there may be elevated FSH levels and azoospermia.

The effects of TBI on reproductive function and sexual development are more predictable—that is, sterility usually occurs. Prepubertal girls experience primary ovarian failure, do not achieve menarche, and do not develop secondary sex characteristics (Sanders and Buckner, 1985). Some prepubertal boys develop secondary sex characteristics, but most will have delayed sexual maturity and permanent azo-

ospermia. Postpubertal women experience primary ovarian failure and early menopause, whereas men have primary gonadal failure and azoospermia (Sanders and Buckner, 1985).

The long-term psychological effects of bone marrow transplantation vary with the complications experienced. Patients with recurrent complications report situational depression and anxiety resulting from continued therapy and prolonged restricted activities following transplantation (Gardner and August, 1977). Some patients report residual psychological effects of the primary illness and fears of its recurrence and of dying, especially when chronic complications occur after transplantation. Patients who are able to resume normal activities and return to work have less anxiety about their quality of life and economic stability. Psychological adjustment following transplantation is very dependent upon the patient's health status.

DRUGS USED IN TRANSPLANTATION

Cyclosporine

Cyclosporine is an immunosuppressive agent that suppresses allograft rejection and hypersensitivity reactions. This agent selectively inhibits T-lymphocytes by interfering with the production of effector T-lymphocytes and lymphokines while impairing the cloning of helper T-cells (Smith, 1986b). Cyclosporine is more effective when used prophylactically than when treating an acute rejection. Therefore, cyclosporine is begun on the day before or the day of transplantation and is continued indefinitely (Klemm, 1985).

Routes of Administration

Oral. Cyclosporine is administered orally in an olive oil–based solution, diluted as one part cyclosporine to ten parts of diluent. Although many patients prefer to use chocolate milk, some dilute the drug with regular milk, orange juice, or Ensure. The mixture should be taken at room temperature and mixed in a glass container because cyclosporine will adhere to the walls of other containers. Once the dose has been taken, the container should be rinsed with additional diluent, and this should then be taken by the patient to ensure that the complete dose is ingested. Food interferes with the absorption of this drug, so it should be taken between meals, i.e., at least 1 hour before or 2 hours after food is ingested.

Intravenous. Cyclosporine is supplied in 2-mL ampules in a concentration of 50 mg/mL (41.5 μmol/mL). This amount is further diluted in 20 to 50 mL of 5% dextrose and water or normal saline and administered over 4 to 6 hours. Too rapid administration has been associated with complaints of burning palms and soles of the feet (Klemm, 1985).

Dosage. Dosages are based on body weight and range from 12.5 mg/kg per day (10 μmol/kg per day) to 25 mg/kg per day (20 μmol/kg per day) (Klemm, 1985). Because this agent has a narrow therapeutic range, peak and trough levels may be determined daily. Daily dosages are adjusted according to the results of these assessments.

Side Effects and Precautions. Table 53–4 summarizes the side effects of cyclosporine and the associated nursing interventions.

NURSING DIAGNOSES AND MANAGEMENT

Patients who have undergone bone marrow transplantation require nursing care, assessment, and management. Hospitalization of these patients is prolonged as they await a return to normal blood count levels. During hospitalization the patient must be carefully monitored for infection and complications of therapy. See the nursing care plan for the recommended nursing interventions for actual and potential complications of bone marrow transplantation.

TABLE 53–4. Nursing Actions for the Identification and Management of Cyclosporine Side Effects

Late Effect	Incidence Rate	Time Post-BMT	Signs and Symptoms	Nursing Management	Diagnostic Tools	Medical Treatment
Cataracts						
Total body irradiation, fractionated	20%	1.5–5 years	Poor vision	Anticipatory teaching of BMT risk factors	Examination with slit lamp microscopy	Intraocular lens replacement
Total body irradiation, single dose	50%	1.5–5 years		Ophthalmologist recommendation		
Neurologic complications						
Leukoencephalopathy	7%	1–5 months	Lethargy Somnolence Dementia Seizures Spastic quadriplegia Coma Personality changes	Early intervention Multidisciplinary approach with special education program Routine neurologic assessments	Periodic head computer-assisted tomography (CAT) and psychometric evaluation	Symptomatic and supportive management
Psychological complications	Unknown	Months to years	Depression, weight change Altered body image Survival syndrome Sibling rivalry	Allow patient/family to verbalize feelings Identify coping mechanisms, personal strengths Refer to mental health resources	Psychological testing	Mental health evaluation and treatment from appropriate source
Impaired growth in children						
Irradiation only	100%	Months to years	Subnormal growth and development	Anticipatory teaching to patients/parents Annual evaluation of growth pattern Serial height/weight	Adrenocortical function Growth hormone Thyroid hormone	Possible appropriate hormone replacement Long-term follow-up

From Klemm, P. (1985). Cyclosporin A: Use in preventing graft versus host disease. *The Oncology Nursing Forum*, 12 (5), 25–32.

Interleukin-2/Lymphokine-Activated Killer Cell Therapy (IL-2/LAK)

It is postulated that people with impaired immune response may develop cancer (Jassak and Sticklin, 1986). Interleukin-2 (IL-2) is believed to augment or modulate the immunologic mechanisms involved in the growth or metastasis of tumor cells. Thus, interleukin-2 is thought to enhance the immune system's ability to destroy cancer cells.

Interleukin-2 is a naturally occurring substance produced by helper T-cells in response to specific antigens. It mediates a wide variety of immunoregulatory phenomena (Jassak, 1986). Specific immune responses include enhanced production of T-lymphocytes, stimulated responses of B- and T-cells, augmented cell-killing activity of natural killer cells and cytotoxic T-cells, and increased production of lymphokine-activated killer (LAK) cells.

Administration of IL-2. The efficacy and toxicity of IL-2 are being studied in phase I clinical trials (see Table 53–5 for a summary). In these trials IL-2 is administered by a variety of routes including intravenous bolus, continuous infusions, subcutaneous injection, and peritoneal infusion. The optimal route of administration and dosage has not been established. The maximum tolerated dose has been 100,000 units/kg given three times a day for 5 days, or 100,000 units/kg per hour by continuous infusion (Jassak, 1986).

Preparation of Lymphokine-Activated Killer Cells. Patients receive boluses of IL-2 to stimulate LAK production. IL-2 is the only lymphokine that has been found to stimulate LAK production. In National Cancer Institute clinical trials patients receive IL-2 intravenously every 8 hours for 3 days (Abernathy, 1987). This results in a rebound effect of higher than normal levels of lymphocytes. These lymphocytes are then collected by leukapheresis. Leukopheresis is accomplished by removing the patient's blood through an intravenous catheter. This blood is circulated through a cell separator that removes the leukocytes. The remainder of the patient's blood is returned through another intravenous catheter.

Once the leukocytes have been removed, the lymphocytes are separated and incubated with IL-2 to enhance LAK cell production. These LAK cells are then infused intravenously with additional boluses of IL-2 to continue to activate the LAK cells.

NURSING DIAGNOSES AND MANAGEMENT

Altered Thought Processes. Mental changes result from CNS toxicity of IL-2/LAK therapy.

Expected Outcomes. Toxic reactions and altered thought processes will be rapidly identified and the patient's safety maintained.

TABLE 53–5. IL-2 Toxicities

Central nervous system
Confusion
Disorientation
Combativeness
Psychoses
Anxiety

Gastrointestinal
Nausea
Vomiting
Diarrhea
Mucositis
↓ Apppetite

Renal
Oliguria
↑ Creatinine
↑ BUN
Proteinuria

Pulmonary
Pulmonary edema
Dyspnea

Cardiovascular
Hypotension
Weight gain
Edema
Ascites
Dysrhythmias

Miscellaneous
Headache
Malaise
Chills, fever
Flu-like syndrome
Nasal congestion
Glossitis
Xerostomia

Integumentary
Erythematous rash
Pruritus
Skin desquamation

Hematologic
Anemia
Thrombocytopenia

Hepatic
↑ Bilirubin
↑ SGOT, ↑SPGT, ↑LDH

Abbreviations: BUN, blood urea nitrogen; SGOT, serum glutamic oxaloacetic transaminase; SGPT, serum glutamic pyruvic transaminase; LDH, lactic dehydrogenase.
From Jassak, P. F., and Sticklin, L. A. (1986). Interleukin-2: An overview. *The Oncology Nursing Forum*, 13 (6), 17–22.

Nursing Interventions. The major CNS effect of IL-2/LAK therapy is severe mental confusion. Disorientation, combativeness, increased anxiety, and psychosis have also been noted (Jassak and Sticklin, 1986). The etiology of this toxicity is unknown. Because of the severe toxicities of IL-2/LAK therapy, these patients must receive the therapy in an intensive care unit. It may be difficult to differentiate the CNS effects of toxicity from those resulting from the stress of being hospitalized in an intensive care unit. Frequent assessment of mental status, orientation, and level of consciousness is necessary (Jassak, 1986). Documentation of mental status should be carefully made to allow evaluation over time. Administration of medications that affect CNS function should be avoided. CNS side effects may require the interruption or discontinuation of the therapy.

Fluid Volume Deficit. A volume deficit results from cumulative doses of IL-2, which are associated with increased capillary permeability, extravasation of fluid, and fluid shifts to the extravascular space.

Expected Outcomes. Significant deviations from the patient's normal vital signs and indicators of fluid shift will be rapidly identified and reported. The patient will not develop complications of fluid voume deficit.

Nursing Interventions. Weight gains of more than 10% of baseline have been reported with IL-2 therapy (Lotze, 1985; Rosenberg, 1985). Fluid retention is shown by peripheral edema, ascites, and, eventually, pulmonary interstitial edema (Jassak, 1986). Patients with decreased oxygenation, dyspnea, and respiratory distress may require intubation. Blood gas results should be carefully monitored. Daily weights should be begun in prone patients. Lung auscultation, abdominal girth measurements, and assessment for peripheral edema should be performed along with the vital signs. Careful intake and output measurements should be taken and recorded. Inform the patient of appropriate symptoms that should be promptly reported, e.g., dyspnea, dyspnea on exertion, shortness of breath, orthopnea, peripheral edema, and abdominal pain.

Hypotension associated with IL-2 is thought to be related to reduced vascular system resistance (Jassak, 1986). Continuous blood pressure monitoring or arterial pressure monitoring is required for these patients. Hypotension may be treated with intravenous colloid solutions, e.g., 5% human serum albumin or 5% plasma protein fraction. Sometimes vasopressors such as dopamine hydrochloride or phenylephrine hydrochloride are needed. Fluid replacement therapy is contraindicated because of the danger of pulmonary edema.

Alterations in Urinary Elimination. Changes in urination are due to toxicities resulting from IL-2.

Expected Outcomes. The patient's urinary output will be over 30 mL per hour or, if less, it will be rapidly identified and reported to the physician.

Nursing Interventions. Urinary complications of IL-2 are dose related and include oliguria, proteinuria, elevations of serum creatinine, and increased blood urea nitrogen (BUN). Renal function usually returns to normal within 48 hours of the cessation of IL-2 therapy. Fluid challenges are generally contraindicated (see above), but diuretics may be used if central venous pressure and blood pressure levels are adequate. Intake and output need to be carefully monitored, and each voided specimen should be assessed for proteinuria. Daily serum creatinine and BUN levels should be monitored.

Alterations in Bowel Elimination. Diarrhea results from the toxicity of IL-2.

Expected Outcomes. Patient will maintain normal bowel habits with formed stool; if diarrhea develops, it is rapidly identified, and complications are avoided.

Nursing Interventions. The patient should be instructed about the potential for diarrhea and asked to report any associated symptoms. If diarrhea develops, a record of stools should be maintained. If more than three liquid stools per day are passed, an antidiarrheal medication should be started. The patient should be instructed about the need to take in additional oral fluids to meet fluid losses (2500 to 3000 mL/day); the patient's fluid preferences are determined. The patient is instructed in the appropriate foods to add to the diet (high bulk) and those to avoid (bowel-irritating foods include caffeine, spices, milk products). If diarrhea continues, the need for associated fluid and electrolyte replacement is assessed. The perianal area is carefully cleansed after each stool and white petroleum jelly applied if irritation develops.

Alterations in Nutrition. Intake of less than bodily requirements occurs due to nausea, vomiting, anorexia, and mucositis resulting from side effects of IL-2 therapy.

Expected Outcomes. Patient is able to maintain adequate fluid and food intake, weight remains stable, and intake and output are in balance and in adequate amounts.

Nursing Interventions. The patient should be carefully assessed for indications of nutritional difficulties at each meal. Abdominal assessments should be performed along with the vital signs. Nausea and vomiting may be dealt with by improving the eating environment (removing odors, serving warm foods warm and cold foods cold, and preventing unpleasant sights). Decreasing the size of meals and providing six feedings a day may be helpful (American Cancer Society, 1974). Oral hygiene before meals may remove foul taste. Orally irritating foods (citrus, spices, and mouthwash with alcohol) should be decreased in patients with stomatitis or mucositis. Gargling with a teaspoon of bicarbonate in 8 ounces of water may reduce oral membrane inflammation. Antiemetics may be necessary. The patient is taught about the need to take in adequate amounts of fluids, and goals for fluid intake are set mutually. Parenteral nutrition may be required in severe cases.

Potential for Injury. Hepatotoxicity may result from toxicity from IL-2.

Expected Outcomes. Patients will be carefully assessed for abnormal liver function, and abnormalities will be rapidly identified and therapy initiated.

Nursing Interventions. Liver function tests (lactic dehydrogenase, serum glutamic oxaloacetic transaminase [AST], serum glutamic pyruvate transaminase [ALT], and alkaline phosphatase) levels should be carefully monitored. The skin and sclera should be assessed for icterus. Urine should be assessed for darkening, and stools should be assessed for pasty, clay color. Abdominal assessments should include careful assessment of the position of the liver to note hepatomegaly. Patient complaints of abdominal fullness, nausea, and pain should be carefully evaluated as indicators of hepatomegaly. Abnormalities should be rapidly identified and reported to the physician, who will make the decision about discontinuing this agent.

Potential for Injury. Anemia and thrombocytopenia may result from toxic reactions to IL-2.

Expected Outcomes. Patient will verbalize understanding of the symptoms that should be reported and the precautions that need to be taken. Complete blood count results will be carefully monitored, and abnormal values will be rapidly reported to the physician.

Nursing Interventions. Patients should be told to report dizziness and abnormal bleeding (epistaxis, bleeding gums, hemoptysis, hematemesis, melena, hematuria, or bleeding from wounds). Monitor laboratory values for hematocrit, hemoglobin, prothrombin time, partial thromboplastin time, fibrinogen, and fibrinogen degradation products (Bindon, 1983; Jassak, 1986). Patients should be discouraged from using safety razors. There is no evidence suggesting that these patients are at risk for disseminated intravascular coagulation (Jassak, 1986).

Potential Impaired Skin Integrity. Skin integrity may be impaired due to toxicity of IL-2.

Expected Outcomes. Patients verbalize an understanding of the potential skin reactions and the need to report any untoward findings rapidly.

Nursing Interventions. Instruct the patient to report potential skin reactions including erythema, rash, pruritus, and desquamation. Assess the skin every 8 hours for problem areas. Application of medicated lotions may control most symptoms. Systemic antihistamines may be required for pruritus.

Potential Alterations in Temperature. Temperature may be elevated due to the side effects of IL-2.

Expected Outcomes. The patient's temperature will remain within normal limits or elevations will be rapidly identified and treated.

Nursing Interventions. Chills and temperature elevations of up to 40.5° C have been reported (Jassak, 1986). The patient should be instructed to report chills or feelings of being too warm. Temperature should be monitored with vital signs every 4 hours. Careful assessments for concurrent infection should be made for each temperature elevation. Forcing fluids, tepid baths, and antipyretics may be necessary.

Alterations in Family Processes. Families may be disturbed by having a family member hospitalized for a prolonged period of time.

Expected Outcomes. The patient and family members demonstrate an appropriate stress response for the situation and do not demonstrate maladaptive behavior (excessive anger, displacement, inappropriate anxiety).

Nursing Interventions. Assess the family for causative and contributing factors. Encourage the family to ventilate their feelings about the situation and acknowledge their feelings. Allow maximum family and patient interaction time. Involve the patient and family in the patient's care and in decision making and goal setting. Assist the family in assessing the situation. Aid them in identifying their strengths and previously successful coping mechanisms. Provide health teaching and referrals to a psychiatric nurse clinician if necessary. (See also Chapters 6 and 7.)

Potential for Infection. Immunosuppression may increase the potential for respiratory tract infection.

Expected Outcomes. Patient will not exhibit indications of respiratory tract infection (e.g., he remains afebrile, lungs clear to auscultation, and normal sputum color and amount). Patient will actively participate in pulmonary hygiene.

Nursing Interventions. A protective environment should be effectively maintained. Patients should be instructed in the need to maintain careful oral and personal hygiene. Instruct the patient about the need to perform pulmonary hygiene exercises (coughing, deep breathing, use of incentive spirometry) every 2 hours. Instruct the patient to report chest discomfort, changes in the color or amount of sputum produced, shortness of breath, and the feeling that he may have a fever. Monitor vital signs every 4 hours. Auscultate breath sounds with the vital signs. Increase fluid intake to 2500 to 3000 mL/day to aid in liquifying secretions and aiding their mobilization.

Body Image Disturbance. Changes in body image may occur due to weight loss and alopecia resulting from IL-2.

Expected Outcomes. The patient will state his or her acceptance of changes and not demonstrate indicators of maladaptation (excessive anger, dwelling on physical appearance).

Nursing Interventions. Discuss the changes that can be expected because of therapy (e.g., weight loss and alopecia). Encourage purchase of a wig prior to the onset of alopecia. When appropriate, encourage use of scarves, cosmetics, hats, or similar devices. Discuss the patient's feelings and allow adequate time for ventilation. If necessary, seek assistance from a psychiatric nurse clinician. (See also Chapter 6.)

Ethical Considerations. IL-2 is an investigational drug, and its use raises some ethical concerns as with other investigational therapies. Patients receiving IL-2 have an advanced disease that has been unresponsive to standard therapies. It is common for patients being treated in clinical trials to view the therapy as a last hope for cure of their disease. The nurse should assess the expectations of the patient and family and ensure that they are provided with realistic information about the potential outcome of the therapy, i.e., guarded optimism.

Nursing responsibilities in treating patients enrolled in clinical trials of IL-2 include accurate and thorough documentation of any toxic reactions (Jassak and Sticklin, 1986). Nurses are in the unique position of assessing and documenting their findings on the complications of this therapy while identifying its long-term effects and looking for appropriate areas of nursing research.

ncp nursing care plan

1. Potential for infection due to

Outcome Criteria		Nursing Interventions
Increased potential for respiratory tract infection	No indicators of infection are noted (e.g., patient is afebrile, lungs clear to auscultation) Patient verbalizes understanding of the indicators of respiratory infection	1. Maintain protective isolation 2. Teach the patient the need for strict personal hygiene 3. Oral hygiene is accomplished every 2 hours while awake 4. Instruct the patient in the indicators of infection that require reporting (e.g., dyspnea, chest pain, shortness of breath, change in the amount or color of sputum) 5. Instruct the patient and family in the need to perform pulmonary hygiene exercises every 2 hours while awake (i.e., coughing and deep breathing, use of an incentive spirometer)

2. Knowledge deficit related to

Outcome Criteria		Nursing Interventions
Treatment with bone marrow transplant	Patient and family verbalize their understanding of the treatment and associated toxic reactions	1. Instruct the patient and family in the expected effects of chemotherapy 2. Teach the patient and family about the hygienic practices and mechanisms of isolation precautions during granulocytopenia 3. Instruct the patient and family in postdischarge precautions

3. Fear due to

Outcome Criteria		Nursing Interventions
Primary diagnosis and need for bone marrow transplant with its attendant life-threatening complications	Patient does not exhibit findings of uncontrolled fear Patient is able to identify useful coping mechanisms	1. Assess the patient and family for contributing factors 2. Discuss procedures and describe the intensive care environment 3. Identify and reduce stress-producing misconceptions of the hospitalization and therapy 4. When necessary, seek referral for a psychiatric nurse clinician to aid in family and patient adjustment

See accompanying text for additional related nursing diagnoses for this patient and family.

SUMMARY

The treatment of cancer has become increasingly more successful and aggressive in recent years. Nurses are challenged to provide patients and their families intensive and holistic support. The care of immunosuppressed patient receiving bone marrow transplants and IL-2/LAK therapy has been discussed. The nurse must be knowledgeable about these therapies and their effects on patients. Nurses must be prepared to intervene as needed to assist patients and families to complete the therapy successfully, both physically and emotionally.

References

Abernathy, E. (1987). How the immune system works. *The American Journal of Nursing*, 87 (4), 456–473.

American Cancer Society (1974). *Nutrition for patients receiving chemotherapy and radiation treatment.*

Atkinson, K., and Meyers, J. D. (1980). Varicella-zoster virus infection after marrow transplantation for aplastic anemia or leukemia. *Transplantation*, 29 (1), 47–50.

Armstrong, D. (1984). Protected environments are discomforting and expensive and do not offer meaningful protection. *The American Journal of Medicine*, 76, 685–689.

Becker, T. M. (1981). *Cancer chemotherapy: A manual for nurses.* Boston: Little, Brown.

Bindon, C. M. (1983). Clearance rates and systemic effects of intravenously administered interleukin-2 containing preparations in human subjects. *British Journal of Cancer, 47* (1), 123–133.

Burns, N. (1982). *Nursing and cancer.* Philadelphia: W. B. Saunders.

Carpenito, L. J. (1983). *Nursing diagnosis: Application to clinical practice.* Philadelphia: J. B. Lippincott.

Champlin, R. E., and Gale, R. P. (1984). Role of bone marrow transplantation in the treatment of hematologic malignancies and solid tumors: Critical review of syngeneic, autologous, and allogeneic transplants. *Cancer Treatment Reports, 68,* 145–161.

Cogliano-Shutta, N. A., and Broda, E. J. (1985). Bone marrow transplantation: An overview and comparison of autologous, syngeneic, and allogeneic treatment modalities. *Nursing Clinics of North America, 20* (1), 49–66.

Corbett, J. V. (1987). *Laboratory tests and diagnostic procedures with nursing diagnoses* (2nd ed.). Norwalk, CT: Appleton & Lange.

Corcoran-Buchsel, P. (1986). Long-term complications of allogeneic bone marrow transplantation: Nursing implications. *The Oncology Nursing Forum, 13* (6), 61–70.

Corey, B. S., and Collins, J. L. (1986). Implementation of an IL-2/LAK cell clinical trial: A nursing perspective. *The Oncology Nursing Forum, 13* (6), 21–36.

Crane, L. R., Emmer, D. R., and Grguras, A. (1980). Prevention of infection on the oncology unit. *Nursing Clinics of North America, 15* (4), 843–856.

Daly, P. A. (1983). Supportive care for the patient with myelosuppression and immunosuppression. *Irish Medical Journal, 76* (11), 466–470.

Deisseroth, A. B., Abrams, R., and Holohan, T. (1982). Blood component replacement, applications of the continuous flow centrifuge, and bone marrow transplantation. In A. S. Levine (Ed.), *Cancer in the young.* New York: Masson Publishing USA.

DeVita, V. T. (1985). *Cancer: Principles and practice of oncology* (2nd ed.). Philadelphia: J. B. Lippincott.

Doney, K. C., and Weiden, P. L. (1981). Treatment of graft versus host disease in human allogeneic marrow graft recipients: A randomized trial comparing ATG and corticosteroids. *American Journal of Hematology, 11,* 1–18.

Espersen, S. (1986). Nursing support of host defenses. *Critical Care Quarterly, 2* (1), 51–56.

Foon, K. A., and Gale, R. P. (1982). Controversies in the therapy of acute myelogenous leukemia. *The American Journal of Medicine, 72,* 963–978.

Gardner, G. G., and August, C. S. (1977). Psychological issues in bone marrow transplantation. *Pediatrics, 60* (4), 625–630.

Garner, J. S., and Simmons, B. P. (1983). Modification of isolation precautions. *Infection Control, 4* (4), 324–325.

Jassak, P. F., and Sticklin, L. A. (1986). Interleukin-2: An overview. *The Oncology Nursing Forum, 13* (6), 17–22.

Klemm, P. (1985). Cyclosporin A: Use in preventing graft versus host disease. *The Oncology Nursing Forum, 12* (5), 25–32.

Levine, A. S., and Siegel, S. E. (1973). Protected environments and prophylactic antibiotics: A prospective controlled study of their utility in the therapy of acute leukemia. *The New England Journal of Medicine, 288* (10), 477–483.

Lokich, J. J. (1976). Managing chemotherapy-induced bone marrow suppression in cancer. *Hospital Practice, 11* (8), 61–67.

Lotze, M. T. (1985). In vivo administration of purified human interleukin-2. *Journal of Immunology, 135* (4), 2685–2875.

McCarron, K. (1986). Fever—the cardinal vital sign. *Critical Care Quarterly, 2* (1), 15–18.

McGlave, P. B. (1985). The status of bone marrow transplantation for leukemia. *Hospital Practice, 20* (11), 97–110.

Nauta, E. H. (1979). Infection in the compromised host. In G. Dick (Ed.), *Immunological aspects of infectious disease.* Baltimore: University Park Press.

Oniboni, A. C. (1985). Understanding and preventing infection in the patient with cancer. *The Oncology Nursing Forum, 12,* 56–64.

O'Reilly, R J. (1983). Allogeneic bone marrow transplantation: Current status and future directions. *Blood, 62,* 941–964.

Reheis, C. E. (1985). Neutropenia: Causes, complications, treatment, and resulting nursing care. *Nursing Clinics of North America, 20* (1), 219–225.

Ristuccia, A. M. (1985). Hematologic effects of cancer chemotherapy. *Nursing Clinics of North America, 20* (1), 235–239.

Rosenberg, S. A. (1985). Special report observations on the systemic administration of autologous lymphokine—activated killer cells and recombinant interleukin-2 to patients with metastatic cancer. *The New England Journal of Medicine, 313* (23), 1485–1492.

Ruccione, K., and Fergusson, J. (1984). Late effects of childhood cancer and its treatment. *The Oncology Nursing Forum, 11* (5), 54–64.

Sanders, J. E., and Buckner, C. D. (1985). Growth and development following marrow transplantation for hematologic malignancy. *Blood, 66* (5) (Suppl. 1), 253a.

Seipp, C. A., and Simpson, C. (1986). Clinical trials with IL-2. *The Oncology Nursing Forum, 13* (6), 25–29.

Smith, S. L. (1986a). Immunosuppressive drugs used in clinical practice. *Critical Care Quarterly, 9* (1), 19–24.

Smith, S. L. (1986b). Physiology of the immune system. *Critical Care Quarterly, 9* (1), 7–13.

Sondel, P. M., and Hank, J. A. (1987). Status and potential of interleukin-2 for the treatment of neoplastic disease. *Oncology, 1* (6), 41–48.

Stewart, F. M., and Thomas, R. M. (1985). Bone marrow transplantation: Three treatments for disease. *ACORN Journal, 42* (2), 196–205.

West, W. H., and Tauer, K. W. (1987). Constant-infusion recombinant interleukin-2 in adoptive immunotherapy of advanced cancer. *The New England Journal of Medicine, 316* (15), 898–905.

Winston, D. J., Winston, G. H., and Gale, R. P. (1982). Therapeutic granulocyte transfusions for documented infections. *Annals of Internal Medicine, 97,* 509–515.

Witherspoon, R. P., and Storb, R. (1981). Recovery of antibody production in human allogeneic marrow graft recipients: Influence of time post-transplantation, the presence or absence of chronic graft-versus-host disease, and antithymocyte globulin treatment. *Blood, 58* (2), 360–368.

Wolcott, D. L., and Wellisch, D. K. (1987, February). Bone marrow transplant recipients report good psychological adjustment. *Oncology Nurse Bulletin,* 2–3.

Patients with HIV-Related Disease and AIDS

Kathleen McMahon Casey
Lucinda H. Cave

HISTORICAL DEVELOPMENT

In 1981 the established health community became aware of the illness that has since become known as AIDS (Gottlieb et al., 1981; Centers for Disease Control, 1981). Young, primarily homosexual men who had been previously healthy and had not been treated with immunosuppressive therapies were seeking medical care for opportunistic infections and a malignancy, Kaposi's sarcoma. This heralded the development of an epidemic. In the major metropolitan areas of the east and west coasts of the United States (primarily New York City, Los Angeles, and San Francisco) there were increasingly frequent reports of this new phenomenon then called GRIDS (gay-related immunodeficiency syndrome), a name that reflected the major risk group and characteristic. Later, when it became clear that other groups were acquiring the disease through other risk behaviors and sexual relations, the name was changed to acquired immunodeficiency syndrome (AIDS). Before the etiologic agent was discovered, it was becoming increasingly evident that an infectious agent was involved. At first, cytomegalovirus was thought to be the causative agent, but questions remained about why the syndrome was a recent development. Transmission data cited blood contacts, sexual behaviors, and perinatal acquisition, which framed hepatitis B as a model for this new and still undiscovered agent. Additionally, because transmission presumptively occurred between persons not obviously ill, a prodromal period of illness or infectivity was probable.

It became clear that the illness was a clinical consequence of infection with a virus. Other co-factors such as recent trends in recreational drug use, use of nitrites as inhalants in sexual pleasure experiences, a scientific experiment gone awry, other viral co-factors, and genocidal sabotage were suggested as possible intervening variables. Table 54–1 summarizes the historical development of the illness in the United States.

EPIDEMIOLOGY

Since its clinical emergence, AIDS has claimed the lives of 122,805 adults and children in the United States (Centers for Disease Control, 1991). With 191,601 known cases diagnosed, another 1,000,000 Americans are estimated to be infected. It is projected that 165,000 to 215,000 more deaths will occur by the end of 1993 (Centers for Disease Control, 1991b).

In terms of sheer numbers of cases, New York and San Francisco continue to be the hardest hit areas. Data summarizing case rates and reported numbers of cases for the leading metropolitan areas are summarized in Table 54–2. Table 54–3 contrasts the situation in metropolitan and nonmetropolitan areas.

AIDS is a leading cause of death for men and women in their late twenties. The data on age and sex distribution of the cases are presented in Table 54–4. Men who have sex with men (MWHSWM) comprise the leading exposure category in adult AIDS cases (59%), with intravenous drug users (22%) second and MWHSWM who also use intravenous drugs (7%) third. In children's cases, the highest risk factor is a mother with or at risk for HIV (84%), followed by receipt of a blood transfusion or blood components or tissue (9%). Minorities are unequally represented compared with their representation in

TABLE 54–1. Historical Development of AIDS: The United States Experience

1969	A mid-1980s retrospective analysis into the causes of death of a teenage boy in St. Louis, Missouri who died in 1969 shows Kaposi's sarcoma and HIV.
1976–1981	Few but significant changes appear in demographics of Kaposi's sarcoma in New York City cancer registry (i.e., never married males, unusual sites of presentation of the illness, geographic clustering of cases in New York City's Greenwich Village).
1978–1981	Physicians, community leaders, and others in contact with vast social network of gay men begin to detect unusually high rate of nonspecific illness. Some public health officials are concerned about the rate of venereal disease and hepatitis.
1981	First AIDS-related publication: *Morbidity and Mortality Weekly Report* (CDC) reports clustering of PCP in homosexual men in Los Angeles. CDC forms task force to undertake surveillance and conduct epidemiologic and laboratory investigations. Makes formal request for all state health departments to report all biopsy-proven Kaposi's sarcoma cases in persons less than 60 years old if not on immunosuppressive treatment *and* all cases of documented opportunistic infections in patients with no known underlying illness or history of immunosuppressive treatment. Total of 159 cases reported with 5 to 6 additional cases being reported weekly.
1981–1983	Emergence of cases in other major metropolitan areas; other risk behaviors and groups identified; general acceptance of a prodromal illness and period of infectivity prior to outright AIDS.
1984	Discovery in France and the United States of a virus as the causative agent.
1985	Blood tests available for detection of HIV in the blood supply.
1986	Name HIV (human immunodeficiency virus) formally endorsed by International Committee on Taxonomy of Viruses (ICTV).
1987	Anti-HIV clinical trials programs started (AIDS Cooperative Trial Group).
1988	A few cases of HIV-2 reported in New Jersey (West African–born patient).
1991	122,905 U.S. deaths reported (cumulative) 191,601 U.S. cases reported (cumulative) 1,000,000 U.S. infected persons (estimated) The approximately 44,000 new cases reported in this year reflect 25% of *all* cases reported in the previous decade.

CDC, Centers for Disease Control; PCP, *Pneumocystis carinii* pneumonia.

the population. In New York, the epicenter of the epidemic in the United States, 90% of children and 85% of women with AIDS are either black or Hispanic. Although 24% of the city is black, 32% of the reported patients are blacks. It is estimated that 60,000 to 70,000 children in New York City will lose at least one parent to AIDS. The high minority representation reflects the impact of culture, economics, power, and health care systems.

INTERNATIONAL STATISTICS

The World Health Organization (WHO) reports 418,403 AIDS cases worldwide, with sub-Saharan Africa and Brazil affected the most (personal communication WHO hotline, Oct 1991). WHO also estimates the actual number of cases as 1.5 million because of frequent underreporting due to discrimination, scarcity of medical care, lack of public health resources, and other social causes.

It is postulated that human immunodeficiency virus (HIV)-1 first emerged in central Africa as a new disease, originating from a recent simian-to-human retrovirus transmission (Kanski et al., 1985). The virus was probably transported to the western hemisphere in the 1970s and began infecting Americans

around 1978 (Osborn, 1986). HIV-2 is believed to be endemic in West Africa. Several well-documented cases of HIV-2 infection have been reported in Europeans and among West Africans residing abroad. There have been a few cases reported in New Jersey.

Many countries owe acquisition of HIV infection in their population to contact with American blood products that were exported prior to the 1985 HIV

TABLE 54–2. AIDS Case Rates per 100,000 Population by Metropolitan Area with 500,000 or More Population, September 1990–August 1991, with Cumulative Case Totals by Age Group

City	Rate	Adults/ Adolescents	Children <15 Years
San Francisco, CA	146.2	10,827	18
Miami, FL	90.2	5,429	188
New York, NY	80.6	34,080	816
Jersey City, NJ	74.2	1,980	56
Ft. Lauderdale, FL	69.2	3,108	62
San Juan, PR	66.7	3,656	115
Newark, NJ	49.3	4,805	154
Atlanta, GA	39.0	4,006	31

Centers for Disease Control. (1991). *HIV/AIDS Surveillance Report*, September, 6–7.

TABLE 54–3. AIDS Cases and Rates September 1990–August 1991 in Metropolitan Areas versus Suburban/Rural Areas

	Number	Rate	Adult Cases	Children Cases
Metropolitan areas[a]	37,223	25.0	160,256	2,710
All other areas	7,491	7.1	28,092	543
Total	44,714	17.5	188,348	3,253

[a]500,000 or more population
Centers for Disease Control. (1991). *HIV/AIDS Surveillance Report*, September, 6–7.

screening procedures or to sexual transmission (Osborn, 1986).

Worldwide epidemiologic studies indicate that there are three broad but distinct geographic patterns of AIDS transmission. In pattern I, typical of industrialized countries with large numbers of reported cases, most cases occur among homosexual or bisexual males and among urban intravenous (IV) drug users. Only a small percentage of cases is attributed to heterosexual transmission, but this percentage is increasing. Transmission due to exposure to HIV-contaminated blood or blood products occurred between the late 1970s and 1985, but this has since been largely controlled through routine blood screening procedures. The ratio of male-to-female patients ranges from 10:1 to 15:1, and perinatal transmission is relatively rare. The overall population seroprevalence is less than 1%, but this is significantly higher (up to 50% higher) in high-risk behavior groups such as IV drug users and men with multiple male sex partners (Centers for Disease Control, 1988a).

Pattern II is seen in areas of central, eastern, and southern Africa and in some Caribbean countries. Most cases occur among heterosexuals, and the male-to-female ratio is approximately 1:1. Perinatal transmission is relatively more common than in other areas. Transmission through intravenous drug use and homosexual transmission either does not occur or occurs at a very low rate. The overall population seroprevalence is estimated to be over 1%, and in a few urban areas up to 25% of all sexually active people are infected. Transmission through contaminated blood and blood products remains a significant problem (Centers for Disease Control, 1988a).

Pattern III occurs in areas of eastern Europe, the Middle East, Asia, and most of the Pacific basin. It appears that HIV has been introduced to these areas only since the mid-1980s, and only small numbers of cases have been reported. Generally, cases have occurred among those who have traveled to endemic areas or who have had sexual contact with individuals from endemic areas, such as homosexual men and prostitutes. Only a small number of cases has been reported due to receipt of imported HIV-contaminated blood (Centers for Disease Control, 1988a). The exception to pattern III in eastern Europe is the large-scale nosocomial transmission of HIV in Rumania associated with lack of needle and syringe sterilizations and blood and blood product screening prior to transfusion (Beldescu and associates, 1990). This transmission rate is elevated due to the common national medical practice of microtransfusion for newborns. Other developing countries also have a substantial risk of disease transmission owing to the lack of testing and sterilization capabilities and to cultural attitudes toward needles in disease treatment.

HUMAN IMMUNODEFICIENCY VIRUS

Immunopathogenesis

It has become evident that AIDS is the most severe form of a spectrum of clinical consequences resulting from the immunologic reaction to HIV infection. A working knowledge of the virus' morphology, characteristics, and immune system response assists the clinician in preparing interventions.

Morphologic Features

HIV is a piece of RNA surrounded by a lipid envelope that measures slightly over 100 mm in diameter. Electron microscopy reveals a characteristic dense cylindrical nucleoid containing core proteins, genomic RNA, and an enzyme, reverse transcriptase (RT), that classifies it as a retrovirus (Ho et al., 1987). HIV selectivity infects the T4 (or CD4+) cell (Bowen et al., 1985; Gallo, 1987; Lawrence, 1985; Margolick et al., 1987; Urba and Longo, 1985), but infects other

TABLE 54–4. AIDS Cases by Sex, Age at Diagnosis, Reported Through August 1991, United States

	Age at Diagnosis (Yr)	Percentage
Males	<5	1
Total cases	25–29	15
170,823	30–34	24
	35–39	22
	40–44	15
Females	<5	6
Total cases	25–29	18
20,778	30–34	25
	35–39	19
	40–44	10

Centers for Disease Control. (1991). *HIV/AIDS Surveillance Report*, September, 12.

cell types as well, which may also possess the CD4 receptor molecule. These cell types include monocytes-macrophages, transformed B-cells, dendritic cells, microglial cells, endothelial cells, astrocytes and oligodendrocytes, transformed colon cells, neurons, and CD8+ and CD4− cells (Koenig and Fauci, 1988). Very little cell-free virus is found in HIV-infected persons (Ho et al., 1987).

HIV Replication Cycle in Human T4-Lymphocytes

HIV enters the host and then attaches to a particular surface molecule receptor on the T4 cell membrane (McDougal et al., 1986). T4 cell glycoprotein is essential for HIV binding, but additional factors may be required for penetration (Isobe et al., 1986). HIV enters the cell and becomes uncoated. Viral RNA is then transcribed into DNA by the enzyme reverse transcriptase, is circularized, and then becomes integrated into the host T4 genome (Ho et al., 1987). The HIV replication cycle is restricted at this stage until the infected cell is "activated." In vitro, activation takes place through mitogenic, antigenic, or allogenic stimulation. In vivo, potential activators include other pathogens (i.e., hepatitis B virus, cytomegalovirus, herpes virus) and allogenic exposure to semen, blood, or allografts (Ho et al., 1987). Upon activation, transcription occurs, and then protein synthesis. Viral proteins and genomic RNA are then assembled at the cell surface, and mature virions are formed by budding. With HIV replication, the T4 cell is killed (Ho et al., 1987).

Immunologic Abnormalities

HIV has been found in only a few types of cells in infected persons. The cell population most profoundly affected is the helper subset of T-lymphocytes that express the cell surface (leu 3/T4) molecule. In vitro studies allow the detection of HIV genes in infected cells in tissues of AIDS- and HIV-infected patients at a rate of 1 in 10,000 to 1 in 1,000,000 lymphocytes. Both acute and chronic effects are demonstrated after successful HIV infection (Lane and Fauci, 1985). The most devastating effect, however, is the gradual, progressive depletion of the helper T-lymphocytes, which leads to irreversible immunodeficiency. Table 54–5 summarizes the immunologic abnormalities.

T-CELL ABNORMALITIES

HIV eventually destroys human T4-lymphocytes, reducing their overall number and function (Bowen et al., 1985; Lane and Fauci, 1985; Lawrence, 1985; Margolick et al., 1987; Seligmann et al., 1987). Table 54–5 cites the major immunologic abnormalities. Sev-

TABLE 54–5. *Immunologic Abnormalities in AIDS*

T-Cell Number	Low T4 Cell Number—Lymphopenia
T-cell function	Decreased ability to release lymphokines Decreased cytotoxicity Decreased B-cell help Decreased proliferation in mixed lymphocyte culture Decreased responsiveness to specific antigen
B-cell number	Normal
B-cell function	Polyclonal activation with increased Ig levels and increased circulating complexes Inability to respond to new antigen by antibody production
Macrophage number	Normal
Macrophage function	Decreased intracellular killing during phagocytosis Decreased chemotaxis Decreased expression of class II HLA antigens

From Grady, C. (1989). The immune system and AIDS/HIV infection. In J. H. Flaskerud (Ed.), *AIDS/HIV infection: A reference guide for nursing professionals* (p. 45). Philadelphia: W. B. Saunders.

eral mechanisms for this process have been proposed: (1) direct cytopathic effect of HIV, (2) putative autoimmune mechanism, or (3) T4 expression of HIV antigen, which includes other cytotoxic mechanisms (Seligmann et al., 1987).

In vitro, a major mechanism of T-cell death involves cell-cell fusion and the formation of multinucleated giant cells, which die within 24 to 48 hours. The HIV envelope glycoprotein, gp 160, binds with the CD4 (leu 3/T4) molecule on an uninfected T-cell and initiates fusion.

Immunologically normal people have 600 to 1200 T4 cells/mm^3, whereas persons with HIV may have only 0 to 500. Decreased T4 cell counts are associated with an increase in clinical problems, especially infection (Lane and Fauci, 1987). The cytotoxic T-cell subpopulation is responsible for attaching virally infected and malignant cell populations and removing them from the body. The overall lymphocyte count is low, and the T4/T8 cell ratio is also decreased (Bowen et al., 1985; Lane and Fauci, 1985; Lawrence, 1985; Margolick, 1987).

Besides having fewer T4 cells, a person with AIDS has absent or depressed T4 cell function. In AIDS there is (1) decreased ability to release lymphokines, (2) decreased cytotoxicity, (3) decreased T-cell to B-cell mediation necessary for antibody production, (4) decreased ability of T-cells to proliferate in mixed lymphocyte cultures, and (5) lack of antigen-induced T-cell function (Bowen et al., 1985; Lane and Fauci, 1985; Margolick, 1987). Clinically, a person with AIDS is lymphogenic, especially if there is a low T4-cell count, has a decreased T4/T8 cell ratio, and is anergic (Grady, 1989). Due to the central role of T4 cells in

TABLE 54–6. Risks and Benefits of HIV Testing

Risks	Benefits
Relationship problems	Protection of blood supply
Blaming	Protection of organ recipients
Sexual dysfunction	Support for medical diagnosis
Disrupted ability to make plans as a couple	Avoiding medical mismanagement of asymptomatic patients
Employment problems	Examination of cerebrospinal fluid in asymptomatic persons with syphilis
Insurance problems	infection of more than 1 year's duration
Spiritual distress	Interpretation of a PPD test as positive if it shows at least 5 cm of induration
Stigmatization, discrimination	(and stated prophylaxis with longer duration of treatment)
Self-imposed social withdrawal	Administration of influenza and pneumovax vaccines and use of inactivated
Preoccupation with bodily symptoms, fear	oral polio vaccine
Desire for revenge, homicidal thoughts	Help women decide about pregnancy, giving birth, and breast feeding
Psychological impairment	Access to clinical trials
Anxiety	Identification of contacts
Nightmares	
Depression	
Suicidal ideology	

Adapted from McMahon, K. M. (1988). The integration of HIV testing and counseling into nursing practice. *Nursing Clinics of North America* 23(4), 814.

the normal immune response, any defect in T4 cell function consequently reduces the activity of other immune cell types (Seligmann et al., 1987).

B-CELL ABNORMALITIES

B-cell abnormalities in AIDS patients are due perhaps to the aforementioned T-cell abnormalities; to direct B-cell activation by HIV, CMV, or another virus; or possibly to excessive secretion of B-cell stimulating lymphokines (Bowen et al., 1985; Lane and Fauci, 1985; Margolick et al., 1987). B-cells in patients with AIDS are polyclonal activated, resulting in oversecretion of IgG, IgA, and IgM (hypergammaglobulinemia) and increased levels of circulating immune complexes and autoantibodies (Lane and Fauci, 1985). B-cells, however, will not mount an antibody in response to a new antigen. Therefore, a patient with AIDS will not respond to immunization with appropriate antibody production (Lane and Fauci, 1985), and most patients should not be vaccinated with a live virus vaccine (Amman, 1984). An exception is made, however, for HIV-infected children, who are vaccinated for measles, mumps, and rubella (MMR). Following reports of severe measles in symptomatic HIV-infected children, and no report of serious or unusual adverse effects of MMR vaccination, the Immunization Practices Advisory Committee recommended MMR vaccination for all HIV-infected children (Centers for Disease Control, 1988b).

MACROPHAGE ABNORMALITIES

Monocyte-macrophage abnormalities (see Table 54–5) may be due to a lack of gamma-interferon and other monocyte-stimulating lymphokines from the T-cell as well as to direct infection of monocytes-macrophages with HIV. Frequent infections may result from these monocyte-macrophage abnormalities (Bowen et al., 1985; Margolick et al., 1987).

In addition, monocytes and macrophages may serve as important reservoirs for the persistence of HIV in the host and are possibly the vehicles that transport HIV across the blood-brain barrier and into the central nervous system (Ho et al., 1987).

Testing for HIV

Testing for HIV is useful for personal health maintenance and for early medical intervention and public health considerations. Table 54–6 shows the risks and benefits of testing. Very serious issues of confidentiality, occupational and public safety, civil liberties and rights, and ethics are involved. Background information on the purposes, possible outcomes, and types of testing are central to handling HIV testing issues well.

The risk that testing may impede a person's ability to function emotionally and socially is one of the components of counseling required during the pretest session. Others include information on the tests, the clinical significance of positive results, potential difficulties (legal, insurance, relational, health care), and review of the benefits. Informed consent is required in most situations, with laws governing practice in some states. Table 54–7 lists the components of the counseling sessions.

Testing serum for antibodies to HIV is currently the most cost-effective and accurate method of screening for infection. Since March 1985, when the first serologic assay became available, many more methods have become commercially available. Others are primarily research tools without clear commercial uses. A venipuncture specimen of 5 to 7 mL of sterile, whole clotted blood is sufficient for performing repeated tests as well as any needed supplemental tests. Specimens should be refrigerated but can be transported at ambient temperatures. They can be frozen.

TABLE 54–7. Essential Components of HIV Counseling and Testing Sessions

Pretest Session

Review of meaning and significance of test, positive or negative results; time frames; testing procedures

Identification of client's motive for testing

Elaboration of risk reduction behaviors; availability of education and supportive counseling

Description of confidentiality and limits

Discussion of possible psychological, emotional, social, legal, spiritual, and medical consequences and benefits

Exploration of coping strengths and support; availability of anonymous test sites

Informed consent

Post Test Sessions

Interpretation of results

Recommendations for medical follow-up

Referral for education and counseling services

Education about transmission and partner or contact notification

Discussion of discrimination, social and psychological crisis needs

Review of immediate post-test counseling session plans for safety and confidentiality

Appointment for medical care

Adapted from McMahon, K. M. (1988). The integration of HIV testing and counseling into nursing practice. *Nursing Clinics of North America* 23(4); 814–815.

ENZYME-LINKED IMMUNOSORBENT ASSAY (ELISA)

ELISA for HIV antibody is a highly specific (98.6%) and highly sensitive (97.3%) test. It has become a useful screening tool for blood donors and populations at risk for AIDS and helps in diagnosing cases in which AIDS is suspected. When a person is adequately exposed to HIV, an antibody is made that is usually detectable by ELISA within 3 months of exposure. A positive result does not, however, mean that the person has AIDS. It is estimated that approximately 54% of all people who test positive for HIV antibody will develop AIDS within 10 years (Pedersen et al., 1989). The test is widely available through private physicians, health departments, clinics, and other health care providers.

WESTERN BLOT ANALYSIS

Because ELISA is very sensitive, a positive result is confirmed by several repetitions and by the more specific Western blot analysis. Western blot analysis detects various antibodies made in response to HIV proteins of particular molecular weights. A person who tests positive on both ELISA and Western blot analysis is believed to be infected and is considered infectious.

RAPID LATEX AGGLUTINATION ASSAY

Quinn and associates (1985) described a test for HIV antibodies that uses latex beads coated with a purified polypeptide (antigen CVre3) derived from the middle portion of the HIV envgenome. Human serum to be tested is diluted and mixed with a suspension latex antigen and allowed to react for 2 to 5 minutes. A positive reaction (presence of HIV antibodies) consists of agglutination that is visible in bright light, and a negative reaction reveals no such agglutination. Of 1220 laboratory-tested serum samples, the rapid latex agglutination assay was 99.3% sensitive and 100% specific compared with Western blot regardless of geographic location or clinical phase of HIV infection. Advantages include its rapid results and relative ease of performance. It is more likely to produce false positive results, however.

Rapid latex agglutination assay has been suggested for use in blood transfusion and organ donation screening programs for its quick results. Its most likely use occurs in developing countries where facilities capable of testing for HIV antibody are scarce, even in blood bank screening programs.

HIV Antigen Testing

Commercial tests are available to detect HIV p24 antigen in the serum, plasma, and cerebrospinal fluid of infected individuals as well as in the supernatant media of viral cultures. These assays also have clinical application in evaluating the virologic efficacy of antiretroviral therapy.

p24 Antigen Capture Assay. The p24 antigen capture assay is another test, used primarily by researchers, that measures the amount of p24, an actual piece of HIV referred to as core antigen. Monoclonal antibody to p24 is reacted with the patient's serum and will "capture" any p24 present. A second labeled antibody is then added to detect captured p24 through color change. Initial studies suggest that p24 antigenemia precedes the development of clinical symptoms or opportunistic infections and is associated with a depletion of T4 cells (Rosenberg and Fauci, 1989).

Assay for HIV Nucleic Acid. HIV nucleic acid may be the only molecular sign of infection in a number of circumstances: early in the HIV infection process during latency, when HIV replication occurs at a very low rate, or during infancy when maternally derived HIV antibody from an infected mother is present. Antibody tests are not capable of detecting these infections, HIV antigen assays are not sensitive enough, and cultures are limited by cost, training, and lack of mass application capability (Cohen et al., 1990).

POLYMERASE CHAIN REACTION

One disadvantage of the assays previously mentioned is that they test for HIV antibodies, not for the presence of the virus itself. An HIV-infected person may not produce detectable antibody levels

TABLE 54–8. Sexual Practice: Risk Categories for HIV Transmission

Safe	Moderate to Low	High Risk
Fantasy	French kissing	Unprotected anal receptive intercourse
Hugging	Cunnilingus	Unprotected vaginal intercourse
Massage	Fellatio with ingestion	Unprotected anal insertive intercourse
Social kissing	Fisting (manual-anal intercourse)	Blood contact during sex
Mutual masturbation	Intercourse using a latex condom	
Nonshared sex toys		

for at least 4 months, and HIV isolation methods require up to 3 or 4 weeks for a result. Detection of disease in such cases is possible by use of "gene amplification" techniques.

By means of a selective DNA amplification technique called the polymerase chain reaction (PCR), HIV proviral sequences can be identified directly in DNA isolated from peripheral blood mononuclear cells of seropositive persons (Ou et al., 1988). A single viral DNA molecule can be detected among a million white blood cells. Results are generally available within 3 days. Potential uses of PCR technology include HIV detection in research settings, for early diagnosis, or as a prognostic indicator (Cohen et al., 1990).

HIV Isolation and Culture Isolation

The first isolate of HIV was derived from in vitro cultures made from an individual with lymphadenopathy syndrome. Since then, HIV has been isolated from a wide variety of sources. It has been frequently obtained from human peripheral blood lymphocytes obtained from HIV seropositive individuals. Rarely, it has been isolated from seronegative individuals with a history of HIV exposure (Mayer et al., 1986). HIV has also been isolated from lymph nodes, serum, brain, saliva, semen, breast milk, urine, tears, cerebrospinal fluid, cervical secretions, pericardial and pleural fluids, and blood (McMahon and Sutterer, 1988).

Cultivation

HIV can be isolated through in vitro cultivation of suspected infected T-lymphocytes with the T-cell growth factor, interleukin-2 (IL-2). Fluid suspected of containing free HIV can be added to cultures of normal T-lymphocytes, which will replicate to provide progeny virus. A high ELISA antibody test result correlates best with viral culture isolation. The percentage of blood sample response to culture depends upon the clinical status of the source patient: 70% in AIDS or Kaposi's sarcoma patients and those with symptomatic but not frank AIDS versus 30% to 50% in AIDS or opportunistic infection patients or those who are asymptomatic HIV-positive. Most results are available in 3 weeks; however, certain body fluids,

including tears and cervical secretions, have cultured viruses at 60 days (Wofsky et al., 1986). Cultures cannot be used to quantify the extent of HIV infection because lymph nodes and other structures may harbor HIV, reflecting the true status of the disease not present in peripheral blood lymphocytes. Because of cost, laboratory skill, quality assurance, and time factors, viral isolation is not used to analyze large numbers of samples for general clinical use (Cohen et al., 1990).

MODES OF TRANSMISSION

Blood and blood products, semen, vaginal secretions, and breast milk have been linked to HIV transmission. Contact with saliva and tears containing HIV has not been shown to result in infection. HIV has not been documented to be transmitted by casual contact (Centers for Disease Control, 1988c). Exposure to the virus does not always result in infection.

Sexual Contact

HIV transmission through sexual contact occurs when infected semen, blood, or vaginal fluid is exchanged between partners. Posing the highest risk of infection is anal receptive intercourse followed by vaginal intercourse. Table 54–8 reviews sexual behaviors with categories of risk.

Risk is reduced through use of the latex condom. For the wearer, condoms provide a mechanical barrier limiting penile exposure to infectious cervical, vaginal, vulvar, or rectal secretions or lesions. For the wearer's partner, proper condom use should prevent semen deposition, contact with urethral discharge, and exposure to lesions on the head or shaft of the penis. Oil-based lubricants may make condoms ineffective, so should not be used. Water-soluble lubricants are considered safe. Natural membrane condoms (made from lamb cecum) contain small pores and do not block HIV passage in laboratory studies (Centers for Disease Control, 1988d).

The HIV virus is found in greater concentrations in semen than in vaginal fluids, which supports the hypothesis that transmission occurs more readily from male to female than from female to male. Animal studies have demonstrated infection occurring through vaginal and urethral viral swabs, thereby demonstrating that transmission can occur despite the lack of trauma.

Rates of sexual transmission vary among groups, reflecting the role of co-factors. Co-factors include sexually transmitted diseases, genital ulcerations, lack of circumcision, and use of oral contraceptives. Multiple partners and frequent exposure also raise the risk of transmission.

Abstinence from sexual intercourse is the sole safe way to prevent transmission. Over a period of time precautions tend to fail due to breakage of condoms or failure to maintain precautions. Sexual activity in a mutually monogamous relationship in which neither partner is HIV-infected and no other risk factors are present is considered safe.

Blood

It has been estimated that an HIV-infected drop of human blood contains 1 to 100 live virus particles. In comparison, a drop infected with hepatitis B virus has 100 million to 1 billion organisms (Favero, 1987). Even so, blood transmission of HIV does occur, primarily through sharing of contaminated needles among IV drug users and through blood transfusion. With the implementation in March 1985 of a donor screening program of the nation's blood supply, blood transfusion is now even safer; the current risk of transmission of AIDS through this route is estimated to be 1 in 100,000 to 1 in 1,000,000. It is possible that prior to blood screening implementation up to 12,000 persons were infected. A large percentage of hemophiliacs acquired HIV in this manner. Donor screening, HIV testing, and heat treatment of clotting factor have greatly reduced the risks. To further decrease the possibility of HIV transmission through transfusion of blood and blood products, patients scheduled to undergo elective surgery are increasingly advised to make predeposited blood donations for intraoperative autotransfusion.

Needlesticks and Splashes

Transmission due to occupational exposure of health care workers has occurred in needlestick accidents and blood splashes to the oral mucosa (McMahon and Sutterer, 1988). Needlestick is the most common route. Thousands of health care workers who were so exposed have been studied, and only about 20 cases of well-documented infection have been reported worldwide. The risk of infection through this route is estimated to be 0.02%, and every effort should be made to decrease the exposure rate. Educational efforts, implementation of engineering controls in needled and sharp-edged medical devices, the use of hard plastic needle disposal units where these devices are most frequently used, and the development of procedural details to avoid blood

and body fluid contact would greatly reduce the exposure rate (Jagger, 1990b). Health care workers must apply universal precautions to all activities to avoid contact with potentially HIV-infected human fluids. Safer medical equipment, particularly needled and sharp-edged devices, must be redesigned.

Needle-Sharing

Transmission of HIV among intravenous drug users (IVDUs) occurs primarily through contamination of injection paraphernalia with infected blood. Behaviors such as needle-sharing, "boosting" the injection with blood, using a shooting gallery, and performing frequent injections increase the risk. Sharing of equipment is common due to legal and financial restrictions and cultural norms. Geographically, the rate of infection varies: 80% of New York City addict needle-sharers are infected as opposed to much lower rates in other metropolitan area clusters. Secondary transmission occurs to women, children, and sexual partners.

Maternofetal Transmission

HIV is transmitted to infants by transplacental spread from mother to fetus in utero, during parturition, or through breast feeding after birth (Ziegler et al., 1985). Because infants have underdeveloped natural resistance systems, they are highly susceptible to many infections, including HIV. In vivo transmission is the most common route. Studies of infected mothers reflect a 0 to 65% rate of transmission with a mean about 30%. Both uninfected and infected infants have been born to mothers who have previously borne an infected infant. Though once hypothesized as probable, pregnancy has not been shown to accelerate the disease in the mother.

Artificial Insemination and Organ Transplantation

Because these procedures are much less common than other transmission-related activities, there have been very few case reports of HIV acquisition by this route. HIV has been transmitted via the kidneys, liver, heart, pancreas, bone, and, possibly, skin grafts and through artificial insemination (Osborn, 1986). HIV testing is used in these circumstances to rule out infection (Centers for Disease Control, 1988e).

NATURAL HISTORY AND CLASSIFICATION OF HIV INFECTION

The system of classification of HIV infection, which applies only to patients who have been diagnosed with the disease, divides manifestations of the disease into four mutually exclusive groups. The groups are not intended to have prognostic significance, nor do they indicate severity. They are hierarchical, however, in that persons classified in one group have met the criteria for the preceding group. Refer to Table 54–9 for a summary of the Centers for Disease Control classification system.

Group I: Acute HIV Infection

Group I includes patients who have signs and symptoms that appear transiently at the time of, or shortly after, the initial HIV laboratory diagnosis. All group I patients are reclassified into another group following resolution of the acute syndrome. Descriptions of illness include a mononucleosislike ailment lasting a few days to a few weeks, during which malaise, fever, a maculopapular rash, diarrhea, and lymphadenopathy predominate. One study (Pedersen et al., 1989) described a correlation between the length of the "seroconversion" illness and an accelerated progression along the spectrum of HIV infection. Of those with a primary illness of more than 14 days duration, 78% progressed to group IV of the CDC classification within 3 years. Of those with a minor illness, less than 10% progressed as fast.

Group II: Asymptomatic HIV Infection

Group II includes patients who have no signs or symptoms of HIV infection and have not had previous clinical findings that would classify them into group II or group IV. They may be subclassified on the basis of a laboratory evaluation that includes a complete blood count with differential white blood cell count and a platelet count. Immunologic tests, such as the T-lymphocyte helper and suppressor cell

---

TABLE 54–9. Summary of Classification System for Human Immunodeficiency Virus (HIV) Infection

Group I. Acute infection
Group II. Asymptomatic infection[a]
Group III. Persistent generalized lymphadenopathy[a]
Group IV. Other disease
  Subgroup A. Constitutional
  Subgroup B. Neurologic disease
  Subgroup C. Secondary infectious diseases
    Category C-1. Specified secondary infectious disease listed
                  in the CDC surveillance definitions for AIDS[b]
    Category C-2. Other specified secondary infectious diseases
  Subgroup D. Secondary cancers[b]
  Subgroup E. Other conditions

---

[a]Group II and III may be subclassified on the basis of a laboratory evaluation.
[b]Includes those patients whose clinical presentations fulfills the definitions of AIDS used by the CDC for national reporting.
From Centers for Disease Control. (1986). Classification system for human T-lymphotrophic virus III/lymphadenopathy associated virus infections. *Morbidity and Mortality Weekly Report*, 35, 335.

counts, are also an important part of the overall evaluation. Patients with test results that are within normal limits and those who have not yet had complete evaluations should be differentiated from patients whose test results are consistent with HIV-associated defects—lymphopenia, thrombocytopenia, and a decreased number of T-helper (T4) lymphocytes.

Group III: Persistent Generalized Lymphadenopathy

Group III includes patients with persistent generalized lymphadenopathy (PGL) but without further disease findings that would classify them into group IV. PGL is defined as palpable lymph node enlargement of 1 cm or greater at two or more extralinguinal sites that persists for more than 3 months in the absence of a concurrent illness or condition other than HIV infection to explain the findings.

Group IV: Other HIV Disease

Group IV disease includes patients with signs and symptoms of HIV infection other than or in addition to PGL. Patients are assigned to one or more subgroups based on the clinical findings. Subgroups include (a) constitutional disease; (b) neurologic disease; (c) secondary infectious disease; (d) secondary cancer; and (e) other conditions resulting from HIV infection. These subgroups are not hierarchical based on severity and are not mutually exclusive. Each subgroup may include patients who are minimally symptomatic as well as those who are severely ill.

Subgroup A: Constitutional Disease. Patients in this subgroup have one or more of the following: fever persisting more than 1 month, involuntary weight loss of greater than 10% of baseline, diarrhea persisting for more than 1 month, and an absence of a concurrent illness or condition other than HIV infection to explain the findings. The condition was formerly called AIDS-related complex, a term used infrequently now.

Subgroup B: Neurologic Disease. Patients in this subgroup have one or more of the following: dementia, myelopathy, or peripheral neuropathy and an absence of any concurrent illness or condition other than HIV to explain the findings.

Subgroup C: Secondary Infectious Diseases. Patients in this subgroup have been diagnosed with an infectious disease that is either associated with HIV infection or is at least moderately indicative of a defect in cell-mediated immunity. This subgroup is further divided into two categories.

Category C-1. This category includes patients with symptomatic or invasive signs of one of 12 specified secondary infectious diseases listed in the CDC surveillance definition of AIDS: *Pneumocystis carinii* pneumonia, chronic cryptosporidiosis, toxoplasmosis, extraintestinal strongyloidiasis, isosporiasis, candidiasis (esophageal, bronchial, or pulmonary), cryptococcosis, histoplasmosis, mycobacterial infection with *Mycobacterium avium* complex or *M. kansasii*, cytomegalovirus infection, chronic mucocutaneous or disseminated herpes simplex virus infection, and progressive multifocal leukoencephalopathy.

Category C-2. This category includes patients with symptomatic or invasive signs of one of six other specified secondary infectious diseases: oral hairy leukoplakia, multidermatomal herpes zoster, recurrent *Salmonella* bacteremia, nocardiosis, tuberculosis, or oral candidiasis (thrush).

Subgroup D: Secondary Cancers. Patients in this subgroup have been diagnosed with one or more kinds of cancer known to be associated with HIV infection as listed in the CDC surveillance definition of AIDS and at least moderately indicative of a defect in cell-mediated immunity: Kaposi's sarcoma, non-Hodgkin's lymphoma (small, noncleaved lymphoma or immunoblastic sarcoma), or primary lymphoma of the brain.

Subgroup E: Other Conditions in HIV Infections. Patients in this subgroup have other clinical findings or diseases, not classifiable above, that may be attributable to HIV infection or may be indicative of a defect in cell-mediated immunity. Included are patients with chronic lymphoid interstitial pneumonitis or those with other clinical illnesses whose course or management is complicated or altered by HIV, and patients with infectious diseases not listed in subgroup C or neoplasms not listed in subgroup D.

DEFINITION OF AIDS

The definition of AIDS has undergone several revisions as the clinical syndromes and diseases associated with HIV expanded. The latest definition is scheduled to go into effect in 1992. It labels AIDS patients as those HIV-infected individuals who have T4 cell counts of 200 or less. This change in definition may be delayed, since T4 cell studies are not readily available for all patients.

OPPORTUNISTIC ILLNESSES FREQUENTLY ASSOCIATED WITH AIDS

Opportunistic infections (OIs) are caused by a diverse spectrum of infectious agents that rarely cause disease in persons with normal intact immune systems. They reflect the specific immune defects

related to HIV, geographical clustering (i.e., New York City and tuberculosis, south central states and histoplasmosis), age-appropriate illnesses, a relationship to life-style, and an impressive consistency of the clinical presentations of certain infections. The morbidity and mortality of AIDS are chiefly an effect of the major OIs. The most common infections and malignancies are listed in Table 54–10.

Opportunistic Infections—Protozoal

***Pneumocystis carinii* pneumonia (PCP).** PCP is the most common opportunistic infection seen in patients with AIDS, occurring in at least 60% and recurring in many (Kovacs and Masur, 1988). Patients generally present with an insidious onset of fever, dyspnea on exertion, and a nonproductive cough. Respiratory rate is slightly increased, PA_{O_2} is decreased, and chest x-ray reveals diffuse interstitial infiltrates (Kovacs and Masur, 1988). A high degree of suspicion for PCP should accompany the clinical evaluation of any HIV-positive patient with fever and cough. Diagnosis is usually made from identification of pneumocysts from induced sputum specimens or from tissue examination following bronchoscopy with bronchial lavage and transbronchial biopsy.

With treatment, 72% of patients with AIDS with *P. carinii* infection survive their first episode. Without treatment, PCP can progress to a fulminant and life-threatening infection. This mortality risk has changed, however, as prevention efforts have improved and clinical treatment expertise has developed.

Early detection of PCP improves survival and the course of illness dramatically. AZT (zidovudine) and aerosolized pentamidine prophylaxis or sulfatrimethoprim (Bactrim) can greatly reduce the severity and

---

TABLE 54–10. Opportunistic Infections and Malignancies Commonly Associated with HIV Infection

A. Infections
  1. Protozoal
      a. *Pneumocystis carinii*
      b. *Toxoplasma gondii*
      c. *Cryptosporidium*
  2. Bacterial
      a. *Mycobacterium avium intracellulare*
      b. *M. tuberculosis*
  3. Fungal
      a. *Candida albicans*
      b. *Cryptococcus neoformans*
      c. *Histoplasma capsulatum*
  4. Viral
      a. Herpes simplex
      b. Varicella zoster
      c. Cytomegalovirus

B. Neoplastic diseases associated with HIV infections
  1. Kaposi's sarcoma
  2. Non-Hodgkin's lymphoma
  3. Primary central nervous system lymphoma

frequency of PCP. Most patients do require hospitalization for treatment with sulfatrimethoprim or pentamidine. Others can be successfully treated at home if the illness is caught early enough.

Toxoplasma gondii. Toxoplasmosis is a common source of CNS disease in patients with AIDS. Presenting symptoms include fever, headache, seizures, lethargy, and focal neurologic findings. Some patients have personality or cognitive changes (Kovacs and Masur, 1988). Diagnosis is usually difficult; however, most patients display multiple space-occupying lesions on brain CT scan (Kovacs and Masur, 1988). Definitive diagnosis is made upon brain biopsy of an accessible lesion and identification of the *Toxoplasma* trophozoite (Kovacs and Masur, 1988). Patients often require adjuvant therapy with Dilantin, folinic acid, and decadron. Clindamycin is used for patients who cannot tolerate sulfa drugs. Most patients respond well to therapy but need to be treated indefinitely.

A standard prophylactic therapy has not been established. Patients should avoid contact with cat feces and should cook meat well to avoid contact with *T. gondii* cysts if they have no serologic evidence of prior infection. Reactivation and dissemination of latent toxoplasmosis cannot yet be prevented.

Cryptosporidium. Cryptosporidiosis is an intestinal infection manifested by watery diarrhea that occasionally causes severe dehydration and wasting (Kovacs and Masur, 1988). Common symptoms include anorexia, malaise, weight loss, and abdominal cramping. Malabsorption is frequently present. No therapy has yet been shown to be consistently effective, and the AIDS patient with *Cryptosporidium* gastroenteritis is at great risk for severe weight loss, fluid and electrolyte imbalance, malnutrition, and debility.

The disease is highly infectious; it is transmitted from person to person or from animal to person and has an incubation period of 5 to 14 days. In AIDS patients, although cryptosporidiosis is typically associated with a severe, profuse, usually chronic diarrhea, the degree of symptomatology is highly variable. Symptoms of cryptosporidiosis can be exactly mimicked by another parasite, *Isoporra belli.*

Diagnosis is established through stool testing, biopsy of the large or small bowel, and serologic techniques. Response to treatment has been very poor. Treatment most often has been somewhat effective using spiramycin, trimethoprim-sulfamethoxazole, or SMS 201-995, a long-acting somatostatin analog. Supportive care, nutritional repletion, and hydration are used to combat the effects of cryptosporidiosis. There is currently no prophylactic therapy, and enteric precautions and infection control measures are the key to controlling nosocomial transmission. Cryptosporidiosis has been known to regress spontaneously as the patient's T-cells increase in number. Diarrheal disease can also be caused by other parasites, bacteria, and malabsorption (Kotler, 1989).

Mycobacterial Infections

MYCOBACTERIUM AVIUM–INTRACELLULARE

Infection with *Mycobacterium avium–intracellulare* (MAI) has developed in 50% of patients with AIDS (Gold and Armstrong, 1989) and is usually a disseminated disease. It occurs evenly in all risk groups and is a late complication of AIDS. Symptoms include fever, rigor, diarrhea, weight loss, and abdominal cramping. Enlarged lymph nodes and positive blood cultures indicate illness. Medical treatment with four or five drug regimens has been somewhat successful. Patients remain debilitated, however.

Patients are taught to refrain from cleaning fish tanks. Some physicians require patients even to avoid taking showers because the infection is thought to be aerosolized in water. The organism is ubiquitous. There is no evidence of human to human transmission.

MYCOBACTERIUM TUBERCULOSIS

One hundred years ago, tuberculosis (TB) was the leading cause of death from infectious diseases in America. Although evidence of TB has been found in neolithic and pre-Columbian skeletons (Des Prez and Heim, 1990), it was not until the crowded living conditions of the Industrial Revolution that transmission occurred so easily among the population. Treatment programs consisting of various pulmonary surgeries, prolonged rest, and fresh air were implemented, and sanitariums to house sick TB patients were developed. With the advent of INH in 1952, the rate of TB infection declined substantially. It was even anticipated that TB might be eradicated. However, since the mid-1980s there has been a rise in the anticipated number of cases. This infection rate is fueled by poverty, the immigration of people from endemic areas, and underlying HIV infection.

Mycobacterium tuberculosis is an aerobic, obligate parasitic, acid-fast bacillus. Infection is spread by inhalation of droplet nuclei, which are produced when the source patient talks, coughs, or sneezes. A cough can produce 3000 infectious droplet nuclei, and particles remain suspended in the air for a long time (Des Prez and Heim, 1990). Infection occurs when inhaled particles settle in the peripheral lung and multiply. Chance and the underlying diseases of malnutrition, alcoholism, HIV, and immunologic disorders combined with long-term exposure create a high-risk situation. In HIV-infected patients, most new cases reflect reactivation of a latent infection, but the risk of progression to clinical illness is greater. Secondary spread of infection occurs among social contacts of these patients and others who share their air space.

Because AIDS patients may become anergic, Mantoux testing for TB should be done early in the course of the patient's disease. The clinical presentation of tuberculosis (afternoon fevers, weight loss, cough, fatigue, night sweats) is hard to distinguish from that of other HIV-related ailments. In AIDS patients extrapulmonary sites of TB can be common; these include lymph nodes, bones, genitourinary tract, miliary sites, and bone marrow. Diagnosis is usually made from the Mantoux test, chest x-ray, and sputum cultures for acid-fast-bacillus in a patient with clinically suspicious signs. HIV patients with TB need to be treated more aggressively and for a longer period of time than non-HIV infected patients.

Infection control efforts are challenged by the presence of droplet nuclei in the area (Nardell, 1990) and by the fact that a laboratory may take 6 to 8 weeks to culture the TB organism. Use of disposable particulate respirators, engineering controls in room design, ultraviolet lighting, air ducts, room air flow, and cough suppression or avoidance mechanisms is critical. Case finding in HIV-infected patients with early therapy is very important (Ungvarski, 1990). Additionally, interventions that assist patients to comply with the prolonged treatment regimen are necessary. Failure to take medication as prescribed permits development of resistant strains of TB that may be lethal (Division of Tuberculosis Control et al., 1990).

Fungal Infections

CANDIDIASIS

Candida albicans is the most common fungal infection in AIDS patients. The fungus is a commensal organism that in humans exists in the gastrointestinal tract, the female genital tract, the oropharynx, and on diseased skin. Most AIDS patients develop *Candida* infection, although the exact relationship of this organism to T-cell depletion is not understood. Patients develop mucocutaneous disease that is rarely systemic.

Thrush is characterized by creamy, curdlike patches on the tongue and buccal mucosa. Diagnosis is established by inspection and oral scrapings treated with potassium oxide. Clotrimazole troches, nystatin, and ketoconazole are used medically for treatment.

Candidal esophagitis should be suspected in AIDS patients with thrush, odynophagia, and substernal chest pain. It is usually diagnosed presumptively by contrast radiology, and definitely by esophagoscopy. Other infectious agents can cause esophagitis (herpes, CMV). Candidal esophagitis is often difficult to treat. Topical antifungals, troches, and suspensions may fail because swallowing does not allow sufficient time for the antifungal agent to act on the esophageal infection. Oral ketoconazole is often needed. Patients at times require low-dose treatment with amphotericin B.

CRYPTOCOCCOSIS

Cryptococcosus neoformans occurs in about 7% of AIDS patients (Kovacs and Masur, 1988), meningitis being the most common presentation. In the normal host, the initial pulmonary infection is usually asymptomatic. The onset of cryptococcal meningitis in AIDS patients is usually subtle with nonspecific complaints of fever, headache, nausea, vomiting, and malaise. The headache is usually frontal or temporal, and close associates of the patient notice subtle personality and behavioral changes.

Diagnosis is established by detection of fungal infection in CSF fluid, detection of cryptococcal antigen, or fungal culture. Treatment is fluconazole or amphotericin B. Relapse is so common that continued suppressive therapy is warranted.

Viral Infections

HERPES SIMPLEX VIRUS

Most herpes simplex virus (HSV) infections in AIDS patients are reactivations of latent infection. The principal mode of transmission is contact with oral secretions (for HSV-1) or genital secretions (for HSV-2). HSV-1 can occur in the genital or perirectal area by means of oral-sexual contact or by autoinoculation (hands). The same is true of HSV-2 if it occurs orally. Higher rates of HSV-2 infection are seen in patients with higher numbers of sexual partners, in prostitutes, with lack of condom use, in adults of lower socioeconomic class, in persons attending sexually transmitted disease clinics, and in homosexual men (Corey and Spear, 1986).

After the initial HSV infection resolves, it becomes dormant within the nerve ganglia. The severity of an acute attack of reactivated infection is related to the patient's degree of immunosuppression. Oral and labial infections may be mild or may involve pain, fever, and cervical lymphadenopathy. Illness in a patient with HIV infection may last for weeks. Genital or perianal lesions also demonstrate a prolonged healing time and carry a risk of dissemination. Intervention in the form of topical, oral, or intravenous acyclovir is initiated when the prodromal symptoms of burning, tingling, and itching begin. Lesions usually occur in the same place as the prior infection. A rare presentation of HSV in AIDS patients is acute encephalitis. Mental status change, fever, headache, and nausea are associated with it. A diagnosis of HSV is made by culture of the lesion. If acyclovir treatment fails, vidarabine or foscarnet is used.

HERPES ZOSTER

The development of herpes zoster (shingles) may signal the progression of HIV illness in an HIV-infected patient. Herpes zoster produces characteristic painful, red lesions in the skin region of the affected dermatome. Disseminated lesions may appear in the hands and feet. A biopsy to establish the diagnosis is usually not needed, and treatment with intravenous acyclovir is begun. Strict isolation, avoidance of infection, and measures to prevent dissemination and afford pain relief are implemented quickly.

CYTOMEGALOVIRUS

CMV, like the herpes family viruses, begins with an initial infection (though it is often unnoticed), and a life-long infection, though usually dormant, results. CMV causes disease by directly destroying organ tissue, impairing immunologic responses, and aiding neoplastic transformation. The initial infection is usually a result of in vitro birth canal or breast milk infection, childhood contact with other children who are infected (via respiratory secretions), or sexual intercourse (vaginal or anal).

In AIDS patients, CMV is the most common opportunistic pathogen detected at autopsy. It causes over 95% of the chorioretinitis seen in AIDS patients. The patient complains of blurred vision, decreased visual acuity, or floaters. Intravenous ganciclovir is used as a suppressive therapy in patients with sight-threatening CMV retinitis. Neutropenia is a common dose-limiting toxic reaction. In some cases, intravitreal injections are used instead with good results (Heinemann, 1989). In 1991, foscarnet was also made available as a treatment. Foscarnet does not cause neutropenia, but renal toxicity is a common side effect.

CMV also infects and affects all parts of the gastrointestinal tract. CMV colitis is associated with weight loss, anorexia, fever, and diarrhea (Kotler et al., 1991). Kotler and colleagues (1989) found that intravenous ganciclovir treatment for CMV colitis repleted body cell mass and body fat, raised the serum albumin level, and allowed patients to gain weight.

CMV pneumonia most frequently occurs in the setting of other pneumonias concurrently with another pneumonia.

PROGRESSIVE MULTIFOCAL LEUKOENCEPHALOPATHY

Progressive multifocal leukoencephalopathy (PML) is a subacute demyelinating disease of the central nervous system. Multiple lesions develop in the white matter of the cerebrum, brain stem, or cerebellum, resulting in focal neurologic deficits. The disease progresses rapidly to dementia with blindness and paralysis. Death usually occurs within 1 year.

PML is caused by infection with the JC virus, named after the first patient diagnosed with the illness. By adulthood most persons are infected. It is

not clear whether PML in AIDS patients is a reactivation of a latent infection or a newly acquired infection. Only 1% of all AIDS patients have been diagnosed with PML.

Initial symptoms of extremity weakness, gait disturbance, speech disturbance, and visual loss are compounded by altered mentation. A diagnosis is established by a brain biopsy, although magnetic resonance imaging, CT scans, electroencephalography, and other studies to rule out CNS lymphoma, toxoplasmosis, and cryptococcal meningitis contribute heavily to the diagnosis. There is no clear treatment.

Malignancies

KAPOSI'S SARCOMA

Kaposi's sarcoma (KS) is the most common type of malignancy seen in AIDS patients. It occurred in approximately 30% of all AIDS patients diagnosed in 1981 but now occurs in 10% of patients at the time of AIDS diagnosis. Before AIDS was discovered, forms of KS had occurred in various clinical settings. The disease was first described in an 1872 report published by Dr. Moriz Kaposi entitled "Idiopathic multiple pigmented sarcoma of the skin" (Friedman-Kien et al., 1989). The original disease described by Kaposi is referred to as classic KS, whereas many other authors have described an indolent disease mainly confined to the lower extremities and frequently occurring in men from the Mediterranean area (Friedman-Kien et al., 1989; Volberding, 1990).

In 1984 Breimer reviewed the original paper and uncovered striking similarities between this "classic" KS and our "epidemic" KS (usually described as being much more aggressive and largely affecting the gastrointestinal tract, skin, and upper extremities). According to Breimer's review, Kaposi described an incurable, rapidly lethal (death within 2 to 3 years) generalized illness composed of lesions affecting the gastrointestinal tract and liver. Before the era of AIDS, KS was considered very rare, and most cases were distinctly clustered among the following groups: elderly men of Mediterranean or eastern European Jewish descent, young black males and children in equatorial Africa, and organ transplant patients who receive immunosuppressive therapy.

KS is believed to originate from the endothelial cell wall. There has been extensive investigation into the possible co-factors (nitrite inhalers, CMV, genetic factors, other infectious agents) that may predispose an HIV-infected person to develop KS. The latest medical thinking is that KS is caused by an as yet unidentified sexually transmitted agent. Although in this country KS is firmly associated with men who have sex with men (MWHSWM), primarily in California and New York, it also occurs commonly in adults who acquire HIV heterosexually in Puerto

Rico, Haiti, Mexico, Central America, and Africa. Women who acquire HIV heterosexually from men who have sex with men have a fourfold incidence of KS compared to women who acquire HIV from heterosexual partners (Beral et al., 1990). Friedman-Kien and co-workers (1990) even reported KS in six homosexual men without HIV. Kumar and associates (1989) reported a fatal case of KS in a white heterosexual male without HIV.

KS generally develops in multicentric fashion in asymptomatic nodules, which range in color from red-brown to violet, pink, and dark purple. KS invades other organs besides the skin. The most common extracutaneous sites are the gastrointestinal tract, lymph nodes, and lungs. KS causes both structural and functional damage, with internal organ involvement signaled by weight loss, emaciation, hemorrhage, and diarrhea (Safai, 1989).

When KS is localized to the skin, cryosurgery, laser therapy, and surgical excision have been used, but radiotherapy is the most promising treatment (Myskowski, 1989). Radiotherapy is also useful for palliative or cosmetic purposes. Various chemotherapy regimens and zidovudine with interferon have also been used.

NON-HODGKIN'S LYMPHOMA

The case definition of AIDS was expanded in 1987 to include patients with HIV who have an intermediate or high-grade lymphoma. In patients with AIDS, the lymphoma is usually of B-cell origin. Approximately 4% to 10% of all AIDS patients develop lymphoma (Levine, 1988). The earliest sign is usually a unilateral, painless, enlarged lymph node. As the condition progresses, it spreads through the lymphatic channels to nearby nodes and organ systems, especially the spleen, liver, gastrointestinal tract, skin, lungs, CNS, and bone marrow. Fevers, weight loss, and night sweats commonly occur.

A biopsy of affected tissue clearly makes the diagnosis. Patients with persistent generalized lymphadenopathy (PGL) have an 850-fold rate of lymphoma based upon incidence rates in America, age adjusted for lymphoma. Because of this, PGL patients should have serial biopsies to monitor for malignant conversion.

Much of the non-Hodgkin's lymphoma that occurs in AIDS patients is confined to the central nervous system. The most frequent presenting symptoms are hemiparesis, aphasia, seizures, cranial nerve palsies, and headache (Kaplan, 1990). The second most common site is the gastrointestinal tract, with tumors arising in the mouth, esophagus, stomach, duodenum, and other sites. Bone marrow involvement is also commonly seen.

Staging of the illness requires bone marrow aspiration and biopsy bilaterally, lumbar puncture, chest x-ray, CT scans of the chest and abdomen, and assorted blood work. Treatment is initiated with intent to cure. Lymphoma is very responsive to chemotherapy, but if the patient has had a prior opportunistic infection, control or palliation can be the only realized goal. A rapid remission can be achieved, but neutropenia may delay subsequent courses of therapy. Colon-stimulating factors are used to combat this time loss. Successful treatment has been associated with methotrexate, bleomycin, doxorubicin, cytoxan, vincristine, and dexamethasone (M-BACOD modified).

HIV-RELATED CONDITIONS
Wasting Syndrome

Wasting syndrome in patients with HIV-related disease has a myriad of presentations because there are several mechanisms by which persons with HIV disease might become malnourished, including oral lesions that affect food intake, carcinomatosis, disseminated infections, and, possibly, endocrine malfunction (Moore, 1991). Studies have shown that protein-energy malnutrition (PEM) is a common problem in patients with AIDS (Kotler et al., 1985). Deficiencies in macronutrients and micronutrients have adverse effects upon immunologic function, and studies have strongly suggested that the timing of death may be influenced by the extent of tissue depletion (Kotler et al., 1989b). The debilitation caused by starving and malnutrition probably also contributes to hospitalization, diminished quality of life, poor functional living habits, and absence of clear mentation.

Several studies have documented the ability of malnourished AIDS patients to be repleted (Kotler et al., 1989a; Tierney et al., 1991; Von Roenn et al., 1991). Repletion has been successful using various methods depending on the reason for the malnutrition. Home total parenteral nutrition, home enteral feedings through a percutaneous feeding tube, oral diet change to an elemental diet if the patient is a malabsorber, use of megace to stimulate appetite, and aggressive counseling by a dietitian early in the course of illness are among the methods that have been used successfully. A key consideration is that, in the presence of an active opportunistic infection, most forms of nutritional support will not lead to nutritional repletion. If the patient is put into a positive caloric balance, the excess calories are deposited as fat, not protein (Moore, 1991). The point is that AIDS patients require aggressive evaluation and prompt treatment of opportunistic diseases (Task Force on Nutritional Support in AIDS, 1989). Innovative therapies such as intralesional and oral steroid therapy for CMV esophageal ulcers and thorough examinations to detect the parasite causing enteropathy are necessary. HIV patients should have routine consultations with a dietitian.

Feeding the patient enterally or parenterally may also slow the psychomotor retardation seen in these patients. It is possible that some of the slowing of thought processes thought to be related to a patient's dementia or CNS infection may be a profound effect of malnutrition on personality (Moore, 1991).

Presently, the tools needed to evaluate nutritional status in ill patients are lacking. Weight can be confounded by hydration; caliper skinfold measurements do not have generalized inter-rater reliability and take time; caloric counts measuring intake do not provide data on a patient's use of the calories to make protein stores. Body cell mass can be estimated by determining body potassium content, nitrogen content, and total body water. However, these calculations are not widely available. Newer equipment such as the portable Xitron-4000 multifiguring bioelectrical impedance analyzer, which can measure fat-free mass and estimate total body water, could provide this clinical information.

A few years ago, AIDS patients were not placed on total parenteral nutrition for several reasons: fear of line sepsis, fear of not being able to stop treatment once it was started, and judgments about prolonging life. Now there is a much more aggressive effort to feed patients as developments in long-term venous access, patient and physician contracts on treatment goals, and longer life expectancy have been achieved. This development, coupled with more treatment options for opportunistic infections and a growing sophistication about nutritional support for patients with HIV illness (Bradley-Springer, 1991), has wrought substantial change in a few short years.

AIDS Dementia Complex

At least 65% of AIDS patients undergo clinically significant progressive dementia (Navia, Jordan and Price, 1986) and changes consistent with dementia are present in 90% of autopsied patients (de la Monte, 1987). AIDS dementia complex (ADC) is thought to be a direct result of HIV infection of the brain. Although the brain is infected by HIV from the time of the patient's initial seroconversion from HIV neg-

TABLE 54–11. Major Signs and Symptoms of AIDS Dementia Complex

Early	Late
Cognitive	Cognitive
Impaired concentration	Global dementia
"Memory loss"	Confusion
Mental slowing	Disorientation
	Disinhibition
Motor	Motor
Unsteady gait	Paralysis
Loss of coordination	Hemiparesis
Tremor	Incontinence
Leg weakness	Psychomotor slowing
Behavioral	Behavioral
Apathy	Mutism
"Depression"	
Withdrawal	
Hallucinations (rare)	

TABLE 54–12. Staging System for AIDS Dementia Complex

Stage	Features
0	Normal function
0.5	Equivocal or subclinical
1	Mild Able to work and perform activities of daily living Unequivocal evidence of functional, intellectual, or motor impairment
2	Moderate Able to do basic self-care Unable to work or maintain more demanding activities of daily living Ambulatory
3	Severe Major cognitive and motor incapacity
4	Nearly vegetative

ative to HIV positive, patients are asymptomatic until their T4 cell levels drop. ADC may be the first manifestation of AIDS but usually occurs with other AIDS-defining ailments. It is a progressive disease that waxes and wanes. Table 54–11 lists the major signs and symptoms, and Table 54–12 highlights the functional staging system. A battery of neuropsychiatric tests labels the deficits that are not adequately assessed by the standard minimental status examination. Sensitive neuropsychiatric tests include the timed gait test and the nondominant finger tapping test.

Not all patients develop moderate to severe dementia. Patients who have clinical symptoms have improved on antiretroviral therapy such as zidovudine and psychostimulants.

PATIENT CARE PLANNING

The care of HIV-infected patients is complex and multifaceted. Patients exhibit a myriad of diseases and symptoms related to HIV itself and to the multiple infections, cancers, and conditions associated with it. Tables 54–13 through 54–15 provide highlights of selected care considerations.

SUMMARY

This chapter has outlined the historical development of HIV, its definition, classification system, testing, and many manifestations. It is an evolving illness, epidemic in nature, requiring tremendous financial, research, care, and social resources. Imposing a relentless assault on the immune system, its attacks become ever stronger if it is given time to ravage—physically, psychologically, financially, and socially—the diseased person and those he loves. The human toll cannot be adequately conveyed. However, many patients are living well and living longer. Much of this benefit is due to devoted

Text continued on page 1162

TABLE 54–13. Health Appraisal Specific for HIV Infection and Related Illnesses

A. Social history
    1. Sexual activities
        a. Absolutely safe behavior: abstinence or mutually monogamous with a noninfected partner
        b. Very safe behavior: noninsertive sexual practices
        c. Probably safe behavior: insertive sexual practices with the use of condoms and spermicide
        d. Risky behavior: everything else
        e. Use of condoms including application, removal, and use of lubricants
        f. Engaging in sex with multiple partners
        g. Use of mood-affecting drugs before sexual activities
        h. Whether AIDS has developed in anyone with whom client has had sex
    2. Use of mood-affecting drugs
        a. Drugs such as alcohol, marijuana, cocaine, crack, LSD, Quaalude, amphetamines, barbiturates, tranquilizers, amyl or butyl nitrate (called "poppers"), heroin
        b. Route of administration: oral, inhalation (including sniffing, snorting, and smoking), intravenous
        c. Any current or previous treatment for substance abuse
    3. Needle exposure
        a. Use of drugs via intravenous route, sharing of needles, syringes, and other drug paraphernalia
        b. Other needle-exposure activities such as tattoos, acupuncture, treatment by unlicensed individuals or "folk doctors," or sharing prescribed drugs between friends
        c. Whether AIDS has developed in anyone with whom client has shared needles
    4. Occupational history
        a. Client's occupation and responsibilities in relation to risk potential for HIV exposure
        b. Whether client has experienced any exposures
        c. What type of health care follow-up the client has pursued since exposure
        d. Client's knowledge level regarding the signs and symptoms or seroconversion and need for follow-up
    5. Travel
        a. Within the past 10 years
        b. Sexual activities when traveling in areas where the number of AIDS cases is high, such as New York, California, New Jersey, Texas, Florida, or countries such as Haiti or Zaire
B. Medication history: Current or previous use of medication that suppresses the immune system, such as steroids; current treatment for drug addiction if applicable
C. Medical history
    1. Major disease including (but not limited to) tuberculosis; hepatitis A or B or non A/B; mononucleosis; and hemophilia; receiving treatment with clotting replacements such as factor VIII
    2. Treatment for psychiatric or emotional disorders
    3. Transfusion donor or recipient
D. Surgical history
E. Childhood illnesses, including but not limited to varicella
F. Sexually transmitted diseases (STDs), including (but not limited to) syphilis; gonorrhea; amebiasis; herpes simplex (oralis or genitalis); *Giardia lamblia* enteritis, and lymphogranuloma venereum
G. Review of systems
    1. General: a comment from the client concerning a self-appraisal of current state of health should be elicited
    2. Skin: eruptions, lesions, itching, dryness, redness, rashes, lumps, color changes, changes in hair or nails
    3. Head: headaches, lightheadedness, or other sensations
    4. Eyes: blurred vision or diploplia
    5. Ears: impaired hearing or tinnitus
    6. Nose and sinuses: obstruction, pain, discharges, or nosebleed
    7. Mouth and throat: creamy white patches, lesions, bleeding gums, dysphagia, odynophagia, changes in taste, or sore throat
    8. Respiratory: dyspnea with or without certain activities, coughing, wheezing, chest pain, "cold" or "flulike" symptoms, as well as the date of last chest x-ray examination and tuberculin test and results
    9. Cardiovascular: chest pain, palpitations, edema, and known hypertension or hypotension
   10. Gastrointestinal: changes in appetite, involuntary weight loss, abdominal pain or cramping, changes in bowel habits, diarrhea, blood in stool, rectal or perianal pain or itching
   11. Genitourinary: dysuria, nocturia, pain, itching, discharges, or lesions
   12. Gynecologic: changes in menstruation, dyspareunia, vaginal discharge, breast problems, obstetrical history, and contraception
   13. Musculoskeletal: arthralgia or myalgia
   14. Neurologic and emotional: problems with memory, nervousness, personality changes, confusional states, stiff neck, photophobia, tremors, paresthesias, seizures, or syncope
   15. Endrocrine: polyuria, polyphagia, polydipsia, fevers, or night sweats
   16. Hematopoietic: lymphadenopathy, bruising or bleeding, history of anemia

TABLE 54–13. Health Appraisal Specific for HIV Infection and Related Illnesses Continued

A. Neurologic examination
   1. Cerebral functions: impaired cognitive functions, decreased level of consciousness, anger, inattentiveness, depression, denial
   2. Cranial nerve (CN) examination
      a. CN II (optic nerve): papilledema, cotton-wool patches (exudate); visual field deficiencies, blurred vision
      b. CNs III, IV, VI (oculomotor, trochlear, abducens nerves): impaired extraocular movements, unequal pupils, diplopia, ptosis, nystagmus
      c. CN V (trigeminal nerve): photophobia
      d. CN VII (facial nerve): hemiparesis
      e. CN VIII (acoustic nerve): tinnitus, vertigo, impaired hearing
      f. CNs IX, X (glossopharyngeal and vagus nerves): dysphagia, dysarthria
   3. Motor examination: hemiparesis, paraparesis
   4. Sensory examination: dysesthesias, paresthesia, areas of anesthesia
   5. Cerebellar examination: ataxia, dysmetria, intention tremors
   6. Reflexes: abnormal reflexes, positive Babinski's sign
   7. Meningeal signs: nuchal rigidity, Brudzinski's sign, Kernig's sign
B. Mouth and throat examination: lesions, discoloration, exudates
C. Cardiovascular examination
   1. Heart: disturbances in cardiac rate, rhythm and presence of pericardial friction rub
   2. Peripheral vascular: edema, decrease in peripheral pulse(s)
D. Respiratory examination: tachypnea, lag of excursion on palpation, dullness to percussion, presence of rales (crackles) or rhonchi (wheezes)
E. Lymphatic examination: lymphadenopathy
F. Abdominal examination: masses, tenderness, hepatomegaly, splenomegaly, hyperactive bowel sounds
G. Examination of genitalia and perianal region: lesions or discharges
H. Musculoskeletal examination: pain on range of motion
I. Skin examination
   1. Lesions or discolorations
   2. Dryness
   3. Thinning of hair or alopecia

From Ungvarski, P. J. (1992). Nursing management of the adult client. In J. H. Flaskerud and P. J. Ungvarski (Eds.), *HIV/AIDS: A guide to nursing care* (2nd ed., pp. 149–151). Philadelphia: W. B. Saunders.

TABLE 54–14. Drugs Used to Treat HIV Infection and AIDS-related Conditions

Generic Name (Trade Name)	Route of Administration	Indications	Side/Adverse Effects
*Adenine arabinoside (Vidarabine) (Vira-A)	IV	Herpes simplex virus infection, herpes zoster infection, progressive multifocal leukoencephalopathy, varicella infection	Anorexia, nausea, vomiting, diarrhea, tremors, dizziness, confusion, hallucinations, ataxia, psychosis, leukopenia, thrombocytopenia, elevated SGOT and bilirubin levels, anemia
Amikacin (Amikin)	IV, IM	*Mycobacterium avium* complex infection	Increase/decrease in frequency of urination or amount of urine, increased thirst, loss of appetite, nausea, vomiting, muscle twitching, numbness, tingling, any loss of hearing, ringing or buzzing, clumsiness, dizziness, unsteadiness, difficulty in breathing
Amphotericin B (Fungizone)	IV	Candidiasis, coccidioidomycosis, cryptococcosis, histoplasmosis	Fever, chills, hypokalemia (irregular heartbeat, muscle cramps or pain, extreme fatigue), pain at site of infusion, anemia, blurred or double vision, renal failure (increased or decreased urination), paresthesias, impaired hearing, tinnitus, seizures, shortness of breath, skin rash or itching, agranulocytosis or leukopenia, thrombocytopenia
Ampicillin (Omnipen) (Omnipen-N) (Polycillin) (Polycillin-N) (Principen) (Totacillin) (Totacillin-N)	PO, IM, IV	Salmonellosis	Anaphylaxis, serum sickness, neutropenia, platelet count dysfunction, skin rash, fever, hives, itching, pseudomembranous colitis, seizures, diarrhea, nausea, vomiting, thrush, abdominal pain or cramps
*AS-101	IV	HIV infection	Garlic smell of breath, rash, nausea, vomiting, diarrhea, lightening of hair color, Stevens-Johnson syndrome
Azidouridine (AzdU)	PO	HIV infection	Nausea, headaches, leukopenia
Bleomycin (Blenoxane)	IV	Kaposi's sarcoma, non-Hodgkin's lymphoma	Cough, shortness of breath, pneumonitis, fever, chills, stomatitis, confusion, syncope, diaphoresis, changes in skin color and texture, rashes, swelling of fingers, nausea, vomiting and anorexia, weight loss, hair loss
*CD4, recombinant soluble (Receptin)	IV, IM	HIV infection	Local reactions at injection site, fever
Chloramphenicol (Anocol) (Chloromycetin)	PO, IM, IV	Salmonellosis	Blood dyscrasias, abdominal distention, blue-gray skin color, low body temperature, difficulty breathing, coma, cardiovascular collapse, skin rash, fever, confusion, delirium, headache, loss of vision, paresthesias, extremity weakness, diarrhea, nausea, vomiting, pale skin, sore throat, bleeding
Ciprofloxacin (Cipro)	PO	*Mycobacterium avium* complex infection	Restlessness, tremors, seizures, crystalluria (blood in urine, dysuria, low back pain), skin rash, itching, redness, swelling of face or neck, joint pains, stiffness, visual disturbances, photosensitivity, dizziness, headache, abdominal pain, diarrhea, nausea, vomiting, insomnia, unpleasant taste in mouth
Clindamycin (Cleocin)	PO, IM, IV	Toxoplasmosis, pneumocystosis	Pseudomembranous colitis, skin rash, neutropenia, thrombocytopenia, abdominal pain, nausea and vomiting, diarrhea, fungal overgrowth

TABLE 54–14. Drugs Used to Treat HIV Infection and AIDS-related Conditions Continued

Generic Name (Trade Name)	Route of Administration	Indications	Side/Adverse Effects
Clofazimine (Lamprene)	PO	*Mycobacterium avium* complex infection	Colicky or burning abdominal or stomach pain, nausea, vomiting, pink or red to brownish black discoloration of skin (two suicides have been reported as a result of mental depression secondary to skin discoloration), visual changes, gastrointestinal bleeding, hepatitis or jaundice, dry rough scaly skin, anorexia, dizziness, drowsiness, dryness, burning, itching or irritation of eyes, skin rash, photosensitivity
Clotrimazole (Mycelex Troches)	PO	Candidiasis (oropharyngeal)	Abdominal or stomach cramping or pain, diarrhea, nausea or vomiting
Cyclophosphamide (Cytoxan) (Neosar)	PO, IM, IV	Non-Hodgkin's lymphoma	Missing menstrual cycles, darkening of skin and fingernails, loss of appetite, nausea, vomiting, diarrhea, stomach pain, flushing and redness of face, headache, increased sweating, swollen lips, skin rash, hives, loss of hair
Cycloserine (Seromycin)	PO	*Mycobacterium avium* complex infection, *Mycobacterium tuberculosis*	Anxiety, confusion, dizziness, drowsiness, increased irritability, increased restlessness, mental depression, muscle twitching or trembling, nervousness, nightmares, other mood or mental changes, speech problems, skin rash, numbness, tingling or burning pain or weakness in the hands or feet, headache, seizures
Cytarabine (Ara-C) (Cytosine arabinoside) (Cytosar-U)	PO, IM, IV	Non-Hodgkin's lymphoma, progressive multifocal leukoencephalopathy	Fever, chills, cough, hoarseness, lower back/side pain, difficult urination, diarrhea, sores in mouth or on lips, unusual bleeding/bruising, numbness or tingling in fingers, toes, or face, unusual tiredness, swelling of feet or lower legs, pain at injection site, skin rash, reddened eyes, chest pain, shortness of breath, itching of skin, headache
Dapsone (Avlosulfon) (DDS)	PO	Pneumocystosis	Hemolytic anemia, Stevens-Johnson syndrome, agranulocytosis (fever and sore throat), hepatic damage, methemoglobinemia (bluish fingernails, lips, or skin, fatigue, dyspnea), mood changes, peripheral neuritis
*Didanosine (formerly known as ddI) (Videx)	PO	HIV infection	Diarrhea, abdominal pain, pancreatitis, peripheral neuropathy, seizures, headaches, abnormal bone marrow function, abnormal liver function, electrolyte abnormalities, cardiac arrhythmias, allergic reactions
*Didehydrodide-oxythymidine (d4T)	PO	HIV infection	Peripheral neuropathy, elevated liver function tests, headaches, nausea
*Dideoxycytidine (ddC)	PO	HIV infection	Peripheral neuropathy, oral aphthous ulcers, fever, rash, stomatitis
*Diethyldithiocarbamate (DTC) (Imuthiol)	PO, IV	Immunomodulation	Metallic taste, abdominal pain, fatigue, nausea, inability to concentrate, increased energy levels after IV infusion, Antabuse-like effect when alcohol is ingested
Doxorubicin hydrochloride (Adriamycin)	IV	Kaposi's sarcoma, non-Hodgkin's lymphoma	Leukopenia or infection (fever, chills, sore throat), stomatitis, esophagitis, flank, stomach, or joint pain, pain at infusion site, peripheral edema, fast or irregular heartbeat, shortness of breath, gastrointestinal bleeding, thrombocytopenia (unusual bleeding or bruising), changes in skin color, diarrhea, nausea, vomiting, skin rash or itching, hair loss, reddish color to urine

Table continued on following page

TABLE 54–14. Drugs Used to Treat HIV Infection and AIDS-related Conditions Continued

Generic Name (Trade Name)	Route of Administration	Indications	Side/Adverse Effects
*Eflornithine hydrochloride (DFMO) (Ornidyl)	PO, IV	Cryptosporidiosis, pneumocystosis	Diarrhea, thrombocytopenia, anemia, hearing loss
Epoetin alfa, recombinant (Epogen) (Eprex) (Procrit)	IV, SC	Anemia associated with HIV infection or zidovudine therapy	Chest pain, edema, tachycardia, headache, hypertension, polycythemia, seizures, shortness of breath, skin rash, arthralgias, asthenia, diarrhea, nausea, fatigue, influenza-like syndrome after each dose. NOTE: should be temporarily discontinued if the hematocrit reaches or exceeds 36%
Ethambutol (Myambutol)	PO	*Mycobacterium avium* complex infection, *Mycobacterium tuberculosis*	Acute gout, chills, pain and swelling of joints, skin rash, fever, arthralgias, numbness, tingling, burning pain, weakness of hands/feet, blurred vision, eye pain, red-green color blindness, any loss of vision, abdominal pain, anorexia, nausea, vomiting, headache, mental confusion
Ethionamide (Trecator-SC)	PO	*Mycobacterium avium* complex infection, *Mycobacterium tuberculosis*	Yellow skin/eyes, tingling, burning or pain in hands or feet, mental depression, clumsiness/unsteadiness, confusion, mood or mental changes, changes in menstrual periods, coldness, decreased sexual ability, dry puffy skin, weight gain, hyperglycemia, blurred vision or loss of vision, skin rash
Etoposide (VePesid)	IV	Kaposi's sarcoma, non-Hodgkin's lymphoma	Leukopenia, thrombocytopenia, stomatitis, ataxia, paresthesias, tachycardia, shortness of breath or wheezing, pain at site of injection, nausea, vomiting, loss of appetite, diarrhea, fatigue, loss of hair
Fluconazole (Diflucan)	PO, IV	Candidiasis, cryptococcosis	Abnormal liver function, Stevens-Johnson syndrome, nausea, headache, skin rash, vomiting, abdominal pain, diarrhea
Flucytosine (Ancobon) (5-Fluorocytosine) (5FC)	PO	Candidiasis, cryptococcosis	Anemia, yellow eyes/skin, skin rash, redness, itching, sore throat, fever, unusual bleeding/bruising, confusion, sensitivity of the skin to sunlight, abdominal pain, diarrhea, loss of appetite, nausea, vomiting, dizziness, lightheadedness, drowsiness, headache
*Foscarnet sodium (Foscavir)	IV	Cytomegalovirus infection, herpes simplex virus infection, HIV infection	Increased thirst, headaches, nausea, anorexia, flank pain, muscle twitching, elevated creatinine, mild proteinuria, renal failure, decrease in hemoglobin, both increase and decrease in calcium hyperphosphatemia, fatigue, irritability, tremors, seizures, genital ulcers
Ganciclovir (Cytovene) (formerly known as DHPG)	PO, IV	Cytomegalovirus infection	Granulocytopenia, thrombocytopenia, anemia, mood changes, tremor, nervousness, fever, skin rash, abnormal liver function, phlebitis, abdominal pain, loss of appetite, nausea, vomiting
*Granulocyte, macrophage-colony stimulating factor-E (GM-CSF) (LEUCOMAX) (rGM-CSF)	IV, SC	Neutropenia associated with HIV infection or zidovudine or ganciclovir therapy	Hypersensitivity reactions (urticaria, angioedema, bronchoconstriction, anaphylaxis), fever, chills, rigors, bone pain, arthralgias, adult respiratory distress syndrome, rash, pericarditis, local erythema at site of injection, hypoxia

TABLE 54–14. Drugs Used to Treat HIV Infection and AIDS-related Conditions Continued

Generic Name (Trade Name)	Route of Administration	Indications	Side/Adverse Effects
Interferon alfa recombinant (Intron-A) (Roferon-A)	PO, IM, SC	HIV infection, Kaposi's sarcoma	Parenteral: flulike syndrome (fever, myalgias and malaise), leukopenia, elevation in liver enzyme levels, weight loss, hair loss, fatigue, proteinuria, reversible congestive cardiomyopathy (weight gain and signs of right- or left-sided congestive heart failure) Oral: no side effects have been reported with low-dose oral alfa interferon
*Interleukin-2 recombinant (IL-2) (Proleukin)	IV	HIV infection	Fluid retention, hypotension, fever, chills, elevated creatinine, elevated BUN, oliguria, anuria, azotemia, fatigue, weight gain, tachycardia, nausea, vomiting, transient changes in liver function studies, headache, lightheadedness, dizziness, mental changes, pulmonary symptoms, anemia, leukocytosis, skin rash, myalgia, arthralgia
Isoniazid (INH) (Izonid) (Laniazid) (Nydrazid) (Teebaconin)	PO, IM	*Mycobacterium avium* complex infection, *Mycobacterium tuberculosis*	Loss of appetite, nausea, vomiting, diarrhea, unusual tiredness or weakness, dark urine, yellow eyes/skin, clumsiness or unsteadiness, numbness, tingling, burning or pain in hands or feet, fever, sore throat, unusual bleeding/bruising, skin rash, pain at injection site, arthralgia, seizures, depression, psychosis, blurred vision with or without eye pain
*Intraconazole (Sporanox)	PO	Maintenance therapy for cryptococcosis or histoplasmosis	Nausea, headaches, fatigue, abdominal cramps, rash, loss of potassium, edema
Ketoconazole (Nizoral)	PO	Candidiasis	Hepatitis, nausea, vomiting, diarrhea, dizziness, drowsiness, gynecomastia, headache, skin rash, itching, impotence, insomnia, photophobia
Leucovorin (Citrovorum) (Folinic Acid) (Wellcovorin)	PO, IM, IV	Prophylaxis and treatment of toxicity related to: methotrexate, pyrimethamine, or trimethoprim	Skin rash, hives, itching, wheezing
*Megestrol acetate (Megace)	PO	HIV wasting	Alteration of menstrual pattern with unpredictable bleeding, pain in chest, visual disturbances, headache, insomnia, pain in abdomen, groin, calf or leg, loss of coordination, slurred speech, weakness or numbness in extremities, yellow eyes/skin, depression, skin rashes, peripheral edema, brown spots in skin, acne, increased body hair, increased breast tenderness, loss of scalp hair
Methotrexate (Folex) (Folex PFS) (Mexate) (Mexate-AQ)	PO, IM, IV	Non-Hodgkin's lymphoma	Gastrointestinal ulceration or bleeding, enteritis, intestinal perforation, leukopenia, bacterial infections, septicemia, thrombocytopenia, stomatitis, renal failure, azotemia, hyperuricemia, nephropathy, cutaneous vasculitis, hepatotoxicity, pulmonary fibrosis, pneumonitis, central nervous system toxicity, anorexia, nausea, vomiting, acne, boils, skin rash
Miconazole (Micatin) (Monistat Derm) (Monistat IV)	PO, IM, IV, topical	Candidiasis, coccidioidomycosis, cryptococcosis	Fever, chills, skin rash, itching, redness, swelling at injection site, unusual tiredness, weakness, unusual bleeding/ bruising, anorexia, diarrhea, nausea, vomiting
Nystatin (Mycostatin) (Nilstat) (Nystex)	PO	Candidiasis (oropharyngeal)	Diarrhea, nausea, vomiting, stomach pain

Table continued on following page

TABLE 54–14. Drugs Used to Treat HIV Infection and AIDS-related Conditions Continued

Generic Name (Trade Name)	Route of Administration	Indications	Side/Adverse Effects
*Octreotide (Sandostatin)	SC	HIV-related diarrhea	Hyperglycemia, hypoglycemia, abdominal pain, diarrhea, nausea, vomiting, pain at injection site, headache, fatigue, dizziness, lightheadedness, edema, flushing of face, hepatic dysfunction
*Paromomycin sulfate (Humatin)	PO	Cryptosporidiosis	Nausea, vomiting, diarrhea, renal damage
Pentamidine isethionate (Nebupent, inhalation) (Pentam parenteral)	IM, IV, inhalation	Pneumocystosis	Parenteral: blood dyscrasias, rapid irregular pulse, diabetes mellitus, skin rash, hyperglycemia, hypoglycemia, hypotension, pain or tenderness at site of injection, redness or flushing of the face, metallic taste in mouth Inhalation: chest pain, congestion, coughing, dyspnea, pharyngitis, wheezing, skin rash, metallic taste in mouth, pneumothorax
*Pentosan polysulfate sodium (Elmiron) (PPS)	PO, IV	HIV infection, Kaposi's sarcoma	Bone marrow suppression, bruising, bleeding, headache, dizziness, nausea, diarrhea, dyspepsia, peripheral edema, skin rash, anemia, thrombocytopenia, abdominal pain, appetite change, tremors, night sweats, impaired concentration, fatigue, confusion, stomatitis, shortness of breath, peripheral neuropathy
*Piritrexim isethionate	PO, IV	*Mycobacterium avium* complex infection, *Pneumocystis carinii* infection, toxoplasmosis	Mucositis, myelosuppression, anemia, leukopenia, thrombocytopenia, nausea, vomiting, phlebitis
*Polyribonucleotide (Ampligen)	IV	HIV infection	Mild flulike symptoms including transient headache, fever, myalgia, malaise, flushing of face and chest, shortness of breath, nausea, diarrhea, photophobia, rash, transient visual disturbances
Pyrazinamide (PZA)	PO	*Mycobacterium tuberculosis*	Joint pain, loss of appetite, unusual tiredness or weakness, yellow eyes/ skin, swelling of joints, itching, rash
Pyrimethamine (Daraprim)	PO	Pneumocystosis, toxoplasmosis	Folic acid deficiency (loss of taste, glossitis, diarrhea, sore throat, dysphagia, ulcerative stomatitis), fever, bleeding, bruising, fatigue, skin rash, trembling, unsteadiness or clumsiness, seizures, anorexia, vomiting
*Rifabutin (Ansamycin)	PO	*Mycobacterium avium* complex infection	Increase in both liver enzymes and creatinine, rash, fever, leukopenia, gastrointestinal distress, hemolysis, arthralgias
Rifampin (Rifadin) (Rifadin IV) (Rimactane)	PO, IV	*Mycobacterium avium* complex infection, *Mycobacterium tuberculosis*	Chills, difficult breathing, dizziness, fever, headache, muscle and bone pain, shivering, rash, itching, skin redness, sore throat, yellow eyes/skin, unusual bleeding/bruising, loss of appetite, nausea, vomiting, unusual tiredness or weakness, bloody or cloudy urine, stomach cramps, diarrhea, sore mouth or tongue, discoloration of urine, feces, saliva, sputum, sweat or tears
*Spiramycin (Rovamycine)	PO, IV	Cryptosporidiosis	Parenteral: paresthesias, irritation at injection site, dysesthesia, giddiness, pain, stiffness, burning sensation, hot flashes Oral: nausea, vomiting, diarrhea, fatigue, indigestion, sweating, heaviness in chest, cool sensation in mouth or pharynx

TABLE 54–14. Drugs Used to Treat HIV Infection and AIDS-related Conditions Continued

Generic Name (Trade Name)	Route of Administration	Indications	Side/Adverse Effects
Sulfadoxine and pyrimethamine (Fansidar)	PO	Pneumocystosis	Stevens-Johnson syndrome, toxic epidermal necrolysis, fulminant hepatic necrosis, agranulocytosis, aplastic anemia, photosensitivity, bleeding and/ or bruising, folic acid deficiency (loss of taste, glossitis, diarrhea, sore throat, dysphagia, ulcerative stomatitis), skin rash, fatigue, aching in joints or muscles, hematuria, dysuria, goiter, tremors, seizures, headache, dizziness, nausea, vomiting
Sulfamethoxazole and trimethoprim (Bactrim) (Bethaprim) (Cheragan W/TMP) (Cotrim) (Septra) (Sulfamethoprim) (Sulfaprim) (Sulfatrim) (Sulfoxaprim) (Triazole) (Uroplus)	PO, IV	Isosporiasis, pneumocystosis, salmonellosis, toxoplasmosis	Skin rash, itching, Stevens-Johnson syndrome (myalgia, arthralgia, redness, blistering, peeling, or loosening of the skin, extreme fatigue), dysphagia, fever, leukopenia (sore throat), thrombocytopenia (unusual bleeding or bruising), hepatitis (dark urine, pale stools, yellow skin and/or sclera), cystalluria, hematuria, diarrhea, dizziness, headache, anorexia, nausea, vomiting
Sulfamethoxazole (Gantanol)	PO	Toxoplasmosis	Fever, itching, skin rash, hepatitis, photosensitivity, blood dyscrasias, difficulty swallowing, redness, blistering, peeling of skin, hematuria, crystalluria, thyroid dysfunction, dizziness, headache, anorexia, nausea, vomiting, diarrhea
Sulfisoxazole (Gantrisin)	PO	Toxoplasmosis	Fever, itching, skin rash, hepatitis, photosensitivity, blood dyscrasias, difficulty swallowing, redness, blistering, peeling of skin, hematuria, crystalluria, thyroid dysfunction, dizziness, headache, anorexia, nausea, vomiting, diarrhea
Trimethoprim (Proloprim) (Trimpex)	PO	Salmonellosis	Blood dyscrasias (bleeding), headache, methemoglobinemia, skin rash, itching, alteration in taste, sore mouth or tongue, anorexia, diarrhea, nausea, vomiting, abdominal pain, cramping
*Trimetrexate glucuronate	IV	Pneumocystosis	Decrease in neutrophil and platelet counts, nausea, vomiting, diarrhea, reversible liver function abnormalities, skin rash, fever
Vinblastine (Velban) (Velsar)	IV	Kaposi's sarcoma	Fever, chills, cough, hoarseness, lower back pain, side pain, painful or difficult urination, pain or redness at site of injection, sores in mouth and on lips, rectal bleeding, dizziness, difficulty in walking, double vision, drooping eyelids, headache, jaw pain, mental depression, numbness or tingling in fingers and toes, pain in fingers or toes, pain in testicles, weakness, nausea, vomiting, loss of hair

Table continued on following page

TABLE 54–14. Drugs Used to Treat HIV Infection and AIDS-related Conditions Continued

Generic Name (Trade Name)	Route of Administration	Indications	Side/Adverse Effects
Vincristine (Oncovin) (Vincasar PES) (Vincrex)	IV	Kaposi's sarcoma, non-Hodgkin's lymphoma	Constipation, stomach cramps, bed wetting, decrease or increase in urination, dizziness, lightheadedness, dysuria, lack of sweating, joint pain, lower back or flank pain, visual changes, ataxia, drooping eyelids, headache, jaw pain, numbness or tingling in fingers or toes, pain in testicles, weakness, hyponatremia, leukopenia, thrombocytopenia, stomatitis Syndrome of inappropriate antidiuretic hormone (SIADH) evidenced by agitation, confusion, dizziness, hallucinations, anorexia, mental depression, seizures, insomnia, loss of consciousness
Zidovudine (Retrovir) (formerly known as AZT)	PO, IV	HIV infection	Anemia, leukopenia, neutropenia, platelet count changes (either increased or decreased), anorexia, asthenia, diarrhea, dizziness, fever, headache, nausea, insomnia, malaise, myalgia, pain in abdomen, rash, somnolence, taste alteration
Zovirax (Acylovir)	PO, IV, topical	Herpes simplex virus infection, herpes zoster infection, varicella infection	Parenteral: skin rash, hives, hematuria, lightheadedness, headache, diaphoresis, confusion, tremors, abdominal pain, difficulty breathing, decreased frequency of urination, nausea, vomiting, unusual thirst, extreme fatigue Oral: changes in menstrual period, skin rash, diarrhea, dizziness, headache, joint pain, nausea, vomiting, acne, anorexia, somnolence Topical: mild pain, burning, itching, skin rash

*Investigational as of March 1991.
From Flaskerud, J. H., and Ungvarski, P. J. (Eds.) (1992). *HIV/AIDS: A guide to nursing care* (2nd ed., pp. 461–475). Philadelphia, W. B. Saunders.

TABLE 54–15. AIDS-Associated Symptoms and Nursing Care

Sensory-Perceptual Alterations

Many symptoms may be associated with this nursing diagnosis. They include impaired memory, "slowed" thinking, impaired concentration, dementia, headache, obtundation, confusion, lethargy, impaired vision, blindness, peripheral neuropathy, social isolation, social withdrawal, forgetfulness, or confusion. Etiologic factors to be considered include opportunistic CNS malignancies and infections, HIV infection of the CNS or peripheral nervous system, site-specific opportunistic infection such as CMV retinitis or herpes zoster, the adverse effects of medications, fluid and electrolyte imbalances, metabolic and vascular disruptions, social ostracism, discrimination, and malnutrition.

Blindness/Decreased Visual Acuity

Probable Cause	Special Features	Nursing Interventions
CMV retinitis	May develop suddenly Antiviral intervention should be started as soon as possible to prevent extension of visual loss	Instruct on symptoms Ensure prompt ophthalmic consult upon development of initial symptoms

Rare causes of visual disturbances
Toxoplasma gondii
Cryptococcus neoformans
Mycobacteria/fungi
	Many patients cannot remain on Ganciclovir due to neutropenia
	Many patients dread the development of blindness
	Full rehabilitation is frequently not a realistic goal. The use of a guide dog or proficiency at Braille may never be achieved
	Medical treatment is life-long
	Foscarnet therapy was approved by the FDA in 1991
		Provide psychosocial and spiritual support
		Combat social isolation and withdrawal
		Focus on anxiety and frustration management
		Arrange for outpatient or home care infusion therapy
		Active referrals as appropriate to blind organizations—i.e., association for the blind occupational retraining programs, home care agencies, Meals on Wheels, mental health professionals
		Promote assistive devices
		  Talking clocks, books, newspapers, cane, traveling with a sighted person, tactile identification markers
		Teach measures enhancing independence and safety
		  Fire prevention and response
		  Hygiene and grooming
		  Meal preparation
		  Communication
		  Transportation
		  Housekeeping and laundry

Dementia

Probable Cause	Special Features	Nursing Interventions
HIV *Other causes in a differential diagnosis* CNS malignancy CNS infection Metabolic complications Cerebrovascular complications Adverse effects of medications Malnutrition	Many patients and care partners dread the development of dementia Diagnosis may be difficult to establish. It involves a thorough assessment The vast majority of AIDS patients have some evidence of early-stage dementia ADC patient's symptoms can wax and wane. Progression ensues at a variable rate	Assist with neuropsychiatric assessment and medical evaluation Provide support, guidance for families/friends. Refer for home care, "buddy" volunteer, day care residential living, or respite care as appropriate Patient may need to move to more structured living arrangements Assess need for medication. Administer and supervise—i.e., Haldol, Ativan—as prescribed. Promote timed drug dosage, pill box alarms, checklists Obtain physical therapy consult for gait, assistive devices Use reminder devices: telephone calls, appointment book, "to do" lists, checklists, maps of food store Advocate antiviral research therapy as appropriate Model interactive techniques. Simplify communications and logistics

Table continued on following page

TABLE 54-15. AIDS-Associated Symptoms and Nursing Care Continued

Altered Breathing Patterns

Many symptoms may be associated with this nursing diagnosis. The most common are the constellation of signs and symptoms that patients who are developing PCP demonstrate. They include a fever with a dry, nonproductive cough; chills; exercise intolerance; and dyspnea.

There are other etiologic agents that cause altered breathing patterns in patients with AIDS. The symptoms include productive coughs, wheezing, and dyspnea. These other underlying concerns include bacterial endocarditis with resulting valvular disease, congestive heart failure, CMV pneumonia, KS lesions in the main lung structures, pleural effusion, pneumothoraxes, recurrent bacterial respiratory infections, or tuberculosis.

Cough

Probable Cause	Special Features	Nursing Interventions
PCP	Those HIV-infected patients, whose T-cell count is below 400, are most at-risk for PCP	Instruct ARC and AIDS patients on initial symptoms and signs of PCP
Other common causes of cough	Symptoms may worsen during first days of treatment for PCP	Instruct patient on PCP prophylaxis therapy. Ensure compliance
Bacterial, mycobacterial, or CMV pneumonia	Bactrim and aerosolized pentamidine treatments are used to prevent PCP episodes	Encourage patient to seek urgent treatment at the initiation of symptoms of PCP
KS lesions in the lungs		Assist in diagnostic work-up—i.e., sputum induction cultures, bronchoscopy
Pneumothorax		Administer Bactrim, pentamidine, dapsone, fansidar, Solu-Medrol, or other experimental agent as ordered for PCP

Potential Fluid Volume Deficit: Impaired Tissue Integrity

Many symptoms may be associated with these diagnoses. They include anorexia, nausea, vomiting, candidiasis, oral warts, weight loss, perirectal infections, inability to sustain or gain weight, oral hairy leukoplakia, diarrhea, stomatitis, gingivitis, and marked change in taste. Etiologic factors to be considered include malabsorption, opportunistic cancers or infections, underlying viral infections (CMV, Epstein-Barr, herpes simplex virus), the unrelenting wasting syndrome, and complications due to CNS disease or noncompliance.

Altered Mucous Membranes

Probable Cause	Special Features	Nursing Interventions
Oral Candidiasis	The development of candidiasis in the asymptomatic, HIV-infected patient signifies progression of illness	Normal saline mouth rinses; tub baths.
Vaginal Candidiasis		Vitamin A&D ointment to lips.
		Avoid agents that are drying—i.e., contain alcohol, hydrogen peroxide, Betadine
Other common causes of impaired membranes	The development of esophageal candidiasis establishes an AIDS diagnosis	Use oral irrigation and suction if unable to adequately rinse mouth
Kaposi's sarcoma		Administer prescribed oral, vaginal, or systemic antifungal, antiviral, or analgesic medications
Herpes virus		
Inadequate mouth care		Oral powder sprays to mildly débride and stimulate circulation if necessary
Malnutrition		Use rigid oral suction catheter if patient is having difficulty swallowing

Moderate to Severe Diarrhea

Probable Cause	Special Features	Nursing Interventions
Infections, parasitic and viral	Despite aggressive use of antidiarrheals, diarrhea can be unrelenting	Assist in aggressive work-up for causative agents
Other common causes of diarrhea	Various agents are in clinical trials to address diarrhea	Contain diarrhea. Use panty liners, sanitary napkins, adult diapers, ostomy equipment, soft rectal tube, or bed with chamber pot opening ("cholera" bed), depending on severity. Consult with physician before using rectal tube
Malabsorption	Extreme diligence in making a diagnosis of a GI infection is warranted	
Kaposi's sarcoma		
Other infections (cryptosporidiosis, *Salmonella, Shigella, Isospora belli*)	Nutritional repletion is a vital component of treatment	Institute caloric and volume intake and volume output investigation
		Instruct to clean, rinse, and dry perirectal area after bowel movements
		Protect perianal skin integrity using Vitamin A & D ointment, Skin Prep, and other skin barriers. Avoid using Stomadhesive-like barriers
		Reinstruct patient to avoid anal sexual practices
		Avoid orthostatic hypotension–related syncope
		Promote hydration

TABLE 54-15. AIDS-Associated Symptoms and Nursing Care Continued

Impaired Skin Integrity

Many symptoms may be associated with this diagnosis. They include pruritus, lesions, dryness, rash, skin breakdown with decubitus ulcer formation, wounds, impetigo, psoriasis, xerosis, folliculitis, vasculitis, and dermatitis. Etiologic factors to be considered include HIV, HIV seroconversion-associated illness, drug reactions, and infections—i.e., candidiasis, varicella zoster, molluscum contagiosum, *Staphylococcus*, syphilis, herpes simplex virus, and malignancies.

Ulcerative KS Lesions

Probable Cause	Special Features	Nursing Interventions
Terminal-stage illness of AIDS/KS	Lesions are unsightly Healing of wound is not a realistic goal Lymphadenopathy with edema complicates healing process Radiation may assist in palliative and cosmetic improvements	Inform patient to discontinue using make-up to hide KS lesions once they open Clean nondraining, noninfected open lesions. Cover lightly or leave open to air and light Clean open, draining, infected lesions with potassium permanganate soaks followed by normal saline rinse daily. Betadine foam with hydrogen peroxide can be used in place of potassium permanganate If malodorous, use air purifier, air freshener, spirits of peppermint, activated charcoal, vinegar, baking soda, or hospital trash odor control agent, depending on severity Use strips of iodoform nugauze to pack deep wounds. Use Kerlix to avoid tape contact with skin Maintain wound and skin precautions Simplify dressing technique as much as possible and teach skill to patient or care partner Consult with dermatologist about other measures used Avoid the use of occlusive barrier dressings—i.e., Stomadhesive—which depend on mature neutrophils to clear infection Refer patient to enterostomal therapy nurse's caseload

Pruritus

Probable Cause	Special Features	Nursing Interventions
Infections and underlying systemic, advanced disease	Often complaints of pruritus have to be solicited	Inform patient that scratching enhances itching. It also leads to escoriated skin with a resultant medium for infection Question patient about the development of pruritus, since it may be a symptom of an underlying infection, drug reaction, or disease Promote hydration, frequent use of emollient creams, i.e., Nivea, Eucerin, tepid water in bathing, and a mild soap—i.e., Dove Add oil to bath water toward the end of bathing or to moist skin after a shower—i.e., Aveeno Provide humidified air Use distraction, relaxation, guided imagery, music at night, when pruritus usually worsens Aggressively assist in the treatment of underlying disease to lessen pruritus. Administer antihistamines, antibiotics, or corticosteroids as prescribed

Table continued on following page

TABLE 54–15. AIDS-Associated Symptoms and Nursing Care Continued

Body Images Disturbance; Impaired Social Interaction

Many symptoms may be associated with these diagnoses. They may include social isolation, social withdrawal, fearfulness, and body image changes. Etiologic factors to be considered include anxiety; discrimination; stigmatization; generalized weakness; HIV transmission; visible signs of illness; and reaction of family, friends, or society in general.

Body Image Changes

Common Causes	Special Features	Nursing Interventions
KS lesions Premature aging Substantial weight loss	Be sensitive to age of patient May be helpful to compare "before" and "after" photographs in order to grasp amount of change	Provide psychosocial and spiritual support Discuss the handling of uncomfortable social situations, questions from acquaintances, and stares Facilitate the use of make-up cover for KS lesions if desired Promote the wearing of loosely fitting clothing, turtlenecks, long sleeves, caps, and other camouflaging means if desired Attune yourself to patient's grieving process and feelings of loss

Decreased Socialization

Common Causes	Special Features	Nursing Interventions
Fear of transmission Feelings of uncleanliness Stigmatization Rejection of others Continued substance abuse	Behavior change in these areas is difficult to attain and maintain Group and social network support is advantageous to maintenance of behavior change Education and reinforcement must be ongoing Health care professionals often need professional supervision in these areas due to low knowledge base, cultural insensitivity, and countertransferance issues	Reinforce safer sex and drug use teaching Discuss with patient and loved ones specifics of body substance isolation Advocate pregnancy avoidance Refer patient's contacts for HIV testing and counseling Promote the participation in HIV/AIDS support groups. Initiate such a group if needed Encourage maintenance of predisease activities, routine, schedule, network if feasible Confront and guide patient to drug treatment service as needed. Refer to a Twelve Step anonymous program Familiarize patient with local AIDS-advocacy group, governmental departments on discrimination, other community services Form multidisciplinary team to meet patients' and loved ones' needs

Adapted from McMahon, K. M. and Coyne, N. (1989). Symptom Management in Patients with AIDS. *Seminars in Oncology Nursing* 5(4); 294–298.

clinicians and tireless researchers who have prevailed. There remains much pioneering clinical work to be done to put a dent into the needs that are evident. Satisfying intellectual challenge, participation in our century's great human drama, the ability to integrate spiritual, psychological, and biophysical care in alternative practice settings, and an opportunity to contribute on many levels to relieve suffering and help frightened but proud and courageous persons with AIDS await these pioneers.

References

Amman, A. J. (1984). Immunodeficiency disease. In D. P. Sites, J. D. Stobo, H. H. Fudenberg, et al. (Eds.) *Basic and Clinical Immunology.* Los Angeles, Lange Medical Publications.

Beldescu, N., Apetrei, R., and Calumfirescu, A. (1990). Nosocomial transmission of HIV in Romania. *Sixth International Conference on AIDS (Abstracts)*. TH. C.104, 159.

Beral, V., Peterman, T. A., Berlkelman, R. L., et al. (1990). Kaposi's sarcoma among persons with AIDS: A sexually· transmitted infection? *Lancet*, 2, 123–128.

Bowen, D., Lane, H. and Fauci A. (1985). Immunopathogenesis of the acquired immunodeficiency syndrome. *Annals of Internal Medicine*, 5, 103, 704–709.

Bradley-Springer, L. (1991). Nutritional support in HIV infection: A multilevel analysis. *Image*, 23(3), 155–160.

Breimer, L. H. (1984). Did Moriz Kaposi describe AIDS in 1872? *Clio Media*, 19(1–2), 156–158.

Centers for Disease Control. (1981). *Pneumocytis pneumoniae*—Los Angeles. *MMWR*, 30, 250–252.

Centers for Disease Control (1988a). Quarterly report to the domestic policy council on the prevalence and rate of spread of HIV and AIDS in the United States. *MMWR*, 37, 181–183.

Centers for Disease Control (1988b). Immunization of children infected with human immunodeficiency virus—supplementary ACIP statement. *MMWR*, 37, 181–183.

Centers for Disease Control (1988c). Update: Acquired immunodeficiency virus and human immunodeficiency virus infection among health care workers. *MMWR*, 37:229–232.

Centers for Disease Control (1988d). Condoms for prevention of sexually transmitted diseases. *MMWR*, 37, 133–137.

Centers for Disease Control (1988e). Semen banking, organ and tissue transplantation and HIV antibody testing. *MMWR*, 37, 57–58.

Centers for Disease Control. (1991). *HIV/AIDS Surveillance Report,* September, 1–18.

Cohen, P. T., Sande, M. A., and Volberding, P. A. (Eds). (1990). *The AIDS knowledge base.* Waltham, MA: Medical Publishing Group.

Corey, L. and Spear, P. G. (1986). Infection with herpes simplex virus. *New England Journal of Medicine,* 314 (11), 686–691.

de la Monte, S. M., Ho, D. D., Schooley, R. T. et al. (1987). Subacute encephalomyelitis of AIDS and its relation to HTLV-III infection. *Neurology* 37, 562–569.

Des Prez, R. M., Heim, C. R. (1990). Mycobacterium tuberculosis. In G. L. Mandell, R. G. Douglas, Jr, and J. E. Bennett (Eds.), *Principles and practices of infectious disease* (3rd ed., pp. 1877–1906). New York, Churchill Livingstone.

Division of Tuberculosis Control, Centers for Disease Control and American Thoracic Society. (1990). *National tuberculosis training initiative: Core curriculum on tuberculosis.* New York, American Lung Association.

Favero, M. (1987). *AIDS.* Paper presented at 18th National Symposium, American Nephrology Nurses Association (May), New York.

Friedman-Kien, A. E., Ostreich, R., and Saltzman, B. (1989). Clinical manifestations of classical, endemic African, and epidemic AIDS-associated Kaposi's sarcoma. In A. E. Friedman-Kien (Ed.), *Color Atlas of AIDS* (pp. 11–48). Philadelphia, W. B. Saunders.

Friedman-Kien, A. E., Saltzman, B. R., Mirabile, M., et al. (1990). Kaposi's sarcoma in HIV-negative homosexual men [letter]. *Lancet* (335), 168–169.

Gallo, R. C. (1987). The AIDS Virus. *Scientific American,* 256 (1), 46–56.

Gold, J. W. M., and Armstrong, D. (1989). Opportunistic infections in AIDS patients. In P. Ma, and D. Armstrong (Eds.), *AIDS and infections of homosexual men* (2nd ed., pp. 325–335). Boston, Butterworths.

Gottlieb, M. S., Schroff, R., Schranker, H. M., et al. (1981). *Pneumocystis carinii* pneumoniae and mucosal candidiasis in previously healthy homosexual men. *New England Journal of Medicine,* 305, 1425.

Grady, C. (1989). The immune system and AIDS/HIV Infection. In J. H. Flaskemd, (Ed.). AIDS/HIV Infection: A Reference Guide for Nursing Professionals (p. 45). Philadelphia, W. B. Saunders.

Heinemann, M. H. (1989). Long term intravitreal ganciclovir therapy for cytomegalovirus retinopathy. *Archives of Ophthalmology,* 107 (12), 1767–1772.

Ho, D. D., Pomerantz, R. J., and Kaplan, J. C. (1987). Pathogenesis of infection with human immunodeficiency virus. *New England Journal of Medicine,* 317, 278–286.

Isobe, M., Huebner, K., Madden, P. J., et al. (1986). The gene encoding the T-cell surface protein T4 is located on human chromosome 12. *Proceedings of the National Academy of Science, USA,* 83 (12), 4399–402.

Jagger, J., Hunt, E. H., Brand-Elnagger, J., et al. (1990a). Rates of needlestick injury caused by various devices in a university hospital. *New England Journal of Medicine,* 319(5), 284.

Jagger, J., Hunt, E. H., and Pearson, R. D. (1990b). Sharp object injuries in the hospital: Causes and strategies for prevention. *American Journal of Infection Control,* 18(4), 227.

Kanski, P. J., Alroy, J., and Essex, M. (1985). Isolation of T-lymphotropic retrovirus related to HTLV-III/LAV from wild-caught African monkeys. *Science,* 230, 951–954.

Kaplan, L. D. (1990). The malignancies associated with AIDS. In M. A. Sande, and P. A. Volberding (Eds.), *The Medical Management of AIDS* (2nd ed., pp. 335–364). Philadelphia, W. B. Saunders.

Koenig, S., and Fauci, A. S. (1988). Immunology of the acquired immunodeficiency syndrome. *Kansenshgaku Zasshi March,* 62 (Supple)., 252–263.

Kotler, D. P., Wang, J., and Pierson, R. N. (1985). Body composition studies in patients with the acquired immunodeficiency syndrome. *American Journal of Clinical Nutrition,* 42, 1255–1265.

Kotler, D. P. (1989). Diarrhea in AIDS: Diagnosis and management. *Medical Times,* 117(3), 101–108.

Kotler, D. P. (1991). Cytomegalovirus colitis and wasting. *Journal of the Acquired Immune Deficiency Syndrome,* 4 (Suppl. 1), 536–541.

Kotler, D. P., Tierney, A. R., Altilio, D., et al. (1989a). Body mass repletion during ganciclovir therapy of cytomegalovirus infections in patients with acquired immunodeficiency syndrome. *Archives of Internal Medicine,* 149, 901–905.

Kotler, D. P., Tierney, A. R., Ferraro, R., et al. (1991). Enteral alimentation and repletion of body cell mass in malnourished patients with acquired immunodeficiency syndrome. *American Journal of Clinical Nutrition,* 53, 149–154.

Kotler, D. P., Tierney, A. R., Wang, J., et al. (1989b). The magnitude of body cell mass depletion determines the timing of death from wasting in AIDS. *American Journal of Clinical Nutrition,* 50, 444–447.

Kovacs, J. A., and Masur, H. (1988). Opportunistic infections. In V. T. De Vita, S. Hellman, and S. A. Rosenberg (Eds.), *AIDS: Etiology, diagnosis, treatment, and prevention* (2nd ed., pp. 199–225). Philadelphia, J. B. Lippincott.

Kumar, S., Schade, R. R., Peel, R., et al. (1989). Kaposi's sarcoma with visceral involvement in a young heterosexual male without evidence of acquired immune deficiency syndrome. *American Journal of Gastroenterology,* 84(3), 318–321.

Lane, H. C., and Fauci, A. S. (1985). Immunodeficiency abnormalities in the acquired immunodeficiency virus. *Annual Review of Immunology,* 3, 477–500.

Lawrence, J. (1985). The immune system in AIDS. *Scientific American,* 253, 84–93.

Levine, A. M. (1988). Reactive and neoplastic lymphoproliferative disorders and other miscellaneous cancers associated with HIV infection. In V. T. De Vita, S. Hellman, and S. A. Rosenberg (Eds.), *AIDS: Etiology, diagnosis, treatment, and prevention* (2nd ed., pp. 263–265). Philadelphia, J. B. Lippincott.

Mayer, K. H., Stoddard, A. M., McCuster, J., et al. (1986). Human T-lymphotropic virus type III in high risk, antibody negative homosexual men. *Annals of Internal Medicine,* 104, 194–196.

McDougal, J. S., Kennedy, M. S., Sligh, J. M., et al. (1986). Binding of HTLV III/LAV to T4 and T-cells by a complex of the L10 K viral protein and the T4 molecule. *Science,* 231, 382–385.

McMahon, K. M., and Sutterer, M. G. (1988). Safety precautions and hospital practices in dealing with seropositive individuals. In V. T. De Vita, S. Hellman, and S. A. Rosenberg (Eds.), *AIDS: Etiology, diagnosis, treatment, and prevention* (2nd ed., pp. 396–420). Philadelphia, J. B. Lippincott.

Margolick, J., Lane, H., and Fauci, A. (1987). Immunopathogenesis of HTLV III/LAV infection. *Viruses and human cancer* (pp. 56–70). New York, Alan R. Liss.

Moore, M. (Ed.) (1991). *Wasting syndrome in HIV disease: Transcript of panel proceedings from first annual conference: Clinical care options for HIV disease.* Westborough, MA: Criticial Care America.

Myskowski, P. (1989). Treatment of Kaposi's sarcoma. In P. Ma, and D. Armstrong (Eds.), *AIDS and infections of homosexual men* (2nd ed., pp. 317–327). Boston, Butterworth.

Nardell, E. A. (1990). Dodging droplet nuclei [letter]. *American Review of Respiratory Disease,* 142, 501.

Navia, B. A., Jordan, B. D., and Price, R. N. (1986). The AIDS dementia complex I. clinical features. *Ann Neurol,* 19, 517–524.

Osborn, J. E. (1986). AIDS, social sciences, and health education: A personal perspective. *Health Education Quarterly,* 13, 287–299.

Ou, C., Kwok, S., Mitchell, S. M., Mach, D. H., et al. (1988). DNA amplification for direct detection of HIV-1 in DNA of peripheral blood mononuclear cells. *Science,* 239, 295–297.

Pedersen, C., Lindhardt, B. O., Jensen, B. L., et al. (1989). Clinical course of primary HIV infection: Consequences for the subsequent course of the infection. *Abstracts volume: Fifth International AIDS Conference* (Abstracts). No. TAO 30, 60.

Quinn, T. C., Mann, J. R., and Curran, J. W. (1986). AIDS in Africa: An epidemiologic paradigm. *Science,* 234, 955–963.

Rosenberg, Z. and Fauci, A. (1989). The immunopathogenesis of HIV Infection. *Advances in Immunology,* 47, 377–431.

Safai, B. (1989). Clinical manifestations of Kaposi's sarcoma. In P. Ma, and D. Armstrong (Eds.), *AIDS and infections of homosexual men* (2nd ed.). Boston, Butterworth.

Seligmann, M., Pinching, A. J., Rosen, F. S., et al. (1987). Immunology of human immunodeficiency virus infection and the acquired immunodeficiency syndrome: An update. *Annals of Internal Medicine,* 107, 235–242.

Task Force on Nutritional Support in AIDS. (1989). Guidelines for nutrition support in AIDS. *Nutrition,* 5(1), 39–46.

Tierney, A. R., Cuff, P., and Kotler, D. P. (1991). The effect of megestrol acetate (megace) on appetite, nutritional repletion, and quality of life in AIDS cachexia. *Proceedings: Seventh International Conference on AIDS*, MB 2263.

Ungvarski, P. J. (1990). Human immunodeficiency virus (HIV) and *Mycobacterium tuberculosis* (TB). *Journal of the New York State Nurses Association*, 21(4), 7.

Urba, W. J., Longo, D. L. (1985). Clinical spectrum of human retroviral-induced diseases. *Cancer Research* 45(a)(Suppl), 4637s–4643s.

Volberding, P. A. (1990). Non-HIV Kaposi's sarcoma: Classic KS and KS associated with immunosuppression. In P. T. Cohen, M. A. Sande, and P. A. Volberding (Eds.), *The AIDS knowledge base* (pp. 712.1–712.2). Waltham, MA: Medical Publishing Group.

Von Roenn, J., Roth, E., Murphy, R., et al. (1991). Controlled trial of megestrol acetate for the treatment of AIDS related anorexia and cachexia. *Proceedings: Seventh International Conference on AIDS*, WB 2392.

Wofsky, C. B., Cohen, J. B., Haver, L. B., et al. (1986). Isolation of AIDS-associated retrovirus from genital secretions of women with antibodies to virus. *Lancet*, 1, 527.

Ziegler, J. B., Cooper, D. A., Johnson, R. O., Gold, J. (1985). Postnatal transmission of AIDS-associated retrovirus from mother to infant. *Lancet*, 1(8434), 896–898.

Integumentary System

55

Wound Healing

Nancy A. Stotts
JoAnne D. Whitney

Healing after injury is a central concept in care of patients in the critical care unit. Injured tissue is repaired or replaced and tissue continuity is restored. Disruption in the physiologic function of various systems occurs frequently in the critically ill patient and has potential for disruption of normal wound healing. Impairment in wound healing in critically ill patients has serious consequences, including localized wound infection, delayed healing, dehiscence, and sepsis.

Early identification of the patient at risk for impaired healing, manipulation of factors that place the patient at increased risk of impaired healing, support of therapies to facilitate healing, and mitigation of the effects of impairment are the responsibility of the critical care nurse. Often there are staff members of many medical subspecialties caring for the critically ill patient, each with his or her own focus of concern. The critical care nurse frequently is the person who acts to coordinate the prescribed treatments to maximize the therapeutic effects, to suggest medical treatments that have been overlooked, and to initiate nursing interventions to facilitate healing; thus, the critical care nurse's role in supporting healing is central to the patient's welfare. A substantial scientific foundation is essential to enactment of this role and to the care of critically ill patients with wounds.

This chapter addresses the physiology of wound healing; pathophysiology, which results in disrupted healing; clinical presentation of normal and disrupted healing; and care of patients with disrupted tissue integrity and impaired healing. Throughout the chapter, the emphasis is on healing of acute injuries in the critically ill; chronic wounds seen in the critically ill are addressed but in less detail.

PHYSIOLOGY OF WOUND HEALING

Classically, wound healing has been divided into three phases and presented as having sequential but overlapping processes (Table 55–1). Although this paradigm is correct for full thickness injuries, it does not address those wounds that are partial thickness. Advances in the field of wound healing have led investigators to describe wound healing by the type of tissue being formed (e.g., epithelium, collagen) or by the cells involved in the healing process (e.g., fibroblasts, endothelial cells, macrophages). Application of research on the physiology of healing to clinical care might best be approached by using the model of partial thickness and full thickness injuries, in which the focus is on the type of tissue involved in healing. This approach allows the clinician to examine the full range of wounds seen in critically ill patients and to examine differences in the healing processes in various types of wounds. Partial thick-

---

TABLE 55–1. Phases of Wound Healing

Inflammatory phase: healing initiated
Hemostatic responses
Vascular responses
Cellular responses

Proliferative phase: major repair phase
Collagen synthesis
Angiogenesis
Epithelialization

Remodeling phase: repair process completed
Changes in collagen

---

ness injuries involve the epidermal layer of the skin and may extend to the dermis. They include tape burns, abrasions, and the donor site for a skin graft. Full thickness injuries involve the epidermis and the dermis of the skin and may extend into the subcutaneous fat, muscle, and bone.

Anatomy of the Skin

The skin is composed of an epidermal and a dermal layer separated by the basement membrane (Fig. 55-1). The outer layer of the skin, the epidermis, is composed of the stratum corneum and the stratum germinativum. The stratum corneum provides external protection, whereas the stratum germinativum is important because of its intense mitotic activity during healing. The dermis is composed of elastic fibers; collagen; fibroblasts; ground substance; blood vessels and adnexal structures; hair follicles; and sebaceous, eccrine, and apocrine glands, all of which are a rich reservoir of keratinocytes to replace damaged epidermis (Jakubovic and Ackerman, 1985). The dermis is critical to epidermal function because it provides blood flow and structural support. In addition, the primary cell of the dermis is the fibroblast, a cell that is essential for synthesis of connective tissue.

The skin is a major epithelial structure; however, the epithelia of the tracheobronchial tree, the gastrointestinal tract, and other tissues and organs respond in the same way to injury and repair as does the skin. Variations in rates of mitosis, migration, and healing are related to the type of epithelial cell involved (Jakubovic and Ackerman, 1985).

Repair of Partial Thickness Injuries

Partial thickness injuries involve the epidermal layer of the skin and may extend into the dermis. With injury, mitosis of epithelial cells is stimulated. The epithelial cells at the wound edge migrate toward the open wound; mitosis and differentiation into mature epidermal cells then take place. In a partial thickness injury, epithelial cells move from the adnexal structures as well as from the wound edges. Migration goes on until epithelial cells reach other epithelial cells and undergo contact inhibition. Epithelial migration continues until the area denuded of epithelial cells is entirely recovered; then migration ceases and the epithelium is built in layers until it reaches its original thickness. When the injury involves loss of part of the epithelium, plasma is lost onto the surface. When drying of the wound fluid occurs and a scab is formed, epidermal cells must migrate under the scab, and this requires more energy than unimpeded migration.

Epidermal cells migrate, undergo mitosis, and differentiate most efficiently in a moist, well oxygenated environment (Winter and Scales, 1963; Hinman and Maibach, 1963). Adequate nutrients for cell function must be present in order for cellular activities to take place (Young, 1988).

Repair of Full Thickness Injuries

Closure of full thickness injuries occurs by primary, secondary, or tertiary intention (Table 55-2). These three approaches to wound closure all involve the development of a blood supply across the injured tissue, filling of the tissue defect with scar tissue, and covering of the scar tissue with epithelial cells. Differences exist among these three types of healing, but the differences are primarily in the size of the defect requiring repair and the time required for healing.

Healing occurs in a predictable fashion (see Table 55-1). At the time of injury, blood vessels in the area vasoconstrict, the coagulation cascade is initiated, and platelet factors are released, which result in hemostasis at the site. After a few minutes, vasodilatation occurs and vessels proximal to the injury dilate and capillary permeability increases. Fluid and cells leak out of the injured vessels into the interstitium, resulting in edema. The edema is localized by fibroblasts that plug the lymphatics.

Chemotactic substances released at the site of injury attract white blood cells (WBCs) and complement to the area. The WBCs present in the greatest quantity at this time are polymorphonucleocytes (poly), and the neutrophil is the poly that is preponderant. Neutrophils phagocytose foreign material and bacteria and are a major factor in removing debris in the new injury. However, neutrophils have a short half-life (about 24 hours) and are not replaced at the wound site after their death. Monocytes, the preponderant WBCs at the wound site after 24 to 48 hours, are transformed into macrophages and become the most prevalent WBC present in the wound on a long-term basis. Macrophages are essential for phagocytosis, stimulating angiogenesis, replication of fibroblasts, and release of collagen from fibroblasts. Wounds will heal in the absence of neutrophils; however, without macrophages, wounds will not heal. Another important factor in wound cleansing is complement. Complement functions to lyse some bacteria and mark other bacteria for later phagocytosis by WBCs (Clark, 1985; Orgill and Demling, 1988).

Growth factors are important to angiogenesis and the development of scar tissue. Angiogenesis is stimulated by a substance from platelets called platelet-derived angiogenesis factor and by a substance from macrophages called angiogenesis factor (Hunt et al., 1984; Knighton et al., 1982; Ross, 1987). The stimulus for angiogenesis is not entirely understood but seems to be some combination of the mitogenic factors, lactate, and hypoxia. When these factors are present in the wound space, capillary buds come out from the opposing edges of the wound space and grow until they reach a capillary bed from the opposite

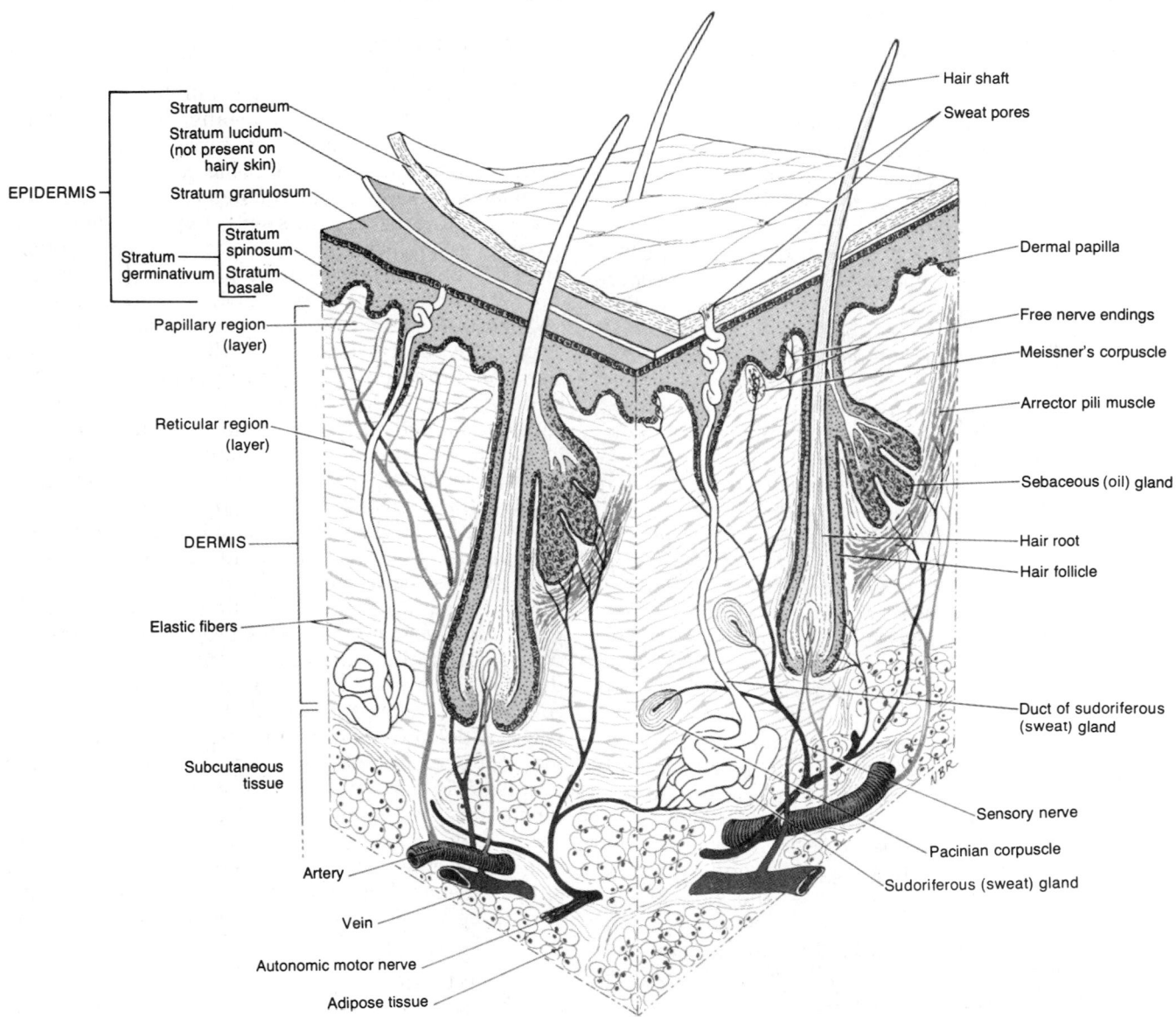

FIGURE 55–1. Structure of the skin and underlying subcutaneous layer. (Figure from PRINCIPLES OF HUMAN ANATOMY, 4th edition, by Gerald J. Tortora. Copyright © 1986 by Leonard Dank, 1986 by Biological Sciences Textbooks, Inc. Reprinted by permission of HarperCollins Publishers.)

TABLE 55–2. Wound Closure Techniques

Primary intention
Edges of wound well approximated and closed with suture, clips, or tape

Secondary intention
Left open to close by formation of granulation tissue, covered by epithelial tissue, and undergo contraction

Tertiary intention
Left to heal by secondary intention until bacteria count falls and then wound edges approximated

---

wound edge. As the new capillaries stretch out into the hypoxic acidotic wound space, intravascular cells and plasma are pushed into the advancing capillary bed. When the two ends of the capillary meet, flow occurs across the capillary. As the bed of capillaries is built, the amount of plasma and red blood cells traversing the new capillary bed in the wound space increases and over time, the hypoxia abates, the acidotic wound fluid is absorbed into the circulation, and the stimulus for angiogenesis ceases (Clark, 1985; Orgill and Demling, 1988).

Collagen formation also is dependent on growth factors. Among the substances recognized as growth factors that stimulate collagen formation are platelet-derived growth factor and macrophage-derived growth factor (Knighton et al., 1982; Ross, 1987). Collagen is synthesized and released by fibroblasts. There is a continual turnover of collagen as the scar tissue matures, and the tensile strength of the wound increases as the biochemical nature of the collagen changes over time. Collagen formation is a complex process; oxygen, vitamin C, zinc, iron, and alpha-ketoglutarate are critical to this formation (Goodson and Hunt, 1988).

Wounds healing by secondary intention undergo the process of wound contraction, in which wound size decreases. The controls for this process are not entirely understood, but the myofibroblast is thought to be a critical factor in this process.

To close the wound healing by secondary intention, epithelial cells migrate across the base of the wound. Epithelial tissue formation and migration also depend on growth factors to stimulate the epithelial cells to migrate, undergo mitosis, and differentiate as previously described.

DETERMINANTS OF HEALING

Factors in the internal and external environment of the patient affect healing (Fig. 55–2). The internal environment is that within the patient's own body; the external environment is outside the patient. Dimensions of the internal environment important to healing are tissue perfusion, oxygenation, nutrition, concurrent disease, and constitutional factors. Aspects of the external environment that affect healing are local wound treatment and systemic drugs and

treatments. Some of these factors can be manipulated to provide an environment favorable to healing. Other factors need to be recognized so that appropriate monitoring can be initiated and realistic goals can be established about the rate and nature of healing.

Internal Environment

TISSUE PERFUSION

Adequate perfusion of tissue is important to bring substances to the injury for healing. Sufficient intravascular volume is needed to carry the substances for healing to the wounded tissue as well as dispose of metabolic wastes. Hypovolemia results in impaired healing, and most patients with hypovolemia show classic signs of increased heart rate, decreased blood pressure, and decreased urinary output (Heughan et al., 1974; Chang et al., 1983). Chang and coworkers (1983) found a small proportion of subjects who had impaired wound perfusion and did not show clinical signs of decreased intravascular volume; currently, these patients cannot be identified using standard clinical parameters. Data indicate that support needs to be provided to assist in maintaining the circulating volume in all patients and that frank hypovolemia needs to be aggressively avoided.

In addition to decreased volume, edema increases the space across which substrates must move to get from the vasculature to the tissue, and thus has been accepted as a deterrent to healing (Reed and Clark, 1985). The mechanism by which the edema formation occurs is complicated and not entirely understood at this time (Hargens and Akeson, 1986). Hunt and colleagues (1986) proposed that edema may not always be deleterious to wound healing and therefore may not need to be treated. They suggest that when perfusion is disrupted, it is obvious that edema is deleterious and needs to be treated. On the other hand, they suggest that when edema is the result of fluid replacement, its harmful effects are not as clear cut and it is not known at this time whether attempts should be made to remove edema of this etiology.

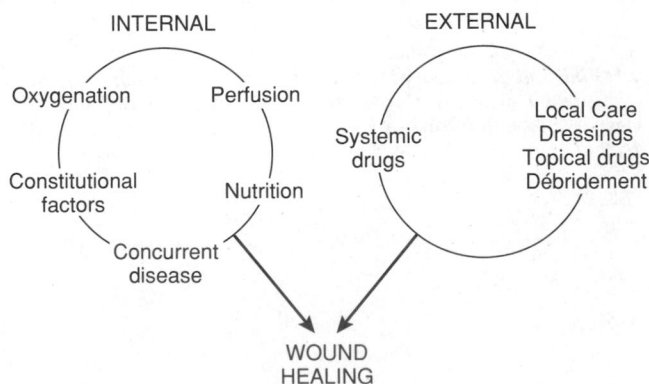

FIGURE 55–2. Environmental factors critical to healing.

These investigators acknowledge that additional data are needed to understand this process.

OXYGEN

Oxygen is critical to wound healing. It is an essential component in the transport of collagen from the fibroblast and in the cross-linking of collagen. In the absence of oxygen, the synthesis of collagen is halted but the action of the collagenases is not hindered, such that in a hypoxic environment, collagen lysis exceeds synthesis.

Oxygen also is important for the function of WBCs. WBCs remove debris and bacteria from wounds by phagocytosis and degranulation. When WBCs phagocytose foreign material and bacteria, they have a respiratory burst and use up to 20 times as much oxygen as in their resting state. During the respiratory burst, they use additional oxygen, ingest bacteria, and produce high-energy radicals such as superoxides, hypochlorite, hydroxyl radicals, peroxides, and aldehydes. Radicals are toxic to foreign cells and host cells and are responsible for some of the bactericidal action of the WBCs as well as some local tissue damage; however, enzymes present in healthy tissue quickly inactivate radicals, so that their action in healthy tissue is short lived (Knighton et al., 1984). Once phagocytosis has taken place, bacteria are killed by degranulation when intracellular enzymes are released. In the absence of oxygen, WBCs do not function as efficiently; bacteria may proliferate at a rate greater than phagocytosis, and infection may develop (Knighton et al., 1984).

Anemia also has been linked to impaired healing. Yet when concomitant conditions such as decreased volume are controlled, anemia has not been shown to be implicated in impaired healing except when the hematocrit drops below about 20 mg/dL (Heughan et al., 1974; Jensen et al., 1986).

Tobacco smoking also may affect oxygenation and wound healing. The carbon monoxide that is produced binds to the hemoglobin, leaving fewer sites available for binding of oxygen. In addition, platelets of long-term smokers are altered, so that aggregation occurs more frequently; the full implications of these effects on wound healing are not entirely understood.

Research data at this time do not provide the direction about which interventions will support oxygenation in the wound. Until such research data are available, measures used to support systemic oxygenation need to be applied to these patients (e.g., inspiratory maneuvers, early mobilization and activity, positioning of the patient to support an optimal ventilation-perfusion ratio, secretion clearing techniques, manipulation of ambient oxygen and/or ventilation as needed).

NUTRITION

Nutrients are critical to all of the processes that take place during healing. Angiogenesis, collagen formation, and epithelialization all require energy, vitamins, and minerals (Goodson and Hunt, 1988; Young, 1988).

Energy substrates include proteins, fats, and carbohydrates. The need for all of them is increased by injury; however, the most significant increase is in protein (Long et al., 1979). Protein is needed to provide the nitrogenous structure for new cell formation. The new cells and biologic factors of importance are those in the wound module itself (macrophages, fibrobasts, endothelial cells) and those that provide immunologic protection (WBCs, complement, prostaglandins). Deficiencies of protein result in decreased fibroblast proliferation, proteoglycan and collagen synthesis, angiogenesis, and remodeling (Fitzpatrick and Fisher, 1982; Williamson and Fromm, 1955; Rhodes et al., 1942; Irvin, 1978; Temple et al., 1975).

Carbohydrates are an important source of energy for the body, and in times of stress, the need for energy is increased. Fats provide the substrate from which the intracellular structures and cell walls are made. They also provide an important source of concentrated calories, especially important in situations such as massive trauma when energy needs are great and the patient's ability to manage large volumes of high protein–high carbohydrate fluid is limited. The effects of deficiencies are seen only in prolonged starvation, when fat stores become a primary source of energy for the body.

Vitamins also are important to healing. All of the vitamins play a role in wound healing. Water-soluble vitamins especially important to healing are vitamins B and C. The B vitamins serve as cofactors in the enzyme system. Vitamin B_1 (thiamine) is necessary for the strength of collagen (Alvarez and Gilbreath, 1982). Vitamine B_5 (pantothenic acid) deficiency is associated histologically with decreased fibroblasts and experimentally with decreased tensile strength (Grenier et al., 1982). Vitamin C is critical to collagen formation and angiogenesis. In addition, needs are increased with injury because vitamin C is required for efficient WBC function. When vitamin C intake is depressed, improper sequencing of amino acids occurs, such that collagen formation is disrupted. In addition, because collagenases continue to function even during starvation, lysis of collagen may exceed synthesis. New wounds may not heal well, and old wounds may come apart. Administration of vitamin C rapidly restores this dimension of collagen formation and healing.

Vitamins A, D, E, and K are fat-soluble vitamins. Deficiencies related to healing occur only in prolonged starvation and/or severe injury, as there are reserves of them in the body fat. Vitamin A is important to the inflammatory response and is a cofactor in collagen synthesis and cross-linking as well as in epithelialization (Pollack, 1979). Vitamin A also reverses the stabilizing effect of steroids on lysosomal membranes (Ehrlich and Hunt, 1968; Bark et al., 1984).

Vitamin D is needed for bone repair, as it is an

essential component in calcium absorption and excretion. Liver stores of vitamin D are often adequate in patients with uncomplicated injuries, but patients with multiple long bone fractures may require supplementation (Hey et al., 1982).

Vitamin E is an important component in normal fat metabolism. Scientific data indicate that supplemental vitamin E retards healing and fibrosis (Ehrlich et al., 1973; Kagoma et al., 1985).

Vitamin K is needed for coagulation, one of the first responses to tissue injury. Inadequate levels of vitamin K may result in bleeding into the wound space with hematoma formation and delay of the healing process. However, coagulation is one of the most fundamental of the body processes and factors needed for coagulation are not decreased unless severe and/or prolonged depletion of vitamin K occurs. Only in prolonged starvation, acute life-threatening hemorrhage, or feeding with total parenteral nutrition does vitamin K supplementation become a consideration.

Minerals also are important to healing; however, very small quantities of them are needed for normal bodily function and deficits related to healing have not often been reported. Zinc, iron, and manganese are important to collagen formation. Zinc is important in nucleic acid formation and protein synthesis. Deficiencies of serum zinc have been documented to impair healing, and impairment has been shown to be reversed by supplemental zinc (Sandstead et al., 1982; Pories et al., 1967; Barcia, 1970). Zinc deficiency is especially a threat in the elderly, the malnourished, and those with chronic metabolic stress and chronic diarrhea. Zinc is widely distributed in the body and is protein bound; therefore, measurement of serum zinc is not a sensitive measure of decreased intake and deficiencies are not seen until intake has been restricted for a long period.

Iron deficiency has been noted as a factor in impaired healing; however, only in children have deficiencies been related to impaired healing. Theoretically, the elderly may have iron deficiency secondary to changes in absorption of iron, increasing their risk for healing impairment, but clinically this has not been reported. Manganese functions as a cofactor in collagen formation. Deficiencies of this mineral have not been reported, but it must be considered when supplementation is provided.

CONCURRENT CONDITIONS

Patients with diabetes, perfusion problems, fluid and electrolyte disruptions, cancer, malnutrition, immunologic suppression, and infection are all at risk for impaired healing. The mechanism of impairment is different in each case.

Diabetics are a population known to be at risk for impaired healing. They have small vessel disease and experience periods of excessive hyperglycemia with injury (Goodson and Hunt, 1977). Increased glucose levels impair WBC function and often result in wound infection (Bagdale et al., 1974). If glucose levels can be kept to below 200 mg/dL in the first 72 hours after injury, healing will progress with fewer problems (Goodson and Hunt, 1977). Neuropathy that accompanies long-standing disease probably also is of importance. The neuropathy may play a part in the initial cause of wounds. With decreased peripheral sensation, the patient may not feel pain as damage occurs and therefore the source of injury may not be relieved, leading to more severe injury. The neuropathy may also predispose the patient to iatrogenic injury during his stay in the critical care unit. Excessive pressure or mechanical trauma may lead to tissue damage, and because it is not perceived, pressure-relieving strategies may not be initiated.

Patients in the critical care unit with problems of perfusion also are at risk for impaired healing. Commonly, these patients have cardiac disease with its central pump problems or have vascular disease that results in decreased tissue blood flow. The mechanism by which impaired healing occurs is related directly to impaired delivery of substrates to the injury and wastes not being removed in a timely manner. In many critical care units, patients with actual or potential perfusion problems are the primary population and the potential for impaired wound healing needs to be considered when nursing diagnoses for these patients are generated.

Fluid and electrolyte disorders seen in the critically ill may impair healing. Normal sodium and potassium levels are important to cell function. Sodium excess and hyperosmolarity are seen in dehydrated patients and in patients with hemoconcentrations. Potassium loss often occurs with gastrointestinal fluid losses. In addition, the aldosterone secretion that occurs with stress may result in a period of potassium loss and sodium retention. Phagocytosis is inhibited by high glucose levels and serum osmolarity of greater than 300 mmol/liter. Acid-base balance affects healing. Acidosis reduces the inflammatory response to healing, and alkalosis inhibits wound contraction (Schilling, 1976).

Cancer patients are immunologically impaired and at risk for impaired healing. In addition, the radiation therapy and chemotherapy that they often receive disrupt the cell, so that cancer patients have multiple factors that place them at risk for impaired healing.

Other major groups of patients who are at risk for impaired healing are those who have malnutrition and those who are immunosuppressed. In malnutrition, substrates needed for healing are not present in sufficient quantities and the processes of angiogenesis, collagen formation, and epithelialization are slowed. When substrate stores are entirely depleted, healing cannot progress and/or infection develops. Among the patients who are immunosuppressed are transplant patients, those being treated for inflammatory disorders such as arthritis and inflammatory bowel disease, those with AIDS, patients with severe metabolic stress, and patients who have undergone anesthesia. They cannot mount a cellular defense to heal tissue and are at risk for infection.

Infection impairs healing because energy substrates needed for healing are used to support the life of the foreign organisms. In the process, complement factors and leukocytes are depleted, energy needed for repair is consumed, and, unless other events intervene, healing is delayed. The byproducts of bacterial action also are toxic and inhibit activities of healthy cells. Immunocompetence is the critical determinant of whether an infection can be controlled and healing returned to its usual rate.

CONSTITUTIONAL FACTORS

The very young and the very old are at risk for impaired healing. In the very young, the immunologic support system is immature and in the presence of heavy bacterial contamination, they cannot provide efficient protection against infection. Older patients do not replicate cells as rapidly as younger ones do; the rate of cell formation decreases the ability of these patients to mount an inflammatory response, fight infection, and produce new tissue. The inflammatory response and classic signs of infection may not be as marked as in the younger adult (e.g., redness, warmth, and temperature). This requires that the nurse look for the more subtle changes in the patient's wound status and act on those. Because cell production is slowed in the elderly, the ability to make macrophages and complement is decreased, so that these patients are at increased risk of infection. Concomitantly, the rate of epithelialization is delayed; therefore, the wound is not healing from external contamination as rapidly in the elderly.

In the older population, development of connective tissue and scar tissue in wounds healing by primary intention also is delayed and tensile strength builds slowly, increasing the length of time that these wounds are at risk for dehiscence. In wounds healing by secondary intention, development of a healthy bed of granulation tissue takes longer in the elderly than in the younger critically ill patient; until this bed of tissue is robust, the wound is at increased risk of infection. Knowledge of this risk is translated into increased efforts to prevent cross-contamination and aggressive local and systemic care that will support healing. The activities involved in the care of the elderly are the same as those with any other population, yet they differ because the elderly require greater protection and more prompt and aggressive treatment for less overt signs and symptoms of wound impairment.

External Environment

LOCAL TREATMENT

Local treatment of wounds is an important determinant of healing or a significant deterrent to it. The principles of therapy and available therapies are discussed in detail later in the chapter.

SYSTEMIC DRUGS AND TREATMENTS

Steroids are anti-inflammatory agents that affect healing. Their most potent effects are seen when they are given in the first few days after injury because they inhibit the inflammatory response, which is critical to all phases of healing. Administration of steroids immediately after injury inhibits the migration of the WBCs and the extent of the inflammatory response. The anti-inflammatory effects of steroids also result in suppression of the immunologic response to bacteria. Thus, patients receiving steroids may have only subtle signs of infection when the bacterial load in the wound is very great. The immunosuppression mutes the inflammatory response, and fairly advanced infection may be present before signs and symptoms are overt (e.g., suppuration, increased temperature). Small changes in signs and symptoms of infection in immunosuppressed patients demand attention and exploration to determine whether they are related to the wound. In addition, it should be recognized that steroids impair all phases of healing, interfering with angiogenesis, collagen formation, epithelialization, and wound contraction (Ehrlich and Hunt, 1969; Sandberg, 1964).

Vitamin A is used as an inflammatory agent to reverse all of the effects of steroids except wound contraction. It is prescribed in an aqueous form or ointment base and is applied topically for 7 to 10 days to stimulate healing (Ehrlich et al., 1973; Hunt, 1986). Topical use confines the majority of the effects of vitamin A to the local wound and does not disrupt the systemic effects of steroids prescribed for other therapeutic purposes.

Radiation and chemotherapy slow wound healing. Both interrupt the cell cycle of tumor and healthy cells. In the patient undergoing elective surgery, these therapies may be withheld for a period prior to the procedure to allow the body to restore cells critical to the cellular response to healing. In patients with recent exposure to these therapies or for whom these therapies are continued, the inflammatory response is depressed. Clinically, this results in delayed healing and also in muting of the signs and symptoms of infection. Thus, the patient receiving chemotherapy or radiation therapy bears a double burden: he is not replicating cells in the wound module, and he also is immunosuppressed.

CLINICAL PRESENTATION OF IMPAIRED TISSUE

Integrity in Partial Thickness Wounds

Partial thickness wounds heal primarily by epithelialization. Epithelial cells arise from the adenyl structures of the skin, and closure of these defects usually occurs rapidly. Normal epithelialization is seen in pink tufts of epithelial cells arising around the adenyl structures.

In critical care patients, partial thickness injuries in themselves are not usually a problem because they rarely become infected. Impairment most commonly becomes manifested when these areas do not close in a timely manner and/or epithelial cells dehydrate and scabs form. They are, however, a serious concern because they are a site for entry of foreign organisms into the body because the skin, the body's first line of defense, is disrupted.

Full Thickness Wounds

Impairment in healing may manifest itself in several different ways because full thickness wounds are closed by varying methods. Closure of full thickness wounds occurs by primary, secondary, or tertiary intention (see Table 55–2).

PRIMARY INTENTION

Immediately after injury, wounds closed by primary intention generally have an initial inflammatory response seen at the wound site as redness, induration, and warmth. Pain and loss of function may be seen, depending on the extent of injury and the body part that is involved. The incision line normally is well approximated.

Epithelialization begins soon after injury, and in the patient with an uncomplicated injury, the epithelial layer seals the wound from external contamination within 24 to 48 hours. If wound drainage along the incision line is allowed to dry, a scab will form. The scab eventually falls off, revealing pink scar tissue below. Connective tissue needed to bridge the wound space is limited in wounds healing by primary intention. A sign that connective tissue repair is proceeding normally is the presence of a healing ridge by days 7 to 9 after injury. The healing ridge is palpable collagen and is an expected finding in all patients except those undergoing cosmetic surgery. Wound closure techniques used in patients having cosmetic surgery minimize scar formation and the associated healing ridge.

Impairment in the wound closed by primary intention is characterized by three alterations: drainage along the incision (in the absence of a drain) that continues after the first 48 hours, lack of a normal

---

TABLE 55–3. Abnormal Findings in Wounds Healing by Primary Intention

Drainage from the incision line 48 or more hours after wound closure
Severely decreased or absent inflammatory response
No healing ridge by days 7–9

---

inflammatory response, and absence of a healing ridge by days 7 to 9 (Table 55–3). Drainage along the incision line indicates that the wound has not been sealed by epithelialization. Lack of a normal inflammatory response is described as edema and redness 0.5 cm on both sides of the incision line. When the inflammatory response is depressed, WBCs and growth factors are not brought to the area and healing cannot occur at its normal rate. Absence of a healing ridge by the seventh to ninth day indicates that dehiscence and evisceration may occur.

SECONDARY INTENTION

Assessment and management of wounds healing by secondary intention provide the nurse with a challenge. The size and location of these wounds must be assessed. Size needs to be measured across several dimensions of the wound, and depth of the wound at the deepest area is measured perpendicularly with a sterile swab. Each time size and depth are measured, it is important that the patient be in the same position because shift of tissues with different positions will alter the size and depth of the wound. The wound is examined for the presence of tracts or tunnels that extend into the tissue. The number and location of the tracts are noted, and the size of each tract is measured and recorded. Tracts vary in area, and it is important to obtain an accurate measure so that changes can be appraised over time.

The wound itself then is examined. The granulation tissue is first examined, and then the exudate. Expected findings in wounds that are healing normally include the presence of granulation tissue that initially is pink and progresses to bright red. The change in the color of the tissue reflects the vascularization of the wound. As angiogenesis proceeds, capillary buds connect with similar buds from the opposite side of the wound and RBCs traverse the new capillaries, increasing the red color in the wound. This bright red color has been called "beefy red" because the color is that of a fresh beefsteak. When the tissue color does not progress from pink to red, the nurse needs to be concerned that healing is delayed. Granulation tissue normally is moist, and moisture needs to be maintained so that cells remain hydrated and do not have their cellular processes disrupted. When granulation tissue becomes dry, healing is delayed.

The presence of exudate in the wound then is assessed. Exudate is the byproduct of bacteria. The color and odor of the exudate are related to the specific organism involved. Colors frequently seen are serosanguineous, yellow, brown, and green. Black indicates that the tissue is necrotic. However, color may be deceptive because topical agents affect the color of the exudate; for example, povidone-iodine stains exudate yellow. Also, color becomes darker when it gets drier. Exudate may have no odor or may be musty, sweet, or foul smelling.

The wound edges are surrounded by pink epithelial tissue that normally is continuous around the wound. Over time, it becomes pearly white and extends down into the wound. When healing is abnormal in wounds closing by secondary intention, the epithelial edge may not be present or it may not be continuous around the wound. In addition, over time it may not extend down into the wound. Table 55–4 lists the abnormal findings in wounds healing by secondary intention.

Pressure Ulcers: Additional Evaluation of Wounds Healing by Secondary Intention

Pressure ulcers are a special case of wounds healing by secondary intention. A pressure ulcer is a localized area of tissue necrosis that develops when soft tissue is compressed between a bony prominence and a firm surface. Intrinsic factors that determine susceptibility to pressure ulcers are malnutrition, sensory loss, impaired mobility, altered mental status, incontinence, and old age. Extrinsic factors that contribute to ulcer formation are excessively high or prolonged tissue pressure, shear force, friction, and moisture (Macklebust, 1987). Ulcers are graded, or classified, according to depth, as well as assessed as described previously. Grading of ulcers helps the health care team predict when the ulcer will heal and determine whether the ulcer will heal with conservative medical treatment or whether it will require surgical treatment. Grades III and IV ulcers are the most serious. Grade III ulcers extend into subcutaneous tissue and muscle. Grade IV ulcers involve tissue down to the bone and are the most problematic, often requiring surgical intervention. Table 55–5 lists a frequently used grading system.

Documenting Clinical Status

Although the format each institution uses to organize data may vary, the content important to accurate documentation should be present in any system used, e.g., organization according to a nursing theory, nursing diagnosis, concepts, or problems.

TABLE 55–4. Abnormal Findings in Wounds Healing by Secondary Intention

Granulation tissue
  Very pale or not progressing from pink to beefy red
  Excessively moist or excessively dry
Wound size
  Unchanged or increasing after it is exudate free
Tracts
  Unchanged or increasing in size or number
Exudate
  Present; thick with or without an odor
Epithelial edge
  Not present or continuous around the wound

TABLE 55–5. Grading of Pressure Ulcers

I: Skin is red; capillary refill is delayed

II: Superficial skin damage is present; skin may be open or closed

III: Damage extends into the fat and/or muscle

IV: Damage extends to the bone

For wounds healing by primary intention, assessment parameters previously discussed are documented. Guidelines for documenting the status of wounds healing by secondary intention are found in Table 55–6.

External Environment: Local Treatment

Wound treatment is planned so that an environment that supports granulation tissue formation and re-epithelialization is maintained while contamination and dehydration are kept to a minimum. The characteristics of wounds help to direct treatment.

The treatment for wounds healing by primary intention requires a gauze dressing and in some cases an absorbent dressing as a cover for 2 to 3 days until the wound surface is sealed with a layer of epithelial cells.

Treatment for wounds healing by secondary intention is based on assessment to establish whether the wound is clean, exudative, or necrotic. Clean wounds are usually healthy with a bed of red granulation tissue and an edge of new epithelial tissue. Clean wounds with mature granulation tissue resist infection and generally heal well. Exudative wounds may have patches of granulation tissue but are preponderantly covered with exudate and debris. Characteristics of exudate color, odor, and viscosity vary with the type of organism present in the wound (Table 55–7). The exudate serves to enhance bacterial growth and retard tissue regeneration. Necrotic wounds are covered completely or in part with hard black eschar, which must be removed before healing can proceed.

Local treatment of wounds includes the use of dressings, topical application of antiseptics and drugs, débridement, and experimental treatment with growth factors (Knighton et al., 1988). Within each of these therapies there exist a myriad of treat-

TABLE 55–6. Guidelines for Documentation of Wounds Healing by Secondary Intention

Use a consistent protocol to describe the wound
Assess the wound rather than its dressing
Assess granulation tissue, exudate, and epithelialization
Record wound length, width, and depth at multiple locations
Use the same terminology as other members of the staff to describe the wound

TABLE 55–7. Characteristics of Wound Exudate

Organism	Color	Consistency	Odor
Streptococcus	Pink	Thin, watery	None
Clostridia	Brown	Thick	Sweet
Staphylococcus aureus	Serosanguineous/ creamy	Thin/thick	None
Endogenous bacteria (e.g., Bacteroides fragilis, Escherichia coli, Bacteroides oralis)	Purulent	Thick	Foul

Data from Alexander, J. W. (1983). Infection, host resistance, and antimicrobial agents. In American College of Surgeons, *Manual of preoperative and postoperative care* (3rd ed., pp. 106–136). Philadelphia: W. B. Saunders.

ment choices. Decisions about which therapy to use involve understanding the physiologic events of healing, establishing the state of the wound in the progression of healing, and having knowledge of the therapy and its influence on the physiologic processes of healing.

DRESSINGS

Biosynthetic Dressings

Traditionally, dressings have been used to protect and stabilize the wound; more recently, it has been recognized that dressings help to create an environment that supports healing. Research findings in the 1960s documented the beneficial effects of a moist environment for healing, demonstrating an increased rate of re-epithelialization (Hinman and Maibach, 1963; Winter, 1962; Winter and Scales, 1963). Wounds epithelialize twice as fast in a moist environment without the presence of a scab (Winter and Scales, 1963). Epithelial cell migration across a wound is impeded by the presence of dehydrated wound fluid that forms a scab. Recognition of the influence of a moist environment on healing has led to the development of many types of wound dressings, which vary in their permeability to gas or fluids and are generally classified as biosynthetic dressings. Biosynthetic dressings can be further categorized as semipermeable films, also called transparent polymer dressings; semiocclusive hydrogels; occlusive hydrocolloids; absorbent bead dressings; and foam dressings (Cuzzell, 1990). Definitions of these dressing categories and the properties of the dressings are summarized in Tables 55–8 and 55–9. Indications for the use of these dressings and their advantages and disadvantages are found in Tables 55–10 and 55–11.

GENERAL EFFECTS OF BIOSYNTHETIC DRESSINGS

The semipermeable, semiocclusive, and occlusive dressings support healing of open and primary wounds through varying mechanisms. They protect the wound's new epithelial edge from injury due to friction, prevent desiccation of tissue and allow epi-

dermal cell migration, promote autolytic digestion of necrotic material by polymorphonuclear leukocytes and macrophages in the wound fluid, and stimulate fibroblasts to synthesize collagen (Witkowski and Parish, 1986).

Relief of pain is associated with all of the biosynthetic dressings, particularly for wounds such as dermabrasions and skin graft donor sites. Hydrogel dressings may provide the most comfort because of their cooling effect. The mechanism for the relief of wound pain with occlusive dressings is not clear. A possible explanation is offered by the fact that some prostaglandins cause pain and these products may be limited by this type of dressing. Specifically, the prostaglandin synthetase system, which participates in the formation of prostaglandin E_2 (PGE_2), is oxygen dependent. Less PGE_2 may result from the reduction in oxygen under the occlusive dressing with less oxygen available for use in synthesizing these prostaglandins (Silver, 1985).

The wound fluid contained under biosynthetic dressings has antibacterial components such as complement, immunoglobulins, and lysozymes (May, 1984; Buchan et al., 1981). Along with the active WBCs in wound fluid, the presence of these factors and an acidic environment created by the dressings may help to explain the infrequent reports of infections associated with these dressings. However, biosynthetic dressings should be used cautiously in the presence of gram-negative bacteria, which thrive in a moist environment and increase after 48 hours (Mertz et al., 1985), and in patients who are immunosuppressed. It also has been shown that although occlusive dressings provide physical barriers to exogenous bacteria, once pathogens are introduced, the local environment will support their growth (Katz et al., 1986). Thus, gauze dressings are more appro-

TABLE 55–8. Categories of Biosynthetic Dressings

Category	Definition
Semipermeable films	Polyurethane sheets that are permeable to water vapor, oxygen, and other gases but impermeable to water. Nonabsorbent, maintain moisture
Semiocclusive hydrogels	Polyethylene oxide gel that is permeable to oxygen and water vapor. Absorbent, cooling, and maintain moist environment
Occlusive hydrocolloids	Gelatin, pectin, and hydroactive particles. Impermeable to gas and moisture. Absorbent, maintain moisture, contour to wound
Absorbent dressing	Dextran polymer beads or alginates. Oxygen and water permeable. Absorbent
Foam dressing	Polyurethane. Impermeable to gas and moisture. Maintains contour

TABLE 55–9. Properties of Biosynthetic Dressings

Category	Permeability		Absorbent	Excludes Bacteria	Damage to New Epidermis
	Gas	Fluid			
Polymers	Yes	No	No	Some	Yes
Hydrogels	Yes	Yes	Yes	No	No
Hydrocolloids (HCDs)	No	No	Yes	Yes	No
Absorbent dressing	?	?	Yes	No	No
Foam dressing	No	No	Yes	Yes	No

priately used in patients whose cultures show gram-negative organisms than the occlusive or semiocclusive dressings.

Depending on the patient's general condition, occlusive and semiocclusive dressings can be used for clean, seminecrotic, and exudative wounds. The schedule for changing the dressing will vary. More frequent changes are indicated in critically ill individuals, who are more likely to be colonized with pathogens, and in cases in which gram-negative organisms are present or suspected. Heavily exudative wounds will require more frequent dressing changes.

The higher cost of the biosynthetic dressings compared with gauze or other traditional dressings is often raised as a concern. Determination of the cost of wound treatment should include not only the cost of the product but also the time associated with dressing changes. The frequency of wound care, the rate of healing, and associated complications, if any occur, also need to be evaluated. For instance, the biosynthetic dressings do not need to be changed as often as gauze dressings and may significantly reduce time required for wound care (Kurzuk-Howard et al., 1985). Because the dressings are associated with faster epithelialization and stimulation of reparative

cells, healing may be achieved more quickly. When these factors are considered, the use of biosynthetic dressings may provide a cost-effective alternative for wound care.

The major categories of dressings are discussed in the following sections.

SEMIPERMEABLE TRANSPARENT DRESSINGS

Transparent polymer dressings are composed of polyurethane and are marketed as thin, transparent sterile sheets (e.g., Opsite, Tegaderm, Bioclusive, Ensure). They are permeable to gases such as oxygen and carbon dioxide and also transmit moisture vapor. It was thought that a dressing's ability to increase

TABLE 55–10. Clinical Indications for Dressings

Type of Wound	Appropriate Dressing(s)
Partial Thickness Wounds	
Blisters; dermabrasions; stage I and II ulcers; skin graft donor sites	Transparent films; hydrogels; hydrocolloids; wet to wet gauze
Exudative	Hydrogels; hydrocolloids; absorbent dressing; wet to damp gauze
Necrotic	Hydrocolloids; wet to damp gauze
Full Thickness Wounds	
Primary intention	Dry gauze
Secondary intention:*	
Healthy, granulating	Wet to damp or wet to wet fine mesh gauze; hydrocolloid granules
Exudative	Absorbent dressing; damp coarse mesh gauze
Necrotic	Wet to dry or wet to damp coarse mesh gauze

*Includes stage III and IV ulcers.

TABLE 55–11. Advantages and Limitations of Dressings

Dressing	Advantages	Limitations
Wet to damp or wet to wet gauze	Keeps tissue moist; vehicle for application of solutions; absorbs exudate; inexpensive	Damage to new tissue if removed when dry; may require frequent changing; can macerate new tissue
Transparent films (e.g., Tegaderm)	Keep tissue moist; preserve wound fluid; relieve pain; easy to apply	Nonabsorbent; can damage new tissue on removal; aspiration may be needed for excessive fluid; do not exclude all bacteria
Hydrogels (e.g., Vigilon)	Keep tissue moist; no damage to new tissue; relieve pain; easy to apply	Require frequent changing; not bacteria resistant; can macerate normal tissue
Hydrocolloids (e.g., Duoderm)	Keep tissue moist; absorb some exudate; relieve pain; easy to apply	Cannot assess wound directly, due to opacity
Absorbent beads	Highly absorbent; dressing relieves pain; reduces bacteria	May dehydrate tissue excessively
Foam dressing	Insulating; relieves pain	Opaque, so cannot directly assess wound

oxygen tension at the wound surface enhances the rate of re-epithelialization (Silver, 1972). However, this has not been substantiated in more recent studies that show that even though these dressings are gas permeable, oxygen tensions at the wound surface are very low (Varghese et al., 1986; Eaglstein, 1985).

The semipermeable transparent dressings are fluid impermeable and have no absorptive properties, so that pooling of fluid under the dressing occurs. The dressings adhere to intact epithelium surrounding the wound but not to the denuded wounds. However, as healing progresses and the wound has less exudate, the dressings may adhere to the wound surface and damage new epithelium during their removal (Witkowski and Parish, 1986). Transparent dressings have been used to cover decubitus and stasis ulcers, surgical incisions (in animal and human studies), and skin graft donor sites (Linsky et al., 1981; Barnett et al., 1983). Donor sites covered with transparent dressings have healed faster than those covered with fine mesh gauze (6.9 days compared with 10.5 days) (Barnett et al., 1983). A reduction in wound pain also has been associated with the transparent dressings (Witkowski and Parish, 1986). The effects of these dressings on surgical incisions in humans when compared with gauze dressings included faster re-epithelialization, less eschar formation, less inflammation, and better wound apposition in 70% of 19 cases. In an animal study of incisions closed by primary intention, transparent dressing–treated wounds demonstrated diminished influx of fibroblasts, less collagen synthesis, and a decreased breaking strength when compared with wounds exposed to air (Linsky et al., 1981). Partial thickness wounds dressed with polyurethane have shown increased collagen synthesis compared with wounds exposed to air and wounds dressed with wet to dry gauze. However, the increase in collagen does not ensure that bursting strength is greater (Alvarez et al., 1983). This finding can be understood by remembering that breaking strength is related to maturity of collagen with the cross-linking of fibers. Hence, polyurethane dressings provide moist environments that promote wound comfort and re-epithelialization of primary and secondary wounds. Their effect on fibroblast activity and ultimate scar strength raises questions about their use for incisions closed primarily. Further research on the effects of these dressings beyond 7 days is needed to answer questions about the long-term effects of polyurethane dressings on wound strength.

HYDROGEL DRESSINGS

Hydrogel dressings (e.g., Vigilon, Spenco Second Skin, Geliperm) are a mixture of 96% water and 4% polyethylene oxide suspended between two sheets of polyethylene, providing a semitransparent dressing. Like transparent dressings, they are permeable to oxygen and water vapor; however, they do not adhere well to either intact or wound tissue and a gauze cover and/or tape is required to secure them. The hydrogel material has absorbent properties and can absorb nearly its own weight in wound exudate (Mandy, 1983). The hydrogel material is placed on the wound after removing one of the encasing polyethylene sheets. If desired, the top sheet also can be removed and a gauze dressing applied so that exudate moves from the wound bed to the outer dressing layers. In addition to their absorptive qualities, hydrogel dressings produce a cooling sensation, a reduction in pain, and rapid re-epithelialization, making them an ideal choice for dermabrasion and friction blisters with exudate and fluid production (Wheeland, 1987).

Bacterial proliferation has been shown to occur under hydrogel dressings in an animal model in which wounds were inoculated with *Staphylococcus aureus*, *Escherichia coli*, or *Pseudomonas aeruginosa* (Leaper et al., 1984). Wounds inoculated with *S. aureus* or *E. coli* did not have delayed wound contraction. In these wounds, the numbers of organisms increased for about a week but were decreasing after 10 days. However, wounds with *Pseudomonas* did have delayed healing and a large increase in organisms after 10 days of occlusion. These results suggest that hydrogel dressings should be changed frequently in order to avoid bacterial growth, especially if *Pseudomonas* is present.

HYDROCOLLOID DRESSINGS

Hydrocolloid dressings (HCDs) such as DuoDerm, Comfeel, and Granuflex consist of hydroactive particles, gelatin, pectin, and carboxymethylcellulose in a hydrophobic polymer base. The dressing is applied after removal of the silicone release paper that covers one side of the dressing. It adheres to intact epithelium, but over the wound, fluid interacts with the dressing materials and forms a semisolid gel that expands into the wound cavity (Turner, 1985). Hydrocolloid dressings are opaque, are impermeable to gases or fluid, and are absorbent to the extent that there is gel available. The wound fluid–gel formation keeps the wound bed moist, supporting epithelial cell migration and also protecting newly formed tissue from injury when the dressing is removed. Angiogenesis has been shown to be significantly greater after 7 days of healing in wounds dressed with hydrocolloid as compared with gauze dressings (Cherry and Ryan, 1985). The HCD wounds had a 29% decrease in size compared with 23% for gauze-covered wounds. This finding is explained by the fact that hydrocolloid dressings are impermeable to oxygen, and the authors hypothesized that a hypoxic stimulus for angiogenesis may be produced by the dressings (Cherry and Ryan, 1985).

Hydrocolloid dressings are appropriate coverings for skin graft donor sites and also may prove to be useful for incisions closed by primary intention. Comparisons of healing time for skin graft donor sites covered with HCDs or saline gauze have been reported (Biltz et al., 1985; Madden et al., 1985). Both reports show that re-epithelialization was significantly faster for HCDs, and those patients with HCDs had significantly less pain at the donor site in both reports. HCDs have also been used as an alternative to conventional postoperative dressings for incisions closed by primary intention. Young and Weston-Davies (1985) compared comfort, convenience, incidence of complication (skin sensitivity or infection), and cosmetic appearance of the wound for HCDs and standard postoperative dressings. There were no differences in complications associated with either dressing, and the researchers reported that HCDs were easier to apply and required less changing; they also reported how HCDs affect collagen synthesis and strength in incisions closed by primary intention.

Bacterial proliferation of normal skin flora (micrococci, diphtheroid bacilli, and *S. aureus*) in normal volunteers decreased over a 4-day period of occlusion with an HCD (Lawrence and Lilly, 1985). In another study of venous leg ulcers treated either with an HCD plus compression or a double-layer bandage (inner layer impregnated with zinc oxide paste), *S. aureus* and other pathogenic bacteria decreased as healing progressed with both dressings (Eriksson, 1985).

ABSORBENT DRESSINGS

Absorbent dressings (e.g., Debrisan) are hydrophilic dextran polymer porous beads. The beads are useful for exudative wounds because of their ability to absorb wound fluid. They are placed into the wound dry or in combination with anhydrous glycerin and then covered with a polymeric transparent dressing. The beads act to draw wound exudate into the interspaces between beads by capillary action; the fluid is then absorbed by the beads. Substances in wound fluid also are absorbed into the beads, depending on molecular weight and size. Larger molecules and bacteria are not absorbed into the beads but become trapped in the interspaces between beads. The effect of the beads is to draw fluid and bacteria away from the surface of the wound and into the upper gel layer that forms as the beads swell. The use of absorptive beads for chronic leg ulcers, pressure sores, surgical sites, and chemical necrosis wounds has been associated with decreased wound inflammation, decreased exudate, and an improved granulation bed in the wound (Jacobsson et al., 1976a; Jacobsson et al., 1976b; Pace, 1978). These effects have been helpful in reducing the time to prepare a wound or ulcer for split thickness skin grafting (Jacobsson et al., 1976a). Although it is not clear whether the beads expedite the healing process, they have improved healing in patients with wounds resistant to other treatments (Pace, 1978). The beads have also been noted to reduce pain associated with skin graft donor sites (Jacobsson et al., 1976b). In one report, excessive dehydration of several wounds treated with absorptive beads occurred in patients

with decreased arterial blood supply, suggesting the need for cautious use in some patients, particularly the elderly (Pace, 1978). The primary action of absorptive beads is to reduce bacterial load on the wound surface and absorb exudate effectively, reducing mediators of inflammation or infection. There is no evidence that they débride wounds, and although the beads draw bacteria away from the wounds, there is proliferation of bacteria within the dressing after 24 hours (Jacobsson et al., 1976b). They seem to be most beneficial for treatment of heavily exudative wounds or those unresponsive to other therapies.

Alginate dressings are another type of absorbent dressing. They are made from the salts of alginic acid, a polymer that is a critical component of the cell wall of brown seaweed. These dressings come as a fiber and display their hydrophilic properties when in contact with the small amount of sodium that is present in wound exudate. An ion exchange results in the formation of a gel. The gel wicks exudate into the dressing and away from the wound while maintaining an ambient environment that is moist and physiologic. The dressing is removed with saline irrigation, and so dressing change does not interfere with the new granulation tissue that has been formed.

Alginate dressings have been used for a variety of purposes over time, e.g., as a hemostatic agent (Oliver and Blaine, 1950). After refinement, they were reintroduced in the wound market in Europe to be used in the management of exudating wounds such as pressure ulcers, vascular ulcers, diabetic ulcers, and superficial wounds. They have been shown to augment the rate of wound closure and to reduce pain to the wound site (Gilchrist and Martin, 1983; Thomas, 1985; Odugbesan and Barnett, 1987). Reports also indicate that they have been used in cavity wounds (Dealey, 1989). Dressings initially are changed several times per day, and as exudate abates the frequency may move to as infrequently as every 4 days before another product replaces it.

Foam Dressings

Foam dressings are a two-surfaced dressing with a nonabsorbable polyurethane that faces the wound and a foam that provides the outer layer. Thus foam dressings combine the properties of an absorption control dressing that maintains a moist environment with those of an insulating and protecting dressing (Cuzzell, 1990; Krasner, 1991). The value of the insulation has not been established with empirical studies, but temperature variations among parts of the body long have been associated with the rate of healing—i.e., warmer areas heal faster.

The foam dressings are designed for use with more superficial types of wounds (Cuzzell, 1990); e.g., radiation reactions, first and second degree burns, pressure ulcers, vascular ulcers, and dermabrasion.

Some are self-adhesive, whereas others require sealing with tape. All are opaque, making observation of the wound possible only when the dressing is changed.

Gauze Dressings

Gauze dressings, especially for full thickness open wounds, provide a moist healing environment when dampened with solutions such as physiologic saline or antimicrobial agents. Selection of the type of gauze (coarse or finer mesh) depends upon the characteristics of the wound. The use of coarse gauze is recommended for exudate removal and is based on the principle that exudate and wound fluids will move away from the wound into the interstices of gauze and be absorbed and removed when the dressing is changed (Noe and Kalish, 1976). A finer gauze with smaller interstices is appropriate for wounds that are clean and granulating. When gauze dressings are applied to wounds that are healing by secondary intention, the dressing should first be opened completely and then moistened with normal saline or another solution as prescribed. The gauze is then placed into the wound cavity so that a layer of gauze is in contact with all of the wound surface. Other layers of dressings are then added as necessary, care being taken to avoid packing the wound too tightly, which might apply unwanted pressure to the healing tissues.

Gauze "wet to dry" or "wet to damp" or "damp to damp" dressings are inserted into wound cavities; the damp layer keeps the granulating tissue and wound margin moist. The outer layers of these gauze dressings protect the wound from external contamination. Wet to damp dressings are removed before the dressing has dried completely and while the inside layer is still damp. This allows the removal of exudate and wound debris without disrupting new tissue. Wet to wet dressings are not permitted to dry and therefore require frequent changing. These dressings maintain a moist environment for the wound that appears to promote cleansing and offer a small amount of débridement (Rudolph and Noe, 1983).

Controversy exists as to whether the gauze should be allowed to dry before removal as in wet to dry dressings, but current thinking on the subject supports removal of the dressing when it is moist and not stuck to the tissue (Sawyer et al., 1980). Dressings that are removed when still moist, or moistened before removal, will be less likely to disrupt and damage fragile new granulation and epithelial tissue. Bleeding that occurs with the removal of a dressing indicates that capillaries have been injured and will have to undergo repair. Continual damage to new tissue by removal of dressings needs to be avoided.

TOPICAL SOLUTIONS AND OINTMENTS

Topical treatment of wounds often includes the use of antiseptic solutions and antimicrobial oint-

ments employed to limit the growth of microorganisms. Although many of the agents are recognized for their efficacy as antibacterial agents, their effects on wound healing are less clear and thus controversial (Table 55–12).

Antiseptic Solutions

Bacterial contamination of wounds to the extent of producing infection delays healing. However, the prolonged use of antiseptics on healing wounds has been debated because of their effects on physiologic processes of healing. Antiseptics are toxic to microbes as well as to host cells. Topical antiseptics aid healing only through bacterial control and are probably more detrimental than helpful to processes of cellular repair unless a wound is heavily contaminated or infected (Goodman and Gilman, 1985). They are absorbed irregularly and unpredictably, particularly when the skin is not intact, and can have adverse systemic effects. Popular antiseptic solutions used in wound care include sodium hypochlorite, povidone-iodine, acetic acid, and hydrogen peroxide.

Sodium hypochlorite (0.5%), povidone-iodine (1%), acetic acid (0.25%), and hydrogen peroxide (3%) are common solutions used in wound care and have been shown to be toxic to human fibroblasts and to retard epithelialization in animal wounds (Lineaweaver et al., 1985). Hypochlorite solutions are intended for disinfecting contaminated wounds (Goodman and Gilman, 1985). Sodium hypochlorite, a component of Dakin's solution, is a bleaching agent that kills bacteria by the release of free chlorine into the wound. It is recommended that half-strength (0.25%) Dakin's solution be applied using wet to wet coarse mesh gauze dressings that are not allowed to dry (Rudolph and Noe, 1983). Studies have shown that hypochlorite solutions have damaging effects on wound healing. One study documented less collagen synthesis and prolonged inflammatory response in animal wounds treated with 1% hypochlorite containing solutions compared with wounds treated with normal saline (Brennan et al., 1986). A solution of 1% hypochlorite applied directly to granulation

TABLE 55–12. Adverse Effects of Antiseptic Solutions

Solution	Effect on Wound
Sodium hypochlorite (Dakin) (0.5%)	Decreased epithelialization; toxic to fibroblasts, new granulation tissue
Povidone-iodine (1%)	Toxic to fibroblasts; decreased epithelialization; increased susceptibility to infection
Hydrogen peroxide (3%)	Damage to new epithelium
Acetic acid (0.25%)	Toxic to fibroblasts; may delay healing time

tissue was also found to be toxic to the new vessels of granulation tissue (Brennan and Leaper, 1985). These results suggest that chlorine containing solutions be used with caution and that their use in healthy granulating wounds be avoided.

Iodine is complexed with polyvinylpyrrolidone to produce povidone-iodine, which liberates free iodine in solution. Its mechanism of killing bacteria and spores is unknown, but it is considered an effective germicide when used on intact skin (Goodman and Gilman, 1985). Its use in wounds healing by secondary intention is controversial and has been described as indiscriminate (Rodeheaver, 1989). Reports on the effects of povidone-iodine on healing are variable. When used on full and split thickness wounds in animals or human skin graft donor sites, it has not produced a delay in mean healing time (Gruber et al., 1975). Rodeheaver and associates (1982) reported that wounds exposed to the scrub form of povidone-iodine actually had increased susceptibility to infection, probably due to cytotoxic action of the detergent on leukocytes. Furthermore, povidone-iodine antiseptic solution treated wounds did not differ from saline treated wounds in terms of bacteria counts. Another study of patients with contaminated pressure ulcers showed povidone-iodine to be the least effective agent in reducing bacterial load when compared with saline and silver sulfadiazine (Kucan et al., 1981). Wounds treated with 1% povidone-iodine also have been reported to be significantly weaker than control wounds when irrigated three times per day for a 4-day period (Lineaweaver et al., 1985). On the other hand, when 1% povidone-iodine was used once as a wound soak for 15 minutes prior to surgical closure, there was no difference in development of wound strength compared with control wounds (Mulliken et al., 1980).

The use of povidone-iodine in cases in which large areas of tissue are exposed to the solution merits careful consideration. Iodine can be absorbed from dressings into the systemic circulation. This absorption has been associated with metabolic acidosis and renal failure (Aronoff et al., 1980). Povidone-iodine should be used cautiously not only because of its potentially damaging effects to reparative cells and questionable efficacy for bacterial control but also because of its documented systemic consequences.

Hydrogen peroxide is an oxidizing agent; contact with tissues releases oxygen, producing a short period of antimicrobial action (Goodman and Gilman, 1985). It acts as a surface cleanser and is often used in solution with normal saline as a wound irrigant. Wounds treated with a solution of 3% hydrogen peroxide showed shorter healing times in one study; however, the solution produced bullae on skin graft donor sites, suggesting damage to new epithelium (Gruber et al., 1975). Because of this effect, Gruber and colleagues (1975) recommended that hydrogen peroxide not be used on newly epithelialized wounds. In addition, hydrogen peroxide (0.3% and 3% solutions) is toxic to fibroblasts and therefore

would have deleterious effects on collagen formation (Lineaweaver et al., 1985).

Acetic acid as an antimicrobial agent is effective against gram-negative organisms, especially *Pseudomonas aeruginosa* (Goodman and Gilman, 1985). In one study, a solution of 0.25% acetic acid had no significant effects on healing time or microscopic findings (Gruber et al., 1975). Conversely, a solution of 0.25% acetic acid has been shown to be toxic to fibroblasts (Lineaweaver et al., 1985).

Antimicrobial Agents

Treatment of wounds with topical antimicrobial agents has not demonstrated as many negative effects on healing as antiseptic solutions; however, reports are limited. Three antimicrobial agents were investigated for their effect on epidermal wound healing (Eaglstein and Mertz, 1981). Neosporin ointment (a mix of neomycin, polymyxin, and bacitracin-zinc) promoted healing by 25% compared with untreated controls. Furacin-soluble dressing (nitrofurazone) slowed healing by 30%, and Silvadene (silver sulfadiazine) produced the fastest healing rate, 28% greater than nontreated control wounds. It is possible that the medium containing the antimicrobial agents plays a role in altering the rate of re-epithelialization, since antimicrobial agents of the different ointments alone did not account for the healing differences (Eaglstein and Mertz, 1981).

Summary of Topical Agents

The available data indicate that topical antimicrobial solutions and ointments need to be used with caution, due to documented adverse effects on healing. They are indicated for wounds that are necrotic and/or heavily contaminated and may in fact assist in the débridement and sloughing of necrotic material and debris (Leaper and Simpson, 1986). Once the wound is clean, these agents are no longer necessary, and a change to a moist saline gauze, occlusive, or semiocclusive type dressing is preferable.

DÉBRIDEMENT

Necrotic tissue that is left undisturbed in a wound acts to encourage infection in the wound and delay the healing process. Infection is promoted by necrotic tissue through its action as a culture medium and through its inhibiting effect on leukocyte phagocytosis and function (Edlich et al., 1977). Removal of devitalized tissue is critical for healing to proceed and can be accomplished through several methods.

Surgical Débridement

Surgical débridement is often the treatment of choice and most quickly rids the wound of the necrotic debris. However, sometimes the patient's condition or the involvement of specialized tissues such as tendons or nerves in the necrotic wound limits the extent to which surgical débridement can be used. Other methods include mechanical débridement using irrigation or gauze dressings; chemical débridement with topical enzymes; and biologic débridement, described as autolysis occurring with biosynthetic dressings.

Chemical Débridement

Proteolytic enzyme products (e.g., Travase, Elase, Collagenase) are available for use in wound débridement. This type of product is often selected for the treatment of necrotic pressure ulcers and vascular ulcers of the lower extremities. There is little research documenting the efficacy of these products in removing necrotic tissue. These enzymes can be used as an adjunct to surgical débridement or alone as a wound treatment. They are tissue-specific enzymes that act by digesting denatured and undenatured collagen and by dissolving fibrinous exudates and clots without damaging healthy tissue (Reuler and Cooney, 1981).

Débriding enzymes are applied topically to the wound eschar and are covered with a moist dressing. Because they do not penetrate eschar well, it is recommended that the eschar be crosshatched first to promote their effectiveness (Fowler, 1987). Results are usually obtained within a 14-day period. Manufacturer recommendations need to be followed closely to obtain the best results; some enzymes are inactivated by acidic environments and should not be used. Wound solutions such as acetic acid may interact with metals and cannot be used with products containing chlorine, iodine, or silver (Alterescu, 1984).

Mechanical Débridement

Wound irrigation, usually in combination with dressings, is used to clean and débride exudative or necrotic wounds mechanically. Debris and necrotic material present in the wound are removed when the irrigation pressure exceeds the adhesive forces of the contaminants (Edlich et al., 1977). High-pressure irrigation, defined as pressure that is 8 or more pounds per square inch (psi), has been found to be more effective than low-pressure irrigation for wound débridement (Brown et al., 1978; Hamer et al., 1975; Rodeheaver et al., 1975). High-pressure irrigation producing 8 psi can be accomplished using an 18-gauge plastic catheter attached to a 35-mL syringe (Edlich et al., 1977; Stevenson et al., 1976). Although pulsatile high-pressure irrigation is more effective in cleansing wounds compared with continuous low-pressure irrigation, it damages the wound's resistance to infection (Wheeler et al., 1976). These studies suggest that high-pressure, continuous irrigation using a syringe will provide effective cleaning that does not compromise host resistance.

NURSING OF PATIENTS WITH WOUNDS

Nursing care of patients with wounds is based on data from the patient's history and physical examination and knowledge of the patient's underlying disease and how it is being treated. The history gives the nurse data about risk factors that the patient has brought to the critical care unit (e.g., diabetes, age, steroid therapy). The physical examination provides data about the patient's wound status as well as about his general status (e.g., oxygenation, volume of nutrition). These data, together with knowledge of the patient's underlying disease state, allow the nurse to develop a plan of nursing care that addresses local and systemic support for healing in the context of the multitude of other clinical problems that patients in the critical care unit experience. Table 55–13 lists the nursing diagnoses commonly seen in patients with wounds. A nursing care plan is found at the end of the chapter.

Systemic support is provided for the patient with wounds. Major concerns include adequate tissue perfusion, normal acid-base status and electrolyte levels, fluid balance, good control of glucose, sufficient oxygenation, and adequate nutrients. To the best of our knowledge, critically ill patients with wounds need care directed at establishing and maintaining normal laboratory values and usual amounts of intravascular volume, oxygen, and nutrients for healing.

Intravascular volume in patients with wounds is maintained most often through intravenous fluids, with the goal being good circulating volume without having the patient develop congestive heart failure or hypovolemia. Strategies used for balancing volume status are consistent with those used for any patient in the critical care unit.

Research has shown that tissue oxygenation is consistently higher than wound oxygen levels

---

TABLE 55–13. Nursing Diagnoses for Patients with Healing Wounds

Major Diagnostic Category*
Potential impaired skin integrity
Impaired skin integrity
Impaired tissue integrity

Related Factors
Fluid volume deficit
Impaired perfusion, oxygen supply
Inadequate nutrition
Infection
Immune system incompetence
Impaired physical mobility

*Data from North American Nursing Diagnosis Association (NANDA), 1988.

(Chang et al., 1983); however, data are not currently available that indicate whether specific nursing activities influence wound oxygenation (e.g., coughing, deep breathing, ambulation, positioning). Until such data are available, activities that support systemic oxygenation as seen in Pa_{O_2} levels and oxygen saturations need to be pursued in patients with wounds.

Similarly, nutritional support based on patients' metabolic needs should be adequate to meet the energy and substrate needs of critically ill patients with wounds. Attention also needs to be given to vitamin and mineral support, but specific prescriptive guidelines for patients with varying types and severity of wounds have not yet been developed. Until such guidelines are available, vitamin and mineral support is formulated pragmatically based on knowledge of metabolic need and estimated losses through wounds, diarrhea, and fistula drainage.

The local and systemic effects of drugs also need to be factored into the care of patients with wounds. Patients receiving steroids are at increased risk for impaired healing because these drugs inhibit all phases of healing. The use of vitamin A to reverse all the effects of the steroids except contraction has been recommended by some investigators but has not been recommended universally as an approach to mitigation of steroid effects. Chemotherapeutic drugs also delay healing. When these medications cannot or are not stopped prior to wounding, nursing care needs to focus on increased support of aseptic technique to minimize wound contamination and the possibility of infection. In wounds that have been closed by primary intention, additional splinting of the incision line needs to be provided to support the tensile strength of the wound and prevent dehiscence. Anticoagulants are another group of drugs that may impair healing. Their effects are prominent in patients in the early post-injury period, when the coagulation cascade participates most fully in stopping bleeding into the wound. Awareness of the possibility of this complication will allow the nurse to assess wounds for continued bleeding and/or oozing so that early intervention can be undertaken to reverse the effects of anticoagulants, use measures to stop the bleeding (e.g., pressure to the area), and/or provide local evacuation of wound hematomas so that the site does not become a nidus for infection.

Local wound care is based on the appearance of the wound and knowledge of the patient's underlying disease and its treatment. Fundamentally, wounds healing by primary intention need treatment aimed at providing moisture to support epithelialization, preventing external contamination, and mitigating mechanical trauma. For these wounds, a dry sterile dressing is most frequently used. When in contact with the patient's skin, this dressing traps skin moisture and promotes epithelialization. If the wound is in an area where it may be threatened by external contamination (e.g., tracheostomy secretion), a hydrophobic layer such as Vaseline gauze may be used next to the incision to prevent contamination of the wound. Similarly, if the area may be

subject to trauma, as is seen in lateral thoracic incisions with turning, extra padding may be needed to prevent mechanical damage to the tissue. Although the newer dressings at times have been used on wounds closed by primary intention, because they delay early development of tensile strength along the incision, they probably cannot be recommended as routine treatment until research establishes their safety, especially for use in the critically ill, who frequently experience multiple confounding factors that increase the risk of impaired healing. For the most part, wounds healing by primary intention seal within 48 hours of closure and risk of impairment in healing is more related to the success of the intraoperative intervention and support of systemic factors than to very sophisticated, unusual, or newer approaches to local wound care.

Wounds healing by secondary intention can be a challenge to the critical care nurse. Many products and approaches have been developed to treat these wounds. A paradigm has been developed to aid the nurse in determining the type of local care required by wounds healing by secondary intention (Stotts, 1990). This approach, called the *three color concept*, provides guidelines for therapy based on the color of the wound. Although untested, this approach uses principles of care established over time in care of patients with all types of wounds. The paradigm is based on knowledge of healthy granulating tissue, the ideal for this type of wound. Optimal tissue appearance is beefy red, and healing is supported when the wound is kept moist. Delay in healing is seen when the wound surface is yellow or black. Yellow and all of its shades from a very pale creamy yellow to the yellows with more green in them indicate that exudate is present and the wound is contaminated. Yellow exudate needs to be removed from the wound by cleansing. A black appearance to a wound indicates that necrotic tissue is present. Necrotic tissue is an ideal medium for growth of bacteria and is treated by débridement.

The paradigm indicates that red wounds are kept moist, yellow wounds are cleansed, and black wounds are débrided. These three principles guide care, yet do not dictate the specific product or approach that is to be used (Table 55–14). For example, débridement may be performed with enzymes or moist to moist dressings, mechanically (high-pres-

TABLE 55–14. Three Color Concept

Color	Goal of Treatment	Examples
Red	Keep moist	Transparent dressings; hydrogel
Yellow	Clean	Irrigation; Moist to moist dressings
Black	Débride	Enzymes; whirlpool

Data from Stotts, 1990.

sure irrigation or a whirlpool), surgically (with a scalpel), or by auto-débridement (patient's own body cleans area). Similarly, cleansing may be accomplished with hydrophilic beads, with hydrogel polymers, mechanically (high pressure irrigation), with antibiotic ointment, or with moist to moist dressings. Maintaining moisture of the wound can be facilitated by a number of methods; approaches such as transparent dressings, hydrogels, moist to moist dressings, and drug impregnated dressings have been used.

To use the three color approach, the critical care nurse must know the products and therapies that are available in her institution, the advantages and limitations of each, and how those therapies fit with the overall goals for the patient. Such an approach will allow the nurse to plan local wound care that is based on current scientific knowledge, maximizes use of available products and therapies (which vary among settings), and provides local care in the context of the overall goals of care for the patient.

Recent nursing research in the care of patients with healing wounds has focused on the effect of the environment on healing. Studies have examined the effects of noise on healing in a rat model (Wysocki, 1986) and the use of guided imagery to reduce stress and enhance wound healing in patients with surgical incisions (Holden-Lund, 1988). Although these studies were not conducted in the critical care unit with critically ill patients, they laid the foundation for research that addresses these concepts with critical care patients. In addition, the concept of pain management during dressing changes of patients with wounds healing by secondary intention has received attention. Music has been used to augment narcotics in pain management during dressing changes of surgical patients with wounds healing by secondary intention (Angus and Faux, 1989). Also, pain control during dressing changes of similar wounds has been shown to be augmented with the use of transcutaneous electrical nerve stimulation (Hargreaves and Lander, 1989). Although additional research is reported that establishes the value of these approaches to pain management and wound healing during dressing changes, such strategies might also be considered for individual patients who present especially difficult or complex management problems.

In the future, wound care will continue to focus on manipulation of the patient's surroundings to provide an optimal environment for healing and, in addition, probably will involve the application of growth factors to influence cell growth and tissue repair. Several growth factors that stimulate fibroblasts and endothelial and epithelial cells have been isolated, e.g., platelet-derived growth factor (PDGF), epidermal growth factor (EGF), and insulin-like growth factor 1 (IGF-1). The sources of the factors include cells such as platelets and macrophages, and organs such as the brain and liver, with delivery of the factors to responding cells by endocrine, paracrine, and autocrine pathways (Nemeth et al., 1988). The growth factors are present in wound fluid and act to attract cells necessary for repair and stimulate proliferation of cells. Research in this area is expanding rapidly, providing a better understanding of the effects of growth factors on healing, the normal growth environment, and whether there is a role for the use of these substances in wounds with impaired healing (Hunt, 1988).

A study by Knighton and colleagues (1988) illustrates the potential benefit of growth factors in treating poorly healing wounds. In a double-blind, crossover clinical trial, 32 patients with wounds that had not healed in 8 or more weeks were randomized between a control group and an experimental group for treatment with platelet-derived wound healing formula (PDWHF), which is produced from the patient's blood. Patients were treated for 8 weeks; at that time, the control group "crossed-over" to receive the experimental treatment of PDWHF. In the original experimental group all wounds were completely epithelialized in an average of 6 weeks, whereas in the control group only 25% of wounds healed in 8 weeks. When the control patients received the PDWHF, all of the unhealed wounds epithelialized in an average of 6.5 weeks. Although one clinical trial, with a relatively small sample, does not constitute a basis for general treatment, the study provides an example of the possible clinical use and benefits that growth factors may hold for wound healing in the future.

PHYSICIAN AND NURSING COLLABORATION

Physicians and nurses in critical care units often work together to determine the best treatment for the patient systemically as well as to establish a plan for local care of wounds. With the patient who is admitted to a unit primarily for prevention or treatment of wound healing impairment, the physician often takes the lead in determining the nature of treatment the wound is to receive locally as well as the appropriate supportive care. However, probably more common is the patient who is admitted to a unit for another problem and happens to have a wound. Often in fact, the wound in such a patient is a secondary concern and may be neglected in the more immediate needs of perfusion, oxygenation, and maintenance of organ viability that characterize the critically ill population. In this case, the nurse often takes the initiative to assess the wound and recommend therapy. Probably the third category of patients with wounds seen in critical care units are those who develop iatrogenic wounds such as pressure ulcers, fistulas, or skin tears. These are situations in which the nurse often is the first to diagnose the problem and recommend a plan of care or seek to develop one cooperatively with the physician. In all cases, the institution's standards of care and unit protocol establish route nursing therapies that are employed independently and those treatments that require prescription by the physician.

ncp nursing care plan

1. Impaired tissue integrity related to:

Inadequate perfusion	Fluid and electrolyte disturbances
Insufficient tissue oxygenation	Cancer
Malnutrition	Immunosuppression
Diabetes	Infection

Outcome Criteria	Nursing Interventions

Partial thickness wounds will be healing as evidenced by:
  Presence of new epithelium.
  Decrease in wound size.
Full thickness wound closed by primary intention will be healing as evidenced by:
  Well-approximated wound edges.
  Inflammation present for about 3 days after injury seen as redness, induration, warmth, pain, and loss of function.
  Inflammatory response abated after 3 days.
  No drainage from incision line after 48 hours (in wound with no drain present).
  Healing ridge present 7–9 days after closure.
Full thickness wound healing by secondary intention will be healing as evidenced by:
  Granulation tissue is present and moist and is progressing from a light pink to a beefy red.
  Decrease in wound size.
  Decrease in the number and size of tracts.
  Decreasing or absent exudate.
  Epithelial tissue is forming around edge of wound and migrating into the wound.
	Monitor patient for signs of impaired healing:
	  Wound edges in primary healing wound not well approximated.
	  Lack if an inflammatory response with first 3 days of injury *or* inflammation persisting after day 5.
	  Drainage present 48 or more hours after primary closure (when no drain is present).
	  No healing ridge by day 7–9 after closure.
	  For open wounds, measure size of wound (length, width, depth) and presence and size of tracts; also note location of wound.
	  If pressure ulcer, determine grade of ulcer.
	  Evaluate presence, color, moisture, and texture or granulation tissue.
	  Evaluate the presence, color, consistency, odor of exudate; evaluate whether epithelial tissue is progressing over open wound and entirely surrounds it.
	Apply gauge or absorbent dressing to wounds healing by primary intention for 2–3 days.
	Keep granulating wounds healing by secondary intention moist with a dressing such as moist gauze moistened with normal saline or Duoderm.
	Clean exudative wounds with products such as coarse, moist gauze; topical antiseptics; and/or high-pressure irrigation.
	Remove necrotic tissue using débridement performed with a scalpel, enzymes, moist gauze, or other dressings.
	Maintain perfusion to wound by optimizing fluid balance and mitigating edema.
	Maximize oxygenation with usual measures—e.g., maximal inspiratory efforts, increased ambient oxygen, removal of secretions.
	Provide nutrients sufficient to meet metabolic need through enteral or parenteral route; special attention to protein, energy sources, vitamins B and C, zinc, and iron for healing.
	Mitigate stress response by intervening to prevent pain of dressing changes, maximize opportunities of sleep, and provide a quiet environment.

References

Alterescu, V. (1984). Debriding enzymes. *Journal of Enterostomal Therapy*, 11 (3), 122–124.

Alvarez, O. M., and Gilbreath, R. L. (1982). Thiamine influence on collagen during the granulation of skin wounds. *Journal of Surgical Research*, 32, 24–31.

Alvarez, O. M., Mertz, P. M., and Eaglstein, W. H. (1983). The effect of occlusive dressings on collagen synthesis and re-epithelialization in superficial wounds. *Journal of Surgery Research*, 35, 142–148.

Angus, J. E., and Faux, S. (1989). The effect of music on adult postoperative patients' pain during a nursing procedure. In S. G. Funk, et al. (Eds.), *Key aspects of recovery* (pp. 116–172). New York: Springer-Verlag.

Aronoff, G. R., Friedman, S. J., Doedens, D. F., and LaVelle, K. J. (1980). Increased serum iodide concentration from iodine absorption through wound treated topically with povidone-iodine. *American Journal of Medical Science*, 219, 173–176.

Bagdale, J. D., Root, R. K., and Bulger, R. J. (1974). Impaired leukocyte function in patients with poorly controlled diabetes. *Diabetes*, 23, 9–15.

Barcia, P. J. (1970). Lack of acceleration of healing with zinc sulfate. *Annals of Surgery*, 172, 1048–1050.

Bark, S., Rettura, G., Goldman, D, et al. (1984). Effect of supplemental vitamin A on the healing of colon anastomosis. *Journal of Surgical Research*, 36, 470–474.

Barnett, A., Bekowitz, R. L., Mills, R., and Vistnes, L. M. (1983). Comparison of synthetic adhesive moisture vapor permeable and fine mesh gauze dressings for split-thickness skin graft donor sites. *American Journal of Surgery*, 145, 379–381.

Biltz H., Kiessling, M., and Kreysel, H. W. (1985). Comparison of hydrocolloid and saline gauze in the treatment of skin graft donor sites. In T. J. Ryan (Ed.), *An environment for healing: The role of occlusion* (pp. 125–128). London: The Royal Society of Medicine.

Brennan, S. S., and Leaper, D. J. (1985). The effect of antiseptics on the healing wound: A study using the rabbit ear chamber. *British Journal of Surgery*, 72 (10), 780–782.

Brennan, S. S., Foster, M. E., and Leaper, D. J. (1986). Antiseptic toxicity in wounds healing by secondary intention. *Journal of Hospital Infections*, 8 (3), 263–267.

Brown, L. L., Shelton, H. T., Bornside, G. H., and Cohn, I. (1978). Evaluation of wound irrigation by pulsatile jet and conventional methods. *Annals of Surgery*, 187, 170–173.

Buchan, I. A., Andrews, J. K., and Lang, S. M. (1981). Clinical and laboratory investigation of the composition and properties of human skin wound exudate under semi-permeable dressing. *Burns*, 7, 326–334.

Chang, N., Goodson, W. H. III, Gottrup, F., and Hunt, T. K. (1983). Direct measurement of wound and tissue oxygen tensions in postoperative patients. *Annals of Surgery*, 197, 470–478.

Cherry, G. H., and Ryan T. J. (1985). The physical properties of a new hydrocolloid dressing. In T. J. Ryan (Ed.), *An environment for healing: The role of occlusion* (pp. 61–68). London: The Royal Society of Medicine.

Clark, R. A. (1985). Cutaneous tissue repair: Basic biological considerations. *Journal of the American Academy of Dermatology*, 13 (1), 701–725.

Classification of Nursing Diagnoses: Proceedings of the Eighth

Conference (1988). R. M. Carroll-Johnson (Ed.). Philadelphia: J. B. Lippincott.

Cuzzell, J. Z. (1990). Choosing a wound dressing: A systematic approach. *AACN Clinical Issues in Critical Care Nursing*, 1 (3), 566–577.

Dealey, C. (1989). Management of cavity wounds. *Nursing*, 3(39), 25–27.

Eaglstein, W. H. (1985). Experiences with biosynthetic dressings. *Journal of the American Academy of Dermatology*, 12 (2), 434–439.

Eaglstein, W. H., and Mertz, P. M. (1981). Effect of topical medicaments on the rate of repair of superficial wounds. In P. Dineen and G. Hildlick-Smith (Eds.), *The surgical wound* (pp. 150–170). Philadelphia: Lea & Febiger.

Edlich, R. F., Rodeheaver, G. T., Thacker, J. G., and Edgerton, M. (1979). Technical factors in wound management. In T. K. Hunt and J. E. Dunphy (Eds.), *Fundamentals of wound management* (pp. 408–413). New York: Appleton-Century-Crofts.

Ehrlich, H. P., and Hunt, T. K. (1968). Effects of cortisone and vitamin A on wound healing. *Annals of Surgery*, 167, 324–341.

Ehrlich, H. P., and Hunt, T. K. (1969). The effects of cortisone and anabolic steroids on the tensile strength of healing wounds. *Annals of Surgery*, 170, 203.

Ehrlich, H. P., Traver, H., and Hunt, T. K. (1973). Effect of vitamin A and glucocorticoids upon inflammation and collagen synthesis. *Annals of Surgery*, 177, 222.

Eriksson, G. (1985). Comparative study of hydrocolloid dressing and double layer bandage in treatment of venous stasis ulceration. In T. J. Ryan (Ed.), *An environment for healing: The role of occlusion* (pp. 111–113). London: The Royal Society of Medicine.

Fitzpatrick, D. W. and Fisher, H. (1982). Carnosine, histidine and wound healing. *Surgery*, 91, 56–60.

Fowler, E. M. (1987). Equipment and products used in management and treatment of pressure ulcers. *Nursing Clinics of North America*, 22 (2), 449–461.

Gilchrist, T., and Martin, A. M. (1983). Wound treatment with Sorbsan: An alginate fibre dressing. *Biomaterials*, 4, 317–320.

Goodman, A. G., Gilman, L. S., Rall, T. W., and Murad, F. (Eds.), (1985). *Pharmacologic basis for therapeutics* (7th ed.). New York: Macmillan.

Goodson, W. H. III, and Hunt, T. K. (1977). Studies of wound healing in experimental diabetes mellitus. *Journal of Surgical Research*, 22, 221–227.

Goodson, W. H. III, and Hunt, T. K. (1988). Wound healing. In J. M. Kinney, K. N. Jeejeebhoy, G. L. Hill, and O. E. Owen (Eds.), *Human metabolism and nutrition in patient care* (pp. 635–642). Philadelphia: W. B. Saunders.

Grenier, J. F., Aprahamian, M., Genot, C., and Dentinger, A. (1982). Pantothenic acid (vitamin B₅) efficiency on wound healing. *Acta Vitaminologica et Enzymologica*, 4, 81–85.

Gruber, R. P., Vistnes, L., and Pardoe, R. (1975). The effect of commonly used antiseptics on wound healing. *Plastic Reconstructive Surgery*, 55 (4), 472–476.

Hamer, M. I., Robson, M. C., Krizek, T. J., and Southwick, W. O. (1975). Quantitative bacterial analysis of comparative wound irrigations. *Annals of Surgery*, 181, 819–822.

Hargens, A. R., and Akeson, W. H. (1986). Stress effects on tissue nutrition and viability. In A. R. Hargens (Ed.), *Tissue nutrition and viability* (pp. 1–24). New York: Springer-Verlag.

Hargreaves, A., and Lander, J. (1989). Use of transcutaneous electrical nerve stimulation for postoperative pain. *Nursing Research*, 38 (3), 159–161.

Heughan, C., Chir, B., Grislis, G., and Hunt, T. K. (1974). The effect of anemia on wound healing. *Annals of Surgery*, 179, 163–167.

Hey, H., Lund, B., Sørensen, O. H., and Lund, B. (1982). Delayed fracture healing following jejunoileal bypass surgery for obesity. *Calcified Tissue International*, 34, 13–15.

Hinman, C. D., and Maibach, H. (1963). Effect of air exposure and occlusion on experimental human skin wounds. *Nature (London)*, 200, 377–378.

Holden-Lund, C. (1988). Effects of relaxation with guided imagery on surgical stress and wound healing. *Research in Nursing & Health*, 11, 235–244.

Hunt, T. K. (1986). Vitamin A and wound healing. *Journal of the American Academy of Dermatology*, 15 (4), 817–821.

Hunt, T. K. (1988). Prospective: A retrospective perspective on the nature of wounds. In A. Barbul, E. Pines, M. Caldwell, and T. K. Hunt (Eds.), *Progress in clinical and biological research. Growth factors and other aspects of wound healing* (Vol. 266, pp. xiii–xx). New York: Alan R. Liss.

Hunt, T. K., Knighton, D. R., Thakral, K. K., et al. (1984). Studies on inflammation and wound healing: Angiogenesis and collagen synthesis stimulated in vivo by resident and activated macrophages. *Surgery*, 96, 48–54.

Hunt, T. K., Rabkin, J., and von Smitten, K. (1986). Effects of edema and anemia on wound healing and infection. *Current Studies in Hematology & Blood Transfusion*, 53, 101–111.

Irvin, T. T. (1978). Effects of malnutrition on wound healing. *Surgery, Gynecology and Obstetrics*, 146, 33–37.

Jacobsson, S., Jonsson, L., Rank, F., and Rothman, U. (1976a). Studies on healing of Debrisan-treated wounds. *Scandinavian Journal of Plastic and Reconstructive Surgery*, 10 (2), 97–101.

Jacobsson, S., Rothman, U., Arturson, G., et al. (1976b). A new principle for the cleansing of infected wounds. *Scandinavian Journal of Plastic and Reconstructive Surgery*, 10 (1), 65–72.

Jakubovic, H. R., Ackerman, A. B., Pochi, P. E., et al. (1985). Structure and function of the skin. In S. L. Moschella and H. J. Hurley (Eds.), *Dermatology* (pp. 1–103). Philadelphia: W. B. Saunders.

Jensen, J. A., Goodson, W. H. III, Vasconez, L., et al. (1986). Wound healing in anemia: A case study. *Western Journal of Medicine*, 144, 465–467.

Kagoma, P., Burger, S. N., Seifter, E., et al. (1985). The effect of vitamin E on experimentally induced peritoneal adhesions in mice. *Archives of Surgery*, 120, 949–951.

Katz, S., McGinley, K., and Leyden, J. J. (1986). Semipermeable occlusive dressings. *Archives of Dermatology*, 22 (1), 58–62.

Knighton, D. R., Doucette, M., Fiegel, V. D., et al. (1988). The use of platelet derived wound healing formula in human clinical trials. In A. Barbul, E. Pines, M. Caldwell, and T. K. Hunt (Eds.), *Progress in clinical and biological research. Growth factors and other aspects of wound healing* (Vol. 266, pp. 313–329). New York: Alan R. Liss.

Knighton, D. R., Halliday, B., and Hunt, T. K. (1984). Oxygen as antibiotic: The effect of inspired oxygen. *Archives of Surgery*, 119, 199–204.

Knighton, D. R., Hunt, T. K., Thakral, K. K., and Goodson, W. H. III (1982). Role of platelets and fibrin in the healing sequence. *Annals of Surgery*, 196 (4), 379–388.

Krasner, D. (1991). Resolving the dressing dilemma: Selecting wound dressings by category. *Ostomy/Wound Management* 35, 62–70.

Kucan, J. O., Robson, M. C., Heggers, J. P., and Ko, F. (1981). Comparisons of silver sulfadiadene and physiologic saline in the treatment of chronic pressure ulcers. *Journal of the American Geriatric Society*, 29, 232–235.

Kurzuk-Howard, G., Simpson, L., and Palmieri, A. (1985). Decubitus ulcer care: A comparative study. *Western Journal of Nursing Research*, 7 (1), 58–75.

Lawrence, J. C., and Lilly, H. A. (1985). Bacteriological properties of a new hydrocolloid dressing on intact skin of normal volunteers. In T. J. Ryan (Ed.), *An environment for healing: The role of occlusion* (pp. 51–53). London: The Royal Society of Medicine.

Leaper, D. J., and Simpson, R. A. (1986). The effect of antiseptics and topical antimicrobials on wound healing. *Journal of Antimicrobial Chemotherapy*, 17 (2), 135–136.

Leaper, D. J., Brennan, S. S., Simpson, R. A., and Foster, M. E. (1984). Experimental infection and hydrogel dressings. *Journal of Hospital Infection*, 5 (Suppl. A), 69–73.

Lineaweaver, W., Howard, R., Soucy, D., et al. (1985). Topical antimicrobial toxicity. *Archives of Surgery*, 120 (3), 267–270.

Linsky, C. B., Rovee, D. T., and Dow, T. (1981). Effect of dressing on wound inflammation and scar tissue. In P. Dineen and G. Hildick-Smith (Eds.), *The surgical wound* (pp. 377–378). Philadelphia: Lea & Febiger.

Long, C. L., Schaffel, N., Grieger, J. W., et al. (1979). Metabolic response to injury and illness: Estimation of energy and protein needs from indirect calorimetry and nitrogen balance. *Journal of Parenteral and Enteral Nutrition*, 3 (6), 452–456.

Macklebust, J. (1987). Pressure ulcers: Etiology and prevention. *Nursing Clinics of North America*, 22 (2), 359–377.

Madden, M. R., Finkelstein, J. L., Hefton, J. M., and Yurt, R. (1985). Optimal healing of donor site wounds with hydrocolloid dressings. In T. J. Ryan (Ed.), *An environment for healing: The role of occlusion* (pp. 133–136). London: The Royal Society of Medicine.

Mandy, S. H. (1983). A new primary wound dressing made of polyethylene oxide gel. *Journal of Dermatologic Surgery*, 9 (2), 153–155.

May, S. R. (1984). Physiology, immunology and clinical efficacy of an adherent polyurethane wound dressing: Op-site. In D. L. Wise (Ed.), *Burn wound coverings* (Vol. 2, pp. 54–78). Boca Raton, FL: CRC Press.

Mertz, P. M., Marshall, D. A., and Eaglstein, W. H. (1985). Occlusive wound dressings to prevent bacterial invasion and wound infection. *Journal of the American Academy of Dermatology*, 12 (4), 662–668.

Mulliken, J. B., Healey, N. A., and Glowacki, J. (1980). Povidone-iodine and tensile strength of wounds in rats. *Journal of Trauma*, 20 (4), 323–324.

Nemeth, G. G., Bolander, M. E., and Martin, G. R. (1988). Growth factors and their role in wound and fracture healing. In A. Barbul, E. Pines, M. Caldwell, and T. K. Hunt (Eds.), *Progress in clinical and biological research. Growth factors and other aspects of wound healing* (Vol. 266, pp. 1–17). New York: Alan R. Liss.

Noe, J. M., and Kalish, S. (1976). The mechanism of capillarity in surgical dressings. *Surgery, Gynecology and Obstetrics*, 143, 454–456.

Odugbesan, O., and Barnett, A. H. (1987). Use of a seaweed-based dressing in management of leg ulcers in diabetics. *Practical Diabetes*, 4, 46–47.

Oliver, L. C., and Blaine, G. (1950). Haemostasis with absorbable alginates in neurological practice. *British Journal of Surgery*, 174, 1.

Orgill, D., and Demling, R. H. (1988). Current concepts and approaches to wound healing. *Critical Care Medicine*, 16 (9), 899–908.

Pace, W. E. (1978). Beads of a dextran polymer for the local treatment of cutaneous ulcers. *Journal of Dermatology, Surgery, and Oncology*, 4 (9), 678–682.

Pollack, S. V. (1979). Wound healing: A review. *Journal of Dermatology, Surgery, and Oncology*, 5 (6), 477–481.

Pories, W. J., Henzel, J. H., Robb, C. G., et al. (1967). Acceleration of wound healing in man with zinc sulphate given by mouth. *Lancet*, 1, 121–124.

Reed, B. R., and Clark, R. A. F. (1985). Cutaneous tissue repair: Practical implications of current knowledge. *Journal of the American Academy of Dermatology*, 13, 919–941.

Reuler, J. B., and Cooney, T. G. (1981). The pressure sore: Pathophysiology and principles of management. *Annals of Internal Medicine*, 94, 661–666.

Rhodes, J. E., Fliegelman, M. T., and Panzer, L. M. (1942). The mechanism of delayed wound healing in the presence of hypoproteinemia. *Journal of the American Medical Association*, 118, 21–25.

Rodeheaver, G. (1989). Controversies in topical wound management. *Wounds*, 1, 19–27.

Rodeheaver, G., Bellamy, W., Kody, M., et al. (1982). Bactericidal activity and toxicity of iodine-containing solutions in wounds. *Archives of Surgery*, 117 (2), 181–186.

Rodeheaver, G. T., Pettry, D., Thacker, J. G., et al. (1975). Wound cleansing by high pressure irrigation. *Surgery, Gynecology and Obstetrics*, 141, 357–362.

Ross, R. (1987). Platelet derived growth factor. *Annual Review of Medicine*, 38, 71–79.

Rudolph, R., and Noe, J. M. (1983). *Chronic problem wounds*. Boston: Little, Brown.

Samela, K., and Ahonen, J. (1981). The effect of methylprednisolone and vitamin A on wound healing. I. *Acta Chirurgica Scandinavica*, 147, 307–312.

Sandberg, N. (1964). Time relationship between administration of corticosterone and wound healing in rats. *Acta Chirurgica Scandinavica*, 127, 446.

Sandstead, H. H., Henricksen, L. K., Greger, J. L., et al. (1982). Zinc nutrituse in the elderly in relation to taste acuity, immune response and wound healing. *American Journal of Clinical Nutrition*, 36, 1046–1059.

Sawyer, P. N., Bergan, J., Dagher, F. J., et al. (1980). Treatment alternatives for pressure sores. *Modern Medicine*, 48, 49–56.

Schilling, J. A. (1976). Wound healing. *Surgical Clinics of North America*, 56, 859–874.

Silver, I. A. (1972). Oxygen tension and epithelialization. In H. I. Maibach and D. T. Rovee (Eds.), *Epidermal wound healing* (pp. 291–305). Chicago: Year Book Medical Publishers.

Silver, I. A. (1985). Oxygen and tissue repair. In T. J. Ryan (Ed.), *An environment for healing: The role of occlusion* (pp. 15–21). London: The Royal Society of Medicine.

Stevenson, T. R., Thacker, J. G., Rodeheaver, G. T., et al. (1976). Cleansing the traumatic wound by high pressure syringe irrigation. *Journal of the American College of Emergency Physicians*, 5, 17–21.

Stotts, N. A. (1990). Seeing red . . . and yellow . . . and black: The three-color concept of wound care. *Nursing '90*, 20 (2):59–61.

Temple, W. J., Voitk, A. J., Snelling, C. F. T., and Crispin, J. S. (1975). Effect of nutrition, diet, and suture material on long-term wound healing. *Annals of Surgery*, 182, 93–97.

Thomas, S. (1985). Use of a calcium alginate dressing. *The Pharmaceutical Journal*, 235, 188–190.

Turner, T. D. (1985). Semiocclusive and occlusive dressings. In T. J. Ryan (Ed.), *An environment for healing: The role of occlusion* (pp. 5–14). London: The Royal Society of Medicine.

Varghese, M. C., Balin, A. K., Carter, M., and Caldwell, D. (1986). Local environment of chronic wounds under synthetic dressings. *Archives of Dermatology*, 122, 52–57.

Wheeland, R. G. (1987). The newer surgical dressings and wound healing. *Dermatologic Clinics*, 5 (2), 393–407.

Wheeler, C. B., Rodeheaver, G. T., Thacker, J. G., et al. (1976). Side-effects of high pressure irrigation. *Surgery, Gynecology and Obstetrics*, 143, 775–778.

Williamson, M. B., and Fromm, H. J. (1955). The incorporation of sulfur amino acids into the proteins of regenerating wound tissue. *Journal of Biological Chemistry*, 212, 715–712.

Winter, G. D. (1962). Formation of the scab and the rate of epithelization of superficial wounds in the skin of the young domestic pig. *Nature (London)*, 193, 293–294.

Winter, G. D., and Scales, J. T. (1963). Effect of air drying and dressings on the surface of a wound. *Nature (London)*, 197, 91–92.

Witkowski, J. A., and Parish, L. C. (1986). Cutaneous ulcer therapy. *International Journal of Dermatology*, 25 (7), 420–426.

Wysocki, A. B. (1986). The effect of intermittent noise exposure on the rate of wound healing in albino rats. Unpublished dissertation, University of Texas at Austin.

Young, M. E. (1988). Malnutrition and wound healing. *Heart & Lung*, 7 (1), 60–69.

Young, R. A. L., and Weston-Davies, W. H. (1985). Comparison of a hydrocolloid with a conventional island dressing as a primary surgical wound dressing. In T. J. Ryan (Ed.), *An environment for healing: The role of occlusion* (pp. 153–156). London: The Royal Society of Medicine.

56

Patients with Burns

Randy M. Caine
Nancy D. Lefcourt

Burns are immediately or potentially life-threatening traumatic injuries. In the United States alone, more than 2 million persons suffer burn injuries each year, approximately 61,000 of whom are hospitalized. Despite the advances in burn treatment and intervention that have been made, more than 8000 of these people will die as a result of their burns (Frank et al., 1987). Prevention as well as emergency care and critical care interventions for burns is necessary.

Burn nursing is both complex and challenging. Nurses involved in the emergent, acute, or rehabilitative aspects of burn care must be knowledgeable about the pathophysiologic and psychosocial changes that occur in the burned patient. These patients are traumatically injured, have multisystem organ involvement, and therefore present with an abundance of difficulties and special challenges. It is for these reasons that the care of the burned patient, as well as the family, cannot be provided by critical care nurses alone but must involve a team effort.

TYPES OF BURN INJURIES

Thermal Injuries

Thermal injuries, or heat-related injuries, range from hot water scalds to flame burns to direct contact with a heat source. Because of the diverse mechanisms of injury, treatment must be tailored to the specific etiologic agent.

When we think of thermal injuries, we most often think of house fires. Only 5% of all burn victims, however, are injured as result of house fires. Smoke inhalation from house fires causes the largest number of burn-related deaths. Hot water scalds account for approximately 22% of all burns, with most victims under the age of 4 (Choctaw et al., 1987). Flammable liquids, grease, vehicle fires, and explosions also account for thermal injuries. Despite the cause of injury, all thermal burns are classified according to the depth of injury.

Chemical Injuries

Chemical agents generally do not "burn" in the sense that they destroy tissue through the effect of heat, although some chemicals can act in this manner. Tissue damage and destruction result from the chemical coagulation of protein, precipitation of chemical compounds in the cell, severe cellular dehydration, and protoplasmic poisoning or complete dissolution of tissue proteins (Hersperger and Dahl, 1978). The effects of chemical damage on tissues are determined by the following factors: (1) strength or concentration of the chemical; (2) length of contact with tissue; (3) quantity; (4) extent of tissue penetration; and (5) mode of action of the chemical.

It should be remembered that the skin and the underlying structures will continue to be injured until the chemical source is removed or inactivated by reaction with cellular components. Very few chemicals cannot be washed off the skin with water.

Several types of chemical agents that cause burns include oxidizing agents, reducing agents, corrosive agents, protoplasmic poisons, desiccants, and vesicants. *Oxidizing agents* such as sodium hypochlorite, chromic acid, and potassium permanganate become oxidized on contact with body tissue. *Reducing agents*, including nitric acid and hydrochloric acid, cause tissue damage through a denaturing effect on the cellular proteins. *Corrosive agents* are phenols, white phosphorus, sodium metals, and lyes. *Protoplasmic poisons* such as tannic acid, picric acid, formic acid, oxalic acid, and hydrofloric acid produce tissue damage by forming salts with the cellular cations, resulting in protein coagulation. *Desiccants* such as sulfuric acid and muriatic acid are mineral acids that produce tissue damage through extreme cellular dehydration and generate considerable heat when in contact with tissue fluids. *Vesiccants* include cantharides, dimethyl sulfoxide, and mustard gas. Their burn mechanism of action is not known; however, tissue ischemia and anoxia are the end results of this chemical reaction.

Gasoline burns due to prolonged contact of gasoline with tissue (without ignition) are well documented (Simpson and Cruse, 1981). Unleaded gasoline contains 0.5% to 3% benzene, an absorbable, potentially toxic agent. Gasoline can cause central nervous system depression with the potential for further injury (Edelman, 1987).

Management of chemical injuries depends upon the type of agent involved. In general, all chemicals should be flushed with copious amounts of water until definitive therapy can be provided. Regional poison centers maintain specific guidelines and should be contacted immediately. Once tissue damage is complete, standard burn care is instituted.

Electrical Injuries

Approximately 1000 people die each year in the United States as a result of electric shock (Uehara et al., 1986). Electrical injuries occur less frequently than scald injuries but are potentially life-threatening. Tissue damage due to electricity may be caused by either direct contact with the current or the flash caused by electrical arcing. Although actual damage to the body depends on the current passing through the body, a number of other factors influence the severity of the injury as well, including (1) amperage, the amount of resistance applied to the voltage; (2) voltage, a measure of force of the flow of current; (3) type of current, alternating current (AC) or direct current (DC) (alternating current is found in homes and most industries, whereas direct current is used in chemical and metallurgic industries and street car systems, and on board ships; (4) duration of contact—the greater the duration of contact, the more severe the damage; (5) surface area of contact, that is, the larger the surface area, the greater the damage; and (6) tissue resistance, because the body conducts current as a result of its electrolyte content. In declining order, the human tissues may be listed according to the resistance they offer: skin, bone, fat, nerve, muscle, blood, body fluids (Somogyi and Tedeschi, 1977). This means that a given current flowing through bone will generate more heat in the local tissues than will the same current in blood. The resistance of skin also varies with the thickness and moisture content of the skin.

Electrical current may cause death directly by ventricular fibrillation, asphyxiation secondary to tetanic contractions of the muscles of respiration, or respiratory arrest. Indirect causes of death are severe thermal injury, nervous system damage, vascular injury, and renal failure (Hersperger and Dahl, 1978). Electrical current may also cause long bone fractures resulting from tetanic contractions as well as associated injuries from falls.

Radiation Burns

Ionizing radiation burns are significantly different from burns caused by flame, steam, chemical agents, or electricity. These burns have long-term biologic effects that result in chronic health care concerns that may be seen years after the initial injury. The critical care nurse will most likely care for these patients, however, as an immediate result of ionizing radiation exposure or a catastrophic nuclear disaster or accident.

The term ionizing radiation includes alpha and beta particles, gamma rays, and roentgen or x-rays. The intracellular destruction of DNA molecules and the resultant loss of genetic information is a significant consequence of radiation injuries. This loss is shown most prominently in the altered replicative ability of the cell (Nicosia and Petro, 1983). For example, mucosal cells of the intestine, which normally reproduce rapidly, demonstrate cellular changes earlier as a result of radiation injury.

Acute radiation injury caused by localized irradiation appears much like the initial stages of thermal injury with erythema, edema, pain, and tissue ischemia. The potential for acute and chronic infection and necrosis is apparent. Whole body irradiation, on the other hand, causes systemic symptoms, termed radiation sickness, which are dose dependent. Death may result in as little as hours or days with high radiation doses, whereas lower doses of radiation may cause chronic ulceration, osteoradionecrosis, skin changes, or malignancy. Treatment of whole body irradiation is primarily supportive in terms of skin care, pain management, infection control, and emotional support.

Tar Injuries

Hot tar burns account for approximately 5% of all burn injuries in adults. When tar is in its liquid form it may be as hot as 500 °F. After coming in contact with the skin, the tar quickly cools, solidifies, and becomes enmeshed in the hair. The cooling process should be expedited by the addition of cool water. The literature states that the tar can be removed with any petroleum-based ointment; however, removal of the tar has been shown to be of a lesser concern than the cooling process (Hill et al., 1984). Once the tar has been cooled, the burning process has ended, and the tar can be slowly removed in a matter of days as it is lifted with silver sulfadiazine cream. No increased incidence of bacterial colonization has been shown by leaving the tar in place (Hill et al., 1984).

Once the tar has lifted, the burn is treated like any other burn.

PATHOPHYSIOLOGY

Anatomy and Physiology of Skin

The skin comprises the largest organ of the body. It is composed of three layers—the thin, nonvascular outer layer termed the epidermis, the middle tissue layer termed the dermis or corium, and the subcutaneous fat layer (Fig. 56–1). The epidermis consists of stratified epithelial tissue, whereas the dermis consists of fibrous connective tissue. Subcutaneous tissue is made up of loose areolar and, in some cases, adipose tissue.

The epidermis has five layers, which include the stratum corneum, stratum lucidum, stratum granulosum, stratum spinosum, and stratum germinativum. Two of these layers, the stratum corneum and the stratum germinativum, figure prominently in an understanding of burn wound healing. The stratum corneum is composed of keratin fibers surrounded by a monolipid layer that is water repellent. This layer functions as a vapor barrier that prevents fluid loss. Thus, in extensive burn injuries involving this layer, large fluid losses occur. The stratum germinativum is also important because it is constantly producing new cells that move to the surface to replace other epidermal layers that are continually being sloughed off. Melanin may also be found in this layer; it affects the color of the skin.

The dermis or corium serves as both a supportive and a nutritional basis for the epidermis. The complex dermis is composed of blood vessels, sensory receptors for touch, pain, and pressure, and the epidermal appendages that include the hair follicles, sebaceous glands, and sweat glands. Collagen fiber is also found in the dermis. Scattered throughout the collagen are connective tissue cells called *mast cells*, which are responsible for secretion, phagocytosis, and repair. Increased amounts of histamine are re-

leased by these mast cells in patients with burn injury. When burn injuries destroy the epidermis, epithelial cells from the epidermal appendages begin to form new epithelium.

The subcutaneous fat layer contains the roots of the hair follicles and the sweat glands. Collagen fibers from the dermis extend to this layer to ensure adhesion of the dermis to the subcutaneous tissue. The collagen found here plays a significant role in burn injury because it is collagen that anchors the eschar in place, thus making removal of eschar difficult.

The largest of the skin arteries are found in the subcutaneous tissue just beneath the dermis. Thus, in burn injury, plasma leaking from the arteries may cause edema and blistering.

The skin plays an active role in the prevention of infection as the first line of defense. In addition, it conserves body fluids, regulates body temperature, produces vitamin D when exposed to ultraviolet light, secretes oil to lubricate and soften skin, allows excretion of excess water and waste products, and serves as a sensory organ for touch, pain, and pressure.

Classification of Burn Depth

Burns have commonly been described in terms of degree—first-, second-, third-, and fourth-degree. More recently, first- and second-degree burns have been described as superficial (first-degree) and partial-thickness (second-degree); any burn deeper than the dermis is described as full-thickness (third-degree). Classification of fourth-degree burns includes injuries extending into the subcutaneous fat, muscle, and bone. These injuries are now included in the full-thickness classification (Table 56–1).

Superficial Burns. These burns result either from prolonged exposure from low-intensity heat (e.g., sunburn) or from a short-duration flash exposure to a high-intensity heat source. Erythema of the skin with local edema is the result. Superficial burns do not require treatment other than local pain relief and are not calculated in the amount of body surface area burned when determining the extent of a burn. Comfort measures include aspirin, fluids, local topical pain relief, and frequent application of water-soluble lotion. Superficial burns heal in 3 to 5 days following desquamation and do not cause scarring or require further treatment.

Partial-Thickness Burns. A superficial partial-thickness burn is equal to the classic second-degree burn characterized by fluid-filled blisters appearing immediately after injury and by pain when the blisters are removed and the burn is exposed to air. The blister membrane, in its intact condition, forms a sterile environment that prevents excessive water loss from the burn wound.

Since the dermal layer of the skin is for the most

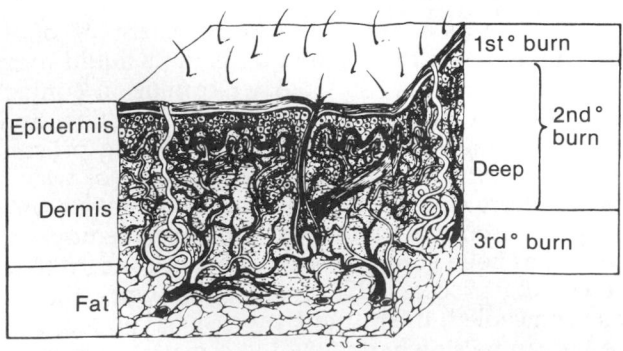

FIGURE 56–1. Cross section of the skin. (From Demling, R.H. (1989). In W.C. Shoemaker et al. (Eds.), *The society of critical care medicine textbook of critical care* (2nd ed., p. 1301). Philadelphia: W.B. Saunders.)

TABLE 56–1. Depth of Injury

	Superficial	Partial-Thickness	Full-Thickness
Morphology	Destruction of epidermis only	Destruction of epidermis and some dermis	Destruction of epidermis, dermis and underlying subcutaneous tissue
Function	Intact	Absent	Absent
Appearance after initial débridement	Reddened, desquamates after 3–5 days	Pink, moist, may be mottled	White, cherry-red, black; thick, leathery appearance; dry, visible thrombosed vessels
Healing time	3–7 days	7–28 days	30 days to many months; may close secondarily from edges if wound is small; generally requires surgery.
Scarring	None	Minimal to severe influenced by genetic predisposition	Minimal to severe; depends on time to grafting and surgical techniques used

Adapted from Kravitz, M. (1988). Thermal injuries. In V. D. Cardona, et al. (Eds.), *Trauma nursing: From resuscitation through rehabilitation*. Philadelphia:. W. B. Saunders.

part intact, healing takes place between 10 and 14 days after injury, and scarring is minimal. In some cases, there is a significant loss of melanocytes, which can result in a minor and sometimes permanent color change.

The deep partial-thickness burn consists of a disruption of the epidermis and most of the dermis, sparing the appendages such as hair follicles and sweat glands. This sparing of appendages is what allows the wound potentially to regenerate (thus it is a partial-thickness burn). Blistering of the wound may occur as in the more superficial partial-thickness burn, but this is not an essential component. The wound is more often characterized by eschar formation. Deep partial-thickness burns exhibit massive fluid losses because the cellular barrier that normally protects against bacterial invasion and wound sepsis is no longer present.

Sensation is usually present in deep partial-thickness burns but may be decreased because of actual destruction of nerve endings in the dermal layer of the skin. Wound healing takes longer at this depth, usually 21 to 28 days, and more scar is formed.

Full-Thickness Burn. In a full-thickness burn the epidermis, dermis, and all the dermal appendages are destroyed. The burn may extend into the subcutaneous fat, muscle, or bone. A thick, leathery eschar forms that allows copious amounts of fluid loss through the wound and fails to protect against bacterial invasion and wound sepsis. Because dermal appendages have been destroyed by the burn, the wound will heal by contraction and epithelial growth from the edges. If allowed to heal by this means, the scar will be deformed and unstable; therefore, in clinical practice, skin grafts are applied to promote function and stability.

If the full-thickness burn extends into the muscle, myoglobinuria can become a significant problem. This may lead to renal failure in poorly hydrated patients.

Most experienced burn practitioners can determine burn depth correctly by visual inspection only approximately 50% of the time. Visual inspection tends to be very subjective. Objective means for determining burn depth such as the use of lasers, fluorescein, and magnetic resonance imaging have been studied for some time. Determination of burn depth by the laser Doppler technique is relatively new and has the highest reliability at this time. A laser beam looks at the flow of blood through burn tissue, providing information about the circulatory physiology of the burn wound. Normal skin has a relatively low basal blood flow, whereas burn tissue increases blood flow remarkably in response to local heating. Full-thickness burn wounds that fail to heal have low blood flow and minimal or no increase of flow in response to local heating. Partial-thickness burns that do heal have elevated blood flow, which may increase even further with local heating (Waxman et al., 1989).

Fluorescein has also been used to attempt to determine the depth of injury. Fluorescein is injected intravenously. If the drug is present in the burn wound, it means that blood flow is adequate to allow the wound to heal. Results of fluorescein injection have been found to be less accurate than those achieved with Doppler study and close to those characteristic of visual inspection.

Magnetic resonance imagery (MRI) is a relatively new tool that is now being used to assess the level of injury in patients with electrical burns, in which there can be significant internal damage. MRI remains in very limited use, however, due to its high cost and the requirement that the patient must be stable to be transported to an MRI center.

Severity of Burn Injury

Both the American Burn Association (ABA) and the American College of Surgeons (ACS) rate the severity of burns as minor, moderate, or major (Table

TABLE 56–2. Criteria of Burn Injury Severity

| | American Burn Association | | American College of Surgeons | |
	Adults Degree %	Children Degree %	Adults Degree %	Children Degree %
Minor	2nd—<15 3rd —<2	2nd 3rd } <10	2nd 3rd } <15	2nd 3rd } <10
Moderate	2nd—>15–25 3rd —<10	2nd—>10–20 3rd —<10	2nd 3rd } 15–25	2nd 3rd } 10–20
Major	2nd—>25 3rd —>10	2nd—>20 3rd —>10	2nd—>25 3rd —>10	2nd—>20 3rd —>10

From Achauer, B. M. (Ed.) 1987. *Management of the burned patient.* Norwalk, CT: Appleton & Lange; Prentice-Hall.

56–2). Both the ABA and the ACS agree that minor burns can be treated on an outpatient basis. Moderate burns can usually be cared for in a general hospital if a burn center is unavailable; however, all major burns should be cared for in a burn center. In addition, moderate burns of the hands, feet, eyes, ears, face, and perineum should also be cared for in a burn center because of the high risk of either infection or functional disuse in these areas.

Calculation of Total Body Surface Area Burned. ABA standards require that the extent of burn injury be calculated upon entry to the health care system. Two methods are used for calculating the amount of total body surface area (TBSA) burned. The first is the rule of nines (Fig. 56–2), which is commonly used in the emergency department and in the field. It is a simple and quick method of estimating the extent of injury. There is a rule of nines for adults and another for children. Because infants and small

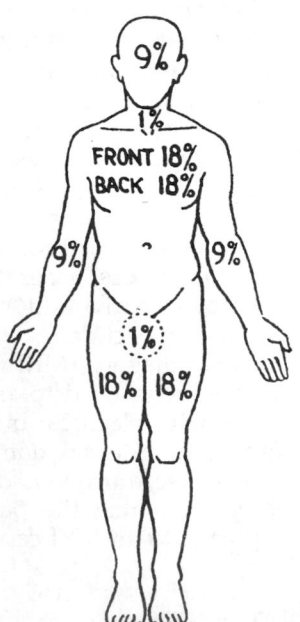

FIGURE 56–2. Rules of nines for calculating the total body surface area burned. (Adapted from Wallace, A.B. (1951). The exposure treatment of burns. *Lancet,* 1, 501.)

children have larger heads and smaller legs than adults, the Lund and Browder formula (Fig. 56–3) is commonly used for them. The Lund and Browder chart is also a more specific method of estimating burn extent in the adult. This method, however, is more time consuming to calculate than the rule of nines.

When estimating TBSA burned, only partial- and full-thickness burns are included. Superficial burns are not part of this calculation nor of the amount of fluid needed for fluid resuscitation, which is based on the concept that superficial burns have intact skin that still functions normally.

PHASES OF BURN PHYSIOLOGY AND PATIENT CARE MANAGEMENT

When burns cause major destruction in the skin's integrity, numerous physiologic and hemodynamic changes occur throughout each of the body systems. The primary physiologic changes occur in the cardiovascular system in terms of the phases of fluid shifts. Other systemic changes become evident in the immediate period following burn trauma, and, as time from burn injury progresses, these systems undergo additional physiologic alterations. Three general phases in burn physiology and patient care management have been identified; these include the *emergent* or *shock phase*, the *acute* or *fluid remobilization phase*, and the *rehabilitation* or *recovery phase*. For each of these phases, a discussion of the physiology, including the multisystemic effects, and patient care management will be provided.

Emergent (Shock) Phase

PHYSIOLOGY

The emergent phase of burn pathophysiology is characterized primarily by capillary permeability and a shift of fluid from the plasma into the interstitial space as well as loss of plasma through the skin. Along with the shifting fluid goes debris from hemolyzed blood cells, proteins, and electrolytes. In

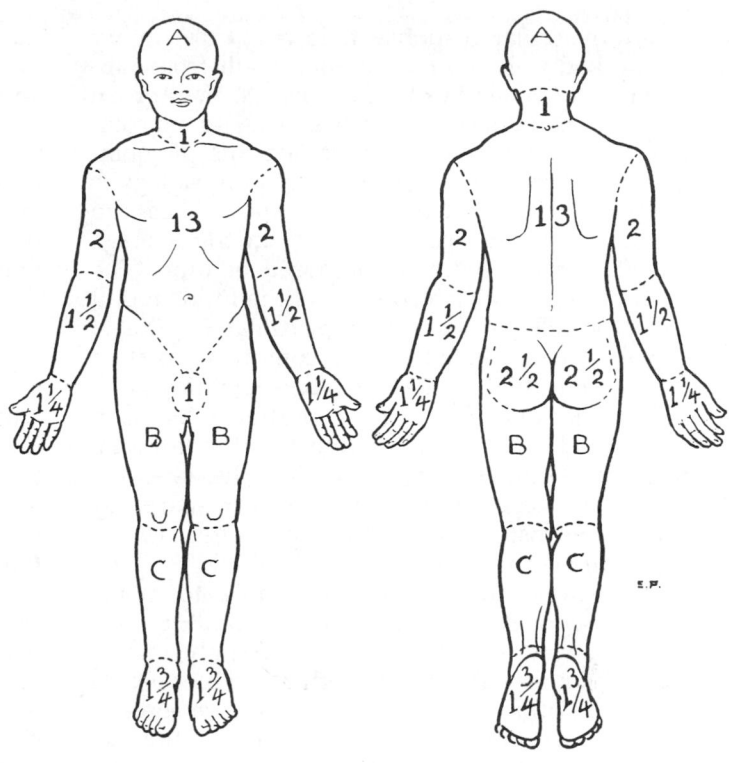

Age	Birth	1	5	10	15	Adult
Area						
Head	19	17	13	11	9	7
Neck	2	2	2	2	2	2
Anterior trunk*	13	13	13	13	13	13
Posterior trunk‡	13	13	13	13	13	13
Buttocks	5	5	5	5	5	5
Genitalia	1	1	1	1	1	1
Upper arms	8	8	8	8	8	8
Forearms	6	6	6	6	6	6
Hands	5	5	5	5	5	5
Thighs	11	13	16	17	18	19
Legs	10	10	11	12	13	14
Feet	7	7	7	7	7	7
Total	100	100	100	100	100	100

*Without neck or genitalia.
‡Without neck or buttocks.

FIGURE 56–3. Lund and Browder chart for estimation of areas of burns. *Abbreviations:* A, one-half of head; B, one-half of thigh; C, one-half of leg (A, B, and C refer to areas affected by growth). (Modified from Lund, C.C., and Browder, N.C. (1944). The estimation of areas of burns. By permission of SURGERY, GYNECOLOGY & OBSTETRICS, 79, 353.)

major burns, the fluid loss results in decreased cardiac output and hypovolemic shock. To compensate, vasoconstriction occurs. Capillary permeability occurs within 30 minutes of the burn injury, but the most significant changes begin to occur 6 to 8 hours following the burn. This phase generally lasts from 36 to 48 hours after the burn but may last as long as 96 hours depending on the extent of total body surface area burned and when fluid resuscitation was initiated. Hypovolemic shock now occurs less frequently in burn patients because of improved early resuscitation efforts.

Every system is affected by the devastating nature of burn injury. The critical care nurse must be aware of the effect of burn injury on each of the primary systems to provide knowledgeable care of the patient.

MULTISYSTEMIC EFFECTS

Patients with burn injuries experience massive physiologic trauma. The mortality rate in patients with extensive burn injuries is high, not only because of the consequences of burn injuries themselves and the resulting sepsis, but also because of the effects of the injury on all major systems of the body. The following section describes the systemic effects of burn injuries during the emergent phase.

Cardiovascular System Effects. The most significant cardiovascular response following burn injury is the marked fluid alterations that result from capillary damage. When burn injury occurs, the normal equilibrium maintained among the various fluid compartments is disturbed. To appreciate this phenomenon, an understanding of the normal physiology is necessary. Fluid is normally compartmentalized into intracellular and extracellular areas. In the average adult, 60% of the body is composed of fluid. The intracellular fluid, which consists of the fluids found in all body cells, makes up approximately 40% of that total. The extracellular fluid, comprising plasma and interstitial fluid, constitutes the remaining 20%. Of the extracellular fluid, three-fourths is found in the interstitial spaces and one-fourth in the intravascular space. Equilibrium is maintained between the fluid in the interstitial and intravascular spaces by balancing hydrostatic and osmotic pressures. *Hydrostatic pressure* is the driving force of a liquid pushing against a surface that causes the liquid to move. *Osmotic pressure* is a counterbalancing, pulling force that causes water to move from low to high concentrations of solute particles through a semipermeable membrane. Within the circulatory system, as a result of arterial blood pressure that is higher than the pull of plasma proteins, hydrostatic pressure at the proximal end of the capillaries is normally greater, resulting in fluid being pushed into the interstitial spaces. Capillaries are not normally permeable to plasma proteins. Osmotic pressure, however, is greater at the distal end of the capillaries because blood pressure here is lower than the pull of the plasma proteins. This results in fluid being pulled back into the blood vessels. When capillary integrity is lost in the immediate postburn period, osmotic pressure is negative (Jacoby, 1974).

Lymph is also responsible for maintaining fluid balance. Lymphatic vessels are particularly numerous in the skin and contain terminating valves that open into the interstitial spaces and absorb excess fluid. Eventually, these vessels empty into the larger venous channels (Minar, 1978).

Fluid balance also is maintained between the interstitial and intracellular compartments through the distribution of sodium, potassium, and proteins. Sodium is the chief cation of extracellular fluid and is present in both the intravascular and interstitial spaces in approximately the same amounts. Potassium is the chief cation in intracellular fluid. The relative distribution of sodium and potassium is maintained by a pump mechanism that normally pushes sodium from the cell in exchange for potassium. Protein, found in large quantities within the cell in the form of protoplasm, exerts osmotic pressure to attract and maintain fluid inside the cell. This pull is counterbalanced by the sodium in the extracellular fluid, thus contributing to the balance between the interstitial and intracellular fluid compartments.

In burn injuries, the major physiologic alteration in the fluid compartments involves the extracellular compartment, in which a shift of fluid occurs from the intravascular into the interstitial space as a result of the disruption in balance between the hydrostatic and osmotic pressures. Capillary damage results in increased permeability and decreased selectivity. The increased permeability allows fluid to pass more rapidly and freely from the intravascular into the interstitial space. The decreased selectivity allows the plasma protein to leave the interstitial space. Because these proteins, or *colloids* as they are also called, are the main solutes responsible for exerting osmotic pressure, there is a resulting decrease in osmotic pressure within the blood vessels and an increased osmotic pressure in the interstitial spaces. Thus, while hydrostatic pressure continues to drive fluid into the interstitial space, osmotic pressure is unable to pull the excess fluid back into the intravascular space. Ultimately, the major loss of fluid from the intravascular compartment results in retention of fluid in the tissues in the form of massive edema. If patients have circumferential burns or if a large body surface area has been burned, the fluid under the overwhelming eschar results in a tourniquet effect on the underlying structures, causing increased interstitial pressure, destruction of nerve endings, and circulatory collapse. To relieve this pressure, escharotomy or fasciotomy may be required.

After a burn, more sodium than water is drawn into the interstitial spaces. The sodium pump becomes less efficient, and more water and sodium enter the intracellular spaces. To attempt to compensate for the loss of water and sodium from the intravascular space, increased secretion of aldosterone and antidiuretic hormone occurs, further contributing to the retention of sodium and water. Following a major burn, several liters of fluid may be retained.

Fluid losses in patients with burn injuries may also result from water evaporation, blistering, or wound drainage. Approximately 20 times as much fluid is lost through evaporation when the skin is destroyed as when the skin is intact (Busby, 1979; Hayter, 1978). Both sodium and potassium, essential electrolytes, are lost through burned skin as well. Potassium is released from injured tissue and cells and escapes into the extracellular fluid, resulting in a temporary increase in serum potassium levels.

Proteins from the injured cells or from the intravascular fluid freely pass through the injured capillaries into the interstitium. However, this protein is not lost as quickly as electrolytes and water. Therefore, the protein concentration initially increases, in turn increasing the osmotic pressure gradient. This pulls fluid from the interstitial spaces throughout the body to maintain cardiac output and adequate circulating fluid volume. When the interstitial fluid is depleted, the intracellular fluid is used next. If these events are untreated, death of the patient follows.

In addition to massive fluid volume changes, the cardiovascular system is further compromised because of decreased myocardial perfusion. Circulating myocardial depressant factors, liberated as a result of the shock, cause an increase in production of lactic acid and endotoxins. Although thought to occur only in patients with very significant or extensive body surface area burns, this view is controversial (Jacoby, 1974).

Serial electrocardiograms (ECG) are indicated in all victims of electrical injuries and in any patient over age 40 years with a history of cardiovascular disease. ECGs, although not diagnostic of the burn injury, can be diagnostic of other problems, and a baseline ECG can be invaluable later in the patient's course of treatment.

Lysis and entrapment of red blood cells as well as alterations in coagulation and fibrinolysis, sometimes resulting in disseminated intravascular coagulation (DIC), can occur in patients with burn injuries (Ohura, 1988). These events may cause anemia or, in extreme cases, thrombi may form in the capillaries as a result of stasis or heat from the burn. The ischemia or necrosis of tissue that results is sometimes treated with anticoagulant therapy (Zawacki, 1974). More recently, anticoagulant therapy using heparin with antithrombin III (AT-III) is reserved for severely burned victim unless DIC is documented (Ohura, 1988).

Anemia in the burn patient may be masked by the initially high hematocrits caused when fluid is lost from the intravascular space. If the patient's hematocrit is within normal values, the critical care nurse should suspect anemia, particularly if the patient has suffered other traumatic injuries. If bleeding from these traumatically injured sites remains undetected or untreated, the anemia may progress.

Pulmonary System Effects. Following burn injury, pulmonary sequelae such as the loss of respiratory cilia, development of a chemical pneumonitis, destruction of respiratory cell protein, and atelectasis as a result of inhalation injuries are common. Inhalation injuries are caused by a variety of substances toxic to the respiratory passages. Inhalation injuries should be suspected in the patient who has obvious burns to the face, neck, or chest. Patients found burned in an enclosed space should also be assessed for inhalation injury; however, inhalation injuries should not be ruled out in patients burned in open areas.

Inhalation burns may be classified according to the relationship of the burn to the glottis (i.e., supraglottic or subglottic). Burns to the respiratory tract below the glottis are extremely rare; if present, they are usually the result of inhalation of live steam. The trachea is an excellent heat exchanger, effectively cooling hot inspired air. In addition, hot air causes a reflex closure of the vocal cords, further protecting the lower airways from direct heat injury. The usual signs associated with inhalation injury are listed in Table 56–3.

Bronchospasm, alveolar damage, or carbon monoxide poisoning may be responsible for respiratory distress in the burn patient. These pulmonary complications of inhalation injury can be complex and

TABLE 56–3. Signs and Symptoms of Smoke Inhalation

Burned in an enclosed space
Chest, face, or neck burns
Singed nasal hair or eyebrows
Carbonaceous material in the mouth
Carbonaceous sputum
Carboxyhemoglobin > 10%
Wheezing
Hoarseness of the voice
Deep, labored respirations
Altered level of consciousness

may constitute a major threat to the patient's survival.

Acute airway obstruction can also result from severe facial, oral, or laryngeal edema. Most cases of airway obstruction occur within 24 to 48 hours following burn injury (Wiener and Barrett, 1986). Edema may be a direct result of heat injury in patients with orofacial burn trauma, or it may result from fluid administration.

Smoke is a suspension of small particles in hot air or gas. This particulate matter becomes trapped in the nose, mouth, and throat, and, during inhalation, the gaseous fraction of the particulate matter enters the respiratory passages. Carbon monoxide and hydrogen cyanide, known to be toxic substances, are present in this gaseous fraction of the smoke. Another major concern with smoke inhalation is the possibility of subsequent inhalation of lung-damaging and highly toxic gases that result from the burning of plastic material (e.g., polyvinyl chloride). Polyvinyl chloride alone has been shown to produce 75 toxic gases when burned, the most lethal of which is hydrogen chloride (Dyer and Esch, 1976). Upon entering the lungs, these gases react to form strong acids or alkalis that ultimately destroy the pulmonary epithelium and cilia. Inhaled carbon monoxide binds with hemoglobin, thereby displacing the oxygen-carrying capacity of the hemoglobin and causing a rise in the carboxyhemoglobin (COHb) level to greater than 10% and a shift to the left of the oxygen dissociation curve. Less oxygen is transported, and cerebral hypoxia results, even though the Pa_{O_2} may be normal. Carboxyhemoglobin levels of over 10% are definitely diagnostic of carbon monoxide poisoning, and early intubation is required (Desai, 1984); COHb levels of less than 10% do not rule out carbon monoxide poisoning because of the short half-life of carboxyhemoglobin (Fig. 56–4). It is therefore imperative that carboxyhemoglobin levels be monitored judiciously.

Arterial blood pH and gases should be tested periodically because they have the greatest diagnostic clinical value for the majority of patients. When inhalation injury is suspected, fiberoptic bronchoscopy, periscope-type laryngoscopy, or a xenon-133 scan is performed to confirm the diagnosis. Bronchoscopy aids in the diagnosis of smoke inhalation and is indicated whenever there is a question of

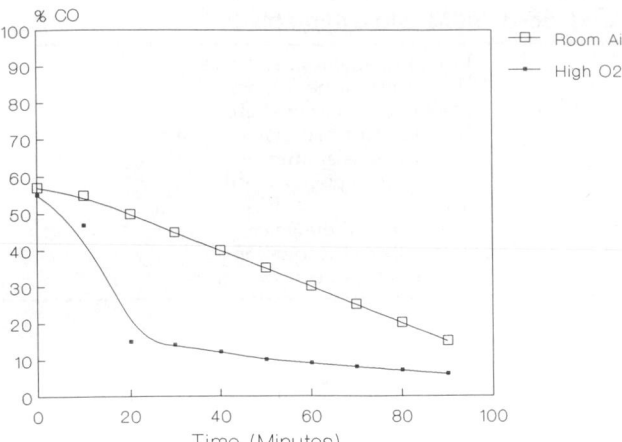

FIGURE 56–4. Half-life of carboxyhemoglobin.

whether a patient should be intubated. The vocal cords can be visualized along with other structures at this time. The presence of carbonaceous material or edema around the vocal cords is an indication for immediate intubation. If there is no carbonaceous material but slight edema is seen around the vocal cords, the physician may choose to perform serial bronchoscopies every 6 to 8 hours to follow the edema. Carbonaceous sputum at or below the larynx may suggest the need for pulmonary lavage during bronchoscopy. Ventilation-perfusion lung scans involve the intravenous administration of a small bolus dose of ^{133}Xe. Since this isotope is poorly soluble in water, it is almost entirely excreted in the alveoli. If the xenon fails to clear the lung in 90 seconds, the test is abnormal and strongly indicates inhalation injury in the absence of previous pulmonary pathology. In the patient with inhalation injury, washout of the ^{133}Xe is delayed. Patients with red and swollen vocal cords or supraglottic area should have a nasogastric tube inserted before edema of the hypopharynx and larynx makes intubation difficult (Wiener and Barrett, 1986).

The consequences of gaseous and thermal injury are typically time dependent, and the immediate effects of burn injury are related to the combination of gases and the temperature involved. Relatively mild inhalation injuries, if left untreated, may progress to adult respiratory distress syndrome (ARDS). Table 56–4 lists the early and late pulmonary symptoms associated with pulmonary injury.

All of the pulmonary manifestations, when accompanied by an increased percentage of total body surface area burned, result in a decreasing functional residual capacity, atelectasis, ventilation-perfusion ($\dot{V}/\dot{Q}$) mismatch, progressive hypoxemia, and eventual death. Chest x-rays are often normal in the early postburn period following inhalation injury and therefore are unreliable early indicators for assessment. X-rays first become abnormal approximately 24 hours following the injury.

Patient care management of pulmonary sequelae

involves administration of warm humidified O_2, use of bronchodilators, postural drainage, percussion, incentive spirometry, intermittent positive pressure breathing, and use of ultrasonic nebulizers. A decreasing Pa_{O_2} may require nasotracheal intubation and the use of positive end-expiratory pressure (PEEP) in patients with upper airway injuries. Management of lower airway injuries may involve intubation accompanied by humidification, bronchodilation, and aggressive pulmonary hygiene.

Even in the absence of inhalation injuries, burn patients with circumferential full-thickness injuries to the upper chest and neck also are at risk for respiratory complications. The inelastic eschar formation that results from these injuries impedes adequate respiratory excursion, causing hypoxia, hypoxemia, and respiratory distress. Immediate lifesaving escharotomy permits the chest wall to expand and decreases the respiratory distress.

Other respiratory complications can arise from a decreased cough reflex and the patient's inability to expectorate pulmonary secretions. Arterial blood gas changes can be caused by hyperventilation associated with fear or anxiety. In addition, preexisting pulmonary pathology, such as bronchitis, pulmonary emphysema, or asthma can affect the patient's survival. A compromised respiratory status can ultimately lead to death, and therefore an astute critical care nurse continues to monitor the patient to prevent compromised respiratory status.

Immunologic System Effects. The burned patient has an altered host defense response. The granulocytic functions of chemotaxis, phagocytosis, and destruction of ingested bacteria are abnormal, and breakdown of the skin and the mucosal barriers is often responsible for infection in the patient with burns. Infection has long been recognized as potentially the most lethal complication of burn injuries. More recently, however, it has become clear that the increased incidence of fatal sepsis following major burn insult is associated with the immune system (Wardenn, 1987). Of importance is the active cell-mediated suppression of the antigen-specific immune response to burn injury. The cellular events that precipitate this response are unknown; however, research has suggested a relationship between postburn immunosuppression and prolonged exposure to burn eschar. Suppression of the cell-mediated

TABLE 56–4. Symptoms Associated with Pulmonary Injury

Early Symptoms	Late Symptoms
Laryngeal edema	Parenchymal infection
Stridor	Hypoxemia
Hoarseness	Atelectasis
Bronchospasm	$\dot{V}/\dot{Q}$ mismatch
	Adult respiratory distress syndrome

immune response in thermally injured patients is associated with significantly compromised biologic activity of helper T-lymphocytes. Research studies by Teodorczyk-Injeyan and colleagues showed that interleukin-2 (IL-2) can promote the synthesis of immunoglobulin M (IgM) by human B-lymphocytes in the presence of functional T-lymphocytes. T-lymphocytes respond to IL-2 by releasing other soluble mediators of the humoral immune response (Teodorczyk-Injeyan et al., 1989). Steroids increase mortality and infection rates in burn patients and are therefore nearly always contraindicated (Jacobson et al., 1988).

Gastrohepatic System Effects. The gastrohepatic system is primarily responsible for providing a continual supply of nutrients, fluids, and electrolytes for tissue building and repair. The mouth, pharynx, esophagus, stomach, and small intestines are primarily responsible for ingestion and movement of products through the system, the secretion of essential enzymes and electrolytes to break down the materials ingested, and the absorption of the end products of digestion into the blood. The liver, an accessory organ, is responsible for the metabolism of proteins, carbohydrates, and fats. During stress, such as that occurring following a burn, these functions are compromised. Increased glucose is released from the pancreas, resulting in an increase in some plasma proteins and in nonesterified fatty acid concentration. Hyperglycemia may also be due to an altered storage of glycogen in the liver, muscle, and brain or to the sympathoadrenal stress response that alters glucose production and breakdown through the effects of the catecholamines on alpha- and beta-adrenergic receptors. A decrease in serum albumin, plasma amino acids, and liver and muscle glycogen also occurs (Jacoby, 1974) in burn injuries. Storage and filtration of blood are other essential activities assumed by the liver. In the burn patient, because a functioning liver is critical to the patient's successful recovery, liver function tests are performed routinely. In particular, the critical care nurse should be alert to a prolonged prothrombin time, elevated serum transaminases and serum bilirubin, and retention of sulfobromophthalein as a result of liver reserve functions. It must be noted that in the presence of associated traumatic injuries, these values may also become abnormal. Other factors contributing to abnormal liver function include infectious processes, poor nutrition, blood transfusions, drugs, and anesthesia.

Redistribution of hepatic blood flow was once considered the primary reason for alterations in gastrointestinal and hepatic function in burn patients. Because these alterations continue to occur in the presence of adequate fluid replacement, it is felt that three factors may contribute to gastrohepatic alterations in the burn patient: (1) decreased mucosal mass; (2) decreased rate of DNA synthesis; and (3) enhanced permeability of the small intestine to bacteria (Carter et al., 1988).

The use of narcotic analgesics accompanied by prolonged bedrest or inadequate fluid intake predisposes the patient to constipation, whereas antibiotic therapy or hypertonic enteral tube feedings may cause diarrhea. These bowel problems create a constant challenge for the critical care nurse requiring diligent assessment and intervention.

Genitourinary System Effects. The kidney responds immediately to the decreases in circulating blood volume, cardiac output, and blood pressure that occur with burns. With these decreases, renal vasoconstriction also occurs, giving rise to a decrease in the glomerular filtration rate. Antidiuretic hormone (ADH), secreted by the posterior pituitary, controls water reabsorption through active transport at the distal tubules. Release of ADH causes retention of water as a compensatory mechanism resulting in oliguria. Blood urea nitrogen and creatinine levels become elevated. Glomerular filtration may be reestablished if adequate fluid resuscitation measures are undertaken and monitored. This reaction may occur on a temporary or permanent basis. If decreased glomerular filtration is treated with adequate fluid resuscitation, it will return to normal; however, if the patient has a history of kidney disease, it may not. Tubular damage is a likely possibility if glomerular filtration is untreated.

Myoglobin, a pigment released when muscle tissue is damaged and found following massive flame and electrical injuries, sludges in the kidney along with hemolyzed red blood cells. The urine in patients with myoglobinuria or hemoglobinuria has a characteristic rust or burgundy color. It is imperative that these substances are flushed from the kidney before acute tubular necrosis occurs. Patients may be diuresed by flushing with fluids or osmotic diuretics such as mannitol (Osmitrol) or urea. During the initial period following burn injury, when edema is most acute, a Foley catheter is essential to monitor fluid resuscitation efforts regardless of the potential infection risk associated with catheterization. Dialysis is not usually necessary if adequate fluid resuscitation is employed.

Glycosuria may occur initially as a result of pseudodiabetes related to the stress of the burn injury. This usually clears spontaneously.

Neuroendocrine System Effects. Neurologic effects usually occur as later sequelae to burn injuries. If manifested early, two major effects may be seen. Although rare, direct nerve injury may occur following electrical injury because the low resistance of nerve tissue conducts the electrical current. This nerve injury generally resolves, and partial or complete recovery of nerve function occurs. The major goal is to prevent further injury to the nerve (Achauer, 1987). The other immediate effect of burn injury is encephalopathy, which may occur as a result of other systemic alterations such as hypoxemic states.

Loss of skin integrity is accompanied by profound metabolic responses. Catabolic negative nitrogen balance is the primary characteristic associated with the metabolic response to burn injuries. Because of the large urinary nitrogen losses, progressive wasting of skeletal muscle mass and muscle weakness occur, accompanied by loss of skeletal muscle protein.

The neuroendocrine response to stress is activated immediately following a burn injury. The hypothalamic-pituitary system attempts to stabilize the body by activating the target organs. All major burns are accompanied at various times by exaggerated endocrine and metabolic responses. In particular, increases in ACTH, ADH, cortisol, aldosterone, catecholamines, glucagon, immunoreactive insulin, calcitonin, parathyroid hormone, renin, angiotensin II, 17-ketosteroids, 17-ketogenic steroids, and 17-hydroxycorticosteroids are found. Decreased levels of triiodothyronine (T_3), thyroxine (T_4), testosterone in males, follicle-stimulating hormone (FSH), and progesterone are also found (Dolecek, 1985). Increased ACTH is produced as a result of anterior pituitary stimulation. The adrenal cortex is then stimulated to produce increased amounts of corticoids, which increase glucose production.

The adrenal medulla, under sympathetic response, secretes the catecholamines epinephrine and norepinephrine, which assist in the "fight or flight" response to stress. The increased epinephrine increases heart rate, constricts the vessels in the skin and kidney, and may depress pancreatic and insulin production. Cardiac output rises along with blood pressure and a subsequent decrease in peripheral resistance. The bronchi and bronchioles dilate, and the individual becomes hyperpneic. Blood supply is increased to the heart, muscles, and nervous system. These increased circulating catecholamines in the emergent phase of burn physiology cause an increase in circulating white blood cells and a decrease in circulating eosinophils.

Burn injuries, more than any other traumatic injury, cause increased stress on the human body. The burn patient sustains a hypermetabolic state from the time of injury usually until the time of wound closure. The increased metabolic activity leads to loss of weight and a negative nitrogen balance. Energy and protein reserves are quickly used up, depleting the body of necessary resources for tissue repair and building. In an effort to supply the tissues with available energy, the body undergoes gluconeogenesis and ureagenesis. The catabolism that occurs as a result of these activities is related to the extent and severity of burn injury. The caloric needs of burn patients are staggering. Calculations to determine the caloric and protein requirements following massive thermal injury are usually based on body weight in kilograms and total body surface burned. Nomograms to calculate nutritional requirements use age, sex, total body surface burned, and basal metabolic rate to determine caloric and nitrogen requirements. The increased nutritional requirements mandate enteral or parenteral hyperalimentation.

Decreased nutritional intake, particularly proteins, increases the patient's risk of poor wound healing because insufficient nutrients will be available for tissue repair. Loss of one-fourth to one-third of the protein mass from the body is predictably fatal in the absence of nutritional support (Kravitz, 1988).

Other Associated Systemic Changes. Burn-related infection presents an acute risk to the burn patient and a challenge to the entire health care team. Pneumonia, burn wound infection, urinary tract infection, and septicemia caused by fungi, bacteria, or viruses are only a few of the potentially lethal infections that may occur.

Joint function is a major challenge in the rehabilitation of the burn patient. Preservation of joint mobility begins early in the care of the patient to permit a return to functional use. Active participation by physical and occupational therapists begins during the emergent phase of burns.

Corneal abrasions may result following facial burns. Ectropion or exposure keratitis may result from eyelid contractures. Chronic complications of electrical burns may involve cataracts or glaucoma. Ophthalmic examination is necessary in patients with burns to the face. Fluorescein strips can aid in the diagnosis of corneal abrasions or burns.

Burns of the face, hands, feet, and genitalia need special consideration in the emergent phase of burn care. Special care often involves shaving the hair if necessary, preventing pressure on these sites, exposure of the area, elevation (e.g., scrotum), and frequent cleaning and use of topical agents.

PATIENT CARE MANAGEMENT DURING THE EMERGENT PHASE

Initial patient care management during this emergent phase primarily involves stabilization of the patient with fluid resuscitation and support of the cardiovascular, pulmonary, and renal systems.

Physical Assessment. Assessment of the burn victim begins in much the same way as that of any other trauma victim; in fact, a burn injury is one of the greatest traumas the body can suffer. Airway, breathing, and circulation must first be established. A secondary trauma survey should then be performed because the burn victim may present with concomitant traumatic injuries. Special attention should be paid to respiratory assessment, even though the patient may not be obviously compromised.

A verbal history from the patient should be taken immediately upon arrival in the emergency department because the burn victim is generally lucid and able to provide pertinent information about the event and about preexisting health problems. If the history is delayed until a more convenient time, the nurse may find the patient intubated, sedated, or in a state of shock.

In taking a history from the patient who is burned, specific emphasis should be placed on the history of the accident, including the time and location of the incident, how the incident occurred, whether it was indoors or outdoors, and whether drugs or alcohol were involved. The nurse should also obtain a history of preexisting health problems such as allergies, diabetes, or heart or lung disorders that could interfere with fluid resuscitation and wound healing.

The burn victim should be weighed as soon as possible after arrival at the hospital because the preburn weight is of vital importance in providing adequate fluid resuscitation, nutrition, and drug dosages. Table 56–5 is a sample of admission orders used for the burned patient.

Other orders may relate to hemodynamic parameters, nutritional guidelines, respiratory support, consultations, and depth determination studies. Standard orders for admission such as these can shorten the admission process and assist in ensuring that important areas of care are not overlooked.

Laboratory Tests. Alterations in laboratory values are carefully monitored during this critical time. The following laboratory tests are usually performed upon admission and monitored throughout the patient's recovery:

Arterial blood gases
Carboxyhemoglobin level
Chemistry panel
Complete blood count (with differential)
Clotting studies (prothrombin time [PT] and partial thromboplastin time [PTT])
Type and crossmatch
Drug and alcohol screen (if indicated)
Urine analysis
Other tests as indicated, such as HIV titer

Metabolic acidosis develops after a major burn injury. This is easily correctable with adequate fluid resuscitation and normalization of the cardiac output. Even in the presence of smoke inhalation, if the patient is adequately oxygenated, blood gases may be abnormal. Elevated carbon monoxide levels should not be depended upon to indicate smoke inhalation injuries. Metabolic acidosis also occurs when mafenide acetate (Sulfamylon) is applied topically over a large portion of the body surface area.

Acid-base derangements also occur secondary to shock states, renal failure, and pulmonary failure. The primary causes of the acid-base imbalance should be treated when possible.

Carboxyhemoglobin levels of more than 10% are diagnostic of carbon monoxide poisoning, and early intubation is required (Desai, 1984). It is important to remember, as stated previously, that the opposite does not hold true, and the absence of an elevated COHb does not rule out an inhalation injury.

Following the burn injury the intracellular sodium concentration increases. This creates an osmotic pressure gradient that pulls water into the cell. In exchange, potassium leaves the cell and concentrates in the serum. This, in addition to the hemolysis of

---

TABLE 56–5. Sample Admission Orders for the Severely Burned Patient

1. Diagnosis: _____ % TBSA _____ % full-thickness
2. Condition:
3. Vital signs (T, BP, P, R) every _____ min
4. Daily weight
5. Intake and output every 1 hour
6. Foley to gravity drainage
7. IV fluids: Ringer's lactate at _____ mL/hour for _____ hours, then _____ mL/hour for _____ hours. 5% albumisol at _____ mL/hour for _____ hours; then _____ mL/hour for _____ hours
8. Titrate IV fluids to maintain urine output at _____ mL/hour, CVP _____ mm Hg, PAP _____ mm Hg
9. Neurovascular checks of circumferential extremity burns every 1 hour
10. Humidified oxygen by face mask at 6 liters/hour
11. Chest x-ray now and daily for _____ days
12. Hydrotherapy every _____
13. Wound care with silver sulfadiazine dressings every _____
14. Physical and occupational therapy consults
15. Morphine sulfate IV push 2–20 mg/hour prn. Begin continuous drip if needed
16. Laboratory studies: CBC now and every _____ hour, electrolytes now and every _____ hour, PT/PTT now and every _____ hour
17. Place NG tube to low suction
18. Begin supplemental feedings at _____
19. Other laboratory studies _____

Abbreviations: TBSA, total body surface area; T, temperature; BP, blood pressure; P, pulse; R, respirations; CVP, central venous pressure; PT, prothrombin time; PTT, partial thromboplastin time; NG, nasogastric.

red blood cells, leads to hyperkalemia, which is often seen early following the burn injury.

Serum electrolyte values are also affected by the fluid status of the patient. Sodium and chloride ions are often increased secondary to the hemoconcentrated state of the patient. The actual number of ions has not changed, but the percentage of solute has decreased.

The patient who has sustained a major burn injury is also unable to regulate the loss of electrolytes through the skin. Sodium is often lost through the skin and requires replacement. Chlorides, on the other hand, are reabsorbed by the kidney.

Alterations in the complete blood count (red blood cells [RBC], white blood cells [WBC], and platelets) occur in response to burn injury. There is some cellular destruction of red cells (<10%), which occurs as a response of the local heat damage to the burned area. The burn patient initially experiences an increase in hematocrit due to a loss of plasma volume into the interstitial space and hemoconcentration. Hematocrit values are usually obtained every 2 to 4 hours during the first 48 hours after the burn and as needed thereafter to assess fluid status. Anemia often develops during hospitalization due to the progressive hemolysis of RBCs.

Leukocytosis occurs early in the postburn period, the WBC count often going as high as 30,000/mm³. This situation generally resolves within 24 to 48 hours. Persistent leukocytosis may indicate infection. Leukopenia often occurs as a side effect of topical therapy with silver sulfadiazine but it generally resolves within 24 to 48 hours without withdrawal of the therapy or other treatment (Fuller and Engler, 1988).

Thrombocytopenia is often seen during the first 72 hours after the burn. This temporary decrease in platelets may result from the dilutional effects of fluid resuscitation and some degree of microvascular thrombosis or DIC.

Clotting studies are often abnormal in the initial period as well. The PT and PTT are often elevated during the first 72 hours after the burn. As plasma leaks out of the vascular space and into the interstitial space, clotting factors follow. Clotting factors generally return to normal during the first week and need not be treated as long as active bleeding is not observed.

The kidneys perform a major role in regulating the fluid and electrolyte balance and in excreting waste products. Hourly measurements and testing of urine output are required to determine how well the kidney is functioning. During the first 48 hours post burn, an output of 50 to 100 mL of urine/hour indicates adequate renal perfusion. After the first 48 hours, 30 mL of urine/hour is acceptable in the adult. Urine output in children should equal 1 mL/kg per hour during the first 48 hours and 0.5 to 1 mL/kg per hour thereafter.

Specific gravity should be maintained within normal values (1.002 to 1.035). Elevated specific gravity

may indicate decreased intravascular fluid volume and dehydration.

A urinalysis that is positive for protein indicates that the body is using protein stores rather than food, an indicator that the patient is in a negative nitrogen balance. Urine that is positive for glucose may indicate that the body is not utilizing ingested glucose, or it may indicate either diabetes or pseudodiabetes, which is often associated with the stress of this major injury. Glucose intolerance is also a sign of sepsis and should be reported and followed. Insulin may be required to assist the body to utilize glucose. Acetone is normally negative on urinalysis. A positive reading may indicate that the body is burning its own fats and proteins and is in a state of starvation.

The color of the urine should normally be yellow or straw-colored. A rust or burgundy appearance indicates myoglobinuria due to the breakdown of muscle tissue secondary to a deep burn injury. Green urine may indicate a *Pseudomonas* infection; a urine culture is indicated.

Urine that tests positive for blood may indicate RBC breakdown, which is secondary to hemolysis from the initial injury or from septic shock.

A blood alcohol level may be indicated upon admission if the patient has an overwhelming odor of alcohol or if the circumstances surrounding the accident are suspicious. Drug screens are also indicated if the patient is behaving in an inappropriate manner or if the injury is more severe than might be expected. Screening the patient's HIV status is controversial at the present time and may have legal ramifications in some states but can be useful. If there is reason to suspect a positive HIV titer, the reason for the test should be discussed with the patient and his consent obtained if possible. Patients with a positive HIV titer who have major burns usually do not respond to treatment as would be expected because their immune system is compromised, causing infection and nonhealing of wounds. It is important to discuss this subject with the patient early in the course of treatment because it may influence treatment plans and outcomes.

Alterations in laboratory values are carefully monitored during this critical time. Table 56–6 lists the typical laboratory findings found in burn patients in the emergent phase.

TABLE 56–6. Expected Emergent Phase Laboratory Values

Serum potassium elevated
Serum sodium elevated
Hematocrit elevated
Serum glucose elevated
Bicarbonate deficit
Prolonged PT and PTT
Metabolic acidosis
Thrombocytopenia
Leukocytosis

Fluid Resuscitation. In 1952 Evans published the first successful surface area/weight formula for calculating fluid resuscitation in the burn-injured patient. Since that time various other formulas have been developed. In general, patients with a burned area of greater than 20% of the total body surface area require intravenous fluid resuscitation because of the physiologic fluid shifts. Time is the major factor in determining fluid management of the burned patient. Administration of fluids is calculated from the time of the initial burn injury, not from the time the patient enters the facility or resuscitation is commenced. All fluids must be infused using a large-bore needle or subclavian or subclavicular lines (Dressler et al., 1988). If at all possible, these lines should not be placed through burned tissue to prevent the possibility of infection.

Each patient presents a unique challenge in that fluid requirements must be estimated correctly to ensure adequate cardiac output while preventing shock. The type and amount of fluid to be used in fluid resuscitation remain extremely controversial (Williams and Porvaznik, 1989). Fluid resuscitation therapy for children with burns depends on careful matching of the selected therapy with the patient's tolerance to injury and subsequent treatment (Graves et al., 1988).

Although there is no standard formula for all patients, neither is there a standard for the type of solution chosen for fluid resuscitation or the parameters used to monitor the efficacy of fluid therapy. Most clinicians agree, however, that the burn patient requires electrolyte solutions during the first 24 hours post burn. Crystalloid solutions chosen most frequently include a balanced salt solution such as lactated Ringer's solution without dextrose or normal saline. Free water, given as a 5% dextrose in water solution, is administered to replace insensible water loss. Additional electrolytes may be added to this solution. Colloids are added anywhere from 6 to 24 hours after injury (Williams and Porvaznik, 1989) when capillary integrity begins to be restored. Some clinicians suggest the use of hypertonic saline (250 mEq sodium/liter of water) as the resuscitation or back-up fluid. Advocates of this therapy state that this solution delivers less free water, acts to draw extravascular fluid into the vascular compartment, lessens edema away from the burn site, decreases the need for escharotomy, increases cardiac output, eliminates ileus, and decreases intrapulmonary water in the inhalation-injured patient, but others argue that this solution poses a risk of severe electrolyte disturbances (Williams and Porvaznik, 1989).

The fluid regimens presented in Table 56–7 and the measurements commonly monitored to determine fluid resuscitation efficacy (Table 56–8) are therefore intended as guides and should be geared toward the individual patient's needs and responses. Children with massive burn injuries require a greater volume of fluid relative to body weight and burn size than the average adult (Graves et al., 1988). Often, burn size may have been underestimated in

children who initially fail to respond to fluid resuscitation.

The modified Baxter formula is based on the concept that colloid molecules do not remain in the intravascular space during the first 24 hours after a burn; thus the formula recommends giving only crystalloid solution during the first 24 hours and colloid thereafter. This formula has been adopted by the American College of Surgeons based on its ease of use, the fact that it is readily available, and its reduced cost (Aharoni et al., 1989).

Colloid solutions such as salt-poor albumin or fresh frozen plasma are used infrequently during the first 24 hours post burn; however, some burn units currently use colloid solutions (Brigham formula) exclusively in the first 24 hours (University of California, Irvine Medical Center, 1989). These solutions are usually costly, and their efficacy compared with crystalloid in the critical first 24 hours has not been proved (Robertson et al., 1985). After the first 24 hours, other fluid regimens recommend colloid to increase the intravascular oncotic pressure.

A typical burn patient receives large volumes of fluid. Using the Parkland formula, for example, a 70-kg patient with a 40% TBSA would require 11,200 mL (11.2 liters) of fluid during the first 24 hours post burn. Although the volume of fluid administered seems high, the critical care nurse must remember that unless the patient has cardiovascular compromise because of prior cardiovascular disease, all fluid infused into such a hypovolemic patient will diffuse through the capillary sieve as quickly as it is infused. Regardless of the solution chosen, it must be emphasized that careful titration of the fluid is necessary to prevent shock and maintain the adequacy of urine output, vital signs, acid-base balance, tissue perfusion, and level of consciousness.

Fluid resuscitation in burn patients is not without hazards. Over-resuscitation with fluids becomes a priority, as pulmonary morbidity requires vigilance on the part of the critical care nurse to avoid a life-threatening event. Over-resuscitation may also cause increased peripheral edema, which can impede wound blood flow, in turn altering healing or converting burn injury from a partial- to a full-thickness injury (Graves et al., 1988).

Pain Management. Pain control is of major concern during all phases of burn treatment. The pain of a burn injury is more intense and longer lasting than any other acute injury or illness. The pain is often both physical and emotional. Any victim of a burn injury should be continually assessed for pain, whether in the field or in the outpatient unit. No member of the burn team should assume that the patient does not have pain because he or she is not complaining of pain. Patients with full-thickness burns do have pain, even though by definition viable nerve endings are not exposed in full-thickness burns and therefore do not hurt. Pure full-thickness burns are rare; more often these burns are mixed with areas of partial-thickness burns.

TABLE 56–7. Fluid Resuscitation Formulas

Formula Name	Electrolyte	Colloid	Water	First 24 Hours*	Second 24 Hours
Artz	Ringer's lactate: 3.0 mL × kg weight × %TBSA			Half of total given in first 8 hours; balance over remaining 16 hours	
Brigham		5% albumin: 10% body weight	80 mL/hour D$_5$W	Half of total given during first 8 to 12 hours; balance over following 36 hours	
Brooke	Ringer's lactate: 1.5 mL × kg weight × %TBSA	0.5 mL × kg weight × %TBSA	2000 mL D$_5$W	Half of total in first 8 hours; balance over remaining 16 hours	Half of colloids and electrolyte solutions and all water
Burn Budget of F.D. Moore	Ringer's lactate: 1000 mL titrating to 4000 mL 0.45 normal saline: 1200 mL	7.5% kg weight	1500–5000 mL D$_5$W	All electrolyte, colloid, and water	All electrolyte, colloid = 2.5% of kg weight and all water
Evans	Normal saline (0.9%): 1.0 mL × kg weight × %TBSA	1.0 mL × kg weight × %TBSA	2000 mL D$_5$W	All electrolyte, colloid, and water	Half electrolyte, half colloid
HALFD (hypertonic, albuminated fluid-demand resuscitation)	Hypertonic saline (240 mOsm sodium, 120 mOsm Cl, 120 mOsm lactate) to maintain urine output > 40 mL/hour and MAP at 60 mm Hg	1.5 g albumin/liter	0	All electrolytes and colloid	
Hypertonic formula	300 mEq Na, 200 mEq dextrose, 1 liter lactate, 100 mEq Cl to maintain urine output > 30 mL/hour in adults	0	0		One-third to one-half of first day's requirements
Hypertonic saline solution (New Mexico formula)	250 mEq Na/L: Volume to maintain urine output > 30 mL/hour	0	0	All electrolyte	One-third of sodium solution up to 3500 mL orally
Modified Brooke	Ringer's lactate: 2.0–3.0 mL × kg weight × %TBSA, titrating to 4 mL/kg per %TBSA	0	0		
Parkland	Ringer's lactate: 4.0 mL × kg weight × %TBSA	0	0	Half of total in first 8 hours, balance over remaining 16 hours	No formula
Rambam†	Ringer's lactate: 2000 mL	Plasma: 75.0 mL × kg		All electrolytes and plasma over 36 hours	

*Fluid requirements for the first 24 hours are calculated from time of injury, not entry into the facility.
†Aharoni et al., 1989.

TABLE 56–8. Monitored Parameters in Thermal Injury

1. Level of consciousness
2. Arterial blood pressure
3. Pulse rate and rhythm
4. Central venous pressure
5. Pulmonary artery and capillary wedge pressures
6. Cardiac output including cardiac index, stroke index, systemic vascular resistance, left ventricular stroke index, right ventricular stroke index, pulmonary vascular resistance
7. Arterial blood gases
8. Hematocrit and hemoglobin
9. Urine output including specific gravity, and urine sodium concentration
10. Electrolyte values

During the emergent phase of burn care patients with massive burns often suffer pain continuously, and because of the increased metabolic rate, they metabolize drugs very rapidly. Normal doses of narcotics given intravenously every 1 to 2 hours may not offer enough relief to the patient. During this emergent phase, the nurse must remember that after care of the airway, breathing, and circulation, pain relief has a high priority. Intramuscular injections are usually not given during this phase of care. Altered capillary permeability and muscular blood flow leave drug absorption rates during this phase questionable. Intravenous medications are the route of choice during the emergent phase. Often patients suffering large burn injuries are placed on a titrated morphine drip to make them relatively comfortable yet allow them to remain alert. An analog pain assessment scale is useful and can be done frequently along with vital signs.

Patients who have a history of drug or alcohol abuse may require unusually high doses of morphine before they state that relief has been achieved. Often 60 to 100 mg of morphine are administered intravenously upon admission with little or no reported pain relief. Often the addition of an antianxiety medication such as Ativan is useful.

Nutritional Support. Major thermal injuries result in a hypermetabolic response that is proportional to the burn injury. Basal metabolic needs may be increased as much as 100% above normal in patients with burns exceeding 50% TBSA (Giel, 1987). Nutritional support for the burned patient can be started as soon as the patient is stabilized in the intensive care unit, usually within 24 hours post burn. Careful attention is paid to the nutritional needs of the patient, including an estimate of preburn nutritional status. Enteral feedings are always preferred over parenteral feedings because the latter require large amounts of calories that necessitate a central line through which high concentrations of glucose are given, thus increasing the patient's risk of infection. Enteral feedings are usually successful if they are started slowly and increased progressively until the patient's caloric needs are met.

The Curreri formula (Table 56–9) is most com-

monly used to estimate the caloric needs of adult burn patients, and a similar formula developed by Sutherland is used to estimate the caloric needs of children under 12 years of age (Giel, 1987). Additional calories are sometimes given to compensate for calories not provided during the initial hours of fluid resuscitation and before and after surgical procedures.

Nursing Diagnoses. The critical care nurse systematically assesses various phenomena in order to classify information about the patient with burn injuries. Based on this assessment, as well as on previous knowledge and experience and an ability to think critically, the nurse categorizes the information into diagnostic statements. Table 56–10 provides a list of approved nursing diagnoses that could potentially be selected during the emergent phase of a burn injury.

Goals and Expected Outcomes. During the emergent phase of burn injury, the critical care nurse identifies goals and expected, measurable outcomes. The major goals in the emergent phase of burn injury are to maintain adequate pulmonary function; maintain intravascular volume and cardiac output; maintain renal function; preserve joint function and mobility; preserve self-concept; and prevent complications associated with the emergent phase of burn injury. Although it is generally desirable to collaborate with the patient in the formulation of goals, this is usually not possible in patients with burns; however, the nurse should attempt to have the patient and the family participate in this process as much as possible. The nursing care plan provides suggested goals, expected outcomes based on those goals, and nursing interventions for both the emergent and the acute phases of burn injury, since they are similar for both phases.

Acute (Fluid Remobilization) Phase

The acute phase is characterized by eschar separation and fluid remobilization. This phase lasts until spontaneous healing of the burn wound occurs or until autografts are in place. Primary patient care management involves removal of burn eschar, wound coverage, and prevention of complications. It is during this phase that patients are most likely to develop complications such as septicemia and cardiovascular collapse. This phase may last weeks to months depending on the severity of the burn

TABLE 56–9. Estimating Caloric Needs

Curreri formula: 25 kcal x weight (kg) + 40 × TBSA burn
Sutherland formula for children: 60 kcal × kg + 35 × TBSA burn

Abbreviations: TBSA, total body surface area.

TABLE 56–10. Nursing Diagnoses: Emergent Phase of Burn Injury

Ineffective airway clearance
Anxiety
Altered body temperature, potential for
Ineffective breathing pattern
Decreased cardiac output
Pain
Impaired verbal communication
Ineffective coping, family: Disabling
Ineffective coping, individual
Fear
Fluid volume deficit: Actual
Impaired gas exchange
Anticipatory grieving
Hopelessness
Hyperthermia
Hypothermia
Potential for infection
Potential for injury
Knowledge deficit
Impaired physical mobility
Altered nutrition: Less than body requirements
Post trauma response
Powerlessness
Body image: Disturbance
Personal identity: Disturbance
Self-esteem: Disturbance
Sensory perceptual alterations: Visual, kinesthetic, tactile
Impaired skin integrity: Actual
Sleep pattern disturbance
Impaired thermoregulation
Altered thought processes
Impaired tissue integrity
Altered oral mucous membranes
Altered tissue perfusion: Renal, cerebral, cardiopulmonary,
    gastrointestinal, peripheral
Altered patterns of urinary elimination

---

injury and resultant treatment protocols. Again, as during the emergent phase, multisystemic effects occur during the acute phase of burn injuries.

Cardiovascular System Effects. In this phase, the capillary leak begins to resolve and the intravascular fluid volume begins to stabilize. There is a decrease in capillary permeability that results in stabilization of the fluid shifts. The large amounts of fluids required for resuscitation in the emergent period are no longer necessary during the acute phase other than for maintenance of hydration and electrolyte balance. In addition, the lymphatic tissue is better able to withstand the fluid load, restoring equilibrium. It is during this phase that the intravascular oncotic pressure must be maintained to preserve physiologic function. This may be achieved through the judicious use of colloids such as salt-poor albumin or fresh frozen plasma. Care must be maintained in this process, particularly in elderly patients and patients with a history of cardiovascular pathology.

Decreased tissue perfusion as a result of edema in the emergent phase causes aggregation of cellular byproducts in the microcirculation during the acute phase. This debris prevents adequate blood flow, which is necessary for healing. Septicemia is also a major concern during this phase. Wound infections as well as other systemic infections such as bacterial infections of the heart may occur; such infections may result from the collection of debris or the administration of steroids.

Pulmonary System Effects. If the patient survives the respiratory distress that occurs during the early phases of smoke inhalation, increased cellular permeability in the alveoli results in noncardiogenic interstitial and intra-alveolar edema, which interferes progressively with gas exchange. Infusion of large amounts of crystalloid solutions in the fluid resuscitation of the burn patient may further compound the pathogenesis of pulmonary edema. Bronchopneumonia may occur during the acute phase as a result of imposed immobility, increased fluid volume infusions, changes in pulmonary capillary permeability, and pulmonary parenchymal damage. Respiratory failure in this stage is a poor prognostic sign.

Patients may continue to be intubated during the acute phase, and this is associated with the risk of infection. Patients with endotracheal tubes are at risk of nosocomial infections. In addition, nasotracheally intubated patients are at risk of sinus infections.

Immunologic System Effects. During the acute phase of burn injury, critical interventions include removal of necrotic or devitalized tissue and coverage of the wound with grafts to prevent infection leading to septicemia. Because the patient continues to be immunosuppressed, infectious organisms are more easily able to invade the body, further compromising the patient's condition.

Gastrohepatic System Effects. Approximately 90% of burned patients have erythema, punctate hemorrhages, and erosion of the duodenal and gastric membranes (Wiener and Barrett, 1986). Curling's ulcer, a duodenal ulcer, is a devastating source of gastrointestinal hemorrhage and perforation and can occur during the acute phase of burn injury. Gastric dilatation and paralytic ileus may also occur, caused by fear, anxiety, or sepsis. Paradoxically, these ulcers are not associated with gastric acid secretion but arise from the gastric mucosa, which is altered as a result of back-diffusion of H+ ions, ischemia, and inadequate mucosal cell proliferation (McAlhany et al., 1979). These ulcers can be prevented by providing adequate nutritional support, gastric intubation, and pH monitoring, and by administering histamine blockers and antacids.

The presence of blood in the nasogastric aspirate, emesis, or stool should be carefully monitored. Early in the postburn period it may be caused by gastric irritation, whereas later it may be duodenal in origin. Early congestion in the gastric mucosa may be a factor in the development of this phenomenon, which may be caused by hemoconcentration, neurohumoral stimulation, or infection (Jacoby, 1974). Colon ulcers may also occur in the presence of hypovolemia, sepsis, or multiple organ failure. These ulcers serve as a source of bacteremia.

Although rare, bacteremia may also cause acalculous cholecystitis. Patients may complain of acute upper right quadrant pain and may present with jaundice. Ultrasonography and radioisotopic scans confirm the diagnosis (Wiener and Barrett, 1986).

Genitourinary System Effects. Renal failure can occur during any phase of burn injury. During the acute phase, it may be the result of infection, sepsis, or pharmacologic agents. Knowledge of the route of excretion of drugs accompanied by careful monitoring of renal function may prevent further renal damage.

Neuroendocrine Effects. Severe metabolic strain continues in the acute phase of burn injury. Symptoms of adrenal insufficiency are found occasionally in the first week following burn injury and may occur anytime until the burn wound is healed. If adrenal insufficiency occurs, the nurse assesses for hypotension, hyponatremia, hyperkalemia, elevated urine sodium, decreased urine potassium, alterations in temperature, leukopenia, and anorexia.

PATIENT CARE MANAGEMENT DURING THE ACUTE PHASE

Assessment and prevention of complications during this phase cannot be minimized because the patient is always susceptible to them. It is important for the nurse to be vigilant with respect to assessment parameters and laboratory data.

Laboratory Studies. During the acute phase laboratory values are followed periodically for changes from normal. When necessary, daily laboratory studies may be ordered, and when the patient is more stable they may be ordered once or twice a week. Generally, if the patient is undergoing a surgical procedure or is septic, laboratory studies are required more often. Table 56–11 lists the expected laboratory findings in the acute phase.

Wound Care. It is important to remember that the skin is the largest organ in the body and the first line of defense against outside elements. If the skin is broken, it is unable to protect the body against bacterial invasion. The burn may be sterile initially due to the heat causing the burn; however, soon after the injury the normal flora from adjacent areas

can invade the burn wound. The burned patient is at risk for wound sepsis until the wound is either healed or has been grafted during the acute or rehabilitative phases of care. To prevent bacterial invasion of the wound until that time, hydrotherapy is performed at least once a day. During hydrotherapy the wound is cleansed either in a whirlpool-type bath or a shower. Cleansing solutions such as povidone-iodine (Betadine), chlorhexidine (Hibiclens), or a 1:240 sodium hypochlorite solution is added to the bath or shower water (Martin, 1989).

Burn wounds are débrided to rid the wound of necrotic tissue and to remove previously applied topical agents. Débridement can be either surgical, mechanical, or enzymatic. Mechanical débridement takes place daily when the patient receives hydrotherapy. This is accomplished using a washcloth with long, firm strokes. At times this procedure must be done with the aid of an anesthetic agent because of the degree of pain it causes.

Surgical débridement is done in the operating room under a general anesthetic. Guarded knives are used to remove burn eschar. Devitalized skin is removed in layers until viable tissue is observed. If the tissue bed is healthy and clean, the patient can be grafted immediately; if an infection is present, the wound is dressed, and grafting takes place at a later date.

Enzymatic débridement to remove eschar has been used effectively in some burn centers. To be effective, the burn eschar must be soft and moist. These enzymatic agents include Elase and Travase. Travase has been known to sting upon application to the burn, causing patients increased pain. The enzymatic débridement process usually takes a minimum of a week and will débride only through the layers of the skin. If the burn eschar extends into the subcutaneous fat, this tissue will remain undigested. These agents are generally used after mechanical débridement and rarely after surgical débridement. One disadvantage of these agents is that wound sepsis is difficult to manage because topical enzymatic agents are not antimicrobial. If the patient has signs of wound-related sepsis, enzymatic débridement is discontinued, and appropriate topical antimicrobial therapy is begun.

After débridement a topical antimicrobial agent is applied to the burn. Table 56–12 lists the most commonly used topical agents, their advantages, disadvantages, and method of use.

After débridement down to healthy tissue has been performed, grafting, if necessary, can be performed. Split-thickness skin grafts (STSG) are most common and can be either meshed or sheet. STSGs can be taken from any donor site but usually are not taken from cosmetic areas such as the arms, upper chest (if possible), or face. Ideal donor sites are the scalp, thighs, and buttocks. Full-thickness skin grafts (FTSG) are also possible. The donor site for these grafts is most commonly the groin, and because this forms a full-thickness deficit from the donor site, it is closed by primary intention. FTSGs are never

---

TABLE 56–11. Expected Initial Acute Phase Laboratory Values

Serum potassium decreased
Serum sodium decreased
Hematocrit decreased
Bicarbonate decreased

TABLE 56–12. Topical Antimicrobial Therapy of Burns

Topical Preparation	Indication for Use	Advantages	Disadvantages
Mafenide acetate (Sulfamylon)	Deep burns (i.e., electrical, ear burns)	Wide-spectrum antimicrobial coverage	Painful on application and for 20 to 30 minutes afterwards; potent carbonic anhydrase inhibitor causing decreased renal bicarbonate production; metabolic acidosis is a problem, especially if patient already has respiratory compromise; potassium is also lost in the urine; does not adhere to burn well and requires frequent reapplication
Silver sulfadiazine (Silvadine)	Partial- and full-thickness thermal injuries	Wide-spectrum antimicrobial action; painless on application; eschar remains soft, pliable, easily debridable	Not effective against fungal organisms; may cause leukopenia (self-limiting); resistant organisms can occur with prolonged use
Silver nitrate	Partial- and full-thickness burns	Chemoprophylactic; no reported sensitivities; painless on application	Depth of penetration is only 1 to 2 mm of eschar; hypotonicity of solution will pull Na, Ca, K, and Cl from the burn wound—these effects are seen when larger surface areas are treated; dressings must be kept wet. Dry silver nitrate can injure tissue when allowed to concentrate by evaporation. Range of motion is limited by thick dressings. Silver nitrate stains everything black (clothing, floors, skin, linens)
Acetic acid	Infected partial-thickness burns, post grafting	Sensitive to *Pseudomonas* infection; débridement of grafts by bacterial lysis of eschar; inexpensive	Must be a wet to dry dressing; range of motion is limited by thick dressings; removal of dressings may be painful
Sodium hypoclorite (Dakins)	Débridement of grafts	Drys "soupy" wounds; inexpensive	Must be a wet to dry dressing; range of motion is limited by thick dressings; removal of dressings may be painful

meshed because this would defeat the purpose of being full thickness.

Grafts may be meshed (expanded) to one and a half to one, three to one, or six to one times their original size. Meshing is prepared using a mechanical meshing device. The greater the mesh, the less the initial wound is covered, but within 1 to 2 weeks the graft epithelializes into the interstices of the mesh with new epidermis. The larger the mesh the greater the amount of scarring because as the wound matures there is more wound contracture. For this reason, the smallest amount of meshing possible is used.

Sheet STSGs are used for cosmetic areas such as the hand or face as well as for highly functional areas. Sheet grafts contract less than meshed grafts and therefore are excellent for grafting the hands and neck. Once healed, sheet grafts blend into the normal skin better than meshed grafts.

FTSGs are used for cosmetic areas such as the eyelid. Skin taken from the groin is applied directly to the defect. Once grafted, both the donor site and the recipient area require wound care. Biobrane or Xeroform gauze, among others, is frequently applied to the donor site.

The method of care of the recipient site varies from institution to institution. Graft take should be expected to be 90% to 100%. Although some burn centers inspect the grafted site every 4 to 8 hours (University of California, Irvine Medical Center, 1989), others leave one dressing intact for 5 to 7 days. Each burn center has its own dressing protocols.

For burns that do not require grafting or are waiting to be grafted there are two types of dressing techniques, open and closed. In the open dressing a topical agent is applied to the burn, but no gauze dressings are placed over the topical agent or the burn. Closed dressings consist of layers of gauze dressings over the burn plus topical agents, virtually excluding outside elements from the burn. A semi-open method combines elements of both. Usually one layer of gauze is placed over the burn together with a topical agent. This method permits the burn to "breathe" while providing a means to hold the topical agent in place.

Biologic dressings consist primarily of viable tissues used to cover the burn temporarily as a substitute for conventional dressings or for leaving the burn wound exposed. The benefits of these materials are reduced loss of fluid, electrolytes, and protein, decreased pain, inhibition of bacterial growth, and faster healing of the burn wound. Materials used include allograft (cadaver skin), porcine xenografts (pig skin), and amniotic membrane.

In the past few years allograft has become the most popular biologic dressing. Skin harvest should always be considered when organ donation is being considered from a cadaver. Skin banks are able to store harvested skin indefinitely. Cyclosporine has been used in skin allografts to increase the likelihood of adherence. Although allografts are considered a temporary wound covering, one case has been reported in which permanent coverage was achieved with the use of cyclosporine (Achauer et al., 1986). Generally, lower doses of cyclosporine are used than in other organ grafts. The risk of sepsis is omnipresent and must be evaluated continuously. Although no permanent synthetic wound covering is currently available, there are several materials that can be advantageous in the treatment of both minor and moderate burns. The first is Biobrane. Biobrane is an ultrathin, polydimethyl-siloxane rubber-like membrane that is bonded to a mixture of hydrophilic collagen peptides. This flexible, nylon-like fabric is used to cover clean partial-thickness burns or to cover temporarily clean, excised full-thickness burns. Biobrane will actually adhere to a partial-thickness burn and acts as an artificial skin until the patient's own skin reepithelializes.

Synthetic dressings such as Opsite or Duoderm are also used on burn wounds. Opsite is permeable to oxygen and carbon dioxide, but not to water or bacteria. Hydron, another barrier-type dressing, is made into a paste at the time of application and is applied directly over the burn. Hydron allows drainage through the material and may remain in place for up to 7 days.

A synthetic dressing, Sildimac, is a newly developed drug delivery system composed of polyethylene glycol, poly-2-hydroxyethyl methacrylate, dimethyl sulfoxide, and silver sulfadiazine. When these components are mixed they form an elastic, flexible sheet that is adherent to dry surfaces and conforms closely to body contours. When incorporated into the delivery system, silver sulfadiazine is released in a sustained fashion. Studies have shown that Sildimac dressings on partial-thickness burns can be left in place for 5 to 7 days while bacterial levels are controlled and twice daily dressings with silver sulfadiazine are continued (Deitch et al., 1989).

Skin generally provides a barrier to outside agents and prevents foreign bacteria from entering the body. When the layers of the skin are destroyed, this barrier is lost. Inspection of the wound takes place at least daily, looking for signs of infection, odors, and exudate. There is much controversy over what isolation techniques should be required for burn patients. Some burn centers use strict isolation techniques, including hats, masks, caps, shoe covers, and scrub attire. Other centers require only scrub attire and universal isolation precautions. The type of isolation used should be decided in consultation with the epidemiologists at each institution. Culture results should be obtained at least weekly and followed for trends. Although some burn centers have serious cross-contamination and infection problems, others have none.

Pain Management. Pain management remains a priority during the acute phase of recovery. Without adequate pain relief the patient cannot be expected to participate in his own care or to tolerate necessary procedures and therapies. During this phase the patient usually participates more in activities, is more aware of his surroundings, and generally has little to concentrate on other than his burn care. There are many options for managing pain, including drugs, guided imagery, and relaxation techniques. During the early part of the acute phase the patient is generally weaned off the morphine drip and can be placed on patient-controlled analgesia (PCA) if he is free of handsplints and able to understand and use the equipment. PCA sometimes provides the patient with the only independence he experiences. Time-released oral morphine preparations, oral Dilaudid, methadone, and vicodin are among the countless other drugs that have been shown to work well in patients with burns. Often the addition of an antianxiety medication (e.g., Ativan) will enhance the narcotic effects of these drugs and provide better relief for the patient.

Guided imagery can be used by the bedside nurse after minimal training. This technique is especially useful during painful procedures such as hydrotherapy. A conversation with the patient beforehand is useful to establish rapport and to assess the activities and places the patient finds relaxing and calming. It is to those activities or places that the patient is taken during guided imagery.

Relaxation techniques can also be taught to the patient during this phase. Deep breathing with cleansing breaths, relaxation audio tapes, and audio tapes of calm, relaxing music work well with some patients. Others can be taught techniques to use with imagery. Quiet times should be provided for the patient so that he can achieve adequate rest.

Nutritional Support. Nutritional support during this phase is one of the top priorities of care. The patient with massive burns continues to receive enteral feedings, which can be supplemented with oral feedings until the patient is able to take in enough calories orally to meet his needs. Generally, this situation occurs when the patient has only 30% to 40% TBSA left unhealed. Patients are often provided with oral supplements (e.g., Ensure Plus) to assist in attaining adequate caloric intake.

If the patient becomes septic and develops ileus during the acute phase, nutrition continues to remain a high priority. A duodenal tube can be inserted, either through gravity or by gastroscopy, and feedings can continue despite ileus; otherwise, total parenteral nutrition (TPN) must be started through a central venous line. TPN carries an additional risk of intravenous line sepsis, given the large concentrations of glucose that must be administered to meet the patient's high caloric needs.

During the acute phase of recovery periodic urine tests for nitrogen may be done to assess the patient's nitrogen balance. Maintenance of a positive nitrogen balance is important, as is assessment of other nutritional parameters such as serum protein and serum albumin levels.

Nursing Diagnoses. Table 56–13 presents nursing diagnoses that may be applicable during the acute phase of burn injury.

Goals and Expected Outcomes. There is a substantial degree of overlap in nursing care during the emergent and acute phases of burn injury. The major goals during the acute phase of burn injury are to maintain intravascular pressure, volume, and cardiac output; maintain electrolyte balance; maintain nutritional support; promote continued joint function and mobility; promote continued autonomy and self-concept; and prevent complications associated with the acute phase of burn injury. The goals and outcome criteria presented in the nursing care plan outline the care planning data pertinent to both phases.

Rehabilitation Phase

Rehabilitation actually begins immediately following burn injury. This process is managed by a multidisciplinary network of professionals who contribute to the patient's eventual return, functionally and cosmetically, to his usual roles and responsibilities. The major goals of this phase of burn injury include enabling the patient to adapt emotionally to the burn injury, achieve maximum function of the involved body parts, and achieve rehabilitation within the limits of the disabilities.

PATIENT CARE MANAGEMENT DURING THE REHABILITATIVE PHASE OF BURN INJURY

Pain Management. Most patients continue to experience pain until the burn is totally healed and for some time thereafter. Pain medications are prescribed during this phase, although they tend to be less

potent than the PCA and oral medications prescribed earlier. Tylenol with codeine is often used.

Pruritus is also a major complaint during this phase of recovery but is a normal part of the healing process. Benadryl and Atarax are often prescribed to help control the symptoms. Lanolin-based skin lotions assist in maintaining lubrication for the healed skin, something that is not always present after a burn injury. Applications of lotion as frequently as every 2 hours may be necessary.

Nutritional Support. During this phase of recovery the patient is generally able to take in his caloric needs orally and is weaned from enteral feedings. It is important for the patient to continue to ingest a high-protein, high-calorie diet until the burns are completely healed. After healing has occurred, the patient's caloric intake should revert back to his preburn level.

Psychosocial Assessment and Support. The skin is the defining feature of each person and serves to influence an individual's identity as well as his body image and concept of self. The nurse must be cog-

---

TABLE 56–13. Nursing Diagnoses: Acute Phase of Burn Injury

Ineffective airway clearance
Anxiety
Potential for altered body temperature
Constipation
Diarrhea
Bowel incontinence
Pain
Ineffective family coping: Compromised
Altered family process
Fear
Dysfunctional grieving
Hopelessness
Hyperthermia
Potential for infection
Potential for injury
Knowledge deficit
Impaired physical mobility
Noncompliance
Altered nutrition: Less than body requirements
Post trauma stress
Powerlessness
Self-care deficit: Feeding
Body image: Disturbance
Personal identity: Disturbance
Self-esteem: Disturbance
Sensory perceptual alterations: Kinesthetic, tactile
Impaired skin integrity: Actual
Sleep pattern disturbance
Social isolation
Impaired thermoregulation
Altered thought processes
Impaired tissue integrity
Altered oral mucous membrane
Altered tissue perfusion: Renal, cardiopulmonary, gastrointestinal, peripheral
Altered patterns of urinary elimination

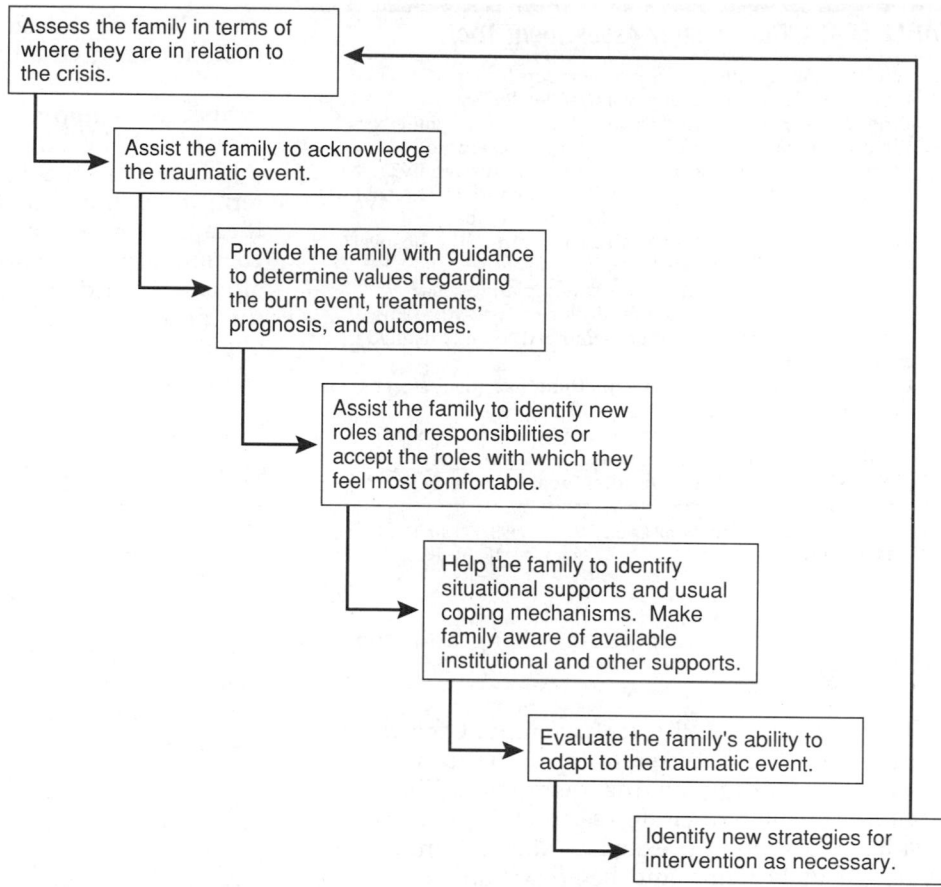

Assess the family in terms of where they are in relation to the crisis.

Assist the family to acknowledge the traumatic event.

Provide the family with guidance to determine values regarding the burn event, treatments, prognosis, and outcomes.

Assist the family to identify new roles and responsibilities or accept the roles with which they feel most comfortable.

Help the family to identify situational supports and usual coping mechanisms. Make family aware of available institutional and other supports.

Evaluate the family's ability to adapt to the traumatic event.

Identify new strategies for intervention as necessary.

FIGURE 56-5. Framework for care of families of critically ill patients. (Adapted from Caine, R.M. (1989). Families in crisis: Making the critical difference. *Focus on Critical Care,* 16 (3), 188.)

nizant of the importance of the relationship between the burn patient's appearance and his attitudes and behavior toward care.

It should be noted that increasing numbers of patients are being admitted with burns resulting from abuse or are self-inflicted. Patients with self-inflicted burns fall into two categories, those with burns suffered without suicidal intent and those who are suicidal (Klasen et al., 1989).

The burn patient and the family are unprepared for the traumatic nature of the devastating injury. They may be unable to manage both internal and external stressors as a result of compromised resources. This inability may continue well into the rehabilitation phase following burn injury, and thus the critical care nurse plays a key role in the assessment and early intervention to aid the patient and family. Most burn-related suicide patients are between 20 and 40 years of age and attempt suicide at home (Klasen et al., 1989). This fact points to the need for family intervention for this group in particular.

The most frequent psychological responses encountered after burn trauma include loss, pain, and fear of physical discomfort, disfigurement, mutilation, or death. Disequilibrium caused by inability to manage the stressful event of the burn along with a distorted perception of the event may precipitate a psychological crisis. In addition, patients may dem-

onstrate concerns about abandonment, reliance on life-support equipment, surgical procedures, loss or change of role, and a lengthy convalescence. These concerns may be grounded in reality or unfounded. Resolution in either event may take several weeks to months or years depending on the severity of the burn, the course of recovery, and individual response to treatment (Caine and Bufalino, 1987, 1988, 1991).

Individual patients react differently to the actual and perceived disfigurement associated with burn injuries. The importance of providing support and assisting with adaptive coping cannot be minimized. Others who have had similar experiences can provide a valuable resource in the adjustment of both burn patients and families.

The problem of overwhelming helplessness for both the patient and family (Caine and Bufalino, 1988) and dependency in the early stages of postburn psychological processes (Flashman and Shapiro, 1983) needs to be taken seriously by the critical care nurse. The nurse must assess both the patient and family comprehensively to plan for psychological equilibrium. A framework for assessment of the patient and family is given in Figure 56–5 and suggestions for questions that may assist in the family assessment may be found in Table 56–14. Social support is important for the adjustment of burn-injured patients. The presence of caring and knowledgeable individuals rather than the performance of

TABLE 56–14. Burn Family Assessment Tool

1. Who are the significant family members?
2. Who does the family identify as the leader?
3. Who makes health care decisions for the family members?
4. What is the family's spiritual/religious and ethnic orientations? How important are these to the family?
5. What is the developmental level of the patient? The family?
6. What is the educational level of family members?
7. Where does the family live in relationship to the hospital? How far must they travel?
8. What time of the day does the family plan to visit?
9. What information does the family need or want to know?
10. Which significant family members need to be consulted in decision making?
11. Has the family experienced something like this before? How did they cope? What resources did they use?
12. What emotional support do the family members need?
13. What are the family members' expectations regarding the patients' outcome? What are their goals for the patient?

Adapted with permission from Caine, R. M. (1989). Families in crisis: Making the critical difference. *Focus on Critical Care*, 16 (3), 186.

selected activities is important (Cheng and Rogers, 1989).

Occupational and Physical Therapy. Considerable overlap may exist between occupational and physical therapy, depending on the institution. These two disciplines usually include assisting the patient with positioning, splinting, exercise, ambulation, and activities of daily living and begin within 24 hours of the patient's admission to the burn center. The goal of these therapies is to maintain and regain optimal functioning at the earliest possible time.

Because the rehabilitative process begins at admission, the therapists provide once or twice daily passive and active range of motion exercises. Although both active and passive range of motion exercises are difficult during the emergent phase, the patient's recovery is thought to progress faster and with less initial edema if exercises are instituted then.

Hand splints are custom made to fit each patient and are used in patients with circumferential burns of the wrist and burns of the dorsal surface of the fingers involving the joints. Initially, splints are worn 23 hours a day, but as the burns heal the patient is allowed to wear the splints at night only.

Pain often deters the inexperienced therapist from performing the needed range of motion exercises. Careful coordination with the nursing staff is necessary to ensure that the patient is adequately medicated, and each form of therapy is allotted a space of uninterrupted time during the day. This therapy may be difficult while the patient's condition is extremely critical, but even 5 minutes at a time is useful.

The occupational therapist is specially trained to assist with the management of scars as the wounds heal. Pressure garments can be fitted for any part of the body and are worn for 6 months to 1 year. They provide pressure on the burn scar, helping to keep it flat and thin. Without the pressure garment, burn scars become raised and thick. Each garment is custom measured and created to fit that one patient.

Speech Therapy. The speech therapist is another member of the burn team. Although most patients do not require this therapy, those who require long-term intubation and tracheostomy will. The speech therapist can assist in helping the patient develop communication techniques, either by means of an alphabet board or other techniques depending on the needs of the patients. When both hands are splinted, the patient may even have difficulty in pointing.

Nursing Diagnoses. A list of nursing diagnoses appropriate to the rehabilitation phase of burn injury is presented in Table 56–15.

RELEVANT RESEARCH

During the past two decades tremendous improvements in burn care and survival have occured, including improved quality of life. Ongoing research has been vital in these improvements. Research ranges from pain management and wound care to immunologic concerns. Three current research topics include tissue culturing, use of hyperbaric oxygenation for patients with carbon monoxide poisoning, and use of cyclosporine in patients with skin transplants.

Cultured epithelium (CE) is not a new idea; however, the ability to perform the procedure in a clini-

TABLE 56–15. Nursing Diagnoses: Rehabilitation Phase of Burn Injury

Activity intolerance
Potential for activity intolerance
Impaired adjustment
Anxiety
Constipation
Diarrhea
Bowel incontinence
Chronic pain
Diversional activity deficit
Fear
Knowledge deficit
Noncompliance
Powerlessness
Bathing hygiene: Self-care deficit
Dressing-grooming: Self-care deficit
Feeding: Self-care deficit
Toileting: Self-care deficit
Body image: Disturbance in self-concept
Personal identity: Disturbance in self-concept
Self-esteem: Disturbance in self-concept
Sensory perceptual alterations: Kinesthetic, tactile
Altered sexuality patterns
Impaired skin integrity, actual
Sleep pattern disturbance
Impaired social interaction
Social isolation
Potential for violence: Self-directed

cally practical way is new. CE is used in patients with extensive burns when available donor sites are minimal and would not provide the patient with adequate skin coverage. Generally, a skin biopsy of 1 cm² is taken from an available donor site and grown under careful laboratory methods in agar dishes into a thin sheet of epithelium of 1 m² in approximately 6 weeks time (Compton et al., 1989).

Although this method of "growing skin" is still very new, the possibilities seem enormous. Some successes have been reported with CE; however, the long-term implications of this skin are not known, such as its durability, or its ability to heal normal injuries.

Hyperbaric oxygenation continues to be a controversial treatment in the care of the burn patient. Administration of hyperbaric oxygen to patients with carbon monoxide (CO) poisoning to prevent acute and delayed neurologic symptoms is also an option, but its benefits have not been proved (Grube et al., 1988).

Cyclosporine has been used for a number of years in patients with transplants of a variety of organs with increasing success. Skin, the largest organ of the body, is commonly transplanted (allograft) from a cadaver to burn victims and is considered a temporary wound covering until donor sites from the patient himself are available to provide autografts. Ongoing studies with cyclosporine suggest that it may be possible to cover a burn wound permanently with allografted skin using this drug. In 1986, B. M. Achauer reported a child with extensive burns who was given cyclosporine to extend the survival of cadaver allografts from numerous unmatched donors until adequate autografts were available. No evidence of allograft rejection was seen during the time cyclosporine was used or subsequently after it was withdrawn.

Interest in the use of cyclosporine increased after this report, and research is continuing to investigate the possibility of using cyclosporine and allografts as a substitute for normal autografts to prevent the need for harvesting at donor sites, the blood loss that occurs during the procedure, and the presence of a donor site scar.

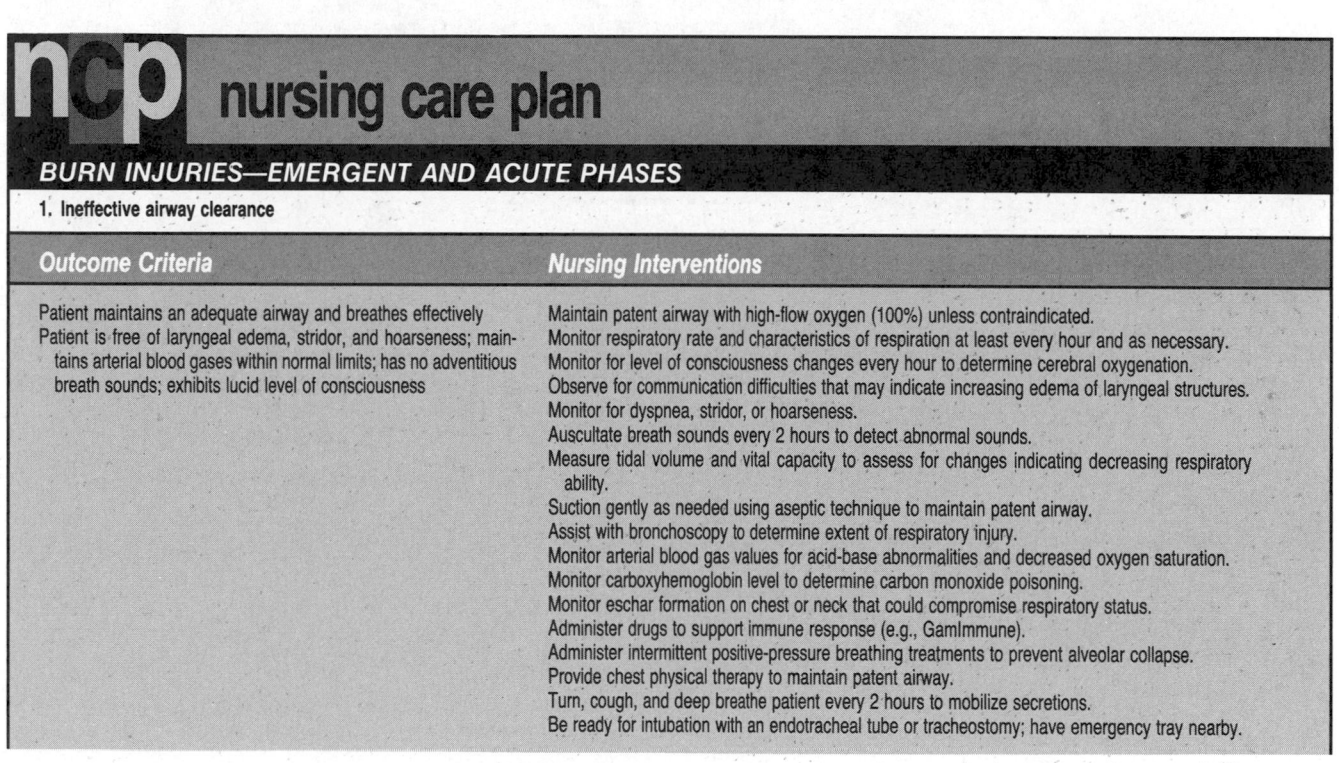

nursing care plan

BURN INJURIES—EMERGENT AND ACUTE PHASES

1. Ineffective airway clearance

Outcome Criteria	Nursing Interventions
Patient maintains an adequate airway and breathes effectively Patient is free of laryngeal edema, stridor, and hoarseness; maintains arterial blood gases within normal limits; has no adventitious breath sounds; exhibits lucid level of consciousness	Maintain patent airway with high-flow oxygen (100%) unless contraindicated. Monitor respiratory rate and characteristics of respiration at least every hour and as necessary. Monitor for level of consciousness changes every hour to determine cerebral oxygenation. Observe for communication difficulties that may indicate increasing edema of laryngeal structures. Monitor for dyspnea, stridor, or hoarseness. Auscultate breath sounds every 2 hours to detect abnormal sounds. Measure tidal volume and vital capacity to assess for changes indicating decreasing respiratory ability. Suction gently as needed using aseptic technique to maintain patent airway. Assist with bronchoscopy to determine extent of respiratory injury. Monitor arterial blood gas values for acid-base abnormalities and decreased oxygen saturation. Monitor carboxyhemoglobin level to determine carbon monoxide poisoning. Monitor eschar formation on chest or neck that could compromise respiratory status. Administer drugs to support immune response (e.g., GamImmune). Administer intermittent positive-pressure breathing treatments to prevent alveolar collapse. Provide chest physical therapy to maintain patent airway. Turn, cough, and deep breathe patient every 2 hours to mobilize secretions. Be ready for intubation with an endotracheal tube or tracheostomy; have emergency tray nearby.

Nursing Care Plan continued on following page

2. Fluid volume deficit: Actual

Outcome Criteria	Nursing Interventions
Patient maintains adequate blood volume; fluid and electrolyte balance; cardiac output; urinary output; and tissue perfusion Patient maintains CVP between 5 and 15 cm water; is hemodynamically stable; maintains electrolytes within normal limits; excretes at least 0.5 to 2.0 mL/kg per hour	Record weight of patient as soon as possible after admission. Monitor vital signs at least every hour and as needed; observe for trends. Record accurate fluid intake (e.g., oral, IV) and output (e.g., urine, nasogastric [NG] suction) every hour. Start IV with large-bore needle (No. 14 or No. 16). Insert Foley catheter utilizing aseptic technique. Titrate fluid replacement based on urine output, central venous pressure (CVP), level of consciousness, or other parameters used in your institution. Administer crystalloid and/or colloid fluid per hospital protocol. Observe hemodynamic parameters for changes in stability caused by fluid overload or hypovolemia. Assess for signs and symptoms of inadequate fluid replacement/impending shock (e.g., restlessness, disorientation, excessive thirst, increased pulse, decreased blood pressure, decreased urine output, CVP less than 5 cm water). Assess for signs and symptoms of excessive fluid replacement/pulmonary congestion/pulmonary edema (e.g., dyspnea, venous engorgement, moist rales, increased blood pressure, CVP greater than 15 cm water). Assess ECG for dysrhythmias that may result from electrical burn injury or hemodynamic instability. Monitor laboratory results and report those that directly reflect a fluid and electrolyte imbalance (most frequent laboratory requests include electrolytes, hemoglobin, hematocrit, glucose, serum proteins, serum potassium, serum sodium, blood urea nitrogen [BUN], creatinine, and urinalysis). Administer potassium-restricted foods/fluids if patient is hyperkalemic. Measure circumference of burned areas to determine if edema is increasing. Prepare for escharotomy and/or fasciotomy if circumferential edema or constriction of burn eschar compromises circulation. Elevate, if possible, all burned areas to allow for venous return. Monitor distal peripheral pulses utilizing a Doppler if necessary; notify physician immediately and prepare for fasciotomy if pulses are unobtainable. Observe urine for hematuria or brownish red color indicative of intravascular hemolysis related to thrombosis/hemomyoglobinuria.

3. Altered comfort: Pain

Outcome Criteria	Nursing Interventions
Patient maintains an adequate level of comfort Patient verbalizes decreasing levels of pain on a rating scale; participates in care as able	Determine level of discomfort, considering depth and extent of injury, areas of involvement, age, other pathology present, and previous treatment. Assess the level of discomfort using a 0–10 point self-rating scale to obtain an objective measure of the pain. Maintain an accurate record of amount, time, and type of medication utilized (too much medication, too soon, can cause respiratory difficulties); chart effect. Administer sedation/pain medication IV to increase adequate absorption; give 30 minutes–1 hour prior to treatments, débridement procedure, and application of topical agents to ensure patient comfort and adequate relaxation. Administer pain medication cautiously, judiciously, and conservatively, ensuring that patient is given adequate relief but is not overmedicated. Provide diversional activity to distract patient from the pain experience. Maintain environmental temperature at approximately 76°–82°F to ensure warmth and comfort of patient. Monitor patient temperature every hour.

4. Potential for infection

Outcome Criteria	Nursing Interventions
Patient is free of infection and maintains normothermia Patient has negative findings on wound and blood cultures; is free of wound drainage or odor; exhibits acceptance of grafts and absence of edema or decreased viability of recipient graft site; maintains normothermia	Determine the type of isolation techniques to be used; wear gowns, gloves, and masks to help keep the bacterial count to a minimum. Maintain an aseptic environment using sterile equipment and supplies. Observe for signs and symptoms of infection (e.g., malodorous wound drainage, elevated leukocyte count, elevated temperature). Use strict sterile technique when changing dressings. Administer antibiotics and observe response. Prepare for hydrotherapy treatments and eschar débridement (tangential excision, enzymatic débridement). Explain importance. Encourage participation. Apply topical antimicrobials and bacteriostatic agents. Prepare for grafting procedures, maintaining asepsis of donor and recipient sites. Obtain cultures from wounds, preventing contamination from skin flora. Prevent skin surfaces from touching to prevent autocontamination. Assess the necessity to continue isolation techniques; monitor laboratory data. Shave or clip body hair that may harbor bacteria. Provide special site care for face, eyes, ears, or perineum. Observe for signs and symptoms of septicemia (e.g., positive blood cultures, hemodynamic changes). Discourage visits from family or friends with infections. Administer tetanus immunization prophylactically. Use strict sterile technique when changing a dressing. Administer antibiotics and medications to support immune response, and observe patient response. Apply topical antimicrobials and bacteriostatic agents; evaluate and document effectiveness. Prepare for tangential excision, enzymatic débridement by explaining procedures, providing preoperative care. Prepare for grafting procedures, maintaining asepsis of donor and recipient sites; utilize wet soaks to injured tissue; observe viability of donor and recipient sites during dressing changes; identify patient concerns and questions regarding the procedure. Know about various skin grafts that may be used, including allograft, autograft, and xenograft.

5. Altered nutrition: Less than body requirements

Outcome Criteria	Nursing Interventions
Patient maintains adequate nutrition; demonstrates adequate gastric motility Patient is within 10% of preburn weight; is free from paralytic ileus; has no occult blood in gastric aspirate; has pink and moist oral mucous membranes	Insert NG tube; attach to low intermittent suction. Administer hyperalimentation. Administer tube feedings. Monitor pH of gastric aspirate for a decrease indicating hyperacidity. Administer antacids through the NG tube, clamping tube following administration. Administer high-calorie, high-protein tube feedings or oral diet when tolerated; establish small, frequent feedings interspersed with high-calorie, high-protein snacks; work with patient/family regarding food likes and dislikes; refer to dietician as necessary. Provide an environment conducive to eating (e.g., remove soiled dressings, bedpans, and other distractors; eliminate offensive odors). Assess ongoing nutritional status; observe oral mucous membranes; assess skin turgor. Provide oral hygiene every 4 hours. Provide adequate rest to ensure that patient is not too tired to eat. Weigh patient daily. Maintain accurate intake and output records. Auscultate bowel sounds every 4 hours. Monitor bowel evacuation for constipation or diarrhea.

Nursing Care Plan continued on following page

6. Body image disturbance

Outcome Criteria	Nursing Interventions
Patient and family verbalize feelings about changes in body image; will cope with the extent and number of losses Patient experiences minimum anxiety; states realistic appraisal of burn injury; expresses grief, fears, anxieties, and feelings about self or family; communicates needs as able; utilizes family for support; uses situational support for adaptation	Give as much information as patient/family want to help decrease fear and anxiety. Encourage to talk about current situation and feelings; provide empathic listening. Encourage participation and cooperation in care. Continue to help to express feelings about current status, fears; listen actively; incorporate other health care personnel as appropriate. Reinforce use of adaptive defenses while patient/family moves through grieving stages. Plan experiences for the patient to control, manipulate, and succeed in to decrease feelings of powerlessness (e.g., allow to make some decisions regarding own care, schedule). Refer patient for cosmetic counseling as appropriate, since an enhanced physical appearance may improve patient's body image. Assess importance and impact of appearance changes; discuss with patient/family. Provide careful explanation of procedures to dispel fears. Organize care to prevent undue pain and anxiety. Inform patient/family of any signs of progress. Project calm, unhurried attitude while performing procedures. Demonstrate respect for patient/family. Allow for privacy when visitors are with patient. Provide for financial and spiritual counseling as desired.

7. Impaired physical mobility

Outcome Criteria	Nursing Interventions
Patient is free from complications associated with immobility Patient participates in range of motion exercises of all joints at minimum of once daily; participates in activities of daily living to extent possible	Provide for proper positioning and immobilization of burn wound/graft site using splints, traction, etc.; consult with physical or occupational therapist to plan adaptive devices for patient use; encourage patient/family participation in planning. Provide active and passive range of motion (ROM) exercises at least daily; utilize hydrotherapy as necessary. Turn patient at least every 2 hours to prevent formation of pressure areas. Provide diversional therapy; encourage visits from family and friends; place a clock and calendar within patient's field of vision; reorient to surroundings as necessary.

Adapted with permission from Caine, R. M., and Bufalino, P. (1987). *Nursing care planning guides for adults*; and Caine, R. M., and Bufalino, P. (1988). *Critically ill adults: Nursing care planning guides*. © 1987, 1988, The Williams & Wilkins Co., Baltimore.

SUMMARY

The consequences of burn injury can be devastating for the patient and his family. Physiologic changes following burn injury are life-threatening if left untreated. The initial phase following burn injury is characterized by a massive fluid shift from the intracellular to the interstitial compartment. This emergent period has a short duration and is followed immediately by a period of fluid remobilization, during which fluid shifts back. It is during these first two phases that the most critical changes occur and the critical care nurse must be most alert. The rehabilitation phase is the final phase following burn injury and can last months to years. The psychologic changes that occur after burn injury cannot be minimized, and the astute critical care nurse balances the physiologic care of these traumatically injured patients with the intense psychological care that must also occur.

References

Achauer, B. M. (1987). Extremities. In B. M. Achauer (Ed.), *Management of the burned patient* (pp. 121–131). Norwalk, CT: Appleton & Lange.

Achauer, B. M., Black, K. S., Waxman, K. S., et al. (1986). Long-term skin allograft survival after short-term cyclosporin treatment in a patient with massive burns. *Lancet*, 1, 14–15.

Aharoni, A., Abramovici, D., Weinberger, M., et al. (1989). Burn resuscitation with a low-volume plasma analysis of mortality. *Burns*, 15(4), 230–232.

Busby, H. C. (1979). Acute burn patient and nursing management of optimal burn recovery. *The Journal of Continuing Education in Nursing*, 10 (4), 16–30.

Caine, R. M. (1989). Families in crisis: Making the critical difference. *Focus on Critical Care*, 16 (3), 184–189.

Caine, R. M., and Bufalino, P. (1987) (1991). *Nursing care planning guides for adults*. Baltimore: Williams & Wilkins.

Caine, R. M., and Bufalino, P. (1988). *Critically ill adults: Nursing care planning guides*. Baltimore: Williams & Wilkins.

Carter, E., Tompkins, R. G., and Burke, J. F. (1988). Hepatic and intestinal blood flow following thermal injury. *Journal of Burn Care and Rehabilitation*, 9 (4), 347–350.

Cheng, S., and Rogers, J. C. (1989). Changes in occupational role performance after a severe burn: A retrospective study. *American Journal of Occupational Therapy*, 43 (1), 17–24.

Choctaw, W. T., Eisner, M. E., and Wachtel, T. L. (1987). Causes, prevention, prehospital care, evaluation, emergency treatment, and prognosis. In B. M. Achauer (Ed.), *Management of the burned patient* (pp. 3–19). Norwalk, CT: Appleton & Lange.

Compton, C. C., Gill, J. M., Bradford, D. A., et al. (1989). Skin regenerated from cultured epithelial autografts on full thickness burn wounds from six days to five years after grafting. *Laboratory Investigation*, 60 (5), 600–612.

Deitch, E., Sittig, K., Heimbach, D., et al. (1989). Results of a multicenter outpatient burn study on the safety and efficacy of

DIMAC-SSD. A new delivery system for silver sulfadiazine. *Journal of Trauma*, 29 (4), 430–434.

Desai, M. H. (1984). Inhalation injuries in burn victims. *Critical Care Quarterly*, 7 (3), 1–6.

Dolecek, R. (1985). The endocrine response after burns: Its possible correlations with the immunology of burns. *Journal of Burn Care and Rehabilitation*, 6 (3), 281–294.

Dressler, D. P., Hozid, J. L., and Nathan, P. (1988). *Thermal injury*. St. Louis: C. V. Mosby.

Dyer, R., and Esch, V. (1976). Polyvinyl chloride toxicity in fires. *Journal of the American Medical Association*, 235 (4), 293–297.

Edelman, P. E. (1987). Chemical and electrical burns. In B. M. Achauer (Ed.), *Management of the burned patient* (pp. 183–202). Norwalk, CT: Appleton & Lange.

Flashman, A., and Shapiro, E. (1983). Emotional care of the burned patient. In J. E. Nicosia, and J. A. Petro (Eds.), *Manual of burn care*. New York: Raven Press.

Frank, H. A., Berry, C., Wachtel, T. I., et al. (1987). The impact of thermal injury. *Journal of Burn Care and Rehabilitation*, 8 (4), 260–262.

Fuller, F. W., and Engler, P. E. (1988). Leukopenia in nonseptic burn patients received topical 1% silver sulfadiazine cream therapy: A survey. *The Journal of Burn Care and Rehabilitation*, 9 (6), 606–609.

Giel, L. C. (1987). Nutrition. In B. M. Achauer (Ed.), *Management of the burned patient* (pp. 135–148). Norwalk, CT: Appleton & Lange.

Graves, T. A., Cioffi, W. G., McManus, W. F., et al. (1988). Fluid resuscitation of infants and children with massive thermal injury. *Journal of Trauma*, 28 (12), 1656–1659.

Grube, B. J., Marvin, J., and Heimbach, D. M. (1988). Therapeutic hyperbaric oxygenation: Help or hindrance in burn patients with carbon monoxide poisoning. *Journal of Burn Care and Rehabilitation*, 9 (3), 249–252.

Hayter, J. (1978). Emergency nursing care of the burn patient. *Nursing Clinics of North America*, 13 (2), 223–234.

Hersperger, J. E., and Dahl, L. M. (1978). Electrical and chemical injuries. *Critical Care Quarterly*, 1 (3), 43–49.

Hill, M. B., Achauer, B. M., and Martinez, S. (1984). Tar and asphalt burns. *Journal of Burn Care and Rehabilitation*, 5 (4), 271–274.

Jacobson, B. K., Cuono, C. B., Kupper, T. S., et al. (1988). Immunologic alterations following excisional wounding and immediate repair with syngeneic or allogeneic skin grafts. *Journal of Burn Care and Rehabilitation*, 9 (4), 354–358.

Jacoby, F. G. (1974). *Nursing care of the patient with burns* (2nd ed.). St. Louis: C. V. Mosby.

Klasen, H. J., van der Tempel, G. L., and Sauer, E. W. (1989). Attempted suicide by means of burns. *Burns*, 15 (2), 88–92.

Kravitz, M. (1988). Thermal injuries. In V. D. Cardona, P. Hurn, P. J. B. Mason, et al. (Eds.), *Trauma nursing: From resuscitation through rehabilitation*. Philadelphia: W. B. Saunders.

Martin, L. M. (1989). Nursing implications of todays burn care techniques. *RN*, 52 (5), 26–33.

McAlhany, J. C., Czaja, A. J., and Rosenthal, A. (1979). Acute gastroduodenal disease after burns. In C. P. Artz, J. A. Moncrief, and B. A. Pruitt (Eds.), *Burns: A team approach* (pp. 512–522). Philadelphia: W. B. Saunders.

Minar, V. (1978). Fluid resuscitation of the burn patient. *Journal of Emergency Nursing*, 4, 39–43.

Nicosia, J. E., and Petro, J. A. (1983). *Manual of burn care*. New York: Raven Press.

Ohura, T. (1988). The Everett Idris Evans Memorial Lecture, 1987: Twenty-five years experience treating burns. *Journal of Burn Care and Rehabilitation*, 9 (1), 106–117.

Robertson, K. E., Cross, P. J., and Terry, J. C. (1985). CE burn care: The crucial first days. *American Journal of Nursing*, 1, 30–45.

Simpson, J. B., and Cruse, C. W. (1981). Gasoline immersion injury. *Journal of Plastic and Reconstructive Surgery*, 67 (1), 54–57.

Somogyi, E., and Tedeschi, C. G. (1977). Injury by electrical force. In C. G. Tedeschi, W. G. Eckert, and L. G. Tedeschi (Eds.), *Forensic medicine*. Philadelphia: W. B. Saunders.

Teodorczyk-Injeyan, J. A., Sparkes, B. G., and Peters, W. J. (1989). Regulation of IgM production in thermally injured patients. *Burns*, 15 (4), 241–247.

Uehara, D. T., Baumgartner, E. A., and Eisner, R. F. (1986). Burns. In S. H. Cahill, and M. Balskus (Eds.), *Interventions in emergency nursing: The first 60 minutes* (pp. 225–240). Rockville, MD: Aspen Publications.

University of California, Irvine Medical Center (1989). *Standing admission orders: Burn Unit*.

Wardenn, G. (1987). Immunology. In B. M. Achauer (Ed.), *Management of the burned patient* (pp. 49–63). Norwalk, CT: Appleton & Lange.

Waxman, K., Lefcourt, N., and Achauer, B. (1989). Heated laser Doppler flow measurements to determine depth of burn injury. *American Journal of Surgery*, 157 (6), 541–543.

Wiener, S. L., and Barrett, J. (1986). *Trauma management*. Philadelphia: W. B. Saunders.

Williams, R., and Porvaznik, J. (1989). Initial resuscitation of major burn patients. *Journal of Family Practice*, 28 (4), 449–456.

Zawacki, B. (1974). Reversal of capillary stasis and prevention of necrosis in burns. *Annals of Surgery*, 180 (1), 98–102.

S · E · C · T · I · O · N

13

Multisystem Disorders

57

Patients with Trauma

*Gary Sparger**
Sheila Sanning Shea
Judy Selfridge

WHAT MAKES THE TRAUMA PATIENT UNIQUE

The trauma patient creates unique challenges for the health care team and critical care nurse. The incidence of trauma is unpredictable. Little if any information is available about the actual mechanism of injury or about the patient's previous health status, current medications, allergies, and usual vital signs. The injured individual may arrive at the hospital unexpectedly or with only a few minutes' advance warning. Care of the trauma patient requires immediate availability of specialized personnel, equipment, and supplies, a staffed surgical suite, and critical care space. Depending on the transport time from the scene of the incident to the hospital and the qualifications of prehospital personnel, the patient may or may not have undergone initial stabilization.

To accomplish the essential life-saving interventions and diagnostic procedures in a timely manner, a trauma team—surgeon, emergency physician, anesthesiologist, registered nurses, and ancillary staff—must function together in carrying out an organized approach to the trauma patient. This implies that a large number of health professionals will perform preestablished roles to provide care for an undiagnosed individual, frequently an individual experiencing life-threatening injury to one or more body systems.

*Deceased 1991.

Scope of Trauma

The incidence of trauma in the United States is a major health care and economic issue. Trauma continues to be the fourth leading cause of death for all ages. Statistics indicate that over 140,000 deaths resulted from trauma in 1983 and that one person in three suffered a nonfatal injury (Committee on Trauma Research, 1985). Only heart disease, cancer, and strokes result in a higher death rate. Trauma is the leading cause of death in persons between the ages of 1 and 44 years, the peak incidence occurring in the 15- to 24-year-old age group, thereby affecting otherwise healthy and productive members of society. Trauma is the greatest killer of children. It is the most common cause of hospitalization among individuals less than 45 years of age and is the leading cause of physician contacts in the United States (Committee on Trauma Research, 1985).

Epidemiology of Trauma

Over half of all traumatic incidents involve the use of alcohol, drugs, or other substance abuse. Frequently the substance abuser kills someone else besides himself. Injury results in both short-term and long-term disability. More than 75,000 Americans sustain head injuries that result in long-term disability each year. In 1981, 144 million days were spent in bed because of traumatic injury (Committee on Trauma Research, 1985). It has been estimated that over 4 million years of future worklife are lost to injury annually in the United States alone (Committee on Trauma Research, 1985).

Economic factors are important from the standpoint of the direct and indirect costs associated with trauma. It is estimated that trauma costs society $83.5 billion annually or $228 million each day. Other nations have assessed the impact of trauma on their gross national product and have found it economically feasible to finance national trauma systems. Because trauma is predominantly a disease of the young and carries the potential for permanent disability, it is evident that trauma is responsible for the loss of significant productive work years. Unlike cardiovascular disease, cancer, and cerebrovascular accidents, trauma is thought to be preventable. Advocates of trauma systems identify prevention as an essential component of an organized approach to trauma. Monies used to educate society about the preventive aspects of injury and to initiate activities designed to remove injury risk factors from the environment are estimated to be lower than the monies actually spent on the direct and indirect costs associated with trauma.

SYSTEMS APPROACH TO TRAUMA CARE

Historical Perspective

A systems approach to trauma care is not necessarily a new or unique idea. In many settings, often large, county-based teaching facilities, a trauma team concept has existed for a number of years. The concept of regionalization has similarly been applied already to transplantation, cardiac surgery, burn care, neonatal centers, and other patient populations requiring specialized and organized care.

It is possible that in the future hospitals and medical centers will become increasingly specialized, to such an extent that acute care and critical care services will be available in only a few selected facilities. Such hospitals will likely consist of only emergency receiving and resuscitation areas, surgical suites, and critical care beds, with all the sophisticated support services and personnel these services require. The majority of hospitals may not receive emergency and critically ill patients and therefore would not be expected to maintain highly sophisticated and costly equipment and personnel. This type of specialization might therefore result in a significant reduction in health care costs outside of the critical care phase.

Accidental Death and Disability: The Neglected Disease of Modern Society, a landmark National Research Council report in 1966, presented data demonstrating that injury was a national public health problem. This document identified the need for an organized approach to trauma care, the development of trauma systems, implementation of community education and prevention activities, and further research in the

area of trauma and prevention of injury. A more recent document, *Injury in America* (Committee on Trauma Research, 1985), indicated that slow progress has been made in the prevention of injury and the development of trauma systems. Specific recommendations from this report included the following:

1. Establishment of a center for injury control within the federal government.

2. Provision of funding for research on injury commensurate with the importance of injury as the largest cause of death and disability of children and young adults in the United States.

3. Establishment of effective injury surveillance systems that have the capacity to identify and control outbreaks of specific injuries.

4. Education and persuasion of persons at risk of injury to alter their behavior to provide increased self-protection.

5. Enactment of laws or administrative rules requiring individuals to change their behavior.

6. Provision of automatic protection by requiring changes in product and environmental design.

7. Coordination of a multidisciplinary approach to injury biomechanics research to provide a clearer understanding of the mechanisms of injury.

8. Development of specialized centers to provide immediate care and rehabilitation of injured individuals.

9. Establishment of programs designed to train professionals in the research and care of injuries.

10. Establishment and provision of support for research programs in the areas of mechanics of injury, prevention of injury, immediate care and rehabilitation of injured individuals, and model systems designed to provide optimal trauma care (Committee on Trauma Research, 1985).

Role of Professional Organizations or Agencies

Professional organizations have been involved in the development and implementation of trauma systems and trauma care standards that are specific to this particular field of practice. The American College of Surgeons (ACS) in 1976 organized a Task Force on Trauma, later to become the Committee on Trauma (ACSCOT), to address trauma care from a surgical perspective. In 1976, ACSCOT published *Guidelines for the Care of Trauma Patients*, delineating the specific staff, equipment, supplies, education, and resources that are essential for trauma care. This document was the first effort by a professional organization to establish standards and list the actual requirements needed for the delivery of trauma care within a trauma system. ACSCOT continues to be a leader in establishing trauma standards for prehospital care and triage, resuscitation and stabilization, rehabilitation, systems monitoring and evaluation, and specialized care such as that required for injured children, burned patients, and patients with spinal cord injury. The ACS additionally provides resources for developing trauma systems and centers through actual consultation and on-site surveys.

The Advanced Trauma Life Support (ATLS) Course, developed by the American College of Surgeons, provides a standardized plan of care for the surgical management of the trauma patient. This course represents the first national educational program that presents a systematic approach to the care of the injured individual. ACS has also developed a trauma course for prehospital personnel that provides advanced training in the care of victims of major trauma.

The American College of Emergency Physicians (ACEP) has also recognized the need to become involved in trauma systems development and maintenance, standards of care, and patient care. ACEP has taken a highly organized approach to the legislative issues of trauma care, including legislation to provide funding at various levels for care of the injured individual and the development of trauma care systems. ACEP developed and implemented a trauma course for prehospital personnel. Through this course ACEP has played an instrumental role in establishing national standards for the field care and appropriate triage and transport of the trauma patient.

The Emergency Nurses Association (ENA) has long realized the need to establish standards related specifically to the nursing aspects of the initial resuscitation of the trauma patient. In 1981, ENA began to develop a national trauma course for emergency nurses. After several attempts, the Trauma Nursing Core Course was published and implemented in 1987. Through this course a national standard of practice has been established for emergency nurses and other registered nurses involved in the early phases of trauma care. A national Standing Committee: Trauma was formally initiated in 1989 with the goals of monitoring the trauma problem as related to emergency nursing, identifying areas of possible involvement by ENA, and recommending activities to the ENA Board of Directors. The committee also plans to suggest activities related to community education and prevention projects.

Professional organizations play an important role in the political and legislative arena. Professional experts are frequently responsible for educating local and national politicians, increasing their awareness of trauma issues, and initiating desired legislation. Financial support from either a county, state, or federal agency is frequently the goal of these political efforts. Various governmental agencies are currently involved in assessing trauma care needs and developing plans for dealing with trauma. The development, implementation, and financial support for a national trauma system may provide an opportunity to decrease the mortality and morbidity resulting from injury.

Other professional organizations, such as the American Association of Critical-Care Nurses (AACN), provide education for their members specific to the needs of the trauma patient through annual meetings and the National Teaching Institute. As the knowledge base about trauma care continues to expand, other nursing groups will probably become involved, such as those interested in rehabilitation and orthopaedics.

The Joint Commission for Accreditation of Health Organizations (JCAHO) is an example of another type of agency that is involved in developing trauma systems and trauma care. JCAHO implemented minimal trauma care standards as a component of its accreditation process in 1991. Currently, a committee composed of physicians, registered nurses, and hospital administrators is developing standards to be used by JCAHO. Although JCAHO accreditation is a voluntary process, it is often a requirement for facilities seeking governmental funding for certain aspects of health care. It is the intention of JCAHO to survey all hospitals in relation to specific trauma care capabilities. Should a hospital elect not to comply with the established minimum standards the expectation is that trauma patients will be transferred to a facility with an institutional commitment to meeting their special needs.

Trauma System Components

Table 57–1 lists the essential components of a trauma system, which includes all aspects of care from point of injury through rehabilitation and return to society. During the 1970s and early 1980s most trauma systems centered around a facility that had developed its trauma care capabilities because of the large volume of major trauma cases received at the hospital. Frequently a surgeon with special interest and skill in trauma care was identified as the expert and was responsible for the level of trauma care provided. Trauma systems in this setting often involved only expertise in the care of patients routinely received in such a facility. A "system" did not actually exist except from an internal operations point of view.

The concept of a trauma system does not necessarily imply that a designated trauma center is a "better" hospital. The designation of a hospital as a trauma center does imply that an institutional com-

TABLE 57–1. Components of a Trauma System

Triage and in-field treatment
Communications network
Air and ground transportation
Trauma team concept (in-hospital patient management)
Rehabilitation facilities organized for trauma care
Education of health care personnel and community about trauma care and prevention
Systems evaluation and monitoring
Political and community support of systems approach to trauma care
Financial support of trauma care for medically indigent patients

mitment to trauma care exists. Commitment at an institutional level consists of a demonstrated interest in trauma care and the availability of essential staff and resources, including fiscal resources. It should be remembered that the designated trauma center is only one component of a trauma system.

Trauma Team Concept

The concept of a trauma team is especially important to health care personnel. The term trauma team refers to health care professionals who respond immediately to participate in the initial resuscitation and stabilization of the trauma victim. Table 57–2 lists the composition of a typical trauma team. Figure 57–1 indicates one view of placement of the team within the resuscitation area. Essential to the team approach is the fact that each team member is preassigned and understands the specific responsibilities inherent in a particular team role. The trauma surgeon is ultimately responsible for the activities of the trauma team and acts as "team leader" in establishing resuscitation, stabilization, and intervention priorities. Other physician members may have specific

---

TABLE 57–2. Multidisciplinary Trauma Team

Typical Composition
Trauma surgeon (team leader)
Emergency physician
Anesthesiologist
Trauma nurse team leader (TNTL)—emergency nurse
Trauma resuscitation nurse (TRN)—critical care nurse
Trauma scribe—emergency nurse
Trauma surgical nurse
Laboratory phlebotomist
Radiologic technologist
Respiratory technologist
Social worker/pastoral services
Hospital security officer
Physician specialists as necessary
   (neurosurgeon, orthopaedic surgeon, urologic surgeon)

Inner-Core–Outer-Core Approach
Inner-Core Team
Trauma surgeon (team leader)
Emergency physician
Anesthesiologist
Trauma nurse team leader (TNTL)—emergency nurse
Trauma resuscitation nurse (TRN)—critical care nurse
Trauma scribe—emergency nurse

Outer-Core Team
Nursing supervisor (team leader)
Laboratory phlebotomist
Radiologic technologist
Respiratory technologist
Social worker/pastoral services
Hospital security officer
Registration/emergency clerk
Physician specialist as necessary
   (neurosurgeon, orthopaedic surgeon, urologic surgeon)

(This concept alleviates congestion during initial
   resuscitation efforts.)

---

responsibilities or may receive direction from the trauma surgeon.

Nursing members of the trauma team may all come from the emergency department, as often occurs in large teaching facilities that have adequate numbers of emergency nurses in the department 24 hours each day. In many trauma centers nurses are asked to respond from other areas of the hospital such as the surgical unit or the trauma intensive care unit. Inclusion of a critical care nurse as a member of the initial response team increases continuity of care for the trauma patient and often enhances certain trauma team capabilities such as hemodynamic monitoring. A surgical nurse may also be included in the trauma team. This individual's responsibility includes assessment of the patient's potential surgical needs and assistance if an emergency thoracotomy or other surgical procedure is required in the resuscitation area.

Levels of Trauma Care

Levels of trauma care in various hospitals have been difficult to ascertain. The American College of Surgeons Committee on Trauma devised a system that could be used to identify a trauma center's expected level of care (American College of Surgeons, 1987). Table 57–3 lists the various levels of care available according to trauma center status. In most trauma systems, level I and level II trauma centers are capable of providing the same level of care. The most frequent difference between the two is that a level I center is a teaching facility that maintains surgical resident training and is involved in trauma-related research. A level II center receives surgical leadership and care through an in-house surgeon with no involvement of surgical residents. Some areas of the country allow level II centers to be staffed by surgeons that are immediately available from outside the hospital, although this system is not widely accepted.

Level III centers serve communities that lack the resources necessary to provide level I or level II trauma care. A sparsely populated community may not receive an adequate volume of major trauma victims or may not have adequate physician staffing to achieve level II status. This type of trauma center does not have in-house surgical capability and often lacks neurosurgical coverage. Therefore, level III centers should develop transfer agreements with hospitals providing a higher level of care.

The concept of a systems approach to trauma care, or regionalization, limits the number of identified trauma centers, depending instead on the incidence of major trauma within a region. Many regions find that more hospitals are interested in seeking trauma center status than are actually needed to provide optimal trauma care. As in other highly specialized care situations, a certain patient volume is necessary to enable a facility to provide optimal trauma care.

EMERGENCY ROOM CHARGE NURSE
1. Initiates Trauma Team activation.
2. Coordinates activities.
3. Maintains communications with Trauma Control Nurse.

TRAUMA CONTROL NURSE
1. Readies room.
2. Communicates with MICN re: field treatment.
3. Relates information to Trauma Surgeon.
4. Communicates with ED Charge Nurse.
5. Orders all tests.
6. Documents all patient information—"Scribe."

ED TRAUMA NURSE
1. Assists Trauma Control Nurse with set-up.
2. Obtains MICU report.
3. Initiates patient assessment report and reports to Trauma Control Nurse for documentation.
4. Monitors ECGs and vital signs.
5. Assists with equipment and procedures from right side of table.
6. Administers medications.
7. Inserts nasogastric tube.
8. Accompanies patient with transfer process.

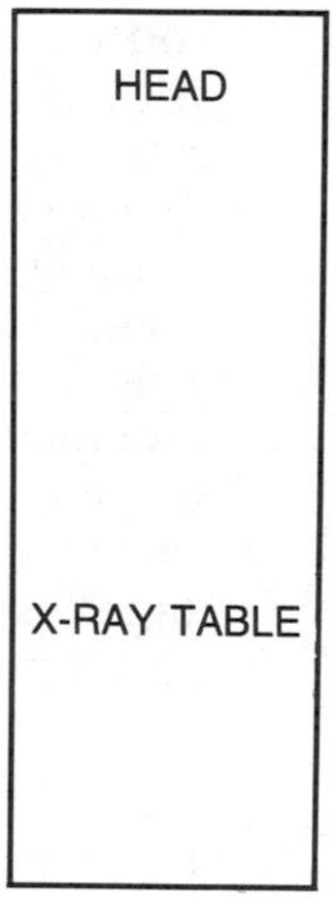

```
┌─────────────┐
│             │
│    HEAD     │
│             │
│             │
│             │
│             │
│ X-RAY TABLE │
│             │
└─────────────┘
```

ICU TRAUMA NURSE
1. Assists ED Nurse.
2. Vital signs.
3. IV management.
4. Performs CPR.
5. Assists with drugs.
6. CVP readings.
7. Inserts Foley and records output.
8. Assists with transfer.
9. Assists with airway maintenance.

OR TRAUMA NURSE
1. Assists with minor procedures.
2. Becomes scrub nurse for operating procedures.

TRAUMA NURSE COORDINATOR
1. Evaluates.
2. Back-up support person.

FIGURE 57–1. Trauma team placement resuscitation area.

TABLE 57–3. Characteristics of Various Trauma Center Levels

Level I Trauma Center

Regional resource trauma center
Provides the most sophisticated care as an acute and tertiary center
Provides educational programs for physicians, nurses, paramedics, and other trauma personnel
Conducts major outreach programs, including prevention and public education
Conducts clinical or basic science research related to trauma care

Level II Trauma Center

Community trauma center (the most prevalent)

Level III Trauma Center

Rural trauma hospital
Maximum commitment to trauma care commensurate with its local resources
Plans for care of the injured include transfer agreements and protocols

---

Data from the American College of Surgeons, Committee on Trauma (1990). *Resources for optimal care of the injured patient.* Chicago: American College of Surgeons.

The American College of Surgeons recommends that a level I trauma center treat 600 to 1000 patients and a level II center 350 to 600 patients each year.

Experience indicates that approximately 1 severe injury occurs annually for each 1000 population. Additionally, overtriage of patients into a trauma system of as much as 30% to 70% may occur to prevent missing those individuals with potentially life-threatening injuries. Therefore, a community with a population of 1,000,000 can expect to treat 1000 major trauma patients each year, with an additional volume of 300 to 700 patients resulting from overtriage. Such a community might require one level I and one or two level II specialized centers to achieve optimal trauma care.

Recognition of Trauma Capabilities

An institution may be recognized as a trauma center through various processes. Currently, such recognition is decided at a county, regional, or state level, although the potential does exist for a national trauma system. Additionally, an institution can designate itself as possessing special capabilities in trauma care. Self-designation is likely to occur only in areas where no trauma plan has been developed; it does not necessarily imply that a trauma system exists, only that an institution provides an organized approach to the care of trauma patients. Recognition

of trauma centers may occur through a designation or verification process. Designation means that an authorized agency has assessed an institution's trauma care capabilities and has identified or appointed it as a trauma center. A verification process includes a similar assessment process by an authorized agency but merely confirms an institution's compliance with specified criteria and trauma care standards. The surveying agency does not officially appoint or identify such a facility as a trauma center.

Maryland was the first state to approach trauma care from a statewide perspective. In this system, designated trauma centers are strategically located throughout the state. Mandatory triage criteria identify which patients should be transported to a trauma center. Other states have taken a similar approach—Oregon, Nevada, Tennessee, Washington, D.C., and West Virginia. Although the systems are similar, components such as mandatory triage criteria and systems monitoring may differ.

In other parts of the country state trauma plans have been devised but the development of trauma systems within a particular county or region of the state has not been mandated. For example, California has legislated a state trauma plan that identifies minimum requirements for trauma centers. A county or regional agency is obligated to comply with the state plan only if trauma system development and trauma center designation occurs within that area.

Some states have elected not to address the trauma issue, and therefore local systems may be developed. This situation allows a local agency, often the county Emergency Medical Services (EMS), to develop, implement, and monitor a trauma system. This occurred in several Southern California counties (Orange, San Diego, and Los Angeles) prior to the development of a state trauma plan.

Trauma Triage

Triage of an injured individual to the appropriate care facility is another essential component of a trauma system. Triage in a trauma system means sorting the patients to determine which individuals need specialized care for either actual or potential injuries. Determination of which patients require transport to a trauma center rather than a basic emergency care facility occurs according to established protocols, policies, and procedures. Triage decisions are often made by prehospital personnel based on knowledge of the mechanisms of injury and rapid assessment of the patient's clinical status. Medical direction of this process occurs through radio contact with a base station hospital and medical review of triage decisions.

Trauma, injury resulting from an external force, may be accidental, self-inflicted, or the result of an act of violent aggression. Trauma may be classified

TABLE 57–4. Trauma Score

	Rate	Codes	Score
A. Respiratory rate	10–24	4	
Number of respirations	25–35	3	
in 15 seconds;	>35	2	
multiply	<10	1	
by 4	0	0	A. _____
B. Respiratory effort			
Retractive: Use of	Normal	1	
accessory muscles or	Retractive	0	B. _____
intercostal retraction			
C. Systolic blood pressure	≥90	4	
Systolic cuff pressure:	70–89	3	
either arm, auscultate	50–69	2	
or palpate	<50	1	
No carotid pulse	0	0	C. _____
D. Capillary refill			
Normal: Forehead or	Normal	2	
lip mucosa color refill			
in 2 seconds			
Delayed: More than 2	Delayed	1	
seconds capillary refill			
None: No capillary	None	0	D. _____
refill			

E. Glasgow Coma Scale

		Total GCS Points	Score
1. Eye opening			
Spontaneous	___ 4	14–15	5
To voice	___ 3	11–13	4
To pain	___ 2	8–10	3
None	___ 1	5–7	2
		3–4	1 E. _____

2. Verbal
   response
   Oriented ___ 5
   Confused ___ 4
   Inappropriate
   words ___ 3
   Incomprehensible
   sounds ___ 2
   None ___ 1

3. Motor response
   Obeys
   commands ___ 6
   Purposeful
   movements
   (pain) ___ 5
   Withdraw (pain) ___ 4
   Flexion (pain) ___ 3
   Extension (pain) ___ 2
   None ___ 1

Total GCS points (1+2+3)___   Trauma Score _____

(Total points A + B + C + D + E)

Trauma score ≤ 12 = major trauma

as major or minor depending upon the severity of injury. Minor trauma refers to single system injuries that do not pose a threat to life or limb and can be appropriately treated in a basic emergency facility. Major trauma refers to serious multiple system injuries that require immediate intervention to prevent disability, loss of limb, or death. Major trauma pa-

tients and individuals with the potential for major injury are those requiring triage to a trauma center.

Various methods are used to determine which individuals might be classified as major trauma patients and which may benefit from an organized approach to trauma care. Triage decisions may be based upon abnormal findings in the patient's physiologic functions, the severity of the mechanism of injury, the anatomic area of injury, or evidence of risk factors such as age and preexisting disease.

Figure 57–2 adapted from the American College of Surgeons (1987), presents a triage decision scheme. Various trauma scoring tools may also be used to determine triage to the trauma center. The Trauma Score (Table 57–4) is widely used to determine the severity of injury. A Trauma Score of 12 or less is usually considered justification for transporting a patient to a trauma center. Another scoring tool, the CRAMS (Circulation, Respirations, Abdomen, Motor Speech) scale (Table 57–5), is less commonly used. A score of 8 or less on the CRAMS scale justifies transporting the trauma victim to a trauma center. The Glasgow Coma Scale is an appropriate method for assessing and reporting the patient's neurologic status.

The development of and adherence to established triage criteria are essential for maintaining an effective system of optimal care of the trauma patient. Some of the identified triage criteria, such as a systolic blood pressure of less than 90 mm Hg in an adult trauma patient, are considered absolute and should always result in transport to a trauma care facility. Other criteria, such as passenger space intrusion and a 30-inch deformity of an automobile, may be guidelines for considering triage to a trauma center. Because prehospital personnel can actually visualize the situation surrounding a specific trauma

TABLE 57–5. Crams Scale

Circulation	
Normal capillary refill and BP > 100	2
Delayed capillary refill or 85 < BP < 100	1
No capillary refill or BP < 85	0
Respirations	
Normal	2
Abnormal (labored or shallow)	1
Absent	0
Abdomen	
Abdomen and thorax nontender	2
Abdomen or thorax tender	1
Abdomen rigid, flail chest, or penetrating wounds	0
Motor	
Normal	2
Responds only to pain other than decerebrate	1
No response or decerebrate	0
Speech	
Normal	2
Confused	1
No intelligible words	0

Score ≤ 8 = Major trauma; score ≥ 8 = minor trauma.

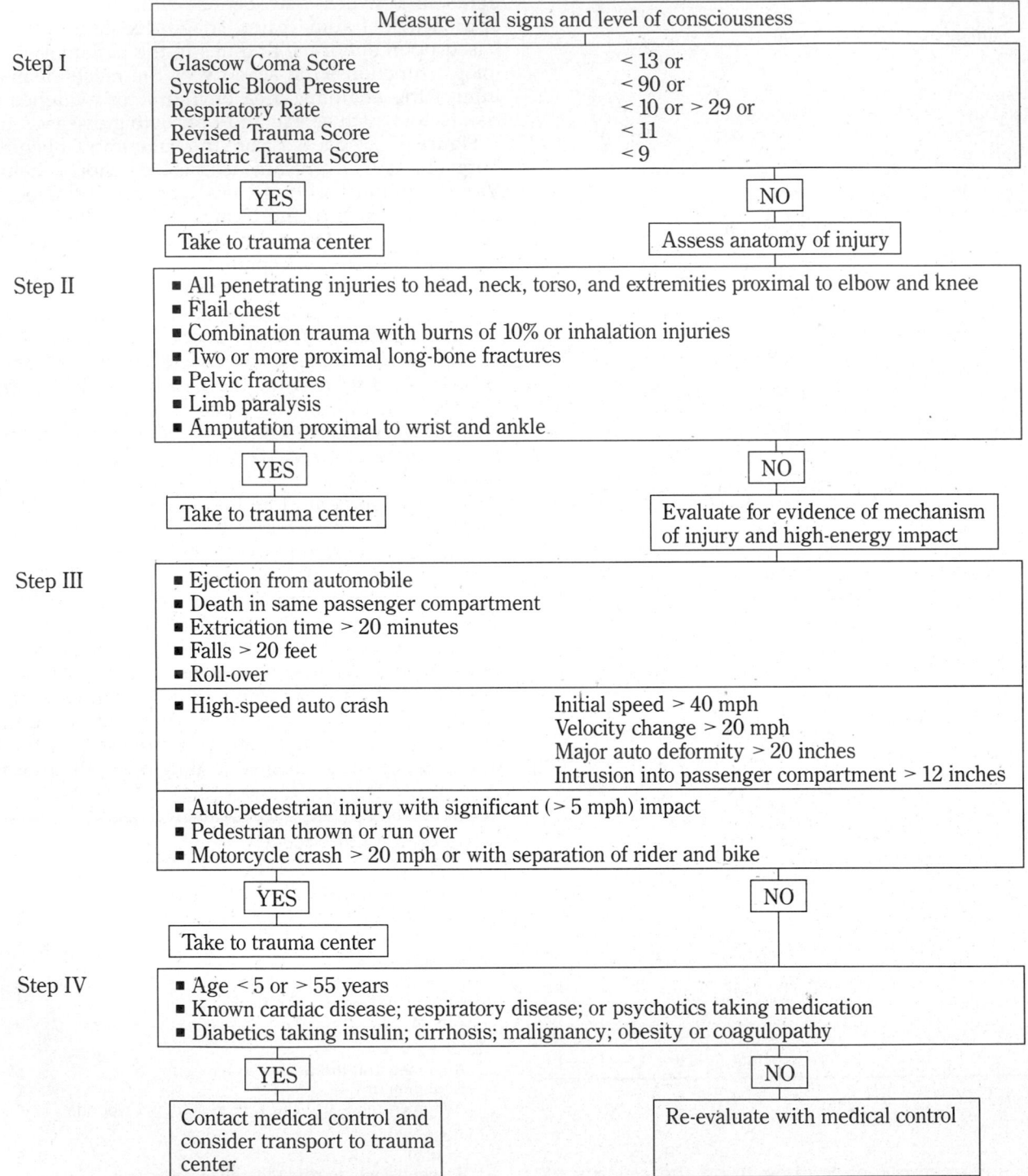

FIGURE 57–2. Triage decision scheme. *Notes to figure appear on page 1244.* (From the American College of Surgeons, Committee on Trauma (1990). *Resources for optimal care of the injured patient.* Chicago: American College of Surgeons.)

incident and the patient's clinical condition, they often elect to transport the patient to a trauma center even though none of the accepted triage criteria are evident.

MECHANISM OF INJURY

Injury to the body occurs when an uncontrolled source of energy comes into contact with the body. Energy may be kinetic (mechanical), thermal, chemical, electrical, or radiating. The absence of oxygen may result in injury, as in drowning or suffocation. The severity of injury is related to the amount of energy released (the force of impact), duration of impact, body part involved, injuring agent, and the presence of associated risk factors such as alcohol or substance abuse, gender, and age of patient. Injury and death result from both unintentional events such as vehicle collisions and sports activities and from deliberate events such as violent aggression and suicide. Because only uncontrolled energy causes injury, it may be assumed that injuries are preventable if the energy source is controlled.

As identified in Table 57–6, adapted from *Injury in America* (1985), kinetic energy accounts for the majority of injury-related deaths and nonfatal injuries. Kinetic energy is defined as mass times velocity squared, divided by 2. Therefore, the greater the mass and velocity (speed), the greater the kinetic energy that must be dissipated to the body structures.

Trauma may be either blunt or penetrating. The incidence of blunt trauma is usually greater in rural and suburban areas, whereas penetrating trauma occurs more frequently in inner-city urban areas.

Blunt Trauma

Blunt trauma most frequently results from motor vehicle crashes but may also result from assaults with blunt objects, falls from heights, and sports-related activities. As previously stated, the severity of injury depends on the amount of kinetic energy dissipated to the body and its underlying structures.

Vehicular trauma, as well as some other forms of blunt trauma, results from an acceleration-deceleration type of event. The vehicle in which the body is carried, and therefore the body itself, travels or is accelerated at a certain speed. In normal circumstances, stopping occurs in a timely manner, and the body slows to a stopped state. When the vehicle stops abruptly, however, as in collision with a stationary object, the body continues to travel forward until it comes into contact with a stationary object, frequently the dashboard, windshield, or steering column. Further injury occurs in the presence of rapid deceleration, when the body contents continue to travel within an enclosed space or compartment such as the cranium. At the point of impact between the vehicle and a stationary object, the body continues to move until it strikes a stationary object. Once the body strikes a stationary object it also stops abruptly. At this point the brain may strike the cranium and be thrown back against the opposite side of the cranial vault. This results in a coup-contrecoup type of injury. Rapid deceleration causes tearing and disruption of vessels and tissues.

The severity of injury resulting from a blunt force is also contingent upon the duration of impact and the body part involved. The longer the force of impact is in contact with the body, the more kinetic energy dissipates to the body and underlying structures. Various body tissues and structures respond to kinetic energy in different ways. Low-density, porous tissues and structures such as the lungs tolerate energy transference and often experience little damage. Conversely, high-density solid organs such as the heart, spleen, and liver tolerate energy transference poorly. Additionally, some body structures are encapsulated, and force or pressure applied to these organs actually causes rupture or fragmentation.

TABLE 57–6. Major Categories of Injury Deaths in 1982 in the United States

Injury Category	Unintentional	Suicide	Homicide	Undetermined	Total
Motor vehicles (traffic)	44,713	57	*	16	44,786
Firearms	1,756	16,575	14,117†	540	32,988
Falls and jumps	12,077	797	12	127	13,013
Drowning	6,351	530	85	387	7,353
Poisoning by solids or liquids	3,474	2,943	22	787	7,226
Fires and burns	5,364‡	147	242	151	5,904
Suffocation, hanging, and strangulation	881	4,061	977	81	6,000
Cutting	118	409	4,365*	36	4,928
Poisoning by motor-vehicle carbon monoxide	596	2,032	2,528	163	2,791
Other	18,752	691	22,348	924	22,895
TOTAL	94,082	28,242		3,212	147,884

*Not separately identified in mortality statistics.
†Includes 276 firearm deaths termed "legal intervention."
‡Includes 4200 deaths from housefires, primarily attributable to carbon monoxide poisoning, rather than burns.
Reprinted with permission from *Injury in America: A Continuing Public Health Problem*, 1985. Published by National Academy Press, Washington, DC.

Blunt trauma requires expert clinical judgment to assess and diagnose actual and potential injury. Because an injurious impact may leave no external signs on the body, an awareness of the mechanism of injury is of great importance in the care of the blunt trauma patient.

Penetrating Trauma

Penetrating trauma results from objects that are impaled in the body, such as stabbings, or from ballistic injuries. Penetrating injuries are frequently more easily diagnosed and treated because of the availability of obvious signs of injury.

Stab wounds are low-velocity injuries because the velocity is equal only to the speed with which the object is thrust into the body. Important considerations in stabbings are the length and width of the impaling object and the presence of vital organs in the area of the stab wound. A direct path of injury occurs with an impaled object, resulting in damage only to those vessels and tissues that come into contact with the object.

Ballistic trauma in a civilian environment may consist of either low- or high-velocity injuries. Low-velocity weapons deliver bullets at approximately 1200 to 1500 feet/second and include guns such as the .22 caliber pistol. High-velocity injuries result from missile speeds approximating 2000 feet/second and may be caused by .45 caliber semiautomatic weapons. Obviously, the greater the velocity, the more kinetic energy is dissipated in the body. A high-velocity missile causes cavitation as it passes through body tissues. Depending upon the range, distance from the weapon to the point of impact, and velocity of the missile, cavitation may be as great as 20 to 30 times the diameter of the bullet. Although the bullet itself does not come into direct contact with tissues outside its path, cavitation can result in tearing and disruption of tissue and vessels.

Missiles that come into contact with internal structures, thus causing a change in pathway, release more energy and result in more damage than missiles passing through the body in a direct path. Bullet design is important in determining the injuring capability of a gunshot wound. Solid point bullets remain intact, whereas hollow point bullets tend to break apart or fragment, resulting in multiple missiles instead of one missile traveling through the body.

As a missile or bullet enters the body and travels to its point of impact, it may pass through clothing, glass, wood, or other objects. These foreign objects are carried into the body and may result in additional injury and potential for infection. In addition, the missile itself may result in further complications such as a bullet embolus (Shea, 1986).

PREHOSPITAL CARE AND TRANSPORT

Reduced morbidity and mortality can be achieved with rapid assessment in the field by prehospital personnel and immediate transport of the trauma victim to an appropriate care facility. Care of the trauma patient is unique in the prehospital care setting because early efforts at field care were centered around the care of cardiac patients, who required extensive resuscitation and stabilization prior to transport. Unlike the cardiac patient, the trauma patient cannot be resuscitated and stabilized by the interventions available to emergency medical technicians and paramedics. Stabilization of the trauma patient often occurs only after surgical intervention and resuscitation from the hypovolemic shock state. Prehospital care in the past has sometimes been detrimental to the outcome of the injured patient. Attempts to stabilize the patient in the field caused delays in transport and in definitive surgical intervention to control hemorrhage. Education and training in this area have resulted in more appropriate field care for trauma victims.

Once prehospital personnel arrive at the scene of a traumatic incident, they immediately begin to control the situation, preparing the patient for transport and frequently contacting a base station hospital for medical direction of field care. In some parts of the country prehospital personnel perform according to very strict protocols and are not required to make base station contact. Medical direction is provided by a physician or registered nurse with special education and qualifications in prehospital and emergency care, often a mobile intensive care nurse (MICN). Together the prehospital personnel and the professional providing medical direction determine appropriate field treatment, mode of transport, and final patient destination.

"Scoop and run" or "load and go" are terms that appropriately describe the most beneficial prehospital care for trauma victims. Today, advocates of trauma systems recommend that prehospital personnel not delay transport while establishing intravenous lines and infusing large volumes of fluid. Instead, only minimal care should be rendered at the scene, paying attention to the airway with cervical spine immobilization, breathing, and circulation. Prehospital personnel establish or maintain a patent airway with cervical spine immobilization, provide high-flow supplemental oxygen, and assist ventilation as necessary. Large-bore venous access and administration of crystalloid solution may be done during transport. Additional interventions, depending upon predetermined protocols, may include application and inflation of the pneumatic antishock garment (PASG) and life-saving treatment of injuries affecting airway, breathing, or circulation. This includes treatments such as placing an occlusive dressing over an open chest wound, needle thoracostomy to relieve a tension pneumothorax, endotracheal intubation, or cricothyroidotomy.

Transport to the appropriate care facility may involve travel past a hospital with a basic emergency care capability. Previous experience both in military and civilian settings indicates that increased survivability results with transport to a hospital where a trauma team concept is in place. Only in situations involving traumatic arrest or inability to establish and maintain a patent airway is transport to a basic emergency facility beneficial to the major trauma patient.

Either ground or air transport is appropriate for the transport of the trauma patient from the scene of the injury to the trauma center. Considerations in the choice of method of transport should include travel time, terrain, availability of air and ground units, capabilities of transport personnel, and weather. In San Diego County, California, as many as 75% of all major trauma victims are transported by helicopter because of lengthy ground transport times and the immediate availability of helicopter transport.

Once the decision is made to transport a patient to a trauma center, the health care professionals composing the trauma team are notified. In most trauma centers the initial resuscitation and stabilization of the trauma patient occur in a designated resuscitation area, usually within the emergency department. The trauma team responds, optimally prior to patient arrival, and begins preparations based on the report of the patient's actual injuries and clinical status.

EMERGENCY CARE PHASE

Preparation for Patient Admission

Data obtained during the prehospital phase provide valuable information that is essential to ensure a coordinated, life-saving approach to the trauma patient. While the patient is in transit to the hospital, the trauma nurse plays a vital role in ensuring that adequate preparations for the patient have been made (Cardona and associates, 1988). Preparations include notification of the appropriate hospital personnel and verification that the necessary equipment for resuscitation is present and ready for use. Most trauma events are considered "scoop and run" situations with short transport times, but other patients may come to the hospital by private car. For these reasons, the resuscitation area must always be in a state of readiness for the next trauma patient. Delays in implementing definitive critical interventions will adversely affect patient outcomes and may increase mortality to more than 15% for every hour of delay (Cowley and Dunham, 1982). Equipment needed for management of the airway with cervical spine immobilization, breathing, circulatory support, and hemorrhage control must be immediately available and easily accessible.

Most trauma resuscitations take place in a specific area in traditional emergency department settings. Some facilities utilize a separate resuscitation unit located outside the emergency department and staffed with critical care nurses. Unstable trauma patients may be admitted directly to the operating room for resuscitation and immediate surgical intervention (Butler and Campbell, 1988).

No single intervention is as vital to patient survival as airway management, and therefore measures to ensure the patency of the airway and support of ventilation are the first priorities of care. Knowledge of the mechanism of injury and the patient's clinical condition will provide information about additional or specialized equipment that may be required during the resuscitation phase. Technical tasks such as turning on oxygen and suction, assembling endotracheal intubation equipment, flushing intravenous lines, and opening sterile trays are performed prior to the patient's arrival. Testing intercoms or telephone lines to verify open communications to the blood bank and the operating room may be considered.

Initial Patient Assessment

Patient survival after a serious traumatic event depends on prompt, rapid, and systematic assessment in conjunction with immediate resuscitative interventions. Priorities of care must be determined based on the patient's clinical presentation, physical assessment, and history of the traumatic event. Evaluation of airway patency, ventilation, and venous access with circulatory support are of prime importance and take precedence over other diagnostic or definitive interventions. Adherence to established protocols for patient assessment and intervention is essential to ensure that management priorities are addressed in an appropriate manner.

PRIMARY SURVEY

The primary survey is the most crucial assessment tool in trauma care. This rapid (1- to 2-minute) evaluation of the patient's airway, breathing, and circulation (ABCs) is completed by the first medical responder at the scene of the injury and again by the trauma surgeon (team leader) on the patient's arrival at the resuscitation area. It is designed to identify life-threatening injuries accurately, establish priorities, and provide simultaneous therapeutic interventions. The primary survey is a systematic survey of airway patency (with cervical spine immobilization), breathing presence and effectiveness, circulatory status, and gross overview of neurologic disabilities. Table 57–7 details the critical assessment parameters included in the primary survey.

SECONDARY SURVEY

The secondary survey is initiated after the primary survey has been accomplished and all actual or potential life-threatening injuries have been identified and resolved. The secondary survey is a methodical head-to-toe evaluation of the patient utilizing the assessment techniques of inspection, palpation, percussion, and auscultation. After the

TABLE 57-7. Primary Survey

Assessment		Observations Indicating Impaired ABCs
Airway:	Open and patent Maintain cervical spine immobilization	Shallow, noisy breathing Stridor Cyanosis Nasal flaring Accessory muscle use Inability to speak Drooling Anxiety Decreased level of consciousness Trauma to face, mouth, neck Debris or foreign matter in mouth or pharynx
Breathing:	Presence and effectiveness	Asymmetric rise and fall of chest Absent, decreased, or unequal breath sounds Open sucking chest wounds Blunt chest injury Dyspnea Cyanosis Respiratory rate <8 to 10/ minute or >40/minute Accessory muscle use Anxiety Tracheal shift Distended neck veins Paradoxical chest wall motion
Circulation:	Presence of major pulses External hemorrhage	Weak, thready pulse >120 Moisture, color, temperature of skin Capillary refill >2 seconds Obvious external hemorrhage Decreased level of consciousness Distended neck veins
Disability:	Gross neurologic status Pupil size, equality, and reactivity to light	GLASGOW COMA SCALE

anterior portion of the body has been evaluated, the trauma team logrolls the patient to each side and the posterior side is examined for hidden injuries (Table 57–8).

Prior to the secondary survey, the patient's clothes are removed to facilitate a thorough examination. Clothing may be cut off to prevent delays in assessment and to avoid movement of the patient. Warming measures such as warmed blankets, heated intravenous solutions, or overhead radiant warmers are instituted to prevent hypothermia. Temperature, heart rate, respiratory rate, and auscultated blood pressure are obtained at this time and documented as a baseline for analysis of trends during the resuscitation phase. Application of an automatic blood pressure monitor and oxygen saturation device may be done to provide ongoing assessments. Insertion of an indwelling urinary catheter and nasogastric tube is done at this time if not contraindicated by the patient's condition. These interventions facilitate the ongoing assessment and also provide diagnostic data about occult problems such as hematuria.

Information about actual and potential injuries is noted and used to establish diagnostic and treatment priorities. Radiologic and laboratory studies may be done according to a standardized trauma protocol or may be based on assessment of suspected injuries. The sequence of diagnostic procedures is influenced by the stability of the patient's condition, mechanism of injury, and identified injuries. As data are obtained, the team leader determines the need for consultation with specialty physicians such as neurosurgeons, orthopaedists, urologists, or others. Supportive interventions such as splinting of extremities, wound care, and administration of tetanus prophylaxis and antibiotics are done at this time. Finally, the secondary survey provides data that enable the team leader to establish priorities for definitive care and ongoing management of the trauma patient. Table 57–9 presents a mnemonic to guide performance of the initial assessment, including the primary and secondary surveys.

NURSING DIAGNOSES, ACTUAL AND POTENTIAL

The trauma nurse plays an instrumental role in the initial assessment, resuscitation, and ongoing evaluation of the trauma patient. Assessment findings are formulated into an individualized plan of care using the priority nursing diagnoses. The complexity of the trauma patient's injuries makes it possible to apply many approved nursing diagnoses to a patient with multiple trauma. However, during this critical phase, the nurse focuses interventional measures on the nursing diagnoses that are considered emergent in nature. These diagnoses are listed in Table 57–10.

The trauma resuscitation nurse also makes clinical judgments based on nursing diagnoses concerned with potential problems or needs facing the trauma patient and his or her significant others. These additional nursing diagnoses address the less emergent physical, psychosocial, and spiritual needs of the trauma patient. The care of each patient is guided by care plans designed to meet specific needs. Additional nursing diagnoses that may apply to trauma patients are listed below:

Physical Alterations
Potential for infection
Altered comfort
Impaired physical mobility
Hypothermia
Altered bowel elimination
Altered nutrition
Impaired tissue integrity

Psychosocial or Spiritual Alterations
Fear
Grieving
Powerlessness

TABLE 57–8. Secondary Survey

Area	Inspection	Palpation	Percussion	Auscultation

Head:
  Scalp
  Skull
  Face
  Eyes/ears
  Nose
  Mouth
	Soft tissue injury
	Deformities
	Edema
	Asymmetry of face
	Open bite
	Periorbital
	Edema
	Otorrhea
	Rhinorrhea
	Bloody drainage
	Extraoccular movements
	Subcutaneous air
	Gross vision
	Eye injuries
		Bony deformities of facial
		  bones or skull
		Scalp wounds
		Subcutaneous air
		Crepitus
		Pain
		Decreased sensation of face		

Neck	Soft tissue injury
	Tracheal, position
	Distended neck veins
	Ask about pain, hoarseness,
	  dysphagia
		Crepitus
		Subcutaneous air
		Tracheal position
		Cervical spine tenderness or
		  deformities		

Chest	Soft tissue injury
	Open sucking wound
	Subcutaneous air
	Intercostal retractions
	Symmetry of chest
	Respiratory rate, effort
	Seatbelt marks
	Impaled objects
		Crepitus
		Subcutaneous air
		Bony deformities
		Chest wall excursion
			Dullness
			Hyperresonance
				Absent or diminished
				  breath sounds
				Distant heart or gastric
				  sounds

Abdomen and
  flanks*
	Soft tissue injury
	Distention
	Seatbelt marks
	Impaled objects
	Contour
	Discolorations
		Rigidity
		Distention
		Pain: diffuse or localized
			Dullness
			Hyperresonance
				Bowel sounds in all four
				  quadrants

Pelvis or perineum	Soft tissue injury External genitalia injury Blood at urinary meatus Vaginal bleeding Rectal bleeding Suprapubic masses Priapism	Pelvic instability Femoral pulses Rectal sphincter tone Prostate position Vaginal integrity Open fractures		
Extremities	Soft tissue injury Amputation Crush injury Deformity: open or closed Motor/sensory	Diminished or absent pulses Crepitus Pain or tenderness		

Back	Soft tissue injury
	Buttock
	Posterior thighs
	Flanks
		Thoracic, lumbar sacral spine
		  pain, tenderness,
		  deformity		

*Note: The sequence of examination of the abdomen is inspection, auscultation, palpation, and percussion

Ineffective coping
Body image
Altered sensory perception

INTERVENTIONS

Ineffective Airway Clearance. Airway obstruction, whether it occurs at the time of injury or develops during resuscitation, is a potential problem for every trauma patient. Maintaining a patent airway and adequate ventilation is an essential element of trauma management. The tongue, due to posterior displacement, frequently obstructs the airway. Other causes of obstruction are foreign debris such as blood clots or vomitus, and maxillofacial fractures with bleeding or secretions. Patients with a depressed sensorium and an absent gag reflex also require interventions for airway management. Injury to the throat or neck can result in damage to vital airway structures. Control of the airway in the trauma patient is based on the need for protection, ventilation, and oxygenation (Baxt, 1985). Basic airway interventions are listed in Table 57–11.

Manual Techniques of Airway Clearance. Because posterior displacement of the tongue commonly re-

TABLE 57–9. Initial Assessment Tool

A	Airway	Assess and maintain patency
B	Breathing	Assess presence and effectiveness
C	Circulation	Assess presence and effectiveness
D	Disability	Assess gross neurologic disability and pupillary status
E	Expose	Remove all clothing
F	Freezing	Institute warming measures to prevent hypothermia
G	Get vital signs	Obtain temperature, heart rate, respiratory rate, blood pressure
H	Head to toe inspection	Systematic assessment
I	Inspect the back	Posterior assessment

Unpublished material developed by California Emergency Nurses Association State Trauma Committee, 1987.

sults in airway obstruction, opening the airway is often easily accomplished by the simple manual technique of a jaw thrust or chin lift. These maneuvers do not hyperextend the neck or compromise the integrity of the cervical spine. These are temporary interventions that serve to move the mandible anteriorly and create a patent airway.

The airway must be cleared of any foreign material such as blood, vomitus, bone fragments, or teeth. A rigid, large-bore suction device such as a tonsillar suction catheter is used to remove debris. Suction of the nares with a soft suction catheter should be performed with caution in patients with midfacial trauma and potential cribriform plate fractures. Suction should be limited to 15- to 20-second intervals to prevent hypoxemia associated with the procedure. Oxygenation with 100% concentrations prior to suctioning is recommended to limit hypoxia.

Artificial Airways. Oropharyngeal and nasopharyngeal airways are the simplest artificial airway adjuncts used in patients with spontaneous respirations and adequate ventilatory effort. Both devices help maintain a patent airway by preventing posterior displacement of the tongue. Although relatively easy to insert, these adjuncts are not without disadvantages. The oropharyngeal airway may create further airway obstruction if it is too small. It may also be placed incorrectly and positioned against the tongue, pressing it onto the posterior wall of the pharynx. Too large an oropharyngeal airway may stimulate the gag reflex and cause vomiting with possible aspiration. The oropharyngeal airway is not to be used in awake patients with a gag reflex.

The nasopharyngeal airway, or nasal trumpet, is relatively contraindicated in patients with midfacial trauma and suspected fractures of the cribriform plate. This device is well tolerated in the awake patient.

Esophageal Obturator Airway and Esophageal Gastric Tube Airway. The esophageal obturator air-

way (EOA) and its modification, the esophageal gastric tube airway (EGTA), are blind-ended, cuffed airway tubes that are inserted into the esophagus. The cuff is inflated and the patient is ventilated through a face mask. Air passes into the trachea through holes located in the proximal end of the tube. Advantages of these airways are that they are easy to insert and do not require hyperextension of the neck. A disadvantage is that incorrect placement of the tube in the trachea results in lack of oxygenation. Death will occur if incorrect placement is not recognized immediately and corrected. The use of the EOA-EGTA remains controversial in airway management (Baxt, 1985).

Tracheal Intubation. Tracheal intubation is the ideal nonsurgical airway management technique and allows for complete control of the airway. Tracheal intubation may be achieved by either the oral or nasal route. However, for the patient in distress, priority must be given to oxygenation before intubation is attempted. Immediate ventilation with 100% oxygen by a bag-valve-mask (BVM) device is vital in the hypoxic patient and should be initiated simultaneously with preparation for intubation.

In the presence of documented or suspected cervical spine injury, oral tracheal intubation is avoided to prevent possible manipulation of the neck. However, for apneic patients without midfacial trauma, oral tracheal intubation can be performed with in-line manual immobilization of the neck provided by an assistant. Disadvantages of oral tracheal intubation include possible manipulation of the cervical spine, incorrect tube placement in the esophagus or right mainstem bronchus, vocal cord trauma, or trauma to the intraoral structures.

Nasal tracheal intubation is performed in breathing trauma patients, particularly when the urgency of the resuscitation procedure does not allow time to obtain preliminary cervical spine x-rays. Spontaneous respirations are required to perform nasal tracheal intubation successfully because the absence of respirations creates a difficult "blind" intubation situation. The nasal route is contraindicated in patients with maxillofacial trauma or suspected basilar skull

TABLE 57–10. Emergent or Primary Nursing Diagnoses

Airway
  Ineffective airway clearance

Breathing
  Ineffective breathing pattern
  Impaired gas exchange

Circulation
  Altered cardiac output: Decreased
  Actual fluid volume deficit
  Potential fluid volume deficit
  Altered tissue perfusion: Cardiopulmonary, cerebral

Disability (Neurologic)
  Potential for injury: Spinal cord injury
  Altered tissue perfusion: Cerebral

TABLE 57–11. Basic Airway Interventions

Goal	Process	Expected Outcome
Maintain patent airway Avoid manipulation of cervical spine and stimulation of gag reflex	Open airway by performing jaw thrust or chin lift Gently suction with tonsillar tip catheter or finger sweep oral cavity Maintain open airway with appropriate artificial airway adjunct Provide 100% oxygen by mask Ventilate with bag-valve-mask device if indicated Prepare to assist with oral/nasal intubation, crico/trach Control secretions, bleeding, vomiting Prepare for nasogastric tube insertion Monitor airway status frequently for evolving or recurring problems	Improved airway clearance evidenced by: No stridor Clear bilateral breath sounds Decreased accessory muscle use No cyanosis

fractures. Disadvantages of nasal intubation are epistaxis, injury to the nasal turbinates, and introduction of infection. Topical use of a vasoconstrictive agent such as Neo-Synephrine prior to nasal tracheal intubation may decrease the incidence of bleeding (Grande, 1988).

Postintubation ventilation with 100% oxygen is initiated immediately after placement of the tube. Correct position of the tube is verified by auscultation of bilateral breath sounds and chest film.

Selection of the appropriate size of endotracheal tube is an important consideration. The tube with the largest diameter that can be easily inserted is the best size. In general, the recommended size is 7.0 to 8.0 mm internal diameter (ID) for women and 8.0 to 9.0 mm ID for men. Advantages of the 7.0 mm ID or larger tube include improved oxygenation and the ability to perform fiberoptic bronchoscopy through the tube.

Cricothyroidotomy. Inability to intubate the trauma patient is an indication for surgical intervention to control the airway. Conditions that may require a cricothyroidotomy are maxillofacial trauma, laryngeal fractures, facial or upper airway burns, and severe oropharyngeal hemorrhage. The anatomic position of the avascular cricoid membrane makes this a relatively bloodless, safe, and rapid procedure. The adult cricothyroid membrane is located inferior to the thyroid cartilage and above the cricoid cartilage. Access to the trachea through the cricothyroid membrane can be accomplished by either needle cricothyroidotomy or surgical cricothyroidotomy.

Needle cricothyroidotomy is a percutaneous technique that entails insertion of a 12- to 14-gauge needle into the trachea below the level of the obstruction. Intermittent transtracheal ventilation is then carried out using a 50-psi oxygen source. This temporary method is useful for only 30 to 45 minutes before the accumulation of carbon dioxide reaches unacceptable levels.

Surgical cricothyroidotomy is an alternative method of tracheal access in which an incision is made through the skin into the cricothyroid membrane. The incision is dilated and secured with a tracheostomy tube of 5.0 to 7.0 mm ID.

The choice of airway management technique is based on familiarity with the procedures, the clinical condition of the patient, and hemodynamic stability. The resuscitation nurse has an important responsibility in assessing and maintaining ongoing monitoring of airway patency. A patent airway is the cornerstone of a successful trauma resuscitation.

Pharmacologic Agents. Combative critical trauma patients with an altered level of consciousness may require the use of a paralytic agent to facilitate intubation. The two most frequently used agents in the emergent phase of airway management are succinylcholine (SCh) and pancuronium bromide (Morris, 1988). These medications are used with caution and only if the practitioner is prepared to provide ventilatory assistance through a BVM device or cricothyrotomy if attempts at intubation are unsuccessful.

SCh is a commonly used, short-acting depolarizing muscle relaxant that causes complete flaccid paralysis within 1 minute of intravenous administration. Depolarization rapidly causes fasciculations, or muscle contractions, of the upper torso, followed by paralysis of the extremities. As the muscles become refractory to stimulation, the intercostal muscles and diaphragm are finally paralyzed. It is possible to achieve intubation within 1 to 2 minutes after intravenous administration of SCh. Duration of the effects of SCh is a brief 8 to 10 minutes. The dosage for intravenous SCh is 1.0 to 1.5 mg/kg.

Pancuronium bromide is a long-acting, nondepolarizing neuromuscular blocking agent that causes flaccid paralysis. The onset of action occurs within 45 to 60 seconds after intravenous administration and lasts up to 45 to 60 minutes. The peak effect for intubation occurs 3 minutes after administration of the usual dosage of 0.5 to 2.0 mg/kg. Pancuronium bromide does not cause the muscle fasciculations associated with SCh and may be desirable in patients when increased intracranial, intraocular, or intragastric pressure is of concern (Hochbaum, 1986). The prolonged duration of action may be contraindicated in selected trauma situations.

The short duration of effect of SCh may make it the paralytic agent of choice in the resuscitation phase. Pretreatment with pancuronium is one method of preventing SCh-induced fasciculations that may be detrimental to the patient's clinical condition. The dosage for pretreatment with pancuronium is 0.01 to 0.03 mg/kg given 1 to 3 minutes prior to the administration of SCh (Morris, 1988).

There is some evidence that intravenous lidocaine may decrease the rises in intracranial pressure and blood pressure that occur during intubation (Grande, 1988). The pharmacologic properties of lidocaine may decrease the systemic vascular response that occurs during intubation, provide prophylaxis against ventricular dysrhythmias in the hypoxic patient, and cause beneficial cerebral vasoconstriction. For the head-injured patient, the dosage of lidocaine is 1.5 mg/kg given intravenously 3 to 5 minutes prior to intubation.

In some instances rapid-sequence induction of general anesthesia is used to control the airway. This method of administering anesthesia is a useful technique for preventing aspiration in the head-injured patient. Rapid-sequence induction requires prior preparation of medications, suction, and intubation and ventilatory equipment. Preoxygenation with 100% oxygen for 1 to 2 minutes is a critical first step in the process. A defasciculating dose of pancuronium is administered to limit increases in intracranial and intragastric pressures. General anesthesia is then induced using either thiopental 3 to 4 mg/kg or ketamine 2 mg/kg intravenously. At least 3 minutes after administration of pancuronium, the patient is given SCh 1 to 2 mg/kg (Morris, 1988; Strange, 1987). As consciousness is lost, cricoid pressure compresses the esophagus and inhibits aspiration of gastric contents.

Ineffective Breathing Patterns. Interventions to restore normal breathing patterns are directed toward the specific injury or underlying cause of respiratory distress, with the goal of improving ventilation and gas exchange. Basic nursing interventions for patients with ineffective breathing patterns include application of supplemental oxygen with ventilatory assistance if needed, preparation for intubation, and evaluation of specific interventions.

Evaluation of interventions and ongoing monitoring of these patients are performed frequently to assess respiratory rate and effort, heart rate and rhythm, breath sounds, skin signs, tracheal position, and neck vein distention. Fluid intake and output is monitored to guide the resuscitation process. The nurse also assists in obtaining diagnostic studies such as arterial blood gases and chest films to ensure the effectiveness of specific interventions. Etiologies of traumatic injuries that result in ineffective breathing patterns and specific interventions for them are listed in Table 57–12.

Impaired Gas Exchange. Impaired gas exchange follows airway obstruction as the most crucial problem of the trauma patient. Etiologies of impaired gas exchange include a decrease in inspired air, retained secretions, lung collapse or compression, atelectasis, or accumulation of blood in the thoracic cavity.

Fluid volume deficit secondary to hemorrhage also affects adequate gas exchange. Patients with multiple systemic injuries or trauma to the central nervous system or chest and victims in hemorrhagic shock are all at risk for impaired gas exchange.

Interventions are directed toward maintaining a patent airway and optimizing gas exchange. Trauma patients require high-flow supplemental oxygen to promote optimal gas exchange. Specific nursing actions include monitoring the patient's respiratory status for respiratory rate, ventilatory effort, and alterations in breathing patterns and assisting with removal of secretions. Other interventions include preparation for intubation, mechanical ventilation, and other measures used to improve gas exchange such as needle thoracostomy, chest tube insertion, and restoration of circulating blood volume.

Altered Cardiac Output: Decreased. The most common etiology of impaired cardiac output in the trauma patient is hypovolemic shock due to acute blood loss. The causes may be external, as with hemorrhage, or internal, as with hemothorax, hemoperitoneum, or massive pelvic fractures. Other etiologies that may cause a decrease in cardiac output are tension pneumothorax, resulting in compression of the heart and great vessels, and pericardial tamponade, resulting in impairment of cardiac filling and ventricular ejection. Table 57–13 demonstrates the predictability of stages of hemorrhagic shock (American College of Surgeons, 1984).

The trauma nurse must maintain a high index of suspicion for the development of hemorrhagic shock and carefully monitor the patient to prevent the vicious cycle of cellular death and organ failure that occurs if successful resuscitation is not accomplished. Adequate fluid resuscitation is of critical importance. Other interventions are directed toward the specific cause of impaired cardiac output, tension pneumothorax and pericardial tamponade.

Tension Pneumothorax. Tension pneumothorax is a rapidly fatal emergency that is easily resolved with early recognition and intervention. It occurs when an injury to the chest allows air to enter the pleural cavity but not to escape. Air accumulates in the pleural space with each inspiration and as intrathoracic pressure increases, the lung collapses. The increased pressure then causes compression of the heart and great vessels toward the unaffected side as evidenced by mediastinal shift and distended neck veins. The resulting decreased cardiac output and impaired gas exchange are manifested by severe respiratory distress and signs of shock.

On recognition of a tension pneumothorax, the immediate intervention is a needle thoracostomy using a 12- to 16-gauge needle in the second intercostal space in the midclavicular line on the injured side to relieve intrapleural pressure. In evaluating

TABLE 57–12. Specific Interventions for Ineffective Breathing Patterns

Etiology	Interventions
Tension pneumothorax	Prepare for decompression by needle thoracostomy with a 12- to 16-gauge needle in second intercostal space in midclavicular line on affected side Prepare for chest tube insertion
Pneumothorax	Prepare for chest tube insertion on affected side
Open sucking wound	Seal wound with occlusive dressing and monitor chest for signs of tension pneumothorax Remove one corner of dressing if respiratory distress develops. Prepare for chest tube insertion
Massive hemothorax	Establish two 14- to 16-gauge IV lines with normal saline or Ringer's lactate Obtain blood for type and cross-match Prepare for large chest tube insertion Prepare autotransfusion device Administer blood or blood products as ordered Anticipate and prepare for emergency open thoracotomy
Pulmonary contusion	Prepare for early intubation and mechanical ventilation Administer intravenous normal saline or Ringer's lactate TKO if no signs of shock present to avoid fluid overload
Flail chest	Stabilize chest wall: may position on affected side with head of bed elevated or apply manual pressure while preparing for definitive internal stabilization Prepare for early intubation and mechanical ventilation Prepare for chest tube insertion Administer intravenous normal saline or Ringer's lactate TKO if no signs of shock present to avoid fluid overload Administer analgesics as ordered Assist with intercostal nerve block
Tracheobronchial injury	Elevate head of bed to facilitate breathing Prepare for chest tube insertion Anticipate bronchoscopy
Spinal cord injury	Avoid hyperextension or rotation of neck Maintain complete spinal immobilization Prepare for application of cervical traction tongs or halo device Monitor motor and sensory function Monitor for signs of neurogenic shock
Decreased level of consciousness	Position head midline with head of bed elevated Administer osmotic diuretics, steroids, anticonvulsants, or paralytic agents as ordered Anticipate CT scan

patients with open sucking chest wounds that have been covered, care is taken to monitor the possible development of a tension pneumothorax. If this occurs, the occlusive dressing is immediately removed. A chest tube is placed after decompression of the chest by needle thoracostomy, and a chest film is then obtained. Definitive intervention is never delayed in order to confirm the presence of a tension pneumothorax by radiologic film.

Pericardial Tamponade. Pericardial tamponade is a life-threatening condition caused by rapid accumulation of fluid (usually blood) in the pericardial sac. As the intrapericardial pressure increases, cardiac output is impaired due to decreased venous

TABLE 57–13. Estimated Fluid and Blood Requirements* (Based on Patient's Initial Presentation)

	Class I	Class II	Class III	Class IV
Blood loss (mL)	up to 750	750–1500	1500–2000	2000 or more
Blood loss (%BV)	up to 15%	15–30%	30–40%	40% or more
Pulse rate	<100	>100	>120	140 or higher
Blood pressure	Normal	Normal	Decreased	Decreased
Pulse pressure (mm Hg)	Normal or increased	Decreased	Decreased	Decreased
Capillary blanch test	Normal	Positive	Positive	Positive
Respiratory rate	14–20	20–30	30–40	>35
Urine output (ml/hr)	30 or more	20–30	5–15	Negligible
CNS-mental status	Slightly anxious	Mildly anxious	Anxious and confused	Confused-lethargic
Fluid replacement (3:1 rule)	Crystalloid	Crystalloid	Crystalloid + blood	Crystalloid + blood

*For a 70-kg male.

Data from the American College of Surgeons, Committee on Trauma. (1984). *Advanced trauma life support course: Instructors manual.* Chicago, American College of Surgeons.

return and compression of cardiac activity. Blood, if unable to flow into the right side of the heart, causes increased central venous pressure and distended neck veins. Classic signs of this injury are profound shock, muffled or distant heart sounds, and distended neck veins. All three signs of this condition (Beck's triad) may not be present in each case of pericardial tamponade.

Pericardial tamponade is generally caused by penetrating trauma to the chest. However, it should be suspected in any patient with blunt trauma and multisystem injuries who is in shock and does not respond to aggressive resuscitation. Pericardial tamponade is often difficult to diagnose in the presence of other injuries that may also be the source of decreased cardiac output.

Diagnosis of pericardial tamponade is achieved by performing a pericardiocentesis. This procedure may also provide therapeutic intervention by decompressing the pericardium. Needle aspiration of the pericardial sac is done with a 14- to 18-gauge catheter over a needle, such as a spinal needle, attached to a 35- to 50-mL syringe with a three-way stopcock. Aspirated pericardial blood usually will not clot unless the heart itself has been penetrated. Arterial blood pressure may dramatically improve with removal of as little as 20 to 30 mL of blood.

Equipment for an emergency thoracotomy must be immediately available if cardiac arrest occurs. After stabilization, the patient is transferred to the operating room for definitive surgical intervention.

Actual or Potential Fluid Volume Deficit

Altered Tissue Perfusion: Cardiopulmonary. Early recognition and aggressive management of hemorrhagic shock are essential for successful resuscitation of the multiply injured patient. Therapeutic interventions are directed toward arresting the hemorrhage and replacing circulating blood volume to restore adequate tissue perfusion.

As always, a patent airway and adequate ventilation are priority interventions. Efforts to correct loss of circulating blood volume are addressed next. Continued blood loss due to obvious external hemorrhage is controlled with direct pressure, elevation of an extremity, or compression of pressure points. Tourniquets are avoided to prevent compromise of circulation to the extremity and possible loss of the limb.

The pneumatic antishock garment (PASG) is a pneumatic counterpressure device that is used to control hemorrhage by tamponading intra-abdominal, pelvic, and lower extremity bleeding. It also provides splinting and stabilization of pelvic and leg fractures. The PASG increases vascular resistance and prevents further blood loss into the abdomen and legs and may provide translocation of a small amount (150 to 300 mL) of blood into the central circulation. The use of the PASG is contraindicated in patients with signs and symptoms of pulmonary edema. It is controversial in patients with the poten-

tial for increased intracranial pressure or thoracic injuries (Baxt, 1985; Cardona, 1988).

Venous Access. Venous access and infusion of volume is the key to optimal resuscitation in the patient with hemorrhagic shock. At least two large-bore (14- to 16-gauge) peripheral intravenous lines are necessary. The antecubital fossa is an accessible site; vessels may be cannulated by either percutaneous or cutdown methods. Central line placement for resuscitation is often time-consuming and should not be considered as a primary resuscitation line but may be necessary in situations of severe vascular collapse. Such a line is more beneficial as a resuscitation monitoring tool and is indicated after the initial resuscitation phase. In general, the most appropriate venous access route is the largest one that can be established rapidly.

Fluid Resuscitation. Rapid infusion of fluids is done through large internal diameter blood tubes with a short catheter to facilitate flow. Lines placed by cutdown may use an 8-F catheter, and pressure bags are helpful. Rapid infusion devices are available that facilitate fluid infusion of 1000 to 1500 mL/minute.

A universal problem involved in rapid infusion of fluids is that of hypothermia. Blood or fluid warming devices frequently cannot infuse fluid rapidly enough to allow adequate resuscitation. It is desirable to warm any fluid infused above the diaphragm to prevent the hazardous effects of cold fluid on the myocardium. Small warming ovens are available to store limited amounts of crystalloid solutions.

Hemorrhage causes blood loss from the intravascular space and fluid loss from the extravascular space as fluid shifts occur. Volume resuscitation is directed toward replacing both losses. Although agreement on replacing red blood cell depletion seems to be universal, the choice of an asanguineous fluid remains very controversial (Bant, 1985; Cardona, 1988; Conn, 1988). Colloids are better maintained initially in the intravascular space due to their oncotic properties. Administration of crystalloids requires approximately three times as much volume and will also replace losses in the extravascular spaces. The expense and complications associated with the use of each solution remain the basis for debate.

Fluid resuscitation is guided by the patient's physiologic response to the therapy. If signs of class I or class II shock are present, rapid infusion of crystalloid solution is given at a ratio of 3 mL for every 1 mL of suspected blood loss (Baxt, 1985). Plasma expanders such as hetastarch may be used to augment crystalloids in patients who do not show signs of immediate improvement with crystalloids alone. Close continuous monitoring of hemodynamic status, including capillary refill time, central venous pressure, and urinary output, is necessary to direct further efforts in volume resuscitation and prevent harmful unnecessary fluid overload. Ideally, fluid replacement is measured by monitoring mean arterial pressure (MAP), pulmonary capillary wedge pressure

(PCWP), pulmonary artery pressure (PAP), and cardiac output (CO).

Continued signs and symptoms of shock such as falling hematocrit, deteriorating arterial Pa_{O_2} and pH, decreasing urinary output (less than 30 mL/hour), and increasing arterial lactate levels indicate the need for more aggressive measures. It is important to remember that hemoglobin and hematocrit values may be unreliable in gauging the degree of shock initially because it may be up to 4 hours before changes are evident. As metabolic acidosis worsens, decreasing Pa_{O_2} and pH demonstrate the body's response to anaerobic metabolism.

Blood products are administered using a formula of 1 mL for each 1 mL of blood loss (Baxt, 1985) to maintain a hemoglobin concentration above 10 to 12 g/100 mL and a hematocrit of 30%. Type-specific or group O negative blood is used in cases of exsanguination. Fully cross-matched blood is administered as soon as it is available. Preparation of type and cross-matched blood takes 30 to 60 minutes and is appropriate only for patients who have been stabilized with crystalloids and colloids.

Autotransfusion of shed blood, or autologous blood, is an alternative method of blood replacement that can be used in the patient with hemorrhage caused by hemothorax or other intrathoracic injuries. This inexpensive, safe, and rapid technique involves accumulation of the patient's own blood into a suction device. The blood is then anticoagulated and filtered and is immediately available for reinfusion. Autotransfusion is an excellent way to provide fresh, warm blood that carries no risk of antibody problems and eliminates the risk of transmittable infectious diseases.

Diagnostic peritoneal lavage (DPL) may be done during the resuscitation phase to determine whether the intraperitoneal space is the source of the fluid volume deficit. If the patient responds to fluid replacement and abdominal injury is suspected, the diagnostic study of choice is computed tomography (CT) scan of the abdomen.

Potential for Injury: Spinal Cord Injury. Appropriate immobilization and management of the patient with multisystem trauma will aid in preventing further possible injury. Field measures of immobilization should be maintained during the initial assessment and resuscitation efforts. Interventions at this time are directed toward maintaining vital function and attempts to restore neurologic functions. Chapter 35 includes a discussion of specific spinal cord injuries and interventions. Conscious patients are reassured and alerted not to move. All patient assessment and intervention activities are performed by the resuscitation team under the direction of the team leader.

A complete neurologic examination is completed after evaluation of the airway, breathing, and circulation has been completed. Portable lateral films of the cervical spine are obtained, and the patient is prepared for possible spinal CT scan to rule out occult injury. Dislocations of the spine are reduced as soon as possible by means of postural reduction or by either cervical traction tongs or halo traction devices. Surgical open reduction is not usually necessary during the first 24 hours. Other current modalities include the administration of methylprednisolone intravenously in a 30 mg/kg bolus followed by an intravenous drip infusion of 8 to 10 mg/kg over the subsequent 23 hours.

Ongoing assessment includes evaluation of airway and ventilatory function, heart rate and rhythm, blood pressure, and urinary output. Frequent documentation of motor and sensory status of all extremities is important.

Altered Cerebral Tissue Perfusion. Cerebral perfusion pressure depends on adequate blood flow and oxygenation of the brain. It is important to consider whether protection of the brain from further insult during the initial resuscitation phase is needed. Cerebral ischemia is associated with increased mortality, and interventions are directed toward providing appropriate levels of blood flow, oxygen, and glucose to the brain (Gennarelli, 1984).

Aggressive volume resuscitation is necessary to return the hemorrhagic shock patient to a normotensive state quickly. Care must be exercised, however, to avoid overhydration and increased intracranial pressure (ICP). Supplemental oxygen is essential, and tracheal intubation with mechanical ventilation is often required to optimize arterial oxygen content.

Increased ICP causes further cerebral ischemia and requires prompt attention. Hyperventilation to a Pa_{CO_2} of between 26 and 30 mm Hg is an effective method of decreasing intracerebral blood volume by regulating cerebral vessel size. Osmotic diuretics such as mannitol to decrease brain water are recommended for serious or deteriorating head injuries (Gennarelli, 1984).

The initial resuscitation and stabilization of the major trauma patient will result in a tentative diagnosis by the trauma surgeon (team leader). In most situations, the patient will require further diagnostic evaluation, CT scan, or angiography or will be transported to the surgical suite for immediate surgical intervention. A systems approach to the care of the trauma patient requires the immediate availability of a staffed operating room 24 hours a day and a readily available and appropriately staffed critical care bed, either in a surgical, neurologic, or trauma intensive care unit.

Once in the critical care unit, care of the major trauma patient is similar to that of any other patient requiring continual monitoring, evaluation, and intervention. A major difference is that other patients have a definitive diagnosis and have not undergone severe and sudden injury. Often, the previous medical history and other valuable information is not available to the critical care nurse.

Care of the victim of trauma should include consideration of the mechanism of injury and an awareness of concurrent injuries frequently associated with a specific mechanism of injury. The potential for significant additional injuries is a priority during the initial critical care phase. Recent experience indicates that late trauma deaths, those occurring days and even weeks after the initial insult, frequently are a result of specific complications.

CRITICAL CARE PHASE

Once the trauma patient has entered the critical care phase for continued stabilization and recovery, the critical monitoring of hemodynamic parameters, analysis of assessment trends, and the institution and evaluation of therapeutic interventions become the focus of patient care. Patient assessment data are collected using a systems approach. This involves continued assessment of the neurologic, respiratory, cardiovascular, gastrointestinal, renal, and skin and extremity systems. Additional information on the individual patient's metabolic, pain response, and psychosocial needs must also be gathered. Continual assessment data help to guide therapies aimed at correcting identified problems or injuries and preventing or minimizing actual or potential postinjury complications.

Nursing care of the trauma patient in the critical care phase continues to be directed toward maintenance of the patient's airway, breathing, and circulatory functions along with interventions consistent with the specific injury. Care of specific traumatic injuries, such as neurologic, orthopaedic, abdominal, and other issues including pain management are addressed in other chapters throughout this book.

The patient with multisystem injuries is, however, at risk for developing a myriad of complications due to the body's compromised condition, prolonged immobility, and the long-term rehabilitation associated with trauma care. The most common secondary complications encountered during this critical phase of care are related to impaired gas exchange, potential for infection, altered patterns of urinary elimination, and altered nutrition with less than body requirements. Abnormalities of coagulation that can occur are discussed in detail in Chapter 50. These secondary complications are often sequelae to the severe shock state that is associated with major blood loss resulting from traumatic injury (Koziol and associates, 1988).

Impaired Gas Exchange

According to an early study completed by Blaisdell and Schlobohm (1973), respiratory complications contribute to 75% of hospital deaths of trauma patients. These complications are related most commonly to causes such as respiratory distress syndrome, pulmonary thromboembolism, and fat embolism syndrome. Critical nursing assessment skills requiring observation for often subtle and discrete changes in trends are needed to identify patients developing actual or potential gas exchange complications.

RESPIRATORY DISTRESS SYNDROME

Respiratory distress syndrome (RDS) is a complication that has been discussed in the literature since World War II. The syndrome gained greater recognition during the postresuscitation treatment of soldiers in the Vietnam War. Today, the syndrome continues to carry a 50% to 60% mortality (Slotman and colleagues, 1988). Factors directly linked to the development of RDS are closely related to the medical problems of hypovolemic shock, traumatic injury, traumatic shock, and sepsis. The syndrome is manifested by a cluster of symptoms that may occur physiologically 12 to 48 hours after a traumatic injury. However, recognizable clinical symptoms may not occur for 5 or more days after injury.

In the beginning stages of the syndrome, increases in pulmonary hydrostatic pressure or pulmonary vessel permeability occur. The exact cause of this occurrence continues to be investigated, but theories have centered around neutrophilic infiltrates in the lung (Hallgren and colleagues, 1984), the formation of thromboxane A_2 (Slotman and colleagues, 1988), and the release of bradykinin (DeOleveira, 1988). These substances are known to cause changes in the membrane integrity of the pulmonary microvascular or alveolar systems. As membrane permeability increases, pulmonary interstitial and alveolar edema occur. The normal alveolar surfactant action decreases due to this edema formation, and functional lung units begin to collapse. The end result is a ventilation-perfusion (V/Q) deficit or mismatch, pulmonary shunting (Qs/Qt), an increase in physiologic dead space, and development of lung consolidation (Cardona and others, 1988).

It is important for the critical care nurse first to identify those patients at risk for developing this syndrome because early initiation of therapy is crucial for successful recovery. Knowledge of the types of traumatic injuries that lead to the development of RDS is vital. Patients who have suffered a flail chest, pulmonary contusions, cardiac contusions, prolonged hypovolemic shock, major head injuries, or sepsis are at high risk for developing RDS. Overinfusion of balanced salt solutions during the resuscitative phase of care also contributes to the development of RDS.

Symptomatology of the development of RDS usually occurs in the critical care phase. Indicators may include low pulmonary wedge pressure, continued low arterial oxygen content, rising carbon dioxide levels, increased respiratory distress, and new diffuse bilateral chest infiltrates (Table 57–14).

Treatment interventions for RDS are directed toward correcting the underlying cause, maintaining ventilatory support, decreasing pulmonary congestion, and supporting the patient's cardiovascular system. Any specific chest injury or fluid overhydra-

TABLE 57-14. Respiratory Distress Syndrome Indicators

Pulmonary wedge pressure less than 18 mm Hg
Continued low arterial oxygen content—less
   than 75 mm Hg with oxygen administration at 0.50 FI_{O_2}
Radiologic evidence of diffuse bilateral chest infiltrates
Increasing Pa_{CO_2} levels
Acidotic arterial pH

tion must be corrected. Mechanical ventilation, if not instituted during the resuscitative phase, is required in a majority of patients with RDS. Positive end-expiratory pressure (PEEP) is used to increase the patient's Pa_{O_2} levels while using a lower inspired concentration of oxygen. PEEP is usually set at a low to moderate level of less than 15 cm H_2O. The higher levels of PEEP, above 25 cm H_2O, are reserved for patients who demonstrate pulmonary shunting problems (Qs/Qt) and associated hypoxemia (Cardona and associates, 1988). Positive end-expiratory pressure can be delivered to the patient by either controlled or intermittent mechanical ventilation.

Cardiovascular compromise can result from the use of PEEP, leading to a decrease in cardiac output. It is imperative that cardiac output be maintained to prevent further patient deterioration. Manipulation of preload, contractility, and afterload functions of the heart through administration of pharmacologic agents may be necessary to support a stable hemodynamic system.

Cardiac contractility is enhanced by the use of dopamine, dobutamine, and occasionally digoxin. These medications augment cardiac output through inotropic actions while maintaining the lowest possible increased myocardial oxygen consumption. Dopamine 2 to 5 μg/kg per minute and dobutamine 3 to 5 μg/kg per minute increase cardiac output. Higher doses of dopamine, 8 to 10 μg/kg per minute, produce vasoconstriction that can lead to other detrimental effects. Digoxin administered at 75% of the normal dosage exerts an inotropic effect, thereby increasing cardiac output. However, for digoxin to produce desirable effects, the patient's serum potassium level must be maintained at a minimum of 4 mmol/liter. Digoxin has been shown to be helpful in maintaining cardiac output, particularly in the elderly population. Isoproterenol at a dosage of 0.25 to 1.00 mg/kg per minute is another pharmacologic agent that augments cardiac output.

The afterload function of the heart can be altered by the use of nitroprusside. Nitroprusside improves left ventricular filling pressures and stroke volume. However, nitroprusside may worsen pulmonary shunting through its vasodilatory effects. Vasoconstriction in response to hypoxia is a compensatory mechanism that can actually help preserve the V/Q perfusion ratio. The arterial vasodilating effect of nitroprusside can reverse this compensatory mechanism.

Fluid therapy in the trauma patient with RDS or with the potential for developing RDS, requires careful monitoring. A balanced electrolyte solution (BES) is the most common type of fluid used to correct the hypovolemia associated with trauma patients. The amount of infused fluid must be sufficient to maintain the patient's cardiac output and intravascular volume without increasing intrapulmonary edema. Continual monitoring of the patient's mean PAP, PCWP, and central venous pressure (CVP) is important because these pressures are critical response indicators that further guide fluid therapy.

Transfusion of red blood cells may be required not only to provide cardiovascular support but also to augment oxygen delivery and minimize cellular oxygen debt. Ideally, the patient's hemoglobin should be maintained at a minimum of 10 to 12 g/100 mL and the hematocrit should be between 30% and 35%.

A new approach in the treatment of RDS has centered around the use of the pharmacologic agent ketoconazole, an imidazole-based antifungal compound that is generally used in the treatment of systemic mycosis. However, this medication also inhibits thromboxane synthetase, which is a necessary product in the formation of thromboxane A_2 (Slotman and associates, 1988). Thromboxane A_2 has been suspected as a cause of RDS. The suggested daily oral dose of ketoconazole is 200 mg.

PULMONARY THROMBOEMBOLISM

The complication of pulmonary thromboembolism (PTE) is frequently a result of musculoskeletal trauma, particularly injury to the lower extremities or pelvis. Clot formation in the peripheral veins of the lower extremities or pelvis is a common occurrence following injury. Sudden changes in blood flow and the increased pressure changes that accompany quick movements can dislodge formed clots, or clots may be dislodged spontaneously (Cardona and others, 1988). The dislodged clot becomes an embolus and travels through the body's vasculature until it lodges in either the pulmonary artery or its smaller branches. Once the embolus becomes lodged, blood flow is obstructed distally. Tissues distal to the obstruction become hypoxic, and vasoactive substances are released from the hypoxic tissue. These vasoactive substances lead to an increase in pulmonary resistance, a concurrent right ventricular strain or failure, and possible systemic shock (Cardona and colleagues, 1988).

High-risk patients need to be continually monitored for the development of the signs and symptoms associated with PTE. These symptoms include new-onset dyspnea, changes in respiratory rate and effort, and changes in cerebral and systemic tissue perfusion (Table 57-15). Symptoms of pulmonary tissue infarction comprise the above assessment findings in addition to hemoptysis, pleuritic pain, and fever.

Supporting laboratory data demonstrate changes in the patient's arterial blood gas concentrations. Hypoxemia, Pa_{O_2} levels of less than 60 mm Hg, hypocarbia, decreased oxygen saturation, and an alkalotic

TABLE 57–15. Pulmonary Thromboembolism (PTE) Assessment Findings

Dyspnea—sudden onset
Chest pain—sudden onset
Rapid, shallow respiratory rate
Increasing shortness of breath
Auscultation of bronchial breath sounds
New onset of loud S_2 heart sound
Pale, dusky, cyanotic skin coloring
Increased anxiety
Decreased level of consciousness
Other signs of hypovolemic shock
  Decreasing systolic blood pressure
  Narrowing pulse pressure
  Tachycardia

pH are associated with the development of PTE. Additional abnormal laboratory data reveal increases in leukocytes and serum enzyme elevations of lactic dehydrogenase (LDH), creatine kinase (CK), and SGOT. Electrocardiographic changes include development of tachycardia, peaked T waves, a widened QRS complex, ST- and T-wave changes, and right axis deviation. Chest radiologic films may be normal initially with later evidence of atelectasis or infarction. A lung scan may be either normal or may indicate a perfusion defect. The most definitive objective test is a pulmonary angiogram defining the area of obstruction.

Therapy for PTE is directed toward improving gas exchange and pulmonary tissue perfusion. Positioning the patient in a high Fowlers position facilitates breathing and increases diaphragmatic excursion. Administration of supplemental oxygen provides additional oxygen to correct impaired gas exchange and enhance tissue perfusion. Suctioning to prevent airway clearance problems may be necessary. Patients with severe PTE require additional interventions of intubation, mechanical ventilation, and institution of PEEP. Dissolution of the embolus itself using anticoagulant heparin therapy is desirable. Initial therapy consists of intravenous administration of 5000 to 10,000 units of heparin as a loading dose. Subsequent doses are delivered intravenously at 1500 units/hour or 25 units/kg per hour. Clotting times are then maintained at 2 to 2½ times normal to prevent the future development of clots. Other interventions include cardiovascular support with vasopressors, inotropic agents, and volume expanders. Interventions for pain control are an important consideration.

Prophylactic surgical insertion of a caval filter or umbrella into the jugular vein and then advancing it into the inferior vena cava is being implemented in some institutions. With this device, flow of emboli is impeded by entrapping them in the opened umbrella, thus preventing emboli from becoming lodged in the pulmonary vasculature.

FAT EMBOLISM

Development of the fat embolism syndrome (FES) is a risk factor that accompanies traumatic injury of the long bones, pelvis, and multiple skeletal fractures. The syndrome develops between 24 and 48 hours postinjury. One theory of the development of FES focuses on a mobilization mechanism. As a bone is stressed or injured, bone marrow fat globules from the fracture site are released into torn vessels and the systemic circulation. A second theory, the physiochemical theory, revolves around the production and release of free fatty acids in abnormal amounts following skeletal injury. These free fatty acids are implicated in the destruction of pulmonary endothelial tissue. Microvascular permeability within the pulmonary vessels then occurs, resulting in pulmonary edema. Whichever theory is correct, bone marrow fat has been recovered by biopsy or at autopsy within the systemic microvessels.

Hallmark clinical signs that accompany FES begin with development of a low-grade fever followed by a new-onset tachycardia, dyspnea, increased respiratory rate and effort, and abnormal arterial blood gas concentrations (Table 57–16). If pulmonary distress continues, the patient will begin to demonstrate symptoms of cerebral hypoxia such as changes in level of consciousness or coma. Electrocardiographic findings include development of a right bundle branch block, S waves of prominent size in lead I, Q waves in lead III, T-wave inversion, depressed RST segments, and dysrhythmias. Upper body, oral mucosa, or conjunctival petechiae are pathognomonic indicators of the development of FES, although these are uncommon findings. The exact etiology of the development of petechiae is unknown, however it has been postulated that fat globules cause superficial capillary obstruction and rupture.

Treatment for FES is directed toward the preservation of pulmonary function and maintenance of cardiovascular stability. Administration of supplemental oxygen, intubation, mechanical ventilation, and the use of PEEP may be required to restore or maintain pulmonary perfusion and ventilation. Monitoring of the patient's cardiovascular stability must be continued throughout the critical care phase, paying attention to the development of electrocardiographic and hemodynamic changes.

A study by Schonfeld and colleagues (1983) examined the use of prophylactic cortical steroids in patients who are at high risk for the development of FES. Their study indicated that the administration of cortical steroids prior to the development of FES was effective in decreasing the effects of fat emboli. However, cortical steroids administered after development of FES were found to be less effective.

TABLE 57–16. Fat Embolism Syndrome (FES) Indicators

Tachycardia—pulse greater than 100 beats/minute
Dyspnea—new onset
Tachypnea—respiratory rate greater than 24/minute
Decreasing levels of Pa_{CO_2}
Alkalotic arterial pH
Radiologic evidence of pulmonary infiltrates

Ideally, prevention of FES is the best treatment. Stabilization of fractures of the extremities to minimize both bone movement and the release of fatty products from the bone marrow must be accomplished as early as possible. Either internal or external fixation devices are used depending upon the location and extent of the fractures.

Potential for Infection

Trauma patients are at high risk for development of a transient bacteremia or the more extreme form of septic shock. Patients at greatest risk for development of septic shock are those who have sustained open wounds, open fractures, massive tissue injury, or significant head injury. Development of septic shock is associated with both gram-negative bacilli and gram-positive organisms. The most common gram-positive organisms responsible for the development of septic shock are staphylococci, pneumococci, and fungi. Sequential or multiple organ failure is a sequela of septic shock.

Initially septic shock produces a systemic hyperdynamic state demonstrated by increased cardiac output and decreased vascular resistance. This hyperdynamic state is maintained while the body mobilizes its defenses against the offending organisms. However, this state is maintained for only a limited period of time. Eventually myocardial depression occurs followed by high cardiac output failure. A subsequent fall in cardiac index along with decreased left ventricular ejection fraction results in a systemic hypodynamic state. As cardiac output continues to decrease, the arteriovenous oxygen consumption difference widens in response to an increased extraction of oxygen. This change from a hyperdynamic to a hypodynamic state is a poor prognostic sign for patient survival (Cardona and associates, 1988).

Other systemic pathophysiologic changes that occur with septic shock include hematologic and pulmonary disturbances along with cellular metabolic dysfunction. Circulating bacterial endotoxins activate the complement cascade along with two anaphylotoxin protein fragments, C3a and C5a (Littleton, 1988). Normally, these protein fragments assist in protecting the body against bacterial invasion. However, in the overwhelming global response of sepsis, these complement fragments can cause detrimental reactions. Mast cells become degranulated, causing the release of histamine. Histamine release is implicated as a cause of the vasodilation and increased capillary permeability associated with septic shock (Littleton, 1988). Platelet abnormalities, evidenced by thrombocytopenia, and systemic coagulation disorders can develop.

Pulmonary hypertension, thought to be caused by increased neutrophil infiltration of lung tissue and thromboxane A_2 synthesis, is present in patients with septic shock. Neutrophilic infiltration leads to increased capillary permeability, alveolar fluid accu-

mulation, and decreased lung compliance. Thromboxane from the lung parenchymal cells is released, leading to vasoconstriction of the pulmonary vasculature, hypoxia, and development of RDS (Littleton, 1988).

Development of lactic acidosis secondary to increased oxygen debt from abnormal cellular metabolism is a common finding in patients with septic shock. Increased cellular metabolic demands lead to proteolysis, increased gluconeogenesis, increased serum insulin concentrations, and lipolysis.

Early identification of septic shock and initiation of appropriate therapies may decrease the mortality associated with this complication. Interventions are directed toward decreasing the cellular oxygen debt, maintaining cardiovascular stability, and reducing bacterial endotoxins. Supplemental oxygen can be administered by either nasal cannula or face mask. Endotracheal or nasotracheal intubation with mechanical ventilation and PEEP may be required to maintain Pa_{O_2} levels and decrease pulmonary shunting. A patient on PEEP must be monitored for the development of decreased pulmonary compliance or pneumothorax. Increased respiratory effort, pain, deterioration of arterial blood gas concentrations, decreased oxygen saturation levels, increased peak inspiratory pressures, and abnormal changes in breath sounds indicate these complications.

Cardiovascular hemodynamics need to be maintained and supported. Administration of the pharmacologic agents dobutamine or dopamine may be required to increase myocardial contractility and systemic vascular resistance. Adequate fluid replacement, avoiding overhydration, with a balanced electrolyte solution is critical for maintaining tissue perfusion. Continual monitoring of arterial blood pressure, mean arterial pressure, central venous pressure, pulmonary artery pressure, and pulmonary capillary wedge pressure and calculation of cardiac output and cardiac index are mandatory measures in the evaluation of hemodynamic status. Administration of beta-endorphin inhibitors such as naloxone to counter the effects of hypotension caused by endogenous opioid peptids released by septic organs has been studied. Naloxone has proved effective in producing short-term reversal of hypotension but has not yet significantly changed patient survival (Gaudette and Browne, 1986).

Administration of appropriate antibiotic therapy to reduce circulating endotoxins must be started as early as possible. Such therapy may be done prophylactically in the resuscitation phase of care or following development of an increase in body temperature. Utilization of sterile technique for dressing changes, care of drains, line insertion sites, or other invasive procedures is mandatory to minimize bacterial introduction into an already compromized trauma patient.

Altered Patterns of Urinary Elimination

Renal function may be impaired in the trauma patient due to either the systemic effects of trauma or actual injury to the renal system. Acute renal failure is a sequela of sustained circulating volume loss (prerenal failure), direct injury to the kidney (intrarenal failure), or obstruction in the drainage system (postrenal failure). The trauma patient is at risk for the development of acute renal failure from any of these causes.

Trauma patients who have experienced a shock state or low cardiac output have experienced a significant reduction in renal blood flow. This decreased blood flow reduces the normal glomerular filtration rate as well as other functions of the kidney, thereby leading to prerenal failure.

Intrarenal failure is caused by actual renal tissue damage, nephrotoxicity resulting from administration of nephrotoxic antibiotics, or development of rhabdomyolysis. When large muscles are damaged, as often occurs with traumatic injury, myoglobin is released into the systemic circulation. As the blood passes through the renal structures, myoglobin becomes trapped in the tubules, causing rhabdomyolysis and intrarenal failure.

Postrenal failure may be the result of injury, increased pressure, or displacement of postrenal structures. Administration of medications, such as ganglionic blocking agents or antihistamines, can interrupt the autonomic nervous supply to the postrenal structures, thereby causing obstruction.

Assessment data must be continually monitored to analyze the trends of renal function. Urinalysis provides information about specific gravity and the presence of substances such as protein, myoglobin, and white or red blood cells. Creatinine and blood urea nitrogen (BUN) levels are indicators of renal function. Elevated levels of creatinine and BUN are indicative of decreased renal function. Total urine output measurements provide additional information about renal function.

Three phases occur in patients with acute renal failure. These phases are related to the amount of urine produced by the patient in 24 hours. Oliguria is the first phase. Urine output decreases to less than 600 mL/24 hours. Patients experience fluid retention and electrolyte imbalances. This phase usually lasts from 10 to 21 days (Cardona and associates, 1988). The second phase is diuresis. Urine output now increases to 1000 to 6000 mL/24 hours. However, even though the total urine output has increased, the kidneys' ability to concentrate urine is nonspecific or nonfunctioning (Cardona and associates, 1988). Recovery marks the third phase. This phase may last anywhere from 3 to 12 months. Urine output and renal function return to normal. However, some patients may later develop chronic renal failure (Cardona and colleagues, 1988).

Treatment for trauma patients with acute renal failure depends on the cause and severity of the failure. Some patients may recover fully after removal of the underlying cause, whereas others may require treatment with hemodialysis.

Altered Nutrition: Less Than Body Requirements

Nutritional demands of the trauma patient are significantly increased due to alterations in metabolism. The healthy, noninjured person normally maintains a nutritional balance between the anabolic and catabolic processes that exist in the body. Because of the high energy demands and metabolic alterations that often are present in critically injured patients, the catabolic process tends to predominate, thereby increasing a nutritional imbalance.

Carbohydrates are the preferred energy source within the body. The final transport compound of carbohydrate metabolism is glucose, which provides energy in the form of adenosine triphosphate (ATP). Excess amounts of carbohydrates or glucose are stored in the liver, muscle, and fat in the form of glycogen. If necessary, in time of stress or increased metabolic demands, glycogen is released from these storage areas to meet energy or metabolic demands. Proteins, a second energy source, are also stored in the body and provide supplemental calories when necessary. Proteins function in the body's transport system and chemical reactions. Osmotic pressure gradients are maintained by available proteins. However, the main function of proteins is related to tissue synthesis. Fats, the third energy source, serve as a major energy reservoir. Fats act as an insulating and protective component for the body.

Once an injury occurs, systemic energy demands are increased. The body's metabolism is increased by activation of the sympathetic response. Other conditions such as hypoxia, pain, decreased fluid volume, anxiety, tissue injury, and decreased resistance to infection further stimulate the sympathetic response, and a hypermetabolic stress state is induced. Available glucose is used rapidly as the provider substrate for energy, followed by initiation of glycogenolysis, the metabolism of glycogen stores. As high energy demands continue, formation of glucose from stored protein and fats (gluconeogenesis) occurs. This period of metabolic response to injury has been termed the ebb or shock phase and encompasses a period of time during the first 24 to 48 hours after injury (Richardson and colleagues, 1987). During the ebb phase there may actually be an overall weight gain due to fluid retention.

The second, or flow phase, begins at the end of the ebb phase and lasts until recovery (Richardson and colleagues, 1987). This phase is the catabolic phase. The patient's metabolic rates increase and usually peak 5 to 10 days post injury. The average increase in metabolic rate (above the basal metabolic rate) ranges from 12% to 20% (Richardson and associates, 1987). During the flow phase, protein catabolism is continuous, and fat often acts as the main energy substrate. Nutritional imbalances easily occur due to the body's increased caloric and protein needs and the patient's inability to ingest nutritional supplements. Patients may demonstrate decreased body mass, increased metabolic needs, increased oxygen consumption, increased carbon dioxide production, delayed wound healing, and a weakened immune system (Cardona and associates, 1988).

Baseline nutritional assessments are done early in the critical care phase. Assessment data should include a history of the patient's previous caloric and protein intake, weight-height ratios, anthropometric measures of the triceps skin fold or midarm circumference, and biochemical measures such as creatinine-height index, serum proteins, nitrogen balance, total lymphocyte count, and metabolic rate (Cardona and associates, 1988).

Nutritional replacement for the trauma patient should be instituted no later than 3 to 4 days post injury. Patients who are kept NPO (nothing by oral route) for a prolonged period of time are susceptible to the development of stress ulcers. This complication can delay the healing process. Decisions on the route of administration and the rate and concentration of nutritional replacement are best accomplished using a team approach. This team should include the physician, nurse, and nutritional support personnel. Nutritional support may be administered by the oral, enteral, or parenteral route; the oral route is indicated in noncomplicated cases.

The enteral route includes the use of an oral-nasal gastric feeding tube, a jejunostomy tube, or, for long-term use, a gastrostomy tube. If the oral-nasal gastric route is used, care must be taken to place the tube correctly. This can be accomplished by visualizing the feeding tube in the stomach on radiologic film. A soft Silastic tube in a small French size is ideally used because it will prevent unnecessary pressure on the nostrils and esophagus. Patients who are receiving nutritional support through the enteral route need to be monitored for tolerance to the supplements; those receiving concentrated hyperosmolar feeding solutions may experience diarrhea. Intolerance to nutritional formulas is demonstrated by patient complaints of nausea or vomiting, abdominal distention, diarrhea, or abdominal pain. Prior to administration of nutritional feedings, the head of the bed should be elevated to 45 degrees to facilitate infusion of the solution and prevent aspiration. Feedings may be administered by either bolus or continuous infusion. Osmolality of the feeding formula may range from 300 mOsm (isotonic) to 850 mOsm (hypertonic). The starting formula osmolality is usually isotonic or a diluted (one-half to one-fourth) hypertonic strength (Cardona and associates, 1988).

Parenteral nutritional support is administered by either partial (PPN) or total (TPN) methods. Partial parenteral nutritional support is infused through the peripheral veins. It is a short-term administration method and must be used in conjunction with administration of lipids. The dextrose concentration is usually between 5% and 10% (Cardona and colleagues, 1988).

Total parenteral nutritional support is instituted in patients who are unable to resume gastrointestinal

nutritional intake for a minimum of 5 days. Total parenteral nutritional support is infused through tubing placed in the superior vena cava. The glucose content is a hyperosmolar concentration. The insertion site and the TPN line itself must be given meticulous care to prevent infection related to the presence of the hyperosmolar formula. Lipid administration should also occur in conjunction with TPN nutritional support. The patient must be monitored for tolerance to TPN as well as serum and urine osmolality levels. Urine is monitored for increased glucose and acetone levels, which indicate glucose intolerance. Liver function tests must be monitored because TPN can cause alterations in liver function.

Decisions about nutritional support for the trauma patient are made on an individual basis. The goal is to provide the patient with balanced nutritional support. Excess replacement can produce physiologic stress on the body by increasing oxygen consumption and carbon dioxide production. Additionally, fatty infiltrates may develop in the liver, producing other complications. Inadequate replacement often results in body protein loss, delayed wound healing, and decreased resistance to infectious processes (Richardson and associates, 1987).

CONTINUING CARE

Trauma patients require very specialized nursing care during their critical care hospitalization. The majority of these patients were young, healthy, productive citizens prior to injury. MacKenzie and associates (1988) studied the functional ability of 479 trauma patients 1 year after injury. This study indicated that, of head- or brain-injured patients (the most common type of traumatic injury), 5% were still convalescing 1 year post injury, and 75% of those that had been employed in full-time work prior to injury had returned to full-time employment (MacKenzie and colleagues, 1988). This, however, leaves a significant percentage of trauma patients that were unable to return to preinjury levels of function. The psychosocial aspects of trauma patient care need to be incorporated into the critical care phase of hospitalization. This again is best accomplished by a multidisplinary approach involving the physician, nursing staff, social service personnel, physical therapists, occupational therapists, and family members.

References

American College of Surgeons, Committee on Trauma (1976). Optimal hospital resources for care of the severely injured. *Bulletin of American College of Surgeons*, 61, 15–22.
American College of Surgeons, Committee on Trauma (1984). *Advanced trauma life support course: Instructors manual*. Chicago: American College of Surgeons.
American College of Surgeons, Committee on Trauma (1986). *Hospital and prehospital resources for optimal care of the injured*

patient and appendices A through J. Chicago, American College of Surgeons.

Barach, E., Tomlanovich, M., Nowak, R. (1986). Ballistics: A pathophysiologic examination of the wounding mechanism of firearms: Part I. *Journal of Trauma*, 26(3), 114–124.

Baxt, W. G. (1985). *Trauma: The first hour.* Norwalk, CT: Appleton-Century-Crofts.

Bires, B. A., and Sparger, G. (1988). Trauma. In N. M. Holloway (Ed.), *Nursing the critically ill adult* (3rd ed.). Menlo Park, CA: Addison-Wesley Publishing Company.

Blaisdell, F., and Schlobohm, R. (1973). The respiratory distress syndrome: A review. *Surgery*, 74, 251–262.

Butler, V., and Campbell, S. (1988). Resuscitation in the operating room. *Trauma Quarterly*, 5(1), 57–61.

Cales, R. H., and Heilig, R. W. (1986). *Trauma care systems: A guide to planning, implementation, operation, and evaluation.* Rockville, MD: Aspen Publishers.

Cardona, V. D., Hurn, P. D., Mason, P. J. B., et al. (1988). *Trauma nursing: From resuscitation through rehabilitation.* Philadelphia: W. B. Saunders.

Champion, H. R., Sacco, W. J., Carnazzo, A. J., et al. (1981). Trauma score. *Critical Care Medicine*, 9, 672–676.

Committee on Trauma Research, Commission of Life Sciences, National Research Council and the Institute of Medicine (1985). *Injury in America: A continuing public health problem.* Washington, D. C.: National Academy Press.

Conn, A. (1985). Hypovolemic shock. *Emergency Care Quarterly*, 1(2), 37–46.

Cowley, R. A., and Dunham, M. (1982). *Shock trauma/Critical care manual.* Baltimore: University Park Press.

DeOleveira, G. (1988). Adult respiratory distress syndrome (ARDS): The pathophysiological role of catecholamine-kinin interactions. *Journal of Trauma*, 28(2), 246–253.

Fackler, M. L. (1986). Wound ballistics. In D. D. Trunkey, and F. R. Lewis (Eds.), *Current therapy of trauma* (Vol. 2). Burlington, CA: Decker.

Gaudette, R., and Browne, B. (1986). Use of naloxone in septic shock. *Journal of Emergency Nursing*, 12(2), 81–84.

Gennarelli, T. A. (1984). Emergency department management of head injuries. *Emergency Medicine Clinics of North America*, 2(4), 749–760.

Grande, C. M. (1988). Airway management of the trauma patient in the resuscitation area of the trauma center. *Trauma Quarterly*, 5(1), 30–49.

Hallgren, R., Borg, T., Venge, P. et al. (1984). Signs of neutrophil and eosinophil activation in adult respiratory distress syndrome. *Critical Care Medicine*, 12, 14–18.

Hillery, T. (1988). Infectious complications in patients with severe head injury. *Journal of Trauma*, 28(11), 1575–1577.

Hochbaum, S. R. (1986). Emergency airway management. *Emergency Medicine Clinics of North America*, 4(3), 411–425.

Horowitz, M. D., Dove, D. B., Eismont, F. J., et al. (1985). Impalement injuries. *Journal of Trauma*, 25, 914–916.

Kelley, M. (1987). Unmasking pulmonary embolism. *Diagnosis*, 9(12), 46–60.

Koziol, J., Rush, B. F., Smith, S. M., et al. (1988). Occurrence of bacteremia during and after hemorrhagic shock. *Journal of Trauma*, 28(1), 10–16.

Littleton, M. (1988). Pathophysiology and assessment of sepsis and septic shock. *Critical Care Nursing Quarterly*, 11(1), 30–47.

MacKenzie, E., Siegel, J. H., Shapiro, S., et al. (1988). Functional recovery and medical costs of trauma: An analysis by type and severity of injury. *Journal of Trauma*, 28(3), 281–297.

Morris, I. R. (1988). Pharmacologic aids to intubation and the rapid sequence induction. *Emergency Clinics of North America*, 6(4), 753–768.

National Academy of Sciences, National Research Council (1966). *Accidental death and disability: The neglected disease of modern society.* Washington, D. C.: U. S. Government Printing Office.

Ordog, G. J., Wasserberger, J., and Balasurbramanium, S. (1984). Wound ballistics: Theory and practice. *Annals of Emergency Medicine*, 13, 1113–1122.

Ornato, J., Mlinek, E. J., Craren, E. J., et al. (1985). Ineffectiveness of the trauma score and the CRAMS scale for accurately triaging patients to trauma centers. *Annals of Emergency Medicine*, 14, 1061–1064.

Rea, R. (1987). *Trauma nursing core course: Instructors manual.* Chicago: Award Printing Corp.

Richardson, J. (1987). *Trauma: Clinical care and pathophysiology.* Chicago: Year Book.

Saba, T. (1983). Potential value of fibronectin in the treatment of organ failure with septicemia following trauma. *Current Concepts in Trauma Care*, 8–15.

Schonfeld, S. A., Ploysongsang, Y., DiLisio, R., et al. (1983). Fat embolism prophylaxis with corticosteroids: A prospective study in high-risk patients. *Annals of Internal Medicine*, 99, 438–443.

Shea, S. S. (1986). Bullet embolism. *Journal of Emergency Nursing*, 11(6), 300–303.

Slotman, G. J., Burchard, K. W., DArezzo, A., et al. (1988). Ketoconazole prevents acute respiratory failure in critically ill surgical patients. *Journal of Trauma*, 28(5), 648–654.

Strange, J. M. (1987). *Shock trauma care plans.* Springhouse, PA: Springhouse Corporation.

Swan, K. G., and Swan, R. C. (1980). *Gunshot wounds: Pathophysiology and management.* Littleton, MA: PSG Publishing.

Thompson, J. M., McFarland, G. K., Hirsch, J. E., et al. (1986). *Clinical nursing.* St. Louis: C. V. Mosby.

Trunkey, D. (1983). Trauma. *Scientific American*, 249, 28–35.

West, J. G. (Ed.) (1983). *Trauma care systems: Clinical, financial, and political considerations.* New York: Praeger.

NOTES TO FIGURE 57-2 (p. 1226)

Step I Physiologic status thresholds are values of the Glasgow Coma Score, blood pressure, and respiratory rate from which further deviations from normal are associated with less than a 90 percent probability of survival. Used in this manner, prehospital values can be included in the admission trauma score and the quality assessment process.

A variety of physiologic severity scores have been used for prehospital triage and have been found to be accurate. The scores contained in the triage guidelines, however, are believed to be the simplest to perform, and provide an accurate basis for field triage based on physiologic abnormality.

Step II Even in the presence of normal physiology, it is important to evaluate the likely presence of injuries that should be treated in a trauma center. A patient who has normal vital signs at the scene of the accident may still have a serious or lethal injury. Accurate diagnosis of life-threatening injury at the accident scene is unlikely. Thus, it is essential to look for indications that significant forces were applied to the body.

Evidence of damage to the automobile can be a helpful guideline to the change in velocity ($^\wedge$V). A $^\wedge$V of 20 mph will produce an ISS of greater than 15 in 90 percent of automobile crash occupants. $^\wedge$V can be estimated if one inch of vehicular deformity is equated to approximate one mph of $^\wedge$V.

Step III Certain other factors that might lower the threshold at which patients should be treated in trauma centers must be considered in field triage. These include the following:

A. Age Patients over age 55 have an increased risk of death from even moderately severe injuries. Patients younger than age 5 have certain characteristics that may merit treatment in a trauma center with special resources for children.

B. Co-morbid Factors The presence of significant cardiac, respiratory, or metabolic diseases are additional factors that may merit the triage of patients with moderately severe head injury to trauma centers.

Step IV It is the general intention of these triage guidelines to select patients with an ISS of greater than 15 for trauma center care. Patients with this level of ISS have at least a 10 percent risk of dying from a single severe or multiple serious injuries. When there is doubt, the patient is often best evaluated in a trauma center.

CHAPTER 58

Patients with Sepsis

Cynthia Allen
John M. Clochesy

During the past 40 years, the most common cause of death in many intensive care units is shock secondary to sepsis (Parrillo, 1989b). Sepsis is a physiologic response to a systemic inflammatory process. Extensive tissue damage and necrosis, the invasion of microorganisms or various cellular byproducts from these conditions trigger the human body's inflammatory response system. Sepsis with its causative factors creates perfusion and metabolic abnormalities. Manifestations of sepsis syndrome include tachycardia, fever or hypothermia, tachypnea, and inadequate organ perfusion (shock) or organ failure (Bone and colleagues, 1989).

SIGNIFICANCE

Yearly, an estimated $200 million and 1.4 million hospital days are expended due to nosocomial bacteremias (Hoyt, 1990). In the 1950s, nosocomial infections were not well understood. However, as the use of indwelling urinary catheters associated with the management of dysfunctional urinary bladder syndromes became more common in the late 1940s, mechanisms of catheter-associated urinary tract infections became evident. The use of various invasive devices has proven that any microorganism, given a port of entry, can produce an infection.

In the past, the circulatory instability seen in septic shock was attributed solely to circulating microorganisms (bacteria, viruses, fungi, rickettsia, spirochetes, protozoa, parasites). However, current research attributes the pathogenesis of septic shock to various chemical mediators produced during the body's inflammatory response (Parrillo, 1989a).

Neither sepsis nor septic shock is a reportable disease. Therefore, an accurate estimate of the current incidence is not available (Parrillo, 1989b). How-

ever, baseline data can be estimated from the complications associated with gram-negative bacteremia. The Centers for Disease Control estimates that 140,000 cases of gram-negative bacteremia occur annually in the United States (Roach, 1990). Yet bacteremia does not always create systemic complications. Complications occur when patients' cardiovascular systems are compromised by circulating chemical mediators released from the inflammatory response. Regardless of the cause, mortality statistics for all septic conditions remain high. When the diagnosis of sepsis is followed by prompt therapy, mortality ranges from 40% to 60%. However, if management is delayed or ineffective, mortality increases to 90% to 95%.

Approximately 1 out of 100 hospitalized patients develops sepsis, and 40% of these experience septic shock. The reasons for this are multifactorial (Parrillo, 1989b). First, invasive devices or procedures increase the risk of microbial invasion. Second, the use of antineoplastic and immunosuppressive therapies decreases patients' immune response, allowing bacterial cells to infect the circulatory system. Third, the widespread use of antimicrobial therapy creates drug-resistant pathogens. Last, modern technology, in all aspects of health care, has lengthened the lifespan of our society to the point where individuals are living longer with chronic diseases.

SUSCEPTIBILITY

To delineate a single causative factor of septic shock is often impossible. Signs and symptoms of the inflammatory response can result from a vast array of problems including infection, hematoma formation, dehydration, drug or transfusion reactions, atelectasis, or tissue necrosis. Infections result from many factors. The probability of infection is related to the number of organisms present, their ability to cause disease (virulence), and patients' degree of resistance. Any direct access for microbial invasion or condition that compromises tissue perfusion can devitalize tissue and foster the environment in which microorganisms flourish. Microorganisms produce various toxic substances that play an important role in triggering the inflammatory response. Gram-negative bacteria (*Escherichia coli, Klebsiella* sp., *Enterobacter* sp., *Serratia* sp., *Pseudomonas aeruginosa, Bacteroides* sp., and *Proteus* sp.) produce endotoxin. *Staphylococcus aureus*, a gram-positive bacillus, produces an endotoxin known as leukocidin (Massanari, 1989). Leukocidin damages the circulating white blood cells, especially neutrophils, which are essential for the removal of cellular debris and bacteria. These endotoxins activate several components of the complement, coagulation, kallikrein-kinin, and plasminogen-plasmin cascade systems.

Resistance to microbial invasion and systemic complications depends on a range of host-related and treatment-related risk factors listed in Table 58–1. Many of the interventions used to support organ function in critically ill patients interfere with normal defense mechanisms. For example, the benefits of a nasogastric tube can become unbalanced when sinusitis or gastric colonization of microorganisms develops. When integrated with other risk factors, such as histamine-2 blocking agents, excessive antacid therapy, gastric lavage and suctioning, or development of stress ulcers, this common device can foster infection by disturbing patients' protective gastric acid and mucosal barrier.

A debilitated individual is susceptible to colonization of microorganisms in the lungs. The presence of a nasal or oral endotracheal tube impedes the normal defense mechanisms of mucosal clearing and glottic closure. Thoracic or abdominal surgical procedures can create limitations in chest wall function. A reduction in inspiratory and expiratory forces can foster the accumulation of secretions and create an optimal environment for microbial colonization. At the other extreme, barotrauma from excessive positive end-expiratory pressure or tidal volumes during mechanical ventilation can also increase the potential for developing pneumonia and empyema. The function of the central nervous system's sensory and motor components form an integral defense mechanism. A paralyzed patient, as a result of neuromuscular blockade or a transected spinal cord, is more susceptible to infection due to compromised protective mechanisms such as coughing and withdrawal reflexes. Bedridden and immobilized patients are at risk for developing pneumonia due to gravitational forces that create pooling of secretions in the dependent lung area and atelectasis.

Trauma patients are extremely susceptible to infection for many reasons. The conditions of the accident, extent of the injury and physiologic characteristics, and the disturbance in the anatomic defense mechanisms that result from injury or therapy trigger multiple pathologic events (Hoyt, 1989). Operative procedures and diagnostic tests requiring cannulation into the vascular system interrupt the protective barrier of intact skin.

Coagulase-negative staphylcocci, coagulase-positive staphylcocci, aerobic and anaerobic streptococci, diphtheroids, and *Bacillus* are species of the skin's normal flora (Hoyt, 1990). These organisms regulate the pH of the skin and prevent colonization of pathogenic organisms. However, normal flora become pathogenic when the delicate balance between the normal flora and defense mechanisms is disturbed. Failure to resolve the inflammatory response or eliminate the causative organism creates the grave prognosis associated with sepsis.

STIMULUS-RESPONSE SYSTEMS PRECIPITATING SEPTIC SHOCK

The body's immunologic surveillance system and inflammatory response direct immunogenic cells to sites of injury and infection. Any type of cellular damage or microbial infection initiates an acute inflammatory response. This response results in increased blood flow and vascular permeability to allow immunogenic cells to reach the sites of injury or infection. One of the immunogenic cells that travels to the site of injury or infection is the macrophage. Macrophages, mononuclear phagocytes derived from bone marrow, are capable of (1) adhering to foreign cells to initiate an antibody response, (2) engulfing particulate matter, and (3) recognizing, attaching to, and destroying foreign cells. Granulocytes, another type of white blood cell, are further differentiated into basophils, eosiniphils, and neutrophils. Activation of granulocytes is thought to amplify various

---

TABLE 58–1. Factors Decreasing Resistance to Microbial Invasion and Systemic Complications of Sepsis

Host-Related
Burns
Trauma
Malnutrition
Leukemia
Age over 70 years
Debilitating disease states, especially chronic lung disease, cardiovascular disease, diabetes mellitus, renal or liver failure
Pregnancy
Immunocompromised state

Treatment-Related
Foreign body insertion, including difficulty with insertion and emergency insertion
Drugs, especially immunosuppressives, cytotoxics, and antibiotics
Artificial airways (endotracheal and tracheostomy tubes)
Surgery
Immobility

TABLE 58–2. Chemical Mediators of Sepsis

Endotoxin
Oxygen radicals
Interleukin-1 (IL-1) and interleukin-2 (IL-2)
Tumor necrosis factor (TNF)
Arachidonic acid cascade
   Prostaglandins
   Thromboxane
   Prostacyclin
   Leukotrienes
Complement cascade
Coagulation and fibrinolytic cascades
Bradykinin
Myocardial depressant factor
Beta-endorphin

physiologic responses in patients with sepsis (Stroud and colleagues, 1990).

The second aspect of the inflammatory response involves the release of numerous chemotactic factors from immunogenic cells or microbes. The chemical mediators currently identified in sepsis are listed in Table 58–2. Several others may be undiscovered at this time (Parrillo, 1989a). The chemical mediators involved in the development of sepsis create major alterations in the peripheral vasculature and heart (Parrillo, 1989a).

CHEMICAL MEDIATORS

Endotoxin

Endotoxins, lipopolysaccharides, are a component of gram-negative microbes' cell membranes. Microbial cells lysis or reperfusion of the microcirculation following ischemia due to various shock states, hypoxemia, ischemia, radiation injury, vasoconstriction therapy, burns, trauma and graft rejection can liber-

ate endotoxins into the systemic circulation (Stroud and associates, 1990). Circulating endotoxins activate several protein systems that create many pathophysiologic alterations, displayed in Figure 58–1.

Oxygen Radicals

Endotoxins activate macrophages that release monokines. In addition, in the response that endotoxins are capable of activating, macrophages release toxic oxygen-free radicals and proteolytic enzymes. The released superoxide ions or single oxygen molecules form hydrogen peroxide. In the presence of iron, these oxygen radicals create extremely destructive hydroxyl radicals. Under normal circumstances, the body's antioxidant system limits the destructive nature of this reaction. However, septic patients have depleted their antioxidant defense mechanisms (Stroud and associates, 1990). In sepsis, alveolar epithelial cells are especially vulnerable to the destructive effects produced by this reaction. Other toxic products released by macrophages include interleukin-1 (IL-1) and tumor necrosis factor (TNF).

Interleukin-1 and Interleukin-2

When macrophages are stimulated they secrete a substantial amount of the glycoprotein called interleukin-1. A smaller amount of IL-1 is produced by endothelial cells, epithelial cells, dendritic cells, neutrophils, and B-lymphocytes. All cells capable of synthesizing IL-1 can be stimulated by (1) other inflammatory mediators, (2) cells of the immune system, (3) agents that induce DNA synthesis and proliferation of cells, and (4) various latex or silica particles (Coleman and colleagues, 1989).

Interleukin-1 produces a series of chemotactic

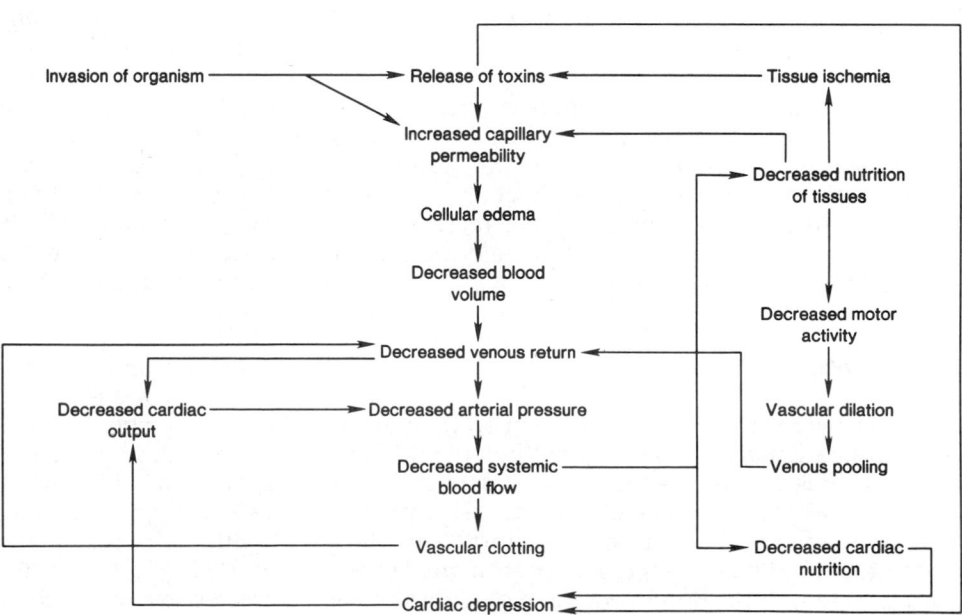

FIGURE 58–1. Schematic diagram of the feedback mechanisms in progressive shock. (Reprinted from Critical Care Nursing Quarterly, Vol. 7, No. 4, p. 63, with permission of Aspen Publishers, Inc., © 1985.)

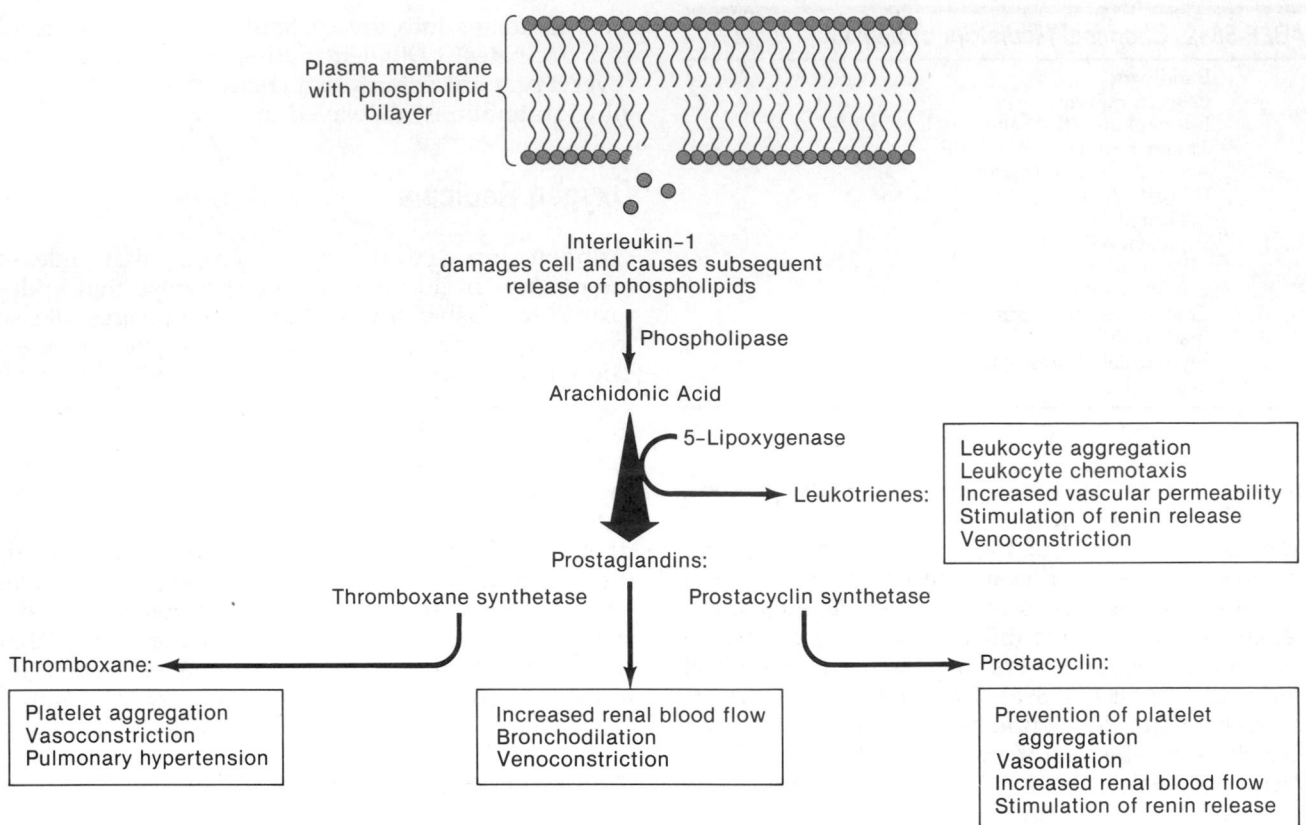

FIGURE 58–2. Arachidonic acid cascade and role of mediators in sepsis.

events. During an inflammatory response this chemical mediator is responsible for facilitating the movement of white blood cells toward injured, ischemic, or infected cells. IL-1 stimulates the release of arachidonic acid from phospholipids located in plasma membranes. Administration of IL-1 during experimental animal studies produces fevers, hypotension, and a decrease in systemic vascular resistance (Parrillo, 1989a). In addition to these responses, IL-1 and its metabolite, proteolysis-inducing factor, break down muscle protein.

Interleukin-1 and other components of cellular immunity activate the production of interleukin-2 (IL-2). IL-2 plays a role in the decreased blood pressure, decreased systemic vascular resistance, decreased left ventricular ejection fraction, increased left ventricular end-diastolic volume, increased cardiac output, and increased heart rate that occur during sepsis (Parrillo, 1989a).

Tumor Necrosis Factor

Tumor necrosis factor, also known as cachexin or cachectin, is a macrophage-derived polypeptide hormone. TNF is capable of stimulating platelet-activating factors as well as prostaglandin and IL-1 production. The role of TNF as a mediator is not fully understood, but it appears to have detrimental effects during sepsis. Protection from organ dysfunction has

been noted to occur in animals receiving TNF monoclonal antibodies 2 hours prior to experimental bacteremia (Tracey and associates, 1987).

Arachidonic Acid Cascade

The discovery of 3 of the currently identified 87 arachidonic acid metabolites (leukotriene, thromboxane, prostacyclin) collectively known as eicosanoids began in the late 1970s. Arachidonic acid, the fatty acid precursor present in membrane phospholipids, can be liberated by endotoxins, cellular agitation, or hypoxia. The arachidonic acid cascade is activated and controlled by specific enzymes, as shown in Figure 58–2. Once arachidonic acid is released from the cell membrane, it can be metabolized by two major pathways, one resulting in the prostaglandin family and the other in the leukotriene family of compounds.

Prostaglandin. Fatty acid cyclo-oxygenase metabolizes arachidonic acid into prostaglandins and other stable metabolites such as thromboxane and prostacyclin. During an overwhelming inflammatory response, arachidonic acid metabolites and damaged vascular endothelium often inhibit prostaglandin synthesis. Prostaglandins are potent vasodilators, and they attempt to balance the adverse effects created by other chemical mediators in the arachidonic acid cascade. For instance, prostaglandins create cerebral vasodilation to balance the cerebral vasoconstricting property of thromboxane. An imbalance in thromboxane and prostaglandin levels creates the central nervous system, pulmonary, and fibrin-fibrinolysis disturbances seen in sepsis (Reines and Haluska, 1989).

Thromboxane. This chemical mediator plays an important role in the clinical manifestation and sequence of events seen during sepsis. The maldistribution of blood flow during sepsis is attributed to thromboxane's potent vasoconstricting and platelet-aggregating effect. Tissue ischemia is a consequence of hypoperfusion initiated by this mediator.

Prostacyclin. One clinical manifestation of septic shock is largely due to the release of prostacyclin from the walls of blood vessels. Prostacyclin is a potent vasodilator and antiaggregant. The initial decrease in the patient's systemic vascular resistance is due to the widespread production of this mediator by the vascular endothelium (Littleton, 1988). The production and quantity of chemical mediator release depends on the specific tissue of origin.

Leukotrienes. The other major pathway in the arachidonic acid cascade leads to the production of the slow-reacting substances of anaphylaxis, collectively referred to as leukotrienes. Several authors hypothesize that leukotrienes are associated with increased capillary endothelial permeability (Reines and Haluska, 1989; Vane and Botting, 1989). Leukotrienes produce increased tissue permeability, bronchoconstriction, and a chemical response activating more neutrophils. The cyclic nature of the disease develops through the actions of neutrophils, free oxygen radicals, IL-1, and TNF as well as antigenic substances capable of activating neutrophils in an immunocompetent individual and synthesizing leukotrienes.

Complement Cascade System

An important defense mechanism against foreign cells is achieved through activation of a group of serum proteins that constitutes the complement system. A deficiency of complement components can increase a patient's susceptibility to infection. An inflammatory response can disturb the complement system's delicate balance of cellular destruction and clearance. The biologic effects of this cascade include cell lysis, stimulation of smooth muscle contraction, mast cell degradation, neutrophil chemotaxis, and activation of phagocytosis.

There are two mechanisms by which the complement cascade can be activated, the classic and the alternative pathways. The classic pathway is activated by immunocompetent cells as a result of an antibody binding to a cell surface or forming an antibody-antigen complex. In contrast, the alternative pathway does not require immunocompetent cells and is activated by the carbohydrate portion of a microbe's cell membrane. Regardless of the initiating pathway, the process generates a cascade of active molecules that initiate inflammatory and lytic reactions.

The complement cascade's biologic activity is not limited entirely to cell lysis. Various intermediate components in the complement cascade are important factors in the pathogenesis of sepsis (Fig. 58–3). For example, one component of the cascade, known as C5a, is an anaphylotoxin that produces mediator release by mast cells and, when bound to macrophages, releases IL-1. The amount of histamine released from mast cells during sepsis may not account for the increased vascular permeability and decreased systemic vascular resistance seen in this condition (Parrillo, 1989a). Nevertheless, C5a plays a significant role in sepsis because neutrophilic aggregation, formation of multiple microemboli, hypoperfusion, and tissue necrosis augment the disease process. Another component of the complement cascade, C3a, binds to lymphokines secreted by suppressor T-lymphocytes, decreasing the amount of antibody produced. The complement system also contains specific components that amplify and inhibit the cascade. The sequential, controlled activation of complement components creates lysis targeted toward the activation stimulus. Yet during an overwhelming systemic inflammatory response the binding of complement components to target cells becomes less specific and controlled. This chaotic lysis of all cells further increases the release of other chemical mediators.

Coagulation and Fibrinolysis Cascade

Injury to the vascular endothelium initiates the formation of fibrin. The toxic effects of chemical mediators on blood vessels and cell membranes stimulate the release of the Hageman factor and tissue thromboplastin (Kirchner, 1982). Fibrin clot formation attempts to stabilize the site of injury. To keep the extent of clotting under control, the coagulation cascade also activates fibrinolysis. During sepsis, consumption of various factors in both systems creates mediator-induced disseminated intravascular coagulation (DIC).

Bradykinin

Kinins, polypeptides with vasodilatory properties, are normally inactive. Activation of the Hageman factor in the coagulation cascade or complement activation stimulates the prekallikrein system to release a potent vasodilator, bradykinin. The volume depletion characteristic of sepsis is a consequence of bradykinin's ability to create vasodilation and capillary leak.

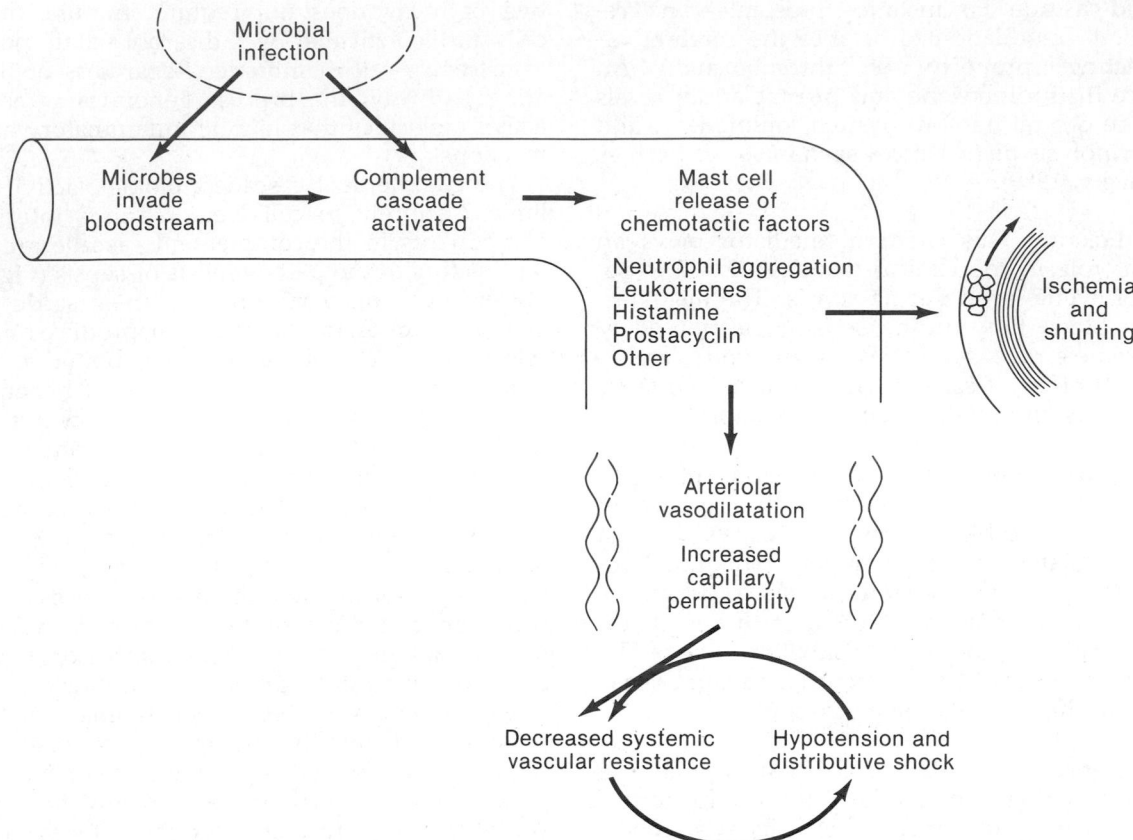

FIGURE 58–3. Activity of components.

Myocardial Depressant Factor

The prominent maldistribution of blood flow in patients with sepsis adversely affects tissue perfusion. An ischemic pancreatic cell releases a serum protein known as myocardial depressant factor (MDF). MDF has been found in at least 40% of patients with septic shock. It has not been found in nonseptic critically ill patients (Parrillo, 1989a). MDF causes a decrease in the degree and velocity of contractions of myocardial cells. The decrease in left and right ventricular ejection fractions is proportional to the amount of circulating MDF present (Parrillo, 1989a). Lactate production, respiratory decompensation, and pulmonary capillary wedge pressure increase in the presence of circulating MDF.

Beta-Endorphins

It is hypothesized that beta-endorphins, endogenous opiates located in the pituitary and hypothalamus, are released during the early phase of septic shock (Parrillo, 1989b). Maldistribution of blood flow, vasodilation, and cellular alterations precipitate the release of beta-endorphins. Once this opiate attaches to its receptor site within the central nervous system, inhibition of sympathomedullary transmission oc-

curs. Research further postulates that beta-endorphins may excite the parasympathetic efferent fibers of the heart (Schumann and Remington, 1990). Combined, these two actions produce peripheral vasodilation and a decrease in cardiac contractility, leading to the destructive pathogenic process of septic shock (Faden, 1980).

Other Chemical Mediators

Since septic shock is a multifactorial disease entity, no single mediator explains all of the responses resulting from the septic insult. In reviewing the published literature pertaining to this disease, it is understood that other mediators remain to be discovered and understood in the progression of septic shock.

PATHOPHYSIOLOGY

As the septic insult continues to stimulate various chemical inflammatory mediators, the body loses its characteristic homeostasis, and septic shock evolves. The severity and duration of the systemic inflammatory response determine a patient's clinical course. Manifestations of cardiovascular dysfunction are complex and often differ from patient to patient depending on the types of mediators released, the amount of mediator released, and the timing of mediator synthesis and release in combination with the host's ability to compensate (Parrillo, 1989b). In general, the chemical mediators of septic shock create three major effects within the cardiovascular system, specifically (1) vasodilation, (2) maldistribution of blood flow, and (3) myocardial depression.

Peripheral Vasodilation

Peripheral vasodilation is a result of activation of the arachidonic acid and complement cascades with subsequent release of vasoactive substances. Dilation in the arterial and venous circulation increases the diameter of the blood vessels, which in turn decreases systemic vascular resistance and preload. Initially, septic patients attempt to compensate by developing an increase in cardiac output. Yet tissue perfusion continues to decrease because of coinciding factors that create maldistributions of blood flow and cardiac dysfunction.

Maldistribution of Blood Flow

Although septic shock is usually associated with vasodilation, not all vessels experience this form of instability. The release of sympathetic catecholamines, angiotensin, and thromboxane creates pulmonary, renal, and splenic vasoconstriction. As a result, perfusion to some organs becomes compromised while other organs receive additional flow depending on the intravascular fluid status. Inadequate tissue perfusion also occurs due to vascular occlusion. The direct effects of microbial invasion and mediator release damage the vascular endothelium. Migration and aggregation of neutrophils and platelets to the damaged cells create thrombosis and potential embolic events. Maldistribution of blood flow is also a consequence of blood volume displacement. Histamine and bradykinin increase capillary permeability, allowing serum to migrate into the interstitial space. This fluid shift depletes the circulating volume and increases blood viscosity. The end result is irreversible cellular dysfunction secondary to inadequate tissue perfusion.

Cellular dysfunction results from disturbances within the cell membrane and inadequate blood flow. As cells are invaded by microorganisms or are traumatized, their membranes lose the ability to maintain a normal balance of intracellular and extracellular components. Disturbances of membrane integrity allow sodium and water to enter the cell freely. Electrolyte imbalances and cellular swelling alter the function of the cell. As a consequence, the cell becomes dysfunctional and eventually ruptures, releasing intracellular enzymes and membrane components that activate chemical mediators. Endotoxins create metabolic derangements by altering chemical

reactions in the cell's mitochondria. During an inflammatory response, the demand for oxygen exceeds the supply. As intracellular oxygen depletion occurs, anaerobic metabolism begins. Excessive amounts of lactic acid and minimal levels of adenosine triphosphate (ATP) are produced. A deficiency of ATP decreases the utilization of glucose and oxygen and disturbs the cell's selective membrane. Cell death and multiple organ system failure become inevitable as tissue destruction and energy depletion progress.

Myocardial Depression

A cell that is not directly attacked by inflammatory chemical mediators can experience cellular dysfunction as a result of selective vasoconstriction or microemboli within the circulatory system. For example, the liver and spleen become ischemic as blood is shunted to vital organs during septic shock. When pancreatic cells die, they release pancreatic enzymes such as lipase, amylase, and the chemical mediator MDF into the lymphatic and systemic circulations. As a result of the volume depletion and myocardial dysfunction that occur in this disease, most authors classify septic shock as a prototype of both cardiogenic and distributive shock. The cardiovascular pattern of patients who recover from septic shock consists of a high cardiac index (CI), low systemic vascular resistance (SVR), decreased left ventricular ejection fraction (LVEF), a dilated left ventricle, and a normal stroke volume (Parrillo, 1989a). Nonsurvivors of septic shock generally die from any of the following syndromes: hypotension due to a perpetual decrease in SVR, hypotension due to a decrease in CI, or multiple organ system failure (Parrillo, 1989a).

SIGNS AND SYMPTOMS

Nurses who maintain a vigilant awareness and are able to recognize trends in a patient's status play an extremely pivotal role in the course of this disease because proper early management often limits the destructive cyclic nature of septic shock. Septic shock is a syndrome that can create and maintain irreversible tissue damage until it or another disease claims the patient's life. Therefore, an understanding of the pathophysiologic changes, indicative clinical symptoms or laboratory results, and treatment modalities during the progression of this disease is imperative for providing optimal nursing care.

During the onset of sepsis, the patient shows the signs and symptoms of a systemic inflammatory response without any apparent profound cardiovascular changes. As microorganisms and toxic products enter the patient's bloodstream, a stress response is elicited, and energy expenditure increases. Stimulation of the patient's sympathetic nervous system creates an increase in heart rate and cardiac index.

During the stress response, glucagon is also released. Glucagon, a hormone produced by alpha cells in the islets of Langerhans, stimulates the conversion of glycogen to glucose in the liver. Under normal conditions (homeostasis), glucose is capable of supplying the body with energy.

The early cardinal signs of a systemic infection and an inflammatory response—tachycardia, tachypnea, and mental cloudiness—are due to circulating endotoxins (Rice, 1984). As the cells become infected with endotoxins, their ability to metabolize glucose diminishes, and metabolic alterations develop. As intracellular lactic acid increases during sepsis, neurons within the pons and medullary areas of the brain sense the increase in hydrogen ion concentration, causing the patient to begin to hyperventilate. Other mediators that create microemboli or vasoconstriction in the pulmonic or cerebral vessels increase the vascular resistance, thereby decreasing tissue perfusion.

Despite sympathetic stimulation, the septic patient's level of consciousness continues to deteriorate during an impending shock state. This clinical manifestation is often an indication of the severity of the disease. Cerebral blood flow is a reflection of cerebral perfusion pressure (CPP), and CPP is calculated from the mean arterial pressure (one-third of the pulse pressure plus the diastolic pressure) minus the intracranial pressure. As circulatory volume is redistributed during sepsis, systemic filling pressures are reduced. Therefore, indications of mediator-induced peripheral vasodilation may be shown by a declining trend in mean arterial pressure and noted clinically by the compromised perfusion pressure to the brain as well as other organs.

Another manifestation of sepsis can be noted by observing the appearance of the patient's skin. In the early stages of the disease, vasoactive mediators create a flushed appearance due to peripheral vasodilation. During an inflammatory response, activation of the white blood cells (WBCs) stimulates the release of endogenous pyrogens. Leukotrienes, prostaglandins, and interleukin-1 are endogenous pyrogens that are capable of circulating to the hypothalamus. Once at this location, the mediators signal the chemoreceptors in the thermoregulatory center to increase the set point of the body temperature as a protective mechanism to destroy microbes thermally. As the set point becomes elevated, the skeletal muscles shiver to generate heat, circulation to the skin decreases to minimize heat loss, and fever develops as a consequence. Depending on the temperature gradient (core vs. environmental temperatures) and the degree of peripheral vasodilation, body heat may dissipate. Therefore, although fever is often described as one of the cardinal signs of an infection, a patient can experience hypothermia (core temperature below 35°C) during sepsis. Elderly patients and patients who have sustained burns, spinal cord injuries, or extensive soft tissue injuries also lose the skin's thermoregulatory function, and a hypothermic set point develops (Hoyt, 1989). Again, the impor-

tance of observing trends in a patient's condition remains crucial.

As an inflammatory response develops, leukopenia (WBC count less than 5000/mL) is an early finding in a septic immunocompetent patient. As endotoxins and chemical mediators adhere to the surface of WBCs, these WBCs become "tagged" and removed from circulation by the reticuloendothelial system (macrophages, Kupffer cells of the liver, reticular cells of the lungs, bone marrow, spleen, and lymph nodes). This clearance process initially reduces the patient's serum WBC count. As sepsis progresses, the septic insult develops a synergistic effect with the patient's immune system because the inflammatory response signals the bone marrow to accelerate leukocyte synthesis and release. Consequently, more WBCs are released into the circulation, and some cells, especially neutrophils, are immature. This process is reflected in a complete blood count, in which the WBC count will be greater than 10,000/mm³ and a shift to the left is present.

Approximately one-third of patients with septicemia experience manifestations of septic shock (Rice, 1984). The clinical manifestations and progression of septic shock depend on the patient's circulatory volume (Hoyt, 1989). The initial cardiovascular pattern of septic shock consists of a high cardiac index and a low systemic vascular resistance (Parrillo, 1989a). There is a discrepancy in the literature about whether septic patients can be divided into two groups, hyperdynamic and hypodynamic, during the initial onset of septic shock. The category of hyperdynamic, or warm septic shock, denotes a septic patient who has bounding pulses, warm skin, an elevated cardiac index, and a reduced systemic vascular resistance. Hypodynamic, or cold septic shock, describes a septic patient who has thready pulses, cool skin, decreased cardiac index, and an elevated systemic vascular resistance. Prior to the 1970s, septic patients generally were inadequately hydrated (Parrillo, 1989a). At that time, inadequate fluid replacement was assumed to be a method for preventing pulmonary edema and the consequences of respiratory distress during sepsis. As knowledge of adult respiratory distress syndrome (ARDS) and its causes increased, this assumption that fluid overload was the sole contributing factor in ARDS was disregarded. Researchers have reevaluated the historical data that originally formed these two categories, and they now believe that volume depletion and a reduction in preload were factors that contributed to the patient's low cardiac index. Today, aggressive volume replacement and vasoactive therapy are used in the management of septic shock because a patient's survival is jeopardized within the first hour of shock (Hoyt, 1989).

A common indicator in all forms of shock (cardiogenic, extracardiac obstructive, oligemic, and distributive) is reduced blood flow to several tissues (Parrillo, 1989b). The chemical mediators of septic shock produce profound effects on the peripheral vasculature and myocardium. As mediators impair the host's normal vasomotor reflexes, autoregulation of the capillary perfusion pressure becomes impaired (Parrillo, 1989a). As a result, some organs are hypoperfused and others receive an abundance of blood flow. Shunting of blood increases as the microvasculature becomes occluded with fibrin or aggregates of leukocytes, platelets, and damaged cells during the inflammatory response. Gross peripheral maldistribution of blood flow is also due to an increase in capillary membrane permeability. Although the predominant vascular effect precipitating septic shock is vasodilation, some vascular beds develop severe vasoconstriction. In either case, tissue perfusion ultimately becomes deranged despite the presence of a high CI, and the organs most frequently affected are the kidneys, liver, brain, and lungs.

The kidney is an organ with an abundant eicosanoid supply and cyclo-oxygenase activity. Renal blood flow, excretion of sodium and water, creatine clearance, and renin release are all affected by the production of thromboxane and prostaglandins during sepsis. As renal blood flow in the patient in septic shock is reduced, urine output decreases, and the body is unable to eliminate waste products. As chemical mediators continue to shunt blood to various organs, the patient's liver becomes hypoperfused. Hyperbilirubinemia and jaundice are common clinical indicators that this organ is becoming adversely affected during the systemic inflammatory response.

As a septic patient's mean arterial pressure falls below 60 mm Hg, irreversible tissue damage occurs due to the compromised cerebral and pulmonary perfusion pressures. A multitude of factors in the neurologic sensorium change in the septic shock patient, but one imbalance specific to the sequence of events in this disease is that between thromboxane and prostacyclin. The lungs also are a target organ throughout the progression of septic shock. As the patient's serum lactate level increases, the respiratory system attempts to compensate. Circulating endotoxins further debilitate the pulmonary status of the patient because the initial pulmonary response to endotoxins creates bronchoconstriction (Luce, 1987). Consequently, an increase in airway resistance requires the patient's respiratory muscles to generate a greater degree of negative inspiratory force or pressure to allow optimal ventilation. During the progression of septic shock, a ventilation-perfusion mismatch develops as chemical mediators create pulmonary interstitial edema and maldistributions in pulmonic blood flow. As pneumocytes experience a decrease in perfusion, surfactant synthesis diminishes and lung compliance decreases. The risks of developing ARDS from sepsis alone or in combination with the occurrence of septic shock are cited to be, respectively, 4% to 10% and 40% to 60% (Luce, 1987).

Septic shock is a generalized process that involves many organs. In addition to vasomotor dysfunction, several authors relate the occurrence of myocardial depression to the development of septic shock (Ellrodt and colleagues, 1985; Parrillo and associates,

1985; Parker and associates, 1984). Intracellular disturbances, namely, the reduction of calcium ions within the sarcoplasmic reticulum, limit the excitation-contraction mechanism that is vital for proper functioning of myocardial cells. Effective myocardial contractility is also reduced by the presence of circulating myocardial depressant substances or factors (MDF), which decrease LVEF (Parrillo, 1989a). Experimental data link early myocardial depression to circulating MDF and have recognized a pattern in the recovery from septic shock in that these patients experience a normal LVEF and an absence of circulating MDF 10 days after the onset of shock (Parrillo, 1989b). As stated earlier, many septic shock patients experience cardiac dysfunction with ventricular dilatation and a decrease in ejection fraction. The exact cause of these phenomena is not known. It was once believed that a reduction in coronary blood flow and myocardial ischemia precipitated the development of myocardial depression. To date, however, there is no evidence supporting a reduction in coronary blood flow or ischemia as the cause of early myocardial depression in septic shock (Parrillo, 1989b).

The compensatory mechanism of an increase in CI to maintain perfusion may be attributed to five factors: (1) left ventricular dilatation, (2) decreased ejection fraction, (3) increased left ventricular end-diastolic volume index (EDVI), (4) decreased SVR, and (5) an increase in heart rate (Parrillo, 1989a). The ability to calculate a patient's EDVI is important because the measurements represent ventricular volume or preload. Institution of therapy that reflects these hemodynamic patterns, a decrease in LVEF and an increase in EDVI, increases a septic shock patient's chances of survival because it allows simultaneous increases in CI, HR, and normal or elevated stroke volume.

MANAGEMENT

The principles involved in the management of sepsis and septic shock are based on the pathogenic mechanisms and degree of organ dysfunction present. Early diagnosis of septic shock is usually possible from the clinical manifestations. Prompt recognition of a systemic inflammatory response is imperative in that early recognition and prompt management often prevent the progression of the disease. The nurse's highest priority in caring for a suspected septic patient is continual observation of trends in the patient's condition. The priorities of care become twofold because indicative trends, or other diagnostic results, confirm the diagnosis of sepsis or an impending shock state. Aggressive management is required to augment tissue perfusion and prevent metabolic derangements and tissue death. The goals of therapy focus on eradicating the precipitating septic insult, maintaining blood pressure and organ perfusion, and reducing serum lactate levels (Parrillo, 1989b).

Intervention

CRITICAL CARE ENVIRONMENT

The cardiovascular and metabolic abnormalities involved in septic shock can produce hemodynamic changes in unpredictable ways and time frames. Therefore, monitoring the septic patient in a critical care setting is important for a variety of reasons. First, the patient's chances of survival are increased when hemodynamic monitoring guides the initiation and duration of treatment. Second, the insidious and progressive nature of sepsis and septic shock mandates hemodynamic monitoring for noting trends and guiding management. Continuous electrocardiographic monitoring is important because septic patients are at risk for developing atrial tachycardia with occasional episodes of ventricular tachycardia. Invasive pressure devices (arterial blood pressure and the hemodynamic parameters obtained from a pulmonary artery thermodilution catheter) provide serial measurements relating to the cardiovascular status of the patient. Because of the fluctuations in blood pressure and the inaccuracy of cuff pressures during septic shock, arterial blood pressure monitoring provides the most accurate method of measurement. The diagnosis of septic shock is made or confirmed by the patient's hemodynamic profile obtained from a thermodilution pulmonary artery catheter. For example, if a patient presents with a decreased SVR, an increased or decreased CI, and a narrow arterial-venous mixed venous oxygen content difference, he is experiencing distinguishable characteristics of septic shock. By implementing nursing measures for infection control, arterial lines remain beneficial in managing septic patients because the catheter provides access for diagnostic testing (arterial blood gas analysis, serum lactate and electrolyte levels) without augmenting the cascade of chemical mediator release that occurs through excessive venipunctures.

ANTIMICROBIAL THERAPY

Due to the cascade of events that can trigger the sepsis syndrome, a single definitive cause of the inflammatory response may be unidentifiable. It is important to realize that a causative microorganism cannot be detected in 50% of cases of sepsis (Parrillo, 1989b). Clinical manifestations of sepsis with negative blood cultures may be a result of improper culture technique, failure to locate any specific site of infection, intermittent invasion of the bloodstream by microorganisms, or chemical mediators leaking into the bloodstream from a secluded origin of infection or tissue necrosis. Because sepsis syndrome can develop from other causes besides microorganism invasion, a definitive diagnosis is not solely dependent on culture results. However, in a patient in whom sepsis is suspected, specimens (urine, blood, sputum, cerebral spinal fluid, or wound drainage) should be analyzed for culture and antibiotic sensi-

tivity results. Once cultures have been obtained, initial antibiotic therapy should be based on consideration of the antibiotic susceptibilities and resistance patterns within the institution (Roach, 1990). Administration of a broad-spectrum third-generation cephalosporin is also recommended in combination with an aminoglycoside to provide coverage against all of the pathogens harbored within some settings (Parrillo, 1989b; Roach, 1990). Diagnostic viewing of internal body organs and cavities may also be helpful in locating a nidus of infection. After interpreting the results of all of the diagnostic tests, the goal of management is to select the antimicrobial drug that is sensitive to the identified microbe and capable of circulating to the infected body site. But it is important to remember that sepsis is a "toxic" syndrome and antibiotic therapy is often ineffective in preventing the consequences of the inflammatory response. Due to the complex pathophysiology of sepsis antimicrobial therapy is a limited "cure-all" for the disease because (1) a microbe may fail to be identified during a culture; (2) a microbe can develop resistance to antimicrobial therapy; (3) superinfection is a risk of antimicrobial therapy; and (4) hemodynamic instability can develop from the progression of the disease or as a consequence of endotoxin release during antimicrobial therapy. Therefore, during the first 48 to 72 hours of septic shock, other treatment modalities are imperative to reverse or limit hemodynamic instability.

VOLUME REPLACEMENT

Restoration of adequate intravascular volume is an important aspect of patient care during episodes of hypotension. The combination of vasodilation and third-spacing during sepsis produces a dramatic decrease in preload and afterload pressures. Indicators of low contractility, such as a decreased left ventricular stroke work index (LVSWI) or right ventricular stroke work index (RVSWI), can result from the reduction in preload or from circulating MDFs. The amount and type of fluids administered to a septic patient depend on the pulmonary artery wedge pressure (PAWP) and the composition of the intravascular fluid. One author (Parrillo, 1989b) recommends the following: (1) If the patient's hematocrit is less than 30%, administer blood as a volume expander; (2) if the patient's albumin concentration is less than 2.0 g/dL, administer 50 to 100 g of albumin; (3) if neither of the two previous conditions is present, a crystalloid solution chosen to correct any existing electrolyte abnormalities should be administered. There is no definite guide to what type of fluid resuscitation is superior to ensure adequate cardiovascular performance or a favorable outcome. Yet choice of the appropriate amount of fluid is very important during therapy. During an infusion the patient's arterial blood pressure can be used as a guide to fluid requirements if (1) the arterial pressure rapidly responds to the fluid replacement and maintains a MAP of 60 mm Hg or greater, (2) there is no question about the definitive diagnosis of septic shock, and (3) there is no evidence of heart failure. If the patient fails to meet these criteria, the PAWP and LVEF are useful guides for estimating volume requirements. During an infusion the PAWP should be maintained at 12 to 18 mm Hg. The decision to increase a PAWP from 12 to 16 to 18 mm Hg depends on ventricular function and other goals of therapy. A Starling curve can be plotted from the values obtained from hemodynamic parameters. Simultaneous plotting of the patient's LVSWI, PAWP, and CI will show the degree to which the myocardial cells are functioning in relation to the progression or management of the disease. Other criteria indicating the therapeutic success of volume replacement and eradication of the septic insult include (1) a MAP greater than 60 mm Hg, (2) a blood flow that remains adequate for normal CNS, kidney, and lung function (evidenced by indirect measurements such as urine output greater than 20 mL/hour and adequate arterial blood gas values) and arterial blood lactate levels of below 2.2 mmol/dL (Parrillo, 1989a).

VASOPRESSOR THERAPY

Vasopressor therapy is generally not used during the initial management of septic shock but is indicated when fluids fail to restore intravascular volume and adequate tissue perfusion (Parrillo et al., 1990). Therefore, if the septic patient remains hypotensive when fluid replacement has increased the PCWP to 18 mm Hg, vasopressor therapy is generally instituted. Some clinicians prefer to maintain preload pressures at normal levels and support the circulation with vasoactive drugs, the rationale for this being that elevated filling pressures do not improve the cardiac output for all patients, and excessive filling pressures may increase edema formation and oxygen requirements.

Several authors (Parrillo, 1989b; Parrillo et al., 1990; Luce, 1987) recommend the following guidelines relating vasoactive support during septic shock. In general, dopamine is the initial vasopressor of choice because the type of stimulation that it produces is dependent on the infusion rate, and dopamine can be combined with other agents to achieve various therapeutic effects. At low doses, 2 to 4 μg/kg per minute, dopamine increases renal blood flow and in some individuals will create a moderate pressor effect by increasing cardiac performance. Heart rate and contractility increase as the beta-adrenergic effects of dopamine predominate at doses of 5 to 10 μg/kg per minute. Alpha-adrenergic (vasoconstrictive) effects predominate at levels above 10 μg/kg per minute. If dopamine is ineffective at raising the patient's MAP above 60 mm Hg with an infusion rate of 20 μg/kg per minute, a more potent vasopressor is administered. Levarterenol (Levophed), a powerful alpha-adrenergic agonist with moderate beta-adrenergic activity, is useful during septic shock when loss of vasomotor tone predominates. This drug is usually infused at a rate of 2 to 8 μg/minute and is titrated to maintain blood pressure. Due to its potent vasoconstrictor effect, dopamine at low doses is often employed to enhance renal blood flow when the renal vasculature is adversely affected (Schaer and colleagues, 1985). Epinephrine and phenylephrine are also potent vasopressors used to maintain arterial pressure with an infusion rate of 1 to 8 μg/minute and 20 to 200 μg/minute, respectively. If the patient is experiencing tachyarrhythmias, phenylephrine is a useful vasoconstrictor because it is a pure alpha-adrenergic drug and therefore does not directly stimulate the heart.

VASODILATOR THERAPY

Theoretically, the use of vasodilators to enhance perfusion through vasoconstricted vessels during septic shock seems rational. Yet due to the unpredictable pharmacologic activity of vasodilation on the systemic vessels, the benefits of improving the maldistribution of blood flow by this method during septic shock are limited. Nonspecific vasodilation is potentially harmful when the patient's blood pressure is low. Therefore, until vasodilator therapy can focus on specific pathologically constricted vessels, this group of drugs is generally not beneficial in the treatment of septic shock (Parrillo, 1989a).

OXYGEN THERAPY

Patients with septic shock may suffer from a variety of adverse effects, including (1) bronchoconstriction, (2) compensatory mechanisms placing an increased workload on respiratory muscles, (3) pulmonary hypertension, (4) destruction of lung tissue, and (5) increased capillary permeability, with resultant respiratory failure. Ventilatory therapy with positive end-expiratory pressure (PEEP) or continuous positive airway pressure (CPAP) is often beneficial for oxygenation. Positive pressure fails to decrease the amount of extravascular fluid in the lungs, but it does improve the systemic arterial oxygen tension by increasing the alveolar diameter or redistributing the intra-alveolar fluid into the interstitial spaces of the lung (Luce, 1987). The risk of barotrauma is potentiated by the occurrence of parenchymal lung disease in sepsis; therefore, the lowest amount of positive pressure that adequately saturates the patient's hemoglobin is generally used.

CORTICOSTEROIDS

In the management of septic shock, the difference between the dosage of corticosteroids needed to produce a beneficial result and the margin of safety remains controversial. The fundamental principles that justify the use of corticosteroids as an adjunctive therapy in sepsis are based on investigational data demonstrating that corticosteroids (1) inhibit complement activation, (2) prevent complement-induced neutrophil aggregation, (3) stabilize lysosomal membranes, and (4) inhibit prostaglandin and thromboxane synthesis through membrane stabilization. One drawback to this list of benefits is that, because this drug is administered over an extended period of time, the possibility of superinfection increases because the drug inhibits leukocyte function. (*Note*: Corticosteroid use is controversial, and the administration of this drug should be reserved for septic patients with suspected or documented adrenal insufficiency [Parrillo et al., 1990].) Therefore, a septic patient does not generally benefit from this drug because it may prolong the course of illness.

NUTRITIONAL SUPPORT

During the initial phase of shock, nutrition is not a priority. But once the septic patient is hemodynamically stable, nutritional support is a necessity because the patient experiences increased energy demands due to the stress, fever, shock state, and inflammatory process. In choosing nutritional support one must consider whether the supplement will benefit the host or the inflammatory process. If feasible, it is recommended that a high-protein source of enteral feedings with an iso-osmotic content be instituted. Due to the nature of sepsis, shunting of blood away from the gut may limit the possibility of this route of nutritional support, and parenteral therapy may be required. In the event that parenteral feedings become necessary, glucose content is minimized in the early phase of the disease and advanced during recovery. Lipids are generally limited to 10% to 15% of the patient's total caloric requirements. Lipids or fat emulsions provide a source of neutral triglycerides, unsaturated fatty acids, glycerol, and egg yolk phospholipids. Because the destructive properties of sepsis can be triggered by the arachidonic acid cascade and consumption of dietary linoleic acid (which is a derivative of arachidonic acid) as well as other complex lipids, the concentration of fat emulsions may be crucial in preventing excessive amounts of fatty acid administration from potentiating mediator release.

Experimental Therapies

NALOXONE (NARCAN)

The mechanism of action of naloxone in septic shock is not fully understood, but it is thought to reverse the endogenous opiate-induced hypotension and decreased cardiac contractility that occur during the onset of septic shock (Schumann and Remington, 1990). The results obtained from various research studies in which naloxone was administered during endotoxic shock are inconsistent. The use of naloxone in conjunction with other therapies, the timing of naloxone administration, and the amount given dif-

fer, posing questions about the validity of the results. Therefore, the clinical use of naloxone during septic shock is under investigation, and one author feels that this disease may be a challenge to the present effective pharmacologic actions due to the fact that acidosis, hypothermia, and serum glucose imbalances, all of which are common manifestations of sepsis, antagonize naloxone (Schumann and Remington, 1990).

INHIBITORS OF PROSTAGLANDIN SYNTHESIS

With the discovery of various arachidonic acid metabolites, the metabolic pathways and enzyme intermediates have also been revealed. Anti-inflammatory steroids, namely corticosteroids, prevent the formation of prostaglandin, thromboxane, and leukotriene metabolites because of the agents' ability to block the site of action that converts membrane phospholipids into arachidonic acid in the presence of phospholipase (Vane and Botting, 1989). Nonsteroidal anti-inflammatory drugs such as aspirin, ibuprofen, indomethacin, and meclofenamate also inhibit prostaglandin biosynthesis by blocking the activity of cyclo-oxygenase. This inhibits the formation of thromboxane, prostacyclin, and prostaglandin metabolites, but leukotriene metabolism is not affected. Since one pathway is blocked, it is possible that an accumulation of the precursor is present for activity through the other pathway as lipo-oxygenase converts arachidonic acid into leukotrienes. Therefore, even though the biosynthesis of some chemical mediators is reduced, the overall effect from this process may not be totally beneficial.

IMMUNE SUBSTRATES

Fortunately, as the pathogenesis of sepsis is becoming better understood, researchers are developing investigational therapies to eradicate the causative mediator activity. Therapies that appear to be most promising focus on agents that are capable of blocking either the pathogens responsible for sepsis or the body's immune response. Monoclonal antibodies to the endotoxin lipid A core, found in all gram-negative bacteria, have been developed (Zeigler and colleagues, 1982), and an increase in survival and improvement in organ system failure has been documented with various other specific serum immunoglobulins (Lachman and colleagues, 1984; Collins and Dorsey, 1984). Antiserum cachectin or tumor necrosis factor (TNF) is also undergoing investigational study. Experimental data suggests that the prophylactic use of this antibody in patients at risk for sepsis could deter the progression of any consequences. Survival is thought to be enhanced by the antibody's ability to improve cardiac output and limit the role of TNF in sepsis-associated myocardial depression (Tracey and colleagues, 1987). Future management incorporating antibodies or other pharmacologic inhibitors of endotoxins and the various inflammatory mediators will play a vital role in reversing the pathogenetic cascade of events in sepsis.

SUMMARY

Sepsis and its consequences require prompt recognition and early treatment to prevent its rapidly progressive and destructive consequences. Managing the septic patient is often a challenge, and effective nursing care requires an ability to identify and respond to various trends in the clinical course of the disease. By relating the patient's response and knowledge of the condition's pathophysiology to the sequence of events, the nurse can formulate measures that remain effective and are directed at eradicating the cause of the disease.

References

Bone, R. C., Fisher, C. J., Clemmer, T. P., et al. (1989). Sepsis syndrome: A valid clinical entity. *Critical Care Medicine*, 17(5), 389–393.

Bowton, D. L., Bertels, N. H, Prough, D. S., et al. (1989). Cerebral blood flow is reduced in patients with sepsis syndrome. *Critical Care Medicine*, 17(5), 399–403.

Burns, K. M. (1990). Vasoactive drug therapy in shock. *Critical Care Nursing Clinics of North America*, 2(2), 167–177.

Coleman, R. M., Lombard, M. F., Sicard, R. E., et al. (1989). *Fundamental Immunology*. Dubuque, IA. William C. Brown.

Collins, M. S., and Dorsey, J. H. (1984). Comparative anti–*Pseudomonas aeruginosa* activity of chemically modified and native immunoglobulin G (human), and potentiation of antibiotic protection against *Pseudomonas aeruginosa* and group B streptococcus in vivo. *American Journal of Medicine*, 30, 155–160.

Desjars, P., Pinaud, M., Bugnon, D., et al. (1989). Norepinephrine therapy has no deleterious renal effects in human septic shock. *Critical Care Medicine*, 17(5), 426–429.

Ellrodt, A. G., Riedinger, M. S., Kimchi, A., et al. (1985). Left ventricular performance in septic shock: Reversible segmental and global abnormalities. *American Heart Journal*, 10, 402–409.

Faden, A. L., and Holaday, J. W. (1980). Experimental endotoxin shock: The pathophysiologic function of endorphins and treatment with opiate antagonists. *Journal of Infectious Disease*, 142(2), 229–238.

Houston, M. C. (1990). Pathophysiology of shock. *Critical Care Clinics of North America*, 2(2), 143–149.

Hoyt, N. J. (1989). Host defense mechanisms and compromises in the trauma patient. *Critical Care Nursing Clinics of North America*, 1(4), 753–762.

Hoyt, N. J. (1990). Preventing septic shock: Infection control in the ICU. *Critical Care Nursing Clinics of North America*, 2(2), 287–296.

Keely, B. R. (1985). Septic shock. *Critical Care Nursing Quarterly*, March, 59–67.

Kirchner, C. W., and Reheis, C. (1982). Two serious complications of neoplasia—sepsis and disseminated intravascular coagulation. *Nursing Clinics of North America*, 17(4), 595–606.

Kuhn, M. M. (1990). Nutritional support for the shock patient. *Critical Care Nursing Clinics of North America*, 2(2), 201–220.

Lachman, E., Pitsoe, S. B., and Gaffin, S. L. (1984). Antilipopo-lysaccharide immunotherapy in management of septic shock of obstetric and gynaecological origin. *Lancet*, 1, 981–983.

Littleton, M. T. (1988). Pathophysiology and assessment of sepsis and septic shock. *Critical Care Nursing Quarterly*, 11(1), 30–47.

Luce, J. M. (1987). Pathogenesis and management of septic shock. *Chest*, 91(6), 883–888.

Massanari, R. M. (1989). Nosocomial infections in critical care units: Causation and prevention. *Critical Care Nursing Quarterly*, 11(4), 45–57.

Parker, M. M., Selhamer, J. H., and Bacharach, S. L. (1984). Profound but reversible myocardial depression in patients with septic shock. *Annals of Internal Medicine*, 100, 483–490.

Parrillo, J. E. (1989a). The cardiovascular response to human septic shock. In B. P. Fuhrman and W. C. Shoemaker (Eds.), *Critical Care: State of the Art* (pp. 285–314). Fullerton, CA: Society of Critical Care Medicine.

Parrillo, J. E. (1989b). Septic shock in humans: Clinical evaluation, pathophysiology & therapeutic approach. In W. C. Shoemaker, W. L. Thompson, P. H. Holbrook, et al. (Eds.), *Textbook of Critical Care* (2nd ed., pp. 1006–1023). Philadelphia: W. B. Saunders.

Parrillo, J. E., Burch, C., Shelhamer, J. H., et al. (1985). A circulating myocardial depressant substance in humans with septic shock. *Journal of Clinical Investigations*, 76, 1539–1553.

Parrillo, J. E., et al. (1990). Septic shock in humans: Advances in the understanding of pathogenesis, cardiovascular dysfunction, and therapy. *Annals of Internal Medicine*, 113(3), 227–242.

Rackow, E. C., Mecher, C., and Astiz, M. E., (1989). Effects of pentastarch and albumin infusion on cardiorespiratory function and coagulation in patients with severe sepsis and systemic hypoperfusion. *Critical Care Medicine*, 17(5), 394–398.

Rackow, E. C., et al. (1989). Systemic response to sepsis. *Critical Care Medicine*, 17(5), 483.

Reines, D. H. and Haluska, P. V. (1989). Arachidonic acid metabolites—the eicosanoids. In W. C. Shoemaker, W. L. Thompson, P. H. Holbrook, et al. (Eds.), *Textbook of Critical Care* (2nd ed., pp. 1028–1034). Philadelphia: W. B. Saunders.

Rice, V. (1984). The clinical continuum of septic shock. *Critical Care Nurse*, Sept.-Oct., 86–108.

Roach, A. C. (1990). Antibiotic therapy in septic shock. *Critical Care Nursing Clinics of North America*, 2(2), 179–186.

Schaer, G. L., Fink, M. B., and Parrillo, J. E. (1985). Norepinephrine alone versus norepinephrine plus low-dose dopamine: Enhanced renal blood flow with combination pressor therapy. *Critical Care Medicine*, 13, 492.

Schumann, L. L., and Remington, M. A. (1990). The use of naloxone in treating endotoxic shock. *Critical Care Nurse*, 10(2), 63–71.

Stroud, M., Swindell, B., and Bernard, G. R. (1990). Cellular and humoral mediators of sepsis syndrome. *Critical Care Nursing Clinics of North America*, 2(2), 151–160.

Tracey, K. J., Fong, Y., Hesse, D. G., et al. (1987). Anti-cachectin/TNF monoclonal antibodies prevent septic shock during lethal bacteraemia. *Nature*, 330(17), 662–664.

Vane, J. R., and Botting, R. M. (1989). Prostaglandins, prostacyclins, thromboxane, and leukotrienes: The arachidonic acid cascade. In B. P. Fuhrman and W. C. Shoemaker (Eds.), *Critical Care: State of the Art*, (pp. 1–23). Fullerton CA: Society of Critical Care Medicine.

Vincent, J. L., Roman, A., Kahn, R. J. (1990). Dobutamine administration in septic shock: Addition to a standard protocol. *Critical Care Medicine*, 18(7), 689–693.

Zeigler, E. J., McCutchan, J. A., Fierer, J., et al. (1982). Treatment of gram-negative bacteremia and shock with human antiserum to a mutant *Escherichia coli*. *New England Journal of Medicine*, 307, 1225–1230.

59

Patients with Shock

Jeremiah Suhl

Shock is the classic critical illness. Early recognition and prompt treatment are vitally important. Skillful management requires knowledge of sophisticated monitoring and support technology as well as an appreciation of the many devastating physiologic derangements that make shock so lethal. Despite advancing understanding and technologic development, mortality from most forms of shock is high, and care of patients with shock remains a most demanding and challenging task. This chapter deals with the mechanisms of shock, the varied diseases that result in shock, the clinical presentations of shock, and the general and specific treatments available.

DIAGNOSIS OF SHOCK

Shock is not a disease but the end result of many differing disease processes. For practical purposes, shock can best be defined as a condition in which systemic blood pressure is inadequate to provide perfusion to vital organs. This definition identifies two requirements for the diagnosis of shock. First, there must be a reduction in mean systemic blood pressure, usually to levels below 70 mm Hg. Second, there must be evidence of hypoperfusion of vital organs. The most important signs of this are altered mentation and low urine volume. Increased levels of lactic acid are also suggestive of the global ischemia resulting from shock.

MECHANISMS OF SHOCK

On a cellular level, shock is a condition of inadequate perfusion, that is, insufficient delivery of oxygenated blood and nutrients. Blood flow through a vascular bed is directly related to the perfusion pressure, that is, the difference between arterial and venous pressure. Therefore, as arterial pressure drops, blood flow drops, resulting in shock.

A large number of distinct diseases can cause shock, but each causes blood pressure to fall as a result of one or more basic physiologic mechanisms:

1. Cardiogenic shock: Failure of the heart as a pump.
2. Hypovolemic shock: Inadequate blood volume.
3. Obstructive shock: Obstruction in the central arteries or veins.
4. Distributive shock: Excessively rapid run-off of blood through the vascular beds.

Cardiogenic Shock

The heart may fail in its pumping function in a number of ways. The contractile elements may be unable to generate sufficient force. This occurs when at least 40% of the left ventricle has been damaged by infarction or diffusely injured by myositis. The contractility of the heart can be reversibly impaired by a variety of metabolic derangements such as severe hypoxemia, acidosis, hypoglycemia, or hypocalcemia.

Disturbances of heart rate can result in inadequate pump function. Because cardiac output is the product of heart rate and stroke volume, very slow rhythms (e.g., sinus bradycardia or heart block) reduce cardiac output despite a normal or even increased stroke volume. Very fast rhythms can reduce stroke volume because of insufficient diastolic filling time, resulting in a reduction in cardiac output despite the rapid heart rate.

Cardiac output may be severely impaired despite normal muscle function if the heart valves malfunction. Regurgitant or stenotic valve lesions can result in abrupt onset of shock and congestive heart failure.

Hypovolemic Shock

The normal heart can pump only the blood that returns from the systemic vasculature; therefore, a severe reduction in venous return will result in decreased cardiac output and shock. The volume of blood ejected from the ventricles is dependent on their "preload," which is the amount of stretch of the muscle fibers at the onset of contraction. Preload is represented most closely by the volume of blood present in the ventricle at the onset of contraction. Preload is mainly influenced by systemic venous pressure and ventricular compliance.

Systemic venous pressure is the pressure tending to force blood into the ventricles during diastolic filling. It is determined by the amount of systemic venous tone and the total volume of blood in the circulation, most of which is in the veins. Any condition reducing the venous tone or reducing intravascular volume can cause a decrease in venous return and hypovolemic shock. For example, central venous pressure is reduced in septic or anaphylactic shock in part because of mediators that cause venodilation are released into the circulation.

Compliance refers to the elasticity of the ventricles during diastolic filling. Compliance is reduced by myocardial ischemia or fibrosis and increased by infarction and some medications.

A loss of vascular volume can result from a loss of whole blood, plasma, or water. Blood may be lost externally, as in penetrating injuries; however, internal losses are common. Large quantities of blood may be lost into the gastrointestinal tract with no bleeding apparent at first. Several units of blood may hide in the thigh or pelvis or in the peritoneal, retroperitoneal, or pleural space. Loss of plasma can be significant in patients with extensive burns. Profound losses of water and electrolytes commonly accompany diabetes mellitus, severe diarrhea, or vomiting.

Obstructive Shock

Obstruction in the vascular tree can cause shock if the obstruction occurs in a central artery or vein that has no collateral route for blood flow.

Pulmonary Artery. The classic cause of obstructive shock is pulmonary thromboembolism (PE). Shock due to PE occurs in a small percentage of patients, usually when a large clot lodges in the main pulmonary artery at its first division ("saddle" embolus), thus obstructing blood flow to both lungs.

Aorta. The aorta may become obstructed by an acute dissection, in which a flap of the inner layer of the artery (the intima) occludes the true lumen.

Obstruction to Systemic Venous Return. Complete occlusion of either the superior or inferior vena cava does not itself result in shock because the collateral circulation is sufficient to provide venous return. Both vena cavae can be obstructed if the pressure surrounding them rises abnormally, thus compressing them and preventing venous return. This occurs in tension pneumothorax. The mechanism of shock in pericardial tamponade is often categorized as obstructive for similar reasons. When pressure surrounding the heart rises above systemic venous pressure, venous return ceases. The amount of increase in pericardial pressure depends on the amount of time in which the fluid accumulates. As little as 100 mL of rapidly accumulated pericardial fluid can cause tamponade, yet the pericardium can eventually stretch to accommodate liters of fluid. Most commonly, acute tamponade results from hemorrhage into the pericardium due to myocardial infarction, rupture or penetrating injury, or fluid accumulation due to inflammation, infection, renal failure, or tumor.

Distributive Shock

As discussed above, blood pressure depends on the balance between the blood added to the arterial tree with each heart beat and the blood that runs out of the arteries through the vascular beds. The run-off is generally controlled by smooth muscle cells surrounding the small precapillary arterioles. These "sphincters" regulate the distribution of the cardiac output to the vascular beds that are in need of blood supply. Normally, some smooth muscle tone in most arterioles is necessary to provide adequate arterial pressure.

NORMAL REGULATION OF ARTERIOLAR TONE

Arteriolar tone in each vascular bed is normally regulated by four known mechanisms: neural input, circulating mediators, autoregulation, and local mediators.

Neural Input. The arteriolar muscles are innervated by the sympathetic nervous system by means of two types of receptors. Alpha-adrenergic receptor stimulation results in vasoconstriction, whereas beta-adrenergic receptor stimulation results in vasodilation.

Circulating Mediators. A variety of blood-borne substances influence the arteriolar smooth muscle tone. Glucocorticoid hormones increase the sensitivity of muscle cells to catecholamines. Circulating catecholamines, angiotensin, and many inflammatory mediators directly affect vascular tone.

Autoregulation. Many vascular beds can regulate their blood flow within limits, despite fluctuations in arterial pressure, by means of a myogenic reflex. As pressure in the arterioles rises or falls, the smooth muscle contracts or relaxes, respectively, thus altering local vascular resistance to restore blood flow

TABLE 59–1. Vasoactive Mediators in Infectious Shock

Mediator	Source	Actions
Vasodilators		
Histamine	Mast cells, basophils	Decrease systemic vascular resistance
		Increase vascular permeability
		Augment GI motility
Prostaglandin E_2	Arachidonic acid	Decrease systemic vascular resistance
		Inhibit platelet aggregation
		Increase vascular permeability
		Activate production of cAMP
		Potentiate leukotriene effects
		Increase GI smooth-muscle contraction
Prostacyclin	Arachidonic acid	Decrease systemic vascular resistance
		Decrease pulmonary vascular resistance
		Increase vascular permeability
		Inhibit platelet aggregation
Endorphins	Autonomic system and CNS	Decrease systemic vascular resistance
		Reduce cardiac output and blood pressure
		Diminish GI motility
		Relieve pain and alter mood
		Enhance parasympathetic, inhibit sympathetic nervous system
Vasoconstrictors		
Thromboxane A_2, B_2	Arachidonic acid	Pulmonary and systemic vasoconstriction
		Enhance platelet aggregation
Leukotrienes C, D, E	Arachidonic acid	Promote smooth-muscle contraction
		Increase vascular permeability
		Increase systemic vascular resistance
Catecholamines	Adrenal gland and sympathetic outflow	Increase systemic vascular resistance

From Shoemaker, W. C., Ayres, S. M., Grenvik, A., et al. (Eds.). (1989). *Society of Critical Care Medicine: Textbook of Critical Care.* (2nd ed.). Philadelphia: W. B. Saunders.

toward normal. This is an important mechanism of blood flow regulation in the brain and kidneys.

Local Mediators. Perhaps the finest mechanism of control of blood flow to individual vascular beds is through the response of arteriolar smooth muscle to the products of metabolism generated by the tissues adjacent to the arteriole. Substances such as potassium, hydrogen ion, adenosine, carbon dioxide, and lactic acid are released from actively metabolizing cells and cause local vasodilation, resulting in delivery of greater blood flow to the vascular beds with higher metabolic activity.

In various disease states, abnormal substances released into the circulation can have powerful and widespread effects on arteriolar tone and thereby on regional blood flow. Considering that blood pressure is determined by cardiac output and systemic vascular resistance (SVR), if the cardiac output is unchanged, a drop in SVR will result in a reduction in blood pressure. In most cases, the cardiac output actually rises but not enough to compensate for the profound reduction in vascular resistance.

It may not be apparent at first glance why a patient in distributive shock is in trouble because his overall cardiac output may in fact be above normal despite a low arterial pressure. The answer lies in where that cardiac output goes. Inappropriate vasodilation occurs largely in vascular beds that normally receive a small amount of blood flow such as the skin and nonexercising muscles. Flow may also occur through arteriovenous anastomoses, which are direct connections from arteries to veins that allow blood to bypass capillary beds, leaving relatively less blood flow for the metabolically active vital organs.

CAUSES OF DISTRIBUTIVE SHOCK

The most frequent cause of distributive shock is sepsis, particularly gram-negative bacterial sepsis (Barnett and Sanford, 1969; Corrin, 1980; Shubin et al., 1977; Weil, 1977). The presence of bacteria and bacterial products in the circulation results in the activation of a large variety of mediators (Table 59–1), which are capable of interfering with the normal regulation of arteriolar tone (Luce, 1987). As a result, arteriolar tone is reduced inappropriately, and shock occurs. Shock occurring in sepsis is associated with a very high mortality.

Other conditions can cause distributive shock and should be considered in patients who have a shock state resembling that seen in sepsis. A variety of endocrine abnormalities can result in shock. It is important to recognize these because proper treatment can be life-saving. Adrenal insufficiency (Dorin, 1988), hyperthyroidism, and hypothyroidism can result in shock.

Anaphylactic shock is the most severe manifestation of allergy and can occur after exposure of sensitized individuals to drugs, foods, insect venoms, or other allergens. The mechanism of shock is largely distributive because release of histamine and other

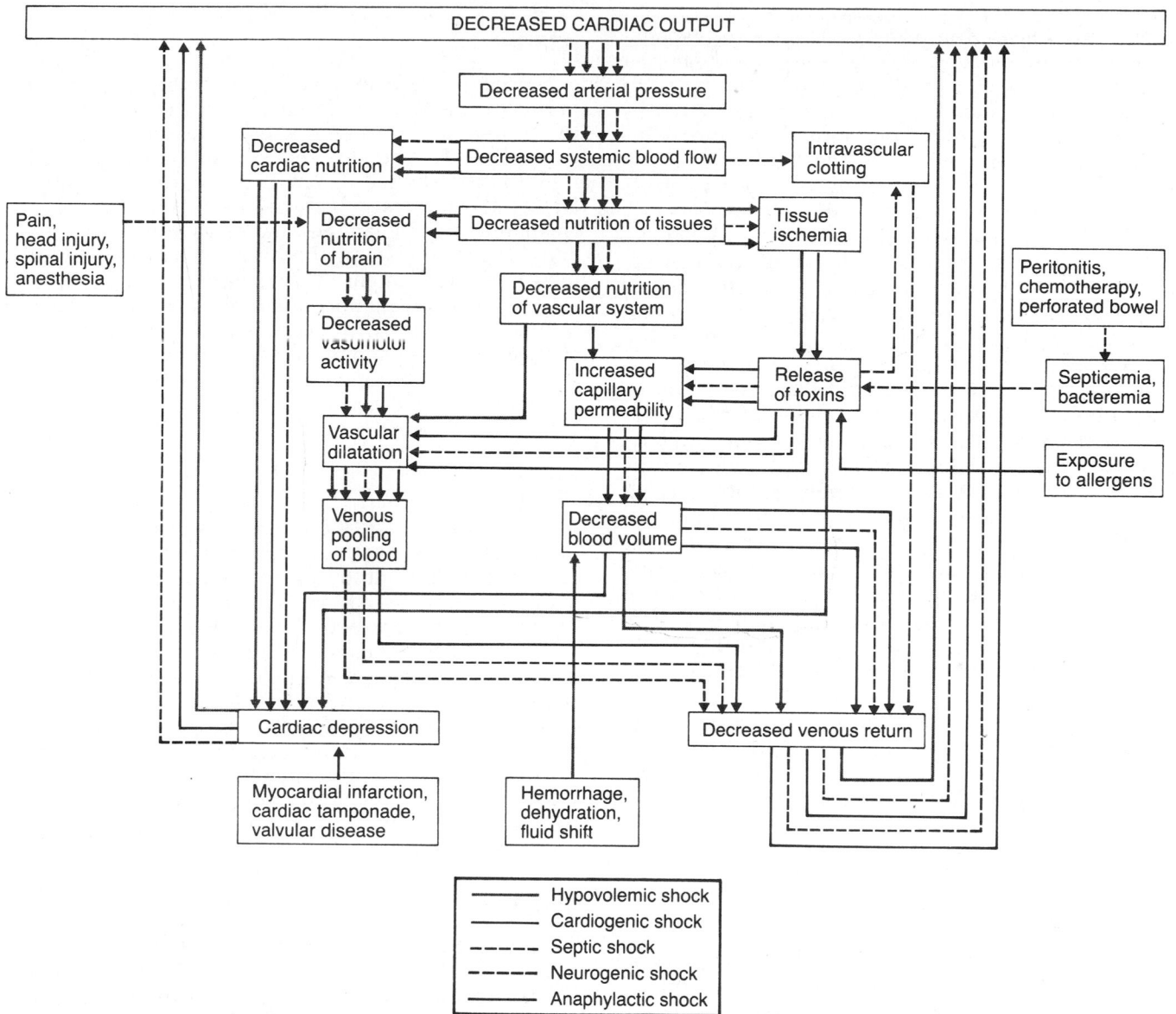

FIGURE 59-1. Initiators of shock and the futile cycles of physiologic compensation. (Modified from Guyton, A. C. (1986). *Textbook of medical physiology* (7th ed.). Philadelphia: W. B. Saunders; in Ignatavicius, D. D., and Bayne, M. V. (Eds.) (1991). *Medical-surgical nursing: A nursing process approach* (p. 404). Philadelphia: W. B. Saunders.)

vasoactive compounds from mast cells results in vasodilation and capillary leak. Anaphylactic shock is often accompanied by an urticarial rash, wheezing, or stridor. Drug or toxins such as opiates, barbiturates, and heavy metals can impair vascular tone. Metabolic derangements such as uremia, hepatic failure, respiratory failure, hypoglycemia, or severe acidosis can present with a similar picture of vasodilation and shock.

STAGES OF SHOCK

Compensated Shock

Early in the course of an illness that results in shock the body attempts to maintain homeostasis

and supports the blood pressure by a variety of mechanisms. (Fig. 59-1). Although perfusion is threatened, compensatory mechanisms can maintain arterial pressure, if only briefly.

Neural Response. The drop in blood pressure is sensed in the aortic and carotid bodies, which signal an increase in sympathetic nervous system activity to the heart and vessels. Contractility and heart rate are increased, thereby increasing cardiac output. Increased venous tone causes increased venous pressure for the same vascular volume, thus increasing venous return to the heart. In addition, arteriolar tone is increased, which decreases arterial run-off of blood, thus increasing arterial pressure.

Hormonal Response. In addition, a variety of hormones are released into the circulation in response to a drop in blood pressure. *Antidiuretic hormone (ADH)* is released from the posterior pituitary and results in vasoconstriction and retention of water by the kidneys. When blood pressure is low, the reduction in perfusion pressure to the kidney results in release of the renal hormone *renin*, which catalyses the transformation of renin substrate to *angiotensin-I*. Angiotensin-I is converted to *angiotensin-II* by angiotensin-converting enzyme (ACE) in the vascular epithelium of the lungs as well as other tissues including the heart, adrenals, kidneys, and brain. Angiotensin-II is a powerful vasoconstrictor. It also stimulates the production of *aldosterone* by the adrenal gland, which results in salt and water retention by the kidneys. Shock stimulates release of *adrenocorticotropic hormone (ACTH)* from the anterior pituitary, which stimulates the adrenal glands to release *cortisol*. Cortisol sensitizes the arteriolar smooth muscle to the effects of catecholamines. The adrenal medulla releases *epinephrine* and *norepinephrine*, which increase myocardial contractility, heart rate, and vascular resistance and help to regulate the distribution of blood flow to vital organs. The vasoconstriction and retention of water and salt induced by these hormones tend to restore blood pressure toward normal.

Autoregulation. Blood flow to vital organs is regulated by the myogenic reflex, as previously discussed. The brain, for example, is able to maintain an adequate blood flow with mean arterial pressures as low as 50 mm Hg.

Decompensated Shock

If the disease process continues, the blood pressure will eventually drop. At this stage, all vital organs have inadequate blood flow and become injured. Rapid correction of the underlying process is necessary to prevent death.

Irreversible Shock

If uncorrected, overt shock will lead to a complex spiral of cell injury giving rise to multiple organ failure and inevitable death. At this point, correction of the primary disorder will not prevent death.

COMPLICATIONS OF SHOCK

Although the shock state may be initiated by a specific disease process affecting only one organ, for example, hemorrhage from a duodenal ulcer, the resulting drop in organ perfusion causes secondary insults to all vital organs. These "innocent bystanders" become sufficiently injured to perpetuate the shock state even if the original cause is corrected.

Heart

The heart is jeopardized by shock because shock produces an unfavorable change in the balance between myocardial oxygen supply and demand. Decreased arterial pressure reduces the coronary blood flow and thereby reduces myocardial oxygen supply. Demand is increased because the reflex increase in circulating catecholamines increases the heart rate and contractile state of the heart. Afterload may be increased due to intense vasoconstriction. Reversible, segmental wall motion abnormalities have been found in patients with septic shock, suggesting ischemia. In many shock states, circulating "myocardial depressant factors" are released, which decrease contractility. Myocardial damage is frequently detected by isoenzymes following shock states.

Lung

Shock of any variety often results in injury to the lungs, manifest by progressive hypoxemia and diffuse pulmonary infiltrates called adult respiratory distress syndrome (ARDS). The mechanism for lung injury may involve activation of complement proteins, especially C3a and C5a, which promote aggregation of granulocytes in the lung. The granulocytes release proteolytic enzymes and toxic oxygen radicals that injure the lung. The resulting gas exchange abnormalities decrease oxygen delivery to the vital organs. Pulmonary capillaries become plugged with granulocytes and microthrombi, increasing pulmonary vascular resistance. This results in compromised right heart performance.

Intestine

An intact intestinal mucosa excludes gut bacteria and bacterial toxins from entering the circulation. Shock impairs the intestinal barrier, causing increased entry of bacteria or bacterial toxins into the bloodstream, thus further compromising the patient.

Liver

Shock frequently results in severe liver damage, with very high transaminase enzyme levels and centrilobular necrosis seen on biopsy. The liver is a key organ in the removal of drugs and toxins as well as in the synthesis of serum proteins and clotting factors, so hepatic dysfunction during shock can contribute to the coagulopathy and accumulation of toxins that can further perpetuate the shock process.

Humoral Factors

Shock of any cause can activate the complement and coagulation cascades and stimulate the release of bradykinin, beta-endorphins, myocardial depressant factors, tumor necrosis factor, prostaglandins, and other molecules that may further compromise the circulation (Stroud, et al., 1990).

It should be apparent by now that even if the

cause of shock is focal, for example, a bleeding duodenal ulcer, shock soon becomes a process of multisystem organ failure that itself prevents recovery. Recognition of shock in its earlier and reversible stages followed by prompt, aggressive, general, and specific treatments are the keys to successful management.

APPROACH TO THE PATIENT IN SHOCK

Recognition of Compensated Shock

The above mentioned compensation mechanisms may allow restoration of blood pressure temporarily, but if the disease process is not recognized and corrected promptly, the compensation mechanisms will be insufficient, and blood pressure and blood flow will drop. It is therefore important to become aware of the clinical signs that are the forerunners of overt shock, so that the disease process can be recognized and treated *before* the onset of overt shock.

Most of the signs and symptoms of compensated shock are due to an excess of catecholamines and other vasoconstricting hormones and an increased sympathetic neural activity to the heart and vasculature. The heartbeat is rapid. Ventilation becomes rapid and shallow. The skin is cold and clammy, especially in the extremities. Urine volume is reduced. The patient becomes restless and agitated. There may be a fine tremor of the hands or tongue.

In patients with septic shock or other forms of distributive shock in which hypotension is primarily due to inappropriate vasodilation, the extremities may remain warm. There may be a lacy blue appearance to the extremities, livedo reticularis, which is due to venodilation and slow flow of blood. The kneecaps may be cool.

Assessment of the Patient in Shock

Assessment of the patient should be done rapidly, almost simultaneously with initiation of appropriate treatment. This is necessary because the shock process is well underway by the time blood pressure is observed to drop, thanks to the body's compensatory mechanisms. It may be useful to narrow the spectrum of diseases that might cause shock to a few categories, which can be distinguished on the basis of two very simple physical observations: the distention of the neck veins and the warmth of the extremities. In patients with shock due primarily to a distributive mechanism, vasoconstriction will not occur appropriately in response to the shock stimulus, and therefore the skin will be inappropriately warm, especially over the legs and feet. Patients with the other physiologic mechanisms of shock will have an intact adaptive vasoconstriction response and will therefore have cold and often diaphoretic skin. Patients with

primarily hypovolemic shock will have flat neck veins, whereas those with obstructive or cardiogenic shock will have noticeably distended neck veins. Although these findings are by no means constant, this "quick and dirty" way to identify the mechanism of shock may help to focus on the likely cause. Although general therapy may be started immediately, a thorough history and physical examination will often provide the clues to the specific diagnosis and thus to specific therapy.

History. The patient may have complaints of pain, bleeding, or other localizing symptoms, such as dyspnea, which might pinpoint the cause. For example, tearing pain between the shoulder blades could signify an aortic dissection. The patient may have a past or present condition that is capable of causing shock. For example, a patient undergoing treatment for deep venous thrombosis who develops shock may have had a hemorrhage or pulmonary embolism. A patient with a history of drug allergy might be in shock from an anaphylactic reaction to a new drug he has received. Family members and friends may provide useful supplementary or confirmatory information.

Vital Signs. Fever or hypothermia may be a clue to sepsis. Hypothermia may also be seen in severe hypothyroidism, some types of drug intoxication, such as alcohol or barbiturate toxicity, or exposure. Ventilation may be labored in patients with pneumonia, sepsis, or severe metabolic acidosis such as diabetic ketoacidosis. On the other hand, quiet ventilation is seen in other types of drug intoxication, especially intoxication with narcotics, tranquilizers, or barbiturates. The change in systolic blood pressure during the respiratory cycle (pulsus paradoxus) may be abnormal (more than 10 mm Hg) in pericardial tamponade. An irregular pulse may be seen in patients with cardiac disease or pulmonary embolism.

General Inspection. There may be obvious evidence of trauma, bleeding, or infection. The aroma of the patient's breath may suggest a cause of shock, such as ketoacidosis (fruity), uremia (urine), hepatic failure (musky), or pulmonary infection (foul).

Skin. Cool skin is a sign of intact vasoconstriction. It may be associated with livedo reticularis, a lacy purple appearance of the skin in the extremities due to sluggish venous flow. This may be an early warning sign of impending shock. Cyanosis of the extremities or lips (acrocyanosis) signifies intense vasoconstriction and poor blood flow, whereas generalized cyanosis suggests severe hypoxemia due to poor gas exchange in the lungs. Skin turgor may be poor in patients with hypovolemic shock. It is best to check turgor in nonsun-damaged skin, such as the chest or buttocks, rather than the arms, where thinning of the skin may give the impression of poor tissue turgor. If the skin tents easily and does not return to its normal appearance immediately after release, turgor is reduced. The presence of urticaria may signify anaphylaxis, whereas petechiae suggest infection, especially meningococcemia or rickettsial infection, or severe thrombocytopenia. Jaundice or pallor denotes hepatic failure or anemia, respectively.

Head and Neck. Assessment of the neck veins is crucial. Because of the presence of venous valves, the external jugular vein may be unreliable. The internal jugular vein is a more reliable measure of central venous pressure. Neck stiffness might signify meningitis. A goiter or neck scar might suggest hypothyroidism. Tracheal shift may be a clue to tension pneumothorax.

Lungs. Unilaterally decreased breath sounds, together with a tracheal shift away from the affected lung and increased resonance to percussion, are classic findings in tension pneumothorax. Findings of basilar crackles are consistent with heart failure, whereas localized rales with dullness to percussion and bronchial breath sounds are found in patients with pneumonia. Wheezes may signify anaphylaxis, heart failure, or pulmonary embolism.

Heart. Massive pulmonary embolism may be evidenced by a right ventricular heave felt over the left sternal margin, or a loud second component of the second heart sound (P_2). Tamponade may be accompanied by a pericardial rub and heart failure by a third heart sound (S_3). Heart tones may be diminished in patients with cardiogenic shock, pneumothorax, or pericardial tamponade.

Abdomen. An abdominal site of sepsis or hemorrhage may be accompanied by guarding, rigidity, rebound tenderness, absent bowel sounds, or evidence of ascites.

Extremities. Half of patients with pulmonary embolism have some evidence of swelling, venous thrombosis (cord), or pain in the calves or thighs. In trauma patients and the elderly, the hips should be checked for ecchymosis, deformity, or enlargement because a considerable amount of blood can hide in the thigh following a hip fracture.

Neurologic. Most often, irritability and agitation are the earliest neurologic signs of impending shock, but as arterial pressure drops, patients most often become obtunded or unresponsive. Pupillary signs may be helpful: Constricted pupils are seen with opiate overdose or pontine strokes, whereas a unilaterally dilated pupil is seen with brain herniation.

Laboratory Findings. A battery of laboratory tests is mandatory to complement the physical assessment. They should include a complete blood count with cell differential and platelet count; electrolyte measurements, including calcium, phosphorus, and magnesium; arterial blood gases; liver and kidney function tests, and creatine kinase.

For many patients, sepsis cannot be immediately excluded, and therefore cultures of blood and urine as well as any wounds or abnormal body fluids such as sputum, ascites, or joint fluid should be obtained. Cultures of indwelling catheters, cerebrospinal fluid, stool, or other sites may also be obtained. Chest radiographs, an electrocardiogram, urinalysis, stool, and nasogastric aspirates for blood are required in most cases. Additional diagnostic procedures depend on the clinical circumstances.

General Treatment of Shock

Treatment of shock is both simple and complex. General measures for most patients include rapid fluid administration, followed by vasopressor therapy, if necessary. Specific therapies are many and are directed by the suspected or proven cause of shock, as uncovered by ongoing and intensive investigations.

FLUIDS

In general, most patients in shock can benefit from an increase in intravascular volume. The clear exception is the patient who already has pulmonary edema due to cardiogenic shock. If the patient's fluid status is uncertain, the risk of giving extra vascular volume to a patient who is already fluid-overloaded is less than the risk of not giving enough fluid to a patient in shock who may need it. As the Persian proverb goes, "the drowning man is not troubled by rain."

Hypovolemic Shock. In these patients, the primary defect is a reduced vascular volume, so fluid replacement is the key.

Distributive Shock. The effect of uncontrolled arteriolar and venular dilation is to distribute the bulk of the vascular volume away from the central veins. Dilation of the venous capacitance vessels will cause a decrease in venous pressure despite a constant total vascular volume. In addition, most causes of distributive shock, such as sepsis and anaphylaxis, will result in increased permeability of the capillaries to fluids and proteins, resulting in a loss of vascular volume into the extravascular fluid spaces. Because heart function is impaired during shock because of the circulating myocardial depressant factors, stroke volume of the heart may be increased by raising the left ventricular end-diastolic volume (preload) above normal with added fluids.

Obstructive Shock. The benefits of volume expansion in obstructive shock are not as certain as they are in patients with hypovolemic or distributive shock. In pericardial tamponade there may be no benefit and yet no harm in increasing preload. In patients with pulmonary embolism with acute right ventricular (RV) failure, volume may be beneficial because the reduced RV stroke volume due to the sudden increased RV afterload can be compensated by an increased RV preload.

Cardiogenic Shock. Patients with primarily right ventricular infarction may need a much higher systemic venous pressure to provide adequate preload to the left ventricle (LV) in the absence of an effective RV pump. Therefore, fluids may be indicated to correct cardiogenic shock due to this uncommon cause. Even in the more frequent left ventricular infarction with shock, administration of fluids may restore cardiac output by optimizing LV preload. Of course, such attempts should be made cautiously, with careful hemodynamic monitoring.

Initial methods of fluid resuscitation include "autotransfusion" methods such as use of the modified-Trendelenburg position, leg elevation, or application of a pneumatic compressive garment to the lower extremities. All of these methods result in reversible increase in central venous pressure by shifting vascular volume from the extremities to the central circulation. The advantage of these methods is that they are rapid and reversible and restore the circulation with an oxygen-carrying fluid, the patient's own blood. The amount of venous pressure restored is limited, however, and these methods must be followed by infusion of exogenous fluids as soon as possible.

The Rapid Fluid Challenge. This simple step should represent the next therapeutic intervention in all patients in shock who are not in obvious pulmonary edema. It involves rapid administration of a small bolus of 0.9% saline intravenously, with reassessment of the blood pressure and pulse immediately afterward. If an increase in blood pressure is noted, a second bolus is given, and this is repeated until no further increment in blood pressure is noted. The recommended starting volume is 400 mL of normal saline, infused over 5 minutes, followed by repeated boluses of 200 mL infused over 5 minutes each.

There are several advantages of this simple procedure:

1. It allows a very rapid restoration of vascular volume in patients who are volume depleted.
2. After optimal volume is reached, the risk of volume overload is small because of the frequent reassessment of the patient.
3. In patients whose shock is not volume responsive, it allows a transition to further treatment very early, i.e., within a few minutes.
4. It may allow avoidance of vasopressors in patients with hypovolemic shock, in whom such therapy may be either not necessary or potentially harmful.

5. It does not require pulmonary artery monitoring, which may delay necessary therapy.
6. It does not require equipment that is not already available in any nursing unit.
7. The use of an electrolyte solution for initial fluid challenge allows room for error, in that saline rapidly equilibrates within the extracellular fluid space, and thus any intravascular fluid overload is soon corrected. It is also readily available and inexpensive.

Do not delay fluid resuscitation to place a pulmonary artery catheter. Physicians order fluids "wide open," yet this may be a mere trickle if the fluid is gravity-fed through a small-diameter catheter into a peripheral vein.

Although the fluid challenge is given in small increments, the *rate* of infusion is very fast: up to 5000 mL/hour. This greatly exceeds the capacity of most IV pump systems, so old-fashioned methods such as direct pressure on the saline bag, and use of macro-drip tubing are preferred. If necessary, a stopcock and large syringe may be inserted into the fluid line and pumped manually to achieve the rapid infusion rate necessary. Generally, multiple large-bore intravenous lines are needed.

Choice of Fluids. Although some controversy remains about the most appropriate fluid for volume resuscitation in shock, there is even more general agreement (Shine, 1980). The fluid choices include (1) electrolyte ("crystalloid") solutions, such as saline, Ringer's lactate, or dextrose in water 5%; (2) colloid solutions such as albumin, hydroxyethyl starch, dextran, and plasma; (3) blood, whole blood or packed red blood cells (RBCs).

The choice of fluid may be influenced by many factors:

Oxygen-Carrying Capacity of the Blood. In conditions resulting in reduction of functioning RBCs from the circulation (e.g., massive hemorrhage, carbon monoxide poisoning, hemolysis, sickle cell crisis, or methemoglobinemia), the appropriate replacement fluid is blood. As hematocrit rises, however, the viscosity of blood increases, reducing the stroke volume. Because delivery of oxygen is the product of oxygen content and cardiac output, the effect of hematocrit on oxygen delivery becomes nonlinear, and a plateau is reached at a hematocrit of about 30%. Increase of hematocrit above this point does not appreciably contribute to oxygen delivery but does contribute to the risks of blood transfusion therapy.

Volume of Distribution. The fluids listed above are distributed throughout the body in different fluid spaces. The total body water is about 60% of body weight, in liters. Of this, two-thirds is intracellular and one-third is extracellular. About one-fourth of the extracellular fluid is intravascular, the rest being interstitial fluid. Therefore, the blood volume represents only one-twelfth of the total body water. Dextrose in water 5% (DW5%) remains within the vascular space for only a few minutes as it redistributes throughout the total body water. An hour after an infusion of 1 liter of DW(5%), only 80 mL remain in the vascular space where it can contribute to venous return. Saline or Ringer's lactate is distributed within a few minutes throughout the extracellular space, so after a few minutes, only 25% of administered saline remains in the vascular space.

Colloidal solutions remain in the vascular space for a longer period. Albumin remains in the vascular space for several hours before it is redistributed into the extracellular space. Because of these differences, patients who are treated with large doses of electrolyte solutions are more likely to be resuscitated slowly and to develop peripheral edema and a decrease in plasma oncotic pressure and increased pulmonary edema than are patients resuscitated with colloidal solutions (Rackow et al., 1983).

Transfused red blood cells remain within the (intact) vascular space. Blood is the only fluid available that is capable of carrying oxygen. Artificial oxygen-carrying solutions such as fluorinated hydrocarbons and stroma-free hemoglobin are currently under investigation.

Toxicity. Blood carries an unavoidable risk of transmission of infectious agents, especially hepatitis viruses, cytomegalovirus, and, rarely, human immunodeficiency virus (HIV). In addition, transfusion reactions, both hemolytic and febrile, and leukoagglutination, can complicate or confuse the patient's course. Colloids are free of infectious risks but can cause other toxicities. Dextran can induce renal failure and coagulopathy. Hydroxyethyl starch can cause coagulopathy in high doses as well.

In general, it seems reasonable to treat patients with the fluid that appears to be lost. For hypovolemic shock due to losses of fluids and electrolytes such as diabetic crises, severe diarrhea, or vomiting, replacement fluids should be electrolyte solutions. For patients with hemorrhage, adequate blood replacement is indicated, as is correction of any coagulopathy with fresh frozen plasma. For patients with sepsis who are already depleted of serum proteins, such as those with malnutrition or liver disease, colloids are justified.

CATECHOLAMINES

If shock persists after adequate fluid challenges have corrected any component of hypovolemia, the next step in general treatment is the use of catecholamines by continuous infusion (Hoffman and Lefkowitz, 1990). These act by stimulating specific receptors in the heart (beta) and arterioles (alpha and beta). Beta receptors in the heart promote increased heart rate and contractility. Alpha receptors in the arterioles cause vasoconstriction, whereas beta receptors cause vasodilation.

The most widely used catecholamine by far is dopamine. The net effect of dopamine depends on the dosage. At very low doses, only dopamine receptors in the renal and mesenteric circulations are stimulated to dilate, thereby preserving blood flow to these organs. At higher doses, the force of heart contractions increases, and a drop in peripheral vascular resistance occurs. At moderate doses, inotropy increases, along with increasing vascular resistance and preservation of renal blood flow. At high doses, renal blood flow is reduced, and vasoconstriction becomes more intense. The dose at which these effects occur varies between individuals. Local extravasation of dopamine causes such intense vasoconstriction that tissue necrosis may occur. Direct subcutaneous injection of an alpha blocker such as phentolamine 10 mg into the site of dopamine infiltration can prevent tissue necrosis if the problem is identified and treated promptly. Other catecholamines are less commonly used but may be preferred in some circumstances.

Norepinephrine (levarterenol) is a strong alpha receptor agonist in the peripheral vessels and a beta agonist in the heart, resulting in increased inotropy and vasoconstriction. For patients with distributive shock who do not benefit from high doses of dopamine, norepinephrine may be helpful. The intense vasoconstriction does not spare the renal circulation, so it may be beneficial to give low dose dopamine at the same time (Schaer, 1985).

Epinephrine is a strong beta agonist in the heart. In low doses it vasodilates the arterioles, whereas in higher doses it causes vasoconstriction. Epinephrine is particularly useful in anaphylactic shock, especially when bronchoconstriction and tissue edema may play a role.

Isoproterenol is a particularly hazardous catecholamine and should be used only when its strong chronotropic effect is needed. It causes beta stimulation of the heart and arterioles, resulting in increased heart rate and contractility, but it also causes peripheral vasodilation, which can result in further reduction in blood pressure or distribution of blood flow away from the brain and heart.

Dobutamine has mainly inotropic effects, with minimal direct effect on the peripheral vessels. It is useful in patients with heart failure without shock; however, if shock develops, the support of blood pressure is paramount, and dopamine should be used.

OTHER GENERAL THERAPIES

Empirical therapy for highly treatable potential causes of shock should also be given unless these causes can be specifically excluded.

Dextrose. For any patient who could be hypoglycemic, blood for glucose determination by Dextrostix and laboratory investigation should be obtained. If results are not available within a few minutes, a bolus of 50 g dextrose (100 mL of 50% dextrose) should be given. Patients at particular risk for hypoglycemia are those who are known to have diabetes and are taking oral hypoglycemic agents or insulin, those with suspected liver failure, and those with concomitant seizures.

Antibiotics. Septic shock should be presumed unless another cause of shock has been determined at the outset. Early appropriate coverage with intravenous antibiotics is an important factor in successful treatment of infection. When a septic focus (e.g., urinary tract or lung) has been identified, the antibiotic should be tailored to the organism(s) identified. In general, coverage for gram-positive, gram-negative, and anaerobic organisms is recommended. Before the patient can develop too much trouble from antibiotic toxicity, the cultures will guide a change to a less toxic therapy, or antibiotics can be discontinued when a noninfectious cause of shock is determined.

Naloxone. In any patient in shock for whom narcotic overdose cannot be excluded, 0.8 mg of naloxone should be given intravenously. Patients with a prior history of drug abuse or findings of needle tracks or pinpoint pupils should be considered at risk. The suspected diagnosis may be confirmed by urine testing for opiates.

Glucocorticoids. Although rare, adrenal insufficiency is fatal unless specific therapy with glucocorticoids is given. Patients at risk include those with a history of chronic steroid use within the preceding 6 months, those at risk of adrenal hemorrhage (anticoagulation and stress), those with known or suspected hypothyroidism, and those with meningococcemia. Glucocorticoids should not be used as adjunctive therapy in septic shock because recent controlled trials have shown no survival benefit (Bone et al., 1987).

Mechanical Ventilation. Patients who have shock may hyperventilate due to stimulation of the respiratory center by hypotension and metabolic acidosis. The work of breathing in these patients will be increased. It may be appropriate, therefore, to place the patient on mechanical ventilation to reduce the work of breathing and decrease the proportion of cardiac output directed to the muscles of breathing.

Monitoring the Patient in Shock

Patients in early or overt shock should be observed in the intensive care unit because of the need for frequent nursing assessment, continuous invasive and noninvasive monitoring, and, frequently, continuous infusions of vasoactive medications, such as dopamine.

ELECTROCARDIOGRAPHY

Continuous monitoring of rhythm is essential in all shock patients because of the frequent occurrence of fatal dysrhythmias, especially in patients in cardiogenic shock. As mentioned earlier, the heart may also be an "innocent bystander" and may be injured secondarily in any shock state. In addition, dopamine

and other catecholamine infusions can induce significant ischemia and dysrhythmias. Some modern monitoring systems are equipped with continuous ST segment monitoring, which can provide an early warning to silent ischemia.

PRESSURE MONITORING

All patients in shock need frequent assessment of arterial pressure, preferably continuously. Auscultation or Doppler methods can significantly underestimate true arterial pressure in patients who are vasoconstricted. In addition, frequent blood drawing for arterial blood gas measurements and other laboratory tests are needed. For these reasons, an indwelling arterial catheter for continuous pressure monitoring is recommended in most patients whose shock state is not readily reversed with fluids. The preferred sites are the radial and ulnar arteries because of their collateral circulation. The brachial, femoral or dorsalis pedis artery may also be used.

URINE OUTPUT

Catheterization of the urinary bladder with hourly determinations of urine volume is a simple but important means of monitoring the adequacy of renal blood flow. The risk of renal shutdown following severe hypotension is high. Urine volume of less than 30 mL/hour suggests the possibility of acute tubular necrosis and should be managed aggressively because this complication increases overall mortality.

PULMONARY ARTERY CATHETERIZATION

The advent of bedside pulmonary artery catheterization has greatly enhanced our ability to diagnose causes of shock and has allowed a more controlled guide to fluid and drug therapy.

Diagnostic Uses of the Pulmonary Artery Catheter. Although clinical examination is often revealing, at times the cause of shock may be obscure. Many specific diseases and physiologic categories of shock have characteristic hemodynamic findings.

Hypovolemic Shock. Right atrial (RA) and pulmonary artery wedge (PAW) pressures are very low.

Distributive Shock. Some reduction in RA and PAW pressures is usually found. The cardiac output (CO) is high despite a low mean arterial pressure (MAP), resulting in a very low calculated SVR, which is diagnostic of this mechanism of shock.

Cardiogenic Shock. RA and PAW pressures are high, CO is low, SVR is high. With an RV infarct, the RA is high but the PAW may be low.

Pericardial Tamponade. RA and PAW pressures are high. The characteristic finding here is a flat Y descent, with diastolic equalization of pressures throughout the chambers of the heart.

Pulmonary Embolism. In a patient with no prior severe lung disease, the finding of high PA systolic and diastolic pressures with a low PAW is very suggestive of massive pulmonary embolism. In acute pulmonary embolism, the PA systolic pressure rarely exceeds 50 mm Hg because the right ventricle is normally thin and is not capable of generating very high pressures. Other conditions producing a similar pattern are severe emphysema and other pulmonary vascular diseases such as primary pulmonary hypertension. These, however, often result in higher PA systolic pressures because the gradual onset of pulmonary vascular obstruction allows the right ventricle to hypertrophy, thereby generating higher pressures.

Mitral Regurgitation. Acute onset of mitral regurgitation can result in severe pulmonary edema and hypotension. A characteristic V wave is usually seen in the PAW tracing.

Therapeutic Uses of the Pulmonary Artery Catheter. Information obtained with the PA catheter can provide a safer passage through the hazardous straits of fluid management. Patients in shock need sufficient fluid to provide optimum cardiac output, yet they are at higher risk of formation of pulmonary edema. It is important to be able to restore vascular volume aggressively without risking fluid overload. This can be accomplished with careful use of the PA catheter.

The PA catheter allows repeated measurement of cardiac output and vascular resistance, which are important guides to therapy of afterload reduction in patients with heart failure. It also allows calculation of oxygen delivery and oxygen extraction, which are useful for determining the effects of mechanical ventilation and the optimal use of positive end-expiratory pressure (PEEP).

Specific Therapies in Shock

Certain causes of shock deserve emphasis because of their unique modes of treatment.

Cardiogenic Shock. When vasopressor and inotropic agents fail to restore arterial pressure, Mechanical Cardiac Assist Devices may be used (see Chapter 11). The most frequently used device is the intra-aortic balloon. Briefly, a balloon is passed through a femoral artery into the aorta. It is inflated during diastole and deflated just before systole. This method increases coronary and systemic blood flow by increasing diastolic aortic pressure, and reduces left ventricular afterload by reducing systolic aortic pressure (McEnany et al. 1978; Bolooki, 1984) Mortality from cardiogenic shock has been reduced with long-term use of the intra-aortic balloon, especially when it is combined with coronary revascularization surgery (Kanter et al., 1988).

Anaphylactic Shock. Anaphylactic shock is due to a severe, generalized allergic reaction. It is most often seen in those with a history of allergies and can result from exposure to any allergen to which the patient is highly sensitized. Laryngeal edema with stridor or an urticarial rash (hives) may accompany shock and are clues to the diagnosis. Shock occurs because of arteriolar and venular dilation and increased capillary leak. Epinephrine is the catecholamine of choice (Barach et al., 1984). In addition, fluids, antihistamines, and corticosteroids should be given. Identification and removal of the allergen are important.

Septic Shock. Broad-spectrum antibiotic therapy should be given promptly, based on the suspected site of infection or organism, and should be adjusted to the most effective and least toxic regimen once culture results are available. For patients with suspected gram-negative sepsis and septic shock, treatment with anti-endotoxin antibodies reduces mortality, and such preparations are now available for clinical use (Ziegler, 1991; Greenman, 1991).

Toxic Shock. This form of shock is due to a staphylococcal exotoxin. Although tampon use is the most common risk factor, any focus of staphylococcal infection can give rise to toxic shock. Associated symptoms and signs that may be a clue to toxic shock include fever, nausea, diarrhea, and an erythematous rash with subsequent desquamation of palms and soles. Treatment includes antistaphylococcal antibiotics such as methicillin, cephalothin, or vancomycin, fluids, and control of the focus of infection.

Adrenal Insufficiency. Insufficiency of adrenal corticosteroids occurs in patients who have recently stopped taking therapeutic corticosteroids or patients with diseases affecting the adrenal glands such as meningococcemia, tuberculosis, or adrenal hemorrhage. A significant number of patients entering the intensive care unit have relative adrenal insufficiency, that is, they are unable to boost their output of cortisol in response to stress. This can result in overt adrenal insufficiency when the patient is stressed by a serious illness. Adrenal hemorrhage sufficient to cause acute adrenal insufficiency is uncommon. It occurs generally in stressed, anticoagulated patients and often is not associated with other sites of bleeding. Clinical findings are similar to those of septic shock and include fever, confusion, abdominal pain, and hypotension. Adrenal insufficiency is fatal if unrecognized, yet it is readily treated by administering glucocorticoids. Any patient in shock with suspected adrenal insufficiency should have the cortisol level tested, followed by intravenous hydrocortisone until the diagnosis is ruled out.

Pulmonary Embolism. Pulmonary embolism causes shock in a small percentage of patients. Almost always, patients have a recognized risk factor such as immobilization, tissue injury, or conditions causing hypercoagulability such as pregnancy, estrogen therapy, recent surgery, or carcinoma. When shock is due to massive pulmonary embolism, thrombolytic therapy should be used. Agents available are streptokinase, urokinase, and tissue plasminogen activator. Contraindications to thrombolytic therapy include recent stroke or surgery or active uncontrolled bleeding.

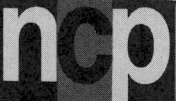 **nursing care plan**

---

1. Fluid volume deficit related to blood loss
Patient will maintain adequate fluid volume.

Outcome Criteria	Nursing Interventions

Maintains an IV or PO fluid intake of at least 1000 mL per shift (8 hours).
Maintains an hourly fluid intake within 30 mL of the hourly fluid output from urine, wound drainage, or blood loss.
Avoids weight fluctuations of greater than 5%.
	1. Administer fluid and electrolytes as well as blood and blood products as ordered.
	  a. Fluids and electrolyte solutions are given for the replacement of fluid and plasma loss.
	  b. Blood is given for replacement of blood loss.
	  c. Blood products, such as plasma protein fraction (Plasmanate), are given to replace blood and fluid loss.
	2. Evaluate the patient's response to therapy.
	3. Obtain daily weights and maintain a day-to-day comparison chart.
	4. Monitor fluid intake and output, including loss from GI tract, wounds, drains, or bleeding.

Patient will demonstrate adequate oxygen-carrying capability.
  Says he or she feels well and exhibits signs of adequate oxygen carrying capabilities, as evidenced by pink skin with adequate turgor and capillary refill.
  Maintains a hemoglobin level of 12 to 14 g/100 mL and a hematocrit of 30% or greater.
	1. Assess the patient for signs of fluid and electrolyte imbalance.
	  a. Poor skin turgor.
	  b. Weakness.
	  c. Irritability or confusion.
	  d. Nausea or vomiting.
	2. Monitor hemoglobin and hematocrit levels daily.

Patient will maintain hemodynamic stability.
  Maintains a blood pressure of 90 to 120/60 to 80 and a heart rate of 70 to 110 beats/minute.
  Maintains a urinary output of at least 30 mL/hour.
	1. Monitor the patient's vital signs and fluid status.
	  a. Evaluate blood pressure, pulse, and urinary output.
	  b. Monitor cumulative fluid intake and output.
	  c. Note and report variations from baseline.

---

2. Decreased cardiac output related to: decreased venous return
Patient will reestablish hemodynamic stability.

Outcome Criteria	Nursing Interventions

Maintains a blood pressure of 90 to 120/60 to 80.
Has a regular heart rate of 70 to 110 beats/minute.
  Has warm and dry skin and is free of discomforts associated with diminished venous return to the heart.
Patient will have increased cardiac output.
  States that he or she is feeling well.
  Reports a sense of feeling rested and calm.
Patient will take medications prescribed for improving cardiac output and decreasing the workload of the heart
	1. Obtain and monitor the patient's vital signs.
	  a. Monitor the blood pressure level for declining trends.
	  b. Monitor the pulse for increasing rate and irregularity.
	  c. Assess all body systems for the effects of diminished cardiac output.
	1. Reduce the workload of the heart by
	  a. Restricting the client to bed rest in a Fowler position.
	  b. Providing a calm, quiet atmosphere conducive to rest.
	1. Administer medications that increase the contractility of the heart and document their effects on the patient's blood pressure and heart rate.

---

3. Altered thought processes related to: decreased cerebral perfusion
Patient will experience improved cerebral circulation.

Outcome Criteria	Nursing Interventions

States that she or he feels alert and well oriented to the environment.
Communicates needs.
	1. Assess each patient for baseline behavior patterns.
	  a. Response to verbal and tactile stimuli.
	  b. State of orientation.
	2. Note changes in the patient's behavior indicative of cerebral hypoperfusion.
	  a. Restlessness.
	  b. Confusion.
	  c. Lethargy.
	  d. Somnolence.
	  e. Unresponsiveness.
	  f. Seizures.
	3. Notify the physician of significant findings.

Patient will experience decreased vasoconstriction.
  Reports warm extremities without tingling or pain.
  Maintains full active range of movement.
Patient will experience no hypoxia.
  Remains alert and exhibits equal pupillary responses to light.
  Is free from abnormal neurologic manifestations, such as seizures.
  Maintains all protective reflexes.
	1. Assess the patient for the presence of cool, moist extremities often associated with pain.
	2. Assess the patient for spontaneous and equal movement of all extremities.
	1. Assess each patient for baseline neurologic status and document deficits. Evaluate
	  a. Level of consciousness.
	  b. Pupillary response to light.
	  c. Presence of protective reflexes, such as a blink and cough reflex.
	  d. Presence of tremors or seizures.

From Ignatavicius, D. D., and Bayne, M. V. (Eds.) (1991). *Medical-surgical nursing: A nursing process approach* (pp. 416–417). Philadelphia: W. B. Saunders.

SUMMARY

Shock, the state of global ischemia due to inadequate arterial pressure, has been described as the "reversible stage of dying" and as "a rude unhinging of the machinery of life." These descriptions convey the severity and urgency of the problem. Shock can be the result of a great number of separate illnesses that cause reduced arterial pressure by one or more of four mechanisms: (1) reduced heart function, (2) reduced vascular volume, (3) obstruction in the circulation, and (4) uncontrolled vasodilation. Early in the course of shock, the arterial pressure is preserved due to neural and hormonal responses, but as the process continues, arterial pressure drops, and all vital organs suffer a reduced blood flow. Overt shock can be tolerated for a very brief time before irreversible damage to multiple vital organs dooms the patient to die. General treatment involves rapid fluid resuscitation in all patients except those in overt pulmonary edema, followed, if necessary, by vasopressor infusion. Specific treatment depends on the specific diagnosis uncovered. All patients in shock should be treated and monitored in an intensive care unit because of their high mortality, their need for a high level of nursing attention, and their need for sophisticated monitoring and therapeutic technology.

References

Barach, E. M., et al. (1984). Epinephrine for treatment of anaphylactic shock. *Journal of the American Medical Association*, 251(16), 2118–2122.

Barnett, J. A. and Sanford, J. P. (1969). Bacterial shock. *Journal of the American Medical Association*, 209, 1514–1517.

Bolooki, H., (1984). *Clinical application of intra-aortic balloon pump* (2nd ed.). Mt. Kisco, NY: Futura.

Bone, R. C., et al. (1987). A controlled clinical trial of high-dose methylprednisolone in the treatment of severe sepsis and septic shock (1988). *New England Journal of Medicine*, 317(11), 653–658.

Corrin, B. (1980). Lung pathology in septic shock. *Journal of Clinical Pathology*, 33, 891–894.

Dorin, R. I., and Kearns, P. J. (1988). High output circulatory failure in acute adrenal insufficiency. *Critical Care Medicine*, 16(3), 296–297.

Greenman, R. L., et al. (1991). A controlled clinical trial of E5 murine monoclonal IgM antibody to endotoxin in the treatment of gram-negative sepsis. *Journal of the American Medical Association*, 266(8), 1097–1102.

Hoffman, B. B., and Lefkowitz, R. J. (1990). Catecholamines and sympathomimetic drugs. In A. G. Gilman, T. W. Rall, A. S. Nies, and P. Taylor (Eds.), *Goodman and Gilman's The Pharmacological Basis of Therapeutics* (8th ed., pp. 187–207). New York: Pergamon Press.

Kanter, D. R., et al. (1988). Follow-up of survivors of mechanical circulatory support. *Journal of Thoracic and Cardiovascular Surgery*, 96, 72–80.

Luce, J. M. (1987). Pathogenesis and management of septic shock. *Chest*, 91(6), 883–887.

McEnany, M. T., Kay, H. R., Buckley, J. M., et al. (1978). Clinical experience with intra-aortic balloon pump in 728 patients. *Circulation*, 58 (Suppl. I), I-124–I-132.

Rackow, E. C., et al. (1983). Fluid resuscitation in circulatory shock: A comparison of the cardiorespiratory effects of albumin, hetastarch, and saline solutions in patients with hypovolemic and septic shock. *Critical Care Medicine*, 11, 839.

Schaer, G. L., Fink, M. P., and Parrillo, J. E. (1985). Norepinephrine alone versus norepinephrine plus low-dose dopamine: Enhanced renal blood flow with combination pressor therapy. *Critical Care Medicine*, 13(6), 492–496.

Shine, K. I. (moderator) (1980). Aspects of the management of shock. *Annals of Internal Medicine*, 93, 723–734.

Shubin, H., Weil, M. H., and Carlson, R. W. (1977). Bacterial shock. *American Heart Journal*, 94, 112–114.

Stroud, M., Swindell, B., and Bernard, G. R. (1990). Cellular and humoral mediators of sepsis syndrome. *Critical Care Nursing Clinics of North America*, 2, 151–160.

Weil, M. (1977). Current understanding of mechanisms and treatment of circulatory shock caused by bacterial infections. *Annals of Clinical Research*, 9, 181–191.

Zeigler, E. J., et al. (1991). Treatment of gram-negative bacteremia and septic shock with HA-1A human monoclonal antibody against endotoxin: A randomized, double-blind, placebo-controlled trial. *New England Journal of Medicine*, 324, 429–436.

60

Patients with Chemical Dependency

Paula J. Rabinowitz
Norlee K. Manley

At one time or another, every nurse encounters patients who test the nurse's confidence. Substance abuse patients in critical care are a prime example. Typically, patients are admitted to critical care units for overdoses or physical complications related to their addiction. They pose unique problems for nurses who are not familiar with substance abuse and specific issues related to addictions.

This chapter provides an overview of commonly encountered substance abuse problems: alcohol, cocaine, narcotics or opioids, barbiturates, and benzodiazepines (e.g., diazepam). These are the most frequently encountered addictive substances that cause management problems for the health care team. The chapter discusses assessment of the patient, signs and symptoms of toxicity and withdrawal for each drug, drug-seeking behaviors, implications of drug and alcohol antagonists, pain management, and interpersonal issues.

Generally, substance abuse occurs when an individual uses a particular substance in excess to create a euphoric state of consciousness. When a person abuses a substance continuously for a long period of time, he or she will need more of the substance to create the same euphoric state. This process is referred to as tolerance. Eventually, people develop physical or psychological dependence on the substance, and this constitutes addiction. Many drugs are both physically and psychologically addictive and can result in life-threatening problems. Many patients abuse multiple substances. The most common combination is cocaine and alcohol, both of which are extremely lethal substances. Although chemical dependency is the most current term used to describe this problem, we will refer to these patients as substance abusers because this term more accurately describes their self-image.

Substance abusers who require treatment in a critical care unit are extremely anxious. In addition to worries about their presenting problem, they are afraid that their addiction may not be identified or handled appropriately. If the addiction is not identified, the patient will begin the painful and sometimes life-threatening withdrawal process. Another problem is pain management. A patient addicted to narcotics or opioids will not experience pain relief from standard doses of morphine. The health care team is often afraid to use analgesics in the extreme doses required by the addicted patient from fear that they will depress the respiratory center or contribute to the addiction.

Patients fear that staff have a negative attitude toward them because they are substance abusers. Many care givers misunderstand substance abuse, retaining long-held beliefs and attitudes. Many people believe that these patients have a moral defect or weakness that caused the addiction or that they chose to become addicted. These people do not understand that the addiction affects every aspect of their physical being and their lifestyle and pervades their thoughts. Many care givers are also affected by negative thoughts or experiences they have had in their personal lives with family or friends who have abused substances. A supportive, nonjudgmental approach is essential to dispel these fears and initiate a therapeutic environment.

The health care team also have a unique set of fears when caring for substance abuse patients. They fear that these patients will be difficult to care for or may become agitated, hostile, or aggressive. Another concern is that these patients will continuously ask for medication or display other manipulative behaviors to satisfy their needs. Also, the health care team is unsure of the effects of needed medications on these patients.

ASSESSMENT OF CHEMICALLY DEPENDENT PATIENTS

A thorough substance abuse assessment does not infringe on an individual's right to privacy. It can be one of the most comforting aspects of the initial assessment for the substance abuser. The key to ensuring valid results is the manner in which it is conducted. If the nurse approaches the patient, or the significant other of an unconscious patient, in a nonjudgmental, professional manner, the patient is given permission to disclose information that will be essential in planning treatment. The nurse's nonjudgmental, confident approach provides comforting assurance to the patient that members of the health care team are knowledgeable about all of his or her needs.

A substance abuse assessment form can be used as a general guideline. It is a simple, direct method for ensuring inclusion of this vital information and implies that all patients are routinely assessed for substance abuse (Table 60–1). Many patients understate or exaggerate their illicit drug use. It is important to ask pertinent questions and then reframe them to obtain the most accurate information. If it is necessary to conduct this assessment with a significant other because of the patient's inability to communicate, separate the person from the group of concerned family and friends and provide privacy for the interaction. To determine which person would be the most appropriate selection for this interview, consider the most often reported supportive persons in the substance abuser's life: spouse, siblings, mother, and lastly, the father.

In the interview with the conscious patient or a significant other of an unconscious one, begin by explaining that you are assessing the possibility of substance abuse in order to collect vital information that is necessary to interpret observable signs and symptoms accurately. Explain further how these data can be life-saving in terms of allowing the health care team to act quickly and prevent complications. Most substance abuse patients wear Medic-alert bracelets or carry drug identification or information if they are taking an alcohol or drug antagonist treatment modality. The implications of this information for treatment are included later in this chapter in the sections on alcohol and narcotics.

Because people from different strata of our society have different thoughts and beliefs about addictive substances, it is important to use terms familiar to them. One example is the belief that drinking beer or wine daily is not the same as drinking "hard liquor." Another example involves the addiction to cough syrup containing narcotics. Most addicts believe that the addictive component, which is responsible for their sickness when they cease drinking it, is the narcotic. Actually, the alcohol content of cough syrup is 40% and is far more detrimental to the patient and important for the treatment team who must manage the abstinence syndrome.

Components of a good assessment form include the following: Does the patient use any drugs, prescribed by a physician or otherwise? In order of importance, according to the patient, which drugs are used? If the list does not include marijuana, ask specifically if the patient uses marijuana. Likewise, if the patient does not list alcohol, ask specifically about the use of alcohol, beer, and wine. Then, for each drug listed and in the order presented, ask the following questions: How often do you use it (daily, weekly, monthly)? When did you first begin using it? Have you ever attempted to stop using it? When and what happened? How long have you been using it this time? How do you use it (snorting, injecting, smoking, and so on)? If the patient is injecting, ask him to show you the sites of injection. Then ask, how much do you use each time? How many times do you use it in a 24-hour period? When did you last use the substance and how much did you use then?

Once you have adequate, in-depth information about all of the substances used, begin asking about the patient's history of overdose. Then ask how he feels when he does not have access to the substance and what he does to relieve any uncomfortable feelings during that time. Sort out physical, life-threatening symptoms from those of less immediate importance. Specifically ask the alcohol abuser if he or she has experienced delirium tremens, blackouts, tremors, or seizures. Ask if he needs a drink in the morning to relieve shaking.

When you have enough information to determine the severity of current usage, ascertain if the patient is being treated with methadone, naltrexone (Trexan), or disulfiram (Antabuse) (patients may not remember the generic names of these drugs). If so, obtain the name of the program in which he or she is enrolled. Ask the patient if he knows the current dosage. However, be aware that many programs do not inform patients about specific dosages to discourage them from fixating on that aspect of treatment. Ask the patient when he received the last dose.

Once the assessment is completed, call the program to verify the patient's information. Even though treatment for substance abuse is strictly confidential, program staff are obligated to reveal information when their patients are hospitalized or are in other emergency situations. Contact with the program is also viewed in a positive manner by the patient, who will be very concerned about having an explanation for his or her absence from the program relayed to the program's staff.

Other assessment data, which are vital in terms of validating the patient's information, include toxicology reports. Blood level determinants are the most accurate and desirable data in critical care for deter-

TABLE 60–1. Substance Abuse Assessment Form

Client's Name *John Doe*   Date   *1-1-92*

Source of Information   *Mary Doe, Spouse*

1. Do you use any drugs, prescribed by a physician or otherwise?
   Yes

2. In order of importance, list the drugs that you use:

Drug	Frequency	Method	Started	Amount	Last Use
A.					
Cocaine	*2-3 ×/wk.*	*Smoke*	*June 1988*	*Variable*	*Today*
B.					
Marijuana	*3-4 ×/wk.*	*Smoke*	*Feb. 1988*	*2-3 joints*	*Today*
C.					
Beer	*Daily*	*Drink*	*Dec. 1987*	*12 cans/day*	*Today*

3. Describe what happens when you stop using the substance:
"He has to drink beer to mellow out after a coke run."

4. Have you ever experienced the following:

Delirium tremens *No*   When was the last time *N/A*

Blackouts *Yes*   When was the last time *Christmas Day*

Seizures *No*   When was the last time *N/A*

Drinking in A.M. *Yes*   When was the last time *Today*

5. Have you ever used the following:

Antabuse *No*   When? *N/A*

Methadone *Yes*   When? *June 1979—December 1981*

Trexan? *No*   When? *N/A*

6. If currently using any drug listed in #5:
Name of program *N/A*

Current dose *N/A*   Last dose *N/A*

7. Do you have any "tracks"? *Yes*   Location *Left forearm (old)*

8. Are there any areas on your body where you have injected drugs?
No   Location *No evidence of recent injection*

---

mining alcohol and barbiturate levels. Serum concentrations of other drugs may be too low to measure. Mass screening to detect a variety of drugs in urine samples is therefore crucial.

Some general information about drug testing is helpful when considering laboratory reports to validate the patient's information. There are a number of urinalysis techniques in use today that determine drug content. A common error made by persons assessing the validity of a drug test is a failure to consider the type of test used. The following information on laboratory testing has been extracted from the work of Eric Wish (1988).

Thin layer chromatography (TLC) is a general test that can screen for a variety of drugs in a short period of time. It is widely used because it is economical. It is an extremely subjective process and requires experienced technicians to interpret the results.

The enzyme multiplied immune test (EMIT) involves a chemical reaction of the specimen with an antibody to react to a specific drug. The chemical reaction causes a change in the specimen's transmission of light. This change in transmissibility is detected by a machine that provides a quantitative reading that is compared with the reading from a standard solution containing a known concentration of the drug. If the reading is higher than that of the standard, the specimen is positive for that drug.

Because the determination of a positive specimen is based on specific numbers, the level of subjectivity involved in the EMIT is less than that for TLC.

TLC appears to be more economical because as many as 20 different drugs can be tested for approximately $2.00. EMITs are specific to one drug and cost between $1.00 and $5.00 for each drug tested. The TLC test fails to detect common street drugs by almost two-thirds compared with the EMIT. Many laboratories use a two-test approach to the identification of drugs. They screen first by using the TLC and apply a confirmatory test to positive results by using the EMIT. False negative results are reported more frequently when using the TLC method. Therefore, many laboratories are using the EMIT instead of the TLC.

The EMIT is not without its own set of problems. Because of its extreme sensitivity, false positive results are frequently reported. Some common licit drugs can cross-react with the test's reagents to produce a positive result. Ingestion of poppy seeds, used in baking, can produce positive results for opiates, and cold medications containing pseudoephedrine can result in a false positive result for amphetamines.

There are other urinalysis techniques available for detecting drugs, including radioimmunoassay and gas chromatography–mass spectrometry (GC/MS). The GC/MS is costly and time-consuming and is used infrequently as an initial test in large-scale screening programs. It has been used as a confirmatory test and is considered the most accurate technique currently available for identifying drugs in the urine; however, it costs between $70.00 and $100.00 per specimen. If a patient has been involved in some criminal act prior to being admitted to the critical care unit, this method of testing for drugs is justified, because the courts have ruled on its validity (Wish, 1988).

For mass screening many laboratories use the TLC method, which may not pick up marijuana, ethanol, or benzodiazepines. Special requests for these substances must be ordered in addition to the general drug screen. The presence of quinine also deserves some consideration along with other assessment data. Heroin is frequently "cut" with quinine, which gives the user an added "rush." Since the half-life of quinine is considerably longer than that of heroin, it remains positive in urine drug screens for up to 14 days following use. Tonic water, Triple Six ("666") and Bromoquine will also test positive for quinine.

The primary goal of the health care team is the stabilization of the presenting patient problem. The presence of chemical dependency does not alter this goal but may complicate the process. After the initial assessment is completed, the type and extent of dependency is estimated. The goal is now to fulfill the dependency requirements and to manage the associated problems. It is not appropriate to withdraw patients from their dependency at this time. Withdrawal alone can create life-threatening problems that complicate the presenting problem. If the presenting problem is an overdose or a toxic state, the goal is to stabilize the life-threatening complications. After this, the patient can be transferred to a detoxification or medical unit for withdrawal.

Sifting through a patient's polysubstance abuse appropriately is critical at this stage. It is necessary to determine which drugs may create a lethal situation and ensure that this does not occur. Drugs that are less potent and do not have lethal complications are not addressed immediately but are considered in the overall treatment plan.

The patient assessment data presented in Table 60–1 exemplifies this approach. This patient presented with acute cocaine intoxication and underlying alcohol dependency as well as occasional use of marijuana. The immediate concern was to monitor the complications due to the cocaine intoxication. However, the amount of alcohol consumed regularly indicated that the patient was dependent on alcohol. Untreated alcohol withdrawal can be lethal, especially in conjunction with acute cocaine intoxication. Therefore, both the complications of cocaine intoxication and prevention of alcohol withdrawal had to be addressed by the health care team. On the other hand, since the patient's spouse reported only occasional use of marijuana, and withdrawal from marijuana does not present life-threatening symptoms, withdrawal from marijuana was not of primary importance.

The North American Nursing Diagnosis Association (NANDA) has identified 26 diagnoses that are commonly used for addictions (American Nurses Association [ANA] and National Nurses Society on Addictions, 1988). The diagnoses in Table 60–2 were chosen from the current NANDA listing, with modifications made for addicted patients. The diagnoses are grouped according to types of patient responses to addictions. They include four groups: biologic, cognitive, psychosocial, and spiritual. Table 60–2 lists a few nursing diagnoses that are pertinent to acutely intoxicated patients or patients with medical complications of their addiction (Carpenito, 1983).

In summary, a thorough substance abuse assessment, nursing care plan, and basic understanding of toxicology tests are highly beneficial to all concerned.

TABLE 60–2. Selected Nursing Diagnoses and Expected Outcomes Related to Addictions

Nursing Diagnosis	Expected Outcome
Sensory perceptual alteration	The patient will stabilize in a safe environment
Alteration in comfort: Pain	The patient achieves relief of pain
Alteration in thought process	The patient exhibits resolution of impaired thinking and disorientation
Anxiety: (Specify level)	The patient experiences decreased anxiety
Powerlessness	The patient recognizes loss of control of addiction

TABLE 60-3. Effects of Blood Alcohol Levels

Blood Alcohol Level	Effects
50 mg/dL	Difficulties with balance
	Impaired ability to concentrate
	Decreasing awareness of stimuli
100–150 mg/dL	Marked decline of cognitive and motor functioning
	Ataxia
	Slurred speech
	Impaired short-term memory and judgment
200 mg/dL	Loss of ability to respond to stimuli
250 mg/dL	Loss of consciousness
500 mg/dL	Death

They provide vital information for the health care team, allay the patient's fears and apprehension concerning treatment, and set the stage for successful management of the substance abuser in a critical care unit.

ALCOHOL ABUSE

Ethyl alcohol is a widely abused substance. It is frequently used in conjunction with other drugs such as cocaine. Most people in our society consume some amount of alcohol on an occasional basis. This alone does not constitute a problem. Individuals who consume large amounts of alcohol over an extended period of time often develop a physical dependence as well as chronic alcohol-related health problems. Physical dependence on alcohol and associated medical complications are problematic when an individual is admitted to a critical care unit.

The acute effects of alcohol are directly related to blood alcohol levels in the body. Table 60–3 describes the effects of increasing blood alcohol levels (Barry, 1979). Individuals who drive an automobile after drinking are considered to be driving under the influence (DUI) if blood levels are 100 mg/dL or higher (Hunt, 1983). The blood alcohol levels established by the National Council on Alcoholism (1972) necessary for a diagnosis of alcoholism are as follows: a blood alcohol level greater than or equal to 300 mg/dL on any occasion; a blood alcohol level of 100 mg/dL on routine clinical examination; a blood alcohol level greater than 150 mg/dL in a patient who does not appear to be grossly intoxicated. Determination of the patient's blood alcohol level will permit the health care team to estimate the time necessary for the patient to attain sobriety. Blood alcohol levels decline at a rate of 12 to 50 mg/dL per hour (Mc-Micken, 1983). Novice drinkers and children exhibit altered consciousness with blood alcohol levels that barely reach legally intoxicated limits. Chronic drinkers, on the other hand, can maintain remarkable degrees of alertness and ambulation at profound blood alcohol levels (Jackimczyk and Roberts, 1984).

Acute alcohol withdrawal can begin anywhere from a few hours to 14 days after the last consumption of alcohol. Most often, symptoms appear within 6 to 12 hours after the last drink. The severity of withdrawal symptoms differs greatly among patients. Patients who have consumed larger amounts of alcohol over longer time periods experience more severe withdrawal symptoms. Other associated health factors create differences as well. Patients with a poor nutritional status and those over age 40 experience more severe symptoms. Those who have related medical problems, for example, hepatic, renal, or psychological problems or a previous history of severe withdrawal or seizures are also at high risk (Meyers, 1988a).

Symptoms of alcohol withdrawal are currently classified in two stages and can be life-threatening in either stage. The first stage consists of early or minor withdrawal symptoms (Table 60–4). Major or latent symptoms can occur if the early signs of alcohol withdrawal are untreated. Major symptoms can also develop from the onset of withdrawal without earlier symptoms. This is most likely if there is a late onset of withdrawal, 48 to 72 hours after the last drink, or if there is concurrent use of other drugs (Meyers, 1988a). Major or latent symptoms of withdrawal are referred to as delirium tremens. Table 60–4 describes the major and minor symptoms of alcohol withdrawal (Meyers, 1988a, 1988b; Tabakoff and Rothstein, 1983; Wolfe and Victor, 1971).

Since alcohol is a central nervous system depressant, management of acute withdrawal is accomplished by using agents with similar effects. Benzodiazepines are the drugs of choice because of their antianxiety, sedative, and anticonvulsant effects (Meyers, 1988b). An exception is a patient who uses a combination of barbiturates and alcohol. In this case a long-acting barbiturate (e.g., phenobarbital) is preferable because it manages the withdrawal symptoms from both drugs (Tabakoff and Rothstein, 1983). The patient must have adequate hepatic function if this regimen is initiated.

The goal of treating patients with benzodiazepines is to prevent an abrupt withdrawal from alcohol by substituting a similarly addictive substance and then

TABLE 60-4. Symptoms of Alcohol Withdrawal

Minor or Early Symptoms	Major or Latent Symptoms (Delirium Tremens)
Nausea or vomiting	Dehydration
Other gastrointestinal disturbances	Hallucinations
Mild diaphoresis	Visual
Pruritus	Auditory
Visual disturbances	Tactile
Time disorientation	Delirium
Tremulousness	Delusions
Psychomotor agitation	Tonic-clonic seizures
Anxiety	Hyperthermia
Sleep disturbances	Marked tachycardia
Mild tachycardia	Marked hypertension
Mild hypertension	
Tonic-clonic seizures	

gradually taper it while monitoring the dose needed to alleviate withdrawal symptoms. Continuous IV infusions of diazepam or a similar agent are given, and the dosage is titrated to alleviate withdrawal symptoms (Tabakoff and Rothstein, 1983).

Patients who experience alcohol withdrawal may exhibit tonic-clonic seizures. Patients without other seizure disorders may have withdrawal seizures. Because some of these patients may have had prior head trauma related to their alcohol abuse, it is important to assess whether any seizure activity is related to alcohol withdrawal. Focal seizures are not associated with alcohol withdrawal (Tabakoff and Rothstein, 1983). Patients with symptoms of severe tremulousness, blackouts, or hallucinations and those who have had prior withdrawal seizures are at greatest risk.

Most withdrawal seizures occur within 72 hours of the last ingestion of alcohol. Alcohol decreases the body's transportation and metabolism of thiamine, which lowers the seizure threshold (Hoyumpa, 1980). As a result, the standard treatment includes daily doses of thiamine, and the initial dose should be given as soon as possible. Unless the patient experiences extreme withdrawal symptoms, the thiamine can be replaced by a multivitamin pill after 3 days. The use of magnesium sulfate to decrease tremors, withdrawal seizures, and cardiac arrhythmias is currently considered to be of no proven benefit (Meyers, 1988b). Management of symptoms with benzodiazepines as well as adequate hydration will assist in preventing seizures. Beyond these preventive measures, seizures are managed as they occur. Usually, diazepam is given to terminate seizure activity. Other safety measures that address the potential for injury include placement of a padded tongue blade at the bedside, prevention of aspiration, and protection of the extremities. The use of phenothiazines to control nausea and vomiting should be avoided because they also lower the seizure threshold and may decrease blood pressure (Tabakoff and Rothstein, 1983).

Because alcohol is a diuretic, most patients exhibit varying levels of dehydration. As mentioned earlier, adequate hydration assists in the prevention of withdrawal seizures. Because alcohol is a water-soluble substance, good hydration helps not only in the excretion of alcohol but also addresses the fluid volume deficit (Tabakoff and Rothstein, 1983). If the patient is able to take oral fluids, nonacidic, noncarbonated beverages can be placed at the bedside. These fluids will not aggravate any gastrointestinal disturbances. In patients who are unconscious, nauseated, or vomiting, parenteral fluids are indicated. Electrolyte imbalances are also commonly associated with dehydration, and electrolytes need to be monitored closely with appropriate supplements given to correct any deficits.

Temperature monitoring is also critical because hyperpyremia is a major cause of death during withdrawal. Access to a cooling blanket is an essential part of the emergency equipment needed for this condition (Meyers, 1988b).

Several complications of the hematologic system, including leukopenia, macrocytosis, and coagulation disorders, are associated with alcohol withdrawal. Leukopenia increases the potential for infection in these patients. Folic acid therapy is often necessary in response to macrocytosis (Van Thiel, 1983). In patients with chronic liver disease, decreases in circulating levels of clotting factors, dependent on vitamin K, occur. If such patients are admitted for treatment of an acute gastrointestinal hemorrhage, this can be a life-threatening complication. If prothrombin times are significantly prolonged, vitamin K is indicated (Van Thiel, 1983).

Since alcohol affects every body system, the medical complications of alcohol abuse are numerous. The most common problems of consequence include metabolic acidosis, hepatic cirrhosis, pancreatitis, hemorrhage, cardiac myopathy, infarction, Wernicke's encephalopathy, Korsakoff's syndrome, anemias, infections, and respiratory failure (Van Thiel, 1983).

Antabuse (disulfiram) has been commonly used in the treatment of alcoholism (Hald and Jacobsen, 1948). It is a nonaddicting, prescription medication that causes a strong physical reaction if the patient drinks while taking the drug. Disulfiram blocks the usual metabolic process of alcohol. The exact mechanism is not known, but some research indicates that it interferes with the breakdown of acetaldehyde, a component of alcohol. During a disulfiram-ethanol reaction (DER), blood levels of acetaldehyde are very high, and it is hypothesized that this accounts for many of the symptoms of the disulfiram-ethanol reaction (Deitrich and Peterson, 1983; Kitson, 1977). Patients with advanced liver disease are not candidates for disulfiram therapy.

The disulfiram-ethanol reaction occurs within 5 to 15 minutes of ingestion or topical use of alcohol or a therapeutic agent with a significant alcohol content. In 20 to 30 minutes, symptoms of the DER peak, and the reaction usually subsides within 2 hours. However, mild symptoms may persist as long as alcohol remains in the blood. Signs and symptoms of the DER can occur after ingesting small amounts of alcohol and can be fatal at this point (Linden and associates, 1984). Effects of disulfiram persist after the medication is discontinued. In most patients, effects dissipate after 5 days. However, it is possible for a patient to experience a DER up to 2 weeks after disulfiram has been discontinued. Table 60–5 describes the signs and symptoms of a disulfiram-ethanol reaction (Linden and associates, 1984).

Patients taking disulfiram are given Medic-alert necklaces or bracelets for easy identification. They usually also carry a card in their wallet that lists the signs and symptoms of a DER. Family members are also knowledgeable about disulfiram. All patients complete a thorough informed consent process prior to starting the drug and are extremely fearful of experiencing a DER. If they are able to speak, patients can often tell the health care team what specific agents to avoid that may interact with disulfiram or

TABLE 60–5. Signs and Symptoms of the Disulfiram-Ethanol Reaction (DER)

Mild or Moderate	Advanced
Flushing (face and trunk)	Respiratory distress
Headache	Crushing chest pain
Red eyes	Myocardial ischemia
Diaphoresis	Dysrhythmias
Dyspnea	Shock
Tachycardia	Seizures
Orthostatic hypotension	Death from cardiovascular
Nausea or vomiting	collapse

cause a DER. It is imperative for the health care team to be aware of these agents. Disulfiram potentiates the effects of many drugs such as digitalis, anesthetics, and anticoagulants (Martin, 1978). Other drugs or agents can create a DER. When a patient on disulfiram is admitted, the pharmacy should be consulted about the appropriateness of all proposed drug therapies. Iodine prep solutions are used in lieu of alcohol prep for these patients.

It is not necessary to continue disulfiram in the critical care unit. Upon transfer, the health care team in the new unit should be made aware of the patient's disulfiram therapy. Discharge planning includes the need to plan for continued disulfiram therapy.

COCAINE ABUSE

Cocaine is the most frequently abused illicit drug today. It is estimated that 22 million Americans have at least tried cocaine. Its use has reached epidemic proportions in the major cities in the form of "crack" cocaine. Crack is made by heating cocaine hydrochloride solution with baking soda. This process yields a solid chunk, which can be divided into hundreds of small "rocks." Five to six rocks are placed to a vial and sold for $15 or $20. Sometimes crack cocaine is altered during the heating process with amphetamines or lidocaine. A vial containing a couple of rocks is sold for $5.

Because of its availability, rapid onset of addiction, and ease of transport, dealers are able to make large amounts of money in a short period of time. Teenage street dealers make hundreds of dollars a day, and children as young as 6 to 8 years old are used as runners and lookouts. All of these factors have implications for critical care nurses. Gunshot and stabbing wounds are more likely to occur now than ever before, with a resulting increase in emergency admissions for people of all ages.

Cocaine is classified as a local anesthetic and sympathomimetic drug. It has been compared with amphetamines in terms of its sympathomimetic effects, which explains why drug abusers frequently use amphetamines with cocaine to heighten the effect or in place of cocaine when their supply is depleted.

Although the mucous membrane of the nose is a favored site for some cocaine abusers, smoking or injecting the drug intravenously produces a greater "high" because there is an immediate peak in blood levels. A number of studies suggest that the behavioral effects of cocaine are mediated by an increase in concentration of the neurotransmitter dopamine in synapses of the brain (Woolverton and Kleven, 1988).

Frequent use of cocaine can result in a drug-induced psychosis requiring close observation or the use of restraints. Tactile hallucinations, such as the perception that something is crawling under the skin, seem so real that addicts may inflict damage to the skin as they scratch incessantly. Visual hallucinations occur and are frequently reported as seeing things in miniature. For people around them, one of the most disturbing effects of cocaine abuse is the paranoid thought disorders of the addict. These thoughts are very real to the addict, and because they feel threatened, they frequently become violent toward others (Cohen, 1985).

Polydrug abuse is common among chronic cocaine abusers. Alcohol, benzodiazepines, barbiturates, and heroin are used to relieve insomnia and to soften the "crash" when they cease using cocaine. Therefore, a coexisting dependence on a substance that can produce physical withdrawal symptoms during the abstinence period must be considered. Signs and symptoms of early to latent intoxication, the toxic effects of overdose, and the abstinence stage are described in Table 60–6.

The main cause of cocaine-related deaths is the drug's cardiovascular effects. The heart rate accelerates, ectopic beats can occur, and ventricular fibrillation can result in death. Respiratory arrest has also been reported as a cause of death. At first, respirations increase and then become shallow and later irregular. Gross pulmonary edema develops, followed by a paralysis of the medullary brain center and then death (Cohen, 1985). Idiosyncratic cardiovascular reactions to cocaine have been related to myocardial oxygen imbalances associated with adrenergic stimulation of heart rate and coronary vasoconstriction, electrocardiographic conduction defects, and hypertension (Loveys, 1987).

Acute hypertension can cause a cerebral blood vessel to rupture, resulting in hemiplegia or death. Increased systemic blood pressure due to cocaine use in patients with chronic hypertension has resulted in rupture of the ascending aorta. Hyperthermia, to a level that requires aggressive cooling measures, can also occur. This is due to cocaine's direct action on the temperature-regulating centers of the brain, vasoconstriction, and increased muscular activity. Infrequently, seizures occur and, if neglected, can lead to death from status epilepticus (Cohen, 1985).

Successful treatment of cocaine toxicity requires prompt recognition of patients who are experiencing the more advanced stages of intoxication (e.g., hallucinations and hyperthermia). Treatment goals are to minimize nervous system stimulation and support ventilation and circulation. Intravenous propranolol is used to block beta-adrenergic stimulation of heart

TABLE 60–6. Cocaine Signs and Symptoms

Intoxication	Overdose	Withdrawal
Early	Flaccid paralysis	Depression
Euphoria	Coma	Anhedonia
Sudden headache	Fixed, dilated pupils	Intense craving for drug
Cold sweats	Ventricular fibrillation	Irritability
Muscle jerks	Circulatory failure	Irregular sleep patterns
Bradycardia	Cyanosis	Aches and pains
Increased blood pressure	Gross pulmonary edema	Increased appetite
Tachypnea	Respiratory failure	Poor concentration
Dyspnea	Loss of reflexes	Suicide
Psychotic behavior	Cardiac arrest	
	Death	
Advanced		
Decreased level of consciousness		
Generalized hyperreflexia		
Seizures		
Incontinence		
Status epilepticus		
Increased, weak, irregular pulse		
Increased blood pressure, then rapid decrease		
Irregular respirations		

rate and blood pressure (Rappolt and colleagues, 1977). Some authors recommend the use of alpha-adrenergic blocking agents such as phentolamine or afterload-reducing agents such as sodium nitroprusside to counteract the alpha-adrenergic effects of vasoconstriction (Benowitz and colleagues, 1979).

Benowitz and co-workers (1979) reported an increase in survival rate, decreased hyperthermia, and decreased cardiotoxicity with the use of chlorpromazine in these patients. Liberal doses of diazepam have been used to reduce anxiety, relieve skeletal muscle spasm, and prevent or control seizures. Compazine is used to reduce the incidence of vomiting. Hypothermic therapy should be instituted for the treatment of hyperthermia. To aid urinary excretion of cocaine, intravenous ammonium chloride should be administered. Protein and vitamin B deficiencies can be expected, and therefore replacement therapy is indicated (Loveys, 1987).

Although cocaine does not produce a stereotypical abstinence syndrome as with the opioids and barbiturates, abrupt cessation of chronic high doses can result in a variety of symptoms. Intense craving for the drug can reach a point where the addict ceases to eat or sleep and is consumed by depression. It is this intense craving to abort the dysphoric aspects of abstinence that drives the patient back to using cocaine. This reinforcing behavior is not seen to this extent with any other psychoactive agent (Cohen, 1985). Because intravenous cocaine abusers inject so frequently, they are the most at-risk population for contracting AIDS (Battjes and Pickens, 1988).

Once the initial crisis that brought the patient to the critical care setting is under control, the major concern of the health care team is the need to be aware that the patient's severe depression can assume suicidal proportions. If this depressive state is prolonged, antidepressant therapy should be considered post-cocaine. Patients need to be informed that during the postcocaine period they may lose the capacity to enjoy pleasurable events. This anhedonia will persist until dopamine homeostasis is restored, and the reward centers in the brain regain sensitivity to pleasurable activities without the use of cocaine (Cohen, 1985). Referral to a chemical dependency treatment center is vital for these patients.

BARBITURATE ABUSE

Barbiturates are classified as sedative-hypnotics, which are used to treat insomnia and anxiety. They are also used in the management of seizures. They have a high risk of toxicity and dependence, and when misused they can be deadly.

There are four types of barbiturate abusers. Those seeking relief from emotional distress may carry their use to such an extreme that it interferes with the activities of daily living. These individuals become oblivious to their surroundings and live in a somewhat permanent stupor (Levine, 1973).

Those whose tolerance has developed because of continued use of high doses experience a reinforcing paradoxical reaction that includes excitation and a feeling of well-being. In some people, this stimulating effect has been observed in the absence of long-term use. In these individuals, the stimulating effect is due to the release of inhibitions by the drug. These people take the drug for its exhilarating and animating effect and to bring about "increased efficiency" (Levine, 1973).

The third group of barbiturate abusers includes those who use it in combination with other illicit drugs such as cocaine. The barbiturate counteracts the effects of the stimulant, or both a stimulating and a sedative effect are achieved simultaneously (Levine, 1973).

The fourth group of abusers uses barbiturates concurrently with other substances such as alcohol or opiates. These individuals seek the potentiating effect of barbiturates on alcohol and opiates (Levine, 1973).

Short-acting barbiturates are the most widely abused. Taken orally, they produce a "high" shortly after ingestion and require no paraphernalia, needles, or syringes. The onset and duration of action of the various barbiturates cover a wide range, as summarized in Table 60–7.

Tolerance develops even when relatively low doses are taken repeatedly. In contrast to narcotics, however, there is a limit to the dose level at which a person can become tolerant. Therefore, the difference between a tolerated dose and a lethal one is marginal. This factor is responsible for a number of accidental deaths in barbiturate-dependent persons (Smith and Wesson, 1975).

Management of a patient with an overdose of barbiturates includes maintenance of an adequate airway, assistance with ventilation, and administration of oxygen as needed. If the patient is awake, vomiting is induced with the use of syrup of ipecac rather than lavage. Vomiting is preferable to lavage in a conscious patient because the first part of the small intestine is also emptied with vomiting, whereas gastric lavage clears only the stomach contents. The gastric contents should undergo toxicologic analysis to determine exactly which drugs were ingested. If concomitant alcohol consumption is suspected, a breath analyzer test can rapidly determine the blood alcohol level. Vital signs should be taken every 15 minutes and the patient observed to determine whether the overdose will progress to a stuporous or comatose state (Smith and Wesson, 1975).

If the patient is semicomatose, vomiting should not be induced. Careful gastric lavage with 10 to 15 liters of fluid is indicated if it can be determined that the drug was ingested within 4 hours of treatment. Activated charcoal may be left in the stomach to slow absorption of any material not removed by lavage. The advantage of removing the unabsorbed drug must be weighed against the possibility of pulmonary aspiration, which can occur during lavage. Because of the danger of impending respiratory failure, arterial blood gas levels must be determined to evaluate the degree of respiratory depression. Vital signs and ventilation are monitored until the patient is stable and has regained consciousness (Smith and Wesson, 1975).

If the patient is comatose upon arrival, he is in an immediate life-threatening situation. A brief history and physical examination should be done and the patient's airway evaluated. Vital signs are taken, and an endotracheal tube is passed rapidly to guard the airway. Gastric lavage should be performed with fluid containing activated charcoal to remove any remaining drugs from the stomach and for toxicology analysis. An intravenous line should be established to assist in maintaining the cardiovascular system and in the rapid administration of drugs. Arterial blood gas concentrations should be determined to evaluate the degree of respiratory acidosis that results from depressed ventilation with retained carbon dioxide and a low blood pressure. These two signs indicate the approach of respiratory failure and cardiovascular collapse. Life support measures, including assisted ventilation, parenteral fluids, cardiovascular monitoring, and careful monitoring of urinary output are critical at this point (Smith and Wesson, 1975).

The use of stimulants (to overcome central nervous system depression), hemodialysis, or osmotic diuresis is not recommended. When stimulants are used to counteract the depressive effects of sedative-hypnotics, the stimulants' side effects create more problems than they solve (Smith and Wesson, 1975).

Once the emergency situation brought on by the overdose is under control, attention must be given to management of the withdrawal syndrome. Onset of withdrawal begins within 72 hours after the last dose and can produce a second life-threatening crisis for the patient. Minor withdrawal symptoms begin to appear within 8 to 12 hours in the following order: anxiety, muscle twitching, tremor of hands and fingers, progressive weakness, dizziness, distortion in visual perception, nausea, vomiting, insomnia, and orthostatic hypotension (Physicians' Desk Reference, 1991).

It is imperative that replacement drug therapy begin as soon as possible once the patient is stabi-

TABLE 60–7. Barbiturates: Onset and Duration of Action

Classification	Onset	Duration of Action
Ultra short-acting (thiopental)	Immediate (IV)	15 minutes to 3 hours
Short-acting (Amobarbital) (Pentobarbital) (Secobarbital)	10–15 minutes when taken orally	3 hours or less
Intermediate-acting (Butabarbital)	10–30 minutes when taken orally	3–6 hours
Long-acting (Phenobarbital)	30–60 minutes when taken orally	6 or more hours

lized. Failure to do so will result in the need to administer larger doses of phenobarbital initially to combat withdrawal symptoms. Phenobarbital is the drug of choice in the management of withdrawal because it maintains a constant blood level without producing a "high." If replacement therapy has been delayed and acute withdrawal symptoms are present, phenobarbital sodium should be administered intravenously. The nurse should wait after each dose to determine its full effect because the drug may take 15 minutes or longer to attain peak levels in the brain. Too rapid administration may cause vasodilation and decreased blood pressure, respiratory depression, apnea, or laryngospasm. During intravenous administration, blood pressure, respirations, and cardiac function are monitored and preparations are made for resuscitation and assisted ventilation if necessary.

To calculate the amount of phenobarbital needed to cover the amount of short-acting street drug used by the patient, add the total amount of street drug reportedly used in a 24-hour period. Thirty milligrams of phenobarbital will adequately cover 100 mg of the short-acting drug; therefore, substitute 30 mg of phenobarbital for every 100 mg of street drug. Divide the amount of phenobarbital into four equal doses to be administered every 6 hours. Because the accuracy of the amount of street drug use reported by the patient is always questionable, a PRN dose of 5 to 10 mg should be ordered in case withdrawal symptoms occur between regular doses (Smith and Wesson, 1975). Signs and symptoms of barbiturate intoxication, overdose, and withdrawal are presented in Table 60–8.

Stabilization is the goal while the patient is in the critical care unit. Therefore, management of the detoxification process by gradual reduction of phenobarbital will not be addressed.

BENZODIAZEPINE ABUSE

The benzodiazepines—chlordiazepoxide, chlorazepate, diazepam, flurazepam, lorazepam, midazolam, and oxazepam—have found wide acceptance as antianxiety agents. They reduce anxiety without inducing sleep, and most have muscle-relaxant and anticonvulsant properties as well. They produce nonspecific central nervous system depression and closely resemble sedative-hypnotic drugs (barbiturates) in pharmacologic properties.

Because of its widespread use and abuse, diazepam warrants specific mention in this chapter. According to the Drug Abuse Warning Network (DAWN), diazepam was among the top three drugs reported in emergency episodes in 1985 (Drug Enforcement Agency Report, 1987). Like the barbiturates and opioids, diazepam produces physical and psychological dependence. Diazepam has a prompt onset of action, about 1 hour, and its effects have a 24-hour duration. Tolerance develops rapidly, thus requiring increasing doses to achieve the desired effect (Cohen, 1985).

Individuals who abuse diazepam fall into three main categories. Some receive the drug legitimately by prescription for its antianxiety properties. With months of continued use, they begin to build tolerance to the prescribed dose. Attempts to discontinue its use are met with distinct physiologic symptoms such as agitation, nausea, vomiting, depression, tremors, and seizures. These individuals return to using diazepam to prevent the progression of symptoms without considering the abuse-dependency properties of the drug.

The second group of abusers use diazepam in conjunction with other drugs such as methadone (Dolophine) and alcohol to potentiate the euphoric effect of the latter agents. These combinations are particularly dangerous because they heighten central nervous system or respiratory depression.

The third group uses diazepam alone as a drug of choice. They describe a euphoria that is soothing and similar to a narcotic-induced state of intoxication.

Regardless of how an individual develops dependence on diazepam, it is one of the most difficult drug dependencies to overcome. A suicide attempt should

TABLE 60–8. Barbiturates: Signs and Symptoms

Intoxication	Overdose	Withdrawal
Slurred speech	Seizures	Anxiety
Incoordination	Oliguria	Muscle twitching
Ataxia	Cyanosis	Tremors of hands, fingers, tongue, and eyelids
Impaired memory or attention span	Moist skin	
Lateral nystagmus	Hypotension	Dizziness
Euphoria	Respiratory and CNS depression	Distortion in visual perception
Drowsiness	Absent reflexes	Nausea
Depression	Slight miosis to paralytic dilation	Vomiting
Irritability	Tachycardia	Insomnia
Lethargy	Hypothermia	Orthostatic toxic hypotension
Seizures	Apnea	Tachycardia
Psychosis	Circulatory collapse	Diaphoresis
	Respiratory arrest	Seizures
	Death	Amnesia
		Anorexia
		Delirium
		Death

always be suspected when an individual who has overdosed on diazepam is being treated.

Management of a benzodiazepine overdose is essentially the same as that used for a barbiturate overdose and includes immediate emptying of the stomach by gastric lavage. Monitor vital signs, maintain an adequate airway, and administer fluids. Hypotension may be managed with norepinephrine. Dialysis is of limited value (Geffner, 1984).

Signs and symptoms of benzodiazepine intoxication, overdose, and withdrawal are presented in Table 60–9. Paradoxical reactions such as a hyperexcited state, anxiety, hallucinations, increased muscle spasticity, and insomnia can occur. Benzodiazepines and barbiturates should not be given for management of excitation because they will potentiate the paradoxical reaction. In general, alcohol, narcotic analgesics, sedative-hypnotics, and other central nervous system depressant drugs are contraindicated for the management of a benzodiazepine overdose. They increase central nervous system depression, hypotension, and muscular weakness. Cimetidine is contraindicated because it decreases clearance of diazepam (Geffner, 1984).

As with the barbiturates, it is imperative to begin planning for management of the withdrawal syndrome as soon as the patient is stabilized. Abrupt cessation of diazepam can be life-threatening for the chronic abuser of diazepam. The drug of choice in the management of withdrawal symptoms is diazepam. Although some authors report using it, phenobarbital substitution for detoxification generally offers no pharmacologic advantage over slow withdrawal with diazepam (Smith and Wesson, 1975). For replacement therapy, oral administration is desired; however, if it is absolutely necessary to give diazepam intravenously, it should be administered slowly, no faster than 5 mg (1 mL)/minute. Because diazepam is barely soluble, slow injection through infusion tubing as close as possible to the vein insertion is preferred (Geffner, 1984). Apnea and cardiac arrest can occur during administration of intravenous diazepam; therefore, one should be prepared for resuscitation and assisted ventilation.

Once again, the goal of the health care team in the critical care unit is stabilization of the patient. Detoxification can be safely accomplished in a less acute setting.

NARCOTICS AND OPIOIDS

Narcotics and opioids are classified as controlled substances because of their high abuse potential. They have both sedative and analgesic properties, produce insensitivity to pain, and have a depressant effect on the central nervous system. Heroin, morphine, and codeine are derived from opium. They, along with the popular synthetic narcotics (meperidine, hydromorphone, methadone, oxycodone) are among the most widely abused drugs in this category. Collectively, we refer to this group of drugs as narcotics.

Intravenous injection is the most popular route of administration of narcotics. It is preferred because it delivers a "rush." For some patients, the sight of a needle can produce an overwhelming craving for narcotics. Repeated injection into one vein causes sclerosis of the vein and is referred to as a track. Prolonged injection into one area may result in tissue necrosis requiring surgical intervention. These visible signs of drug abuse provide valuable information about the length and severity of the patient's dependence. Because chronic use of narcotics creates

---

TABLE 60–9. Signs and Symptoms Associated with Benzodiazepines

Intoxication	Overdose	Withdrawal
Slow reflexes	Confusion	Seizures
Decline in mental acuity	Coma	Tremor
Drowsiness	Cardiovascular collapse	Abdominal and muscle cramps
Fatigue	Dyspnea	Vomiting
Ataxia	Hypotension	Diaphoresis
Confusion	Laryngospasm	Agitation
Depression	Somnolence	Nausea
Dysarthria	Diminished reflexes	Depression
headache	Depressed respirations	Anxiety
Slurred speech	Apnea	Impaired memory
Syncope	Cardiac arrest	Depersonalization
Vertigo		Loss of appetite
Hallucinations		Headache
Bracycardia		Metallic taste
Blurred vision		Photophobia
Diplopia		Incoordination
Nystagmus		Vertigo
Tremor		Flulike illness
		Paranoid reactions
		Visual hallucinations
		Hypersensitivity to touch and pain
		Paresthesias

physical and psychological dependence, narcotic intoxication, overdose, and withdrawal states produce well-defined signs and symptoms. These are presented in Table 60–10.

Emergency management of a narcotic overdose consists of supporting or restoring vital functions and administering a narcotic antagonist. Pinpoint pupils, depressed respirations (2 to 4/minute), and shallow coma form a classic triad of narcotic overdose. However, the pupils may be dilated if the patient's overdose is due to meperidine or if he has used phenothiazines. Pupils will also be dilated if anoxia has been severe (Senay, 1983).

Pulmonary edema is frequently observed in the overdose state. The addict's friends may have complicated this condition by administering coffee, milk, salt solutions, and so on, thereby inducing an aspiration pneumonia. A differential diagnosis is made by determining the respiratory rate. It will be elevated if the patient is suffering from aspiration pneumonia, and depressed or normal if narcotic-induced pulmonary edema is present (Senay, 1983).

The treatment of choice for narcotic overdose is naloxone. Unlike nalorphine, it does not have agonist effects that can cause further respiratory depression if the overdose is due to other classes of drugs such as barbiturates or alcohol (Senay, 1983). Naloxone is administered intravenously, usually in a dose of 0.4 to 2 mg. It should be administered slowly to avoid too rapid a return to consciousness with the possibility of disorientation, hyperactivity, extreme dysphoria, and possible violence. Response is indicated by reversal of respiratory depression within minutes. An increase in the level of consciousness and a widening of the pupils is also generally seen. Repeated doses may be given every 2 to 3 minutes if necessary. The respiratory rate usually increases within 1 to 2 minutes following a therapeutic dose, and the effects last 1 to 4 hours. Side effects of naloxone include nausea, vomiting, and narcotic withdrawal symptoms (Potter, 1984).

If withdrawal symptoms do appear, they may be severe but should last only as long as the effect of the naloxone. Because the narcotic may have a longer duration of action than naloxone, serious respiratory depression and coma can recur. The patient should be carefully observed and naloxone readministered as required. Patients should remain in the critical care unit for at least 24 hours following an acute overdose to ensure full recovery.

As with barbiturates, once stabilized, the patient is at risk for withdrawal symptoms. Generally, the narcotic abstinence syndrome begins 8 to 12 hours after the last dose. It subsides gradually over a period of 7 to 10 days. Methadone is an exception. Its long-lasting properties delay the abstinence syndrome for 24 to 48 hours after the last dose, with peak intensity occurring on the third day. Symptoms gradually subside over a period of 3 weeks or longer (Physicians' Desk Reference, 1991).

The withdrawal syndrome can be relieved by using methadone in its oral form. The key to successful management is to provide medication prior to the onset of late withdrawal symptoms, using the least amount of methadone necessary to control symptoms. Usually 5 mg given orally or by nasogastric tube three times in a 24-hour period as needed is sufficient. Once the patient has been stabilized, the dosage can be reduced gradually until detoxification is safely completed. This is usually done in a less acute care unit. If further hospitalization is not necessary, referral to a drug treatment program is indicated.

In addition to patients who are admitted to the critical care unit for management of a narcotic overdose, drug-dependent patients receiving legitimate medications for their dependency may be admitted for other reasons. The critical care team should be aware of two such treatment modalities. If not assessed adequately, the patient could suffer needlessly. Both medical and behavioral complications can arise.

One modality, methadone maintenance, consists of administration of a carefully determined dose of methadone daily. The dose may be as low as 5 mg or as much as 100 mg; however, experience has proved 60 mg to be the maximum therapeutic dose. At 60 mg or less, patients are not obsessed with drug-seeking activities. They are free of physical symptoms and are able to engage in therapy. Patients should be maintained on their current therapeutic dose throughout the acute stage of their illness. Ongoing communication with the patient's treatment program is vital to provide continuity of care after

TABLE 60–10. Signs and Symptoms Associated with Narcotics

Intoxication	Overdose	Withdrawal	
		Early	*Late*
Pupils: constricted	Pupils: pinpoint	Drug-seeking behavior	Insomnia
Respirations: decreased	Respirations: severely depressed	Respirations: increased	Nausea
Euphoria	Coma	Diaphoresis	Vomiting
Somnolence	Death	Lacrimation	Diarrhea
Hypotension		Yawning	Abdominal cramps
Bradycardia		Rhinorrhea	Tachycardia
Hypothermia		Piloerection	Hypertension
Clouded sensorium		Restlessness	Involuntary muscle spasms

they are discharged from the hospital. Refer to the section on pain management in this chapter for recommendations concerning the concurrent use of analgesics and methadone maintenance.

The other treatment modality, which is used less frequently but deserves mention, is naltrexone (Trexan). In contrast to methadone, which is a substitute for illicit narcotics, naltrexone is used to eliminate the reinforcing properties of narcotics. Naltrexone's antagonist actions block the usual euphoric effect of narcotics by competitively occupying the brain receptor sites that interact with narcotics. Research indicates that naltrexone does not cause physical or psychological dependence. Patients do not develop tolerance to the narcotic antagonist. Naltrexone will cause withdrawal symptoms if it is given to a person who has any trace of narcotic in his system. Therefore, chemical dependency treatment programs are extremely careful to detoxify their patients completely prior to starting treatment with naltrexone.

Once the patient is on a maintenance dose, naltrexone antagonizes physical effects such as respiratory depression in patients taking doses of narcotics as large as 25 mg of heroin. They can, however, surmount this antagonism by taking even larger doses of narcotics. In such cases, profound respiratory depression and death may occur (Du Pont de Nemours, 1985).

Naltrexone also blocks the analgesic effects of narcotics. Therefore, patients on naltrexone maintenance will not obtain relief from the usual doses of narcotic analgesics. In an emergency situation that requires analgesia that can only be achieved with narcotics, the amount required will be greater than usual and the resulting respiratory depression will be deeper and more prolonged. In addition, if narcotic analgesics that lead to histamine release are given, facial swelling, itching, and generalized erythema may occur. Whenever an analgesic is used to reverse naltrexone's blockade properties, the patient should be monitored closely for adverse effects. Patients may discontinue naltrexone without experiencing withdrawal symptoms. It will take up to 3 days to neutralize its antagonistic effect on narcotics (Physicians' Desk Reference, 1991).

PAIN MANAGEMENT

Pain management in a chemically dependent patient is one area of treatment that can be problematic for the health care team. Several issues contribute to the difficulties. The first is that the staff are afraid they will "feed the addiction" or create a greater need for drug use. This is not true. The patient with an addiction has already created a life pattern that requires drugs. In an acute treatment situation, the patient's pain must be relieved in the most effective manner possible in spite of a preexisting addiction. Prolonged experience of pain will only increase the patient's anxiety and create an atmosphere of mis-

trust that will heighten the patient's drug-seeking behavior. Another issue is that the health care team may feel inadequate in assessing the level of pain and determining the amount of pain relief needed. A good, therapeutic relationship between the patient and the health care team is the basis of appropriate pain management.

Since each patient's perception of pain is unique, pain management must be individualized. One method of obtaining accurate baseline assessments of a patient's pain is to ask him or her to rate the pain on a scale of one to ten, one representing no pain and ten representing the worst pain ever felt. This gives the patient a way of measuring and expressing pain and actively involves him in the assessment, which has the added benefit of reducing anxiety. This activity will also provide a baseline for future pain assessments (Potter, 1985).

The National Institute on Drug Abuse (NIDA) has been a forerunner in supporting research aimed at developing nonaddicting analgesics. Through their efforts, naturally occurring substances in the central nervous system, endogenous opioids, were identified as having pain-relieving properties. These substances, endorphins and enkephalins, seem to have functions similar to those of adrenaline. That is, these chemicals are released under conditions of stress. This fact may account for the remarkable lack of pain perception on the battlefield and the reduced pain perceived during childbirth (Israel and associates, 1978).

Researchers have further demonstrated that when exogenous supplies of narcotics are administered repeatedly, as in drug abuse, there is a decreased rate of synthesis and a decreased release of endogenous opioids. The central nervous system then becomes dependent on exogenously supplied narcotics (Rapaka, 1986). This may account for the narcotic-dependent person's decreased tolerance of pain. It would then follow that narcotic addicts are in greater need of pain-relieving medications than the general population.

Senay (1983) states that the health care team should not add stress to stress. If an addict has a gunshot wound, a broken bone, or a diabetic crisis, he has enough stress, and adding the stress of detoxification is not advisable. Dependence on narcotics should be maintained until the medical or surgical problem is resolved. Once that is accomplished, medical management of detoxification can be considered if the patient consents. Senay (1983) further states that it is sound practice to discharge street addicts back to the street without detoxifying them if that is what they want.

Analgesic needs and narcotic maintenance are independent issues. Narcotics given to substitute for street drug dependence have little or no analgesic effect. If a patient who is being maintained on methadone is admitted to a critical care unit, his usual daily dose of methadone should be maintained throughout the period of hospitalization. For pain management, analgesics in the usual doses and frequencies should be given in addition to the regular dose of methadone (Senay, 1983).

Sedation and relaxation observed in an addict indicate that analgesia is probably present. If the patient continues to request medication, it is usually because he is seeking an intoxicating dose rather than a pain-relieving one. Talking to him or her about the observed responses and displaying an attitude of concern and competence will reduce this drug-seeking behavior.

In narcotic dependent patients, the use of drugs that have antagonist as well as agonist effects (pentazocine, nalbuphine, and butorphanol) should be avoided. The antagonist effects are strong enough to produce withdrawal symptoms (Senay, 1983).

In summary, maintenance of narcotic addiction and relief of pain are two distinct, separate issues. Both require individual assessment and intervention.

INTERPERSONAL ISSUES

The interpersonal issues that surface with substance abuse patients can create disruption for the health care team. Therefore, it is critical to establish and maintain a therapeutic approach in the critical care unit. One key element of the therapeutic approach is maintaining good and consistent communications among the health care team, the patient, and the family.

Some basic components are involved in establishing a therapeutic style of communication. The first and most important requirement is that all team members must participate in establishing effective communication. If this does not happen, the patient and the family will not feel that they can be honest and candid and will withhold information that could be critical. A nonjudgmental attitude is mandatory for the establishment of trust with the patient and family.

Once a nonjudgmental atmosphere has been established, the next step is to develop a supportive relationship with the patient. This will help the patient to view the health care team as an ally instead of an adversary. Again, this increases the level of trust between the patient and the team. Keep in mind that this supportive relationship must be grounded in good therapeutic judgment. The effect of a supportive relationship is to make the patient feel that the team is concerned and willing to meet his or her needs, thus decreasing the patient's need to manipulate or use other disruptive behaviors to ensure that these needs are met.

An assertive style of communication is appropriate with this population. This is the model of communication that is advocated in substance abuse rehabilitation settings (Wilford, 1987). Patients and their families respond well to this style and are often more assertive with the health care team in return. Because of the fear and anxiety that patients and family members have about the crisis of receiving treatment

in a critical care unit, it is also helpful to be directive in communication. Establishing expectations and relating other treatment parameters will help to decrease the patient's concerns.

Manipulative, hostile, and aggressive behaviors are common patient reactions that are feared by the health care team. When hostile and aggressive behavior is a result of an acute toxic state, the patient is not able to respond to verbal direction. In these cases, it is necessary to use chemical and physical restraints to manage the behavior. Outside of these situations, the patient usually responds well to a firmly assertive, directive style.

Another typical scenario is the whining, manipulative patient who is continuously demanding the nurse's attention in whatever manner possible (call-bell, setting off monitor, or verbal comments). These are the patients that the nurse would like to ignore, so these behaviors are not reinforced. Actually, these are the patients that need to be talked with the most. This situation is common with narcotic addicts. The best response is to spend some time with the patient as soon as this behavior begins, or on admission as a prophylactic measure. During this initial discussion, the nurse states her plan to assess the patient's needs diligently on a routine, ongoing basis and sets some limits. Inform them that their attention-seeking behavior is disruptive and not necessary. Then follow up by routinely assessing and enforcing these limits and sharing this approach with the entire treatment team.

The key to preventing disruptive behavior is meeting the patient's needs. The patient's and family's perception is crucial in this respect. If they feel their needs are not being addressed, many disruptive behaviors will follow.

The final interpersonal issue that can be potentially disruptive and explosive is related to the management of visitors in the unit. Remember that it is extremely possible that family members or friends are also substance abusers. As such, they can be as much or more disruptive than the patient because they are verbal and ambulatory. The entire treatment team must be alert to this potential management problem. To avert potentially dangerous situations, certain precautions should be instituted routinely. First, visitors should be required to submit any items brought for the patient to a check by the staff. This is to ensure that drugs or other substances that could be dangerous are not given to the patient. Also, the health care team should observe the visit in case the visitor tries to offer drugs to the patient. Another possibility is that the visitor may try to obtain drugs, syringes, or other drug paraphernalia that is commonly available in the unit. The staff should remove these items from the bedside and observe supply areas containing these items. If a visitor presents in an intoxicated state, security should be notified to remove the visitor immediately. This is an extremely unsafe situation that can result in aggressive or violent behavior. An understanding of addiction and of all the dynamics surrounding those who are addicted will help the health care team manage these patients without adversity.

RESOURCES AND REFERRALS

Depending on the size and scope of the hospital, there are numerous potential resources available to assist in the assessment and treatment of these patients. Many hospitals have inpatient units or outpatient programs specializing in the treatment of addictions. If the patient or family states that the patient has been treated in a specific substance abuse program, or that the patient has a specific outpatient counselor, the program or counselor, if contacted, can offer valuable treatment information and support. If pain management is a problem, a pain management specialist should be consulted when a substance abuse program is not available.

In smaller facilities in which substance abuse programs are not available, resources may be more difficult to locate. Since substance abuse is often a problem for psychiatric or mental health patients, staff in these settings may be able to offer assistance. They can help with management of the behavioral and interpersonal problems that may arise. Another alternative is to contact a local Alcoholics or Narcotics Anonymous office or counselor for information.

For current publications on individual substances and treatment issues contact the National Institute of Drug Abuse. Each year NIDA publishes numerous books that contain excellent reference material.

Referring substance abuse patients for further treatment is a major discharge planning issue that must be addressed. When a physical crisis related to substance abuse occurs, such as a gastrointestinal bleed, overdose, or toxic reaction, it can break through the patient's normal denial of the addiction. Often such a patient verbalizes his realization of the addiction and acknowledges the need for treatment. Referral to a substance abuse treatment program can be incorporated into the discharge plans. The receiving unit can follow through with this plan.

SUMMARY

Management of substance abuse patients is facilitated by a basic knowledge of chemical dependency and the consistent use of this knowledge to guide treatment interventions by the health care team. The information presented in this chapter is only a brief synopsis of the most critical treatment issues that arise.

It is wise to be aware of the illicit drugs that are popular in one's own community and to become familiar with the basic management of those drugs in a treatment setting. It is always necessary for nurses to update their knowledge about which drugs are in vogue. Use of specific drugs can change very rapidly as new drugs become available.

These patients often exhibit obnoxious and disruptive behaviors that mask their fear and anxiety. It is important to look beyond these obnoxious behaviors and not to reject patients for this reason. Instead, the team's confident, knowledgeable demeanor and willingness to meet the patient's needs can decrease or eliminate the need for the behavior.

Another important point to remember is that these patients do not fit any particular profile. All age groups from the elderly to children and infants may have substance abuse problems. Men and women from all socioeconomic groups may be chemically dependent.

The most important need is to address the issues related to substance abuse from the onset of treatment and throughout the hospitalization. Chemical dependency does create a unique set of problems and can complicate other aspects of treatment. However, with consistent application of a basic knowledge of chemical dependency, these problems can be minimized.

References

American Nurses Association and National Nurses Society on Addictions (1988). *Standards of addictions nursing practice with selected diagnoses and criteria.* Kansas City: American Nurses Association.

Barry, H., III. (1979). Behavioral manifestations of ethanol intoxication and physical dependence. In E. Majchrowicz and E. P. Noble (Eds.), *Biochemistry and pharmacology of ethanol.* New York: Plenum.

Battjes, R. J., and Pickens, R. W. (1988). *Needle sharing among intravenous drug abusers: National and international perspectives.* National Institute on Drug Abuse Research Monograph Series 80. Rockville, MD: National Institute on Drug Abuse.

Benowitz N. L., Rosenberg, J., and Becker, C. E. (1979). Cardiopulmonary catastrophes in drug-overdosed patients. *Medical Clinics of North America, 63,* 267.

Carpenito, L. J. (1983). *Nursing diagnosis: Application to clinical practice.* Philadelphia: J. B. Lippincott.

Clouet, D., Asghar, K., and Brown, R. (1988). *Mechanisms of cocaine abuse and toxicity* (p. ix). National Institute on Drug Abuse Research Monograph Series 88. Rockville, MD: National Institute on Drug Abuse.

Cohen, S. (1985). *The substance abuse problems.* Vol. 2. *New issues for the 1980's.* New York: Haworth.

Deitrich, R. A., and Peterson, D. R. (1983). Interactions of ethanol with other drugs. In B. Tabakoff, B. Sutker, and C. L. Randall (Eds.), *Medical and social aspects of alcohol abuse* (pp. 247–272). New York: Plenum.

Drug Enforcement Administration (1987). *Drug profile series report.* Washington, D. C.: Office of Diversion Control: Drug Control Section.

Du Pont de Nemours (1985). *Trexan in opioid addiction.* Wilmington: Du Pont Pharmaceuticals.

Geffner, E. S. (1984). *The psychiatrists' compendium of drug therapy.* New York: Biomedical Information Corporation.

Hald, J., and Jacobsen, E. (1948). A drug sensitizing the organism to ethyl alcohol. *Lancet, 2,* 1001–1004.

Hoyumpa, A. M., Jr. (1980). Mechanisms of thiamine deficiency in chronic alcoholism. *American Journal of Nutrition, 33,* 2750–2761.

Huff, B. B. (1988). *Physicians' Desk Reference.* Oradell, NJ: Medical Economics Company.

Hunt, W. A. (1983). Ethanol and the central nervous system. In B. Tabakoff, P. Sutker, and C. L. Randall (Eds.), *Medical and social aspects of alcohol abuse* (pp. 133–155). New York: Plenum.

Israel, Y., Glaser, F. B., Kalant, H., et al. (1978). *Research advances in alcohol and drug problems*. Vol. 4. New York: Plenum.

Jackimczyk, K. C., and Roberts, M. R. (1984). Approach to the intoxicated patient. *Topics in Emergency Medicine*, 6(2), 9–13.

Kitson, T. M. (1977). The disulfiram-ethanol reaction. A review. *Journal Studies on Alcohol*, 38, 96–113.

Levine, S. F. (1973). *Narcotics and drug abuse*. Cincinnati: W. H. Anderson.

Linden, C. H., Kulig, K. K., and Rumack, B. H. (1984). Disulfiram. *Topics in Emergency Medicine*, 6(2), 30–37.

Loveys, B. J. (1987). Physiologic effects of cocaine with particular references to the cardiovascular system. *Heart & Lung*, 16(2), 175–180.

Martin, E. W. (Ed.). (1978). *Hazards of medication*. Philadelphia: J. B. Lippincott.

McMicken, D. B. (1983). Alcohol-related disease. In P. Rosen, F. Baker, G. R. Braen, et al. (Eds.), *Emergency medicine: Concepts and clinical practice*. St. Louis: C. V. Mosby.

Meyers, M. (1988a). Withdrawal: Stages I and II. *Professional Counselor*, 2(6), 16.

Meyers, M. (1988b). Withdrawal: Stages III and IV. *Professional Counselor*, 3(1), 16.

National Council on Alcoholism (1972). Criteria for the diagnosis of alcoholism. *American Journal of Psychiatry*, 129, 127–135.

Potter, D. O. (Ed.). (1984). *Drugs. Nurse's reference library*. Springhouse, PA: Springhouse Corporation.

Potter, D. O. (Ed.). (1985). *Emergencies. Nurse's reference library*. Springhouse, PA: Springhouse Corporation.

Rapaka, R. S. (1986). Frontiers of research in the medicinal chemistry and molecular pharmacology of opioid peptides. In R. S. Rapaka, G. Barnett, and R. L. Hawks (Eds.), *Opioid peptides: Medicinal chemistry* (pp. 3–20). National Institute on Drug Abuse Research Monograph Series 69. Rockville, MD: National Institute on Drug Abuse.

Rappolt R. T., Gay, G. R., and Inaba, D. S. (1977). Propranolol: A specific antagonist to cocaine. *Clinical Toxicology*, 10, 265.

Senay, E. C. (1983). *Substance abuse disorders in clinical practice*. Boston: John Wright, PSG.

Smith, D. E., and Wesson, D. R. (1975). *Diagnosis and treatment of adverse reactions to sedative-hypnotics*. Rockville, MD: National Institute on Drug Abuse.

Tabakoff, B., and Rothstein, J. (1983). Biology of tolerance and dependence. In B. Tabakoff, B. Sutker, and C. L. Randall (Eds.), *Medical and social aspects of alcohol abuse* (pp. 187–217). New York: Plenum.

Van Thiel, D. H. (1983). Effects of ethanol on organ systems. In B. Tabakoff, P. B. Sutker, and C. L. Randall (Eds.), *Medical and social aspects of alcohol abuse* (pp. 79–120). New York: Plenum.

Wilford, B. B. (1987). *Review course syllabus: American medical society on alcoholism and other drug dependencies*. New York: American Medical Society.

Wish, W. D. (1988). Identifying drug-abusing criminals. In C. G. Leukefeld and F. M. Tims (Eds.), *Compulsory treatment of drug abuse: Research and clinical practice* (pp. 139–159). National Institute on Drug Abuse Research Monograph Series 86. Rockville, MD: National Institute on Drug Abuse.

Wolfe, V. M. and Victor, M. (1971). The physiological basis of alcohol withdrawal syndrome. In N. K. Mello and J. H. Mendelson (Eds.), *Recent advances in studies of alcoholism: An interdisciplinary symposium*. Publication No. (HSM) 71-9045. Washington, D. C.: U. S. Government Printing Office.

Woolverton, W. L., and Kleven, M. S. (1988). Multiple dopamine receptors and the behavioral effects of cocaine. In D. Clouet, K. Asghar, and R. Brown (Eds.), *Mechanisms of cocaine abuse and toxicity* (pp. 160–184). National Institute on Drug Abuse Research Monograph Series 88. Rockville, MD: National Institute on Drug Abuse.

Patients After Near Drowning

Susan Joy Nelson

Drowning is the third leading cause of death in the United States (Baker, 1984). Submersion injury alters pulmonary, acid-base, cardiac, neurologic, renal, and hematologic system function. A victim experiencing any loss of consciousness or respiratory embarrassment following submersion will be hospitalized for at least 6 hours (Robinson and Seward, 1987). Consequently, submersion victims are admitted to critical care or observation units. The purpose of this chapter is to acquaint the reader with the factors that contribute to drowning and discuss the pathophysiology, complications, and interventions associated with victims of near drowning.

EPIDEMIOLOGY

Drowning, the third leading cause of accidental death in the United States, is the second leading cause of death in individuals between the ages of 1 and 25 (Robinson and Seward, 1987). The incidence of submersion injury peaks twice in the population by age. The first peak occurs in children under 4 years old, and the second occurs in individuals aged 15 to 25. Submersion injury in the female population peaks once, at the age of 1 year, then sharply declines and does not rise again. At all ages, male drowning victims greatly outnumber female drowning and near

drowning victims (Robinson and Seward, 1987; Orlowski, 1987).

Drowning occurs in private swimming pools, natural bodies of water, bathtubs, and household water receptacles. The place of submersion injury differs for toddlers and adolescents. Toddler immersion accidents occur predominantly in swimming pools, whereas adolescent episodes occur most frequently in lakes, rivers, ponds, and canals (Table 61–1) (Wintemute et al., 1987). Factors that contribute to submersion accidents are inadequate adult supervision, inadequate barriers around pools, unfamiliarity with the body of water, alcohol consumption, lack of flotation device usage, and epilepsy (Orlowski, 1987; Wintemute et al., 1987).

Substance use is a predominant factor in many teen and adult drownings (Orlowski, 1987). Alcohol alters the protective cardiovascular responses associated with the diving reflex. Heart rate does not slow as much as it does in the sober state, and stroke volume fails to increase. Peripheral vascular resistance decreases when submersion occurs after alcohol consumption (Wittmers et al., 1987). These alterations reduce the supply of oxygen and nutrients to the heart and brain. Alcohol also impairs mentation and coordination of respiratory and swallowing reflexes. Forty to fifty per cent of diving accident victims have consumed alcohol (Orlowski, 1987). The victim is usually not acquainted with the area where

TABLE 61–1. Contribution of Submersion Media to Drowning Accidents

	Toddlers 1 to 4 Years (%)	Adolescents 15 to 25 Years (%)	Total Population (%)
Salt water			1–2
Fresh water			98
Pools	74		53
Natural bodies of water		70	20
Household receptacles	25		10

his dive is to be made. The most serious injuries sustained in diving accidents are death, spinal cord injury, and head injury. In most cases the diver is removed from the water by friends who are unaware of the spine injury and do not use a spine board.

People with seizure disorders are another important risk group for drowning and near drowning. Drowning and near drowning are four to five times more frequent in people with known epilepsy (Orlowski, 1987). Seizures can be elicited by visual and auditory environmental stimulants (Daniele et al., 1987; Kasteleijn-Nolst Trenite et al., 1987; Vergnes et al., 1986). The rhythmic reflection of light from water or the sound of wave motion can provide separate or synergistic stimulants that trigger seizure activity. These risks are further increased when epilepsy is poorly controlled or when these people have had recent changes in medication or are mentally subnormal.

Weekends, warm climates, and weather are associated with an increased incidence of drowning and near drowning accidents. Approximately fifty per cent of submersion injuries occur during summer, and 40% occur on weekends. Drowning rates are generally highest in southern and western states (Table 61–2) (Orlowski et al., 1987). Alaska is an exception; it has the highest rate for the United States. Occupational exposure to very cold water is thought to elevate Alaska's drowning rate (Orlowski et al., 1987; Wintemute et al., 1987).

Prevention is the most important intervention because even short-term submersion injury has devastating consequences. Education should focus on pool fencing, close toddler supervision, abstinence from alcohol and drugs around water, and close supervision or observation of medically ill individuals (Pitt, 1986; Davis et al., 1985).

PATHOPHYSIOLOGY

Submersion accidents are described in terms that communicate the sequence of events and expectations of outcome to health care providers. The primary terms used for submersion incidents are (1) drowning, and (2) near drowning. Drowning is defined as death by suffocation following submersion in a liquid, whereas near drowning denotes survival or temporary survival following an asphyxia-producing submersion episode. Death occurring more than 24 hours after a submersion episode results from complications of near drowning. The term secondary

TABLE 61–2. Regional Drowning Rates (per 100,000 population)

United States (average)	3.5
Alaska	10
California	5
Louisiana	5

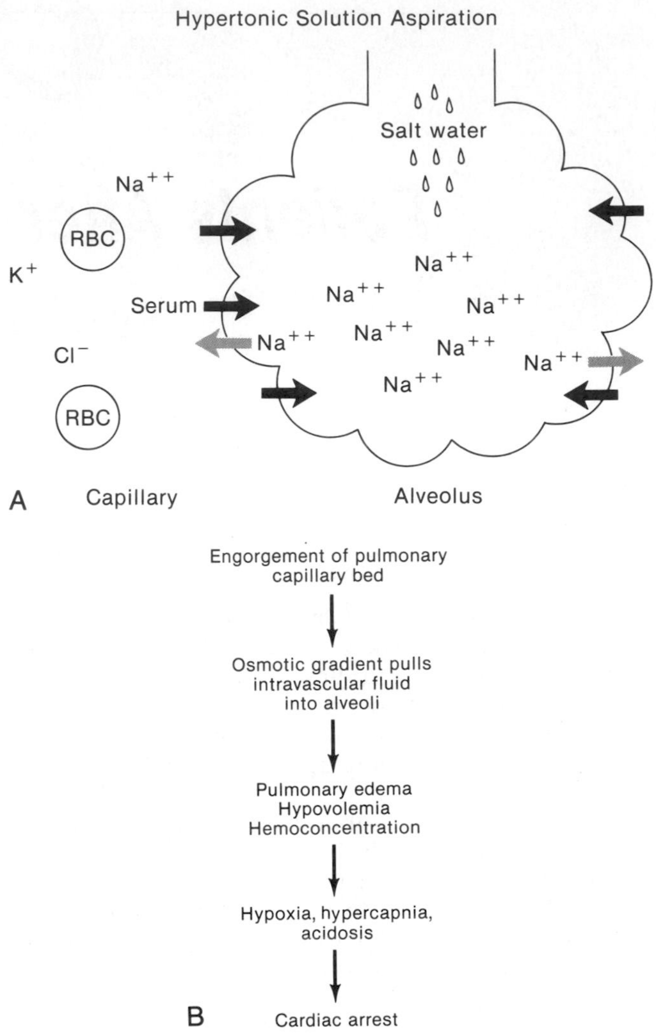

FIGURE 61–1. *A,* Osmosis pulls intravascular fluid into the alveoli, producing fulminating pulmonary edema. A significant loss of fluid from the circulatory system may result in hypovolemia, hemoconcentration, and elevated electrolyte levels. Serum sodium may be additionally elevated by diffusion of sodium from the alveoli into the circulatory system. *B,* Sequence of events in aspiration of hypertonic solutions.

drowning has been used to describe death from near drowning complications and will not be referred to again to eliminate possible confusion.

Submersion injury is not limited to pulmonary insult but also includes multisystem dysfunction. The complications of drowning are primarily related to hypoxia. Sustained laryngospasm and damaged pulmonary tissue impair gas exchange. Hypoxia reduces mentation, consciousness, muscle work capacity, and cellular survival. Blood flow to various organs is diminished in an effort to meet the oxygen and nutrient requirements of the heart and brain. Hypoxia induces anaerobic metabolism, which produces acidic byproducts and predispose to clotting abnormalities. Consequently, irreversible damage to all organs may occur.

Unexpected submersion in a liquid medium results in aspiration of a small amount of fluid initially.

Laryngospasm immediately occurs and may continue for 2 minutes (Orlowski, 1987). Increasing hypoxia and panic precipitate swallowing and additional aspiration of liquid.

The terms dry and wet are used to describe the volume of fluid aspirated and denote a separate sequence of events in drowning and near drowning incidents. Victims that experience dry drowning and near drowning aspirate a second, small amount of liquid, which results in recurrence of severe laryngospasm. The second episode of laryngospasm persists and results in severe hypoxia, seizures, and death. Wet drowning and near drowning victims aspirate large volumes of fluid, which occurs when hypoxia produces muscle relaxation, thus relieving laryngospasm.

Salt water and fresh water aspiration are expected to present different pathologic findings (Martin, 1984; Karch, 1986). Sea water is hypertonic. Aspiration of a large amount of salt water causes body fluid to be drawn from the interstitial and intravascular compartments into the alveoli. The pulmonary arteries contract, and the pulmonary veins dilate, causing capillary bed engorgement and sludging of red blood cells. Alveolar type I cells separate from their capillary basement membranes (Mathur and Mathur, 1986). Extravasation of fluid into the alveoli results in fulminant pulmonary edema with progressive hypovolemia, hemoconcentration, and increased serum electrolytes in addition to hypoxia, hypercarbia, acidosis, and eventual cardiac arrest (Fig. 61–1*A*, *B*) (Modell, 1986).

Fresh water, a hypotonic media, is rapidly absorbed from the alveoli into the intravascular space. The resulting hypervolemia causes hemodilution and lowers serum electrolyte concentrations. Red blood cells may swell and rupture (Fig. 61–2*A*) (Karch, 1986). Potassium is liberated as red blood cells are destroyed. Increased serum potassium coupled with anoxia precipitate ventricular fibrillation and death (Fig. 61–2*B*) (Mathur and Mathur, 1986).

These dramatic physiologic changes may occur with aspiration of large amounts of salt or fresh water and are seen predominantly in experimental animals who die of drowning. Severe responses are not common in near drowning victims. Most of these victims aspirate minimal fluid, if any (Modell, 1986). Even when relatively large, nonlethal amounts of fresh water are aspirated, the circulating intravascular volume returns to normal within 60 minutes. Serum electrolyte concentrations that are abnormal enough to require treatment are rarely seen and are primarily limited to victims who have aspirated extremely concentrated salt solutions, such as water in the Dead Sea (Modell, 1986). Hypoxemia is the major physiologic abnormality seen, and electrolyte disturbances play only a minor role.

Clinical experience, however, has shown little difference between fresh and salt water drowning or near drowning. Patients who survive long enough to be transported to the hospital have probably inhaled a small amount of fluid and suffer from hypoxemia, metabolic acidosis, and transient hypercarbia. The severity of respiratory compromise depends on the amount of liquid aspirated, the pathogens in the liquid, and the duration of submersion.

Studies show that aspiration of both fresh and salt water produces similar ultrastructural and microscopic changes (Karch, 1986; Torr et al., 1983). Lung tissue is edematous but equally expanded. There may be widespread focal hemorrhages in the lower lobes. The pulmonary vascular endothelium is swollen, with more than half the mitochondria swollen to twice their normal size (Fig. 61–3). Emphysematous changes with thinning of the alveolar septa and bleb formation have been demonstrated but are not widespread (Fig. 61–4) (Karch, 1986).

Fresh water aspiration has been shown to cause greater hypoxia than saline solutions. Hypoxia is more prolonged with fresh water aspiration, and carbon dioxide retention is more marked. Aspiration of fluid into the alveoli is thought to produce hypoxia because blood flows through perfused but nonventilated lung tissue. Both salt and fresh water complicate the ventilation-perfusion mismatch by lowering the surface tension of surfactant, causing alveolar collapse and decreased lung compliance (Karch, 1986).

A massive release of catecholamines accompanies the victim's response to drowning and near drowning. High levels of catecholamines can cause severe myocardial necrosis and possibly the pulmonary endothelial damage associated with near drowning. Catecholamines are released in panic situations to prepare for flight or fight. Blood flow is consequently increased to the heart, brain, and muscles to supply oxygen and vital nutrients. However, oxygen utilization increases during the struggle and, coupled with aspiration or laryngospasm, produces profound hypoxemia. Hypoxia reduces mental activity, decreases the work capacity of muscles, and may progress to coma. Hypoxia increases acidosis and can cause tissue death in all organs.

Acidosis is a common finding in near drowning victims. Metabolic acidosis is primarily due to tissue hypoxia, but a respiratory component may be present following aspiration (Mathur and Mathur, 1986). Aspiration of water or gastric contents increases ventilation-perfusion mismatch. Fluid or debris impedes gas exchange across the alveolar capillary membrane. In addition, laryngospasm and the reduced blood flow through various tissues prevent normal removal of carbon dioxide. Exchange of carbon dioxide and oxygen may continue to be abnormal following reestablishment of ventilation. The metabolic component of acidosis may create additional challenges.

Lactic acid is produced during hypoxia-induced anaerobic glycolysis (Guyton, 1986). Blood flow, reduced to nonessential organs such as the liver, kidneys, and gut, becomes sluggish and predisposes to clot formation. Acids and products of deterioration from ischemic tissue traumatize the red blood cells, triggering the intrinsic clotting mechanism (Guyton, 1986). Blood clots begin to form in the microvascu-

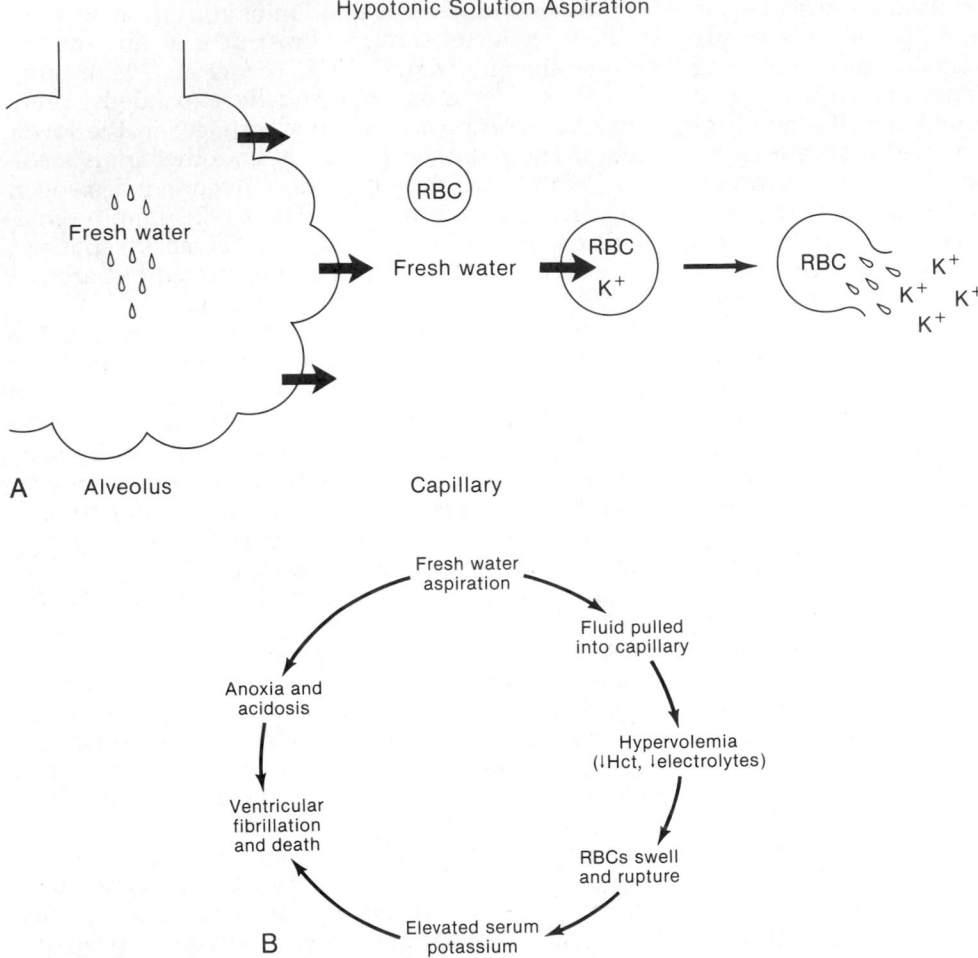

Hypotonic Solution Aspiration

FIGURE 61–2. *A,* Osmotic pressure causes fresh water to flow into the capillary from the alveoli. Fluid also enters the red blood cells, causing cellular swelling with subsequent rupture. Red blood cells contain high concentrations of potassium, which is liberated on cell destruction. Serum potassium may become high enough to produce ventricular fibrillation and death. *B,* Sequence of events in hypotonic solution aspiration.

lature and may progress to disseminated intravascular coagulation.

Cellular function relies on ATP to meet energy requirements. Anaerobic metabolism is inefficient in ATP generation but can produce sufficient quantities for several minutes (Guyton, 1986). During this process, intracellular and extracellular acids increase rapidly, reducing cell function. Active transport of sodium and potassium through the cell membrane diminishes as ATP availability drops. Eventually the ATP supply is exhausted, and cellular integrity deteriorates further (Guyton, 1986). Consequently, sodium and chloride accumulate in the cells, and po-

tassium is lost. Increased sodium concentration leads to intracellular edema and eventual cell destruction (Henneman, 1986). These changes affect many organs of the body, particularly the liver, heart, kidney, and brain. Complications that may be seen include hypoxic encephalopathy, renal failure, myocardial dysrhythmias and infarction, and altered liver function.

Hypoxia and acidosis act as myocardial depressants and precipitate circulatory collapse. The primary problem in circulatory arrest is to prevent brain injury. Four to five minutes without cerebral perfusion will result in some permanent brain damage.

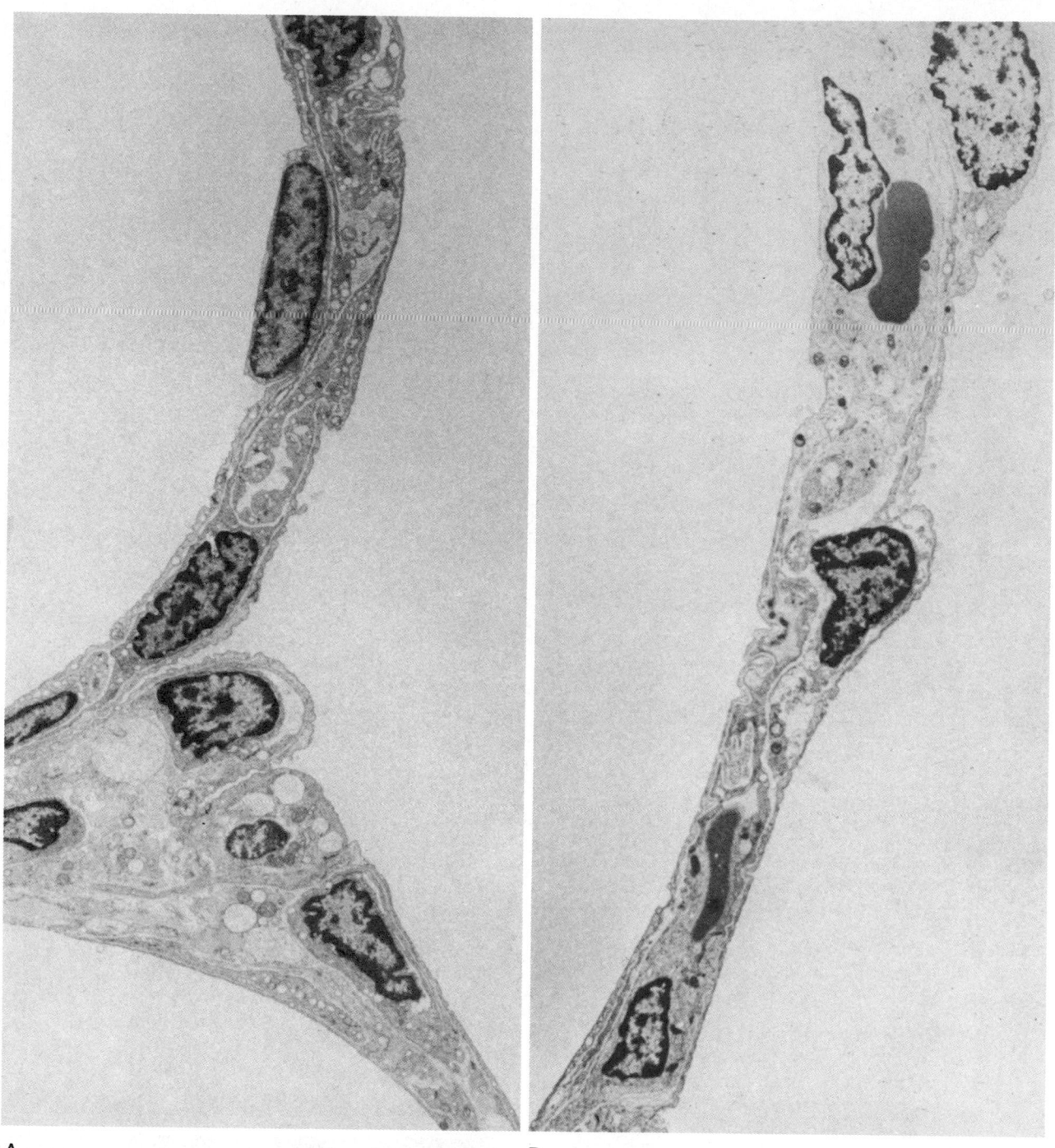

A   B

FIGURE 61–3. *A*, Normal pulmonary vessels and endothelium of a control rabbit. *B*, Nearly drowned rabbit pulmonary blood vessels show swelling of subendothelial, endothelial, and mitochondria (× 3852). (From Karch, S. (1986). *American Journal of Emergency Medicine*, 4 (1), 4–9.)

Cerebral hypoxia was formerly assumed to be responsible for this brain damage. However, studies have shown that up to 30 minutes of circulatory arrest in dogs will lead to no permanent brain damage "if the blood is removed from the brain prior to the arrest." Based on the findings of these studies, circulatory arrest is postulated to cause diffuse vascular clots that result in permanent or semipermanent ischemic brain areas (Guyton, 1986). Cerebral reperfusion demand and supply mismatch is thought to play an important role in the cerebral insult that occurs following cardiac resuscitation and near drowning.

HYPERVENTILATION SUBMERSION INJURY

Typically, hyperventilation submersion injury involves good swimmers and is preceded by intentional

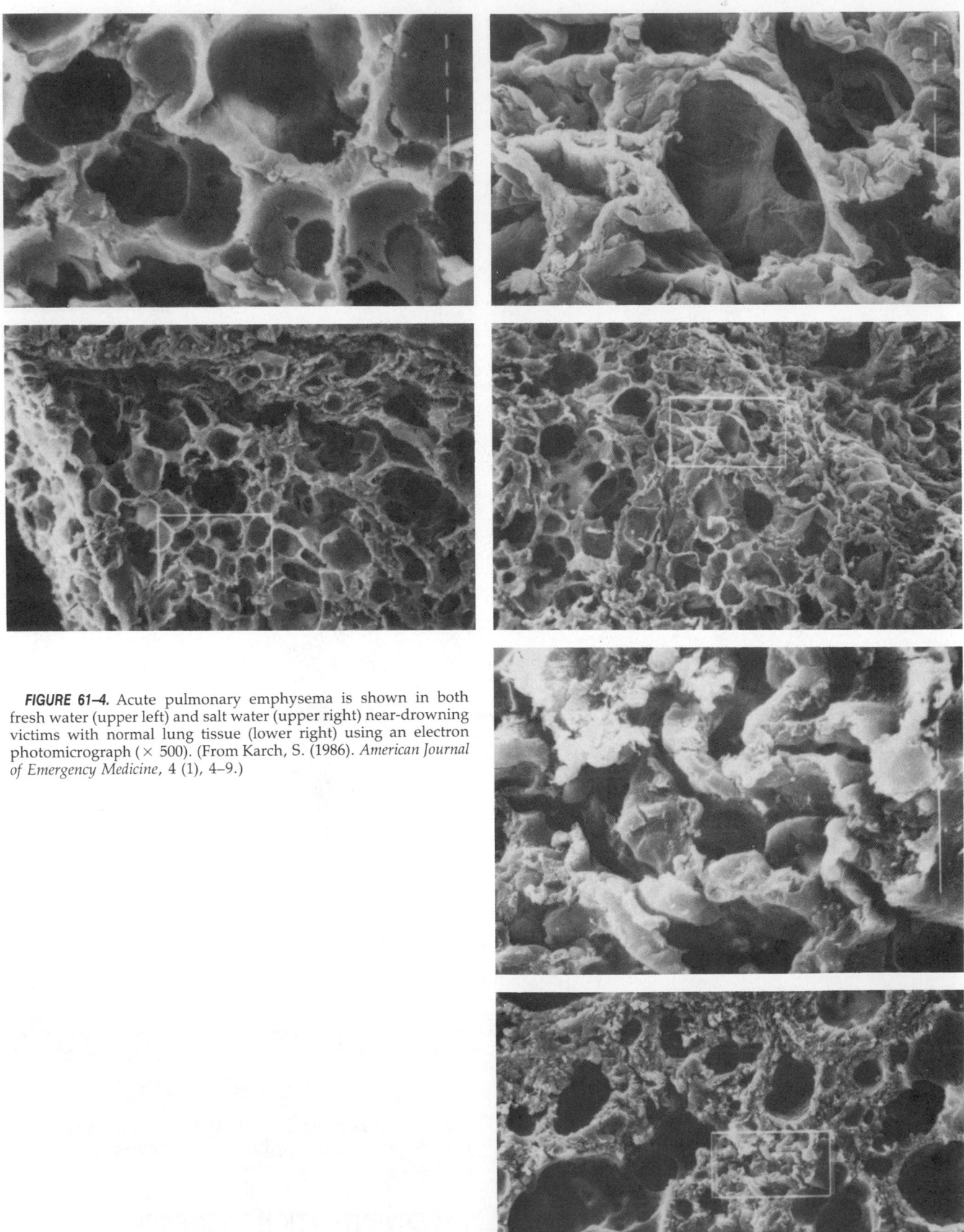

FIGURE 61–4. Acute pulmonary emphysema is shown in both fresh water (upper left) and salt water (upper right) near-drowning victims with normal lung tissue (lower right) using an electron photomicrograph (× 500). (From Karch, S. (1986). *American Journal of Emergency Medicine*, 4 (1), 4–9.)

hyperventilation in an effort to increase underwater time (Gonzales-Rothi, 1987). Hyperventilation reduces carbon dioxide levels, resulting in hypocapnia. Since carbon dioxide is the primary central stimulus for breathing, hyperventilation-induced hypocapnia will suppress respiratory drive even when severe hypoxemia, resulting from breath holding, occurs (Gonzales-Rothi, 1987). Often the victim loses consciousness before recovering spontaneous respiratory effort. Immediate rescue and resuscitation must be implemented to ensure survival.

COLD WATER IMMERSION

As water temperature decreases, survival from immersion is reduced because of man's limited ability to tolerate hypothermia. Survival generally depends on heat production and heat conservation. Heat is produced by oxidative metabolism, physical exertion, and shivering. The thermoregulatory center is located in the hypothalmus. Cold stimulates the central and peripheral nervous system to produce vasoconstriction. Direct cooling below 12°C causes paralysis of the vascular smooth muscle and subsequent vasodilation (Martin, 1984; Guyton, 1986). Exercise and shivering are less effective in producing heat in cold water than in cold air. Exercise and shivering also increase both blood flow to the muscles and conductive heat loss. Convective heat loss is also increased as a result of stirring the water. Exhaustion from exercise may accelerate collapse and subsequent drowning in cold water (Martin, 1984).

A continued decrease in core temperature may be observed for a period of time following removal of the hypothermic victim from the water. The explanation proposed is that peripheral vasodilation shunts cooler blood from the extremities to the body core (Martin, 1984). Additional cooling of the myocardium increases the potential for lethal dysrhythmias.

Immersion in cold water may lead to drowning related to hypothermia-induced dysrhythmias and altered consciousness. Atrial fibrillation and sinus bradycardia are the most common dysrhythmias. However, ventricular fibrillation and asystole occur at core temperatures below 28°C (Martin, 1984; Clochesy, 1984). Additional electrocardiographic (ECG) findings in hypothermia may include prolongation of the PR, QT, QRS, and T-wave intervals. Atrial pacing is not effective due to the prolonged atrioventricular (AV) conduction time, and ventricular pacing is contraindicated because it may induce ventricular fibrillation. Immersion syndrome, in which sudden death results instead of the protective diving reflex, may occur on contact with cold water. Sudden death occurs from vagally mediated bradyasystolic cardiac arrest or ventricular dysrhythmias (Gonzales-Rothi, 1987).

Infants and children have a greater likelihood of surviving prolonged cold water submersion. It is thought that their increased survival is due to a stronger diving reflex (Martin, 1984). In addition, the larger surface area of children facilitates more rapid cooling. A more quickly lowered metabolic rate and a stronger circulation shunting response improves the survival rate for children in cold water (Orlowski, 1987).

PULMONARY BAROTRAUMA

Barotraumatic cerebral air embolism is second to drowning as the most frequent cause of death among divers (Neuman, 1980). Divers who use a compressed air supply for deep diving are the only people at risk for air embolus. According to Boyle's Law, the product of pressure and volume of gas must remain constant at a given temperature (Neuman, 1980). More simply, a given volume of gas at a constant temperature must expand as pressure is reduced. A submerged diver fills his lungs with compressed gas. As the diver rises to the surface, water pressure is reduced, and the gas expands. If the air is not allowed to escape during ascent, as happens with breath holding, rupture of the intrapulmonary blood vessels may occur. The gas then enters the pulmonary venous circulation, flows to the left myocardial chambers, and is pumped to the systemic circulation. Cerebral air embolism may occur. The expanding air may dissect through the interstitium of the lung to the hila. In this case, although it is less common, pneumomediastinum, pneumopericardium, subcutaneous emphysema, or pneumothorax may result (Neuman, 1980).

Submersion injury is associated with multisystemic complications that range from negligible to severe. Table 61–3 summarizes the complications of submersion injury and the findings that accompany them. The pulmonary system receives the initial insult, which causes hypoxemia. Injury may produce immediate or delayed findings on examination. Pulmonary complications may include pulmonary edema, adult respiratory distress syndrome (ARDS), interstitial pulmonary fibrosis, aspiration pneumonia, atelectasis, empyema, and pulmonary barotrauma. Prolonged hypoxia alters multisystemic function causing varying degrees of damage to all tissues and organs. The liver, heart, kidneys, and brain are particularly susceptible to injury. Severity of compromise is related to the amount of fluid aspirated, the infective nature of the fluid, and the duration of submersion.

INITIAL TREATMENT

Submersion injuries range from asymptomatic injury to cardiopulmonary arrest. Initial findings on assessment reflect the extent of hypoxic injury to the cardiopulmonary and cerebral systems. It is important to remember that injury to the head, spine, and

TABLE 61–3. Complications and Clinical Findings in Cases of Drowning and Near Drowning

Complication	Signs and Symptoms
Hypoxemia	Pallor, increasing respiratory distress, use of accessory muscles in respiration, acidosis, restlessness, headache, gasping, lethargy or drowsiness, disorientation, tachycardia followed by bradycardia, dysrhythmias, cyanosis, and Pao_2 less than 50 mm Hg
Acidosis	Metabolic: Tachypnea, pallor, lethargy, hypotension Respiratory: Tachypnea, wheezing, rhonchi, decreased breath sounds, copious secretions, use of accessory muscles in breathing, nasal flaring, restlessness, grunting, coughing, cyanosis, and dysrhythmias
Atelectasis and pneumonia	Decreased breath sounds, change in pitch or quality of breath sounds, egophony and whispering pectoriloquy, reduced or absent vocal fremitus over area of involvement, adventitious breath sounds—fine, high-pitched rales at end inspiration. Less chest motion on affected side of chest, affected side retracted with ribs appearing closer together, increased ventilation-perfusion mismatch, tachypnea, shallow respirations, and fever Chest x-ray demonstrates a scattered white fluffy area, usually limited to one lobe. An air bronchogram may have been taken; it allows visualization of the bronchi as intrapulmonary black tubes due to collapsed alveoli around the bronchi. Occasionally obliteration of the cardiac silhouette occurs. Large atelectatic areas pull the diaphragm up toward the collapsed alveoli.
Bronchospasm	Prolonged expiratory time, wheezing, tachypnea, use of accessory muscles in breathing, decreased air movement, cyanosis, fatigue, hypoxemia, generalized hyperinflation of lungs visualized on chest x-ray
Pulmonary edema	Wheezing, rhonchi, grunting, decreased breath sounds, copious frothy secretions that may be pink-tinged, nasal flaring, use of accessory muscles in breathing, jugular venous distention, restlessness, tachypnea or apnea, tachycardia followed by bradycardia, and mental confusion. On chest x-ray the pulmonary veins become bilaterally prominent near the hila and may produce a butterfly appearance
Adult respiratory distress syndrome (ARDS)	Rapid onset and progression (within hours) produce hypoxemia, decreasing lung compliance, and diffuse multilobular, hazy infiltrates on chest x-ray. Decreased breath sounds, tachypnea, use of accessory muscle in breathing, tachycardia, restlessness, agitation, and cyanosis may be present
Pneumothorax	Decreased breath sounds, change in pitch of breath sounds, hyper-resonance of chest to percussion, decreased chest expansion during inspiration, tachypnea, use of accessory muscles, decreased compliance, and tachycardia. Chest x-ray demonstrates an area near the chest wall that has no vascular markings, the lung border is visible well away from the chest wall, and mediastinal shift toward the pneumothorax may occur
Tension pneumothorax	Worse respiratory distress occurs than in pneumothorax, also restlessness, agitation, and tracheal deviation away from the affected side. Cardiac sounds are displaced, jugular venous distention may be present, as may cyanosis, hypotension, and cardiac arrest. The chest x-ray demonstrates an area without vascular markings, the lung border is visible well away from the chest wall, and mediastinal shift occurs toward the fully expanded lung, away from the deflated lung tissue
Pneumomediastinum	Symptoms range from none (asymptomatic) to varying degrees of apprehension, tachypnea, tachycardia, cyanosis, hypotension, cardiac arrest, or a mediastinal shift with decreased tissue density in the mediastinal-hilar area on chest x-ray
Pneumopericardium	Pulsus paradoxus more than 15 mm Hg, electrical alternans on ECG, hypotension, jugular venous distention more than 3 cm above sternal angle with the patient sitting at a 45-degree angle, diaphoresis, angina, pallor, tachycardia, cold extremities, decreased tissue density around heart on chest x-ray. Heart sounds may become accentuated or muffled depending on the position of the heart and the amount of air in the pericardium. Signs and symptoms are similar to those characteristic of cardiac tamponade
Subcutaneous emphysema	Crepitus of skin on upper chest, neck, and head, bloated appearance; neck appears to shorten and disappear
Hypothermia	Pink flushing of skin, rectal temperature (T) less than 35°C (95°F) T 34° to 36°C—Confusion, disorientation, and shivering T 33° to 34°C—Amnesia, cardiac dysrhythmias, and persistent muscle rigidity T 30° to 33°C—Semiconscious T <30°C —Unconscious, pupils dilated, absent tendon reflexes T 28°C —Profound bradycardia, ventricular fibrillation possible, especially with physical manipulation of body T 20° to 25°C—Spontaneous ventricular fibrillation T 15° to 20°C—Refractory ventricular fibrillation and asystole until warmed
Disseminated intravascular coagulation	Petechial or purpuric body rash; diffuse bleeding from any venipuncture site; decreased fibrinogen level, platelets, and factors II, V, and VII; prolonged PT and PTT; fibrin degradation products (FDP), hemoptysis, and hematuria may be present
Hypoxic cerebral encephalopathy	Decreased level of consciousness, seizures, and motor or sensory deficits. Pupils may dilate with sluggish response to light or may be unequal; reflexes are decreased; headache, emesis, hypertension, brady- or tachycardia, altered respiratory pattern, decreased rate or depth of breathing, and death may occur.
Renal dysfunction	Oliguria, anuria, hematuria, urine output that exceeds intake, urine osmolality and specific gravity that do not increase when urine output decreases, and elevated potassium, creatinine and blood urea nitrogen levels
Liver dysfunction	Malaise, irritability or lethargy, forgetfulness, slurred speech, reversal of sleep and wake cycles, decreased clotting factors VII and VIII, prolonged PT, ecchymosis, petechiae, elevated concentrations of direct serum bilirubin, transaminases, alkaline phosphatase, ammonia, SGOT, SGPT, lactic dehydrogenase, creatine phosphokinase, and creatinine. Hypokalemia, hypocalcemia, hypoglycemia, decreased albumin, anemia, and leukopenia occur with severe necrosis

other areas may occur with submersion injury (Orlowski, 1987). Core temperature should be determined to identify the presence of hypothermia. Pulmonary assessment may demonstrate multiple adventitious sounds. Copious frothy sputum or cyanosis indicates severe respiratory embarrassment and impending respiratory arrest. Cardiac rhythm monitoring may reveal dysrhythmias. Decreased mental status may be due to many factors: cerebral hypoxia, intracranial injury, drug overdosage, postictal state, or hypoglycemia.

The victim must be removed from the water as soon as possible. Caution must be exercised to prevent injury to the rescuers. The water environment should be checked for electrical hazards. Rescuers must have protective equipment available to provide protection in cold water and weather. The victim's cervical spine must be protected during treatment and removal from the water, in case spinal injury has occurred (Pearn, 1985).

Once the patient is on a stable surface, the ABCs (airway, breathing, circulation) of resuscitation are instituted. Airway patency must be obtained while cervical spine precautions are maintained. High-flow oxygen and adequate suctioning should be used for all submersion victims. Inability to maintain an airway or handle secretions or the presence of copious frothy sputum or cyanosis are indications for prehospital intubation (Robinson and Seward, 1987). Intubation of hypothermic individuals must be performed gently to avoid producing intractable ventricular dysrhythmias (Pearn, 1985).

Empirical evidence does not support use of postural drainage (Robinson and Seward, 1987) or Heimlich maneuvers to remove fluid from the trachea (Heimlich et al., 1986). These maneuvers increase the risk of loss of airway control, interrupt CPR, and aggravate spinal injuries (Robinson and Seward, 1987). Cardiac monitoring and intravenous access should be instituted. Shock may be present, related to hemorrhage, hypovolemia, or neurogenic factors. Treatment of shock includes application of a MAST suit, initiation of an intravenous fluid bolus, and rapid transport (Robinson and Seward, 1987). A second intravenous access route should be established en route to the hospital. Severe metabolic acidosis may persist regardless of adequate ventilation by endotracheal or esophagotracheal tube. Symptoms of severe acidosis include altered mental status, cyanosis, persistent hypotension despite volume replacement, and cardiac dysrhythmias. Naloxone and 50% dextrose may be administered when mental status is altered. Children may have taken drugs, and young children become hypoglycemic quickly under stress. Submersion of a child requires adherence to some basic principles:

■ Initial resuscitative efforts should never be withheld. Ten to twenty per cent of children with fixed, dilated pupils who are comatose recover fully (Robinson and Seward, 1987; Orlowski, 1987).
■ Tranport delay to initiate an IV is not advisable.

■ Transportation to the hospital should be carried out regardless of clinical symptoms (Robinson and Seward, 1987; Orlowski, 1987; Mathur and Mathur, 1986).
■ Further heat loss should be prevented by removing wet clothing.
■ Inspection for evidence of additional injuries should be made (Robinson and Seward, 1987; Orlowski, 1987).

The hypothermic heart is relatively unresponsive to pharmacotherapy and electrical stimulation (Orlowski, 1987). If ventricular fibrillation occurs, a single countershock attempt should be made if the rectal temperature is greater than 29.5°C (Orlowski; 1987). Unsuccessful attempts at defibrillation can be followed with bretylium administration, which may restore sinus rhythm (Orlowski, 1987). CPR should be continued if this is unsuccessful.

HOSPITAL TREATMENT

The patient history of submersion is usually incomplete on admission to the hospital. Information can be valuable in assisting with correct identification and differentiating between injury or complications from injury and the victim's preimmersion health status. Information can be obtained during a period of a few hours from bystanders, rescuers, police, and ambulance staff. Table 61–4 lists data that are helpful. Frequently, drowning results from other medical problems.

Treatment of the patient is directed by clinical assessment and the results of tests performed after arrival at the hospital. Cardiopulmonary support is continued during assessment, if required. The following problems must be assessed: hypoxia, pulmonary injury, metabolic acidosis, hypothermia, concomitant injuries, volume status, and cerebral resuscitation (Robinson and Seward, 1987).

Airway effectiveness, oxygenation, and ventilation must be evaluated. Patients receiving 100% oxygen by mask who have an arterial P_{O_2} of less than 50 mm Hg or P_{CO_2} of more than 50 mm Hg also require endotracheal intubation (Robinson and Seward, 1987). A chest x-ray must be obtained as soon as

---

TABLE 61–4. *Data Collection for History of Submersion and Resuscitation*

1. Estimated time of accident
2. Type of fluid aspirated: i.e., salt, fresh, chemicals, gastric
3. Estimated water temperature
4. Degree of water contamination
5. Estimated duration of submersion
6. Details of rescue
7. Was CPR performed? If so, by a trained person?
8. Occurrence of emesis
9. Time until first gasp after rescue
10. CPR maintained with or without interruptions
11. Past health of victim (i.e., epilepsy, asthma, etc.)

possible. Initial findings on x-ray may vary from normal to signs of pulmonary edema. Follow-up x-rays may reveal a deteriorating pulmonary status, compared with that on admission, as late as 12 hours later in normal individuals (Orlowski, 1987). Additional injuries such as pneumothorax, hemothorax, pneumopericardium, and pneumomediastinum may also be revealed. Chest tube insertion may be indicated for hemothorax and significant pneumothorax. Pericardial or mediastinal tap may also be necessary.

Pulmonary edema occurs over a number of hours following submersion injury. Patients with normal arterial blood gas (ABGs) levels while receiving oxygen may have abnormal ABGs while breathing room air. Occasionally, adequate oxygenation can be accomplished with high-flow oxygen. Patients may benefit from continuous positive airway pressure (CPAP) by mask or mechanical ventilation with positive end-expiratory pressure (PEEP). Results of steroids to improve pulmonary outcome vary. Bronchospasm may be present; it can be treated with beta-antagonists. Bronchoscopy may be required if a large amount of particulate matter, such as mud or gastric contents, has been aspirated (Orlowski, 1987).

A nasogastric tube should be inserted early in persistently symptomatic patients. Gastric dilatation is common and may interfere with ventilation by preventing full descent of the diaphragm. Nasogastric tube insertion will prevent emesis and further aspiration of gastric contents (Robinson and Seward, 1987).

Initial vital signs should include a core temperature to assess the degree of hypothermia (Robinson and Seward, 1987). Pulmonary artery, tympanic membrane, bladder, or rectal temperature may be used to record core temperature. Resuscitation efforts for cardiac arrest continue until the patient has warmed to at least 30°C and preferably to 36°C. A rectal temperature of below 29.5°C places the patient at great risk for ventricular dysrhythmia, and rewarming should be accomplished rapidly (Orlowski, 1987).

Concomitant injuries must be considered in all accident victims. The most common injuries associated with swimming and diving accidents are intracranial and cervical spine trauma (Robinson and Seward, 1987). Victims of scuba diving accidents may have a dysbaric air embolism, which requires emergent transport to a hyperbaric chamber. Unexplained shock is frequently due to concealed hemorrhage.

Assessment of intravascular volume status can be accomplished by monitoring vital signs, urinary output via Foley catheter, serial ABGs, and central venous pressure. Central line placement may lead to intractable dysrhythmias in hypothermic patients.

Cerebral resuscitation is facilitated by rapid stabilization and correction of the problems previously discussed. Attention should be given to the possibility of drug overdose and intracranial injury. Toxicology studies and an emergent CT scan may be indicated.

Cerebral hypoxic injury should be suspected in all individuals who have had a cardiovascular arrest. The degree of hypoxic injury may be influenced by the length of resuscitation efforts needed and the degree of hypothermia. Treatment modalities that should be implemented for suspected hypoxic insult are (1) hyperventilation to achieve a Pa_{CO_2} of between 25 and 30 mm Hg, (2) elevation of the head to 30 degrees if vital signs are stable and there is no indication of spine injury, (3) administration of diuretics, (4) control of seizure activity by use of diazepam initially followed by phenobarbital, and (5) muscle relaxation and sedation. Agitation and pain increase intracranial pressure and cerebral metabolism. Muscle relaxation can be achieved with pancuronium bromide every hour. The use of steroids, mannitol, high-dose barbiturates, and hypothermia remains controversial (Robinson and Seward, 1987; Waquier et al., 1987).

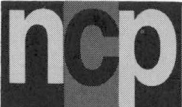 **nursing care plan**

1. Impaired gas exchange related to:

Atelectasis	Pneumomediastinum
Aspiration pneumonia	Pulmonary edema
Bronchospasm	Adult respiratory distress syndrome
Pneumothorax	Inadequate ventilation support

Outcome Criteria	*Nursing Interventions*

Outcome Criteria

Adequate and equal lung expansion and bilateral equal aeration without adventitious breath sounds; pH 7.35 to 7.45 Pa_{CO_2} less than 45 mm Hg, P_{O_2} 80 to 100 mm Hg, and O_2 saturation greater than 90%.

Nursing Interventions

1. Assess and record heart rate, respiratory rate, blood pressure, temperature, expansion, breath sounds, and lung compliance every 2 to 4 hours.
2. Observe for evidence of atelectasis, aspiration pneumonia, bronchospasm, pneumothorax, tension pneumothorax, pneumomediastinum, pulmonary edema, and adult respiratory distress syndrome every 2 to 4 hours.
3. Evaluate chest x-ray for evidence of complications daily.
4. Insert nasogastric sump tube in intubated, lethargic, or comatose patients to minimize risk of aspiration of gastric contents.
5. Assess adequacy of ventilatory support:
   a. Assess ABGs after every change in ventilation parameters or condition of patient.
   b. Initiate use of pulse oximetry and capnography if available (Nelson, 1988).
   c. Verify patency of endotracheal (ET) tube and its position by auscultation and chest x-ray. Bilateral breath sounds should be heard to ensure proper position and patency of the ET tube. On chest x-ray the tip of the ET tube should be 5 to 7 cm above the carina in adults and 1 to 2 cm above the carina or at the level of the third rib in a child. Malposition usually places the tip of the ET tube in the right mainstem bronchus and may cause hypoventilation of the left lung (visualized on x-ray).
   d. Verify the proper position of the nasogastric tube by intragastric pH or observe it on the chest x-ray. Follow the tube down the esophagus. The tip of the nasogastric tube should extend 2 to 3 inches into the stomach, and there should be no kinks along its course. Make sure the nasogastric tube is not in the bronchi; there, it would worsen hypoxemia.
   e. Perform lavage and suction through the ET tube every 2 to 4 hours. Lavage stimulates cough and thins secretions, facilitating their removal. Suctioning will also assist in maintaining a clear, unobstructed tube.
   f. Verify and record the fraction of oxygen being delivered and all other ventilatory parameters hourly. The oxygen setting on the equipment may be inadvertently changed or may not be returned to the proper setting following suctioning. Percentage of oxygen delivery controls on equipment are not accurate and must frequently be adjusted using an oxygen analyzer for accurate delivery.
   g. A manual resuscitation bag and mask must be at the bedside with a mask and an oxygen supply in readiness for mechanical failure, accidental extubation, suctioning or a cardiac arrest.
   h. Perform percussion and postural drainage every 2 to 4 hours to facilitate mobilization of secretions.
   i. Turn the patient every 2 hours to facilitate secretion mobilization.
   j. If patient is not intubated, use incentive spirometry, turning, coughing, and deep breathing every 2 hours and PRN.
   k. Elevate head of bed to 30 degrees to allow maximal diaphragmatic excursion (Guyton, 1986; Hazinski, 1984). Blood flow is increased to the dependent lung areas (Guyton, 1986). Elevating the head redirects blood flow to the more anterior areas of lung tissue. The anterior alveoli usually contain fever secretions and atelectasis, which improves ventilation-perfusion matching (Guyton, 1986).
6. Notify the physician promptly of all changes in the patient's condition.
7. A chest tube may be inserted for treatment of pneumothorax and tension pneumothorax. Observe and record the color, consistency, and amount of drainage, and the presence of an air leak.
8. A mediastinal tap may be required for pneumomediastinum. Gather the required equipment, assist with the sterile procedure, and monitor the patient.
9. Bronchospasm requires nebulized bronchodilators and possibly IV or PO aminophylline to prevent air trapping and decrease airway resistance (Robinson and Seward, 1987). Observe and record the patient's response to treatment and the duration of relief from symptoms. Watch for drug-induced dysrhythmias.

Nursing Care Plan continued on following page

2. Altered cardiac output
Decreased cardiac output, related to
pneumopericardium and tension pneumothorax

Outcome Criteria	Nursing Interventions
Mean systemic blood pressure more than 60 mm Hg; capillary refill less than 3 seconds; jugular venous distention (JVD) less than 3 cm above the sternal angle with head of bed (HOB) elevated to 45 degrees; no air visible on chest x-ray between the cardiac silhouette and lung tissue or diaphragm.	1. Monitor electrocardiogram (ECG) continuously for myocardial infarction and pericarditis, both of which cause ST segment elevation greater than 1 mm above baseline. 2. Monitor and record vital signs every 1 to 2 hours. 3. Observe and record capillary refill time, JVD, and skin temperature of extremities (for coolness) every 2 to 4 hours. 4. Observe for pulsus paradoxus of more than 15 mm Hg with each blood pressure determination. Notify the physician immediately if it is over 15 mm Hg because this indicates possible tamponade and may progress to cardiac arrest if not corrected. Pericardiocentesis may be required. Assemble equipment, prepare patient, assist with procedure, and monitor patient. 5. Auscultate heart sounds for change in loudness and presence of rub every 2 to 4 hours. 6. Evaluate chest x-ray daily. 7. Notify physician promptly if signs of pneumopericardium or deterioration in patient condition occurs.

3. Hypothermia related to:
Exposure to cold water

Outcome Criteria	Nursing Interventions
Core temperature of more than 35°C, normal sinus rhythm, absence of dysrhythmias, normal reflexes, normal mentation and level of consciousness (LOC), skin warm and dry.	1. Monitor core temperature continuously using an indwelling probe. 2. Monitor LOC hourly without inducing noxious stimuli while core temperature remains below 35°C. 3. Administer heated, humidified oxygen. 4. Warm all IV solutions continuously. 5. Perform nasogastric lavage with warmed fluid every 15 minutes until rectal temperature remains above 29.5°C.

4. Altered tissue perfusion: Cerebral compromise related to:
Hypoxemia
Decreased perfusion
Increased intracranial pressure (ICP)

Outcome Criteria	Nursing Interventions
Cerebral perfusion pressure (CPP) of more than 50 mmHg, normal LOC, pupils equal and briskly reactive to light, and no seizure activity.	1. Seizure precautions: bed rails up and padded with bed in low position. Nasopharyngeal airway available at bedside. 2. Observe and document seizure activity—location, duration, and type. Notify physician immediately if seizures occur. 3. Monitor ICP and blood pressure hourly. Calculate the cerebral perfusion pressure. 4. Determine the range for ICP and CPP. Initiate prescribed treatment if CPP drops below the desired range. 5. Monitor urine hourly to check for an output in excess of intake without diuretics. Notify physician immediately if this occurs.

5. Potential for injury: Bleeding related to:
Stimulation of the intrinsic clotting mechanism
Hypoxemia
Metabolic acidosis

Outcome Criteria	Nursing Interventions
Hematocrit of more than 30%, no new development of petechiae or purpuric rash; absence of bleeding; normal clotting factors II, V, and VIII; platelet count more than 60,000; prothrombin time (PT) 11 to 15 seconds; partial thromboplasted time (PTT) 30 to 45 seconds; and fibrinogen 200 to 330 mg/100 mL.	1. Monitor secretions, urine, and stool for evidence of bleeding. 2. Observe venous and arterial puncture sites for active bleeding. 3. Monitor clotting factors, platelet level, PT, PTT, fibrinogen, and hematocrit every 4 hours as ordered. 4. Administer blood products as ordered. 5. Observe skin for petechiae and purpuric rashes. 6. Administer heparin infusion to maintain PTT and clotting time as ordered by physician. 7. Notify physician if evidence of bleeding occurs.

6. Altered tissue perfusion: Renal related to:
Hypotension
Clot formation

Outcome Criteria	Nursing Interventions
Urine output more than 1 to 2 mL/kg/hour, urine osmolality and specific gravity consistent with normal urine volume variations (urine osmolality and specific gravity rise with low output), BUN less than 80 mL/dL (Hazinski, 1984). Creatinine less than 1.5 mL/dL, and serum K⁺ less than 5.0.	1. Monitor and record urine output hourly. Notify physician immediately if urine output falls below 1 mL/kg/hour or if intake greatly exceeds output. 2. Monitor color and turbidity of urine hourly. A rusty color indicates hemolized RBCs, which may contribute to low urine output (Whittaker, 1985). 3. Monitor osmolality and specific gravity every 4 hours. 4. Monitor electrolytes and acid-base balance. 5. Monitor serum and urine osmolality, sodium, BUN, and creatinine. If prerenal failure is present, serum BUN will begin to rise before serum creatinine. When hypovolemia is present and is responsible for prerenal failure, urine sodium content will be less than 20 mEq/liter and urine osmolality will be more than 500 mOsm/liter. 6. Maintain patency of Foley catheter, irrigate with 25 mL of bacteriostatic water if catheter is thought to be obstructed and subtract the instilled amount of fluid from the urine output. 7. Tape the Foley catheter in place and position it so that traction on the catheter is avoided, drainage is facilitated, and the dependent loop is eliminated.

References

Baker, S. P. (1984). Drowning. *Injury fact book* (pp. 155–165). Lexington, MA: D.C. Heath, Lexington Books.

Clochesy, J. M. (1984). Profound hypothermia. *Focus on Critical Care*, 11, 19–21.

Daniele, O., Mattaliano, A., and Natale E. (1987). Bimodal sensory stimulation-induced seizures. *Acta Neurologica Scandinaveia* 76, 297–301.

Davis, S., Ledman, J., and Kilgore, J. (1985). Drowning of children and youth in a desert state. *Western Journal of Medicine*, 143, 196–201.

Gonzales-Rothi, R. J. (1987). Near drowning: Consensus and controversy in pulmonary and cerebral resuscitation. *Heart & Lung*, 16, 474–481.

Guyton, A. C. (1986). *Text book of medical physiology* (7th ed.). Philadelphia: W. B. Saunders.

Hazinski, M. F. (1984). *Nursing care of the critically ill child*. St. Louis: C. V. Mosby.

Heimlich, H. J., Ornato, J. P., and Moxley, J. H. (1986). The Heimlich maneuver and the resuscitation of near drown victims. *Journal of the American Medical Association*. 256, 2960–2961.

Henneman, E. A. (1986). Brain resuscitation. *Heart & Lung*, 15, 3–11.

Karch, S. (1986). Pathology of the lung in near-drowning. *American Journal of Emergency Medicine*, 4, 4–9.

Kasteleijn-Nolst, D. D., Trenite, D. G., Binnie, C. D., Meinardi, H. (1987). Photo-sensitive patients: Symptoms and signs during intermittent photic stimulation and their relationship to seizures in daily life. *Journal of Neurology, Neurosurgery and Psychiatry*, 50, 1546–1549.

Malasanos, L., Barkauskas, V., Moss, M., et al. (1986). *Health assessment* (3rd ed.). St. Louis: C.V. Mosby.

Martin, T. G. (1984). Near-drowning and cold water immersion. *Annals of Emergency Medicine*, 4, 263–273.

Mathur, G. P., and Mathur, S. (1986). Drowning and near drowning. *Indian Pediatrics*, 23 (Suppl.), 189–194.

Menn, S. J. and Stool E. W. (1980). Mechanical ventilation: Weaning and complications. In R.A. Bordow (ed.), *Manual of clinical problems in pulmonary medicine* (pp. 264–269). Boston: Little, Brown.

Modell, J. H. (1986). Near drowning. *Circulation*, 74 (Suppl. 4), 27–28.

Nelson, S. J. (1988). Pulse oximetry. In J. M. Clochesy (Ed.), *Advanced technology in critical care*. Frederick, MD: Aspen Publishers.

Neuman, T. (1980). Near drowning—diving and decompression. In R.A. Bordow (ed.), *Manual of clinical problems in pulmonary medicine* (pp. 374–377). Boston: Little, Brown.

Orlowski, J. P. (1987). Drowning, near-drowning, and ice-water submersions. *Pediatric Clinics of North America*, 34, 75–92.

Pearn, J. (1985). The management of near drowning. *British Medical Journal*, 291, 1447–1452.

Pitt, W. R. (1986). Increasing incidence of childhood immersion injury in Brisbane. *Medical Journal of Australia*, 144, 683–985.

Robinson, M. D., and Seward, P. N. (1987). Submersion injury in children. *Pediatric Emergency Care*, 3, 44–49.

Spragg, R. G. (1980). Adult respiratory distress syndrome. In *Manual of clinical problems in pulmonary medicine* (pp. 252–253). Boston: Little, Brown.

Torr, C., Varetto, L., and Tappi, E. (1983). Scanning electron microscopic ultrastructural alterations of the pulmonary alveolus in experimental drowning. *Journal of Forensic Science*, 28, 1008–1012.

Vergnes, M., Kiesmann, M., Marscaux, C., et al. (1986). Kindling of audiogenic seizures in the rat. *International Journal of Neuroscience*, 36, 167–176.

Waquier, A., Edmonds, H. L., and Clincke H. C. (1987). Cerebral resuscitation: Pathology and therapy. *Neuroscience Biobehavior Review*, 11, 287–306.

Whittaker, A. A. (1985). Acute renal dysfunction: Assessment of patients at risk. *Focus on Critical Care*, 12, 12–17.

Wintemute, G. J., Kraus, J. F., Teret, S. P., et al. (1987). Drowning in childhood and adolescence: A population-based study. *American Journal of Public Health*, 77(7), 830–832.

Wittmers, L. E., Pozos, R. S., Fall, G., et al.: (1987). Cardiovascular responses to face immersion (the diving reflex) in human beings after alcohol consumption. *Annals of Emergency Medicine*, 16, 1031–1036.

Special Clinical Situations

62

Preventing Postanesthesia Complications

Ginger Schafer Wlody

Prevention of complications in the immediate post-anesthesia period is a vital and complex aspect of critical care nursing. Major physiologic derangements occur because general anesthesia and surgery result in the release of neurohormonal substances and endogenous catecholamines (Stoelting, 1980). These substances are released in conjunction with the stress response as well as the effects of specific anesthetic agents. This combination of factors results in physiologic alterations in the cardiovascular, pulmonary, central nervous, metabolic, renal, and gastrointestinal systems. In a study of 183 men and 242 women undergoing general anesthesia (Vaughan, 1982), 24% of the sample experienced at least one critical incident in the operating room. Thirty-one per cent experienced at least one critical incident in the postanesthesia care unit (PACU). Of these, prolonged airway management accounted for 39% and dysrythmias for 16%. PACU critical incidents were defined as occurrences requiring nursing or medical intervention. Table 62–1 describes the most common critical incidents in the PACU. In a more recent study, Eichorn (1989) found that among 1,001,000 patients with American Society of Anesthesiologists (ASA) physi-cal status 1 and 2 there were 11 major intraoperative accidents "solely attributable to anesthesia." These included five deaths, four cases of permanent CNS damage, and two cardiac arrests with eventual recovery. Review of these untoward anesthetic events revealed that unrecognized hypoventilation, found in seven patients, was the most common cause.

Critical care nurses caring for patients in the immediate postanesthesia period must anticipate, assess, and manage these physiologic derangements. In addition to the stress of anesthesia and surgery, preoperative, intraoperative, and postoperative factors contribute to both physiologic and emotional complications. It is imperative for the nurse to consider all the stressors that may contribute to complications in this potentially hazardous period.

In this chapter, complications that may occur subsequent to general anesthesia and related drug therapy are explored. Regional anesthesia (spinal, epidural, and local) will not be discussed because the majority of critical care patients receive general anesthesia or a combination of general and regional anesthesia. The discussion will identify factors that may lead to postanesthesia complications and will target nursing interventions to prevent them in the critically ill patient. Specific anesthetic agents, skeletal muscle relaxants, and considerations for nursing interventions are identified and discussed. Nursing assessments and interventions that focus on the postanesthetic needs of the critically ill patient are presented.

IDENTIFYING PREOPERATIVE RISK FACTORS

The critical care nurse assesses the patient for preoperative risk factors that may influence the post-

---

TABLE 62–1. Most Common Critical Incidents in the Postanesthesia Care Unit

Dysrhythmias
Hypotension (30% below preoperative systolic BP)
Hypoxemia
Hypercarbia
Electrolyte disturbances
Airway maintenance
Hypothermia ($<34°C$ core)

Data from Vaughan (1982).

TABLE 62-2. Preoperative Factors That May Lead to Complications in the Postoperative Period

Age	Immunologic compromise
Preexisting cardiovascular disease	Presence of infection
Preexisting respiratory disease	Disease of the blood-forming organs
Endocrine disorders	Hepatic disease
Obesity	Renal disease
Diabetes	Genetic factors
Porphyria	Hypothermia
Drug addiction	Prolonged response to anectine
Psychological state/psychiatric disorders	Nutritional state

operative course. As described in Table 62-2, this preoperative evaluation focuses on detection and subsequent correction of abnormal states. The nursing role includes visiting elective surgery patients preoperatively for nursing assessment, teaching, and emotional support. Risk factors that should be considered include age, cardiovascular disease, respiratory status, nutritional status, infection, immunologic compromise, hepatic disease, renal failure, and genetic factors.

The anesthesiologist classifies the patient preoperatively according to the American Society of Anesthesiologists (ASA) classification system and records this classification on the patient record. The critical care nurse utilizes this information in the overall plan of care in conjunction with the nursing assessment. The ASA classification system categorizes patients preoperatively to define risk. The classification is as follows (Norman, 1980):

Class 1 Normal healthy patient
Class 2 Mild systemic disease
Class 3 Severe systemic disease limiting activity, but not incapacitating
Class 4 Incapacitating due to systemic disease with a constant threat to life
Class 5 Moribund, not expected to live 24 hours with or without surgery

Risk Factors

Age. Age is a risk factor that increases perioperative complications, thereby placing pediatric and geriatric patients at higher risk. In one study the primary mortality of patients aged 70 or more in major operations was 9.2% (Palmberg and Hirsjarvi, 1979). Many physiologic changes in the elderly patient affect the perioperative course and perioperative management. These physiologic changes are summarized in Table 62-3.

Cardiovascular Status. The presence of preexisting cardiovascular disease is another important risk factor. Patients who have had previous myocardial infarction, history of dysrhythmias, valvular problems, congestive heart failure, or hypertension are considered to be at greater risk (Goldman et al., 1977). It is recommended that elective surgery be delayed until 6 months after myocardial infarction because of the chance of reinfarction during or after anesthesia and surgery (Tarhan, 1981).

Respiratory Status. Patients who have a history of respiratory disease or impaired pulmonary function and those who smoke present an increased surgical risk (Hybels, 1981). This includes patients with chronic obstructive pulmonary disease (COPD), chronic bronchitis, asthma, and past lung operations. The incidence of pulmonary complications in cigarette smokers is 26 times the normal rate (Forestner, 1981).

Endocrine Function. The most common endocrine disorder that poses a threat to the surgical patient is diabetes mellitus (Stoelting, 1980). Studies have shown that, compared with the general population, the diabetic patient has an increased risk of surgical morbidity and mortality. The risk is thought to result from the high incidence of cardiovascular disease, impaired response to infection, impaired wound healing, and increased protein breakdown that occur in patients with diabetes mellitus (Walts, 1983). Patients with hyperthyroidism also require careful perioperative management. Severe circulatory and metabolic changes may complicate the surgical and anesthetic management of the thyrotoxic patient (Snow, 1977). Proper preoperative control of thyrotoxicosis reduces the likelihood of postoperative thyroid storm. Because of the possible development of thyroid storm, atropine is not given as a preanesthetic medication to these patients (Dripps et al., 1988). Patients with adrenal insufficiency and patients on chronic corticosteroid therapy also are at increased surgical risk. Stress doses (300 mg/day) of intravenous cortisol must be administered during the perioperative period (Siperstein, 1988). These patients also are prone to urinary salt wastage. Fluid and electrolyte levels must be closely monitored in the perioperative period.

Nutritional Status. Nutritional status is another factor that affects postoperative complications in the surgical patient. Any patient with depleted glycogen

TABLE 62-3. The Geriatric Patient: Physiologic Changes That Affect the Perioperative Course and Perioperative Management

Decreased metabolic rate
Decreased central nervous system function
Diminished airway reflexes
Decreased serum protein levels
Increased percentage of body fat in relation to lean body mass
Decreased cardiovascular reserve
Decreased pulmonary reserve
Decreased hepatic and renal function

Data from Fraulini (1987).

stores is at risk (Shelby, 1967). This may occur in malnourished or emaciated patients, chronic alcoholics, or extremely obese patients. Albumin levels below 3.0 gm/100 mL are associated with moderate malnutrition, and levels below 2.1 gm/100 mL indicate severe malnutrition (Hybels, 1981).

Immunologic and Hematologic Function. The presence of infection prior to surgery greatly increases perioperative risk and enhances the possibility of generalized sepsis. When possible, the operation should be delayed until the infection is resolved (Forestner, 1981). Immunologic compromise results from systemic disease or the use of immunosuppressive agents. For example, steroids suppress the normal adrenal response. These patients must be given a "steroid prep" and observed carefully for adequate adrenal response (Bass, 1973). Anemia, thrombocytopenia, coagulation disorders, and other diseases of the hematopoietic system predispose the patient to complications. Coagulopathy should be suspected in patients with liver disease or those who have had massive transfusions.

Hepatic Disease. The liver detoxifies most general anesthetic agents and barbiturates. Recovery from general anesthesia will be prolonged in patients with hepatic disease.

Renal Failure. Patients with acute or chronic renal failure may present problems in the postanesthetic period. Preoperatively, the patient may be hypertensive or anemic or may have abnormal electrolyte levels. Volume overload and severe electrolyte imbalances can occur rapidly in the surgical patient with renal failure (Burke and Gulyassy, 1979).

Medication History. It is important to recognize that the patient's current medications may cause postanesthesia complications. Chronic or preoperative drug therapy may modify organ function directly and may also alter patient response to anesthetic agents or adjuvants (Muravchick, 1980). For example, individuals taking quinidine who then receive curariform drugs during surgery may have prolonged postoperative apnea (Caranasos, 1979). Ethanol, tranquilizer, or narcotic abuse also increases the possibility of altered physiologic responses to anesthesia.

Genetic Factors. There are several known genetic factors that affect surgical risk. Malignant hyperthermia is a severe, life-threatening, postanesthetic complication that occurs in genetically susceptible individuals (Arens and McKinnon, 1971). Another group with genetic risk with surgery includes patients with sickle cell disease. In these patients there is an increased risk of a vaso-occlusive crisis during or immediately after the operation. A third genetic defect that increases risk is the presence of an abnormal anectine response. One of every 3000 patients

has an abnormal response to anectine (Snow, 1977), resulting in decreased pseudocholinesterase activity. When this occurs, the metabolism of anectine is greatly prolonged, and ventilatory support is needed. The patient's susceptibility to malignant hyperthermia can be evaluated in several ways. A careful anesthetic history, taken by the anesthesiologist, reveals a family history of malignant hyperthermia or relatives who have experienced hyperpyrexic reactions secondary to anesthesia. Electrophysiologic and muscle biopsy studies may be carried out to identify a suspected susceptibility to malignant hyperthermia. Evidence of muscle abnormalities is usually evident on physical examination (Marchildon, 1982).

Psychological Factors. Preoperative anxiety or psychological stress may profoundly affect patients. Past experiences or negative information influences the way the patient views the surgical experience. Studies have shown that fear or stress influences the outcome of surgery as well as the way the patient deals with pain and discomfort. Fears related to the unfamiliar environment of the surgical suite, the anesthesia itself, the outcome of the procedure, pain, prolonged illness, and lack of general medical knowledge are added stressors and further disturb the patient's normal equilibrium. Identification of a patient's potential for ineffective coping triggers supportive measures by the critical care nurse or the entire team. Preoperative teaching and counseling in conjunction with targeted preoperative medication and nursing support are usually effective in assisting patients to manage their stress.

INTRAOPERATIVE FACTORS

The critical care nurse must recognize intraoperative factors that may precipitate postanesthesia complications. Anesthetic agents (Table 62–4) and skeletal muscle relaxants (Table 62–5) have specific actions that can have deleterious effects upon the patient. Nursing assessments and actions are based on the intraoperative factors described in this section. In assessing the effects of anesthetic agents the critical care nurse considers the physiologic effects of the preoperative medication, the method of induction, and the use of muscle relaxants, narcotics, anesthetics, and "reversal agents." Knowledge of which drugs were administered intraoperatively (e.g., anticoagulants, antibiotics), which mechanical devices were utilized (e.g., intra-aortic balloon pump), and the occurrence of any problems encountered during surgery are vital.

The type of operation also influences what postoperative complications occur. For example, fat embolism can occur after multiple, severe injuries, especially in the long bones. Fat droplets are released into the circulation, and these fat emboli spread widely, possibly causing abnormalities in many or-

TABLE 62–4. Common Anesthetic Agents, Characteristics and Considerations for Nursing Interventions

Route	Official Generic or Chemical Name	Commercial Name or Synonym	Characteristics	Considerations for Nursing Interventions
Inhalation Liquids with volatile vapor	Ether (diethyl oxide)	Diethyl ether Ethyl ether	Explosive; used for poor-risk patients due to minimal cardiovascular effects; safe	Side effects: increased secretions, nausea, vomiting, prolonged recovery period
	Trichloroethylene	Trilene	Nonflammable; used widely in obstetrics	Tachypnea, ventricular arrhythmias, bradycardia
	Halothane	Fluothane	Nonexplosive, inflammable; Incomplete muscle relaxation, rapid induction; overdosage easily possible (potent agent); relaxes the uterus; is a halogenated substance	Possible cause of hepatic necrosis; myocardial and respiratory depressant; causes vasodilation, hypotension and shivering; parasympathetic-like effect on the heart (AV and junctional arrhythmias); highly soluble in fatty tissue
	Methoxyflurane	Penthrane	Nonexplosive, inflammable; slow induction compared to halothane; good muscle relaxation; is a halogenated substance	Hepatotoxic myocardial and respiratory depressant; causes vasodilation, hypotension and shivering; may have increased urinary output postoperatively; longer recovery period than Fluothane; has analgesic properties; highly soluble in fatty tissue; sympathetic-like effect on heart
	Enflurane	Ethrane	Potent, halogenated ether, nonexplosive, inflammable	Vasodilation, parasympathetic-like effect on heart, nephrotoxic, nausea, vomiting, may cause abnormal EEG in normal patient; avoid use with seizure patients; currently popular agent used in balanced anesthesia, does not seem to sensitize myocardium
	Isoflurane	Forane	Smooth, rapid induction; halogenated ether, nonexplosive, inflammable; approved for use Spring 1981; provides good muscle relaxation with CNS excitation	Seems to have no hepatic or renal toxicity, does not seem to cause arrhythmias; causes respiratory depression, reduced BP ulterine relaxation; is equal to halothane and Ethrane in potential to trigger malignant hyperthermia
Gaseous anesthetics	Nitrous oxide	Laughing gas	Nonflammable, supports combustion; induction may be accompanied by dreams; recovery rapid; poor muscle relaxation; is rapidly reversible; more soluble than nitrogen in blood	Causes diffusional hypoxemia postoperatively; causes vasoconstriction and increased BP; laryngospasm may occur
	Cyclopropane	None	Explosive, inflammable; rapid induction and recovery; rarely used due to explosive properties	Increases irritability of myocardium; causes vasoconstriction and increased BP; emergent excitement; bronchospasm may occur; nausea, vomiting, increased intracranial pressure

TABLE 62–4. *Common Anesthetic Agents, Characteristics and Considerations for Nursing Interventions* Continued

Route	Official Generic or Chemical Name	Commercial Name or Synonym	Characteristics	Considerations for Nursing Interventions
Intravenous				
	Thiopental sodium	Sodium pentothal (known as Thiopentone in England)	Ultrashort-acting barbiturate; rapid induction and recovery; given with another anesthetic to produce relaxation and anesthesia; may be used to control certain convulsive states	May cause respiratory depression, laryngospasm (restlessness, stridor, cyanosis), generalized muscle twitching; liver and renal damage have occurred; vasodilation may cause shivering with pooling of blood; decreased venous return; causes respiratory depression, nausea, vomiting, urinary retention
	Morphine sulfate	Same	Is a narcotic analgesic; used for open-heart and vascular surgery; does not affect cardiac reserve; contraindicated in convulsive states; used in conjunction with nitrous oxide and muscle relaxants	
	Fentanyl and droperidol	Innovar	Combination fentanyl (narcotic analgesic) and droperidol (a neuroleptic); combination increases pain threshold, decreases reflex excitability, allays anxiety; droperidol is longer acting than fentanyl	Causes respiratory depression, decreases intraocular pressure; fentanyl has vasodilator effects, may occasionally cause muscle rigidity and cause respiratory and cardiovascular depression; droperidol causes dissociation and drowsiness; patients "forget" to breathe; when given without an analgesic, droperidol causes dystonic reactions
	Ketamine	Ketalar	Dissociative anesthetic; rapid onset, short duration; usually used for superficial operations in children when no muscle relaxation is required	Causes hallucinatory emergence, more so in adults; quiet environment and absence of stimulation minimizes this; arterial pressure and pulse may be elevated; may cause or precipitate laryngospasm when surgery about mouth or lips is performed; causes increased intracranial pressure

From Wlody, G. S. (1982). Postoperative complications. In American Association of Critical-Care Nurses: *The NTI proceedings book—1982* (pp. 279–280). Newport Beach, CA: AACN.

gan systems (Drain and Shipley, 1979). Fat embolism usually occurs 12 to 24 hours after injury or surgery.

Effects of Anesthetic Agents

Anesthetic agents, whether volatile, gaseous, intravenous, regional, spinal or epidural, all affect the body systems. To anticipate complications, the critical care nurse must view the process of surgery and anesthesia as a planned assault upon the patient. It is a physical and metabolic attack upon the body systems.

Myocardial Depression. The currently used volatile or gaseous anesthetic agents (forane, ethrane, nitrous oxide, and so on) and intravenous narcotics

are myocardial depressants. The clinical expression of this myocardial depressant effect is usually intraoperative hypotension. In the postoperative period, myocardial depression manifests as congestive heart failure. The most feared cardiovascular morbidity in the perianesthetic period is that of myocardial infarction (Briggs, 1980). About 0.15% of adult patients experience myocardial infarction with general anesthesia and operation.

Alterations in Respiratory Function. General anesthesia results in impaired gas exchange leading to an increase in venous admixture and alveolar dead space. A primary determinant of this impaired function is an alteration in the distribution of ventilation during anesthesia leading to increased ventilation/perfusion (V_A/Q) imbalance, which then results

TABLE 62–5. Effects of Skeletal Muscle Relaxants on the Cardiovascular System

Muscle Relaxant	Action*
Tubocurarine (Tubarine)	Lowers arterial blood pressure (principally by blocking transmission at autonomic ganglia)
Pancuronium bromide (Pavulon)	Does not have histamine-releasing or ganglion-blocking effects; has weak vagolytic action which can increase heart rate slightly and may raise arterial pressure and cardiac output; very useful in the high risk patient, especially if long period of relaxation is required
Suxamethonium (Anectine)	Has a cholinergic effect; potentiation action of cardiac glycosides; in patient not completely digitalized, it may cause prolongation of P-R interval, depression of S-T segment and T wave flattening or inversion

*In patients with severe cardiac decompensation, it is often preferable not to attempt reversal of the muscle relaxant but to continue ventilation postoperatively until cardiorespiratory function has become more stable.

From Wlody, G. S. (1982). Postoperative complications. In American Association of Critical-Care Nurses. *The NTI proceedings book—1982* (p. 280). Newport Beach, CA: AACN.

in hypoxemia (Otto, 1980). There is a decrease in functional residual capacity (FRC), which leads to airway closure with gas trapping and microatelectasis.

Decreased Renal Blood Flow. Renal blood flow is decreased due to sympathetic activity and other factors. Renal vascular resistance and the filtration fraction increase while the glomerular filtration rate (GFR), urine output, and renal blood flow fall (Tonneson, 1980). The types and amounts of fluids administered intraoperatively play an important role in the patient's fluid volume status during the postanesthetic period.

Central Nervous System Alterations. Inhalation and intravenous anesthetics have profound effects on the cerebral metabolic rate, cerebral blood flow, and intracranial pressure dynamics. Cerebral vasodilation results from all the commonly used volatile anesthetics. This may result in an increase in intracranial pressure, which in turn results in decreased cerebral blood flow. Intravenous anesthetics act as cerebral metabolic depressants and cerebral vasoconstrictors (Drain and Shipley, 1979).

Neuromuscular Blockade. Neuromuscular blocking agents (anectine, pavulon, tubarine, flaxedil, and so on) are routinely administered as adjuncts to anesthesia to induce skeletal muscle relaxation and to facilitate intubation (Emerson et al., 1979). These neuromuscular blocking agents interfere with the physiology of neuromuscular transmission and produce muscle weakness or paralysis. The sensitivity of different muscle groups varies. The muscles of the eyelids are most sensitive and are paralyzed first, then the extremities, the jaw, intercostal muscles, and finally the diaphragm (Snow, 1977). The critical care nurse must be aware of the type of muscle relaxant used and its mechanism of action.

Drug Interactions. Many of the drug interactions that contribute to anesthetic risk result from impaired neuromuscular function or prolonged action of neuromuscular blocking agents (Muravchick, 1980; Caranosos, 1979). For example, when aminoglycoside antibiotics are administered parenterally or used to irrigate body cavities intraoperatively, neuromuscular blockade and subsequent paralysis are enhanced (Goodwin, 1982). This effect carries over to the postanesthesia period and prolongs muscle paralysis or weakness, so that mechanical ventilation may be required. Other drugs interact with neuromuscular blocking agents to produce prolonged apnea. Commonly used drugs that produce this effect include lithium, phospholine iodide (eye drops used in glaucoma), monoamine oxidase (MAO) inhibitors, and phenothiazines (Caranosos, 1979).

Thermal Regulation—Temperature Monitoring During Anesthesia. Temperature monitoring during anesthesia is routinely carried out to prevent hypothermia or hyperthermia by means of simple electronic devices that utilize a ceramic bead. Resistance to electrical current in the thermometer incorporating the ceramic bead may be found at various body sites. The site of temperature monitoring in the operating room varies according to the anesthesiologist's specific monitoring objectives. Esophageal temperature measures temperature at the level of the right heart and is a good indicator of average body temperature. Tympanic, bladder, and rectal sites are also utilized. The esophageal temperature is not influenced by the temperature of inhaled gases and is responsive to changes in body heat stores. The esophageal site for temperature monitoring may be uncomfortable for the patient if he or she is in the awake or semiconscious state. Rectal temperature is an indicator of core temperature but changes slowly in relation to other parts of the body. The temperature that most closely reflects that of the hypothalamus, or thermoregulatory center, is measured at the tympanic membrane. This site has quick access for use by the anesthesiologist.

Hypothermia. Hypothermia (temperature below 34°C) is a frequently recognized problem during prolonged surgery and particularly affects the very young, the elderly, and patients with hypothyroidism (Atkinson et al., 1987). In a sample of 312 adult surgical patients, 71.6% of intubated patients were hypothermic on admission to the PACU (Fraulini et al., 1985). Vaughn and colleagues (1981) studied 198 adults postoperatively and found that 13% were hypothermic on discharge from the PACU.

Normally, the body seeks to maintain its temperature within a certain range through the use of a strict set point that controls the temperature of the blood perfusing the posterior hypothalamus. When there is a deviation from this set point, mechanisms are activated to bring the temperature of the blood back to the preset level. For example, fever sets the thermostat at a higher level, and the body attempts to reach that new set point by increasing metabolism.

Maintenance of normal temperature during surgery is generally difficult. Several factors act in combination to make the patient susceptible to accidental hypothermia in the operating room suite. Ambient temperature is usually cool to keep the surgeon and staff comfortable. The modern operating room environment is maintained at 19° to 23°C with controlled humidity at about 45%. During surgery a large portion of the patient's body surface area is exposed to the cool environment and to cool solutions during the skin preparation.

Anesthetic agents alone do not induce hypothermia or hyperthermia in a normal patient (Flacke et al., 1982). Temperature is controlled by the thermoregulatory center in the hypothalamus through the mechanisms of conduction, convection, radiation, and evaporation. Anesthetic agents depress the thermoregulatory system, and therefore the response of the body depends upon the direction of temperature change in the environment. In addition, most anesthetic techniques result in vasodilation, which causes cooling of the blood.

Hypothermia may depress all body activity and, if uncontrolled, may be fatal. Hypothermia that results in myocardial depression and vasoconstriction is sometimes accompanied by shivering, restlessness, and an unstable cardiovascular state (Vale, 1981). Oxygen consumption is increased during rewarming, causing additional stress on the cardiovascular and pulmonary systems. Rebound shivering during the recovery period has been shown to increase oxygen consumption by 400% (Flacke et al., 1982; Vaughan et al., 1981). As consciousness returns in the anesthetized patient, the temperature-sensitive neurons in the anterior hypothalamus become aware of cold, releasing 5-hydroxytryptamine (5-HT), which stimulates the posterior hypothalamic heat production center (Vale, 1981). The production of heat requires additional oxygen consumption during the rewarming period. This excessive oxygen demand initiates increased minute ventilation to facilitate oxygen uptake, and cardiac output must increase simultaneously to ensure oxygen delivery. Ventilatory embarrassment or fixed low cardiac output during shivering represents a potentially hazardous situation (Goldman et al., 1977).

Hyperthermia. Malignant hyperthermia (MH) is a fulminant, hypermetabolic crisis that is usually triggered by volatile anesthetics or neuromuscular blocking agents. It is a rare disorder that occurs in susceptible individuals when they are exposed to specific anesthetic agents. MH occurs most often in the operating room environment and is characterized by a rapid temperature rise. The temperature rise results from a hypermetabolic state of skeletal muscle caused by an increase in the concentration of calcium ion in the sarcolemma (Flacke et al., 1982). Even though MH may respond to treatment with dantrolene sodium, hyperthermia may recur, and these patients must be monitored for 24 to 36 hours postoperatively. The nursing care plan at the end of the chapter presents nursing diagnoses and interventions pertinent to the surgical patient experiencing malignant hyperthermia.

Positioning. Hemodynamic stability is affected by the position of the patient on the operating room table (Smith, 1987). For example, rapid change from the lithotomy to the supine position can bring about a significant fall in blood pressure (Martin, 1987). The prone position may exert pressure against the inferior vena cava and the femoral veins, resulting in decreased venous return and hypotension (Smith, 1987). Venous return from the head may be obstructed when the head is turned to one side. Engorged eye vessels, eyelid edema, postoperative headache, and subglottic edema may result.

Other hazards associated with position of the operating room table include peripheral nerve damage (Berkebile, 1973), reduction of ventilation (Forestner, 1981), and air embolism to the brain. Air embolism may occur when the sitting position is utilized, as in neurosurgical procedures (Snow, 1977). The position of the patient during surgery is recorded on the intraoperative record.

Other Factors. In addition to anesthetic agents, narcotics, skeletal muscle relaxants, and positioning, other factors affect surgical risk. Duration of anesthesia and the length and complexity of the surgical process affect the incidence of postanesthetic complications (Minckley, 1969; Otto, 1980). Specific operative procedures affect the type and placement of the incision used, which in turn affect the potential for pulmonary complications. Research has documented that the transverse incision used in thoracic and abdominal surgery is associated with fewer pulmonary complications than is the vertical incision (Strauss and Wise, 1987).

In summary, intraoperative factors that must be considered by the critical care nurse in preventing postanesthetic complications include the following: preoperative condition of the patient, anesthetic agents and their physiologic effects, drug interactions, thermal regulation, fluids administered, patient positioning, and the specific surgical procedure used and its effects. Intraoperative factors that may lead to complications in the postoperative period are summarized in Table 62–6.

PREVENTING POSTANESTHESIA COMPLICATIONS

Because intraoperative events directly affect complications occurring in the postanesthesia period

TABLE 62–6. Intraoperative Factors That May Lead to Complications in the Postoperative Period

Anesthetic agents utilized
Adjunctive drug therapy utilized
Duration of anesthesia and surgery
Position of patient during operative procedure
Type of operation
Type of incision
Use of irrigants
Amount and type of fluid replacement
Thermal regulation

(Forestner, 1981), the critical care nurse receives a detailed and comprehensive report from the anesthesiologist and the circulating nurse at the time of the patient's arrival from the surgical suite. This report includes a summary of the patient's overall condition, type of surgery performed, fluid status, anesthetic agents used, muscle relaxants and narcotics used, duration of anesthesia, and unusual events. The critical care nurse focuses on assessment and monitoring of vital body functions in the immediate postoperative period. Maintenance of the airway and oxygenation, monitoring of cardiopulmonary and renal function, wound care, body position, and fluid and electrolyte balance are critical. The critical care nurse must be aware of factors that precipitate complications.

The most common postanesthesia complications occur in the respiratory, central nervous, and cardiovascular systems. However, significant postanesthesia complications also may occur in the renal and gastrointestinal systems as well.

Respiratory Complications

General anesthesia results in an altered pattern of ventilation as well as a diminution in lung volumes. In addition, respiratory depression results from the use of narcotics or muscle relaxants (Forestner, 1981). The sequence of hypoventilation, atelectasis, and pneumonia occurs in 20% to 40% of postsurgical patients. Because the incision site affects chest wall motion, patients subjected to thoracic or upper abdominal surgery have the greatest chance of developing pulmonary complications (Harmon and Lillington, 1979).

Airway Obstruction. Airway obstruction may occur postoperatively in the oropharynx, nasopharynx, or tracheobronchial tree. Upper airway obstruction is most common. Anesthetics and related medications depress the patient's reflexes, resulting in muscular flaccidity. Secretions, blood, or vomitus may be present, thereby increasing the hazard of aspiration and laryngospasm. Laryngospasm usually results from irritation or bleeding in the throat or mouth and may be life-threatening unless promptly recognized and treated.

Hypoventilation. Hypoventilation secondary to anesthesia is a frequent postoperative complication. If uncorrected, hypoventilation may lead to hypercapnia and hypoxia. A moderate amount of hypoventilation leads to atelectasis and pneumonitis, which frequently occurs in surgical patients.

Muscle relaxants used intraoperatively lead to hypoventilation if they have not worn off or are not reversed chemically with agents such as physostigmine, neostigmine, pyridostigmine, or edrophonium. These reversal agents prevent metabolism of acetylcholine (Dripps et al., 1988). The most frequently encountered complication of muscle relaxants is unsuccessful reversal of neuromuscular blockade (Lebowitz and Savarese, 1980). Depolarizing muscle relaxants such as succinylcholine are shorter acting and cannot be reversed chemically. Respiratory support is needed until the effects wear off.

Other causes of hypoventilation include restrictive casts or dressings around the thorax, abdominal distention, and excessive accumulations of adipose tissue in thoracic and abdominal areas (Cullen, 1980). Pain, particularly in the upper abdominal or thoracic area, is a major contributing factor to hypoventilation (Otto, 1980). If hypoventilation is narcotic induced, narcotic antagonists such as naloxone may be administered. Hypoventilation resulting from barbiturates responds only to respiratory support until the agent is detoxified and the effects wear off.

Pulmonary Edema. Circulatory overload may result from massive fluid resuscitation or blood administration (Berkebile, 1973). A shift of blood and fluid from the periphery to the pulmonary vascular bed occurs. Pulmonary edema results from elevated left atrial and pulmonary artery blood pressure in combination with decreased myocardial contractility.

Diffusion Hypoxia. Diffusion hypoxia follows breathing of room air by a patient at the close of anesthesia in which a gaseous agent is used in high concentration (e.g., nitrous oxide). Nitrous oxide is about 30 times more soluble than nitrogen, so that at the end of anesthesia the volume of nitrous oxide coming out of the blood greatly exceeds the volume of nitrogen being absorbed. Tissues are saturated with the agent, resulting in a steep pressure gradient from the tissues to the zero partial pressure of gas in room air. This favors a rapid diffusion of the gas from the tissues to the bloodstream and then to the alveoli when air is substituted for the inspired anesthetic mixture. The resultant dilution of alveolar oxygen by the gas leads to varying degrees of hypoxemia and cyanosis lasting 3 to 10 minutes, depending upon the patient's minute ventilation. Medical treatment consists of administration of 100% oxygen for 5 to 10 minutes (Forestner, 1981).

Pneumothorax. Postoperative pneumothorax may be present due to trauma to the lung or thoracic cavity, such as central line placement. Patients with chronic obstructive lung disease are prone to pneumothorax due to rupture of blebs on the lung.

Nursing Management of Respiratory Complications. Nursing care during the postoperative period is directed toward maintaining airway patency and facilitating adequate gas exchange. Specific nursing goals and interventions are described in the nursing care plan.

Ineffective Breathing Patterns. Nursing care of the postanesthetic patient includes assessment and support of ventilation. Evaluation of respiratory rate, tidal volume, character of ventilation, presence of obstruction, and chest and diaphragmatic movements is done frequently to assess the adequacy of the patient's breathing pattern. Breath sounds are auscultated bilaterally to assess the adequacy of air flow. If the patient is intubated, artificial airways and oxygen are utilized in conjunction with the physician's prescriptions. The nurse checks the patient's ability to lift his head and neck and also checks handgrip strength and tidal volume prior to extubation (Lebowitz and Savarese, 1980). The patient is observed for signs of increased restlessness. Restlessness is a key sign of inadequate oxygenation. Restrictive dressings are adjusted to permit maximum chest expansion.

Adequate pain control is necessary to facilitate deep breathing. The nurse administers pain medication and monitors the patient for evidence of narcotic-induced hypoventilation. Narcotic-induced hypoventilation can be prevented by reducing the narcotic dosage and by using the intravenous route for quick action, uptake, and distribution. Narcotic antagonists are utilized as ordered.

Impaired Gas Exchange. Gas exchange may be impaired due to airway obstruction, atelectasis, or pneumothorax. Proper positioning of the patient to prevent occlusion of the airway by the tongue is vital. Nursing measures are used to prevent vomiting. These include moving the patient gently, using antiemetic medications, and ensuring that gastric drainage tubes are functioning properly. Suction equipment is kept readily available to assist in airway clearance should the patient vomit.

Nursing measures to facilitate alveolar ventilation and gas exchange include assisting the patient to perform coughing and encouraging deep breathing exercises and the use of incentive spirometry. The lungs are auscultated for diminished breath sounds and the presence of adventitious sounds.

Cardiovascular Complications

The risk of harmful cardiovascular events in the perioperative period most likely arises from impairment of cardiac function by the altered metabolic state associated with the operative procedure and anesthesia. Hypertension, hypotension, and arhythmias are the most frequent cardiovascular complications. Disturbances of myocardial energetics can result from increased cardiac oxygen demand, diminished oxygen supply to the heart, or both (Fig. 62–1). The two major effects of anesthesia and surgery are myocardial depression and a tendency toward arhythmias. Myocardial depression may result in myocardial infarction.

Myocardial Infarction. Almost all currently used inhalational agents are myocardial depressants. A combination of factors may lead to myocardial ischemia or infarction in the high-risk patient during or after general anesthesia. These include increased myocardial oxygen demand, decreased oxygen delivery, and decreased coronary blood flow.

Factors that decrease oxygen delivery include arterial hypoxemia, a shift of the oxyhemoglobin dissociation curve to the left, and decreased body temperature. Myocardial oxygen demand is increased by hypertension, tachycardia, increased preload, and increased myocardial contractility. Factors that decrease coronary blood flow include hypotension, tachycardia, and coronary artery spasm. A decreased coronary blood flow coupled with decreased oxygen delivery and increased oxygen demand may lead to myocardial ischemia (Emerson et al., 1979). Monitoring of pulmonary capillary wedge pressure will give an indication of left ventricular function. Nitrous oxide has been used with other agents (i.e., narcotics) for anesthesia in patients with severe coronary artery disease because it produces minimal cardiovascular depression (Calahan et al., 1987).

Hypotension. One of the first indications of myocardial depression is hypotension. Hypotension may also result from hypovolemia, hypoxia, respiratory or metabolic acidosis, sepsis, or vasodilation due to the effects of anesthetic agents. Rapid positional change, pain, dysrhythmias, and mechanical interference in venous return may also result in hypotension. Table 62–7 summarizes the causes of postanesthesia hypotension.

Hypertension. Hypertension is defined as an elevation in the systolic or diastolic pressure of 25% to 30% over the baseline preoperative blood pressure. This level of hypertension should at least arouse concern. Precipitating causes of hypertension include the presence of pain, which results in increased levels of circulating catecholamines. Drugs given in the perioperative period may result in an elevation of blood pressure. Respiratory insufficiency results in hypercarbia and hypoxia and subsequently in hypertension resulting from the release of catecholamines. Hypertension may also be caused by excessive fluid or blood administration resulting in hypervolemia. Other causes of hypertension include postoperative shivering due to decreased body temperature and restlessness such as occurs in emergence delirium. The causes of postanesthesia hypertension are summarized in Table 62–8.

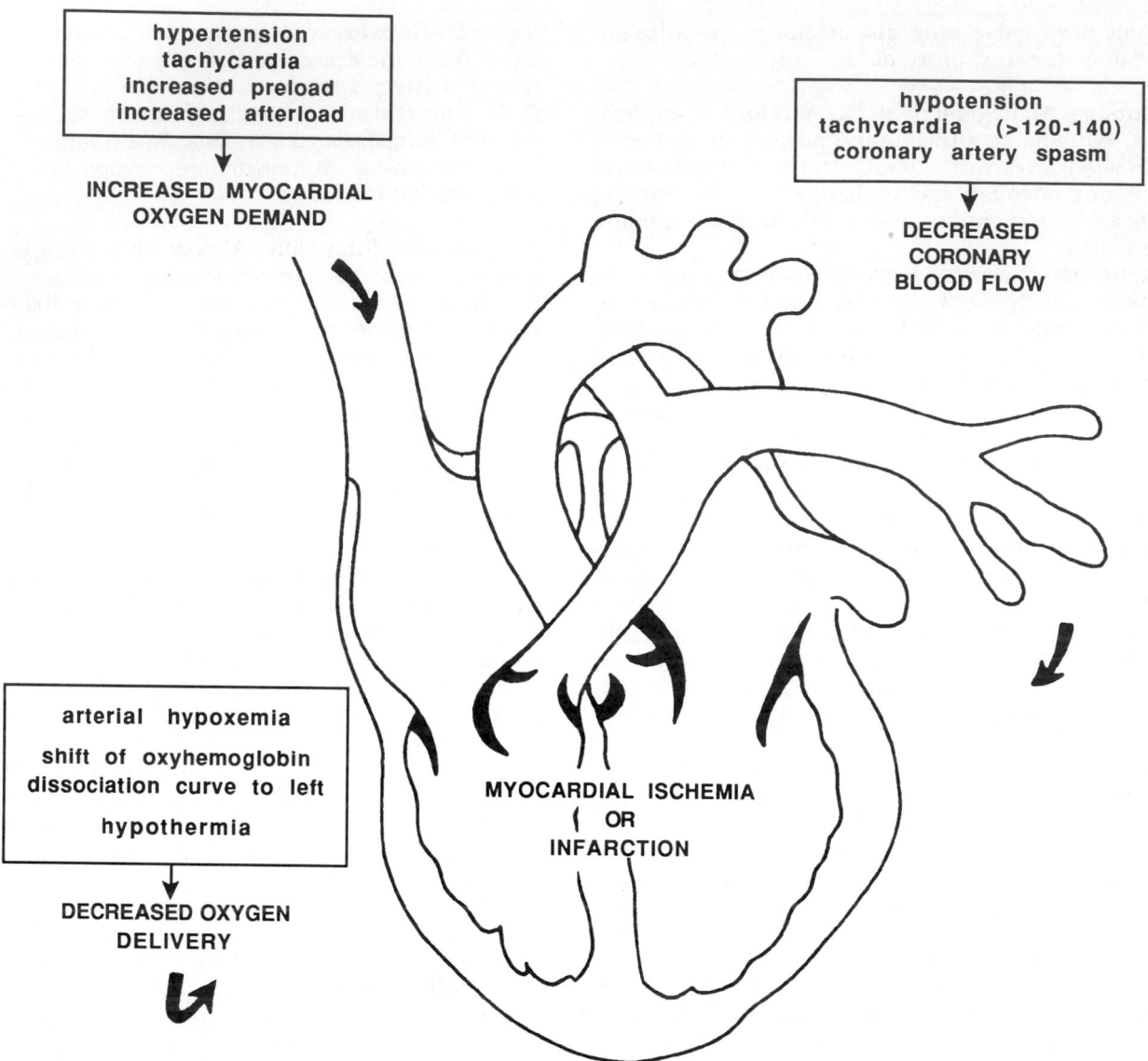

hypertension
tachycardia
increased preload
increased afterload

INCREASED MYOCARDIAL
OXYGEN DEMAND

hypotension
tachycardia (>120-140)
coronary artery spasm

DECREASED
CORONARY
BLOOD FLOW

arterial hypoxemia
shift of oxyhemoglobin
dissociation curve to left
hypothermia

MYOCARDIAL ISCHEMIA
OR
INFARCTION

DECREASED OXYGEN
DELIVERY

FIGURE 62–1. Postanesthesia causes of myocardial ischemia or infarction in the high risk patient. (Adapted from Wlody, G.S. (1982). Postoperative complications. In the *NTI proceedings book—1982* (p. 283). Newport Beach, CA: AACN. Computer enhancement courtesy of Mr. Turner McGehee. M.A., Hastings College.)

Dysrhythmias. Dysrhythmias are precipitated by factors that cause myocardial irritability in the postoperative period (Fig. 62–2). The incidence of dysrhythmias during anesthesia is 15% to 30% (Snow, 1977). Many of the intraoperative causes of dysrhythmias are also precipitating causes in the recovery period. These include intubation or extubation, specific anesthetic agents, duration of operation, and hypothermia. Premature ventricular contractions are the most frequent type of dysrhythmia. Sinus bradycardia may result from vagal stimulation during the operation.

Nonperfused ventricular beats lower cardiac output and can lead to ischemia in vital organs. The critical care nurse must determine if the dysrhythmia is caused by a primary cardiac disease process or is secondary to coincidental or associated abnormalities. Some causes of secondary dysrhythmias include increased sympathetic tone due to fever, anxiety,

pain, or stress, hypoxia and acidosis, and electrolyte abnormalities. Left ventricular failure and complications of antidysrhythmic therapy may also result in secondary dysrhythmias (Philbin and Hutter, 1979).

Cardiac dysrhythmias occur frequently during reversal of neuromuscular blockade. The muscarinic action of anticholinesterase drugs delays atrioventricular conduction and can cause bradycardia and atrioventricular block (Lebowitz and Savarese, 1980). Atropine is usually given with anticholinesterase drugs to prevent bradycardia, but it must be used judiciously to prevent tachycardia.

Cardiac arrest is more likely to occur in geriatric patients because of their diminished cardiac reserve and decreased tolerance of stress (Latz and Wyble, 1987). Factors associated with cardiac arrest include heart block, digitalis toxicity, congestive heart failure, myocardial infarction, electrolyte imbalance, dehydration, and massive hemorrhage (Snow, 1977).

TABLE 62–7. Causes of Postoperative Hypotension/ Shock

Anesthesia and drugs/cardiovascular effects
Myocardial infarction
Cardiac dysrhythmias
Position changes
Impaired venous return
Hypovolemia
Hypoxia
Acidosis—Respiratory/metabolic
Hypercarbia
Pulmonary embolism
Sepsis
Steroid dependency
Anaphylaxis

Nursing Management of Cardiac Complications.
Nursing assessments of postanesthetic patients are directed toward monitoring vital signs and preventing complications. The nursing care plan provides specific nursing interventions for the postoperative critically ill patient.

Decreased Cardiac Output. Since anesthetic agents produce myocardial depression, the postoperative patient may experience alterations in cardiac output and tissue perfusion. Arterial lines, pulmonary artery catheters, central venous pressure lines, and cardiac output determinations provide valuable hemodynamic information. Assessment for hypovolemia is made, and blood, colloids, and crystalloids are replaced as needed. Dressings, tubes, and catheter insertion sites are observed for drainage or bleeding. Cardiac rhythm is monitored, and heart sounds are assessed and evaluated for the appearance of S_3 and S_4 sounds, rubs, and murmurs. Peripheral pulses are checked, and jugular venous distention is noted. Prolonged pain should be prevented by the judicious administration of narcotics. Blood pressure is supported when necessary by the use of vasopressors or beta-adrenergic drugs. The patient is checked for any mechanical interference of venous return. Postoperative myocardial infarction may be difficult to recognize because chest pain may be obscured by the anesthetic or by the narcotics given. Because the most common cause of dysrhythmias in the immediate postoperative period is hypoxemia, the nurse must ensure that oxygenation is adequate to protect the myocardium.

Potential Fluid Volume Excess or Deficit. Fluid volume alterations are related to intraoperative changes in renal blood flow or to the administration or loss of fluids during surgery. The nurse assesses the amount of fluid being lost through gastrointestinal drainage, wound drainage, and urinary output. Fluid losses are replaced in conjunction with physician prescriptions. Use of medications that alter renal function is noted, and the patient is monitored for the anticipated effect. Changes in cardiac output, preload, and afterload are carefully evaluated.

The patient's electrolyte levels are monitored. Careful attention is paid to potassium, calcium, and sodium levels because imbalances in these electrolytes may precipitate dysrhythmias.

Central Nervous System Complications

During general anesthesia depression of the central nervous system occurs in descending order as follows: (1) cortical and psychic centers, (2) basal ganglia and cerebellum, (3) spinal cord, and (4) medullary centers (Snow, 1977). The reverse order occurs during emergence from anesthesia. General anesthesia causes depression of consciousness and of the medullary centers that control the respiratory, cardiac, and temperature functions. Emergence delirium, prolonged recovery, abnormal neurologic signs, shivering, hypothermia, and malignant hyperthermia are central nervous system (CNS) complications that may occur.

Emergence Delirium. Emergence delirium is a state of CNS excitation that occurs in the patient emerging from anesthesia. The patient may be disoriented and exhibit uncoordinated movements, agitation, convulsions, or even psychotic reactions (Heller, 1981). This state may be due to sudden wakefulness without adequate analgesia having been achieved. Delirium may also be a result of central cholinergic toxicity, referred to as the central anticholinergic syndrome (Borchardt and Fraulini, 1987), which may occur after administration of anticholinergic agents such as scopolamine. The central anticholinergic syndrome is characterized by excitement, thought impairment, drowsiness, or coma. In the excitement stage patients thrash about in bed and may hallucinate. Anticholinergic-induced emergence delirium responds dramatically to treatment with physostigmine (Cullen, 1980). Physostigmine is effective because it is the only cholinergic drug that crosses the blood–brain barrier (Nursing '82, 1982).

Prolonged Unconsciousness. Delayed or prolonged return to consciousness after anesthesia is most often caused by prolonged effects of anesthetic agents or by an actual overdose of anesthetic agents. Prolonged unconsciousness may also be caused by drug interactions, respiratory insufficiency, intraoperative untoward events (e.g., hemorrhage, cardiac arrest), allergic or atypical drug responses, or a

TABLE 62–8. Causes of Postoperative Hypertension

Anesthesia and drugs
Pain
Hypoxemia
Hypervolemia
Central nervous system lesions
Shivering
Surgical procedure
Restlessness
Preexisting disease—daily medications not given

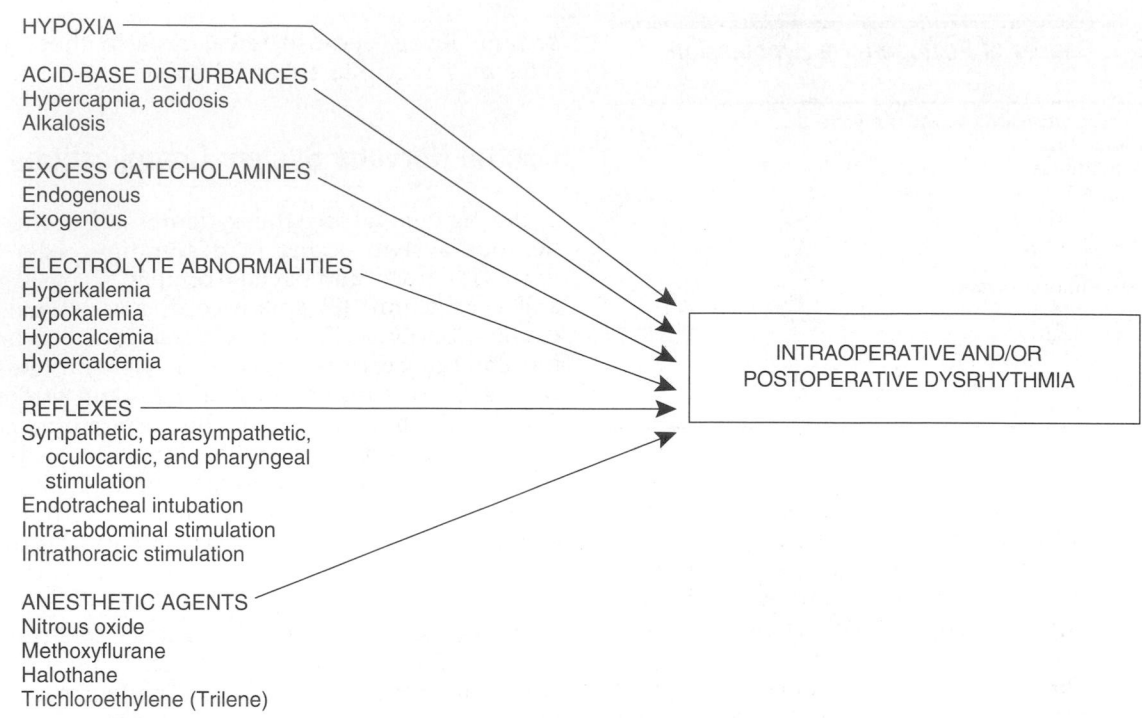

HYPOXIA

ACID-BASE DISTURBANCES
Hypercapnia, acidosis
Alkalosis

EXCESS CATECHOLAMINES
Endogenous
Exogenous

ELECTROLYTE ABNORMALITIES
Hyperkalemia
Hypokalemia
Hypocalcemia
Hypercalcemia

REFLEXES
Sympathetic, parasympathetic,
   oculocardic, and pharyngeal
   stimulation
Endotracheal intubation
Intra-abdominal stimulation
Intrathoracic stimulation

ANESTHETIC AGENTS
Nitrous oxide
Methoxyflurane
Halothane
Trichloroethylene (Trilene)

INTRAOPERATIVE AND/OR
POSTOPERATIVE DYSRHYTHMIA

FIGURE 62–2. Etiologic factors in the production of intraoperative and postoperative dysrhythmias.

preexisting pathologic condition (Frost, 1983). Treatment is usually supportive and includes maintenance of cardiovascular stability, oxygenation, correction of acid-base balance, and temperature regulation. Reversal agents (e.g., neostigmine with atropine) may be used if skeletal muscle relaxants are still in effect. Naloxone is given if narcotics are suspected as the cause of the delayed awakening.

Nursing Management of CNS Complications
Altered Consciousness. During the immediate postanesthetic period, nursing assessments are directed toward monitoring the patient's neurologic signs and preventing CNS complications. The patient's level of consciousness is assessed at frequent intervals. The nurse observes the patient for signs of excitation and agitation that may be indicative of emergence delirium. The nurse controls the patient's environment to prevent overstimulation. The environment is kept as quiet as possible. During the awakening period, the nurse frequently reorients and reassures the patient. The nursing care plan contains specific nursing interventions directed toward management of CNS complications in the postanesthetic patient.

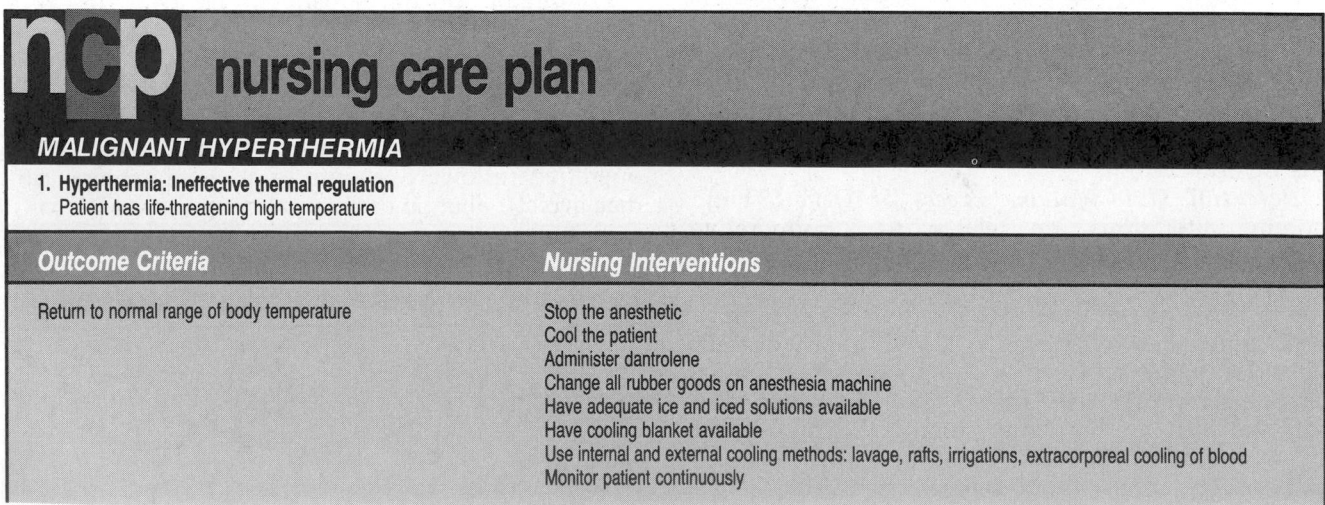

ncp nursing care plan

MALIGNANT HYPERTHERMIA

1. Hyperthermia: Ineffective thermal regulation
Patient has life-threatening high temperature

Outcome Criteria	Nursing Interventions
Return to normal range of body temperature	Stop the anesthetic Cool the patient Administer dantrolene Change all rubber goods on anesthesia machine Have adequate ice and iced solutions available Have cooling blanket available Use internal and external cooling methods: lavage, rafts, irrigations, extracorporeal cooling of blood Monitor patient continuously

2. Alteration in acid–base balance resulting in
Respiratory and metabolic acidosis (hyperventilation, acute renal failure, high BUN, oliguria)

Outcome Criteria	Nursing Interventions
pH 7.35 to 7.45	Correct acidosis, $NaHCO_3$ (acidosis will be severe) Administer insulin or dextrose 50% to decrease hyperkalemia Hyperventilate the patient, using 100% O_2 Provide ventilatory support

3. Alteration in cardiac output, decreased, secondary to
Arrythmias (unstable blood pressure, edema)

Outcome Criteria	Nursing Interventions
Normal cardiac rhythm; normal range of vital signs	Administer procainamide, 15 mg/kg over 60 minutes; may repeat dose Insert Swan-Ganz catheter, arterial line, central venous pressure line Monitor heart rate and rhythm

4. Alteration in fluid volume, excessive, secondary to
Impaired renal function (pulmonary edema, cerebral edema, oliguria, anuria)

Outcome Criteria	Nursing Interventions
Normal fluid volume status; maintenance of intravascular volume	Administer fluids at a rapid rate: 1 liter over 10 minutes × 30 minutes Insert bladder catheter Keep accurate intake and output records

5. Alteration in vascular integrity secondary to
Coagulopathy (bleeding from multiple sites, many hematomas, red or red-brown urine)

Outcome Criteria	Nursing Interventions
Return to normal coagulation values	Keep pressure on needle-stick sites Observe wound sites

6. Alteration in consciousness, decreased
Decreased consciousness, persistent coma, decreased DTR's, seizures

Outcome Criteria	Nursing Interventions
Return to conscious state Avoidance of cerebral edema	Protect patient's reflexes Observe for seizures

7. Impaired tissue integrity secondary to
Neurologic deficit and fever potential for skin breakdown

Outcome Criteria	Nursing Interventions
Prevention of skin breakdown	Use cooling measures Keep sheets dry Assess peripheral pulses Change position, frequent skin care Assess motor and sensory functions

Nursing Care Plan continued on following page

PREVENTION OF POSTANESTHESIA COMPLICATIONS

1. Breathing patterns, ineffective related to
Anesthesia
Hypoventilation
Hypoxia
Surgical incision site or type

Outcome Criteria	Nursing Interventions
Normal breathing patterns; PaO_2 within normal limits	Maintain close observation of breathing patterns
	Assess ventilation, rate, character, tidal volume, movements of chest, diaphragm
	Auscultate breath sounds bilaterally
	Position patient properly to prevent airway occlusion
	Utilize artificial airways and oxygen prn
	Prevent narcotic-induced hypoventilation by reducing narcotic dosage and administering medication intravenously for quick action, update, and distribution; utilize narcotic antagonists as ordered (i.e., Narcan)
	Adjust restrictive dressings
	Administer pain medication to facilitate deep breathing

2. Impaired gas exchange, related to
Airway obstruction
Aspiration of vomitus
Atelectasis
Pneumothorax
Laryngospasm

Outcome Criteria	Nursing Interventions
A clear airway and ventilatory tree; effective gas exchange as evidenced by adequate tissue perfusion and oxygenation; absence of pulmonary infection	Prevent airway obstruction; assess as above
	Prevent vomiting, aspiration by moving patient gently, emptying stomach contents, using medications prn
	Utilize deep breathing techniques

3. Altered cardiac output, decreased related to
Hypotension or shock   Hypoxemia
Dysrhythmias   Respiratory and/or metabolic acidosis
Anesthetic agents   Mechanical interference with venous return

Outcome Criteria	Nursing Interventions
Normal cardiac output, normal range of vital signs, normal cardiac rhythm	Monitor vital signs, intake and output
	Replace blood; administer crystalloids, colloids prn; use warm solutions when replacing large amounts
	Observe catheters, tubes for bleeding
	Use hemodynamic monitoring to determine fluid needs
	Observe patient for signs of shock
	Assess and monitor heart sounds, appearance of S_3, S_4, jugular venous distention
	Check peripheral pulses, monitor cardiac rhythm
	Monitor arterial blood gases; observe for hyperventilation as well as hypoventilation
	Check for tight abdominal dressings
	Administer pressors as indicated

4. Altered cardiac output, decreased related to
Hypertension
Pain
Hypervolemia
Increased circulating blood volume due to excess fluid/blood administration. Seen with halothane anesthesia due to peripheral vasodilator effects during anesthesia and peripheral vasoconstriction after anesthesia is stopped
Shivering

Outcome Criteria	Nursing Interventions
Normal cardiac output, normal vital signs for patient Systolic/diastolic pressures within 25% to 30% of baseline	Assess pain, medicate judiciously in small increments (IV). Use intercostal blocks, epidural medications
	Monitor intake and output
	Use vasodilators or antihypertensives as needed (nitroglycerin, Nipride, etc.)
	Prevent shivering by careful temperature monitoring and using warm solutions, blankets, and so on

5. Altered consciousness, decreased, related to
Anesthetics and drugs
Sensory perceptual changes, visual or auditory; prolonged somnolence; loss of memory (temporary)

Outcome Criteria	Nursing Interventions
Return to conscious state within 2 hours	Assess somnolence; determine anesthetic agents and narcotics used; support ventilation prn; assess pupils, motor and sensory activity and response to stimuli Maintain quiet environment, avoid overstimulation if patient exhibits sensory perceptual changes; during awakening process reorient patient frequently

6. Altered fluid volume: Potential for excess or deficit, related to
Administration of or loss of fluids during surgery

Outcome Criteria	Nursing Interventions
Maintain normal physiologic fluid balance throughout perioperative period	Assess use of medications that alter renal function (i.e., diuretics, antibiotics) Prevent GI, nasogastric or wound fluid losses or replace prn Monitor intake and output hourly; monitor vital signs, and continue frequent total patient assessments; assess breath sounds for crackles/rales Assess patient for normal electrolyte levels, especially potassium, calcium, sodium; monitor electrocardiogram for changes indicating electrolyte imbalance Assess cardiac output, preload and afterload, central venous pressure

7. Altered temperature: Potential for hypothermia, related to
Cold operating room environment, exposure of body surface areas, administration of large amounts of cold fluids or blood

Outcome Criteria	Nursing Interventions
Return to or maintenance of normothermia	Assess temperature on admission. Warm patient as needed to prevent or reduce hypothermia. Prevent shivering, which increases oxygen consumption

8. Potential for wound infection related to
Interruption of skin integrity by surgical incision

Outcome Criteria	Nursing Interventions
Healing; absence of signs of infection (i.e., redness, pus, temperature, etc.)	Assess all wounds. New infections will be manifest 24 to 48 hours postoperatively. Utilize good handwashing and aseptic techniques. Change dressings prn and protect skin surrounding wound

9. Fear, actual or potential related to
Anesthesia, surgery, and the ICU. Fear may be related to outcome of surgery, anesthesia, or being left alone
Fear may be related to pain.
Related Nursing diagnoses:
1. Ineffective coping
2. Sensory perceptual alteration: visual/auditory

Outcome Criteria	Nursing Interventions
A postoperative state of calm because fears have been allayed, discussed. Verbal expression by patient	Visit patient preoperatively. Allow patient to verbalize. Clarify concerns and questions. Discuss problems as needed with surgeon or other team members. Postoperatively, maintain calm, supportive environment. Administer pain medication as necessary

10. Alteration in drug utilization/effectiveness, related to
Anesthetic agents. Potential for untoward effects, allergic responses, prolonged somnolence

Outcome Criteria	Nursing Interventions
Normal metabolic state	Identify anesthetic agents utilized and ascertain potential problems (see text). Anticipate emergency actions. Assess all body systems every 15 minutes or more often as needed. Take appropriate actions as identified

SUMMARY

Anesthesia and surgery impose certain inescapable risks and stressors on the critically ill patient. Many patients return to the critical care unit directly from the surgical suite, thereby bypassing the postanesthetic recovery unit. This chapter has provided information about complications related to anesthesia that may occur in the critical care unit. The nurse must understand the pharmacologic and kinetic effects of anesthetic agents, multiple risk factors, and the actual or potential stressors that affect critically ill patients prior to their arrival in the critical care unit.

Anesthetic agents profoundly affect the pulmonary, cardiovascular, neurological, and renal systems. In addition, intraoperative environmental factors place the patient at risk. By utilizing a systematic assessment, predicting potential outcomes, making sharp observations, and communicating with the multidisciplinary team members, the nurse will provide high-quality care to the patient in the postanesthesia period. Nursing diagnoses and a nursing care plan for postanesthesia recovery have been presented.

References

Arens, J. F., and McKinnon, W. M. (1971). Malignant hyperpyrexia during anesthesia. *Journal of the American Medical Association*, 215, 919–922.

Atkinson, R. S., Rushman, G. B., and Lee, J. A. (1987). *A symposium of anesthesia* (pp. 311–317). Bristol: Wright.

Bakutis, A. (1972). Anesthetic reactions. *Nursing 72*, 9/72, 16–20.

Bass, B. F. (1973). Steroids. *Clinical Anesthesia*, 10 (1), 249.

Berkebile, P. (1973). Postoperative care. *International Ophthalmology Clinics*, 13 (2), 189–214.

Borchardt, A. C., and Fraulini, K. E. (1987). Postanesthetic problems. In K. E. Fraulini (Ed.), *After anesthesia*. Norwalk, CT: Appleton & Lange.

Briggs, B. A. (1980). Perioperative cardiovascular morbidity and mortality. *International Anesthesiology Clinics*, 18 (3), 71–83.

Burke, G., and Gulyassy, P. (1979). Surgery in the patient with renal disease and related electrolyte disorders. *Medical Clinics of North America*, 63 (6), 71–83.

Calahan, M. K., Prakash, O., Evert, N., et al. (1987). Addition of nitrous oxide to fentanyl anesthesia does not induce myocardial ischemia in patients with ischemic heart disease. *Anesthesiology*, 76, 925–929.

Caranasos, G. (1979). Drug reactions and interactions in the patient undergoing surgery. *Medical Clinics of North America*, 63 (6), 1245.

Cullen, D. (1980). Recovery room care of the surgical patient. *International Anesthesiology Clinics*, 18 (3), 39–52.

Drain, J. H., and Shipley, S. (1979). *The recovery room*. Philadelphia: W. B. Saunders.

Dripps, R., Eckenhoff, J., and Vandam, L. (1988). *Introduction to anesthesia: The principles and safe practice* (7th ed.). Philadelphia: W. B. Saunders.

Eichorn, J. H. (1989). Prevention of intraoperative anesthesia accidents and related severe injury through safety monitoring. *Anesthesiology*, 70, 572–577.

Emerson, C., Davis, R., and Philbin, D. A. (1979). Anesthetic management of patients with coronary artery disease. *International Anesthesiology Clinics*, 17 (1), 97–127.

Flacke, W., Flacke, J., Ryan, J., et al. (1982). Altered temperature regulation. In F. Orkin and L. Cooperman (Eds.), *Complications in anesthesiology*. Philadelphia: J. B. Lippincott.

Forestner, J. (1981). Complications of anesthesia. In J. Hardy (Ed.), *Complications of surgery and their management* (4th ed.). Philadelphia: W. B. Saunders.

Fraulini, K. E., Borchadt, A. C., Randall Andrews, D. T., et al. (1985). Mean body temperature of recovery room adults. *Anesthesia and Analgesia* 64 (2), 213.

Fraulini, K. E. (1987). *After anesthesia: A guide for PACU, ICU and Medical-Surgical Nurses*. Norwalk, CT: Appleton & Lange.

Frost, E. A. (1983). Differential diagnosis of postoperative coma. *International Anesthesiology Clinics*, 21 (1), 13–30.

Goldman, L., Caldera, D. L., Nussbaum, S., et al. (1977). Multifactorial index of cardiac risk in noncardiac surgical procedures. *New England Journal of Medicine*, 297, 845.

Goodwin, S. (1982). Drug interactions. *Current Reviews for Recovery Room Nurses*, 4, 15.

Harmon, E., and Lillington, G. (1979). Pulmonary risk factors in surgery. *Medical Clinics of North America*, 63 (6), 1289.

Heller, F. (1981). Recovery from anesthesia. In M. Goldin (Ed.), *Intensive care of the surgical patient* (2nd ed.). Chicago: Year Book.

Hybels, R. (1981). Preoperative evaluation. *Otolaryngolic Clinics of North America*, 14 (3), 557–577.

Latz, P. A., and Wyble, S. (1987). Elderly patients' perioperative nursing implications. *AORN Journal*, 46 (2), 238–252.

Lebowitz, P., and Savarese, J. J. (1980). Complications involving neuromuscular pharmacology. *International Anesthesiology Clinics*, 18 (3), 139–156.

Marchildon, M. (1982). Malignant hyperthermia: Current concepts. *Archives of Surgery*, 117, 349–351.

Martin, J. T. (1987). General aspects of safe positioning for the surgical patient. In J. T. Martin (Ed.), *Positioning in anesthesia and surgery* (2nd ed., pp. 5–12). Philadelphia: W. B. Saunders.

Minckley, B. B. (1969). Physiologic hazards of position changes in the anesthetized patient. *American Journal of Nursing*, 69 (12), 2606–2611.

Muravchick, S. (1980). Preoperative pharmacology and anesthetic risk. *International Anesthesiology Clinics*, 18 (3), 62–66.

Norman, J. (1980). Use of anesthesia: Preoperative assessment of patients. *British Medical Journal*, 28, 1507–1508.

Nursing 82. (1982). *Drug handbook*. Springhouse, PA: Intermed Communications.

Otto, C. (1980). Respiratory morbidity and mortality. *International Anesthesiology Clinics*, 18 (3), 85–106.

Palmberg, S., and Hirsjarvi, E. (1979). Mortality in geriatric surgery. *Gerontology*, 25, 103–112.

Philbin, D., and Hutter, A. (1979). Intraoperative cardiac arrythmias. *International Anesthesiology Clinics*, 17 (1), 55–65.

Shelby, E. (1967). Preoperative evaluation of the poor risk patient. *International Anesthesiology Clinics*, 5 (3), 614–629.

Siperstein, M. D. (1988). Endocrine disease and the surgical patient. In L. W. Way (Ed.), *Current surgical diagnosis and treatment* (8th ed.). Norwalk, CT: Appleton & Lange.

Smith, B. (1987). Physiological changes in the normal conscious human subject on changing from the erect to the supine position. In J. T. Martin (Ed.), *Positioning in anesthesia and surgery* (2nd ed., pp. 13–32). Philadelphia: W. B. Saunders.

Snow, J. (1977). *Manual of anesthesia*. Boston: Little, Brown.

Stoelting, R. (1980). Metabolic effects of anesthetics. *International Anesthesiology Clinics*, 18 (3), 53–69.

Strauss, R. J., and Wise, L. (1987). Operative risks of obesity. *Surgery, Gynecology and Obstetrics*, 146, 286–291.

Tarhan, S. (1981). Risk of anesthesia in patients with heart disease. *Cleveland Clinic Quarterly* 48 (1), 50–54.

Tonneson, A. (1980). Acute renal failure. *International Anesthesiology Clinics*, 18 (3), 107–121.

Vale, R. (1981). Monitoring of temperature during anesthesia. *International Anesthesiology Clinics*, 19 (1), 61–83.

Vaughan, M. S. (1982). When should anesthesia monitoring stop? In *Selected Abstracts for the 8th Postanesthesia Symposium for Recovery Room Nurses*. Chicago: Illinois Society of Anesthesiologists, May 6–8.

Vaughan, M. S., Vaughan, R., and Cork, R. C. (1981). Postoperative hypothermia in adults: Relationship of age, anesthesia and shivering to rewarming. *Anesthesia and Analgesia*, 60 (10), 746–751.

Wade, J., and Stevens, W. (1981). Isoflurane: An anesthetic for the eighties. *Anesthesia and Analgesia*, 60 (9), 666–682.

Walts, L. F. (1983). Managing diabetics during surgery. *AORN Journal*, 37 (5), 928–941.

63

Patients with Obstetric Crises

Becky Hull

Pregnancy and childbirth are considered to be normal physiologic events for the vast majority of women. However, a small number of women experience serious complications during pregnancy. These complications can be life-threatening to both mother and fetus.

The critically ill obstetric patient poses a unique challenge to the critical care nurse. This chapter focuses on severe preeclampsia and amniotic fluid embolism, two life-threatening complications of pregnancy.

PREGNANCY-INDUCED HYPERTENSION (SEVERE PREECLAMPSIA)

Several different terms have been used to describe the complication of hypertension in pregnancy. Historical terms such as toxemia of pregnancy coexist with the current nomenclature of pregnancy-induced hypertension (PIH) and descriptions of clusters of symptoms regarding severe preeclampsia (the HELLP syndrome). PIH has three distinct subsets: (1) hypertension without edema or proteinuria; (2) hypertension with edema and proteinuria (preeclampsia); and (3) hypertension, edema, proteinuria, and seizures (eclampsia). For purposes of clarity, the terms and definitions used in this discussion are those of the Committee on Terminology of the American College of Obstetricians and Gynecologists (Table 63–1), with the inclusion of the HELLP syndrome (Table 63–2).

Preeclampsia complicates from 5% to 7% of all pregnancies (Pritchard et al., 1985; Roberts, 1989). In rare instances (1 in 1000 to 1500 pregnancies), eclampsia develops (Pritchard et al., 1985). Extremes

of age seem to be associated with the development of preeclampsia with women older than age 40 being at higher risk than teenagers (Roberts, 1989). There does seem to be a strong familial tendency toward the development of preeclampsia. Chesley (1984) followed the female family members of women with a history of preeclampsia-eclampsia. His findings indicate that the daughters of women with eclampsia have a 48% incidence of developing preeclampsia, and that sisters of women who were eclamptic have a 55% incidence. Six per cent of the daughters-in-law control group developed preeclampsia, which

---

TABLE 63–1. Terms Used in Discussions of Pregnancy-Induced Hypertension

Pregnancy-induced hypertension (PIH): The development of hypertension without edema or proteinuria during pregnancy

Preeclampsia: The development of hypertension with proteinuria, edema, or both, after the twentieth week of pregnancy

Eclampsia: The occurrence of seizures/convulsions, not caused by coincidental neurologic disease, in a woman whose condition fulfills the criteria for preeclampsia

Superimposed preeclampsia or eclampsia: The development of preeclampsia or eclampsia in a woman with chronic hypertension or renal disease

From the Committee on Terminology of the American College of Obstetricians and Gynecologists (1972).

TABLE 63–2. The HELLP Syndrome

Hemolysis
Elevated liver enzymes
Low platelets

would be expected in the general population. Issues of racial predilection are less clear. From 1960 to 1970, the incidences of preeclampsia, eclampsia, and preeclampsia superimposed on chronic hypertension were equal for black and white women, even though the incidence of chronic hypertension in black women is twice that of white women (Chesley, 1984). Similar findings were reported for the years 1979 to 1986 (Saftlas et al., 1990). Incidence of preeclampsia among non-white women was slightly higher until 1986, when the rate for white women exceeded that of non-whites. Preeclampsia during one pregnancy does put the woman at increased risk for the development of preeclampsia in subsequent pregnancies (Roberts, 1989b). A woman with preeclampsia is not at increased risk for developing hypertension in later life. However, if preeclampsia was in reality superimposed on chronic hypertension, the chance of developing worsening hypertensive problems increases. In those women who do go on to develop hypertension, it is felt that the preeclampsia was an unmasking of underlying, preexisting hypertension (Roberts, 1989).

Morbidity and mortality are of significance for both the mother and the fetus or newborn. The mortality rate in women with preeclampsia-eclampsia is very low. Early but cautious interventions have improved maternal mortality figures over the past several decades (Roberts, 1989). Fetal death is still relatively high, with the cause of fetal demise being inadequate placental perfusion and abruptio placentae. Neonatal morbidity and mortality are most commonly related to complications of prematurity.

In most instances, women with preeclampsia are adequately cared for by obstetricians and obstetric nurses. A small percentage of women with preeclampsia develop severe preeclampsia, which is manifested by failure of many organ systems. These women may require intensive nursing and medical care to reverse complications and prevent further deterioration.

Pathophysiology

During pregnancy, profound physiologic changes occur that affect all body systems. The most significant of these changes occur in the cardiovascular and hematologic systems. In order to fully understand the changes seen in preeclampsia, these normal adaptations to pregnancy must be recognized.

NORMAL ADAPTATION TO PREGNANCY

Cardiac output increases during pregnancy as a result of an increase of 40% to 50% in blood volume

and a slight increase (10 to 15 beats/minute) in pulse rate. The increase in blood volume begins in the first trimester and continues throughout pregnancy (Ueland, 1976).

Blood pressure decreases slightly in a normal pregnancy, returning to prepregnant levels by approximately 36 weeks' gestation. Normal ranges of blood pressure are 112 to 122 systolic and 68 to 75 diastolic (Roberts, 1989). The drop in blood pressure is accomplished by a decrease in peripheral vascular resistance and the growth of the placenta, a low-resistance vascular bed.

The use of hemodynamic monitoring in pregnancy is not extensive, but data are now available on the effects of pregnancy on common hemodynamic parameters (Table 63–3). Some degree of caution must be used in interpreting hemodynamic data obtained during pregnancy. The effects of maternal position must be taken into consideration, and the effects of labor on normal readings is not well documented. With these caveats in mind, however, it does appear that in the normal pregnancy central venous pressure, pulmonary capillary wedge pressure, and mean pulmonary artery pressure do not change from the nonpregnant state (Kirshan and Cotton, 1987).

Renal blood flow increases in pregnancy by 60% to 70% in mid-pregnancy, causing a 50% increase in the glomerular filtration rate (Davison, 1985). This increased renal efficiency is reflected in changes in normal laboratory measures of renal function (Table 63–4).

Uterine blood flow is also increased in pregnancy, with blood going to the muscle of the uterus itself as well as through the placenta. Adequate placental blood flow is necessary for the oxygenation and nourishment of the fetus. Indirect means of measuring placental perfusion indicate a blood flow of 500 to 700 mL/minute (Pritchard et al., 1985).

The laboratory values seen in Table 63–4 reflect the dilutional effect of the increase in plasma volume over red cell mass and the increased activity of the kidneys. Changes in liver function and coagulation studies are not observed in a normal pregnancy. The majority of these parameters are affected by preeclampsia, especially severe preeclampsia.

TABLE 63–3. Hemodynamic Parameters in Pregnancy

	Nonpregnant	Pregnant
Central venous pressure (mm Hg)	1–7	Unchanged
Pulmonary capillary wedge pressure (mm Hg)	6–12	Unchanged
Mean pulmonary artery pressure (mm Hg)	9–16	Unchanged
Systemic vascular resistance (dynes/second/cm)	800–1200	600–900 (25% decrease)
Pulmonary vascular resistance (dynes/second/cm)	20–120	15–90 (25% decrease)
Cardiac output (liters/minute)	4–7	5.6–9.8 (30–45% increase)

TABLE 63–4. Laboratory Values in the Nonpregnant and Pregnant State

Parameter	Normal Nonpregnant	Normal Third Trimester
Hemoglobin (g/dL)	11.5–16.0	11.2–15.0
Hematocrit (%)	35.1–46.0	28.6–38.4
Platelets (1000s/mm³)	166–264	132–276
Burr cells and schistocytes	Absent	Absent
Blood urea nitrogen (mg/dL)	7–18	5–8
Aspartate aminotransferase (U/mL)	8–40	Unchanged
Alanine aminotransferase (U/mL)	1–36	Unchanged
Prothrombin time (seconds)	10–14	Unchanged
Partial thromboplastin time (seconds)	30–45	Unchanged
Fibrinogen (mg/dL)	200–400	393–539

PATHOGENESIS OF PREECLAMPSIA

The cause of preeclampsia is unknown. Numerous theories have been proposed, but none have been definitively proved. Nutritional theories associating decreased serum albumin with inadequate dietary protein have been explored. One current focus of research is on a possible immunologic cause of preeclampsia (Scott and Beer, 1976). The most promising area of current study is in the role of prostaglandins. The effects of prostacyclin, a potent vasodilator, and thromboxane A_2, a potent vasoconstrictor, are balanced during a normal pregnancy. In preeclampsia, however, the amount of prostacyclin is decreased and thromboxane A_2 is increased. These changes may allow vasospasm, vascular permeability, and platelet aggregation to occur (Worley, 1984; Friedman, 1989). The presence of a factor released by poorly perfused placental tissue, which may cause endothelial cell damage, is also being investigated (Roberts et al., 1989).

Vasospasm is the underlying physiologic cause for the signs and symptoms seen in preeclampsia (Pritchard et al., 1985). Although the cause of the vasospasm is unknown, the effects are observed throughout all body systems. A tendency toward vascular hypersensitivity occurs before any indication of preeclampsia can be seen. Studies of the hypertensive effects of angiotensin II indicate an increased sensitivity to this agent as early as 14 weeks' gestation in women who subsequently became preeclamptic (Gant et al., 1973).

Cardiac output in the preeclamptic patient usually remains in the normal range for pregnancy (Clark and Cotton, 1988). Plasma volume has been shown to be increased over the nonpregnant state, but to a lesser amount than in an uncomplicated pregnancy. It is surmised that the lack of hemodilution may be due to vasoconstriction or due to decreased oncotic pressure allowing the extravasation of fluid (Pritchard et al., 1984).

Because vasospasm causes a profound increase in peripheral vascular resistance, systemic hypertension in severe preeclampsia can reach significant levels. Pulmonary vascular resistance is not affected (Clark and Cotton, 1988).

Renal blood flow is decreased as a result of vasospasm. Renal arteriospasm is thought to be responsible for the proteinuria seen in preeclampsia (Roberts, et al., 1989). Glomerular damage does occur in preeclampsia, but in the majority of cases it is limited to the duration of the disease itself. Glomerular lesions are only rarely present by 5 to 10 weeks' postpartum (Roberts et al., 1989).

Uterine blood flow is apparently two to three times less in preeclamptic pregnancies than in normal pregnancies (Pritchard et al., 1984). Histologic examination of the placenta shows the spiral arteries, which carry blood through the myometrium to the placenta, to be constricted. These arteries, which are maximally dilated in a normal pregnancy, are reduced in diameter by as much as 60% (Roberts, 1989).

Cerebral blood flow may also be affected by vasospasm, resulting in headaches and visual disturbances. Cerebral vasospasm may be the cause of the seizures of eclampsia. The only evaluations of brain tissue have been from autopsy findings, and the cerebral edema reported in the past may have been related to edema that occurred after death (Pritchard et al., 1985).

The pathophysiologic processes found in the type of severe preeclampsia known as the HELLP syndrome are also related to vasospasm. Microangiopathic hemolytic anemia is the primary feature of the HELLP syndrome. Microscopic lesions are created in the microvasculature throughout the body from the alternating dilation and vasospasm of the arterioles. As the intima is torn, platelets aggregate at the site of the damage, resulting in platelet consumption, which is manifested by thrombocytopenia, ecchymosis, and petechia (Weinstein, 1982). The platelets form a sieve-like structure in the microvasculature. The red blood cells are lysed when they are forced through these areas of platelet aggregation. This results in a falling hematocrit and the presence of schistocytes and burr cells in peripheral blood smears (Brain et al., 1962; Weinstein, 1982).

Associated with these changes are indications of hepatic tissue damage. At cesarean section, the liver may be noted to be very edematous. Autopsy findings may reveal subcapsular hemorrhage and localized areas of necrotic damage. In rare cases the liver may rupture, almost invariably leading to the patient's death (Weinstein 1986; Pritchard et al., 1985).

A summary of the physiologic changes occurring in severe preeclampsia, including the associated physical findings, can be seen in Figure 63–1 and Table 63–5.

Clinical Presentation

The patient with severe preeclampsia may present with a very clear "textbook" picture of her disease

TABLE 63–5. Characteristics of Preeclampsia

Mild Preeclampsia

Hypertension	140/90 mm Hg or >30/15 over baseline
Proteinuria	>1+ on two specimens obtained by catheterization at 6-hour intervals
Edema	Clinically evident swelling or rapid weight gain

Severe Preeclampsia

Hypertension	>160/>110 mm Hg
Proteinuria	>5 g/24 hours
Oliguria	<500 mL/24 hours
Headache	
Hyper-reflexia	
Scotomata	
Anasarca	
Epigastric or right upper quadrant pain	
Pulmonary edema	

Other Factors Associated with Severe Preeclampsia

Thrombocytopenia
Elevated AST/ALT
Elevated blood urea nitrogen/creatinine
Fetal growth retardation

or with a confusing combination of laboratory and physical findings that may lead to an erroneous diagnosis. When a pregnant woman is given a diagnosis of acute renal disease, acute hepatic disease, idiopathic thrombocytopenic purpura, or other medical disease, the diagnosis of severe preeclampsia must be given serious consideration as well (Goodlin, 1976).

PHYSICAL FINDINGS

Significant hypertension will be noted in the typical patient with severe preeclampsia. A blood pressure of 140/90 mm Hg or an increase of 15 points in the diastolic or 30 points in the systolic reading above prepregnancy levels is considered a sign of mild preeclampsia. In severe preeclampsia, the systolic blood pressure is often greater than 160 mm Hg and the diastolic greater than 110 mm Hg.

Edema is another characteristic of preeclampsia. Often, the associated weight gain is rapid and may be in excess of 5 pounds in a week. The typical edema associated with normal pregnancy is due to hydrostatic pressure and is limited to dependent areas. The edema associated with preeclampsia is thought to be due to sodium retention and to decreased oncotic pressure. Therefore, it is not limited to dependent areas. Edema of the hands and face is characteristic of fluid retention in severe preeclampsia (Roberts et al., 1989). Anasarca may also occur.

Proteinuria is the third typical finding of preeclampsia. In severe preeclampsia, proteinuria may be 3+ to 4+ on dipstick or more than 5 g/24 hours and will vary in amount over a 24-hour period. Alternating periods of renal vasospasm are thought to be responsible for the variation in proteinuria (Roberts et al., 1989).

Oliguria or anuria may develop in severe preeclampsia. It appears that there may be three different causes of the decreased urinary output. In patients with oliguria who were invasively monitored, one subgroup was found to have low pulmonary capillary wedge pressures indicating hypovolemia. A second group was found to have significantly elevated systemic vascular resistance and inadequate cardiac output. The third group was found to have high cardiac output, normal or slightly increased systemic vascular resistance, and adequate preload. In this last group, it was felt that the oliguria was due to severe renal arteriospasm (Lee et al., 1987; Clark et al., 1986a).

Hemodynamic parameters in severe preeclampsia are confusing at best. It is difficult to generalize the information from current case reports because the patients were often managed differently, with fluid restriction, fluid loading, sodium restriction, or the use of antihypertensive agents prior to invasive monitoring. Any of these treatments may affect hemodynamic parameters. One review indicates that most severe preeclamptic patients will present clinically as if they are hypovolemic and will have low to normal pulmonary capillary wedge pressures. They usually have elevated systemic vascular resistance with normal pulmonary resistance, normal cardiac output, and hyperdynamic left ventricular function (Clark and Cotton, 1988).

Worsening preeclampsia is often characterized by headache, which is probably related to decreased cerebral blood flow. Another ominous sign is right upper quadrant or epigastric pain, thought to be caused by hepatic distention. The development of either or both of these signs is associated with the onset of seizure activity and is a definite sign that the patient's condition is deteriorating (Pritchard et al., 1985).

Hyper-reflexia has historically been associated with an increased risk of seizure activity. Although reflexes continue to be assessed, the association with seizures is weak (Pritchard et al., 1985).

Decreased uteroplacental perfusion, another finding in severe preeclampsia, may cause fetal growth retardation, fetal death, or the development of signs of fetal hypoxia during labor. Although these findings are not usually a part of critical care nursing practice, the critical care staff must realize that the patient and her family may be very concerned about fetal loss or prematurity.

LABORATORY FINDINGS

Laboratory findings in severe preeclampsia support the physical findings. In the presence of the HELLP syndrome, the hematocrit may fall as a result of the lysing of red cells. Thrombocytopenia, associated with platelet consumption in the microvasculature, may reach levels below 50,000/mm³. Other factors in the coagulation panel will almost always remain normal, unless true disseminated intravas-

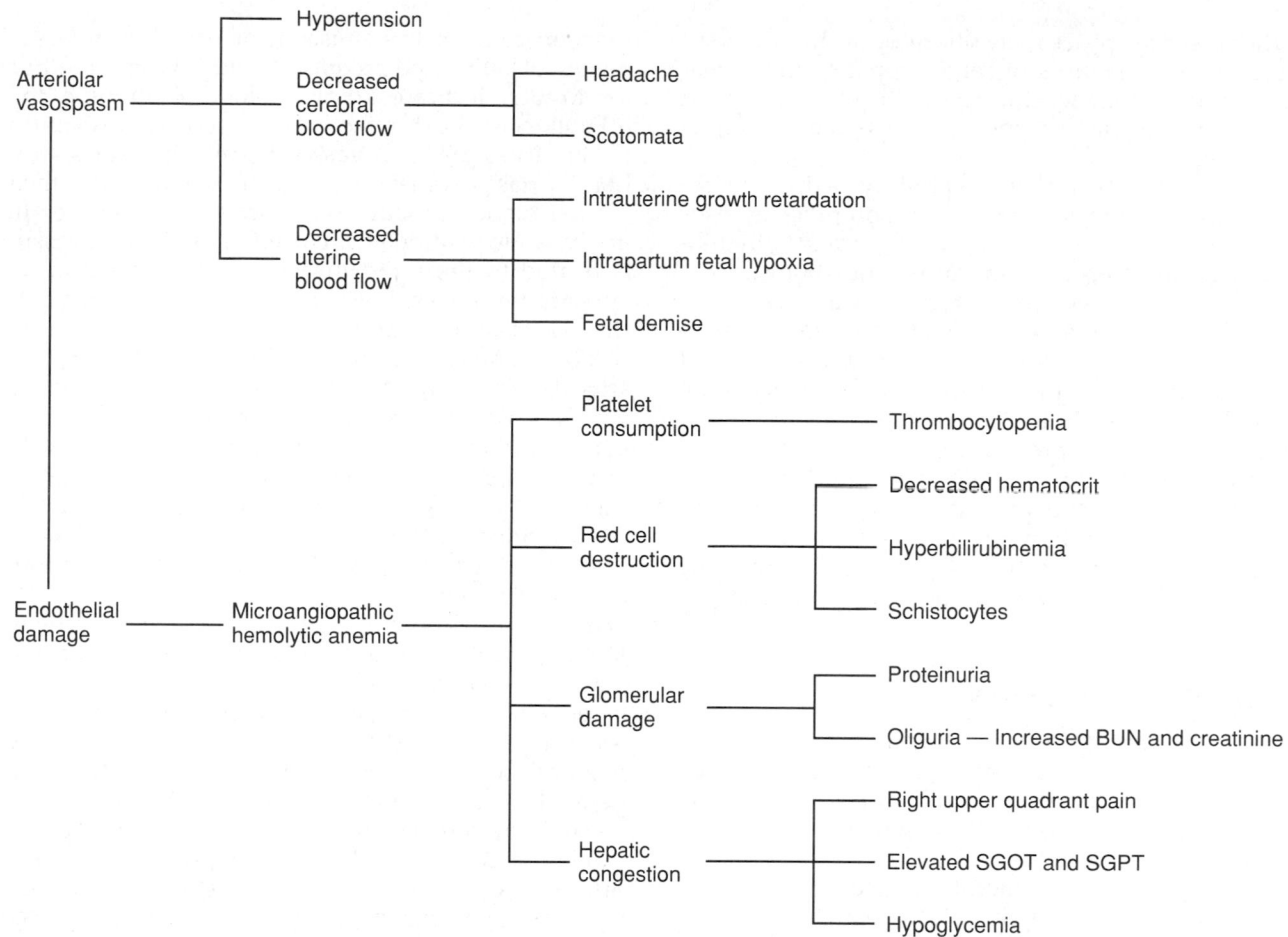

FIGURE 63–1. Pathophysiology of severe preeclampsia. *Abbreviations*: BUN, blood urea nitrogen; SGOT, serum glutamic-oxaloacetic transaminase; SGPT, serum glutamic-pyruvic transaminase. (Adapted from Whittaker, A.A., Hull, B.J., and Clochesy, J.M. (1986). *Heart & Lung*, 15 (4), 402–410.)

cular coagulation (DIC) develops. Table 63–6 summarizes the differences in clinical and hematologic findings in DIC and HELLP. Elevations of the alanine amentransferase (ALT) and aspartate aminotransferase (AST) confirm hepatic damage. Hyperbilirubinemia may also be present and is most likely related to

TABLE 63–6. Differential Diagnosis Between Disseminated Intravascular Coagulation (DIC) and the HELLP Syndrome

	DIC	HELLP
Clinical findings	Oozing from puncture sites, petechiae, ecchymosis	Oozing from puncture sites, petechiae, ecchymosis
Platelet count	Mild to moderate decrease	Moderate to marked decrease
Fibrinogen level	Low	Normal to high
Prothrombin time, partial thromboplastin time	Elevated	Usually normal
Red blood cells	Slight to moderate fragmentation	Mild to moderate fragmentation (burr cells, schistocytes)

the rapid destruction of red cells rather than another indication of hepatic failure. Significant hypoglycemia, with blood glucose levels less than 40 mg/dL, is associated with very high maternal mortality.

Laboratory findings of elevated blood urea nitrogen (BUN), uric acid, and creatinine confirm the diagnosis of renal damage in severe preeclampsia. Because the kidneys are usually more effective in pregnancy, normal values for these laboratory tests are lower than in the nonpregnant individual. Thus, a small elevation in the BUN to greater than 11 mg/dL is significant in the pregnant patient.

Medical Management

To provide a complete picture of the management of the preeclamptic patient, a review of antepartum and intrapartum decision-making and management will be presented. Postpartum management in the critical care unit is an extension of the therapy initiated during the antepartum and intrapartum periods.

ANTEPARTUM MANAGEMENT

Antepartum management of the mild preeclamptic patient is referred to as "expectant." The progression of the disease process is monitored by frequent laboratory assessments of renal, hepatic, and hematologic functions; monitoring of the patient's blood pressure and urinary output; and assessment of fetal well-being.

Hypertension is initially treated by bedrest, without sodium or fluid restriction. If blood pressure rises to a diastolic value greater than 110 mm Hg, hydralazine is administered as an intravenous bolus.

Delivery is delayed until fetal maturity is established or until the maternal or fetal condition worsens to the extent that delivery is necessary to prevent further deterioration or death. Vaginal delivery is the delivery route of choice whenever possible, as patients with severe preeclampsia are placed at increased risk when surgical delivery is undertaken. In most cases when the patient is not close to term, induction of labor will not be successful and delivery will be by cesarean section. Figure 63–2 shows the decision-tree approach to managing the preeclamptic patient.

INTRAPARTUM MANAGEMENT

The only cure for preeclampsia is delivery. The obstetric goals of intrapartum management include prevention of seizures, control of blood pressure, maintaining appropriate intravascular volume, and safe delivery of the infant.

Seizure prevention is accomplished by the use of magnesium sulfate ($MgSO_4$). The usual dosage for $MgSO_4$ is listed in Table 63–7. $MgSO_4$ is the anticonvulsant of choice because it has been proved to be safe in pregnancy and is effective in preventing eclamptic seizures. $MgSO_4$ acts at the neuromuscular

junction to slow transmission of nerve impulses. A review of published recommended dosage schedules for $MgSO_4$ indicates that a blood level of 4 to 6 mEq/liter is most effective for seizure prevention (Sibai et al., 1981). Invasive monitoring shows that $MgSO_4$ has a transient effect of lowering the mean arterial blood pressure but does not alter other hemodynamic parameters. The effect on blood pressure is related to the rapid infusion bolus dose and disappears within an hour when the continuous infusion is sustained (Cotton et al., 1984). Because the risk of eclamptic seizures continues for 24 to 48 hours after delivery, the $MgSO_4$ infusion is continued during this period or until a significant diuresis takes place (Sibai et al., 1981). $MgSO_4$ toxicity may develop in the patient who is oliguric or anuric, as $MgSO_4$ is excreted by the kidneys. The presence of at least 1+ deep tendon reflexes indicates a blood level below the toxic range. If reflexes are lost, the $MgSO_4$ should be discontinued.

If seizures do occur when the patient is receiving $MgSO_4$, another anticonvulsant such as diazepam may be given. Additional bolus doses of $MgSO_4$ may be effective, but the risk of toxicity exists. Once the seizure has stopped (usually 1 to 2 minutes), serum magnesium levels can be determined and the therapeutic level achieved (Roberts et al., 1989).

Antihypertensive therapy is begun if the patient exhibits a consistent diastolic pressure greater than 110 mm Hg, because the risk of stroke is increased by pressure of this level. The first-line drug choice is hydralazine because of its vasodilating effect and because it has been proved safe for the fetus. Hydralazine has the additional benefit of increasing cardiac output, which, presumably, will increase

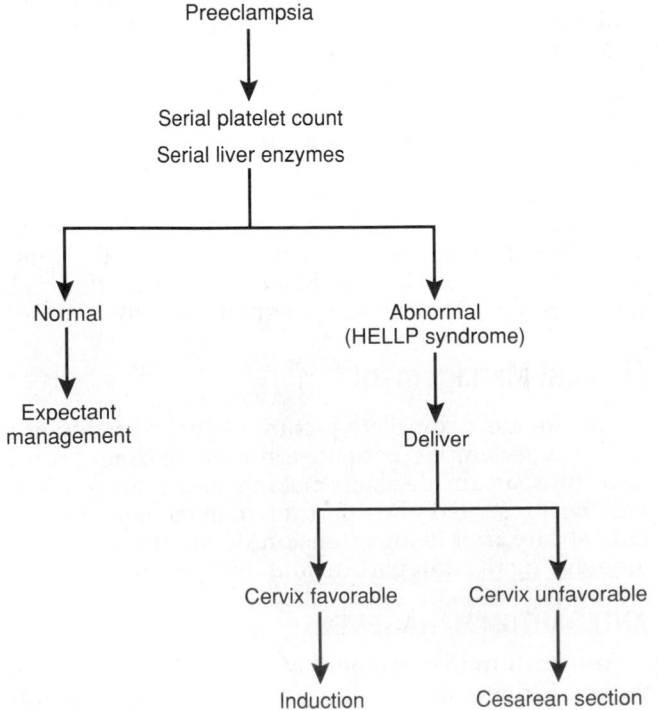

FIGURE 63–2. Medical management of the preeclamptic patient.

TABLE 63–7. Dosage Schedule for Magnesium Sulfate

Loading dose: 4 g of 10% MgSO₄ in 250 mL D5W intravenously over 15–20 minutes
Maintenance: 1–3 g/hour of MgSO₄ by continuous intravenous infusion

Data from Sibai et al., 1981.

uterine perfusion. Hydralazine is best given as intravenous bolus doses rather than by continuous infusion.

More potent antihypertensive agents are rarely needed in severe preeclampsia. Sodium nitroprusside has been used only rarely in pregnant patients. Concerns regarding fetal cyanide toxicity, and results of studies in animal models indicating that improved placental perfusion was not accomplished, leave obstetricians reluctant to choose this drug (Stempel et al., 1982).

The maintenance of intravascular volume is another goal of obstetric management; however, there is as yet no consensus regarding the type of fluid best used in preeclampsia. Studies indicating that plasma oncotic pressure is lower in preeclampsia than in normal pregnancies cause some authorities to recommend the judicious use of colloids to maintain circulating volume (Benedetti and Carlsen, 1979). Others feel that colloids may cause an increase in ventricular preload by pulling too much extravascular fluid back into circulation (Moise and Cotton, 1986). Most authorities continue to recommend the use of crystalloids at rates of 80 to 125 mL/hour (Pritchard et al., 1985; Roberts et al., 1989).

The use of invasive monitoring is not advised for most patients with preeclampsia, even most patients with severe preeclampsia. Invasive monitoring is not without risk and, therefore, is reserved for patients with pulmonary edema or oliguria, patients unresponsive to antihypertensive therapy, and those who need conduction anesthesia (Clark and Cotton, 1988). Oliguria in the preeclamptic patient, as previously stated, is usually but not always related to decreased intravascular volume. Even without the use of invasive monitoring, it is considered reasonable to infuse 500 to 1000 mL over an hour if urinary output has fallen below 30 mL/hour (Clark and Cotton 1988; Roberts, 1989). If oliguria persists for 3 hours, or is unrelieved by fluid challenge, invasive monitoring will be necessary to safely continue fluid therapy. It is noted, however, that if delivery is anticipated within 2 to 3 hours, permanent renal damage will not take place even if oliguria persists (Clark and Cotton, 1988). Pulmonary edema, a rare management problem in the patient with severe preeclampsia, presents another challenge related to intravascular fluid volume. Pulmonary edema may be caused by iatrogenic fluid overload, by left ventricular failure, by decreased colloid oncotic pressure and altered pulmonary capillary integrity, or by all three mechanisms at once (Clark and Cotton, 1988). In patients

with pulmonary edema, the use of invasive monitoring will allow the physician to tailor therapy based on wedge pressures, cardiac output and systemic vascular resistance.

Diuretic agents are rarely used during antepartum or intrapartum management of severe preeclamptic patients because of the dangers inherent in reducing intravascular volume. Once the patient delivers the baby and the risk of decreasing placental perfusion is past, furosemide or other diuretic agents may be employed.

Safe delivery of the infant is the final goal of intrapartum management of the severely preeclamptic patient. Labor will often need to be induced because of worsening maternal or fetal condition. Unless the cervix is "ripe" (3 to 4 cm dilated, 60% to 70% effaced, and of a soft consistency), induction of labor may take 24 hours or more (Bishop, 1964). In most cases of severe preeclampsia with delivery being undertaken because of maternal or fetal deterioration, a brief labor induction of 6 to 12 hours is all that is recommended. After that time, unless delivery is imminent, cesarean section is performed (Weinstein, 1982).

Analgesia during labor and anesthesia for delivery represent another area in which there is no consensus. Epidural anesthesia, which is widely used during labor and for cesarean section in normal pregnancies, has added risks when used in the preeclamptic patient. Vasodilation occurring below the level of the sympathetic blockade can lead to a significant fall in blood pressure. To counteract this effect in a normal pregnancy, a 1000-mL fluid load is given prior to beginning the block. In the preeclamptic patient, two problems are presented: (1) a 1000-mL fluid load may not be tolerated by the woman with a decreased intravascular space, with pulmonary edema being the result; and (2) the block may decrease diastolic pressures below 90 mm Hg (the level considered necessary for placental perfusion in the hypertensive patient), and fetal distress may occur.

The use of general anesthesia for cesarean section poses additional problems because acute hypertension frequently accompanies induction of anesthesia. In the normotensive patient this is usually well tolerated, but in the severe preeclamptic woman additional elevations of blood pressure are not without risk. It is recommended by some investigators that epidural anesthesia be the method of choice, provided that invasive monitoring can be performed. With arterial blood pressures and wedge pressures monitored, initial fluid bolusing may be used safely and blood pressure kept at adequate levels for placental perfusion (Wheeler and Harris, 1982). Other authorities in obstetrics advise against the use of conduction anesthesia and recommend meperidine for pain relief in labor, local anesthesia for vaginal deliveries, and the usual array of general anesthetic agents for cesarean section (Pritchard et al., 1985).

POSTPARTUM MANAGEMENT

The goals of medical management in the postpartum period include continued seizure prevention, control of hypertension, and prevention of pulmonary edema. Although the cure for preeclampsia is delivery, the pathophysiologic processes are not immediately reversed. However, the physician does have a wider scope of interventions available when the potential fetal effects are no longer of concern.

It is estimated that up to one-third of all eclamptic seizures occur in the first 24 hours postpartum. Any anticonvulsant therapy can be used, but, because of its effectiveness and ease of use, $MgSO_4$ is usually continued until the patient's condition is improved, or for 24 hours after delivery (Roberts et al., 1989).

Women may remain hypertensive for several weeks after delivery. If blood pressures reach dangerous levels postpartum, the more potent vasoactive agents like diazoxide or sodium nitroprusside can be used because fetal effects no longer are of concern. Diuretic agents to help control pressures can also be utilized. In most cases, a significant diuresis (200 mL/hour) will begin spontaneously within 24 to 36 hours post delivery. This is a clear indication that the patient is improving (Roberts et al., 1989).

The risk of pulmonary edema continues during the postpartum period until the expected diuresis begins. Extravascular fluids return to the intravascular space during the first 24 hours after delivery. If colloid rather than crystalloid fluids have been used during the intrapartum period, additional extravascular fluid may be pulled into circulation. If this additional volume is not tolerated, pulmonary edema may result (Moise and Cotton, 1986).

Nursing Management

Several nursing diagnoses are used to guide nursing management of the patient with severe preeclampsia. During the antepartum and intrapartum periods, nursing care includes measures to assess and protect the fetus as well as the mother. After delivery, nursing management continues as before with the emphasis on assessment and protection of the mother. The ensuing discussion focuses primarily on the nursing care of the postpartum patient.

POTENTIAL FOR INJURY

Seizure Activity

From the time the patient is admitted to the hospital with the diagnosis of preeclampsia until at least 24 to 48 hours postpartum, the patient must be assessed for increased risk of seizures and be protected from injury if seizures should occur. Assessment parameters include evaluation of mentation, evaluation of headache, and deep tendon reflexes. Unfortunately, there is no one sign that adequately predicts the onset of seizures. Measures to decrease

the potential for seizure activity are the direct responsibility of the nurse. Decreasing stimulation from light and noise is important. Indirect room lighting is preferred. Enough light is needed to allow assessment of the woman's skin color without having lights shine directly into her eyes. If she needs to be moved from room to room, her eyes can be covered to avoid the strobe-light effect from passing under a series of ceiling lights. Noise levels are reduced as much as possible, with monitor sound indicators turned to a low level. Nursing care and medical procedures should be coordinated whenever possible to allow for periods of rest.

In addition to the complications of aspiration and physical injury when tonic-clonic seizures occur, abruptio placenta and precipitous delivery may be caused by the extremes in muscle activity. When seizure activity has ceased and respiratory status is ensured, the nurse should prepare the patient for a vaginal examination. The physician will perform a vaginal examination to assess cervical dilation, effacement, and station of the fetal presenting part.

Magnesium Sulfate Toxicity

The dosage schedule for magnesium sulfate ($MgSO_4$) is detailed in Table 63–7. Key aspects of nursing care include the assessment of deep tendon reflexes. These are performed hourly or more frequently as the patient's condition dictates. Although reflexes are reported on a scale of 1+ to 4+, the most significant finding is that reflexes are either present or absent. Toxic levels of magnesium, which may suppress respirations, will not be achieved until deep tendon reflexes have been ablated. The patellar reflexes are most commonly assessed. If the patient has received epidural anesthesia, the patellar reflexes will be absent and antecubital reflexes will need to be determined.

Urinary output is also an important assessment parameter when magnesium is being infused. Magnesium is excreted by the kidneys, and prolonged periods of oliguria can allow toxic levels to develop. While urinary output is low, it is especially important to monitor deep tendon reflexes, as they provide the best information about magnesium levels between laboratory determinations of blood levels.

Respiratory patterns and rate will be assessed hourly. Calcium gluconate is recommended as the antidote for respiratory depression from magnesium toxicity and should be kept at the patient's bedside. If the respiratory rate falls below eight breaths per minute, 10 mL of 10% calcium gluconate may be given as an intravenous push over 3 minutes (Roberts et al., 1989).

Electrocardiographic changes of prolonged P–R intervals and widening of the QRS complexes are not seen until the blood level of magnesium reaches 15 to 25 mEq/liter (Zuspan and Zuspan, 1981). Although nursing care certainly includes assessment of

ECG patterns, initial recognition of magnesium toxicity will not be made from ECG changes.

Hemorrhage

Nursing care during the immediate postpartum period will include assessment of the uterus and lochia every 15 minutes for the first 2 hours and then hourly. Blood loss at the time of delivery is estimated. A 300- to 500-mL loss is usual in a vaginal delivery. The usual amount estimated after cesarean section is 1000 mL. Preeclamptic patients are at risk for hemorrhage because one effect of $MgSO_4$ is to relax the uterine muscle, allowing increased bleeding. The uterine fundus is palpated for position and tone. The fundus should be firm, at or below the level of the umbilicus, and centered in the midline. If the fundus is relaxed or boggy, it should be massaged to increase the muscle contraction. Fundal massage is performed by placing one hand above the symphysis pubis to support the uterus and placing the other hand around the top of the uterus. Gentle rotation of the hand over the surface of the fundus should make the uterus become firm. Urinary bladder distention is a cause of uterine atony. The postpartum patient without an indwelling Foley catheter in place is encouraged to void hourly. The bladder should be emptied if the uterus becomes displaced from the midline or if a full bladder is palpable. Palpation of the uterus after cesarean section is difficult. The uterus should remain under the area covered by the abdominal dressing. Gentle palpation around the edges of the dressing will enable the nurse to detect the fundus if it has become displaced. Very gentle palpation of the uterus through the dressing can be performed, but vigorous massage will be painful to the patient.

The lochia seen after delivery should be dark red. Bright red bleeding may be indicative of a vaginal or cervical laceration that has gone undetected and therefore unrepaired. Bright red bleeding or heavy bleeding (saturating more than one peripad per hour) must be reported to the obstetrician immediately.

Medications to control uterine atony are limited to oxytocin rather than ergotrate derivatives in the patient with preeclampsia. Ergonovine maleate derivatives are contraindicated because they cause a rise in blood pressure. Oxytocin is usually added to the intravenous infusion in amounts of 10 to 40 units/liter. The infusion is commonly run at 125 mL/hour. Oxytocin can be given intramuscularly, but the infusion approach is most common. Direct intravenous push of oxytocin is not recommended because it can cause a transient but significant drop in arterial blood pressure (Secher et al., 1978).

Severe postpartum hemorrhage may be treated with 15-methyl prostaglandin $F_{2\alpha}$ (Hemabate, Upjohn Company, Kalamazoo, MI). The dosage schedule for 15-methyl-$F_{2\alpha}$ is 0.25 mg intramuscularly every 90 minutes. Dosage is not to exceed 2.0 mg. The nurse observes for side effects, including gastrointestinal upset, fever, and flushing. The diastolic blood pressure may increase in preeclamptic patients, but research studies indicate that there is no need to increase antihypertensive agents for these patients (Hyashi et al., 1984).

Assessment for the development of petechiae, ecchymoses, oozing from puncture sites, and hematuria will complete the nurse's physical assessment for signs of increased risk of hemorrhage. Laboratory values for hemoglobin and hematocrit may vary, related to the influx of fluids into the circulation, as well as in response to bleeding, and must be carefully evaluated.

The patient's blood pressure and heart rate are closely monitored during the immediate postpartum period. A fall in blood pressure is always evaluated in terms of hemorrhage rather than simply accepted as a sign that the patient is improving.

ALTERED TISSUE PERFUSION (RENAL, HEPATIC)

Hourly assessment of renal function is a key nursing role in caring for the patient with severe preeclampsia. Proteinuria is a sign of renal damage, but hourly changes are rarely significant. Although most nurses will check for proteinuria in preeclamptic patients hourly, it is not absolutely necessary. Protein levels may be recorded every 4 hours.

Specific gravity will be assessed hourly along with the measurement of urine volume. Specific gravity measurements provide important information about the woman's fluid status when more direct measurements are not available. If urine output is falling and specific gravity is rising, it may indicate that the patient is becoming hypovolemic. Decreasing urinary output may be related to inadequate fluid volume or to increasing renal damage and is usually a problem in the antepartum or intrapartum periods. Because the use of diuretics is contraindicated while the patient is pregnant, nursing measures to improve urinary output are important. Positioning the patient on her left side will promote venous return via the inferior vena cava, thus increasing circulating volume. If a fluid challenge is ordered, careful management by the nurse will be important, as the risk of fluid overload is always present.

During the first 24 hours postpartum, most patients will experience a mobilization of extravascular fluid and urinary output will reflect this increase in circulating volume. A profound diuresis usually takes place, with hourly outputs commonly in the range of 200 mL/hour. This is a very reassuring sign that the patient's condition is improving.

Signs of hepatic tissue hypoperfusion will be reflected in abnormal laboratory values and in patient complaints of right upper quadrant or epigastric pain. In addition, elevated AST and ALT and falling blood glucose levels are bad prognostic signs. If blood glucose determinations are not part of the ordered laboratory profile, the astute nurse may perform a blood glucose determination at the bedside with a reflection glucometer. Levels below 80 mg/dL should be reported to the physician for follow-up. Hepatic rupture may occur in severe preeclamptic patients (Weinstein, 1982). Because this complication is life-threatening, the nurse carefully evaluates the patient for changes in abdominal pain, the appearance of other abdominal signs, and the onset of hemodynamic instability.

IMPAIRED GAS EXCHANGE

During the postpartum period, fluid that had been in the extravascular space returns to circulation, putting the woman at risk for fluid volume overload and development of pulmonary edema. Nursing assessment includes auscultating for the presence of rales, inspecting the neck veins for distention, and being alert to the development of dyspnea or a cough. In the patient with a flow-directed pulmonary artery catheter, trending the pulmonary capillary wedge pressure (PCWP) measurements provides additional information regarding fluid volume status. The temptation to overhydrate the woman should be resisted until the expected hemodynamic changes of the first 24 to 72 hours postpartum have been realized (Hankins et al., 1984).

ANXIETY

The patient and her family are often unprepared for the critical illness accompanying her pregnancy. What is usually considered to be a most joyous occasion has become life-threatening for both mother and infant. The patient and family members will have many questions and concerns. The nurse who is calm and unhurried and provides easily understandable information will be most therapeutic for the family. Listening to their fears and concerns and providing support will be a continuing necessity. A social service consultation may be beneficial for the family during the critical illness and after the patient has left the critical care environment.

POTENTIAL FOR ALTERED PARENTING

The critically ill mother will be separated from her infant. In most cases of severe preeclampsia, the neonate will also require observation and care in a neonatal intensive care unit. In many instances, this will mean that the infant will be transported to another hospital, adding to the concerns of the mother and other family members. Frequently, family members will divide their time between different hospitals during the first critical days.

The family can be encouraged to take pictures of the newborn for the mother to keep with her, making the birth experience more real. The nursery staff can be contacted several times each day for progress reports on the infant's condition. If the infant is in the same hospital, nursery staff can be encouraged

to give reports directly to the mother. A family member can also be encouraged to interact with the newborn and tell the mother of the infant's temperament and appearance. If the infant is seriously ill, a social worker should be assigned to both the mother and the infant to provide continuity and long-term support.

AMNIOTIC FLUID EMBOLISM

Amniotic fluid embolism (AFE) is a very rare, but almost invariably fatal, complication of pregnancy in which amniotic fluid enters the maternal circulation leading to circulatory collapse and coagulopathies. AFE remains an enigma after over 50 years of study, because of its unanticipated onset, its inconsistent manifestations, and its infrequency.

The term amniotic fluid embolism was coined by Steiner and Lushbaugh (1941). These two pathologists studied eight sudden deaths in laboring women at the Chicago Lying-In Hospital and found squamous cells and mucin, presumably of fetal origin, in the maternal pulmonary vasculature. They compared these findings with a control group of 34 maternal deaths attributed to other causes and found no fetal debris in the vasculature of these latter women. Subsequently, they published their findings using the term "amniotic fluid embolism" to replace the term "obstetric shock," which had previously been used to explain sudden maternal deaths during labor.

AFE occurs in approximately 1 in 20,000 to 30,000 pregnancies (Sperry, 1986). The mortality rate is very high for both mother and fetus, with the maternal mortality rate being as high as 80% (Clark, 1990). The fetal mortality rate is approximately 40% (Duff, 1984). Twenty-five to fifty per cent of deaths occur in the first 60 minutes, as a result of irreversible cardiopulmonary arrest (Duff, 1984). After the first hour, death is attributed to coagulopathies that result in irreversible hemorrhage (Clark et al., 1985).

AFE can occur early in pregnancy, during labor, or even several hours postpartum. It is not possible to define specific criteria that definitely put a woman at risk for the development of AFE. Table 63–8 lists events often associated with AFE. The relatively high incidence of these events, when compared with the incidence of AFE, is indicative of the futility in attempting to develop a profile of the patient at risk.

Pathophysiology

AFE is identified by the presence of squamous cells, lanugo, fetal fat cells, mucin from the fetal respiratory tract, and meconium in the woman's pulmonary vasculature (Clark, 1986). Amniotic fluid is thought to enter the maternal circulation through small tears in the uterine or cervical veins. Once the fluid containing fetal debris enters the pulmonary circulation, embolization occurs with resultant car-

TABLE 63–8. Factors Associated with Amniotic Fluid Embolism

Pregnancy termination
    Suction curettage
    Sharp curettage
    Saline injection
    Prostaglandin F2$_a$ injection
    Urea injection
    Hysterotomy
Uterine rupture
Amniocentesis—third trimester
Vaginal delivery
    High parity
    Hypertonic uterine contractions
    Macrosomic infant
    Meconium stained amniotic fluid
Cesarean section

Data from Duff, 1984.

diopulmonary collapse. Fetal debris is found not only in the pulmonary vasculature but also in the microcirculation throughout the body.

It is not known what substance in amniotic fluid causes the profound shock and subsequent hemorrhage experienced by patients with AFE. In studies using animal models, pure amniotic fluid and amniotic fluid with various quantities of meconium have been injected into an animal's circulation. A clear relationship has not been demonstrated between the type of injectate and the degree of pathologic change (Clark, 1986). Amniotic fluid contains substances other than particulate matter. These other substances, such as prostaglandins, leukotrienes, and trophoblastic material, have vasoactive properties that may lead to the initial cardiovascular response. These substances also have some hematologic properties that may contribute to coagulation defects (Clark, 1986).

Clinical Presentation

The immediate findings with AFE are dyspnea and cyanosis, followed by shock and coma. The most consistent descriptions of women with AFE describe a woman in labor who suddenly becomes short of breath, cyanotic, hypotensive, and loses consciousness. Seizure activity develops in 10 to 20% of cases. If the woman survives these initial events for an hour or more, she is likely to develop a coagulopathy (Clark, 1986). Fetal loss occurs as a result of hypoxia secondary to maternal circulatory collapse.

HEMODYNAMIC FINDINGS

Hemodynamic findings are becoming more widely published as the use of invasive monitoring becomes more common in critically ill obstetric patients. In most cases, however, catheters are not in place at the time the embolus occurs and are often not inserted for at least an hour after the initial event.

Consequently, immediate hemodynamic findings are rarely available (Clark, 1986).

Based on available hemodynamic data, it appears that there is a biphasic response to AFE. It is postulated that when the amniotic fluid and fetal debris enter the pulmonary circulation, there is a relatively short period of intense vasoconstriction, pulmonary hypertension, and hypoxia. Because the time period for these events is thought to be brief (30 to 60 minutes), invasive monitoring data are not yet available in humans to support this hypothesis. This acute onset of pulmonary hypertension and hypoxia may account for the 50% of patients who die in the first hour after the amniotic fluid embolus occurs (Clark, 1986; Clark, 1990).

If the patient survives the initial insult, the second phase of left ventricular failure ensues. The PCWP is elevated, and the left ventricular stroke work index is depressed. The elevation of pulmonary artery pressure and pulmonary vascular resistance are similar to readings found in patients with left-sided heart failure alone. Pulmonary edema is found in 70% of patients and is thought to be noncardiogenic, similar to the findings in adult respiratory distress syndrome (ARDS) (Clark, 1986).

HEMATOLOGIC FINDINGS

In the patients who survive the profound cardiopulmonary effects of AFE, 40% will develop disseminated intravascular coagulation (DIC), which often leads to fatal hemorrhage. DIC may present within minutes to hours of the initial event. The clinical findings include frank hemorrhage from the uterus and persistent oozing from incision sites or venipunctures. Laboratory findings will include the presence of fibrin split products, prolonged prothrombin and partial thromboplastin times, and thrombocytopenia (Clark, 1986; Clark, 1990). (For a more in-depth discussion of the clinical findings and management of DIC, the reader is referred to Chapter 50.)

Medical Management

Medical management of the patient with AFE is initiated in the labor and delivery suite by available medical and nursing staff. The outline of therapy presented in this discussion incorporates the care started in the labor and delivery area and care that may be continued in the critical care unit.

For the patient in cardiopulmonary arrest, cardiopulmonary resuscitation (CPR) is the first response. If the patient is still conscious and breathing, high concentrations of oxygen may be given by mask. If necessary, the patient should be intubated and ventilated with 100% fractional inspired oxygen (Fi_{O_2}). Positive end-expiratory pressure (PEEP) will be required for the patient in severe respiratory failure (Clark, 1986; Duff, 1984).

Crystalloid intravenous fluids will be used for initial correction of hypotension. Dopamine may be administered to stimulate cardiac function and promote vasoconstriction (Clark, 1986). A flow-directed pulmonary artery catheter will be inserted as soon as possible to provide data necessary for fluid management. Blood can be withdrawn from the right side of the heart and placed in a heparinized tube for laboratory examination to confirm the presence of fetal debris (Clark, 1986).

Once the patient has been successfully resuscitated, left ventricular failure should be anticipated. Rapid digitalization may be necessary (Clark, 1986). Inotropic drugs may be infused to support the failing ventricle. If the systemic vascular resistance is elevated, afterload reduction with vasodilators will be initiated.

The development of adult respiratory distress syndrome (ARDS) should be anticipated. Once the initial hypotension is corrected, fluid volume is carefully restricted to avoid pulmonary edema. If the patient is intubated, PEEP and Fi_{O_2} can be balanced to achieve a partial pressure of oxygen (P_{O_2}) of 50% to 60% (Balk and Bone, 1983).

Blood products will be ordered and immediately available in anticipation of DIC. Whole blood, packed red cells, and fresh frozen plasma can be used to replace clotting factors. Platelets can be given to correct thrombocytopenia. Heparinization is not universally recommended following AFE (Clark, 1986; Duff, 1984).

When it becomes clear that resuscitative efforts are failing, immediate cesarean delivery of the infant is indicated. If the patient is responding to supportive treatment, the fetus can be delivered when both the mother and fetus are stable.

Nursing Management

Unfortunately, for the majority of patients with AFE nursing care will involve unsuccessful resuscitative efforts and immediate crisis intervention for the family members who have just lost a young, healthy mother-to-be, and often the infant as well. For those women who are successfully managed during the acute event, skilled nursing care will be necessary and these patients will be cared for in a critical care environment.

ALTERATION IN TISSUE PERFUSION

The labor and delivery nurse or the critical care nurse who responds to the emergency resuscitation call will be active in assisting with cardiopulmonary resuscitation. Once airway management and chest compressions are established, the nurse will ensure patency of two large-bore peripheral intravenous infusions and begin fluid resuscitation.

While the pregnancy is still viable, a nurse will monitor the fetal status. Preparations will be made for an immediate cesarean delivery and the potential need for infant resuscitation.

IMPAIRED GAS EXCHANGE

A key aspect in improving gas exchange in the lungs is positioning the patient to allow the best respiratory effort. Although it is difficult to turn patients who have several peripheral IV sites and hemodynamic monitoring catheters and are being ventilated, it is still necessary to do so. Positioning will need to be individualized, and the effects of position changes monitored using blood gas results, pulse oximetry data, and cardiac outputs (Bradley, 1987).

One of the nurse's major responsibilities is to follow the patient's fluid status to prevent fluid overload and pulmonary edema. The central venous pressure and PCWP will be trended and all intake and output recorded and monitored. Lungs will be auscultated frequently to assess the patient's ability to tolerate fluid volume.

For more detail regarding the nursing management of the patient with ARDS, the reader is encouraged to read Chapter 26.

POTENTIAL FOR INJURY

Once the patient has been stabilized, she will be at increased risk of hemorrhage. Assessment of the skin for petechiae and oozing from venipuncture sites may provide early warning of the development of DIC and impending hemorrhage. Blood may be placed in a non-heparinized blood tube and timed for clot formation.

If the patient has delivered, she will be at risk of hemorrhage from an atonic uterus. Assessment of uterine tone must be performed regularly. (For more information regarding assessment of uterine tone and medications used to treat uterine atony, see the previous section of this chapter.)

ANTICIPATORY FAMILY GRIEVING

As in any instance of sudden death or potential for death, family members will need assistance in coping with this tragic situation. It is easy to forget the family during resuscitative efforts and during the critical period after successful resuscitation. As soon as possible, the nurse should delegate someone to communicate with the family, help the family summon clergy, or arrange for a social worker to provide support. If the infant has survived, encouraging the family to spend time with the newborn may be helpful. However, the family may react to the infant as the cause of the woman's death or illness. The nurse must be prepared to assist the family members to deal with their grief.

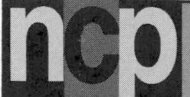 nursing care plan

1. Potential for injury related to:
Seizure activity, magnesium sulfate toxicity, and hemorrhage secondary to severe preeclampsia

Outcome Criteria	Nursing Interventions

Seizures will be prevented.
Patient will be free from injury if seizures do occur.
Magnesium sulfate toxicity will be prevented.
Postpartum blood loss will not exceed 1 peripad/hr.
	Assess the patient for increased risk of seizures from the time of admission for preeclampsia until at least 24 to 30 hours postpartum.
	Include evaluation of mentation, headache, and deep tendon reflexes in ongoing assessments.
	If patient is on magnesium sulfate: perform deep tendon reflex assessments using patellar or antecubital reflexes every hour or more frequently as the patient's condition dictates.
	Assess urinary output and monitor deep tendon reflexes more frequently while urinary output is low.
	Decrease stimulation from light and noise
	  Provide indirect room lighting.
	  Cover patient's eyes if movement to another room is necessary.
	  Decrease volume on monitors with sound indicators.
	Coordinate nursing and medical procedures to allow for periods of rest.
	Protect from injury if seizures do occur.
	When seizure activity has ceased and respiratory status is stable, prepare patient for a vaginal examination.
	Assess the uterus and lochia every 15 minutes for the first 2 hours and then hourly.
	  Palpate uterine fundus for position and tone. If the fundus is relaxed or boggy, it should be massaged.
	  Encourage the patients without indwelling Foley catheter to void hourly or perform intermittent catheterization to ensure an empty bladder.
	  Administer oxytocin intravenously with fluids to control uterine atony as prescribed.
	  Lochia should be dark red. Report bright red bleeding or heavy bleeding (saturating more than one peripad per hour) immediately.
	  Treat severe postpartum hemorrhage with 15-methyl prostaglandin $F_{2\alpha}$ as prescribed and monitor for side effects of GI upset, fever and flushing.
	Assess for the development of petechiae, ecchymosis, oozing from puncture sites, and hematuria.
	Monitor laboratory values of hemoglobin and hematocrit.
	Monitor blood pressure and heart rate.

2. Altered tissue perfusion: Renal and hepatic related to:
Vasospasm secondary to preeclampsia

Outcome Criteria	Nursing Interventions
Urine output and fluid volume status will remain at baseline levels. Factors indicating hepatic damage will be recognized.	Record urine protein levels every 4 hours. Measure urine output and specific gravity every hour. Position patient on her left side to promote venous return via the inferior vena cava. Carefully monitor for fluid overload if fluid challenge is ordered. Monitor for complaints of right upper quadrant or epigastric pain. Monitor hepatic laboratory values. Perform blood glucose measurements. Closely monitor for changes in abdominal pain, the appearance of other abdominal signs, and the onset of hemodynamic instability.

3. Impaired gas exchange related to:
Fluid volume overload and pulmonary edema secondary to severe preeclampsia

Outcome Criteria	Nursing Interventions
Signs of impending pulmonary edema will be recognized.	Ausculate for the presence of rales. Inspect neck for jugular distention. Be alert to the development of dyspnea or cough. Trend the pulmonary capillary wedge pressure measurements in patients with a flow-directed pulmonary artery catheter. Avoid overhydration for at least 24 to 72 hours.

4. Anxiety related to:
Unexpected critical illness

Nursing Care Plan continued on following page

Outcome Criteria	Nursing Interventions
Patient and family will discuss concerns and fears.	Interact in an unhurried manner and provide easily understandable information. Listen to patient's and family's fears and concerns and provide continuing support. Consider a social service consultation.

5. Potential for altered parenting related to:
   Physical separation from infant in neonatal intensive care unit

Outcome Criteria	Nursing Interventions
Mother will maintain contact with infant.	Encourage family to take pictures of the newborn for the mother to keep with her. Contact or encourage the mother to contact the nursery staff several times a day for progress reports on infant's condition. Encourage a family member to interact with the newborn and tell the mother of the infant's temperament and appearance. Consider the involvement of a social worker if the infant is seriously ill.

6. Alteration in tissue perfusion related to:
   Cardiopulmonary collapse secondary to amniotic fluid embolism

Outcome Criteria	Nursing Interventions
Mother and child will survive delivery.	Assist with cardiopulmonary resuscitation as needed. Ensure patency of two large-bore peripheral intravenous infusions and begin fluid resuscitation. Monitor fetal status while the pregnancy is still viable. Prepare for an immediate cesarean delivery and the potential need for infant resuscitation.

7. Impaired gas exchange related to:
   Amniotic fluid in maternal pulmonary circulation secondary to amniotic fluid embolism

Outcome Criteria	Nursing Interventions
Pulmonary status will remain within baseline levels.	Position patient to allow best respiratory effort. Monitor blood gas results, pulse oximetry data, and cardiac outputs to determine optimal positioning. Follow fluid status to prevent fluid overload and pulmonary edema. Evaluate trends of the central venous pressure, PCWP, and intake and output records. Auscultate lungs frequently.

8. Potential for injury related to:
   Hemorrhage and disseminated intravascular coagulation (DIC)

Outcome Criteria	Nursing Interventions
Hemorrhage will be prevented or quickly detected.	Assess skin for petechiae and oozing from venipuncture sites. Evaluate blood for clot formation by placing it in a non-heparinized tube and observing. Assess uterine tone regularly.

9. Anticipatory family grieving related to:
   Sudden death or potential death secondary to amniotic fluid embolism

Outcome Criteria	Nursing Interventions
Family will be periodically informed of patient's status. Support will be available to family.	During resuscitation efforts, delegate someone to communicate with the family, summon clergy, or arrange for a social worker to provide support. Encourage the family to spend time with the newborn if the infant has survived. Prepare to assist the family members to deal with their grief.

SUMMARY

Life-threatening complications arising from pregnancy are rare. When they occur, however, they present a major challenge to the critical care nurse. Nursing care of the critically ill obstetric patient must take into account the physiologic as well as the psychological condition of the patient and her family. The special needs of the critically ill obstetric patient require a nursing team approach. The obstetric nurses seek consultation and help from the critical care nursing specialists when hemodynamic monitoring and mechanical ventilation are required during the intrapartum period. The critical care staff members request obstetric nursing help in assessing the usual postpartum parameters of uterine involution and lochia. The nursing staff of the newborn nursery/ICU may also be called upon to provide information about the infant's condition. This nursing team approach maximizes professional nursing care and provides the best possible care for the woman and her family.

References

Balk, R., and Bone, R. (1983). The adult respiratory distress syndrome. *Medical Clinics of North America*, 67 (3), 685–700.

Benedetti, T. J., and Carlson, R. W. (1979). Studies of colloid osmotic pressure in pregnancy-induced hypertension. *American Journal of Obstetrics and Gynecology*, 135 (3), 308–311.

Bishop, E. H. (1964). Pelvic scoring for elective induction. *Obstetrics and Gynecology*, 24 (2), 266–268.

Bradley, R. B. (1987). Adult respiratory distress syndrome. *Focus on Critical Care*, 14 (5), 48–59.

Brain, M. C., Dacie, J. V., and Hourihane, D. O. B. (1962). Microangiopathic hemolytic anemia: The possible role of vascular lesions in pathogenesis. *British Journal of Haematology*, 8, 358–374.

Chesley, L. C. (1984). History and epidemiology of preeclampsia-eclampsia. *Clinical Obstetrics and Gynecology*, 27 (4), 801–819.

Clark, S. L. (1986). Amniotic fluid embolism. *Clinics in Perinatology*, 13 (4), 801–811.

Clark, S. L. (1990). New concepts of amniotic fluid embolism: A review. *Obstetrical and Gynecological Survey*, 45 (6), 360–368.

Clark, S. L., and Cotton, D. B. (1988). Clinical indications for pulmonary artery catheterization in the patient with severe preeclampsia. *American Journal of Obstetrics and Gynecology*, 158 (3), 453–458.

Clark, S. L., Greenspoon, J. S., Aldahl, D., and Phelan, J. P. (1986a). Severe preeclampsia with persistent oliguria: Management of hemodynamic subsets. *American Journal of Obstetrics and Gynecology*, 154 (3), 490–494.

Clark, S. L., Montz, F. J., and Phelan, J. P. (1985). Hemodynamic alterations associated with amniotic fluid embolism: A reappraisal. *American Journal of Obstetrics and Gynecology*, 151 (5), 617–621.

Clark, S. L., Pavlova, Z., Greenspoon, J., et al. (1986b). Squamous cells in the maternal pulmonary circulation. *American Journal of Obstetrics and Gynecology*, 154 (1), 104–106.

Cotton, D. B., Gonik, B., and Dorman, K. F. (1984). Cardiovascular alterations in severe pregnancy-induced hypertension: Acute effects of intravenous magnesium sulfate. *American Journal of Obstetrics and Gynecology*, 148 (2), 162–165.

Davison, J. M. (1985). The physiology of the renal tract in pregnancy. *Clinical Obstetrics and Gynecology*, 28 (2), 257–265.

Duff, P. (1984). Defusing the danger of amniotic fluid embolism. *Contemporary OB/GYN*, 24 (2), 127–149.

Friedman, S. (1989). Preeclampsia: A review of the role of prostaglandins. *Obstetrics and Gynecology*, 71 (1), 122–137.

Gant, N. F., Daley, G. L., Chand, S., et al. (1973). A study of angiotensin II pressor response throughout primigravid pregnancy. *Journal of Clinical Investigation*, 52, 2682–2685.

Goodlin, R. C. (1976). Severe pre-eclampsia: Another great imitator. *American Journal of Obstetrics and Gynecology*, 125 (6), 747–753.

Hankins, G. D., Wendel, G. D., Cunningham, F. G., and Leveno, K. J. (1984). Longitudinal evaluation of hemodynamic changes in eclampsia. *American Journal of Obstetrics and Gynecology*, 150 (5), 506–512.

Hyashi, R. H., Castillo, M. S., and Noah, M. L. (1984). Management of severe postpartum hemorrhage with a prostaglandin $F_{2\alpha}$ analogue. *Obstetrics and Gynecology*, 63 (6), 806–808.

Kirshan, B., and Cotton, D. B. (1987). Invasive hemodynamic monitoring in the obstetrical patient. *Clinical Obstetrics and Gynecology*, 30 (3), 579–590.

Lee, W., Gonik, B., and Cotton, D. B. (1987). Urinary diagnostic indices in preeclampsia-associated oliguria: Correlation with invasive hemodynamic monitoring. *American Journal of Obstetrics and Gynecology*, 156 (1), 100–103.

Moise, K. J., and Cotton, D. B. (1986). The use of colloid osmotic pressure in pregnancy. *Clinics in Perinatology*, 13 (4), 827–842.

Pritchard, J. A., Cunningham, F. G., and Pritchard, S. A. (1984). The Parkland Memorial Hospital protocol for treatment of eclampsia: Evaluation of 245 cases. *American Journal of Obstetrics and Gynecology*, 148 (7), 951–963.

Pritchard, J. A., et al. (1985). *William's obstetrics* (17th ed.) New York: Appleton-Century-Crofts.

Roberts, J. M. (1989). Pregnancy-related hypertension. In R. K. Creasy and R. Resnik (Eds.), *Maternal-fetal medicine: Principles and practice* (2nd ed., pp. 777–823). Philadelphia: W. B. Saunders.

Roberts, J. M., Taylor, R. N., Musci, T. J., et al. (1989). Preeclampsia: An endothelial cell disorder. *American Journal of Obstetrics and Gynecology*, 161 (5), 1200–1204.

Saftlas, A. F., Olson, D. R., Franks, A. L., et al. (1990). Epidemiology of preeclampsia and eclampsia in the United States, 1979–1986. *American Journal of Obstetrics and Gynecology*, 163 (2), 460–465.

Scott, J. R., and Beer, A. A. (1976). Immunologic aspects of preeclampsia. *American Journal of Obstetrics and Gynecology*, 125 (3), 418–427.

Secher, N. J., Arnsbo, P., and Wallin, L. (1978). Haemodynamic effects of oxytocin (Syntocinon) and methyl ergometrine (Methergine) on the systemic and pulmonary circulation of pregnant anesthetized women. *Acta Obstetrica et Gynecologica Scandinavica*, 57, 97–103.

Sibai, B. M., Lipshitz, J., Anderson, G. D., and Dilts, P. V. (1981). Reassessment of intravenous $MgSO_4$ therapy in preeclampsia-eclampsia. *Obstetrics and Gynecology*, 57 (2), 199–202.

Sperry, K. (1986). Amniotic fluid embolism: To understand an enigma. *Journal of the American Medical Association*, 255 (16), 2183–2186.

Steiner, P. E., and Lushbaugh, C. C. (1941). Maternal pulmonary embolism by amniotic fluid as a cause of obstetric shock and unexpected deaths in obstetrics. *Journal of the American Medical Association*, 117, 1245–1254; 1341–1345.

Stempel, J. E., O'Grady, J. P., Morton, M. J., and Johnson, K. A. (1982). Use of sodium nitroprusside in complications of gestational hypertension. *Obstetrics and Gynecology*, 60 (4), 533–538.

Ueland, K. (1976). Maternal cardiovascular dynamics. VII. Intrapartum blood volume changes. *American Journal of Obstetrics and Gynecology*, 126 (6), 671–677.

Weinstein, L. (1982). Syndrome of hemolysis, elevated liver enzymes, and low platelet count: A severe consequence of hypertension in pregnancy. *American Journal of Obstetrics and Gynecology*, 142 (2), 159–167.

Weinstein, L. (1986). The HELLP syndrome: A severe consequence of hypertension in pregnancy. *Journal of Perinatology*, 5 (4), 316–320.

Wheeler, A. S., and Harris, B. A. (1982). Anesthesia for pregnancy-induced hypertension. *Clinics in Perinatology*, 9 (1), 95–111.

Whittaker, A. A., Hull, B. J., and Clochesy, J. M. (1986). Hemolysis, elevated liver enzymes, and low platelet count syndrome: Nursing care of the critically ill obstetric patient. *Heart & Lung*, 15 (4), 402–410.

Worley, R. J. (1984). Pathophysiology of pregnancy-induced hypertension. *Clinical Obstetrics and Gynecology*, 27 (4), 821–834.

Zuspan, F. P., and Zuspan, K. H. (1981). Strategies for controlling eclampsia. *Contemporary OB/GYN*, 18 (1), 135–144.

Patients with Oncologic Emergencies

Marcia Rostad

Oncologic crises are emergency events that occur during the course of the cancer experience. Unmanaged, these critical events diminish the patient's quality of life and carry high morbidity and mortality. Because many cancers are responsive to treatment and are potentially curable, medical management of oncologic emergencies is of great importance. Even when the cancer is considered incurable, most oncologic crises are aggressively managed to extend an already limited life span.

PATHOPHYSIOLOGY OF CANCER

Neoplasms are classified according to the tissue from which they originate. Sarcomas are tumors that derive from embryonic tissue, or so-called connective tissue. Carcinomas are those tumors of epithelial cell origin. Carcinomas account for nearly 80% of human cancers (Hupchella and Burton, 1988). As a means of more definitively identifying the aberrant cells, tumors are further defined by their histologic characteristics. Squamous cell carcinoma and adenocarcinoma are two examples of tumors whose histologic appearance has been confirmed. The confirmation of tissue histology assists in identifying the best treatment for the cancer.

Four major theories attempt to explain the causation of cancer. Although none by itself has been successful in accounting for all the aspects of cancer, each supports the basis for today's approach to treatment (Upton, 1982).

The first theory attributes neoplasia to genetic abnormalities that can occur at any time during life. This disruption in the regulation of cellular growth and differentiation may account for the development of certain cancers in families, such as breast cancer

or leukemia in identical twins. In contrast, the second theory suggests that the development of cancer may be epigenetic, that is, changes in the regulation of genes and not their structure may account for the development of certain cancers. The carcinogenic action of diethylstilbestrol on the human vagina is one example. The viral theory attempts to link DNA and RNA oncogenic viruses to the transformation of malignant cells. Burkitt's lymphoma is almost certainly due to infection by the Epstein-Barr virus (EBV). The last theory hypothesizes that malignant cells in early development may lie dormant until, if ever, the appropriate stimulus comes along. Only then does a malignancy occur. This theory may explain why immunodeficiency often increases susceptibility of the host to neoplasia.

Once the neoplastic process has begun, the aberrant cell continues unregulated and uncontrolled proliferation without regard for the needs of the host. The malignant cells may double at amazing speed, allowing a tumor to quickly occupy its immediate space and eventually invade nearby structures. This local extension may lead to regional extension via metastasis to the lymph nodes. Metastasis occurs when tumor emboli detach from the tumor and are carried to the lymph nodes by the downstream flow of lymph (Hupchella and Burton, 1988).

Distant metastasis primarily occurs by the spread of cancer through the bloodstream. It is generally believed that the more aggressive cancer cells reach the bloodstream through direct invasion of the capillaries and veins (Hupchella and Burton, 1988). While in the bloodstream, the cancer cells interact with other cancer cells, blood components, and the elements of the immune system. This interaction allows the cell to develop additional complex characteristics, which aid in its eventual relocation and growth in other tissues of the body.

Eventually the cancer cells come to rest and establish neoplastic growth. It is unclear why there is a tendency for certain cancers to metastasize to certain sites, particularly the liver, lymph nodes, bones, lung, and brain. The mechanics of circulation may explain where metastasis occurs and where it does not. In tissues where there is a high blood flow rate, it is believed that cancer cells cannot lodge long enough to become attached (Hupchella and Burton, 1988). It is also suggested that metastasizing cells, because of their genetic make-up, prefer specific tissue types, or "congenial soil." The presence of a receptor on the cancer cell may cause it to associate with particular tissues or organs (Hupchella and Burton, 1988; Fidler and Hart, 1982). Regardless of the cause for metastases, it is the effect of the spreading cancer that causes concern.

Chemotherapy, radiation, surgery, and biotherapy are currently the four treatment choices for cancer. These interventions may be used as a singular approach to treatment or in combination. Surgery, the oldest treatment for cancer, is used for diagnosis and treatment. The surgical role in diagnoses is to obtain a tissue sample of the tumor for exact histologic diagnosis. Surgery is also used to evaluate the effectiveness of other treatments in eliminating the tumor. An exploratory laparotomy is one example of surgery being used to evaluate the effectiveness of chemotherapy for lymphoma.

Surgery can be an effective treatment for a tumor that is resectable. If the tumor is not entirely resectable, surgery is employed to debulk (reduce the size of) the tumor so that radiation or chemotherapy can be more effective. Surgery is also useful in relieving a growing tumor that may be compressing other organ structures, causing pain or obstruction.

At times surgery can be radical, involving the removal of normal as well as malignant tissue, muscle, and parts of or entire organs or limbs. Radical surgery may eventually be followed by restorative, reconstructive, or plastic surgery.

Chemotherapy is a successful systemic approach to treating most malignancies. However, chemotherapy is limited in its usefulness because of the myelosuppression it causes and the development of tumor resistance to the antineoplastic agents. The aim of chemotherapy is to reduce the number of cancerous cells by affecting their ability to reproduce. To best accomplish this, chemotherapy agents have their most toxic effect against rapidly proliferating cells. Unfortunately, many rapidly proliferating normal cells—leukocytes, platelets, hair follicles, cells lining the gastrointestinal tract—will also be destroyed. Until chemotherapy is further refined to be cancer cell specific, the complications of chemotherapy will limit its therapeutic effectiveness.

The development of drug resistance by malignant cells also hinders the success of chemotherapy. Because drug resistance develops after subsequent doses, the first dose of chemotherapy has the best chance of being effective. Maximum doses of combination chemotherapy are usually carefully calculated to provide the patient with the highest cell kill while preventing life-threatening complications.

Radiation therapy damages cellular DNA and RNA, which results in impaired cellular function or cell death. As with chemotherapy, radiation therapy is not specific for malignant cells. Radiation will have its devastating effects on all cells, normal or malignant, within the path of ionization.

Radiation may be delivered as an external beam treatment. The beam of ionization is aimed exactly at the site and depth of the tumor and is delivered in such a way as to minimize its effect on normal tissue. Radiation may also be delivered as a sealed source of cesium, iodine, iridium, or radium that is surgically implanted directly into or immediately surrounding the tumor.

Radiation may be used as a curative therapy, as in Hodgkin's disease, or as adjunctive treatment for uterine cancer. Radiation may also be used palliatively to relieve symptoms, such as bone pain or superior vena cava obstruction, associated with incurable advancing disease.

There has been increasing focus on the treatment arena of biotherapy. In the past, bacille Calmette-Guérin (BCG) vaccine has been used to stimulate the patient's own immune system to counteract the cancer. Through a greater understanding of the immune system and the development of technologic advances, biologic response modifiers (BRMs) have surfaced as the newest weapon against cancer. BRMs are defined by the National Cancer Institute as "those agents or approaches that modify the relationship between tumor and host by modifying the host's biological response to tumor cells with resultant therapeutic effects" (Abernathy, 1987). A list of biologic response modifiers and what they do is presented in Table 64–1.

There are many side effects associated with the use of BRMs. Hematologic and gastrointestinal reactions are similar to those that result from conventional therapy. The unique side effects of BRMs include cardiovascular and neurologic reactions. The neurologic effects from BRMs may be subtle. Cognitive changes and lethargy may be difficult to assess if the patient is critically ill (Irwin, 1987). Significant toxicities involving the cardiovascular, pulmonary, renal, and other organ systems are frequently associated with the use of interleukin-2 (IL-2). Because of these toxic side effects, it is common for the patient to require an intensive care setting and the skills of a critical care nurse during treatment. Table 64–2 summarizes the findings and clinical implications for the patient receiving IL-2 therapy.

As the development and spread of cancer are better understood, treatment modalities can be refined to improve their effectiveness. Until that occurs, cancer patients will continue to receive treatment that affects normal as well as malignant cells. Health care professionals will be challenged to support patients through life-threatening complications.

TABLE 64–1. Biologic Response Modifiers

Colony-stimulating factor	A monokine that stimulates production of leukocytes by stem cells in the bone marrow
Interferon (INF)	A family of glycoproteins made by mammalian cells in response to viral infections and other types of inducers
Interferon inducer	Agents capable of inducing the release of various types of interferon from the body
Interleukin-2 (IL-2)	A lymphokine essential to the growth of T-lymphocytes; it augments various T-cell functions and supports the growth and augmentation of natural killer cells
Lymphokine	A protein secreted by lymphocytes that is capable of directing the function of other cells
Lymphokine-activated killer cells	Lymphoid cells capable of lysing either autologous or allogeneic tumor cells
Monoclonal antibody	An antibody produced by one single clone of a B-lymphocyte directed against an antigen on tumor cells
Monokine	A protein secreted by mononuclear phagocytes capable of directing the function of other cells
Tumor necrosis factor	A monokine capable of directly killing tumor cells by inducing hemorrhagic necrosis in tumor cells without harming normal tissues

Data from Abernathy, E. (1987). *Oncology Nursing Forum,* 14 (6), 14.

Some oncologic crises—spinal cord compression, superior vena cava syndrome, carotid artery rupture—are unique complications of cancer. These complications are discussed in detail in this chapter. The development of other pathophysiologic states is not necessarily limited to the cancer population. The progression of the malignancy or the complications of cancer treatment may lead to hemorrhage, disseminated intravascular coagulation (DIC), or septic shock secondary to myelosuppression. Electrolyte imbalances develop as a result of hypercalcemia, tumor lysis syndrome, or the syndrome of inappropriate antidiuretic hormone (SIADH). Bowel obstruction results from tumor growth or from the neurotoxic effects of some chemotherapy agents. Table 64–3 briefly describes these pathophysiologic states as they appear in oncologic patients.

SPINAL CORD COMPRESSION

Spinal cord compression (SCC) is a complication of metastasizing solid and hematologic malignancies.

Without prompt medical intervention, the inevitable neurologic damage truly makes SCC an oncologic emergency (Kornblith and Cassady, 1985). Even in incurable cancers, the disruption in quality of life caused by SCC encourages most practitioners to aggressively treat this complication at its earliest detection.

Pathophysiology

The spinal cord has both motor and sensory functions. The spinal cord receives and transmits signals from 31 pairs of spinal nerves. Every spinal nerve contains a dorsal (afferent) and ventral (efferent) root. The afferent root serves as the sensory division of the peripheral nervous system. The somatic afferent fibers carry impulses from the skin, skeletal muscles, joints, and tendons to the central nervous system. The central nervous system receives impulses from the viscera via the visceral afferent fibers (Henze, 1984).

The efferent division responds to the sensory input with motor activity. The visceral efferent system innervates through the autonomic nervous system, of which the sympathetic and parasympathetic divisions belong. The somatic efferent system innervates the muscles, tendons, and joints through the pyramidal (upper motor neurons) and extrapyramidal (lower motor neurons) systems (Henze, 1984).

Disruption of the sensory and/or motor functions of the spinal cord can be the result of an extramedullary tumor, intramedullary tumor, extradural tumor within the spinal canal, or bony metastasis to a vertebra outside of the spinal canal. In cancer, SCC is usually the result of a primary tumor metastasizing to the epidural space. The lesion is most frequently extramedullary, with only 5% occurring within the spinal column. Solid tumors have the highest overall chances of metastatic SCC. Cancers of the lung, breast, and prostate carry the highest risk. SCC may also be the result of metastatic hematologic malignancies such as multiple myeloma and lymphoma. The most common site of metastasis is the thoracic vertebrae (68%), with cervical and lumbar involvement equally less affected (15% each) (Kornblith and Cassady, 1985; Bruckman and Bloomer, 1981).

Tumor impairment of the neurons will disrupt reflexes and motor function. Spastic paralysis below the level of the tumor will occur if the upper motor neuron or corticospinal tract is affected. Lower motor neuron damage affects voluntary muscle movement and will result in flaccid paralysis and sensory disturbance below the level of the tumor (Couillard-Getreuer, 1985).

The prognosis for SCC varies. The prognosis is good if the onset is slow, the duration of motor dysfunction is less than 24 hours, sphincter control remains present, and the patient is able to maintain an ambulatory status. Location of the tumor within the posterior epidural space and in the lumbar or

TABLE 64–2. Interleukin-2 (IL-2)

Interleukin-2 (IL-2) is a lymphokine naturally produced by helper T-cells that plays a variety of immunoregulatory roles. Studies have discovered that IL-2 enhances natural killer cell function, augments alloantigen responsiveness, activates lymphokine-activated killer cells, and improves the recovery of immune function. This biologic response modifier also causes a marked redistribution of lymphoid cells to specific tissues, including the lungs, liver, and mesentric lymph nodes (Jassak and Sticklin, 1986).

IL-2 is used in clinical trials as one means to restore or "boost" the host's own immune system. Augmenting the patient's immune system through the use of IL-2 hypothetically will control the growth or metastasis of tumor cells (Jassak and Sticklin, 1986).

The use of IL-2 is investigational. It may be administered by a variety of routes, including intravenous, subcutaneous, and peritoneal. As clinical trials continue, the maximum tolerated dose, by the various routes of administration, will eventually be determined. It is also hoped that clinical trials will identify medical and nursing interventions that will improve the management of the toxic side effects of IL-2. The major dose-limiting toxic effect of IL-2 is the development of a capillary-leak syndrome. A release of vasoactive factor facilitates the flow of protein-containing plasma water out of the vascular compartment and into the interstitial space of many organs. This results in hemodynamic instability and renal dysfunction. Toxic effects associated with the clinical use of IL-2 are summarized as follows (Jassak and Sticklin, 1986; Padavic-Shaller, 1988; Oncology Nursing Society, 1989.

Organ System	Clinical Findings	Clinical Implications
Central nervous system	Confusion Altered mentation	Sleep deprivation, unfamiliar sights and sounds, etc., may exacerbate CNS toxicity of IL-2 Patient must be protected from harm Patient is frequently assessed for continued deterioration of mental status IL-2 therapy may be interrupted if confusion is severe
Renal	Elevated blood urea nitrogen (BUN) Elevated serum creatinine Proteinuria Oliguria	Urine output must be monitored hourly Urine is tested for protein Daily BUN and creatinine levels are determined during IL-2 treatment An infusion of 2–5 µg/kg/minute of dopamine may be used to increase renal perfusion Loop diuretics (furosemide) may be prescribed to increase urine flow through the renal tubules
Pulmonary	Interstitial pulmonary edema Dyspnea Hypoxemia	Intubation and mechanical ventilation may be required The patient is carefully assessed for signs of increasing dyspnea, restlessness Arterial blood gases (ABGs) are monitored for decreasing oxygen saturation
Cardiac	Decreased pulmonary capillary wedge pressure Decreased central venous pressure Hypotension Peripheral edema Transient dysrhythmias ST–T wave changes Elevated creatine kinase (CK) levels	Fluid shifts (as much as 10%) from the vascular space into the interstitium Large amounts of crystalloid and colloid fluid may be needed to maintain intravascular volume Vasopressors may be required to maintain blood pressure
Gastrointestinal	Nausea/vomiting Diarrhea	Antiemetics and antidiarrheal medications may be helpful in controlling symptoms
Integument	Erythematous rash Pruritus Skin desquamation	Meticulous skin care is essential Topical ointments may be prescribed to relieve discomfort
Hematologic	Thrombocytopenia Anemia Fever Chills Flu-like syndrome	Hemoglobin, hematocrit, and platelets are monitored closely. Transfusion of red blood cells and/or platelets may be required Fever and chills may be alleviated by the administration of an antipyretic (acetaminophen), an antihistamine (diphenhydramine hydrochloride), and a narcotic analgesic (meperidine hydrochloride)

sacral areas is an additional favorable sign. A poor prognosis is associated with rapid onset, motor dysfunction of greater than 48 hours, absent sphincter control, and if the patient experiences paralysis. Prognosis is less favorable when the tumor is located in the anterior epidural space and lies in the thoracic or cervical areas (Couillard-Getreur, 1985; Bruckman and Bloomer, 1981).

Clinical Presentation

The clinical presentation of SCC is divided into prodromal and compressive phases (Couillard-Getreuer, 1985; Bruckman and Bloomer, 1981). Progressive back pain from local bony involvement characterizes the prodromal phase. The back pain is usually

TABLE 64–3. Common Pathophysiologic States Occurring in Oncologic Patients

Myelosuppression

Etiology:	Replacement of bone marrow by primary or metastatic cancer
	Effects of myelosuppressive treatment
Clinical findings:	Infection secondary to granulocytopenia
	Bleeding secondary to thrombocytopenia
	Anemia secondary to erythropenia
Management:	Support host defense mechanisms
	Avoid damage to protective body barriers (e.g., invasive procedures)
	Reduce exposure to new potential pathogens
	Suppress colonizing organisms

Tumor Lysis Syndrome

Etiology:	Cellular death and lysis after chemotherapy releases large amounts of intracellular electrolytes and metabolites into the circulation
Clinical findings:	Elevated serum phosphate, potassium, uric acid levels
	Decreased serum calcium level
Management:	Prevent renal failure by hydration, administration of allopurinol, diuretics
	Monitor and treat electrolyte imbalances as they occur

SIADH (Syndrome of Inappropriate Antidiuretic Hormone [ADH] Secretion)

Etiology:	Ectopic production of ADH by certain tumors (small or oat cell carcinoma of the lung, duodenal and pancreatic carcinoma, others)
Clinical findings:	Fluid retention, fluid volume overload
	Dilutional hyponatremia
Management:	Fluid restriction
	Diuresis with hypertonic saline
	Drug therapy: demeclocycline, urea, furosemide, lithium carbonate

Hypercalcemia

Etiology:	Acceleration of bone resorption, bone destruction, and release of calcium into the extracellular fluid as a result of bony metastases
Clinical findings:	Gastrointestinal disturbances (e.g., anorexia, nausea, vomiting, constipation)
	Neuromuscular and cardiac symptoms reflecting interference with normal contractility of muscle
	Polyuria, precipitation of calcium salts in urine resulting in acute renal failure
	Metabolic alkalosis
	Bone pain, pruritus
Management:	For serum calcium levels of 6.0 mEq/L or greater: hydration, diuretics to increase urine flow
	Drug therapy to inhibit bone resorption: mithramycin, calcitonin, glucocorticoids, oral phosphates
	Mobilization of patient
	Hemodialysis

Bowel Obstruction

Etiology:	Primary tumor occlusion of the lumen of the bowel
	Secondary tumor obstruction
	Bands of adhesions or scar tissue from prior abdominal surgery
	Tissue changes secondary to radiation treatments
	Neurotoxicity from chemotherapy with vinca alkaloids
	Chronic use of narcotics that inhibit peristalsis leading to bowel impaction
Clinical findings:	Abdominal pain, distention
	Vomiting, change in elimination pattern
	Dehydration, hypovolemia
	Electrolyte, acid-base disturbances
Management:	Surgical intervention to eliminate/reduce the source of obstruction
	Decompression by nasogastric drainage tube
	Hydration and electrolyte therapy

Data from Johnson, B. L., and Gross, J. (Eds.) (1985). *Handbook of oncology nursing.* Bethany, CT: Fleschner.

localized to the involved spinal segment with or without radicular pain to the chest, abdomen, or extremities. The pain usually begins 6 months or less before the diagnosis of SCC is eventually made. The pain may be aggravated by motion or by lying down.

Invariably, pain is followed by the development of other symptoms (Bruckman and Bloomer, 1981). The compressive phase is the result of motor and sensory dysfunction from the growing tumor compressing the cord. In the compressive phase, sensory dysfunction begins with extremity parethesia, numbness, tingling, and coolness. As the lesion enlarges, these symptoms tend to ascend the body. Motor dysfunction may occur concomitant with or after sensory dysfunction. As described in Figure 64–1, the degree of motor dysfunction depends on whether complete or incomplete upper motor neuron (UMN) or lower motor neuron (LMN) dysfunction has occurred (Couillard-Getreuer, 1985).

In addition to pain and numbness, 75% of patients will also complain of weakness (Kornblith and Cassady, 1985). Footdrop and difficulty in maintaining balance may also be noted (Bruckman and Bloomer, 1981). Disturbances in micturition and sensory impairment commonly occur together if the site of compression involves the lower lumbar portion of the spinal cord. Bowel or bladder dysfunction are unfavorable prognostic signs. Two-thirds of patients with bowel and bladder dysfunction become nonambulatory from the progression of the disease (Kornblith and Cassady, 1985).

Respiratory depression is a possibility if the lesion is located at cervical level 5 or above. In addition to progressive paresis of diaphragmatic and intercostal muscles, the small muscle groups of the hands, forearms, and arms may also waste (Couillard-Getreuer, 1985).

Medical Management

SCC is medically managed by surgery, surgery followed by radiation, or radiation alone. The decision as to therapy depends on the type of tumor, the level of block, and the rapidity of onset or duration of symptoms (Kornblith and Cassady, 1985).

SURGICAL DECOMPRESSION

Surgical decompression may be the first line of treatment in complete block with rapidly progressing neurologic defects, and in cervical lesions with risk of respiratory failure. Surgery is also indicated in patients who fail to respond to radiation. A laminectomy can achieve prompt decompression of the spinal cord, but rarely can it remove all of the tumor. Significant surgical morbidity and mortality may occur, making this choice of treatment unlikely in patients with a short life expectancy (Kornblith and Cassady, 1985).

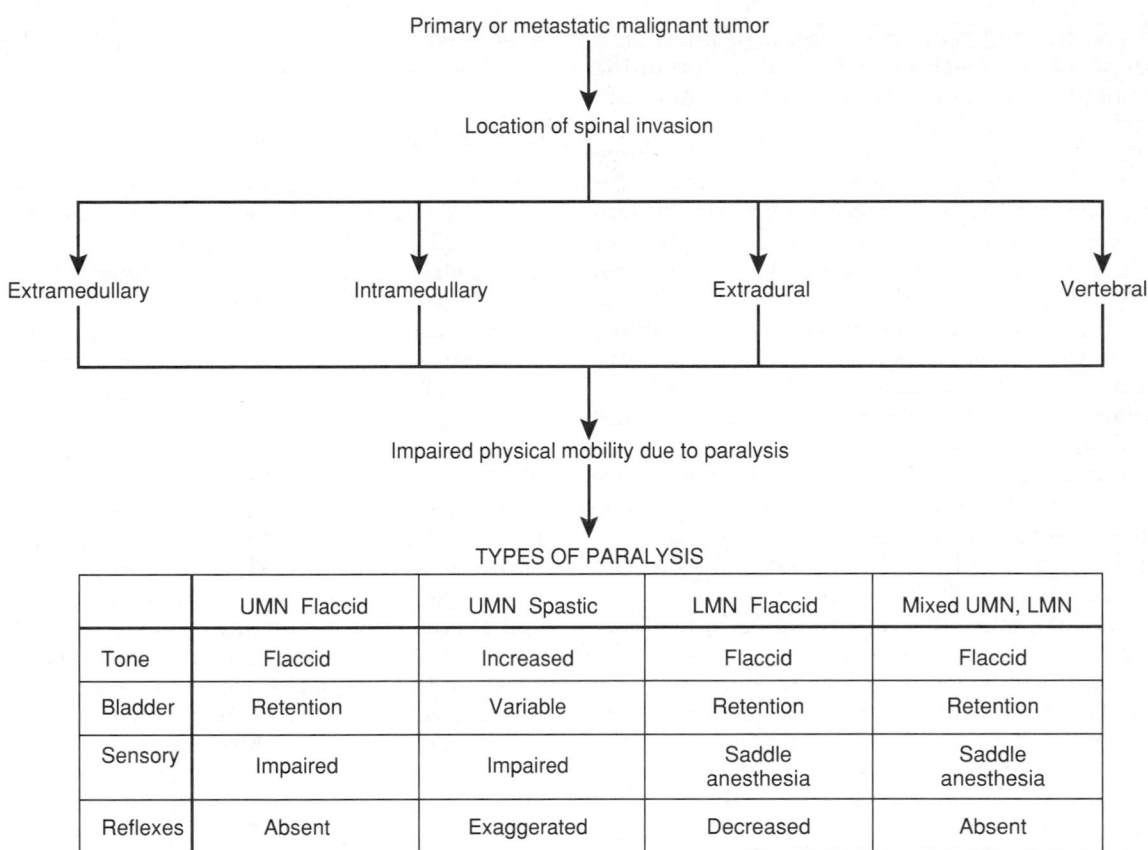

Primary or metastatic malignant tumor

Location of spinal invasion

Extramedullary   Intramedullary   Extradural   Vertebral

Impaired physical mobility due to paralysis

TYPES OF PARALYSIS

	UMN Flaccid	UMN Spastic	LMN Flaccid	Mixed UMN, LMN
Tone	Flaccid	Increased	Flaccid	Flaccid
Bladder	Retention	Variable	Retention	Retention
Sensory	Impaired	Impaired	Saddle anesthesia	Saddle anesthesia
Reflexes	Absent	Exaggerated	Decreased	Absent

FIGURE 64–1. Paralysis in acute spinal cord compression. *Abbreviations*: UMN, upper motor neuron; LMN, lower motor neuron.

RADIATION THERAPY

Radiation treatment after surgical decompression prevents tumor regrowth and reduces the size of the remaining tumor. More patients experience a return in ambulation than those treated with surgery alone (Kornblith and Cassady, 1985; Bruckman and Bloomer, 1981).

The primary treatment of choice remains local irradiation and corticosteroids. Fractionated irradiation doses range from 3000 rad to 4000 rad delivered over 2 to 4 weeks. The radiation port includes the affected vertebra plus the two vertebral bodies above and below. The therapy is begun immediately upon diagnosis (Kornblith and Cassady, 1985).

Corticosteroids are concomitantly administered in high doses. One common dosage regimen is 100 mg dexamethasone daily for 3 days with tapering as tolerated. Corticosteroids are given to decrease inflammation, improve neurologic function, and relieve pain (Couillard-Getreuer, 1985; Kornblith and Cassady, 1985).

Nursing Management

The nursing management of patients with SCC is based on the patient's actual and potential problems. Nursing interventions are implemented to prevent the development of secondary complications, prevent further injury, and detect the progression of the neurologic symptoms while still in an early and manageable state.

ACUTE PAIN

The destruction of the spinal column and damage to the cord and spinal nerve roots lead to acute, agonizing pain. The critical care nurse assesses the patient for pain with each contact and records the location, severity, and characteristics of the pain. Basic pain management principles include an effective analgesic protocol. Assisting the patient to achieve a position of comfort may be in direct conflict with maintaining a stable spinal position. If this is the case, a quiet environment, behavioral techniques, or soothing touches can help distract the patient from the pain experience.

IMPAIRED PHYSICAL MOBILITY

Upper or lower motor neuron damage results in muscle weakness, reflex alterations, or paralysis. The critical care nurse conducts neurologic assessments every 1 to 2 hours. The nurse compares these assessments with previous baseline findings to determine if the cord compression is improving, stablizing, or progressing. Because the patient's prognosis is directly correlated with the amount of neurologic impairment, early detection of a deterioration in the patient's neurologic status can prevent further injury (Couillard-Getreuer, 1985).

Specific neurologic assessments to detect a change in the patient's motor pathways include a testing for hand grip, arm and leg strength, and finger to thumb coordination. Reflexes to be tested include the biceps, triceps, upper and lower abdominal, knee, ankle, and plantar (Babinski). Additional observations include the presence of muscle atrophy, fasciculations, involuntary movement, lack of voluntary movement, or abnormal positions (Couillard-Getreuer, 1985). These findings help to define and further pinpoint the spinal nerves affected.

The nurse should consider a patient's spine unstable until proved otherwise (Couillard-Getreuer, 1985). If the vertebrae's skeletal integrity has been severely compromised by the invading lesion, the patient may be placed in an immobile position to prevent cord damage. In preparation for immobilizing the patient, the critical care nurse evaluates the need for a Stryker frame or other position-maintaining beds. Crutchfield tongs may be necessary if the cervical vertebrae are involved. If absolute immobilization is not required, the critical care nurse sees that spinal alignment is maintained during turning and positioning of the patient in bed (e.g., log roll). When the patient is in the supine position, the nurse maintains the patient's ideal spinal alignment by avoiding the use of pillows and by placing a footboard at the end of the bed. The use of a footboard or other special devices will help to counteract the irreversible effects of footdrop.

In addition to maintaining the patient in a stable position, the nursing plan of care includes interventions that prevent further patient injury from immobility. Respiratory exercises and a skin care protocol are necessary. If possible, range of motion exercises are performed to prevent development of deep vein thrombosis.

POTENTIAL FOR IMPAIRED SKIN INTEGRITY

The loss of normal sensory and motor function and the possible need for immobilization to prevent further damage to the spinal cord threaten the integrity of the patient's skin. The status of the skin is assessed every 2 hours, special attention being paid to bony prominences and areas of pressure. Nursing interventions include massaging the areas of greatest pressure to promote circulation, padding pressure points to prevent skin breakdown, and keeping the patient and bedding clean and dry.

Because cancer patients may be in negative nitrogen balance due to the nutrition-robbing effects of their disease, the maintenence of skin integrity becomes a critical element of nursing care. Supporting the nutritional status as a mechanism to preserve skin integrity is much easier than trying to promote the healing of pressure ulcers. The critical care nurse

may need to collaborate with the dietitian to identify effective means of maintaining nutritional status.

INEFFECTIVE BREATHING PATTERN

Spinal cord lesions at cervical level 5 or above will affect both diaphragmatic and intercostal musculature. Lesions below cervical level 5 will paralyze the intercostals (Mitchell, 1981). A thorough patient assessment will identify how much of the respiratory musculature is affected by the motor and sensory impairment. Patients with lesions below thoracic level 4 will maintain adequate voluntary respiratory function, whereas patients with lesions above thoracic level 4 will require frequent evaluation of respiratory function (Mitchell, 1981).

Bedside spirometry can easily measure the patient's vital capacity (VC). By monitoring VC, the critical care nurse will detect whether the patient is losing respiratory muscle function secondary to spinal edema or advancing tumor. The patient may require ventilatory assistance if the VC is below one-third of the predicted value or less than 600 cm^3. Respiratory patterns, signs and symptoms of respiratory insufficiency, arterial blood gases, and lung sounds assist the nurse in assessing the patient's ability to ventilate satisfactorily (Mitchell, 1981).

ALTERATION IN BOWEL ELIMINATION

Lesions above the sacral cord result in the loss of voluntary control and in sphincter dysfunction of the bowel. The loss of gastric motility from higher lesions may manifest as paralytic ileus.

Upon admission of the patient to the critical care unit, signs and symptoms of paralytic ileus and impaction are assessed. In addition, the patient is assessed for abdominal distention, decreased or absent bowel sounds, and nausea and vomiting. If a paralytic ileus is suspected, intestinal decompression should begin.

The critical care nurse immediately initiates a daily bowel evacuation program to prevent impaction and obstipation. Gentle manual removal of rectal contents or enemas may be needed until rectal reflexes return (Couillard-Getreuer, 1985). Oral intake is withheld until bowel sounds and the passing of flatus have returned. In the meantime, nutritional support of the patient must be maintained through alternative feeding routes such as total parenteral nutrition. Intravenous solutions can provide the fluids necessary for optimal bowel elimination.

URINARY RETENTION

The disruption of the innervation of the bladder from spinal lesions above the sacral cord results in the loss of voluntary bladder elimination of urine (Mitchell, 1981). An indwelling catheter is necessary during the initial course of SCC as a means of avoiding bladder distention. Throughout the period of continuous bladder catheterization, the nurse monitors temperature trends and the characteristics of the urine for any signs of possible bladder infection. Later, in preparation for bladder retraining, the nurse initiates intermittent catheterizations to check for residual urine (Couillard-Getreuer, 1985). Between intermittent catheterizations, the patient is assessed for bladder distention. Because the patient is lacking the sensation to void, the urinal or bedpan is offered at regular intervals.

DECREASED CARDIAC OUTPUT

Acute spinal cord injury may result in spinal shock. During the period of spinal shock, somatic and autonomic reflex activity below the level of the lesion is lost. With the loss of sympathetic function and the predominance of parasympathetic function, the cardiovascular system and viscera slow down. Bradycardia and arrhythmias can occur because the vagal influence is unopposed (Mitchell, 1981). Hypotension becomes problematic because with the loss of the sympathetic nervous system, peripheral vascular resistance can no longer be maintained. Adjusting the patient's position from side to side carries a risk of hypotension because the heart has lost the reflexes to adjust blood pressure in response to a change in position. The loss of peripheral vascular tone impairs venous return to the heart and promotes venous stasis. Not only do these accentuate the problem of hypotension, they also lead to the development of deep vein thrombosis (Mitchell, 1981).

When caring for the patient in spinal shock, the critical care nurse monitors the patient's cardiac rate and rhythm to detect serious arrhythmias or bradycardia. The nurse monitors the blood pressure before and after turning to assess the patient's cardiovascular tolerance to a change in position. Circulatory fluid volume is maintained through the cautious use of intravenous fluids. Throughout volume replacement, the nurse carefully monitors the patient for the development of pulmonary edema (Mitchell, 1981).

The patient in spinal shock is unable to maintain an appropriate body temperature because the peripheral vessels have remained dilated from the loss of sympathetic function. As a result, the body temperature takes on the temperature of the environment. In the typical air-conditioned unit, the patient's temperature will drop. If the patient's body temperature cannot be maintained through the usual application of warm blankets, a heating blanket may be necessary. A cooling blanket may be utilized if the patient's temperature is too high. Because the patient cannot feel the temperature of the device, the nurse needs to assess the functioning of the equipment and the condition of the patient's skin (Mitchell, 1981).

SUPERIOR VENA CAVA SYNDROME

Superior vena cava syndrome (SVCS) commonly is associated with bronchogenic carcinoma and ma-

lignant lymphomas. The syndrome has also been increasingly reported as a complication of the use of central venous catheters. SVCS occurs when the thin walled superior vena cava is obstructed resulting in systemic congestion and increased pressure. An obstruction of the superior vena cava may retard the flow of blood from the head, neck, and upper thorax, leading to the development of signs and symptoms classic for this acute oncologic emergency (Varricchio, 1985). In most situations, these patients will be cared for in ambulatory settings or general care units. However, if the patient presents with a severe decrease in cardiac output and ineffective breathing patterns, admission to a critical care unit is appropriate. Supporting the patient throughout the initial work-up and initiation of treatment to relieve the obstruction is the primary focus of the critical care nurse.

Pathophysiology

The superior vena cava is located in the superior mediastinum and is surrounded by solid structures including the trachea, vertebral bodies, sternum, and lymph nodes. As a thin walled, low-pressure vessel, the superior vena cava is particularly vulnerable to compression. Benign as well as malignant causes contribute to the development of this complication. Benign causes usually occlude the vessel by extrinsic pressure, whereas malignant diseases occlude the vessel by extrinsic pressure or direct invasion (Simpson et al, 1981). A third cause of SVCS is intraluminal thrombosis. Central venous catheters and even pacemakers have been associated with the development of this complication. A central venous catheter will irritate the wall of the vein, causing local injury and thrombus formation. The pacemaker may stimulate an inflammatory reaction and tissue fibrosis, which may contribute to the development of an obstruction near the right atrium (Sculier and Feld, 1985).

A significant obstruction of the superior vena cava will interfere with the return of blood from the head, neck, upper extremities, and upper thorax. Other routes or vessels are used to bypass the obstruction and return the blood to the heart. The development of this collateral circulation depends upon the location of the obstruction. If the obstruction of the superior vena cava has occurred above the azygos vein, the blood flow will return to the heart through the subclavian vein and proximal superior vena cava. An obstruction proximal to the superior vena cava–azygos vein junction will result in blood flow being redirected through the inferior vena cava. Most problematic is the obstruction that occurs directly at this junction. More distal routes must be utilized and collateral channels developed to assist in the return of the blood from the upper torso back to the heart (Miller, 1987). It is in these obstructions that the more dramatic and classic signs and symptoms of SVCS occur.

Clinical Presentation

The clinical manifestations of SVCS are the result of increased venous pressure and stasis of blood flow. The developing signs and symptoms are reflective of the vascular congestion in the cerebrum, pulmonary complications, and thrombogenic sequelae (Miller, 1987). Clinical symptoms include dyspnea (43%), cough (20%), and chest pain (20%). Dysphagia, visual disturbances, hoarseness, dizziness, and a feeling of facial fullness are also frequently reported. Among the physical findings are prominent collateral veins of the upper thorax, including the distention of the thoracic veins (67%), and neck vein distention. As shown in Figures 64–2 and 64–3, tachypnea, facial swelling, swelling of the upper torso, plethora of the face, edema of the conjunctivae, and increased jugular venous pressure are also observed (Simpson et al, 1981; Miller, 1987). These symptoms worsen when the patient is recumbent. Left untreated, SVCS can progress into laryngeal edema; severe upper airway obstruction; cyanosis of the upper body due to venous stasis; and altered consciousness, including coma (Miller, 1987).

Medical Management

The medical management of SVCS includes disease management, resolution of the obstruction, and application of comfort measures.

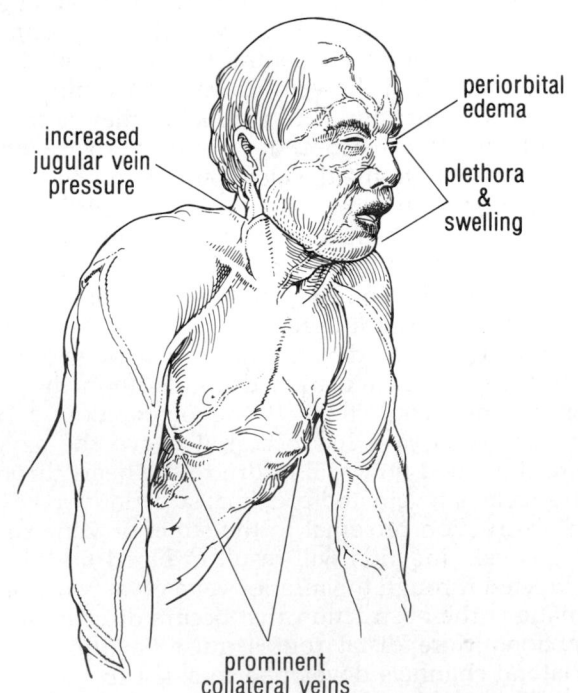

FIGURE 64–2. Signs of superior vena cava obstruction. (From Miller, S.E. (1987). Super vena cava syndrome. In R.C. Polomano and S.E. Miller (Eds.), *Understanding and managing oncologic emergencies* (p. 28). Adria Laboratories, Division of Erbamont Inc.)

DIAGNOSIS

Patients who present with SVCS may or may not have a previous cancer diagnosis. Because up to 90% of all cases are associated with a malignant disease, of which bronchogenic carcinoma is most prevalent, medical attention will be directed toward obtaining an accurate diagnosis. Diagnostic proceedings usually are concentrated on obtaining a tissue biopsy specimen. In addition to tissue diagnosis, sputum cytology, bronchoscopy, transbronchial biopsy, percutaneous biopsy, cervical mediastinal exploration, and thoracotomy may also be performed (Simpson et al, 1981). A chest x-ray will show a mediastinal widening, a mass, distention of the azygous vein, or associated pleural effusion (Miller, 1987). After an accurate tissue diagnosis has been made, appropriate treatment for the underlying disease may begin.

Controversy surrounds the issue of establishing a tissue diagnosis in patients presenting with SVCS. Traditional practice has been to treat the worrisome complication and reduce the severity of obstruction before obtaining biopsy specimens. In addition, patients were considered at high risk for bleeding if invasive procedures were conducted. However, current literature suggests that diagnostic procedures can be conducted safely in the presence of SVCS. Mortality is considered to be more directly attributed to the underlying disease rather than to the complication itself (Ahmann, 1984).

DISEASE MANAGEMENT

Radiation therapy is the treatment of choice for SVCS. Generous chest portals, including the mediastinum hila and any adjacent pulmonary lesions, are irradiated. The total dose of irradiation usually reaches 4000 to 5000 rad fractionated into daily treatments of 180 to 200 rad. Total irradiation doses may reach 6000 rad. Subjective relief of symptoms may be experienced 3 to 4 days after the first dose of radiation (Simpson et al, 1981; Miller, 1987).

As radiation treatments continue, the patient will experience adverse effects as the underlying tissues become damaged. Esophagitis, dysphagia, hoarseness, dry cough, loss of appetite, and lethargy occur. Although most of these adverse effects resolve after treatment is completed, they are nevertheless distressful to the patient.

Chemotherapy is a useful treatment for SVCS if the underlying disease is small cell carcinoma of the lung or lymphomas (Simpson et al, 1981; Miller, 1987). These malignancies are very responsive to the effects of chemotherapy, and the patient will experience rapid relief of the symptoms. Following the administration of chemotherapy, radiation treatment may or may not be needed for further control of the disease.

Anticoagulants and fibrinolytic therapy are appropriate treatments if the underlying cause of the complication is thrombosis, as seen with the use of

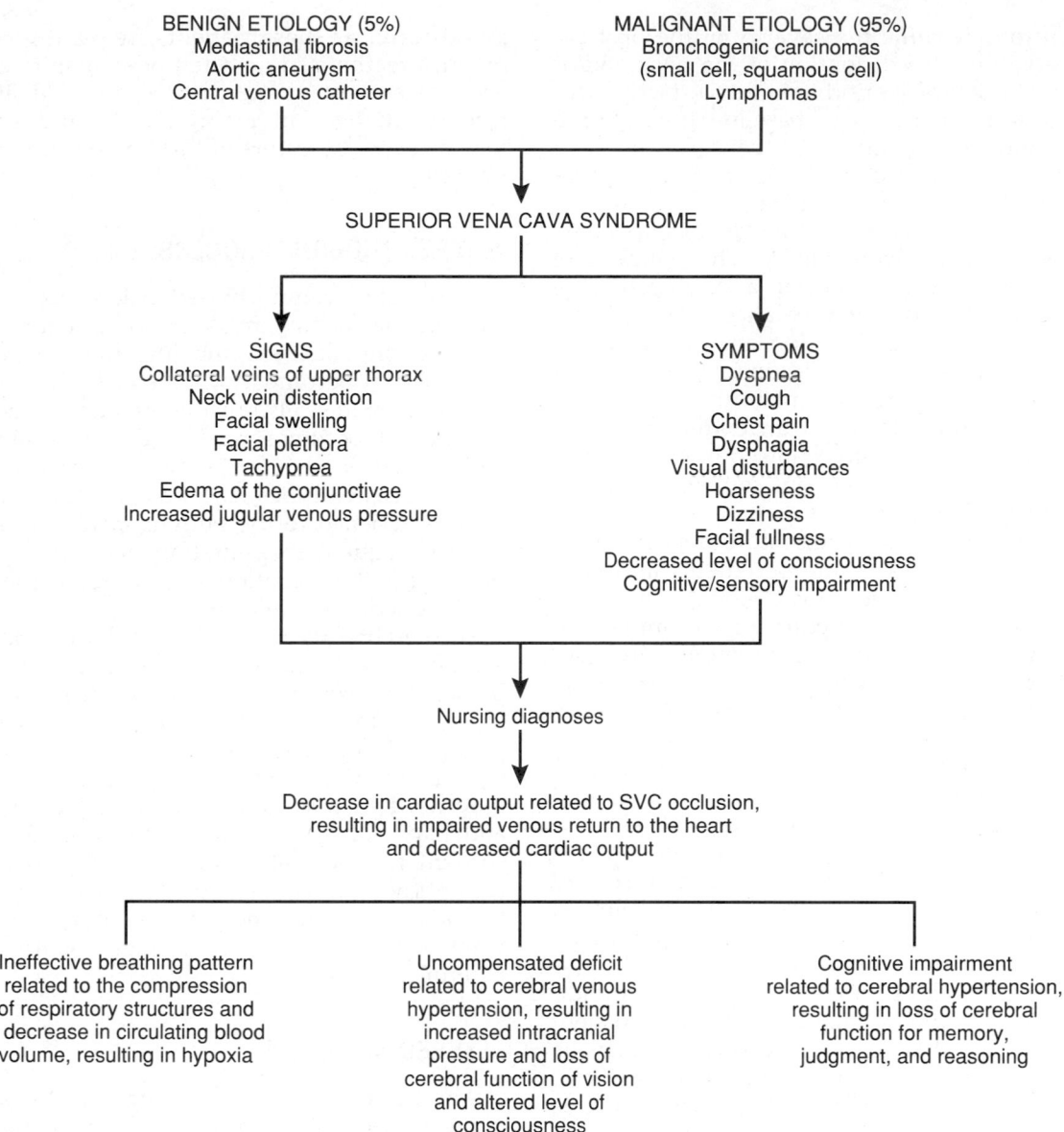

BENIGN ETIOLOGY (5%)
Mediastinal fibrosis
Aortic aneurysm
Central venous catheter

MALIGNANT ETIOLOGY (95%)
Bronchogenic carcinomas
(small cell, squamous cell)
Lymphomas

SUPERIOR VENA CAVA SYNDROME

SIGNS
Collateral veins of upper thorax
Neck vein distention
Facial swelling
Facial plethora
Tachypnea
Edema of the conjunctivae
Increased jugular venous pressure

SYMPTOMS
Dyspnea
Cough
Chest pain
Dysphagia
Visual disturbances
Hoarseness
Dizziness
Facial fullness
Decreased level of consciousness
Cognitive/sensory impairment

Nursing diagnoses

Decrease in cardiac output related to SVC occlusion,
resulting in impaired venous return to the heart
and decreased cardiac output

Ineffective breathing pattern
related to the compression
of respiratory structures and
a decrease in circulating blood
volume, resulting in hypoxia

Uncompensated deficit
related to cerebral venous
hypertension, resulting in
increased intracranial
pressure and loss of
cerebral function of vision
and altered level of
consciousness

Cognitive impairment
related to cerebral hypertension,
resulting in loss of cerebral
function for memory,
judgment, and reasoning

FIGURE 64–3. Superior vena cava syndrome.

central venous catheters. Removal of the catheter may be required. The literature has reported surgical bypass procedures using Dacron prosthesis or the patient's own saphenous vein (Sculier and Feld, 1985; Miller, 1987).

SYMPTOM MANAGEMENT

Supportive therapy promotes comfort and helps reduce the patient's level of distress. Diuretics may be used to reduce edema, but they must be used with caution. Diuretic induced dehydration may potentiate thrombus formation or the development of hypovolemic shock (Varricchio, 1985). Steroids may be appropriately prescribed if the patient exhibits respiratory insufficiency. Supplemental oxygen may be indicated for dyspnea (Miller, 1987).

Nursing Management

Nursing care of the patient diagnosed with SVCS focuses on symptom management and the prevention of acute complications. Though not the life-threatening complication it was originally believed to be, SVCS requires an intensive nursing approach to the management of the distressful signs and symptoms that the patient may experience (Ahmann, 1984).

DECREASED CARDIAC OUTPUT

As presented in Figure 64–3, obstruction of the superior vena cava results in impaired venous return to the heart and decreased cardiac output. The critical care nurse conducts an initial physical assessment of the patient to determine the severity of the obstruction. Observations for distention of the neck and/or chest veins, facial and periorbital edema, tachypnea, and cyanosis are made. The baseline findings are recorded, and the observations continue every 4 hours throughout the acute phase of this complication (Chernecky and Ramsey, 1984).

A decrease in cardiac output makes these patients susceptible to hypovolemic shock. The critical care nurse monitors the urinary output and calculates the intake:output ratio for fluid balance. The maintenance of an intravenous infusion ensures adequate hydration of the patient in addition to providing a vascular route for emergency medications. It is important for the nurse to select an extremity whose circulation has not been compromised by the obstruction before insertion of the venous catheter. In severe cases of SVCS, the location of a site for the venous catheter may become quite difficult to determine.

Central venous pressure measurements and neck vein distention measured in centimeters help the critical care nurse assess the patient's current cardiovascular condition. These measurements are conducted every 1 to 2 hours (Chernecky and Ramsey, 1984). To detect the early development of circulatory problems, the peripheral pulses are assessed for bilateral quality and the nailbeds tested for blanching. The skin is assessed for color, temperature, and moisture. The head of the bed is kept at 45 to 60 degrees to promote the return of the blood to the heart and to prevent further edema (Spross and Stern, 1979). Bedrest is essential, as even minimal activity may overtax the cardiovascular system's ability to meet the increased need for oxygen.

A change in the level of consciousness is an indication of failing cardiovascular function in the patient with SVCS. The change in consciousness may be due, in part, to cerebral hypertension (Varricchio, 1985). With this in mind, the critical care nurse is required to assess all possible causes of the presenting signs and symptoms and plan nursing interventions accordingly.

INEFFECTIVE BREATHING PATTERN

The compression of respiratory structures by growing or bulky tumors and the decrease in circulating blood volume result in hypoxia. Bedrest, high Fowler position, and minimal activity are nursing measures that conserve the patient's need for oxygen (Spross and Stern, 1979). In addition, the critical care nurse frequently assesses breath sounds for the early detection of adventitious sounds. With each patient contact, it is also important to assess for dyspnea and respiratory distress and to initiate supplemental oxygen at 2 liters/minute or as prescribed. The critical care nurse supplements the physical assessments by monitoring arterial blood gas values and adjusting the patient's nursing plan of care as indicated (Chernecky and Ramsey, 1984).

Other nursing interventions include meticulous mouth care, as these patients frequently convert to mouth breathing in an attempt to inspire additional air. Assessment of the client's voice quality is performed; changes in pitch, clarity, and hoarseness may be early indicators of further compression of the trachea.

ALTERED THOUGHT PROCESSES

The cerebral venous hypertension and oxygen deprivation that occurs in SVCS account for an altered level of consciousness and impaired vision. Patient safety issues become a prime concern for the critical care nurse. Side rails must be up and padded in case the patient becomes restless and disoriented. The patient may inadvertently damage intravenous tubing, nasogastric tubes, endotracheal tubes, and other devices attached to the body or bed. These patients require frequent reorientation from the critical care nurse and the initiation of protective measures to prevent accidental injuries.

The cerebral hypertension results in a loss of cerebral function for memory, judgment, and reasoning. Before all procedures, the critical care nurse will need to explain the purpose and technique in terms the patient will understand. Simple commands may be difficult for the patient to understand. The patient may need to have information frequently repeated and may not be able to reliably provide informed consent for medical treatments. It is essential that the critical care nurse be able to assist the family with bedside visits and meetings with the health care team so that a mutually beneficial plan of care can be implemented.

ALTERED NUTRITION

Another nursing care problem in SVCS is inadequate nutritional support. The patient may be too breathless to eat or may experience difficulty in swallowing. Malignant disease and the patient's increased breathing activity require additional sources of nutrition if a positive nitrogen balance is to be maintained. If oral nutritional support is inadequate, tube feedings usually are implemented. The critical care nurse is responsible for maintaining the feedings, supplementing them with water to maintain hydration, and monitoring for any adverse effects from the feedings. Depending on the type of adverse effect, the nurse modifies the formula or rate of infusion so that the feedings can continue.

PAIN

Pain management is important for the patient with SVCS. High doses of narcotics may depress the respiratory rate or further impair the senses. Therefore, the critical care nurse carefully assesses the patient's degree of pain before administering narcotics. A low dose of narcotics plus other comfort measures may be all that is needed to provide the patient with adequate pain relief.

CAROTID ARTERY RUPTURE

Carotid artery rupture is a complication associated with head and neck cancers. A 1980 study reported that carotid artery rupture was the mechanism of death in 11% of patients with advanced head and neck cancer (Shedd et al, 1980). Improved surgical techniques and modified irradiation protocols may help reduce the incidence of this devastating complication.

Pathophysiology

The common carotid arteries supply nearly all the blood to the head and neck. As each carotid artery nears the level of the thyroid cartilage, it bifurcates into the internal and external carotid arteries. The internal carotid enters the skull, where it branches out and supplies blood to the brain. The external carotid artery has 11 different branches, which supply blood to the face, jaw, and scalp (Kane, 1983).

The arteries are composed of three layers: the intima, the media, and the adventitia. The outer layer, the adventitia, supports and gives shape to the vessel. The middle layer, the media, regulates the diameter of the vessel. The inner coat, the intima, provides a smooth passageway for blood (Bullock, 1984; Kane, 1983).

The carotid artery may become exposed to the drying effects of the atmosphere during radical head and neck operative procedures. The integrity of the carotid artery is also threatened as the result of infection, formation of fistulas, or skin necrosis. Destruction of the outer wall of the artery may begin 6 to 10 days following injury and is manifested by eschar formation. Eventually the eschar sloughs off, exposing the inner medial layer. As the process of eschar formation and eschar sloughing continues, the fragile inner or intima layer becomes exposed (Keith, 1979).

Contributing to poor local wound healing in the head and neck cancer patient are the continuous growth of the tumor, poor nutritional status, local tissue damage from previous irradiation, disruption of normal local blood supply due to the radical dissection of tissue, and infection (Kane, 1983).

Clinical Presentation

Patients at risk for carotid artery rupture are those who demonstrate poor local wound healing, are in overall poor health, and have had a radical neck dissection. Local signs that suggest a high risk for carotid artery rupture are listed in Table 64–4. There are only two known possible forewarnings of carotid

TABLE 64–4. Local Signs Suggestive of High Risk for Carotid Artery Rupture

Pale or black skin color
Unilateral temperature change (cool)
Presence or increase of edema
Increase in size and shape of the wound
Changes in the type, amount, or odor of drainage
Evidence of bleeding, pulsations, or arterial exposure

artery rupture. Patients may complain of sternal or high epigastric pain several hours before the event. In some cases, a small bleed may be noted at the wound site 24 to 48 hours before the rupture (Kane, 1983).

Medical Management

Expert surgical technique minimizes the time the carotid artery is exposed to the atmosphere. The use of reconstructive skin flaps to cover the wide defect created by the removal of the malignant tumor provides a protective barrier over the vulnerable carotid artery (Keith, 1979).

Maintenance of a viable skin flap is the key in protecting the artery from exposure. A wound drain is inserted at the time of closure to keep the flap free of pressure. The site is protected from drying with a fine mesh petroleum gauze. The patient's head may have to be immobilized to prevent pulling and tension on the healing wound and skin flap (Keith, 1979).

If the wound is draining, the dressings are changed frequently to reduce bacterial growth (Kane, 1983). The site is assessed for drainage, redness, and swelling, which indicate local infection. Cultures of the drainage are obtained, and antibiotic therapy is initiated. The dressing is replaced with a petroleum impregnated gauze to keep the wound moist.

If the flap shows signs of necrosis, débridement is initiated. Débridement is conducted carefully by the surgeon because of the relative closeness of the underlying carotid (Keith, 1979).

If the carotid artery does rupture, there are two choices of medical intervention. The first choice is to intervene aggressively by applying pressure to the bleeding site, maintaining the airway, and replacing fluid volume. The patient is taken to the operating room for emergency ligation of the bleeding artery. The second choice is to support the patient compassionately through this terminal event. All members of the health care team as well as the patient and family should be aware of the risk of bleeding. The treatment of choice must be predetermined by discussion between the health care team, the patient and family members. Even when aggressive treatment is initiated, mortality rates may be as high as 46% (Coleman, 1985).

Nursing Management

Nursing interventions are primarily focused on prevention of carotid artery injury. Preplanned protocols must be in place should a bleed occur.

IMPAIRED SKIN INTEGRITY

A dry, edematous, infected wound is more likely to expose the carotid artery. To prevent this from occurring, the critical care nurse performs gentle, meticulous dressing changes. Old dressings are removed carefully so as not to disturb the fragile healing tissue. Normal saline may help loosen old dressings. The amount of drainage determines the frequency of dressing changes. A large amount of drainage may require a dressing change every 8 hours in order to reduce the bacterial growth. Dressings are reapplied following aseptic technique using petroleum impregnated gauze. Occlusive dressings promote the growth of yeast and fungus and are inappropriate for this situation.

POTENTIAL FOR INJURY

Internal pressure may threaten the integrity of the fragile carotid artery. To prevent a rise in internal pressure, the critical care nurse restricts the patient's activity in several areas.

The critical care nurse instructs the patient in alternative pulmonary exercises, including deep, sustained inhalations. Deep coughing and the strenuous use of the thoracic muscles in respiratory movements are avoided because they generate high intrathoracic pressures. Nasotracheal or tracheal or oral-pharyngeal suction may be the chosen treatment to remove pulmonary secretions rather than forceful coughing (Kane, 1983).

The critical care nurse also implements a bowel program to prevent constipation, since the stress and straining of defecation can raise the intrathoracic pressure. This pressure can rupture the fragile carotid artery. If the patient is able to eat, a fiber-rich diet is indicated. Stool softeners and plenty of fluids will help maintain adequate elimination.

Vomiting raises the intra-abdominal pressure, which in turn increases the intrathoracic pressure. Controlling vomiting and preventing further epi-

sodes through the administration of antiemetics become part of the critical care nursing plan.

FLUID VOLUME DEFICIT

If carotid artery rupture does occur, the nursing actions will be either aggressive or supportive.

If aggressive management is preplanned, the critical care nurse will have maintained a large-bore needle kept open to a continuous infusion. Several units of typed and cross-matched blood are kept readily available in the blood bank (Kane, 1985).

Upon discovery of the ruptured carotid artery, the critical care nurse immediately applies pressure to the area and signals for assistance. The airway is maintained by inserting an oral airway or, if a cuffed tracheostomy tube is in place, the tracheostomy cuff is inflated to prevent aspiration of blood. The airway is suctioned free, and oxygen is administered. Maintaining an open airway in the presence of hemorrhage may not always be possible.

The patient is placed in the Trendelenburg position. Vital signs are obtained frequently throughout the emergency. The cardiovascular status is stabilized through the rapid infusion of intravenous fluids and the administration of blood. As the patient is prepared for emergency surgery for ligation of the vessel, the patient and family will require comforting. By acting in a calm, organized manner, the nurse reassures the patient and family that all that can be done is being done (Kane, 1985).

ANTICIPATORY GRIEVING

Supportive management of carotid artery rupture is much different (Kane, 1983). Airway maintenance is attempted by inflating the tracheostomy cuff or by turning the patient's head to the side and suctioning the oral cavity free of blood. An oral airway is usually not inserted. The free flowing blood is absorbed with gauze or towels.

The nurse remains with the patient and gives family members the opportunity to leave or stay as they wish. Emotional support is provided to the patient and to the family throughout the frightening experience. Morphine is often given to the patient in this situation because it diminishes attention and anxiety (Kane, 1983). The nurse remains with the patient throughout the terminal process.

ncp nursing care plan

1. Acute pain related to:
Destruction of the spinal column and damage to the spinal cord

Outcome Criteria	Nursing Interventions
Patient will state an increase in comfort.	Assess the patient for pain with each contact and record the location, severity, and characteristics of the pain. Manage pain using an effective analgesic protocol. Assist patient in achieving a position of comfort if not in direct conflict with maintaining a stable spinal position. Provide a quiet environment, behavioral technique, or soothing touches if positioning for comfort is contraindicated.

2. Impaired physical mobility related to:
Upper or lower motor neuron damage secondary to spinal cord compression

Outcome Criteria	Nursing Interventions
Deterioration in patient's neurologic status will be detected quickly. Further injury to spinal cord will not occur. Injuries due to immobility will not occur.	Conduct neurologic assessments every 1 to 2 hours and compare with baseline findings. Observe for presence of muscle atrophy, fasciculations, involuntary movement, lack of voluntary movement, and abnormal positions. Evaluate the need for a Stryker frame or other position-maintaining bed. Ensure that spinal alignment is maintained during turning and positioning of patient. Maintain ideal spinal alignment by avoiding the use of pillows and by placing a footboard at the end of the bed. Provide respiratory exercises and initiate a skin care protocol. Perform range of motion exercises if possible.

3. Potential for impaired skin integrity related to:
Loss of sensory and motor function and immobilization

Outcome Criteria	Nursing Interventions
Patient's skin will remain intact.	Assess skin status every 2 hours, paying special attention to bony prominences and areas of pressure. Massage areas of greatest pressure. Pad pressure points. Keep patient and bedding clean and dry. Collaborate with the dietitian to identify effective means of maintaining nutritional status.

4. Ineffective breathing pattern related to:
Spinal cord lesions

Outcome Criteria	Nursing Interventions
Patient will be free of respiratory complications.	Assess the patient's ability to ventilate satisfactorily by monitoring respiratory patterns, signs and symptoms of respiratory insufficiency, arterial blood gases, and lung sounds. Monitor patient's vital capacity using bedside spirometry.

5. Alteration in bowel elimination related to:
Loss of voluntary control, sphincter dysfunction, and paralytic ileus

Outcome Criteria	Nursing Interventions
Bowel routine will remain within baseline.	Assess for signs and symptoms of paralytic ileus and impaction upon admission. Assess for abdominal distention, decreased or absent bowel sounds, nausea or vomiting. Begin intestinal decompression if a paralytic ileus is suspected. Initiate a daily bowel evacuation program. Consider gentle manual removal of rectal contents or an enema until rectal reflexes return. Withhold oral intake until bowel sounds and the passing of flatus have returned. Maintain nutritional support through alternative feeding routes such as total parenteral nutrition.

6. Urinary retention related to:
Loss of voluntary bladder elimination

Nursing Care Plan continued on following page

Outcome Criteria	Nursing Interventions
Urinary elimination will return to baseline.	Maintain an indwelling urinary catheter. Monitor temperature trends and the characteristics of the urine for signs and symptoms of infection. Initiate intermittent catheterizations to check for residual urine in preparation for bladder retraining. Assess for bladder distention between catheterization. Offer the urinal or bedpan at regular intervals.

7. Decreased cardiac output related to:
   Spinal shock

Outcome Criteria	Nursing Interventions
Bradycardia, dysrhythmias, and hypotension will not occur.	Monitor the patient's cardiac rate and rhythm. Monitor blood pressure before and after turning. Maintain circulatory fluid volume through cautious use of intravenous fluids. Carefully monitor the patient for the development of pulmonary edema throughout volume replacement. Maintain patient's body temperature through use of blankets, a heating blanket, or a cooling blanket. Assess the condition of the patient's skin and the functioning of the equipment used to maintain body temperature.

8. Decreased cardiac output related to:
   Impaired venous return secondary to superior vena cava syndrome

Outcome Criteria	Nursing Interventions
Patient will not experience hypovolemic shock.	Conduct an initial assessment to determine the severity of the obstruction. Observe for distention of the neck and/or chest veins, facial and periorbital edema, tachypnea, and cyanosis. Record baseline findings and assess every 4 hours throughout acute phase. Monitor urinary output and calculate the intake:output ratio for fluid balance. Maintain an intravenous infusion for hydration and vascular access. Monitor central venous pressure and measure neck vein distention in centimeters every 1 to 2 hours. Assess peripheral pulses for bilateral quality and test nailbeds for blanching. Assess skin for color, temperature, and moisture. Keep the head of the bed at 45 to 60 degrees. Ensure patient complies with bedrest and minimal activity. Assess all possible causes of changes in consciousness.

9. Ineffective breathing pattern related to:
   Compression of respiratory structures by growing or bulky tumors and decreased circulating blood volume.

Outcome Criteria	Nursing Interventions
Patient will not experience hypoxia.	Conserve the oxygen demand by ensuring bedrest, high Fowler position, and minimal activity. Frequently assess breath sounds. Assess for dyspnea and respiratory distress with each patient contact. Administer oxygen as prescribed. Monitor arterial blood gas values and adjust the nursing plan of care as indicated. Provide meticulous mouth care. Assess patient's voice for changes in pitch, clarity, and hoarseness.

10. Altered thought processes related to:
   Cerebral venous hypertension and oxygen deprivation

Outcome Criteria	Nursing Interventions
Patient will be free of injury.	Place side rails up and provide padding. Frequently reorient the patient and initiate protective measures to prevent accidental injuries from intravenous tubes, nasogastric tubes, endotracheal tubes, and other devices attached to the body or bed. Explain the purpose and technique of all procedures prior to performing. Frequently repeat information as necessary. Assist the family with bedside visits and meetings with the health care team so that mutually beneficial plan of care can be implemented.

11. Altered nutrition related to:
   Dysphagia or respiratory distress

Outcome Criteria	Nursing Interventions
If oral nutritional support is inadequate, implement tube feedings. Supplement tube feedings with water to maintain hydration and monitor for any adverse effects from the feedings. Modify the formula or rate as necessary.	

12. Pain related to:
   Superior vena cava syndrome

Outcome Criteria	Nursing Interventions
Patient will state an increase in comfort.	Carefully assess patient's degree of pain prior to the administration of narcotics. Consider the smallest effective dose of narcotics to prevent respiratory depression or further impairment of the senses.

13. Impaired skin integrity related to:
   Surgical incision, poor local wound healing

Outcome Criteria	Nursing Interventions
A dry, edematous, or infected wound will be prevented.	Perform gentle, meticulous dressing changes. Remove old dressings carefully, using normal saline if necessary. Change dressing every 8 hours or as needed. Reapply dressings following aseptic technique and petroleum-impregnated gauze. Avoid occlusive dressings.

14. Potential for injury related to:
   Internal carotid pressure

Outcome Criteria	Nursing Interventions
A rise in internal pressure will be prevented.	Instruct the patient in alternative pulmonary exercises including deep, sustained inhalations. Avoid deep coughing and strenuous use of the thoracic muscles. Remove pulmonary secretions through nasotracheal, tracheal, or oral-pharyngeal suction rather than forceful coughing. Implement a bowel program to prevent the stress and strain of defecation. Provide a fiber-rich diet, stool softeners, and plenty of fluids. Administer antiemetics to control vomiting as necessary.

15. Fluid volume deficit related to:
   Carotid artery rupture with aggressive management

Outcome Criteria	Nursing Interventions
Rupture will be quickly detected and patient will remain viable throughout preparations for surgery.	Keep several units of typed and crossmatched blood readily available. Upon discovery of carotid artery rupture, immediately apply pressure to the area and signal for assistance. Maintain an airway by inserting an oral airway or inflate the tracheostomy cuff if applicable to prevent aspiration. Suction airway and administer oxygen. Place patient in Trendelenburg position. Obtain vital signs frequently throughout the emergency. Stabilize the cardiovascular status through the rapid infusion of intravenous fluids and the administration of blood. Provide comfort for the patient and family as the patient is prepared for emergency surgery. Calmly reassure patient and family that all possible interventions are being performed.

16. Anticipatory grieving related to:
   Carotid artery rupture with supportive management only

Outcome Criteria	Nursing Interventions
Patient will remain comfortable to a peaceful death. Family will receive emotional support.	Attempt to maintain airway by inflating tracheostomy cuff or by turning the patient's head to the side and suctioning the oral cavity free of blood. Absorb the free flowing blood with gauze or towels. Remain with the patient and give family members the opportunity to leave or stay with the patient as they wish. Provide emotional support to the family. Administer morphine to the patient.

SUMMARY

Oncologic emergencies are critical events that complicate the course of cancer treatment and rehabilitation. They are frequently viewed as setbacks and are discouraging, frustrating experiences for the patient and family as well as the health care provider. Regardless of the patient's prognosis or chance for cure or remission, oncologic emergencies are usually treated aggressively to preserve some semblance of quality of life.

Unless one personally experiences cancer, it is difficult to understand why one would submit to such aggressive treatment in light of a progressing disease. Knowing that the patient and/or family have opted for this treatment, the nurse must support the patient and the family through the crisis with the best professional, technical, and compassionate nursing care.

References

Abernathy, E. (1987). Biotherapy: An introductory overview. *Oncology Nursing Forum*, 14 (6) (Suppl.), 13–15.

Ahmann, F. R. (1984). A reassessment of the clinical implications of the superior vena caval syndrome. *Journal of Clinical Oncology*, 2 (8), 961–969.

Bullock, B. L. (1984). Normal circulatory dynamics. In B. L. Bullock and P. P. Rosendahl (Eds.), *Pathophysiology: Adaptations and alterations in function*. Boston: Little, Brown.

Bruckman, J. E., and Bloomer, W. D. (1981). Management of spinal cord compression. In J. W. Yarbro and R. S. Bornstein (Eds.), *Oncologic emergencies*. New York: Grune & Stratton.

Chernecky, C. C., and Ramsey, P. W. (1984). Critical nursing care of the client with cancer. E. Norwalk, CT: Appleton-Century-Crofts.

Coleman, J. J. (1985). Treatment of the ruptured or exposed carotid artery: A rational approach. *Southern Medical Journal*, 78 (3), 262–267.

Couillard-Getreuer, D. L. (1985). Spinal cord compression. In B. L. Johnson and J. Gross (Eds.), *Handbook of oncology nursing*. Bethany, CT: Fleschner.

Fidler, I. J., and Hart, I. R. (1982). Principles of cancer biology: Biology of cancer metastasis. In V. T. DeVita, Jr., S. Hellman, and S. A. Rosenberg (Eds.), *Cancer: Principles and practice of oncology*. Philadelphia: J. B. Lippincott.

Henze, R. (1984). Normal structure and function of the central and peripheral nervous systems. In B. L. Bullock and P. P. Rosendahl (Eds.), *Pathophysiology: Adaptations and alterations in function*. Boston: Little, Brown.

Hupchella, C. E., and Burton, R. M. (1988). Cellular biology of cancer. In B. L. Groenwald (Ed.), *Cancer nursing: Principles and practices*. Boston: Jones and Bartlett.

Irwin, M. M. (1987). Patients receiving biological response modifiers: Overview of nursing care. *Oncology Nursing Forum*, 14 (6) (Suppl.), 32–37.

Jassak, P. F., and Sticklin, L. A. (1986). Interleukin-2: An overview. *Oncology Nursing Forum*, 13 (6), 17–22.

Kane, K. K. (1983). Carotid artery rupture in advanced head and neck cancer patients. *Oncology Nursing Forum*, 10 (1), 14–18.

Kane, K. K. (1985). Infiltrative emergencies. In B. L. Johnson and J. Gross (Eds.), *Handbook of oncology nursing*. Bethany, CT: Fleschner.

Keith, C. F. (1979). Wound management following head and neck surgery. *Nursing Clinics of North America*, 14 (4), 761–778.

Kornblith, P. L., and Cassady J. R. (1985). Central nervous system emergencies. In V. T. DeVita, Jr., S. Hellman and S. A. Rosenberg (Eds.), *Cancer: Principles and practice of oncology* (2nd ed.). New York: J. B. Lippincott.

Miller, S. E. (1987). Superior vena cava syndrome. In R. C. Polomano and S. E. Miller (Eds.), *Understanding and managing oncologic emergencies*. Columbus, OH: Adria Laboratories.

Mitchell, P. H. (1981). Neurologic disorders. In M. R. Kinney, C. B. Dear and D. P. Packa (Eds.), *AACN's clinical reference for critical-care nursing*. New York: McGraw-Hill.

Oncology Nursing Society. (1989). *Biological response modifiers*. Pittsburgh.

Sculier, J. B., and Feld, R. (1985). Superior vena cava obstruction syndrome: Recommendations for management. *Cancer Treatment Reviews*, 12, 209–218.

Shedd, D. P., Carl, A., and Schedd, C. (1980). Problems of terminal head and neck cancer patients. *Head and Neck Surgery*, 2, (6), 476–481.

Simpson, J. R., Perez, C. A., Presant, C. A., and Van Amburg, A. L. (1981). Superior vena cava syndrome. In J. W. Yarbro and R. S. Bornstein (Eds.), *Oncologic emergencies*. New York: Grune & Stratton.

Spross, J., and Stern, R. (1979). Nursing management of oncology patients with superior vena cava obstruction syndrome. *Oncology Nursing Forum*, 6 (3), 3–5.

Upton, A. C. (1982). Principles of cancer biology: Etiology and prevention of cancer. In V. T. DeVita, Jr., S. Hellman, and S. A. Rosenberg (Eds.), *Cancer: Principles and practice of oncology*. Philadelphia: J. B. Lippincott.

Varricchio, C. (1985). Clinical management of superior vena cava syndrome. *Heart & Lung*, 14, (4), 411–416.

65

Elderly Patients

Teresa L. Britt

The segment of the United States' population that is 65 years and older is growing at an unprecedented rate. By the year 2050, an average of one out of every three persons is expected to be 55 years or older and one in five will be over age 65 (U.S. Senate Special Committee on Aging, 1985–1986). The 85-plus age group is the fastest growing segment of the population. Between 1980 and 2050, it is estimated that this age group will increase seven times (U.S. Senate Special Committee on Aging, 1985–1986).

The elderly constitute the most cost-intensive health consumer group. Older adults account for 29% of all hospital discharges and one-third of the country's personal care expenditures, although they constitute only 11% of the total population (U.S. Senate Special Committee on Aging, 1985–1986). In a study on elderly patients in intensive care units, it was found that 24.1% of the patients admitted to critical care units (n = 792) were 65 and older (Nicolas et al., 1987). As people age, changes occur in multiple body systems, increasing the complexity of care required.

Elderly persons present a growing challenge to the critical care nurse, not only in terms of these compelling demographics, but also due to the sophistication of knowledge required to provide comprehensive nursing care for this special population. This chapter presents an overview of age-related changes in the older adult. Specific clinical implications for critical care nursing are discussed.

SYSTEMS OVERVIEW OF AGE-RELATED CHANGES

Aging represents a new frontier for research and practice. The research literature contains much debate regarding the "normal" changes of aging. Until recently, very little research was done regarding the process of aging. Part of the reason for the dearth of available research is the fact that people are now living to much older ages than in the past. Coupled with the increased longevity of older adults is the fact that increased control over infectious disease, improved nutrition, and generally more favorable economic conditions have tended to diminish problems once thought to be normal consequences of aging. Exactly what constitutes normal aging is still in the process of being defined. Thus, the term "age-related changes" is used throughout this chapter.

There is general consensus that the organ systems age at different rates. This is, of course, influenced considerably by genetic predisposition, nutritional status, physical conditioning, environmental exposures, and physical and/or psychological challenges. The diversity of the elderly population has made rigorous research into age-related changes difficult. Technologic and methodologic advances as well as the use of animal models have provided some inroads to better understanding physiologic changes.

The Cardiovascular System

Although heart disease continues to be the leading cause of death among older adults, it should be recognized that these diseases represent pathology, not age-related changes (U.S. Senate Special Committee on Aging, 1985–1986). The aging process does create a milieu in which pathophysiologic changes may occur, especially if the individual has a predisposing risk.

Several significant changes occur in the cardiovascular system during the aging process. The three most important include alterations in blood pressure, decreased myocardial function, and diminished baroreceptor sensitivity (Rebensen-Piano, 1989). Table 65–1 provides an overview of age-related changes in the cardiovascular system.

TABLE 65–1. Age-Related Changes in the Cardiopulmonary System

Structure	Age-Related Change	Clinical Manifestation
Arterioles	Arteriosclerosis	Decreased arterial compliance
	Atherosclerosis	Hypertension
		Left ventricular hypertrophy
Myocardium	Decreased pumping efficiency	Decreased stroke volume
	Decreased contractile strength	Decreased cardiac output
		Decreased cardiac reserve
Baroreceptors	Decreased receptor sensitivity	Postural hypotension
Lung	Decreased elastic recoil	Increased residual volume
	Decreased chest wall compliance	Impaired alveolar-capillary oxygen diffusion
	Alveolar hyperinflation-destruction	Arterial hypoxemia
	Decreased cilia	Impaired airway clearance
	Decreased cough	
	Diminished alveolar macrophage function	Increased susceptibility to infection

ALTERATIONS IN BLOOD PRESSURE

Arteriosclerosis results in a thickening of the vascular lumen as a consequence of collagen and calcium deposition. Atherosclerosis results from the accumulation of fibrinous products and lipoproteins within blood vessels (Rebensen-Piano, 1989; Ross, 1986). In the elderly, these two processes combine to result in a decreased radius of the arterial lumen and decreased compliance of the large and small vessels (Ross, 1986). Clinically, this means that a small increase in intravascular volume results in a disproportionately large rise in systolic blood pressure and may result in pressure-induced ventricular hypertrophy (Walsh, 1987). Hypertension affects approximately half of the elderly population (Davidson, 1989). In the Framingham Study, hypertensive elderly aged 65 to 74 had a tripled risk of cardiovascular disease, a doubled risk of cardiovascular mortality, and a doubled risk of cardiovascular accidents when compared with normotensive control subjects (Kannel and Gordon, 1978).

Sodium excretion and glomerular filtration rate decrease with advancing age, thus affecting sodium homeostasis. Increased serum sodium concentration results in increased intravascular volume, thus elevating blood pressure (Rose, 1984). Older persons also have a delayed natriuretic response following sodium loading and plasma volume expansion (Luft et al., 1979).

DECREASED MYOCARDIAL FUNCTION

With aging, the pumping efficiency and contractile strength of the heart diminish. The result is a decreased stroke volume and subsequent decrease in cardiac output. The heart rate remains unchanged or may be slightly decreased at rest. Along with the diminished stroke volume, the decrease in heart rate results in a decreased cardiac reserve. Therefore, the elderly patient may not be able to increase cardiac output sufficiently to meet the increased demand for oxygen during periods of stress. Cardiac reaction to stress is slower and the degree of increase in heart rate is also smaller than in a younger adult. The time it takes the heart to recover after stress is also substantially longer in the elderly (Esberger and Hughes, 1989; Yurick et al., 1980).

Under normal circumstances, cardiac performance is not significantly affected by age-related changes. However, in the face of critical illness or surgery, the cardiac reserve may be unable to meet the demands of the body. Congestive heart failure is a common sequela, as the body's compensatory mechanisms attempt to maintain adequate perfusion (Yurick et al., 1980).

Two other important age-related changes occur in the myocardium. The first is a weakened inotropic response to cardiac glycosides (e.g., digitalis) (Lakatta et al., 1975). The second alteration is a decreased inotropic response to endogenous catecholamines. Other studies have demonstrated that the aged heart requires a higher dosage of beta-adrenergic medication to elevate the heart rate (Vestal et al., 1979).

BARORECEPTOR SENSITIVITY

The loss of arterial compliance leads to decreased baroreceptor sensitivity in older adults (Gribbin et al., 1971; Collins, 1980). This decrease in baroreceptor sensitivity results in an increased incidence of postural hypotension after prolonged bedrest (Rebensen-Piano, 1989).

CLINICAL IMPLICATIONS OF AGE-RELATED CARDIOVASCULAR CHANGES

Assessment of the critically ill adult is based on the recognition of the changes in vascular compliance, myocardial function, and baroreceptor sensitivity that occur in the elderly patient. Increased peripheral resistance is manifested as cold, pale hands and feet; slow capillary refill; and weak pedal pulses. Mottling of the extremities may be present. Because the patient's tolerance of cold may be weakened, extra blankets or increases in ambient temperature may be appropriate. Blood samples to determine arterial blood gases (ABGs) may be difficult to draw even though the pulse is easily palpated, due to rigidity and tortuosity of the arteries. Sclerotic changes in the aortic valve lead to diastolic murmurs that are best heard at the base of the heart. The apical heart beat may be displaced due to kyphoscoliosis. There may also be an increase in benign premature beats. Premature ventricular contractions increase with age and occur in 10% of electrocardiograms and in 30% to 40% of Holter monitored elderly patients (Kane et al., 1989). There is controversy regarding whether these premature ventricular beats should be treated.

Decreased Tissue Perfusion. Changes in peripheral resistance and myocardial function may lead to impaired tissue perfusion in the critically ill elderly patient. Also, immobility predisposes the critically ill older adult to reduced tissue perfusion due to an obstruction (e.g., thrombus) in the vasculature (Matteson and McConnell, 1988). Deep vein thrombosis and pulmonary emboli are the leading cause of morbidity and mortality in hospitalized elderly patients (Lee, 1980). The goals of nursing care include obtaining a baseline assessment of the peripheral vasculature and prevention of deep venous thrombosis (DVT) formation. Prevention of dehydration and immobility is important because these factors substantially increase the risk of DVT formation (Matteson and McConnell, 1988). Warning signs of DVT include pain; dependent edema; and cyanosis, pallor, or rubor of the extremity. There may be no clinical warning signs at all; conversely, one-third of the patients exhibiting warning signs have no venous pathology, thus making diagnosis difficult (MacLennan et al., 1984). Treatment consists of medical anticoagulation, pain control, and bedrest. Because elderly people are more sensitive to oral anticoagulants (warfarin sodium), lower doses are usually given. Clotting studies must be monitored carefully (Matteson and McConnell, 1988).

Decreased Cardiac Output. Diminished cardiac reserve and altered response to inotropic medications place the elderly patient at risk of developing congestive heart failure or cardiogenic shock. The aged patient's response to endogenous catecholamines may be manifested as a decreased and slower cardiac response to stress. Because the heart rate may be an unreliable indicator of stress, the nurse observes for other signs such as mental status changes, agitation, and random or purposeless movements.

Nursing goals are centered on optimizing the availability of oxygen to tissues, maximizing cardiovascular function, and minimizing fear and anxiety and making an accurate nursing diagnosis (Bumann and Speltz, 1989; Kelly, 1989). Nursing actions include administering supplemental oxygen and positioning the patient with the head of the bed elevated if blood pressure is stable. The blood pressure, heart rate, and hemodynamic parameters are closely monitored until stable. Urine output is measured hourly, and electrolytes and ABGs are monitored frequently.

Positive inotropic agents (dopamine, dobutamine, calcium chloride) may be administered intravenously as ordered. Beta-adrenergic infusions are carefully

monitored. The nurse anticipates that the elderly patient may require a higher dosage to achieve the desired inotropic effect. Vasodilators may be ordered to decrease preload. The elderly patient's attenuated response to cardiac glycosides must be carefully monitored. Stepwise increases in doses of digitalis preparations should be anticipated.

Loss of baroreceptor sensitivity may lead to dizziness or even fainting when the patient rises after being supine. Prolonged bedrest in the critical care unit further exacerbates this problem. Thus, early ambulation of the elderly patient is extremely important. The goal is to increase the patient's activity level gradually. The patient's response to activity is carefully assessed. Lying, sitting, and standing blood pressure measurements are documented.

The Respiratory System

Age-related changes in the respiratory system can be divided into three categories: structural alterations, defense mechanisms, and respiratory control. These changes do not usually affect the healthy older adult. However, when critical illness is present, these alterations place the elderly patient at risk of developing devastating complications. Age-related changes in the respiratory system are enhanced by factors such as environmental pollution, smoking, and infections. Table 65–1 summarizes the age-related changes that take place in the respiratory system.

STRUCTURAL ALTERATIONS

The elastic recoil of the lung structures lessens with aging (Krumpe et al., 1985). Thus, when the older adult exhales, it is more difficult for the lung to return to its normal resting size (Esberger and Hughes, 1989). This loss of elastic recoil may be due to a generalized decrease in strength of the respiratory muscles (Murray, 1986; Pierson and Hudson, 1981). Chest wall compliance decreases, leading to decreased respiratory excursion (Levitzky, 1984). Kyphosis and increased abdominal girth may also decrease thoracic excursion (Rebensen-Piano, 1989). The result of these changes is a tendency to trap air due to the inability to exhale fully. The total lung capacity remains the same, but the residual volume and the functional residual capacity increase (Levitzky, 1984). The vital capacity is slightly decreased.

In the elderly person, the number of small airways that remain closed during restful breathing increases. Some alveolar tissue is replaced by fibrotic tissue. The decrease in functional alveoli is accompanied by a diminished number of pulmonary capillaries (Pierson and Hudson, 1981). These three mechanical changes make alveolar-capillary diffusion of oxygen more difficult. The arterial oxygenation (Pa_{O_2}) decreases approximately 4 mm Hg per decade. By age 80, the "normal" arterial oxygenation level is

70 mm Hg (Pierson and Hudson, 1981; Sorbini et al., 1968). Carbon dioxide levels and pH remain stable in the healthy older adult. Breath sounds may be decreased in the bases of the lung fields due to decreased lung expansion (Kidd and Murakami, 1987).

DEFENSE MECHANISMS

Cell-mediated immunity and formation of humoral antibodies decline with aging (King and Schwartz, 1982; Pierson and Hudson, 1981). Macrophage activity is less effective, resulting in impaired phagocytic destruction of foreign particles on the alveolar surface (Bowles et al., 1981). Macrophage function is particularly weakened in elderly individuals with a significant smoking history (Matteson and McConnell, 1988).

The volume, force, and flow rate of the cough reflex are diminished in the elderly (Matteson and McConnell, 1988). Older adults have fewer cilia, and the remaining cilia are less functional than in youth. Thus, the movement of particles out of the body is impaired (Bowles et al., 1981). The secretory immunoglobulin A (IgA) is decreased, and its neutralizing effect against viruses is diminished (King and Schwartz, 1982).

RESPIRATORY CONTROL

Ventilation is controlled by centers in the brain that receive and process information from central and peripheral chemoreceptors. The central chemoreceptor is located in the medulla and is responsible for 75% of the response to carbon dioxide (Matteson and McConnell, 1988). That is, it stimulates ventilation in response to increased Pa_{CO_2}, thereby lowering the arterial carbon dioxide level. The central chemoreceptor acts slowly relative to the peripheral chemoreceptors that are located in the carotid bodies and the aorta. The peripheral chemoreceptors respond to a decrease in arterial Pa_{O_2} and pH by increasing ventilation. The peripheral receptors are solely responsible for the increase in ventilation triggered by hypoxemia (King and Schwartz, 1982). Both the central and peripheral chemoreceptors function less effectively in elderly persons (Mauderly, 1981).

CLINICAL IMPLICATIONS OF AGE-RELATED CHANGES IN THE RESPIRATORY SYSTEM

The age-related changes in pulmonary structure, immune defenses, and respiratory control have a number of clinical implications for the critically ill elderly patient. It is important to recognize that the elderly patient's Pa_{O_2} is lower than that of the younger adult. Older patients also respond more gradually to oxygen therapy (Matteson and McConnell, 1988). Therefore, it is essential that oxygen deprivation be identified and treated as quickly as possible so that the patient has the extra time needed to respond.

Ineffective Airway Clearance–Potential for Infection. The loss of cilia, impaired macrophage activity, and diminished cough reflex that occur with aging make the elderly patient more susceptible to respiratory infection. Keeping the airway free of secretions is an important nursing goal for the critically ill elderly patient.

The elderly patient is at risk of retaining secretions due to the decreased cough reflex. An ineffective cough can result in inhalation of secretions that have been incompletely coughed out of the airways. Coughing in a cascade, i.e., several times during exhalation, helps to move secretions up and out of the airway. The older patient may need to be suctioned more frequently because of the diminished cough reflex.

Suctioning and chest physiotherapy are performed after the use of a bronchodilator so that the airways are as open as possible. Because these procedures are often very tiring for elderly patients, they are scheduled to allow for adequate rest periods. If the patient is able to eat, chest physiotherapy should be performed no less than 45 minutes before meals or 1 hour after meals (Esberger and Hughes, 1989).

Pneumonia is the most frequently missed diagnosis in the elderly (Fox, 1988). One reason for this may be that the signs of respiratory infection are much more subtle in the elderly individual. For example, an elevated white blood cell count, temperature spikes, and a productive cough may be completely absent. The first signs of respiratory infection in the aged patient may be mental status changes, tachypnea, and signs of dehydration (Cohen, 1989; Matteson and McConnell, 1988). The atypical presentation of infection may lead to delayed treatment and/or misdiagnosis (Fox, 1988).

Narrow-spectrum antibiotics are the preferred pharmacologic agents because of the specificity of their effects. The narrow-spectrum agents cause fewer alterations in other systems; thus, risk of superinfections is decreased (Fox, 1988). Sputum cultures are necessary to isolate the microorganism responsible so that the appropriate medication can be ordered. Community acquired pneumonia is often caused by *Haemophilus influenzae* or *Streptococcus pneumoniae*. Nursing home–acquired pneumonia is often due to *Klebsiella pneumoniae* (Berk and Smith, 1983; Cohen, 1989).

Treatment also entails rest, humidification of inspired gases, hydration, and chest physiotherapy. Supplemental oxygen is often utilized. Because administration of oxygen may alter taste and smell, the patient's appetite is often diminished. If the patient is able to take food or fluid by mouth, all attempts are made to honor special dietary requests because nutrition is such an important factor in improving health.

The elderly patient is vigorously monitored for

adverse reactions to therapy. Adverse reactions are 2 to 7 times more likely in elderly patients than in patients in their twenties (Mostow, 1983).

Impaired Breathing Pattern. The elderly patient may develop significant arterial hypoxemia from a relatively small pulmonary incident (Block, 1979). Retained secretions, excessive sedation, or positioning that impairs chest expansion may result in significant changes in the older patient's oxygenation status.

Age-related changes in the respiratory and other systems alter the elderly patient's response to hypoxemia. The usual signs of hypoxemia (e.g., increased respiratory rate, tachycardia, elevated blood pressure) may be blunted in the elderly (Wahba, 1983). Other indicators such as restlessness or mental status changes are of increasing significance to the nurse.

In general, management of mechanical ventilation for the older adult without pulmonary disease is very similar to management of the younger ventilated patient. Structural changes in the lungs and decreased muscle strength have implications for the weaning process. Usual predictors of successful weaning were developed for younger populations and do not have as much discriminating potential for older individuals. Thus, general weaning protocols may not be appropriate for certain elderly individuals. Weaning must be tailored to the specific needs of the patient (Krieger et al., 1989).

Weakness of the respiratory muscles is one age-related change that plays an important role when the elderly patient is being weaned from mechanical ventilation. The critical care nurse assesses the patient's activity level and energy expenditure and provides for adequate rest periods during the weaning process. When possible, activities such as bathing should be done well before weaning begins. Explanations of the activity are verbalized clearly, both well before the procedure is underway and during the procedure.

The Nervous System

Age-related changes in the nervous system can be categorized as structural, chemical, and functional alterations. Table 65–2 describes the age-related changes occurring in the nervous system.

STRUCTURAL ALTERATIONS

Age-related changes vary in the different parts of the nervous system. There is a general decrease in neuronal cells and a proliferation of glial cells (Davis-Sharts, 1989). Neuronal loss occurs only in certain areas (e.g., the locus ceruleus), but glial cell increase occurs throughout the entire nervous system (Curcio et al., 1982; Duara et al., 1985). Cell loss in the basal ganglia and cerebellum is thought to play a role in

TABLE 65–2. Age-Related Changes in the Nervous System

Structure	Age-Related Change	Clinical Manifestation
Central nervous system	Decreased neurons	Impaired motor control
	Increased glial cells	Decreased reaction time
	Brain atrophy Neurotransmitter alterations Decreased synthesis Increased degradation Decreased binding at receptor sites	
Peripheral nervous system	Degeneration of axons	Slowed nerve conduction velocity

the progressive loss of coordinated motor control in the elderly (Davis-Sharts, 1989). The number of dendritic spines and length of the dendrites decrease. There is also an increase in lipofuscin, neuritic plaques, and neurofibrillary tangles (Duara et al., 1985). Gross observations show brain atrophy, an increase in cranial cavity dead space, and an asymmetrical quality of the ventricles (Lytle and Altar, 1979).

In the peripheral nervous system, there is a decrease in the number and density of nerve fibers (Davis-Sharts, 1989). A degeneration of axons and an increase in the connective tissue content of neurons are observed. These changes lead to a slowing of nerve conduction velocity (Dorfman and Bosley, 1979). Slowed nerve conduction velocity may account for decreased sensations of vibration and touch in the extremities. Deep tendon reflexes in the wrist and ankle are also decreased (Davis-Sharts, 1989).

CHEMICAL CHANGES

Age-related biochemical alterations in the nervous system include neurotransmitter imbalance; membrane changes; and alterations in neurotransmitter precursors, receptors, and degradation products.

Acetylcholine. No overall change in acetylcholine is demonstrated in animal studies of aging. Age-related reductions in choline (an acetylcholine precursor) uptake and choline acetyltransferase (an enzyme used in acetylcholine formation) activity have been observed. There is also a decrease in acetylcholine release and degradation in aging (Rebensen-Piano, 1989; Rogers and Bloom, 1985). This is an excellent example of the following hypothesis: "With aging, alterations in neurotransmitter function appear to be the result of an imbalance between neurotransmitters rather than an increase or decrease of a single chemical" (Davis-Sharts, 1989, p. 757).

Dopamine. The activity of tyrosine hydroxylase, an enzyme that is essential for the synthesis of dopamine, decreases in aging human and rat brains. There is also an increase in dopamine degradation and a build-up of the catabolic byproducts. At the receptor, dopamine binding also declines (Rebensen-Piano, 1989; Rogers and Bloom, 1985).

Norepinephrine. Because dopamine is a precursor for norepinephrine synthesis, the reduction in available dopamine also results in a decrease in norepinephrine synthesis. However, the rate of norepinephrine inactivation also decreases with age. Thus, depending on the section of the brain under examination, norepinephrine levels have been found to be unchanged or decreased (Rogers and Bloom, 1985).

Serotonin. Serotonin levels are found to be either decreased or unchanged in the elderly. Presynaptic reuptake of serotonin is unaltered with age. There may be a reduction in serotonin receptor binding, but data are scarce (Rebensen-Piano, 1989; Rogers and Bloom, 1985).

FUNCTIONAL ALTERATIONS

Reaction Time. The time between stimulation and the initiation of a response increases with age (Gottsdanker, 1982). Reaction time is further delayed with increasing complexity of the stimulus or the necessary response. Elderly individuals tend to sacrifice speed and therefore respond more slowly yet more accurately than younger adults (Botwinick, 1978). Patient teaching may take longer, and the ICU nurse may have to repeat information in both written and verbal form. The section on sensory alterations discusses this topic more fully.

Maintenance of Posture. Maintenance of an upright posture requires balance, proper alignment of body parts, and the control of equilibrium in movement (Matteson and McConnell, 1988). Elderly persons may receive incorrect or insufficient information from the environment as a result of altered vision, vestibular sensation, proprioception, hearing, and touch-pressure sensory integration. The effect of this is that these individuals may experience dizziness, lightheadedness, or vertigo. Dizziness includes a sense of impending loss of consciousness that may be due, in part, to inadequate blood flow to the brain. Disequilibrium is due to an alteration in motor system control and results in loss of balance when standing or walking. Lightheadedness is the result of sensory impairment, vestibular alterations, or auditory dysfunction. Vertigo is the sensation that the individual is spinning or the room is rotating. Vertigo is usually caused by disorders in the vestibular system (Matteson and McConnell, 1988).

Other age-related changes in posture and movement include slowing of motor activity, decrease in

reflexes, joint rigidity, tremors, and difficulty in fine motor movement (Matteson and McConnell, 1988).

Thermoregulation. Elderly persons are at increased risk of developing both hypothermia and hyperthermia.

Hypothermia (rectal temperature $\leq 35°$ C.) is usually due to environmental exposure. Usually exposure is a result of social factors such as inadequate housing or insufficient income to maintain a warm environment. Physiologic alterations such as loss of body fat or the inability to sense cold may also be the cause of hypothermia. Alcohol abuse, confusion, and falls also contribute to hypothermia in the elderly (Exton-Smith and Overstall, 1979).

Heat stroke is the most dangerous heat regulation disorder among the aged. Heat stroke is caused by an impairment of the thermoregulatory system in which heat cannot be effectively dissipated from the body. Impaired peripheral circulation decreases the body's ability to move heat away from the core. Impaired peripheral circulation coupled with decreased perspiration in the older adult increases the risk for heat stroke. Individuals taking phenothiazines are at even higher risk, as these medications decrease sweat gland activity (Matteson and McConnell, 1988).

Sleep Changes. The elderly have an increase in wakefulness relative to the total time spent in bed (Fig. 65–1). In particular, there are more frequent awakenings and the awakenings last longer. In addition, there is an increased latency to sleep onset (Zepelen, 1983). The most evident age-related change in human sleep is the decreased amplitude of the sleep EEG delta activity. Stages 3 and 4, referred to as "deep sleep," decrease with age. Some individuals

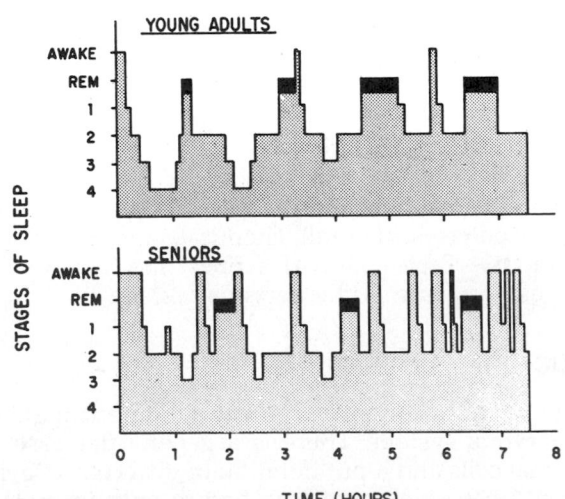

FIGURE 65–1. Normal sleep cycles. With aging, it takes longer to fall asleep and there is less deep sleep, more awakenings and less rapid eye movement (REM) sleep. (From Ancoli-Israel, S., and Kripke, D. F. (1986). Sleep and aging. In E. Calkins, et al. (Eds.), *The practice of geriatrics*, p. 242. Philadelphia: W. B. Saunders.)

completely lose stage 4 sleep in late adulthood (Miles and Dement, 1980). Large decreases in rapid eye movement (REM) sleep are not usually seen until extreme old age (Williams et al., 1974).

CLINICAL IMPLICATIONS OF AGE-RELATED CHANGES IN THE NERVOUS SYSTEM

Sleep-Pattern Disturbance. Fragmented sleep patterns and feelings of fatigue, which occur at baseline, may be worsened by numerous factors in the critical care unit. These include pain, depression, severe stress, urinary frequency, respiratory distress, and medications. The environment of the critical care unit, with its bright lights, equipment and personnel noise, and ambient temperature alterations, also affects the elderly patient's ability to sleep. Nursing assessment includes both patient factors and environmental factors. Attention is paid to relieving patient factors, such as pain, as well as altering the environment to promote a quiet and restful atmosphere.

Signs of sleep deprivation differ somewhat based on the stage of sleep the person is missing. For example, signs of non-REM sleep deprivation include apathy, slurred speech, lethargy, impaired judgment, ptosis, and lack of facial expression. Deprivation of REM sleep may be manifested as agitation, confusion, impaired control of impulses, emotional lability, and hyperactivity (Lukasiewicz-Ferland, 1987).

Nursing actions to promote sleep include providing the patient with reminders of the time of day. For example, a window with the shades partially open or, if no window is available, varying the intensity of artificial lighting according to the time of day is helpful. This provides external cues that may help maintain the elder's sense of circadian rhythm (Monk, 1989). Scheduling procedures to provide rest periods in between is important for all ICU patients, but especially in the elderly because their sleep pattern is more interrupted at baseline than younger adults. If at all possible, the patient's normal bedtime regimen is followed and may be augmented by a back or foot massage.

Noise is a major cause of sleep disruption in hospitalized patients and can be modified, at least in part, by nurses (Webster and Thompson, 1986). Noises from equipment and talking by staff members are primary offenders (Bentley et al., 1977). By reducing unnecessary noises, the nurse provides a more optimal level for sleep not only to be initiated, but to be extended for a period of time.

A study of ICU patients found that patients who complained of a lack of sleep identified the inability to get comfortable (due to a different bed, tubing, invasive procedures) and pain as two contributing factors (Jones et al., 1979). By reducing the barriers to comfort and by relieving pain, the ICU nurse provides an environment more conducive to sleep.

Sleep is very difficult to assess visually. Using polygraphic recordings compared with nursing notes, Aurell and Elmquist (1985) found that surgical ICU nurses consistently overestimated the amount of sleep their patients got. Because sleep is so elusive in the ICU and because it is so difficult to evaluate, all attempts are made to provide daytime-nighttime cues, extended rest periods, comfort measures, and a quiet and restful environment.

Cardiac dysrhythmias and pulmonary hypertension have been associated with periods of apnea that occur during REM sleep (Davis-Sharts, 1989). The nurse carefully observes the patient's electrocardiogram, respiratory rate, and pulmonary artery pressures during sleep and documents the occurrence of any abnormalities.

The Endocrine System

The production of some hormones and receptivity of some target tissues are altered with advanced age. There is also a change in the degradation and elimination of hormones (Eckel and Hofeldt, 1982). The plasma levels of aldosterone, renin, estrogen, calcitonin, growth hormone, somatomedin C, and prolactin are decreased with age. Conversely, plasma levels of follicle-stimulating hormone, luteinizing hormone, and norepinephrine increase with age (Davis and Davis, 1983). Adrenal secretion of cortisol is stable; therefore, there are no significant changes in the hypothalamic-pituitary-adrenal axis and the stress response (Davis and Davis, 1983).

The basal metabolic rate decreases with age. Because lean body mass also decreases with age, the ratio between basal metabolic rate and lean body mass remains relatively constant (Matteson and McConnell, 1988; Rock, 1985).

The endocrine functions of the kidney are also affected by aging. Plasma renin and aldosterone levels decrease in the normotensive older adult, leading to alterations in sodium regulation. Hyperkalemia may occur as a consequence of impaired renin and aldosterone secretion and decreased glomerular filtration rate. The conversion of 1-OH-cholecalciferol to 1-25-$(OH)_2$ cholecalciferol is diminished, leading to decreased calcium absorption from the intestine. Erythropoietin production is also slowed, thus contributing to anemia (Matteson and McConnell, 1988). Table 65–3 summarizes the age-related changes in the various endocrine organs.

CLINICAL IMPLICATIONS OF AGE-RELATED CHANGES IN THE ENDOCRINE SYSTEM

Endocrine system changes associated with aging usually do not affect the older adult's daily functioning. However, illness places a greater stress on all body systems and may enhance these changes.

Potential for Acute Complications and Alterations in Glycemic Control. One very common endocrine

TABLE 65–3. Age-Related Changes in the Endocrine System

Organ	Changes Related to Aging	Clinical Implication
Pituitary	Atrophy Decreased size and cell mass Fibrosis Decreased vascularity	
Thyroid	Decreased mass, increased fibrosis Increased incidence of nodules and small goiters Increased plasma level of inorganic iodide Plasma T_4 level unchanged Plasma T_3 level decreased	Decreased basal metabolic rate
Adrenal cortex	Cortisol secretion unchanged Aldosterone secretion decreased	Stress response intact Decreased renal reabsorption of sodium in response to activity changes and dietary sodium restrictions
Parathyroid	Effect on PTH secretion is undetermined	
Pancreas	Decrease in glucose tolerance Decreased insulin secretion Decreased receptor site sensitivity	Hyperglycemia Glucosuria

Abbreviations: T_4, thyroxine; T_3, triiodothyronine; PTH, parathyroid hormone.

disorder occurring in later life is diabetes mellitus. Approximately 17% of 65-year-olds and 26% of 85-year-olds have diabetes (Williams, 1978). Signs of diabetes may be very subtle in elderly persons. Leg cramps, numbness, weakness, impotence, vaginal itching, urinary incontinence and cool extremities may be the first clinical manifestations of the disease (Eliopoulous, 1978; Zimmerman, 1981). Two of the hallmarks of diabetes mellitus are polyuria and polydipsia, but these symptoms may be absent in older adults (Fonesca, 1981). Because the renal threshold for glucose increases with age, the spilling of glucose in the urine may not happen until blood glucose levels are 300 mg/dL or higher (Marchesseault, 1983).

Diabetic ketoacidosis (DKA) is not as prevalent in older adults because fat is seldom used for energy and older adults usually continue to produce some insulin (Hayter, 1981). Hyperosmolar hyperglycemic nonketotic coma (HHNK) is a more common problem for elderly diabetics and can be life-threatening (Gioiella and Bevil, 1984). The average age of HHNK

presentation is 60, and the fatality rate is 40% to 70% (Goldberg, et al., 1985; Nasr, 1983). Both DKA and HHNK can be precipitated by the stress of any acute illness (Gioiella and Bevil, 1984; Goldberg et al., 1985).

Nursing management of HHNK includes replacing the fluid volume deficit; administering insulin and potassium as ordered; and monitoring the patient's cardiac status, electrolytes, and clinical presentation closely (Holloway, 1988). Because nursing goals for the diabetic patient are long term (weight control, diet, exercise, medical management), discharge planning is initiated as soon as possible. If the critical care nurse identifies areas of patient need, appropriate referrals are initiated.

Gastrointestinal System

There are very few changes in the gastrointestinal (GI) system that are a part of normal aging. There is evidence to suggest that changes in the GI system are the result of disease processes and other organ system changes rather than related to aging. The age-related changes in the GI system are described in Table 65–4.

MOUTH

Elderly persons retain more of their natural teeth than in generations past (Baum, 1981). There may be a decrease in saliva production, but it is not considered an inevitable effect of aging (Baum et al., 1984). Frequently, problems arise in coordinating chewing with the initiation of swallowing (Krumpe et al., 1985). For instance, the process of chewing followed by smooth swallowing is often disrupted and may take more time and energy than in a younger individual.

TABLE 65–4. Age-Related Changes in the Gastrointestinal System

Structure	Age-Related Change	Clinical Manifestation
Esophagus	Presbyesophagus	Difficulty in swallowing
	Achalasia	Risk of aspiration
Stomach	Thinning of gastric mucosa	Ulcer formation
	Hiatal hernia	Heartburn–sternal pain
Colon	Decreased colonic motility	Constipation
Pancreas	Decreased pancreatic lipase	Altered fat absorption
Liver	Decreased hepatic enzymes	Altered drug metabolism
	Decreased albumin synthesis	Altered drug-protein binding

ESOPHAGUS

There is much controversy in the literature about whether esophageal function declines with aging. Vierling and Reichen (1982) maintain that alterations in esophageal motility in older adults are due to the high prevalence of vascular, metabolic, and neurologic diseases in the elderly.

Some common disorders seen in the elderly include presbyesophagus and achalasia. Presbyesophagus is abnormal esophageal motility due to nonperistaltic contractions (Soergel et al., 1964). Achalasia is the failure of the lower esophageal sphincter to relax completely during swallowing (Krumpe et al., 1985). Both presbyesophagus and achalasia result in difficulty in swallowing, and some patients may experience gastric reflux. Achalasia increases the risk of aspiration (Krumpe et al., 1985).

STOMACH

Aging adults exhibit atrophy of the gastric mucosa, resulting in a weakened capacity for the release of hydrochloric acid (Vierling and Reichen, 1982). There is also a thinning of the gastric mucosa. When the stomach is exposed to stress, alcohol, or other drugs, there is an increased risk of ulcer formation (Matteson and McConnell, 1988). Motility and emptying of the stomach contents have not been well studied in the elderly.

Hiatal hernia is more common in older adults. Sixty per cent to ninety per cent of elders develop a hiatal hernia by the age of 70 (Reynolds, 1982). Symptoms include heartburn, dysphagia, and sternal pain. Because symptoms often mimic cardiac warning signs, these individuals are frequently admitted to critical care units to rule out myocardial infarction.

SMALL INTESTINE

Very little is known about the age-related changes in the small intestine; therefore, no conclusions can be made about alterations in motility (Rebensen-Piano, 1989). There is evidence of atrophy in the villi of the duodenum and jejunum in aging rats (Hoehn et al., 1978). Segmentation and peristalsis are stimulated by the presence of food in the intestine. Changes in dietary intake and physical activity may decrease intestinal motility.

LARGE INTESTINE

Blood flow to the colon may be reduced due to twisting of blood vessels in elderly persons. There is a decrease in colonic motility and an increased tendency to develop outlet obstruction (Rebensen-Piano, 1989). One of the most common complaints of elders is constipation. This problem may be a result of decreased stool bulk, altered transit time, or an increased volume of rectal distention necessary to stimulate the defecation response (Vierling and Reichen, 1982).

PANCREAS

The incidence of dilation and distention of the pancreatic ducts increases 8% per decade after the age of 60 years (Matteson and McConnell, 1988). There is a decrease in the production of lipase, which results in abnormalities of fat absorption.

LIVER

Liver mass declines after age 50 (Sato et al., 1970). Blood flow in the liver is also diminished. Hepatic protein synthesis is weakened, and there are changes in some microsomal drug metabolizing enzymes (e.g., NADPH–cytochrome c reductase) (Kato, 1986). These changes are especially important in the metabolism of some drugs. The attenuation of microsomal drug metabolizing activity and decrease in liver blood flow make drug toxicity a danger for older adults (Rebensen-Piano, 1989). Research has shown no age-related abnormalities in liver function tests, including bilirubin, alkaline phosphatase, and aspartate aminotransferase (Kampmann et al., 1975).

The production of serum albumin decreases with age. This may affect drug distribution of highly protein-bound drugs, such as phenytoin, warfarin, thyroxine, non-steroidal anti-inflammatory drugs, aspirin, and oral hypoglycemic agents (Kane et al., 1989). The result is an increased susceptibility to adverse side effects and drug toxicity at what would typically be considered therapeutic doses.

CLINICAL IMPLICATIONS OF AGE-RELATED CHANGES IN THE GASTROINTESTINAL SYSTEM

Alterations in gastrointestinal function have a number of important implications for the critically ill elderly patient. Impaired intestinal absorption may result in suboptimal nutrition. Constipation or diarrhea result from changes in bowel function.

Nutrition Less than Body Requirements. There is a slight decrease in the rate of absorption of carbohydrates, proteins, and lipids with aging (Rebensen-Piano, 1989). Of these, decreased absorption of lipids is the most clinically significant. Accompanying the decreased absorption of lipids is a diminished rate of absorption of fat-soluble vitamins. Because vitamin K is lipid soluble, bleeding tendencies and clotting abnormalities may occur. The patient is carefully assessed for evidence of bleeding, bruising, and petechiae. Coagulation studies are monitored for abnormalities. Parenteral vitamin K may be administered as a supplement.

Elderly patients are at increased risk for malnutrition (Bienia et al., 1982). Furthermore, the stress of being in the critical care atmosphere coupled with the demands of life-threatening illness also increases protein and calorie requirements (Champagne and Ashley, 1989). Assessment of nutritional status in the ICU is based on laboratory values, height and weight, and the patient's appearance. A serum albumin of 3.0 to 3.4 mg/dL indicates mild protein depletion; 2.1 to 2.9 mg/dL indicates moderate depletion, and 2.0 mg/dL or less indicates severe depletion (Champagne and Ashley, 1989). A total lymphocyte count of less than 1500 cells may indicate risk, and counts less than 900 signal severe protein depletion (Champagne and Ashley, 1989). When low serum albumin and low total lymphocyte counts occur together, the risk of complications and death increases (Seltzer et al., 1982).

Nursing goals center on providing the patient with adequate nutrition, an especially challenging task because many patients in the ICU cannot eat or drink. The nurse is often the first to recognize the need for enteral or parenteral feedings. As a guide, critically ill elderly patients who are expected to be unable to take nutrition by mouth for 5 days or more should be started on parenteral or enteral nutrition as soon as possible (Champagne and Ashley, 1989).

Enteral feedings have several benefits. The intestinal villi grow in size; enzyme production is stimulated; and when used in combination with histamine H_2-receptor blocking drugs or antacids, enteral feedings decrease the incidence of duodenal ulcers in patients on ventilators (American Society for Parenteral and Enteral Nutrition, 1987; Pingleton and Hadzima, 1983). Because milk-based formulas are not well tolerated by some elders, lactulose-free complete formulas are the enteral feeding of choice. Soft, small-bore nasointestinal tubes are the safest for patients who have impaired swallowing or gag reflexes. Infusion pumps are used so that the feeding can be regulated to prevent complications such as diarrhea, dehydration, and hyperglycemia. Adequate hydration is essential before enteral feedings are started, to prevent electrolye imbalances and dehydration. Intake and output, weight, calorie counts, electrolytes, and glucose levels are monitored closely (Champagne and Ashley, 1989).

If the GI tract cannot be used as a route for nutrition, total parenteral nutrition (TPN) is instituted. Because TPN solutions are hypertonic, metabolic balance is carefully monitored. In the elderly patient, TPN is started slowly (1 liter per 24 hours) so as not to overcome the patient's physiologic response to increased fluid, glucose, and protein loads (Champagne and Ashley, 1989).

In mechanically ventilated patients, excessive caloric intake is avoided. When glucose exceeds metabolic requirements, the surplus glucose is converted to fat, a process that releases CO_2. This release of CO_2 increases the respiratory quotient to greater than 1, and may interfere with weaning (Deitel et al., 1983; Grossman, 1985).

Early identification of the older patient requiring tube feedings or TPN is an important nursing function. Although the ICU nurse may not be in contact with the patient long enough to see malnutrition corrected, adequate nutrition can decrease complications and enhance recovery (Champagne and Ashley, 1989).

Constipation. Constipation is not a normal result of aging and should be carefully evaluated and treated. In the critically ill patient, constipation may impede abdominal assessment. The patient's discomfort related to constipation may mask other physical problems. Straining during defecation, accompanied by the Valsalva maneuver, may result in cardiac dysrhythmias.

Causes of constipation include dietary factors, medications, decreased physical mobility, obstruction, lesions, neurologic disorders, and psychological problems (Altman, 1983). Treatment may include increased fluid intake, increased fiber intake, initiation of active or passive range of motion, and administration of stool softeners or laxatives.

Diarrhea. Whereas constipation is frequently a concern of older adults, diarrhea is a very common problem for elders in the critical care unit. The causes of diarrhea include foods, medications, infections, malabsorption, neoplasms, stress, and fecal impaction (White, 1983; Anderson, 1986). Drugs that may cause diarrhea include antibiotics, aminophylline, digitalis, antiarrhythmics, and potassium (Kane et al., 1989; Malseed, 1983). The nurse monitors intake and output, mental status, tissue turgor, and electrolytes. Nursing actions include isolating the causative agent(s), slowing enteral feedings, and supporting the elderly patient who may be having difficulty controlling episodes of diarrhea. Frequent and gentle perineal care decreases anal excoriation. Commercial washes and powders are available and should be used according to product instructions.

Genitourinary System

A number of age-related changes occur in the genitourinary system. These changes have significant implications, as they result in altered elimination of wastes and drugs from the body. Age-related changes in the urinary system are summarized in Table 65–5.

TABLE 65–5. Age-Related Changes in the Urinary System

Structure	Age-Related Change	Clinical Manifestation
Kidney	Decreased number of nephrons	Decreased glomerular filtration rate
	Diminished renal blood flow	Altered sodium excretion
	Altered tubular function	Impaired drug excretion
Bladder	Muscle weakening	Incomplete emptying
	Decreased capacity	Incontinence
		Increased risk of infection

KIDNEY

Age-related changes in the kidney can be categorized by their structural and functional aspects.

Structural Alterations. With increasing age, there is a loss of nephrons, loss of renal mass, increase in interstitial tissue, and decrease in the number of glomeruli. Progressive decreases are seen in both proximal tubular length and volume. There is a thickening of both the tubular basement membrane and the small arteries of the parenchyma (Rowe, 1982; Darmady et al., 1973). Renal perfusion is decreased as a result of sclerotic changes in the renal arterioles (Hollenberg et al., 1974).

Functional Alterations. Aging results in a smaller filtering surface area in the glomerulus, accompanied by a decreased renal blood flow and lower glomerular filtration rate (Rowe, 1982). The creatinine clearance also decreases with age. The older adult has a diminished ability to concentrate urine and conserve sodium. This does not present a problem to the healthy individual. However, if there is an acid challenge, as in metabolic acidosis, there is a reduced rate and quantity of net acid secretion (Rebensen-Piano, 1989). Excretion of drugs and glucose may also be impaired (Hickler, 1985; Feinstein, 1986).

BLADDER

With age, fibrous connective tissue replaces some of the smooth muscle and elastic tissue of the bladder. The bladder muscles weaken. Subsequently, bladder capacity decreases and incomplete emptying occurs. Thus, frequency of urination increases. Changes in the bladder outlet may cause obstruction (benign prostatic hypertrophy) in the male. In females, incontinence may occur due to relaxation and weakening of the pelvic muscles (Matteson and McConnell, 1988). These changes may also lead to difficulty in starting the urinary stream.

Incomplete emptying and possible outlet obstruction place elderly patients at higher risk of developing urinary tract infections.

REPRODUCTIVE ORGANS

Male. Prostatic hypertrophy occurs in the majority of men by age 60. To compensate for the obstruction of urine flow posed by the prostate, the bladder wall muscle hypertrophies to increase the pressure to empty the bladder. This may result in residual urine, overflow incontinence, and even obstructive renal damage (Matteson and McConnell, 1988).

Testicular volume diminishes in aging males. Spermatogenesis slows, and there is some sclerosis of the tubules (Matteson and McConnell, 1988). A reduction in blood flow to the penis may lead to diminished erectile capacity. Impotence may occur, but not usually as a direct effect of aging. Rather, as in other times of life, psychological factors, disease, and medications are the major causes of impotence (Matteson and McConnell, 1988).

Female. The length and width of the vagina decrease in the older female. The vaginal lining becomes thinner and less elastic, and vaginal pH rises. These effects are the result of estrogen deficiency.

CLINICAL IMPLICATIONS OF AGE-RELATED CHANGES IN THE GENITOURINARY SYSTEM

The age-related changes in the genitourinary system have both physiologic and psychosocial implications for the critically ill elderly patient.

Fluid Volume Deficit. Alterations in urine production place the elderly patient at risk of developing extracellular fluid volume deficit. The impaired concentrating ability and reduced level of aldosterone may lead to urinary sodium and water losses in the face of a contracted extracellular fluid volume.

The circadian rhythm of urine production may be lost in advanced age, resulting in nocturia (Matteson and McConnell, 1988). Dehydration is a common problem in the elderly due to loss of the thirst perception mechanism, difficulty in obtaining and swallowing fluid, and a reluctance to drink fluids due to subsequent urgency to void and incontinence. If large volume losses, such as vomiting or diarrhea, occur in addition to the underlying state of mild dehydration, the result can be marked hypovolemia.

Dehydration often results in acute confusion in the older adult. It is important that critical care nurses obtain a baseline of the elderly patient's mental status and continually monitor the patient for evidence of confusion or decreased mentation. Mental status changes frequently provide the first indication of a physiologic alteration. If three or more of the following behaviors are exhibited, further assessment is required: restlessness, agitation, personality changes, disorientation, decreased cognitive functioning, impaired judgment, incoherent communication, and inability to integrate cues into a meaningful pattern. Further assessment includes vital signs as compared with baseline; a medication review; assessment of neurologic, cardiovascular, respiratory, and peripheral vascular status; and evaluation of environmental factors and laboratory work (BUN-creatinine, ABGs, complete blood count with differential, electrolytes, and glucose). Fluid volume deficit is one cause of confusion in the elderly, but other etiologic factors include respiratory insufficiency, sepsis, alterations in temperature, hyperglycemia, hypoglycemia, and drug toxicity. Further evaluation and treatment are tailored to the underlying pathology (Foreman, 1984).

Potential for Injury. The creatinine clearance decreases with age. However, because of a generalized decrease in muscle mass, the elderly person's serum creatinine concentration may remain relatively unchanged. For this reason, the creatinine clearance is utilized as an index of renal function when drug dosages are determined (Matteson and McConnell, 1988). The serum creatinine and blood urea nitrogen (BUN) levels are monitored closely when the patient is receiving aminoglycoside antibiotics. Maintenance of adequate hydration is an important factor in preventing nephrotoxicity in the elderly patient. The patient's fluid volume status is carefully assessed. Intravenous fluids are administered as prescribed. If the patient is taking oral liquids, the nurse encourages the patient to drink.

Urinary Incontinence. Up to 43% of acute care patients experience urinary incontinence (Lincoln and Roberts, 1989). Incontinence may result from many factors, including neurogenic disease, medication, and stress. An increase in intra-abdominal pressure due to coughing, sneezing, or laughing may also result in incontinence.

Hospitalization may initiate or exacerbate urinary incontinence. For instance, many elderly people schedule their medications (e.g., diuretics) and fluid intake so that voiding will not interrupt planned activities or sleep. Older adults may not take in fluids after 6 P.M. so that they can avoid trips to the bathroom at night. However, in the ICU these patients may be receiving intravenous fluids, enteral feedings, or medications at times that disrupt their normal pattern of voiding and may result in a lack of bladder control.

Medications that depress the central nervous system can cause confusion in older adults, which may result in decreased control over external sphincter function as well. Imposed bedrest and physical restraints decrease mobility, and the patient may not be familiar with how to express the need to void or how to estimate the length of time it will take to get assistance.

Many patients in the ICU have indwelling urinary catheters. Narrowing of the urethra may make catheterization difficult. Often it is necessary to change the position of the patient and use extra lubrication when inserting catheters. In some elderly female patients, the external genitalia appear distorted due to childbirth or loss of elasticity. Adequate lighting and maintenance of a sterile field are essential to a successful noncontaminated catheterization. Problems may occur for the patient when the catheter is removed. The bladder may have decreased tone, and residual urine may be retained. Frequent, small voids may occur, and the risk of a urinary tract infection is increased (Lincoln and Roberts, 1989).

Nursing goals for bladder training programs are long-term interventions that are discussed in discharge planning. Depending on the cause of incontinence, it may be easily treated with Kegel exercises, surgery, medication, or behavioral modification. Because incontinence is a very important factor in determining placement of elders after hospitalization, every attempt is made to accurately assess and treat the cause of incontinence.

Altered Self-Concept. Stereotypes about older people being asexual must be eliminated. When the older adult is admitted to the critical care unit, his or her sexual identity may not be acknowledged as readily as would a younger person's. It is important that the older patient be treated with dignity and respect. Privacy and modesty should be afforded the elderly whenever possible.

Sexual self-concept involves one's image of the self as masculine or feminine and one's perceived adequacy in gender roles. Sexual self-concept includes body image as well as an evaluation of how that image compares with personal or societal standards (Woods, 1987). Sexual function is often more gradual in older adults. The sexual self-concept must be adjusted to accept this slowed response without feelings of inadequacy. The sexual role may change as new ways of sharing intimacy are developed or as the elderly person learns to live with the loss or illness of a partner (Mims and Swenson, 1980). Surgery, illness, or injuries may alter the elderly person's self-concept even further.

Nursing goals for altered self-concept include talking to the patient about what bodily changes can be expected as a result of illness or surgery. Also, helping the patient prepare to talk with his or her partner is of assistance. Verbal validation about the importance of expressing sexual concerns or questions enhances self-concept and increases self-efficacy (Woods, 1987). The nurse may teach the patient that slowed sexual response is an expected part of aging and that additional lubrication, patience, and extra time can enhance sexual relations between older adults. Although the ICU milieu often precludes long discussions dealing with self-concept, many of these interventions can be done while other care is given.

The Immune System

There are three lines of defense against invading pathogens: the integument, the digestion of invading agents by macrophages, and the humoral response. Age-related changes in the latter two mechanisms are examined in this section.

Elderly people are more susceptible to infectious diseases, perhaps due to a decline in antibody production and a weakening of cell-mediated immunity (Wekster, 1983). The level of circulating antibodies declines, and there is also a corresponding decline in antibody responsiveness with age. Delayed-type hypersensitivity reactions are also depressed with aging. Thus, the older individual is at even higher risk for developing certain diseases, including tuberculosis (Cohen, 1989; Sternberg, 1988).

Autoimmune disorders occur when antibodies or cytotoxic T-lymphocytes are produced to combat the body's own tissue. When this happens, the tissues that are not recognized as "self" come under attack. Autoimmune disorders related to aging include rheumatoid arthritis, systemic lupus erythematosus, and chronic hepatitis (Sternberg, 1988; Cohen, 1989).

Interestingly, it has been found that there is a decrease in immunologic rejection of tissue grafts with aging. Therefore, in some cases, the aging immune system may be an advantage to the patient (Sternberg, 1988).

Whereas the spleen and lymph nodes do not change much with age, the thymus begins to involute and thymic weight declines (Kay and Baker, 1979; Good and Gabrielson, 1964). The thymus secretes polypeptide substances that are vital for thymocyte maturation into T-cells and generalized immune function. Thus, with aging, several thymic factors are diminished. This may prove to be a major factor in the decline of the immune system with age (Sternberg, 1988).

TUMOR GROWTH

With age, the immune system's ability to detect and respond to tumor cells is decreased. There is a higher incidence of tumor growth in elderly persons, perhaps because of age-related changes in the components of the immune system that are responsible for tumor surveillance. There is an increased incidence of leukemia and breast, lung, prostate, stomach, colon, and pancreas cancer in older adults (Sternberg, 1988).

AIDS IN THE ELDERLY

There is a dearth of research literature concerning human immunodeficiency virus (HIV) infection in older persons. The oldest reported patient with acquired immune deficiency syndrome (AIDS) was 82 years old (Moss and Miles, 1987). People over age 60 with an AIDS diagnosis fall primarily into the risk groups of hemophiliacs, transfusion recipients, heterosexuals, and undetermined categories (Cohen, 1989; Moss and Miles, 1987). AIDS dementia may be the first major manifestation of HIV infection in an elderly patient. Symptoms of behavioral, cognitive, and motor abnormalities can easily mimic Alzheimer's disease, Parkinson's disease, or other disorders associated with advanced age (Navia and Price, 1987; Sabin, 1987).

CLINICAL IMPLICATIONS OF AGE-RELATED CHANGES IN THE IMMUNE SYSTEM

Potential for Infection. In elderly patients, the signs and symptoms of infection can be quite different from those of the young adult. The respiratory tract and urinary tract are the most common sites of infection in older adults (Fox, 1988). Some indicators of infection in the elderly are increased dependency upon care providers, falls, postural instability, immobility, confusion, and incontinence of urine or feces. Often these problems or their complications are what brings the person to the ICU. Unfortu-

nately, the presenting problem may be treated while the underlying infection goes undiagnosed. Because there is a loss of reserve in many body systems in aging, the development of infection in one system may produce negative consequences in many other systems (Fox, 1988).

Clinical assessment includes recording of body temperature, although there is less of a febrile response to illness in elderly persons (Finklestein et al., 1983). Temperature should be recorded rectally at least every 6 hours to identify subtle trends (Berman et al., 1987; McAlpine et al., 1986). With infection, the white blood cell count will be elevated (>11,000/μL) in two-thirds of elderly patients and the erythrocyte sedimentation rate (ESR) is usually elevated above 50 mm/hour (Fox, 1988; Crawford et al., 1987). Antibiotics, hydration, and nutrition are the hallmarks of treatment. The nurse evaluates the effectiveness of treatment not only by the laboratory values but also by improvements in functional impairments such as confusion, decreased mobility, and fatigue.

Musculoskeletal System

The musculoskeletal system is composed of the bones, muscles, and joints. All of these structures are affected by the aging process.

BONES

The bony skeleton is relatively resistant to deterioration when compared with the rest of the musculoskeletal system. However, bones do tend to become weaker with age (Matteson and McConnell, 1988). The skeleton also decreases in mass due to an imbalance between rates of bone formation and bone resorption.

One of the primary metabolic functions of bone is to maintain calcium balance in the extracellular fluid. In fact, bone tissue is a major storage site of calcium. When serum calcium levels are low, parathyroid hormone is released, which stimulates the release of calcium from the bone into the blood. Parathyroid hormone and vitamin D promote absorption of dietary calcium from the gastrointestinal tract and reabsorption through the kidneys. Conversely, when serum calcium is high, calcitonin is released from the thyroid to promote storage of calcium in the bone (Ganong, 1987).

In later adulthood, there is a decreased calcium absorption through the gastrointestinal tract. This may be due either to a diminished calcium intake or to decreased calcium absorption efficiency (Giansiracusa and Kantrowitz, 1981).

MUSCLES

There is a decrease in the number of muscle fibers along with a decrease in muscle strength in older age. Individual muscle fibers become smaller and more diverse in size. Lipofuscin, fat, and fibrous tissue may be deposited within the muscle tissue (Matteson and McConnell, 1988; Davis-Sharts, 1989; Larsson, 1982). Along with changes in muscle fibers, there are also age-related alterations at the neuromuscular junction. These alterations are not consistent among junctions. As the amount of acetylcholine decreases, the junction can no longer sustain transmission of nerve impulses (Davis-Sharts, 1989). The velocity of nerve conduction slows, and, in general, movement of the older person is slowed. The older person may exhibit diminished facial expressions and decreased blinking, which may be due to impaired extrapyramidal and motor neuron function (Matteson and McConnell, 1988; Larsson et al., 1979). In addition, involuntary movements may be exacerbated by fatigue and loss of sodium chloride (Matteson and McConnell, 1988).

"Restless legs" syndrome is common in old age. This syndrome is characterized by continuous leg movement in order to avoid the pain of paresthesias when the legs are still (Matteson and McConnell, 1988).

There may be a decrease in deep tendon reflexes with age due to atrophy and sclerosis of muscles and tendons. Increased extensor responses (e.g., a positive Babinski sign) are not normal and should be further evaluated (Matteson and McConnell, 1988; Grob, 1978; Carter, 1986).

JOINTS

The joints, especially the wrists, elbows, knees, hips, neck, and vertebrae, tend to become slightly more flexed with age. This is due in part to tendon and muscle rigidity and decreased movement (Matteson and McConnell, 1988). Joint changes also involve the progressive roughening of cartilage surfaces, as well as thickening and loss of elasticity of the cartilage (Davis-Sharts, 1989; Armstrong and Gardner, 1977). Changes at the heads of long bones also occur, and there is a tendency to develop bone spurs (Byers et al., 1970). These changes result in a decreased latency of fatigue and an increased risk of osteoarthritis.

CLINICAL IMPLICATIONS OF AGE-RELATED CHANGES IN THE MUSCULOSKELETAL SYSTEM

The critically ill older adult is at great risk for alterations in mobility by virtue of these age-related changes, their disease process, and the critical care environment (Davis-Sharts, 1989). Medications, physical restraints, tubing and other equipment, anxiety, and many other iatrogenic factors, when superimposed upon age-related changes, can certainly place the elderly person at even greater risk.

Impaired Physical Mobility. The ability to move freely is often taken for granted until it is lost. The body functions best when it changes positions often.

For example, when the body is upright, all but the lower calices of the kidney drain and the axes of the bronchioles, with the exception of the middle lobes, are in the vertical plane. The joints, muscles, and tendons are all dependent on the stress of movement for their function (Milde, 1981).

Assessment of the patient with impaired mobility is focused on the possible complications of immobility. The muscles may have decreased tone, size, and endurance, and range of motion in the joints may be restricted. Hypercalciuria and hypercalcemia may occur. The rate at which this bone mineral loss occurs depends on the length of immobility. Excretion of calcium increases rapidly from the third day to the third week of immobility and levels off during the fifth or sixth week (Dietrick et al., 1948; Heath and Earl, 1972; Rose, 1966).

Respiratory consequences of immobility due to decreased endurance and loss of muscle strength include abnormal or adventitious breath sounds, reduced arterial oxygen level, and change of percussion from resonant to dull as fluid consolidates. The supine position reduces the vital capacity by approximately 4% (Browse, 1965). Gravitational forces and position alter the shape of the chest and impair movement of the chest wall. Prolonged low volume breathing decreases the production of surfactant and places the patient at increased risk for atelectasis (Bendixen et al., 1963; Clements et al., 1951).

Cardiovascular complications of impaired mobility include thromboembolism and orthostatic intolerance. Also, the heart of a healthy person works 20% harder when the body is in a flat, supine position. In individuals with disease, the heart works 40% harder in a recumbent position than when sitting (Coe, 1954). This increased work load is due to the blood volume being redistributed to the thorax from the legs, thus increasing preload, resistance, and afterload (Sjostrand, 1952).

The goals of nursing care include maintenance of muscle strength and endurance by isometric and isotonic exercises. Skeletal strength is enhanced by ambulation, resistive exercises, range of motion exercises, and a diet with adequate calcium. Flexibility and joint mobility can be maintained through range of motion exercises and correct positioning. Elevation of the head of the bed and prevention of the Valsalva maneuver help to maintain adequate venous circulation (Milde, 1981). Maintenance of bowel and bladder function has been described elsewhere in this chapter. For the elderly person, the ultimate goal is to maintain pre-immobilization functions and abilities while preventing complications.

Integumentary System

Age-related changes in the integument are perhaps the most visible indicators of senescence. Wrinkled skin and gray hair are hallmarks of passing years. The changes in the integument are not due to aging process alone. Environmental factors also play a large part in the changes that occur. Because elderly people have been exposed to the sun for many years, solar damage is far more prevalent in the elderly than in other age groups (Timiras, 1988; Forbes et al., 1979).

EPIDERMIS

In aging, there is a decrease in height and surface area of epidermal cells. The moisture content of the superficial layer of cells, the stratum corneum, is decreased. The result is a dryness or roughness of the skin. There is an increased incidence of benign and malignant neoplasms in the aging skin. The junction between the epidermis and the dermis becomes flattened, reducing the junction's total surface area. For this reason, older adults are much more prone to blister formation and abrasions (Timiras, 1988). Shear-type injuries are also quite prevalent. This is of concern when one considers the shearing force of the bed linens over the coccyx when the patient is supine with the head of the bed elevated.

The turnover rate of epidermal cells slows, which means that cells are present at the surface for longer periods of time before they are exfoliated. This places the cells at increased risk of contacting carcinogens and plays a role in delayed wound healing (Timiras, 1988).

Irregular pigmentation in aging skin may be due to a reduction in the number of melanocytes. Melanocytes serve as protectors, waging an inflammatory warning signal when insults, such as sunburn, are present. There is also a decrease in Langerhans cells, which may contribute to the skin's impaired cell-mediated immune response associated with aging. Exposure to ultraviolet rays also decreases Langerhans cells (Timiras, 1988).

DERMIS

The dermal layer decreases in density and has fewer blood vessels. This may be accompanied by prolonged time necessary for dermal clearance of topical drugs and other substances. Collagen becomes thicker and less soluble. The total amount of collagen decreases linearly after age 20. Due to the loss of elasticity, older skin is more susceptible to tears, wrinkles, and damage to underlying tissues after trauma (Timiras, 1988).

SUBCUTANEOUS TISSUE

With age, there is a decrease in the thickness of the subcutaneous layer. There is also a decrease in the number and patency of the blood vessels in the skin. Therefore, thermoregulation is impaired. The decrease in subcutaneous fat leaves bony prominences less protected from wear and tear.

GLANDS

Sebaceous glands show little structural change with aging, but their functional capabilities decline and they decrease in number. Sebum secretion decreases, which results in drier, coarser skin (Pochi et al., 1979).

Sweat glands decrease in number, size, and efficiency with age. Diminished capacity for perspiration has a deleterious effect on thermoregulation (Matteson and McConnell, 1988). Because the body cannot use perspiration as a mechanism of cooling, the tendency to overheat is increased.

SENSORY END-ORGANS

The number of pacinian and Meissner corpuscles decrease with age, leading to diminished sensation of pressure and light touch. This loss of sensation predisposes elderly persons to injury and may interfere with fine motor movements in the hands (Timiras, 1988).

HAIR AND NAILS

There is a decrease in the number of hair follicles. The loss of functional melanocytes in hair bulbs as well as genetic factors plays a role in the graying of hair.

The rate of linear nail growth decreases with age. The thickness of nails, especially toenails, may increase. Longitudinal cracks may occur, leading to infection or further injury.

CLINICAL IMPLICATIONS OF AGE-RELATED CHANGES IN THE INTEGUMENT

Age-related changes in the integument place the critically ill elderly patient at high risk of developing skin breakdown and related infections.

Nail care is especially important in the older diabetic patient, since peripheral neuropathy, impaired circulation, and slowed wound healing are all superimposed upon the changes inherent in the aging process.

Impaired Skin Integrity. Pressure ulcers are a complication of immobility and are a common problem for hospitalized elderly patients. The presence of pressure ulcers significantly increases the patient's risk for morbidity and mortality (Goode, 1989). The primary cause of ulceration is pressure, but shearing forces, friction, nutrition, and moisture are also intervening variables (Goode, 1989).

Preventive nursing interventions are focused on decreasing these factors. For example, repositioning individuals frequently is basic nursing care, but for the critically ill elder, frequency of positioning must be quite individualized. When soft tissue is compressed between a bony prominence and an external surface for a short period of time, after the pressure is relieved the skin will be red but will blanch quickly when pressed gently (blanchable erythema). However, when pressure is prolonged, the skin will not blanch when pressed, indicating tissue damage (Goode, 1989). Critical care nurses assess common sites of pressure in elderly patients (sacrum, greater trochanters, ischial tuberosities, heels, and lateral malleoli) and tailor the frequency of position changes to fit the individual.

Shearing forces are present in the sacral area when a patient sits up in bed or in a chair and then slides downward. Shearing forces lower the amount of pressure needed to cause compression of blood vessels (Bennett and Ouslander, 1989). Furthermore, these shearing forces are greater in elderly individuals than in young people (Bennett and Ouslander, 1989).

Friction is generated when a patient is pulled across bed linens. Friction results in intraepidermal blisters, which, when broken, result in superficial erosions (Goode, 1989). Therefore, turning sheets should be used in repositioning. Moisture from urinary or fecal incontinence further increases the risk for pressure ulcer development. Additional reasons that elderly patients are at risk for pressure ulcer development include increased immobility; age-related decreases in ascorbic acid levels, which may increase blood vessel fragility; and the decreased number of dermal blood vessels in aged skin (Gilchrest, 1982; Taylor et al., 1974).

When a pressure ulcer is examined, only a small part of the damage can be visualized. Injury due to pressure usually begins in deeper tissue and spreads toward the skin (Daniel et al., 1981). Thus, when an ulcer is visible (as blanchable erythema), immediate intervention is necessary. First, the ulcer is assessed for size, color, drainage, odor, location, and classification. Because there are a number of staging tools in use for classifying ulcers, documentation of which system was used is necessary. The most important intervention in healing pressure ulcers is removing the pressure. Without doing this, all other therapeutic interventions are futile (Daniel et al., 1981). Special beds and antipressure devices may be utilized. Vitamin C supplementation and increased calories and protein may be indicated. Antibiotics will be ordered if infection is present. Local care includes cleansing with a topical disinfectant-antibiotic. Various solutions have been used and are still being evaluated for effectiveness.

The Senses

VISION

Table 65–6 describes the structural changes that occur in the eye during the aging process. There is a gradual decline in visual acuity, which may be due to altered light refraction, decreased accommodation, constriction of pupils, decreased number and func-

TABLE 65–6. Age-Related Changes in the Eye

Structure	Age-Related Change	Clinical Manifestation
Cornea	Thickening Decreased curvature Arcus senilis (gray ring around outer edge of cornea)	Altered refraction Greater risk of astigmatism
Iris	Loss of pigmentation	Iris appears to be lighter color
Pupil	Senile miosis (reduced pupil size)	Average baseline pupil size Age 20—8 mm Age 60—6 mm Age 90—5 mm
Lens	Hardening Increased opacity	Changes in refraction Altered color perception Sensitivity to glare Changes in accommodation Increased distance required for near vision Cataract development
Retina	Thinning around edges Decreased number of rods	Altered dark-light adaptation

tion of receptor cells, or central neural changes (Meisami, 1988). Light scattering in the cornea and lens produces an increased sensitivity to glare. The dark-adapted eye utilizes rods as opposed to cones. Therefore, as the number of rods decrease with age, dark and light adaptation takes longer in the elderly. Changes in refraction may alter color perception.

Changes in accommodation occur primarily for near vision, that is, "the minimal distance between the object and the eye for formation of a clear image" (Meisami, 1988, pp. 158–159). The distance required increases 10-fold during the life span. Most people over 55 need eyeglasses for near-vision tasks.

Loss of peripheral vision is common in the elderly. Older persons may not be able to see other people or objects in their peripheral fields.

HEARING

Although old age does not mean an inevitable loss of hearing, impairments in hearing do affect more than one-third of those 65 years of age and older (Meisami, 1988). Presbycusis is the term used to identify age-related hearing loss. Presbycusis is characterized by a loss of hearing sounds in the high-frequency range. This hearing loss is exacerbated in persons from urban versus rural communities, indicating that exposure to loud noise may contribute to hearing loss (Rosen et al., 1962). Exposure to work-related noise is one possible cause of the increased hearing loss in men as compared with women (Spoor, 1967). If this is true, the incidence of hearing loss in women will increase as more women are employed in loud environments. Spencer (1973) reported an increased incidence of hearing loss in patients with high cholesterol levels, possibly due to atherosclerotic changes.

With age, there is also a decreased ability to ascertain the location of sounds. Localization of high-frequency sounds is dependent upon the gradient of sound intensity between the two ears. Localization of low-frequency sounds hinges on the time difference between when the sound is heard in each ear. The older patient has the most difficulty localizing the high-frequency sounds.

Presbycusis affects discrimination of speech in that consonants are not heard as well as vowels. Consonants make speech meaningful, whereas vowels are linked to the volume of speech. For this reason, many elders complain of not being able to understand speech even though they may hear it (Meisami, 1988).

Elderly persons may also have trouble masking sounds, that is, they have difficulty sorting the background noise from the stimuli to which they wish to attend. In addition, loud noises may irritate elderly persons. Furthermore, because more time is necessary for processing stimuli at the higher auditory centers, accelerated speech is more difficult for the older person to understand (Matteson and McConnell, 1988; Meisami, 1988).

OLFACTION

With age, the olfactory mucosa loses receptor neurons (Nakashima et al., 1984; Meisami, 1988). In some individuals, there is complete loss of the olfactory neurons (Naessen, 1971). There is also a loss of neurons at the higher nerve centers, the olfactory bulbs, which lie just below the frontal lobes (Smith, 1942; Bhatnagar et al., 1987; Meisami, 1988). All of these changes lead to a decreased ability to identify or detect odors.

Some studies report that the severity of olfactory degeneration is not correlated with increasing age and may be more a function of environmental factors such as pollution or smoking (Corso, 1971; 1975; Matteson and McConnell, 1988).

TASTE

There is a gradual decline in the number of taste buds as well as an atrophy of the remaining taste buds with age. These losses do not affect discrimination of the four taste qualities—sweet, sour, salt, bitter—until the sixth decade, if at all (Corso, 1971; Matteson and McConnell, 1988; Engen, 1977). Results of research on age-related changes in taste are conflicting, but it appears that loss of gustatory sensation, if it occurs, is less marked than that of other senses.

TOUCH

There is some decline in tactile sensitivity with age. For example, elderly adults tend to have increased thresholds to touch stimuli, decreased vibratory sensitivity, decreased corneal sensitivity, and decreased sensitivity on the palate (Bruce, 1980; Meisami, 1988; Newman, 1979). The decreased sensation in the palate increases the risk of aspiration. This risk is further increased by the elder's decreased cough reflex.

Two-point discrimination declines with age, as does stereognosis (Meisami, 1988). Of potential danger is the loss of pain and thermal sensitivity associated with aging. This loss cannot be attributed solely to tactile losses. Affective, cognitive, and environmental factors are thought to play a large role in this alteration (Meisami, 1988).

Elderly persons have far less acuity relative to the perception of pain. In addition, many elderly persons and their health care providers tend to accept pain and discomfort as normal accompaniments to aging. This fallacy may lead to under-reporting and/or delayed treatment of injury or illness (Kligman et al., 1985).

CLINICAL IMPLICATIONS OF AGE-RELATED CHANGES IN THE SENSORY ORGANS

Sensory Alterations. Maintaining sensory equilibrium for the critically ill elder can make a substantial difference in the patient's experience and outcome. The ICU environment is typically saturated with noises, smells, sights, and multiple tactile cues. The nurse is in the position to change the environment in a way that enhances patient care. The nursing goal is to balance sensory deficits often experienced by older patients with sensory overload often characteristic of the ICU.

Unnecessary equipment is placed out of sight to reduce the number of visual stimuli. The colors of walls, floors, and curtains should be soothing, yet different enough from one another so that the person can distinguish the horizontal and vertical boundaries of the room. Pastel uniforms or scrubs provide pleasing visual cues, whereas white uniforms may appear frightening, especially when seen in the dark.

Elderly persons have particular difficulty distinguishing blues and greens. Therefore, using yellow, orange, and red contrasting colors can be very helpful to older adults (Matteson and McConnell, 1988). For example, the older person's medications may be dispensed in the colors seen best.

Elderly persons may not be able to see other people or objects in their peripheral fields. When speaking to an older adult in the critical care unit, the nurse should validate that the person can see him or her. Alarms and other noises that may originate out of the elder's field of vision should be explained. Fluorescent lighting and uncovered windows produce glare on floors, walls, and objects, which may alter the older person's perception of his or her environment while in the ICU.

Because red light stimulates only the cones, elderly people can see well enough to function by red light in the dark. Also, the time needed for dark adaptation is reduced in red light. Therefore, a red light may be placed at the bedside at night to improve the rate of dark adaptation and to increase visibility (Matteson and McConnell, 1988; Hilgard et al., 1975).

Awareness of the changes in hearing experienced by older adults will enable the nurse to minimize communication problems by speaking in lower tones in a voice of normal volume, allowing the patient to visualize the nurse's lips, and speaking at a slightly slower rate. When background noise is apparent, as in the critical care unit, messages may need to be repeated or also conveyed in simple written form. Getting the patient's attention before speaking and allowing the person adequate time to respond are very important due to the increased time needed for processing verbal stimuli. Only one question is asked at a time. If it is necessary to repeat the inquiry, it is repeated verbatim to decrease the complexity of the stimuli. Any attempt to decrease background noise is also helpful. Documenting the most effective interventions assists other professionals working with the patient (Bernardini, 1985).

To decrease olfactory stimulation, personnel do not wear heavy perfume or aftershave. Meals are served promptly and are taken away from the patient care area as soon as possible. Charcoal filters are used for air purification instead of scented room deodorizers. Linen and drainage apparatus are changed frequently to decrease odors (Bernardini, 1985).

At a time when perception of touch is reduced by aging, the opportunities for nurturing touch are also decreased due to losses of friends and loved ones. In the ICU, when many people and objects may be touching the patient as part of therapeutic interventions, this task-oriented touching is not perceived in the same way as empathetic, caring touch. Cultural and personal interpretations of touch vary widely, so that the ICU nurse assesses the meaning of touch to the patient before using it as a therapeutic intervention. When touch is used appropriately, it can be a powerful therapeutic tool. The nurse may take the hand of the patient and put it on hers or his while speaking to focus the attention on the conversation. Use of nonverbal communication is especially important to the elder, who is likely to be feeling anxious, depressed, and/or isolated (Bernardini, 1985).

TABLE 65–7. Pharmacologic Considerations in the Elderly

Drug	Route of Elimination	Clinical Implications
Analgesics		
Acetaminophen	Hepatic	No substantial age-related change in kinetics
Aspirin	Renal	Highly protein-bound; half-life may be prolonged
Narcotics	Hepatic	Blood levels higher; pain relief longer
		Lower doses are usually effective
		Constipation is major side effect in elderly patient
Antimicrobials		
Aminoglycosides	Renal	Prolonged half-life may require increased dosage intervals (e.g., q 12 hrs, q 24 hrs)
		Nephrotoxicity and ototoxicity are major problems; monitor blood levels, serum creatinine, creatinine clearance
		Formula for calculating age-referenced interval in men:
		[140 − age × kg body wt]/72 × serum creatinine; women: 85% of this
Cephalosporins	Renal	Half-life prolonged
Penicillins	Renal	Half-life prolonged
	Hepatic	Some are highly protein bound
Tetracycline	Renal	Half-life prolonged
Amphotericin	Nonrenal	Nephrotoxicity a major problem in elderly with underlying renal dysfunction
Cardiovascular Drugs		
Beta-adrenergic effect	Renal	Elderly patients may require increased dosage to achieve
Digoxin	Renal (15–40% nonrenal)	Decreased clearance; half-life prolonged
Lidocaine	Hepatic	Volume of distribution is increased; half-life prolonged; clearance unchanged
Procainamide	Renal	Clearance decreased; highly protein bound
		Half-life prolonged; steady-state levels higher
Quinidine	Nonrenal	Highly protein bound; clearance decreased
		Half-life prolonged
Verapamil	Hepatic	Clearance decreased
		Effects more pronounced and prolonged
Antihypertensives		
Diltiazem	Hepatic	Clearance decreased; used cautiously in sinus node dysfunction
Hydralazine	Hepatic	Highly protein bound
Propranolol	Hepatic	Highly protein bound
		Half-life prolonged; clearance decreased; blood levels higher
		Sensitivity to effects decreased
Diuretics		
Furosemide	Renal	Highly protein bound
		Elderly patients at high risk of dehydration and electrolyte imbalance

PHARMACOGERIATRICS

There are many physiologic changes associated with aging that are relevant to medication use and administration. The pharmacologic parameters that are altered by aging include absorption, distribution, metabolism, excretion, and tissue sensitivity (Kane et al., 1989; Kidd and Murakami, 1987). Table 65–7 outlines special considerations for drugs commonly used in the elderly patient in the critical care area.

Drug absorption is affected by decreases in the absorptive surface of the gut and blood vessels and a reduction in splanchnic blood flow. Increased gastric pH, as well as altered gastrointestinal motility, also may alter drug absorption (Kane et al., 1989).

Changes in drug distribution may occur in the elderly patient as a result of decreases in total body water and lean body mass and a lower serum albumin concentration. Changes in protein binding have been demonstrated, but the clinical relevance of these changes has not been established (Kane et al., 1989).

Reduced liver blood flow, diminished hepatic enzyme activity, and decreased enzyme inducibility may change the actual metabolism of drugs. The results of research related to drug metabolism and aging are inconclusive as far as being able to predict metabolic alterations linked to specific drugs (Kane et al., 1989).

Changes in excretion of drugs may be due to diminished renal blood flow, decreased glomerular filtration rate, and impaired tubular secretion function. Tissue sensitivity is altered due to changes in the number of receptors and receptor affinity for certain drugs. In addition, there may be cellular and nuclear responses that change with aging (Kane et al., 1989).

The drug dosing rate is adjusted downward to prevent excessive drug accumulation, side effects, and potential toxicity. Patients are started at lower doses, and the doses are increased more gradually than in younger people. Drug interactions are prevalent due to polypharmacy in the elderly, so there is ongoing consultation with the clinical pharmacist to monitor for side effects and to evaluate effectiveness of drug regimens (Chapron, 1988).

SUMMARY

Many changes accompany the aging process. The physiologic changes depicted in this chapter are of both structural and functional decline. However, it is important for the nurse to recognize that with every stage of life, old capabilities are lost as new ones are gained. Although the elderly individual may be declining in some physiologic parameters, other areas of his or her life are growing in strength and complexity. New strengths may include wisdom, capability for higher abstraction of thought, and an ability to transcend the physical pain and limitations of the body (Reed, 1983). Perhaps the most important developmental challenge the older person faces is the inevitability of death (Erikson, 1963). This issue becomes even more salient in the face of critical illness. Certainly, the critically ill elderly patient represents a complex interaction of many dynamic systems and requires nursing care based on diverse and sound clinical knowledge.

References

Altman, D. F. (1983). Gastrointestinal diseases in the elderly. *Medical Clinics of North America, 67,* 435.

American Society for Parenteral and Enteral Nutrition (ASPEN) Board of Directors (1987). Guidelines for the use of enteral nutrition in the adult patient. *Critical Care Nursing Quarterly, 12* (1), 15–25.

Anderson, B. J. (1986). Tube feeding: Is diarrhea inevitable? *American Journal of Nursing, 6,* 706.

Armstrong, G. G., and Gardner, D. L. (1977). The thickness and distribution of human femoral head articular cartilage changes with age. *Annals of Rheumatoid Disease, 36,* 407.

Aurell, J., and Elmquist, D. (1985). Sleep in the surgical intensive care unit: Continuous polygraphic recording of sleep in nine patients receiving post-operative care. *British Medical Journal, 290,* 1029–1032.

Baum, B. J. (1981). Characteristics of participants in the oral physiology component of the Baltimore longitudinal study of aging. *Community Dental and Oral Epidemiology, 9,* 128–134.

Baum, B. J., Costa, P. T., Jr., and Izutsu, K. T. (1984). Sodium handling by aging human parotid glands is inconsistent with a two-stage secretion model. *American Journal of Physiology, 246,* R35–R39.

Bendixen, H., Hedley-Whyte, M. B., Chir, B., and Laver, M. B. (1963). Impaired oxygenation in surgical patients during general anesthesia with controlled ventilation. *New England Journal of Medicine, 269,* 991.

Bennett, R. G., and Ouslander, J. G. (1989). Air-fluidized bed treatment of nursing home patients with pressure sores. *Journal of the American Geriatric Society, 37,* 235–242.

Bentley, S., Murphy, F., and Dudley, H. (1977). Perceived noise in surgical wards and an intensive care unit: An objective analysis. *British Medical Journal, 2,* 1503–1506.

Berk, S. L., and Smith, J. K. (1983). Infectious diseases in the elderly. *Medical Clinics of North America, 67,* 273–293.

Berman, P., Hogan, D. B., and Fox, R. A. (1987). The atypical presentation of infection in old age. *Age and Ageing, 16,* 201–207.

Bernardini, L. (1985). Effective communications as an intervention for sensory deprivation in the elderly client. *Topics in Clinical Nursing, 4,* 72–81.

Bhatnagar, K. P., Kennedy, R. C., Baron, G., and Greenberg, R. A. (1987). Number of mitral cells and the bulb volume in the aging olfactory bulb: A quantitative morphological study. *Anatomical Record, 218,* 73–87.

Biena, R., Ratcliff, S., and Barbour, J. (1982). Malnutrition in the hospitalized geriatric patient. *Journal of the American Geriatric Society, 30,* 433–436.

Block, E. R. (1979). Pitfalls in diagnosing and managing pulmonary diseases. *Geriatrics, 34* (2), 70–79.

Botwinick, J. (1978). *Aging and behavior* (2nd ed.). New York: Springer.

Bowles, L. T., Portnoi, V., and Kenney, R. (1981). Wear and tear: Common biological changes of aging. *Geriatrics, 36* (4), 77–86.

Browse, N. L. (1965). *The physiology and pathology of bedrest.* Springfield, IL: Charles C Thomas.

Bruce, M. F. (1980). The relation of tactile thresholds to histology in the fingers of the elderly. *Journal of Neurology, Neurosurgery and Psychiatry, 43,* 730–734.

Bumann, R., and Speltz, M. (1989). Decreased cardiac output: A nursing diagnosis. *Dimensions of Critical Care Nursing, 8,* 6–15.

Byers, P. D., Contempomi, C. A., and Farkas, T. A. (1970). A post mortem study of the hip joint, including the prevalence of the features of the right side. *Annals of Rheumatoid Disease,* 19, 15.

Carter, A. B. (1986). The neurological aspects of aging. In I. Rossman (Ed.), *Clinical geriatrics* (3rd ed., pp. 326–351). Philadelphia: J. B. Lippincott.

Champagne, M. T., and Ashley, M. L. (1989). Nutritional support in the critically ill elderly patient. *Critical Care Nursing Quarterly,* 12 (1), 15–25.

Chapron, D. J. (1988). Influence of advanced age on drug disposition and response. In J. C. Delafuente and R. B. Stewart (Eds.), *Therapeutics in the elderly* (pp. 107–120). Baltimore: Williams & Wilkins.

Clements, J. A. (1951). Surface tension of lung extracts. *Procedures in Social and Experimental Biology & Medicine,* 95, 170.

Coe, W. S. (1954). Cardiac work and the chair treatment of acute coronary thrombosis. *Annals of Internal Medicine,* 40, 42.

Cohen, F. L. (1989). Immunologic impairment, infection, and AIDS in the aging patient. *Critical Care Nursing Quarterly,* 12 (1), 38–45.

Collins, K. J. (1980). Functional changes in autonomic nervous responses with aging. *Age and Ageing,* 9, 17–20.

Corso, J. F. (1971). Sensory processes and age effects in normal adults. *Journal of Gerontology,* 26, 90–105.

Corso, J. F. (1975). Sensory process in man during maturity and senescence. In J. M. Ordy and K. R. Brizzer (Eds.), *Neurobiology of aging* (pp. 119–143). New York: Plenum Press.

Crawford, J., Eye-Boland, M. K., and Cohen, H. J. (1987). Clinical utility of erythrocyte sedimentation rate and plasma protein analysis in the elderly. *American Journal of Medicine,* 82, 239–246.

Curcio, C. A., Buell, S. J., and Coleman, P. D. (1982). Morphology of the aging central nervous system: Not all downhill. In J. A. Mortimer, F. J. Pirozzolo, and G. J. Maletta (Eds.), *The aging motor system* (pp. 7–35). New York: Praeger.

Daniel, R. K., Priest, D. L., and Wheatley, D. C. (1981). Etiological factors in pressure sores: An experimental model. *Archives of Physical Medicine and Rehabilitation,* 62, 492–498.

Darmady, E. M., Offer, J., and Woodhouse, M. A. (1973). The parameters of the aging kidney. *Journal of Pathology,* 109, 195–207.

Davidson, R. A. (1989). Hypertension in the elderly. *Medical Clinics of North America,* 73 (6), 1471–1481.

Davis, P. J., and Davis, F. B. (1983). Endocrinology and aging. In W. Reichel (Ed.), *Clinical aspects of aging* (2nd ed., pp. 396–410). Baltimore: Williams & Wilkins.

Davis-Sharts, J. (1989). The elderly and critical care: Sleep and mobility issues. *Nursing Clinics of North America,* 24 (3), 755–767.

Deitel, M., Williams, V., and Rice, T. (1983). Nutrition and the patient requiring mechanical ventilatory support. *Journal of the American College of Nutrition,* 2, 25–32.

Dietrick, J. E., Whedon, G. D., and Shorr, E. (1948). Effects of immobilization upon various metabolic and physiologic functions of normal men. *American Journal of Medicine,* 4, 3.

Dorfman, L., and Bosley, T. (1979). Age-related changes in peripheral and central nerve conduction in man. *Neurology,* 29, 38.

Duara, R., London, E. D., and Rapoport, S. I. (1985). Changes in structure and energy metabolism of the aging brain. In C. E. Finch and E. L. Schneider (Eds.), *Handbook of the biology of aging* (pp. 595–616). New York: Van Nostrand Reinhold.

Eckel, R. H., and Hofeldt, F. D. (1982). Endocrinology and metabolism in the elderly. In R. W. Schrier (Ed.), *Clinical internal medicine in the aged* (pp. 222–255). Philadelphia: W. B. Saunders.

Eliopoulous, C. (1978). Diagnosis and management of diabetes in the elderly. *American Journal of Nursing,* 78, 884–886.

Engen, T. (1977). Taste and smell. In J. E. Birren and K. W. Schaie (Eds.), *Handbook of the psychology of aging* (pp. 554–561). New York: Van Nostrand Reinhold.

Erikson, E. (1963). *Childhood and society.* New York: W. W. Norton.

Esberger, K. K., and Hughes, S. T., Jr. (Eds.) (1989). *Nursing care of the aged.* Norwalk, CT: Appleton & Lange.

Exton-Smith, A. N., and Overstall, P. W. (1979). *Geriatrics.* Lancaster, England: MIP Press.

Feinstein, E. I. (1986). Renal disease in the elderly. In I. Rossman (Ed.), *Clinical Geriatrics* (3rd ed. pp. 352–363). Philadelphia: J. B. Lippincott.

Finklestein, M. S., Petkun, W. M., Freedman, M. L., and Antopol, S. C. (1983). Pneumococcal bacteremia in adults: Age-dependent differences in presentation and outcome. *Journal of the American Geriatric Society,* 31, 19–27.

Fonesca, V. (1981). Sulphonylurea and insulin combination in the treatment of diabetes (letter). *British Medical Journal,* 283, 797.

Forbes, P. D., Davies, R. E., and Urbach, F. (1979). Aging, environmental influences and photocarcinogenesis. *Journal of Investigative Dermatology,* 73, 131–134.

Foreman, M. D. (1984). Acute confusional states in the elderly: An algorithm. *Dimensions in Critical Care Nursing,* 3, 209–215.

Fox, R. A. (1988). Atypical presentation of geriatric infections. *Geriatrics,* 43 (5), 58–65.

Ganong, W. F. (1987). *Review of medical physiology* (13th ed.). Los Altos, CA: Lange Medical Publications.

Giansiracusa, D. F., and Kantrowitz, F. G. (1981). *Rheumatic and metabolic diseases in the elderly.* Lexington, MA: The Collamore Press.

Gilchrest, B. A. (1982). Age-associated changes in the skin. *Journal of the American Geriatric Society,* 30, 139–143.

Gioiella, E. C., and Bevil, C. W. (1984). *Nursing care of the aging client: Promoting healthy adaptation.* Norwalk, CT: Appleton-Century-Crofts.

Goldberg, A. P., Andes, R., and Bierman, E. L. (1985). Diabetes mellitus in the elderly. In R. Andres, E. Bierman, and W. Hazzard (Eds.), *Principles of geriatric medicine* (pp. 750–763). New York: McGraw-Hill.

Good, R. A., and Gabrielson, A. B. (Eds.) (1964). *Thymus in immunobiology.* New York: Hoeber-Harper.

Goode, P. S. (1989). The prevention and management of pressure ulcers. *Medical Clinics of North America,* 73 (6), 1511–1524.

Gottsdanker, R. (1982). Age and simple reaction time. *Journal of Gerontology,* 37, 342–348.

Gribbin, B., Pickering, T. G., Sleight, P., and Peto, S. (1971). Effect of age and high blood pressure and baroreceptor sensitivity in man. *Circulation Research,* 29, 424–431.

Grob, D. (1978). Prevalent joint diseases in older persons. In W. Reichel (Ed.), *Clinical Aspects of aging* (pp. 161–175). Baltimore: Williams & Wilkins.

Grossman, G. (1985). Nutritional assessment of critically ill patients. *Respiratory Care,* 30, 463–469.

Hayter, J. (1981). Diabetes and the older person. *Geriatric Nursing,* 1, 32–36.

Heath, H., and Earl, J. M. (1972). Serum ionized calcium during bedrest in fracture patients and normal men. *Metabolism,* 21, 633.

Hickler, R. B. (1985). The physiology of aging: Implications for drug therapy. In E. P. Hoffer (Ed.), *Emergency problems in the elderly* (pp. 1–17). Oradell, NJ: Medical Economics Books.

Hilgard, E. R., Atkinson, R. C., and Atkinson, R. L. (1975). *Introduction to psychology* (6th ed). New York: Harcourt Brace Jovanovich.

Hoehn, P., Gabbert, H., and Wagner, R. (1978). Differentiation and aging of the rat intestinal mucosa, II. Morphological, enzyme histochemical and disc electrophoretic aspects of the aging of the small intestinal mucosa. *Mechanics of Aging and Development,* 7, 217.

Hollenberg, N. K., Adams, D. F., Solomon, H. S., et al. (1974). Senescence and the renal vasculature in normal man. *Circulation Research,* 34, 309–316.

Holloway, N. M. (1988). *Nursing the critically ill adult.* Menlo Park, CA: Addison-Wesley.

Jones, J., Hoggart, B., Withey, J., et al. (1979). What the patients say: A study of reactions to an intensive care unit. *Intensive Care Medicine,* 5, 89–92.

Kampmann, J. P., Sindling, J., and Moller-Jorgensen, I. (1975). Effect of age on liver function. *Geriatrics,* 30, 91–95.

Kane, R. L., Ouslander, J. G., and Abrass, I. B. (1989). *Essentials of clinical geriatrics* (2nd ed). New York: McGraw-Hill.

Kannel, W. B., and Gordon, T. (1978). Evaluation of cardiovascular risk in the elderly: The Framingham study. *Bulletin of the New York Academy of Medicine,* 54, 573–591.

Kato, R., and Takanaka, A. (1986). Metabolism of drugs in old rats II. *Japanese Journal of Pharmacology,* 18, 389–396.

Kay, M. M. B., and Baker, L. S. (1979). Cell changes associated with declining immune function in aging series. In A. Cherkin, C. E. Finch, N. Kharasch, et al. (Eds.), *Physiology and cell biology of aging* (pp. 27–49). New York: Raven Press.

Kelly, D. J. (1989). The identification and clinical validation of the defining characteristics of the nursing diagnosis alteration in tissue perfusion: Cardiac. (Unpublished Masters Thesis, University of Arizona, Tucson.)

Kidd, P. S., and Murakami, R. Y. (1987). Common pathologic conditions in elderly persons: Nursing assessment and intervention. *Journal of Emergency Nursing*, 13 (1), 27–32.

King, T. E., and Schwartz, M. I. (1982). Pulmonary function and disease in the elderly. In R. W. Schrier (Ed.), *Clinical internal medicine in the aged* (pp. 124–148). Philadelphia: W. B. Saunders.

Kligman, A. M., Grove, G. L., and Bakin, A. K. (1985). Aging of human skin. In C. E. Finch and E. L. Schneider (Eds.), *Handbook of the biology of aging* (2nd ed., pp. 820–841). New York: Van Nostrand Reinhold.

Krieger, B. P., Ershowsky, P. F., Becker, D. A., and Gaserogly, H. B. (1989). Evaluation of conventional criteria for predicting successful weaning from mechanical ventilatory support in the elderly. *Critical Care Medicine*, 17 (9), 858–861.

Krumpe, P. E., Knudson, R. J., Parsons, G., and Reiser, K. (1985). The aging respiratory system. *Clinics in Geriatric Medicine*, 1, 143–175.

Lakatta, E. G., Gerstenblith, G., Angell, C. S., et al. (1975). Diminished inotropic response of aged myocardium to catecholamines. *Circulation Research*, 36, 262–269.

Larsson, L. (1982). Aging in mammalian skeletal muscle. In J. A. Mortimer, F. J. Pirozzolo, and G. J. Maletta (Eds.), *The aging motor system* (pp. 60–94). New York: Praeger.

Larsson, L., Grimby, G., and Karlsson, J. (1979). Muscle strength and speed of movement in relation to age and muscle morphology. *Journal of Applied Physiology*, 46, 451–456.

Lee, B. Y. (1980). Non-invasive detection and prevention of deep-vein thrombosis in the geriatric patient. *Journal of the American Geriatric Society*, 28, 171–175.

Levitzky, M. G. (1984). Effects of aging on the respiratory system. *Physiologist*, 27, 102–107.

Lincoln, R., and Roberts, R. (1989). Continence issues in acute care. *Nursing Clinics of North America*, 24 (3), 741–753.

Luft, F. C., Grim, C. E., Fineberg, N., and Weingerber, M. C. (1979). Effects of volume expansion and contraction in normotensive whites, blacks and subjects of different ages. *Circulation*, 59, 643–650.

Lukasiewicz-Ferland, P. (1987). When your ICU patient can't sleep. *Nursing*, 17 (11), 51–53.

Lytle, L. D., and Altar, A. (1979). Diet, central nervous system, and aging. *Federation Proceedings*, 38, 2017–2022.

MacLennan, W. J., Shepherd, A. N., and Stevenson, I. H. (1984). Disorders of the vascular system. In *The elderly* (pp. 42–58). New York: Springer-Verlag.

Malseed, R. T. (1983). *Pharmacology: Drug therapy and nursing considerations*. Philadelphia: J. B. Lippincott.

Marchesseault, L. C. (1983). Diabetes mellitus and the elderly. *Nursing Clinics of North America*, 18 (4), 791–798.

Matteson, M. A., and McConnell, E. S. (1988). *Gerontological nursing*. Philadelphia: W. B. Saunders.

Mauderly, J. L. (1981). Lung-thorax system. In E. J. Masaro, R. C. Adelmon, and G. S. Roth (Eds.), *CRC handbook of physiology in aging* (pp. 197–214). Boca Raton, FL: CRC Press.

McAlpine, C. H., Martin, B. J., Lennox, I. M., and Roberts, M. A. (1986). Pyrexia in infection in the elderly. *Age and Ageing*, 15, 230–234.

Meisami, E. (1988). Aging of the nervous system: Sensory changes. In P. S. Timiras (Ed.), *Physiological basis of geriatrics* (pp. 156–178). New York: Macmillan.

Milde, F. K. (1981). Physiological immobilization. In L. Hart, G. Reese, and R. Fearing (Eds.), *Concepts common to acute illness* (pp. 67–109). St. Louis: C. V. Mosby.

Miles, L., and Dement, W. (1980). Sleep and aging. *Sleep*, 3, 119–200.

Mims, F., and Swenson, L. (1980). *Sexuality: A nursing perspective*. New York: Appleton-Century-Crofts.

Monk, T. H. (1989). Sleep disorders in the elderly: Circadian rhythm. *Clinics in Geriatric Medicine*, 5 (2), 331–346.

Moss, R. J., and Miles, S. H. (1987). AIDS and the geriatrician. *Journal of the American Geriatric Society*, 35, 460–464.

Mostow, S. R. (1983). Infectious complications in the elderly COPD patient. *Geriatrics*, 38 (10), 42–48.

Murray, J. F. (1986). *The normal lung* (2nd ed., pp. 339–360). Philadelphia: W. B. Saunders.

Naessen, R. (1971). An inquiry on the morphological characteristics and possible changes with age in the olfactory region of man. *Acta Otolaryngologica*, 71, 49–62.

Nakashima, T., Kimmelman, P., and Snow, J. B., Jr. (1984). Structure of human fetal and adult olfactory neuroepithelium. *Archives of Otolaryngology*, 10, 641–646.

Nasr, H. (1983). Endocrine disorders in the elderly. *Medical Clinics of North America*, 67, 481–495.

Navia, B. A., and Price, R. W. (1987). The acquired immunodeficiency syndrome dementia complex as the presenting or sole manifestation of human immunodeficiency virus infection. *Archives of Neurology*, 44, 65–69.

Newman, H. F. (1979). Palatal sensitivity to touch: Correlation with age. *Journal of the American Geriatric Society*, 27, 319.

Nicolas, F., LeGall, J. R., Alperovitch, A., et al. (1987). Influence of patients' age on survival, level of therapy and length of stay in intensive care units. *Intensive Care Medicine*, 13, 9–13.

Pierson, D. J., and Hudson, L. D. (1981). Pulmonary problems. *Geriatrics*, 36 (4), 45–47.

Pingleton, S., and Hadzima, S. (1983). Enteral alimentation and gastrointestinal bleeding in mechanically ventilated patients. *Critical Care Medicine*, 11, 13–16.

Pochi, P., Strauss, J. S., and Downing, D. T. (1979). Age-related changes in sebaceous gland activity. *Journal of Investigative Dermatology*, 73, 108–111.

Rebensen-Piano, M. (1989). The physiologic changes that occur with aging. *Critical Care Nursing Quarterly*, 12 (1), 1–14.

Reed, P. G. (1983). Implications of the lifespan developmental framework for well-being in adulthood and aging. *Advances in Nursing Science*, 6 (3), 18–25.

Reynolds, J., Guyang, A., and Cohen, S. (1982). Recent advances in diagnosis and treatment of esophageal disease. *Geriatrics*, 37 (6), 91–93; 97; 101–104.

Rock, R. C. (1985). Interpreting thyroid tests in the elderly: Updated guidelines. *Geriatrics*, 40, 61–68.

Rogers, J. R., and Bloom, F. E. (1985). Neurotransmitter metabolism and function in the aging central nervous system. In C. E. Finch and E. L. Schneider (Eds.), *Handbook of the biology of aging* (pp. 645–691). New York: Van Nostrand Reinhold.

Rose, B. D. (1984). *Clinical physiology of acid-base and electrolyte disorders*. New York: McGraw-Hill.

Rose, G. A. (1966). Immobilization osteoporosis. *British Journal of Surgery*, 53, 769.

Rosen, S., Bergman, M., Plester, D., et al. Presbycusis study of a relatively noise-free population in the Sudan. *Annals of Otology*, 71, 727–743.

Ross, R. (1986). The pathogenesis of atherosclerosis—an update. *New England Journal of Medicine*, 314, 488–500.

Rowe, J. W. (1982). Renal system. In J. W. Rowe and R. W. Besdine (Eds.), *Health and disease* (pp. 165–183). Boston: Little, Brown.

Sabin, T. D. (1987). AIDS: The new "great imitator." *Journal of the American Geriatric Society*, 35, 467–468.

Sato, T. G., Iwa, T., and Tauchi, H. (1970). Age changes in the human liver of the different races. *Gerontologia*, 16, 368–380.

Sjostrand, T. (1952). The regulation of the blood distribution in man. *Acta Physiologica Scandanavica*, 26, 312.

Smith, C. G. (1942). Age incidence of atrophy of olfactory nerves in man: A contribution to the study of the process of aging. *Journal of Comprehensive Neurology*, 77, 589–596.

Soergel, K. H., Zboralske, F. F., and Amberg, J. R. (1964). Presbyesophagus: Esophageal motility in nonagenarians. *Journal of Clinical Investigation*, 43, 1472–1479.

Sorbini, C. A., Grassi, Z., Solinas, E., and Muiesan, G. (1968). Arterial oxygen tension in relation to age in healthy subjects. *Respiration*, 25, 3–13.

Spencer, J. T., Jr. (1973). Hyperlipoproteinemia in the etiology of inner ear disease. *Laryngoscope*, 83, 639–678.

Spoor, A. (1967). Presbycusis values in relation to noise induced hearing loss. *International Audiology*, 6, 148–157.

Sternberg, H. (1988). Aging of the immune system. In P. S. Timiras (Ed.), *Physiological basis of geriatrics* (pp. 103–122). New York: Macmillan.

Taylor, T. V., Timmers, S., and Day, B. (1974). Ascorbic acid supplementation in the treatment of pressure sores. *Lancet, 2,* 544–546.

Timiras, M. L. (1988). Aging of the skin and connective tissue. In P. S. Timiras (Ed.), *Physiological basis of geriatrics* (pp. 371–379). New York: Macmillan.

U.S. Senate Special Committee on Aging (1985–1986 ed.). *Aging of America: Trends and projections.*

Vestal, R. E., Wood, A. J., and Shand, D. G. (1979). Reduced beta-adrenoreceptor sensitivity in the elderly. *Clinical Pharmacology and Therapeutics, 26,* 181–186.

Vierling, J. M., and Reichen, J. (1982). Physiology and diseases of the digestive system in the aged. In R. W. Schrier (Ed.), *Clinical internal medicine in the aged* (pp. 149–166). Philadelphia: W. B. Saunders.

Wahba, W. M. (1983). Influence of aging on lung function—clinical significance of changes from age twenty. *Anesthesia and Analgesia, 62,* 764–776.

Walsh, R. A. (1987). Cardiovascular effects of the aging process. *American Journal of Cardiology, 82,* 34–40.

Webster, R. A., and Thompson, D. R. (1986). Sleep in hospital. *Journal of Advanced Nursing, 11,* 447–457.

Wekster, M. E. (1983). Senescence of the immune system. *Medical Clinics of North America, 67* (2), 263–272.

White, E. H. (1983). Problems of absorption and elimination. In S. M. Lewis and I. C. Collier (Eds.), *Medical-surgical nursing: Assessment and management of clinical problems.* New York: McGraw-Hill.

Williams, R., Karncan, I., and Hursch, C. (1974). *EEG of human sleep: Clinical applications.* New York: John Wiley and Sons.

Williams, T. (1978). Diabetes mellitus in the aged. In R. Greenblatt (Ed.), *Geriatric endocrinology* (pp. 103–114). New York: Raven Press.

Woods, N. F. (1987). Toward a holistic perspective of human sexuality: Alterations in sexual health and nursing diagnosis. *Holistic Nursing Practice, 1* (4), 1–11.

Yurick, A. G., Robb, S. S., Spier, B. E., and Ebert, N. J. (1980). *The aged person and the nursing process.* New York: Appleton-Century-Crofts.

Zepelen, H. (1983). Normal age related changes in sleep. In H. Zepelen, *Sleep disorders: Basic and clinical research* (pp. 431–444). SP Medical and Scientific Books.

Zimmerman, F. (1981). Type II diabetes mellitus in the senior citizen. *Nurse Practitioner, 6,* 31–32.

15

Advocacy

C · H · A · P · T · E · R

66

Ethics in Critical Care

Barbara J. Daly

Critical care has become a well-recognized and respected specialty within modern health care. Paralleling the growth of this specialty, new problems have developed related to the decisions involved in providing care to critically ill persons. Bioethics has emerged as a growing field of inquiry that seeks to answer questions about the appropriateness of what we can do, the proper way of distributing scarce resources, and the meaning of what is being done in health care.

NURSING ETHICS

Ethics is a branch of moral philosophy that attempts to address questions about right conduct. In clinical practice, ethical study generally focuses on specific rules, principles, and approaches that can be used to guide decision making. As shown in Figure 66–1, it rests on a broader philosophical base that examines the fundamental meaning of such terms as right, goodness, moral, and duty. Bioethics may be defined as the study of the "moral and conceptual problems associated with health care and the biomedical sciences" (Englehardt, 1986). Nursing ethics is a branch of bioethics and is different and distinct from other branches, such as medical ethics or research ethics, only in the sense that the responsibilities, constraints, and particular questions nurses face are inextricably related to the role of the nurse in modern health care. The term nursing ethics should not be interpreted to mean that there are

FIGURE 66–1. Derivation of the study of ethics.

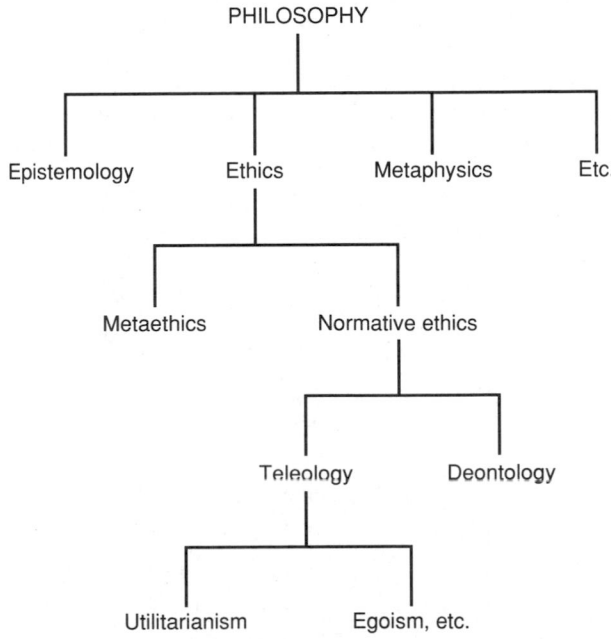

1375

necessarily different principles or moral rules that apply only to nurses.

Critical care nursing is, first and foremost, the actual provision of care to critically ill patients. It is based on a body of knowledge established through ongoing investigation. As a specialty within a practice discipline, the primary concern of critical care nurses is effectiveness. With this as an assumption, the purpose of this chapter is not to provide an indepth analysis of the many theories and principles that may underlie moral responsibility but rather to offer the reader some guidance in developing an articulated moral intuition that can be further refined and applied in clinical practice.

A further assumption is that the majority of nurses have some degree of moral intuition. Benner and Tanner, in their extensive studies of expert nurses, described nurses' clinical intuition as "understanding without a rationale" (Benner and Tanner, 1987). Experienced practitioners are often able to respond to cues in an ethical dilemma, identify the situation as similar or dissimilar to others, and attain a commonsense grasp of the whole. Yet, at the same time, they may be unable to articulate the elements and provide a rationale that convinces others of the validity and "rightness" of their views. Thus, a situation is created that is often associated with frustration on the part of the nurse and unresolved conflicts among the health care team. Just as intuitive clinical judgment skills can be taught and fostered, moral intuition and the ability to act effectively upon it can be developed.

In the acquisition of most skills, the initial stages involve learning steps in a process using certain facts and principles as tools. In the case of ethics, many authors recommend a multistep process of ethical reasoning that can be used by the novice in learning (Krekeler, 1987; Fowler, 1987b; Curtin, 1982). Although there is some variation in the exact components and number of steps, the processes recommended are very similar. A five-step process, described in Figure 66–2, will be used as the organizing framework for the rest of this chapter. It is important for the reader to keep in mind that this process is most helpful when one is first beginning to pursue ethical inquiry seriously. It is less helpful as the practitioner becomes more fully involved in analyzing ethical dilemmas and is able to use moral intuition. Regan (1986) points out that, like the scientific method, any standard method for answering moral questions will not *in itself* contain the answer to the problem. Rather, it may prove to be a reliable way to get to the answer.

ETHICAL REASONING

Review the Facts

Although a thorough review of the facts may seem to be an obvious step in any problem-solving situation, the importance of it in ethical deliberation is often underestimated. There are two reasons why it is helpful to start this process with a formal review of the exact facts of the situation. First, we often assume the existence of more unanimity about the facts of a case than is actually warranted. This is particularly true of data and opinion regarding prognosis or patient and family wishes. What seems to be an ethical dispute may be a difference in assessment or in data base. This situation very often occurs with issues related to the withdrawal of life support, involving appraisal of the usefulness or futility of treatment, the probable outcome, and the choice the patient would make in light of these predictions. When caregivers disagree with each other about the proper course of action because they differ in their assessments of the likely benefits, the disagreement is one of fact, not morals. The following case study illustrates how these different data bases may lead to apparently different ethical choices.

CASE HISTORY

Mr. T is a 54-year-old widower with two sons. He was diagnosed 10 months ago with small cell carcinoma of the lung and underwent a lobectomy, followed by a course of radiation therapy that he did not complete. Several weeks ago he began complaining of memory loss, headaches, and bouts of confusion that were becoming worse. He was readmitted to the hospital, and a series of diagnostic tests were ordered. A large space-occupying mass was found in the temporal area. The neurosurgeon recommended a craniotomy and resection of the tumor, which was thought to be a metastatic lesion. Mr. T has refused the surgery. His son is supporting this decision. The medical and nursing staff disagree about the best course of action.

The neurosurgeon believes that the patient is not competent to make an informed choice because, on examination, the patient could not consistently state the correct date or where he was. He was not able to solve the standard number or sentence interpretation tests (e.g., performing serial 7s). The neurosurgeon believes that the surgical procedure presents a relatively low risk, could relieve the patient's symptoms of lethargy and confusion, and could extend his life at least 6 months to 1 year. He

---

ETHICAL REASONING

1. Review the facts
2. Define the problem
3. List the choices
4. Decide on an action
5. Evaluate the choice

FIGURE 66–2. Steps in the process of ethical reasoning.

has never spoken to the patient's son but feels that the son does not have the right to make a decision for an incompetent parent unless he has been declared Mr. T's guardian by the courts. He believes that the best course of action is to petition the court to appoint a legal guardian, who may be willing to consent to what is clearly the "best medical care."

The patient's primary nurse has had several conversations with Mr. T's son. He has consistently stated that his father did not want aggressive treatment and that he had not finished the radiation therapy because he did not like the side effects and just "didn't see any reason to put himself through that." He is aware that his father is not now competent but believes that if he were he would definitely not agree to the surgery. Both of Mr. T's sons are concerned about their father's welfare and have asked the nurse for advice. Both are unmarried and do not feel they would be able to care for their father in their homes but are willing to pay jointly for whatever kind of nursing home or extended care he may need. The nurse feels that, given the circumstances, the best option is to arrange for hospice care for Mr. T.

The patient's internist also agrees that Mr. T. is not now competent to make his own decisions. However, she remembers several conversations she had in the past with Mr. T. after his lobectomy. He repeatedly stated that he regretted having the surgery, that it was terribly painful, and that he would never go through that again. She thinks that Mr. T. might agree to treatment but not if it involved surgery. Consequently, she would like to keep Mr. T. in the hospital and explore the possibility of enrolling him in an experimental chemotherapy protocol.

This case illustrates how several caregivers may come to very different conclusions about the best course of action. The differences arise, not from any disagreement about important ethical principles or values but from different responses to different facts. At this point, the disagreement here is not an ethical problem. It may be possible to resolve it by sharing all of the facts and then discussing the ethical components.

The second reason that it is useful to start with a formal review of the facts is that such a review identifies which of the many immediate elements of the situation the players are responding to. As opposed to a philosophical problem, ethical dilemmas are significantly affected by the details of the situation. Jonsen and Toulmin (1988) point out that the biomedical sciences have a tradition of relying on the rules and formal principles of the biological sciences, even though the aesthetic components of the art of medicine are also recognized. This is especially true in areas of health care where technology is heavily used. Critical care is one such area. To match principles to cases, one must not forget that these principles are "general rules invoked to support *practical* decisions that require *specific* actions affecting *personal* circumstances of *individual* human beings" (Jonsen and Toulmin, 1988). Starting the process by a review of these personal, individual facts grounds the deliberations in the here and now and guards against making a sterile and unrealistic although "principled" decision.

Define the Problem

The next step in the process is to define the problem. An ethical dilemma is a situation in which a choice must be made between various courses of action, and the conflict between these choices involves fundamental concepts of good and evil. Ethical choices are not matters of different appraisals of facts or a difference in opinion about the most effective care or treatment approach. Ethical dilemmas almost always involve the concepts of rights, duties, and responsibilities.

The purpose of defining the problem, using one or two clear sentences, is to focus one's own attention on the specific aspect or choice of action that must be addressed to resolve the dilemma. In some situations, this step also brings to light different dilemmas faced by other care givers. For example, in the case described earlier, suppose that, after sharing all of the facts and discussing the options, some care givers still felt that it would be wrong to allow Mr. T. to be discharged without treatment, whereas others felt that it would be wrong to initiate treatment against his previous wishes to refuse it. In this situation, the problem might be described as follows: "This adult patient, who is not now fully competent, is, with his family's agreement, refusing therapy that has been deemed the preferred medical therapy. The question is what course of action at this point is indicated?" Stating the problem in this way leads naturally to consideration of how to address the problem by specifying the issues involved. Is there any justification for violating this person's expressed wishes, such as a serious doubt about the validity of those wishes or the likelihood that he will change his mind if given a better explanation of facts or more time to think about it? Conversely, are the health care professionals justified in refraining from providing the indicated therapy for this patient's health problem? That is, is it certain that a valid indication of patient choice exists? Have the benefits and risks of the offered therapy been clearly described? Has the situation been explored on several different occasions with all interested parties?

List the Choices

The third step in ethical reasoning is to list all of the possible options. This step ensures that some options are not eliminated due to invalid assumptions. Options in Mr. T's case might include: (1) Discharge the patient home; (2) discharge the patient to a hospice or other facility; (3) keep the patient in the hospital and reevaluate the situation in another few days, continuing discussions with him and his sons; (4) begin legal proceedings to have a guardian appointed. Performing this step also ensures that an action is chosen in an ethical dilemma, rather than a principle or a theory.

Decide on the Action

The next step is to make a choice from the list of possible options, using theories, principles, and intuitions for reference or direction. There is a tendency to jump to this step first rather than waiting until the earlier steps have been completed. It is this step that is sometimes considered the most formal aspect of ethical analysis.

Theories and Principles. There are several levels of analysis in ethics. On the most general level are theories that direct our method or criteria for determining right actions. The two theories most widely discussed are utilitarianism (also called the consequentialist or teleological approach) and deontology.

Utilitarianism looks to the consequences of an action in judging its goodness. The best action is that which results in the greatest benefit with the least harm for the greatest number of people. In making a choice between conflicting actions, the utilitarian would attempt to compute a kind of moral calculus in comparing the net effects, both short- and long-term, of one action with the net effects of another. Act utilitarians limit their analysis to the effects of the specific acts in question, whereas rule utilitarians examine the effects of acting according to one rule versus another.

Deontologists analyze possible courses of action in terms of their adherence to moral imperatives or rules. This theory is also referred to as a duty-based theory (Benjamin and Curtis, 1981). Assessment of the particular consequences of an act plays no part in the analysis. The rules may take various forms, ranging from the most general prescriptions to more specific provisions such as those found in modern professional codes of ethics. Some philosophers, like Immanuel Kant, believe that there is only one guiding principle or rule. Others are pluralists, identifying several principles such as beneficence and justice that should in all cases direct our actions (Frankena, 1973).

The major difference between these two theories lies in the justification for the methods and rules employed in making decisions regarding right action. As can be seen, both involve the use of rules and principles. Although it is helpful to have some familiarity with the major forms of utilitarianism and deontology, these theories do not in themselves provide useful direction without further discussion of the specific values and principles they utilize. A value may be defined simply as something of worth or importance to us. Values include both nonmoral goods, such as a nice house, job, or leisure time, and moral goods, such as freedom and justice. Values are, however, closely linked to principles that delineate fundamental laws or codes of conduct and entail obligation or an "ought" clause (e.g., we are obligated to [ought to] respect all persons). As can be seen, principles usually reflect the things—beings, objects, or concepts—we value and equate with "the good."

Many values and principles underlie the moral traditions of nursing. Several clearly have such an important influence on daily practice that they warrant more discussion. These are the principles of autonomy and beneficence.

Autonomy. Autonomy refers to the right of self-determination. It is grounded in one's status as a rational human being and closely allied to the concepts of liberty and freedom. In western culture, we believe that all persons have the right to make their own decisions, to choose freely, and to act on that choice, limited only by the restriction that we do not infringe upon the rights of others.

In the health care arena, the belief in the importance of autonomy is seen as the requirement to obtain informed consent before we act upon others. Because man is essentially free and has the right to make his own decisions, we have the obligation not to constrain his decision making through withholding of information or presuming consent where none may exist. Respect for the individual's autonomy is a prima facie principle; that is, we must act according to the dictates of this principle unless another, overriding principle, such as beneficence, intervenes.

Beneficence. This is the obligation to do good or to prevent or minimize harm. Closely related is the principle of nonmaleficence, which imposes the duty to avoid or refrain from inflicting harm. Beneficence and nonmaleficence are probably the strongest principles underlying professional ethics in health care. The Hippocratic oath, the oldest of all codes, specifies: "I will apply dietetic measures for the *benefit* of the sick according to my ability and judgment: I will keep them from *harm and injustice*" (emphasis added) (Beauchamp and Walters, 1978). The first sentence in the International Council of Nurses Code for Nurses states, "The fundamental responsibility of the nurse is fourfold: to promote health, to prevent illness, to restore health and to alleviate suffering" (Benjamin and Curtis, 1981). In the most recent revision of the American Nurses Association Code for Nurses (1976), the preamble reads:

Nursing encompasses the protection, promotion, and restoration of health; the prevention of illness; and the alleviation of suffering in the the care of clients . . . . When making clinical judgments, nurses base their decisions on consequences and universal moral principles . . . The most fundamental of these principles is respect for persons. Other principles stemming from this basic principle are autonomy, beneficence, nonmaleficence, veracity, confidentiality, fidelity, and justice.

Both the medical and nursing codes utilize the concept of benefit, referring to the good towards which our professional activities are directed. This statement raises the question of what that good is—how we determine it and how we resolve conflicts between opposing goods. The conflicting directions we receive from these two crucial principles, autonomy and beneficence, illustrates that merely having a clear idea of important principles does not always solve dilemmas.

Paternalism. When a patient wishes to make a choice that is in agreement with our assessment of what is "good" or beneficial or in his best interests, we find it easy to believe in autonomy. Likewise, when a patient wishes us to administer the treatment or service that is in his best interests, we find it easy to believe that beneficence is of primary importance in meeting our professional obligations. The difficulty arises when a patient does not choose what we believe to be clearly and definitely in his own interests. Similarly, a conflict arises when we seem to be in a situation in which the only way to help a patient and thus meet our obligations, is to go against his wishes.

Although any two principles may conflict in this way, this particular struggle, between autonomy and beneficence, is very common in health care and is at the heart of the problem of paternalism. Paternalism is an action deemed to be in the client's or patient's best interest without or regardless of that person's completely voluntary and informed consent (Bayles, 1981). Some authors use the term weak or justified paternalism to refer to situations in which informed consent is impossible (Veatch, 1981), such as emergency situations or when a patient is incompetent. Those who defend some limited forms of paternalism cite the impossibility of ensuring that lay persons possess the meaningful understanding needed to meet the requirements of true informed consent. Also cited is the conscious willingness of many patients to give decision-making responsibility to trusted professionals. Opponents warn against the dangers of chipping away at respect for individual autonomy. They point to the inconsistency of any form of paternalism with the principle of liberty.

Pelligrino (1985), discussing ethics in critical care medicine, suggests an approach that may be helpful in sorting out these conflicting obligations. He believes that acting for the patient's good is, indeed, the central principle of medical ethics. However, there are several possible components of "good":

■ The ultimate good as defined by the patient's most considered, enduring judgment
■ The good of the patient as a person
■ The patient's perception of the good at that moment
■ The biomedical or technical good of the patient

Although all four are appropriate aims of the practitioner and serve as the reference standard for choices, in situations of conflict we can order them by rank. They are presented in the order of their importance, with the first "good" being the good of last resort, or the one to which we must look in final decisions.

Evaluation of Choice

As can be seen from this brief discussion of theories and principles, a mere understanding of the meaning of the terms does not automatically provide direction in moral debate. To use these tools, one must have some individual system of morality that orders these principles and provides guidelines for applying them in real-life situations. The fifth step in the process of ethical reasoning provides a check on the degree to which one's decision is consistent with other similar decisions and coherent with one's overall moral scheme.

A very practical problem faced by all of us in dealing with moral dilemmas is the sorting out of the conflicting feelings or emotions that inevitably arise. The pace, the demands, and the stresses of critical care generate strong emotions in most nurses. These can easily influence decision making. We may have very valid desires to see a patient's suffering end, to have fewer patients admitted, to not have to deal with a noncompliant patient who keeps returning to the intensive care unit (ICU) for treatment, to avoid conflicts with physicians, administrators, or coworkers. It can be difficult to separate the influences of these forces from stringent moral considerations. One way to make this more likely, however, is to examine our choices in terms of their consistency and coherence.

Consistency refers to the criterion of universalizability. A valid moral decision should reflect principles and values that are consistently important guides in all similar situations. That is, if in a particular case we believe we are making a decision to refrain from providing a certain treatment for a patient because the patient has made a competent choice to refuse the treatment and we must respect his autonomy, then we should expect to apply this principle consistently in all similar cases. Most importantly, we should apply this principle even when we do not agree with the patient's choice.

Coherence refers to the degree to which our moral principles fit together in an overall pattern. For example, it is unlikely that we could regard the principle of autonomy as very important if, in addition, we did not have a clear belief in the worth and dignity of all human beings. As part of our ongoing development as moral agents, we must assess how a given choice reflects basic principles and if we would be willing, or have been willing in the past, to adhere to this same principle in other similar situations. We must ask if the most important of our principles and beliefs fit together into a logical, compatible whole.

MYTHS AND HANDICAPS IN ETHICAL REASONING

Use of the process just outlined can be helpful in approaching ethical dilemmas in a rational, orderly fashion. However, the process does not ensure that the outcome will be the right or best decision because a number of myths and handicaps play a part in constraining our ability to make reasoned ethical decisions.

The term myth, as used here, indicates beliefs that, although untrue, persist in the minds of many. They may stem simply from misunderstanding, or they may reflect a less conscious bias. The most profound of these is the belief that there is no right or wrong in ethics, that ethics are a matter of personal choice, and one person's ethical beliefs are just as valid and sound as another's. There are actually two components to this belief: an acceptance of ethical relativism and an assumption that there can be no changes in ethical belief systems based on considered review of facts and principles. Ethical relativism is the belief that whatever customs, actions, and mores are believed to be right by any one culture or society are right, and that there are no basic, fundamental, or absolute moral principles that apply to all peoples. This is not just the recognition that different people *think* different acts are right but the belief that, because the acts are thought right, they in fact *are* right.

The variations in both practice and moral systems that exist in the world and even within one hospital unit may seem, on first consideration, to support the idea of relativism. In addition, it is very difficult and requires considerable study to find and support a foundation on which absolute morality can rest. On the other hand, most philosophers recognize that we do in fact have a very strong intuitive belief that there are some absolute rights and wrongs. More important, if we were to accept the belief that ethical relativism is true, then there would be no reason for any ethical inquiry at all. In fact, concepts such as right and wrong and good and evil would have no meaning outside of the individual.

Another myth or misunderstanding is the belief that establishing the legality or illegality of an action answers the moral question. Although laws are assumed to represent the will and mores of the people, many acts that are quite legal, such as violating confidentiality or breaking promises between friends, are quite immoral. The legal system is designed, in theory, first and foremost to uphold the principle of justice. Although this may be a relevant principle in many situations, it is inadequate for determining the moral action in *all* cases.

A similar error in moral reasoning is to mistake expertise in one area for expertise in moral debate. This is a particular danger in critical care units, where medical and nursing professionals are accustomed to acting decisively and to being deferred to and treated by others as experts. Knowledge of the biomedical sciences, obviously important in its own right, is unrelated to the ability to make sound ethical judgments. The most accomplished professional is no more capable, by virtue of clinical expertise, of sound moral reasoning than the least prepossessing of lay persons.

The last common myth or handicap in resolving ethical dilemmas is one that is particularly relevant to nurses. Perhaps the most important practical constraint on moral inquiry by a nurse is the belief that nurses are powerless to affect the outcome of a moral dilemma because they lack formal authority in the health care system. There are many factors that contribute to the perception that nurses cannot affect moral decisions. These include unfamiliarity with the process of ethical reasoning, which leads to a lack of confidence in their own decisions and intuitions. In addition, many people, not just nurses, are confused about the distinction between legal and moral issues. This leads to a perception of constraints where none exist. Last, there are very real institutional and personal constraints imposed on nurses by virtue of their status as employees. Many people still hold the traditional view of nurses as "order followers" rather than professionals who have an independent code of conduct that takes precedence over institutional policies and procedures.

The existence of bureaucratic constraints does pose barriers and obstacles. The nurse who chooses to implement a moral decision that is in conflict with either institutional policy or the wishes or decisions of others, particularly supervisors or physicians, may encounter very real consequences. However, the reality of nonmoral consequences, such as conflict, censure, or disciplinary action, do not make the nurse powerless. They do present the need to add to the moral equation the evaluation of whether or not the principle or issue at hand is important enough for the nurse to risk the consequences.

MAKING ETHICAL DECISION MAKING OPERATIONAL

Because there are very real constraints against moral inquiry by nurses, it is equally important to consider how we can facilitate this process. The making of an isolated decision by a nurse, regardless of how valid or sound it is, is of limited value unless nurses are empowered to implement it.

Education is, of course, the first step. This should include both learning about the actual process of moral reasoning and learning about resources and methods for addressing issues of concern. The popularity of continuing education offerings in the area of ethics attests to both the recognized importance of this area and the willingness of practitioners to engage in active study. The effectiveness of educational programs in the hospital setting depends on a planned, well-designed ethics curriculum. The curriculum should begin with basic orientation classes and proceed throughout the professional development program, regardless of whether it is provided on a centralized or unit-based basis. Sporadic, single classes that are not integrated within the entire educational plan are less likely to have a lasting impact on the development of moral reasoning skills.

A number of pragmatic considerations can be helpful to nurses in the practice setting. Even before the nurse has developed clear ideas on an issue, it is helpful to discuss the situation with colleagues. It is very difficult if not impossible to resolve these thorny issues and sort through the many considerations without help from others, even if it is just in the form of listening and validating the data base or the logic of the process. Although it may be ideal to have an ethicist or nurse philosopher help the staff in these investigations, it is not necessary. It is more important for some dialogue and exchange of views to take place among coworkers.

Ethics committees can be of great assistance to all care givers when ethical dilemmas occur. These are multidisciplinary groups that serve an advisory function. They generally meet at the request of a care giver and review the facts of the case, discuss the relevant ethical considerations, and provide recommendations about possible courses of action (Cohen 1988a, b). Such meetings provide care givers with a chance to talk with other clinicians who are knowledgeable about clinical ethics and often provide the support necessary to implement a difficult decision. Although many hospitals have implemented ethics committees within the past few years, they are still underutilized, particularly by nurses.

Situations that are most difficult for nurses are those in which there is disagreement among care givers about what action is proper or those in which the nurse perceives an improper action on the part of another care giver. Under these circumstances formal administrative support for intervention and resolution is essential. This can take many forms. Formal policies outlining the chain of command to be used in addressing ethical issues provide nurses with guidance as to procedure. A formal policy is also a tangible sign of the appropriateness and importance attached by the administration to the right and the responsibility of every care giver to address ethical concerns. Ethics grand rounds and ethics nursing care conferences serve the same function in an even more public fashion.

When formal administrative support is absent, there are still some guidelines that can be helpful to individual nurses facing ethical dilemmas. In addition to discussing the issue with colleagues, it is usually more effective to pursue the desired course of action with at least one other person, if not a small group. Groups provide support, and it is less likely that the concerns of a group will be ignored. Paying attention to the chain of command is always important, especially when issues of proper performance are concerned. Gaining the support of at least one person in the administrative hierarchy is useful. Putting concerns in writing at some stage can be helpful, both in assisting the nurse to lay out the issue in a clear, concise, and logical format and in beginning a process of documentation that may be needed if the concerns are not addressed.

In critical care, unfortunately, some issues arise that need to be dealt with immediately, and the options discussed above cannot be utilized. In these cases it is obviously important for nurses to have the knowledge needed to analyze complex situations and come to decisions quickly. It is vital for them to know that the nursing department, if not the hospital bureaucracy as a whole, will support them in these endeavors.

THE ETHICAL AGENDA OF CRITICAL CARE NURSING FOR THE 1990s

In addition to the preceding discussion of theoretical issues and practical guidelines, the future direction or agenda for critical care nursing as a practice discipline needs to be considered. Three items are significant enough to warrant special consideration.

Help the Patient to Own His or Her Care

If we accept autonomy as one of the primary values, if not the most important, then we must take active steps to ensure that patients are capable of acting autonomously. This is particularly important in the very foreign environment of the critical care unit. We must routinely talk with patients about their goals for health care, the measures we can offer, the priorities that we recommend. Obviously, this cannot be done in emergency situations, with patients who are incompetent by virtue of their physical condition, or abruptly in the midst of an ICU admission. Because there are so many practical limitations on these kinds of discussions, it is all the more imperative to take advantage of the opportunities we do have to move away from the rigid care practices so common in critical care.

In considering how we can help the patient to own his care, the concept of advocacy may be relevant. Given the highly complex nature of most hospitals today, it is easy to see why the patient may need someone to speak for him, to represent his interests, and to safeguard his rights. Nowhere does this seem more necessary than in the very technical, foreign environment of the intensive care unit. Nurses are, in many ways, uniquely qualified for the role of advocate because of their continual presence at the bedside and their special relationship to and knowledge of patients and their families. However, there are two considerations that may limit the usefulness of the advocate role for nurses.

First, by definition, the first duty of the person whose goal is to protect patients' rights is to promote informed consent. This includes and may even start with enabling the patient to choose his or her own advocate. Patients may or may not choose a nurse. It is unlikely that patients will see nurses as candidates for this role in environments where a different nurse is assigned to the patient each day and no attempt is made by the nurse to involve the patient and family in discussions about care routines and options. All care givers—physicians, social workers, respiratory therapists, nurses—would insist that their actions are guided by a concern for patient welfare and that their role is to benefit the patient. If we believe that nurses have an additional role as patient advocates, then we must pay attention to the characteristics of the environment and the health care delivery system that foster or hinder this role.

The second limit on the advocacy role for nurses lies in focusing too narrowly on the role of advocate. Patients may always need a member of the health care team to act as a guide through the bureaucratic maze and as a counselor in decision making. It may be far more valuable, however, for nurses to concentrate some of their energies on changing at least some small part of the system in order to minimize the need for an advocate in the first place.

As part of this process, nurses can actively evaluate the routine practices used in critical care nursing, which they accept without question, in terms of their effect on patient autonomy. For example, is it really necessary to limit visiting hours, to restrict the family's access to the patient? Most individuals are certainly more at ease in discussing their concerns with their friends and family, yet the restrictive visiting policies of many ICUs may have the unintended effect of making it more difficult for the patient to express his wishes. Similarly, would it really be impossible to let the patient choose the routine for the day, such as when to have a bath, when to get out of bed, when to eat? The actual practice is less important than the nurse's willingness to provide opportunities for the patient to have choices, or, at the very least, to make explicit which routines are negotiable and which must be prescribed.

Avoid Having to Solve Ethical Dilemmas in Crisis Situations

As with any problem, the best approach is prevention. Although we cannot hope to prevent ethical dilemmas from arising, we can be alert to the beginnings of situations that herald a dilemma. We can intervene before we are in a forced-choice situation. For example, when a patient with a clearly poor prognosis is admitted to the ICU, that is the time to clarify with all care givers involved which discussions about aggressive treatment and resuscitation have taken place—not when the patient develops a cardiopulmonary arrest. If there are practice issues that are repeatedly problematic, such as do not resuscitate (DNR) orders, allocation of scarce ICU beds, or utilization of experimental protocols, these should be addressed proactively, not in the heat of a specific patient problem.

Participate in Policy-Making Decisions

This item refers to activities that do not generally take place at the bedside yet affect each nurse's

practice. As mentioned earlier, one of the very important ways in which we can support and foster ethical inquiry is in establishing formal policies governing the procedure to be used for ethical debate and guidelines for managing problematic issues such as DNR orders. Engelhardt (1985) pointed out the importance of the joint decision making that is used in today's pluralistic society to reach mutual agreements on moral issues. We can no longer rely on a predominant religious view or a predominant social value system; therefore, "if authority cannot be derived from the grace of God or from a successful rational argument, it can be derived from . . . the consent of all involved . . . in a project" (Engelhardt, 1985). Nurses, as the primary implementers of many of the decisions affecting patient care, must be among those involved in reaching a consensus.

On another level, nurses must be active participants in social policy development that affects the health care of individuals and groups. We will continue to face new and puzzling dilemmas as technology continues to expand the limits of our knowledge. Mandatory testing for AIDS, the status of fetuses conceived in vitro, selective reduction of the number of fetuses in cases of multiple-fetus pregnancies, and the use of human organs and tissues for commercial purposes are just a few of the new issues presented by advances in technology. Nurses can play a crucial role in these issues but can affect the outcome only if they are willing to become involved in the legislative process. Involvement may occur through participation in professional nursing associations or individually in local community councils or legislative offices. The most essential factor is that critical care nurses recognize the unique knowledge and perspective they can bring to these complex human problems and invest themselves in working toward solutions.

SUMMARY

This chapter has reviewed selected principles and concepts that are relevant to the practice of critical care nursing. A process for addressing ethical dilemmas was suggested, recommending the following steps: review the facts, define the problem, list the choices, decide on the proper action, and evaluate the choice.

Although many principles are relevant to ethical inquiry in nursing, autonomy and beneficence were selected as illustrative of these principles. Autonomy reflects a fundamental value placed on human beings and requires us to respect each individual's right of self-determination. As a prima facie duty, it obligates us to ensure that patients have the necessary information and the opportunity to give informed consent before we act upon them. Beneficence directs us to aim for the good and further requires us to evaluate and define the meaning of this good, giving priority to the patient's own conception of good.

Practical considerations were also discussed. Because the ethics of nursing as a practice discipline must involve the active engagement of nurses in addressing moral questions, an agenda for the future was offered. This agenda includes helping the patient to own his own care, avoiding the need to solve ethical dilemmas in crisis situations, and participating in policy-making decisions. These steps were suggested as a means of both developing a more effective ethical practice and improving the moral environment in which this practice takes place.

References

American Nurses Association (1976). *Code for nurses with interpretive statements*. Kansas City, MO: American Nurses Association.

Bayles, M. D. (1981). *Professional ethics*. Belmont, CA: Wadsworth Publishing.

Beauchamp, T. L., and Walters, L. (Eds.) (1978). *Contemporary issues in bioethics* (p. 138). Encino, CA: Dickenson Publishing.

Benjamin, M., and Curtis, J. (1981). *Ethics in nursing*. New York: Oxford University Press.

Benner, P., and Tanner, C. (1987). Clinical judgment: How expert nurses use intuition. *American Journal of Nursing 87*, 1, 23–31, 1987.

Bowie, N. E. (1986). *Making ethical decisions*. New York: McGraw-Hill.

Cohen, C. B. (Ed.) (1988a). Birth of a network. *Hastings Center Report*, 18 (1), 11–13.

Cohen, C. B. (Ed.) (1988b). Is case consultation in retreat? *Hastings Center Report*, 18 (4), 23–24.

Curtin, L. (1982). No rush to judgment. In L. Curtin, and M. J. Flaherty (Eds.), *Nursing ethics—theories and pragmatics* (pp. 57–66). Bowie, MD: Robert J. Brady Company.

Engelhardt, H. T. (1985). Moral tensions in critical care medicine: "Absurdities" as indications of finitude. In J. C. Moskop, and L. Kopelman (Eds.), *Ethics and critical care medicine* (pp. 23–34). Boston: D. Reidel Publishing.

Engelhardt, H. T. (1986). *The foundations of bioethics*. New York: Oxford University Press.

Fowler, M. D. (1987a). Introduction to ethics and ethical theory: A road map to the discipline. In M. D. Fowler, and J. Levine-Ariff (Eds.), *Ethics at the bedside* (pp. 24–38). Philadelphia: J. B. Lippincott.

Fowler, M. D. (1987b). Piecing together the ethical puzzle: Operationalizing nursing's ethics in critical care. In M. D. Fowler, and J. Levine-Ariff (Eds.), *Ethics at the bedside* (pp. 182–212). Philadelphia: J. B. Lippincott.

Frankena, W. K. (1973). *Ethics* (2nd ed.). Englewood Cliffs, NJ: Prentice-Hall.

Fry, S. T. (1987). Autonomy, advocacy, and accountability: Ethics at the bedside. In M. D. Fowler, and J. Levine-Ariff (Eds.), *Ethics at the bedside* (pp. 39–49). Philadelphia: J. B. Lippincott.

Gert, B. (1988). *Morality*. New York: Oxford University Press.

International Council of Nurses (1981). Code for nurses. In M. Benjamin, and J. Curtis, *Ethics in nursing* (p. 153). New York: Oxford University Press.

Jonsen, A., and Toulmin, S. (1988). *The abuse of casuistry*. Berkeley: University of California Press.

Krekeler, K. (1987). Critical care nursing and moral development. *Critical Care Nursing Quarterly*, 10 (2), 1–8.

Pelligrino, E. D. (1985). Moral choice, the good of the patient, and the patient's good. In J.C. Moskop, and L. Kopelman (Eds.), *Ethics and critical care medicine* (pp. 117–138). Boston: D. Reidel Publishing.

Regan, T. (Ed.) (1986). *Matters of life and death* (2nd ed., pp. 3–34). New York: Random House.

Reich, W. T. (1985). Moral absurdities in critical care medicine: Commentary on a parable. In J. C. Moskop, and L. Kopelman (Eds.), *Ethics and critical care medicine* (pp. 12–22). Boston: D. Reidel Publishing.

Toulmin, S. (1981). *The tyranny of principles*. Hastings Center Report, 11 (6), 31–39.

Veatch, R. M. (1981). *A theory of medical ethics*. New York: Basic Books.

67

Legal Issues in Critical Care

Ginny Wacker Guido

As society has become more litigious, increasing numbers of nurses are being named as defendants in medical malpractice lawsuits. Understanding and applying a few legal principles will help critical care nurses to protect themselves against these growing numbers of lawsuits.

Until the present time, few lawsuits originated within critical care settings. Several factors may account for this phenomenon: (1) the competency and accountability of critical care nurses, (2) the advanced technologic skills required in all aspects of critical care medicine and nursing, and (3) the relatively low nurse–patient ratios in critical care areas. Perhaps the single most significant factor is the open communication that occurs in the critical care setting between health care givers and patients and family members. Patients and families are much less apt to file lawsuits when they perceive the potential defendants as open, honest, and caring (Murchison et al., 1982).

Despite the factors mitigating the risk of lawsuits against health care providers in critical care settings, increasing consumer knowledge and "malpractice fever" in general mean that the possibility of lawsuits cannot be ignored. Two factors that may help to keep the numbers of lawsuits low are the increased education of consumers about the limitations of medicine and realistic ideas about the benefits that can be expected from medical care, and the increased involvement of patients and their families in the decision-making process. Perhaps the best means of reducing the risk of a potential lawsuit is for nurses to gain a working knowledge of the basic principles of law underlying their professional practice. Table 67–1 summarizes the various torts discussed in this chapter.

STANDARDS OF CARE

Standards of care or standards of practice define the minimum level of care provided by a given profession that is considered adequate. In other words, standards of care are the skills and knowledge commonly possessed by members of a given profession. Standards of care are used daily in all aspects of health care delivery. Standards form the basis for high-quality health care and serve as the criteria for determining whether less than adequate care was delivered to a specific patient. Thus, the concept of standards of care is a basic legal issue that critical care nurses must understand and deal with in their everyday practice.

The legal system views standards of care as the pivotal point in a malpractice action. Nurses have a duty to use reasonable care in interactions with patients. The minimum or reasonable level of care that should be given is the care that would be given by a prudent critical care nurse under similar circumstances. The question to be asked is, "How would a reasonably prudent critical care nurse with the same skills, experience, and educational level as the defendant critical care nurse have acted under the same or similar circumstances?" If the reasonable, prudent critical care nurse would have acted in the same manner as the defendant nurse did, then the defendant nurse may not be legally liable to the injured patient.

Standards of care are derived from various sources and may be classified into two broad categories: internal and external. Internal standards are those established by the nurse's background and role and include the nurse's specific job description and the institution's policies and procedures. External standards are established by professional nursing organizations, the state nurse practice act, federal guidelines and policies, precedent court decisions, current textbooks and journal articles, and certification standards.

The most important internal standard is the standard of care set by a particular nurse's education and experience. The more education a nurse has and the greater the nurse's professional skills, the more po-

TABLE 67–1. Negligent, Intentional, and Quasi-Intentional Torts

Elements of the Tort	Nursing Examples
Negligence	
1. Duty owed the patient	Failure to monitor the patient as ordered
2. Breach of duty owed	
3. Foreseeability	Failure to communicate a change in the patient's status
4. Causation	
5. Injury	Failure to prevent the patient from falling
6. Damages	
a. General	Failure to provide patient education
b. Specific	
c. Emotional	Failure to provide safety for the patient
d. Punitive or exemplary	
Intentional Torts	
Shared elements of all intentional torts	
1. There must be a volitional action by the defendant	
2. The person so acting must intend to bring about the consequences	
3. There must be causation: The act must be a substantial factor in bringing about the consequences	
Assault	
1. Shared elements plus:	Threatening the patient with an injection or an intravenous line
2. Placing another person in apprehension of being touched in an offensive or insulting manner	
Battery	
1. Shared elements plus:	Forcing a patient to ambulate
2. Actual contact with another person without his or her consent	
False Imprisonment	
1. Shared elements plus:	Refusing to allow a patient to leave against medical advice
2. Unjustifiable detention or confinement of a person	
Quasi-intentional Torts	
Invasion of Privacy	
1. An act that intrudes or pries into another's seclusion	Taking unauthorized pictures of a patient
2. The intrusion must be objectionable to a reasonable person	Releasing confidential information to others without consent
3. The intrusion must concern private facts	Allowing unauthorized persons to witness patient procedures
4. There must be public disclosure of private information	
Defamation	
1. Use of language that adversely affects one's reputation	Making false chart entries about the patient's lifestyle
2. Use of false language about or concerning a living person	Falsely accusing staff members in front of other staff or patients
3. Publication of false information to a third person	
4. Damage to one's reputation	

tentially liable the nurse becomes for failure to perform at an acceptable level of care. Thus, the definition of "acceptable care" changes as the nurse gains education and experience.

In the legal system, standards of care are established during court trials by the use of expert witnesses. The expert witness aids the judge and jury in determining the acceptable standard of care in a given case. The expert witness explains the actual care that was given and describes what the acceptable level of care should have been. The judge and jury then decide whether the defendant acted according to the appropriate standard of care. Thus, an expert witness testifying in a lawsuit that involves a critical care nurse's performance must have a thorough understanding of the skills and clinical expertise needed at the time of the alleged malpractice. The expert would then establish, for the court, the standard of care for which the defendant nurse is accountable.

NEGLIGENCE AND MALPRACTICE

Most of the lawsuits or potential lawsuits encountered in clinical practice involve negligence or malpractice. Although frequently used interchangeably, these two terms are not synonymous. Negligence is either an act or a failure to act that leads to the injury of another. In its simplest definition, negligence is carelessness. Negligence may be attributed to either a professional or a nonprofessional person. Anyone who fails to perform to the standard of care that a reasonable person would meet in a particular set of circumstances may be liable for negligence. Malpractice is a specific type of negligence that includes the status of the care giver as well as the standard of care owed. Courts have defined malpractice as any professional misconduct, unreasonable lack of skill or fidelity in professional duties, or illegal and immoral conduct (*Napier v. Greenzweig*, 1919; *Forthofer v. Arnold*, 1938). In a more modern definition, malpractice is the failure of a professional person to act in accordance with prevailing professional standards or a failure to foresee consequences that a professional person, who has the necessary skills and education, should foresee.

The most common areas of negligence or malpractice in critical care settings include medication errors, patient falls, failing to assess the patient for changes in health status, and failing to notify the primary health care provider of changes in patient status.

In accusations of either malpractice or negligence, the person bringing the lawsuit (plaintiff) must prove to the court that the health care professional or health care institution was truly at fault. To do so, the plaintiff must establish six legal elements: the duty owed the patient, breach of the duty owed the patient, foreseeability, causation, injury, and damages.

Duty Owed the Patient

Establishing that a duty was owed the patient requires the plaintiff to demonstrate that a professional relationship existed between the nurse and the plaintiff and that the nurse owed the patient a specific standard of care. Historically, the relationship between a nurse and a patient is the easiest element to prove in a court of law. This is certainly true of critical care nurses who work in hospital settings. Since the nurse works for the hospital and the patient is the hospital's patient, a nurse–patient relationship is readily established. Some courts also refer to this relationship as a reliance relationship because the patient is relying upon the nurse for his or her professional expertise.

The second step under duty owed the patient is establishment of the standard of care that was owed. This is accomplished through the use of expert witnesses.

Breach of Duty Owed the Patient

This legal element involves showing a deviation from the standard of care owed the patient. For example, if the acceptable standard of care involves taking and recording vital signs every 5 to 15 minutes, then recording vital signs every 30 minutes is below the acceptable standard of care. The nurse has breached the duty owed the patient.

Usually a deviation from a standard of care is called ordinary or mere negligence, implying professional negligence either in performing an action or in omitting a required action. However, a nurse may be liable for gross negligence if he or she willingly or consciously ignores a risk known to be significantly harmful to a given patient. For example, if the nurse assesses vital signs every 30 minutes in a patient who has just been placed on potent vasopressors and the patient then suffers a stroke, the nurse may be considered grossly negligent.

Foreseeability

The third element of malpractice that must be shown by the plaintiff is foreseeability, defined as the recognition that certain events are expected to cause certain outcomes. In the previous example, it is foreseeable that an elevated blood pressure might result in a stroke and that infusion of potent vasopressors could cause a significantly elevated blood pressure.

Foreseeability is judged on the facts known at the time of the occurrence or happening, not at the time the case finally comes to court. The question asked is, "Could the reasonable, prudent critical care nurse have foreseen a particular result based upon the level of medical knowledge available to practitioners at the time of the occurrence?" Journal articles and text-

books aid in establishing the level of medical and nursing knowledge available to professionals at the time of the happening.

Causation

Demonstration of causation requires proof that the injury resulted directly from a negligent action or omission of a required action. The injury itself is not sufficient proof. Nor does the failure to meet appropriate standards of care result in liability. The injury must be a direct outcome of the negligence.

The legal system uses two different approaches in establishing cause. If a single defendant is involved in the lawsuit, the court asks the "but for" question: "Would this injury have resulted but for the action or omission of the defendant?" "Would the patient have fallen and broken his hip but for the nurse's negligence in failing to put the side rail in its up position?" When two or more defendants are involved in the lawsuit, the court uses the substantial factor test. Each defendant's action is examined to see if it was a substantial factor in the resultant injury. For example, "Was the failure of a nurse to verify the physician's order a substantial factor in the overdosing of the patient with a given medication?" If the answer is yes to the substantial factor question, then causation has been established.

Injury

The plaintiff must demonstrate that some type of physical, financial, or emotional injury resulted from the breach of duty owed the patient. For example, a critical care nurse may be at fault for failing to raise the side rails on the bed of a combative, disoriented patient, but unless some injury results (e.g., the patient falls and sustains a broken hip), there is no liability in a court of law for the negligent care.

Generally speaking, the courts do not allow damages for emotional injuries unless they are accompanied by physical injuries. For example, damages for pain and suffering are allowed when there is physical injury but not when no physical injury can be shown.

Damages

Damages compensate the injured person for the cost of medical care for injuries sustained and for restoring the patient to his or her original state, as far as financially possible. Damages are not necessarily meant to punish the wrongdoer for the negligent action. For example, the awarded damages are greater if the patient requires prolonged hospitalization and future medical care than if the patient has failed to survive the negligent act.

Damages are grouped into four categories: general,

special, emotional, and punitive or exemplary. General damages are those inherent to the injury itself. Included in this category are pain and suffering and any permanent disability or disfigurement. Special damages include all losses and expenses incurred as a result of the injury. These include medical bills, lost wages, and expenses incurred for hiring medical personnel at home or for mechanical alterations needed at home (e.g., wheelchair ramps, safety rails for bath tubs, and so on). Emotional damages are those allowed for counseling and for pain and suffering of the spouse. Punitive damages are allowed only if the action has been willful or conscious and if gross negligence has been found by the court. Punitive damages are meant to punish the wrongdoer and set an example for the remainder of the profession, thus deterring future misconduct.

INTENTIONAL TORTS

A tort is a civil wrong committed against a person or a person's property. Civil law, the body of law dealing with the rights of private citizens, is based upon fault. The accountable person has either failed to meet his or her responsibility or has performed an action below acceptable standards. Once fault has been shown, the person harmed may be awarded compensation.

Intentional torts committed by nurses differ from negligence and malpractice in several ways. Intent is necessary for an intentional tort. The nurse must intend to do a particular action or appear to intend a particular action that brings about a consequence. For example, the nurse must *intend* to hold or restrain a patient in order to give the patient an injection. Likewise, an action must take place for an intentional tort to occur. An omitted action can never be an intentional tort. In the previous example, the nurse *held* the patient to administer the injection. An intentional tort need not involve actual injury. That is, the plaintiff must show that the tort occurred, not that an injury or damage occurred. Using the same example, the patient would need to show that the nurse held him or her against his or her will, not that the injection caused any physical injury. Intentional torts most commonly seen in critical care settings include assault, battery, and false imprisonment. Though commonly pled together, assault and battery are two separate torts.

Assault and Battery

An assault is any action by one person that makes another person fear that he or she will be touched without consent in an offensive, insulting, or physically injurious manner. Actual touching is not required; the action or motion alone creates the fear. For example, if a nurse approaches a patient with a syringe as if to administer an injection without the patient's consent, no contact has occurred, yet the patient could successfully show that an assault has taken place.

Battery is harmful or unwarranted contact with a person without his permission. The person need not be injured by the contact, nor does he need to be aware that the contact has taken place. For example, a battery occurs when a patient is restrained for the purpose of giving some type of necessary nursing care, whether or not the patient knows about the contact. It is the contact, not the knowledge of the contact or the manner of the contact, that results in the commission of a battery.

In most situations, assault and battery are averted because the health care provider has the prior consent of the patient to proceed with the treatment or therapy. Also, self-defense may be a valid defense in a lawsuit brought by a patient for assault and battery. The health care provider may use necessary force to prevent patients from harming either themselves or others in their immediate area.

False Imprisonment

False imprisonment is the unjustifiable detention of a person without a legal right to detain that person. A nurse falsely imprisons a patient when she or he confines or restrains the patient within a confined, bounded area with the intent of limiting the patient's freedom. Refusing to return the patient's clothing, car keys, or other personal belongings may also be considered false imprisonment.

To prove liability of the health care provider for this action, the patient must show that he or she was aware of the confinement. Confused and disoriented persons who are restrained for their own or other people's protection will not be successful in bringing a lawsuit for false imprisonment. Care, caution, and reasonableness are prerequisites in the use of restraints.

QUASI-INTENTIONAL TORTS

Quasi-intentional torts are those that lack the intent that is so crucial to intentional torts. Because action and causation must be shown, these torts involve more than mere negligence. The two quasi-intentional torts seen most frequently in critical care settings are invasion of privacy and defamation of character.

Invasion of Privacy

The right of protection against unreasonable and unwarranted interference with one's solitude is well recognized in the legal system. This tort is frequently encountered in critical care settings when confidential information is given to persons not entitled to it.

For example, pictures may be taken of a patient with a particularly interesting diagnosis and used without the patient's consent. More commonly, information about a patient's diagnosis and status may be given over the telephone to interested callers without the patient's permission.

Nurses must be cautious when releasing information about patients. Even family members do not have a right to information about the adult patient without the patient's permission. Before releasing information over the telephone, the nurse should verify that the patient has consented to the release of the information and that the caller is entitled to receive the information. A simple notation on the Kardex listing who is authorized to receive information should be made at the time of the patient's admission. If the caller is not entitled to the information, the caller should be referred to the patient's spouse or other family member.

Invasion of patient privacy rights may also occur during shift reports, particularly if the institution utilizes walking reports or walking rounds. Frequently, nurses relay information about patients to other health care providers at the patient's bedside or in a central location. Because other patients and family members may overhear such reports, the potential for invasion of privacy is great. Nurses should either ask family members to leave during reports or give the reports in a more secluded area.

Defamation

Defamation is a tort of wrongful injury to a living person's reputation. Such wrongful injury may consist of either written or oral communication to someone other than the defamed person. A claim of defamation may arise from the release of inaccurate or inappropriate medical information or from untruthful statements made about a patient.

Caution is the key advice in preventing this tort. Nurses must be careful about making comments about patients, especially when making entries in the patient's chart or medical record. For example, writing in the chart that a patient is "crazy" may be defamation; describing the actual behaviors or statements of the patient is not.

LIABILITY AND THE CRITICAL CARE NURSE

The hospital or employing institution may incur liability for the actions of its employees under the doctrine of respondent superior, or "let the master respond." According to this legal doctrine, the employer has the right to both hire and fire the individual employee and thus becomes accountable for negligence occurring during the employee's work day. In other words, the nurse would not have been in a position to allow harm to come to a patient if the hospital had not hired the nurse and allowed the patient to come into contact with that nurse. For the hospital to be liable for the negligent action, the nurse must be acting within the course and scope of employment at the time of the incident. For example, if a nurse allows a patient to fall, the employing hospital as well as the nurse may be found liable in a subsequent lawsuit. If the nurse is acting outside of his or her job description or against hospital policy and procedure, the hospital may escape liability. For example, a hospital may have a policy that forbids nurses to remove invasive lines (e.g., pulmonary artery balloon catheters, external pacemaker wires) from patients. If a nurse harms a patient by negligently removing an external pacemaker wire, the hospital will argue that the nurse was acting outside the course and scope of his or her employment. The nurse, thus, remains liable but the hospital is not.

The hospital and the supervising physician may jointly be liable for a nurse's actions. Termed dual servant role, this type of situation is most often encountered in critical care settings during cardiopulmonary resuscitation. Because one person is directly in charge of the resuscitation efforts, the nurse may be said to be acting as an employee of the directing physician as well as an employee of the institution. In this type of situation, a negligent action on the part of the nurse could potentially make the nurse, the physician, and the hospital liable to the injured party.

Always to be remembered is that the person directly responsible for a negligent action will retain accountability for that action. The law may make others liable for a given employee's actions, but the employee always retains some individual liability.

Supervisor Liability

If a staff nurse in a critical care setting performs a required nursing action negligently or fails to assess a given patient accurately and the patient sustains an injury, the staff nurse may be liable for that injury. But what about the charge nurse and the supervisor nurse? Is the charge nurse or supervisor potentially liable merely because he or she assigned the staff nurse to care for that particular patient? What is the potential liability of the manager or supervisor who assigned the staff nurse to that unit?

The answer to these questions depends upon several factors. If the staff nurse is consistently competent and has the necessary education and experience required to care for critically ill patients, then the supervisor and charge nurse would incur no liability merely by assigning the staff nurse to work in the unit and care for the patient. Also, if the staff nurse does nothing, either in words or actions, to alert the supervisor or charge nurse that he or she is not competent to care for the patient, then the supervisor and charge nurse are not liable. For example, suppose the supervisor and charge nurse have frequently observed a staff nurse caring for critically ill patients in a competent manner, and the staff nurse has said nothing to either of them about personal problems or about feeling unable to care for a specific patient. Should an untoward occurrence happen and the patient be injured, there is no vicarious liability on the part of either the supervisor or the charge nurse.

The situation is different, however, if at the beginning of the shift, the staff nurse had talked with the supervisor about a personal crisis at home and asked to be assigned only to stable patients. Or, perhaps the supervisor and charge nurse had noted that the staff nurse was consistently giving care below the accepted standard of care and had said nothing to the staff nurse. In these cases, the supervisor and charge nurse would incur some liability for the untoward happening that injured the patient. They knew or should have known that there was a problem and did nothing to protect the patient from harm. A supervisor may also incur liability if he or she continues to employ a nurse who does not meet the requirements of the unit. Any incompetent action by that nurse that results in harm to a patient could then be imputed to the supervisor.

An issue that frequently arises is that of the float nurse in a critical care setting. What is the standard of care required of the float nurse, who typically works in other areas of the hospital and who is unfamiliar with the policies and procedures of the unit? Generally speaking, the float nurse is held to the same standard of care required of all critical care nurses if the float nurse accepts responsibility for patients within this very specialized setting. Some points that will help protect the float nurse from liability in these settings include the following. The float nurse's expertise and general nursing skills must be ascertained before the nurse is assigned to a specific patient. Patient assignments should always be made on the basis of the type of care the float nurse is capable of giving. The charge nurse serves as a resource person to answer questions and reassign the float nurse if it becomes apparent that his or her expertise has been exceeded. Implementation of classes to cross-educate nurses to the critical care unit will assist the float nurse to give the same standard of care that is required of all nurses working within the setting.

Expanded Roles in Nursing

As the scope of nursing and of medicine become more intertwined, the question is raised whether critical care nurses are indeed practicing medicine rather than nursing. This question is especially pertinent in situations that require expert clinical skills and immediate action. For example, a patient in the coronary care unit may begin to have frequent paired multifocal premature ventricular contractions (PVCs) and short bursts of ventricular tachycardia. Lidocaine is readily available in its intravenous form. If the coronary care nurse acts upon this medical diagnosis by administering 100 mg of lidocaine through a previously ordered and placed intravenous line, is that nurse practicing medicine? Or, as Roth and Daze (1984) contend, is the nurse, who has accepted an increased level of responsibility through advanced education and experience, merely practicing good nursing?

To answer this question, several factors must be addressed. First, the courts have long recognized the duty of a nurse to use individual judgment when caring for patients and have held nurses accountable for using this independent judgment (*Fraijo v. Hartland Hospital*, 1979; and *Cooper v. National Motor Bearing Company*, 1955). This type of court interpretation provides the basis for interpreting the legal liability of expanded nursing roles.

The state nurse practice acts also provide guidance for interpreting acceptable nursing roles and practices. Several of these practice acts now allow nurses to make nursing diagnoses and to treat patients based upon these diagnoses. If the acceptable standard, according to the state nurse practice act, is that intensive care nurses may institute appropriate measures to alleviate a patient's presenting symptoms in emergency situations, then to take such measures is considered the practice of nursing, not medicine. A nurse so acting may be said to be making a nursing assessment of the patient and responding accordingly.

Hospital policies and protocols may also give guidance to nurses. If the protocol of the unit is to act upon presenting symptoms in emergency situations, then the coronary care nurse is acting within the scope of nursing when he or she administers lidocaine to a patient with multiple PVCs and short runs of ventricular tachycardia. Such hospital protocols should be established by a joint committee representing both nursing and medicine. The joint committee must take the state nurse and medical practice acts into consideration when establishing the protocols. The guidelines for standards of care published by the Joint Commission for the Accreditation of Health Organizations should also be reviewed. These published standards are unit-specific and nationally based. They provide evidence of reasonable nursing care. The protocols should be reviewed and updated regularly to allow their recommendations to remain current in the light of changing technology and standards of care and to ensure that they are within the guidelines of the state practice acts for both professions.

The presence of an emergency may give the experienced critical care nurse legal standing to initiate immediate therapy. It is important for the nurse to ensure that the situation is an appropriate emergency based upon the following criteria: (1) the patient's life or physical well-being is imminently threatened; (2) the nurse's level of expertise and skill is not exceeded by taking the appropriate actions; and (3) there is no one more qualified in the immediate situation to take control and initiate therapy. A judgment on what is allowable under a true emergency situation is usually based upon whether the nurse acted in a reasonable manner and whether sound nursing practices were followed.

In the example cited above, the nurse giving lidocaine to a patient with multiple PVCs should document in the patient's record how the patient's life or physical well-being was threatened. In this case, rhythm strips can be permanent documentation of the life-threatening nature of the event. Before proceeding, the nurse must ensure that his or her skills and level of expertise will not be exceeded by taking the actions required. In this example, the nurse was well versed in the effects of lidocaine, the proper dosage, and the rate of administration. Suppose, however, that the patient required immediate oral intubation and the critical care nurse was the only health care provider available. Unless the nurse had received training and had had experience in intubating patients, proceeding with the emergent intubation would exceed the nurse's level of expertise.

Certification is the process of granting recognition to individuals who have attained a specific level of knowledge and expertise in a given field of a profession. Certification may aid nurses in showing that they have the necessary skills and expertise to proceed in an emergency situation. Such advanced credentials may weigh favorably in the event of a subsequent lawsuit.

Another criterion of the emergency situation is that no one more qualified is present to take control and initiate therapy. This means that the nurse may not proceed if a person with more authority under the medical practice act is present. In the lidocaine example, suppose that a medical resident had walked into the coronary care unit just as the nurse was deciding to give the lidocaine, and, when asked, had said to give an alternative drug instead of the lidocaine. If the nurse had proceeded to administer the lidocaine in that situation, he or she could be liable to the charge of practicing medicine without a license. The nurse could be liable even if the patient responded in the desired manner.

Suppose, on the other hand, that no physician was available and the nurse had administered the intravenous lidocaine. Despite the nursing action, the patient experienced cardiac arrest and could not be successfully resuscitated. Does the unfavorable outcome increase the nurse's liability? No. Liability is not increased if the nurse met the three criteria previously stated and acted reasonably and in accordance with sound nursing judgment.

What if the nurse has the necessary skills and expertise but fails to respond to an emergency situation, and the patient dies because immediate action was not taken? Does the failure of the nurse to respond in accordance with his or her education and experience result in liability to the patient's family? Recent literature suggests that such a failure to act might be the basis of a successful malpractice lawsuit against the nonresponding nurse (Dean, 1985). A current California lawsuit seems to indicate that the nurse in such a situation was not acting as a patient advocate and might be held liable for the result (*Bardenilla v. Kaiser Foundation Hospital*, Cal-LA Superior Ct, 1988).

SPECIFIC LEGAL CONCERNS IN CRITICAL CARE

Critical care nurses face several specific legal concerns in their day-to-day clinical practice. Some of the more commonly encountered concerns include issues relating to patient consent, do-not-resuscitate orders, life support, withdrawal of "ordinary" care, and staffing.

Informed Consent

All patients have the right to be consulted and to give consent before health care providers proceed with ordered treatments and interventions. Once the patient or his or her legal representative gives informed consent, the health care provider may proceed without fear that a lawsuit for battery will be filed.

Informed consent, a concept of the late 1950s, ensures that the patient or his or her legal representative has been given sufficient information upon which to base an informed choice. This means that the person has been told about the nature of the proposed therapy or procedure, the risks inherent in the procedure or therapy, any alternatives to the therapy or procedure, and the complications that might arise with the proposed therapy or procedure. Table 67–2 summarizes the criteria that are necessary to establish informed consent. The patient or legal representative, once aware of these facts, may refuse to give consent. At law, such refusal is termed "informed refusal" because the person is fully aware of what is being refused.

Informed consent is usually obtained from the patient or legal representative as a signature on a consent form. Other valid legal means of obtaining

---

TABLE 67–2. Elements of Informed Consent

The Person(s) Giving Consent Must Fully Comprehend
The procedure or therapy to be performed
The risks involved in the procedure or therapy
The expected or desired outcomes of the procedure or therapy
Any complications or undesired side effects
Alternative therapies, including no therapy at all

The Consent Is Given by One Who Has the Legal Capacity for Giving the Consent
Competent adult
Legal guardian or representative for the incompetent adult
Emancipated, married minor
Mature minor (if applicable)
Parent or legal guardian of a minor
Minor (for diagnosis and treatment of specific disease states or conditions)
Court order

consent include oral consent, apparent consent, and implied consent. Oral consent is consent given freely by word of mouth. Unless the institution has a policy that no verbal consent will be accepted, verbal consent is just as valid as written consent. It differs in that verbal consent is more difficult to prove.

Apparent consent is inferred by the patient's conduct. The foundation for apparent consent is an 1899 lawsuit, *O'Brien v. Cunard Steamship Company*. In that case, a female passenger joined a line of people receiving vaccinations. She neither questioned nor refused the vaccination but merely held out her arm for the injection. Examples of apparent consent may be found in most critical care settings today. The reasonable practitioner infers by the patient's actions that the patient both understands and consents to the therapy or intervention.

Implied consent normally is involved in true emergency situations. The patient is unable to make his or her consent known, is incapable of refusing the procedure or therapy, and a delay in providing care would result in loss of life or permanent injury to the patient. The law of implied consent allows the health care provider to proceed in emergency situations as if valid consent had been obtained. Areas of the hospital where implied consent is most often relied upon include the emergency department and the critical care unit.

The duty to see that informed consent is obtained prior to initiating therapy or interventions usually falls upon the physician or primary health care practitioner. The nurse's role in this area of the law is still evolving. Some hospitals by policy make the nurse accountable for seeing that the patient or legal representative signs the informed consent form. Other hospitals have policies mandating that valid informed consent forms be obtained by the primary health care provider and that the nurse may sign only as a witness to the patient's signature. Some institutions require a separate signed form for each procedure and therapy, whereas others rely on documentation of the patient's consent in the medical record.

Generally, the nurse is responsible for informing the physician and hospital administration if there is a problem with informed consent. For example, the patient may ask a nurse about the surgical procedure scheduled for the next day. It then becomes clear to the nurse that the patient has not been informed by the physician or that the information given was incomplete. The nurse now has a duty to see that valid consent is obtained prior to the scheduled surgery. This may be done by talking with the primary physician, notifying the nursing supervisor, or alerting the operating room staff.

Just as important as conveying necessary information upon which to base informed consent is the acquisition of the proper signature on the informed consent form. The competent adult patient presents no problem in this area of the law. For minors and persons who are incompetent to sign a consent form, the various states' statutes mandate who may legally sign for the patient and when a court-appointed guardian is necessary.

Durable Power of Attorney for Health Care

A newer concept in substituted decision-making authority is the power of attorney, also referred to as a durable power of attorney for health care. Legally, this concept allows patients to give valid authorization for informed consent or informed refusal to a person of their choosing. The authorization must be made while the patient is still competent and capable of authorizing a substitute decision maker.

Durable power of attorney has become a popular concept in states that do not recognize family consent laws. Under the current informed consent doctrines, the competent adult is the proper person who either gives or refuses informed consent. What happens, though, if that competent adult sustains a severe head injury in an accident or becomes comatose due to metabolic derangements? Under current law in most states, a relative or friend would be required to obtain the court's permission to become guardian for the now incompetent adult. Using the durable power of attorney doctrine, the competent adult signs a document declaring that a certain named person has his or her authorization to provide informed consent should the adult in question not be able to give consent due to injury, disease, or disability.

Use of the durable power of attorney is frequent in two situations. Many nonmarried couples use the durable power of attorney to ensure that if anything should happen to one partner, the other partner would be able to give valid informed consent for necessary medical care. The durable power of attorney is also used by elderly widows or widowers to ensure that one of their children can give valid consent for medical care. In these cases, the durable power of attorney is often used when there are several children and the mother or father desires that a prenamed child serve as his or her substituted decision maker. This designation avoids the chance that family members will be unable to agree on what medical care the parent would have wanted.

To protect health care providers from liability, all durable power of attorney documents should be verified with the hospital's legal department prior to implementation. This procedure simply verifies the fact that the document is in accordance with state laws. Once a person holding a valid power of attorney is identified, health care providers can avoid allegations of invasion of privacy, breach of confidentiality, and negligence based upon lack of informed consent.

Do-Not-Resuscitate Issues

Since the mid 1960s, the use of cardiopulmonary resuscitation has been fairly standard for all hospitalized patients unless other orders exist. The problem at issue for nursing has generally not been whether one could or should obtain a "no code" order for a given patient but rather whether a verbal order is sufficient and whether the manner in which the code is implemented is correct.

It has always been the best course of action for nurses to obtain a written and documented "do not resuscitate" order. Most hospital policies require the attending physician to write such an order before resuscitation efforts will be withheld. In the absence of policy or state statute, a verbal "no code" order is legally enforceable, although it may be more difficult to prove the existence of such in a court of law. It is also recommended that written or verbal orders be reevaluated and revalidated every 24 to 72 hours. This measure is thought to ensure that the patient's status will be closely followed by the primary health care provider (Greenlaw, 1982).

If cardiopulmonary resuscitation is to be initiated, a "slow" or "partial" code, in which the nurses move slowly or fail to respond in a timely manner, should never be permitted. Such actions always fall below the minimum standard of care and open the nursing staff to liability. The patient should either be resuscitated in a competent manner or a valid "no code" order should be obtained so that no resuscitation efforts need be initiated.

A newer concept, the "chemical" code, is a valid order today and may be carried out by nurses without fear of liability. This type of code involves the use of drug interventions only. If the patient has a respiratory or cardiac arrest, he or she is allowed to die without chest compressions or intubation. Many families feel that this type of intervention prevents unnecessary suffering in their loved one, yet allows the person to die with some dignity.

Living Wills and Natural Death Acts

To ensure that a patient's wishes in regard to life-support measures are respected, living wills and natural death acts have become popular. A living will is a document made by a competent individual and directed to medical personnel and family members regarding the type of treatment the individual wishes to receive if a diagnosis of terminal illness is made. The living will is not necessary if the person, once diagnosed, remains competent, but becomes vital if the person has become incompetent at the time of the terminal diagnosis. Natural death acts, also called medical treatment decision acts, are in reality statutory enactments of living wills.

The great majority of states in the United States have enacted natural death acts. The statutory provisions of these acts vary greatly from state to state. All ensure that practitioners who, in good faith, follow the dictates of the natural death act will be immune from civil and criminal lawsuits. Requirements for witnesses of the living will, for a signature on the document as opposed to an oral wish, and

for the consequences of noncompliance with the act vary according to the state or territory.

Withdrawal of Ordinary Care Measures

Perhaps one of the only areas in medicine in which the state courts have concurred in their opinions is the withdrawal of ordinary care measures. These ordinary care measures include supplemental oxygen therapy, tube feedings, and nutritional and hydration support. The question of removing such ordinary care devices usually arises in the patient who is terminally ill or who is in a persistent vegetative state. Although agreeing that there should be strict guidelines for decision making in this area, all courts have allowed the removal of such devices in the terminally ill and in patients who remain in a persistent vegetative state. Even the President's Commission in 1983 concluded that "no particular treatments—including such ordinary hospital intervention as parenteral nutrition or hydration, antibiotics, and transfusions—are universally warranted and thus obligatory for a patient to accept." (President's Commission, 1983).

SUMMARY

This chapter has explored various legal doctrines applicable to critical care, the legal definition of standards of care, the basis for nursing liability, and some specific concerns of critical care nurses. Because individual state laws may vary, the nurse is cautioned to read this chapter in conjunction with his or her individual nurse practice act and to explore the state statutes, particularly in the areas of informed consent, living wills and natural death acts, and personal injury actions. Knowledge of the interplay between nursing and the law not only helps to prevent the nurse from becoming involved in a potential lawsuit but also ensures professional growth and improved clinical practice.

References

Bardenilla v. Kaiser Foundation Hospital. (1988). Cal-LA Superior Court.
Cooper v. National Bearing Motor Company. (1955). 288 F 2d 581 (California).
Dean, K. (1985). Parameters of nursing practice. *Focus on Critical Care*, 12(1), 48–50.
Forthofer v. Arnold. (1938). 60 Ohio App 436, 21 NE 2d 869.
Fraijo v. Hartland Hospital. (1979). 160 Cal Rept 246, 99 Cal App 3d 331.
Greenlaw, J. (1982). Orders not to resuscitate: Dilemma for acute care as well as long term care facilities. *Law, Medicine, and Health Care*, 10 (1), 29–31, 45.
Murchison, I., Michols, T., and Hanson R. (1982). *Legal Accountability in the Nursing Process*. (2nd ed.). St. Louis: C. V. Mosby.
Napier v. Greenzweig. (1919). 256 F 196 (2d Cir).
President's Commission. (1983). *Deciding to Forego Life-Sustaining Treatment*. Washington, D.C.: author.
Roth, M. D., and Daze, A. M. (1984). Are nurses practicing medicine in the ICU? *Dimensions of Critical Care Nursing*, 3 (4), 230–237.

68

Patient Education

Patria E. Constancia

Patient education is an important aspect of comprehensive patient care. Patients receiving health care expect to receive information about their illness and about the measures being taken to improve their condition and promote their health status. Traditionally, most critically ill patients have been viewed as "too sick" to benefit from patient education. However, with increasing consumer demand for health care information and the decreased length of patient hospitalization, it is apparent that nursing care for critically ill patients must include both expert technical care and a plan for effective patient education.

This chapter will review the concept of patient education and the teaching-learning process. The development of teaching strategies and the selection of appropriate teaching methods for critically ill patients will be discussed.

EVOLUTION OF CONCEPT AND PRACTICE IN PATIENT EDUCATION

Evolution of Patient Education

The importance of health education was recognized following World War II, coinciding with an increased incidence of chronic diseases and an increased lifespan of those with long-term disabilities. At that time, the focus of health education expanded from disease prevention to include patient and family education about living with chronic illness. Government-supported pilot projects were implemented to teach patients about their diseases. Patient education programs were established to target specific disease conditions such as diabetes, rheumatic fever, cancer, renal disease, and stroke.

During the 1960s consumers became aware of their right to be informed about the product or service they were receiving. In response to the consumer movement, a number of health care agencies adopted a patients' bill of rights. These documents specified the patient's right to obtain information about his or her diagnosis, treatment, and prognosis in terms that the patient could understand. During the 1960s patient education was described as a process of disseminating information to patients with specific disease conditions. Information was aimed toward increasing the patient's knowledge of the disease process and the treatment regimen.

In 1973 the American Hospital Association Committee on Health Education concluded that health care institutions have an obligation to provide educational programs to patients. These programs were to be established with the goals of improving the quality of patient care, utilizing outpatient facilities more effectively, decreasing the length of hospital stay, and reducing health care costs (American Hospital Association, 1974).

At present, patient education is considered a patient right and a legal responsibility of health care professionals who provide patient care (Falvo, 1985). Appropriate patient education is necessary for quality health care. It is recognized as a factor that has the potential to increase the efficiency of the health care delivery system. Patients realize that knowledge about illness and medical care is not the exclusive property of health professionals (Storlie, 1973). As they recognize their right to know, health care consumers have become more vocal in asserting that right. The growing number of malpractice suits alleging a failure to disclose sufficient information to the patient is evidence that patients seek recompense when they feel their right to information has been abused.

Patient Education as Part of Quality Patient Care

The need for patient education as a structured, organized activity has been recognized formally by a variety of health care professions. Statements by various professional groups acknowledge their commitment to the concept and implementation of patient education. The American Nurses Association (ANA) recognizes patient teaching as an integral part of quality patient care (American Nurses Association, 1973). The ANA has outlined the professional nurse's responsibility and accountability in providing the patient and family with the relevant facts about specific health care needs and in supporting appropriate modification of patient behavior.

Nurse practice acts in several states specifically define the practice of nursing as including teaching (Connecticut, 1978; New Jersey, 1978). Nurses are statutorily authorized to instruct their patients concerning health problems. In other states where patient education is not authorized by statute, patient education is placed under the guidance and prescription of the physician.

PATIENT EDUCATION: THE TEACHING-LEARNING PROCESS

Andragogy is the theory of education of how adults learn. Knowles (1984) has identified four key attributes of the adult learner: (1) possession of an independent self-concept and of self-direction in learning; (2) possession of a wealth of life experiences on which to base learning; (3) a motivation for learning that arises from a need to solve problems; and (4) a need for immediate applicability of the learned material.

These attributes of the adult learner may be significantly altered in the critically ill patient. Critical illness or injury greatly decreases the patient's independence and self-direction. The patient loses control of daily activities and even the most basic bodily functions. The patient and family may not have had prior experience with hospitalization and the health care system. They cannot rely on past experiences to provide cues for their current learning needs. The fear and anxiety that frequently accompany critical illness may result in a "here and now" focus, which interferes with patient education. The effects of critical illness and the critical care environment have important implications for patient education that will be discussed in the following sections.

Assessment of the Learner

A thorough assessment of the patient as learner is the most important factor in successful teaching. The nurse is expected to provide thorough and accurate teaching to a wide variety of patients. The critical care nurse may begin teaching a 75-year-old retired accountant about his home care following cardiac surgery while at the same time reviewing and reinforcing prior instruction on diabetes with a noncompliant 21-year-old patient recovering from diabetic ketoacidosis. The challenge is to teach these diverse patients in such a manner that optimum reception and retention of the information occur. The patient's ability to receive and retain information depends upon his or her readiness, willingness, and ability to learn. These three factors must be considered and incorporated in the teaching plan.

Readiness to Learn. To determine the patient's readiness to learn, the nurse assesses the patient's emotional state, motivation, stage of adaptation to illness, maturational level, and past life experiences. The patient's emotional state affects the way he or she looks at the world. Patients who feel good about themselves and the progress of their disease and treatment are more likely to be ready to learn than patients who have low self-esteem, extensive health problems, and multiple complications. Decreased self-confidence and feelings of lack of control may leave the patient depressed and uninterested in learning.

Adults learn best when they are motivated. Motivation affects the patient's readiness to learn in several ways. First, the patient's basic physiologic and safety needs must be satisfied before he can engage in higher cognitive functions (Maslow, 1970). For example, a patient experiencing status asthmaticus will not be interested in learning a new medication regimen until he or she is not acutely short of breath. During the critical event, this patient's primary motivation is achieving adequate air exchange. Similarly, the patient will be most motivated to learn when he can see the direct applicability of the information on the treatment or prevention of the disease process.

Patients progress through several stages of adaptation in the course of illness. These stages include disbelief, awareness, acceptance, reorganization, identity change, and finally, successful adaptation. Each stage involves various patient coping mechanisms. The nurse must be aware of the patient's current stage of adaptation in order to plan an effective teaching strategy. For example, a myocardial patient who is in the stage of disbelief may deny the seriousness of the illness. This patient will not be receptive to teaching about risk factor modification. Table 68–1 presents an example of the stages of adaptation to illness for the patient with myocardial infarction.

Maturational level affects the patient's ability to cope with the stress of illness and hospitalization and influences the motivation to learn and try out new behaviors. As a person matures, he acquires certain skills and experiences that assist in learning new tasks. A patient's experience, not only with health care but also with hobbies and work, can increase his readiness to learn by making learning more meaningful and familiar.

Willingness to Learn. The patient's health beliefs, sociocultural background, and religious beliefs are

TABLE 68–1. Assessment of Patient's Adaptation to Myocardial Infarction

Stage of Adaptation	Assessment/ Description	Implication for Nurse
Disbelief	Denies seriousness of MI	Focus on present
	Refuses to accept diagnosis	Integrate teaching into routine care
	Avoids expression of feelings about MI	Explain procedures clearly
Awareness	Expresses anger	Focus on present needs
	Resists dependency and life-style changes	Explain care as it relates to present patient needs
		Avoid lectures and long presentations of facts
Reorganization	Accepts diagnosis and increased dependence	Begin teaching with the content patient identifies as most important
	Acknowledges changes that have occurred	
Identity change	Defines changes and difference in life style because of MI	Answer patient's questions as they arise
Successful adaptation	Lives comfortably with limitations and modifications of life style following MI	Nurse may act as a consultant to patient

Data from Crate, M.A. (1965). Nursing functions in adaptation to chronic illness. *American Journal of Nursing, 65*(10), 72.

important considerations in planning patient education. Certain beliefs affect a person's health and response to illness. These beliefs also affect the person's ability to accept and profit from health education. Theories such as the health belief model attempt to explain and correlate a variety of factors that influence a person's willingness to obtain health care and to comply with the resulting recommendations (Rosenstock, 1975; Devon and Powers, 1984). The health belief model suggests that individuals take action relating to health care if (1) they believe themselves to be susceptible to the disease; (2) they believe that the disease will have serious effects on their life; (3) they believe that taking certain actions will reduce the risk or severity of the disease; and (4) they believe that the threat presented by taking action will be less than the threat presented by the disease (Becker, 1974).

The nurse must also assess the patient's sociocultural background for factors that influence the response to illness. The values and customs of different groups have an impact on a patient's life style and thus influence the patient's ability to learn and modify certain behaviors. For example, if the patient's sociocultural background defines an ill person as

someone who should be passive and cared for by others, then that person will not respond positively to patient education that promotes active self-care.

The nature and strength of the patient's religious beliefs can also influence his or her attitude toward treatment and cure of disease. Patients who strongly believe that health or illness is the will of God may not see a need for active participation in their treatment. Restrictions against blood transfusions and dietary restrictions are other examples of religious beliefs that influence the patient's attitude toward treatment of disease.

Ability to Learn. The patient's ability to learn depends on his or her current physical and intellectual status. The nurse must assess for any physical or mental problems that could interfere with the patient's ability to learn. For example, the presence of severe incisional pain may prevent the patient-learner from understanding and responding to teaching about postoperative respiratory exercises. Electrolyte imbalances, azotemia, or hypoxemia may decrease the patient's ability to concentrate on and comprehend the information presented. Sleep deprivation and disorientation also block the learning process.

The patient's ability to learn can be estimated by his or her vocabulary and use of language. Other indicators include the patient's knowledge of the illness and his understandings of and compliance with previous medical instructions. Learning barriers such as language difficulties, physical handicaps, senility, and mental retardation must be given special attention.

Educational level and current job status should also be considered. Patients with financial difficulties may experience greater anxiety levels during hospitalization. High anxiety levels are associated with decreased learning. Similarly, the patient will respond less favorably to teaching if he or she cannot afford to purchase the supplies and equipment required to carry out the teaching plan.

Assessment data related to the patient's readiness, willingness, and ability to learn are utilized in the formation of the teaching plan. Based on the assessment information, the nurse modifies the teaching plan and selects the appropriate strategies to ensure that learning takes place.

Assessment of the Patient's Learning Needs

Once the assessment of the patient as learner has been completed, a learning needs assessment is performed to identify specifically what needs to be taught to the patient. The nurse should have a clear idea of what the patient needs to know in order to cope with the illness, to promote optimum wellness, or to prevent further debilitation.

Careful assessment of learning needs saves the

TABLE 68–2. Teaching Plan for a Cardiac Surgery Patient: Preparation for Discharge

Topic	Learning Objectives	Teaching Resources	Teaching Activity	Date/Initial
Medication	The patient/family will identify the purpose of all discharge medications The patient/family will describe the effect of all discharge medications The patient/family will properly administer all discharge medications	Staff nurse Pharmacist Medication sheets	Give patient medication sheet to read Evaluate patient's knowledge of medication purpose, dose, and toxic effects Provide medication schedule sheet Provide information about Medi-Alert bracelet Teach patient to take pulse if applicable	
Diet	The patient/family will identify foods allowed on home diet The patient/family will identify foods not allowed on home diet The patient family will describe ways in which current food preferences can be adapted	Staff nurse Dietitian AHA pamphlets	Contact dietitian to provide initial diet teaching with patient/family Provide patient with appropriate AHA pamphlets Evaluate patient/family knowledge of diet by: 1. Asking them to list foods not allowed on diet 2. Asking them to develop a new menu that is compatible with diet 3. Asking them to discuss ways of adapting current food preferences to diet	
Care of incisions	The patient/family verbalize and demonstrate how to care for incisions at home	Staff nurse Discharge booklet	Have the patient read the discharge booklet Demonstrate/return demonstrate bathing, cleansing, etc. Demonstrate/return demonstrate application of antiembolic stockings	
Activity at home	The patient/family will describe the normal progression of activity and exercise at home	Staff nurse Physical therapist Discharge booklet	Give patient booklet to read With physician's assistance, develop an individualized plan for regular exercise and recreation	
Sleep and rest	The patient/family will discuss the importance of adequate sleep and regular rest periods following cardiac surgery	Staff nurse	Give patient discharge booklet to read Reinforce with patient/family the importance of frequent rest periods during the day	
Sexual activity	The patient/family will identify guidelines for sexual activity following cardiac surgery	Staff nurse Discharge booklet	Have patient read booklet Encourage patient/family to ask questions and verbalize concerns about sexual activity postoperatively	
Risk factor modification	The patient/family will identify the cardiac risk factors that affect him The patient/family will identify ways to control cardiac risk factors that affect him	Staff nurse AHA pamphlets AHA film on risk factors	Have patient read discharge booklet Have patient/family view film Assist patient/family to identify controllable risk factors Explore means of controlling each risk factor with the patient	

Courtesy of Leslie Kern, RN, MN, Los Angeles, CA.

nurse valuable teaching time. It helps to pinpoint specific learning needs. Learning needs assessment also facilitates teaching by allowing the nurse to identify physical, emotional, mechanical, and environmental barriers that may interfere with teaching and learning.

A variety of sources of information can be utilized in a learning needs assessment. The nurse may interview the family members to ascertain what they feel are important learning needs. If the patient is intubated or so ill that adequate information cannot be obtained from him or her, the family may be able to provide information about learning needs. If the family is to be involved in the patient's care or treatment plan, their learning needs should be carefully assessed as well. Such interviews also provide clues to patient and family concerns and to their level of understanding about the disease process and treatment plan. The patient's medical record is an excellent source of information about the patient's learning needs. The medical record contains the medical treatment plan as well as interdisciplinary notes that reflect the patient's response to treatment. These can be used to identify specific areas in which patient knowledge is deficient. The nursing care plan can be used to identify additional problems that require patient education. Interdisciplinary patient care conferences are beneficial in identifying patient learning needs and in facilitating a team approach to patient education.

Developing and Implementing a Plan for Patient Teaching

Once assessment of the patient's learning needs has been accomplished, content areas for teaching are identified. The nurse then develops learning objectives and a teaching plan based on these content areas.

Formulation of Learning Objectives. Learning objectives give direction to patient teaching. They are statements of intended outcomes or the results that are to be achieved by the patient. Objectives serve as a base on which to focus teaching efforts. For a learning objective to be effective, it must be learner centered. It should involve a single task that is easily achievable. Learning objectives are written as expected behaviors. Multiple learning objectives may be required for complex content areas such as medication administration. Table 68–2 provides examples of learning objectives for a cardiac surgery patient who is being discharged.

Developing a Teaching Strategy. Chatham and Knapp (1982) categorized learning needs and objectives into four general learning areas: knowledge, attitudes, skills, and practices. When choosing a teaching strategy, the nurse must decide which area is most closely related to the learning need. The

knowledge learning area consists of information, facts, concepts, and generalizations that need to be incorporated into the patient's concept of health. Skills are tasks or activities that must be learned by the patient or family. Because attitudes are learned, emotion-based predispositions to react in a particular way to an object, idea, or person, the attitude learning area involves changing these previously held tendencies. Practices are patterns of behavior that occur regularly over time. Health practices are visible syntheses of the patient's health-related knowledge, skills, and attitudes.

There are many teaching methods available to the nurse for use in patient education. The challenge for the nurse is to match the learning area with the appropriate teaching method. Table 68–3 provides a guide to the selection of teaching methods based on the area of the identified learning need. A number of teaching methods can be effectively utilized within each learning area. The teaching strategy chosen will depend on the characteristics of the patient-learner, the skills and preference of the nurse, the time available, and the patient's learning needs. Table 68–4 describes the advantages and disadvantages of the most common teaching methods.

Since teaching-learning is a process, it should not be viewed as a single event. This is particularly important in the critical care unit. As described in Table 68–1, many patients in the critical care unit will be in the early stages of adaptation to the illness (disbelief or awareness). These patients are not interested in formal teaching. The best approach to

TABLE 68–3. Teaching Methods of Choice

Learning Area	Teaching Methods of Choice
A. Knowledge	Discussions Lectures Audiovisual aids Printed materials Dialogues Question and answer sessions (interviews)
B. Skills	Demonstrations Guided practice Step-by-step self-instruction guides Problem-solving Audiovisual demonstrations Drills
C. Attitudes	Group discussions Listening/feedback sessions Role-playing Sharing experiences Case examples Dramatizations/simulations
D. Practices	Behavioral contracting Behavior modification Brainstorming Problem-solving Counseling (listening/feedback)

From Chatham, M., and Knapp, B. (1982). *Patient education handbook* (p. 112). Bowie MD: Prentice-Hall.

TABLE 68–4. Teaching Methods: Advantages and Disadvantages

Method	Description	Advantages	Disadvantages
Audiovisuals	Films, slide-tape programs, video programs, models, charts, posters	1. A large amount of information is provided in a simple manner 2. Makes efficient use of nursing time 3. Retention and understanding are increased when both visual and audio messages are used	1. Requires equipment purchase, storage, and maintenance 2. May be expensive 3. Difficult to measure effectiveness 4. Content cannot be readily changed
Behavioral contracting	Negotiation between the nurse-teacher and patient to effect change in an identified behavior or practice	1. Patient is more likely to change behavior due to the contractual nature of agreement 2. Progress toward target behavior can be easily evaluated 3. Facilitates communication between nurse and patient 4. Provides a clear statement of expectations of both nurse and the patient	1. Patient may not identify the same problems as the nurse 2. Benefits resulting from changing present behavior may not be obvious to patient 3. Patient may not comply with contract
Case examples/story telling	Anecdotes about health experiences help to demonstrate to patients that they are not alone in their ailments. Permits sharing of insight into health problems	1. Provides information and different solutions that are applicable to patient's problem 2. Encourages patients to express their feelings about their health and health care practices 3. Minimal time is required	1. Must maintain confidentiality of case examples 2. Patients may misunderstand message or become sidetracked on other issues
Demonstrations	Skills are taught to the patient through demonstration, guided practice, and supervision	1. The patient can see the skill performed 2. Information can be presented during demonstration 3. The patient is an active part of the demonstration	1. Supplies/equipment may be expensive 2. Return demonstration is not a guarantee that the patient will perform the skill at home
Individual/group discussions	Conversations between nurse and patient or groups of patients in which ideas and information are exchanged	1. Informal, flexible format 2. Patients and nurse can suggest solutions to problems 3. Inexpensive to implement	1. Must be conducted in a relatively stable ongoing group 2. Nurse must have good communicatin skills 3. Group discussions tend to be time-consuming 4. Difficult to evaluate results
Drills	Repetitious practice of a skill or information set	1. Rapid method of learning a skill or set of information 2. Improves retention of skill 3. Patient is actively involved	1. Special equipment may be required 2. Patient must cooperate 3. Not applicable to more complex skills

teaching these patients is to provide them with bits of relevant information during and related to routine care. Much of this information will have to be repeated several times. It is important for the critical care nurse to recognize this ongoing process of teaching and to continue it throughout the patient's stay in the critical care unit.

Barriers to Teaching-Learning Process

Certain factors in any teacher-learner interaction can interfere with successful teaching. These barriers to learning can be influenced by the nurse, the patient, the family, or the learning environment.

Barriers to Teaching

Time. Lack of time is usually considered the greatest barrier to effective teaching. Lack of appropriate planning, inadequate teaching skills, and selection of the wrong teaching methods may contribute to the perceived lack of time.

Communication. Poor communication among the different members of the health care team can result in a disorganized and ineffective patient education effort. Confusion between the patient and his teachers results when the patient's needs and learning

TABLE 68–4. Teaching Methods: Advantages and Disadvantages Continued

Method	Description	Advantages	Disadvantages
Lectures	One-way communication from speaker to audience; used when teaching a large group	1. Large amount of information can be covered in a short time 2. More than one teacher can participate 3. Audiovisuals or demonstrations can be used to enhance lecture	1. Nurse needs time to prepare for lecture 2. Learners may lose interest 3. Only information acquisition can be evaluated 4. Little or no patient participation
Printed materials	Books, pamphlets, brochures, handouts	1. Little nursing time required 2. Wide variety of topics and presentations available 3. Can reinforce verbal teaching	1. Patient must be able to read 2. Information may not be used if no reinforcement occurs 3. May be expensive
Problem-solving technique	Structured analysis of problems and solutions	1. Used with individuals or groups 2. Inexpensive 3. Can be used in conjunction with other methods such as demonstrations 4. Encourages the patient to take responsibility for own health care	1. Nurse must avoid making judgments and expressing opinions 2. Nurse must possess good listening and feedback skills 3. Patient may not implement solutions
Question and answer	Questions phrased to stimulate new ideas or elicit information. May be used to determine if learning has occurred	1. Formal or informal structure 2. Used with individuals or groups 3. Informative, flexible format	1. Cannot stand alone as a teaching method 2. Patient may not ask the right questions 3. Only patient knowledge can be evaluated
Role-playing	Spontaneous enactment of an event or situation. Allows patient to try out new behaviors and receive feedback from nurse	1. Most effective with groups 2. Used to present examples of behavior that are not easily demonstrated in other ways 3. Used to clarify problems and solutions	1. Requires a large amount of time 2. Groups must build trust level to be effective 3. Group members may sabotage the process
Self-instructional materials	Collections of information, facts, concepts presented in a step-by-step format. The learner completes the material individually	1. Patient learns at own pace 2. Information is broken down into small learning units 3. Minimal nursing time required 4. Contain built-in reinforcement for learning and provide immediate feedback	1. Patient must be motivated to use materials 2. Patient may lose interest 3. Patient must be able to read 4. Requires a fair amount of patient time 5. May be expensive

Adapted from: Chatham, M., and Knapp, B. (1982). *Patient education handbook.* Bowie, MD: Prentice-Hall.

progress are not communicated from one teacher to another. Documentation becomes a barrier to the teaching-learning process when the nurse does not document the teaching plan and the entire content that is taught to the patient. Without appropriate communication and documentation, some information may be duplicated while other learning needs may be neglected.

Language. Use of medical terminology is confusing to the patient and can increase anxiety. The teaching-learning interaction will be most effective when information is conveyed in simple, easily understood words. When possible, teaching should be done in the patient's primary spoken language.

Family Involvement. Family members can be helpful in reinforcing the teaching effort and preparing the patient to make the transition from hospital to home. Lack of family support can hamper patient teaching.

Attitudes and Values. Both the patient and the nurse possess a set of values and beliefs. Value judgments by either interfere with communication and destroy trust and rapport.

Barriers to Learning

Stress of Hospitalization. The adult learner is independent, self-directing, and self-sufficient. Illness and hospitalization interrupt this normal pattern and place physical and psychological restrictions on the patient. These restrictions result in increased anxiety, which may interfere with the patient's ability to learn.

Motivation. The patient must be motivated to learn. The nurse may be able to influence motivation positively by pointing out the benefits to be gained by learning and the potential problems that may result from ignoring the teaching.

Intensive Care Unit Environment. The environment in the critical care unit is not conducive to effective learning. Lack of privacy and constant activity around the unit may distract the patient from learning. Noise from staff, equipment, and various monitor alarms may also detract from the presentation of information. Every effort must be made to minimize distractions and provide privacy during patient teaching.

Physical Condition. The disease process, sensory impairment, pain, and other physiologic abnormalities affect the patient's ability to learn. Modified teaching efforts—that is, a time frame or a lower level of difficulty—must be considered for the patient in poor health.

Age. Declining memory, poor eyesight, slower thought process, and slower movements affect the learning ability of the elderly. Consideration of these factors will increase the effectiveness of teaching the elderly patient.

Socioeconomic Status. Religious beliefs, values, ethnic customs, and family traditions have the potential to interfere with or enhance patient teaching. The economic status of the patient is also a consideration when one is teaching home care that involves the purchase of supplies and equipment.

Evaluation of the Teaching-Learning Process

Evaluation of patient education is a means of measuring the effectiveness and efficiency of the teaching intervention. The teacher examines whether or not the learning objectives were met and whether further teaching is needed. Evaluation is an objective method of measuring patient learning. It focuses on the achievement of learning objectives and on whether the target behaviors have changed.

What to Evaluate. Evaluation must examine both the effects and the results of the patient teaching program. If the learning objectives are written correctly, the nurse will have little difficulty in evaluating what the patient has learned. For example, the nurse could evaluate the teaching program for the cardiac surgery patient by ascertaining whether the patient is able to describe the purpose and effect of the discharge medications. The nurse might also evaluate the patient's ability to self-administer these medications properly by observing him take his own medications prior to discharge.

Evaluation of the nurse as a teacher is also important. The selection of teaching strategies and the method used to carry them out reveal the teacher's strengths and weaknesses. All teaching methods must be evaluated for appropriateness and effectiveness in accomplishing the stated learning objectives.

With the increasing emphasis on reducing health

care costs, patient education is viewed as a means of decreasing complications, achieving shorter hospital stays, providing for continued care at home, and decreasing readmissions to the hospital. Teaching strategies must be examined to determine whether these outcomes are realized in terms of the time, money, and resources invested.

When to Evaluate. Evaluation does not occur only at the end of a teaching activity. Patient evaluation should be planned and initiated early in the teaching process. By measuring both the successes and failures, the strengths and weaknesses of teaching methods prior to the end of the teaching plan, changes can be made before an unfavorable outcome occurs. Observation of the patient's participation, enthusiasm, interest, resistance, or indifference provides a valuable indication of end results.

How to Evaluate. Several types of evaluation techniques can be used in patient education. As described in Table 68–5, these include written methods, observation, and verbal techniques. Written methods are relatively easy to assemble and administer. They are best used to evaluate patient learning of the knowledge conveyed by the teacher. Written tests may be anxiety-provoking for some patients. Observations may be used to evaluate patient performance of learned skills. The nurse can also utilize observation techniques to evaluate patient participation, coping, and other actions. Verbal communication, using nonthreatening open-ended questions, elicits much information about the patient's knowledge and attitudes. "What if . . ." scenarios can be used to evaluate the patient's ability to synthesize newly gained knowledge.

Documentation of Patient Teaching-Learning

Documentation of the patient teaching and learning that have occurred is important from several perspectives. First, documentation of teaching and learning in the medical record is an important com-

TABLE 68–5. Evaluation Techniques in Patient Education

Method	Example
Written	Questionnaires
	Checklists
	Fill-in-the-blank tests
	Multiple choice tests
	Lists
Observation	Patient demonstration of skill
	Patient participation in group
Verbal	Question and answer session
	Open-ended questions
Problem solving	Hypothetical scenarios

munication tool. Documentation promotes patient education as a process. Concise documentation of what was taught, the patient's and family's response and attainment of learning, and identification of additional learning needs assists other health care team members in evaluating patient learning and in following through appropriately with the teaching-learning plan.

Documentation of teaching-learning also serves to demonstrate that the standard of care was met for that particular patient (Bille, 1981). This is useful from a quality assurance standpoint. Documentation of teaching-learning may also provide an important defense in the event of litigation.

THE FAMILY IN PATIENT EDUCATION

The patient can be viewed as an individual interacting with and forming an integral part of a social group known as the family. Depending on the patient's sociocultural background, the patient's family may be defined as the nuclear family, the extended family, or the augmented family composed of close friends. Regardless of the composition, the family plays an important role in the patient's recovery from or adaptation to illness. The family is the support system to which the patient turns for comfort and information to help him or her cope with illness. The presence of a strong support system reduces stress, improves self-esteem and self-confidence, and allows the patient to concentrate on learning.

Health Care and the Family

One basic family function is to protect its members' health and promote their physical well-being. The family is a personal care system within which health is organized and provided.

The illness of a family member frequently results in reorganization of the family structure. Such reorganization can lead to role impairment or role disruption in other family members. For example, the wife may be forced to assume the leadership role in the family following her husband's myocardial infarction and cardiac surgery. This situation can be very stressful for the family.

The patient and family's ability to adapt to role reorganization plays a major role in their willingness to accept teaching and make any necessary behavioral changes. If successful adaptation to role reorganization does not occur, the family may not be able to support the patient's learning efforts. Therefore, it is important for the nurse to assess family functioning. When planning patient education activities, it is vital for the nurse to be aware of the influence of the family on the patient's prescribed health regimen. Assessment data can be used to develop strategies to support the family as well as the patient.

Family-Centered Teaching

Because the needs and function of the family may have a negative influence on patient education, it is imperative to view the family within the framework of total patient care. Assessment of the family's learning needs can be achieved by interviewing family members. The nurse looks specifically for past and present information about health status, family perceptions of the illness, their feelings, and their adaptation to previous illness. Family roles and relationships, communication patterns, resources, and support systems must also be identified. Key questions to be asked include:

Who will be the primary caregiver for the patient at home?
Who is the head of the family or who will assume the position of head of the family?
How will decisions be made within the family?
Which family member appears most capable of organizing support systems and resources?

Individualized teaching activity for the family is planned using a multidisciplinary approach. Contributions of specific knowledge and skills will come from various members of the health care team—the physician, the nurse, the pharmacist, the dietitian, the physical therapist, the social worker, and other health care professionals. Teaching may be done using an individual or group strategy or a combination of both, and will be based on the identified needs of the patient and the family. Hospital routines and treatment schedules may need to be modified to accommodate family participation in patient education.

ETHICAL CONSIDERATIONS IN PATIENT EDUCATION

The concepts of patient autonomy and paternalism may come into conflict in the patient education process. Autonomy can be defined as the right of self-determination or self-governance. The nurse supports the patient's autonomy by respecting the patient's individuality and by acknowledging that the patient is defined by his or her own values. Paternalism occurs when the health care professional, in the best interests of the patient, makes all the decisions to do good for that patient, even though the patient would ordinarily make those decisions (Fromer, 1981). Nurses as teachers practice paternalistic behavior to some degree. In the process of patient education, the nurse may force or manipulate the patient and family to acquire certain knowledge and skills. Attempts may be made, through patient education, to change attitudes and practices that the nurse views as undesirable. Although the goals of such changes may be to prevent exacerbation of illness and promote restoration of health, they are in conflict with the patient's autonomy. The patient's individuality must be respected even when he or she refuses to change behaviors that result in illness. An example of this situation is the patient who continues to abuse alcohol despite numerous ICU admissions for bleeding esophageal varices.

Leff (1986) suggests that the patient's sense of self-worth is undermined when the nurse ignores the patient's values or replaces them with his or her own. There are two reasons why the principle of autonomy is ignored in patient education. First, nurses are convinced that they are the best authorities for determining what the patient needs to learn. Second, nurses feel a sense of professional responsibility for teaching the patient. This sense of responsibility arises from the nurse's professional education, legal accountability, and the ethical duty to promote the well-being of patients.

Respect for the patient's autonomy requires the nurse to begin the teaching process by assessing the patient's needs from the patient's perspective. The nurse's relationship with the patient includes respect for his or her individuality and self-determination as well as a willingness to help the patient adapt health practices to his or her own life style (Connelly, 1984). This is an important aspect of patient teaching, especially if the patient's health beliefs and practices conflict with the nurse's own values.

SUMMARY

Patient education is considered an integral part of high-quality patient care. The teaching-learning process consists of assessment of patient needs, assessment of learning needs, formulation of learning ob-

jectives, selection and implementation of teaching methods, and ongoing evaluation of teaching effectiveness. Important nursing considerations in patient teaching include incorporating the family into the teaching plan and maintaining respect for the individuality and autonomy of the patient.

References

American Hospital Association. (1974). *The role of hospitals and other health care institutions in personal and community health education.* Chicago: author.

American Nurses Association. (1973). *Standards of nursing practice.* Kansas City: author.

Becker, M. H. (Ed.) (1974). *The health belief model and personal health behavior.* Thorofare, NJ: Charles B. Slack.

Bille, D. (1981). *Practical approaches to patient teaching.* Boston: Little, Brown.

Chatham, M., and Knapp, B. (1982). *Patient education handbook.* Bowie, MD: Prentice-Hall.

Connecticut General Statute Annals. (1978). 20–78a, Supplement.

Connelly, C. (1984). Economic and ethical issues in patient compliance. *Nursing Economics,* 1, 342–347.

Crate, M. A. (1965). Nursing functions in adaptation to chronic illness. *American Journal of Nursing,* 65, 72.

Devon, H. A., and Powers, M. J. (1984). Health beliefs, adjustment to illness and control of hypertension. *Research in Nursing and Health,* 7 (1), 10–16.

Falvo, D. (1985). *Effective patient education.* Rockville, MD: Aspen Systems.

Fromer, M. (1981). Paternalism in health care. *Nursing Outlook,* 29: 284–290.

Knowles, M. S. (1984). *Andragogy in action.* San Francisco: Jossey-Bass.

Leff, E. (1986). Ethics and patient teaching. *Maternal Child Nursing,* 11, 375–378.

Maslow, A. (1970). *Motivation and personality.* New York: Harper & Row.

New Jersey Statute Annals. (1978). 45, 11–23.

Rosenstock, J. M. (1975). Patients' compliance with health regimens. *Journal of the American Medical Association,* 234, 402–403.

Storlie, R. (1973). Some latent meanings of teaching of patients. *Heart & Lung,* 2, 506.

69

Optimizing Patient Recovery (Inpatient Cardiac Rehabilitation)

Patricia McCall Comoss

High-tech: the one word picture of a 1990 critical care unit. High-touch: a modern descriptor of the long-standing tradition of nursing. The preceding terms, popularized by Naisbitt in 1982, in the now classic *Megatrends,* dramatize the differences between science and art in health care. The warning of *Megatrends* is that the two must coexist. The more technology that surrounds us, the greater the need for human touch (Naisbitt, 1982).

In critical care settings, nurses strive to balance complex technology with personalized care (Sinclair, 1988). A holistic philosophy is the driving force behind such nursing efforts (Dossey and Guzzetta, 1984). It is the successful blend of art and science in the practice of nursing that ensures the optimal recovery of critically ill patients.

Opportunities for providing high-touch nursing in cardiac care settings have grown with the advent of structured programs of cardiac rehabilitation. Cardiac rehabilitation is the process of actively assisting the known cardiac patient to achieve and maintain optimal health (Comoss et al., 1979). The process begins with the acute event and ideally continues through life-long maintenance of wellness. The program sequence is divided into three major parts: inpatient, outpatient, maintenance.

Inpatient cardiac rehabilitation takes place in the critical care unit (CCU) and the intermediate coronary care unit (ICCU) or on the general medical floor. The purpose of cardiac rehabilitative nursing care while the patient is in the hospital is twofold: to minimize actual or potential problems from the acute event and to promote optimal recovery. Optimal recovery is the first step toward the ultimate rehabilitation goal of optimal health. Therefore, inpatient cardiac rehabilitation is the vital beginning in a long-term

process that applies equally to both medical and surgical cardiac patients.

Although a number of health care professionals may participate in caring for recovering cardiac patients, the most common providers of cardiac rehabilitative care in community hospitals are critical care nurses. In keeping with their holistic philosophy, critical care nurses integrate elements of cardiac rehabilitation with daily patient care. Holistic nursing goals that address physical, psychosocial, and health educational needs of patients are listed in Table 69–1, which provides an overview of the program structure.

The purposes of this chapter are to review the basic elements of an inpatient cardiac rehabilitation program, to discuss how programs can be designed for the shorter stays characteristic of the 1990s, and to emphasize the role of critical care nurses in CCU/ICCU settings in providing cardiac rehabilitative care. Earlier chapters of this text have addressed the psychosocial needs of patients in critical care units. Therefore, only the physical and educational elements of an inpatient cardiac rehabilitation program will be discussed here. Although this chapter discusses the cardiac patient, the underlying philosophy and structure of the program can be applied to a variety of patient populations requiring rehabilitation.

NURSING ROLES IN THE RECOVERY PROCESS

Historical Overview

In the 1950s Levine and Lown promoted armchair treatment of recovering cardiac patients (Levine and

---

TABLE 69–1. Program Structure:
Inpatient Cardiac Rehabilitation

Purpose:
1. To minimize actual/potential physical or psychological complications from an acute cardiac event and its treatments, AND
2. To optimize recovery through facilitation of self-care and activities of daily living
THEREBY providing a head start toward long-term rehabilitation and behavior change to a heart-healthy life style

Structure
Event/Intervention
Critical Care Unit
    Rehabilitation introduced (time permitting)
    Stay = 1 to 2 days (in uncomplicated cases)
    Rehabilitation begins as soon as patient is stable
    Use routine CCU activities (see also Table 69–5)

Stable/Transfer
Intermediate Care/Medical Floor
    Rehabilitation emphasized (shared nursing responsibility)
    Stay = 5 to 6 days for most patients with myocardial infarction or coronary artery bypass graft (patients who have had percutaneous transluminal coronary angioplasty stay 2 to 3 days after the procedure)
    Activity increases progressively daily according to guidelines
    Use progressive activity protocol (see Table 69–5)

Discharge/Outpatient Cardiac Rehabilitation Follow-up

Nursing Goals
Physical
To minimize deconditioning and prevent complications from bedrest, and to promote self-care and activities of daily living

Psychosocial
To minimize the anxiety of sudden illness and the stress of a strange environment and to provide support to both patient and significant others

Educational
To explain the event, its treatment and implications and to offer information to address the patient's/family's priority questions and concerns

---

Lown, 1952). In the 1960s Wenger and colleagues documented the safety of early ambulation (Wenger, 1973). But with the exception of a few medical centers involved in research, organized programs for inpatient cardiac rehabilitation did not emerge in community hospitals until the early 1970s (Wilson, 1988). With growing acceptance and the increasing need to refer to cardiac-related rehabilitation services, the term "cardiac rehab" became common. As an increasing number of hospitals introduced the new service around mid-decade, a specialty nursing role evolved to provide or coordinate cardiac rehabilitation care. And, with the wider acceptance and frequent reference to rehabilitation services, the name shortened, and "rehab" became the accepted term. The cardiac rehabilitation nurse specialist saw patients on referral to advance their activities or to provide cardiac education. Rehabilitation services were slowly advanced over a 2-week hospital stay.

The advantages of employing one nurse (more in larger facilities with greater patient volume) in such a specialty role included the development and utilization of that nurse's expert knowledge and the assurance that all patients in the program would receive the same quality care. These strengths contributed to the acceptance and growth of the new rehabilitation programs. Among the disadvantages of the single (or several) specialist approach were lack of availability on late shifts and weekends and, from an administrative perspective, the cost of an "extra" nurse. Efforts to decrease the costs of health care near the end of the decade resulted in some hospitals eliminating nurse specialty positions, including those covering inpatient cardiac rehabilitation.

In the early 1980s, an emphasis on primary nursing coupled with efforts at cost containment resulted in staff nurses assuming responsibility for providing inpatient cardiac rehabilitation services. The disadvantages of this primary or bedside approach to rehabilitation were immediately obvious. Nurses in CCU and intermediate care areas had little time for and less expertise in providing rehabilitation care. However, when time and knowledge deficits were addressed, the advantages of the primary care approach became clear. Because of a more continuous therapeutic relationship with patients, bedside nurses were able to capitalize on rehabilitation opportunities—they were able to teach at the time questions were asked and to schedule activities at times that best fit the patient's schedule. Patients appreciated the timeliness of services. Nurses reported greater job satisfaction giving holistic care. Rehabilitation services progressed over a 10-day hospital stay.

Passage of the prospective payment law in 1983 and the shorter hospital stays that followed raised questions about how to modify inpatient cardiac rehabilitation programs appropriately. In the late 1980s, the problem of shorter stays was compounded by the worst nursing shortage in history. The combined impact of too little time and too few nurses rendered some existing inpatient cardiac rehabilitation programs inoperative and aborted the start of those still in the planning stages.

Current Recommendations

At the present time, many programs are in a state of transition; some are trying to salvage the best parts of the old system and others are planning to start over with a new design for the 1990s. One approach that builds on the strengths of the past while recognizing the constraints of the present is the plan suggested in this chapter for sharing responsibility for cardiac rehabilitation care between critical care nurses in CCU and ICCU and cardiac rehabilitation nurses from outpatient programs. Shared responsibility recognizes the time limitations of bedside caregivers while tapping the expertise of outpatient rehabilitation specialists. This collaborative effort of nurses from different departments has the common goal of promoting optimal recovery of cardiac patients.

Subsequent sections of this chapter detail how such a plan can be designed and implemented to address the nursing diagnoses of knowledge deficit and potential activity intolerance that are commonly seen in cardiac inpatients. Table 69–2 provides a sample of the distribution of nursing responsibilities that might occur using the suggested shared approach.

NURSING STRATEGIES FOR OPTIMIZING CARDIAC REHABILITATION IN CRITICAL CARE UNITS

Minimizing complications and optimizing recovery are the dual goals of an inpatient cardiac rehabilitation program. The overall process of rehabilitating a cardiac patient begins as soon as the diagnosis of coronary artery disease is made, and the specific components of the program are implemented as soon as the patient's condition stabilizes after the acute event. Although emergency room and mobile intensive care unit (ICU) staffs often provide patient care that contributes to rehabilitation goals, critical care nurses are usually the first providers of planned rehabilitation care. Thus, the critical care unit is recognized as the site of origin of cardiac rehabilitation efforts.

The structure of cardiac rehabilitation in the critical care unit is directly related to the patient's length of stay. In the past, when patients remained in the unit for 2 to 3 days after being stabilized, activity and teaching components of the program were highly structured, and most nurses followed a strict schedule of planned care on each CCU day.

TABLE 69–2. A Model of Shared Nursing Responsibilities for Inpatient Cardiac Rehabilitation

Critical Care Nurses	Cardiac Rehabilitation Nurses
Exercise	
Supervise progressive activities of daily living per activity protocol (e.g., showering, hall ambulation)	Perform specific exercise routines per activity protocol (e.g., upper body exercises, stair climbing)
Education	
Teach basic cardiac lessons per patient-selected priorities (e.g., what is a heart attack? why did it happen to me?)	Teach predischarge lessons per research results (e.g., emergency planning, activity guidelines)
Follow-up	
Review case with cardiac rehabilitation nurse	Schedule patient for outpatient cardiac rehabilitation follow-up

As CCU stays have become shorter, previously used rehabilitation protocols have become obsolete. Currently, most cardiac patients, both medical and surgical, are being transferred from the critical care unit as soon as they are stable. As a result, the time available for critical care nurses to provide structured cardiac rehabilitation care has been reduced to a minimum. However, although less time in the unit changes the structure of the CCU phase of rehabilitation, it does not alter the need for involvement of CCU nurses. More than ever, the nursing care a patient receives in the critical care unit is the vital first step toward optimal recovery.

Nursing Diagnosis: Potential Activity Intolerance Due to Bedrest

Recognizing the Problem. Bedrest, accepted for many years as the treatment of choice for recovering cardiac patients, is now recognized as the cause of more problems than the solution (Caplin, 1986; Rubin, 1988; Winslow, 1985). The inactivity typical of bedrest results in a general decline in oxygen transport and cardiovascular function known as deconditioning (Rowell, 1986). Specifically, complications range from annoyances like joint stiffness to life-threatening events like pulmonary emboli (Caplin, 1986). Muscular disuse plays a role in the development of deconditioning. However, recent research indicates that the major factor contributing to the negative effects of bedrest is the shift of body fluids caused by the gravitational changes that occur when a person lies down (Convertino, 1983; Rowell, 1986; Winslow, 1985).

Deconditioning begins within a few hours of confinement to bed and progresses at a rapid rate during the early days of immobility (Rowell, 1986). The longer the duration of bedrest, the more severe the deconditioning and the greater the likelihood of major cardiovascular complications. In their classic study, Saltin and colleagues showed a 25% decrement in maximal oxygen uptake in healthy young men after 3 weeks of bedrest (Saltin et al., 1968).

The medical and nursing care needed to stabilize a patient who has had an acute coronary event necessarily involves confinement to bed. Recognizing the risks to which a patient in a non-weight-bearing supine position is subjected, the critical care nurse should diagnose potential activity intolerance in all acute cardiac patients and plan CCU interventions to minimize deconditioning and prevent complications arising from bedrest. If nurses do not recognize the serious threat presented by inactivity and if patients are allowed to remain in bed longer than is medically necessary, the result will be orthostatic intolerance. Assumption of the upright position and attempts to perform ordinary movements will result in increased heart rate, decreased blood pressure, and reduced cardiac output. Such orthostatic stress may be enough to precipitate angina or myocardial infarction in patients with an already restricted coronary blood flow (Convertino, 1983).

Designing the Activity Plan. The nursing answer to the problem of bedrest is the obvious one: Get the patient up and moving as soon as the acute condition is stabilized. Techniques for mobilizing cardiac patients in critical care units have evolved from in-bed passive range of motion exercises in the early 1970s (Lavin, 1973) to standing upper body warm-up exercises in the late 1980s (Marshall and Hawrysio, 1988).

From their inception, cardiac rehabilitation activity plans have been based on two basic principles of exercise physiology: oxygen demand and dynamic exercise. These two concepts remain the foundation of today's aggressive activity protocols.

An awareness of oxygen demand at rest is the basis of understanding the activity-oxygen relationships used to construct progressive activity plans for inpatient cardiac rehabilitation. The body needs to take in, transport, and use 3.5 mL of oxygen/kg body weight per minute to accomplish the task of being awake, alert, and sitting upright (American College of Sports Medicine, 1986). Any task more vigorous than this relative resting state requires more oxygen than the baseline level. For example, casual walking in hospital hallways demands approximately 7 mL of oxygen/kg per minute or twice the resting metabolic requirement, whereas outdoor jogging needs about 35 mL/kg per minute, 10 times more than the resting rate. These multiples of resting oxygen demand are referred to as metabolic equivalents or METs (American College of Sports Medicine, 1986). Using the equation of 1 MET = 3.5 mL oxygen/kg body weight per minute, activities can be described by either their oxygen demand or their MET conversion. Exercise scientists working in human performance laboratories have measured and documented the oxygen demands of numerous activities (American College of Sports Medicine, 1986; American Heart Association, Committee on Exercise, 1975; Shephard, 1987). Availability of such data enables clinicians to select the appropriate levels of activity for recovering cardiac patients.

Dynamic or isotonic exercise involves repetitive movements of the muscles and joints in contrast to the static muscular contractions called isometric exercise (Dehn, 1980). Walking, cycling, swimming, and rhythmic calisthenics such as jumping jacks are examples of isotonic exercises. Exercises that involve pushing, pulling, lifting, or carrying, including calisthenics such as push-ups, are predominantly isometric. Dynamic exercise is the preferred approach to activities for cardiac patients because it stimulates oxygen transport and elicits a heart rate response that is proportional to the intensity of effort expended (or MET level). In contrast, the tension state characteristic of isometric exercise has a greater impact on blood pressure and may evoke a sudden increase that could result in chest pain, dysrhythmia, or other

cardiac ischemic responses (Dehn, 1980; Wenger, 1981, 1984).

The design of an activity plan for use in critical care units, then, needs to incorporate upright posture, dynamic movement, and known levels of oxygen demand. Specific activities selected for use with the plan should allow the patient to progress from 1 to 2 METs before transfer from the critical care unit (Wenger, 1981). In an innovative approach to activity plans for today's shorter CCU stays, many critical care units are adopting "routine CCU activities" for use as soon as the cardiac patient is stable.

This new approach includes the use of patient care services that emphasize self-care and activities of daily living while meeting the physiologic guidelines recommended for early cardiac rehabilitation. Usually included in these routine activities are out-of-bed, upright activities such as use of a bedside commode, meals taken in a chair, partial bath at bedside, and self-grooming. Simple in design compared to earlier editions of activity plans, this streamlined activity approach is practical for use by critical care nurses and is effective in accomplishing the goal of minimizing deconditioning. Table 69–3 shows a sample of the patient care activities routinely performed in the CCU along with corresponding MET levels and heart rate responses. With the exception of the shower, the activities shown are close enough to the planned 1 to 2 MET range to be allowed during this early stage of recovery.

Implementing the Activity Plan. Planned activity for recovering cardiac patients is considered therapy and thus requires a physician's order to be implemented. Given a medical order, critical care nurses can initiate routine CCU activities as soon as a patient is clinically stable. Nurses and physicians involved with planning the inpatient cardiac rehabilitation program need to collaborate on developing a working definition of "stable" that is clear to all parties caring for the patient and is easy to assess.

In the context of cardiac rehabilitation, a stable condition has been defined as being free of pain and

TABLE 69–3. Metabolic Demands of Patient Care Activities

Activity	Method	METs	Heart Rate
Toileting	Bedpan	1.4	Average: 10 beats above resting HR
	Commode	1.5	
	Urinal (in bed)	1.3	
	Urinal (stand)	1.4	
Bedmaking	Occupied	1.2	Average: 5 beats above resting HR
	Unoccupied	1.3	
Bathing	Bed bath	2.5	Little or no change
	Tub bath	2.5	
	Shower	3.7	Significant increase

Data from Johnston et al., 1981; Lane and Winslow, 1987; Winslow et al., 1984.

having cardiac complications under control (Wenger, 1984). Patients with major dysrhythmias, heart failure, and cardiogenic shock are obviously not stable and therefore would not be considered for participation in rehabilitation-related activities until the crisis is resolved.

Because cardiovascular assessment is a routine part of critical care nursing, CCU nurses are in a position to know when a patient becomes stable and when activities should commence. Some units have found it helpful to use an assessment checklist to help ensure consistent interpretation of the term "stable cardiac condition" preceding implementation of activities. Checkpoints include:

Vital signs within normal limits

No new or recurrent chest pain during last 8 hours

No new or major dysrhythmias or other electrocardiographic (ECG) changes

No signs of congestive heart failure, including dyspnea, edema, crackles, or gallops

Complications that destabilize the patient's condition and produce any of the above signs or symptoms are contraindications to beginning or proceeding with an activity program. When properly implemented, the critical care component of progressive activity accomplishes its purpose of minimizing deconditioning and thus provides the patient with a head start toward achieving optimal recovery from an acute cardiac event.

Nursing Diagnosis: Knowledge Deficit Due to Recent Cardiac Event

Patient education is an integral part of modern nursing practice. Legally, most state nurse practice acts mandate health teaching as an obligation of licensure as a professional nurse. Professionally, standards of nursing practice express peer expectations of teaching (American Nurses' Association, 1981). Philosophically, most nurses embrace teaching and learning opportunities as a means of involving patients in their own care and promoting optimal recovery. A survey by Bille (1984) reported that cardiovascular nurses share common beliefs about patient education, including the belief that education is synonymous with nursing care and that the patient has the right to know what is being done. Patient education is a high-touch element of nursing practice within the high-tech environment of critical care.

Assuming the Teaching Role. Although critical care nurses want to teach, they often feel ill prepared to be health educators. Specialty training provides critical care nurses with a strong background in *what* to teach cardiac patients, but they are less certain of *how* to do the teaching. Structured inservice programs

designed to prepare CCU and ICCU nurses for cardiac rehabilitation teaching roles have been shown to improve both teaching performance and related learner outcomes (Murdaugh, 1980).

Mistakenly, teaching and learning are often thought of as cause and effect. In fact, they are separate and distinct events that do not always occur in tandem. The teaching and learning process is an interpersonal interaction, a communication designed to stimulate change (Redman, 1980). In the cardiac rehabilitation setting, the patient-learner needs guidelines and information that he can use to understand and handle changing health circumstances. The nurse-teacher has such information to give. Exchanging that information efficiently and effectively is the challenge.

The best known framework for use with adult education efforts such as cardiac teaching is the andragogy theory of Malcolm Knowles (Knowles, 1973). Andragogy, derived from the Greek word *andros*, pertaining to man or adult, is based on four major assumptions about how adults learn. A working knowledge of these principles is fundamental for patient teaching (Murdaugh, 1988). Table 69–4 summarizes the principles of adult learning and provides examples of how they can be applied to cardiac teaching. Effective teaching builds on the principles governing adult education. Ineffective teaching usually results from failure to follow the principles or failure to recognize obstacles to learning.

Assessing Readiness to Learn. The nursing literature has identified a number of barriers to or reasons why patients don't learn as well as nurses might expect (Murdaugh, 1982a; Ward, 1986). Two problems are most evident in the critical care setting. First, lack of nursing time is an obvious problem. Shortened CCU stays coupled with the high-tech responsibilities of today's critical care nurses leave little time for nurses to sit and teach as was done in the past. To find time for their teaching role, CCU nurses must learn to integrate teaching into all aspects of patient contact and nursing care (Murdaugh, 1982b). To capitalize on teaching opportunities critical care nurses must be prepared to teach at any time.

The second and biggest obstacle to learning in the CCU is lack of patient readiness. Readiness to learn can be defined as both psychological willingness and physical ability to learn (Narrow, 1979). All nurses involved with teaching encounters must determine whether the patient is ready to learn when the nurse is ready to teach. Many nurses feel compelled to teach because a clock or calendar says it's time. However, to proceed with teaching with no awareness of patient readiness is inappropriate and ineffective.

A checklist of the major elements of readiness can be used to ensure consistent assessment. For example:

TABLE 69-4. Adult Learning Theory in Cardiac Teaching

Principle	Application
Adults need to be self directing, to participate in decisions about their own health and treatment, to be actively involved in the learning process	Plan teaching activities to include as much patient participation and decision making as possible.
	Offer choices of *when* to teach, i.e., "Mr. Smith, I can be available at either 11 A.M. or 2:15 P.M. today to discuss the blood pressure information you requested earlier."
	Suggest alternative learning experiences, i.e., "Would you prefer to go to this afternoon's class on heart-healthy eating or have a private appointment with the dietitian when your wife can be here?"
Adults have cumulative past experience that acts as a resource by either helping or hindering learning	Assess what exposure, if any, the patient has had to the subject matter and what is his current understanding. Is the patient receptive or resistant to new learning? "Mr. Smith, last evening you mentioned that your brother died of a heart attack while having sex; that story has probably raised many questions in your mind. I suggest we set aside some time today to talk about guidelines for sexual activity to clear up any doubts you may have."
Adults have a problem-solving orientation and best learn material that can be used in the immediate time frame	Plan to teach cardiac topics according to the patient's priorities and concerns. As a cardiac teacher, remind yourself often that what you want to teach is not necessarily what the patient wants to learn right now (see text for further priorities).
Adults learn *only* if and when they are ready to learn	Assess patient's readiness to learn before each teaching encounter (see text for suggested criteria).
	If patient is not ready, do not proceed with the planned teaching; instead, document the assessment of lack of readiness to learn as the reason for deferral of the teaching.

1. Is the patient physically able to learn at this time?
   a. Is his or her physical condition stable?
      Obviously, a patient in pain or in the midst of complex treatment of complications is not ready to receive educational information.
   b. Does he or she have adequate energy with which to learn?
      Learning is a dynamic event requiring the output of effort and energy. It is common for cardiac patients to be tired and inattentive during their first few days in the hospital. In addition to the fatigue from the acute event, energy and alertness may be further depleted by sleep deprivation, visits from other health professionals, or by medications given for pain, sleep, and anxiety while the patient is in the CCU.
2. Is the patient psychologically willing to learn at this time?
   a. Is he or she in an appropriate emotional state?
      Anxiety, the most common emotional reaction to an acute cardiac event, is typically observed in CCU patients. Although mild to moderate anxiety can facilitate learning, severe anxiety results in reduced perception and inability to focus attention (Budan, 1986).
   b. Has he or she expressed awareness or acceptance of the new cardiac problem?
      Denial also occurs early in the acute experience. When a patient is still unable to face the situation, he or she is best helped by non-threatening reminders of reality. Teaching is not effective until the patient has acknowl-

edged the problem. Acknowledgment can usually be recognized by questions or actions that help the patient examine what has occurred and explore what needs to be done in the future (McHatton, 1985).

There is no guarantee that teaching will be effective even when all of the conditions of readiness are met. However, the more ready the patient is, the more likely it is that learning will result from the nurse-patient educational exchange. Therefore, before attempting to teach, CCU nurses must assure themselves that patients are prepared to learn. Use of a checklist can help document that a nursing assessment was made and that an appropriate decision was made to teach or not to teach at this time.

Communicating Essential Information. Although lack of readiness may defer structured teaching, it does not eliminate the need to give basic information to the patient. Efforts at communication that explain the patient's condition and treatment and maintain the patient's orientation are imperative throughout the CCU stay. Most CCU nurses are expert at describing procedures as they perform them and at offering reality-based reassurance. During this early stage of recovery, the nurse should concentrate on answering questions, reducing anxiety, and building rapport.

Critical care nurses should also keep in mind that although the patient may not yet be ready to learn, family members may be eager to receive education while the patient is in the CCU (Keeling, 1988). Small

TABLE 69–5. Sample Activity Progression Plan, Inpatient Cardiac Rehabilitation Program

Critical Care Unit—1–2 METs
Begin routine CCU activities as soon as patient is stable; emphasize out-of-bed upright activities of daily living including use of bedside commode, meals taken in chair, partial bath, and self-grooming

Intermediate Cardiac Care Unit—2–4 METs
Level 1
Continue ADL activities as in CCU; chair sitting as desired (and all meals taken in chair), walking in room, and bathroom privileges

Level 2
Upper body exercises—head and neck ROM and stretching exercises (perform standing), 5 minutes; walk in hall at comfortable pace for 5 minutes twice this day (first time with supervision); shower with seat or tub bath (nurse nearby)

Level 3
Upper body exercises—arm and shoulder ROM and stretching (perform standing) for 5 minutes; walk in hall at comfortable pace for 10 minutes twice this day (first time with supervision); bathing as above

Level 4
Upper body exercises—torso and waist ROM and stretching exercises (perform standing) for 5 minutes; walk in hall at comfortable pace for 15 minutes twice this day (first time with supervision); shower standing (with nurse nearby)

Level 5
Upper body exercises—any combination of above routines (perform standing) for 10 minutes; walk in hall by self 15 minutes, once today; walk DOWN one flight of stairs (10 to 14 steps) with supervision (return by elevator); shower as above

Level 6
Upper body exercises as above; walk in hall as above; walk UP one flight of stairs with supervision; shower as above

Near Discharge
Low-level treadmill test to obtain prognostic information and evaluate function

Abbreviations: ADL, activities of daily living; ROM, range of motion.

group classes are a practical way to offer education to family members and have the added advantage of providing a supportive environment for ventilating feelings (Fournet and Schaubhut, 1986) (also see Chap. 7).

The nursing care plan given in this chapter addresses the rehabilitation-related diagnoses of knowledge deficit and potential activity intolerance as discussed in this section of the text. As the patient progresses from acute to intermediate care, these diagnoses are adjusted slightly and the interventions are expanded throughout the remainder of the hospital stay.

NURSING STRATEGIES FOR OPTIMIZING CARDIAC REHABILITATION IN INTERMEDIATE CORONARY CARE UNITS

Nursing Diagnosis: Potential Activity Intolerance Due to Restricted Activity

Just as the patient who remains in bed too long in the critical care unit can develop complications, so too an inactive patient in the intermediate care unit can slide back into a deconditioned state. Like their CCU colleagues, intermediate care nurses need to recognize potential activity intolerance in cardiac patients and have a plan available for gradually

increasing activities safely and effectively to prevent complications and encourage an optimal recovery. The plan should build on what was started in the CCU.

Increasing the Plan of Activities. In the critical care unit activities are focused on getting the patient up, moving, and participating in basic self-care. Although self-care participation continues to expand in ICCU, the emphasis in rehabilitation shifts toward providing more specific exercises. Walking is used as the major leg activity. Calisthenics are introduced for the arms and upper body, and trial walks on stairs and treadmills are included shortly before discharge.

Table 69–5 provides a recommended protocol for increasing these new activities through six steps or levels. Six levels are appropriate for the current average length of stay for both medical and surgical cardiac patients with no complications. In the past, not only were programs longer but also many facilities used different protocols for medical and surgical patients (Fletcher, 1982; Meyer, 1980; Pollock, et al., 1986). Typically, patients who had had coronary artery bypass graft surgery were advanced more rapidly than those recovering from myocardial infarctions. The rationale for the different pace was that patients with infarction were disadvantaged by loss of some myocardial function whereas bypass patients had the advantage of revascularization (Alling-Berne, 1987; Marshall, 1985). However, as a result of recent aggressive medical interventions, differences between these two groups of patients are no longer as dramatic, and the same progressive activity protocol serves as the core program for both patient groups.

The sample activity protocol included here is designed to take the patient from the 2-MET level achieved with routine CCU activities to a 4-MET capability by the time of discharge. Since most daily activities fall in the range of 3 to 5 METs (American College of Sports Medicine, 1986), achievement of a 4-MET goal helps to ensure that most patients are physically capable of carrying out the usual activities of daily living when they get home. For rehabilitation professionals, a documented performance of 4 METs or more provides a bench mark that can be used to provide discharge advice. Table 69–6 lists the major activities used in the protocol along with supporting metabolic and response data.

Two specific activities included in the plan may challenge nursing resourcefulness. Level two introduces showering but specifies use of a seat in the shower. As shown in Table 69–3, taking an upright shower requires 3.7 METs. The higher demand compared to other types of bathing is due to a combination of upright posture, increased arm movement, and body flexion (Johnston et al., 1981). Because the MET level of showering is near the high end of the desirable range of activities for intermediate care and because standing still in a hot environment promotes venous pooling and adds to orthostatic problems, a seat is suggested to reduce cardiac demand and minimize risk during the first few showers (Riegel, 1988). Level four progresses to a standing shower to prepare the patient gradually for home activities. At this level, nurses need to caution patients to move their feet frequently and shift their weight while standing in the shower and to use warm instead of hot water. Until more hospitals have access to waterproof telemetry for use in showers, nurses should arrange to remain within earshot of cardiac patients while they shower.

Stair climbing is recommended prior to discharge to provide the patient and family with physical demonstration and psychological reassurance that this activity can be performed safely (Cornett and Watson, 1984). In the sample protocol, stairs are introduced during level five by having the patient walk down a flight. Walking downhill or downstairs places a lower metabolic demand on the body than walking upstairs because body weight is being carried toward gravity (American College of Sports Medicine, 1986). On level six, the patient progresses to walking upstairs.

In some hospitals the physical design of stairwells consists of two flights of stairs between floors, which interferes with the proposed sequence. If a patient is not able to walk one flight and then ride the elevator in the opposite direction, a modification of the plan is necessary. For example, on level five the patient could walk down half a flight of stairs, pause briefly, and then walk up. Performance on level six could consist of the reverse sequence. Wooden physical therapy steps or mechanical stair climbing machines are other options.

In addition to the details of performing activities, attention must be paid to appropriate amounts of rest between performances. Back-to-back activities, such as stair climbing and upper body stretches, should not be attempted in an effort to save time. Nurses must be cautious about combining activities to prevent excessive cardiovascular response. Alteri (1984) demonstrated that a minimum of 10 minutes of rest is needed between most activities of daily living for cardiovascular responses to stabilize (Alteri, 1984). One notable exception is showering. Patients studied required 30 minutes of rest after taking an upright shower for their responses to return to baseline.

Use of any activity plan requires an order from a physician. The physician may write a continuing order to "start cardiac activity program and progress daily per guidelines," or exact levels of the program may be specified with a new order needed on each

TABLE 69–6. Metabolic Demands of Progressive Activity

Activity	Method	METs	Heart Rate (average beats/minute)
Walking	Flat surface		
	2 mph	2–2.5	10 beats above resting level
	2.5 mph	2.5–2.9	
	3 mph	3–3.3	
Upper body exercise	While standing:		
	Arms	2.6–3.1	19
	Trunk (leg calisthenics)	2–2.2	11
		2.5–4.5	24
Stairs	One flight = 12 steps:		
	Down one flight	2.5	10 beats above resting level
	Up one flight	3.5	
	Up two flights	5.0	

Data from American College of Sports Medicine, 1986; Green et al., 1980; Silvidi et al., 1982.

day of the patient's stay. Most patients are likely to progress at a rate of one level per day, although in some cases it will be necessary to hold steady at a particular level, advance several levels, or start in the middle. Patients who have had balloon angioplasty are an example of patients needing the latter adjustment. Many patients who undergo this procedure were never acutely ill and have been hospitalized only for the treatment (Lanoue et al., 1986). They do not require the gradual buildup in performance of activities that is necessary with healing medical and surgical patients, and many are discharged within 48 hours after percutaneous transluminal coronary angioplasty (PTCA). Some of these patients can be placed directly on level five and six activities for the 2 postprocedure days in intermediate care.

Evaluating Patient Responses. The safety of early ambulation programs for cardiac patients has been extensively studied and documented (Wenger, 1984a, b). There is no doubt that programs that follow established principles and response guidelines are safe for both medical and surgical cardiac patients (Dion et al., 1982; Silvidi et al., 1982). The nursing role in helping to maintain patient safety during these activities involves two specific areas of patient assessment.

First, critical care and intermediate care nurses are responsible for performing daily assessments of their cardiac rehabilitation patients to determine that they have remained stable. In critical care units, stabilization of the patient's acute condition is required to start activities. In intermediate care, continued stability is a prerequisite for maintaining progression. The cardiac rehabilitation nurse needs to determine and document that no new problems indicating destabilization have developed. Should signs or symptoms indicating a complication appear, exercise is contraindicated, the progression of activities is put on hold until the patient is medically treated and again stabilized.

The second safety-related assessment occurs during exercise performance itself. The patient's performance must be supervised not only to ensure that it is executed properly, but also, and more important, to monitor and evaluate the patient's responses to the exercise. Heart rate, blood pressure, and cardiac rhythm are the three parameters routinely assessed before, during, and after each activity. Research findings have firmly established that the gradual, low-level exercises that comprise inpatient activity protocols do not cause excessive change in any of these three responses.

Heart rate should not increase by more than 10 to 20 beats above resting rate, and systolic blood pressure should not change by more than about 10 mL (Wenger, 1984a). Early upright activities may cause systolic blood pressure to fall slightly due to orthostatic changes. Such changes can usually be minimized by emphasizing standard orthostatic precautions, such as changing positions slowly and flexing the leg muscles while standing. As an added safety check, exercise blood pressures should be closely observed in patients who are taking vasodilators because these medicines increase the likelihood of orthostatic problems such as lightheadedness and fainting due to venous pooling (Kendrick et al., 1987).

Other than a slight increase in heart rate, the cardiac rhythm should remain stable. There should be no rhythm disturbance and no ST-segment change. Observation of the ST segments is a critical exercise assessment. The ST segment is the part of the ECG complex that reflects coronary perfusion during diastole. Exercise-induced ischemia produces ST-segment depression. Occurrence of ST-segment depression during low-level activity such as inpatient rehabilitation exercises is an ominous prognostic sign (Ellestad, 1986).

High-tech equipment is now available that can provide diagnostic quality telemetric tracings so that ST-segment analysis is possible from the ECG strips produced during exercise. The introduction of portable telemetric monitors has solved past problems of how to monitor the stair climbing sequence. Nurses can now lead a patient with one hand while holding a small telemetry monitor in the other, directly observing both subjective and objective responses to performance of the activity. Should any of the patient's responses exceed the expectations described or should new symptoms develop, the activity should be discontinued and medical consultation requested.

Sharing Responsibility. As each hospital designs a new activity plan or revises an old one, supporting policies must address the professional roles involved in carrying out the plan. As discussed in an earlier section of this chapter, the current trend in cardiac rehabilitation is for bedside nurses in CCU and ICCU to share responsibilities with outpatient cardiac rehabilitation nurses. The exact division of care is done in such a way that the time, talent, and other resources of each nursing group are used to the best advantage.

For example, with the activity plan proposed in Table 69–5, ICCU nurses could be responsible for supervising showers and hall ambulation. Because these activities are a part of routine patient care, little additional time is demanded of busy staff nurses. Outpatient cardiac rehabilitation nurses, with their knowledge and expertise in exercise parameters, could assume responsibility for teaching upper body exercises and supervising stair climbing. Working with patients prior to hospital discharge provides the cardiac rehabilitation nurse with the opportunity to evaluate the need for outpatient follow-up (Wagner and Williams, 1987).

Nursing Diagnosis: Knowledge Deficit Due to Coronary Artery Disease

Like their colleagues in critical care units, nurses in intermediate cardiac care units must assume the role of cardiac teachers. To be successful in their teaching efforts, they must have a general understanding of the principles of adult education and must be specifically skilled at assessing readiness to learn as discussed in the CCU section of this chapter (see also Chap. 68).

Unlike CCU nurses, nurses in intermediate care areas usually find that their patients are ready to learn. Once transfer anxiety has passed, a check of the readiness criteria suggested previously often produces "yes" answers. Most patients are both physically and psychologically ready to learn during their ICCU stay. The challenge for the nurse-teacher at this stage of patient recovery is deciding what to teach first.

Setting Learning Priorities. The average length of hospital stay for a cardiac patient in 1990 is 7 days with about 5 of those days spent in the post-acute unit. Assuming that about 30 minutes of teaching per patient per day is possible, then 150 minutes, or a total of 2.5 hours is available for teaching during each patient's ICCU stay. Obviously, everything the nurse wants a patient to know about heart disease cannot be taught in such a limited amount of time. Nurse-teachers must plan their few teaching hours to address the individual concerns of patient-learners. Priority must be given to what each patient wants to learn, not necessarily to what a nurse wants to teach.

Determining learning priorities involves the patient actively. The patient is asked to identify major questions or concerns and to rank them in order of priority. For many patients, a written tool listing the lesson choices helps them put their concerns into words (Miller, 1985). This participative assessment procedure makes use of the adult education principle that learners are self-directing and are focused on problem solving. Results provide the teacher with a plan for what to teach first, second, and so on. Table 69–7 shows a sample of a patient priority checklist.

The priority approach to cardiac teaching is a logical one given the time constraints imposed by shorter hospital stays. However, it has found slow acceptance by nurses because, in the author's experience, some nurses still believe that there is a specific beginning and definite sequence through which teaching must proceed. Two factors seem to contribute to the reluctance of nurses to vary their order of teaching. First, inexperienced nurse educators are most comfortable teaching their lessons in a predictable order. Often the material is organized to be taught to patients in the same way it was learned by nurses. For example, a new nurse-teacher may feel that it is essential for the first lesson with a cardiac patient to cover cardiac anatomy and physiology. In fact, a complete lesson on heart structure and function is seldom necessary when teaching cardiac patients. Nurse-teachers need to increase their awareness that, in general, it is more important for patients to understand their symptoms, problems, and ther-

apies than to have a detailed pathophysiologic understanding of their disease process (Sivarajan and Newton, 1984).

The second reason why use of a variable sequence of teaching has been slow to catch on is simple habit. Cardiac teaching programs established 10 or more years ago prescribed teaching sequences. Protocols listing what topic to teach on each day of the hospital stay were common (Wenger, 1978; Wilson, 1988). Shorter hospital stays have made such rigid instructional formats obsolete. In the 1990s, cardiac educational programs are designed to be flexible in meeting the highest priority learning needs of each patient (Hellerstein et al., 1986).

A growing volume of nursing research supports the priority lesson approach. Gerard and Peterson (1984) clearly showed that much of what nurses wanted to teach was *not* what patients wanted to learn. In that study, fortunately, patients and nurses independently identified chest pain management as the most important lesson. Unfortunately, there was little agreement about priorities among the remaining topics! CCU nurses thought it very important to teach material relating to anatomy and physiology, medications, and congestive heart failure, whereas patients wanted to learn how to recognize the signs and symptoms of heart disease and how to control risk factors to prevent recurrence. Other studies, including one that recently replicated the research of Gerard and Peterson, have confirmed that what patients want to learn is different from what nurses would choose to teach (Karlik and Yarcheski, 1987). Therefore, it is recommended that lessons be taught in the order preferred by the patient-learner rather than that designed by the nurse-teacher.

Investigations of the learning needs and priorities of patients recovering from coronary artery bypass surgery also show a divergence between the information patients want and the material nurses present. Grady and colleagues (1988) documented that patients who have undergone cardiac bypass wanted to know more about the side effects of their medications, specific diet guidelines, and available posthospital follow-up. Perhaps surprising to many nurse-teachers, Grady's group felt that they had received excessive information about sexual activity and emotional changes after surgery.

Newton and Killien (1988) studied the learning needs of both bypass patients and their spouses. According to their results, more than 50% of cardiac surgical patients went home with unanswered questions. Patients and wives had concerns about identifying symptoms, handling complications, and resuming activity. In contrast to the findings reported by Grady and colleagues, patients in this study group wanted more information on sexual activity and emotional changes.

The learning needs of spouses of cardiac patients have also been studied separately. Sikorski (1985) reported that the most troubling questions among wives of convalescing coronary artery bypass surgery

TABLE 69–7. Sample Assessment Form: Patient Learning Priorities

Dear Patient:

Like most people with heart problems, you probably have many questions. During the next few days we want to address those concerns that are uppermost in your mind. So, to help plan the best sequence for our discussions, please place the numbers 1 through 3 in front of the topics for which you would like more information:

_____CCU machines and treatments
_____Heart structure and function
_____Coronary arteries normal/abnormal
_____Activity progression during hospital stay
_____What to do for chest pain
_____*_____Emergency planning for home
_____Heart attack and healing
_____Your risk factors
_____How to take your pulse
_____High blood pressure
_____High blood cholesterol
_____Your medicines
_____Fitness and health
_____Eating for a healthy heart
_____Sexual activity and your heart
_____Emotional changes after heart problems
_____Development of heart disease
_____Stress and your heart
_____Smoking and your heart
_____Alcohol and your heart
_____*_____Guidelines for activities at home
_____Activity/exercise precautions
_____Heart catheter procedure
_____Bypass graft surgery
_____Heart balloon procedure
_____Heart failure
_____Heart rhythms
_____Cardiac rehabilitation program
_____Treadmill exercise test
_____Effects of heart problems on families
_____Return to work questions

Other questions you would like to have answered:

_____
_____
_____

*These topics will be discussed by the cardiac rehabilitation nurse a day or two before you go home.

patients concerned the resumption of physical activity and the possibility of future problems.

As exemplified by these results, most studies that have looked at patient or spouse learning priorities have documented the need for early and definitive information about recognizing signs and symptoms and managing future cardiac crises. Based on this common need to know "what to do if," some programs have adjusted their teaching sequence to emphasize "survival skills" first among cardiac topics (Shank, 1987). Activity guidelines are a frequent second priority (Steele and Ruzicki, 1987). Thereafter, there is little agreement about what should be taught; in whatever amount of time remains for teaching, priority should be given to what the patient wants to learn.

Effective implementation of such an individualized approach to cardiac teaching requires comprehensive program planning and specific patient assessment.

As cardiac educators, critical care nurses must be fully prepared to address whatever cardiac topic a patient requests. A collection of "lesson plans," each outlining a common cardiac topic, is a helpful guide for refreshing a teacher's memory about the content to be included in the selected lesson. Additionally, structured lesson plans specify learner outcomes for evaluation and help to ensure that the material taught is consistent among all nurses on the unit. With a broad range of lessons to choose from, nurse-teachers can quickly match their educational presentations to the priorities identified by patient-learners.

Selecting Teaching Aids. Lesson plans, as suggested above, provide the core curriculum for cardiac teaching. Development of each lesson includes the selection of teaching aids, such as handouts or audio-visual materials, used to supplement the nurse-patient educational exchange. A countless array of educational materials for cardiac teaching is available, ranging from traditional handout brochures to innovative computer programs. It is easy for a nurse-teacher to become overwhelmed by the quantity of choices.

To avoid impulsive and sometimes inappropriate decisions about what should be given or shown to patients, a deliberate procedure is recommended to critique this educational material. First, each educational aid must be reviewed to determine that its content is correct, current, and compatible with what the patient is being told by his or her health care providers (Scalzi and Burke, 1982). Because printed material becomes outdated quickly, and treatment methods may vary in different parts of the country, a booklet printed 2 years ago or in another part of the country may be inappropriate. For example, it is increasingly routine for cardiac patients to be advised that they may return to full sexual activity when they are capable of performing 5 METs of activity on a treadmill. Many patients, having successfully completed a predischarge treadmill test, leave the hospital with no restrictions on sexual activity. If a booklet for cardiac patients states that most patients resume sexual activity at about 6 weeks after the acute event, it is obviously old information not compatible with local standards of practice and should not be used as a patient handout.

The second step in reviewing teaching aids is to evaluate the reading level of the material presented. The importance of reading level of patient materials has often been overlooked. In 1983, Boyd and Citro enlightened nurse-teachers by reporting that 90% of the cardiac educational materials in common use was beyond the eighth grade reading ability of the patients receiving it. That study impressed many cardiac educators with the need for careful analysis of reading level of all printed materials as well as scripts of content from other media. Formulas that can be used to determine reading level are available (Miller, 1985). Simplifying the reading level of patient educational material to the range of fifth through eighth grade is necessary if nurse-teachers expect the majority of cardiac patients to comprehend what is given to them. Although the technology used to assist educational efforts (e.g., closed-circuit television, videotapes, and interactive computers) is becoming more sophisticated and increasingly available, the need for simplicity of information remains paramount.

Sharing Educational Responsibilities. Critical care nurses working in CCU and ICCU want to be involved in teaching their cardiac patients (American Hospital Association, 1982). In support of that desire, nursing research has shown that patients prefer to be taught on a one-to-one basis (Boyd and Feldman, 1984) and that learning is most effective when patients are taught by their primary nurse (Knapp et al., 1985). But even when critical care nurses are properly prepared for the teaching role and provided with the necessary guidelines and tools, there still remains the problem of limited time. As suggested earlier, the solution of sharing responsibilities for cardiac teaching between bedside nurses in CCU and ICCU on the one hand and outpatient cardiac rehabilitation nurses on the other hand makes the best use of the time and expertise of each nursing group in a cooperative effort. Bedside nurses are in the best position to know whether and when a patient is ready to learn and could be responsible for daily education based on patient priorities. Cardiac rehabilitation nurses could assume the responsibility for specific components of predischarge teaching such as the high-priority lessons of chest pain management and home activity guidelines. Both of these lessons emphasize what the patient needs to do at home, and the content can be subsequently reinforced through the outpatient program.

Inpatient cardiac teaching should be viewed as a head start program that helps patients begin to learn how to live with their heart problem. Unlike programs in the past, when longer hospital stays made it possible to finish a structured cardiac teaching program, current nursing emphasis must be directed toward merely starting the educational process while the patient is still in the hospital. A nursing care plan is presented for addressing the cardiac patient's knowledge deficit and potential activity intolerance during the post-acute hospital stay. By making use of the interventions listed in this plan, critical care nurses working in acute and intermediate critical care units deliver cardiac rehabilitative care, thus optimizing patient recovery.

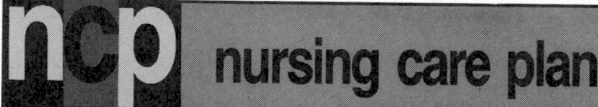

nursing care plan

OPTIMIZING CARDIAC REHABILITATION IN THE CRITICAL CARE UNIT

1. Knowledge deficit due to recent cardiac event

Outcome Criteria	Nursing Interventions

Upon transfer from CCU the patient will
1. Express less anxiety about cardiac event
2. Express satisfaction with support of nurse
3. Acknowledge that questions were answered appropriately when asked
4. Demonstrate increased knowledge:
  a. *General*—express awareness of event, purpose of treatments, and plan for recovery and rehabilitation
  b. *Specific*—perform objectives listed on lesson plan for each lesson taught (or family member)
	1. Assume teaching role, follow principles of adult education
	2. *Assess* readiness to learn, including physical ability and psychological willingness
	3. *Implement* teaching if patient is ready (see next section of nursing care plan for optimizing recovery in the ICCU)
	  a. Formal: keep teaching separate
	  b. Informal: teach during routine care
	4. *Document* teaching efforts
	5. Defer teaching if patient is not ready; *document* lack of readiness
	6. Provide frequent, supportive communication to
	  a. Answer questions
	  b. Explain status and treatments
	  c. Maintain orientation
	  d. Reduce anxiety
	7. *Teach* family on one-to-one basis if they are ready, or small groups if available
	8. *Evaluate* learning according to lesson objectives; *document* responses

2. Potential activity intolerance due to bedrest

Outcome Criteria	Nursing Interventions

Patient will
1. Exhibit no complications from bedrest
2. Perform basic self-care without excessive cardiovascular responses
	1. *Assess* stability of acute problem:
	  a. Patient should be pain free
	  b. Complications should be under control
	  c. Vital signs should be within normal limits
	2. Confirm physician's order for activities
	3. *Implement* routine CCU activities:
	  a. Upright position
	  b. Dynamic large muscle movements
	  c. Effort level at 1 to 2 METs
	  d. Emphasis on self-care in activities of daily living
	4. *Monitor and document* patient's responses to each new activity

OPTIMIZING CARDIAC REHABILITATION IN THE INTERMEDIATE CRITICAL CARE UNIT

1. Knowledge deficit due to coronary artery disease

Outcome Criteria	Nursing Interventions

Upon discharge the patient will demonstrate increased knowledge by
1. Performing objectives of specific lessons taught
2. Expressing a decision to take responsibility for healthy living
3. Discussing need for follow-up care, including visits to the physician and attending an outpatient cardiac rehabilitation program
	1. Assume a teaching role using principles of adult education
	2. Assess readiness to learn based on physical ability and psychological willingness
	3. Defer teaching if patient is not ready (see nursing care plan for optimizing recovery in CCU)
	4. Implement teaching if patient is ready:
	  a. Present lessons in order of patient-selected priorities
	  b. Use teaching by the primary nurse on a one-to-one basis for most daily sessions
	  c. Follow content outline on standardized lesson plans
	  d. Use critiqued printed handouts (or other communication media) at an appropriate reading level to supplement teaching
	  e. Involve the family when possible
	5. Document teaching efforts
	6. Refer special lessons to other professionals—e.g., heart-healthy guidelines may be taught by the dietitian
	7. Consult the cardiac rehabilitation nurse to teach priority discharge lessons, i.e., emergency planning and activity guidelines
	8. Evaluate learning according to lesson objectives and document patient responses

Nursing Care Plan continued on following page

2. Potential Activity Intolerance due to restricted activity	
Outcome Criteria	**Nursing Interventions**

The patient will
1. Exhibit no major signs of deconditioning or orthostatic intolerance
2. Perform activities of daily living (ADL) without excessive cardio-vascular responses
3. Begin to compare levels of activity performed in the hospital to usual daily activities at home
4. Describe precautions to minimize circulatory side effects
	1. Assess for continued cardiovascular stability
	2. Confirm daily physician orders or protocol progression
	3. Implement the activity protocol: progress 2 to 4 METs
	  a. Bedside nurse: expand ADL (e.g., walking in the hall, showering)
	  b. Rehabilitation nurse: teach upper body exercise, supervise stair climbing
	4. Monitor and document patient responses to each new activity:
	  a. Heart rate = 10 to 20 beats above resting level
	  b. Systolic blood pressure = 10 mm Hg change
	  c. Electrocardiogram = stable rhythm, no ST changes
	5. Enforce adequate rest between activities; at least 30 minutes rest after showering
	6. Teach general orthostatic precautions:
	  a. Avoid sudden changes of posture
	  b. Dangle legs and do ankle circles, plantar flexion and dorsiflexion before getting out of bed
	  c. Take a warm, *not hot*, shower; keep legs moving while showering

SUMMARY

As inpatient cardiac rehabilitation programs have grown during the past 20 years, the effectiveness of the two major program elements, progressive activity and cardiac education, have been extensively studied. Structured cardiac teaching programs have been shown to decrease anxiety, increase knowledge, promote a quicker return to one's usual activities (Hogan and Neill, 1982; Murdaugh, 1980; Raleigh and Odtohan, 1987), and result in shorter hospital stays (Hellerstein et al., 1986; Stanton et al., 1987). Early mobilization programs improve emotional status, promote early discharge, and result in an earlier and more complete return to work (Wenger, 1984b). Combining mobilization and teaching efforts into an organized program of inpatient cardiac rehabilitation creates a potent force for optimizing the recovery of cardiac patients. There is even some evidence to suggest that patients who participate in both education and exercise programs have a reduced mortality rate (Hellerstein et al., 1986).

Although the collective results of inpatient programs are impressive, a program's value is best measured in terms of its results with individual patients. Sample patient outcomes for activity progression and for cardiac education are shown in the nursing care plan at the end of the chapter. Results of activity progression can be evaluated both subjectively and objectively. Subjective feedback should be sought from the patient to evaluate his or her awareness of the purposes of the activity and the guidelines for it. Objectively, review of data from activity flowsheets should verify the patient's level of capability, and descriptions in nurses' notes should indicate whether any unusual responses or complications occurred. Additionally, when predischarge treadmill testing is ordered and performed by the physician, it provides a more formal method of evaluating functional capability and obtaining medical prognostic information before the patient goes home.

Educational outcomes are best evaluated by asking patients to perform the objectives of the specific cardiac lessons that were taught. Written tests are not as useful for evaluating patients' knowledge when the new priority approach is used as they were when all patients were taught the same content during longer hospital stays. However, if written feedback is desired, short quizzes could be developed for each cardiac lesson, and patients could be asked to complete the quizzes for the particular lessons they received. Because several of the projected educational outcomes are related to personal decisions and future plans, verbal feedback from the patient must be solicited.

Patients who leave the hospital physically capable of performing their usual daily activities and intellectually aware of their role and their responsibility for self-care have achieved a solid start in the long-term rehabilitation process. Enrollment in an outpatient program is the logical next step. Part of the discharge planning for cardiac patients should include collaboration with the patient's physician to arrange referral to an available outpatient program so that cardiac rehabilitation efforts can continue without interruption.

In response to the shorter hospital stays of recent years, most outpatient cardiac rehabilitation programs now offer an immediate post-discharge or low-level phase designed to receive patients within 1 to 2 weeks after hospital discharge. This low-level program component continues the rehabilitation care that was started in the hospital. The emphasis is on cardiac teaching based on changing priorities as patients adjust to being at home and attempt to make life-style changes. Activities are expanded to include a progressive walking program and more upper body calisthenics. Perhaps most important, early outpatient involvement provides support and encouragement at a time when many patients need it most. Sharing nursing responsibilities for inpatient cardiac rehabilitation as discussed throughout this chapter strengthens the link between the two programs and enhances the continuity of patient care.

Given the changing environment of cardiac care, successful inpatient cardiac rehabilitation programs of the future must be built on realistic expectations, offer flexible applications, and share rehabilitation responsibilities between cardiac rehabilitation nurses and the patient's primary caregiver in the hospital, the critical care nurse in CCU/ICCU. This chapter has attempted to present timely, practical strategies for designing and delivering services comprising inpatient cardiac rehabilitation. Cardiac rehabilitation involvement provides critical care nurses with an opportunity to add high-touch nursing to high-tech cardiac care to promote optimal recovery of cardiac patients.

References

Alling-Berne, L. (1987). The nurse's role: Early supervised exercise following coronary artery bypass surgery. *Focus on Critical Care,* 14(6), 11–16.

Alteri, C. A. (1984). The patient with myocardial infarction: Rest prescription for activities of daily living. *Heart & Lung,* 13(4), 355–360.

American College of Sports Medicine. (1986). Exercise prescription for cardiac patients. In S. Blair, L. Gibbons, P. Painter, et al. (eds.), *Guidelines for exercise testing and prescription* (pp. 157–172). Philadelphia: Lea & Febiger.

American Heart Association, Committe on Exercise. (1975). *Exercise testing and training of individuals with heart disease or at high risk for its development—Handbook for physicians.* Dallas, American Heart Association.

American Hospital Association. (1982). *Managing cardiac patient education.* Chicago: author.

American Nurses Association and American Heart Association. (1981). *Standards of cardiovascular nursing practice.* Kansas City: American Nurses Association.

Bille, D. A. (1984). Teaching the person with cardiovascular dysfunction. In C. E. Guzzetta and B. M. Dossey (Eds.), *Cardiovascular nursing—Bodymind tapestry* (pp. 863–877). St. Louis: Mosby.

Boyd, M. D., and Citro, K. (1983). Cardiac patient education literature—can patients read what we give them? *Journal of Cardiac Rehabilitation,* 3(7), 513–516.

Boyd, M. D., and Feldman, R. H. L. (1984). Health information seeking and reading and comprehension abilities of cardiac rehabilitation patients. *Journal of Cardiac Rehabilitation,* 4(8) 343–347.

Budan, L. J. (1986). Cardiac patient learning in the hospital setting. *Focus on Critical Care,* 10(5), 16–22.

Caplin, M. (1986). Early mobilization of uncomplicated myocardial infarction patients. *Focus on Critical Care,* 13(2), 36–40.

Commonwealth of Pennsylvania. (1985). *The professional nursing law.* Act No. 109, PL 409. December 20.

Comoss, P. M., Burke, E. A. S., and Swails, S. H. (1979). A philosophy and a model for nursing practice in cardiac rehabilitation. In P. M. Comoss, E. A. S. Burke, and S. H. Swails (Eds.), *Cardiac rehabilitation: A comprehensive nursing approach* (pp. 2–5). Philadelphia: J. B. Lippincott.

Convertino, V. A. (1983). Effect of orthostatic stress on exercise performance after bed rest: Relation to inhospital rehabilitation. *Journal of Cardiac Rehabilitation,* 3, 660–663.

Cornett, S. J., and Watson, J. E. (1984). Management of the patient's restorative rehabilitative needs in the convalescent phase of illness. In *Cardiac rehabilitation: An interdisciplinary team approach* (pp. 132–141). New York: Wiley.

Dehn, M. M. (1980). Rehabilitation of the cardiac patient: The effects of exercise. *American Journal of Nursing,* 80(3), 435–439.

Dion, W. F. Grevenow, P. Pollock, M. L., et al. (1982). Medical problems and physiologic responses during supervised inpatient cardiac rehabilitation: The patient after coronary bypass grafting. *Heart & Lung,* 11(3), 248–255.

Dossey, B. M., and Guzzetta, C. E. (1984). Cardiovascular nursing—bodymind tapestry. In C. E. Guzzetta and B. M. Dossey (Eds.), *Cardiovascular nursing—bodymind tapestry* (pp. 863–877). St. Louis: Mosby.

Ellestad, M. H. (1986). *Stress testing: Principles and Practice* (3rd ed., pp. 278–298). Philadelphia: F. A. Davis.

Fletcher, G. F. (1982). Exercise in secondary prevention and rehabilitation of subjects with coronary disease. In G. F. Fletcher (Ed.), *Exercise in the practice of medicine* (pp. 147–175). New York: Futura.

Fournet, K., and Schaubhut, R. M. (1986). What about spouses—SOS. *Focus on Critical Care,* 13(1), 14–18.

Gerard, P. S., and Peterson, L. M. (1984). Learning needs of cardiac patients. *Cardiovascular Nursing,* 20(2), 7–11.

Grady, K. L., Buckley, D. J., Cisar, N. S., et al. (1988). Patient perception of cardiovascular surgical patient education. *Heart & Lung,* 17(4), 349–355.

Greer, M., et al., (1980). Physiological responses to low intensity cardiac rehabilitation exercises. *Physical Therapy,* 60(9), 1146–1151.

Hellerstein, H. K., Bruce, R. A., Hackett, T. P., et al. (1986). State of the art in education of the cardiac patient in the United States. In N. K. Wenger (Ed.), *The education of the patient with cardiac disease in the twenty-first century* (pp. 338–363). New York: LeJacq.

Hogan, C. A., Neill, W. A. (1982). Effects of a teaching program on knowledge, physical activity, and socialization in patients disabled by stable angina pectoris. *Journal of Cardiac Rehabilitation* 2(5), 379–385.

Johnston, B. L., Watt, E. W., and Fletcher, G. F. (1981). Oxygen consumption and hemodynamic and electrocardiographic responses to bathing in recent post myocardial infarction patients. *Heart & Lung,* 10(4), 666–671.

Karlik, B. A., and Yarcheski, A. (1987). Learning needs of cardiac patients—a partial replication study. *Heart & Lung,* 16(5), 544–551.

Keeling, A. W., (1988). Health promotion in coronary care and step-down units: Focus on the family—linking research to practice. *Heart & Lung,* 17(1), 28–34.

Kendrick, Z. V., Cristal, N., and Lowenthal, D. T. (1987). Cardiovascular drugs and exercise interactions. *Cardiology Clinics,* 5(2), 227–244.

Knapp, D., et al. (1985). Education of cardiac surgery patients—a comparison of the effectiveness of nurse educators and primary nurses. *Journal of Cardiopulmonary Rehabilitation,* 5(9), 429–434.

Knowles, M. (1973). *The adult learner: A neglected species.* Houston: Gulf Publishing.

Lane, L. D., and Winslow, E. H. (1987). Oxygen consumption, cardiovascular response, and perceived exertion in healthy adults during rest, occupied bedmaking, and unoccupied bedmaking activity. *Cardiovascular Nursing,* 23(6), 31–36.

Lanoue, A. S., Snyder, B. A., and Galan, K. M. (1986). Percutaneous transluminal coronary angioplasty: Nonoperative treatment of coronary artery disease. *Journal of Cardiovascular Nursing,* 1(1), 30–44.

Lavin, M. A. (1973). Bed exercises for acute cardiac patients. *American Journal of Nursing,* 73(7), 1226–1227.

Levine, S. A., and Lown, B. (1952). Armchair treatment of acute coronary thrombosis. *Journal of the American Medical Association,* 1365–1369.

Marshall, J. A. R. (1985). Rehabilitation of the coronary bypass patient. *Cardiovascular Nursing,* 21(4), 19–23.

Marshall, J. A. R., and Hawrysio, A. (1988). Inpatient recovery following myocardial infarction and coronary artery bypass graft surgery. *Journal of Cardiovascular Nursing,* 2(3), 1–12.

McHatton, M. (1985). A theory for timely teaching. *American Journal of Nursing,* 85(7), 798–800.

Meyer, G. C. (1980). Exercises for the inpatient. In P. S. Fardy, J. L. Bennett, N. L. Reitz, et al. (Eds.), *Cardiac rehabilitation—Implications for the nurse and other health professionals* (pp. 110–120). St. Louis: Mosby.

Miller, A. (1985). When is the time ripe for teaching? *American Journal of Nursing,* 85(7), 801–804.

Murdaugh, C. L. (1980). Effects of nurses knowledge of teaching learning principles on knowledge of coronary care unit patients. *Heart & Lung,* 9(6), 1073–1078.

Murdaugh, C. L. (1982a). Barriers to patient education in the coronary care unit. *Cardiovascular Nursing,* 18(6) 31–36.

Murdaugh, C. L. (1982b). Using research in practice. *Focus on Critical Care*, 9, 11–14.

Murdaugh, C. L. (1988). The nurse's role in education of the cardiac patient. In L. S. Kern, *Cardiac critical care nursing*. Rockville, MD: Aspen.

Naisbitt, J. (1982). From forced technology to high tech/high touch. In *Megatrends* (pp. 39–53). New York: Warner Books.

Narrow, B. W. (1979). Assessment of readiness to learn. In *Patient teaching in nursing practice*. New York: Wiley.

Newton, K. M., and Killien, M. G. (1988). Patient and spouse learning needs during recovery from coronary artery bypass. *Progress in Cardiovascular Nursing*, 3 (April-June), 62–69.

Pollock, M. L., Pels, A. E., Foster, C., et al. (1986). Exercise prescription and rehabilitation of the cardiac patient. In M. L. Pollock, and D. H. Schmidt (Eds.), *Heart disease and rehabilitation* (pp. 477–499). New York: Wiley.

Raleigh, E. H., and Odtohan, B. C. (1987). The effect of a cardiac teaching program on patient rehabilitation. *Heart & Lung*, 16(3), 311–317.

Redman, B. K. (1980). Teaching—definition, theory, and interpersonal techniques. In *The process of patient teaching in nursing* (pp. 117–137). St. Louis: Mosby.

Riegel, B. (1988). Acute myocardial infarction: Nursing interventions to optimize oxygen supply and demand. In L. S. Kern (Ed.), *Cardiac critical care nursing* (pp. 59–77). Rockville, MD: Aspen.

Rowell, L. B. (1986). Cardiovascular adaptations to chronic physical activity and inactivity. In *Human circulation: Regulation during physical stress*, New York: Oxford University Press.

Rubin, M. (1988). The physiology of bedrest. *American Journal of Nursing*, 88(1), 50–57.

Saltin, B., Blomquist, G., Mitchell, J. H., et al. (1968). Response to exercise after bedrest and after training. *Circulation*, 38(Suppl. 7), 1–78.

Scalzi, C. C., and Burke, L. E. (1982). Education of the patient and family. In S. L. Underhill, S. L. Woods, E. S. Sivarajan, et al. (Eds.), *Cardiac nursing* (pp. 582–591). Philadelphia: J. B. Lippincott.

Shank, J. M. (1987). Inpatient education in cardiac rehabilitation—the role of the clinical nurse specialist. In R. C. Cantu (Ed.), *The exercising adult* (2nd ed., pp. 133–141). New York: Macmillan.

Shephard, R. J. (1987). *Exercise physiology* (pp. 136–137). Toronto: B.C. Decker.

Sikorski, J. M. (1985). Knowledge, concerns, and questions of wives of convalescent coronary artery bypass graft surgery patients. *Journal of Cardiac Rehabilitation*, 5(2), 74–85.

Silvidi, G. E., et al. (1982). Hemodynamic responses and medical problems associated with early exercise and ambulation in coronary artery bypass graft surgery patients. *Journal of Cardiac Rehabilitation*, 2(5), 355–362.

Sinclair, V. (1988). High technology in critical care: Implications for nursing's role and practice. *Focus on Critical Care*, 15(4), 36–41.

Sivarajan, E. S., and Newton, K. M. (1984). Exercise, education, and counseling for patients with coronary artery disease. *Clinics in Sports Medicine*, 349–369.

Stanton, B. A., Jenkins, C. D., Savageau, J. A., et al. (1987). Perceived adequacy of patient education and fears and adjustments after cardiac surgery. *Heart & Lung*, 16(3), 525–531.

Steele, J. M., and Ruzicki, D. (1987). An evaluation of the effectiveness of cardiac teaching during hospitalization. *Heart & Lung*, 16(3), 306–311.

Wagner, E., and Williams, R. S. (1987). Rehabilitation after myocardial infarction. In K. G. Andreoli, D. P. Zipes, A. G. Wallace, et al. (Eds.), *Comprehensive cardiac care* (6th ed., pp. 399–402). St. Louis: Mosby.

Ward, D. B. (1986). Why patient teaching fails. *RN* January, 45–47.

Wenger, N. K. (1973). Coronary care: Rehabilitation after myocardial infarction. Dallas: American Heart Association.

Wenger, N. K. (1978). *Exercise and the heart* (pp. 107–115). Philadelphia: F. A. Davis.

Wenger, N. K. (1981). Rehabilitation of the patient with symptomatic coronary atherosclerotic heart disease. Dallas: American Heart Association.

Wenger, N. K. (1984a). Early ambulation physical activity: myocardial infarction and coronary artery bypass surgery. *Heart & Lung*, 13(1), 14–17.

Wenger, N. K. (1984b). Early ambulation after myocardial infarction: Rationale, program components, and results, In N. K. Wenger, and H. K. Hellerstein (Eds.), *Rehabilitation of the coronary patient* (2nd ed., pp. 97–113). New York: Wiley.

Wilson, P. K., Fardy, P. S., and Froelicher, V. F. (1981). *Cardiac rehabilitation, adult fitness, and exercise testing* (pp. 199–223). Philadelphia: Lea & Febiger.

Wilson, P. K. (1988). Cardiac rehabilitation: then and now. *The Physician and Sports Medicine*, 16(9), 75–80.

Winslow, E. H. (1985). Cardiovascular consequences of bed rest. *Heart & Lung*, 14(3), 236–246.

Winslow, E. H., Lane, L. D., and Gaffney, F. A. (1984). Oxygen uptake and cardiovascular response in patients and normal adults during in-bed and out-of-bed toileting. *Journal of Cardiac Rehabilitation*, 4(8), 348–354.

Index

Note: Page numbers in *italic* refer to illustrations; page numbers followed by t refer to tables.